PRINCIPLES OF

AMBULATORY MEDICINE

SIXTH EDITION

Editors

L. Randol Barker, M.D., Sc.M.
Professor of Medicine
Johns Hopkins University School of Medicine
Co-Director, Division of Internal Medicine
Johns Hopkins Bayview Medical Center
Baltimore, Maryland

John R. Burton, M.D.
Mason F. Lord Professor of Medicine
Director, Division of Geriatric Medicine and Gerontology
The Johns Hopkins University School of Medicine
Director, Division of Geriatric Medicine
Johns Hopkins Bayview Medical Center
Baltimore, Maryland

Philip D. Zieve, M.D.
Professor of Medicine
The Johns Hopkins University School of Medicine
Vice President for Medical Affairs
Johns Hopkins Bayview Medical Center
Baltimore, Maryland

Associate Editors

Nicholas H. Fiebach, M.D.
Associate Professor of Medicine
The Johns Hopkins University School of Medicine
Director, General Internal Medicine Residency Program
Division of General Internal Medicine
Johns Hopkins Bayview Medical Center
Baltimore, Maryland

David E. Kern, M.D., M.P.H.
Associate Professor of Medicine
Johns Hopkins University School of Medicine
Co-Director, Division of General Internal Medicine
Johns Hopkins Bayview Medical Center
Baltimore, Maryland

Patricia A. Thomas, M.D.
Associate Professor of Medicine
Deputy Director of Education
Department of Medicine
Johns Hopkins University School of Medicine
Baltimore, Maryland

Roy C. Ziegelstein, M.D.
Associate Professor of Medicine
The Johns Hopkins University School of Medicine
Executive Vice Chairman, Department of Medicine
Director, Residency Program in Internal Medicine
Johns Hopkins Bayview Medical Center
Baltimore, Maryland

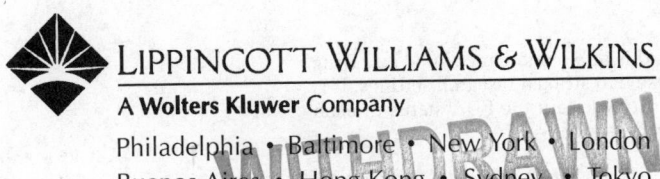
LIPPINCOTT WILLIAMS & WILKINS
A Wolters Kluwer Company
Philadelphia • Baltimore • New York • London
Buenos Aires • Hong Kong • Sydney • Tokyo

Acquisitions Editor: Tim Hiscock
Developmental Editor: Leah Hayes
Production Editor: Robin E. Cook
Manufacturing Manager: Tim Reynolds
Cover Designer: Christine Jenny
Compositor: TechBooks
Printer: Quebecor World

530 Walnut St.
Philadelphia, PA 19106 USA
www.LWW.com

Printed in the USA

Library of Congress Cataloging-in-Publication Data

Principles of ambulatory medicine / editors, L. Randol Barker, John R. Burton, Philip D. Zieve ; associate editors, Nicholas H. Fiebach, David E. Kern, Patricia A. Thomas, Roy C. Ziegelstein—6th ed.
p. ; cm.
Includes bibliographical references and index.
ISBN 0-7817-3486-X
1. Family medicine. 2. Ambulatory medical care. I. Barker, L. Randol (Lee Randol), 1939– II. Burton, John R. (John Russell), 1937– III. Zieve, Philip David, 1932–
[DNLM: 1. Ambulatory Care. WX 205 P957 2002]
RC46 .P894 2002
616—dc21 2001050739

Care has been taken to confirm the accuracy of the information presented and to describe generally accepted practices. However, the authors, editors, and publisher are not responsible for errors or omissions or for any consequences from application of the information in this book and make no warranty, expressed or implied, with respect to the currency, completeness, or accuracy of the contents of the publication. Application of this information in a particular situation remains the professional responsibility of the practitioner.

The authors, editors, and publisher have exerted every effort to ensure that drug selection and dosage set forth in this text are in accordance with current recommendations and practice at the time of publication. However, in view of ongoing research, changes in government regulations, and the constant flow of information relating to drug therapy and drug reactions, the reader is urged to check the package insert for each drug for any change in indications and dosage and for added warnings and precautions. This is particularly important when the recommended agent is a new or infrequently employed drug.

Some drugs and medical devices presented in this publication have Food and Drug Administration (FDA) clearance for limited use in restricted research settings. It is the responsibility of the health care provider to ascertain the FDA status of each drug or device planned for use in their clinical practice.

10 9 8 7 6 5 4 3 2 1

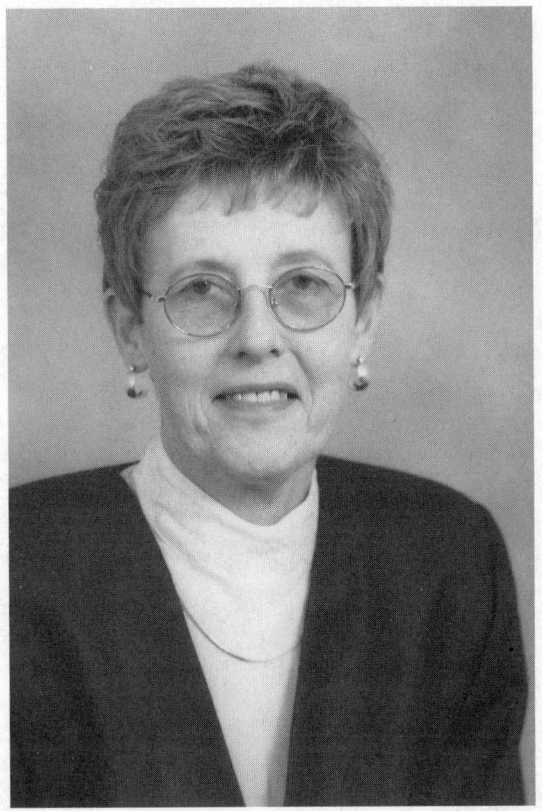

It is with great pride and deep admiration that we dedicate this edition of *Principles of Ambulatory Medicine* to Carole Messman. An analogy has been made that creating a textbook is like creating a play. It is behind the scenes where a play begins and is sustained. For each of the 6 editions of this book, over 23 years, Carole Messman has been the administrative assistant to its editors. She has done much of the manuscript typing, retyping, organizing, and logistical work that goes into creating a large, multiauthored textbook. Only through her absolute dedication to this effort were we able to ensure that this book was fully developed with all of the myriad of details fully addressed and ready on time for publication. Anyone who has edited a text of this complexity will appreciate what this effort has meant to us and to the quality of the textbook.

CONTRIBUTING AUTHORS

Unless otherwise indicated, hospital appointments are at Johns Hopkins Bayview Medical Center, Baltimore, Maryland, and faculty appointments are at the Johns Hopkins University School of Medicine

John E. Anderson
Assistant Professor of Medicine

Ross E. Andersen, Ph.D.
Associate Professor of Medicine

Andrew F. Angelino, M.D.
Assistant Professor of Psychiatry and Behavior Sciences
Medical Director, Acute Psychiatric Services

Michael A. Ankrom, M.D.
Assistant Professor

Frank C. Arnett, Jr., M.D.
Professor and Chairman
Department of Internal Medicine
University of Texas-Houston Health Science Center

Bimal H. Ashar, M.D.
Assistant Professor of Medicine

Paul G. Auwaerter, M.D.
Assistant Professor of Medicine
Staff Physician

L. Randol Barker, M.D., Sc.M.
Professor of Medicine
Co-Director, Division of General Internal Medicine

William H. Barker, M.D., F.R.C.P., Edin.
Professor of Community and Preventive Medicine
University of Rochester Medical Center
Rochester, New York

Linda F. Barr, M.D.
Assistant Professor of Medicine and Oncology

John G. Bartlett, M.D.
Professor
Director, Division of Infectious Disease

Michele F. Bellantoni, M.D.
Associate Professor of Medicine and Gerontology
Medical Director, Long-Term Care
Johns Hopkins Geriatrics Center

Jeffrey S. Bender, M.D., F.A.C.S.
Professor of Surgery
Oklahoma University Health Science Center
Oklahoma City, Oklahoma

Richard G. Bennett, M.D.
Raymond and Anna Lublin Professor of Medicine

George E. Bigelow, Ph.D.
Professor of Psychiatry

Marc R. Blackman, M.D.
Professor of Medicine
National Institutes of Health
Bethesda, Maryland

David G. Borenstein, M.D., F.A.C.P., F.A.C.R.
Clinical Professor of Medicine
George Washington University Medical Center
Washington, D.C.

Gary R. Briefel, M.D.
Associate Professor of Medicine
Acting Chief
Division of Renal Medicine

Anne E. Burke, M.D.
Assistant Professor of Obstetrics and Gynecology

Arthur L. Burnett, M.D.
Associate Professor of Urology

Ronald P. Byank, M.D.
Associate Professor of Orthopedic Surgery

Hugh Calkins, M.D., B.A.
Professor of Medicine
Director of Electrophysiology

Peter H. Cheng, M.D.
Instructor of Medicine

Lawrence J. Cheskin, M.D.
Associate Professor of Medicine

Karan A. Cole, Sc.D.
Assistant Professor of Medicine

Eugene C. Corbett, Jr., M.D.
Associate Professor of Medicine
University of Virginia
Charlottesville, Virginia

J. Raymond DePaulo, Jr., M.D.
Henry Phipps Professor of Psychiatry
Director, Department of Psychiatric and Behavioral Sciences

Adrian S. Dobs, M.D.
Professor of Medicine and Oncology

Mark D. Duncan, M.D., F.A.C.S.
Associate Professor of Surgery
Chief of Surgical Oncology

Christopher J. Earley, M.D., Ph.D.
Associate Professor of Neurology

Rodrigo Erlich, M.D.
Assistant Professor
Chief, Division of Medical Oncology

Peter J. Fagan, M.D.
Associate Professor of Psychiatry

Rita A. Falcone, M.D.
Assistant Professor of Medicine
Director, Comprehensive Vascular Center

Nicholas H. Fiebach, M.D.
Associate Professor of Medicine
Director, General Internal Medicine Residency Program

Michael I. Fingerhood, M.D.
Associate Professor of Medicine

Thomas E. Finucane, M.D.
Professor of Medicine

Paul S. Fishman, M.D.
Professor of Neurology
University of Maryland Medical School
Baltimore, Maryland

John A. Flynn, M.D.
Associate Professor of Medicine

Howard W. Francis, M.D.
Assistant Professor of Otolaryngology–Head and Neck Surgery

David S. Friedman, M.D., M.P.H.
Assistant Professor of Ophthalmology

Steve N. Georas, M.D.
Associate Professor of Medicine
Director, Respiratory Therapy

Sheldon H. Gottlieb, M.D.
Associate Professor of Medicine

Robert I. Gregerman, M.D.
Professor of Medicine
University of Texas Health Science Center at San Antonio
Audie Murphy V.A. Medical Center
San Antonio, Texas

Constance A. Griffin, M.D.
Associate Professor of Medicine

Richard J. Gross, M.D., Sc.M.
Assistant Professor of Medicine

David B. Hellmann, M.D., F.A.C.P.
Mary Betty Stevens Professor of Medicine
Assistant Professor of Orthopedic Surgery
Chairman, Department of Medicine

George R. Huggins, M.D.
Professor of Obstetrics and Gynecology

Nathaniel W. James IV, M.D.
Outpatient Department
Maine Medical Center
Portland, Maine

Constance J. Johnson, M.D.
Clarksville, Tennessee

Calvin E. Jones, Jr., M.D.
Associate Professor of Surgery

Peter W. Kaplan, M.B., B.S., F.R.C.P.
Associate Professor, Department of Psychology
Chairman, Department of Neurology

Philip O. Katz, M.D.
Associate Professor of Medicine
Medical College of Pennsylvania-Hahneman University
The Graduate Hospital
Philadelphia, Pennsylvania

Mark D. Kelemen, M.D.
Assistant Professor of Medicine

David E. Kern, M.D., M.P.H.
Associate Professor of Medicine
Co-Director, Division of General Internal Medicine

Edward S. Kraus, M.D.
Associate Professor of Medicine

Ralph W. Kuncl, M.D., Ph.D.
Professor of Neurology

Brian E. Lacy, M.D., Ph.D.
Assistant Professor of Medicine

Bruce S. Lebowitz, D.P.M.
Instructor and Chief of Podiatry
Department of Orthopedic Surgery

Frederick A. Lenz, M.D., Ph.D.
Professor of Neurosurgery and Neurosurgeon

Mark C. Liu, M.D.
Associate Professor of Medicine

Douglas K. Macleod, M.D.
Raleigh, North Carolina

Alan K. Matsumoto, M.D.
Assistant Professor of Medicine

Una D. McCann, M.D.
Associate Professor of Psychiatry and Behavioral Sciences
Associate Program Director
General Clinical Research Center

Simon C. Mears, M.D.
Assistant Professor of Orthopedic Surgery
University of Maryland

Esteban Mezey, M.D.
Professor of Medicine

Redonda G. Miller, M.D.
Assistant Professor of Medicine

Francis Mark Mondimore, M.D.
Assistant Professor of Psychiatry and Behavioral Sciences

Ali Moshirfar, M.D.
Chief Resident
Department of Orthopedic Surgery

Patrick A. Murphy, M.D.
Professor of Medicine
Chief, Division of Infectious Disease

David N. Neubauer, M.D.
Assistant Professor of Psychiatry

John K. Niparko, M.D.
Professor of Otolaryngology

Irina Petrache, M.D.
Instructor of Medicine

Gregory P. Prokopowicz, M.D., M.P.H.
Assistant Professor of Medicine

Michael J. Purtell, M.D., Ph.D.
Assistant Professor of Medicine

Peter V. Rabins, M.D., M.P.H.
Professor of Psychiatry

Cynthia S. Rand, Ph.D.
Associate Professor of Medicine

Darius A. Rastegar, M.D.
Assistant Professor of Medicine

Robert P. Roca, M.D., M.P.H.
Associate Professor of Psychiatry
Vice President and Medical Director
Sheppard Pratt Health System
Baltimore, Maryland

Annabelle Rodriguez, M.D.
Assistant Professor of Medicine

Linda Rogers, C.R.P.N.
Assistant
Department of Psychiatry

Gary J. Romano, M.D., Ph.D.
Clinical Assistant Professor of Neurology and Neuromuscular Disease
Medical College of Pennsylvania-Hahnemann University
Wynnewood, Pennsylvania

Alvin M. Sanico, M.D.
Assistant Professor of Medicine

Andrew P. Schachat, M.D.
Professor of Ophthalmology

Lawrence N. Scherzer, M.D.
Assistant Professor of Pediatrics
University of Connecticut
Hartford, Connecticut

Chester W. Schmidt, Jr., M.D.
Professor of Psychiatry
Chairman, Department of Psychiatry

Stephen D. Sears, M.D.
Infectious Disease Specialist
Maine General Medical Center
Augusta, Maine

Edward P. Shapiro, M.D.
Professor of Medicine

Stephen D. Sisson, M.D.
Assistant Professor of Medicine

Jeffrey M. Smith, M.D., M.P.H.
Assistant Professor of Obstetrics and Gynecology

Philip L. Smith, M.D.
Professor of Pulmonary and Critical Care Medicine

Maria Elena Soler, M.D.
Instructor of Obstetrics and Gynecology

Jennifer E. Sollenberger, M.S.
Genetic Counselor
Cancer Risk Assessment Program

Robert J. Spence, M.D.
Associate Professor of Surgery
Chief of Plastic Surgery

David A. Spector, M.D.
Associate Professor of Medicine

Kerry J. Stewart, Ed.D.
Associate Professor of Medicine
Director, Johns Hopkins Heart Health

Nisha Chandra Strobos, M.D.
Professor of Medicine

Ray E. Stutzman, MD.
Associate Professor of Urology

Patricia A. Thomas, M.D.
Associate Professor of Medicine
Deputy Director of Education

Catherine S. Todd, M.D.
Instructor of Obstetrics and Gynecology

Alexander S. Townes, M.D.
Professor of Medicine Emeritus
Vanderbilt University School of Medicine
Nashville, Tennessee

Varsha K. Vaidya, M.D.
Assistant Professor
Director, Consult Psychiatry Service
Departments of Psychiatry and General Internal Medicine

Martin D. Valentine, M.D.
Professor of Medicine

Mark F. Walker, M.D.
Assistant Professor of Neurology

Larry Waterbury, M.D.
Associate Professor of Medicine
Director, Division of Hematology/Oncology

Robert S. Weinberg, M.D.
Associate Professor and Chief of Ophthalmology

Laura S. Welch, M.D.
Adjunct Professor of Environmental Health
George Washington University School of Public Health
Washington, D.C.

Karen A. Wendel, M.D.
Assistant Professor of Medicine

James F. Wenz, M.D.
Assistant Professor and Director
Department of Orthopedic Surgery

S. Elizabeth Whitmore, M.D.
Assistant Professor of Dermatology

Mark F. Williams, M.D.
Assistant Professor and Chief
Department of Otolaryngology

Robert A. Wise, M.D.
Professor of Medicine

James M. Wong, M.D.
Assistant Professor of Surgery

E. James Wright, M.D.
Assistant Professor of Urology

Scott M. Wright, M.D.
Assistant Professor of Medicine

Jonathan M. Zenilman, M.D.
Associate Professor of Medicine

Roy C. Ziegelstein, M.D.
Associate Professor of Medicine
Executive Vice Chairman
Department of Medicine

Philip D. Zieve, M.D.
Professor of Medicine
Vice President for Medical Affairs

Acknowledgments

The Editors wish to acknowledge the helpful suggestions of many colleagues, both generalists and specialists, who provided feedback on the fourth edition and who reviewed chapters for the fifth and sixth editions. Two persons, Mrs. Carole Messman (to whom this book is dedicated) and Ms. Susan McFeaters, provided excellent administrative and typographic assistance throughout the preparation of all six editions of this book.

CONTENTS

Section 4: Allergy and Infectious Diseases 385

Section 5: Gastrointestinal Problems 569

Section 6: Renal and Urologic Problems 661

Section 7: Hematologic Problems 745

Section 8: Pulmonary Problems 787

Section 9: Cardiovascular Problems 857

Section 10: Musculoskeletal Problems 1019

Section 11: Metabolic and Endocrinologic Problems 1181

Section 12: Neurologic Problems 1355

Section 13: Selected General Surgical Problems 1475

Section 14: Gynecology and Women's Health 1555

Section 15: Selected Problems of the Eyes 1651

Section 16: Selected Problems of the Ears, Nose, Throat, and Oral Cavity 1683

Section 17: Common Disorders of the Skin 1725

PREFACE

This book is directed to practitioners who care for ambulatory adult patients. The purposes of the book are (a) to provide an in-depth account of the evaluation, management, and long-term course of common clinical problems that are addressed in the ambulatory setting, and (b) to provide guidance for recognizing problems that require either referral for specialized care or hospitalization and for appreciating the expected course of those problems.

Three principles have guided the preparation of each edition of *Principles of Ambulatory Medicine.*

1. Practitioners working in a busy practice need to know about *probabilities* related to the occurrence course, evaluation, and treatment of their patients' problems.
2. The patient makes most decisions in ambulatory care, and the quality of those decisions depends on the *patient–practitioner relationship* and *patient education.*
3. The practitioner and the patient should incorporate a *preventive point of view* into all actions taken to address the patient's health.

With the sixth edition, the senior editors, L. Randol Barker, John R. Burton, and Philip D. Zieve, welcome four colleagues as associate editors. They are: Nicholas H. Fiebach, David E. Kern, Patricia A. Thomas, and Roy C. Ziegelstein. In preparing the sixth edition, the editorial team expanded the number of chapters from 101 to 118. Most are new chapters. Some integrate material from multiple chapters in previous editions. Many of the changes in the content of the sixth edition are reflected in five new or revised sections:

- Section 1: Issues of General Concern. This section was expanded from 9 to 13 chapters and now includes a new chapter on complementary and alternative medicine, a separate chapter on practicing evidence-based medicine, a chapter that integrates all aspects of care at the end of life, and two chapters that integrate approaches from multiple specialties: "Sexuality and Sexual Disorders" and "Sleep Disorders."
- Section 2: Preventive Care. This five-chapter section includes new chapters on nutrition, exercise in healthy patients, and genetic screening and counseling.
- Section 14: Gynecology and Women's Health. This eight-chapter section has an overview of women's health issues across the life span. It includes reproductive health, breast disease, and has separate chapters on menstrual disorders, osteoporosis, and menopause and beyond.
- Section 16: Selected Problems of the Ears, Nose, Throat, and Oral Cavity. This section contains a new chapter, "Epistaxis, Snoring, Anosmia, Hoarseness, and Hiccups."
- Section 17: Common Disorders of the Skin. This section has been expanded from one chapter to six chapters, beginning with "Approaches to the Diagnosis and Treatment of Skin Disorders."

In addition to changes denoted in these five sections, a practical section on the care of immigrant patients has been incorporated into Chapter 41, "International Medicine: Care of the Traveler and of the Immigrant Patient."

All updating and revising have been based on evidence from recent clinical trials, on current consensus-based recommendations for many conditions, and on the comments of those who have used the book. Bold print (general references) and bold numerals (specific references) denote the published reports of randomized controlled clinical trials, meta-analyses, and consensus-based recommendations that have guided the writing of each chapter. Useful websites are included in the general reference section of many chapters.

Principles of Ambulatory Medicine is extensively cross-referenced both to avoid redundancy and to facilitate access to useful information contained elsewhere in the book. In addition, for easy reference, the key topics in each chapter are presented in outline form at the beginning of the chapter.

SECTION 1

Issues of General Concern in Ambulatory Medicine

CHAPTER 1

Ambulatory Care: Domain and Core Proficiencies

L. RANDOL BARKER, MD, ScD

A fundamental tenet of this book is that ambulatory care has distinctive characteristics that should shape practitioners' approaches to patients. This chapter describes the territory of ambulatory care in the United States. It also describes some of the proficiencies that are central to ambulatory practice.

DOMAIN OF AMBULATORY CARE

Who provides ambulatory care? What patients make ambulatory care visits? What problems do patients present at their visits? What ambulatory care is provided for these problems? To answer these questions, the United States National Ambulatory Medical Care Survey (NAMCS), started in 1973, has collected information periodically from a representative sample of physicians' offices.

Office-Based Practitioners

Table 1.1 shows the distribution by specialty of the approximately 757 million visits to physicians' offices in the United States during 1999. Of these visits, 18% were to the offices of internists and 23% were to the offices of general or family practitioners; 3% of all visits were to physician's assistants or nurse practitioners (1). This book is directed primarily to those physicians and other practitioners who provide primary care for adult patients.

Ambulatory Patients

The NAMCS *definition of an ambulatory patient* is "an individual presenting for personal health services who is neither bedridden nor currently admitted to any health care institution." A critical expansion of this definition is that ambulatory or homebound patients (or members of their households) have most of the responsibility for carrying out their own care: They must administer treatments, monitor symptoms and functional status, adapt to the constraints imposed by illness, and decide how to deal with new problems when they arise. These characteristics have important implications for the care of ambulatory patients, as discussed later in this chapter and throughout this book.

The age and sex distribution of the patients who made ambulatory visits to physicians' offices in 1999 is shown in Table 1.2. In that year, the annual number of office visits by adults ranged from 1.6 for people 15 to 24 years old to 6.8 for people aged 75 and older (1).

Problems of Ambulatory Patients

What types of problems are seen in ambulatory practice? Using the *International Classification of Diseases, 9th Revision, Clinical Modification* (ICD-9-CM), participants in NAMCS were asked to name the principal reasons for the visits by patients. Table 1.3 lists the most common responses given by internists and by general/family practitioners, respectively. Because comorbidity, especially the coexistence of physical and mental morbidity, is very common in ambulatory patients, this list of principal reasons for visits tells only part of the story. Furthermore, at least half of ambulatory care visits are for symptoms, and a diagnosis that explains these symptoms is frequently not found (2). Ongoing research on common symptoms will contribute critical information for addressing the needs of ambulatory patients (see Kroenke and Laine, *Investigating Symptoms,* in General References).

Ambulatory Care

In 1999, visits by adults to the offices of general/family practitioners and to internists had the following general characteristics (1):

	General/Family Practice Offices	Internal Medicine Offices
Average time with physician	17.7 min	20.7 min
Status of patient (% of visits)		
Old patient	90.1%	92.2%
New patient	9.9%	7.8%
Drug mentions (% of visits)	75%	81%
Average number of drug mentions per visit	1.7 drugs	2.2 drugs

In the decade 1989–1999, the time spent with primary care practitioners increased by an average of

Table 1.1. Number, Percent Distribution, and Annual Rate of Office Visits by Selected Physician Practice Characteristics: United States, 1999

Physician Practice Characteristics	Number of Visits in Thousands	Percent Distribution	Number of Visits per 100 Persons per Year
All visits	756,734	100.0	278.5
General and family practice	170,571	22.5	62.8
Internal medicine	135,607	17.9	49.9
Pediatrics	74,045	9.8	27.2
Obstetrics and gynecology	59,518	7.9	21.9
Ophthalmology	51,165	6.8	18.8
Orthopedic surgery	40,516	5.4	14.9
Dermatology	32,704	4.3	12.0
Psychiatry	22,346	3.0	8.2
General surgery	21,174	2.8	7.8
Urology	17,415	2.3	6.4
Cardiovascular diseases	16,566	2.2	6.1
Otolaryngology	16,369	2.2	6.0
Neurology	8,298	1.1	3.1
All other specialties	90,440	12.0	33.3

From Cherry DK, Burt CW, Woodwell DA. National Ambulatory Medical Care Survey: 1999 Summary. Advance Data for Vital and Health Statistics No. 322. Hyattsville, MD: National Center for Health Statistics, July 17, 2001.

Table 1.2. Number and Percent Distribution of Office Visits by Patient's Age, Sex, and Race: United States, 1999

Patient's Age (Years), Sex, and Race	Number of Visits in Thousands	Percent Distribution
All visits	756,734	100.0
Age		
<15	116,904	15.4
15–24	59,706	7.9
25–44	186,022	24.6
45–64	201,911	26.7
65–74	92,642	12.2
≥75	99,548	13.2
Sex and Age		
Female	445,566	58.9
<15	55,247	7.3
15–24	38,521	5.1
25–44	119,084	15.7
45–64	119,424	15.8
65–74	51,669	6.8
≥75	61,621	8.1
Male	311,168	41.1
<15	61,658	8.1
15–24	21,185	2.8
25–44	66,938	8.8
45–64	82,487	10.9
65–74	40,973	5.4
≥75	37,926	5.0
Race		
White	654,712	86.5
Black	73,972	9.8
Asian/Pacific Islander	25,477	3.4
American Indian/Alaska Native	1,319	0.2

From Cherry DK, Burt CW, Woodwell DA. National Ambulatory Medical Care Survey: 1999 Summary. Advance Data for Vital and Statistics No. 322. Hyattsville, MD: National Center for Health Statistics, July 17, 2001.

2.0 minutes for prepaid visits and 2.6 minutes for nonprepaid visits (3).

In addition to office visits, *telephone encounters and house calls* are important in the care of ambulatory patients. Telephone encounters enable physicians and patients to handle many problems efficiently. (See Reisman and Stevens, General References.) They constitute approximately 25% of all patient contacts for internists and 19% for family physicians (4). Most telephone encounters are patient initiated, but NAMCS data indicate that telephone follow-up is scheduled at the end of about 2.3% of all visits (1). Home visits are helpful for providing care to patients who are too frail to make office visits and for learning facts about patients' home conditions that may facilitate management of their problems at future office visits.

Table 1.3. Reasons for Ambulatory Visits to Generalists: United States, 1985

Rank	Internists	General and Family Practitioners
	25 Most Common Reasons for Visit (by ICD-9-CM Categories)	
1	Essential hypertension	Essential hypertension
2	Diabetes mellitus	General medical examination
3	Other forms of chronic ischemic heart disease	Acute upper respiratory tract infections
4	Acute upper respiratory tract infections	Diabetes mellitus
5	General medical examination	Normal pregnancy
6	Osteoarthrosis and allied disorders	Suppurative and unspecified otitis media
7	General symptoms	Acute pharyngitis
8	Chronic airway obstruction	Bronchitis
9	Asthma	Chronic sinusitis
10	Bronchitis	Certain adverse effects not elsewhere classified
11	Neurotic disorders	Health supervision of infant or child
12	Angina pectoris	Sprains and strains
13	Chronic sinusitis	Others disorders of urethra and urinary tract
14	Acute pharyngitis	Obesity and other hyperalimentation
15	Cardiac dysrhythmias	General symptoms
16	Other disorders of soft tissue	Contact dermatitis and other eczema
17	Symptoms involving respiratory system	Neurotic disorders
18	Heart failure	Osteoarthrosis and allied disorders
19	Peripheral enthesopathies	Other and unspecified arthropathies
20	Other and unspecified arthropathies	Other disorders of soft tissues
21	Diseases of esophagus	Other noninfectious gastroenteritis
22	Other noninfectious gastroenteritis	Asthma
23	Other disorders of urethra and urinary tract	Sprains and strains of sacroiliac region
24	Allergic rhinitis	Acute tonsillitis
25	Hypertensive heart disease	Disorders of external ear

ICD-9-CM, International Classification of Diseases, 9th Rev., Clinical Modification.

From National Ambulatory Medical Care Survey. Hyattsville, MD: National Center for Health Statistics, 1985.

Self-Care and Alternative Care

Before making visits to physicians, patients usually attempt to diagnose and treat their own symptoms. Additionally, each year 42% of patients in the United States report using one or more of the several types of alternative care that are described in Chapter 5 (5).

Studies of self-care in a number of countries have shown that at any one time approximately 30% of persons are taking nonprescribed medications or are engaged in self-care for a problem for which they have not consulted a physician (6). The frequency distribution of conditions managed by self-care was estimated by Fry (7), on the basis of many years of general practice in a community well known to him, as 25% upper respiratory tract infections, 20% musculoskeletal symptoms, 20% emotional problems, 10% acute gastrointestinal symptoms, 5% skin rashes, and 20% miscellaneous other symptoms. Both the changing status of drugs from prescription to over-the-counter formulations (Table 1.4) and the availability of herbal remedies without a prescription (see Chapter 5) have expanded the "formulary" that patients can access for self-care.

The time interval between the onset of a new problem and the decision to go to a physician (i.e., the duration of self-care) is shown for a number of common conditions in Table 1.5, adapted from NAMCS data. Not surprisingly, patients with lacerations presented within 1 day, patients with symptoms of acute infection and chest pain tended to present within 1 week, and patients with most other problems tended to present after at least 1 week of self-care.

Table 1.4. Examples of Drugs Previously Available in the United States Only by Prescription and Now Available over the Counter

Histamine H_1–receptor antagonists
Diphenhydramine
Histamine H_2–receptor antagonists
Cimetidine
Ranitidine
Famotidine
Nonsteroidal antiinflammatory drugs
Ibuprofen
Naproxen
Ketoprofen
Smoking-cessation aids
Nicotine (gum and patches)
Hair-growth stimulants
Minoxidil (2% and 5%)
Antifungal drugs
Clotrimazole
Ketoconazole
Antidiarrheal drugs
Loperamide
Decongestants
Pseudoephedrine

From Bass EP. Changing the status of drugs from prescription to over-the-counter availability. N Engl J Med 2001;345:810.

Self-care before professional care is an important way in which the patient, not the practitioner, makes the decisions in the domain of ambulatory medicine. The patient's primary role in carrying out the plan of care after an office visit has already been emphasized. These two features confirm the primacy of the patient's actions in determining the course of events in ambulatory medicine.

Temporal Dimension of Ambulatory Medicine

The information from the NAMCS does not illuminate the longitudinal nature of ambulatory care. Table 1.6 shows the 5-year profile of care for an elderly woman. This patient's story illustrates each of the following important questions, for which only the passage of time provides the answers:

- *What is the significance of a recent symptom* (e.g., the temporal headache for 1 year reported in 1975, subsequently not a serious problem)?
- *What is the advisability of initiating a referral for a problem* (e.g., cataract identified but asymptomatic in 1975, evaluated when more symptomatic in 1978 and classified as not mature)?
- *How well will the patient adhere to recommended treatment* (e.g., the digoxin prescribed in 1975 for heart failure, taken reliably for 5 years)?
- *What is the impact of a new treatment on the patient's health* (e.g., addition of a diuretic in 1978, with heart failure gradually improving during the next month)?
- *What is the impact of intercurrent medical problems on the patient's functional status?* (The answer to this question varied over time depending on intercurrent problems: During the 5 years the patient's ambulation deteriorated greatly, but other valued activities, such as crocheting and canning, did not.)
- *What is the impact of the patient's illness on family members in the same household?* (The answer to this question also varied over time; "exhaustion" at one point did not predict transfer to a long-term care facility.)

Table 1.5. Percentage Distribution of New Problem Office Visits by Time Since Onset of Complaint or Symptom, According to Selected Principal Reasons for Visit: United States, 1977

Principal Reason for Visit	Total	Time Since Onset of Complaint or Symptom (days)					
		1	1–6	7–21	30–90	>90	Not Applicable
All new problem visits	100.0	8.2	37.3	15.6	10.3	13.9	14.8
Symptoms of throat	100.0	6.9	77.9	10.6	2.3	1.9	0.4
Cough	100.0	3.3	73.0	18.6	2.9	2.1	0.2
Head cold, upper respiratory tract infection	100.0	6.2	72.5	16.5	3.0	1.1	0.7
Fever	100.0	17.6	76.4	4.7	0.2	1.0	
Headache	100.0	5.1	35.6	19.0	16.5	19.7	3.2
Back symptoms	100.0	6.5	37.6	26.4	11.8	16.2	1.5
Chest pain	100.0	7.6	45.8	22.6	9.3	13.6	1.2
Laceration, upper extremity	100.0	70.4	15.4	7.8	3.0	2.1	1.3

From National Ambulatory Medical Care Survey: 1977 Summary. Hyattsville, MD: National Center for Health Statistics.

Table 1.6. Profile of 5 Years in the Care of an Elderly Patient (each problem *italicized*)

Feature	1975	1976	1977	1978	1979
Encounters	Initial visit, four office visits, many phone calls	Three office visits, many phone calls	Five office visits, two hospital admissions, one home visit, many phone calls	Four office visits, many phone calls	Four office visits, many phone calls
Principal medical problems	*Acute myocardial infarction* (mild congestive heart failure; digitalized; home management by patient's choice)	Stable (digoxin)	Stable (digoxin)	Congestive heart failure (diuretic added)	Stable (digoxin, diuretic)
	Degenerative joint disease (knees for years; cervical spine for years)	Waxes and wanes (aspirin, Motrin)	Same (coated aspirin)	Same (coated aspirin)	Same (coated aspirin)
	Temporal headaches for 1 year (erythrocyte sedimentation rate, 30)	Rarely	Rarely	Rarely	Rarely
	Hearing loss (ear, nose, and throat examination: senile high frequency deficit, no prescription)	Stable	Stable	Stable	Stable
	Bilateral cataracts	Stable	Stable	Referred (not mature)	Stable
	Leukoplakia, mouth (biopsy: not malignant)	Stable	Stable	Stable	Referred for change in appearance (biopsy: not malignant)
	Hematocrit, 35 (guaiac-negative)	Stable	Stable Stable	Stable	Stable
	Constipation (for years)	Waxes and wanes (OTC laxative as needed)	Same (OTC laxative as needed)	Same (OTC laxative as needed and stool softener)	Same (OTC laxative as needed and stool softener)
		Leg cramps (quinine at bedtime)	Minimal (quinine at bedtime)	Same (quinine at bedtime)	Same (quinine at bedtime)
		Left cerebral *transient ischemic attack*	*Left CVA* (hospital, physical therapy)	Stable (right hemiparesis)	Recurrent left CVA (home management)
			Dog bite (cellulitis)	No recurrence	No recurrence
			Rectal bleeding (hospital, negative workup)	No recurrence	No recurrence
			Dysuria (culture negative)		
				Family (temporarily "exhausted"; Visiting Nurses Association)	Family doing well
				Painful toe	Persists (codeine)
				Appetite lost temporarily	No recurrence
Overall profile	87-year-old widow living with daughter's family, ambulatory and independent in the home, mentally intact, crochets and cans food; weight, 166; multiple medical problems identified at initial visit	88 years old, status the same; weight, 160; two new problems	89 years old, ambulation with walker assistance after CVA; weight, 151; four new problems, hospitalized twice	90 years old, status the same; weight, 140; three new problems	91 years old; ambulation more impaired after second CVA; mentally intact, crochets and cans food; weight, 139; no new problems

CVA, cerebrovascular accident; OTC, over-the-counter.

Goals of Ambulatory Care

Patient Expectations

The goals of ambulatory care are strongly influenced by the expectations of patients who reside in the community. When they make office visits for stated medical reasons, ambulatory patients are seeking help to relieve symptoms, to cure, to ameliorate or prevent illness, or to be able to maintain or resume valued activities. Depending on the severity of their problems, outpatients may be greatly, moderately, or not at all constrained from attaining these expectations. By virtue of living in the community, they (or other caregivers) play an active role in how these expectations are addressed, in contrast to the passive role played by hospitalized patients.

Implications for Practice

To determine how any patient is doing, it is helpful to be aware of that person's particular expectations and how well he or she is meeting them. This usually involves learning about the makeup of the patient's current household and his or her usual role in the family, the patient's occupation and level of formal education, and valued activities. It is also helpful to be aware of the developmental tasks that may be relevant to a patient's family. Tasks that are typical of the various stages in the *life cycle of a family* are listed in Table 1.7. The significance of this information can be illustrated by a common example: a middle-aged man who has had an uncomplicated myocardial infarction. After 3 months, the patient might be assessed as "status post-myocardial infarction—doing well." If he has resumed work and other valued activities, then he is probably "doing well." If he is not back at work, is financially stressed, and his wife reports that he has become irritable, then he is not doing well and the situation requires evaluation.

Awareness of a patient's life circumstances is also important in preventive care (see Chapter 14), in which the patient's degree of wellness rather than degree of illness is assessed. Assessing wellness means learning whether a patient engages in health-promoting behaviors and determining what health risks the patient has. For example, a 45-year-old mother who is happily married, is free of chronic disease, has stopped smoking, has had periodic negative Pap smears, and drinks alcohol only socially would be assessed as very well. If everything were the same except that the patient smoked two packs of cigarettes daily, she would be assessed as only moderately well because of the major risk posed by heavy tobacco exposure. If she were recently divorced, had stopped seeing friends, and was smoking and drinking heavily, she would be assessed as not very well, even though she might not complain of any particular symptoms or have objective evidence of any disease.

Table 1.7. Factors to Consider in the Family Life Cycle State of One's Patient

Family Life Cycle State	Developmental Tasks
Leaving home	Differentiate self in relation to family Develop intimate peer relationships Establish oneself in work
Couples and pairing	Form a committed relationship Realign relationships with extended family to include partner
Pregnancy and childbirth	Make room for children in the family Become parents while remaining spouses
Family with young children	Form a parent team Negotiate relationships with extended family to include parenting and grandparenting roles
Family with adolescents	Shift parent–child relationship to permit adolescent to move in and out of system
Adulthood and middle years	Refocus on marital and career issues Deal with disabilities and death in grandparents Deal with own aging and mortality
Graying of the family	Maintain functioning in face of physiologic decline
Death and grieving	Deal with loss of spouse, siblings, and peers Prepare for own death

Adapted from Carter CA, McGoldrick M, eds. The family life cycle: a framework for family therapy. New York: Gardner Press, 1980.

CORE PROFICIENCIES FOR AMBULATORY PRACTICE

Information such as that provided by the NAMCS (discussed earlier) has implications for several core proficiencies needed in the practice of ambulatory medicine. These include proficiency in clinical pharmacology, documentation of care, coordination of care, discharge planning, cost containment, evidence-based decision-making, patient-centered communication, patient education and promotion of healthy behavior, and integration of prevention into practice. Chapters 2, 3, 4, and 14, respectively, address in depth the latter four areas of proficiency.

Clinical Pharmacology

Clinical pharmacology is the source for the many details needed for appropriate prescribing of medications. Apart from the impact of a medication on a patient's condition, it is important to be aware of the following aspects of each drug that one prescribes:

- *Practical information about initiating the drug:* appropriate starting dosage and schedule; modifications in dosage and schedule dictated by patient age, concurrently administered drugs, and the presence of diseases affecting drug metabolism; time interval for the effects of the drug to become apparent; duration of a course of the drug (when not a maintenance drug); how to assess the impact of the drug; potential interaction with other drugs the patient is taking; approximate cost to the patient of the drug; and whether the patient can afford it.
- *The major side effects of the drug:* when to anticipate them and how to detect, monitor for, and manage them.

Table 1.8. Number and Percent Distribution, of Drug Mentions at Office Visits by Therapeutic Classification: United States, 1999

Therapeutic Classification[a]	Number of drug Mentions in Thousands	Percent Distribution
All drug mentions	1,136,686	100.0
Cardiovascular-renal drugs	176,839	15.6
Drugs used for relief of pain	122,469	10.8
Respiratory tract drugs	118,241	10.4
Hormones and agents affecting hormonal mechanisms	112,902	9.9
Antimicrobial agents	106,226	9.3
Central nervous system	100,148	8.8
Metabolic and nutrient agents	74,794	6.6
Skin/mucous membrane	65,027	5.7
Gastrointestinal agents	50,526	4.4
Immunologic agents	48,310	4.3
Other and unclassified	161,204	14.2

[a]Based on the standard drug classification used in the *National Drug Code Directory,* 1995 edition.

From Cherry DK, Burt CW, Woodwell DA. National Ambulatory Medical Care Survey: 1999 Summary. Advance Data for Vital and Health Statistics No. 322. Hyattsville, MD: National Center for Health Statistics, July 17, 2001.

- *The major reasons for inadequate response to a drug:* nonadherence, insufficient dosage of drug, antagonism of the drug by patient behavior or use of concurrent drugs, and primary refractoriness to the drug; how to recognize and manage each of these problems.
- *Practical information about adjusting the dosage:* minimum and maximum dosages that can be tried and the time intervals that are appropriate for adjusting dosages and assessing impact.

Because administration or prescription of medications is the single most common action taken by nonsurgical clinicians in ambulatory practice, rapid access to this practical information through published or electronic resources is particularly important (Table 1.8).

Documentation of Care

Documentation of care in the ambulatory record serves several purposes: to provide for practitioners rapid access to the information they need for clinical decision-making at serial visits; to justify the level of care for which payers are billed; to make data accessible for quality-of-care audit; and to stand as legal evidence of a practitioner's actions. Both paper and electronic records can be designed to meet these purposes.

A well-structured primary care record includes the following components:

- *A primary care front sheet* (Fig. 1.1) that includes a social profile (information about the patient's living situation, marital status, family makeup, occupation, education, social and recreational environment), a problem list that is prominently displayed and facilitates awareness of the patient's problems, and other information that should be readily findable, such as the patient's allergic history, past hospitalizations and operations, and the status of advance directives.
- *A treatment and clinical/laboratory flow sheet* that is prominently displayed and makes important past and current information accessible for decision-making (see Fig. 1.2).
- *A preventive care profile and flow sheet* that documents the patient's risk factors and promotes the appropriate provision of periodic preventive care (see example, Fig. 14.3 in Chapter 14).
- *Encounter forms,* including forms for telephone encounters, that allow clear documentation of information, thinking, and plans.
- Dividers, color-coded forms, and *standardized locations for various types of information* such as consultants' letters and laboratory reports, to increase the accessibility of clinical data.

To document patient education, prescriptions, and work slips, it is helpful to use forms that make duplicates for mounting in the patient's record.

Coordination of Care

Another proficiency important in ambulatory medicine is skill in coordinating the patient's care. Coordination of care refers to referral for and interpretation of the services that a patient may need or receive. The availability of many diagnostic and consultative services requires generalists to be prudent in recommending them and in using the information they provide and to be aware of the cost of a service, the nature of the experience the patient will undergo, and the likelihood that the service will be of value to the patient.

The services recommended for patients may involve permanent, temporary, or partial transfer of responsibility for the patient's care (e.g., to a surgeon), or they may be strictly consultative, meaning that they provide information to be used by the referring physician (ranging from diagnostic test results to a consultant's suggestions).

Approximately 4.4% of office visits include *referral of the patient to another physician* (1). The following general guidelines are important in coordinating the care of a patient who is referred for consultation:

- Whenever a patient is referred for a service, the necessary information should be transmitted to the person who will provide the service. For example, there should be clear communication of the facts generally needed by consultants (Table 1.9).
- Ensure that the patient understands the reason for services that are recommended, arrange to obtain information promptly after a service has been performed, and ensure that the patient learns, as soon as it is appropriate, the meaning of this information.

Patients sometimes obtain services for medical problems without referral by their personal physician. These most often include visits to emergency departments, to specialists such as ophthalmologists, or to alternative practitioners (5). Being aware of these visits is another way in which generalists coordinate their patients' care. When they obtain services elsewhere,

Johns Hopkins Bayview Medical Center

PRIMARY CARE FRONT SHEET

Jane Doe

Date of Birth: 7/23/44

PRIMARY PROVIDER	DATE INITIATED / UPDATED
Jones	6/00 / 8/00, 10/00

ADVANCED DIRECTIVES	ORGAN DONER
TYPE & DATE: 10/00 DPA, LW	DATE: 6/00 ☑ YES ☐ NO

ALLERGIC / DRUG REACTIONS (YEAR)

☑ NONE KNOWN

SOCIAL PROFILE

MARITAL STATUS: married	LIVES WITH: husband
OCCUPATION: accountant	RELIGION: Catholic
HIGHEST EDUCATION: 4 yrs. college, B.A.	PERMANENT IMPAIRMENTS: None

OTHER (CHILDREN, SUPPORT SYSTEM, ACTIVITIES, MAJOR LIFE EVENTS)
John b. 1966, married, 2 children
Charlotte b. 1969, divorced, 1 child
reading, quiltmaking
active @ church

OPERATIONS AND HOSPITALIZATIONS (YEAR)

☐ NONE

1. Pneumonia 1971
2.
3.
4.
5.
6.
7.
8.
9.
10.
11.
12.
13.
14.
15.

G2/P2/Ab0 1966, 1969

☐ T&A ( ) ☐ Appx ( )
☑ GB (1994) ☐ TURP ( )
☑ Hys (1990) ☐ BRL SO ( )
☐ BTL ( ) ☐ Vas ( )

PROBLEM LIST

Onset	First Note	#	Problem & Comments (Key Tests / Consults)	Resolved (Check)
2000	6/00	1	HM (Health Maintenance)	
1966	6/00	2	Smoker	
2000	6/00	3	Hypertension	
2000	6/00	4	Diabetes mellitus Type 2	
2000	8/00	5	Hypercholesterolemia	
2000	8/00	6	Atypical Chest Pain 8/00 EKG nl. 8/00 stress test nl.	

See back for Instructions

☐ See continuation flow sheet

Figure 1.1. Example of a primary care front sheet.

Johns Hopkins Bayview Medical Center
CLINICAL FLOW SHEET
(over for guidelines)

Jane Doe
Date of Birth: 7/23/44

Height (Date) 5'5", 170cm (6/00)

CHRONIC MEDICATIONS & NON-DRUG THERAPY

Date	6/00	8/00	10/00	1/01	5/01	11/01						
Pill Size, Dose, & Schedule (Insert R for refill, specific # disp. for DEA Rx; Insert Y, N, +/- for compliance)												
cong. estrogens	0.625 mg/d	→	→	→	→	Y→						
metformin 6/00		500mg qd	500mg bid	Y→	→	Y→						
lisinopril 8/00			10mg qd	10mg bid	→	Y→						
atorvastatin 8/00			10mg qd	Y→	→	Y→						
smoking	1PPD	1PPD	1PPD	½PPD	⊖	2-3 cigs/d						
exercise	⊖	walks T.I.W.	+/-→	Y→	→	Y→						
low salt, low chol, low sat fat, diabetic diet		→	+/-→	→	→	+/-→						

CLINICAL & LABORATORY DATA

RESULTS →

Weight lb/kg	185/84	186/85	184/84	182/83	181/82	179/81						
BP	154/95	158/100	142/88	134/79	130/65	127/75						
BMI / HgbA1C	29/8.2	/7.5	/7.2	/6.9		28/6.8						
fasting/random glucose	210/	160/	135/	127/		129/						
Cholesterol/fasting triglyceride	265/230	258/208	179/182	164/175	194/190	176/182						
HDL/LDLc	45/174	48/168	46/97	46/83	43/113	47/93						
Microalbumen/U/A	18/NL											
BUN/Cr	18/0.8				19/0.7							
Foot Exam	NL				NL							
Eye Exam			9/00 NL			9/02 NL						
AST/ALT / CK		28/19	24/26	26/21 / 76	/18	/24						

130-656-186N (10/00)

☐ **Check if Clinical and Laboratory Data Flow Sheet continued on reverse**

Figure 1.2. Example of a clinical flow sheet, which aligns treatments and clinical/laboratory parameters.

Table 1.9. Information that Subspecialty Consultants Generally Need from the Referring Physician

The specific reason for the consultation
Relevant current medical problems
Relevant current medications
Relevant diagnostic tests already completed
What the patient has been told about the referral
The patient's attitude about the problem (if relevant)
Patient's address or telephone number

patients can play an essential role by requesting that information be sent to their personal physicians.

Discharge Planning

Admission of the patient to the hospital follows approximately 0.3% of office visits (1). For each admission, hospital discharge usually means the return of the patient to ambulatory care by the patient's primary physician. Each of the generic proficiencies described earlier is especially important when patients make the transition from dependence on hospital personnel to dependence on themselves or their families for management of their medical problems. Beginning with the implementation of the federal prospective payment systems in the 1980s and continuing with the growth of managed care in the 1990s, very short hospital stays have become the norm in the United States. This situation has drawn attention to the elements of effective discharge planning, such as ensuring good understanding of the plan of care by patients and their families, ensuring that a concise discharge summary goes promptly to the practitioner or to the setting responsible for postdischarge care, and using home health services or other community-based services to help patients complete care that was previously carried out during prolonged hospital stays. Chapter 9 provides detailed information about home health services.

Cost Containment and Managed Care

Because of the extraordinary increase in available medical services in the past three decades and because of the parallel increase in the cost and the use of these services, cost containment in medical care is generally recognized as a national imperative. Managed care—that is, health care in which delivery and financing of care are linked in a variety of models—has emerged as a major strategy for containing costs. Managed care plans make arrangements with physicians ranging from directly employing them (staff-model health maintenance organizations [HMOs]) to contracting with them (group-model, network-model, and independent practice association–model arrangements) (8).

Table 1.10 shows for the year 1999 the proportion of ambulatory care visits reimbursed by each of the primary sources of payment in the United States. HMO-type payment accounted for 40% of private insurance visits, 9% of Medicare visits, and 17% of Medicaid visits (1).

Table 1.10. Number and Percent Distribution of Office Visits by Expected Primary Source of Payment: United States, 1999

Expected Source of Payment	Number of Visits in Thousands	Percent Distribution
All visits	756,734	100.0
Private insurance	417,620	55.2
Medicare	156,720	20.7
Medicaid	56,809	7.5
Self-pay	40,658	5.4
Worker's compensation	15,639	2.1
No charge	7,194	1.0
Other	35,616	4.7
Unknown/blank	26,478	3.5

From Cherry DK, Burt CW, Woodwell DA. National Ambulatory Medical Care Survey: 1999 Summary. Advance Data for Vital and Health Statistics No. 322. Hyattsville, MD: National Center for Health Statistics, July 17, 2001.

The goals of containing costs while providing high-quality care have critical implications for generalist physicians in office practice, because it is they who coordinate much of the medical care provided in our society. Practitioners can address these goals in a number of ways:

- Taking a history carefully and allowing some time to pass before embarking on an extensive diagnostic workup of a new symptom
- Keeping well informed about the impact on health outcomes of costly diagnostic procedures and therapies
- Avoiding additional tests that will not alter one's decisions
- Devoting sufficient time to educating patients about their conditions (especially about conditions that often lead to inappropriate and costly doctor shopping by the patient)
- Prescribing only necessary medications and selecting the least expensive preparations
- Using home health services and other community services to forestall the need for hospital admission or to shorten the length of hospitalization

In the past, fee-for-service reimbursement tended to foster excessive use of laboratory tests and costly procedures. There were few external incentives for practitioners to engage in the inquiry, observation, counseling, and decision-making that would have obviated much inappropriate use of health services. Managed care, on the other hand, may foster inappropriately low use of laboratory tests and costly procedures. Fortunately, direct incentives to practitioners to reduce the use of such services have been banned in many settings. To the extent that managed care rewards physicians for cognitive services—and does not overburden them with administrative hurdles or force upon them unreasonable productivity expectations—it has the potential both to promote the health of patients and to reduce the unnecessary use of costly technical services.

General References*

Fry J, Light D, Rodnick J, et al. Reviving primary care: a US-UK comparison. New York: Radcliffe Medical Press, 1995.

Analysis of the revival of primary care in both the United States and the United Kingdom. It addresses the resurgence of interest in primary care, the strengths of the discipline, and the weaknesses that remain to be addressed.

Kroenke K, Laine C, eds. Investigating symptoms: frontiers in primary care research. Ann Intern Med 2001;134:801.

Special supplement that summarizes the current status of research on symptoms and recommends strategies for needed future research.

National Ambulatory Medical Care Survey. [Reports issued periodically]. Washington, DC: U.S. Department of Health and Human Services.

Nationwide study of a probability sample of office-based physicians from all medical specialty areas, using physician- and patient-generated information to delineate the ambulatory care activities of physicians and patients, starting in 1973.

Reisman AB, Stevens DL. Telephone medicine: A guide for the practicing physician. Philadelphia: American College of Physicians, 2002.

Comprehensive, practical, evidence-based text.

Starfield B. Primary care: concept, evaluation, and policy. New York: Oxford University Press, 1992.

Comprehensive monograph that defines primary care, describes in detail its components, reviews the evidence of effectiveness of primary care in the United States and in ten other countries, and delineates options for expanding the role of primary care in the United States.

Specific References

1. Cherry DK, Burt CW, Woodwell DA. National Ambulatory Medical Care Survey: 1999 Summary. Advance Data for Vital and Health Statistics No. 322. Hyattsville, MD: National Center for Health Statistics, July 17, 2001.
2. Kroenke K. Studying symptoms: sampling and measurement issues. Ann Intern Med 2001;134:844.
3. Mechanic D, McAlphine DD, Rosenthal M. Are patients' office visits with physicians getting shorter? N Engl J Med 2001;344: 198.
4. Curtis P. The practice of medicine on the telephone. J Gen Intern Med 1988;3:294.
5. Eisenberg DM, Davis RB, Ettner SL, et al. Trends in alternative medicine use in the United States, 1990–1997. JAMA 1998;280: 1569.
6. Kohn R, White KL, eds. Health care. New York: Oxford University Press, 1976.
7. Fry J. Common diseases: their nature, incidence and care. 2nd ed. Philadelphia: Lippincott, 1979.
8. Gold MR, Hurley R, Lake T, et al. A national survey of the arrangements managed-care plans make with physicians. N Engl J Med 1995;333:1678.

*Bold print (general references) and bold numerals (specific references) denote published clinical trials, meta-analyses, or consensus-based recommendations.

CHAPTER 2

Practicing Evidence-Based Medicine in the Ambulatory Care Setting

SCOTT M. WRIGHT, MD
DARIUS A. RASTEGAR, MD

GENERAL APPROACH

Clinicians are increasingly asked to provide both scientifically sound and cost-effective medical care. These pressures have given rise to the term "evidence-based medicine." Evidence-based medicine (EBM) is the conscientious, explicit, and judicious use of current best evidence in making decisions about the care of individual patients (1). EBM focuses on issues integral to day-to-day patient care: diagnosis, screening, prognosis, treatment, assessment of risks, prevention, and management of the increasing amount of medical information that confronts health care practitioners.

Evidence-based decision-making is especially important in ambulatory practice because this is the setting where patients are most likely to present with undifferentiated problems. It is also the setting where most clinical decisions are made.

The following steps are considered to be indispensable to practicing EBM:

Step 1: Formulate specific questions that are relevant to a patient's care and identify the type of information that is needed (e.g., efficacy or harm of a treatment, accuracy of a diagnostic test).

Step 2: Identify and retrieve the relevant sources of data.

Step 3: Critically appraise the clinically important information.

Step 4: Apply the valid information back to the patient whose presentation initiated the inquiry.

The importance of *step 1,* formulating specific questions, can be understood by considering two similar questions that might be generated when a practitioner sees a patient with hepatitis C who asks about whether antiviral therapy, which the patient has read about in the newspaper, should be initiated:

Question A: How good is the interferon/ribavirin combination for the treatment of hepatitis C?

Question B: For Mr. B, the 48-year-old man with hepatitis C whose transaminases and liver function tests have been normal during the last 9 months, what is the evidence regarding the efficacy and safety of interferon/ribavirin in preventing cirrhosis?

The second question is more specific and will better help to tailor the search effort (step 2) to the clinical outcomes that are most relevant to the practitioner and the patient.

The skills necessary for the successful completion of *step 2,* efficient searching, are currently being taught in medical school and during residency training. Most medical libraries also offer brief hands-on tutorials to teach clinicians how to search databases such as MEDLINE as well as the Internet to find the current best evidence. The National Library of Medicine (see General References) provides access to PubMed (MEDLINE) and multiple health and science databases. It also offers full-text versions of many articles, eliminating the need for additional steps to retrieve the desired manuscripts.

Step 3, critical appraisal, is likely to be most difficult and time-consuming for clinicians. The two components of this step are (a) *deciding whether the results are valid* and (b) *deciding whether the results are important* with respect to the specific question being asked.

It is most efficient to resolve the second component first, which can usually be done fairly quickly. If the results are not clinically important or relevant, then one can avoid the time and effort spent judging the validity and quality of the information. Numerous books and articles published in the medical literature (e.g., the Users' Guides to the Medical Literature series published by the *Journal of the American Medical Association*) aim to teach clinicians the core skills of critical appraisal. Having confidence in one's ability to critically appraise manuscripts that are related to a wide variety of topics (e.g., diagnosis, treatment, cost-effectiveness) and that use a myriad of study designs may take time, practice, and perhaps even additional training. Such training in the form of continuing medical education is frequently offered in workshops at regional and national meetings or through medical libraries.

Step 4 involves integrating the important and valid, newly found information into the care of one's patient. This represents the most satisfying component of practicing EBM. Educating patients, like other medical learners, that a particular diagnostic approach or treatment is supported by current medical research may instill a sense of confidence in patients about the practitioner's knowledge and expertise in keeping abreast with and finding new data.

It would be impractical to assume or recommend that primary care practitioners embark on these fundamental steps of EBM every time a clinical question comes up. However, when critical queries arise that are likely to recur or are particularly important to an individual patient, this version of "self-directed continuing medical education" is likely to be helpful to both practitioners and patients. Some barriers to practicing EBM include skepticism by practitioners, information overload and feeling overwhelmed by the growth of medical knowledge, lack of time, and lack of appropriate resources, skills, or motivation to implement EBM (2).

All dedicated and committed clinicians, however, practice EBM to some degree. To counterbalance the barriers to practicing EBM, several facilitating behaviors have been proposed: (a) reading and keeping up-to-date with the medical literature (see Keeping Up), (b) refining one's EBM skills (practice makes perfect!), (c) collaborating with colleagues so that valuable clinical evidence is shared among practitioners, (d) writing down the specific clinical question (step 1) when it comes up so that the process can continue when time permits, (e) setting up one's computer (e.g., bookmarking relevant websites) and one's office (e.g., acquiring access to high-quality information) to help find information efficiently, and (f) making friends with the librarian at the closest hospital library.

The goal of the remainder of this chapter is to discuss core principles of EBM that apply to issues most relevant to primary care practice: diagnosis, prognosis, treatment, risk or potential harm, and cost-effectiveness. Strategies for keeping up are also discussed. Principles that apply to prevention and screening are discussed in Chapter 14.

DIAGNOSIS

How Clinicians Formulate a Diagnosis

Diagnostic assessment begins the moment one meets a patient. Behavioral scientists have described at least four ways in which clinicians formulate diagnoses: pattern recognition, algorithm, exhaustion, and hypothesis-deduction.

Pattern Recognition

Many diagnoses are made instantly because clinicians have learned to recognize patterns specific to certain diseases, such as the face of a patient with Down's syndrome or the elbows of a patient with psoriasis. The certainty of these types of diagnoses is so great that further testing often is unnecessary.

Algorithm

Algorithms are growing more common as a result of the growth of clinical practice guidelines, which, when grounded scientifically, can be extremely helpful. The drawbacks of algorithms are that they must be constructed before the patient is seen, and they must account for every possibility in a workup. For example, the algorithm for polycythemia must consider cigarette smoking, high-altitude living, and other causes, as well as polycythemia vera.

Exhaustion

As Sackett pointed out (see Sackett et al., *Clinical Epidemiology,* in General References), medical students should be taught how to do a complete history and physical examination, and then be taught never to do one again. However, on occasion, clinicians do resort to comprehensive histories and examinations, as much to buy time to think as to uncover hidden disease.

Hypothesis-Deduction

On most occasions, clinicians diagnose by forming hypotheses and testing them, as is done in scientific experimentation. On hearing that a patient has chest pain, the practitioner builds a short list of hypotheses, invites further description, and then asks focused questions that help confirm or rule out the hypotheses. The questions in the interview and each maneuver in the examination are as much diagnostic tests as the electrocardiogram or the chest radiograph. Studies of clinicians' behavior reveal that the short list of hypotheses usually does not exceed three or four diagnoses. Typically, new hypotheses are added as others are discarded, but the eventual goal is to narrow the list and reduce the uncertainty about which diagnosis is most likely. Studies of clinicians in ambulatory practice showed that hypotheses were generated, on average, 28 seconds into the interview and that correct diagnoses of standard problems were made 6 minutes into 30-minute workups; the correct diagnoses were made in 75% of the encounters (3).

The hypothesis-deduction model reveals a truth common to all methods of diagnosis: A clinician can rarely be absolutely certain of any diagnosis. Clinicians live with uncertainty, and the role of all diagnostic tests—the interview, the physical examination, the laboratory evaluation, trials of empiric treatments, allowing time to pass (expectant observation)—is to narrow the uncertainty enough to place a diagnostic label on a patient's problem. How narrow the uncertainty must be depends on the practitioner's and the patient's tolerance of uncertainty, the severity of the suspected disease, the "treatability" of the suspected disease, and the benefits and risks of possible treatments.

Steps in the Hypothesis-Deduction Process

Evidence shows that clinicians implicitly use common sense and their medical knowledge to reach a diagnosis with adequate certainty. Explicitly, the diagnostic process follows certain steps:

Step 1: Form a Hypothesis and Estimate Its Likelihood

The estimate of likelihood is called the *pretest probability* (or *prior probability*); it simply represents the estimate of prevalence of the disease in a group of people similar to the patient at hand. Each hypothesized diagnosis and the estimate of its likelihood comes initially from evidence collected during the interview and physical examination and from the practitioner's fund of knowledge from sources such as other patients, colleagues, textbooks, and journals. More recently, computer programs have been developed to aid clinicians in making this estimate, and these have the potential to become a powerful tool in clinical decision-making.

Step 2: Decide How Certain the Diagnosis Must Be

If the hypothesized disease is easily and safely treated, one might have to be less certain than if the disease has an ominous prognosis or demands complex, risk-laden treatment. For example, a 75% certainty that a patient has streptococcal pharyngitis might be sufficient to prescribe an antibiotic, whereas a much higher level of certainty would be needed before diagnosing and treating a patient with suspected leukemia. If the pretest probability is above the threshold for a hypothesized disease (e.g., greater than 75% for streptococcal pharyngitis), then further tests are unnecessary and treatment is prescribed. Conversely, if one is adequately certain that the patient does not have the hypothesized disease (e.g., 90% probability that the patient does not have streptococcal pharyngitis), then no further tests are required and the patient can be reassured and educated. However, if the level of uncertainty remains between these two extremes, further testing (e.g., a throat culture) can help move the case toward one extreme or the other. Diagnostic testing usually is most helpful between the two extremes of certainty, whereas further testing usually has little impact on the posttest probability if the pretest probability is very high or very low.

Step 3: Choose a Diagnostic Test

Which test to choose depends on many factors: its safety, its *accuracy* (e.g., how closely an observation or a test result reflects the true clinical state of a patient), how easily it can be done, its cost, and, not least, the patient's preferences and values regarding tests, especially those that carry risks. Accuracy includes both reliability and validity. *Reliability* of a test, also called reproducibility or precision, is the extent to which repeated measurements of a stable phenomenon give results close to one another. *Validity* is the degree to which a test measures what it is supposed to measure. A test can be reliable but not valid (i.e., it reliably measures the wrong phenomenon), or it can be valid but not reliable (i.e., it measures the phenomenon of interest, but with wide scatter).

When considering a test, one needs to reflect on each of these factors. Practical guidelines to assess and critically appraise reported studies of diagnostic tests are summarized in Table 2.1. When selecting a test for a patient, the crucial questions to ask are, "Will the results of the test change my plan?" and "Will my patient be better off from having had the test?" (*the utility of the test*). If the answer to these questions is "No," the test should not be performed.

Step 4: Be Aware of the Test's Performance Characteristics

Every diagnostic test has a sensitivity and specificity for each disease it tests for. For example, if one is checking for anemia caused by hemolysis, a hematocrit is very sensitive but not very specific. However, if one is trying simply to diagnose anemia, the same test becomes 100% specific, because anemia is defined as a low hematocrit.

Table 2.1. Guidelines for Assessing a Study of a Diagnostic Test

Was there an independent blind comparison with a gold standard?
Was the test evaluated in a sample of patients that included an appropriate spectrum of disease (mild and severe, treated and untreated) plus patients with different but commonly confused disorders?
Was the setting for the evaluation adequately described?
Were the reproducibility of the test result (precision) and its interpretation (observer variation) determined?
Was the term *normal* defined sensibly?
Were the methodologies for conducting the test described well enough for their exact replication?
Was the utility of the test determined (i.e., were the patients better off for having had the test)?

Adapted from Sackett DL, Haynes RB, Guyatt GH, et al. Clinical epidemiology: a basic science for clinical medicine. 2nd ed. Boston: Little, Brown, 1991.

Sensitivity and *specificity* have become common terms in medical discussion, but they are commonly misunderstood. The 2×2 table in Fig. 2.1 reveals much about these and other terms. A fundamental fact about sensitivity and specificity is that they are determined by researchers, not by clinicians. Researchers study groups of patients with or without disease, and they go about measuring how well tests perform when applied to those two known groups. The sensitivity of a test (the *true positive rate*) is equal to the number of study subjects with a given disease who have a positive test divided by all study subjects with the disease. The specificity of a test (the *true negative rate*) is the number of study subjects without the disease who have a negative test divided by all those without the disease. "Diseased" and "not diseased" are labels that reflect a best test or a definition of a certain disease: the so-called *gold standard.* For pulmonary embolus, for

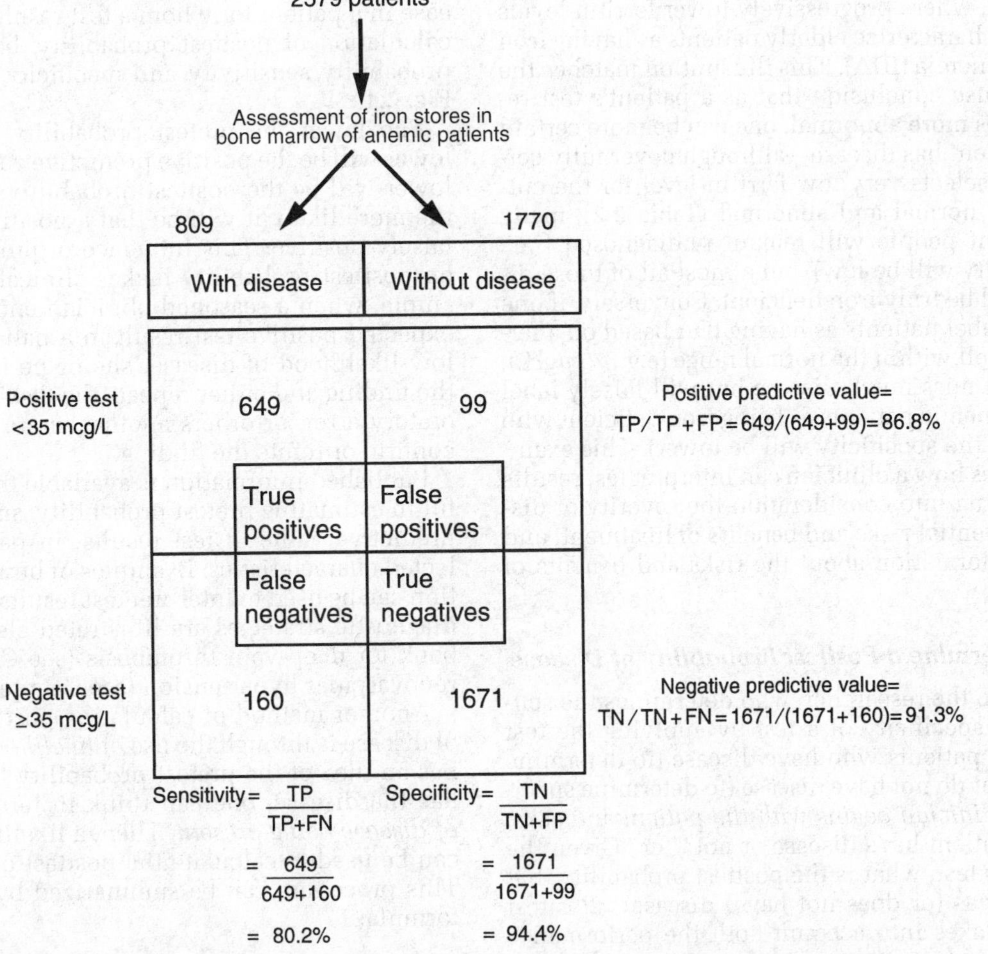

Figure 2.1. Test performance determined by research. Researcher identifies diseased and nondiseased patients using a gold standard and then determines the performance characteristics (sensitivity and specificity) of another test. *Example:* Iron deficiency anemia determination using bone marrow aspirate/biopsy as the gold standard and serum ferritin measurement as the screening test. (Data from Guyatt GH, Patterson C, Ali M, et al. Diagnosis of iron deficiency in the elderly. Am J Med 1990;88:205.)

Table 2.2. Tradeoff Between Sensitivity and Specificity When Diagnosing Iron Deficiency Anemia: Likelihood Ratios

Serum Ferritin Level to be Used as the Cutoff Value (μg/L)	Sensitivity (%)	False Negative Rate (1 − sensitivity, %)	Specificity (%)	False Positive Rate (1 − specificity %)	Positive Likelihood Ratio (sensitivity/false positive rate)	Negative Likelihood Ratio (false negative rate/specificity)
<15	58.6	41.4	98.9	1.1	53.3	0.42
<35	80.2	19.8	94.4	5.6	14.3	0.21
<65	90.4	9.6	84.7	15.3	5.9	0.11
<95	94.1	5.9	75.3	24.7	3.8	0.08

Adapted from Guyatt GH, Patterson C, Ali M, et al. Diagnosis of iron deficiency in the elderly. Am J. Med 1990;88:205 and from Sackett DL, Haynes RB, Guyatt GH, et al. Clinical epidemiology: a basic science for clinical medicine. 2nd ed. Boston: Little, Brown, 1991.

example, the gold standard is the pulmonary angiogram. For angina, there is no sure test, so a case definition becomes the gold standard. Skepticism must be used in evaluating gold standards. For example, when gallbladder ultrasonography was tested for use in the diagnosis of cholelithiasis, it initially seemed to be a poor test in comparison with the gold standard (oral cholecystogram), not because of problems with the new test, but because the gold standard was itself a poor test, as was later shown (4).

Sensitivity and specificity are not static properties of a test. As the cutoff value for an abnormal result is made more extreme, the test's sensitivity decreases and its specificity increases. This principle is illustrated in Table 2.2, where progressively lower ferritin levels are used to characterize elderly patients as having iron deficiency anemia (IDA). This illustration matches the common-sense conclusion that as a patient's test result becomes more abnormal, one can be more certain that the patient has disease—although never fully certain. If one selects very low ferritin level for the cutoff between normal and abnormal (Table 2.2), many iron-deficient people will remain undiagnosed (i.e., the sensitivity will be low), but almost all of those diagnosed will be truly iron deficient. Conversely, if one decides to label patients as having IDA based on a ferritin level well within the normal range (e.g., 75 μg/L), one will not miss much disease but will falsely label numerous anemic patients as being iron deficient who are not (i.e., the specificity will be lower). This example illustrates how a clinician can interpret test results flexibly, taking into consideration the severity of disease, the potential risks and benefits of treatment, and changing information about the risks and benefits of treatment.

Step 5: Determine a Posttest Probability of Disease

In contrast to the researcher, who determines the sensitivity and specificity of a test by applying the test to groups of patients who have disease (to determine sensitivity) or do not have disease (to determine specificity), *the clinician begins with the patient* and asks, "Does my patient have disease or not?" or "Given the result of this test, what is the posttest probability that my patient has (or does not have) disease?" Posttest probability takes into account both the performance characteristics (sensitivity and specificity) of the test and the pretest (prior) probability of disease in a group of patients similar to the patient in question.

One method for determining posttest probability is through the use of *predictive values.* Predictive values can be calculated from the known sensitivity and specificity of a test and the estimated pretest probability of disease. Sensitivity and specificity usually are transferable from study to practice settings, provided the diseased and nondiseased populations in the study and in the practice settings are similar. Sensitivity and specificity usually are not influenced by the prevalence, or pretest probability, of disease. However, predictive values must be recalculated for each patient or population based on the estimated pretest probability or prevalence of disease in that particular group. Positive predictive value is the probability of disease in a patient who has an abnormal test result. Negative predictive value is the probability of no disease in a patient for whom a test result is normal. The calculation of posttest probability, based on pretest probability, sensitivity, and specificity, is illustrated in Fig. 2.1.

The lower the pretest probability of disease, the lower will be the positive predictive value of a test, the lower will be the posttest probability of disease, and the more likely it will be that a positive test result is falsely positive. This influence of pretest probability on posttest probability makes clinical sense. For example, when a seasoned clinician encounters an unexpected positive test result in a patient with a very low likelihood of disease, she or he is suspicious of the finding and either repeats the test, suspecting laboratory error, or orders another, more specific test to confirm or refute the finding.

Published information is available that can be helpful in estimating pretest probability, and therefore the predictive value of test results, in patients with selected characteristics. Examples of how such information can be used to interpret test results and determine diagnostic strategies are illustrated elsewhere in this book for deep vein thrombosis (see Chapter 57) and renovascular hypertension (see Chapter 67).

Another method of calculating posttest probability of disease is through the use of *likelihood ratios.* If one has an idea of the pretest probability that the patient has the disease, one can think in terms of the *odds of disease being present.* Then, a likelihood ratio (LR) can be used to calculate the posttest odds of disease. This procedure can be summarized by the following formula:

$$\text{Posttest odds} = \text{Pretest odds} \times \text{Likelihood ratio}$$

LRs combine the relationships of sensitivity and specificity into a single number. The positive LR is the sensitivity divided by the false positive rate, and the negative LR is the false negative rate divided by the specificity (see calculated LRs for various cutoff points to screen for IDA in Table 2.2). The use of LRs requires the conversion of probabilities to odds for the calculation, then back to probabilities after the calculation. This can easily be performed with the use of the following equations:

$$\text{Odds} = \text{Probability} \div (1 - \text{Probability})$$

$$\text{Probability} = \text{Odds} \div (1 + \text{Odds})$$

For example, suppose the clinician is faced with a 67-year-old male patient who has increasing fatigue and decreasing energy. He has not seen a clinician for 10 years, and he does not recall ever having had any blood tests. A thorough review of systems is unremarkable; the patient has no past medical history and takes no medications. The physical examination is also within normal limits. Laboratory testing is normal except for the following findings: hemoglobin, 11.0 g/dL (normal, 13.9 to 16.3 g/dL); hematocrit, 29% (normal, 41% to 53%); mean corpuscular volume, 82 fL (normal, 80 to 100 fL); mean corpuscular hemoglobin concentration, 32.0 g/dL (normal, 31.0 to 37.0 g/dL); and a red cell distribution width of 13.5% (normal, 11.5% to 14.5%). Knowing that the baseline prevalence (pretest probability) of IDA among anemic elderly patients has been found to be 31% (5), one might consider this man's pretest probability for IDA to be 33%, for an odds of 1 to 2, or 0.5. On learning the results of the initial blood test, the clinician asks the laboratory to add a serum ferritin test, and the result is 33 μg/L (normal, 20 to 200 μg/L). If one considers this level to be a positive result,

$$\text{Posttest odds of IDA} = \text{Pretest odds} \times (+)\text{LR} = 0.5 \times (0.802 \div 0.056) = 0.5 \times 14.3 = 7.16$$

So the patient has 7:1 odds of having IDA based on this test result. Converting back to probability, the patient has a posttest probability of IDA of about $7 \div (1 + 7) = 7 \div 8 = 88\%$. Given this posttest probability, further diagnostic workup (e.g., colonoscopy) to identify the cause of the IDA would be appropriate.

Figure 2.2 provides a nomogram that allows one to convert pretest to posttest probabilities, given a known LR, without having to convert back and forth between odds and probabilities. This alternative is quick, is easy to use, and decreases the chances of calculation error.

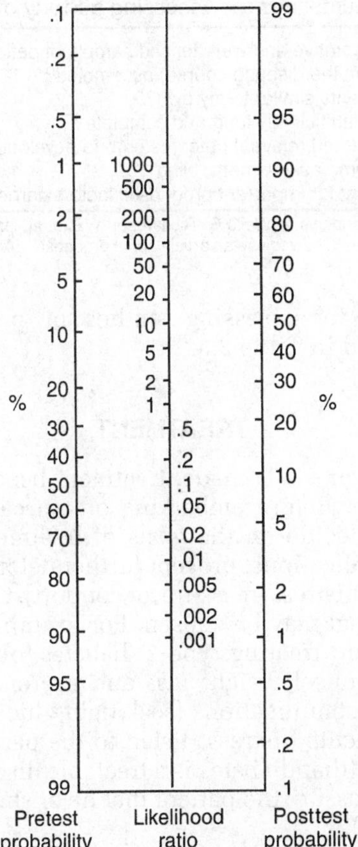

Figure 2.2. Nomogram for interpreting test results using likelihood ratios (LRs). *Example from text:* An elderly male patient with anemia has a pretest probability of having iron deficiency anemia (IDA) equal to 33%. His serum ferritin level is 33 μg/L, which is associated with a positive LR of 14.3. Extending a straight line through the pretest probability of 33% and the LR of 14.3 results in a posttest probability of 88%. (Adapted from Fagan TJ. Nomogram for Bayes' theorem. N Engl J Med 1975;293:257).

PROGNOSIS

Often, the information that is most important to a patient who has a new diagnosis is the prognosis ("What is going to happen to me?"). In choosing therapy, one decides what one can do for the patient's disease. Yet, predicting what will happen to a particular patient usually is not possible, and clinicians must rely on probabilities. Sometimes, specific characteristics ("prognostic factors") such as demographic factors, disease-specific factors, and comorbidities can help further delineate a patient's prognosis. Clinical prediction rules that take these factors into account can help practitioners arrive at more accurate estimates of prognosis.

Prognosis can be addressed in two ways: the *natural history* of a disease and the *clinical course* of a disease. Because few diseases today progress without medical intervention, less is being learned about natural history and more is being learned about clinical course. For example, the natural history of diabetes in the late 20th century is unknown because virtually no diagnosed patients go without some type of therapy. But, through many studies, more is known about the course of treated diabetes (6).

Most information about prognosis comes from prospective cohort studies, in which patients with a disease are monitored over time. Cohort studies may include only untreated subjects (natural history of a disease), only treated subjects, or a combination of both treated and untreated subjects (clinical course of a disease). Cohort studies are simple in design, yet they are often costly in time and money. They are susceptible to biases, such as *sampling bias,* in which the group of patients being monitored is not representative all patients with that condition. Suggested

Table 2.3. Guidelines for Assessing a Study of Prognosis

Was a representative and well-defined sample of patients (at a similar point in the disease course) assembled?
Are these patients similar to my own?
Was follow-up sufficiently long and complete?
Were objective and relevant outcome criteria developed and used?
Was the outcome assessment "blind"?
Was adjustment for important prognostic factors carried out?

Adapted from Laupacis A, Wells G, Richardson WS, et al. User's guides to the medical literature. V: how to use an article about prognosis. JAMA 1994:272:234.

guidelines for assessing studies of prognosis are summarized in Table 2.3.

TREATMENT

Once a diagnosis is made, treatment becomes the focus of care. Before embarking on a treatment plan, one must decide on the goals of treatment (to cure, delay complications, prevent further deterioration, relieve acute distress, reassure, or comfort). Clearly, more than one goal may be chosen. For example, when diagnosing and treating type 2 diabetes, one may seek to cure (counsel weight loss and exercise), to delay or prevent complications (seek tight glucose control), to relieve acute distress (listen to the patient's fears), to reassure (that diabetes is a treatable disease), and to comfort (reassure the patient that he or she will not be abandoned).

Once the goals have been set, treatments are chosen. Unfortunately, many treatments have never been tested scientifically to answer the questions of interest to clinicians and their patients (e.g., probability of benefit, size of benefit, onset time and duration of response, frequency of complications of treatment), and many aspects of treatment are difficult to measure through scientific experiments. These situations are changing as drugs and procedures are increasingly being subjected to clinical trials and measures of quality of life are being included in the evaluation of therapies.

The *clinical trial* is the current standard for assessment of drugs and therapeutic procedures. The strongest clinical trials are randomized, double-blinded controlled trials. The strength of a *randomized controlled trial* (RCT) is that the study groups are likely to be similar with respect to known determinants of outcome, as well as those determinants that are unknown. However, randomization is often difficult to accomplish in the real world, where patients are free to join or refuse to join a clinical trial and where money to support research is limited. Theoretically, in a trial that is *double-blinded* (meaning that neither the patient nor the researcher knows who is receiving the experimental treatment) the researchers' and patients' assessment of outcome is not biased by prior knowledge of their assignment (e.g., to placebo or to active treatment). However, studies are seldom truly blinded; for example, a trial of beta-blockers against placebo for hypertension cannot be truly blinded because patients and clinicians can measure pulse rates. Nonetheless, the clinical trial is the least biased method currently available for researchers to test how well drugs and other interventions work in ideal situations (*efficacy*) and in the real world (*effectiveness*). Table 2.4 lists guidelines that clinicians can use when assessing the results of a treatment trial for patients in their practice. As illustrated in the table, there are important questions to ask of a clinical trial that reports benefits to treated subjects. Were clinically relevant outcomes, such as measures of patient health (e.g., morbid events, functional status) reported, and not just surrogate end points (e.g., reduction of blood pressure)? Was all-cause mortality, not just mortality due to the disease in question (e.g., colon cancer), reported? In addition to reporting the statistical significance of findings (the probability that the findings are true), did the study discuss or clarify the clinical significance of the findings (whether the benefits were clinically meaningful as well as statistically significant)? As the size of a study increases, there is an increased likelihood that clinically small or nonmeaningful benefits, which are nonetheless statistically significant, will be demonstrated (see example in the next paragraph). *Intention-to-treat* analysis is a strategy for analyzing data in which all study participants are analyzed in the group to which they were assigned, regardless of whether they dropped out, were noncompliant, or crossed over to another treatment or nontreatment group. Such an analysis may weaken the ability of a study to demonstrate the effect of a treatment, but it prevents selection biases caused by differences in participants who drop out from a treatment compared with those who remain.

Table 2.4. Guidelines for Assessing a Study of Treatment (Clinical Trials)

Was the assignment of patients to treatments really randomized?
Were all clinically relevant outcomes reported?
Were the study patients recognizably similar to my own?
Were both statistical and clinical significance considered?
Is the treatment feasible for patients in my practice?
Was the analysis performed on an intention-to-treat basis?
Were all patients who entered the study accounted for at its conclusion?

Adapted from Sackett DL, Haynes RB, Guyatt GH, et al. Clinical epidemiology: a basic science for clinical medicine. 2nd ed. Boston: Little, Brown, 1991.

Researchers often report the relative risk reduction of a treatment or the relative risk of adverse events. The *relative risk reduction* (RRR) is the difference in the event rate between a control and an experimental group of patients expressed as a proportion of the event rate in the control group: RRR = (control event rate − experimental event rate) ÷ control event rate. *Relative risk* (RR) is a way to present excess risk; it can be calculated by dividing the incidence of disease in the exposed group by the incidence of disease in the unexposed group. A benefit (decreased risk) will be seen if the exposure is protective in relation to the disease in question. Although these measures are useful, they can be misleading when applied to individual patients. For example, yearly mammography examinations for women between the ages of 50 and 74 years was reported in one study to reduce the risk of death from breast cancer by 33% (RR, .67); however, the *absolute risk reduction* (ARR) over 7 years was only 0.06% (7). The ARR (also known as "risk difference") simply represents the difference in event rates between the two groups of patients: ARR = control event rate − experimental event rate. This example demonstrates that these numbers give very different impressions of the impact of an intervention.

Clinically helpful information can usually be extracted by a careful reading of the original report of a clinical trial. *Number needed to treat* (NNT) (also called "number needed to test") is a very useful concept in practice. It refers to the number of persons who need to be treated (or tested) for one person to benefit (or be diagnosed or harmed). The calculation for NNT is simply 1/ARR, with ARR presented as a fraction (e.g., .10 for an ARR of 10%).

The concepts just described can be demonstrated using data from the Diabetes Control and Complications Trial (8), which reported the clinical results of "tight control" of glucose in patients with type 1 diabetes. In considering progression to neuropathy, the researchers reported an RRR of 71% over 5 years among patients using "tight control" (three or more insulin injections per day or use of an insulin pump), compared with those receiving "usual care" (one to two insulin injections per day). This also can be expressed as an RR of 3.4 for those in usual care compared with patients in tight control (RR = 1 ÷ [1 − RRR]). But in analyzing the study's data, one can estimate the ARR and therefore the NNT with intensive insulin therapy to prevent one case of neuropathy. Table 2.5 explains this estimate. In this example, the ARR is 6.8%, and about 15 patients with type 1 diabetes would have to be aggressively treated for 5 years to prevent one case of neuropathy. As for any therapeutic intervention, one should also consider the potential for harm, which can be described as the NNT to produce one episode of severe hypoglycemia (in this case, two patients per year). Armed with this information about benefit and harm, patients and clinicians can together make appropriate decisions for the best care of an individual patient.

There are a few caveats about clinical trials. Although the RCT is the best study design for assessing the value of a treatment, one should be cautious about relying on the results of any single study, even one that was done well. Systematic reviews and meta-analyses, which combine the results a number of studies, are discussed later in this chapter (see Keeping Up). Sometimes clinical trials have not been performed. In this situation, the clinician may need to rely on cohort, case-control, or cross-sectional studies that assess treatment instead of, or in addition to, harm. These types of studies are discussed in the following section.

RISK OR POTENTIAL HARM

Practitioners are frequently called on to make assessments and judgments regarding risk or potential harm resulting from either medical interventions or environmental exposures. Some guidelines for assessing evidence of harm are summarized in Table 2.6. Ideally, these questions would be answered in an RCT; however, for obvious reasons, RCTs are rarely undertaken with the intent of studying a harmful exposure. Sometimes, a potentially beneficial intervention is unexpectedly found to be harmful in a clinical trial; in other trials, there may be both benefits and harms associated with the intervention.

More commonly, harm is addressed through cohort studies. In *cohort studies,* exposed and unexposed patients are identified and monitored for a period of time, and outcomes in the two groups are compared. For example, a cohort of cigarette smokers and nonsmokers could be monitored and the incidence of lung cancer in both groups measured. In these studies, the two groups may be different with respect to important determinants of outcome other than the exposure being studied. Researchers often can statistically adjust for these factors, but there may be other contributing factors of which they are unaware.

Another method of assessing harm is through *case-control studies.* In these studies, patients with an outcome of interest (cases) are identified and compared with others who are similar in respects other than the outcome (controls). Exposure rates in the case and control groups are then compared to look at the association

Table 2.6. Guidelines for Assessing a Study of Harm

What type of study was reported: a prospective cohort study, with or without a comparison group; a retrospective case-control study; a cross-sectional study; a case series; or a case report?
Were comparison groups clearly identified and similar with respect to potential determinants of outcome, other than the one of concern? If not, were differences in potential determinants controlled for in the analysis of data?
Were outcomes measured the same way in the groups compared (and was the assessment objective and blinded)?
Was follow-up sufficiently long and complete?
Was there a temporal relationship between exposure and harm?
Was there a dose-response gradient?
What was the magnitude of the risk, and how precise is this estimate?

Adapted from Levine M, Walter S, Lee H, et al. User's guides to the medical literature. IV: How to use an article about harm. JAMA 1994;271:1615.

Table 2.5. Use of Data to Estimate Clinical Consequences of Treatment: The Diabetes Control and Complications Trial

Occurrence of Neuropathy at 5 yr Among Type 1 Diabetic Patients		RRR	ARR	NNT to Benefit One Patient
CER: Usual Insulin	EER: Intensive Insulin	(CER − EER) ÷ CER	CER − EER	1 ÷ ARR
9.6%	2.8%	(9.6% − 2.8%) ÷ 9.6% = 71%	9.6% − 2.8% = 6.8%	1 + 6.8% = 15 patients, for 5 years, with intensive treatment

ARR, Absolute risk reduction; CER, control event rate; EER, experimental event rate; NNT, number needed to treat; RRR, relative risk reduction.

From The Diabetes Control and Complications Trial Research Group. The effect of intensive treatment of diabetes on the development and progression of long-term complications in insulin-dependent diabetes mellitus. N Engl J Med 1993; 329:977.

between the exposure and the outcome. For example, a group of patients with lung cancer may be compared with a group of patients of similar age and gender, with the smoking rate in each group compared. These studies, like cohort studies, are limited by the possibility of differences in other unidentified risk factors between the groups. In addition, they are subject to *recall bias*: patients with an illness may be more likely to recall or report an unusual exposure than those who are not ill.

Cohort and case-control studies can also be used to assess medical interventions, as was done in studies that have demonstrated a cardiovascular benefit of hormone replacement therapy. However, this benefit was not demonstrated when studied in an RCT (9), calling the purported benefit into question.

Weaker designs for identifying risk or harm include cross-sectional studies, case series, and case reports. *Cross-sectional studies* can establish associations but not causal links. They are strengthened by statistical methods that control for confounding variables (potential determinants of harm other than the one of concern). Temporal relationships, however, are usually not established. In *case reports* or *case series,* adverse outcomes associated with a particular exposure are reported in a single patient or group of patients. These reports are useful for identifying potentially harmful exposures to be studied further, but they are weak evidence for a causal relationship by themselves. However, if the outcome is very harmful and otherwise rare, this kind of evidence may be sufficient to take action. This might occur, for example, when severe adverse reactions associated with a particular medication are reported, especially if safer alternatives exist. A recent example is troglitazone, which was taken off the market after case reports of severe hepatotoxicity associated with its use.

COST-EFFECTIVENESS

In ambulatory practice, cost considerations arise frequently. Cost-effectiveness analyses evaluate health care outcomes in relation to cost. The primary goals are to determine the most efficient use of resources and to minimize the costs associated with the achievement of health goals and objectives. A common strategy for cost-effectiveness studies is to compare a novel approach or therapy with the current practice or standard of care. The time frame of the study should be long enough to allow for costs and long-term benefits to be realized. The perspective of the analysis takes into account who benefits from the intervention as well as who pays for it (society, the payer, or the patient).

Whether decisions are being made for a population (e.g., frequency of screening colonoscopy, drugs to be added to a formulary) or for a particular patient (e.g., choice of antihypertensive medicine), the potential benefits should be weighed against the resources used and money spent. Some guidelines for assessing evidence in studies performing economic analyses are summarized in Table 2.7.

Table 2.7. Guidelines for Assessing a Study with an Economic Analysis of Clinical Practice

Did the analysis provide a full economic comparison of health care strategies?
Were the costs and outcomes appropriately measured and valued?
Were the estimates of costs and outcomes related to the baseline risk in the treatment population?
Was a sensitivity analysis performed that included a range of estimates for important assumptions? Are the findings consistent across reasonable ranges of assumptions, or do they change as the assumptions vary within reasonable ranges?
What were the incremental costs and outcomes of each strategy?
Are treatment benefits worth the harms and costs?

Adapted from Drummond MF, Richardson WS, O'Brien BJ, et al. User's guides to the medical literature. XIII: How to use an article on economic analysis of clinical practice. JAMA 1997;277:1552.

In *cost-effectiveness analyses,* costs usually are measured in monetary units (e.g., dollars) and a single clinical outcome is considered (e.g., mortality). In *cost-utility analyses,* multiple clinical outcomes, including quality of life, are represented and result in the calculation of "quality-adjusted life years." In both types of analyses, alternative diagnostic or therapeutic approaches are studied with a primary emphasis placed on economic considerations.

KEEPING UP

One of the major challenges to clinicians is keeping one's personal fund of medical knowledge current. For primary care practitioners who are expected to know about a wide array of clinical topics ("jacks of all trades"), keeping up to date can be particularly difficult. It has been suggested that each practitioner should develop a personal mission as to the extent of "up-to-datedness" he or she hopes to achieve and maintain. Two questions that may help to better define this territory are (a) "What information do I need to have in my head to be satisfied with my knowledge base for the performance of my job?" and (b) "What information would I be embarrassed not to know?" (10).

One author estimated that if clinicians tried to keep up with the medical literature by reading one article each day, they would be 55 centuries behind in their reading after 1 year (see Sackett et al., *Clinical Epidemiology,* in General References). In a seminal study, experienced clinicians in ambulatory practice who said they had about two clinical questions per week that went unanswered, were found, when shadowed in day-to-day practice, to actually have about two unanswered questions for every three patients seen (11). Moreover, although these clinicians said that their main sources of information were textbooks and journals, their behavior showed that they got most of their clinical information from colleagues and drug detailers. Fortunately, in ambulatory medicine, there exist some *high-quality secondary or abstracting publications* that produce abstracts and often provide expert commentary on clinical articles believed to be of particular importance (approximately 2% to 3% of articles screened from hundreds of journals) (12).

Table 2.8. Elements of an Information Plan

Browse at least one general journal regularly.
Maintain surveillance on new information.
Establish reliable ways of looking up common facts.
Identify a set of ways to look up obscure facts.
Develop critical appraisal skills.
Set aside high-quality time regularly to deal with information needs.
Invest time to discover new sources of useful information.

From Fletcher RH, Fletcher SW. Keeping clinically up-to-date. J Gen Intern Med 1997;12:S5.

Examples are the *ACP Journal Club* and *Evidence-Based Medicine.*

Scheduling of time to obtain and find relevant reading material is a critical step in keeping up to date. The actual reading of the pulled material can occur either in the scheduled time or when a lull presents itself (e.g., a patient no-show). *Proactive* scanning or browsing through a small number of peer-reviewed journals that regularly yield articles relevant to one's clinical practice is an integral part of keeping up. *Reactive* learning (also called problem-focused learning) is stimulated by clinical encounters or questions from patients or medical learners and requires searching to find the appropriate materials (steps 1 and 2 of the core EBM skills described at the beginning of the chapter). Sackett described the *"educational prescription"* as a means of phrasing and keeping track of questions as they arise with the goal and intent of searching for the best available evidence to answer these queries at some time later. A combination of proactive and reactive approaches is thought to represent the ideal balance for dealing with the evolution of medical knowledge. Several additional ideas have been suggested by insightful authors who are keenly aware of the challenge of keeping clinically up to date (Table 2.8) (13).

Although original research articles continue to be an excellent source for new information, other types of publications can also be helpful in the quest to stay current. One common source of medical information is the *overview.* The chapters of this book (and other textbooks) are one example of an overview; review articles in medical journals are another. These types of overviews are easy to access (especially if the textbook is at hand) and easy to use; they require little work or effort to obtain needed information. However, they are limited by the biases and limitations of the authors and typically do not explain how the information was gathered or how conclusions were reached.

Systematic reviews and meta-analyses published in peer-reviewed journals with detailed methods describing specifically the literature search and the inclusion/exclusion criteria of the original articles can be invaluable. Critical appraisal methods for these two article types have been developed and can be applied to evaluate the quality of the work (14). These methods are summarized in Table 2.9. Some of the limitations that still need to be considered include the heterogeneity of studies (with regard to populations studied and outcomes assessed) and the fact that small studies with negative results are less likely to be published than those with positive results (*publication bias*). Authors often try to correct for these limitations, but meta-analyses have sometimes yielded results and conclusions that were discordant with subsequent large RCTs (15). Nevertheless, meta-analysis can be a powerful tool to synthesize the available evidence in an unbiased fashion. In addition to those published in medical journals, the *Cochrane Collaboration* (and the Cochrane Library—see General References) represents an international endeavor to develop, maintain, and disseminate systematic reviews on clinical and health related topics.

Table 2.9. Guidelines for Assessing a Review Article

Are the results of the study valid?
Did the review address an explicitly described, focused clinical question?
Were appropriate criteria used for selecting studies for review?
Were inclusion and exclusion criteria appropriate?
Were search strategies explicitly described, thorough, and appropriate? Is it unlikely that important, relevant studies were missed?
Was the validity of the included studies appraised and accounted for?
Were assessments of the studies reproducible?
Were results similar from study to study?
If data from different studies were combined quantitatively, were the methods of synthesizing the data explicit and reasonable?
What are the results?
What are the overall results of the review?
How precise are the results?
Are the results presented in a clear manner that permits comparison of and synthesis of the key features and findings of the studies reviewed?
Will the results help me in caring for my patients?
Can the results be applied to my patient care?
Were all clinically important outcomes (benefits and harms) considered?
Are the benefits worth the harms and costs?

Adapted from Oxman AD, Cook DJ, Guyatt GH. Users' guides to the medical literature. VI: How to use an overview. Evidence-Based Medicine Working Group. JAMA 1994;272:1367.

Guidelines are systematically developed statements that offer recommendations to assist with decision-making in specific situations. It has been found that clinicians often do not employ interventions that have been shown to be effective (e.g., prescribing beta-blockers to patients after a myocardial infarction) (16). Guidelines serve the dual purpose of offering easily accessible recommendations for practitioners and publicizing these recommendations to practitioners and the general public. Guidelines typically are developed by expert panels. They are best when they employ explicit criteria for gathering the evidence and making recommendations and acknowledge the level of evidence for each recommendation. Guidelines may be biased by the composition of the expert panel, and sometimes conflicting guidelines are disseminated by different organizations. For example, the American Cancer Society recommends offering digital rectal examination and prostate-specific antigen determinations to screen for prostate cancer, whereas the United States Preventive Services Task Force recommends against them. Some suggestions for evaluating practice guidelines are listed in Table 2.10.

Table 2.10. Guidelines for Assessing a Practice Guideline

Was a recent, reproducible and comprehensive review of the literature carried out?
Were the methods of the review explicit and strong? Specifically, were inclusion and exclusion criteria explicit and reasonable? Were methods of synthesizing the data explicit and reasonable? Was each recommendation assigned a level of evidence supporting it and a strength based on an explicit synthesis of all considerations?
How does this guideline compare to other existing guidelines? Do the groups or organizations issuing this or other related guidelines have biases or conflicts of interest?
Have important large-scale studies been conducted subsequent to the guideline that would alter the recommendations in the guideline?
Does the burden of the problem addressed warrant implementation of the guideline?
Would implementation of the guideline be cost-effective and feasible?

Adapted from Sackett DL, Straus SE, Richardson WS, et al. Evidence-Based Medicine: how to practice and teach EBM. 2nd ed. Edinburgh: Churchill Livingstone, 2000.

Each information source has strengths and weaknesses. Colleagues may be misinformed. Drug detailers have a product to sell, making them biased. Textbooks are often out of date by the time they are printed. Traditional continuing medical education courses have been shown to have virtually no effect on practice and provide variable degrees of evidence-based education.

Because "keeping up" with the medical literature represents a colossal challenge, some authors have provided some direction for how optimize the chance that one's time investment will result in a reasonable return (17,18). They suggest that the usefulness of medical information for a given provider is proportional to its relevance, validity, and accessibility. *Relevance* relates to the frequency with which the provider encounters the topic. *Validity* refers to the quality of the information and the likelihood that the information is true. *Accessibility* connotes the ease with which the information source can be retrieved. These authors recommend that practitioners pay particular attention to information sources that are relevant, valid, and easily accessible.

Finally, *medical librarians* can be extraordinary helpful in keeping clinicians in touch with changes in the medical literature, and they most are happy to meet with clinicians to make them aware of new resources. For example, our librarian recently informed us about PubMed's feature called "cubby" that allows one to store a search strategy and run it periodically to see what has been added since the last run. Befriending one's medical librarian is a critical component of a "keeping up" strategy and can pay huge dividends in the pursuit of evidence-based medical practice.

General References*

ACP Journal Club. Philadelphia: The American College of Physicians.

An abstracting journal published since 1991.

Black ER, Bordley DR, Tape TG, et al. Diagnostic strategies for common medical problems. 2nd ed. Philadelphia: American College of Physicians, 1999.

Contributors take on 51 common problems in internal medicine, from pharyngitis to cancer, and apply clinical epidemiologic principles to them.

Center for Evidence-Based Medicine, Oxford, England, website. Available at: http://cebm.jr2.ox.ac.uk/. Accessed December 2, 2001.

A core website for EBM. It includes numerous tools to practice EBM, databases of current clinical evidence, links to evidence-based journals and Internet-based journals, and links to other EBM sites, such as the Cochrane Collaboration, the NHS Center for Reviews and Dissemination at the University of York, and McMaster University's EBM site.

Cochrane Library website. Available at: http://www. cochrane.org/. Accessed December 2, 2001.

The Cochrane Collaboration has been developed to prepare, maintain, and disseminate systemic reviews of health care–related topics.

Evidence-Based Medicine. Philadelphia: The American College of Physicians.

An abstracting journal published since 1995.

Fletcher RH, Fletcher SW, Wagner EH, eds. Clinical epidemiology: the essentials. 3rd ed. Baltimore: Williams & Wilkins, 1996.

All important points are simply and accurately illustrated. The book focuses on study design and its importance to the clinician, with special attention to newer developments such as meta-analysis and clinical guideline development.

Gray JAM. Evidence-based healthcare: How to make health policy and management decisions. Edinburgh: Churchill Livingstone, 1997.

The book explains how evidence can be applied to health policy and management decisions for populations, rather than for individual patients.

Kassirer JP, Kopelman RI, eds. Learning clinical reasoning. Baltimore: Williams & Wilkins, 1991.

The authors examine how physicians think and sometimes err in diagnostic logic.

National Library of Medicine (NLM) website. Available at: http://www.nlm.nih.gov. Accessed December 2, 2001.

PubMed and other NLM databases are freely accessible to users worldwide to help those in search of health-related information.

Phillips CL, ed. Logic in medicine. 2nd ed. Belfast: BMJ Publishing Group, 1996. (Distributed in the United States by the American College of Physicians.)

A British book that looks at the philosophical underpinnings of why practitioners behave as they do. It does not address day-to-day practice, but it is an excellent review for those who seek the deeper meanings of clinicians' behavior as they work with patients.

Sackett DL, Haynes RB, Guyatt GH, et al. Clinical epidemiology: a basic science for clinical medicine. 2nd ed. Boston: Little, Brown, 1991.

Based on the evidence-based medicine curriculum at McMaster University, this book uses the same principles to demonstrate that clinical epidemiology is truly a bedside (office) science.

Sackett DL, Straus SE, Richardson WS, et al. Evidence-based medicine: how to teach and practice EBM. 2nd ed. New York: Churchill Livingstone, 2000.

A pocket handbook that helps learners (students or experienced clinicians) take patient problems, develop answerable questions, efficiently search out evidence, and assess whether the current evidence is adequate to direct practice.

Specific References

1. Sackett DL, Rosenberg WM, Gray JAM, et al. Evidence-based medicine: what it is and what it isn't. BMJ 1996;312:71.
2. Wilkinson EK, Bosanquet A, Salisbury C, et al. Barriers and facilitators to the implementation of evidence-based medicine in general practice: a qualitative study. Eur J Gen Pract 1999;5:66.
3. Barrows HS, Norman GR, Neufeld VR, et al. The clinical reasoning of randomly selected physicians in general medical practice. Clin Invest Med 1982;5:49.
4. Shea JA, Berlin JA, Escarce JJ, et al. Revised estimates of diagnostic test sensitivity and specificity in suspected biliary tract disease. Arch Intern Med 1994;154:2573.

*Bold print (general references) and bold numerals (specific references) denote published clinical trials, meta-analyses, or consensus-based recommendations.

5. Guyatt GH, Patterson C, Ali M, et al. Diagnosis of iron deficiency in the elderly. Am J Med 1990;88:205.
6. Wang PH, Lau J, Chalmers TC. Meta-analysis of effects of intensive blood-glucose control on late complications of type I diabetes. Lancet 1993;341:1306.
7. Tabar L, Fagerberg CJ, Gad A, et al. Reduction in mortality from breast cancer after mass screening with mammography. Lancet 1985;8433:829.
8. The Diabetes Control and Complications Trial Research Group. The effect of intensive treatment of diabetes on the development and progression of long-term complications in insulin-dependent diabetes mellitus. N Engl J Med 1993;329:977.
9. Hulley S, Grady D, Bush T, et al. Randomized trial of estrogen plus progestin for secondary prevention of coronary heart disease in postmenopausal women. Heart and Estrogen/progestin Replacement Study (HERS) Research Group. JAMA 1998;280:605.
10. Laine C. How can physicians keep up to date? Annu Rev Med 1999;50:99.
11. Covell DG, Uman CG, Manning PR. Information needs in office practice: are they being met? Ann Intern Med 1985;103:596.
12. Wyatt JC. Reading journals and monitoring the published work. J R Soc Med 2000;93:423.
13. Fletcher RH, Fletcher SW. Evidence-based approach to the medical literature. J Gen Intern Med 1997;12:S5.
14. Oxman AD, Cook DJ, Guyatt GH. Users' guides to the medical literature: VI. How to use an overview. Evidence-Based Medicine Working Group. JAMA 1994;272:1367.
15. Borzak S, Ridker PM. Discordance between meta-analyses and large-scale randomized controlled trials: examples from the management of acute myocardial infarction. Ann Intern Med 1995;123:873.
16. Kennedy HL. Current utilization trends for beta-blockers in cardiovascular disease. Am J Med 2001;[Suppl 5A]:2S.
17. Smith R. What clinical information do clinicians need? BMJ 1996;313:1062.
18. Shaughnessy AF, Slawson DC, Bennett JH. Becoming an information master: a guidebook to the medical information jungle. J Fam Pract 1994;39:489.

C H A P T E R 3

The Practitioner–Patient Relationship and Communication During Clinical Encounters

L. RANDOL BARKER, MD, ScD

Each practitioner–patient relationship is established through person-to-person interactions in which the practitioner's goals are to obtain accurate and critical information from the patient and reach a valid formulation of the patient's problem or status, to provide information and ensure that the patient comprehends it, to decide on a management plan with the patient, to facilitate patient adherence to agreed-on plans, to attain mutual satisfaction with the relationship, and to alleviate the patient's symptoms. Achievement of these goals depends on the practitioner's knowledge of medicine, respect for the patient's participation in the interaction, and skills in communication and patient education. This chapter and Chapter 4 address the latter two issues.

THE PRACTITIONER–PATIENT RELATIONSHIP

Types of Relationships

Our society's concept of the practitioner–patient relationship has evolved through the years. In 1951,

Parsons described the patient's role as essentially passive (1). Later Szasz and Hollender (2) outlined the following three types of interactions between practitioner and patient: the *active–passive relationship,* in which the practitioner has all authority (similar to Parson's conceptualization); the *guidance–cooperation relationship,* in which the practitioner still is somewhat authoritarian and the patient cooperates; and *mutual participation,* in which there is active collaboration between patient and practitioner and patients assume more responsibility for their care. The consumer movement of the 1960s and 1970s promoted the mutual participation relationship between practitioners and patients.

In the 1990s, the term *patient-centeredness* was introduced to emphasize the primacy of the patient in the mutual participation model. Authors pointed out that the following are indicators of patient-centeredness (3–5):

- Practitioner's goals that include learning and valuing the patient's personal illness story and reaching agreement with the patient on the meaning of the illness and on the management plan.
- Grounding of the law and medical ethics in the concept of patient autonomy.
- Quality assessment that includes the patient's perspective as a fundamental component.
- Consideration of these factors in planning health care education and research.

More recently, the term *relationship-centeredness* has been promulgated to emphasize more explicitly a relationship that depends equally on the participation of the patient and that of the practitioner (6).

Ethical Aspects of the Relationship

The mutual participation model is central to *the principles of medical ethics that have been delineated in the past two decades* (7). These principles define a practitioner–patient relationship in which the practitioner respects the sanctity of the individual person and believes that that person's goals should be the basis for medical decisions. In practice, these principles require that practitioners learn what their patients' expectations and goals are and that patients (or their surrogates) participate as fully as possible in decisions about their health care. Such participation requires several conditions: that the patient be competent to consider a specific decision; that the patient receive sufficient information regarding available options, demonstrate comprehension of that information, and be given sufficient time to consider the options; and that the patient's decision be voluntary, that is, free from constraints imposed by the interests of other persons. Additional ethical principles that are critical in a respectful practitioner–patient relationship are truthfulness and protection of confidentiality.

Adherence to each of the principles of patient-centered medical ethics is not always possible or appropriate in ambulatory practice. For example, although patients generally want to be well informed, many still prefer to have their practitioner recommend choices for them (8). In addition, a practitioner's personal beliefs and standards of practice must be considered. If a patient requests a course of action that is contrary to the practitioner's beliefs or standards or that endangers others, the practitioner must indicate this to the patient, and, if the patient's wishes cannot be accommodated, care should be transferred to another practitioner or to the court system. Challenging situations such as these are not uncommon in ambulatory practice (9).

For situations that involve patient competence, truth telling, confidentiality, and patient behaviors that may harm others, a practitioner–patient relationship that has been developed over time may make both prevention and resolution of problems more feasible. For example, an elderly patient may agree to discontinue driving and propose satisfactory alternatives in the context of a trusting relationship.

Problems caused by *external factors,* particularly the ground rules governing services covered under managed care plans, may also be amenable to resolution through the practitioner–patient relationship. Encouraging patients to become informed about the processes and guidelines of their health care insurance and offering other options when patients make unreasonable requests are examples of ways to include the patient in addressing such externally imposed challenges (see Managed Care and the Practitioner–Patient Relationship).

Involvement with Family Members and Significant Others

Commonly, a spouse, family members, or friends—especially those who are close to the patient during a period of illness—want to know about the patient's condition and are affected by the patient's illness. Significant others may play an important role in determining the course of the patient's illness by sharing in decision-making, providing support, or, at times, creating barriers. Developing a relationship with those close to the patient is therefore a predictable and important aspect of the care of many patients. A practitioner's involvement with others may range from the brief exchanges that occur at the beginning or end of office visits to interactions during a planned family meeting (9a). The skills for use in the traditional practitioner–patient dyad, described later, are the skills appropriate when others are included.

Special considerations for relating to family members and friends include the following:

- Recognizing the impact on the patient's illness of patient–family dynamics and practitioner–family dynamics.
- Avoiding breach of confidentiality by ensuring that the patient consents and, when feasible and appropriate, holding meetings with others in the presence of the patient.

- Learning about and acknowledging the distress that the patient's illness has caused for those close to the patient.
- Providing information and engaging in problem solving that will facilitate the roles of others in promoting the patient's health.
- When appropriate, including family members in decision-making.

Additional details about the positive and negative influences of family on a patient's health are found elsewhere in this text (see Social Support in Chapter 4).

Planned Family Meetings

There are a number of situations in which it is helpful to convene the members of a patient's family and, at times, others such as a nurse or social worker. Common examples include diagnosis of and plans for addressing a terminal illness; poor control of chronic illness; decisions regarding a long-term care plan; substance abuse (see Family Intervention in Chapter 28); and marital or sexual difficulties or other family dysfunction (see Family Counseling in Chapter 20). Table 3.1 describes specific tasks that one should consider when planning and conducting a family meeting.

Sociocultural Diversity and the Practitioner–Patient Relationship

A classic paper published in 1978 points out that there usually are differences in the ways in which a practitioner and a patient think about and respond to the patient's medical problems (10). The sources of these differences range from the unique ideas of individual patients, not infrequently based on transgenerational family stories of illness (11), to ideas and behaviors particular to the social or cultural groups to which patients belong. The late 20th-century composition of the United States population, summarized in Table 3.2, indicates that patients with diverse cultural traditions are likely to make up an important proportion of the patients cared for by most practitioners. Many of these patients will be recent immigrants. Chapter 41 provides information about the regulations related to health assessment of new immigrants to the United States and about important considerations

Table 3.1. Tasks to Consider for Planning and Conducting a Family Meeting

Premeeting Tasks

Clarify the purposes for the meeting.
Establish which family members, friends, or professionals should attend.
Set up the appointment, specifying the planned duration and location.
Develop a strategy for conducting the meeting, including specific questions, observations, or tasks that will facilitate addressing the purpose of the meeting.

The Five Phases of a Family Meeting

Phase 1: Socialize (Approximately 5 Minutes)

Greet each person attending the meeting.
State the purpose for the meeting, provide any crucial information that all need to know up front, and check briefly with each family member about themselves, their work, their relation to the patient, etc.

Phase 2: Set the Goals (Approximately 5 Minutes)

Ask the group, "What would you like to make sure we accomplish today?"
Restate each goal so it is clear, concise, and realistic; propose any important goals that the family has not mentioned.
Set priorities among the goals.

Phase 3: Discuss the Illness or Issue (Approximately 15 Minutes)

Elicit each participant's view of the illness or issue. Ask about past experiences or recent changes that could have an impact on the issue of concern, such as moves, occupational changes, other illness, or deaths. Observe repetitive family interactional patterns. Final plans should not go against these patterns, unless specifically negotiated.
Encourage the patient and family to ask questions.
Ask how the family has dealt with similar illness or issues in the past.

Phase 4: Identify Resources and Ideas (Approximately 10 Minutes)

Identify family strengths and resources of all kinds.
Identify medical resources and community resources.

Phase 5: Establish a Plan (Approximately 10 Minutes)

Include resources and ideas that family members have suggested.
Negotiate a formal or an informal contract with the family. Have each person state what he or she will do.
Discuss any referrals, if relevant, at this point.
Offer to write down key information for family members.
Ask for any final questions.
Summarize the plan.
Thank everyone for coming and participating in the meeting.

Postmeeting Tasks

Write up a report of the meeting, including the attendance, the problem list, a global assessment of individual and family functioning, the family's strengths and resources, and the plan (both the medical regimen and the roles to be played by the patient and family members).

Adapted from McDaniel S, Campbell T, Seaburn D. Family oriented primary care: a manual for medical providers. New York: Springer-Verlag, 1990.

related to the health care experiences, traditions, and expectations of immigrants.

In a number of ways, the effectiveness of the practitioner–patient relationship may be enhanced, or diminished, depending on awareness of and response to *differences between patient and practitioner.* General approaches that can enhance the relationship are the following:

- Learning and inquiring explicitly about the beliefs, values, and behaviors of the sociocultural group to which one's patient belongs. Common sources of group-determined beliefs and behaviors are religious tenets related to illness, traditional roles of family members in medical decisions, and folk healers. It has been pointed out that culture-based values regarding the following five factors may be fundamental to a person's health-related behavior: status bestowed on practitioners or family members, personal privacy, fatalism, importance of the individual and the group, and access to information. Additionally, patients may bring cultural preferences regarding communication content (e.g., topics appropriate to discuss, nonverbal cues) and style (e.g., directness, distance, touch, degree of formality, forms of address, pace, voice pitch) (see Gardenswartz and Rowe, *Managing Diversity in Health Care*, in General References).
- Recognizing and reflecting about one's own beliefs, biases, and emotional reactions toward cultural and individual differences, and suspending judgment when possible.
- Ensuring that an interpreter is present when there is a language barrier (see Chapter 41 for information about telephone access to interpreters).
- Including culture-friendly objects and patient materials in medical offices, such as artwork that reflects different races, ethnicities, or sexual orientations and patient instructional or educational materials written in different languages.
- Ensuring that patients who are illiterate have access to someone, ideally a family member, who can read information that is important to the patient's medical care.
- Learning about, explicitly inquiring about, and accommodating patients' explanatory models for their illnesses.

Patients' explanatory models for their illnesses address the same issues as practitioners' explanatory models: etiology, name of the illness, pathophysiology ("what is wrong"), expected course, treatment, and response to treatment (10). Often, there are differences in the two models based on the difference in perspective between patients and practitioners (Table 3.3). Both parties may inhibit the development of an effective

Table 3.2. Profile of General Demographic Characteristics: United States, 2000

Subject	Number	Percent
Total population	281,421,906	100.0
Sex		
Male	138,053,563	49.1
Female	143,368,343	50.9
Race[a]		
One race	274,595,6768	97.6
White	211,460,626	75.1
Black or African American	34,658,190	12.3
American Indian and Alaska Native	2,475,956	0.9
Asian	10,242,998	3.6
Native Hawaiian and other Pacific Islander	398,835	0.1
Some other race	15,359,073	5.5
Two or more races	6,826,228	2.4
Hispanic or Latino (of any Race)	35,305,818	12.5

[a]The concept of race as used by the Census Bureau reflects self-identification by people according to the race or races with which they most closely identify. These categories are sociopolitical constructs and should not be interpreted as being scientific or anthropological in nature. Furthermore, the race categories include both racial and national-origin groups.

From U.S. Census Bureau, Census 2000.

Table 3.3. Summary of Common Differences in Explanatory Models Between Western-Trained Practitioners and Traditional Ethnic Patients

Aspect of Model	Western Practitioner	Ethnic Patient
Etiologic Beliefs		
Social causes of illnesses	Usually limited to stress model or attributed to paranoia	Many social indiscretions can cause illness; blaming of self or others for symptoms is common
Environmental causes of illnesses	Exposure to known pathogens, toxins, and social stress may cause symptoms	"Hot–cold" imbalance in the body caused by dietary indiscretions or drafts may cause symptoms
Belief that conditions of the blood cause illness	Limited to specific hematologic disorders or hypertension	Many "conditions" of blood can cause illness (e.g., "too thick," "too slow," "too little")
Symptom Interpretation and Presentation		
Altered states of consciousness (trance, visions, etc.)	Usually considered abnormal	Often considered normal, desirable
Attitudes toward pain expression	Stoicism expected unless complaints are congruent with clear organic pathology	Either total stoicism or emotional expression of pain is healthy and expected
Focus on physical symptoms (somatization)	May be considered as a psychiatric syndrome	Expected, proper way of expressing distress
Treatment Expectations		
Who is the patient?	Individual is the focus of decision-making and care	Family must be involved in decision-making
Beliefs about self-medication and alternative practitioners	Considered potentially dangerous, undesirable	Common

From Johnson TM, Hardt EJ, Kleinman A. Cultural factors in the medical interview. In: Lipkin M Jr, Putnam SM, Lazare A, eds. The medical interview: clinical care, education, and research. New York: Springer-Verlag, 1995.

Table 3.4. The Effects of Managed Care on the Physician–Patient Relationship

Potential Improvements	Potential Threats
Choice	
Expanded choice of managed care plans, particularly in areas with low managed care penetration	"Cherry picking" increasing the number of uninsured Americans
Expanded choice of preventive and pediatric services	Employers restricting patients' choice of managed care plans and physicians
	Price competition forcing patients to choose between continuing with their current physicians or switching to a cheaper plan
	Financial failures of managed care plans forcing change in managed care plan without choice
	Restrictions by managed care plans of choice of specialists and particular services
Competence	
Development and use of measures to assess quality of physicians and managed care plans	Underuse of specialists and specialized facilities
Greater use of preventive medical care	Unreliable and non–risk-adjusted quality measures providing a distorted view of competence
Communication	
Increased number of generalists and primary care providers	Productivity requirements creating shorter office visits, reduced telephone access, and other access barriers to physicians
Creation of physician–nonphysician provider teams to provide a broader range of providers knowledgeable about the patient's condition	Advertising creating inflated patient expectations
Compassion	
	Less time for interaction with patients during stressful decisions
Continuity	
	Price competition forcing patient choice of continuity at a higher price vs the cheapest plan
	"Deselection" of physicians disrupting existing physician–patient relations
	Frequent changes by employer of managed care plans forcing changes of physician
(No) Conflict of Interest	
No incentive to overuse or overtreat as exists in fee-for-service environment	Linking practitioner salary incentives and bonuses to reduced use of tests and procedures for patients

Adapted from Emanuel EJ, Dubler NN. Preserving the physician–patient relationship in the era of managed care. JAMA 1995;273:323.

relationship—practitioners by focusing only on abstract disease formulations to address each of these issues, and patients by dwelling on their own formulation of what is wrong and resenting their practitioner's apparent inattention to that formulation. By recognizing or exploring patients' own explanatory models (and, at times, learning of conflicting beliefs about the illness held by others close to the patient), then coming up with mutually acceptable ways of accounting for and addressing the illness, practitioners are more likely to help patients who bring strongly held personal or cultural beliefs to the encounter.

Racial and language concordance between patient and practitioner appears to correlate with more collaborative relationships (12) or better health care outcomes (13). This finding points to the importance of more diversity in the make-up of the practitioner workforce as well as the need for all practitioners to enhance their commitment and skills for relating to patients in the context of sociocultural differences.

Managed Care and the Practitioner–Patient Relationship

The ways in which managed care may affect the practitioner–patient relationship have received much attention. Table 3.4 contains a summary of potential improvements and threats to the relationship that are associated with managed care. The authors considered the impact on factors key to the relationship (the six Cs): patient *choice,* practitioner *competence,* practitioner–patient *communication,* practitioner *compassion* for the patient, *continuity* of practitioners, and *avoidance of conflict* of interest (14).

Shorey captured much about the change that managed care has brought to the practitioner–patient relationship: From the need to build trust in the context of a dyad (practitioner and patient), practitioners need now to inspire trust in a context (managed care) in which they value dyadic relationships but also consider the health of all patients in their panels (15). A number of other authors have written helpful analyses of this topic (see General References).

COMMUNICATION DURING CLINICAL ENCOUNTERS

The Three Functions of the Medical Interview

The following three functions, delineated by Lazare, Putnam, and Lipkin (16), are widely accepted as ways to describe what happens in medical interviews:

- *Determining and monitoring the nature of the patient's problems*
- *Developing, maintaining, or concluding the therapeutic relationship*
- *Carrying out patient education and implementing a treatment plan*

More recently, an overarching fourth function, *partnership-building*, has been delineated (17). Partnership-building refers to the many ways in which the patient's input is enlisted and respected in information-gathering and decision-making during a practitioner–patient interaction. One or more of these functions is central to all of the skill for practitioner–patient communication described in this chapter and in Chapter 4.

Importance of Effective Communication

The importance of effective communication has been confirmed in a variety of studies of the practitioner–patient relationship. A large body of published research has shown that effective communication skills are correlated with obtaining valid information, getting patients to disclose fully the reasons for their visits, reported satisfaction with the practitioner, improved patient adherence to medical regimens, and reduced risk of being sued for malpractice (see Lipkin et al., *The Medical Interview,*' in General References). A smaller body of literature also exists in which experimental studies, using control and intervention subjects, have documented the positive impact of effective communication skills on patient outcomes including emotional health, symptom resolution, patient function, blood pressure and glucose control, and pain control (18).

Although gathering and providing of information may appear to be the primary reason for direct communication with patients, the *therapeutic nature of the interaction* is perhaps the factor that is most important to the health of the patient. As summarized by Reiser and Schroder (19):

> Repeatedly, practitioners will feel the power of something intangible, yet unmistakable, in the nature of the practitioner–patient relationship that helps a sick person to get better. It is hard to overestimate the potency and curative potential of this very unique and special relationship. For all our technical advances, this relationship remains one of medicine's most powerful therapeutic tools.

The skills that establish the therapeutic nature of *every* medical encounter are described here and in Chapter 4. Chapter 20 describes the important phenomenon of transference and additional skills that are useful when the primary purpose of the encounter is to deal with psychosocial problems.

The Patient's Experience During Ambulatory Encounters

The impact of communication during an ambulatory encounter is determined by the way that both parties think about the encounter in advance and afterwards and by the communication skills used during the encounter. The latter can be seen as skills that are useful for organizing the flow of the visit and skills that are useful throughout the visit (see next section).

Recognizing What the Patient Experiences

An interaction with a patient is likely to be more effective when, as much as possible, the practitioner recognizes the feelings and concerns that the patient brings to the visit. As discussed earlier (see Sociocultural Diversity and the Practitioner–Patient Relationship), this may include being aware of traditional beliefs and behaviors of patients from diverse cultural backgrounds (10).

In is important to realize what it is like for a patient to go to a practitioner. The general way in which patients think about a visit to the practitioner has been described as "expectant trust" (see Chapter 20). Patients may come with anxieties concerning what the practitioner will find wrong with them; they may come expecting the practitioner to solve a broad array of problems; or they may have any of a number of other types of expectations of the visit. Patients know that their practitioners have busy schedules, and some may be reluctant to ask what they think the practitioner will regard as trivial questions. Social distance often exists between practitioner and patient and, when combined with the practitioner's special knowledge, gives the practitioner considerable authority. As a result, patients may be reluctant to contradict or correct their practitioners' statements, may misrepresent their thoughts or feelings to provide answers they think the practitioner wants to hear, or may not ask for clarification despite being confused by medical terminology. During the physical examination, some patients feel embarrassment at being exposed, and this may further inhibit disclosure of important concerns. Most patients, even those who have had a long-standing relationship with their practitioner, experience some of these types of discomfort during an office visit. It can help to ask oneself, "If I were this patient, how would I be feeling during this visit?" It is equally telling to ask oneself, after a visit, "If I were that patient, how would I be feeling about the visit when I have reached home?"

As discussed later (see Challenging Situations and Practitioner Self-Care), practitioners also bring expectations and vulnerabilities to encounters with patients. Awareness of these factors can be seen as an important skill that may determine the quality of communication during a visit.

Rapport

An aspect of the practitioner–patient relationship that especially facilitates disclosure of concerns by patients and readies them to make decisions is the development and maintenance of rapport. Rapport is a mixture of harmony and affinity felt between two or more people. Rapport is fostered with a knowing look or by voicing awareness of the patient as someone unique (e.g., "How's everything going since you moved from your house to an apartment?"). Rapport also develops when a patient feels that his or her input is *respected* and that the practitioner has *empathy* for the patient (see Addressing Emotions).

Skills for Organizing the Flow of the Visit

Given the limited time available for ambulatory visits, it is important to have a scheme for organizing the flow of a visit. The scheme described here emphasizes patient-centered skills that are useful for each of the stages of a visit. The section after this one describes skills that may be helpful in any part of the visit.

Planning the Visit

It is helpful to review critical information in the patient's record before starting the visit. For an established patient, record review could include checking on the patient's social history, on preventive care due at this visit, or on issues addressed at the previous visit. This can be done before seeing the patient or just after the greeting ("Before we start, let me take a minute to get right up to the date with what is in your chart"). This planning ensures that the practitioner knows information that will help set the agenda for the visit, and it limits the need to look through the chart in the presence of the patient.

Opening the Interaction

Greeting a patient, shaking the patient's hand, using the patient's name, and, if it is a first visit, introducing oneself all make the patient feel welcome. The first few moments of first or second encounters are crucial because the practitioner and the patient are sizing up one another, and nonverbal behavior often takes precedence over what is being said. Both practitioner and patient are paying attention to physical features, type of handshake, voice tone and pitch, age, dress, and overall demeanor.

The *seating arrangement* of the office can affect the development of rapport. When the patient's and the practitioner's chairs are arranged so that the two are facing one another without the full breadth of a desk interposed, some patients are less intimidated than when facing a practitioner across a desk.

Exploratory Information Gathering

For gathering information about a patient's problems, it helps to begin with an *exploratory approach* and to ensure that the patient knows that this is one's intent. Exploratory interviewing combines *open-ended phrasing of questions* and *allowing a patient to respond without being interrupted.* An exploratory approach is the most efficient way to learn what the patient knows, and it indicates interest in the patient from the outset. Asking the patient, "How have you been doing since your last visit?" is an appropriate open-ended question for a planned follow-up visit. For a new-patient visit or a visit requested by the patient, the practitioner will want to explore the reason for the visit by saying, "Please tell me what brings you in today." This type of phrasing provides an opportunity for the patient to describe the reasons for the visit and does not imply that there is a problem.

Agenda Setting. In response to the opening inquiry, an example of the patient response might be, "Well, I haven't been doing so well lately. My shoulder has been giving me a problem." Before exploring the first problem mentioned, it is helpful to establish whether there are any other problems that the patient wants to have addressed during the visit. If one assumes that the patient wishes to discuss only one problem and proceeds to explore that problem, the patient may mention other problems whenever there is an opportunity, often when one is preparing to close the visit. The practitioner should also name items to be added to the agenda (e.g., "I also want to get up to date on your smoking"), then restate the issues to be addressed during the visit. If too many issues are identified, it is appropriate to ask, "Which problems seem to be bothering you the most?" and mutually to prioritize those issues to be addressed at the visit.

Getting the Patient's Story. After agreement on the agenda for the visit, the practitioner continues to explore the problems one at a time. "Tell me about the shoulder pain" would be a clear invitation to the patient to describe the problem in his or her own words. When patients give the history in their own words, the length of the interview does not increase (20) and they are more likely to explain why a problem concerns them (e.g., "With spring coming, I'm thinking that I might have to give up tennis altogether because of the pain").

If an exploratory approach is maintained, a patient's medical problem usually emerges as part of a meaningful personal story (4,21). For example, the patient's concern that a shoulder pain means that he or she will never play tennis again may be founded in the experience of the patient's father years before—a personal story that would clarify the importance of the symptom to the patient and would be crucial to consider in the closing part of the visit (see later discussion). In addition to bringing out important information, an interview that allows emergence of a patient's personal story invariably contributes to the development of rapport.

Exploratory questions can be used throughout the interaction. When the patient produces information that needs clarifying, additional exploratory questions are helpful to establish a common meaning. For example, if the patient has named "constipation" as a new concern, it helps to explore what this means to the patient (e.g., "Tell me what you mean by constipation?"). One may discover that the patient has a bowel movement every other day and yet believes that this means constipation.

Clarifying and Hypothesis Testing

Not visible to the patient, but constantly operating during an interview, is hypothesis testing by the practitioner. Because exploratory inquiry rarely provides all of the information needed to evaluate a problem, it is

Table 3.5. Generic Information Important in Assessing Most Problems

Chronology of symptoms
Onset of problem: since when?
Frequency
Duration of an episode
Temporal trend: unchanging, better, worse
Past history of similar problem: when, etc.?
Quality of symptoms
Severe to not severe
Quality consistent or variable
Location, radiation (if pertinent)
Patient's own words to describe quality
Description of one episode (for recurring symptom)
Associated additional symptoms
Factors, circumstances that aggravate symptoms
Factors, circumstances that alleviate symptoms
Remedies or measures tried
Impact of symptoms on valued activities
Patient's explanatory model for symptoms[a]
Fears or concerns caused by symptoms

[a]See page 26 and Table 3.3.

usually necessary to use focused questions to fill in gaps and narrow the differential diagnosis. Table 3.5 lists generic information that is important in assessing most problems.

Direct or focused questions are questions phrased to clarify specific facts, such as, "When did you first notice the pain?" or "What words would you use to describe the pain?" or "Can you show me with your hand where the pain is?" When seeking such specific information, it is important to *avoid asking leading questions*—questions that tend to elicit predetermined answers, usually in the form of a simple "yes" or "no." An example would be the following question, presumably related to a hypothesis that has occurred to the practitioner: "You don't have the pain every day, do you?" This leading question gives the message to the patient that the practitioner does not expect the pain to occur every day. Patients who are somewhat passive may agree to whatever their practitioner suggests, even if the answer is inaccurate. Once a patient has responded inaccurately, the patient may become distracted and forget to report important information.

When a patient cannot provide needed information, it helps sometimes to offer a number of *choices from which to select*. For example, if the patient reports chest pain but is unable to provide accurate information about whether the pain radiates, the practitioner might ask, "Does the pain seem to go anywhere else, such as to your back, one of your arms, your neck, or your legs?" Although the practitioner may have an idea of the likely response, this will not be obvious to the patient because the patient is given several choices. In contract, a question such as, "Does the pain move to your left arm?" is a leading question, giving the patient the impression that this is the correct answer.

A patient will at times give a vague, aggregate description of an episodic symptom. In this situation, it is helpful to have the patient *describe in detail a single episode:* "Tell me about the last time you felt the nausea and crampy pain," for example. This technique clarifies the nature of the symptoms, and, importantly, it often brings to light social or environmental factors important to the problem (e.g., "Well, the last bad headache was Saturday ... yeah, my teenage son had stayed out all night").

When asking direct questions, it is important to *ask only one question at a time* and to phrase each question so that it refers to one piece of information. Thus, when the patient responds, the practitioner knows what the patient is referring to. For example, to questions such as, "Are you having any problems sleeping or eating?" or "Are you constipated or do you have diarrhea?" a positive response may not reveal which is the problem. Conversely, a negative response may refer to only one of these problems.

While responding to questions, the *patient may give verbal cues* related to the discussion or concerning other issues that need exploration. At times it is appropriate to pursue a verbal cue when it is mentioned; at other times it is more appropriate to acknowledge it and let the patient know that you will return to it later. If a verbal cue is pertinent to the present discussion, it is helpful to repeat the patient's words or to explore what the patient means. For example, in response to a question about pain, a patient may respond, "Well, it seems to have gotten worse lately, but maybe it's just my nerves." Here, an appropriate response would be an open-ended question such as "Your nerves?" or "What do you mean?" An example of a verbal cue that one would explore separately would be the following response to a question about sleep quality in a patient with pain: "Sometimes I wake up in the middle of the night, but it isn't because of the pain." Depending on the hypothesis that one is testing regarding the patient's pain, it might be more appropriate to pursue the sleep problem later in the interaction.

A patient's *nonverbal cues* may provide important information. A patient's *vocal message*—including pitch, tone, and tempo—may confirm or contradict the content of the patient's verbal message. Nonverbal cues also include *body language*. Elements of body language that can be observed are the patient's sitting position (e.g., sitting on the edge of the chair suggests apprehension, facing away from the practitioner suggests mental discomfort), head position (e.g., held back in defiance, anxiety, or fear; held down or turned away in sadness, shame, or denial), facial expression (eyes, eyebrows, and forehead show the greatest range of emotions, including surprise, fear, anger, happiness, disgust, sadness), hands (wringing or rubbing of hands can show anxiety; clenched fists may signify anger), and arms and legs (crossing of the legs, and especially the arms, can signify resistance or defensiveness). At times, incongruity between what the patient says and the patient's voice quality or body language is the only indicator of an important problem that the patient is hesitant to disclose.

Carrying Out Patient Education, Choosing a Treatment Plan, and Closing

Telling the patient one's formulation of a medical problem and reaching consensus on next steps are the final phases of an ambulatory encounter. Because ambulatory patients are by definition autonomous, the skills needed in these phases are uniquely important in ambulatory care. Chapter 4, in the section entitled "Patient Education and Promotion of Healthy Behaviors," describes in detail the principles and skills for addressing this part of the visit.

At the close of a visit, it is important to accomplish a number of concrete tasks:

- Schedule a follow-up visit after a mutually agreed interval.
- Instruct the patient to telephone back (or tell the patient that you or someone from the office will telephone) when this is indicated.

At this point, the physician should reemphasize his or her interest in the patient. Actions such as shaking the patient's hand or touching the patient on the shoulder, using the patient's name, ensuring that the patient has one's professional card, and encouraging telephone contact for interval problems convey the physician's interest to the patient.

Skills Useful Throughout the Visit

A number of communication skills, described here, may be useful in any part of an ambulatory visit.

"Road Signs," Summarizing, Vocabulary

"Road signs," summarizing, and affirmative vocabulary help patients participate effectively in the visit. These may include:

- *Using orienting and transitional statements* to ensure that the patient understands when the focus of the interview is changing (e.g., "At this point, I would like to learn more about your day-to-day activities")
- Naming, then addressing, *one problem or issue at a time* (e.g., "Now, about your shoulder pain ..." or "The medicine that I will prescribe ...")
- *Summing up and checking periodically* (e.g., "So far, what I understand about your trouble sleeping is that ..."), which lets patients know that one has heard what they said and gives them the chance to clarify or expand on important information
- Using *vocabulary consistent with the patient's background* and avoiding formulations that may confuse the patient (e.g., telling a patient that test results are "negative" may convey to the patient that something is wrong).

Noting the Patient's Educational Needs

Patient education can be addressed most efficiently by *ascertaining the patient's educational needs throughout the interview*—by hearing or asking what the patient knows or wants to know about issues as they come up—but *deferring the process of providing information and working out a plan* to the latter part of the visit. It helps to give the patient a road sign (e.g., "When we finish up your visit, we will go over several things you can do to lose the weight you have gained"). (See details in the schemes described in Chapter 4.)

Using Eye Contact

The eyes are a primary medium of expression, and they often tell more about a person's message than words do. Maintaining eye contact and communicating with one's eyes at the same level as the patient's (e.g., both parties seated) are basic to patient comfort. Looking at one's watch or at the chart while discussing a patient's problem may indicate to the patient that the practitioner is not listening, is not interested, or is too busy to answer questions that he or she may already be reluctant to ask. Although eye contact is one of the best ways to convey interest, staring can be uncomfortable and should be avoided.

Addressing Emotions

Predictably, patients experience one or more emotions before, during, and after visits to the practitioner. During visits, patients may or may not disclose their feelings. Empiric studies have shown that patients usually do not express emotions directly but through verbal or nonverbal clues (e.g., "It's been kind of different for me lately"; looking down or away when emotions are present) (21,22). A number of communication skills can facilitate disclosure and addressing of emotions (Table 3.6). Three basic reasons for addressing emotions are that patients usually feel better when they know that the practitioner is aware of their feelings; patients may be more able to concentrate and make decisions after an emotional state such as anxiety, sadness, or anger has been addressed even briefly; and expressing emotions may be therapeutic for a patient.

Skills Related to Physical Examination and Documentation

Physical Examination

Appropriate communication during the physical examination includes describing what one is doing, obtaining further history when examining the location of a symptom, and avoiding the tendency to give important information (diagnosis and plan) during the physical examination or when the patient is getting dressed; in both instances the patient is distracted and cannot be expected to focus on the practitioner's message or to formulate questions as well.

Note Taking

Dictating or writing a visit note can be done in a way that does not diminish rapport with the patient. It is helpful to point out that one will be making a few notes during the visit. It is equally helpful to suspend the interaction briefly while focusing on one's note, because this is a time that requires thought as well as writing or dictating.

Challenging Situations

All practitioners have been faced with challenging patients in medical practice. Patients may be challenging

Table 3.6. Skills for Addressing a Patient's Emotions

Skills for Facilitating Disclosure of Feelings

Explicitly Ask or Encourage Patient to Express/Clarify Feelings/Concerns.
Restate patient's words about how he/she feels (e.g., "You feel down. . .?" repeated immediately after the patient says these words).
Acknowledge or probe feelings that seem to be present or just under the surface (e.g., "I notice you're getting tearful" or "How do you feel about. . .?").
Clarify or check feelings that patient has disclosed (e.g., "Let me see if I can better understand what you are feeling").

Allow Patient to Express Feelings/Concerns.
Be attentive, do not interrupt.
Allow silence while patient prepares response or experiences emotional reaction.

Skills for Responding to and Supporting Patient

Convey Concern for and Interest in the Patient.
Explicitly by saying so (e.g., "My concern is to help you get well.").
Implicitly by remaining attentive, facilitating disclosure, indicating that the patient has been heard (e.g., by mentioning aspects of patient's life affected by an illness or by changing facial expression and vocal tone).

Communicate Understanding of Patient's Feelings (Empathize).
Name patient's feelings/situation (e.g., "Sounds as if you are pretty angry").
Check accuracy of naming (e.g., "Is this the way you experience it?").
Use facilitative utterances (e.g., lower voice, use appropriate utterances such as "uh huh" that indicate that the patient is being attended to).

Legitimize Patient's Feelings/Thoughts/Actions.
Indicate that patient's emotions/thoughts/actions are understandable and "normal" under the circumstances (e.g., "It's understandable that you feel this way," "Many would have done as you did.").

Convey Respect for the Patient's Efforts, Ideas.
Compliment patient for whatever patient is doing well or plans to do (e.g., "Your decision to join Weight Watchers sounds good to me," "I can see that you have given a lot of thought to. . .").

Respond Nonjudgmentally.
Do not impose own bias, values, or assumptions on patient characteristics or actions that evoke negative stereotypes or disappointment.
Nonverbally: Do not give negative message (e.g., nodding head disapprovingly, sighing in frustration, when a patient reports noncompliance).
Verbally: Do not imply that patient is "flawed or bad" (e.g., "That's alcoholism for you..." or "Didn't you realize that if you ate crabs you'd put yourself into heart failure again?"). Instead, acknowledge that you have heard the patient's story.

Respond Nondefensively.
Do not respond to patient anger or criticism by defense of performance but acknowledge anger/criticism and try to address the reasons for the patient's behavior and concerns.
Admit mistakes, apologize when appropriate, be open to considering second opinions, and avoid self-righteousness.

Use Self-Disclosure Effectively.
Reveal information about self, when appropriate, to convey support, empathy to patient (e.g., "I felt the same way after I lost my mother.").

Assure Partnership/Support.
Make statements, using the first person, that assure support to the patient and convey the sense of partnership (e.g., "I will be with you throughout this illness.").

to care for because of their style of communicating, because of the overwhelming nature of their problems, because of their failure to adhere to appropriate treatment or behavior, because they present psychosocial distress through somatic symptoms, because they do not respond positively to the practitioner's efforts, or because they have lifelong maladaptive personalities. Approaches to dealing with situations that may be difficult for practitioners are covered in Section 2 of this book, "Psychiatric and Behavioral Problems," and in chapters describing patients who are noncompliant (Chapter 4); adolescent and geriatric patients (Chapters 11 and 12, respectively); patients who have illnesses that create major psychosocial stress, such as cancer (Chapter 10), terminal illness (Chapter 13), human immunodeficiency virus infection (Chapter 39), diabetes (Chapter 79), or epilepsy (Chapter 88); and patients with myocardial infarction (Chapter 63) or stroke (Chapter 91).

Practitioners predictably react emotionally to difficult patients and situations. Often, these reactions are evoked by patients' feelings that seem to be directed personally at the practitioner; at times they are caused by recapitulation of aspects of the practitioner's own relationships (see discussion of countertransference, Chapter 20). Awareness of these feelings sometimes provides clues to a patient's diagnosis (e.g., sadness or feeling drained—depression, frustration—somatoform disorder) and provide the opportunity for reflection and behavior adjustments that can improve practitioner–patient rapport and optimize management.

Table 3.7 summarizes common negative responses of practitioners to patients and strategies for dealing

Table 3.7. Common Negative Responses of Physicians to Difficult Patients and Strategies to Cope with These Responses

Physician's Emotional or Behavioral Reaction	Coping Strategies[a]
Avoidance	Analyze why; attempt to understand and master feelings that lead to avoidance; stay with the patient; discuss with colleagues.
Identification with patient	Recognize, avoid tendency to deny seriousness of disease or to give way to despair; stay with the patient.
Hostility/rejection	Acknowledge and analyze; do not attempt to like the unlikable patient; use behavioral approaches; if situation is intolerable, transfer patient to another physician.
Feelings of impotence, inadequacy (e.g., in caring for dying patient)	Discover areas in which help and comfort can be rendered, both physical and emotional; be realistic about limitations to medicine; give the patient time to go through the stages of dying or bereavement.
Feelings of loss of control or threatened authority	Acknowledge and analyze; be realistic about personal limitations and actual range of influence and authority; be aware that patient's need for control over his or her own body may conflict with physician's urge to control the situation.
Frustration, confusion, uncertainty about dealing with the patient; coping strategies not effective	Request psychiatric consultation/referral.
Anxiety, guilt, frustration about meeting patient's recognized emotional needs	Allocate time realistically according to need; request consultation/referral.

[a]See also skills in Table 3.6 and Psychosocial Treatment Techniques in Chapter 20.

From Gorlin R, Zucker HD. Physicians' reaction to patients. N Engl J Med 1983;308:1059.

with these responses. Most of the strategies require one to take time for self-exploration, one of several strategies that practitioners identify as healthy adaptations to stress (see next section).

PRACTITIONER SELF-CARE

An unstated assumption about the practitioner–patient relationship is that a practitioner is always ready to respond with skill and concern to a patient's distress. Because of the extraordinary needs of sick patients and the demands of running a practice, most practitioners are at risk for experiencing excessive stress themselves, beginning during training and spanning their professional careers. Substance abuse, mental illness, family dysfunction, and loss of satisfaction are well-recognized accompaniments of practitioner stress. To counterbalance the risk of excessive stress and to increase the likelihood that they will be skillful, caring, and satisfied in their professional relationships, practitioners need to address the care of themselves.

When asked about their healthy approaches to stress, practitioners identify the following personal strategies, each of which should be available to most practitioners (23,24).

Values Clarification and Time Management. This strategy, although it is implicitly present in each person's life, can be especially helpful when it is undertaken explicitly by professionals such as practitioners, whose working days often bring more demands than they can reasonably meet. The process of thinking about and writing down one's core values can help to identify activities that do or do not reflect those core values and to rearrange one's priorities. A common example of the impact of value clarification would be the decision of an overcommitted professional to refuse, delegate, or discontinue low-priority activities so that more time can be allocated to valued family activities and personal life.

Self-Awareness and Sharing Feelings with Others. These strategies may be important for addressing stressful situations, which may range from patient care encounters that evoke negative responses (Table 3.7) to family tension caused by the demands of one's professional life. One can incorporate these strategies by reserving time to reflect privately or to write a personal journal. And, if one has a group of like-minded colleagues, one can schedule regular meetings at which to share, in confidence, one another's dilemmas and joys (25) and to better recognize feelings and responses such as those listed in Table 3.7. The latter strategy is especially helpful for dealing with the negative effects of reflecting alone on stressful issues.

Personal Health Care. The strategies in this section can be seen as ways to promote and protect one's mental well-being. It is equally important for practitioners to identify goals for their physical health and to address these goals with concrete measures such as exercising regularly, getting adequate sleep, avoiding harmful health habits, selecting and visiting a personal practitioner, and taking sick time when not well enough to work.

A 1997 multiauthor paper provides extensive information related to practitioner self-awareness and self-care (24).

General References

American Academy on Practitioner and Patient (AAPP) website. Available at: http://www.physicianpatient.org. Accessed December 2, 2001.

National organization that offers a wide variety of courses and learning materials, including a quarterly journal, *Medical Encounter on the Practitioner–Patient Relationship.*

American College of Physicians ethics manual, 2nd ed. Ann Intern Med 1989;111:245; 3rd ed. Ann Intern Med 1992;117:949; and 4th ed. Ann Intern Med 1998;128:576.

Helpful descriptions and discussions of ethical principles governing practitioner–patient, practitioner–practitioner, and practitioner–society relationships.

Cross-cultural medicine. West J Med 1983;139(6). Cross-cultural medicine: a decade later. West J Med 1992;157(3).

Two special issues, covering major problems that are generic to cross-cultural medicine in the United States and containing articles on most of the major immigrant populations in the United States.

Gardenswartz L, Rowe A. Managing diversity in health care. San Francisco: Jossey-Bass Publishers, 1998.

Readable, brief monograph that describes the entire spectrum of practitioner–patient differences that affect health care behaviors and communication.

Lipkin M, Putnam SM, Lazare A. The medical interview: a textbook on medical interviewing. New York: Springer-Verlag, 1994.

Multiauthored text with extensively referenced chapters on all of the uses of the interview in medical practice and research supporting them.

Novack DH. Therapeutic aspects of the clinical encounter. J Gen Intern Med 1987;2:346.

Thorough, well-referenced review, focusing largely on ordinary medical encounters.

Quill TE. Recognizing and adjusting to barriers in practitioner–patient communication. Ann Intern Med 1989;111:51.

Delineates common barriers and practical ways to address them.

Rolland JS. Families, illness, and disability: an integrative treatment model. New York: Basic Books, 1994.

Monograph that draws on the literature and on the author's experience to describe the impact on families and the range of ways to assess and assist families of patients with chronic illness.

Smith RC. Patient-centered interviewing: An evidence-based method. Philadelphia: Lippincott Williams & Wilkins, 2001.

Monograph. Describes the comprehensive approach to patient interviews with excellent examples; designed for use by teachers of medical interviewing.

Smith RC, Hoppe RB. The patient's story: integrating the patient- and physician-centered approaches to interviewing. Ann Intern Med 1991;115:470.

Well-referenced description, with concrete illustrations, of ways to ensure active patient involvement in an exploratory interview.

"Tell me about yourself": the patient-centered interview. Ann Intern Med 2001;134:1079.

The first in a series of articles ("Words That Make a Difference") developed under the sponsorship of the AAPP. Identifies and illustrates words and expressions that have proved particularly effective in practitioner–patient communication.

vom Eigen KA, Inui TS. Special issue: medical care and the physician–patient relationship. Med Encounter 1997;13(2).

Thoughtful essays by ten authors on the challenges that managed care brings to the practitioner–patient relationship.

Specific References

1. Parsons T. The social system. New York: Free Press, 1951.
2. Szasz T, Hollender MH. A contribution to the philosophy of medicine: the basic models of the practitioner–patient relationship. Arch Intern Med 1956;97:585.
3. Laine C, Davidoff F. Patient-centered medicine. JAMA 1996; 275:152.
4. Smith RC, Hoppe RB. The patient's story: integrating the patient- and physician-centered approaches to interviewing. Ann Intern Med 1991;115:470.
5. Stewart M, Brown JB, Weston WW, et al. Patient-centered medicine: transforming the clinical method. Beverly Hills, CA: Sage, 1995.
6. Roter D. The enduring and evolving nature of the patient-physician relationship. Patient Education and Counseling 2000;39:5.
7. Arnold R, Forrow L, Barker LR. Medical ethics and practitioner–patient communication. In: Lipkin M, Putnam SM, Lazare A, eds. The medical interview: a textbook on medical interviewing. New York: Springer-Verlag, 1994.
8. Ende J, Kazis L, Ash A, et al. Measuring patients' desire for autonomy. J Gen Intern Med 1989;4:23.
9. Connelly JE, DalleMura S. Ethical problems in the medical office. JAMA 1988;260:812.

9a. Doherty WJ, Baird MA. Developmental levels in family-centered medical care. Fam Med 1986;18:153.

10. Kleinman A, Eisenberg L, Good B. Culture, illness, and care: clinical lessons from anthropologic and cross-cultural research. Ann Intern Med 1978;88:251.
11. Seaburn DB, Lorenz A, Kaplan D. The transgenerational development of chronic illness meanings. Fam Syst Med 1992;10: 385.
12. Cooper-Patrick L, Gallo JJ, Gonzales JJ, et al. Race, gender, and partnership in the patient-physician relationship. JAMA 1999;282:583.
13. Napoles-Springer A, Perez-Stable EJ. The role of culture and language in determining best practices. J Gen Intern Med 2001;16:493.
14. Emanuel EJ, Dubler NN. Preserving the physician–patient relationship in the era of managed care. JAMA 1995;273:323.
15. Shorey JM. Research in practitioner–patient communication within a managed care era: a physician's perspective. Med Encounter 1997;13(2).
16. Lazare A, Putnam SM, Lipkin M Jr. Three functions of the medical interview. In: Lipkin M Jr, Putnam SM, Lazare A, eds. The medical interview: clinical care, education, and research. New York: Springer-Verlag, 1995.
17. Roter D. The medical visit context of treatment decision-making and the therapeutic relationship. Health Expectations 2000;3:17.
18. Stewart MA. Effective physician–patient communication and health outcomes: a review. Can Med Assoc J 1995;152:1423.
19. Reiser DE, Schroder AK. Patient interviewing: the human dimension. Baltimore: Williams & Wilkins, 1980.
20. Putnam SM, Stiles WB, Jacab MC, et al. Teaching the medical interview: an intervention study. J Gen Intern Med 1988;3:38.
21. Suchman A, Markakis K, Beckman HB, et al. A model of emphatic communication in the medical interview. JAMA 1997;277:678.
22. Levinson W, Goraware-Bhat R, Lamb J. A study of patient clues and physician responses in primary care and surgical settings. JAMA 2000;284:1021.
23. Quill TE, Williamson PR. Healthy approaches to physician stress. Arch Intern Med 1990;150:1857.
24. Novack DH, Suchman AL, Clark W, et al. Calibrating the physician: personal awareness and effective patient care. JAMA 1997;278:502.
25. Williamson PR. Support groups: an important aspect of physician education [Editorial]. J Gen Intern Med 1991;6;179.

CHAPTER 4

Patient Education and the Promotion of Healthy Behaviors

KARAN A. COLE, ScD
DAVID E. KERN, MD, MPH

One meaning of the word *doctor* is "teacher." Teaching is an important practitioner function that can help patients understand their conditions, relieve anxieties, and enhance adoption of treatment regimens. Most of the elements of communication during a visit, described in Chapter 3, contribute to the process of patient education, a process that depends as much on developing trust, identifying the patient's information needs and psychosocial context, and involving the patient in developing a plan as on giving information.

PATIENT EDUCATION

Definition

Patient education can be defined as a patient learning experience during which the heath practitioner uses a combination of educational assessment and intervention strategies that influence the patient's knowledge, attitudes, or health behaviors. *Health behaviors* encompass a wide range of activities that relate to health, including seeking health advice; keeping health care appointments; taking medications; undertaking preventive measures; modifying existing patterns of eating, exercising, or substance use; and solving problems. Patient education sometimes is completed during one practitioner–patient interaction, but more often it is an ongoing process that occurs over the course of several visits.

The Practitioner–Patient Relationship

Patient education takes place in the context of a practitioner–patient relationship, which influences the nature of the educational process. As discussed in Chapter 3, the relationship between practitioner and patient can be conceptualized as a spectrum that ranges from active–passive to mutual participation. In an *active–passive relationship,* the practitioner as expert is responsible for explaining and prescribing and the patient is responsible for following orders. This type of relationship presumes an *authoritative approach* to patient education and behavior change. In a *mutual participation relationship,* the patient and practitioner actively collaborate and patients take more responsibility for their care. This type of relationship assumes that most patients are capable of participating with the practitioner in the development of their own management plans. It incorporates an *empowerment approach* to patient education and behavior change, during which the practitioner facilitates patient involvement in goal identification, problem solving, and planning (1,2). Practitioners assume the role of mentor, consultant, and expert in medical knowledge.

Effective patient education does not involve the exclusive use of either an authoritative or an empowerment approach. Often, approaches are combined, and the balance of authoritative and empowerment approaches within a given practitioner–patient interaction is determined by practitioner and patient attitudes and skills and by patient needs.

Empowerment versus Compliance

Ambulatory patients are responsible for implementing most of the management strategies developed in practitioners' offices. To implement a management plan, not only do patients have to be ready for it, believe it is in their best interest, and believe that they can accomplish it; they also have to do it. Empowerment is the facilitation of active self-management by patients. The more complex and behaviorally demanding a management plan, the greater the challenge for the patient who must integrate it into the demands of day-to-day living. Patients are more likely to succeed if they are provided with the specific information and skills necessary to achieve negotiated goals, rather than a general directive. Such education requires the assessment of patients' needs and interventions that address the knowledge, attitudes, and skills that underlie relevant motivation, goal-setting, behavioral change, problem-solving, decision-making, stress management, coping, access to resources, and development of social support (see later sections, Assessment and Intervention).

Ideally, therefore, the goal of patient education is to provide patients with the knowledge, attitudes and skills that will empower them to make informed decisions and adopt healthy behaviors, rather than simply comply with or adhere to practitioner-dictated treatment plans (3). The terms *compliance, adherence,* and *noncompliance,* used for many years to describe the extent to which patients follow through with medical advice or agreed-upon plans, are now believed to be problematic, because they exaggerate the importance of the clinician, describe behavior inaccurately, and do not address motivation (4).

Importance

Regardless of terminology, it is well established that many patients fail to adopt healthy behaviors or follow through with agreed-upon treatment plans. The result may be poor health outcomes. If practitioners are unaware of their patients' health behaviors, they may falsely attribute poor outcomes to failure of a treatment approach, inadequate dosage, or incorrect diagnosis and subsequently take inappropriate action. When patients do not adopt healthy behaviors, the utilization of health care services may increase. For example, such patients are more likely to be hospitalized, or, if elderly, to be placed in nursing homes. The cost and frequency of use of outpatient services, including emergency room care, may be increased (5,6). Overall, the cost of medical care may rise while its effectiveness declines. An approach to patient education that helps patients to adopt healthy behaviors is, therefore, a fundamental skill for the medical practitioner.

EDUCATIONAL AND BEHAVIORAL CHANGE PRINCIPLES

An empowerment approach to patient education and behavioral change requires an understanding of certain principles that guide the assessment of educational needs and the planning of educational interventions.

Adult Learning

As people age, they become less dependent and more *self-directed* (7–9). They are more likely to make changes and to learn, when they perceive a need or desire to do so, rather than when they are told to do so. They prefer to be actively, rather than passively, involved with their learning. They tend to be *problem-oriented* rather than subject-oriented. And, increasingly with age, they define themselves by their experience. A practitioner who defines a goal and management strategy for a patient, therefore, is less likely to be successful than one who pursues a more *learner-centered* approach. The latter practitioner starts with the patient's perceived needs and expectations and then develops, with the patient, achievable goals and management strategies that take account of the patient's past experiences, expectations, and strengths and that address barriers through mutual problem-solving.

Single versus Multilevel Interventions

Clinical experience and research support the principle that *knowledge is necessary, but not sufficient* when patients are expected to make lifestyle changes. Such changes may range from fitting a medication regimen into a patient's daily routine to altering long-standing patient habits such as overeating or smoking. *Educational interventions that are targeted at several levels, including knowledge, attitudes, behavior, and environment, are most effective.* Studies of the impact of patient education on a number of conditions confirm this principle (10).

Readiness for Change

Matching the practitioner intervention to patient readiness for change predicts patients' success in achieving behavioral change (11). There are *five stages of readiness for change: precontemplation, contemplation, preparation, action, and maintenance* (Fig. 4.1). A patient may move back and forth on this cycle many times before successfully adopting a new habit. *Relapse* is the term applied when patients regress to an earlier stage. Successfully identifying the stage of readiness for change helps the practitioner target appropriate strategies to move the patient to the next phase. If a patient has not even considered a specific behavior change, such as stopping smoking (*precontemplation*), the goal might be to pursue strategies that would help the patient move toward *contemplation*, such as exploring the patient's existing knowledge

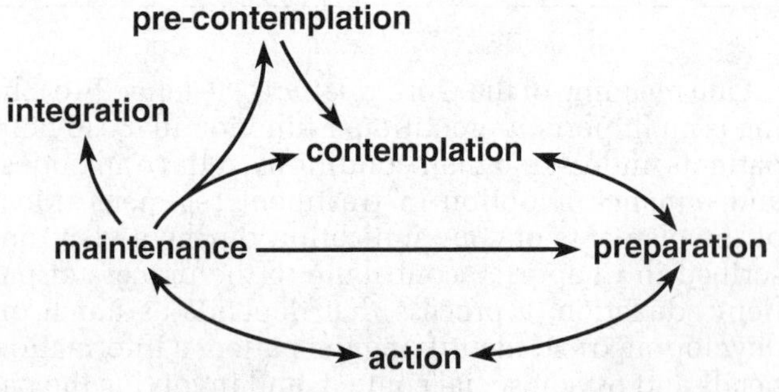

Figure 4.1. The readiness for change cycle.

and attitudes toward smoking and providing an understanding of the hazards of smoking or reasons why the patient might want to stop smoking. If the patient is contemplating a behavioral change, the goal might be to begin to identify potential facilitators or barriers to achieving that change and to make a commitment for a change (*preparation*). In the *action* phase, specific goal setting, anticipatory problem solving, and skills-building would occur, and strategies to support the behavioral change would be identified. In the *maintenance* phase, reactive problem-solving, together with evaluation of existing and implementation of alternative skills-building and support strategies, is appropriate to prevent relapse. Although it is not considered a separate stage, *integration* occurs when the new behavior patterns are fully incorporated into the patient's life.

Self-Efficacy

According to social learning theory (12), the strongest factor in predicting whether a behavior will occur is the level of self-efficacy, or the individual's *confidence in performing the behavior.* Self-efficacy can be increased through the acquisition of skills that make it more likely that the behavior will occur. For example, a patient may increase his or her confidence in making dietary changes by becoming skilled at reading and interpreting ingredient labels on packages. Success with a new behavior increases a patient's confidence. The remembering of past successes can be used to boost a patient's current sense of self-efficacy. Finally, observing others successfully perform a behavior can increase a patient's confidence in his or her own capacities. Numerous studies have identified the relationship between self-efficacy and behavior and demonstrated the effectiveness of interventions targeted toward increasing an individual's self-efficacy (13).

Locus of Control

Individual beliefs regarding who controls one's health status reflect a patient's orientation to control (i.e., internal, external, or chance locus of control) (14). Patients' perceptions of locus of control, self-efficacy, and behavioral change are complexly interrelated, and to a significant degree, they are specific to a given situation (15,16). A patient's beliefs about locus of control are relevant in that they help determine whether an authoritative or an empowerment approach will be most effective.

Patients who believe that their health is a consequence of their own efforts have an *internal locus of control.* These patients believe in mastery and control over the natural environment and prefer to take a high level of responsibility for their health care; for them, a collaborative practitioner–patient relationship and an empowerment approach to patient education and behavioral change are most appropriate.

Those who believe that their health is a consequence of others' efforts, particularly of practitioners' efforts, have an *external locus of control.* They may have experienced frustration when previously attempting to control life events, or they may come from a culture that delegates the responsibility to certain societal roles. These patients prefer explicit directions from their practitioner; an active–passive practitioner–patient relationship and an authoritative approach to patient education are most appropriate. However, a patient's locus of control specific to any health behavior can shift from external to internal if the patient has success as the result of his or her own efforts. Therefore, it is beneficial to gradually include empowerment approaches in order to help patients take more responsibility for their own health over time.

Finally, patients who have a *chance locus of control* believe that health-related outcomes are determined by fate and are therefore uncontrollable. When this belief is inappropriate to the situation (e.g., in a patient with uncontrolled hypertension), the practitioner may wish to explore and address the belief.

Health Beliefs and Explanatory Models

Most patients come to a health practitioner with their own ideas about their health and health problems, which are grounded in their own experiences, social interactions, and culture. Their *explanatory models* may include ideas about etiology, pathophysiology, susceptibility, severity, prognosis, treatment, and prevention (17). The following have been shown to influence a patient's health-related behavior (18):

- Perceived *severity of a disease,* condition, or consequences of not changing one's behavior
- Perceived *vulnerability or susceptibility* to the disease, condition, or consequences of certain behaviors
- Perceived *effectiveness* of the therapy or change in behavior
- Perceived *benefits* of the therapy or change in behavior
- Perceived *potential risks* of the therapy or change in behavior.

It is important to remember that patients' health beliefs and explanatory models are affected by cultural as well as individual factors. The former include family, friends, social network, ethnicity, education, religion, and socioeconomic status. A practitioner who understands a patient's social milieu will, therefore, have clues that may be helpful in exploring the patient's health beliefs.

Practitioners who provide explanations and negotiate management plans that make sense in the context of patients' own health belief systems are more likely to satisfy patients and influence their behavior (19). Likewise, the degree to which patients and practitioners are able to achieve congruence of beliefs about causality and treatment predicts patient satisfaction and patient success in following treatment recommendations (20–23).

Behavioral Intention

There is a positive relationship between patients' intention to adopt or change behaviors and their actually performing the behaviors. Such intention is often a consequence of the aforementioned principles. Patients who are ready to make a behavior change, have high self-confidence in their ability to make the change, agree with the explanation provided by the practitioner, and believe that they will experience benefits if they make the behavior change and consequences if they do not, are likely to have a greater intention to adopt or change a behavior than patients who do not have these characteristics. Also, patients who have been part of the process of decision-making are more likely to have a greater intention to adopt or change a behavior than those who have simply been told to make a change.

Social Support

Social support is defined as external resources that assist efforts of the patient to meet internal and external demands (24). A substantial body of literature explores the effectiveness of social support in preventing illness. Positive relationships have also been documented between social support and adherence to medical recommendations (25), adjustment after myocardial infarction (26,27), and cessation of smoking (28). The *quality,* as well as the quantity, of support is important. For instance, perceptions of the lack of needed assistance predicts negative health outcomes in patients with coronary artery disease (29). An unsatisfying marriage may be worse than no marriage for health outcomes (30). The overinvolvement of spouses, characterized as misguided helping, can have negative effects (31,32). When family members exhibit harmful behaviors that patients are trying to change, such as smoking or eating a high-fat diet, patients have a particularly difficult time changing their own behaviors. On the other hand, if family members can be enlisted to support patients in facilitative and positive ways, patients are more likely to make healthy changes in their behaviors. Family involvement is influenced by culture, which, for example, may determine who makes decisions in a family, whether a family member should be present when negotiating a treatment plan, and how a family responds to a negotiated plan. No matter how many potential supports are available, patients need to be asked about their own perception of them, because the available supports may not be resources but actually barriers to behavioral change. In addition, patients may need to develop skills to communicate their need for support and negotiate for appropriate support.

ASSESSMENT

Importance

Patient education can be conceptualized as successive cycles of assessment and intervention (Fig. 4.2). The

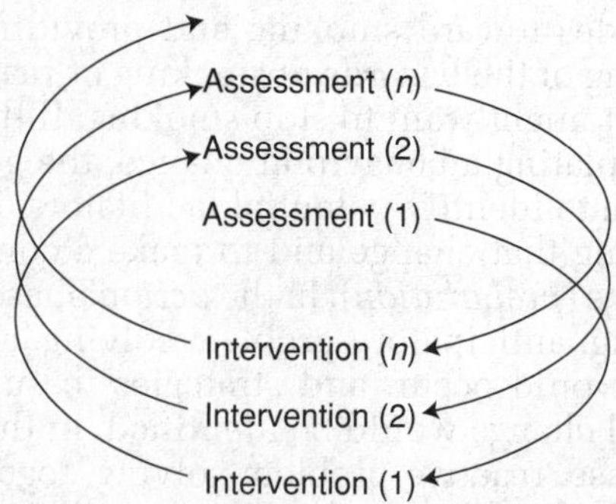

Figure 4.2. The assessment–intervention spiral.

effectiveness of an educational intervention depends on the accuracy of the educational assessment as well as the practitioner's skill in using specific instructional, behavioral, motivational/empowerment, mechanical, and organizational strategies (see Intervention). Patient education, therefore, should begin with an assessment of (a) background information that defines the patient's educational needs, the patient's capacities to adopt new behaviors, and environmental facilitators and barriers and (b) the patient's current health-related behaviors, such as medication taking and nondrug treatments.

Knowing or Obtaining Background Information

There are many factors known to be associated with adherence to medical recommendations (Table 4.1) that should be considered before making an educational diagnosis and developing an educational intervention. Knowledge of this background information about a patient makes it possible to individualize an explanation or a management plan in a way that is likely to be effective.

Patient Characteristics

Patients come to health practitioners with a rich *past.* The meaning they attribute to their health or an illness; their current beliefs, concerns, and behaviors; and the way they relate to health care practitioners are likely to be influenced by their own past experiences, the experience of others in their social circle, and cultural factors. They may already be using alternative health care resources. They may face barriers to accessing mainstream health care such as cost, accessibility, and, in the case of refugees and immigrants, language barriers, the potential for the restimulation of traumatic stress reactions, and the fear of deportation (33). These factors can affect patients' receptivity to health care practitioners and their recommendations.

As noted previously, patients' *knowledge, attitudes, and beliefs* about a condition and its management influence their health-related behaviors. As distinguished from disease, which is an objective entity based on the presence of independently verifiable findings, a patient's explanation and experience of illness is a subjective state that is shaped by personal,

Table 4.1. Assessment: Factors Associated with Adherence to Medical Recommendations

Patient Characteristics
Personal knowledge, attitudes, and beliefs, including
  Explanatory model, fears, concerns
  Past experience
  Locus of control: internal or external vs chance
  Readiness for change
  Perceived self-efficacy
  Behavioral orientation
Cultural/ethnic models of disease and treatment
Value systems: personal and cultural/ethnic
Self-care/self-management skills
Ability to pay for treatment
Previous or concurrent adherence to medical recommendations
Psychological factors (e.g., immaturity, impulsivity, paranoia, hostility, fear of dependence, denial, commitment to a bad decision, type A personality)
Language barriers

Disease Features
Symptomatic vs asymptomatic condition
Comorbid conditions
  Cognitive impairment
  Psychiatric illness (e.g., depression, mania, schizophrenia, paranoia, antisocial or paranoid personality disorders)
  Alcoholism/drug addiction

Treatment Factors
Complexity of treatment regimen (number of medicines or treatments, frequency of dosage or treatment)
Duration of therapy
Requirement for significant behavior change
Delayed benefit or lack of obvious benefit
Side effects, actual and perceived
Expense (to patient)

Environmental Factors
Family/social support
Cultural norms
Residential stability
Experience of similar illness among family/friends
Individual vs block appointments[a]
Convenience (location, quality of transportation, flexibility and accessibility of appointment times)[a]
Waiting time[a]
Referral to specific doctors rather than clinics[a]
Communication skills of support staff (respectfulness, friendliness, caring)[a]

Practitioner–Patient Relationship
Effective communication of information and instructions
Explanations that make sense from patient's perspective
Doctor–patient congruence in understanding of problem and its management
Fulfillment of patient's expectations; addressing of patient's concerns
Accommodation to patient's cultural norms
Patient participation/involvement in development of treatment plan
Empathetic understanding by physician
Positive, friendly, confident approach by physician
Transference/countertransference reactions
Patient trust, confidence in physician
Patient satisfaction
Level of physician supervision
Continuity of provider

[a]Refers to appointment keeping.

interpersonal, and cultural factors. It is the patient's perceptions of an illness and its treatment (see Health Beliefs and Explanatory Models) that correlate with adopting healthy behaviors, rather than the objective realities. An extreme example occurs in patients who deny illness. Patients who have had a myocardial infarction but answer "No" or "Maybe" rather than "Yes" when asked whether they have experienced a heart attack are less likely to follow the practitioner's instructions regarding activity level and smoking cessation (34).

Patients often have their own *models of disease and treatment.* If these models conflict with recommended regimens, patients may not follow the regimens. For example, the commonly held perception of hypertension as an intermittent, symptomatic, stress-related condition encourages an erratic approach to medication taking. Some patients with clearly diagnosable soft tissue injuries may think that their evaluation was incomplete without a radiograph and therefore mistrust the practitioner's diagnosis. Ethnic concepts of disease and treatment can also conflict with the practitioner's approach to diagnosis and management. Such concepts are more prevalent among ethnic group members who experience a language barrier, are generationally close to immigration, live in segregated neighborhoods, are lower in education level and socioeconomic class, experience barriers to receiving personalized medical care, or lack experience with a Western health care system—that is, those who are least integrated into the mainstream culture. For example, some patients might change practitioners or refuse treatment if they are told they have both "high blood pressure" and a "low blood count" (anemia). According to some folk beliefs, these diagnoses are mutually exclusive, so the practitioner making them may be regarded as untrustworthy.

Patient *values* may be congruent with or conflict with those of the practitioner and affect adherence with practitioner recommendations. For example, elderly patients may value the quality of living and dying more highly than the simple preservation of life. They, therefore, may prefer to accept an increased risk of death rather than endure an inconvenient, impersonal hospitalization that separates them from home and family. Patients may also value certain ways of interacting with the world more highly than others. Patients with an *individualistic* orientation believe in self-sufficiency, individual responsibility, and personal autonomy. Those with a *collective* orientation believe in relational interdependence, group harmony, and in-group collaborative spirit. *Power orientation* involves acceptance of power distribution and determines whether patients will question authority. *Risk-taking orientation* determines the extent to which patients feel threatened by unknown situations and the extent to which they try to avoid them. *Gender role orientation* influences the degree to which patients follow rigid versus flexible gender-identified behaviors. Recognition and accommodation of such values and orientations should help practitioners negotiate health management plans that are acceptable to patients.

Self-care and self-management skills are important factors that vary among patients and affect their ability to adopt healthy behaviors. These include general problem-solving, decision-making, and coping skills, as well as condition-specific skills such as changing wound dressings, self-monitoring of blood pressure or blood sugar, and the mixing and injecting of insulin.

Other important patient characteristics that are often overlooked are *patients' feelings and beliefs about themselves.* As previously mentioned, an internal or external (as opposed to chance) locus of control is usually associated with adopting healthy behaviors. Frequently, ethnic minorities do not experience an internal locus of control, due to past experience in not being able to control events determined by the dominant culture. Also previously described, patients who have a high level of self-efficacy, as it relates to the regimen in question, are more likely to be adopt healthy behaviors than those who are not confident in their ability to perform the recommended behaviors. Patients' readiness for change, as well as their behavioral intentions, are usually found to be associated with adopting healthy behaviors. Other feelings, such as dislike of taking medication, the desire not to depend on or be controlled by others, and the need to be seen by self or others as normal, may also interfere with patients' adoption of appropriate treatment regimens.

Surprisingly, *sociodemographic variables* such as age, sex, race, education, occupation, income, and marital status usually do not correlate with adherence behavior. However, elderly patients have been shown to have difficulty in opening childproof medication containers and are at increased risk for diseases that cause cognitive impairment, which in turn can affect comprehension, memory, and execution of a treatment plan. *Inability to pay* for visits, medication, or transportation can be an important barrier for some patients. In some studies, older age, retired status, married status, patient initiation (as opposed to provider initiation) of an appointment, and third-party payment, prepayment, or lack of copayment have been associated with improved appointment-keeping behavior, whereas lower education, lower socioeconomic status, and language barriers have been negatively correlated with appointment keeping.

Previous or concurrent adoption of one aspect of a treatment plan usually correlates with adoption of other aspects of the regimen.

Psychological factors, such as immaturity, impulsivity, hostility, fear of dependence, denial, commitment to a bad decision, and type A personality have been found to correlate with nonadherence in some studies. Moreover, some patients who come to practitioners are experiencing considerable anxiety, which may interfere with cognitive functioning, of which comprehension is one element. Other patients may experience a period of grief in reaction to a diagnosis, such as diabetes or coronary artery disease, and such grief may interfere with their ability to master the demands of a new treatment regimen. Understanding may be further hampered by the tendency of many patients to ask few questions of their practitioners even when they desire information (35).

Disease Features

Patients who are *experiencing symptoms* such as pain, lethargy, and palpitations are more likely than asymptomatic patients to follow treatment recommendations, especially if the symptoms are relieved by the treatment. On the other hand, patients may be so overwhelmed and debilitated by their symptoms that are unable to follow through with aspects of the regimen.

Comorbidity may either create problems for patients or provide the patient with a set of self-management skills that are easily applied. For example, a patient with hypertension and diabetes who has recently had a myocardial infarction may either have trouble following recommendations because of the multiple demands or may actually have an easier time as the result of having learned self-management skills with the hypertension and diabetes. Patients with depression or certain *psychiatric illnesses,* such as mania, schizophrenia, paranoia, or antisocial or paranoid personality disorder, are less likely to follow a treatment regimen. Factors that affect the patient's *ability to comprehend* or to organize and initiate deliberate behavior, such as dementia or mental retardation, should also be expected to impair the patient's ability to follow a treatment regimen. *Alcoholism and drug addiction* correlate highly with failure to follow prescribed regimens.

Treatment Factors

The *complexity* of medical regimens correlates inversely with adherence to them. Adherence decreases as the number of medications or the number of daily doses per medication increases. Unsynchronized schedules (e.g., one drug every 4 hours and another every 6 hours) should also be expected to affect medication-taking behavior adversely. The *duration* of therapy and the requirement for significant *behavioral change* (e.g., weight reduction, smoking cessation) are negatively correlated with adoption of healthy behaviors. *Side effects* of medications may result in failure to follow a medication regimen if they cause significant symptoms or interfere with an important function in the individual's life (e.g., impotence secondary to an antihypertensive drug in a young, sexually active man). *Medication class* is related to medication-taking behavior, with higher adherence rates for seemingly more important drugs (e.g., cardiac and diabetic agents—more than 70% adherence in cross-sectional studies) than for seemingly less important medicines (e.g., antacids, sedatives, and drugs prescribed for symptomatic relief—less than 50% adherence) (36–39). The reason for these differences is unknown; it could relate to sound patient judgment or to increased practitioner emphasis, supervision, and teaching. The relationship between independently audited medication need and medication-taking behavior remains unexplored. Other aspects of the treatment regimen that may influence medication-taking behaviors include *delayed or not obvious benefits* of the therapy, the degree of *lifestyle interference,* and the *expense* to the patient.

Environmental Factors

Patients who have stable *support systems* and stable *family situations* are more likely to adopt healthy behaviors than those who do not. A spouse's concern about a patient's illness can encourage medication taking, appointment keeping, and behavior changes (e.g., diet, smoking cessation). Advice and reinforcement from other family, friends, and lay practitioners can also encourage adoption. Nursing and office staff may promote healthy behaviors by demonstrating enthusiasm and positive attitudes about a treatment regimen. On the other hand, an overly protective family member can sabotage a plan for progressive return to normal function. Disinterested or poorly informed family members or friends may actually discourage patients from following a treatment plan. Family dysfunction or high levels of dependence on the patient (e.g., when the patient is a caretaker) can create a burden that makes adopting healthy behaviors difficult.

The *cultural norms* of social group, ethnicity, family, age, and gender also are important. Adherence to these norms is likely to supersede adherence to the norms of the medical profession when the two are in conflict. Patients may have *competing priorities or environmental obstacles* to adopting healthy behaviors, such as child care problems, crime, poverty, or transportation difficulties.

It should be remembered that patients' *previous experiences of similar disease* among relatives or friends can profoundly affect their beliefs about their own illnesses and influence their health-related behaviors.

Appointment keeping is positively correlated with *appointment scheduling systems* that reduce waiting time, give individual rather than block appointments, minimize the time between scheduling and the actual appointment date, and make referrals to specific practitioners rather than to clinics. *Convenience* in terms of location or hours of operation of a practitioner's practice and *support staff* who are respectful, friendly, and helpful may also encourage appointment keeping and discourage dropping out.

Practitioner–Patient Relationship

Establishment of a good practitioner–patient relationship is well recognized as an important determinant of patients' adherence to treatment plans. Although *effective communication* is a prerequisite to the establishment of such a relationship and affects health care outcomes (23,40–42) as well as the adoption of health-promoting behaviors (19–21,23,43–47), studies show that practitioners commonly communicate poorly with their patients (19,48–50). The necessary skills (see Chapter 3) can be learned and are being taught with increasing frequency in medical schools, residencies, and continuing education courses (50–52).

Effective transfer of information is important (53,54) because patients must understand their regimens before they can be expected to follow them (see Intervention Instructional Strategies). Because patients may already have some ideas and concerns about their problems, explanations that justify a treatment regimen, correct or accommodate misconceptions, and make sense to the patient are most likely to promote adoption of the regimen.

Differences may exist between practitioner and patient *styles of communication.* These include implicit versus explicit, direct versus indirect, self-enhancement versus self-effacement, person-based versus status-based, and verbal-based versus silence-based styles. Practitioners' adjustment of their styles of communication to meet the needs of different patients and different situations may enhance the effectiveness of interactions.

Language barriers are particularly pertinent to multicultural interactions between practitioners and patients. Even with the use of a translator, there may be mistranslation of concepts and errors of omission. Interactions can be optimized by using short and direct sentences; avoiding technical or professional jargon, idioms, and metaphors; avoiding complex questions; and allowing enough time (33).

In some cross-cultural interactions, it may be essential to *accommodate to the norms of the patient's culture.* For example, in traditional Navajo culture, it is important to present important medical information, such as information about a procedure that involves risk, in positive and not negative ways (55). In some cultures it is important to communicate directly with a patient's family member, rather than the patient. This applies to cultures where there are strict gender or generational roles that should be observed in the making of medical decisions.

Other features of the communication process that correlate with patient adherence to treatment regimens include the following (19–21,23,40,41,44,46,47,56):

- *Fulfillment of patient expectations* (requires detection of and attention to the patient's underlying concerns)
- Practitioner *friendliness* and use of a *positive, confident approach*
- Practitioner *response to patient complaints*
- *Encouragement of patient questions*
- A *supportive, nonjudgmental method of eliciting and responding to patient reports of unhealthy behaviors*
- Communication to patients of a genuine and accurate *empathetic understanding* of their perspectives and feelings
- *Encouragement of patients to become actively involved* in their own care
- *Active patient participation* as opposed to practitioner dominance
- *Negotiation rather than dictation of a treatment plan*
- *Identification and resolution of barriers to adopting healthy behaviors*
- *Congruence* between patient and practitioner in their understanding of a problem and its management
- *Practitioner effort to motivate* the patient
- *Patient satisfaction*

Transference, or the subconscious redirection to one person (the practitioner) of feelings and attitudes for others (e.g., parents, siblings, authority figures), may further influence patients' relationships to their practitioner. Depending on their nature, transference reactions, which are based on previous experiences, can promote adoption of healthy behaviors (e.g., the patient who finds it rewarding to please authority figures) or impede it (e.g., the patient who distrusts authority figures). *Countertransference,* the redirection toward the patient of previously developed practitioner attitudes and feelings, can also be detrimental or beneficial to the practitioner–patient relationship (see Chapter 20).

Close supervision of the patient by the practitioner (or an assistant) has proved to be a consistent and significant correlate of adherence to therapeutic regimens. In most studies, *continuity in provider care* has also contributed.

Many of the features just described contribute to the development of *patient trust in the practitioner,* and trust is one of the most important factors in any approach to helping people change. A key element of trust is self-disclosure. Because self-disclosure exposes the patient to possible rejection, ridicule, shame, or exploitation, it is important to elicit and respond to admissions of unhealthy behaviors in a nonjudgmental manner, in the context of a positive and supportive relationship. In cross-cultural interactions, additional aspects related to trust include respecting differences between the practitioner and patient in regard to comfort with personal distance, the amount and placement of touch, perceptions of privacy, and the use of informal or formal communication. With certain ethnicities, trust-building may take additional time and effort on the part of the practitioner owing to the patient's feeling intimidated by the practitioner, difficult past experiences with health care providers, or feelings of powerlessness.

Some practitioners prefer patients who do not ask too many questions and who simply follow instructions. Although this active–passive relationship may be appropriate for some patients, to be effective with other ambulatory patients, practitioners must enter into a relationship of *mutual participation* in which they listen to, educate, and negotiate with patients (40,41,57). It should not be assumed in cross-cultural interactions that patients who do not ask questions are passive or apathetic. They may feel intimidated, or they may be observing cultural norms related to authority, status, and control. A mutual participation approach need not be time-consuming. It is the quality of the interaction, not the amount of time spent, that correlates with patient adoption of healthy behaviors and satisfaction (48,50).

Methods for Assessing Background Information

Much of the information detailed previously may already be known to the practitioner who has an ongoing relationship with a patient. *Review of the primary care and other front sheets* (see Chapter 1) in a well-maintained patient record is an efficient method of obtaining relevant information. A *focused medical and social history* can also elicit important background information. Whenever patients present with new problems or difficulty managing old ones, it is helpful to *inquire* about their understandings, beliefs, feelings, past experiences, and readiness for change related to the problem, as well as their expectations for the practitioner–patient encounter. The information-gathering skills described in Chapter 3 and demonstrated in the following examples pertain to this task.

EXAMPLES

Practitioner: Mrs. Smith, tell me your understanding of hypertension... what it is and how it should be treated [understanding].

or

Practitioner: Mr. Jones, it seems like you have been troubled by this back pain for some time now. What would you most like me to do for you today? [expectations].

or

Practitioner: Ms. Jackson, tell me how you feel about stopping smoking? [readiness for change].

Some patients may not expect, or may feel awkward about, such open inquiry as to their opinions. They may be embarrassed to reveal their ideas or fear being ridiculed for them by the practitioner. Therefore, they may initially avoid answering the questions. In these situations, it is helpful to be gently persistent while conveying genuine interest in and respect for the patient.

EXAMPLE

Practitioner: Mr. Johnson, you seem worried about your sore throat. What do you think might be causing it?

Patient: I don't know. That's what I came here for . . . to find out [possible avoidance].

Practitioner: Well, I have some ideas, but its also helpful for me to hear about my patients' concerns so that I can make sure I address them [gentle persistence].

Patient: Well, I really don't know. I just wanted to make sure it wasn't something serious, since it's been hanging on. You know I'm a smoker, and so was my dad. He died of throat cancer.

Practitioner: Well, that's a very understandable concern [nonjudgmental, supportive, and respectful response].

Result: The practitioner proceeds to explain that there is no reason to suspect cancer on the basis of the history or physical examination and uses the opportunity to explore the patient's readiness to stop smoking.

Assessing Health-Related Behaviors

Knowledge of a patient's medication-taking and other health-related behaviors is a prerequisite to evaluating the effectiveness of current regimens and determining whether there is a need for behavioral change or reinforcement. This section focuses on general assessment strategies. Subsequent chapters address the measurement of some specific health-related behaviors (substance use, Chapters 27 through 29; exercise, Chapters 16 and 63; obesity, Chapter 83) and problem-solving styles (Chapters 19, 20, and 23).

Explicit assessment of health-related behaviors is important because studies have shown that practitioners are poor at subjectively predicting patients' adherence to treatment regimens, sometimes performing no better than expected by chance (58–61). There are several approaches to assessing health behaviors in patients (Table 4.2). Because each method has some limitations, it is often necessary to use more than one method to arrive at a reasonably valid estimate of such behaviors in an individual patient.

Asking

The simplest and most practical method of assessing health-related behavior is to ask the patient. With straightforward questioning, however, only 40% to 80% of patients will acknowledge that they are not following treatment plans (poor sensitivity). On the other hand, self-reports by patients that they are not following desired regimens are generally valid (high specificity). There is even some evidence that patients who admit to not following recommendations may be more amenable to intervention than those who do not (62).

The manner of asking influences the accuracy of patient response and the degree of patient comfort. Certain interview methods can provide reasonably valid estimates of patient health-related behaviors (63). It is generally agreed that patients should be questioned about their behavior in an *open-ended, facilitative, nonthreatening, nonjudgmental, yet detailed and specific* way. Questioning should continue until the patient has provided information about what medicines are being taken and how often, how often doses are missed, and what nonpharmacologic modes of treatment are being used. Patients should specifically be asked about health-related behaviors on the day of and the day preceding their visit. (For example, some diabetic patients routinely omit all drugs, including insulin, at the time of a morning visit; *24-hour recalls* are more accurate than general reports, which tend to be idealized.) Using such techniques, the practitioner will be able to identify 50% or more of those patients who are not following a negotiated regimen (and all of those who have not followed through because they did not understand the regimen). On occasion, more accurate information may be obtained by asking family or household members. In certain cross-cultural interactions, the practitioner may need to use an implicit or indirect approach to determining patient behavior.

EXAMPLE: INEFFECTIVE METHOD

Practitioner: Now, Mrs. Smith, are you taking your medications as prescribed? [judgmental and leading question, permits a Yes/No answer and promotes a Yes answer, confines response to medications].

Patient: Yes, every day.

Result: The practitioner raises the dosage or adds a new medication because the patient's blood pressure is still not adequately controlled. The patient becomes frustrated.

Table 4.2. Assessment of Health-Related Behaviors

Asking: open-ended, facilitative, nonjudgmental, detailed, and specific questioning of patient or family regarding nonpharmacologic as well as medication-taking health-related behaviors; 24-hour recalls (see text example)
Frequency of patient-requested prescription renewals or medication counts
Inspection of all pill bottles
Drug assays
Achievement of expected therapeutic and physiologic outcomes (e.g., blood pressure, weight, heart rate)
Review of longitudinal relationship between therapeutic and outcome measures
Direct observation by physician or staff (office or hospital)
Observations reported by others (e.g., family, visiting nurses)

Example: Effective Method

Practitioner: Now, Mrs. Smith, can you tell me what you are doing to control your blood pressure? [open-ended, nonjudgmental, focuses responsibility on the patient, does not confine response to medications].

Patient: Well, I've stopped adding salt to my food and have pretty much cut out all salted snacks. I do occasionally have a frozen dinner when I'm alone. And, of course, I'm taking the medication.

Practitioner: Uh, huh . . . . [facilitative].

Patient: Yes, that blue pill.

Practitioner: And how are you taking it? [directive, not leading].

Patient: Twice a day.

Practitioner: Any other medications? [directive, not leading].

Patient: No. I stopped the fluid pill when we started the blue one.

Practitioner: And did you take the blue one this morning? [directive].

Patient: No, I never take my medicine the day I come to the office!

Practitioner: What about yesterday? [directive, not leading].

Patient: Yes . . . at least in the morning. Yesterday afternoon was so hectic! You know how busy my days are!

Practitioner: I guess it's hard to take that afternoon dose? [facilitative, empathetic, nonjudgmental].

Patient: Yes, because my schedule varies so much.

Practitioner: What did you decide about starting on an exercise program? [directive, nonjudgmental, focuses responsibility on the patient].

Patient: Thought about it, but haven't done anything yet. Do you really think it's important?

Result: The practitioner congratulates (positively reinforces) the patient on salt restriction, tailors a medication regimen to the patient's schedule, explains why the patient should take her medication on the day of an office visit, provides more information on the value of regular exercise, and provides written instructions and a contract to which both agree. The practitioner decides not to restart the diuretic because the patient has restricted her salt and because the current blood pressure reading does not reflect the effect of the patient's current medication regimen. If the dietary history had been less convincing or the patient had gained weight, the patient might have been asked for a 24-hour diet recall (which is more accurate than general questioning) on this and subsequent visits.

Medication Counts

Medication counts (pill counts) are a form of indirect behavioral monitoring that provides a more objective measure of how patients are following prescribed medication regimens than does simply asking. They have been used to demonstrate the lack of reliability of patient-reported medication-taking behavior. Results are usually expressed in terms of percentages. The ability to measure sequential behavior depends on the use of short intervals between counts, which is usually not feasible. Although more accurate than reported behavior, medication counts also have limitations. If patients are suspicious of being monitored, they can remove medicines from containers without ingesting them. Overestimates of medication usage can also occur if other people are using medicine from the same container. Medication usage may be underestimated if the patient is using two or more medication containers but makes only one available for counting. Furthermore, many patients do not bring their medication containers with them to the practitioner's office, despite reminders. Finally, some patients might take offense at having their medications counted, resulting in deterioration of the practitioner–patient relationship.

The medication count can be approximated by the more practical and less intrusive method of prescribing quantities of medication that should be consumed within a reasonable interval of time, and then observing the *frequency with which prescription renewals are requested.*

Ingenious medication dispensers have been devised that monitor not only the amount but also the regularity with which medicine is removed (64). They are emerging as a new gold standard for the assessment of medication-taking behavior, but currently they are used primarily in research trials, are expensive, and are not generally available for use in clinical practice.

Assays

An objective but indirect method of assessing medication-taking behavior involves testing drug levels in blood, urine, breath, or saliva. Drug levels have been shown to correlate with compliance determined by other methods as well as by outcome. Marked variation in drug levels may reflect inconsistencies in medication taking. Monitoring drug levels and relaying results to the patient may also improve medication-taking behavior.

However, there are limitations to the method. Assays can be expensive. For accurate assessment, multiple measurements are required over an extended period. There is the possibility that patients who know they are being monitored may take medicine immediately before the collection of specimens but not at other times. More important may be differences in drug absorption, distribution, metabolism, and excretion among individuals, which make it impossible in the individual patient to decide whether a low level represents ineffective medication-taking behavior or inadequate dosage. The absence of any drug in the specimen suggests failure to take any of the medication, assuming the specimen has been collected appropriately. The practitioner should have a working knowledge of the pharmacokinetics of the medicine being assayed so that the collection of specimens can be timed correctly. Short-acting drugs, which are rapidly cleared from the blood and excreted, are difficult to monitor by assay techniques because of the difficulty in collecting specimens at appropriate times. Finally, assays are not available for many medications.

Assays can also be used to assess *abstention* from alcohol, drugs, and smoking (see Chapters 27 through 29).

Outcomes

Another objective but more indirect method of assessing health-related behaviors is to monitor expected therapeutic or physiologic outcomes. For example, blood pressure can be monitored in a patient who is taking antihypertensive medication, weight in a patient on a weight reduction diet, and pulse rate in a patient prescribed a β-blocker. *Review of the longitudinal relationship between a specific therapeutic regimen and outcome measures* can provide clues to health-related behaviors (e.g., the review may disclose widely varying blood pressures on a constant regimen). Such a review can be expedited by the presence and maintenance of a treatment versus outcome flow sheet (see Chapter 1). Feedback about outcomes to patients can also serve to motivate them to change their behavior or positively reinforce changes they have made.

Many of the limitations of drug assays also pertain to assessment of health-related behaviors by the monitoring of outcomes. Outcomes can be influenced by variations in drug bioavailability, absorption, distribution, and excretion; multiple measurements are required. Furthermore, additional factors can influence outcome. For example, a reduction in stress may lower blood pressure, or the presence of concomitant heart disease might be responsible for bradycardia.

Observation

An additional approach to assessing health-related behaviors is to observe patients directly, or indirectly through others, such as family members, household members, or visiting nurses. Patient self-monitoring reports can also serve as a form of indirect monitoring. They have the additional benefit of providing feedback to the patient, which can motivate the patient to change behaviors or positively reinforce changes that have been made.

An extension of this approach involves the *comparison of drug levels or outcomes of therapy during observed versus unobserved periods of a targeted behavior* such as medication consumption. Observations and measurements can be accomplished either in the office, at home, or during hospitalization, depending on the pharmacokinetics of a medication, insurance coverage, and the availability of home care resources. A specific example of this methodology is the 5-hour office blood pressure check in patients who have resistant hypertension, during which the patients take their medication under supervision, then have their blood pressure measured at regular intervals for several hours (65).

Inspection of all pill bottles is a commonly used and important form of observation. When the patient appears confused or is unable to provide sufficient information, having the patient bring all medication containers to the office (including those for both prescribed and over-the-counter medications) may provide invaluable information. For example, it may be discovered that a patient is still taking a discontinued medication or is taking two different preparations of the same drug. Selected patients, such as those with cognitive impairment and those on complicated medication regimens, should be encouraged to bring their medication containers with them at every visit.

Table 4.3. Intervention: General Principles

Start with a practitioner–patient relationship that promotes patient trust in the practitioner.
Target the educational intervention to Address patient-identified readiness to change (Fig. 4.1) Meet the patient's specific educational needs
Use specific measurable objectives to focus each interaction; use instructional, behavioral, and motivational/empowerment strategies, mechanical aids, and resources within and beyond the practice as a menu of options to achieve objectives.
Prioritize and limit objectives and material to be covered at each interaction.
Remain patient-centered and interactive.
Avoid premature education before relevant information has been collected and synthesized.
Check for patient comprehension and agreement.

INTERVENTION

General Principles

Once an educational assessment has been made, the practitioner is well positioned to help the patient acquire the information, attitudes, skills, and behaviors needed to deal with the medical problem. It is helpful to keep in mind some general principles (Table 4.3) when designing and implementing an educational intervention for a given patient.

- Whenever possible, *ground the educational intervention in a practitioner–patient relationship that promotes patient trust in the practitioner* (see Practitioner-Patient Relationship earlier in this chapter and Chapter 3 for the characteristics of and methods for developing such a relationship). The successful past management of problems will also enhance trust in the practitioner.
- *Target the intervention* to:
  - Address the stage of the patient's readiness for change, which has been identified as part of the educational assessment process described earlier (Fig. 4.1).
  - Meet the patient's educational needs, including knowledge, attitudinal, behavioral, and environmental needs, which have been identified with the use of assessment approaches described earlier (see Background Information).
- *Develop specific, measurable objectives* that can be used to focus the educational strategies. Then, the numerous instructional, behavioral, and motivational/empowerment strategies; mechanical aids; and resources within and beyond one's practice, which are discussed later, can be viewed as a menu of options that can be used to help achieve the objectives.

EXAMPLES

Objective: Between this visit and the next, the patient will adhere to a medication regimen, agreed upon by him and me.

or

Objective: By the end of this visit, the patient will be reassured that her malaise and weight loss are unlikely to be caused by cancer (her fear) and will entertain the possibility of depression as a cause.

- *Prioritize and limit the objectives and material to be covered* at each interaction, so that they do not overwhelm the patient and can be accomplished within available time limits.
- *Remain patient-centered and interactive* (e.g., by accommodating or addressing the patients' routines, beliefs, values, and expectations and involving them in the plan). This permits the practitioner to continually adapt educational strategies to meet the patient's needs. It enhances patient understanding, retention, and adoption of treatment regimens and agreed-upon lifestyle changes.
- *Avoid premature education.* Except for simple responses to answerable questions, it is generally preferable to provide patient education *after* relevant historical and physical examination data have been collected, information synthesized, an educational assessment made, and a tentative plan formulated. Premature education can result in the giving of misinformation, which will later have to be corrected. It can be ineffective or inefficient if it is not based on adequate assessment or not appropriately focused and prioritized. It is also inefficient because it provides information early in an encounter that will usually be repeated at the close of the encounter.
- *Check for patient comprehension and agreement* with explanations and management plans. Checking helps the practitioner gauge the success of an intervention.

EXAMPLES

Practitioner: I know we covered a lot today. It would help if you could tell me in your own words what you are going to do between now and the next visit.

or

Practitioner: Last visit we discussed treatment options for your angina. I also gave you a handout on angina. I wonder what your thoughts are now on the options and my recommendations?

Applying these general principles to practitioner–patient educational interactions should enhance patients' understanding, satisfaction, and adoption of desired health-related behaviors. Specific educational and behavioral change methods are discussed later in this chapter. They should be viewed as a menu of options that can be used in implementing the general principles that have been discussed in this section and summarized in Table 4.3.

Efficacy of Educational and Behavioral Change Interventions

Educational and behavioral change interventions can be classified as instructional, behavioral, motivational/empowerment, or organizational strategies or mechanical aids. Successful interventions have increased adherence rates by amounts that range from less than 10% to almost 70%, averaging between 25% and 30% (percentage change equals percentage of adherent patients in the experimental group minus percentage of adherent patients in the control group). Adherence-improving interventions can also be cost-effective (5,6). A combination of instructional and behavioral/motivational interventions is more effective than instruction alone.

Instructional Strategies

Some sort of explanation or communication of information is a part of almost every practitioner–patient interaction. Sometimes the explanation is an end in itself (e.g., explaining to a patient the expected course of a condition for which there is no treatment, clarifying a patient's unfounded fears about a laboratory test). In other situations, it promotes adherence by providing patients with a rationale for treatment and clarifying a treatment regimen (53,54). The patient education content related to specific problems and diagnostic procedures is described in later chapters of this book (see especially the Patient Experience sections). Instructional strategies that enhance understanding, retention, and adherence are displayed in Table 4.4 and discussed next.

Information is most effective when it is *targeted* to the needs of the patient, provides an *explanatory framework* understandable and acceptable to the patient, and *addresses misconceptions and potential barriers* to compliance. The use of medical jargon should be avoided, and the use of language should be tailored to the educational and cultural background of the patient.

To improve retention, verbal instructions should be *clear, concise, and explicit,* with *important features emphasized and repeated.* When there is a large or complex body of information to be conveyed, it is helpful to break it down into understandable categories, as in "I am going to tell you what I think is causing your symptoms, what tests I am going to suggest, and the treatment that should help you. Now, what I think is causing these symptoms . . . ." This technique has been shown to improve retention of information when compared with a less organized recitation of facts (66).

An *interactive* as opposed to monologue approach to communicating information encourages patients to ask questions and have their questions answered. It

Table 4.4. Intervention: Instructional Strategies

Target information to meet educational needs.
  Provide explanatory framework understandable and acceptable to patient.
  Address misconceptions, fears, and barriers.
Use language appropriate to educational and cultural background of patient; avoid medical jargon.
Use verbal communication methods that increase understanding and retention.
  Be clear
  Be concise
  Be explicit
  Repeat important content
  Categorize
  Use dialogue, as opposed to monologue
Test for comprehension.
Give written instructions.
Give printed educational material.

permits ongoing targeting of the educational message and assessment of patient understanding. It should also increase retention.

Because patient factors such as anxiety and reluctance to ask questions may interfere with understanding, it is useful to *check for patient understanding and retention* of the essentials of the information that has been communicated. Furthermore, because it has been found that patients tend to recall the diagnosis better than the treatment plan (66), it is important to ascertain retention of the essentials of the treatment plan. For example, for a streptococcal throat infection, determine whether the patient understands that penicillin will be taken for a full 10 days (not the exact dosage or schedule, which will be transcribed onto the pill bottle). In order not to offend the patient when checking for comprehension, it is helpful to use an approach such as, "We covered a lot today, and I'm not sure whether I have explained things clearly. It would help me if you would tell me what you understand to be the plan," rather than directly ordering the patient, "Now tell me what the plan is."

Written instructions further enhance adherence (53) and are an important adjunct to verbal instruction. They can be documented on self-duplicating forms (Fig. 4.3). The duplicate portion can be attached to a visit note or a specially constructed educational flow sheet for documentation and future reference. Providing patients with understandable charts that list medications and display the schedule for each medication enhances adherence to prescribed regimens (67). Legible written or printed instructions provide a remedy for forgetfulness and can be reviewed at leisure in the less stressful environment of the patient's home.

Because it usually requires time to make sense out of information about one's condition (e.g., newly diagnosed hepatitis), because patients retain only about one-half of the essential information communicated at a visit (48,66), and because practitioner–patient communication is usually focused and time-limited, *printed educational materials* can be used to reinforce and expand on what the patient has been told. When printed materials are given to a patient, the practitioner can personalize them by underlining important points, writing down additional important information, and writing the day's date on it. A large collection of printed educational handouts is available in the periodically updated book and CD-ROM, *Griffith's Instructions for Patients* (see General References). Condition-specific publications that are widely available (e.g., from the American Heart Association or National Cancer Institute) are cited in later chapters of this book.

Behavioral Strategies

Communication of information is necessary but often insufficient to ensure the adoption and maintenance of health-related behaviors by a patient. This is particularly true in the setting of chronic disease, probably because most patients have already learned their prescribed regimen and have learned something about their disease. Behavioral strategies (Table 4.5) attempt to directly influence the adoption or maintenance of certain behaviors. Strategies that incorporate various combinations of patient involvement, alterations in the treatment regimen (simplification, tailoring, shaping), use of behavioral stimuli and reinforcements, and supervision have been shown to improve patient adherence to chronic and short-term therapeutic regimens.

Mechanisms of *enhancing patient involvement* include facilitating patient question-asking, negotiating a treatment plan with the patient (rather than dictating

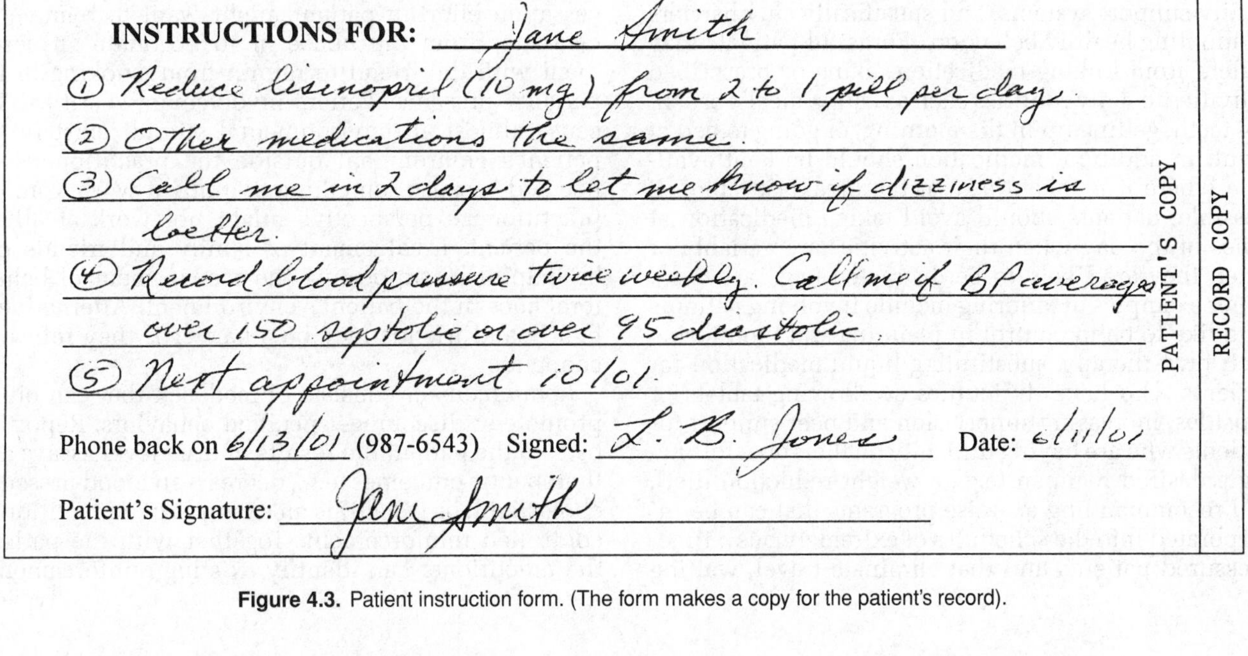

INSTRUCTIONS FOR: Jane Smith

① Reduce lisinopril (10 mg) from 2 to 1 pill per day.
② Other medications the same.
③ Call me in 2 days to let me know if dizziness is better.
④ Record blood pressure twice weekly. Call me if BP averages over 150 systolic or over 95 diastolic.
⑤ Next appointment 10/01.

Phone back on 6/13/01 (987-6543) Signed: L. B. Jones Date: 6/11/01

Patient's Signature: Jane Smith

PATIENT'S COPY

RECORD COPY

Figure 4.3. Patient instruction form. (The form makes a copy for the patient's record).

Table 4.5. Intervention: Behavioral Strategies

Involve patients in
Developing management plans
Self-monitoring
Simplify treatment regimen.
Tailor treatment regimen to fit patient's characteristics and environment.
Implement complex treatment regimen in a stepwise or graduated manner (shaping).
Manage behavioral stimuli (cues).
Use reinforcements.
Enlist support from family, friends, workplace.
Increase supervision.

a treatment plan to the patient), signing a contract with the patient, and encouraging patient self-monitoring, such as the measuring of glucose levels or taking of blood pressure readings at home. All of these measures increase patients' responsibility for their own care, increase patient confidence, and enhance patient motivation to adopt healthy behaviors. They have been shown in several studies to improve health outcomes (40–42,57,68). Self-monitoring may also move patients from precontemplation to contemplation to action in the readiness for change cycle (Fig. 4.1) and may motivate problem solving in cases in which the patient is not following through with a treatment plan.

Simplification of the treatment regimen refers to minimizing the number of medications, minimizing the duration of treatment (for short-term regimens), minimizing the frequency of dosing (e.g., once instead of three times daily), and synchronizing the dosing (e.g., three medicines twice daily instead of one medicine twice daily, the second medicine three times daily, and the third medicine four times daily). The less complex the regimen, the greater the adherence rate. This is a particularly important strategy both because of its effectiveness and its ease of implementation.

Tailoring is a process whereby the therapeutic regimen is fitted to the patient's characteristics and environment. Effective tailoring requires knowledge of patients as persons—their beliefs, lifestyles, social and family support systems, and specifically, any barriers to adopting healthy behaviors. Forgetful patients may benefit from linking medication taking or prescribed activities to daily routines such as eating meals, brushing teeth, getting up in the morning, or going to bed at night. In addition, medication should be kept available where it is taken (e.g., at the breakfast table). If possible, patients should avoid taking medication at times of the day when their activities are variable or when they are likely to be distracted (e.g., at work). Other examples of tailoring include involving patients who like to be in control in planning and monitoring their own therapy, substituting liquid medication for patients who have difficulties swallowing tablets or capsules, increasing supervision and peer support for patients who are having difficulty on their own following a desired regimen (e.g., a weight reduction diet), and recommending exercise programs that can be incorporated into the schedules of extremely busy, time-pressured patients and that eliminate travel, waiting time, and the need for special scheduling. When cost is a factor, less expensive regimens can be prescribed or financial assistance sought. When a patient's health belief or explanatory model of disease interferes, it can sometimes be accommodated. For example, Hispanic patients who subscribe to the hot–cold theory of health and disease avoid the use of hot substances during pregnancy and therefore may refuse to take hot medications such as iron and vitamins. Adherence in this situation may be obtained by encouraging the patient to neutralize the hot properties of these medications with cool substances such as fruit juices or herb teas. *Language barriers* can be addressed by using written, computerized, or automated voice messaging systems that match patients' languages.

When a regimen is particularly complex or difficult, behavior change may be facilitated by *graduated regimen implementation, or shaping,* whereby parts of the regimen are implemented and the patient is initially rewarded for adhering to only part of the regimen. Once the first part has been achieved, additional components of the regimen are added in stepwise fashion, with rewards being given when there is adherence to both previously accomplished and newly added components. Patient involvement in identifying the steps and the rewards further facilitates the process.

In addition to adjusting the therapeutic regimen to meet the patient's needs, patient and practitioner can work together to identify and manage *behavioral stimuli (cues) and reinforcements* that promote or diminish desired behaviors. Watching television, for example, may be an environmental cue for patients who have learned the habit of eating when they watch television, even when they are not hungry. To eliminate this behavior, the practitioner and the patient might reach an agreement whereby a patient eats only at the dining room table with the television off. Another behavioral cue might be the presence of cigarettes or a friend smoking. In preparation for a smoking cessation effort, a patient might want to remove all cigarettes from the house or to negotiate an agreement with the friend to refrain from smoking in the patient's presence. Patient involvement is critical, because almost all environmental stimuli exist in the patient's environment outside the practitioner's office and because something that might work from the practitioner's perspective might not work at all for the patient. Involvement of family and friends can be helpful in supporting the management of behavioral cues in the patient's environment. Alternatively, family and friends may be a barrier if they refuse to cooperate.

Reinforcement consists of feedback that can either promote or discourage specified behaviors. Reporting back to the patient the results of drug level assays and therapeutic outcomes (e.g., decrease in blood pressure, cholesterol, or weight) is an example of a practitioner-controlled reinforcement. Together with the patient, the practitioner can identify existing reinforcements,

Table 4.6. Intervention: Motivation and Empowerment Strategies

Help patients adopt appropriate new beliefs, attitudes, and values.
- Target education to fill gaps in knowledge base, correct misconceptions, provide explanations that are understandable and acceptable to patients, and motivate patients in the context of their value systems.
- Use fear and benefit messages appropriately (relevant, accurate, connected to treatment plan that is effective and feasible for patient).
- Point out current/past patient beliefs, attitudes, behaviors that are congruent with the desired new beliefs, attitudes, and values.

Set agreed-upon goals.

Enhance patient self-perceptions (self-efficacy, locus of control).
- Project a positive attitude about patient's abilities to change.
- Emphasize past and present behaviors that demonstrate self-control.
- Help patients take credit for changes that have been accomplished.
- Reframe "failures" as successes.

Facilitate new skill development.
- Involve the patient in the development of management strategies.
- Facilitate problem solving by the patient.
- Facilitate the development of specific, achievable behavioral objectives by the patient.
- Facilitate the development of self-monitoring skills.

support or initiate those that promote, and attempt to eliminate or diminish those that discourage desired behaviors. Because positive feedback is more effective than punishment in helping patients adopt new behaviors, measures and outcomes that indicate adoption of desired behaviors should be praised, otherwise rewarded, or viewed by the patient as rewards in themselves. When measures or outcomes suggest that the patient is not following the regimen, the problem should be discussed. Rewards should be appropriate to the goals (e.g., eating an ice cream cone would be an inappropriate reward for having followed a diet) and can be increased as the patient gets closer to achieving the goals.

Education and the use of *family, friends, and employers* may be required to optimize rewards for desired behaviors or to reduce the rewards for undesired behaviors at home and in the community. Two common indications for such an intervention are reversal of reinforced psychosocial disability in the physically capable patient after myocardial infarction and maintenance of abstention in the detoxified alcoholic patient.

Increased supervision is a specific form of stimulus management and reinforcement that has been shown to improve adherence. It includes the scheduling of more frequent provider–patient contacts, the use of reminders, the use of drug assays, the use of automated voice messaging, and the eliciting of family or community support to assist in administering and monitoring treatment. For example, the practitioner may request more frequent blood pressure values in a hypertensive patient. The blood pressure readings can be taken by either a nurse at the practitioner's office, a nurse at work, a family member, or the patient. The direct supervision of medication administration is an option that is especially helpful for ensuring adherence in situations where it is known to be low, such as with patients who are forgetful or unreliable, have impaired intellectual or psychological functioning (e.g., patients with alcoholism, dementia, or schizophrenia), or have challenging psychosocial situations. Examples include the use of a single intramuscular long-acting penicillin dose rather than 10 days of an oral preparation, intermittent supervised oral antituberculosis therapy, and use of long-acting parenteral drugs in the ambulatory management of schizophrenia.

Motivation and Empowerment Strategies

Adoption of healthy behaviors tends to decay toward baseline after the cessation of many successful interventions. One explanation for the failure of most adherence-improving interventions to have enduring impact is their reliance on actions and supports that are *external* to the patient. Based on reviews of the relevant adherence, psychological, sociologic, and behavioral literature, DiMatteo and colleagues suggested *approaches that promote internalization of the patient's motivation and ability to adhere* (see DiMatteo and DiNicola, *Achieving Patient Compliance,* in General References). These approaches include helping patients to adopt new beliefs, attitudes, or values; setting agreed-upon goals; enhancing patients' perceptions of their self-efficacy; and facilitating new skill development in patients (Table 4.6).

Patients may have to adopt new beliefs, attitudes, or values and abandon others. Because practitioners are the major source of health information for most Americans (48), they can assist in this process. They are more likely to succeed if they have earned the patient's trust and if they incorporate empowerment strategies that involve the patient in setting goals, solving problems, and planning for the intervention (see Practitioner–Patient Relationship). As previously mentioned, the first step in promoting change in health attitudes is to explore the patient's present knowledge, beliefs, attitudes, and values, as well as social and cultural norms. Education about the patient's diseases and regimens can then be tailored to correct misconceptions, fill in gaps in the patient's knowledge base, provide explanations that are understandable and acceptable to the patient, and motivate the patient in the context of his or her value, social, and cultural systems. Simply taking time for discussion will raise the salience in the patient's mind of the issue being discussed. Threat or fear messages can motivate behavioral change, but they should not be too strong (i.e., so as to cause patient denial or paralysis) or too weak. Furthermore, they should be combined with a positive message about a feasible (for the patient) and effective therapeutic regimen. Because patients are often more present-oriented than future-oriented, short-term as well as long-term benefits of any regimen should be stressed. Because behavior can influence attitudes, and vice versa, the practitioner should point out the patient's own behaviors that support the attitude being promoted. One can help integrate the new attitude into the patient's total system of beliefs by noting how it correlates with other beliefs the patient has. One can also note how the new attitude adheres to cultural and social norms. Of course, new attitudes and beliefs need positive reinforcement, as previously discussed.

Mutually negotiating agreed-upon goals can be motivational and can provide direction for the patient. Patient involvement in, and preferably initiation of, goal setting is a crucial component of this step. For goals to be most effective, they must be "owned" by the patient. Goals should be set at two levels. The first level is long-term goals—such as, "I want to quit smoking in 6 months". The second level is short-term, or proximal, goals. These goals refer to the specific actions that will be required to meet the long-term goal—such as, "I will begin using Nicorette gum at a 4-mg dosage next Monday, and I will reduce this to 2 mg in 6 weeks." These goals are actually more helpful to the patient in that they are easier to achieve and can be measured more directly. To be effective, they should be specific, measurable, realistic, and achievable. Having the patient sign a contract can further increase the likelihood of success.

Patients with unhealthy *self-perceptions* or perceived low self-efficacy may need to be convinced that they can indeed effect a change in their lives (a process sometimes called *cognitive restructuring*). The practitioner can help by emphasizing the patient's past and present behaviors that demonstrated self-control, by enhancing the patient's feelings of responsibility for accomplished changes, by pointing out inaccuracies in the patient's negative self-perceptions, and by having and projecting a positive attitude to the patient about his or her ability to change.

Examples

Practitioner: On one hand, you say you have no self-control. On the other, you tell me you stopped smoking for the entire period of your second pregnancy. That demonstrates to me that you can exhibit tremendous self-control.

Practitioner: Two months ago you told me that you would never be able to manage insulin. Now you are monitoring your own blood sugars and calling me to propose changes in your insulin schedule. What does that tell you about yourself?

Patients and their practitioners often view partial successes as failures (e.g., the patient who has started drinking or smoking after a period of abstinence, the patient who has cut caffeine intake in half). In the office, practitioners can promote patients' self-esteem and sense of self-efficacy by *reframing these "failures" as successes,* as important steps along the way to accomplishing important health goals.

Example

Practitioner: It's great you were able to stop smoking for a month! That really increases your chances of being able to quit for good. Did you know that most people who stop smoking require more than one attempt?

In addition, patients can learn how to shift their own self-perceptions during vulnerable moments at home, when negative thoughts may interfere with following through with a plan. In anticipation, patients can be asked about potential "sticking points." In response to having experienced these sticking points, they can be encouraged to reflect on and contrast their thoughts during the times they have been successful versus the times they have not. Using these awarenesses, they can reframe a failure into a partial success in the moment, or they can use positive self-statements that have been previously effective (e.g., "I can do this"). Patients can take this one step further by *posting positive statements or images as reminders* where they can often see them or at places where they are likely to be tempted to not follow through with a treatment plan. Family members can be enlisted as verbal sources of positive statements or to help patients reframe their negative thoughts. However, it is essential that patients consider this as helpful and not as overinvolvement or an attempt by the family to control their behaviors.

New skills can also be taught to patients, an empowerment approach that enhances their ability, as well as motivation, to initiate and maintain adherence to a difficult regimen. Patients can learn problem-solving skills by analyzing, with the practitioner, the health problem, treatment alternatives, and the advantages and disadvantages of potential actions. They can participate in the development of overall treatment goals. They can be tutored in developing specific, feasible, and measurable behavioral objectives for themselves and in breaking down large tasks into several small, manageable steps. When patients have adopted new attitudes, beliefs, or behaviors, they can be taught to anticipate and prepare themselves for likely challenges by enhancing their decision-making capabilities.

Examples

Practitioner to the recovering alcoholic: What challenges do you expect to your new sobriety? How are you going to handle it when people try to get you to drink at your niece's wedding this weekend?

Practitioner to the hypertensive patient who is sensitive to being viewed as ill by others: How are you going to respond when one of your colleagues at work sees you taking your medication and says "Oh, you have to take medicine now! What's wrong with you?"

Patients can also be taught to analyze and learn from past failures to enhance the likelihood of future success.

EXAMPLES

Practitioner: Why has it been difficult for you to take the second dose?

Practitioner: Exactly how did it occur, when you started smoking again? What does that tell you?

Practitioner: If you could overcome that problem, your chances for success would be really high! Any ideas?

Efforts to help patients adopt appropriate health-promoting beliefs, attitudes, values, skills, and behaviors can be integrated into ongoing care and should usually span several office visits. Once patients have experienced success in implementing changes in one health-related behavior, their sense of efficacy increases, and they are more likely to be successful in changing other behaviors.

Mechanical Aids

Medication-taking behavior can also be improved by the use of a number of mechanical aids. These include well-labeled medication containers (69), medication charts (67), pill calendars (devices on which patients keep track of their medication taking), special pharmaceutical packaging designed to aid memory (e.g., the packaging of birth control pills), and pill dispensers (devices that can be purchased for laying out medications in advance by day and, when necessary, by time of day). Well-designed forms can promote the use and effectiveness of written instructions (Fig. 4.3) (67) and patient adherence to self-monitoring (e.g., by providing patients with flow sheets for recording blood pressure or blood sugar values and asking the patients to bring the sheets with them to their next visit).

Appointment Keeping

A number of factors have been shown to improve appointment keeping by patients (45). Table 4.7 lists the strategies that can be used to improve appointment-keeping behavior.

Telephone and mail reminders, in which patients receive messages several days before their scheduled visits informing them of the dates and times of their appointments or messages inviting patients to reschedule after missed appointments, have consistently improved adherence, usually by 10% to 20%. The impact of the reminders may attenuate over time, however (70), and it may be possible to discontinue reminders without a subsequent increase in missed appointments (71). Wording of the message may be influential. In one study of high-risk patients (72), postcards with a persuasive educational message resulted in a significantly higher adherence rate for influenza vaccination than those with a neutral message simply announcing the availability of the vaccine.

The introduction of *individual instead of block appointment systems* and the *substitution of a single provider for multiple providers* have resulted in decreased waiting time and improved appointment keeping. Individual appointment systems give each patient a precise time for an appointment; block systems schedule several or all patients for the same time, usually at the beginning of office hours.

Techniques that the practitioner can use to improve appointment keeping for individual patients include logically *"bridging" to the next visit* by discussing its purpose with the patient (e.g., monitoring for recurrence, review of test results, decision about therapy); *negotiating a visit interval* that is mutually acceptable; *tailoring the appointment time* to the patient's needs; *obtaining a verbal agreement* from the patient to follow through; and *scheduling the appointment* instead of asking the patient to call for an appointment. Bridging and scheduling have been tested in a successful clinical trial (73).

Because *missed appointments* could presage dropouts from treatment, the charts or names of patients who miss their appointments should be reviewed daily by the patient's practitioner or by a nurse familiar with the patient. When indicated, the patient can be contacted by telephone, letter, or postcard. This review method helps prevent dropping out by patients given a follow-up appointment at the time of the previous visit, but it fails to identify dropouts who were instructed to call for their next appointment.

If referral is required, *educating the patient about the purpose of referral, minimizing the elapsed time* between the referral and the referral appointment, providing secretarial assistance to *facilitate scheduling and transportation,* and *referring the patient to a specific practitioner* and not simply to a specialty group or clinic have also been shown to improve appointment keeping for diagnostic studies and specialty consultations.

Table 4.7. Intervention: Improving Appointment Keeping Behavior

Logically "bridge" to the next appointment.
Negotiate appointment time and interval with patient.
Refer to specific doctors rather than to clinics.
Educate patient about purpose of referral.
Reach agreement with or obtain verbal commitment from patient.
Schedule appointment for patient rather than having patient call for one.
Use individual, as opposed to block, appointment systems.
Minimize waiting time.
Use telephone or mailed reminders.
Establish review system for missed appointments.

Organizing a Practice for Patient Education

Patient education and adoption of healthy behaviors can be further enhanced through the implementation of effective practice operations. *Practice support staff* often have considerable interest in patient education, and involving them in this effort can save practitioner time and enhance the effectiveness of care. Many office practices involve nursing staff in educating patients about preventive measures such as immunizations, breast cancer screening, and family planning and in working with patients who have newly diagnosed chronic illnesses such as diabetes mellitus, asthma, or hypertension. In these instances, it is important to agree in advance which aspects of patient education will be covered by the practice's support staff and which will be covered by the practitioner.

Mailing test results or providing this information to patients through the use of automated voice messaging are services that can be incorporated into routine office operations. Depending on the situation, one may include additional information (e.g., norms and goals for test results, changes in regimen based on test results).

A collection of preselected *printed patient educational materials* can be maintained in an office file or on an office computer and distributed at the discretion of the practitioner or nursing staff. The materials should be available in languages and reading levels that are appropriate for the patient populations that the practice serves.

A certain amount of general patient education can be promoted in the *waiting room* by setting up a *pamphlet rack* containing 10 to 15 of the most commonly applicable printed materials. These might include pamphlets on age- and gender-appropriate preventive measures, smoking cessation, weight reduction, low-salt diets, exercise, and other topics of interest to patients and their families. Some practices have found it helpful to have a *bulletin board* with newspaper clippings about current health topics.

Other possibilities include the *delivery of health messages* to patients on telephone hold and the use of practice newsletters, audiovisual materials, and computerized interactive programs (74). Automated voice messaging can be use to send patients messages, as well as to receive and respond to their questions (75).

Finally, *medical records and related forms* can be structured in ways that promote the education and monitoring of patients. As mentioned earlier, self-duplicating forms for written instructions (Fig. 4.3) facilitate the provision of written instructions to the patient and follow-up by the practitioner at the next visit. Preprinted forms can be used to facilitate or to assist the practitioner in the mailing of diagnostic test results to patients. A flow sheet that chronologically aligns chronic medications and nondrug therapies with clinical and laboratory data (see Chapter 1) facilitates review of the relationship between a specific therapeutic regimen and associated clinical or laboratory parameters. A *method for keeping track of prescription renewals* can be incorporated into the patient record, such as the attachment of duplicate copies of all written prescriptions to a flow-carrier sheet. Such a method allows the practitioner to ascertain quickly when the patient is due for a refill. This is especially helpful when prescriptions are filled by more than one practitioner in the practice.

Using Resources Beyond the Practice

Resources beyond the practitioner's practice can provide information, support, and skills training for patients. The use of such resources is particularly helpful when the practitioner's practice has limited resources or when the educational task is time-consuming or complex. In such situations, the practitioner efforts should be supplemented by referral to:

- *Health professionals who specialize in disease-specific management* (e.g., health educators for diabetic or asthma management)
- *Those who specialize in treatment-specific management* (e.g., nutritionists, physical therapists, trainers, exercise physiologists)
- *Specific treatment programs* (e.g., postmyocardial infarction rehabilitation, smoking cessation programs)
- *Organizations* that provide education and support for specific problems (e.g., American Diabetes Association, Alzheimer's Associations)
- *Support groups* that expose patients to others with similar problems (e.g., community or internet asthma, postmyocardial infarction, ostomy, and mastectomy groups; Alcoholics Anonymous).

Volunteer patients who are followed regularly in one's practice or provided by outside organizations and who have successfully managed their chronic illness can serve as important resources to patients newly diagnosed with the same condition. *Telephone hotlines,* which can provide immediate access to patients who are in distress or in need of immediate information (76) (e.g., patients who are victims of domestic violence). Patients can also be referred to specific *internet sites* or provided with *audiovisual or CD-ROM interactive tutorials.* These have the advantages of availability, a private learning environment, and immediate reinforcement of learning (74).

Combining Strategies (Case Example)

Strategies that combine two or more methods are generally much more effective than single interventions (22,77,78). For example, such combination strategies have been shown to improve adherence in patients with asthma (79), congestive heart failure (80,81), diabetes (82), and hypertension (83) and after myocardial infarction (43). In the last study, patient involvement was accomplished by having patients set their own goals and monitor their own behavior. Frequent contact with the practitioner allowed reinforcement, modification of goals on a negotiated basis, and discussion of problems with the regimen. Involvement of the spouse led to increased supervision and support. In the asthma study, adherence and functional status were better after 1 year in a group of patients with asthma who received an instructional workbook and one-on-one counseling, participated in self-monitoring and an asthma support group, and were asked to identify an asthma control partner, compared with a group given standard informational pamphlets on asthma.

The following is an example of how instructional, behavioral, and motivational/empowerment strategies can be integrated into an office visit (continuation of a previous example).

Example

Practitioner: Well, Mrs. Smith, your blood pressure is 150/100 today, which, as you can see on this flow sheet, is better than when we started but not as low as we'd like it. Do you remember the goal we agreed on? [The word "we" implies shared responsibility. The practitioner focuses the patient's attention on a specific, measurable objective. The practitioner points out that some progress has been made, using a clinical flow sheet.]

Patient: I believe it was less than 140 on the top and less than 90 on the bottom.

Practitioner: Right. What do you think you could do to bring it down further? [The practitioner further involves and transfers responsibility to the patient.]

Patient: Well, as you said, part of the problem with today's blood pressure could be my not taking the medicine this morning. So I'll be sure to take it from now on, including the days I come to see you. Also I've been thinking about enrolling at the athletic club. I like dancing. The club has convenient hours and is on my way to work. I'd prefer not to take any more medicines.

Practitioner: The athletic club is an excellent idea. Regular exercise not only has a direct effect that lowers blood pressure, but it might also indirectly lower your pressure by helping you to lose weight. [The practitioner provides positive reinforcement and notes an added benefit that relates to another goal the patient has for herself.]

Patient: That would be nice.

Practitioner: Does the club have a trainer? A trainer could help ensure that your work out is aerobic and individualized to your needs. [The practitioner enlists the help of a resource external to the practice.]

Patient: I think so. That's a good idea.

Practitioner: I am still concerned about the difficulty you have getting the second dose of medication into your schedule. Blood pressure pills work best when you can take them almost 100% of the time. [The practitioner provides a rationale for this concern.] Would dinner time be a good time for you? [The practitioner initiates the negotiation process.]

Patient: My meal times are irregular and I don't always eat at home.

Practitioner: How about bedtime?

Patient: Sometimes I'm so exhausted, I just fall to sleep while I'm reading, before I've brushed my teeth or anything. Don't you have a pill that can be taken just once a day?

Practitioner: As a matter of fact, that is a possibility. When would you take it?

Patient: With my morning coffee. I never miss that!

Practitioner: Fine, I'll give you a prescription for a pill that you can take once a day with your morning coffee, 100% of the time, even the mornings you come to my office. Is that a deal? [Repetition and emphasis to increase retention].

Patient: Yes! [Solution and verbal contract achieved through tailoring and negotiation].

Practitioner: The side effects for this medicine are the same as for the other. Since you experienced none with the other, you should tolerate this one well.

Patient: Good.

Practitioner: Together with the salt restriction and exercise program, this medicine alone may be enough to control your blood pressure. [The practitioner provides further motivation for salt restriction and exercise.] Of course, we'll start with a low dosage, so we may have to increase it. Can you come back in 2 weeks?

Patient: How about 2 months?

Practitioner: Well, I'd really like to see you more often until your blood pressure is controlled. Of course, if you monitored your own blood pressure at home, you could call the results in to me and there would be less need for frequent office visits. (The practitioner prefers not to yield on the follow-up interval and uses the opportunity to motivate the patient to become further involved in her own management and to create a new environmental reinforcement.]

Patient: How can I do that?

[The practitioner proceeds to explain the process of getting a blood pressure cuff, coming to the office to have it checked, and learning how to use it; to test the patient for her understanding of her responsibilities; to get her verbal commitment; and to write down for her the new management plan.]

FOLLOW-UP

Education can involve the adoption of new beliefs, attitudes, or values; the development of a patient's sense of self-efficacy and self-management skills; the setting of agreed-upon goals; the adoption of new or cessation of old behaviors; and the maintenance of successfully changed behaviors (e.g., the taking of a chronic medication, the cessation of smoking). In the process, patients move forward in the readiness for change cycle (Fig. 4.1). Sometimes, as in the case of diabetes, the required cognitive and behavioral changes are both numerous and complex (see Chapter 79) and are best implemented in incremental steps (see earlier discussion) over the span of several visits. Commonly, patients successfully implement only part of a prescribed or agreed-upon regimen. Often, periods of successful implementation are followed by periods of relapse (Fig. 4.1). Therefore, *follow-up is a crucial component of patient education.* Repetitive cycles of assessment and intervention (Fig. 4.2) are associated with increased success in helping patients adopt and maintain healthy behaviors and should therefore be integrated into ongoing care. The following example illustrates this principle.

Example

A patient with hypertension, diabetes, and hypercholesterolemia was also a heavy smoker. Over the course of 2 years, he gradually succeeded in accepting and understanding his medical conditions; reliably taking his antihypertensive, oral hypoglycemic, and lipid-lowering medications; altering his diet to one low in cholesterol, saturated fats, salt, and concentrated sweets; inspecting his feet regularly; and having yearly eye examinations. Initially, however, he was very resistant to the suggestion that he stop smoking [precontemplation stage]. However, his practitioner listed smoking as a problem on his medical problem list and let him know that smoking cessation was probably the single most effective thing he could do to improve his health [instruction].

On successive visits, the practitioner explored with the patient his feelings about smoking, the pros and cons of his stopping, the barriers to his stopping [assessment, raising the problem to the level of contemplation], and the role of nicotine use in smoking cessation [instruction]. She expressed confidence in his ability to stop when he was ready and indicated her interest in helping him [promotion of the patient's sense of self-efficacy and support]. She checked on his smoking behavior and readiness to stop periodically [maintenance of contemplation].

The patient made one attempt to stop after 2 years [action] and succeeded for 2 months, but then resumed smoking during a period of stress at work [relapse]. His practitioner congratulated him on his success and told him that it proved he was capable of quitting. She noted that most patients who successfully quit require more than one attempt [reframing a "failure" as a success].

Two months later, after discussing his brother's death from a myocardial infarction with his practitioner [additional stimulus, moving the patient from contemplation to action], the patient set a quit date, removed all cigarettes from his home and work environment, elicited support for his quitting from family and friends, and planned for his responses to stressful situations. With the additional help of a nicotine patch and periodic encouragement from his practitioner, he succeeded in stopping for good.

ETHICAL CONSIDERATIONS

It has been suggested that the following three conditions be met before attempting to improve adherence: (a) the diagnosis should be correct; (b) the therapy should be proven to be efficacious and the benefits should outweigh the adverse effects; and (c) the patient should be an informed and willing partner in the intervention (84).

Although the first two conditions are probably applicable to interventions directed toward populations, they may be too rigid for application to individual patients. In some circumstances, it may be reasonable to prescribe an efficacious treatment as a therapeutic trial when the diagnosis is in question. Furthermore, many treatments have not been unequivocally proven to be efficacious, although some evidence supports their usefulness. The practitioner is justified in encouraging the use of such therapies in an attempt to determine whether they relieve symptoms or improve functional status. How else will the practitioner know whether a given antiarrhythmic or analgesic, for example, is effective for a given patient?

In individual practice, therefore, the first two conditions might be replaced with the following requirements: (a) that the therapy be rational and based on sound medical knowledge, and (b) that the potential risks of therapy be less than the likely benefits.

The third condition is that of an informed and willing partner in the intervention. In medical practice one may encounter patients who understand their regimen but fail to adhere against their own best interest. Is the practitioner justified in increasing supervision or attempting to elicit familial support to improve adherence, without obtaining explicit consent from the patient? On one hand, the patient has come to the practitioner's office, voluntarily entered into the patient–practitioner relationship, and accepted a prescribed regimen, suggesting implicit consent. On the other hand, the patient is willfully not adhering to the regimen, suggesting a rejection of the regimen at some level. The dilemma may be somewhat artificial, because most adherence-improving strategies require participation of the patient and therefore require implicit consent. Going beyond the patient–practitioner relationship to enroll family help, however, requires consideration of the patient's feelings with respect to this intervention. Some patients are mentally or psychologically impaired in their ability to understand or make sound decisions regarding their situation. An example might be the symptomatic schizophrenic patient who fails to follow through with taking oral antipsychotic medication; the introduction of long-acting parenteral therapy could reduce symptoms, the rate of relapse, and rehospitalizations. There are no definitive guidelines in these situations, but the following suggestions may be helpful:

- The practitioner should attempt to *determine the patient's own best interest,* considering not only the disease but also the patient's desires, values, psychological makeup, and social environment, and should use this information as a guide to action.
- The practitioner should *weigh the relative benefits versus the risks of intervention* (e.g., self-monitoring of blood pressure in some individuals might markedly increase their anxiety).
- The practitioner should *respect the patient's autonomy and legal rights.*
- When patients are incapable of understanding or making reasonable decisions related to their situation, the practitioner should *consult with responsible family members or guardians* before deciding on a course of action. (See Chapter 19 for determination of mental competence.)
- In particularly difficult situations, the practitioner should *seek advice from others.*

Finally, there is the question of where the patient's responsibilities begin and those of the practitioner end. Is the practitioner ethically bound to check for behaviors that compromise and to facilitate behaviors that promote the health of a patient? Once a patient–practitioner relationship has been established, it is certainly the practitioner's responsibility to work with the patient to improve his or her health status to the best of the practitioner's ability, taking into consideration the severity of the problem, economic constraints, time constraints, and competing obligations to other patients. Not infrequently, we believe, the practitioner's responsibility extends beyond the traditional methods of diagnosing diseases and recommending treatments to facilitating the adoption of healthy behaviors.

General References*

Cross-cultural medicine. West J Med 1983;139(6). Cross-cultural medicine: a decade later. West J Med 1992;157(3).

Two special issues covering major problems that are generic to cross-cultural medicine in the United States, containing articles on most of the major immigrant populations in the United States.

DiMatteo MR, DiNicola DD. Achieving patient compliance: the psychology of the medical practitioner's role. New York: Pergamon, 1982.

Important classic contribution that describes an in-depth social-psychological approach to the understanding, prevention, and management of noncompliant behavior.

Haynes RB, Taylor DW, Sackett DL, eds. Compliance in health care. Baltimore: Johns Hopkins University Press, 1979.

Excellent classic reference with annotated bibliography.

---

*Bold print (general references) and bold numerals (specific references) denote published controlled clinical trials, meta-analyses, or consensus-based recommendations.

Meichenbaum D, Turk DC, eds. Facilitating treatment adherence: a practitioner's guidebook. New York: Plenum, 1987.

A book, written by two leading clinical researchers in cognitive-behavioral therapy, that provides a useful analysis of the adherence literature. It is clinically oriented and full of suggestions for the health care practitioner on how to increase patient adherence by enhancing the practitioner–patient relationship and by use of effective patient education, behavioral modification, and motivational strategies.

Moore SW. Griffith's instructions for patients. 6th ed. Philadelphia: WB Saunders, 1998.

Softbound collection of one- and two-page information sheets on more than 600 conditions. The sheets can be photocopied and distributed to patients. Includes anatomic sketches of most organ systems, which are useful for instructing patients. The sixth edition features a fully updated section on diet and comes with a CD-ROM that enables practitioners to customize instruction sheets for patients.

Sackett DL, Haynes RB, Guyatt GH, et al. Helping patients follow the treatments you prescribe. In: Clinical epidemiology: a basic science for clinical medicine. 2nd ed. Boston: Little, Brown, 1991:249.

Fun, very practical clinical epidemiologic approach to evaluating and improving patient compliance adherence.

Spector RE. Cultural diversity in health & illness. 5th ed. Upper Saddle River, NJ: Prentice Hall Health, 2000.

Useful reference on ethnic health beliefs and practices that complements *Western Journal of Medicine* citations above.

Specific References

1. Feste C, Anderson RM. Empowerment: from philosophy to practice. Patient Educ Couns 1995;26:139.
2. Rodwell CM. An analysis of the concept of empowerment. J Adv Nurs 1996;23:305.
3. Funnell MM, Anderson RM. Patient education for decision-making. Pract Diabet 1997;16:55.
4. Steiner JF, Earnest MA. The language of medication-taking. Ann Intern Med 2000;132:926.
5. Smith M. The cost of noncompliance and the capacity of improved compliance to reduce health care expenditures. In: Improving Medication Compliance: Proceedings of a Symposium. Reston, VA: National Pharmaceutical Council, 1985:35.
6. Mar J, Rodriguez-Artalejo F. Which is more important for the efficiency of hypertension treatment: hypertension stage, type of drug or therapeutic compliance? J Hypertens 2001;19:149.
7. Brookfield S, ed. Self-directed learning: from theory to practice. San Francisco: Jossey-Bass, 1985.
8. Cross KP. Adults as learners. San Francisco: Jossey-Bass, 1988.
9. Knowles MS. Introduction: the art and science of helping adults learn. In: Knowles MS, ed. Andragogy in action. San Francisco: Jossey-Bass, 1984:1.
10. **10.** Roter DL, Hall JA, Merisca R, et al. Effectiveness of interventions to improve patient compliance: a meta-analysis. Med Care 1998;36:1138.
11. Prochaska JO, Velicer WF. The transtheoretical model of health behavior change. Am J Health Promot 1997;12:38.
12. Bandura A. Self-efficacy theory: toward a unifying theory of behavior change. Psychol Rev 1977;84:191.
13. Strecher VJ, Devellis BM, Becker MH, et al. The role of self-efficacy in achieving health behavior change. Health Educ Q 1986;13:73.
14. Wallston KA, Wallston BS, DeVillis R. Development of the multidimensional health locus of control scales. Health Educ Monogr 1978;6:160.
15. Shapiro DH Jr, Swartz CE, Astin JA. Controlling ourselves, controlling our world: psychology's new role in understanding positive and negative consequences of seeking and gaining control. Am Psychol 1996;51:1213.
16. Wallston KA. Hocus-pocus, the focus isn't strictly on locus: Rotter's social learning theory modified for health. Cognit Res Ther 1992;16:183.
17. Johnson TM, Hardt EJ, Kleinman A. Cultural factors and the medical interview. In: Lipkin M Jr, Putnam SM, Lazare A, eds. The medical interview: clinical care, education and research. New York: Springer-Verlag, 1995:153.
18. Janz NK, Becker MH. The health belief model: a decade later. Health Educ Q 1984;11:1.
19. Svarstad BL. Practitioner-patient communication and patient conformity with medical advice. In: Mechanic D, ed. The growth of bureaucratic medicine. New York: Wiley, 1976:243.
20. Francis V, Korsch BM, Morris MJ. Gaps in doctor–patient communication: patients' response to medical advice. N Engl J Med 1969;280:535.
21. Garrity TF. Medical compliance and the clinician–patient relationship: a review. Soc Sci Med 1981;15E:215.
22. **22.** Theis SL, Johnson JH. Strategies for teaching patients: a meta-analysis. Clin Nurs Spec 1995;9:100.
23. Uhlmann RF, Inui TS, Pecoraro RE, et al. Relationship of patient request fulfillment to compliance, glycemic control, and other health care outcomes in insulin-dependent diabetes. J Gen Intern Med 1988;3:458.
24. Lazarus RS, Folkman S. Stress, appraisal and coping. New York: Springer, 1984.
25. Becker MH, Green LW. A family approach to compliance with medical treatment: a selective review of the literature. Int J Health Educ 1975;18:173.
26. Ben-Sira Z, Eliezer R. The structure of readjustment after heart attack. Soc Sci Med 1990;30:523.
27. **27.** Burgess AW, Lerner DJ, D'Agostino RB, et al. A randomized control trial of cardiac rehabilitation. Soc Sci Med 1987;24:359.
28. Cohen S, Lichtenstein E. Partner behaviors that support quitting smoking. J Consult Clin Psychol 1990;58:304.
29. Woloshin S, Schwartz LM, Tosteson ANA, et al. Perceived adequacy of tangible social support and health outcomes in patients with coronary artery disease. J Gen Intern Med 1997;10:613.
30. Coyne JC, Delongis A. Going beyond social support: the role of social relationships in adaptation. J Consult Clin Psychol 1986;54:454.
31. Coyne JC, Ellard JH, Smith DAF. Social support, interdependence, and the dilemmas of helping. In: Sarason BR, Sarason IG, Pierce G, eds. Social support: an interactional view. New York: John Wiley & Sons, 1990:129.
32. Coyne JC, Wortman CB, Lehman DR. The other side of support: emotional overinvolvement and miscarried helping. In: Gottlieb BH, ed. Marshaling social support: formats, process and effects. Newbury Park: Sage, 1988:305.
33. Rothschild S. Cross-cultural issues in primary care medicine. Dis Mon 1998;44:298.
34. Croog SH, Shapiro DS, Levine S. Denial among heart patients: an empirical study. Psychosom Med 1971;33:385.
35. Hackett TP, Cassem NH. White-collar and blue-collar responses to heart attack. J Psychosom Res 1976;20:85.
36. Closson RG, Pharm D, Kikuwaga CA. Noncompliance with drug class. Hospitals 1975;49:89.
37. Hemminki E, Heikkila J. Elderly people's compliance with prescriptions, and quality of medication. Scand J Soc Med 1975;3:87.
38. Hulka BS, Kupper LL, Cassel JC, et al. Medication use and misuse: physician-patient discrepancies. J Chronic Dis 1975;28:7.
39. Inui TS, Carter WB, Pecoraro RE, et al. Variations in patient compliance with common long term drugs. Med Care 1980;18:986.
40. **40.** Greenfield S, Kaplan SH, Ware JE, et al. Patients' participation in medical care: effects on blood sugar control and quality of life in diabetes. J Gen Intern Med 1988;3:448.
41. Kaplan SH, Greenfield S, Ware JE. Assessing the effects of practitioner-patient interactions on the outcomes of chronic disease. Med Care 1989;27:S110.
42. Stewart MA. Effective practitioner-patient communication and health outcomes: a review. Can Med Assoc J 1995;152:1423.
43. Baile WF, Engel BT. A behavioral strategy for promoting treatment compliance following myocardial infarction. Psychosom Med 1978;40:413.
44. **44.** Hall JA, Roter DL, Katz NR. Meta-analysis of provider behavior in medical encounters. Med Care 1988;26:657.
45. Macharia WM, Leon G, Rowe BH, et al. An overview of interventions to improve compliance with appointment keeping for medical services. JAMA 1992;267:1813.
46. Rost K, Carter W, Inui T. Introduction of information during the initial medical visit: consequences for patient follow through

with practitioner recommendations for medication. Soc Sci Med 1989;28:315.

47. Squier RW. A model of empathetic understanding and adherence to treatment regimens in practitioner-patient relationships. Soc Sci Med 1990;30:325.
48. DiMatteo MR, DiNicola DD. Practitioner–patient relationships: the communication of information. In: DiMatteo MR, DiNicola DD, eds. Achieving patient compliance: the psychology of the medical practitioner's role. New York: Pergamon, 1982:29.
49. Fletcher C. Listening and talking to patients. I: The problem. BMJ 1980;281:845.
50. Kern DE, Grayson M, Barker LR, et al. Residency training in interviewing skills and the psychosocial domain of medical practice. J Gen Intern Med 1989;4:421.
51. Smith RC, Marshall AA, Cohen-Cole SA. The efficacy of intensive biopsychosocial teaching programs for residents: a review of the literature and guidelines for teaching. J Gen Intern Med 1994;9:390.
52. Smith RC, Lyles JS, Mettler J, et al. The effectiveness of intensive training for residents in interviewing: a randomized, controlled trial. Ann Intern Med 1998;128:118.
53. Ley P. Cognitive variables and non-compliance. J Compliance Health Care 1986;1:171.
54. Mazzuca SA. Does patient education in chronic disease have therapeutic value? J Chronic Dis 1982;35:521.
55. Carrese JA, Rhodes LA. Western bioethics on the Navajo reservation. Benefit or harm? JAMA 1995;274:826.
56. Steele DJ, Blackwell B, Gutmann MC, et al. Beyond advocacy: a review of the active patient concept. Patient Educ Couns 1987;10:3.
57. Golin CE, DiMatteo MR, Gelberg L. The role of patient participation in the doctor visit: implications for adherence to diabetes care. Diabetes Care 1979;19:1153.
58. Caron HS, Roth HP. Patient's cooperation with a medical regimen: difficulties in identifying the non-cooperator. JAMA 1968;203:120.
59. Charney E, Bynum R, Eldredge D, et al. How well do patients take oral penicillin? A collaborative study in private practice. Pediatrics 1967;40:189.
60. Gilbert JR, Evans CE, Haynes RB, et al. Predicting patient compliance with a regimen of digoxin therapy in family practice. Can Med Assoc J 1980;123:119.
61. Mushlin AI, Appel FA. Diagnosing potential noncompliance: physicians' ability in a behavioral dimension of care. Arch Intern Med 1977;137:318.
62. Johnson AL, Taylor DW, Sackett DL, et al. Self-recording of blood pressure in the management of hypertension. Can Med Assoc J 1978;119:1034.
63. Steele DJ, Jackson TC, Gutman MC. Have you been taking your pill? The adherence monitoring sequence in the medical interview. J Fam Pract 1990;30:294.
64. Cramer JA, Mattson RH, Prevey ML, et al. How often is medication taken as prescribed? A novel assessment technique. JAMA 1989;261:3273.
65. Barker LR. Five-hour blood pressure check to assess hypertension not responding to conventional therapy. Md Med J 1986;35:94.
66. Ley P. Memory for medical information. Br J Soc Clin Psychol 1979;18:245.
67. Raynor DK, Booth TG, Blenkinsopp A. Effects of computer generated reminder charts on patients' compliance with drug regimens. BMJ 1993;306:1158.
68. Lahdensuo A, Haahtela T, Herrala J, et al. Randomized comparison of guided self-management and traditional treatment of asthma over one year. BMJ 1996;312:748.
69. Morrow D, Leirer V, Sheikh J. Adherence and medication instructions: review and recommendations. J Am Geriatr Soc 1988;36:1147.
70. Gates SJ, Colborn DK. Lowering appointment failures in a neighborhood health center. Med Care 1976;14:263.
71. Morse DL, Coulter MP, Nazarian LF, et al. Waning effectiveness of mailed reminders on reducing broken appointments. Pediatrics 1981;68:846.
72. Larson EB, Bergman J, Heidrich F, et al. Do postcard reminders improve influenza vaccination compliance? A prospective trial of different postcard cues. Med Care 1982;20:639.
73. Waggoner DM, Jackson EB, Kern DE. Physical influence on patient compliance: a clinical trial. Ann Emerg Med 1981;10:348.
74. Lewis D. Computer-based approaches to patient education: a review of the literature. JAMA 1999;6:272.
75. McBride CM, Rimer BK. Using the telephone to improve health behavior and health service delivery. Patient Educ Couns 1999;37:3.
76. Soet JE, Basch CE. The telephone as a communication medium for health education. Health Ed Behav 1997;24:759.
77. Bartlett EE. The contribution of consumer health education to primary care practice: a review. Med Care 1980;18:862.
78. Haynes RB, McKibbon KA, Kanani R. Systematic review of randomized trials of interventions to assist patients to follow prescriptions for medications. Lancet 1996;348:383.
79. Bailey WC, Richards JM Jr, Brooks CM, et al. A randomized trial to improve self-management practices of adults with asthma. Arch Intern Med 1990;150:1664.
80. Rich MW, Beckham V, Wittenberg C, et al. A multidisciplinary intervention to prevent the readmission of elderly patients with congestive heart failure. N Engl J Med 1995;333:1190.
81. Rich MW, Gray DB, Beckham RN, et al. Effort of a multidisciplinary intervention on medication compliance in elderly patients with congestive heart failure. Am J Med 1996;101:270.
82. Campbell EM, Redman S, Moffitt PS, et al. The relative effectiveness of educational and behavioral instruction programs for patients with NIDDM: a randomized trial. Diabet Educ 1996;22:379.
83. Morisky DE, Levine DM, Green LW, et al. Five year blood pressure control and mortality following health education for hypertensive patients. Am J Public Health 1983;73:153.
84. Sackett DL. Introduction. In: Sackett DL, Haynes RB, eds. Compliance with therapeutic regimens. Baltimore: Johns Hopkins University Press, 1976:1.

CHAPTER 5

Complementary and Alternative Medicine

BIMAL H. ASHAR, MD

Over the past decade, the use of alternative medicine in the United States has skyrocketed. In 1997, an estimated 42% of patients reported using at least one type of alternative medicine therapy during the previous year. This translated to approximately $27.0 billion dollars' being spent by the public for such services (1). *Alternative medicine* is broadly defined as approaches not routinely used by conventional practitioners. The term *complementary medicine* evolved in an effort to foster a positive relationship between allopathic and nonallopathic medicine. The idea that nonconventional therapies can serve as an adjunct to established Western medical practices has received increasing attention from patients, physicians, and governmental agencies. The 1993 National Institutes of Health (NIH) classification, currently being revised complementary and alternative medicine (CAM) practices into seven major categories that encompass hundreds of individual modalities (Table 5.1) (2). These categories were designed to direct future research initiatives. This chapter is designed to provide the clinician with an overview of some of the more popular CAM modalities currently used by patients. It is hoped that it will serve as a guide to enhance discussion between physicians and their patients.

UNDERSTANDING USE OF COMPLEMENTARY AND ALTERNATIVE MEDICINE

The Patient's Perspective

Before a discussion of specific CAM modalities is undertaken, a general understanding of some of the factors that may be responsible for the patient-driven alternative medicine movement is necessary (Table 5.2). A general theme underlying a majority of CAM therapies is their emphasis on "natural" modes of healing. Acupuncture, chiropractic, massage therapy, and homeopathy are purported to stimulate and invigorate the body's natural potential for preventing and treating disease. Similarly, herbs serve as natural supplements that are assumed by many patients to be milder and safer than human-derived medications. This desire of the public to return to nature has been bolstered by media hype, product advertising, and the widespread availability of information (and misinformation) over the Internet.

Additionally, the status of the conventional physician has changed over the past 20 years. A distrust in the medical profession has developed, in part because of conventional medicine's failure to provide effective and safe therapies for a number of common ailments. Diseases such as chronic fatigue syndrome, fibromyalgia, and other pain syndromes have been defined with little understanding of pathophysiology or disease-specific therapy. Patients with these conditions represent a large subset of seekers of alternative modalities of care.

The Physician's Role

Despite the widespread prevalence of CAM use among the general population, most patients do not inform their physicians of such use (1). It is imperative that clinicians incorporate an "alternative medicine" history into their routine patient evaluations. Information regarding the types of therapies employed as well as the reasons for choosing such therapies should

Table 5.1. National Institutes of Health Original Classification of Complementary and Alternative Therapies

Category	Examples
Mind–body interventions	Meditation, biofeedback, prayer, aromatherapy
Alternative systems of medical practice	Homeopathy, ayurveda, acupuncture
Manual healing methods	Chiropractic, massage, physical therapy
Herbal medicine	*Ginkgo biloba*, saw palmetto, ginseng
Diet and nutrition	Vitamin therapy, mineral therapy, Ornish diet
Bioelectromagnetics	Transcutaneous electrical nerve stimulation
Pharmacologic and biologic treatments	EDTA chelation therapy, shark cartilage

From Alternative medicine: expanding medical horizons. Washington, DC: Government Printing Office, 1993.

Table 5.2. Reasons for Use of Complementary and Alternative Therapies

Belief that natural is better and safer
Failure of conventional medicine
Distrust in conventional medicine
Time constraints on the conventional physician
Media hype
Product advertising
Dissemination of information via the internet

initially be sought. Further discussions should center on patients' experiences (positive or negative), efficacy data (if available), cost, and potential toxicity. Physicians should encourage correspondence with CAM providers in an attempt to develop referral networks. These steps should serve to strengthen the patient–physician relationship and ensure monitoring of potential untoward effects. Specific approaches to obtaining a CAM history have been described elsewhere (3).

ACUPUNCTURE

Technique

Acupuncture is a system of medicine derived primarily from ancient Asian practices. It involves the insertion of fine needles into the skin in order to restore the balance of energy, or *qi* (pronounced "chee"), in the body. Qi flows through channels called meridians that are distinct from neurologic dermatomal patterns.

Patient Experience. An initial acupuncture evaluation begins with the history and physical examination. Conventional allopathic techniques are combined with an in-depth musculoskeletal examination designed to identify potential sensitive areas (trigger points). Additional parts of the examination may include detailed inspections of the tongue, radial pulse, and ear. Once a treatment plan has been developed, the patient is placed in the supine or prone position on a flat table. Thin needles ranging from 0.1 to 3.5 mm in diameter (Fig. 5.1) are then inserted into defined points to affect the flow of qi. The needles traverse to a depth of 0.5 to 8 cm, depending on their location. Additional modalities, such as

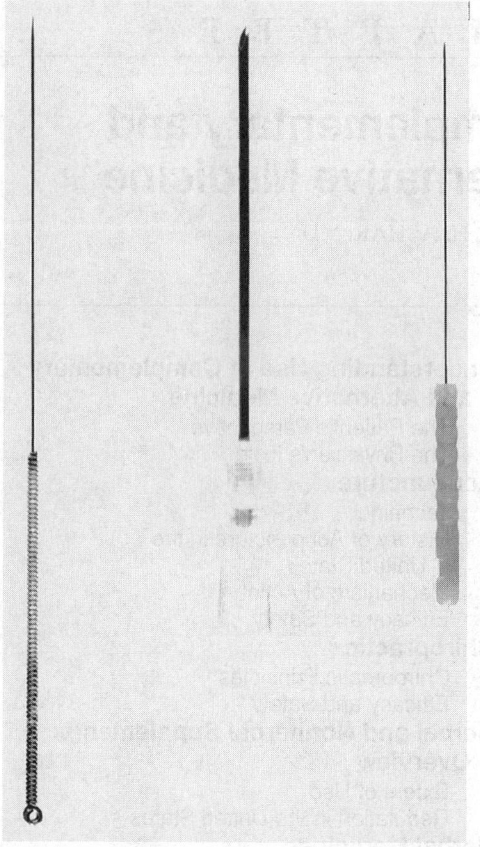

Figure 5.1. A 20-gauge needle *(center)* compared with two typical acupuncture needles *(left and right).*

manual manipulation of the needles, heating of the needles with mugwort (moxibustion), or electrical stimulation, may be employed to assist in the movement of energy (4). The pain experienced by the patient depends on the skill of the practitioner, the thickness of the needle, the depth of insertion, the needle location, and patient sensitivity. Determination of a patient's response usually requires 8 to 12 weeks of therapy. The need for maintenance therapy usually is determined by the chronicity and severity of the underlying condition.

History of Acupuncture in the United States

Although the acupuncture movement seems to have only recently gained popularity, its origins in the United States date back to the 19th century. In the first edition of *Principles and Practice of Medicine,* Sir William Osler described acupuncture as the "most efficient treatment" for acute lumbago (5). In more modern editions of that text, however, references to acupuncture do not appear, reflecting a subsequent lack of confidence in acupuncture as a treatment modality. In 1971, reporter James Reston described how the use of acupuncture successfully relieved his postoperative pain after an appendectomy (6). His article served to stimulate interest among physicians, the public, and the government. More recently, the NIH released a consensus statement that validated the use of acupuncture for certain conditions and strongly encouraged further research (7).

Mechanism of Action

The reluctance of Western medicine to accept acupuncture as a therapeutic tool stems from lack of knowledge regarding the pathophysiology of the acupuncture response. Studies have shown alterations in a number of biologic mediators, including endorphins, neurotransmitters, and neurohormones (7). Functional magnetic resonance imaging studies have suggested a correlation between specific acupuncture points and regionally specific brain cortical activation (8). Blood flow has also been shown to be affected by acupuncture needling (9). Despite these studies, no unifying mechanism has arisen to completely explain the purported benefits of acupuncture.

Efficacy and Safety

More than 7,500 articles are presently indexed in Medline under the search term "acupuncture." Yet, only a few of these papers describe clinical trials on the efficacy of acupuncture therapy. Most of the trials that have been done suffer from small sample sizes and methodologic flaws. Many challenges exist to the performance of meaningful acupuncture research. One major study barrier is the lack of standardization of the acupuncture field. There are many different types of acupuncture practiced today. Traditional Chinese acupuncture, auricular acupuncture, five-elements acupuncture, and hand acupuncture are just a few examples that would use unique points for similar conditions. Even among individuals who practice the same type of acupuncture, great variation may exist in actual point selection based on the practitioner's history, physical examination, and personal style. In the United States, many physician-acupuncturists have been instructed in a more disease-oriented approach that attempts to standardize treatments. Acupuncturists trained in the Chinese tradition typically spend 3 years learning to individualize treatments. In addition, they frequently use Chinese herbs in combination with acupuncture techniques to obtain a response. A major criticism of negative acupuncture studies by traditionalists is the abandonment of holism and individualization of care. Another major obstacle to acupuncture research is the difficulty in blinding practitioners and subjects. The use of "sham" acupuncture (needling inactive points) has been used in many trials but has also been criticized, because the flow of qi is still theoretically affected.

Despite their limitations, randomized controlled trials have been performed for a number of clinical conditions. The NIH consensus report stated that there is strong evidence to support the use of acupuncture for postoperative and chemotherapy-induced nausea and vomiting (7). Additional evidence exists for its efficacy in acute dental pain (10). Systematic reviews of the literature suggest the potential for positive effects on idiopathic headache, fibromyalgia, and osteoarthritis of the knee (11–13). Equivocal evidence exists for the use of acupuncture for chronic pain, low back pain, and asthma (14–16). There is also strong evidence *against* the use of acupuncture for conditions such as smoking cessation and tinnitus (17,18).

The use of acupuncture has been associated with very few serious adverse effects. There are case reports linking acupuncture therapy with pneumothorax, organ puncture, hepatitis, and skin infections; however, these events were usually attributable to improper sterilization of needles or practitioner negligence. Side effects such as needle pain, tiredness, localized bleeding, and vasovagal syncope are more commonly seen but without serious sequelae (19).

CHIROPRACTIC

Chiropractic is a branch of Western medicine that has fought for professional respect since its inception in the late 1890s. Today, it is probably incorrect to classify chiropractic as a form of "alternative" medicine. Between 10% and 20% of the population are estimated to have sought out chiropractic care for an underlying ailment, usually musculoskeletal in origin (1,20). Chiropractors are licensed in all 50 states. Most third-party payers, including Medicare, cover many of the services chiropractors provide.

Chiropractic Principles

Chiropractic philosophy places the nervous system at the center of health and well-being. Disease is considered to be fostered by imbalances in the neurophysiology of the body. This imbalance can be corrected by diagnosing and correcting mechanical abnormalities or subluxations in the spine. Although much variation exists in technique and adjunctive treatments, spinal manipulation remains at the core of the chiropractic approach to disease. It is a holistic form of health care in that it relies on the body's ability to ultimately restore physiologic balance after manipulation.

Patient Experience. A careful history and physical examination is performed by the chiropractor. Specific emphasis is placed on diagnosing spinal dysfunction. Areas along the spine are inspected and palpated for abnormalities in symmetry, tenderness, tone, and temperature. Passive and active range of motion are assessed carefully. Radiographs, ultrasound, heat-sensing devices, and other tests may be employed to aid in diagnosis. After the diagnosis of a spinal abnormality, the patient may be placed with the side of the spinal restriction upward. The doctor's hands are then placed on certain points of the body in order to deliver a high-velocity, short-amplitude thrust to that spinal joint. This is typical of manipulation by direct contact (short-lever technique). In the long-lever technique, the spine is manipulated by thrusts to areas linked to the spine (e.g., a thrust to the thigh moves the vertebrae in the lower spine). Frequently, the patient experiences a cracking or popping noise.

Possible adjuncts to therapy include massage, heat application, and trigger-point deactivation (21,22).

Efficacy and Safety

The most common condition treated by chiropractors is low back pain. Similar to the trials on acupuncture, chiropractic research generally suffers from methodologic flaws and difficulties in design. A meta-analysis of randomized controlled trials suggested that spinal manipulation offers a potential benefit to patients with acute, uncomplicated low back pain (23). Such studies provided enough evidence for the Agency for Health Care Policy and Research (now called the Agency for Healthcare Research and Quality) to include spinal manipulation as an appropriate therapeutic option for acute low back pain of less than 1 month's duration (24). A more recent analysis, however, questioned this recommendation and suggested that current data were not sufficient to draw conclusions regarding spinal manipulation for acute or chronic low back pain (25). Similarly, a clinical trial comparing physical therapy, chiropractic manipulation, and provision of an educational booklet for the treatment of low back pain showed only marginally improved outcomes with chiropractic and physical therapy. However, patient satisfaction was much greater with the manual therapies (26).

Chiropractic has been used for a number of other conditions, including neck pain and headache syndromes. The data on efficacy are contradictory and are based on few well-designed clinical trials. Some patients also turn to their chiropractor for the treatment of other disorders, such as menstrual pain, hypertension, asthma, and fibromyalgia. Again, no definitive conclusions regarding efficacy can be drawn due to the lack of research.

A number of serious adverse effects of chiropractic have been reported. Vertebrobasilar vascular accidents with subsequent infarction, vertebral fracture, diaphragmatic paralysis, internal carotid artery dissection, and tracheal rupture have all been described and attributed primarily to cervical manipulation (22,27). The incidence of such severe complications is unknown. Estimates have ranged from 1 in 120,000 (28) to fewer than 1 in 1 million cervical manipulations (29). Serious complications of lumbar spine manipulation are estimated to be quite rare and to consist primarily of cauda equina syndrome (22). Minor complications such as localized pain are common but transient.

It is important for the primary physician to recognize *contraindications to spinal manipulation.* Patients with a coagulopathy, whether from illness or from medication, should be advised to refrain from chiropractic treatments. Additionally, patients with osteoporosis, rheumatoid arthritis, spinal infections, spinal neoplasms, spinal instability, or an absent odontoid process should avoid such therapy (27). Open communication between the chiropractor and the primary physician is vital to avoid serious complications.

HERBAL AND NONHERBAL SUPPLEMENTS: OVERVIEW

Extent of Use

Of all the fields encompassed by the category CAM, none has grown more rapidly in recent years than the use of over-the-counter supplements. An estimated 12% of the population used over-the-counter herbal products in 1997 (1). Billions of dollars are spent each year by consumers searching for natural substances to foster and maintain their health. The reasons for the popularity of supplements are easy to understand. These are easily accessible, relatively inexpensive, "natural" substances that are purported to improve a number of conditions. Many patients use them to fill the void created by the dearth of available preventive medications. Others see them as a quick, hassle-free cure to an underlying problem. There is potential for gain without the need for practitioner visits, lifestyle changes, or unpleasant procedures. To many physicians, however, supplements are unproven, unregulated, potentially dangerous "drugs" that offer limited benefits to their patients. The roles of various supplements in allopathic medicine will most likely change rapidly as issues of safety, efficacy, and regulation are settled.

Regulation in the United States

The U.S. Food and Drug Administration (FDA) historically regulated dietary supplements as foods, to ensure premarket safety and truthful labeling. In 1994, Congress passed the Dietary Supplements Health and Education Act (DSHEA), which served to expand the definition of "dietary supplements" and to deregulate the industry to meet the concerns of consumers and manufacturers. Vitamins, minerals, amino acids, herbs, and other botanicals are now all considered dietary supplements. Premarket testing for safety or efficacy is no longer required. Supplements are assumed to be safe unless proven otherwise by the FDA. The DSHEA attempted to place restrictions on labeling, however. Manufacturers can make claims only regarding the supplement's effects on a "structure or function" of the body (e.g., "for prostate health"). They cannot claim that their product is "intended to diagnose, treat, cure, or prevent any disease" (e.g., "for the treatment of benign prostatic hyperplasia"). Claims regarding structure and function are not required to be approved by the FDA before marketing. Despite the media attention given to the DSHEA, approximately one third of Americans who use dietary supplements regularly believe that supplements are currently regulated by the government (30). In addition, the majority of Americans believe that such regulation is not enough to ensure that supplements are safe, that contents are pure and doses consistent, and that advertising claims are true.

The lack of regulation of herbal and nonherbal supplements poses a number of problems. There are presently no standards in place to guarantee homogeneity among different products. For example, a patient may wish to take ginkgo biloba to potentially improve his memory. At the store he may choose from a number of different ginkgo products that vary tremendously in their composition. There is no assurance that the active ingredient or ingredients from the plant are even present in a given preparation. Variation also exists among batches from the same manufacturer owing to differences in plant composition, handling, and preparation. In many instances, the active ingredients are unknown, making standardization impossible.

The sale and distribution of herbs depends on proper identification of plants. A number of case reports have described breakdowns in this process. More than 40 cases of Chinese herb-nephropathy were caused in Belgium by the inadvertent substitution of the nephrotoxic herb *Aristolochia fangchi* for *Stephania tetranda,* an herb used in weight-reduction pills. Many of the affected patients went on to develop urothelial carcinoma (31). Cases of adulteration of Chinese herbal products with steroids, benzodiazepines, nonsteroidal anti-inflammatory drugs, and diuretics have also been described. Reports of contamination of herbal products with heavy metals also exist (32).

HERBAL MEDICINES

In general, adequate evidence is lacking to support many of the herbs marketed today. A number of herbal products rely on anecdotal evidence to support their use. Many of the clinical trials in the literature are small-scale, nonrandomized, and/or nonblinded. Large-scale randomized controlled trials are not cost-efficient for manufacturers because herbs are not patentable. Organizations like the Cochrane Collaboration have attempted to pool study data to draw conclusions from meta-analyses. Many of the analyses have been equivocal. The herbs listed in this section and in Table 5.3 represent a few of the more popular herbs used by Americans today. The suggested dosage usually is based on historical usage rather than specific safety or toxicity testing and may be quite variable.

Cranberry

Folklore has for years perpetuated the use of cranberry for the treatment of urinary tract infections. Basic science research has suggested that the proanthocyanidins present in cranberries may inhibit the adherence of *Escherichia coli* to urinary tract epithelial cells. To date, no clinical trials have been done to suggest efficacy of cranberry juice or cranberry extract for the treatment of urinary tract infections. One large, double-blind, placebo-controlled trial has been done and suggested a role in the prevention of urinary tract infections. In that study, a significant reduction in the frequency of bacteriuria with pyuria in elderly women consuming cranberry juice cocktail was seen (33). The quality of this trial, however, has been questioned (34). Although cranberry supplementation is generally accepted to be quite safe, recent studies suggest the potential for nephrolithiasis (35).

Ephedra

Traditional Chinese medicine has for centuries touted the use of ephedra for the treatment of asthma, congestion, and bronchitis. Also known as ma huang, it consists predominantly of two alkaloids, ephedrine and pseudoephedrine. In the United States, ephedra has become a popular ingredient in over-the-counter weight loss preparations. When combined with caffeine, ephedrine has been shown to cause significant weight loss (about 3.4 kg) over a 6-month period (36). However, no long-term data currently exists.

Ephedrine is a sympathomimetic drug, structurally similar to amphetamines. Its effects on the body include central nervous system stimulation, cardiac stimulation (ionotropic and chronotropic), bronchodilation, and blood pressure elevation. Reported side effects have included hypertension, nephrolithiasis, hepatitis, insomnia, arrythmias, myocardial infarction, and stroke. Cases of death and permanent disability have also been reported (37). This potential for toxicity had incited the FDA to propose limitations on dosing and labeling of all products containing ephedrine. To date, these limitations have

Table 5.3. Common Herbal Medications

Common Name	Indications for Use	Suggested Dosage*	Potential Toxicity
Cranberry	Urinary infections	300 mL of juice daily; 400-mg/capsule daily	Nephrolithiasis
Ephedra	Asthma, congestion, weight loss	15–300 mg daily	Hypertension, arrythmias, stroke, death
Echinacea	Upper respiratory, tract infections	Varies: e.g., 900 mg/d *E. purpurae* root	Hypersensitivity reactions
Feverfew	Migraine prophylaxis	50–100 mg of dried leaf preparation	Hypersensitivity reactions
Garlic	Cardiovascular protection	900 mg/day of 1.3% allicin content product	Gastrointestinal upset, bleeding
Ginkgo biloba	Dementia, claudication, tinnitus	40 mg t.i.d.	Gastrointestinal upset, headache, bleeding, seizure
Ginseng	Fatigue, exercise performance, diabetes	100–200 mg/day of standardized extract of 4–7% ginsenosides	Mastalgia, insomnia, vaginal bleeding, hypertension
Kava-kava	Anxiety	60–120 mg of kava lactones/day	Rash, sedation, hepatitis
Saw palmetto	Prostatic hyperplasia	160 mg b.i.d.	Mild gastrointestinal effects
St. John's wort	Depression, anxiety	300 mg t.i.d.	Headache, dry mouth, insomnia, fatigue, photosensitivity

*Dosage highly valuable based on product composition.

not been enacted. It should be noted that pseudoephedrine, a product found in a number of over-the-counter decongestants, is a much weaker stimulant of alpha- and beta-receptors. Concomitant use of ephedra and other stimulant medications should be avoided.

Echinacea

Echinacea is one of the most popular herbs in use today. It is used primarily to prevent and treat upper respiratory tract infections. Although the plant genus *Echinacea* consists of a number of different species, medicinal use has centered predominantly on three of them (*Echinacea purpurea, Echinacea augustifolia,* and *Echinacea pallida*). These herbs have been thought to boost the immune system by stimulating cytokine activity (38). A number of clinical trials have demonstrated a positive effect on prevention and treatment of upper respiratory tract infections. Yet, definitive conclusions regarding efficacy have been difficult to make owing to study limitations. There exists great variation in species of plant studied, parts of the plant used (root, leaf, flower, seed), and extraction methods. Additionally, many of the products use combinations of herbs (39). Echinacea is thought to be quite safe for short-term use. No serious side effects have been reported, although hypersensitivity reactions can occur. Because of its ability to stimulate the immune system, echinacea is not recommended for patients with autoimmune disease or human immunodeficiency virus infection for fear of worsening disease. This concern remains a theoretical risk rather than an established fact. No long-term data on the safety of chronic use are presently available.

Feverfew (*Tanacetum parthenium*)

Feverfew has been used for centuries for a variety of conditions. Presently it is commonly used for the prevention of migraine headaches. It is thought to inhibit prostaglandin synthesis, histamine release from mast cells, and degranulation of platelets. Additionally, it may have direct vasodilatory effects (40). A few clinical trials have suggested that feverfew may be effective in preventing recurrent migraines (41). If the leaves of the plant are chewed directly, mouth ulceration may occur. Otherwise, it is considered safe. Because of its effects on platelets, a theoretical concern about bleeding exists, although no cases have been reported to date.

Garlic (*Allium sativum*)

Garlic is one of the most highly studied herbal medications available. It has been thought to possess antimicrobial, anti-inflammatory, antifungal, antiprotozoal, antioxidant, and antineoplastic properties that make its use as a general tonic attractive. More recently, focus has shifted to garlic's effects on cardiovascular diseases and risk factors. A meta-analysis suggested that garlic supplementation may decrease levels of total cholesterol and low-density lipoproteins modestly, but only in the short-term. Platelet aggregation is significantly reduced, but the clinical importance of this finding remains elusive. No significant effects on blood pressure or glucose levels have been noted (42). Additionally, garlic has not been shown to improve symptomatic peripheral vascular disease (43). Garlic toxicity is usually mild and consists of gastrointestinal upset and body odor. Case reports of spontaneous bleeding and interactions with anticoagulants have been described (32).

Ginkgo biloba

Ginkgo biloba use has skyrocketed over the last few years based on reports and claims of its use for improving memory and treating dementia, peripheral vascular disease, and tinnitus. It is thought to have a number of biologic effects, including increasing blood flow, inhibiting platelet activating factor, altering neuronal metabolism, and working as an antioxidant (44). Mild improvements in cognitive performance and social functioning in patients with Alzheimer's disease or multi-infarct dementia have been seen with the use of ginkgo extract Egb 761 (45). However, there is currently no evidence that ginkgo biloba is effective for the *prevention* of memory loss or dementia. Ginkgo has been shown to have a modest effect on symptoms of intermittent claudication (46) but little effect on tinnitus (47). Side effects are rare and usually consist of gastrointestinal complaints or headaches. Cases of spontaneous bleeding (48) and seizures (49) have been reported. Because of the possible potentiation of anticoagulant effects, ginkgo biloba use should be avoided in patients who are taking warfarin.

Ginseng (*Panax* Species)

Ginseng is thought of by many as a virtual panacea. Asian ginseng (*Panax ginseng*) has been used for centuries as a general tonic, stimulant, and stress reliever. In Chinese medicine, American ginseng (*Panax quinquefolius*) has been used, but it is thought to possess less stimulant activity. Siberian ginseng (*Eleutherococcus senticosus*) has also gained popularity but belongs to a different plant species. The mechanism of action for ginseng is unknown but is thought to involve the concentration of ginsenosides, which are believed to act as an antioxidant and on a number of tissue receptors. Although small studies have suggested some improvement in mental performance and diabetic control, a systematic review of clinical trials failed to provide compelling evidence for advocating ginseng for improving physical performance, psychomotor performance, cognitive function or for treating diabetes (50). In general, ginseng is considered safe. Reports of hypertension, insomnia, vomiting, headache, vaginal bleeding, Stevens–Johnson syndrome, and mastalgia have been cited (51). The possibility of an interaction with warfarin (reduced international normalized ratio [INR]) has also been raised (52). Care should be taken in patients who are taking anticoagulants.

Kava-kava (*Piper methysticum*)

Kava has been used for thousands of years by inhabitants of the South Pacific islands. It has usually been ingested as a mildly intoxicating beverage distinct from alcohol. Current interest in kava has centered on its use as an anxiolytic agent. Its mechanism of action on the central nervous system is unknown. Its effects seem to be independent of benzodiazepine binding sites (53). A review of randomized, double-blind, clinical trials suggested that kava extract is superior to placebo for the treatment of anxiety (54). Undesired effects have usually consist of mild gastrointestinal upset and allergic skin reactions. Eye irritation and a yellow, scaly dry rash (kawaism) has been described with heavy, chronic use (51). Hepatitis and fulminant hepatic failure have also been reported (55). Concomitant use with other anxiolytics or alcohol should be avoided to protect against excess sedation.

Saw Palmetto (*Serenoa repens*)

Benign prostatic hyperplasia is a common clinical condition among elderly men. Despite numerous conventional treatment options, many men chose against therapy because of the potential for adverse effects. This has led to the popularity of saw palmetto as an agent to treat symptoms associated with an enlarged prostate. A number of short-term studies have shown it to be effective in improving urologic symptoms and flow measures (56). Its exact mechanism of action is unknown but may be related in part to inhibition of 5-alpha-reductase (57). In a head-to-head trial, saw palmetto was shown to be equivalent to finasteride in improving symptoms associated with benign prostatic hyperplasia. Fewer sexual side effects and no change in levels of prostate-specific antigen were seen in the group receiving the herbal treatment (58). Side effects reported with the use of saw palmetto have been mild and rare, although adequate data on long-term use are lacking. It should noted that there is no known clinical evidence to date to support its use for the prevention of benign prostatic hyperplasia or prostate cancer.

St. John's Wort (*Hypericum perforatum*)

St. John's wort has been used extensively by Americans for self-diagnosed depression and dysphoria. In Germany, it is the most widely prescribed antidepressant medication. Its mechanism of action and active ingredients have yet to be conclusively defined. However, data suggest that preparations of *Hypericum* extract may inhibit monoamine oxidase activity as well as synaptic neurotransmitter reuptake (59). Systematic reviews of available trials on the efficacy of St. John's wort have suggested a positive effect on mild to moderate depression (60,61). However, many of the trials evaluated in these analyses have had methodologic limitations. A randomized controlled trial that attempted to control for many of those limitations suggested that there may be no significant effect on major depression (62). In general, side effects of St. John's wort are mild and infrequent. The most commonly reported reactions include gastrointestinal irritations, allergic reactions, fatigue, dizziness, dry mouth, and headache. Reports of photosensitization have also been documented (59). Rare cases of serotonin syndrome have been reported with the combined use of St. John's wort and selective serotonin reuptake inhibitors (32). Therefore, caution must be exercised in patients taking prescription antidepressants.

NONHERBAL SUPPLEMENTS

A number of nonherbal supplements have gained popularity over the past decade. These products consist predominantly of molecules normally found in the body. Vitamins, minerals, amino acids, and metabolic intermediates are just a few of the substances encompassed within this category. A manipulation of the concentrations of these molecules is thought to produce beneficial effects toward the prevention and treatment of disease. The efficacy, safety, and regulatory issues that surround herbal medications similarly apply to these supplements. The following paragraphs describe a few of the more popular products in this category.

Coenzyme Q10 (Ubiquinone)

Coenzyme Q10 is a substance produced by the body (and found in some foods) that is structurally similar to vitamins E and K. It is considered to be an antioxidant and has also been shown to also play a major role in mitochondrial oxidative phosphorylation. It has gained popularity as a treatment for various cardiac disorders. To date, interest in coenzyme Q10 has predominantly focused on its use in the treatment of congestive heart failure. A large Italian study showed a reduction in hospitalizations and serious complications in patients with New York Heart Association class III and class IV heart failure treated with coenzyme Q10 (63). However, a more recent study on similar patients failed to show improvement in ejection fraction, peak oxygen consumption, or exercise duration (64). No definitive data on cardiac mortality exist to date. Additionally, there is presently no evidence to support the its use for the primary prevention of cardiac disease. The most commonly reported side effects with coenzyme Q10 administration are nausea, heartburn, and diarrhea. Its structural similarity to vitamin K has been suggested as the cause of a decrease in responsiveness to warfarin when administered concurrently (65,66). Typical doses for the treatment of cardiac disease are 50 to 200 mg/day.

Glucosamine Sulfate and Chondroitin Sulfate

Glucosamine and chondroitin are two of the most widely accepted supplements currently available. Even though they have not lived up to their initial claims as a "cure" for arthritis (67), they have provided many patients with some degree of relief from chronic joint pain. Glucosamine is a amino sugar that is a substrate for the production of glycosaminoglycans and proteoglycans, which are essential building blocks of connective tissue. Chondroitin is a glycosaminoglycan that may inhibit enzymatic destruction of synovial tissue and serve as an anti-inflammatory agent in addition to its role in structural cartilage formation (68). An analysis of clinical trials done to date suggested that glucosamine and/or chondroitin preparations probably have some effect on the symptoms of osteoarthritis of the knee and hip (69). Enthusiasm for the supplements was tempered by methodologic problems with many of the studies reviewed. A recent 3-year trial of glucosamine sulfate alone suggested that it may halt the progression of osteoarthritis as determined by radiography (70). Both glucosamine and chondroitin are generally well tolerated. Mild gastrointestinal side effects are rarely seen. The recommended doses of glucosamine sulfate and chondroitin sulfate are, respectively, 500 mg three times daily and 400 mg three times daily. Treatment effect may not be seen for up to 8 weeks after beginning therapy. No significant drug interactions have been noted, although a theoretical risk of bleeding with concurrent administration of chondroitin sulfate and anticoagulants exists owing to chondroitin's structural homology with a small component of certain heparinoids (71).

SAMe (*S*-Adenosylmethionine)

S-Adenosylmethionine (SAMe) is a common metabolic intermediary produced in the body through the interaction of methionine and adenosine triphosphate (ATP). It is considered to be vital to appropriate cellular functioning and survival. Because of its role in numerous metabolic pathways, it is has been proposed to be of benefit for a wide array of diseases, the best studied of which is osteoarthritis. A number of small clinical trials have suggested that its ability to improve the symptoms of osteoarthritis is equivalent to that of nonsteroidal anti-inflammatory drugs but with fewer side effects (72). SAMe has also been touted for use in depression, although there is insufficient evidence to support this claim (73). Conclusive data to support its use in fibromyalgia and liver disease are also lacking. Nausea and abdominal discomfort have been described rarely with the use of SAMe. In a number of depression trials, subsets of patients experienced hypomania (73). Additionally, there is concern for interactions with tricyclic antidepressants (74,75). Therefore, concomitant use should be avoided. A major limitation to the use of SAMe is its cost. At its suggested dose of 400 to 1,600 mg/day, 1-month supply can amount to well over $200 in out-of-pocket expense.

Supplement–Drug Interactions

It has been estimated that one of every five adults taking prescription medications is also using over-the-counter supplements (1). Given that many of the supplements in use today have not been rigorously studied, little is known about their potential interactions with prescription medications. A number of case reports have appeared to suggest that some herbal and nonherbal products may directly interact with certain drugs to inhibit or enhance their effects. Additionally, supplements may indirectly potentiate or oppose medication effects through independent mechanisms. Table 5.4 lists some potential cautions when mixing prescription medications and supplements. Most of the cited warnings are based on case reports and theoretical concerns. It is imperative that physicians discuss the possibility of interactions with their patients and report any suspected cases to the FDA. The MedWatch program has been set up to monitor the safety of drugs, devices, biologicals, and dietary supplements. Physicians should report any significant adverse reactions or supplement–drug interactions to this program. Reporting can be completed over the Internet (at the MedWatch website, http://www.fda.gov/medwatch) or by telephone (1-800-FDA-1088).

HOMEOPATHY

The principles of homeopathy were first publicized by Samuel Hahnemann in the late 1700s. Since that time, it has had generated much controversy and experienced waxing and waning popularity. Common diagnoses currently treated by homeopaths include otitis media, depression, allergy, hypertension, arthritis, and headache. In the United States, an estimated 3.4% of the population presently uses homeopathic remedies (1). This has occurred despite criticism from many scientists who believe that the homeopathic effect is nothing more than a placebo response. Much of the opposition stems from the inability to scientifically validate the basic tenets of this unique medical treatment system.

Homeopathic Principles and Medicines

The basis of homeopathy relies on two concepts: the law of similars and the use of dilutions. The law of similars suggests that a patient with certain sets of symptoms can be cured of their ailments by administration of a drug that induces those symptoms in a healthy individual. An example of this principle in conventional medicine would be the use of digoxin to treat arrythmias that it is capable of causing (93). The principle of dilutions suggests that substances retain their biologic activity even when they are diluted to levels at which no molecules of the original substance remain.

Table 5.4. Supplement–Drug Cautions

Supplement	Drug	Reaction (Ref. No.)
Astragalus membranaceus	Cycolsporine	Interference with immune suppression (77)
Capsaicin (chili pepper)	ACE inhibitors	Induce cough (79)
Chondroitin sulfate	Anticoagulants	Theoretic increased risk of bleeding
Coenzyme Q10	Warfarin	Decreased INR (65,66)
Dong quai	Warfarin	Increased INR (76)
Mahuang (ephedra)	MAO inhibitors	Theoretic increased risk of hypertensive crisis
	Theophylline	Increased toxicity (78)
	Stimulants	Potentiation of effect and toxicity
Feverfew	Anticoagulants	Increased risk of bleeding
Garlic	Anticoagulants	Increased risk of bleeding
Ginkgo biloba	Anticoagulants	Increased risk of bleeding
Ginseng (*Panax*)	MAO inhibitors	Headache, tremor (80), mania (81)
	Warfarin	Decreased INR (52)
Kava-kava	Benzodiazepines	Increased sedation and lethargy (83)
Licorice	Oral contraceptives	Hypokalemia, hypertension, edema (84)
SAMe	Tricyclic antidepressants	Potentiation of effect and toxicity (74,75)
Siberian ginseng	Digoxin	Increased digoxin level (82)
St. John's wort	Cyclosporine	Decreased cyclosporine levels (85)
	Digoxin	Decreased digoxin levels (86)
	Indinavir	Decreased indinavir levels (87)
	Oral contraceptives	Breakthrough bleeding (88)
	SSRIs	Serotonin syndrome (89)
	Theophylline	Decreased theophylline levels (90)
	Warfarin	Decreased INR (88)
Yohimbe	MAO inhibitors	Potentiation of effects (91)
	Tricyclic antidepressants	Hypertension (92)

ACE, angiotensin-converting enzyme; INR, international normalized ratio; MAO, monoamine oxidase; SAMe, *S*-adenosylmethionine; SSRIs, Selective Serotonin reuptake inhibitors.

Homeopaths tend to focus on subjective symptoms and sensations rather than objective medical diagnoses. Therefore, a wide variety of medications can be used for the same diagnosis, depending on the clinical presentation. Various encyclopedias of homeopathic remedies exist (called *materia medica*) that describe symptoms produced by various diluted medications when administered to healthy individuals (provings). The patient's symptom complex is matched with the drug provings to determine the optimal therapeutic regimen. Treatment frequency can range from one or two doses to chronic daily dosing. Typically, patients are observed weeks later to determine progress and the need for alterations in the treatment plan.

Homeopathic medicines are typically derived from plant, mineral, or animal sources. They are regulated by the FDA under the Food, Drug, and Cosmetic Act of 1938. Most remedies are sold over the counter and require labeling information that includes ingredients, recommended dose, indications for use, and dilution. Homeopathic medications are typically exempt from requirements related to expiration dating and finished product testing because they contain little or no active ingredients. Additionally, these remedies are not restricted to the 10% alcohol limit of conventional drugs (94).

Efficacy and Safety

A number of clinical trials have been done on a variety of homeopathic remedies. Many of them, however, are of low methodologic quality. Meta-analyses of more than 100 of these trials have suggested that the effects of homeopathy are superior to those of placebo (95,96). Yet, analysis of individual conditions and treatments are less supportive (96). Recent reviews of homeopathic remedies for the treatment of osteoarthritis (97) and asthma (98) were inconclusive. An examination of eight trials done on a specific homeopathic medication (Arnica montana) failed to show efficacy beyond that of placebo (99). As with most other CAM therapies, systematic and rigorous research is needed to definitively prove effect.

Although serious toxicity from the use of homeopathic medicines is rare, unpleasant effects are quite common. "Aggravation reactions" occur when a patient's symptoms worsen acutely after starting a remedy. Homeopathic physicians view these reactions as desirable and as prognostic of a favorable outcome. Patients, however, may equate aggravations with side effects. As with herbal products, the potential for contamination and adulteration of homeopathic medications exists because these preparations are exempt from standard finished product testing.

A more serious problem exists when patients chose to defer effective conventional therapy for an unproven homeopathic remedy. Such cases have occurred with a number of CAM therapies. Additionally, some homeopaths discourage the use of conventional drugs because they are thought to hinder the effectiveness of homeopathic remedies. Many homeopathic physicians are also opposed to immunization and may influence patients against proven preventive health measures (100).

Table 5.5. Techniques Used in Swedish Massage

Technique	Description
Effleurage	Deep or superficial stroking along the length of a muscle
Friction	Deep muscle stimulation applied by compression with fingertips or palm of hand
Petrissage	Kneading of muscles in a circular pattern
Tapotement	Light slapping, beating, or chopping movements
Vibration	Rapid, to-and-fro, shaking movements of fingers by the hands

MISCELLANEOUS COMPLEMENTARY AND ALTERNATIVE THERAPIES

Massage Therapy

Therapeutic massage is defined as the manipulation of soft tissues in order to improve the overall health of the body. It is commonly used to relieve stress and anxiety, to promote relaxation, and to treat certain pain disorders. There are a number of different types of massage (e.g. Swedish, deep-tissue, neuromuscular, shiatsu). Massage therapists commonly combine various methods during a typical session. Swedish massage is the most common form currently practiced. It consists of a number of different techniques (Table 5.5) designed to relieve muscle tension and improve circulation. Aromatic oils are frequently employed as lubricants during treatments. Acupressure or shiatsu massage consists of the application of heavy pressure for extended periods at particular pressure points on the body. It is designed to affect the flow of energy and consequently to restore balance to the body. In deep-tissue massage, increasing amounts of pressure are applied to structurally align the body. Rolfing (structural integration) is a form of deep-tissue massage designed to improve muscular function through manipulation of fascial planes.

Efficacy and Safety

Massage therapy is used primarily as a relaxation technique. It has been shown subjectively and objectively to assist in stress reduction, although the intensity and duration of the response can be quite variable. Small studies have supported the use of massage for a number of conditions, including low back pain, fibromyalgia, chronic fatigue, anxiety, and depression, but there is currently insufficient evidence to make definitive recommendations for its routine use. Massage is generally considered to be safe. Care needs to be taken in patients with coagulation disorders, especially with the use of deep-tissue techniques.

Aromatherapy

Most people experience pleasant and unpleasant smells on a daily basis. Some odors may make us happy, while others may be irritating. The impact that these odors have on our bodies as a whole forms the basis for aromatherapy. In this CAM therapy, plant-derived essential oils are used to induce changes in emotion and health. Jasmine, chamomile, and lavender are just a few of the oils used to induce a positive relaxation response. Aromatherapy has been used alone or in combination with massage therapy for stress reduction. Evidence for its use for specific medical conditions, including anxiety, is presently inconclusive (101). No serious adverse effects are attributed to this therapy, although allergic responses may occur.

General References*

Blumenthal M. Herbal medicine: expanded Commission E monographs. Austin: American Botanical Council, 2000.

A comprehensive translation of the German guide on herbal medicine published by the American Botanical Council.

Cochrane Library's field group in CAM website (CD-ROM available also). Available at: http://www.cochranelibrary.com.

Fugh-Berman A. Alternative medicine: what works. Baltimore: Williams & Wilkins, 1997.

An overview of a number of alternative therapies written for laymen and physicians.

Jonas W, Levin JS. Essentials of complementary and alternative medicine. Philadelphia: Lippincott Williams & Wilkins, 1999.

A concise review of CAM modalities with a specific focus on safety issues.

National Center for Alternative and Complementary Medicine website. Available at: http://www.nccam.nih.gov.

Research Council for Complementary Medicine, U.K., website. Available at: http://www.gn.qpc.org.

Specific References

1. Eisenberg DM, Davis RB, Ettner SL, et al. Trends in alternative medicine use in the United States, 1990–1997. JAMA 1998;280:1569.
2. Alternative medicine: expanding medical horizons. Washington, DC: Government Printing Office, 1993.
3. Eisenberg DM. Advising patients who seek alternative medical therapies. Ann Intern Med 1997;127:61.
4. Helms JM. An overview of medical acupuncture. Altern Ther Health Med 1998;4:35.
5. Osler W. Principles and practice of medicine. New York: D. Appleton & Co, 1892.
6. Reston J. Now about my operation in Peking. New York Times 1971;July 26:1,6.
7. **7.** National Institutes of Health. Consensus statement. 1997 Nov 3–5;15(5):1–34.
8. Cho ZH, Chung SC, Jones JP, et al. New findings of the correlation between acupoints and corresponding brain cortices using functional MRI. Proc Natl Acad Sci USA 1998;95:2670.
9. Yuan X, Hao X, Lai Z, et al. Effects of acupuncture at fengchi point (GB 20) on cerebral blood flow. J Tradit Chin Med 1998;18:102.
10. Ernst E, Pittler MH. The effectiveness of acupuncture in treating acute dental pain: a systematic review. Br Dent J 1998;184:443.
11. **11.** Linde K, Melchart D, Fischer P, et al. Acupuncture for idiopathic headache (Cochrane Review). In: The Cochrane Library, Issue 2, 2001. Oxford: Update Software.
12. Berman BM, Ezzo J, Hadhazy V, et al. Is acupuncture effective in the treatment of fibromyalgia? J Fam Pract 1999;48:213.
13. Ezzo J, Hadhazy V, Birch S, et al. Acupuncture for osteoarthritis of the knee: a systematic review. Arthritis Rheum 2001;44:819.
14. Ezzo J, Berman B, Hadhazy VA, et al. Is acupuncture effective for the treatment of chronic pain? A systematic review. Pain 2000;86:217.
15. **15.** Tulder MW van, Cherkin DC, Berman B, et al. Acupuncture for low back pain (Cochrane Review). In: The Cochrane Library, Issue 2, 2001. Oxford: Update Software.

*Bold print (general references) and bold numerals (specific references) denote published clinical trials, meta-analyses, or consensus-based recommendations.

16. Linde K, Jobst K, Panton J. Acupuncture for chronic asthma (Cochrane Review). In: The Cochrane Library, Issue 2, 2001. Oxford: Update Software.

17. White AR, Rampes H, Ernst E. Acupuncture for smoking cessation (Cochrane Review). In: The Cochrane Library, Issue 2, 2001. Oxford: Update Software.

18. Park J, White AR, Ernst E. Efficacy of acupuncture as a treatment for tinnitus: a systematic review. Arch Otolaryngol Head Neck Surg 2000;126:489.

19. Ernst E, White AR. Prospective studies of the safety of acupuncture: a systematic review. Am J Med 2001;110:481.

20. Astin JA. Why patients use alternative medicine. JAMA 1998;279:1548.

21. Lawrence DJ. Chiropractic medicine. In: Jonas WB, Levin JS, eds. Essentials of alternative and complementary medicine. Philadelphia: Lippincott Williams & Wilkins, 1999;275.

22. Kaptchuk TJ, Eisenberg DM. Chiropractic: origins, controversies, and contributions. Arch Intern Med 1998;158:2215.

23. Shekelle PG, Adams AH, Chassin MR, et al. Spinal manipulation for low-back pain. Ann Intern Med 1992;117:590.

24. Bigos S, Bowyer O, Braen B, et al. Clinical practice guideline no. 14: acute low back problems in adults. AHCPR publication 95-0642. Rockville, MD: US Dept of Heath and Human Services, Agency for Health Care Policy and Research, 1994.

25. Koes BW, Assendelft WJ, van der Heijden GJ, et al. Spinal manipulation for low back pain: an updated systematic review of randomized clinical trials. Spine 1996;21:2860.

26. Cherkin DC, Deyo RA, Battie M, et al. A comparison of physical therapy, chiropractic manipulation, and provision of an educational booklet for the treatment of patients with low back pain. N Engl J Med 1998;339:1021.

27. Ernst E. Adverse effects of spinal manipulation. In: Jonas WB, Levin JS, eds. Essentials of alternative and complementary medicine. Philadelphia: Lippincott Williams & Wilkins, 1999;176.

28. Klougart N, Leboeuf-Yde C, Rasmussen LR. Safety in chiropractic practice. Part II: Treatment to the upper neck and the rate of cerebrovascular incidents. J Manipulative Physiol Ther 1996;19:563.

29. Hurwitz EL, Aker PD, Adams AH, et al. Manipulation and mobilization of the cervical spine: a systematic review of the literature. Spine 1996;21:1746.

30. Blendon RJ, DesRoches CM, Benson JM, et al. Americans' views on the use and regulation of dietary supplements. Arch Intern Med 2001;161:805.

31. Nortier JL, Martinez MC, Schmeiser HH, et al. Urothelial carcinoma associated with the use of a Chinese herb (*Aristolochia fangchi*). N Engl J Med 2000;342:1686.

32. Fugh-Berman A. Herb-drug interactions. Lancet 2000;355:134.

33. Avorn J, Monane M, Gurwitz JH, et al. Reduction of bacteriuria and pyuria after ingestion of cranberry juice. JAMA 1994;271:751.

34. Jepson RG, Mihaljevic L, Craig J. Cranberries for preventing urinary tract infections (Cochrane Review). In: The Cochrane Library, Issue 2, 2001. Oxford: Update Software.

35. Terris MK, Issa MM, Tacker JR. Dietary supplementation with cranberry concentrate tablets may increase the risk of nephrolithiasis. Urology 2001;57:26.

36. Astrup A, Breum L, Toubro S, et al. The effect of an ephedrine/caffeine compound compared to ephedrine, caffeine and placebo in obese subjects on an energy restricted diet: a double blind trial. Int J Obes 1992;16:269.

37. Haller CA, Benowitz NL. Adverse cardiovascular and central nervous system events associated with dietary supplements containing ephedra alkaloids. N Engl J Med 2000;343:1833.

38. Burger RA, Torres AR, Warren RP, et al. Echinacea-induced cytokine production by human macrophages. Int J Immunopharmacol 1997;19:371.

39. Melchart D, Linde K, Fischer P, et al. Echinacea for preventing and treating the common cold (Cochrane Review). In: The Cochrane Library, Issue 2, 2001. Oxford: Update Software.

40. Rotblatt MD. Cranberry, feverfew, horse chestnut, and kava. West J Med 1999;171:195.

41. Ernst E, Pittler MH. The efficacy and safety of feverfew (*Tanacetum parthenium* L.): an update of a systematic review. Public Health Nutr 2000;3:509.

42. Ackermann RT, Mulrow CD, Ramirez G, et al. Garlic shows promise for improving some cardiovascular risk factors. Arch Intern Med 2001;161:813.

43. Jepson RG, Kleijnen J, Leng GC. Garlic for peripheral arterial occlusive disease (Cochrane Review). In: The Cochrane Library, Issue 2, 2001. Oxford: Update Software.

44. Kleijnen J, Knipschild P. Ginkgo biloba. Lancet 1992;340:1136.

45. LeBars PL, Katz MM, Berman N, et al. A placebo-controlled, double-blind, randomized trial of an extract of *Ginkgo biloba* for dementia. JAMA 1997;278:1327.

46. Pittler MH, Ernst E. Ginkgo biloba extract for the treatment of intermittent claudication: a meta-analysis of randomized trials. Am J Med 2000;108:276.

47. Drew S, Davies E. Effectiveness of *Ginkgo biloba* in treating tinnitus: double-blind placebo controlled trial. BMJ 2001; 322:1.

48. Rowin J, Lewis SL. Spontaneous bilateral subdural hematomas associated with chronic *Ginkgo biloba* ingestion. Neurology 1996;46:1775.

49. Gregory PJ. Seizure associated with *Ginkgo biloba*? Ann Intern Med 2001;134:344.

50. Vogler BK, Pittler MH, Ernst E. The efficacy of ginseng: a systematic review of randomized clinical trials. Eur J Clin Pharmacol 1999;55:567.

51. Miller LG. Herbal medicinals: selected clinical considerations focusing on known or potential drug-herb interactions. Arch Intern Med 1998;158:2200.

52. Janetzky K, Morreale AP. Probable interaction between warfarin and ginseng. Am J Health Syst Pharm 1997;54:692.

53. Davies LP, Drew CA, Duffield P, et al. Kava pyrones and resin: studies on GABBA, GABAB and benzodiazepine binding sites in rodent brain. Pharmacol Toxicol 1992;71:120.

54. Pittler MH, Ernst E. Efficacy of kava extract for treating anxiety: systematic review and meta-analysis. J Clin Psychopharmacol 2000;20:84.

55. Escher M, Desmeules J, Giostra E, et al. Hepatitis associated with kava, a herbal remedy for anxiety. BMJ 2001;322:139.

56. Wilt TJ, Ishani A, Stark G, et al. Saw palmetto extracts for the treatment of benign prostatic hyperplasia: a systematic review. JAMA 1999;280:1604.

57. Bayne CW, Donnelly F, Ross M, et al. *Serenoa repens* (Permixon): a 5 alpha-reductase types I and II inhibitor—new evidence in a coculture model of BPH. Prostate 1999;40:232.

58. Carraro JC, Raynaud JP, Koch G, et al. Comparison of phytotherapy (Permixon) with finasteride in the treatment of benign prostate hyperplasia: a randomized international study of 1,098 patients. Prostate 1996;29:231.

59. Greeson JM, Sanford B, Monti DA. St. John's Wort (*Hypericum perforatum*): a review of the current pharmacological, toxicological, and clinical literature. Psychopharmacology 2001;153:402.

60. Linde K, Mulrow CD. St. John's wort for depression (Cochrane Review). In: The Cochrane Library, Issue 2, 2000. Oxford: Update Software.

61. Gaster B, Holroyd J. St John's wort for depression: a systematic review. Arch Intern Med 2000;160:152.

62. Shelton RC, Keller MB, Gelenberg A, et al. Effectiveness of St John's wort in major depression. JAMA 2001;285:1978.

63. Morisco C, Trimarco B, Condorelli M. Effect of coenzyme Q10 therapy in patients with congestive heart failure: a long-term multicenter randomized study. Clin Invest 1993;71:S134.

64. Khatta M, Alexander BS, Krichten CM. The effect of coenzyme Q10 in patients with congestive heart failure. Ann Intern Med 2000;132:636.

65. Landbo C, Almdal TP. Interaction between warfarin and coenzyme Q10. Ugeskr Laeger 1998;160:3226.

66. Spigset O. Reduced effect of warfarin caused by ubidecarenone. Lancet 1994;344:1372.

67. Theodasakis J, Adderly B, Fox B. The arthritis cure. New York: St. Martin's Press, 1997.

68. Ronca F, Palmieri L, Panicucci P, et al. Anti-inflammatory

activity of chondroitin sulfate. Osteoarthritis Cartilage 1998;6(SA):14.
69. McAlindon TE, LaValley MP, Gulin JP, et al. Glucosamine and chondroitin for treatment of osteoarthritis. JAMA 2000;283:1469.
70. Reginster JY, Deroisy R, Rovati LC, et al. Long-term effects of glucosamine sulphate on osteoarthritis progression: a randomised, placebo-controlled clinical trial. Lancet 2001;357: 251.
71. Acostamadiedo JM, Iyer UG, Owen J. Danaparoid sodium. Expert Opin Pharmacother 2000;1:803.
72. Di Padova C. *S*-adenosylmethionine in the treatment of osteoarthritis: review of the clinical studies. Am J Med 1987;83(5A):60.
73. Echols JC, Naidoo U, Salzman C. SAMe (*S*-adenosylmethionine). Harvard Rev Psychiatry 2000;8:84.
74. Iruela LM, Minguez L, Merino J, et al. Toxic interaction of *S*-adenosylmethionine and clomipramine. Am J Psychiatry 1991;148:705.
75. Berlanga C, Ortega-Soto HA, Ontiveros M, et al. Efficacy of *S*-adenosyl-L-methionine in speeding the onset of action of imipramine. Psychiatry Res 1992;44:257.
76. Page RL, Lawrence JD. Warfarin potentiation by dong quai. Pharmacotherapy 1999;19:870.
77. Chu DT, Wong WL, Mavligit GM. Immunotherapy with Chinese medicinal herbs. II: Reversal of cyclophosphamide-induced immune suppression by administration of fractionated *Astragalus membranaceus* in vivo. J Clin Lab Immunol 1998; 25:125.
78. Weinberger M, Bronsky E, Bensch GW, et al. Interaction of ephedrine and theophylline. Clin Pharmacol Ther 1975;17:585.
79. Hakas JF. Topical capsaicin induces cough in patient receiving ACE inhibitor. Ann Allergy 1990;65:503.
80. Shader RI, Greenblatt DJ. Phenelzine and the dream machine: ramblings and reflections. J Clin Psychopharmacol 1985;5:65.
81. Jones BD, Runikis AM. Interaction of ginseng with phenelzine. J Clin Psychopharmacol 1987;7:201.
82. McRae S. Elevated serum digoxin levels in a patient taking digoxin and Siberian ginseng. CMAJ 1996;155:293.
83. Almeida JC, Grimsley EW. Coma from the health food store: interaction between kava and alprazolam. Ann Intern Med 1996;125:940.
84. de Klerk GJ, Nieuwenhuis MG, Beutler JJ. Hypokalemia and hypertension associated with use of liquorice flavoured chewing gum. BMJ 1997;314:731.
85. Mai I, Kruger H, Budde K, et al. Hazardous pharmacokinetic interaction of Saint John's wort (*Hypericum perforatum*) with the immunosuppressant cyclosporin. Int J Clin Pharmacol Ther 2000;38:500.
86. Johne A, Brockmoller J, Bauer S, et al. Pharmacokinetic interaction of digoxin with an herbal extract from St. John's wort (*Hypericum perforatum*). Clin Pharmacol Ther 1999;66: 338.
87. Piscitelli SC, Burstein AH, Chaitt D, et al. Indinavir concentrations and St John's wort. Lancet 2000;355:547.
88. Yue QY, Bergquist C, Gerden B. Safety of St John's wort (*Hypericum perforatum*). Lancet 2000;355:576.
89. Lantz MS, Buchalter E, Giambanco V. St. John's wort and antidepressant drug interactions in the elderly. J Geriatr Psychiatry Neurol 1999;12:7.
90. Nebel A, Schneider BJ, Baker RK, et al. Potential metabolic interaction between St. John's wort and theophylline. Ann Pharmacother 1999;33:502.
91. McGuffin M, Hobbs C, Upton R, et al: Botanical safety handbook. Boca Raton, FL: CRC Press, 1997.
92. Lacomblez L, Bensimon G, Isnard F, et al. Effect of yohimbine on blood pressure in patients with depression and orthostatic hypotension induced by clomipramine. Clin Pharmacol Ther 1989;45:241.
93. Eskinazi D. Homeopathy re-revisited: is homeopathy compatible with biomedical observations. Arch Intern Med 1999;159:1981.
94. Stehlin I. Homeopathy: real medicine or empty promises? FDA Consumer 1996;30. Available at http://www.fda.gov/fdac/096_toc.html. Accessed December 2, 2001.
95. Kleijnen J, Knipschild P, ter Riet G. Clinical trials of homeopathy. BMJ 1991;302:316.
96. Linde K, Clausius N, Ramirez G, et al. Are the clinical effects of homoeopathy placebo effects? A meta-analysis of placebo-controlled trials. Lancet 1997;350:834.
97. Long L, Ernst E. Homeopathic remedies for the treatment of osteoarthritis: a systematic review. Br Homeopath J 2001;90:37.
98. Linde K, Jobst KA. Homeopathy for chronic asthma (Cochrane Review). In: The Cochrane Library, Issue 2, 2001. Oxford: Update Software.
99. Ernst E, Pittler MH. Efficacy of homeopathic arnica: a systematic review of placebo-controlled clinical trials. Arch Surg 1998;133:1187.
100. Lee AC, Kemper KJ. Homeopathy and naturopathy: practice characteristics and pediatric care. Arch Pediatr Adolesc Med 2000;154:75.
101. Cooke B, Ernst E. Aromatherapy: a systematic review. Br J Gen Pract 2000;50:493.

CHAPTER 6

Sexuality and Sexual Disorders

PETER J. FAGAN, PhD
ARTHUR L. BURNETT, MD
LINDA ROGERS, CRNP
CHESTER W. SCHMIDT, Jr., MD

In the past decade, the major change in the management of sexual disorders has been the rapid and highly publicized development of effective somatic treatments, especially for sexual dysfunctions. In this environment, the common error of arguing from treatment to etiology and the biogenic versus psychogenic dichotomy continue to thrive as media and sex researchers give more attention to biogenic factors in sexual disorders. In this social context, we urge the clinician to jettison any strict biogenic versus psychogenic dichotomy in favor of a clinical position that expects both somatic and psychological factors to be involved in the development and maintenance of the sexual disorder. Sexual problems accompany physical illness or surgery; are secondary to side effects of medication or abuse of drugs; and are expressions of interpersonal or intrapsychic distress. Frustration, fatigue, and self-doubt can complicate the sexual life of a person who is ill or recovering from surgery, and relational tensions and distrust can interfere with the sexual response in a generally healthy but aging adult.

The task of the primary clinician is to ensure that the sexual disorder of the patient is treated comprehensively, weighing the biogenic and psychogenic factors that are present. For many patients, these conditions can be addressed in the office of the primary care clinician with the counseling techniques that rely heavily on catharsis, reassurance, and education (see Chapter 20)—albeit requiring more time than usual. However, if the psychological or somatic factors are complex, the primary care clinician will most likely have to refer the patient to a specialist. This is a fine art when the problem is sexual in nature. A good working relationship with the urologist, gynecologist, or mental health professional is a prerequisite.

The encouraging news is that, although data documenting results of treatment for these types of problems in the primary care setting are limited, clinical experience suggests that the outcome for sexual problems related to reversible conditions is usually good, with improvement rates approaching 75%.

HUMAN SEXUAL RESPONSE CYCLE

To assess these disorders rapidly and accurately, it is helpful to be familiar with the human sexual response (HSR) cycle and the major physiologic factors that mediate each phase of the cycle. The HSR cycle is divided into four phases: desire, arousal, orgasm, and resolution. It is important to view the HSR as a construct to understand sexual behavior. In practice, many of the dysfunctions are coexisting and do not occur in the neat sequential order implied by the HSR cycle construct. Among women especially, there is reason to suspect that problems of arousal may be primary even if another dysfunction is the chief complaint.

The Four Phases

The *first phase is one of desire* and consists of fantasies and wishes to engage in sexual activity. This response is psychic in origin, but the psychic stimulation is mediated, at least in men, by circulating androgens.

The *second phase is the arousal phase.* It consists of a number of physiologic changes plus the subjective sense of sexual pleasure. In both sexes there is an increase in heart rate, an increase in breathing rate, and development of muscular tension throughout the body which is most pronounced in the pelvic area and thighs. For both sexes, the major physiologic change is the development of vascular congestion in the genital area. For females, the manifestations of vasocongestion are vaginal lubrication and swelling of the external genitalia. In males, vasocongestion leads to erection. Vasocongestion may occur via either of two neurologic pathways. (a) A local reflex pathway is initiated by tactile stimulation of the penis or clitoris and mediated by sensory fibers entering the dorsal root ganglia at S2 through S4 and by parasympathetic fibers from these ganglia to the perivesicular, prostatic, and cavernous plexuses; postganglionic fibers from these plexuses go to the blood vessels of the corpora cavernosa. (b) A cortical pathway is initiated by psychic stimuli and mediated by sympathetic fibers that originate at the T10–L2 level of the spinal cord. Each of these pathways promotes rapid inflow and retention of blood in the penis and the vulva.

The presence of these two spinal centers governing erection has important clinical implications. Patients with complete cord transection above the sacral center but below the thoracic center may still be capable of psychogenic penile or clitoral erections mediated by impulses descending from higher centers and exiting the cord at T10–L2. With a cord lesion above both spinal centers, psychogenically produced erections are blocked, but the patient may still be capable of reflexogenic erections from direct tactile stimulation of the penis or clitoris even though he or she is unable to experience the sensation.

In addition to neurologic pathways, erection in the male and vasocongestion of the vulva and vagina in the female depend on intact arterial blood flow from the right and left internal pudendal arteries.

The third phase is orgasm. Subjectively, for both sexes orgasm is a peaking of sexual pleasure accompanied by a sense of release from sexual tension. Physiologically in the male, the most obvious manifestation of orgasm is ejaculation. Ejaculation is mediated by the sympathetic nervous system and consists of two processes: emission, resulting from contraction of the vas deferens, prostate, and seminal vesicles; and actual ejaculation, resulting from rhythmic contraction of the muscles of the pelvic floor and from closure of the internal sphincters of the bladder (preventing retrograde ejaculation). In the female, the rhythmic contractions take place within the musculature of the outer third of the vagina and in the perineal muscles. The subjective component of orgasm is a cortical sensory phenomenon; it can be experienced without peripheral correlates such as ejaculation or bladder neck closure in men and vaginal contractions in women.

The fourth phase is called resolution, which subjectively is accompanied by a sense of pleasure, warmth, well-being, and relaxation. Physiologically there is a gradual return of heart rate, breathing rate, and muscle tension to the baseline state. Most men are refractory to entering another cycle of sexual activity for some time (minutes in younger men, an hour or longer in middle-aged and older men). Women are not subject to this refractory period and may have multiple orgasms after continued or additional stimulation.

Alternative Model for Women

A less sequential model of sexual response may more accurately reflect the experience of women, especially those in long-term relationships. Many sexually satisfied women report that they seldom have spontaneous thoughts about sex but are able to be responsive to sexual cues from their partner. Desire for them is experienced after arousal, and then has a positive impact on their arousal. The motivational force is a desire for intimacy with the partner, rather than a "drive." Men may also frequently fit this model. Patients that are concerned about their lack of spontaneous desire may find this model reassuring (1).

COMMON SEXUAL DISORDERS

The nomenclature and criteria used to classify sexual disorders in this chapter are based on the American Psychiatric Association's *Diagnostic and Statistical Manual of Mental Disorders,* 4th edition (DSM-IV) (2). The assessment and management of sexual desire disorders, sexual arousal disorders, orgasmic disorders, sexual pain disorders, and sexual dysfunction caused by general medical conditions or substance use are discussed here.

Organic Causes

As is pointed out in the criteria for each of these disorders, the impact of a medical condition should be considered before attributing a disorder solely to psychological factors. Because sexual functioning involves neural, vascular, and endocrine physiologic mechanisms, as well as cellular receptor activity, many medical conditions and drugs can impair normal function. To make matters more complicated, these pathologic conditions can adversely affect one or more phases of the sexual response cycle (Tables 6.1 through 6.4).

General Characteristics

Frequency

Table 6.5 suggests that the prevalence of sexual disorders in the general population of the United States, and even more in clinical and older populations, is such that it deserves screening attention by the primary care physician. The table describes the prevalence of sexual dysfunction in surveys conducted in the United States that asked about the presence of *problems similar to the dysfunctions* within the past 12 months or less. The primary source is the National Health and Social Life Survey (NHSLS) conducted with a randomly selected and stratified sample of 18- to 59-year-old participants in 1992 (3).

Age at Onset of Common Sexual Disorders

Psychological and behavioral antecedents of sexual disorders can sometimes be found in both adolescent and childhood sexual behaviors and fantasies; however, the common age at onset is early adulthood.

Table 6.1. Medical Conditions that May Affect Sexual Response in Either Sex

Organic Factor	Sexual Disorders
Alcoholic neuropathy	Hypoactive arousal, hypoactive orgasm
Angina pectoris or recent myocardial infarction	Hypoactive desire
Any chronic systemic disease	Hypoactive desire, hypoactive arousal
Chronic pain	Hypoactive desire
Degenerative arthritis and disc disease of lumbosacral spine	Hypoactive desire, hypoactive arousal
Diabetes mellitus	Hypoactive arousal, retrograde ejaculation (men); hypoactive orgasm (women)
Endocrine disorders (thyroid deficiency states, Addison's disease, Cushing's disease, hypopituitarism, hyperprolactinemia)	Hypoactive desire, variable effect on arousal
Multiple sclerosis	Hypoactive desire, hypoactive arousal, hypoactive orgasm
Cord lesions	
Low lesion	Hypoactive reflex arousal (psychogenic arousal and reflex ejaculation may be preserved)
High lesion	Hypoactive psychogenic arousal (reflex arousal and ejaculation may be preserved)
Radical pelvic surgery	Hypoactive arousal, hypoactive orgasm
Temporal lobe lesions	Hypoactive or increased desire
Vascular disease	
Large vessel (Leriche syndrome)	Hypoactive arousal
Small vessel (pelvic vascular insufficiency)	Hypoactive arousal

Table 6.2. Medical Conditions that May Affect Sexual Response: Men Only

Organic Factor	Sexual Disorders
Dyspareunia (genital pain during intercourse)	Hypoactive desire, hypoactive arousal, and hypoactive orgasm
Disturbed penile anatomy (chordee, Peyrone's disease, traumatic fracture, traumatic amputation)	
Penile skin infections	
Prostatic infections	
Testicular disease (orchitis, epididymitis, tumor, trauma)	
Urethral infections (gonorrhea, nonspecific urethral infections)	
Hypogonadal androgen-deficient states (Klinefelter's syndrome, testicular agenesis, Kallman's syndrome, testicular tumors, orchitis, hyperprolactinemia, castration)	Hypoactive desire, hypoactive arousal, hypoactive orgasm
Mechanical problems (inguinal hernia, hydrocele)	Hypoactive arousal
Surgical procedures	
Abdominoperineal bowel resection	Hypoactive arousal
Lumbar sympathectomy	Hypoactive orgasm
Radical perineal prostatectomy	Hypoactive arousal

Table 6.3. Medical Conditions that May Affect Sexual Response: Women Only

Organic Factor	Sexual Disorders
Complications of surgery	Hypoactive desire, hypoactive arousal, hypoactive orgasm, and vaginismus may occur with any of the organic factors listed at the left
Ovarian approximation to vagina	
Posthysterectomy scarring	
Shortened vagina	
Dyspareunia (painful intercourse)	
Agenesis of the vagina	
Clitoral phymosis	
Imperforate hymen, rigid hymen, tender hymenal tags	
Infections of external genitalia: herpes genitalis, labial cysts, furuncles, Bartholin cyst infections	
Infections of the vagina: herpes genitalis, *Candida albicans, Trichomonas*	
Injuries due to birth trauma: episiotomy scars, tears, uterine prolapse	
Irritations of the vagina: chemical dermatitis (douches), atrophic vaginitis, intercourse with insufficient lubrication	
Miscellaneous pelvis problems	
Cystitis, urethritis, urethral prolapse	
Endometriosis, ectopic pregnancy, pelvic inflammatory disease, ovarian cysts and tumors, pelvic tumors	
Intrauterine device complications	

Table 6.4. Common Drugs and Substances That May Affect Sexual Response[a]

Drugs	Sexual Disorders Reported
Alcohol and sedatives (high dose)	Hypoactive desire, hypoactive arousal, delayed orgasm
Amiodarone	Hypoactive desire
Androgens	Increased desire (women); hypoactive or increased desire, and/or hypoactive arousal
Anticonvulsants	
Carbamazepine	Hypoactive arousal
Phenytoin	Hypoactive desire, hypoactive arousal
Antidepressants	
Selective serotonin reuptake inhibitors	Hypoactive desire, hypoactive orgasm
Tricyclics	Hypoactive or increased desire and/or hypoactive arousal
Antihypertensives	
Centrally acting (β-blockers, clonidine, guanabenz, methyldopa, reserpine)	Hypoactive desire, hypoactive arousal, (?) hypoactive orgasm
β-Blockers, hydralazine	Hypoactive arousal
Peripherally acting (guanethidine, guanadrel)	Retrograde ejaculation, hypoactive desire
Antipsychotics	Hypoactive or increased desire, hypoactive arousal, retrograde ejaculation (Mellaril)
Digoxin	Hypoactive desire, hypoactive arousal
Disopyramide	Hypoactive arousal
Disulfiram	Hypoactive arousal, delayed ejaculation
Diuretics	Hypoactive arousal
Estrogens, progesterone	
Men	Hypoactive desire, hypoactive arousal, hypoactive orgasm
Women	Hypoactive desire
H_2 blockers (cimetidine, famotidine, ranitidine)	Hypoactive desire, hypoactive arousal
L-Dopa	Increased desire (elderly men)
Lithium	Hypoactive desire, hypoactive arousal
Marijuana (high dose)	Hypoactive arousal (low dose may produce increased desire in men)
Metoclopramide	Hypoactive desire, hypoactive arousal
Narcotics	Hypoactive desire, hypoactive arousal, hypoactive orgasm
Stimulants, high dose (cocaine, amphetamines)	Hypoactive desire, hypoactive arousal, hypoactive orgasm (low dose may produce increased desire)
Verapamil	Hypoactive arousal

[a]See also Crenshaw TL, Goldberg JP, Sexual pharmacology: drugs that affect sexual function, New York: WW Norton, 1996.

Table 6.5. Prevalence Ranges of Sexual Dysfunctions among Women and Men

Sexual Dysfunction	Prevalence	Source (Ref. No.)
Women		
Hypoactive sexual desire disorder	33% last 12 mo	U.S. random sample, 1994 (3)
Female sexual arousal disorder	19% last 12 mo	U.S. random sample, 1994 (3)
Female orgasmic disorder	24% last 12 mo	U.S. random sample, 1994 (3)
Dyspareunia	14% last 12 mo	U.S. random sample, 1994 (3)
Vaginismus	0.5% to 1% last 12 mo	Two large population samples in Europe, 1998 (4), 1999 (5)
Men		
Hypoactive sexual desire disorder	16% last 12 mo	U.S. random sample, 1994 (3)
Male sexual arousal disorder	10% last 12 mo	U.S. random sample, 1994 (3);
	Current: minimal, 17%; moderate, 25%; complete, 10%	Older (range, 40–70 yr; median, 54 yr) community samples, 1994 (6)
Premature ejaculation	29% last 12 mo	U.S. random sample, 1994 (3)
Male orgasmic disorder	8% last 12 mo	U.S. random sample, 1994 (3)
Dyspareunia	4% last 6 mo	Medical clinic sample, 1998 (7)

Onset can occur at any time during adult life, especially for dysfunctions associated with medical conditions or use of drugs or other substances and for those dysfunctions that are situational or transient.

Predisposing Personality Factors

In general, competent and satisfying sexual function is considered to be associated with a healthy and adaptive personality development. Therefore, defects in personality structure accompanied by maladaptive personality traits (see Chapter 23) or psychopathology may affect sexual function. However, a study involving 288 patients referred because of a diagnosis of a sexual dysfunction revealed that only 30% of the sample fulfilled criteria for an additional psychiatric disorder (8). Negative attitudes toward sexuality caused by particular experience, internal psychic conflicts, or adherence to rigid cultural values can predispose patients to the development of these dysfunctions.

Course and Severity

The course of sexual dysfunctions varies. Dysfunctions may develop after a period of normal functioning or they may be lifelong. They may be generalized, occurring with all partners, or situational, limited to certain partners. There are differing degrees of impairment, from partial or intermittent to total and unremitting. Usually, early age at onset and total impairment indicate chronicity and predict a poor treatment outcome. Conversely, a history of prior adequate sexual function, situational symptoms, and partial impairment are predictive of a self-limited course and a favorable treatment outcome.

Complications

The major complications of sexual dysfunctions are disrupted marital or sexual relationships. In addition, presence of the dysfunction may give rise to a variety of symptoms such as depression, anxiety, guilt, shame, frustration, and anger. These symptoms not only affect the patient but also may intrude into most of his or her relationships.

General Approach to the Patient

Because patients often have difficulty initiating discussion about sexual activities and problems, it is important to inquire about sexual orientation and function as part of the primary care of each patient. In a study in a general medicine practice, 90% of patients appreciated being asked about sexual function (4). Table 6.6 outlines interviewing approaches that may be useful in this inquiry. One should not presume exclusive heterosexuality in a new patient but should ask questions that are gender neutral until orientation has been established. In patients who name a problem, the history of the present problem may be imprecise. Therefore, sufficient time should be set aside with the patient to obtain a clear account of the problem. Occasionally, more than one scheduled session is necessary. The setting for the discussion should be private. For patients whose difficulties involve a partner or a spouse, it is important to have the partner's view of the problem. Sometimes the more functional partner will seek help to gain support for bringing the less functional partner into the evaluation.

The evaluation should be organized to obtain information about the onset and duration of the problem; about factors that make the problem better or worse; about concurrent events such as birth of children, changes in relationships or vocation, or onset of physical or emotional illness; and about use of new medications. It is always important to elicit from patients their ideas about the cause of sexual problems and their expectations of treatment.

If it is determined that a referral to a psychiatrist or mental health specialist in sexual disorders is appropriate, the clinician should advise the patient to consult with his or her health insurance program to ascertain whether such treatment of sexual dysfunction or disorders is a covered benefit. Most plans do not cover marital therapy, and many exclude sexual therapy (especially nonmedical) as a covered benefit.

Sexual Desire Disorders

Diagnostic Classification

Medical conditions or medications that cause decreased sexual desire should be specifically diagnosed. Predominantly psychogenic disorders have been classified as follows in DSM-IV (2):

Table 6.6. Suggested Questions Regarding Sexual Practices and Problems

Suggested Opening (Legitimizing Statement)
"Something that I ask each of my patients about is sexual activity. Is that all right with you?"

Suggested Initial Question
(Open-ended question) "Can you tell me about your present sexual activity (practices)?"
or
(Closed, somewhat leading question) "Have you noticed any problem in your ability to have and enjoy sexual relations?"
or
(Closed but facilitative question) "Do you have any problems or questions related to your current sexual activities?"

Screening Questions for Sexual Dysfunction (Ask for Clarification of any Positive Response)
(Both sexes) "Have you noticed any loss of interest in having sex?"
(Men) "Any problems having an erection?"
(Women) "Any problems with lubrication or swelling of the vagina when you are sexually aroused?"
(Both sexes) "Any problems having an orgasm?"
(Both sexes) "Any pain during intercourse?"

Screening Questions Regarding Sexual Orientation
(Both sexes) "Have you ever had sex with men, women, or both?"
or
(Men) "Do you ever have sex with another man?"
(Women) "Do you ever have sex with another woman?"

Screening Questions for Risk of or History of Sexually Transmitted Disease[a]
(Both sexes) "In the past few years about how many partners have you had for sexual relations?"
(Both sexes) "Have you ever had any kind of infection that you got from having sex?"

Open Question to Obtain Additional Information
"Is there any other information or any other questions about your sexual activities that you would like to discuss with me?"

[a]See list of safe and unsafe sexual practices and instructions for use of a condom (Table 39.2).

Hypoactive Sexual Desire Disorder (Loss of Libido)

A. Persistently or recurrently deficient (or absent) sexual fantasies and desire for sexual activity. The judgment of deficiency or absence is made by the clinician, taking into account factors that affect sexual functioning, such as age, sex, and the context of the person's life.
B. The disturbance causes marked distress or interpersonal difficulty.
C. It does not occur exclusively during the course of another axis I disorder (except another sexual dysfunction) and is not caused exclusively by the direct physiologic effects of a substance (e.g., drugs of abuse, medication) or a general medical condition.

Sexual Aversion Disorder

A. Persistent or recurrent extreme aversion to and avoidance of all or almost all genital sexual contact with a sexual partner.
B. The disturbance causes marked distress or interpersonal difficulty.
C. The sexual dysfunction is not caused by another axis I disorder (except another sexual dysfunction).

Assessment

As seen in Tables 6.1 through 6.4, many medical conditions and drugs have the potential for decreasing sexual desire. In practice, most of these conditions are known to or easily diagnosed by the patient's physician. Only a few conditions may result in a presentation with the initial complaint of decreased or absent desire.

Congenital or acquired *hypogonadism* is associated with decreased sexual interest in men. Because the testosterone level needed to maintain libido is usually lower than that needed for full stimulation of the prostate and seminal vesicles, the patient may also complain of a decrease or absence of emission when loss of sexual desire is caused by hypogonadism. Hypogonadism that occurs before puberty results in eunuchoidism (lack of development of secondary sex characteristics). Similar striking physical findings are not present in patients who acquire hypogonadism after puberty, but subtle physical changes do occur: decrease in beard growth, tendency to female body habitus, and decrease in size of testes. An evaluation for hypogonadism should be undertaken in any male with persistent loss of libido (see Chapters 85).

In both sexes, *prolactin-secreting microadenomas* of the pituitary can cause loss of sexual interest. In men this caused in part by a prolactin-mediated decrease in gonadotropin output, accompanied by a low testosterone level. Hyperprolactinemia causes amenorrhea and galactorrhea in women, but galactorrhea is rare in affected men. Diagnosis can be made in both sexes by measuring serum prolactin levels (normal, less than 15 mg/mL) (see Chapter 85.)

In both sexes, *alcohol or other substance abuse* can cause decreased sexual desire. Patients who abuse drugs are usually guarded or untruthful about their habits; therefore, persistence and use of collateral interviews are often necessary to diagnose the primary problem (see Chapters 28 and 29).

Depression is a common cause of loss of sexual desire. Even mild depressive states can result in decreased sexual desire, but in patients with severe depression this loss is universally observed. The relationship between loss of sexual desire and the presence of depression may be recognized by noting the patient's mood and by obtaining a history of depressive symptoms (see Chapter 24). Life stresses (e.g., loss of a job, death of a family member or friend, birth of a new family member, recent illness such as myocardial infarction) are common sources of decreased sexual desire related to depression or anxiety.

In married couples, decreased sexual desire in one or both partners is often the result of *marital strife*. Arguments between partners create anger that eventually interferes with their sexual relationship. Although spouses may be aware of their anger toward each other, they may fail to draw a connection between loss of sexual interest and their mutual differences. Assessment requires a history taken from the couple together and then separately. Review of their current life situation usually elicits the precipitating stresses and highlights the conflicts. The uncovering of extramarital relationships during the assessment requires careful handling. If both partners are aware of the relationship, it can be discussed openly. If the extramarital relationship is revealed to a physician during the individual interviews, the physician should ask what the partner intends to do about the relationship and with the secret information now shared with the physician. The responsibility for telling the other partner should be left to the patient. In some cases the extramarital relationship is a peripheral issue, and airing it could be destructive to an otherwise salvageable relationship.

Low sexual desire in women is one of the most common sexual complaints encountered by primary care providers. Patients often blame hormonal problems, whereas depression and interpersonal problems are actually much more commonly to blame.

Finally, decreased or absent sexual desire may be caused by the anxiety and frustration of *repeated sexual failure* associated with one of the other sexual disorders discussed in the following sections.

Sexual Aversion Disorder

Certain patients may give a history of *aversion to or avoidance of all forms of genital contact* with a sexual partner, in contrast to a history of gradual or sudden loss of sexual desire. The complaint is often of long standing but may be of recent onset. The aversion may be so severe as to be associated with panic attacks should the patient find himself or herself confronted with a sexual experience.

Treatment of Hypoactive Sexual Desire

Depending on the cause, hypogonadism in men may be treated by surgery, radiotherapy, hormone replacement, or hormone suppression (in the case of hyperprolactinemia). These treatment modalities are discussed in Chapter 85.

In both sexes, if a drug (Table 6.4) is suspected of interfering with sexual desire, it should be discontinued when possible as a diagnostic-therapeutic test. If loss of sexual drive is secondary to alcohol or substance abuse, treatment should be aimed at controlling the abuse (see Chapters 28 and 29).

Patients with coronary artery disease, especially those who have had a myocardial infarction, have particular problems associated with sexual function. The treatment of these patients is discussed as part of the overall approach to rehabilitation after infarction in Chapter 63.

Transient hypoactive sexual desire disorders secondary to *psychological factors* such as stress, anger, or other interpersonal problems can be managed effectively with short-term counseling. When alcoholism, depression, or another psychosocial disorder is the primary problem, specific treatment for that disorder should accompany the counseling. The design of a counseling program should include an agreement between the patient or couple and the physician to meet for a specified number of sessions (usually two to five) for approximately 30 minutes per session.

Example

A couple in their mid-twenties presents with a history of recent loss of sexual desire on the husband's part and a decrease in the frequency of their sexual relationships. Assessment reveals a history of mutually satisfying sexual experiences until 1 month ago, when the husband was threatened with a job layoff. Although the husband still has his job, the layoff is still a possibility. The wife reports that the husband has become quiet, sullen, and generally less interested in activities he usually enjoys. They report fighting frequently over small issues. The assessment is that the husband has an adjustment disorder with depressive features (see Chapter 24). During the initial counseling session, the physician suggests that a relationship exists between changes in the husband's behavior and the threatened layoff. The wife indicates that the husband has refused to discuss his concerns because it is unmanly. During the next counseling session, the physician assists the couple in sharing their anguish with each other and developing contingency plans to cope with the potential layoff. As they are drawn into the discussions of planning, the couple's anger with each other subsides and a collaborative relationship is reestablished. The third session is used to review what contingency plans they have made. As an aside, they report that they have resumed their sexual relationship. During the final session the physician reviews the relationship between stress, anger, and the change in sexual functioning; points out that anger subsided when they worked together and that good sex is difficult to experience when they are angry with each other; and encourages the couple to use what they have learned when stresses arise in the future.

Patients and their physicians often attempt to treat decreased sexual desire with drugs such as testosterone, alcohol, antianxiety compounds, or stimulants. There is no scientific basis for prescribing drugs for sexual desire disorders, except testosterone for the treatment of confirmed hypogonadism and bromocriptine for treatment of hyperprolactinemia (15), as discussed in Chapter 85.

The possibility that androgens may have a role in the treatment of desire disorders in women has generated extreme controversy in recent years. Some studies have found that testosterone levels in women are related to sexual functioning, but other studies have failed to find a relationship.

In the female, androgens are produced in the ovary, in the adrenal cortex, and from the conversion of androgen precursors in the liver, adipose tissue, skin, and elsewhere. Testosterone levels peak when a woman is her twenties and then begin a gradual decline that is related to age and not to menopausal status. In fact, levels of bioavailable testosterone increase at the menopause because of a decrease in the levels of sex hormone–binding globulin (SHBG) secondary to a decrease in estrogen. However, when estrogens are given exogenously, there is a significant increase in SHBG, and a decrease in bioavailable testosterone.

The possibility that there may be an *androgen deficiency syndrome* in women is also controversial. Current assays for androgen levels are unreliable at the lower levels of normal because they were developed to measure levels in men, so it has been difficult to reliably define abnormally low levels. Because about 50% of a woman's testosterone production is lost when a bilateral oophorectomy is done, patients who have undergone this procedure have been a logical group to study for this syndrome. Other possible causes of insufficient androgen production include adrenal insufficiency, Addison disease, hypopituitarism, corticosteroid therapy, estrogen therapy, and chronic illness. About 30% of women complain of impaired sexual function after a bilateral oophorectomy, and several studies have compared the effects of supplementing estrogen alone with estrogen–androgen combinations in these patients and have found significant benefits (9,10). Most of the studies that have found a benefit have used testosterone preparations that resulted in levels above the normal range for women, so the benefit may have been a pharmacologic action of the hormone rather than a physiologic benefit. There is also some confusion regarding whether the benefit from testosterone is due solely to testosterone, because significant conversion of testosterone to 17-beta-estradiol occurs. It may be that androgen supplementation affects sexual function indirectly, through a positive effect on the patient's general sense of well-being that has been observed in most of the studies.

The safety of androgen supplementation, especially in the long term, has not been well studied. Concerns include side effects such as acne, hirsutism, voice changes, and male-pattern baldness. Safety concerns include unknown effects on cardiovascular risk factors, breast cancer risks, and possible liver toxicity. Androgens of any sort, including dehydroepiandrosterone (DHEA), are contraindicated in women at risk for pregnancy, because of the possibility of masculinization of the fetus.

Treatment of Sexual Aversion Disorder

Treatment usually requires a course of individual and couple treatment by a skilled sex therapist. The treatment goal is to replace the negative affect and avoidant behaviors associated with phobic-like stimuli with relaxation and pleasure in mutual sexual expression. The treatment of any associated panic attacks may be augmented with low-dosage antidepressant medication (see Chapter 22).

Sexual Arousal Disorders

Diagnostic Classification

An arousal disorder that is secondary to a medical condition or medication should be diagnosed as a symptom associated with the condition or medication.

Psychogenic disorders have been classified as follows in DSM-IV (2).

Female Arousal Disorder

A. Persistent or recurrent inability to attain or to maintain until completion of sexual activity an adequate lubrication–swelling response of sexual excitement.
B. The disturbance causes marked distress or interpersonal difficulty.
C. The sexual dysfunction is not better accounted for by another axis I disorder (except another sexual dysfunction) and is not caused by the direct physiologic effects of a substance (e.g., drugs of abuse, a medication) or a general medical condition.

Male Erectile Disorder

A. Persistent or recurrent inability to attain or maintain an adequate erection until completion of sexual activity.
B. The disturbance causes marked distress or interpersonal difficulty.
C. The dysfunction is not better accounted for by another axis I disorder (other than a sexual dysfunction) and is not caused exclusively by the direct physiologic effects of a substance (e.g., a drug of abuse, a medication).

Assessment

An initial history usually leads to a formulation that the patient's problem is either organic or predominantly psychogenic. The general features in the history of a male patient that are listed in Table 6.7 are helpful in making this important distinction.

Organic Dysfunction. In both sexes, partial or complete failure to begin and maintain genital vasocongestion can be caused by a large number of medical conditions and drugs. Importantly, when sexual desire is intact, a male erectile disorder is unlikely to be caused by a hypogonadal condition, because libido is typically diminished in patients with hypogonadal conditions (see Chapter 85). In younger patients, drugs are the most common cause of erectile disorders (Table 6.4). In older men, new onset of a erectile disorder is usually caused by vascular or neurologic disease. The other conditions that may cause sexual arousal disorders (Tables 6.1 to 6.3) usually result in other manifestations before the patient complains of this problem.

It is estimated that 25% to 60% of male patients with *diabetes mellitus* will eventually develop an erectile disorder (5). Because some patients present with erectile disorder as the initial symptom of diabetes, a fasting blood glucose determination is indicated for any male patient who presents with a chief complaint of erectile disorder that is not caused by an obvious psychosocial stressor or a recently started medication. There is no consensus in the literature about the prevalence of sexual dysfunction among women with diabetes; however, given no other negative relational or psychological factors, the disease may be presumed to play a significant role in disorders of arousal and orgasm that have emerged with the diabetes (11,12).

Two conditions in women may contribute to arousal disorders: *vaginitis* and *atrophic vaginal changes* secondary to estrogen deficiency (see Chapter 106). Surprisingly, some women do not associate the presence of vaginitis or atrophic changes with the discomfort or pain these conditions can cause when intercourse is attempted. Therefore, the history should include questions to determine whether pain occurs during intercourse, and the physical examination should include a pelvic examination to look for evidence of atrophy (see Chapter 106).

Occlusive vascular disease causing diminished blood flow to the internal pudendal arteries is more likely to affect men than women. Female arousal disorders have been described with large vessel disease (Leriche syndrome) as well as with medium and small vessel disease. If it is suspected that there is a vascular basis for male erectile disorder, the patient should be offered a referral to a vascular surgeon for evaluation (see Chapter 94). The diagnostic techniques that may be used include angiography of the medium-size

Table 6.7. Clinical Features Differentiating Predominantly Psychogenic from Predominantly Organic Erectile Dysfunction

Feature	Psychogenic	Organic
Onset	Usually abrupt, with temporal relationship to specific stress (e.g., marital difficulties, loss of job, bereavement, fatigue)	Usually insidious decline from previous competency (90%–95% of cases)
Course	Selective, intermittent, episodic, transient	Usually persistent, with progressive deterioration
Degree of impairment	Evidence of potential to respond to erotic stimuli and fantasies, with masturbation, other partner	Unable to obtain erection with masturbation, erotic stimuli, other partner
Nocturnal or morning erection	Generally present	Generally absent or reduced in frequency, intensity

Vliet LW, Meyer JK. Erectile dysfunction: progress in evaluation and treatment. Johns Hopkins Med J 1982;151:246.

vessels of the corpora cavernosa, Doppler measurement of penile blood flow, and nocturnal penile tumescence (NPT) studies (13).

The *hypogonadal* states that cause hypoactive desire (discussed earlier) can also cause arousal disorders, and the approach to diagnosis is the same (see Chapter 85).

Psychogenic Arousal Dysfunction. If the assessment for an organic cause, which often includes a trial of a potentially offending drug, does not yield a convincing diagnosis, a psychogenic basis should be considered, and further inquiry followed by appropriate brief counseling (see later discussion) should be used as a diagnostic-therapeutic trial.

Inability to attain and maintain levels of arousal that permit a smooth and trouble-free progression from the beginning of a sexual experience to its completion can be caused by any external or internal psychological events that interfere with the patient's ability to focus on the physical and psychological stimuli that maintain the sexual arousal. A dramatic example of an external event is the ringing of a telephone during the sexual experience. An internal psychological event might be a recurring thought about how one is performing. The history and assessment should be structured to uncover the presence of external events and the specific content of the psychological events when present. A common finding is a persistent preoccupation and anxiety about performing successfully. This problem may be primary, or it may occur as a secondary response to the frustration associated with organic dysfunction. Worry about a successful performance becomes more and more absorbing during the course of the sexual experience, so that the psychological activity crowds out the patient's capacity to focus on the sexual stimuli that maintain the arousal response. When such patients realize they are losing arousal, they try all the harder, shutting off completely their ability to respond to sexual stimuli. This process is called *spectatoring*, a termed coined by William Masters and Virginia Johnson (14). The term describes a process whereby patients, through observation of their performance, psychologically take themselves out of the experience. The mental process is guaranteed to result in loss of sexual arousal. Typically this process may begin after one or two failed experiences secondary to external events or stresses. Once the process begins, it becomes internally reinforcing, leading to further worry and further failure. When this process is suspected, the history should focus on the patient's mental experiences during sexual intercourse. Such information is difficult for most patients to describe, and more than a single interview may be required.

Other common causes of psychologically inhibited sexual arousal are *stressful life situations.* Patients who have recently lost a job, lost a relative, are concerned about retirement, or have developed an illness may be unable to clear their minds of their worries during a sexual experience and therefore cannot respond. Similarly, feelings of anger or resentment directed toward the sexual partner can interfere with the ability to become sexually aroused.

Nocturnal Penile Tumescence Testing. If the patient with suspected psychogenic impotence does not respond to brief counseling (discussed later), management may then proceed either with further diagnostic assessment or with an empirical trial of oral pharmacotherapy (see later discussion). Conventionally, NPT studies have been offered based on the precept that this modality will distinguish psychogenic from organic causes and direct patients to receive appropriate therapy. As a noninvasive and inexpensive diagnostic technique, NPT monitoring assumes that during sleep the psychological factors that impede erectile function during wakefulness are no longer operative, allowing a demonstration of the integrity of one's physiologic capacity. Organic deficits, however, persist during sleep and therefore interfere with the number and duration of erectile episodes. Research has tended to confirm this assumption, with three exceptions: (a) in certain psychiatric disorders (e.g., endogenous depression) in which rapid eye movement (REM) sleep patterns are also disrupted; (b) in some men with organically proven erectile failure who occasionally have an episode of full erection during sleep—such as patients with lower body spasms caused by spinal cord injury or patients with a vascular steal syndrome; and (c) in a previously unrecognized syndrome of impaired penile tumescence in the presence of sleep apnea, hypoventilation with decreased oxygen saturation, myoclonic jerks, and bradycardia. Approaches that have been applied to accomplish NPT monitoring include sleep laboratory testing with polysomnography and at-home evaluation using Rigiscan (Timm Medical Technologies, Eden Prairie, MN) or electrobioimpedance volumetric assessment (NEVA).

The contemporary role of NPT studies has been significantly reduced, mostly as a consequence of the recent introduction of first-line oral therapies for erectile dysfunction that have been used in many instances even for diagnostic trials. Accordingly, responses to treatment irrespective of etiologic diagnosis of erectile dysfunction constitute therapeutic successes and obviate the need for etiologic distinction as a practical matter. On the other hand, NPT studies conducted at a sleep center (see Chapter 7) may be preferred for a pharmacologic trial or for noninvasive diagnostic evaluation in certain circumstances, such as for the patient for whom more invasive testing procedures seem excessive (e.g., an adolescent male with concerns of erectile dysfunction) and for medicolegal purposes. Additional evaluations for vascular or neurologic disorders may be carried out as prerequisites to the initiation of second- or third-line therapies that are considered to be at least semi-invasive and possible irreversible.

Arousal in Women. Problems with sexual arousal are common in women and may actually be at the root of many other sexual disorders. Orgasmic dysfunction and low libido are frequently secondary to difficulty with arousal. It is also possible that coitus with insufficient arousal is a large factor in the etiology of vulvar pain syndromes and vaginismus.

Traditionally the focus was on genital changes in the arousal process in women, as a corollary of the erection process in men. More recently, there has been a recognition that arousal in women is much more complex. Because women's genital changes are less obvious than men's, women may be completely unaware of them. They may attend far more to other somatic changes, such as heart rate, muscle tension, or breast sensations, or to their own subjective state of arousal (1).

There are now several research methodologies that reflect changes in blood flow in the vaginal walls or labia and are used to study women's genital reactions to sexually arousing stimuli. The studies have consistently found a lack of correlation between women's feelings of subjective arousal and the genital changes associated with arousal. For instance, women frequently react to a sexual stimulus with changes in genital blood flow, but they may be unaware of the changes, often do not feel aroused subjectively, and may in fact feel negatively about the stimulus (15).

Treatment for Organic Causes of Arousal Disorder

When a disease process has caused *permanent impairment* of neural, vascular, or anatomic aspects of penile erection, a series of effective, minimally invasive treatment options may be explored (Table 6.8). Generally, these options are considered in consultation with a urologist or gynecologist, although nonspecialist

Table 6.8. Pharmacotherapies for Erectile Dysfunction

Drug	Trade Name	Usual Dose Range	Available Strengths	Selected Side Effects and Comments	Efficacy[a]
Oral Route					
Phosphodiesterase Type 5 Inhibitors					
Sildenafil	Viagra	25, 50, or 100 mg, 1 hr before sexual activity	25, 50, 100 mg	Headaches (16%), flushing (10%), dyspepsia (7%), nasal congestion (4%), visual disturbances (3%) Presence of sexual stimulation is required for efficacy. Contraindicated for men receiving nitrate therapy in any form that in combination may produce severe hypotension. Age, hepatic impairment, renal impairment, and use of drugs that are concurrently metabolized by the cytochrome P450 3A4 isoenzyme pathway in the liver necessitate lower dosing.	46%–69%
α-Adrenoceptor Antagonists					
Yohimbine	Yocon	5.4 mg t.i.d., for 1 mo	5.4 mg	Anxiety, nausea, palpitations, nervousness, hypertension, headache. Modest results suggest its role to be limited to men with psychogenic erectile dysfunction.	~30%
Intraurethral Route					
Alprostadil	MUSE	125, 250, 500, or 1,000 μg, on demand	125, 250, 500, 1,000 μg	Local urogenital pain (29%), minor urethral bleeding (5%), dizziness (4%), hypotension (3%). In-office instruction and titration is highly recommended. Contraindicated for patients with priapism histories.	~40%
Intracavernosal Route				Priapism (1%), penile fibrosis (5%–10%), penile pain (10%). In-office instruction and titration is highly recommended. Contraindicated for patients with histories of priapism and severe coagulopathy.	
Alprostadil	Caverject, Edex	10 or 20 μg, on demand	5–60 μg		~70%
Alprostadil + phentolamine	Bi-mix	20 μg/mL + 0.5 mg/mL, on demand	Variable		~90%
Papaverine + phentolamine	Bi-mix (Androskat)	30 mg/mL + 0.5 mg/mL, on demand	Variable		~90%
Alprostadil + papaverine + phentolamine	Tri-mix	10 μg/mL + 30 mg/mL + 1.0 mg/mL, on demand	Variable		~90%

[a]The outcome measure pertains to the degree of success with sexual intercourse subjectively using patient and partner questionnaires.

clinicians with appropriate qualifications may proceed with treatments after completion of an appropriate basic assessment of the problem.

Somatic Treatment for Men

Oral Pharmacotherapy. Effective, safe, and convenient oral therapies have now emerged as a first-line option for most male patients. Sildenafil citrate (Viagra), a phosphadiesterase inhibitor that facilitates blood flow to the corpora cavernosa, has shown significant promise, and other oral therapies are under development.

An early pivotal study using the rate of successful sexual intercourse as an end point measure reported that almost 70% of men using sildenafil responded, compared with 22% of those using placebo (16). Similar findings were reported in clinical investigations carried out after U.S. Food and Drug Administration (FDA) approval of the medication (17,18). The medication has shown efficacy irrespective of erectile dysfunction etiology, and successes even in patients with apparently severe forms of erectile dysfunction indicate that the medication should be administered to any man presenting with erectile dysfunction as a therapeutic trial as long as the contraindications to its use (discussed later) do not exist.

Treatment dosages of Viagra include 25, 50, and 100 mg. The medication should be taken approximately 1 hour before intended sexual intercourse and in the presence of sexual stimulation, because the medication functions to augment erections and not to induce them. In healthy men, peak serum levels of the medication after oral ingestion are achieved within 1 hour and the drug is metabolized with a mean half-life of 4.5 hours (19). Because sildenafil is metabolized by the cytochrome P450 3A4 isoenzyme pathway in the liver, a lower dose should be prescribed initially for patients who are taking medications that are also metabolized by this pathway (e.g., cimetidine, erythromycin, ketoconazole, nifedipine, saquinavir/ritonavir, and the statins). Because age, hepatic impairment, and renal impairment are also associated with increasing serum levels of the medication, a lower starting dose should also be prescribed in these instances as well.

Reported adverse systemic effects with the medication have been transient and have included headache, nasal congestion, and dyspepsia (20). Current analyses indicate that the cardiovascular risks associated with use of sildenafil relate to the inherent risk factors for adverse cardiovascular events in patients with erectile dysfunction and the risk of an event's occurring during any strenuous exercise, including sexual activity (21). Treadmill testing is recommended for assessment of cardiac ischemia before sildenafil treatment in patients who are considered to be at risk for a major cardiovascular event (e.g., myocardial infarction) with sexual exertion (22). An absolute contraindication is the coadministration of sildenafil and organic nitrates (e.g., nitroglycerin, amyl nitrate "poppers"), because the blood pressure–lowering effects of this combination may be so severe that resuscitation cannot be achieved (22). A precaution only is given regarding the possibility of sildenafil-induced hypotension in patients using antihypertensive medications.

A long-touted erectogenic and aphrodisiac agent, *yohimbine* (Yocon) has been rigorously evaluated to establish its role as an orally delivered agent for the treatment of erectile dysfunction (23–25). The medication is an alkaloid derived from the bark of the yohimbe tree and is reported to exert central effects on the medication of penile erection as an alpha-2-adrenergic receptor antagonist (26). Conventionally, the medication is used at an oral dosage of 5.4 mg three times daily with clinical observation for at least 1 month to assess improvement. Although some evidence suggests that the medication may be more effective then placebo (25), its efficacy beyond placebo has not been affirmed in patients with confirmed organic erectile dysfunction (23,24). Adverse effects appear to be relatively infrequent but include hypertension, anxiety, tachycardia, and headache (23–25). Although yohimbine may be well tolerated, its modest results suggest that the medication may be best limited to men with psychogenic erectile dysfunction.

Local Pharmacotherapies. When oral pharmacotherapy is ineffective or contraindicated, patients may be best directed to consider other nonsurgical treatments, such as intraurethral therapy, intracavernosal therapy, and vacuum constriction devices.

The administration of *vasoactive drugs via the urethral channel* of the penis has been evaluated as a potentially less invasive procedure than intracavernosal needle injections to induce erection. A synthetic formulation of prostaglandin E_1 (alprostadil) can be delivered through a novel transurethral drug delivery system know as Medicated Urethral System for Erection, or MUSE (27,28). Several technical points optimize the success of the treatment, including the patient's properly depositing and manually distributing the medication into the penis and then standing for several minutes after its application to increase penile engorgement. A final responder rate to the medication is documented at approximately 40%, with typical responses including tumescence without full rigidity (27). The combined use of an adjustable penile constriction band (ACTIS), designed and FDA approved to enhance the local retention and effect of the medication, has been shown to improve responses to this treatment (14,29). The most common side effects of MUSE included local urogenital pain associated with metabolism of the medication and minor urethral bleeding associated with traumatic delivery of the medication (13,27).

Intracavernosal pharmacotherapy also employs vasoactive medications, with three that are regularly used: papaverine, phentolamine, and prostaglandin E_1. These vasoactive substances are administered through a single injection to the corpus cavernosum and induce erection by relaxation of the smooth muscle–containing erectile tissue (30). The medications may be used individually or in combination. In-office titration is recommended to determine the dosage that yields an erection of sufficient rigidity for sexual intercourse yet lasts no more than 1 hour. Rates of successful sexual intercourse range between 70% and 90% (16,31).

Intracavernosal pharmacotherapy is contraindicated for men with psychological instability, a history of or risk for priapism (e.g., sickle cell disease, locally advanced pelvic or hematologic malignancy), histories of severe coagulopathy or unstable cardiovascular disease, or reduced manual dexterity (although the partner can be trained in the injection technique) (32). Risks of complications include priapism (1% of men), penile fibrosis at the penile injection site (5% to 10% of men), local trauma such as hematoma (10% of injections), and penile pain (10% of men) (31).

Vacuum constriction devices apply a nonpharmacologic, mechanical means to produce an erection (33). A cylinder is temporarily placed externally around the penis with a seal that allows the creation of negative pressure for blood engorgement of the penis. The erection is maintained by placement of a constricting elastic ring around the base of the penis, after which the cylinder is removed and the erection-like state allows sexual intercourse to occur. The treatment is generally pursued with instructional videotape or in-office teaching. The erection-like state is achieved in at least 95% of applications (34). Significant complications are rare, with typical concerns related to cumbersomeness, coldness of the erect penis, and local penile trauma such as petechiae and ecchymosis (34).

Penile prostheses represent a surgical alternative that ideally should be considered only after nonsurgical options have been found ineffective or unacceptable (35). The devices are surgically implanted within the corporal bodies of the penis. The two main varieties of devices are semirigid malleable devices and hydraulic inflatable devices. Use of the devices requires basic instruction. They reliably produce penile rigidity permitting sexual intercourse. Potential complications (less than 5% at 5 years) include infection, erosion, and malfunction of the device and usually necessitate device removal or replacement (36). Penile revascularization surgery is beneficial to a minority of patients with a confirmed vascular lesion of probable traumatic origin amenable to vascular bypass techniques (35).

Somatic Treatment for Women. The somatic treatment of biogenic arousal disorder in women follows the three-fold goals of stabilizing the disease process, reversing medication side effects, and improving the genital environment (11). Any form of estrogen therapy will benefit atrophic vaginal tissue, but local applications (creams or a vaginal ring) are particularly effective. Women receiving estrogen replacement therapy may also benefit from the addition of vaginal estrogen, especially in the early menopausal years. Estrogen improves lubrication, makes the vaginal epithelium thicker, and may improve vaginal sensitivity. Absorption from the vaginal mucosa is good, so if the uterus is intact a progestin must be used either continuously or cyclically to protect the endometrium.

Concerns relating to hysterectomy are that it may affect sexual functioning. However, the lack of certainty of such effects remains substantial. Clinical investigations have suggested that hysterectomy either produces no change in sexual function for the majority of women or possibly even enhances sexual functioning (37). Nonetheless, theoretical concerns that radical extirpative pelvic surgery in women may compromise the nerve supply involved in optimal sexual functioning have led to the development of techniques to preserve genital innervation.

Vasoactive medications have been extremely effective for erectile problems in men. Research has shown that women's erectile tissue also undergoes age-related vascular changes, which may be associated with arousal problems. There are case reports of women who obtained benefit from sildenafil, but controlled studies have had mixed results. Other vasoactive drugs are also being studied for use in women. In April 2000, the FDA approved a new device for the treatment of arousal problems in women known as Eros-CTD (Urometrics, St. Paul, MN). This is a battery-operated suction device that applies suction to the clitoris and improves sensation, lubrication, and orgasmic capacity. The erectile tissue of the clitoris has recently been found to be more extensive than previously described in anatomy books, through research by a Australian group who performed a series of cadaver dissections on women at various ages (38).

Treatment for Psychogenic Causes of Arousal Disorder

The strategy for management of psychologically based sexual arousal disorders in both sexes depends on whether the patient has had the dysfunction for a sustained period or whether the dysfunction has appeared recently and there is a history of competent sexual functioning. As discussed earlier, transient inhibition of sexual excitement is often secondary to stressful life situations or marital discord (adjustment disorders). These clinical situations often respond to brief counseling. The elements of counseling are similar to those described in the previous example of the couple with sexual desire disorders. The role of the therapist is to help the couple recognize the effect of the stress on their relationship as well as the effect of their feelings (often anger) on their ability to relate sexually. Encouragement of collaborative contingency planning for resolving problems reduces anxiety and anger, often helping the couple to return to their baseline level of sexual function. The same principles and steps are applicable to an individual patient.

When spectatoring (described previously) is a major factor and does not remit after open discussion, referral to a professional skilled in sex therapy usually brings excellent results. Sensate focus therapy, first developed by Masters and Johnson, combines cognitive and behavioral techniques to replace spectatoring with appropriate sexual focus and behavior.

The following factors favor a *good prognosis* after treatment for psychogenic impotence: history of adequate prior sexual functioning, acute versus insidious onset, short duration of sexual impairment, stable social situation, motivation for treatment, presence of sexual desire, partner willing to participate in treatment, absence of severe marital conflicts, and absence of significant concurrent psychopathy.

Even in patients for whom excellent function can be expected, return to normal sexual arousal may be impaired by worry and hesitation. This is especially true when impaired arousal has been present for more than a few weeks, which is often the case. Such patients may be invited to discuss this situation freely and given permission and encouragement to experiment with their partner in one or more ways (e.g., masturbation, erotic pictures or movies, new techniques) in order to test or promote their sexual functions. Of course, such advice should be consistent with the patient's personal beliefs.

Patients who have experienced a sexual arousal disorder over a long period or have never functioned competently may be given a trial of short-term counseling (see Chapter 20). If the counseling does not result in reasonable improvement, referral for more expert help should be considered.

Orgasm Disorders

In the NHSLS, 61% of women in the 18- to 24-year-old age group reported being usually or always orgasmic during sex, as opposed to 78% of women in the 40- to 49-year-old age group. The study also found that only 29% of women overall reported always having an orgasm during sex, but that 40% of women reported feeling extremely physically pleased and 39% reported feeling extremely emotionally satisfied (3).

Approximately one third of men may experience premature ejaculation; fewer than 5% have anorgasmic disorders, unless they are taking medications (e.g., see Antidepressant-Related Side Effects).

Diagnostic Classification

Orgasm disorders caused by medical conditions or medications should be diagnosed as symptoms associated with the responsible conditions or medications (Tables 6.1 through 6.4). Psychogenic disorders have been classified as follows in DSM-IV (2).

Female Orgasmic Disorder

A. Persistent or recurrent delay in or absence of orgasm following a normal sexual arousal phase. Women exhibit wide variability in the type and intensity of stimulation that triggers orgasm. The diagnosis of female orgasmic disorder should be based on the clinician's judgment that the woman's orgasmic capacity is less than would be reasonable for her age, her sexual experience, and the adequacy of sexual stimulation she receives.
B. The disturbance causes marked distress or interpersonal difficulty.
C. The orgasmic disorder is not better accounted for by another axis I disorder (except another sexual dysfunction) and is not caused exclusively by the direct physiologic effects of a substance (e.g., a drug of abuse, a medication) or a general medical condition.

Male Orgasmic Disorder

A. Persistent or recurrent delay in or absence of orgasm following a normal sexual excitement phase during sexual activity that the clinician, taking into account the person's age, judges to be adequate in focus, intensity, and duration.
B. The disturbance causes marked distress or interpersonal difficulty.
C. The orgasmic disorder is not better accounted for by another axis I disorder (except another sexual dysfunction) and is not caused exclusively by the direct physiologic effects of a substance (e.g., a drug of abuse, a medication) or a general medical condition.

Premature Ejaculation

A. Persistent or recurrent ejaculation with minimal sexual stimulation before, upon, or shortly after penetration and before the person wishes it. The clinician must take into account factors that affect duration of the arousal phase, such as age, novelty of the sexual partner or situation, and recent frequency of sexual activity.
B. The disturbance causes marked distress or interpersonal difficulty.
C. The premature ejaculation is not caused exclusively by the direct effects of a substance (e.g., withdrawal from opioids).

Assessment

The organic conditions that affect orgasm comprise for the most part neurologic disorders, drugs that affect the autonomic system, and surgical or traumatic interruptions of the involved neural pathways (Tables 6.1 through 6.4). History taking and physical examination should focus on these possibilities. In women, diabetic autonomic neuropathy is probably the most common organic cause of orgasm disorders, although certainly other neurologic diseases have sexual effects in women (11). Men who are experiencing retrograde ejaculation often state that they have lost their ability to have orgasms. If the history reveals that the patient has the subjective sensations of orgasm but has no ejaculate, and he is not taking a drug that can cause retrograde ejaculation (Table 6.4), the patient should have a urologic evaluation of the function of the internal sphincter of the bladder.

Psychogenic anorgasmia in men is a rare disorder associated with personality disturbances. Obsessive-compulsive, avoidant and, infrequently, sadomasochistic traits are seen in men with psychogenic anorgasmia. It is common that the anorgasmia is restricted to penile-vagina intercourse while other forms of sexual stimulation (e.g., masturbation) produce orgasm.

Premature ejaculation is the most common male orgasmic disorder. Its prevalence may indicate that rapid ejaculation is merely an extreme of the normal distribution of ejaculatory time. However that may be, it is a condition that disrupts greatly the sexual satisfaction of the couple. The psychological assessment of this dysfunction should begin with a clear description of the behavior. Whereas some men recognize that orgasm regularly occurs too soon for their partner to enjoy intercourse fully, others do not; therefore, both partners should be interviewed in order to make the diagnosis. Typically, the couple report that the male experiences orgasm as he is attempting to penetrate, just after he has penetrated, or within several thrusts after penetration.

Men usually have had the dysfunction since they became sexually active. Although occasionally patients report a recent onset of premature ejaculation, these men have invariably experienced this disorder for a sustained period in the past. Another variation is the patient who reports good control with a girlfriend but premature ejaculation with his spouse.

There is no particular personality structure associated with premature ejaculation, although the man who presents clinically with this condition often is an individual who has very high energy or who is anxious and avoidant. One should not presume causal direction in personality features and premature ejaculation; however, the personality features are important in the management of treatment. Some men who are sufficiently frustrated by the disorder may develop a sexual arousal disorder secondarily.

Psychologically caused orgasm disorder is a common problem in women. Studies estimate that up to one quarter of the female population have orgasm problems, and 30% to 50% of all women are occasionally anorgasmic with intercourse. Assessment should focus on the duration of the problem, a history of sexual functioning, the status of the relationship with the spouse or partner, and the presence of a stressful situation. A history of recent onset, competent past functioning, and identifiable precipitating stresses predicts a good response to treatment. Patients who have been anorgasmic for many years and are seeking help because of a change in their relationship or life situations are more difficult to treat.

Some women complain of anorgasmia but evaluation reveals that the patient is actually experiencing a sexual arousal disorder. Because treatment may differ for these disorders, clarification of the phase in which the dysfunction is operating may be important.

Treatment for Orgasm Disorders

Antidepressant-Related Side Effects. Sexual dysfunction caused by treatment with a selective serotonin reuptake inhibitor (SSRI) antidepressant is a frequent complaint. Decreased libido and orgasmic dysfunction are the most common problems, but erectile and arousal difficulties are also reported. The incidence ranges from about 35% to 75% of patients treated. SSRIs probably impair sexual function because of a blockade of the 5-hydroxytryptamine$_2$ (5-HT$_2$) receptor, which is believed to inhibit dopaminergic function in the areas of the brain that are involved with sexual function. Peripheral mechanisms have also been postulated, such as effects on cholinergic receptors or on nitric oxide (39).

In a review article by Zajecka, the common strategies for dealing with antidepressant-related sexual dysfunction were evaluated (40). Gradual reduction of the dose of the SSRI may be helpful, but the patient must be observed closely for the re-emergence of depressive symptoms. Some clinicians wait for tolerance to develop, but only 19% of patients reported any improvement over 4 to 6 months (39). Skipping doses of the antidepressant for 48 hours was helpful in improving sexual function for 50% of patients on the shorter-acting SSRIs such as sertraline or paroxetine (41). Patients at risk for noncompliance should not be encouraged to try this strategy. Many agents have been used as antidotes for sexual dysfunction, but little well-controlled research has been done, and most recommendations are based on case reports or observational studies (Table 6.9). One placebo-controlled trial found that 59% of patients receiving buspirone augmentation had improved sexual function, as opposed

Table 6.9. Antidotes for Selective Serotonin-Reuptake Inhibitor–Related Sexual Dysfunction

Drug	Trade Name	Usual Dose	Available Strengths	Comments
Cyproheptadine	Periactin	4–12 mg q.h.s.	4 mg	Sedating antihistamine
Amantadine	Symmetrel	100 mg b.i.d.	100 mg	Dopaminergic; caution with patients with psychosis
Methylphenidate	Ritalin	5–40 mg/d	5, 10, 20, 20 SR	May also be used prn; abuse potential
Bethanecol	Urecholine	10–50 mg p.r.n.	5, 10, 25, 50 mg	Cholinergic
Granisitron	Kytril	1 mg p.r.n.	1 mg	5-HT$_3$ antagonist
Yohimbine	Yocon Yohimex	5.4 mg t.i.d.	5.4 mg	Can be anxiogenic; α2-adrenergic antagonist
Sildenifil	Viagra	25–100 mg p.r.n. 0.5–4 hr before intercourse	25, 50, 100 mg	Contraindicated with nitrates
Ginkgo biloba	No FDA approved products	40–80 mg t.i.d.	Active ingredient varies with brand	Can increase clotting time, flatulence
Buspirone	Buspar	7.5–30 mg b.i.d.	5, 10, 15, 30 mg	May potentiate antidepressant efficacy
Buproprion	Wellbutrin	75–150 mg q.d. or b.i.d.	75, 100 mg IR; 100, 150 mg SR	May potentiate antidepressant efficacy
Nefazadone	Serzone	50–100 mg/d	50, 100, 150, 200, 250 mg	Blocks 5-HT$_2$ postsynaptic receptor
Mirtazapine	Remeron	15–45 mg/d	15, 30, 45 mg	Blocks 5-HT$_2$ postsynaptic receptor

to 30% of patients receiving placebo, but another study found no difference in improvement in patients augmented with buspirone, amantadine, or placebo (42). Another strategy is to switch the patient to an antidepressant that does not block reuptake at the 5-HT_2 receptor, such as nefazodone, buproprion, or mirtazapine.

Antidepressant-related sexual dysfunction is frequently a difficult problem and can lead to early discontinuation of antidepressant therapy. Because there are potential problems associated with all of the strategies mentioned, the best approach may be to choose an antidepressant that is less likely to cause sexual dysfunction in patients for whom this is an important concern (see Chapter 24). It is critical, when initiating antidepressant therapy, to assess baseline sexual functioning and to consider the potential impact of sexual dysfunction on that patient's recovery. If the patient is warned about the possibility of sexual dysfunction when started on an SSRI, it may be easier for the patient to bring it up if it does occur.

Treatment of Orgasmic Disorders in Men. Men rarely experience loss of orgasmic capacity because of organic factors while retaining the capacity for erection. In fact, it is more common for men to lose their potency while retaining the capacity for emission and some of the subjective sensations associated with orgasm. Most of the physical conditions, diseases, and drugs listed in Tables 6.1, 6.2, and 6.4 affect the capacity for erection before orgasmic function is impaired. There may be isolated instances of side effects of drugs in which men report loss of ability to experience orgasm but retained capacity for erection. In these instances, it is important to distinguish retrograde ejaculation from anorgasmia. Retrograde ejaculation can occur with some drugs, including thioridazine (Mellaril) and guanethidine (Ismelin), while the other components of orgasm remain intact.

Men with psychogenic orgasmic disorder (in contrast to premature ejaculation) usually have longstanding disorders requiring expert sexual or psychotherapy to effect improvement.

There are several *behavioral methods of treatment for premature ejaculation.* The key to helping the man with premature ejaculation is to teach him to become aware of his progression through the HSR cycle and then, with his partner, to practice one of two control techniques. Patients without regular partners cannot readily use this behavioral method. The techniques are the squeeze technique and the stop-and-go technique. The squeeze technique requires the partner to place her thumb and first two fingers around the coronal ridge of the penis and press firmly for 10 seconds. The pressure results in a 10% to 25% loss of erection and a decrease in the subjective sense of arousal. The technique teaches the couple a method of control that can be practiced well before the patient reaches high levels of sexual arousal. The stop-and-go method accomplishes the same result by discontinuing all forms of stimulation. The patient and his partner alternately stimulate and practice control with these techniques until they are confident of their ability to exercise control. At this point they progress to coitus, interrupting the experience as necessary with the squeeze or stop-and-go technique (43,44).

Somatic treatments of premature ejaculation encompass efforts to reduce sensory input to the penis, prevent penile detumescence after ejaculation, and suppress apparent ejaculatory reflex mechanisms. Topical anesthetics ideally serve to attenuate genital sensory input, reducing the likelihood of triggering the ejaculatory reflex. Creams containing prilocaine–lidocaine or other local anesthetics, applied at the time of sexual activity, have shown some efficacy and offer a role, particularly given their simplicity and low cost. Pharmacostimulation of erection (e.g., intracavernosal pharmacotherapy) enables a prolonged erection even after ejaculation has occurred but does not really delay ejaculation *per se* (see Table 6.8). Oral retardants of ejaculation constitute the most common pharmacologic approach. Most of the currently used medications are centrally acting antidepressant drugs that may delay or inhibit ejaculation (see earlier discussion). In particular, SSRIs (e.g., fluoxetine, paroxetine, sertraline) are used as well-tolerated agents with a low incidence of anticholinergic side effects.

Somatic Treatment of Emission and Ejaculation Disorders. The ejaculatory disorder in which there is failure of ejaculation is referred to as "anejaculation." The classic case of anejaculation associated with disruption of the sympathetic nerve supply to the accessory male reproductive tract structures actually represents a failure of emission rather than ejaculation, and patients may experience orgasm because the somatic innervation of the striated musculature of the pelvic floor remains intact (45). Accordingly, remaining somatic and central neuroregulatory interactions remain intact.

Causes of sympathetic denervation include surgical lumbar sympathectomy occurring as a complication of retroperitoneal lymph node dissection for malignant disease, radical extirpative surgery of the pelvis, and even nonsurgical causes such as diabetes mellitus and pharmacologic therapies that interfere with the neurotransmission of the sympathetic nervous system (45).

Treatment of anejaculation, implying failure of emission, is indicated to restore fertility. Adrenergic receptor agonists (e.g., ephedrine sulphate, pseudoephedrine hydrochloride, phenylpropanolamine hydrochloride, imipramine hydrochloride) have been explored for this purpose. However, their variable success and limitations from their sympathomimetic side effects, including dizziness, weakness, nausea, and sweating, have relegated these treatments to a lesser role at this time (46). Electroejaculation and other assisted reproductive techniques are currently applied to an increasing degree (46). Penile vibratory stimulation also has been described as a technique to treat idiopathic orgasmic dysfunction (26,47).

Pharmacologic therapy that interferes with perceived central neurotransmission of ejaculation and the orgasmic response (e.g., SSRIs) dictates other approaches for management, as discussed previously.

Treatment of Orgasmic Disorders in Women. As with biogenic arousal disorder, the somatic treatment of biogenic orgasmic disorder in women follows the three-fold goals of stabilizing the disease process, reversing medication side effects, and improving the genital environment (11). In patients with known neuronal damage, including diabetic neuropathy, when maximum sexual response has been attained in therapy and mindful of the premorbid level of functioning, the goal of therapy should be to help the patient adjust to the permanent loss or decrease of sexual responsiveness. This can be done by assisting the patient to value the role of sensual pleasuring, as distinct from sexual pleasuring that has as its single goal intercourse and orgasm.

Transient forms of anorgasmia caused by psychogenic factors are amenable to treatment with counseling. A history of previous orgasmic response is a good prognostic indicator. The block in orgasmic response is often caused by the process of spectatoring, described earlier. The interfering process is usually secondary to stressful life situations or marital discord. Counseling for married women and others who have a regular sexual partner should include the partner, provided that this is agreeable to the patient. Counseling should be aimed primarily at resolving the dominant problems, which are usually life stresses or interpersonal strife. With the single patient, counseling should be directed at helping the patient suppress or remove the psychological events (i.e., spectatoring) that are occurring at a critical time, when the patient has reached a high plateau level of excitement and is prepared for orgasmic release. The interfering psychological events may be removed by having the patient focus to the best of her ability on the physical stimuli that she is experiencing during the excitement phase.

Women with anorgasmia of long duration can be given a trial of counseling. If counseling does not result in substantial improvement, referral for additional evaluation and treatment should be made.

Directed Masturbation. Orgasmic difficulty in women can be regarded as a skill deficit, and books are available that give women instructions on how to learn to have an orgasm, using masturbation or a vibrator, and then to "bridge" this ability to coitus with a partner. This method is described well in two commonly used books, which can be recommended to patients (48,49). Success rates reported with this method are high; in one study, 95% of patients were able to achieve orgasm through masturbation, 85% with the direct stimulation of a sexual partner, and 40% with penile-vaginal intercourse (50).

Sexual Pain Disorders

Diagnostic Classification

The diagnosis of psychogenic dyspareunia should be made only after all physical causes have been ruled out (Tables 6.2 and 6.3). The DSM-IV diagnostic criteria for sexual pain disorder are listed as follows (2):

Dyspareunia

A. Recurrent or persistent genital pain associated with sexual intercourse in either a male or a female.
B. The disturbance causes marked distress or interpersonal difficulty.
C. The disturbance is not caused exclusively by vaginismus or lack of lubrication, is not better accounted for by another axis I disorder (except another sexual dysfunction), and is not caused exclusively by the direct physiologic effects of a substance (e.g., a drug of abuse, a medication) or a general medical condition.

Vaginismus

A. Recurrent or persistent involuntary spasm of the musculature of the outer third of the vagina that interferes with sexual intercourse.
B. The disturbance causes marked distress or interpersonal difficulty.
C. The disturbance is not better accounted for by another axis I disorder (e.g., somatization disorder) and is not caused exclusively by the direct effects of a general medical condition.

Assessment

The common causes of genital pain during intercourse (dyspareunia) are listed in Tables 6.2 and 6.3. In both sexes, the complaint of discomfort or pain during intercourse requires a careful history, physical examination, and laboratory testing. The most common causes are infections or atrophic vaginitis in women, and urethral or prostatic infection in men. Psychogenic dyspareunia is uncommon, and this diagnosis should be made only after organic causes have been excluded.

Female Sexual Pain Disorders

Dyspareunia. Pain with vaginal intercourse is characterized as introital, vaginal, or deep (pelvic pain with penile thrusting). Deep dyspareunia can be caused by many types of pelvic pathology or by insufficient arousal. Women frequently recognize the lack of lubrication with insufficient arousal, and may use a lubricant, but are unaware of the vaginal changes that accompany arousal. As a result of adequate arousal, there is ballooning in the apex of the vagina and elevation of the uterus. If this does not occur, the penis may hit the cervix, or the back of the uterine fundus if the uterus is retroverted, and cause pain. In addition, engorgement of erectile tissue in the distal part of the vagina may improve the rigidity of the vagina to facilitate penetration. It is important, when recommending a vaginal lubricant, to caution women and their partners not to abbreviate the arousal phase, because lubrication often is not enough to prevent pain with coitus. The experience of pain can then lead to the expectation of pain, which causes muscle tension and less arousal, creating a painful cycle.

Introital dyspareunia is quite common, with prevalence rates as high as 15% of women presenting to a gynecologist's office. The pain may be from tenderness in the introitus, from muscle tension in the pelvic floor, or from a combination of these conditions. When there is introital tenderness, a careful examination should be done to look for vaginal infections or dermatologic conditions. A common cause of vulvar irritation is excessive washing or irritant reactions from the perfumes or antibacterial agents in soaps. Some women have a hypersensitivity to *Candida albicans* or to some element that is present in bacterial vaginosis. Dermatologic conditions that affect vulvar tissue can be subtle, so any skin changes may need to be biopsied for an accurate diagnosis.

Vulvodynia. Vulvodynia is defined as "severe pain on vestibular touch or attempted vaginal entry, tenderness to pressure located within the vulvar vestibule, and physical findings confined to vestibular erythema of various degrees" (51). There are many theories on the etiology of this disorder, but the most accepted theory currently is that most of these cases involve neurologically mediated pain. An older theory was that there was inflammation in the minor vestibular glands, but histologic studies have revealed inflammation only around the vestibular glands. Many patients identify a history of frequent candidal infections, laser treatment for condyloma, or other injury that preceded the onset of pain. Tissue injury causes the release of inflammatory neuropeptides, and nociceptors in the region become sensitized, causing hyperesthesia or allodynia in the area.

Vulvodynia is very similar to neuropathic pain syndromes that occur in other areas in the body, such as reflex sympathetic dystrophy. The vulva may be especially prone to this type of pain because of the density or the type of nerve endings in this area. It is not known why some individuals develop chronic pain from tissue injury and others do not, but the pain often begins during times of stress, so it is possible that hypothalamo-pituitary-adrenocortical axis disruptions may contribute to the process. Genetic factors probably also play a role.

The muscles of the pelvic floor frequently play an important role in the perpetuation of pain in vulvodynia. Muscle splinting begins as a response to localized pain but then becomes chronic. Physical therapists with experience in pelvic floor evaluation and therapy can be invaluable in the treatment of vulvodynia and should be consulted whenever there is tenderness in the muscles around the vagina. In one study, improved muscle strength from biofeedback was highly effective for patients with vulvodynia, resulted in lower resting pressure, decreased muscle instability, and an 83% decrease in subjective pain (52).

Patients with vulvodynia typically see multiple providers before being accurately diagnosed, and they are often highly distressed or depressed at presentation. Studies have consistently found that these women do not differ from controls in underlying psychopathology or incidence of sexual abuse (53,54). Patients who attribute their disorder to psychological causes actually experience higher levels of pain than those who attribute their disorder to physical causes (55). Most vulvodynia patients are Caucasian, and they have higher rates of allergies and skin sensitivities. Almost half of these patients have other comorbid conditions, such as interstitial cystitis, irritable bowel syndrome, fibromyalgia, or migraine headaches.

In the early stages of vulvodynia, patients often continue to have intercourse despite the discomfort. Arousal becomes difficult because of anxiety and pain, and this contributes further to the pain. Women should be counseled not to ignore their own needs, and they may need help in explaining the problem to their partners. As the pain becomes more severe, many women are unable to participate in coitus at all. Mental health counseling should be used early in the treatment process, if possible, to help patients identify maladaptive behaviors and to help the couple cope with the problem.

Treatment of this condition is aimed at breaking the cycle of pain, inflammation, sensitization, muscle tension, and maladaptive behaviors. The level of tenderness around the introitus can be assessed at each visit by touching a cotton-tipped swab to various locations around the vulva and recording the patient's rating of the level of pain. Any potential causes for vulvar irritation should be eliminated and then reassessed periodically during treatment. A short course of a topical steroid is often helpful, but the patient must be watched carefully for rebound dermatitis. Topical applications of estrogen creams or a 5% to 10% lidocaine preparation in a bland cream are also frequently used. Some patients benefit from discontinuing oral contraceptives or from changing to a more estrogenic pill formulation.

The medications that are used to treat neuropathic pain in other areas of the body are used to treat vulvodynia as well (e.g., tricyclic antidepressants, anticonvulsants) (see Chapter 92). These patients are often very somatically focused, so they are quite sensitive to the side effects of medication, which can be minimized by starting with a low dose and increasing slowly. It is important to explain to the patient that these drugs are used for their effects on the pain pathways rather than for depression.

Finally, the patient can be referred to a gynecologist for a surgical procedure, such as a perineoplasty, if more conservative techniques are ineffective. Most patients prefer to avoid an invasive procedure, if possible, but success rates of about 85% are reported for surgical treatments (56).

Vaginismus. Vaginismus can be difficult to differentiate from vulvodynia, and many women have both conditions. Women with involuntary vaginal muscle contractions often have hyperesthesia at the introitus as well. There are no good estimates of the prevalence of this disorder, and most of the research that has been done has involved clinic populations and has not included control groups. Vaginismus is a difficult disorder to study because women are reluctant to come in for treatment due to fear and shame about the condition. The diagnosis is made by palpating the tightened muscles at the vaginal introitus, but women with the disorder are frequently phobic about having a pelvic examination. Diagnosis is further complicated by the fact that the muscle tightening can be situational, so it may be present during coitus but not with a pelvic examination.

The cause of vaginismus is unknown. Many of the older theories have now been discredited, including unconscious conflicts, extreme religiosity, and history of sexual abuse. Many women with severe vaginismus have satisfactory relationships with their partners, and they frequently have satisfactory sexual relationships with noncoital sex. Many have no orgasmic difficulties. Theories about the etiology of other chronic pain syndromes may provide the best explanations for this disorder; these include central sensitization, catastrophization, and illness attribution (55).

Success rates of 80% to 100% are reported for the treatment of vaginismus in most studies. However, dropout rates are frequently high, and very few studies actually consider coital pleasure after treatment. Success in treatment is highly dependent on the motivation of the woman, and the desire for pregnancy may be a more effective motivator than the desire to function sexually.

Treatment usually begins in the office, so that the patient can be taught to insert vaginal dilators. Silicone vaginal dilators can be purchased or plastic syringes can be used with the needle tips cut off. Relaxation techniques and Kegel exercises are also taught. The patient is then instructed to practice inserting progressively larger dilators at home. The vagina is not actually "dilated" during this process, but rather there is a deconditioning of the vaginal response to penetration. These patients are often very uncomfortable with their vaginas and may need help finding the introitus. They often are reluctant to touch their own vaginas without gloves. Follow-up visits in the office are important to motivate the patient to practice consistently. She should be re-examined periodically for introital tenderness or muscle tenderness, because recovery will necessitate treatment of these problems as well.

Dilation exercises can be done by women themselves, or they can be incorporated into the couple's sexual activity. Both methods are highly effective. Couples are provided with a series of exercises to be performed in the privacy of their home. After a relaxing bath, the couple engages in general body touching, excluding the genitals. Next, they repeat general touching but include the genitals, avoiding any touching that is erotically stimulating. At later sessions, they repeat the touching but add the passage of graded-sized dilators, still avoiding stimulation or efforts to attain orgasm. When dilators have reached the size approximating the size of the penis, then the penis can be substituted as a dilator.

Sexual Disorders Resulting from Medical Conditions or Substance Abuse

There are two additions to the diagnostic nomenclature in the DSM-IV (2) for sexual dysfunction: Sexual Dysfunction due to a General Medical Condition and Substance Induced Sexual Dysfunction (2). As one might expect from the labels, these two diagnostic categories address a somatic etiology of a sexual dysfunction, the former based on findings of direct physiologic effects of a general medical condition, the latter on findings of a causal connection between a sexual dysfunction and substance intoxication or medication use. The DSM-IV sets the following criteria:

Sexual Dysfunction due to . . . (Indicate the General Medical Condition)

A. Clinically significant sexual dysfunction that results in marked distress or interpersonal difficulty predominates in the clinical picture.
B. There is evidence from the history, physical examination, or laboratory findings that the sexual dysfunction is fully explained by the direct physiologic effects of a general medical condition.
C. The disturbance is not better accounted for by another mental disorder (e.g., Major Depressive Disorder).

Substance-Induced Sexual Dysfunction

A. Clinically significant sexual dysfunction that results in marked distress or interpersonal difficulty predominates in the clinical picture.
B. There is evidence from the history, physical examination, or laboratory findings that the sexual dysfunction is fully explained by substance use as manifested by either (1) or (2):
   (1) The symptoms in criterion A developed during, or within 1 month of, substance intoxication.
   (2) Medication use is etiologically related to the disturbance.
C. The disturbance is not better accounted for by a sexual dysfunction that is not substance induced. Evidence that the symptoms are better accounted for by a sexual dysfunction that is not substance induced might include the following: the symptoms precede the onset of the substance use or dependence (or medication use); the symptoms persist for a substantial period of time (e.g., about 1 month) after what would be expected given the type or amount of the substance used or the duration of use; or there is other evidence that suggests the existence of an independent non–substance-induced sexual dysfunction, such as a history or recurrent non–substance-related episodes.

GENDER IDENTITY DISORDERS

The essential feature of the gender identity disorders is cross-gender identification. The hallmark is the desire to be, or the insistence that one is, the opposite gender and significant, persistent distress about one's biologic sex. There are childhood and adult forms of the disorder. Children manifest symptoms by rejecting stereotypical dress, play activities, and behaviors associated with being a "boy" or a "girl." The adoption of cross-gender roles is persistent, and attempts by parents to change the behaviors are met with strong resistance and emotional displays of anger and tearfulness.

Adolescents and adults are generally more circumspect about revealing or expressing their cross-gender identification, at least early in the process of coming to an understanding about their cross-gender desires. The consequences of expressing a cross-gender identification in childhood can be significantly adverse, especially for boys who are teased, physically abused, and ostracized by their peers. Coping with the disorder in adulthood has the potential of being extraordinarily disruptive to relationships, education, and professional/vocational development as the desire for cross-gender living, hormonal/surgical reassignment, and social acceptance in the cross-gender role becomes the central focus of the patient's existence. In the past decade, individuals with gender identity disorder have presented wanting to be a blend of both male and female phenotype, presumably to match the gender-blending identity they strive to assume.

Etiology and Prevalence

No known genetic or biologic predisposing factors have been elucidated as yet. There is limited evidence from studies of families that cross-gender identification in children can be reinforced within the context of the parent–child relationship. Clinical studies of adults continue to reveal no specific pathologic personality features or psychiatric symptom clusters associated with the disorder.

The disorders are rare. European epidemiologic studies reveal that 1 in every 30,000 adult males and 1 in every 100,000 adult females seek treatment for these disorders.

Course

Parents usually seek evaluation when the affected child enters school because the cross-gender identification and behaviors become public. One prospective study (57) found that almost three quarters of the boys with this disorder reported a homosexual or bisexual orientation by adolescence or early adulthood without any signs or symptoms of a gender identity disorder. One or two percent reported a gender identity disorder, and the remainder were heterosexual without evidence of a gender identity disorder. The course for girls is not known.

The course in adults is variable. For some it is chronic and unremitting, with the persistent, dedicated drive for living and functioning in the cross-gender role with or without hormonal and surgical reassignment. The ability to achieve the goal of surgical reassignment is usually more dependent on the intellectual and professional competencies and financial resources of the individual than on the influence of medical decision-making. For the majority of adults, the combination of limited resources and a waxing-and-waning intensity of the desire to live and function in the cross-gender role leads to an on again–off again course.

Complications

The problems associated with the childhood form of the disorder have been noted. Adults who are thwarted in their attempts to achieve cross-gender living may become depressed; some have committed suicide, and males, on rare occasion, have attempted self-castration. The more common problems for adults are the disruption of marriage, social relationships, and vocational function associated with a change in gender role.

Assessment and Treatment

Assessment

For both children and adults, a complete medical and psychiatric evaluation is recommended. No specific laboratory tests are indicated. Adult patients may benefit from a personality assessment, such as the NEO-PI-R (58), more for treatment planning purposes than for diagnosis. The psychiatric or psychological component of the evaluation is best performed by professionals who have experience with patients with gender identity disorders.

Treatment

Children and adults who express dissatisfaction with their gender should be referred to professionals with expertise in these disorders. Therapy with children is family oriented, with the goal of treatment being the reduction or elimination of the cross-gender behaviors. The treatment of adults combines aspects of psychotherapy (for consideration of the decision to pursue reassignment), counseling (logistics of cross-gender living, referred to as "the real life test"), endocrinology management (cross-gender hormone therapy), and surgical management (surgical reassignment). The latter two medical interventions are available when the patient meets criteria, such as those of the Harry Benjamin International Gender Dysphoria Association (www.hbigda.org), which set minimum thresholds for access to services that are more or less accepted by most physicians in the United States. Because relatively few patients have the emotional and financial resources to stick with a reassignment program to the ultimate end point, management of these conditions is similar to long-term management of a chronic disorder.

PARAPHILIAS

The paraphilias are sexual disorders with the following essential features in DSM-IV (2): recurrent, intense sexually arousing fantasies, sexual urges, or behaviors involving nonhuman objects, the suffering or humiliation of oneself and/or one's sexual partner, or children or other nonconsenting persons that occur over a period of at least 6 months.

Exhibitionism

Exhibitionism involves the displaying of one's genitals to a nonconsenting person. Sometimes the individual masturbates during the episode; more commonly he later employs the memory of the episode as a masturbatory stimulus. There usually is no attempt to have contact, sexual or otherwise, with the victim.

Fetishism

Fetishism is the use of objects for sexual arousal. Common fetishistic objects are women's underpants, bras, slips, stockings, shoes, or certain textures such as silk or rubberized material. The person usually masturbates while fondling or smelling the object. Some fetishistic behaviors involve body parts such as feet.

Frotteurism

Frotteurism involves touching or rubbing up against a nonconsenting person, usually in a crowded space. The person attempts to rub his genitals or hand against the breast, genitals, or buttocks of the victim. Orgasmic release usually occurs after the episode, with the fantasy of the experience being the sexual stimulus.

Pedophilia

Pedophilia involves sexual activity with prepubescent children. Individuals diagnosed with pedophilia must be at least 16 years of age, and their victim must be at least 5 years younger. Most individuals diagnosed with pedophilia are male, although there are cases of females who sexually abuse children. In most states, the discovery by health providers of sexual abuse of children mandates reporting to local child protective services.

Sadism and Masochism

Sadism and masochism involve sexual activities during which arousal and gratification depend on either inflicting psychological and/or physical pain (sadism) or experiencing it (masochism). These paraphilias include a broad range of fantasies and behaviors, from awareness of potential cruelty or suffering to extreme physical injury and murder. Aspects of both sadism and masochism are often found in the same person, even though one or the other paraphilia is dominant.

Voyeurism

The essential feature of voyeurism involves the act of observing (peeping) unsuspecting victims disrobing or engaging in sexual activity. Orgasmic releases usually achieved through masturbation during or just after the episode of "peeping."

Transvestitic Fetishism

The focus of this paraphilia involves cross-dressing by males in female attire accompanied by sexual arousal and orgasmic release through masturbation. Middle-age transvestites often experience a decrease or disappearance of sexual arousal and report a "calming" or "anxiety reduction" effect associated with cross-dressing. The paraphilia can be differentiated from the cross-dressing associated with gender identity disorders and from the dramatic displays of homosexual "drag queens," which usually do not result in sexual arousal. The transvestite experience often includes the fantasy that the patient is a woman, with singular focus on specific body parts (e.g., legs, breasts, lips). The term now used to denote these fantasies is "autogynephilia"—loving oneself as a woman (59).

Treatment of Paraphilia and Nonparaphilic Sexual Compulsion

The goal of any therapeutic intervention is ideally the elimination of the paraphilic behavior. Achievement of that goal is difficult because these behaviors are enjoyable or are positively reinforced by sexual gratification, or both. Often the best that can be done is continuous control of the behaviors using pharmacotherapy (antiandrogens) in combination with individual (cognitive/behavioral) psychotherapy and/or group therapy. Reports (60) have indicated that the SSRI antidepressants may be helpful in some cases in combination with individual or group therapy, especially among those with nonparaphilic sexually compulsive behaviors. Based on the concept of paraphilia as similar to a sexual addiction, 12-step treatment programs are available for the control of paraphilias. Although these behaviors were once considered untreatable, combinations of the interventions described have demonstrated that they can be controlled in compliant patients.

SEXUALITY AND SPECIAL POPULATIONS

Homosexuality

General Characteristics

The American Psychiatric Association removed homosexuality from its list of mental disorders in 1973. The diagnostic term Sexual Disorder, Not otherwise Specified may be used for patients who experience persistent and marked distress about their sexual orientation.

The NHSLS population-based study of sexual practices in the United States (3) reported that 2.8% of men and 1.4% of women identified themselves as homosexual or bisexual. These numbers are at variance with Kinsey's historic percentages of 10% male and 5% female self-reported homosexuality. The authors of the more recent study are quick to point out there are no easy answers to questions about the prevalence of homosexuality.

Predisposing Factors

Various attempts to relate homosexuality to abnormal pituitary and sex hormone function have been unsuccessful. The evidence to support the contention that homosexuality is genetically determined is scant.

Many theories about the cause of homosexuality involving psychosocial predisposition have been proposed. However, no studies have clearly demonstrated psychosocial precipitants. At this time, it is prudent to consider a multifactorial model in the genesis of homosexual behaviors.

Development

Most people who accept a homosexual orientation continue that orientation throughout life. Some homosexuals are socially open about their lifestyle; many are covert, largely because of negative attitudes (homophobia) that are common in American communities. Aspects of life as a homosexual that are predictably stressful include the process of discovering one's sexual orientation, disclosure to others (coming out), and the threat of hate crimes.

Psychosocial Consequences

In the past, but possibly to a lesser degree at the present time, the principal risk to homosexual individuals (aside from human immunodeficiency virus infection in men) was the social stigma. More recently, many American communities have enacted or are considering legislation that explicitly protects homosexuals from job, housing, and other discrimination. On the other hand, some jurisdictions and many fundamentalist religious groups support legal and moral discrimination against homosexuality. In most states, but not all, criminal penalties for homosexual acts have been eliminated for consenting adults. The principal legal difficulty currently is for people who are promiscuous and who use public facilities for their sexual activities. Homosexuality is entirely compatible with the development of sustained, affectionate, long-term relationships. A series of recent studies do suggest, however, that young homosexuals are at greater risk for mood disorders, anxiety disorders, substance abuse, and suicidal symptoms including suicide attempts (61–63).

Assessment and Management

Most gay men prefer their personal physician to know of their homosexuality and indicate that they are more satisfied with the care they obtain when their physician is aware of their orientation (64). Studies of lesbians have shown that many are reluctant to disclose their sexual orientation to their physicians because of fear of judgmental attitudes (65). Obviously those who do not disclose at-risk sexual behaviors pose a difficult management problem for the physician.

Homosexual men require special considerations in their routine medical care. Those who have multiple partners should always be asked about their knowledge of safe sex practices (see Chapter 39) and of symptoms of sexually transmitted diseases including human immunodeficiency virus infection (see Chapter 39), and they should be screened periodically for type B hepatitis (Chapter 47), syphilis (chapter 37), and gonorrhea (Chapter 37). Men who practice receptive anal intercourse are subject to both infectious and traumatic anorectal conditions (see Chapter 98).

Most sexually transmitted diseases occur less frequently in *lesbian patients*, with the exception of three forms of vaginitis—candidiasis, trichomoniasis, and nonspecific vaginitis—each of which should be considered when a known lesbian patient has a vaginal discharge (65) (see Chapter 37). It is possible that the risk of breast cancer is increased in lesbians. In the absence of adequate information, cancer-screening recommendations for lesbians should be the same as those for other women according to age group (65) (see Chapter 14).

Assessment of patients who express concerns about homosexual fantasies or experiences should focus on the frequency of the experience, on the patients' decisions to continue with homosexual experiences, and on whether they feel comfortable with those decisions. Patients who ultimately identify with a homosexual orientation and are comfortable with that identity do not present problems. However, patients who are anxious or depressed about their homosexual inclinations may need therapy. Adolescents or adults who anxiously report isolated episodes of homosexual experiences or fantasies may need brief supportive counseling (see Chapter 20).

Elderly Patients

Aging people do not lose their capacity for sexual function on the basis of the aging process alone. It is important to invite questions regarding sexual function in the general care of older patients, because they are often embarrassed to bring up this aspect of their health. Patients who have any of the sexual disorders discussed previously should be evaluated in the same manner as a younger patient. The predictable changes associated with aging are slower arousal phase, increased ability to stay at plateau levels of arousal, and, in men, a longer refractory period. Women commonly experience dyspareunia as a result of atrophic vaginitis after menopause; management of this treatable problem is described in Chapter 101.

Dementia is more often marked by decreased sexual desire than by occasional inappropriate sexual behavior. Partners of demented individuals report that the sexual interaction has lost most of its intimate quality and the partner has become impersonal and mechanical in sexual activity.

With 1.6 million elderly persons residing in 20,000 nursing homes in the United States, there is need of institutional sensitivity to their sexual needs as well as appropriate strategies when sexual behaviors become problematic. A growing body of literature addresses these two seemingly contradictory issues (66).

Children

It is unusual for children to complain of sexual difficulties. However, parents occasionally ask their own physicians questions about the developing sexuality of their children. Parents may express concern about the appearance of sexual behavior in children, such as mutual exploration of playmates' genitalia or masturbation. The parents can be reassured that such behaviors are normal and should be discouraged in a nonpunitive fashion. Failure to control the behavior may require further evaluation of both the child and the family. Sexual behavior that is coercive, inflicts pain, or involves a significant discrepancy in age should receive professional attention (67).

Occasionally, a physician recognizes the presence of *sexual abuse within a family,* either on the basis of physical findings or from information disclosed by a child during a medical visit. If someone outside the family has committed the abuse, both the child and the parents may require supportive counseling to help them vent their fear and anger about the experience. Discovery of sexual abuse within a family should be fully evaluated. This procedure should be initiated by reporting the problem to the division of protective services of the local department of social services. The health care professional should be cognizant of the requirements of the reporting laws within his or her jurisdiction and of the limitations of those laws as they have been interpreted and implemented.

Adolescents

Adolescents with sexual difficulties (see Chapter 11) may be brought to the attention of the physician by either the adolescent or the adolescent's parents. Adolescents who are sexually active may have questions about their sexual function, birth control, venereal disease, or abortion. In most states, a physician may provide services for sex-related problems to an adolescent with or without parental consent.

Adolescents may request consultation about *isolated homosexual experiences* or homosexual fantasies. In most cases, the physician's role is to inform the adolescent that these experiences are not necessarily indicative of the development of lifelong homosexuality but may be expressions of adolescent sexual exploration. Adolescents who have developed a homosexual orientation or who are in the process of doing so may be brought to the physician by parents who are disturbed at the discovery of homosexual activities. In these instances, counseling should be given to the parents to help them accept the adolescent's orientation. Adolescents who are older than 17 years of age are unlikely to change their orientation. Younger adolescents have not yet consolidated their personality development and should be offered referral for psychiatric evaluation and possible treatment.

General References*

Fagan P, Osborne C, Gotlib DA. Sexual disorders information sites on the web—recommended resources. Available at: www3.sympatico.ca/dgotlib/meanstreets.html. Accessed December 2, 2001.

A website of sexual information resources to be found on the Internet.

*Bold print (general references) and bold numerals (specific references) denote published controlled clinical trials, meta-analyses, or consensus-based recommendations.

American Psychiatric Association. **Diagnostic and statistical manual of mental disorders. 4th ed.** Washington, DC: American Psychiatric Association, 1994.

Diagnostic criteria and epidemiologic information for all recognized psychiatric disorders.

Crenshaw L, Goldberg JP. Sexual pharmacology: drugs that affect sexual function. New York: WW Norton, 1996.

The definitive reference about the effects of drugs on sexual function.

Laumann EO, Gagnon JH, Michael RT, et al. The social organization of sexuality: sexual practices in the United States. Chicago: The University of Chicago Press, 1994.

The most comprehensive and best designed study of sexual behaviors of 18- to 59-year-olds in the United States. Excellent resource for sexual data.

Leiblum SR, Rosen RC, eds. Principles and practice of sex therapy. 3rd ed. New York: Guilford Press, 2001.

Comprehensive textbook with topic chapters written by recognized leaders in field.

Masters WH, Johnson VE. Human sexual inadequacy. New York: Little, Brown, 1970.

A classic text that provided the foundation for behavioral sex therapy.

Maurice WL. Sexual medicine in primary care. St. Louis: Mosby, 1999.

A very accessible reference guide for the primary care clinician.

Wincze JP, Carey MP. Sexual dysfunction: a guide for assessment and treatment. 2nd ed. New York: Guilford Press, 2001

Guide to recent psychological and somatic approaches to treatment of sexual dysfunction.

Specific References

1. Basson R. The female sexual response: a different model. J Sex Marital Ther 2000;26:51.
2. American Psychiatric Association. Diagnostic and statistical manual of mental disorders. 4th ed. Washington, DC: American Psychiatric Association, 1994.
3. Laumann EO, Gagnon JH, Michael RT, et al. The social organization of sexuality: sexual practices in the United States. Chicago: The University of Chicago Press, 1994.
4. Ventegodt S. Sex and the quality of life in Denmark. Arch Sex Behav 1998;27:295.
5. Fugl-Meyer AR, Sjogren Fugl-Meyer K. Sexual disabilities, problems, and satisfaction in 18–74 year old Swedes. Scand J Sexol 1999;3:79.
6. Feldman HA, Goldstein I, Hatzichristou DG, et al. Impotence and its medical and psychosocial correlates: results of the Massachusetts Male Aging Study. J Urol 1994;151:54.
7. Fass R, Naliboff B, Fullerton S, et al. Sexual dysfunction in patients with irritable syndrome and non-ulcer dyspepsia. Digestion 1998;59:79.
8. Fagan PJ, Schmidt CW, Wise TN, et al. Sexual dysfunction and dual psychiatric diagnoses. Compr Psychol 1988;29(3):278.
9. Sherwin BB, Gelfand MM. The role of androgen in the maintenance of sexual functioning in oophorectomized women. Psychosom Med 1987;49:397.
10. Shifren JL, Braunstein GD, et al. Transdermal testosterone treatment in women with impaired sexual function after oophorectomy. N Engl J Med 2000;343:682.
11. Yang CC. Female sexual function in neurologic disease. J Sex Res 2000;37:205.
12. Herslag A, Peterson CM. Endocrine disorders. In: Berek JS, Adashi EY, Hillard PA, eds. Novak's gynecology. Baltimore: Williams and Wilkins, 1996:833.
13. Lue TF. Erectile dysfunction. N Engl J Med 2000;342:1802.
14. Masters WH, Johnson VE. Human sexual inadequacy. New York: Little, Brown, 1970.
15. Laan E, Everaerd W. Determinants of female sexual arousal: psychological theory and data. Annu Rev Sex Res 1995;6:32.
16. Goldstein I, Lue TF, Padma-Nathan H, et al. Oral sildenafil in the treatment of erectile dysfunction. N Engl J Med 1998;338:1397.
17. Jarow JP, Burnett AL, Geringer AM. Clinical efficacy of sildenafil

citrate based on etiology and response to prior treatment. J Urology 2001;162:722.

18. Steers WD. Meta-analysis of the efficacy of sildenafil (Viagra™) in the treatment of severe erectile dysfunction [Abstract]. J Urology 1998;159:238.
19. Boolell M, Allen MJ, Ballard SA, et al. Sildenafil: an orally active type 5 cyclic GMP-specific phosphodiesterase in the treatment of penile erectile dysfunction. Int J Impot Res 1996;8:47.
20. Morales A, Gingell C, Collins M, et al. Clinical safety of oral sildenafil citrate (Viagra) in the treatment of erectile dysfunction. Int J Impot Res 2001;10:69.
21. Muller JE, Mittleman A, Maclure M, et al. Triggering myocardial infarction by sexual activity: low absolute risk and prevention by regular physical exertion. Determinants of Myocardial Infarction Onset Study Investigators. JAMA 1996;275:1405.
22. Nehra A, Colreavy F, Khandheria BK, et al. Sildenafil citrate—a selective phosphodiesterase type 5 inhibitor: urologic and cardiovascular implications. World J Urol 2001;19:40.
23. Teloken C, Rohden EL, Sogari P, et al. Therapeutic effects of high dose yohimbine hydrochloride on organic erectile dysfunction. J Urol 1998;159:122.
24. Montague DK, Barada JH, Belker AM, et al. Clinical guidelines panel on erectile dysfunction: summary report on the treatment of organic erectile dysfunction. J Urol 1996;156:2007.
25. Ernst E, Pittler MH. Yohimbine for erectile dysfunction: a systematic review and meta-analysis of randomized clinical trials. J Urol 1998;159:433.
26. Clark JT. Suppression of copulatory behavior in the male rats following central administration of clonidine. Neuropharmacology 1991;30:373.
27. Padma-Nathan H, Hellstrom WJ, Kaiser FE, et al. Treatment of men with erectile dysfunction with transurethral alprostadil. Medicated Urethral System for Erection (MUSE) Study Group. N Engl J Med 1997;336:1.
28. Hellstrom WJ, Bennett AH, Gesundheit N, et al. A double-blind, placebo-controlled evaluation of the erectile response to transurethral alphrostadil. Urology 1996;48:851.
29. Lewis RW. Transurethral alprostadil with MUSE (Medicated Urethral System for Erection) vs intracavernous alprostadil: a comparative study in 103 patients with erectile dysfunction. Int J Impot Res 2001;10:61.
30. Virag R. Intracavernous injection of papaverine for erectile failure. Lancet 1982;2:938.
31. Barada JH, McKimmy RM. Vasoactive pharmacotherapy. In: AH Bennett, ed. Impotence. Philadelphia: WB Saunders, 1994: 229.
32. Sharlip ID. Evaluation and nonsurgical management of erectile dysfunction. Urol Clin North Am 1998;25:647.
33. Witherington R. Vacuum constriction device for management of erectile impotence. J Urol 1989;141:320.
34. Hellstrom WJ, Salvatore FT. Vacuum constriction devices: are they useful? In: TF Lue, ed. World book of impotence. London, UK: Smith-Gordon, 1992:169.
35. Jonas U, Evans C, Krishnamurti S, et al. Surgical treatment and mechanical devices. In: Jardin A, Wagner G, Khoury S, et al., eds. Erectile dysfunction. Plymouth, UK: Health Publication Ltd, 1999:357.
36. Lewis RW. Long-term results of penile prosthetic implants. Urol Clin North Am 1995;22:847.
37. Rhodes JC, Kjerulff KH, Langenberg PW, et al. Hysterectomy and sexual functioning. JAMA 1999;282:1934.
38. O'Connell HE, Huston JM, Anderson CR, et al. Anatomical relationship between urethra and clitoris. J Urol 2001;156:1892.
39. Montejo-Gonzalez AL, Llorca G, Izquierdo JA, et al. SSRI-induced sexual dysfunction: fluoxetine, paroxetine, sertraline, and fluvoxamine in a prospective, multicenter, and descriptive clinical study of 344 patients. J Sex Marital Ther 1997;23:176.
40. Zajecka J. Strategies for the treatment of antidepressant-related sexual dysfunction. J Clin Psychol 2001;62[Suppl 3]:35.
41. Rothschild AJ. Selective serotonin reuptake inhibitor-induced sexual dysfunction: efficacy of a drug holiday. Am J Psychiatry 1995;152:1514.
42. Michelson D, Bancroft J, Targum S, et al. Female sexual dysfunction associated with antidepressant administration: a randomized, placebo-controlled study of pharmacologic intervention. Am J Psychiatry 2000;157:239.
43. Leiblum SR, Rosen RC, eds. Principles and practice of sex therapy. 3rd ed. New York: Guilford Press, 2001.
44. Wincze JP, Carey MP. Sexual dysfunction: a guide for assessment and treatment. 2nd ed. New York: Guilford Press, 2001.
45. Vale J. Ejaculatory dysfunction. BJU Int 2001;83:557.
46. Master VA, Turek PJ. Ejaculatory physiology and dysfunction. Urol Clin North Am 2001;28:363.
47. Mulhall JP, Ahmed A, Valenzuela R, et al. An analysis of the utility of penile vibratory stimulation in restoring orgasmic function in men with idiopathic retarded orgasm [Abstract]. J Urol 2001;165:225.
48. Barbach LG. For yourself: the fulfillment of female sexuality. New York: New American Library, 1991.
49. Heiman J, Lopiccolo J. Becoming orgasmic: a sexual and personal growth program for women. New York: Simon and Schuster, 1988.
50. Lopicollo J, Stock WE. Treatment of sexual dysfunction. J Consult Clin Psychol 1986;54:158.
51. Friederich EG. Therapeutic studies on vulvar vestibulitis. J Reprod Med 1988;33:514.
52. Glazer HI, Rodke G, Swencionis C, et al. The treatment of vulvar vestibulitis syndrome by electromyographic biofeedback of the pelvic floor musculature. J Reprod Med 1995;40:283.
53. Meana M, Binik YM, Khalife S, et al. Biopsychosocial profile of women with dyspareunia. Obstet Gynecol 1997;90:583.
54. Van Lankveld JJ, Weijenborg PT, Ter Kuile MM. Psychological profiles of and sexual function in women with vulvar vestibulitis and their partners. Obstet Gynecol 2001;88:65.
55. Binik YM, Meana M, Berkley K, et al. The sexual pain disorders: is the pain sexual or is the sex painful? Annu Rev Sex Res 1999;10:210.
56. McCormack WM, Spence MR. Evaluation of the surgical treatment of vulvar vestibulitis. Eur J Obstet Gynecol Reprod Biol 1999;86:135.
57. Green R. The "sissy boy syndrome" and the development of homosexuality. New Haven, CT: Yale University Press, 1987.
58. Costa PT, McCrae RR. The NEO-PI-R: professional manual. Odessa, FL: Psychological Assessment Resources, 1992.
59. Blanchard R. The concept of autogynephilia and the typology of male gender dysphoria. J Nerv Ment Dis 1989;177:616.
60. Kafka M. Psychopharmacologic treatments for nonparaphilic compulsive sexual behaviors. CNS Spectrums. *The International Journal of Neuropsychiatric Medicine* 2000; 49.
61. Fergusson DM, Horwood LJ, Beautrais AL. Is sexual orientation related to mental health problems and suicidality in young people? Arch Gen Psychiatry 1999;56:876.
62. Herrell R, Goldberg J, True WR, et al. Sexual orientation and suicidality: a co-twin control study in adult men. Arch Gen Psychiatry 1999;56:867.
63. Sandfort TG, de Graaf R, Bijl RV, et al. Same-sex sexual behavior and psychiatric disorders: findings from the Netherlands Mental Health Survey and Incidence Study (NEMESIS). Arch Gen Psychiatry 2001;58:85.
64. Dardick L, Grady KE. Openness between gay persons and health professionals. Ann Intern Med 1980;93:115.
65. White J, Levinson W. Primary care of lesbian patients. J Gen Intern Med 1993;8:41.
66. Kamel HK. Sexuality in aging: focus on institutionalized elderly. Ann of Long Term Care 2001;9:64.
67. Johnson TC. Assessment of sexual behavior problems in preschool-aged and latency-aged children. Child Adolesc Psychiatr Clin North Am 1993;2:431.
68. Vleit LW, Meyer JK. Erectile dysfunction: Progress in evaluation and treatment. Johns Hopkins Med J 1982;151:246.

C H A P T E R 7

Sleep Disorders

DAVID N. NEUBAUER, MD
PHILIP L. SMITH, M.D.
CHRISTOPHER J. EARLEY, MD, PhD

EPIDEMIOLOGY AND OVERVIEW

In recent years, disorders of sleep and wakefulness have been recognized increasingly as pervasive throughout our society. The magnitude of the public health implications was emphasized in the 1992 report of the National Commission on Sleep Disorders Research (1). It noted that about 40 million Americans have chronic sleep–wake disorders, and that many of those people are undiagnosed and untreated. Furthermore, the report emphasized the vital role of primary care physicians in recognizing, treating, and helping educate the vast majority of those patients experiencing symptoms related to their sleep–wake cycles. Even though sleep-related complaints are common in general medical practice, a 1991 Gallup survey (2) showed that only a small minority of sleep-disturbed people bring their concerns to the attention of their physicians.

The sleep disorders represent a wide spectrum of symptoms. The inability to sleep at the desired time and the inability to remain awake during appropriate hours make up the majority of patient concerns. Abnormal behaviors and movements also may be associated with sleep. The nosology (3) developed by the American Academy of Sleep Medicine in collaboration with other international sleep associations recognizes more than 70 individual sleep disorders, involving intrinsic and extrinsic processes, as well as sleep disturbances associated with other medical and psychiatric illnesses.

Appropriate diagnosis and effective treatment of sleep disorders can result in significant improvement in quality of life for patients. In addition, it may allow a reduction in the tremendous morbidity and mortality associated with excessive sleepiness. An exploration of sleep–wake patterns and possible sleep disorders is an important component of any general review of systems. Sleep disturbances can exacerbate other medical conditions, and, conversely, many medical illnesses and medications can affect sleep patterns.

BASIC SLEEP PHYSIOLOGY

Daytime alertness and nighttime sleepiness are natural drives for most people leading normal lives. The fundamental sleep–wake cycle is maintained by at least two physiologically distinct control processes:

The *homeostatic mechanism* represents the balance between wake and sleep time over several days. This time balance varies greatly with species, but for adult humans is set at about one third sleep and two thirds waking. Sleep deprivation leads to increased sleepiness; however, the relationship is not exactly linear. Many people have had the experience of getting a second wind of alertness the morning after a night without sleep. This phenomenon is caused by the prominent circadian rhythm driving sleepiness and alertness.

The *circadian oscillator* establishes a sleep propensity variation over the normal 24-hour day. This oscillator also modulates core temperature and the activity levels of a large number of physiologic functions (e.g., certain neurotransmitters and hormone levels). Without time cues, especially the day–night, light–dark cycle, this circadian mechanism has a periodicity slightly greater than 24 hours and therefore must be reset daily. Light exposure during the daytime and darkness at night synchronize the rhythm. Neural pathways including the retina, suprachiasmatic nucleus, and pineal gland are well established.

These mechanisms promote the cycle of sleepiness and alertness and usually are in stable harmony. Although homeostatic sleepiness increases throughout the day, circadian alertness peaks in the evening. Under normal circumstances these rhythms allow one to remain alert for 16 hours and then fall asleep rapidly at one's habitual bedtime.

Normal sleep includes two major physiologically distinct states: *rapid eye movement* (REM) sleep and *non–rapid eye movement* (NREM) sleep. Initially, sleep may consist of the four successively deeper stages of NREM sleep. During each of these four stages, there is decreased fluctuation in heart rate, blood pressure, and respiration. This contrasts with REM sleep, where greater lability is noted. The presleep wake stage and the NREM sleep stages have additional distinctive clinical and electroencephalographic (EEG) characteristics.

- Presleep Wake Stage (Sleep Latency Period). As a person begins to fall asleep, eye blinks, limb movements, and moderate tone in skeletal muscles are accompanied by either low-voltage, mixed-frequency EEG signals or the characteristic alpha pattern (basic posterior rhythm).
- Stage 1. This represents light sleep with slow rolling eye movements. The alpha pattern disappears with lower frequency and usually higher voltage than the wake EEG. Sudden limb jerks normally may occur episodically, particularly during early stage 1 sleep.
- Stage 2. Eye movements become infrequent or absent and muscle tone usually is reduced. The EEG shows the stage-defining sleep spindle bursts, vertex sharp waves, K complexes, and some slow waveforms.
- Stages 3 and 4. EEG high-voltage, slow-wave activity predominates. These stages are defined according to the percentage of slow-wave activity present. Muscle tone is variable. Arousal is difficult from these deeper sleep stages.
- Rapid Eye Movement Sleep. At 1 to 2 hours after sleep onset, the first period of REM sleep occurs, with a characteristic marked decrease in muscle tone and bursts of rapid eye movements. During REM sleep there is a paralysis of major skeletal muscles punctuated by occasional episodes of muscle twitches. Hypercapnic and hypoxic respiratory drive are decreased, thermoregulation is decreased, heart rate and blood pressure are extremely variable, and penile erections occur. Dreaming is also most closely related to REM sleep, but it may occur, usually less vividly, at other times.

On a typical night, a subject passes through three to five cycles of NREM and REM sleep. Typical sleep patterns for healthy young adults and elderly people are shown in Fig. 7.1. With aging, there generally is a decrease in slow-wave sleep (stages 3 and 4), with an earlier sleep onset and waking time and more frequent awakenings during the night. The apparently decreased arousal threshold in older people is the most prominent difference between sleep at age 50 and that at age 80. During the day, young adults require 10 to 15 minutes to fall asleep for a nap; older adults fall asleep more easily. As discussed later in this chapter, the recognition and deviations from the normal sleep cycles are helpful at times in establishing the correct diagnosis for a sleep disorder.

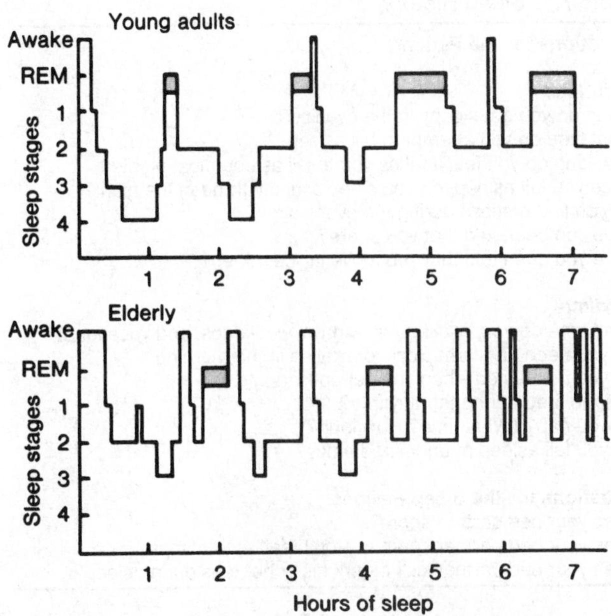

Figure 7.1. Normal sleep cycles in healthy young and elderly subjects.

CLINICAL PRESENTATIONS OF SLEEP DISORDERS

The full evaluation of sleep complaints requires a general consideration of the patient's sleep–wake cycle, as well as specific questions that focus on the presenting symptoms. Table 7.1 lists questions that may yield information that supports a diagnostic hypothesis.

INSOMNIA

Insomnia is the perception of not sleeping well, and it is the most common sleep complaint. It is estimated that 10% to 15% of the adult population in the United States have frequent or chronic difficulty with insomnia. Almost everyone experiences some degree of insomnia during his or her lifetime. People of all ages may experience disrupted sleep; however, there is a general increase in frequency with age. Men and women are affected equally until middle age. From their mid-forties on, women are much more likely to complain of difficulty sleeping (2).

Insomnia may involve difficulty falling asleep, awakening too early, or experiencing disrupted sleep throughout the night. The presentation also may include the report of unrefreshing sleep. Often, the

Table 7.1. Sleep History

Questions for the Patient
Nighttime
When do you get sleepy in the evening?
What time do you attempt to fall asleep?
How long do you feel it takes you to fall asleep most nights?
Once you fall asleep, do you sleep soundly through the night?
Do you feel restless during the evening?
Have you been told that you snore?
Have you been told that you move in your sleep?
Daytime
What time do you awaken (work days, weekends, and vacations)?
Do you need an alarm clock to awaken in the morning?
Do you feel rested when you get up?
Are you tired during the daytime?
Do you nap? (What time? How long?)
Do you fall asleep at undesired times?
Questions for the Sleep Partner
Does your bed partner snore?
Does your bed partner seem to stop breathing at times?
Does your bed partner kick or jerk his or her legs during sleep?

patient complains of fatigue, poor concentration, and low productivity.

In properly diagnosing complaints of poor sleep, it is important to realize that insomnia is a symptom that may result from a wide variety of processes. An important initial consideration is the duration of the disturbance.

Transient insomnia, by definition, lasts a few days and often is associated with a recognizable stimulus, such as anxiety, grief, or anticipation. Changes in the sleep schedule caused by travel or work also can promote brief sleep disturbances.

A sleep disturbance of up to 3 weeks in duration is considered *short-term insomnia.* Again, environmental stressors may be evident, but typically the stimulating factors are more severe, such as the loss of a loved one, loss of a job, or a physical or emotional problem.

Chronic insomnia lasts longer than 3 weeks. An initial precipitant often is recognizable in the history, but other perpetuating factors promote the persistent symptoms (4). Complaints of marked sleep difficulty that have continued for several years are not uncommon. Although the cause of chronic insomnia is often multifactorial, it is useful to consider the individual factors that may be associated with long-standing symptoms (Table 7.2).

Most *psychiatric disorders* can cause disturbed sleep. Symptoms of depression and anxiety often are associated with insomnia and may be precipitating and perpetuating causes. Early morning awakening is a characteristic of major depressive disorder; however, difficulties falling and staying asleep commonly are present as well. Difficulty sleeping is typical of patients with generalized anxiety disorder, posttraumatic stress disorder, panic disorder, schizophrenia, personality disorders, and dementia. Acute sleep changes often are seen with adjustment disorders. Each of these psychiatric disorders is described in detail in Section 2 of this book.

Table 7.2. Causes of Chronic Insomnia

Poor sleep hygiene and behavioral patterns
Circadian rhythm disturbances
Psychiatric disorders
Medical and neurologic illnesses
Sleep disorders (e.g., sleep-disordered breathing)
Medications
Substance abuse
Environmental factors

A broad range of *physical conditions* can cause difficulty sleeping. Pain and discomfort are common factors; however, other pathophysiologic processes may play important contributory roles. The more common medical problems associated with chronic insomnia are arthritic disorders, peptic ulcer disease and gastroesophageal reflux, asthma and chronic obstructive pulmonary disease, cardiovascular disease, hyperthyroidism, and renal failure. Orthopnea and nocturia cause fragmented sleep. Patients with fibromyalgia (see Chapter 74) often complain of unrefreshing sleep. Insomnia is common during normal physiologic stress such as pregnancy, especially during the first and third trimesters.

Among the *neurologic disorders* more commonly associated with insomnia are Parkinson disease and other movement disorders, stroke, epilepsy, and cerebral degenerative processes. Head trauma can cause long-standing sleep disturbance.

Several hundred *medications* can cause insomnia. Stimulants, ranging from caffeine to amphetamines, predictably decrease the ability to sleep. Correspondingly, withdrawal from sedating medications, including hypnotics, can be associated with a temporary sleep disruption. Long-term use of sedatives may cause tolerance and a worsening of insomnia. Bronchodilators, corticosteroids, and some antihypertensives, antiarrhythmics, calcium channel blockers, antiparkinson agents, anticonvulsants, antidepressants, and nonsteroidal anti-inflammatory drugs can cause insomnia. It is important to consider over-the-counter preparations as causes of disrupted sleep, particularly diet and cold or allergy products, because they may contain stimulating compounds such as caffeine or other stimulants.

Substance abuse can promote acute and chronic disturbances of sleep. Cocaine and other stimulants inhibit or fragment sleep. Paradoxically, narcotics such as heroin and morphine can have arousing effects that disturb sleep. The acute sedating effect of alcohol is well known; however, although sleep onset may be enhanced, the withdrawal-related catecholamine release often causes sleep disruption. This may occur after a single episode of moderate drinking. Heavier drinking can impair sleep markedly. Symptoms may persist during months to years of abstinence.

The influence of *circadian rhythms* on the sleep–wake cycle most readily is apparent transiently with acute changes in the sleep schedule. Rapid transmeridian travel causes symptoms of jet lag, and changes in shift-work schedules may promote acutely disturbed sleep. Constantly changing work shifts or permanent night work schedules often inhibit effective entrainment and thereby cause chronic insomnia.

Delayed sleep phase syndrome is a disorder of circadian rhythms characterized by great difficulty attaining sleep until about 3 to 6 a.m. The natural tendency of affected people is to sleep until late morning or into the afternoon. Occupational or educational requirements may demand a more socially acceptable wake-up time that effectively truncates the sleep period and causes chronic sleep insufficiency. These people feel out of synchronization with the rest of society and usually come to the physician because of their inability to fall asleep at a more conventional hour. At the opposite end of the spectrum are people with *advanced sleep phase syndrome*. They may experience sleepiness from 6 p.m. until 2 a.m., then complain of an inability to remain asleep throughout the night. Generally, the delayed pattern is more common among young people, whereas the advanced pattern occurs more often in the elderly. A rare circadian rhythm disturbance occurs in some completely sightless people who are not entrained to a 24-hour cycle. They move in and out of phase with the day–night cycle and therefore have periodic symptoms of insomnia every few weeks.

Symptoms of insomnia may be associated with other sleep disorders in which the primary problems are breathing irregularity or excessive body muscle movements during sleep (see later discussions).

Consideration of the *sleeping environment* is an important component of the evaluation of patients with insomnia. Excessive light or disruptive noise can be arousing. Living near an airport or another source of loud noise may be detrimental to sleep in vulnerable patients. Temperature extremes can disrupt sleep continuity. Discomfort in bed may result from a poor mattress or a snoring bed partner. Household and neighborhood characteristics (e.g., loud televisions, city noises) also may be significant. A sense of insecurity or fear may promote sleeplessness.

Issues related to sleep hygiene (Table 7.3) are important for all patients with insomnia complaints. Even when there is another reason that sleep is disturbed, behavioral patterns that affect sleep commonly play a role in perpetuating the disorder. Irregularity of bedtime and wake time may undermine the underlying circadian drive for sleepiness and alertness at the appropriate hours. Patients may have unrealistic expectations of their ability to change their sleep schedule markedly and then sleep effectively. Some patients nap in the daytime to make up for lost nighttime sleep and thereby further diminish their propensity to fall asleep at the desired hour.

Chronic insomniacs may spend excessive amounts of time in bed in the hope of maximizing their total sleep time, thereby further fragmenting their sleep. Remaining in bed during extended sleepless periods may reinforce the association between being in bed and being awake. Often, frustration and anxiety are integral to this repeated experience and further prolong wakefulness. Subsequently, sleep becomes less attainable.

Table 7.3. Sleep Hygiene Measures

Try to maintain a regular sleep–wake schedule. It is particularly important to get up at about the same time every day.
Avoid afternoon or evening napping if you have difficulty getting to sleep at night.
Allow yourself enough time in bed for adequate sleep duration (e.g., 11 p.m. to 7 a.m.).
Develop a relaxing evening routine for the hours as bedtime approaches.
Spend some idle time reflecting on the day's events before going to bed. Make a list of concerns and how some might be resolved.
Reserve the bed for sleep and sex. Do not do homework, pay bills, or engage in serious domestic discussions in bed.
Avoid evening alcohol.
Avoid caffeine in the afternoon and evening.
Minimize annoying noise, light, or temperature extremes.
Consider a light snack before bedtime.
Exercise regularly, but not late in the evening.
Do not try harder and harder to fall asleep. If you are unable to sleep, do something else out of bed and in another room, if possible.
Avoid smoking.

In *psychophysiologic insomnia*, perpetuating factors predominate after the initial stimulating precipitants have subsided. A conditioned pattern of anxiety and tension has become established. The patient may report increasing tiredness during the evening but tortured wakefulness on getting in bed. Alternatively, what might have been a minor nighttime awakening becomes an exaggerated emotional response that further inhibits a rapid return to sleep.

In summary, the history may identify one or more precipitating or perpetuating conditions that promote chronic insomnia. Practical approaches to the management of these conditions are described later in this chapter (see Management of Sleep Disorders).

EXCESSIVE DAYTIME SLEEPINESS

Clinical Features

Up to 5% of the population have problems with excessive daytime sleepiness (EDS) or related symptoms (Table 7.4). The younger and older age groups tend to experience more EDS than the middle-age group. Also, shift workers complain more of being tired and of various other problems associated with EDS than nonshift workers do. Some people do not perceive that their problems are sleep-related and therefore may not mention being sleepy during the day. The degree or severity of reported sleepiness can be judged by identifying which situations are most likely to produce sleep, by determining how often and how pervasively sleepiness occurs throughout the day, and by learning how disruptive this situation is to family, job, and personal well-being.

In determining the severity of sleepiness, one needs to ask patients under what conditions they are most likely to fall asleep. Table 7.5 sleepiness severity according to the situations in which sleep may occur. If the situations listed are not associated with falling asleep, it is unlikely that EDS is the problem. If patients awaken from sleep feeling tired, further questioning

Table 7.4. Complaints Associated with Excessive Daytime Sleepiness

Sleepiness
Tiredness, fatigue
Poor concentration
Forgetfulness
Decreased motivation
Irritability
Depressed mood
Workplace mistakes
Vehicular accidents or near-accidents

Table 7.5. Sleepiness Severity

Severity	Falls Asleep While
Mild	Watching television
	Reading
	Attending lectures
	Riding in a car
	Sitting in church
Moderate	Socializing with family and friends
	During the working day
	During extended driving
Severe	During local driving or at a stop light
	During conversation
	Eating a meal

about their nighttime sleep habits is needed. Patients' perceptions of sleepiness vary and depend on the environment, level of activity, and degree of motivation. Sitting in a dark room or listening to an uninteresting lecture may unmask sleepiness. Some people may be so busy and active all day that they have no sense of tiredness despite the fact they have not slept in more than 36 hours. As noted in Table 7.4, such people may not complain of being tired but may have problems with concentration or stamina. They may be fatigable or forgetful or have decreased motivation. They may have accidents either on the job or on the highway. Their job performance may suffer. Increased irritability or depression may be noted by family or friends.

Animal and human studies show that with insufficient sleep the EEG identifies brief but frequent disturbances in the ongoing wakeful state. If frequent, these brief intrusions may lead to inattention and poor concentration before sleepiness is perceived. The problems of EDS often are insidious. However, EDS can be identified if the subject is specifically explored by appropriate direct questioning.

Differential Diagnosis

Once it is established that the patient has EDS, the cause must be identified. One first needs to determine whether drugs (e.g., alcohol, benzodiazepines, antidepressants, neuroleptics, antihistamines, some antihypertensive drugs) or medical conditions (e.g., chronic renal failure, cirrhosis, hypothyroidism) might be the cause of the EDS. After considering these causes, one should attempt to identify patients with disturbed nocturnal sleep. Disorders that are likely to cause sleep disruption and therefore EDS were discussed earlier (see Insomnia). Chronic insufficient sleep, chronic fatigue, narcolepsy, and idiopathic hypersomnia are discussed in this section; the sleep apneas are discussed in the next section.

A common cause of transient daytime fatigue is cessation of caffeine consumption (5). The *caffeine withdrawal syndrome* may occur after the discontinuation of even relatively low daily amounts of caffeine, such as 100 mg from one cup of coffee or two to three sodas. Withdrawal effects are more likely at higher doses but can occur after short-term use. The average daily caffeine consumption in adults in the United States is about 250 to 300 mg. Because caffeine use is so widespread, it often is not considered as influencing alertness, sleepiness, and fatigue. The caffeine withdrawal syndrome typically evolves over 12 to 24 hours, and it can persist for several days. It is alleviated by resumed caffeine consumption, even at considerably lower levels. The withdrawal effects can be minimized with a gradual reduction in the daily intake. Aside from fatigue, caffeine withdrawal most typically is associated with headache. Other effects may include irritability, nausea, and flu-like symptoms.

Chronic Insufficient Sleep

The most common cause of EDS is chronic insufficient sleep. The primary problem is that the patients do not have enough sleep to satisfy their body's requirement. The most common causes are personal lifestyles (e.g., shift workers, medical/surgical residents) and poor sleep habits (e.g., watching television until midnight and then getting up for work at 6 am). Such people rarely have problems falling asleep or staying asleep. They may wake up feeling tired and may have symptoms of EDS. A detailed history of the amount of sleep per night over the past several months is important. If someone is getting 7 hours of sleep each a night and is tired, 8 or 9 hours may be needed on a regular basis. Questioning patients about weekend or holiday patterns of sleep, or about how they slept when they were younger or had a different lifestyle, may help determine what the normal amount of sleep is for them. To establish the diagnosis and treat the problem, an 8-hour sleeping pattern must be established. Patients need to *keep a written record* of when they go to sleep (not when they go to bed but when they think they fall asleep) and when they awaken. This should be done for at least 1 month, after which the patient, with the diary in hand, should return for reassessment. If the patient is feeling better after the forced 8-hour sleep schedule, the diagnosis of chronic insufficient sleep is established. If the patient still complains of EDS and the diary indicates 8 or more hours of sleep per night, a referral to a sleep specialist should be offered.

Chronic Fatigue

Psychiatric disorders, especially depression and certain life events (e.g., death of family member, divorce, job loss, marital discord) often are associated with insomnia. Occasionally there is no clear-cut insomnia but only what appears to be symptoms of EDS. The patient may complain of increased fatigue, lack of motivation, poor concentration, or feeling tired all the time. These patients may sleep in the afternoon, but if they consistently sleep for long periods during the day, they invariably will have disturbed sleep at night and thus experience insomnia. The severity of sleepiness (Table 7.5) is important in differentiating fatigue from sleepiness. Although there may be complaints of tiredness, often there are no clear and consistent episodes of falling asleep. More often, the complaints are more severe than the actual degree of reported sleepiness. Finally, when lack of motivation overshadows all other complaints, one should consider chronic fatigue syndrome (see Chapter 58) or depression (see Chapter 24). There is no defined treatment for chronic fatigue other than treating the underlying problem. If a clear distinction between sleepiness and fatigue cannot be made, referral to a sleep specialist is appropriate.

Narcolepsy

The prevalence of narcolepsy in the United States is approximately 0.05% to 0.09%. The disorder may start in childhood, but the peak incidence is in the second decade. The diagnosis is made on clinical grounds; however, a daytime sleep laboratory study (the multiple sleep latency test [MSLT], discussed later) may be valuable when the clinical picture is not clear. Objective support for the diagnosis of narcolepsy is established by an average sleep latency on the MSLT of less than 5 minutes and the presence of two or more naps with REM activity (6). Normal results from this testing include an average sleep latency period of longer than 15 minutes and no REM sleep during these brief daytime naps.

Several clinical features constitute the syndrome of narcolepsy (Table 7.6). The most common of these are problems of attention and concentration and episodes of falling asleep. People with narcolepsy often have little difficulty related to sleepiness when they are physically active. It is when they are engaged in sedentary activities and repetitive or boring tasks that they experience great problems with attention and concentration and uncontrolled bouts of sleepiness. The degree of inattention may be so severe that the individual carries out complex tasks (e.g., driving) and has no recollection of the behaviors. This is referred to as an *automatic behavior*, and is it rarely associated with other disorders. In contrast with individuals who have chronic sleep insufficiency, those with narcolepsy usually benefit greatly from brief naps.

Table 7.6. Clinical Features of Narcolepsy

Altered Levels of Alertness and Attentiveness
Sleepiness
Poor concentration
Memory difficulty
Automatic behavior
Blurred or poorly focused vision

REM-Related Disturbances
Cataplexy
Sleep paralysis
Hypnagogic hallucinations

Sleep Disturbance
Frequent awakenings
Vivid dreams
Sleep terrors

REM, rapid eye movement sleep.

Cataplexy and sleep paralysis are present in some patients with narcolepsy. Both of these conditions are associated with paralysis in the context of full consciousness. Cataplexy occurs when the patient is awake. There is a sudden onset of paralysis that always is precipitated by an acute emotional response. Although fear, anger, and excitement can cause a cataplexy, the most reliable historical indicator is its occurrence during laughter. It can affect any muscle group in the face, trunk, or limbs but is symmetric in its effect. The simplest type of cataplexy is a drop of the jaw, which can affect speech. Cataplexy may make it difficult to hold one's head up for several minutes. Most dramatic are the episodes associated with loss of tone throughout the postural musculature. As the episode evolves, people with cataplexy usually are able to lower themselves to a chair or to the floor, but injury may occur. There is full alertness during these episodes, but occasionally a patient falls asleep during the cataplexy. The cataplexy resolves spontaneously within a few minutes. Sleep paralysis occurs just before falling asleep or just after awakening. The patient cannot move and usually cannot speak, but breathing is not disturbed. There may be a high degree of anxiety or terrifying hallucinations. The paralysis lasts seconds or minutes and resolves spontaneously. Cataplexy occurs only with narcolepsy. Accordingly, a history of cataplexy and excessive daytime sleepiness leads to the diagnosis of narcolepsy. Sleep paralysis may occur alone as an idiopathic condition and therefore does not confirm the presence of narcolepsy. In fact, sleep paralysis is more likely to be seen in patients who are chronically deprived of sleep.

Another cardinal feature of narcolepsy is *hallucinations.* These are vivid and sometimes very realistic sensory experiences that occur before one falls asleep (hypnagogic) or on awakening (hypnopompic). The experiences may be in any sensory modality (e.g., visual, auditory, tactile) and may range from simple to complex in presentation. For example, there may be a sense of something crawling on the legs, a well-formed visual hallucination, or an out-of-body experience. The phenomenon is comparable to dreaming with one's eyes open and being fully alert. Some patients have hypnagogic hallucinations and no other components of the narcolepsy syndrome. This symptom also may exist independently of EDS.

Disturbed nocturnal sleep often is seen with narcolepsy. The most common complaint is that after sleeping for 3 to 4 hours, the patient awakens fully alert. After about 45 to 60 minutes, the patient again becomes tired and falls back to sleep. Sometimes there are multiple awakenings throughout the night. Patients may experience vivid dreams or hallucinations with these awakenings. The vivid dreams can be terrifying and nightmarish in content. The patient starts the day tired and unrested, and this only worsens the underlying daytime problems. The management of narcolepsy is described later (see Management of Sleep Disorders).

Idiopathic Hypersomnia

This syndrome manifests as excessive daytime sleepiness; however, the REM-related clinical features seen with narcolepsy (Table 7.6) are absent in this disorder. The symptoms are similar to those experienced by anyone who has chronic sleep insufficiency; however, these individuals sleep much more. They wake up tired and remain tired. They may be very difficult to arouse and, when awake, may stumble around in a semistuporous state, sometimes called sleep drunkenness. Naps are long and unrefreshing, which is the opposite of what is seen in narcolepsy. Daytime sleep studies (see discussion of the MSLT later in this chapter) demonstrate very short sleep latencies, as is seen with narcolepsy, but there are no REM episodes during these naps. The management of idiopathic hypersomnia is described later (see Management of Sleep Disorders).

SLEEP-DISORDERED BREATHING (SLEEP APNEA)

The sleep apneas are relatively common disorders, with profound potential consequences, which may involve physiologic and psychological functioning. They are characterized by breathing abnormalities that vary from reduction (hypopnea) to complete cessation (apnea) of airflow associated with either an arousal or desaturation in blood oxyhemoglobin, or both. The sleep apneas include central apnea, which is associated with cessation of respiratory effort, and obstructive apnea, which is associated with occlusion of the upper airway and continued respiratory effort. The number of apneas and hypopneas are collated as the number of events per hour of sleep and are reported in various forms, such as the apnea–hypopnea index (AHI), the sleep-disordered breathing (SDB) index, and the respiratory disturbance index (RDI). The assessment of patients with non-apneic snoring is described in Chapter 111.

Epidemiology

A 1993 study of working men and women 30 to 60 years old reported a prevalence of clinically significant SDB of 9% among women and 24% among men (7). The authors estimated that about 2% of the women and 4% of the men met criteria for the sleep apnea syndrome. The prevalence may even be higher among obese people. Because of increased public awareness and the availability of diagnostic facilities, breathing problems during sleep are now being recognized in the very young and very old.

The typical patient who presents with obstructive sleep apnea is a middle-age, mild to moderately obese man. However, it is important to recognize that severe obstructive sleep apnea may be diagnosed in individuals of all ages and body types. Obstructive apneas occasionally are associated with specific abnormalities of the upper airway or with various medical conditions (Table 7.7). In general, patients with medical disorders contributing to the development of obstructive SDB present with relatively overt symptoms and signs of their underlying medical problem. For example, patients with cardiomyopathy present with typical signs of severe congestive heart failure associated with ejection fractions of 30% or less. Patients with renal failure and SDB are usually on dialysis. Patients with the acquired immunodeficiency syndrome also appear to be at increased risk for development of obstructive sleep apnea. There are exceptions to this general rule. Patients with hypothyroidism often go undetected because their complaints of fatigue and sleepiness are ignored. Importantly, even mild obesity (e.g., body mass index [BMI] of 26 to 30) continues to be recognized as a major contributor to the development of sleep apnea. This is especially true with adiposity of the visceral (trunchal) distribution that is frequently seen in patients taking steroids.

In contrast with obstructive sleep apnea, *central sleep apnea* occurs most commonly in infants or patients older than 65 years of age (8). Central apnea may occur as a result of major cerebral disease, brainstem and spinal disorders, or cardiovascular disease (Table 7.7). The Cheyne-Stokes respiratory pattern is one example of central sleep apnea.

Presentation

Characteristically, patients with obstructive SDB present with significant snoring or daytime hypersomnolence, or both (9). The snoring is loud, intermittent, and often punctuated by respiratory efforts unaccompanied by obvious airflow. A *bed partner* may observe that the apneas are associated with a struggling effort (obstructive apnea) or a lack of effort (central apnea).

Table 7.7. Disorders Associated with Sleep-Disordered Breathing

Obstructive sleep apnea
Upper airway abnormalities
Oral (tonsillar hypertrophy, acromegaly)
Bony (micrognathia)
Medical conditions
Obesity
Cardiovascular (congestive heart failure)
Renal failure, dialysis
Acquired immunodeficiency syndrome
Hypothyroidism
Steroid treatment
Central sleep apnea
Cerebral disorder (stroke)
Brainstem-spinal disorder (polio, infarction, neoplasia, surgery)
Congestive heart failure (increased circulation time)

Because apnea, or any form of periodic breathing, usually is associated with both oxyhemoglobin desaturation and a brief arousal, sleep becomes fragmented, leading to daytime sleepiness. Initially, the patient may experience a subtle decrease in alertness toward the end of the day or when engaged in sedentary activities. As the apnea progresses in severity because of weight gain or age, more obvious signs of hypersomnolence, such as napping in the daytime, difficulties driving a car, and even severe sleepiness during normal waking activities, may occur (Table 7.5). Because most patients are unaware of their breathing pattern and often underestimate the severity of daytime hypersomnolence, it is essential that a bed partner or other observer be questioned regarding the patient in whom sleep apnea is suspected. Additional clinical features, such as choking or gasping episodes at night, evidence of systemic or pulmonary hypertension, and, in severe cases, cor pulmonale may also suggest the underlying diagnosis. In general, the presenting symptoms of patients with both obstructive and central apnea are indistinguishable. Patients seldom have pure central or pure obstructive apneas.

The *physical examination* usually is not diagnostic in patients with obstructive apnea, although patients with narrowing of the upper airway are at significantly higher risk. In particular, this disorder should be suspected in children and adults who demonstrate a compatible history and marked tonsillar hypertrophy or retrognathia. The BMI should be calculated and recorded (see Chapter 83), because visual estimation of whether someone is overweight or obese will lead to significant underestimation of the severity of obesity. In elderly patients with central apnea, the physical examination is normal, whereas patients with neurologic or cardiovascular pathology usually demonstrate obvious localizing neurologic signs (e.g., stroke) or cardiomegaly.

Course

The course of obstructive SDB is chronic and progressive because of the typical weight gain seen in a sedentary aging population. Some patients develop progressive cardiopulmonary decompensation manifested by worsening hypercarbia and hypoxemia, which can be associated with cor pulmonale and life-threatening arrhythmias. Nevertheless, these complications are the exception and tend to occur in the more severely obese patients (BMI greater than 40) after many years of disease. By contrast, the course of central apnea is determined by the underlying pathologic process. Therefore, if reversible central nervous system or cardiovascular disease exists, central apnea may resolve entirely. In normal elderly patients with central apnea, the course and prognosis are unknown.

Diagnosis

A working diagnosis of SDB can be made by direct observation of the patient during sleep, either at home or in a general hospital. However, even with ideal observation, clinically significant apnea may not be appreciated. The occurrence of five or more SDB events per hour constitutes an abnormal number of events. Although an SDB rate of more than five events per hour and daytime sleepiness are the minimal criteria that define the sleep apnea syndrome, there is good evidence that the sleepiness is correlated with the severity of the SDB rate and the degree of hypoxemia (10). Definitive diagnosis requires a sleep study (see later discussion) that quantitates the severity of SDB, including the degree of desaturations and the alteration in sleep architecture.

Other laboratory studies, such as determination of arterial blood gases and routine pulmonary function studies, provide information about mechanical abnormalities or problems with waking gas exchange that may be useful in therapy but not in diagnosis. Awake flow-volume curves (see Fig. 60.2 in Chapter 60) may demonstrate fluttering during expiration associated with evidence of variable extrathoracic obstruction in patients with obstructive apnea. However, this test is neither specific nor sensitive; therefore, it is not recommended for screening purposes. Although computed tomography or magnetic resonance imaging may demonstrate narrowing of the upper airway in patients with obstructive sleep apnea, it is unclear at present how this information can best be used in management. The management of SDB is described later (see Management of Sleep Disorders).

RESTLESS LEGS SYNDROME AND PERIODIC LEG MOVEMENTS IN SLEEP

Restless legs syndrome (RLS) is a disorder of sensation of unknown etiology. It occurs in 2% to 5% of the adult population, and in 10% to 15% of individuals 65 years of age or older. The prevalence is increased in conditions of iron deficiency, pregnancy, chronic renal failure, or peripheral neuropathy. It may be induced or aggravated by dopamine antagonists.

RLS is a clinical diagnosis based on the following criteria. First, there is a sensation that usually is characterized as a deep, uncomfortable feeling. This offending sensation occurs in one or both legs, either independently or concomitantly. Occasionally the sensation additionally involves the hands, arms, or trunk. The feeling may be reported as aching, as something moving, as little insects, as crazy legs, or in other ways. The description of the feeling is highly variable but is usually not that of pain. If pain is a prominent component, an alternative or coexisting disorder is suggested, such as a neuropathy. Along with this deep, uneasy feeling is a compulsion or urge to move. The urge to move may be so strong that the legs will seemingly jump on their own. Therefore the patient is constantly moving or rubbing the legs or walking to relieve the sensation. The second feature is that the sensation is brought on with sitting or lying. The third component is that the uncomfortable sensation is relieved with movement and should be absent during walking. The sensation may return as soon as the individual sits or lies down again. The fourth feature is that the sensation is the worst in the late evening or at bedtime. Commonly, it is not present at all during the early morning. However, as the disorder progresses with time, symptoms appear earlier in the daytime, sometimes to the point that RLS symptoms exist throughout the day. Most commonly, the symptoms appear as soon as the person tries to relax in the late evening or gets into bed at night. Because of this sensory disturbance, the affected person cannot rest comfortably. He or she often cannot travel by any means that would limit movement. The patient commonly cannot relax long enough to sit through a movie or to read without having to shuffle or pace compulsively. At night, the sensation prevents sleep. Some patients spend several hours at night pacing, until finally they are exhausted enough to fall asleep.

An associated component of RLS is the presence of semi-involuntary leg movements while awake or semi-rhythmic leg movements during sleep. On observation of the patient during sleep, brief leg and foot movements occurring periodically are evident. They may occur in one or both legs, either independently or simultaneously. These leg movements are called periodic leg movements of sleep (PLMS), and they occur in association with many other conditions (Table 7.8). Occasionally, there is no clear cause for the PLMS and no RLS symptoms. In this situation the condition is referred to as periodic leg movement disorder (PLMD); it is considered to be a variant of RLS and is treated similarly. The major problem created by the periodic leg movements is repeated arousals from sleep. The person usually has no awareness of the arousals but complains of having awakened feeling tired and of being excessively sleepy during the day. Sometimes the leg kicks cause complete awakening several times throughout the night. These patients rarely know that it is the leg movements that are awakening them.

RLS is diagnosed on the basis of the clinical history, whereas PLMS is identified either by the history given by the bed partner or by polysomnographic recording (discussed later). The polysomnographic recording is needed to make the diagnosis of PLMS or PLMD, but not that of RLS. The deep, uneasy feelings of RLS must be differentiated from arthralgia, myalgia, or sensory neuropathy. The absence of frank pain, the history of relief with movement, the compulsion to move, and normal results on neurologic, muscle, and joint examination should help in the differential diagnosis. The presence of an initial sensory component and the voluntary nature of the movements should differentiate the secondary movements of RLS from those of myoclonus or dyskinesia. Nocturnal seizures, sleep-related dystonia, myoclonus, sleep apnea, primary insomnia, and PLMS are part of the differential diagnosis when a patient presents with a history of disturbed sleep associated with movements during sleep. If the clinical history is insufficient to establish the diagnosis, the person should be referred to a sleep disorder clinic. The management of RLS is described later (see Management of Sleep Disorders).

Table 7.8. Causes of Periodic Leg Movements of Sleep

Restless legs syndrome
Sleep-disordered breathing
Antidepressant medications
Aging
Neurodegenerative disorders
Narcolepsy
Idiopathic (PLMD)

ABNORMAL BEHAVIORS EMANATING FROM SLEEP (PARASOMNIAS)

Restful sleep may be punctuated by behaviors that may or may not awaken the patient. These behaviors can range from the benign to the dramatic and may be violent. Several distinct syndromes have been recognized. Factors that can help distinguish the causes include the timing of the behavior, the likelihood of awakening from the episode, the degree of confusion present, and the patient's memory of the events. Sleep laboratory recordings may associate the various types of episodes with different sleep stages. The parasomnias tend to occur in fewer than 10% of the population.

Arousal Disorders

Three types of sleep-related behaviors are classified as arousal disorders (3): sleepwalking, sleep terrors, and confusional arousals. They share an association with *slow-wave sleep* and thereby tend to occur during the first third of the night. The prevalence is greatest in childhood, but the disorders may persist in adulthood. A familial association has been noted in some cases. The frequency of episodes may range from several times per night to less than once a year. Commonly there is *amnesia for the event.* Typically the individual does not awaken spontaneously and is difficult to arouse. The person may become aware of the events because of residual evidence such as relocated furniture or food left out on a table. Resistance to full awakening is characteristic, and marked confusion may be evident. Behaviors may be inappropriate, such as urinating in a closet or searching for nonexistent intruders.

Sleepwalking most commonly is simple, in that the person typically walks around the room or house but rarely goes outside. Generally sleepwalkers do not put themselves or others in a dangerous situation; however, dramatic exceptions have been reported. In some cases, there is an overlap with sleep terror symptoms, in which the person aggressively attempts to escape from, or protect against, an imagined threat.

By definition, *sleep terrors* are dramatic events. Evidence of autonomic discharge may be pronounced. Often, the person sits up and screams loudly and commonly is unarousable. The patient may return to sleep after several minutes and have no recollection of the incident the following morning. People who do awaken report an intense sense of fear. They may describe a distinct threat but generally do not offer a lengthy, dreamlike narrative. The sleep terror may lead to forceful escape behavior, which can cause injury to the patient or to someone else perceived to be an obstacle. Injury may result from leaping out of bed or colliding with furniture. Rarely, people have jumped through windows in an attempt to escape.

Confusional arousals involve persistent disorientation and incomplete awakening after an arousing stimulus that occurs while the person is in slow-wave sleep. Behaviors and speech content may be meaningless or inappropriate. A typical example would be a person responding to a ringing telephone 1 hour after sleep onset. The person may reach for other objects or may make little sense when talking. Amnesia for these episodes is common. Factors promoting deeper sleep increase the likelihood of such incomplete awakening. These may include sleep deprivation and use of sedating substances such as alcohol and central nervous system depressants.

Nightmares

Nightmares usually result in full awakenings and generally are not associated with prolonged confusion or sleep-related behaviors. Typically the patient can recount an extended dream narrative and can describe the frightening aspects of the story. In contrast to arousal disorders, nightmares are most common during REM sleep and tend to occur during the latter part of the night. Nightmares also are more likely to be remembered in the morning.

Dreams may be related to physical activity during sleep in the rare *REM behavior disorder* (3). Normally there is skeletal muscle atonia during REM sleep; however, in this disorder, the active inhibition of motor impulses is incomplete. The dreamer may physically act out dream content. Physical activity may include kicking or punching, and the person may leap from the bed. Violent behaviors causing injury to the patient or to his or her bed partner have been reported. This disorder is more common in elderly persons. Most cases are idiopathic; however, neurologic diseases, toxic and metabolic processes, and medications have been implicated in promoting the symptoms.

In summary, sleep-related behaviors usually can be divided into the slow-wave sleep and REM-associated symptom complexes. *Nocturnal enuresis*, discussed later, is not associated with a particular sleep stage. In rare instances, sleep-related behaviors can be shown to be complex partial seizures (see Chapter 88).

Management of the parasomnias is discussed in the next section.

MANAGEMENT OF SLEEP DISORDERS

Insomnia

A comprehensive sleep history from a patient with insomnia establishes the duration of the symptoms and explores possible predisposing, precipitating, and perpetuating factors. *Multifactorial causes are common* with insomnia. Treatment of the primary cause of the insomnia may be important, but reinforcing factors should also be addressed. Identified medical and psychiatric illnesses must be treated. Attention to sleep hygiene, behavioral programs, relaxation techniques, psychotherapy, environmental manipulations, and the use of hypnotic medications can play important roles in management. The objective of treatment is development by the patient of new behaviors and routines that allow a renewed sense of confidence in the ability to sleep effectively. This is achieved by a therapeutic alliance wherein the patient plays an active role in exploring potential sleep-inhibiting factors. Considerable experimentation may be necessary.

Although the quality of clinical studies has been highly variable, critical reviews of the published literature support the conclusion that both behavioral and pharmacologic approaches reduce the time it takes to fall asleep by 15 to 30 minutes and the number of awakenings by one to three per night (see Kupfer and Reynolds, *Management of Insomnia,* in General References).

Sleep Hygiene Measures

Recommendations about sleep hygiene are beneficial to most patients with insomnia, regardless of the duration of their symptoms (Table 7.3). These basic guidelines address factors that directly cause disturbed sleep and inhibit recovery. They take into account fundamental physiologic and psychological understanding of the sleep process.

It is important to *take full advantage of the underlying circadian rhythm,* described previously, that promotes nighttime sleepiness and daytime alertness. Attempts to sleep at various times throughout the 24-hour cycle may perturb the rhythm. Daytime or evening napping can inhibit the onset of sleep at night. A consistent wake-up time is important because this is when the system is most sensitive to daily reinforcement.

Some people with insomnia spend excessive time in bed (e.g., 9 p.m. to 9 a.m.) in the hope of getting a little more sleep. Generally this is counterproductive. Physiologically there may be less effective support of the circadian pattern. Because continuous sleep is unlikely, the person is creating a situation in which failure is inevitable. Extended wakeful periods may be self-reinforcing. Sleep restriction therapy (see later discussion) is a treatment modality that specifically addresses this problem.

It is useful to consider the extent to which a patient develops *negative associations with the bed and bedtime routines.* Good general advice includes reserving the bed for sleeping and sexual relations. Anxiety-provoking activities performed in bed may promote residual tension when sleep is attempted. Stressful behaviors may include studying for tests, paying bills, having domestic discussions, or watching violent television drama or news programs. These negatively stimulating activities should be replaced with relaxing behaviors.

Some people find significantly improved sleep with the *elimination of stimulants* such as nicotine and caffeine. This especially is true during the hours leading up to bedtime. Late evening alcohol consumption should be avoided because of the potential for stimulation related to withdrawal later in the night.

A *comfortable bedroom environment* is important. Temperature extremes, particularly a warm room, can promote sleep disruption. Outside noises may be blocked out by white noise machines or wax ear plugs. Generally people should not try to fall asleep with the television or radio playing. This tends to inhibit deep sleep and can cause awakenings.

Dietary habits may need to be addressed. Late heavy meals may produce abdominal discomfort or reflux symptoms. On the other hand, hunger may interfere with sleep onset. A light snack may be an appropriate solution.

Regular exercise (see Chapter 16) is recommended to promote improved sleep at night (11). However, aerobic exercises should be avoided in the hours leading up to bedtime to prevent excessive stimulation. For this reason, patients should be warned against trying to wear themselves out at night in the hope of falling asleep quickly.

Behavioral Management

Behavioral approaches are the primary treatment for chronic insomnia.

Relaxation Techniques

Relaxation techniques may have a permissive effect by reducing arousal and thereby allowing sleep onset (4). Relaxation may be achieved through the use of progressive relaxation, meditation, or biofeedback (see Chapter 22). Two other techniques, stimulus control therapy and sleep restriction therapy, involve specific instructions regarding nighttime routines and sleep–wake schedule hours.

Stimulus Control Therapy

Conditioned arousal is an important perpetuating factor in many people with chronic insomnia (12). The goal of stimulus control therapy is to reestablish the connection between the bedroom and sleeping. The fundamental strategy is to eliminate the nightly reinforcement of the anxiety and arousal that have become associated with the act of going to bed or awakening during the night. Basic sleep hygiene measures (Table 7.3) are pointed out as the necessary elements in a stimulus control plan. The purpose of these measures is to minimize the time that the patient is sleepless in bed. Chronic insomniacs often overvalue their time in bed and find the prospect of being out of bed abhorrent. They do not want to miss the opportunity for any potential sleep. The prescription of this technique should be framed positively so that the patient can view the time out of bed as an investment in better future sleep. Considerable discipline in following the guidelines is required for a positive result, but many patients respond very well to this approach.

Sleep Restriction Therapy

The excessive time some chronic insomniacs spend in bed can undermine their recovery. Sleep may occur intermittently over a long period. Maximal reinforcement of the circadian influence is reduced. Sleep restriction therapy (13) attempts to consolidate sleep by limiting time in bed to specific hours. The schedule depends on the patient's perception of total sleep time. For example, patients who report only 5 hours of sleep at night are told that they may be in bed only from 3 a.m. until 8 a.m. As sleep efficiency increases during this restricted time, the bedtime hour gradually is advanced. The wake-up time remains constant to promote regularity in the circadian pattern. The efficacy of this method has been confirmed in at least one clinical trial (14).

Circadian Manipulations

Successful treatment of insomnia may require paying attention to fundamental circadian principles. Transient insomnia secondary to *jet lag* can be minimized with the appropriate timing of activity and bedtime before and after the travel. Generally it is advisable to begin following the day–night pattern of the new time zone as quickly as possible. This allows more rapid entrainment as advantage is taken of external reinforcing stimuli, particularly sunlight. In some cases, problems associated with shift work also can be decreased to a limited extent with strategic manipulation of sleeping hours and light exposure (15).

Basic recommendations include regularity in timing of the sleep–wake cycle to maximize circadian reinforcement. Specific guidelines about bedtime, wake-up time, and bright light exposure are advisable in selected cases. *Delayed sleep phase syndrome* (discussed earlier) may be treated with varying degrees of success by a program of gradually advancing the wake-up time. Exposure to bright light (sunlight or therapeutic light boxes) soon after the wake-up time should help in resetting the underlying circadian clock. Bright light late in the day should be avoided. *Advanced sleep phase syndrome* may be treated with evening bright light exposure and the avoidance of bright light around dawn.

Hypnotic Medications

Hypnotic medications may play a valuable role in the treatment of selected patients. The use of hypnotics should always be part of an integrated approach that includes measures to promote sleep hygiene and psychotherapeutic support. The hypnotics may be used to help the patient during a stressful period and thereby hasten a return to a normal sleep–wake pattern. Hypnotics also may be beneficial in re-establishing a regular sleep cycle after time zone and work schedule shifts. A meta-analysis of clinical trials confirmed the efficacy of benzodiazepines and zolpidem for the short-term treatment of insomnia in adults younger than 65 years of age (16).

All prescription hypnotics share the class labeling indication "for short-term use" (e.g., no more than 3 or 4 weeks), although selected patients may continue to benefit from longer-term use. The hypnotics are helpful mostly for patients with transient and short-term insomnia. The lowest effective dosage should be prescribed for the shortest possible duration. These medications may be used nightly from several days to 3 weeks; however, intermittent use (e.g., 2 to 4 nights per week) should be encouraged for most patients. Rarely is it necessary to recommend a dosage higher than the standard available strengths.

Medications from several classes have been used for their hypnotic effects. The predominant ones have been the barbiturates (secobarbital, amobarbital, and pentobarbital) and related compounds (chloral hydrate, ethchlorvynol, and methyprylon); the benzodiazepines and related compounds (Table 7.9); sedating antidepressant medications (see Chapter 24); and over-the-counter antihistaminic preparations (17).

The *barbiturates* were the mainstay of prescription hypnotic use until the introduction of the benzodiazepines in the 1960s and 1970s. The *benzodiazepines* are much safer (decreased toxicity and potential for lethal overdose, less residual sedation, fewer and less severe withdrawal effects, and reduced potential for abuse and dependence). There is no reason to use barbiturates in the routine management of insomnia. Of the older prescription *nonbenzodiazepine, nonbarbiturate hypnotic agents,* chloral hydrate (500-mg tablet) has the best safety profile, but tolerance and toxicity limit its use.

Sedating antidepressants with minimal anticholinergic action, such as trazodone and nefazodone, and also mirtazapine have been used successfully as hypnotics. They are especially helpful for depressed patients who have markedly disturbed sleep. Some nondepressed patients with insomnia respond well to low dosages of these medications. Characteristics of these drugs are described in Chapter 24.

Table 7.9. Benzodiazepine and Related Hypnotic Medications

Generic Name	Brand Name	Available Strengths and Dosage Ranges (mg)
Shorter-Acting		
Triazolam	Halcion	0.125–0.25
Zaleplon	Sonata	5–10
Zolpidem	Ambien	5–10
Intermediate-Acting		
Estazolam	ProSom	1–2
Lorazepam	Ativan	0.5 to 1–2
Temazepam	Restoril	7.5 to 15–30
Longer-Acting		
Flurazepam	Dalmane	15–30
Quazepam	Doral	7.5–15

There is a confusing array of products now available in the over-the-counter sleep aid market. While some include *antihistaminic agents* (diphenhydramine, hydroxyzine, doxylamine, and pyrilamine), others contain no ingredients with demonstrated sedative characteristics. Among the antihistamine preparations, diphenhydramine is the most common and is present in various pill forms with doses of 25, 38, and 50 mg. Their hypnotic efficacy is limited compared with that of the benzodiazepines. The antihistamines may promote anticholinergic side effects, so they should be used cautiously in elderly individuals and people taking other medications with anticholinergic activity (e.g., some antidepressants). The relatively long antihistamine elimination half-lives commonly promote residual sedation the morning after bedtime use.

Benzodiazepine hypnotics, zolpidem, and zaleplon (positive allosteric modulators of the gamma-aminobutyric acid A receptor complex) are among the most widely prescribed of all medications. All are classified as schedule IV drugs under the federal Controlled Substance Act. Their proper use requires knowledge of their onset and duration of action. All benzodiazepines marketed as hypnotics are rapidly absorbed and therefore have an acceptable onset of action. The duration of action depends on several factors, including volume of distribution, solubility in fat, elimination half-life, and presence of active metabolites. The age of the patient also may be a factor; elderly patients generally have extended elimination periods, as may patients with liver impairment.

The benzodiazepines and related hypnotics can be categorized according to their duration of action (Table 7.9). The advantages and disadvantages of the shorter- and longer-acting medications should be considered in selection of a hypnotic.

Shorter-acting hypnotics (i.e., those of short and intermediate duration) have the advantage of producing minimal *residual daytime sedation.* Excessive daytime sleepiness can be a major problem with longer-acting agents, particularly flurazepam. In addition, impairment of daytime performance and an increased propensity for falls in elderly patients may be associated with the longer-duration hypnotics. On the other hand, the longer-acting medications may be useful when a daytime anxiolytic or sedative effect is desired.

Less common side effects of benzodiazepines include dizziness, headache, and disinhibited or bizarre behaviors. Ataxia, slurred speech, or confusion may be seen at higher dosages. Interdose anxiety and anterograde amnesia have been reported with triazolam in rare cases. Caution is advised in using benzodiazepines for patients with hepatic, renal, or respiratory impairment. Additionally, they should be avoided during pregnancy and lactation. Cumulative effects with other central nervous system depressants always must be considered.

A gradually tapered dosage often is useful when discontinuing a benzodiazepine hypnotic to minimize *withdrawal symptoms.* This helps reduce patient discomfort after extended use of hypnotic agent. Patients may confuse physiologically predictable symptoms of discontinuation insomnia with the belief that they inherently are unable to sleep without the sleeping pill. Patient education is vital to successful treatment. The *longer-acting hypnotics* tend to be associated with less pronounced withdrawal symptoms than are the shorter-duration compounds. An exception may be the reported minimal withdrawal symptoms associated with the short-acting nonbenzodiazepine agents. When withdrawal insomnia is present, it tends to occur earlier with the shorter-acting agents. Withdrawal from longer-acting hypnotics may be delayed for several days after discontinuation. A pronounced *rebound insomnia syndrome* has been reported with sudden discontinuation of triazolam, which has an especially short half-life.

The question of abuse often influences the decision to initiate hypnotic treatment. This issue was examined in a task force report by the American Psychiatric Association (18). It was concluded that most patients who take benzodiazepines do so for limited periods, according to the prescription guidelines. It was noted that benzodiazepine abuse occurs most commonly in patients who are concurrently abusing alcohol and/or other substances (see Chapters 28 and 29). Accordingly, particular caution is recommended with such patients.

In summary, benzodiazepines and related hypnotics can be used effectively in selected patients when they are prescribed as part of an overall treatment plan. The pattern of the patient's sleep disturbance helps guide selection of a hypnotic agent. *Sleep-onset insomnia* may respond well to a short-acting agent. A *sleep continuity problem* may be helped more by a medication of short or intermediate duration.

Narcolepsy and Idiopathic Hypersomnolence

In the management of narcolepsy there are pharmacologic and nonpharmacologic approaches to excessive daytime sleepiness (6). Nonpharmacologic treatments (Table 7.10) should be used by all narcoleptic patients whenever possible. The first of these approaches is *activity*. As long as narcoleptic patients continue some level of physical activity, a reasonable degree of alertness usually can be maintained. Adding exercise to the daily schedule further enhances the alertness. Brief *naps* (10 to 30 minutes), preferably taken on a scheduled basis (e.g., work breaks, lunchtime), are a valuable strategy for maintaining alertness throughout the day. *Caffeinated beverages* may be used for a short and quick pick-me-up, whereas food may attenuate alertness. These various approaches may be used alone or in combination for the best effect. For example, at lunchtime a light meal may be taken or avoided altogether. This may be followed by a brief nap and 30 minutes of mild to moderate activity. A brief nap followed by consumption of a caffeinated beverage may be used just before a conference or just before driving to or from work. In fact, narcoleptic patients should be *instructed about the dangers of driving*. If they feel tired while driving, they should not push themselves but should pull off the road as soon as possible. They can take a brief nap, get out of the car and walk around, or get a cup of coffee. The final concern is *nocturnal sleep*. Extra nighttime sleep has no effect on daytime alertness and sleepiness. However, disturbed sleep at night produces greater problems during the day. Narcoleptic patients need to maintain normal sleep habits when possible. Staying out late at night, working two jobs, doing shift work, or living on 4 or 5 hours of sleep does not work for most people and it definitely does not work for narcoleptic patients.

Table 7.10. Nonpharmacologic Treatment of Narcolepsy

Remain active, when possible
Brief daytime naps (scheduled and/or as needed)
If sleepy, get up, walk around, take a break
Add exercise to the daily routine
Use caffeine beverages as needed
Light meals during the daytime
Avoid sedative medication

The pharmacologic treatment of daytime sleepiness and diminished alertness involves the use of *stimulant medication* (Table 7.11). Attempts to completely normalize a patient with narcolepsy are fraught with many problems, often leading to marked frustration and frequent failure. It is important to identify specific difficulties for targeted use of stimulants (e.g., falling asleep while driving or during meetings, inability to concentrate while at work or during the afternoon). The patient should understand that the ideal of full alertness throughout a 16-hour waking period should not be the ultimate goal of the medication management. Specific times and activities for maximum alertness should be planned. Both pharmacologic and nonpharmacologic treatment must be structured to suit the problems that have been identified. The same amount of medication does not need to be given every day or at the same time each day. Drug holidays on weekends with amphetamine and methylphenidate should be established as often as possible. A persistent increase in heart rate and blood pressure is not uncommon with these medications. Addiction to amphetamine or methylphenidate may occur in rare cases. Weight loss, agitated behavior, tachycardia, hypertension, diaphoresis, end-of-dose depression, and high expectation or strong social pressure to be normal are characteristics of psychophysiologic dependence. In patients who exhibit these characteristics, efforts should be made to withdraw the medication under optimal conditions. This might include support from a chemical dependence service and a specialist in narcolepsy.

The *cataplexy* of narcolepsy may improve when either pharmacologic or nonpharmacologic therapies are used in the management of excessive daytime somnolence. Many people with cataplexy make adaptive changes in their personal and social lifestyles. These changes may reduce or eliminate emotional precipitants in the environment. However, even with the therapies previously described and lifestyle adaptations, cataplexy may remain a significant problem. Frequent

Table 7.11. Stimulant Medication[a,b]

Generic Name	Brand Name	Starting Dose	Maximum Daily Dose (mg)	Divide Daily Dose
Pemoline[c]	Cylert	18.75 mg q.d.	150	b.i.d.
Modafanil	Provigil	100 mg q.d.	400	q.d.
Methylphenidate	Ritalin	5 mg t.i.d.	80	t.i.d./q.i.d.
- extended	Ritalin SR[d]	10 mg b.i.d.	80	b.i.d./t.i.d.
- extended	Concerta[d]	18 mg b.i.d.	72–90	b.i.d./t.i.d.
Dextroamphetamine	Adderall[e]	5 mg b.i.d.	80	b.i.d./t.i.d.
	Dexedrine			
- extended	Dexedrine Spansule	5 mg b.i.d.	80	b.i.d./t.i.d.
Methamphetamine	Desoxyn	5 mg b.i.d.	80	b.i.d./t.i.d.

[a]Pemoline and modafanil are class IV restricted drugs, which means they may be ordered over the telephone and a 6-mo refill may be given. The other stimulants are class II restriction, which means a written prescription is required every month.

[b]It is recommened that dose increases occur no faster than every 1 to 2 weeks for methylphenidate and the amphetamines, and 2 to 3 weeks for pemoline and modafanil. Each incremental increase should not be greater than the initial starting dose.

[c]Pemoline is associated with a high incidence of liver toxicity in children and therefore should be used with caution (see Physicians' Desk Reference for guidelines). The occurrence of liver toxicity in adults appears to be uncommon. However, frequent evaluation of liver function should be made.

[d]The process whereby the half-life of methylphenidate is extended is different for Ritalin SR and Concerta. Patients may respond differently to these two formulations.

[e]Adderall is a mixture of four different D-amphetamine salts and appears to be metabolized differently than D-amphetamine sulphate alone.

and severe cataplexy usually warrants a pharmacologic approach. Previously, tricyclic antidepressants were the primary medication used for this problem. Now, the selective serotonin reuptake inhibitors (SSRIs) should be the first choice for treatment of cataplexy. The standard antidepressant doses often are sufficient (see Chapter 24). If several SSRIs have been tried and have not proved to be completely effective, then a trial on venlafaxine (Effexor) should be considered. The use of a tricyclic antidepressant may be necessary if these initial approaches are unsuccessful. The FDA recently has approved sodium oxybate (Xyrem) for the treatment of cataplexy in patients with narcolepsy. Evidence also suggests that this medication benefits nighttime sleep quality and daytime alertness for those with narcolepsy.

The tricyclic antidepressants can be used to treat *sleep paralysis* and *hypnagogic hallucinations.* Protriptyline, 5 mg, can be given about 1 hour before bedtime if the paralysis or hallucinations occur near sleep onset. Otherwise, the medication can be given at bedtime.

The *management of idiopathic hypersomnia* is less clear-cut than that for narcolepsy. The stimulant medications outlined in Table 7.11 are used, but with less predictable benefits. The use of nonpharmacologic methods, as outlined for narcolepsy, is even less beneficial in this condition. These patients have moderate to severe disabilities related to their excessive daytime tiredness.

Sleep-Disordered Breathing

The treatment of *obstructive sleep apnea* continues to evolve. Usually patients are referred for management of abnormal breathing events that are associated with daytime sleepiness or fatigue. Although SDB may occur in the absence of sleepiness, there is increasing evidence that even 5 to 10 SDB events per hour may predispose to increased cardiovascular risk (19,20) and thus warrant some form of treatment. Patients with comorbid conditions such as diabetes, cardiopulmonary disease, or underlying neurologic disease should be considered a high priority for treatment to reduce further exacerbations of their underlying disease.

Recent epidemiologic studies (19,20) have offered strong support to the hypothesized association between SDB and hypertension. The Sleep Heart Health Study evaluated more than 6,000 individuals age 40 years and older for multiple factors including sleep characteristics and hypertension. This cross-sectional, community-based, multicenter study demonstrated an independent relationship between increasing SDB measures and hypertension. In comparing the groups with the most and the least SDB, an odds ratio for hypertension of 1.37 was calculated. Similarly, the Wisconsin Sleep Cohort Study, a prospective analysis of middle-aged working individuals, analyzed the strength of the association between SDB and hypertension in follow-up assessments with more than 700 participants. Odds ratios for the presence of hypertension in increasingly severe SDB groups were 2.03 and 2.89.

Management options for an individual patient often are recommended by the consultant who has evaluated the patient with a formal sleep study (see Management of Sleep Disorders). Initial management should emphasize correction of associated medical conditions such as hypothyroidism (21), severe tonsillar hypertrophy, and obesity. Central nervous system depressants, if prescribed, should be discontinued. Although the mechanism is still unknown, it is clear that loss of as little as 10% to 15% of body weight may markedly improve the severity of the sleep apnea (22). Because most patients are 30% to 40% above ideal body weight, the minimal amount of weight reduction expected does not represent an unrealistic goal (see Practical Approaches in Chapter 83).

Continuous positive airway pressure (CPAP) remains the mainstay of therapy for symptomatic patients with moderate to severe disease (23). The patient is fitted with a cuplike mask that forces air, usually from a small stationary unit in the bedroom, into the nasal airway. The pressure from the continuous airflow prevents upper airway collapse during sleep. Careful adjustment of pressure is important because patient compliance depends on elimination of apnea and symptom improvement. Patients experience a pressure sensation in the upper airway and the ears when first using the mask. Drying of the mucosal membranes and rhinorrhea can be reduced by adding a humidifier to the inspired air, and nasal congestion is improved by the addition of decongestants. Most patients experience immediate and dramatic improvement in their daytime sleepiness. If fact, there often is a significant impact on the patient's mood and quality of life. If this does not occur, compliance may be inadequate; otherwise, inadequate sleep or another concomitant sleep disorder should be suspected (24). It is expected that successful treatment of SDB with CPAP will decrease associated risks, such as cardiovascular morbidity.

Selection of *surgical measures* to alter upper airway anatomy requires consultation with an otolaryngologist. Although tracheostomy was used regularly in the past for the treatment of this syndrome, it is performed now only when other forms of therapy fail. Palatopharyngoplasty usually is considered after medical therapy has been tried, because the rate of treatment success approaches 40% to 50%. Presently there are limited data to support the use of oral devices, somnoplasty, or laser surgery.

Patients with significant cor pulmonale appear to benefit from *oxygen therapy*. These patients usually have evidence of hypoxemia both when awake and when asleep; therefore, continuous 24-hour oxygen therapy usually is indicated. When central sleep apnea is recognized, the patient should be evaluated for signs and symptoms of congestive heart failure. As a general rule, use of drugs or oxygen reduces, but does not eliminate, episodes of obstructive sleep apnea. The use of oxygen does not have a primary independent role in the treatment of SDB, but it may be beneficial with underlying pathology.

Currently, no therapies for central apnea consistently reduce the frequency of events. However, administration of oxygen may reverse any associated hypoxemia and bradyarrhythmias. CPAP and various respiratory stimulants have produced conflicting results. However, the central sleep apnea associated with Cheyne-Stokes respiration appears to respond to CPAP or theophylline as well as treatment of the underlying heart failure that commonly is associated (25,26). The management of non-apneic snoring is described in Chapter 111.

Restless Legs Syndrome

Nonpharmacologic methods to improve the symptoms of RLS have not been consistently effective (27). Exercise and prolonged soaking in a hot bath usually eliminate the symptoms, and there may be attenuation of the symptoms for a brief period after the patient stops exercising or gets out of the hot bath. This reprieve may be sufficient to allow the patient to fall asleep, but it has little effect on subsequent development of nighttime leg movements.

For patients who ask for treatment, a *pharmacologic approach* to symptom management is the most consistently successful strategy. The medication strategies outlined here may be beneficial for PLMD also. Currently, for the treatment of most RLS cases, the dopamine agonists (Table 7.12) are the first choice, even before levodopa, a dopamine precursor. At best, patients may experience a dramatic improvement or complete disappearance of both the uncomfortable daytime and evening sensations as well as the sleep-related limb movements. There may be rapid improvement soon after initiation of the dopamine agonist, although maximum effectiveness many not be evident for several weeks. For many patients, experimentation with different medications and doses is necessary for an optimal response.

The single most common side effect of the dopaminergic agents is an augmentation of the symptoms. RLS augmentation is seen as a temporal redistribution of the underlying symptoms: The late night symptoms become early evening symptoms. If the dosage is increased further, RLS symptoms may begin in the early afternoon, or, worse become an all-day-long problem. With RLS augmentation, symptoms may extend well beyond the legs and involve the shoulders, hands, arms, and trunk. Augmentation can be so severe as to

Table 7.12. Dopamine Agents for Restless Legs Syndrome (RLS)[a,b,c]

Generic Name	Brand Name	Starting Dose (# tablets)	Increase Dose by # tablets	Maximum Daily Dose
Carbidopa/levodopa[d]	Sinemet	½ (25/100 mg)	½	50/200 mg
Pergolide	Permax	½ (0.05 mg)	½	0.5–0.75 mg
Pramipexole	Mirapex	½ (0.25 mg)	½	1.5–2.0 mg
Ropinirole	Requip	1 (0.25 mg)	1	2.0–3.0 mg

[a]All agents can be increased every 3 days, if necessary. The primary reason to allow 3 days is to avoid side effects.

[b]The maximum daily dose reflects the dose above which RLS augmentation is likely to develop rapidly.

[c]Common side effects seen with these medications in RLS patients are nausea, headache, fluid retention, nasal congestion, hypotension, insomnia, and hypersomnia. Except for the hypersomnia, the other side effects will occur during initial treatment. The hypersomia may occur months to years after medication initiation, and it may result in acute uncontrollable sleep attacks.

[d]Carbidopa/levodopa has a rapid onset (15 to 20 minutes) when taken on an empty stomach. The three dopamine agonists are very slow in onset, with a peak dose time of 2 hours. Therefore, the agonist should be started 2 hours before bedtime to make sure symptoms are relieved by bedtime.

cause a condition indistinguishable from neuroleptic-induced akathisia. At this stage, progressive increments in the daily dose lead to a worsening of symptoms between doses and a shortening of the duration of the medication effectiveness. If augmentation occurs, the choice is to make no further increments in the medication or to change to a nondopaminergic agent.

The opiates are probably the next most effective agents for the treatment of RLS. Opiate effectiveness for RLS does not necessarily parallel analgesic potency. Relatively mild analgesics, such as propoxyphene and tramadol, may be more effective than oxycodone. Several different opiates should be tried before considering this medication class ineffective. Patients who have responded well to opiates and are taking the medication three or more times per day may benefit from changing to a longer-acting preparation or perhaps to methadone. The management of RLS may be sufficiently complicated that referral to a sleep disorder center is warranted. Practical details regarding all classes of dopaminergic medications are found in Chapter 90.

Benzodiazepines and gabapentin may provide another line of treatment if opiates and dopamine agonists fail. However, at this stage, the patient should be assessed by a sleep disorder specialist. If the patient's symptoms are associated with pain or other painful conditions (e.g., neuropathy, back pain, arthritis), then gabapentin or opiates may be employed as first-line agents.

Sleepwalking, Sleep Terrors, and Confusional States

These arousal disorders are viewed as emanating from slow-wave sleep. Sleep deprivation for any reason enhances slow-wave sleep on recovery nights and increases the likelihood of these events in vulnerable people. Accordingly, appropriate recommendations always include minimizing situations that increase sleep loss. Vulnerable people also are more likely to experience episodes during stressful periods. Stress reduction techniques may be helpful for some patients, and psychotherapy may be indicated in selected cases. In some cases, presleep suggestions are beneficial. In a relaxed state at bedtime, the patient can focus on anticipated sleep-related behavior and can reaffirm that he or she will be safe and will do no harm. The sleepwalker can gradually limit the boundaries of wandering in this manner.

The severity in these disorders may be reflected in the frequency of the events and the dangerousness of the behaviors. Particularly severe cases (e.g., multiple episodes per week or less frequent incidents resulting in injury) may be appropriate for *pharmacologic treatment*. In theory, substances that decrease the intensity and duration of slow-wave sleep should decrease the symptoms. This seems to be the case with the benzodiazepines. Successful extended treatment has been accomplished with clonazepam 0.5 mg at bedtime. Some individuals with frequent arousal disorders benefit from nightly zolpidem, although this is not within the scope of FDA approval for this medication. Patients with REM behavior disorder, although it is not associated with slow-wave sleep, often responds well to treatment with clonazepam.

Enuresis

Primary enuresis in the adult, which is not associated with a particular sleep stage, warrants urologic evaluation. The absence of demonstrable organic pathology should not discourage treatment attempts. Several strategies used in children also may be beneficial for adults. Behavioral management is the initial treatment of choice. Conditioning of the urge to urinate and going to the bathroom can be developed with pad and alarm systems (Wet-Stop, Palco Laboratories, Santa Cruz, CA). Standard medication trials have included tricyclic antidepressants. Intranasal desmopressin has been used successfully in many cases (28).

SLEEP CENTER REFERRAL

For a number of the problems discussed in this chapter, referral for expert evaluation and management is recommended. The evaluation of patients with sleep disorders often includes consideration of referral for sleep laboratory evaluation. Because sleep laboratories are now more accessible, it is possible to refer the patient either directly to a laboratory for specific sleep studies or to an expert at a sleep center who may be useful in determining the specific type of sleep test to be conducted. Often, a consultant recommends adjustments in medications or in the sleep–wake cycle before suggesting a sleep study. More importantly, interpretation of the sleep laboratory results and an explanation to the patient must be made by someone familiar with these studies. Currently there are more than 250 sleep disorders centers accredited by the American Academy of Sleep Medicine (AASM). The AASM (6301 Bandel Road NW, Suite 101, Rochester, MN 55901; or on the World Wide Web at www.aasmnet.org) can supply the locations of these centers.

Patient Experience. When patients are evaluated at a sleep center, they undergo a careful historical review of their sleep problem and a general physical examination. An all-night sleep study (polysomnogram) may be scheduled to evaluate sleep objectively. The polysomnogram is performed using noninvasive simultaneous measurements of a number of physiologic activities during sleep: eye movements, brain activity by EEG, submental and anterior tibialis muscle activity, respiratory air flow and effort, cardiac rhythm, and continuous blood oxyhemoglobin saturation. Sometimes additional parameters are recorded, such as rectal temperature, esophageal pH, and penile circumference.

A *multiple sleep latency test* (MSLT), a day test involving four or five 20-minute naps spaced 2 hours apart, may also be scheduled. For this nap test, patients stay in their usual sleeping clothes and are asked to stay awake between the naps. A full-sleep EEG is recorded as for the polysomnogram; however, respiration and oxygen saturation measurements either are not made or are used in a limited form, because the primary question addressed by this test is the degree of excessive sleepiness. The time required for the patient to fall asleep (sleep latency) during these naps provides the measure of the patient's sleepiness. The nap test usually is scheduled for the day after the nighttime polysomnogram. A typical schedule for the patient in the sleep laboratory is 9:30 p.m. to 8 a.m. for the polysomnogram and 8 a.m. to 4:30 p.m. for the nap tests.

General References*

Diagnostic Classification Steering Committee, Thorpy MJ, Chairman. **International classification of sleep disorders: diagnostic and coding manual.** Rochester, MN: Sleep Disorders Association, 1990.

This classification manual lists all recognized sleep disorders. Clinical features and diagnostic criteria are outlined.

Kryger M, Roth T, Dement WC, eds. Principles and practice of sleep medicine. 3rd ed. Philadelphia: WB Saunders, 2000.

This comprehensive textbook covers basic science and clinical issues in sleep disorders medicine.

Kupfer DJ, Reynolds CF III. Management of insomnia. N Engl J Med 1997;336:341.

Up-to-date review. Authors' summary assessments of clinical trials of published behavioral and pharmacologic interventions are included.

Strollo PJ Jr, Rogers RM. Current concepts: obstructive sleep apnea. N Engl J Med 1996;334:99.

Recent well-referenced review article.

Specific References

1. National Commission on Sleep Disorders Research. Report of the National Commission on Sleep Disorders Research. DHHS Publication. Washington, DC: US Government Printing Office, 1992.
2. The Gallup survey: sleep in America. Princeton, NJ: The Gallup Organization, 1991.
3. Diagnostic Classification Steering Committee. International classification of sleep disorders: diagnostic and coding manual. Rochester, MN: Sleep Disorders Association, 1990.
4. Spielman AJ, Caruso LS, Glovinsky PG. A behavioral perspective on insomnia treatment. Psychiatr Clin North Am 1987;10:541.
5. Silverman K, Evans SM, Strain EC, et al. Withdrawal syndrome after the double-blind cessation of caffeine consumption. N Engl J Med 1992;327:1109.
6. Aldrich MS. Narcolepsy. Neurology 1992;42[Suppl 6]:34.
7. Young T, Palta M, Dempsey J, et al. The occurrence of sleep-disordered breathing among middle-aged adults. N Engl J Med 1993;328:1230.
8. Guilleminault C, Eldridge FL, Dement WC. Insomnia with sleep apnea: a new syndrome. Science 1973;181:856.
9. Smith PL. Evaluation of patients with sleep disorders. In: White DP, ed. Seminars in respiratory medicine. New York: Thieme Stratton, 1988:534.
10. Punjabi NM, O'Hearn DJ, Neubauer DN, et al. Modeling hypersomnolence in sleep-disordered breathing. Am J Respir Crit Care Med 1999;159:1703.
11. King AC, Oman RF, Brassington GS, et al. Moderate-intensity exercise and self-rated quality of sleep in older adults. JAMA 1997;277:32.
12. Bootzin RR, Nicassio PM. Progress in behavioral modification. Vol 7: behavioral treatments for insomnia. San Diego: Academic Press, 1978.
13. Spielman AJ, Saskin P, Thorpy MJ. Treatment of chronic insomnia by restriction of time spent in bed. Sleep 1987;10:45.
14. Friedman L, Bliwise DL, Yesavage JA, et al. A preliminary study comparing sleep restriction and relaxation treatments for insomnia in older adults. J Gerontol Psychol Sci 1991;46:1.
15. Czeisler CA, Kronauer RE, Allan JS, et al. Bright light induction of strong (type 0) resetting of the human circadian pacemaker. Science 1989;244:1328.
16. Nowell PD, Mazumdar S, Buysse DJ, et al. Benzodiazepines and zolpidem for chronic insomnia: a meta-analysis of treatment efficacy. JAMA 1997;278(24):2170.
17. Drugs used for anxiety and sleep disorders. In: Drug evaluation subscription. Chicago: American Medical Association, I/PSY-1, Spring 1993.
18. Task Force on Benzodiazepine Dependency. Benzodiazepine dependence, toxicity, and abuse: a task force report of the American Psychiatric Association. Washington, DC: American Psychiatric Association, 1990.
19. Nieto FJ, Young TB, Lind BK, et al. Association of sleep-disordered breathing, sleep apnea, and hypertension in a large community-based study. Sleep Heart Health Study. JAMA 2000;283:1880.
20. Peppard PE, Young T, Palta M, et al. Prospective study of the association between sleep-disordered breathing and hypertension. N Engl J Med 2000;342:1378.
21. Rajagopal KR, Abbrecht PH, Derderian SS, et al. Obstructive sleep apnea in hypothyroidism. Ann Intern Med 1984;101:491.
22. Smith PL, Gold AR, Myers DA, et al. Weight loss in mildly to moderately obese patients with obstructive sleep apnea. Ann Intern Med 1985;103:850.
23. Pack AI, Maisin G. Who should get treated for sleep apnea? Ann Intern Med 2001;134:1065.
24. Kribbs NB, Pack AI, Kline LR, et al. Objective measurement of patterns of nasal CPAP use by patients with obstructive sleep apnea. Am Rev Respir Dis 1993;147:887.
25. Granton JT, Naughton MT, Benard DC, et al. CPAP improves inspiratory muscle strength in patients with heart failure and central sleep apnea. Am J Respir Crit Care Med 1996;153:277.
26. Javaheri S, Parker TJ, Wexler L, et al. Effects of theophylline on sleep-disordered breathing in heart failure. N Engl J Med 1996;335:562.
27. Montplaisir J, Lapierre O, Warnes H, et al. The treatment of the restless leg syndrome with or without periodic leg movements in sleep. Sleep 1992;15:391.
28. Nino-Murcia G, Keenan SA. Enuresis and sleep. In: Guilleminault C, ed. Sleep and its disorders in children. New York: Raven Press, 1987.

*Bold print (general references) and bold numerals (specific references) denote published controlled clinical trials, meta-analysis, or consensus-based recommendations.

CHAPTER 8

Occupational and Environmental Disease*

LAURA S. WELCH, MD

As we enter a new century, we continue to have widespread proliferation of new and potentially toxic chemicals. These hazardous exposures are encountered in homes, schools, the general environment, and especially the workplace. The extent to which such exposures may be causing health problems is a grave concern. Few communities in the United States have escaped public concern over the health hazards of pesticide spraying, asbestos in school buildings, contaminated drinking water, electromagnetic radiation, or toxic waste disposal.

This chapter provides an overview of how environmental diseases occur and outlines an approach for recognizing and addressing them. It emphasizes the workplace, where environmentally induced illness is most commonly recognized. Each year in the United States more than 100,000 people die and more than 400,000 become ill as a direct result of occupational disease. Hazardous exposures and resulting illness also occur in the home or community environment. The same principles that apply to workplace exposure apply to home and community exposure as well.

*James P. Keogh, MD authored this chapter in the first five editions of this book.

VITAL ROLE OF PRIMARY PRACTITIONERS

Primary practitioners are often the first professionals to recognize the hazards of occupational exposure and to document the link between their patients' illnesses and their patients' work. The task of controlling the hazards usually involves public health specialists, but it is vitally important that primary practitioners take the time to report and follow up suspected occupational diseases.

Although the United States has for three decades had the Occupational Safety and Health Administration (OSHA) to ensure workplace safety, there are only enough inspectors to visit every workplace once every 200 years. Each year still brings efforts in Congress to weaken the program that does exist. Locked fire exits, exploitation of immigrants, child labor, and sweatshop conditions persist decades after the New Deal took steps to abolish them. Many workers are unaware of their right to request investigation of potential hazards at work, and concerns for job security deter them from raising complaints about safety with supervisors. Public health surveillance of occupational and environmental disease has been improved in the past decade by the efforts of the National Institute for Occupational Safety and Health (NIOSH) working with state health agencies, but it remains limited in scope and coverage. For all these reasons, if a patient has an occupational health problem or is exposed to a dangerous situation at work, his or her physician may be the single most important factor in protecting the patient's and the community's health.

PATHOGENESIS OF OCCUPATIONAL DISEASE

The pathogenesis of occupational disease is complex and involves not only the interaction between the host and a toxic exposure but also a complex set of social interactions.

Toxin–Host Interaction

For an occupational disease to occur, there must be a triad consisting of a toxic agent, a host, and an environment in which the host is exposed. The illness that may result depends on the toxic properties of the substance or energy source, its route of entry, the dosage received by the host, and the susceptibility of the host to the toxin.

Toxic agents can be inhaled, ingested, or absorbed through the skin. With *inhalation,* the dosage received depends on whether the substance is present as gas, a fume, or a dust. Deposition of dust in the lungs depends to a great extent on particle size and distribution, because smaller particles can more easily enter the alveoli and become trapped. The concentration of the substance in the air (which is related to room ventilation, temperature, and humidity), the rate at which the worker is exercising and breathing, and protective factors such as special clothing or respirator use are other factors that affect the amount of toxin absorbed.

Once the toxic substance is absorbed, there may be an instantaneous effect (as in the case of carbon monoxide poisoning), a brief latent period (as in the case of occupational asthma), or a latent period of years or decades (as in the pneumoconioses). A brief, high-dose exposure may cause serious illness and death and be easy to recognize. Prolonged exposure to a low dosage of a toxin may not cause symptoms at the outset but may produce disease years later.

Impact of Economic and Social Factors

Thousands of new chemicals are introduced into industrial processes every year, and few have been tested to determine their potential toxicity. Even when toxicologic screening tests are done on a compound, they may not predict human disease. Despite the implementation of the Toxic Substances Control Act (TOSCA), which gave the U.S. Environmental Protection Agency (EPA) authority to require pretesting of chemicals, in too many cases, the hazard of a chemical is recognized only after an outbreak of illness. Economic factors play a major role in determining how safe a workplace is. Industrial hygiene programs to monitor exposure are common only in the largest plants. Important decisions, such as improving ventilation or decreasing exposure to noise, may involve significant expense. Workers may be reluctant to complain about working conditions for fear of losing their jobs. This is especially likely during periods of high unemployment, when acceptance of unpleasant and potentially unhealthy working conditions may be the price of having a job. Even when workers are strongly organized, the desire for a safer workplace may be balanced by a concern that increased production costs may result in the decision of a company to relocate its plant to areas where unions are less effective or do not exist. Such anxieties have been heightened by the passage of the North American Free Trade Agreement (NAFTA) and the globalization of manufacturing. Stringent health and safety regulations, with strong enforcement, can put competitors on a more equal footing and protect responsible businesses from being undercut by irresponsible ones.

DIAGNOSING WORK-RELATED DISEASE

Although episodes of illness caused or exacerbated by the patient's work are often seen in ambulatory practice, they frequently are not recognized as such. Misdiagnosis of an occupational disease means that the patient does not benefit from correct diagnosis and management and there is no correction of the poor working conditions that may subsequently injure others or even result in death. Two cases illustrate these points.

Case Study: A Teenager with Bronchitis

An 18-year-old woman complained to her physician of a severe cough and some wheezing. The physician treated her with erythromycin and fluids and advised her to stay in bed for a few days. She recovered and returned to work feeling well. Several days later she had a severe recurrent cough with wheezing and dyspnea and saw her physician again. The physician again prescribed erythromycin and rest. She remained off work for a week. She felt better and returned to work. After 2 days she became extremely short of breath and was brought to the emergency room. She had severe bronchospasm and was admitted, improving on bronchodilators and corticosteroids after a few days. An occupational history on admission disclosed that her work involved grinding drill bits made of tungsten carbide containing a small amount of cobalt, a known pulmonary sensitizer. Once the patient was sensitized, each fresh exposure to the dust caused symptoms after a shorter incubation period. Had the first physician considered the diagnosis of extrinsic asthma and inquired about occupational exposures, the patient's subsequent deterioration could have been prevented.

Case Study: A Man with Severe Abdominal Pain

A 28-year-old man presented to the emergency room of a community hospital with a chief complaint of severe abdominal pain. There was significant abdominal tenderness with a question of guarding. He reported having seen his family physician on two occasions during the preceding 2 weeks, with severe cramping pain felt around the umbilicus. His physician had prescribed a histamine$_2$ blocker and tried to schedule a gastroenterologic consultation, which the patient had not set up because of difficulties with his work schedule. The pain that had been intermittent had now become constant, more in the lower quadrants, and more severe for longer than 6 hours. Blood work showed a normal amylase level and a leukocytosis. A surgical consultant suggested the possibility of an appendiceal abscess but believed that the patient was stable enough to await the results of a computed tomography scan. A gastroenterologist was consulted and was the first physician to take an occupational history. The patient had been a painter for several years and was currently working for a contractor repainting the elaborate metal cornices of a building. For more than a month he had been using a vibrating tool to remove old paint, and this created a lot of dust. He did not know whether lead was in the paint. The gastroenterologist suggested a determination of the patients blood lead level and watchful waiting. The computed tomography scan was normal and the blood lead concentration was elevated. Several coworkers were also poisoned, and the patient's son had an increased blood lead concentration from the contaminated work clothes his father had brought home.

To avoid the pitfalls these cases demonstrate, the following three strategies are fundamental in evaluating a patient:

- Ask every patient about his or her job.
- Consider the possibility that the patient's illness is related to the work or home environment.
- Follow up on one's suspicions. Others may be in danger.

Table 8.1. Components of an Occupational History

Description of the job
Physical exertion
Body mechanics
Pace of work
Repetitive tasks
Job stress
Exposure to hazards
Risk of trauma
Noise and vibration
Heat and cold
Ionizing and nonionizing radiation
Dusts, fumes, mists
Contamination of skin and clothing
Protective measures
Ventilation and respiratory protection
Protective clothing
Medical surveillance
Effects of exposure
Temporal relationship of any symptoms to work (e.g., relationship to time of day, day of week, change of symptoms on vacation, weekends)
Similar symptoms in coworkers

Taking an Occupational History

Inquiring about a patient's job not only helps identify occupational disease but also provides other information useful in caring for a patient. Clearly the physical demands of the job are important when advising a patient about a health problem such as coronary artery disease or diabetes mellitus. Knowing the patient's work schedule is also important, because shift work affects medication schedules, diet, and family life. Medications can dramatically affect the patient's comfort or safety at work (e.g., diuretics in an interstate truck driver, antihistamines in a construction worker who works at elevation). Financial and psychological stress may result from layoffs, whereas regular overtime may bring about chronic fatigue and psychological problems of its own. Usually, a brief discussion of the current job, including a brief description of how the patient spends the working day, is sufficient. This rarely takes more than 3 minutes. The major points to cover in this inquiry are summarized in Table 8.1.

When some aspect of the medical or occupational history has raised suspicions of a work-related condition, further questioning flows naturally. The inquiry should focus on a temporal relationship between symptoms and possible exposure, exposure to an agent known to cause disease, or a pattern of similar illness among coworkers. Because every patient, every job, and every medical presentation is different, there is no single way of taking a history. If the patient uses jargon or job titles that are unfamiliar, it is important to ask for clarification.

The screening history sometimes reveals the need to take a *lifelong work history.* An account of previous jobs and exposures is especially important when the patient has a chronic illness or the possibility of work-related neoplasia. In such cases, the following approach is recommended (it may save time to have the patient bring this information, written out, to a follow-up visit after the initial evaluation):

1. Begin with parents' jobs and childhood exposures.
2. Review each of the patient's jobs in chronological order.
3. Elicit relevant aspects of each period of employment (Table 8.1).

Diseases That Are Commonly Related to Work

The occupational diseases that physicians encounter depend on the industry in the immediate vicinity and the demographic makeup of their practice. For example, practitioners caring for the elderly may see retired workers with previous exposure in all types of industry. Any organ system can be affected by hazardous exposures. Table 8.2 lists clinical problems grouped according to the organ system affected.

Dermatitis and pneumoconiosis are the most commonly reported occupational illnesses. This probably reflects both true incidence (skin and pulmonary epithelium being most in contact with the outside environment) and the greater likelihood of recognition of these disorders as occupational in origin.

The number of chemicals that are toxic to the liver and kidney is so great that a careful exposure history should be taken from all patients with unexplained hepatitis or hepatic or renal failure. Many chemicals can affect the gastrointestinal tract and cause functional disturbances that may be misdiagnosed as peptic disease or irritable bowel syndrome.

Low-level exposure of the respiratory organs to a variety of substances may result in the production of nonspecific upper respiratory tract syndromes that the patient may describe as an intractable cold or as sinus trouble.

Occupational diseases sometimes manifest with striking and unusual signs (e.g., acro-osteolysis in vinyl chloride workers, nasal septal perforation in patients exposed to chromates). More commonly they cause vague systemic symptoms typical of early intoxication or manifest as a disease of ordinary life, such as asthma or eczema.

A few specific clinical situations should always raise the consideration of an occupational or environmental cause:

- *Any unexplained change in personality or behavior.* Poisoning with mercury, lead, pesticides, and a wide variety of other central nervous system toxins may be the cause.
- *New onset of asthma in an adult.* There is usually a temporal relationship between exposure and symptoms of asthma, but because of the time lapse when an immunologic mechanism is involved, wheezing and dyspnea may not be noted until after the workday is over.
- *Any case of pulmonary fibrosis.* A prolonged latent period between exposure and disease onset means that abnormalities that appear on radiographs may be the result of a job the patient had decades ago.

Table 8.2. Common Medical Problems with Examples of Environmental Causes

Clinical Problem	Causative Agent
Skin	
Cyanosis	Methemoglobin formers
	Aniline
	Anisidine, *ortho-* and *para-* isomers
	Dimethylaniline
	Dinitrobenzene, all isomers
	Dinitrotoluene
	Monomethylaniline
	p-Nitroaniline
	Nitrobenzene
	p-Nitrocholorobenzene
	Nitrogen trifluoride
	Nitrotoluene
	Perchloryl fluoride
	n-Propyl nitrate
	Tetranitromethane
	o-Toluidine
	Xylidine
Contact dermatitis	Many chemicals with irritant or sensitizing properties
Chronic eczematous dermatitis	Solvents
	Detergents
Folliculitis	Oil exposure
	Grease exposure
Acne	Polychlorinated biphenyls
	Chlorinated naphthalenes
	Paraffin
	Coal tar
	Dioxin
Photosensitization	Coal tar
	Pitch
	Asphalt
	Anthracene
	Creosote
	Fluorescein
	Phenanthrene
Granulomas	Beryllium
Corns	Asbestos
	Fiberglass
Punctate ulcers	Chromic acid
Painful burns	Hydrofluoric acid (deep pain out of proportion to appearance of burn)
Skin cancer	Soots
	Tars
	Arsenic
	Coke oven emissions
	Cutting oils
	Sunlight
Nervous System	
Central Effects	
Altered consciousness	Hundreds of chemicals have CNS-depressant properties and other CNS effects
Headaches	Carbon monoxide
	Nitrites
	Nitrates
	Alcohols
	Lead
	Organic lead compounds
	Methemoglobin formers (see Cyanosis)
Behavioral change	Mercury
	Lead
	Carbon disulfide
	Carbon monoxide
	Methyl chloride
	Methyl bromide
Peripheral Effects	
Ataxia, tremor, spasticity	Manganese
	Organic lead compounds
	Organic tin compounds
Hyperreflexia, micrographia	Mercury
	Dichlorodiphenyltrichloroethane (DDT)
Peripheral neuropathy	Peripheral neurotoxins
	Acrylamide
	Arsenic and compounds
	Calcium arsenate
	Carbon disulfide
	n-Hexane
	Lead and inorganic lead compounds
	Dimethylaminopropionitrile
	Lucel-7 (2-*t*-butylazo-2-hydroxy-5-methyl hexane)
	Mercury
	Methyl bromide
	Methyl butyl ketone
	Thallium, soluble compounds
	2,4,6-Trinitrotoluene
	Tri-*o*-cresyl phosphate
Auditory	
Decreased acuity and tinnitus	Noise exposure, especially >85 db
Acoustic neuritis	Aniline
	Arsenic
	Carbon monoxide
	Hypoxia
	Lead
	Organic mercury
	Phosphorus
	Sodium nitrate
Otitis externa	Contamination of earplugs used for noise protection
Ear pain	Acute shifts in pressure
Respiratory	
Nasal septal perforation	Chromic acid and other chromates
Laryngeal carcinoma	Asbestos
Laryngitis, bronchitis tracheitis, pneumonitis	Many irritants, including the following:
	Ammonia
	Chlorine
	Oxides of nitrogen
	Ozone
	Phosgene
	Sulfur dioxide
	Vanadium pentoxide
	Mercury
	Manganese
	Cadmium dust
Bronchiolitis obliterans	Nitrogen dioxide
Allergic alveolitis	Many different antigens
Bagassosis	*Thermoactinomyces vulgaris* and *Micropolyspora* sp.
Bird-breeder's lung	Avian proteins
Byssinosis	Cotton, flax, and soft fiber hemps
Cheese-washer's lung	*Penicillium caseil*
Detergents	*Bacillus subtilis*
Farmer's lung	*Micropolyspora faeni* and *Thermoactinomyces vulgaris*
Feathers	Feather proteins
Furrier's lung	Keratinized particles of hair
Malt-worker's lung	*Aspergillis clavatus*
Maple bark-stripper's disease	*Cryptostroma corticale*
Paprika-splitter's lung	*Mucor stolinifer*

Table 8.2—*continued.* **Common Medical Problems with Examples of Environmental Causes**

Clinical Problem	Causative Agent
Respiratory—cont'd	
Bronchospasm	Pulmonary sensitizers (any list is incomplete, because new agents are reported each year)
	Castor bean pomace
	Cobalt, metal fume and dust
	Enzymatic detergents
	Grain dusts
	Maleic anhydride
	Methylene bisphenyl isocyanate
	Methyl isocyanate
	Nickle, metal
	p-Phenylenediamine
	Phthalic anhydride
	Platinum salts
	Polyvinyl chloride (fume from heated film: meat-wrapper's asthma)
	Toluene 2,4-diisocyanate
	Tungsten carbide
	Western red cedar
	Plicatic acid
Pulmonary fibrosis	Asbestos
	Silica
	Beryllium
	Talc
	Coal dust
	Cobalt
	Hematite
	Kaolin
Benign pneumoconiosis deposits in lung without fibrosis	Aluminum powder
	Barium
	Graphite
	Iron oxide
	Tin
	Cerium oxide
	Silver
	Titanium
Pleural effusion	Asbestos
	Paraquat
	Talc
Gastrointestinal	
Gingivitis and gum pigmentation	Mercury
	Lead
	Bismuth
Dental erosion	Acetic acid
	Hydrochloric acid
	Lactic acid
	Nitric acid
	Nitrogen dioxide
	Sulfuric acid
Tongue paresthesias	Furfural
	Rotenone
	Crosol
Green tongue	Vanadium
Nausea and vomiting	Many chemicals including the following:
	CNS depressants
	Cholinesterase inhibitors
	Methemoglobin formers
Constipation	Lead
	Barium sulfate
	Thallium
	Tellurium
	Vanadium
	Fluorides

Clinical Problem	Causative Agent
Hepatomegaly	Hepatotoxins
	Acetylene tetrabromide
	Carbon disulfide
	Carbon tetrachloride
	Chlorodiphenyl
	Chloroform
	p-Dichlorobenzene
	Dimethylacetamide
	Dimethylformamide
	Dioxane
	Ethylene chlorohydrin
	Ethylene dibromide
	Ethylene dichloride
	Hexachloronaphthalene
	Kepone
	Nitroethane
	Octachloronaphthalene
	Pentachloronaphthalene
	Picric acid
	Tetrachloroethane
	Tetrachloroethylene
	Tetrachloronaphthalene
	Trichloronaphthalene
	2,4,6-Trinitrotoluene
Jaundice	Hepatotoxins (see Hepatomegaly)
	Hemolytic agents
	Arsine
	Butyl cellosolve
	Naphthalene
	Phenylhydrazine
	Stibine
Angiosarcoma of liver	Vinyl chloride
Abdominal pain	Antimony
	Arsenic
	Bromine
	Cadmium
	Lead
	Mercury
	Nicotine
	Organophosphates
	Thallium
	Many other chemicals when ingested
Cardiovascular	
Myocardial damage	Antimony
	Arsine
	Carbon disulfide
	Cobalt
Ischemic disease	Nitroglycerin
	Nitroglycol
	Other vasodilating nitrates
Hypertension	Noise exposure
	Aminopyridine
	Arsenic
	Barium
	Boron hydride
	Carbon disulfide
	Cobalt
	Diphenyl
	Lead
	Mercury
	Thallium
Vasospastic disorders—"White finger"	Vibrating tools
Raynaud's phenomenon	Vinyl chloride

Continued

Table 8.2—*continued.* Common Medical Problems with Examples of Environmental Causes

Clinical Problem	Causative Agent
Genitourinary	
Renal disease	Nephrotoxins
	4-Aminodiphenyl
	Cadmium
	Carbon disulfide
	Carbon tetrachloride
	Chloroform
	Dioxane
	Ethylene chlorohydrin
	Ethylene dibromide
	Lead
	Mercury
	Oxalic acid
	Picric acid
	Tetrachloroethane
	2,4,6-Trinitrotoluene
	Turpentine
	Uranium
Renal carcinoma	4-Aminodiphenyl
	Auramine
	Benzidine
	β-Naphthylamine
	4-Nitrodiphenyl
	Magenta
Urinary retention	Dimethylaminopropionitrile
Reproductive	
Female sterility	Lead
Male sterility	Glycolethers
	Carbon disulfide
	Dibromochloropropane (DBCP)
	Lead
	Microwaves to testes (radar workers)
	Stilbestrol
Hematologic	
Anemia	Lead
	Hemolytic agents
	Arsine
	Butyl cellosolve
	Naphthalene
	Phenylhydrazine
	Stibine
	Marrow depressants
	Benzene
	Dinitrophenol
	Tetryl
	2,4,6-Trinitrotoluene
Leukemia	Benzene
	Radiation
	Styrene-butadiene
	Ethylene oxide
Musculoskeletal	
Osteonecrosis	Phosphorus
Osteomalacia	Cadmium
Osteosclerosis	Fluorine
Acro-osteolysis	Vinyl chloride

- *Peripheral neuropathy.* A toxic neuropathy may be recognizable by an unusual pattern of presentation, but in most cases, only careful history taking will reveal the cause.
- *Overuse syndromes in the extremities.* Tendonitis, epicondylitis, and shoulder bursitis often are the result of a pattern of overuse. This can result from occupational or recreational activities. When they are work related, modification of the job is essential.
- *Hearing loss.* Noise-induced hearing loss occurs gradually and usually in older workers, so it is rarely recognized in time to prevent severe damage.
- *Inability to conceive.* Workers often question whether hazardous exposures at work cause infertility. Several toxins do reduce sperm count or increase time to conception.
- *Lung cancer.* Exposures to asbestos and cigarette smoke are very common throughout the United States. Other lung carcinogens may be important in certain parts of the country.
- *Other cancers.* Specific carcinogens are identified in Table 8.3.

Determining Work Relatedness

The key to identifying occupational disease is to be sure that a toxic or environmental etiology is at least considered. In addition, the patient should always be asked, "Do you think this problem could have anything to do with your work?" and, "Does anyone else at work have this same problem?" Very often, if there is a connection, the patient will be able to identify it.

If neither the physician nor the patient knows whether a syndrome is occupational in origin, resources are available that identify toxic causes of a given symptom complex, toxic exposures of given occupations, and the potential hazards of exposure to given substances (Table 8.4).

FOLLOW-UP OF OCCUPATIONAL DISEASE

Physician's Role

If there is suspicion that a patient became ill from an occupational exposure, it is the physician's responsibility to follow up. Not only does diagnosing an occupational disease affect therapy and eligibility for compensation for a patient, but it may indicate that the health of others is also in danger. Often physicians overcome their own uneasiness about a patient's job by advising the patient to change jobs. Then, instead of the potentially hazardous job being made safe, another unsuspecting person is brought in to take the risk.

In some circumstances, occupational disease is recognized but the original hazard has been eliminated (e.g., in a patient with asbestosis who worked in a now-closed shipyard). Even in these circumstances, former coworkers need to be informed of the risk resulting from previous exposure.

It is not necessary to wait for absolute proof of etiology before beginning an investigation of a possible workplace hazard. The least severely affected member of a group of workers may be the one who seeks attention. Moreover, for most occupationally induced diseases, proof of a relationship rests on epidemiologic data rather than on diagnostic study of the individual patient. Often the most practical way to learn whether a patient's problems are caused or exacerbated by his

Table 8.3. Cancers Known to Be Caused by Environmental Agents

Site/Cell Type	Toxic Agent	Industry/Occupation
Liver/hemangiosarcoma	Vinyl chloride monomer	Vinyl chloride polymerization industry
	Arsenical pesticides	Vintners
Nose	Hardwood dusts	Woodworkers, cabinet and furniture makers
	Radium	Radium chemists and processors, dial painters
	Chromates	Chromium producers, processors, users
	Nickel	Nickel smelting and refining
	Unknown agent	Boot and shoe industry
Larynx	Asbestos	Asbestos product manufacture, shipbuilding, construction and maintenance work
Lung	Asbestos	Asbestos product manufacture, shipbuilding, construction and maintenance work
	Coke oven emissions	Topside coke oven workers
	Radon daughters	Uranium and fluorspar miners
	Chromates	Chromium producers and processors, users
	Nickel	Nickel smelters, processors, and users
	Arsenic	Smelters
	Silica	Foundries, abrasive blasting
	Mustard gas	Mustard gas formulators
	Bis(chloromethyl) ether, chloromethyl methyl ether	Ion exchange resin makers, chemists
Pleura and peritoneum/mesothelioma	Asbestos	Asbestos product manufacture, shipbuilding, construction and maintenance work
Bone	Radium	Dial painters, radium chemists and processors
Scrotum	Mineral/cutting oils	Automatic lathe operators, metalworkers
	Soots and tars, tar distillates	Coke oven workers, petroleum refiners, tar distillers
Bladder	Benzidine, α- and β-naphthylamine, auramine, magenta, 4-aminobiphenyl, 4-nitrophenyl	Rubber and dye workers
Esophagus	Asbestos	Asbestos product manufacture, shipbuilding, construction and maintenance work
Stomach	Asbestos	Asbestos product manufacture, shipbuilding, construction and maintenance work
Colon	Asbestos	Asbestos product manufacture, shipbuilding, construction and maintenance work
Kidney	Coke oven emissions	Coke oven workers
Hematopoietic/lymphoid leukemia, acute	Unknown	Rubber industry
	Ionizing radiation	Radiologists
Myeloid leukemia, acute	Benzene	Refining, chemical, and manufacturing industries
	Ionizing radiation	Radiologists
Erythroleukemia, acute	Benzene	Refining, chemical, and manufacturing industries

Table 8.4. How to Determine the Potential Hazards of an Exposure

Identify the chemical (*Shortcut:* Call local poison center for help)	Employers are required to provide Material Safety Data Sheets (MSDS) on all materials containing potentially hazardous chemicals. Check with the manufacturer, using the phone numbers on the MSDS. For energy exposure, ask employer about equipment specifications or measurements of wavelength and intensity.
Clarify potential health effects (*Shortcut:* Call NIOSH helpline at 513-533-8326 or ATSDR helpline at 404-488-4100)	Use one of the general references listed at the end of this chapter for an overview. Use your medical library or Grateful Med to access Medline and Toxnet at the National Library of Medicine to check newer information.
Synthesize Information (*Shortcut:* Involves a consultant through AOEC, 202-347-4976)	Organize what you have learned from patient history about the exposure: identity of the chemical or mixture, source and wavelength of the energy source, intensity, duration, and time course of exposure. Compare with dosages known to cause human health effects or animal effects.

AOEC, Association of Occupational and Environmental Clinics; ATSDR, Agency for Toxic Substances and Disease Registry; NIOSH, National Institute for Occupational Safety and Health.

or her occupation is to find out whether coworkers are similarly affected. If the physician identifies a possible occupational illness, assistance from others can be sought.

Investigative and Enforcement Agencies

State Level

Many states have a health department unit for investigation of occupational disease. Some states require physicians to report all cases of suspected occupational disease. Such laws should and probably will become more widespread. Reporting any suspected occupational disease problem to the local health department can be the first step in follow-up. In many states, NIOSH assists the health department in surveillance and control of specific occupational diseases.

Federal Level

If there is difficulty in clarifying the potential relationship of illness to environment or if the concerns raised are not addressed by a specific OSHA regulation (see later discussion), it may be helpful to request assistance from NIOSH. This institute is the part of the United States Public Health Service (USPHS) Centers for Disease Control and Prevention that conducts research on occupational disease. An employer, a union, or any three employees can request a formal health hazard evaluation (HHE) of a workplace. Furthermore, NIOSH now has educational resource centers (where consultants are available to help physicians, employers, and workers) in each region of the United States. These centers can provide literature searches and information on available publications and current areas of research and can refer a physician to others who are experts in the field. Access to regional centers can be provided by the central office.

In addition to its investigative function, NIOSH can assist a physician directly in investigating a patient's exposure. Its clearinghouse responds to practitioners' inquiries with information about the hazards of particular trades and toxic substances. (Physicians can contact NIOSH by telephone at 1-800-35-NIOSH or 513-533-8326.)

Enforcement Agencies

Although health departments generally have authority to investigate occupational diseases, regulation of workplace conditions is usually the responsibility of a separate state agency or the local OSHA office in the United States Department of Labor (the telephone number is listed under *United States Government, Labor Department, OSHA*). When a state takes over OSHA enforcement, its regulations are required to be as strict as the federal regulations. In every state, every employer is obligated to report workplace-related injuries and illnesses to OSHA.

If other workers may be in imminent danger of being made ill, the physician should communicate this urgently to OSHA and request an immediate investigation. In most cases, OSHA enforcement officers can determine easily whether regulations are being violated at a workplace, and they provide a follow-up report to the referring physician. In some cases, the inspection suggests that the patient's illness was job related but that at the time of the inspection no specific OSHA regulation was being violated. If a continuing hazard does exist, OSHA can force changes by invoking the employer's general duty to maintain a safe workplace. Especially in these situations, physicians may need to be patient but persistent to see that appropriate action is taken.

The Mine Safety and Health Agency (MSHA) is the specific federal agency with responsibility for safety inspection and enforcement of occupational health standards for the mining industry.

Consultants

Consultants who are particularly knowledgeable about specific problems are increasingly available to help practicing physicians. *Poison centers,* through their national network of contacts, can usually identify an appropriate expert for telephone consultation about an acute problem. *The Association of Occupational and Environmental Clinics* (AOEC), a national network of primarily university-based clinics, can be contacted to identify resources available in most parts of the United States (telephone 202-347-4976).

WORKERS' COMPENSATION PROGRAMS

Every state has a worker's compensation act that provides a system to pay for medical expenses related to occupational disease and injury and for employees' lost earnings. These acts were passed to provide a no-fault system of compensating workers injured on the job and to provide employers with statutory protection from being sued for negligence by their employees.

Although the system sometimes works well for on-the-job injuries, it does not respond well to the needs of a worker with an occupational disease. Here the burden of proof that the disease is work related falls on the worker, and the process of obtaining compensation is often slow and difficult. Because most small employers insure themselves with an insurance company, the insurer may delay action on a claim even when the employer believes the illness was caused by the job. Usually the worker can obtain legal assistance without having to pay an attorney directly, because provision is made for cases to be taken on a contingency basis (i.e., attorneys receive no fee unless the claim is upheld, and then a fixed percentage). Because illness claims are usually complex, the worker will often need a lawyer.

If a physician concludes or even strongly suspects that a patient has an illness caused by or made worse by his or her job, the patient should be encouraged to file for workers' compensation (through the employer, the workers' compensation local office, or a lawyer).

Table 8.5. Responsibilities for the Part-Time Occupational Health Physician

Responsibilities	Regulations to Be Familiar With	Source of Information and Training
Preplacement and fitness-for-duty examinations	Americans with Disabilities Act Federal Aviation Administration, Department of Transportation (DOT) requirements	Equal Employment Opportunity Commission *Technical Assistance Manual* ACOEM training courses[a]
Testing for substance abuse	DOT regulations	Medical review officer course[a] Substance-specific regulations
Surveillance	Occupational Safety and Health Administration (OSHA) regulations	
Care of injured or ill workers	Worker's compensation procedures for one's state Rules governing access to medical records	

[a]American College of Occupational and Environmental Medicine (telephone 847-818-1800).

Table 8.6. Ethical Responsibilities of the Occupational Health Physician

The primary responsibility of the physician is to the individual patient, no matter who is paying the bill.
The physician may reveal nothing to others, including management, about the patient without his or her permission. Reports should be limited to a statement about the patient's fitness to work and any specific limitations of activity.
The physician must acquire all available information about the workplace that may be relevant to a patient's health.
Everything that the physician learns or may deduce about the safety of the workplace must be explained to those whose health may be affected.
The physician should report occupational disease to the local health department or state Occupational Safety and Health Administration (OSHA).
The physician should not take sides in any dispute between the management, the workers, or the government, but should only provide accurate information and honest opinion to all concerned.

If a claim is pursued and won (even though it takes time), the patient is usually guaranteed lifetime *medical coverage from workers' compensation funds for that illness.* Compensation may lift some of the financial burdens from the patient and his or her family, particularly in cases of chronic or fatal illness.

To some extent, the workers' compensation system has failed because of inadequate physician diagnosis and follow-through. For example, a 1980 Department of Labor survey showed that only 3% of workers disabled by occupational respiratory disease were receiving compensation. The remaining 97% were living on Social Security or welfare payments, and their medical bills were being paid by health insurance, Medicare, or state welfare funds. Therefore, most of the economic and social costs of industrial disease are borne not by the companies that may have acted irresponsibly but by the victims and the taxpayers, including businesses that are trying to protect their employees properly.

Physicians are often reluctant to become involved with workers' compensation, believing that a claim may tie them up in court. This is an unsubstantiated fear, because the medical record usually provides sufficient medical evidence and the physician does not have to appear at the hearing. If the record does not provide adequate information, the attorneys involved are almost always willing to take a statement at the physician's convenience.

PART-TIME OCCUPATIONAL HEALTH PHYSICIAN

A primary care practitioner may become involved in a workplace at the invitation of the employer or the union representing the employees. Many small- and medium-sized workplaces need the assistance of part-time physicians to conduct effective programs to detect and prevent occupational disease. A physician who takes on an occupational health role should become thoroughly acquainted with the goals and procedures of the proposed program, as well as the applicable regulations. Table 8.5 lists the principal responsibilities that an occupational physician might be asked to assume and the sources of regulations that guide these physician responsibilities. The American College of Occupational and Environmental Medicine (ACOEM) sponsors regular training sessions to keep its members and interested physicians up to date in these roles.

Some physicians in occupational medicine regard themselves as responsible to the management of the company that pays them, rather than to the patients they serve. In some instances, physicians have withheld information from patients about work-related diseases. In other cases, physicians modify their therapy for illnesses and injuries to meet the needs of production rather than the needs of the patient. This role of the company physician as a servant of management rather than of the patient has had tacit acceptance in the past. In the last decade, the ACOEM has called for adherence to ethical practice, and many abuses have been ended. Today, physicians who apply a different standard of practice while acting as plant physicians may face professional discipline and malpractice suits. Table 8.6 summarizes the principal ethical responsibilities of an occupational health physician.

PHYSICIANS AND HEALTH CARE INSTITUTIONS AS EMPLOYERS

Promulgation of the OSHA Blood-Borne Pathogens Standard has reminded physicians and health care organizations of their responsibilities to those they employ and supervise. Most hospitals and state and local medical societies have available information and instructional material to simplify compliance with the requirements for protective equipment, immunization, and education. The basic components of universal precautions to protect health workers from infected body fluids are summarized in Table 39.16, and postexposure actions to address the risk of acquiring hepatitis or human immunodeficiency virus infection are summarized in Tables 18.5 and 39.17, respectively.

HAZARDS AT HOME AND IN THE COMMUNITY

Exposures at Home

The average American home is a Pandora's box of potentially harmful exposures. Between kitchen, bathroom, garage, and garden, family members may have access to caustics, a variety of aerosols, pesticides, solvents, paint removers, adhesives, and electrical equipment. These types of exposure should be considered when warning about childproofing for toddlers and when evaluating dermatoses and allergic reactions. Exposures at home may also produce illness in ways that come less readily to mind (Table 8.7). Case reports have documented poisoning from inappropriate use of cosmetics and vitamin supplements. Many hobbies can involve exposure to chemicals with fewer protections than workers in industry enjoy. For example, lead poisoning has been documented from ceramics, stained glasswork, and cosmetics; paint strippers containing methylene chloride can produce carbon monoxide poisoning sufficient to aggravate angina and precipitate infarction; and injudicious combinations of cleaning materials can release hazardous fumes. Homes themselves may have hazards. For example, lead-containing paints are a risk to both children and do-it-yourself enthusiasts, and formaldehyde-urea foam insulation can release sensitizing fumes. In cases of illness caused by such exposures, physicians need to take a careful history to recognize the cause.

Heating and ventilation systems deserve special mention. Even up-to-date heating systems can produce carbon monoxide poisoning if flues are blocked or inadequate air for combustion is provided. Because symptoms of early carbon monoxide poisoning are nonspecific and mimic those of stress and depression, a high level of suspicion is critical, especially early in the heating season. With the current emphasis on increased insulation and barriers to air infiltration, houses are often poorly ventilated by fresh air. The increasing use of wood, coal, and kerosene heaters may make matters worse. Use of scrap lumber treated with chemical preservatives is an additional hazard.

Table 8.7. Common Hazards at Home

Heating and air conditioning
Water damage and mold
Insulation and lack of ventilation
Vitamins and health foods
Cleaning chemicals
Lead-containing paint
Electric appliances
Water supply
Hobbies
Home repair
Neighborhood pollution sources

Leaking roofs and windows can lead to water damage to ceilings and walls. Condensation onto concrete slabs under carpet also can cause damp conditions. Water damage is the major cause of disruption of lead-containing paint and can give rise to significant growth of mold.

Office and commercial buildings are also increasingly tight, as heated or cooled air is recycled. Many epidemics of illness caused by chemical or biologic agents circulated through the air are being reported. Building-associated illness can be caused by exposure to particulates, chemical fumes from cleaning materials and office equipment, and mold spores or other biologic antigens. Because symptoms are often nonspecific, diagnosis may depend on recognizing a temporal pattern or symptoms in coworkers. Evaluation of the ventilation system often reveals inadequacies, and in many situations, improved ventilation may be all the therapy that is needed.

Exposures from Sources in the Community

Physicians are increasingly being asked for advice relating to concerns about contaminated drinking water and air and the cleanup of toxic wastes. Many communities dependent on groundwater have had their supplies threatened by illegal dumping of chemicals or by leakage from licensed landfills.

There is no substitute in such situations for enlisting the assistance of appropriate experts, and physicians in a community may be expected to take the lead in getting help from state and local agencies. Often there is a continuing role for practitioners to play in facilitating the resolution of problems. In many cases, knowledgeable specialists have difficulty in translating what they have to say into language that the lay public can understand. Physicians, who spend a good part of their days translating medical science into advice for their patients in the office, are well suited to serve in this role. At the same time, community members may need someone who can represent their acute personal concerns to the authorities in a reasoned way. A physician can serve as advocate and critical reviewer for the community, making sure that the statements and positions of all of those involved are supported by factual evidence and calling on independent expertise when appropriate. The Agency for Toxic Substances and Disease Registry of the USPHS has made a commitment to support physicians in communities affected by environmental contamination with information and assistance. Emergency help is available 24 hours a day by telephone at 404-488-4100.

Table 8.8. Checklists for Physicians and Others Involved in Hazardous Materials Incidents

What toxic and hazardous substances have been identified?
What are the concentrations in air, water, and soil?
What are the known health hazards at these concentrations?
What are the potential hazards of fire, explosion, or chemical interactions?
How many people have been exposed and how many are likely to become exposed in the near future?
What groups in the exposed population are likely to be most susceptible to health effects?
How many exposures are resulting in hospital admissions? Outpatient visits?
What clinical findings, if any, are being observed?
What technical resources are available on short notice to assist in evaluation and control? Is there a local Hazardous Materials Team?
Is the community adequately handling the casualties?
What is the capacity of local hospitals, clinics, and physicians to absorb the additional caseload?
Should hospital disaster plans be mobilized?
Are intensive care or specialty services adequate or available to the degree needed?
Are local physicians experienced and knowledgeable about this kind of problem? If not, what is the best way to obtain expert help quickly?
Is this community covered by a repository (such as a tumor registry of population-based research study) that could be used to monitor the exposed population in the future?

Air Pollution

Patients with respiratory disease are especially concerned about the effects of air pollution. Patients often develop symptoms of respiratory tract irritation during periods of severe pollution, and patients with cardiac or respiratory disease may suffer exacerbations. Prudent advice is in order in such situations. Advice to move to less polluted areas is rarely practical, and such advice should be given only after a great deal of thought about the impact of a move on the patient's entire life. Durable solutions to problems caused by air pollution depend on efforts to limit industrial discharges and, importantly, the emissions of automobiles. Pollution of indoor air in workplaces and in public facilities from cigarette smoking is an equally important challenge to the medical profession and to each community. In recent years, the increase in smoke-free public places has significantly reduced exposure to this form of air pollution. In most states, the American Lung Association is leading the struggle for clean air.

Hazardous Materials: Accidents and Disposal

Physicians with no special background in toxicology or public health may be pressed into service in cases of accidental emissions of toxic fumes or accidents involving transport of hazardous materials.

In responding to such emergencies, a practitioner should clarify immediately that the hazard is being contained as effectively as possible, that people not needed at the scene are not being exposed, and that orderly procedures for the care of casualties are being set up. Many communities have developed a coordinated plan for response to hazardous materials incidents. Usually the local emergency response system (fire department or 911 system) will alert a hazardous materials (HAZMAT) team. A checklist is provided in Table 8.8.

General References

Baxter PJ, Adam PH, eds. Hunter's diseases of occupations. 9th ed. Oxford: Arnold, 2000.

Excellent descriptions of clinical syndromes, updated from a classic textbook.

McCunney RJ. A practical approach to occupational and environmental medicine. Boston: Little, Brown, 1994.

Has good material for the part-time occupational physician.

Paul M. Occupational and environmental reproductive hazards. Baltimore: Williams & Wilkins, 1993.

The best available text about reproductive health and the environment.

Rosenstock L, Cullen MR. Clinical occupational medicine. Philadelphia: WB Saunders, 1994.

A good text organized by both organ system and type of hazard.

Sullivan JB, Kreiger GR, eds. Clinical environmental health and toxic exposures. Baltimore: Lippincott: Williams & Wilkins, 2001.

Excellent source for information on specific environmental toxins.

Zenz C. Occupational medicine. Chicago: Mosby–Year Book Medical Publishers, 1994.

Especially good for physicians involved in providing occupational health services.

CHAPTER 9

Selected Special Services: Disability Insurance, Vocational Rehabilitation, and Home Health Services

L. RANDOL BARKER, MD, ScD

Maintenance of a patient's overall health often requires efforts beyond those of the physician and the patient. Often, assistance comes from community-based programs to which physicians may refer their patients. Many of these programs provide services for patients with specific types of illnesses; the roles of such categorical community services are described in the appropriate chapters in this book. Other services are designed to assist patients regardless of their type of illness. This chapter describes three services of this kind: Social Security programs for disabled people, vocational rehabilitation, and home health services. The purpose of this chapter is to explain eligibility for these services, the nature of the benefits, and the role of physicians in enabling their patients to receive these services. Chapter 8 provides similar information about another noncategorical program, worker's compensation, which is designed to provide coverage for health care costs and income support to people with work-related diseases.

SOCIAL SECURITY PROGRAMS FOR DISABLED PEOPLE

Loss or decrease of a person's ability to earn a living accompanies many illnesses. Beginning with 1954 amendments to the Social Security Act, income support for medically disabled people has been available in the United States. Further modifications since 1954 have led to the program that exists today. Three fundamental benefits are currently available through the Society Security Administration: disability insurance (DI), Supplemental Security Income (SSI), and Medicare (health insurance for DI recipients). Medicaid is a federally and state-administered health insurance program that is available automatically in many states for people who receive SSI and for mothers of dependent children whose incomes are below the poverty level. Detailed information about each of these services is available from any local Social Security office.

Definition of Medical Disability

The Social Security Act defines disability as the "inability to engage in any substantial gainful activity by reason of a medically determinable physical or mental impairment that can be expected to result in death or has lasted or can be expected to last for a continuous period of not less than 12 months."

Disability Insurance (Title II of the Social Security Act)

Eligibility

To be eligible for DI payments, a disabled worker must have paid into the Social Security program for a minimum period of time before becoming disabled; in addition, there is a requirement for coverage during 5 of the 10 years before the onset of disability. Today, 9 of 10 workers and their employers pay the Social Security tax (Federal Insurance Contributions Act, or "FICA"). For younger workers (up to age 31), there are modified requirements to meet insured status.

Disabled dependents of a fully insured worker who is retired, disabled, or deceased may be eligible for DI payments in two situations: *a child* who became disabled before age 22 (eligible for DI payments at the time that the child's parent retires, becomes disabled, or dies; payments may begin as early as age 18 and continue as long as the child's disability lasts) and *a widow or widower* who is between 50 and 59 years of age and who did not work under Social Security but who became medically disabled before or within 7 years of the death of a fully insured spouse.

Benefits

DI payments go to disabled workers before the age of 65 (after 65, Social Security Retirement Income replaces disability payments) and to eligible children, widows, or widowers as long as they remain disabled. The first monthly DI check is not paid for the first 5 months after the onset of the worker's disability (e.g., a patient who is certified as disabled 6 calendar months after becoming disabled immediately becomes eligible for a check covering the 1 month in excess of the required 5-month wait). SSI (see below) is often awarded to people who are found to be "presumptively disabled," effective the first day of the month that follows the month in which they apply for benefits. Income from DI for a disabled worker is the same amount as the retirement income the worker would receive if he or she were 65.

In 1999, the average monthly payments were $754 to disabled workers and $775 to nondisabled widows and widowers. In that year, 4.9 million disabled workers and 1.6 million spouses and children were receiving DI benefits. The leading causes of disability for disabled workers were mental disorders (27%) that do not involve retardation and musculoskeletal conditions (23%). About 11% had circulatory conditions, and 10% had diseases of the nervous system (1).

In addition to income support, disabled people under age 65 receive Medicare (Social Security Health Insurance) after they have been eligible for disability benefits for 24 months. Patients with end-stage renal disease receive Medicare coverage effective when they begin long-term dialysis.

Process of Disability Determination

There are a number of steps in the process of determining medical disability.

- The patient completes a detailed application at a local social security office. The patient must not be gainfully employed at the time of application. In 2001, *gainful employment* was defined as an activity that yields a monthly income of $740 for those with impairments other than blindness and $1,240 for people who are blind (2). Most patients initiate disability claims by themselves, but at times a physician or social worker suggests application to a patient who is not aware that his or her condition qualifies as a medical disability.
- The patient's physician receives a request for medical information and returns this report to the state Disability Determination office. The report sent by the patient's physician should be succinct and precise and should provide objective data regarding the condition for which disability is being claimed. It should be divided into the following subheadings: history, physical, laboratory reports, diagnosis, treatment, and response. The report should also describe the individual's ability to perform work-related activities (e.g., sitting, standing, walking, lifting, carrying, handling objects, hearing, speaking, traveling; for mentally-impaired persons, the ability to understand, to remember instructions, or to respond appropriately to supervision). The information provided should permit claim reviewers to determine both the severity and the duration of the patient's condition. If malingering is suspected, the report should describe the circumstances that raise doubts rather than recording this assessment without supporting information. The most helpful guide for completing these medical reports is the booklet *Disability Evaluation Under Social Security* (available free from any Social Security office or the state Disability Determination office). This manual, which was most recently revised in 2001, lists, with criteria that must be met, most conditions that are so severe they automatically qualify an individual for DI. These are referred to as Medical Listings. Tables 9.1 through 9.4 illustrate the criteria listed for four common conditions: chronic obstructive pulmonary disease, cerebrovascular accident, epilepsy due to major motor seizures, and arthritis of a major weight-bearing joint. The conditions in the Medical Listings are the basis for most DI allowances made by disability claim reviewers. Since 1980 the Social Security Administration has paid a small fee to physicians for medical reports for the DI program; a small fee has also been paid for SSI reports since the inception of that program in 1974. Previously, patients were expected to pay for these reports. In some states, doctors also have access to a free teledictation service for dictating their reports.

Table 9.1. Impairments Qualifying a Person with Chronic Obstructive Pulmonary Disease for Medical Disability Under Social Security

Height Without Shoes (cm)	Height Without Shoes (inches)	FEV_1 Equal to or Less Than (L)
154 or less	60 or less	1.05
155–160	61–63	1.15
161–165	64–65	1.25
166–170	66–67	1.35
171–175	68–69	1.45
176–180	70–71	1.55
181 or more	72 or more	1.65

Chronic obstructive pulmonary disease due to cause, with the FEV_1 equal to or less than the values specified in this table corresponding to the person's height without shoes. (In cases of marked spinal deformity, see 3.00E.)

FEV_1, forced expiratory volume in 1 second.

From Disability Evaluation Under Social Security, 2001, with permission.

Table 9.2. Impairments Qualifying a Person with Central Nervous System Vascular Accident for Medical Disability Under Social Security

Central nervous system vascular accident, with one of the following more than 3 months postvascular accident:

A. Sensory or motor aphasia resulting in ineffective speech or communication, or

B. Significant and persistent disorganization of motor function in two extremities, resulting in sustained disturbance of gross and dexterous movements or gait and station.

From Disability Evaluation Under Social Security, 2001, with permission.

Table 9.3. Impairments Qualifying a Person with Epilepsy Due to Major Motor Seizures for Medical Disability Under Social Security

Major motor seizures (grand mal or psychomotor), documented by EEG and by detailed description of a typical seizure pattern, including all associated phenomena: occurring more frequently than once a month, despite at least 3 months of prescribed treatment[a] with

A. Daytime episodes (loss of consciousness and convulsive seizures), *or*

B. Nocturnal episodes manifesting residuals that interfere significantly with activity during the day.

[a]Adherence to therapy must be objectively confirmed by measurements of drug levels that are in the therapeutic range.

EEG, electroencephalogram.

From Disability Evaluation Under Social Security, 2001, with permission.

Table 9.4. Impairments Qualifying a Person with Arthritis of a Major Weight-bearing Joint for Medical Disability Under Social Security

Arthritis of a major weight-bearing joint (due to any cause) with history of persistent joint pain and stiffness with signs of marked limitation of motion or abnormal motion of the affected joint on current physical examination with
A. Gross anatomic deformity of hip or knee (e.g., subluxation, contracture, bony or fibrous ankylosis, instability) supported by x-ray evidence of either significant joint space narrowing or significant bony destruction *and* markedly limiting ability to walk or stand, *or*
B. Reconstructive surgery or surgical arthrodesis of a major weight-bearing joint and return to full weight-bearing status did not occur, or is not expected to occur, within 12 months of onset

From Disability Evaluation Under Social Security, 2001, with permission.

- The information provided by the patient and the physician (the disability claim) is reviewed by the state Disability Determination Service (DDS) by a team comprised of a disability claims examiner and a physician. If deemed necessary, an independent medical examination is purchased by the DDS. In keeping with the 1974 Freedom of Information Act, patients may have access to their disability claim files.

If an insured worker has an impairment that does not meet the standard criteria for disability but nevertheless claims inability to do his or her usual job, the DDS obtains additional information to determine the claimant's residual functional capacity to perform past work despite the impairment(s). If the past work was such that the impairment would prevent performing the work, DDS proceeds to a last step to determine if the claimant can do other work. Limitations of age, education, training, and work experience are considered by the DDS team in establishing whether a worker is able to perform "other work."

Appeals Process

If the initial claim of disability has been denied, the claimant may file for reconsideration within 60 days of receiving a denial notice. The case is then reevaluated by a different DDS team. If the claim is denied at this reconsideration, the claimant has 60 days to file a request for a hearing. Hearings are conducted by administrative law judges. If the claim is again denied, the claimant may make an additional appeal for review by the Appeals Council. After that, the case may be taken to the United States District Court.

A patient's personal physician can be instrumental in ensuring that the patient gets the fullest consideration throughout the Disability Determination process. If the physician believes there are aspects of the patient's illness that make it more severe than the criteria indicate, the physician should communicate this information in writing, together with support for this opinion, to the Disability Determination office.

Periodic Review and Return to Work Incentives

All claims are reviewed for referral to vocational rehabilitation (see below) at the time the disability decision is made. In addition, every person with a permanent impairment is reevaluated every 5 to 7 years. Those expected to improve are reviewed 6 to 8 months after the DI decision is made, and those in whom improvement is possible but less predictable are reviewed about every 3 years. Even if the original impairment is judged not to be severe on review, payments are continued for those who have started a vocational rehabilitation program because of improvement in their medical condition; benefits continue until the rehabilitation services are completed or until the person stops receiving these services. The purpose of these processes, and the following conditions, is to encourage disabled people to return to work:

- Disabled beneficiaries may test their ability to work for 9 months while continuing to receive benefits. After this trial work period, a determination is made about whether the work constitutes substantial gainful activity (defined in 2001 as an activity that yields a monthly income of $740 or more); if it does, benefits are suspended after an additional 3-month adjustment period (2).
- If a person who still has a disabling impairment stops work again within 36 months after Social Security payments have been suspended because of substantial gainful activity, the monthly DI benefits can be resumed, usually without a new application.
- A worker can usually continue to have Medicare coverage for at least 39 months after his or her DI benefits stop because of return to substantial gainful activity. If a worker starts receiving DI benefits again within 5 years after the DI was stopped and if the patient was previously entitled to Medicare, that protection resumes immediately.
- Work expenses related to the impairment that are paid for by a disabled person may be deducted from the patient's earnings in determining whether these constitute substantial gainful activity. This is true even if these expenses also apply to needs for daily living (e.g., a wheelchair).

In addition to disabled workers, workers' children who became disabled before the age of 22 and disabled widows and widowers can also have a trial work period.

The *Red Book on Employment Status,* available from Social Security, provides details about all aspects of the return to work process (2).

Supplemental Security Income

SSI is a federal program introduced in 1974 under Title XVI of the Social Security Act. It is paid for out of general funds rather than Social Security funds, but it is administered by the same state agencies that administer the Disability Determination program. The application process is similar to that described above for Social Security DI. Applications are filed at a local Social Security office, and the same criteria are used to evaluate SSI disability claims as are used for DI claims.

The basic differences between SSI and Social Security benefits are as follows:

- *Eligibility.* SSI is available for two groups of people when they are not insured by Social Security: those under age 65 who are medically disabled and all uninsured people over the age of 65. SSI for people over age 65 is similar in purpose to Social Security retirement income. In addition to these two groups, people who have presumptive disability (claim for total disability being processed) and disabled people who are in the 5-month waiting period for their DI payments to begin may be eligible for SSI. Eligibility in all these groups is based on need (total resources found to be below a certain defined level) and the absence of gainful employment (defined as earned monthly income of $740 or more).
- There is no waiting period. A person becomes eligible for the first SSI payment the first day of the month after he or she files a disability claim.

In most states, people approved for SSI are also eligible for Medicaid and other social services provided by their state. All people receiving SSI are reviewed once each year to determine whether their income and other resources still make them eligible to receive SSI. Like DI recipients, they are reviewed every 3 or 7 years to establish whether their disability is still present (see above).

The maximal monthly income from SSI was increased in 2000 to $500 for an individual and $769 for a couple. In 1999 there were 6.6 million recipients of SSI, on the basis of disability, blindness, and age (over age 65 and without Social Security). Most had a mental disorder: 24% mental retardation and 34% another mental disorder (1).

As described for DI, the report of a patient's physician must be received before income support under SSI can be initiated.

VOCATIONAL REHABILITATION

State vocational rehabilitation agencies existed before the federal Disability Determination program was created in 1954. In many states, these agencies administer the Disability Determination program in addition to providing vocational rehabilitation services.

Eligibility

To be eligible for vocational rehabilitation, a person must have an impairment that interferes with his or her capacity to obtain suitable employment or that is a threat to his or her present career; this does not mean that the person has to meet the criteria for medical disability discussed earlier. The person must have a reasonable chance of being able to engage in a suitable occupation after vocational rehabilitation services are provided. A suitable occupation would include being a homemaker provided that vocational rehabilitation would enable the person to remain in his or her own home instead of requiring institutional care.

Services

The services provided by vocational rehabilitation agencies vary among states. However, they usually include the following:

- *A medical examination.* A complete medical examination is provided to determine the extent of a person's disability.
- *Counseling and guidance.* A trained rehabilitation counselor is assigned to guide each client through the rehabilitation process.
- *Physical aids.* Items such as artificial limbs, braces, hearing aids, eyeglasses, and wheelchairs may be provided if needed.
- *Job training.* Training for the proper job is provided when necessary. This may be given at a vocational school, college or university, rehabilitation facility, or in the home.
- *Help with transportation expenses.*
- *Equipment and licenses.* Tools, equipment, and licenses necessary for getting started in the right job may be provided.
- *Job placement.* Placement in the right job is an important part of the rehabilitation process. The abilities of each client are carefully matched to job requirements.
- *Follow-up.* The counselor follows up on each placement to make sure that the client's job is suitable.

Physician's Role

As noted earlier, all people applying for Social Security disability benefits are screened for referral to vocational rehabilitation. For those people, the report of the patient's physician (see above) may be used by the vocational rehabilitation agency. For people who are not applying for medical disability, the physician is often asked to provide a general medical report for the vocational rehabilitation agency. An important role of physicians is to encourage patients to apply for vocational rehabilitation and to maintain continued interest in their progress. It has been estimated that every $1,000 spent for vocational rehabilitation increases by $35,000 the lifetime earnings of those who are rehabilitated.

HOME HEALTH SERVICES

A consequence of illness as distressing to the patient as the loss of the ability to earn an income is the temporary or permanent loss of the ability to remain at home. Most people require acute hospital care one or more times in their adult lives, and a small proportion also require long-term institutional care. The principal objectives of home health services are to minimize the need for admission to acute or long-term care facilities and to decrease length of stay and associated costs in these facilities.

National Trends

Home health care is the sector of the health care industry that grew the most in the past decade (3). Growth in home health initially accelerated after passage of the Omnibus Reconciliation Acts of 1980 and 1981, which increased funding for home health services by Medicare and Medicaid. Between 1980 and 1995, the number of patients served per year grew from about 0.9 million to approximately 3.6 million for Medicare and from about 0.4 million to approximately 1.4 million for Medicaid. More recently, cost-effectiveness initiatives from the managed care industry have further promoted home care as an alternative to hospital care.

Range of Services and Providers

Home health services provided include basic care provided by informal caregivers (family members and friends), home food services available at a nominal cost to the patient (Meals-on-Wheels), care provided by physicians or their associates who make home visits, services provided by the personnel of home health agencies, specimen collection and performance of diagnostic procedures such as radiographs and electrocardiograms by clinical laboratories, and delivery/rental by medical suppliers of infusion equipment, medications, and durable medical equipment such as hospital beds. Even when professional help is involved, most of the responsibility for carrying out care is assumed by the patient or a member of the patient's family; as noted in Chapter 1, it is the assumption of responsibility by patients and their families that most distinguishes ambulatory care from institutional care.

Overall coordination of the home care provided by home health agencies is usually provided by a nurse case manager. A substantial proportion of the care is often carried out by home health aides, analogous to nursing aides on hospital wards, under the supervision of the nurse. In recent years, nurse practitioners, enterostomal therapists, and clinical pharmacy consultants have been added to the staffs of many home health agencies, so that more sophisticated care can be provided. In addition to nursing, home care services may include physical, occupational, and speech therapy; nutritional, behavioral, and social work counseling; and mental health services. Home health agencies provide the professional services of *hospice programs* (see Chapter 13) in many communities or may have their own hospice programs. In addition, *maternal and child health programs* have been developed to respond to the needs created by rapid discharge of mothers and newborns.

In recent years, home health agencies and suppliers have added services that require skilled use of equipment traditionally used only in hospitals. These services include the administration of *intravenous therapies,* ranging from short-term normal saline and electrolyte infusions to courses of antibiotics, cancer chemotherapy, cardiac medications, and total parenteral nutrition, and the care of *ventilator-dependent patients* at home. These initiatives have emerged in response to efforts to reduce the length of costly hospitalization for patients who prefer home care to hospital care for parenteral therapy that may have to be administered for 1 week or more. Day-to-day supervision of the overall care of patients receiving in-home parenteral therapy or ventilator support is usually not provided by the company that supplies and monitors the equipment; therefore, this responsibility is assumed by a nurse case manager who knows the physician's comprehensive plan for the patient and is in close contact with the supplier.

The types of clinical problems most commonly referred to home health agencies are listed in Table 9.5.

Criteria for Third-Party Reimbursement

Any patient or patient's family may purchase services from a home health agency. During the past 25 years, much of the cost of home care has been covered by Medicare, Medicaid, other third-party payers, and managed care organizations. The number and types of services authorized are being more tightly controlled today as part of cost-containment efforts. Effective 2001, Medicare changed from a cost-based to a prospective payment approach, similar to the diagnosis-related group approach to paying for hospital care. These changes have promoted the development of detailed care guidelines and increased focus on instructing patients and family members to carry out care plans. Patients must meet the generic criteria listed in Table 9.6 for services to be reimbursed by Medicare and other third-party payers.

Medicare pays for "intermittent" home care services, defined as no more than 35 hours per week. There must be a documented goal of care that has a finite

Table 9.5. Problems Most Commonly Referred for Home Health Services

Postsurgical wound care (teach or provide dressing changes)
Orthopedic problems (rehabilitation after hospitalization)
Congestive heart failure (monitor for change in status, provide dietary counseling, assess medication compliance)
Diabetes (e.g., supervise insulin technique, provide dietary counseling, teach blood or urine monitoring of glucose, care of the lower extremities)
Incurable cancer and AIDS (provide dietary counseling, intravenous therapies, psychological support, and other aspects of hospice care)[a]
Stroke and other incapacitating neurologic problems (provide physical and occupational therapy)
Decubitus and stasis ulcers (teach or provide debridement and dressing changes)
Dementia in an older person living alone (assess environment for health hazards)
Chronic obstructive pulmonary disease (assess home for oxygen therapy, teach energy conservation strategies)

[a]See details in Chapter 13.

AIDS, acquired immunodeficiency syndrome.

Table 9.6. Criteria for Third-party Reimbursement for Home Health Services

Medicare[a,b]
Part A pays 100% for all covered services (skilled nursing, home health aide, social work, physical, occupational, and speech therapy). Care must be provided by a certified home health agency and must be medically necessary. The following conditions must be met to qualify for reimbursement:
1. Patient is *homebound* (i.e., the patient's condition interferes with the normal ability to leave the home or leaving the home would require a considerable effort).
2. Need for *intermittent* skilled nursing, physical therapy, or speech therapy. (One of these three services must be needed to qualify for reimbursement for the other services provided by home health agencies, i.e., social work, occupational therapy, home health aide, and nutrition services.)
3. Physician must sign renewal of orders every 60 days.

Medicaid
Coverage for home health services varies by state.
Veterans Administration
Home care from hospital-based programs
Blue Cross and other private health insurance
Coverage for home health services varies by plan.

[a]Note that since 1981, Part A Medicare has covered patients even if they have not been recently hospitalized.
[b]See Chapter 13 for details regarding hospice criteria and benefits.

end point. Because of the Medicare criterion that the patient must have a medical problem requiring skilled care, payment for the services of a home health aide is often denied after the active problem becomes stable, even when the home health aide's services are important in maintaining the patient's health. In some instances, Medicaid funding is available for ongoing personal care services, provided in lieu of nursing home care.

Physician's Role

For home health services that are reimbursed, the patient's physician must approve and sign orders for all services and revisions of services. Medicare requires an extensive report and newly signed orders every 2 months.

The quality of the communication between physicians and home care providers often determines how much the patient will benefit from home health services. When physicians provide clear and complete initial information and both physicians and home care providers can reach each other easily when needed, patients who would otherwise require in-hospital care can receive excellent care in their homes.

The American Academy of Home Care Physicians (website: www.aahcp.org) is an organization of physicians and other home care professionals, founded in the late 1980s, that is dedicated to improving the quality of home care. The organization's newsletter, other publications, and annual meeting focus on the evaluation of and education about home health care ideas and programs.

General References

Disability evaluation under Social Security SSA Publication No. 64-039. January 2001. *www.ssa.gov/disability/professionals/bluebook/AdultListings*.htm.

Gives criteria for impairments that qualify a person for medical disability under Social Security (available free from local Social Security Office and State Disability Determination Service).

Rothkopf MM, ed. Standards and practice of homecare therapeutics, 2nd ed. Baltimore: Williams & Wilkins, 1997.

A practical resource for physicians who authorize home care for their patients. Contains separate chapters on each of the sophisticated modes of care now available through home health agencies.

Social Security Administration Office of Program, Policy, and Evaluation and Communications. Understanding SSI. SSA Publication No. 17-008, ICN 443175, May 1996.

Explains all aspects of SSI. Useful for patients and providers.

Specific References

1. Social Security Administration Annual Statistical Supplement 2000 (website: www.ssa.gov/statistics/Supplement/2000/).
2. Social Security Administration. 2001 Red book on employment support: a summary guide to employment support available to people with disabilities under the Social Security Disability Insurance and Supplemental Security Income Programs. SSA Publication No. 64-030, ICN 436900, January 2001.
3. Basic statistics about home care 1996. Washington, DC: National Association for Home Care, October 1996.

CHAPTER 10

Care of the Patient with Cancer

LARRY WATERBURY, MD
MICHAEL J. PURTELL, MD, PhD

The purpose of this chapter is to examine the role of the generalist in caring for patients who have cancer. Common cancers are discussed in other chapters (breast, Chapter 105; gastrointestinal, Chapter 45; gynecologic, Chapter 104; lung, Chapter 61; prostate, Chapter 53; skin, Chapter 114). The estimated distribution of newly diagnosed cancers and cancer deaths for 2001 is depicted in Fig. 10.1. After initial diagnostic evaluation, the location of the primary cancer is unidentified in some patients with metastatic disease. The most common primary cancers that are eventually identified in such patients are cancers of the pancreas, lung, kidney, and colon (1).

GENERAL ASPECTS OF CARE

Communicating the Diagnosis

A patient's primary care provider is the one who is most likely to initiate diagnostic evaluation for cancer and to communicate the diagnosis to the patient. During these initial steps, the following elements are important: promptly scheduling tests and notifying the patient of results; communicating clearly; allowing the patient ample time to react to bad news; promptly explaining options/recommendations, based on the type and extent of the cancer; checking patient's understanding of and questions about information that has been given; and including family members that the patient selects in all discussions regarding diagnosis, options, and prognosis. Chapters 3 and 4 discuss in detail approaches to communication with patients and their family members.

Initial Referral and Treatment

When possible, one should refer patients to oncologists whom one trusts and knows to be helpful, considerate clinicians. Multimodality treatment regimens involving the combined efforts of surgical, medical, and radiation oncologists may result in a bewildered patient without a clinician who accepts the primary responsibility for care. The patient's primary care practitioner should either coordinate care or identify who will be the coordinator for the patient's care and who will be accessible to the patient to answer questions, provide support, and ensure that necessary information is communicated. By receiving up to date and complete information about the diagnostic and therapeutic plans and the patient's evolving status, the primary care practitioner may be able to assess the overall picture and, as time goes on, identify when problems resulting from treatment (e.g., side effects, expense, family disruption, and deteriorating psychological status of patient) outweigh the likely benefits of continued therapy.

Follow-Up Care

Most oncologists welcome participation of the patient's primary care practitioner in continuing care. This is particularly important when treatment is given in an oncology center in a distant city. Some less toxic ambulatory treatment regimens and particularly symptom management strategies may even be handled by the primary care practitioner under the direction of the specialist.

The follow-up of treated patients requires knowledge of the common sites and manifestations of tumor recurrence and the appropriate timing of follow-up examinations and tests and a great deal of sensitivity in recognizing the feelings of the patient and the patient's family. Chapters elsewhere in this book on specific cancers discuss what is known and what is not known about the utility of follow-up assessments. Some patients function better if they are scheduled to be seen less frequently, not to be constantly reminded of the possibility of recurrence. Others require the constant reassurance of a negative examination and normal tests and are more comfortable with frequent follow-up visits. Usually there is room for considerable flexibility in a follow-up plan without jeopardizing the health of the patient.

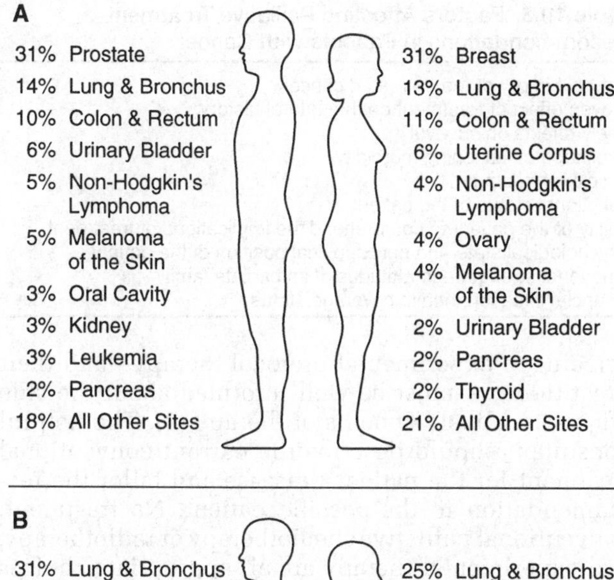

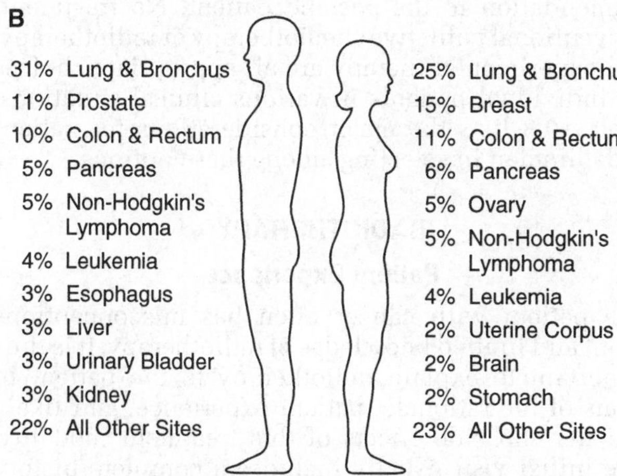

Figure 10.1. Estimated new cancer cases **(A)** and estimated cancer deaths **(B)** in 10 leading sites by sex, United States, 2001; excludes basal and squamous cell skin cancer and carcinoma *in situ* except bladder. (From Greenlee RT, Hill-Harmon MB, Murray T, Thun M. Cancer statistics 2001. CA Cancer J Clin 2001;51:15, with permission.)

Whenever a patient with cancer is seen in follow-up, it is important to explain carefully the meaning of symptoms or physical findings and the rationale for tests. If tests will take several days to return, that should be explained and a time for a telephone follow-up arranged.

It is possible in the future that *tumor markers* measured in the patient's serum—either to screen for cancer or to monitor therapy in patients with disseminated cancer—may be shown to have important utility in patient care. A critical analysis published in 1991 (2) and a more recent National Cancer Institute report (3) described potential roles for tumor markers in clinical decision-making. Although tumor markers can be useful in monitoring the progress of known disease and the response to therapy, these are uses that benefit patients chiefly as part of the care plan of an oncologist or other specialist who is treating them. The routine use of tumor markers to screen for cancer in the asymptomatic patient remains potentially harmful, and there is no current consensus regarding any of the available markers, including the prostate specific antigen (see discussion in Table 14.2 and Chapter 53). Generally, it is inappropriate to monitor tumor markers routinely as part of the follow-up of patients with cancer who are potentially cured after primary and adjuvant therapy. This issue has been particularly well studied in patients with breast cancer (4).

Family Concerns

The crises attending evaluation for possible cancer and the diagnosis and care for cancer profoundly affect the spouses and families of patients. Common dilemmas for family members include emotional strain, physical demands in caring for the patient, altered roles and life-styles, finances, and uncertainty about prognosis (5). In addition, there may be questions about the likelihood of cancer occurring in other members of the family. Each of these issues may require consideration by the patient's primary care practitioner (for details, see chapters on specific cancers and Chapters 13, 17, and 20).

Support from the American Cancer Society

The American Cancer Society has chapters in each state and can provide a variety of services to patients and their families. Services vary among states but may include loan of supplies (e.g., hospital beds), transportation to treatment facilities, reduced costs for chemotherapy, respite coverage for caregivers, and a wide range of information about support groups and other help available in the patient's community.

NONOPERABLE CANCERS IN WHICH TREATMENT MAY PROLONG SURVIVAL

Table 10.1 lists a number of nonoperable cancers in which survival may be prolonged by modern treatment regimens; patients with such cancers need ongoing follow up with cancer specialists. These patients often benefit from multimodality treatment. Even within this group of cancers, when specialty help is needed, the primary care practitioner continues to play an important role, especially if the relationship with the patient or the family has been a lengthy one.

Table 10.1. Some Nonoperable Cancers in which Treatment May Be Curative or Dramatically Prolong Survival

Acute leukemia
Hodgkin disease
Lymphoma
Metastatic testicular cancer
Metastatic ovarian cancer
Small cell carcinoma of the lung
Metastatic breast cancer
Chronic myelocytic leukemia
Chronic lymphocytic leukemia
Multiple myeloma

Patients with these cancers require specialized multimodality therapy. Bone marrow and stem cell transplantation have a role in the treatment of some of these cancers.

CANCERS POORLY RESPONSIVE TO TREATMENT

Table 10.2 lists a number of cancers less responsive to therapy, where the impact of therapy on survival is unproven or minimal. Diagnosis and initial therapy usually require surgery, but when metastasis is proven, the effect of systemic therapy, radiotherapy, or both is at most palliative. In such situations, patients often expect their primary care practitioners to help them select or to actually recommend treatment plans. Several questions come up at this juncture.

Should palliative chemotherapy be recommended? Although it is difficult to generalize, several factors must be considered in attempting to help patients and their families decide whether the patient is likely to benefit from palliative chemotherapy. More than age, the functional status of the patient must be considered in such therapeutic decisions. The infirm, ill, poorly functional patient with widely disseminated and rapidly progressive disease may be more harmed than benefited by the side effects and discomforts of palliative treatment, especially if response rates are small and toxicity of treatment is high. Weight loss before therapy correlates closely with poor response rates in clinical chemotherapy trials in these less responsive cancers (6). Other patients, even if elderly, in good functional status are much more suitable candidates for attempts at palliation (7). The patient who believes that any chance of response is worth the price of toxicity and who cannot feel comfortable unless attempting some therapy should generally be offered treatment.

If some attempt at palliative treatment seems worthwhile, should it be conventional therapy or experimental protocol therapy? Every oncology center has current protocols for the metastatic cancers listed in Table 10.2. Clinical protocols designed to seek improved methods of treatment are important for advances that may improve the outlook and the comfort of future patients. However, experimental therapy may have undesirable consequences for the individual patient. Sometimes, such protocols involve the investigation of treatments with more toxicity than current conventional therapies. They may require more frequent visits to the clinician and more frequent diagnostic tests, because of the necessity to document precisely the objective response. They may therefore also involve increased expense to the patient. The patient's insurance may or may not cover the specific experimental therapy being considered. Patients agreeing to experimental protocol therapy—and their practitioners—must be well informed about the side effects and likely benefits of therapy (8). The helpful consultant should describe the current conventional treatment for the patient's disease and tailor the recommendation to the specific patient. No treatment, conventional palliative chemotherapy or radiotherapy, and experimental therapy are all appropriate choices for individual patients in various clinical situations. Table 10.3 lists the major considerations for patient and clinician in selecting among these options.

Table 10.2. Some Cancers in which Treatment May Provide Palliation or a Modest Effect on Survival

Non-small cell lung cancer (unresectable)
Metastatic large bowel cancer
Metastatic stomach cancer
Metastatic pancreatic cancer
Metastatic malignant melanoma
Metastatic soft tissue sarcomas
Metastatic cervical cancer
Metastatic endometrial cancer
Metastatic hypernephroma
Hormone refractory metastatic prostate cancer

Table 10.3. Factors Affecting Palliative Treatment Recommendations in Patients with Cancer

Natural history of the untreated cancer
Proven effect of treatment on the natural history
Likely effects on survival
Likelihood of lessening morbidity
Toxicity of treatment
Functional status of the patient
Ability of the patient to comprehend the implications of treatment
Psychological state and philosophical position of the patient
Emotional strength and attitudes of immediate family
Financial situation, health coverage status

RADIOTHERAPY

Patient Experience

The patient with cancer often has misconceptions about and limited knowledge of radiotherapy. It is thus important to explain radiotherapy to the patient in terms of the rationale, patient experience, and likely benefits and side effects of this treatment modality. The initial visit usually includes a complete history and physical examination by the radiotherapist. Further diagnostic tests (e.g., radiographs and computed tomography) may be obtained. If the therapist agrees that treatment is appropriate and urgent, the radiotherapy ports may be determined at the first visit and the patient may receive his or her first treatment at that time. The patient is told that skin tattoos may be placed to facilitate the uniformity of subsequent treatments. It is important to explain that the therapy machines are bulky and somewhat overwhelming in appearance. Some patients are frightened by the experience; if the referring clinician appreciates this, it is useful to contact the radiotherapist and to explain the particular fears of the patient ahead of time. Therapists often give patients and their families a tour of the radiotherapy treatment rooms before starting therapy and spend extra time answering questions about the treatment and its benefits and complications. The patient should be aware that the treatments themselves are not painful. The initial consultation is usually time-consuming (several hours), but subsequent treatments are usually scheduled precisely and frequently require only a small amount of time (15 to 30 minutes). Treatments are usually given several days a week, and the entire course may take several weeks to complete. The patient usually does not see the radiotherapist at the time of each treatment but is seen by a radiotherapy nurse or technician. The patient therefore needs to know precisely with whom to communicate to address side effects or questions during radiotherapy.

Time Until Symptomatic Response

In addition to the timing and types of side effects that may be experienced, it is important for the patient to know that the response to treatment is often delayed and that sometimes the maximal effect is noted a few weeks after the course of radiotherapy is completed. For example, radiotherapy is useful in the palliation of pain secondary to local bony metastases, but 2 to 3 weeks may elapse before improvement occurs and improvement may not be maximal until a few weeks after treatment is discontinued. Some responses are more rapid, occurring after only a few days of therapy (e.g., relief of superior vena caval obstruction and neurologic deficits from spinal cord obstruction or central nervous system metastasis).

An excellent booklet, *Radiation Therapy and You: A Guide to Self-Help During Treatment,* is available free from the National Institutes of Health to patients undergoing radiotherapy (see General References). It is helpful to have copies of this booklet available for patients and families to read when radiotherapy is being considered.

Side Effects

Table 10.4 describes important side effects of radiotherapy. The patient will be most concerned by the common side effects that occur during treatment and by those that may remain for a few weeks after treatment is discontinued.

Dermatitis secondary to radiotherapy is less common than it used to be because of the use of the modern high-energy machines. Severe burning requiring specialized treatment is uncommon; however, skin discoloration may occur. The patient should be told that the radiation field should not be exposed to sunlight or extreme cold and that total but temporary hair loss will usually occur in the areas being radiated and that complete return of hair, after high-dose radiation, may take many months or may not occur.

The most troublesome side effects that occur during radiotherapy are *gastrointestinal.* Patients receiving radiation to the chest or upper back often experience symptoms of radiation esophagitis (odynophagia and sometimes reflux symptoms that may respond to elevation of the head of the bed and to antacids). Severe esophagitis is more likely to occur when radiotherapy has been used in patients who have had prior chemotherapy, especially with such agents as doxorubicin, bleomycin, or *cis*-platinum. *Candida* superinfection of the irritated esophagus is not unusual, especially in patients who are receiving steroids. This usually responds well to treatment with fluconazole (100 mg daily). Patients should improve with a 1-week course of therapy. Abdominal irradiation can cause diarrhea that may persist to some degree during the entire course of treatment. In addition to replacing fluids and electrolytes, some dietary maneuvers may minimize diarrhea; these are listed in Table 10.5. Nausea and anorexia are the most troublesome side effects of abdominal irradiation and are discussed separately later in this chapter.

Patients who receive radiotherapy to the head or neck are subject to *oral and dental complications.* Before treatment, all patients should have a complete

Table 10.4. Important Side Effects of Radiotherapy

Dermatitis: Less common with newer high-energy machines; avoid sunlight and extreme cold.
Acute radiation pneumonitis: Transient, usually occurring 6–12 wk after treatment; precipitated by corticosteroid withdrawal, concomitant chemotherapy; clinical manifestations include nonproductive cough, dyspnea, fever, leukocytosis with parenchymal infiltrates on radiograph in the area of the radiation ports; may respond to steroid treatment.
Pulmonary fibrosis: Occurs 6–12 mo after treatment; not responsive to steroids.
Esophagitis: Usually occurs during treatment; particularly severe when radiotherapy and chemotherapy are administered together.
Nausea, vomiting, and diarrhea: Occur during treatment with most abdominal radiotherapy, usually self-limited.
Enteritis: Rare, more likely with very high-dose treatment; small bowel more sensitive than large bowel and stomach; occurs weeks to years after radiotherapy; manifestations include obstruction, bleeding, perforation; pelvic irradiation (e.g., in the treatment of bladder or prostate cancer) may cause acute *proctitis,* which occasionally becomes chronic, sometimes leading to bleeding or stricture formation.
Pericarditis: Occurs months to years after radiation, usually resolves, occasionally progresses to constrictive pericarditis or tamponade requiring pericardiectomy. There is also an increased incidence of coronary artery disease seen years after mediastinal irradiation.
Neurologic side effects: Transverse myelitis, very rare; side effects from CNS irradiation in adults are rare. Lhermitte sign (the sensation of electric shocks passing down the body when the head is flexed) seen in 10% of patients undergoing mantle irradiation for Hodgkin disease; after radiotherapy herpes zoster is common.
Hypothyroidism: Common in patients treated for Hodgkin disease with mantle field; may develop years after treatment.
Sterility: Usually temporary.
Growth retardation in children: Occurs both from direct skeletal effects and from hypopituitarism from CNS irradiation.
Oral and dental side effects: Dry mouth and partial or complete loss of taste or smell are common. Severe dental problems are common after head and neck irradiation because of decrease in saliva formation, increased sensitivity to caries. Osteonecrosis is a rare but serious side effect of head and neck irradiation
Cystitis: Occurs during treatment with pelvic irradiation; clinical manifestations include urgency dysuria and hematuria occurring usually during the third and fourth weeks of treatment; usually self-limited and treated symptomatically with fluids and phenazopyridine (Pyridium), 200 mg four times a day; chronic bladder fibrosis is a rare late complication manifested usually by painless hematuria.

CNS; Central nervous system.
See Refs. 11,16–20.

Table 10.5. Dietary Maneuvers for Therapy-induced Diarrhea

Clear liquids (warm or at room temperature)
Avoid fiber (roughage) in the diet
Take smaller amounts of food more often
Avoid fatty foods
Avoid highly spiced foods
Avoid carbonated drinks, beans, cabbage, broccoli, cauliflower, and corn

dental examination by a dentist experienced in the treatment of patients who have undergone radiotherapy. Damage to the teeth, gums, and bone, plus the xerostomia that results from high-dosage radiotherapy to the oral mucous membranes and salivary glands, may result in severe problems. Many of these can be prevented by appropriate prophylaxis (aggressive treatment of periodontal disease and infected teeth before radiation) and an ongoing program during and after radiotherapy, which should be strictly followed. The use of artificial saliva (Saliva Substitute, Roxane Laboratories) may be helpful for patients with xerostomia.

Corticosteroids and Radiotherapy

The patient's primary care practitioner may sometimes be involved with the early treatment of central nervous system metastases or spinal cord compression, using corticosteroids in conjunction with radiotherapy. Multiple regimens are used. A common regimen consists of dexamethasone (Decadron), 4 to 25 mg four times a day, continued until the patient has received several courses of radiotherapy and then slowly tapered over 2 to 3 weeks. Steroids decrease the local edema that occurs in these situations and help protect against radiation-induced edema during the first few days of therapy.

Cumulative Dosage

A maximal cumulative dosage of radiotherapy can safely be given to any one site without the risk of significant permanent tissue damage. This dosage varies for each organ system. If ports do not overlap, definitive full-dose radiotherapy can be given to multiple sites either concomitantly or sequentially. Problems occur when ports are contiguous or overlapping. For example, it is often more beneficial to give palliative total spine irradiation to patients with several isolated spine metastases than to treat only focal symptomatic areas, which may preclude later palliative radiotherapy to symptomatic contiguous areas.

CHEMOTHERAPY

Patient Experience

The chemotherapy experience for the patient is so varied (depending on the disease being treated) that it is hard to give a general description. The medical oncologist giving therapy can best explain to the patient the specifics of treatment, including how it is administered, the frequency of treatment, the hoped-for response, and the side effects. The most common troublesome side effects for the patient are hair loss and nausea and vomiting. The frequency and degree of hair loss vary with the treatment regimen, but it is helpful for the patient to know that hair will regrow once the treatment is discontinued. The treatment of nausea and vomiting is discussed later in this chapter. Table 10.6 lists other acute and chronic side effects of various chemotherapeutic agents. Knowledge of the long-term side effects of various agents is particularly important for the primary care practitioner, who may be responsible for follow-up care of patients with good prognoses after chemotherapy.

Table 10.6. Common Side Effects of Chemotherapy (21)

Hair loss: Alkylating agents, vincristine, vinblastine, adriamycin, mithramycin daunomycin, taxanes, gemcitibine. Hair regrowth occurs once chemotherapy is discontinued.
Hypercalcemia: Estrogens, antiestrogens (tamoxifen).
Fluid retention: Estrogens, androgens, steroids.
Skin darkening: Adriamycin (nails), 5-FU, bleomycin, busulfan, methotrexate. May improve slowly over time.
Dermatitis: Methotrexate, alkylating agents, vinblastine, 6-MP, 6-thioguanine bleomycin (may be delayed).
Marrow depression: Almost all chemotherapy agents, except for vincristine and bleomycin. Nitrosoureas may be associated with delayed thrombocytopenia.
Neurologic: cis-Platinum (deafness), vincristine, vinblastine, methotrexate, hexamethylmelamine, 5-FU (ataxia), procarbazine, ifosphamide (encephalopathy seizures), taxanes, vinorelbine. Neurologic deficits occur during treatment and sometimes gradually improve, but sometimes are permanent.
Diarrhea: Vinorelbine, 5-FU, leukovorin, irinotecan.
Gastrointestinal ulcerations: Methotrexate, 5-FU, bleomycin (mucocutaneous), adriamycin, leukovorin.
Cardiomyopathy: Adriamycin, daunorubicin, mitoxantrone, infusional 5-FU, Herceptin.
Pulmonary fibrosis: Bleomycin, alkylating agents, mitomycin-C. Occurs gradually during treatment or may be delayed.
Renal damage: cis-Platinum, methotrexate, streptozotocin, ifosphamide, nitrosoureas.
Red urine: Adriamycin, daunomycin.
Hepatic toxicity: Mithramycin, methotrexate, nitrosoureas, cytosine arabinoside, 6-MP, taxanes.
Sexual and gonadal dysfunction: Many drugs and regimens.
Secondary neoplasm: Alkylating agents, especially when combined with radiotherapy. Occurrance is delayed years.
Flulike symptoms, malaise: Biologics (IL-2, interferon, monoclonal antibodies) gemcitabine, taxanes, cladribine.
Fever: Bleomycin, biologics.
Hypersensitivity reaction: Taxanes, etoposide, monoclonal antibodies.

5-FU, 5-fluorouracil; 6-MP, 6-mercaptopurine; IL-2; interleukin-2.

An excellent free booklet, *Chemotherapy and You: A Guide to Self-Help During Treatment,* written for patients, is available through the National Institutes of Health (see General References). It is helpful to have this booklet available for patients and families to read when chemotherapy is being considered.

Chemotherapy-Induced Granulocytopenic Fever

The most common side effect of cytotoxic chemotherapy is myelosuppression and the associated risk of systemic infection (9). Granulocytopenia is defined as an absolute neutrophil count of less than 1,000 cells/mm^3. However, a significant risk of infection is not incurred until the level falls below 500/mm^3. In particular, the incidence of culture-proven septicemia correlates best with the number of days a patient remains with a neutrophil count below 100/mm^3. The nadir of the white count, and hence the largest risk of serious infection, usually occurs 10 to 14 days after chemotherapy is administered. It is the responsibility of the treating oncologist to monitor the neutrophil counts and instruct patients when to check their temperatures and when to seek help if a fever or other signs (e.g., malaise, chills, cough) of infection develop. However, there may be circumstances when the patient's primary care practitioner may be contacted by the patient.

It has been dogma that any granulocytopenic patient is at great risk for gram-negative bacteremia, especially *Pseudomonas,* and that all febrile neutropenic patients need immediate hospitalization with appropriate empiric antibiotic coverage. For the primary care practitioner, who may not have the patient's latest hemogram and may not have followed the recent course of the patient, this still may be the best guideline. On admission the patient should have blood and urine cultures and a chest radiograph. A history of new symptoms and an examination guided by symptoms, but always including attention to the mouth, skin, and perirectal area, may reveal a source. Unlike unimpaired patients, immunocompromised patients can have a life-threatening septicemia with few or no focal signs or symptoms. Therefore, instead of watching and waiting at the time of admission, one should initiate treatment with broad-spectrum antibiotics such as a semisynthetic penicillin and an aminoglycoside or third or fourth-generation cephalosporin to which *Pseudomonas* is sensitive. In recent years, the incidence of *Pseudomonas* bacteremia has markedly decreased in these patients; *Escherichia coli* and *Klebsiella pneumoniae* remain the most common infections, and the incidence of gram-positive infections, especially coagulase-negative staphylococci, has risen, probably because of the increased use of indwelling venous access devices. On occasion, when the patient is not sick and the expected length of neutropenia is short, the experienced oncologist may elect to treat the febrile neutropenic patient as an outpatient. The quinolones are most commonly used. When gram-positive infections are suspected, clindamycin and amoxicillin/potassium clavulanate are frequently used.

NAUSEA, VOMITING, AND ANOREXIA

Nausea and vomiting can be the most troublesome side effects of radiotherapy and chemotherapy. In the past, the symptomatic treatment of nausea was only moderately effective, and vomiting was particularly troublesome with therapies containing *cis*-platinum. However, antiemetic regimens combining corticosteroids (dexamethasone, 10 to 20 mg intravenously) with a serotonin blocker (e.g., ondansetron, 15 to 30 mg intravenously) have greatly reduced the incidence of nausea and vomiting in the first 24 hours after therapy with *cis*-platinum and other strongly emetic regimens (10). Oral serotonin blockers can be helpful for ongoing nausea from radiotherapy and chemotherapy. Lorazepam may have a role in relaxing the anxious patient before chemotherapy, and because of its interference with short-term memory, it may also lessen the chance of a patient developing anticipatory nausea (11). The nausea of less emetigenic regimens usually can be controlled with a 10- to 20-mg dose of dexamethasone supplemented with prochlorperazine (either 10 mg intravenously or 5 to 10 mg by mouth). Nausea that begins a day or 2 after the administration of the chemotherapy and lasts up to a week or more is still a difficult problem to treat, especially after administration of *cis*-platinum. Attempts to treat with a short course of oral dexamethasone (8 to 12 mg/day) or with prochlorperazine (one or two 10-mg capsules orally or 25-mg suppository every 4 to 6 hours) are only moderately successful. An oral serotonin blocker may also be helpful (12). In addition to pharmacologic palliation, the patient with marked nausea will find that it is often helpful to be extremely still, lying down in a quiet room without external stimuli. Even with the improvements in therapy for chemotherapy-induced nausea, patients still consider nausea and vomiting among the most troublesome side effects of chemotherapy (13).

A number of *dietary maneuvers* may be helpful to the patient experiencing nausea and vomiting after therapy. The patient who experiences severe nausea and vomiting after therapy should probably drink only clear liquids until the symptoms are decreased. In general, it is more helpful to take smaller portions of food frequently than to take larger meals less often, to take foods that are low in fat, and to avoid overly sweet foods. Mild nausea, especially that experienced before therapy or in anticipation of therapy, may be helped by taking dry toast or crackers in small quantities. It is recommended that patients not lie down just after eating. Some patients find also that it is helpful not to drink liquids with their food (because this may increase their feeling of bloating and subsequent nausea). Many patients become nauseated at the smell of food cooking, and it may be helpful for them to go to another part of the house or to stay out of the house when food is being prepared. Greasy and fried foods seem to be the worst offenders in this regard and are best avoided.

One of the major problems with intensive cancer therapy is *general anorexia* often associated with alterations in taste and smell, which may result in considerable nutritional problems and weight loss (14). Consultation with a dietitian may be helpful in such a situation. Oral progesterone (Megace) in large doses (300 to 800 mg/day) may be helpful for the patient with persistent anorexia (15).

An excellent free booklet, *Eating Hints: Recipes and Tips for Better Nutrition during Cancer Treatment,* is available through the National Institutes of Health (see General References). It contains all sorts of dietary advice for patients with cancer, including many recipes.

TERMINAL CARE

The primary care practitioner who has participated in various phases of cancer care and who has an ongoing relationship with the patient and his or her family is often in the best position to help during a patient's terminal illness. The practitioner who develops some expertise in this regard can find enormous gratification from this role. Chapter 13 deals with many of the issues important in caring for terminally ill patients and their families, including the very important issues of pain control, hospice care, and bereavement. An excellent publication, *Coping with Cancer: A Resource for the Health Professional,* is available free of charge from the National Institutes of Health (see General References). In addition to other useful information, it lists organizations and agencies that provide useful services that may aid the practitioner in providing support for the dying patient.

General References

Abeloff MD, Armitage JO, Lichter AS, et al., eds. Clinical oncology, 2nd ed. New York: Churchill Livingstone, 2000.

Exhaustive textbook.

Loescher LJ, Welch-McCaffrey D, Leigh SA, et al. Surviving adult cancers. Part I. Physiologic effects. Ann Intern Med 1989;111:411.

Welch-McCaffrey D, Hoffman B, Leigh SA, et al. Surviving adult cancers. Part 2. Psychosocial implications. Ann Intern Med 1989;111:517.

Companion critical review articles that summarize knowledge and knowledge gaps regarding physiologic and psychosocial aspects of long-term survival in treated patients with cancer.

Booklets from the National Institutes of Health cited in this chapter are available free of charge from the Office of Cancer Communications, Department of Health and Human Services, NIH, Bethesda, MD 20205. Telephone 301-496-4070.

Useful websites and phone number for patients and families:
National Cancer Institute
http://www.nci.nih.gov
Cancer Information Service (CIS) 1-800-4-CANCER
American Cancer Society (ACS)
http://www.cancer.org
American Society Clinical Oncology (ASCO)
http://www.asco.org

Specific References*

1. Le Chevalier T, Cvitkovic E, Caille P, et al. Early metastatic cancer of unknown primary origin at presentation: a clinical study of 302 consecutive autopsied patients. Arch Intern Med 1988;148:2035.
2. Bates SE. Clinical applications of serum tumor markers. Ann Intern Med 1991;115:623.
3. ASCO Breast Cancer Surveillance Expert Panel. Recommended breast cancer surveillance guidelines. J Clin Oncol 1997;15: 2149.
4. National Cancer Institute. Tumor markers. National Cancer Institute CancerWEB. www.graylab.ac.uk/cancernet/600518.html.
5. Lewis FM. The impact of cancer on the family: a critical analysis of the research literature. In: Patient education and counseling. Limerick: Elsevier Scientific Publishers Ireland, 1986: 269.
6. Dewys WD. Prognostic effect of weight loss prior to chemotherapy in cancer patients. Am J Med 1980;69:491.
7. Yancik R, Ganz A, Varricchio GA, et al. Perspectives on comorbidity and cancer in older patients: approaches to expand the knowledge base. J Clin Oncol 2001;19:1147.
8. Penman DT. Informed consent for investigational chemotherapy: patients' and physicians' perceptions. J Clin Oncol 1984; 2:849.
9. Hughes WT, Armstrong D, Bodey GP, et al. Guidelines for the use of antimicrobial agents in neutropenic patients with unexplained fever. Clin Infect Dis 1997;25:551.
10. Hainsworth JD, Hesbeth PJ. Single-dose ondansetron for the prevention of cisplatin induced emesis: efficacy results. Semin Oncol 1992;19[Suppl 15]:14.
11. Franzen P, Nyman J, Hagberg H, et al. A randomized placebo controlled study with ondansetron in patients undergoing fractionated radiotherapy. Ann Oncol 1996;7:587.
12. Gralla RJ, Osoba D, Krfis MG, et al. Recommendations for the use of antiemetics: evidence-based, clinical practice guidelines. J Clin Oncol 1999;17:2971.
13. Griffin AM, Butow PN, Coates AS, et al. On the receiving end—patient perception of the side-effects of cancer chemotherapy, 1993. Ann Oncol 1996;7:189.
14. Ottery FD. Supportive nutrition to prevent cachexia and improve quality of life. Semin Oncol 1995;22[Suppl 2]:98.
15. Bruera E, Ernst S, Hagen N, et al. Effectiveness of megestrol acetate in patients with advanced cancer: a randomized, double-blind, crossover study. Cancer Prev Control 1998;2:74.
16. Myer JL, Jerome MV. Radiation injury: advances in management and prevention. In: Myer JL, ed. Frontiers of radiation therapy and oncology. Vol. 32. Basel: Karger, 1999.
17. Zimmerman RP, Mark RJ, Tran LM, et al. Concomitant pilocarpine during head and neck RT is associated with decreased posttreatment xerostomia. Int J Radiat Oncol Biol Phys 1997;37:571.
18. Berk L. An overview of radiotherapy trials for the treatment of brain metastases. Oncology 1995;9:1205.
19. Blayney DW, Longo D. Radiation induced pericarditis. N Engl J Med 1982;306:550.
20. Gross NJ. Pulmonary effects of radiation therapy. Ann Intern Med 1997;86:81.
21. Perry MC, ed. Toxicity of chemotherapy. Semin Oncol 1992;19: 453.

*Bold print (general references) and bold numerals (specific references) denote published clinical trials, meta-analyses, or consensus-based recommendations.

CHAPTER 11

Adolescent Patients: Special Considerations

LAWRENCE N. SCHERZER, MD

From a developmental perspective, adolescence is a time of dynamic changes, with tremendous physical, sexual, psychologic, and intellectual growth. This chapter describes the normal changes and the major problems associated with each of these four spheres of development and delineates practical approaches to the office care of the adolescent patient.

ADOLESCENT MORTALITY AND MORBIDITY

Adolescence should be the healthiest period of life; morbidity and mortality rates are low compared with other age groups, but the absolute number of adolescents who die or have chronic illnesses is considerable. Because the number of productive years at stake for a teenager with a significant illness is large, adolescent health is a special priority.

Accidents are by far the leading cause of death among adolescents and young adults. The victims of accidental death usually have bypassed preventive measures, and in many instances behavioral problems underlie those deaths. For example, alcohol is implicated in more than 50% of automobile accidents, and there may be an element of suicidal intent in some of them.

The second and third leading causes of death in older adolescents (and an important problem in young adolescents) are *homicide* and *suicide*, respectively, problems that are discussed later in this chapter.

The fourth leading cause of death among adolescents and young adults is *neoplasia*. The most common diagnoses are acute leukemia (both lymphocytic and myelogenous), lymphomas (including non-Hodgkin lymphoma and Hodgkin disease), central nervous system tumors (especially supratentorial and infratentorial gliomas), bone tumors (especially osteogenic sarcomas and Ewing sarcomas), and solid organ tumors (especially of genital organs).

As medical treatment improves, conditions that were previously fatal in childhood are frequently seen in adolescents and young adults. It is common for patients with cystic fibrosis, nephritis, congenital heart disease, and leukemia to survive into adolescence and young adulthood.

Most visits to a practitioner by adolescents are for preventive care or minor problems (Table 11.1). However, a number of more severe medical problems are limited chiefly to the adolescent period or are problems of adulthood that begin during adolescence (Table 11.2). The data in Tables 11.1 and 11.2 do not depict the significant distress that many adolescent patients (and their physicians) experience. This distress is often related to the pressures unique to the several chronologic stages of adolescence.

The *young teen* (11 to 15 years old), who typically has special concern over physical development, may have anxieties about mutilation and death. Hostility toward an illness may be expressed in a fantasy of invincibility, leading to an uncooperative noncompliant patient. Other young adolescents become greatly depressed by their illnesses and become annoying, complaining, whiny patients, often regressing to a childlike dependence on adult caretakers.

The *middle adolescent* (14 to 19 years old) who is seriously ill suffers from the loss of valued contact with friends and schools. Illness may interrupt important aspirations and shatter dreams. Body image is at a critical developmental stage in mid-adolescence, and the teen may be more worried about a cosmetic defect resulting from an illness than about the disease or its therapy. Such fears must be faced early and dealt with honestly.

The *older adolescent* (18 to 21 years old) shares many adult concerns. For example, the patient may express anxiety over the cost of an illness, the length of hospitalization, and the burdens these place on the family.

Table 11.1. Number of Office Visits Made by Adolescents and Percentage Distribution by the 15 Most Common Diagnoses (by ICD-9-CM Categories), According to Age: United States, 1985

Principal Diagnosis[a]	No. of Visits (Thousands)	Percentage Distribution	Principal Diagnosis[a]	No. of Visits (Thousands)	Percentage Distribution
Aged 11–14 yr			**Aged 15–20 yr**		
Total	58,996	100.0	Total	39,637	100.00
General medical examination	1,433	7.40	Normal pregnancy	3,391	8.56
Acute pharyngitis	709	3.66	Diseases of sebaceous glands	2,487	6.27
Acute upper respiratory infections of multiple or unspecified sites	637	3.29	General medical examination	1,942	4.90
Certain adverse effects, not elsewhere classified	555	2.87	Acute upper respiratory infections of multiple or unspecified sites	1,169	2.95
Allergic rhinitis	553	2.86	Acute pharyngitis	1,105	2.79
Health supervision of infant or child	527	2.72	Other diseases caused by viruses and chlamydias	965	2.43
Contact dermatitis and other eczema	475	2.46	Allergic rhinitis	803	2.03
Suppurative and unspecified otitis media	473	2.44	Disorders of refraction and accommodation	722	1.95
Other diseases caused by viruses and chlamydias	459	2.37	Suppurative and unspecified otitis media	668	1.68
Disorders of refraction and accommodation	458	2.37	Acute tonsillitis	585	1.48
Diseases of sebaceous glands	401	2.07	Other disorders of urethra and urinary tract	547	1.38
Curvature of spine	311	1.61	Contact dermatitis and other eczema	535	1.35
Acute tonsillitis	308	1.59	Contraceptive management	510	1.29
Streptococcal sore throat and scarlet fever	300	1.55	Certain adverse effects, not elsewhere classified	483	1.22
Asthma	297	1.53	Specific investigations and examinations	464	1.17
All other diagnoses	11,464	59.21	All other diagnoses	23,208	58.55

[a]Based on Public Health Service and Health Care Finance Administration. International classification of diseases, 9th revision, clinical modification (ICD-9-CM). Washington, DC: Public Health Service, 1980.

From Nelson C. Office visits by adolescents: National Ambulatory Medical Care Survey, 1985. Advance Data from Vital and Health Statistics of the National Center for Health Statistics, No. 196, April 11, 1991, with permission.

Table 11.2. Selected Medical Problems Limited to Adolescence or Persisting into Adulthood

Limited Chiefly to Adolescence	Chronic Problems that May Begin in Adolescence
Slipped epiphysis	Obesity
Distortion of body image	Hypertension
Delinquency[a]	Diabetes mellitus
Anorexia nervosa	Hypercholesterolemia
Primary amenorrhea	Duodenal ulcer
School or learning problems[b]	Inflammatory bowel disease
	Irritable bowel syndrome
	Dental caries
	Drug abuse
	Alcoholism
	Personality disorders
	Somatization disorder
	Depressive neurosis

[a]May begin earlier.
[b]Often develop earlier.

PHYSICAL DEVELOPMENT

Normal Patterns and Concerns

Physical maturation is an important feature of the second decade of life. Although the rate and the timing of maturation may vary, they follow the hormonal changes of puberty in a given individual. A notable *growth spurt* occurs during the adolescent years, with a 20% to 25% increase in height over 2 to 3 years. This spurt usually occurs earlier in the female than in the male (as does sexual maturation). During puberty, there is an average twofold increase in both lean and nonlean body mass. The ratio of lean to nonlean body mass is greater in males than in females. Fat accumulation tends to be greatest when growth ceases and may extend into adulthood.

The *musculoskeletal system* has special characteristics during adolescence. To accommodate growth, the ligaments and tendons become lax and elastic, often giving the teen a slouched-over appearance. Similarly, there is an increase in skeletal growth, particularly in long bones, and metaphyseal-epiphyseal junctions remain soft. Thus, the actively growing teen, who may not have developed muscle mass to correspond to skeletal growth, may be prone to some special injuries, particularly joint dislocations and fractures along epiphyseal plates.

As with all areas of development, the adolescent may have particular concerns about growth and weight. The principal reason for this is that adolescents often base judgment of each other's adequacy and acceptability on size or (for males) on athletic ability, and adult criteria of social status based on other standards (or prejudices) are less important.

Children called "squirt" or "runt" are given various types of parental advice, much of it unhelpful. Some children adapt by engaging in an activity in which height is unimportant (e.g., debating, chess, fencing, swimming, or body building). Occasionally, normal children with a familial basis for their short stature require psychological counseling to promote effective adaptation to their stature. Some teens who are very sensitive about height and strength limitations may try radical and potentially harmful solutions such as self-injections of purported growth stimulants.

The concern of the adolescent about height may be generalized to many other aspects of appearance, including body habitus, beauty (or lack of beauty), and skin condition. It is important to recognize when concern about body image is the patient's primary concern and to provide reassurance that he or she is medically and biologically normal. The physician can promote such reassurance by suggesting books in which the adolescent can learn more about normal growth (see General References).

Short Stature

Short stature is discussed under Short Stature and Delayed Sexual Maturation, below.

Obesity

A practical definition of *obesity* is a weight of 20% or more over ideal body weight (see Chapter 83). This can be estimated by determining the weight that corresponds to the growth chart height percentile for the age and sex of the child and dividing this into the actual weight (Fig. 11.1). A result of greater than 1.2 would be suspect. This ratio should be compared with the clinical appearance of the child because the fat distribution changes at puberty in boys, when extra weight may be transformed into musculature, and in girls, who normally increase their storage of fat. Obesity remains a clinical diagnosis. Adolescent obesity is usually caused by overeating. Most estimates place the prevalence between 4% and 10%, with the highest frequency among lower socioeconomic groups. Often, obesity begins in early childhood but becomes a concern in adolescence because of desires to conform to peer standards.

Obese teens should be screened for other cardiovascular risk factors, such as positive family history, high blood pressure, elevated serum cholesterol or triglyceride, diabetes mellitus, and smoking. If multiple risk factors are present, the patient should be monitored more frequently and risk modification should be encouraged.

Obesity in adolescence will generally continue into adulthood and will be a risk factor for cardiovascular

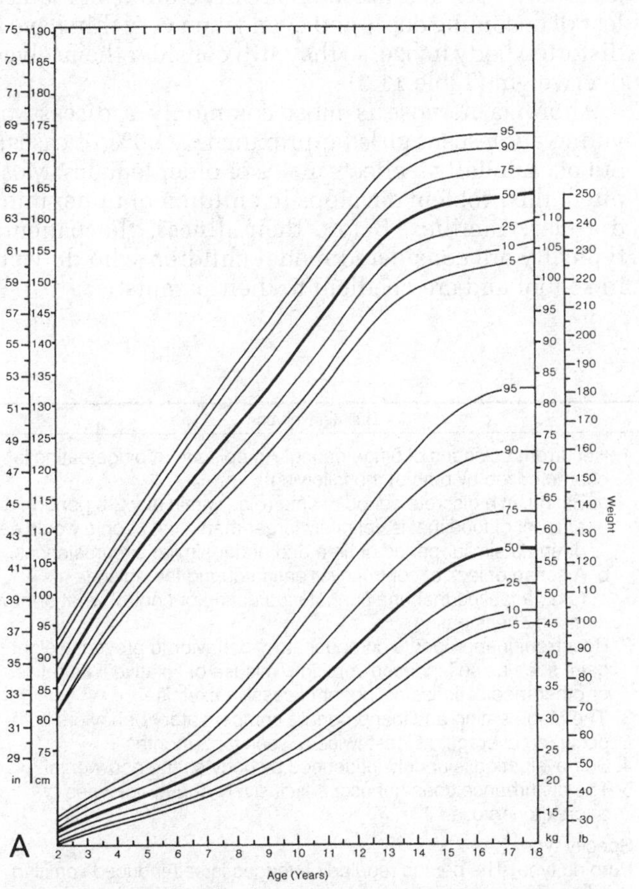

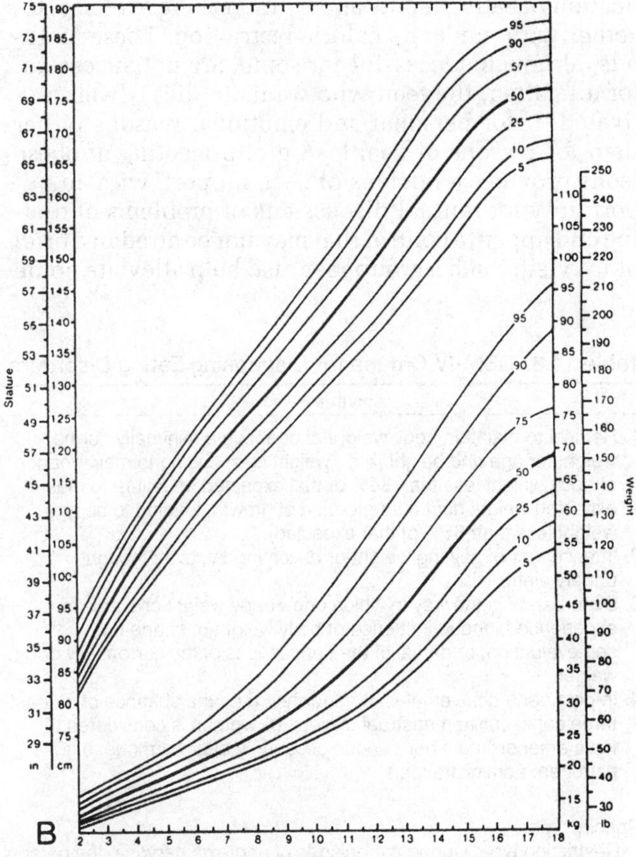

Figure 11.1. A: Physical growth in girls. Plot height and weight against age at each encounter. The curve so obtained should parallel percentile lines within the clear area (growth patterns of 90% of children/adolescents). If the curve deviates from percentile lines, an abnormal growth pattern is likely. The upper series of curves represents the normal range of height at various ages and the lower series of curves, the normal range of weight at various ages. (From National Center for Health Statistics. NCHS growth charts, 1976. Monthly vital statistics report. Vol. 25, no. 3, suppl. [HRA] 76-1120. Rockville, MD: Health Resources Administration, June 1976, with permission.) **B: Physical growth in boys.**

disease, type II diabetes mellitus, and earlier mortality. To treat adolescent obesity successfully, the teen must be motivated to accept the physician's assessments and recommendations. Often, the patient has attempted to cope with the problem by him- or herself. Certain fad diets, such as fasting and water diets, may yield rapid weight loss but will deplete the strength of the child. Generally, because no modification of long-term eating habits is attempted, the weight is regained upon cessation of the diet. Occasionally, serious biologic complications are associated with prolonged adherence to highly restrictive diets. Macrobiotic diets have been associated with symptoms of protein and vitamin deficiencies, and liquid protein diets have cardiotoxic effects that have resulted in deaths (see details in Chapter 83). Severely calorie-restricted diets lead to a cessation of linear growth and may cause menstrual irregularities.

Medications are of no value in weight control. In particular, amphetamines and methamphetamines are contraindicated because of their potential for abuse. Surgical treatment (e.g., jejunoileal bypass or gastric stapling) of obesity is rarely indicated, particularly in the adolescent years.

One is left with methods of dietary control by modification of eating habits and by increasing exercise, together with moderate calorie restriction. These methods, although successful for some, are not successful for all. Often, the teen who wants to diet is well motivated, if for personal and emotional reasons rather than for reasons of health. A group meeting of obese teens provides a nucleus of peer support, with an opportunity for mutual discussions of problems of dieting and appetite control that may not be aired in a brief office visit. Such a group may also help alleviate home pressures. Parental coercion and control of diet in the context of a normally antagonistic parent–teen relationship may result in an angry rebellious youngster who is gaining rather than losing weight.

For overweight young to mid-adolescents, a reasonable goal is to maintain their current body weight because excess caloric restriction may result in a loss of lean body weight. For the late adolescent, the goal may be weight loss. For all obese patients, one wishes to achieve a change in long-term eating patterns.

Some adolescents overeat because of unresolved psychological difficulties. If there are expressions of problems in peer, school, or parental relationships, these should be explored further. However, obesity alone is not an indication of psychopathology.

Anorexia Nervosa and Bulimia

Anorexia nervosa is an uncommon but serious disorder of growth in adolescents. It is marked by extreme loss of appetite and weight (at least 15% of the baseline weight) that is not attributable to a medical or psychiatric illness ordinarily associated with weight loss (i.e., inflammatory bowel disease or a major affective disorder). Patients characteristically exhibit an intense fear of becoming obese and even when very thin have a distorted body image, so they still consider themselves overweight (Table 11.3).

Anorexia nervosa is most commonly a disease of young adolescent girls (approximately 90% of cases), but occasionally it affects males or older females. Most often, the problem develops in children of upper middle class families. Before their illness, the patients typically are considered model children who do well in school and are obedient to their parents.

Table 11.3. DSM-IV Criteria for Diagnosing Eating Disorders

Anorexia Nervosa	Bulimia Nervosa
1. Refusal to maintain body weight at or above a minimally normal weight for age and height (e.g., weight loss leading to maintenance of body weight less than 85% of that expected, or failure to make expected weight gain during period of growth, leading to body weight less than 85% of that expected). 2. Intense fear of gaining weight or becoming fat, even though underweight. 3. Disturbance in the way in which one's body weight or shape is experienced, undue influence of body weight or shape on self-evaluation, or denial of the seriousness of the current low body weight. 4. In postmenarchal females, amenorrhea (i.e., the absence of at least three consecutive menstrual cycles). (A woman is considered to have amenorrhea if her periods occur only after hormone, e.g., estrogen, administration.)	1. Recurrent episodes of binge eating. An episode of binge eating is characterized by both of the following: a. Eating, in a discrete period of time (e.g., within any 2-h period), an amount of food that is definitely larger than most people would eat during a similar period of time and under similar circumstances. b. A sense of lack of control over eating during the episode (e.g., a feeling that one cannot stop eating or control what or how much one is eating). 2. Recurrent inappropriate compensatory behavior to prevent weight gain, such as self-induced vomiting, misuse of laxatives, diuretics, or other medications; fasting; or excessive exercise. 3. The binge eating and inappropriate compensatory behaviors both occur, on average, at least twice a week for 3 months. 4. Self-evaluation is unduly influenced by body shape and weight. 5. The disturbance does not occur exclusively during episodes of anorexia nervosa.
Specify type Restricting type: During the episode of anorexia nervosa, the person does not regularly engage in binge eating or purging behavior (i.e., self-induced vomiting or the misuse of laxatives or diuretics). Binge eating/purging type: During the episode of anorexia nervosa, the person regularly engages in binge eating or purging behavior (i.e., self-induced vomiting or the misuse of laxatives or diuretics).	Specify type Purging type: The person regularly engages in self-induced vomiting or the misuse of laxatives or diuretics. Nonpurging type: The person uses other inappropriate compensatory behaviors, such as fasting or excessive exercise, but does not regularly engage in self-induced vomiting or the misuse of laxatives or diuretics.

From Diagnostic and statistical manual of mental disorders, 4th ed. (DSM-IV). Washington, DC: American Psychiatric Association, 1994, with permission.

The cause of the disease is unknown. Although many theories have been proposed to explain it, none is entirely satisfactory. Often, there has been some stress in the family (divorce, death, change of location) before the onset of the illness.

No simple treatment can be recommended for patients with anorexia nervosa. Help should be sought from a psychiatrist who has experience with eating disorders. The best results seem to be achieved by involving the patient and the patient's family in an intensive program in which counseling and behavior modification are used to restructure the patient's eating habits and attitude toward food. Very ill patients should be hospitalized so that a proper program of nutrition can be instituted.

Complete remission of anorexia nervosa is unusual, but approximately 75% of patients achieve an acceptable improvement in both their physical and emotional states. The rest remain chronically undernourished and maladapted. With current treatment, mortality has been reduced to 2% to 8%. Cause of death is equally attributable to overt suicide and medical complications of starvation. Poor prognosis has been associated with long duration of illness, disturbed parent–child relationships, concomitant personality disorder, and the presence of vomiting (more common in bulimia). The degree of weight loss generally is not related to prognosis (1).

Bulimia is a second eating disorder seen in adolescents and young adults. Most bulimic patients are female; bulimic symptoms have been reported by up to 10% of young women interviewed in community surveys (2). Characteristically, patients with bulimia periodically gorge themselves, only to follow this by self-induced vomiting and by further self-reprisals through abstinence from food (Table 11.3). As the disease progresses, patients may become withdrawn and depressed, leading to further appetite suppression. Amenorrhea is common in these patients, and it may be the presenting complaint. Some patients have a history of both anorexia and bulimia. Treatment of a patient with severe bulimia requires the help of a professional skilled in the management of eating disorders. Self-help groups such as Overeaters Anonymous may play an important role in the patient's long-term handling of bulimia.

SEXUAL DEVELOPMENT

Normal Patterns and Concerns

A major difference between the child and the adolescent is the development of the teen into a sexual being. The onset of puberty is associated with an intensification of sexual feelings and desires that lead to sexual exploration. With the liberalization of sexual mores in recent years, the problems of adolescent pregnancy and venereal diseases have grown to epidemic proportions.

The *staging of physical sexual development* of adolescents established by Tanner is a widely accepted method of following the physical changes of puberty (Tables 11.4 and 11.5 and Fig. 11.2). As the adolescent enters puberty, he or she also assumes a role as a sexual being who must begin to meet expectations of society, family, and peer group and who is

Table 11.4. Typical Progression of Female Adolescent Sexual Development (see also Fig. 11.2)

Stage 1
There is no pubic hair present, and there is no breast development.
The ovaries have begun to enlarge. The external genitalia are preadolescent or those of a child.

Stage 2
Breast bud formation usually begins before pubic hair growth. A small mound is formed by the elevation of the breast and papilla. Areolar diameter increases. The adolescent height spurt begins, and there is an acceleration in the deposition of total body fat. The adult female habitus emerges as the breasts enlarge and the hips widen.

Stage 3
There is further spread of pubic hair and further enlargement of breasts and areola, with no separation of their contours. The vagina enlarges and the vaginal epithelium, responding to estrogen stimulation from the maturing ovaries, increases in thickness, with considerable deposition of glycogen. The height spurt usually reaches a peak early in stage 3, before menarche.

Stage 4
If menarche has not occurred late in stage 3, it should occur during stage 4. Axillary hair appears just before or after menarche, usually in early stage 4. There is a projection of the areola and papilla to form a secondary mound above the level of the breast. The areolar mound may be absent (25% of females). The breasts and pubic hair progress. The ovaries continue to enlarge. Ovulation may occur just after menarche, but it is usually delayed until stage 5.

Stage 5
Pubic hair and breast development resemble those of the adult female; the areola has recessed to the general contour of the breast. Height increase has decelerated since menarche; height may increase 2 to 4 inches after menarche. By 2 years after menarche, regular ovulation may be expected.

Stage 6
In 10% of females there is a further spread of pubic hair.

From Tanner JM. Growth at adolescence. New York: Appleton-Century-Crofts, 1966, with permission.

Table 11.5. Typical Progression of Male Adolescent Sexual Development

Stage 1
The male has no pubic hair or increase in size of the penis.
This describes the male as a preadolescent or child. However, the testes are beginning to mature. Usually there is considerable acceleration in height and weight gain along with changes in body composition (especially more body fat).

Stage 2
There is early growth of the testes and scrotum before pubic hair appears. The height spurt accelerates; the male physique begins to change as fat and muscle are added, and the areola of the breast increases in size and darkens slightly.

Stage 3
There is further enlargement of the testes and scrotum, enlargement of the penis (mainly in length), and spreading and darkening of the pubic hair. Facial hair first appears at the corners of the upper lip. The height spurt accelerates further; there is broadening of the shoulders relative to the hips and generalized increased molding of the body, with considerable increase in muscle mass relative to fat. Hair appears in the perineum. Facial expression is significantly altered and appears more adult. The cartilage of the larynx enlarges, and the voice may begin to deepen. There is transient gynecomastia with slight projection of the areola.

Stage 4
Axillary hair first appears. There is continued enlargement of the scrotum, testes, and penis (the last, mainly in breadth). The pubic hair begins to appear adult. Facial hair is still limited to upper lip and chin. The first ejaculation, indicating considerable growth of the prostate gland, occurs early in stage 4. Sebaceous glands are approaching adult size and function. The voice deepens further.

Stage 5
Genital size and pubic hair distribution are adult in appearance. Hairs are present on the sides of the face. Gynecomastia has disappeared. The height spurt has decelerated and the physique is that of the mature male.

Stage 6
Some adolescents have a further spread of pubic hair up the linea alba, which may be described as stage 6. This later development, often not reached until the early twenties, occurs in 80% of males.

From Tanner JM. Growth at adolescence. New York: Appleton-Century-Crofts, 1966, with permission.

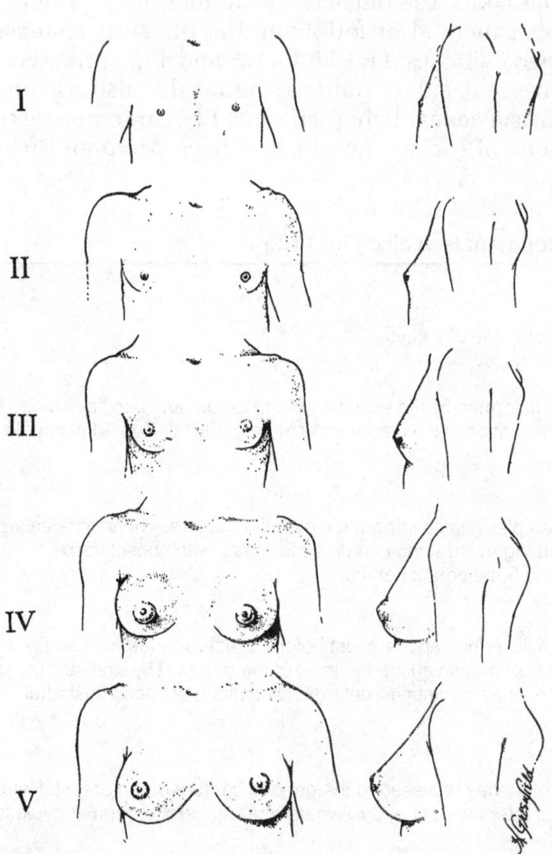

Figure 11.2. Diagrammatic representation of Tanner stages I to V of human breast maturation. (Adapted from Marshall WA, Tanner JM. Variations in pattern of pubertal changes in girls. Arch Dis Child 1969;44:291, with permission.)

pushed into sexual propriety and conformity. These expectations are transmitted to the teen by multiple messages that are often conveyed poorly, and many teens remain ignorant and insecure about sexual issues.

Early adolescence is characterized by a bisexual period, in which close friendships are formed with members of the same sex but heterosexual attitudes develop. Young teens often develop best-buddy relationships. These relationships may even be physically intimate, but they are not considered characteristic of adult homosexuality. However, the teen (particularly male) may fear being a homosexual, and the frequent name calling of this period (in which people are called “gay” or “queer” with little provocation) may be taken too seriously. Boys who have developed noticeable gynecomastia may be particularly confused about their sexual identity. Such boys need to be reassured of the normality of these concerns. Masturbation tends to be a frequent practice in this period, and there may be associated guilt that increases as the sex drive stimulates the teen to continue the practice. Again, where appropriate, problems associated with masturbation should be met with reassurance of its normality.

In mid to late adolescence, dating and heterosexual activities begin in earnest. By age 15, one in four females and one in three males have had sexual intercourse (3). Often, teens rush into sexual activity before they fully understand their own feelings about it. It is often part of the dating relationship—a prerequisite to communication, rather than vice versa. It may be part of thrill-seeking behavior for some teens, and others use it to escape from loneliness and depression.

Short Stature and Delayed Sexual Maturation

A common problem that comes to the attention of physicians is the teenager with short stature or delayed puberty. These two symptoms are often interrelated, and the medical investigation is similar, so they are discussed together. However, the presence of one does not necessarily indicate a problem with the other.

Most of these patients simply are at one end of the spectrum of normal development (4). Many teenage boys may not appreciate the fact that some people fall into the 10th percentile of a normal curve, and they may not accept a cursory dismissal of their concerns about size. Some may be helped by looking at normal growth curves that indicate the predicted ultimate height for people in their percentile (Fig. 11.1). Patients may need detailed discussion to comprehend fully and to cope with normal findings.

Assessment of short stature and delayed puberty by the generalist consists of the following steps:

1. A history of the onset of puberty and of the height of siblings, parents, and grandparents should be obtained. In particular, a history of several short family members (males under 5′6″, females under 5′0″) should be noted.
2. Growth records of the patient should be reviewed. Heights and weights should be plotted on an appropriate growth curve (Fig. 11.1). If a child has followed a single curve throughout life, a significant metabolic reason for this short stature is unlikely. However, if there is a falling away from a growth line, a metabolic problem is more likely.
3. The medical history should be reviewed, including a prenatal and neonatal history. A history of operations, head injuries, or chronic medical conditions that could predispose the patient to failure to thrive should be noted. If the child had a low birth weight, a review of underlying factors may disclose a possible chromosomal abnormality or toxic exposure (e.g., maternal cigarette smoking or alcohol use) that could produce long-term growth delay.
4. A developmental and psychosocial history may indicate possible familial problems or emotional neglect that could predispose to constitutional growth delay (so-called psychosocial dwarfism).
5. Inquiries into the teen's general health and daily habits may reveal problems needing investigation, such as poor appetite, frequent infections, drug abuse, chronic abdominal pain, or general fatigue and listlessness.

A *physical examination* is essential, including an accurate height and weight and Tanner stage assessment (Tables 11.4 and 11.5). If the testes are softening and show enlargement or if breast budding is present, there usually will be a normal sexual development. Unusual facies or ears, unusual hand creases, clinodactyly (deviation or deflection of the fingers), obesity, or delayed intellectual development may suggest a recognizable hereditary syndrome.

The initial *laboratory investigation* should include urinalysis; measurement of serum urea nitrogen, creatinine, and electrolytes; and radiographs of the hands and wrists to assess skeletal growth. More *specific laboratory investigations* may be suggested by the history and physical examination. Examples are thyroid enlargement (testing for hypothyroidism); normal physical examination and appearance but markedly short stature that is falling away from growth lines (testing for growth hormone deficiency); girls with delayed puberty, heights under the third percentile, associated with a short webbed neck, a systolic murmur, or widely spaced nipples (buccal smears performed to rule out Turner syndrome, i.e., X-O chromosomes); and striking pubertal delay without a history of similar delay in other family members (testing for gonadal failure including measurement of serum follicle-stimulating and luteinizing hormones, estradiol or testosterone, and urinary 17-ketosteroids and 17-hydroxysteroids; vaginal smear for maturation index and buccal smear for sex chromatin analysis or blood chromosome analysis).

Definitive diagnosis and planning for adolescents with suspected endocrine, metabolic, genetic, or psychological reasons for maturation delay require referral to an appropriate specialist. Patients with hereditary disorders may benefit from genetic counseling, particularly those who will be unable to bear children (e.g., patients with Turner syndrome). The availability of biosynthetic growth hormone has raised possibilities for the management of teens with familial short stature. It is unclear whether growth hormone will increase the final adult height of normal children, although for some the rate of growth increases. Weighed against its questionable efficacy, growth hormone treatment is very expensive (often costing $5,000 to $10,000 per year).

Sexually Transmitted Disease

Sexually transmitted diseases (STDs) are epidemic in 15 to 19 year olds. For example, more than 500,000 adolescents contract gonorrhea each year (3). The high frequency of STDs is partially caused by more casual attitudes toward sex, with frequent changes of sex partners. Sex education programs have had little impact on the problem. Fear of infection apparently does not deter some teens, who seem irresponsible, impulsive, and emotionally insecure and who appear to have little respect for others. Often, parents fail to provide basic information about sex and the risks of infection and pregnancy that accompany it.

In most states, adolescents have a legal right to receive treatment for STDs without the parents' knowledge; it is important to be receptive to the teen seeking treatment. Visits for treatment should also be used to explain the mechanism of acquiring venereal infection and to explain and encourage the use of condoms to prevent reinfection. The diagnosis and treatment of various STDs are discussed elsewhere in this book (see Chapter 37).

The high rates of sexual intercourse and adolescent pregnancy in the 1980s and 1990s have raised concerns about acquisition of infection with the human immunodeficiency virus (HIV) in this age group. Given the long incubation period of HIV infection, data showing that 21% of all acquired immunodeficiency syndrome cases occur in people 20 to 25 years of age suggest strongly that adolescence is an important period of acquisition of HIV infection (5). Other data suggest that a frequent route of spread of the virus in adolescence is by heterosexual transmission, rather than intravenous drug abuse, blood products, or homosexual contacts. Furthermore, many cases of HIV infection in infants may be linked to maternal acquisition of the virus during adolescence. It is imperative that teenagers, especially sexually active teens, are counseled about high-risk behaviors that may expose them to HIV infection and about safe sex practices. This information and details about the ambulatory care of HIV-infected patients are described in Chapter 39.

Pregnancy

By age 18, 1 in 4 female adolescents has had a pregnancy, and this number increases to more than 4 in 10 by age 20. Each year more than a million women under the age of 20 become pregnant, half of them out of wedlock (3). Many of these pregnancies are associated with serious medical risks for the mother and the fetus. Mothers under 14 have particularly high risks of toxemia, anemia, prematurity, infants with low birth weight, prolonged labor, and postpartum complications. Many of these problems can be prevented by good obstetric care, so that the first goal in adolescent pregnancy should be early diagnosis and entry into a comprehensive treatment program.

There are multiple social and behavioral reasons for the high number of teenage pregnancies. For many adolescents, pregnancy may be part of a maladaptive attempt to solve psychological issues, such as independence from a clinging mother or manipulation of a boyfriend. Such patients may have previously engaged in other maladaptive activities, such as drug abuse or delinquency. They may also be ignorant about methods and availability of birth control (see Chapter 100), including emergency contraception (see below).

The teenager herself may be ambivalent about her pregnancy. Often, the manipulations that led to the pregnancy (e.g., the promise of a prolonged relationship) have not succeeded and the patient feels abandoned. Furthermore, the pregnancy may result in hostility from the family when the teenager is in greatest need of help from her parents.

Clearly, the teenager about to make important decisions about herself and her pregnancy needs counseling. It can be provided by her primary physician or, commonly, by a staff member of a counseling agency such as Planned Parenthood. In either case, the patient's primary physician should be aware of programs in the community, including public schools that accommodate the needs of teenagers who choose to have their babies, and should be available for any problems that a pregnant teenager may wish to discuss. In many states, adolescents have the right to treatment for pregnancy-related events, including abortion, without parental consent or knowledge. If the teenager decides to continue with the pregnancy, she should be prepared to assume a parenting role. Furthermore, she should be educated about future pregnancies and given medical assistance for the pediatric care needed for her infant. If possible, daycare, vocational, and educational services should be available for the mother so that she may continue her education after the birth of her child. As an integral part of counseling, a stable caring person should be identified (a parent, if possible) who can assist the teen emotionally and financially and who can help her see the future for herself and her baby in a realistic manner.

Rape

Rape is a sexual act, usually intercourse, with a nonconsenting victim. The most common type of adolescent rape has been called acquaintance rape, and it is probable that most instances are never reported. Acquaintance rape occurs when the victim is sexually misused by a boyfriend during a date or by a casual friend or when a trusting teen accompanies her friends to a strange place where she is gang raped.

Teens, in exploring sexuality, may not have set limits to their petting, or if limits have been set unilaterally, they may afford little protection for the victim, especially when the assailant is an adolescent for whom limit setting has not been successful in other areas. Some teens may also, in their uncertainty, present themselves in provocative pseudo-mature ways (e.g., by wearing clothing that may be viewed as sexually inviting by male acquaintances).

There is a tendency in dealing with adolescent rape victims to imply that the victim may have invited the assault. This viewpoint inappropriately diverts attention from the fact that rape should always be treated as a very serious problem for the victim who reports it.

Initial care for the rape victim should be handled by a physician, with follow-up by a rape counseling service if one exists in the community. Often, a physician who is already acquainted with the patient can provide the best care.

There are several important considerations in caring for the rape victim:

- Rape is a crime of violence, as well as a sexual act.
- Above all else, the adolescent reporting rape has usually had a very frightening experience and needs short-term counseling either by her regular physician (see Chapter 20) or, ideally, through the auspices of a rape victims' support program. She will usually have a number of questions about the physical meaning of her experience, and it is important to ensure that she obtains answers to them.

- She should be examined carefully for evidence of trauma, both to the pelvic organs and to the rest of her body, and the information should be carefully recorded.
- She must decide whether she wishes to report the rape to the police. In this instance, it is essential to obtain a wet and fixed smear of the vaginal contents as early as possible to confirm the presence of spermatozoa.
- Most rape victims will need ongoing counseling by their physician or a counselor for a number of months to discuss persisting anxieties and questions.
- When it is not possible to exclude (by identifying and testing the rapist) exposure to HIV, the rape victim should be offered surveillance for HIV infection following a protocol similar to that described in Chapter 39 for accidental needlesticks in health care personnel.
- If sexual intercourse occurred within 72 hours of the examination, the rape victim should be offered emergency STD prophylaxis and contraception.
- *STD prophylaxis* in adolescents and adults after sexual assault is as folllows:

  Ceftriaxone 125 mg intramuscularly in a single dose, *plus*
  Metronidazole 2 g orally in a single dose, *plus*
  Doxycycline 100 mg orally twice a day for 7 days.
  Consider Hepatitis B vaccination if nonimmune.
- *Pregnancy prophylaxis* (emergency contraception) in adolescents and adults after sexual assault is as follows:

  Norgestrel or levonorgestrel plus ethinyl estradiol pills (oral contraception pills) within 72 hours of assault and again 12 hours later.

Brand	Color	First Dose	Second Dose
Ovral	White	2 pills	2 pills
Lo/Ovral	White	4 pills	4 pills
Levlen	Light orange	4 pills	4 pills
Nordette	Light orange	4 pills	4 pills
Tri-Levlen	Yellow	4 pills	4 pills
Triphasil	Yellow	4 pills	4 pills

- Serum pregnancy test should be obtained and proven negative. If a woman is pregnant, there is a risk of fetal urogenital malformations if emergency contraception fails.
- Nausea is a common side effect of treatment.
- Informed consent should be obtained.

PSYCHOSOCIAL DEVELOPMENT

Normal Patterns and Concerns

The major psychosocial developmental task for the adolescent as adulthood approaches is to increase independence from their parents and to establish a positive identity congruent with social norms. In early adolescence, the young teen is faced with the dilemma of seeking independence from parents while at the same time relying on them for emotional and physical support. The conflict over independence is evidenced by contradiction and ambivalence. For example, a teen may refuse to listen to parents' suggestions about study habits but blame mediocre grades on the fact that the parents did not help with homework assignments.

As teens enter middle and late adolescence, they demonstrate a remarkable resourcefulness in coping with anxiety over separation and in learning more mature behavior. Much assistance comes through peer relationships. Teens support each other by experimenting with adult roles that mirror societal expectations of behavior; a sense of moral responsibility begins to take shape. In this period, individual identity tends to be blunted by the seeking of independence from the family. Peers tend to look alike, dress alike, date alike, and experiment with drugs and sex alike. Later, as teens address their concerns about careers, a greater differentiation of personalities takes shape and individual identities emerge.

Normal development also requires the example of secure healthy parents in an environment in which the teen can feel secure. Thus, parents who are preoccupied with their own psychological problems at work, in their marriage, or with their own families may have difficulties helping and coping with the development of their adolescent offspring. Often such parents have not previously succeeded at their own adolescent tasks and so are unable to proceed with the task of adulthood—they have not developed the ability for intimacy, close personal feelings, the sharing of feelings and thoughts with others, and adhering to reasonable limits.

One clear fact about adolescent development is that its *emotional course is variable,* even among normal adolescents. The idea that adolescence is usually a time of crisis, in which persistent neurotic behavior is essential for development of a personal identity, has not been borne out by longitudinal research. On the other hand, it has been found that at least 20% of first-year college students have psychological problems, usually personality disorders of the compulsive, schizoid, or passive-aggressive type (see details Chapter 23) expressed as difficulties in academic, social, and psychosexual functioning (6). Furthermore, adolescents are more likely than people in other age groups to be hospitalized for psychiatric conditions (7). A longitudinal study of teenage boys (8) points out that achievement of identity is a long-term process. Subjects were first studied in the first year of high school and were followed for 7 years. At the end of this interval, most subjects had yet to consolidate their identities to the point where they could develop an intimate relationship, one of the best indicators of progress to adulthood. Despite this, self-satisfaction and parental satisfaction were the norm. For many, adolescence is a crisis, but an internalized noiseless one.

Generally, the teen must succeed in the other spheres of development to meet tasks in the psychosocial sphere successfully. In children with retardation, physical disabilities, or chronic illness, the dependence–independence struggle may persist, impairing the development of self-esteem needed to develop a sense of identity.

Juvenile Delinquency

Juvenile delinquency is a legal term for youthful behavior that violates the law and would be adjudicated and punished if it had been committed by an adult. It is a major social problem and is sometimes brought to the attention of the practitioner, who is asked whether there is an underlying psychological cause for the delinquent behavior. To deal with this issue, it is necessary to distinguish between three broad categories of delinquency, described by Weiner (9) as sociologic delinquency, characterologic delinquency, and neurotic delinquency.

Sociologic delinquency refers to illegal acts organized by a subcultural group (i.e., street gang). The delinquent acts are adaptive in that the teen receives the approval of his or her peers. The following four features of the clinical history suggest sociologic delinquency: first, the delinquent acts are performed with valued companions, rather than alone or with strangers; second, these teens see themselves as accepted and integral members of their peer group and rarely exhibit feelings of alienation or inadequacy; third, sociologic delinquents give little evidence of neurotic symptom formation or basic character flaws; and fourth, these delinquents often have had supportive family relationships during early childhood, although there may have been more recent problems that have led to their current activities. Often, involvement in other positive group activities changes the delinquent orientation of these teens.

Characterologic delinquents reflect a basically antisocial attitude toward life. Their acts do not evoke in them any guilt or remorse. Such teens are often loners who have not established a strong relationship of basic trust in their life. Their history suggests a series of problems, with a flurry of destructive acts such as fighting, fire setting, and cruelty to animals preceding their more destructive delinquent activity. Such children often require long-term psychiatric treatment. Chapter 23 provides additional details about the course and management of patients with an antisocial personality.

The *neurotic delinquent* commits destructive acts as an atypical (for him or her) behavior pattern to illustrate and emphasize certain needs. These acts may reflect feelings of being ignored by family or peers or indicate that the teen is suffering from some form of psychological distress, most often depression. The acts are committed in such a way that the teen is caught in the process or gives himself or herself away soon after; generally, if concealment of illegal acts is repetitive and successful, a neurotic basis of the delinquency is unlikely. There is rarely a history of early behavioral problems, and typically the delinquent has enjoyed a loving relationship with parents and family members. Occasionally, however, some recent family stress may trigger the delinquent act. In general, neurotic delinquency may be treated through short-term counseling (see Chapter 20).

Violence and Violence Prevention

Recent shootings in schools in the United States by children and adolescents have brought to the forefront the issue of youth aggression and violence. Professionals that work with youth must work to define their roles and develop skills to address the risk factors and warning signs of violent behavior.

Violence (homicide and suicide) is the major cause of death and morbidity, outside of accidents, for teens and young adults. Youth have continuing exposure to violence, sex, and drug use through television, movies, and music videos; one estimate suggests that young people may view 10,000 acts of violence a year (10). Research suggests that a cause and effect relationship exists between media violence and aggression (11). Of deeper concern is the exposure of young teens to actual violence and aggression. One large cross-sectional study stated that almost 30% of 6th to 10th graders reported that they have participated in bullying, been bullied, or both (12). This study went on to suggest that bullies and those who are bullied both have a range of concurrent conduct, school, emotional, and physical problems. As adults, bullies are likely to exhibit criminal behavior, and those who have been bullied have higher rates of depression and poor self-esteem. It is disturbing that the perpetrators of the violence in Littleton, Colorado, Pearl, Mississippi, and Santee, California may have been bullying victims.

The American Academy of Pediatrics Task Force on Violence has suggested a number of age-appropriate interventions (13). These include promoting appropriate parenting skills by querying and counseling about discipline at home, substance abuse, violence and abuse exposure—physical, sexual, and verbal—at school and home, dating and dating behavior, and how conflicts have been resolved at home. Most importantly, practitioners should have knowledge of community- and school-based resources where at-risk youth may be referred. Practitioners who are very interested in violence prevention may work with communities to help design curricula, advocate for increased services, promote preventive activities, and foster community attitudes that affect the risk and incidence of violence. These may include promoting gun safety and reducing child access to guns, working with child abuse teams, and designing school curricula that include violence prevention. Practitioners can also work through advocacy groups to affect laws and regulations that are pertinent to violence prevention, such as gun safety requirements, prohibition of corporal punishment in schools, visitation programs for isolated families and new parents, and after-school programs for children and teens.

Substance Abuse

Although substance abuse, including tobacco use, is a major problem of adult life, it often begins during the adolescent years (see statistics in Table 29.2). By age 11, 1 in 5 adolescents has smoked cigarettes and approximately 1 in 11 adolescents has had his or her first drink of alcohol; by the age of 15, 1 in 7 adolescents smokes on a daily basis and more than 1 in 3 adolescents has drunk excessively at least once (3). Experimenting with substances of abuse may be viewed as a rite of passage bridging the gap between childhood and adulthood or as a condition for belonging to peer groups or organizations. Advertising or exposure to images that appear to link the use of cigarettes and alcohol to life successes, popularity, and sex can be important inducements for adolescents to try alcohol or tobacco. A major concern is to identify the adolescent abuser—one whose life is being disrupted by aberrant activities. This teenager is most likely to continue to abuse alcohol or drugs in adult life.

The routine evaluation of a teen should include questioning about the use of alcohol and of drugs. Substance use should be explored using nonthreatening questions such as those listed in Table 11.6. The presence of drug abuse and its impact on a teenager can also be uncovered by asking the parents questions such as those in Table 11.7. If the use of a substance is excessive and hazardous, factors that might have led to abuse should be explored. Drugs and alcohol are often abused as a response to some psychosocial problem, and it is only by identifying the problem that the abuse may be stopped. Lecturing on the dangers of alcohol, drugs, or tobacco seems to have little impact on adolescents. Unfortunately, teens who drive and use alcohol and drugs may endanger others, so it still behooves practitioners to discuss substance abuse with teens who deny personal drug use.

Occasionally, the serious abuser of hazardous substances develops physiologic symptoms that are dramatic enough to come to the physician's attention.

Table 11.6. Sample Questions Concerning Drug Use for Adolescents

I know that many schools have drug problems. Does your school have such a problem?
Do most of your friends drink alcohol or smoke marijuana at parties?
Do any of your friends use drugs other than alcohol or marijuana?
Where do most young people obtain drugs?
Do you smoke cigarettes? How many per day?
Have you ever tried alcohol? Marijuana? Other drugs?
Have you ever been ill as a result of using drugs or drinking?
Have you ever been in trouble with the law as a result of drugs or alcohol?
Do your parents know that you've used alcohol or drugs?
What would (did) they say?
Have you ever worried about your alcohol or drug use?
Have you ever been drunk or stoned and driven a car (or motorcycle)?

From Schonberg SK, ed. Substance abuse: a guide for health professionals. Elk Grove Village, IL: American Academy of Pediatrics, 1988, with permission.

Table 11.7. Questions for Interviewing the Parents of the Adolescent Suspected of or Known To Be Abusing Drugs or Alcohol

1. Does your son/daughter spend many hours alone in his/her bedroom apparently doing nothing?
2. Does your son/daughter resist talking to you or persistently isolate himself/herself from the family?
3. Has your daughter's/son's taste in music had a dramatic change to hard rock music?
4. Has there been a definite change in your son's/daughter's attitude at school? With his/her friends? At home?
5. Has your daughter/son shown recent pronounced mood swings with increased irritability and angry outbursts?
6. Does your son/daughter always seem to be unhappy and less able to cope with frustration than he/she used to be?
7. Has your daughter's/son's personality changed from being a considerate and caring person to being selfish, unfriendly, and unsympathetic?
8. Does your son/daughter always seem to be confused or "spacey"?
9. Have money or valuable articles recently disappeared from your home?
10. Has your daughter/son begun to neglect household chores or homework?
11. Has there been a change in your son's/daughter's friends from age-appropriate friends to older "unacceptable" associates?
12. Has there been a change in your daughter's/son's appearance (i.e., sloppy dress and poor grooming and hygiene)?
13. Have there been excuses and alibis made and has there been lying to avoid confrontation or not to get caught?
14. Do you feel you have lost control of your son/daughter?
15. Has your daughter/son begun lying to cover up sources of money and possessions?
16. Have there been episodes of "ditching" or "skipping" school? Has your son/daughter lied to cover up bad report cards?
17. Have there been stealing, shoplifting, or encounters with the police?
18. Has your daughter/son become a "con artist"?
19. Have you noticed a marked increase in your son's/daughter's interest in drugs, drug literature, and the drug "culture" (i.e., clothing and accoutrements, paraphernalia, belt buckles, and tee shirts with a drug theme)?
20. Has your daughter/son recently quit a sport or dropped out of school clubs or social groups, stopped music lessons, quit the band or orchestra, or lost interest in a hobby?
21. Has there been a deterioration of school performance, frequent truancy, or conflict with coaches or teachers?
22. Do you feel your daughter/son has become untrustworthy, insincere, and distrustful ("paranoid")?
23. Has he/she become unpredictable or rebellious?
24. Has your son/daughter been verbally abusive to you or your spouse?
25. Has your daughter/son been physically abusive to you or your spouse?
26. Has your son/daughter tried to introduce any of your other children to drugs or alcohol?
27. Has your daughter/son talked about suicide or running away?
28. Is your son/daughter more argumentative lately? Does he/she tend to blame others for his/her problems?
29. Is there a paranoid flavor to all of your daughter's/son's relationships with adults, siblings, and authority figures?

From Schonberg SK, ed. Substance abuse: a guide for health professionals. Elk Grove Village, IL: American Academy of Pediatrics, 1988, with permission.

Hospitalization for observation is almost always indicated for the teenager presenting with drug intoxication, even if emergency room evaluation indicates no immediate medical risks. The possibility of attempted suicide may be real and must be explored. Even if this is not a factor, there is still concern about the teen's ability to control his or her own drug abuse behavior.

How to intervene in teenage drug abuse behavior is a difficult question. Practical approaches to patients with substance abuse are contained in Chapters 27, 28, and 29.

Depression and Suicide

A behavioral hallmark of adolescents is mood shifts, from the peaks of elation to the depths of despair. Depressive symptoms are normal parts of psychosocial development. The quest for identity is balanced by a sense of loss once independence is achieved. Similarly, rejections by peers (e.g., first loves) may be felt very deeply. It is not unusual, as part of these depressions, for the adolescent to contemplate suicide. More than 1 in 4 adolescents in grades 9 through 12 has thought seriously about suicide, and 1 in 12 adolescents has actually attempted suicide (3).

Mattsson (14) describes *five depressive states of adolescence*:

1. Normal depressive mood swings represent transient reactions to personal disappointments or family difficulties. They rarely affect other life functions.
2. Acute depressive reactions are more severe states, often lasting weeks or months. They are normal reactions, similar to states of grief (see Chapter 24), often related to separation or loss of a close friend, relative, or teacher.
3. The adolescent who does not successfully work through grief and who becomes increasingly depressed and incapacitated by loss suffers from a depressive neurosis. Such teens withdraw from their normal functioning, are chronically sad, and begin to entertain suicidal ideation. This is a fairly severe level of depression and demands professional intervention.
4. The masked depressions of adolescence can be viewed as a subgroup of the depressive neuroses. Such teens cannot tolerate their painful feelings and express them through a variety of somatic or behavioral complaints. They may be frequent visitors to the primary care physician, suffering from ill-defined atypical symptoms without a clear organic basis. Their behavior may include overeating, delinquent acts, exhibitionist acts resulting in accidental self-destruction, and drug and alcohol abuse.
5. Psychotic depressive disorders are marked by impaired reality testing, thought disorders, paranoia, and suicidal intention, in addition to depressive symptomatology.

Primary care physicians are sometimes asked to evaluate depressed or suicidal adolescents. In taking the history, one should try to uncover recent events that may have precipitated the depressive disorder: any long-standing family, school, or peer problems; possibilities of organic brain disease or drug abuse that may mimic depressive symptoms; symptoms of cognitive or reality disturbances, suggesting a psychosis; and symptoms suggesting a masked depression. Openness in inquiry about depression usually puts the adolescent at ease and conveys that the physician truly understands what he or she may be feeling. A physical examination helps to rule out physical problems, and communication with the school may provide additional observations about the teen's current level of functioning.

Adolescents with depressive symptoms need some counseling. If one believes medication is necessary and is unfamiliar with the use of psychoactive drugs in adolescents, conjoint treatment with a psychiatric consultant may prove helpful. Patients with long-standing depressive symptoms, which suggest thought disturbances, and possible suicide attempts should be referred for psychiatric intervention. Additional details about the office assessment and management of depression are contained in Chapter 24.

INTELLECTUAL DEVELOPMENT

Normal Patterns and Concerns

In adolescence, a major change occurs with respect to education and intellect. Schools differentiate students, placing them into vocational or academic tracks. The emphasis shifts from the learning of tasks (e.g., basic reading, writing, and arithmetic) to the accumulation of facts and the ability to think abstractly. As teens prepare for college, learning becomes a competitive task. For some teens and families with high aspirations, the competitive nature of academic rankings and the pressure to be admitted into very selective colleges may isolate the child and interfere with social development. Career choices become limited as an individual's abilities and talents become manifest. Upon entering college, a greater amount of independence and responsibility is expected. Symbolically, the university begins to resemble the workplace in terms of both potential rewards and potential pressures.

Scholastic Failure

Academic achievement is strongly related to parental aspirations, socioeconomic status, and intellectual ability. Occasionally, a child cannot meet parental expectations, and the resultant crisis may lead to a visit to the physician. Failure in school may also be a symptom of a physical impairment, mental retardation, substance abuse, specific learning disabilities, or emotional stress. By making an accurate diagnosis of the underlying problem, a caring practitioner can help such children.

First, a history is necessary to determine the nature of the school difficulties. When did they begin? Has educational achievement been a problem throughout a school career, as with a global intellectual deficit, or is it specific to certain subjects or tasks, as with learning disorders? Is there a family history of poor school performance, as is seen with familial dyslexics? How does the teen act with family and peers? Is there evidence of disturbed behavior outside school, as with emotional disorders? Is the family structure stable or has there been separation, divorce, or death of a parent or grandparent? Is there evidence of substance abuse or physical abuse on the part of the teen or a member of the family? Is there daytime hypersomnolence that suggests a sleep disorder? What has the family done to try to work through problems?

Second, a physical examination, including neurologic examination, is indicated, with emphasis on signs of minimal cerebral dysfunction, such as difficulty with right–left discrimination or spatial orientation, or overt signs of cerebral palsy (14). In such patients, there may be suggestions of a neurologic problem in the medical history, the birth may have been abnormal, or the patient may have shown hyperactivity or attention deficits as a child. Vision testing and office assessment for slight or moderate hearing loss (see Chapter 110) are also particularly important.

Third, some specific intelligence testing is indicated. Children with mental retardation tend to show low intelligence quotient scores, and achievement tests show a delay of several grades in math and reading levels. Children with dyslexia have a normal intelligence quotient but show a wide scatter of scores on subtests, indicating a nonglobal deficit. Achievement tests may also show a difference between abilities in reading and mathematics.

Some learning problems may appear late in a school career (15). The recent criticism of the ability of some college students to write well has given credence to the notion of expressive language disorders, which may not become manifest until adolescence. Some people with fine perceptual problems may not reveal difficulties until geometry or drafting is studied in high school.

In 1974, Congress passed Federal Law 94-142, ensuring a free appropriate educational placement for all children up to age 21. Thus, adolescents with specific learning problems, retardation, or emotional difficulties are entitled to be placed in a classroom setting where they will learn. The physician who suspects an unrecognized problem in one of these spheres may help by referring the teen and the teen's parents for evaluation, usually available through the school or the local education system. Unfortunately, problems remain unrecognized for many children and, out of frustration, they drop out of school.

Attention Deficit/Hyperactivity Disorder

Attention deficit/hyperactivity disorder (AD/HD) may be one of the most common disorders of childhood, with prevalence rates ranging from 3% to 6% of prepubertal children. Although data on prevalence and persistence in adolescents and adults are limited, long-term follow-up studies show that critical symptoms of AD/HD—impairment of attention and regulation of activity and poor impulse control—often persist into adulthood, and many adults with AD/HD remain distractible, impulsive, inattentive, and disruptive throughout life. On average, symptoms of AD/HD diminish by about 50% every 5 years between the ages of 10 and 25 years. Adolescents with AD/HD may have impaired school performance, a disorganized approach to tasks, limited participation in extracurricular activities, increased risk of delinquency, and harmful social relationships and family interactions. In adults, AD/HD is often linked with psychiatric illness, incarceration, job failures, marital discord, and divorce (16).

Diagnosis

AD/HD is diagnosed, usually at serial visits using information from multiple sources. Criteria for the diagnosis are listed in Table 11.8. The diagnostic challenge in adolescents and adults is to detect the more subtle presentations of symptoms in these stages of life. For example, in teens and adults, symptoms of hyperactivity may be confined to fidgetiness or an inner feeling of jitteriness or restlessness. Current nomenclature differentiates AD/HD into three types: predominantly inattentive, predominantly impulsive, and combined.

The physical examination usually is noncontributory in diagnosing AD/HD but may be useful to rule out other conditions that are characterized by hyperactivity or short attention spans (see below). In teens, it is helpful to examine results of intellectual testing and academic achievement testing. A symptom checklist (Connor scale, Child Behavior Checklist) that can be completed by teachers and parents is also helpful to identify and quantify symptoms that teens may be demonstrating in their classrooms and homes.

Comorbidity

Up to 65% of adolescents with AD/HD have one or more comorbid conditions, such as learning disabilities, mood disorders (10% to 20%), substance abuse, and alcoholism, and may also be confused with other conditions that have hyperactivity as a feature, such as hyperthyroidism, Gilles de la Tourette syndrome, adjustment or oppositional disorders, affective disorders with manic features, social or personality difficulties, and medication-induced attention problems (e.g., substance abuse) (16). These patients have difficulty in the workplace, in school, and in social relations. They have more cognitive difficulties, poor performance in school, and significant difficulties with social skills and appropriate behavior. As a result, they tend to be underachievers with personalities that may be intrusive, immature, or negative.

Treatment

AD/HD is treated best with a multimodal combination of medication and counseling. On the basis of placebo-controlled trials, it has been found that stimulant drugs

Table 11.8. Diagnostic Criteria for Attention Deficit/Hyperactivity Disorder

A. Either 1 or 2
1. Six (or more) of the following symptoms of inattention have persisted for at least 6 months to a degree that is maladaptive and inconsistent with developmental level.
Inattention
a. Often fails to give close attention to details or makes careless mistakes in schoolwork, work, or other activities.
b. Often has difficulty sustaining attention in tasks or play activities.
c. Often does not seem to listen when spoken to directly.
d. Often does not follow through on instructions and fails to finish schoolwork, chores, or duties in the workplace (not because of oppositional behavior or failure to understand instructions).
e. Often has difficulty organizing tasks and activities.
f. Often avoids, dislikes, or is reluctant to engage in tasks that require sustained mental effort (such as schoolwork or homework).
g. Often loses things necessary for tasks or activities (e.g., toys, school assignments, pencils, books, or tools).
h. Is often easily distracted by extraneous stimuli.
i. Is often forgetful in daily activities.
2. Six (or more) of the following symptoms of hyperactivity–impulsivity have persisted for at least 6 months to a degree that is maladaptive and inconsistent with developmental level.
Hyperactivity
a. Often fidgets with hands or feet or squirms in seat.
b. Often leaves seat in classroom or in other situations in which remaining seated is expected.
c. Often runs about or climbs excessively in situations in which it is inappropriate (in adolescents or adults, may be limited to subjective feelings of restlessness).
d. Often has difficulty playing or engaging in leisure activites quietly.
e. Is often "on the go" or often acts as if "driven by a motor."
f. Often talks excessively.
Impulsivity
a. Often blurts out answers before questions have been completed.
b. Often has difficulty awaiting turn.
c. Often interrupts or intrudes on others (e.g., butts into conversations or games).

B. Some hyperactive–impulsive or inattentive symptoms that caused impairment were present before age 7 years.
C. Some impairment from the symptoms is present in two or more settings (e.g., at school [or work] and at home).
D. There must be clear evidence of clinically significant impairment in social, academic, or occupational functioning.
E. The symptoms do not occur exclusively during the course of a pervasive developmental disorder, schizophrenia, or other psychotic disorder and are not better accounted for by another mental disorder (e.g., mood disorder, anxiety disorder, dissociative disorder, or a personality disorder).

Diagnosis is:
Attention deficit/hyperactivity disorder, combined type if both criteria A1 and A2 are met for the past 6 months.
Attention deficit/hyperactivity disorder, predominantly inattentive type if criterion A1 is met but criterion A2 is not met for the past 6 months.
Attention deficit/hyperactivity disorder, predominantly hyperactive–impulsive type if criterion A2 is met but criterion A1 is not met for the past 6 months.
For individuals (especially adolescents and adults) who currently have symptoms that no longer meet full criteria, "in partial remission" should be specified.

From Diagnostic and statistical manual of mental disorders, 4th ed. (DSM-IV). Washington, DC: American Psychiatric Association, 1994, with permission.

greatly reduce the core symptoms of AD/HD, hyperactivity, impulsivity, and inattentiveness (16). It is estimated that 70% to 80% of children and 60% of adults have improvement in academic and social behaviors and in cognition and a reduction of disruptive and negative behaviors. Long-term improvement in academic outcome has not been found, however. Most patients with AD/HD are treated pharmacologically with psychostimulant medications, such as methylphenidate or dextroamphetamine, although a small number respond well to antidepressant agents, such as desipramine. Practical information regarding these medications is summarized in Table 11.9. Medication should be titrated carefully and should be used on school or work days and other days where focus and attention may be needed (e.g., for long-distance drives). Medication should be prescribed to cover learning and work-related needs, such as homework and examination preparation times. With short-acting stimulant medications such as methylphenidate, holiday periods off medication may be permitted. Counseling interventions include psychoeducational counseling, behavioral management, school-based interventions, family therapy, and social competence training. The following support groups for AD/HD patients and their families, respectively, exist in many communities: Children and Adults with AD/HD and the AD/HD Association.

APPROACH TO THE ADOLESCENT PATIENT IN THE OFFICE SETTING

When interviewing teens, it is helpful to keep in mind that the transitional nature of adolescence makes it a time of great experimentation and risk taking (see Sexual Development and Substance Abuse, above).

Each adolescent approaches the developmental pressures of this period of life with his or her particular skills and emotions. From a health perspective, adolescents can be responsible partners in maintaining their well-being and complying with medical care, or they can be infantile, dependent, uncommunicative, aggressive, or irresponsible. It is important to interview adolescents in private. Adolescents need to believe they are the patient and that their problems are

Table 11.9. Medications for Attention Deficit Disorder with Hyperactivity (AD/HD) in Adolescents and Adults

Drug	Available Strengths (mg)	Dosage	Comments
Methylphenidate (Ritalin, Concerta)	Tabs: 5, 10, 20 Slow-release tabs: 20 (6- to 8-h duration) Concerta: 18, 36, 54 (8- to 12-h duration)	Initial: 0.25 mg/kg/dose given with breakfast and lunch Maintenance: 1–2 mg/kg/24 h Maximum: 60 mg daily	Begin with initial dose. May double dosage weekly until desired clinical effect is achieved or maintenance dosage is reached. Stop if no improvement in 1 month. May give after-school dose for homework. Use cautiously in patients with HTN, epilepsy. Contraindicated in patients with glaucoma, Gilles de la Tourette syndrome, MAO inhibitor use. Commonly causes insomnia, anorexia. If full day medication needed (e.g., afterschool activities, homework) can use Concerta, releases methylphenidate for up to 12-h period, usually start with 36 or 54.
Dextroamphetamine (Dexedrine or Adderall, combination of dextroamphetamine with d, amphetamine)	Tabs: 5, 10 Elixir: 5 mg/5 mL Sustained-release caps: 5, 10, 15 Caps: 15 Adderall: 5, 10, 20, 30	Initial: 10 mg/24 h in morning Maximum: 60 mg daily	Begin with initial dose. May increase by 10 mg/wk until maximum dose. Same guidelines as methylphenidate. Side effects more common than with methylphenidate because of longer duration of action. Adderall may start 5 b.i.d. and work up by 5 per dose.
Desipramine (Norpramine)	Tabs: 10, 25, 50, 100, 150	Initial: 10 mg/24 h in morning Maximum: 100 mg daily	Begin at lowest dose for adolescent. Increase according to tolerance and response. Usual dosage 25–50 mg/day for adolescents. Must obtain ECG when using medication to look for signs of prolongation of QRS and QT intervals. For this reason, a poor choice in patients with cardiovascular disease, congenital heart disease, hypertension, etc. Occasional behavioral side effects noted, especially if manic–depressive illness not recognized. May cause leukopenia, especially during febrile illness.

being listened to and taken seriously. It is often useful to talk to the parents separately as well.

Interviewing the Patient

Some adolescent patients are difficult to interview. An uncommunicative patient may have been sent to a physician involuntarily or may lack verbal skills needed for coherence. One must be verbally active with such patients and watch for any nonverbal cues to use as wedges in trying to get the patient to speak. Examples of nonverbal cues are a look of interest or initiation of eye contact when a subject is mentioned that the patient would like to discuss, a clenched fist when an anger-provoking subject is raised, and frequent position change and fidgeting when the patient is anxious about a specific subject or about the visit to the physician in general. Because adolescents are often reticent about their major concerns, open-minded invitations to share information (e.g., "Is there anything else you wanted to talk about?") should be included in each office contact. The initial comprehensive interview may require several sessions. At the first visit, warmth and interest in the adolescent may open the way to better communication in future sessions.

Some adolescents respond more honestly to *written questionnaires* rather than interviews. It may be a useful strategy to preface an interview with a form questionnaire for both the adolescent and the parent. As part of this questionnaire, ground rules can be outlined, such as assurances of confidentiality. In general, an adult-oriented questionnaire, with reviews of systems, is not appropriate for younger teens and should be reserved for teens aged 18 years or older. The questionnaire should not take the place of the personal interview but can guide the interview to address issues of concern of the patient in greater detail.

Many adolescents continue to go to a pediatrician for medical care until they enter college, take a job, or marry. Because of this long-term association, their relationship may be almost like that of a parent and child: warm, intense, and comradely. These feelings cannot be transferred easily to a new physician, and it is unwise to attempt to transfer them.

Practitioners can most effectively surmount problems in communicating with adolescents by explaining their modus operandi in advance, emphasizing that they will be primarily the adolescent's physician rather than an agent of the patient's parents, as had been the case previously. The adolescent should also be encouraged to initiate patient–practitioner contacts. It is important to guard against paternalistic advice giving and to avoid showing disapproval or surprise when the adolescent attempts to impress one with tales of sexual exploits or the use of vulgar language. *Sexuality* is an important topic to address with teens, but one should not impose judgment on a teen's sexual activities, gender preferences, or other characteristics. Instead, one should address how a teen's sexuality may create health risk and focus screening and health education efforts on these risks.

It is wise to *establish certain ground rules* with adolescents. Patient–doctor confidentiality, for example, can be assured to adolescents only insofar as they do not reveal that they are contemplating harmful acts, such as running away or committing suicide.

However, certain privileged communications should be kept confidential from parents. In particular, adolescent minors have the right to be seen for STDs or for sex offense-related examinations without the prior consent of a parent. The teen may also wish to keep some health-related or emotional problems, such as drug experimentation, from a parent's knowledge.

Interviewing the Parents

Whenever possible, parents should be involved with and concerned about the health of the teen. A separate interview with parents, immediately before or after the examination, may prove helpful and can emphasize particular concerns downplayed or denied by the patient. The parents of adolescent patients may be useful in providing emotional support and ensuring compliance with therapy; therefore, informing them about the adolescent's problems and needs is important.

Some parents ask physicians to take on the role of health educator or counselor for their adolescent child. Usually, these requests are for anticipatory guidance about birth control or drug usage. At times, the physician is asked to help the teen work through an upcoming family crisis, such as divorce, serious illness, or death. Often, adolescents welcome the opportunity to discuss these issues in private. Their knowledge in these areas is often found wanting, and a sensitive physician may help the adolescent grasp realities and make intelligent decisions. A number of books on these subjects are directed to an adolescent and young adult audience, and it may be useful to make these titles available (see General References).

Parents often have questions about specific adolescent behavior. A particular episode or issue may come to the parents' attention, and they may ask the physician whether they should exert control over it. In such instances, one should not offer specific advice but should try to discern any moral or behavioral conflicts between the parents and the adolescent. When the parents' behavior is inconsistent with the parents' own stated values, adolescents often act in opposition to those values. Miller (17) suggests that parents are not helped in this instance by being told how to behave. Advice either increases the parents' uncertainty when faced with later difficulties or implies that the parents' own opinions are inappropriate. Adolescents probably turn out mentally healthier when presented with models of adult behavior with which their parents are comfortable, whether consistent with societal norms or not. However, parents must be prepared to make allowances so that their children have freedom to make their own mistakes. Family counseling is a technique that a general physician can use when several members of a household are involved (see Chapter 20).

Health Assessment and Preventive Care

The initial interview(s) should be comprehensive enough to ensure that the adolescent is meeting *appropriate developmental tasks.* Inquiries should be made into teenagers' relationships and functioning with their families, at school, and with peers. It is important to determine whether teenagers are establishing positive personal identities (Do they have hobbies? Do they voice their own opinions? Can they choose their own friends or must friends be approved by the parents? Do they have plans for the future?), whether they are accepting their sexuality and adjusting to adult sexual roles (Do they date? Are they sexually active? Do they have a knowledge of contraception? Is contraception used?), whether they are establishing independence from the family (Do they drive? Do they earn money on their own? What sort of hours do they keep?), whether they are working toward a career (What are their plans after high school? What subjects in school do they like? What are their grades? Do they plan to go to college? Are their goals realistic and are they supported by the family?), whether they have established good health habits (What are their views about nutrition? Do they have an adequate source of calcium and iron in their diet [see Chapter 15]? Do they eat breakfast? Is eating done on the run, in isolation, or with friends and family? Have they experimented with alcohol, tobacco, or other recreational drugs? What drugs? Have they ever been drugged or high when driving or when attending school?), and whether affective swings are interfering with functioning (Do they often feel down? What makes them happy? Have sad feelings ever made them consider harming themselves?).

As part of the *review of systems before examination,* a self-administered medical questionnaire may be useful and time saving. Such a questionnaire should be brief, with language simple enough to be understood by teens with poor reading skills. Positive answers must be explored further.

A *physical examination* should be performed in the absence of parents. Teenage girls examined by male physicians may be more comfortable with a female adult in the room with them. Some parts of the physical examination occasionally omitted by physicians but essential for adolescent patients include blood pressure measurement and examination of the entire integument, the spine (for scoliosis), and the external genitalia (for signs of venereal disease and for assessment of sexual development using Tanner staging [Tables 11.4 and 11.5]). All sexually active adolescent girls should have a pelvic examination, including gonorrheal cultures and a Pap smear (see Chapter 104). If one is uncomfortable doing this examination, the teen should be referred to a gynecologist (preferably female) who is used to dealing with adolescents.

There are *several important adjuncts to the physical examination of the healthy adolescent,* including testing for myopia and hyperopia (using a Snellen chart) and screening for deafness (by pure tone audiometry). Adolescence is a period marked by noise pollution in the form of loud music that can cause permanent damage to the eighth nerve (see Chapter 110). Adolescents who have difficulty in school should be screened for learning disorders. Having a teenager read a newspaper paragraph out loud or do some simple

Procedure	Early				Middle			Late			
Age of adolescent	11	12	13	14	15	16	17	18	19	20	21
Health guidance											
Parenting*	—	—	■	—	—	■	—				
Development	■	■	■	■	■	■	■	■	■	■	■
Diet & physical activity	■	■	■	■	■	■	■	■	■	■	■
Healthy lifestyles**	■	■	■	■	■	■	■	■	■	■	■
Injury prevention	■	■	■	■	■	■	■	■	■	■	■
Screening history											
Eating disorders	■	■	■	■	■	■	■	■	■	■	■
Sexual activity***	■	■	■	■	■	■	■	■	■	■	■
Alcohol & other drug use	■	■	■	■	■	■	■	■	■	■	■
Tobacco use	■	■	■	■	■	■	■	■	■	■	■
Abuse	■	■	■	■	■	■	■	■	■	■	■
School performance	■	■	■	■	■	■	■	■	■	■	■
Depression	■	■	■	■	■	■	■	■	■	■	■
Risk for suicide	■	■	■	■	■	■	■	■	■	■	■
Physical assessment											
Blood pressure	■	■	■	■	■	■	■	■	■	■	■
BMI	■	■	■	■	■	■	■	■	■	■	■
Comprehensive exam	—	—	■	—	—	■	—	—	—	■	—
Tests											
Cholesterol	—	—	1	—	—	1	—	—	—	1	—
TB	—	—	2	—	—	2	—	—	—	2	—
GC, Chlamydia, Syphilis & HPV	—	—	3	—	—	3	—	—	—	3	—
HIV	—	—	4	—	—	4	—	—	—	4	—
Pap smear	—	—	5	—	—	5	—	—	—	5	—
Immunizations											
MMR	—	■									
Td	—	■									
HepB	—	■			—	6	—	—	—	6	—
HepA	—	—	7	—	—	7	—	—	—	7	—
Varicella	—	—	8	—	—	8	—	—	—	8	—

1. Screening test performed once if family history is positive for early cardiovascular disease or hyperlipidemia.

2. Screen if positive for exposure to active TB or lives/works in high-risk situation, e.g., homeless shelter, health care facility.

3. Screen at least annually if sexually active.

4. Screen if high-risk for infection.

5. Screen annually if sexually active or if 18 years or older.

6. Vaccinate if high risk for hepatitis B infection.

7. Vaccinate if at risk for hepatitis A infection.

8. Vaccinat if no reliable history of chicken pox.

* *A parent health guidance visit is recommended during early and middle adolescence.*

** *Includes counseling regarding sexual behavior and avoidance of tobacco, alcohol, and other drug use.*

*** *Includes history of unintended pregnancy and STD.*

Figure 11.3. Preventive health services for adolescents by age and procedure. (American Medical Association. AMA guidelines for adolescent preventive services [GAPS]. http://www.ama_assn.org/ama/pub/category/1980.html. Updated April 2001, with permission.)

Table 11.10. Sports Participation Health History

This evaluation is only to determine readiness for sports participation. It should not be used as a substitute for regular health maintenance exams.

Name____________ Grade________ Sports________

	YES	NO
1. Have you ever had an illness that		
a. Required you to stay in the hospital?	____	____
b. Lasted longer than a week?	____	____
c. Caused you to miss 3 days of practice or a competition?	____	____
d. Is related to allergies? (i.e., hay fever, hives, asthma, insect stings)	____	____
e. Required an operation?	____	____
f. Is chronic? (i.e., asthma, diabetes)	____	____
2. Have you ever had an injury that		
a. Required you to go to an emergency room or see a doctor?	____	____
b. Required you to stay in the hospital?	____	____
c. Required x-rays?	____	____
d. Caused you to miss 3 days of practice or a competition?	____	____
e. Required an operation?	____	____
3. Do you take any medication or pills?	____	____
4. Have any members of your family under age 50 had a heart attack or heart problems, or died unexpectedly?	____	____
5. Have you ever		
a. Been dizzy or passed out during or after exercise?	____	____
b. Been unconscious or had a concussion?	____	____
6. Are you unable to run ½ mile (2 times around the track) without stopping?		
7. Do you		
a. Wear glasses or contacts?	____	____
b. Wear dental bridges, plates, or braces?	____	____
8. Have you ever had a heart murmur, high blood pressure, or a heart abnormality?	____	____
9. Do you have any allergies to any medicines?	____	____
10. Are you missing a kidney?	____	____
11. When was your last tetanus booster?	________	
12. For women		
a. At what age did you experience your first menstrual period?	________	
b. In the last year, what was the longest time you have gone between periods?	________	

EXPLAIN ANY "YES" ANSWERS

Signature of parent____________

Signature of athlete____________

Date____________

INTERIM HEALTH HISTORY

This form should be used during the interval between participation evaluations. Positive responses should prompt a physical exam.

1. Over the next 12 months, I wish to participate in the following sports:
   a. ____________
   b. ____________
   c. ____________
   d. ____________
2. Have you missed more than 3 consecutive days of participation in usual activities because of an injury this past year?
   YES____ NO____
3. Have you missed more than 5 consecutive days of participation in usual activities because of an illness, or have you had a medical illness diagnosed that has not resolved in the past year?
   YES____ NO____
   If yes, please indicate type of illness:________
4. Have you had a seizure or concussion, or been unconscious for any reason in the last year?
   YES____ NO____
5. Have you had surgery or been hospitalized in this past year?
   YES____ NO____
   If yes, please indicate
   a. Reason for hospitalization________
   b. Type of surgery________
6. List all medications you are currently taking and what condition the medication is for.
   a. ____________
   b. ____________
   c. ____________
   d. ____________
7. Are you worried about any problem or condition at this time?
   YES____ NO____
   If yes, please explain: ________

Signature of athlete____________

Signature of parent____________

Date____________

From Committee on Sports Medicine and Fitness, American Academy of Pediatrics. Sports medicine: health care for young athletes, 2nd ed. Elk Grove Village, IL: American Academy of Pediatrics, 1991, with permission.

arithmetic may reveal a previously undetected learning disability.

Laboratory screening tests for healthy adolescents are remarkably few. Screening for anemia with a hematocrit or hemoglobin determination may be limited to menstruating young women. Tuberculosis screening with purified protein derivative should be performed only if there are family or community risk factors. Screening for hyperlipidemia is controversial during adolescence. The chance of diagnosing a problem severe enough to require pharmacologic therapy is small, whereas the benefits of a diet low in total fat and cholesterol may be universal. The decision to screen adolescents may be influenced by family history of myocardial infarction or stroke under the age of 55 or by personal opinion about whether an abnormal lipid profile may influence a patient's dietary practices. Urinalysis, blood chemistry screens, chest radiographs, and electrocardiograms are not indicated in healthy adolescents.

Healthy adolescents may require tests, immunizations and/or physical examinations for special needs, such as travel, sports, camp, and college entry. In addition, there may be optional vaccines or tests that will need to be coordinated with the routine health schedule, such as meningococcus or varicella vaccine for students entering college or chest x-rays for students who have had BCG vaccine.

Recommended Preventive Services

Figure 11.3 summarizes the consensus American Medical Association Guidelines for Adolescent Preventive

Table 11.11. Medical Conditions and Sports Participation

Condition	May Participate?	Explanation[a]
Atlantoaxial instability	Qualified yes	Condition common with Downs' syndrome. Athlete needs evaluation to assess risk of spinal cord injury during sports participation.
Bleeding disorder	Qualified yes	Athlete needs evaluation.
Cardiovascular diseases[b]		
Carditis	No	Carditis may result in sudden death with exertion.
Hypertension	Qualified yes	With essential hypertension, avoid weight and power lifting, body building, and strength training. Those with secondary hypertension or severe essential hypertension need evaluation.
Congenital heart disease	Qualified yes	Those with mild forms may participate fully. Those with moderate or severe forms, or who have undergone surgery, need evaluation.
Arrhythmia	Qualified yes	Athlete needs evaluation because some types require therapy or make certain sports dangerous, or both.
Mitral valve prolapse	Qualified yes	Those with symptoms (chest pain, symptoms of possible arrhythmia) or evidence of mitral regurgitation on physical examination need evaluation. All other may participate fully.
Heart murmur	Qualified yes	If the murmur is innocent, full participation is permitted. Otherwise, the athlete needs evaluation.
Cerebral palsy	Qualified yes	Athlete needs evaluation.
Diabetes mellitus	Yes	All sports can be played with proper attention to diet, hydration, and insulin therapy. Particular attention is needed for activities that last 30 min or more.
Diarrhea	Qualified no	Unless disease is mild, no participation is permitted because diarrhea may increase the risk of dehydration and heat illness. See "Fever."
Eating disorders Anorexia nervosa Bulimia nervosa	Qualified yes	These patients need both medical and psychiatric assessment before participation.
Eyes: functionally one-eyed athlete, loss of any eye, detached retina, previous eye surgery or serious eye injury	Qualified yes	A functionally one-eyed athlete has a best-corrected visual acuity of less than 20/40 in the worse eye. These athletes would suffer significant disability if the better eye were seriously injured, as would those with loss of an eye. Some athletes who have undergone eye surgery or had a serious eye injury may have an increased risk of injury because of weakened eye tissue. Availability of eye guards approved by the American Society of Testing Materials (ASTM) and other protective equipment may allow participation in most sports, but this must be judged on an individual basis.
Fever	No	Fever can increase cardiopulmonary effort, reduce maximum exercise capacity, make heat illness more likely, and increase orthostatic hypotension during exercise. Fever may rarely accompany myocarditis or other infections that make exercise dangerous.
Heat illness, history of	Qualified yes	Because of the increased likelihood of recurrence, the athlete needs individual assessment to determine the presence of predisposing conditions and arrange a prevention strategy.
Human immunodeficiency virus infection	Yes	Because of the apparent minimal risk to others, all sports may be played that the state of health allows. In all athletes, skin lesions should be properly covered, and athletic personnel should use universal precautions when handling blood or body fluids containing visible blood.
Kidney, absence of one	Qualified yes	Athlete needs individual assessment for contact/collision and limited contact sports.
Liver, enlarged	Qualified yes	If the liver is acutely enlarged, participation should be avoided because of the risk of rupture. If the liver is chronically enlarged, individual assessment is needed before collision/contact or limited contact sports are played.
Malignancy	Qualified yes	Athlete needs individual assessment.
Musculoskeletal disorders	Qualified yes	Athlete needs individual assessment.
Neurologic conditions		
History of serious head or spine trauma, severe or repeated concussions or craniotomy	Qualified yes	Athlete needs individual assessment for collision or limited contact sports and for noncontact sports if there are deficits in judgment or cognition. Recent research supports a conservative approach to management of concussion.
Convulsive disorder, well controlled	Yes	Risk of convulsion during participation is minimal.
Convulsive disorder, poorly controlled	Qualified yes	Athlete needs individual assessment for collision or limited contact sports. Avoid the following noncontact sports: archery, riflery, swimming, weight or power lifting, strength training, or sports involving heights. In these sports, occurrence of a convulsion may be a risk to self or others.
Obesity	Qualified yes	Because of the risk of heat illness, obese athletes need careful acclimatization and hydration.
Organ transplant recipient	Qualified yes	Athlete needs individual assessment.
Ovary, absence of one	Yes	Risk of severe injury to the remaining ovary is minimal.
Respiratory		
Pulmonary compromise including cystic fibrosis	Qualified yes	Athlete needs individual assessment, but generally all sports may be played if oxygenation remains satisfactory during a graded exercise test. Patients with cystic fibrosis need acclimatization and good hydration to reduce the risk of illness.

Continued

Table 11.11—*continued.* **Medical Conditions and Sports Participation**

Condition	May Participate?	Explanation[a]
Asthma	Yes	With proper medication and education, only athletes with the most severe asthma must modify their participation.
Acute upper respiratory	Qualified yes	Upper respiratory obstruction may affect pulmonary function. Athlete needs individual assessment for all but mild disease. See "Fever."
Sickle cell disease	Qualified yes	Athlete needs individual assessment. In general, if status of the illness permits, all but high-exertion collision/contact sports may be played. Overheating, dehydration, and chilling must be avoided.
Sickle cell trait (AS)	Yes	It is unlikely that athletes with sickle cell trait have an increased risk of sudden death or other medical problems during athletic participation except during the most extreme conditions of heat, humidity, and possibly increased altitude. These patients, like all athletes, should be carefully conditioned, acclimatized, and hydrated to reduce any possible risk.
Skin: boils, herpes simplex, impetigo, scabies, molluscum contagiosum	Qualified yes	While the patient is contagious, participation in gymnastics with mats, martial arts, wrestling, or other collision/contact or limited contact sports is not allowed. Herpes simplex virus is probably not transmitted via mats.
Spleen, enlarged	Qualified yes	Patients with acutely enlarged spleens should avoid all sports because of risk of rupture. Those with chronically enlarged spleens need individual assessment before playing collision/contact or limited contact sports.
Testicle, absent or undescended	Yes	Certain sports may require a protective cup.

[a]"Needs evaluation" means that a physician with appropriate knowledge and experience should assess the safety of a given sport for an athlete with the listed medical condition. Unless otherwise noted, this is because of the variability of the severity of the disease or the risk of injury among specific sports.

[b]Cardiac causes of sudden death in sports: hypertrophic cardiomyopathy, aortic rupture secondary to Marfan syndrome, congenital coronary artery anomalies, atherosclerotic coronary artery disease, and aortic stenosis. Most are rarely diagnosed during routine physical examination, although presence of marfanoid body habitus or characteristic heart murmur could aid early detection. Examiner needs to be alert to patients with positive family histories of early heart disease, hyperlipidemia, early sudden death, and Marfan syndrome.

From Andrews JS. Making the most of the sports physical. Contemp Pediatr 1997;14:183–205, and American Academy of Pediatrics, Committee on Sports Medical Fitness. Medical conditions affecting sports participation. Pediatrics 1994;94:757, with permission.

Services. Some offices find it useful to keep this table, as a prompt and for documenting completed actions, in the records of adolescent patients.

Examining the Adolescent Athlete

The examination of adolescent athletes requires an evaluation of their health and consideration of their functional ability, growth, and maturation. The purpose of the preparticipation health evaluation is to identify medical conditions that might preclude safe and effective athletic participation, including those that might become worse by participation in sports activities. A brief screening questionnaire (Table 11.10) along with information already known to the physician will identify most conditions that may disqualify an adolescent from participation in various types of sports (Table 11.11).

As athletes become more experienced, the most commonly encountered problems are residuals of previous sports injuries, most of them musculoskeletal problems. Common exercise-related musculoskeletal injuries that can be managed in the office are described in Chapter 72.

General References*

American Academy of Pediatrics. Care of the young athlete. Elk Grove Village, IL: American Academy of Pediatrics, 2000.

Developed by the American Academy of Pediatrics and the American Academy of Orthopedic Surgery, a single source reference for all aspects of childhood athletics.

American Academy of Pediatrics. Practicing adolescent medicine. A collection of resources. Elk Grove Village, IL: American Academy of Pediatrics, 1998.

American College of Physicians. **Position paper: Health care needs of the adolescent**. Ann Intern Med 1989;110:930.

Consensus recommendations, with references.

American Medical Association. **AMA guidelines for adolescent preventive services (GAPS): recommendations and rationale**. Baltimore: Williams & Wilkins, 1994.

A set of guidelines, updated periodically by an expert panel, addressing recommendations for the delivery of health services, health guidance, screening, and immunizations for adolescents. Updates may be found on the American Medical Association website for GAPS: www.ama_assn.org/ama/pub/category/1980.html.

American Academy of Pediatrics, Committee on Adolescence. Care of the adolescent sexual assault victim. Pediatrics 2001;117:1476.

A condensed knowledge base for primary care physicians who care for adolescent patients who have been sexually assaulted.

D'Angelo JD, Farrow J. Clinical problems in adolescent medicine. J Gen Intern Med 1989;4:64.

Brief review of selected problems of adolescents (growth and development, substance abuse, eating disorders, sexual problems, and violence).

Erickson EH. Identity, youth and crisis. New York: W.W. Norton, 1994.

The most widely used theoretical model of adolescent psychosocial development.

McAnarney ER, Kreipe RE, Orr DP, et al. Textbook of adolescent medicine. Philadelphia: W.B. Saunders, 1992.

An excellent comprehensive textbook with large sections on practice applications, psychologic issues, and medical problems as they present and are managed in teens.

Tanner JM. Growth at adolescence, 2nd ed. Springfield, IL: Charles C Thomas, 1962.

A classic system for describing the physiologic changes of adolescents. www.aap.org (website for the American Academy of Pediatrics—go to section on policy statements). www.adolescenthealth.org (website for the society of adolescent medicine).

Two websites for updates on adolescent medicine topics and guidelines.

*Bold print (general references) and bold numerals (specific references) denote published controlled clinical trials, meta-analyses, or consensus-based recommendations.

Books and Materials that May Be Helpful for Adolescents to Read

Pamphlets such as the following titles are available from the American Academy of Pediatrics, Division of Publications, 141 Northwest Point Boulevard, P.O. Box 927, Elk Grove Village, IL 60009-0927.

Better Health Through Fitness
Important Information for Teens Who Get Headaches
Acne Treatment and Control
Making the Right Choice: Facts Young People Need to Know About Avoiding Pregnancy
Striving: Coping with Adolescent Depression and Suicide

Alexander RB, ed. Changing bodies, changing lives. New York: New York Times Books, 1998.

Otis CL, Goldingay R. Campus health guide. The college student's handbook for healthy living. New York: College Entrance Examination Board, 1989.

A guide for teens living away from home for the first time.

www.chbucto.ns.ca/Health/TeenHealth/index.html

A website for teens looking for links to health topics, designed and maintained by medical students from Dalhousie University.

Resources for Parents

Alexander-Roberts C. ADHD and teens: a parent's guide for making it through the tough years. Dallas: Taylor, 1995.

A learning tool to help parents understand the heightened difficulties of transition faced by teens with AD/HD.

American Academy of Child and Adolescent Psychiatry. In: Pruitt DN, ed. Your adolescent. Emotional, behavioral, and cognitive development from early adolescence through the teen years. New York: Harper Collins, 1999.

An excellent, balanced, and brief review of normal teenage development and developmental and emotional disorders of adolescence, written for concerned parents.

Dinkmeyer D, McKay GD. Parenting teenagers: systematic theory for parenting of teens. Circle Pines, MN: American Guidance Service, 1998.

A STEP guide with helpful exercises and improvement insights regarding communication skills for parents with teens in trouble.

Elkind D. Parenting your teenager. New York: Ballantine, 1994.

A set of columns and contributions to Parents Magazine. Strong on normal development and everyday problems of normal teens.

Fenwick E, Smith T. Adolescence: the survival guide for parents and teenagers. New York: D.K. Publishing, 1996.

A good general source book, including teen milestones, talking to teens, and helping teens deal with their growing independence.

Philadelphia Child Guidance Center. Your child's emotional health: adolescence. New York: Macmillan, 1995.

Directive style to help parents deal with a number of common teen issues.

Weiss L. Give your ADD teen a chance. A guide for parents of teenagers with attention deficit disorder. Colorado Springs: Pinon, 1996.

Wolf E. Get out of my life, but first could you drive me and Cheryl to the mall? A parent's guide to the new teenager. New York: Noonday Press, 1992.

Strategies for parents to address teenage behavior issues, written in a jargon-free style by a clinical psychologist.

www.fenichel.com/adolhealth.shtml

A website created and maintained by Michael Fenichel, PhD, with resources and links to adolescent behavior topics.

Specific References*

1. Kreipe RE. Eating disorder among children and adolescents. Pediatr Rev 1995;16:370.
2. Pope HG, Hudson JI, Yurgelun-Todd D. Anorexia nervosa and bulimia among 300 suburban women shoppers. Am J Psychiatry 1984;141:292.
3. American Medical Association. AMA guidelines for adolescent preventive services (GAPS): recommendations and rationale. Baltimore: Williams & Wilkins, 1994.
4. Kogut MD. Growth and development in adolescents. Pediatr Clin North Am 1973;20:789.
5. Hein K. Commentary on adolescent acquired immune deficiency syndrome: the next wave of the human immunodeficiency virus epidemic? J Pediatr 1989;114:144.
6. Kysar JR, Zaks MS, Schuchman HP, et al. Range of psychological functioning in normal late adolescents. Arch Gen Psychiatry 1969;21:515.
7. Burns BJ, Taube CA. Mental health service for adolescents: assessment background paper for U.S. Congress, Office of Technology Assessment. In: Adolescent health I: summary and policy options. OTA-H-468. Washington, DC: U.S. Government Printing Office, 1991.
8. Offer D, Marcus D, Offer JL. A longitudinal study of normal adolescent boys. Am J Psychiatry 1970;126:917.
9. Weiner IB. Delinquent behavior. In: Psychological disturbance in adolescence. New York: Wiley, 1992.
10. Donnerstein E, Slaby R, Eron L. The mass media and youth aggression. In: Eron L, Gentry J, Schlegel P, eds. Reason to hope: a psychological perspective on violence and youth. Washington, DC: American Psychological Association, 1995.
11. Strassburger V, Donnerstein E. Children, adolescents and the media: issues and solutions. Pediatrics 1999;103:129.
12. Nansel T, Overpeck M, Pilla R, et al. Bullying behaviors among US youth. Prevalence and association with psychosocial adjustment. JAMA 2001;185:2094.
13. American Academy of Pediatrics Task Force on Violence (Spivak H, chair). The role of the pediatrician in youth violence prevention in clinical practice and at the community level. Pediatrics 1999;103:173.
14. Mattsson A. Adolescent depression and suicide. In: Hockelman RA, Blatman S, Bounell PA, et al, eds. Principles of pediatrics. New York: McGraw-Hill, 1978.
15. Levine MD, Zallen BG. The learning disorders of adolescence: organic and non-organic failure to thrive. Pediatr Clin North Am 1984;31:345.
16. Goldman LS, Genel M, Bezman RJ, et al. Diagnosis and treatment of attention-deficit/hyperactivity disorder in children and adolescents. JAMA 1998;279:1100–1107.
17. Miller D. Adolescent crisis: challenge for patient, parent, and internist. Ann Intern Med 1973;79:435.

CHAPTER 12

Geriatric Medicine: Special Considerations

PETER H. CHENG, MD
THOMAS E. FINUCANE, MD

OVERVIEW

Geriatrics is formed from two Greek root words meaning "old age" and "healing" or "physician." Related words are *gerontology,* which refers generally to the study of aging, and *iatrogenic,* which literally means "caused by a physician or healer."

In 2000 there were approximately 35 million people in the United States 65 years or older; by 2030 this number is expected to double. Ambulatory adult medicine in the United States is already geriatric medicine to a great extent, and it is likely to become increasingly geriatric in the next several decades. These observations result from two distinct phenomena. First, at every age, life expectancy is increasing (Table 12.1). In 1980, a 65-year-old American could expect on average to live another 16.4 years. By 1997, this number has increased to 17.6 years. An 85-year-old woman today has a life expectancy of 6.6 years, 1 more year than a man at the same age. These "oldest old," over age 85, are a special challenge to society as a whole and to physicians in particular. They are predominantly women, and as a group they are exceedingly frail, requiring a great deal of medical and social support. Of people 65 years old in 1980, 25% are expected to survive to age 90. By the year 2050, more than 40% will survive to age 90, based on moderately optimistic assumptions about mortality rates (1,2).

The second important phenomenon is the postwar baby boom of children born between 1945 and 1965. From 2010 to 2030, the U.S. population aged 65 to 84 will increase 80%, whereas the population under 65 will increase only 7%. Thereafter, baby boomers will become "old old," above age 85. In 1990 there were 3 million old old Americans. In 2010 there will be 6 million, and in 2050, 19 million people will be over age 85 (1).

The challenge for physicians will be sharpened by two additional effects: the rates of disability and poverty among the elderly. Disability arises from concomitant chronic medical illnesses, memory deficits, and depressive symptoms, in addition to underlying frailty. The percentage of people who need assistance with everyday activities rises steeply with age. Among the "young old," aged 65 to 75 years, approximately 10% require assistance, whereas among the old old, nearly half do. These figures are higher for African-American and Hispanic elders. Thus, large numbers of caregivers will be needed. Defining poverty in the United States is arbitrary, but 1992 Census Bureau data showed that 10% of men and 20% of women aged 75 and over were poor. Of African-Americans over age 75, 35% of men and 43% of women were poor, and of Hispanics, 19% of men and 32% of women were poor. On the average, out of pocket health care spending totaled $1,654 per year (13% of income) in the lowest income quintile of households headed by an older person. The relative burden of this expenditure is much greater in this group when compared with those in the top income brackets (2).

Care of the old, and especially the very old, requires special awareness of the progressive socioeconomic and physiologic vulnerability of old age. More than knowledge of specific disease states, awareness of the extreme frailty of the very old defines clinical geriatrics.

PUBLIC POLICY

Medicare

Medicare was intended as hospital insurance for the elderly, regardless of income, covering a period of acute illness and subsequent convalescence. Eligibility depends on age or other qualifying condition (e.g.,

Table 12.1. Life Expectancy of Older Americans: in 1900, 1950, and 1997

	1900	1950	1997
Life expectancy at birth (yr)			
Total	49.2	68.1	76.5
Men	47.9	65.5	73.6
Women	50.7	71.0	79.4
Life expectancy at age 65 (additional years)			
Total	11.9	13.8	17.7
Men	11.5	12.7	15.9
Women	12.2	15.0	19.2
Life expectancy at age 85 (additional years)			
Total	4.0	4.7	6.3
Men	3.8	4.4	5.5
Women	4.1	4.9	6.6

Adapted from Federal Interagency Forum on Aging-Related Statistics. Older Americans 2000: Key Indicators of Well-Being.

end-stage renal disease) but not on income. In general, Part A pays institutions for hospital inpatient care, brief posthospital care (whether institutional or provided by a home health agency), and Medicare hospices. Part B pays physicians and providers of outpatient services such as independent laboratories, mental health services, and rehabilitation services. Durable medical equipment is also covered by Part B. Some preventive services are covered under Medicare, including influenza and pneumococcal vaccines, screening mammograms every 2 years, screening Pap smears every 3 years, colonoscopy every 10 years, and dual-energy x-ray absorpimetry (DEXA) bone mineral density measurements every 2 years. Discussions among public policy makers continue regarding future coverage of prescription drugs.

In 1996 Medicare indicated that it would cover inpatient hospital admissions for symptom palliation in terminally ill patients (3). For their services, hospice programs receive a prearranged payment to cover medical care, medications, and supplies related to the terminal diagnoses in the dying patient. Much debate about the most recent reform proposals has been driven by the escalating costs of health care; this is emphasized by the name Balanced Budget Act of 1997. This Act has had widespread fundamental effects on medical care in America. Its implementation has meant changes to Medicare support of graduate medical education, attempts at increasing choices for health care plans (Medicare health maintenance organizations), and the restructuring of reimbursement schedules for physician services and home health care (4). On the other hand, long-term care will likely remain beyond Medicare's purview. Chronically ill patients in nursing homes are generally not covered. Short-term stays for rehabilitation after hospitalization are reimbursed, but Medicare coverage ends, as a rule, once the patient stops improving.

Medicare has grown in size (to more than 34 million beneficiaries) and in complexity since its inception in 1965. More changes are anticipated in the coming years. Effective care of the geriatric population entails continual efforts at keeping up to date with these and future amendments to Medicare. Detailed information on Medicare benefits for individuals is available from the Federal government (see Preretirement Counseling and Planning later in this chapter).

Medicaid

Both Medicare and Medicaid are federally funded with oversight from the Center for Medicare and Medicaid Services (formally Health Care Financing Administration). However, unlike Medicare, Medicaid administration is left largely to the individual states. Each state sets its own policies within certain federal guidelines. To be eligible for Medicaid, it is necessary, but not sufficient, to be impoverished; age and other criteria such as disability must be met. In general, Medicaid offers more benefits than those covered by Medicare and traditional insurance plans. These benefits may include prescription drugs, prosthetics, hearing aids, and both inpatient and outpatient services. Although more than 41.3 million Americans participate in this program, with many now enrolled in Medicaid managed-care plans, less than half of poor Americans are actually covered by Medicaid. In 1997 alone, $159.9 billion dollars were spent for its services (5).

Most Medicaid dollars are spent on long-term care in nursing homes, and about half of nursing home revenue comes from Medicaid. Eligibility for nursing home placement is defined by the states and depends on functional disability and medical illness. Medicaid pays for nursing home care only if the person is indigent. Thus, a person with assets may qualify in one of two ways. He or she may spend the assets on nursing home care until impoverished or divest the assets by giving them to adult children. Rules about divestment are changing, but a "look back" period is common: Any assets given away in the previous 30 months, for example, may be counted as current assets. The issue of divestment is extremely divisive, as it is mainly the well off who can plan ahead to this extent. Increased authority and responsibilities have been parceled to the states since welfare reform. Because the program is in a period of change, practitioners should seek specific advice about nursing home placement and Medicaid eligibility from state and local sources.

Home Health Care

Home health care refers liberally to care, formal or informal, provided in the home. Nonetheless, this term is often used to refer to a specific Medicare benefit.

Part A Medicare certifies home health agencies and pays them for in-home care, primarily by nurses and aides. In keeping with Medicare philosophy, the program was intended to facilitate hospital discharge planning and to manage episodes of acute illness at home, thus shortening or even preventing some hospital admissions. Traditionally, spouses, adult children, other relatives, and sometimes friends assumed most of the caregiving responsibilities for disabled community-dwelling adults. In recent years, families have shared more of these tasks with help from paid formal home care. Increased caregiver stress, increased family and occupational responsibilities of caretakers, and perhaps some overall increase in the financial resources of older adults may have played roles in this trend.

From 1988 to 1997, home health agency reimbursements grew from $2 billion to more than $17 billion. By 1997, 1 in 10 Medicare recipients had received home health care, accumulating an average of 80 home visits (4). Although the intent of the home health care program was to substitute or complement acute hospital care, 61% of all visits were to enrollees receiving services for 6 months or more. In fact, geographic areas with high rates of home care use do not have lower rates of hospitalization or shorter lengths of stay. The need for chronic care among community-dwelling elderly, along with several other factors, simply was not foreseen in the original design of Medicare (6). The criteria for Medicare coverage for homebound patients with unstable medical conditions and for hospice patients are summarized in Chapters 9 and 13, respectively.

Public policy about medical care of the elderly, especially the poor and frail elderly, is in flux. Out of pocket costs are rising, as are government expenditures. Federal scrutiny and demands on provider documentation will continue as definitions of eligible services become more refined. A broad-based plan for efficacious health care in the home may one day inspire more physician house calls (already reimbursable under Medicare) and perhaps usher in the concept of the home-based hospital (7).

Agencies on Aging

The Administration on Aging was born in 1965 out of President Johnson's Great Society Program, with an intent to establish federal legislative agendas to serve the needs and improve the quality of life of Americans age 60 and older. Through the Older American Act and its subsequent amendments, the Administration on Aging has since mandated the establishment of Units on Aging within all states. These Units allocate federal moneys to local area Agencies on Aging. There are local area Agencies on Aging, each receiving federal moneys allocated by the state Units on Aging. Today there are 57 Units on Aging; they oversee more than 655 local Agencies on Aging and 223 tribal organizations. The challenge has been to provide appropriate guidance to an increasingly diverse elderly population. For the more functional elders, services have included assistance with employment placement and the establishment of senior activities centers. For the frail elderly and their families, help has come from services such as home delivered meals, advice on planning for long-term care, and support for caregivers. It is likely that comprehensive primary care of elderly patients will increasingly rely on referrals to the local Agencies on Aging (8).

EVALUATING OLDER PATIENTS

General Issues

Several aspects of the clinical evaluation of older patients deserve emphasis. *Old records* should be obtained before the first visit, when possible. If not, they should be requested at the first visit. Patients should routinely bring all their medications to appointments, including over the counter medications and herbal supplements.

Attention should be paid to the *physical environment*. Bright direct light is often uncomfortable for patients with cataracts. Prolonged sitting on a backless examining table or in a chilly room can be uncomfortable. Making a patient comfortable probably improves the quality of the medical history. For patients with presbycusis, it is more important to face the patient and speak slowly and clearly than it is to speak loudly. Also, the practitioner should have an assistive listening device (see Chapter 110) available for use by the patient when needed. Patients with marked kyphosis can often lie down more comfortably if a rolled-up sheet is placed on the pillow under the occiput.

Some form of *mental status examination* should be included in the initial evaluation of every older patient (see Chapter 26). Clinicians' impressions have been shown to be insensitive in detecting mild cognitive impairment (9). Cognitive impairment is extremely common, with prevalence rates of 30% to almost 50% among the very old (10). Becuase symptoms of disease in the elderly may be absent, atypical, or ignored by the physician, subtle deterioration of cognitive or functional capacity may be the only indication of a serious pathologic condition.

In general, *more time* is needed for the evaluation of an elderly patient than for a younger patient. The former often has multiple problems, including sensory and mobility impairments that require a slower evaluation. Diagnostic testing should be highly selective. Stressful tests (which may include radiographic studies for a frail person with a mobility disorder) should have an expected therapeutic implication and should be explained thoroughly to the patient and, when applicable, to the caregiver. Extensive evaluation may require several visits. The highly streamlined evaluations so characteristic of modern medicine are simply too stressful for many ill elderly patients. Empathy and compassion are essential in high quality care for a frail older patient. Several 30- or 60-minute visits may be more easily tolerated than a single longer encounter, provided it is not too difficult for the patient and family to come to the office. However, too short an encounter (e.g., 10 to 20 minutes) is disappointing, inadequate for proper care, and difficult for many elders.

Standardized Approaches to Functional Assessment

The traditional problem-oriented approach to medical care focuses primarily on medical diagnoses. Functional assessment is intended to measure the impact of disease and aging on a patient's ability to care for him- or herself, to live in the community, and to accomplish goals that are meaningful to the patient. Problems in constructing valid and useful measures have been carefully described (11).

Frailty

The syndrome of frailty has many descriptions, including decreased resilience in the face of external stress, difficulty in maintaining homeostatic conditions, and vulnerability to adverse events. Declines in lean body mass, strength, endurance, balance, and walking performance and lower levels of activity are observed in frail older adults.

Research has identified an individual as frail if three or more of the following specific criteria are met (Table 12.2): unintended weight loss of 10 or more pounds over the previous 12 months, poor grip strength, self-reported poor endurance and exhaustion, slow walking time, and low physical activities level (12). Frail individuals have higher rates of disability, hospitalization, and mortality and are more likely to have coexisting cardiovascular diseases. A phenotype for frailty representing a unique physiologic syndrome has been proposed. Related biochemical markers and immunologic correlates of frailty are being sought. Targeted interventions that improve outcomes in frail patients may emerge (12).

Disability

Living independently requires the performance of certain essential activities. Essential goals of caring for an elderly person are to identify and minimize his or her dependence on others for these activities. The *Katz index of activities of daily living* (ADLs) outlines tasks that are fundamental to independent living (Table 12.3). A patient's ability to bathe, dress, toilet, transfer, feed, and maintain continence enables a clinician to deploy targeted interventions that meet the patient's current functional needs. Comparing ADL scores obtained before and after certain interventions (e.g., physical and occupational therapy for a patient after a stroke) allows the clinician to track the degree of functional improvement. Improvement in ADL scores, however, is not realistic in some patients. In fact, poor performance of the Katz ADLs has been correlated with increased mortality, nursing home placement, and inadequate recovery from hip fracture (13,14). The *Barthel index* is another instrument with well-documented reliability and validity that has been used to quantify (via a 0 to 100 scoring scale) degrees of disability. Scores from the Barthel index correlate with recovery from stroke. Dependency in ADLs is part of the determination of nursing home eligibility and has been an entry criterion for many of the long-term care plans proposed in the debate over health care reform. Despite this, physicians caring for ambulatory patients often underestimate or overlook important disabilities in their patients (15).

Instrumental ADLs require a higher level of function and include abilities to travel outside the home, shop, prepare meals, do housework, or handle finances (16). The evidence basic for the assessment, natural history, demography, impact of disability, and interventions to prevent disability has been elegantly summarized (17).

Overall understanding of a patient's level of functional ability, as well as his or her capability to function in home, can enrich a physician's understanding of the goals of treatment for that patient.

Table 12.2. Characteristics of Frailty[a]

Trait	Measure
Shrinking Weight loss (unintentional) Sarcopenia (loss of muscle mass)	>10-lb weight loss (loss of ≥5% of body weight over the previous year)
Weakness	Grip strength: lowest 20% of population at baseline, adjusted for gender and body mass index
Poor endurance	Self-report of exhaustion
Slowness	Walking time/15 feet: slowest 20% of population (by gender, height)
Low activity	Lowest 20% of population in terms of energy expenditure: <383 kcals/wk (males) <270 kcals/wk (females)

[a]Presence of three or more of above in an individual points to presence of the frailty phenotype. Adapted from Fried LP, Tangen CM, Walston JB, et al. Frailty in older adults: evidence for a phenotype. J Gerontol 2001;56A:M146–M156, with permission.

Table 12.3. Areas and Levels of Assessment in the Katz Index of Independence in Activities of Daily Living

Bathing	Receives no assistance Receives assistance in bathing only one part Receives assistance in bathing more than one part
Dressing	Gets clothes and dresses without assistance Needs assistance in tying shoes only Needs assistance greater than above or stays undressed
Toileting	Needs no assistance Needs assistance only in getting to toilet room or in cleaning self Does not go to toilet room
Transferring	Needs no assistance from another person Needs assistance with transferring Does not get out of bed
Continence	Continent Occasional accident Needs supervision, uses catheter, or is incontinent
Feeding	Needs no assistance Needs assistance in cutting meat or buttering bread Needs more assistance or is tube or intravenously fed

From Katz S, Ford AB, Moskowitz RW, et al. Studies of illness in the aged: the index at ADL: standardized measures of biological and psychosocial function. JAMA 1963;185:94, with permission.

Geriatric Assessment

Comprehensive *geriatric assessment* is usually a multidisciplinary and always a multidimensional assessment of frail elderly patients and their support systems. It is occasionally confused with functional assessment, described in the prior section. Although it has received a great deal of favorable attention, geriatric assessment lacks a precise definition, and data supporting its usefulness are sketchy. The referral source and initial characteristics of patients, the nature of interventions (e.g., whether inpatient, in the office, or in the home and whether consultation or ongoing therapy), and the measured outcomes have varied from study to study. Furthermore, caregivers and clinicians often do not agree on perceived goals of care for frail elderly patients (18).

There is no doubt that certain frail elderly patients and their caregivers would benefit from assessment by a careful and competent social worker, a nurse who has the time and desire to teach, or perhaps a visit with a pharmacist, nutritionist, or therapist. On the other hand, it is difficult to imagine how this multidisciplinary approach would cause a 50% reduction in mortality in treated subjects compared with randomized controls in 1 year, as reported in an early and influential article on inpatient geriatric assessment (19). A subsequent large randomized study of inpatients from the same institution showed no clinically meaningful difference on any of the measured outcomes (20). A more recent randomized study found that inpatient assessment followed by postdischarge home intervention resulted in shortening of initial and subsequent (if any) hospital stay, rate of immediate nursing home placement, and functional status. No survival benefits were found (21). Another recent outpatient randomized control trial also found no mortality benefit. Though some measures of functional independence were improved, no differences were seen in Medicare expenditures or use of health services (22). Assessment of elderly patients in their homes has definite benefits. Studies of case finding and surveillance (23), postdischarge assessment (24), and pharmacy assessment (25) done in the home have demonstrated significantly improved outcomes.

Table 12.4 lists the central elements of geriatric assessment. Assessments performed in the above-cited studies generally contain these elements. Medicare currently does not provide specific compensation for multidisciplinary comprehensive geriatric assessment.

Table 12.4. Some Important Components of the Initial Geriatric Assessment

- Cognitive Assessment
  - History from family often vital
  - Mental status screening may involve Folstein Mini-Mental State Examination (see Table 26.1) (77)
- Functional Assessment
  - Inventory of functional status may include
    - Katz activities of daily living (Table 12.3)
    - Instrumental activities of daily living
  - Fall risk assessment
    - Assessing history of falls, usual activity level
    - Observing patient rise unassisted from chair, walk several paces, turn, and return to the chair
- Psychosocial assessment
  - Depression screening may include Yesavage Geriatric Depression Scale (78)
  - Consider assessment of
    - Driving skills
    - Risk for elder abuse
    - Available social support system
    - Adequacy of current living situation
    - Other barriers to ability to safe living
    - Caregiver stress
- Outlook assessment
  - Raise the issue of advanced directives (see elsewhere in the book)
- Medications review
  - Explicitly justify each prescription drug to ensure benefits exceed risks
  - Evaluate the utility of alternative/complementary medicines based on available data
- Preventive health care
  - Recommend appropriate vaccinations
  - Perform dental, vision, and hearing screen
  - Recommend appropriate cancer screening

MEDICATION USE IN THE ELDERLY

One way of conceptualizing the aging process is as a gradual decline in the organism's ability to respond to perturbation and stress. At rest, for example, the body temperature, serum sodium, glucose, and heart rate of healthy younger patients are about the same as those of older patients. When stressed by environmental temperature extremes, free water load, glucose challenge or exercise, however, the older patient will have a wider excursion from normal, will take longer to recover equilibrium, and is more likely to get sick, even in the absence of underlying disease. Medications can be seen as a perturbation: Most younger people can recover from this perturbation safely, but the elderly are more likely to have adverse effects as a result.

Elderly Americans take large numbers of drugs. Although some drugs are clearly beneficial, many others have little or no evidence of efficacy. Risks to the elderly patient from imprecise drug use can be substantial. A majority of physicians are inaccurate in reporting what medications their patients are taking, even when questioned in clinic or if they use the clinic chart to determine the medication regimen (26,26a). In an epidemiologic study in the United States, 87% of independent elderly were taking at least one over the counter medication and 6% were taking five or more (27). Complementary and alternative medications are popular (see Chapter 5). A useful clinical strategy is to insist that all medications, including over-the-counter and complementary medications, are brought to each visit and then to consider the justification for each drug.

Studies of drug disposition in the elderly demonstrate wide heterogeneity in several important physiologic functions. Although drug absorption is unimpaired in general, distribution within the body compartments may be different in older than in younger subjects. In older subjects, muscle mass, bone mass, body water, and some serum proteins are lower, whereas body fat content is higher. Hepatic drug clearance, in simplest terms, depends on hepatic blood flow, serum protein binding, and the intrinsic capacity of the hepatocyte mass. The first two of these factors may decrease with age, resulting in impaired drug metabolism in some patients. Renal glomerular filtration rate can fall approximately 30% from the third decade to the eighth. The fall in glomerular filtration rate may not be accompanied by a rise in serum creatinine because muscle mass is falling concomitantly. Because of variability among subjects, prediction of drug levels from dosage is unreliable.

In many cases, *very low dosages* of medication may be effective, such as 12.5 mg of hydrochlorothiazide per day and beginning dosages of 0.25 mg haloperidol or 10 mg imipramine or nortriptyline per day. Unless the clinical situation requires otherwise, drugs should be started at low dosages in the elderly and titrated carefully upward during frequent early follow-up. When available, drug levels are useful in monitoring the patient.

New drugs pose particularly serious risks for the elderly. In general, the U.S. Food and Drug Administration approves new drugs after safety has been demonstrated in relatively small trials (28). Once the drugs are released, however, they are often used widely by the frail elderly, and serious but uncommon toxicities become apparent. Benoxaprofen (Oraflex), zomepirac (Zomax), suprofen (Suprol), nomifensine (Merital), and temafloxacin (Omniflox) have been heavily promoted and then withdrawn from the market after reports of serious injury or death of patients. More recently, bromfenac (Duract), terfenadine (Seldane), mibefradil (Posicor), alosetron (Lotronex), cisapride (Propulsid), cerivastatin (Baycol), troglitazone (Rezulin), phenylpropanolamine, and several diet pills have also been withdrawn. Tramadol (Ultram), zolpidem (Ambien), linezolid (Zyvox), and the antifungal drugs itraconazole (Sporanox) and terbinafine (Lamisil) are examples of drugs whose early advertising campaigns touted safety but later demonstrated unexpected toxicities. New drugs should be tried carefully in older patients only after more standard drugs have been tried unsuccessfully. Older drugs have more well-established safety profiles and are generally less expensive. Prescribing a new drug means entering a patient into the postmarketing surveillance phase. Claims about the safety or the lack of side effects of newly released drugs should be viewed simply as advertising techniques.

Some specific drugs, selected because of their widespread use in the elderly, are considered here.

Neuroleptics

These drugs are associated with increased risk of falls, hip fracture (29), and tardive dyskinesia. They are sometimes efficacious in treating the behavioral complications of dementia. Of 100 demented patients treated with neuroleptics, 18 could be expected to benefit beyond placebo, according to a meta-analysis. No one neuroleptic has been shown to be more effective than another (30). For example, the average wholesale price of risperidone (Risperdal) is 91 times that of generic haloperidol (31). If these drugs are prescribed, evidence of good effect should be sought. If they provide nothing more than sedation (assuming sedation is desirable), other drugs should be used instead, such as short-acting benzodiazepines. The properties of available antipsychotic drugs are described in Chapter 25, and the practical use of psychoactive drugs in the elderly is discussed fully in Chapter 26.

Nonsteroidal Anti-Inflammatory Drugs

For treatment of inflammatory conditions, nonsteroidal anti-inflammatory drugs (NSAIDs) are an excellent choice. When they are used as analgesia for noninflammatory chronic pain, their considerable toxicities may outweigh their benefit. Current users of NSAIDs are almost five times more likely to have a fatal upper gastrointestinal hemorrhage when compared with former users or subjects who have never used them (32). Frail, elderly, white women are especially at risk. Renal and central nervous system toxicities are well known (see Chapter 77 for a full discussion on NSAIDs). In many cases of pain without underlying inflammation, acetaminophen may have a superior risk-to-benefit profile. In middle-aged women with osteoarthritis of the knee, for example, 4 g of acetaminophen daily was as good as low dosage (1,200 mg daily) or high dosage (2,400 mg daily) ibuprofen for pain relief (33).

The cyclooxygenase-2 (COX-2) specific NSAIDs are heavily advertised, widely prescribed, and extremely expensive. They may be slightly safer than older NSAIDs, but their true safety profile is as yet unclear.

Cold Remedies

There is no cure for the common cold, but there is a multimillion-dollar market in remedies. Common treatments bring the risk of antihistaminic or narcotic sedation, sympathomimetic stimulation, or a combination of the two. Substantial amounts of alcohol are often included: Vicks NyQuil is 50 proof, for example. Many common combinations are irrational, even contradictory. Clinicians should discourage their elderly patients, who are likely to be susceptible to anticholinergic and sympathomimetic effects, from buying these nostrums, many of which contain a variety of useless ingredients. Treatments for the common cold are discussed in Chapter 33. As mentioned above, decongestants and antihistamines are occasionally discovered to have fatal toxicities, as with phenylpropanolamine and terfenadine.

Sleeping Pills

Disrupted sleep is common in old age (see Fig. 7.1), and the electroencephalogram of a normal elderly patient looks very different from that of a normal younger patient. In addition, some of the cognitive changes that occur in old age resemble the changes of sleep deprivation, such as slowed reaction time and slower learning of new material. It is not reasonable to expect, nor is it true, that any sedative hypnotic can convert the blunted and simpler sleep electroencephalogram of an older person to the complex and delicate electroencephalogram of a younger person. In fact, no sleeping pill has been shown to improve alertness or daytime problem solving when given to patients with insomnia. The side effects can be very serious. A randomized trial showed that teaching about sleep hygiene is as effective as giving sleeping pills and has more long-lasting effect (34). Cognitive behavioral therapy may be even more effective (35). When insomnia is a symptom of depression, sleep quality does improve with treatment of the depression.

Drug–Drug Interactions

Elderly patients who take many medications are at high risk for drug–drug interactions. Selegiline (Eldepryl) taken with a selective serotonin reuptake inhibitor can cause delirium and death. An industry publication has compiled 1,231 pages of drug–drug interactions and 250 pages of side effects (36). Physicians should become familiar with and use a small number of medications. Coumadin is increasingly used in elderly patients and its effect on coagulation can be affected by many drugs (see Chapter 57).

NEGLECT AND ABUSE IN THE ELDERLY

Most dependent elderly live in the community and are cared for by relatives. In most of these cases, excellent loving care is provided. In some cases, however, there is frank abuse or neglect, and in some the situation is ambiguous. The number of older Americans who are abused is likely to increase. This is thought to be partly due to the national trend toward smaller families, as well as the rapidly increasing numbers of the very old, who are no longer wage earners and are more likely to be frail and dependent. Clear-cut examples of physical and emotional violence, sexual abuse, financial exploitation, and harmful neglect of frail elderly people have been reported.

The definition of abuse can be difficult, in large part because the victims are presumably competent adults who choose to continue the relationship, leading to putative abuse. Neglect is also often difficult to define, especially in a relationship in which the caregiver has no legally defined responsibility. Furthermore, some situations offer only tragic options. If a single working mother cares for her demented mother who repeatedly wanders or urinates in closets, is it abuse if the daughter uses physical restraints? Suppose neither mother nor daughter will accept a nursing home and employment of professional caregivers is not financially feasible.

Diagnosis is difficult because both abuser and victim may deny or minimize abuse. Therefore, diagnosis is often inferential. Treatment may be problematic in all but extreme cases. Remedies might include an alternative environment that is healthy, supportive, and acceptable to the victim or the provision of services that can relieve a stressed caregiver. Such treatment is often unavailable. Risk factors for abuse are shown in Table 12.5 (37,38).

Table 12.5. Risk Factors for Elder Abuse

Characteristics of the victim
Lives with related relative, not spouse
Severely demented
Behavior problem
Medically ill
Characteristics of the abuser
Has provided long-term care
Stressed significantly by care of the victim
Under severe external stress
Abused as a child
Expresses frustration
Uses recreational drugs, including alcohol

Clinicians may be reluctant to become involved in a situation in which there is little reward, poor reimbursement, and potential liability. State statutes vary in defining the physician's responsibility and liability. The Council on Scientific Affairs of the American Medical Association has published a useful report on this subject. The report outlines several strategies for prevention and intervention (37). (The full report may be obtained by writing to the Council on Scientific Affairs, AMA, 535 N. Dearborn St., Chicago, IL 60610.) In severe cases, however, legal advice should be sought and state and local agencies such as Adult Protective Services should be involved.

FALLS

Falls are common in the elderly and often have serious consequences, including death. It has been estimated that 35% to 40% of community-dwelling adults 65 years and older have at least one fall annually.

The risk of frequent or severe falls accompanies many geriatric syndromes. Etiology is often multifactorial and hard to define. Caregivers, the environment, medications, sensory impairment, dementia, and deconditioning—as well as specific neurologic, cardiovascular, or musculoskeletal diseases—often contribute to the problem. Progress in research about falls has been steady. More risk factors have been identified, such as impaired cognition, abnormal reaction to a push, history of palpitations, abnormal stepping, slow timed chair stands, decreased arm strength, vision or hearing impairment, and high anxiety or depression scores (39).

At least once yearly assessment of falls has been advocated. Evaluation should focus on the number of falls, events leading up to and after the falls, and environmental circumstances surrounding the falls. Moreover, potential factors that may have led to the falls ought to be reviewed. This includes an assessment of prescription and alternative medicines; examination of vision, gait, balance, strength and flexibility of lower extremity; and evaluation of cardiovascular, neurologic, and other medical problems that may have caused the patient to fall. Mobility function may be determined by observing the patient as he or she stands up from a chair without assistance, walks several steps, turns, and returns to sit in the chair (40,41). Environmental factors such as dim lighting, steep stairs, loose carpeting, or small pets should be sought and, when possible, remedied.

Those at risk for recurrent falls are candidates for further interventions. For example, some exercise programs, particularly those including balance exercise (e.g., tai chi), have been shown to reduce risk of falls by 10% to 17% (42). Home environmental assessments and subsequent modifications have also been shown to be effective, as have reviewing and modifying medication profiles of those who have fallen (especially if they take more than four medications). A multifactorial intervention program targeting four specific risk factors in a vulnerable population reduced falls during 1 year of follow-up from 47% to 35%. The risk factors are postural hypotension, use of sedatives, use of four or more prescription medications, and impairment in arm or leg strength or range of motion, transfer skills, or gait skills (43). Finally, hip protectors are helpful adjuncts in preventing potentially serious fractures. In a randomized controlled study that recruited ambulatory frail elderly persons, those who wore hip protectors had their risk for hip fractures after a fall reduced by 66% over an 18-month period. Once convinced to wear them, study participants kept them on 50% of the possible time (74% had them on during the falls). These protectors are becoming commercially available (44).

Falls in elderly outpatients are carefully reviewed by King and Tinetti (45).

NUTRITION

For a variety of reasons, precise definition of dietary requirements for ambulatory elderly people is difficult. The elderly are physiologically and metabolically an extremely diverse group with a variety of illnesses, taking a variety of medicines. Absorptive function in the aging gut is poorly studied. However, recommended daily allowances for the elderly are extrapolated from data collected in studies of younger people. Recommended daily allowances based on age alone are imprecise. More complicated calculations will probably replace them. Basic principles of nutrition for persons of all ages are covered in Chapter 15.

Two general principles have been demonstrated. First, most elderly Americans who seek medical attention are not undernourished. Second, desirable body weight for the elderly may be somewhat heavier than previously determined on the basis of insurance company tables of mortality and body mass index (BMI). These tables do not consider age. Based on independent analysis of insurance company data, Andres (46) calculated mortality ratios in various age groups according to BMI. This analysis suggests that the BMI associated with the lowest mortality rate varies with age. The older the age group, the higher the best BMI. For example, the BMI associated with the lowest mortality among 25-year-old men is 21.4. For a 6-foot-tall man, this corresponds to a weight of 158 pounds. For a 65-year-old man, the best BMI is 26.6, 196 pounds for the same 6-foot-tall man. Roughly speaking, these tables allow a gain of approximately 1 pound per year throughout adult life. Several studies of long-term weight change tend to confirm that modest weight gain during adult life is associated with lower mortality (47). These tables do not apply to patients with diseases that are related to weight. For patients with type II diabetes mellitus, hypertension, and hyperlipidemia, weight loss is often an essential part of treatment.

The pattern of body fat distribution has been shown to be associated with several important diseases and with mortality. High waist-to-hip circumference ratio has been shown to be more strongly associated with death than is BMI in women (see Chapter 83) (48).

A variety of psychosocial factors (e.g., isolation, alcoholism, depression, low income) and physiologic changes (e.g., diminished taste and smell sensation, dental problems, dementia, dysphagia, acid peptic disease) may contribute to a diminished intake of nutritious meals. Although difficult to demonstrate except in extreme cases, malnutrition may occur in these situations. The effects of multivitamin supplements are unknown. Trials of supplementation with specific vitamins (carotene and tocopherol) have shown no benefit (49,50). Although risks are low when vitamins are taken in moderation, costs can be high. Data are inconclusive about canned "complete" nutritional products provided to alert patients as a supplement to or substitute for regular food.

Weight loss can result from a variety of causes, some trivial and some lethal. In general, the known causes of weight loss can be classified as decreased intake, reduced absorption, and increased use. Involuntary weight loss can be troubling in the elderly. In approximately 25% of cases, no cause is discovered despite intensive evaluation (51). Almost all the remaining causes can be found with a careful history and physical examination and judicious use of the laboratory. In the elderly, decreased intake should be carefully sought. The search for malignancy during a careful history and physical examination and the exclusion of hyperthyroidism with appropriate laboratory investigation are also an important part of the evaluation.

When inflammatory illness and cachexia are present, there are very few data to show that increasing nutrient intake benefits the patient. So-called markers of nutritional status may simply signal the presence of inflammatory illness.

EXERCISE AND THE ELDERLY

Benefits from exercise are now incontrovertible and include improvements in bone density, sleep (52), risk of falls (53), disability and pain from knee arthritis (42), cardiovascular risk factors and disease (54), weight reduction (55), and rate of disability (12). Moderate levels of resistive and aerobic exercises confer benefit. In fact, leisure time physical activities ranging from walking to yard work and tai chi or calisthenics may suffice. Nonetheless, as with other age groups, older Americans as a whole maintain a relatively sedentary lifestyle. Barriers to attaining the above goals range from real (i.e., unsafe neighborhood, fear of exacerbating underlying illness) to perhaps merely conceptual (i.e., lack of time). Exploring these barriers in the sedentary older person and assessing the level of motivation seem to be reasonable initial steps in encouraging exercise in the sedentary older adult. Adherence to a prescription of exercise may also correlate with activities that are enjoyable to the individual, take place in a preferred setting, and fit into his or her schedule.

For those who are inactive, it is reasonable to begin by finding ways to reduce inactivity (such as reduce television watching) and suggesting some ways to augment baseline activities (i.e., taking stairs rather than escalator, establishing habit of taking walks). Gradually, the intensity and duration of physical activities may be increased. The adage for medications applies here as well: start low, go slow. Two suggestions may be useful. First, the pace of walking should be slow enough that the elderly person can converse comfortably. Second, competition between walkers should be specifically discouraged. Shopping malls are good places to walk. The goal for the initially sedentary person is 30 *cumulative* minutes a day of moderately intense activities on most days of the week (55,56). This may be achieved, for example, by several 10-minute walks. For older adults who exercise already, emphasis might be placed on injury prevention and proper exercise techniques (i.e., such as avoidance of inadvertent Valsalva maneuvers that may induce hypotension) and benefits of both aerobic and resistive (strength training) programs. Fruitful follow-up visits usually incorporate continual encouragement, assessment and reassessment of attainable goals, careful questioning for symptoms of ischemic heart disease, and attention to any concerns of pain and injuries (55).

Patients with cardiac risk factors or established cardiovascular disease require careful evaluation, and perhaps in part for medicolegal reasons, a stress test should be considered. Those with an abnormal cardiac response to exercising (abnormally high blood pressure: greater than 250/120, decrease in systolic blood pressure of more than 20 mm Hg, repeated heart rate increase more than 90% of age-specific maximum) are not suited for moderate or vigorous exercise programs (57). The risk of an exercise-related cardiac event has been evaluated in those over age 70 (58). As expected, the rate of myocardial infarction occurrence is higher after vigorous exercise than moderate exercise in those over 75. Although vigorous exercise does incur a higher relative risk of ensuing myocardial infarction than moderate exercise in those older than 70, this relative risk was not significantly different from those who were younger than 70. Nonetheless, most previously sedentary older seniors (i.e., 75 and older) do not begin and seldom end up with a high intensity aerobic program (59).

The value of *exercise testing* for apparently healthy elderly patients who want to begin an exercise program remains uncertain. Routine testing of all healthy older persons wanting to exercise may prove to be expensive, and the cost may be an unexpected barrier to starting an exercise program. Both the American Heart Association and the American College of Sports Medicine recommend exercise stress testing for sedentary older people before starting a *vigorous* exercise program, even in the absence of suspected or known underlying cardiovascular disease. In the case of moderate exercise for these individuals, the American College of Sports Medicine recommends testing if certain symptoms and signs suggestive of underlying cardiovascular disease (but otherwise relatively nonspecific) are present (60). However, neither addresses the utility of exercise stress testing before *resistive* exercise programs. Meaningful interpretation of treadmill testing is often undermined by the resting electrocardiogram abnormalities commonly seen in older persons. Moreover, the ability to successfully complete the exercise stress test diminishes with age; compared with 30% of those between ages 75 and 79, only 9% of those older than 85 who agreed to undergo exercise stress testing completed the test. If available guidelines were followed, one might expect a high rate of additional follow-up cardiac testing, potentially exposing patients to the inherent risks and costs of these procedures (55).

A reasonable *approach to preexercise assessment* starts with a complete history and physical. The physician should first screen for patients with overt cardiac disease or potential contraindications to exercising outside of a monitored setting (i.e., overt congestive heart failure, uncontrolled hypertension, angina, or myocardial infarction within the previous 6 month). This may be followed by an assessment of resting electrocardiogram (for new Q waves, ST-T abnormalities) and cardiac reserve before prescribing exercise regimens. Simple office-based maneuvers have previously been proposed to evaluate cardiac reserve, including getting up and down from the clinic examination table, walking a distance of 15 m, climbing a flight of stairs, and cycling in the air for 60 seconds while sitting or lying on the examination table. In the absence of worrisome findings, a prescription for an exercise program may then be given, tailored to the interested individual (55).

ELDERLY DRIVERS

Physicians are increasingly asked to provide guidance on the issue of driving to older adults and their families. Driving keeps elderly persons connected to friends and resources. It may connote a sense of independence. For some (especially rural dwellers), driving may be the sole means of transportation. Public transportation may be limited, unreliable, or unsafe for others.

Drivers older than age 65 can be a potential safety concern. They are involved in 8% of all nonfatal traffic accidents and account for 12% of traffic fatalities. Rather than high speed and alcohol intoxication as in younger drivers, the causes of accidents at the hands of older drivers are frequently related to turning (especially left handed), lane changes, backing up, and nonobservance of traffic signs. The per mile fatality rate of those older than 75 is higher than any other adult age group; this rate is highest in drivers older than 85, exceeding even that recorded for teens. Older drivers who sustain similar injuries as their counterparts also are more likely to die from them. Unlike those involving younger drivers, accidents with older drivers occur at intersections, close to home, and usually take place during the day in good weather (60).

Potential barriers for the older driver include age-associated physiologic changes such as slower reaction time, lower visual acuity, and decreased joint mobility. Use of alcohol and some medications also leads to some accidents. Burdens of common chronic illnesses (such as Alzheimer dementia, depression, arthritis, diabetes mellitus, and cerebrovascular accidents) increase the likelihood of motor vehicle accidents in the elderly (61). Many older adults avoid accidents by driving shorter distances, stopping more on longer trips, and picking less busy thoroughfares. Some may avoid driving during rush hour, night time, and inclement weather. Others simply stop driving voluntarily. Women are more likely than men to do this. Those who no longer drive tend to be older, nonwhite, and have vision and/or functional impairments (62).

An office assessment of the older driver should elicit data to identify risks for underlying driving impairment. This may include screening for alcohol or substance abuse, causes of daytime somnolence (some medications, sleep apnea), and predisposition to hypoglycemic episodes, seizures, and syncopal events. Moreover, one should note that visual acuity below 20/50 falls below legal limits in most state. Predictors of adverse driving outcomes include impaired ability to copy a design on the Mini Mental State Examination, walking less than a block per day, foot and leg abnormalities (toe deformities, bunions, knee contractures, slowed toe tapping, or impaired toe walk), heart disease, and hearing deficit (62–64). The use of long-acting benzodiazepines has been associated with an increased risk of motor vehicle crash among the elderly (65). Concerns about driving ability are often first voiced by family members rather than patients. Asking them and the patient to recount specific incidences of problematic driving and traffic violations add to the understanding of the issues at hand. Seat belt use, whether as a driver or passenger, should be encouraged.

Some physicians have used office- or hospital-based computerized simulators to help tailor their assessment. Unfortunately, there is yet no available standardization of these models, and they cannot realistically be expected to gauge all necessary skills required on the road. Other physicians screen for higher risk drivers and send them to occupational therapy-based assessment programs when available. These Medicare reimbursable programs attempt to assess the impact of physical or cognitive deficits on driving. Therapies are then tailored with the goal of modifying underlying deficits via rehabilitation and fitting of adaptive equipment (60).

Which 90-year-old drivers are more dangerous than 16-year-old drivers? When should the freedom to drive be coercively limited? These are complex questions. Medical, legal, and ethical considerations interact, and laws vary from state to state. The American Geriatrics Society and the American Association of Retired Persons cosponsor the 55 Alive/Mature Drivers Program. Information is available at AARP 55 Alive, 601 E. Street NW, Washington, DC 20049 (website: www.aarp.org).

HOSPITALIZATION

In planning a course of care for a sick elderly patient, hospitalization is often an option. However, the incidence of adverse events in hospitalized patients is well documented, and elderly patients are at particular risk. Patients over age 65 have more than twice the risk of adverse effects in the hospital compared with those aged 16 to 44. These patients also have the highest rates of adverse effects caused by negligence among all age groups (66). Moreover, rates for every category of procedure-related and drug-related adverse event are highest in patients over age 65 (67,68). In one study, iatrogenic causes comprised 11% of the admissions to an intensive care unit, with older age and higher number of drugs being the main risk factors (69).

The in-hospital *effects of prolonged immobilization* on ventilation, bone metabolism, plasma volume, and muscle strength and the risks of sensory deprivation, physical restraints, and sensory deprivation have been well described (70). Bed sores, diminished functional status, nosocomial infection, delirium, malnutrition from hospital diets, and trauma are all further risks of hospitalization (71). Falls are common, and commonly harmful, immediately after hospital discharge (72). Efforts to take care of many moderately ill elderly patients at home are likely to develop further, independent of payer considerations.

PREVENTIVE GERIATRICS

Rowe and Kahn distinguish usual from successful aging (73). In a group of usual aging Americans, for example, bone and muscle mass fall and glucose tolerance worsens with age. However, regular exercise is associated with improved glucose metabolism, increased bone mass, and muscle strength and thus modifies "usual" aging.

Although available data do not permit clear-cut recommendations, most authorities believe that the well elderly should receive periodic testing similar to that of younger patients (see Chapter 14). Elderly patients with marked cognitive impairment or severe chronic diseases make up a separate group of patients for whom the value of screening is uncertain. Decisions about cancer screening for very frail elderly people are particularly complex. Life expectancy, quality of life, and burdens of testing should be factored into the decision whether or not to initiate screening. Moreover, one should also consider the impact of the target disease if diagnosed late versus the overall effects of treatment regimens if the target disease is diagnosed early. Consent for screening from a cognitively impaired patient is a particularly vexing problem.

Data show that although elderly women visit physicians more often than younger women, they are less likely to have a pelvic examination and Pap smear and less likely to be diagnosed with uterine, ovarian, or cervical cancer in a localized (and potentially curable) stage (74). The prevalence of abnormal Pap smears among elderly women was 13.5 per 1,000 in one study, and the death rate from cervical cancer is highest in women over 65 (75). Chapter 104 provides guidelines for gynecologic cancer screenings. A discussion of the controversy concerning screening for prostate disease in men is provided in Chapter 53.

In patients at high risk for vertebral compression or hip fracture and for those with established kyphosis, a survey of the house for environmental hazards is recommended; such patients also should not lift heavy objects, including grandchildren. Adjunctive DEXA scanning may confirm osteoporosis, which can be treated with pharmacologic and nonpharmacologic interventions. Prevention of falls is discussed earlier in this chapter, and specific treatment of osteoporosis is discussed in Chapter 103. Screening for and treating hyperlipidemia in elderly patients is a controversial topic discussed in Chapter 82. Screening methods for visual loss and hearing loss are discussed in Chapters 107 and 110, respectively.

The benefits of discontinuing cigarette smoking among the elderly are probably substantial. Although several studies of smoking cessation among the elderly show little effect on primary prevention of coronary heart disease, in those with established disease, smoking cessation reduces the risk of myocardial infarction and death (76). Cessation is a key step in the primary prevention of lung and other cancers and the primary or secondary prevention of obstructive lung disease, peripheral vascular disease, and peptic ulcer disease. A full discussion of strategies for smoking cessation is presented in Chapter 27.

The routine use of aspirin and estrogens in older women continues to provoke considerable scrutiny (see Chapters 57 and 106, respectively). Both agents may provide valuable benefits to certain elderly people, but each has associated risks. Immunization information is provided in Chapter 18.

PRERETIREMENT COUNSELING AND PLANNING

Several problems of the elderly can be minimized if they are anticipated and planned for well in advance. Books are available to help the older person in planning (see General References). Large corporations, senior citizen centers, and several colleges offer courses in preretirement counseling and planning. Fee for service care management services are mushrooming across the country, touting their expertise in coordinating home services; serving as a conduit between patients, families, and care providers; and helping with the search for appropriate senior housing and institutions. The American Association of Retired Persons has a wide range of materials to assist in such planning. Information is available by writing to the AARP Fulfillment Department, 601 E Street NW, Washington, DC 20049 (website: www.aarp.org).

Important topics for the older person to consider include anticipated economic changes, preparation of wills and estate planning, changes in tempo and nature of activities, the importance of developing hobbies and activities for leisure time, health care resources, and systems of health care and social support. As noted in Chapter 13, advance directives guiding medical therapy in the event of debilitating illness can be extremely valuable and are important for every adult to consider. Long-term care insurance is becoming more available, although there are disparities in cost, eligibility, and scope of coverage from one company policy to the next. A useful publication on the Medicare insurance program, Medicare and You 2001 (publication number 10050), is available to patients and physicians (Superintendent of Documents, U.S. Government Printing Office, Washington DC 20402, telephone 202-783-3238; website: www.medicare.gov.). This concise booklet explains services and provides definitions of terms used by Medicare (e.g., skilled nursing facility care). An understanding of the Medicare program is important for every elderly citizen. However, Medicare covers only 44% of total health expenditures for the elderly, so the aging patient and his or her family will need sound advice to plan properly for potential health care needs. The physician should encourage young elderly patients to investigate all these resources before they attain the age at which frailty is more common.

SPECIAL HOUSING AND OTHER COMMUNITY-BASED PROGRAMS

Housing programs primarily for the elderly are increasingly available. Many states or local governments have developed programs in the setting of a congregate facility in which support services such as eating programs or housekeeping are provided. These programs may be called *sheltered housing* or *elder housing* and are generally available only to people who are able to satisfy an economic means test. Information regarding such programs can be obtained through the state or regional office on aging.

Continuing care retirement communities are increasingly available. These require that an elder move (usually while still functionally independent) to a community that provides a variety of resources and usually includes primary medical care, access to nursing home care and personal care such as meal preparation and transportation, and social programs. Several types of retirement communities exist. Some provide comprehensive services, including nursing home and medical service, meals, and programs for an inclusive entrance and monthly fee. Others provide only housing and access to additional services that may be purchased on an a la carte basis. Cost varies tremendously. Patients who ask about entering such a community should be advised to carefully analyze the services included in the fee, review the record of the community with the state office on aging, and review the contract with a lawyer before agreeing to sign it. Some people are exuberant about such retirement communities, arguing that they provide excellent socialization and the reassurance that providing care in the event of dependency will never be a direct burden to one's family members. Others reject these arguments, claiming that these retirement communities are simply ghettos for the frail elderly. Because of the expense, only a small portion of the elderly population could ever consider such an option.

In part because of the high cost of community care retirement communities, programs are being developed to provide similar support services while patients remain in their own homes. Such programs, typically called *social health maintenance organizations* or *life care at home programs*, are still experimental. One such model, On Lok, developed in the late 1970s in San Francisco, is now being replicated at a number of sites around the country. This *Program for All-Inclusive Care for the Elderly* provides comprehensive care on a capitated basis featuring adult medical day-care and, in many sites, special housing programs.

Medical and social day-care centers are available in many communities. The state, county, or city area office of aging will have information about these programs. Generally, such programs provide an opportunity for daytime socialization or medical care and surveillance. Importantly, they also provide an opportunity for caregivers to have a respite from their care responsibilities. Unfortunately, medical day-care programs are not covered by most private insurance programs or Medicare (except for those who receive it under a Medicare/Medicaid waiver, e.g., via the Program for All-Inclusive Care for the Elderly). Medicaid does provide reimbursement for medical day-care services in some states, but it is means tested. For others, medical day-care is an out of pocket expense that, although expensive, is usually about half the cost of nursing home care. Social day-care programs (sometimes known as senior centers) are less expensive but usually require that a person is functionally totally independent. Social day-care programs (as opposed to medical day-care) are often sponsored by churches, local government, or other organizations, which usually help offset the cost.

Assisted living facilities have become a popular option for seniors in recent years. In addition to housing arrangements, they usually offer some additional services such as transportation, social activities, and prepared meals. Basic nursing support is sometimes available. Some facilities are built with the intention of serving cognitively impaired seniors. All 50 states have some form of regulations and licensure requirements for these facilities, and proposals for a national standard for quality are being devised. Quality of care and scale of operation vary greatly. Well-run operations may be found in a variety of settings, from modified homes operated by individual providers to gated communities with a multitude of amenities constructed by large corporations. As a whole, residents of assisted living facilities have multiple medical problems yet wish to maintain some levels of independence in a residential type of community. These facilities may increasingly become a viable arena for physicians interested in providing home-based medical care to the elderly.

Table 12.6. Some Helpful Internet Resources

Websites	Agency or Organization
http://www.aoa.gov	U.S. Administration on Aging
Helpful information on area agencies on aging, statistics on the elderly population, and descriptions of some national programs related to care of the elderly	
http://www.aoa.dhhs.gov/naic	National Aging Information Center
Programs and public policies concerning older Americans; helpful information on locating community resources for the elderly	
http://www.medicare.gov	Center for Medicare and Medicaid Services
Official U.S. Government site on Medicare; relevant material on coverage, participating providers, updates on policies, and contact numbers (available in English, Spanish, and Chinese)	
http://www.americangeriatrics.org	American Geriatrics Society
Information of interest for practicing geriatricians	
http://www.ama-assn.org	American Medical Association
Separate sections for physicians, medical students, other health professionals, and the general public	
http://www.aarp.org	American Association of Retired Persons
Designed for the public; outlines issues related to senior living and health	
http://www.alz.org	Alzheimer's Association
Sections for patients, caregivers, medical communities, and the media	
http://www.arthritis.org	The Arthritis Foundation
Resources, educational materials, and available discussion groups for those with arthritis	

OTHER IMPORTANT PROBLEMS OF THE ELDERLY PATIENT

The following problems are discussed in detail elsewhere in this book: constipation (Chapter 42), diverticular disease (Chapter 46), musculoskeletal problems (Section 10), menopause (Chapter 106), osteoporosis (Chapter 103), hearing loss (Chapter 110), skin problems (Section 17), dental problems (Chapter 112), disorders of the feet (Chapter 73), hypertension (Chapter 67), cataracts and macular degeneration (Chapter 107), psychiatric illnesses of old age such as dementia and delirium (Chapter 26), depression (Chapter 24), bereavement (Chapters 13 and 24), and urinary problems such as infection (Chapter 36) and retention (Chapter 53) and incontinence (Chapter 54).

ADDITIONAL INFORMATION AND RESOURCES

Table 12.6 lists some governmental agencies and other organizations that offer information and resources to health care providers, caregivers, and the elderly.

General References*

Cassel CK, Cohen HJ, Larson EB, et al., eds. Geriatric medicine, 3rd ed. New York: Spring-Verlag, 1997.

Hazzard WR, Bierman EL, Blass JP, et al., eds. Principles of geriatric medicine and gerontology, 3rd ed. New York: McGraw-Hill, 1994.

Jahnigen DW, Schrier RW, eds. Geriatric medicine, 2nd ed. Cambridge: Blackwell Science, 1996.

Three comprehensive texts.

Specific References

1. Hobbs FB, Damon BL. U.S. Bureau of the Census. Current Population Reports, Special Studies, P23-190, 65+ in the United States. Washington, DC: U.S. Government Printing Office, 1996.
2. Federal Interagency Forum on Aging Related Statistics. Older Americans 2000: Key Indicators of Well Being. Washington, DC: US Government Printing Office, August 2000.
3. Cassel CK, Vladeck BC. ICD-9 code for palliative or terminal care. N Engl J Med 1996;335:1232.
4. Iglehart JK. The American health care system: Medicare. N Engl J Med 1999;340:403.
5. Iglehart JK. The American health care system: Medicaid. N Engl J Med 1999;340:327.
6. Welch HG, Wennberg DE, Welch WP. The use of Medicare home health care services. N Engl J Med 1996;335:324.
7. Oldenquist GW, Scott L, Finucane TE. Home care: what a physician needs to know. Cleve Clin J Med 2001;68:433.
8. Stupp H. Area agencies on aging: a network of services to maintain elderly in their communities. Care Manage J 2000;2:54.
9. Klein LE, Tovs RP, McArthur J, et al. Diagnosing dementia: univariate and multivariate analysis of the mental status examination. J Am Geriatr Soc 1985;33:483.
10. Evans DA, Funkenstein HH, Albert MS, et al. Prevalence of Alzheimer's disease in a community population of older persons: higher than previously reported. JAMA 1989;262:2551.
11. Fries J, Singh G, Morfeld D, et al. Running and the development of disability with age. Ann Intern Med 1994;121:502.
12. Fried LP, Tangen CM, Walston JB, et al. Frailty in older adults: evidence for a phenotype. J Gerontol 2001;56:M146.
13. Katz S, Stoud MW. Functional assessment in geriatrics: a review of progress and directions. J Am Geriatr Soc 1987;37:267.
14. Lichtenstein MJ, Federspiel CF, Schaffner W. Factors associated with early demise in nursing home residents: a case-control study. J Am Geriatr Soc 1985;33:315.
15. Calkins DR, Rubenstein LV, Cleary PD, et al. Failure of physicians to recognize functional disability in ambulatory patients. Ann Intern Med 1991;114:451.
16. Fillenbaum GG. Screening the elderly: a brief instrumental activities of daily living measure. J Am Geriatr Soc 1985;33:698.
17. Fried LP, Guralnik JM. Disability in older adults: evidence regarding significance, etiology, and risk. J Am Geriatr Soc 1997;45:92.
18. Bogardus ST, Bradley EH, Williams CS, et al. Goals for the care of frail older adults: do caregivers and clinicians agree? Am J Med 2001;110:97.
19. Rubenstein LZ, Josephson KR, Wieland GD, et al. Effectiveness of a geriatric evaluation unit: a randomized clinical trial. N Engl J Med 1984;311:1664.
20. Reuben D, Borok G, Wolde-Tsadik GD, et al. A randomized trial of comprehensive geriatric assessment in the care of hospitalized patients. N Engl J Med 1995;332:1345.
21. Nikolaus T, Specht-Leible N, Bach M, et al. A randomized trial of comprehensive geriatric assessment and home intervention in the care of hospitalized patients. Age Ageing 1999;28:543.
22. Boult C, Boult LB, Morishita L, et al. A randomized clinical trial of outpatient geriatric evaluation and management. J Am Geriatr Soc 2001;49:351.
23. Pathy MS, Bayer A, Harding K, et al. Randomized trial of case finding and surveillance of elderly people at home. Lancet 1992;340:890.
24. Hansen FR. Geriatric follow-up by home visits after discharge from hospital: a randomized controlled trial. Age Ageing 1992;21:445.
25. Der EH, Rubenstein LZ, Choy GS. The benefits of in-home pharmacy evaluation for older persons. J Am Geriatr Soc 1997;45:211.
26. Anderson DN, Prunty N, Partridge M, et al. Does anyone know what medication the patient should be taking? Int J Geriatr Psychiatry 1994;9:573.
26a. Bikowski RM, Rispin CM, Lorraine VL. Physician-patient congruence regarding medication regimens. *J Am Geriatr Soc* 2001;49:1353.
27. Stoehr GP, Ganguli M, Seaberg EC, et al. Over-the-counter medication use in an older rural community: the MoVIES Project. J Am Geriatr Soc 1997;45:150.
28. Kessler DA. The regulation of investigational drugs. N Engl J Med 1989;3:81.
29. Ray WA, Griffin MR, Schaffner W, et al. Psychotropic drug use and the risk of hip fracture. N Engl J Med 1987;316:363.
30. Schneider LS, Pollock VE, Lyness SA. A meta analysis of controlled trials of neuroleptic treatment in dementia. J Am Geriatr Soc 1990;38:553.
31. Medical Letter. New York: The Medical Letter. 2001;Issue 1106,43:51.
32. Griffin MR, Ray WA, Schaffner W. Non-steroidal anti-inflammatory drug use and death from peptic ulcer in elderly persons. Ann Intern Med 1988;22:82.
33. Bradley JD, Brandt KD, Katz BP, et al. Comparison of an anti-inflammatory dose of ibuprofen, an analgesic dose of ibuprofen and acetaminophen in the treatment of patients with osteoarthritis of the knee. N Engl J Med 1991;325:87.
34. Morin CM, Colecchi C, Stone J, et al. Behavioral and pharmacological therapy for late-life insomnia: a randomized controlled trial. JAMA 1999;281:991.
35. Edinger JD, Wohlgemuth WK, Radtke RA, et al. Cognitive behavioral therapy for treatment of chronic primary insomnia: a randomized controlled trial. JAMA 2001;285:1856.
36. PDR guide to drug interactions, side effects, indications, contraindications. Montvale, NJ: Medical Economics Company, 1997.
37. Council on Scientific Affairs, American Medical Association. Elder abuse and neglect. JAMA 1987;257:966.
38. Jones J, Dougherty J, Schelble D, et al. Emergency department protocol for the diagnosis of geriatric abuse. Ann Emerg Med 1988;17:1006.

*Bold print (general references) and bold numerals (specific references) denote published controlled clinical trials, meta-analyses, or consensus-based recommendations.

39. Tinetti ME, Inouye SK, Gill TM, et al. Shared risk factors for falls, incontinence, and functional dependence: unifying the approach to geriatric syndromes. JAMA 1995;273:1348.
40. Executive summary of the American Geriatrics Society, British Geriatrics Society, and the American Academy of Orthopaedic Surgeons. Clinical practice guideline: the prevention of falls in the older persons. J Am Geriatr Soc 2001;49:664.
41. Feder G, Cryer C, Donovan S, et al., on behalf of the Guidelines Development Group. Guidelines for the prevention of falls in people over 65. Br Med J 2000;321:1007.
42. Ettinger WH, Burns R, Messier SP, et al. A randomized trial comparing aerobic exercise and resistance exercise with a health education program in older adults with knee osteoarthritis: the Fitness, Arthritis and Seniors Trial (FAST). JAMA 1997;277:25.
43. Tinetti ME, Baker DI, McAvav G, et al. A multifactorial intervention to reduce the risk of falling among elderly people living in the community. N Engl J Med 1994;331:821.
44. Kannus P, Parkkari J, Niemi S, et al. Prevention of hip fracture in the elderly people with the use of a hip protector. N Engl J Med 2000;343:1506.
45. King MB, Tinetti ME. Falls in community-dwelling older persons. J Am Geriatr Soc 1995;43:1146.
46. Andres R. Mortality and obesity: the rationale for age-specific height-weight tables. In: Hazzard WR, et al., eds. Principles of geriatric medicine and gerontology. New York: McGraw-Hill, 1990.
47. Shimokata H, Andres R, Coon PJ, et al. Studies in the distribution of body fat. II. Longitudinal effects of change in weight. Int J Obesity 1989;13:455.
48. Folsom AR. Body fat distribution and 5-year risk of death in older women. JAMA 1993;269:483.
49. Hennekens CH, Buring JE, Manson JE, et al. Lack of effect of long-term supplementation with beta carotene on the incidence of malignant neoplasms and cardiovascular disease. N Engl J Med 1996;334:1145.
50. Rapola JM, Virtamo J, Ripatti S, et al. Randomized trial of α-tocopherol and β-carotene supplements on incidence of major coronary events in men with previous myocardial infarction. Lancet 1997;349:1715.
51. Thompson MP, Morris K. Unexplained weight loss in the ambulatory elderly. J Am Geriatr Soc 1991;39:497.
52. King AC, Oman RF, Brassington GS, et al. Moderate-intensity exercise and self-rated quality of sleep in older adults. JAMA 1997;277:32.
53. Province MA, Hadley EC, Hornbrook MC, et al. The effects of exercise on falls in elderly patients: a preplanned meta-analysis of the FICSIT trials. JAMA 1995;273:1341.
54. National Institutes of Health. Physical activity and cardiovascular health. JAMA 1996;276:241.
55. Christmas C, Andersen RA. Exercise and older patients: guidelines for the clinician. J Am Geriatr Soc 2000;48:318.
56. U.S. Department of Health and Human Services. Physical activity and health: a report of the surgeon general. Atlanta: U.S. Department of Health and Human Services, Centers for Disease Control and Prevention, National Center for Chronic Disease Prevention and Health Promotion, 1996.
57. Gill TM, DiPietro L, Krumholz HM. Role of exercise stress testing and safety monitoring for older persons starting an exercise program. JAMA 2000;284:3.
58. Mittleman MA, Maclure M, Tofler GH, et al. for Determinants of Myocardial Infarction Onset Study Investigators. Triggering of acute myocardial infarction by heavy physical exertion: protection against triggering by regular exertion. N Engl J Med 1993;329:1677.
59. Hollenberg M, Ngo LH, Turner D, et al. Treadmill exercise training in an epidemiologic study of elderly subjects. J Gerontol A Biol Sci Med Sci 1998;53A:B259.
60. American College of Sports Medicine. Guidelines for exercise testing and prescription, 5th ed. Baltimore: Williams & Wilkins, 1995.
61. Messinger-Rapport BJ, Rader E. High risk on the highway: how to identify and treat the impaired older driver. Geriatrics 2000;55:32.
62. Koespell TD, Wolf ME, McCloskey L, et al. Medical conditions and motor vehicle collision injuries in older adults. J Am Geriatr Soc 1994;42:695.
63. Gallo JJ, Rebok GW, Lesikar SE. The driving habits of adults aged 60 years and older. J Am Geriatr Soc 1999;47:335.
64. Marottoli RA, Cooney LM Jr, Wagner DR, et al. Predictors of automobile crashes and moving violations among elderly drivers. Ann Intern Med 1994;121:842.
65. Stutts JC. Do older drivers with visual and cognitive impairments drive less? J Am Geriatr Soc 1998;46:854.
66. Hemmelgarn B, Suissa S, Huang A, et al. Benzodiazepine use and the risk of motor vehicle crash in the elderly. JAMA 1997;278:27.
67. Brennan TA, Leape' LL, Laird NM, et al. Incidence of adverse events and negligence in hospitalized patients: results of the Harvard Medical Practice Study I. N Engl J Med 1991;324:370.
68. Thomas EJ, Brennan TA. Incidence and types of preventable adverse events in elderly patients: population based review of medical records. Br Med J 2000;320:741.
69. Leape LL, Brennan TA, Laird N, et al. The nature of adverse events in hospitalized patients: results of the Harvard Medical Practice Study II. N Engl J Med 1991;324:377.
70. Darchy B, Le Miere B, Figueredo B, et al. Iatrogenic diseases as a reason for admission to the intensive care unit: incidence, causes, and consequences. Arch Intern Med 1999;159:71.
71. Creditor MC. Hazards of hospitalization of the elderly. Ann Intern Med 1993;118:219.
72. Mahoney JE, Palta M, Johnson J, et al. Temporal association between hospitalization and rate of falls after discharge. Arch Intern Med 2000;160:2788.
73. Rowe JW, Kahn RL. Human aging: usual and successful. Science 1987;237:143.
74. Grover SA, Cook EF, Adam J, et al. Delayed diagnosis of gynecologic tumors in elderly women: relation to national medical practice patterns. Am J Med 1989;86:151.
75. Mandelblatt J, Bopaul I, Wistreich M. Gynecologic care of elderly women: another look at Papanicolaou smear testing. JAMA 1986;256:367.
76. Hermanson B, Omenn GS, Kormal RA, et al. Beneficial six-year outcome of smoking cessation in older men and women with coronary artery disease: results from the CASS registry. N Engl J Med 1988;319:1365.
77. Folstein MF, Folstein SE, McHugh PR. Mini-Mental State: a practical method for grading the cognitive state of patients for the clinician. J Psych Res 1975;12:189.
78. Yesavage JA, Brink TL. Development and validation of a geriatric depression screening scale: a preliminary report. J Psych Res 1983;17:37.

CHAPTER 13

Care at the End of Life

THOMAS E. FINUCANE, MD
LARRY WATERBURY, MD
MICHAEL J. PURTELL, MD, PhD

Family practitioners traditionally took care of their patients from cradle to grave, and then they managed the grief and bereavement of the survivors. They provided implicit guidance during the interval of severe illness and dying. For several reasons this situation has changed dramatically in the last 40 to 50 years. Society has become more mobile. Clinicians have become more specialized. Burdensome treatments have developed, about which meaningful decisions must be made. And autonomy has become the preeminent principle in American biomedical ethics. Recently, interest in the care of dying patients has grown steadily, stimulated in part by the growth of the hospice movement. It is likely that because of this interest the primary care practitioner again will be able to treat many dying patients in their own homes. In this chapter we discuss advance care planning, communicating with patients during severe eventually fatal illness, symptom management, and the management of grief and bereavement.

WHO IS DYING?

Most patients die of the exacerbation of a chronic illness, and it is usually impossible to give a precise estimate of when death will occur. Two studies from the Study to Understand Patient Preferences for Outcomes and Risks of Treatment outline the difficulty (1,2). One study looked at patients with heart, lung, or liver failure who survived to hospital discharge and used a variety of models to identify who would meet the hospice criteria for an expected survival of 6 months or less. With the strictest criteria, fewer than 1% of patients were identified as terminal, and yet over half of the rigorously selected group were still alive at 6 months. Using the most lenient criteria, 70% of the patients identified as terminal were still alive at 6 months and 58% of patients who were not identified as terminal had died in that interval. These authors concluded that most of these chronically ill patients "never experience a time during which they are clearly dying of their disease" (1).

A second study reviewed 1,976 patients who died in the hospital during the Study to Understand Patient Preferences for Outcomes and Risks of Treatment and for whom sophisticated estimates of likelihood of survival had been made in the days before death. For patients dying of heart failure, the average chance of living 6 more months, calculated 3 days before death, was 60%. Two days before dying of chronic obstructive pulmonary disease, the corresponding figure was 50% (2). Lubitz and Riley (3) found that of the most expensive 1% of Medicare patients in a given year, half die and half survive. It is the inability to identify those who are "dying" that leads to at least some of the lavish spending on patients in their last year of life.

GLOSSARY OF TERMS

Several concepts and terms are used very imprecisely in discussions about care at the end of life. As just discussed, a central ambiguity arises in the use of terms such as "terminal," "end of life," and "the dying process." The ability to know who was going to die soon would greatly simplify decision making for the gravely ill.

- *Palliative care:* The word "palliative" comes from a Latin word for "cloak" or "cover." In general it refers literally to treatments aimed mainly at the control of symptoms. The word has acquired an additional connotation, however, that treatments with curative intent are being foregone. In this latter usage, morphine for a leg broken in football would not be palliative, whereas morphine for malignant fracture in a patient dying of cancer would be, particularly if disease-specific treatment was being withheld.
- *Hospice:* "Hospice" refers both to a philosophy of care and to a Medicare benefit. In the former sense, patients are said to receive hospice treatment when the goals of treatment have become palliative rather than curative. The Medicare hospice benefit, discussed below, is a well-defined formal program.
- *Surrogate, proxy, and substitute:* Gravely ill patients often lose the ability to make complex medical decisions for themselves. These decisions must then be made by others. A substitute may make decisions because he or she had been designated by the patient at an earlier time. If the incapacitated patient has not designated a substitute, a substitute must be identified by default. The default decision maker is usually next of kin, but states vary in their definitions of default decision makers and the order in which default decision makers are accorded authority. In some

states the designated substitute is called a proxy, and the default substitute is called a surrogate. In other states, the opposite is true; proxies are default substitutes and surrogates are those who have been designated. "Health care agent" and "durable power of attorney" are common usages, generally referring to a designated substitute. Other terms are used as well. Different states have different rules about how much authority will be granted to any substitute decision maker and different rules for designated versus substitute decision makers. Some authors use these terms quite loosely. Because of the variation in and ongoing changes in state laws, practitioners should become familiar with the relevant terms and laws for their locality.

- *Advance directives:* This term generally refers to directives made by a capable patient to leave guidance about treatment in the future if the patient by then has become incapable of making decisions. Designating a health care agent is one way of doing this. The other way involves describing particular scenarios of illness and stating whether treatment should or should not be provided in each. The best-known example of this type of advance directive is the living will. The term is also occasionally used to refer to plans made by others on behalf of an already incapacitated person. Decisions made in advance of severe illness by family and staff on behalf of an incapacitated nursing home resident, for example, are sometimes called advance directives.

ADVANCE DIRECTIVES

The cornerstone task in establishing advance directives requires the patient to imagine two hypothetical circumstances. First, the patient imagines that he or she has become so ill that decisions about life-sustaining treatment have become necessary, that he or she has not made these decisions in advance, and that he or she has become incapable of making these decisions. As stated above, the patient can address this hypothetical situation by naming a *health care agent.* Doing this is probably the optimal solution for many patients.

Second, the patient may try to imagine particular scenarios and to specify what treatments should or should not be given. *Living wills* are examples of this type of advance directive, but are subject to extreme limitations in almost every state. In particular, they are ineffective by statute unless the patient has a qualifying condition. In Maryland for example, life-sustaining treatment may not be withheld on the basis of a living will unless the patient is either terminally ill or in a persistent vegetative state. Most other states have similar limitations. A few states have created categories where severe dementia serves as a qualifying condition, and the scenario-based document can be invoked. With a few exceptions (4), most studies show that many patients do not want to do living wills (5) and that when living wills are done they have little effect on the subsequent process of care (6). Nonetheless, they are commonly included in discussions about improving care at the end of life.

Do not resuscitate orders to withhold cardiopulmonary resuscitation (CPR) deserve special mention. Although they can be seen easily as scenario-based advance directives ("If I were to suffer cardiac arrest, I direct that CPR not be performed"), the laws in most states treat them as real-time decisions about a proposed course of treatment. A patient may refuse CPR just as she or he may refuse surgery or chemotherapy. If this were not so, and in-hospital do not resuscitate orders were treated as advance directives, their use would be restricted to patients with the requisite qualifying conditions.

A more difficult problem arises for patients who are outside the hospital, either at home or in a nursing home. Almost every state has specific legislation designed to guide emergency medical service providers in cases where the patient wishes to decline CPR. Most states require a particular form to be completed, and many require an easily recognizable symbol, which indicates to emergency medical service providers that CPR may be withheld in the emergency setting.

In ambulatory practice, a general approach that works for most patients is to give them information on advance directives during one encounter and then to discuss their preferences regarding advance directives with them and their families during subsequent encounters. In most states, the most useful and effective form of advance directive is the designation of a substitute decision maker. This person is broadly authorized in most states to make real-time decisions that balance burdens and benefits of treatment on behalf of a person who has become incapacitated, using their knowledge of what they believe would have been the person's wishes. Advance directives that outline specific preferences to decline treatment are generally not enforceable by statute unless the person has a "qualifying condition," such as terminal illness or persistent vegetative state. Discussions about these preferences are valuable, nonetheless, because they help family members, substitute decision makers, and the clinician to develop a picture of the patient's values in balancing longer life versus lesser suffering. It is important to realize, in discussing advance directives, that cultural differences may exist (7–9).

SUBSTITUTE DECISION MAKING

In principle, substitute decision makers, whether designated or by default, should be guided by the ethical idea of "substituted judgment." This means that the substitute should be trying to act as a conduit, to bring to the health care team what the patient would have said or how he or she would have decided if that patient was still able to make decisions about the question at hand. The substitute should only use a "best interests" standard if there is no realistic way to understand what the patient would have wanted. In brief, the provider should ask "What would he or she tell us to do for him or her?" (substituted judgment) in preference to "What do I think would be best for him or her?" (best interests). In practice, of course, complex judgments are often made on behalf of patients who arrive in circumstances that are beyond anything they ever could have imagined.

In many cases there is no correct answer to questions about life-sustaining treatment for incapacitated patients. What is important is that the way in which the decision is reached is fair, well intentioned, and, ideally, consensual. Different states have evolved different techniques for resolving conflicts among substitute decision makers. The educational organization Partnership for Caring provides helpful information regarding living wills and other ways to protect the autonomy of a dying person (see Resources for Patients and Their Loved Ones at the end of the chapter).

EMOTIONAL REACTIONS IN THE FACE OF DEATH

Terminally ill patients often go through a series of five stages in accepting the reality of their impending death (10). The duration of these stages and the intensity and sequence with which they are experienced are highly variable from one patient to the next. The stages are

1. Shock and denial
2. Anger
3. Bargaining
4. Depression
5. Acceptance

During the first stage, when patients are informed of their diagnosis and poor prognosis, they are usually unable to "hear" it. Some patients may be shocked and surprised temporarily, but a profound sense of disbelief in the practitioner's pronouncements keeps them calm. They may go from practitioner to practitioner to find someone to tell them what they would like to hear—that their condition is not serious. This denial of illness can be best summed up in a phrase: "No, not me." Eventually, such attempts are futile, and the patient has to face reality.

During the stage of anger it may be difficult to deal with patients. They complain about their care, and as a result, family, friends, and health care providers may avoid them. This rejection further increases their rage. They are likely to ask "Why me?" They often feel cheated and envious of others. If one does not feel guilty and lose one's self-esteem, he or she is likely, after this period of anger, to move on to the stage of bargaining. On the other hand, if one feels that he or she deserves punishment for past doings as an explanation of one's illness, he or she is likely to become depressed. From being very mad, the patient moves to being very sad.

During the stage of bargaining the dominant theme is "Yes, it is me, but . . . ." With the realization of an impending death, patients offer to do things that they did not do before or to live their lives differently in exchange for the prolongation of their life. A number of patients go through a religious experience, and some of them believe they are "born again." Often at this stage the patient looks comfortable and peaceful, but that sense of well-being is short lived. As the illness advances and suffering is compounded, the patient becomes depressed.

During the stage of depression the reality of impending death sinks even deeper. Patients may have already gone through many real (and imagined) losses by this time, such as loss of a body organ, missing important events in the lives of their family members, or loss of their job or savings. Depression at this stage is not so much compounded by anger as it is colored with resignation. Patients begin to separate from everyone and everything they loved before. At this time they do not want any false hopes. It is a very private and personal time in their lives. They may not want any visitors and may not even say much to their own immediate family members. They want their family's love, affection, and respect but may not be able to give them anything in return. They may exhaust their caregivers by developing regressive behavior patterns, such as failing to accomplish activities of daily living of which they are capable, making many small demands, and becoming incontinent. This stage is very difficult for the family.

Finally, when patients have experienced anger and grief, they move to the *stage of acceptance.* If patients have the strong support of their family, they go through all stages to arrive at a final stage of equanimity characterized by tranquillity, in which the patient is neither happy nor sad. At this stage, a patient may simply say "My time is coming close," "It is all right," or "I am ready."

CARE OF A DYING PERSON

Most patients who experience prolonged but predictable dying are patients in the terminal stage of cancer or, currently, acquired immunodeficiency syndrome (AIDS). This discussion focuses on terminal care for such patients, much or all of which can be provided out of hospital. Chapters 10 and 39, respectively, describe the care of patients with cancer and patients with AIDS before the terminal stage.

Throughout the care of a patient with terminal illness, it is important to determine the physical stage of the illness but also the patient's psychologic stage of accepting impending death (see above) and the patient's concerns regarding family or business affairs. Terminally ill patients' needs differ widely, and every effort should be made to provide care that is adapted to these unique needs.

Communication

Communication of Diagnosis, Treatment Plan, and Prognosis

People have different opinions about the need for and importance of communication about the diagnosis, treatment plan, and prognosis of terminally ill patients. A common practice in the past, which still prevails in some societies (11), was to maintain a conspiracy of silence in which the patient's practitioner in collusion with family members covered up the diagnosis of a terminal illness to "protect" the dying patient from emotional shock. This practice may lead to isolation of the patient from family, friends, and health care providers. Honesty and sincerity toward the patient usually make dealing with terminal illness more bearable for patient, family members, and health care providers. Although most patients become temporarily demoralized in the face of this news, in the long run, they usually appreciate the truth. Moreover, it is then easier for their families to relate to them in an open and honest manner. Families participating in a conspiracy of silence may have greater emotional difficulties than do families in situations in which truth has prevailed. Occasionally, patients indicate that they do not want to know the unpleasant truth; in that case, one should respect that wish. However, invariably these patients, and those whose clinician and family withhold the diagnosis from them, come to know the nature of their illness even if it has not been told directly to them.

The *giving and discussing of bad news* with a patient and family is challenging, important, and helped by the use of specific communication skills (12,13). Before delivering bad news it is important to be certain of the diagnosis and to anticipate and be prepared to answer commonly asked questions regarding prognosis, referral, and treatment. When one is ready to discuss the diagnosis and expected course of the illness with a terminally ill patient, it is important to sit down with the patient and the family in a private place. One should avoid lengthy introductions, be precise and concise but not hurried, pay attention to the emotional reactions of the patient and of the family members, and respond with silent pauses, followed by verbal acknowledgment of the patient's emotional reactions. It is also important not to use euphemisms (e.g., *swelling, tumor,* or *lump*) but to acknowledge the presence of cancer or malignant disease, to pledge to help reduce suffering as much as possible, and to affirm that you will be involved and supportive to the very end. Most patients do not hear the bad news when it is first delivered and must be told the truth in small doses in the course of several interviews. Details about the patient's disease and management options should be paced and given at times when the patient or family is receptive, often in response to their questions.

A *caveat* is that the above recommendations pertain to the dominant American culture. When appropriate, the practitioner may need to accommodate to the norms of patients with a different cultural heritage. In some cultures, for example, is it customary to communicate directly with the patient's family member rather than the patient. Some cultures observe strict gender or generation roles in making health care decisions. In other cultures, such as traditional Navajo (9), where it is important to present information in a positive and not negative way, the giving and discussing of bad news should be approached thoughtfully, and when one is not experienced, with consultation.

Staying Connected

Often terminally ill patients receive attention during the early stages of their illness, but that attention wanes as their disease progresses. This occurs largely because of the helplessness that others feel when confronting the patient's plight. The stages of denial, anger, and depression often cause a withdrawal of family, friends, health care practitioners, and other caregivers, and these behaviors establish a vicious cycle; that is, the more the patient is ignored, the more unmanageable and inaccessible the patient becomes. For these reasons, a most important principle of the care of a terminally ill patient is for all parties to maintain a consistency of involvement. The clinician should counsel family members in this regard and should plan regular contacts with the patient, either by scheduling office visits or by making visits to the home. These actions can reduce patients' anguish, making it easier for them to express feelings and ask questions. During these ongoing contacts, the physician can ascertain and respond to the patient's desires and concerns regarding end-of-life care. A recent qualitative study of advance care planning in predominantly white renal dialysis patients, human immunodeficiency virus-infected patients, and residents of a long-term care facility revealed the following concerns regarding end-of-life care: receiving adequate pain and symptom management, avoiding inappropriate prolongation of dying, achieving a sense of control, relieving burden, and strengthening relationships with loved ones (14). Again racial and ethnic differences may play a role. Black Americans, for example, are more likely than white Americans to desire aggressive treatment at the end of life (7,8). Continued and consistent involvement of practitioner, family, and other caregivers not only provides the opportunity to ascertain and respond to patient concerns, it provides the opportunity for important communication between parties to occur and gives dignity to a dying person. The patient continues to feel like a person until the very end.

Communication With the Patient's Family

The emotional problems of the family of the dying person need attention. Family members go through stages of emotional adjustment and have difficulties in accepting the diagnosis and projected course of a terminal illness, just as the patient does. By encouraging open communication between the patient and the family, the practitioner can make an important contribution in the care of the dying person. Each family member will react differently to the impending death of a relative, depending on his or her age, personality, role, and relationship with the dying relative and the rest of the family. To be effective, the practitioner must be aware of these factors and allocate time to meet the needs of individual family members. Caregivers may be stressed by trying to balance their personal needs and the needs of their own family with those of the loved one. Not infrequently patients and their caregivers face economic and other burdens related to a terminal illness; simply listening to and acknowledging these concerns can be helpful (15). It may be helpful to convene a *family meeting* one or more times to deal with decisions (see the practical approach to this in Chapter 3).

Important advice to family members includes the fact that a dying person has a great need to have access to his or her children and that children have a great need to be close to their dying parent. The same is true for other loved ones. The practitioner should encourage these necessary contacts. In addition, the family should be urged to find ways to gratify small needs of the patient. Removing restrictions from food, alcohol, and cigarettes is not only humane but sensible. Considerations such as these are described in an excellent booklet for families, *Taking Time: Support for People with Cancer and the People Who Care About Them,* available free from the National Cancer Institute (see Resources for Patients and Their Loved Ones at the end of the chapter). It was prepared by patients with terminal cancer and their families to help others deal with many draining and awkward experiences they will face. For elderly patients near death, the 80-page booklet, *Hard Choices for Loving People* (see Resources for Patients and Their Loved Ones at the end of the chapter), can be useful. It is written by a chaplain and provides a nontechnical presentation about the decision whether to prolong life with greater suffering or accept a shorter life with less suffering.

Management of Pain, Anxiety, Depression, Delirium, Dyspnea, and Hydration

Pain

A large number of patients with cancer have significant pain during the terminal stage of their illness. Therefore, a basic principle in the care of these patients is to provide adequate relief of pain. This often requires the administration of narcotic analgesics. Because of fear of inducing addiction, patients may receive dosages of narcotics that are too small or too infrequent to relieve pain adequately. In fact, the risk of addiction in this setting is slight; narcotics should be given on schedule (not as needed), including at night, when it is often better to disturb patients for their medication than to wait for pain to waken them.

Another misconception about narcotic use in patients with cancer concerns tolerance. Many patients with cancer who take narcotics do not develop tolerance and are able to remain on the same dosage of medication for prolonged periods. When tolerance does occur, it usually manifests itself as a decrease in the duration of analgesia and can be treated by shortening the dose interval or increasing the dosage or both. When the requirement for medication increases, this is often caused by disease progression rather than the development of tolerance. *Physical dependence* (abstinence syndrome occurring at the time of abrupt withdrawal of narcotics) develops within 2 weeks of the initiation of narcotic therapy in most patients.

Important considerations in *selecting medication* for pain are effectiveness, route of administration (e.g., the cachectic patient may have few sites for injections), available forms for oral administration (e.g., some patients may be able to take only liquids easily; liquid morphine is especially useful for such patients), and duration of pain relief. Table 13.1 summarizes practical information about a number of narcotics that are used in controlling pain.

It is usually preferable to *assess the adequacy of pain relief* after a given regimen has been in place for 24 hours. For constant pain, it is important to use dosages that control the pain and regular (rather than as needed) dosing intervals to prevent the pain from resurfacing. Appropriate intervals may be as frequent as hourly for oral liquid morphine. In evaluating pain control over time, it is helpful to use a visual analog scale, such as the scale illustrated in Fig. 13.1, to provide an ongoing record of the effectiveness of pain treatment (16).

Sometimes pain control is inadequate with orally achievable dosages or is impractical when a patient refuses intramuscular injections. Many times adequate blood levels of analgesics can be achieved through *buccal, rectal, or cutaneous absorption.* For these purposes opiate suppositories or fentanyl as patches or lozenges can be used. Fentanyl patches provide constant narcotic blood levels (achieved 8 to 12 hours after initial application) for 48 to 72 hours. The patches are expensive (two to four times the cost of equianalgesic doses of oral narcotics), and one usually needs to supplement with as needed oral narcotics when the patches are initially applied and for breakthrough pain. Blood levels remain constant at the time of changing the patch (usually after 72 hours), because when the old patch is removed the skin depot continues to release drug as the new depot accumulates. One should start low and slowly build up the dosage, supplementing with oral analgesics as needed. If a patient is overmedicated, the drug will be in the blood for hours after the patch is removed.

Parenteral administration is usually reserved as a last resort. Intermittent parenteral administration usually is impractical in the home setting. *Constant infusion of narcotics*, however, may provide even and satisfactory pain relief (17). Morphine or hydromorphone is usually prescribed, and the medication is delivered via a small portable pump. The pump allows an infusion of a constant dose plus a periodic bolus programmed to allow the patient to better control the degree of analgesia (*patient-controlled analgesia*). The subcutaneous route is far preferable to the intravenous route because of ease of care (family members can be taught how to change the subcutaneous site). Medicare and other third-party payers will pay for constant infusion of narcotics for cancer pain, making this an important option for patients without prescription plans.

All narcotic analgesics may cause the following *side effects*: sedation, respiratory depression, nausea and vomiting, suppression of cough, constipation, bladder spasm, or urinary retention. In the terminally ill patient, rarely, there may be a need to reverse narcotic effect because of respiratory depression. When possible, one should simply withhold the next dose. If reversal is needed, this can be achieved with small doses of

Table 13.1. Selected Drugs for Treating Pain

Constituents	Trade Name	Available Preparations	Usual Dose Range[a]	Approximate Equivalent IM Dose of Morphine	Peak Effect (h)	Duration (h)	Federal Narcotic Schedule
Moderately potent							
Codeine phosphate		Tablets, 30, 60, mg	30–120 mg	1–6 mg	2	3–4	II
		Injectable, 10 mg/5 mL					
Codeine-acetaminophen[b]	Tylenol No. 3	Tablets, 30 mg codeine	1–2 tablets	1–2 mg	2	3–4	III
	Tylenol No. 4	Tablets, 60 mg codeine	1 tablet	2 mg	2		
		Elixir, 12 mg codeine/5 mL	15–30 mL				
Oxycodone	Roxicodone	Tablets, 5 mg	1–3 tablets	1–5 mg	1	3–4	II
		Liquid, 5 mg/5 mL	5–15 mL	1–5 mg	1	3–4	
	Oxycontin[c]	Controlled-release tablets 10, 20, 40 mg	10–80 mg	2–16 mg	3	12	
Oxycodone aspirin-phenacetin-caffeine	Percodan	Tablets, 5 mg oxycodone	1–3 tablets	1–5 mg	1	3–4	II
Oxycodone acetaminophen	Tylox[d]	Capsules, 5 mg oxycodone	1–2 capsules	1–3 mg	1	3–4	II
	Percocet[b] Roxicet[b]	Tablets, 5 mg oxycodone	1–3 tablets	1–5 mg	1	3–4	
Most potent							
Morphine sulfate[e]		Injectable, 10 mg/mL	10–30 mg	10–30 mg	0.5	3–4	II
		Constant infusion[e]	1–20 mg/h	NA	NA	NA	
		Liquid, multiple concentrations	20–200 mg	4–40 mg	1	2–3	
		Tablets 30, 60 mg	30–90 mg	6–20 mg	1	3–4	
	MS Contin[c]	Controlled release 15, 30, 60, 100 mg	30–200 mg	6–40 mg	3	8–12	
	RMS suppos	Suppository, 5, 10, 20, 30 mg	30–90 mg	6–20 mg	1	3–4	
Methadone[f]	Dolophine	Tablets, 5, 10 mg	2.5–20 mg	1–10 mg	2	4–5	II
		Injectable, 10 mg/mL		10 mg			
Meperidine	Demerol	Tablets, 50, 100 mg	50–300 mg	2–10 mg	2	3–4	II
		Syrup, 50 mg/5 mL					
		Injectable, 25, 50, 75, 100 mg/mL	50–150 mg	6–20 mg	1	2–4	
Hydromorphone	Dilaudid	Tablets, 1, 2, 3, 4 mg	2–8 mg	4–10 mg	1	3–4	II
		Suppository, 3 mg					
		Injectable, 1, 2, 3 mg/mL	1–2 mg	10 mg	0.5	3	
Levorphanol[f]	Levo-Dromoran	Tablets, 2 mg	2–4 mg	5–10 mg	2	4–5	II
Fentanyl transdermal patch[e]	Duragesic[c]	Patch, 25, 50, 75, 100 μg/h	50–300 μg/h	30–360 mg/day	12	48–72	II

[a]Higher doses are needed in patients who develop tolerance. (oral/parenteral ratio = 6 to 1 for one dose, 3 to 1 for multiple doses).
[b]Each tablet contains 300–325 mg acetaminophen; elixir contains 120 mg (Perocet) or 325 mg (Roxicet) acetaminophen per 5 mL.
[c]Controlled-release treatment may need to be supplemented with short-acting oral narcotics.
[d]Each capsule contains 500 mg acetaminophen.
[e]See text for further details.
[f]The plasma half-life of methadone and levorphanol in long ($\geq$15 h) and cumulative effects may occur with continual use of these drugs.

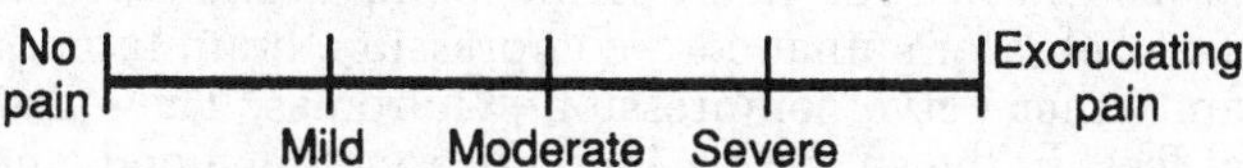

Figure 13.1. Visual analog scale for rating pain severity.

naloxone (0.1 to 0.2 mg intravenously every few minutes), but with the use of naloxone one runs the risk of acute withdrawal and severe pain.

Nausea is extremely common in terminally ill patients, especially as a side effect of narcotic usage, and should be treated *aggressively*. Phenothiazines are usually helpful for narcotic-induced nausea. Prochlorperazine (Compazine, 5 to 10 mg orally or 25 mg by suppository every 4 to 6 hours, or 15-mg spansules every 6 to 8 hours) causes less sedation and hypotension than chlorpromazine. Opioid rotation can also be very helpful. Changing to another opioid at comparable doses can eliminate nausea. Haloperidol (0.5 to 2 mg orally or subcutaneously every 6 to 8 hours) is useful for nausea in the agitated patient. Methylprogesterone (Megace) 160 to 800 mg/day can help nausea and stimulate appetite. It has no effect or an adverse effect on quality of life or survival. Autonomic failure is very common in the dying patients. Metoclopramide (Reglan, 10 to 20 mg orally or intramuscularly every 6 hours) is useful if gastric fullness is a common complaint. Dexamethasone (4 mg every 8 to 24 hours) may also be helpful in the nauseated patient and may potentiate the antiemetic effects of metoclopramide. Hyoscyamine (Levsin tablets, 1 or 2 tablets every 4 hours) is useful for controlling upper airway secretions. Octreotide may be useful in patients with intestinal obstruction by decreasing gastrointestinal secretions (18). Other causes of nausea and vomiting are also common in terminally ill patients, such as that caused by chemotherapy, radiotherapy, or the disease itself. The treatment of nausea and vomiting

Table 13.2. Adjuvant Analgesic Drugs for Adults and Children Weighing 50 kg or More

Class and Drug	Approximate Dosage Range	Administration	Use
Corticosteroids			
Dexamethasone	16–96 mg/day	Oral or intravenous	For pain associated with brain metastases and epidural spinal cord compression
Prednisone	40–80 mg/day	Oral	
Anticonvulsant agents			
Carbamazepine	200–1,600 mg/day	Oral	For neurophatic pain
Gabapentin	900 mg–1 g/day	Oral	
Phenytoin	300–500 mg/day	Oral	
Antidepressant agents			
Amitriptyline	25–150 mg/day	Oral	For neuropathic pain
Doxepin	25–150 mg/day	Oral	
Imipramine	20–100 mg/day	Oral	
Neuroleptic agents			
Methotrimeprazine	40–80 mg/day	Intramuscular	For analgesia, for sedation, as antiemetic agent
Antihistamines			
Hydroxyzine	300–450 mg/day	Intramuscular	As adjuvant to opioids for postoperative and other types of pain; for relief of complicating symptoms including anxiety, insomnia, and nausea
Local anesthetic and antiarrhythmic agents			
Lidocaine	5 mg/kg per day[a]	Intravenous or subcutaneous	For neuropathic pain
Mexiletin	450–600 mg/day	Oral	
Tocainide	20 mg/kg per day[a]	Oral	
Psychostimulants			
Dextroamphetamine	5–10 mg/day	Oral	To improve opioid analgesia and decrease sedation
Methylphenidate	10–15 mg/day	Oral	

[a]The dosage given is per kilogram of body weight per day.

Adapted from Agency for Health Care Policy and Research (AHCPR). Management of cancer pain: clinical practice guideline, Publication No. 94-0592, 1994, with permission.

due to chemotherapy and radiotherapy is discussed in Chapter 10.

Constipation is a universal problem in the terminally ill patient who is taking narcotics, and it may contribute to nausea; it should be treated prophylactically. Bulk laxatives require an adequate intake of food and fluid to be effective and may have little use in the terminally ill patient with poor oral intake. A stool softener alone is rarely effective for narcotic-induced constipation. More useful sequential strategies are the following:

1. Use daily a preparation that combines a stool softener and a mild stimulant laxative such as dioctyl sodium sulfosuccinate plus casanthranol (Peri-Colace, 1 daily to 2 three times daily) or docusate sodium plus senna (Senokot-S, 1 daily to 4 three times daily).
2. If no success, add bisacodyl (Dulcolax, 5 mg by mouth at bedtime to 15 mg three times daily) or milk of magnesia (30 to 60 mL once or twice daily).
3. If still unsuccessful, add sorbitol or lactulose (Chronulac, 10 g/15 mL, 30 to 45 mL at bedtime or twice a day).
4. If constipation continues, check for impaction. If present, with a hard stool, try glycerine suppositories or olive oil retention enemas. If there is no impaction, add bisacodyl suppositories (Dulcolax, 10 mg) or Fleet enema.

Poor pain control often results from inadequate dosage of narcotic, too infrequent administration, and failure to use adjuncts such as nonsteroidal anti-inflammatory drugs. *A number of adjunctive pharmacologic and nonpharmacologic measures may help the terminally ill patient with pain.* Aspirin and other nonsteroidal anti-inflammatory drugs at dosages similar to those used for musculoskeletal pain are often helpful for many types of pain, especially bone pain caused by metastases (see Chapter 77 for nonsteroidal anti-inflammatory drug table). Table 13.2 summarizes practical information and indications for other nonnarcotic drugs to control pain. Tricyclic antidepressants may be helpful for neuropathic pain, especially if the pain is associated with insomnia or depression. Gabapentin is also useful for neuropathic pain. Corticosteroids are useful for spinal cord compression, brain tumors, and other nerve compression syndromes. They also, at least in the short run, increase appetite, mood, and general sense of well-being. Methylphenidate (Ritalin) may be useful to combat the lethargy of analgesics. Transcutaneous nerve stimulation may be helpful temporarily for localized (particularly neuropathic) pain. A number of psychologic approaches (hypnosis, relaxation training, guided imagery, distraction techniques) are also useful for the cancer patient with pain (see practical approaches described in Chapter 22).

Nerve damage, as might occur from tumor infiltration or radiation fibrosis, can produce a neuropathic pain that is difficult to control. Studies of the pathophysiology of neuropathic pain suggest that this refractoriness to treatment is partly a consequence of repeated pathologic afferent inputs from the damaged peripheral nerves onto the secondary pain receptors in the spinal cord. This causes a phenomenon termed "windup," a condition in which the secondary afferent pain receptors become permanently turned on. Because these receptors are relatively insensitive to the inhibitory effects of morphine, customary analgesics may prove ineffective. For instance, methadone with its ability to decrease windup more efficiently than morphine becomes a more appropriate choice of analgesic in this condition. Similarly, ketamine, dextromethorphan, or topiramate, which act directly to inhibit the secondary receptors, should be considered in refractory cases. Adjuncts, such as tricyclic antidepressants or gabapentin, should nearly always be used in patients with neuropathic pain because they potentiate inhibitory central inputs to these secondary receptors and serve to assist in turning down windup (19).

Anxiety

The family's and practitioner's concern and accessibility may be all that are necessary to relieve the anxiety of the dying patient. Anxiolytic drugs also can be of some help in the management of these patients (see Chapter 22). When insomnia is also a major problem, a benzodiazepine hypnotic can be used to induce sleep (see Chapter 7). The sedating antihistamine hydroxyzine (Atarax, Vistaril), 25 to 50 mg by mouth three times daily, may also help patients who have anxiety associated with pain.

Depression

Most patients who go through the depressive stage of dying do not require antidepressant medications, although periodically some may require antianxiety medications. The family's and the practitioner's support is most therapeutic for this kind of depression. Some patients develop severe depression, particularly after a brief stage of anger, when they conclude they are being punished for their sins. Loss of self-esteem, guilt feelings, psychomotor retardation, early morning awakening with a diurnal variation in mood, and even suicidal thoughts may appear in this setting. When a number of these and other indicators of a major depression are present, antidepressants may bring relief. There is a detailed discussion of the use of these drugs in Chapter 24. Discussion of suicide, even in a terminally ill and suffering patient, should raise the question of depression.

Delirium

Periodic or persistent delirium (inattentiveness, inaccessibility, inability to recognize loved ones, gross confusion) is very common in the final days or weeks of terminal disease (20,21). In fact, most terminal cancer patients die in delirium (21). Most of these patients do not have an agitated delirium, and their course is characterized by increasing withdrawal and somnolence. Some patients continue in a state of agitated delirium and require chronic medication. Haloperidol, in a controlled study, was more useful than benzodiazepines and phenothiazines in the treatment of agitated delirium (a very small study, done in AIDS patients) but should be used temporarily while other treatable causes are addressed (22). The cause is almost always an identifiable metabolic derangement, infection, excess analgesic or psychotropic medication, tumor metastasis to the brain, or a combination of these factors. Loss of clear communication as a result of delirium may be distressing to the patient's family. Management of easily reversible causes is therefore important except in the patient whose death is imminent. A list of the principal causes of delirium is found in Chapter 26.

Dyspnea

Dyspnea is a common and distressing symptom for the dying patient. In terms of treatment, it is important to focus on the patient's symptom and not the observer's interpretation of physical findings. Patients who are tachypneic may not feel dyspneic, and patients breathing calmly may feel dyspneic. Physical impediments to breathing and psychologic fears and discomfort are often combined when a patient is near death. In this situation, a number of measures can help. If patients have rapidly recurring pleural effusions, a small-diameter tube can be placed in the radiology suite, left in for days to weeks, and managed at home without the discomfort associated with chest tube placement and sclerosis. Positioning the patient upright in bed or in a chair and administering oxygen (if the patient is hypoxic) are useful (23). Patients may feel better if air is circulated past them from a fan or an open window. If the patient and caretaker can be taught relaxation techniques (see Chapter 22) and calming strategies, this can be very useful.

Low dosages of opiates (e.g., morphine 2 mg intravenously or oral liquid morphine 5 to 10 mg every 1 to 2 hours as needed) may be helpful for the terminally ill dyspneic patient and when carefully titrated can calm without leading to respiratory depression The beneficial effect on dyspnea does not usually last as long as the effect on pain, and one may have to administer morphine in small doses hourly or by continuous infusion. The usefulness of nebulized morphine has been examined in a few studies. Many believe it is helpful especially in patients who benefit from nebulizer treatment However, randomized trials have failed to find it more useful than placebo (24). There is evidence that physicians underuse bronchodilator therapy in dying patients (24).

Practitioner worry about respiratory depression is a major impediment to helping dying patients with dyspnea. Most patients, especially if they are not narcotic naive, do not develop significant respiratory depression, and if they do, tolerance to that effect usually develops quickly. Other medications that may be helpful for dyspnea include steroids (for radiation pneumonitis, lymphangitic pulmonary metastases, or chemotherapy-induced hypersensitivity lung disease) and phenothiazines (chlorpromazine and promethazine have been shown to decrease dyspnea in patients with chronic lung disease, probably because of their sedative effects, as has buspirone).

Hydration

Whether or not to supplement oral fluid intake in the dying patient is a complex issue. Families are frequently uncomfortable about letting loved ones become dehydrated. Data demonstrate a weak relationship between the experience of thirst and the patient's actual state of hydration (25). Thirst occurs in some patients who are dying of cancer and can almost always be alleviated by good oral hygiene and a modest amount of oral fluids (26). It does not appear that thirst is a reason to consider parenteral fluids. Delirium may be another matter because there are data that dehydration (decreased renal perfusion) may affect drug clearance, potentiating the central nervous side effects of medications such as opioids (21). When the patient is truly terminal, it may be undesirable to prolong the dying process by reversing the patient's delirium. If assisted parenteral hydration is determined to be useful for symptom management or to address family wishes, it can be easily accomplished without intravenous access by short subcutaneous infusions (500 mL over 1 hour twice daily is usually adequate to maintain hydration in most dying patients) (27).

Hospice Care

In most communities, patients and their families can be cared for by their primary care practitioner in cooperation with a hospice, a program designed to provide terminal care, including relief of pain, to the dying patient and to provide support to the family. Services are delivered either in the patient's home, a hospital, a nursing home, or other hospice facility by a multidisciplinary team under the direction of the health care practitioner.

In hospice care, the primary focus changes from curing and caring to simply caring, and the overall goal changes from prolongation of life to the enhancement of the quality of life during the patient's final days. Since the introduction of the hospice movement in the United States and the founding of the first hospice here in 1974, hospice programs have been developed in most communities, and most third-party payers now provide hospice benefits. *Eligibility criteria* for hospice benefits under Medicare are the following: The patient must be terminally ill with a life expectancy of 6 months or less, must be unable to benefit from or have refused further aggressive (curative) therapy, must be able to receive most care at home, and have a caregiver (relative or friend) who will assume the responsibility for custodial care of the patient and be the decision maker in the event the patient becomes incompetent to make decisions. Table 13.3 summarizes in detail the processes and services included in Medicare hospice benefits.

The mushrooming of hospice programs may create an erroneous impression that hospice-type care can be provided only in hospices. Comprehensive humanistic treatment for the dying patient and the family can be offered by any health care practitioner. Home health agencies can play a pivotal role in this care (see Chapter 9). The essentials for the delivery of hospice-type care at home are practitioner knowledge and skill in prescribing for symptom relief, practitioner availability, willingness and ability to work with a multidisciplinary team, and willingness to spend extra time and effort to foresee and alleviate the problems faced by the dying patient and the family.

Table 13.3. Medicare Hospice Benefits

The Medicare hospice benefit is divided into benefit periods:
- An initial 90-day period
- A subsequent 90-day period
- An unlimited number of 60-day periods

The beneficiary must be recertified as terminally ill at the beginning of each benefit period. The following covered hospice services are provided as necessary to give palliative treatment for conditions related to the terminal illness: nursing care; services of a medical social worker, physician, counselor (including dietary, pastoral, and other), and home care aide and homemaker; short-term inpatient care (including both respite care and procedures necessary for pain control and acute and chronic system management); medical appliances and supplies, including drugs and biologicals; physical and occupational therapies; and speech–language pathology services. Bereavement service for the family is provided for up to 13 months after the patient's death.

Dying patients and their families especially appreciate the assurance that the place of care can be changed at appropriate moments from acute medical services to hospice services, inpatient or at home, and families appreciate the health care practitioner's willingness to continue to be involved with the care of the dying patient at home when the patient has voiced a preference for death at home.

Families need to know ahead of time what to do when the patient dies at home. The family does not need to call the police. If in hospice care, the family calls the hospice nurse on call who will come to the home to provide support. Many clinicians who manage hospice home care patients ask the family or the hospice nurse to call them so they can provide support. It is helpful to have already made contact with a funeral home so that a simple call to inform the funeral home that the patient has died at home is all that is needed at this frequently stressful time. In most states the funeral home has 72 hours to bring the death certificate to the health care practitioner to sign.

Information on hospice care in the United States is provided by both the National Hospice and Palliative Care Organization and the Hospice Association of America (see Resources for Patients and Their Loved Ones at the end of the chapter).

MANAGEMENT OF GRIEF

If death of a loved one has been unexpected, grief usually begins with an initial stage of shock and disbelief accompanied by a general numbing of all affect. If death has been anticipated, however, this stage is less prominent. There is often a feeling of relief that the dead person's suffering has ended. Soon afterward (within hours to a few days) there is a more demonstrative phase characterized by protest and anguish, often accompanied by tears. These feelings come in waves and may be precipitated by even an indirect reference to the lost person; ordinarily, they do not persist for more than 1 or 2 months. Other symptoms of mourning normally occur throughout the first year after the death of a loved one. During this year, survivors are continuing to grieve while they reorient their lives. As time passes there often is a preoccupation with memories of the lost person. Guilt feelings for not having done enough for the deceased are very common. In some cases, this guilt may be expressed as hostility toward the health care practitioner. Bereaved people often have the experience of seeing the dead person in a crowd or in some other individual fleetingly, which is then followed by the reality of permanent loss. The bereaved person is likely to visit the grave during the first year of loss more frequently than in later years. Sometimes, there is a dramatic change in personality, and the manners and the terminal symptoms of the dying patient are assumed by the bereaved person. This is another way of resolving grief, by attempting to make the lost person a part of the survivor.

Approximately 80% of bereaved people are depressed and have disturbed sleep; 40% have a poor appetite, weight loss, difficulty in concentrating, and general loss of interest in daily life (28). Depression is especially common in spouses in the middle or later years of their lives; about one-third of spouses have symptoms that meet the criteria for the diagnosis of a major depression (see Chapter 24) (29). Although depression may last for many months, 80% of individuals show improvement within 10 weeks. However, two-thirds of bereaved spouses at the end of the first year of bereavement continue to have some symptoms of apathy, aimlessness, and a disinclination to look to the future. Only a small fraction of these survivors develop complicated or atypical mourning.

The *management of normal grief* during the first year of bereavement should be individualized, depending on the patient's personal, family, and social background. All bereaved people need to be reminded that their grief and its psychophysiologic concomitants are normal. This has to be done with special care, acknowledging the irreparable loss while encouraging them to lead a full life without feeling guilty. Bereavement support groups exist in many communities and are usually known to clergy and social workers. Sharing feelings with others who have lost a loved one may be particularly helpful during this lonely time. A practitioner's encouragement can be important in helping a grieving person decide to seek such support. When severe emotional reactions become prolonged, pastoral counseling or psychotherapy may be necessary.

Bereaved persons may have new somatic symptoms or amplification of preexisting symptoms. When evaluation reveals no change in physical status, the management strategies suggested for adjustment disorders are appropriate (see Chapter 21). In time, with the completion of their grieving reaction, those patients give up their physical symptoms and again become actively engaged in a new life.

Some bereaved persons may need short-term medication for the relief of insomnia and anxiety. A benzodiazepine hypnotic (see Chapter 7) at bedtime if needed for sleep or one of the anxiolytic benzodiazepines (see Chapter 22) as needed for anxiety should be considered for 1 to 2 weeks in the management of normal grief. On the other hand, many patients may be satisfied with an empathetic and supportive health care practitioner.

Additional ways in which a clinician can be supportive early after a patient's death are to visit the funeral home and to telephone or write to the family, acknowledging one's own sense of loss, supporting the family in what they have done to help in the terminal care of the patient, and inviting contacts at a later time. The latter idea is suggested by a finding that more than half of bereaved spouses report that they had unanswered questions about their spouse's death 1 year later (30).

During the first year of bereavement, special attention should be paid to the grieving person during holidays, anniversaries, or on other important dates. Some symptoms of acute grief are likely to resurface around these times. Supportive therapy at such times usually controls the symptoms.

The primary care practitioner is in a good position to detect the early signs of pathologic mourning, when a person either shows no signs of grieving or shows the exaggerated features of grieving characterized by excessive or prolonged (longer than a year) social isolation, unmoderated guilt or anger, panic attacks, and physical symptoms without any clear-cut organic etiology. In such cases, short-term counseling by the primary care practitioner (see Chapter 20) or consultation with a mental health professional is appropriate to help remove obstacles that have inhibited the mourner from undergoing a normal grief reaction (31). Antidepressant medication should be considered when anxiety or depressive features are prominent, particularly if the patient satisfies criteria for major depression (see Chapters 22 and 24).

General References*

Agency for Health Care Policy and Research (AHCPR). **Management of cancer pain: clinical practice guideline.** U.S. Public Health Service, AHCPR Publication No. 94-0592. Washington, DC: U.S. Department of Health and Human Services, 1994.

A 200-page document providing critical assessment and practical guidelines. Companion guides for patients and families are also available (free copies available on request by telephone: 1-800-4-CANCER).

Care at the end of life. Ann Intern Med.

A series of journal articles on care at the end of life, focusing on symptom control and communication skills. It was inaugurated by the editorial Lo B, Snyder L, Sox HC. Care at the end of life: guiding practice where there are no easy answers. Ann Intern Med 1999;130:772–774.

Caring for the dying: identification and promotion of physician competency. American Board of Internal Medicine, Philadelphia, 1996.

This publication (two booklets: one an education resource document and the other personal narratives by physicians) provides information for the practitioner on professionalism related to end-of-life care, epidemiology and control of symptoms, clinical competencies, hospice care, and the role of the health care team, psychiatric issues, the role of religion, and the role of literature.

*Bold print (general references) and bold numerals (specific references) denote published controlled clinical trials, meta-analyses, or consensus-based recommendations.

Cherny NI, Foley KM, eds. Pain and palliative care. Hematol Oncol Clin North Am 1996;10.

Contains excellent reviews of hospice care and management of pain and other symptoms.

Council on Scientific Affairs, American Medical Association. Good care of the dying patient. JAMA 1996;276:474.

Standards of excellence in supportive care of the terminally ill.

Creagan ET. Psychosocial issues in oncologic practice. Mayo Clin Proc 1993;68:161.

Excellent review of many of the practical issues in the care of terminally ill patients and their families.

Kaye P. Symptom control in hospice and palliative care. Essex, CT: Hospice Education Institute, 1989.

Practical tips used in an English hospice.

Kubler-Ross E. On death and dying. New York: Macmillan, 1969.

A classic work on the subject of death and dying.

Levy MH. Pharmacologic treatment of cancer pain. N Engl J Med 1996;335:1124.

Very readable review of the management of cancer pain.

Zimmerman JM, ed. Hospice: complete care for the terminally ill, 2nd ed. Baltimore: Urban & Schwarzenberg, 1986.

Well-referenced and practical book that covers all aspects of the hospice approach to terminal care.

Resources For Patients And Their Loved Ones

Dunn H. Hard choices for loving people. Herndon, VA: A and A Publishers, 2001.

Eighty-page booklet, written by a chaplain, provides a nontechnical presentation about the decision whether to prolong life with greater suffering or accept a shorter life with less suffering. Hospice Care Information in the United States:

National Hospice and Palliative Care Organization, 1700 Diagonal Road, Suite 300, Alexandria, VA 22314, 703-837-1500, www.nhpco.org

Hospice Association of America, 228 7th Street SE, Washington, DC, 202-546-4759.

National Cancer Institute. Taking time, support for people with cancer and the people who care about them. Bethesda, MD: National Cancer Institute; phone 1-800-422-6237, website http://www.cancer.gov.

An excellent booklet for the patient, their families, and loved ones. It provides guidance and advice on emotional and practical issues related to cancer care, with insights from patients, family members, and loved ones.

Nelson T. It's your choice, the practical guide to planning a funeral. Glenview, IL: Scott, Foresman, 1982.

A practical paperback on making funeral plans in the face of impending death.

Partnership for Caring, Inc., America's Voices for the Dying. National Office: 1620 Eye Street NW, Suite 202, Washington, DC 20006; Phone: 202-296-8071; Fax: 202-296-8352; Hotline: 800-989-9455 (option 3); e-mail: pfc@partnershipforcaring.org; website: http://www.partnershipforcaring.org

A national nonprofit organization that partners individuals and organizations in a collaboration to improve how people die. Among other services, Partnership for Caring operates a crisis and informational hotline dealing with end-of-life issues and provides state-specific living wills and medical powers of attorney.

Specific References

1. Fox E, Landrum-McNiff K, Zhong Z, et al., for the SUPPORT investigators. Evaluation of prognostic criteria for determining hospice eligibility in patients with advanced lung, heart, or liver disease. JAMA 1999;282:1638.
2. Lynn J, Harrell F, Cohn F, et al. Prognoses of seriously ill hospitalized patients on the days before death: implications for patient care and public policy. New Horiz 1997;5:56.
3. Lubitz JD, Riley GF. Trends in Medicare payments in the last year of life. N Engl J Med 1993;328:1092.
4. Teno JM, Lynn J, Wenger N, et al. Advance directives for seriously ill hospitalized patients: effectiveness with the Patient Self-Determination Act and the SUPPORT intervention. J Am Geriatr Soc 1997;45:500.
5. Hofmann JC, Wenger NS, Davis RB, et al. Patient preferences for communication with physicians about end-of-life decisions. Ann Intern Med 1997;127:1.
6. Teno JM, Stevens M, Spernak S, et al. Role of written advance directives in decision making: insights from qualitative and quantitative data. J Gen Intern Med 1998;13:439.
7. Hopp FP, Duffy SA. Racial variations in end-of-life care. J Am Geriatr Soc 2000;48:658.
8. Mebane EW, Oman RF, Kroonen LT, et al. The influence of physician race, age, and gender on physician attitudes toward advance care directives and preferences for end-of-life decision-making. J Am Geriatr Soc 1999;47:579.
9. Carrese JA, Rhodes LA. Western bioethics on the Navajo reservation: benefit or harm? JAMA 1995;274:826.
10. Kubler-Ross E. On death and dying. New York: Macmillan, 1969:38.
11. Thomsen OO, Wulff HR, Martin A, et al. What do gastroenterologists in Europe tell cancer patients? Lancet 1993;341:473.
12. Ptacik JT, Eberhardt TL. Breaking bad news. JAMA 1996;276:496.
13. Girgis A, Sanson-Fisher RW. Breaking bad new: consensus guidelines for medical practitioners. J Clin Oncol 1995;13:2449.
14. Singer PA, Martin DK, Kelner M. Quality end-of-life care: patients' perspectives. JAMA 1999;281:163.
15. Emanuael EJ, Fairclough DL, Slutsman J, et al. Understanding economic and other burdens of terminal illness: the experience of patients and their caregivers. Ann Intern Med 2000;132:452.
16. Portenoy RK. Pharmacologic management of cancer pain. Semin Oncol 1995;22[Suppl 2]:112.
17. Kerr IG, Sone M, DeAngelis C, et al. Continuous narcotic infusion with patient-controlled analgesia for chronic cancer pain in outpatients. Ann Intern Med 1988;108:554.
18. Mercadante S. The role of octreotide in palliative care. J Pain Symptom Manage 1993;9:406.
19. Foley KM. Advances in cancer pain. Arch Neurol 1999;56:413.
20. Massie MJ, Holland J, Glass E. Delirium in terminally ill cancer patients. Am J Psychiatry 1983;140:1048.
21. Pereira J, Hanson J, Bruera E. The frequency and clinical course of cognitive impairment in patients with terminal cancer. Cancer 1997;79:835.
22. Breitbart W, Marotta R, Platt MM, et al. A double-blind trial of haloperidol, chlorpromazine, and lorazepam in the treatment of delirium in hospitalized AIDS patients. Am J Psychiatry 1996;153:231.
23. Bruera E, de Stoutz N, Velasco-Leiva A, et al. Effects of oxygen on dyspnoea in hypoxaemic terminal cancer patients. Lancet 1993;342:13.
24. Ripamonti C, Fulfaro F, Bruera E. Dyspnoea in patients with advanced cancer: incidence, causes and treatments. Cancer Treat Rev 1998;24:69.
25. Musgrave CF, Bartal N, Opstad F. The sensation of thirst in dying patients receiving i.v. hydration. J Palliat Care 1995;11:17.
26. McCann RM, Hall WJ, Groth-Juncker A. Comfort care for terminally ill patients. The appropriate use of nutrition and hydration. JAMA 1994;272:1263.
27. Steiner N, Bruera E. Methods of hydration in palliative care patients. J Palliat Care 1998;14:6.
28. Clayton PJ, Halikas JA, Maurice WL. The bereavement of the widowed. Dis Nerv Syst 1971;32:597.
29. Clayton PJ, Halikas JA, Maurice WL. The depression of widowhood. Br J Psychiatry 1972;120:71.
30. Tolle SW, Bascom PB, Hickam DH, et al. Communication between physicians and surviving spouses following patient deaths. J Gen Intern Med 1986;1:309.
31. Melges FT, DeMaso DR. Grief-resolution therapy: relieving, revising, and revisiting. Am J Psychother 1980;34:51.

SECTION 2

Preventive Care

CHAPTER 14

Integrating Prevention into Ambulatory Practice: An Overview

DAVID E. KERN, MD, MPH
GREGORY P. PROKOPOWICZ, MD, MPH

Prevention has become a central part of patient care (1). Medical organizations, government agencies, insurance companies, and patients themselves expect practitioners to offer preventive services (2,3). Practitioners are in an important position to help reduce the burden of disease that affects society and its members. Evidence suggests that a health practitioner's advice is the single most influential factor in patients' decisions to reduce their risk of future disease (4,5). Increasingly, practitioners are being trained to interpret risks to health, to effectively communicate this information to patients, and to assist patients in desired behavior changes.

Three characteristics distinguish preventive from curative care:

1. *Preventive care aims to protect health prospectively.* In contrast to treatment, which tries to return a patient to a previous state of health, prevention attempts to maintain an existing state of health. This is true even for a chronically ill patient, for whom prevention might mean maintaining a sedentary existence at home rather being admitted to a hospital or nursing home for a preventable worsening of illness.
2. *The practitioner, not the patient, usually initiates preventive care.* Although patients increasingly request preventive services, more often it is the practitioner who is aware of the need for such interventions.
3. In preventive care, *the practitioner must be more certain that an intervention is effective than in the care of established disease or symptomatic conditions.* Uncertainty is inherent in medicine. When ill patients seek treatment, the practitioner often must make a best guess regarding treatment. In prevention, however, patients are usually healthy and will remain so in the proximate future regardless of whether they undertake preventive measures. Therefore, there is an ethical obligation for the practitioner to have a high degree of certainty that suggested preventive interventions are likely to result in more good than harm (6).

Several considerations underlie the importance of prevention in routine office practice. First, approximately 50% of mortality from the 10 leading causes of death in the United States can be traced to alterable behavior (life-style) (7). Second, early detection and treatment of a number of common disorders, such as cervical carcinoma *in situ* and hypertension, effectively reduce mortality and morbidity from these conditions. Third, although infectious diseases have, to a large extent, been controlled in developed countries by public health measures, including immunization, outbreaks continue to occur, especially among the poor, elderly, and immunocompromised. For example, tuberculosis is reemerging as a major cause of death, and influenza remains a major preventable cause of death (8). Fourth, the value of a comprehensive approach to prevention is suggested by the reduction in maternal and perinatal deaths that has been attributable to prenatal care (9,10). In addition, a comprehensive preventive approach to care has been shown to reduce mortality, acute hospitalizations, and nursing home placement in high-risk elderly patients, while improving their functional status and morale (11–15).

TERMINOLOGY

Depending on when the effort is made, prevention can be divided into three stages (Fig. 14.1). *Primary prevention* prevents disease from occurring. For example, smoking cessation decreases the likelihood that a patient will develop coronary artery disease or lung cancer; barrier contraception and abstinence prevent the development of cervical dysplasia; immunization prevents various infectious diseases. *Secondary prevention* detects disease once it has begun but before it has appeared clinically. Breast, cervical, and colon cancer screening to identify occult malignancies (in which early intervention leads to better outcomes) represents secondary prevention. *Tertiary prevention* seeks to stop further complications after a disease has become clinically evident. Cholesterol reduction and beta-blockers given after myocardial infarction represent tertiary prevention.

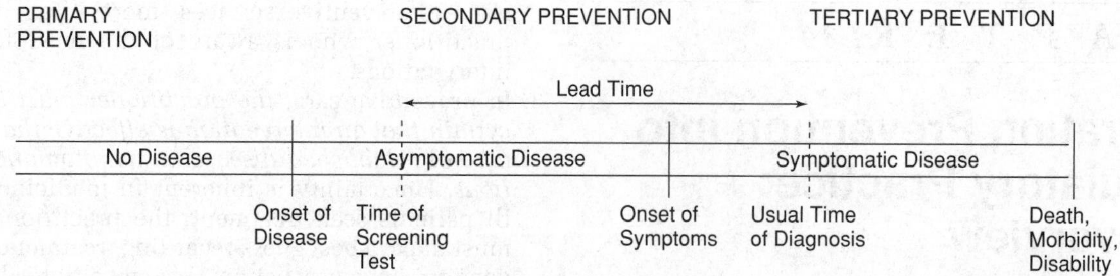

Figure 14.1. Primary, secondary, and tertiary prevention in the spectrum of a disease (see text for definitions).

Although conceptually useful, the distinctions between primary, secondary, and tertiary prevention can become blurred in clinical practice. The early detection and treatment of asymptomatic hypertension, for example, would be considered tertiary prevention if one considers hypertension a disease and considers congestive heart failure, stroke, and renal failure complications of that disease. On the other hand, hypertension can be considered a risk factor for congestive heart failure, stroke, and renal failure, so that detection and treatment of hypertension to prevent these diseases from occurring can be considered primary prevention. Smoking cessation, as another example, represents primary prevention in the healthy patient but tertiary prevention in the patient with atherosclerotic cardiovascular or chronic obstructive pulmonary disease.

Several other terms are relevant to the practice of prevention. *Screening* is the process of identifying patients with unrecognized diseases or risk factors by the application of examinations, tests, or other procedures. A positive test is usually not diagnostic but requires further testing. *Mass screening* is screening applied to a large group, and *multiphasic screening* is simultaneous screening for various diseases, such as blood pressure and cholesterol measurement done at health fairs. *Case finding* occurs in a practitioner's practice when the clinician screens for disease unrelated to the symptom for which the patient has come.

Table 14.1. Questions to Ask in Evaluating a Recommended Preventive Measure

What is the burden of suffering attributable to the targeted condition?
What is the prevalence and/or incidence of the condition?
What is the size of the attributable morbidity?
What is the mortality rate?
Do efficacious screening tests exist?
Do they have acceptable sensitivity, specificity, and predictive value?[a]
Are they reliable?[a]
Are they practical and reasonably priced?
Are the side effects of screening acceptable?
Is preventive intervention efficacious in research settings?
Is the intervention efficacious in study groups?
Are compliance levels in study situations acceptable?
Are side effects acceptable?
Is intervention in the asymptomatic stage more beneficial than intervention after onset of symptoms?
Would use of the measure be effective in routine office practice?
Have suitable field trials been conducted?
Is the measure effective in reducing morbidity and mortality in nonstudy situations?
Are the compliance levels in nonstudy situations acceptable?
Are side effects in nonstudy situations acceptable?
What are the reliability, sensitivity, specificity, and predictive value of screening tests in one's own setting?[a]
Is the measure cost-effective?

[a]See Chapter 2 for a discussion of reliability, sensitivity, specificity, and predictive value.

EVALUATING PREVENTIVE MEASURES FOR USE IN AMBULATORY PRACTICE

The first step in integrating preventive care into office practice is deciding which measures to offer patients routinely. In deciding which measures to recommend, one should consider the burden of suffering attributable to each preventable condition, in terms of its prevalence and severity; the efficacy, cost, and safety of available screening tests; the efficacy and complications of treatment; and the effectiveness of each measure in routine office practice (Table 14.1). Recommendations that are periodically published by organizations such as the U.S. Preventive Services Task Force (USPSTF), Canadian Task Force on Preventive Health Care (CTF), the American Cancer Society, the American College of Physicians–American Society of Internal Medicine, the American Medical Association, the Centers for Disease Control and Prevention, and others can be consulted. For some measures, however, the recommendations are conflicting. The reports of the USPSTF and the CTF are firmly grounded in clinical epidemiology and provide the most scientific least biased framework to date for evaluating which preventive health measures should be included in routine care (see General References).

In evaluating a given measure, it is important to be aware of certain terms, concepts, pitfalls, and special considerations. The terms *sensitivity, specificity, prevalence,* and *predictive value,* which help define the value of a screening test, are defined in Chapter 2. *Efficacy* describes how well a test or maneuver performs under ideal circumstances. *Effectiveness* describes how well a test or maneuver performs under real-world circumstances. The effectiveness of a test or maneuver is usually somewhat less than its efficacy. *Efficiency* describes how well the test or maneuver optimizes the use of limited resources. A *risk factor* is anything that, if present, increases the likelihood of disease. The proportion of a specific disease that can be accounted for by a risk factor is called the *attributable risk.*

Lead time (Fig. 14.1) is the period between the early detection of disease and its usual time of diagnosis. In the evaluation of the efficacy of early detection and treatment, lead time must be subtracted from overall survival time in screened patients to avoid *lead time bias.* Otherwise, early detection might appear to increase survival time, when in reality it is only increasing the duration of patients' awareness of their disease. Numerous cancer screening procedures have been thought to improve survival until lead time was addressed (16). A related bias in screening is *length-time bias* (also called length bias, time-linked biased sampling, and length-biased sampling). Most types of tumors have variable rates of growth. Screening tests may selectively find slow-growing tumors, which have long presymptomatic stages and better prognoses, but miss fast-growing cancers, which have short presymptomatic stages, develop and become clinically manifest between screening intervals, and have worse prognoses. Thus, survival is better for patients detected by screening because of the characteristics of their tumors (less aggressive, lower grade), whereas overall mortality in screened and unscreened populations remains identical. *Selection bias* occurs when patients undergoing a preventive measure differ from those with whom they are compared in a manner that affects the likelihood of their developing disease or the natural history of their disease, once acquired. Volunteers, for example, may have more healthful life-styles than those who do not volunteer. It is because of these biases that randomized controlled trials are important in evaluating preventive interventions.

The process of screening itself can cause morbidity. The test itself may carry a risk of complications (e.g., perforation from colonoscopy). The test may label some people as having a disease when they are in fact healthy (*false positives*), thereby causing anxiety or other suffering in the absence of disease. False positives are particularly likely if the disease is rare or if the screening test does not have a high specificity (see Chapter 2). For this reason, positive screening tests are usually followed by more specific diagnostic tests, which may carry additional risks. Furthermore, if a screening test does not have a high sensitivity (see Chapter 2), some patients with the disease may be inappropriately reassured that they are healthy (*false negatives*) and may not seek care promptly when they become symptomatic. Even when a test correctly identifies patients with a disease, evidence suggests that undue suffering can occur from the *labeling effect* (17–19). For example, one study showed that absenteeism from work increased after workers were found to be hypertensive (18). A disadvantage of mass screening is that a significant proportion of labeled people will not seek follow-up with a practitioner. Practitioners can minimize problems of labeling by confirming that a problem is present, usually through repeated or additional observations; taking time to explain the meaning of a problem to a patient and answering his or her questions (effective patient education); screening only for conditions for which early detection is likely to benefit the patient; and ensuring follow-up.

Caution should be used in adopting recommendations or guidelines that are based on proof of efficacy in highly controlled situations. Costs and conditions may be different in office practice. For example, before deciding to screen for carotid artery disease, it is important to know the level of expertise and complication rate associated with carotid endarterectomy at one's institution. Before recommending routine sigmoidoscopy or colonoscopy to all patients over the age of 50 (recommendations based on less than conclusive evidence in study situations), the clinician should assess the cost, availability of diagnostic services, and complication rates in the local setting. Although colon perforation rates of less than 0.1% have been reported for sigmoidoscopy among trained gastroenterologists, the rates for trained and untrained generalists are less well established. The availability and insurance coverage for screening colonoscopy will vary from setting to setting, as may the complication rate (from 0.1% to 0.4% without and from 0.3% to 1.0% with polypectomy in reported studies).

Despite these precautions, there is sufficient evidence to support the integration of a number of primary and secondary preventive measures into office practice. Failure to do so reflects an inadequacy in the provision of primary care.

COMPONENTS OF PREVENTIVE CARE

General Examination and Baseline Data

Most practitioners perform a baseline general examination (history, physical, and selected laboratory tests) for some or all of their ambulatory patients. In addition, some practitioners update all or part of this examination on a periodic basis. As contrasted to the provision of selected preventive care measures discussed below, no firm scientific evidence links most of the general examination to reductions in morbidity and mortality. However, most clinicians would agree that knowledge of a patient's past hospitalizations and operations; past and present illnesses; medication and allergic history; and diet, habit, social, and family history is indispensable to the provision of effective preventive, symptomatic, and curative care. Periodic general examinations are sometimes required and may be of use for people upon whom others' lives depend (e.g., airline pilots).

Provision of Selected Measures for Asymptomatic Patients (Primary and Secondary Preventive Care)

It is generally recommended that practitioners offer asymptomatic patients certain preventive care measures, selected on the basis of their likely benefits versus harm (see above and Table 14.1). Preventive measures that are often considered for inclusion in the care of asymptomatic nonpregnant adults are summarized in Table 14.2. For each preventive measure, the

Table 14.2. Preventive Measures to Consider in the Care of Asymptomatic Nonpregnant Adults

Preventive Measure	Patient Population (Age, Sex, Risk Status)	Time Interval	Year of Recommendation	Strength of Recommendation	Chapter to See for Details
Good Evidence to Include					
Blood pressure	All M, F	1–2 yr	1996[a], 1994[b]	A[a], B[b]	67
Cervical cytology (Pap test)	All F, onset of sexual activity or age 18 (whichever comes earlier) to age 60 or 70 (assuming past normal cytology)	1 yr × 2, then 3 yr[c]	1996[a], 1994[b]	A[a], B[b]	104
Chlamydia screening	High-risk F[d]	Discretionary, recommend at time of Pap smears[e]	2001[a], 1996[b]	A[a], B[b]	37
Cholesterol, nonfasting total cholesterol (TC) and HDL cholesterol levels with further evaluation and treatment of those found to be have high TC or low HDL[f]	All M ≥ 35 All F ≥ 45	5 yr	2001[a]	A[a]	82
Colorectal cancer screening: fecal occult blood testing	All M, F ≥50, normal risk	1 yr	1996[a], 2001[b]	B[a], A[b]	45
Folate prophylaxis	F, previously affected pregnancy (neural tube deficit) or planning pregnancy	Beginning 1–3 mo before conception through 1st trimester	1996[a], 1994[b]	A[a,b]	100
Gonococcal culture, screening	High-risk M, F[g]	Discretionary	1996[a], 1994[b]	B[a], A[b]	37
Hepatitis B vaccination	All young adults not previously immunized and high-risk M, F of all ages[h]	Three doses, at 0, 1, and 6 mo	1996[a]	A[a]	18,47
HIV antibody testing	High-risk M, F[i]	Discretionary	1996[a], 1994[b]	A[a,b]	39
Influenza vaccination	All M, F ≥65 High-risk M, F of all ages[j] Health providers for high-risk patients	1 yr	1996[a], 1994[b]	A[a], B[b]	18
Mammography, with (preferable) or without clinical breast examination by health care practitioner	All F 50–69	1–2 yr	2001[a], 1998[b]	B[a,y], A[b,y]	105
Measles, mumps, rubella (MMR) vaccination (live)	All M and nonpregnant F born after 1956 who lack evidence of immunity to measles[k]	Once, or 2 doses ≥1 month apart[k]	1996[a]	A[a]	18
Pneumococcal vaccination	High-risk M, F[l] (see below for others)	Once, consider repeat dose at 5 yr	1996[a], 1998[b]	B[a], A[b]	18
Smoking/tobacco use, counseling	All M, F	1–5 yr	1996[a], 1994[b]	A[a,b]	27
Syphilis (serology), screening	High-risk M, F[g]	Discretionary	1996[a]	A[a]	37,38
Tetanus/diphtheria vaccination	All M, F	10 yr or once after 50 (boosters), primary series at 0, 2, and 6–14 mo if not previously immunized	1996[a]	A[a]	18
Tuberculin skin test	High-risk M, F[m]	Discretionary	1996[a], 1994[b]	A[a,b]	34,39
Travel to developing countries: immunization, prophylactic medications, counseling regarding preventive health practices	At-risk M, F	Varies		A[c]	41
Fair Evidence to Include					
Alcohol use, screening, with counseling of patients with problem drinking and counseling/referral of alcohol dependent patients	All M, F	Discretionary	1996[a], 1994[b]	B[a,b]	28

Table 14.2—*continued.* **Preventive Measures to Consider in the Care of Asymptomatic Nonpregnant Adults**

Preventive Measure	Patient Population (Age, Sex, Risk Status)	Time Interval	Year of Recommendation	Strength of Recommendation	Chapter to See for Details
Birth control counseling to reduce unwanted pregnancies	All sexually active M, F of childbearing age, especially adolescents	Discretionary	1996[a], 1994[b]	B[a,b]	100
Cholesterol, nonfasting TC and HDL cholesterol levels, with further evaluation and treatment of those found to be have high TC or low HDL[f]	M 20–35 F 20–45 with risk factors[n]	5 yr	2001[a]	B[a]	82
	M 20–35 F 20–45 without risk factors[n]	5 yr	2001[a]	C[a]	82
Colorectal cancer screening: sigmoidoscopy	All M, F ≥50, normal risk	3–10 yr	1996[a], 2001[b]	B[a], B[b]	45
Dietary					
Limit dietary fat	All M, F	Ongoing	1996[a], 1994[b]	A[a], B[b]	82
Limit dietary cholesterol	All, M, F	Ongoing	1996[a]	B[a]	82
Increase fruits, vegetables, grain products containing fiber	All M, F	Ongoing	1996[a], 1994[b]	B[a,b]	15,45,82
Maintain caloric balance through diet and exercise	All M, F	Ongoing	1996[a]	B[a]	15,16
Maintain adequate calcium intake	All M, F	Ongoing	1996[a]	B[a]	81,85,106
Dietary counseling by					
Specially trained educators	All M, F	Discretionary, follow-up important	1996[a]	B[a]	15
Primary care practitioner	All M, F	Discretionary, follow-up important	1996[a], 1994[b]	C[a], B[b]	15
Hearing impairment, screening	All M, F >65	Discretionary	1996[a], 1994[b]	B[a,b]	110
Hormone replacement therapy, counseling[o]	Perimenopausal and postmenopausal women	Discretionary	1996[a], 1994[b]	B[a,b]	103,106
Mammography with or without clinical breast examination by healthcare practitioner	All F 40–49	1–2 yr	2001[a,b]	B[a,y], C[b]	105
Pneumococcal vaccination	All M, F ≥65 (see above for others)	Once	1996[a], 1998[b]	B[a], C[b]	18
Rubella vaccination (or MMR) or rubella antibody screening and vaccination of those susceptible[p]	All nonpregnant F of childbearing age without documentation of previous rubella vaccination	Once, or 2 doses ≥1 month apart[p]	1996[a], 1994[b]	B[a,b]	18
Seatbelt use, counseling	All M, F	Discretionary	1996[a], 1994[b]	B[a,b]	—
Skin inspection to detect skin cancer	High-risk M, F[q]	Discretionary	2001[a], 1994[b]	I[a], B–C[b]	114
Varicella vaccination	Susceptible adolescents and adults	2 doses given 4–8 wk apart	2001[b]	B[b]	18
Visual acuity testing	All M, F >65	Discretionary	1996[a], 1995[b]	B[a,b]	107
Insufficient Evidence to Include or Exclude					
Abdominal aortic aneurysm, screening: physical examination or ultrasonography	All M, F ≥60	Discretionary	1996[a], 1994[b]	C[a,b]	94
Aspirin therapy for the primary prevention of cardiovascular disease	All M 40–84 All F 50–84	Not applicable	1996[a], 1994[b] 1996[a], 1994[b]	C[a,b] C[a,b]	57,62
Bone densitometry	Postmenopausal F	Discretionary	1996[a], 1994[b]	C[a], D[b]	103
Breast self-examination, teaching/encouraging	All F ≥20	1 mo	2001[a,b]	I[a], D[b]	105
Carotid artery stenosis, screening					91
Auscultation	All M, F >40–60 or at high risk for atherosclerotic cardiovascular disease	Discretionary	1996[a], 1994,[b]	C[a], D[b]	
Auscultation or ultrasound		Discretionary	1996[a]	C[a]	

Continued

Table 14.2—*continued.* **Preventive Measures to Consider in the Care of Asymptomatic Nonpregnant Adults**

Preventive Measure	Patient Population (Age, Sex, Risk Status)	Time Interval	Year of Recommendation	Strength of Recommendation	Chapter to See for Details
Clinical breast examination by healthcare practitioner	All F ≥40	1–2 yr	2001[a]	I[a]	105
Colorectal cancer, screening: colonoscopy[r]	All M, F ≥50	5–10 yr	1996[a], 2001[b]	C[a,b]	45
Dementia (cognitive impairment) screening	All M, F ≥65–75	Discretionary	1996[a], 2001[b]	C[a,b]	26
Dental hygiene, primary care practitioner screening (for periodontal disease) or counseling (regarding brushing, flossing, fluoride, diet, and regular dental visits)[s]	All M, F	Discretionary	1996[a], 1994[b], 1995[b]	C[a,b]	112
Depression, screening	All M, F	Discretionary	1996[a], 1994[b]	C[a], D[b]	24,26
Diabetes mellitus, screening (with plasma glucose or glycosylated hemoglobin)	All M, F	Discretionary	1996[a], 1994[b]	C[a], D[b]	79
Domestic violence, screening	All F and elderly	Discretionary	1996[a], 1994[b]	C[a,b]	28
Driving while impaired by alcohol or drugs, counseling	All M, F	Discretionary	1996[a], 1994[b]	C[a,b]	28,29
Drug abuse, screening	All M, F	Discretionary	1996[a]	C[a]	29
Electrocardiography, resting or exercise	All M, F ≥50	Discretionary	1996[a]	C[a]	62
Exercise, inquiry and counseling[t]	All M, F	Discretionary	1996[a], 1994[b]	C[a,b]	12,16,63,83,103
Falls prevention, counseling[u]	All M, F ≥70–75	Discretionary	1996[a], 1994[b]	C[a,b]	12
Firearms at home, counseling[v]	All M, F	Discretionary	1996[a], 1994[b]	C[a,b]	—
Helmets,[w] bicycle or motorcycle, counseling	All M, F	Discretionary	1996[a], 1994[b]	C[a,b]	—
Homocysteine, screening with fasting or postmethionine load plasma total homocysteine to detect and treat patients with high levels	M ≥ 35 F ≥45 at normal or high risk for coronary artery disease	Once	2000[b]	C[b]	62
Mammography, with (preferable) or without clinical breast examination by health care practitioner	All F ≥70		1996[a]	C[a]	105
Obesity					83
Screening (weight and height, BMI calculation)	All M, F[x]	Periodic	1996[a], 1996, and 1999[b]	B[a], C[b]	
Counseling	All M, F[x]		1994[b]	C[b]	
Sexually transmitted diseases, counseling	All sexually active M, F	Discretionary	1996[a]	C[a]	37,39
Thyroid function tests (TSH) or clinical examination to diagnose occult hyper- and hypothyroidism	All F, postmenopausal	Discretionary	1996[a], 1994[b]	C[a,b]	80
Tonometry and ophthamoscopy to detect glaucoma	All M, F ≥40	Discretionary	1996[a], 1995[b]	C[a,b]	108
Fair to Good Evidence to Exclude					
Breast cancer chemoprophylaxis	All F, low to normal risk	Ongoing	2001[b]	D[b]	105
Lung cancer screening					61
Chest radiograph	All smoking M, F	4 mo–1 yr	1996[a], 1994[b]	D[a], E[b]	
Sputum cytology		4 mo	1996[a], 1994[b]	D[a,b]	
Gonococcal culture	All sexually active M, F	Discretionary	1996[a], 1994[b]	D[a,b]	37
Electrocardiography, resting	All M, F ≤50	Discretionary	1996[a]	D[a]	62

Table 14.2—*continued.* **Preventive Measures to Consider in the Care of Asymptomatic Nonpregnant Adults**

Preventive Measure	Patient Population (Age, Sex, Risk Status)	Time Interval	Year of Recommendation	Strength of Recommendation	Chapter to See for Details
Prostate cancer screening					53
Digital rectal examination	All M ≤40–50	1–2 yr	1996[a], 1994[b]	D[a], C[b]	
Prostate specific antigen (PSA)				D[a,b]	
Transrectal ultrasound				D[a,b]	

This table is organized into four major categories, based on the *strength of the recommendation* for including or excluding a preventive measure, as rated by the U.S. Preventive Services Task Force (USPSTF) and the Canadian Task Force on the Periodic Health Examination (CTF) (see text for explanation of ratings). When ratings differ between the USPSTF and CTF, a preventive measure is placed in one of the four categories based upon its highest rating. Preventive measures are listed in alphabetical order under each category.

[a]Rated by the USPSTF. See text for explanation of ratings.

[b]Rated by the CTF. See text for explanation of ratings.

[c]Recommended intervals vary. When screening is initiated, it is often recommended that the first two to three smears are obtained 1 yr apart to compensate for possible practitioner error in collection or laboratory error. The best trade-off between yield and use of resources for the general population seems to occur at a screening interval of 3 yr. Risk factors such as early onset of sexual intercourse, history of multiple sexual partners, and low socioeconomic status may warrant more frequent testing. More frequent intervals are recommended for HIV-infected patients (currently every 6 mo until two successive normals, then every year).

[d]High-risk group includes sexually active female ≤25; new sexual partner; multiple sexual partners; history of sexually transmitted disease; cervical friability, ectopy, or mucopurulent discharge; unmarried status; inconsistent use of barrier contraceptives; other settings where prevalence is known to be high.

[e]Rated by the authors on the basis of USPSTF, CTF, or other reports.

[f]Because of biologic variation and measurement error, two blood tests are often recommended to provide a more accurate measure for classification of risk. When total cholesterol concentration is >200 mg/dL (>5.2 mmol/L) or HDL is low (<40 mg/L), a fasting determination of total cholesterol, triglyceride, and HDL cholesterol levels with calculation of LDL cholesterol level is recommended to more precisely determine risk and direct treatment (see Chapter 82). The National Cholesterol Education Program recommends a fasting lipid profile every 5 years in all adults ≥20 (see Chapter 82).

[g]High-risk groups include persons with multiple sexual partners or a partner with multiple sexual contacts, sexual contacts of persons known to have a sexually transmitted disease, persons with repeated episodes of gonorrhea, and prostitutes.

[h]High-risk groups include homosexually active men, injection drug users and their sex partners, persons who have a history of sexual activity with multiple partners in the previous 6 mo or who have recently acquired another sexually transmitted disease, international travelers to countries where hepatitis B virus is of high or intermediate endemicity, and persons in health-related jobs with frequent exposure to blood or blood products.

[i]High-risk groups include homosexual and bisexual men, prostitutes and their sex partners, injection drug users and their sex partners, people with sexually transmitted diseases, people who received blood products between 1978 and 1985, sexual contacts of HIV-positive people, and people from countries with a high prevalence of HIV infection.

[j]High-risk groups include residents of chronic care facilities and other institutions and persons with chronic cardiopulmonary disorders, metabolic diseases (including diabetes mellitus), hemoglobinopathies, immunosuppression, or renal dysfunction.

[k]Evidence of immunity can include receipt of two doses of live vaccine after first birthday, laboratory evidence of immunity, or practitioner-diagnosed disease. Contraindicated in immunosuppressed and pregnant patients. Women should be advised not to become pregnant for 1–3 mo after vaccination. Patients vaccinated before 1967 are likely to have received inactivated vaccine or have been vaccinated before the age of 12 mo. Two doses may be required ≥1 mo apart to ensure long-term efficacy. One dose is about 95% effective in achieving seroconversion.

[l]High-risk groups include patients with sickle cell disease, patients postsplenectomy; institutionalized patients ≥50, people in epidemic or endemic settings. Antibody levels may fall after 5 yr, and revaccination at 5 yr is recommended in certain populations (see Chapter 18).

[m]High-risk groups include household/close contacts of patients with tuberculosis (e.g., staff members of tuberculosis clinics, homeless shelters); recent immigrants from countries with high tuberculosis prevalence; migrant workers and other populations with high prevalence of tuberculosis; residents of nursing homes, correctional institutions, and homeless shelters; persons with certain underlying medical disorders (e.g., HIV infection); alcoholics; and injection drug users.

[n]Risk factors include hypertension, cigarette smoking, HDL <40 mg/dL (subtract one risk factor if HDL is ≥60 mg/dL), age ≤40 (men) or ≤55 (women), family history of coronary artery disease (before 55 in male first-degree relative or before 65 in a female first-degree relative).

[o]Patients should receive information on the benefits and risks of hormonal therapy. Concerns about actual and potential complications of treatment prevented a higher level recommendation. The presence of postmenopausal symptoms, a high risk of fracture (thin, Caucasian premature or surgical menopause), and the absence of a uterus increase the likelihood of benefit in individual patients. Cardiovascular benefits have recently been called into question. Hormonal replacement therapy is contraindicated in patients with breast cancer. See Chapters 103 and 107 for details.

[p]For prevention of congenital rubella. Contraindicated in immunosuppressed and pregnant patients. Women should be advised not to become pregnant for 1–3 mo after vaccination. One dose is about 95% effective in achieving seroconversion.

[q]High-risk groups defined as persons of high risk for cancer of skin, such as outdoor workers, fair-skinned men and women, those in contact with polycyclic aromatic hydrocarbons, those with atypical or >50 moles, and those with family history of melenoma.

[r]There is fair (B) evidence to support a recommendation for routine colonoscopy in patients with familial adenomatous polyposis (FAP) and hereditary nonpolyposis colon cancer (HNPCC). A strong family history of colon cancer (e.g., >2 first-degree relatives with colorectal cancer) will likely influence the patient and clinician toward colonoscopy as a screening strategy. It is a standard of care for patients with inflammatory colon disease (ulcerative colitis or Crohn disease), usually at intervals of 1 to 2 yr.

[s]Efficacy of primary care practitioner screening or counseling to change behaviors has not been adequately evaluated. There is fair (B) to good (A) evidence, however, based on level I, II-1, and II-2 evidence to support water fluoridation, tooth brushing with fluoride-containing toothpaste, and professionally applied topical fluorides (for high-risk patients) to prevent caries and to support regular brushing and flossing, professional scaling and prophylaxis, and use of chlorhexidine or phenolic antiseptic (e.g., Listerine) oral rinses as an adjunct to tooth cleaning to prevent gingivitis/periodontal disease.

[t]Efficacy of counseling by primary care practitioner is unproven. There is good (A) to fair (B) evidence, based on II-1 and II-2 level evidence, to suggest that regular physical activity can prevent all-cause mortality coronary artery disease, hypertension, diabetes mellitus, obesity, and other diseases. Physical activity is also associated with improvements in self-esteem, stress management, lipoprotein levels, and physical fitness.

[u]Efficacy of practitioner counseling to patients to address risk factors for falls is unproven. There is good (A) to fair (B) evidence, based on I, II-1, and II-2 level evidence, to support multidisciplinary assessment and intervention to prevent falls in the elderly.

[v]Efficacy of practitioner counseling is unproven. There is fair (B) evidence, based on level II-2, II-3, and III evidence, to support removal of guns from or safe storage of guns in the home (USPSTF).

[w]Efficacy of practitioner counseling is unproven. There is good (A) evidence, based on level II-2 and II-3 evidence, to support wearing approved helmets.

[x]In 1999, the CTF gave a "B" rating for measuring weight, height, and BMI in obese patients with obesity related diseases: diabetes mellitus, hypertension, coronary artery disease, hyperlipidemia, and obstructive sleep apnea.

HDL, high density lipoprotein; HIV; human immuno deficiency virus; BMI, body mass index.

[y]A recent meta-analysis has called into question the efficiency of screening mammography (50,51) and precipitated controversy (52,53). The USPSTF subsequently issued recommendations, downgrading the strength of their recommendation from A to B after critiquing the above meta-analysis and extending their recommendation to women 40–49. The USPSTF does note that the evidence is strongest for women 50–69 and weaker for women 40–49. The CTF has not yet responded to the above meta-analysis.

table provides the following information:

1. The *patient population* to which the measure should be applied (age, sex, risk status);
2. Recommended *time interval between preventive interventions*;
3. *Year of the recommendation*;
4. *Strength of the recommendation* for including or excluding the preventive measure in the care of asymptomatic patients, classified using rating systems developed by the CTF and the USPSTF. Both the CTF (personal communication, Nadine Wathen, CTF) and the USPSTF (20) revised their rating systems in 2002.

The revised CTF ratings for their recommendations are as follows:

A. The CTF concludes that there is *good* evidence to recommend the clinical preventive action.
B. The CTF concludes that there is *fair* evidence to recommend the clinical preventive action.
C. The CTF concludes that the existing evidence is *conflicting* and does not allow making a recommendation for or against use of the clinical preventive action; however, other factors may influence decision making.
D. The CTF concludes that there is *fair* evidence to recommend against the clinical preventive action.
E. The CTF concludes that there is *good* evidence to recommend against the clinical preventive action.
I. The CTF concludes that there is *insufficient* evidence (in quantity and/or quality) to make a recommendation; however, other factors may influence decision making.

The revised USPSTF ratings for their recommendations are as follows:

A. The USPSTF strongly recommends that clinicians routinely provide the service to eligible patients. (The USPSTF found good evidence that the service improves important health outcomes and concludes that benefits substantially outweigh harms.)
B. The USPSTF recommends that clinicians routinely provide the service to eligible patients. (The USPSTF found at least fair evidence that the service improves important health outcomes and concludes that benefits outweigh harms.)
C. The USPSTF makes no recommendation for or against the service to eligible patients. (The USPSTF found at least fair evidence that the service can improve health outcomes but concludes that the balance of the benefits and harms is too close to justify a general recommendation.)
D. The USPSTF recommends against routinely providing the service to asymptomatic patients. (The USPSTF found at least fair evidence that the service is ineffective or that harms outweigh benefits.)
I. The USPSTF concludes that the evidence is insufficient to recommend for or against routinely providing the service. (Evidence that the service is effective is lacking, of poor quality, or conflicting, and the balance of benefits and harms cannot be determined.)

Both task forces rate the *quality of evidence* using a hierarchy of *research design:*

I. Evidence obtained from at least one properly randomized controlled trial.
II-1. Evidence obtained from well-designed controlled trials without randomization.
II-2. Evidence obtained from well-designed cohort or case-control analytic studies, preferably from more than one center or research group.
II-3. Evidence obtained from comparison between times or places (CTF) or from multiple time series (USPSTF) with or without the intervention. Dramatic results in uncontrolled experiments (such as the results of the introduction of penicillin treatment in the 1940s) could also be regarded as this type of evidence.
III. Opinions of respected authorities, based on clinical experience, descriptive studies, or reports of expert committees.

In addition, both task forces explicitly rate the *quality of evidence* based on the *internal validity of each study* reviewed as "good," "fair," or "poor."

The USPSTF explicitly rates the quality of the *body of evidence* (good, fair, or poor), which in turn is based on assessments of aggregate internal validity, aggregate external validity (generalizability from the various studies to primary care practice settings), and the coherence/consistency of the body of evidence. The USPSTF explicitly rates the magnitude of benefit, harm, and net benefit for each service as "substantial," "moderate," "small," or "zero/negative." The USPSTF uses a synthesis of its ratings and the CTF a less explicit synthesis to arrive at their recommendations. The CTF uses two primary reviewers for each topic; the USPSTF involves expert external reviewers before finalizing recommendations. Although both bodies place special emphasis on the strength of the evidence regarding the effectiveness of preventive intervention, consideration is also given to the burden of suffering caused by the target condition and to the characteristics of the intervention (e.g., cost [21], availability, and acceptability). Most of this information is available in the publications and full text reviews available at the CTF and USPSTF websites (see General References).

Recommendations in Table 14.2 that precede mid-2001 are rated by the *old rating system* used by both the CTF and USPSTF, which is listed below:

A. There is good evidence to support the recommendation that the condition is specifically considered in a periodic health examination.
B. There is fair evidence to support the recommendation that the condition is specifically considered in a periodic health examination.
C. There is insufficient evidence to recommend for or against the inclusion (USPSTF) or poor evidence regarding the inclusion or exclusion (CTF) of the

condition in a periodic health examination, but recommendations may be made on other grounds.

D. There is fair evidence to support the recommendation that the condition is excluded from consideration in a periodic health examination.
E. There is good evidence to support the recommendation that the condition is excluded from consideration in a periodic health examination.

When recommendations are not available from the CTF or USPSTF, the authors provide their own recommendation using the USPSTF rating system.

The preventive measures summarized in Table 14.2 pertain to average and high-risk asymptomatic nonpregnant adults. Factors that may dictate expanded or more limited surveillance for the individual patient may not be included. Characteristics that should always be considered when planning preventive care for an individual patient include the average remaining life expectancy for a person of the patient's age, comorbidity that is likely to affect the patient's life expectancy, and the time to benefit for the preventive measure being considered. Thus, a 55-year-old male patient with inoperable lung cancer should receive influenza and pneumococcal vaccines but should not receive most of the other preventive care appropriate for his age and sex. On the other hand, a 50-year-old male patient who has survived an uncomplicated myocardial infarction at the age of 48 has a reasonable life expectancy and should be offered all the preventive care appropriate for his age group. Life expectancies for elderly patients are included in Table 12.1. Another characteristic that may influence decisions about preventive care is the presence of certain diseases. For example, in the presence of hereditary polyposis or ulcerative colitis, endoscopic screening should be encouraged because of the increased risk of colorectal cancer.

Preventive Care for Established Conditions (Tertiary Preventive Care)

Preventing complications of chronic diseases is a major part of office practice. By careful practice of tertiary prevention, practitioners may minimize or postpone the poor outcomes of diabetes mellitus, congestive heart failure, degenerative joint disease, and other conditions. Of course, appropriate preventive care for an established disease depends on the disease and the patient. Examples include appropriate education and monitoring of foot care and screening for retinopathy in diabetic patients, taking steps to enhance compliance and prevent rehospitalization in a poorly compliant elderly patient with congestive heart failure, prescribing aspirin and controlling cholesterol in a hypercholesterolemic patient after myocardial infarction, and providing short-term counseling for a survivor of a myocardial infarction who is showing early symptoms of depression. The strategies for optimal preventive management of established conditions are discussed in later chapters.

Extending Prevention to the Family and the Community

Practitioners should extend preventive care beyond the individual when this is appropriate. In some instances, preventive treatment should be recommended for members of a *patient's family and other close contacts*. Immunoglobulin prophylaxis for the family of a patient with infectious hepatitis A and treatment of sexual contacts of patients with sexually transmitted diseases are classic examples. In other situations, the practitioner should recommend evaluation of the relatives of patients with certain chronic diseases that show a tendency to occur in families. For example, relatives of patients with familial hypercholesterolemia should have plasma lipid levels determined, and routine screening should be encouraged for at-risk relatives of patients with breast and colon cancers. For some conditions and some patients, genetic testing and counseling may be advisable (see Chapter 17).

Prevention should be extended to the *community at large* when *a notifiable communicable disease* is diagnosed in an individual patient (Table 14.3). Similarly, any suspected *occupational disease* in an individual worker should be reported to local health authorities and/or a regulatory agency, such as the Occupational Safety and Health Administration or the Environmental Protection Agency. In some states, laboratories are required to report abnormal findings of public health significance (e.g., elevated levels of heavy metals). Such reporting may be critical in protecting the health of others in the same community, work, or home environments (see Chapter 8).

These extensions of the role of the practitioner from treating individual patients to interventions at the family and community levels may raise important questions about patient confidentiality. Although practitioners are bound to protect confidentiality, some states and some courts have ruled that society's welfare occasionally outweighs the patient's right to privacy. Some states require reporting of all patients with newly diagnosed human immunodeficiency virus infection, and some protect practitioners who break confidentiality to notify exposed individuals at risk. Most courts agree that practitioners have a duty to warn individuals when patients make threats to harm them. Primary care practitioners should become acquainted with local and state rules regarding reporting.

Finally, some practices are situated to address the *preventive care needs of defined populations and not just the patients who visit the practice*. Examples of defined populations might be all enrollees in a managed care plan assigned to one's practice or people living in a geographic area related to one's practice. Ideally, practices should develop processes by which the health problems and preventive care needs of such defined populations are systematically identified and addressed. This approach to health care, called *community-oriented primary care*, combines principles of primary care medical practice, clinical

Table 14.3. Reportable Diseases and Conditions[a]

Acquired immunodeficiency syndrome (AIDS)[b]	Meningitis (viral, bacterial, parasitic, and fungal)
Amebiasis	Meningococcal disease[b,c]
Animal bites[c]	Mumps[b]
Anthrax[b,c]	Mycobacteriosis, other than tuberculosis and leprosy
Botulisum[b,c]	Occupational disease
Brucellosis[b]	Pertussis[b,c]
Cancer, most types	Pertussis vaccine adverse reactions
Chancroid[b]	Plague[a,b]
Chlamydia trachomatis, genital infection[b]	Poliomyelitis, paralytic[b,c]
Cholera[b,c]	Psittacosis[b]
Coccidiomycosis[b]	Rabies, human or animal[b,c]
Cryptosporidiosis[b]	Rocky Mountain spotted fever[b]
Cyclosporiasis[b]	Rubella (German measles)[b,c]
Diphtheria[b,c]	Rubella congenital syndrome[b,c]
Ehrlichiosis, human granulocytic[b]	Salmonellosis[b]
Ehrlichiosis, human monocytic[b]	Septicemia in newborns
Encephalitis	Shigellosis[b]
Encephalitis, California serogroup viral[b]	Streptococcal disease, invasive, group A[b]
Encephalitis, eastern equine[b]	*Streptococcus pneumoniae*, drug resistant, invasive disease[b]
Encephalitis, St. Louis[b]	Streptococcal toxic shock syndrome[b]
Encephalitis, western equine[b] *Escherichia coli* 0157:H7[b]	Syphilis[b]
Gonocorrhea[b]	Syphilis, congenital[b]
Haemophilus influenzae, invasive disease[b,c]	Tetanus[b]
Hantavirus pulmonary syndrome[b]	Trichinosis[b]
Heavy metal poisoning (e.g., tests showing elevated levels of lead, mercury, arsenic, cadmium must be reported by the laboratory in Maryland)	Toxic shock syndrome[b]
	Tuberculosis[b]
	Tularemia
Hemolytic-uremic syndrome, postdiarrheal[b]	Typhoid fever[b,c]
Hepatitis, viral (A,[b] B,[b] C, non-A, non-B,[b] D, E, G, undetermined)	Varicella (chickenpox)[d]
Human immunodeficiency virus (HIV) infection, adult[b]	Varicella deaths[b]
HIV infection, pediatric[b]	Yellow fever[b]
Kawasaki syndrome	
Legionellosis[b]	An outbreak of disease of known or unknown etiology that may be a danger to public health[c]
Leprosy (Hansen disease)[b]	
Leptospirosis	A single case of a disease of known or unknown etiology that may be a danger to public health
Lyme disease[b]	
Malaria[b]	An unusual manifestation of a communicable disease
Measles (rubeola)[b,c]	

[a]Determined at the state and federal levels. Reportable to local health department. This list was developed based on information obtained from the Maryland Department of Health and Mental Hygiene and Department of the Environment and from Summary of Notifiable Diseases, United States, 1999 MMWR 2001;48(53):101–102. Other diseases may be reportable in other states.

[b]Notifiable Diseases, United States (reported by state or local health departments to the Centers for Disease Control and Prevention, Atlanta, Georgia).

[c]Reportable immediately by telephone to the local health department.

[d]Although varicella is not a nationally notifiable disease, the Council of State and Territorial Epidemiologists recommends reporting of cases of this disease to the CDC.

epidemiology, and public health (22). Increasing computerization, health care databases, and opportunities for the linkages of databases are enhancing the feasibility of such approaches. However, limited financial support is an important current barrier to widespread implementation (23).

PUTTING PREVENTION INTO PRACTICE

Practitioner Performance

Despite sound evidence that supports the routine provision of selected preventive measures, studies show that practitioners often fail to provide them (24–27). This is so even in academic centers (28–33). Results from the Centers for Disease Control and Prevention's Behavioral Risk Factor Surveillance System reported that Pap tests had been obtained within the last 3 years for 77% of eligible women and clinical breast examinations and mammography in 65% within the last 2 years (34). The *Healthy People 2010* report targets a goal of 90% for Pap smears and 70% for mammography. Additionally, fecal occult blood testing is to be increased from 35% in 1998 to 50% by 2010 (1).

Barriers to Optimal Performance

While the American Medical Association has promoted the periodic health examination since the 1920s, only recently have both practitioners and the public come to accept the value of prevention (3). Practitioner attitudes toward prevention predict performance (24), and negative attitudes remain a barrier. Training of medical residents in clinical prevention may be inadequate (32,33,35). Although coverage of preventive services by insurance companies is improving and reimbursement is available from most managed care organizations and private insurers, confusion remains in the minds of practitioners and patients alike regarding the value of specific preventive services. The promotion of innumerable preventive measures by special interest medical groups can be overwhelming and confusing to practitioners and the public alike, because the guidelines are often short-lived, conflicting, and based on incomplete analysis and inadequate evidence. The publishing of guidelines based on clearly defined rules of evidence by the USPSTF and the CTF has helped alleviate the situation (see above and Table 14.2). Nonetheless, some practitioners disagree with the recommendations of these organizations and choose not to follow them (36,37). An additional barrier is time; a 1992 study of one family practice setting showed that implementation of all relevant USPSTF recommendations at that time would have required assessment of 15.4 risk factors and implementation of 13 screening recommendations, 10.5 counseling recommendations, and 1.1 immunization recommendations per adult patient (38). Perhaps the most important barrier to providing preventive services is the failure of practitioners to organize their practices for the efficient reliable provision of selected indicated preventive services.

Improving Performance in One's Practice

It is generally agreed that preventive care must be planned carefully if it is to be offered routinely and effectively to patients in a busy office practice. First, agreed upon and feasible guidelines must be developed that outline which measures are to be offered to which patients. Second, a plan must be developed to implement the guidelines. Third, assessment of the effectiveness of implementation should be performed.

The guidelines can be made accessible to practitioners by posting them, in abbreviated form, for quick reference in each examining and consulting room (Fig. 14.2). Methods that may cue practitioners to provide indicated preventive care include health maintenance as a problem at the top of each patient's problem list (see Fig. 1.1) and a risk profile on the front sheet or on a preventive care profile (Fig. 14.3) in the chart of each patient. Documentation of preventive care is often inadequate (39). Maintenance of a preventive care flow sheet (Fig. 14.3) will help the practitioner efficiently determine which measures are due and which have already been done. Otherwise, much time may be spent trying to retrieve relevant information that has become buried in the text of the chart. Office computers can be programmed or available computer software can be used to produce preventive care reminders for each visit, which can appear in patients' electronic patient records or can be attached to their paper charts (26,40–43). Nurses (44) or midlevel practitioners also can be trained to monitor and provide preventive care within the office. Audit and feedback can result in improvements in practitioner performance that can be transferred from one setting to another and persist after

JOHNS HOPKINS BAYVIEW MEDICAL CENTER
GUIDELINES FOR ROUTINE HEALTH MAINTENANCE OF NONPREGNANT ADULTS

	INTERVAL	PATIENTS		INTERVAL	PATIENTS
BASELINE DATA			PHYSICAL EXAM		
Complete H&P	Baseline	All	Blood pressure	At least q2yr	All
			Breast examination	q1yr	All F≥40 (↑risk, younger)
LIFESTYLE COUNSELING			Hearing	Discretionary	↑risk (all ≥65)
Advance directives	Once, w.f/up	All	Height	Once	All
Alcohol/drug use	q1–5yr	All	Visual assessment	Discretionary	All ≥65
Birth control	q1–5yr	Childb. age	Weight	q1–2yr	All
Exercise	q1–5yr	All			
Hormone replacement	Once	All F postmenop	LABORATORY PROCEDURES		
Overweight status	q1yr	All BMI 25–30	Chlamydia	At time of Pap	↑risk F
Obesity status	q1yr	All BMI >30	Total and HDL cholesterol (nonfast)	q5yr	All M≥35, All F≥45 All M,F with ≥1 RF>20
Sexual practices	Discretionary	All			
Tobacco use	q1–5yr	All			
			Colon cancer (fecal occult blood) or	q1y	All ≥50 (↑risk ≤50)
IMMUNIZATIONS			Colon cancer (sigmoidoscopy)	q5yr	All ≥50 (↑risk ≤50)
Hepatitis B vac.	Once (0, 1, 6 m)	↑risk (all <25)	or Colon cancer (colonoscopy)	q10yr	All ≥50 (↑risk ≤50)
Influenza vac.	q1yr	↑risk (all ≥65)	GC culture, cervix	q 1yr	↑risk F
Measles vac. (MMR)	Once, or 2 doses ≥1 month apart	All born after 1957, without immunity	HIV antibody	Discretionary	↑risk M,F
Pneumococcal vac.	Once, booster at 5yrs	↑risk (all ≥65)	Mammogram	q1–2yr	All F 50–69 ↑risk ≥35
Rubella vac. (MMR)	Once, or 2 doses ≥1 month apart	F childb. age, without immunity, ≥3 m **before** pregnancy	Pap (pt w/ cervix)	1yr x 2, then q3yr, after 2nl	All F 18–60 stop at 60 assuming 2 normal Paps
Tet/diphth toxoid	Primary (0, 1, 6–14m)	All			
	Booster q10yr, or once after age 50	All	PPD	Discretionary	↑risk
			STS	Discretionary	↑risk
PREVENTION FLOW SHEET		All			
PROBLEM LIST		All	MEDICATION FLOW SHEET		All

Figure 14.2. Sample of abbreviated preventive care standards available as wallet-size cards and posted in each examining room in the medical clinic. (Courtesy of Johns Hopkins Bayview Medical Center, Baltimore, MD.)

Johns Hopkins Bayview Medical Center
PREVENTIVE CARE PROFILE & FLOWSHEET

Jane Doe
Date of Birth: 7/23/44

Dates of Baseline History & Physical Examination: 6/00

FAMILY HISTORY

Dates Performed: 6/00 Other: DM, mother, in 40's, alive 79

ASHD: N ☐ Y ☒ (fa d. MI age 62, pat uncle died MI age 58)

Breast Ca: N ☒ Y ☐ ( )

Colon Ca: N ☒ Y ☐ ( )

HABIT HISTORY

Dates Performed: 6/00 Seatbelt: N ☐ Y ☒ ( )

Smoking: N ☐ Y ☒ (1PPD, onset 1966) Sexual Activity: ☐ Never ☐ Past, Now inactive ☒ Active

ETOH: N ☐ Y ☒ (occ. wine w/ dinner) If Active: ☒ 1 partner ☐ > 1 partner (past 1 year)

CAGE: 0 of 4 ( ) Birth Control/Safe Sex Method: post-menopausal or ☒ None

Drug Use: N ☒ Y ☐ ( ) Other:

Exercise: N ☒ Y ☐ ( )

OCCUPATIONAL EXPOSURES

☒ NONE

FLOW OF PREVENTIVE MEASURES

YEAR:	2000	2001	2002								
PAP 1996, 99 nl	s/p hys										
Breast Exam	6/00 ⊖	5/01 ⊖									
Mammogram	7/00 ⊖	8/01 ⊖									
Stool Occult Blood	7/00 ⊖ x3	7/01 ⊖ x3									
Sigmoid/Colonscopy	sig ⊖ 11/00										
Vision/Glaucoma	SEE CLINICAL FLOW SHEET										
Hearing	6/00 NL										
Cholesterol* / TG *	SEE CLINICAL FLOW SHEET										
IMMUNIZATIONS:											
Influenza	10/00	11/01									
Pneumococcal	10/00										
Tetanus / Diptheria	6/00										
MMR	NA										
Hepatitis B	NA										
OTHER:											

* Screening Only; if hyperlipidemia use clinical flowsheet. See back for Instructions.

Figure 14.3. Sample preventive care profile and flow sheet. (Courtesy of Johns Hopkins Bayview Medical Center, Baltimore, MD.)

cessation of the intervention (28,31,45). Financial reimbursement in fee-for-service settings and financial incentives in managed care settings may also motivate improved practitioner performance (46).

Although it is desirable to schedule special time for a baseline history and physical examination for patients new to a practice, ongoing preventive care is best incorporated into routine office visits. This is so because few visits to the practitioner are purely preventive and because attendance rates are lower for preventive than for problem-based visits (47). For otherwise healthy patients who see their practitioners infrequently, however, health maintenance visits should be scheduled and appointment reminders sent to increase attendance rates.

Motivating Patients

Unfortunately, simply recommending a preventive measure to a patient is not sufficient to ensure compliance. When the preventive measure involves an unpleasant procedure (e.g., sigmoidoscopy or pelvic examination) or requires active participation (e.g., collection and return of stool samples or the long-term taking of medication), poor compliance is likely. It is most likely to be a problem when the preventive intervention requires a major change in behavior on the part of the patient (e.g., dietary change or smoking cessation).

Motivating patients to comply with recommendations requires considerable skill on the part of the practitioner. Increasing patients' knowledge and understanding is a necessary but often insufficient prerequisite for behavioral change. Important additional ingredients for success include the establishment of a trusting, friendly, and supportive patient–practitioner relationship (see Chapters 3 and 4); involvement of patients in planning and monitoring their own health maintenance plan (see Chapter 4); use of motivational and behavioral strategies to enhance compliance (see Chapters 4 and 27); and the promotion of healthy positive beliefs, attitudes, values, and self-perceptions in one's patients (see Chapter 4). Patients who have confidence and truly believe they can affect their health are more likely to do so than those who do not. This perceived self-efficacy or expectation for success may be the best predictor of whether patients will initiate and persist in an activity (48,49). It should be remembered that a patient's motivation to comply may be different from the practitioner's motivation in wanting them to comply. For example, patients tend to be less impressed than practitioners with long-term and more impressed with short-term benefits. Accordingly, the practitioner should stress the factors that seem to motivate the patient. Conversations related to prevention provide opportunities for patients to share their life goals with practitioners and may increase the satisfaction of both with the practitioner–patient relationship.

The USPSTF recommends the *following strategies for promoting behavioral change*:

1. Match the teaching to the patient's perceptions. It is important to understand the patient's beliefs and concerns and to focus the teaching accordingly (e.g., "What gets in the way of your exercising regularly?"). The same "sales pitch" will not work on everyone.
2. Fully inform patients about the purposes and expected effects of an intervention (e.g., a cholesterol lowering medication) and when to expect the effects.
3. Suggest small changes rather than large ones.
4. Be specific (e.g., suggest walking for more than 20 minutes three or more times per week, reading labels for fat or salt content when shopping, or not cooking with salt).
5. Consider adding a new behavior, which is easier to accomplish, before eliminating an established one (e.g., suggesting that a sexually promiscuous patient use condoms rather than observe abstinence, or that a patient begin moderate physical activity before changing established dietary patterns).
6. Link new behaviors to old ones (e.g., suggest that a patient use her treadmill while watching the evening news or take prescribed medicine with her morning coffee).
7. Use the power of the profession. A direct simple message such as "I want you to stop smoking" may be effective simply because it is coming from a health professional.
8. Try to get an explicit commitment from the patient as to how they will achieve mutually agreed-upon health goals.
9. Use a combination of strategies. Interventions that use more than one strategy are most likely to be successful.
10. Involve the entire office staff; a team approach can facilitate improved patient education.
11. Use available resources, such as voluntary health organizations (e.g., the American Diabetes Association) and patient support groups (e.g., a smoking cessation group).
12. Monitor progress through follow-up contact.

Mechanical aids may assist this process. Printed education materials can provide information on preventive care measures for patients. Easy-to-use forms for recording and monitoring their own preventive care may promote patients' involvement in their own care, thereby prompting patients to achieve and practitioners to address recommended preventive measures.

General References*

Canadian Task Force

The Canadian Task Force on the Periodic Health Examination. **The Canadian guide to clinical preventive health care.** Ottawa: Minister of Supply and Services Canada, Canada Communication Group, 1994.

*Bold print (general references) and bold print (specific references) denote published controlled clinical trials, meta-analyses, or consensus-based recommendations.

Critical evaluations of 81 preventive measures and recommendations regarding their use in periodic health examinations.

Canadian Task Force on Preventive Health Care (name changed 2001) **website:** http://www.ctfphc.org

Excellent website that contains description of CTF history and methods; quick access to all recommendations and full text reviews, including a list and access to all publications since 1994; and quick summary tables.

For additional information, contact Nadine Wathen, Coordinator at St. Joseph's Health Centre–Parkwood Site, Room A-575, 801 Commissioners Rd. East, London, Ontario, Canada N6C 5J1. Tel: (519) 685-4292 ext. 42327, Fax: (519) 685-4016, E-mail: Nwathen@ctfphc.org.

United States Preventive Services Task Force

Guide to clinical preventive services: report of the United States Preventive Services Task Force, 2nd ed. Baltimore: Williams & Wilkins, 1996.

Reviews of 70 preventive measures that include Task Force recommendations, recommendations of others, analysis of the burden of suffering caused by the condition being considered, efficacy of screening tests, evidence of effectiveness of preventive intervention, discussion, and references. In-depth reviews of specific measures have also been published. Third edition due 2002.

United States Preventive Services Task Force website: http://www.ahrq.gov/clinic/uspstfix.htm

Excellent website that contains background information on the USPSTF; quick access to all recommendations, the 1996 Guide, and new publications; and links to other useful websites such as the Canadian Task Force, Healthy People 2010, National Guideline Clearing House, and Put Prevention into Practice.

For additional information, contact Barbara Gordon at 301-594-4024 or E-mail: bgordon@ahrq.gov.

Other Publications

American Medical Association. **Guidelines for adolescent preventive services (GAPS).** http://www.ama-assn.org/ama/pub/category/1980.html

This website includes 24 recommendations that were developed in collaboration with a GAPS Scientific Advisory Board. It provides a model and related resources that enable physicians and other health care providers to provide comprehensive clinical preventive services for adolescents between 11 and 21 years of age. It provides information on ordering implementation materials.

CDC Travelers' Health website: http://www.cdc.gov/travel/

This website of the Centers for Disease Control and Prevention provides up-to-date and comprehensive information on immunization requirements and health recommendations for international travelers. One can also phone the CDC at 404-639-3311 (general number) or 404-332-4555 (voice information system).

Epidemiology and prevention of vaccine-preventable diseases, 6th ed. Waldorf, MD: Public Health Foundation, 2001.

A comprehensive resource developed for practitioners by the National Immunization Program of the CDC. The book contains chapters on all the major vaccine-preventable diseases and their vaccines, as well as several useful appendices, including immunization schedules, implementation strategies, vaccine information statements, handling instructions, and safety guidelines.

Morbidity and Mortality Weekly Report. Atlanta: Centers for Disease Control and Prevention, U.S. Department of Health and Human Services. Website: http://www.cdc.gov/mmwr

A weekly report containing very current information about disease incidence (e.g., regional incidence of influenza) and updated recommendations for disease prevention (including immunizations).

Healthy People 2010

U.S. Department of Health and Human Services. Healthy people 2010, 2nd ed. Volume I: Understanding and improving health objectives for improving health (Part A); Volume II: Objectives for improving health (Part B); and Appendices. Washington, DC: U.S. Government Printing Office, November 2000.

These and other Healthy People 2010 publications set out the health goals and objectives for the U.S. population, document the statistical basis for the initiative, and provide guidance for its implementation. They are available in print and online at: http://www.health.gov/healthypeople.

Put Prevention Into Practice

Put prevention into practice: clinician's handbook of preventive services, 2nd ed. McLean, VA: International Medical Publishing, Inc., 1998. Website: http://www.ahrq.gov/clinic/ppipix.htm, also reachable through USPSTF website (see above)

A national program, designed by the U.S. Office of Disease Prevention and Health Promotion, to increase the appropriate use and delivery of clinical preventive services, such as screening tests, immunizations, and counseling, based on U.S. Preventive Services Task Force recommendations. PPIP is now part of the Agency for Healthcare Research and Quality's (AHRQ's) integrated program in clinical prevention. Each chapter includes a description of the target condition and risk factors for the condition, information about the effectiveness of the preventive service, a list of relevant recommendations by major authorities, instructions for performing the service, and listings of patient and provider resources. In addition, PPIP provides office posters, timeline charts for guidelines, preventive flow sheets to be used for individual patients, postcard reminders, and patient education materials in English and Spanish.

Woolf SH, Jonas S, Lawrence RS, eds. Health promotion and disease prevention in clinical practice. Baltimore: Williams & Wilkins, 1996.

Multiauthor book that focuses on the practical implementation of preventive measures in office practice, with numerous examples, sample forms, tables, and lists of resources.

Specific References

1. U.S. Department of Health and Human Services. Healthy people 2010, 2nd ed. Vol. I: Understanding and improving health objectives for improving health (Part A); Vol. II: Objectives for improving health (Part B); and Appendices. Washington, DC: U.S. Government Printing Office, November 2000.
2. Richmond R, Kehoe L, Heather N, et al. General practitioners' promotion of healthy life styles: what patients think. Aust N Z J Public Health 1996;20:195.
3. Han PK. Historical changes in the objectives of the periodic health examination. Ann Intern Med 1997;127:910.
4. Li VC, Coates TJ, Ewart CK, et al. The effectiveness of smoking cessation advice given during routine medical care: physicians can make a difference. Am J Prev Med 1987;3:81.
5. Russell MAH, Wilson C, Taylor C, et al. Effects of general practitioners' advice against smoking. BMJ 1979;2:231.
6. Holland WW. Screening: reasons to be cautious. BMJ 1993;306:1222.
7. McGinnis JM, Foege WH. Actual causes of death in the United States. JAMA 1993;270:2207.
8. Moran WP, Nelson K, Wofford JL, et al. Increasing influenza immunization among high risk patients: education or financial incentive? Am J Med 1996;101:612.
9. Committee to Study the Prevention of Low Birth Weight. Preventing low birth weight. Washington, DC: Institute of Medicine, National Academy Press, 1985:132.
10. Fiscella K. Does prenatal care improve birth outcomes? A critical review. Obstet Gynecol 1995;85:468.
11. Burns R, Nichols LO, Graney MJ, et al. Impact of continued geriatric outpatient management on health outcomes of older veterans. Arch Intern Med 1995;155:1313.
12. Naylor M, Brooten D, Jones R, et al. Comprehensive discharge planning for the hospitalized elderly: a randomized trial. Ann Intern Med 1994;120:999.
13. Stuck AE, Siu AL, Wieland GD, et al. Comprehensive geriatric assessment: a meta-analysis of controlled trials. Lancet 1993;342:1032.
14. Stuck AE, Aronow HU, Steiner A, et al. A trial of annual in-home comprehensive geriatric assessments for elderly people living in the community. N Engl J Med 1995;333:1184.
15. Gillespie LD, Gillespie WJ, Cumming R, et al. Interventions for preventing falls in the elderly [Systematic Review]. Cochrane

Musculoskeletal Injuries Group. Cochrane Database of Systematic Reviews, Issue 2, 2001.
16. Bailar JC III, Smith EM. Progress against cancer? N Engl J Med 1986;314:1226.
17. Hampton ML, Anderson J, Lavizzo BS, et al. Sickle-cell nondisease: a potentially serious public health problem. Am J Dis Child 1974;128:58.
18. Haynes RB, Sackett DL, Taylor DW, et al. Increased absenteeism from work after detection and labeling of hypertensive patients. N Engl J Med 1978;299:741.
19. Quill TE, Lipkin M Jr, Greenland P. The medicalization of normal variants. The case of mitral valve prolapse. J Gen Intern Med 1988;3:267.
20. Harris RP, Helfand M, Woolf SH, et al. Current methods of the U.S. Preventive Services Task Force: a review of process. Am J Prev Med 2001;20:21.
21. Saha S, Hoerger TJ, Pignone MP, et al. The art and science of incorporating cost effectiveness into evidence-based recommendations fro clinical preventive services. Am J Prev Med 2001;20:36.
22. Nutting PA, Green LA. Community-oriented primary care. In: Rakel RE, ed. Textbook of family practice, 5th ed. Philadelphia: W.B. Saunders, 1995:225.
23. Longlett SK, Kruse JE, Wesley RM. Community-oriented primary care: critical assessment and implication for resident education. J Am Board Fam Pract 2001;14:141.
24. Dietrich AJ, Goldberg H. Preventive content of adult primary care. Do generalists and subspecialists differ? Am J Public Health 1984;74:223.
25. Lurie N, Manning WG, Peterson C, et al. Preventive care: do we practice what we preach? Am J Public Health 1987;77:801.
26. McPhee SJ, Bird JA, Fordham D, et al. Promoting cancer prevention by primary care physicians: results of a randomized controlled trial. JAMA 1991;266:538.
27. Smith HE, Herbert CP. Preventive practice among primary care physicians in British Columbia: relation to recommendations of the Canadian Task Force on the Periodic Health Examination. Can Med Assoc J 1993;149:1795.
28. Kern DE, Harris WL, Boekeloo BO, et al. Use of an outpatient medical record audit to achieve educational objectives: changes in residents' performance over six years. J Gen Intern Med 1990;5:218.
29. Kosecoff J, Fink A, Brook RH, et al. General medical care and the education of internists in university hospitals: an evaluation of the Teaching Hospital General Medicine Group Practice Plan. Ann Intern Med 1985;102:250.
30. McPhee SJ, Richard RJ, Solkowitz SN. Performance of cancer screening in a university general internal medicine practice: comparison with the 1980 American Cancer Society guidelines. J Gen Intern Med 1986;1:275.
31. Winickoff RN, Coltin KL, Morgan MM, et al. Improving physician performance through peer comparison feedback. Med Care 1984;22:527.
32. Keim DB, Gomez CF, Wolf AM. The level of preventive health care in an internal medicine residency clinic: still only an ounce of prevention? South Med J 1998;91:550.
33. Sharma VK, Corder FA, Raufman JP, et al. Survey of internal medicine residents' use of the fecal occult blood test and their understanding of colorectal cancer screening and surveillance. Am J Gastroenterol 2000;95:2068.
34. Blackman DK, Bennett EM, Miller DS. Trends in self-reported use of mammograms (1989–1997) and Papanicolaou tests (1991–1997)—Behavioral Risk Factor Surveillance System. Morb Mortal Wkly Rep CDC Surveill Summ 1999;48:1.
35. Borum ML. Medical residents' colorectal cancer screening may be dependent on ambulatory care education. Dig Dis Sci 1997;42:1176.
36. Woo B, Woo B, Cook EF, et al. Screening procedures in the asymptomatic adult. Comparison of physician's recommendations, patients' desires, published guidelines, and actual practice. JAMA 1985;254:1480.
37. Zyzanski SJ, Stange KC, Kelly R, et al. Family physicians' disagreement with the US Preventive Services Task Force recommendations. J Fam Pract 1994;39:140.
38. Meddar JD, Kahn NB Jr, Susman JL. Risk factors and recommendations for 230 adult primary care patients, based on US Preventive Services Task Force guidelines. Am J Prev Med 1992;8:150.
39. Dresselhaus TR, Peabody JW, Lee M, et al. Measuring compliance with preventive care guidelines: standardized patients, clinical vignettes, and the medical record. J Gen Intern Med 2000;15:782.
40. Burack RC, Gimotty PA, George J, et al. Promoting screening mammography in inner-city settings: a randomized controlled trial of computerized reminders as a component of a program to facilitate mammography. Med Care 1994;32:609.
41. Litzelman DK, Dittus RS, Miller HE, et al. Requiring physicians to respond to computerized reminders improves their compliance with preventive care protocols. J Gen Intern Med 1993;8:311.
42. McDonald CJ, Sui LH, Smith DM, et al. Reminders to physicians from an introspective computer medical record. A two-year randomized trial. Ann Intern Med 1984;100:130.
43. Demakis JG, Beauchamp C, Cull WL, et al. Improving residents' compliance with standards of ambulatory care: results from the VA Cooperative Study on Computerized Reminders. JAMA 2000;284:1411.
44. Davidson RA, Fletcher SW, Retchin S, et al. A nurse-initiated reminder system for the periodic health examination. Implementation and evaluation. Arch Intern Med 1984;144:2167.
45. Korn JE, Schossberg LA, Rich EC. Improved preventive care following an intervention during an ambulatory care rotation: carryover to a second setting. J Gen Intern Med 1988;3:156.
46. Gold MR, Hurley R, Lake T, et al. A national survey of the arrangements managed-care plans make with physicians. N Engl J Med 1995;333:1678.
47. Sackett DL, Snow JC. The magnitude of compliance and noncompliance. In: Haynes RB, Taylor DW, Sackett DL, eds. Compliance in health care. Baltimore: Johns Hopkins University Press, 1979:11.
48. Bandura A. Self-efficacy: toward a unifying theory of behavior change. Psychol Rev 1977;84:191.
49. Wilson GT. Cognitive factors in life style changes: a social learning perspective. In: Davidson PO, Davidson SM, eds. Behavioral medicine: changing health lifestyles. New York: Brunner/Mazel, 1980.
50. Gøtzsche PC, Olsen O. Is screening with mammography justifiable? Lancet 2000;355:129.
51. Olsen O, Gøtzsche PC. Screening for breast cancer with mammography. The Cochrane Library, issue 4, 2001.
52. deKoning H. Commentary: assessment of nationwide cancer-screening programs. Lancet 2000;355:80.
53. Correspondence related to ref. 50. Lancet 2000;355:747.

CHAPTER 15

Principles of Nutrition in Ambulatory Care

EUGENE C. CORBETT, Jr., MD

As much as any behavior, eating reflects the complexities and variability of human life. What and how we eat derives from our tastes, our habits, our psychological milieu, our culture, and what is presented to us at the table or at the grocery store. Yet fundamentally, food is *nutrient.* It serves the biologic need for the growth, development, and maintenance of tissue structure and function. What is eaten, combined with individual variation in absorption and metabolism, determines whether nutrients fulfill their varied purposes optimally or cause harm to the individual. When nutrient consumption, absorption, and metabolism result in deficiency or excess, pathologic consequences may ensue. Although historically, and in certain parts of the world even now, diseases of undernutrition have been more common, in Western culture diseases of nutrient excess have become epidemic. It has been estimated that diet and activity patterns account for at least 14% of the causes of death in the United States through their influence, particularly on the development of cancer, cardiovascular disease, and diabetes mellitus (1). By implication, the morbid effects are even greater. In clinical care, an understanding of and attention to the essential aspects of human nutrition is therefore important so that when aberrations in health occur, appropriate efforts to modify nutritional influences can be undertaken.

Food to the consumer is more than nutrient. It is also the source of important and pleasurable experiences that motivate eating beyond that which biologic need dictates. Thus, excessive or, at times, deficient intake of nutrient on a day to day basis is more likely the rule than the exception. Fortunately, the body has the capacity in many instances to eliminate nutrients that are consumed in excess of need and the ability to store others in physiologically neutral depots for use when intake may be insufficient. Vitamin B_{12}, for example is used at a rate of about 1 μg/day, whereas the capacity for hepatic storage is approximately 1,500 times that much. When B_{12} intake exceeds these metabolic needs and storage capacities, the excess is eliminated by the kidney, a process made easy because of the water-soluble nature of this vitamin. Caloric nutrient, however, which is maximally absorbed and generally not excreted, increases disease risk when accumulation begins to exceed 120% of ideal body weight. Vitamin A, because of its fat-soluble nature and the body's more limited storage and elimination capacity, causes a variety of pathologic consequences when consumed in sufficient excess. In the final analysis, and despite the many influences that motivate what and how people eat, the essential clinical concern is the health risk associated with either a sustained *deficit* or *excess* of nutrient in the diet.

In this chapter, we emphasize *an approach* to assessing nutrition and those situations when nutritional advice is appropriate in the care of the ambulatory patient. Special attention is given to selected nutrients, consensus dietary recommendations, and contemporary dietary patterns. For easy reference, much of the information is provided in table form.

STANDARD NUTRITION INFORMATION AND RECOMMENDATIONS

Generally speaking, nutritional information should be considered approximate when compared with more objective data that are often available for evaluating health status. For example, nutritional studies show that dietary intake reported by the patient often understates and only occasionally overestimates actual nutrient intake (2). Similarly, nutrient intake values included in many of the tables and charts in this chapter are approximations of food values derived from standard references. Understanding of general amounts is given priority over focusing on smaller differences that might be attributed to variable food portion sizes, the chosen example of a certain food group, or the variability that is generally assigned to differences in gender. Variability in labeled and reported nutrition data is due to many factors, including differences in food packaging, growing environments, and manufacturing. Nutrient intake also varies from individual to individual depending on food preferences, genetic endowment, body size, gastrointestinal function, physical activity, and, most of all, eating habit and even bite size. For most clinical thinking about nutrition in day to day practice, average values suffice for general assessment and advising purposes.

Guidelines for Americans

The availability and standardization of nutritional information has increased in recent years because of both consumer demand and governmental influence upon food consumption recommendations and food labeling. Since 1980, the U.S. Departments of Agriculture (USDA) and Health and Human Services have published dietary guidelines for Americans every 5 years, most recently in 2000 (3). These represent consensus recommendations for food consumption in the United States and provide the basis for federal nutrition policy. They are based on the work of a committee of nutrition experts who regularly review existing published literature. The guidelines include the *food guide pyramid* (Fig. 15.1), which is widely used to educate the consumer about ideal food consumption choice. The pyramid depicts, in terms understandable to the average lay person, *daily recommended amounts from each major food group.* Table 15.1 provides the details needed to apply the food guide pyramid to daily eating selections. Table 15.2 lists the daily number of servings from each food group recommended for types of people according to their approximate daily expenditure of calories.

Nutritional Labeling

Uniformity in *nutrition labeling* accelerated in the United States with the passage of the Nutrition Labeling and Education Act in 1990 (Public Law 101-535). This federal mandate preempted all existing state and federal laws and regulations and stimulated a planned schedule to achieve uniformity in the way that food content is named and quantified on all food products, including water (4). Food labels contain standardized information on serving size, caloric content, and ingredients (Fig. 15.2). Reference is also made to the amount of certain ingredients in comparison with recommended daily values (5). There are 10 *mandatory* components of the nutrition label: total fat, saturated fat, cholesterol, sodium, total carbohydrate, dietary fiber, vitamin A, vitamin C, calcium, and iron.

Percent of recommended daily values for specific nutrients as used by the USDA/Health and Human Services is required in food labeling (Fig. 15.2). The daily value is based on an average caloric intake of 2,000 calories per day for an adult who performs at a light to moderate activity level. Although exact definitions are not used, this designation generally refers to an individual who is not sedentary in life-style and who does not perform specific daily exercise. The actual daily value may be higher or lower depending on physical activity level. Food labels always list, in the footnote, the actual daily value for each major nutrient for both a 2,000- and 2,500-calorie diet.

In 1996, new U.S. Food and Drug Administration (FDA) regulations required relabeling of 2% low-fat

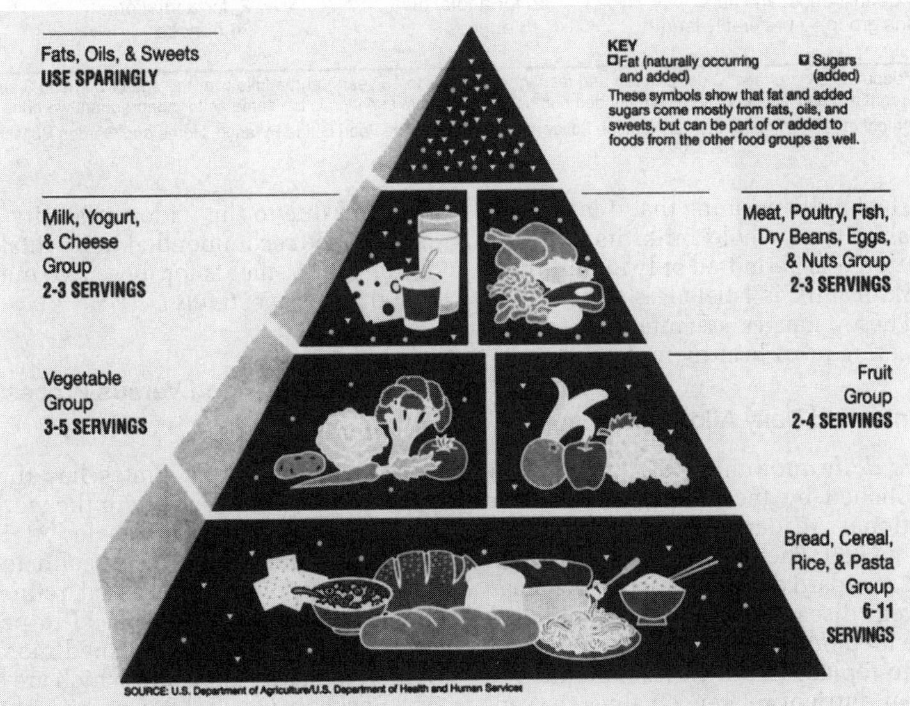

Figure 15.1. Food guide pyramid: a guide to daily food choices. (From U.S. Department of Agriculture, U.S. Department of Health and Human Services, with permission.) See sample serving components in Tables 15.1 and 15.2.

Table 15.1. Food Selection Guide

Food Group	Major Macronutrients and Micronutrients (Vitamins and Minerals)	Daily Servings Recommended[a]	Sample Serving
Fats, oils, and sweets	Fat, sugar, vitamins	Use sparingly	• 2 tbsp olive or pufa oil • 1 can of soda
Milk, yogurt, and cheese	Protein, calcium, vitamin D, fat, lactose	2–3	• 1 cup milk • or 1 cup yogurt • or 2 oz. cheese
Meat, poultry, fish, dry beans, eggs, and nuts	Protein, fat, vitamin B_{12}, other vitamins, iron, minerals	2–3	• 3.5 oz cooked lean meat, poultry, fish (about the size of a deck of cards) • or count each of the following as 1 oz meat: 1 egg, ½ cup cooked beans, 2 tbsp peanut butter, 1 cup raw tofu
Vegetable	Fiber, carbohydrate, vitamins A and C, folate, potassium, magnesium, minerals	3–5	• 1 cup raw or leafy or ½ cup chopped or cooked
Fruit	Carbohydrate, fiber, vitamins A and C, folate, potassium, minerals	2–4	• 1 raw fruit • 3/4 cup fruit juice • ½ cup canned fruit • 1/4 cup dried fruit
Bread, cereal, rice, and pasta	Carbohydrate, vitamins, minerals, fiber	6–11	• 1 slice bread or • 1 cup cereal or • ½ cup cooked rice, pasta, or cereal

[a]See Table 15.2 for recommendations according to daily calorie needs.

Adapted from U.S. Department of Agriculture, Human Nutrition Information Service, with permission. (See General References.)

Table 15.2. How Many Servings Do You Need Each Day?

Food Group	Children Ages 2 to 6 years, Women, some Older Adults (about 1,600 calories)	Older Children, Teen Girls, Active Women, Most Men (about 2,200 calories)	Teen Boys, Active Men (about 2,800 calories)
Bread, cereal, rice, and pasta group, (grains group)—especially whole grain	6	9	11
Vegetable group	3	4	5
Fruit group	2	3	4
Milk, yogurt, and cheese group (milk group)—preferably fat free or low fat	2 or 3[a]	2 or 3[a]	2 or 3[a]
Meat, poultry, fish, dry beans, eggs, and nuts group (meat and beans group)— preferably lean or low fat	2, for a total of 5 ounces	2, for a total of 6 ounces	3, for a total of 7 ounces

[a]The number of servings depends on your age. Older children and teenagers (ages 9 to 18 years) and adults over the age of 50 need 3 servings daily. Others need 2 servings daily. During pregnancy and lactation, the recommended number of milk group servings is the same as for nonpregnant women.

Adapted from U.S. Department of Agriculture, Center for Nutrition Policy and Promotion. The Food Guide Pyramid, Home and Garden Bulletin Number 252, 1996, with permission.

milk as "reduced-fat" milk, meaning that it must have at least 25% less fat than whole milk. Its previous "low-fat" designation was permitted only for milk containing 1% fat. Skim milk is labeled as "fat-free" or "non-fat" milk. These changes are intended to help consumers in selecting heart healthy milk products.

Recommended Daily Allowances

The *recommended daily allowance* (RDA) for specific nutrients is established by the Food and Nutrition Board of the National Academy of Sciences. RDAs were last revised in 1989. They represent a nutrient intake value that is 2 standard deviations above the mean necessary to prevent disease in a healthy population (6). The *recommended daily intake* has more recently been introduced to replace the RDA. It is intended to incorporate a set of nutrient reference values that encompass the RDA and various Canadian and European value systems. Because the occurrence of sodium and potassium deficiency in the healthy U.S. population is rare and due to the wide variability in intake and excretion, the recommended daily intake tables list *minimum* requirements for these two nutrients (2,400 and 3,500 mg, respectively).

Natural Food Versus Processed Food

Organic Food

Although the United States has the most abundant and available food supply in the world, there is growing concern that it is unsafe. At issue is whether proper nutrition requires "health food" (natural, organic) as opposed to processed, refined or "junk food," or food that has been exposed to pesticides or additives. This debate has assumed moralistic overtones: Which foods are good and which are bad? (See Corbett and Becker in General References, from which this section is adapted.)

It is difficult to define organic or natural food. Most foods are grown or raised, and in the chemical sense,

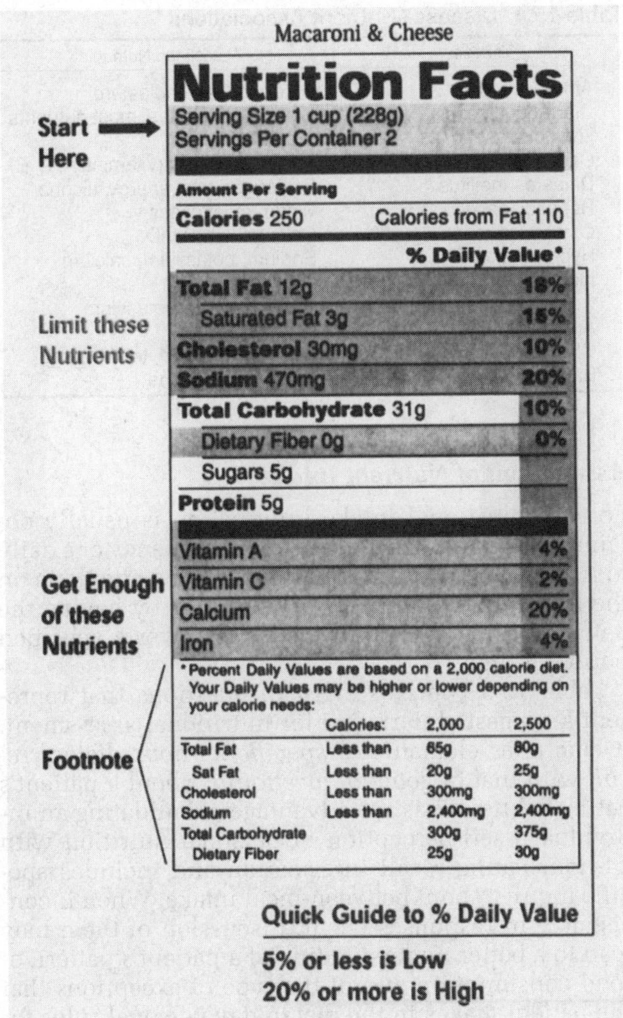

Figure 15.2. How to read a nutrition facts label. (From Dietary guidelines for Americans, 2000, with permission.)

manufactured foods consist of organic compounds. Nevertheless, organic or natural foods are relatively free from fertilizers, pesticides, additives, and commercial processing. In this sense, such foods are pure but not necessarily better. Of necessity, production of organic foods is limited. In contrast, modern agriculture and food science manage to make it possible to feed huge urban populations. As food is processed on its way from farm to store shelf, does it become less nutritious and less natural? How toxic are the various chemicals that increase productivity and retard spoilage?

Organic and natural foods can be compared with the foods that are generally available in stores and restaurants. Such comparisons should examine nutritional value, cost, and toxicity. It appears, for example, that an organic apple is as nutritious as a nonorganic apple, but it costs more (7).

The nutritional content of "fast foods" has been examined in detail. Perhaps surprisingly, examples of fast-food meals conform closely to modern dietary standards in terms of carbohydrate, fat, protein, vitamins, and minerals. Although the sodium content of fast food meals is high, it is no higher than that of the traditional American meal purchased at a restaurant (steak, French fries, salad with dressing) (8).

Pesticides and Additives

Although it is relatively easy to defend the nutritional value of processed food, the question of toxicity from pesticide contaminants and food additives is more difficult to answer. Although hazards from pesticide residues are of concern, review of the experience in the United States has not disclosed injuries or deaths related to their presence in foods (9). It is difficult, if not impossible, to produce food absolutely free of pesticides. Pesticide residues are commonly found even in organic produce. There are certainly environmental and occupational risks associated with the pesticide industry, but their potential ill effects as food contaminants have been prevented by policies enforced by the FDA and the USDA. On the other hand, there have been instances in which environmental and other industrial toxins (mercury, polybrominated biphenyls) have tragically contaminated the food chain.

Certain food additives concern the public, such as nitrates, synthetic antioxidants, food colors, mold inhibitors, monosodium glutamate, diethylstilbestrol, refined sugar, and salt. All additives are scrutinized by the FDA for reproductive, teratogenic, mutagenic, carcinogenic, and toxic effects. Many synthetic food dyes have been replaced by natural compounds, such as carotene, with inherent food value. Because of public feeling about "chemicals" in food, mold inhibitors (propionates and sorbates) and synthetic antioxidants (butylated hydroxyanisole and butylated hydroxytoluene) are used less frequently now by food manufacturers.

Survey Data on Nutritional Patterns

Because the study of nutrition and its relationship to health status have become increasingly important, national nutritional surveillance surveys were begun in the United States in 1970 (10). *National Health and Nutrition Examination Surveys* have been conducted three times (1971, 1976, and 1988) by the National Center for Health Statistics of the Centers for Disease Control and Prevention. These population-based surveys use a probability sample of 25 to 35 thousand individuals using 24-hour dietary recall and food frequency questionnaires. Physical examination and a battery of clinical measurements and tests are also performed on all individuals in the sample. The National Health and Nutrition Examination Survey data are used to establish food consumption patterns and nutritional status by both demographic and nutrient-specific criteria.

NUTRITIONAL ASSESSMENT

Although clinicians in ambulatory practice may refer patients to nutritionists for detailed assessments of dietary habit and for assistance in managing patients with nutritionally related disease such as obesity, atherosclerosis, diabetes, or renal failure, much general dietary counseling can be done by a patient's primary care provider. Useful dietary counseling requires a practical approach to nutritional assessment that helps to identify dietary deficiencies and excesses. The two steps of a practical approach to assessment include taking a nutritional history and recognizing manifestations of nutritional deficiency or excess.

Table 15.3 lists the more important macronutrients and micronutrients that should be considered in dietary assessment. Table 15.1 shows the food group(s) that contain each of the important macronutrients and micronutrients. Macronutrients are consumed in readily observed forms. Micronutrients, on the other hand, are less visible constituents of the major food groups. They include *vitamins* (organic compounds that are required in small amounts) and *minerals*.

The *serving sizes* used in this chapter (see examples in Table 15.1), which may vary considerably from individual to individual, are based on a standard reference that is widely used by nutrition professionals (11).

Taking a Nutritional History

Importance

The initial step in identifying dietary influence in the routine care of the patient is to collect information that provides a database for each individual with respect to important nutrients. From this, a judgment can then be made about whether these nutrients are deficient or excessive in the patient's diet. The nutrient history can be obtained by the physician directly or by another staff member. A physician-directed history has the advantage that the doctor can simultaneously assess the patient's willingness to discuss their eating habits and make a judgment as to the veracity of the information. Additionally, the patient is more likely to conclude that personal nutrition has value comparable with other data that one seeks in the clinical interview. Given the major impact that diet has on the etiology, pathogenesis, and course of many diseases, such a dialogue is important in current prevention and treatment strategies. Table 15.4 lists nutrients associated with the most common contemporary diseases of humans (12,13).

Table 15.3. Important Nutrients

Macronutrients	Micronutrients
Total carbohydrate	Calcium
Fiber	Folate
Starch[a]	Iron
Sugar	Magnesium
Alcohol	Potassium
Total fat	Sodium
Saturated	Vitamin A
Unsaturated	Vitamin B_{12}
Cholesterol	Vitamin C
Protein	Vitamin D
Water	Vitamin E

[a]Starch refers to foods (e.g., corn) that contain polymers of glucose and that are generally resistant to digestion until they are cooked. Cooking ruptures cell membranes and makes carbohydrate available for enzymatic breakdown.

Table 15.4. Disease–Nutrient Associations

Disease	Associated Nutrients
Atherosclerosis	Saturated fat, cholesterol
Diarrheal disease	Water, electrolytes, most nutrients
Liver disease	Alcohol
Cancer	Fat, antioxidants (vitamins A, C, E)
Diabetes mellitus	Fat, sugar, total energy, alcohol
Renal disease	Water, electrolytes
Osteoporosis	Calcium, vitamin D
Hypertension	Sodium, potassium, calcium
Malnutrition	Many nutrients
Congestive heart failure	Sodium, water, potassium
Anemia	Iron, folate, B_{12}
Obesity	Fat, carbohydrate, total energy
Breast disease	Vitamin E, caffeine

Assessment of Nutrient Intake

Formal nutritional intake information is usually obtained with the use of either a food frequency or a daily food intake questionnaire. The latter may be done on the basis of a 24-hour dietary recall or by having the patient complete a daily food diary over a specified period of time.

Table 15.5 contains a list of questions that represent a suggested narrative for nutritional assessment. It combines elements of *specific 24-hour dietary recall* with that of *general questioning* about a patient's eating habits. It has the advantage of validating an individual's self-perception of personal nutrition with 24-hour eating recall information and includes specific inquiry about between-meal intake. When inconsistency in responses occur, discussion of them may lead to a better understanding of a patient's pattern of food consumption and of the type of exceptions that the patient makes in the day to day personal rules for eating. Although a single 24-hour dietary recall may be atypical, repeated 24-hour recalls can provide a fairly reliable assessment of average dietary intake.

An alternative more time-efficient way to assess 24-hour intake is to give the patient a readable table of information about food groups such as Table 15.1 and have the patient fill in the number of servings of each food group consumed in the prior day. Because food intake reporting methods have been shown to collect information that often underestimate actual food consumption (2), it is wise to interpret any food intake report as representing *minimal food consumption.* Nevertheless, such information is essential in developing a starting point for discussion of an individual's food consumption behavior.

Once information about the average daily food intake is collected, an estimate of actual macronutrient and micronutrient element consumption can be made, using basic information in Table 15.1.

Micronutrient intake is generally assessed by an analysis of food type consumption (Table 15.1). It can also be inferred from levels measured in the laboratory (Table 15.6); however, these levels may reflect not only intake but absorption and loss related to disease states (e.g., pernicious anemia) or medical treatments (e.g., diuretics). Table 15.7 contains additional information about selected micronutrients pertinent to assessment

Table 15.5. Sample Clinical Nutrition History that Combines Specific Dietary Recall and General Information

Meal-oriented questioning

1. How many meals do you generally eat on a daily basis? How many *yesterday* or today?
2. What do you generally eat for breakfast? What did you eat *this morning*?
3. What do you generally eat for lunch? What did you actually eat for lunch *today or yesterday*?
4. Do you ever eat or drink anything between breakfast and lunch? What might you have had between breakfast and lunch *today or yesterday*?
5. What do you generally have for dinner/supper? What did you have *today or yesterday*?
6. Do you normally eat or drink between lunch and dinner/supper? If so, what do you have? Did you do so *today or yesterday*?
7. What do you generally eat or drink between dinner/supper and bedtime? What did you have then either *today or yesterday*?
8. Do you generally snack? If so, what are your preferred snacks? How often do you snack?

Selected nutrient questioning

1. What liquids do you generally consume? What and how much did you drink in the past 24 hours? Do you drink water by itself? How often/how much?
2. Do you add salt to your food at the table? Do you cook with salt?
3. What fats do you generally cook with? What did you use *yesterday*?
4. Do you ever eat sweets? Daily? How often? What do you usually reach for in a snack? Do you add sugar to coffee or tea?
5. Do you consume foods with caffeine? Coffee? Tea? Soda? Chocolate? Quantities?
6. Do you know what fiber containing foods you eat on a daily basis? Fresh vegetables? Fresh fruits? Salad? Fiber supplements?
7. Do you know how much cholesterol related foods you eat on a daily basis? Red meat? Saturated fats?
8. What and how much dairy products do you eat daily? Dark greens? Calcium supplements?

Table 15.6. Micronutrient Laboratory Tests

Nutrient	Test	Normal Range[a]
Calcium	Serum calcium	8.2–10.0 mg/dL
	Bone mineral density	Radiologic reference
Folate	Serum folate	2.6–17.0 ng/mL
	Red cell folate	150–450 ng/mL
Iron	Serum iron	40–160 μg/dL
	% saturation	20%–55%
	Transferrin	213–360 mg/dL
	Ferritin	18–311 ng/mL
Magnesium	Serum Mg	1.9–2.7 mg/dL
Potassium	Serum K+	3.6–5.0 mEq/L
	24-hr urinary excretion	25–125 mEq/d (varies with diet)
Sodium	Serum sodium	135–145 mEq/L
	24-hr urinary excretion	20–250 mEq/d (varies with diet)
Vitamin A	Serum retinol	35–70 μg/dL
Vitamin B_{12}	Serum B_{12}	251–911 pg/mL
Vitamin C	Serum ascorbic acid	0.6–2.0 mg/dL
Vitamin D	25-OH vitamin D	15–80 ng/mL
	1,25$(OH)_2$ vitamin D	18–62 pg/mL
Vitamin E	Serum tocopherol	0.5–1.2 mg/dL

[a]Reference values vary between laboratories.

regarding sufficient intake. It includes the RDA, the type of food that generally provides each nutrient (vegetable, meat, dairy), and the food servings that would provide the total RDA. The amount of each micronutrient contained in a standard over-the-counter multivitamin or pill supplement is also shown. Finally, when considering micronutrient dietary adequacy, it is helpful to know the amount that is stored in the body, the duration of the body's storage, and amount lost daily (Table 15.8) (6).

Recognizing Clinical Manifestations of Nutritional Deficiency and Excess

In addition to the nutrition history, the physical examination and some laboratory tests offer important clues to both macro- and micronutrient abnormalities. Tables 15.9 and 15.10 summarize the major clinical manifestations of nutrient deficiency and excess.

Dietary Recommendations According to Caloric Expenditure

In addition to assessing the nutrition of patients, it is important to provide basic information and counseling regarding healthy nutrition. The U.S. Preventive Services Task Force includes dietary counseling by primary care providers as a recommended preventive measure (see Chapter 14). Strategies and skills helpful in motivating healthy behavior are described in detail in Chapter 4.

An appropriate diet is one that maintains body weight and provides sufficient daily nutrient intake so that deficiency and excess are avoided. The guidelines in Table 15.2 summarize recommended diets for individuals according to their average caloric expenditure. When individualizing recommendations, additional energy intake requirements should be estimated depending on the patient's level of physical activity. Table 15.11 provides a guide for estimating additional caloric expenditure for a variety of common activities.

Multivitamins

Despite the absence of clinical trials, there is enough suggestive evidence for health benefit and lack of harm to recommend that healthy adults should take an inexpensive multivitamin daily (13a). Multivitamins contain 100% of the RDA for each constituent vitamin.

CONSIDERATIONS RELATED TO SELECTED NUTRIENTS

Certain nutrients are particularly important in their relationship to health and disease: some because they constitute the basic components of a selective diet (e.g., a vegetarian diet), some because of their influence on caloric intake, some because of refinement in the processing of foods in the past century; and others because they contribute to commonly experienced symptoms.

Vegetarian Diets

Vegetarian diets are becoming more popular. One reason for this is the increasing awareness that the current epidemic of hypercholesterolemia and atherosclerosis is related to saturated fats and the cholesterol content of animal protein foods. Second, evidence that vegetal sources of protein contain sufficient amounts of

Table 15.7. Micronutrient Dietary Sources

Nutrient	Recommended Daily Allowance	Food Source	Food Servings	Over the Counter Preparation
Calcium	1200 mg	Dairy, vegetal	1 qt milk	200–1000 mg
Folate	400 μg	Vegetal	5	400 μg
Iron	15 mg	Meat, vegetal	6	15 mg
Magnesium	350 mg	Vegetal > meat	6	100 mg
Potassium	2,000 mg	Most foods	8	80 mg
Sodium	500 mg	Most foods	8	None
Vitamin A	1,000 RE	Vegetal, dairy, liver	4 <1	1,000 RE
Vitamin B_{12}	2 μg	Meat, fish	1	6 μg
Vitamin C	60 mg	Vegetal	2	60 mg
Vitamin D	400 IU	Dairy	1 qt milk	400 IU
Vitamin E	10 mg	Vegetal oil Most foods	3 tblsp 6	10 mg

RE, retinol equivalents.

From Food and Nutrition Board, National Research Council. Recommended daily allowances, 10th ed. Washington, DC: National Academy Press, 1989, with permission.

Table 15.8. Micronutrient Storage Capacity and Daily Losses

Nutrient	Storage Capacity	Supply Duration	Average Daily Loss
Calcium	1,200 g (1% extraskeletal)	Years	200 mg
Folate	5000 μg	60 days	60 μg
Iron	500 mg	>1 yr	1 mg male, 1.5 mg female
Magnesium	2,500 mg	100 days	150 mg
Potassium	180,000 mg (4,500 mEq)	~1 wk	800 mg (20 mEq)
Sodium	>100,000 mg (>4,400 mEq)	Years	<230 mg (10 mEq)
Vitamin A	500,000 μg	>1 yr	1,000 μg
Vitamin B_{12}	>2,000 μg	>3 yr	2 μg
Vitamin C	1,500 mg	30 days	>30 mg
Vitamin D[a]	?	Unknown	100 IU (2.5 μg)
Vitamin E[b]	?	?	?

[a]Vitamin D is one of the nonessential vitamins.

[b]Vitamin E deficiency is rare.

From Food and Nutrition Board, National Research Council. Recommended daily allowances, 10th ed. Washington, DC: National Academy Press, 1989, with permission.

Table 15.9. Clinical Manifestations Related to Macronutrients

Macronutrient	Manifestations of Deficiency	Manifestations of Excess
Carbohydrate, total	Weight loss, asthenia, urinary ketosis	Obesity, weight gain
Carbohydrate, fiber	Constipation	Frequent stooling, abdominal bloating
Carbohydrate, starch	Weight loss, asthenia	Obesity, weight gain
Carbohydrate, sugar	None	Obesity, weight gain, halitosis, dental caries
Carbohydrate, alcohol	None	Facial plethora, alcoholic breath, large parotid glands, hepatitis, cirrhosis
Total fat	Weight loss, asthenia, vitamin D deficiency	Obesity, weight gain, xanthelasma, atherosclerosis
Saturated fat	Unknown	Hypercholesterolemia, atherosclerosis, corneal arcus
Cholesterol	Unknown	Hypercholesterolemia, atherosclerosis, corneal arcus
Protein	Weight loss, edema, infection, lethargy, hypoalbuminemia (kwashiorkor)	None
Water	Dehydration, high urine specific gravity	Hyponatremia (unusual)

the 10 essential amino acids has debunked the long held myth that vegetarian eating does not provide as complete a protein source as animal meats (14). An important example is the demonstration that soybeans contain an amino acid content equivalent to that of egg albumin, the long held standard referent for an ideal protein source (15).

Finally, it is becoming increasingly appreciated that vegetarian eating not only can sustain health, but may lead to improved health status. For example, studies show that vegetarian diets are consistently associated with lower rates of ischemic heart disease (16–18). In addition, studies of Seventh-Day Adventists reveal that their vegetarian-oriented life-style is also associated with decreased rates of cancer and all-cause mortality (19). Vegetarian diets contain higher amounts of fiber, antioxidants, folic acid, and phytochemicals, all of which are receiving increasing attention in modern dietary recommendations.

The vegetarian tradition is Asian in origin, particularly among Hindu populations. It currently includes a number of variations along a continuum of vegetarian purity. A *vegan* diet is considered the strictest diet. It excludes all forms of animal products, including dairy and honey. A *lactovegetarian* diet includes dairy products, and *ovolactovegetarian* allows for the inclusion of both eggs and dairy. Many individuals use the term *partial vegetarian* to indicate they occasionally use animal products. *Pescovegetarianism* refers to a diet that includes fish but no other animal products. A *macrobiotic* diet derives from Japanese traditions and in its most traditional form involves the practice of a gradual change from a balanced vegetarian diet to one that primarily consists of grain, all in the interest of progressive nutritional and spiritual purity. Generally, it emphasizes brown rice, fruits, and vegetables. Cooking is

Table 15.10. Clinical Manifestations Related to Micronutrients

Micronutrient	Manifestations of Deficiency	Manifestations of Excess
Calcium	Osteoporosis, kyphosis, hypocalcemia	Constipation, hypercalcemia, hypercalciuria, urolithiasis
Folate	Macrocytic anemia, neurologic birth defects	None
Iron	Microcytic anemia	Manifestations of hemachromatosis (cirrhosis, diabetes, etc.)
Magnesium	Muscle weakness, low serum Mg, hypokalemia, long QT interval	None
Potassium	Neuromuscular symptoms, ECG U-wave prominence	Cardiac arrhythmia, ECG peaked T waves
Salt	Neuromuscular symptoms, hyponatremia, hypotension	Hypertension, edema
Vitamin A	Impaired night vision, xerophthalmia, follicular hyperkeratosis, dry skin	Headache, desquamation, alopecia, osteosclerosis, splenomegaly
Vitamin B_{12}	Macrocytic anemia, glossitis, peripheral neuropathy	None
Vitamin C	Scurvy, malaise	Diarrhea
Vitamin D	Hypocalcemia, rickets, osteomalacia	Hypercalcemia, hypercalciuria, calcinosis
Vitamin E	Reproductive failure, neuromuscular dysfunction (chronic malabsorption states)	Unknown

ECG, electrocardiogram.

Table 15.11. Physical Activity and Caloric Expenditure

Physical Activity	Calories Expended (kcal/h)[a]
Rest	90
Sitting	120
Stand and move	252
Walk 2 mph	198
Walk 4 mph	396
Cycle 5 mph	180
Cycle 10 mph	396
Swim 20 yd/min	294
Swim 40 yd/min	594
Run 5 mph	564
Run 10 mph	1128
Hike with pack	420
Tennis, singles	468
Basketball	462
Raquetball	606

[a]Calculated from Appendix C tables in Williams MH. Nutrition for health, fitness and sport, 5th ed. Boston: McGraw-Hill, 1999:425–431, with permission.

preferred over raw foods. Processed foods are avoided, as are tomatoes and potatoes. Fish is permitted.

The food guide pyramid (Fig. 15.1) includes vegetarian eating in its general design and recommended food selections. The U.S. Department of Agriculture website contains more detailed information on vegetal choice (see General References). Complete sources of amino acids are obtained in diets that combine legumes (beans, peas, lentils, or soybeans) and grain. Tofu is a particularly versatile soybean-based product, used in the preparation of many vegetarian dishes.

In addition to alternative protein sources, vegetarian diets differ from meat-based diets in that they contain lower fat content and little saturated fat. They also have less iron, little if any vitamin B_{12}, and less vitamin D, calcium, and zinc. However, they contain more fiber and antioxidant vitamins, magnesium, and folate (20,21). In addition, they potentially limit vitamin D availability in wintry months when sun exposure is limited. Although years can pass before people who become vegans develop B_{12} deficiency, breast-fed infants of strict vegetarian mothers have been reported to develop B_{12} deficiency (22). As well, milk-free diets can lead to rickets in young children (23). Significant nutrient deficiency is unusual in nonvegan vegetarian individuals. When eggs and dairy are avoided. however, supplementation with vitamin B_{12}, calcium, and vitamin D is recommended.

Caloric Nutrient

Caloric nutrient excess has reached epidemic proportions in the United States today. Obesity rates approach 40% of the adult population in this country and are increasing in many other countries (see Chapter 83). The increasing availability of energy-dense foods coupled with more sedentary life-styles together contribute to this phenomenon. The epidemic of type II diabetes associated with chronic caloric excess leading to obesity has many of the same implications for life-style as obesity.

The word *calorie* is derived from the Latin word *calor*, meaning warm. The term is used as a measure of heat energy in food. Specifically, it refers to the amount of heat required to raise the temperature of 1 kg of water 1°C. In common food-related usage calorie is used, although technically *kilocalorie* is the more correct designation. The caloric value of the four major energy-containing nutrients is shown in Table 15.12.

Once ingested, over 99% of caloric foods are absorbed. Very little of ingested caloric content is excreted in urine or stool under normal conditions. An exception is alcohol, which can be excreted unmetabolized in the urine. Ketones, which represent the incompletely metabolized combustion products of fat breakdown, are the other exception to this rule. Thus, most caloric intake is destined for either immediate metabolic use or storage as either glycogen (liver, muscle) or triglyceride (adipose cells).

The absorption and metabolic processing of caloric nutrients require energy. The incremental amount of caloric energy required in providing for metabolic processing varies from nutrient to nutrient (24,25). Table 15.13 shows average estimates for the metabolic cost of caloric macronutrient processing and storage. The net amount of calories stored for an equivalent

Table 15.12. Energy Contained in Caloric Nutrients

Nutrient	Energy (kcal/g)
Protein	4
Carbohydrate	4
Alcohol	7
Fat	9

(100 calories) amount of ingested carbohydrate, fat, or protein is shown. The last column of the table gives an estimate of the comparative annual weight that might be gained if an *extra 100 kcal/day* were eaten for each nutrient.

Salt

Sodium chloride is the major osmotic constituent of the extracellular vascular and interstitial spaces. It is also the major component of intravenous fluids. From a dietary perspective, it is also a nutrient that can be deficient or excessive in the diet. Excessive salt can contribute to expansion of the extracellular space and influence the development of hypertension and congestive heart failure. In an otherwise healthy individual, diet-related salt deficiency is rare.

The normal human is capable of adapting to a very wide range of salt intake. Under conditions of limited salt intake, the kidney will excrete less than 230 mg (10 mEq) of sodium per day. This represents about one-tenth of a teaspoon of salt. On the other hand, among certain Oriental cultures, an intake and excretion of over 25 g/day has been documented. The renin-angiotensin-aldosterone system adjusts salt excretion to match salt intake.

In U.S. surveys, daily sodium intake ranges from 3.8 to 7.5 g (26). In a workplace study of urinary 24-hour sodium excretion, a large range (4 to 24 g) was observed (27). Approximately 50% of salt intake is that added by the consumer for seasoning. For example, one teaspoon of salt contains 1.8 g of sodium. Because of its importance in common health problems, quantitative information about the amount of sodium is required for standard nutritional labeling (Fig. 15.2). A daily value (the maximum amount recommended) of 2.4 g is used. Table 15.14 lists the sodium and salt content of selected intake sources. One gram of sodium is found in 2.5 g of salt (NaCl).

Table 15.13. Caloric Processing and Storage

Caloric Nutrient	% Calories Expended in Processing and Storage	Net Calories Stored[a] From 100 Ingested	Weight Gain per Year[b] in Pounds
Fat	3	97	9.7
Carbohydrate	25	75	7.5
Protein	25–50	50–75	5–7

[a]Assuming calories eaten exceed those needed for metabolic use.
[b]Weight gain if an extra 100 calories per day is eaten of nutrient = net calories stored per day × 365 days/3,500 calories per pound as stored triglyceride.

Table 15.14. Sodium and Salt Equivalents in Various Sources of Sodium

Intake	Sodium	Sodium (mEq)	Salt
Minimal intake	0.250	11	0.625
Low sodium diet	0.5	22	1.5
1 tsp salt	1.8	78	4.5
Daily value	2.4	104	6.0
Average U.S. intake	5.0	217	12.0
1 L lactated Ringer's	3.1	134	7.75
1 L normal saline solution	3.5	154	8.75
125 mL/h of normal saline solution × 24 h	10.6	462	26.25

1 mEq Na = 23 mg; 2.5 mg NaCl contains 1 mg Na.

Sugar

The consumption of sugar in the American diet increased throughout the 20th century, continuing a trend that began in the 19th century when inexpensive methods of sugar production developed. The average annual per capita consumption was estimated to be 75 pounds in 1909, rising to approximately 130 pounds today. Sugar comprises approximately 25% of the total energy consumption in the U.S. diet. As an energy-dense nutrient that is easily consumed, it contributes to excess caloric intake and therefore influences the development of obesity and diabetes. It also contributes to the development of dental caries.

Three-fourths of dietary sugar is sucrose, the type found in refined sugars; the remaining dietary sugars (fructose, maltose, lactose) come from natural foods such as in fruit, honey, and milk. Sugar is added to many manufactured foods, including products not thought of as "sweet," such as salad dressings, mayonnaise, catsup, bread, crackers, and chips. Table 15.15 lists the sugar and caloric content of a variety of modern foodstuffs.

Fiber

Since the 1960s, the importance of fiber in the diet has become more appreciated. It had been considered an inert ingredient until clinical studies revealed an association between colonic disease and the lack of fiber in the diet, and the favorable effect of fiber on blood sugar control in diabetes was recognized.

There are six vegetal fiber constituents: gum, mucilage, pectin, hemicellulose, lignin, and cellulose. All but the latter two are at least partially digested by human colonic bacteria. *Bran* generally refers to the form of fiber that mostly passes unaltered through the digestive tract, usually consisting of cellulose, hemicellulose, and lignin. Dietary fiber has hydrophilic activity and increases the water content of small intestinal and colonic stool. These factors explain why fiber increases stool bulk and diminishes bowel transit time (28). Dietary fiber also slows gastric emptying time and moderates carbohydrate absorption rates (29). Fiber can increase the fecal loss of nutrients, but this effect has

Table 15.15. Sugar Content of Selected Foods

Food Item	Sugar Content (g)	Total Sugar (cal)	Total Serving (cal)[a]
Teaspoon of sugar	4.5	18	18
Soda, 12 oz[b]	40	160	160
Ice cream, 1 cup	32	128	340
Yogurt, 4 oz	29	116	130
Juice, 8 oz	26	104	104
Chocolate bar, 1.6 oz	22	88	230
Cookie, 1 oz	21	84	120
Crackers, 5	16	64	70

[a]Includes sugar and nonsugar calories.
[b]Diet sodas contain less than 10 calories per 12 oz.

not been associated with overt nutritional deficiency. The fiber content of common foods is discussed in Chapter 42.

General References*

Bendich A, Deckelbaum R. Preventive nutrition: the comprehensive guide for health professions, 2nd ed. Totowa, NJ: Humana Press, 2001.

A one-source evidence-based reference for preventive nutrition information.

Corbett G, Becker DM. "Nutrition" in prevention in clinical practice. New York: Plenum Medical Book Company, 1988.

Addresses all facets of nutrition in the context of preventive health care.

Katz DL. Nutrition in clinical practice. Philadelphia: Lippincott Williams & Wilkins, 2001.

A concise and well-referenced review of nutrition organized by clinical condition. Contains excellent information about nutritional counseling and detailed profiles on each of the micronutrients in the Appendix.

Pennington JAT. Bowes & Church's food values portions community used, 17th ed. Philadelphia: Lippincott Williams & Wilkins, 1998.

A comprehensive and detailed source for the nutritional contents of all foods.

Shils ME, Olson JA, Shike M. Modern nutrition in health and disease, 8th ed. Philadelphia: Lea & Febiger, 1994.

A traditional and very comprehensive nutrition text in two volumes that contains epidemiologic and biochemical information as well as clinically relevant discussion of all known nutrients.

The Second International Congress on Vegetarian Nutrition. Am J Clin Nutr 1994;59[Suppl 5s].

The Third International Congress on Vegetarian Nutrition. Am J Clin Nutr 1999;70[Suppl 3s].

These two references contain a variety of summary articles on the science of vegetarian nutrition.

U.S. Department of Agriculture Food & Nutrition Info Website: http://www.nal.usda.gov/fnic/

Excellent resource for accessing all sources of data and standards regarding nutrition in the United States.

Williams SR. Nutrition and diet therapy, 8th ed. St. Louis: Times Mirror/Mosby College Publishing, 1998.

A comprehensive text on clinically oriented nutrition written in a style appropriate for health professionals generally as well as for interested public readers.

Specific References

1. McGinnis JM, Foege WH. Actual causes of death in the United States. JAMA 1993;270:2207.
2. National Research Council. Nutrient adequacy: assessment using food consumption surveys. Report of the Subcommittee on Criteria for Dietary Evaluation, Food and Nutrition Board, Commission on Life Services. Washington, DC: National Academy Press, 1986.
3. Nutrition and your health: dietary guidelines for Americans, 2000. USDA/USDHHS, 5th ed., 2000, Home and Garden Bulletin no. 232.
4. Food and Nutrition Board, Institute of Medicine. Food labeling, toward national unity. Washington, DC: National Academy Press, 1992.
5. Code of Federal Regulations, Food and Drugs, title 21, part 101.9, Nutrition Labeling of Food, 1996.
6. Food and Nutrition Board, National Research Council. Recommended daily allowances, 10th ed. Washington, DC: National Academy Press, 1989.
7. Jukes TH. Organic food. CRC Crit Rev Food Sci Nutr 1977;9:395.
8. Appledorf H. Nutritional analysis of foods from fast food chains. Food Technol 1974;28:50.
9. Jukes TH. How safe is our food supply? Arch Intern Med 1978;138:772.
10. National Center for Health Statistics, National Health and Nutrition Examination Survey, www.cdc.gov/nchs/about/major/nhanes.htm.
11. Pennington JAT, ed. Bowes & Church, food values of portions commonly used, 17th ed. Philadelphia: Lippincott Williams & Wilkins, 1998.
12. Murray CJL, Lopez AD. Mortality by cause for eight regions of the world: global burden of disease study. Lancet 1997;349:1269.
13. Murray CJL, Lopez AD. Global mortality, disability, and the contribution of risk factors: global burden of disease study. Lancet 1997;349:1436.

13a. Willett WC, M Stampfer MJ. What vitamin should I be taking doctor? NEJM 2001;345:1819.

14. Young VR, Pellett PL. Plant proteins in relation to human protein and amino acid nutrition. Am J Clin Nutr 1994;59:1203S.
15. Young VR. Soy protein in relation to human protein and amino acid nutrition. JADA 1991;91:823.
16. Key TJ, Fraser GE, Thorogood M, et al. Mortality in vegetarians and non-vegetarians: detailed findings from a collaborative analysis of five prospective studies. Am J Clin Nutr 1999;70:516S.
17. Appleby PN, Thorogood M, Mann JI, et al. The Oxford Vegetarian Study. Am J Clin Nutr 1999;70:525S.
18. Joshipura KJ, Hu FB, Manson JE, et al. The effect of fruit and vegetable intake on risk for coronary heart disease. Ann Intern Med 2001;134:1106.
19. Fraser GE. Associations between diet and cancer, ischemic heart disease and all-cause mortality in non-Hispanic white California Seventh-Day Adventists. Am J Clin Nutr 1999;70:532S.
20. Dwyer JT. Vegetarian eating patterns: science, values and food choices—where do we go from here? Am J Clin Nutr 1994;59:1255S.
21. Haddad EH, Berk LS, Kettering JD, et al. Dietary intake and biochemical, hematologic and immune status of vegans compared to non-vegetarians. Am J Clin Nutr 1999;70:586S.
22. Higginbottom MC, Sweetman L, Nyhan WL. A syndrome of methylmalonic aciduria, homocystinuria, megaloblastic anemia and neurologic abnormalities in a vitamin B12-deficient breast-fed infant of a strict vegetarian. N Engl J Med 1978;299:317.
23. Dwyer JT, Dietz WM, Huss G, et al. Risk of nutritional rickets among vegetarian children. Am J Dis Child 1979;133:134.
24. Anderson GH, Rolls BJ, Steffen DG. Nutritional implications of macronutrient substitutes. Ann N Y Acad Sci 1997;819:51.
25. Westerterp-Plantenga MS, Fredix EWHM, Steffens AB, et al. Food intake and energy expenditure. pp. 247–250.
26. Fregley MJ. Attempts to estimate sodium intake in humans. In: Horan M.J, Blaustein M, Dunbar JB, eds. National Institute of Health workshop on nutrition and hypertension. New York: Biomedical Information Corp., 1985:93.
27. Dahl LK, Love RA. Etiological role of sodium chloride intake in essential hypertension in humans. JAMA 1957;164:397.
28. Burkitt DP, Walker ARP, Printer NS. Effect of dietary fiber on stools and transit times, and it's role in the causation of disease. Lancet 1972;2:1408.
29. Holt S, Heading, RC, Carter DC, et al. Effect of gel, fibre or gastric emptying on absorption of glucose and paracetamol. Lancet 1979;1:636.

* Bold print (general references) and bold numerals (specific references) denote published controlled clinical trials, meta-analyses, or consensus-based recommendations.

CHAPTER 16

Exercise for the Healthy Patient

ROSS E. ANDERSEN, PhD
KERRY J. STEWART, EdD

The purpose of this chapter is to describe the health benefits of regular exercise, to describe the major types of exercise, and to provide practical information for helping individuals to engage in exercise. The role of exercise in the management of a number of chronic diseases is described in other chapters.

The health benefits of regular exercise are well documented (1). Increased levels of physical activity and exercise are associated with increased longevity and with a decreased incidence of coronary artery disease, serum lipid abnormalities, hypertension, and non–insulin-dependent diabetes. Unfortunately, the scientific knowledge about the benefits of exercise among both the public and health professionals has not translated into a more active population. Presently, only about 23% of adults in the United States engage in levels of activity sufficient to produce health benefits and 40% do not participate in any regular physical activity (1). Activity levels remained essentially unchanged throughout the 1990s despite large-scale public health education campaigns. Furthermore, people with chronic disease are more likely to report a sedentary life-style (2), as are minorities and individuals in lower socioeconomic classes (3). By adding a sedentary life-style to its list of controllable risk factors for coronary artery disease, the American Heart Association has made regular exercise a major focus for preventive medicine (4).

The physical activity goal in *Healthy People 2010* is to increase the proportion of adults who engage in regular exercise, preferably daily moderate activity for at least 30 minutes per day (1). This goal matches the Surgeon General's 1996 recommendation that all Americans should accumulate at least 30 minutes of activity throughout the day on most days of the week (5). It should be noted that those meeting these standards may derive additional health and fitness benefits by further increases in frequency or intensity of exercise.

OVERALL HEALTH BENEFITS OF EXERCISE

Several studies suggest a *dose–response relationship* between the amount of physical activity performed and health risk (6,7). Thus, the most fit individuals have the best risk profiles. For example, men and women who were healthy but less fit by treadmill testing had a higher risk of death from any cause over an 8-year follow-up (6). As shown in Fig. 16.1, only a moderate increase in fitness above the lowest levels produced substantial mortality risk reduction. Further increases in fitness produced relatively modest additional benefits. Thus, individuals do not need to attain high levels of fitness to accrue substantial health benefits from exercise.

EFFECT OF CHANGING FITNESS LEVELS ON RISK PROFILES

In 1994, a large-scale prospective study carried out in 10,269 Harvard alumni reported the impacts of changes in physical activity and other life-style characteristics on mortality (8). Using mail-back questionnaires sent between 1962 and 1977, the investigators were able to examine life-style changes over an 11- to 15-year follow-up. The effects of these changes were assessed in relation to mortality in the period from 1977 to 1985. The investigators reported that men who were initially sedentary but started to participate in moderately vigorous sports had a 23% lower risk of death than those who remained inactive. Interestingly, improving any of four risk indicators (smoking, obesity, hypertension, physical inactivity) appeared to have the same relative impact on risk reduction.

The relationship of change in activity to mortality was also evaluated in 9,777 men who underwent two preventive medicine examinations (9). The effects of changes in physical activity levels were assessed in relation to mortality over an average 5.1-year follow-up. There were 223 deaths during this time. Men who were unfit at both assessments had the highest death rates, whereas those who were fit at both times had the lowest death rates, and those who improved fitness status had intermediate rates. Those individuals who became fit had a 44% lower age-adjusted risk of all-cause mortality than did their sedentary counterparts. Each of these studies provides a strong rationale for encouraging sedentary patients to become more active.

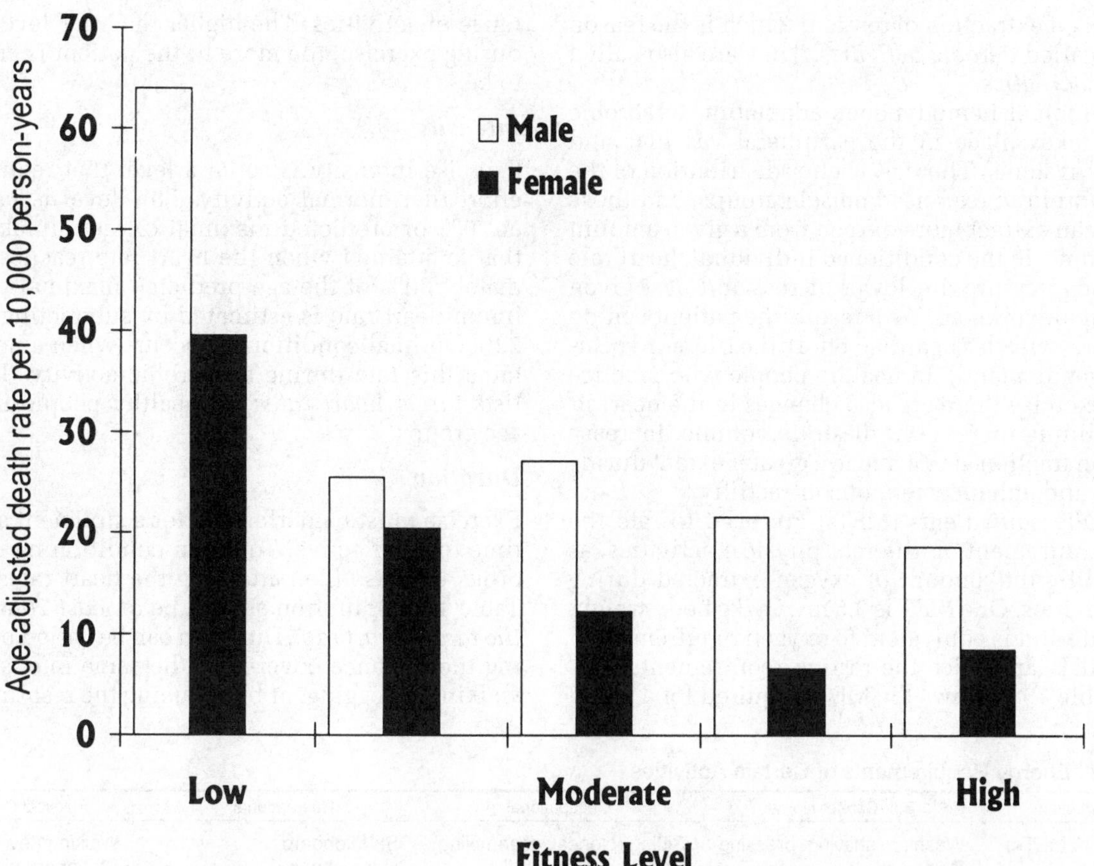

Figure 16.1. Relationship between fitness and all-cause mortality. Fitness levels were based on maximum treadmill performance. (Adapted from Blair SN, Kohl HW, Paffenbarger RS. Physical fitness and all-cause mortality: a prospective study of healthy men and women. JAMA 1989;262:2395, with permission.)

MUSCULAR AND CARDIOVASCULAR EFFECTS OF EXERCISE

The body responds and adapts to the kind and amount of physical demands placed on it. The response is *specific,* meaning that the greatest changes are observed only in the areas on which demands are placed. For exercise to bring about an improvement in physical fitness, it must *overload* the muscles or organ system involved in the exercise. To overload is to exercise at a greater intensity than the intensity to which one is accustomed. The overload must be applied gradually, in stages, for maximal effectiveness and safety. *Threshold of training* is the amount of exercise that must be done to produce fitness improvements.

A consequence of the above principles is that the *type of exercise* engaged in must match the body function one wants to improve. Thus, if the objective is to improve cardiovascular endurance, exercise that increases heart rate and peripheral oxygen consumption is required. If the objective is to improve strength, exercise with increasing amounts of resistance is. There is little carryover of the effects of an exercise from one component of fitness to another.

The factors that must be considered when establishing a plan for physical conditioning differ for each of three types of exercise described below: cardiovascular conditioning, moderate-intensity exercise, and resistance exercise.

VIGOROUS EXERCISE LEADING TO CARDIOVASCULAR CONDITIONING

Vigorous exercise, with the goal of attaining the physiologic adaptation known as the *conditioning effect,* is beneficial for healthy people and patients with most chronic diseases. *Moderate-intensity exercise* that does not produce a full conditioning effect is also associated with health benefits (see below). Cardiovascular principles related to vigorous exercise are described here. The importance of stretching exercises and of not increasing the stress on the musculoskeletal system too rapidly is described in Chapter 72.

Aerobic Activities

Activities for cardiovascular fitness entail rhythmic repetitive movements of large muscle groups against small resistance. Such activities can be performed for a relatively long time. They include walking, jogging, swimming, cycling, rowing, jumping rope, skating, running, and cross-country skiing. These activities increase the demand for oxygen, and the muscles adapt by enhanced extraction of oxygen, which is the reason they are called *aerobic activities*. They are also called *dynamic activities*.

The principal hemodynamic adaptation to aerobic exercise takes place in the peripheral vascular and muscular systems. There is a better distribution of the cardiac output to exercised muscle groups, and those muscles can extract more oxygen from a given amount of blood flow. In the conditioned individual, heart rate and blood pressure are lower at rest and at a given submaximal workload. As a result, the patient can do more work with less cardiac effort (i.e., less myocardial oxygen demand). In healthy people who practice aerobic exercise there are also changes in the heart itself, including increase in diastolic volume, increase in ejection fraction at rest and to a greater extent during exercise, and enhancement of contractility.

Metabolic equivalents (METs) are used to rate the energy requirement of different physical activities, as indicated by the amount of oxygen extracted during those activities. One MET is 3.5 mL O_2/kg body weight per minute and is equivalent to oxygen requirement at rest; 2 METs are twice the resting requirements, and so on. Table 16.1 shows the METs required for a broad range of activities. The higher the MET level attained during exercise, the more fit the patient is considered to be.

Intensity

Exercise intensity is set at a level that requires more effort than normal activity. This level is usually set at 70% of predicted maximal oxygen uptake, a level that is attained when the heart rate reaches approximately 80% of the age-predicted maximal rate. Maximum heart rate is estimated by subtracting age from 220. Optimal conditioning occurs when a person sustains this rate during an aerobic activity. Table 16.2 lists *target heart rates* for healthy people in various age groups.

Duration

Exercise must be performed for a sufficient amount of time to be effective. To attain conditioning using vigorous exercise (i.e., attaining the heart rates listed in Table 16.2), duration should be *at least 20 minutes at the target heart rate*. Duration can be varied by increasing the distance covered at the same rate, such as in walking or jogging, or by reducing the rest time during

Table 16.1. Energy Requirements of Certain Activities

Activity Level	Self-Care or Home	Occupational	Recreational	Physical Conditioning
Very light (≤3 METs)	Washing, shaving, dressing Desk work; writing, washing dishes Driving car[a]	Sitting (clerical, assembling) Standing (store clerk, bartender) Driving truck[a] Crane operator[a]	Shuffleboard Horseshoes Bait casting Billiards Archery[a] Golf (cart)	Walking (level, at 2 mph) Stationary bike (very low resistance) Very light calisthenics
Light to moderate (3–5 METs)	Cleaning windows Raking leaves Weeding Power lawn moving Waxing floors (slowly) Painting Carrying objects 15–30 lb[b]	Stocking shelves (light objects)[b] Light welding Light carpentry[b] Machine assembly Auto repair Paper hanging[b]	Dancing Golf (walking) Sailing Horseback riding Volleyball Tennis (doubles) Sexual intercourse[a] (see details in the text)	Walking (3–4 mph) Level bicycling (6–8 mph) Light calisthenics
Moderate (5–7 METs)	Easy digging in garden Level hand lawn mowing Climbing stairs (slowly) Carrying objects 30–60 lb[b]	Carpentry (exterior home building)[b] Shoveling dirt[b] Pneumatic tools[b]	Badminton (competitive) Tennis (singles) Snow skiing (downhill) Light backpacking Basketball Football Skating (ice and roller) Horseback riding (gallop)	Swimming (breast stroke)
Heavy (7–9 METs)	Sawing wood[b] Heavy shoveling[b] Climbing stairs (moderate speed) Carrying objects 60–90 lb[b]	Tending furnace[b] Digging ditches[b] Pick and shovel[b]	Canoeing[b] Mountain climbing[b] Fencing Paddleball Touch football	Jogging (5 mph) Swimming (crawl stroke) Rowing machine Heavy calisthenics Bicycling (12 mph)
Very heavy (9 METs)	Carrying loads upstairs[b] Carrying objects 90 lb or more Climbing stairs (quickly) Shoveling heavy snow[b] Shoveling for 10 min (16 lb)	Lumber jack[b] Heavy laborer[b]	Handball Squash Ski touring over hills[b] Vigorous basketball	Running (6 mph) Bicycling (13 mph or steep hill) Rope jumping

[a]May cause added psychologic stress that will increase load on the heart.

[b]May produce disproportionate myocardial demands because of use of arms or isometric exercise. See further discussion regarding isometric (resistive) exercise in physical conditioning section of this chapter.

METs, metabolic equivalents.

From Haskell WL. Design and implementation of cardiac conditioning programs. In: Hellerstein HK, ed. Rehabillitation of the coronary patient. New York: John Wiley & Sons, 1978:203, with permission.

Table 16.2. Target Heart Rates for Healthy People by Age Approximately 80% Maximal Predicted Heart Rate)

Age (yr)	Heart Rate (beats/min)
20–29	170
30–39	160
40–49	150
50–59	140
60–69	130

From Parmley JF Jr, Blair S, Gazes PC, et al., eds. Proceedings of the National Workshop on Exercise in the Prevention, Evaluation, and Treatment of Heart Disease. J South Carolina Med Assoc 1969;65(12): Suppl 1: i, with permission.

a rest period. Studies in exercise physiology suggest that the total work done during an exercise session (i.e., duration times intensity) may be more important in eliciting improvements than intensity or duration alone. Therefore, a long moderate-intensity workout in which heart rate reaches 40% to 60% of the age-predicted maximum may be equivalent to a shorter high-intensity workout if the total work is the same. A long moderate-intensity workout (e.g., long period of sustained walking) may be more suitable for beginners and for middle-aged or older patients because it would reduce the risk of injury.

Frequency

This factor refers to the number of times per week exercise is to be done. Exercise must be performed regularly, and for most types of exercise three to five times per week is desirable. However, two to three times per week is probably more sensible for the beginner because musculoskeletal injuries can occur at the start of a program from overuse. Exercise can then be increased to three to five times per week as adaptation takes place.

Hormonal and Metabolic Effects

In addition to the effect of training on the cardiovascular and muscular systems, aerobic exercise is associated with beneficial changes in a number of other systems; there is increased vagal tone, lowering of catecholamines, decrease in serum triglycerides, increase in the ratio of high- to low-density lipoprotein, reduction in adipose tissue, slowing of loss of bone mass, augmentation in plasma fibrinolytic activity, and enhanced endogenous opiate activity (may add to sense of well-being). A comprehensive review (see Peterson, General References) distinguishes exercise (planned, structural, repetitive physical activity that leads to physical conditioning) from all other physical activity and summarizes benefits and risks that accompany both and the specific instructions that can be given to patients.

Initiating a Vigorous Exercise Program

Healthy people can develop their own physical conditioning programs, using a self-instruction program (see references in Table 16.3). The objective of conditioning programs is to reach an exercise level at which the body achieves 70% of maximal predicted oxygen uptake, a level that is attained when the heart rate reaches approximately 80% of the maximal predicted rate (Table 16.2). As stated previously, optimal conditioning in healthy people occurs with aerobic activity at the target heart rate for 20 minutes at least three times per week. Lower levels of aerobic exercise also produce a partial conditioning effect in healthy people.

Selected people should consult their physicians before beginning a vigorous exercise program. In general, men over the age of 40, women over the age of 50, and those with major risk factors for atherosclerosis should have a physical examination and a resting electrocardiogram. Exercise stress tests should be considered for some people in these categories, as summarized in Table 16.4. Nondiagnostic fitness tests for apparently healthy people are usually available at health clubs, YMCAs, wellness centers, and community colleges. When supervised and interpreted by qualified allied health professionals, these tests can provide the basis for the exercise prescription. Fees are usually nominal and are included in the overall package for exercise sessions.

Long-Term Maintenance of Cardiovascular Conditioning

Long-term compliance with formal exercise programs is often poor. It is necessary to exercise regularly at the proper intensity, frequency, and duration if physical fitness is to be maintained. Measurable deterioration in the conditioning effect occurs after missing only a few weeks. The time required to retrieve lost ground seems to be directly related to the length of time without exercise and the degree of physical fitness achieved before cessation of exercise.

MODERATE INTENSITY EXERCISE

For years, exercise scientists recommended that in order for exercise to "count," it had to be conditioning-level exercise, as described above. Unfortunately, as previously noted, only a small proportion of adults engage in regular vigorous physical activity. Although most people recognize that regular exercise plays an important role in promoting a healthy life-style, the sedentary majority are not able participate in vigorous activity, do not enjoy it, or do not prioritize it highly enough to allocate time for it. Recent studies have shown that many of the health benefits of physical activity can be obtained from moderate intensity exercise (e.g., activities such as those that require 3 to 5 METS, as listed in Table 16.1) (10–12). Both the accumulation of bouts of activity throughout the day and a single extended exercise session can benefit health. For example, a recent study found that women in weight loss programs who accumulated a series of short bouts of exercise throughout the day had slightly greater weight loss than those who exercised for the same total amount of time daily in one continuous session (13). Persons with sedentary occupations may find it easier to fit these shorter bouts of

Table 16.3. Suggested Patient Readings

Websites

The American Council on Exercise has an excellent website with lots of fitness information. They also offer information on how to select a personal trainer. http://www.acefitness.org.

The American College of Sport Medicine offers a list of certified personal trainers as well as its position stands on a variety of topic related to exercise. http://www.acsm.org.

The American Heart Association offers several options for people who are initiating an exercise program. They also publish their position stand on exercise for both adults and children. http://www.americanhear.org.

The International Health and Racquet Sports Association is the association of quality health clubs. This site can help patients learn about current fitness-related news and to locate a quality health club in their area. http://www.inrsa.org.

This site has an online exercise diary for patients to track their training sessions. They also offer a virtual personal trainer. http://www.justmove.org.

Publications

Advil forum on Health Education: *Fit over 40: your doctor's prescription.* Advil forum on Health Education, 1500 Broadway, New York, NY 10036 (Free; mail orders only). http://www.advil.com.
Offers sensible suggestions for older patients to begin an exercise program.

American Heart Association. *Exercise diary.* American Heart Association, 7272 Greenville Ave., Dallas, TX 75231, (800) 242-8721 (Free).
This is a nice log book for tracking changes in physical activity. http://www.americanheart.org.

American Heart Association, *Your heart: an owner's manual.* Prentice Hall, Englewood Cliffs, NJ, 07632 ($27.95).
This text contains a thorough explanation of the cardiovascular system in lay terms. http://www.americanheart.org.

Blair SN. *Living with exercise: improving your health through moderate activity.* The Learn Education Center, Box, Dallas, TX, (800) 736-7323 ($18.95). http://www.learneducation.com.
This manual suggests a practical approach to help sedentary persons adopt a more physically active life-style.

Kennedy WL, ed. *American College of Sports Medicine fitness book.* Human Kinetic, Box 5976, Champaign, IL 61825-5076, (800) 747-4457 ($11.95). http://www.acsm.org.
This book outlines each of the components of fitness and suggests strategies for improving overall health.

Stanford Center for Research and Disease Prevention. *The walking kit and the jogging kit.* Health Promotion Resource Center, 1000 Welch Rd., Palo Alto, CA 94304-1885, (415) 723-0003 ($2.75 each).
These kits offer walkers and joggers a systematic approach to increasing their levels of activity and fitness. http://www.prevention.stanford.edu/publications.

Table 16.4. People for Whom Stress Testing Should Be Considered when Beginning Vigorous Exercise Programs

Status	Test or Training Mode
Healthy, men < 40 yr, women < 50 yr	No special test
Healthy, men ≥ 40 yr, women ≥ 50 yr	Consider stress test[a]
Coronary prone, all ages	Stress test
Coronary stricken, all ages	Stress test

[a]Tests performed by paramedical personnel to assess baseline exercise capacity.

Note: Age-related criteria adapted from Gibbons RJ, Balady GJ, Beasley JW, et al. ACC/AHA guidelines for exercise testing: executive summary. A Report of the American College of Cardiology/American Heart Association Task Force on Practice Guidelines (Committee on Exercise Testing). Circulation 1997;96:345, with permission.

life-style activities into busy schedules. For example, 30 minutes of activity could be accumulated throughout the day by taking the stairs in lieu of elevators or escalators, walking instead of driving short distances, using fewer labor-saving devices, and doing house or yard work (12,14,15). The theoretical model of the activity options for sedentary persons in Fig. 16.2 shows the equivalent energy expenditures of multiple bouts of life-style activity exercise and planned vigorous exercise (16).

A *physical activity* log can be used to help individuals identify times they spend in sedentary activities. The log may also identify times where bouts of physical activity could be worked into a person's life-style. This offers people who dislike vigorous activity another approach to increasing their activity levels. Moreover, for people who are unable to set aside 30 minutes for physical activity, shorter episodes are clearly better than none.

Inexpensive pedometers can offer a simple way for patients to monitor their changes in activity levels. These small devices are available in most sports stores. Many of them can estimate distance walked or even energy expended by entering the stride length and body weight. Pedometers work best when placed firmly on the belt or waist band of a skirt. Many individuals enjoy logging the number of steps taken each day and use the device to ensure that they are indeed accumulating more activity.

The beneficial effects of low intensity and/or accumulated exercise are the basis for the Surgeon General's guidelines for people who get little or no physical activity: "All children and adults should accumulate at least 30 minutes per day of moderate intensity physical activity on most, preferably all, days of the week" (5). The 1995 document *Physical activity and public health: a recommendation from the Centers for Disease Control and Prevention and the American College of Sports Medicine* (see General References) promotes this approach and stresses that two other components of fitness—flexibility and muscular strength—should not be overlooked. The report advises that people who maintain or improve their strength and flexibility may be better able to perform daily activities, less likely to develop back pain, and better able to avoid disability, especially as they advance into older age.

RESISTANCE EXERCISE

Resistance exercise has long been used to enhance muscle size and strength, and its beneficial relationship to health has only recently been recognized. In 1990, the American College of Sports Medicine added resistance training to their guidelines for exercise training in healthy adults (17). Regular resistance

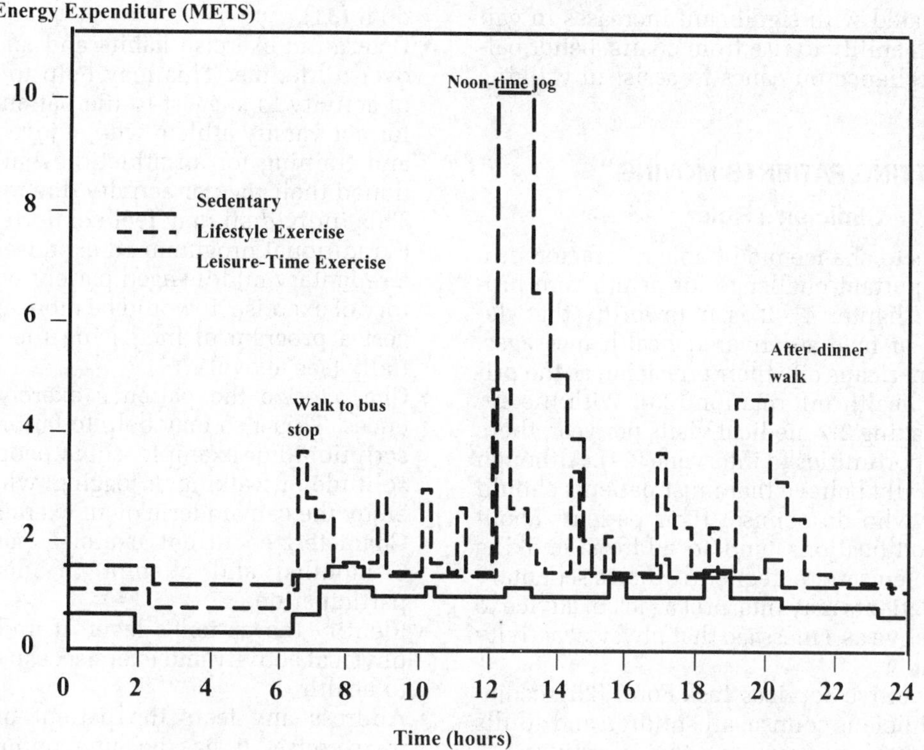

Figure 16.2. Theoretical model of activity options for sedentary persons. The *solid line* indicates the energy expenditure over the course of a day for a sedentary person. The *dashed line* represents the energy expenditure of an individual who engages in planned vigorous exercise during leisure time (such as a jog during lunchtime) but is otherwise sedentary. The *dotted line* illustrates energy expenditure for an individual with a sedentary job who seeks opportunities to accumulate short bouts of physical activity throughout the day. (Adapted from Blair SN, Kohl HW, Gordon NF. Physical activity and health: a lifestyle approach. Med Exerc Nutr Health 1992;1:54, with permission.)

training can result in increased bone mineral density, lean body mass, and muscle strength (18). Moreover, it may lead to improved quality of life and promote independence in the frail elderly patient (19).

Sustained slow-movement activity, often involving small muscle groups against high resistance, is known as *static activity* or *resistive exercise*. Examples are weight lifting, pushups, sit-ups, carrying heavy packages, and hand grips. Most activities requiring lifting and straining, such as shoveling, have a large static component. In such activities there is increased peripheral vascular resistance, with subsequent increase in blood pressure but little increase in heart rate or cardiac output. Such exercises do not bring about enhancement in oxygen extraction, so they are generally not aerobic. Some aerobic-type conditioning is attained when one uses repetitive resistive exercise equipment and sequentially completes 10 to 15 repetitions on a variety of exercise machines, each designed to exercise a different group of muscles (4).

In the healthy person, gradual involvement in activities such as weight lifting may be beneficial and desirable, especially in those whose jobs require static efforts. Brief episodes of moderate resistive exercise occasionally aggravate or cause musculoskeletal symptoms but do not have adverse cardiovascular effects. Recently, the American Heart Association issued a scientific advisory on resistance exercise in individuals with and without cardiovascular disease (see General References). These guidelines note that after careful screening and risk stratification, and when appropriately prescribed, resistance training is an effective method for improving muscular strength and endurance, preventing and managing a variety of chronic medical conditions, modifying cardiac risk factors, and enhancing psychosocial well-being. It is suggested, however, that a resistance training program should complement, rather than replace, an individual's aerobic exercise regime.

Resistance training may be especially beneficial in preserving health in older persons. Muscle dysfunction and atrophy, common among the elderly, increase the risk of falls (a major cause of mortality), bone fractures, and functional dependency. For example, low dynamic quadriceps strength has been found to be associated with difficulties in standing from a seated position in a chair and a shorter distance covered in a 6-minute walk test (20). A number of studies have confirmed the benefits of resistance training in older subjects. An 8-week high intensity resistance training program increased muscle strength and mass and functional mobility among frail nursing homes residents who were on average 90 years of age (19). Other studies have shown that strength gains in the elderly are associated with significant increases in gait speed, improved ability to rise from chairs, better balance, and less reliance on canes to assist in walking (19,21,22).

GETTING PATIENTS MOVING

Clinician's Role

Helping patients to change modifiable risk factors is a difficult but important challenge for health care professionals (see Chapter 4). It is noteworthy that despite a barrage of media-delivered health messages, fully 80% of Americans cite their physician as the primary source of health information (23). With the average patient making 2.7 medical visits per year, there are multiple opportunities to intervene (24). Although clinicians generally believe that most patients should exercise, many who do counsel their patients about health-habit modifications tend to address smoking and weight problems more frequently than a sedentary life-style (23). Patients may interpret a lack of advice to become more active as a message that physical activity is not important.

The U.S. Preventive Services Task Force (25) recommended that clinicians counsel all children and adults to engage in a program of regular physical activity tailored to the individual's health status and life-style. Tailoring messages to meet patients' needs in primary care settings has been found to improve dietary behaviors (26,27), smoking cessation outcomes (28), and activity levels in sedentary patients (29). Many physicians, however, do not feel adequately prepared in the detail of tailoring an exercise prescription for their patients (30).

Prescribing Exercise

A systematic approach to prescribing exercise is essential if one's effort is to be successful.

Exercise/Activity History

To help a patient adopt a more active life-style, it is critical to listen carefully to the patient's description of what barriers exist to increasing their physical activity level and then to build on the patient's preferences. To illustrate how these principles can be applied consider the following case.

Joe is a 51-year-old male who is basically healthy. He works at an office job and was successful in quitting smoking (30 pack-years) but has gained 10 kilograms since. He comes for a checkup. Aside from the usual evaluation, the following series of questions and recommendations should be considered:

- Broach the subject of physical activity, for example, "It must be hard to stay physically active with all the time you need to spend at a desk job."
- Obtain information on the patient's attitudes and beliefs about exercise and establish a desire to begin an exercise program. Many sedentary patients would like to become more active but do not know how to do it (31).
- Determine exercise habits and sports participation over a lifetime. This may help to identify the type of activity to suggest to the patient. For example, a former varsity athlete who enjoyed regular exercise and training for an athletic event may have abandoned their regular activity due to time constraints. This individual may feel comfortable and welcome a traditional programmed exercise prescription. For a sedentary middle-aged patient with no formal history of exercise, it would be more appropriate to suggest a program of increasing life-style activity initially (see above).
- Characterize the patient's exercise/activity preferences. This also may help to tailor the exercise prescription. For example, some people may enjoy the solitude of walking or jogging, whereas other could enjoy the camaraderie of an exercise class.
- Characterize current exercise patterns (past 3 to 6 months) and attempt to identify barriers to participation.
- Identify the patient's level of understanding about physical activity and exercise, especially as it relates to health.
- Address any fears the patient may voice related to exercise. It has become popular for the press to dwell on exercise-related tragedies in elite athletes, in presumably excellent physical condition, who succumbed to sudden cardiac death. Jim Fixx, Johnny Kelly, and Hank Gathers are typical examples of highly fit individuals who died suddenly during exercise. Patients should understand that in reality regular physical activity is associated with lower risks of heart disease. Furthermore, the cardiac risks of moderate intensity activity are considerably less than more intense vigorous exercise (32).

Specifics of an Exercise Prescription

Setting small goals for a patient to achieve between office visits is the best way to start. For example, after establishing baseline levels of physical activity, a first step for a sedentary person could be to prescribe increased life-style activities. The prescription should be very specific, achievable, and realistic. Writing the recommendation on a prescription pad may increase the likelihood of the activity being followed (Fig. 16.3). Table 16.5 lists information useful for planning and writing down exercise prescriptions according to a person's baseline activity profile.

A sequential approach to assessing and recommending physical activity is presented in the flow diagram in Fig. 16.4. Each patient will fit one of three profiles: adequately active, inadequately active, or sedentary. The first step involves assessing current activity levels. For sedentary patients, an exercise history should explore potential strategies to initiate activity as well as the willingness to augment levels of

BAYVIEW MEDICAL CLINIC PATIENT INSTRUCTIONS

Seek to increase your level of activity by 30 minutes each day. This may be done by accumulating your activity throughout the day.
Also reduce the time you spend doing sedentary activities (such as T.V. watching).

Phone back on Oct 1, 2001 550-0530 Signed Ross Andersen Date Aug 1, 2001

*Second copy to be attached to visit note by clerk.

I understand the above instructions: Signed ______________________ (Patient)

PATIENT'S COPY

6731-004 REV. 6/88 ED 6-80

Figure 16.3. Simple written exercise prescription with specific achievable life-style activity goals.

Table 16.5. Exercise Prescription Principles for the Apparently Healthy Adult Based on Current Levels of Physical Activity.

Baseline Activity Profile	Sedentary	Inadequately Active (Irregular Physical Activity)	Adequately Active (Regular Exerciser)
Goals	Decrease health risks Become more active	Improve adherence/become regular exerciser Optimize aerobic fitness	Health maintenance Sports participation or competition
Activity modes	Walking, life-style activity,[a] cycling, low impact aerobics, circuit weight training	Individual aerobic exercise, group exercise classes, resistance training, life-style activity	Individual and group aerobic exercise, competitive games and sports, resistance training
Exertion level	Moderate	Moderate to vigorous	Vigorous
Aerobic exercise	40–60% max HR	50–65% max HR	65–85% max HR
Intensity	Keep constant	Gradually increase	Keep constant
Duration	15–20 min uninterrupted or accumulate 30 min of activity	20–60 min	30–60 min
Frequency	Most days of the week (5–7 days)	3 days or more per week	3–5 days per week
Progression	Start slow, progress gradually Increase duration by 5% per week	Increase frequency by 1 day per week	Maintain or increase current activity and training goals, consider injury risk
Counseling style	Empathic listening/ supportive/encouraging	Praising accomplishments and problem solving with the patient	Informative

[a]Activity that can be incorporated into a person's existing life-style (e.g., using stairs, walking instead of driving short distances).

Adapted from Andersen RE, Blair SN, Cheskin L, et al. Encouraging patients to become more physically active: the physicians role. *Ann Intern Med* 1997;127:395, with permission.

activity. During follow-up visits, exercise participation should routinely be readdressed, commended, and/or encouraged anew.

Exercise Adherence

Despite the best intentions, half of all adults who begin or renew an exercise program will fail to maintain it at the level they intended (33). In a typical supervised setting, about 50% of the clients will drop out within 6 months to a year (34). Thus, the focus of an exercise or activity program should be not only to decrease sedentary living but also to focus on long-term adherence to the program.

A list of barriers and predictors of regular exercise adherence is shown in Table 16.6. A sincere recommendation from one's primary care practitioner to begin an activity program may be one of the strongest predictors of long-term exercise (35). During subsequent office visits, showing interest in and encouraging the patient's physical activity can be very helpful in increasing adherence. Even small steps in the right direction are helpful and worthy of approval.

It is also important to capitalize on the fact that persons who are aware of the health benefits of exercise are more likely to become regular exercisers (36). Printed materials and list of suggested reading can help the patient to self-educate and may also enhance adherence (Table 16.3).

A *lack of time* is one of the most common reasons cited by adults for not exercising. Let patients know that three programmed workouts per week for minimum of 20 minutes is optimal but that doing something is much better than no activity at all because the greatest gains to health, as described earlier, are derived by moving from being totally sedentary to a moderate level of fitness. In many cases, patients are able to find more time for exercising once they become active and notice results from the program.

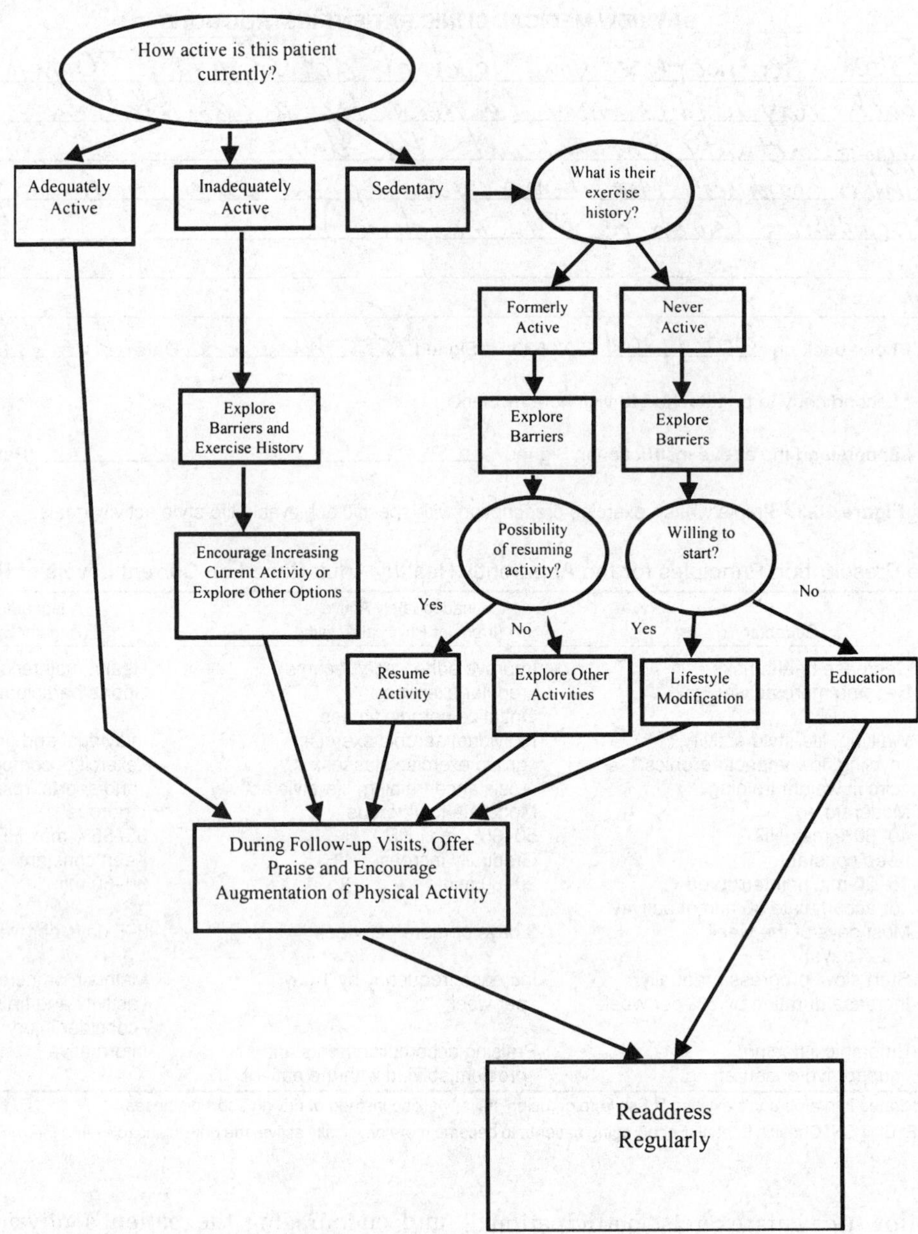

Figure 16.4. A framework for physicians to initiate discussion about exercise and physical activity. (From Christmas C, Andersen RE. Exercise and older patients: guidelines for the clinician. J Am Geriatr Soc 2000;48:318, with permission.)

Table 16.6. Barriers and Predictors of Exercise Adherence

Predictor	Barrier
Physician's suggestion	Time interruption
Time-efficient routine	Lack of interest in exercise
Freedom from injury	Musculoskeletal injury
Instruction	Lack of knowledge
Feedback on fitness progress	Inadequate leadership
Spouse and peer approval	Lack of spousal support
Group participation	Poor progress awareness
Past participation	Boredom
Risk of disease	High intensity exercise
Regular routine	Inclement weather

Periodic *feedback* on health improvements related to life-style improvement can lead to renewed enthusiasm. Recording prescribed physical activity in patient charts can help with follow-up office visits and exercise-related discussions. Reductions in resting heart rate, blood pressure, body weight, and waist circumference are all findings that can be pointed out as evidence of success. Improved serum lipid profiles may also accompany a moderate intensity exercise program.

Choosing the intensity level is important. Sedentary persons who begin exercising at moderate intensities are more likely to adhere to their programs than those who begin vigorously. Excessive frequencies (e.g., more than 5 days per week) or intensities that the patient perceives as being "hard" may also lead to higher dropout rates (34,36). The Borg Rating of Perceived Exertion scale can be used to help patients understand and select the appropriate exercise intensities (37). When beginning an exercise program, sedentary adults should perceive that they are working "somewhat hard" but not "very hard" on the 20-point Borg Scale (see scale, Fig. 63.7). As noted above (Table 16.2), heart rate can be used in the healthy adult as an indication of aerobic level activity.

To *reduce the risk of injury*, patients should be encouraged to warm up, stretching the muscles they will be exercising at the beginning of an exercise session. Progression should be moderate as well, because many overzealous new exercisers injure themselves when increasing the intensity of their workouts too quickly. A 5% per week increase in the duration or intensity of training sessions will help to reduce the risk of injury. Individuals who use exercise equipment should also be encouraged to learn how to adjust the equipment to minimize injury risk. For example, a bicycle seat that is set too low may result in knee pain. Patients should be encouraged to seek out advice on proper equipment adjustment and body alignment during exercise from the home fitness stores where equipment is purchased or from local health clubs.

A deconditioned patient who is unaccustomed to regular activity risks an overuse injury from starting out too vigorously. Exercise-related injuries predictably increase the risk of dropping out of exercise programs.

Appropriate footwear is important for all individuals who exercise, but even more so for those who are overweight or who suffer from joint or bone problems. High quality shoes can dramatically reduce the risk of overuse injuries. Selecting appropriate footwear can be somewhat daunting for many beginning exercisers because there are hundreds of shoes to pick from. Encouraging patients to purchase their shoes from a vendor that specializes in athletic footwear will ensure that they receive a "sport-specific" shoe that is properly fitted. Popular running magazines and fitness magazines publish annual ranking of the top footwear for each type of shoe on the market. For persons whose main activity will be walking, the features of appropriate shoes are illustrated in Chapter 73.

Patients who choose walking or jogging as a mode of activity should be encouraged to exercise on appropriate terrain. Hard surfaces should be avoided when possible. For example, walking or running on concrete walks can cause ankle, knee, and hip injuries. Uneven or canted surfaces (e.g., beaches or crowned roads) may result in knee problems as well. Cross-training or performing different types of activity may also help to reduce risk of injury and boredom.

Long-term exercise adherence has been found to be related to *support* from spouses, friends, exercise leaders, and family (33,34,38). Physicians can also become a vital link in their patient's social support network, even if contact is not frequent.

General References*

Blair SN. Living with exercise. Dallas, TX: American Health Publishing, 1991.

This book shows the reader how to look for opportunities to be more physically active.

Cotton RT, Andersen RE, eds. Clinical exercise specialist manual: ACE's source for training special populations. San Diego, CA: American Council on Exercise, 1999.

This textbook has 27 chapters that outline how people with various chronic diseases can adopt a more active life-style.

Dunn AL, Andersen RE, Jakicic JM. Lifestyle physical activity interventions: history, short- and long-term effects, and recommendations. Am J Prev Med 1998;15:398.

This review paper examines the literature on physical activity intervention trials.

Dunn AL, Marcus BH, Kampert JB, et al. Comparison of lifestyle and structured interventions to increase physical activity and cardiorespiratory fitness: a randomized trial. JAMA 1999;281:327.

This is largest intervention done comparing the comparable effects of life-style activity to aerobic exercise.

Peterson DM. **Exercise and physical activity in the adult population: a general internist's perspective.** J Gen Intern Med 1993;8:149.

Review of benefits and risks of physical activity. Contains specific instructions for patients for whom the primary physician recommends exercise.

Physical activity and cardiovascular health. NIH Consensus Statement 13(3):1–33, Dec. 18–20, 1995.

Expert panel review of data recommending physical activity as a major focus for prevention.

Physical activity and public health: a recommendation from the Centers for Disease Control and Prevention and the American College of Sports Medicine. JAMA 1995;273:4.

Summary statements by organizations heading effort to promote increasing physical activity as a means of prevention.

Pollock ML, Franklin BA, Balady GJ, et al. **Resistance exercise in individuals with and without cardiovascular disease (American Heart Association Science Advisory).** Circulation 2000;101:828.

Well-referenced article on benefits, exercise modalities, and safety of resistance exercise in persons with or without cardiovascular disease.

1996 Surgeon General's report on physical activity and health (S/N 017-023-01196-5). U.S. Department of Health and Human Services, Centers for Disease Control and Prevention, National Center for Chronic Disease Prevention and Health Promotion, The President's Council on Physical Fitness and Sports.

Reviews and summarizes the benefits of life-style changes.

Specific References*

1. U.S. Department of Health and Human Services. Healthy People 1020, 2nd ed. 2 vols. Washington, DC: U.S. Government Printing Office, November 2000.
2. Crespo CJ, Keteyian SJ, Snelling A, et al. Prevalence of no leisure-time physical activity in persons with chronic disease. Clin Exerc Physiol 2000;1:68.
3. Crespo CJ, Smit E, Andersen RE, et al. Race/ethnicity, social class and their relation to physical inactivity during leisure time: results from the Third National Health and Nutrition Examination Survey, 1988–1994. Am J Prev Med 2000;18:46.
4. **4.** Fletcher GF, Balady G, Blair SN, et al. Statement on exercise: benefits and recommendations for physical activity programs for all Americans. A statement for health professionals by the Committee on Exercise and Cardiac Rehabilitation of the Council on Clinical Cardiology, American Heart Association. Circulation 1996;94:857.

*Bold print (general references) and bold numerals (specific references) denote published controlled clinical trials, meta-analyses, or consensus-based recommendations.

5. U.S. Department of Health and Human Services. Physical activity and health: a report of the Surgeon General. Atlanta, GA: U.S. Department of Health and Human Services, Centers for Disease Control and Prevention, National Center for Chronic Disease Prevention and Health Promotion, 1996.
6. Blair SN, Kohl HW, Paffenbarger RS. Physical fitness and all-cause mortality: a prospective study of healthy men and women. JAMA 1989;262:2395.
7. Paffenbarger RS, Hide RT, Wing AL, et al. Physical activity, all-cause mortality, and longevity of college alumni. N Engl J Med 1986;314:605.
8. Paffenbarger RS Jr, Kampert JB, Lee I-M, et al. Changes in physical activity and other lifestyle patterns influencing longevity. Med Sci Sports Exerc 1994;26:857.
9. Blair SN, Kohl HW III, Barlow CE, et al. Changes in physical fitness and all-cause mortality: a prospective study of healthy and unhealthy men. JAMA 1995;273:1093.
10. Andersen RE, Wadden TA, Bartlett SJ, et al. Effects of lifestyle activity vs structured aerobic exercise in obese women. JAMA 1999;281:335.
11. Dunn AL, Marcus BH, Kampert JB, et al. Comparison of lifestyle and structured interventions to increase physical activity and cardiorespiratory fitness: a randomized trial. JAMA 1999;281:327.
12. Dunn AL, Andersen RE, Jakicic JM. Lifestyle physical activity interventions: history, short- and long-term effects, and recommendations. Am J Prev Med 1998;15:398.
13. Jakicic JM, Winters C, Lang W, et al. Effects of intermittent exercise and use of home exercise equipment on adherence, weight loss, and fitness in overweight women: a randomized trial. JAMA 1999;282:1554.
14. Blair SN. 1993 C.H. McCloy Research Lecture: physical activity, physical fitness, and health. Res Q Exerc Sport 1993;64: 365.
15. Blair SN. Living with exercise. Dallas, TX: American Health Publishing, 1991.
16. Blair SN, Kohl HW III, Gordon NF. Physical activity and health: a lifestyle approach. Med Exerc Nutr Health 1992;1: 54.
17. American College of Sports Medicine. Recommended quantity and quality of exercise for developing and maintaining cardiorespiratory and muscular fitness in healthy adults. Med Sci Sports Exerc 1990;22:265.
18. Pollock ML, Wilmore JH. Exercise in health and disease: evaluation and prescription for prevention and rehabilitation. Philadelphia: W.B. Saunders, 1997.
19. Fiatrone MA, O'Neill EF, Ryan ND, et al. Exercise training and nutritional supplementation for physical frailty in very elderly people. N Engl J Med 1994;330:1769.
20. Cress ME, Schechtman KB, Mulrow CD, et al. Relationship between physical performance and self-perceived physical function. J Am Geriatr Soc 1995;43:93.
21. Fiatrone MA, Marks EC, Ryan ND, et al. High-intensity strength training in nonagenarians. JAMA 1990;263:3029.
22. Nelson ME, Fiatarone MA, Morganti CM, et al. Effects of high-intensity strength training on multiple risk factors for osteoporotic fractures. A randomized controlled trial. JAMA 1994;272:1909.
23. Weaver FJ, Herrick KL, Ramirez AG, et al. Establishing a community data-base for cardiovascular health education programs. Health Values 1978;2:249.
24. Shappert SM. National ambulatory medical care survey: 1991 summary, advance data from Vital and Health Statistics. 1993; no. 230.
25. Harris SS, Caspersen CJ, DeFriese GH, et al. Physical activity counseling for healthy adults as a primary preventive intervention in the clinical setting: report for the U.S. Preventive Services Task Force. JAMA 1989;261:3590.
26. Kramish-Campbell M, DeVellis BM, Strecher VJ, et al. Improving dietary behavior: the effectiveness of tailored messages in primary care settings. Am J Public Health 1994;84:783.
27. Strecher VJ, O'Malley MS, Villagra VG, et al. Can residents be trained to counsel patients about smoking? J Gen Intern Med 1991;6:9.
28. Strecher VJ, Reuter M, Boer DJ, et al. The effects of computer tailored smoking cessation messages in family practice settings. J Fam Pract 1994;39:262.
29. Strecher VJ, Seijts GH, Kok GJ, et al. Goal setting as a strategy for health behavior change. Health Educ Q 1995;22:190.
30. Patrick K, Sallis JF, Long B, et al. A new tool for encouraging activity: Project PACE. Phys Sports Med 1994;22:245.
31. Pollock ML. Prescribing exercise for fitness and adherence. In: Dishman RK, eds. Exercise adherence: its impact on public health. Champaigne, IL: Human Kinetics, 1988:259.
32. Kohl HW III, Powell KE, Gordon NF, et al. Physical activity, physical fitness, and sudden cardiac death. Epidemiol Rev 1992;14:37.
33. Dishman RK. Determinants of participation in activity. In: Bouchard C, Shephard RJ, Stephens T, et al., eds. Exercise, fitness, and health: a consensus of current knowledge. Champaigne, IL: Human Kinetics, 1990:75.
34. King AC, Blair SN, Bild DE. Determinants of physical activity and interventions in adults. Med Sci Sports Exerc 1992;24:S221.
35. Marcus BH, Pinto BM, Clark MM, et al. Physician-delivered physical activity and nutrition interventions. Med Exerc Nutr Health 1995;4:325.
36. Rohm-Young D, King AC. Exercise adherence: determinants of physical activity and applications of health behavior change theories. Med Exerc Nutr Health 1995;4:335.
37. Borg GAV. Psychological bases of perceived exertion. Med Sci Sports Exerc 1982;14:377.
38. Dishman RK. Supervised and free-living physical activity: no differences in former athletes and nonathletes. Am J Prev Med 1988;4:153.

CHAPTER 17

Genetic Testing and Counseling

JENNIFER E. SOLLENBERGER, MS
CONSTANCE A. GRIFFIN, MD

Numerous genes present in normal-appearing individuals can affect an individual's susceptibility to disease or contribute to the way an individual metabolizes particular drugs. Generalist physicians need to be able to recognize genetic syndromes that may have a significant impact on their patients' future health. The goal of this chapter is to provide an overview of basic genetics, to summarize currently recognized genetic syndromes important in the practice of adult medicine, and to describe the role of genetic testing and counseling in today's medical practice.

PRIMER OF BASIC GENETICS AND INHERITANCE

Genetic Code

The genetic code is spelled out in our DNA. DNA is built of a combination of nucleotides, including purines (adenine [A], guanine [G]) and pyrimidines (cytosine [C], thymine [T]). DNA is further arranged in a double helix, held together by hydrogen bonds between the complementary bases (A pairs with T, C pairs with G). The 20 amino acids found in the proteins of humans are spelled out using the four nucleotide bases. A sequence of three bases is called a *codon;* each codon codes for a specific amino acid. Because 64 combinations of bases are possible ($4 \times 4 \times 4$), the code is redundant, meaning that some amino acids are coded for by several different combinations of bases. The gene specified by the DNA is transcribed into messenger RNA and via the action of RNA is translated into specific proteins. Not all DNA codes for proteins. Some DNA codes for "worker" RNA. Other DNA has structural functions at parts of the chromosomes called centromeres. The function of much of the DNA is unknown. The process of translating the code from our DNA to the specified gene product (i.e., protein) is complex and requires editing functions that are specified in the code itself.

DNA is packaged into *chromosomes,* which are physical structures in the cell nucleus consisting of DNA and associated proteins. Humans have 46 chromosomes, arranged in 23 pairs. Twenty-two of these pairs are *autosomes,* meaning they are found in both males and females. The 23rd pair, consisting of XX or XY, specifies the individual's sex. During production of germline cells, namely eggs or sperm, the chromosomes undergo a reduction to haploidy, or a single set of chromosomes. When fertilization occurs, diploidy (two sets) is restored by the combination of one set of chromosomes from the mother and one set from the father.

In the process of duplicating our DNA, copy changes can occur. *Polymorphisms* are alterations that occur in the genetic code for a protein but that do not result in loss of function of the protein. The term *mutation* is generally reserved for changes in DNA sequence, which alter the coded protein significantly. Types of mutations observed range from single base pair substitutions, insertions or deletions of one or a few bases, to mutations that cause a shift in the DNA reading frame resulting in a premature stop of protein translation.

Types of Inheritance

Gregor Mendel described the basic types of inheritance, and from his name comes the term "Mendelian inheritance." This term describes single-gene inheritance. Individuals have two copies (alleles) of each gene and receive one copy of each gene from the germ cells of each parent. *Autosomal dominant disease* requires only a single abnormal copy of the gene to manifest disease. Examples of autosomal dominant diseases include Huntington disease and many of the recognized cancer predisposition syndromes. *Autosomal recessive diseases* require the inheritance of an abnormal copy of the gene from both the mother and the father. Cystic fibrosis is a well-known example in which phenotypically normal parents are only recognized to be carriers of a mutant allele when they have a child who has inherited the dysfunctional forms of the gene from both parents. *Sex-linked disease* means that the disease gene is located on a sex chromosome. Most sex-linked diseases are linked to the X chromosome. With X-linked inheritance, women typically do not manifest disease even when they inherit a mutant gene because the normal copy of the gene on their other X chromosome compensates. Men, with only a single copy of the X chromosome, are not protected by a normal gene copy and therefore manifest disease. Duchenne muscular dystrophy and hemophilia A are examples of sex-linked diseases.

Other disorders, including common diseases such as diabetes mellitus and hypertension, may involve the interactive effects of multiple genes. This is referred to as *polygenic or multifactorial inheritance,* and simple rules of Mendelian inheritance seem not to be in play here. *Mitochondrial inheritance* describes yet another form of inheritance, because mitochondria, and therefore the genome of the mitochondria, are inherited only from the egg of the mother. Mitochondrial diseases include oxidative phosphorylation disorders, and widely varying manifestations can include specific types of cardiomyopathy, deafness, skeletal myopathy, and renal tubular acidoses, to name just a few.

The term *genotype* describes the genetic composition of an individual, whereas the term *phenotype* refers to the physical manifestations of a given genetic blueprint. Similar phenotypes can result from mutations in different genes presumably in related pathways; the specific molecular alteration in a gene may also relate to the phenotype observed. *Penetrance* of a gene refers to the likelihood that an abnormal form of a gene will be observed to cause an abnormal phenotype during an individual's lifetime. Some genes are high penetrance, such as those causing the hereditary forms of breast and ovarian cancer. Such individuals have a lifetime risk of developing breast cancer that is as high as 85%. Other genes are of relatively low penetrance, such as the I1307K mutation in the *APC* gene. This mutation is found in approximately 6% of the Ashkenazi Jewish population and is correlated with a lifetime colon cancer risk estimated to be between 10% and 30%. The interaction of environmental exposure, mutation repair, and the presence of other modifier genes presumably combine to affect the expression of disease.

CORE COMPETENCIES IN GENETICS

Health care professionals ordering genetic testing must be adequately trained to provide genetic counseling, obtain informed consent, and correctly interpret test results. Because availability of specialized genetics services is still limited, the generalist may be called upon to provide genetic counseling as part of routine care. The Core Competency Working Group of the National Coalition for Health Professional Education in Genetics has proposed a set of core competencies in genetics, of which the major components are listed here. The original publication describes the competencies in their entirety (1).

All health professionals should understand the following:

- The basic patterns of biologic inheritance and variation within families and populations;
- How identification of disease-associated genetic variations facilitates development of prevention, diagnosis, and treatment options;
- The difference between clinical diagnosis of disease and identification of genetic predisposition to disease;
- The influence of ethnicity, culture, related health beliefs, and economics in the client's ability to use genetic information and services;
- The potential physical and/or psychosocial benefits, limitations, and risks of genetic information for individuals, family members, and communities;
- The ethical, legal, and social issues related to genetic testing and recording of genetic information;
- The resources available to assist clients seeking genetic information or services;
- One's own professional role in the referral to genetic services or provision, follow-up, and quality review of genetic services.

All health professionals should be able to:

- Gather genetic family history information, including an appropriate (minimum three generations) family history;
- Identify clients who would benefit from genetic services;
- Explain basic concepts of probability and disease susceptibility and the influence of genetic factors in maintenance of health and development of disease;
- Seek assistance from and refer to appropriate genetics experts and peer support resources;
- Obtain credible current information about genetics for self, clients, and colleagues;
- Recognize the importance of delivering genetic education and counseling fairly, accurately, and without coercion or personal bias;
- Seek coordination and collaboration with an interdisciplinary team of health professionals;
- Recognize the limitations of their own genetics expertise.

The need for these competencies is illustrated in a study by Giardiello et al. (2), who examined physicians' ordering and interpretation of genetic testing for familial adenomatous polyposis (FAP). Eighty-three percent of tests were ordered for valid indications, but only 18.6% of patients received genetic counseling, only 16.9% of patients provided written consent, and 31.6% of test results were misinterpreted by the ordering physician.

IDENTIFYING PATIENTS AT RISK FOR GENETIC DISORDERS

In contrast to genetic diseases recognized in childhood, such as cystic fibrosis or Duchenne muscular dystrophy, a number of other genetic disorders, in addition to hereditary cancer, may not be recognized until one is an adult. Many, such as Marfan syndrome or neurofibromatosis types 1 and 2, have major clinical phenotypic manifestations and very specific

Table 17.1. Examples of Genetic Diseases with Specific Phenotypic Features for Which Genetic Testing Is Available

Disease	Characteristics	Gene(s) Involved	Type of Inheritance	Clinical Management	Comments
Marfan syndrome	Systemic disorder of connective tissue; high variability. Tall, thin, with long limbs, hands, feet	*FBN1*	AD	At risk for dislocated lens, aortic root dilitation, mitral valve prolapse, scoliosis	Clinical molecular testing by linkage analysis; 25% of cases are new mutations (no history of disease in family)
Fragile X syndrome	Moderate mental retardation in males; mild mental retardation in affected females; abnormal faces	*FMR* (triple repeat expansion)	X-linked dominant	Supportive care; genetic counseling for family members	Prevalence about 20/100,000 males; mothers of affected individuals carry presymptomatic gene expansion
Huntington disease	Progressive motor, cognitive, psychiatric disorder	*HD* (triple repeat expansion)	AD	Only symptomatic treatment; genetic counseling of family members	Presymptomatic genetic testing preceded by extensive genetic counseling
Neurofibromatosis type 1	Multiple café au lait spots, neurofibromas, axillary/ inguinal freckling; extreme clinical variability	*NF1*	AD	Annual physical exam with attention to features of NF1, especially hypertension and malignant tumors	One of most common AD-inherited disorders; prevalence 1/3,000; 50% of cases are new mutations
Neurofibromatosis type 2	Bilateral vestibular schwannomas	*NF2*	AD	About 1/2 also develop meningiomas; 2/3 develop spinal tumors	Prevalence 1/37,000. Main role of DNA-based testing is early detection of at-risk children of affected parents

AD, autosomal dominant.

Table 17.2. Examples of Genetic Diseases Without Specific Phenotypic Features for Which Genetic Testing Is Available

Disease	Characteristics	Gene(s) Involved	Type of Inheritance	Clinical Management	Comments
Hereditary hemochromatosis	Excessive iron storage in liver, heart, pancreas, other organs. Penetrance >90% for homozygotes.	*HFE*	AR	Removal of excess iron	Diagnosis of clinical disease requires clinical, biochemical, histologic, and gene studies. Carrier frequency estimated at 1/9.
Factor V Leiden	Increased risk for venous thrombosis.	*F5* ("Leiden" mutation is specific single base change)	AD	Prolonged anticoagulation following thrombotic event	Mutation found in 20% of patients with venous thrombosis.
Platelet glycoprotein IIIA	Risk factor for coronary thrombosis.	*PLA2* mutation	AD	May benefit from statin or specific antithrombotic therapy	Mutation prevalence three times higher in individuals <60 with myocardial ischemia.

AD, autosomal dominant disease; AR, autosomal recessive disease.

diagnostic criteria (see Online Mendelian Inheritance in Man, General References). Genetic testing is available for many of these disorders, a subset of which is illustrated in Table 17.1. In contrast, a number of inherited diseases lack specific phenotypic features but may present with abnormal laboratory values or with common clinical events such as venous thrombosis (see examples in Table 17.2).

Profile of a Common Inherited Disease: Hemochromatosis

Hereditary hemochromatosis is a genetic disease with significant implications for the generalist. It is an autosomally recessively inherited disease, in which early diagnosis and treatment can lead to a normal to near-normal lifespan; the phenotypic manifestations are not usually apparent before significant iron overload has occurred. Because one in nine individuals in the population carries a mutant *HFE* allele, the prevalence of individuals with two disease-causing mutations is high, estimated at approximately 1 in 400. Mutations in the *HFE* gene result in inappropriately high absorption of iron by the gastrointestinal tract. Excess iron stores in the liver, pancreas, heart, skin, and other organs first produce only nonspecific symptoms, but left untreated, ultimately patients develop hepatic fibrosis or cirrhosis, diabetes mellitus, congestive heart failure, and other problems. Symptoms usually develop between ages 40 and 60 in males and somewhat later in females, after menopause.

Diagnosis in patients with symptoms is usually based on a serum transferrin iron saturation of more than 60% for men and more than 50% for women on at least two different determinations, in the absence of other causes of primary and secondary iron overload disorders. *Heterozygotes* (individuals carrying one copy of normal allele and one copy of mutant allele) do tend to have serum iron and ferritin and transferrin saturation levels that exceed normal but do not develop clinical iron overload. Confirmatory tests after the elevated transferrin iron saturation then

Table 17.3. Examples of Hereditary Cancers for Which Genetic Testing Is Available

Disease	Characteristics	Gene(s) Involved	Type of Inheritance	Clinical Management	Comments
Hereditary nonpolyposis colon cancer (HNPCC)	Early onset colon cancer, uterine cancer, other cancers; 80% penetrance	Mutation in one of several mismatch repair genes (*MLH1, MSH2, PMS1, PMS2, MSH3, MSH6*)	AD	Yearly colonoscopy minimizes chance of developing invasive colon cancer	Accounts for about 5% of colon cancer
Familial adenomatous polyposis (FAP)	Colonic polyposis results in early age colon cancer, 100% penetrance	Mutations in *APC* gene	AD	Prophylactic colectomy	Accounts for about 1% of colon cancer
I1307K predisposition to colon cancer	10%–30% lifetime risk of colon cancer	Single base pair change in *APC* gene	AD	Biyearly colonoscopy	Mutation limited to Ashkenazi Jewish population
Hereditary breast cancer	Early onset breast/ovarian cancer; male breast cancer	Mutations in *BRCA1, BRCA2*	AD	Frequent breast and ovarian surveillance	Carriers have 50%–85% lifetime risk of breast cancer
Multiple endocrine neoplasia (MEN) type 1	Parathyroid, pancreatic islet, and pituitary tumors; parathyroid adenomas in 90% of patients	*MEN1*	AD	Screening in family with MEN1 begins at ages 5–10 yr	Multicentricity of tumor suggests familial syndrome
MEN type 2a, 2b	Medullary thyroid cancer, pheochromocytoma, parathyroid hyperplasia	*RET*	AD	Screening and prophylactic thyroidectomy as early as age 5	Genetic testing is now gold standard for MEN2a screening

AD, autosomal dominant disease; AR, autosomal recessive disease.

include liver biopsy or genetic testing for the two mutations that have been observed. Between 60% and 90% of patients with hereditary hemochromatosis (varies with the population) are *homozygotes* (individuals in whom both alleles of a gene are mutant) for the missense mutation C282Y. About 3% are *compound heterozygotes:* they have one copy of the C282Y mutation and their second copy of the *HFE* gene contains a different missense mutation (H63D). The remainder of individuals with clinical manifestations of hereditary hemochromatosis have other mutations in the *HFE* gene or no identifiable mutation in the *HFE* gene. Molecular identification of the type(s) of mutations present in an affected individual is important, because C282Y homozygotes have greater degrees of iron overload than do compound heterozygotes. Identification of mutation in affected individuals allows predictive testing in their at-risk siblings and children. Treatment of hereditary hemochromatosis is by phlebotomy at regular intervals.

Identifying Patients at Risk for Hereditary Cancer

Most cancers are sporadic or nonhereditary in origin. However, approximately 5% to 10% of all cancers are believed to be caused by inherited mutations in cancer-related genes. The characteristics of hereditary cancer include one or more of the following:

- Two or more family members affected with the same type of cancer;
- More than one person in a single generation affected with the same type of cancer;
- Relatives in more than one generation affected with the same type of cancer;
- Ages at diagnosis younger than those seen in the general population;
- A single individual with more than one primary cancer;
- Clustering of two or more types of cancer known to be linked to a particular syndrome (e.g., breast and ovarian; colon and uterine);
- Male breast cancer.

Table 17.3 contains information about selected cancers for which genetic testing is available. Several excellent reviews describe the currently recognized cancer predisposition syndromes (3,4). Those identified thus far are those that are strongly influenced by a single gene. The role of additional genes, each of which might contribute a more moderate risk for cancer development, will undoubtedly be elucidated in the future.

GENETIC COUNSELING AND TESTING

The impact of genetic testing on the health of patients has not yet been subjected to extensive clinical trials. In the coming decade, it is likely that much will be learned about this evolving area of preventive medicine. The approach to testing for genetic susceptibility to disease begins with genetic counseling. The flow diagram in Fig. 17.1 illustrates the decisions in this process, beginning with the generalist physician's recognition of a possible genetic disorder and the decision to offer referral for genetic counseling. Because much of the currently available genetic testing and counseling in adults is cancer related, Fig. 17.1 and the following sections describe the approach to an individual or family in which there may be a hereditary predisposition to cancer. The same approach would pertain to evaluation of other inherited diseases, infertility, and in prenatal diagnostics.

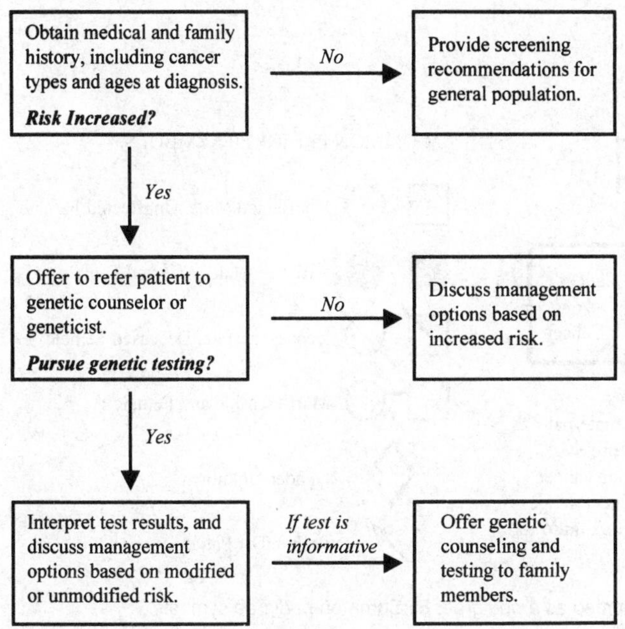

Figure 17.1. Recommended approach for a patient contemplating genetic testing for hereditary cancer.

Overview of Genetic Counseling for Hereditary Cancers

To ensure that genetic tests are ordered appropriately and interpreted accurately, it is important, whenever possible, to enlist the help of a practitioner trained in cancer genetics. *Genetic counselors* are health care professionals who typically hold a masters level graduate degree in the field of genetics. The American Board of Genetic Counseling currently certifies approximately 1,500 genetic counselors (not limited to cancer). Genetic counselors who specialize in hereditary cancer syndromes are typically located in larger cities, but some may be involved in outreach clinics to less populated areas. The National Society of Genetic Counselors maintains a directory of genetic counselors and their affiliated institutions. The cost of a genetic counseling visit usually ranges from $150 to $300. Depending on the problem, patients may need to return for one or more visits.

Genetic counseling is generally undertaken in a nondirective fashion (5). Because the decision to undergo genetic testing has family, societal, and insurance implications, it must be an informed decision made by the person who will be tested. Except for hereditary cancer syndromes that have onset in childhood and for which treatment is available, testing is not performed on children. These exceptions currently include FAP, which requires colon screening beginning at puberty, and multiple endocrine neoplasia type 2, for which thyroidectomy at a very young age is standard of care.

When a patient schedules a genetic counseling session, a detailed medical history is obtained. Often the patient is asked to return background information in advance. If the patient has been diagnosed with cancer, relevant information includes type and location of the cancer, age at diagnosis, how the cancer was diagnosed, stage at diagnosis, whether or not the cancer was bilateral, history of other cancers, history of other chronic medical conditions, and history of exposures to carcinogens. Pathology reports are extremely useful when obtaining personal or family history, because patients often have difficulty distinguishing specific cancer types, such as uterine and ovarian or colon and prostate, or distinguishing between primary cancers and recurrences or metastases.

The *proband* is the individual who comes for consultation. The *consultand* identifies the parent(s) who comes for consultation when the proband is a minor. The family history is the key to identifying a hereditary pattern of cancer within a family. Information about the proband and his or her parents, aunts, uncles, cousins, siblings, and children is obtained and diagramed into a three-generation *pedigree* (6) (Fig. 17.2). This diagram makes traits inherited in a Mendelian manner easier to recognize. Included is information about unaffected as well as affected relatives. For each family member, the same information collected on the proband is necessary. It is important to recognize that in some diseases, such as FAP, the rate of new germline mutations is high (approximately 30%), and there may be no family history of disease. However, an individual with a new germline mutation can still pass on the disease to his or her children.

If the medical and family history is suspicious for inherited cancer susceptibility, this is discussed with the patient. The patient is educated on the characteristics of hereditary cancer, basic information regarding genetics, and various patterns of disease inheritance. Specific hereditary cancer syndromes are discussed, and if applicable genetic testing is explained in detail. The risks, benefits, and limitations of genetic testing are overviewed, and the most informative approach to testing is determined. In addition, the patient is told about possible discrimination and about the most current legal decisions regarding genetic testing.

Management of cancer risk is then discussed, both with patients interested in genetic testing and those who prefer not to pursue such an analysis. Management options include increased surveillance, chemoprevention, prophylactic surgery, and life-style alterations. For some disorders, such as FAP or inherited forms of breast or ovarian cancer, consideration of prophylactic surgery may be indicated, whereas for others, a specific surveillance regimen is more appropriate. Because the genes that cause cancer syndromes have been identified only recently, there is virtually no evidence-based data regarding the impact of preventive behaviors, such as low-fat diet, exercise, and so forth, on the development of cancer in mutation-positive individuals. Because the disorders most often discussed are hereditary, some patients also seek information regarding various reproductive options.

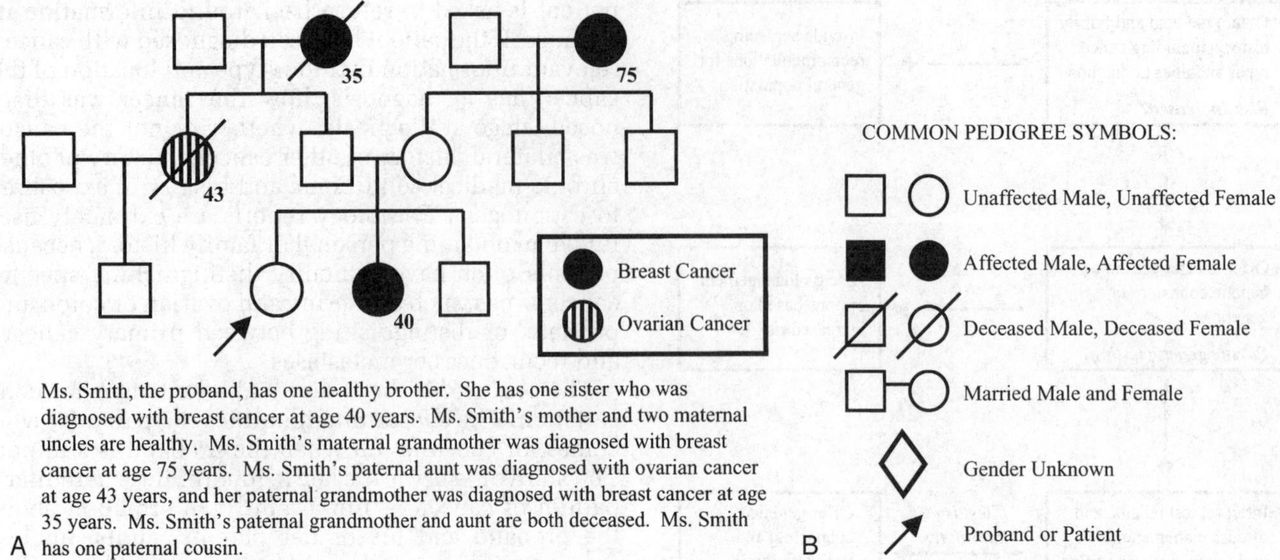

35
75
43
40
Breast Cancer
Ovarian Cancer
Ms. Smith, the proband, has one healthy brother. She has one sister who was diagnosed with breast cancer at age 40 years. Ms. Smith's mother and two maternal uncles are healthy. Ms. Smith's maternal grandmother was diagnosed with breast cancer at age 75 years. Ms. Smith's paternal aunt was diagnosed with ovarian cancer at age 43 years, and her paternal grandmother was diagnosed with breast cancer at age 35 years. Ms. Smith's paternal grandmother and aunt are both deceased. Ms. Smith has one paternal cousin.
A
COMMON PEDIGREE SYMBOLS:
Unaffected Male, Unaffected Female
Affected Male, Affected Female
Deceased Male, Deceased Female
Married Male and Female
Gender Unknown
Proband or Patient
B

Figure 17.2. A: Example of a patient's family history diagrammed as a pedigree. **B:** Common pedigree symbols.

Genetic test results may be positive, negative, or inconclusive (see below). Therefore, if a patient chooses to undergo genetic testing, he or she usually must return to the genetic counselor to receive an accurate interpretation the results of the test. At this visit, previous management recommendations may be altered based on the genetic test results. In addition, if there are genetic testing recommendations for other family members, they are often outlined during this visit.

Overview of Genetic Testing for Hereditary Cancers

Peripheral blood is usually the specimen of choice for genetic testing. Although some specific testing can be performed on paraffin-embedded formalin-fixed pathology specimens, the preservation of DNA in the specimen may be inadequate for the technical requirements of many of the analytical processes currently in use. The specific type of laboratory test that is performed is related to the type of alteration being sought. Some disease-causing mutations tend to occur in one area or a limited number of areas of a gene, and testing can be confidently limited to those regions (Table 17.3). An example is multiple endocrine neoplasia type 2b, where over 90% of cases have the same mutation. For other genetic disorders, such as hereditary nonpolyposis colon cancer (HNPCC) and *BRCA*-linked breast cancer, mutations in the relevant genes can occur over many thousands of bases. These mutations must be sought using screening techniques to identify portions of the gene that subsequently must then undergo DNA sequencing. For this reason, genetic testing ideally begins with an affected individual, so that one can define the mutation being sought. If testing detects a specific disease-causing mutation in an affected individual, this is termed *positive.* Individuals in that family can then be tested for that specific mutation if they wish and receive definitive (*positive* or *true negative*) results. The test is deemed *inconclusive* if an affected individual is tested but no mutation is found. It is also inconclusive if an affected individual is not available for testing and testing of the at-risk unaffected individual does not identify a known disease-causing mutation. One cannot exclude a specific mutation in tested family members unless one knows this mutation is definitely present in a family. Test results are also considered inconclusive if the laboratory detects an alteration in the DNA but is unable to classify it as clearly disease causing or as a polymorphism. This is termed a "variant of uncertain significance." Typically, at-risk relatives are not tested for these variants.

Genetic testing for cancer syndromes may cost as little as $250 or more than $3,000. There may only be one laboratory in the world that performs a specific analysis, or there may be as many as 10 or 12 that offer testing for the same disorder. Very often, test availability is a function of patents or licenses on particular genetic tests. Some testing techniques are more sensitive than others, again based primarily on the type(s) of genetic abnormalities being sought. Depending on whether a single base pair change is sought or an entire gene must be sequenced, days to months may elapse before a genetic test result is reported. A genetic test is classified as a high-complexity test under current Public Health Service Clinical Laboratory Improvement Act of 1988 guidelines. Quality control programs for genetic testing are under development, but at this time, these tests are not specifically regulated. Therefore, choice of a testing laboratory is best left to professionals with experience with specific laboratories.

Psychosocial Issues

Genetic testing not only impacts the individual patient but other family members as well. Therefore, patients may experience emotions different from those regularly encountered in the clinical setting (7). Positive results can evoke fear, anxiety, uncertainty, and an impression that such a result is a "death sentence." Patients who have children may also feel guilt at having potentially passed a mutation to a child or anger for having inherited the mutation from a parent in the first place. Negative results can lead to such feelings as relief and happiness. However, these individuals may also experience survivor's guilt over having been "spared" from the disease that affected so many family members. This is more often noted in families where some relatives are positive whereas others are negative, and such results may lead to strained familial relationships. Some patients report a feeling of relief from uncertainty, regardless of whether the result is positive or negative, because there is a sense that, at the least, the cancer risk is better able to be defined and managed.

It should be noted that each individual has a different perception of high risk versus low risk. To some patients, a 45% risk is still viewed as a better chance of not having cancer than having it. To others, however, a 5% to 10% risk is frighteningly high. Therefore, before embarking on genetic testing, it is important to explore the patient's viewpoints. Particular attention should be paid to risk perception, ability to handle a positive or negative result, and the patient's interpretation of his or her relatives' opinions regarding genetic testing. It is also advantageous to discuss which management options the patient seems to prefer, knowing that decisions may ultimately be shaped by the results of the genetic testing.

Laws, Insurance, and Employment Concerns

When involved in genetic testing, it is important to be familiar with ethical, social, and legal issues. One such issue is the necessity for informed consent. Proper informed consent includes a thorough discussion of the risks, benefits, and limitations of testing. Among other details, the patient should be made aware of what information can and cannot be obtained by the particular test in question. The sensitivity of the test must be clearly explained as well, and the patient should understand that the test may not be informative, meaning that it may not provide information that is useful for risk modification. The patient should also be aware that genetic testing is a personal decision and he or she should not be pressured into obtaining such testing.

As previously addressed, genetic testing provides information about other family members in addition to the individual seeking testing. Therefore, a second issue that arises is the ethical dilemma of "duty to warn." In short, this dilemma encompasses the question of whether or not a health care professional is required to notify relatives of a patient if a genetic disorder is detected in the family. Thus far, legal decisions on this matter have conflicted, because disclosure of information may violate confidentiality, whereas failure to disclose may be viewed as endangerment. Therefore, it is important that patients are informed of the impact of genetic information on other individuals as well.

A third issue is potential discrimination by insurance companies or employers. Currently, the concern is that genetic information will be viewed as evidence for a preexisting condition that insurers will refuse to cover or that will render an individual unemployable. Federal laws, such as the Health Insurance Portability and Accountability Act, provide some protection for individuals who are covered under a group health insurance plan. Many states have enacted protective laws as well. As of now, however, there is no federal legislation regarding patients who have individual health insurance coverage. There is also no protection from discrimination relating to life insurance or disability insurance.

In practice, genetic counseling is often recommended and used before testing for mutations in cancer-predisposition genes, as discussed above. In contrast, informed consent and extensive counseling before ordering tests for alterations in coagulation predisposition genes, such as factor V Leiden, are uncommon. This may reflect a decreased perception of risk for discrimination or the fact that the mutation in factor V is a simpler, less expensive, more widely available test.

FUTURE ROLES OF GENETICS IN PATIENT CARE

Testing for genetically determined responses to drugs and screening for a broad array of genetic susceptibility to disease may soon be available for use in clinical decision making. As is true of all tests used in clinical preventive medicine, expanded genetic testing and counseling will require critical assessment of their impact on patients' health before they become standards of care.

Pharmacogenomics describes the concept of individualized choice of drug therapy based on knowledge of the differences in drug absorption, metabolism, and excretion as determined by variation in the relevant genes (8). For example, a polymorphism in the gene *NAT2* (*N*-acetyltransferase 2) determines whether an individual is a rapid or slow acetylator of many drugs such as hydralazine and isoniazid. Adverse drug reactions, such as the increased risk for peripheral neuropathy caused by isoniazid, occur more frequently in individuals who are slow acetylators. Identification of increasing numbers of polymorphisms in genes that affect drug metabolism will allow physicians to prescribe some drugs on the basis of the genetic profile of individual patients. This will only occur if testing for such genetic alterations can be performed quickly and inexpensively.

Technologic advances, such as the development of *microarray technology*, offer a way to screen for multiple genetic changes quickly and cheaply. Commonly known as "chips," these are high-density assemblies of oligonucleotides or complementary DNAs on a membrane or glass substrate. Specific DNA sequences can be sought by annealing with fluorescent-dye labeled RNA or DNA in solution and read with the assistance of computer programs. The Human Genome Project, which completed the sequencing of the human genome in 2001, is providing the information needed to develop such diagnostic technology. The day may not be far off when an individual with high blood pressure can be rapidly screened for specific genetic changes that affect blood pressure and the drugs that could be used to treat it, resulting in prescription of individualized rational drug therapy.

To introduce widespread use of genetic information for clinical decision making, it will be necessary not only to develop efficient and affordable technologies but also to address concerns discussed above regarding privacy and potential discrimination.

General References*

Useful Websites

http://www.nsgc.org
National Society of Genetic Counselors. Phone: 610-872-7608.

http://www.hopkins-coloncancer.org
The Johns Hopkins Hereditary Colorectal Cancer Program provides a comprehensive review of hereditary colorectal cancer and associated syndromes.

http://www.macgn.org
Mid-Atlantic Cancer Genetics Network is a research registry that provides information about hereditary cancer and promotes research for hereditary cancer syndromes.

http://www.geneclinics.org
Gene Clinics maintains a detailed list of genetic syndromes, including diagnostic characteristics, testing options, and treatment recommendations.

http://www.genetests.org
Gene Tests maintains a list of clinical and research laboratories that provide genetic testing.

http://www3.ncbi.nlm.nih.gov/omim
Online Mendelian Inheritance in Man is a comprehensive overview of known genetic syndromes and is searchable by disease name or symptom.

http://www.guideline.gov
National Guideline Clearinghouse contains up to date surveillance and management guidelines for various hereditary and nonhereditary syndromes.

http://www.geneticalliance.org
Genetic Alliance provides information about genetic syndromes and maintains a list of genetic syndrome support groups.

http://www.cancer.nci.nih.gov
CancerNet is a comprehensive overview of cancer and includes information about diagnosis, surveillance, and treatment, as well as ongoing clinical trials.

http://www.nchpeg.org
National Coalition for Health Professional Education in Genetics provides information to facilitate integration of genetic knowledge for health care professionals.

Published References

Aerssens J, Armstrong M, Gilissen R, et al. The human genome: an introduction. The Oncologist 2001;6:100.

Collins FS, McKusick VA. Implications of the human genome project for medical science. JAMA 2001;285:540.

Holtzman NA, Watson MS. Promoting safe and effective genetic testing in the United States. Baltimore, MD: Johns Hopkins University Press, 1998.

Institute of Medicine. Assessing genetic risks: implications for health and social policy. Washington, DC: National Academy Press, 1994.

Four resources that offer critical appraisal and commentary on the current and future roles for genetics in medicine.

Resource document for curriculum development in cancer genetics education. J Clin Oncol 1997;15:2157.

Describes curriculum on role of cancer predisposition testing developed by the Ad Hoc Task Force of the American Society of Clinical Oncology.

Specific References*

1. Recommendations of core competencies in genetics essential for all health professionals. Genet Med 2001;3:155.
2. Giardiello FM, Bresinger JD, Petersen GM, et al. The use and interpretation of commercial APC gene testing for familial adenomatous polyposis. N Engl J Med 1997;336:823.
3. Eng C, Hampel H, de la Chapelle A. Genetic testing for cancer predisposition. Annu Rev Med 2000;52:371.
4. Lindor NM, Greene MH. Mayo Familial Cancer Program. Special article: the concise handbook of family cancer syndromes. J Nat Cancer Inst 1998;90:1039.
5. Johnson KA, Brensinger JD. Genetic counseling and testing: implications for clinical practice. Nurs Clinic North Am 2000;35:615.
6. Bennett RL, Steinhaus KA, Uhrich SB, et al. Recommendations for standardized human pedigree nomenclature. Pedigree Standardization Task Force of the National Society of Genetic Counselors. Am J Hum Genet 1995;56:745.
7. Grady C. Ethics and genetic testing. Adv Intern Med 1999;44: 389.
8. Rusnak JM, Kisabeth RM, Herbert DP, et al. Pharmacogenomics: a clinician's primer on emerging technologies for improved patient care. Mayo Clin Proc 2001;76:299.

*Bold print (general references) and bold numerals (specific references) denote published controlled clinical trials, meta-analyses, or consensus-based recommendations.

CHAPTER 18

Immunization to Prevent Infectious Disease

WILLIAM H. BARKER, MD, FRCP Edin

Protection against infectious diseases can be conferred by active immunization with vaccines and by passive immunization with immune globulin (IG) preparations. Additional vaccines will become available in the next few years, and additional information will be generated to improve our understanding of the mechanisms of immune response to vaccines. Therefore, it can be expected that recommendations appropriate today will be revised in the future. This chapter describes vaccines and IG preparations available in the United States, focusing on several questions commonly considered in practice: Who should receive what specific immunization? When should they receive it? What are the common side effects or adverse reactions? Chapter 41 provides similar information on immunization for travelers to developing countries.

PATIENT ASSESSMENT

History

A history of immunizations should be obtained from all patients. In young adults, this information may be readily available, but in older persons, it is often hard to obtain. Patients may or may not keep personal records that are of use. People who have served in the military will have received routinely recommended immunizations and several additional vaccines not generally administered to the general population. People who travel abroad frequently should have this information recorded on their International Vaccination Card. Immunization history is particularly important in determining whether to give tetanus toxoid or antitoxin after an injury, whether diphtheria should be seriously considered in the diagnosis of acute pharyngitis (see Chapter 33), and what immunizations are needed by patients who plan to travel outside the United States (see Chapter 41).

A history of *allergic reactions* or other untoward reactions to vaccines or their components should always be excluded before giving an immunization. Most modern vaccines are highly purified, and allergic reactions after their use are rare. However, a history of a severe adverse reaction to a vaccine is a contraindication to its further use. Anyone with a history of severe allergic reactions after eating eggs should not receive vaccines made in eggs (e.g., influenza and yellow fever vaccines). Viral vaccines prepared in tissue culture often contain small amounts of antibiotics (especially neomycin) to which some patients may be allergic. For patients with previous allergic reactions to any vaccine, the contents of each vaccine should be determined from the package insert before administration.

Immunization with live virus vaccines is generally contraindicated in patients with known *immunodeficiency syndromes* or recent treatment with *immunosuppressive drugs*. Patients known to be infected with the human immunodeficiency virus (HIV) may be at increased risk when receiving live vaccines, although adverse effects have been documented infrequently. Current recommendations for vaccines in HIV-infected persons are outlined in Chapter 39. *Pregnant women*, in whom a vaccine virus might pose a risk to the fetus, should generally not be given live vaccines. In addition to ascertaining by history that a woman of childbearing age is not pregnant, it is important to counsel the patient to use contraceptive practices to prevent pregnancy for 3 months after immunization with a live vaccine (see Chapter 100). Prophylactic use of IG and the various hyperimmune globulin preparations is considered safe in pregnancy. Pregnancy is not a contradiction to administering live vaccine to children with whom a pregnant woman (e.g., mother or classroom teacher) will come in contact.

Recent administration of IG preparations requires that the use of live virus vaccines be postponed because passively acquired immunity can interfere with the active response to the vaccine (1). IG preparations should not be administered earlier than 2 weeks after live virus vaccine so that the vaccine virus can stimulate an active immune response. Yellow fever and oral polio vaccines are exceptions because interference does not occur. These vaccines can be given without regard to IG administration.

Minor illness (e.g., upper respiratory infection with or without a low-grade fever) is not a contraindication to necessary immunization. A patient with moderate or *severe acute illness* should generally not be immunized until after the illness has resolved, both because vaccine side effects might add to the patient's morbidity and because the effectiveness of the vaccination may be diminished.

Physical and Laboratory Evaluation

When immunization is contemplated, physical examination and laboratory testing usually add little to the assessment of the patient. Pregnancy or an acute illness (see above) may be confirmed on examination if the history suggests one of these, and findings suggestive of an immunodeficiency syndrome should be pursued with appropriate clinical laboratory studies.

Serologic tests are useful in deciding whether to immunize adults in selected situations. When considering the use of rubella vaccine in a woman of childbearing age, the presence of antibodies to rubella virus obviates the need for vaccination. When considering the use of hyperimmune globulin preparations or hepatitis B vaccine for protection against hepatitis B, the demonstration of preexisting antibody to hepatitis B makes additional protection superfluous. The decision regarding screening for antibodies before vaccination should be based on the estimated prevalence of markers for hepatitis B infections in the population from which the patient comes and the cost of serologic testing (see below).

IMMUNIZATION PROCEDURES

The package insert for a vaccine always includes information about dosage, route, site of administration, interval between immunizations, common and uncommon side effects, contraindications, potential trace contaminants that may cause hypersensitivity reactions, and appropriate storage conditions for the vaccine.

Many widely used vaccines can be given simultaneously. The Advisory Committee on Immunization Practices (ACIP) of the Centers for Disease Control and Prevention lists the following guidelines for simultaneous vaccine administration: Inactivated vaccines can be administered simultaneously at separate sites or at the same site with combination preparations. Tetanus and diphtheria toxoids (Td) are most effectively given together as a combined vaccine. However, when vaccines commonly associated with side effects are given together, the side effects may be accentuated and consideration should be given to vaccinating on separate occasions. An inactivated vaccine and a live attenuated virus vaccine can be administered simultaneously at separate sites. Some live virus vaccines, such as measles, mumps, and rubella (MMR), are routinely given in combination.

Patients should be informed of the risks and benefits associated with any vaccine in understandable lay terms. The range of common side effects and appropriate symptomatic therapies should be explained. Because of the rare possibility of anaphylactic reactions, patients receiving any immunization should be observed for about 15 minutes after vaccine administration. Finally, patients should be clearly informed of the name of the immunizations they have received and encouraged to keep a written record of them. Official immunization cards are available in every state for this purpose.

Physicians and health care providers are required to maintain permanent records of immunizations and to report certain adverse effects to the U. S. Department of Health and Human Services (2). These recording requirements are summarized in the U.S. Food and Drug Administration Drug Bulletin (3). A preventive care flowsheet, kept in the patient's office record, is an ideal location for vaccine history (see Fig. 14.3).

CURRENT RECOMMENDATIONS FOR VACCINES AND IMMUNE GLOBULINS

Table 18.1 summarizes the major and commonly used vaccines and IG preparations available in the United States. The following sections provide practical information on selected infectious diseases for which immune protection of adults is most likely to be undertaken in ambulatory practice.

INFORMATION FOR PATIENTS ABOUT VACCINATION SCHEDULES

Table 18.2, furnished by the National Coalition for Adult Immunization, provides a quick reference that can be provided to adults so that they are aware of appropriate scheduling of recommended vaccines. Chapter 11 provides similar information for adolescents. A *new strategy for ensuring vaccination of adolescents* recommends routine preventive care visits to health care providers for patients 11 to 12 years of age to vaccinate adolescents who have not been previously vaccinated with varicella virus vaccine, hepatitis B vaccine, or the second dose of MMR vaccine; to provide a booster dose of tetanus and diphtheria toxoids; to administer other vaccines that may be recommended for certain adolescents; and to provide other recommended preventive services (4).

DELIVERY SYSTEMS AND CONTINUING MEDICAL EDUCATION FOR PROVIDERS

Underutilization and missed opportunities to provide indicated vaccination among adults enrolled in medical practices have been repeatedly documented, particularly among minority groups (5). A variety of

Table 18.1. Characteristics and Administration of Commonly Used Vaccines and Immune Globulin Preparations (See Details in Text)

Vaccine or Immune Globulin	Type of Preparation	Population to be Immunized[a]	Usual Age and Immunization Schedule[b]	Common Adverse Reactions[c]
Diphtheria toxoid	Toxoid	All	Series of 3 primary injections (day 0, 1 mo, 6–12 mo) with boosters every 10 yr[d]	Local pain and swelling
Tetanus toxoid	Toxoid	All	Series of 3 i.m. injections (day 0, 1 mo, 6–12 mo) with boosters every 10 yr[d]	Local pain and swelling
Tetanus immune globulin (TIG)	High-titered human immune globulin	Unimmunized person with wound	Single i.m. injection (250 units)	Not significant
Acellular pertussis vaccine	Fractionated killed bacteria and toxoid	All children	2, 4, 6 mo, 15–18 mo, and 4–6 yr	Mild fever, fretfulness
Measles vaccine as MMR	Live attenuated virus[a]	All children	12–15 mo and 4–6 yr or 11–12 yr	Fever, rash
Rubella vaccine as MMR	Live attenuated virus[a]	All children and unimmunized women	12–15 mo and 4–6 yr or 11–12 yr, women through childbearing age with measles vaccine as MMR	Arthralgias, fever
Mumps vaccine as MMR	Live attenuated virus[a]	All children and young adults without history of mumps	12–15 mo and 4–6 yr or 11–12 yr with measles vaccine as MMR	Not significant
Polio vaccine, IPV	Killed virus	All	Ages 2, 4 mo, 12–18 mo, and 4–6 yr Children, adults; primary series of 3 doses, each separated by a minimum of 4 mo	Not significant
Haemophilus influenzae type B	Conjugated purified polysaccharide	All children, high-risk adults (e.g., asplenic)	Children, some adults; series of 3 injections beginning at 2 mo	Not significant
Hepatitis B vaccine	Recombinant proteins from yeast	All (eventually)	Childhood, adolescents 11–18 yr, selected adults; 3 injections (0 time, 1 mo, 6 mo in adolescents and adults; birth, 1–2 mo, third dose at 6–12 mo in children)	Not significant
Hepatitis B immune globulin	High-titered human γ-globulin	Persons exposed to hepatitis B	0.06 mL/kg at time of exposure and again 1 mo later	Not significant
Hepatitis A vaccine	Killed virus	Selected children and adults with high risk of exposure, travelers to hepatitis A endemic lands	Initial dose followed by booster dose 6–18 mo later	Local soreness
Influenza vaccine	Killed virus (whole virus and "split virus") preparations of virus components change yearly	All persons $\geq$50 years old or chronically ill persons of all ages	Adults: single injection (whole virus) repeated yearly Children under 12: split virus preparation, 2 doses at 4-week intervals	Fever, local tenderness
Immune globulin (IG)	Pooled human γ-globulin	Persons exposed to hepatitis A or B or measles	Usually adults Hepatitis A: 0.02 mL/kg, once Hepatitis B: 0.06 mL/kg, twice Measles: 0.25 mL/kg, once	Pain
Meningococcal vaccine	Purified polysaccharide (serogroups A, C, Y, W135)	During epidemic disease; those at high risk	All ages; young adult military; college freshmen Single injection	Erytherma at injection site
Rabies vaccine	Killed virus	Persons bitten by possibly rabid animal or at high risk of exposure Unimmunized persons with indication	Any age; postexposure: 5 doses of vaccine i.m. (days 1, 3, 7, 14, 28) Any age; preexposure: 3 doses of vaccine i.m. (days 0, 7, 21 or 28)	Pain, rare neurologic reactions, urticaria
Rabies immune globulin (HRIG)	High-titered human γ-globulin	Unimmunized persons with suspicious animal bite	Any age; single injection, up to ½ infiltrated into wound	Not significant
Pneumonococcal vaccine	Polyvalent purified polysaccharide (23 serotypes)	Persons with asplenia, or chronic illness, elderly	Any age (>2 yr); single injection, booster after $\geq$5 years (high-risk only) (see text)	Erythema at injection site
Bacillus Calmette–Guérin vaccine (BCG)	Live attenuated bacteria	Newborns in developing countries and persons with high risk of developing multiple drug-resistant tuberculosis	Infants and children; single injection, intradermal	Prolonged granuloma or ulcer at injection site, lymphadenitis
Varicella vaccine	Live attenuated virus	All children, susceptible persons $\geq$13 yr (especially if in contact with immunosuppressed persons)	Children 1–12 yrs: single dose at 12–18 mo Persons $\geq$13 yr: 2 doses 4–8 weeks apart	Erythema soreness at injection site
Varicella zoster immune globulin (VZIG)	High-titered human δ-globulin	Immunocompromised people without history of varicella who are exposed to varicella	125 units/10 kg once, within 96 hr of exposure	Not significant

[a]Populations cited represent general ambulatory patients. Certain subsets (HIV-infected, other immunocompromised persons) may benefit from specifically tailored immunization programs (see Chapter 39).

[b]All injections are intramuscular unless otherwise specified. Schedules given are for adults unless the vaccine is used solely in pediatric age group.

[c]Reactions listed are most common and/or serious. This listing is *not* exhaustive. Allergic hypersensitivity is possible with almost any vaccine, but is rare.

[d]Boosters of diphtheria and tetanus are particularly important for those traveling to underdeveloped countries. Diphtheria and tetanus vaccines should be given in a combined (Td) preparation. (See also Table 18.3).

[e]Given as the combination mumps, measles, and rubella vaccine (MMR). (See additional details about measles vaccine in Table 18.6).

Table 18.2. Information About Immunization Schedules that Can Be Provided to Adults

Infection Prevented	Timing of Immunizations			
Adult				
Hepatitis A (Hep A) for those at risk[a]	Two doses are recommended for long-term protection.			
	First dose		Second dose 6–12 mo later	
Hepatitis B (Hep B) for those at risk[a]	First dose	Second dose 1 mo later	Third dose 5 mo after second dose	
Measles, Mumps, Rubella (MMR)[b]	First dose	Second dose 28 days or more after first dose		
Tetanus, diphtheria (Td) if initial series not given during childhood	First dose	Second dose 1 mo later	Third dose 6 mo after second dose	Booster shot every 10 yr
Varicella[c] for susceptible individuals[d]	First dose	Second dose 28 days or more after first dose		
Older adults and those with chronic illnesses				
Influenza (flu)	Given yearly in the fall to people age 50 or older. Also recommended for people younger than 50 who have medical problems such as heart disease, lung disease, and other conditions, and for others who work or live with high-risk individuals.[a]			
Pneumococcal	One dose given to those ≥65 years of age.			
	First dose for those 2–64 years of age with chronic illness/at high risk[a]	One "booster" dose given 5 yr after the first dose (only applies to persons who were 2–64 yr of age at the time of the first dose).		

[a]Consult your doctor to determine your level of risk.
[b]Should not be given to pregnant women; pregnancy should be avoided for 3 months following receipt of MMR vaccine.
[c]Should not be given to pregnant women; pregnancy should be avoided for 1 month following receipt of varicella vaccine.
[d]Susceptible individuals include adults who have not been immunized previously and who do not have a reliable history of chickenpox.
Modified from the National Coalition for Adult Immunization.

simple techniques for improving vaccination delivery, including reminder mailings, standing orders, staff nurse roles, and tracking systems, has been shown to be effective in both private office and clinic settings (6–9). A novel strategy for tracking and promoting provision of annual influenza immunization to target patients in a practice population is illustrated in Fig. 18.1 *Continuing medical education* on such techniques for use in adult vaccination may be accessed from the Association of Teachers of Preventive Medicine (202-463-0550) (www.atpm.org) and the National Coalition for Adult Immunization (301-656-0003).

PROTECTION AGAINST SELECTED INFECTIONS

Diphtheria

Fewer than five cases of diphtheria are reported each year in the United States. People who have never received diphtheria toxoid should be immunized, and diphtheria toxoid should be given as booster doses with tetanus toxoid (Td) whenever tetanus toxoid is indicated (10).

For unimmunized school-aged children and adults, *adult type* (Td) tetanus and diphtheria toxoids are used. This preparation contains only approximately 25% of the diphtheria toxoid contained in the pediatric diphtheria and tetanus toxoids and pertussis vaccine and no pertussis antigen to minimize the risk of local reactions in sensitized adults. Primary immunization in these age groups consists of an initial dose, a 1-month dose, and a third dose at 6 to 12 months. A Td booster is recommended every 10 years to ensure protection. In adults, there is a 25% to 50% incidence of local soreness, swelling, and itching after Td injections; fever occurs in less than 10% and urticaria in approximately 2% of individuals. Serious reactions (swelling of the whole arm or anaphylaxis) occur rarely.

For *asymptomatic unimmunized contacts of patients with diphtheria*, management includes prophylactic antibiotics (600,000 units of benzathine penicillin intramuscularly or a 7-day course of erythromycin, 250 mg four times daily), primary vaccination as outlined above, and daily surveillance for 7 days for clinical evidence of diphtheria (see Chapter 33).

Tetanus

Approximately 50 cases of tetanus are reported each year in the United States. Although natural immunity to tetanus has been found in some adult populations, everyone should be regarded as susceptible unless

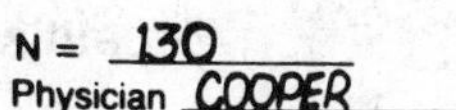

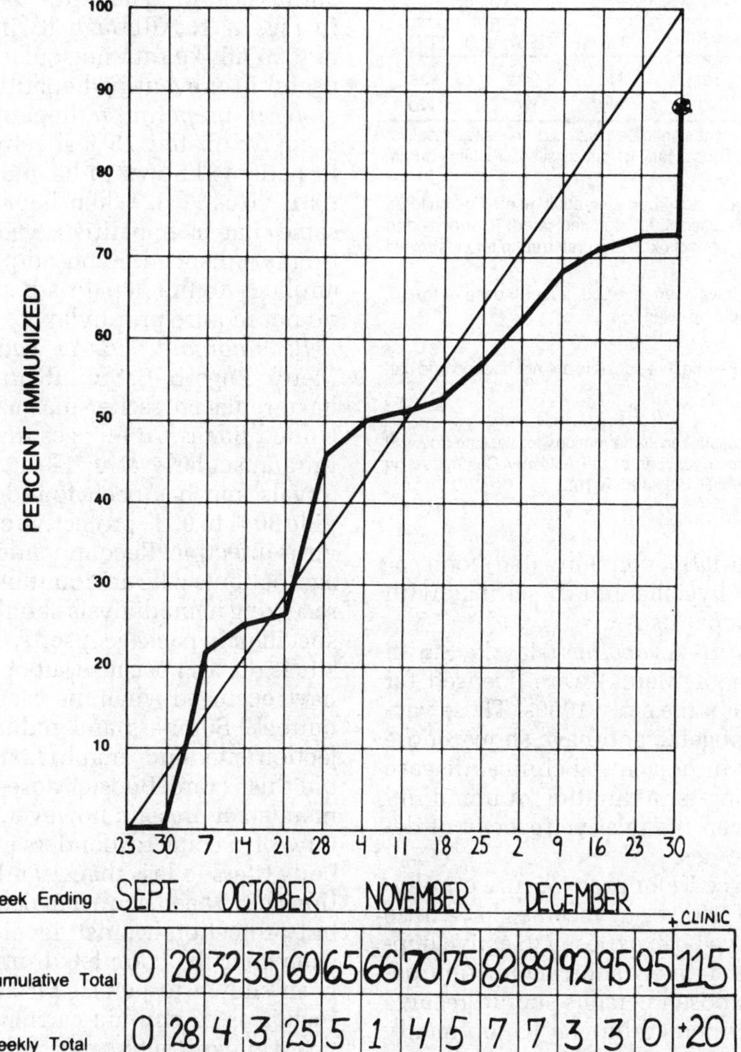

Figure 18.1. Completed poster displayed in an office practice. Year refers to the immunization season and *N* is the target population of patients 65 years old or older. The weekly and cumulative numbers of immunizations are tallied below the graph, and the percentage of the target population immunized is plotted weekly. (From Buffington J, Bell KM, LaForce FM, and the Genesee Hospital Medical Staff. A target-based model for increasing influenza immunizations in private practice. J Gen Intern Med 1991;6:204, with permission.)

actively immunized (10). This includes individuals who recover from clinical tetanus, because this illness does not evoke durable immunity to reinfection. Most cases of tetanus in the United States occur in people over age 60, primarily in those who were never immunized. Tetanus usually occurs after penetrating wounds from accidents and animal bites (see Chapter 32). The incubation period is 4 to 21 days with an average of 10 days.

In those who have received a primary series of three doses of toxoid at any time in their life, an injection of adsorbed toxoid (Td) once every 10 years is sufficient to boost antitoxin titers to protective levels. The need for booster doses of combined diphtheria–tetanus toxoids (Td) in people with wounds depends on the number of previous doses of tetanus toxoid received and the type of wound (Table 18.3). Only alum-adsorbed toxoids should be used. Fluid toxoids are still available in the United States, but these preparations are less immunogenic than alum-adsorbed preparations.

Patients who require *tetanus IG* because they have not been adequately immunized (Table 18.3) should be given 250 units intramuscularly. This preparation is made from human serum; therefore, hypersensitivity reactions do not occur. Patients who require tetanus IG should at the same time (but at a different site) be given their first dose of toxoid, followed by repeated doses of toxoid 1 month and 6 to 12 months later.

Hepatitis A

Hepatitis A is primarily transmitted by the fecal–oral route and constitutes a significant risk for people living

Table 18.3. Summary Guide to Tetanus Prophylaxis in Routine Wound Management (United States)

History of Adsorbed Tetanus Toxoid Doses	Clean Minor Wounds		All Other Wounds[a]	
	Td[b]	TIG	Td[b]	TIG
Uncertain or <3	Yes	No	Yes	Yes
≥3[c]	No[d]	No	No[e]	No

[a]Such as, but not limited to, wounds contaminated with dirt, feces, and saliva; puncture wounds; avulsions; and wounds resulting from missiles, crushing, burns, and frostbite.

[b]Td, tetanus and diphtheria toxoids, adsorbed (for adult use). For children <7 years old, DTP (DT, if pertussis vaccine is contraindicated) is preferred to tetanus toxoid alone. For persons ≥7 years old, Td is preferred to tetanus toxoid alone.

[c]If only three doses of fluid toxoid have been received, a fourth dose of toxoid, preferably an adsorbed toxoid, should be given.

[d]Yes, >10 years since last dose.

[e]Yes, >5 years since last dose. (More frequent boosters are not needed and can accentuate side effects.)

TIG, tetanus immune globulin.

From Diphtheria, tetanus, and pertussis: recommendations for vaccine use and other preventive measures. Recommendations of the Advisory Committee on Immunization Practices (ACIP). MMWR 1991;40(RR-10):1.

in settings with potentially contaminated food or water or poor personal hygiene and in settings with high endemic rates of hepatitis A.

Two inactivated hepatitis A vaccines (Havrix, Smith Kline Beecham, and Vaqta, Merck) were licensed for use in the United States in the early 1990s. These vaccines are highly immunogenic and have shown more than 90% effectiveness in preventing clinical disease in field experiences. Long-term duration of immunity has not been tested, given the relative recency of development of these vaccines.

Vaccines should replace IG for preexposure prophylaxis against hepatitis A. However, vaccines have little to offer patients who have been exposed to active hepatitis A because of the relatively short incubation period of 2 to 8 weeks. Exposed persons should receive passive protection with pooled human IG, optimally within 2 weeks of exposure (11). The usual dose is 0.02 mL/kg intramuscularly.

Active immunization with hepatitis A vaccine is recommended for international travelers to regions with poor sanitation and endemic hepatitis, children living in communities with known high endemic rate of hepatitis A, homosexually active men, users of illicit injectable drugs, people working closely with nonhuman primates, and patients who receive clotting factor replacement concentrates.

Vaccine should be administered intramuscularly in the deltoid muscle, generally in a two-dose schedule, with the second dose given at 6 to 12 months; the dosage of vaccine antigen varies by patient age and by specific product. Side effects include soreness and redness at injection site, usually within 3 days, and occasional headache. Serious adverse events have not been observed. Protective antibody levels develop in over 90% of recipients within 1 month after the first dose and in virtually 100% of the second dose of vaccine. These are sustained for at least 10 years.

Hepatitis B

The timing and patterns of appearance of antigens and antibodies after hepatitis B infection are illustrated in Fig. 47.1. Although IG in large doses (two doses of 0.06 mL/kg intramuscularly 4 weeks apart) may be useful in preventing hepatitis B (12), a *hyperimmune globulin preparation* (hepatitis B IG) is preferred and is approximately 75% effective in preventing hepatitis in patients known to have direct exposure to hepatitis B virus (13). When hepatitis B IG is given at the same time as hepatitis B vaccine (see below), protection is enhanced. Exposed patients who already have antibody to the hepatitis B surface antigen (anti-HBs) do not require prophylaxis.

Recombinant HBsAg vaccines (Recombivax HB, Merck; Engerix-B, SmithKline Beecham) made in yeast have replaced earlier plasma-derived vaccines in the United States. At all ages the vaccine is administered intramuscularly at 0, 1- to 2-, and 4- to 6-month intervals and has been found in clinical trials to provide 80% to 95% protective efficacy against hepatitis B virus infection. Recommended doses vary according to age; patients who are immunocompromised or who are receiving hemodialysis should be given larger doses as specified in package inserts. The preferred vaccination site is the arm because suboptimal antibody responses have occurred when the vaccine was injected into the buttock. Soreness and redness may occur at the injection site, and anaphylaxis has been documented, but this is rare. Booster doses are not routinely recommended at present; however, after 5 to 8 years, 30% to 60% of vaccine responders experience decline in antibody titers to less than 10 mIU/mL. Subclinical infections have been shown to occur in vaccinated persons, but protection against developing the chronic carrier state after the completed immunization schedule has been shown to persist for at least 15 years. The few instances of chronic carrier state developing several years after an active antibody response have occurred in immunocompromised individuals, primarily people with HIV infection.

Table 18.4 summarizes the current recommendations of the ACIP for postexposure prophylaxis for infants born to mothers with acute or chronic hepatitis B

Table 18.4. Recommended Prophylaxis After Perinatal, Sexual, or Household Exposure to Hepatitis B Virus

Type of Exposure	Type of Infection in Contact	Type of Prophylaxis
Perinatal	Acute or chronic	Vaccination + HBIG[a]
Sexual contact	Acute	HBIG[b] + vaccination
	Chronic	Vaccination
Household contact	Chronic	Vaccination
	Acute	
	No exposure	None
	Known exposure	HBIG[b] ± vaccination
	Infant (<12 mo)	Vaccination
		HBIG[a] if not vaccinated

[a]0.5 mL.

[b]0.06 mL/kg.

From CDC 1997.

Table 18.5. Recommendations for Hepatitis B Prophylaxis After Percutaneous or Permucosal Exposure

	Treatment When Source Is Found To Be		
Exposed Person	HBsAg Positive	HBsAg Negative	Source Not Tested or Unknown
Unvaccinated	HBIG × 1[a] and initiate HB vaccine[b]	Initiate HB vaccine[b]	Initiate HB vaccine[b]
Previously vaccinated			
Known responder	No treatment	No treatment	No treatment
Known nonresponder	HBIG × 2 *or* HBIG × 1 and initiate revaccination	No treatment	If high-risk source, treat as if HBsAg positive
Response unknown	Test exposed for anti-HBs 1. If inadequate[c] HBIG × 1 plus HB vaccine 2. If adequate, no treatment	No treatment	Test exposed for anti-HBs 1. If inadequate,[c] initiate revaccination 2. If adequate, no treatment

[a]HBIG dose, 0.06 mL/kg i.m.
[b]Adult dose, product specific.
[c]Adequate anti-HBs is ≥10 mIU/mL by radioimmunoassay or positive by electroimmunoassay.
From CDC 1997.

infection and for sexual contacts or household contacts of persons with hepatitis B infections. Table 18.5 summarizes recommendations for postexposure prophylaxis for people who have had percutaneous, ocular, or mucous membrane exposure to blood from patients with known or suspected acute or chronic hepatitis B infections.

The American Academy of Pediatrics and the ACIP have recommended routine three-dose hepatitis B vaccine for all infants, beginning preferably before the newborn is discharged from hospital, and routine vaccination of adolescents through age 18, if not previously vaccinated. Hepatitis B vaccine is also recommended for others who are at increased risk of exposure: health care professionals exposed frequently to blood or blood products (e.g., laboratory and blood bank personnel, operating room staff, surgeons, dentists, endoscopists, pathologists, staff in oncology, and dialysis units and emergency room staff), homosexually active men, family members or sexual partners of chronic HBsAg carriers, prostitutes, patients who frequently receive transfusions of blood or blood products, patients in hemodialysis units, inmates and staff of institutions for the mentally retarded, inmates of long-term correctional institutions, users of illicit injectable drugs, selected international travelers (see Chapter 41), people from countries with high endemic rates of hepatitis B virus infection, and members of a family that adopt HBsAg-positive children. The vaccine is not routinely recommended for individuals who come in contact with HBsAg carriers at work or school. Screening for antibodies to hepatitis B virus before immunization is cost effective only in populations in which the prevalence of such antibodies is high (e.g., intravenous drug abusers). Vaccination of individuals who have anti-HBs from previous infection does not result in increased adverse effects.

People at high risk of repeated exposure to blood or blood products should consider *testing for anti-HBs* 1 to 3 months after the third dose of vaccine to ensure they have responded (Table 18.5, footnote c). Testing at intervals of 1 year or more after vaccination may not accurately determine whether some people have responded to the vaccine. The need for booster doses for adults who receive a primary series in infancy remains to be assessed.

Hepatitis C and Non-A, Non-B Hepatitis

There is no IG preparation known to be protective against the multiple agents of non-A, non-B hepatitis, which are now the most common cause of posttransfusion hepatitis (14). Most non-A, non-B infection is caused by hepatitis C. All blood donors are now screened for hepatitis C. Hepatitis in ambulatory patients is discussed in Chapter 47.

Influenza

Inactivated virus vaccines have been available for the prevention of influenza for many years. Earlier vaccines often led to fever and malaise, but current preparations are highly purified (15); in carefully controlled placebo studies side effects are limited to short-lived soreness at the site of the injection in approximately one in five vaccinees. Specifically, there is no evidence of increased frequency of flulike upper respiratory illness after vaccination (16). Patients with egg allergy should not receive influenza vaccination. Whole and split virus vaccines are available; either may be used in adults. The vaccine recommended each year is polyvalent, which means that it contains antigens from the type A and B strains that are expected to prevail during that season. The efficacy of the vaccine depends on the closeness in matching between the vaccine strains and the viruses circulating that year. Influenza vaccine has had consistently high (70% to 80%) protective efficacy against acute influenza among healthy young adults in most years. Although somewhat less protective against acute upper respiratory tract influenza in older patients, influenza vaccine is generally 50% to 70% protective against life-threatening pneumonia and other cardiovascular complications in this vulnerable age group (17). A protective antibody response occurs within 2 to 3 weeks of vaccination. This response is not impaired in patients with chronic pulmonary disease who are on maintenance systemic cortico steroids.

The *recommendation* (15) is an annual immunization with the current year's vaccine between September and December, before influenza season, for those in whom influenza causes the highest morbidity and mortality. This includes all individuals over age 50 (officially modified in 2000 from previous ACIP recommendation, which targeted age 65 and above) and patients of any age with significant heart, lung, metabolic, immunocompromising disease, or chronic debilitating conditions and women who will be in the second or third trimester of pregnancy during the influenza season (December through April). The vaccine is also recommended for those involved in critical jobs in which absenteeism may be detrimental (e.g., firemen, policemen); for medical personnel or other staff of medical institutions; close contacts and or caregivers interacting with the above groups; and for children or teenagers receiving chronic aspirin therapy because they are at risk of Reye syndrome. Trivial intercurrent illnesses, such as mild upper respiratory tract infections, should not be viewed as contraindications to timely influenza immunization of high-risk individuals. Medicare now reimburses physicians for influenza vaccination of patients over 65 and in younger disabled persons enrolled in Medicare.

The diagnosis and management of influenza in ambulatory patients, including the use of antiviral agents, is discussed in Chapter 33.

Pneumococcal Disease

Purified polyvalent polysaccharide vaccine is available for the prevention of disease caused by *Streptococcus pneumoniae.* Protective efficacy is estimated to be in the range of 50% to 80% against bacteremic illness with the pneumococcal serotypes in the vaccine that has been manufactured since 1983 (23 serotypes that are responsible for 80% to 90% of invasive pneumococcal disease in the United States, including the 6 serotypes responsible for most penicillin-resistant pneumococcal disease). The vaccine is given as a single 0.5-mL dose, administered intramuscularly or subcutaneously, and produces few untoward effects (18). It may be administered simultaneously with influenza vaccine, preferably in the opposite arm, without diminishing antibody response. It is recommended for all people 65 or older and for people aged 2 to 64 years with immunocompromising disease, chronic cardiac or pulmonary disease, diabetes, alcoholism, or functional (e.g., sickle cell disease) or anatomic asplenia.

One-time revaccination after 5 years or more is now recommended for the following two groups: people less than 65 years of age at high risk (e.g., immunocompromised persons, because they have relatively rapid decline in antibody titer) and people 65 years of age or older who received their initial dose before they were 65 years of age. This recommendation is based on the finding that postvaccination antibody levels and/or protective efficacy may not be lifelong (19). Patients who are revaccinated are more likely to report a local reaction at the injection site than those receiving a first vaccination. In a study population the incidence was 11% and 3%, respectively, and the reaction usually resolved within 3 days (20). Physicians may administer a booster dose to those initially vaccinated after age 65, with no increased risk of side effects, although such boosters are not recommended by the ACIP (18).

Pneumococcal pneumonia in ambulatory practice is discussed in Chapter 33.

Lyme Disease

Lyme disease, first recognized in the United States in the early 1980s, is most common in the middle Atlantic, northeast, and upper Midwestern parts of the country; occurs predominately in spring and summer months; and is mainly transmitted to humans by ticks that have initially become infected from deer or rodents (see Chapter 38).

In April, 2002, the vaccine described in the following paragraphs was withdrawn from the market. For more information, see Chapter 38.

Lyme disease vaccine (LYMErix, SmithKline and Beecham), licensed for use in the United States in 1998, is a recombinant-derived vaccine comprised of the *Borrelia burgdorferi* outer surface protein OspA. The vaccine is administered intramuscularly in the deltoid muscle as a three-dose regimen, with second and third doses given at 1 and 12 months after the initial dose (21). In randomized clinical trials, involving subjects between 15 and 70 years of age, three doses attained 76% protective efficacy against occurrence of laboratory-confirmed clinical Lyme disease. Common side effects consist of soreness at injection site; a small percent of subjects experience short-lived fever and myalgia. The duration of protection and need for booster inoculation of this recently released vaccine remain to be determined.

The ACIP recommends the vaccine for persons aged 15 to 70 years who live in regions of high Lyme disease endemicity and who engage in frequent occupational, property maintenance, recreational, or leisure activities in tick-infested habitats. For persons with history of previously uncomplicated Lyme disease who are at continued high risk of exposure, vaccination should be considered; however, such persons who have treatment-resistant Lyme arthritis should not be vaccinated because of the association between this condition and immune reactivity to OspA antigen.

Measles

Measles is a moderately severe illness in most people (22) and has been associated with an overall case fatality rate of 3 per 1,000 in recent years. Case fatality rates are higher in young infants and adults than in school-aged children. Since 1963, inactivated, and subsequently live, attenuated measles vaccines have been available. From the 1960s, when measles vaccination of children was introduced generally in the United States, the number of cases reported annually fell from more than 400,000 to less than 1,500. However, from 1989 to 1991, more than 55,000 cases were reported, including 11,000 hospitalizations and 130 deaths (23). Although most cases in recent years have occurred in unvaccinated preschool children, measles continues to cause disease in adolescents and adults, especially in schools and other group settings. Recent data show

Table 18.6. Current Recommendations for Measles Vaccination

	Criteria for Adequate Protection
Routine childhood schedule, United States	
Most areas	Two doses,[a,b] first dose at 12–15 mo second dose at 4–6 yr (entry to kindergarten or first grade)[c]
High-risk areas[d]	Two doses,[a,b] first dose at 12 mo second dose at 4–6 yr (entry to kindergarten or first grade)[c]
Colleges and other educational institutions after high school	Documentation of receipt of two doses of measles vaccine after the first birthday[b] or other evidence of measles immunity[e]
Medical personnel beginning employment	Documentation of receipt of two doses of measles vaccine after the first birthday[b] or other evidence of measles immunity[e]

[a]Both doses should preferably be given as combined measles, mumps, rubella (MMR) vaccine.

[b]No less than 1 mo apart. If no documentation of any dose of vaccine, first dose of vaccine should be given at the time of school entry or employment and second dose no less than 1 mo later.

[c]Some areas may elect to administer the second dose at an older age or to multiple age groups.

[d]A county with more than five cases among preschool-aged children during each of at least 5 yr, a county with a recent outbreak among unvaccinated preschool-aged children, or a county with a large inner-city urban population. These recommendations may be applied to an entire county or to identified risk areas within a county.

[e]Prior physician-diagnosed measles disease, laboratory evidence of measles immunity, or birth before 1957.

From CDC 1997.

that a single dose of measles vaccine does not confer lifelong immunity in a small proportion of people.

In response to the evidence that immunity wanes in some vaccine recipients, the following two-dose vaccine schedule, preferably using MMR vaccine (see below), is now recommended: initial dose at 12 to 15 months of age and second dose at 4 to 6 years of age (Table 18.6). For students entering college after high school who do not have documentation of two doses, a second dose is recommended. Measles vaccine is associated with transient fever (103°F or greater) or rash 7 to 12 days after vaccination in approximately 5% of vaccines recipients. Special attention should be directed toward ensuring immunity in all health care providers and providing measles vaccine to adolescents and young adults.

Unimmunized household contacts of persons with measles, especially infants born to nonimmune women, should be given IG 0.25 mL/kg (up to 15 mL maximum). Immunocompromised children and adults exposed to measles should receive 0.5 mL/kg (maximum dose 15 mL) of IG.

Mumps

From 1967 to 1995, the number of cases of mumps reported annually in the United States fell from more than 100,000 to less than 1,000 because of the widespread use of mumps vaccine in children. Live attenuated mumps virus vaccine, preferably given as MMR (see below), is recommended routinely for children and for unvaccinated young adults with no history of physician-diagnosed mumps (22). Most people born before 1957 can be considered immune. Because the mumps virus can cause severe illness in adults (orchitis, meningitis, or pancreatitis), there is good reason to provide protection to young adults who may be susceptible. Outbreaks of mumps have been reported among college and university students, and this group merits special attention. A single dose of mumps vaccine, alone or in MMR, yields durable protection in approximately 90% of recipients.

Rubella

Since 1970, live attenuated rubella virus vaccine has been administered routinely to children 1 year of age and older (22). The major rationale for use of this vaccine is prevention of the spread of rubella virus to pregnant women and thus reduction of the incidence of the congenital rubella syndrome. From 1972 to 1996, the number of cases of rubella reported annually in the United States fell from more than 56,000 to less than 200. Reported cases of congenital rubella syndrome remained constant at 50 to 60 from 1970 to 1980 and then fell dramatically to 13 in 1983 and 1 in 1988. In 1990 and 1991, a resurgence of rubella was observed, and there were more than 40 cases of documented congenital rubella syndrome reported in the United States.

Anyone working in a medical facility who does not have documentation of past rubella vaccination or serologic evidence of immunity should be vaccinated against rubella (MMR vaccine, see below) (22). Adults, and especially nonpregnant adolescent girls and women in the childbearing age group, should be offered rubella vaccine if they have not received vaccine or are not known to have serologic evidence of immunity. Serologic testing before vaccination is unnecessary because prior immunity does not increase the risks of vaccination. Vaccinated women should be cautioned against becoming pregnant (see Chapter 100) for the 3 months after receiving rubella vaccine because of the theoretical possibility of fetal damage. However, no cases of congenital abnormalities have been observed in more than 300 susceptible women who received rubella vaccine just before or during pregnancy, and the theoretical risk is less than 1%. Approximately 25% of postpubertal women receiving rubella vaccine experience arthralgias in the first 1 to 3 weeks after immunization. Frank arthritis is much less common and all symptoms are usually mild and transient.

Measles, Mumps, and Rubella Vaccine

In most cases, MMR is the vaccine of choice when any of its components is indicated, although the three vaccines are available separately. *A two-dose schedule is now highly recommended for all children* (22). The first dose of MMR should be administered at 12 to 15 months of age; the second dose is now recommended at 4 to 6 years, before school entry, but may be given at 11 to 12 years of age. The measles component is associated with the occurrence of fever or mild rash within 7 to 12 days after injection. MMR or its component vaccines should not be given to pregnant women. Anaphylaxis or other serious systematic adverse reactions are rare with MMR or any of the three individual component vaccines.

Most adults born before 1957 are assumed to be immune to mumps, measles, and rubella. *Adults born in 1957 or later* who do not have a medical contraindication should receive at least one dose of MMR vaccine unless they have documentation of vaccination with at least one dose of MMR-containing vaccine or other acceptable evidence of immunity to these three diseases: laboratory evidence of immunity or physician documented diagnosis of the disease. Serosurveys document a lack of identifiable antibody to measles, mumps, or rubella among 15% to 20% of young adult Americans (24). It is now recommended that adolescents and college students who have no documentation of live MMR vaccinations or other acceptable evidence of immunity should receive a two-dose course of MMR vaccine, with the second dose administered no sooner than 1 month after the initial dose. Students with medical contraindications to vaccination with MMR and any of its component vaccines should be given a letter of explanation to present to the health officials of their educational institution.

Meningococcal Disease

Meningococcal disease is a serious potentially fatal infection that usually occurs sporadically, with the highest incidence in infants. Occurrence is relatively rare among the general population, but the incidence is increased among healthy young adults living in congregated circumstances, particularly military recruits in barracks and college students in dormitories. A quadrivalent meningococcal polysaccharide vaccine (Menomune, Aventis Pasteur) for serotypes A, C, Y, and W-135 is available and is administered as a single 0.5-mL subcutaneous injection that elicits protective antibody within 2 weeks. *Vaccination is recommended to control community outbreaks* (25), defined as three or more cases within less than 3 months that result in an attack rate of 10 or more per 100,000 population at risk. College freshmen should be made aware of their modest increase in risk and should be offered vaccination.

Polio

Wild poliovirus and new-onset poliomyelitis have been eradicated from the Western hemisphere, and global eradication is anticipated within several years. Vaccine-associated paralytic polio among primary vaccinees with oral polio vaccine (OPV) or their household contacts remains a rare but real risk in the United States, where 125 cases occurred between 1980 and 1994—approximately 1 case per 750,000 first doses of OPV. Polio does not occur after inactivated polio vaccine (IPV). During the latter half of the 1990s with a view to eliminating vaccine-associated paralytic polio, which was accounting for all new domestically acquired polio in the United States, the ACIP and other advisory groups recommended transitioning, effective 1997, to a sequential IPV-OPV vaccination schedule (two doses given to children at 2, 4, and 6 to 18 months and 4 to 6 years of age) (26).

Polio vaccination for adults in the United States is recommended for travelers to remaining polio endemic parts of the world (see Chapter 41), unvaccinated adults whose children will be receiving OPV, and laboratory workers who handle specimens that may contain polioviruses.

The recommended schedule for unvaccinated adults consists of three doses of IPV, with the second dose administered 4 to 8 weeks after the first and a third dose at 6 to 12 months. For adults at increased risk of exposure to wild poliovirus (travelers, laboratory workers) who have previously completed a primary OPV or IPV series, a single booster dose of IPV may be administered.

Rabies

Indigenously acquired human rabies is rare in the United States. Theoretically, all clinical cases of rabies are preventable if protective treatment is given promptly after exposure. The incubation period is usually 2 to 8 weeks, but it may be as short as 10 days or as long as 1 year or more.

Since 1982, inactivated rabies virus vaccine produced in human diploid cells has been in use in the United States. It causes fewer and milder reactions than the older duck embryo-derived vaccine. Formulations for intramuscular or intradermal injection are available, as is a hyperimmune globulin derived from human sera (HRIG).

For *postexposure prophylaxis* after an animal bite (see Chapter 32), the recommended treatment schedule is as follows (27): on day 1, simultaneous administration of HRIG (20 IU/kg, up to half infiltrated into the wound and the remainder intramuscularly), and the first dose of vaccine, also given intramuscularly; additional vaccine doses are given on days 3, 7, 14, and 28. The effectiveness of this regimen in protecting humans from rabies has been well established. Adverse reactions (urticaria, anaphylaxis, transient headache, and fever) occur in less than 0.5% of persons receiving this vaccine.

For *preexposure prophylaxis*, people working in areas where rabies is enzootic or in occupations where potential for rabies exposure is high (e.g., veterinarians) should be vaccinated before exposure. In this situation, the appropriate formulation may be given intradermally in 0.1-mL doses or intramuscularly in 1.0-mL doses on days 0, 7, and 21 or 28 with booster doses every 2 years (see Chapter 41 for details regarding frequency of vaccine for those living in high-risk areas outside of the United States). Preexposure immunization does not eliminate the need for postexposure prophylaxis, but it obviates the need for HRIG and decreases the number of vaccine doses required to two (days 0 and 3).

Tuberculosis

Efforts to control tuberculosis in the United States are based on early identification and treatment of active disease and on isoniazid prophylaxis of the contacts of tuberculous patients and other groups at increased risk (see Chapter 34). Because most new tuberculosis cases are reactivation of disease in older individuals and because efficacy has been questioned in the past, indications for immunization with bacillus Calmette–Guérin (BCG) vaccine in the United States have been limited (28). However, the recent spread of multiple drug-resistant tuberculosis, unresponsive to isoniazid and rifampin, and a recent meta-analysis indicating up to 50% reduction in the risk of tuberculosis in BCG-vaccinated individuals (29), have prompted reconsideration of the use of BCG in the United States.

At present, BCG should be considered for the following two groups:

- Infants and children who have a negative tuberculin skin test and (a) who have repeated exposure to persistently untreated or unsuccessfully treated sputum-positive pulmonary tuberculosis and cannot be separated from the presence of the infectious patient or reliably receive isoniazid or (b) who have repeated exposure to active disease caused by multiple drug-resistant tuberculosis organisms and cannot be separated from the infectious patient.
- Health care workers who have negative tuberculin skin tests and work in settings with recurrent transmission of multiple drug-resistant tuberculosis.

BCG is a live attenuated vaccine derived from *Mycobacterium bovis*. The Tice strain (Organon, Inc.) is the only BCG vaccine licensed in the United States. It is administered percutaneously through multiple punctures in the upper arm, with doses differing by age of recipient. A small ulcerating postule typically occurs at the vaccination site several weeks after receiving the vaccine. BCG vaccine is contraindicated in people receiving immunosuppressive therapy or who have immunocompromising conditions, including HIV infection.

Varicella

Varicella (chickenpox) is a highly contagious generally self-limited disease of childhood caused by varicella zoster virus. Although varicella occurs infrequently among adolescents and adults, it is more severe among these groups and among immunocompromised people in all age groups. Complications include pneumonia, encephalitis, and occasionally death. In 1995, a live attenuated varicella virus vaccine (Varivax, Merck) was licensed for use in people 12 months of age or older in the United States.

Although primarily intended for children, varicella vaccination is recommended for everyone 12 years of age or older, particularly those who are susceptible (those with negative or unknown history of varicella) and who have close household or occupational (health care workers) contact with immunocompromised people or others at high risk of serious complications (30). Because 70% to 90% of adults without a reliable history of varicella are actually immune, serologic testing before vaccination is likely to be cost effective in these subjects.

Vaccination of children between 12 months and 12 years of age consists of a single dose, whereas vaccination of persons more than 12 years old consists of two doses, with the second dose administered subcutaneously 4 to 8 weeks after the initial dose. Adverse effects have been limited to pain and redness at the injection site.

For *postexposure prophylaxis,* varicella zoster IG, available from American Red Cross distribution centers, is indicated for immunocompromised adolescents and adults who are susceptible to varicella (i.e., have negative history for chickenpox and no history of receiving varicella vaccine) and have been exposed to an active varicella case. It is effective in preventing or suppressing varicella if given within 96 hours of exposure. Healthy adults and pregnant women who are susceptible to varicella (see above) are at increased risk of varicella complications and may also be given varicella zoster IG for postexposure prophylaxis. Recommended prophylactic dosage of varicella zoster IG is 125 units/10 kg (22 lb), administered intramuscularly. The major adverse reaction is discomfort at the injection site; anaphylactic shock is rare.

General References*

ACP Task Force on Adult Immunization and Infectious Diseases Society of America. **Guide for adult immunization**, 4th ed. Philadelphia: American College of Physicians, 2001.

Contains all standard recommendations in a single source with critical discussions of efficacy, indications, administration, and adverse effects of vaccines and IG preparations and new section on practice strategies for maximizing vaccine delivery.

Periodic Reports of the Advisory Committee on Immunization Practices (ACIP) at **www.cdc.gov/nip/publications/ACIP**.

ACIP reports include current recommendations for specific vaccine preventable disease and for selected population subgroups, including children, adolescents, adults, pregnant woman, immunocompromised persons, and health care workers.

Immunization Action Coalition at www.immunize.org.

Public and private funded clearinghouse for wide variety of current immunization information for professional and consumer.

Red book 2000: report of the Committee on Infectious Disease. Elk Grove Village, IL: American Academy of Pediatrics. Contact: www.aap.org.

Comprehensive sourcebook for vaccine preventable disease of children.

Chen J, ed. Control of communicable diseases in man, 17th ed. Washington, DC: American Public Health Association, 2000.

A concise summary of epidemiology, prevention, and management of virtually all communicable diseases, updated at 5-year intervals.

Centers for Disease Control and Prevention National Immunization Program and National Center for Infectious Disease. **Prevention and control of vaccine-preventable disease in long-term care facilities**. J Am Med Directors Assoc 2000;5:S1.

*Bold print (general references) and bold numerals (specific references) denote published controlled clinical trials, meta-analyses, or consensus-based recommendations.

Provides practical guidelines for implementing immunization and surveillance programs for vaccine preventable diseases in long-term care facilities.

Humiston SG, Good C. Vaccinating your child. Questions and answers for the concerned parent. Atlanta: Peachtree Publishers Ltd., 2000.

Clearly written and very informative in addressing concerns of lay public.

Jordan Report 2000 at www.nih.gov/Report/NIAID.

Prepared by the National Institute of Allergy and Infectious Disease (NIAID), the report highlights recent advances in vaccinology and offers a comprehensive overview of vaccine development against some 60 disease caused by bacteria, viruses, fungi, and parasites.

Recommendations of the Advisory Committee on Immunization Practices (ACIP). **Use of vaccines and immune globulins in persons with altered immunocompetence**. MMWR Morb Mortal Wkly Rep 1993;42(RR-4):1.

Recommendations of the Advisory Committee on Immunization Practices (ACIP). **Vaccine side effects, adverse reactions, contraindications and precautions**. MMWR Morb Mortal Wkly Rep 1996;45(RR-12):1.

Recommendations of the Advisory Committee on Immunization Practices (ACIP) and the Hospital Infection Control Practices Advisory Committee (HICPAS). **Immunization of health care workers**. MMWR Morb Mortal Wkly Rep 1990;46(RR-1):1.

Recommendations of the Advisory Committee on Immunization Practices (ACIP). **Adult immunization programs in nontraditional settings: quality standards and guidance for program evaluation and use of standing order programs to increase adult vaccination rates**. MMWR Morb Mortal Wkly Rep 2000;49(RR-1):1.

Specific References

1. Siber GR, Werner BG, Halsey NA, et al. Interference of immune globulin with measles and rubella immunization. J Pediatr 1993;122:204.
2. Chen RT, Rastogi SC, Mullen JR, et al. The vaccine adverse event reporting system (VAERS). Vaccine 1994;12:542.
3. Food and Drug Administration. New reporting requirements for vaccine adverse events. FDA Drug Bull 1988;18:16.
4. Recommendations of the Advisory Committee on Immunization Practices (ACIP), the American Academy of Pediatrics, the American Academy of Family Physicians, and the American Medical Association. Immunization of adolescents. MMWR Morb Mortal Wkly Rep 1996;45(RR-13):1.
5. Williams WW, Hickson MA, Kane MA, et al. Immunization policies and vaccine coverage among adults. The risk for missed opportunities. Ann Intern Med 1988;108:616.
6. Gyorkos W, Tannenbaum TN, Abrahamowicz M, et al. Evaluation of the effectiveness of immunization delivery methods. Can J Public Health 1994;85[Suppl]:S14.
7. Szilagyi PG, Bordely C, Vann JC, et al. Effect of patient reminder/recall interventions on immunization rates a review. JAMA 2000;284:1820.
8. Briss PA, Rodewald LE, Hinman AR, et al. Reviews of evidence regarding interventions to improve vaccination coverage in children, adolescents, and adults. Am J Prev Med 2000;18(IS):97.
9. Association of Teachers of Preventive Medicine. What works. Computer assisted instruction on strategies to improve adult vaccination rates. For information contact www.atpm.org.
10. Recommendations of the Advisory Committee on Immunization Practices (ACIP). Diphtheria, tetanus, and pertussis: recommendations for vaccine use and other preventive measures. MMWR Morb Mortal Wkly Rep 2000;40(RR-10):1.
11. Recommendations of the Advisory Committee on Immunization Practices (ACIP). Prevention of hepatitis A through active or passive immunization. MMWR Morb Mortal Wkly Rep 1999;48(RR-12):1.
12. Recommendations of the Advisory Committee on Immunization Practices (ACIP). Hepatitis B virus infection: a comprehensive immunization strategy to eliminate transmission in the United States. MMWR Morb Mortal Wkly Rep 1991;40:1.
13. Stevens CE, Taylor PE, Tong MJ, et al. Yeast-recombinant hepatitis B vaccine. Efficacy with hepatitis B immune globulin in prevention of perinatal hepatitis B virus transmission. JAMA 1987;257:2612.
14. Lemon SM, Thomas DL. Vaccines to prevent viral hepatitis. N Engl J Med 1997;336:196.
15. Recommendations of the Advisory Committee on Immunization Practices (ACIP). Prevention and control of influenza. MMWR Morb Mortal Wkly Rep 2001:50(RR-4):1. (Note: Update for each year issued by ACIP.)
16. Margolis KL, Nichol KL, Poland GA, et al. Frequency of adverse reactions to influenza vaccine in the elderly. JAMA 1990;264:1139.
17. Gross PA, Hermogenes AW, Sacks HS, et al. The efficacy of influenza vaccine in elderly persons. A meta-analysis and review of the literature. Ann Intern Med 1995;123:518.
18. Recommendations of the Advisory Committee on Immunization Practices (ACIP). Prevention of pneumococcal disease. MMWR Morb Mortal Wkly Rep 1997;46(RR-8):1.
19. Shapiro ED, Berg AT, Austrian R, et al. The protective efficacy of polyvalent pneumococcal polysaccharide vaccine. N Engl J Med 1991;1453.
20. Jackson LA, Benson P, Sneller VP, et al. Safety of revaccination with pneumococcal polysaccharide vaccine. JAMA 1999;281:243.
21. Recommendations of the Advisory Committee on Immunization Practices (ACIP). Recommendations for the use of Lyme disease vaccine. MMWR Morb Mortal Wkly Rep 1999;48(RR-7):1.
22. Recommendations of the Advisory Committee on Immunization Practices (ACIP). Measles, mumps, and rubella: vaccine use and strategies for measles, rubella, and congenital rubella syndrome elimination and control of mumps. MMWR Morb Mortal Wkly Rep 1998;47(RR-8):1.
23. Atkinson WL, Orenstein WA, Krugman S. The resurgence of measles in the United States, 1989–1991. Annu Rev Med 1992;43:451.
24. Kelly PW, Petrucelli BP, Stehr-Green P, et al. The susceptibility of young adult Americans to vaccine preventable infections. JAMA 1991;266:2724.
25. Recommendations of the Advisory Committee on Immunization Practices (ACIP). Prevention and control of meningococcal disease and meningococcal disease and college students. MMWR Morb Mortal Wkly Rep 2000;49(RR-7):1.
26. Recommendations of the Advisory Committee on Immunization Practices (ACIP). Poliomyelitis prevention in the United States. MMWR Morb Mortal Wkly Rep 2000;49(RR-5):1.
27. Recommendations of Immunization Practices Advisory Committee (ACIP). Human rabies prevention: United States. MMWR Morb Mortal Wkly Rep 1999;48(RR-1):1.
28. Advisory Council for Elimination of Tuberculosis and Advisory Committee on Immunization Practices (ACIP). The role of BCG vaccine in the prevention and control of tuberculosis in the United States. MMWR Morb Mortal Wkly Rep 1996;45(RR-4): 1.
29. Brewer TF. Preventing tuberculosis with bacillus Calmette-Guérin vaccine: a meta-analysis of the literature. Clin Infect Dis 2000;3:S64.
30. Recommendations of the Advisory Committee on Immunization Practices (ACIP). Prevention of varicella. MMWR Morb Mortal Wkly Rep 1996;45(RR-11):1.

SECTION

3

Psychiatric and Behavioral Problems

C H A P T E R 19

Evaluation of Psychosocial Problems

VARSHA K. VAIDYA, MD
CHESTER W. SCHMIDT, Jr., MD

Patients with psychological and social problems often consult their general physicians, usually complaining of not feeling well in some physical sense. The problems these patients present range from temporary distress to enduring and disabling conditions.

The temporary disturbances that are most often seen by the generalist are anxiety regarding the meaning of a new symptom (e.g., cancer fear), frustrations attending an illness that interrupts valued activities (e.g., recovery phase after myocardial infarction), and dysphoric mood related to recent social stress (e.g., anxiety in the mother of a teenager who has run away from home). Such problems are common in people with excellent previous mental health. These disturbances usually resolve when the interviewing and counseling skills discussed in Chapters 3, 4, and 20 are used in conjunction with management of the patient's medical problem.

Patients with more persistent psychosocial problems need to be evaluated and treated for common psychosocial syndromes. This chapter and Chapter 20 provide general approaches for the evaluation and treatment of such patients. Later chapters cover the specific psychosocial syndromes seen by generalists.

EPIDEMIOLOGY

The publication, *Mental Health: A Report of the Surgeon General,* completed and disseminated in 1999, describes the importance and the challenges of mental health problems in the United States (1). The report defines mental health as "the successful performance of mental function, resulting in productive activities, fulfilling relationships with other people, and the ability to adapt to change and to cope with adversity." It points out that mental disorders account for more than 15% of the overall burden of disease from all causes. And it recommends a combination of population-focused and patient-focused initiatives as the most important ways to prevent, identify, or treat mental illness.

The Epidemiologic Catchment Area (ECA) Survey, conducted in 1980 to 1982, identified the frequency of common psychosocial syndromes in a *representative sample of American communities* (1). Table 19.1 lists the four most common disorders in major sex and age subgroups. Approximately 12% of adults reported symptoms of a diagnosable mental disorder during the previous 6 months, and 25% had had a mental illness at some time in their lives. Of subjects meeting criteria for disorders other than alcohol or other drug abuse or dependence, approximately 30% had more than one disorder; of those with alcohol or drug abuse/dependence, 45% and 72%, respectively, had coexisting mental disorders (2). These figures probably underrepresent the true prevalence of mental disorders because the study instrument did not identify patients with two common syndromes: adjustment disorder and generalized anxiety disorder. More than half of those persons with mental illness reported that the only health care providers they saw were generalists, and of these people, the majority had not discussed their mental illness with their health care providers (3).

In one multi-institutional study of American primary care settings, one in four patients met full criteria for a specific psychosocial disorder. However, in these settings, 50% to 75% of those patients suffering from a common mental disorder were not diagnosed or treated (4). A World Health Organization (WHO) survey of 14 countries found a similarly high rate of mental disorders among primary care patients; the rates of both occupational and physical disability were higher in patients with mental illness than in other patients (5). These findings, combined with the ECA community-based data, point to the importance of evaluating patients for mental illness.

SYNDROMAL DIAGNOSIS

Accurate diagnosis of a psychosocial problem is essential for prognosis and management. The *Diagnostic and Statistical Manual of Mental Disorders,* 4th edition TR (DSM-IV TR), published in 2000 by the American Psychiatric Association, is a particularly useful resource because it provides diagnostic criteria, epidemiologic information, and prognostic profiles for most of the psychosocial syndromes encountered in office practice. DSM-IV PC, also published by the American Psychiatric Association, is a useful tool in the diagnosis of psychiatric disorders in the primary care

Table 19.1. Four Most Common Psychiatric Disorders by Sex and Age Based on 6-Month Prevalence Rates[a]

Rank	18–24 Yr	25–44 Yr	45–64 Yr	65+ Yr	Total
Men					
1	Alcohol abuse/ dependence	Alcohol abuse/ dependence	Alcohol abuse/ dependence	Severe cognitive impairment	Alcohol abuse/ dependence
2	Drug abuse/ dependence	Phobia	Phobia	Phobia	Phobia
3	Phobia	Drug abuse/ dependence	Dysthymia	Alcohol abuse/ dependence	Drug abuse/ dependence
4	Antisocial personality	Ant social personality	Major depressive episode without grief	Dysthymia	Dysthymia
Women					
1	Phobia	Phobia	Phobia	Phobia	Phobia
2	Drug abuse/ dependence	Major depressive episode without grief	Dysthymia	Severe cognitive impairment	Major depressive episode without grief
3	Major depressive episode without grief	Dysthymia	Major depressive episode without grief	Dysthymia	Dysthymia
4	Alcohol abuse/ dependence	Obsessive-compulsive disorder	Obsessive-compulsive disorder	Major depressive episode without grief	Obsessive-compulsive disorder

[a]Dysthymia included. The basis for ranking was the mean 6-month prevalence rates for New Haven, Baltimore, and St. Louis combined.

From Myers JK, Weissman MM, Tischler GL, et al. Six-month prevalence of psychiatric disorders in three communities. Arch Gen Psychiatry 1984;41:959.

setting. DSM-IV criteria are stated wherever relevant in the chapters that follow.

Despite the availability of diagnostic criteria, reaching an accurate psychosocial diagnosis in general medical practice can be difficult for several reasons:

- When the presenting symptoms are somatic, physical illness must always be considered, even when the patient's presentation suggests a psychosocial problem.
- Often psychosocial symptoms or findings are not specific for one syndrome.
- The necessary information is different from that needed to evaluate a physical symptom; the most salient information is subjective, obtained by inquiring about or observing thoughts, feelings, behaviors, events, and relationships.

After initial information gathering about mental symptoms, it is usually possible to decide which general phenomenon is the dominant problem (e.g., anxiety, depression, somatization, cognitive impairment, maladaptive behavior). To refine the diagnosis, additional information is needed. For example, consider a patient with a depressed mood. With a systematic approach, the diagnosis of depression may be more accurately formulated as one of the following:

- Adjustment disorder with depressed mood
- Major depression
- Dysthymic disorder (depressive neurosis)
- Depression related to a recently prescribed drug
- Alcoholism presenting as depression

INFORMATION GATHERING

The order in which information is gathered and the particular information gathered vary depending on the style one has developed with previous patients and the diagnosis being considered. With a minimal amount of prompting, many patients volunteer information that would otherwise require systematic questioning. Both the efficiency and the accuracy of the interview are probably enhanced when this occurs. Other interviewing skills useful in eliciting a psychosocial history are described in Chapter 3.

Building on the patient's initial account, one should assess relevant aspects of the social history, the patient's mental status, the patient's personality and coping styles, the chronology of the patient's problem, and the family history of psychosocial problems. Given the time limitations, it may not be possible to get all the information at one time. However, it is important not to miss the following (remembered with the mnemonic "SHAPES"): *s*uicidal ideas, *h*omicidal ideas, problems with *a*ctivities of daily living, *p*sychotic symptoms, *e*mergency medical conditions, and *s*ubstance abuse.

With the patient's permission, additional information should be obtained from family members, other physicians, and previous medical records whenever possible. Current medications should be identified, because psychological disturbances can be caused or worsened by a large number of drugs (6). Tables in other chapters list drugs that can cause anxiety (Table 22.1), depression (Table 24.4), psychotic symptoms (Table 25.2), delirium (Table 26.3), or sexual dysfunction (Table 6.4).

Social and Developmental History

The history should always include a profile of the patient's current life situation (e.g., marital status, family structure, household makeup, educational level, occupation, recreational activities, substance use). At times, it is also helpful to know the principal patterns and events that have characterized a patient's development from childhood until the present (e.g., family makeup, interactions, conflicts, losses, relationships in school, service in the armed forces, jobs) and to have patients depict their view of the type of person they are and have been. Some of this information is known already to the patient's personal physician, which makes the assessment of a new psychosocial problem simpler

Table 19.2. Common Social Factors Related to Psychological Symptoms

Loss: (a) Personal loss—loss of a loved one through death or desertion. (b) Loss of things—imposed loss of home, cherished possession, or job.
Conflict: (a) Interpersonal—conflict within family, with neighbors, or at work, where hostility is recognized. (b) Intrapersonal—role conflict or conflicting demands on the patient (as in a working mother).
Change: (a) Development—where time of life is the major problem (as in adolescence, menopause, or senescence). (b) Geographic—where a move to an unfamiliar environment is the major problem (as in immigration).[a]
Maladjustment: (a) Interpersonal—problems between people with no overt conflict (as in failure to achieve a satisfactory sexual relationship without hostility between partners). (b) Personal—failure to adjust to the environment (home or job) in the absence of the above-mentioned loss, conflict, or change.
Stress: (a) Acute—unexpected event not covered under loss, conflict, or change (for example, the sudden illness of self or of a family member or friend). (b) Chronic—long-term situation not included in loss, conflict, or change (e.g., the presence of a handicapped child in the family).
Isolation—not from any recent loss, change, or conflict (as in an elderly widow).
Failure or frustrated expectations—when the patient's goals in life are not fulfilled and when there is no evidence of an intervening event covered by loss, conflict, or change (e.g., failure at school or failure to achieve occupational promotion).

[a]See Table 1.7 (shows developmental challenges at each stage in family life cycle).

From McWhinney IR. Beyond diagnosis: an approach to the integration of behavioral science and clinical medicine. N Engl J Med 1972;287:384.

at times. When a psychosocial problem seems likely, the presenting symptom should be re-explored in the context of social interactions (e.g., "Tell me just where you were and who was there the last time you noted the nausea and quivering in your stomach"). The patient should be asked to describe any recent changes in life situation and to discuss the nature of critical relationships (e.g., with spouse, children, work associates). If substance abuse or domestic violence, which is often related to substance abuse, is suspected, skillful inquiry is needed to make a diagnosis (see Chapter 28 on alcoholism and domestic violence and Chapter 29 on illicit drugs).

Much psychosocial illness is related to *stressors and maladjustments* that are disclosed by the patient during this inquiry. The social factors most commonly related to psychosocial distress were summarized by McWhinney (Table 19.2). The significance of a report of one of these factors becomes clear when it is integrated into the rest of the history. For example, an interpersonal conflict may be the stress causing an adjustment disorder, or it may be a symptom of alcoholism, depression, or sexual dysfunction.

In addition to providing clues to the diagnosis, the social history usually discloses important assets and liabilities in the patient's life. This information is useful in planning treatment for a psychosocial problem.

Mental Status

When the patient's behavior is the principal problem or when psychological symptoms are causing a great deal of subjective distress (e.g., marked anxiety or depression) or suggest a major psychiatric disorder (e.g., dementia, schizophrenia, manic-depressive illness), a brief mental status examination should be performed.

The mental status examination is a systematic assessment of the patient's current mental functioning. The elements of the mental status examination most useful for the general physician are the following:

- *Appearance:* Grooming, attention to dress, motor activity (quiet versus agitated).
- *General level of consciousness:* Alert, sleepy, stuporous, obtunded.
- *Orientation:* The patient knows who he or she is, where he or she is, and the date (day, month, and year).
- *Speech:* Ability to use customary syntax. Note slurring, inability to find the right word, pressured speech, flight of ideas, looseness of association, muteness.
- *Memory:* Recent memory, or knowledge of recent events, capacity to remember names of current treating physicians. Remote memory, or ability to give history and present illness in proper historical sequence.
- *Attention and concentration:* Ability to understand and follow questions or instructions.
- *Intelligence:* Can be estimated from level of schooling achieved, vocational history, use of language.
- *Mood:* A pervasive, sustained emotion described by the patient (depressed, euphoric, neutral).
- *Affect:* An observable and immediately expressed emotion (e.g., anger, anxiety, sadness, fear, humor, lability). Note whether display of affect is consistent with the content of speech, thoughts, and behavior.
- *Abnormal perceptions:* Presence of hallucinations (i.e., visual, auditory, or somatic perception occurring in the absence of appropriate external stimuli).
- *Abnormal thoughts:* Presence of delusions (fixed beliefs that are false), paranoid ideas, obsessional thoughts (recurrent intrusive thoughts), compulsive behaviors (repetitive behaviors), or persistent phobias (fears directed toward specific objects or situations).
- *Suicidal thoughts:* Statement or actions that indicate the patient wishes to harm or kill himself or herself.
- *Homicidal or violent thoughts:* Statements or actions that indicate the patient wishes to harm or kill others.
- *Judgment:* Capacity of the patient to understand his or her current situation or to demonstrate appropriate compliance with instructions for care.

Most of the data needed for a brief mental status examination are observable while the patient gives the history. Depending on the cues the patient provides, the practitioner should question the patient more about his or her mental status and other features of the syndromes suggested by the history. For patients whose mental status suggests focal or global cognitive impairment, a more formal cognitive examination can be administered in a few minutes (see Table 26.1 in Chapter 26). For those who describe cardinal symptoms of anxiety, affective disorders, or psychotic disorders, focused interviewing is necessary (see Chapters 22, 24, and 25, respectively).

Personality

Personality is the enduring attitudes and patterns of behavior that typify an individual. Generally a physician becomes acquainted with a patient's personality, particularly the patient's behavior pattern in the face of illness, through caring for that patient during months or years. Some patients exhibit the features of a maladaptive personality, and recognition of this fact may be helpful in planning the patient's care, as discussed in more detail in Chapter 23.

Coping Responses

Coping responses are unconscious intellectual maneuvers that people assume in adapting to life stresses. There are several common coping responses that should be recognized because patients may use them to avoid confronting a problem for which help is needed. When maladaptive coping is recognized, the physician can often help the patient to disclose the primary problem and to reach a healthier adaptation to it.

Denial is a common response by which a distressing problem is avoided. Denial may be silent (e.g., a patient with bloody stools may withhold this information to avoid confronting the fear of cancer), or it may be voiced openly (e.g., a man who greatly fears sudden death during convalescence from a myocardial infarction may boast of robust health and deny angina or other symptoms he is experiencing).

Rationalization serves the same function as denial. It is a process in which a patient gives plausible explanations for behavior designed to avoid unpleasant realities (e.g., a relapsing alcoholic explains that demands at work increased so much lately that it was impossible to continue to go to Alcoholics Anonymous meetings).

Regression is reversion to dependent behavior typical of childhood. Regressive behavior is a common response to major illness or other circumstances that threaten a person's autonomy (e.g., a man who is recovering slowly from a hip fracture complains excessively about small problems at home, gets upset when his son cannot continue to visit daily, and expects his wife to order for him when they go out to a restaurant on the weekend).

Projection is a process in which an unpleasant aspect of one's self is ascribed to another person (e.g., a teenager who is angry about limits set by her mother criticizes her older sister for being hostile to their mother).

Displacement is a process in which feelings toward one person are directed toward another (e.g., a researcher who is furious at a colleague who has beaten him to an important finding becomes irritable toward his wife for no apparent reason).

Chronology

Accurate information about the chronology of a psychosocial problem is important for diagnosis, prognosis, and management. Therefore, as the interview is closing, one should ensure that the patient has provided the following essential information: duration of the present episode; the times and circumstances during which the current symptoms have either improved or worsened (if temporal relationships are unclear, it is helpful to have the patient keep a log of symptoms and events for 1 week or longer); the patient's optimal level of functioning during the past year (when was it and how long did it last?); and the time and circumstances of any previous episode of similar symptoms or of previous mental illness and any previous treatments.

Family History

In the family of a patient with a chronic psychosocial disorder, occurrence in others of the same disorder or of other psychiatric problems is common. Information about psychiatric illness in the family and related beneficial treatments may strengthen one's diagnostic hunches, influence the choice of treatment, and help the patient to recognize the nature of his or her own problem.

OVERALL FORMULATION OF THE PROBLEM

When the essentials of a patient's psychosocial history have been collected, a useful way to formulate the problem is the five-axis approach recommended by the American Psychiatric Association.

- *Axis I:* Clinical psychiatric and/or substance abuse disorders, plus conditions not attributable to a formal mental disorder that are a focus of attention (e.g., psychological factors affecting medical condition, malingering, uncomplicated bereavement, noncompliance with medical treatment, academic or occupational problems)
- *Axis II:* Personality disorders or styles and specific developmental disorders
- *Axis III:* General medical conditions
- *Axis IV:* Psychological and environmental stressors that may be recent or of long standing (Table 19.3).
- *Axis V:* Global assessment of functioning (GAF)—current level and highest level for at least a few months during the past year (Table 19.4).

Case Study

Mr. J, a 60-year-old married security guard, underwent coronary artery bypass graft (CABG) surgery in January 1998. His postoperative hospital course was uneventful. Shortly after discharge, he came twice in the same day to the emergency

Table 19.3. Axis IV: Categories for Psychosocial and Environmental Problems

Problems with primary support group
Problems related to the social environment
Educational problem
Occupational problem
Housing problem
Economic problem
Problems with access to health care services
Problems related to interaction with the legal system/crime
Other psychosocial problem

Reprinted with permission from Diagnostic and statistical manual of mental disorders. 4th ed. Washington DC: American Psychiatric Association, 1994.

department complaining of severe chest pain and cold upper extremities. Evaluation revealed mild tenderness at the location of his sternotomy scar. The next day he returned, this time describing inability to sleep in addition to the previous symptoms. A thorough evaluation, including an exercise stress test, did not disclose a physical basis for his symptoms.

The patient's wife described regressive behavior since the patient returned home (e.g., he wanted her to bring his meals to him in bed, asked her to pick his clothes for him each day, was having occasional urinary incontinence, and had put her in charge of dispensing all of his medicines). He was not sleeping well and awakened his wife whenever he could not sleep. Additional inquiry and observation revealed a somewhat diminished sense of self-worth and some doubts regarding his future. He was worried specifically that he would not return to work, as he had expected to preoperatively, and his calculations suggested that his income would be significantly lower if he applied for Social Security benefits.

The patient eventually disclosed that he was sure that he had been on the pump too long and that he feared that his incision would break down (this had happened to a friend after CABG).

Mr. J had always seemed to be a self-reliant man. He had worked as a security guard, while receiving medical therapy for his angina, for several years. The CABG was recommended when his angina worsened in November 1997, making it difficult for him to walk the distances required at his job. He had never developed markedly regressive behavior in the past, although he had depended on his wife to make decisions about almost all purchases they made, had never been separated from her for a full day during their long and tranquil marriage, and often referred to her as "Mother." There was no history of significant psychiatric illness in his family.

Based on this story and additional inquiry, the formulation of Mr. J's illness was as follows:

- *Axis I:* Adjustment disorder, with depressed mood and physical complaints
- *Axis II:* No personality disorder; history of dependency that made him vulnerable to the behavior he exhibited after CABG
- *Axis III:* (a) Coronary artery disease; (b) status postcoronary artery bypass graft, with good technical result
- *Axis IV:* Economic problems
- *Axis V:* Current GAF = moderate symptoms and functional impairment (code 60 in Table 10.4); past year GAF = slight symptoms and functional impairment (code 80 in Table 10.4)

COMORBID SUBSTANCE ABUSE

In a patient with comorbid substance abuse, it is often difficult to tease out which came first: Is the patient depressed or hypomanic because he or she is using drugs, or is the patient using drugs to "self-medicate" his or

Table 19.4. Global Assessment of Functioning (GAF) Scale

Consider psychologic, social, and occupational functioning on a hypothetical continuum of mental health–illness. Do not include impairment in functioning caused by physical (or environmental) limitations.

Code	
100–91	Superior functioning in a wide range of activities, life's problems never seem to get out of hand, is sought out by others because of his or her many positive qualities. No symptoms.
90–81	Absent or minimal symptoms (e.g., mild anxiety before an examination), good functioning in all areas, interested and involved in a wide range of activities, socially effective, generally satisfied with life, no more than everyday problems or concerns (e.g., an occasional argument with family members).
80–71	If symptoms are present, they are transient and expectable reactions to psychosocial stressors (e.g., difficulty concentrating after family argument); no more than slight impairment in social, occupational, or school functioning (e.g., temporarily falling behind in schoolwork).
70–61	Some mild symptoms (e.g., depressed mood and mild insomnia) OR some difficulty in social, occupational, or school functioning (e.g., occasional truancy, or theft within the household), but generally functioning pretty well, has some meaningful interpersonal relationships.
60–51	Moderate symptoms (e.g., flat affect and circumstantial speech, occasional panic attacks) OR moderate difficulty in social, occupational, or school functioning (e.g., no friends, unable to keep a job).
50–41	Serious symptoms (e.g., suicidal ideation, severe obsessional rituals, frequent shoplifting) OR any serious impairment in social, occupational, or school functioning (e.g., no friends, unable to keep a job).
40–31	Some impairment in reality testing or communication (e.g., speech is at times illogical, obscure, or irrelevant) OR major impairment in several areas, such as work or school, family relations, judgment, thinking, or mood (e.g., depressed man avoids friends, neglects family, and is unable to work; child frequently beats up younger children, is defiant at home, and is failing at school).
30–21	Behavior is considerably influenced by delusions or hallucinations OR serious impairment in communication or judgment (e.g., sometimes incoherent, acts grossly inappropriately, suicidal preoccupation) OR inability to function in almost all areas (e.g., stays in bed all day; no job, home, or friends).
20–11	Some danger of hurting self or others (e.g., suicide attempts without clear expectation of death, frequently violent, manic excitement) OR occasionally fails to maintain minimal personal hygiene (e.g., smears feces) OR gross impairment in communication (e.g., largely incoherent or mute).
10–1	Persistent danger of severely hurting self or others (e.g., recurrent violence) OR persistent inability to maintain minimal personal hygiene OR serious suicidal act with clear expectation of death.
0	Inadequate Information.

Reprinted with permission from Diagnostic and statistical manual of mental disorders. 4th ed. Washington, DC: American Psychiatric Association, 1994.

Figure 19.1. PRIME-MD (Primary Care Evaluation of Mental Disorders) one-page patient questionnaire that is to be completed by the patient before seeing the physician. (From Spitzer R, Williams J, Kroenke K. Utility of a new procedure for diagnosing mental illness in primary care: the PRIME-MD 1000 Study. JAMA 1994;272:1749. Reproduced with permission of the American Medical Association.)

PATIENT QUESTIONNAIRE

NAME: ____________ **TODAY'S DATE:** ____________

INSTRUCTIONS: This questionnaire will help your doctor better understand problems that you may have. Your doctor may ask you more questions about some of these items. Please make sure to check a box for every item.

*During the **PAST MONTH**, have you **OFTEN** been bothered by...*	Yes	No		Yes	No	*During the **PAST MONTH**...*	Yes	No
1. stomach pain	☐	☐	12. constipation, loose bowels, or diarrhea	☐	☐	22. have you had an anxiety attack (suddenly feeling fear or panic)	☐	☐
2. back pain	☐	☐	13. nausea, gas, or indigestion	☐	☐	23. have you thought you should cut down on your drinking of alcohol	☐	☐
3. pain in your arms, legs, or joints (knees, hips, etc)	☐	☐	14. feeling tired or having low energy	☐	☐	24. has anyone complained about your drinking	☐	☐
4. menstrual pain or problems	☐	☐	15. trouble sleeping	☐	☐	25. have you felt guilty or upset about your drinking	☐	☐
5. pain or problems during sexual intercourse	☐	☐	16. the thought that you have a serious undiagnosed disease	☐	☐	26. was there ever a single day in which you had five or more drinks of beer, wine, or liquor	☐	☐
6. headaches	☐	☐	17. your eating being out of control	☐	☐	Overall, would you say your health is:		
7. chest pain	☐	☐	18. little interest or pleasure in doing things	☐	☐	Excellent ☐		
8. dizziness	☐	☐	19. feeling down, depressed, or hopeless	☐	☐	Very good ☐		
9. fainting spells	☐	☐	20. "nerves" or feeling anxious or on edge	☐	☐	Good ☐		
10. feeling your heart pound or race	☐	☐	21. worrying about a lot of different things	☐	☐	Fair ☐		
11. shortness of breath	☐	☐				Poor ☐		

her symptoms? It is important to obtain a history of substance abuse, as detailed in Chapter 29. Information from the patient about how long he or she was abstinent from drugs is of special relevance. If the patient had symptoms during a reasonably long "clean" or drug-free period and relapsed when depressed, then he or she is more likely to need and benefit from psychotropic medication. There will remain a subgroup of patients for whom the chronology is unclear or who have had no clean time; it may be reasonable to treat the symptoms if they persist beyond the initial withdrawal dysphoria (7,8).

COMORBIDITY IN THE PATIENT'S FAMILY

Psychosocial problems create substantial stress for the spouse, children, and other people with close ties to the affected patient. This is particularly true of chronic problems such as alcoholism, affective disorders, anxiety disorders, and the somatoform disorders. The impact of the patient's illness on others should always be considered in the evaluation of psychosocial problems. As pointed out in other chapters in this section, there are important ways in which the comorbidity of the family can be alleviated as part of the overall approach to these trying problems. Chapter 3 describes how to conduct a family meeting that focuses on a specific problem, and Chapter 20 describes the process for formal family counseling.

SCREENING FOR MENTAL ILLNESS IN PRIMARY CARE SETTINGS

The questionnaire known as PRIME MD (Primary Care Evaluation of Mental Disorders) is a useful and well-validated tool that can be used to screen patients in primary care settings. It is relatively brief and covers the spectrum of psychiatric disorders inclusive of alcoholism (Fig.19.1).

ASSESSMENT OF COMPETENCE, DECISION-MAKING CAPACITY, AND NEED FOR COMMITMENT

The three situations covered here require input by a physician or multiple physicians who know or have examined the patient. A physician assesses the patient's competence and decision-making capacity implicitly at every medical encounter. At times, the assessment must be done explicitly.

Competence and *incompetence* are legal terms, and their use should generally be restricted to situations in which a formal determination has been made. Under the law, people are presumed competent to manage their own affairs until a judicial determination has been made. A physician may be called on to provide evidence to be used in such a determination. Common civil issues that require determination of mental competence include competence to accept or refuse medical care, commitment to hospitals, contesting of wills, and guardianship decisions. In the ambulatory setting, perhaps the most common problem presented by marginally competent patients is unreliable self-care; here, the assistance of a reliable household member or visiting nurse is essential, in addition to the measures needed to obtain a legal decision about competence.

Decision-making capacity is a clinical term referring to the capacity of the patient to make a particular decision. It is also called *clinical competency.* Judgments regarding such capacity are made by clinicians every day, particularly when informed consent is sought for performing medical procedures. Decision-making capacity is said to be present when the patient demonstrates the following:

- Capacity to comprehend information relevant to the decision
- Capacity to deliberate about the choices in accordance with personal values and goals
- Capacity to communicate (verbally or nonverbally) with caregivers

Patients may have the capacity to make one decision (e.g., to assign power of attorney to a relative) but not another (e.g., to decide whether to undergo an experimental surgical procedure), so decision-making capacity must be addressed each time a decision is required. The presence of a psychiatric or neurologic disorder does not necessarily imply incapacity. Although patients who are demented, delirious, delusional, or hallucinating often lack decision-making capacity, they may actually be able to make some decisions themselves. Therefore, they require the same assessment as patients without these disorders or symptoms.

Commitment laws in most states require examination by a physician and do not specify examination by a psychiatrist. Therefore, the patient's primary physician is occasionally required to assist in a commitment determination. A complete psychiatric evaluation, including a complete mental status examination, is necessary to determine whether a patient is dangerous to himself or herself or to others, which is the usual test for commitment.

General References*

American Psychiatric Association. **Diagnostic and statistical manual of mental disorders.** 4th ed., Text Revision. (DSM-IV TR). Washington, DC: American Psychiatric Association, 2000.

Diagnostic criteria and epidemiologic information for all recognized psychiatric disorders.

American Psychiatric Association. **Diagnostic and statistical manual of mental disorders.** 4th ed., Primary Care Version (DSM-IV PC). Washington, DC: American Psychiatric Association, 2000.

Easy to use diagnostic tool with disorders grouped by presenting symptoms seen in primary care, with algorithms for the nine most common presenting symptoms. Comes with a 15-minute video guide to describe the algorithms.

Spitzer R, Williams J, Kroenke K. Utility of a new procedure for diagnosing mental illness in primary care: the PRIME-MD 1000 Study. JAMA 1994;272:1749.

An excellent screening tool for psychiatric disorders in primary care.

Specific References

1. U.S. Department of Health and Human Services. Mental health: a report of the Surgeon General—executive summary. Rockville, MD: U.S. Department of Health and Human Services, Substance Abuse and Mental Health Services Administration, Center for Mental Health Services, National Institutes of Health, National Institute of Mental Health, 1999.
2. Myers JK, Weissman MM, Tischler GL, et al. Six-month prevalence of psychiatric disorders in three communities. Arch Gen Psychiatry 1984;4:959.
3. Regier DA, Farmer ME, Rae DS, et al. Comorbidity of mental disorders with alcohol and other drug abuse: results from the Epidemiologic Catchment Area (ECA) study. JAMA 1990;264: 2511.
4. Ford DE, Kamerow DB, Thompson JW. Who talks to physicians about mental health and substance abuse problems? J Gen Intern Med 1988;3:363.
5. Spitzer R, Williams J, Kroenke K. Utility of a new procedure for diagnosing mental illness in primary care: the Prime -MD 1000 Study. JAMA 1994;272:1749.
6. Ormel J, VonKorff M, Ustun B, et al. Common mental disorders and disability across cultures: results from the WHO collaborative study on psychological problems in general health care. JAMA 1994;272:1741.
7. Drugs that cause psychiatric symptoms. Med Lett 1998;40:21.
8. Brooner RK, King VL, Schmidt CW. Bigelow Psychiatric and Substance Abuse comorbidity among treatment seeking opiod users. Arch Gen Psychiatry 1997;54:71.

*Bold print (general references) and bold numerals (specific references) denote published controlled clinical trials, meta-analyses, or consensus-based recommendations.

CHAPTER 20

Psychotherapy in Ambulatory Practice

ROBERT P. ROCA, MD, MPH
L. RANDOL BARKER, MD

Psychotherapy consists of verbal and behavioral processes that are used for the purpose of relieving symptoms and resolving intrapersonal and interpersonal conflicts. Although many different techniques have been described, there are fundamental principles that are common to all. Generalist physicians have many opportunities to use psychotherapy, both formally and informally.

GENERAL PRINCIPLES

Demoralization

Most candidates for office psychotherapy suffer from *demoralization,* a painful sense of disappointment and personal inadequacy in the face of life circumstances. By the time such patients acknowledge their distress to the doctor, their usual problem-solving methods have failed and their usual sources of support have been exhausted. Demoralization can be formulated as the product of *interactions between environmental stressors and personal vulnerabilities.* Environmental stressors may be remediable (e.g., temporary unemployment) or irremediable (e.g., conjugal bereavement). Personal vulnerabilities may be constitutional (e.g., mental retardation) or learned (e.g., excessive dependency or perfectionism). Particular personal vulnerabilities make individuals susceptible to particular stressors. For example, an exceedingly dependent person may be especially sensitive to the death of a spouse; rigid, controlling parents may be especially distressed by the rebelliousness of their adolescent children.

Psychotherapy may be viewed as an interactive process intended to restore morale. It involves both cognitive and relational tasks. The primary *cognitive task* is to develop a working formulation of patients' difficulties as products of environmental stressors and personal vulnerabilities, to appreciate the personal strengths and resources available to patients for problem-solving and amelioration of emotional distress, and to help patients apply these strengths and resources to regain a sense of mastery over life problems. Some strategies useful for these purposes are described in later sections of this chapter (see Psychosocial Treatment Techniques and Forms of Counseling).

The *relational task* is to promote in patients what Jerome Frank has called "*expectant trust*" (see Frank, 1968, in General References). This describes an attitude on the part of patients that their physician cares about them, is competent to help, is confident of their recovery, and is committed to remain available until relief is obtained. Expectant trust is an important element in psychotherapeutic success, and it is enhanced by several of the techniques described in this chapter. Its effective mobilization also requires an understanding of the concepts of transference and countertransference.

Transference

Patients' expectations of their doctors have complex psychosocial roots. In part, they grow out of patients' experiences with their parents in circumstances of fear, pain, and other forms of distress. As a result of these experiences, patients consciously and unconsciously may come to expect that new people in their lives, particularly caretakers such as physicians, will treat them as their parents did. These expectations are known as transference phenomena: *patients transfer expectations onto their physicians.* When the transferred expectations are positive (*positive transference*), physicians have at their disposal a powerful resource in their work to help their patients feel better. Positive transference may partly explain placebo responses and must be borne in mind when the effects of new therapeutic interventions are being evaluated.

Not all transference phenomena are positive. Everyone experiences anger, frustration, and other painful emotions in response to the disappointments and deprivations that invariably accompany growing up. These experiences sometimes leave emotional residua that may contaminate the relationship of the patient with caretakers or authority figures such as physicians. For example, patients who were abandoned by their parents may unconsciously expect that their physician will also abandon them and may therefore cling to the doctor with pathologic dependency. Other sorts of early life experiences may lead to passivity, hostility, compulsiveness, and other maladaptive responses. Negative expectations (negative transference), as well as positive expectations, may be transferred onto physicians and may give rise to maladaptive reactions that complicate the physician–patient relationship and interfere with therapeutic success if not properly managed.

In psychotherapy, transference phenomena are regarded as tools and opportunities as well as potential obstacles. Psychological distress is often the result of interpersonal problems with family, friends, and associates. Transference phenomena create, in the presence of the psychotherapist, modified but reasonably accurate representations of patients' current and past relationships. As patients, through transference, begin to treat the therapist as a significant person from the past, the therapist gains valuable insight into the roots of patients' interpersonal difficulties and may ultimately use these insights to help patients improve their relationships.

The type and intensity of the transference and the opportunities for its use in treatment vary with the intensity of the therapeutic relationship and the frequency of visits. In short-term counseling, intense therapeutic relationships generally do not develop, and the transference is predominantly positive.

Countertransference

Physicians, like their patients, must endure the trials and tribulations of childhood and adolescence and may thereby develop positive and negative *expectations that are transferred onto other people, including patients.* These expectations, called countertransference, may compromise the ability of the physician to care for particular patients. For example, the physician son of an abusive alcoholic father may have such a personal emotional stake in promoting the abstinence of his male alcoholic patients that he becomes enraged and ineffective with them when they relapse. It is the responsibility of the physician to be aware of countertransference phenomena and to resist their intrusion into the doctor–patient relationship, particularly in the context of counseling. The physician may find psychotherapy helpful for this purpose.

PSYCHOSOCIAL TREATMENT TECHNIQUES

Because the simple disclosure of emotional distress and its causes may bring considerable relief to patients, the process of psychosocial evaluation often has therapeutic value in itself. General aspects of evaluation for psychosocial problems are described in Chapter 19. This section describes the principal techniques used in counseling, and the following section describes the forms of planned counseling useful in office practice.

Establishing a Therapeutic Relationship

As noted earlier (see Transference), the therapeutic relationship recapitulates to some extent the parent–child relationship. Several elements are generic to an effective therapeutic relationship. The patient must trust the physician. Physicians earn trust by showing interest consistently, accepting sensitive information without being judgmental, taking the patients' concerns seriously, and controlling inappropriate reactions to difficult patients (see Table 3.7 in Chapter 3). In addition to establishing trust, physicians should ensure that their patients understand how to gain access to them and recognize limits regarding access during ongoing treatment. It is useful to reflect on whether these trust-promoting and condition-setting actions have been accomplished before embarking on counseling.

Identifying and Addressing Information Needs

Misinformation or lack of information causes much distress. Patients often come to the office with a unfounded fear of dread illness or a significant misunderstanding of an established condition. At times, a patient's own "explanatory model" for what is wrong dominates the picture (see Chapter 4). When careful interviewing reveals the need for information and explanation, physicians provide a vital service by tailoring their teaching to patients' needs and taking care to confirm that the information has been received and understood. Clear explanations of normal physiology, disease processes, and treatment regimens are often overlooked as powerful aids in counseling. Besides providing information, such explanations draw patients into collaborative relationships with their physicians.

The following interventions are often therapeutic in themselves:

- Identification or clarification regarding a *feared or existing physical disorder.* For example,

  The son of a recently deceased diabetic patient thinks he also has diabetes and is greatly relieved by a negative workup for diabetes and a brief explanation of the implications of the result.

  A woman with mitral valve prolapse who has adopted unnecessary activity limitations is reassured by teaching regarding the benign course of her condition and by advice that she should resume valued activities. Her physician gives her the American Heart Association booklet, *Mitral Valve Prolapse*, to reinforce the clarification.

- Identification or clarification regarding a *psychophysiologic basis for somatic symptoms.* For example,

  A man with panic disorder obtains partial relief from an explanation of how hyperventilation leads to central nervous system symptoms.

- Identification or clarification of the *role of a psychosocial stressor in producing symptoms.* For example,

  A man with an anxiety disorder is helped to recognize that his symptoms are being intensified by an expected job layoff, alleviating his fear that he is "going crazy."

- Identification of a working *diagnosis, the plan, and the likely prognosis.* For example,

A woman with major depression is encouraged when she is told the diagnosis, the plan to use gradually increasing doses of antidepressants, and the likelihood of significant improvement after a few weeks.

A man with hypochondriasis reaches a truce with his physician when he is informed that he will probably continue to have some minor symptoms but that he is not seriously ill and may resume valued activities from which he has withdrawn.

Eliciting and Responding to Feelings

It is critical for physicians to be skillful in the management of emotions. Central to emotional management are a willingness to allow patients to discuss feelings in the office and an ability to listen empathically.

Empathic Listening

Patients find it reassuring when physicians pay close attention to what they are saying and to the feelings that they are experiencing. Granting the patient time to reflect, remembering details of the history, responding with appropriate affect to situations described by the patient, and indicating what one has observed or heard about the patient's feelings are actions that demonstrate concern, diminish the isolation that accompanies unexpressed feelings, and enhance the patient's self-esteem. For example,

A man with generalized anxiety disorder feels better after a visit to his physician at which the physician listened attentively, summarized what the patient said, and told him that he understood how distressing it must be for the patient to have tension headaches and difficulty concentrating on his work when he is plagued by worries.

Legitimizing Feelings

Patients often feel embarrassed or isolated by their reactions to a situation. One way to help alleviate those feelings is to point out that anyone in the patient's situation might have similar reactions. For example,

A college professor who is confronting surgery for breast cancer is troubled by nagging feelings of anger; she was preparing to move to another city when she discovered the lump in her breast. She says that it helped when her physician acknowledged the anger and stated, "Your anger is very understandable. Anyone in your situation would feel the same way."

Ventilation of Feelings

Patients who have "held in" strong feelings about past or current experiences usually feel better after giving voice to these feelings. The physician can encourage a therapeutic expression of feelings by stating that the patient looks tense, angry, or depressed or by commenting that the experience that the patient has just described must have made the patient feel upset. For example,

A middle-aged woman with chronic depression (dysthymic disorder) feels better when she cries in the presence of her physician about feelings of guilt caused by the anger she develops toward members of her family in response to day-to-day domestic frustrations.

Problem-Solving

Demonstrating Respect and Facilitating Choice

When counseling a patient, one should avoid a condescending, patronizing, or overbearing tone. As noted earlier (see Demoralization), patients usually attempt to resolve their problems on their own before seeking professional help. Furthermore, they may describe themselves as usually able to handle problems. Inquiring about and acknowledging previous efforts, even when they have been inept or unsuccessful, and supporting any voiced characterization of themselves as problem-solvers can help ready patients for addressing a current problem. The fundamental strategies for facilitated problem-solving involve helping the patient recognize assets (e.g., supportive people, enjoyed activities), identify options, and make choices that favor resolution of current problems. It is occasionally necessary to be more directive.

Contingency Planning

Stressful life situations can often be made more manageable by simple practical measures. Distressed patients sometimes cannot see these opportunities. Once the particular facts of a patient's dilemma are known, the physician may be able to help the patient develop specific plans for dealing with anticipated problems. In making contingency plans, it is useful to present hypothetical situations and to have the patient decide how to handle them. For example,

A woman who lives alone is distraught because her only child, a grown daughter who recently moved to another city, has hinted that she may not be able to get home for Christmas. The woman's physician encourages her to make alternative Christmas plans so that she will not be alone for the holiday if her daughter is in fact unable to come to visit. She telephones later in the week to say that she still does not know whether her daughter will be able to come for Christmas but has invited friends to her home for Christmas dinner (contingency plan) with her and feels much better.

Advice (Persuasion)

The physician is considered by the patient to be an expert and should be willing to take advantage of that status under appropriate circumstances. Concrete recommendations may be especially helpful for patients whose decision-making ability may be impaired. For example,

A middle-aged man with major depression who is unrealistically dissatisfied with his job performance is tactfully persuaded to defer his decision about early retirement until his mood has improved.

Advice may also be used confrontationally to force patients to acknowledge dangerous or destructive behavior. The shock of the confrontation may challenge complacency and facilitate behavioral change.

MANAGING ABNORMAL ILLNESS BEHAVIOR

Abnormal illness behavior is present when the patient's symptoms or impairments, and associated health-care seeking behavior, are disproportionate to detectable disease. Although such behavior is commonplace in medical practice, abnormal illness behavior forms the core of the *somatoform disorders* (see Chapter 21), conditions in which patients express their emotional distress mainly in terms of somatic complaints and convictions that they have serious illness. The following general strategies are useful for patients whose psychosocial problems present mainly as abnormal illness behavior:

1. *Do not facilitate or reinforce abnormal illness behavior.*
   A. Avoid unnecessary testing.
   B. Avoid unnecessary prescribing.
   C. Avoid unnecessary referral to specialists.
   D. *Schedule regular visits* (i.e., do not make visits contingent on a new or worsening symptom) and stay within a time frame agreed upon for visits.
2. *Permit the patient to have some symptoms* (do not view elimination of symptoms as an essential goal).
3. *Encourage the patient to talk about his or her life situation instead of about somatic symptoms.* For example,

A patient with somatization disorder (see Chapter 21) and an unremarkable recent urinalysis states that she plans to see the urologist who took care of her friend's bladder problem. She is instead persuaded to come for brief weekly visits to her primary physician. At the weekly visits, the physician focuses chiefly on the patient's efforts to keep her teenage daughter in school and commends her for any success that she reports in handling these and other domestic problems. Her urinary complaints gradually resolve.

Involving Family, Friends, and Environment

Family members, close friends, and the environment are potentially valuable clinical resources. When including family members and others in the care of a patient, it is vital to respect the patient's right to confidentiality. It is important to obtain the patient's permission to speak with others and, when appropriate, to include the patient in meetings with family members (see Table 3.1 in Chapter 3). The following are common interventions that may enhance the usefulness of these meetings.

Meeting the Family's Information Needs. Family and close friends often suffer greatly because of their loved one's illness and often have the same information needs as the patient (see earlier discussion). If they are to understand the patient's feelings and behavior and handle appropriately their own feelings and behavior toward the patient, these needs must be addressed. For example,

A 70-year-old man who has a major depression tells his physician that his son will probably telephone the physician to ask for information. The son telephones the physician and expresses the concern that his father has been angrily criticizing his young grandchildren for all kinds of petty reasons and that this is not the way he used to treat the children. Furthermore, the son is worried that his father must have an ulcer because he leaves the table rubbing his stomach and shaking his head after eating a few bites. The physician empathizes with the patient's son and explains that the behavior change is typical for a depressed man, that the antidepressant medication that has just been started should lead to some improvement within 2 to 3 weeks, that the history and physical examination did not reveal evidence for anything like an ulcer, and that it is likely that his father will recover entirely within 2 to 4 months. The son is relieved and expresses the hope that things will go the way the physician predicts.

Enlisting the Family's Help. For some conditions in which the patient demonstrates a failure to make choices favoring improvement, the family may be instrumental in promoting such choices. For example,

The family of an alcoholic patient agrees to participate in a family intervention (see Chapter 28) to get the patient to accept treatment.

Facilitating Healthy Choices Regarding the Patient's Environment. For example,

The mood of a woman with a long-standing depression (dysthymic disorder) improves after she is encouraged to take a job as a companion and housekeeper for an elderly woman who had a stroke.

Knowing and Using Community Resources

Support groups, recreational or vocational programs, and home health services are among the community resources that may be helpful to patients. A physician's awareness of and enthusiasm about a community resource can be instrumental in determining its impact on a patient. For example,

The depressed and anxious wife of an alcoholic man experiences marked improvement in her symptoms after she becomes active in Al-Anon, a resource suggested by her physician.

An elderly woman attends a medical day care program, which provides supervised activity for her 5 days a week. This resource, suggested by her physician, enables the patient's family to continue to have her live with them and alleviates the patient's feelings of anger and guilt toward family members who felt compelled to check on her frequently during the day.

FORMS OF COUNSELING

The treatment techniques described earlier in this chapter help at times in the care of all patients. Several forms of planned counseling, each of which integrates a number of these treatment techniques, are helpful in the care of selected patients.

Supportive Therapy

The purpose of supportive therapy is to help a patient cope with both ongoing medical problems and stressful life circumstances. Unlike short-term counseling (see next section), the duration of supportive therapy is open ended, and it is often incorporated into the routine management of a chronic disease.

Example: Supportive Therapy

A physician decides that supportive psychotherapy will be helpful in the long-term treatment of a diabetic patient with a history of poor compliance and multiple family problems. The patient is seen once a month for 20 minutes to monitor the patient's diabetes, enhance compliance, and review family problems. The verbal exchange during the visits includes a review of the medical regimen and glucose monitoring, check for new symptoms, brief review of what has occurred in the patient's life since the last visit, elicitation and acknowledgment of feelings, and discussion of ways to cope with existing family problems. In this manner, a significant supportive service is provided in the context of management of the patient's chronic disease.

Short-Term Counseling

This form of intervention is especially useful in the treatment of the patient who accepts a psychological formulation for symptoms and who wants help in resolving a crisis related to those symptoms. The goals of treatment are to strengthen the defenses of the patient and to relieve symptoms without attempting to deal with long-standing intrapsychic conflicts.

It is usually important at the outset of counseling to establish a *therapeutic contract,* specifying the purpose, length, frequency, and cost of the sessions. These details form the boundaries within which the treatment will take place and may become significant during the course of treatment. Patients often react to the boundaries as part of the transference phenomenon (described previously) by objecting to them or by attempting to change or violate them. Although there are exceptions, the boundaries should not be modified because of a change in the relationship between the patient and the physician that arises as a result of transference. The contractual agreements should remain stable throughout the course of treatment.

The practical realities of practice usually require that sessions be brief (15 to 20 minutes) and limited in number (5 to 10). The short-term nature of treatment helps limit the emergence of negative transference reactions and inappropriate dependency. Patients are usually seen individually, although at times, couples and families may be treated together (see Family Counseling). The aim of such short-term treatment is restoration of morale and relief of emotional distress, not personality change. Treatment should focus on problems that are conscious (i.e., readily accessible, not repressed) and current; one should gently divert patients from repeated recitations of past experiences and injuries. The interactive style should be natural and conversational rather than remote and analytical, and it should be tailored to enhance expectant trust (see earlier discussion). When appropriate, one should point out that the patient's emotional state is an understandable and valid reaction to difficult life circumstances and then, having validated the feelings of distress, express confidence that they will improve. The physician's role is to facilitate problem-solving, usually not to prescribe solutions. To promote problem-solving, one should be prepared to help patients identify their strengths and resources, praise their demonstrations of adaptiveness, and help them explore how they might build on their strengths to solve problems. Patients should be encouraged to try options identified in the sessions by means of homework assignments carried out between sessions.

Throughout the course of short-term counseling, it is important to listen and screen for evidence of a complicating major psychiatric disorder, such as panic disorder, major depression, or alcoholism, because in these conditions, psychotherapy may need to be supplemented by pharmacotherapy or other interventions (see Chapters 22, 24, and 28).

Example: Short-Term Counseling

A 25-year-old woman came for evaluation because of severe leg pain. She had suffered a severe burn injury 1 year before and had experienced leg pain intermittently since then. The physician commented that she appeared tired and tense. At this, she became tearful and said that she and her husband had separated and that, although she felt this was for the best, she was extremely anxious and uncertain that she could manage on her own. She had frightened herself during the previous week by thinking that she might be better off dead.

The history revealed that she was not suicidal and did not meet criteria for major depression or panic disorder. The physician viewed the patient as demoralized and sought to identify the pertinent personal vulnerabilities and environmental stressors. On the basis of a long relationship, the physician knew the patient to be a quiet, self-conscious woman who depended on attractiveness as a source of self-esteem. She was also ambitious and hard-working and had enjoyed considerable occupational success. Her major stressor had been the burn injury. She had been spared facial disfigurement but had considerable scarring on her trunk and lower extremities, which she kept covered at all times. Another stressor was the dissolution of her marriage. She regarded this as a positive development, yet she became tearful when discussing it. When the physician pointed this out, she revealed that she was apprehensive about dating again. She felt certain that the scarring from her burns would make her unattractive to men and that she would therefore remain alone, unable to remarry and have children.

The physician responded that her distress was very understandable in view of the problems she had identified, especially her fears of future loneliness. The physician also told her that these fears might be premature and needed to be examined and proposed meeting weekly for five visits, 20 minutes each, to talk about her choices and assumptions. She agreed.

During the next session she complained about her dissolving marriage. After 5 to 10 minutes the physician praised her for having stuck with it as long as she had and for managing to hold a demanding job so successfully at the same time. She then spoke of compliments given her by coworkers, one of whom had always paid special attention to her. She was grateful for this now but insisted that no one would take an interest in her if he knew of her injuries. The physician asked her how she knew this, reiterated the position that her assumptions warranted exploration, and asked how she might comfortably undertake such an exploration. She considered some options and over the course of several weeks tried several of them, initially simply discussing her injury with others to assess people's responses to the news and finally allowing some friends to see her scarring. The physician praised her for her courage as she proceeded with these explorations and empathized with her as she dealt with feelings generated by recalling the accident and risking rejection by testing people's responses to her.

By the end of the allotted 5 weeks, she was no longer convinced that the future was hopeless. Although still anxious about the ongoing separation and her potential opportunity to date again, she was no longer feeling overwhelmed and believed herself capable of overcoming her self-consciousness about the injury. The physician acknowledged her progress and offered future support.

Family Counseling

The goals of this form of counseling are to facilitate effective communication among family members, bring to their awareness maladaptive patterns of behavior that may be destructive to one or more members of the family, and have family members develop more constructive patterns of behavior. The specific techniques are similar to those used in individual counseling.

Example: Family Counseling

A couple asked their family physician for help in dealing with their adolescent daughter, who was continually misbehaving at school and at home. Evaluation of the problem revealed that the parents had been inconsistent in limit-setting for their daughter and that the family considered the girl to be the "black sheep" of the family. Counseling for the whole family was recommended. During the first session family members demonstrated their usual conflictual pattern of interaction in the presence of the physician: both parents and the other siblings attacked the daughter, blaming her for all of the family's troubles. The physician interrupted the attack and proposed that this exchange must resemble what goes on at home, indicated that the situation seemed uncomfortable for all who were present, and ventured that they would probably like to do something about it. After everyone concurred with these points, the physician shifted the focus to the development of a contract between the parents and their daughter designed to define the rules they expected her to follow and the consequences of violating the rules. The next session was a review of the parents' and daughter's adherence to the contract. The parents reported that the daughter broke the contract by misbehaving, but one of the older siblings pointed out that the parents were inconsistent in their application of the agreed-upon limit-setting rules. This revelation confronted the family with the fact that the girl's behavior was a shared responsibility within the family. Over the remaining sessions, the physician continued to encourage the family to establish fair rules to which all could adhere consistently. By focusing on the behavior of the entire family, the pressure on the daughter was relieved, destructive patterns of interacting were interrupted, and new, constructive patterns were introduced.

Behavior Modification

The impact of office psychotherapy and the impact of the strategies for managing many medical problems described in this book depend on the elements essential to any change in a patient's behavior: being concerned about one's problem, becoming motivated to make a change, taking action to make a change, and maintaining the change. The conceptual bases for promoting behavior change and skills for facilitating behavior change are described in detail in Chapter 4. Skills and interventions useful for addressing specific conditions are described in most of the chapters of this book.

General References

Frank J, Frank J. Persuasion and healing. 3rd ed. Baltimore: Johns Hopkins University Press, 1993.

Presents a model of the patient in distress and the components of practical psychotherapy. Commonalities among Western and non-Western societies are described in this monograph.

Frank JD. The influence of patients' and therapists' expectations on the outcome of psychotherapy. Br J Med Psychol 1968;41:349.

A classic paper on the effect of expectations on treatment outcome.

Jacobson GF. In: Arieti S, ed. American handbook of psychiatry. 2nd ed. New York: Basic Books, 1974.

A concise review of the subject of crisis theory and technique.

McDaniel SH, Campbell TL, Seaburn DB, eds. Family-oriented primary care: a manual for medical providers. New York: Springer-Verlag, 1990.

Helpful for improving one's grounding in theoretical and practical aspects of family involvement in the care of patients with medical and psychosocial problems.

Stuart MR, Lieberman JA. The fifteen-minute hour: applied psychotherapy for the primary care physician. 2nd ed. New York: Praeger, 1993.

Provides an overview of rationale for short-term counseling and describes empirically validated techniques for use in a primary care practice.

CHAPTER 21

Somatization

ROBERT P. ROCA, MD, MPH

ILLNESS BEHAVIOR AND SOMATIZATION

People who consult health care practitioners are expected to have discernible pathologic or pathophysiologic abnormalities (i.e., disease) accounting for their symptoms. The magnitude of their complaints and the associated disability are expected to be proportional to the disease diagnosed. They are supposed to pursue and cooperate with medical care and to resume normal social functioning as soon as possible. This sequence of responses is called *normal illness behavior* (1).

Sometimes there is a discrepancy between diagnosable disease and the magnitude and duration of symptoms and disability. Patients may complain of weakness or pain in the absence of objective findings. They may have pseudoseizures. They may visit their health care practitioners repeatedly with fears of having acquired immunodeficiency syndrome (AIDS) despite several negative human immunodeficiency virus (HIV) serology results and normal physical examinations. Such responses are examples of *abnormal illness behavior.*

Patients exhibiting abnormal illness behavior are often manifesting *somatization,* a phenomenon in which unexplained or amplified physical symptoms are linked to psychological factors or conflicts. Somatization is a feature of many formal psychiatric disorders. Its causes are incompletely understood, but factors promoting somatization can often be discovered in individual cases.

WHY PATIENTS SOMATIZE

Explanations of somatization come from at least four distinct perspectives (2): Somatization may be viewed as a symptom of a disease, a manifestation of personality, a modeled or reinforced behavior, or an understandable product of a patient's life story. Each perspective calls for different observations and illuminates different aspects of the phenomenon of somatization.

Somatization as a Symptom of Disease

Somatization may occur as a symptom of a psychiatric disorder, particularly major depression, panic disorder, schizophrenia, or dementia. Sometimes somatic symptoms are the only complaints that patients with these conditions present to their health care practitioners (3).

Unexplained physical symptoms may also be caused by undiagnosed physical disease, even when the symptoms seem to be expressing a psychological conflict or need. Studies of one subset of somatizing patients—those originally diagnosed as hysterics—have shown that up to 30% may ultimately be found to have medical or neurologic disorders that, in retrospect, explain the presenting hysterical symptoms (4). On the other hand, a general tendency to complain of somatic symptoms may be *negatively* correlated with the presence of particular specific pathologic entities (e.g., coronary artery disease) (5).

Somatization as a Manifestation of Personality

The concept of personality implies enduring attitudes and habitual patterns of response. Personalities may be viewed as approximations of ideal prototypes (e.g., histrionic, obsessive-compulsive), as discussed in Chapter 23, or as clusters of individual traits (e.g., dependency, assertiveness). Somatization has been associated with personality viewed both ways. Patients with a histrionic or an obsessive-compulsive personality type may be predisposed to develop, respectively, somatization disorder or hypochondriasis (see later discussion). Furthermore, patients who are highly introspective (i.e., tend to devote diffuse attention to thoughts and feelings about the self) (6) or neurotic (i.e., emotionally unstable, vulnerable to stress, and self-conscious) (7) tend to experience and report unexplained physical symptoms.

Somatization as Reinforced Behavior

Somatization may be viewed as behavior modeled or reinforced by the patient's environment (8). This perspective prompts exploration for a history of similar symptoms in the patient or a close contact and encourages a search for evidence of social benefit associated with the patient's current symptoms.

CASE EXAMPLE

A 20-year-old woman was evaluated in the office for back pain. The physical examination was unimpressive, and an extensive workup was unrevealing. Discussions with the family disclosed that the patient's father was about to lose his disability income and that financial hardship was expected. Environmental reinforcements related to possibly becoming eligible for disability, thereby ameliorating the family's anticipated financial crisis, probably contributed to the continuation of this patient's symptoms.

Somatization and the Life Story

Somatization may be viewed as a maladaptive but understandable expression of difficulties originating in early life experiences. Although particular formulations can never be proven, they may help clinicians comprehend illness behavior that is otherwise irritating and baffling. For example, patients who suffer parental deprivation and neglect often carry into adulthood potent admixtures of hostility and dependency that may be activated in relationships with health care practitioners. Such patients may develop physical symptoms without diagnosable disease and pursue unrevealing medical evaluations. Often hostile and demanding, they demean the competence and the commitment of their health care practitioners, even as they crave medical attention and insist on even more care. Such behaviors may be seen as expressions of angry disappointment with their earliest caretakers, who did not adequately meet their dependency needs, now displaced onto the practitioner. Other patients, when they were children, may have experienced attention and caring only when they were ill, or they may have come from families or cultures in which it was customary to express emotional distress as physical symptoms. Such formulations may help clinicians respond to such patients with empathy and permit the development of a workable doctor–patient relationship. Other formulations of this type are discussed elsewhere (9,10).

Reaching a Working Formulation

The development of a working formulation requires consideration of the relative merits of the four distinct explanatory points of view in a particular case. There are four fundamental questions:

1. Does the patient have a mental illness of which somatization is a symptom?
2. Does the patient have personality traits or a personality type associated with somatization?
3. Is the patient's abnormal illness behavior modeled or reinforced by some aspect of the patient's environment?
4. Is this behavior understandable when one considers the patient's unique life history and current predicament?

Table 21.1. Psychiatric Disorders Associated with Somatization

Mental disorders
Mood disorders, especially major depression
Anxiety disorders, especially panic disorder
Schizophrenia
Personality disorders, especially histrionic, dependent, and obsessive-compulsive
Reactive emotional states
Adjustment disorder with anxiety or depression
Psychological factors affecting physical conditions
Somatoform disorders
Somatization disorder
Undifferentiated somatoform disorder
Hypochondriasis
Conversion disorder
Somatoform pain disorder
Body dysmorphic disorder
Disorders with voluntary symptom production
Factitious disorder with physical symptoms
Malingering

As shown later, the working formulation often carries specific therapeutic implications.

Somatizing patients often fall into defined diagnostic groups. The psychiatric disorders associated with somatization are listed in Table 21.1. This chapter describes patients in three groups: those with reactive emotional states, those with primary somatizing disorders (see Somatoform Disorders), and those in whom symptom production is deliberate. Mood disorders (Chapter 24), anxiety disorders (Chapter 22), schizophrenia (Chapter 25), and personality disorders (Chapter 23) are discussed in detail elsewhere in this book.

REACTIVE EMOTIONAL STATES

Adjustment Disorders

Description

Adjustment disorders are reactive emotional states resulting from difficulty meeting the demands of life (11). Patients feel overwhelmed by illness, marital discord, or other problems and become demoralized. Their distress may be expressed in somatic terms, both because somatic complaints legitimize a visit to the doctor and because emotional distress can cause somatic symptoms such as light-headedness, fatigue, nausea, urinary frequency, palpitations, precordial pain, and breathlessness. When such symptoms arise in response to psychosocial problems, a diagnosis of adjustment disorder may be made (see Table 24.1 in Chapter 24).

CASE EXAMPLE

A shy 26-year-old parochial school teacher was evaluated for dizziness, abdominal cramps, nausea, excessive urination, and a sensation of fullness in the bladder. When physical examination and laboratory tests revealed no physiologic disturbance, a more detailed history was taken. It showed that the patient's symptoms began shortly after a confrontation with his school principal over his attempt to organize a teacher's union and his criticism of school policies. (Diagnosis: adjustment disorder with anxiety and physical symptoms.)

Patients such as this one are often unaware of the relationship between their psychological distress and somatic symptoms. As illustrated in the following example, diagnosis may be difficult when the symptoms precipitated by psychosocial stress resemble those of a patient's established disease process.

Case Example

A 54-year-old widowed white woman recovering from a myocardial infarction complained to her primary care practitioner of fatigue, breathlessness, and pleuritic-like chest pain unrelated to exertion. Her physical examination and electrocardiographic findings were unchanged. Questioning revealed that the patient was forced to leave her job after her heart attack and was barely able to afford necessary medications. She tearfully revealed that, although her son had offered to help pay for her medications, her daughter-in-law hinted that they could not really afford to help. This proud and formerly self-sufficient woman, who was initially reluctant to accept any help, now felt even more vulnerable and inadequate, and she acknowledged that the periodic symptoms in her chest invariably occurred while she was thinking about these difficulties. (Diagnosis: adjustment disorder with mixed emotional features and physical symptoms.)

In this case, emotional distress produced symptoms suggesting cardiac disease. The correct diagnosis was made when the appropriate history was elicited.

Three strategies are important in evaluating patients who may have adjustment disorders:

1. *Elicit the relevant history.* Asking the patient open-ended questions such as, "How are things at home (or at work)?" invites patients to expand on their history and often reveals potential sources of psychosocial distress. Most patients are grateful for a clinician's interest, respect time limits, and go on to solve the precipitating problem themselves. Even before the practitioner has taken a psychosocial history, patients may provide verbal and nonverbal cues suggesting distress (e.g., saying "Things aren't the way they used to be," wringing hands and looking away when describing a new somatic symptom) (12). Many patients who are initially reluctant to acknowledge psychosocial distress eventually open up in response to gentle, persistent encouragement from a trusted clinician.
2. *Rule out major depression.* Patients who attribute their low mood to identifiable psychosocial stressors do not necessarily have an adjustment disorder. Such symptoms as persistently depressed mood, loss of interest in usual activities, poor concentration, reduced energy, diminished appetite, and disturbed sleep suggest a major depressive disorder for which antidepressant medication usually is indicated (see Chapter 24). The presence of an apparent psychosocial precipitant should never deter the physician from inquiring about such symptoms.
3. *Temper the workup.* Patients should be examined and appropriate laboratory tests ordered; however, extensive workups to exclude improbable diagnoses should be undertaken only after careful consideration and after allowing some time to elapse, because such workups may imbed patients in the sick role and prolong their disability.

Management

The identification of a psychosocial basis for patients' somatic complaints is often sufficient to allow them to marshal their own resources for coping (13). When these measures fail, the patient may need goal-focused short-term counseling (see Chapter 20). In selected cases, short-term prescription of anxiolytic or hypnotic medications may be helpful.

There have been only a few reports of outcomes of minor mood disturbances managed by generalists (13–16). From these studies, the following tentative conclusions can be stated:

- A large proportion of patients get better after just one office visit. Most often, this visit includes empathic listening, a partial physical examination, and reassurance that the patient does not have a serious physical problem.
- Short-term prescribing of drugs for anxiety or insomnia may not increase the proportion of patients who show significant improvement (about two thirds of patients) on re-evaluation after 1 month (14). This conclusion derives from a single careful study in which patients with minor mood disturbances were allocated at random to receive brief counseling plus a benzodiazepine drug or brief counseling only.

Several practical considerations regarding longitudinal management are suggested by these findings:

- It is generally prudent to determine the impact of an initial visit on a patient's distress (by a brief telephone or office follow-up visit within 1 week) before considering a psychotropic drug for an adjustment disorder.
- About one third of patients who seem to have an adjustment disorder do not respond to the aforementioned strategies. At follow-up visits, such patients should be interviewed systematically to look for evidence of panic disorder (see Chapter 22), major depression (see Chapter 24), alcoholism, chemical dependency, domestic violence affecting themselves or a member of their household (see Chapters 28 and 29), or one of the somatoform disorders described later in this chapter. For all of these problems, specific treatment in addition to office psychotherapy is indicated.

Psychological Factors Affecting Medical Conditions

Description

Psychological factors can exacerbate somatic symptoms caused by a concurrent physical disorder. The resulting symptoms are sometimes called

Table 21.2. Common Conditions in Which Psychophysiologic Symptoms Are Important

Physiologic System	Symptomatic Condition	Chapters with Further Information
Cardiovascular	Migraine headache	87
	Vasovagal syndrome (fainting)	89
	Hypertension (usually asymptomatic)	67
	Supraventricular tachycardia	64
	Angina	62
Gastrointestinal	Irritable bowel syndrome	44
	The following symptoms may occur singly or together: anorexia, nausea, vomiting, abdominal cramps, diarrhea, constipation, aerophagia, acid-peptic symptoms	42–46
Genitourinary	Menstrual disturbance	101
	Difficulties in micturition: frequency (in both sexes), retention (females), hesitancy (in males)	
	Sexual disorders	6
	Dyspareunia	
	Anorgasmia	
	Inhibited sexual excitement	
	Delayed ejaculation, premature ejaculation	
Musculoskeletal	Pain secondary to increased muscle tension: occipital or bitemporal headaches, backaches, myalgia in various muscle groups	71, 74, 87
	Fatigue	
	Tremor	90
	Rheumatoid arthritis	77
Respiratory	Hyperventilation syndrome	22
	Bronchospasm	60
	Dyspnea	59
Skin	Hyperhidrosis	
	Pruritus	

Table 21.3. Diagnostic Criteria for Psychological Factors Affecting Physical Condition

A. A general medical condition (coded on axis III) is present.
B. Psychological factors adversely affect the general medical condition in one of the following ways:
1. The factors have influenced the course of the general medical condition as shown by a close temporal association between the psychological factors and the development or exacerbation of, or delayed recovery from, the general medical condition.
2. The factors interfere with the treatment of the general medical condition.
3. The factors constitute additional health risks for the individual.
4. The factors elicit stress-related physiologic responses that precipitate or exacerbate symptoms of a general medical condition (e.g., chest pain or arrhythmia in a patient with coronary artery disease).

psychophysiologic. Table 21.2 lists the most common conditions in which such symptoms may occur. When the features listed in Table 21.3 are present, the diagnosis from the *Diagnostic and Statistical Manual of Mental Disorders,* 4th ed. (DSM-IV), is Psychological Factors Affecting Medical Condition.

Most of the conditions listed in Table 21.2 may occur with or without a significant psychological component; detailed descriptions of most of these conditions are found elsewhere in this book, as indicated in the table. For a patient's symptoms to be interpreted as psychophysiologic, they should bear a temporal relationship to a stressful life situation and should subside when the stressful situation abates.

Conversion symptoms (see later discussion) are differentiated from psychophysiologic symptoms by the absence of a pathophysiologic condition in the former. Psychophysiologic problems are closely related to adjustment disorders, but they are distinguishable from them in that the somatic symptoms are caused by a recognized pathophysiologic condition and the same symptoms may occur in the absence of psychosocial stressors. This diagnosis is also used when psychological factors interfere with the treatment of a general medical condition (e.g., when strong denial of illness interferes with adherence to medication regimens).

Management

When initiation or exacerbation of a physical condition is related to environmental stressors, management is the same as that described for adjustment disorder.

SOMATOFORM DISORDERS

As a group, the somatoform disorders are characterized by the occurrence of physical symptoms that lack an organic basis and are linked, by positive evidence or strong presumption, to psychological factors or conflicts. They may be acute or chronic, mild or severely disabling. Because patients with these disorders believe themselves to be physically ill, they are treated primarily by nonpsychiatrists and generally do not accept psychiatric referral. In addition to the management strategies described here, the strategies for managing abnormal illness behavior, described in Chapter 20, usually are helpful.

Somatization Disorder

Description

The best-studied disorder in this group is somatization disorder, formerly known as hysteria or Briquet syndrome. This is a chronic disorder beginning before 30 years of age in which the patient seeks treatment for multiple, widely distributed symptoms lacking any known pathologic basis or pathophysiologic mechanism. To meet DSM-IV criteria for this disorder, the patient must have a history of at least eight such symptoms, drawn from the four symptom subgroups listed in Table 21.4: Pain symptoms (at least four), gastrointestinal symptoms (two or more), sexual symptoms (at least one), and pseudoneurologic symptoms (at least one). Accurate diagnosis often requires review of old records and careful history-taking to determine that a sufficient number of unexplained symptoms have been presented for evaluation and treatment or have caused the patient to take over-the-counter remedies or alter his or her lifestyle. *Seven symptoms are especially useful in screening*: shortness of breath without exertion, dysmenorrhea, burning sensations in sexual organs, difficulty swallowing (lump in throat), amnesia, vomiting, and pain in extremities. The presence of three of these symptoms without adequate physical explanation identifies somatization disorder with a sensitivity of 87% and specificity of 95% (17). Symptoms are often described in dramatic and colorful terms, but details tend to be vague and contradictory.

Somatization disorder occurs in 0.2% to 2.0% of women in the general population, but it is much more common among women seen in clinical settings (18). It is rare in men. Histrionic personality traits may be present. Somatization disorder occurs in 10% to 20% of female first-degree relatives of women with somatization disorder; alcoholism and antisocial personality disorder occur frequently along their male relatives.

Common complications include substance abuse and iatrogenic illness. One classic study found that women with hysteria undergo more than three times as many operations as control women and lose, by weight, more than three times the mass of organs (19).

The disorder is chronic. In a retrospective study of 49 patients, almost 70% of women were still symptomatic 15 years after diagnosis (20). However, the mortality rate of women with somatization disorder is the same as that of normal women (21), and the likelihood of developing another medical or psychiatric disorder explaining the symptoms is only 10% in long-term follow-up (22).

Case Example

A 43-year-old married white woman was referred for psychiatric evaluation by her internist who, noting her presentation with ill-defined symptoms, was requesting help with management. She complained of generalized muscle aching and periodic sensations throughout her body described as "how you feel when someone scratches his fingers on a blackboard." She also complained of skin lesions on her back and stated that she was hypothyroid and suffered from a chronic urinary tract infection. Her history included tonsillectomy, groin lymph node biopsy (twice), hysterectomy, bladder suspension (twice), rectocele repair, removal of abdominal adhesions, multiple cystoscopies, appendectomy, and removal of a tongue papilloma. The patient stated she had Meniere disease and episodes of sudden shortness of breath. She also carried a diagnosis of fibrositis, for which she had taken steroids in the past, and restless legs syndrome. She had stopped having sexual intercourse with her husband because of "pain that 10 gynecologists could not cure." Her current medicines included a benzodiazepine, a nonsteroidal anti-inflammatory agent, and a belladonna alkaloid. She mentioned that she had always been ill and that she hated men. Her psychosocial history included marriage to an alcoholic who abused her and a positive family history of suicide. In presenting her symptoms, the patient was extremely vague and interjected facts about her emotional life with an inappropriate laugh. She believed that her symptoms were caused by food allergy. She had stopped eating and at the time of her initial visit to her internist had ingested only distilled water for 4 days. Physical examination and laboratory test results were normal.

Table 21.4. Diagnostic Criteria for Somatization Disorder

A. History of many physical complaints beginning before 30 years of age, occurring over a period of several years, and resulting in treatment being sought or significant impairment in social or occupational functioning.

B. Each of the following criteria must have been met at some time during the course of the disorder.
  1. Four pain symptoms: A history of pain related to at least four different sites or functions (such as head, abdomen, back, joints, extremities, chest, rectum, during sexual intercourse, during menstruation, or during urination)
  2. Two gastrointestinal symptoms: A history of at least two gastrointestinal symptoms other than pain (such as nausea, diarrhea, bloating, vomiting other than during pregnancy, or intolerance of several different foods)
  3. One sexual symptom: A history of at least one sexual or reproductive symptom other than pain (such as sexual indifference, erectile or ejaculatory dysfunction, irregular menses, excessive menstrual bleeding, vomiting throughout pregnancy)
  4. One pseudoneurologic symptom: A history of at least one symptom or deficit suggesting a neurologic disorder not limited to pain (conversion symptoms such as blindness, double vision, deafness, loss of touch or pain sensation, hallucinations, aphonia, impaired coordination or balance, paralysis or localized weakness, difficulty swallowing, difficulty breathing, urinary retention, seizures; dissociative symptoms such as amnesia, or loss of consciousness other than fainting)

C. Either of the following must have been met:
  1. After appropriate investigation, each of the symptoms in criterion B cannot be fully explained by a known general medical condition, or the direct effects of a substance (e.g. a drug of abuse, a medication).
  2. When there is a related general medical condition, the physical complaints or resulting social or occupational impairment are in excess of what would be expected from the history, physical examination, or laboratory findings.

D. The symptoms are not intentionally produced or feigned (as in Factitious Disorder or Malingering).

Reprinted with permission from Diagnostic and statistical manual of mental disorders, 4th ed. Washington, DC: American Psychiatric Association, 1994.

Management

Because these patients adhere vigorously to the idea that they are physically ill, they usually do not accept psychiatric referral, and their treatment lies largely in the hands of nonpsychiatrists. Guidelines for management include the following:

1. *Review past medical records* to determine the range of symptomatic complaints brought to health care practitioners and the adequacy of documented evaluations.
2. *Respond to physical symptoms appropriately* by taking a careful history and doing the appropriate physical examination. Recognize that the history, as a diagnostic test, will have comparatively low specificity for physical disease (see Chapter 2) and that questioning techniques that diminish the likelihood of false positive findings, such as the use of open-ended and nonleading questions (see Chapter 3), are particularly important for such patients. Avoid hospitalizations, specialty consultations, and invasive laboratory tests unless objective indications exist (see Managing Abnormal Illness Behavior in Chapter 20).
3. *Review the four explanatory perspectives* (see Why Patients Somatize) for factors that might be promoting the development of somatization: psychiatric disease (especially major depression), personality disorder (especially histrionic type), behavioral model (e.g., sick family members), and environmental reinforcers (e.g., increased attention from parents) supporting the sick role, as well as aspects of the patient's life story (e.g., poor attention to early childhood dependency needs) that make his or her symptoms (e.g., endless recitation of complaints that keep the patient under very close medical scrutiny) understandable. When possible, address the apparently etiologic factors in the treatment plan (e.g., treat major depression with antidepressants; counsel family members to give attention for healthy behavior but to refrain from rewarding illness behavior).
4. Do not expect symptoms to remit entirely, and *do not promise cure or complete resolution of symptoms.*
5. *Promote the performance of normal function despite symptoms,* and praise the patient for carrying out specific activities and for being productive in the face of discomfort.
6. Assure the patient of your continuing availability, and *schedule regular, brief visits* so that access to medical attention does not require the development of new symptoms.
7. *Do not tell the patient that the symptoms are psychological,* but point out that emotional factors worsen physical distress and attempt to direct the patient to discuss life problems. Praise evidence of coping with the demands of daily life despite illness and discomfort.
8. *Help the family* of the patient recognize that, despite the abundance and persistence of symptoms, no serious disease has been found, and encourage them to support a strategy that de-emphasizes expensive and elaborate diagnostic tests and stresses maintenance of function in the face of symptoms.
9. *Try "mining for gold"* (23). Because these patients focus on physical symptoms, which usually are not explained by physical disease and do not resolve with treatment, the clinician is likely to spend each visit investigating the physical symptoms of concern, performing unrevealing diagnostic tests, and becoming frustrated. By spending some time during each visit "mining for gold"—which involves getting to know in depth the person who is the patient—the clinician may find admirable and likeable aspects of the patient, forge a mutually satisfactory practitioner–patient relationship, and be able to facilitate more effectively the patient's maintenance of health and functional status despite symptoms.

The usefulness of measures such as these in the management of somatization disorder has been demonstrated in a randomized, controlled study (24).

Undifferentiated Somatoform Disorder and Multisomatoform Disorder

Undifferentiated somatoform disorder is a residual category designed to accommodate patients who do not fully meet criteria for somatization disorder (Table 21.5). Symptoms must be present for at least 6 months for the diagnosis to be made. There need be no identifiable precipitant. Although the disorder has not been well studied, it is believed to be much more

Table 21.5. Diagnostic Criteria for Undifferentiated Somatoform Disorder

A. One or more physical complaints (e.g., fatigue, loss of appetite, gastrointestinal or urinary complaints)
B. Either of the following:
   1. After appropriate investigation, the symptoms cannot be explained by a known general medical condition or pathophysiologic mechanism (e.g., the effects of injury, medication, drugs, or alcohol).
   2. When there is a related general medical condition, the physical complaints or resulting social or occupational impairment are grossly in excess of what would be expected from the physical findings.
C. The symptoms cause clinically significant distress or impairment in social, occupational, or other important areas of functioning.
D. The duration of the disturbance is at least 6 months.
E. The disturbance is not better accounted for by another mental disorder (e.g., another somatoform disorder, sexual dysfunction, mood disorder, anxiety disorder, sleep disorder, or psychotic disorder).
F. The symptoms are not intentionally produced or feigned (as in Factitious Disorder or Malingering).

Reprinted with permission from Diagnostic and statistical manual of mental disorders, 4th ed. Washington, DC: American Psychiatric Association, 1994.

common than somatization disorder. Its prognosis and clinical course are unknown.

Multisomatoform disorder is a term that does not appear in DSM-IV. It has been proposed as an alternative to "undifferentiated somatoform disorder" for patients with a 2-year history of apparent somatoform symptoms and at least three current somatoform symptoms, reported from a 15-symptom checklist (25). Of 1,000 participants in the Primary Care Evaluation of Mental Disorders (PRIME-MD) (26) study, 82 (8.2%) met criteria for this condition. These patients had significantly greater numbers of disability days and doctor visits as well as impairments in health-related quality of life and were far more likely than patients with other psychiatric conditions to be judged "difficult" by their physicians.

Although there are no studies of treatment for these specific disorders, there is evidence that techniques useful in full-fledged somatization disorder (described previously) are helpful for long-term somatizing patients who do not meet all of the diagnostic criteria for somatization disorder (27).

Conversion Disorder

Description

Conversion disorder is a disorder in which an unexplained loss or alteration of body functioning develops in the presence of evidence that the symptoms solve or express a psychological conflict or need (Table 21.6). The symptoms often simulate neurologic disease but conform to the patient's notion of body function rather than to the rules of neuroanatomy, and medical evaluation yields no evidence of diagnosable disease. Amnesia, aphonia, blindness, paralysis, numbness, and seizures are among the most common conversion symptoms. The disorder probably occurs more often in women than in men, and it usually begins in adolescence or early adulthood. Patients may have histrionic or dependent personalities and may exhibit remarkable serenity (*"la belle indifference"*) in the face of their impairments.

Conversion disorder is unique among DSM-IV somatoform disorders in that the definition not only describes the diagnostic criteria but also proposes psychological mechanisms as explanations. A mechanism called *secondary gain* is invoked when unexplained symptoms allow the patient to avoid onerous tasks or undesirable duties (see Somatization as Reinforced Behavior).

Case Example

A 15-year-old girl with a history of migraine headache and transient visual field cuts was evaluated for a new visual field cut that had developed without headache over the previous 24 hours. On examination, the visual defect was found to split the macula. At the time of psychiatric interview she revealed that she expected her visual problems to prevent her from obtaining a driver's license when she turned 16. She went on to say that she was afraid to drive, that no other woman in her family drove, and that she would be called upon by everyone to provide transportation. She was referred to a pediatric neurology service, where she received physical therapy and daily psychotherapy. Her field defect resolved.

A second mechanism, *primary gain,* is invoked when conversion symptoms appear to resolve an internal conflict created by a feeling, impulse, or wish that the individual finds frightening or morally unacceptable.

Case Example

A 50-year-old man was admitted to the hospital because of amnesia. He spoke normally and was otherwise neurologically intact, although he could not remember his name or any other details of personal history. After about 24 hours he began speaking freely about anger related to the recent dissolution of his marriage. Particularly upsetting had been news that his boss was dating his wife. Immediately before the development of amnesia he had thought that he might be provoked to violence if he discovered them together. His amnesia completely resolved in 2 days, and he was discharged from the hospital. He briefly participated in outpatient psychotherapy. The working formulation was that the amnesia had served to remove unacceptable violent intentions from his awareness and to protect him from acting on them.

Acute conversion symptoms have a good prognosis for recovery, especially if the patient has no other psychiatric disorder.

Management

Guidelines for the treatment of patients with conversion disorder include the following:

1. Be certain that the patient has had an *adequate medical evaluation,* because some patients with conversion symptoms have an undiagnosed medical disorder (4).

Table 21.6. Diagnostic Criteria for Conversion Disorder

A. One or more symptoms or deficits affecting voluntary motor or sensory function suggesting a neurologic or general medical condition.
B. Psychological factors are judged to be associated with the symptom or deficit because the initiation or exacerbation of the symptom or deficit is preceded by conflicts or other stressors.
C. The symptom or deficit is not intentionally produced or feigned (as in Factitious Disorder or Malingering).
D. The symptom of deficit cannot, after appropriate investigation, be fully explained by a neurologic or general medical condition, and is not a culturally sanctioned behavior or experience.
E. The symptom or deficit causes clinically significant distress or impairment in social, occupational, or other important areas of functioning; or warrants medical evaluation.
F. The symptom or deficit is not limited to pain or sexual dysfunction, does not occur exclusively during the course of somatization disorder, and is not better accounted for by another mental disorder.

Reprinted with permission from Diagnostic and statistical manual of mental disorders, 4th ed. Washington, DC: American Psychiatric Association, 1994.

2. *Review the various explanatory perspectives for factors that might be promoting the development of conversion symptoms*: psychiatric illness (especially major depression), personality disorders (especially dependent and histrionic types), behavioral models (e.g., sick family members), or environmental reinforcers supporting the sick role (e.g., increased attention from family members), and aspects of the patient's life story (e.g., violent feelings toward an abusive alcoholic father) that make the symptoms understandable (e.g., paralysis of the hand when the patient considers violent revenge against the father). When possible, address specific interventions to the etiologic factors identified (e.g., treat major depression with antidepressants; counsel family members to reward healthy behavior instead of illness behavior; refer the angry child of an alcoholic to Al-Anon).
3. Emphasize the evidence that no serious disease is present, and express optimism about the prospect of full recovery. Consider physical therapy or some other physical rehabilitative intervention to *help the patient save face* during recovery.
4. *Do not bluntly confront the patient with the psychological origins of the symptoms,* but stress that emotional factors can exacerbate such problems. Review the patient's current life circumstances and difficulties, and consider undertaking a course of short-term counseling (see Chapter 20).

Hypochondriasis

Description

Hypochondriasis is a chronic disorder in which unrealistic interpretation of physical symptoms leads the patient to fear the presence of a serious illness in the face of repeated reassurances based on adequate medical evaluation (Table 21.7). Onset is usually in the third decade but may occur later. Both sexes are equally affected. Obsessive-compulsive personality traits are often observed. Anxiety, depression, drug dependence, and iatrogenic disease are common complications. The disorder tends to be chronic, with waxing and waning intensity. Symptomatic exacerbations occur in response to psychosocial stresses and to stimuli that provoke bodily preoccupation and fear of disease.

Case Example

A 30-year-old accountant had always been self-conscious about his physical appearance, a concern that he attempted to allay by weight lifting. After his father died of a heart attack, he became concerned that he might have heart disease and was fearful about the implication of insignificant chest pains. He also worried about his blood pressure, which was transiently elevated at the time of his yearly physical examinations. His most recent examination revealed insignificant liver enzyme elevations, a finding over which he fretted for weeks. Despite these concerns, he rarely missed a day of work. He was not sure that he did not have a serious disease but thought he had best trust his health care provider.

Management

Because patients with hypochondriasis believe that they are physically ill, they often refuse psychiatric treatment. Guidelines for management by generalists are similar to those for other chronic somatoform disorders and include the following:

1. *Review past medical records* to determine the range of symptomatic complaints brought to health care practitioners and the adequacy of documented evaluations.
2. *Respond to physical symptoms appropriately* by taking a careful history and doing the appropriate physical examination. Reassurances cannot be given to the patient if the physical complaints are not investigated. At the same time, recognize that the history, as a diagnostic indicator, may have comparatively low specificity for physical disease (see Chapter 2), and that questioning techniques that diminish the likelihood of false positive findings, such as the use of open-ended and nonleading questions (see Chapter 3), are particularly important in such patients. Avoid hospitalization, inappropriate specialty consultations, and invasive laboratory tests unless objective indications exist (see Managing Abnormal Illness Behavior in Chapter 20).
3. *Review the four explanatory perspectives* (see Why Patients Somatize) for factors that might be promoting hypochondriasis: psychiatric illness (especially major depression and anxiety disorders), personality disorder (especially obsessive-compulsive type), behavioral models or environmental reinforcers supporting the sick role (e.g.,

Table 21.7. Diagnostic Criteria for Hypocondriasis

A. Preoccupation with fears of having, or the idea that one has, a serious disease based on the person's misinterpretation of bodily symptoms.
B. The preoccupation persists despite appropriate medical evaluation and reassurance.
C. The belief (in criterion A) is not of delusional intensity (as in Delusional Disorder, Somatic type) and is not restricted to a circumscribed concern about appearance (as in Body Dysmorphic Disorder).
D. The preoccupation causes clinically significant distress or impairment in social, occupational, or other important areas of functioning.
E. The duraton of the disturbance is at least 6 months.
F. The preoccupation does not occur exclusively during the course of generalized anxiety disorder, obsessive-compulsive disorder, panic disorder, major depressive episode, separation anxiety, or another somatoform disorder.

Specify if with poor insight: if, for most of the time during the current episode, the person does not recognize that the concern about having a serious illness is excessive or unreasonable.

Reprinted with permission from Diagnostic and statistical manual of mental disorders 4th ed. Washington, DC: American Psychiatric Association, 1994.

family members who were excessively concerned about patient's childhood health and lavished attention in response to minor ailments), and aspects of the patient's life story (e.g., religious upbringing with particular emphasis on sexual morality and punishment of sinners) that make the symptoms empathically understandable (e.g., hypochondriacal fear of AIDS in a man with repeatedly negative HIV antibody tests who had a single extramarital encounter 5 years before). When possible, address specific interventions to etiologic factors identified (e.g., counsel family members to give attention for healthy behavior but refrain from rewarding illness behavior). It is especially important to consider treating concurrent major depression and anxiety disorders with antidepressant medications, because the amelioration of major mood and anxiety symptoms often greatly improves the receptivity of hypochondriacal patients to reassurance about their physical health.

4. Do not expect symptoms to remit entirely, and *do not promise cure or complete resolution of symptoms* (see Managing Abnormal Illness Behavior in Chapter 20).
5. *Promote the performance of normal functions despite symptoms,* and praise patients for carrying out specific activities and being productive in the face of discomfort.
6. Reassure the patient of your continuing availability, and *schedule regular, brief visits* so that access to medical attention does not depend on the development of new symptoms.
7. *Do not tell the patient that the symptoms are psychological,* but point out that emotional factors worsen physical distress and attempt to direct the patient to discuss life problems.
8. *Help the family* of the patient recognize that despite the persistence of symptoms no serious disease has been found, and encourage them to support a strategy de-emphasizing expensive and elaborate diagnostic tests and stressing maintenance of function in the face of symptoms.
9. *Try "mining for gold"* (23). Because these patients focus on physical symptoms, which usually are not explained by physical disease and do not resolve with treatment, the clinician is likely to spend each visit investigating the physical symptoms of concern, performing unrevealing diagnostic tests, and becoming frustrated. By spending some time during each visit "mining for gold"—which involves getting to know in depth the person who is the patient—the clinician may find admirable and likeable aspects of the patient, forge a mutually satisfactory practitioner–patient relationship, and be able to facilitate more effectively the patient's maintenance of health and functional status despite symptoms.
10. Some patients may accept *short-term counseling* (see Chapter 20). Formal cognitive-behavioral therapy has been shown to be effective, at least when provided to willing patients by experienced therapists (28). "Explanatory therapy," a similar but less technical approach originally described by Kellner (29), has also been shown to reduce hypochondriacal fears, emotional distress, and health care utilization, but it is not presently of proven benefit when administered by nonspecialists (30).

Pain Disorder

Description

Somatoform pain disorder is a chronic disorder characterized by unexplained or amplified complaints of pain (Table 21.8). It usually has its onset in the fourth or fifth decade and is associated with marked functional disability. The diagnosis is most useful when psychological factors can be linked to the onset and maintenance of pain. A typical scenario begins with lower back pain, which often develops on the job and is initially diagnosed as a sprain. The patient may see his or her primary care practitioner and attempt to return to work. Soon thereafter the pain recurs, sometimes after apparent reinjury. Specialty consultations (e.g., orthopedic, neurosurgical) ensue. Conservative treatments (e.g., physical therapy) are ineffective. Surgery may be performed, perhaps with transient benefit, but soon there is a resurgence of symptoms described as worse than ever. After 6 to 12 months of illness the patient is out of work, socially isolated, physically inactive, dependent on narcotic analgesics, angry, and demoralized. He or she may believe that health professionals and family members do not regard the pain as real.

Management

Treatment of somatoform pain disorder is similar to the management of other somatoform disorders:

1. *Review past medical records* to determine the timing and extent of prior evaluations and treatments.
2. Respond to pain complaints with a *thorough history and physical examination* and determine that adequate medical, surgical, and neurologic evaluations have been done, but avoid procedures and hospitalization in the absence of clear indications.
3. *Review the four explanatory perspectives* (see Why Patients Somatize) for factors that might be promoting unexplained or amplified pain complaints,

Table 21.8. Diagnostic Criteria for Pain Disorder

A. Pain in one or more anatomic sites is the predominant focus of the clinical presentation and is of sufficient severity to warrant clinical attention.
B. The pain causes clinically significant distress or impairment in social, occupational, or other important areas of functioning.
C. Psychological factors are judged to have an important role in the onset, severity, exacerbation, or maintenance of the pain.
D. The symptoms are not intentionally produced or feigned (as in Factitional Disorder or Malingering).
E. The pain is not better accounted for by a mood, anxiety, or psychotic disorder and does not meet criteria for dyspareunia.

Reprinted with permission from Diagnostic and statistical manual of mental disorders, 4th ed. Washington, DC: American Psychiatric Association, 1994.

and design a treatment plan that addresses specific etiologic factors identified: major psychiatric disease (especially major depression and chemical dependency, both of which are common in patients with somatoform pain), personality traits (especially exaggerated dependency), environmental reinforcers (e.g., financial compensation, relief from work responsibility, sympathy from family and friends), and aspects of life history that make the pain complaints empathically understandable (e.g., abusive or negligent parenting leading to a yearning to be cared for in a passive-dependent way that is often hidden behind a defiant facade).

4. Convey optimism that improvement is likely, but *do not promise cure or complete resolution of symptoms.*
5. *Promote the performance of functions that are reasonable for the patient to perform despite symptoms,* and praise patients for carrying out specific activities and being productive in the face of discomfort.
6. Reassure the patient of your continuing availability, and *schedule regular, brief visits* so that access to medical attention does not require exacerbation of symptoms.
7. *Consider topical treatments and physical therapy* because of their intrinsic value, safety, and symbolic value as indicators that the physical reality of the patient's pain is recognized.
8. In general, *avoid prescribing benzodiazepines and narcotic analgesics,* and persuade addicted patients to pursue detoxification. In selected patients who are functional on a stable opioid regimen, it is reasonable to maintain the regimen as part of a contractual plan for the management of chronic pain (see Chapter 29). Antidepressant medication may be of use in some patients, especially if the pain is neuropathic in nature (see Chapters 13 and 84) or if there is concomitant anxiety (see Chapter 22) or depression (see Chapter 24).
9. *Do not tell the patient that the symptoms are psychological,* but stress that emotional factors undoubtedly worsen physical distress, and attempt to direct the patient to discuss life problems, especially interpersonal conflicts and disappointments.
10. *Enlist the support of the patient's family* in an effort to reinforce maintenance of function in the face of symptoms rather than persistence of disability.
11. Consider referral to a center specializing in the *multidisciplinary care* of patients with chronic pain syndromes.
12. *Try "mining for gold"* (23). By getting to know in depth the person who is the patient, the clinician may find admirable and likeable aspects of the patient, forge a mutually satisfactory practitioner–patient relationship, and be able to facilitate more effectively the patient's maintenance of health and functional status despite pain.

Table 21.9. Diagnostic Criteria for Body Dysmorphic Disorder

A. Preoccupation with an imagined defect in appearance. If a slight physical anomaly is present, the person's concern is markedly excessive.
B. The preoccupation causes clinically significant distress or impairment in social, occupational, or other important areas of functioning.
C. The preoccupation is not better accounted for by another mental disorder (e.g., dissatisfaction with body shape and size in Anorexia Nervosa).

Reprinted with permission from Diagnostic and statistical manual of mental disorders, 4th ed. Washington, DC: American Psychiatric Association, 1994.

Body Dysmorphic Disorder

Description

Body dysmorphic disorder is a disorder characterized by an excessive or completely unfounded preoccupation with a defect in personal appearance (Table 21.9). The prevalence of the disorder is unknown, but it may be common. Onset typically occurs between adolescence and age 30 years. Perceived facial imperfections, such as the shape of the nose or jaw, are the most common sources of concern.

Case Example

A 60-year-old man entered into psychiatric treatment for chronic depression. He reported long-standing attitudes and patterns of behavior suggesting obsessionality and extreme self-consciousness. He also reported a preoccupation beginning in adolescence with the shape of his jaw. He had undergone elaborate surgical treatment for this but continued to feel that other people were put off by his appearance, a belief contributing to his social discomfort. The examining psychiatrist found nothing remarkable about the appearance of his face. The patient's preoccupation with this perceived defect was partially ameliorated by antidepressant treatment, but he continued to regard himself as misshapen.

Management

Little is known about the treatment and prognosis of the disorder. Some authors believe it should be regarded as a symptom, not as a distinct condition. In general, patients should be discouraged from pursuing surgical solutions, especially when their concerns are entirely unfounded. Otherwise, many of the management guidelines described earlier for other chronic somatoform disorders are applicable. In particular, it is useful to review the four explanatory perspectives for factors promoting the development and maintenance of the symptoms and to treat any specific etiologic factor identified: an associated major psychiatric illness (usually major depression), personality types predisposing to the disorder (especially obsessive-compulsive and avoidant types—see Chapter 23), behavioral models for these concerns (e.g., parents who were dissatisfied with similar physical attributes in themselves), and aspects of the life story that make the symptoms empathically understandable (e.g., early experiences with critical parents leading the patient to feel unwanted or unacceptable).

DISORDERS WITH VOLUNTARY SYMPTOM PRODUCTION

The fundamental feature of disorders with voluntary symptom production is the deliberate simulation of physical symptoms. This characteristic distinguishes patients with these disorders from those with chronic somatoform disorders, described earlier, in whom symptom genesis is not apparently voluntary.

Factitious Disorder with Physical Symptoms

Description

Factitious illness is characterized by the deliberate simulation of physical symptoms for the sole purpose of assuming the role of patient. When this behavior is chronic and leads to multiple hospitalizations, it is known as chronic factitious disorder with physical symptoms (Table 21.10) or *Munchhausen's syndrome.* When there is deliberate simulation of a psychiatric syndrome, it is designated as Factitious Disorder with Psychological Symptoms.

Patients may report invented symptoms (e.g., severe right lower quadrant abdominal pain), or they may deliberately produce physical signs by heating thermometers, tying tourniquets around their legs, or ingesting anticoagulant drugs. The history may be dramatic but vague in medically relevant detail. Onset is usually in early adulthood, often shortly after hospitalization for a *bona fide* physical illness. Job stability, family life, and other interpersonal relationships suffer profoundly as a result of multiple lengthy hospitalizations.

Management

The main goals of management are to prevent unnecessary hospitalizations and to avoid invasive procedures. The management of the hospitalized patient may be facilitated by early psychiatric consultation to assist in diagnosis, determine whether other treatable psychiatric disorders are present, help plan tactful confrontation of the patient with the diagnosis, and attempt to persuade the patient to accept psychiatric hospitalization.

Malingering

Description

Malingering is the deliberate simulation of physical (or psychological) symptoms to achieve a specific benefit. It is an important and common problem in settings where sickness is rewarded with certain benefits (e.g., avoidance of military service or court appearances, financial compensation for injuries). Malingering comprises three types (see Ford, *The Somaticizing Disorders,* in General References):

1. Pure malingering, in which there is deliberate deception by the description or production of nonexistent symptoms or signs (rare)
2. Partial malingering, which involves the conscious and voluntary exaggeration of symptoms of a real disease
3. Deliberate attribution of an actual disability to an injury or accident that did not cause it.

The diagnosis of malingering should be suspected whenever symptoms or disabilities greatly exceeding objective disease are accompanied by obvious social or financial benefit. Other observations suggesting the diagnosis include inconsistency of symptoms (e.g., a blind person detected reading), unusually vague or markedly exaggerated reports of symptoms, and the expression of indignant anger in response to gentle confrontation.

Malingering must be distinguished from factitious disorders, in which the patient has no goal aside from achieving patienthood, and from conversion disorders, in which symptom production is not conscious or intentional.

Management

The goal of management is to persuade malingering patients to give up their symptoms. Patients should gradually and tactfully be made aware that malingering is suspected, and the gratifications associated with the sick role should be removed. Reports of symptoms should be given minimal attention. Because serious psychiatric disorders may underlie apparent malingering, psychiatric consultation should be obtained if possible.

Table 21.10. Diagnostic Criteria for Factitious Disorder with Physical Symptoms

A. Intentional production or feigning of physical or psychological signs or symptoms.
B. The motivation for the behavior is to assume the sick role.
C. External incentives for the behavior (such as economic gain, avoiding legal responsibility, or improving physical well-being, as in Malingering) are absent.

Reprinted with permission from Diagnostic and statistical manual of mental disorders, 4th ed. Washington, DC: American Psychiatric Association, 1994.

General References*

American Psychiatric Association. **Diagnostic and statistical manual of mental disorders**. 4th ed. (DSM-IV). Washington, DC: American Psychiatric Association, 1994.
Diagnostic criteria and epidemiologic information for all recognized psychiatric disorders.

Ford CV. The somatizing disorders: illness as a way of life. New York: Elsevier, 1983.
Practical, well-referenced monograph covering all disorders in which somatization is the principal feature.

Kaplan CK, Lipkin M, Gordon GH. Somatization in primary care: patients with unexplained and vexing medical complaints. J Gen Intern Med 1988;3:177.
Review article focusing on origins of somatization and on diagnosis and management by the primary care practitioner.

Specific References

1. Mechanic D. The concept of illness behavior: culture, situation, and personal disposition. Psychol Med 1986;16:1.

*Bold print (general references) and bold numerals (specific references) denote published controlled clinical trials, meta-analyses, or consensus-based recommendations.

2. McHugh PR, Slavney PR, eds. The perspectives of psychiatry, 2nd edition. Baltimore: Johns Hopkins University Press, 1998.
3. Simon GE, VonKorff M, Piccinelli M, et al. An international study of the relation between somatic symptoms and depression. N Engl J Med 1999;341:1329.
4. Lazare A. Conversion symptoms. N Engl J Med 1983;305:745.
5. O'Malley PG, Jones DL, Feuerstein IM, et al. Lack of correlation between psychological factors and subclinical coronary artery disease. N Engl J Med 2000;343:1298.
6. Hansell S, Mechanic D. Introspectiveness and adolescent symptom reporting. J Hum Stress 1985;11(Winter):165.
7. Costa PT, McCrae RR. Hypochondriasis, neuroticism, and aging. Am Psychol 1985;40:19.
8. Lipowski ZJ. Somatization: the concept and its clinical application. Am J Psychiatry 1988;145:1358.
9. Barsky AJ. Patients who amplify bodily sensations. Ann Intern Med 1979;91:63.
10. Barsky AJ, Klerman GL. Overview: hypochondriasis, bodily complaints, and somatic styles. Am J Psychiatry 1983;140:273.
11. Stoeckle J, Zola IK, Davison GE. The quantity and significance of psychological distress in medical patients. J Chronic Dis 1964;17:959.
12. Drossman DA. The problem patient: evaluation and care of medical patients with psychosocial disturbances. Ann Intern Med 1978;88:366.
13. Johnstone A, Goldberg D. Psychiatric screening in general practice. Lancet 1976;1:605.
14. Catalan J, Bath D, Edmonds G, Ennis J. The effects of nonprescribing of anxiolytics in general practice: I. Controlled evaluation of psychiatric and social outcome. Br J Psychiatry 1984;144:593.
15. Catalan J, Bath D, Bond A, et al. The effects of nonprescribing of anxiolytics in general practice: II. Factors associated with outcome. Br J Psychiatry 1984;144:603.
16. Thomas KB. Temporarily dependent patient in general practice. BMJ 1974;1:625.
17. Othmer E, DeSouza C. A screening test in somatization disorder (hysteria). Am J Psychiatry 1985;142:1146.
18. Manu P, Lane TJ, Matthews DA. Screening for somatization disorder in patients with chronic fatigue. Gen Hosp Psychiatry 1989;11:294.
19. Cohen ME, Robins E, Purtell JJ, et al. Excessive surgery in hysteria. JAMA 1953;151:977.
20. Coryell W, Norten SG. Briquet's syndrome (somatization disorder) and primary depression: comparison of background and outcome. Compr Psychiatry 1981;22:249.
21. Coryell W. Diagnosis-specific mortality. Primary depression and Briquet's syndrome (somatization disorder). Arch Gen Psychiatry 1981;38:939.
22. Perley MJ, Guze SB. Hysteria: the stability and usefulness of clinical criteria. N Engl J Med 1962;266:421.
23. Levinson W. Mining for gold. J Gen Intern Med 1993;8:172.
24. Smith GR, Monson RA, Ray DC. Psychiatric consultation in somatization disorder: a randomized controlled study. N Engl J Med 1986;314:1407.
25. Kroenke K, Spitzer RL, deGruy FV, et al. Multisomatiform disorder: an alternative to undifferentiated somatoform disorder for the somatizing patient in primary care. Arch Gen Psychiatry 1997;54:352.
26. Spitzer RL, Williams JBW, Kroenke K, et al. Utility of a new procedure for diagnosing mental disorders in primary care: the PRIME-MD 1000 study. JAMA 1994;272:1749.
27. Smith GR, Rost K, Kashner TM. A trial of the effect of a standardized psychiatric consultation on health outcomes and costs in somatizing patients. Arch Gen Psychiatry 1995;52:238.
28. Warwick HMC, Clark DM, Cobb AM, et al. A controlled trial of cognitive-behavioural treatment of hypochondriasis. Br J Psychiatry 1996;169:189.
29. Kellner R. Psychotherapeutic strategies in hypochondriasis: a clinical study. Am J Psychother 1982;36:146.
30. Fava GA, Grandi S, Rafanelli C, et al. Explanatory therapy in hypochondriasis. J Clin Psychiatry 2000;61:317.

C H A P T E R 22

Anxiety and Anxiety Disorders

UNA D. MCCANN, MD
ROBERT P. ROCA, MD, MPH

Anxiety is the term applied to a psychophysiologic state characterized by worry (apprehensive expectation), muscle tension, autonomic hyperactivity, and hypervigilance. Anxiety may improve performance in response to danger or challenge and thus may serve an adaptive function. However, when excessive or inappropriate in form or context, it leads to subjective distress and impairment in social and occupational functioning. Anxiety can be caused by a number of medical illnesses (e.g., hyperthyroidism, pheochromocytoma), and the presence of anxiety can prolong or exacerbate medical conditions (e.g., irritable bowel syndrome). There is also some evidence that anxiety, like depression, may be an independent risk factor for the development of certain conditions, such as cardiovascular disease, hypertension, irritable bowel syndrome, and migraine headaches (1,2).

NORMAL ILLNESS-RELATED ANXIETY

Patients visiting their health care providers or awaiting the results of tests are often anxious. Although such anxiety may be understandable and realistically related to concerns about the meaning of symptoms and consequences of disease, it nonetheless requires recognition and management because it may interfere with medical care. For example, it has been found that survivors of myocardial infarction and their spouses recollect little of the information given to them during in-hospital convalescence, partly as a result of anxiety (3). Such findings highlight the importance of detecting normal illness-related anxiety and treating it skillfully. The following approaches are helpful:

- Assume that patients with new symptoms have concerns about serious illness. It is helpful to ask patients for their ideas about the causes of their symptoms. Often, a relative or friend has had a similar symptom related to a serious disease.
- Avoid comments or jargon that might sensitize or frighten patients (e.g., commenting, while examining a skin lesion, "It's been a long time since I've seen one like that.").
- Prepare the patient for painful or unfamiliar procedures with explanations. Assume that any procedure may be frightening to a patient.
- Assume that any patient recovering from serious illness is anxious about the future; determine whether any unnecessary disability in such patients is caused by fear or inadequate education. Hospitalized patients often get incomplete explanations of their illnesses at the time of discharge.

DRUG-RELATED ANXIETY

When evaluating patients with symptoms of anxiety, it is important to identify all medications or substances taken during or just before the onset of symptoms of anxiety. Prescribed drugs, over-the-counter preparations, caffeine, ephedra-containing cold medications or dietary supplements, "herbal" preparations, alcohol, and other substances can all cause symptoms similar to those found in the primary anxiety disorders described later in this chapter. Licit and illicit stimulants, such as methylphenidate, amphetamine, cocaine, and 3,4-methylenedioxymethamphetamine (MDMA or "ecstasy") can produce symptoms indistinguishable from those of idiopathic anxiety disorders. Common examples of such compounds are listed in Table 22.1.

When considering the role of *caffeine* in producing anxiety, it is helpful to know the approximate amount of caffeine in commonly consumed beverages and substances:

- Coffee (1 cup): brewed, 60 to 180 mg; instant, 30 to 120 mg; decaffeinated, 2 to 5 mg
- Tea (1 cup): brewed U.S. brands, 20 to 90 mg; imported brands, 25 to 100 mg
- Soft drinks (6 oz): 15 to 23 mg
- Dark chocolate (1 oz): 5 to 35 mg

Patients who experience prominent anxiety, panic attacks, obsessions, or compulsions in relation to the ingestion of these substances are classified by the American Psychiatric Association (APA) as having a substance-induced anxiety disorder. However, because individuals with an anxiety disorder, particularly panic disorder, are more susceptible to the anxiogenic effects of stimulants (4), the clinician should be vigilant for an underlying idiopathic pre-existing anxiety disorder in patients with substance-induced anxiety.

Table 22.1. Drugs and Other Substances that May Exacerbate (or Produce) Anxiety

Anticholinergic drugs
Coricosteroids
Drugs of abuse[a]
Amphetamines and amphetamine derivatives
Cocaine
Hallucinogens
Inhalants
Marijuana and other drugs that alter perception
Methylenedioxymethamphetamine (MDMA, "Ecstasy")
Phencyclidine (PCP)
Sympathomimetic Agents
β_2 bronchodilators
Decongestants (found in most over-the-counter cold remedies)
Ephedra-containing dietary supplements and "energy boosters"
Weight-reduction agents
Thyroid hormone
Xanthine-containing drugs, foods, and beverages
Bronchodilators with theophylline
Caffeine (use and discontinuation)[b]
Many over-the-counter cold and arthritis remedies
Withdrawal symptoms
Alcohol
Sedative-hypnotics
Tobacco

[a]See Chapter 29.

[b]See text for approximate amount of caffeine in common beverages.

ANXIETY DISORDERS

The anxiety disorders are a group of distinct psychiatric conditions in which anxiety is the predominant symptom. Anxiety causes distress and dysfunction because it is *excessive, unrealistic,* or *inappropriate in form or context.* The five major anxiety disorders are panic disorder, obsessive-compulsive disorder (OCD), phobia (specific or social), posttraumatic stress disorder (PTSD), and generalized anxiety disorder (GAD). As a group, the anxiety disorders are the most common psychiatric illnesses in the United States, affecting an estimated 19 million American adults (5); information is available from the National Institute of Mental Health (NIMH) website (available at: www.nimh.nih.gov/anxiety/anxiety.cfm). In addition to existing in their "pure" forms, anxiety disorders are frequently comorbid with other psychiatric conditions, including affective disorders (Chapter 24), somatoform disorders (Chapter 21), substance abuse (Chapters 28 and 29), and eating disorders (Chapter 11). Although adjustment disorder with anxiety is not classified as an anxiety disorder, this condition is frequently encountered by primary physicians and should be considered in the differential diagnosis of anxiety. Therefore, a brief description of adjustment disorder with anxiety is provided here before the anxiety disorders are reviewed.

Adjustment Disorder with Anxiety

Description

The term *adjustment disorder with anxiety* is used when excessive and maladaptive anxiety occurs in response to a recent, identifiable stressor. This "reactive" anxiety resolves when the stressor remits or when the patient reaches a new level of adaptation or adjustment. APA criteria are listed in Chapter 24, Table 24.1.

Case Study

A 55-year-old married man presented to the office because of nonexertional chest pain, dizziness, and breathlessness. He had suffered a heart attack 3 months before but had recovered uneventfully. A recent stress test had shown no signs of coronary insufficiency or serious arrhythmia. His wife reported that the patient had not been himself since leaving the hospital and that "every little thing gets on his nerves." Although he had formerly been "on the go all of the time," he was now afraid to go out of the house. Physical examination now showed no evidence of heart failure, and the electrocardiogram (ECG) was unchanged. The physician reviewed the encouraging results of the ECG and treadmill test, reassured the patient about his symptoms, explained that anxiety is common after myocardial infarction, and asked the patient to enroll in a cardiac rehabilitation program, to telephone in 1 week to report on his symptoms, and to return to the office in 2 weeks for follow-up examination and a review of his progress. The physician also demonstrated some simple relaxation techniques (see later discussion) and gave the patient a small supply of lorazepam to be used on an as-needed basis.

Epidemiology, Origins, and Natural History

Estimates of the prevalence of adjustment disorder are highly variable, ranging from 5% to 20%. Adjustment disorder is believed to be equally common in males and females. By definition, an adjustment disorder with anxious mood must begin within 3 months of a precipitating stressor and last no longer than 6 months after the stressor (or its consequences) ceases.

Treatment

Management includes the following steps:

- Advise the patient to moderate or eliminate use of caffeine and other stimulants.
- Consider short-term counseling (see Chapter 20) to meet the patient's informational needs, assist in problem-solving, provide encouragement, and restore morale.
- Offer training in relaxation and other techniques of self-regulation (see later discussion).
- Consider instituting a time-limited (1 to 2 weeks) course of anxiolytic medication, usually a benzodiazepine (see later discussion).

Panic Disorder

Description

The hallmark feature of panic disorder is the occurrence of panic attacks—discrete episodes of extreme anxiety—accompanied by a variety of physical and emotional symptoms. To meet the criteria for a *panic attack,* the episode must comprise at least four symptoms in addition to intense fear or discomfort. Symptoms of panic include palpitations, sweating, trembling, shortness of breath, feeling of choking, chest pain or discomfort, nausea or abdominal distress, dizziness, derealization (feelings of unreality) or depersonalization (feeling detached from oneself), paresthesias, chills or hot flushes, fear of losing control or going crazy, and fear of dying. In addition to the involvement of panicky feeling and physical/emotional symptoms, panic attacks must reach peak intensity within 10 minutes after their onset.

The presence of repeated, unexpected panic attacks is necessary but not sufficient for the diagnosis of *panic disorder.* As described later, a number of other anxiety disorders as well as mood disorders are sometimes associated with panic attacks. In contrast to other disorders, panic disorder requires that, after the experience of a panic attack (or attacks), the affected individual is persistently (for at least 1 month) worried about having another panic attack or concerned about the significance or consequences of the panic attack.

Patients with panic disorder have significantly increased *utilization* of both outpatient and inpatient general medical services. *Utilization of primary care services* by patients with panic disorder is approximately three times higher than that of the average patient and is higher than that of patients with other psychiatric illnesses, such as major depression (2,6). The prevalence of panic disorder may be increased in several medical conditions, including labile hypertension (7), mitral valve prolapse (8), asthma (9,10), chronic obstructive pulmonary disease (11), and migraine headache (12,13).

Approximately one third of individuals with panic disorder develop *agoraphobia,* or fear and avoidance of places and situations where a panic attack might occur or escape would be difficult (14). If the agoraphobia is left untreated, the number and extent of avoided situations can expand and generalize, rendering the patient housebound. Agoraphobia occasionally occurs in the absence of panic attacks (agoraphobia without history of panic disorder in *Diagnostic and Statistical Manual of Mental Disorders,* 4th edition), but this is apparently rare, at least in clinical samples (15). Among patients with panic disorder, those most likely to develop agoraphobia are women who have persistent panic attacks (i.e., no history of clinical remissions), a high degree of interpersonal sensitivity, and a history of anxiety or depression in childhood (15). APA diagnostic criteria for panic disorder without and with agoraphobia are summarized in Table 22.2.

Case Study

A 24-year-old graduate student was referred by the emergency department for recurrent episodes of substernal chest pain, some of which had occurred during sleep. Chest pain was associated with abdominal pain, shortness of breath, and dizziness. Medical work-up had revealed no cardiac or endocrine source for the patient's symptoms. The patient reported that during the last semester of graduate school she began experiencing these episodes "out of the blue." Her first episode took place when she was "pulling an all-nighter studying for her dissertation presentation." She acknowledged drinking quite a bit of coffee during that period, but since then she had experienced panic attacks while not using caffeine heavily. Although she admitted to some life stressors, such as starting a new job and moving to a new city, she viewed these stressors as positive. The patient reported that since she first began to have panic

Table 22.2. Diagnostic Criteria for Panic Disorder Without and With Agoraphobia

Without Agoraphobia

A. Both 1 and 2:
   1. Recurrent unexpected panic attacks.
   2. At least one of the attacks has been followed by a month or more of (a) persistent concern about having additional attacks, (b) worry about the implications of the attack or its consequences (e.g., losing control, having a heart attack, "going crazy"), or (c) a significant change in behavior related to the attacks.

B. Absence of agoraphobia (defined below).

C. The panic attacks are not due to the direct effects of a substance (e.g., drugs of abuse, medication) or a general medical condition (e.g., hyperthyroidism).

D. The anxiety is not better accounted for by another mental disorder, such as Obsessive-Compulsive Disorder (e.g., fear of contamination), Posttraumatic Stress Disorder (e.g., in response to stimuli associated with a severe stressor), Separation Anxiety Disorder, or Social Phobia (e.g., fear of embarrassment in social situations).

With Agoraphobia

A. Both 1 and 2:
   1. Recurrent unexpected panic attacks.
   2. At least one of the attacks has been followed by a month or more of (a) persistent concern about having additional attacks, (b) worry about the implications of the attack or its consequences (e.g., losing control, having a heart attack, "going crazy"), or (c) a significant change in behavior related to the attacks.

B. The presence of agoraphobia, that is, anxiety about being in places or situations from which escape might be difficult (or embarrassing) or in which help may not be available in the event of having an unexpected or situational predisposed panic attack. Agoraphobic fears typically involve characteristic clusters of situations that include being outside the home alone, being in a crowd or standing in a line, being on a bridge, and traveling in a bus, train, or car. Note: Consider the diagnosis of Specific Phobia if limited to one or only a few specific situations, or Social Phobia if the avoidance is limited to social situations.

C. Agoraphobic situations are avoided (e.g., travel is restricted), or else endured with marked distress or with anxiety about having a panic attack, or require the presence of a companion.

D. The panic attacks are not due to the direct effects of a substance (e.g., drugs of abuse, medication) or a general medical condition (e.g., hyperthyroidism).

E. The anxiety or phobic avoidance is not better accounted for by another mental disorder, such as Specific Phobia (e.g., avoidance limited to a single situation like elevators), Separation Anxiety Disorder (e.g., avoidance of school), Obsessive-Compulsive Disorder (e.g., fear of contamination), Posttraumatic Stress Disorder (e.g., avoidance of stimuli associated with a severe stressor), or Social Phobia (e.g., avoidance limited to social situations because of fear of embarrassment).

attacks she had become "obsessed" with the thought that she had some sort of heart condition that would kill her.

The patient stated that she would be agreeable to both medication treatment and "talking therapy." She was started on a low dose of a selective serotonin reuptake inhibitor (SSRI) and was referred to a cognitive behavioral therapist for short-term (12-week) symptom-focused therapy. Within 6 weeks the patient reported that her anticipatory anxiety had diminished significantly, as had the intensity and frequency of her panic attacks. Within 3 months, she was panic free. She continued taking the SSRI for 18 months, after which it was slowly tapered.

Epidemiology, Origins, and Natural History

The case study illustrates a number of characteristic features of panic disorder. It typically begins in late adolescence or early adulthood, with the median age at onset of 24 years (16). It has a prevalence of 1% to 2% and is twice as common in women as in men (14,16). Many patients with panic disorder experience panic-free remissions, particularly after treatment. However, panic disorder is typically a chronic, lifelong condition, and those patients who achieve remission often experience relapses (15). Frequently associated psychiatric conditions include major depression, social phobia, PTSD, GAD, agoraphobia, OCD, and substance abuse (14,17–19).

Patients with panic disorder present special differential diagnostic challenges to generalists and cardiologists. Although panic symptoms are often difficult to distinguish from angina and may lead to unnecessary cardiac catheterization (20), patients with panic disorder have an increased cardiovascular mortality rate (21–23). Other studies, which were limited by the fact that they included male subjects only, revealed that the risk of sudden cardiac death in patients with panic-like symptoms is as much as six times higher than in patients with low anxiety levels, even when known risk factors for cardiac death (e.g., cholesterol level, tobacco use, family history) are taken into account (2). In addition, panic symptoms may be simulated by a number of noncardiac medical disorders, including alcohol and sedative-hypnotic drug withdrawal, marijuana use, pheochromocytoma, hyperthyroidism, hypoglycemia, and temporal lobe epilepsy.

Studies support the view that panic disorder is *primarily a biologic disorder.* Genetic factors have been implicated by family studies demonstrating a tenfold increase in panic disorder among first-degree relatives of panic probands (24) and a markedly higher concordance rate for panic disorder among monozygotic than among dizygotic twins (25). Lactate infusion (26) and hyperventilation (27) may stimulate panic attacks in people with panic disorder, suggesting the existence of specific biologic triggers. Pharmacologic treatments may by themselves dramatically reduce the frequency of panic episodes (see later discussion). Although the neurobiology of panic disorder is not clearly established, preclinical models of conditioned fear, in concert with clinical pharmacologic and neuroimaging studies, have implicated a number of brain regions and neurotransmitters or neuromodulators in the symptoms of anxiety and panic. With regard to brain regions, there are considerable data suggesting that the central nucleus of the amygdala, the orbitofrontal cortex/anterior insula, and the anterior cingulate cortex are involved in the expression of fear and anxiety. Among the endogenous neural substances that are believed to be involved in anxiety are norepinephrine, serotonin, corticotrophin-releasing factor, gamma-aminobutyric acid (GABA), and substance P.

There are also *learning (or conditioning) theories* to explain panic disorder. These propose that panic attacks develop when physical sensations occurring at times of stress are interpreted as signs of grave illness, giving rise to panic. The physical sensations of arousal become conditioned phobic stimuli, provoking the panic symptomatology (conditioned response) (28). Conditioning models have been particularly persuasive in accounting for the development and maintenance of agoraphobia (29).

Evaluation and Treatment

A systematic approach to the evaluation and treatment of panic disorder includes the following steps:

- Take a history and perform a focused physical examination, looking for evidence of a medical disorder that could simulate panic disorder (e.g., insulin-induced hypoglycemia, temporal lobe seizures, cardiac ischemia or dysrhythmias).
- Inquire about the use of caffeine-containing beverages, stimulant drugs, alcohol, marijuana, and other substances associated with anxiety or panic symptoms (Table 22.1).
- Inquire about sleeping habits. Studies have demonstrated that the symptoms of panic disorder worsen with sleep deprivation, so erratic sleep–wake schedules should be avoided.
- Inquire about life stressors, and facilitate the patient's solving of problems (see Chapter 20). Although this may not eliminate panic attacks, it will help reduce the levels of generalized anxiety that often develop in patients with panic disorder.
- *Use pharmacologic means* to reduce the frequency and intensity of panic attacks. The first-line treatment for new-onset idiopathic panic disorder is the use of an SSRI (30,31). Although most antidepressants are effective in the treatment of panic disorder, the SSRIs have a favorable side effect profile compared with either the tricyclic antidepressants or the monoamine oxidase inhibitors. A number of new-generation antidepressants with excellent side effect profiles appear also to be effective in the treatment of panic disorder but do not yet have the track record established by the SSRIs. High-potency benzodiazepines used to be a popular method for treating panic disorder, and they have the advantage of rapid onset of action compared with the antidepressants. However, given the potential risks of tolerance and dependence, they should not be considered a first- or second-line treatment option.

Regardless of the type of antidepressant used for treatment, patients with panic disorder are notoriously sensitive to a variety of medications. It is quite common for a patient with panic disorder, if treated with a "typical" starting dose of an antidepressant (e.g., 50 mg of sertraline or 20 mg of fluoxetine) to develop what is commonly referred to as the "jitteriness syndrome." Patients report feeling keyed up, or on edge, or as if they had consumed excessive amounts of caffeine. Some patients actually note an increase in the number of panic attacks early in the course of treatment. To avoid severe jitteriness and consequent noncompliance, it is important to educate the patient about this phenomenon in advance and to initiate dosing at lower than typical dosages (i.e., 25 mg sertraline or 10 mg fluoxetine). Doses should not be increased until jitteriness totally resolves. Some patients experience an increase in jitteriness each time the dose is increased, but typically this is a short-lived phenomenon (1 to 2 weeks).

Panic disorder is a chronic, recurring illness. In new-onset panic disorder, it is generally accepted that pharmocotherapy should continue for at least 1 year, at which time medications can be tapered over a 4- to 6-month period for a drug-free trial period (32). It is clear, however, that many patients relapse after medications are discontinued. Patients who have experienced more than one previous relapse should be considered for long-term antidepressant treatment, which has been shown to be effective in preventing relapse (33,34).

Once widely accepted as a first-line therapy for the treatment of panic disorder, benzodiazepines now are generally viewed as a short-term adjunct to therapy by most anxiety disorder experts in this country. Patients who are significantly impaired by their symptoms of anxiety during the period before stabilization on antidepressant are sometimes treated with benzodiazepines as a "bridge" (35). However, this strategy is not always fully successful, because more than 50% of patients have difficulty discontinuing benzodiazepines (36).

Controlled clinical research studies have also demonstrated the efficacy of cognitive behavioral therapy (CBT) in the treatment of panic disorder (37). Indeed, CBT has been found, in most studies, to be equally or more efficacious than medication treatment alone, and it can be quite cost-effective. The biggest drawback to CBT, assuming that the patient is willing to make the time commitment to participate, is the paucity of well-trained therapists skilled in administering CBT effectively. As suggested by its name, CBT comprises both cognitive and behavioral therapeutic techniques and is typically administered in 12 sessions over a 12-week period. During this time, patients systematically learn to recognize and correct cognitive distortions associated with their panic attacks (e.g., "When I feel my heart beat quickly it means that I have a fatal cardiac illness") and master relaxation methods to use in the face of mounting anxiety. Because hyperventilation is a frequent feature of panic attacks that exacerbates some panic symptoms (and can lead to acrothesia), most CBT programs for panic involve breathing retraining, wherein patients learn diaphragmatic breathing techniques and how to decrease their respiratory rate when anxious. Finally, CBT often involves interoceptive exposure (i.e., producing physical symptoms, such as dizziness, that are associated with panic and distorted cognitions). If a patient has concomitant agoraphobia, the therapist may also employ exposure therapy techniques, gradually exposing the patient to feared situations as he or she learns to employ cognitive and behavioral methods of panic control.

As with most psychiatric illnesses, an important aspect of the treatment of panic disorders is education of the patient and significant others regarding the nature of panic disorder. Usually, patients are relieved to learn that panic disorder is a common, treatable disease with a biologic basis. Education by the clinician, supplemented by readily available books written for the lay person, may help reduce the patient's sense of isolation and embarrassment and provide practical advice about managing panic symptoms. The National Institutes of Health (NIH) has an up-to-date website with comprehensive information about all of the anxiety disorders as well as a list of books, web links, and national organizations suitable for professionals and laypersons (available at: http://www.nimh.nih.gov/anxiety/anxietymenu.cfm).

Obsessive-Compulsive Disorder

Description

As suggested by its name, the essential features of OCD are obsessions—recurrent, persistent, intrusive thoughts (e.g., "Touching this doorknob will give me a disease")—and compulsions—purposeful but senseless behaviors or rituals (e.g., washing hands 17 times each morning). The obsessive thoughts are distressing to the patient, who usually is aware that the thoughts are illogical and unreasonable. In an individual patient, obsessions and compulsions are often related, and the compulsive behaviors are conducted in an effort to reduce the anxiety brought on by the obsessive thoughts. However, it is not uncommon for a patient to have a variety of obsessions that have no thematic relationship. It is the presence of obsessions and compulsions that distinguishes OCD from obsessive-compulsive *personality* disorder (see Chapter 23), a personality type characterized by meticulousness, perfectionism, and rigidity. The APA diagnostic criteria for OCD are listed in Table 22.3.

Case Study

An 83-year-old widow was referred for evaluation because of disabling fears of contamination. She was a retired mathematics teacher who liked her subject because 1 and 1 always equal 2: "I like the certainty." A practicing Catholic, she recalled that during adolescence she had once delayed disposing of a sanitary napkin because she had sneezed over it after returning home after Mass and worried that bits of the communion wafer might have lodged in it. She had received psychiatric treatment several times for obsessive-compulsive symptoms but had recently been doing well until she was forced to change apartments. After the move she became preoccupied with worries about contamination with germs. Especially vexing was deciding when she had adequately washed her hands after defecating; she was consumed by uncertainty about how long she should wash and how she could safely dispose of the towel after drying her hands. Her main fear was that others might be contaminated and become ill as a result of her carelessness. As a result of these ideas, she washed her hands excessively, did not leave her apartment, ate poorly (so that she would defecate less), and was unable to engage in normal conversation. Treatment consisted of a form of CBT called "response prevention" and the use of an SSRI (see later discussion). Within 2 weeks she showed improvement, and by the end of 8 weeks she was able to dispel obsessive ideas effortlessly and felt no compulsion to wash excessively.

Table 22.3. Diagnostic Criteria for Obsessive-Compulsive Disorder

A. Either obsessions or compulsions:

Obsessions as defined by 1, 2, 3, and 4:

1. Recurrent and persistent thoughts, impulses, or images that are experienced, at some time during the disturbance, as intrusive and inappropriate, and cause marked anxiety or distress.
2. The thoughts, impulses, or images are not simply excessive worries about real-life problems.
3. The person attempts to ignore or suppress such thoughts or impulses or to neutralize them with some other thought or action.
4. The person recognizes that the obsessional thoughts, impulses, or images are a product of his or her own mind (not imposed from without as in thought insertion).

Compulsions as defined by 1 and 2:

1. Repetitive behaviors (e.g., handwashing, ordering, checking) or mental acts (e.g., praying, counting, repeating words silently) that the person feels driven to perform in response to an obsession, or according to rules that must be applied rigidly.
2. The behaviors or mental acts are aimed at preventing or reducing distress or preventing some dreaded event or situation; however, these behaviors or mental acts either are not connected in a realistic way with what they are designed to neutralize or prevent, or are clearly excessive.

B. At some point during the course of the disorder, the person has recognized that the obsessions or compulsions are excessive or unreasonable. Note: This does not apply to children.

C. The obsessions or compulsions cause marked distress, are time-consuming (take more than an hour per day), or significantly interfere with the person's normal routine, occupational functioning, or usual social activities or relationships with others.

D. If another axis I disorder is present, the content of the obsessions or compulsions is not restricted to it (e.g., preoccupation with food in the presence of an eating disorder, hair pulling in the presence of trichotillomania, concern with appearance in the presence of body dysmorphic disorder, preoccupation with drugs in the presence of a substance use disorder, preoccupation with having a serious illness in the presence of hypochondriasis, or guilty ruminations in the presence of major depressive disorder).[a]

E. Not due to the direct effects of a substance (e.g., drugs of abuse, medication) or a general medical condition.

[a]See Chapter 19 for definition of axis I and axis II disorders.

Reprinted with permission from Diagnostic and statistical manual of mental disorders. 4th ed. Washington, DC: American Psychiatric Association, 1994.

Epidemiology, Origins, and Natural History

One to two percent of people in the community (38) and in the general medical clinic (39) meet criteria for OCD. Its prevalence is slightly higher among women and tends to decline with age. Symptoms usually have their onset in adolescence or early adulthood. In one study of patients with OCD (40), the most common obsessions were fear of contamination (55%), fear of acting aggressively (50%), and fear of performing unacceptable sexual activities (32%). Somatic obsessions were present in 34% of patients, including a woman performed breast self-examinations 100 times per day to reassure herself that she had not developed breast cancer (40), and 36% had obsessive thoughts involving the need for symmetry. The most common compulsions involved checking, cleaning, and counting. In most cases the symptoms were chronic and continuous, with some tendency for symptomatic worsening during times of stress. Associated psychiatric diagnoses included major depression (30%), simple phobia (7%), and panic disorder (5%).

Explanations for OCD have been advanced from several perspectives. Psychoanalytic writers have viewed obsessive-compulsive symptoms as products of reaction formation against unacceptable wishes and impulses, often related to aggression and sexuality. Behavioral theorists and practitioners have stressed the anxiety-reducing effects of compulsive rituals and have proposed that compulsions are maintained precisely because of their positively reinforcing ameliorating effects on conditioned anxiety. The importance of personality traits in the development of OCD is suggested by data showing that preexisting obsessive traits (e.g., meticulousness, perfectionism, indecisiveness) are very common in clinical samples of patients who go on to develop OCD (40) and that people who are obsessional, anxious, or self-conscious may be especially vulnerable to the emergence of OCD in response to life change (41).

Other research suggests that OCD has *biologic origins*. The importance of genetic factors is supported by studies showing high concordance for OCD among monozygotic twins (42) and increased risk for OCD among first-degree relatives of probands with Gilles de la Tourette syndrome (43). Clinical studies linking OCD with head trauma (44) and other neurologic disorders (45) add support to the conception that OCD may be a manifestation of brain disease. Of all the anxiety disorders, OCD has been most extensively studied with neuroimaging techniques. Available neuroimaging data, considered together, implicate abnormalities within the cortico-striato-thalamo-cortical network (46). In particular, patients with OCD tend to have hyperactive orbitofrontal, anterior cingulate, and caudate activity that is further activated during symptom provocation and that is attenuated with treatment (47). It has been proposed that the primary lesion of OCD is located in the corpus striatum (48), an hypothesis that is supported by the finding that autoimmune processes known to damage the striatum can be associated with new-onset OCD (49). Results of functional neuroimaging studies, considered together with genetic, epidemiologic, and pharmacologic data, have led to the hypothesis that prefrontal–basal ganglia–thalamic–prefrontal circuits are particularly important in the pathophysiology of OCD (50). Of great theoretical and practical importance is the demonstration that numerous antidepressants that prevent uptake of serotonin into presynaptic neurons are effective in the treatment of OCD (51). This observation strongly implicates a role for central serotonergic neuronal systems in the pathophysiology of this disorder.

Evaluation and Treatment

A systematic approach to the evaluation and treatment of OCD involves the following steps:

- In the history and physical examination, look for evidence of medical conditions, medications, or dietary practices that may simulate or exacerbate symptoms of anxiety. It has been found that some individuals develop OCD after a streptococcal infection and subsequent autoimmune damage to the corpus striatum (49), so the relationship between symptom onset and a possible streptococcal infection should be explored.
- Consider *use of cognitive behavioral therapy.* Most experts recommend CBT as a first-line treatment for every patient who is willing to participate (52). This suggestion follows from the view that compulsions are maintained by their temporary amelioration of conditioned anxiety. Patients are taught to control their obsessive ruminations by commanding themselves to stop ruminating when obsessive ideas arise (thought stopping), and they are exhorted to resist carrying out their compulsive acts so that they can learn that there are no dire consequences associated with nonexecution of the rituals (response prevention). These techniques are often helpful if patients can be persuaded to practice them.
- Consider use of *antidepressant medications* that have been shown to have specific efficacy in OCD. First-line drugs, all of which are significantly more effective than placebo, include the tricyclic clomipramine and the SSRIs (53–55). As with all anxiety disorders, when initiating treatment with an SSRI, medication dosages should gradually be titrated upward. Patients should receive treatment for 10 to 12 weeks with an SSRI in adequate doses before alternative therapy is considered (56). For reasons that are not entirely clear, patients with OCD often require dosages of SSRI in excess of those used to treat depression or other anxiety disorders, and even on the highest tolerated dose, up to 25% of patients are unresponsive to treatment (57,58). As with depression and other anxiety disorders, initial responses may not be apparent until 4 to 6 weeks into treatment, and it can take months before optimal treatment effects are reached. Treatment should be continued for at least 6 to 12 months and then tapered slowly, if a drug-free trial is desired. If symptoms of OCD reappear during the course of the drug taper, medication doses should be restored to pretaper levels (56). For patients with chronic severe symptoms, long-term maintenance treatment should be considered, because it has been shown that medications can protect against relapse (59). Practical information about antidepressant drugs is found in Chapter 24.
- Consider short-term *problem-solving counseling* (see Chapter 20). Although this may not bring total relief, it is clear that symptomatic exacerbations of this chronic disorder tend to come at times of stress and change, and short-term counseling may help reduce the impact of such influences. On the other hand, insight-oriented, introspective psychotherapies have generally been ineffective in the treatment of OCD.

Generalized Anxiety Disorder

Description

GAD is characterized by persistent and excessive worry that is present more days than not for at least a

Table 22.4. Diagnostic Criteria for Generalized Anxiety Disorder

A. Excessive anxiety and worry (apprehensive expectation), occurring more days than not for at least 6 months, about a number of events or activities (such as work or school performance).
B. The person finds it difficult to control the worry.
C. The anxiety and worry are associated with at least three of the following six symptoms (with at least some symptoms present for more days than not for the past 6 months):
  1. Restlessness or feeling keyed up or on edge
  2. Being easily fatigued
  3. Difficulty concentrating or mind going blank
  4. Irritability
  5. Muscle tension
  6. Sleep disturbance (difficulty falling or staying asleep, or restless unsatisfying sleep)
D. The focus of the anxiety and worry is not confined to features of an axis I disorder, e.g., the anxiety or worry is not about having a panic attack (as in Panic Disorder), being embarrassed in public (as in Social Phobia), being contaminated (as in Obsessive-Compulsive Disorder), being away from home or close relatives (as in Separation Anxiety Disorder), gaining weight (as in Anorexia Nervosa), or having a serious illness (as in Hypochondriasis), and is not part of Posttraumatic Stress Disorder.[a]
E. The anxiety, worry, or physical symptoms cause clinically significant distress or impairment in social, occupational, or other important areas of functioning.
F. Not due to the direct effects of a substance (e.g., drugs of abuse, medication) or a general medical condition (e.g., hyperthyroidism), and does not occur exclusively during a mood disorder, psychotic disorder, or pervasive developmental disorder.

[a]See Chapter 19 for definition of axis I and axis II disorders.

Reprinted with permission from Diagnostic and statistical manual of mental disorders. 4th ed. Washington, DC: American Psychiatric Association, 1994.

6-month period. In addition to excessive, inappropriate, or unrealistic worry, the patient must experience at least three of six physical symptoms, including restlessness, easy fatigability, difficulty concentrating, irritability, muscle tension, and sleep disturbance. APA criteria are listed in Table 22.4.

Case Study

A 50-year-old woman came to her physician complaining of difficulty swallowing, insomnia, tremor, and loose stools. She reported that she'd been a "worrier" since her twenties, but that this characteristic had increased in the year since her husband died and she became responsible for managing all aspects of the household. Three of her adult children, one of whom had mental retardation, lived at home, and she continued to prepare their meals and do their laundry. She admitted that she was "scared of everything," generally tense ("Little things make me jump"), and often experienced feelings of shakiness, diaphoresis, and fluttering in the chest, usually in response to contemplating driving by herself or engaging in another feared activity. She did not describe discrete intense panic episodes (see later discussion). She did report feeling blue for the past several months, and that she had difficulty enjoying things. Physical examination, ECG, and exercise stress test results were normal. Although she was reluctant to take medications, she agreed to try treatment with venlafaxine XR, beginning at a dose of 75 mg/day. In addition, she agreed to meet with her physician on a monthly basis for 12 months for counseling. During counseling sessions she learned simple relaxation techniques (see later discussion), helped construct a program of systematic desensitization regarding driving, and developed a plan to request that her children participate more consistently in the running of the household. At the end of 1 year she was greatly improved. She was driving regularly to visit friends across town with growing confidence.

Epidemiology, Origins, and Natural History

GAD is one of the more common anxiety disorders, with an estimated lifetime prevalence of 5.1% (60). Patients frequently initially present to their general practitioner with a variety of somatic complaints, for which no medical basis is discovered (61). Like all of the anxiety disorders except OCD, GAD is more common in women and usually begins in the early twenties. GAD is a chronic illness that often persists for several decades (61,62). It is extremely rare for GAD to exist in isolation; the great majority of patients also meet criteria for major depression, another anxiety disorder, or alcohol abuse (63).

The causes of GAD are not fully understood. A number of studies have indicated that there is a mild genetic component to GAD (25,64,65). A recent, large-scale study in female twins suggested that GAD and major depression share a common genetic basis, possibly explaining the frequent comorbidity of these two illnesses (66). Traumatic early life experiences, especially the death of a parent (67), may be a predisposing factor, although patients with this disorder do not characterize their childhoods as more difficult than nonanxious people do (68). Events in later life, especially unexpected events perceived as important and negative (69), may also play a role in the emergence of symptoms.

Evaluation and Treatment

A systematic approach to the evaluation and treatment of the patient with GAD includes the following steps:

- Take a medical history and perform a focused physical examination to look for evidence of medical disorders (e.g., hyperthyroidism, pheochromocytoma, hypoglycemia) that may manifest with concomitant somatic symptoms and anxiety.
- Inquire about consumption of alcohol, caffeine-containing beverages, and other drugs (e.g., diet pills), and counsel the patient to eliminate ingestion of caffeine and other stimulants and to moderate alcohol consumption.
- Inquire about life stresses and encourage the patient to find solutions to problems; anxious patients are often demoralized and benefit from short-term counseling (see Chapter 20) aimed at solving problems and restoring self-esteem.
- Instruct the patient in *self-regulation techniques* such as progressive muscle relaxation (see later discussion), and encourage regular practice.
- Consider a trial of *buspirone.* It is well tolerated and effective in the treatment of GAD, particularly for the core symptoms of worry and apprehensive expectation, although its onset of action is slower than that of benzodiazepines, and it may not be particularly effective in patients with a history of long-term benzodiazepine use. It carries essentially no risk of

tolerance or dependency. Effective therapy is continued for at least 6 to 12 months.

- Consider the use of an *antidepressant medication.* There is growing evidence that a variety of antidepressants may be effective for the treatment of GAD (70–75) (see Table 24.5 in Chapter 24). The newer antidepressants, such as the SSRIs and venlafaxine, have favorable side effect profiles in comparison to tricyclic antidepressants and are a good first-line option, particularly in patients with comorbid depression or another anxiety disorder. In contrast to benzodiazepines, antidepressants must be taken for several weeks before they become effective, and they carry little risk of tolerance or dependence. Patients should be treated for at least 1 year before tapering and discontinuation of medication is considered.
- Be reluctant to prescribe *benzodiazepines.* Unfortunately, many patients receive benzodiazepines as their first treatment for GAD because of their ability to treat symptoms of arousal, autonomic hyperactivity, and muscle tension. Given that there are numerous other medication options, these drugs should not be considered as a first treatment option. Benzodiazepines commonly cause symptoms such as drowsiness and sedation, and they can also cause atazia, dizziness, and uncoordination (76). Because patients with GAD are at increased risk for substance abuse, benzodiazepines should be prescribed only with caution and for the short term.
- No response to treatment or relapse should lead to reassessment of the diagnosis, examination for medical and psychiatric comorbidity (especially major depression), and possible psychiatric referral.

Phobias

Description

As a group, phobias are enduring fears of harmless objects or situations (phobic stimuli) that lead patients to avoid contact with them (phobic avoidance). Patients with *specific phobia* fear discrete objects and situations, such as animals, heights, air travel, needles, and visits to the doctor, whereas patients with *social phobia* have fears of social humiliation and the scrutiny of others. People with *agoraphobia* fear being in situations from which escape is difficult or where help may not be available in the event of an anxiety-provoking episode, such as in open or public spaces (literally, fear of the *agora* or marketplace). Although phobic patients generally recognize their fears to be excessive and unreasonable, they nonetheless seek to avoid the phobic stimulus because exposure provokes intense anxiety. The diagnosis of phobia is made only if avoidance of the feared object or situation leads to social or occupational impairment or if the patient experiences great distress as a result of the symptom.

APA criteria for specific phobia and social phobia are listed in Tables 22.5 and 22.6, respectively. Agoraphobia can be seen in a number of anxiety disorders (e.g., social phobia, PTSD) and is described in the section on panic disorder.

Table 22.5. Diagnostic Criteria for Specific Phobia

A. Marked and persistent fear that is excessive or unreasonable, cued by the presence or anticipation of a specific object or situation (e.g., flying, height, animals, receiving an injection, seeing blood).
B. Exposure to the phobic stimulus almost invariably provokes an immediate anxiety response, which may take the form of a situationally bound or situationally predisposed panic attack. Note: In children, the anxiety may be expressed by crying, tantrums, freezing, or clinging.
C. The person recognizes that the fear is excessive or unreasonable. Note: In children, this feature may be absent.
D. The phobic situation is avoided or else endured with intense anxiety or distress.
E. The avoidance, anxious anticipation, or distress in the feared situations interferes significantly with the person's normal routine, occupational (academic) functioning, or social activities or relationships with others, or there is marked distress about having the phobia.
F. The anxiety, panic attacks, or phobic avoidance associated with the specific object or situation are not better accounted for by another mental disorder, such as Obsessive-Compulsive Disorder (e.g., fear of contamination), Posttraumatic Stress Disorder (e.g., avoidance of stimuli associated with a severe stressor), Separation Anxiety Disorder (e.g., avoidance of school), Social Phobia (e.g., avoidance of social situations because of fear of embarrassment), Panic Disorder with Agoraphobia, or Agoraphobia without history of panic disorder.

Adapted with permission from Diagnostic and statistical manual of mental disorders. 4th ed. Washington, DC: American Psychiatric Association, 1994.

Table 22.6. Diagnostic Criteria for Social Phobia

A. A marked and persistent fear of one or more social or performance situations in which the person is exposed to unfamiliar people or to possible scrutiny by others. The individual fears that he or she will act in a way (or show anxiety symptoms) that will be humiliating or embarrassing. Note: In children, there must be evidence of capacity for social relationships with familiar people and the anxiety must occur in peer settings, not just in interactions with adults.
B. Exposure to the feared social situation almost invariably provokes anxiety, which may take the form of a situationally bound or situationally predisposed panic attack. Note: In children, the anxiety may be expressed by crying, tantrums, freezing, or withdrawal from the social situation.
C. The person recognizes that the fear is excessive or unreasonable. Note: In children, this feature may be absent.
D. The feared social or performance situations are avoided or else endured with intense anxiety or distress.
E. The avoidance, anxious anticipation, or distress in the feared social or performance situation interferes significantly with the person's normal routine, occupational (academic) functioning, or social activities or relationships with others, or there is marked distress about having the phobia.
F. The fear or avoidance is not due to the direct effects of a substance (e.g., drugs of abuse, medication) or a general medical condition, and is not better accounted for by Panic Disorder with or without Agoraphobia, Separation Anxiety Disorder, Body Dysmorphic Disorder, a Pervasive Developmental Disorder, or Schizoid Personality Disorder.
G. If a general medical condition or other mental disorder is present, the fear in criterion A is unrelated to it; for example, the fear is not of stuttering, trembling (in Parkinson disease) or of exhibiting abnormal eating behavior (in Anorexia Nervosa or Bulimia Nervosa).

Adapted with permission from Diagnostic and statistical manual of mental disorders. 4th ed. Washington, DC: American Psychiatric Association, 1994.

Case Study

A 50-year-old married business executive sought treatment because of an addiction to chlordiazepoxide. In his early twenties he had first become aware of his discomfort in large groups, particularly when he was the focus of attention. On occasion, he would experience panic attacks during these large social gatherings. He discovered that regular use of chlordiazepoxide improved his general level of comfort, and by age 50 he was using 80 mg/day routinely. In addition to feeling anxious in large groups, the patient was anxious in small groups when he was the center of attention. He avoided writing checks in public because he was afraid that his hand would tremble or that he would hold up a check-out line, and he had great difficulty dealing with authority figures. His job required that he occasionally make professional presentations before clients and supervisors. In the days preceding a presentation, he would experience great anticipatory anxiety associated with the fear that he would be unable to recall what he wanted to say or that his throat would close up, preventing him from speaking. In response to this fear, he would increase his daily chlordiazepoxide dosage by 50% to 100%. On the day of the presentation he would take 200 to 300 mg and would perform well. He was dissatisfied with this practice because he now felt depressed and believed that the medication might be playing a role. His diagnosis at the time of evaluation was social phobia and benzodiazepine dependence. A slow chlordiazepoxide taper was undertaken and completed within 6 months. At the same time, the patient participated actively in a structured CBT group and was prescribed an SSRI. His social anxiety declined, and his confidence grew as he succeeded in attending parties and giving talks.

Epidemiology, Origins, and Natural History

In recent years, the distinctions among the various types of phobias have received increased scrutiny (77). These include *specific phobia* (e.g., fear of heights, snakes, blood, insects), *circumscribed social phobia* (fear of one type of social situation, such as public speaking) and *generalized social phobia* (fear of a number of different social situations). Of the various types of phobia, generalized social phobia is associated with the greatest impairment and is more likely to be present with other psychiatric disorders.

Specific phobias are characterized by excessive fear of specific objects or situations. When confronted with the feared object or situation, a patient with a specific phobia becomes extremely anxious and may experience a situation-bound panic attack. Most adults with specific phobias recognize that their fear is irrational, but despite this realization, they avoid the object or endure exposure with great difficulty. One survey found that among eight common phobias, the most common fear in women was that of animals, and the most common in men was that of heights (78). Other common phobias include fear of enclosed places, blood, snakes, spiders, and various forms of transportation, such as flying in airplanes. Approximately 8% of the adult population suffer from one or more specific phobias during a 1-year period (79). Most phobias are chronic, and they generally do not remit without treatment.

Social phobia, also known as social anxiety disorder, is characterized by excessive and persistent anxiety in social situations, including performances and public speaking (80). The basis of the anxiety is that patients are afraid that they will humiliate or embarrass themselves. Often patients are concerned that people will notice certain embarrassing physical symptoms, such as perspiration, blushing, trembling, or tremulous voice. When placed in unavoidable social situations, patients with social phobia can have panic attacks. In contrast to panic disorders, the panic attacks in social phobia are not "out of the blue." Further, although patients with panic disorder are concerned about the symptoms of the panic attack (e.g., believe they are having a heart attack), patients with social phobia are concerned that others will notice that they are having a panic attack. Like both panic disorder and specific phobias, social phobia is often characterized by significant anticipatory anxiety for days or weeks before the feared social interaction.

The lifetime prevalence of social phobia is approximately 13.3% (60). This number includes both patients with circumscribed and those with generalized social phobia. Like most anxiety disorders, social phobia is more common in women than in men and typically begins in childhood or adolescence. It is frequently comorbid with other psychiatric illnesses, including the affective disorders (41.4%), other anxiety disorders (56.9%), and substance abuse disorders (39.6%) (79). As with panic disorder, patients with social phobia have an increased risk of certain medical conditions (e.g., peptic ulcers) and make more frequent use of medical resources than the does the general population (81). Generalized social phobia is a chronic, often lifelong condition (81).

Patients with social phobia may become addicted to alcohol or to sedative-hypnotics as a result of self-directed efforts to ameliorate their social anxiety. Furthermore, phobias and phobic anxiety may be risk factors for ischemic heart disease and other forms of cardiovascular morbidity. There is a significant association between measures of phobic anxiety (fears of enclosed spaces, illness, going out alone, heights, and crowds) and the probability of subsequent ischemic cardiac events (82). Such relationships may be mediated by anxiety-related hyperventilation, which has been shown to cause coronary vasospasm and cardiac ischemia (83), or by anxiety-induced arrhythmia (84).

Treatment

Approaches to treatment of specific phobia are based on the notion that this form of anxiety develops as a product of the pairing of an innocuous stimulus with a threatening one. Phobic avoidance emerges and is maintained by the anxiety-preventing consequences of the avoidance. The treatment of phobias has advanced greatly with the development of behavioral therapies aimed at extinguishing phobic anxiety and phobic avoidance. Three commonly used techniques are desensitization, participant modeling, and social skills training.

Systematic *desensitization* begins with the gradual exposure of the patient to increasingly vivid and anxiety-provoking mental images of the phobic stimulus. As anxiety is generated, the patient induces relaxation by use of a relaxation technique (see later discussion). By exercising a response incompatible with anxiety (i.e., relaxation) in reaction to the phobic stimulus, the patient gradually extinguishes the phobic anxiety. This treatment occurs over a series of sessions until the patient is comfortable enough to encounter the stimulus *in vivo.* Related to systematic desensitization is *flooding* or *implosion,* in which the imagery is presented suddenly rather than gradually.

In vivo desensitization involves gradual, stepwise exposure of the patient to the feared stimulus in real life. The patient is often initially accompanied by the therapist or a trained family member. Progress from less to more anxiety-producing tasks is accomplished by mastering anxiety at each level. The basis for the technique is that repeated exposure leads to extinction of phobic anxiety.

Participant modeling is a form of *in vivo* desensitization in which the therapist models the desired interaction with the feared object. This kind of procedure may be useful with patients who have a severe needle phobia and whose avoidance of needles may be potentially life-threatening (e.g., in-patients requiring insulin). Therapy involves the following steps (85):

- Education aimed at providing realistic information about the feared object
- Response modeling, in which the therapist handles the feared object
- Joint performance, in which the patient and therapist are both exposed to the phobic stimulus
- Self-directed practice (e.g., inserting a needle into an orange)

Behavioral techniques such as these have been used successfully to treat phobias related to hemodialysis, needles, and return to work after medical illness. They may be carried out by nonphysicians and are usually effective within 15 sessions or less. Among patients treated by these techniques, phobias, hypochondriacal symptoms, and work adjustment often improve within 6 months, and visits to health care providers decrease markedly (86,87).

Social skills training is not an appropriate treatment for phobias, including social phobia. Cognitive behavioral treatment of social phobia often involves exposure to social situations. The issue is not lack of social competence, however; it is getting over unrealistic anxiety regarding humiliation and embarrassment.

Specific phobias are typically treated with the CBT methods described previously. Some patients with prominent sympathomimetic symptoms (e.g., tremor, diaphoresis, palpitations) in isolated performance situations benefit from treatment with beta-adrenergic blockers, administered the day of the performance situation. These individuals should always initially take low doses (e.g., 25 to 50 mg of atenolol) and should have a test dose days or weeks before use in the performance situation. This "practice" dose serves to reassure the patient that he or she will not experience untoward effects and that the dose is not excessive (e.g., associated with disabling drops in blood pressure). Social phobia can be effectively treated by either use of CBT (individual or group) or medications. CBT for social phobia involves correcting distorted cognitions (e.g., "The audience will see me perspire and blush and will think I am incompetent") and teaching behavioral techniques (e.g., progressive muscle relaxation) to use in the face of social anxiety. As with most forms of CBT, treatment for social phobia is time limited (typically 12 weeks) and focuses on the symptoms of social phobia rather than interpersonal conflicts or long-standing psychological issues.

At present, the first-line treatment for generalized social phobia is an SSRI, although monoamine oxidase inhibitors, high-potency benzodiazepines, and the anticonvulsant gabapentin have also been demonstrated to be efficacious (88–90). Some of the newer-generation antidepressants also show significant promise for the treatment of generalized social phobia, although they have a less well-established track record than the SSRIs do (91).

Posttraumatic Stress Disorder

Description

People who have been exposed to a traumatic event that involved *potential death or serious injury to themselves or another* sometimes develop a syndrome characterized by intrusive recollections or dreams of the event, avoidance of stimuli provoking memories of the event, and a heightened level of arousal. When such symptoms have been present for less than 3 months, a diagnosis of acute PTSD is appropriate. When this syndrome has been present for at least 3 months, the diagnosis of chronic PTSD is made. APA criteria are summarized in Table 22.7.

Case Study

A 45-year-old mechanic sustained burns on the arms and thorax when an engine exploded during repair. He had no history of psychiatric disorder. His surgical treatment was successful, leaving him with little residual physical disability. However, after discharge he experienced marked sleep disturbance, generalized anxiety, and loss of interest in usual activities. He avoided proximity to fire in any form and could not tolerate listening to reports about fires on the radio. Treatment with an SSRI aided sleep, improved his mood, and reduced the frequency of his intrusive memories and recurrent dreams, but it did not affect his avoidance behavior. On the anniversary of his injury he would not leave his room because he could not be persuaded that it was safe to do so.

Epidemiology, Origins, and Natural History

About 3.6% of U.S. adults ages 18 to 54 years (5.2 million people) have PTSD during the course of a given year (NIMH website, 2001). In men, the full syndrome is usually found among Vietnam veterans who were injured in combat; in women, the most common precipitant is physical assault. Individual posttraumatic stress symptoms (particularly nightmares, feelings of jitteriness, and sleep disturbances) are much more common, occurring in approximately 15% of the population. Combat, physical assault, seeing someone being hurt or die, and experiencing a serious threat or close call are the most common traumatic experiences associated with such symptoms (92). The highest rates of poststress disorder are found among women who are

Table 22.7. Diagnostic Criteria for Posttraumatic Stress Disorder

A. The person has been exposed to a traumatic event in which both of the following have been present:
   1. The person has experienced, witnessed, or been confronted with an event or events that involve actual or threatened death or serious injury, or a threat to the physical integrity of oneself or others.
   2. The person's response involved intense fear, helplessness, or horror. Note: In children, it may be expressed instead by disorganized or agitated behavior.

B. The traumatic event is persistently re-experienced in at least one of the following ways:
   1. Recurrent and intrusive distressing recollections of the event, including images, thoughts, or perceptions. Note: In young children, repetitive play may occur in which themes or aspects of the trauma are expressed.
   2. Recurrent distressing dreams of the event. Note: In children, there may be frightening dreams without recognized content.
   3. Acting or feeling as if the traumatic event were recurring (includes a sense of reliving the experience, illusions, hallucinations, and dissociative flashback episodes, including those that occur upon awakening or when intoxicated). Note: In young children, trauma-specific reenactment may occur.
   4. Intense psychologic distress at exposure to internal or external cues that symbolize or resemble an aspect of the traumatic event.
   5. Physiologic reactivity upon exposure to internal or external cues that symbolize or resemble an aspect of the traumatic event.

C. Persistent avoidance of stimuli associated with the trauma and numbing of general responsiveness (not present before the trauma), as indicated by at least three of the following:
   1. Efforts to avoid thoughts, feelings, or conversations associated with the trauma
   2. Efforts to avoid activities, places, or people that arouse recollections of the trauma
   3. Inability to recall an important aspect of the trauma
   4. Markedly diminished interest in participation in significant activities
   5. Feeling of detachment or estrangement from others
   6. Restricted range of affect (e.g., unable to have loving feelings)
   7. Sense of a foreshortened future (e.g., does not expect to have a career, marriage, children, or a normal life span)

D. Persistent symptoms of increased arousal (not present before the trauma), as indicated by at least two of the following:
   1. Difficulty falling or staying asleep
   2. Irritability or outbursts of anger
   3. Difficulty concentrating
   4. Hypervigilance
   5. Exaggerated startle response

E. Duration of the disturbance (symptoms in B, C, and D) is more than 1 month.

F. The disturbance causes clinically significant distress or impairment in social, occupational, or other important areas of functioning.

Acute: if duration of symptoms is less than 3 months
Chronic: if duration of symptoms is 3 months or longer
Delayed Onset: onset of symptoms at least 6 months after the stressor

Reprinted with permission from Diagnostic and statistical manual of mental disorders. 4th ed. Washington, DC: American Psychiatric Association, 1994.

victims of violent crime, especially rape (93). For reasons that are not entirely clear, PTSD is more common in women than men (94,95).

People with PTSD are twice as likely as people without PTSD to have another psychiatric disorder, particularly OCD, dysthymia, substance abuse, bipolar affective disorder, or antisocial personality. There is also an increased risk of PTSD among people with a history of childhood behavioral problems, especially lying, stealing, truancy, vandalism, and school expulsion. Among people with a history of four such behaviors, 6% met formal criteria for PTSD and 29% reported at least one symptom (92).

There are three subtypes of PTSD. The first is the acute subtype. By definition, this includes individuals who meet criteria for PTSD but in whom symptoms persist for less than 3 months following the traumatic event. In contrast, chronic PTSD is the descriptor for those patients whose symptoms last longer than 3 months. Some individuals develop PTSD months or years after the traumatic event; these patients have what is known as delayed-onset PTSD.

Patients who have PTSD are significantly impaired by their symptoms, although they may not attribute their problems to PTSD. National Comorbidity Survey respondents who met criteria for PTSD had 40% elevated odds of high school and college failure, 30% elevated odds of teenage child-bearing, 60% elevated odds of marital instability, and 150% elevated odds of unemployment at the time of the survey, compared with people without PTSD (95,96).

Explanations of PTSD have been advanced from several perspectives. From the behavioral viewpoint, the posttraumatic symptoms (e.g., hyperarousal, intrusive recollections) are viewed as products of classically conditioned linkages between innocuous stimuli (e.g., a news report about a fire) and the original traumatic event (e.g., painful injury in a fire). The avoidance symptoms are explained in terms of operant conditioning: Avoidance of stimuli reminiscent of the traumatic event is reinforced by resulting protection of the patient from the symptoms of phobic anxiety (i.e., hyperarousal). Biologic theorists have proposed explanations involving changes in central adrenergic autonomic arousal (97) and in cerebral mechanisms regulating sleep cycles (98). Neuroimaging studies implicate right cerebral limbic and paralimbic areas in the symptoms of PTSD, with hyperreactivity of the amygdala in response to reminders of the trauma (47). Potential roles for personality traits and early life experiences have been suggested by observations of burn patients and other trauma victims demonstrating relationships between maladaptive personality traits, early life loss, trauma, behavioral problems, and poor posttraumatic adjustment (92,99).

Treatment

Behavioral, psychotherapeutic, and pharmacologic treatment approaches have all been advocated for the treatment of PTSD. *Behavioral treatments* such as desensitization are generally required to help patients overcome the conditioned avoidance of stimuli reminiscent of the traumatic event. *Psychotherapy* is virtually always needed to assist patients in dealing with anger about the injury, guilt about survival, and similar themes common among people with PTSD.

Antidepressant and anxiolytic medications have been used with variable efficacy. Tricyclic antidepressants and monoamine oxidase inhibitors may be effective in ameliorating hyperarousal, intrusion, and avoidance symptoms and in relieving concurrent major depression (100,101). Several studies have demonstrated the utility of SSRIs for the treatment of PTSD, and there is some evidence that anticonvulsants such as gabapentin may be useful (102,103). Benzodiazepines are sometimes used, but there is no empiric evidence for their effectiveness in this setting, and they are relatively contraindicated in patients who are at high risk for chemical dependency. Neuroleptic drugs are almost never indicated (104).

TREATMENT OF ANXIETY DISORDERS: GENERAL MEASURES

Specific treatments and results have been described for each specific anxiety disorder. This section describes nonpharmacologic and pharmacologic measures that may be of use in multiple anxiety disorders.

Nonpharmacologic Approaches

A variety of cognitive and behavioral interventions are useful in the treatment of anxiety disorders, some of which are listed here.

Education and Explanation

Patients with panic attacks, obsessions and compulsions, posttraumatic distress symptoms, and generalized anxiety often feel different, isolated from others, and confused about the nature of their malady. They benefit greatly from learning that they have a diagnosable disorder, that they are not alone in their suffering, and that there are effective treatments. Patients should be encouraged to contact the NIMH (see General References) for free and up-to-date science-based information on the anxiety disorders.

Self-Regulation Techniques

Many patients benefit from learning specific techniques that reduce motor tension, hyperarousal, and autonomic hyperactivity. These self-regulation techniques include muscle relaxation, diaphragmatic breathing, biofeedback, self-hypnosis, and meditation exercises (105). Interested generalists can develop skills in teaching these techniques to their patients. Alternatively, patients can be referred to behavioral therapists for instruction.

In progressive muscle relaxation and diaphragmatic breathing (Table 22.8), patients learn to ameliorate anxiety by sequential contraction and relaxation of muscle groups or by slow inhalation using the diaphragm. With regular practice, patients can apply these techniques in times of distress and achieve considerable relief. Commercially available audiotapes are available to help guide patients through the procedure (see General References); the book, *The Relaxation Response* (106), is written for the layperson and may also be useful.

In *biofeedback* training (107), patients learn to control anxiety with the aid of electromyographic information provided to them in the form of visual or auditory messages. During treatment sessions, electrodes

Table 22.8. Essential Steps in Progressive Muscle Relaxation, Rapid Muscle Relaxation Techniques, and Diaphragmatic Breathing Exercises

A. Progressive muscle relaxation[a]	
Forehead/scalp	Raise the eyebrows high; hold; feel strain; relax.
Forehead	Scowl or frown; bunch eyebrows with nose upward; relax.
Eyes	Squeeze eyes shut; hold; feel strain in temples; relax.
Mouth	Smile broadly until mouth quivers slightly; relax; press lips tightly inward; hold; relax.
Jaw	Grit teeth gently but firmly; hold; relax; part lips slightly.
Neck/arm/shoulder	Press head back against right hand; relax; repeat exercise with left hand.
Neck/arm/shoulder	Press head forward against right hand placed on forehead; relax; repeat with left hand.
Back/legs/abdomen	Sitting, grip chair sides firmly; raise legs slightly; lift buttocks 1 inch from chair; point toes forward, then backward; relax.
Hands/arm	Make fist; clench tightly; relax.

B. Rapid Relaxation[b]
1. Sit or lie down. The quieter the place, the better.
2. Take a deep breath through your mouth, hold it for 10 seconds, and exhale slowly.
3. Mentally repeat the word "relax" 4 times in a calm manner.
4. Gradually space out repeating "relax" until each repetition takes about 7 seconds.
5. Keep practicing until you achieve the level of relaxation you desire.

C. Diaphragmatic breathing—While sitting or lying down with a pillow at the small of your back
1. Breathe in slowly and deeply by pushing your stomach out.
2. Say the word "relax" silently to yourself before exhaling.
3. Exhale slowly, letting your stomach come in.
4. Repeat entire procedure 10 times consecutively, with emphasis on slow, deep breaths.

Practice should take place 5 times per day, 10 consecutive diaphragmatic breaths each sitting. Time for mastery is after 1–2 wk of daily practice.

[a]Subject is instructed to practice this exercise while seated comfortably or reclining.
[b]For immediate relaxation in everyday stressful situations.

are placed in a muscle (e.g., frontalis) or muscle group. Patients then attempt to reduce muscle tension, receive immediate feedback about the effectiveness of their efforts (e.g., reduction in amplitude of a tone fed back to them through earphones), and learn to alter their technique to achieve more complete electromyographic (and clinical) relaxation.

Self-hypnosis training often begins with office-based sessions during which the therapist uses a standard hypnotic induction technique and then, for example, asks the patient to notice a warm, tingling feeling starting in the legs and feet and spreading slowly throughout the body. Pleasant, peaceful mental images might be suggested. Patients are taught to induce these states on their own and are advised to practice them regularly, reinforced by periodic office visits for reassessment and further practice. Clinicians may develop skills in performing hypnosis by attending seminars such as those sponsored by the Society for Clinical and Experimental Hypnosis.

Meditation techniques, such as Zen, yoga, or transcendental meditation, have been practiced for centuries. They have recently become popular treatments for anxiety because they favorably alter anxiety-related physiologic variables such as respiratory rate, oxygen consumption, and galvanic skin response, a measure of autonomic activity. Meditation techniques that are effective in ameliorating anxiety include or encourage the following elements: (108).

- *A mental device:* There should be a constant stimulus, such as a sound, word, or phrase repeated silently or audibly or fixed gazing at an object.
- *Passive attitude:* If distracting thoughts occur during the repetition or gazing, they should be disregarded and attention should be redirected to the chosen stimulus. The patient should not worry about the quality of performance.
- *Decreased muscle tone:* The patient should be in a comfortable position so that minimal muscular work is required.
- *Quiet environment:* An environment with minimal distractions should be chosen. If visual fixation on an object is not used, the patient's eyes should be closed.

Pharmacologic Treatments

Individual pharmacologic treatments for the various anxiety disorders have already been discussed. In general, the SSRIs are a reasonable first-line treatment choice for all of the anxiety disorders, with the possible exception of GAD, for which buspirone may be a better first choice. However, data demonstrating the efficacy of venlafaxine in the treatment of GAD suggest that it may be an excellent first-line choice as well (70). Also, given that GAD is commonly comorbid with depression and other anxiety disorders, the combination of buspirone with an SSRI or other antidepressant may be indicated.

Guidelines for use of SSRIs and antidepressants are described in other elsewhere in this text (see Chapter 24). As noted earlier, when treating new-onset panic disorder or GAD, clinicians often prescribe benzodiazepines as a bridge to help relieve anxiety in patients during the period of upward titration of

Table 22.9. Usual Dosage and Pharmacokinetics of Anxiolytic Benzodiazepines

Drug (Trade Name), Year Introduced	Onset of Effect After Oral Dose[a]	Available Strengths (mg)	Oral Daily Dosage Range Divided Two or Three Times a Day (mg)	Active Metabolites Present	Elimination Half-Life[b] (hr)
Alprazolam[c] (Xanax), 1981	Intermediate	0.25, 0.5, 1 (scored tablets)	0.75–6	No	8–16
Chlordiazepoxide[c] (Librium; Libritabs), 1960	Intermediate	5, 10, 25 (capsules); 5, 10, 25 (tablets)	15–100	Yes	5–30
Clonazepam[d] (Klonopin), 1990	Intermediate	0.5, 1, 2 (tablets)	1.5–20	Yes	18–50
Clorazepate dipotassium[c] (Tranxene; Tranxene SD), 1972	Rapid	3.75, 7.5, 15 (capsules); 11.25, 22.5 (tablets)	15–60 22.5 (single doses are intended for patients stabilized on 3.75 or 7.5 mg t.i.d.)	Yes Yes	36–200 36–200
Diazepam[c] (Valium), 1961	Rapid	2, 5, 10 (tablets)	4–40	Yes	20–50
Diazepam (Valrelease), 1982	Slow	15 (capsules)	15–30 (single dose is equivalent to 5 mg of Valium t.i.d.)	Yes	20–50
Halazepam (Paxipam), 1981	Slow to intermediate	20, 40 (tablets)	80–160	Yes	50–100
Lorazepam[c] (Ativan), 1977	Intermediate	0.5, 1, 2 (tablets)	1–6	No	10–20
Oxazepam[c] (Serax), 1963	Slow to intermediate	10, 15, 30 (capsules) 15 (tablets)	30–120 30–120	No	5–10
Prazepam (Centrax), 1977	Slow	5, 10 (capsules)	20–60	Yes	36–200

[a]Drugs with more rapid onset of action are those more rapidly absorbed.

[b]Elimination half-life of lipophilic activity.

[c]Generic available.

[d]Clonazepam is not approved by the U.S. Food and Drug Administration for treatment of anxiety. It is approved as an anticonvulsant, and for short-term use in panic disorder.

antidepressant therapy. Typically, high-potency benzodiazepines such as lorazepam or clonazepam are used for this purpose. Generally, the initial dosages should be low (e.g., 0.25 mg lorazepam every 8 hours or 0.25 mg clonazepam twice daily). Patients should be warned not to drink alcohol or engage in activities such as driving when first using benzodiazepines. Some patients develop a central nervous system toxicity even at low dosages of these drugs, and patients should be vigilant for this adverse effect. Although pharmaceutical manufacturers and the U.S. Food and Drug Administration (FDA) recommend that benzodiazepines be used only on a short-term basis (i.e., days to weeks) (109), approximately 90% of benzodiazepines sold in the United States in 1990 were used by people reporting daily use for 4 months or longer (110). This may be related to reports indicating that long-term benzodiazepine users have difficulty discontinuing medication and use benzodiazepines to avoid withdrawal (111). Because of the risk of tolerance and dependence, clinicians should limit the duration of benzodiazepine use to the minimal period required for adequate relief of acute anxiety symptoms. Usual dosages and pharmacokinetic properties of the various benzodiazepines are displayed in Table 22.9.

In recent years, the popularity of herbal remedies and "natural" dietary supplements has grown significantly (see Chapter 5). A number of these dietary supplements are purported to relieve symptoms of anxiety, including kava-kava, valerian root, and St. John's wort. Although none of these alternative treatments has yet been proved effective by FDA standards, there is growing acceptance that they may be useful for the treatment of anxiety disorders, particularly in less severe cases. Patients often do not view these substances as "medications" and may not report their use to their primary caregiver. Therefore, the primary care physician should inquire about use of herbal dietary supplements, particularly before initiating treatment with pharmaceutical-grade medications. "Natural" herbal supplements can be psychoactive and are often metabolized by pathways similar to those of pharmaceutical medications. Drug interactions (occasionally severe) and additive effects have been reported in patients who simultaneously used prescription drugs and herbal or nonherbal supplements (see Table 5.4 in Chapter 5). Therefore, caution should be exercised in prescribing drugs to patients who are taking supplements. Patients taking kava-kava who are prescribed anxiolytics and patients taking St. John's wort who are prescribed SSRIs should be advised to taper their herbal supplement before initiating treatment with the prescribed medication.

During the next few years, several new agents may become available for the treatment of anxiety disorders. Among these are corticotropin-releasing factor antagonists and substance P antagonists, both of which have shown great promise in preclinical models of anxiety. Several pharmaceutical companies are developing these agents for potential use in anxiety disorders and depression.

General References*

American Psychiatric Association. **Diagnostic and statistical manual of mental disorders**. 4th ed. (DSM-IV). Washington, DC: American Psychiatric Association, 1994.

Diagnostic criteria and epidemiologic information for all recognized psychiatric disorders.

National Institutes of Mental Health (NIMH) website. Available at: http://www.nimh.nih.gov. Accessed December 5, 2001.

Public inquiries may be directed to NIMH, 6001 Executive Boulevard, Rm. 8184 MSC 9663, Bethesda, MD 20892-9663 U.S.A. (voice mail, 301-443-4513; fax, 301-443-4279).

Information on anxiety disorders is available at: http://www.nimh.nih.gov/anxiety/anxiety.cfm. Accessed December 5, 2001.

Relaxation cassettes. A variety of audiocassette programs that provide self-instruction in relaxation techniques.

Available from Guilford Publications, Inc., 72 Spring St., New York, NY 10003, and from New Harbinger Publications, 5674 Shattuck Ave., Oakland, CA 94609.

Specific References

1. Kubzansky LD, Kawachi I, Weiss ST, et al. Anxiety and coronary heart disease: a synthesis of epidemiological, psychological and experimental evidence. Ann Behav Med 1998;20:47.
2. Zaubler TS, Katon W. Panic disorder in the general medical setting. J Psychosom Res 1998;44:25.
3. Mayou R, Williamson B, Foster A. Attitudes and advice after myocardial infarction. BMJ 1976;1:1577.
4. Gorman JM, Kent JM, Sullivan GM, et al. Neuroanatomical hypothesis of panic disorder, revised. Am J Psychiatry 2000;157:493.
5. **5.** Anxiety Disorders. NIH Publication No. 00-3879. Bethesda, MD: National Institutes of Health, 1994. Reprinted 1995, 1997, and 2000.
6. Katon W. Panic disorder: relationship to high medical utilization, unexplained physical symptoms and medical costs. J Clin Psychiatry 1996;57[Suppl 10]:11.
7. Zaubler TS, Katon W. Panic disorder and medical comorbidity: a review of the medical and psychiatric literature. Bull Menninger Clin 1996;2[Suppl A]:A12.
8. Margraff J, Ehlers A, Roth WT. Mitral valve prolapse and panic disorder: a review of their relationship. Psychosom Med 1988;50:93.
9. Shavitt RG, Gentil V, Mandetta R. The association of panic/agoraphobia and asthma: contributing factors and clinical implications. Gen Hospital Psychiatry 1992;14:420.
10. Yellowlees PM, Haynes S, Potts N, et al. Psychiatric morbidity in patients with life-threatening asthma: initial report of a controlled study. Med J Austr 1988;149:246.
11. Spinhoven P, Ros M, Westgeest A, et al. The prevalence of respiratory disorders in panic disorder, major depressive disorder and V-code patients. Behav Res Ther 1994;32:647.
12. Merikangas KR, Angst J, Isler H. Migraine and psychopathology: results of the Zurich cohort study of young adults. Arch Gen Psychiatry 1990;47:849.
13. Breslau N, Davis GC. Migraine, physical health and psychiatric disorder: a prospective epidemiologic study in young adults. J Psychiatric Res 1993;27:211.
14. Regier DA, Rae DS, Narrow WE, et al. Prevalence of anxiety disorders and their comorbidity with mood and addictive disorders. Br J Psychiatry 1998;[Suppl 34]:24.
15. Aronson TA, Logue CM. On the longitudinal course of panic disorder: developmental history and prediction of phobic complications. Compr Psychiatry 1987;28:344.
16. Robins LN, Regier DA, eds. Psychiatric disorders in America: the Epidemiologic Catchment Area Study. New York: The Free Press, 1991.
17. Breier A, Charney DS, Heninger GR. Major depression in patients with agoraphobia and panic disorder. Arch Gen Psychiatry 1984;41:1129.

---

*Bold print (general references) and bold numerals (specific references) denote published controlled clinical trials, meta-analyses, or consensus-based recommendations.

18. Breier A, Charney DS, Heninger GR. The diagnostic validity of anxiety disorders and their relationship to depressive illness. Am J Psychiatry 1985;142:787.
19. Breier A, Charney DS, Heninger GR. Agoraphobia with panic attacks. Arch Gen Psychiatry 1986;43:1029.
20. Bass C, Cawley R, Wade C, et al. Unexplained breathlessness and psychiatric morbidity in patients with normal and abnormal coronary arteries. Lancet 1983;1:605.
21. Coryell W, Noyes R, Clancy J. Excess mortality in panic disorder: a comparison with primary unipolar depression. Arch Gen Psychiatry 1982;39:701.
22. Kawachi I, Colditz GA, Ascherio A, et al. Prospective study of phobic anxiety and risk of coronary heart disease in men. Circulation 1994;89:1992.
23. Kawachi I, Sparrow D, Vokonas PS, et al. Symptoms of anxiety and risk of coronary heart disease: the Normative Aging Study. Circulation 1994;90:2225.
24. Pauls DL, Slymen P. A family study of panic disorders. Arch Gen Psychiatry 1983;40:1065.
25. Torgersen S. Genetic factors in anxiety disorders. Arch Gen Psychiatry 1983;40:1085.
26. Gorman JM, Dillon D, Fyer AJ, et al. The lactate infusion model. Psychopharmacol Bull 1985;21:428.
27. Clark DM, Salkovskis PM, Chalkley AJ. Respiratory control as a treatment for panic attacks. J Behav Ther Exp Psychiatry 1985;16:23.
28. Barlow DH. Behavioral conception and treatment of panic. Psychopharmacol Bull 1986;22:802.
29. Goldstein AJ, Chambless DL. A reanalysis of agoraphobia. Behav Res Ther 1978;9:47.
30. Zohar J, Westenberg HG. Anxiety disorders: a review of tricyclic antidepressants and selective serotonin reuptake inhibitors. Acta Psychiatr Scand 2000;403[Suppl]:39.
31. Oehrberg S, Christiansen PE, Behnke K. Paroxetine in the treatment of panic disorder: a randomized, double-blind, placebo-controlled study. Br J Psychiatry 1995;167:374.
32. Sheehan DV. Current concepts in the treatment of panic disorder. J Clin Psychiatry 1999;60[Suppl 18]:16.
33. Davidson JRT. Long-term treatment of panic disorder. J Clin Psychiatry 1998;49[Suppl 8]:17.
34. Le Crubier Y, Judge R. Long-term evaluation of paroxetine, clomipramine and placebo in panic disorder. Acta Psychiatr Scand 1997;95:153.
35. American Psychiatric Associating. Practice guideline for the treatment of patients with panic disorder. Am J Psychiatry 1998:155[Suppl 5]:1.
36. Gorman JM. The use of newer antidepressants for panic disorder. J Clin Psychiatry 1997;58[Suppl 14]:54.
37. Otto MW, Pollack MH, Maki KM. Empirically supported treatments for panic disorder: costs, benefits, and stepped care. J Consult Clin Psychol 2000;68:556.
38. Myers JK, Weissman MM, Tischler GL, et al. Six-month prevalence of psychiatric disorders in three communities. Arch Gen Psychiatry 1984;41:959.
39. Van Korff M, Shapiro S, Burke JD, et al. Anxiety and depression in a primary care clinic. Arch Gen Psychiatry 1987;44:152.
40. Rasmussen SA, Tsuang MT. Clinical characteristics and family history in DSM-III obsessive-compulsive disorder. Am J Psychiatry 1986;143:317.
41. McKeon J, Roa B, Mann A. Life events and personality traits in obsessive-compulsive neurosis. Br J Psychiatry 1984;144:185.
42. Carey G, Gottesman II. Twin and family studies of anxiety, phobic, and obsessive disorders. In: Klein DF, Rabkin JG, eds. Anxiety: new research and changing concepts. New York: Raven Press, 1981:116.
43. Pauls DL, Towbin KE, Leckman JF, et al. Gilles de la Tourette's syndrome and obsessive-compulsive disorder. Arch Gen Psychiatry 1986;43:1180.
44. McKeon J, McGuffin P, Robinson P. Obsessive-compulsive neurosis following head injury: a report of four cases. Br J Psychiatry 1984;144:190.
45. Grimshaw L. Obsessional disorder and neurological illness. J Neurol Neurosurg Psychiatry 1964;27:229.
46. Saxena S, Brody AL, Schwartz JM, et al. Neuroimaging and frontal-subcortical circuitry in obsessive-compulsive disorder. Br J Psychiatry 1998;173[Suppl 35]:26.
47. Rauch SL. Neuroimaging research and the neurobiology of obsessive-compulsive disorder: where do we go from here? Biol Psychiatry 2000;47:168.
48. Rauch SL, Whalen PJ, Dougherty DD, et al. Neurobiological models of obsessive compulsive disorders. In: Jenike MA, Baer L, Minichiello WE, eds. Obsessive-compulsive disorders: practical management. St. Louis: Mosby, 1998:222.
49. Swedo SE, Leonard HL, Garvey M, et al. Pediatric autoimmune neuropsychiatric disorders associated with streptococcal infections: clinical description of the first 50 cases. Am J Psychiatry 1998;155:263.
50. Insel TR. Toward a neuroanatomy of obsessive-compulsive disorder. Arch Gen Psychiatry 1992;49:739.
51. Stein DD. Neurobiology of the obsessive-compulsive spectrum disorders. Biol Psychiatry 2000;47:296.
52. March JS, Frances A, Carpenter D, et al. The expert consensus guideline series: treatment of obsessive-compulsive disorder. J Clin Psychiatry 1997;58[Suppl 4]:1.
53. Greist JH, Jefferson JW, Kobak KA, et al. Efficacy and tolerability of serotonin transport inhibitors in obsessive-compulsive disorder: a meta-analysis. Arch Gen Psychiatry 1995;52:53.
54. Thoren P, Asberg M, Cronholm B, et al. Clomipramine treatment of obsessive-compulsive disorder: I. A controlled clinical trial. Arch Gen Psychiatry 1980;37:1281.
55. Turner SM, Jacob RG, Beidel DC, et al. Fluoxetine treatment of obsessive-compulsive disorder. J Clin Psychopharmacol 1985;5:201.
56. Rasmussen SA, Eisen JL. Treatment strategies for chronic and refractory obsessive-compulsive disorder. J Clin Psychiatry 1997;58[Suppl 13]:9.
57. Goodman WK. Obsessive-compulsive disorder: diagnosis and treatment. J Clin Psychiatry 1999;60:S27.
58. Vythilingum B, Cartwright C, Hollander E. Pharmacotherapy of obsessive-compulsive disorder: experience with the selective serotonin reuptake inhibitors. Int Clin Psychopharmacol 2000;15[Suppl 2]:S7.
59. Romano S, Goodman W, Tamura R, et al. Long-term treatment of obsessive-compulsive disorder after an acute response: a comparison of fluoxetine versus placebo. J Clin Psychopharmacol 2001;21:46.
60. Kessler RC, McGonagle KA, Zhao S, et al. Lifetime and 12-month prevalence of DSM-III-R psychiatric disorders in the United States: results from the National Comorbidity Survey. Arch Gen Psychiatry 1994;51:8.
61. Barlow DH, Blanchard EB, Vermylyea JA, et al. Generalized anxiety and generalized anxiety disorder: description and reconceptualization. Am J Psychiatry 1986;143:40.
62. Yonkers KA, Warshaw MG, Massion AO, et al. Phenomenology and course of generalized anxiety disorder. Br J Psychiatry 1996;168:308.
63. Brawman-Mintzer O, Lydiard RB. Generalized anxiety disorder: issues in epidemiology. J Clin Psychiatry 1996;57 [Suppl 7]:3.
64. Noyes R Jr, Clarkson C, Crowe R, et al. A family study of generalized anxiety disorder. Am J Psychiatry 1987;144:1019.
65. Skre I, Torgersen S, Lygren S, et al. A twin study of DSM-III-R anxiety disorders. Acta Psychiatr Scand 1993;88:85.
66. Kendler KS. Major depression and generalized anxiety disorder: same genes, (partly) different environments—revisited. Br J Psychiatry 1996;[Suppl 30]:68.
67. Torgersen S. Childhood and family characteristics in panic and generalized anxiety disorders. Am J Psychiatry 1986;143:630.
68. Hoehn-Saric R. Characteristics of chronic anxiety patients. In: Klein DF, Rabkin J, eds. Anxiety: new research and changing concepts. New York: Raven Press, 1981.
69. Blazer D, Hughes D, George LK. Stressful life events and the onset of a generalized anxiety syndrome. Am J Psychiatry 1987;144:1178.
70. Rickels K, Pollack MH, Sheehan DV, et al. Efficacy of extended-release venlafaxine in nondepressed outpatients with generalized anxiety disorder. Am J Psychiatry 2000;157:968.

71. Rocca P, Fonzo V, Scotta M, et al. Paroxetine efficacy in the treatment of generalized anxiety disorder. Acta Psychiatr Scand 1997;95:444.
72. Hedges DW, Reimherr FW, Strong RE, et al. An open trial of nefazadone in adult patients with generalized anxiety disorder. Psychopharmacol Bull 1996;32:671.
73. Hoehn-Saric R, McLeod DR, Zimmerli WD. Differential effects of alprazolam and imipramine in generalized anxiety disorder: somatic versus psychic symptoms. J Clin Psychiatry 1988;49:293.
74. Rickels K, Downing R, Schweizer E, et al. Antidepressants for the treatment of generalized anxiety disorder: a placebo-controlled comparison of imipramine, trazadone, and diazepam. Arch Gen Psychiatry 1993;50:884.
75. Kahn RJ, McNair DM, Lipman RS, et al. Imipramine and chlordiazepoxide in depressive and anxiety disorders. II: Efficacy in anxious outpatients. Arch Gen Psychiatry 1986;43:79.
76. American Psychiatric Association. Benzodiazepines: dependence, toxicity and abuse. A task force report of the American Psychiatry Association. Washington, DC: American Psychiatric Association, 1991.
77. Kessler RC, Stein MB, Berglund P. Social phobia subtypes in the National Comorbidity Survey. Am J Psychiatry 1998;155:613.
78. Curtis GC, Magee WJ, Eaton WW, et al. Specific fears and phobias: epidemiology and classification. Br J Psychiatry 1998;173:212.
79. Magee WJ, Eaton WW, Wittchen HU, et al. Agoraphobia, simple phobia and social phobia in the National Comorbidity Survey. Arch Gen Psychiatry 1996;53:159.
80. Ballenger JC, Davidson JR, Lecrubier Y, et al. Consensus statement on social anxiety disorder from the International Consensus Group on Depression and Anxiety. J Clin Psychiatry 1998;59[Suppl 17]:54.
81. Davidson JRT, Hughes DL, George LK, et al. The epidemiology of social phobia: findings from the Duke Epidemiological Catchment Area Study. Psychol Med 1993;23:709.
82. Haines AP, Imeson JD, Meade TW. Phobic anxiety and ischaemic heart disease. BMJ 1987;295:297.
83. Rasmussen K, Henningsen P. Provocative testing with prolonged hyperventilation and ergometrine in patients suspected of coronary artery spasm: a comparative study. Int J Cardiol 1987;15:151.
84. Lown B. Mental stress, arrhythmias, and sudden death. Am J Med 1982;72:177.
85. Taylor CB, Ferguson JM, Wermuth BM. Simple techniques to treat medical phobias. Postgrad Med J 1977;53:28.
86. Marks I. Fears and phobias. London: Heinemann, 1969.
87. Marks I. Recent results of behavioral treatments of phobias and obsessions. J Intern Med 1977;5[Suppl 5]:15.
88. Van Ameringen MA, Lane RM, Walker JR, et al. Sertraline treatment of generalized social phobia: a 20-week, double-blind, placebo-controlled study. Am J Psychiatry 2001;158:275.
89. van Vliet IM, den Boer JA, Westernberg HG. Psychopharmacological treatment of social phobia: a double blind placebo controlled study with fluvoxamine. Psychopharmacology 1994;115:.
90. Jefferson JW. Benzodiazepines and anticonvulsants for social phobia (social anxiety disorder). J Clin Psychiatry 2001;62[Suppl 1]:50.
91. Altamura AC, Pioli R, Vitto M, et al. Venlafaxine in social phobia: a study in selective serotonin reuptake inhibitor non-responders. Int Clin Psychopharmacol 1999;14:239.
92. Helzer JE, Robins LN, McEvoy L. Post-traumatic stress disorder in the general population: findings of the Epidemiologic Catchment Area Survey. N Engl J Med 1987;317:1630.
93. Acierno R, Resnick H, Kilpatrick D, et al. Risk factors for rape, physical assault, and posttraumatic stress disorder in women: examination of differential multivariate relationships. J Anxiety Disord 1999;13:541.
94. Breslau N, Kessler RC, Chilcoat HD, et al. Trauma and posttraumatic stress disorder in the community: the 1996 Detroit Area Survey of Trauma. Arch Gen Psychiatry 1998;55:626.
95. Kessler RC, Sonnega A, Bromet E, et al. Posttraumatic stress disorder in the National Comorbidity Survey. Arch Gen Psychiatry 1995;52:1048.
96. Kessler RC. Posttraumatic stress disorder: the burden to the individual and to society. J Clin Psychiatry 2000;61[Suppl 5]:4.
97. Kolb LC. A neuropsychological hypothesis explaining posttraumatic stress disorders. Am J Psychiatry 1987;144:989.
98. Ross RJ, Ball WA, Sullivan KA, et al. Sleep disturbance as the hallmark of posttraumatic stress disorder. Am J Psychiatry 1988;146:697.
99. Andreasen NJ, Noyes R, Hartford CE. Factors influencing adjustment of burn patients during hospitalization. Psychosom Med 1972;34:517.
100. Davidson J, Kudler H, Smith R, et al. Treatment of posttraumatic stress disorder with imipramine and placebo. Arch Gen Psychiatry 1990;47:259.
101. Kosten TR, Frank JB, Dan E, et al. Pharmacotherapy for posttraumatic stress disorder using phenelzine or imipramine. J Nerv Ment Dis 1991;179:366.
102. Alarcon RD, Glover S, Boyer W, et al. Proposing an algorithm for the pharmacological management of posttraumatic stress disorder. Ann Clin Psychiatry 2000;12:239.
103. Brannon N, Labbate L, Huber M. Gabapentin treatment for posttraumatic stress disorder. Can J Psychiatry 2000;45:84.
104. Friedman MJ. Toward a rational pharmacotherapy for posttraumatic stress disorder: an interim report. Am J Psychiatry 1988;145:281.
105. Goldberg RJ. Anxiety reduction by self-regulation: theory, practice, and evaluation. Ann Intern Med 1982;96:483.
106. Benson H. The relaxation response. New York: William Morrow, 1976.
107. Gaarder KR, Montgomery PS. Clinical biofeedback: a procedural manual for behavioral medicine. 2nd ed. Baltimore: Williams & Wilkins, 1981.
108. Benson H, Beary JF, Carol MP. The relaxation response. Psychiatry 1974;37:37.
109. National Institutes of Health. Drugs and insomnia: Consensus Development Conference Summary. Bethesda, MD: National Institutes of Health, 1984;4:1.
110. Giffiths RR, Weerts EM. Benzodiazepine self-administration in humans and laboratory animals: implications for problems of long-term use and abuse. Psychopharmacology 1997;134:1.
111. Romach M, Busto U, Somer G, et al. Clinical aspects of chronic use of alprazolam and lorazepam. Am J Psychiatry 1995;152:1161.

CHAPTER 23

Personality and Personality Disorders

ROBERT P. ROCA, MD, MPH

CONCEPT OF PERSONALITY AND PERSONALITY DISORDER

Definition and Methods of Classification

The enduring attitudes, behaviors, and capacities that distinguish individuals from each other are collectively called personality. Personality is commonly conceptualized categorically or dimensionally.

Categoric approaches specify personality *types* and classify individuals according to the type they most closely resemble. The ancient Greek topology of personality (phlegmatic, melancholic, sanguine, and choleric) was of this sort, and the American Psychiatric Association uses this approach in the classification of personality disorders published in the most recent *Diagnostic and Statistical Manual of Mental Disorders* (DSM-IV) (see later discussion).

Dimensional approaches view personality as a mosaic of *traits,* each possessed by individuals in differing degrees (1). Intelligence, as defined by the *intelligence quotient* (IQ), is a model of such a trait. IQ scores are normally distributed in the population and are highly correlated with academic and occupational achievement. People with above-average IQ scores tend to be successful in school and work, whereas those with below-average IQs often have difficulty meeting the demands of daily life independently. Knowledge of a person's position on the dimension of intelligence thus illuminates strengths and vulnerabilities and allows one to predict circumstances that the person might find overwhelming.

Case Study

A 30-year-old man was admitted to the hospital for cellulitis of the feet. His physician discovered that he had only completed the third grade and that he was unable to read, write, or calculate. Further investigation disclosed that he had recently lost his job in a laundromat and that he had been observed walking barefoot in a dumpster looking for items he needed. His physician explained to him, carefully and repeatedly, the relationship between his infection and his behavior. A social worker was called to help him apply for financial assistance and other entitlements.

Dimensions can be converted into categories, sometimes with misleading consequences. "Mental retardation," for example, is said to be present when the IQ is lower than 70. By this definition, a man with an IQ of 68 is categorized as mentally retarded but one with an IQ of 72 is not, despite the fact that their risk of intelligence-related difficulty is essentially identical. A categoric approach may thus obscure clinically important vulnerability.

Although IQ is by far the best-studied dimension of personality, other personality traits may also be described dimensionally. We use dimensional thinking intuitively when we recognize that some people are more meticulous, more gregarious, or more ambitious than others. Psychologists use this approach technically when they administer standardized tests to describe quantitatively how introverted or neurotic someone is. At some arbitrary point, the meticulous person may be categorized as obsessional or the introverted person as schizoid and thus be said to have a personality disorder; however, it is useful to recognize that certain patients are more meticulous or more introverted than others even when they are not categorically obsessional or schizoid. A dimensional view facilitates the recognition of such traits and prepares the physician to take these attributes into account when dealing with patients.

Development of Personality

Personality evolves out of interactions between constitutional, or inborn, factors and the molding influences of the environment. *Constitutional factors* include capacities, such as intelligence, and aspects of temperament, such as sociability and emotionality, all of which may have neurobiologic correlates and genetic determinants (2). The most important *environmental influences* are interpersonal relationships, particularly with parents. Many theories have been offered to account more specifically for personality development, but none has yet proved fully adequate (3).

Conceptualization of Personality Disorder

Personality disorders are among the most controversial conditions in psychiatry. There is no doubt that some people have enduring patterns of maladaptive attitudes and behaviors that interfere with their ability to work effectively and to develop and sustain gratifying interpersonal relationships. It is also clear that such people are at increased risk for long-term social impairment and for many major psychiatric illnesses (4,5). The controversy lies in how best to conceptualize and subdivide these disorders. This chapter describes three such conceptualizations.

The dominant approach in the United States—that adopted by the American Psychiatric Association in DSM-IV—is prototypical and categoric. In this scheme, the *diagnostic criteria* for the personality disorders are lists of attitudes and behaviors (e.g., self-dramatization) that, in combination, evoke an ideal prototype (e.g., the histrionic personality). Only a person exhibiting the requisite number of such attitudes and behaviors (e.g., at least five of eight, in the case of histrionic personality disorder) is said to have the condition. Personality disorders are relatively uncommon when defined in this way.

Maladaptive personalities can also be conceptualized in terms of quantitative deviations from normal along specific personality dimensions. As mentioned earlier, many clinically important personality traits can be viewed dimensionally, for example, in terms of meticulousness, dependence, or self-confidence. Extreme deviations from "normal" along any of these dimensions may produce special vulnerability, particularly under certain circumstances. For example, excessive meticulousness may lead to great distress when the environment is out of order and out of one's control, and poor self-confidence may predispose one to demoralization in response to criticism from a superior. These examples illustrate that dimensional thinking about personality disturbances calls for consideration of the environmental stresses that play on the vulnerability as well as the trait-based vulnerability itself. Because there are many relevant dimensions, this approach illuminates areas of potential vulnerability in many patients.

Finally, personality disorders may be viewed as incomplete or atypical expressions of schizophrenia, mood disorders, or other major psychiatric illnesses.

Subtyping of Personality Disorder

The DSM-IV describes ten types of personality disorders and groups them into *three clusters:* the dramatic (histrionic, borderline, narcissistic, and antisocial types), the anxious or fearful (obsessive-compulsive, dependent, and avoidant types), and the odd or eccentric (schizoid, schizotypal, and paranoid types) clusters. In the descriptions of the categoric disorders that follow in this chapter, it is clear that many of the disorders may be viewed as manifestations of extreme positions on dimensions of personality such as emotionality, narcissism, trust, sociability, self-esteem, and assertiveness. It is also seen that the types within each cluster tend to share traits and vulnerabilities and, therefore, implications for management. A few disorders are linked to major psychiatric illnesses. It is important to emphasize that a patient with clinically obvious disturbances involving dimensions of personality may meet criteria for several DSM-IV personality disorders or may meet criteria for none.

Personality disorders are axis II diagnoses in the multiaxial assessment system that is recommended in DSM-IV. The estimated population prevalence and sex ratios for the major personality disorders are shown in Table 23.1.

Table 23.1. Estimated Prevalence and Sex Ratios of the Major Personality Disorders

Personality Disorder	Prevalence (General Population)	Sex Ratio
Dramatic cluster		
Histrionic	2%–3%	F > M
Narcissistic	<1%	?
Borderline	1%–2%	F > M
Antisocial	1%–3%	M(~3%) > F(1%)
Anxious cluster		
Avoidant	0.5%–1%	F = M
Dependent	Common	F > M
Obsessive Compulsive	1%	M > F
Passive Aggressive	?	?
Odd/Eccentric cluster		
Paranoid	0.5%–2.5%	M > F
Schizotyped	3%	M > F
Schizoid	Uncommon	M > F

Adapted from Diagnostic and statistical manual of mental disorders. 4th ed. Washington, DC: American Psychiatric Association, 1994.

GENERAL APPROACH TO MANAGEMENT OF PERSONALITY TRAITS AND DISORDERS

Several points are useful to bear in mind when dealing with patients with maladaptive traits or frank personality disorders of any subtype:

Because the patient's maladaptive trait or traits are well established and deeply ingrained, it is doubtful that they will change in response to the physician's efforts. An exception to this rule is when particular aspects of temperament (e.g., harm avoidance) change in response to pharmacologic treatment of concurrent mood disorders that are making these traits more prominent (6). Otherwise, the general approach to primary care management of personality disorders is to recognize these sources of vulnerability, take them into account when interacting with the patient, and minimize their adverse impact on the provision of medical care.

Patients often become angry or depressed when their maladaptive traits are pointed out to them, and these responses defeat the physician's purposes. Yet it is often important to call patients' attention to ways in which they are undermining their medical care. When such action is necessary, it is helpful to refer to specific behaviors rather than to aspects of personality and to present one's observations plainly but compassionately and without criticism (e.g., "It is difficult for us to provide you with the care you need when you curse at us and criticize every effort we make.").

In general, counseling by the general physician, if undertaken at all, is best when it is symptom-focused and short-term (see Chapter 20). For long-term treatment, patients with seriously disturbed personalities should be referred to a mental health professional.

DRAMATIC CLUSTER

Patients with personality disturbances in this cluster tend to occupy extreme positions on the dimensions of emotionality and self-esteem. They are intensely emotional, sometimes acting impulsively, aggressively, or self-destructively. They are also self-absorbed, lacking in empathy for others, and extreme (unrealistically high or low) in their self-regard. They tend to be demanding of others, and their relationships are unstable, tempestuous, and exploitive, qualities that may characterize their interactions with physicians and complicate the provision of medical care.

Histrionic Personality

The essence of the histrionic type *is excessive emotionality, self-dramatization, and attention-seeking.* Patients meeting criteria for the categoric disorder are self-centered, unusually eager for approval and praise, overly concerned with physical attractiveness, and often inappropriately sexually seductive or flattering ("Of all the doctors I've had, you are the first to really listen to me"). Their style of speech is dramatic, impressionistic, and factually imprecise, and their expression of emotions is often exaggerated, rapidly shifting, and apparently shallow. They may manifest an unusually warm and sometimes seductive manner with the physician and present to the office with complaints that are dramatically expressed but vague in medically relevant detail. Histrionic patients may be especially inclined to develop somatization disorder (see Chapter 21).

Narcissistic Personality

The narcissistic personality type is characterized by *an exaggerated sense of self-importance,* intolerance of criticism, and insensitivity to the needs of others. Narcissistic people may exploit others for their own ends, require constant admiration and attention, believe themselves entitled to special treatment, and envy those who are more successful, attractive, intelligent, or otherwise praiseworthy. Such patients are often difficult to care for because they tend to believe that their problems are unique and can be solved only by remarkable physicians. They may challenge the doctor's knowledge, skill, and judgment and expect that their convenience will be the prime consideration in the scheduling of tests and appointments.

Borderline Personality

Extreme instability—in mood, identity, interpersonal relationships, and self-regard—is the essence of the borderline personality. Although this condition was once believed to lie on the "border" of schizophrenia, recent data more strongly support a link with affective disorders. Substance abuse, sexual impulsiveness, poor self-esteem, self-mutilation, recurrent (often manipulative) suicidal threats, and brief bouts of intense depression and rage, superimposed on chronic feelings of emptiness or boredom, characterize the long-term functioning of these patients. A shifting tendency to view other people as all good or all bad and to react to them with extremes of idealization or devaluation creates difficulties in all interpersonal relationships, including those with physicians and other caretakers, who are seen as either good or bad and are pitted against one another (staff splitting).

Antisocial Personality

The antisocial personality type is characterized by a chronic and *pervasive pattern of irresponsible and socially unacceptable behavior.* Truancy, vandalism, fire setting, lying, and theft in childhood give way to impulsiveness, recklessness, aggressiveness, sexual promiscuity, financial irresponsibility, and outright criminality in adulthood. Often complaining of mistreatment themselves, they shamelessly exploit others in their relationships. In medical settings they may be malingerers (see Chapter 21), consciously feigning disease for obvious gain; and in their dealings with medical staff they may be either demanding and abusive or flattering and ingratiating, depending on which approach they perceive to be most expedient.

Management of Dramatic Subtypes

When dealing with dramatic patients one can expect a show of emotional extremes and pressure to bestow emotional and material favors as well as medical care. It is helpful to maintain equanimity in the face of the patient's emotional excesses, to avoid defensiveness when challenged, and to give special attention to professional boundaries. Socializing or becoming unusually familiar with histrionic or borderline patients is particularly risky. Because patients with these traits lack empathy and exploit others, it is often necessary to spell out, firmly but nonpunitively, the limits of acceptable behavior with medical staff, nurses, and other members of the health care team; such limit-setting is most often needed with narcissistic and antisocial patients.

ANXIOUS OR FEARFUL CLUSTER

Patients with personality disturbances in this cluster tend to be self-doubting, timid, and tense. Lacking confidence in themselves, they may seek to avoid making decisions or taking on responsibility, preferring to have others decide or perform for them; however, they are often dissatisfied with and critical of the efforts of others. They tend to be socially unassertive, submitting to the wishes of others and even avoiding friendships in the first place for fear of ultimate rejection. Levels of generalized anxiety are chronically high.

Avoidant Personality

The avoidant person *craves social contact but avoids it* because of intense social discomfort related to expectations of criticism and rejection. These people often complain of loneliness, but they are too shy to make the social contacts required to solve the problem unless they are certain of acceptance. Major depression and social phobia commonly occur. Because physicians are generally viewed as accepting of their patients, avoidant people may feel particularly comfortable in the presence of their doctors and may develop symptoms justifying regular visits to alleviate their loneliness.

Dependent Personality

Dependent people *lack self-confidence and go to great lengths to ensure the availability of others* on whom they can depend for advice and reassurance. Because they feel uneasy and helpless when alone, they may endure abuse and perform unpleasant or demeaning tasks to preserve the dependent relationship. They are exceedingly sensitive to criticism and abandonment. Patients of this type may become quite dependent on their physicians, particularly when other relationships are unsatisfactory, and may use vague, chronic complaints as a means of remaining in close touch, especially in times of stress. Such patients may also become ill before a period of planned unavailability on the part of the physician (e.g., a vacation).

Obsessive-Compulsive Personality

People with obsessive-compulsive personalities are *rigid, parsimonious, morally scrupulous, and emotionally constricted.* Exceedingly committed to work, they are reluctant to delegate duties, convinced that no one else can do things correctly, yet they are also indecisive and at times are rendered ineffective by perfectionism or preoccupation with trivial details. They tend to describe upsetting emotional experiences in a cool, detached manner (isolation of affect). When ill, they often present their physicians with extremely detailed accounts of their symptoms and request lengthy explanations of their disease and its treatment, including very precise instructions about medication use and likely side effects. They are usually aware of hospital rules and routines and are intolerant of lateness and inefficiency. People with obsessive-compulsive personalities may be especially prone to developing hypochondriasis (see Chapter 21) and obsessive-compulsive disorder, a condition characterized by recurrent, resisted thoughts and repetitive, senseless actions (see Chapter 22).

Passive-Aggressive Personality

Although not listed in DSM-IV, passive-aggressive personality disorder warrants brief mention because of its potential impact on the provision of medical care. Passive-aggressive people *do not want to meet the expectations of others but do not want to be held responsible for this decision.* Thus they do not say "no" directly but express hostile resistance in terms of procrastination, intentional inefficiency, and feigned forgetfulness. Usually dependent and lacking in self-confidence, they seek the counsel of others, yet often paradoxically resist following the advice of those whom they consult. In medical settings they insist that they intend to comply with treatment recommendations but then, for example, forget to keep a symptom log required to assess the effectiveness of a new treatment or forget to make it to the laboratory for an important blood test.

Management of Anxious Subtypes

The general guidelines described previously are applicable. Because patients with these types of personality traits tend to develop anxious attachment to their physicians, the management of dependency is a central issue. It may be necessary to allow patients to be excessively dependent, within manageable bounds, during times of unusual stress. It may be helpful to give them regular, brief appointments so that they do not need to develop new symptomatic complaints to gain access to attention (see Chapter 21), and it may be useful to advise them to call weekly at a specified time to provide updates on their status; this may preempt emergency calls at less convenient times. Such patients also generally benefit from advance notice about vacations and may appreciate meeting the covering physician ahead of time. Treatment for generalized anxiety disorder, phobias, and major depression may be indicated in selected cases (see Chapters 22 and 24).

ODD OR ECCENTRIC CLUSTER

Patients with disorders in this cluster occupy extreme positions on the dimensions of trust and sociability. They tend to be highly suspicious and to isolate themselves from other people due to anxious mistrust, awkwardness, or indifference.

Paranoid Personality

Patients with paranoid personalities *tend to perceive threats and insults at every turn.* Expecting to be exploited or harmed by others, they hear veiled threats in neutral remarks and readily question the loyalty of friends and the fidelity of spouses. They are guarded, easily slighted, defensive, and unforgiving. Although their suspiciousness does not carry the intensity or conviction of a true delusion, they have family histories of schizophrenia and delusional disorders more often than other people (2). In medical settings these patients may be reluctant to provide a complete history, especially a social history ("What does this have to do with my medical problem?") and may balk at undergoing laboratory tests ("You doctors are just trying to make money off me").

Schizotypal Personality

People with schizotypal personality type exhibit odd behavior, *have peculiar beliefs, and suffer social isolation*—as a result of their own social anxiety as well as the impact of their beliefs and behavior on others. Their affect is often constricted, their talk vague and digressive, and their appearance unkempt. They tend to be suspicious and superstitious. People with this disorder are generally severely impaired, often meeting criteria for other personality disorders simultaneously (5). There are family links with schizophrenia (7,8), and there is evidence that this disorder should be viewed as belonging to the "schizophrenia spectrum" (7). Schizotypal patients may be guarded and suspicious in medical settings but may also present to physicians with unusual symptoms (e.g., "feelings of electricity in my scalp") or idiosyncratic theories of causation ("Could my neighbors be doing this to me?").

Schizoid Personality

The essential features of the schizoid personality are *indifference to the company of others and constricted emotionality.* These people are loners who seldom marry, prefer solitary activities, and appear cold and aloof. Despite its name, this disorder does not appear to be closely linked to schizophrenia. Schizoid people tend to shun contact with physicians and may appear very uncomfortable when hospitalization thrusts them into close and constant proximity to others.

Management of Eccentric Subtypes

The general guidelines described previously apply here as well. The most important specific principle of management is to work gradually toward the establishment of rapport by meticulous honesty, composure in the face of the patient's suspiciousness and reserve, and a consistent demonstration of sincere concern for the patient's well-being and respect for his or her privacy.

General References*

American Psychiatric Association. **Diagnostic and statistical manual of mental disorders.** 4th ed. (DSM-IV). Washington, DC: American Psychiatric Association, 1994.

Diagnostic criteria and epidemiologic information for all recognized psychiatric disorders.

Specific References

1. McHugh PR, Slavney PR. The perspectives of psychiatry. 2nd ed. Baltimore: Johns Hopkins University Press, 1998.
2. Rutter M. Temperament, personality, and personality disorder. Br J Psychiatry 1987;150:443.
3. Herbst JH, Zonderman AB, McCrae RR, et al. Do the dimensions of the Temperament and Character Inventory map a simple genetic architecture? Evidence from molecular genetics and factor analysis. Am J Psychiatry 2000;157:1285.
4. Rutter M, Quinton D. Parental psychiatric disorder: effects on children. Psychol Med 1984;14:853.
5. Zimmerman M, Coryell W. DSM-III personality disorder diagnoses in a nonpatient sample. Arch Gen Psychiatry 1989;46:682.
6. Hellerstein DJ, Kocsis JH, Chapman D, et al. Double-blind comparison of sertraline, imipramine, and placebo in treatment of dysthymia: effects on personality. Am J Psychiatry 2000;157:1436.
7. Cadenhead KS, Light GA, Geyer MA, et al. Sensory gating deficits assessed by the P50 event-related potential in subjects with schizotypal personality disorder. Am J Psychiatry 2000;157:55.
8. Kendler KS, Gruenberg AM, Strauss JS. An independent analysis of the Danish adoption study of schizophrenia. II. Arch Gen Psychiatry 1981;38:982.

*Bold print (general references) and bold numerals (specific references) denote published controlled clinical trials, meta-analyses, or consensus-based recommendations.

CHAPTER 24

Affective Disorders

FRANCIS MARK MONDIMORE, MD
J. RAYMOND DEPAULO, Jr., MD

Clinically significant depressions often go undetected and undiagnosed in the ambulatory medical setting (1). As a consequence, many depressed patients remain untreated for depression but receive costly and misdirected diagnostic procedures and symptomatic therapies (2). Undiagnosed depressions exact an even bigger toll on patients and families in the form of severe and persistent functional impairments (3). This chapter outlines the public health consequences of depressive conditions, describes the spectrum of mood disorders that afflict patients, and provides an approach to the treatment of these patients by the generalist.

PUBLIC HEALTH IMPACT OF AFFECTIVE DISORDERS

By any measurement, depressive conditions are major public health problems. In a medical outcome study of community-dwelling people, the *poor functioning uniquely associated with depressive symptoms* was comparable to or worse than that uniquely associated with eight major chronic medical conditions (4). The eight conditions compared to depressive symptoms were current arthritis, current advanced coronary artery disease (recent myocardial infarction), current angina, current back problems, current severe lung problems, current gastrointestinal disorders (ulcers or inflammatory bowel disorders), diabetes, and hypertension. The depressed subjects ranked fourth in impairment in physical functioning, third in impairment in role functioning, second (behind advanced coronary disease) in the number of bed days, and worst of all in social functioning and in their sense of well-being about their current health.

Excess deaths attributed to depression are primarily from suicides. Studies of populations of depressed patients show that 15% eventually die by suicide (5). Suicide was the eighth leading cause of death in the United States in 1998, and the third leading cause of death among 19- to 24-year-olds. In this group, illicit substance abuse is a powerful factor thought to account for the recent increase in adolescent suicide (rates increased almost five-fold between the mid-1950s and the mid-1980s among white male adolescents). In the Old Order Amish population, where there is very little if any drug and alcohol abuse, more than 90% of all suicides between 1880 and 1980 were by people with major depression or bipolar disorder (6). It was also observed that these suicides clustered in families who had multiple family members with major depression and bipolar disorder.

Several studies have shown that the *incidence and outcome of other medical disorders are affected adversely by depression.* For example, the incidence of myocardial infarction is increased about fourfold in subjects with a prior episode of major depression (7). The odds of dying in the 18 months after a myocardial infarction are three times greater in patients with concurrent depression than in those without depression (8).

In economic terms, the most recent and systematic study (9) estimated that the annual cost of depressive disorders to the U.S. economy was $44 billion, substantially higher than the estimated annual cost of stroke ($18 billion), about the same as the estimated annual cost of coronary artery disease ($44 billion), and slightly less than half of the estimated annual cost of all cancers ($104 billion) (10).

BEREAVEMENT AND ADJUSTMENT DISORDERS

Some mood disturbances are the normal and expected, perhaps even inevitable sequelae of personal, medical, or financial setbacks. It is important and appropriate to evaluate and help patients in these situations (i.e., those with bereavement or adjustment disorders), not only because they affect the patient's sense of well-being but also because patients with these nonpathologic mood disturbances are at risk for development of significant medical conditions. Bereavement, for example, is associated with increased rates of medical visits, heart attacks, and death in the first year after the loss of a spouse (11). Various medical conditions have been noted to have poor medical outcomes in patients with mild depression (i.e., an adjustment disorder that does not meet criteria for a major depressive disorder) (12).

Bereavement or Grief Reactions

Although grief reactions are individual in their content, they share a number of characteristic features. Their intensity tends to reflect the bereaved person's closeness to the deceased. The reaction tends to proceed in phases, beginning at the time at which the death is made known. The *first phase* is called the numbness or shock phase. Although painful, this first period of about 1 week is remarkable for the organized or calm way in which many bereaved people appear to go through the societal rituals of mourning, funeral, burial, and the visits with close family and friends. In retrospect, patients describe themselves as confused and not fully appreciating their loss during this first week. A *second phase* emerges after completion of the structured rituals of mourning with increasingly intense feelings of sadness, loneliness, and pining for the lost loved one. Wellings of grief, intense feelings of loss that come in waves, initially may be as relentless as ocean surges but they usually begin to come less frequently over a period of several weeks. The waves then progressively and substantially diminish in frequency and intensity over a period of 6 to 12 months, but they may recur from time to time for years, perhaps for a lifetime, especially when reminders of the loved one are encountered. As the wellings of grief diminish in frequency, a *third phase* emerges as the bereaved person returns to his or her normal daily activities such as work, school, and social activities. Apathy, a diminished sense of organization, disinterest in doing a job that was previously engaging, and an inability to enjoy things are the characteristic signs of this period. The feelings of apathy and disengagement usually remit slowly and incrementally over many months as they are replaced by a sense of re-engagement in old and new activities.

Patients may seek out or be brought to primary care clinicians during any of the three phases of bereavement. In the early stages, it is usually because of sleeplessness or agitation. Validating the reasons for distress, normalizing and explaining the grieving process, and instructing family members on how to help are useful responses. Prescribing small amounts of hypnotic or anxiolytic medications may sometimes be necessary. Patients may come on their own during the later phases of grief because they are concerned about their physical health or about persistent problems in functioning at work or at home. These patients benefit from reassurance and from explanations of the phenomenology of the normal bereavement process, emphasizing that 12 months is usually necessary for the substantial completion of "grief work."

The bereavement process may be more lengthy, complex, and difficult if the loss has been totally unexpected, and especially if the death has been violent or the result of a crime. Referral to a grief counselor is often appropriate in such cases. The death of a child is especially difficult. Local chapters of a national organization, *The Compassionate Friends,* provide grief counseling for families who have experienced the death of a child. Local hospices also often have grief counselors on staff or can be a source of referrals.

It is crucial to remember that major depression is often precipitated by the loss of a loved one in susceptible patients. This becomes apparent in the third phase of bereavement when persistent mood symptoms can give way to the full-blown depressive syndrome (see later discussion for differential diagnostic pointers.) Chapter 13 contains additional information about the experience of the family members of dying and deceased patients.

Adjustment Disorder with Depressed Mood

Adjustment disorder with depressed mood is a normal or an exaggerated emotional reaction to a loss or stressful life event that has just occurred or is imminent. Table 24.1 shows the criteria for the diagnosis of adjustment disorder from the *Diagnostic and Statistical Manual of Mental Disorders,* 4th edition (DSM-IV), published by the American Psychiatric Association (APA). The diagnosis of adjustment disorder is usually straightforward and depends on identifying the link between emotional or behavioral symptoms and the precipitating stressors.

The critical and sometimes difficult diagnostic task is the assessment of individuals who present with

Table 24.1. Diagnostic Criteria for Adjustment Disorder

A. The development of emotional or behavioral symptoms in response to an identifiable stressor occurring within 3 months after the onset of the stressor.
B. These symptoms or behaviors are clinically significant as evidenced by either of the following:
   1. Marked distress that is in excess of what would be expected from exposure to the stressor
   2. Significant impairment in social or occupational (academic) functioning
C. The stress-related disturbance does not meet the criteria for any specific axis I disorder and is not merely an exacerbation of a preexisting axis I or axis II disorder.[a]
D. Does not represent bereavement.
E. The symptoms do not persist for more than 6 months after the termination of the stressor (or its consequences).

Acute: if the symptoms have persisted for less than 6 months
Chronic: if the symptoms have persisted for 6 months or longer

[a]See Chapter 19 for definition of axis I and axis II disorders.

Reprinted with permission from Diagnostic and statistical manual of mental disorders. 4th ed. Washington, DC: American Psychiatric Association, 1994.

what seem like unexpected, exaggerated, or prolonged emotional reactions to stressful events. Patients with any form of depression and those with personality disorders are more likely to overreact or to become functionally impaired in the face of a significant stressor. The identification of axis I disorders (e.g., major depression) or of personality disorders becomes a priority in these cases.

Major depressive disorders regularly manifest in the context of an apparent adjustment disorder. Although at the time of presentation the patient's distress is often focused on the stressor, and the doctor needs to help the patient adapt to the stressor, this empathic task is distinct from the diagnostic task of identifying a major depression.

If the history does not suggest a coexisting axis I or II disorder, the appropriate intervention is very similar to the approaches described earlier in this chapter for bereaved patients and to those described in Chapter 20.

EVALUATION OF PATIENTS WITH DEPRESSIVE SYMPTOMS

Depressed patients who seek medical attention usually do not complain of depressed mood as a primary symptom. If they acknowledge depressed feelings, they usually do so in relation to other complaints, which they see as primary. They usually present to generalists with three types of general complaints: (a) vegetative symptoms of depression (loss of energy, inability to concentrate, poor sleep, poor appetite, weight loss, decreased motivation or interests) and autonomic anxiety symptoms (tachycardia, chest discomfort, light-headedness); (b) aches and pains that may have anatomic bases but are out of proportion to what the patient usually experiences (e.g., worsening of migraine headaches, irritable bowel, or back pains) or what is expected (e.g., postsurgical pain that continues to require narcotic analgesics a month after surgery); and (c) nervous complaints such as increased tension and feelings of anxiety, often expressed in relation to stressful life circumstances such as marital distress or job difficulty (13). The presence of a mood disturbance does not explain or invalidate physical complaints. The coexistence of psychiatric and medical disorders is the rule rather than the exception.

Even when they are specifically asked about mood, almost half of depressed patients deny depression or sadness as their predominant mood. They may describe their predominant mood as apathetic (e.g., "blah"), anxious, or even "numb" (i.e., unable to experience normal emotions including sadness, love, and grief). If appropriate inquiries are made, however, it is likely that the classic features of depression will emerge. Changes in mood (sadness, anger), mental sluggishness, decreased physical energy, pessimistic feelings about the future, and negative self-attitude are features central to depressive disorders. Despite the difficulty describing these pathologic states, patients should be asked specifically about them as well as about their sleep, appetite, and libido.

The term *atypical depression* appears in the DSM-IV and refers to depressive states in which hypersomnia, overeating, and lethargy are seen more often than insomnia, anorexia, and psychomotor agitation. These patients seem particularly prone to panic-type anxiety symptoms. Patients with atypical depression have the characteristic depressive changes in self-attitude and vital sense, but they often describe their mood as fatigued rather than as sad. The term *atypical* may not be strictly justified, because all three of the "atypical" symptoms are common among depressed patients. However, the concept of atypical depression serves to remind clinicians of the importance of surveying *both* sides of eating and sleeping behavior. When asked, "How is your appetite?" a depressed patient may respond, "Good," or "Too good," or "No problem." It easy to misinterpret these answers as negative screening responses rather than as clues to overeating associated with depression.

Family members, if available, should be asked to corroborate and augment the information obtained from the patient. With the patient's agreement, the physician also should share with the family the diagnostic assessment, the plans for treatment, and the prognosis. The depressed patient is usually be hard pressed to remember what was said and tends to interpret everything negatively (see Counseling the Family).

DYSTHYMIC DISORDER

Dysthymia is a chronic depressive state (lasting 2 years or longer) in which the number of depressive symptoms experienced is fewer than what is required for the diagnosis of major depressive disorder (Tables 24.2 and 24.3). It has a point prevalence of approximately 3%. The dysthymic state is associated with marked impairment in social functioning, especially in close personal relationships. Dysthymia not infrequently begins in childhood and, because the low mood is so persistent, these patients, their family and friends, and their doctors often judge the problem to be an innate part of a chronically unhappy person's disposition (i.e., a personality disorder). In reality, the unhappy disposition of dysthymic patients depends to a large degree on treatable depression (14).

Diagnosis

Although each patient's sense of what is normal determines why one patient complains to the doctor and another does not, when depressive symptoms cause suffering or interfere with normal functioning they become a disorder warranting detection and intervention. Even milder forms of depression cause serious functional impairments that are as severe as those of chronic medical conditions such as ulcerative colitis or rheumatoid arthritis (4).

Presenting or complicating problems associated with depressed mood in dysthymic patients include suicide attempts or self-injurious behavior (usually

Table 24.2. American Psychiatric Association Diagnostic Criteria for Dysthymic Disorder[a]

A. Depressed mood for most of the day, for more days than not, as indicated either by subjective account or observation made by others, for at least 2 years.
B. Presence, while depressed, of at least three of the following:
   1. Low self-esteem or self-confidence, or feelings of inadequacy
   2. Feelings of pessimism, despair, or hopelessness
   3. Generalized loss of interest or pleasure
   4. Social withdrawal
   5. Chronic fatigue or tiredness
   6. Feelings of guilt, brooding about the past
   7. Subjective feelings of irritability or excessive anger
   8. Decreased activity, effectiveness or productivity
   9. Difficulty in thinking reflected by poor concentration, poor memory, or indecisiveness
C. During the 2-year period of the disturbance, the person has never been without the symptoms in criteria A and B for more than 2 months at a time.
D. No major depressive episode during the first 2 years of the disturbance, that is, not better accounted for by chronic major depressive disorder, or major depressive disorder in partial remission.
E. Has never had a manic episode, or an unequivocal hypomanic episode.
F. Does not occur exclusively during the course of a chronic psychotic disorder, such as schizophrenia or delusional disorder.
G. Not due to the direct effects of a substance (e.g., drugs of abuse, medication) or a general medical condition (e.g., hypothyroidism).

[a]Criteria for children have been omitted from this table.

Reprinted with permission from Diagnostic and statistical manual of mental disorders. 4th ed. Washington, DC: American Psychiatric Association, 1994.

nonfatal but often requiring heroic medical interventions to prevent a fatal outcome); multiple medical complaints and excessive medical care-seeking behavior or abnormal illness behavior (see Chapter 21); serious diagnosable medical disorders; alcohol and drug abuse (see Chapters 28 and 29); family and marital discord; and job difficulties.

Patients with dysthymic disorder usually have the characteristic sustained changes in self-attitude and vital sense seen with major depression (see later discussion). However, these symptoms appear much less prominent, probably because of the chronicity of dysthymia. Hypersomnia, difficulty in getting up, increased appetite and weight gain, and loss of energy and libido are common, as are anxiety symptoms.

Table 24.2 shows the criteria of the APA for making the diagnosis of dysthymic disorder.

Treatment

Since studies have revealed greater similarities between patients with dysthymia and those with major depression, the treatment of dysthymia has increasingly resembled the treatment of major depressive episodes.

Several selective serotonin reuptake inhibitors and tricyclic antidepressants (see later discussion) have been shown to be effective in reducing depressive symptoms (15). In addition, brief psychotherapies are also known to be helpful (see Chapter 20). The major differences in treatment for the two types of depression relate to the increased rate of comorbid behavior, personality, and life problems associated with the more chronic form of depression (dysthymia).

Recognizing that depression plays an important part in their life problems can be helpful for dysthymic patients. However, appreciating the difference between accepting medical regimens to treat mood disorders and making the effort required to overcome maladaptive behavior patterns is equally important.

Prognosis

In contrast to the major affective syndromes, prognosis in dysthymic disorders is more problematic. The disorder typically continues beyond a 2-year period, and the time to remission cannot be estimated with much confidence. There is a high rate of superimposed major depressive episodes among dysthymic patients (so-called "double depression"), and these patients tend to respond well to antidepressants. Poor outcomes are most common among patients with severe social maladjustments and personality disorders (see Chapter 23).

Table 24.3. American Psychiatric Association Diagnostic Criteria for Major Depressive Episode[a]

A. At least five of the following symptoms have been present during the same 2-week period and represent a change from previous functioning; at least one of the symptoms is either (1) depressed mood or (2) loss of interest or pleasure.
   1. Depressed mood most of the day, nearly every day, as indicated by either subjective report (e.g., feels sad or empty) or observation made by others (e.g., appears tearful)
   2. Marked diminished interest or pleasure in all, or almost all, activities most of the day, nearly every day (as indicated either by subjective account or observation made by others)
   3. Significant weight loss or weight gain when not dieting (e.g., more than 5% of body weight in a month), or decrease or increase in appetite nearly every day
   4. Insomnia or hypersomnia nearly every day
   5. Psychomotor agitation or retardation nearly every day (observable by others, not merely subjective feelings of restlessness or being slowed down)
   6. Fatigue or loss of energy nearly every day
   7. Feelings of worthlessness or excessive or inappropriate guilt (which may be delusional) nearly every day (not merely self-reproach or guilt about being sick)
   8. Diminished ability to think or concentrate, or indecisiveness, nearly every day (either by subjective account or as observed by others)
   9. Recurrent thoughts of death (not just fear of dying), recurrent suicidal ideation without a specific plan, or a suicide attempt or a specific plan for committing suicide
B. The symptoms cause clinically significant distress or impairment in social, occupational, or other important areas of functioning.
C. Not due to the direct effects of a substance (e.g., drugs of abuse, medication) or a general medical condition (e.g., hypothyroidism).
D. Not occurring within 2 months of the loss of a loved one (except if associated with marked functional impairment, morbid preoccupation with worthlessness, suicidal ideation, psychotic symptoms, or psychomotor retardation).

[a]Criteria for children have been omitted from this table.

Reprinted with permission from Diagnostic and statistical manual of mental disorders. 4th ed. Washington, DC: American Psychiatric Association, 1994.

EPIDEMIOLOGY AND NATURAL HISTORY OF THE MAJOR AFFECTIVE DISORDERS

Mania and major depression are the two syndromes that give the traditional name *manic-depressive disorder* to this group of disorders. Most patients suffer only recurrent depressive episodes *(the unipolar group)*; a few have only manic episodes (they are grouped with patients with bipolar disorder); and the remainder suffer from both manic and depressive episodes *(the bipolar group).* A national community survey of mental disorders, the Epidemiological Catchment Area Study, estimated that 6% to 12% of women and 2% to 5% of men experience at least one major depressive episode during their adult life, and such an episode may occur at any age. Only 0.6% to 1.2% of adults develop a bipolar disorder; it is equally common in men and in women, and the first manic episode usually occurs before 30 years of age (16).

Both major depressive disorder and bipolar disorder can be highly recurrent illnesses (see Prognosis and Long-term Treatment of Affective Disorders). Many patients with major depressive disorder (recurrent unipolar depression) have frequent relapses of clinical depression as well as prolonged periods of subsyndromal depressive symptoms. A naturalistic, prospective study of 431 patients with unipolar major depressive disorder found that these patients met diagnostic criteria for major depression or for dysthymic disorder or had subthreshold depressive symptoms during 59% of the weeks of the 12-year study. Twenty-seven percent of these patients had no weeks during which they were completely free of symptoms (17). The course of the bipolar disorders is so widely variable as to defy simple description or easy categorization. Some patients enjoy many years of symptom remission with maintenance treatment, and others endure almost unrelenting mood cycling and substantial psychosocial morbidity (18).

MAJOR DEPRESSIVE DISORDER

The most common form of clinical depression is major depressive disorder (Table 24.3). Most depressed people visit a health care facility during the depressive episode, but only about 30% are diagnosed and given treatment for depression (19,20).

Diagnosis

The *differential diagnosis* of symptoms that suggest major depression varies depending on the patient's age, the presenting manifestations, and other associated factors. In *younger patients,* it is important to differentiate major depression from schizophrenia, especially when hallucinations or delusions are part of the presenting picture. In younger adults with none of the features of schizophrenia (see Chapter 25), the differential is between adjustment disorder and major depression in those with recent onset of symptoms, and between adjustment disorder and dysthymia in those with more chronic presentation. In *elderly patients* with memory complaints, the differential diagnosis is more complex, because memory complaints without substantial memory performance problems are common and also because a modest but reversible dementia can result from the depression alone (so-called pseudodementia; see Chapter 26). In addition, depression and dementia syndromes can both be related to underlying neuropathologic disorders, particularly Parkinson disease and stroke (see Chapters 90 and 91).

Stressful life events are common precipitating factors of major depressions, so their presence is not useful for making or excluding the diagnosis. In patients with panic attacks or obsessive-compulsive symptoms, it is important to remember that both panic disorder and obsessive-compulsive disorder (see Chapter 22) can occur in the context of a major depressive syndrome.

Alcohol abuse and abuse of other substances commonly cause mood syndromes that may be indistinguishable from those of the major affective disorders. Substance abuse is a comorbidity common in patients with major affective disorders as well. Therefore, screening for substance abuse should be a routine part of the assessment of the depressed patient.

A variety of *prescribed medications* have been reported to cause mood syndromes (Table 24.4). The lengthy lists of pharmaceutical agents reported to be depressogenic that appear in most textbooks are often based only on case reports and uncontrolled case series and are of questionable utility to the physician who is trying to decide whether to discontinue an effective medication in a patient who becomes depressed while taking it. A survey of more than 2,000 community subjects found that most commonly prescribed medications are not associated with depressive syndromes. In this study, beta-blockers, angiotensin-converting enzyme inhibitors, lipid lowering agents,

Table 24.4. Drugs and Substances that May Cause or Precipitate Mood Syndromes

Agents associated with depressed states
- Alcohol
- Stimulant and cocaine withdrawal
- "Ecstasy" and other "club drug" withdrawal
- Benzodiazepines
- Corticosteroids
- Oral contraceptives
- Tamoxifen
- Interferon
- Digitalis

Agents associated with hypomanic and manic states
- Amphetamines, cocaine, "ecstasy" and "club drugs"
- Levodopa
- Corticosteroids
- Anabolic-androgenic steroids
- Antidepressants (all classes)
- Thyroid hormones

Modified from: Patten SB, Love EJ. Drug-induced depression. Psychother Psychosom, 1997;66:63, and Peet P, Peters S. Drug-induced mania. Drug Saf 1995; 12:1466.

and digoxin—all drugs commonly reported to cause depression—showed no association with the depressive syndrome (21). An association between beta-blockers and depression, touted as a clinical pearl since this class of drugs first became available, remains unproven and controversial despite many years of investigation (22). A more impressive association between depression and treatment with digitalis has been demonstrated, and digitalis intoxication can present as a depressive syndrome (23). Steroid medications have clearly been shown to precipitate both the major depressive syndrome and manic syndrome in some patients (24). Drug-induced depression caused by interferon during treatment for hepatitis C or malignancy, by acute estrogen deficiency during the treatment of breast cancer with tamoxifen, and by naltrexone in the treatment of alcoholism has also been well established. Medication-induced mood syndromes often respond to reduction in dose of the causative agent or to treatment with antidepressant or mood-stabilizing medication (25). The differentiation of affective disorders from drug-induced syndromes and the management of mood symptoms in the medically ill patient who is taking multiple needed medications can be complex and challenging (26). Close coordination with a psychiatric consultant and thoughtful risk-benefit analysis of various medication approaches is the best course for the generalist in these situations.

Finally, it is important to differentiate unipolar from bipolar depressive states, because antidepressants can precipitate manic or mixed manic mood swings in patients with bipolar disorder.

The specific criteria of the APA for major depressive episode (Table 24.3) require the presence of at least five of nine depressive symptoms and related functional impairment for 2 weeks, not caused by the direct effect of a medication or a drug of abuse or of a general medical condition. *Either depressed mood or loss of interest or pleasure in usual activities (anhedonia) must always be present;* these symptoms can be considered core symptoms of major depression and should always be sought. A positive response to either of two questions—(a) "Have you had a down, low, or depressed mood in the past month?" or (b) "Have you been bothered by a loss of interest and pleasure in your usual activities?"—has been reported to have a 96% sensitivity in the diagnosis of major depression (27).

A patient with a history of episodic depressive disorder and the fully developed symptom cluster is not difficult to diagnose. However, patients with major depression who present with a dominant somatic complaint or with a clear "reason" to be depressed, guilty, or hopeless may easily be missed if they are not specifically asked about depressive symptoms. When major depression is strongly suspected, probing inquiry about symptoms from both the patient and those close to the patient usually clarifies the diagnosis.

A *fully developed major depression* is characterized by a sustained alteration in mood, self-attitude, and vital sense. The sustained lowering of mood is impervious to environmental influence once the depression becomes severe. Events that are not usually stressful are perceived as overwhelming by a depressed patient as the syndrome develops. The *change in self-attitude* is usually manifested in expressions of guilt, inferiority, uselessness, and hopelessness. The *changes in vital sense* (i.e., the subjective assessment of one's physical and mental functioning) result in complaints of confusion or poor memory, inability to concentrate, lack of energy, and easy fatigability. Sometimes patients complain only of a vague sense of ill health. This preoccupation with physical symptoms can occasionally reach delusional intensity, and seriously depressed patients can become convinced that they are dying of cancer or of acquired immunodeficiency syndrome when there is no evidence of these diseases.

Marked psychomotor retardation (i.e., slowed speech and movements), *delusions* with depressive content, and *diurnal mood variation* (worst mood in the morning) occur in a minority of patients but are diagnostically useful when present because they are fairly specific to this disorder.

Treatment Overview

Once the diagnosis of major depression is made, treatment consists of explaining the diagnosis to the patient (and family), prescription and monitoring of antidepressant medications, and providing supportive counseling for the patient and family.

Antidepressant Treatment: General Points

For the patient with major depression who is in good physical condition and who is neither overwhelmed with depressive delusions nor suicidal (see Suicide Prevention), antidepressant medication is the appropriate initial treatment. Any antidepressant drug is effective in approximately 70% of patients with major depression, and no antidepressant on the market has been shown to be more effective than the others. In medication trials, "effective" usually means a 50% or greater reduction in symptoms as measured by a standardized rating instrument such as the Hamilton Rating Scale of Depression, the HAM-D (28). Patients who fail to respond to an antidepressant from one class often respond to one from a different class (see Switching Antidepressants). Depressed patients tolerate side effects (and what they perceive to be side effects) poorly and often stop taking antidepressants without completing a full 8-week trial of the medication. Therefore, the selection of the first antidepressant has more to do with convenience of administration and side effects than with the probability of a therapeutic response. The exception to this rule is the patient who has had a prior good (or poor) response to a particular antidepressant. The mechanism of therapeutic action of antidepressant drugs is unknown. Although much indirect evidence suggests that they exert their therapeutic effects by enhancing catecholaminergic and serotoninergic neurotransmission, their clinical use remains empiric.

Depressed patients with delusions, hallucinations, or profound psychomotor retardation tend to be less responsive to drugs than those without these clinical features. Referral for psychiatric consultation and consideration for electroconvulsive therapy (ECT) are appropriate for such patients. Among patients with suicidal intent (see Suicide Prevention), antidepressants, especially tricyclics, should be dispensed in small amounts to avoid providing enough drug for a lethal overdose.

Characteristics of Available Antidepressants

Characteristics of available antidepressant drugs are listed in Table 24.5. *Tricyclic antidepressants* (TCAs), the oldest class, are listed in two subgroups: secondary and tertiary amines. The monoamine oxidase (MAO) inhibitors are not listed. These drugs, which were the main alternatives to tricyclics before 1990, are uncommonly used today even by psychiatrists specializing in the treatment of depression.

There are five *selective serotonin reuptake inhibitors* (SSRIs) on the market in the United States: citalopram, (Celexa), fluoxetine (Prozac and Serafem), fluvoxamine (Luvox), paroxetine (Paxil), and sertraline (Zoloft). They are similar in efficacy and side effect profiles. Fluvoxamine is sedating in large doses and, along with citalopram and paroxetine, is often more sedating than fluoxetine or sertraline. Because of its extremely long half-life (up to 4 days), fluoxetine has been formulated for once-a-week dosing during the maintenance phase of treatment (Prozac Weekly). Although preliminary studies support the efficacy of once-weekly compared with daily dosing of fluoxetine (29), whether it actually improves patient compliance is not known.

Nefazodone (Serzone), is a less sedating relative of the older antidepressant *trazodone* (Desyrel). Nefazodone is well tolerated at therapeutic dosages of 300 to 600 mg/day and is a good second-line antidepressant, joining bupropion. Cases of life-threatening hepatic failure have been reported in patients taking nefazodone. Although trazodone is often too sedating for use as an antidepressant, small doses (e.g., 50 mg each night) are a non–habit-forming alternative to benzodiazepine hypnotics for depressed patients.

Bupropion (Wellbutrin) is an antidepressant of the aminoketone class, unrelated to the tricyclic and SSRI antidepressants but related to the phenylethylamines. It inhibits serotonin, norepinephrine, and dopamine reuptake. An uncommon but serious side effect is seizures, which occur in 0.4% of patients treated at dosages up to 450 mg/day. This is only slightly greater than the rate of seizures with tricyclics. At higher dosages (up to 700 mg) originally approved by the U.S. Food and Drug Administration (FDA), bupropion was associated with a higher rate of seizures; this finding led to the recommended 450-mg limit on total daily dosage. For the same reason, the limit for any single dose is 150 mg, and doses should be separated by at least 4 hours. Therefore, most patients need a two- or three-times-daily dosing schedule to achieve a therapeutic daily dosage of 300 to 450 mg. (The maximum recommended daily dose is only 400 mg for the sustained-release preparation, Wellbutrin SR). Bupropion has also been found to be useful in smoking cessation and is marketed under the brand Zyban for this indication.

Venlafaxine (Effexor), another phenylethylamine antidepressant, is usually given twice daily at a total daily dosage of 150 to 300 mg (the maximum recommended daily dose is only 225 mg for the sustained-release preparation, Effexor XR). Because venlafaxine causes diastolic hypertension in a small fraction of patients, particularly at higher dosages, blood pressure monitoring for 2 weeks after starting the drug and after any dosage elevation is recommended.

Mirtazapine (Remeron) is associated with significant sedation but has a sufficiently long half-life to allow bedtime dosing. A less common but serious side effect is granulocytopenia. Mirtazapine is currently recommended only for patients who have not responded to other antidepressants.

Complementary and Alternative Treatments

A number of nutritional supplements and herbs have been claimed by enthusiasts to be safe and effective for depression (see Chapter 5). Patients may ask about alternative treatment because trials with standard antidepressants have failed or because of the misconception that herbal and nutritional preparations must be safer than the FDA-approved medications for which numerous possible adverse reactions are listed. *St. John's wort* gained considerable attention in the late 1990s after several studies seemed to indicate its effectiveness in depressed patients. However, a randomized, placebo-controlled study found no difference between St. Johns' wort extract and placebo in the treatment of patients with major depression (30). *Omega-3 fatty acids,* administered as fish oil capsules, were proposed as a natural remedy for depression and bipolar disorder after the appearance of several preliminary studies suggesting benefit for some patients. Further studies are needed before omega-3 fatty acids can be recommended over established treatments for affective disorders (31).

Selection and Dosage Adjustment of Antidepressants

Because of their favorable side effect profile and ease of use, the SSRIs have become the drugs of first choice for most depressed patients. Because almost every depressed patient is more prone to or more intolerant of some side effects than others, selection of an antidepressant for a particular patient depends on the fit between the patient's medical history and the antidepressant's side effect profile. The SSRIs have a significant advantage over the TCAs because of their relative safety in overdose (32). Both fluoxetine and the tricyclic nortriptyline have been shown to be safe for use during the first trimester of pregnancy. Although both were associated with a small increase in spontaneous abortions, neither was associated with any increase in fetal abnormalities (33).

Table 24.5. Characteristics of Antidepressant Drugs

Drug	Strengths of Available Oral Preparations (mg)	Low or Starting Dosage Range	Usual Dosage Range	Common Side Effects	Special Considerations
Tricyclics					
Secondary amines					
Nortriptyline[a] (Pamelor, Aventyl, others)	10, 25, 50, 75, 100	25 mg q.h.s.	50–150 mg q.h.s.	Dry mouth, sedation, orthostasis, constipation, weight gain, sexual dysfunction	Titrate to a.m. trough serum level 90–150 ng/dL
Desipramine[a] (Norpramin, others)	10, 25, 50	25–50 mg q.h.s.	150–250 mg q.h.s.	Same as other tricyclics	Titrate to level >150 ng/dL upper limit unclear—?250 ng/dL
Tertiary amines					
Amitriptyline[a] (Elavil, others)	10, 25, 50, 75, 100	25–50 mg q.h.s.	150–250 mg q.h.s.	Same as other tricyclics, but more severe	Titrate to combined amitriptyline plus nortriptyline level >150 ng/dL upper limit unclear—? 250 ng/dL
Doxepin[a] (Sinequan, Adapin, others)	10, 25, 50, 100	25–50 mg h.s.	150–250 mg q.h.s.	Same as amitriptyline	Titrate to level >125–250 ng/dL
Imipramine (Tofranil, others)	10, 25, 50, 100	25–50 mg h.s.	150–250 mg q.h.s.	Same as amitriptyline	Titrate to level >180 ng/dL
Selective serotonin reuptake inhibitors (SSRIs)					
Citalopram (Celexa)	20, 40	20 mg q.d.	20–60 mg q.d.	Insomnia, gastrointestinal discomfort, restlessness, diarrhea, headache, sweating, anxiety, sexual dysfunction	Note: All SSRIs can raise levels of other drugs, including anticonvulsants, tricyclics, thoephylline, digoxin, coumadin, some antiarrhthymics, β-blockers, calcium channel blockers
Fluoxetine (Prozac, Serafem)	10, 20, 40	10–20 mg q.d.	20–40 mg q.d.	Same as citalopram but more activating	Very long half life, available in once-a-week preparation
Sertraline (Zoloft)	25, 50, 100	25–50 mg q.d.	100–200 mg q.d.	Same as citalopram but perhaps more gastrointestinal symptoms	—
Paroxetine (Paxil)	10, 20, 30, 40	10–20 mg q.d.	20–40 mg q.d.	Same as citalopram, sometimes sedation	May be taken at bedtime
Fluvoxamine (Luvox)	50, 100	25–50 mg q.d.	150–200 mg q.d.	Similar to sertraline but more sedating	—
Others					
Nefazodone (Serzone)	100, 150	37.5–75 mg b.i.d.	100–200 mg b.i.d.	Nausea, dry mouth, headache, sedation, occasional orthostasis	"Black box" warning of risk of hepatic failure issued in 2002
Trazodone (Desyrel, others)	50, 150, 300	25–100 mg q.h.s.	300–500 mg q.h.s.	Same as nefazodone but more sedation	Useful in low dose (25–100 mg h.s.) as relatively safe hypnotic without dependence or cognitive impairment
Bupropion				Insomnia, gastrointestinal upset, more reduction of seizure threshold than others; less sexual dysfunction than other antidepressants	Incompatible with ritonavir; new sustained-release preparation for better b.i.d. dosing
(Wellbutrin)	75, 100	75 mg q.d. or b.i.d.	100–150 mg b.i.d. or t.i.d.		
(Wellbutrin SR)	100, 150	150 mg q.d.	100–200 mg b.i.d.		
Venlafaxine				Nausea, insomnia, sedation, sweating, gastrointestinal discomfort	May have more rapid relapse of symptoms with cessation than others, can cause blood pressure increase
(Effexor)	37.5, 75	37.5–75 b.i.d.	100–150 b.i.d.		
(Effexor XR)	37.5, 75,150	37.5–75 mg q.d.	100–225 mg q.d.		
Mirtazapine (Remeron)	15, 30, 45	7.5–15 mg q.h.s.	15–45 mg q.h.s.	Sedation, weight gain, dizziness, rarely granulocytopenia	—

[a]Generic preparation available.

In the otherwise healthy depressed patient, it is reasonable to initiate antidepressant treatment with 20 mg/day of *fluoxetine* or *paroxetine*. These two SSRIs are administered once a day and require no titration of the daily dosage. Studies showed that most responders do as well on the usual starting dosage of 20 mg/day as on higher dosages (34). For patients who are very sensitive to medication side effects, initiating treatment at 10 mg/day and advancing to 20 mg/day after 1 week is a reasonable option.

For patients given *sertraline,* a starting dosage of 25 to 50 mg/day is advisable. The 25-mg dosage can be increased to 50 mg as soon as the patient can tolerate this dosage of medication (usually 1 or 2 days). At the 50-mg daily dosage, some patients need no more upward titration. Therefore, it is advisable to wait 2 weeks before considering the next dosage increase. If the patient appears to be improving rapidly, waiting another 2 weeks is almost always advisable. If there is doubt about the degree of improvement or if no improvement is evident, increasing the dosage by another 25 to 50 mg/day is advisable every 2 weeks until the patient is markedly improved or the dosage has reached 200 mg/day.

The tricyclic *nortriptyline* has fewer side effects than the other TCAs and the most clearly established therapeutically effective serum concentration range. Patients should begin with 25 to 50 mg/day and take 50 mg for 2 weeks before an attempt is made to assess the drug's efficacy. If some improvement is apparent, no change should be considered for another 2 weeks. If improvement is marginal or absent, a plasma TCA level should be obtained. The optimal nortriptyline concentration is 90 to 150 ng/mL. The process of dosage adjustment to produce an effective result is repeated every 2 weeks until the patient is improved greatly or has not responded to 4 weeks of optimal treatment.

Treatment with *imipramine, desipramine, amitriptyline,* or *doxepin* should begin at a dosage of 50 mg/day and be increased in 50-mg increments as tolerated to 150 mg/day. The blood level should be measured after 2 weeks at a stable dosage, and then the dosage should be adjusted to achieve a therapeutic blood level of 150 ng/mL or greater for any of these four TCAs (Table 24.5). Starting dosages of TCAs should be reduced by approximately 50% in *older patients* (especially those with medical illnesses). TCA dosage may be increased every 2 to 4 days in young, physically healthy patients, but weekly increases are safer for older or infirm patients. Giving the total daily dosage at bedtime is desirable for most patients.

Bupropion can be started at 75 mg on day 1 and increased to 75 mg twice daily on day 2. Thereafter, it can be increased in 75-mg increments up to 150 mg three times a day. The usual therapeutic dosage is 300 to 450 mg/day (400 mg/day for Wellbutrin SR). Stopping at 150 mg twice daily is warranted until it is clear that that dosage is insufficient (2 to 4 weeks at that dosage without a substantial improvement).

Antidepressant Side Effects

Patients must be encouraged to tolerate the mild side effects that often occur before the therapeutic effects of antidepressant drugs begin. Many depressed patients tolerate even mild side effects poorly and need frequent reassurance that the treatment is safe and likely to be effective (in 3 to 8 weeks). Emphasizing that side effects are not unusual and that they are benign and usually temporary is very helpful in getting patients through this period.

The common side effects of *all SSRIs* are transient mild nausea, transient insomnia, and transient nervousness and muscular irritability. All SSRIs have good antianxiety properties when taken for 2 weeks or longer at a steady dosage.

The *SSRIs and venlafaxine cause sexual dysfunction* in up to one third of patients, usually decreased interest in sex (decreased libido), delayed orgasm or anorgasmia, and, less commonly, diminished sensation in the genital areas. Erectile function usually is not affected by the SSRIs, but impotence can be caused by TCAs. Strategies for managing SSRI-related sexual dysfunction fall into several categories (35). Monitoring and waiting is appropriate for patients with delayed orgasm, because many patients notice improvement in this side effect after several months. Decreased libido and anorgasmia do not often resolve spontaneously, and other measures are usually necessary to relieve these problems. The section on antidepressant side effects in Chapter 6 provides details about the approaches that can be tried in these patients.

The most common side effects of the *tricyclic antidepressants* are anticholinergic: dry mouth, constipation, and, less often, delayed micturition, blurred vision, and an anticholinergic delirium. Orthostatic hypotension is particularly problematic in elderly patients and in any patient with unsteady gait or balance problems. TCAs may also produce increased appetite with weight gain, granulocytopenia (rarely), hypomania or mania, slowed cardiac conduction, and cardiac arrhythmias.

Because of the *cardiac side effects,* TCAs should be given cautiously to patients with pre-existing conduction abnormalities or any unstable cardiac conditions (e.g., recent myocardial infarction). Nortriptyline has been studied in cardiac patients and can be safely administered to those with pre-existing stable heart disease (36). SSRIs, venlafaxine, and bupropion have few cardiac effects and therefore offer greater safety for the cardiac patient.

Bupropion is contraindicated in patients with a seizure disorder. The FDA recommends that the dosage not exceed 150 mg per dose or 450 mg/day (400 mg/day of Wellbutrin SR) to minimize the risk of seizures.

Drug Kinetics and Interactions

Among the TCAs and SSRIs, fluoxetine has an unusually long half-life (7 days for its active metabolite, norfluoxetine). This property can be advantageous because this antidepressant is less often associated with a withdrawal syndrome when discontinued, compared with other SSRIs and venlafaxine. The long half-life increases the time required to achieve washout before changing to another antidepressant. It is mandatory to await complete washout when the switch is made from an SSRI or venlafaxine to a MAO inhibitor, a distinctly uncommon transition in the primary care setting.

All SSRIs inhibit one or more of the cytochrome P-450 enzymes, but the clinical impact of this property, first reported in 1991, has proved to be modest. In patients taking paroxetine, fluoxetine, citalopram, or sertraline, blood levels of coadministered benzodiazepines, antipsychotics, TCAs, and flecainide-type antiarrhythmic agents may increase (Table 24.6).

Switching Antidepressants

Almost one third of depressed patients fail to respond to an adequate trial of an antidepressant medication. Switching antidepressants is one reasonable approach to the patient with treatment-resistant depression. Naturalistic studies indicate that switching antidepressants results in a treatment response approximately 50% of the time. Most authorities recommend switching to an antidepressant with a mechanism of action different from that of the failed agent, such as switching from an SSRI to venlafaxine or mirtazapine, agents that have actions on both serotonin and norepinephrine transport. Open label studies indicate, however, that switching from one SSRI to another can be effective (37). A medication wash-out is clearly indicated only with a switch from a MAO inhibitor to another antidepressant. Immediate substitution is usually well tolerated when switching within the same medication class (e.g., one SSRI or TCA to another) and has the advantage of avoiding discontinuation symptoms. Immediate substitution of mirtazapine for a SSRI has also been shown to be well tolerated. Gradual introduction of the new agent while gradually tapering the failed one is another well-tolerated strategy (38). The time to treatment response after switching to another agent cannot be estimated with any reliability. Numerous studies indicate that some patients require up to 12 weeks or even longer to have a response to changes in treatment approaches (39).

Table 24.6. Drugs that May Interact with Antidepressants

Antidepressant Drug Class	Interaction
Tricyclics (TCAs)	
Anticholinergic antispasmodics	Enhanced anticholinergic side effects
Anticholinergic antiparkinsonian drugs	Enhanced anticholinergic side effects
Antihypertensive drugs	Enhanced orthostatic hypotension
Selective serotonin reuptake inhibitors (SSRIs)	
TCAs, anxiolytics, hypnotics, neuroleptics	SSRIs block metabolism so blood levels rise; TCA plasma levels may rise twofold or more
Monoamine oxidase inhibitors	Potentially fatal serotonin syndrome

Treatment-Resistant Depression

The management of treatment-resistant depression is challenging and requires a substantial investment of time and considerable patience on the part of both the patient and the clinician. Biweekly or weekly monitoring visits are fairly standard practice in psychiatric settings for such patients during the many weeks, sometime many months, required for adequate new trials of antidepressant agents. Significant psychotherapeutic support in the form of education and encouragement, reassurance, and simple coaching needs to accompany the process as well. Clinicians should consider psychiatric referral of the patient who has not benefited from even an initial antidepressant trial if these time-intensive interventions are not possible in the clinician's own practice.

Duration of Drug Treatment

In a patient with persistent and significant depressive symptoms, an adequate therapeutic trial usually requires 2 months at a therapeutically effective dosage. After recovery from a first or from an infrequently recurrent depressive syndrome, the medication that induced the remission should be continued for 12 months, the time of highest risk for relapse (40). Most patients with a history of episodes and relapses should be advised to continue their antidepressant for a number of years. The terms "indefinite" and "for the rest of your life" may convey a sense of pessimism to patients. The commitment to long-term treatment should rather be an incremental decision, made after comparing 1 and then 2 years of treatment experience with the period before treatment. The use of a lower dosage of the patient's antidepressant for "maintenance" treatment is not recommended. Patients who took half of the acute antidepressant dosage had no better outcome than the placebo group in one controlled study (41). After ECT (see later discussion), maintenance treatment with antidepressants is essential for most patients to reduce the risk of relapse.

Drug Discontinuation

Patients who discontinue antidepressant medications can experience a variety of uncomfortable physical symptoms, especially if they stop a medication abruptly. Symptoms including dizziness, lightheadedness, headache, insomnia, fatigue, nausea, sensory disturbances, and flu-like malaise have been reported after discontinuation of TCAs, SSRIs, and newer antidepressants including venlafaxine (42). Discontinuation symptoms are more common with agents that have a shorter half-life (e.g., paroxetine) and less likely with agents that have a longer half-life (e.g., fluoxetine) (43). The overall incidence of antidepressant withdrawal symptoms is difficult to estimate because of the wide variation among antidepressants and probable variations in patient sensitivity, but discontinuation symptoms have been reported in up to one third of patients within the context of controlled trials of drug efficacy (42). Symptoms can occur within hours or days and may persist for up to several weeks.

When medications must be discontinued, tapering the dosage usually, but not always, prevents discontinuation symptoms from developing. Antidepressants should be tapered over a period of at least 10 days and over a longer period if the drug has been taken at higher dosages. A reasonable approach is to taper by 25% of the patient's dose every 3 to 4 days until the patient has been taking half of the usual starting dose for 3 to 4 days, and then discontinuing altogether. Patients taking low doses of antidepressants can be tapered more rapidly. Other than reassurance, treatment of discontinuation symptoms is rarely necessary. However, discontinuation symptoms can usually be aborted by restarting or increasing the dose of the medication being discontinued, followed by a more gradual taper.

Counseling and Psychotherapy

Counseling Visits

For the first 6 to 8 weeks, the patient with major depression should be seen at least every other week for adjustment of medication and for brief supportive psychotherapy as described in Chapter 20. For patients with major depression, the first priority in supportive counseling is consistent repetition of the answer to the three questions most troublesome to depressed patients: "What is wrong with me?"; "Is this treatment going to work?" (this question may be presented as a concern: "I think this pill is making me worse; I want to stop it."); and "What is going to happen to me (if this doesn't work for me)?" Answers to these questions should be prefaced by a reassuring statement, like, "You have clinical depression. We don't understand how it is caused, but it is not your fault. It is a medical disease. You will get better. We are going to continue to care for you and fight the depression with you until you are better." Supportive counseling is important for members of the patient's family as well.

A second focus of counseling is more directive. It is remarkable how many patients resign jobs and separate from spouses based on distorted depressive perceptions about not being able to do their usual work, not being able to feel love for a spouse, and feeling somehow that "facing this (negative conclusion) reality" will allow them and their loved ones "to move on." It is important therefore that the physician counsel patients not to attempt any *major life decisions* while they are depressed. Job-related and personal relationship changes should likewise be deferred until the patient's ability to maintain a more objective and positive perspective recovers.

Frank discussion of *suicidal feelings*, plans, and intentions should be a routine part of each visit (see Suicide Prevention). Candid discussion of the level of risk and protective measures available is equally important and may require the participation of a family member or loved one.

The patient should be routinely assessed for the *side effects* that are most typical of the antidepressant being used (see previous discussion). The more depressed the patient, the less tolerant he or she will be of minor adverse drug effects and the more likely to give up on the treatment before it has been given an adequate trial. The support of the doctor in encouraging persistence with drug therapy is crucial.

Office Psychotherapy

Traditional or "insight-oriented" psychotherapy has been a two-edged sword for depressed patients. On one hand, it engages depressed patients in an empathic consideration of their feelings and concerns. On the other hand, the theories behind the practice propose that depression results from maladaptive responses to life experiences and can therefore be alleviated through the insights and personal growth that psychotherapy facilitates. Psychodynamic therapy may thus convey the message at times that, when depressive symptoms persist, the patient rather than the treatment has failed—a distinctly inaccurate and even harmful implication for patients with major depression.

The briefer and more present-oriented psychotherapies (*cognitive therapy* and *interpersonal therapy*) can be shown to help patients recover from depressive symptoms, especially when used concurrently with antidepressant pharmacotherapy (44). Some of the more common *cognitive distortions* that depressed patients experience and express are listed in Table 24.7. Even someone who is not trained in cognitive therapy can help patients by gently challenging negative thoughts such as those listed. A supportively offered challenge can help patients access what they already know and what they have experienced, both of which usually argue against the most negative and distorted conclusions of the depressed state. *Interpersonal therapy* emphasizes the social contexts and consequences

Table 24.7. Cognitive Distortions in Depression

All-or-nothing thinking: Thinking occurs in black-and-white terms with no recognition of a middle ground. Things are wonderful or awful. One's actions reflect either perfection or total failure.

Overgeneralization: Words such as "always" and "never" may portray a single negative event as a never-ending pattern of defeat.

Selective abstraction: A single negative detail is focused on and ruminated about until it colors everything.

Disqualifying the positive: Positive experiences are often discounted as not relevant, not real, or not deserved.

Arbitrary inferences: It is assumed that things are or will be negative, regardless of the facts.

Magnification or minimization: One's own failures and others' successes are magnified; one's own successes and others' failures are minimized.

Emotional reasoning: Bad feelings are taken as the litmus test of reality.

"Should" statements: Repetitive "I should/should not" or "I must/must not" statements often contribute to depression, resentment, guilt, and hopelessness.

Labeling and mislabeling: Mistakes or shortcomings become sweeping self-condemnations.

Personalization: Depressed people often assume they are the cause of some unfortunate or unpleasant event for which, in actuality, they are not responsible.

Adapted from Burns DD. Feeling good: the new mood therapy. New York: New American Library, 1980.

of the patient's depression. It includes skills such as identifying and addressing stressors, pointing out assets, and providing alternative choices. These and other skills useful in interpersonal therapy are described in Chapter 20.

Cognitive and interpersonal psychotherapy also can help, in combination with antidepressants, to reduce the risk of relapse during the months following successful treatment (44,45). Even these modes of psychotherapy are not indicated in the most acute depressive states, because psychotherapy requires that the patient be able to concentrate, recall, and maintain a level of objectivity and hopefulness.

Referral for Psychiatric Treatment

General physicians should be able to treat most of the patients in whom they diagnose major depression. However, some depressed patients should be referred to a psychiatrist: Those in whom the diagnosis is not clear enough to allow confident treatment; those who show no improvement after 8 weeks of treatment with therapeutic dosages of antidepressant medications (about one in three patients); those who cannot or will not take antidepressant medications; those who are overtly suicidal; and those with delusions, hallucinations, or depressive stupor (i.e., mute and unresponsive). Hospitalization, more intensive counseling, more aggressive drug therapy, or ECT (see later discussion) is usually suggested for these patients by the psychiatric consultant.

Although many patients initially resist the idea of seeing a psychiatrist, a primary care physician with whom a patient has good rapport can be most persuasive in helping the patient understand the need for and reasons necessitating psychiatric consultation or referral. Patients may interpret psychiatric referral as an indication that their situation is hopeless, or they may feel that they are being shunned by their personal physician (as many depressed patients fear). It is important, therefore, to explain the reasons for referral to the patient, specifically that additional treatments, with which the psychiatrist has more experience, are available.

Electroconvulsive Therapy

ECT is an effective and rapid treatment for major depressive disorder. The decision to use ECT should be made by the psychiatrist with the informed consent of the patient and, when available, the informed consent of the patient's family. This treatment was previously given only to hospitalized patients, but outpatient ECT is increasingly available and suitable for medically and behaviorally stable patients. The indications for ECT involve emergency situations mandating a rapid response (such as the malnourished, dehydrated, or suicidal patient); the presence of medical illness that makes drug therapy excessively risky; the presence of delusions or overwhelming severity of the depression; and failure of drug therapy. The likelihood of marked benefit from ECT is higher than with antidepressants: It is approximately 80% in patients with major depression. The benefit is short term however, lasting anywhere from several weeks to 6 months. Therefore, ECT is an excellent first choice for patients with clearly episodic depressions that are severe but infrequent. The benefit usually requires 6 to 12 treatments given two to three times per week. The procedure involves anesthetization with a short-acting barbiturate, which is administered before a muscle-relaxing agent (usually succinyl choline).

Aside from the small risk of brief anesthesia, the *adverse effects* that follow ECT involve primarily memory. Commonly, retention of new and occasionally old memories is mildly defective for weeks to months after a series of ECT treatments. These memory gaps are usually spotty and involve primarily declarative memories (events, things that were heard or read) as opposed to procedural memories (how to perform a task). Typically, the patient in whom this effect becomes clinically apparent (perhaps 40% of treated patients) has trouble recalling names of recent acquaintances or forgets events that occurred during or just before beginning ECT. Clinically apparent memory defects typically resolve within 2 months. Formal testing has revealed mild defects lasting up to 3 months, but none at 6 months after treatment (46).

MANIA

Diagnosis

The manic syndrome, like major depression, is defined by a sustained change in mood, self-attitude, and vital sense. The manic patient's mood may be euphoric or irritable, or it may alternate between the two. The *self-attitude* is one of overconfidence; in more severe cases, it is reflected in an inflated sense of power, position, and importance. *Heightened vital sense* is manifested in the patient's sense of quickened and totally accurate thinking. The patient has an overconfident ease in decision-making and a sense of heightened perception of sounds, colors, and tastes and sees only continued supreme well-being in his or her future. The patient manifests dramatically increased energy and a decreased need for sleep. In the speeded-up and overconfident state, the patient is observed by his or her family to be very distractible in speech (jumping from topic to topic) and behavior (jumping from one new project to another, completing none). Finally, judgment ranges from poor to catastrophic as patients spend impulsively, including giving away money and personal belongings on the street, and are uncharacteristically disinhibited and provocative in word and deed.

Delusions and hallucinations, when present, are either persecutory or grandiose. Occasionally symptoms thought to be characteristic of schizophrenia occur (see Chapter 25), leading to the clinical rule that "schizophrenic" symptoms are not in themselves diagnostic but should be judged by the company they keep. In the presence of the characteristic manic syndrome, symptoms thought of as first-rank symptoms of schizophrenia would be considered part of a mania if they follow the course of the other manic symptoms, remitting as the mood and behavior normalize. The diagnosis of *schizoaffective disorder–manic type* is reserved for patients in whom the psychotic symptoms persist well beyond the manic syndrome so that the patient is psychotic in the absence of the manic symptoms throughout most of the course of the illness. Whether these patients have an unusually severe form of bipolar disorder or a condition more related to schizophrenia is currently unknown. The specific criteria of the APA for mania are shown in Table 24.8.

Initial Treatment

General Principles

The disruptive and disinhibited symptoms of mania are more difficult to manage in medical terms, and the manic patient's behavior can be quite agitated and out of control. Therefore, manic patients are almost always best referred to psychiatrists, and many of them require inpatient psychiatric treatment.

The referral may be difficult, because acceptance by a manic patient of the need for help is the exception rather than the rule. The patient's personal physician can be a crucial—at times the only—clinician involved with the manic patient in the initial presentation, and by virtue of an already established relationship with the patient or the family, this physician may be able to persuade the patient to take some medication and to accept a referral to a psychiatrist or to a hospital inpatient unit. Basic knowledge about the use of neuroleptic drugs and mood-stabilizing medications (e.g., lithium, sodium valproate) is therefore important for primary care physicians.

Table 24.8. American Psychiatric Association Diagnostic Criteria for a Manic Episode

A. A distinct period of abnormally and persistently elevated, expansive, or irritable mood, lasting at least 1 week (or any duration if hospitalization is necessary).
B. During the period of mood disturbance, at least three of the following symptoms have persisted (four if the mood is only irritable) and have been present to a significant degree:
   1. Inflated self-esteem or grandiosity
   2. Decreased need for sleep (e.g., feels rested after only 3 hours of sleep)
   3. More talkative than usual or pressured to keep talking
   4. Flight of ideas or subjective experience that thoughts are racing
   5. Distractibility (i.e., attention too easily drawn to unimportant or irrelevant external stimuli)
   6. Increase in goal-directed activity (either social, at work or school, or sexually) or psychomotor agitation
   7. Excessive involvement in pleasurable activities that have a high potential for painful consequences (e.g., the person engages in unrestrained buying sprees, sexual indiscretions, or foolish business investments)
C. The mood disturbance is sufficiently severe to cause marked impairment in occupational functioning or in usual social activities or relationships with others, or to necessitate hospitalization to prevent harm to self or others.
D. Not due to the direct effects of a substance (e.g., drugs of abuse, medication) or a general medical condition (e.g., hyperthyroidism).

Reprinted with permission from Diagnostic and statistical manual of mental disorders. 4th ed. Washington, DC: American Psychiatric Association, 1994.

Hypomania, a milder form of the manic syndrome, can sometimes by treated on an outpatient basis but usually indicates the presence of a complex mood disorder that will require specialized care. Close symptom monitoring, discontinuation of antidepressant medication, and prompt psychiatric evaluation usually are indicated. Hypomania can escalate rapidly and dangerously into full-blown mania, and initiation of antipsychotic medication is often appropriate (see later discussion).

Winning the cooperation of the acutely manic patient can be very difficult. The euphoric or irritable manic patient often will not accept the notion that his or her behavior is disturbed, much less that it requires inpatient therapy. Explaining the need for medical treatment in a manner that does not inflame the patient and provoke even more disordered behavior is a valuable skill. If possible, consultation with the family about the diagnosis and plan of treatment should be arranged before, not after, confronting the patient with the diagnosis and treatment plan. Despite the uncontrollable behavior of the manic patient, family members may be afraid to support the doctor's resolve to have the patient treated out of fear of being seen by the patient as betraying his or her trust. The clinician's task is to calm the patient and the family, to persuade the manic patient to accept hospitalization voluntarily if needed, and to resort to civil commitment if necessary.

Although *laws on commitment* vary among states, all states currently have legal provisions to allow the involuntary hospitalization of patients with mental disorders who are clearly dangerous to themselves or others and for whom no less restrictive alternative is appropriate. Physicians should make themselves familiar with commitment laws in the community where they practice and know the steps necessary to initiate commitment procedures. These difficult processes often require the teamwork of the clinician, the family, the staff of an emergency room, and sometimes law enforcement officials to be successful.

Medication for Severe Mania

Severe acute mania requires treatment initially with *neuroleptics* and later with both mood stabilizers, such as lithium, and neuroleptics. For the first week or two, this treatment is usually carried out in the hospital. The generalist's role with such patients many include initial diagnosis, treatment with sufficient medication to get the manic patient to the hospital, and then continued participation in follow-up care.

For acute manic agitation, the use of parenteral fluphenazine (Prolixin) or another high-potency neuroleptic is usually effective. Modest doses (5 to 10 mg intramuscularly) calm most patients with little or no depression of blood pressure and little sedation. Older, more sedating phenothiazines such as chlorpromazine (Thorazine) are more difficult to work with because repeated doses are often necessary to break the agitated manic state and these preparations often produce significant orthostatic hypotension. Within 15 to 20 minutes, intramuscular high-potency neuroleptics usually bring about a calming effect that may last for several hours. This period can be used to get the patient admitted to hospital. Even in this short period, however, patients may develop *extrapyramidal side effects* from the high-potency neuroleptics, most often acute dystonic reactions. This condition is alleviated by 50 mg of intramuscular diphenhydramine (Benadryl) or 1 to 2 mg of trihexyphenidate (Cogentin). Newer neuroleptic agents (e.g., olanzapine) are superior alternatives to standard neuroleptics for patients in the manic state, especially because they have less propensity for inducing extrapyramidal side effects. These preparations have their own troublesome side effects, which include sedation orthostatic blood pressure changes and weight gain.

Maintenance Therapy for Bipolar Disorder

To date, lithium is the only medication for which efficacy has been unequivocally established for preventing relapses in patients with bipolar disorder or mania after acute episodes have remitted (47). Most controlled comparisons of carbamazepine and lithium suggest that they are approximately equivalent in prophylactic efficacy (48). There are as yet no rigorous therapeutic trials comparing lithium with other anticonvulsants that may be useful for maintenance treatment of bipolar disorder. Despite this lack of data, valproate continues to be widely prescribed as a maintenance treatment for patients with bipolar disorder as an alternative to lithium, perhaps because of its lower toxicity. Newer antiepileptics are also increasingly being used to treat patients with bipolar disorder, but only lamotrigine appears to be effective in controlled studies (49). Several other agents, including calcium channel blockers and high-potency benzodiazepines, particularly clonazepam, may also have antimanic utility.

Lithium

Lithium Dosage and Schedule. When lithium is the mood stabilizer selected, it is prescribed in divided doses, beginning with 300 to 600 mg on the first day and increasing in small increments every 3 to 4 days until the therapeutic blood level is achieved. The usual maintenance dosage is 600 to 1,800 mg given in divided doses (two to three times daily with standard preparations and once or twice daily with slow-release preparations). Blood levels, which should be measured 12 hours after a dose (trough levels), should be monitored once or twice per week at first. Even in a compliant patient who is thoroughly stabilized, lithium levels should be checked at least six times per year. In addition, because of the possibility of long-term renal effects, the maintenance dosage should be aimed at maintaining the lowest therapeutic level (probably 0.6 to 0.9 mEq/L) and not necessarily the level required for acute antimanic activity (0.9 to 1.4 mEq/L). Lithium should be used cautiously with other medications, because a number of important drug interactions are associated with its use (Table 24.9).

Side Effects. The early side effects of lithium include nausea and vomiting, diarrhea, mild lassitude, and drowsiness. These effects typically resolve as the serum level stabilizes in the therapeutic range. An accentuated *physiologic (postural) tremor* (see Chapter 90) appears in a large percentage of patients (about 60%) during the maintenance phase of treatment but is rarely severe. Chronic lithium therapy causes nontoxic *goiter and mild alterations of thyroid function tests* (borderline low thyroxin levels or elevated thyroid-stimulating hormone values). Less often, frank hypothyroidism may occur, usually in patients who had subclinical hypothyroidism before receiving lithium. For these reasons, thyroid function should be assessed before lithium treatment is begun. Finally, long-term lithium therapy is associated with a *renal concentrating defect* (partial nephrogenic diabetes insipidus due to vasopressin resistance). This abnormality causes symptoms of polyuria and polydipsia in approximately 10% of patients. The concentrating defect predisposes the patient to dehydration and, therefore, to frank lithium intoxication. Polyuric patients must be counseled to maintain good hydration even under circumstances that might inhibit their interest in adequate water intake (including depression) or that increase water loss (e.g., diarrhea). They should also be instructed to report the onset of polyuria at any time in the course of lithium treatment. A patient's usual daily urine volume and glomerular filtration rate should be assessed (see Chapter 51) before lithium is started and yearly thereafter.

The *toxic effects of lithium* occur uncommonly at normal serum levels but increase in frequency as

Table 24.9. Important Drug Interactions with Lithium

Drugs that may enhance lithium toxicity
- Ace inhibitors[b]
- Amiloride[a]
- Ethacrynic acid[a]
- Furosemide[a]
- Nonsteroidal anti-inflammatory drugs[a]
- Spectinamycin[a]
- Spironolactone[a]
- Tetracycline[a]
- Thiazide diuretics[a]
- Triamterene[a]

Drugs that may increase lithium excretion
- Acetazolamide[c]
- Theophylline[c]

Drugs that may aggravate lithium tremor
- Caffeine[b]
- Neuroleptics[b]
- Theophylline[b]
- Tricyclic antidepressants[b]
- Valproate[b]

[a]Decreased renal excretion.
[b]Mechanism not established.
[c]Increased renal excretion.

serum levels exceed 1.5 mEq/L. Premonitory signs are the recurrence of gastrointestinal side effects and worsening of polyuria and hand tremor, lethargy, and clumsiness. Obvious changes in the level of consciousness are reflected in confusion, delirium, stupor, and finally coma. Focal as well as nonlocalizing neurologic signs are often present. Serum concentrations greater than 4.0 mEq/L are potentially fatal. The toxic syndrome may resolve quite slowly. A 10- to 14-day lapse before the mental state clears is not unusual, even if serum lithium levels have been brought down rapidly (e.g., by renal dialysis). Management of suspected lithium intoxication begins with discontinuation of lithium when the early signs of the disorder appear and an emergency measurement of the serum lithium concentration. If the clinical or laboratory evaluations suggest the likelihood of the toxic syndrome, hospitalization is mandatory.

The most important treatment strategy for lithium intoxication is prevention. Overingestion and inadequate renal excretion (at times, related to one of the drugs listed in Table 24.8) are the only causes of the disorder.

Valproate

Although the clinical research data supporting the use of valproate for the maintenance phase of treatment of bipolar disorder are much less extensive than for lithium, it is widely prescribed for this purpose, and many patients with bipolar disorder seen by primary care providers will be taking it.

Valproate Dosage and Schedule. Therapeutic dosages for valproate in the treatment of bipolar disorder are the same as for epilepsy. Divalproex sodium is the preparation of choice; it is prescribed at 10 to 15 mg/kg per day, or approximately 750 to 2,000 mg/day in most adults. An extended-release preparation has also become available, allowing once-a-day dosing, a factor that enhances compliance. Serum levels of 50 to 100 μg/mL are usually considered therapeutic, although this range has been borrowed from the neurology literature. Serum levels greater than 45 μg/mL have been correlated with symptom improvement in acute mania, whereas adverse effects were disproportionately associated with levels greater than 125 μg/mL (50). Studies correlating serum levels with relapse prevention in bipolar disorder are still lacking. Valproate is extensively metabolized by the liver and inhibits oxidative metabolization. Therefore, significant drug–drug interactions may occur with drugs that share these metabolic pathways. Serum concentrations of drugs that undergo oxidative metabolization (e.g., phenobarbital, tricyclic antidepressants) can increase when they are coadministered with valproate. Drugs that induce hepatic microsomal enzymes (e.g., carbamazepine) decrease the half-life of valproate and lower serum valproate levels. Conversely, agents that inhibit metabolism (e.g., fluoxetine) increase them. Valproate is 90% protein bound, and valproate toxicity can be precipitated by coadministration of other highly protein-bound drugs (e.g., warfarin).

Side Effects. The most common side effects are transient gastrointestinal discomfort, including anorexia, nausea, and vomiting. Less common central nervous system effects include sedation, ataxia, and tremor. Elevation of hepatic enzymes occurs in up to 40% of patients, usually asymptomatically during the first several months of treatment. Transient hair loss often improves with use of a selenium-containing shampoo. Mild, asymptomatic thrombocytopenia and leukopenia occur and usually respond to a reduction in dosage. Weight gain is a more troublesome long-term side effect.

Rare cases of fulminant hepatitis have occurred in patients taking valproate. The hepatic fatalities have occurred largely in children younger than 2 years of age who were taking valproate concomitantly with other antiepilepsy drugs. One 5-year retrospective review found no hepatic fatalities among patients older than 10 years of age who were taking valproate as monotherapy for epilepsy (51). Most psychiatrists monitor liver functions at 6-month intervals in patients who are taking valproate. Patients should also be instructed on the signs and symptoms of hepatic dysfunction.

Polycystic ovaries and hyperandrogenism have been reported in women on long-term valproate therapy for epilepsy. Valproate is teratogenic, and women of childbearing age who take should practice birth control.

Valproate has a high therapeutic index, and unintentional overdose is rare. Signs of overdose include somnolence, heart block, and coma.

PROGNOSIS AND LONG-TERM TREATMENT OF AFFECTIVE DISORDERS

Because of their fundamental similarities, the prognoses of unipolar depression and bipolar disorder are discussed together. Before modern treatment, patients with these disorders tended to recover spontaneously within 6 to 18 months. With modern treatments, remissions usually can be achieved much more quickly. However, approximately 20% of patients with severe major depressions may not recover fully in a 2-year period after entering treatment (52). Manic episodes tend to be briefer and are less likely to become chronic; however, some patients with bipolar disorder have chronic depressions or such frequent cycling of their illness that they are never well and may become completely disabled. *Predictors of poor outcome* include severity sufficient to require hospitalization and long duration of major symptoms (1 year) before treatment. It has also been noted that many patients who do not recover have simply not been aggressively treated after an initial treatment failure, such as failure to respond to a trial of antidepressant medication. Although some patients fail to respond to any treatment, clinical experience teaches that most correctly diagnosed patients in whom initial treatment fails will eventually respond to a second, third, or fourth treatment effort.

Relapse

A hallmark of the course of unipolar and bipolar disorders is the tendency to remit and to *relapse*. The frequency of relapse is variable. However, more than 80% patients with a major affective syndrome relapse at some point. There is a tendency for relapses to become more frequent later in the life of the patient (or later in the course of the illness).

The use of lithium and antidepressants has been shown to be beneficial in preventing recurrent affective episodes. Depressive relapses that occur in patients taking lithium or a TCA are usually less severe and of shorter duration. Lithium is the only treatment demonstrated to reduce the frequency of manic relapses. Other mood stabilizers have been shown to have antimanic activity (see earlier discussion), but current data are insufficient to establish long-term efficacy of these medications.

Maintenance Treatment

Maintenance treatment usually is continued indefinitely in patients with a clearly relapsing disorder. The patient's personal physician can often provide the basic treatment, particularly if that physician is monitoring the patient regularly for chronic medical problems. Brief visits every 2 to 3 months are sufficient when the patient is well. The objective of these visits is to monitor the mood state, the drug therapy, and the social progress of the patient. Recovery of social ease and full functioning lags several months behind the recovery of mood-related symptoms (3).

The patient and his or her family should be educated about the relapsing and remitting course of the illness, and they should know that relapses will probably be fewer, milder, and of shorter duration with drug therapy. Individual aspects of the patient's illness, particularly the early symptoms of relapse, must be remembered by the patient and the family, and there should be a plan for management of these symptoms when they recur.

Counseling the Family

Family members of patients with serious affective disorders often experience feelings of confusion, hopelessness, guilt, and recrimination toward the patient. Not only are these feelings painful, but they impede the family's attempts to support their ill relative. Physicians need to address the family's needs directly through meetings with them. Above all, the family must recognize major affective disorders as diseases and realize that these disorders are not caused by the family, the patient, or even the social predicaments affecting the patient. The family also should know that although the pathophysiology of affective disorders is unknown, empiric treatments are effective and the prognosis for complete recovery from an episode is generally good, although relapses occur frequently. These points usually require some repetition and are best repeated in response to questions that the family should be encouraged to raise in such a meeting or consultation. It is equally important to reassure families and patients with dysthymic and transiently demoralized mood states that the patients are not suffering from a major mental illness.

Educational materials on affective disorders are available from the APA and the National Institute of Mental Health, and a number of accessible and well-written books about the disorders for patients and their families are available (see General References). In addition, patients and families will gain considerable help from patient and family-member support groups (see Sources of Information in General References).

Heritability of Depression

Evidence from many studies of concordance comparing identical and nonidentical twins has established a substantial genetic contribution to major affective disorders, although the relevant genes have not yet been isolated. The modest findings to date support the supposition that genetic heterogeneity underlies these disorders and that the disease genotype comprises an ensemble of genes that act in concert to predispose people to these illnesses. It appears that a sibling or offspring of a patient with a major affective disorder has a 10% chance of developing the disorder. However, in some families this risk may be as high as 50%. Counseling of patients and their families about the genetic risk should be tailored to the needs and relevant history in each family. The major themes of counseling should be that most cases are genetically influenced, that effective treatment is available, and that treatment is greatly enhanced by early detection of the disorder.

CYCLOTHYMIC DISORDER

An episodic bipolar affective disorder that is sufficiently mild or so brief that the episodes fail to meet the APA criteria for major depression or mania (Tables 24.3 and 24.8, respectively) is categorized as a *cyclothymic disorder*. Patients with cyclothymic disorder must be distinguished from patients with the personality traits of emotional lability and self-dramatization (see Chapter 23), who often report rapid but unsustained mood changes. The family histories of cyclothymic patients are similar to those of patients with bipolar affective disorders. The long-term course is also similar to that of bipolar disorder, and 35% of such patients have been found to experience full-blown manic, hypomanic, or depressive episodes in a 2- to 3-year period of follow-up (53).

SUICIDE PREVENTION

The rate of suicide in most countries is low enough (11 per 100,000 in the United States) that successful prediction of an individual suicide at a given point in time is very unlikely.

Practical strategies in this area are to protect those with high risk in the short term and to reduce the risk in these patients over a longer term. *Risk factors for successful suicide* include depressive disorder (greater severity is associated with greater risk), older age, male gender, alcoholism, living alone, previous suicide attempt, and refusal to accept referral for psychiatric treatment. Retrospective studies of patient groups with major affective disorders in the era before affective drugs were available suggest that approximately 15% of the deaths were caused by suicide. In addition, clinical observations suggest that the risk of suicide increases when improvement begins (or just after a depressed patient is discharged from the hospital) or when the depressive ruminations become frankly delusional convictions. Retrospective studies also suggest that there are fewer suicides among patients treated with ECT or long-term lithium therapy (54).

When evaluating any patient with depressed mood, direct and open inquiry should be made regarding suicidal ideas ("Are you having any thoughts of hurting yourself?"), and the patient should be asked about specific plans that he or she may have formulated ("Have you thought about how you might try to harm yourself?"). An assessment of the lethality of the patient's plans and the availability of the means to carry them out should be made. Seriously depressed patients should always be asked about the presence of firearms in the home, and any weapons should be removed, even in the face of a patient's disavowal of plans to use them. One study of adolescent suicide showed that the presence of a firearm in the home increased the risk of completed suicide regardless of whether the weapon was a handgun or a long gun, kept loaded or unloaded, locked up or not (55). Information about the capability and availability of constant family supervision is also helpful in determining whether treatment may be attempted safely on an outpatient basis. Asking patients to "*contract for safety*"—that is, to promise verbally or even in writing to contact a family member or the physician, or to call police or go to an emergency room, if their suicidal impulses should intensify or become difficult to resist—has frequently been recommended in the management of suicidal patients. Obtaining a "*no-harm contract*" helps the physician engage the patient in a discussion of his or her suicidal thinking, emphasizes the physician's concern for the safety of the patient, communicates the physician's assessment of the gravity of the situation, and also requires the development and discussion of an action plan should suicidal thinking worsen. This "contract" does not, however, substitute for a complete assessment of the patient's risk for suicidal behavior, and it is only as effective as the soundness of the underlying therapeutic alliance (56). The suicide risk evaluation should also be guided by the knowledge that delusional depressed patients have a significantly increased risk of suicide and that patients with prior suicide attempts are more likely than others to attempt it again when depressed.

It should be recalled that most people who commit suicide with pills have obtained the lethal dose in a single prescription at a recent visit to a physician (57). Such an amount could represent as little as a 1- to 2-week supply of a TCA. Therefore, small prescriptions and, at times, family supervision of medication use are needed. Finally, short-term protection of patients with suicidal intent via hospitalization, including involuntary commitment, is sometimes required. The most crucial activities of physicians in preventing suicides, however, are the diagnosis, treatment, and prophylaxis of major depressive episodes.

Most patients who present to emergency facilities after an *overdose of pills* do not have major depression but rather an adjustment disorder or personality disorder, and they usually do not die by suicide. However, they should be methodically evaluated in the same manner as noted previously, because many such patients are prone to take overdoses again when stressed. These patients may benefit from brief hospital admissions when social support for them is lacking and suicidal feelings are intense. All should have some outpatient counseling.

General References*

American Psychiatric Association. **Diagnostic and Statistical Manual of Mental Disorders.** 4th ed. (DSM-IV). Washington, DC: American Psychiatric Association, 1994.

Beliles K, Stoudemire A. Psychopharmacologic treatment of depression in the medically ill. Psychosomatics 1998;39:S2.

Montano CB. Primary care issues related to the treatment of depression in elderly patients. J Clin Psychiatry 1999;60:45.

Reeve A. Recognizing and treating anxiety and depression in adolescents: normal and abnormal responses. Med Clin North Am 2000;84:891.

Williams JW, Mulrow CD, Chiquette E, et al. **A systematic review of newer pharmacotherapies for depression in adults: evidence report summary.** Ann Intern Med 2000;132:743.

Wisner KL, Zarin DA, Holmboe ES, et al. Risk-benefit decision making for treatment of depression during pregnancy. Am J Psychiatry 2000;1577:12;1933.

Wollen M, Simon G. Managing depression in medical outpatients. N Engl J Med 2000;343:1942.

Patient Information and Education

American Psychiatric Association. Let's talk facts about depression; Let's talk facts about bipolar disorder–manic depression; Let's talk facts about teen suicide; Let's talk facts about mental health of the elderly.

These pamphlets are available from the American Psychiatric Association, 1400 K St. NW, Washington, DC 20005, or on-line at: http://www.psych.org/public_info/. Accessed December 10, 2001.

National Institute of Mental Health. Depression; Let's talk about depression; Bipolar Disorder; Depression: what every woman should know.

Available from the National Institute of Mental Health, 5600 Fishers Lane, Rockville, MD 20857. Similar information is available on-line at: http://www.nimh.nih.gov/publicat. Accessed December 10, 2001.

DePaulo JR, Ablow KR. How to cope with depression: a complete guide for you and your family. New York: Ballantine Books, 1996.

*Bold print (general references) and bold numerals (specific references) denote published controlled clinical trials, meta-analyses, or consensus-based recommendations.

Mondimore, FM. Depression: the mood disease. Baltimore: Johns Hopkins University Press, 1995.

Mondimore, FM. Bipolar disorder: a guide for patients and families. Baltimore: Johns Hopkins University Press, 1999.

Sources of Information about Support Groups for Depressed Patients and Their Families

Depression and Related Affective Disorders Association (DRADA), Meyer 3-181, Johns Hopkins Hospital, 600 N. Wolfe St., Baltimore, MD 21287-7381 (telephone 410-955-4647), or visit their website at: http://www.hopkinsmedicine.org/drada. Accessed December 10, 2001.

National Alliance for the Mentally Ill (NAMI), 2101 Wilson Blvd., Suite 302, Arlington, VA 22201 (telephone 800-950-6264), or visit their website at: http://www.nami.org. Accessed December 10, 2001.

National Depressive and Manic Depressive Association, 730 N. Franklin St., Suite 501, Chicago, IL 60610 (telephone 800-82-NDMDA), or visit their website at: http://www.ndmda.org. Accessed December 10, 2001.

National Mental Health Association (NMHA), National Mental Health Information Center, 1021 Prince St., Alexandria, VA 23314-2971 (telephone 800-969-6642), or visit their website at: http://www.nmha.org. Accessed December 10, 2001.

Specific References

1. Wells KB, Hays RD, Burnam MA, et al. Detection of depressive disorder for patients receiving prepaid or fee for service care. JAMA 1989;262:3298.
2. Simon GE, VonKorff M, Barlow W. Health care costs of primary care patients with recognized depression. Arch Gen Psychiatry 1995;52:850.
3. Mintz J, Mintz LI, Arruda MJ, et al. Treatments of depression and the functional capacity to work. Arch Gen Psychiatry 1992;49:761.
4. Wells KB, Stewart A, Hays RD, et al. The functioning and well being of depressed patients: results from the medical outcomes study. JAMA 1989;262:914.
5. Guze SB, Robins E. Suicide and primary affective disorders. Br J Psychiatry 1970;117:437.
6. Egeland JA, Sussex JN. Suicide and family loading for affective disorders. JAMA 1985;254:915.
7. Pratt LA, Ford DE, Crum RM, et al. Depression, psychotropic medication, and risk of myocardial infarction. Circulation 1996;94:3123.
8. Frasure-Smith N, Lesperance F, Talajic M. Depression and 18 month prognosis after myocardial infarction. Circulation 1995;91:999.
9. Greenberg PE, Stiglin LE, Finkelstein SN, et al. The economic burden of depression in 1990. J Clin Psychiatry 1993;54:405.
10. Greenberg PE, Stiglin LE, Finkelstein SN, et al. Depression: a neglected major illness. J Clin Psychiatry 1993;54:419.
11. Schaefer C, Quesenberry CP Jr, Wi S. Mortality following conjugal bereavement and the effects of a shared environment. Am J Epidemiol 1995;141:1142.
12. Spitzer RL, Kroenke K, Linzer M, et al. Health-related quality of life in primary care patients with mental disorders. JAMA 1995;274:1511.
13. Wilson DR, Widmer RB, Cadoret RJ, et al. Somatic symptoms: a major feature of depression in a family practice. J Affect Disord 1983;5:199.
14. Markowitz JC, Moran ME, Kocsis JH, et al. Prevalence and comorbidity of dysthymic disorder among psychiatric outpatients. J Affect Disord 1992;24:63.
15. **15.** Williams JW, Barrett J, Oxman T, et al. Treatment of dysthymia and minor depression in primary care, a randomized controlled trial in older adults. JAMA 2000;284:1519.
16. **16.** Robins LN, Helzer JE, Weissman MM, et al. Lifetime prevalence of specific psychiatric disorders in three sites. Arch Gen Psychiatry 1984;41:949.
17. Judd LL, Akiskal HS, Maser JD, et al. A prospective 12-year study of subsyndromal and syndromal depressive symptoms in unipolar major depressive disorders. Arch Gen Psychiatry 1998;55:694.
18. Suppes T, Dennehy EB, Gibbons EW. The longitudinal course of bipolar disorder. J Clin Psychiatry 2000;61[Suppl 9]:23.
19. German PS, Shapiro S, Skinner EA. Mental health of elderly: use of health and mental health services. J Am Geriatr Soc 1985;33:246.
20. Shapiro S, Skinner EA, Kramer M, et al. Measuring need for mental health services in a general population. Med Care 1985;23:1033.
21. Patten SB. Medication use and major depressive symptoms in a community population. Compr Psychiatry 2000;42:124.
22. **22.** Ried LD, McFarland BH, Johnson RE, et al. Beta-blockers and depression: the more the murkier? Ann Pharmacother 1998;32:699.
23. Seiner SJ, Mallya G. Treating depression in patients with cardiovascular disease. Harv Rev Psychiatry 1999;7:85.
24. Brown ES, Suppes T. Mood symptoms during corticosteroid therapy: a review. Harv Rev Psychiatry 1998;5:239.
25. Gleason O, Yates W. Five cases of interferon-alpha-induced depression treated with antidepressant therapy. Psychosomatics 1999;40:510.
26. Beliles K, Stoudemire A. Psychopharmacologic treatment of depression in the medically ill. Psychosomatics 1998;39:S2.
27. Whooley MA, Avins AL, Miranda J, et al. Case-finding instruments for depression: two questions are as good as many. J Gen Intern Med 1997;12:439.
28. Fawcett J, Barken RL. Efficacy issues with antidepressants. J Clin Psychiatry 1997;58[Suppl 6]:3222.
29. Schmidt ME, Fava M, Robinson J. The efficacy and safety of a new enteric-coated formulation of fluoxetine given once weekly during the continuation treatment of major depressive disorder. J Clin Psychiatry 2000;61:851.
30. **30.** Shelton RC, Keller MB, Gelenberg A, et al. Effectiveness of St John's wort in major depression: a randomized controlled trial. JAMA 2001;285:1978.
31. Mascholon D, Fava M. Docosahexanoic acid and omega-3 fatty acids in depression. Psychiatr Clin North Am 2000;23:785.
32. Kapur S, Mieczkowski T, Mann JJ. Antidepressant medications and the relative risk of suicide attempt and suicide. JAMA 1992;268:3441.
33. Pastuszak A, Schick-Boschetto B, Zuber C, et al. Pregnancy outcome following first-trimester exposure to fluoxetine. JAMA 1993;269:2246.
34. **34.** Tignol J. A double-blind, randomized, fluoxetine-controlled, multicenter study of paroxetine in the treatment of depression. J Clin Psychopharmacol 1993;13[Suppl 2]:188S.
35. Zajecka J. Strategies for the treatment of antidepressant-related sexual dysfunction. J Clin Psychiatry 2001;62[Suppl 3]:35.
36. Veith RC, Raskind MA, Caldwell JH, et al. Cardiovascular effects of tricyclic antidepressants in depressed patients with chronic heart disease. N Engl J Med 1982;306:954.
37. Posternak MA, Zimmerman M. Switching versus augmentation: a prospective, naturalistic comparison in depressed, treatment-resistant patients. J Clin Psychiatry 2001;62:135.
38. Thase ME, Blomgren SL, Birkett MA. Fluoxetine treatment of patients with major depressive disorder who failed initial treatment with sertraline. J Clin Psychiatry 1997;58:16.
39. Fava M. Management of nonresponse and intolerance: switching strategies. J Clin Psychiatry 2000;61[Suppl 2]:10.
40. Maj M, Veltro F, Pirozzi R, et al. Pattern of recurrence of illness after recovery from an episode of major depression: a prospective study. Am J Psychiatry 1992;149:795.
41. **41.** Kupfer DJ, Frank E, Perel JM, et al. Five-year outcome for maintenance therapies in recurrent depression. Arch Gen Psychiatry 1992;49:769.
42. Zajecka J, Tracy K, Mitchell S. Discontinuation symptoms after treatment with serotonin reuptake inhibitors: a literature review. J Clin Psychiatry 1997;58:291.
43. Rosenbaum JF, Fava M, Hoog SL, et al. Selective serotonin reuptake inhibitor discontinuation syndrome: a randomized clinical trial. Biol Psychiatry 1998;44:75.
44. Karasu TB. Toward a clinical model of psychotherapy for depression: II. An integrative and selective treatment approach. Am J Psychiatry 1990;147:269.
45. Kupfer DJ, Frank E. Relapse in recurrent unipolar depression. Am J Psychiatry 1987;144:86.

46. Squires LR, Chace PM. Memory functions six to nine months after electroconvulsive therapy. Arch Gen Psychiatry 1975;32:1557.
47. Schou M. Forty years of lithium treatment. Arch Gen Psychiatry 1997;54:9.
48. Dardennes R, Even C, Bange F, et al. Comparison of carbamazepine and lithium in the prophylaxis of bipolar disorders: a meta-analysis. Br J Psychiatry 1995;166:378.
49. Frye MA, Ketter TA, Kimbril TA, et al. A placebo-controlled study of lamotrigine and gabapentin monotherapy in refractory mood disorders. J Clin Psychopharmacol 2000;20:607.
50. Bowden CL, Janiak PG, Orsulak P, et al. Relation of serum valproate concentration to response in mania. Am J Psychiatry 1996;153:765.
51. Dreifuss FE, Santilli N, Langer DH, et al. Valproic acid hepatic fatalities: a retrospective review. Neurology 1987;37:379.
52. Keller MB, Klerman GL, Lavori PW. Long-term outcome of episodes of major depression. JAMA 1984;252:240.
53. Akiskal HS, Djenderejiian AH, Rosenthal RH, et al. Cyclothymic disorder: validating criteria for inclusion in the bipolar affective group. Am J Psychiatry 1977;134:1227.
54. Nierenberg AA, Gray SM, Grandin LD. Mood disorders and suicide. J Clin Psychiatry 2001;62[Suppl 25]:27.
55. Brent D, Perper J, Allman C, et al. The presence and accessibility of firearms in the homes of adolescent suicides: a case control study. JAMA 1991;266:2989.
56. Simon RI. The suicide prevention contract: clinical, legal and risk management issues. J Am Acad Psychiatry Law 1999;27:445.
57. Murphy GE. The physician's responsibility for suicide. I: An error of commission. II: Errors of omission. Ann Intern Med 1975;82:301.

CHAPTER 25

Schizophrenia and Related Psychotic Disorders

ANDREW F. ANGELINO, MD
CHESTER W. SCHMIDT, Jr., MD

Schizophrenia is a mental disorder, or group of disorders, for which the etiology is unknown. The American Psychiatric Association (APA) lists the essential features of the disorder as the presence of certain psychotic features for a significant length of time (i.e., a 1-month period, with some signs persisting for at least 6 months); characteristic chronic symptoms involving multiple psychological processes; deterioration from a previous level of functioning; and median age at onset in the mid-twenties for men and late twenties for women. As noted later (see Diagnosis), none of these symptoms is pathognomonic for schizophrenia, and each is seen in other psychotic states.

Familiarity with schizophrenia is important to the generalist for three reasons: In the prodromal stage, the patient often presents first to a general physician; the interested generalist may provide much of the care for a patient with this lifelong disorder; and patients with schizophrenia have significant medical comorbidity as a result of diminished self-care and adverse effects of psychotropic medications.

EPIDEMIOLOGY

Schizophrenia has been found in all societies throughout the world. The distribution is similar throughout all populations. Epidemiologic studies in Western societies have found the lifetime prevalence of schizophrenia to be slightly less than 1 case per

100 persons. Lifetime incidence rates have been reported to range from 0.6% to 1.9% (1). Studies of incidence and prevalence in Europe using strict and somewhat narrow criteria for schizophrenia have produced case numbers and rates lower than similar studies done in the United States, which used broader criteria. In 1943, Lemkau et al. (2) determined that 15% to 25% of patients with schizophrenia never entered the hospital. Developments in psychopharmacology over the past three decades and the wide availability of ambulatory treatment resources have expanded the number of patients who never enter the hospital and greatly reduced the duration of confinement for those who do require hospitalization.

Schizophrenia is equally common in men and women. Onset is usually during young adulthood, with the first hospitalization usually occurring between the ages of 25 and 34 years. Most schizophrenic patients are single and are members of lower socioeconomic groups. The proposed reason for the clustering of patients in the lower socioeconomic groups is a downward social drift resulting from deterioration of social and vocational function.

CAUSES

The cause or causes of schizophrenia remain unknown. Numerous constitutional, genetic, neurologic, anatomic, biochemical, nutritional, psychosocial, and psychoanalytic theories have been offered. Present evidence strongly suggests some genetic transmission, because schizophrenia has long been known to run in families. The increased risk ranges from 3% for second-degree relatives, to 7% to 15% for siblings and children of one schizophrenic parent, to 40% for children of two schizophrenic parents. Concordance rates are 10% to 15% in dizygotic twins and 45% in monozygotic twins (3). Children born of schizophrenic parents but raised in adoptive families also show a higher incidence of the disease. This evidence indicates that transmission of schizophrenia is not explained by simple mendelian inheritance. Current research is seeking a polygenic mechanism, possibly with incomplete penetrance. Further, the study of "biomarkers," subtle neurologic signs and physical features, is emerging to help determine the precise genes involved.

In regard to the pathology of schizophrenia, many autopsy and neuroimaging efforts have played a significant role in the last decade. As the data emerge, it is becoming evident that schizophrenia is not a disease of one specific brain area but rather a functional disorder of brain systems which affects the developing brain of adolescents and young adults, causing several types of symptoms to emerge gradually. A significant research effort is now being directed at the heteromodal association cortex, a group of related brain structures thought to be involved in the higher, executive functions of the neocortex (4).

Neurochemical mechanisms involved in the production of symptoms of schizophrenia are still being investigated. An important clue emerged from studies of the pharmacologic effects of antipsychotic agents on schizophrenia. These medicines antagonize dopamine-mediated neurotransmission, leading to the speculation that excessive activity of the dopamine systems may be part of a biochemical defect in schizophrenic patients. Research has now shown that cortical serotoninergic systems modify the activity of the mesocortical and mesolimbic dopamine systems (5) and has led to the development of newer medicines that tend to have reduced rates of certain adverse effects.

NATURAL HISTORY OF SCHIZOPHRENIA

Although the first episode of acute psychosis usually occurs in late adolescence or early adulthood, *prodromal manifestations* of the disease are often present for years before the acute episode. During the prodromal phase, patients gradually withdraw from social relationships. They become indifferent to their grooming, ignore social graces and social rituals, and may develop suspicious attitudes about others. They appear different, peculiar, and sometimes bizarre. Timing of the onset of this phase plays a significant role in the achievement of social, educational, and occupational milestones. In some patients, the deterioration of social and vocational skills may be so striking that the patient seems to have a changed personality. In many cases of early-onset schizophrenia, the patient has developed only marginal social and vocational skills, so his or her deterioration appears more insidious.

In one study of the prodromal stage of schizophrenia (10), most patients demonstrated some dysphoria (anxiety or depression) in association with social deterioration, and more than half of them developed vague somatic complaints for which they sought help from a generalist physician.

Psychiatrists classify psychotic symptoms into categories of positive, negative, and disorganized symptoms. *Positive symptoms* include delusions (fixed, false, idiosyncratic ideas) and hallucinations (perceptions without stimuli). Thought disorders—including loosening of associations, illogical or magical thinking, and inability to carry on discourse—and bizarre behavior and emotions make up the *disorganized symptoms.* The *negative symptoms* include apathy, preoccupation with fantasies and an inner psychological world (autism), inability to carry out goal-directed behavior because of preoccupation with consequences of alternatives (ambivalence), and anhedonia (loss of pleasure in activities). Occasionally, patients display catatonic symptoms, which include stereotypical movements, mutism, and sometimes rigid posturing.

Acute psychotic episodes are marked by the development or exacerbation of any of the positive or disorganized symptoms and are often brought on by stressful life events. Before antipsychotic medications were available, these episodes could last from weeks to years. Currently, most episodes are brought under pharmacologic control within several weeks. After treatment, positive and disorganized psychotic symptoms subside and in some cases seem to disappear completely. Some patients, however, develop a more chronic course, with persistent positive and disorganized symptoms. Many patients also suffer from prominent negative symptoms, which may be evident only between acute exacerbations. With each subsequent psychotic episode, the patient may slip further into a dependent, regressed state in which he or she is unable to function and becomes entirely dependent on family or society. Scholastic and vocational ability often diminish. Fewer than 20% of patients work full-time; most are financially supported by welfare programs or federal disability programs. Institutionalization is required in some cases because the patients lose all ability to care for themselves.

Schizophrenia is a lifelong disease consisting of psychotic symptoms that periodically become intense and an arrest or deterioration of social and vocational functioning, probably caused by massive withdrawal of interest in the outside world. The devastation of the disease is supported by the fact that 50% of schizophrenics attempt suicide at least once, and 10% complete suicide (6).

DIAGNOSIS

The diagnosis of schizophrenia, especially during the initial episodes of acute psychosis, is based on clinical judgment and diagnostic criteria that, until recently, were unreliable. No pathognomonic symptoms, signs, or laboratory findings point to the diagnosis. The medical history of the patient does not contribute to the diagnosis, and, as discussed earlier, family history of the disease provides only partial information.

The diagnostic criteria for schizophrenia described in the APA's *Diagnostic and Statistical Manual of Mental Disorders,* 4th edition (DSM-IV), are an excellent synthesis of several recognized diagnostic formulations (Table 25.1). Diagnosis rests on the findings of the symptoms of psychosis elicited by a mental status examination (see Chapter 19) and a history that documents the prodromal phase.

Table 25.1. Diagnostic Criteria for Schizophrenia

A. Characteristic symptoms: Two (or more) of the following, each present for a significant portion of time during a 1-month period (or less if successfully treated):
   1. Delusions
   2. Hallucinations
   3. Disorganized speech (e.g., frequent derailment or incoherence)
   4. Grossly disorganized or catatonic behavior
   5. Negative symptoms, i.e., affective flattening, alogia, or avolition
      (Note: Only one criterion A symptom is required if delusions are bizarre or hallucinations consist of a voice keeping up a running commentary on the person's behavior or thoughts, or two or more voices conversing with each other.)

B. Social/occupational dysfunction: For a significant portion of the time since the onset of the disturbance, one or more major areas of functioning such as work, interpersonal relations, or self-care is markedly below the level achieved before the onset (or when the onset is in childhood or adolescence, failure to achieve expected level of interpersonal, academic, or occupational achievement).

C. Duration: Continuous signs of the disturbance persist for at least 6 months. This 6-month period must include at least 1 month of symptoms (or less if successfully treated) that meet criterion A (i.e., active-phase symptoms), and may include periods of prodromal or residual symptoms. During these prodromal or residual periods, the signs of the disturbance may be manifested by only negative symptoms or two or more symptoms listed in criterion A present in an attenuated form (e.g., odd beliefs, unusual perceptual experiences).

D. Schizoaffective and mood disorder exclusion: Schizoaffective disorder and mood disorder with psychotic features have been ruled out because either (a) no major depressive, manic or mixed episodes have occurred concurrently with the active-phase symptoms, or (b) if mood episodes have occurred during active-phase symptoms, their total duration has been brief relative to the duration of the active and residual periods.

E. Substance/general medical condition exclusion: The disturbance is not due to the direct psychologic effects of a substance (e.g., a drug of abuse, a medication) or a general medical condition.

F. Relationship to a pervasive developmental disorder: If there is a history of autistic disorder or another pervasive developmental disorder, the additional diagnosis of schizophrenia is made only if prominent delusions or hallucinations are also present for at least a month (or less if successfully treated).

Reprinted with permission from Diagnostic and statistical manual of mental disorders. 4th ed. Washington, DC: American Psychiatric Association, 1994.

DIFFERENTIAL DIAGNOSIS

Any kind of psychotic state may resemble acute schizophrenia. However, differences in symptoms permit differentiation and diagnosis. *Delirium, dementia, and amnestic and other cognitive disorders* (see Chapter 26) are marked by disturbances in consciousness (delirium); by disorientation with respect to time, place, and person; and by impairment in intellectual functions (e.g., memory, calculations). In addition, especially in patients younger than 50 years of age, there is usually evidence from the history, physical examination, and laboratory tests of specific organic findings that are etiologically related to the mental condition. *Single psychotic symptoms,* such as persecutory delusions or auditory hallucinations, may occur *de novo* in elderly patients as symptoms of dementia or paraphrenia (see Chapter 26). Effects of illicit drugs, especially amphetamine and phencyclidine (see Chapter 29), may mimic the acute phase of schizophrenia. In addition, a number of *prescription drugs* may occasionally produce hallucinations and other manifestations that suggest psychosis (Table 25.2). History of drug use and absence of the prodromal phase help differentiate these conditions from schizophrenia.

The *psychotic symptoms of major affective episodes* (both mania and depression; see Chapter 24) can also be similar to those seen during acute episodes in the course of schizophrenia. Affective disorders differ from schizophrenia in that psychotic symptoms (e.g., delusions, hallucinations) appear after the development of the affective disturbance (depression or mania) and generally remit when the affective disturbance remits. In schizophrenia, marked depression or mania may appear, but the affective disturbance occurs after the onset of the psychotic symptoms, which often exist as well in the complete absence of affective symptoms. These principles of differential diagnosis are far from perfect, and patients with both types of disorder

Table 25.2. Prescription Drugs that Have Been Reported Occasionally to Cause Hallucinations or Other Manifestations of Psychosis

- Angiotensing converting enzyme inhibitors
- Acyclovir (Zovirax)
- Albuterol (Proventil; Ventolin)
- Amantadine (Symmetrel)
- Amiodarone (Cordarone)
- Amphetamine-like drugs
- Anabolic steroids
- Anticonvulsants
- Antidepressants, tricyclic
- Antihistamines
- Atropine and anticholinergics
- Baclofen (Lioresal)
- Benzodiazepines
- Beta-adrenergic blockers
- Bromocriptine (Parlodel)
- Bupropion (Wellbutrin)
- Caffeine
- Chloroquine (Aralen)
- Ciprofloxacin (Cipro)
- Clonidine (Catapres)
- Cocaine
- Corticosteroids (prednisone, cortisone, adrenocorticotropic hormone, other)
- Cyclobenzaprine (Flexeril)
- Cyclosporine (Sandimmune)
- Deet (Off)
- Digitalis glycosides
- Disopyramide (Norpace)
- Disulfiram (Antabuse)
- Ethchlorvynol (Placidyl)
- Fluoxetine (Prozac)
- Ganciclovir (Cytovene)
- Histamine H_2-receptor antagonists
- Isoniazid (INH, others)
- Levodopa (Sinemet)
- Methyldopa (Aldomet)
- Methylphenidate (Ritalin)
- Metronidazole (Flagyl)
- Nalidixic acid (NegGram)
- Narcotics
- Nonsteroidal anti-inflammatory drugs
- Pantazocine (Talwin)
- Pergolide (Permax)
- Phenelzine (Nardil)
- Phenylephrine (Neo-Synephrine)
- Prazosin (Minipress)
- Procainamide (Pronestyl)
- Procaine penicillin G
- Pseudoephedrine
- Quinacrine (Atabrine)
- Quinidine
- Salicylates
- Selegiline (Eldepryl)
- Sulfonamides
- Tamoxifen (Nolvadex)
- Thyroid hormones
- Trazodone (Desyrel)
- Verapamil
- Zidovudine (Retrovir)

Adapted from Drugs that cause psychiatric symptoms. Med Lett 1993;35:65 (which includes references to reports).

have been mislabeled. Because the prognosis associated with schizophrenia is often worse than of affective disorders, mislabeling has significant consequences, including attitudes toward the patient and actual treatment provided.

Schizoid and schizotypal personality disorders, described in Chapter 23, are personality types that may share some of the features of withdrawal from society, but they are not accompanied by the psychotic features seen in schizophrenia (Table 25.1). There is speculation that these personality types may comprise part of a spectrum of schizophrenic illness, an idea supported by data showing higher rates of these types in families of patients with schizophrenia.

TREATMENT AND PROGNOSIS

Antipsychotic Drugs

The primary treatment of the acute and chronic psychotic manifestations of schizophrenia in ambulatory or hospitalized patients is with the antipsychotic agents. There are several classes of antipychotics, with numerous drugs in each class. The common drugs are listed in Table 25.3, together with available strengths and potency equivalents to chlorpromazine.

Although the structures of the various antipsychotics are well known, the pharmacology is not. Dose–response relationships have not yet been worked out for humans. The drugs generally produce effects within 1 hour after oral administration and within 10 to 15 minutes after intramuscular injection. They are lipid soluble with a high affinity for cell membranes. The drugs and their metabolites are distributed generally throughout the central nervous system with no local or regional accumulation. Metabolites are partially excreted each day, with significant portions retained in lipid-rich tissues and connective tissues. As these tissues become saturated, the drugs undergo slow turnover. The drugs are detoxified and inactivated mainly through oxidation by hepatic microsomal enzymes, and they are excreted through both bile and urine.

There is no evidence that these agents are addicting, although tolerance to some of the side effects (sedation, hypotension, anticholinergic effects, parkinsonian symptoms) has been reported. The drugs are fairly safe but may induce delirium if used in great excess. Further, antipsychotic drugs prolong the QTc (Q-T interval corrected for heart rate) to a varying degree depending on the specific agent, and care should be exercised when prescribing them to patients with cardiac conduction delays, because cases of sudden cardiac death have been reported. If patients are found to have a prolonged QTc interval (longer than 500 μsec), the antipsychotic medicine should be evaluated for discontinuation, and consultation with a cardiologist should be obtained.

The mechanisms of action of the antipsychotics are not fully understood. Although it has been speculated that specific antipsychotic activity may result from the dopamine-antagonist action of these agents, the drugs have a variety of effects on many metabolic processes. Newer, so-called atypical, antipsychotics affect neurotransmitters other than dopamine, especially serotonin, and additional dopamine receptor types compared with the older agents. This is the proposed basis for their lower rates of certain side effects, such as extrapyramidal symptoms, and it may be the mechanism of action of their effect on negative symptoms. These atypicals include clozapine (Clozaril) (16), risperidone (Risperdal) (17), olanzapine (Zyprexa) (18), quetiapine (Seroquel), and ziprasidone (Geodon).

Treatment of Acute Psychotic Episodes

All antipsychotics are equally efficacious for controlling positive psychotic symptoms associated with schizophrenia, but only the atypical antipsychotics have any efficacy in the treatment of negative symptoms. The choice of one drug over another depends on predicted differences in side effects, the history of a particular patient's response, and the clinician's familiarity with the agent. The treatment of acute psychotic episodes should begin with the equivalent of 300 to 1,000 mg of chlorpromazine (Thorazine) per day, in divided doses (usually three times daily). This dose range is equivalent to 2.5 to 10 mg of haloperidol (Haldol), which may be given as a single or divided dose. Only one antipsychotic should be given at a time, because administration of more than one agent increases the probability of side effects.

Table 25.3. Available Strengths and Equivalent Doses of Commonly Used Neuroleptic Antipsychotic Agents

Generic Name	Trade Name	Available Strengths of Oral Preparations (mg)	Approximate Equivalent Dose of Chlorpromazine (mg)
Phenothiazines			
Aliphatic			
Chlorpromazine[a]	Thorazine	10, 25, 50, 100, 200	100
Triflupromazine	Vesprin	10, 25	30
Piperidines			
Mesoridazine	Serentil	10, 25, 100	50
Piperacetazine	Quide	10, 15	12
Thioridazine[a]	Mellaril	10, 15, 25, 50, 100, 150, 200	95
Piperazines			
Fluphenazine[a,b]	Prolixin, Permitil	1, 2.5, 5, 10	2
Perphenazine[a]	Trilafon	2, 4, 8, 16	10
Trifluoperazine[a]	Stelazine	1, 2, 5, 10	5
Thioxanthenes			
Aliphatic			
Chlorprothixene	Taractan	10, 25, 50, 100	65
Piperazine			
Thiothixene[a]	Navane	1, 2, 5, 10, 25	5
Dibenzazepine			
Loxapine	Loxitane, Daxolin	10, 25, 50	15
Butyrophenone			
Haloperidol[a,c]	Haldol	0.5, 1, 2, 5, 10	2
Indolone			
Molindone	Moban	5, 10, 25	10
Atypical			
Clozapine	Clozaril	25, 100	50
Risperidone	Risperdal	1, 2, 3, 4	1–2
Olanzapine	Zyprexa	5, 7.5, 10, 15	2–3
Quetiapine	Seroquel	25, 100, 200	50
Ziprasidone	Geodon	20, 40, 80	20

[a]Generic available.

[b]Long-acting fluphenazine decanoate or enanthate, for injection, comes in a concentration of 25 mg/mL; also available for injection as fluphenazine hydrochloride, a short-acting preparation.

[c]Haloperidol for injection comes in a concentration of 2 mg/mL

Combativeness, hyperactivity, and agitation are usually controlled within 24 to 48 hours after beginning treatment. If these symptoms are not modified within that period, the dosage should be increased, up to the equivalent of 800 to 1,000 mg of chlorpromazine, or 7.5 to 10 mg of haloperidol. It may be necessary to administer the drugs intramuscularly during the acute phase of agitation if the patient is unable to take oral medication. Haloperidol 2 to 5 mg is a good choice for intramuscular injection because of its minimal effects on circulatory regulation. For patients who do not respond to an adequate trial (4 to 6 weeks) of at least one antipsychotic, a trial of clozapine should be considered. Because clozapine causes fatal agranulocytosis in up to 1% of patients, a history of blood dyscrasias and poor compliance are contraindications. Clozapine trials should last at least 3 months at a dosage of 200 to 600 mg/day.

Delusions, hallucinations, associational defects, negativism, and withdrawal begin to subside within 1 to 2 weeks after treatment begins. Continued improvement of these symptoms may take place over an additional 4 to 8 weeks. If very high dosages of antipsychotic agents is initially required, the dosage should be cautiously reduced to the equivalent of 400 to 600 mg of chlorpromazine, because high doses of conventional antipsychotic agents can worsen apathy and negativism. This adjustment in dosage can usually begin 1 to 2 weeks after the peak dosage is reached.

Early Side Effects of Antipsychotics

Antipsychotic drugs with lower potency per milligram, such as chlorpromazine (Table 25.3), produce *sedation,* which can be a useful side effect in treating hyperactive or combative patients but is a disadvantage in regressed, withdrawn patients. The *anticholinergic properties* of all phenothiazines produces annoying symptoms of dry mouth, stuffy nose, blurred vision, and occasional urinary retention in older patients and delirium at high dosages. Side effects often abate or disappear within 2 to 4 weeks. The most worrisome side effect is drug-induced *Parkinson syndrome,* also called *extrapyramidal symptoms.* This occurs with greatest frequency in association with drugs of higher potency per milligram, such as haloperidol, the piperazine class of phenothiazines, thioxanthene, loxapine, and molindone (Table 25.3). The syndrome usually appears within 5 to 30 days after beginning treatment and includes tremor, rigidity, bradykinesia, fixed facies, drooling, and stooped posture. Because this problem commonly causes patients to discontinue antipsychotic treatment, it should be managed properly. In most cases reduction of dosage or addition of small amounts of an antiparkinsonism agent controls these side effects (see Chapter 90). The parkinsonian effects of antipsychotic drugs tend to decrease after 1 or 2 months. Therefore, withdrawal of antiparkinsonism drugs should be attempted after 6 to 12 weeks. Prophylactic treatment of all patients with antiparkinsonism drugs is generally discouraged because of the additional anticholinergic effects of these drugs.

The incidence of extrapyramidal symptoms is lower with the *newer antipsychotic agents* such as olanzapine, quetiapine, and ziprasidone. Risperidone also shows a lower incidence at lower doses, but the symptoms appear at doses greater than 8 to 10 mg with the same regularity as with haloperidol or other potent agents.

Acute dystonias occur in some patients within 1 to 5 days after initiation of any antipsychotic; these effects are most often seen with haloperidol and the piperazine class of phenothiazines. The symptoms are sudden onset of severe, tonic contractions of the musculature of the neck (torticollis), the spine, the heels (opisthotonos), the extraocular muscles (oculogyric crises), the mouth, and the tongue. These symptoms remit promptly after intravenous or intramuscular injection of diphenhydramine (Benadryl, 25 to 50 mg) or benztropine (Cogentin, 1 to 2 mg). Antipsychotic treatment can be continued in these patients; an antiparkinsonism agent should be added for about 1 month to protect against recurrent dystonia. *Akathisia* may also occur early in treatment. This side effect is marked by motor restlessness with pacing, fidgeting, and restless legs. It does not resolve with treatment as predictably as the acute dystonias do. Treatment is the same as that prescribed for drug-induced parkinsonism. In a small, controlled trial the lipophilic beta-blocker, propranolol, in daily doses of 20 to 60 mg, was shown to improve symptoms of akathisia in most patients (7).

A number of *nonneurologic side effects* can result from administration of the antipsychotics. *Cardiovascular toxicity* includes orthostatic hypotension; this problem is most commonly seen with the aliphatic and piperidine classes of phenothiazines and with chlorprothixene. Frank syncope may occur, rarely, after intramuscular administration of low-potency antipsychotics. Many agents have been shown to prolong the QTc to varying degrees. In particular, thioridazine and mesoridazine have been shown to cause significant QTc prolongation, and those drugs contain warnings in their prescription information mandated by the U.S. Food and Drug Administration. Torsades de pointes and ventricular tachycardia are rare side effects; there are no baseline characteristics that help one recognize patients at risk for this problem (see Chapter 64 for a discussion of cardiac arrhythmias). Reversible *cholestatic jaundice* can occur as an allergic response. *Agranulocytosis* is an exceedingly rare side effect.

The *neuroleptic malignant syndrome* is a rare, and occasionally lethal, idiosyncratic complication. It usually occurs within 1 month after the onset of treatment, when the dosage is increased, or when a second drug is introduced. Over 24 to 72 hours, the patient develops confusion, muscle rigidity, hypertension or severe orthostatic hypotension, and a high temperature (as high as 42°C). Patients with this syndrome should be hospitalized immediately in an intensive care unit, because hypoventilation occurs as a consequence of the rigidity of the patient's chest wall muscles. The treatment involves discontinuation of all antipsychotic agents, aggressive intravenous hydration, and, in some cases, the administration of dantrolene or bromocriptine. Patients should remain off all antipsychotic drugs for a minimum of 2 weeks before reintroduction. In the interim period, acute exacerbations of symptoms are common, and patients may require inpatient psychiatric hospitalization.

Because *older schizophrenic patients* are more prone to the development of the common side effects, dosages should be lower for these patients, by the equivalent of 100 to 200 mg of chlorpromazine or 1 to 2 mg of haloperidol. The very high dosages described for treatment of combativeness and hyperactivity should be avoided in elderly patients.

Long-Term Drug Treatment of Schizophrenia

Interested generalists can assume responsibility for the long-term care of schizophrenic patients. Pharmacotherapy is the principal mode of long-term treatment. Many studies show that 60% to 70% of schizophrenic patients relapse within 1 year if they do not receive medication (8). Most patients require antipsychotics indefinitely, but evidence reveals that relapse rates decline significantly if patients are treated for a minimum of 6 months after resolution of an acute episode. Further reduction in relapse rates has been suggested if patients are maintained on medication for 2 years after an acute episode.

The goal of long-term pharmacotherapy is to minimize psychotic symptoms with the lowest dosage of antipsychotic possible. Moderate maintenance dosages appear to be as effective as, and safer than, the larger dosages that have been popular in the United States (9). For most patients a low to moderate dosage is the equivalent of 200 to 400 mg of chlorpromazine (or 1.5 to 4 mg of haloperidol) daily. Patients receiving this dosage often continue to have psychotic symptoms but do not seem to be disturbed by them (e.g., "I still hear the voices, but they don't bother me").

Compliance Problems

Some patients temporarily have difficulty maintaining a regular medication schedule because of psychotic disorganization, negativism, or fear of medication. Inability to comply with the medication regimen may signal the onset of an acute episode. With the first indication of a disruption in medication schedule, the patient should be evaluated, the frequency of visits increased to at least once a week, and the medication dosage increased if warranted. If the patient remains unable to comply, a long-acting intramuscular agent, such as fluphenazine decanoate (Prolixin Decanoate, available in doses of 25 mg/mL), 1 to 2 mL every 2 weeks, or haloperidol decanoate (Haldol Decanoate, available in doses of 50 mg/mL), 2 to 4 mL every 4 weeks, should be used. The patient can be returned to an oral medication when symptom control is reestablished. Long-acting intramuscular agents are also useful for new patients for whom no information is available on compliance in aftercare or ambulatory programs.

Evidence suggests that family therapy and behavioral therapy improve compliance with medication regimens (6). Patients having difficulty with medication compliance should be referred for one of these types of therapy in addition to the previously described measures.

Nonresponders

Between 5% and 25% of schizophrenic patients do not respond to antipsychotics, and a similar number are intolerant of the side effects. Both groups of patients are candidates for treatment with *clozapine* (Clozaril) (11), a tricyclic dibenzodiazepine. The recommended starting dosage is 25 mg once or twice per day, to be increased by 25 mg every other day to 100 mg per dose, then increased by 50 mg every other day to 300 to 450 mg per day by 2 weeks. Clozapine is available in 25- and 100-mg tablets. The risk of agranulocytosis is 1% to 2% and necessitates initial weekly blood monitoring. Because of dose-related incidence of seizures, the dosage should not exceed 600 mg. Common side effects are weight gain, sedation, drooling, and dizziness. There are reports of increased incidence of type 2 diabetes mellitus in patients treated with clozapine.

Late Side Effects of Antipsychotics

Onset of the early-type side effects is uncommon in patients taking maintenance dosages of antipsychotics (see earlier discussion). When an increase in medication is necessary, drug-induced parkinsonism may appear. Patients who experience symptoms of parkinsonism over a long period should try other antipsychotic medications until one is found that does not produce the side effect. As noted previously, long-term use of antiparkinsonism medication is to be avoided if possible (see Chapter 90).

Tardive dyskinesia is an extrapyramidal syndrome that occurs in patients after prolonged (months to years) moderate- to high-dosage antipsychotic treatment. The cumulative prevalence is approximately 24%–27% in women and 22% in men—but is much lower with the newer, atypical antipsychotic agents and is nonexistent for clozapine. The prevalence reaches its peak in men between 50 and 70 years of age but continues to rise after age 70 years in women. Asians have lower prevalence than North Americans, Europeans, or Africans (12). The disorder has been reported in association with long-term treatment with anticonvulsants, and there is a very small incidence among untreated schizophrenic patients. Up to 25% of patients treated with antipsychotics who are evaluated for drug-induced tardive dyskinesia are found to have another disorder causing their dyskinesia. The most common of these is the oral-buccal-lingual dyskinesia that arises in 10% of edentulous patients.

The syndrome of tardive dyskinesia consists of *involuntary or semivoluntary movements* of a choreiform, tic-like nature, sometimes associated with a dystonic component that classically involves the tongue, facial, and neck muscles. Early manifestations include fine, worm-like movements of the tongue at rest, facial tics, and jaw movements. Later symptoms are bucco-lingual-masticatory movements, chewing motions, lip smacking, puffing of cheeks, blinking of eyes, and choreoathetoid movements of the extremities. Younger patients often have significant involvement of the extremities and trunk. Although the syndrome is painless, it can be socially embarrassing and can interfere with patients' ability to feed and care for themselves.

The prognosis for remission of tardive dyskinesia is poor, regardless of treatment, and symptoms last for years if not indefinitely. The emphasis of antipsychotic use should therefore be on prevention of tardive dyskinesia, by careful selection of patients for long-term antipsychotic treatment, trials of atypical agents first, and use of the lowest possible dosage. At the first sign of the disorder, antipsychotics should be tapered and discontinued if possible. Symptoms gradually diminish or disappear over several months in approximately one third of patients who can be taken off drugs early.

Because there is no satisfactory treatment for tardive dyskinesia, understanding support by the physician and family members is especially important in long-term care of the patient. Antiparkinsonism medications usually worsen the symptoms. One short-term effective treatment is the use of more potent antipsychotics to suppress the symptoms, but this usually requires increasing dosages of the suppressing agent, and subsequent withdrawal of antipsychotics often leads to worsening of the symptoms for a period of time. In case reports, benzodiazepines, pure lecithin, lithium, sodium valproate, and vitamin E have been reported to be useful, but there are no well-delineated guidelines for selecting one of these agents. Another strategy is to switch the patient to clozapine, so that antipsychotic therapy is continued with a medication that does not cause tardive dyskinesia; this strategy is best done in consultation with a psychiatrist.

Overall Psychiatric Treatment of the Patient

The schizophrenic patient is sensitive to change or instability in any aspect of his or her life. Whenever possible, a single practitioner should provide continuous care, so that that practitioner becomes a predictable resource for helping the patient to maintain his or her role in the community. Although few schizophrenic patients work full time, patients should be referred for vocational rehabilitation (see Chapter 9) or for sheltered workshops when requested. Most patients determine their own levels of social activity and may not change despite encouragement, but offers and suggestions should be made. The clinician should be available to the patient's family or to foster care providers for periodic review of the patient's progress and expectations. The book, *Surviving Schizophrenia,* should be recommended to the patient's family (see General References).

Ideally, residential facilities are available when there is no family for the patient to live with or when the family is a harmful influence. However, in many communities, such facilities do not exist. For some patients, the clinician and the ambulatory center itself become the sources of the few social contacts that the patient has outside his or her home and inner psychological world.

Regular office visits should be scheduled. Frequency of visits should be determined on the basis of current status of the patient, history of the course of the patient's illness, reliability of the patient in taking medication, and the patient's ability to recognize early signs of onset of acute episodes. Office visits need last only 15 to 20 minutes and should include an interim history, a brief mental status examination, a review of the effectiveness of medications and of significant side effects, and provision of support or advice regarding the ways in which the patient is dealing with day-to-day matters. In other words, these office visits may be defined as supportive therapy, as described in Chapter 20.

In addition to individual office visits, *a family management approach* may be useful for patients who are having difficulties with their families (13). The method involves a two-step process:

1. Sessions devoted to educating the patient and family about the nature, course, and treatment of schizophrenia.
2. Family sessions aimed at reducing existing family tensions and improving problem-solving skills of the family in coping with causes of stress (see Family Counseling in Chapter 20).

Management is enhanced if the clinician has ready access to social services, emergency mental health services, and psychiatric day care and inpatient services. Social services, especially for financial support (e.g., welfare, food stamps, disability payments), are important in the treatment of schizophrenic patients because of their usual dependent status. Many acute episodes of psychosis are precipitated by threatened or actual withdrawal of welfare and disability payments.

The generalist caring for a schizophrenic patient may need to consult with a psychiatrist for confirmation of the initial diagnosis, decisions regarding hospitalization, or treatment recommendations when symptoms respond poorly to antipsychotics or when side effects are intolerable.

Medical Comorbidity in Patients with Schizophrenia

Patients who suffer from schizophrenia may have little contact with primary care physicians unless they are part of a program that mandates medical visits or have family members dedicated to keeping up with general health issues. The number one cause of death for schizophrenic patients is heart disease, and the patients have several risk factors.

First, there is a growing body of evidence that patients with schizophrenia are frequently comorbid with obesity (14). It is as yet unclear how much of this problem is caused by the lifestyle of the diseased patient and how much by side effects of medications used to treat the disorder. In fact, most antipsychotic agents are associated with weight gain, the notable exceptions being pimozide and molindone, two older typical antipsychotics. The mechanism for this effect is still unclear but may involve several factors. First, sedation and rigidity may decrease nonexercise activity thermogenesis (calorie-burning activity associated with daily movements). Second, central histamine blockade may result in increased appetite. Finally, antipsychotic medications have been associated with increases in serum leptin levels, possibly resulting in desensitization of leptin receptors, leading to increased fat storage. In general, weight issues and diet should be addressed in all patients with schizophrenia, and attempts should be made to help obese and overweight patients reduce weight. Attention should be given to possible medication effects, and attempts to alleviate sedation and/or rigidity should be actively pursued. If necessary, patients may try switching to antipsychotics associated with less weight gain, under careful supervision for recurrence of psychotic symptoms.

Second, there is a high rate of comorbidity between schizophrenia and nicotine addiction. Although there are theories about the specific effects of nicotine on schizophrenic brains, suggesting a self-medication model for this behavior, the untoward effects of smoking on the cardiopulmonary system run rampant. In general, although efforts to force schizophrenic patients to quit smoking may be fruitless, all attempts should be made to reduce smoking to the lowest level possible, offering nicotine replacement as necessary and behavioral therapy to address cravings.

Third, there is evidence that diabetes is a more common problem in schizophrenia than in the general population (15). The possible mechanisms are that diabetes and schizophrenia are in some way genetically linked, so that risk genes may be transmitted together due to their proximity on chromosomes, and that antipsychotic medications may cause diabetes by directly impairing glucose handling and by causing obesity, which may impair insulin responsiveness. Diabetes complications arise as the disease takes its toll on the body, and schizophrenics may be poorly compliant with diet and hypoglycemic or insulin regimens. All schizophrenic patients should be regularly screened for diabetes on routine examinations.

In addition to heart, lung, and endocrine diseases, patients with schizophrenia are at increased risk for certain infectious diseases. Tuberculosis is associated with homelessness, a far-too-frequent sad consequence of chronic mental illness. The rates of human immunodeficiency virus infection and viral hepatitis in patients with schizophrenia are frighteningly high.

Sexual transmission of these viruses may be related the a smaller sample of the population with whom patients with schizophrenia have the opportunity for intercourse. There are data to suggest that schizophrenic patients choose sexual partners most often from among other patients in the psychiatric clinic. Further, there is a profound comorbidity of substance use disorders in schizophrenia. The possible mechanisms for this are (a) as a method of self-medication for positive or negative symptoms, (b) as a means of increasing social interaction via a fairly scripted set of rules that patients with schizophrenia can follow, and (c) as a result of increased availability in impoverished areas, to which schizophrenic patients tend to "drift" due to social disenfranchisement. In any case, intravenous drug use may lead directly to infection, and because many schizophrenic patients do not see internists or family practitioners regularly, the illnesses may be overlooked until later stages of infection, when treatment is more difficult and possibly less efficacious. Patients with schizophrenia should be routinely asked about sexual practices and intravenous drug use, and appropriate serologic testing should be performed.

Prognosis for the Treated Patient

Schizophrenia is a lifelong disease that requires an open-ended commitment by the clinician. The patient's life is disrupted by periodic psychosis, sometimes necessitating hospitalization, and by an arrest or deterioration of social function. Some patients are able to work and maintain satisfying interpersonal relationships. Many lead lonely, withdrawn, socially marginal existences. Psychopharmacologic treatment is effective for controlling the symptoms of acute psychosis and suppressing the intensity of psychotic symptoms over long periods. Suppression of psychosis may permit the patient to use his or her intellectual and social talents more effectively in developing and maintaining some role in the community. The atypical antipsychotics (Table 25.3) are reported to have an efficiency in the treatment of the negative symptoms that may impair social function.

General References*

American Psychiatric Association. **Diagnostic and statistical manual of mental disorders. 4th ed. (DSM-IV).** Washington, DC: American Psychiatric Association, 1994.

Diagnostic criteria and epidemiologic information for all recognized psychiatric disorders.

Bleuler E. Dementia praecox or the group of schizophrenias. New York: International Universities Press, 1950.

A classic work on schizophrenia.

Arana GW, Rosenbaum JF, eds. Handbook of psychiatric drug therapy. 4th ed. Philadelphia, PA; Lippincott Williams & Wilkins, 2000.

Concise information on actions and side effects of currently used antipsychotic drugs.

Practice guidelines for the treatment of patients with schizophrenia. Am J Psychiatry 1997;154[4 Suppl].

A current, thorough review of the comprehensive treatment of schizophrenia, including treatment of neuroleptic-induced side effects.

Torrey EF. Surviving schizophrenia: a family manual. New York: Harper & Row, 1995.

A thorough book that contains invaluable information for families of schizophrenic patients and for physicians.

Specific References

1. Regier DA, Boyd JH, Burke JD, et al. One-month prevalence of mental disorders in the United States. Arch Gen Psychiatry 1988;45:977.
2. Lemkau PU, Tietze C, Cooper M. Survey of statistical studies on prevalence and incidence of mental disorder in sample population. Public Health Rep 1943;58:1909.
3. Mowry BJ, Levinson DF. Genetic linkage and schizophrenia: methods, recent findings and future directions. Aust N Z J Psychiatry 1993;27:200.
4. Snyder SH. The dopamine hypothesis of schizophrenia: focus on the dopamine receptor. Am J Psychiatry 1976;133:197.
5. Kapur S, Remington G. Serotonin-dopamine interaction and its relevance to schizophrenia. Am J Psychiatry 1996;153:466.
6. Pearlson GD. Neurobiology of schizophrenia. Ann Neurol 2000;48:56.
7. Lipinski JF, Zubenko GS, Barreira P, et al. Propranolol in the treatment of neuroleptic-induced akathisia [Letter]. Lancet 1983;2:685.
8. Hogarty GE, Goldberg SC, Schooler NR, et al. Drug and sociotherapy in the aftercare of schizophrenic patients: two-year relapse rates. Arch Gen Psychiatry 1974;31:603.
9. Baldessarini RJ, Cohen BM, Teicher MH. Significance of neuroleptic dose and plasma level in the pharmacologic treatment of psychoses. Arch Gen Psychiatry 1988;45:79.
10. Perkins DU. Adherence to antipsychotic medications. J Clin Psychiatry 1999;60[Suppl 21]:25.
11. Meltzer HY. Treatment of the neuroleptic-nonresponsive schizophrenic patient. Schizophr Bull 1992;18:515.
12. Yassa R, Jeste DV. Gender differences in tardive dyskinesia: a critical review of the literature. Schizophr Bull 1992;18:701.
13. Falloon IR, Boyd JL, McGill CW, et al. Family management in the prevention of exacerbation of schizophrenia. N Engl J Med 1982;306:1437.
14. Goldman LS. Medical illness in patients with schizophrenia. J Clin Psychiatry 1999;60[Suppl 21]:10.
15. Mukherjee S, Decina P, Bocola V, et al. Diabetes mellitus with schizophrenic patients. Compr Psychiatry 1996;37:68.
16. Carpenter WT, Conley RR, Buchanan RW, et al. Patient response and resource management: another view of clozapine treatment of schizophrenia. Am J Psychiatry 1995;152:827.
17. Marder SR, Meibach RC. Risperidone in the treatment of schizophrenia. Am J Psychiatry 1994;151:825.
18. Beasley CM, Tollefson G, Tran P, et al. The Olazapine HGAD Study Group. Olanzapine versus placebo and haloperidol acute phase results of the North American double-blind olanzapine trial. Neuropsychopharmacology 1996;14:111.

* Bold print (general references) and bold numerals (specific references) denote published controlled clinical trials, meta-analyses, or consensus-based recommendations.

CHAPTER 26

Cognitive Impairment and Mental Illness in the Elderly

PETER V. RABINS, MD, MPH

Although overall rates of mental disorders are similar across the adult age span, the elderly are the least likely to seek help for mental illness. Those who do are most likely to receive treatment from a primary care provider during a routine medical visit.

GENERAL PRINCIPLES

Importance of Diagnosis

Making the correct diagnosis is a crucial first step in determining proper treatment. The most common mistakes made in assessing psychiatric symptoms in older patients are ascribing them to normal aging, confusing symptoms with syndromes, and not appreciating the frequent interaction between physical and psychiatric disorders. Asking the appropriate questions and attempting to elicit the classic signs and symptoms should lead to the correct diagnosis even when the presentation is unusual.

Relationship Between Physical and Mental States

Physical and psychiatric illnesses commonly coexist in the elderly. A prudent strategy when facing a patient with both physical and psychiatric complaints is to establish a differential diagnosis for each symptom before assuming that either the physical or the psychiatric disorder is primary. The two types of symptoms may be related in a number of ways.

- *Mental distress complicating a primary physical illness.* Demoralization, anxiety, grief, irritability, and frustration are especially common in older patients with significant physical illness. These feelings usually begin after the onset of the physical illness, vary over time, and respond to the techniques for psychotherapy described in Chapter 20.
- *Physical complaints as the primary manifestation of psychiatric disorder.* Particularly in older patients, focused complaints of physical ill health may be the most prominent or only sign of mental illness, especially depression. Although the physical complaint must be appropriately evaluated, a psychiatric cause should be suspected when the somatic complaint is bizarre, seems to be exaggerated, or has been evaluated without a cause being found or when the patient has some symptoms of depression.
- *Psychiatric disorders arising from specific diseases.* Cancer of the pancreas, hypothyroidism, and several structural brain diseases (stroke, Parkinson disease, dementia) are commonly accompanied by a depression. Because the rates of depression are higher in these disorders than in arthritic or orthopedic conditions with similar levels of impairment, it is likely that the medical disorder is the cause of the depression or that the medical and psychiatric disorders share a common etiology. These depressions respond well to antidepressant treatment.
- *Psychiatric syndromes caused by medication and by substance abuse.* Psychiatric syndromes can be precipitated by a variety of medications and by alcohol abuse. Corticosteroids, beta-blockers, and other drugs that affect the adrenergic system can induce depressive symptoms. Anticholinergic compounds, dopaminergic agonist compounds, benzodiazepines, and H_2 blockers can induce delirium. Patients with dementia are more vulnerable to developing cognitive side effects from these compounds than are cognitively normal elderly people. Alcoholism, often hard to recognize in elderly patients, can also cause symptoms of depression and anxiety or cognitive defects (see Chapter 28). Abstinence can lead to resolution of the psychiatric symptoms.

Importance of Psychosocial Factors

Psychosocial factors are important to consider in patients of all ages. They become particularly important in the elderly because reduced physical mobility, isolation from family and friends, and financial limitations are more common and can directly interfere with the treatment of medical and psychiatric disorders. For elderly patients with mental illness, referring the patient to a social service agency or enlisting the help of the patient's family may be especially important in ensuring successful treatment and follow-through. Even when dementia is present, psychosocial interventions provide an important avenue for relieving morbidity.

Importance of Cognitive Assessment

Because dementia and delirium are common disorders of the elderly, it is important to be familiar with

Table 26.1. Components of a Mental Status Examination

Orientation
Person [intact patients will know their complete name]
Date [intact patients should know the date within 3 days]
Place [intact patients will be fully oriented to place]
Memory, registration
Give 3–5 words to remember and ask to recall them in 2 minutes
Attention/Concentration:
Days of the week backward, starting with Sunday, or
Spell a word backwards, e.g. "house", or
Subtraction of 7 serially from 100 for 5 iterations [intact persons should be able to get 4 of 5 of the spelling or math and all of the days of the week]
Memory, recall
Recall the 3–5 words [intact patients should remember 2 of 3 or 4 of 5 words]
Language
Naming: show two common items (e.g. watch, shoe) and one uncommon item (e.g. lapel, shoelace)
Repetition: e.g., repeat "Today is a [sunny] day in [March]."
Reading: e.g., ask "Raise your right hand".
Writing: ask to write a complete sentence.
[Intact patients can do all correctly]
Visual–Spatial
Copy a complex figure, or
Draw a clock, put in numbers, and put in hands at specific time [intact patients will do correctly]
Executive
Ask, "What does this proverb mean: 'Don't cry over spilled milk'?" [correct response, "What is done is done" or similar statement: may be missed because of low education or cultural background]

the assessment of cognitive function. Performance of a mental status examination, which contains the components displayed in Table 26.1, allows the clinician to identify the types of cognitive deficits the patient is experiencing and to provide a comparison for future examinations. The Mini-Mental Status Examination is a reliable, brief, widely used screening tool (1a) that permits standardized scoring and facilitates following patients over time. However, it may be normal in the initial evaluation of mildly demented patients. Formal neuropsychometric testing and/or reevaluation of patients at a later time may be useful in such situations.

SPECIFIC PSYCHOGERIATRIC DISORDERS

Psychiatric disorders in older patients may present with the classic symptoms described in other chapters of this book. The following pages focus on several syndromes that are particularly important in the elderly.

Depression

Depressive Symptoms

Symptoms of depression and sadness become more common in late life even though the syndrome of major depression is less common in the elderly. This dissociation may be caused by both the criteria used to make diagnoses and intrinsic differences between the young and old. The *Diagnostic and Statistical Manual of Mental Disorders,* 4th edition, divides mood disorder into several categories (see Chapter 24). The differences among them depend on both symptom clustering and course. The presentation of these disorders in older patients may differ from the presentation in younger patients in several ways.

An adjustment disorder with depressed mood is characterized by sad or low mood that follows, within 3 months, a clearly identifiable stressor or precipitant. In elderly patients, stressors such as illness, decreases in functional status, isolation, and financial limitations (see Importance of Psychosocial Factors, above) are particularly common. The approaches to office psychotherapy described in Chapter 20 are fully applicable to elderly patients with adjustment disorders.

A dysthymic disorder, conversely, is characterized by the presence of depressive symptoms for more than 2 years. Mood often fluctuates widely but in no discernible pattern. The patient may experience hours, days, or weeks of improved mood, mixed with prolonged periods of unhappiness. In the elderly, a dysthymic disorder should be considered when the patient reports chronic depressive symptoms throughout his or her life and denies the cyclicity and periods of normal mood found in recurrent depressive or bipolar disorder (see Chapter 24). It may require specialty referral because of its chronicity.

Major Depression

The diagnostic criteria of the major affective disorders and their treatment, as described in Chapter 24, are generally applicable to the elderly. Hypochondriacal features, agitation, and suspiciousness or frank paranoia often accompany depression in the elderly and are common sources of diagnostic confusion. A study demonstrated that the elderly with major depressive disorder are less likely to report being sad than the young (1). Therefore, denial of sadness does *not* rule out the diagnosis of major depression.

Elderly patients with a hypochondriacal focus usually deny that their mood is sad but focus on physical symptoms for which there is minimal or no evidence of abnormality on physical examination or laboratory assessment. Depressed hypochondriacal patients often have changes in their vital sense ("something is wrong with me") and a negative self-attitude ("I've done something to deserve this or cause this"). Therefore, the patient should be asked specifically about these cardinal features of major depression when hypochondriasis is present.

Because suspiciousness and paranoia are common in depressed elderly patients, other evidence for a major depression should be sought when these symptoms are present. When paranoia and depression coexist, depression is most commonly the primary disorder.

As in younger patients, major depression in the elderly often requires pharmacotherapy or electroconvulsive therapy. Practical details about these modes of treatment are given in Chapter 24. Selective serotonin reuptake inhibitor antidepressants are the treatment of choice for the initiation of antidepressant pharmacotherapy. Sertraline (Zoloft) should be started at a dosage of 25 to 50 mg in the morning; 200 mg is the maximum dosage. Paroxetine (Paxil) should be started at a dosage of 10 mg in the morning; 30 mg is the maximum dosage. Citalopram (Celexa) should be started at a dosage of 15 mg in the morning. The maximum dose is 45 mg. The long half-life of fluoxetine (Prozac) suggests that it should be used in lower dosages in the elderly than in young patients, starting at a dosage of 10 mg in the morning. The maximum dosage is 40 to 60 mg. Tricyclic antidepressants with the most pronounced anticholinergic properties (e.g., amitriptyline and doxepin) should be avoided. The tricyclics with the highest likelihood of causing orthostatic hypotension (e.g., amitriptyline and imipramine) should also be avoided or closely monitored because elderly patients are at higher risk of falls and are more likely to be receiving antihypertensive drugs or other compounds that also can cause orthostasis. Nortriptyline and desipramine are the tricyclic agents that are least likely to cause these side effects. A usual starting dosage in the otherwise healthy elderly person is 10 to 25 mg at bedtime; however, a dosage of 10 mg should be prescribed in the frail elderly or in patients with the potential for medical complications from the drugs.

Electroconvulsive therapy is sometimes safer than pharmacotherapy for older patients with cardiac disease. It is equally effective in all age groups (see details regarding electroconvulsive therapy, Chapter 24). Low-dose antipsychotic drugs (see Table 25.3) are indicated when *delusions* complicate depression, especially when the suspiciousness is significantly interfering with the patient's function, is life threatening (e.g., the patient will not eat because he or she believes that the food is poisoned), or causes distress for the patient or those close to him or her.

Depression-Induced Cognitive Impairment

Patients with the onset of depression in late life can present with the belief that they are becoming demented. Some depressed patients perform poorly on routine tests of cognitive function. Previously this condition was called *pseudodementia,* but this term has fallen into disfavor because patients with this syndrome perform in the demented range on standardized tests of cognitive function and because up to 50% of these patients eventually develop a progressive dementing illness (2). Nonetheless, recognition of the syndrome is important because both the mood disorder and cognitive function can improve with antidepressant treatment. Depression-induced cognitive impairment should be considered when the onset of cognitive impairment has been subacute (less than 6 months and particularly less than 3 months), when the history of an episode of depression earlier in life is elicited, when a dementia is complicated by hypochondriacal or bizarre delusions (3), when the patient constantly emphasizes his or her cognitive disability (a behavior that is uncommon in Alzheimer disease), or when a cognitively impaired patient reports early morning awakening, lack of energy, self-blame, or guilt. At times it is difficult to determine whether the patient has a primary dementing illness with secondary depression or primary depression with reversible dementia. In such cases a therapeutic trial of an antidepressant (e.g., at least 4 weeks at a therapeutic dosage, as described in Chapter 24) may be the best way to determine which disorder is primary.

Depression Coexisting with Brain Disease

Major depression may complicate primarily organic disorders of the central nervous system. Stroke, Parkinson disease, and Alzheimer disease are three common late-life disorders in which major depressive symptoms occur in 20% to 50% of patients (4). The importance of recognizing these as coexisting disorders is that the physical disorder and the psychiatric disorder may both need to be treated if either problem is to improve. For example, depression has been shown to interfere directly with rehabilitation from *stroke.* Thus, the treatment of depression after stroke improves the degree of recovery from the stroke; at the same time, gains from rehabilitation improve the patient's morale and mood (see details in Chapter 91). In *Parkinson disease,* depressive symptoms and parkinsonian symptoms (e.g., psychomotor retardation) often overlap, and it can be difficult to determine which disorder is causing specific symptoms. In planning treatment, it is best to focus on the depressive or parkinsonian symptoms separately and to treat first the disorder that is causing the worst impairment in function. The treatment of Parkinson disease is described in Chapter 90. The treatment of depression in patients with *Alzheimer disease* or multi-infarct dementia can improve behavior, and mood, although cognitive impairment will persist (5).

Paranoia and Suspiciousness

Suspiciousness is more common among the elderly than in younger people. This becomes clinically relevant when the suspiciousness interferes with the patient's life. Several types of disorders can present with suspiciousness.

Suspiciousness as an Isolated Symptom

Some elderly people become more suspicious as they age but have no accompanying signs or symptoms of other mental illness. It is important to determine whether there is a basis for the patient's suspiciousness because financial abuse of the elderly is not uncommon and concerns about the environment being unsafe can be appropriate. An understandable reaction to difficult circumstances should not be assumed, however, and a review of symptoms that explores other psychiatric conditions is necessary.

Suspiciousness Complicating Depression

As noted above, suspiciousness occurs in some elderly patients with major depression. Depression should be considered primary if the person feels deserving of persecution or punishment or has changes in vital sense and other manifestations of depression (see Chapter 24).

Late-Life Schizophrenia or Paraphrenia

Older patients occasionally develop a syndrome similar to schizophrenia in young people (see Chapter 25). Such patients have *delusions* (fixed, false, idiosyncratic ideas) and *auditory* or *visual hallucinations* and lack symptoms of depression or cognitive impairment.

The treatment of late-life schizophrenia and paranoia is similar to that for younger patients (see Chapter 25) except that significantly lower dosages of antipsychotic drugs are effective. Although no single antipsychotic drug is more efficacious than another, those likely to induce orthostatic hypotension, such as chlorpromazine (Thorazine), or with high anticholinergic effects, such as thioridazine (Mellaril), are less desirable, especially if the patient is taking an antidepressant that also has anticholinergic properties. A starting dosage of 0.5 mg of risperidone (Risperdal) two to three times daily, olanzapine (Zyrexa) 2.5 mg at bedtime, or thiothixene (Navane) 1 mg at bedtime (may be increased to 2 mg twice daily) is recommended. Thiothixene is significantly less expensive than risperidone or olanzapine. Of these drugs, risperidone is least likely to cause parkinsonian side effects or orthostasis at low dosages. Because old age is a risk factor for developing tardive dyskinesia, an attempt should be made to discontinue antipsychotic drug treatment after the patient has stabilized. Chapter 25 describes the use of antipsychotic drugs in detail.

Paranoia and Persecutory Delusions as Symptoms of an Organic Disease

Paranoia can be symptomatic of a focal brain disease (e.g., tumor or stroke), a diffuse brain disease such as Alzheimer disease (6), a systemic condition such as a metabolic disorder (e.g., hyperthyroidism or hypoparathyroidism), or psychoactive substance abuse. Any patient with a persistent suspicious belief should have a clinical assessment for evidence that supports the presence of one of these causes.

Mild Cognitive Impairment

Some older patients complain of memory loss or slower rate of processing information, or members of their families notice these phenomena, but a history from both the patient and family reveals no social or occupational dysfunction and screening cognitive tests reveal minimal impairment in memory. Recent research suggests that 6% to 12% of these individuals develop dementia each year over the next 5 years (7). Those unlikely to have a dementia complain of such things as misplacing keys or having more difficulty remembering names or words than they once did; on questioning they acknowledge that names and words often come to them minutes later and that they have not forgotten important engagements or events. Patients who are especially concerned about memory difficulties and report a decline in function in social, personal, or occupational realms should be referred to a neuropsychologist for *formal neuropsychologic evaluation* to better formulate the problem. Impairments in memory and executive function are the best predictors of subsequent decline (8). Careful attention should be given to the medical status of such patients because they could have a subclinical delirium (see below). When no dysfunction is identified and objective testing makes a progressive dementia unlikely, reassurance and an agreement to reassess the patient in 6 months may help relieve the anxiety associated with this condition.

Dementia

Definition and Epidemiology

Dementia is characterized by a decline in cognitive abilities from a previous level, multiple impairments in cognitive function such as memory (i.e., amnesia) or language (i.e., aphasia), and the presence of clear consciousness. Dementia can have many etiologies, but fewer than 2% of affected patients have dementia caused by a reversible etiology (9).

Moderate to severe dementia affects approximately 8% of people over 65. However, most dementia occurs among the very old; prevalence is 20% in people 80 and older and approximately 30% in people over 90. Prevalence rates are similar in European, North American, and Asian prevalence studies. A recent study from Africa suggests lower rates in Nigeria (10).

Etiologic Evaluation

The assessment of a person with complaints of cognitive decline has three purposes. The first purpose is to identify the probable cause of the dementia, including the identification of treatable disorders. The three most common causes of treatable dementia in elderly patients are medication toxicity, depression, and thyroid disease. In younger patients, acquired immunodeficiency syndrome dementia is now an important cause (see Chapter 39). Commonly used medications that have been associated with global cognitive impairment are the benzodiazepines (most common), H_2 blockers, and anticholinergic drugs. The second purpose of assessment is to identify treatable symptoms and comorbidity. Because few patients have a truly reversible dementia, the treatment of medical and behavioral comorbidity is the main focus of both the assessment and the treatment of almost all patients in the ambulatory setting. The third purpose is to identify issues in the caregiver and environment that are amenable to intervention.

Clinical Characteristics

In considering possible etiologies, it is useful to *determine whether the dementia has the clinical characteristics of a subcortical or cortical dementia.* Most treatable dementias present as subcortical dementias. *Subcortical dementias* are characterized by memory loss, apathy, slowness, and movement disorder with intact language (i.e., the patient is able to name objects, repeat a phrase, and follow a command) and normal visuospatial function (i.e., the patient is able to copy a diagram) (see Table 26.1). Causes of subcortical dementia include hypothyroidism, Parkinson disease, multiple sclerosis, normal pressure hydrocephalus, the dementia syndrome of depression, and most instances vascular dementia. The *cortical dementias* are characterized by memory loss plus multiple defects in higher cortical functions: *aphasic language* (making paraphasic errors such as substituting a letter, as in "tee" instead of "tie," or saying an incorrect word, such as "paper" instead of "pencil"), *apraxia* (inability to perform skilled movements such as showing how to drink with a cup on command), or *agnosia* (inability to recognize common objects or sensory stimuli). Alzheimer disease is the most common cortical dementia, but frontal dementias, Lewy body dementia, and rare dementias such as Creutzfeldt-Jakob disease are included in this category.

Screening Tests

The Agency for Health Care Policy and Research (AHCPR) 1996 Consensus Statement (11) on the differential diagnosis of dementia suggests the following inexpensive screening tests, each targeted at potentially treatable causes, for all patients: complete blood count, serum electrolyte levels, creatinine clearance, liver function tests, calcium and phosphate concentrations, thyroid-stimulating hormone, vitamin B_{12} level, and serologic tests for syphilis. The more recent clinical practice guidelines published by the American Academy of Neurology recommends screening for depression, B_{12} deficiency, and hypothyroidism but, because of its rarity in the United States, recommends against routinely screening for syphilis, except in high prevalence regions or high-risk patients (12). Imaging of the brain is listed as optional by the AHCPR and as appropriate by the American Academy of Neurology. It is reasonable to obtain a noncontrast computed tomography (CT) study on all patients with symptoms of less than 2 years duration, onset before age 70, or focal findings on neurologic examination. CT or magnetic resonance imaging (MRI) can identify focal lesions such as a tumor, subdural hematoma, or abscess; demonstrate findings compatible with hydrocephalus; or provide confirmatory evidence for vascular etiology of the dementia. However, it is impossible to diagnose Alzheimer disease solely by any imaging study. Overreliance on CT or MRI reports of "white matter hyperintensities" has led to an overdiagnosis of vascular dementia. A 1997 consensus statement issued by multiple organizations concurs with the AHCPR recommendations (13).

Alzheimer disease is diagnosed by inclusion and exclusion criteria. The diagnosis should be made when other specific causes of dementia, including vascular disease, have been excluded, when the condition has been slowly progressive, and when the cognitive disorder includes language impairment, apraxia, or agnosia in addition to memory impairment.

Vascular dementia should be diagnosed when the history suggests distinct episodes of worsening (a stair-step course); when evidence of vascular disease and hypertension are present on examination; when the neurologic examination reveals asymmetries in reflexes, strength, or sensation; and when a lesion on CT or MRI correlates with the abnormalities or neurologic examination. Evidence of prior stroke on neurologic examination or imaging study is necessary because a history of stroke without confirming evidence is an unreliable indicator of vascular dementia.

The *frontal dementias* are a group of slowly progressive diseases that present with pronounced changes in behavior and personality early in the disease. They are neuropathologically heterogeneous. On CT, they show disproportionate frontal atrophy.

Lewy body dementia presents in a fashion similar to Alzheimer disease but also has extrapyramidal symptoms (rigidity and parkinsonian tremor), hallucinations, delusions, frequent falls, and episodes of worsening early in the course. Antipsychotic medications should be avoided, if possible, because they can cause marked worsening of the parkinsonian symptoms.

Management

The management of irreversible dementia can be divided into six aspects:

1. *The assessment process.* This is the first step in management. The diagnosis has often been suspected by the family or patient, but at times abnormal behavior has been misinterpreted as purposefully irritating. As specific a *diagnosis* as possible should be made and conveyed to the family. The family may ask about long-term *prognosis.* The average patient with Alzheimer disease lives 7 to 10 years after early symptoms, but life span while demented can be as long as 20 years. In general, a dementia that has progressed slowly will continue to do so, whereas a history of rapid progression predicts rapid decline. Although the patient has the right to know his or her diagnosis, many lack the ability to realize that they have a deficit. Patients who, when asked, deny that they have any problems with their memory usually do not accept that there is a problem when told directly. Some patients, and most families, experience a measure of relief when it is pointed out that the patient's dementia is a medical problem and not just part of getting older or becoming intentionally stubborn.

   The evaluation process should elicit specific *problems in behavior caused by the dementia* (see commonly cited problems, Table 26.2). Difficulty in speaking, dressing, and performing potentially dangerous activities as driving, smoking, and cooking should be inquired about. When present, these problems should be explained as the result of the illness. The family or other caregivers should then

Table 26.2. Behavior Problems of Patients and Problematic Activities of Daily Living Cited by Families of Demented Patients[a]

Behavior	Percentage of Families Reporting Occurrence	Percentage of Families Reporting Behavior as a Problem
Memory disturbance[b]	100	93
Catastrophic reactions[b,c]	87	89
Demanding/critical behavior	71	73
Night walking	69	59
Hiding things	69	71
Communication difficulties	68	74
Suspiciousness[b]	63	79
Making accusations[b]	60	82
Difficulty eating meals	60	55
Daytime wandering	59	70
Difficulty bathing	53	74
Hallucinations	49	42
Delusions	47	83
Physical violence	47	94
Incontinence[b]	40	86
Difficulty cooking	33	44
Hitting[b]	32	81
Impaired driving	20	73
Smoking	11	67
Inappropriate sexual behavior	2	0

[a]Based on an open-ended interview with the primary caregivers of 55 patients with irreversible dementia.

[b]Cited as most serious problem.

[c]See example in text.

Adapted from Rabins PV, Mace NL, Lucas MJ. The impact of dementia on the family. JAMA 1982;248:333, with permission.

try to adapt the environment to the disordered behaviors and should take steps to eliminate dangerous behaviors. Helping caregivers to specifically identify each problem can enable them to institute common-sense solutions they have not otherwise tried. In regard to the patient who continues to drive, the practitioner should instruct the patient to stop driving rather than asking a family member to do so. Most states require periodic relicensure for older people, and some even require health care practitioners to report all patients with dementia. Because these regulations can be helpful, it is important to be aware of them in one's state.

Families needing legal and financial advice should be advised to seek this out early and not wait for a crisis. Guidelines for assessing competence or for obtaining legal guardianship are described in Chapter 19.

2. *Optimizing general medical care.* Medical conditions such as congestive heart failure, urinary tract infection, and respiratory disease can worsen the functioning of patients with dementia if not optimally treated. Drugs that can affect cognition (e.g., cimetidine, beta-blockers, benzodiazepines, methyldopa, digoxin, anticholinergics) should be carefully monitored and all unnecessary medications discontinued. A search for superimposed medical illness should be instituted if there is a sudden deterioration in behavior, cognition, or functional ability.
3. *Addressing environmental problems, behavioral symptoms, and depression.* Not sleeping at night, suspiciousness, easy irritability, and catastrophic reactions (see below) can be more problematic than cognitive impairment. Nonpharmacologic environmental approaches should be tried first. For insomnia, these include keeping the person more active in the daytime (day care centers are a significant help in this regard) and not letting the patient nap during the day. Irritability, suspiciousness, and frustration are usually best managed by eliminating tasks that the patient can no longer do and avoiding situations that frustrate the patient. Ongoing reality orientation can be helpful in improving behavior and cognitive functioning (14). It is prudent to have the demented patient wear a medical alert bracelet that describes his or her condition.

Antipsychotic medications should be used only when other approaches have failed and a specific target symptom (hallucinations, delusions, aggression) is present that presents a danger to the patient or others or is very distressing to the patient. Importantly, these drugs are not indicated for controlling wandering or swearing. The usual dosages for these drugs are listed above (see Late-Life Schizophrenia or Paraphrenia). After target symptoms have been controlled for several months, the dosage can often be lowered, and drugs can be discontinued in about one-fourth of patients. Patients taking these drugs must be monitored for two common side effects, orthostatic hypotension and extrapyramidal symptoms (see details in Chapter 25). If only insomnia is a problem, trazodone, 50 to 100 mg, causes the least paradoxical agitation and the least daytime drowsiness.

Aggressive behavior may be treated with antipsychotic drugs or divalproex sodium (Depakote). The starting dosage of the latter is 125 mg daily, in a pill or sprinkles. The dosage can be increased cautiously to 250 mg twice daily. Dosage should be adjusted based on clinical response and blood levels. Ataxia/delirium or gastrointestinal distress can occur.

Depression is present in at least 20% of patients with dementia (15–17). When it has the characteristics of an adjustment disorder or demoralized state (see above), it is best managed with supportive therapy (see Chapter 20). However, major depressions with symptoms of early morning awakening, anorexia, self-blame, worthlessness, nihilistic attitudes, or morbid hypochondriasis also occur and should be treated with antidepressants. Their treatment is discussed under major depression, above.

In a *catastrophic reaction,* an overwhelming sense of frustration, fear, anger, or anxiety occurs when the patients are brought into a situation in which they are forced to confront their failing aptitudes. These poorly controlled emotions further impair the patient's already limited functional ability, leading to total decompensation of a previously coping patient.

An example is the following case study.

Patient Experience. A 72-year-old woman with a history of several small strokes experienced moderate forgetfulness and confusion but was generally calm and pleasant. Keeping track of the date with a calendar and making copious notes to herself, she managed to maintain an independent existence at home. At the supermarket checkout counter she could not find her wallet but insisted she had money to pay for her food. The clerk grew impatient, and the patient became increasingly agitated, tearful, and accusatory. When the store manager was called, she picked up grocery items and began throwing them.

These catastrophic reactions can have an adverse impact on both the patient and the patient's family. The explanation of their cause and their prevention through avoidance of provoking circumstances can forestall the need for institutionalization. The use of small dosages of an antipsychotic drug (see Late-Life Schizophrenia or Paraphrenia, above) may be beneficial in patients in whom episodes like this recur despite the caregiver's best efforts.

4. *Family support.* Family distress is common. Its treatment begins with the assessment. The problem-solving approach outlined under step 3 above gives families a sense of control and the hope that most problems can be managed despite the irreversibility and probable progression of the underlying disorder (18). Feelings of guilt, anger, discouragement, and demoralization are common, as are concerns about loss of friends, hobbies, and leisure time; family conflicts; and worry that the principal caregiver will become ill. Allowing families time to express these feelings and concerns and acknowledging that they are common can be helpful. Referring them to support groups can also be helpful. There is evidence from one controlled trial that a combination of counseling that addresses caregivers' needs and support group participation can delay the need for nursing home placement of demented patients, in this study for an average of 329 days (19).

   The *Alzheimer's Disease Association* can provide information about nearby resources and has a toll-free telephone number (1-800-621-0379). It is also helpful to recommend a book, such as *The 36-Hour Day* (see General References), which explains dementia and offers practical advice for dealing with the vexing problems created by a demented family member.
5. *Longitudinal care.* Because the dementing illnesses are progressive (new symptoms appear while old symptoms worsen), expected changes should be described to families. It is also prudent to discuss the possibility of eventual nursing home placement soon after the diagnosis is made. Although most families report that they do not want to place their loved one in a nursing home, it is important to urge them not to promise this unconditionally because medical issues or behavioral problems may necessitate placement. The family's emotional needs may change over time. A nonjudgmental listening approach helps family members to feel supported.
6. *Decisions about limiting therapy.* Chapter 13 describes the processes whereby patients and their families may plan in advance the limitation of therapy (living wills and other forms of advance directives) and the delegation of decision-making to others. These processes are especially important in planning the care of a demented patient early in the patient's course of dementia.

Drugs for Dementia

Three cholinesterase inhibitors have been approved for the treatment of cognitive impairment in patients with Alzheimer disease. Their effectiveness is quite modest (about 6 months improvement in some measures of cognitive function on average). All cause gastrointestinal side effects (nausea, vomiting, and diarrhea), anorexia, and gait disorder. The starting dosage of donepezil (Aricept) is 5 mg at bedtime. If no side effects develop it should be increased to 10 mg at bedtime in 4 to 6 weeks. Rivastigmine (Exelon) is started at 2 mg twice daily and increased monthly to 6 mg twice a day. Galanthamine (Reminyl) is started at 4 mg twice a day and increased monthly to a total of 16 or 24 mg daily. Tacrine is not recommended because it has been associated with a high prevalence of reversible hepatotoxicity.

Ginkgo biloba, an herbal alternative, may modestly improve cognitive and social functioning compared with placebo (20,21). Side effects, most commonly gastrointestinal complaints or headaches, are rare (see Chapter 5).

Delirium

Definition and Diagnosis

The essential features of delirium are cognitive impairment, clouding of consciousness, and difficulty sustaining and shifting attention. Delirium usually has rapid onset, brief duration, and marked fluctuation throughout the day. Delirious patients may appear drowsy or hyperalert (hypervigilant), trail off in the middle of sentences, fail to answer questions or ask that questions be repeated, or appear perplexed. Perceptual disturbances such as illusions (misinterpretations of real external stimuli) or hallucinations are common. Delirium is especially common in patients with dementia. Although patients with either dementia or delirium may experience memory impairment, disorientation, hallucinations, delusions, and disturbed thinking, the patient with dementia is alert, whereas the delirious patient is drowsy and fluctuates in alertness over minutes or hours. The abrupt onset of delirium (within hours or days) differs from dementia, which develops over months or years in most instances.

The presence of cognitive impairment and rapid fluctuation distinguishes delirium from schizophrenia and other psychotic disorders. The hallucinations and delusions associated with delirium are often fleeting and poorly systematized in comparison with those of other psychotic disorders, in which they are sustained and well organized. The electroencephalogram (EEG) in the delirious patient often reveals a generalized slowing of background activity, whereas the EEG is generally normal in schizophrenic and depressed patients.

In some patients, the manifestations of delirium may be so subtle that they are not recognized by an examiner who is unfamiliar with the patient's baseline status. At other times the symptoms suggest depression, dementia, or schizophrenia. Older age is a strong risk factor for developing delirium. Delirium can be precipitated by cognitive impairment, sleep deprivation, immobility, visual impairment, hearing impairment, acute medical illnesses, drug toxicity, and dehydration.

The key to accurate diagnosis of delirium is a high index of suspicion in any elderly patient with a history of recent or sudden change in mental status and behavior (22). The EEG shows diffuse slowing in both delirium and dementia. In delirium, the EEG slowing is often marked, even when the cognitive and behavioral impairment is minor; conversely, severe cognitive impairment and a mildly abnormal EEG are most common in dementia.

Etiologic Evaluation

Delirium can result from a wide range of organic causes that adversely affect brain metabolism (Table 26.3). Special attention should be given to medications in the elderly because they may produce a delirium at therapeutic dosages. Beta-blockers, H_2 blockers, benzodiazepines, and the many compounds with anticholinergic activity are common causes of delirium. Although electrolyte disturbances are the most common metabolic cause of delirium, any disorder of metabolic homeostasis can cause delirium. Withdrawal from alcohol or sedatives is often overlooked in the elderly as a possible cause of delirium. Multiple causes are suspected, and no one specific cause is identified in 30% to 50% of cases. When there is no obvious cause for a patient's apparent delirium, an EEG may be helpful in confirming that delirium is present.

The key to treatment is the identification of the underlying causes when they can be identified. The physical, neurologic, and laboratory examination should focus on causes that are likely in a particular patient. Attention to nutrition, fluid intake, and electrolyte balance is crucial (22).

The treatment of the behavioral and emotional complications of delirium can become as urgent as the identification of the underlying cause. Frequent reorientation and reassurance, a well-lighted environment, and avoidance of overstimulation are important aspects of treatment. If the agitation, hallucinations, or delusions do not respond to environmental intervention and are overwhelming to the patient or adversely affecting the patient's safety, then a low dosage antipsychotic drug given by mouth or intramuscularly (e.g., haloperidol, 0.5 to 1.0 mg every 4 hours) can be ordered.

Table 26.3. Etiologic Classification of Delirium

In a medical or surgical illness (no focal or lateralizing neurologic signs; cerebrospinal fluid usually clear)
- Metabolic disorders: hepatic stupor, uremia, hypoxia, hypercapnia, hypoglycemia, porphyria, hyponatremia
- Congestive heart failure
- Pneumonia, septicemia, typhoid fever, other febrile illnesses (especially in elderly)
- Hyperthyroidism and hypothyroidism
- Postoperative and postraumatic states

In neurologic disease that causes focal or lateralizing signs or changes in the cerebrospinal fluid
- Cerebrovascular disease
- Subarachnoid hemorrhage
- Hypertensive encephalopathy
- Cerebral contusion
- Subdural hematoma
- Tumor
- Abscess
- Meningitis
- Encephalitis
- Status epilepticus (by electroencephalogram)

The abstinence states and exogenous intoxications (signs of other medical surgical, and neurologic illnesses absent or coincidental)
- Withdrawal of alcohol (delirium tremens), barbiturates, and nonbarbiturate sedative drugs, following chronic intoxication
- Drug intoxication from benzodiazepines, opiates, neuroleptics, antidepressants, antihistamines, H_2 blockers, centrally acting antihypertensives, anticholinergics, digitalis, illicit drugs (see Chapter 29), etc.

Beclouded dementia
- Any dementing or other brain disease in combination with infective fevers, drug reactions, heart failure, or other medical or surgical disease

Adapted from Adams RD. Delirium and other acute confusional states. In: Isselbacher KJ, Adams RD, Braunwald E, et al., eds. Harrison's principles of internal medicine, 9th ed. New York: McGraw-Hill, 1980:126, with permission.

General References*

Alzheimer's Association telephone number: 800-272-3900; website: http://www.ALZ.ORG.
A resource for professionals and families.

Blazer DG. Depression in late life, 2nd ed. St. Louis: CV Mosby, 1993.
Helpful overview of all aspects of this problem.

Doody RS, Stevens JC, Beck C, et al. Practice parameter: management of dementia (an evidence-based review): report of the Quality Standards Subcommittee of the American Academy of Neurology. Neurology 2001;56:1154.

LaRue A. Aging and neuropsychological assessment. New York: Plenum, 1992.
A readable introduction to geriatric neuropsychology.

Mace NL, Rabins PV. The 36-hour day. Baltimore, Johns Hopkins Press, 1981; 3rd edition, 1999.

*Bold print (general references) and bold numerals (specific references) denote published controlled clinical trials, meta-analyses, or consensus-based recommendations.

A book that provides detailed practical information for the caregiver of persons with dementia. Available in most bookstores for the general public.

Rabins PV, Lyketsos KG, Steele CD. Practical dementia care. New York: Oxford University Press, 1999.

Practice Guidelines

American Academy of Neurology:

Petersen RC, Stevens JC, Ganguli M, et al. **Practice parameter: early diagnosis of dementia: mild cognitive impairment (an evidence-based review). Report of the Quality Standards Subcommittee of the American Academy of Neurology**. Neurology 2001;56:1133.

Knopman DS, Dekosky ST, Cummings JL, et al. **Practice parameter: diagnosis of dementia (an evidence-based review). Report of the Quality Standards Subcommittee of the American Academy of Neurology**. Neurology 2001;56:1143.

Doody RS, Stevens JC, Beck C, et al. **Practice parameter: management of dementia (an evidence-based review): Report of the Quality Standards Subcommittee of the American Academy of Neurology**. Neurology 2001;56:1154.

Website: http://www.aan.com/public/practiceguidelines/

Agency for Health Care Policy and Research (AHCPR), now Agency for Healthcare Research and Quality (AHRQ):

Agency for Health Care Policy and Research. **Recognition and initial assessment of Alzheimer's disease and related dementias**. AHCPR Publication No. 97-0702, 1996.

American Psychiatric Association:

Am J Psychiatry 1997 May; 154 (5 Suppl):1-39 [243 references] Washington (DC): American Psychiatric Press, Inc; 1997 May. 93 p. (**APA practice guidelines; no. 1997**). [243 references] Available at http://www.guideline.gov/index.asp

Consensus guidelines:

Small GW, Rabins PV, Barry PP, et al. **Diagnosis and treatment of Alzheimer disease and related disorders: consensus statement of the American Association of Geriatric Psychiatry, the Alzheimer's Association, and the American Geriatrics Society**. JAMA 1997;278:1363.

Specific References*

1. Gallo JJ, Rabins PV, Lyketsos CG, et al. Depression without sadness: functional outcomes of nondysphoric depression in later life. J Am Geriatr Soc 1997;45:570.

1a. Folstein MF, Folstein SE, McHugh PR. "Mini-mental state": a practical method for grading the cognitive state of patients for the clinician. J Psychiatr Res 1975;12:1975.

2. Alexopoulos G, Meyer BS, Young, RC, et al. The course of geriatric depression with "reversible dementia." Am J Psychiatry 1993;150:1693.

3. Rabins PV, Merchant A, Nesdadt G. Criteria for diagnosing reversible dementia caused by depression: validation by 2-year follow-up. Br J Psychiatry 1984;144:488.

4. Starkstein SE, Robinson RG. Depression in neurological disease. Baltimore: Johns Hopkins Press, 1989.

5. Lyketsos CG, Sheppard J-ME, Steele CD, et al. Randomized placebo-controlled, double-blind clinical trial of sertraline in the treatment of depression complicating Alzheimer's disease: initial results from the depression in Alzheimer's disease study. Am J Psychiatry 2000;157:1686.

6. Burns A, Jacoby R, Levy R. Psychiatric phenomena in Alzheimer's disease. I. Disorders of thought content. Br J Psychiatry 1990;157:72.

7. Petersen RC, Smith GE, Waring SC, et al. Mild cognitive impairment: clinical characterization and outcome. Arch Neurol 1999;56:303.

8. Albert M, Moss MB, Tanzi R, et al. Preclinical prediction of AD using neuropsychological tests. J Int Neuropsychol Soc 2001;7:631.

9. Rabins PV. Does reversible dementia exist and is it reversible? Arch Intern Med 1988;148:1905.

10. Hendrie HC, Ogunnixi A, Hall KS, et al. Incidence of dementia and Alzheimer disease in 2 communities—Yoruba residing in Ibadan, Nigeria and African Americans residing in Indianapolis, Indiana. JAMA 2001;6:739.

11. Agency for Health Care Policy and Research. Recognition and initial assessment of Alzheimer's disease and related dementias. AHCPR Publication No. 97-0702, 1996.

12. Knopman DS, Dekosky ST, Cummings JL, et al. Practice parameter: diagnosis of dementia (an evidence-based review). Report of the quality standards subcommittee of the American Academy of Neurology. Neurology 2001;56:1143.

13. Small GW, Rabins PV, Barry PP, et al. Diagnosis and treatment of Alzheimer disease and related disorders: consensus statement of the American Association of Geriatric Psychiatry, the Alzheimer's Association, and the American Geriatrics Society. JAMA 1997;278:1363.

14. Spector A, Orrell M, Davies S, et al. Reality orientation for dementia. Cochrane Database of Systematic Reviews. Issue 3, 2001.

15. Lyketsos CG, Steinberg M, Tschantz JT. Mental and behavioral disturbances in dementia: findings from the Cache County study on memory in aging. Am J Psychiatry 2000;157:708.

16. Burns A, Jacoby R, Levy R. Psychiatric phenomena in Alzheimer's disease. III. Disorders of mood. Br J Psychiatry 1990;157:81.

17. Rovner B, Broadhead J, Spencer M, et al. Depression and Alzheimer's disease. Am J Psychiatry 1989;146:350.

18. Teri L, Logsdon R, Uomoto J, et al. Behavioral treatment of depression in dementia patients: a controlled clinical trial. J Gerontol Psychol Sci 1997;52B:P159.

19. Mittelman MS, Ferris SH, Shulman E, et al. A family intervention to delay nursing home placement of patients with Alzheimer disease. JAMA 1996;276:1725.

20. Lebars PL, Katz MH, Berman N, et al. A placebo-controlled, double-blind, randomized trial of an extract of Ginkgo biloba for dementia. JAMA 1997;340:1136.

21. Ernst E, Pittler MH. Ginkgo biloba for dementia: a systematic review of double-blind, placebo-controlled trials. Clin Drug Invest 1999;17:301.

22. Inouye SK, Bogardus ST, Charpentier PA, et al. A multicomponent intervention to prevent delirium in hospitalized older patient. N Engl J Med 1999;340:669.

CHAPTER 27

Tobacco Use and Dependence

GEORGE E. BIGELOW, PhD
CYNTHIA S. RAND, PhD

Tobacco use, primarily in the form of chronic cigarette smoking, is the greatest single cause of illness, disability, and death in the United States. Smoking is estimated to cause more than 430,000 deaths annually—almost 20% of all deaths.

The perniciousness of the habit relates largely to its long history of social acceptability and to the failure by society and by health professionals to recognize and respond to smoking as a health-damaging behavior. This situation has been changing, and it continues to change. Within the United States and many other countries, both society and health professionals are now acting to proscribe, prevent, restrict, and treat smoking. Still, much remains to be done. The prevalence and acceptability of smoking remain high in many subgroups and in many countries. The World Health Organization (WHO) estimates that worldwide tobacco-related deaths will increase from 3 million annually in 1990 to more than 8 million annually in 2020.

PREVALENCE OF TOBACCO USE

The decline of smoking prevalence in the United States in recent decades represents an impressive success of public health and prevention efforts. Beginning in 1965, adult smoking prevalence declined by 0.5% to 1.0% per year, from 42% in 1965 to 25% in 1993. The rate of decline has now slowed; total prevalence fell only one more percentage point over the next 5 years, to 24% in 1998. Smoking is becoming concentrated in more resistant individuals. Table 27.1 summarizes the prevalence of adult cigarette smoking in relation to demographic characteristics for the 1998 National Health Interview Survey. There are substantial differences among demographic subgroups. Smoking is more common in poor communities and least common among the highly educated.

Smoking prevalence has been fairly constant in recent years among U.S. adults, but it has been increasing among adolescents since 1992, with 23% of high school students reporting daily smoking in 1999. Adult smoking prevalence is highest among Native Americans, fairly similar among African Americans and whites, but lower among Hispanics (especially Hispanic women). In contrast, adolescent prevalence is appreciably lower among African Americans than whites, with Hispanics intermediate; daily smoking prevalences for high school students in 1999 were 8%, 27%, and 14%, respectively. Other forms of tobacco use occur predominantly in males: pipe and cigar use in approximately 3% and 5%, respectively, and use of smokeless products (snuff, chewing tobacco) in approximately 6%. However, in some locales and subgroups (e.g., young men in rural or southern areas), the prevalence of smokeless tobacco use may approximate that of smoking.

CAUSES AND RISK FACTORS

The development of tobacco dependence can be viewed as a pediatric disorder. Smoking typically begins in the preteen or teenage years; initiation after 18 to 20 years of age is rare. The habit is so widespread that it is not limited to any specific environmental, physiologic, or psychological circumstances. Social influences, such as peer pressures or efforts to display independence and to appear mature and self-confident, are major factors in promoting and sustaining initial smoking experiences. Aversive initial experiences (e.g., coughing, nausea, dysphoria) are described even by people who proceed to chronic dependence. Nicotine is the causative pharmacologic agent responsible for establishing and maintaining tobacco use and addiction. The continued easy availability of nicotine-delivering tobacco products, combined with strong learned behavioral habits, memories, and associations, make tobacco use a truly addictive disorder—with characteristic resistance to change (1).

Table 27.1. Percentage of Adults (Age ≥18 yr) Who Smoke Cigarettes, United States, 1998

Parameter	Men	Women	Total
Race/Ethnicity			
White	26.5	23.6	25.0
African American	29.0	21.3	24.7
Hispanic	24.7	13.3	19.1
Native American	41.7	38.1	40.0
Asian/Pacific	17.9	9.9	13.7
Years of education (for ages ≥25 yr only)			
9–11	39.7	34.3	36.8
12	31.5	24.1	27.4
13–15	26.6	22.8	24.6
≥16	11.5	11.2	11.3
Age (yr)			
18–24	31.3	24.5	27.9
25–44	29.4	25.6	27.5
45–64	27.7	22.5	25.0
≥65	10.4	11.2	10.9
Socioeconomic status			
At or above poverty level	25.7	21.3	23.5
Below poverty level	37.0	29.3	32.3
Total	26.4	22.0	24.1

From Centers for Disease Control. MMWR 2000;49:881–884.

About half of individuals who smoke for 1 month become chronically dependent (2). Certain risk factors are associated with an increased likelihood of becoming a chronic cigarette smoker. Smoking runs in families. An individual with parents and siblings who smoke is four times as likely to become a smoker as is an individual from a nonsmoking family. The familial association results from both genetic and environmental factors. Twin studies indicate an approximately 50% heritability of smoking (3). Smoking is also significantly associated with adverse childhood experiences; violence in the family, childhood abuse, and stressful life events are each associated with a two- to four-fold increase in the probability of being a smoker (4,5). In the past, males were more much likely to smoke than females, but this is no longer the case. There is no distinct personality type that is characteristic of smokers, but on average they tend to be somewhat more extroverted than nonsmokers, more adventuresome or risk taking, and more likely to deviate from social norms or rules. These latter characteristics may, in adolescence, increase the probability of experimentation with smoking, with a consequent increased risk of chronic dependence. Smoking is also more prevalent in individuals with other substance use disorders (e.g., 70% to 90% prevalence in alcoholics and other drug abusers). This relationship may reflect similar or overlapping etiologic influences. Smoking may serve as a conveniently visible risk factor or marker for those at increased risk of other substance use disorders.

PRIMARY PREVENTION

Primary prevention efforts must be directed to preadolescents and adolescents. An important element is changing societal norms about the acceptability of tobacco use. Formal preventive interventions should begin in elementary grades and continue for several years. Effective interventions are not simple fact-based health education, but instead teach specific skills for resisting social pressure and include explicit instructions and rehearsals with peers in vignettes about resisting offers to use cigarettes, alcohol products, and illegal drugs. Children who receive such training have reduced rates of smoking onset (6). As community health leaders, physicians should encourage and support preventive interventions, including bans on tobacco use in public areas, enforcement of prohibitions on tobacco sales to minors, and restrictions on advertising that glamorizes smoking or appeals to youth.

COURSE OF THE HABIT

The health hazards of smoking are now widely recognized, and the social acceptability of smoking has declined. Consequently, most smokers vacillate between defending and justifying their habit and trying to end it. Most smokers would like to quit, and about half attempt to stop in a given year. Adverse health events and advice from physicians are potent forces in promoting increased cessation efforts by patients. In the United States there are now about twice as many former smokers as there are current smokers.

Patterns of Quitting and Relapse

Approximately 60% to 80% of smokers who attempt to quit achieve at least a minimal period of abstinence. However, the relapse rate is high, and much relapse occurs very early (7). Approximately two thirds of quitters resume smoking within 3 to 6 months, many within only a few days. Only 15% to 20% of untreated quitters remain cigarette free for 6 months or longer. Treatment approximately doubles the long-term success rate, but relapse, repeat quit attempts, and repeat treatments are commonplace. Cessation should not be considered successful until abstinence has been sustained for at least 6 months. The probability of relapse after 6 months of abstinence is reduced but still present.

Approximately 95% of smoking cessation occurs as the result of smokers' self-directed personal efforts, without formal treatment. Abrupt ("cold turkey") cessation is more likely to be successful than is gradual reduction. Most successful quitters require more than one attempt before becoming permanent ex-smokers. Repeated quitting and relapsing are characteristic of the normal, successful cessation process. The *risk of relapse is increased* when patients are under emotional stress (e.g., anger, frustration, anxiety, depression), when ex-smokers are exposed to cues associated with prior smoking (e.g., after meals, when consuming alcoholic beverages), and in people whose spouse or friends continue to smoke (8).

HEALTH CONSEQUENCES

Risk of Disease

Although smoking dramatically increases overall population morbidity and mortality, its effects on individual smokers are unpredictable, and some smokers escape major health consequences. Age-adjusted mortality rates for smokers are 70% greater than those for nonsmokers. Life expectancy is significantly shortened by smoking (e.g., 8.1 years less for the 30-year-old two-pack-a-day smoker than for a comparable nonsmoker). Risk is dose related; mortality increases with increasing number of cigarettes smoked, with increasing number of years as a smoker, and with depth of inhalation.

Smoking is associated with increased risk of cancer (especially of the respiratory tract), cardiovascular disease, chronic obstructive pulmonary disease, gastric ulcer, prostate cancer, cervical cancer, postmenopausal osteoporosis, diabetes, and macular degeneration. Smoking by pregnant women reduces fetal growth and birth weight and increases the risk of fetal death; smoking interacts with the use of oral contraceptives by women and increases the risk of myocardial infarction, subarachnoid hemorrhage, and thromboembolic disease.

The *risks of cancer and chronic pulmonary disease* in smokers are ten times those in nonsmokers. The percentage of oral, throat, and lung cancer deaths attributable to smoking exceeds 80%. The *risk of atherosclerotic cardiovascular disease* is approximately doubled in smokers. The percentage of cardiovascular disease deaths attributable to smoking is 20%. Because of the much greater population prevalence of cardiovascular disease, it is in this area that the greatest overall health benefits of smoking cessation occur.

Benefits of Cessation

The greatest immediate benefit of smoking cessation is the reduction of cardiovascular risk. Within hours after smoking cessation, both carbon monoxide and nicotine—the two cigarette products thought to be primarily responsible for cardiovascular disease—are dissipated from the body, with a consequent reduction in cardiac work requirement and a concurrent increase in oxygenation. There is also prompt reduction in the risk of upper respiratory tract infection. Slower to accrue are a reduction in the rate of decline of pulmonary function and a reduction in cancer risk; benefits of cessation are measurable in these domains within 3 and 10 years, respectively, after smoking cessation.

Health benefits of smoking cessation are greater for smokers who quit before the development of symptoms; however, the benefits of cessation also extend to those who have already experienced symptoms of smoking-related disease. For example, individuals who stop smoking after myocardial infarction have improved survival rates compared with those who continue smoking. Similarly, there are pulmonary benefits to smoking cessation even late in life (9).

Low-Yield Cigarettes

Because the risks of smoking are dose related, it is tempting to believe that substantial health benefits might be achieved by switching to low-yield cigarettes. This is no longer the case; the variations in currently marketed tobacco yields have little health impact, and there are negligible correlations between the stated yield values and blood levels of nicotine and its major metabolite, cotinine (10). Biologic yield may differ substantially from stated yield because of behavioral variations in the way the cigarettes are smoked. When nominal yields change, smokers tend to change their behavior so as to keep biologic delivery unchanged (e.g., by smoking more cigarettes, inhaling more smoke). The primary manufacturing technique for producing current low-yield cigarettes is to place ventilation holes in the sides of the filter to dilute the smoke stream with air. With these low-yield brands it is especially likely that biologic delivery will significantly exceed assay delivery, because the smoker's fingers tend to block these ventilation holes (11). Smokers should be cautioned that so-called low-yield cigarettes may still have high biologic delivery.

Physical Dependence and Craving

Chronic tobacco use produces physical dependence on nicotine. On cessation of use, an *abstinence syndrome* typically occurs (12–14). The subjective aspects of the syndrome can be very distressing and include irritability, restlessness, sleep disturbances, difficulty in concentrating, anxiety, gastrointestinal disturbances, hunger, weight gain, and, most important, craving for cigarettes. Most patients feel normal again within approximately 2 weeks of abstinence, except that the craving for tobacco may persist for months or years. Nicotine substitution treatment (see later discussion) is effective in reducing the abstinence syndrome. The physiologic aspects of the tobacco abstinence syndrome are generally inconsequential, consisting of a slight and gradual decline in heart rate and blood pressure.

Craving for tobacco is an extraordinarily persistent obstacle to sustained abstinence. Many ex-smokers report craving years after cessation. The duration of craving is highly variable, but it should be expected to persist for at least 3 to 6 months, with its frequency and urgency diminishing over that interval. Craving may be a learned phenomenon rather than part of an abstinence syndrome, because it is high even among smokers making no attempt to quit or reduce their smoking.

Passive Smoking

Passive smoking-exposure of nonsmokers to air contaminated by the smoking of others is not only an irritant to many nonsmokers; it has definite adverse health effects. Although the levels of smoke products detected in the blood and urine of passively exposed nonsmokers are low compared with those in smokers, there are significant health risks associated with passive smoking (15–18). Passive exposure to the smoke of spouses is associated with impaired pulmonary function, increased lung cancer risk, and increased coronary heart disease risk. Children passively exposed to smoke by parents have increased rates of respiratory infections, slower developmental increases in pulmonary function, and an increased incidence of asthma attacks. Maternal smoking contributes to reduced birth weight, and smokers who stop the habit during pregnancy have significantly heavier babies than do those who continue smoking (19).

Physicians should try to protect nonsmokers from cigarette smoke and should recognize that most indoor ventilation systems simply diffuse and redistribute smoke rather than remove it. Smoking (including employee smoking) should be emphatically prohibited in physicians' offices, and physicians should support similar efforts in all public settings, especially in health care facilities. Legal prohibition of indoor smoking in public or commercial facilities is now common.

RECOGNITION AND DIAGNOSIS

Nicotine dependence is a diagnosable substance use disorder in the American Psychiatric Association's *Diagnostic and Statistical Manual of Mental Disorders,* 4th edition. The diagnostic criteria are identical to those for other substance-related disorders (see Chapter 29), reflecting the growing recognition of extensive commonalities among alcoholism, drug abuse, and tobacco dependence.

There is widespread failure of health professionals to recognize and diagnose tobacco dependence and to maintain it on an active problem list. Tobacco use status should be considered at every visit at the office reception point (20). There should be a clear and prominent chart indication to prompt attention at subsequent visits.

Assessment of smoking status is normally via patient self-report. Objective biologic indices may become more important as the social acceptability of admitting to smoking declines. Smoking status can be assessed by measuring carbon monoxide concentrations in expired breath (concentrations greater than 5 to 8 ppm normally indicate smoking). Urine and saliva test-strips for detection of nicotine or its metabolites have been developed. The potential value of such objective assessment is indicated by the fact that up to 20% to 30% of self-reported quitters show biologic evidence of continuing to smoke.

TREATMENT

Substantial evidence, assistive materials, and pharmacologic modalities are now available for the rational planning and implementation of smoking cessation interventions with patients. They are summarized here. Detailed office approaches are described in the next section.

Role of the Health Care Provider

Concern about health remains the most cited reason smokers quit, and smokers cite physicians as the people most able to influence their decisions to attempt to quit. The optimal role of a physician or other health care practitioner in the treatment of tobacco dependence is to advise and assist all smoking patients to stop. It is a mistake to rely heavily on referral to specialized smoking cessation programs. Results of referral are disappointing when compared with those obtained by devoting equal or less time to brief direct advice.

Brief advice can significantly increase rates of smoking cessation (21,22). A recent rigorous review of more than 30 studies (with more than 27,000 smokers) conducted over the past 25 years found that physician advice resulted in a small but significant increase in the odds of quitting. Although counseling effectiveness is not necessarily directly related to the intensity of advice, direct comparisons of minimal advice versus intensive counseling found a significant improvement in cessation rates (23). Medical economic analyses have shown that smoking cessation advice is as cost-effective as other common interventions, such as treatment of hypercholesterolemia or mild hypertension. An increase in smoking cessation rates of between 1% and 3% can be expected if practitioners simply caution each smoker to quit during routine office visits for other problems. Addition of pharmacologic treatment (discussed later) further increases success. Among certain patients, advice alone can achieve impressive efficacy. For example, the smoking cessation rate after a first myocardial infarction is as high as 50% for patients given directive smoking cessation advice by their physician, compared with approximately 35% for patients receiving usual care. Similarly high rates of cessation are seen in prenatal care settings, where up to 20% to 30% of smokers may quit during a pregnancy (19).

Consistency of Counseling

Despite its known benefits, the frequency and consistency of physician counseling to quit smoking remain disappointing. Fewer than 50% of smokers report receiving smoking cessation advice from their physician (24,25). Patients who are younger, male, African American, uninsured, healthier, or lighter smokers are less likely to report receiving physician advice to quit smoking. This may be related to frequency of patient health care contacts, or physicians' likelihood to counsel may be influenced by patient characteristics (24,26).

Absolute rates of smoking cessation in response to physician advice are likely to remain frustratingly low.

But, it is important to recognize that the overall public health benefit may be very large due to the number of smokers counseled. Routine smoking cessation advice from physicians plays an important role in reducing overall societal smoking rates (27). Further, although patients may not immediately quit smoking as a result of direct physician advice, such counseling may play an important role in increasing readiness to quit smoking in the future (28).

Motivational Communication

The goal of effective doctor–patient communication is to provide advice that maximizes a smoker's motivation and decision to quit. A common error is to rely too much on fact-based health education that implicitly seeks to motivate through fear. Smokers are now well aware of the health risks of smoking and do not respond to that information alone. The five actions described later in this chapter (see Recommended Office Approach) integrate what is known about motivational communication into a practical approach for helping smokers to quit. The approach includes many of the behavioral strategies described in Chapter 4. It focuses on one clear and simple message—"I strongly advise you to quit"—delivered in a manner free of blame or rancor. *The advice should be personally relevant to patients, should describe in a positive way the benefits to be gained, and should prescribe a particular course of action.* These three objectives can be attained by pointing out the association between smoking and the specific symptoms, illnesses, or health risks of the individual patient; by pointing out that smoking cessation can prevent, reverse, or stop the progression of disease (whichever is appropriate); and by stating clearly, simply, and directly the course of action to be taken: stop smoking. A general statement that "Smoking is bad for your health and you can kill yourself if you continue" fails on all three of these points. It is not specifically personal, it describes no benefit, and it is not sufficiently directive. More personalized and directive statements can be more persuasive (e.g., "I strongly advise you to stop smoking; both your coughing and your recurring colds and flus are caused in part by your smoking; I want you to try to quit smoking, and then we should see some improvement").

Patients differ in their readiness and willingness to change their smoking habit. The goal is to move patients along the continuum depicted in Fig. 4.1. When patients are ready to attempt cessation, the goal should be to agree on a cessation date and to provide therapeutic assistance. Patients not yet ready for cessation may become ready in response to repeated nonjudgmental encouragement and motivational advice.

Brochures and Self-Help Materials

Self-help smoking cessation brochures can provide useful motivational advice and specific helpful techniques for smokers. A wide variety are available, and these change periodically. Local offices of the American Cancer Society, the American Heart Association, or the American Lung Association can be contacted to obtain copies of their smoking cessation self-help brochures. The National Cancer Institute offers a *Quit for Good Kit* for physicians that includes patient self-help brochures (telephone, 1-800-4-CANCER). Patients with Internet access can also be referred to a wide range of smoking cessation self-help aids, programs, and support groups available (in multiple languages) on the Internet (see General References).

Pharmacologic Treatments

There have been substantial advances in recent years in the availability of pharmacologic treatments for tobacco dependence. Nicotine chewing gum and transdermal patch products are now available over the counter without prescription. Other types of nicotine replacement treatment products are available by prescription, including nicotine nasal spray and nicotine vapor inhaler. Also, bupropion, the first non-nicotine smoking cessation product, is available by prescription. Characteristics and 2001 costs of these products are summarized in Table 27.2. Additional products are under development, including a lozenge-like oral transmucosal nicotine. Table 27.3 compares *the costs of smoking and the costs of pharmacologic treatment* with available products.

Mechanism and Indication

Smoking cessation medications are intended to aid patients who are making a serious attempt to stop tobacco use. They will not themselves induce such an attempt. They enhance the success of motivated behavior change efforts but do not cause or motivate such behavior change directly. Nicotine replacement products suppress the nicotine abstinence syndrome and reduce subjective desire or craving for tobacco. The mechanism of bupropion's efficacy is uncertain, although it also appears to suppress nicotine withdrawal and craving. Medications are to be used in conjunction with a complete cessation of tobacco use. If tobacco use persists beyond the first couple of weeks of treatment, the medication should probably be discontinued until some future renewed effort at total cessation is attempted.

Efficacy

Strong data support the efficacy of all these marketed treatments, but none is clearly superior (29–32). Meta-analyses quantifying their effectiveness are summarized in the recent clinical practice guideline released by the Surgeon General (29). All have been shown to increase smoking cessation rates by approximately 50% to 100% over placebo comparison conditions. The absolute rates of smoking cessation depend on many factors: patient motivation and setting, intensity of concurrent behavioral counseling, definition of cessation, and time of assessment. Most clinical efficacy

Table 27.2. Summary of Smoking Cessation Products

Type and Brand Name	Dosage	Package	2001 Retail Cost[a]	Comments
Over-the-Counter Products				
Nicotine gum				
Nicorette (also as generic)	2 mg × 9–24 day	108 pieces 48 pieces	\$50 \$29	Give special instructions on how to "chew-and-park" the gum.
	4 mg × 9–24 day	108 pieces 48 pieces	\$56 \$32	Absorption is through oral mucosa. Emphasize importance of adequate use. Target is 9–24 per day for 4–6 weeks, then gradual tapering over 2–4 weeks.
Nicotine patch				
Nicoderm CQ	21 mg/24 hr 14 mg/24 hr 7 mg/24 hr	14 patches 14 patches 14 patches	\$46 \$46 \$46	Target is maintenance for 4–10 weeks, possibly followed by gradual dosage tapering over 2–6 weeks. All may be used for 16 or 24 hr as preferred.
Nicotrol	15 mg/16 hr	14 patches	\$70	
Generics and store brands	22 mg/24 hr	14 patches	\$37	
Prescription Products				
Nicotine nasal spray				
Nicotrol NS	1 mg × 8–40 mg/day 2 sprays = 1 mg	100 mg	\$44	Target is maintenance for 6 or more weeks, possibly followed by gradual tapering of use, up to 12 weeks total. Provides most rapid onset of nicotine effects.
Nicotine vapor inhaler				
Nicotrol inhaler	10 mg/cartridge (delivers 4 mg)	42 cartridges	\$41	Absorption is via oral mucosa, not lungs. Similar in appearance to a cigarette; may simulate sensory/manipulation aspects of smoking. 6 to 16 cartridges per day for up to 12 weeks.
Bupropion SR				
Zyban	150 mg (1/day × 3 days then 2/day)	60 tablets	\$86	Begin 1 week before quit date. No dosage tapering needed. May be combined with nicotine replacement product for possibly greater total effectiveness.

[a]Based on large pharmacy chain in Baltimore, Maryland region, October 2001.

Table 27.3. Cost of Smoking Versus Cost of Treatment

Annual Cost of Smoking		Cigarette Packs Per Day 1/2	1	2
Price per pack[a]				
\$2		\$365	\$730	\$1430
\$3		\$547	\$1095	\$2190
\$4		\$730	\$1460	\$2860
Cost of Treatment[b]				
Nicotine gum	\$200			
Nicotine patch	\$165			
Nicotine nasal spray	\$300			
Nicotine inhaler	\$510			
Bupropion	\$170			

[a]Varies by region and taxation.
[b]Estimates based on current retail prices and typical 8-wk treatment course.

trials described in product labeling are conducted in patients sufficiently motivated to volunteer for smoking cessation treatment and in conjunction with individual or group counseling; success is generally defined as 4 weeks of smoking abstinence during active treatment. Under these conditions cessation success rates of 30% to 50% are often achieved in active medication groups, compared with rates of 10% to 30% in placebo groups. Success rates decline to half of these values when assessed 6 to 12 months after the end of treatment. Despite variations in the absolute rates of success, the relative efficacy of active pharmacologic treatment over placebo is robust and is preserved across different populations, settings, counseling levels, and follow-up periods.

Nicotine Patch

The nicotine transdermal patch is the treatment of choice at present. This preference relates primarily to its ease of use and relatively good patient compliance. Patches may be worn for either 24 or 16 hours/day with equivalent effectiveness. The rationale for 24-hour use is to minimize nicotine withdrawal on waking. The rationale for 16-hour (daytime only) use is to minimize sleep disturbances that may accompany 24-hour use. The most common side effect is skin irritation at the site of patch application. In a placebo-controlled trial, the nicotine patch was shown to be effective and safe for use in a wide spectrum of patients with chronic cardiac problems (30).

Nicotine Chewing Gum

A potential advantage of nicotine gum is the ability to adjust dosage individually and to schedule use as needed in response to situational variations in nicotine withdrawal and craving. Its major disadvantages are the extensive behavioral compliance required for effective use and the common failure of patients to use enough. Patients must be instructed in proper chewing technique; they must understand that the nicotine is absorbed primarily through the oral mucosa but very poorly if swallowed. Proper use involves a few chews until a peppery taste or tingling is felt, parking the gum inside the cheek to allow absorption, then repeating at intervals of about 1 minute. Nicotine absorption is not rapid, so a regularly timed dosing schedule of 1 gum every 1 to 2 hours is usually more successful than self-selected dosing. Acidic beverages (coffee, juices, soda, and wine) should be avoided before or during gum use because their pH reduces nicotine absorption. The 4-mg dosage form is intended for patients with higher levels of nicotine dependence. Convenient indices of dependence level are number of cigarettes smoked per day (25 or more is considered high dependence) and how soon after waking the first cigarette is smoked (smoking within just a few minutes of waking reflects high dependence).

Nicotine Nasal Spray

The nicotine nasal spray more closely simulates the pharmacokinetics of nicotine delivery via tobacco smoking than the other nicotine substitution medications do. It produces a larger and more rapid increase in blood nicotine levels, although still less than that achieved with smoking. The nasal spray may be especially beneficial to highly dependent smokers, who may need more rapid and more substantial nicotine delivery. The nasal spray's more rapid onset makes as-needed dosing more practical than with gum, but regularly scheduled dosing is still the recommended procedure.

Nicotine Vapor Inhaler

The nicotine vapor inhaler is similar in appearance to a cigarette and may be especially useful to patients who desire the physical manipulation and sensory aspects of smoking. There is no heat or combustion; puffs on the inhaler draw air over an internal nicotine-laden plug. Each puff delivers a very small dose of nicotine vapor (approximately 0.013 mg) to the mouth, where the nicotine is absorbed through the oral mucosa.

Bupropion

Zyban is a sustained-release tablet formulation containing 150 mg of the antidepressant drug bupropion. The mechanism of action of bupropion in promoting smoking cessation is unknown, but it probably relates to its inhibition of norepinephrine and dopamine uptake. This is the only marketed non-nicotine smoking cessation medication. It is effective as a sole treatment, but its efficacy can perhaps be further enhanced by combination use with a nicotine replacement product (31). In a controlled trial in patients who were not depressed, bupropion, 300 mg (150 mg twice daily), yielded a 1-year cessation rate of 23.1%, compared with 12.4% in patients treated with placebo (32). Treatment was initiated 1 week before each patient's quit date and discontinued after 7 weeks. For the first 3 days, patients took 150 mg/day, then 150 mg twice daily. All patients received simple smoking cessation counseling.

Bupropion is also marketed as an antidepressant under the brand name Wellbutrin (see Chapter 24); patients should not use the two preparations simultaneously.

Combined Nicotine Replacement Treatments

Some studies suggest that combinations of nicotine replacement products (e.g., patch plus gum) might be more effective than single products. Theoretically, such an approach has some merit, but data are at present insufficient to permit firm recommendation.

Chronic Treatment

Current recommendations are for nicotine replacement medications to be used for no longer than 2 to 3 months, during which time they are tapered gradually and discontinued. However, some patients who succeed at stopping smoking continue to use nicotine replacement products for longer periods and may be at risk for smoking relapse if the medication substitution is stopped. There is no consensus on the appropriate response to this circumstance. However, the health risks of chronic nicotine maintenance are certainly much lower than the risks of smoking.

Potential Medication Interactions

Nicotine substitution treatment typically yields nicotine blood levels well below those achieved during tobacco use. Therefore, potential medication interactions relate primarily to the cessation of tobacco use rather than to the administration of smoking cessation medications. After tobacco cessation, a *dosage decrease* may be required for acetaminophen, adrenergic antagonists (e.g., prazosin, labetalol), caffeine, imipramine, insulin, oxazepam, pentazocine, propranolol and other beta-blockers, and theophylline. After tobacco cessation a *dosage increase* may be required for adrenergic agonists such as isoproterenol or phenylephrine. Bupropion is contraindicated within 14 days of monoamine oxidase inhibitor use.

Weight Gain

Weight gain is a common, distressing consequence of smoking cessation. Weight gain results both from dietary changes (increased snacking and selection of high-calorie foods) and from discontinuation of the metabolic effects of nicotine (33). Weight gain of patients remaining abstinent for 1 year averages 5 to 15 lb. This magnitude of weight gain is medically insignificant relative to the health benefits of smoking cessation. Unfortunately, the anticipated social, cosmetic, and economic (e.g., wardrobe cost) consequences of weight gain deter some smokers from quitting and contribute to relapse in others. Smoking cessation is most successful if patients accept temporary weight gain rather than struggling against it during the early cessation period. Nicotine replacement treatment and bupropion both significantly attenuate weight gain after smoking cessation (34). Recent research suggests that, among women concerned about weight gain, cognitive behavioral therapy can improve smoking cessation outcomes and decrease weight concerns (35). The goals of the cognitive behavioral therapy were to reduce concerns about, and promote acceptance of, modest weight gain; to discourage dietary restraint, dieting, and active resistance to weight gain; and to encourage moderate consumption of healthy foods in between-meal snacks. The important message for patients concerned about possible postcessation weight gain is perhaps counterintuitive: Focusing on weight control concurrent with smoking cessation leads to worse outcomes on both smoking and weight.

Organized Treatment

Health care practitioners often would like to refer smokers to formal cessation programs. For the small minority of smokers who attend them, organized programs at little or no cost are often available through local voluntary service organizations such as the Lung Association or Heart Association. There are also available in some communities self-help peer-counseling programs (e.g., Nicotine Anonymous) modeled after the 12-step approaches used with other addictions. Commercial programs offer no clear advantages. Most organized programs incorporate standard behavioral principles of self-monitoring, control of environmental cues, and scheduling of rewards. These principles are also well represented in various self-help guides and in the patient education materials packaged with cessation medications. Patients often express interest in using alternative strategies for smoking cessation, such as acupuncture, hypnosis, or herbal aids. Although research has found no significant benefit of these often costly approaches, patients who are highly motivated to use such alternative strategies may benefit.

Relapse Prevention

As with most addictive disorders, the likelihood of relapse after cessation is high. Most relapses occur within the first few days or weeks of cessation, although patients are at some risk for relapse even after months of abstinence. New quitters face many urges to smoke again. Anticipation and advance planning can prevent relapse. Self-help educational brochures are useful for this purpose. They provide warnings about relapse risk circumstances and suggest coping strategies. In addition, they help patients recognize the normality of "slips" and the importance of continued commitment to cessation. Slips or brief episodes of relapse are strong predictors of full relapse to smoking; therefore, patients should be carefully counseled that even one cigarette may jeopardize their smoking cessation attempt. Practical aspects of addressing relapse are described in the next section.

RECOMMENDED OFFICE APPROACH

Most health care practitioners advise smoking cessation for patients with obvious smoking-related illnesses, such as the patient with chronic obstructive pulmonary disease or the inpatient recovering from a myocardial infarction. However, too often physicians neglect to give smoking cessation advice in routine office care. Patients with smoking-related diseases obviously require strong smoking cessation interventions, but it is the smoking patient who has not yet experienced negative health consequences of smoking who stands to benefit most from smoking cessation. This section describes the primary care smoking cessation practice developed and recommended in the 2000 *Treating Tobacco Use and Dependence* clinical practice guideline published by the U.S. Public Health Service (http://www.surgeongeneral.gov/tobacco).

Although health care practitioners agree that it is appropriate and important for them to counsel patients to stop smoking, they are inconsistent in providing such advice. Reported barriers to counseling include a belief that such advice is ineffectual, a belief that most smoking patients are uninterested in counseling, a perceived lack of skills, and time constraints. However, studies have repeatedly found that brief, directive smoking interventions delivered during routine care are cost-effective and have the potential for significant public health benefit. A routine office visit for the treatment of eczema, flu, or indigestion can be used successfully to change smoking behavior, in the same way that it may also be used to screen for hypertension. These office-based smoking cessation practices are most effective when the smoking cessation interventions are viewed as essential components of good care. Just as measuring blood pressure at each office visit is now standard practice, so also should smoking status assessment and smoking cessation interventions be systematically integrated into standard office practice (20).

Motivating Smokers to Quit Smoking

Effective motivational counseling for smoking cessation recognizes that smokers cycle through several levels of readiness before attempting smoking cessation (see Fig. 4.1 in Chapter 4). Many factors can influence a smoker's progress through the stages of a change process. Life events, health symptoms, workplace smoking restrictions, and the price of a pack of cigarettes can all move a smoker closer to cessation. Alternatively, stress, weight gain, family problems, and smoking peers can act as barriers to change. The strong, directive advice smokers receive from their health care practitioner regarding the personal importance of quitting smoking is often one of the significant forces that moves smokers closer to quitting.

Health concern is one of the most common reasons smokers cite as a motivation for quitting. Physicians and other practitioners can increase overall motivation for cessation by underscoring the personal *relevance* of quitting for that individual patient. The *risks* of smoking to both the smoker and his or her family can be highlighted, as well as the *rewards* of quitting, such as better health, saving money, improved vitality, and fewer wrinkles. And finally, because developing sufficient motivation for change may take a smoker months or years, the effort to motivate patients should be *repeated* at every clinical contact. Practitioners who consistently and repeatedly use these *4 Rs*—Relevance,

Risks, Rewards, and Repetition (Fig. 27.1)— and provide smoking patients with advice and encouragement to quit smoking over the course of their medical care are most likely to see success. This *4 Rs* strategy should be used in conjunction with the actions outlined in Figures 27.2 to 27.6.

Actions: Ask, Advise, Assess, Assist, and Arrange

The Surgeon General's clinical guidelines (see General References) for treating tobacco use and dependence were derived from rigorous review of approximately 3,000 scientific reports. Those satisfying scientific quality criteria were analyzed by meta-analytic techniques. This permitted the authors to synthesize outcome data from different smoking cessation treatments and to identify effective treatment elements. Based on this review, the authors concluded that brief interventions are effective in promoting smoking cessation; therefore, "Every patient who uses tobacco should be offered at least brief treatment." The resulting guidelines for brief counseling are based on sound scientific evidence, and they recognize the time constraints on practitioners. These recommended practices are designed to require 3 minutes or less. They consist of five actions that are described more fully in the following paragraphs: Ask, Advise, Assess, Assist, and Arrange.

Office-based practitioners should systematically ***ask*** *about tobacco use* at every visit (Fig. 27.2). Clinicians are more likely to intervene with smoking patients when office procedures are designed to identify smokers and document smoking status. Smoking status should be considered a vital sign that is automatically collected, updated, and integrated into the permanent medical record.

The clinician should next ***advise*** *every smoking patient* in a strong, direct, personalized manner of the importance of quitting smoking (Fig. 27.3). Even brief advice to quit smoking (3 minutes or less) will increase smoking cessation rates.

After advising cessation, the clinician should ***assess*** *the smoker's motivation,* identify those patients who are willing to make a quit attempt, and determine the type of treatment they will accept (Fig. 27.4). For the unmotivated smoker, the clinician can attempt to enhance motivation for future cessation.

For patients interested in quitting smoking, the clinician should ***assist*** *in formalizing a quit* plan by setting a quit date within 2 weeks (Fig. 27.5). Brief counseling

ACTION	STRATEGIES FOR IMPLEMENTATION
Relevance	Motivational information given to a patient has the greatest impact if it is relevant to a patient's disease status, family or social situation (e.g., having children in the home), health concerns, age, gender, and other important patient characteristics (e.g., prior quitting experience).
Risks	The clinician should *ask the patient to identify the potential negative consequences of smoking.* The clinician may suggest and highlight those that seem most relevant to the patient. The clinician should emphasize that smoking low-tar/low-nicotine cigarettes or use of other forms of tobacco (e.g., smokeless tobacco, cigars, pipes) will not eliminate these risks. Examples of risks follow. • Acute risks: Shortness of breath, exacerbation of asthma, impotence, infertility, increased serum carbon monoxide. • Long-term risks: Heart attacks and strokes, lung and other cancers (larynx, oral cavity, pharynx, esophagus, pancreas, bladder, cervix, leukemia), chronic obstructive pulmonary diseases (chronic bronchitis and emphysema). • Environmental risks: Increased risk of lung cancer in spouse and children; higher rates of smoking by children of smokers; increased risk for SIDS, asthma, middle ear disease, and respiratory infections in children of smokers.
Rewards	The clinician should *ask the patient to identify the potential benefits of quitting smoking.* The clinician may suggest and highlight those that seem most relevant to the patient. Examples of rewards follow. • Improved health • Improved sense of taste • Improved sense of smell • Cost savings • Improved self-esteem • Better-smelling home, car, and breath • No more worrying about quitting • A good example for children • Healthy babies and children • No worrying about exposing others to smoke • Feeling better physically • Freedom from addiction • Better performance in sports
Repetition	The motivational intervention should be repeated every time an unmotivated patient visits the office setting.

Figure 27.1. The *4 Rs* Strategy: Components of clinical interventions to enhance motivations to quit smoking. (From the Agency for Health Care Policy and Research. Smoking cessation: clinical practice guideline, no. 18. (USDHHS) AHCPR Publication No. 96-0692. Washington, DC: US Government Printing Office, 1996.)

Figure 27.2. ASK—Systematically identify all tobacco users at every visit. (From Fiore MC, Bailey WC, Cohen SJ, et al. Treating tobacco use and dependence: clinical practice guideline. Rockville, MD: U.S. Department of Health and Human Services, Public Health Service, June 2000.)

Action	Strategies for implementation
Implement an office-wide system that ensures that, for EVERY patient at EVERY clinic visit, tobacco-use status is queried and documented. *a*	Expand the vital signs to include tobacco use or use an alternative universal identification system. *b* **Vital Signs** Blood Pressure: ______ Pulse: ______ Weight: ______ Temperature: ______ Respiratory Rate: ______ Tobacco Use: Current Former Never (circle one)

a Repeated assessment is not necessary in the case of the adult who has never used tobacco or has not used tobacco for many years, and for whom this information is clearly documented in the medical record.

b Alternatives to expanding the vital signs are to place tobacco-use status stickers on all patient charts or to indicate tobacco use status using electronic medical records or computer reminder systems.

Figure 27.3. ADVISE—Strongly urge all tobacco users to quit. (From Fiore MC, Bailey WC, Cohen SJ, et al. Treating tobacco use and dependence: clinical practice guideline. Rockville, MD: U.S. Department of Health and Human Services, Public Health Service, June 2000.)

Action	Strategies for Implementation
In a *clear, strong,* and *personalized* manner, urge every tobacco user to quit.	Advice should be: • *Clear*--"I think it is important for you to quit smoking now and I can help you." "Cutting down while you are ill is not enough." • *Strong*--"As your clinician, I need you to know that quitting smoking is the most important thing you can do to protect your health now and in the future. The clinic staff and I will help you." • *Personalized*--Tie tobacco use to current health/ illness, and/or its social and economic costs, motivation level/readiness to quit, and/or the impact of tobacco use on children and others in the household.

Figure 27.4. ASSESS—Determine willingness to make a quit attempt. (From Fiore MC, Bailey WC, Cohen SJ, et al. Treating tobacco use and dependence: clinical practice guideline. Rockville, MD: U.S. Department of Health and Human Services, Public Health Service, June 2000.)

Action	Strategies for Implementation
Ask every tobacco user if he or she is willing to make a quit attempt at this time (e.g., within the next 30 days).	Assess patient's willingness to quit: • If the patient is willing to make a quit attempt at this time, provide assistance. • If the patient will participate in an intensive treatment, deliver such a treatment or refer to an intensive intervention. • If the patient clearly states he or she is unwilling to make a quit attempt at this time, provide a motivational intervention. • If the patient is a member of a special population (e.g., adolescent, pregnant smoker, racial/ethnic minority), consider providing additional information.

can encourage the patient to inform his or her family of the quit date, remove cigarettes from the environment before quitting, review previous quit attempts, identify aids and barriers, and anticipate challenges (e.g., withdrawal symptoms). Nicotine replacement therapy (discussed earlier) should be encouraged for most patients. Patients should be advised that *total abstinence is essential,* that alcohol should be avoided, and that smoking friends and family members should either join the plan to quit or not smoke around the patient.

Finally, for patients who have set a quit date, a *follow-up contact should be* ***arranged,*** preferably within 2 weeks after the quit date (Fig. 27.6). This contact can be used to reinforce success, troubleshoot problems, monitor nicotine replacement therapy, and recommend more intensive smoking cessation assistance if necessary.

Action	Strategies for implementation
Help the patient with a quit plan.	*A patient's preparations for quitting:* • *Set a quit date*--Ideally, the quit date should be within 2 weeks. • *Tell* family, friends, and coworkers about quitting and request understanding and support. • *Anticipate* challenges to planned quit attempt, particularly during the critical first few weeks. These include nicotine withdrawal symptoms. • *Remove* tobacco products from your environment. Prior to quitting, avoid smoking in places where you spend a lot of time (e.g., work, home, and car).
Provide practical counseling (problem solving/training).	• *Abstinence*--Total abstinence is essential. "Not even a single puff after the quit date." • *Past quit experience*--Identify what helped and what hurt in previous quit attempts. • *Anticipate triggers or challenges in upcoming attempt*--Discuss challenges/triggers and how patient will successfully overcome them. • *Alcohol*--Since alcohol can cause relapse, the patient should consider limiting/abstaining from alcohol while quitting. • *Other smokers in the household*--Quitting is more difficult when there is another smoker in the household. Patients should encourage housemates to quit with them or not smoke in their presence.
Provide intra-treatment social support.	• Provide a supportive clinical environment while encouraging the patient in his or her quit attempt. "My office staff and I are available to assist you."
Help patient obtain extra-treatment social support.	• Help patient develop social support for his or her quit attempt in his or her environments outside of treatment. "Ask your spouse/partner, friends, and coworkers to support you in your quit attempt."
Recommend the use of approved pharmacotherapy, except in special circumstances.	• Recommend the use of pharmacotherapies found to be effective. Explain how these medications increase smoking cessation success and reduce withdrawal symptoms. The first-line pharmacotherapy medications include bupropion SR, nicotine gum, nicotine inhaler, nicotine nasal spray, and nicotine patch.
Provide supplementary materials.	• *Sources*--Federal agencies, nonprofit agencies, or local/state health departments (*see website addresses at end of chapter*). • *Type*--Culturally/racially/educationally/age appropriate for the patient. • *Location*--Readily available at every clinician's workstation.

Figure 27.5. ASSIST—Aid the patient in quitting. (From Fiore MC, Bailey WC, Cohen SJ, et al. Treating tobacco use and dependence: clinical practice guideline. Rockville, MD: U.S. Department of Health and Human Services, Public Health Service, June 2000.)

Action	Strategies for implementation
Schedule follow-up contact, either in person or via telephone.	*Timing*--Follow-up contact should occur soon after the quit date, preferably during the first week. A second follow-up contact is recommended within the first month. Schedule further follow-up contacts as indicated. *Actions during follow-up contact*--Congratulate success. If tobacco use has occurred, review circumstances, and elicit recommitment to total abstinence. Remind patient that a lapse can be used as a learning experience. Identify problems already encountered and anticipate challenges in the immediate future. Assess pharmacotherapy use and problems. Consider use or referral to more intensive treatment.

Figure 27.6. ARRANGE—Schedule follow-up contact. (From Fiore MC, Bailey WC, Cohen SJ, et al. Treating tobacco use and dependence: clinical practice guideline. Rockville, MD: U.S. Department of Health and Human Services, Public Health Service, June 2000.)

Dealing with Relapse

Risk of relapse is very high for patients who slip and have even one cigarette. Drinking alcohol, socializing with smokers, and high-stress events can all trigger relapse episodes. Patients should be counseled in advance about factors associated with the risk of relapse and reinforced in the continuing challenge of staying abstinent. If relapse occurs, it is important to reassure the patient that relapse is not an indicator that they cannot quit smoking, but instead a common event that most former smokers have experienced before successful quitting. A relapse experience is discouraging for a patient, but it can provide information on the risks and barriers to be addressed in the next cessation effort. Patients should be encouraged to retry cessation as soon as they are ready, and they should be encouraged to use more intensive interventions (e.g., multisession group programs, longer-duration pharmacotherapy) if acceptable (36).

OTHER FORMS OF TOBACCO USE

This chapter focuses on cigarette smoking because it is the most prevalent form of tobacco use and has the greatest health impact. Other forms of tobacco use—cigars, pipes, snuff, and chewing tobacco—also have deleterious health effects (37). Mortality rates associated for these other forms of tobacco use are intermediate between those of cigarette smokers and those of nonusers of tobacco; for example, the total mortality rate of cigar or pipe smokers is approximately 15% to 20% higher than that of comparable nonsmokers. Site-specific cancer rates in the oral-nasal cavity are five times as great as in nonusers of tobacco, and there is increased risk of cardiovascular disease. Treatment approaches for these other varieties of tobacco dependence are the same as for cigarette smoking.

HEALTH CARE PROFESSIONALS AND PUBLIC POLICY

The likelihood of success in overcoming addiction to nicotine is increased not only by the personal motivation and willpower of the cigarette smoker but also by a social and legal environment that encourages nonsmoking, restricts access to tobacco, and reduces the social acceptability of smoking. An increasing body of evidence supports the value of increased taxation on tobacco, restrictive smoking policies, and antitobacco advertising in reducing smoking prevalence in the community. Just as public policies that ensure clean water and adequate sanitation facilities have made dysentery and cholera rare diseases in this country, emerging public policies designed to restrict and control the use of tobacco may someday make smoking-related diseases rare, rather than the leading cause of preventable death that they are now. Tobacco use is as much a public health risk as the infectious diseases of the past century, and the primary care clinician should be a vocal member of the antitobacco activism within his or her community.

General References: Selected Web-Based Resources and Publications

The Surgeon General's Tobacco Cessation Guideline. Available at: http://www.surgeongeneral.gov/tobacco. Accessed December 10, 2001.

This site includes the full text of the Clinical Practice Guideline, *Treating Tobacco Use and Dependence,* as well as the *Quick Reference Guide for Primary Care Clinicians* (also available by telephone at 1-800-358-9295). Additional resources available on this website include patient brochures (in PDF format) to aid smoking cessation, in both English and Spanish versions.

The Centers for Disease Control and Prevention. Tobacco Information and Prevention Source (TIPS). Available at: http://www.cdc.gov/tobacco/index.htm. Accessed December 10, 2001.

Includes a quitting guide, educational materials for educators and parents, tobacco facts and research data, a smoking and health database, state information, and a publications guide with ordering information.

Action on Smoking or Health (ASH). Available at: http://www.ash.org/. Accessed December 10, 2001.

Includes materials on a variety of smoking and health topics. Focuses on legislative action to protect nonsmokers' health.

QuitNet. Available at: http://www.quitnet.com/qn_main.jtml. Accessed December 10, 2001.

A free smoking cessation support forum moderated by counselors, that offers personalized smoking cessation aids and materials. Operated in association with Boston University.

Fiore MC, Bailey WC, Cohen SJ, et al. **Treating tobacco use and dependence: clinical practice guideline.** Rockville, MD: U.S. Department of Health and Human Services, Public Health Service, June 2000.

This clinical practice guideline provides an authoritative and comprehensive but manageable review of the science supporting both the counseling aspects and the pharmacologic aspects of treating tobacco use and dependence. It provides meta-analyses documenting and quantifying the effectiveness of each of the various nonpharmacologic and pharmacologic approaches to smoking intervention. It also provides meta-analyses and an excellent link to the scientific literature and to current issues in treatment and research.

Rigotti NA. Treatment of tobacco use and dependence. N Engl J Med 2002;7:506.

Well-referenced evidence-based review article.

Specific References

1. Stolerman IP, Jarvis MJ. The scientific case that nicotine is addictive. Psychopharmacology 1995;117:2.
2. Breslau N, Johnson EO, Hiripi E, et al. Nicotine dependence in the United States: prevalence, trends, and smoking persistence. Arch Gen Psychiatry 2001;58:810.
3. Herttema JM, Corey LA, Kendler KS. A multivariate genetic analysis of the use of tobacco, alcohol, and caffeine in a population based sample of male and female twins. Drug Alcohol Depend 1999;57:69.
4. Simantov E, Schoen C, Klein JD. Health-compromising behaviors: why do adolescents smoke or drink? Identifying underlying risk and protective factors. Arch Pediatr Adolesc Med 2000;154:1025.
5. Anda RF, Croft JB, Felitti VJ, et al. Adverse childhood experiences and smoking during adolescence and adulthood. JAMA 1999;282:1652.
6. **6.** Bruvold WH. A meta-analysis of adolescent smoking prevention programs. Am J Public Health 1993;83:872.
7. Ockene JK, Emmons KM, Mermelstein RJ, et al. Relapse and maintenance issues for smoking cessation. Health Psychol 2000;19[1 Suppl]:17.
8. Shiffman S, Paty JA, Gnys M, et al. First lapses to smoking: within-subjects analysis of real-time reports. J Consult Clin Psychol 1996;64:366.
9. Higgins MW, Enright PL, Kronmal RA, et al. Smoking and lung function in elderly men and women. JAMA 1993;269:2741.
10. Benowitz NL, Jacob P. Nicotine and carbon monoxide intake from high- and low-yield cigarettes. Clin Pharmacol Ther 1984;36:265.
11. Kozlowski LT, Frecker RC, Khouw V, et al. The misuse of less-hazardous cigarettes and its detection: hole-blocking of ventilated filters. Am J Public Health 1980;70:1202.
12. Hughes JR. Tobacco withdrawal in self-quitters. J Consult Clin Psychol 1992;60:689.
13. Hughes JR, Hatsukami D. Signs and symptoms of tobacco withdrawal. Arch Gen Psychiatry 1986;43:289.
14. West R, Shiffman S. Effect of oral nicotine dosing forms on cigarette withdrawal symptoms and craving: a systematic review. Psychopharmacology 2001;155:115.

*Bold print (general references) and bold numerals (specific references) denote published controlled clinical trials, meta-analyses, or consensus-based recommendations.

15. Brownson RC, Alavanja MCR, Hock ET, et al. Passive smoking and lung cancer in nonsmoking women. Am J Public Health 1992;82:1525.
16. Chilmonczyk BA, Salmun LM, Megathlin KN, et al. Association between exposure to environmental tobacco smoke and exacerbations of asthma in children. N Engl J Med 1993;328:1665.
17. Fielding JE, Phenow KJ. Health effects of involuntary smoking. N Engl J Med 1988;319:1452.
18. He J, Vupputuri S, Allen K, et al. Passive smoking and the risk of coronary heart disease: a meta-analysis of epidemiologic studies. N Engl J Med 1999;340:920.
19. Sexton M, Hebel JR. A clinical trial of change in maternal smoking and its effect on birth weight. JAMA 1984;251:911.
20. Ahluwalia JS, Gibson CA, Kenney RE, et al. Smoking status as a vital sign. J Gen Intern Med 1999;14:402.
21. Sippel JM, Osborne ML, Bjornson W, et al. Smoking cessation in primary care clinics. J Gen Intern Med 1999;14:670.
22. Ritvo PG, Irvine MJ, Lindsay EA, et al. A critical review of research related to family physician-assisted smoking cessation interventions. Cancer Prev Control 1997;1:289.
23. Silagy C, Stead LF. Physician advice for smoking cessation (Cochrane Review). Cochrane Database Syst Rev 2001;2:CD-000165.
24. Doescher MP, Saver BG. Physicians' advice to quit smoking: the glass remains half empty. J Fam Pract 2000;49:543.
25. Ellerbeck EF, Ahluwalia JS, Jolicoeur DG, et al. Direct observation of smoking cessation activities in primary care practice. J Fam Pract 2001;50:688.
26. Ossip-Klein DJ, McIntosh S, Utman C, et al. Smokers ages 50+: who gets physician advice to quit? Prev Med 2000;31:364.
27. Orleans CT, Cummings KM. Population-based tobacco control: progress and prospects. Am J Health Promot 1999;14:83.
28. Kreuter MW, Chheda SG, Bull FC. How does physician advice influence patient behavior? Evidence for a priming effect. Arch Fam Med 2000;9:426.
29. Fiore MC, Bailey WC, Cohen SJ, et al. Treating tobacco use and dependence: clinical practice guideline. Rockville, MD: U.S. Department of Health and Human Services, Public Health Service, June 2000.
30. Joseph AM, Norman SM, Ferry LH, et al. The safety of transdermal nicotine as an aid to smoking cessation in patients with cardiac disease. N Engl J Med 1996;335:1792.
31. Jorenby DE, Leischow SJ, Nides MA, et al. A controlled trial of sustained-release bupropion, a nicotine patch, or both for smoking cessation. N Engl J Med. 1999;340:685.
32. Hurt RD, Sachs DPL, Glover ED, et al. A comparison of sustained-release bupropion and placebo for smoking cessation. N Engl J Med 1997;337:1195.
33. Ferrara CM, Kumar M, Nicklas B, et al. Weight gain and adipose tissue metabolism after smoking cessation in women. Int J Obes Relat Metab Disord 2001;25:1322.
34. Hays JT, Hurt RD, Rigotti NA, et al. Sustained-release bupropion for pharmacologic relapse prevention after smoking cessation: a randomized, controlled trial. Ann Intern Med 2001;135:423.
35. Perkins KA, Marcus MD, Levine MD, et al. Cognitive-behavioral therapy to reduce weight concerns improves smoking cessation outcome in weight-concerned women. J Consult Clin Psychol 2001;69:604.
36. Smith SS, Jorenby DE, Fiore MC, et al. Strike while the iron is hot: can stepped-care treatments resurrect relapsing smokers? J Consult Clin Psychol 2001;69:429.
37. Council on Scientific Affairs. Health effects of smokeless tobacco. JAMA 1986;255:1038.

CHAPTER 28

Alcoholism and Associated Problems

MICHAEL I. FINGERHOOD, M.D.

Along with cardiovascular disease and cancer, alcoholism ranks among the top three causes of death and disability in the United States. The estimated cost of alcoholism to society in 1998 was $184.6 billion (1), with an untold additional cost in the suffering of people who are close to alcoholics. However, the majority of alcoholics in the United States do not receive treatment for their alcoholism. Many of these people have early alcoholism and would be likely to recover successfully if diagnosed and treated.

Until recently, alcoholism was widely regarded as a hopeless condition with a poor prognosis for recovery. Yet alcoholism is one of the most treatable of all medical and psychiatric conditions, with a high long-term success rate when a disease model of alcoholism is used in diagnosis and treatment.

DEFINITION OF ALCOHOLISM

A useful, broad definition of alcoholism is *recurring trouble associated with drinking alcohol.* The trouble may occur in one or more of several domains, including interpersonal (e.g., valued relationships, especially within the family), educational, legal, financial, medical, and occupational. Although there are many exceptions, trouble caused by alcoholism usually occurs in that order of progression, so that one's health and job are last to be overtly affected. The trouble may include the physiologic manifestations of dependence or addiction: *tolerance* (the need for increased amounts of a substance to achieve intoxication or desired effect) and *withdrawal* symptoms. Characteristics of alcoholism include inability to control one's use of alcohol (always present), drinking alone, avoiding situations where alcohol is not available, drinking before going to a party, gulping drinks, and continuing to drink alcohol despite occupational, psychosocial, or physical problems caused by drinking.

Consensus Definition

In 1992, a multidisciplinary committee of the National Council on Alcoholism and Drug Dependence and the American Society of Addiction Medicine issued its definition of alcoholism: "Alcoholism is a primary, chronic disease with genetic, psychosocial, and environmental factors influencing its development and manifestations. The disease is often progressive and fatal. It is characterized by impaired control over drinking, preoccupation with the drug alcohol despite adverse consequences, and distortions in thinking, most notably denial. Each of these symptoms may be continuous or periodic" (2). Unlike previously issued definitions, this one specifically included denial as a key component of the definition of alcoholism.

Alcoholism is classified by the American Psychiatric Association (APA) under the broad rubric *Substance-Related Use Disorders* (3). In its subclassification for these disorders, the APA has generic criteria for *substance abuse* (abnormal use, with unwanted consequences) and *substance dependence* (more intensive abuse patterns or physiologic manifestations of addiction). The criteria for these two sub-classifications are found in Chapter 29. Another widely used term for these disorders is *chemical dependence.* Many people with chemical dependence abuse multiple psychoactive substances (e.g., an alcoholic patient may also abuse cocaine or a benzodiazepine). Chapter 29 describes polydrug abuse and delineates the characteristics of the specific substance use disorders that are common in the United States.

CAUSES

The causes of alcoholism are multifactorial and poorly understood (4,5). A predisposition to alcoholism appears to be inherited by at least half of all alcoholic patients, and there is some evidence that inherited factors are associated with the inability to control use of alcohol (6,7). Social conditioning, enabling behavior by others close to the individual (see Co-alcoholism), and being a child in a dysfunctional family (see later discussion) are important non-genetic factors. For some alcoholic men, another mental disorder (especially antisocial personality disorder, primary abuse of other substances, or an affective disorder) may play a role. For alcoholic women, there is evidence that preexisting mental illness, especially a phobic disorder or major depression, may play a role. In addition, for elderly alcoholics whose problem began after the 50 years of age, the losses and isolation that accompany aging are often associated with the onset of problem drinking (see Special Populations). These factors do not account for all alcoholism. They only add credence to the concept that alcoholism is a complex disease and not the result of moral turpitude.

ALCOHOLIC BEVERAGES: CONTENT AND METABOLISM

Alcoholic beverages can be divided into non-distilled (wine and beer) and distilled varieties. The concentration of alcohol (ethanol) in wine ranges from 10% to 22% by volume and is 12% to 14% in most wines. Beer usually contains 4% to 5% alcohol by volume, but beers fermented in the bottle contain a higher percentage of alcohol. The distilled alcoholic beverages—whiskey, brandy, rum, gin, and vodka—contain a higher percentage of alcohol. Alcoholic fermentation ceases when the concentration of alcohol exceeds 15% by volume; therefore, to manufacture more potent beverages, distillation or fortification is necessary. In the United States, "*proof*" is double the percentage of alcohol by volume; for instance, 90 proof whiskey contains 45% alcohol by volume. One drink of distilled alcohol (1 fluid oz), one glass of wine (4 oz), and one beer (12 oz) contain approximately the same amount of alcohol.

In a 154-pound (70-kg) person, on an empty stomach, one drink of distilled alcohol (usually 1 fluid oz or 30 mL) produces a peak blood alcohol level (BAL) of approximately 25 mg/dL within 30 minutes after ingestion. Approximately 15 mg/dL is metabolized per hour. For example, the alcohol in 120 mL of whiskey would take about 6 hours to be metabolized. The rate of metabolism is higher (in the range of 20 to 25 mg/dL per hour) in the alcoholic who drinks heavily each day for many months. A BAL of 100 mg/dL is equivalent to 0.08%, in the units commonly used by law enforcement to indicate driving impairment. To reach a BAL of 300 mg/dL, a 70-kg person typically has to consume 14 to 20 drinks over a few hours.

EPIDEMIOLOGY

Prevalence

Alcoholism affects approximately 8% of adult Americans (1). Among the homeless, this figure runs higher, with some estimates running as high as 45%. Studies of teenage students show that the rates of problem drinking (heavy drinking or drinking to get drunk) exceed the rates of alcoholism in adults, even though the purchase of alcohol by teenagers is illegal.

In 1997, yearly consumption of alcohol in the United States was 2.18 gallons of pure alcohol, the equivalent of about 517 twelve-ounce cans of beer, for every person over the age of 15 years (1). Per capita alcohol consumption peaks before age 50 and declines with increasing age. Because about one third of the adult population is abstinent, the consumption of alcohol is concentrated in the approximately 94 million drinking Americans. About one third of that number (30 million) consume approximately 70% of all the alcohol produced. It is this group that uses the health system more often, is most at risk of trauma, and has the recurring problems that constitute alcoholism.

Mortality and Morbidity

Prospective studies show that alcoholic patients have two to four times higher death rates and much higher rates of medical and psychosocial morbidity than do matched controls (8). The most common causes of early death in alcoholics are cirrhosis of the liver, cancers of the respiratory and gastrointestinal tracts, accidents, suicide, and ischemic heart disease. Most alcoholics smoke and, in fact, lung cancer is the most common cancer diagnosed in alcoholics (9). During 1997, alcohol-related motor vehicle accidents resulted in more than 16,000 deaths in the United States (1). Alcohol-related traffic accidents are the leading cause of death for teenagers and young adults. Importantly, it was found that alcoholic men who achieved long-term abstinence did not differ from nonalcoholic men in mortality rate (10). However, relapse was significantly related to mortality.

NATURAL HISTORY OF ALCOHOLISM

The natural history of alcoholism in men has been delineated in retrospective and prospective studies. In Jellinek's classic retrospective study of recovering alcoholic men (4), the majority of subjects identified multiple phases in the progression of their disease: (a) an initial phase, lasting months to years, in which they used alcohol to relieve tension and developed tolerance to alcohol; (b) a phase in which they experienced blackouts (amnesia for drinking-associated events), increasing preoccupation with getting alcohol, and profound loss of control over use of alcohol; (c) a phase in which there were overt psychological and behavioral consequences (rationalization, grandiosity, aggressive behavior, remorse, efforts to abstain); and (d) a stage characterized by chronic intoxication and serious deterioration of health and psychosocial functioning. In Vaillant's more recent prospective study (5), this multiphase course of alcoholism characterized three quarters of men who became alcoholic. Most of the remaining men exhibited abnormal drinking patterns, usually rituals to constrain the uncontrolled drinking that they themselves recognized as abnormal, and had less alcohol-related trouble with family, job, and health. Importantly, in these and other studies of the course of alcoholism, it has been found that periodic abstinence or moderation of use is typical. Although anecdotal information suggests that occasionally a person with what appears to be alcoholism can return to normal drinking, this is very uncommon and is not clinically useful to consider.

MANIFESTATIONS OF ALCOHOLISM

Alcoholism is a protean disease, and it is probably the most common great masquerader today. Table 28.1 lists medical, psychosocial, legal, and other manifestations often associated with alcoholism. Manifestations are ranked in the table according to their strength as diagnostic features, ranging from those that are diagnostic of alcoholism to those that should make one at least consider alcoholism. A number of the most important manifestations of alcoholism are discussed here.

Legal Problems

A history or record of driving while intoxicated (DWI) highly suggests alcoholism. In one study of about 21,000 consecutive people with DWIs (11), approximately 75% of first-time offenders were found to be alcoholic. Of those with two DWI arrests, more than 90% were alcoholic, and of those with three, essentially 100% were alcoholic. A prison record is also strongly suggestive, because most prison inmates have a history of alcoholism or other chemical dependence. Child and spouse or partner abuse is also highly associated with alcoholism.

Behavioral, Psychiatric, and Neurologic Problems

Accidents and trauma, including burns, are often associated with alcoholism; in the majority of patients with severe trauma, alcohol or other psychoactive drug use can be detected. Among patients with symptoms of chronic mental illness, especially symptoms of depression and anxiety, alcoholism is common. Usually alcoholism is the primary problem in these patients, and treatment of mental symptoms is not successful until the alcoholism is treated.

Alcohol Intoxication

The best known acute consequence of alcoholism is alcohol intoxication, which should usually present no diagnostic problem. Because this condition is so common, diagnostic errors are made when it is forgotten that "drunken" behavior—often with evidence of recent alcohol use—may be caused by a host of conditions, such as infection, metabolic disturbance, neurologic disease, or other drug toxicity. Because alcoholics are especially prone to many disorders that may be manifested as deranged behavior, they should be examined systematically before a diagnosis of simple drunkenness is made.

Alcohol intoxication may be characterized by one or more of the following: relaxation and sedation, euphoria, impaired coordination, loudness, lowered inhibitions, poor memory and judgment, labile mood, slurred speech, nausea, vomiting, and obtundation (Table 28.2). An initial period of excitement and euphoria is often followed by depression and sleep, or possibly coma. The duration and magnitude of the intoxication depend on the amount and the rapidity with which the alcohol was drunk and whether the patient drank on an empty stomach (enhancing the rate of absorption). Tolerance is also a significant factor, because an alcoholic may acquire the (reversible) capacity to increase the rate of alcohol metabolism.

Table 28.1. Medical, Psychiatric, Legal, and Other Findings Suggestive (unmarked to *) to Highly Suggestive (to ***) or Diagnostic (****) of Alcoholism**

	Presenting Complaint and History		
****	Drinking problem, recurring[a]	*	Depression
***	Blackouts with drinking	*	Suicide attempt
***	Spouse/other complains of patient's drinking	*	Sexual dysfunction
***	Driving while intoxicated (DWI) record	*	Legal problem
***	Prison record	*	Noncompliance in treatment
***	Change in alcohol or drug tolerance	*	School learning problem
**	Frequent requests for mood-changing drugs	*	Hypertension
**	Gastrointestinal bleeding, especially upper		Headache
**	Traumatic injuries, fracture		Palpitations
**	Parent, grandparent, or relative alcoholic		Abdominal pain
**	Friends alcoholic or other chemical dependence		Amenorrhea
**	Family or other violence		Weight loss
**	Child abuse or neglect		Vague complaints
**	First seizure in an adult		Insomnia
**	Job performance problem		Anxiety
*	Unexplained syncope		Marital discord
			Financial problem
	Alcohol or Other Drug Use History		
****	Alcohol use recurring, interfering with health, job, or social functioning[a]	**	Other drug misuse or dependence
***	Patient says, "I can stop drinking anytime" or the equivalent; or patient gets evasive or angry, or talks glibly during taking of drinking history	*	Cigarette smoker
***	Patient states that he or she has consciously stopped drinking completely for any length of time		
	Physical Examination		
***	Odor of beverage alcohol on breath	*	Borderline tachycardia
***	Parotid gland enlargement, bilateral	*	Thin extremities in proportion to trunk
***	Spider nevi or angioma	*	Splenomegaly
***	Tremulousness, hallucinosis	*	Hypertension
**	Cigarette stains on fingers		Diaphoresis
**	Breath mints odor		Alopecia
**	Many scars or tattoos		Abdominal tenderness
**	Hepatomegaly		Cerebellar signs (e.g., nystagmus)
**	Gynecomastia		
**	Small testicles		
**	Unexplained bruises, abrasions, or cuts		
	Laboratory Abnormalities		
****	Blood alcohol level >300 mg/100 mL[a]	**	Abnormal liver function tests (especially AST > ALT)
***	Blood alcohol level >100 mg/100 mL without impairment	**	Anemia, macrocytic or megaloblastic, microcytic, or mixed
***	High serum ammonia	*	Hyperuricemia
***	Gamma-glutamyl transpeptidase elevation	*	Creatine kinase elevation
**	Blood alcohol level positive, any amount	*	Hypophosphatemia or hypomagnesemia
**	High amylase (nonspecific for pancreas)		Electrolyte imbalance (hyponatremia, hypokalemia)
			Low white blood cell or platelet count
			Hyperlipoproteinemia, type 4 or 5
	Diagnosis		
****	Hepatitis, alcoholic[a]	**	Attempted suicide
***	Pancreatitis, acute or chronic	**	Gastritis
***	Cirrhosis	**	Refractory hypertension
***	Portal hypertension	**	Cerebellar degeneration
***	Wernicke–Korsakoff syndrome	**	Peripheral neuropathy
***	Frequent trauma	**	Aspiration pneumonia
***	Cold injury	*	Gout
***	Nose and throat cancer	*	Cardiomyopathy
**	Other chemical dependence	*	Tuberculosis
**	Drownings	*	Anxiety
**	Burns, especially third degree	*	Depression
**	Leaves hospital against medical advise	*	Marital discord or family problem

ALT, alanine aminotransferase; AST, aspartate aminotransferase.

[a]Major criterian of the National Council on Alcoholism for the diagnosis of alcoholism (see General References).

Table 28.2. Expected Effects According to Blood Alcohol Level for a Person Without Tolerance to Alcohol

Blood Alcohol Level (mg/dL)	Expected Effect	Approximate Location of Physiologic Disturbance
25–50	Relaxation, sedation	—
50–100	Coordination impaired; euphoric; loud conversation; apparent reduction of social inhibitions	Cerebral cortex
100–200	Ataxia; depressed fine motor ability, decreased mentation, attention span, and memory; poor judgment; labile mood; beginning of slurred speech	Limbic system and cerebellum
200–300	Marked ataxia and slurred speech, nausea and vomiting, tremor, irritable	Reticular activating system
300–400	Stage 1 anesthesia (unconsciousness), memory lapse	Reticular activating system
>400	Respiratory failure, coma, death	Medulla oblongata

Moreover, alcoholics characteristically develop substantial central tolerance, so that they appear fairly sober at BALs of 150 mg/dL or more. Most nonalcoholic people become intoxicated at levels between 100 and 200 mg/dL, and some at levels as low as 30 mg/dL. Levels greater than 400 mg/dL can be lethal, with death usually resulting from depressed respiration or from aspiration of vomitus.

Blackouts

Blackouts—amnesia for events that occurred during a period of intoxication—are common. However, 10% to 25% of alcoholics do not have memory blackouts, and some normal drinkers have experienced blackouts after drinking.

Alcohol Idiosyncratic Intoxication

Alcohol idiosyncratic intoxication (pathologic intoxication) is an uncommon syndrome characterized by an extreme, often aggressive or violent reaction to drinking alcohol, which is often followed by amnesia for the episode. The behavior is atypical of the person when not drinking. The duration of this condition is brief (hours), and the person returns to his or her normal state as the BAL falls. Temporal lobe epilepsy, sedative-hypnotic use, and malingering should be ruled out.

Alcohol Amnestic Disorder (Korsakoff Psychosis)

Alcohol amnestic disorder (Korsakoff psychosis) is characterized chiefly by short-term memory impairment, associated with some loss of long-term memory, in the absence of clouded consciousness (delirium) or general loss of intellectual abilities (dementia). (For definitions and detailed discussions of delirium and dementia, see Chapter 26.) Patients with less advanced forms of this disorder may be substantially impaired, but they may appear superficially to be normal, particularly because they often attempt to minimize their impairment and to confabulate in order to fill in memory gaps.

The amnestic disorder often follows an episode of *Wernicke encephalopathy,* a syndrome of global confusion, ataxia, and impaired eye movement, caused by thiamine deficiency, which may occur suddenly or gradually over several days. Parenteral thiamine given during an acute episode of Wernicke encephalopathy may prevent the amnestic syndrome. With abstention from alcohol and good nutrition for several months, some patients recover entirely from the alcohol amnestic syndrome. However, many remain grossly impaired and require institutional care.

Dementia Associated with Alcoholism

When more generalized intellectual impairment develops after years of heavy drinking, the diagnosis of dementia associated with alcoholism is appropriate. An estimated 70% of actively drinking chronic alcoholics have some cognitive impairments, as measured by psychological testing. Perhaps 10% of these have dementia that is sufficiently apparent and noticeable without psychological testing. Because even detoxified alcoholics are likely to show some cognitive impairment for a period after cessation of drinking, this diagnosis should not be made unless dementia persists for at least 1 month after drinking has stopped. Other causes of dementia must be excluded (see Chapter 26). All alcoholics with any signs of dementia should be treated with high-dosage thiamine (100 mg/day) and long-term multivitamin therapy. Some improve over months to years of abstinence.

Other Medical Complications

The various *deficiency states* involved in a diet composed largely of nutritionally empty alcoholic calories (7 cal/g), as well as the *direct toxic actions of alcohol* itself, have been implicated in the pathogenesis of many of the medical consequences of alcoholism. These disorders are legion, sparing no body system, and most are related to the quantity and duration of alcohol consumption. Among the more common medical complications of alcoholism are gastritis; fatty liver, hepatitis, or cirrhosis; pancreatitis; cerebellar ataxia; gout; peripheral neuropathy; rhabdomyolysis; hematologic abnormalities (elevated mean corpuscular volume of red blood cells, anemia, thrombocytopenia); hypoglycemia; ketoacidosis; electrolyte abnormalities (hyponatremia, hypokalemia, hypomagnesemia, and hypophosphatemia); pulmonary infections suggesting aspiration or impaired defenses (tuberculosis and pneumonia); cancers of the liver, respiratory, and gastrointestinal tract; atrial fibrillation; cardiomyopathy; hypertension; and trauma. *Chronic hypertension* is a very common manifestation of alcoholism. Because it often remits within weeks after discontinuation alcohol, it may be the most common reversible cause of hypertension (see Chapter 67).

Because it is both serious and preventable, the *fetal alcohol syndrome* deserves special mention. It is manifested by morphologic abnormalities, low birth weight, and developmental and cognitive impairment. This syndrome is a consequence of alcohol ingestion by the mother during pregnancy. The risk of minor abnormalities (e.g., low birth weight) begins with the consumption of one drink per day; this risk increases with increasingly larger amounts of alcohol consumption. It is prudent to advise women not to drink any alcohol during pregnancy.

Medical Consequences: A Summary View

Almost all of the medical consequences of alcoholism tend to have certain common characteristics:

- Drinking alcohol causes them.
- A poor diet generally makes most of them worse and makes them occur earlier.
- Harmful habits, such as cigarette smoking and the misuse of other drugs, also tend to compound the medical consequences.

If the patient continues to consume alcohol, damage involving major organs progresses slowly, but relentlessly, over the course of a few years, often ending in organ failure. The organs affected by alcohol and the rate of decline in function of these organs vary greatly among patients. Severity of damage is loosely correlated with dosage of alcohol. For the liver, damage is more common in women at any level of alcohol consumption (see Special Populations).

Progression of organic damage occurs no matter what medical or psychological intervention the patient receives, as long as drinking continues. If the patient stops drinking, many of the pathophysiologic processes caused by alcohol reverse rapidly, such as those in the blood and bone marrow (cytopenias), those in the small intestine (malabsorption), hypertension, and fluid and electrolyte imbalance. Other processes do not reverse rapidly with abstinence, but they usually do not progress and often improve over weeks and months. Alcoholic hepatitis, chronic pancreatitis, and cognitive deficits are conditions that tend to improve more gradually.

SCREENING FOR AND DIAGNOSING ALCOHOLISM

Overview

Except when a patient presents with overt behavioral or medical evidence of alcoholism (see Table 28.1), the diagnosis of alcoholism requires skillful interviewing and careful evaluation of other information (12). Such an approach is needed for most alcoholics, whose disease is a private problem experienced by them and those who are close to them. In addition to unwanted psychosocial and physiologic consequences of alcoholism, two cardinal features inevitably emerge when one is obtaining information from an alcoholic or others who know the alcoholic: evidence of inability to control the use of alcohol and denial that a significant problem exists.

Persons who are recognized in the early stages of alcoholism may be helped by *brief interventions* as described in a separate section at the end of this chapter.

Loss of Control

Continuous inability to control the use of alcohol is not always present in alcoholics. Indeed, many can go for periods of a few hours (e.g., at a social gathering) to a few months with apparently normal drinking. Therefore, the absence of overt loss of control for a period of time does not rule out alcoholism. In such patients, the loss of control returns eventually. In addition, some alcoholic patients describe rituals to constrain their intake because of previous trouble with control (e.g., never having a first drink until after dinner). Nonalcoholic people do not describe drinking in these ways, and such information usually indicates that there is a serious problem. Control of alcohol consumption is always an issue for the alcoholic.

Denial

Denial (i.e., the direct or implied message that there is no problem) is present in almost all actively drinking alcoholics. Denial behavior and responses may be caused by one or more of the following mechanisms: (a) conscious lying (one of the least common mechanisms); (b) classic denial (an adaptive coping response to avoid the shame, lowered self-esteem, and distressing inability to overcome the drinking problem that are experienced by most alcoholics); (c) memory blackout caused by drinking; (d) euphoric recall (the patient remembers only the good times experienced when drinking); (e) the fact that no one points out problems related to drinking; (f) wishful thinking; (g) denial on the part of the family and other close people, including helping professionals; (h) ignorance of what an alcoholic is; (i) toxic effects on information processing and memory; (j) stigma related to the term *alcoholic*; and (k) a complex thinking quandary. This last mechanism consists of genuine confusion on the part of the patient; he or she knows that something is wrong but somehow cannot connect it with drinking alcohol.

Denial presents in some of the following ways: rationalizations (e.g., "I drink because my work is more than anyone should try to do"), glibness and humor, hostility ("I came to you about my blood pressure and I would appreciate it if we could stay out of my personal life"), comparison of oneself with a "real problem drinker" ("Now see here, I have a lovely family, a job that I enjoy . . . . I have nothing in common with those poor guys who have lost it; those are your alcoholics"), reticence to discuss drinking, and the assertion that other physicians or family members do not perceive a problem with alcohol. An alcoholic patient's denial responses are usually the result of years of complex adapting to dependence on alcohol. This helps explain why these responses may seem to be refractory and may cause much frustration during screening and diagnostic interviewing and during efforts to get the patient to accept the diagnosis and agree to treatment.

Screening for Alcoholism

Because alcoholism is common and because the evidence for it is usually private information that patients do not volunteer, all patients should be screened for this problem. The goal of screening, and of further inquiry when there are positive responses to screening, is to be confident that one has ruled out alcoholism, has detected definite alcoholism, or must continue to consider alcoholism as a possible diagnosis.

There are a number of ways to screen for the cardinal features of alcoholism. The approach outlined in Fig. 28.1 incorporates the four so-called CAGE questions into the interview (13). In this approach, exploratory inquiry about the use of alcoholic beverages follows inquiries about less sensitive habit information, and the inquiry begins with an open-ended question that prompts patients to respond with more than a simple *Yes* or *No* or with a quantitative reply (e.g., "a few beers"). In patients who report any current or recent use of alcohol and in those with discomfort, glibness, voluntary reporting of heavy use, or other information suggesting alcoholism (Table 28.1), including that from the patient's medical history, there is increased likelihood that a problem exists (14). In the absence of such clues, all patients who report alcohol use should still complete the follow-up questions listed in Fig. 28.1 or other questions that focus on similar content.

1. Integrate alcohol use inquiry into interview so that it follows inquiry about less sensitive habits.

   Example: "We have talked about your usual diet and your smoking. Can you tell me how you use alcoholic beverages?" (or "How about alcoholic beverages . . .?").

   If the patient says that he/she has never used alcohol and shows no sign of discomfort, inquire about problem use in others (e.g., "Anyone in your family or other close persons who have a drinking problem?"). This helps to identify a risk factor for alcoholism and to identify patients who may suffer because of the alcoholism of another person.[a]

2. **General Questions:** For patients who report present or past use of alcohol, screen for evidence of alcoholism, with a general question such as the following:

   "Has (Did) your use of alcohol caused (cause) any kinds of problems for you?" or "Have you ever been concerned about your drinking?"

3. **CAGE Questions:**[b] If the patient has not disclosed a problem with drinking, use these four focused questions and probe for clarification of positive or ambivalent responses.

   "I'd like to ask you a few more questions about alcohol that I ask all of my patients . . ."

   C "Have you ever felt you ought to CUT DOWN on your drinking (use of ___________)?"

   A "Have people ANNOYED you by criticizing your drinking (use of ___________)?"

   G "Have you ever felt bad or GUILTY about your drinking (use of ___________)?"

   E "Have you ever had a drink first thing in the morning (EYE OPENER) to steady your nerves or get rid of a hangover?" (For other substances: "Have you found that you have to take some ___________ most days/some days to feel okay?")

[a]See section on "Co-Alcoholism."

[b]Modifications of questions for substances other than alcohol are shown in parentheses.

Figure 28.1. A recommended approach to the use of interviewing to screen all patients for alcoholism and problems with alcohol in the family.

The approach in Fig. 28.1 is designed to uncover specific data that point to the diagnosis of alcoholism. Lengthier than the CAGE, the Michigan Alcoholism Screening Test (MAST), is a 24-question standardized instrument that has been used extensively for alcoholism screening (Table 28.3) (15). The questions in the MAST may be helpful when one is attempting to uncover occult alcoholism. The questions are best used to gather additional information within the flow of obtaining a history related to drinking, complementing and adding information to positive CAGE answers. Another screening tool, the 10-item Alcohol Use Disorders Identification Test (AUDIT), developed by the World Health Organization, focuses on alcohol consumption and as such can be regarded as a screening tool for problem drinking (Table 28.4) (16,17). The CAGE questions have the advantage of being simple to incorporate into an office interview, being phrased in a nonthreatening way, and focusing on several features that are present in most patients with alcoholism:

- C: *Inability to control* one's drinking, which leads to cutting back or quitting attempts.
- A: *Domestic problems* caused by one's drinking that evoke negative responses from other people. The phrasing of this question places the blame on the one criticizing, so that a positive response is not self-incriminating.
- G: *Bad feelings* that one has about drinking-related actions. The phrasing of this question allows the patient to blame the drinking and not himself or herself.
- E: *Physiologic dependence,* as denoted by the need to drink to suppress withdrawal symptoms.

Studies of the CAGE questions have shown that they are sensitive (70% to 90% of alcoholics respond positively to one or more of the questions, and most have at least two positive responses) and specific (80% to 95% of nonalcoholic people respond negatively to all four questions) (18). These test characteristics of the CAGE questions are superior to those of laboratory tests—gamma-glutamyl transpeptidase (GGT), other liver function tests, and mean corpuscular volume (MCV)—that are often measured in patients with alcoholism (19). However, abnormalities in these specific tests may be helpful in supporting persistent inquiry and in confrontation of the patient with suspected alcoholism (discussed later). A recently developed

Table 28.3. Michigan Alcoholism Screening Test (MAST)[a]

	Yes	No
0. Do you enjoy having a drink now and then?	0	
1. Do you feel you are a normal drinker? (By normal we mean you drink less than or as much as most other people and you have not gotten into any recurring trouble while drinking.)		2
2. Have you ever awakened the morning after some drinking the night before and found that you could not remember a part of the evening?	2	
3. Does either of your parents, or any other near relative, or your spouse, or any girlfriend or boyfriend ever worry or complain about your drinking?	1	
4. Can you stop drinking without a struggle after one or two drinks?		2
5. Do you feel guilty about your drinking?	1	
6. Do friends or relatives think you are a normal drinker?		2
7. Are you able to stop drinking when you want to?		2
8. Have you ever attended a meeting of Alcoholics Anonymous (AA)?	5	
9. Have you gotten into physical fights when you have been drinking?	1	
10. Has your drinking ever created problems between you and either of your parents, or another relative, your spouse, or any girlfriend or boyfriend?	2	
11. Has any family member of yours ever gone to anyone for help about your drinking?	2	
12. Have you ever lost friends because of your drinking?	2	
13. Have you ever gotten into trouble at work or at school because of drinking?	2	
14. Have you ever lost a job because of drinking?	2	
15. Have you ever neglected your obligations, your school work, your family, or your job for 2 or more days in a row because you were drinking?	2	
16. Do you drink before noon fairly often?	1	
17. Have you ever been told you have liver trouble? Cirrhosis?	2	
18. After heavy drinking have you ever had severe shaking, or heard voices or seen things that really weren't there?	2(5 DTs)	
19. Have you ever gone to anyone for help about your drinking?	5	
20. Have you ever been in a hospital because of drinking?	5	
21. Have you ever been a patient in a psychiatric hospital or on a psychiatric ward of a general hospital where drinking was part of the problem that resulted in hospitalization?	2	
22. Have you ever been seen at a psychiatric or mental health clinic or gone to any doctor, social worker, or clergy for help with any emotional problem, where drinking was a part of the problem?	2	
23. Have you ever been arrested for drunk driving, driving while intoxicated, or driving under the influence of alcoholic beverages or any other drug? (If YES, How many times?)	2 each	
24. Have you ever been arrested, or taken into custody, even for a few hours, because of other drunk behavior, whether due to alcohol or another drug? (If YES, How many times?)	2 each	

[a]Interpretation of standard MAST: 0 to 3 points, probable normal drinker; 4 points, borderline score; 5 to 9 points, 80% associated with alcoholism/chemical dependence; ≥10 points, 100% associated with alcoholism. The values assigned to each response are shown.

blood test, carbohydrate-deficient transferrin (CDT), helps identify heavy alcohol intake and may help monitor a male alcoholic's abstinence (20). An increased level may be an indicator of alcohol use and an increase compared with baseline may be an indicator of relapse in someone who has been abstinent. It is not useful in women or in individuals with significant liver disease. As such, it has not yet been shown to be useful in screening of general medical patients for alcoholism.

Screening questions that focus on one common consequence of alcoholism, *trauma,* may be sensitive—especially the question, "Have you ever been injured after drinking?" A positive response to this question, or a history of unexplained repeated trauma or traffic accidents, may be important in patients whose CAGE responses are equivocal and in those who have few of the social contacts that are implied in the CAGE questions. The latter group includes antisocial younger drinkers, older people, and others who commonly become isolated.

Importantly, the approach in Fig. 28.1 does not include direct inquiry about quantity or frequency of alcohol use. Although *quantitative inquiry* may be helpful occasionally for identifying a patient who is ready to discuss problems associated with drinking, its disadvantages are that it does not focus on inability to control use or on adverse consequences of drinking, there is no gold standard for the cutoff quantity below or above which one can confidently exclude or diagnose alcoholism, and problem drinkers usually underreport the amount and frequency of their drinking.

Diagnosis of Alcoholism

The confident diagnosis of alcoholism requires nonjudgmental exploration of any positive information obtained in screening. This may include asking for

Table 28.4. Alcohol Use Disorders Identification Test (AUDIT) Questionnaire[a]

1. How often do you have a drink containing alcohol?
   (0) Never (1) Monthly or less (2) Two to four times a month (3) Two to three times a week (4) Four more times a week
2. How many drinks containing alcohol do you have on a typical day when you are drinking?
   [Code number of standard drinks.]
   (0) 1 or 2 (1) 3 or 4 (2) 5 or 6 (3) 7 to 9 (4) 10 or more
3. How often do you have six or more drinks on one occasion?
   (0) Never (1) Less than monthly (2) Monthly (3) Weekly (4) Daily or almost daily
4. How often during the last year have you found that you were not able to stop drinking once you had started?
   (0) Never (1) Less than monthly (2) Monthly (3) Weekly (4) Daily or almost daily
5. How often during the last year have you failed to do what was normally expected from you because of drinking?
   (0) Never (1) Less than daily (2) Monthly (3) Weekly (4) Daily or daily
6. How often during the last year have you needed a first drink in the morning to get yourself going after a heaving drinking session?
   (0) Never (1) Less than monthly (2) Monthly (3) Weekly (4) Daily or almost daily
7. How often during the last year have you had a feeling of guilt or remorse after drinking?
   (0) Never (1) Less than monthly (2) Monthly (3) Weekly (4) Daily or almost daily
8. How often during the last year have you been unable to remember what happened the night before because you had been drinking?
   (0) Never (1) Less than monthly (2) Monthly (3) Weekly (4) Daily or almost daily
9. Have you or someone else been injured as a result of your drinking?
   (0) No (2) Yes, but not in the last year (4) Yes, during the last year
10. Has a relative or friend or a doctor or other health worker been concerned about your drinking or suggested you cut down?
   (0) No (2) Yes, but not in the last year (4) Yes, during the last year

[a]A score of 8 or more indicates a strong likelihood of harmful alcohol consumption.

clarification ("Can you tell me more about the last time you decided to cut back a bit?" or "Exactly what does she say to annoy you?" and gentle confrontation ("That must have made you feel pretty bad—sounds like the drinking had a lot to do with it") (21).

At times, a *planned interview with a family member or close friend,* by telephone or in person, may be needed to make a confident diagnosis of alcoholism. This entails requesting the patient's permission to discuss his or her drinking with another person. Questions to another person regarding the patient's drinking patterns and consequences of the drinking (asking the same questions contained in the CAGE and MAST instruments, such as, "Has your husband ever felt that he ought to cut down on his drinking?") usually yield abundant evidence for alcoholism when the problem is present. An exception may be the relatives of an elderly alcoholic who have little contact with the patient or have tacitly agreed to ignore or deny a frustrating, seemingly hopeless situation. In this instance, educating the family about the disease concept of alcoholism may be necessary before they are willing to describe the patterns and consequences of the patient's drinking.

Through contact initiated by one or more family members, information will be produced that supports the diagnosis of alcoholism. Family members should be encouraged to tell the patient that they have contacted his or her doctor to describe these concerns. Ways in which the family can influence the treatment of the patient and can get help for themselves are described later in this chapter.

In summary, except for the presence of the diagnostic manifestations of alcoholism (Table 28.1), there is no simple way to diagnose alcoholism. When the problem is not overt, skillful interviewing of the patient and evaluation of multiple pieces of information are needed to make this diagnosis. This process may be accomplished at one or two visits or over weeks to months.

GENERAL PRINCIPLES OF TREATMENT

Definition of Successful Treatment

Alcoholism is a highly treatable disease. Successful treatment depends largely on the skills of those who motivate the alcoholic patient to accept the diagnosis, to undergo detoxification (see later discussion), and to enter and adhere to a long-term treatment process. *Treatment success can be defined as the achievement of abstinence or progressively longer periods of abstinence from alcohol (and other drugs), with improved life functioning for patients and their families.* (A case example is shown in Fig. 28.2.) Factors associated with good and poor outcomes after treatment are summarized later (see Prognosis with Treatment). The appropriate terms for describing an alcoholic in recovery are *recovered alcoholic* (a public or polite term) or *recovering alcoholic* (a personal or clinical term). The terms *ex-, reformed, former, or cured alcoholic* are inappropriate. Despite reports that some alcoholics can learn controlled drinking, this goal of treatment has been shown in careful studies to be unrealistic for most alcoholics and should be avoided.

Avoiding a Psychoanalytic Approach

It has been shown repeatedly that treating alcoholics as though their abnormal drinking behavior is secondary to underlying psychopathology is usually unsuccessful and often counter-therapeutic. Insight-oriented or in-depth psychotherapy early in the treatment of alcoholism is therefore contraindicated. By contrast, supportive and directive psychotherapy, using the

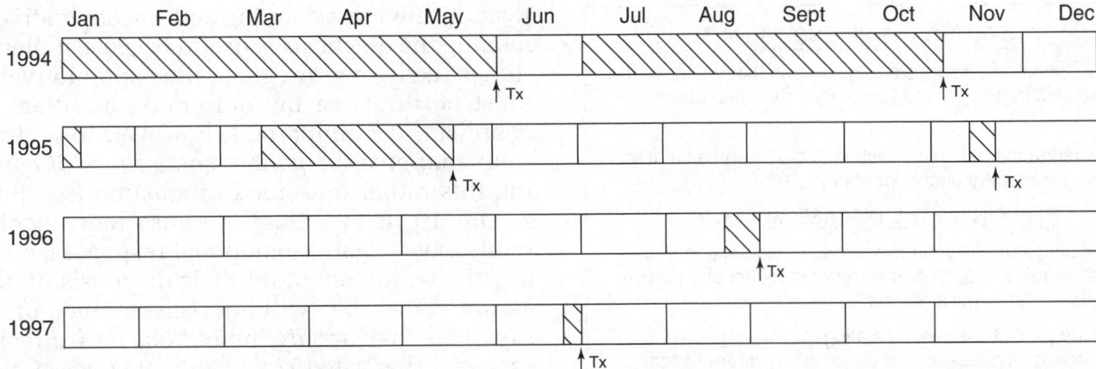

Figure 28.2. Drinking–sober profile of a 53-year-old factory supervisor who had been abusing alcohol for 15 years. The achievement of longer and longer periods of abstinence is typical of the process of recovery from alcoholism. *Hatched areas,* drinking; *clear areas,* abstinence; *Tx,* came in for treatment after having dropped out of treatment.

treatment methods outlined here and focused on the alcoholism as a primary disease, is usually effective in helping the alcoholic patient reach a successful recovery.

Breaking Down Denial and Motivating the Patient

Denial (discussed earlier) is the major obstacle to having a patient accept the diagnosis of alcoholism and agree to treatment. Three motivational techniques are fundamental for breaking down denial in patients and, if necessary, in their family members: confrontation, showing empathy, and offering hope. These techniques are equally important in one-on-one interviews and in the other paths to treatment that are described later. *Confrontation* is telling the person what one observes, including that one has diagnosed the disease alcoholism. The patient usually denies the diagnosis and may even get angry. However, with persistent and nonjudgmental confrontation, most patients eventually admit that they have a problem with alcohol. It is important in a confrontation not to argue with the patient but simply to restate the facts.

Statements that convey empathy and offer hope are important in allaying the person's denial, anxiety, anger, and shame. They should be interspersed with confrontational statements. Empathy is conveyed by stating that one recognizes the patient's feelings ("I can see that this is upsetting you") and by conveying concern ("I am very concerned about you"). Offering hope is crucial. The patient must hear, repeatedly, that there is a way out and that there is relief from the misery and bewilderment of the condition. The way out is through abstinence from alcohol and other psychoactive drugs—one day at a time—and regular use of group treatment, which includes self-help groups and group therapy (see later discussion).

Motivation of the patient is an ongoing process. In a model described by Prochaska and DiClemente (Fig. 28.3), one must first facilitate the patient to move from the state of *precontemplation* to *contemplation.* The patient must seriously be ready for change *(determination),* must *take action* (detoxification and treatment) and, finally, must work toward long-term sobriety (*maintenance*). Unfortunately, because alcoholism is a chronic disease, *relapse* is a likely part of the cycle (22).

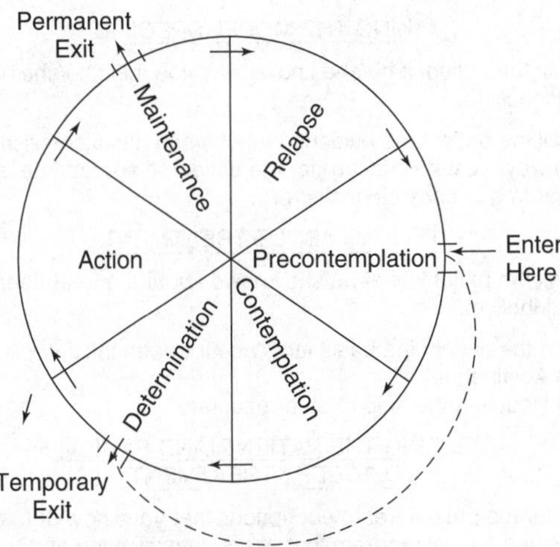

Figure 28.3. A stage model of the process of change. (Adapted from Prochaska JO, DiClemente CC. Transtheoretical therapy: toward a more integrative model of change. Psychother Theory Res Pract 1982;19:276. Reprinted with permission from Miller WR, Jackson KA. Practical psychology for pastors. Englewood Cliffs, NJ: Prentice-Hall, 1985:130.)

After a confident diagnosis of alcoholism has been made, the objectives of care are to have the patient accept the diagnosis and agree to treatment. Specific aspects of this process are described here, beginning with one-on-one confrontation of the patient.

Confrontation

Using the motivational techniques described previously, one can often persuade an alcoholic patient to accept treatment. Several actions are critical in the confrontation of the patient:

- Stating the diagnosis
- Explaining the disease model
- Making the model specific to the patient

STATING THE DIAGNOSIS

1. Tell the patient the diagnosis (e.g., "I think that you have the disease alcoholism . . . and I am very concerned about you").
2. Acknowledge the patient's reaction (e.g., "I can see that this is making you pretty uncomfortable . . .").

EXPLAINING THE DISEASE MODEL

3. Ask the patient to tell you his/her idea of what alcoholism is. (Patient usually describes stereotype model of a skidrow alcoholic . . . "and that's not me!". . .)
4. Clarify the patient's model by stating four basic facts:
   a) Alcoholism is a disease ("a disease like other medical diseases . . . for example diabetes").
   b) Like other diseases, alcoholism has an early stage way before what you described.
   c) Like other diseases, alcoholism is not the patient's fault.
   d) Alcoholism can be treated and the chances of recovery are excellent.

MAKING THE MODEL SPECIFIC

5. Ask the patient if he/she knows why you think he/she has alcoholism.
6. Tell the patient the evidence that he/she has alcoholism. (Always restate concern for the patient; if appropriate, stress features of early alcoholism.)

TELLING ABOUT TREATMENT

7. Ask the patient what he/she knows about the treatment of alcoholism.
8. Tell the patient the basic facts about treatment:
   a) Abstinence
   b) Requires the help of other people

GETTING THE PATIENT (AND FAMILY) TO ACCEPT TREATMENT

9. Offer the patient treatment options that you know of (always include a local program that offers detoxification and Alcoholics Anonymous).
10. Get the patient to select a treatment plan and to make contact promptly (e.g., call available detoxification program, call local AA office and let patient speak with AA representative).
11. With the patient's permission, contact his/her spouse or significant person(s) (tell the diagnosis and plan, and initiate plans for family treatment).

FOLLOWING THROUGH

12. Schedule follow-up appointment in 1 or 2 weeks (consider 1 or 2 days if patient has not agreed to make a treatment decision).

Figure 28.4. A recommended approach for one-on-one confrontation of the patient in whom alcoholism has been diagnosed.

- Telling about treatment
- Getting the patient (and the family) to accept (support) treatment
- Following through

Figure 28.4 summarizes a recommended approach that includes each of these actions. This approach may be incorporated into the interview at a single visit or into interviews at multiple visits. The term *drinking problem* may be used early in the discussion, before the patient's feelings regarding alcoholism are known. Even in the most denying and uncooperative patient, naming the diagnosis is useful because it plants a seed that is likely to grow, given time and motivation. One must be directive in confronting a patient with alcoholism. It is important, however, to include questions that *give the patient some sense of control* during this rather one-sided interaction (see items 3, 5, 7, and 10 in Fig. 28.4). Because most alcoholic patients have negative emotional responses, either overt or private, to being told their diagnosis, it should be assumed that they will not register much of what one says and that *brevity, repetition, and directness* are essential. Repeated *statements of concern, optimism, and support* for the person are as important as statements of fact about the disease. Such statements help patients while they are hearing a diagnosis that inevitably brings shame and help convince them that they have a disease for which they are not to blame. To ensure that patients do not conclude that they cannot avoid further drinking because they have a disease, one should tell them that it is their responsibility to seek treatment.

The first goal of treatment is abstinence from alcohol and other psychoactive drugs. However, it is never sufficient simply to tell the patient to stop drinking. Early in treatment, the patient must accept help in the difficult process of recovery. *This help is multidimensional.* In addition to regular follow-up by a supportive physician who believes the patient can recover, the most important elements are a plan for detoxification, Alcoholics Anonymous (AA) or group therapy, and family involvement (discussed later). Inpatient treatment in a specialized alcoholism treatment facility may be needed. Each of the possible treatment options should be explained to the patient and the family. If the clinician is not familiar with these, an alcoholism counselor should be asked to explain them to the patient. If the patient is in a crisis and not enough time is available during the first visit, a return appointment should be scheduled within a few days or the patient should be immediately referred to a reliable treatment program.

Formal Intervention

All too often, alcoholics with concerned families do not respond to efforts to motivate them to accept treatment. In this situation, the family should be told about the option of using a formal intervention. This consists of a meeting at which people closest to the alcoholic (immediate family members, concerned friends, employer, or other important people) create a crisis that motivates the alcoholic to accept treatment.

The intervention team is composed of as many people as possible who are emotionally important to the alcoholic. Before the actual intervention, this team meets to talk about the alcoholism, to come together in their thinking, and to agree that their purpose is to show the patient in unmistakable terms that there is a problem and that he or she needs treatment. The process is initiated by having each participant put in writing specific dramatic instances of drinking-related incidents that led to anger, fear, disappointment, sadness, embarrassment, or other distress for the team member. The team then rehearses confronting the alcoholic. Each person learns to begin with an expression of concern for the alcoholic, to describe the disturbing event and how it made that person feel, and to name specific measures they will take if the patient does not agree to treatment (e.g., loss of job, no further visits by grandchildren). As part of a formal intervention, arrangements may be made in advance to have the person admitted for alcoholism treatment. Financing of treatment, packing clothes, arranging for absence from work, and other details must all be worked out by the team ahead of time.

Motivating through Employee Assistance Programs

Increasingly, employers have recognized the economic and human costs of alcoholism and have developed employee assistance programs to motivate and assist alcoholics into treatment. Employers threaten to terminate employees who have deteriorating job performance due to alcoholism unless they get treatment and remain in treatment. Physicians asked to write work excuses can often work with employee assistance programs to coerce the denying alcoholic to get appropriate treatment for alcoholism. This approach uses the strong motivation to keep a job as leverage for getting treatment and following through to recovery—leverage the physician alone may not have on the patient. The problem of the impaired professional and the use of measures similar to employee assistance programs are discussed in a later section.

DETOXIFICATION

The majority of alcoholics can be detoxified from alcohol by outpatient procedures (23). With the cost of treatment now a major consideration, the decision between inpatient and outpatient detoxification should be based mostly on medical history and severity of alcohol withdrawal symptoms.

Alcohol Withdrawal Symptoms

The diagnosis of alcohol withdrawal requires a history of recent heavy drinking followed by reduced intake or cessation of use, the absence of other conditions that could cause symptoms mimicking withdrawal, and one or more of the four major manifestations of alcohol withdrawal (tremors, seizures, hallucinosis, and delirium tremens) (24). These occur also in other conditions, ranging from withdrawal from other sedative-hypnotic drugs to meningitis (see list of causes of delirium in Chapter 26, Table 26.5).

Tremulousness usually begins 8 to 12 hours after the patient's last drink and peaks in 24 to 36 hours. *Withdrawal seizures* occur within 8 to 24 hours. Withdrawal seizures may occur independent of other manifestations of alcohol withdrawal. Both seizures and tremulousness can occur before the BAL has reached zero.

The *alcohol hallucination* is almost never the mythical pink elephant. Rather, it is usually one of moving insects, small animals, or threatening voices. In a series of 50 consecutive patients, 58% of their hallucinations were purely visual, 16% were purely auditory, and 26% were mixed (25). In certain patients these hallucinations may not be all negative; that is, the patient becomes used to them and is no longer frightened. Hallucinations may begin up to several days after the patient stops or markedly reduces alcohol use (usually in the first 48 hours). Typically, alcoholic hallucinosis lasts from minutes to days (usually less than 1 week) but in a very small percentage of patients hallucinosis continues for weeks to months or, rarely, as a continuous symptom.

Delirium tremens is a late manifestation of withdrawal, occurring from 48 hours (most common interval) to 14 days (uncommon) after cessation of drinking (26). It may begin after the patient has shown signs of improvement from the early manifestations of withdrawal. Any of the symptoms of delirium, described in Chapter 26, may signal the onset of delirium tremens.

At least half of ambulatory alcoholic patients who stop drinking develop none of the four major manifestations of withdrawal. Additional minor symptoms are common. Anorexia, nausea, and sometimes vomiting are present in varying degrees. Tachycardia, systolic hypertension, and paroxysmal diaphoresis also are common. Generalized weakness may be prominent, and tinnitus, hyperacusis, itching, muscle cramps, and mood and sleep disorders are sometimes experienced. The patient often is hyperalert, startles easily, and has difficulty concentrating and usually craves alcohol or other drugs to quiet symptoms.

Selection of Patients for Inpatient versus Outpatient Detoxification

There are a number of indications for referring a withdrawing alcoholic patient for *inpatient detoxification* (Table 28.5). Inpatient detoxification provides careful 24-hour monitoring and treatment of withdrawal symptoms, evaluation of inter-current medical problems, and removal of patients from the environment that has facilitated their drinking. If medically stable, patients participate in groups (usually AA) and receive individual counseling.

For mildly symptomatic patients with a stable home environment and supportive family and friends, *outpatient detoxification* supervised at daily visits to a treatment program or physician's office is as effective as inpatient detoxification. Patients may contract to attend an AA meeting daily with a friend or family member. For moderately sick patients, the choice of outpatient versus inpatient detoxification should be based on what programs are available. Some outpatient detoxification programs are intensive, requiring patients to spend entire days being monitored, with

Table 28.5. Indications for Referring a Withdrawing Alcoholic for Inpatient Detoxification

Evidence of hallucinations, severe tachycardia, severe tremor, fever, extreme agitation, or a history of severe withdrawal symptoms
History of seizure disorder
Presence of ataxia, nystagmus, confusion, or ophthalmoplegia, which may be indicative of Wernicke encephalopathy
Severe nausea and vomiting that would prevent the ingestion of medication
Evidence of acute or chronic liver disease that may alter the metabolism of drugs used in the treatment of withdrawal
Presence of cardiovascular disease such as severe hypertension, ischemic heart disease, or arrhythmia, for which the sympathetic surge of catecholamines during withdrawal poses particular risk
Pregnancy
Presence of associated medical or surgical condition requiring treatment
Lack of medical or social support system to allow outpatient detoxification

patients receiving medication as needed and participating in group counseling but going home to sleep. Other outpatient detoxification programs consist only of brief daily visits.

Use of Drugs in Detoxification

A useful *tool for making decisions about pharmacologic treatment in the withdrawing alcoholic* is the Clinical Institute Withdrawal Assessment for Alcohol (CIWA-Ar) (Table 28.6) (27). Pharmacologic therapy is not indicated for a score less than 10. For scores of 10 to 20, clinical judgment should determine the need for pharmacologic treatment. For scores greater than 20, treatment with drugs is indicated and should be administered on either an outpatient or an inpatient basis. For scores of 20 to 40, the assessment can be repeated after administration of a dose of medication; patients without improvement need more intensive monitoring as inpatients. Notably, pulse and blood pressure are not part of the CIWA scale. Although elevations of blood pressure and pulse do occur in alcohol withdrawal, the other signs and symptoms are more reliable in the assessment of severity of withdrawal. Therefore, one should not make a decision about whether to prescribe drugs for alcohol withdrawal based solely on blood pressure and pulse measurements.

Detoxification with the use of orally administered psychoactive drugs appears to be most effective when it is combined with the non-pharmacologic techniques described in the next section and when treatment is given early. The safest and most effective drugs for this purpose are the benzodiazepine sedative-hypnotics (28). All of the benzodiazepines are effective. Diazepam has the advantages of having a rapid onset of action, a longer half-life, and a lower cost. Its long half-life permits loading on the first day; that is, 5 to 10 mg every 1 to 4 hours until severe symptoms dissipate, which will reduce or perhaps eliminate the need for further dosing on subsequent days. Lorazepam (Ativan) does not require hepatic metabolism and is safer in patients with severe liver disease (i.e., prolonged prothrombin time). Patient response to a dose of benzodiazepine is unpredictable and is not necessarily related to the amount of drinking. Ideally, patients should be monitored for response after initial dosing to make an assessment of indicated dosage and dosing interval. Dosing should be titrated to effect. Essential to management is early recognition of withdrawal, early treatment, frequent monitoring, and continual treatment. Given the decision to use sedative drugs in the detoxification process, one can choose low or high dosages (Table 28.7). Low dosages of sedative-hypnotic drugs may be tried first for most patients. The advantage of low-dose treatment is that the patient remains more alert. High dosages of these drugs may be indicated when the low dosage does not suppress or prevent symptoms within the first few hours.

The aim of drug treatment is to alleviate the most bothersome symptoms and signs of withdrawal. Symptom-driven therapy, compared to fixed schedule therapy, has been shown to decrease treatment duration and the amount of benzodiazepine used (29). Benzodiazepines should be given in such a manner that withdrawal symptoms are improved without oversedation of the patient. If the patient is being treated as an outpatient, each day's medication should be entrusted to a family member or friend who will be staying with the patient. Most patients need to be medicated for only 24 to 72 hours. Other drugs have been used for management of alcohol withdrawal, most notably clonidine and beta-blockers. Both of these drugs effectively alleviate the sympathetic markers of withdrawal (hypertension and tachycardia) but do little for the more severe aspects of withdrawal (seizures and hallucinosis). For this reason, if a patient is so symptomatic that the use of drugs is deemed appropriate, a benzodiazepine should be the drug of choice. The prevention of withdrawal seizures is discussed later.

Detoxification without Drugs

Candidates for nonpharmacologic outpatient detoxification should be ambulatory and, except for their chronic alcoholism and acute withdrawal, should be otherwise free from serious chronic illness or acute problems. The primary aim in non-pharmacologic detoxification is to provide a non-threatening, positive environment for the patient. The patient should be kept ambulatory when possible and given a regular diet. Except when asleep or resting comfortably, the patient should be encouraged to perform purposeful activities, such as carrying out small duties or attending introductory group education and therapy sessions.

Nonpharmacologic therapy can be just as effective as drug therapy in the detoxification of ambulatory patients in uncomplicated cases (30). The advantages of nonpharmacologic detoxification, compared to traditional detoxification with drugs, are that it can be done largely by non-medical personnel, it is less expensive, and the patient is more likely to remain alert and, consequently, able to participate in treatment. The only

Table 28.6. Addiction Research Foundation Clinical Institute Withdrawal Assessment for Alcohol (CIWA-Ar)[a]

Patient ________ Date |__|__|__| (y m d) Time ____:____ (24-hour clock, midnight = 00:00)

Pulse or heart rate, taken for 1 min: ______ Blood pressure: ______ / ______

NAUSEA AND VOMITING—Ask "Do you feel sick to your stomach? Have you vomited?" Observation.
0 no nausea and no vomiting
1 mild nausea with no vomiting
2
3
4 intermittent nausea with dry heaves
5
6
7 constant nausea, frequent dry heaves and vomiting

TREMOR—Arms extended and fingers spread apart. Observation.
0 no tremor
1 not visible, but can be felt fingertip to fingertip
2
3
4 moderate, with patient's arms extended
5
6
7 severe, even with arms not extended

PAROXYSMAL SWEATS—Observation.
0 no sweat visible
1 barely perceptible sweating, palms moist
2
3
4 beads of sweat obvious on forehead
5
6
7 drenching sweats

ANXIETY—Ask "Do you feel nervous?" Observation.
0 no anxiety, at ease
1 mildly anxious
2
3
4 moderately anxious, or guarded, so anxiety is inferred
5
6
7 equivalent to acute panic states, as seen in severe delirium or acute schizophrenic reactions

AGITATION—Observation.
0 normal activity
1 somewhat more than normal activity
2
3
4 moderately fidgety and restless
5
6
7 paces back and forth during most of the interview, or constantly thrashes about

TACTILE DISTURBANCES—Ask "Have you any itching, pins and needles sensations, any burning, any numbness, or do you feel bugs crawling on or under your skin?" Observation.
0 none
1 very mild itching, pins and needles, burning or numbness
2 mild itching, pins and needles, burning or numbness
3 moderate itching, pins and needles, burning or numbness
4 moderately severe hallucinations
5 severe hallucinations
6 extremely severe hallucinations
7 continuous hallucinations

AUDITORY DISTURBANCES—Ask "Are you more aware of sounds around you? Are they harsh? Do they frighten you? Are you hearing anything that is disturbing to you? Are you hearing things you know are not there?" Observation.
0 not present
1 very mild harshness or ability to frighten
2 mild harshness or ability to frighten
3 moderate harshness or ability to frighten
4 moderately severe hallucinations
5 severe hallucinations
6 extremely severe hallucinations
7 continuous hallucinations

VISUAL DISTURBANCES—Ask "Does the light appear to be too bright? Is its color different? Does it hurt your eyes? Are you seeing anything that is disturbing to you? Are you seeing things you know are not there?" Observation.
0 not present
1 very mild sensitivity
2 mild sensitivity
3 moderate sensitivity
4 moderately severe hallucinations
5 severe hallucinations
6 extremely severe hallucinations
7 continuous hallucinations

HEADACHE, FULLNESS IN HEAD—Ask "Does your head feel different? Does it feel like there is a band around your head?" Do not rate for dizziness or lightheadedness. Otherwise, rate severity.
0 not present
1 very mild
2 mild
3 moderate
4 moderately severe
5 severe
6 very severe
7 extremely severe

ORIENTATION AND CLOUDING OF SENSORIUM—Ask "What day is this? Where are you? Who am I?"
0 oriented and can do serial additions
1 cannot do serial additions or is uncertain about date
2 disoriented for date by no more than 2 calendar days
3 disoriented for date by more than 2 calendar days
4 disoriented for place and/or person

Total CIWA-A Score ______
Rater's Initials ______
Maximum Possible Score 67

[a]This scale is not copyrighted and may be used freely.

routine medication should be vitamins (100 mg of thiamine, 1 mg of folate, and a multivitamin daily). These vitamins should be continued for the first month or more of recovery.

Many communities have established alcoholism facilities that provide a sheltered, supportive environment to care for alcoholics, using a social model for detoxification. Patients are screened and evaluated to detect any obvious medical problems before or shortly after being admitted. Should complications arise, backup hospital/medical support is available. The length of stay varies in each program, from 3 days

Table 28.7. Characteristics of Benzodiazepines Used Orally in the Treatment of Alcohol Withdrawal

Drug	Onset of Action	Rate of Metabolism	Liver Metabolized	Low Dosage (mg/6 hr)	High Dosage (mg/2–4 hr)
Chlordiazepoxide	Intermediate	Long	Yes	25	100
Diazepam	Fast	Long	Yes	2–5	10–20
Lorazepam	Intermediate	Intermediate	No	0.5	2
Oxazepam	Slow	Short	No	10–15	30

to more than 30 days. Most social setting programs use AA extensively, and many of the larger programs use techniques used in other alcoholism treatment centers. These centers can be either day treatment or residential facilities.

For detoxification at home without the use of drugs, a reliable family member or other person should be present to observe the patient for at least 2 full days. The physician supervising such detoxification should be in touch with the patient or the family member daily during the 2 to 4 days required for detoxification. The following is a checklist for home detoxification:

1. The patient should be motivated to achieve detoxification at home.
2. A reliable person should stay with or frequently check on the patient.
3. There should be access to a telephone so that the patient can call the physician or counselor daily for reassurance and for monitoring withdrawal.
4. There should be no active medical problems requiring aggressive treatment and no significant chemical dependence to drugs other than alcohol.
5. There should be arrangements to see a supervising physician, nurse, or counselor each day.
6. The patient should be as active as possible (attend AA, take foods and fluids as desired, and take multivitamins daily).
7. The patient should have arrangements to start an outpatient program on completion of detoxification.

Prevention of Withdrawal Seizures

There is no consensus about whether *phenytoin* (Dilantin) should be included in the detoxification of patients with a history of withdrawal seizures. It has been shown that phenytoin at a dosage of 300 mg/day for 5 days can prevent most withdrawal seizures, even though therapeutic plasma levels of phenytoin are not reached (31). However, in another study, when patients received an intravenous load of phenytoin or placebo within 6 hours after a first alcohol withdrawal seizure, phenytoin provided no benefit in preventing further seizures (32).

There is evidence that a *high-dosage benzodiazepine* regimen for withdrawal can prevent seizures (33). Therefore, patients who are significantly symptomatic and are receiving sufficient pharmacologic therapy with a benzodiazepine do not require phenytoin. However, patients who are only mildly symptomatic and have a history of a withdrawal seizure should receive prophylactic phenytoin if they are not going to be treated with a benzodiazepine. This recommendation is based on the fact that a seizure may occur without the presence of any other manifestations of alcohol withdrawal (34).

NONPHARMACOLOGIC TREATMENT AFTER DETOXIFICATION

Overview

Treatment consists of motivating the patient, initiating a treatment plan, and providing regular follow-up. The clinician who initially motivates an alcoholic to accept treatment may elect not to coordinate the overall treatment but to provide a referral elsewhere. For this important referral, one should select a specialist or a program with demonstrated expertise in helping alcoholics recover. The simplest ways to find such expert help are to call the local National Council on Alcoholism, to ask a colleague who has had experience in referring or treating alcoholics, or to refer the patient to an existing community alcoholism treatment program.

In selecting skilled help, one should look for several characteristics. Effective programs are abstinence-oriented; use AA or group therapy as a mainstay of treatment; offer disulfiram to patients; avoid the use of psychoactive drugs in long-term treatment; refer the spouse to Al-Anon or family therapy; provide close follow-up; and avoid insight-oriented psychotherapy, unless indicated later in the course of recovery. The physician who makes the referral should reinforce participation in the treatment program whenever the patient returns for follow-up.

Alcoholics Anonymous and Group Therapy

Alcoholics and other chemical-dependent people seem to recover best in group treatment settings. Groups effectively break down the denial process and heal the associated guilt and shame through a combination of identification, nonjudgmental acceptance, confrontation, and support. Every alcoholic should be strongly encouraged to attend AA regularly. Studies show that regular AA attendance is strongly correlated with long-term recovery and improved functioning (5,35).

Many patients are reluctant to attend AA or a therapy group. Therefore, when referring a patient, it is important to convey that one is familiar with these programs and has confidence in them. Immediate action, taken while the patient is in the office, may consist of having the patient contact a family member or friend who is active in AA, telephoning the local AA office and having the patient request a contact to take him

Table 28.8. The Process of Alcoholics Anonymous

AA was founded in 1935 by two chronic alcoholics, one a stockbroker and one a physician.

Meetings

AA meetings are held frequently in all communities in the United States and in most other countries. Meetings are either open or closed (most are open and most welcome nonalcoholics interested in treating alcoholism). A published directory of meetings, places, times, and information by telephone are available from each local chapter of AA. By contacting AA, an alcoholic can almost always arrange to be taken to a meeting in his or her community, often on the day he or she makes the request. Many AA members attend meetings several times a week. Some attend at least one meeting per day. Lifelong activity in AA is the basis for maintaining health for many recovering alcoholics.

Meetings are usually 1 hour in length. Most are held in the evening, although there are many daytime meetings as well. Meetings begin with a recitation by one member of the Twelve Steps and the Twelve Traditions and are devoted to examination and interpretation of these, as illustrated in personal experiences described by a number of members. One member of the group chairs the meeting and calls on speakers. Speakers introduce themselves by their first names (e.g., "I'm Joe—I'm an alcoholic"). Meetings end with group recitation of the Lord's Prayer or the Serenity Prayer "God grant me the Serenity to accept the things I cannot change, Courage to change the things I can, and Wisdom to know the difference."

AA on the surface can sometimes look insubstantial and unsophisticated, often turning off newcomers. Often the spiritual overtones of the program are rejected. However, the program is *profound and life changing.* Without an administrative structure, owning no property, and having no dues or fees, it continues to grow because it works and meets human need.

Publications

AA provides printed educational aids in the form of pamphlets (available at meetings) and "the Big Book" (*Alcoholics Anonymous,* a collection of personal stories that illustrate vividly the ways that lives are damaged by alcoholism and the AA path to recovery). One can obtain this book or other literature at meetings, at the local AA office, or by writing AA World Services, Box 459, Grand Central Station, New York, NY 10017.

The 12 Steps

1. We admitted we were powerless over alcohol, that our lives had become unmanageable.
2. Came to believe that a power greater than ourselves could restore us to sanity.
3. Made a decision to turn our will and our lives over to the care of God as we understood Him.
4. Made a searching and fearless moral inventory of ourselves.
5. Admitted to God, to ourselves, and to another human being the exact nature of our wrongs.
6. Were entirely ready to have God remove all these defects of character.
7. Humbly asked Him to remove our shortcomings.
8. Made a list of all persons we had harmed, and became willing to make amends to them all.
9. Made direct amends to such people wherever possible, except when to do so would injure them or others.
10. Continued to take personal inventory, and when we were wrong promptly admitted it.
11. Sought through prayer and meditation to improve our conscious contact with God, as we understood Him, praying only for knowledge of His will for us and the power to carry that out.
12. Having had a spiritual awakening as the result of the Steps, we tried to carry this message to alcoholics, and to practice these principles in all our affairs (note: for this step, Altman substitutes "others" for the word "alcoholics").

Boiled down, these steps mean, simply:

a. Admission of alcoholism.
b. Personality analysis and catharsis.
c. Adjustment of personal relations.
d. Dependence on some higher power.
e. Working with other alcoholics.

The 12 Traditions

1. Our common welfare should come first; personal recovery depends upon AA unity.
2. For our group purpose there is but one ultimate authority—a loving God as He may express Himself in our group conscience. Our leaders are but trusted servants; they do not govern.
3. The only requirement for AA membership is a desire to stop drinking.
4. Each group should be autonomous except in matters affecting other groups or AA as a whole.
5. Each group has but one primary purpose—to carry out its message to the alcoholic who still suffers.
6. An AA group ought never endorse, finance, or lend the AA name to any related facility or outside enterprise, lest problems of money, property, and prestige divert us from our primary purpose.
7. Every AA group ought to be fully self-supporting, declining outside contributions.
8. AA should remain forever nonprofessional, but our service centers may employ special workers.
9. AA, as such, ought never to be organized; but we may create service boards or committees directly responsible to those they serve.
10. Alcoholics Anonymous has no opinion on outside issues; hence the AA name ought never be drawn into public controversy.
11. Our public relations policy is based on attraction rather than promotion; we need always maintain personal anonymity at the level of press, radio, and films.
12. Anonymity is the spiritual foundation of our Traditions, ever reminding us to place principles before personalities.

or her to a convenient AA meeting, or telephoning an alcoholism treatment program and arranging an intake appointment for the patient. The best way for physicians to learn about these programs is to attend one or more AA meetings and, if available, open group therapy meetings. To locate such meetings, one should call the local AA office or the local National Council on Alcoholism. The AA process is summarized in Table 28.8.

Psychotherapy

It is commonly thought that all alcoholic patients have a primary and causative underlying psychological problem. If treatment of this condition is successful, the alcoholism is expected to resolve because it is considered to be chiefly a manifestation of the underlying psychological problem. Although this approach may seem theoretically valid, this therapeutic strategy rarely works unless there happens to be a coexisting psychosis. Patients with alcoholism cannot gain insight into aspects of their lives successfully until they have maintained sobriety. Early psychotherapy may impede maintenance of sobriety and trigger relapse. Even in patients with coexisting psychosis, the alcoholism must also be treated. After rapport is established, therefore, the initial effort in psychotherapy should be to work with the patient toward abstinence and regular participation in group treatment.

Ongoing supportive care by the provider, as described in Chapter 20, is useful for reinforcing the patient's understanding of the disease and the recovery process; for monitoring the patient's functioning in important life areas, such as family, job, and interpersonal relations; and for assisting the patient in change and growth.

Discussions with the Spouse or Closest Family Members

As part of the early treatment of an alcoholic patient, the situation should be discussed with the spouse or person closest to the patient. Such discussions (which should be conducted without breaking the patient's confidentiality) serve to ensure that the family agrees with the goal of abstinence; explore the spouse's own drinking pattern; discern any special problems occurring in any of the close family members, and educate the spouse about the enabling process. *If the family does not change and grow, usually through regular attendance at Al-Anon meetings, it will be more difficult for the patient to recover.* Family treatment and the Al-Anon process are described later (see Co-alcoholism).

PHARMACOLOGIC TREATMENT OF ALCOHOL DEPENDENCE

Disulfiram (Antabuse)

Although controlled studies have not shown that it increases duration of sobriety (36–39), the use of disulfiram to prevent drinking should be considered for some patients. Patients must be in active recovery, including AA and individual or group therapy. Disulfiram should not be used as the focus of treatment but as an adjunct. The risks of prescribing disulfiram have probably been overemphasized. Disulfiram is available, as Antabuse, in the form of scored tablets containing 250 or 500 mg.

Disulfiram–Alcohol Interaction

Alcohol is initially oxidized by the hepatic enzyme alcohol dehydrogenase to acetaldehyde, and disulfiram inhibits acetaldehyde oxidation by interfering with aldehyde dehydrogenase. This effect may persist for up to 2 weeks after cessation of disulfiram. The symptoms of the alcohol–disulfiram reaction are related to *elevated acetaldehyde;* they are usually proportional to the amounts of disulfiram and alcohol ingested. Some people have typical symptoms after drinking as little as 7 mL of alcohol (about half of a drink). A very small percentage of patients seem to be able to drink despite taking disulfiram with no significant symptoms.

The common symptoms of the alcohol–disulfiram reaction usually begin within 10 minutes and include flushing, throbbing in the head and neck, headaches, anxiety, general discomfort, sweating, and respiratory difficulty. The reaction typically lasts between 30 minutes and several hours. Less often, nausea, vomiting, hypotension, thirst, chest pain, palpitation, dyspnea, hyperventilation, tachycardia, syncope, weakness, blurred vision, and confusion can occur.

Office Prescribing of Disulfiram

Patients who are motivated to succeed in recovery and who have experienced relapse or dread the likelihood of relapse are candidates for disulfiram. Table 28.9 summarizes a practical plan that can be used in office practice. This supervised approach is similar in its demands on patients and physicians to the initiation and management of long-term treatment. Patients should carry an identification card that identifies them as taking disulfiram.

Advantages of Disulfiram

Disulfiram has several advantages. Because the drug is taken daily, it is a constant reminder that one cannot drink safely. Additionally, it provides evidence of compliance in the treatment program; it is compatible with other forms of treatment of alcoholism; and it can also provide family and employer with reassurance that as

Table 28.9. The Suggested Approach to Supervised Use of Disulfiram

1. Satisfy the following indications: the patient is willing to take medication several times a week under supervision, the patient can recall making the decision to take the first drink of a relapse, and the patient is actively involved in an organized outpatient treatment program.
2. Rule out contraindications and ask yourself the following question: "Can this patient survive a disulfiram–alcohol reaction?"
3. Ensure sober state before the initiation of treatment.
4. Be sure patient and spouse know how to avoid hidden alcohol in foods, over-the-counter medications, toiletries, etc.
5. Have the patient read, discuss, and sign a consent form before initiating treatment.
6. Begin with a dosage of one tablet (250 mg) daily.
7. *Keep the medication bottle in the office* and have the patient come in three times a week to be dispensed two (or three) doses by the office staff. After 1 month, decrease the visits to twice a week and increase the number of pills dispensed accordingly. After another month, go to weekly visits and continue these for the duration of disulfiram treatment. See the patient at least monthly and repeat laboratory testing every 3 months.
8. If the patient misses more than one or two appointments in a row, have the office staff contact the people on the consent form, and stop administering the medication.

long as it is taken daily, the alcoholic cannot get drunk. Patients should consider four additional advantages: The decision not to drink has to be made only once a day; because of this, patients tend not to worry about whether they can drink; not worrying or thinking about drinking saves considerable energy; and this makes recovery easier.

Side Effects and Contraindications

Disulfiram at recommended dosages of 250 to 700 mg/day is well tolerated by most patients. Some patients complain of drowsiness, fatigability, headaches, a garlic-like or metallic aftertaste, breath odor, or acneform eruptions. To avoid the problem with drowsiness, the disulfiram can be taken at bedtime. The other side effects usually subside within a few days or weeks with continued therapy. More rarely, confusion (particularly in the elderly), optic neuritis, polyneuritis, and peripheral neuritis may occur.

Contraindications for the use of disulfiram include a history of hypertension, diabetes, emphysema, seizures, significant liver or renal disease, coronary artery disease, hypothyroidism, pregnancy, or a history of drinking while taking disulfiram. If alcohol-related liver disease is present, prescribing of disulfiram should be delayed until the levels of serum aspartate aminotransferase (AST) and serum alanine aminotransferase (ALT), two serum markers of liver disease, are less than three times the normal range. Disulfiram may impair the metabolism and *potentiate the effects of caffeine, warfarin, and phenytoin,* and it may interact additively to *potentiate the neurologic side effects of isoniazid* (ataxia, psychosis). It should be used with caution in conjunction with these drugs or with the following other classes of drugs: alpha- or beta-adrenergic antagonists, vasodilators, sympathomimetic amines, monoamine oxidase inhibitors, tricyclic antidepressants, and neuroleptics. Most cough syrups no longer contain alcohol, but an alcoholic patient should avoid medications such as cough syrups and foods (e.g., salad dressings) that name alcohol as an ingredient.

Naltrexone

Naltrexone (ReVia) is a second drug that is potentially useful as an adjunct to a formal treatment program for individuals with alcohol dependence (40,41). Unlike disulfiram, patients do not get sick if they drink while taking naltrexone. Naltrexone has been shown to *reduce alcohol craving* and as a result may be particularly useful in preventing relapse in motivated patients (37,42). Additionally, when patients relapse they tend to drink smaller amounts. However, the numbers of patients in most studies have been small, and there are few long-term data. Most published studies have reported the effectiveness of naltrexone in drinkers for 3 to 6 months.

Naltrexone is an opiate antagonist and therefore cannot be prescribed to patients who are taking opiate analgesics. Furthermore, patients maintained on naltrexone will not obtain pain relief if prescribed an opiate. Naltrexone is well tolerated, with nausea as its main side effect. To avoid nausea, patients should be prescribed 25 mg (one-half tablet) each day for 7 days and 50 mg/day thereafter. Naltrexone can be used in combination with disulfiram. Although there is no clear evidence of hepatotoxicity, the makers of naltrexone advise monitoring of liver function tests (initially at monthly intervals and then less frequently). If naltrexone is tolerated and is successful in aiding abstinence, the recommended initial course of treatment is 3 months. Naltrexone does not cause physical dependence and can be stopped at any time without withdrawal symptoms. If a patient is going to have elective surgery, naltrexone should be stopped at least 72 hours beforehand to allow the use of opiate analgesia.

A decision to stop naltrexone or disulfiram is best made jointly by the physician, the spouse or other close person, the AA sponsor, and the patient. It should be based on the strength of the patient's recovery. Important guidelines in this decision are active AA or group therapy participation, coping with crises without recourse to drinking, improved family relationships, dissolution of denial, social ease (diminution in social anxiety), growth in self-esteem, and prolonged abstinence.

Psychoactive Drugs

Although many alcoholics have symptoms such as anxiety, insomnia, and tremors that might be helped by sedatives, in actuality these drugs usually interfere with successful recovery. Anxiolytic drugs may have a role in acute detoxification (see earlier discussion), and major tranquilizers, antidepressants, and lithium have usefulness in treating, respectively, the schizophrenic, the severe protracted depressive, and the manic-depressive alcoholic (as long as these patients are being treated concomitantly for alcoholism). Apart from these situations, psychoactive drugs should not be prescribed for alcoholics. There are many reasons for this recommendation: (a) all sedatives are cross-tolerant with alcohol and thus have a built-in escalation factor; (b) combining sedatives with alcohol is often dangerously synergistic; (c) inability to control consumption, a cardinal feature of alcoholism, occurs with prescribed sedative drugs; (d) memory blackouts may also occur with other sedatives and minor tranquilizers; (e) patients may alter the prescription to obtain excessive quantities of these drugs; (f) prescribing these drugs reinforces psychoactive substance use as a coping mechanism and impairs development of the patient's own coping mechanisms; and (g) the drugs interfere with learning to relate to others in a healthy manner.

FOLLOW-UP: PREVENTION AND MANAGEMENT OF RELAPSE

Next to dealing with denial and motivating the patient, follow-up is the most difficult part of treatment. One reason is that when an alcoholic recovers there may be an early honeymoon period during which the patient feels and looks so good that one is lulled into believing that regular follow-up is unnecessary. However, because it takes 2 to 3 years of appropriate treatment before recovery can be secure, regular follow-up is indicated.

During the first 6 weeks after stopping drinking, patients need much support and direction, for this is the time when they are most likely to relapse. At least weekly patient contacts are indicated for this time, with a gradually decreasing frequency thereafter. Some of these contacts may be by telephone. Other *high-risk times for relapse* include special days and occasions, such as vacations, holidays, business trips, birthdays, and anniversaries, and crises, such as separation, divorce, death of a close person, or illness in the family. Other relapse danger times are when a patient stops taking disulfiram or stops attending AA or group therapy meetings.

"Dry drunks" are often part of the natural history of recovery. This is the name given by recovering alcoholics to the negative emotions and behaviors reminiscent of those that occurred when the patient was drinking. Dry drunks may last from a few hours to several weeks or even months. Treatment is by recognition, education, and alteration of the diet and other current life habits. Dry drunks are often associated with eating poorly. Regular, well-balanced meals should be recommended, and caffeine intake, including coffee, tea, colas, and chocolate, should be markedly decreased or discontinued. Increased attendance at AA or group therapy meetings at this time is very important. Moderation in the patient's work and recreational activities and rest should be advised.

The *relapse process generally begins long before the person drinks.* It often progresses in the following sequence: reactivation of denial, progressive isolation and defensiveness, building a crisis to justify symptom progression, immobilization, confusion and overreaction, depression, loss of control over behavior, recognition of loss of control, and finally relapse to drinking.

Although it should not be telegraphed to the patient, relapse is part of the natural history of successful recovery for most alcoholics, and one should not become discouraged if it happens (Fig. 28.3). Instead, one should immediately recruit the patient back into treatment using the same motivational techniques used initially. Relapse is a time for both patient and therapist to learn about their mistakes and to correct them by strengthening treatment.

INPATIENT REHABILITATION

Although controlled studies differ regarding the advantage of inpatient rehabilitation versus outpatient treatment, inpatient rehabilitation for 2 to 6 weeks may be especially helpful for selected patients (43). It is always planned for in advance when a formal intervention is used (see earlier discussion). Other indications for inpatient rehabilitation are strong denial, especially if it persists in outpatient treatment; unsuccessful or too slow recovery despite adequate outpatient treatment; weak or unavailable support systems; danger to self or others; severe medical, psychiatric, or other problems related to the alcoholism; and patient's desire for inpatient treatment.

Although treatment goals among inpatient rehabilitation programs vary, some of the major goals include breaking down denial, educating about alcoholism, providing an introduction to group treatment (self-help groups and group therapy), learning how to ask for help, learning how to communicate directly and honestly, learning how to enjoy life while abstinent, beginning family restoration, and developing a specific, appropriate, and structured long-term recovery program.

PROGNOSIS WITH TREATMENT

A number of factors, described here, are associated with a good or poor prognosis for recovery. Even factors traditionally thought to be major barriers to treatment success—a skid row lifestyle or being an unattached young adult—do not always preclude successful recovery.

Factors Associated with a Good Prognosis

The first of the factors associated with a good prognosis is *clinician commitment to facilitating patient motivation.* Most patients are only marginally motivated to get well. Patients are ambivalent: A part of them wants to get well, and another part of them wants to continue drinking and stay sick (patients usually do not know what is wrong with them because no one has told them of the diagnosis in an effective way). Such patients have a good chance of getting into recovery if their physician is committed to the treatment of their alcoholism and consistently uses the motivational techniques described previously.

The *presence of a crisis situation* is also a positive prognostic factor if the crisis is used as a motivational tool. The crisis may be the threat of a job loss, family separation or divorce, a DWI charge, a health-related crisis, an organized formal intervention (described earlier), or some other dramatic event. The physician actually precipitates a crisis when the confrontation approach is used (Fig. 28.4). As in that approach, it is critical to act promptly if a situational crisis is to be used effectively to motivate the patient to accept treatment. If exploitation of this crisis does not work, at least a seed has been planted that may eventually yield results.

A third factor associated with a good prognosis is *appropriate treatment for at least 2 years.* Patients whose alcoholism began before 25 years of age usually require at least 3 years of treatment. Many alcoholics who begin treatment either believe they can do it on their own or return to drinking and drop out of treatment. To recover effectively, most alcoholics need to be with people who are recovering successfully. This favorable environment is found most easily in self-help groups such as AA and in group therapy. Therefore, if patients show any indication of dropping out of treatment, it is important to promptly persuade them against this move.

The prognosis is also better if *family, job, health, and cognitive function are intact.* The status of family, job, health, and cognitive function usually correlates with how far alcoholism has advanced. Making a diagnosis early in the course of the alcoholism generally portends a better prognosis because each of these aspects of the patient's life tends to be more intact early in the illness. Also, in early illness the patient's and family members' denial systems and other defense systems tend not to be as strong. If one or more members of the patient's family is receiving treatment for co-alcoholism (discussed later), the prognosis for the patient usually is better.

Additional factors that increase the likelihood of long-term success are prompt recognition and intervention when relapse occurs (see earlier discussion) and the acceptance by patient and physician of a recovery model that views alcoholism as a physical, mental, and spiritual illness.

Factors Associated with a Poor Prognosis

If the patient has *no perceived threat of loss* from continued drinking, the prognosis for recovery is generally worse. Another factor that may worsen the prognosis is one of the following forms of *inappropriate treatment*: disulfiram alone, psychoanalytically oriented psychotherapy in the first year of alcoholism treatment, controlled drinking treatment, use of sedatives in long-term management, inpatient or outpatient treatment that does not treat alcoholism as a primary illness, and treatment that is too short in duration.

Although many patients who have a continued self-destructive bent do not tend to recover, some do. Often, intensive inpatient alcoholism treatment for 2 months or longer can be helpful for such patients. However, economic restraints most often limit this option. Cognitive impairment or psychosis often makes treatment difficult. However, the presence of these factors alone does not preclude a full attempt at treatment. With abstinence there is often surprising improvement over time.

Acceptance of a *derelict subculture status* by the patient makes the prognosis virtually hopeless. However, it can be helpful to screen for a potentially reversible derelict status by looking at prior career and duration of dereliction. For example, a person who up until 2 years ago was in a productive profession or trade and is now on skid row has potential for recovery. By contrast, a skid row person who has had no constructive activities for many years usually has little chance for reaching a successful long-term recovery. Patients who have *powerful enablers* to deny, cover up, and protect them from the consequences of drinking or drug using (see Co-alcoholism) are less likely to make a successful recovery.

SPECIAL POPULATIONS

Alcoholism in Older Persons

It is estimated that alcoholism is present in 3 to 4 million Americans older than 60 years of age, with prevalence estimates of 2% to 10%. Most elderly alcoholics have not been diagnosed, and even fewer are in treatment (44). This is true despite the fact that the elderly alcoholic is more likely than a younger alcoholic to have seen a physician recently.

The diagnosis of alcoholism can be more difficult in the elderly because they are less likely to face job loss, legal problems, marital problems, or fear of premature death. However, any change in functional status can be an important clue. The CAGE questionnaire, discussed previously, has been validated in a cohort of 323 elderly patients in an outpatient medical practice of an urban university teaching hospital. The sensitivity and specificity were 86% and 78%, respectively, for a score of 1 and 70% and 91%, respectively, for a score of 2. In this population, scores of 2, 3, and 4 yielded positive predictive values of 79%, 82%, and 94%, respectively (45). The CAGE may not be effective in detecting elderly binge drinkers who are at high risk of falling (46). As an adjunct, a geriatric version of the MAST has been developed (Table 28.10) (47).

Older patients with alcoholism tend to fall into two groups: those with early onset and those with late onset. Two thirds of patients fall into the *early-onset group*. These are patients who have had ongoing alcoholism but may have avoided some of the usual sequelae. They are often hidden, functional alcoholics who, as they lose mobility or cognitive abilities, become unable to function normally. The *late-onset patients* are likely to have had a recent stressor (i.e., loss of spouse, retirement, a new impairment in activities of daily living). Occasionally, late-onset alcoholism occurs in a previous teetotaler (48). Compared with younger alcoholic patients, the elderly are more likely to be separated, divorced, or widowed and are more likely to live alone.

Older people are more sensitive to the acute effects of alcohol, with amplification of preexisting deficits. Dysphoria predominates over euphoria. In addition, there is more likely to be interaction with prescribed drugs.

Once an older patient is confronted and agrees to treatment, there are some aspects of treatment specific to the elderly. The elderly patient who experiences significant alcohol withdrawal is best monitored in an inpatient setting. For patients with mild withdrawal treated at home, family or friends should stay with the patient for at least the first week of abstinence. In addition, home health care, if available, should be considered (see Chapter 9). Once the patient is medically stable, treatment toward continued abstinence should be initiated. Treatment must be specifically tailored for the elderly. Because of decreased mobility and an inability to drive, patients may find AA meetings more difficult to reach. Meetings during the day must be found for elderly patients who are afraid to go out

Table 28.10. Michigan Alcohol Screening Test—Geriatric Version (MAST-G)[a]

		Yes	No
1. After drinking have you ever noticed an increase in your heart rate or beating in your chest?	1.	(1)	(0)
2. When talking with others, do you ever underestimate how much you actually drink?	2.		
3. Does alcohol make you sleepy so that you often fall asleep in your chair?	3.		
4. After a few drinks, have you sometimes not eaten or been able to skip a meal because you didn't feel hungry?	4.		
5. Does having a few drinks help decrease your shakiness or tremors?	5.		
6. Does alcohol sometimes make it hard for you to remember parts of the day or night?	6.		
7. Do you have rules for yourself that you won't drink before a certain time of the day?	7.		
8. Have you lost interest in hobbies or activities you used to enjoy?	8.		
9. When you wake up in the morning, do you ever have trouble remembering part of the night before?	9.		
10. Does having a drink help you sleep?	10.		
11. Do you hide your alcohol bottles from family members?	11.		
12. After a social gathering, have you ever felt embarrassed because you drank too much?	12.		
13. Have you ever been concerned that drinking might be harmful to your health?	13.		
14. Do you like to end an evening with a night cap?	14.		
15. Did you find your drinking increased after someone close to you died?	15.		
16. In general, would you prefer to have a few drinks at home rather than go out to social events?	16.		
17. Are you drinking more now than in the past?	17.		
18. Do you usually take a drink to relax or calm your nerves?	18.		
19. Do you drink to take your mind off your problems?	19.		
20. Have you ever increased your drinking after experiencing a loss in your life?	20.		
21. Do you sometimes drive when you have had too much to drink?	21.		
22. Has a doctor or nurse ever said they were worried or concerned about your drinking?	22.		
23. Have you ever made rules to manage your drinking?	23.		
24. When you feel lonely, does having a drink help?	24.		

[a]Scoring: 5 or more "yes" responses indicative of alcohol problem.

at night. The elderly tend to be more comfortable in smaller groups. These can often be found in meetings that run in a senior center. The senior center can also be a source of activities to fill the new void of free time formerly spent drinking.

Because older adults are often taking many medications and are more likely to have other chronic medical illnesses, disulfiram should generally be avoided. Many elderly alcoholics would benefit from a 30-day stay at an inpatient treatment center. Some centers have recovery programs specifically for the elderly alcoholic. Access to this type of treatment is usually related to insurance status and cost.

Alcoholism in Women

Alcoholism is more likely to go unrecognized in women than in men, yet suicide, trauma, and liver disease are more common in female than in male alcoholics (49–51). Women are also more likely to develop alcohol dependence after a lesser duration of drinking. An additional concern is the pregnancy-related complication of fetal alcohol syndrome, mentioned previously. Alcoholism decreases a woman's average life expectancy by 15 years (52). More than 50 case-controlled studies and 7 meta-analyses have shown a direct relationship between alcohol consumption and breast cancer (49,53).

Women tend to drink more subtly and covertly. In part, this is related to society's considering drinking in public, especially in a tavern or bar, less acceptable in women than in men. Women often drink at home. Women who are unmarried, divorced, or unemployed drink more. Alcoholic women are also more likely to have alcoholic spouses.

The techniques discussed previously should be used to screen, diagnose, and confront women with alcoholism. There are some particular obstacles to treatment. Women are more likely to need provision of child care while they are in treatment. In addition, alcoholic women tend to have less spousal support than alcoholic men do. There are treatment programs aimed specifically toward women, including women-only meetings of AA. Alcoholic women, who make up only about 30% of AA participants, should generally seek other women to be their sponsors.

The Impaired Physician or Other Professional

The prevalence among physicians of alcoholism and other chemical dependencies is probably similar to that for the general population (54). Each year, a substantial number of physicians are lost to the profession because of chemical dependence or other treatable illnesses, and many more practice despite being seriously troubled or impaired. Numerous professional organizations have implemented programs to address impairment in colleagues, including organizations of physicians, nurses, dentists, pharmacists, psychologists, social workers, lawyers, and others.

Definitions

Impaired professionals may be defined as those who are troubled by personal difficulties to the extent that they cannot (a) offer reasonable patient care, (b) effectively help others through interpersonal skills, or (c) maintain skills by continuing education. Impairment is also characterized by denial. Intervention with appropriate treatment as soon as alcoholism is recognized is a major goal of the impaired physician movement.

Recognition and Management

The manifestations, symptoms, or signs of impairment from alcoholism or other chemical dependence among professionals are the same as those seen in nonprofessionals. When one is concerned about impairment in a colleague, it is advisable to contact one or more close associates of that colleague to confirm the impairment. Likely reasons for the impairment may be uncovered by this discreet inquiry, and often alcoholism or another chemical dependency is the underlying problem. Persuasion of an impaired physician to accept the existence of a problem and agree to rehabilitation can be attempted by a concerned colleague. Such efforts are likely to be met with intense denial. A second approach is to use the state's physician rehabilitation committee. Each state medical society has a committee and maintains telephone access for confidential reporting of impaired physicians. Subcommittees undertake verification of the problem, followed by confrontation of the troubled physician, similar to the formal intervention technique described earlier in this chapter. The goal of this process is to rehabilitate the physician, usually through intensive treatment in a residential facility.

BRIEF INTERVENTION FOR NONDEPENDENT DRINKERS

Brief interventions are time-limited sessions provided by primary care providers that focus on *reducing alcohol use in the nondependent drinker.* Many targeted people may be in the early stages of alcoholism, having not yet lost control of their drinking. Brief interventions have been found to be effective in reducing alcohol consumption (or achieving treatment referral) of problem drinkers (55–57).

Brief intervention is a process of assessing alcohol use, giving feedback, contracting and goal setting, arriving at a strategy for behavior modification, and providing a plan for follow-up. There must be an emphasis on personal responsibility for change and clear advice to change. Therapeutic empathy describes the recommended counseling style. Typically, the goal of brief intervention is not abstinence. Therefore, patients must receive follow-up assessments to determine whether they are not just problem drinkers but are indeed alcoholics.

The approach to brief intervention parallels the approach previously mentioned for confronting the patient with alcoholism. *Six essential elements* should be included: (a) feedback of personal risk (patient-focused review of the evidence for existing or potential risk related to drinking), (b) emphasis on personal responsibility for change (empowering the patient to take control of the decision for change), (c) clear advice for change ("Based on all we have discussed, you need to make a change"), (d) offering a menu of alternative options ("Here's some ways you can make a change"), (e) therapeutic empathy as an innate part of the intervention ("I know this may be difficult"), and (f) enhancement of patient self-efficacy ("This is not hopeless; with change, things will get better for you"). Chapter 4 describes in detail the concepts that underlie these behavior modification techniques.

The brief intervention procedures used in studies vary, but none involve more than six contacts. No outside referrals are made, but written materials are often helpful. Typical follow-up sessions are usually 15 minutes long. Studies have shown reduction of alcohol consumption in problem drinkers by 10% to 35% at 1-year follow-up. Some showed an impact on drinking with just one interventional session. This further illustrates the importance of addressing alcohol use in all patients, even those who are not alcoholic, because problem drinking, independent of alcohol dependence, plays an enormous role in contributing to trauma, especially automobile accidents.

CO-ALCOHOLISM (CO-DEPENDENCE)

Co-alcoholism can be defined as ill health or maladaptive, problematic, or dysfunctional behavior that is associated with living with, working with, treating, or otherwise being close to a person with alcoholism. Co-alcoholism is a specific example of the more general phenomenon of codependence (i.e., suffering or dysfunction associated with or caused by focusing on the needs or behaviors of others). The long-term sequelae of one type of codependence—growing up in a family dominated by alcoholism or by other unhealthy or dysfunctional abnormal patterns—is described later in this chapter (see Adult Children of Dysfunctional Families).

Co-alcoholism affects not only individuals and families but also helping professionals, communities, businesses, other institutions, and even whole societies. Its signs and symptoms range from passive acceptance and absence of overt problems to the following range of manifestations:

In People Close to an Alcoholic

- Behaviors to protect the alcoholic (enabling)
- Behavioral or psychological symptoms, such as anxiety disorders, depression, insomnia, hyperactivity, aggression, anorexia nervosa, bulimia, or suicidal gestures

Table 28.11. Family Drinking Survey[a]

	Yes	No
1. Does someone in your family undergo personality changes when he or she drinks to excess?	1. ____	____
2. Do you feel that drinking is more important to this person than you are?	2. ____	____
3. Do you feel sorry for yourself and frequently indulge in self-pity because of what you feel alcohol is doing to your family?	3. ____	____
4. Has some family member's excessive drinking ruined special occasions?	4. ____	____
5. Do you find yourself covering up for the consequences of someone else's drinking?	5. ____	____
6. Have you ever felt guilty, apologetic, or responsible for the drinking of a member of your family?	6. ____	____
7. Does one of your family member's use of alcohol cause fights and arguments?	7. ____	____
8. Have you ever tried to fight the drinker by joining in the drinking?	8. ____	____
9. Do the drinking habits of some family members make you feel depressed or angry?	9. ____	____
10. Is your family having financial difficulties because of drinking?	10. ____	____
11. Did you ever feel like you had an unhappy home life because of the drinking of some members of your family?	11. ____	____
12. Have you ever tried to control the drinker's behavior by hiding the car keys, pouring liquor down the drain, etc.?	12. ____	____
13. Do you find yourself distracted from your responsibilities because of this person's drinking?	13. ____	____
14. Do you often worry about a family member's drinking?	14. ____	____
15. Are holidays more of a nightmare than a celebration because of a family member's drinking behavior?	15. ____	____
16. Are most of your drinking family member's friends heavy drinkers?	16. ____	____
17. Do you find it necessary to lie to employers, relatives, or friends in order to hide your spouse's drinking?	17. ____	____
18. Do you find yourself responding differently to members of your family when they are using alcohol?	18. ____	____
19. Have you ever been embarrassed or felt the need to apologize for the drinker's actions?	19. ____	____
20. Does some family member's use of alcohol make you fear for your own safety or the safety of other members of your family?	20. ____	____
21. Have you ever thought that one of your family members had a drinking problem?	21. ____	____
22. Have you ever lost sleep because of a family member's drinking?	22. ____	____
23. Have you ever encouraged one of your family members to stop or cut down on his or her drinking?	23. ____	____
24. Have you ever threatened to leave home or to leave a family member because of his or her drinking?	24. ____	____
25. Did a family member ever make promises that he or she did not keep because of drinking?	25. ____	____
26. Did you ever wish that you could talk to someone who could understand and help the alcohol-related problems of a family member?	26. ____	____
27. Have you ever felt sick, cried, or had a "knot" in your stomach after worring about a family member's drinking?	27. ____	____
28. Has a family member ever failed to remember what occurred during a drinking period?	28. ____	____
29. Does your family member avoid social situations where alcoholic beverages will *not* be served?	29. ____	____
30. Does your family member have periods of remorse after drinking occasions and apologize for his or her behavior?	30. ____	____
31. Please write any symptoms or medical or nervous problems that you have experienced since you have known your heavy drinker. (Write on back if more space is needed.)	31. ____	____

[a]If you answer "Yes" to any two of the above questions, there is a good possibility that someone in your family has a drinking problem.
If you answer "Yes" to four or more of the above questions, there is a definite indication that someone in your family *does* have a drinking problem.
These survey questions are modified or adapted from validated survey instruments such as the Children of Alcoholics Screening Test (CAST) and the Howard Family Questionnaire, and from the Family Alcohol Quiz from Al-Anon.

- Functional or psychosomatic illness
- Family violence or neglect
- Alcoholism or another chemical dependence

In Helping Professionals

- Failure to diagnose alcoholism
- Failure to treat alcoholism as a primary illness
- Treating the alcoholic with sedatives or tranquilizers
- Treating the co-alcoholic with sedatives or tranquilizers

In Society at Large

- Not confronting relatives, friends, and colleagues who are inappropriately intoxicated or are chronically abusing alcohol or drugs
- Placing a positive social value on those who drink
- Stigmatizing those who are alcoholics or those who do not drink

Co-Alcoholism in the Individual

The following is a typical case history of co-alcoholism in an individual.

A 38-year-old white, married woman presented with recurring episodes of upper abdominal pain of about 4 years' duration. During that time she had been evaluated by two internists and had been hospitalized once. After extensive evaluations, the working diagnosis was functional abdominal pain. She was treated with antispasmodics and sedatives but there was no substantial improvement. The pain occurred almost every day. On a follow-up visit 6 months later, the patient said that a friend had suggested that she attend the self-help group Al-Anon because her husband's drinking had been bothering her for at least 5 years. The patient reported that after she attended 12 Al-Anon meetings over 3 months, her abdominal pain gradually abated. On follow-up 2 years later, she had continued to attend Al-Anon and the symptoms had not recurred. In the meantime, the patient's husband had continued to drink.

This case study illustrates a common manifestation of co-alcoholism: a psychosomatic illness that resolved after the patient recognized an alcohol problem in the family and attended Al-Anon regularly.

Recognition and Treatment of the Co-alcoholic Patient

When a patient has unexplained somatic or psychological symptoms, it is helpful to ask whether the patient has ever been concerned about the drinking (or drug use) of anyone close to him or her. If the answer is *Yes,* the patient should be asked to describe the problem. If the patient is vague or doubtful, one can administer some or all of the questions in the *Family Drinking Survey* shown in Table 28.11. One can also ask the possible co-alcoholic to answer CAGE questions (Fig. 28.1) or the questions on the MAST (Table 28.3) as though they were addressed to, and answered honestly by, the potentially alcoholic person to whom he or she is close. A positive score on one of these is a strong indication of co-alcoholism.

Initially, the psychological and behavioral adjustments of the co-alcoholic are normal responses to an abnormal situation. However, these adaptive responses eventually lead to the person's becoming dysfunctional. Co-alcoholism, like alcoholism, is chronic and progressive; it is characterized by denial, ill health, and/or maladaptive behavior and by a lack of knowledge about alcoholism.

The major strategies in treating a patient with co-alcoholism are remarkably similar to those for treating the alcoholic:

- Have the patient accept that he or she is a co-alcoholic.
- Motivate the patient to get help (occasionally by using a coercive intervention, such as the formal intervention described previously).
- Refer the patient to Al-Anon or Alateen (as with AA referrals, enthusiasm for and a good understanding of the Al-Anon process [Table 28.12] on the part of the referring physician are critical to successful referral).
- Provide supportive psychotherapy at follow-up visits (see Chapter 20) and refer the patient or the family for additional therapy, especially group therapy for codependents or adult children of dysfunctional families (discussed later).
- Assist in the process of getting the alcoholics who are the source of the problem into treatment.

Co-alcoholism in the Helping Professions

Co-alcoholism includes behavior on the part of professionals that enables alcoholics to remain enmeshed in their disease. Enabling behavior often coexists with otherwise excellent clinical skills. The *Professional Enablers Screening Test* (Table 28.13) is useful for identifying the various ways in which enabling may occur in the context of medical practice. Societal norms (including one's own approach to the use of alcohol or other drugs), plus a lack of awareness of modern approaches to diagnosis, motivation, and treatment of the alcoholic, are probably the major reasons for co-alcoholism in helping professionals. Several steps are recommended for the professional who wishes to cease being an enabler:

- Update your knowledge of alcoholism.
- Attend some AA and Al-Anon meetings.

Table 28.12. The Al-Anon Process

Al-Anon began in the 1940s as an Alcoholics Anonymous (AA) auxiliary and initially called itself AA Family Groups. In 1952, the wives of the two founders of AA established Al-Anon.

Al-Anon is a fellowship of family members of alcoholics who meet together to share their experiences, strengths, and hopes so that they can achieve health and serenity. The organization is modeled after AA and uses the 12 Steps of AA (see Table 28.8) as its principles for individual recovery. Its focus is not on the alcoholic but on the family members; thus, it powerfully frees families from their dependence on the alcoholic.

Al-Anon meetings are all open to the public and often meet at the same time and location as AA meetings. In most communities, Al-Anon has a telephone listing where meeting information, help, and literature can be obtained. Where there is no local Al-Anon office, the AA office can provide Al-Anon information.

Al-Anon meetings generally last 1 hour and follow the format of AA meetings (see Table 28.8), but they are usually smaller and discussion of topics is often freer than in AA.

Al-Anon is the sponsor of Ala-Teen and Ala-Tots, which are organizations for teenage and young children of alcoholics, respectively. These groups follow the Al-Anon discussion format and in general are not open to the nonalcoholic public, but helping professionals are usually welcome if they request to attend ahead of time. In the last several years in some areas, Al-Anon members have begun groups for adult children of alcoholics. These groups offer help to adults who may no longer live with an alcoholic family member, but whose life continues to be adversely affected by the legacy of growing up in an alcoholic home. These are especially powerful, and many patients with this background can be profoundly helped.

Al-Anon publishes a number of pamphlets that are available at meetings for families. *Al-Anon Faces Alcoholism,* Al-Anon's "Big Book," describes the family's plight with alcoholism through a variety of stories that graphically describe how families become sick in response to the alcoholic. Its other major book, *Living with an Alcoholic,* offers practical suggestions for recovery.

More information can be obtained by writing Al-Anon Family Group Headquarters, Box 182, Madison Square Station, New York, NY 10010.

Table 28.13. Professional Enablers Screening Test[a]

Please check your answer to each question. For medically oriented questions, please check the space to which you would subscribe, even though you may not be a physician.

Question	Yes	No
1. Do you sometimes avoid raising sensitive issues related to drinking because it might offend your patient, or make him or her angry or feel bad?	(2)	
2. Do you generally treat the heavy-drinking person's problems without focusing most of the treatment on the drinking behavior?	(5)	
3. Do you avoid confronting your heavy-drinking patient when there is good evidence that he or she has misinformed you about his or her drinking?	(2)	
4. Do you generally suggest to your alcoholic patients that they cut down on their drinking?	(3)	
5. Do you believe what your heavy-drinking patient tells you about his or her drinking without using other sources such as a spouse, employer, screening test, blood alcohol test, or other laboratory test?	(5)	
6. Do you generally prescribe a sedative or minor transquilizer for the nervous conditions or sleep problems of your alcoholic patients?	(5)	
7. Do you refer most of your alcoholic patients to attend Alcoholics Anonymous meetings regularly?		(5)
8. Do you refer many of your alcoholic patients to an alcoholism therapy group?		(3)
9. Do you prescribe disulfiram (Antabuse) to many of your alcoholic patients?		(3)
10. When your alcoholic patient has a minor crisis requiring hospitalization, do you routinely hospitalize him or her in a community hospital general ward?	(5)	
11. Do you refer most of the spouses of family members of your alcoholic patients to attend Al-Anon meetings regularly?		(5)
12. Do you subscribe to the theory that most alcoholics have an underlying psychologic disorder that is the major cause of the alcoholism?	(5)	
13. Do you believe that most alcoholics will not respond positively to treatment for their alcoholism?	(5)	

[a]Numbers in parentheses are the scores recommended for the corresponding responses. A score of 0 to 3 points indicates a probable nonenabler, 4 to 6 points may indicate a possible enabler, 7 points or more indicates a probable enabler.

- In your own practice, try using skills such as those described in this chapter. The best cure for co-alcoholism in the physician is success in getting a number of alcoholics and their families into the recovery process.

DOMESTIC VIOLENCE

Domestic violence is present in all demographic and socioeconomic strata. It is especially prevalent in women whose partners abuse alcohol or other drugs and in women who themselves abuse substances. It is estimated that 75% of wives of alcoholics have been threatened and 45% have been assaulted by their alcoholic partners (58). *Domestic violence has been defined* by the American Medical Association (see General References) as an ongoing debilitating experience of physical, psychological, or sexual abuse in the home, associated with increased isolation from the outside world and limited personal freedom and accessibility to resources.

In the United States, it is estimated that 2 million women are victims of domestic violence each year and that more than 12 million will be abused at some time during their lives. Most of these women never seek help from health care providers for the consequences of domestic violence. However, studies demonstrate a relationship between domestic violence and medical and psychiatric illness.

Brief screening for domestic violence should be incorporated into the medical interview of all women. Because some women may not initially recognize themselves as victims of domestic violence, questioning should be specific (Table 28.14). The issue should be dealt with sensitively, validating the difficulty most women have in discussing the issue. The patient may be reluctant to disclose information because of shame, humiliation, low self-esteem, or fear of retaliation by the perpetrator. Some women may also believe that they deserve the abuse and do not deserve help or that they need to protect their partner, who is often their only source of affection and support. There may also be a belief on the part of the victim that the medical provider will not understand the problem or will not believe her.

Table 28.14. A Recommended Approach to the Use of Interviewing to Screen Patients for Domestic Violence

Integrating domestic violence inquiry into interview as part of social history:

"Because abuse and violence have unfortunately become a common part of a woman's life, I ask all my patients about it routinely."

We all occasionally fight at home. What happens when you and your partner disagree?

Have you ever been treated badly or threatened by your partner?

Has your partner ever prevented you from leaving the house, seeing friends, getting a job, or continuing your education?

Does your partner ever force you to have sex or force you to engage in sex that is uncomfortable to you?

(if appropriate) You mentioned your partner drinks (uses drugs). How does he (or she) act when he is drinking (using drugs)?

In addition to screening, certain patient problems should alert the practitioner to the possibility of domestic violence (Table 28.15). Problems may range from direct evidence of physical trauma (contusions, abrasions, broken bones) to nonspecific complaints of fatigue and difficulty concentrating. The screening

Table 28.15. Clinical Signs and Symptoms Suggestive of Domestic Violence

Alcohol or drug abuse
Anxiety
Atypical chest pain
Change in appetite
Chronic headaches
Chronic pain of unclear etiology
Depressed mood
Difficulty concentrating
Dizziness
Fatigue
Frequent evidence of minor trauma
Frequent requests for pain medications or tranquilizers
Frequent visits with vague somatic complaints
Gastrointestinal upset, diarrhea, or dyspepsia
Insomnia
Palpitations
Panic attacks
Paresthesias
Pelvic pain
Suicide attempts or gestures

information and medical history related to domestic violence must be well documented in the medical record, because they provide evidence that may be used in a legal case. The record should include detailed descriptions of any injuries and, if possible, photographs of injuries sustained.

Once evidence of abuse is obtained, one must validate the seriousness of the situation to the patient. This must occur even if the patient is not yet ready to leave the abusive spouse. In addition, the immediate safety of the woman should be assessed. Unfortunately, the level of severity of past violence may not be a predictor of the severity of future violence. If safety is in question, the woman (and her children) should be advised to stay with family or friends, or at a shelter that specializes in caring for abused women and their families. Medical attention may also be needed for abused children in the household.

Often, the patient resists taking action. One should continue to show concern and work to motivate the patient toward change. Once the patient has agreed to take action, local community resources that can provide support, safety, and advocacy must be accessed. The *National Domestic Violence Hotline* (1-800-799-SAFE) is a 24-hour service that helps women find a safe place to stay in their community. At times, psychiatric or substance abuse referral may also be appropriate.

General References*

Alcoholics Anonymous. The story of how many thousands of men and women have recovered from alcoholism ("The Big Book"). 3rd ed. New York: Alcoholics Anonymous World Services, 1976.

The nature of alcoholism and the recovery process using AA are illustrated in a large number of personal stories.

American Medical Association. **Diagnostic and treatment guidelines on domestic violence.** Chicago: American Medical Association, 1992.

An excellent brief monograph written for clinicians.

Barnes HN, Aronson MD, Delbanco TL, eds. Alcoholism: a guide for the primary care physician. New York: Springer-Verlag, 1987.

An excellent guide for clinicians.

Bean MH, Zinberg NE, eds. Dynamic approaches to the understanding and treatment of alcoholism. New York: Free Press, 1981.

Detailed description of the denial process and other psychodynamic aspects of the alcoholic's behavior.

Drews T. Getting them sober: a guide for those who live with an alcoholic. Plainfield, NJ: Haven Books, 1980.

Widely available paperback for families of alcoholics; quick reading. Advice regarding numerous practical issues.

Fiellin DA, Reid MC. O'Connor PG. Outpatient management of patients with alcohol problems. Ann Intern Med 2000;133:815.

A thorough recent review of outpatient care for alcohol-related problems.

Gorski TT, Miller M. Staying sober: a guide for relapse prevention. Independence, MO: Independence Press, 1986.

A book that describes in detail the relapse process and how to deal with it. An excellent resource for recovering alcoholic patients.

Jellinek EM. The disease concept of alcoholism. New Haven: College and University Press, 1960.

Landmark monograph reviewing the history of the disease concept.

O'Connor PG, Schottenfeld RS. Patients with alcohol problems. N Engl J Med 1998;338:592.

Well-referenced update on the full spectrum of problems associated with alcohol, focusing on the needs of the generalists.

Rogers RL, McMillin CS, eds. Don't help: a positive guide to working with the alcoholic. New York: Bantam, 1989.

Practical account of techniques for group or individual counseling that, in conjunction with AA, are often effective in long-term treatment of alcoholism.

Specific References

1. Secretary of Health and Human Services. Tenth special report to the U.S. Congress on alcohol and health. Washington, DC: US Department of Health and Human Services, June 2000.
2. Morse RM, Flavin DK. The definition of alcoholism. JAMA 1992;268:1012.
3. American Psychiatric Association. Diagnostic and statistical manual of mental disorders. 4th ed. (DSM-IV). Washington, DC: American Psychiatric Association, 1994.
4. Jellinek EM. Phases of alcohol addiction. Q J Stud Alcohol 1952;13:673.
5. Vaillant GE, ed. The natural history of alcoholism, revisited. Cambridge, MA: Harvard University Press, 1996.
6. Blum K, Noble EP, Sheridan PJ, et al. Allelic association of human dopamine D2 receptor gene in alcoholism. JAMA 1990;263:2055.
7. Conneally PM. Association between the D_2 dopamine receptor gene and alcoholism: a continuing controversy. Arch Gen Psychiatry 1991;48:664.
8. Klatsky AL, Armstrong MA, Friedman GD. Alcohol and mortality. Ann Intern Med 1992;117:646.
9. Hurt RD, Offord KP, Croghan IT, et al. Mortality following inpatient addictions treatment: role of tobacco use in a community-based cohort. JAMA 1996;275:1097.
10. Bullock KD, Reed RJ, Grant I. Reduced mortality risk in alcoholics who achieve long-term abstinence. JAMA 1992;267:668.
11. Fine E. Philadelphia DWI study. U S J Alcohol Drug Abuse 1983;19.
12. Johnson B, Clark W. Alcoholism: a challenging physician—patient encounter. J Gen Intern Med 1989;4:445.
13. Ewing JA. Detecting alcoholism: the CAGE questionnaire. JAMA 1984;252:1905.
14. Cyr MG, Wartman SA. The effectiveness of routine screening questions in the detection of alcoholism. JAMA 1988;259:51.
15. Powers JS, Spickard A. Michigan Alcoholism Screening Test to diagnose early alcoholism in a general practice. South Med J 1984;77:852.
16. Bush K, Kivlahan DR, McDonell MB, et al. The AUDIT alcohol consumption questions (AUDIT-C): an effective brief screening test for problem drinking. Arch Intern Med 1998;158:1789.

*Bold print (general references) and bold numerals (specific references) denote published controlled clinical trials, meta-analyses, or consensus-based recommendations.

17. Saunders JB. Development of the Alcohol Use Disorders Identification Test (AUDIT). Addiction 1993;88:791.
18. O'Connor, Patrick G, Schottenfeld, et al. Medical progress: patients with alcohol problems. N Engl J Med 1998;338:592.
19. Beresford TP, Blow FC, Hill E, et al. Comparison of CAGE questionnaire and computer-assisted laboratory profiles in screening for covert alcoholism. Lancet 1990;336:482.
20. Huseby NE, Nilssen O, Erfurth A et al. Carbohydrate-deficient transferrin and alcohol dependency: variation in response to alcohol intake among different groups of patients. Alcohol Clin Exp Res 1997;21:201.
21. Samet JH, Rollnick S, Barnes H. Beyond CAGE: a brief clinical approach after detection of substance abuse. Arch Intern Med 1996;56:2287.
22. Prochaska JO, DiClemente CC. Toward a comprehensive model of change. In: Miller WR, Heather N, eds. Treating addictive behaviors: process of change. New York: Plenum, 1986.
23. Hayashida M, Alterman AI, McLellan T, et al. Comparative effectiveness and costs of inpatient and outpatient detoxification of patients with mild-to-moderate alcohol withdrawal syndrome. N Engl J Med 1989;320:358.
24. Turner RC, Lichstein PR, Peden JG Jr, et al. Alcohol withdrawal syndromes: a review of pathophysiology, clinical presentation, and treatment. J Gen Intern Med 1989;4:432.
25. Victor M, Hope JM. The phenomenon of auditory hallucinations in chronic alcoholism. J Nerv Ment Dis 1958;126:451.
26. Saunders JB. Delirium tremens: its aetiology, natural history and treatment. Curr Opin Psych 2000;13:629.
27. Sullivan JT, Sykora K, Schneiderman J, et al. Assessment of alcohol withdrawal: the revised clinical institute withdrawal assessment for alcohol scale (CIWA-Ar). Br J Addict 1989;84:1353.
28. Mayo-Smith MF, for the American Society of Addiction Medicine Workshop Group on Pharmacologic Management of Alcohol Withdrawal. Pharmacologic management of alcohol withdrawal: a meta-analysis and evidence-based medicine practice guideline. JAMA 1997;278:144.
29. Saitz R, Mayo-Smith MF, Roberts MS, et al. Individualized treatment for alcohol withdrawal: a randomized double-blind controlled trial. JAMA 1994;272:519.
30. Whitfield CL, Thompson G, Lamb A, et al. Detoxification of 1,024 alcoholics without psychoactive drugs. JAMA 1978;239:1409.
31. Sampliner R, Iber F. Diphenylhydantoin control of alcohol withdrawal seizures. JAMA 1974;230:1430.
32. Alldredge BK, Lowenstein DH, Simon RP. Placebo-controlled trial of intravenous diphenylhydantoin for short-term treatment of alcohol withdrawal seizures. Am J Med 1989;87:645.
33. Sellers EM, Naranjo CA, Harrison M, et al. Diazepam loading: simplified treatment of alcohol withdrawal. Clin Pharmacol Ther 1983; :822.
34. Ng SK, Hauser WA, Brust JC, et al. Alcohol consumption and withdrawal in new-onset seizures. N Engl J Med 1988;319:666.
35. Hoffman NG, Harrison PA, Belille CA. Alcoholics Anonymous after treatment: attendance and abstinence. Int J Addict 1983;18:311.
36. American College of Physicians. Disulfiram treatment of alcoholism. Ann Intern Med 1989;111:943.
37. Garbutt JC, West SL, Carey TS, et al. Pharmacologic treatment of alcohol dependence. JAMA 1999;281:1318.
38. Swift RM.. Drug therapy: drug therapy for alcohol dependence. N Engl J Med 1999;340:1482.
39. Wright C, Moore RD. Disulfiram treatment of alcoholism. Am J Med 1990;88:647.
40. Fiellin DA. Reid MC, O'Connor PG. New therapies for alcohol problems: application to primary care. Am J Med 2000;108:227.
41. O'Connor PG, Farren CK, Rousanville BJ, et al. A preliminary investigation of the management of alcohol dependence with naltrexone by primary care providers. Am J Med 1997;103:477.
42. Volpicelli JR, Alterman AI, Hayashida M, et al. Naltrexone in the treatment of alcohol dependence. Arch Gen Psychiatry 1992;49:876.
43. Walsh DC, Hingson RW, Merrigan DM, et al. A randomized trial of treatment options for alcohol abusing workers. N Engl J Med 1991;325:775.
44. Reid MC, Tinetti ME, Brown CJ, et al. Physician awareness of alcohol use disorders among older patients. J Gen Intern Med 1998;13:729.
45. Buchsbaum DG, Buchanan RG, Welsh J, et al. Screening for drinking disorders in the elderly using the CAGE questionnaire. J Am Geriatr Soc 1992;40:662.
46. Adams WL, Barry KL, Fleming MF. Screening for problem drinking in older primary care patients. JAMA 1996;276: 1964.
47. Blow FC, Brower KJ, Schulenberg JE, et al. The Michigan Alcoholism Screening Test—Geriatric version (MAST-G): a new elderly-specific screening instrument. Alcohol Clin Exp Res 1992;16:372.
48. Atkinson RM, Tolson RL, Turner JA. Late versus early onset problem drinking in older men. Alcohol Clin Exp Res 1990;14:574.
49. Bradley KA, Badrinath S, Bush K, et al. Medical risks for women who drink alcohol. J Gen Intern Med 1998;3:627.
50. Gore-Gearhart J, Beebe DK, Milhorn HT, et al. Alcoholism in women. Am Fam Physician 1991;44:907.
51. Wilsnack SC, Wilsnack RW. Epidemiology of women's drinking. J Subst Abuse Treat 1991;3:133.
52. Roman PM. Biological features of women's alcohol use: a review. Public Health Rep 1988;103:628.
53. Smith-Warner SA, Spiegelman D, Yaun S, et al. Alcohol and breast cancer in women: a pooled analysis of cohort studies. JAMA 1998;279:535.
54. Moore RD, Mead L, Pearson TA. Youthful precursors of alcohol abuse in physicians. Am J Med 1990;88:332.
55. Bien TH, Miller WR, Tonigan JS. Brief interventions for alcohol problems: a review. Addiction 1993;88:315.
56. Fleming MF, Barry KL, Manwell LB, et al. Brief physician advice for problem alcohol drinkers: a randomized controlled trial in community-based primary care practices. JAMA 1997;277:1039.
57. Wilk AI, Jensen NM, Havighurst TC. Meta-analysis of randomized control trials addressing brief interventions in heavy alcohol drinkers. J Gen Intern Med 1997;12:274.
58. Eisenstat, Stephanie A. Bancroft, Lundy. Primary care: domestic violence. N Eng J Med 1999;341:886.

CHAPTER 29

Illicit and Therapeutic Use of Drugs With Abuse Liability

MICHAEL I. FINGERHOOD, MD

DEFINITIONS

Drugs with abuse liability modify mood, feeling, thinking, and perception. Many are commonly prescribed and are useful therapeutic agents. The use and abuse of such substances date back thousands of years. Plant alkaloids, alcohol, and an ever-increasing array of newly synthesized chemicals have also been used in illicit endeavors. Patterns of use and the social acceptance of use of these agents have differed from time to time and from place to place. Successive generations of the same society have held discordant views about which substance to use, at what age, in what amount, and under which circumstances (e.g., attitudes regarding alcohol use in the preprohibition and postprohibition eras in the United States). Neighboring cultures have also differed about the sanctioned use of psychoactive substances. In 20th-century Western society, there are two forms of less problematic use of illicit substances (experimental and social–recreational) and two defined patterns of abnormal use (substance abuse and substance dependence).

Experimental Use

The experimental use of illicit substances is sporadic; the initial trial and experience usually are associated with youthful rites of passage. These experiments usually have little impact on mental health. They are potentially dangerous because of possible dosage errors, because unsterile methods of exposure may occur, because of behaviors that may endanger the user or other people, and because some people may find the drug experience extraordinarily rewarding, leading to repeated use. Incorrect labeling of such drugs (a common problem) increases the risk of these untoward consequences.

Social–Recreational Use

The social and recreational use of illicit substances suggests that they have been used repetitively but that control has been exerted over the dosage and the time of use. The risks of unintended overdosage, improper exposure, and mislabeling are increased by the frequency of use. Recreational use often is not psychologically disabling even though adverse consequences may occur. Adequate social and behavioral function is maintained. Most American use of alcohol and marijuana conforms to this pattern of social–recreational use.

Substance Abuse and Substance Dependence

The 1994 version of the *Diagnostic and Statistical Manual of the American Psychiatric Association* (DSM-IV) delineates two diagnostic categories for substance-related disorders (1). The diagnostic criteria are the same for all psychoactive substances, including alcohol.

The Diagnostic and Statistical Manual, 4th edition, Criteria for Substance Abuse

A. A maladaptive pattern of substance use leading to clinically significant impairment or distress, as manifested by one or more of the following occurring at any time during the same 12-month period:
   1. Recurrent substance use resulting in a failure to fulfill major role obligations at work, school, or home (e.g., repeated absences or poor work performance related to substance use; substance-related absences, suspensions, or expulsions from school; neglect of children or household).
   2. Recurrent substance use in situations in which it is physically hazardous (e.g., driving an automobile or operating a machine when impaired by substance use).
   3. Recurrent substance-related legal problems (e.g., arrests for substance-related disorderly conduct).
   4. Continued substance use despite having persistent or recurrent social or interpersonal problems caused or exacerbated by the effects of the substance (e.g., arguments with spouse about consequences of intoxication, physical fights).

B. Has never met the criteria for substance dependence for this class of substance.

The Diagnostic and Statistical Manual, 4th edition, Criteria for Substance Dependence

A maladaptive pattern of substance use, leading to clinically significant impairment or distress, as manifested by *three or more of the following* occurring at any time in the same 12-month period:

1. Tolerance, as defined by either of the following:
   a. Need for markedly increased amounts of the substance to achieve intoxication or desired effect;
   b. Markedly diminished effect with continued use of the same amount of the substance.
2. Withdrawal, as manifested by either of the following:
   a. The characteristic withdrawal syndrome for substance (refer to the criteria sets for withdrawal from the specific substances);
   b. The same (or closely related) substance is taken to relieve or avoid withdrawal symptoms.
3. The substance is often taken in larger amounts or over a longer period than was intended.
4. There is a persistent desire or unsuccessful efforts to cut down or control substance use.
5. A great deal of time is spent in activities necessary to obtain the substance (e.g., visiting multiple doctors or driving long distances), use the substance (e.g., chain smoking), or recover from its effects.
6. Important social, occupational, or recreational activities are given up or reduced because of substance use.
7. Continued substance use despite knowledge of having had a persistent or recurrent physical or psychologic problem that was likely to have been caused or exacerbated by the substance.

Table 29.1. Categories of Psychoactive Drugs

CNS depressants
Alcohol
Sedative-hypnotics
Benzodiazepines
Barbiturates
Other—meprobromate (Equanil or Miltown), glutethimide, methaqualone (Quaalude)
Inhalants
Nitrous oxide, toluene, volatile hydrocarbons
Opioids
Morphine, hydromorphone (Dilaudid), heroin, oxycodone, meperidine (Demerol), codeine, methadone
Stimulants
Cocaine, amphetamine, methylphenidate (Ritalin), MDMA (Ectstasy), caffeine, nicotine, arecoline, phenmetrazine (Preludin)
Drugs that alter perception (including hallucinogens)
Marijuana, LSD, dimethyltryptamine, psilocybin, mescaline, PCP, MDMA, GHB, belladonna alkaloids (atropine, scopolamine)

CNS, central nervous system; MDMA, methylenedioxymethamphetamine; LSD, lysergic acid diethylamide; PCP, phencyclidine; GHB, gamma hydroxybutyrate.

Classification by Pharmacologic Effect

Later sections of this chapter describe the manifestations and the principles of management for selected substances of abuse common in the United States today (Chapters 27 and 28 describe tobacco and alcohol abuse/dependence, respectively). A list of all drugs that have abuse potential would be extremely long. However, it is possible to group the various substances into broad classes, the members of which share common characteristics and are readily distinguishable from other classes (Table 29.1). Psychoactive substances may thus be generally classified as depressants, opioids, stimulants, and drugs that alter perception (including hallucinogens).

Tolerance and Physical Dependence

Most drugs of abuse share the capacity to induce tolerance. *Tolerance* is defined as the phenomenon whereby with repeated use an increased amount of drug is required to produce a given effect. Alternatively, the same amount of drug produces a lesser effect with repeated administration. The time required for the induction of tolerance ranges from days after repeated intravenous or intramuscular administration of opioids to weeks or months after repeated oral administration of opioids, barbiturates, alcohol, and other sedatives.

Physical dependence is defined as the phenomenon whereby abrupt cessation of a drug results in withdrawal symptoms and signs (the abstinence state). Withdrawal symptoms and signs are often the opposite of the biologic effects exerted by the drug in question (Table 29.2). Physical dependence is not synonymous with addiction. People who are prescribed benzodiazepines may exhibit physical dependence

Table 29.2. Characteristics of Dependence on Drugs of Abuse

Drug	Physiologic Effect	Withdrawal Symptoms and Signs (1–7 Days After Last Dose)	
Opioids	Pupillary constriction Analgesia Constipation Respiratory depression	Pupillary dilation Myalgia Diarrhea Stimulation of respiratory centers ("yawning") Rhinorrhea Gooseflesh Nausea and vomiting Restlessness	
Alcohol, barbiturate, benzodiazepines	Induction of sleep (hypnosis) Sedation Alcohol usually decreases but may increase seizure activity (other sedatives decrease seizure activity)	Insomnia Nausea Tremulousness Anxiety Irritability Autonomic hyperactivity (sweats, tachycardia, hypertension) Delirium Seizures Death (alcohol and barbiturates)	Minor symptoms Onset 24–72 hr after last dose Duration 72–96 hr after last dose Major symptoms Onset 72 hr to 1 wk after last dose Duration up to 2 wk after last dose
Cocaine	Pupillary dilation Tachycardia Hypertension	Bradycardia Hyperphagia Fatigue Hypersomnolence	

(sometimes called therapeutic dependence) but do not fulfill criteria for substance dependence (see DSM-IV criteria above). Similarly, many people exhibit a withdrawal syndrome for caffeine but also do not fulfill criteria for substance dependence.

PRIMARY CARE PRACTITIONER'S ROLE

Background

Since the 1920s, with the exception of small numbers of psychiatrists and substance abuse specialists from other disciplines, practitioners in the United States have been reluctant to become involved in problems of substance abuse and dependence. This is understandable because, since the passage of the Harrison Narcotic Act in 1914, laws prohibit opioid maintenance prescribing. From 1920 to 1940, some physicians, nurses, and pharmacists who persisted in regarding narcotic addiction as a medical problem and in prescribing or dispensing narcotics in violation of the Harrison Act were prosecuted and imprisoned. This campaign led to avoidance of the problems of addiction by physicians and other health care providers. Providers are still reluctant to become involved in problems with addiction because of a lack of knowledge of how to deal with these patients, their own attitudes toward substance abuse, and the understandable response to the difficult behaviors these patients often exhibit. In recent years, substance abuse has been recognized as the major cause of much of the morbidity seen in medical practice—usually a mix of physical, mental, and social consequences—and the responsibility of primary care practitioners to care for the patient with substance abuse has been emphasized. This role may be further expanded with recent federal legislation to allow primary care practitioners to prescribe buprenorphine as opioid replacement therapy.

Specific Roles

For the patient with substance abuse, the role of the primary care practitioner is recognition of the problem, motivation of the patient to accept treatment (see Chapter 4), referral to a treatment program, ongoing care for the patient's other medical problems, and continued motivation to remain in recovery. By prescribing controlled substances wisely, the primary care practitioner can also play an important role in preventing prescription drug abuse.

Recognition/Diagnosis

Discovery of a substance abuse problem starts with a suspicion of the diagnosis if signs, symptoms, and elements of the history suggest the possibility, even in the most unlikely subjects. People from all walks of life abuse drugs. The stereotype of the drug abuser is of a young antisocial male of unkempt appearance who uses drugs for their euphoric effect. Although this is often the case, the abuse of illicit drugs such as marijuana and cocaine also occurs commonly among middle and upper class Americans, and the misuse and abuse of prescription analgesics and anxiolytics by people who are in the mainstream of American society have been recognized for many years. Patients with chronic anxiety, insomnia, or pain are at risk of abusing medications used to treat those conditions. In some instances, escalated use (and sometimes abuse) develops not because the patient is primarily seeking drug-induced euphoria or intoxication but because the tolerance that develops during continued use leads the patient to increase the dosage to inappropriate levels. Elderly patients are at particular risk because they are more likely to be given medications. Changes in the pharmacokinetics of drugs secondary to the aging process also make the elderly more vulnerable to normally prescribed dosages.

Advice on history taking includes the following: do not use the label *addict,* ask questions about drug use in the context of general medical history, develop a nonjudgmental approach, use direct questions, learn to recognize qualified answers, be persistent and friendly, and do not discuss rationalizations. It is often helpful to obtain information from a family member or close friend, with the patient's consent.

Interviewing techniques helpful in screening for alcoholism and motivating the alcoholic to accept treatment are described in Chapter 28. Techniques such as the CAGE questionnaire, as shown in Fig. 28.1, can be adapted to screen patients for the abuse of other drugs and substances.

Urine Testing

Urine testing to establish drug abuse seems a tempting and objective means of cutting through the problems of denial, unreliable histories, and the less than clear-cut signs and symptoms presented to arrive at a diagnosis. In the primary care practitioner's office, however, testing for drug abuse can prove problematic. The patient already knows whether he or she is abusing drugs. The question is whether the patient is willing to share that information with the family or practitioner.

The testing requires informed voluntary consent of any person 18 years of age or older, except in true emergencies. Faced with this requirement, laboratory testing yields no more information than the patient is willing to provide by history. Testing at the request of an employer or school authority, in particular, is fraught with ethical questions. Nevertheless, many employers now require drug testing (which is legal). This often provides evidence of illicit drug use that the patient is not willing to share.

There are problems of sensitivity and specificity in using urine screening tests to identify drug abusers. False negative results occur because of deception in collection and insensitive testing. False positive results occur because of innocent confounding substances, errors in processing samples, and the normal frequency of testing error. Experimental, social, and recreational use of illicit substances is so widely practiced that a positive test by no means establishes abuse or dependency. It also does not provide evidence of intoxication or impairment. Furthermore, prescribed drug use such as a benzodiazepine for anxiety or codeine for pain leads to positive urine tests.

The testing of minors under the age of 18, which theoretically can be authorized by parents and legal guardians regardless of the wishes of the patient, raises issues of patient trust, ethics, and legality if contested. Possible drug use can be explored most productively in the context of the total family relationship, without the referring practitioner appearing to have to take sides.

In most instances, testing should be performed by the consulting specialist or treatment program. Avoiding urine testing in the primary care setting also helps facilitate the doctor–patient relationship. It is hoped that people who relapse will be open and honest and will be more likely to show up for medical visits if they do not have to worry about urine testing.

Prescribing Controlled Drugs

Prescription drug abuse can be best avoided by careful and thoughtful prescribing of medications. Office-based practitioners prescribe large amounts of controlled drugs. A summary description of the various schedules under the Controlled Substances Act is shown in Table 29.3. When prescribing these drugs, it is important to realize that chronic pain, anxiety, and insomnia treated with controlled drugs on a long-term basis will result in physiologic dependence.

Practitioners must be vigilant to avoid being "duped," acquiescing to patient demands by prescribing inappropriately. To avoid possible abuse, medications with abuse liability should be prescribed on a fixed schedule. This strategy improves control of symptoms, minimizes the development of symptoms (rather than reacting to symptoms after they occur), and avoids patient focus on immediate relief. Medications should be prescribed for short periods during treatment of acute problems. Patients should be seen

Table 29.3. Controlled Substances Act

The Controlled Substances Act (Title II of the Federal Comprehensive Drug Abuse Prevention and Control Act of 1970) is designed to improve regulation of the manufacturing, distribution, and dispensing of controlled substances by providing a "closed" system for legitimate handlers of these drugs. If not specifically exempted, every person who manufactures, distributes, *prescribes,* administers, or dispenses any controlled substance must register annually with the Attorney General. Accurate records of drugs purchased, distributed, and dispensed must be maintained and kept on file for 2 years by all persons who regularly dispense and charge for controlled substances in the course of their practice.

Each drug or substance subject to control is assigned to one of five schedules depending on the potential for abuse, medical usefulness, and degree of dependence if abused. The five schedules and the drugs included in them follow:

Schedule I: Drugs and other substances having a high potential for abuse and no current accepted medical usefulness. Included are certain opium derivatives (e.g., *heroin*), some synthetic opioids (e.g., α-methylfentanyl), and hallucinogens (e.g., LSD).

Schedule II: Drugs having a high potential for abuse and accepted medical usefulness; abuse leads to severe psychologic or physical dependence. In general, drugs in this schedule were previously controlled under the Narcotic Acts (e.g., opium and derivatives, other *opioids, cocaine*). Stimulants, such as amphetamine and related compounds, and the short-acting *barbiturates* also are in this schedule.

Schedule III: Drugs having less abuse potential and accepted medical usefulness; abuse leads to moderate dependence. Included in this schedule are certain stimulants and depressants (e.g., barbiturates not included in other schedules), as well as preparations containing *limited quantities of certain opioid drugs.*

Schedule IV: Drugs having a low abuse potential, accepted medical usefulness, and limited dependence. Included in this schedule are certain depressants not in another schedule (e.g., chloral hydrate, phenobarbital, the *benzodiazepines*).

Schedule V: Drugs, including a few *over-the-counter preparations,* having a low abuse potential, accepted medical usefulness, and limited dependence. Mixtures containing limited quantities of opioids with nonopioid drugs are included in this schedule. (e.g., buprenorphine, pediatric narcotic suspensions).

Table 29.4. Generally Inappropriate Prescribing Practices

Combinations of scheduled drugs
Two prescriptions for the same scheduled drug filled on the same or consecutive days
Regular prescriptions of "preferred" drugs of abuse
Prescribing for two or more family members of a family the same drug or combination of scheduled drugs
Multiple scheduled drugs for the same purpose
Prescribing scheduled drugs to family members
Prescription of scheduled drugs from two or more practitioners simultaneously

for reassessment at frequent intervals and telephone refills should be avoided.

There is a definite risk of theft of prescription blanks or alteration of a prescription. All prescription pads should be safeguarded and, ideally, marked "not for scheduled drugs." Prescription blanks for scheduled drugs should be kept locked separately. Prescriptions should be written clearly, and the number of pills to be dispensed and the number of refills should be written out (not just a number). If no refills are to be given, "no refill" should be noted. All prescribing of scheduled drugs should be documented clearly in the chart.

Practitioners should be suspicious of patients who lose prescriptions or medications; obtain prescriptions from multiple practitioners; run out of medication before the time that would be expected; demand one specific drug as the only one that will work; have a sudden deterioration in work, school, or relationships; have a history of substance abuse; have a history of violent behavior; and have slurred speech or unexplained cognitive impairment. Prescribing practices that may be illegal, dangerous, or inappropriate or indicate drug abuse are listed in Table 29.4.

Two classes of controlled drugs, benzodiazepines and narcotics, are the most commonly abused prescription drugs (2). Long-term use of these drugs is sometimes appropriate (see Chapter 22 and Chronic Pain Management, below). However, intermittent use is required to avoid physical dependence. Nonpharmacologic modalities should always be used to increase the interval between doses, decrease the required dosage, and permit intermittent use of these drugs if possible.

Nonscheduled drugs with abuse liability include muscle relaxants, clonidine, and antiemetics. Clonidine, prescribed for hypertension, commonly finds its way onto the streets, where it is sold to opiate addicts to alleviate opiate withdrawal. Muscle relaxants are abused commonly as sleeping pills.

SOCIAL AND EPIDEMIOLOGIC ASPECTS

Social Aspects

Drug abuse has been a dominant public health concern for the past 30 years. Quite apart from toxic effects that may represent specific health threats to the individual abuser (discussed at greater length below under each substance), there are major societal consequences. The loss of impulse control directly associated with drug abuse, especially that caused by depressant intoxication, is clearly recognized as conducive to acts of violence (assault, rape, murder, and suicide). Impaired judgment and performance secondary to intoxication are associated with greatly increased rates of vehicular and workplace accidents and trauma, as well as impaired work performance and attendant economic loss.

Finally, not as a result of pharmacologic effects but as an unintended byproduct of illicit status, substances of abuse are closely linked to crime (3). Illegal status raises the cost of such substances and creates an economic stimulus to hook and then supply consumers. Tens of billions of dollars annually in property crime and robberies are committed by addicts to pay the hugely inflated price of their addiction. Thousands of homicides annually are linked to drug abuse, many by dealers to acquire and police their turf. Many more billions of dollars are spent in the criminal justice system in the apprehension, trial, and imprisonment of addicts and dealers. More than 80% of people in prison in the United States have committed drug-related crimes.

Epidemiology

Although survey data show changes in the use of some illicit substances among important segments of the U.S. population, drug abuse continues to be one of the most serious problems faced by public health and law enforcement authorities. Overall, in 1999 there were an estimated 14.8 million Americans who used an illicit drug at least once (4). This represents 6.7% of the population over age 12. Illicit drug use was limited to marijuana in 57% of the individuals. About 3.5 million Americans were dependent on an illicit drug. Trend indicators for cocaine showed a total of 1.5 million Americans as current users, with decreased use in 18 of 21 metropolitan areas surveyed. Conversely, heroin use increased in 15 of the 21 areas surveyed, with an estimated 200,000 Americans as current users of heroin. In the past 5 years, there has been a tremendous surge in the use of the so-called "rave" drugs—3,4-methylenedioxymethamphetamine (MDMA, Ecstasy), gamma-hydroxybutyrate (GHB, liquid Ecstasy), Rohypnol, and methamphetamine. Abuse of MDMA increased in 17 of 21 metropolitan areas surveyed and in Boston was the most frequently mentioned drug in telephone calls to the Poison Control center.

Drug use and abuse are not evenly distributed throughout various segments of society. The incidence and prevalence of regular use and abuse are greater among inner city populations characterized by low levels of employment and educational achievement. Minorities are over-represented in this population. These groups have not shown as great a decline in drug use as the more middle class populations have (4).

Women are at lower risk of drug abuse than men but still make up about a third of the treatment population. They also are more likely than men to abuse illicit drugs by smoking or snorting rather than injecting. Particular problems include prostitution and consequent high rates of sexually transmitted diseases as well as pregnancy, child care problems, and single-parent status. Access to and acceptance of prenatal care improve pregnancy outcome (perinatal morbidity and mortality). Alcohol is the most teratogenic of the drugs of abuse. Longer term effects for other drugs are less certain. Neonatal opioid withdrawal is common and often requires intensive care monitoring.

The *elderly* are not at high risk for illicit drug use. Addiction to illicit drugs tends to wane over the years in those who survive beyond their fifties or sixties. Most drug problems in the elderly occur with alcohol, tobacco, and prescription drugs (opioids for analgesia and benzodiazepines for insomnia). Occasionally, elderly people are seen in methadone programs, where they tend to do well.

Polydrug use, abuse, and dependence are extremely common. For example, more than 80% of alcoholics are cigarette smokers. Many younger alcoholics also abuse cocaine. Alcoholics, in general, are at greater risk of abusing benzodiazepines when compared with non–drug-abusing populations. People in methadone maintenance programs often abuse cocaine, benzodiazepines, and alcohol, and more than 90% are cigarette smokers. Heroin and cocaine are frequently injected together as a "speedball." Use of a particular drug can be a function of price and availability, as illustrated by geographic differences in the patterns of drug abuse. Sometimes a drug interaction is desired (e.g., anxiolytic effects of alcohol counteract stimulant effects of cocaine). In general, people who find one drug of abuse particularly rewarding are likely to find other drugs of abuse also to be rewarding.

Psychiatric disorders are more common among substance abusers than in the population as a whole. These both precede onset of substance abuse and result from substance abuse. Consequences of substance abuse also mimic psychiatric disorders. For example, patients with anxiety disorders may self-medicate with alcohol or benzodiazepines. Withdrawal from these substances produces anxiety regardless of whether the patient has an anxiety disorder. Stimulants acutely produce psychotic reactions, and depression is seen during withdrawal. Substance abusers are often given personality disorder diagnoses (especially the antisocial type). A low mood state (hypophoria) is common among substance abusers (see Gold and Slaby in General References for a review of psychiatric disorders associated with substance abuse).

CAUSES

Predisposing Factors

Drug abuse as defined above is merely an operational definition. The causes are clearly complex. Some of the factors involved are as follows:

- *Pharmacologic.* Certain drugs, classes of drugs, and routes of administration are consistently reported to be rewarding or reinforcing.
- *Genetic.* Certain individuals appear to be biologically predisposed to the rewarding effects of drugs of abuse and to the acquisition of drug dependence. This is most well recognized for alcohol and tobacco but is increasingly being recognized for other drugs of abuse.
- *Learning and behavior.* Repeated use of drugs (rewarding stimulus) elicits various conditioned responses and behaviors that perpetuate drug use.
- *Personality and psychiatric disorder.* People who have difficulty in deferring gratification seem to be predisposed to drug abuse. Those with mood or anxiety disorders may find that certain drugs of abuse normalize these states.
- *Social, environmental, and cultural.* Different societies have different attitudes and customs regarding use of psychoactive substances (e.g., French attitude toward wine). People who have few other rewarding activities (e.g., gainful employment) may be predisposed toward drug abuse as a rewarding activity.

Models for Understanding and Managing Substance Abuse

These causes do not speak to possible legal consequences or to therapeutic maneuvers. Four models, described here, have been proposed to encompass these concerns. The models, although distinct, are not mutually exclusive, and most people fit into more than one model, illustrating the complexity of their disease.

Moral Failure Model

This view attributes substance abuse to a failure by parents or parental surrogates (e.g., religious training, schools, movies, television, and music) to inculcate values and to the absence of an ongoing morality that would prevent the use and abuse of drugs. From a public health viewpoint the model has utility. When applied to the person already dependent on drugs and with a long criminal record, it is not useful unless there is some religious conversion experience or complete acceptance of a 12-step program (e.g., Alcoholics Anonymous or Narcotics Anonymous).

Legal Model

Proponents define behavior as aberrant only when specific acts violate existing law and then recommend existing legal remedies such as trial, fines, and imprisonment to deal with these infractions. This model counters the disease or illness concept of addiction.

Disease Model

The disease model hypothesizes a host susceptibility to drugs of abuse that is lifelong, progressive, and incapable of modification and hence can be coped with only by total abstinence. It takes as its substrate only those meeting the definitions of substance abuse or dependence (see above) and does not concern itself with social or experimental use. The disease model partially encompasses research advances in psychopharmacology.

The disease model was originally proposed to counter adverse societal attitudes and judgmental views toward alcohol and drug abuse. This model also offers a nonstigmatizing explanation of substance abuse to organizations such as Alcoholics Anonymous and Narcotics Anonymous. These organizations have helped unleash a vast movement for self-improvement that has helped a significant number of abusers. The disease model is the paradigm for the proponents of *methadone maintenance,* developed in the 1960s. Chronic narcotic abuse was seen as a biologic modification of the brain that required supplementation by a narcotic substitute that does not lead to significant dysfunction.

Psychosocial Model

The psychosocial model sees chemical dependency as the inadvertent effect of repeated self-medication by a vulnerable population intent on relieving overwhelming anxiety or psychic pain attendant on loss, hopelessness, boredom, depression, and fear. Drugs of abuse are potent and effective, albeit short-term, chemical alleviators of these symptoms. Vulnerability in this model is not a function of genetic constitution (although this may define an enhanced susceptibility). Rather it is because of membership in at-risk populations who, because of youthful immaturity, socioeconomic disability, and the lack of responsible familial or peer support systems, have not developed the same repertoire of behaviors that the greater part of society uses to cope with adversity. This model has the virtue of defining an at-risk population from among the young, the drop-outs, and the socially and economically disadvantaged that best fits most abusers in our current epidemic. The model helps explain the potential for endemic abuse by people who, although they may be socially and economically advantaged, may also turn to repetitive self-medication in the face of losses or situational anxiety, demoralization, or physical pain. The psychosocial model avoids a simplistic expectation of cure by mere detoxification or by enforced abstinence if release back into the same environment occurs without change in the conditions of vulnerability. The model also relies on support systems and self-help as a condition of remission.

SELECTED DRUGS OF ABUSE

Opioid (Narcotic) Analgesics

Opioids are commonly prescribed drugs and play an essential role in the care of patients. It has been widely observed that the fear of causing opioid addiction has led practitioners to undermedicate in the management of acute pain. This is a common legitimate criticism of practitioners. Less commonly, there has been a tendency in treating patients with chronic pain to continue the use of opioid analgesics when the development of tolerance has rendered them less effective or even countertherapeutic. Patients who have been taking opioid analgesics for long periods may experience little pain relief and may, in fact, confuse incipient withdrawal toward the end of a dosing interval with the onset of pain. An understanding of the tolerance induction, physical dependence, and addiction can ensure more rational prescribing patterns.

The opiate-dependent patient is not generally seen in office practice seeking treatment for drug dependence, although a review of medical histories given by patients entering methadone maintenance programs indicates that they often receive treatment for a range of other medical problems. Patients often appear in office practice settings attempting to obtain prescription drugs when they experience difficulty in obtaining heroin. Morphine, hydromorphone (Dilaudid), oxycodone, and meperidine (Demerol) are the drugs most preferred by addicts, but they will readily use the whole range of less potent opioid and nonopioid analgesics if preferred drugs are unavailable. The term *opioid* refers both to drugs derived from opium (opiates) and to synthetic drugs with similar actions. If analgesics are difficult to obtain, opioid addicts temporarily use virtually any depressant drug. Alcohol, benzodiazepines, and promethazine (Phenergan) are often abused by patients maintained on methadone because of their tendency to potentiate the effects of methadone.

Usual Effects and Therapeutic Use

Opiates are the prototype for managing patients with pain. To prevent abuse, they should be prescribed on a fixed schedule. For a comparison of the different opioids, see Chapter 13. Used for short intervals after an acute pain syndrome, opioids are safe and effective. Abuse liability increases with potency. Heroin, the most commonly abused illicit opioid, is usually injected intravenously but can also be injected subcutaneously (skin-popping), smoked, or sniffed (snorting). Heroin crosses the blood–brain barrier more effectively than other opioids. The effects after use consist of a brief and intense period of euphoria followed by several hours of a pleasant dreamy state in which the user may slowly nod as if falling asleep. Areas of pain feel numbed. The skin may itch (because of histamine release), which leads to characteristic scratching. Other effects include increased talkativeness (soap boxing), increased activity, and conjunctival suffusion (red eye). Stomach turning and vomiting (pleasant sick) occur. Physiologic effects include miosis and respiratory depression.

Acute Adverse Effects

Opioid overdose is characterized by depressed consciousness and respiration. Pulmonary edema, a common complication of opioid overdose, contributes to hypoxia and may cause death. Some opioids, such as propoxyphene (Darvon) and meperidine, cause convulsions at high dosages. The latter has a proconvulsive metabolite (normeperidine) that accumulates in the setting of renal failure.

Chronic Adverse Effects

The adverse effects of chronic heroin abuse result from use of dirty needles (see Complications of Injecting Drugs, below), the adulterants mixed with the heroin, and the associated life-style (poor nutrition, lack of health care, and criminal activity) rather than from the drug itself. Heroin is usually mixed with milk sugar (lactose) and quinine under unsterile conditions. Other more dangerous adulterants may also be included to mask the dilution of the heroin. Heroin nephropathy, a focal glomerulosclerosis, is predominantly reported in African Americans. Its precise cause is unclear, but it is thought to be secondary to an adulterant.

An analogue of meperidine, 1-methyl-4-phenyl-1,2,5,6-tetrahydropyridine (MPTP), which is a commercially available compound, has been used intravenously by drug abusers as a form of synthetic heroin. Some MPTP users have developed a severe form of parkinsonism. Others who have not developed parkinsonism have evidence of nigrostriatal dopamine depletion.

Tolerance (defined above) to heroin develops quickly and can be demonstrated to some degree after only a few days of administration of the drug. The degree of tolerance and the consequent severity of withdrawal symptoms depend primarily on dosage levels and the frequency and duration of use. However, the severity of a patient's addiction to heroin is as much a function of psychologic and social factors as it is a simple consequence of tolerance or of withdrawal symptoms.

Opioid withdrawal is characterized by anxiety, nausea, yawning, diarrhea, sweating, rhinorrhea, dilated pupils, and piloerection (gooseflesh). In the advanced stages of withdrawal, the patient experiences vomiting and muscle spasms that often appear as jerky kicking movements of the legs. Although the untreated addict experiences significant anxiety and discomfort during withdrawal, the process itself presents no serious medical risks. Opioid addicts tend to confuse anxiety with the early symptoms of withdrawal, so the diagnosis of withdrawal should be made on the basis of observable signs rather than solely on subjective reports of anxiety.

Treatment

Opioid overdose must be treated in an emergency room. Emergency treatment requires cardiorespiratory monitoring and support. The opioid antagonist naloxone (Narcan) is safe and effective in countering the central nervous system (CNS) depression caused by opioid overdose but may precipitate withdrawal. The initial dose is 0.4 mg intravenously. This may need to be repeated because naloxone has a shorter duration of action than most opioid agonists.

Any patient who has been abusing heroin or other opioids and is willing to accept help should be referred for treatment. Few addicts voluntarily seek treatment before being faced with the destructive consequences of their drug use.

Detoxification from opiate dependence most often involves the administration of an opiate agonist (methadone, levomethadyl acetate [LAAM]), the nonopiate clonidine, or a partial agonist (buprenorphine). Methadone, the only opiate agonist approved for detoxification, has a long duration of action and is conveniently administered orally. However, federal regulations limit the use of methadone to specially licensed centers. Detoxification may be accomplished by substituting methadone for the opioid previously used by the patient and then gradually reducing the dosage over time (usually at least 7 days). The initial dose should be sufficient to suppress withdrawal symptoms without causing sedation. Methadone detoxification is normally done on an ambulatory basis by specially licensed drug treatment programs.

Clonidine is a nonopioid medication demonstrated effective in suppressing symptoms of opiate withdrawal. A centrally acting alpha-adrenergic agonist, clonidine reduces sympathetic nervous system related effects of opiate withdrawal. It is more effective in suppressing signs than in relieving symptoms of withdrawal (5). Clonidine is dosed at 0.1 mg every 4 to 6 hours for the first day, followed by 0.1 mg every 8 hours the second day, and 0.1 mg every 12 hours on the third day. Dosages are held for systolic blood pressure less than 100. Transdermal clonidine may be an effective adjunct in outpatient treatment. However, it has a delayed onset of action, not crossing the dermis for at least 24 hours after placement. Recent cases of oral ingestion of the clonidine patch resulting in profound hypotension and bradycardia may limit its use in the future. Outpatient use of clonidine is also impacted by diversion for illicit use. Other pharmacologic aids (dicyclomine for abdominal cramps, ibuprofen for bone pain, and loperamide for diarrhea) provide additional treatment for symptoms of opiate withdrawal.

Buprenorphine is a partial mu opiate receptor agonist with a long duration of action. The parenteral formulation has been used to treat opiate withdrawal symptoms in hospitalized medically ill opiate-dependent patients (6). Experimental studies have demonstrated the efficacy of a sublingual preparation of buprenorphine as a maintenance therapy for opiate dependence (7). This preparation has just recently become available for use in the United States and will likely become the drug of choice for outpatient treatment of opiate withdrawal

It is illegal for a care provider to prescribe an opiate for the treatment of opiate withdrawal. As with detoxification from any substance, the patient should be engaged in a program of outpatient chemical dependency counseling during and after detoxification (see sections on detoxification and rehabilitation, below). Even short-term detoxification has been shown to impact positively on future outcomes related to opiate dependence (8).

Cocaine and Other Stimulants

Cocaine, the amphetamines, and methylphenidate are the most commonly abused stimulant drugs. (Nicotine is discussed in Chapter 27.) *Cocaine* is used in several forms. The route for cocaine intake depends on the form used. As the natural water-soluble powder, cocaine hydrochloride, it is either sniffed (snorted) and absorbed through the nasal mucosa or injected intravenously. Forms of cocaine that can be smoked (using a water pipe or in cigarette form) are produced by extracting or freeing the cocaine alkaloid from the hydrochloride salt. When ether is used as the reagent in this process, the resulting product is referred to as freebase. When baking soda and water are used as reagents, the resulting product is crack, so named because of the crackling sound that is produced when the drug is smoked. Although they may differ in appearance and concentration, freebase and crack are pharmacologically the same.

Cocaine use appears in variable patterns. In the early stages, sessions of cocaine use typically last 2 to 4 hours, with intervals of days or weeks between sessions. Some users are able to maintain this pattern of use without progressing further. However, many users follow a pattern of rapidly escalating use in which both the length of sessions and the rate of consumption increase; users of freebase and crack may be more likely to succumb to this pattern than are users who snort cocaine powder.

Chronic abusers typically engage in runs or periods of intensive cocaine use that can last anywhere from a few hours to several days. A run is terminated when the user runs out of cocaine or money or is too physically exhausted to continue. A run may be followed by a crash that lasts 1 or 2 days. During the crash, the user may experience some or all of the following: depression, hypersomnia, hyperphagia, fatigue, anxiety, irritability, and intense craving for cocaine.

Methamphetamine, a synthetic stimulant, is sold as a white powder that is taken orally, intranasally, or intravenously or as a clear "rock" that is heated and smoked. It is known on the street as ice, speed, crystal meth, crank, tina, or glass. It is easily synthesized in illegal small-time laboratories that quickly change location. Methamphetamine is especially popular in nonurban areas that have less influx of cocaine.

Methylphenidate (Ritalin) mimics the effects of naturally occurring stimulants such as cocaine and can be taken orally or intravenously. Legitimately used for the treatment of attention deficit disorder, methylphenidate is sometimes obtained by diversion from family members with the disorder or by seeking refills for reportedly affected family members from unsuspecting practitioners.

Abusers of stimulants develop some tolerance to the euphoric effects of the drugs but may become more sensitive to other effects such as irritability, restlessness, hypervigilance, and paranoia. Users report that in any given session of cocaine use, the duration and intensity of the euphoric effect seem to recede with successive doses, a phenomenon called "chasing the dragon's tail."

Usual Effects and Therapeutic Use

CNS stimulants produce euphoria, increased confidence and energy, increased heart rate and blood pressure, dilated pupils, constriction of peripheral blood vessels, and increased body temperature. Effects are caused by sympathetic stimulation centrally and peripherally. The duration and intensity of effect depend on the dosage and the route of administration. Single oral doses of amphetamines produce effects lasting 2 to 4 hours. The effects of cocaine, when snorted, are rapid in onset but short in duration. Smoking freebase or crack produces an intense short-duration effect (i.e., peak effect in 2 to 3 minutes, duration about 10 minutes) because smoking is an extremely efficient method of drug administration. Intravenous dosing produces similar (or greater) intensity and longer duration of effects. Smoking and intravenous use of methamphetamine results in a pleasurable rush that lasts a few minutes. Oral use results in a muted longer duration effect.

Its capacity to produce euphoria gives cocaine a high abuse potential. In animals, cocaine produces certain reinforcing responses that exceed those of other drugs of abuse. The administration of cocaine in humans is associated with an increased desire for more cocaine (i.e., the presence of the drug itself in the body increases desire for cocaine). Users often delay entry into treatment until they are physically and emotionally exhausted or are faced with serious financial, legal, or medical problems.

Acute Adverse Effects

Very large doses of all stimulants may cause hyperpyrexia, arrhythmias, hypertension, and coronary and cerebral artery vasospasm, leading to myocardial infarction, stroke, convulsion, cardiovascular collapse, and death (9). Large doses of cocaine may also cause respiratory depression with a fatal outcome.

A *reversible organic delusional disorder* that resembles paranoid schizophrenia is occasionally seen. This syndrome may occur in normal subjects with no previous psychiatric history. Subjects who have taken higher dosages of a stimulant (e.g., 10 mg of dextroamphetamine every hour) have developed the disorder within 24 hours, as have high-dose cocaine and methylphenidate users.

Chronic Adverse Effects

The chronic abuser of cocaine, amphetamines, and other long-acting stimulants is typically hyperactive, jittery, and irritable while using and depressed, exhausted, or lethargic afterward. Often, previously stable people may develop unexplained financial problems or uncharacteristic overnight disappearances. With chronic heavy use there is usually a history of sleep disturbance and weight loss. The patient may be emotionally labile, and periods of irritability, depression, and fatigue may alternate with periods of elation and enthusiasm (mania). In addition to acute delusional disorders, cases of persistent psychotic disorders have been reported. Intravenous Ritalin abusers almost uniformly develop talc lung because talc is contained as a filler in the Ritalin tablet.

Physical examination may reveal needle marks; rhinitis; teeth worn from bruxism (grinding of teeth); ulcers on the lips, tongue, or nose; tremor; flushing; cardiac arrhythmias; and excessive sweating. Although cocaine may initially enhance sexual functioning, chronic use often interferes with sexual performance. Extremely heavy users may exhibit rapid, repetitious, and ritualistic body movements.

Treatment

No data at present distinguish stimulant-abusing patients who should be hospitalized from those who may succeed as outpatients. Clearly, patients who present a risk of suicide should be hospitalized, as should patients who are unable to maintain abstinence long enough to begin a program of outpatient treatment. Although virtually all patients experience a moderate mood disturbance after a session of cocaine use, only a small percentage become suicidal. In most cases, sessions of continuous cocaine use do not exceed 12 hours, and episodes of use are often separated by periods of abstinence lasting several days or more. Abstinence may occur because the user is unable to obtain more cocaine, is too exhausted to continue using, or is making an attempt to stop or control use. In many instances these periods of abstinence last several days or more, long enough for the patient to recover from the fatigue and hypophoria that normally follow use.

Motivated patients with appropriate external supports can be engaged in outpatient treatment during such breaks in cocaine use. Treatment preferably involves daily counseling sessions during the first few weeks of abstinence. Necessary external supports include stable employment, a drug-free home environment, and active involvement in Narcotics Anonymous. For such patients, hospitalization should probably be considered only after an initial attempt at outpatient treatment has failed. No specific pharmacologic treatment is indicated for cocaine withdrawal because symptoms are mild. Currently, no drugs have been convincingly demonstrated to be efficacious in maintaining abstinence. A variety of drugs, including fluoxetine, desipramine, and ondansetron, has been studied for their effects in reducing the reinforcing responses to cocaine in humans. To date, none has become clinically useful.

Sedative-Hypnotics and Benzodiazepines

Currently, the most commonly abused sedatives are alprazolam (Xanax), clonazepam (Clonopin), and diazepam (Valium). Rohypnol (flunitrazepam) has recently gained attention for abuse as "the date rape drug." It is not licensed in the United States but is sold illicitly on the street. Rohypnol may cause paradoxical agitation and is not detectable by routine urine toxicology.

Usual Effects and Therapeutic Use

Sedatives cause intoxication similar to that seen with alcohol. Sufficient amounts are often taken to produce a depression of cortical function and to relax social and personal inhibitions. A high, or a state in which mood is elevated and anxiety is reduced, occurs. Normal individuals and those with anxiety disorders do not necessarily find these effects pleasurable or reinforcing. Because of their safety profile, benzodiazepines have become the only sedative-hypnotics prescribed for anxiolytic or sedating purposes. The proper prescribing of benzodiazepines for this purpose is discussed in Chapter 22. This class of medicine should be avoided in all patients with a history of substance abuse. Phenobarbital should be the only prescribed barbiturate, with its indication being for seizure prevention. Shorter acting barbiturates are contained in migraine medicines such as Fiorinal. These medications have a high abuse potential and should be avoided.

Acute Adverse Effects

Overdose may lead to slurred speech, impaired judgment, and unsteady gait. Even greater overdose may lead to stupor, coma, respiratory depression, vasomotor collapse, and death. Benzodiazepines (compared with barbiturates) cause less loss of motor coordination and almost never cause death when taken alone in large doses (unless given rapidly intravenously, e.g., midazolam or diazepam). However, the combination of alcohol and benzodiazepines can be lethal.

Chronic Adverse Effects

Almost no organ toxicity is associated with chronic administration of these drugs. From this standpoint, they are safer than alcohol. Patients should receive prescriptions for sedatives with a clear plan and clear instructions. If prescribed for insomnia, benzodiazepines should be prescribed for short-term treatment (10,11). Otherwise, if patients use the medications on a regular basis, they will induce tolerance and increase the dosage. Such escalation of the dosage is especially common in those with histories of drug or alcohol abuse, particularly patients who are on methadone maintenance. Chronic use of benzodiazepines may go undetected until confusion, irritability, slurred speech, or ataxia are recognized as signs of sedative intoxication.

Physical examination may include ecchymoses from injuries sustained during an intoxicated state. Sedative-hypnotics can also produce anterograde amnesia. This is mostly dosage related and has been most often described with flunitrazepam (Rohypnol), triazolam (Halcion), and diazepam (Valium).

Physical dependence on benzodiazepines and the potential for major withdrawal symptoms may occur in as little as 2 months if dosages substantially above therapeutic levels are used. From a clinical point of view, most patients who abuse and have significant physical dependence on benzodiazepines abuse other drugs concurrently. It has been well established that withdrawal symptoms occur in patients taking therapeutic dosages daily for 6 months or more (12). The risk of withdrawal can be reduced by tapering the dosage. Although chronic use may create the risk of withdrawal symptoms, there is evidence that patients may use benzodiazepines on a chronic basis without developing tolerance to the anxiolytic effects of the medication (10,13,14).

Treatment

Nonbenzodiazepine sedative overdose is a life-threatening occurrence that should be treated in an emergency department. Because of physical dependence (detailed above), patients who use excessive dosages of sedative drugs are at risk of serious withdrawal reactions, including life-threatening seizures. Outpatient treatment for therapeutic dependence can often be managed by tapering the prescribed benzodiazepine or switching to a benzodiazepine with a longer half-life and tapering it over several weeks (15). Onset time of withdrawal symptoms (Table 29.2) is inversely related to the half-life of the benzodiazepine of use. Inpatient treatment is often required for high-dose abuse and can be managed using phenobarbital, which has a long half-life (80 to 100 hours) and provides the pharmacokinetic umbrella to prevent withdrawal symptoms (16).

Marijuana and Hashish

Marijuana consists of the dried leaves of the *Cannabis sativa* plant, which are usually smoked in pipes or cigarettes (joints). *Hashish* is a concentrated resin of cannabis and contains approximately 5 to 10 times the concentration of the principal psychoactive ingredient—9-tetrahydrocannabinol—as compared with *marijuana*. The discussion that follows applies to both marijuana and hashish. Cannabis can also be added to foods such as brownies, but when it is eaten, effects appear less rapidly and are less under control of the user.

Usual Effects and Therapeutic Use

The effects of marijuana from usual smoked doses last from 3 to 6 hours. The more common effects are elation or high, an increased tendency to laughter and silliness, tachycardia, reddening of the eyes, and a later stage of relaxation. At higher dosages these effects are enhanced. The user may misjudge the effects of time, and perception of sound, color, and other sensations may be distorted or sharpened. Short-term memory and logical thinking are impaired, as is the ability to drive a car or perform other complex tasks. Additive effects occur with alcohol or other CNS depressants. Dosages three to five times higher than those producing relaxation and mild euphoria can result in effects similar to those of lysergic acid diethylamide (LSD) and other hallucinogenic substances (depersonalization, auditory, and visual hallucinations). Some of the usual effects of marijuana that might be enjoyable to the experienced user, as well as the more alarming effects associated with high dosage, can be frightening to the inexperienced user. The setting is important in determining the effects of the drug. When smoked in a pleasant and familiar setting, marijuana is less likely to produce a negative response than when used in unfamiliar or threatening surroundings.

Cannabis has effects that are *potentially useful for therapeutic purposes* (e.g., decreased intraocular pressure, antiemetic properties). However, other currently approved drugs are of similar or superior efficacy for these indications and have fewer side effects. Accordingly, there are no strong pharmacologic indications for the introduction of cannabis as a therapeutic agent. The principal psychoactive substance in cannabis is marketed in oral preparations. Dronabinol (Marinol) is a schedule II drug in the United States and nabilone is available in Canada, where they are approved, respectively, for use as appetite stimulants.

Acute Adverse Effects

Considering the large number of regular users in the United States, it is clear that adverse reactions to marijuana requiring medical treatment are rare. The most common adverse response is an *acute anxiety reaction* that is similar to the panic attacks described in Chapter 22. It is different in that it includes paranoid ideation and the usual effects of the drug in exaggerated form, which are not typically features of panic attacks. These reactions are most likely to occur in novice users or in users who unexpectedly receive a much larger than usual dose. Most reactions last only the few hours it takes for the effects of the drug to wear off. Some patients experience persistent anxiety for several days after the initial panic subsides.

There have also been reports of delirium induced by marijuana. A dysphoric reaction characterized by disorientation, catatonic immobility, acute panic, and heavy sedation has also been reported. These conditions tend to remit within 2 to 4 hours as the effects of the marijuana diminish.

Reports of enduring psychotic reactions after heavy marijuana use have appeared, largely in countries where marijuana is used at much higher dosages than in the United States. Reports of confirmed psychotic reactions to marijuana in this country are rare.

Chronic Adverse Effects

There is substantial evidence that marijuana at dosage levels associated with common social usage results in loss of energy and drive, impaired memory, and apathy. This is sometimes called the amotivational syndrome.

Smoking marijuana alone does not appear to affect pulmonary function (17). However, heavy cannabis users tend to be heavy tobacco smokers. The tar content of cannabis smoke is 50% higher than that of tobacco. Accordingly, users have chronic bronchitis and other respiratory diseases. Marijuana smoke contains 70% more carcinogens than does tobacco smoke (18). There have been conflicting findings concerning possible adverse effects of marijuana on the immune system. Some studies report changes in immunologic responsiveness, but the clinical implications of these changes are currently unknown. There is evidence that marijuana reduces testosterone levels in men, although the average level for users remains within normal limits (19).

Regular use induces moderate *tolerance*. High dosages followed by sudden cessation produces a mild *withdrawal* syndrome in both animals and humans. Regular users of marijuana often exhibit restlessness, sleep disturbance, loss of appetite, and irritability when they stopped using marijuana. Because most social use is not regular and of high dosage, neither tolerance nor physical dependence is a major issue.

Treatment

Because they must be closely observed and may take several hours to recover, patients with panic reactions are best managed in a setting such as a drug abuse program, mental health center, or emergency department where continuing observation and supportive contact can be provided. Generally, these patients require simple reassurance and an explanation that they are experiencing a drug reaction that will dissipate as the drug is eliminated from their bodies.

Delusional or delirious patients should be seen in an emergency department because they present more complicated management problems and may require sedation or hospitalization. Furthermore, other causes of delirium should be ruled out. Restraints should be used only when absolutely necessary for the safety of the patient or others. Drugs should also not be used unless the patient is extremely agitated and difficult to control.

Treatment for chronic use should involve the support necessary for abstinence: a drug-free environment, active participation in 12-step meetings of Alcoholics Anonymous or Narcotics Anonymous, and, in some circumstances, group counseling.

3,4-Methylenedioxymethamphetamine (Ecstasy)

MDMA is a synthetic drug that is both a stimulant and hallucinogen (LSD-like). It was originally synthesized as a drug to facilitate communication during psychotherapy (20). Street names for MDMA include Ecstasy, Adam, XTC, hug, beans, and love drug. Most MDMA sold on the street has MDMA in combination with other drugs, including LSD, amphetamine, caffeine, heroin, and lactose. Using MDMA with LSD is termed "candyflipping." MDMA comes in the form of a white powder that is usually pressed into pills, but other routes of use snorting, injecting, and as a rectal suppository have been reported.

Usual Effects

When taken on an empty stomach, oral ingestion of MDMA results in a "rush" within minutes. The rush, consisting of euphoria and an intensification of perceptions, lasts 25 to 30 minutes. Individuals crave the effect and take additional doses. However, repeated doses have diminished effect. After the initial intense phase, a plateau phase occurs during which users report a trance-like feeling that lasts a few hours. A down phase occurs 3 to 6 hours after initial ingestion and is accompanied by feelings of dysphoria and anxiety. Despite feelings of exhaustion, users are unable to fall asleep.

Acute and Chronic Adverse Effects

MDMA is neurotoxic, damaging dopamine and serotonin producing neurons in the brain. Acute use of MDMA results in muscle rigidity, involuntary teeth clenching, nausea, blurred vision, faintness, and cold sweats. Cases of acute rhabdomyolysis have been reported. Heart rate and blood pressure increases may be dose dependent. MDMA can cause confusion, depression, sleep problems, severe anxiety, and paranoia. These effects may linger weeks after use. Hepatotoxicity and an acneform rash occur in many individuals after chronic use. Long-term users of MDMA may suffer permanent deficits in thought and memory (21). Motor disturbances may occur resulting in a syndrome resembling Parkinson disease.

Treatment

The acute toxic effects of MDMA are short lived. It is metabolized in the liver and excreted in the urine. Management of overdose is supportive care in a quiet dark setting. For individuals who are agitated and paranoid, treatment with benzodiazepines will ameliorate symptoms. Intravenous hydration is indicated in cases of overdose accompanied by rhabdomyolysis. Dantrolene may be useful if severe persistent muscle spasms occur.

Long-term treatment for abuse of MDMA is similar to other drugs of abuse, consisting of counseling and 12-step groups. Most users of MDMA are young and should seek treatment centers that have programs specific for adolescents and young adults.

Gamma-Hydroxybutyrate

GHB is a precursor of the neurotransmitter gamma aminobutyric acid. It was developed as an adjunct to anesthesia and has been used clinically for narcolepsy. It is sold in small bottles as a salty clear liquid and goes by the street names liquid ecstasy, easy lay, cherry meth, soap, liquid X, liquid G, and liquid E. After ingestion, the onset of action is within 15 to 30 minutes with effects lasting up to 3 hours. The drug's half-life is about 30 minutes with elimination by expiration as carbon dioxide.

Usual Effects

Acting on the central dopaminergic system, GHB produces euphoria and disinhibition without a subsequent dysphoria.

Adverse Effects

Idiosyncratic responses to GHB occur. These include delusions, aggressive behavior, altered mental status, seizures, nausea, vertigo, ataxia, nystagmus, amnesia, somnolence, and coma. Recovery from somnolence and coma is often characterized by myoclonic jerks and confusion. During intoxication, individuals are at risk for aspiration. In severe cases of intoxication, coma may be accompanied by bradycardia and myoclonus. Adverse effects are potentiated by CNS depressants, including alcohol, benzodiazepines, and opiates. Use of GHB with methamphetamine increases the risk of seizures.

Treatment

Management of acute overdose is supportive. Comatose patients may require intubation for airway protection. Atropine should be prescribed in the presence of symptomatic bradycardia. Because many patients ingest GHB with other drugs, a screen for other drugs should be performed with treatment for toxicity from other drugs as indicated.

Long-term treatment for abuse of GHB is similar to other drugs of abuse, consisting of counseling and 12-step groups. GHB users are at high risk of developing dependence to other drugs. Most users of GHB are young and should seek treatment centers that have programs specific for adolescents and young adults.

Phencyclidine

Phencyclidine (PCP) is a barbiturate-like anesthetic and derivative of ketamine. However, PCP exhibits selective action as an anesthetic, appearing to depress sensory tracts—including proprioception, pain, touch, and temperature—to a greater degree than it depresses cortical function. The resultant state of sensory deprivation and relative cortical wakefulness makes for a peculiar sense of detachment, disembodiment, and weightlessness. These sensations are intensely pleasurable for some, whereas for others they induce intense anxiety and even panic. PCP was developed as an anesthetic but was abandoned for this purpose when it was found to cause disturbing side effects. It continues to be used by veterinarians as an animal tranquilizer or immobilizing agent. Pure PCP is a white powder that dissolves in water. It is usually sprinkled on marijuana, dried parsley flakes, or other organic material and smoked. Less often, it is obtained in powder or tablet form and ingested or snorted. Street names for the drug vary considerably from region to region, but it is most commonly known as angel dust, flakes, crystal, greens, hog, or sheets.

Usual Effects

The effects of PCP are dose related, although both individual responses vary. People who take PCP in the dosages normally associated with street use may experience exhilaration, euphoria, inebriation, tranquilization, and perceptual disturbances. Some unpleasant effects commonly reported include disorientation, hallucinations, anxiety, paranoia, excitability, and irritability. At usual street dosages, most users reach peak intoxication in 5 to 30 minutes and remain high for 4 to 6 hours. It may take 24 hours or more before the user feels completely normal again.

Acute Adverse Effects

Even at low dosages, PCP is capable of occasionally causing severe reactions that may precipitate extreme agitation and acts of violence toward the user and to others. With higher dosages, users are more likely to exhibit delirium, which may include hallucinations.

There is a difference between the delirium that is seen in acute PCP toxicity and what has been called PCP psychosis, a disorder closely resembling schizophrenia that develops after acute intoxication and persists for 24 hours or more. Such psychoses may develop out of the original intoxication or may occur days after the intoxication has cleared.

Ataxia, nystagmus, slurred speech, and ptosis are common features of acute PCP toxicity. Very high dosages of PCP, which are normally the result of oral ingestion rather than smoking, can result in coma, severe respiratory depression, seizures, and death.

Chronic Adverse Effects

Chronic use of PCP may produce persistent changes in personal habits (hygiene or dress), problems with memory or speech, sleep disturbances, mood changes (depression, irritability), delusional thinking, and unusual excitability or lethargy. Little is known about long-term physical effects.

Treatment

Consistent correlation has been found between the patient's initial level of consciousness and the time course of improvement. Patients with delirium clear in 3 to 8 hours, patients who remain stuporous or comatose for 1 to 4 hours clear in 5 to 62 hours, and patients whose stupor or coma lasts 6 or more hours clear in 75 to over 200 hours. Therefore, patients who are delirious at presentation can be treated in an emergency department and do not require hospitalization. Repeated mental status examinations should be performed to ensure that the patient is in a state of clear consciousness for at least 4 hours before discharge. Members of the family should be cautioned that the patient should stay in the company of family members or reliable friends for several days. Patients can have the onset of severe depression or a PCP psychosis for several days after the acute effects of the drug have subsided. Patients who remain comatose or stuporous for more than 2 hours or who develop a PCP psychosis require hospitalization. PCP abuse usually occurs in the setting of polysubstance abuse, and long-term treatment should include traditional 12-step meetings.

Lysergic Acid Diethylamide

LSD is the prototype of a number of alkaloid substances of high potency that predictably cause hallucinations. Others include psilocybin, dimethyltryptamine, and mescaline. All are classified as hallucinogens and are CNS depressants at higher dosages. LSD (acid) is sold illicitly in the form of powder, tablets, or capsules. Sugar cubes, small squares of gelatin (window pane), or paper (blotter acid) that have been impregnated with the drug are also available. LSD is usually ingested orally and its effects appear within 30 to 40 minutes, reaching a peak at about 90 minutes, with physiologic effects gone by 6 hours but subjective effects persisting for 8 to 12 hours.

Usual Effects

LSD usually produces some combination of the following subjective effects: depersonalization, altered time perception, labile mood, perceptual distortions (usually visual), body image distortion, and feelings of increased insight. Physiologic effects include slight rises in blood pressure and heart rate, fever, lack of coordination, dilated pupils, increased salivation and lacrimation, hyperreflexia, and occasionally vomiting.

Acute Adverse Effects

Inexperienced users may have an acute panic reaction that occurs because the normal effects of the drug are unfamiliar or unexpected. In more severe reactions, users of LSD may experience hallucinations (usually visual) and delusions that may persist beyond the time when the drug is circulating in the blood.

Flashbacks, spontaneous recurrences of the original LSD experience, have been estimated to occur in 1 of every 20 users (from days to years later). They are more likely to occur in chronic users (and can occur after the use of any hallucinogenic drug, including marijuana). There have also been reports of prolonged psychotic reactions after the use of LSD, although these are rare.

Patients with acute LSD toxicity can be differentiated from those with PCP toxicity or schizophrenia in several ways. LSD causes dilation of the pupils, which is absent in PCP toxicity and schizophrenia. PCP toxicity usually is characterized by clouding of consciousness, and the patient often exhibits ataxia, nystagmus, and ptosis, which are not features of LSD toxicity or of schizophrenia.

Chronic Adverse Effects

Some degree of tolerance develops with repeated use of LSD, but no withdrawal syndrome has been observed.

Treatment

Adverse reactions to LSD usually remit in 8 to 24 hours, and hospitalization is usually unnecessary. However, the patient should be observed until symptoms clear. Referral to an emergency room or to a drug abuse program that can provide this type of support will usually be necessary. The same supportive measures described earlier for the treatment of adverse reactions to marijuana are appropriate. Extremely agitated patients should be given diazepam (Valium), 20 mg orally or intramuscularly, before being sent to a treatment center.

Inhalants: Solvent Abuse

The inhalation of solvents is a form of substance abuse that is most commonly found among children and adolescents. Because solvents are easily obtainable and inexpensive, they are likely to be preferred by people who lack the money or other resources needed to obtain more desirable drugs. A partial list of specific substances subject to this type of abuse includes gasoline, ignition spray, airplane glue, paint thinner, spray paint, lighter fluid, nail polish remover, cleaning fluid, and shoe polish. Toluene and other similar chemicals are the psychoactive substances. Inhalation is typically accomplished by saturating a rag with the substance and holding it directly over the face or placing it in a bag that is then placed over the nose and the mouth.

Usual Effects

The effects of solvents are immediate and of short duration, usually dissipating in a few hours or less (depending on the dosage). Acute intoxication is similar to alcohol intoxication except for the shorter duration.

Acute Adverse Effects

A hangover, with symptoms of headache and nausea, that is similar but perhaps milder than the hangover produced by alcohol has been observed. Some users experience apparent delirium characterized by tactile hallucinations, spatial distortions, and body image distortions. Sudden sniffing deaths have been described when inhalants were used during strenuous activity or under conditions in which blood oxygen is reduced. Such deaths apparently occur as a result of cardiac arrhythmias. Other deaths have been caused by suffocation when the user loses consciousness with the bag containing the solvent covering the nose and mouth.

Chronic Adverse Effects

The effects of solvents on the CNS, liver, kidneys, and bone marrow are not well understood. Cerebellar damage (which is partially reversible with abstinence) and peripheral neuropathy occur with long-term use. Numerous studies have demonstrated organ damage from long-term exposure to low concentrations of industrial solvents, but it is less clear to what extent these findings can be generalized to the short-term high-concentration exposures experienced by inhalant abusers.

There is evidence that tolerance develops with chronic solvent abuse, but withdrawal symptoms and signs are uncommon, probably because the concentration of the substance in neurons is not sustained.

Treatment

Because the acute effects of solvents are usually of short duration, abusers rarely present for medical treatment. On rare occasions, a patient may be brought in for treatment of a solvent-induced delirium. Chronic solvent abuse requires the same type of intense counseling and rehabilitative intervention indicated for other forms of self-destructive substance abuse (see below).

Anabolic Androgenic Steroids

These drugs are used to enhance athletic performance. They are derivatives of testosterone and promote growth of skeletal muscle and may increase lean body mass. Use is widespread but data are limited. Anabolic steroids are mostly used in cycles of weeks or months. Stacking (use of more than one preparation) and pyramiding (dosages gradually increased and then tapered) are common patterns of administration. Dosages used are much greater than those administered for therapeutic purposes.

Usual Effects and Therapeutic Use

Anabolic steroids are prescribed routinely to individuals with hypogonadism. Acute experimental administration of testosterone to eugonadal individuals produces no acute psychoactive effect (22). Total body weight increases in less than a week, partly because of salt and water retention and also because of a true increase in lean body mass. Some studies have shown anabolic steroids to directly contribute to an increase in strength in trained individuals (23).

Anabolic steroids have therapeutic benefit in people with weight loss related to human immunodeficiency virus (HIV) infection. Both oxandrolone, an oral synthetic anabolic steroid, and testosterone are prescribed for involuntary weight loss and wasting related to medical illness. In these settings they are safe to prescribe, with low abuse potential.

Chronic Adverse Effects

Although it is not clear whether there are any acute adverse effects, there are chronic adverse effects if these drugs are taken in excess. Adverse chronic effects include decrease in sperm count, testicular atrophy, masculinization in women (hoarse voice and clitoral hypertrophy), premature fusion of epiphyses in adolescents, decreased glucose tolerance, an unfavorable lipid profile (increased low-density lipoprotein, decreased high-density lipoprotein), acne, alopecia, hirsuteness, hepatitis, and complications of injecting drug use (see above). There is a tenuous link with malignancy and case reports of myocardial infarction and other vascular events. The best documented psychologic effect is an increase in aggression. Some users fulfill DSM-IV criteria for psychoactive substance abuse and dependence as defined at the beginning of this chapter (24).

Atropinic Drugs

Belladonna derivatives such as atropine (the alkaloid produced by deadly nightshade [*Atropa belladonna*] and also by jimsonweed [*Datura stramonium*]) and scopolamine are acetylcholine antagonists that at high dosages produce hallucinations, delirium, and varying states of excitement, insomnia, or amnesia. These effects may be followed by CNS depression and coma. The undesired pharmacologic effects of these drugs—dryness of the mouth, blurred vision, anhidrosis, and tachycardia—limit their appeal as psychoactive agents. Thus, the rare instances of abuse are mostly by teenagers experimenting with jimsonweed in rural areas or, in the past, by use of over the counter soporifics that contained scopolamine until this was banned by the Food and Drug Administration some years ago. Treatment of toxic overdose is a medical emergency requiring gastric lavage and ingestion of activated charcoal to limit intestinal absorption, maintenance of vital signs, administration of physostigmine, and lowering of body temperature.

Arecoline (Betel/Areca Nuts)

Arecoline is a parasympathomimetic alkaloid somewhat similar in structure to nicotine. It is used for its psychoactive effects by about a billion people, mostly in Southeast Asia and the Indian subcontinent. It is the world's fourth most popular psychoactive drug (after caffeine, alcohol, and nicotine). It is a cholinergic drug, exerting effects similar to acetylcholine, including sweating, salivation, and increase in bladder tone. At low dosages it produces general arousal and is usually classified as a stimulant. Effects are generally a mixture of arousal and depression according to dosage and individual response. The nuts have a bitter taste and produce reddened saliva and stained teeth, and chronic use commonly leads to grinding of the teeth and cancer of the oral cavity. They are usually chewed with lime to enhance absorption. Treatment of arecoline poisoning consists of administration of atropine and cardiorespiratory support.

COMPLICATIONS OF INJECTING DRUGS

Cutaneous complications in chronic injecting drug users include needle marks or scars, usually in the antecubital fossae of both arms, on the forearms and wrists, or on the backs of the hands. The presence of old abscess scars and of bluish phlebitis scars from past injections also indicates chronic use. Long-time users are usually forced to seek new injection sites as old sites become unusable because of scarring, and they may exhibit fresh needle marks on the legs and neck.

Skin and soft tissue infections are extremely common. *Staphylococcus aureus* is the most common pathogen (staphylococcal colonization is universal among injecting drug users). Streptococci (groups A and G) are the next most common pathogens. However, almost every common pathogen (as well as some uncommon ones) is seen. The types of infections include cellulitis, abscess, multiple chronic ulcerations, necrotizing fasciitis, pyomyositis, septic phlebitis, and infected aneurysms. Regional lymphangitis and lymphadenitis are common with all of these conditions. More unusual infections introduced at the site of injection include wound botulism, candidiasis, and tetanus.

When needles are shared, there is a high risk of acquiring viral *hepatitis*. Seroprevalence surveys among injecting drug users reveal positive hepatitis C serology in up to 86% of users (25). Many individuals have chronically elevated aminotransferase levels. Although the natural history of hepatitis C in this population is not yet well described, a recent paper showed injecting drug users infected with hepatitis C were more likely to die from drug overdose than from hepatitis C (26). Hepatitis B virus is also common among injecting drug users with carrier (antigen positive) rates of 4% and previous infection (antibody positive) rates ranging from 30% to 94% (25,27). People who have been infected with hepatitis B virus are at risk for infection with hepatitis D virus (delta virus). Hepatitis B vaccine should be given to seronegative injecting drug users. Chapters 18 and 47 describe hepatitis vaccines and hepatitis in detail.

Approximately 30% of recent cases of acquired immunodeficiency syndrome (AIDS) in the United States and 50% in Europe relate to injecting drug use (28). Prevalence of *HIV infection* among populations of U.S. injecting drug users ranges from less than 10% in Los Angeles to 56% in New York City and San Juan (29). Injecting drug users are the main sources of heterosexual, and subsequent perinatal, transmission of HIV. Compared with homosexuals who are HIV positive, injecting drug users who are HIV positive are more likely to have morbidity related to bacterial infections (endocarditis, pneumonia, and abscesses). In general, studies have found that modest behavior change among injecting drug users has occurred as a result of concern about AIDS. This relates mostly to risk reduction rather than to elimination (smoking or snorting rather than injecting drugs). Multiple simultaneous interventions appear to be needed. These include access to drug abuse treatment (including methadone), education, counseling, social support, and needle and syringe exchange/availability (30). Even with these interventions, many individuals (especially those with antisocial personality) do not significantly change their behavior. Chapter 39 describes HIV infection in detail.

Endocarditis usually caused by bacteria at injection sites, and most often affects the tricuspid valve. *S. aureus* is the most common causative organism. Mitral and aortic valves are not uncommonly involved and are more likely to be affected if there is preexisting pathology. *Streptococci* (enterococcus, viridans, and alpha-hemolytic) are next most common and are more likely to affect left-sided valves. Other offending organisms include gram-negative organisms (*Pseudomonas*) and fungi (*Candida*). Polymicrobial and culture-negative endocarditis also occur. Prognosis is related to size of vegetations and to complications such as heart failure and embolic events. Treatment should be in a controlled inpatient setting. Chapter 40 describes the posthospital management of endocarditis.

Skeletal infections account for a significant number of admissions of injecting drug abusers. Osteomyelitis and septic arthritis occur, mainly by hematogenous, but occasionally from contiguous, spread. The lumbar spine, sternoarticular structures, and the pelvis and its articular structures are commonly involved. Synovial joints (most commonly the knee) and occasionally the appendicular skeleton can be involved. The most common organisms are aerobic gram-negative bacilli (mostly *Pseudomonas aeruginosa*). Tuberculosis and fungal infections are also encountered. Gonococcal arthritis is commonly seen among drug-abusing women who prostitute. Chapter 40 describes the ambulatory aspects of diagnosis and management of osteomyelitis.

Pulmonary complications, other than septic emboli, are mostly related to obtundation and drug intoxication with consequent aspiration pneumonia (or pulmonary edema from opiates), lung abscess, and empyema. Microembolization, talc granulomas, pulmonary fibrosis, and, uncommonly, pulmonary hypertension are sometimes seen. Pneumothorax may occur as a complication of attempted injection in the neck.

Defects in host defense mechanisms (independent of HIV-induced problems) are present in injecting drug users. Cell-mediated immunity is depressed, but the mechanisms involved are not clearly understood. Other factors such as malnutrition and concurrent alcohol abuse complicate the study of this problem. The humoral immune response is not diminished. Polyclonal increases in immunoglobulin, probably related to repeated antigenic exposure, result in elevated total protein levels. Thrombocytopenia commonly occurs as a result of circulating immune complexes reacting with platelets. Up to 25% of drug users have a biological false positive serologic test result for syphilis. Usually, the positive titer is 1:4 or less, and the more specific fluorescent treponemal antibody test is negative.

PHARMACOLOGIC APPROACHES TO TREATMENT OF SUBSTANCE ABUSE

As mentioned above, the roles of the primary care practitioner, generally, are to recognize substance abuse, to nonjudgmentally discuss the problem with patients and manage their other medical problems, to help motivate patients to accept and remain in treatment (see Chapter 4), and to refer patients for treatment. Pharmacologic treatment and rehabilitation are generally managed by specialists in substance abuse in the context of a treatment program.

Detoxification

With the exception of opioid-addicted patients who enter methadone maintenance treatment, rehabilitation usually begins with detoxification. This is the process or set of procedures involved in readjusting the patient to a lower or absent tissue level of the substance of abuse. Where they are available, the specific pharmacologic approaches to detoxification have been described above under descriptions of individual drugs of abuse.

Detoxification is the first and easiest task for the recovering addict. Patients tend to attach too much significance to the task of physiologic withdrawal and too little significance to the behavioral changes that are required to prevent relapse (see Rehabilitation, below).

With proper support, many chemically dependent patients can be detoxified on an outpatient basis. Such patients should be seen on a daily basis throughout the detoxification and should be participating concurrently in an intensive program of counseling and education. Medications should be administered on a daily basis so that the patient has only the dosages needed between visits. Clearly many patients do not have the social support and accessibility to appropriate programs for this to occur. The other conditions needed for successful outpatient detoxification are described in detail in Chapter 28.

In general, *inpatient* detoxification is necessary when (a) the patient is unable to discontinue use of illicit substances on an outpatient basis; (b) the patient has concurrent medical problems that require hospitalization or significant medical problems that would be exacerbated by detoxification (e.g., symptomatic coronary artery disease); (c) the patient has developed an extremely high tolerance and has a history of major withdrawal symptoms such as seizures and delirium tremens; (d) the patient presents a clear risk of suicide or, because of chronic intoxication and impaired judgment, is a danger to self or others; or (e) the patient is dependent on multiple drugs.

For most patients, it is not physical dependence that presents the major obstacle to recovery. Rather, it is the propensity to relapse, and the factors that influence this, that determine the success of the patient's efforts to become drug free.

Methadone Maintenance

Methadone maintenance is the most widely used chemotherapeutic approach to the treatment of opioid addiction. Methadone is a long half-life opioid that is taken orally in a single daily dose. Methadone is substituted for the opioid previously used by the patient at a dosage that prevents withdrawal but causes less sedation or intoxication. The starting dose is usually 30 mg. The methadone dosage is gradually increased, thereby increasing the patient's tolerance for all opioids to a level where the user is less able to experience a significant effect, even from large dosages of illicit narcotics. Although this methadone blockade can be overridden by a sufficiently large dose of another narcotic, the payoff for doing so is small in relation to the cost. Patients taking methadone are partially tolerant to its euphoric–sedative effects and are thus able to function normally in home and work settings.

Numerous studies have shown methadone maintenance to be a cost-effective approach in treating opioid addiction (31). Methadone maintenance produces substantial reductions in crime and increases economic productivity of patients in treatment (32). It has also taken on a new significance because of its potential for reducing the spread of AIDS.

Contingency management treatment has been most often applied to methadone maintenance programs. Attempts are made to change behavior by manipulating consequences. Rewards or punishments are provided as incentives for desirable behavior. For example, take-home privileges are linked to the provision of clean urine tests.

Although demonstrably cost effective, methadone treatment has several limitations. As with other forms of chemical dependency treatment, there is a high turnover and rate of relapse. Patients are required to take methadone under observation at a clinic at least three times a week, and this requirement sometimes conflicts with work and family commitments. Although methadone is effective in suppressing the use of opioids, it has no such effect on alcohol or other drugs, and many methadone-maintained patients develop problems with other substances. Methadone-maintained patients become both physically and psychologically dependent on the drug, and many experience considerable difficulty in making the transition from methadone to abstinence. Some treatment professionals believe that opioid addicts have a biochemical abnormality that is corrected by methadone so that it may be necessary for them to remain on methadone for life. No scientific evidence supports this view at this time. However, it is likely that genetic studies will reveal a biologic predisposition to opioid use, as has been demonstrated with alcohol and tobacco. Some patients who make appropriate changes in life-style and develop good social and emotional support systems are able to detoxify successfully from methadone.

Newer pharmacologic treatments have been introduced in the last few years, including *LAAM* and *buprenorphine.* LAAM has a longer half-life than methadone and can be given three times weekly, thus decreasing the need for take-home medication and decreasing the possibility of diversion. However, recent reports of cardiac arrhythmias related to LAAM have curtailed its use. Buprenorphine, not yet approved for oral use in the United States, is a partial opioid agonist that has a superior safety profile to both methadone and LAAM (with significantly lower chance of respiratory depression). It is as effective as methadone in treating opiate addiction and is likely to become the drug of choice for maintenance opioid treatment (7). Recently passed legislation in the United States will allow primary care providers to prescribe buprenorphine directly to patients for treatment of opiate dependence.

Naltrexone

Naltrexone is an orally administered opioid receptor antagonist that is highly effective in blocking the effects of opioids. It is a long-acting drug that can effectively block the effects of opioids when administered three times a week. Because naltrexone causes an acute withdrawal reaction, candidates for naltrexone treatment must first be detoxified from the opioid to which they are addicted. Unlike methadone, which works by increasing the patient's tolerance for opioids, naltrexone competes with opioids at the receptor site. Another important difference is that naltrexone is not addicting, and patients can discontinue use without difficulty. The major disadvantage of naltrexone is that few patients are willing to use the drug and stay on it for an appropriate length of time. Its effectiveness is thus limited to highly motivated patients or patients who can be required to take the drug. Like methadone, naltrexone is not effective in blocking the use of other substances of abuse. A patch preparation of naltrexone is under development. Equivalents of methadone and naltrexone have not been developed that would allow for the pharmacologic management of other forms of drug abuse, such as cocaine.

REHABILITATION

All forms of drug abuse optimally require both acute and long-term intervention. Acute interventions (see above) include the management of overdose, toxicity, and withdrawal under medical supervision (if this is indicated). However, when the immediate physical consequences of drug abuse have been successfully treated, there remains a need to identify and treat, if possible, any underlying conditions that motivated drug misuse in the first place. Many drug abusers have significant problems of psychologic and social adjustment and may benefit from counseling and rehabilitation over extended periods. As described above, the primary care practitioner's major role in dealing with long-term rehabilitation is to motivate patients to cease drug abuse and to enter and continue in rehabilitation programs.

Effective rehabilitation programs stress the development of practical social and vocational skills and the avoidance of social environments conducive to drug use. Unfortunately, many employers are reluctant to hire someone with a history of substance abuse, whereas at the same time employment is a key aspect of recovery. In recent years, there has been an increasing recognition that families may actually enable drug abuse by one or more members. Family therapy has been used successfully with opiate addicts and appears to be the treatment of choice with drug-abusing teenagers who are still living with their parents.

Because many drug abusers have important deficits in education and vocational preparation, lack basic social and recreational skills, and are handicapped by problems of poor impulse control and low self-esteem, the process of rehabilitation often takes considerable time. Some treatment programs serve as therapeutic workplaces, integrating drug treatment and vocational training.

There is evidence that existing treatment modalities improve the course of substance abuse disorders and reduce the amount of injury to both the individual and the community. There is evidence that treatment reduces the economic costs that result from drug abuse and that these cost reductions substantially exceed the actual cost of providing care (33). However, it must also be acknowledged that definitive treatment methods that result in lasting abstinence from drugs in a significant proportion of patients do not currently exist.

Principal Types of Rehabilitation Programs

Residential Treatment Programs

Two types of residential treatment programs are commonly encountered in the United States.

Therapeutic communities typically require patients to commit themselves to 6 months or more of treatment. Patients are subjected to an intense aggressively confrontational form of group therapy that is intended to facilitate change by stripping away antisocial drug-oriented beliefs and values and replacing them with socially adaptive beliefs and values. Therapeutic communities tend to have high dropout rates in the first few weeks of treatment because many patients are not willing to make the commitment required by this form of treatment. Patients who remain for the duration of treatment, however, often achieve an enduring drug-free adjustment.

A more common form of residential treatment is the *intermediate-term residential program.* These programs are typically 4 weeks in duration and were originally designed to treat alcoholism. Over the last two decades, they have evolved into chemical dependence programs that accept patients with a wide range of substance abuse problems. Intermediate-term residential programs use a more traditional group therapy approach that is less aggressive than the approach used by therapeutic communities. They also place a strong emphasis on education. In most facilities, patients attend lectures and films designed to increase their understanding of the disease of chemical dependency and the nature of the recovery process.

Traditionally, intermediate-term residential programs have been viewed as the treatment of choice for chemical dependency, but in recent years they have come under pressure from a variety of groups concerned about the rising cost of health care benefits. Residential treatment is considerably more expensive than outpatient care, and comparisons of the two approaches for one form of drug abuse—alcoholism—show little difference in outcome for comparable patients (33). There are few data for other drugs of abuse. In response to the demand for more cost-effective treatment approaches, intermediate-term residential facilities now offer flexible lengths of stay rather than admitting all patients for the same 28- or 30-day program.

Intensive Outpatient Treatment Programs

Demands for more cost-effective forms of treatment have led to a greater emphasis on the use of outpatient approaches. Intensive outpatient programs offer a combination of education and group counseling similar to that found in the intermediate-term residential programs, but they provide treatment in the evenings so patients do not have to be absent from home or work. Intensive outpatient programs have patients attend treatment sessions four to six times a week and offer 12 to 20 hours of therapeutic activities each week for 4 to 6 weeks or longer. Traditional individual psychotherapy (rather than counseling) has not proved particularly effective in treating drug dependence.

Urine Testing

Although not generally recommended for use by the primary care practitioner (see above), urine testing is often included in the rehabilitation programs to which patients agree. The goals are to provide motivation for patients and to permit monitoring by program staff.

Self-Help Groups

Self-help groups such as *Alcoholics Anonymous* (AA) and *Narcotics Anonymous* (NA) provide another valuable resource for people seeking help for a substance abuse problem. These 12-step programs provide a clearly defined sequence of steps that the addict must take to recover. They also provide immediate access to the emotional support and encouragement of others who have successfully coped with similar problems. AA and NA both maintain hotlines that are listed in the telephone directories of every major community in the United States and Canada. The NA process is identical to the process of AA, which is described in Chapter 28. Most drug-free treatment programs incorporate the tenets of NA into their approach and encourage patients to get actively involved with a 12-step program.

Nar-anon provides support for members of the addict's family using 12 steps modeled on the 12 steps of Al-Anon (see Chapter 28). Even if the patient refuses to accept treatment or try self-help groups, family members (who may be codependents) can be referred to Nar-anon. Codependents may experience a wide range of physical and emotional stresses as a result of another family member's addiction. Codependents often experience guilt, shame, loss of self-esteem, diminished self-confidence, and social isolation. They often believe that they are in some way to blame for the substance abuser's problems, a belief that is often fostered by the substance abuser, who is more than happy to shift responsibility to others. Codependents often engage in enabling behaviors—actions that are intended to help the substance abuser but only shield the substance abuser from the consequences of his or her behavior and therefore delay serious efforts at recovery. Codependents often resort to a variety of strategies intended to control or prevent access to drugs by the substance abuser. Such efforts are usually unsuccessful. Recovery usually occurs when the substance abuser feels the need for change and is willing to accept full responsibility for making change occur. Substance abusers who recover are motivated to change in large part by the unpleasant and painful consequences of their drug use. Nar-anon helps family members recognize and discontinue enabling behaviors and helps them cope with the physical and emotional stresses that result from living with a substance abuser.

Common Obstacles to Recovery

Many patients, particularly those in the early stages of addiction, have difficulty accepting the requirement of total abstinence. Although they might not admit it, many patients enter treatment with the unstated agenda of gaining control of their drug use rather than stopping it. They are reluctant to give up the pleasurable effects of drugs or they doubt their ability to cope with emotional distress without the relief afforded by drugs. They secretly hope to learn how to enjoy the benefits of drugs while avoiding the problems that have accompanied their drug use in the past. This is part of the process of denial. Other patients enter treatment believing that they have a problem with one type of drug but not with others. Cocaine addicts, for example, often believe that they do not have a problem with alcohol or marijuana and see no reason to give up the use of those drugs. Experience has shown, however, that continued use of non–problem drugs tends to predispose patients to relapse with their problem drug. Furthermore, patients who continue to use other drugs are less likely to make the changes in life-style that are important in maintaining recovery over the longer term.

One of the most important tasks for the patient in early recovery is to sever ties with drug users and to develop new relationships with nonusers, or at least with nonabusers. The relationships with other abusers tend to be superficial and based mainly on the shared activity of getting high. In addition to forming new relationships, the recovering addict must learn to form a new type of relationship, one that involves a level of trust, honesty, and intimacy that may seem alien to some. Such relationships are fundamental to recovery because they are the primary source of support for the addict struggling with the physical and emotional demands of recovery. During their addiction, most addicts learn to use drugs as a quick and effective, though ultimately destructive, method of dealing with physical or emotional distress. In recovery, the addict must learn other strategies to cope with distress.

The active abuse of drugs during adolescence and early adulthood seems to interfere with the development of basic social skills. In addition, addicts are often hampered by diminished self-esteem and self-confidence and by the expectation that they will be rejected by society. Meeting people for the first time and attempting to initiate new relationships generate anxiety for most people under the best circumstances. When normal social anxiety is compounded by the social and emotional deficits that characterize most addicts in early recovery, the task of forming new relationships can become so intimidating that it may be avoided altogether. The recovering addict who feels lonely or isolated is tempted to resume contact with old friends who are still using drugs.

Another important life-style change has to do with the use of leisure time. Drug use is, among other things, a recreational activity. Getting and using drugs provides a daily routine that fills time and provides stimulation and challenge. For some addicts, the enjoyment of certain aspects of the drug-oriented life-style is as important as the reinforcing effects of drug use in maintaining drug involvement. For other users, being high makes it possible to tolerate what would otherwise be a tedious daily routine. It is important for the addict in early recovery to identify new activities that will provide a reasonable amount of stimulation and satisfaction. Boredom greatly increases the risk of relapse, and the recovering addict who fails to find employment that is in some way rewarding or to develop satisfying leisure activities is in danger of relapse.

Self-help groups (see above) are an invaluable resource for people in early recovery. In addition to providing emotional support and guidance, they are the best available forum for meeting nonusers and developing new friendships. They also sponsor social and recreational activities and provide opportunities for addicts in early recovery to learn new ways of managing leisure time from people who are further along in recovery.

In summary, recovery from chemical dependency requires a multitude of changes in beliefs, relationships, and life-style. Some of the required changes are difficult to accomplish, and the need for them is not immediately apparent to many addicts. In early episodes of treatment, most addicts make some of the needed changes but not enough to avoid relapse over the long term. As a result, relapse rates among patients successfully completing treatment run as high as 80% in the year after treatment. Of course, results highly depend on how the population is selected. Socially stable higher socioeconomic groups have a better prognosis. With successive treatment episodes, however, one can hope to see a changing pattern in which periods of abstinence grow longer and periods of active drug use grow shorter. Perhaps it is best to view relapse as an indication that the patient has so far failed to make all the necessary changes needed to support an enduring recovery. Instead of regarding relapse as an indication that the patient's case is hopeless, the patient's practitioner can encourage the patient to identify the reasons for the current relapse and to make changes that will help the patient avoid a recurrence. The approach should not be very different from that of other chronic diseases such as hypertension or diabetes, in which complete cure is uncommon.

CHRONIC PAIN MANAGEMENT

Chronic pain of nonmalignant origin is not a single entity. It has a variety of causes and contributing factors. It may fit best the syndromal formulation of somatoform pain (see details in Chapter 21). Treatment may vary from behavioral and physical therapy approaches to medications, including opioids. Pain is one of the most common reasons patients consult a practitioner, yet it is often inadequately treated. There is much controversy over the long-term use of opioids for nonmalignant pain. Opioids can clearly be of benefit in some patients with chronic pain who have not responded to other pharmacologic therapies, including nonsteroidal anti-inflammatory drugs (NSAIDs), and have no history of substance abuse. Success or benefit should be measured by improvement in quality of life, as measured by greater ability to perform activities of daily life. Side effects such as respiratory depression and sedation tend to be rare in patients with chronic pain and should not prevent the proper prescribing of opioids.

Evaluation of a patient with chronic pain should include the following: (a) a pain history with specific details of the impact of pain on the patient, (b) an assessment of pain in a typical day (worst score, best score, average score, and response of pain score to pharmacologic and nonpharmacologic interventions—use of a visual analog scale, as illustrated in Chapter 13, Fig. 13.1, can be helpful), (c) a directed physical examination, (d) a review of previous diagnostic studies, (e) a review of previous interventions, (f) an alcohol and drug history, and (g) an assessment of coexisting diseases or conditions. Treatment should be based on the findings in this evaluation and the presenting cause of pain.

Patients with chronic pain require frequent visits and phone calls. Many providers view such patients as time-consuming and frustrating and as a result look to refer them to pain centers. However, referral to pain centers is often limited by insurance as a result of their cost. Most studies of the effectiveness of pain centers focus on patients with chronic back pain. A meta-analytic review of 65 studies of pain centers in the management of chronic back pain tended to show beneficial effects of pain treatment centers, but many studies were poorly designed (34). One randomized controlled study in Denmark of 189 patients with chronic pain of nonmalignant origin showed that the patient group treated at a multidisciplinary pain center had better pain relief and quality of life than the comparison group treated by a general practitioner after initial consultation by a pain specialist (35). No time or cost analysis was performed.

Nonpharmacologic therapies, including acupuncture (see Chapter 5), acupressure, exercise, hydrotherapy, biofeedback, relaxation techniques, massage, and physical therapy, should all be considered and prescribed, if appropriate, as adjuncts to the management of chronic pain (36). They provide an opportunity for patients to be active in their approach to overcoming chronic pain. Psychosocial stress and mood have an impact on pain perception and the ability to cope with pain. Patients should not lose their "identity" to their diagnosis of chronic pain, and these nonpharmacologic modalities often contribute to a better sense of well-being.

The relationship between pain and depression is complex because many patients with depression have a history of chronic pain and vice versa. Depression does lower pain tolerance and increase analgesic requirements. There has been a variety of trials using tricyclic antidepressants as adjuncts for pain control (37,38). In addition, when given at bedtime, they enable sleep, which may have a positive impact on pain during the day. Pain improvement may occur at lower than therapeutic blood levels. Nortriptyline at a dosage of 10 or 25 mg at bedtime is a usual starting point, with gradual increase of dosage depending on effect. Other antidepressants have also been found to be useful as pain management adjuncts, with paroxetine (Paxil) deserving particular mention, especially when coupled with a tricyclic antidepressant (39). Details regarding antidepressants are found in Chapter 24.

Other drugs to be considered as adjuncts for pain management include the anticonvulsants gabapentin, phenytoin, and carbamazepine. A recent meta-analysis provides some evidence from randomized controlled trials supporting the efficacy of these agents but recommends that they be withheld until other interventions have been tried (40). Gabapentin in escalating doses up to 3,600 mg/day may be particularly effective for chronic pain of neuropathic origin (41). It may be better tolerated than the other anticonvulsants and can be titrated up in dose with little side effect other than sedation. The above cited meta-analysis, however, found no statistically significant difference in toxicity (numbers needed to harm) among the three agents (40). Capsaicin, a topical substance P inhibitor, is available without prescription and is often useful

PAIN CONTRACT

1. I understand that the aim of pain management is to improve my quality of life and increase the amount of activity I can perform.

2. I understand that it is unlikely that all of my pain will be relieved.

3. I agree to pursue any/all non-medication therapies that may improve my pain.

4. I understand that narcotic pain medications used over long periods of time cause dependence and if stopped abruptly may result in withdrawal symptoms.

5. I agree to have only one provider prescribe all of my narcotic pain medications.

6. I agree to always take my pain medication as prescribed. Any changes in dose **must** be made by agreement with my provider.

7. I am responsible for my prescriptions lasting the appropriate amount of time. I understand I will not receive additional medication ahead of time.

____
Patient Signature

____
Provider Signature

Figure 29.1. Sample pain contract.

as an adjunct for treatment of postherpetic neuralgia, arthritis, diabetic neuropathy, and reflex sympathetic dystrophy. Topical lidocaine is also useful for postherpetic neuralgia.

If a trial of opioids is deemed appropriate, the provider should ensure that the patient is informed of the risks and benefits of opioid use. Most patients should have already been tried on a course of NSAIDs. The provider may choose to continue an NSAID while initiating opioid therapy. Specific conditions under which opioids will be prescribed should be agreed upon (i.e., strict adherence with directions, no telephone refills, and patient responsibility for the prescription and all pills). Only one provider should be responsible for all prescriptions related to chronic pain. A written agreement specifying these conditions may be useful (Fig. 29.1). Prescribing Controlled Drugs, above, provides additional pointers.

In general, long-acting opioids should be used for chronic pain because they reduce the need for frequent dosing, have reduced abuse liability, and alleviate pain while preventing the re-emergence of pain. Both morphine and oxycodone are available as long-acting twice a day preparations for the treatment of pain. Fentanyl is available in a transdermal patch formulation that lasts for 3 days. Transdermal fentanyl should be prescribed only to patients who are already opioid experienced. A recent multicenter controlled study found transdermal fentanyl to be superior to sustain release oral morphine in the treatment of chronic nonmalignant pain (42). Details regarding opioid analgesics are found in Chapter 13. In most patients, the effective opiate analgesic dose for chronic pain will stabilize at a set dose, without need for escalation over time and with sustained pain relief.

Review of treatment efficacy should be an ongoing process. Patients should keep a pain diary with a record of daily activity and pain scores during a typical day. Monthly follow-up visits should include a review of the pain diary, an assessment of functional status, efficacy of analgesia, drug side effects, quality of life, and any sign of medication misuse. All this information should be documented in the patient chart on each visit.

General References*

Aronoff GM, ed. Evaluation and treatment of chronic pain. Baltimore: Williams & Wilkins, 1992.

An in-depth guide to providing care to patients with chronic pain.

Brecher EM, ed. Licit and illicit drugs. Boston: Little, Brown, 1972.

Although dated, still an excellent overview of the history of drug abuse in the United States.

Gold MS, Slaby AE, eds. Dual diagnosis in substance abuse. New York: Marcel Dekker, 1991.

Review of psychiatric disorders and substance abuse.

Marlatt AG, Gordon JR, eds. Relapse prevention. New York: Guilford Press, 1985.

An excellent review of literature on relapse and relapse prevention.

*Bold print (general references) and bold numerals (specific references) denote published controlled clinical trials, meta-analyses, or consensus-based recommendations.

Mendelson JH, Mello NK. Management of cocaine abuse and dependence. N Engl J Med 1996;334:965.

O'Connor PG, Fiellin DA. Pharmacologic treatment of heroin-dependent patients. Ann Intern Med 2000;133:40.

Specific References

1. American Psychiatric Association. Diagnostic and statistical manual of mental disorders, 4th ed. (DSM-IV). Washington, DC: American Psychiatric Association, 1994.

2. Parran T Jr. Prescription drug abuse. A question of balance. Med Clin North Am 1997;81:967.

3. Deitch D. Koutsenok I. Ruiz A. The relationship between crime and drugs: what we have learned in recent decades. J Psychoactive Drugs 2000;32:391.

4. National Institute of Drug Abuse. Infofax—nationwide trends. December 2000. *www.samhsa.gov.*

5. Jasinski DR, Johnson RE, Kocher TR. Clonidine in morphine withdrawal: differential effects on signs and symptoms. Arch Gen Psychiatry 1985;42:1063.

6. Parran TV, Adelman CL, Jasinski DR. Buprenorphine detoxification of medically unstable narcotic dependent patients: a case series. Subst Abuse 1990;11:197.

7. Johnson RE, Chutuape MA, Strain EC, et al. A comparison of levomethadyl acetate, buprenorphine, and methadone for opioid dependence. N Engl J Med 2000;343:1290.

8. Chutuape MA, Jasinski DR, Fingerhood MI, et al. One-, three-, and six-month outcomes after brief inpatient opioid detoxification. Am J Drug Alcohol Abuse 2001;27:19.

9. Mouhaffel AH, Madu EC, Satmary WA, et al. Cardiovascular complications of cocaine. Chest 1995;107:1426.

10. Benzodiazepine dependence, toxicity and abuse. A Task Force Report of the American Psychiatric Association. Washington, DC: American Psychiatric Association, 1990.

11. Kupfer DJ, Reynolds CF 3rd. Management of insomnia. N Engl J Med 1997;336:341.

12. Noyes R Jr, Perry PJ, Crowe RR, et al. Seizures following the withdrawal of alprazolam. J Nerv Mental Dis 1986;174:50.

13. Shader RI, Greenblatt DJ. Use of benzodiazepines in anxiety disorders. N Engl J Med 1993;328:1398.

14. Moller HJ. Effectiveness and safety of benzodiazepines. J Clin Psychopharmacol 1999;19:2S.

15. Sullivan JT, Sellers EM. Detoxification for triazolam physical dependence. J Clin Psychopharmacol 1992;12:124.

16. Sullivan JT, Sellers EM. Treating alcohol, barbiturate and benzodiazepine withdrawal. Ration Drug Ther 1986;20:1.

17. Tashkin DP, Simmons MS, Sherrill DL, et al. Heavy habitual marijuana smoking does not cause an accelerated decline in FEV1 with age. Am J Resp Crit Care Med 1997;155:141.

18. Hollister LE. Health aspects of cannabis: revisited. Int J Neuropsychopharmacol 1998;1:71.

19. Cushman P. Plasma testosterone levels in healthy male marijuana smokers. Am J Drug Alcohol Abuse 1975;2:269.

20. Schwartz RH, Miller NS. MDMA (Ecstasy) and the rave: a review. Pediatrics 1997;100:705.

21. McCann UD, Eligulashvili V, Ricaurte GA. Methylenedioxymethamphetamine ("Ecstasy")-induced serotonin neurotoxicity: clinical studies. Neuropsychobiology 2000;42:11.

22. Fingerhood MI, Sullivan JT, Testa MP, et al. Abuse liability of testosterone. J Psychopharmacol 1997;11:65.

23. Giorgi A, Weatherby RP, Murphy PW. Muscular strength, body composition and health responses to the use of testosterone enanthate: a double blind study. J Sci Med Sport 1999;2:341.

24. Brower KJ, Blow FC, Young JP, et al. Symptoms and correlates of anabolic-androgenic steroid dependence. Br J Addict 1991;86:759.

25. Fingerhood MI, Jasinski DR, Sullivan JT. Prevalence of hepatitis C in a chemical dependence population. Arch Intern Med 1993;153:2025.

26. Thomas DL, Astemborski J, Rai RM, et al. The natural history of hepatitis C virus infection: host, viral, and environmental factors. JAMA 2000;284:450.

27. Machnick MG, Horchang HL, Peteman RR. Liver disease associated with intravenous drug abuse. In: Levine DP, Sobel JD,

eds. Infections in intravenous drug abusers. New York: Oxford University Press, 1991.
28. Centers for Disease Control and Prevention. HIV/AIDS Surveillance Report for the year 2000. www.cdc.gov/hiv/stats.
29. Khabbaz RF, Onorato IM, Cannon RO, et al. Seroprevalence of HTLV-I and HTLV-II among intravenous drug users and persons in clinics for sexually transmitted diseases. N Engl J Med 1992;326:375.
30. Gostin LO, Lazzarini Z, Jones TS, et al. Prevention of HIV/AIDS and other blood-borne diseases among injection drug users. A national survey on the regulation of syringes and needles. JAMA 1997;277:53.
31. Barnett PG. The cost-effectiveness of methadone maintenance as a health care intervention. Addiction 1999;94:479.
32. Gerstein DR, Johnson RA, Harwood H, et al. Evaluating recovery services: the California Drug and Alcohol Treatment Assessment (CALDATA). Sacramento: California Department of Alcohol and Drug Programs, 1994.
33. Miller WR, Hester RK. Inpatient alcoholism treatment: who benefits? Am Psychol 1986;41:794.
34. Flor H, Fydrich T, Turk DC. Efficacy of multidisciplinary pain treatment centers: a meta-analytic review. Pain 1992;49:221.
35. Becker N, Sjogren P, Bech P, et al. Treatment outcome of chronic non-malignant pain patients managed in a Danish multidisciplinary pain centre compared to general practice: a randomised controlled trial. Pain 2000;84:203.
36. Allegrante JP. The role of adjunctive therapy in the management of nonmalignant pain. Am J Med 1996;101:33S.
37. Godfrey RG. A guide to the understanding and use of tricycle antidepressants in the overall management of fibromyalgia and other chronic pain syndromes. Arch Intern Med 1996;156:1047.
38. Sindrup SH, Jensen TS. Efficacy of pharmacological treatments of neuropathic pain: an update and effect related to mechanism of drug action. Pain 1999;83:389.
39. Jung AC, Staiger T, Sullivan M. The efficacy of selective serotonin reuptake inhibitors for the management of chronic pain. J Gen Intern Med 1997;12:384.
40. Wiffen P, Collins S, McQuay H, et al. Anticonvulsant drugs for acute and chronic pain. Cochrane Database Syst Rev 2001; Issue 2.
41. Eckhardt K, Ammon S, Hofmann U, et al. Gabapentin enhances the analgesic effect of morphine in healthy volunteers. Anesth Analg 2000;9:1185.
42. Allan L, Hays H, Jensen NH, et al. Randomised crossover trial of transdermal fentanyl and sustained release oral morphine for treating chronic non-cancer pain. BMJ 2001;322:1154.

SECTION 4

Allergy and Infectious Diseases

CHAPTER 30

Allergy and Related Conditions

ALVIN M. SANICO, MD
MARTIN D. VALENTINE, MD

Acute and chronic conditions attributed to allergy are among the most common afflictions encountered in medical practice. Allergy is a state of increased immunologic reactivity involving immunoglobulin E (IgE) antibodies against an otherwise innocuous foreign substance. Exposure of a susceptible individual to such an allergen leads to the release of chemical mediators that can cause clinical symptoms. The term *atopy*, which is sometimes used interchangeably with allergy, pertains to the genetic predisposition to develop IgE-mediated hypersensitivity.

A genetic basis for chronic allergic disease is supported by findings of increased concordance rates in monozygotic versus dizygotic twins (1) and of familial clustering. Children of parents with allergic disease are significantly more likely to develop the same illness compared with children whose parents are not affected. Indeed, the child's probability of developing an allergic disease increases as the number of affected parent increases from 0 to 2 (2).

The interaction between genetic and environmental factors further determines an individual's likelihood of developing an allergic disease. Changes in the environment associated with a Western life-style have been noted to correlate with the increasing prevalence of atopic disease in the United States and other industrialized nations. It is hypothesized that decreased exposure to microbial antigens due to excessive hygiene early in life promotes a shift of dominance from a type 1 phenotype of helper T (T_H1) lymphocytes toward T_H2 cells (3,4). Whereas T_H1 cells produce interferon-γ, which suppresses the formation of IgE, T_H2 lymphocytes secrete interleukin-4 (IL-4) and other cytokines that induce the production of these antibodies (Fig. 30.1A).

In this chapter, conditions related to IgE-mediated hypersensitivity (except asthma, which is covered in Chapter 60) and similar disorders are discussed.

PATHOPHYSIOLOGIC BASIS FOR THE OCCURRENCE AND MANAGEMENT OF ALLERGIC DISEASE

Allergens and Immunoglobulin E Antibodies

Most clinically relevant allergens are water-soluble proteins with a molecular weight of 10 to 40 kDs that are capable of inducing IgE production and of binding to these antibodies. Examples of common environmental allergens include Amb a 1 from ragweed (*Ambrosia artemisiifolia*), Fel d 1 from cats (*Felis domesticus*), Can f 1 from dogs (*Canis familiaris*), Bla g 1 from cockroaches (*Blattella germanica*), and Der p 1 or Der f 1 from dust mites (*Dermatophagoides pteronyssinus* or *D. farinae*). Most of the animal-derived allergens belong to the lipocalin family of proteins and naturally function as proteases. Low molecular weight substances such as penicillin can be allergenic by acting as haptens that bind covalently with serum proteins to form a complex that can then interact with IgE.

Under the influence of cytokines such as IL-4 from T_H2 lymphocytes and other sources, B cells mature into plasma cells and secrete antigen-specific IgE. The presence of such antibodies is the principal basis for the development of allergic sensitivity.

Inflammatory Cells and Mediators

IgE binds to high-affinity FcϵRI receptors on the surface of mast cells and basophils. Cross-linking of these receptor-bound IgE antibodies by multivalent allergens triggers a cascade of events leading to the release of mediators. These include preformed granule-associated products (e.g., histamine), newly synthesized products of arachidonic acid metabolism (e.g., leukotrienes), cytokines, and chemokines (e.g., IL-3, -4, and -5). Depending on which organ is affected, *histamine* can cause pruritus, sneezing, rhinorrhea, bronchoconstriction, and cutaneous wheal formation. These signs and symptoms develop within minutes of allergen exposure during the *early phase* of an allergic reaction. *Leukotrienes* are more potent than histamine in causing nasal congestion and bronchoconstriction. The various *interleukins* and *tumor necrosis factor-α*,

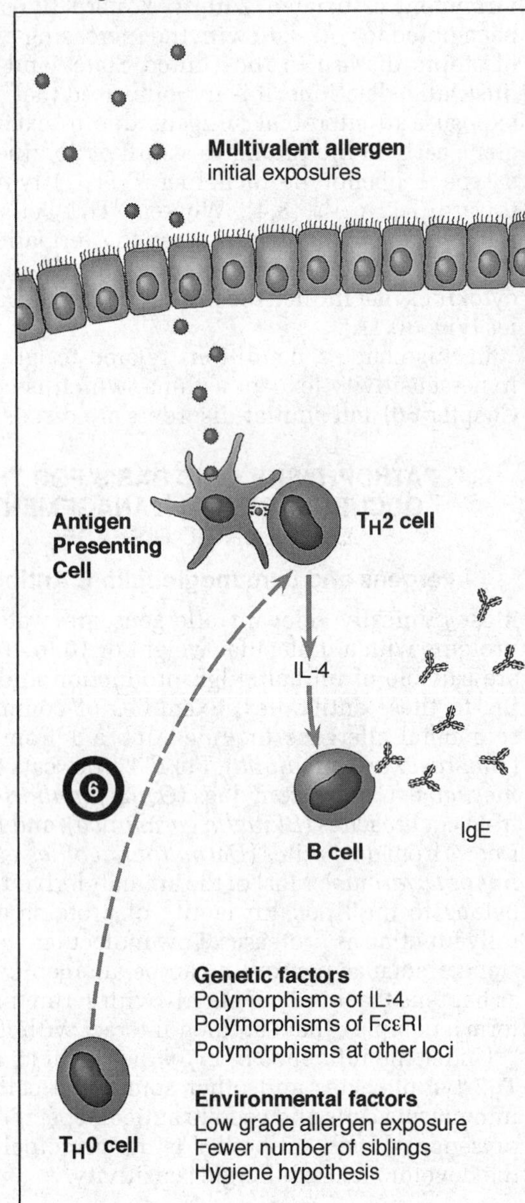

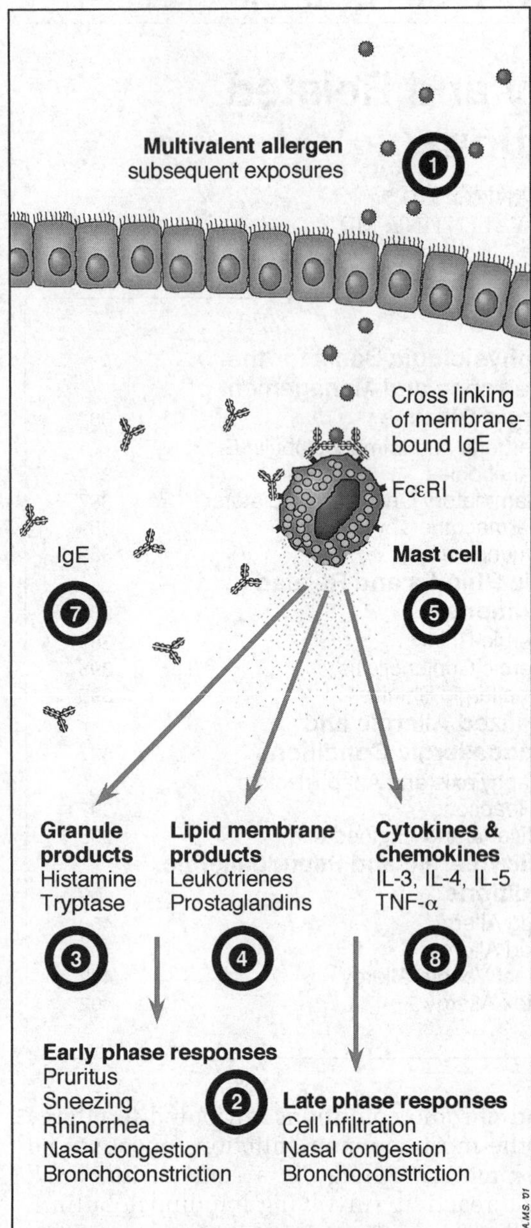

Figure 30.1. Targets for the management of allergic disease. Sensitization to specific allergens **(A)** occurs in an atopic individual, after which allergic inflammation **(B)** can develop upon subsequent re-exposures. The interaction between genetic and environmental factors promotes the development of naïve helper T (T_H0) lymphocytes into T_H2 cells. T_H2 lymphocytes interact with antigen presenting cells and consequently secrete cytokines such as interleukin-4 (*IL-4*), which induce B cells to mature into plasma cells and produce IgE antibodies. Allergic inflammation begins when multivalent allergens cross-link IgE bound to high affinity FcεRI receptors on tissue mast cells or peripheral blood basophils. This initiates a cascade of events leading to the release of granule and lipid membrane-derived products. These mediators, including histamine and leukotrienes, cause various clinical effects during the early and late phases of the allergic response. Various modes of management can be used to target components of this disease pathway. Identification and avoidance of relevant allergens is fundamental (*Target 1*). Pharmacotherapy can be directed toward amelioration of specific symptoms and/or control of the underlying inflammation. Rhinorrhea, nasal congestion, or bronchoconstriction can be specifically relieved by an anticholinergic, sympathomimetic, or beta-agonist agent, respectively (*Target 2*). The effects of histamine or of leukotrienes can be attenuated by their respective receptor antagonists (*Targets 3 and 4*). The number of allergic inflammatory cells and the production of their mediators can be reduced by glucocorticoids (*Target 5*). The shift toward a T_H2 phenotype of helper T cells and consequent production of IgE can be regulated by immunotherapy (*Target 6*). The effects of IgE can be inhibited by a newly developed monoclonal antibody that binds to it (*Target 7*). Other novel forms of treatment such as those directed against cytokines are still being investigated (*Target 8*).

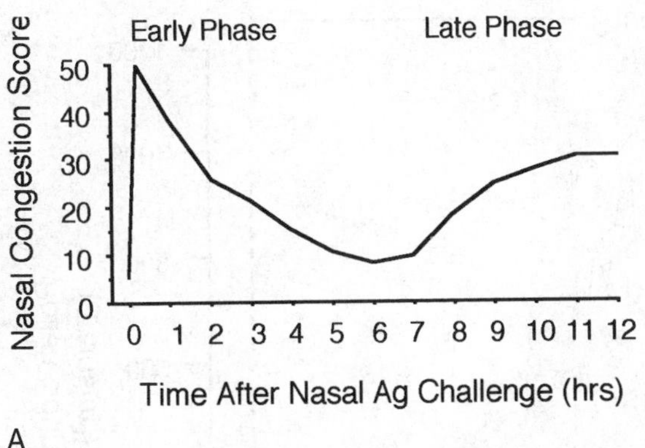

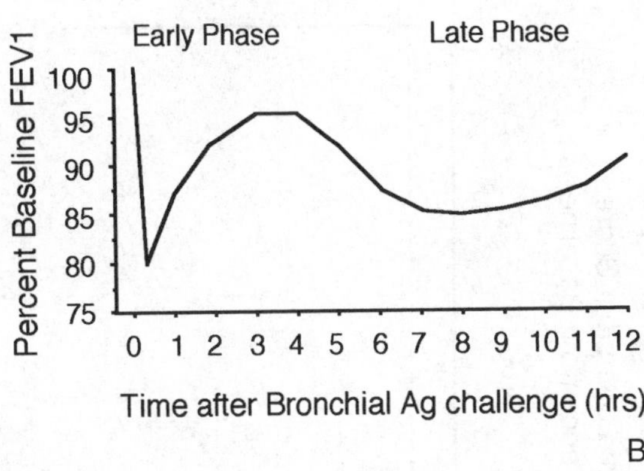

Figure 30.2. Early and late phases of the allergic response. **A:** Within 10 minutes of experimental delivery of allergen (*Ag*) into the nose of subjects with allergic rhinitis, nasal congestion develops and then spontaneously subsides. In 40% to 60% of these individuals, nasal congestion recurs several hours thereafter, during the late phase of the allergic response. **B:** Similarly, inhalation of allergen causes an immediate but transient decrease in forced expiratory volume (FEV_1) in subjects with allergic asthma. In the same proportion of individuals, narrowing of the lower airways may again develop several hours after allergen exposure.

among others, promote local tissue infiltration by cells such as eosinophils 6 to 12 hours after allergen exposure. During this period of the *late phase* response, manifestations of allergy such as nasal congestion and bronchoconstriction may recur (Fig. 30.2).

Pharmacotherapy

Various therapeutic agents can be used to block one or more components of the allergic inflammatory pathway (Fig. 30.1B). Limited symptomatic relief can be achieved by targeting specific end results such as rhinorrhea, nasal congestion, or bronchoconstriction. For example, anticholinergic agents can be used to inhibit mucus secretions, sympathomimetic vasoconstrictors can reduce nasal congestion, whereas beta-adrenergic agonists can reverse bronchoconstriction by activating adenylate cyclase with resultant increase in adenosine 3′,5′-monophosphate. Broader benefits may be attained with antagonists against receptors of mediators such as histamine or leukotrienes. More potent agents such as glucocorticoids have multiple effects, including the reduction of inflammatory cells and of the production or release of their mediators. A monoclonal antibody against IgE recently has been shown in clinical trials to be effective in ameliorating allergic airway disease (5). Cytokine-directed therapies such as antibodies against IL-5 have been developed, but so far they have not achieved significant clinical success (6).

Immunotherapy

Repeated administration of low concentrations of specific allergens has been shown to be highly effective in the management of patients with allergic airways disease or with insect venom hypersensitivity. Immunotherapy induces a shift from a T_H2 to a T_H1 profile of cytokine production with consequent reduction in levels of IgE (Fig. 30.1A), an increase in IgG antibodies that can block the effects of IgE, a decrease in allergen-induced release of mediators, and a reduction in the number of infiltrating allergic inflammatory cells (7).

ALLERGIC RHINITIS AND RELATED CONDITIONS

Allergic Rhinitis

Prevalence, Cost, and Comorbidities

Allergic rhinitis is the most common chronic atopic disease. It is estimated to affect up to 20% of the adult population and up to a total of 40 million people in the United States (8). Its prevalence has been increasing, especially in industrialized countries. Direct and indirect costs associated with this condition amount to several billions of dollars annually (8). While direct costs are related to medications and clinic visits, indirect costs include reduced productivity and quality of life (9). Affected patients have been shown to have decreased cognitive ability, psychomotor speed, verbal learning, and memory during the allergy season (10). These can be due to the disease itself and/or the sedating effects of certain medications used (11). The impact of allergic rhinitis is further magnified by the fact that it contributes to several comorbidities (12). For example, it can predispose a patient to develop recurrent sinusitis, putatively due to impaired clearance of mucus secretions. Allergic inflammation leads to mucosal swelling with resultant obstruction of sinus openings at the ostiomeatal complex (13). In addition, eosinophil-derived products such as major basic protein can disrupt normal ciliary activity (14). In the same manner, uncontrolled allergic rhinitis can contribute to the development of recurrent eustachian tube dysfunction and otitis media in children (15).

Allergic conjunctivitis, commonly seen in conjunction with allergic rhinitis, is addressed later in this chapter.

Association With Asthma

Allergic rhinitis is closely associated with asthma, and together they are becoming more recognized as part of one and the same disease process. Such a condition of concomitant allergic rhinitis and asthma has been named allergic rhinobronchitis by some authors (16). This entity may perhaps be simply termed *chronic allergic respiratory disease.* Up to nine of ten patients

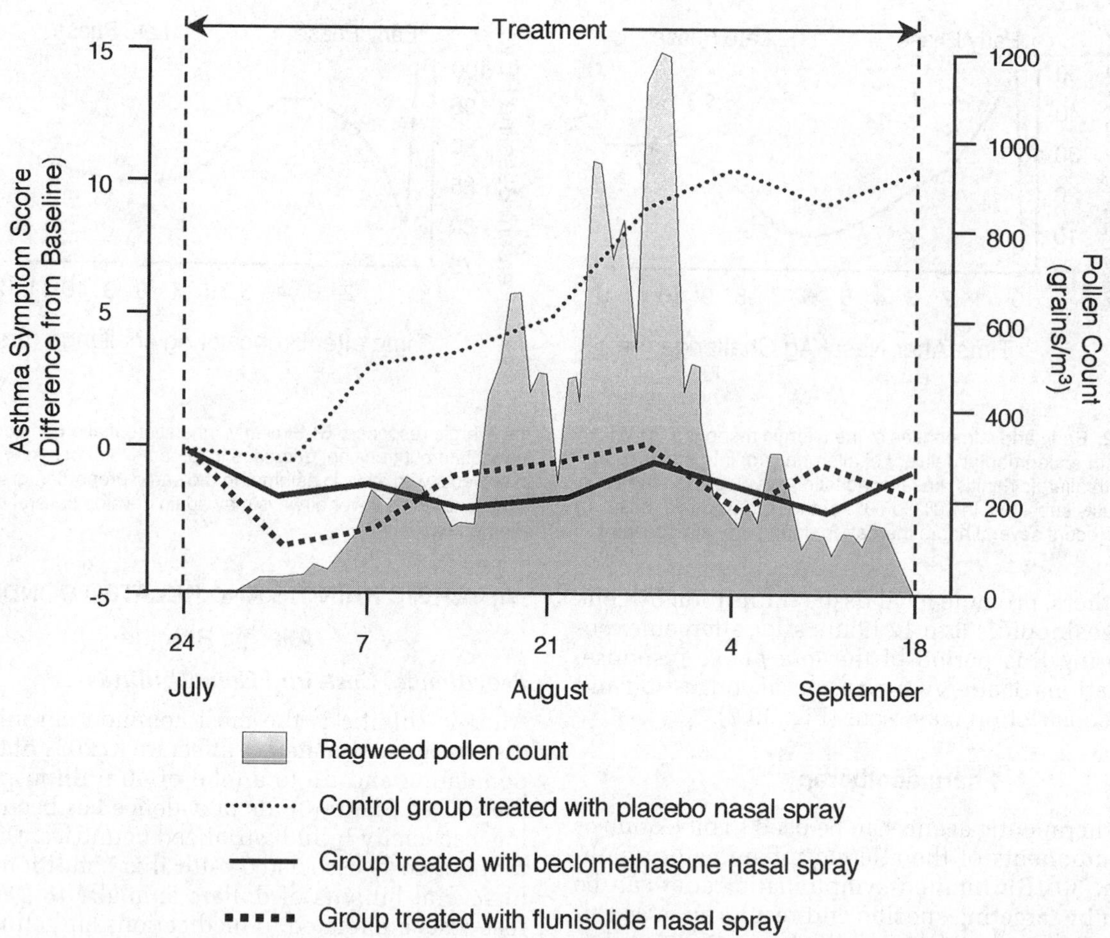

Figure 30.3. Improvement in asthma with treatment of allergic rhinitis. Asthma symptom scores of ragweed-sensitive individuals treated with placebo nasal sprays increase as the pollen count rises during the fall season. In contrast, active treatment of allergic rhinitis with beclomethasone or flunisolide nasal sprays not only improves nasal symptoms but also prevents allergen-induced exacerbation of asthma. (Adapted from Welsh P, Stricker W, Chu C, et al. Efficacy of beclomethasone nasal solution, flunisolide, and cromolyn in relieving symptoms of ragweed allergy. Mayo Clin Proc 1987;62:125.)

with asthma have symptoms of rhinitis (17). Interestingly, even the few asthmatics that deny having upper airway symptoms can be shown to have subclinical evidence of allergic inflammation in nasal tissue biopsies (18). On the other hand, most patients with allergic rhinitis have no symptoms of asthma. This group may represent an earlier and/or milder form of chronic allergic respiratory disease. Of note, some individuals with allergic rhinitis and no apparent asthma exhibit bronchial hyper-responsiveness upon inhalational challenge with methacholine (19). Patients with allergic rhinitis have a significantly greater chance of subsequently developing overt asthma compared with individuals without a history of chronic nasal symptoms. Among asthmatics, those who have more severe allergic rhinitis tend to have worse outcomes. For example, they have more frequent asthma exacerbations and sleep disturbance (20). The effect of rhinitis on asthma may be due to several factors, such as mouth breathing because of significant nasal obstruction. This prevents warming, humidification, and filtering by the nasal passages of air inspired into the lower airways. Furthermore, exposure of the nasal mucosa to relevant allergens can lead to a widespread allergic inflammatory response. Indeed, localized allergen provocation of the nose induces inflammation not only in the nasal mucosa but also in bronchial tissue (21). Corollary to these observations, treatment with intranasal glucocorticoids improves both the nasal and chest symptoms of patients with concomitant allergic rhinitis and asthma (22) (Fig. 30.3). It is thus important to evaluate and manage both the upper and lower airways in such patients.

Manifestations, Etiology, and Evaluation

The typical symptoms of allergic rhinitis include, in decreasing order of frequency, paroxysmal sneezing, nasal pruritus, nasal congestion, rhinorrhea, and postnasal drip. One or more of these symptoms may predominate and may be the focus of therapy. The temporal pattern and chronicity of symptoms, as well as pertinent exacerbating and alleviating factors, should be determined. Our survey of 412 individuals with allergic rhinitis showed that 17% experience symptoms year-round, 41% have strictly seasonal symptoms, and 42% reported perennial symptoms with seasonal exacerbations (Fig. 30.4). *Seasonal symptoms* during spring, summer, or fall may indicate sensitivity

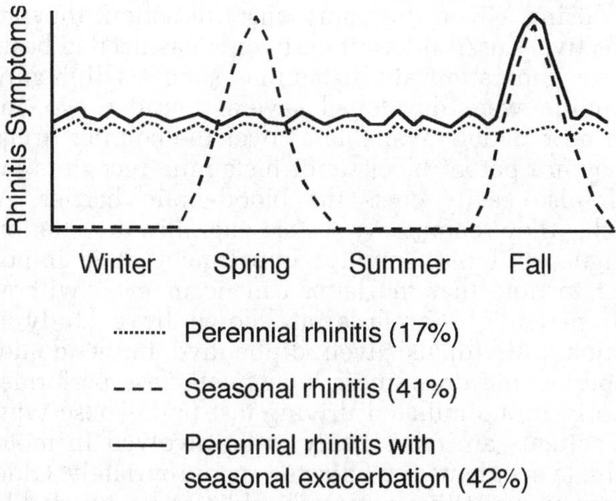

Figure 30.4. Temporal patterns of allergic rhinitis. The temporal pattern of rhinitis symptoms may indicate the environmental allergens to which an individual is sensitive. Our survey of 412 individuals with allergic rhinitis shows that 17% have symptoms year-round, 41% have symptoms only during certain seasons, and 42% have year-round symptoms with seasonal exacerbations.

Table 30.1. Reported Triggers of Allergic Rhinitis Symptoms

Trigger	Patients affected (%)
Pollens	91
Animals	79
Tobacco smoke	71
Other irritants	69
Cold dry air	57

Adapted from Diemer FB, Sanico AM, Horowitz E, et al. Non-allergenic inhalant triggers in seasonal and perennial allergic rhinitis. J. Allergy Clin Immunol 1999;103:S2.

to tree, grass, or weed pollens, respectively. *Perennial symptoms* may be attributable to indoor sources of airborne allergens such as dust mites, fur-bearing pets, cockroaches, or rodents. In addition, irritants such as tobacco smoke and cold dry air can also trigger symptoms of rhinitis (23) (Table 30.1). This could be due to an exaggerated responsiveness of sensory nerves in the nasal mucosa in the setting of allergic inflammation (24).

In evaluating the patient, the temporal pattern of symptoms and details regarding environmental exposure at home and at work should be obtained. Physical examination may reveal boggy nasal turbinates and clear nasal secretions. The peripheral blood typically shows eosinophilia during exacerbations. The presence, if any, of other confounding anatomic abnormalities such as septal deviation or nasal polyps should be noted.

Management

The three main components of the management of allergic rhinitis are allergen avoidance, pharmacotherapy, and immunotherapy. Treatment options are chosen in a stepwise fashion based on the frequency and severity of symptoms (Fig. 30.5). Management of ocular symptoms is described later in this chapter.

Allergen Avoidance. Environmental control measures should be based on a careful assessment of allergen sensitivity. The presence of allergen-specific IgE antibodies can be established through skin testing *in vivo* or *radioallergosorbent testing* of blood samples *in vitro*. During skin testing, small concentrations of various allergen extracts are introduced through superficial punctures or through intradermal injections on the arms or back. Skin testing provides immediate results and is generally more cost effective than *in vitro* testing. Results of these tests should be correlated with the patient's history to determine their clinical relevance. The temporal pattern of symptoms and of exposures should be clarified. For example, a positive skin test with dust mite allergen would be more relevant for an individual with perennial, rather than strictly seasonal, symptoms.

Dust Mites. Allergens of dust mites are contained in their fecal matter (25) and are mostly found in bedding. These arachnids feed on human skin flakes that are normally shed on a daily basis. They are ubiquitous in humid regions but are rare in arid areas. The following measures are clinically effective in reducing exposure to these allergens:

1. Encase pillows and mattresses with dust mite-proof zippered covers that have a pore size $<10\ \mu m$ (26).
2. Wash bedding with hot ($>130°F$) water every 1 to 2 weeks to kill dust mites on the surface and denature their allergens (27).
3. Maintain relative humidity below 50%, with a dehumidifier as needed, to reduce the dust mite population (28).
4. Avoid placement of carpeting, stuffed toys, and other materials in the bedroom that can harbor these creatures.

Because dust mite particles are relatively large and thus do not remain constantly airborne, high efficiency particulate air filters are not effective in eliminating

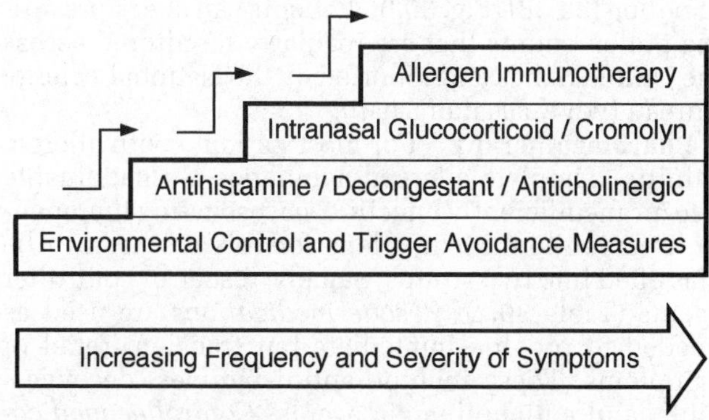

Figure 30.5. Stepwise management of allergic rhinitis. The modes of treatment are chosen based on the frequency and severity of rhinitis symptoms. The first step involves identification and avoidance of relevant allergens and other triggers. Relief of symptoms can be achieved with an antihistamine, decongestant, and/or anticholinergic agent as needed. For persistent disease, control of allergic inflammation can be attained with intranasal glucocorticoids or cromolyn. If these measures do not provide satisfactory improvement, allergen immunotherapy should be considered.

these allergens (29). Likewise, application of so-called acaricides has not been proven to be consistently beneficial on a long-term basis (30).

Pets. Any fur-bearing animal can potentially cause allergic sensitization in a genetically predisposed individual. Cat allergy has been extensively studied in this regard. The allergenic proteins of cats mostly come from their sebaceous and salivary glands and are deposited onto the skin and fur (31). There can be significant variability in the levels of allergen shedding among cats (32). The most effective way to minimize exposure to such allergens in the home unfortunately entails complete removal of the pet. Confining the cat to other parts of the home outside the patient's bedroom and using a high efficiency particulate air filter has been advised empirically. However, a recent study indicates that although these measures can reduce cat allergen levels, a degree of exposure remains that precludes any significant clinical improvement (33). This illustrates that even relatively low levels of allergens are sufficient to cause respiratory symptoms. Washing the cat can reduce levels of airborne allergens, but this effect is not sustained and its clinical benefit has not been proven (34). If and when patients comply with complete removal of the cat, they should be aware that residual allergens could persist up to 6 months later. Elimination of carpeting and thorough cleaning of the walls can facilitate the decline of allergen levels (35). Exposure to animal allergens can also occur outside the home, as shown by findings of significant levels of cat and dog allergens in school buildings (36). Cat allergens in particular tend to adhere to material surfaces and can thus be transported via clothing (37).

Pollens. Complete avoidance of outdoor allergens such as pollens is more difficult to achieve. Keeping the windows closed and using air-conditioning while indoors may help minimize exposure to tree, grass, and weed allergens that are typically prevalent during the spring, summer, and fall seasons, respectively. Multiple studies have documented exacerbation of symptoms among untreated patients in parallel with levels of pollen (22,38) (Fig. 30.6). Patients can check prevailing pollen counts that are regularly monitored across the United States and reported by the National Allergy Bureau (www.aaaai.org/nab).

Pharmacotherapy. For most patients with allergic rhinitis, complete allergen avoidance is unattainable and/or insufficiently effective, necessitating therapeutic intervention. Medications for this disease can be classified into two groups, namely, rescue or controller agents (Table 30.2). *Rescue medications* are used as needed to provide immediate but transient relief of symptoms. These include antihistamines, decongestants, and anticholinergic agents. *Controller medications* are optimally used on a regular daily basis to mitigate the underlying pathology of allergic inflammation. These include topical glucocorticoids and cromolyn sodium.

Histamine-1 Receptor Antagonists. Antihistamines significantly reduce symptoms of paroxysmal sneezing, pruritus, and rhinorrhea within 1 to 3 hours of dosing. Given this rapid onset of action, they are effectively used intermittently on an as-needed basis. Older generation antihistamines such as diphenhydramine were developed several decades ago and are now widely available as over the counter drugs. They are potent blockers of histamine receptors but can also easily cross the blood–brain barrier. As such, they commonly cause significant sedation, fatigue, and psychomotor impairment. It is important to note that the latter can occur even without the patient's awareness, as shown by a study in which individuals given diphenhydramine denied experiencing drowsiness but nonetheless performed poorly in a simulated driving test (39). These types of patients are more likely to be involved in motor vehicle accidents if medicated inappropriately. Older generation antihistamines should also be avoided by anyone operating machinery, because they have been associated with serious work accidents more than any other medication (40). The cost benefit of these agents should thus be weighed against the risk of serious psychomotor impairment and consequent injury. The newer generation antihistamines (Table 30.3) are comparatively more expensive but offer advantages over their older counterparts. They do not readily cross the blood–brain barrier and thus cause little or no central nervous system effects at regular doses (41). Two drugs in this class, terfenadine and astemizole, are associated with the development of cardiac dysrhythmias, particularly when used together with medications such as erythromycin or ketoconazole (42). For this reason, both these antihistamines have been taken off the market in the United States.

Most of the new antihistamines are derivatives of agents developed earlier. For example, cetirizine and fexofenadine are metabolites of hydroxyzine and terfenadine, respectively. The new antihistamines have significantly better safety profiles compared with their parent compounds (42).

Decongestants. Antihistamines readily relieve rhinitis symptoms with the exception of nasal congestion. For this specific condition, oral beta-adrenergic agonists such as pseudoephedrine may be considered. The common side effects of this medication include insomnia, anxiety, restlessness, and tachycardia. It should be avoided in patients with severe hypertension or coronary artery disease. Phenylpropanolamine, another decongestant that has been available for decades, was recently removed from the U.S. market after being implicated in several cases of hemorrhagic stroke (43). Combinations of an antihistamine and pseudoephedrine (Table 30.3) may provide broader symptomatic relief than either agent alone.

Intranasal decongestant sprays such as naphazoline, oxymetazoline, and xylometazoline are available as over the counter medications. These should not be used for more than 3 to 5 days. Otherwise, rebound nasal congestion and rhinitis medicamentosa could develop. Patients with narrow angle glaucoma, hypertension, coronary artery disease, or prostatic hypertrophy should avoid these agents.

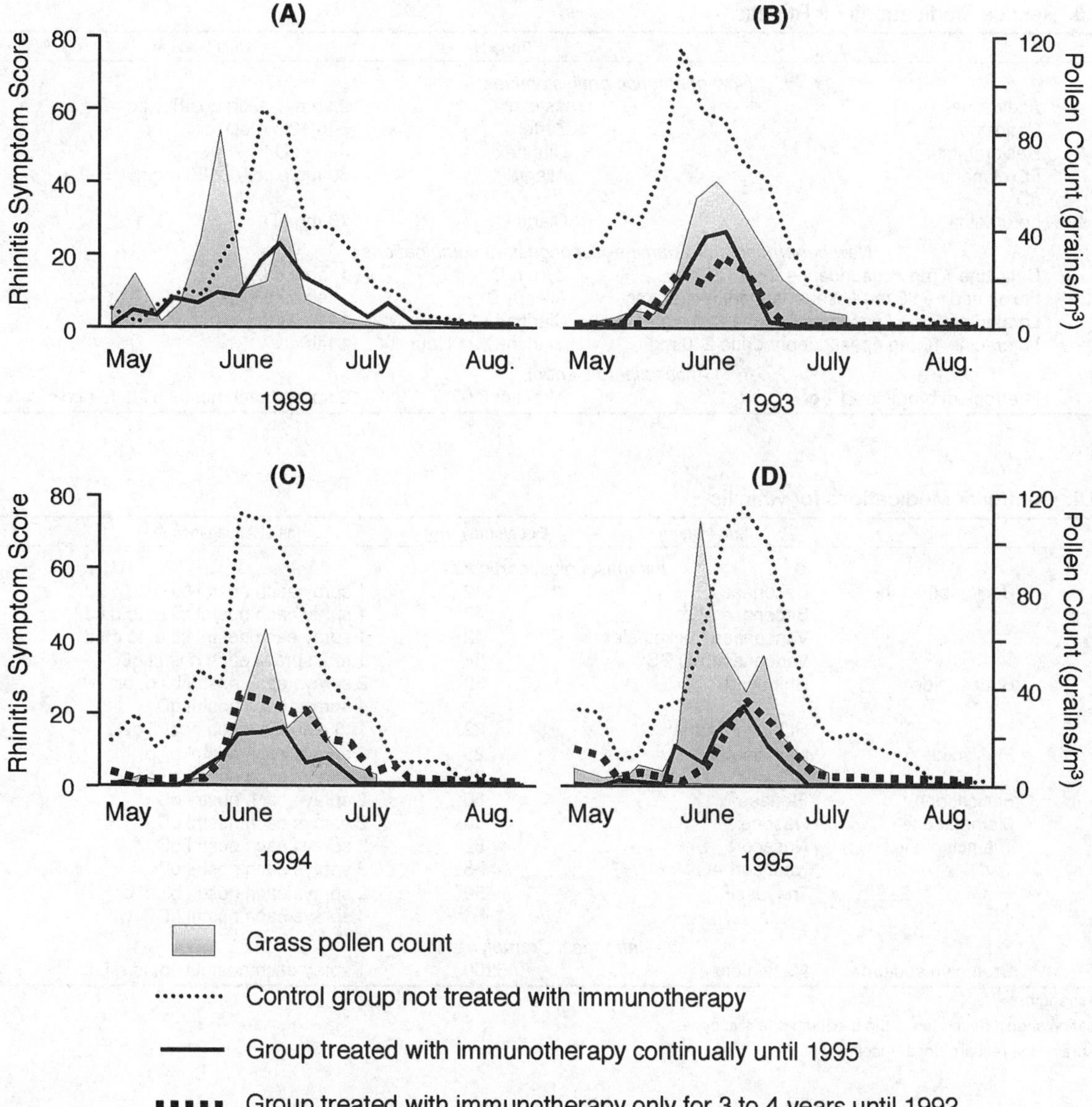

Figure 30.6. Long-term improvement of allergic rhinitis with immunotherapy. Symptom scores of control subjects with seasonal allergic rhinitis increased as grass pollen count rose during the summer season **(A to D)**. In contrast, those who underwent immunotherapy experienced significantly decreased nasal symptoms within 1 year of treatment (A). Those who received continuous immunotherapy consistently had lower rhinitis symptom scores throughout the study (B to D). Interestingly, even those who stopped receiving immunotherapy after 3 to 4 years of treatment experienced extended relief of symptoms (B to D). (Adapted from Durham S, Walker S, Varga E, et al. Long-term clinical efficacy of grass-pollen immunotherapy. N Engl J Med 1999;341:468.)

Table 30.2. Types of Medications for Allergic Rhinitis

Rescue medications taken as needed to relieve symptoms
Oral or intranasal antihistamines
Oral or intranasal decongestants
Oral antihistamine–decongestant combinations
Intranasal anticholinergic agent
Controller medications taken regularly to reduce inflammation
Intranasal glucocorticoids
Intranasal cromolyn

Intranasal Anticholinergic Agent. For patients with persistent rhinorrhea, ipratropium bromide 0.03% intranasal spray may be beneficial (Table 30.3). It can reduce the production of nasal secretions but does not significantly ameliorate other symptoms of rhinitis (44). Possible side effects include excessive nasal dryness and epistaxis.

Intranasal Glucocorticoids. Topical intranasal glucocorticoids are the most effective medications for persistent allergic rhinitis (45). Used prophylactically, they can attenuate the development of inflammation and of nasal symptoms during the early and late phases of the allergic response (46). Their onset of action can be rapidly evident within 1 day of treatment (47–49). As such, studies have demonstrated favorable results even if they are only used intermittently as needed (50). However, these medications are optimally effective when used on a

Table 30.3. Rescue Medications for Rhinitis

Drug	Trade Name	Adult Dosage
New-generation antihistamines		
Azelastine	Astelin	2 sprays each nostril b.i.d.
Cetirizine	Zyrtec	5 to 10 mg qD
Desloratadine	Clarinex	5 mg qD
Fexofenadine	Allegra	60 mg b.i.d. or 180 mg qD
qD		
Loratadine	Claritin	10 mg qD
New-generation antihistamine–decongestant combinations		
Cetirizine 5 mg / pseudoephedrine 120 mg	Zyrtec-D	1 tab b.i.d.
Fexofenadine 60 mg / pseudoephedrine 120 mg	Allegra-D	1 tab b.i.d.
Loratadine 5 mg / pseudoephedrine 120 mg	Claritin-D 12 Hour	1 tab b.i.d.
Loratadine 10 mg / pseudoephedrine 240 mg	Claritin-D 24 Hour	1 tab qD
Anticholinergic agent		
Ipratropium bromide 21 μg	Atrovent 0.03%	2 sprays each nostril b.i.d. to t.i.d.

Table 30.4. Controller Medications for Rhinitis

Drug	Trade Name	Dose/spray (μg)	Initial Adult Dosage[a]
Intranasal glucocorticoids			
Beclomethasone	Beconase	42	1 spray each nostril b.i.d. to q.i.d.
	Beconase AQ[b]	42	1 spray each nostril b.i.d. to q.i.d.
	Vancenase Pockethaler	42	1 spray each nostril b.i.d. to q.i.d.
	Vancenase AQ DS[b]	84	1 to 2 sprays each nostril qD
Budesonide	Rhinocort	32	2 sprays each nostril b.i.d. or 4 sprays each nostril qD
	Rhinocort Aqua[b]	32	1 to 4 sprays each nostril qD
Flunisolide	Nasalide[b]	25	2 sprays each nostril b.i.d.
	Nasarel[b]	25	2 sprays each nostril b.i.d.
Fluticasone	Flonase[b]	50	2 sprays each nostril qD
Mometasone	Nasonex[b]	50	2 sprays each nostril qD
Triamcinolone	Nasacort	55	2 sprays each nostril qD
	Nasacort AQ[b]	55	2 sprays each nostril qD
	Tri-Nasal[b]	50	2 sprays each nostril b.i.d. or 4 sprays each nostril qD
Intranasal Cromolyn			
Cromolyn sodium	Nasalcrom	5200	1 spray each nostril t.i.d. to q.i.d.

DS, double strength.

[a]The medication should be titrated to the minimum effective dose.

[b]Aqueous sprays; the rest are dry aerosol sprays.

regular daily basis. Although the various intranasal glucocorticoids are comparable in terms of clinical efficacy, they have significant differences in their bioavailability (45,51). Nonetheless, they do not cause any significant suppression of the hypothalamic–pituitary–adrenal axis when used at recommended doses (51). As in the case for any nasal spray, they can cause local irritation, particularly in the beginning of treatment when ongoing inflammation makes sensory nerves more sensitive to stimuli. To improve compliance, it may be best to give patients a choice of using either an aqueous solution or a dry aerosolized spray (Table 30.4). Some individuals may find liquid nasal sprays soothing, but others may find it more bothersome than dry sprays. Mild epistaxis can occur, especially when the nasal mucosa becomes too dry, in which case saline nasal sprays may be of benefit. Because anecdotal cases of septal perforation have been reported in association with intranasal sprays, patients should be monitored for the development of any mucosal erosion or incessant bleeding (52). Chronic use of intranasal glucocorticoids itself has not been associated with any detrimental histologic changes such as atrophy (53–55). Intranasal glucocorticoids do not have to be discontinued if the patient incidentally develops an upper respiratory infection, because these medications do not affect the course of such an infection (56).

Chronic or recurrent use of oral or parenteral glucocorticoids for allergic rhinitis is not advisable because of their potential systemic adverse effects.

Intranasal Cromolyn Sodium. Abatement of allergic inflammation can also be achieved with the use of intranasal cromolyn sodium. It typically has to be used up to four times daily to attain optimal benefit (Table 30.4).

Leukotriene Modifiers. The use of leukotriene receptor antagonists and 5-lipoxygenase inhibitors has been shown to provide modest improvement of allergic rhinitis symptoms, especially of nasal congestion (57,58). Cysteinyl leukotrienes are released upon nasal provocation with allergen and cause vasodilatation with resultant nasal mucosal swelling (59). However, their role in the development of other rhinitis symptoms is limited. As expected, the combination of a leukotriene modifier and antihistamine has been shown to be more effective than either agent alone (60). Certain combinations can be comparable in effectiveness with an intranasal glucocorticoid (61). Although allergic rhinitis alone is presently not an indication for the use of leukotriene modifiers, these medications may offer an additional benefit when used for concomitant asthma (see information about available leukotriene modifiers in Chapter 60).

Immunotherapy. Immunotherapy should be considered for patients who do not satisfactorily respond to environmental control measures and pharmacotherapy, can neither tolerate nor consistently comply with the use of medications, or prefer long-term amelioration of their frequent symptoms of allergic rhinitis. The choice of specific allergens used for this mode of treatment should be tailored according to the individual's clinically relevant skin test or *in vitro* test results. Appropriately dosed allergen immunotherapy can be thoroughly effective alone or in combination with medications. Improvement is typically evident within 1 year of beginning treatment, which should then be continued for 3 to 5 years. Data from a long-term study has shown that clinical benefit can endure several years after discontinuation of immunotherapy (38) (Fig. 30.6).

Anaphylactic reactions related to immunotherapy, albeit rare, can occur, particularly during the initial build-up phase. Most such reactions develop within 20 to 30 minutes of the allergen injection (62). This form of treatment should thus be administered only under the supervision of an appropriately trained physician, and patients should remain in the clinic under observation for at least 30 minutes. Personnel, equipment, and medications required for the management of anaphylaxis (discussed later in this chapter) should be readily available. Immunotherapy should not be administered to patients with ongoing cardiac or pulmonary instability. Alternative forms of treatment should also be considered in patients using beta-blockers that could make them less responsive to epinephrine if needed for anaphylaxis. Dosing of allergen extracts should be adjusted accordingly if either systemic or large local reactions develop.

Novel Therapy. Immunomodulation to treat allergic respiratory diseases can also be achieved using novel agents such as omalizumab. This is a humanized monoclonal antibody that links to IgE, thereby preventing the binding of Igϵ to high-affinity FcϵRI receptors on mast cells and basophils. Clinical trials have demonstrated its efficacy in rapidly reducing serum levels of free Igϵ and subsequently ameliorating symptoms of allergic respiratory disease. It is not allergen specific and does not appear to induce anaphylaxis (5). Anti-IgE may thus potentially play a role in the management of allergic rhinitis in the future.

Consultation With an Allergist. In the assessment and care of patients with allergic rhinitis, consultation with an allergist may be considered for several reasons:

- Identification of specific allergens and other factors that are driving the disease process;
- Insufficient and/or adverse response of the patient to medications;
- Need for patient education regarding allergen avoidance measures;
- Consideration of allergen immunotherapy.

Prognosis

A longitudinal study (63) showed that at follow-up after 23 years, about 23% of individuals with allergic rhinitis reported being symptom free, whereas 32% noted improvement in their disease. The condition was reported to be unchanged in 33%, worse in 9%, and in the remaining 3% of patients the data were not available. The probability of improvement tends to increase with younger age at onset of symptoms. There was improvement in 85% of individuals whose symptoms started at ages 1 to 5 years and in only 39% of those whose symptoms started at age greater than 20 years.

Allergic Conjunctivitis

Evaluation

Ocular symptoms often accompany allergic rhinitis. Surveys indicate that up to 88% of patients with nasal symptoms also develop itchy, watery, red, teary, and/or swollen eyes. In parallel with rhinitis symptoms, these can occur on a seasonal or perennial basis. Studies in children indicate that it is also possible to have allergic conjunctivitis as the single manifestation of atopy. On physical examination, hyperemia and edema of the conjunctivae, termed chemosis, may be noted bilaterally.

Management

As in rhinitis, the first step in the management of allergic conjunctivitis is the identification and avoidance of offending factors. Cold compresses may provide symptomatic relief. The application of preservative-free artificial tears may help clear the eyes of allergens. For more persistent symptoms, pharmacotherapy with various ophthalmic solutions can provide benefit. These include antihistamines that reduce ocular itching, topical decongestants that reduce redness and swelling, and mast cell stabilizers and other similar agents that ameliorate the underlying inflammation (Table 30.5). As in allergic rhinitis, immunotherapy has likewise been shown to significantly ameliorate symptoms of allergic conjunctivitis (64).

Nonallergic Rhinitis

Description

Recurrent nasal symptoms can occur independent of IgE, in which case tests for sensitivity to suspected allergens are negative. Various studies in different clinical settings indicate that 17% to 52% of chronic

Table 30.5. Medications for Allergic Conjunctivitis

Classification Drug	Trade Name	Adult Dosage
Ophthalmic antihistamines		
Emedastine	Emadine	1 drop each eye q.i.d.
Levocabastine	Livostin	1 drop each eye q.i.d.
Oral antihistamines		
See Table 30.3		
Mast cell stabilizers		
Cromolyn	Crolom	1 to 2 drops each eye 4 to 6 times daily
Lodoxamide	Alomide	1 to 2 drops each eye q.i.d.
Pemirolast	Alamast	1 to 2 drops each eye q.i.d.
Nedocromil	Alocril	1 to 2 drops each eye b.i.d.
Ophthalmic antihistamines/Mast cell stabilizers		
Azelastine	Optivar	1 drop each eye b.i.d.
Ketotifen	Zaditor	1 drop each eye b.i.d. to t.i.d.
Olopatadine	Patanol	1 drop each eye b.i.d.
Ophthalmic nonsteroidal anti-inflammatory agents		
Ketorolac	Acular	1 drop each eye q.i.d.
Ophthalmic decongestants		
Naphazoline	Vasocon	1 to 2 drops each eye q.i.d.

rhinitis cases have a nonallergic etiology (65). It is difficult to predict whether or not an individual's nasal complaints are IgE mediated simply based on their triggers. Of note, allergic rhinitis symptoms can be triggered not only by allergens but also by nonallergenic irritants such as tobacco smoke and cold dry air (23) (Table 30.1). On the other hand, the age at onset of symptoms can help predict whether a patient has allergic or *nonallergic rhinitis* (NAR). The likelihood of obtaining a positive allergy skin test is greater than 90% if the symptoms began before age 10 years but is less than 40% after age 40 (66). Other details in the history may help differentiate allergic rhinitis from NAR. Symptoms of NAR typically occur year-round, whereas the pattern for allergic rhinitis could be perennial, seasonal, or perennial with seasonal exacerbation (Fig. 30.4). In contrast to allergic rhinitis, NAR is less frequently associated with pruritus, ocular symptoms, concomitant asthma, or a family history of atopy. Gender may also be a risk factor for NAR, as one study showed that 71% of patients with NAR are female compared with 55% in a group with allergic rhinitis (65).

In most cases of NAR, the exact *pathophysiology* is difficult to establish. The commonly used term vasomotor rhinitis may be a misnomer because it suggests an established disease mechanism. Research studies indicate that 15% to 33% of patients with NAR have more than 10% eosinophilia in nasal smears and/or elevated eosinophil cationic protein in nasal fluids and are thus diagnosed with nonallergic rhinitis with eosinophilia syndrome (NARES) (65).

There are several possible *etiologic or contributory factors* for chronic recurrent nasal symptoms in a nonatopic individual (Table 30.6). Rhinorrhea induced by eating spicy foods is termed gustatory rhinitis, which is a reflex response likely involving capsaicin-sensitive and vagal nerve fibers. Nasal obstruction may be related to structural changes due to septal deformities, nasal polyps, granulomatous diseases such as sarcoidosis or Wegener granulomatosis, and benign and malignant tumors of the nasopharynx. Radiographic studies such as sinus computed tomography may be useful in evaluating these possibilities when strongly suspected. Referral to an otorhinolaryngologist is warranted if any of these conditions is discovered. *Pregnancy* may also produce NAR symptoms, which typically increase during the early and late gestational periods and decline postpartum. These develop putatively in association with hormonal and/or vascular physiologic changes. Rhinitis symptoms can commonly occur due to *upper respiratory infection,* which may be characterized by mucopurulent discharge and painful sinuses (see Chapter 33). These are usually self-limited if it is viral or otherwise responsive to appropriate antibiotics if it is bacterial in origin.

Recurrent rhinorrhea and/or nasal congestion can also be associated with certain over the counter and prescription drugs (Table 30.7). For example, prolonged use of intranasal decongestant sprays may lead to rebound congestion and *rhinitis medicamentosa.* This condition is characterized by a hyperemic and edematous nasal mucosa that becomes progressively unresponsive to vasoconstricting agents.

Table 30.6. Possible Causes of Nonallergic Rhinitis Symptoms

Structural
Septal deformities
Granulomatous disease
Nasal polyps
Nasopharyngeal neoplasms
Hormonal
Pregnancy
Hypothyroidism
Infectious
Bacterial upper respiratory infection
Viral upper respiratory infection
Medications
See Table 30.7

Table 30.7. Examples of Medications Reported to Cause Symptoms of Rhinitis

α-Adrenergic antagonists
Prazosin, tamsulosin, terazosin
Angiotensin inhibitors or antagonists
Benazepril, candesartan, lisinopril, losartan, trandolapril, others
β-Adrenergic antagonists
Acebutolol, betaxolol, bisoprolol, carteolol, carvedilol, esmolol, labetalol, nadolol, timolol
Diuretics
Indapamide, torsemide
Other antihypertensive agents
Methyldopa, guanabenz, guanethidine, reserpine
Intranasal decongestants
Naphazoline, oxymetazoline, xylometazoline
Nonsteroidal anti-inflammatory agents
Aspirin, celecoxib, etodolac, felbinac, flurbiprofen, others
Psychoactive agents
Bromperidol, clozapine, femoxetine, fluphenazine, olanzapine, paroxetine, risperidone, trazodone
Other medications
Benzonatate, cilostazol, cisapride, desmopressin, didanosine, nizatadine, pergolide, pilocarpine, sildenafil

Management

The presence of any etiologic or contributory factor for NAR must be addressed. Avoiding exposure to known triggers, particularly irritants such as tobacco smoke at home and in the workplace, may help ameliorate the patient's condition. Empirical use of intranasal glucocorticoids (Table 30.4), such as those used for allergic rhinitis, is the usual mode of treatment. Beclomethasone, budesonide, and fluticasone have Food and Drug Administration-labeled indications for use in NAR. The efficacy of topical steroids, however, tends to be less consistent in NAR compared with allergic rhinitis. Patients with NARES tend to respond more favorably to intranasal glucocorticoids compared with those with other forms of NAR (65). However, the evaluation of nasal smears to detect eosinophilia and diagnose NARES is unnecessary, because patients can alternatively be given a trial of intranasal glucocorticoids. Azelastine nasal spray also has an indication for use in NAR. For patients with *severe rhinitis medicamentosa*, a short course of oral glucocorticoids (prednisone 30 mg/day for 5 to 7 days) minimizes the rebound phenomenon as the decongestant spray is tapered and discontinued. Oral decongestants and/or anticholinergic agents (Table 30.3) can also be used for symptom-directed treatment of NAR. Immunotherapy is not a consideration in these cases because they are not IgE mediated.

GENERALIZED ALLERGIC AND PSEUDOALLERGIC CONDITIONS

Anaphylaxis and Anaphylactoid Reactions

Description

Anaphylaxis is a rapidly evolving systemic allergic reaction that can be life threatening. Although most of these reactions develop at home (67), they also occur in the hospital setting. It is estimated to affect 1 of every 3,000 inpatients in the United States with a 1% risk of a fatal outcome (68). A study in Great Britain indicated that approximately half of fatal anaphylactic reactions are iatrogenic (69).

Anaphylaxis involves IgE-mediated release of mediators from mast cells and basophils upon exposure of a previously sensitized person to a foreign substance. Such mediators can affect multiple organs, resulting in any combination of cutaneous, respiratory, cardiovascular, and/or gastrointestinal manifestations. The frequency of occurrence of these signs and symptoms recorded in a case series of anaphylaxis (70) are listed in Table 30.8. Respiratory distress can be due to upper airway obstruction and/or bronchoconstriction. Hypotension can be due to vasodilatation and/or increased vascular permeability. These developments typically occur within minutes of exposure to the offending agent but can develop up to an hour later. The more rapid reactions tend to be more severe. Various reports indicate that 2% to 23% of affected patients exhibit a biphasic pattern in which signs and symptoms again develop 1 to 8 hours after they initially resolve (67,71). It is thus important to keep them under close observation during this period.

Table 30.8. Signs and Symptoms of Anaphylaxis

Signs and Symptoms	Frequency (%)
Urticaria, angioedema	90
Dyspnea, wheezing	60
Dizziness, near-syncope	29
Flushed skin	28
Diarrhea, abdominal cramps	26
Upper airway obstruction	24
Nausea, vomiting	20
Hypotension	20
Nasal congestion, rhinorrhea	16
Eye swelling	12
Chest pain	6
Headache	5
Generalized pruritus without rash	4
Blurred vision	2
Seizure	2

Adapted from Kemp SF, Lockey RF, Wolf BL, et al. Anaphylaxis: a review of 266 cases. Arch Intern Med 1995;155:1749.

Anaphylactic reactions can be triggered by minute amounts of an allergenic substance. The most commonly implicated factors are certain drugs and foods. Other causes of anaphylaxis include stinging insect venoms and latex. The evaluation and management of allergy to these specific elements are discussed separately later in this chapter. About 6% to 20% of cases have no identifiable cause and are thus termed idiopathic anaphylaxis (67,72).

The term *anaphylactoid* reaction denotes the same clinical picture produced by anaphylaxis but by definition is not mediated by IgE antibodies. Nonetheless, these so-called pseudoallergic reactions may similarly involve bioactive mediators released by mast cells and basophils. These cells can be directly activated, independent of IgE, by opiates (73) or by hyperosmolar agents (74). Other possible mechanisms include activation of the complement cascade and production of anaphylatoxins such as C3a and C5a that can trigger mediator release (75). In contrast to anaphylaxis, these pseudoallergic reactions do not require previous exposure.

Depending on the patient's clinical presentation, the *differential diagnosis* may include vasovagal reaction, acute ischemia, asthma exacerbation, hyperventilation syndrome, carcinoid syndrome, and systemic mastocytosis. The diagnosis of anaphylaxis could be strongly supported by the demonstration of elevated serum histamine or tryptase. However, this could be difficult to achieve given the short half-lives of these mediators. Results of one study indicate that the best time to measure histamine is within 10 minutes to 1 hour and that for tryptase is within 1 to 2 hours of the anaphylactic reaction (76).

Management

Because acute anaphylactic or anaphylactoid reactions are potentially fatal, the patient's cardiopulmonary status and the need for timely intervention must be quickly addressed. Most anaphylaxis deaths due to food allergy are associated with respiratory arrest,

Table 30.9. Medications for the Acute Management of Anaphylaxis

Drug	Adult Dose and Administration
Epinephrine	0.2 to 0.5 mL of 1:1,000 solution i.m. or s.c. every 10–15 min up to 3 doses
Diphenhydramine	2 mg/kg i.m. or i.v. then 25–50 mg i.v., i.m., or p.o. every 4–6 h
Cimetidine	300 mg i.v. then 300 mg p.o. every 6 h
Methylprednisolone	1–2 mg/kg i.v. every 6–8 h or 60 mg p.o. then 60 mg p.o. per day tapered over several days

whereas those due to drugs and stinging insect venoms are associated with cardiovascular collapse. The median time to respiratory or cardiac arrest has been found to be 30 minutes for fatal anaphylactic reactions to foods, 15 minutes for insect venom, and 5 minutes for drugs (69).

Epinephrine is the drug of choice for the acute treatment of life-threatening anaphylaxis in view of its combined alpha- and beta-agonist properties. The alpha component increases peripheral vascular resistance and ameliorates hypotension, urticaria, and angioedema, whereas the beta component has inotropic and bronchodilatory effects. The adult dose is 0.2 to 0.5 mL of a 1:1,000 solution (0.2 to 0.5 mg epinephrine) given subcutaneously or intramuscularly (Table 30.9). The latter route of administration appears to produce faster systemic absorption and higher peak levels of the drug (77). Dosing can be repeated every 10 to 15 minutes as needed for up to three doses. A retrospective study has shown that more than one dose of epinephrine is required in 36% of cases of anaphylaxis (78).

Antihistamines can help reduce the effects of this mediator released from mast cells and basophils. Diphenhydramine is given intramuscularly or intravenously at a dose of 1 to 2 mg/kg and then 25 to 50 mg intravenously, intramuscularly, or orally every 4 to 6 hours to relieve recurrent signs and symptoms (Table 30.9). Studies have shown that additional treatment with an H_2 blocker such as ranitidine or cimetidine can provide further benefit (79).

Bronchodilator therapy with nebulized albuterol should be given if bronchospasm occurs as part of the anaphylactic reaction, especially in asthmatic patients. Intubation or tracheotomy to allow ventilatory support may be required in severe cases of respiratory distress.

Glucocorticoids are not first-line agents for the treatment of anaphylaxis but are commonly used, putatively to attenuate any late-phase reaction. Methylprednisolone is given at a dose of 1 to 2 mg/kg intravenously (Table 30.9).

A detailed history should be taken in an attempt to identify any causative agent so preventive measures can be implemented. Referral to an allergist may be considered for further evaluation and management. Detection of specific IgE against suspected agents can be achieved through skin testing or *in vitro* tests. If future re-exposure is anticipated, desensitization against certain drugs or immunotherapy against insect venom may be applicable, as discussed later in this chapter.

Patient Education

Patients have to be educated about the early recognition of anaphylaxis and the need for immediate action. They should always carry epinephrine for self-administration in case of future life-threatening allergic reaction. A survey has shown that a large percentage of patients with a history of anaphylaxis do not carry epinephrine (70). This should be addressed, because failure to promptly administer this drug increases the risk for fatal anaphylaxis (71). *EpiPen* Auto-Injector, a device that delivers 0.3 mL of 1:1,000 epinephrine (0.3 mg) intramuscularly through a spring-activated concealed needle, can be used for this purpose. For small children, the *EpiPen* Jr. Auto-Injector device delivers 0.3 mL of 1:2,000 epinephrine (0.15 mg). The patient has to be instructed about the proper use of this device to avoid mistakes that lead to ineffective delivery of the drug (80). Epinephrine should be used only in the event of actual or impending cardiovascular or respiratory compromise. In such cases, the patient should seek emergency medical care because additional treatment could be required. Periodic follow-up should be made to ensure that unused epinephrine is replaced before its expiration date (81).

Prognosis

A longitudinal study has shown that at follow-up after an average of 2.5 years, 60% of patients with *recurrent idiopathic anaphylaxis* report resolution of this problem. In 26% of cases, the frequency of anaphylactic episodes decreased, whereas in 6% of cases it increased (82). The prognosis among patients with allergic reactions to known causes such as foods, drugs, or insect venom is discussed later in this chapter.

Urticaria and Angioedema

It is estimated that 16% to 24% of the U.S. population will develop *urticaria* at least once in a lifetime (83). Affected individuals present with pruritic, erythematous, circumscribed superficial wheals or "hives" that can be coalescent. The individual skin lesions usually resolve within 24 hours, but others may develop at additional sites. The hives, which are largely due to local plasma extravasation, typically appear on the trunk and extremities but can arise anywhere on the body. *Angioedema* is swelling of deeper subcutaneous or submucosal tissue that is less circumscribed than urticaria. Unlike other forms of edema, these are often asymmetrically distributed and have no predilection for dependent areas. Urticaria and angioedema occur together in 49% of cases. About 40% of affected patients develop urticaria alone, whereas 11% develop angioedema without hives (83).

Urticaria and angioedema are arbitrarily classified as *acute* if they occur over a period of less than 6 weeks or *chronic* if they last longer. For acute urticaria and/or angioedema an apparent cause may be found, whereas chronic cases rarely have an identifiable cause.

Evaluation

Acute Urticaria and/or Angioedema. Possible causes of acute urticaria and/or angioedema that can be gleaned from the history include drugs, foods, insect bites or stings, physical elements, infections, and topical irritants. Of note, only some of these cases have demonstrable involvement of IgE-mediated allergy. It would be helpful if a temporal relationship between the onset of symptoms and a particular trigger factor could be established. For example, a history of food ingestion or insect sting minutes before the development of urticaria and/or angioedema strongly suggests an allergic reaction. Several nonallergic causes can likewise be identified. A history of exercise or heat exposure preceding the appearance of pinpoint hives suggests *cholinergic urticaria*, a nonallergic state. Other physical elements that can trigger urticaria and/or angioedema include pressure, vibration, and cold temperature (84). Urticaria and/or angioedema have also been associated with various forms of infection, for example, with hepatitis virus or *Helicobacter pylori*. However, reports in this regard have been conflicting (83,85,86).

If allergen sensitivity is suspected as a cause of recurrent acute urticaria and/or angioedema, appropriate skin testing or *in vitro* tests by an allergist may be useful. If physical elements are suspected, diagnostic provocation can be performed. For example, an ice cube may be applied for 5 to 10 minutes on the forearm of a patient with a history of cold-induced urticaria to verify such diagnosis (87). If no specific cause can be identified, a limited workup may be considered to screen for any underlying systemic condition. This includes a complete blood cell count with differential analysis, measurement of erythrocyte sedimentation rate, and liver function tests. Further diagnostic evaluation should be performed if warranted based on findings in the history, physical examination, or screening tests.

Chronic Urticaria and/or Angioedema. For patients with chronic urticaria and/or angioedema, differential diagnoses to consider include connective tissue disease or vasculitis, complement-related disorders, presence of autoantibodies, lymphoproliferative diseases, or mastocytosis with urticaria pigmentosa. A thorough review of systems and physical examination should be performed to evaluate the possibility of these conditions.

The cutaneous lesions associated with *urticarial vasculitis* are different from benign urticaria in that they are purpuric, persist longer than 24 hours, are painful rather than pruritic, and typically leave residual skin pigmentation.

Angioedema, specifically if it is not accompanied by urticaria, can be due to a *C1 esterase inhibitor (C1 INH) deficiency*. This condition may be hereditary or acquired. Laryngeal or gastrointestinal tissue swelling can cause airway obstruction or abdominal discomfort, respectively. Of note, the latter can be the sole manifestation of this disease and can lead to unnecessary exploratory laparotomy (88). *Hereditary angioedema* (HAE) is an autosomal dominant disorder due to several possible defects in the C1 INH gene (89). *Acquired angioedema* has been associated with connective tissue diseases, lymphoproliferative disorders, malignancies, or autoantibodies against the C1 INH protein (90). For patients with chronic angioedema without urticaria, complement C4 levels should be measured. These are persistently low during and between attacks of angioedema due to C1 INH deficiency. In contrast, levels of C2 are low only during episodes of active disease, whereas C3 levels are unaffected. The diagnosis is established by demonstrating low quantitative and/or functional levels of C1 INH. Its quantity is low in type 1 HAE, which accounts for 85% of cases. In the 15% of cases with type 2 HAE, C1 INH is normal in quantity but is functionally impaired (91). To distinguish between hereditary and acquired angioedema, C1q level should be measured. Levels of C1q are normal in HAE but are low in acquired angioedema (90). Resultant elevations in C2 kinin and bradykinin are believed to be the cause of tissue swelling in these patients (90,92). Elevation in bradykinin, which increases vascular permeability, has likewise been implicated in angioedema associated with angiotensin-converting enzyme inhibitors.

Some studies suggest that *autoimmunity* may play a role in subgroups of patients with chronic idiopathic urticaria and/or angioedema. Various investigators have implicated autoantibodies against thyroid peroxidase or thyroglobulin (93) and against IgE or the alpha chain of the IgE receptor (FcϵRIα) (84,94,95). However, the exact role of these various autoantibodies in the pathogenesis of chronic urticaria and angioedema remains unclear. As such, routine measurement of their levels is not cost effective. In recalcitrant cases of urticaria or when vasculitis is suspected, skin biopsy should be considered.

Management

Management of Urticaria and/or Angioedema Without a Known Cause. Management of *idiopathic* urticaria and angioedema is mainly directed toward amelioration of symptoms. For this purpose, various combinations of antihistamines can provide benefit. Older generation antihistamines are quite effective, but they often cause significant psychomotor impairment in contrast to newer agents (Table 30.3). Addition of H_2 receptor antagonists such as cimetidine or ranitidine to treat persistent cases may provide further benefit (96). Tricyclic antidepressants such as doxepin have potent H_1 and H_2 blocking capabilities and may thus play a therapeutic role. However, their use could be limited by side effects such as sedation and psychomotor impairment (97). Chronic use of oral or parenteral glucocorticoids is not advised in view of their known adverse affects. However, brief courses of oral glucocorticoids may be needed occasionally for severe exacerbations. The use of aspirin and similar nonsteroidal anti-inflammatory drugs (NSAIDs) should be discouraged because they can induce exacerbation of chronic idiopathic urticaria and angioedema (98).

Management of Urticaria and/or Angioedema With a Known Cause. For *nonidiopathic* cases wherein a specific cause such as food or drug has been identified, avoidance measures should be implemented. For patients diagnosed with C1 INH deficiency, prophylactic management with anabolic steroids such as stanozolol or danazol can preclude recurrence in cases of life-threatening angioedema. The dosage should be cautiously reduced to the lowest effective level possible. The patient's liver function, serum cholesterol, and iron profile should be monitored. Adverse effects in women can include signs of virilization such as hoarseness, acne, irregular menses, and changes in hair pattern (99). If available, infusion of vapor-heated C1 inhibitor concentrate can be used to treat acute episodes of angioedema (100).

For patients with chronic urticaria and findings of thyroid autoantibodies, treatment with thyroid hormone has been reported to provide benefit in some individuals (93). However, such an effect is neither consistent nor predictable.

Prognosis

A study of patients with chronic idiopathic urticaria or angioedema showed that at follow-up after 1 year, 38% of those with urticaria alone, 20% with angioedema alone, and 60% with combined urticaria and angioedema were symptom free (101). Another study indicated that up to 20% of patients with chronic idiopathic urticaria continue to be affected after 20 years (84).

SPECIFIC ALLERGIC AND PSEUDOALLERGIC CONDITIONS

Drug Allergy

About 10% to 20% of hospitalized patients in the United States experience some form of adverse drug reaction (102), with fatal outcomes in an estimated 100,000 cases a year (103). Although most of these reactions are not IgE mediated, approximately 6% to 10% may have an allergic or immunologic basis (104).

Beta-Lactam Antibiotics

Penicillin is the most common cause of drug-related fatal anaphylaxis. It is estimated that anaphylactic reactions occur in 0.004% to 0.015% of all courses of penicillin (105). Such reactions tend to occur more frequently when penicillin is given parenterally rather than orally (106). Although most cases involve middle-aged adults, elderly patients tend to have more fatal outcomes, probably due to underlying cardiovascular insufficiency.

If patients who give a history of a penicillin-induced allergic reaction require treatment with this drug, *skin testing* should be done first to identify those at risk for anaphylaxis. If the anaphylactic reaction recently occurred, skin testing should be deferred for 1 to 2 weeks; otherwise, the result could be unreliable (107). Skin testing should be performed using major and minor antigenic determinants of this drug. Benzylpenicilloyl polylysine (Pre-Pen) is considered the major determinant because it represents 95% of haptenated penicillin. The minor determinants include benzylpenicillin (penicillin G), which is commercially available, and benzylpenicilloate and benzylpenniloate, which are available only in certain medical centers. It is believed that the minor determinants are responsible for more severe hypersensitivity reactions. Of note, skin testing does not predict adverse effects that are not IgE mediated such as delayed cutaneous rash, erythema multiforme, Stevens-Johnson syndrome, and toxic epidermal necrolysis. Skin testing is not required if there is no personal history of adverse reaction to this drug, even if there is a family history of penicillin allergy. At present, there is no reliable *in vitro* test for hypersensitivity to this antibiotic.

Only 10% to 20% of patients who give a history of reaction to penicillin are truly allergic to this drug based on skin testing (105). About 97% to 99% of patients with negative skin tests using the major and minor determinants will tolerate penicillin. On the other hand, patients with a positive history and positive skin test have at least a 50% probability of developing an immediate hypersensitivity reaction if they receive penicillin (108). Alternative antibiotics should therefore be used in these cases. If administration of penicillin is mandatory, the patient should first undergo desensitization. This entails administration of incremental doses of the drug in a carefully monitored setting until therapeutic levels are reached to achieve immunologic tolerance.

About 98% of patients with a history of penicillin allergy will tolerate treatment with cephalosporins, especially the second and third generations of this class of antibiotics. However, the 2% who do react will likely have life-threatening anaphylaxis. There is no validated skin test available for cephalosporins, because their antigenic determinants remain to be established. For these reasons, patients with a history of anaphylactic reaction to penicillin and a positive penicillin skin test should either avoid cephalosporins or undergo desensitization (102,109).

Carbapenems such as imipenem can be cross-reactive with penicillin and should be avoided by penicillin-allergic patients (110). In contrast, the monobactam aztreonam rarely cross-reacts with penicillin (111).

Ampicillin and amoxicillin are known to cause *morbilliform rashes*, which are not life threatening, in 5% to 10% of patients. These effects are not IgE mediated, so skin testing is not warranted.

Although some patients maintain their hypersensitivity for long periods of time, in the majority the penicillin skin test becomes negative within 10 years (112). This may partially explain why 80% to 90% of patients who give a past history of allergy to penicillin have no evidence of sensitivity to this drug upon testing.

Table 30.10. NSAIDs that Should Be Avoided by Patients with Aspirin Sensitivity

Drug	Trade Name
Diclofenac	Voltaren
Diflunisal	Dolobid
Etodolac	Lodine
Fenoprofen	Nalfon
Flurbiprofen	Ansaid
Ibuprofen	Advil, Motrin
Indomethacin	Indocin
Ketoprofen	Orudis
Ketorolac	Toradol
Meclofenamate	Meclomen
Mefenamic acid	Ponstel
Nabumetone	Relafen
Naproxen	Aleve, Anaprox, Naprosyn
Oxaprozin	Daypro
Piroxicam	Feldene
Sulindac	Clinoril
Tolmetin	Tolectin

NSAIDs, nonsteroidal anti-inflammatory drugs.

Aspirin and Nonsteroidal Anti-Inflammatory Drugs

Aspirin ranks second to penicillin as a frequent cause of adverse drug reactions. Affected patients typically experience exacerbation of their pre-existing rhinoconjunctivitis, asthma, urticaria, and/or angioedema. However, these side effects are largely unrelated to IgE-mediated mechanisms. In addition to aspirin sensitivity, some patients can have concurrent asthma and nasal polyposis. These three conditions constitute the so-called Samter triad.

Patients with sensitivity to aspirin similarly develop adverse reactions to NSAIDs such as those listed in Table 30.10. Furthermore, a study has shown that up to 34% of aspirin-sensitive asthmatic patients can have mild reactions to acetaminophen at high doses of 1,000 mg or greater (113). As such, patients with aspirin sensitivity should avoid both NSAIDs and high doses of acetaminophen. However, these individuals can tolerate lower doses of acetaminophen.

There is no skin test or *in vitro* test for the diagnosis of aspirin or NSAID intolerance. An oral challenge with aspirin is the only definitive way to establish the presence of sensitivity to this medication.

Desensitization should be considered if the benefit outweighs the risk of an adverse reaction. One example is the use of aspirin in patients with myocardial infarction. Patients who successfully undergo aspirin desensitization are also expected to tolerate NSAIDs. Once tolerance is achieved, administration of therapeutic doses of the drug should be continued on a daily basis. Otherwise, full sensitization may recur if the medication is discontinued for up to 7 days.

Radiographic Contrast Material

The incidence of adverse reactions to radiocontrast material is estimated to be 5% to 8%. These can occur with intravascular administration or during hysterosalpingograms, myelograms, and retrograde pyelograms. Although these effects are believed to be unrelated to IgE-mediated hypersensitivity, the reaction is clinically similar to anaphylaxis. The acute treatment of anaphylactoid reactions to radiocontrast media is also similar to the management of anaphylaxis. Individuals who have a history of reactions to this agent have a greater risk of experiencing adverse effects upon re-exposure. The reported probability of a recurrent anaphylactoid reaction upon repeat exposure ranges from 16% to 44%. This risk can be lowered to approximately 1% by pretreating the affected patient with glucocorticoids and antihistamines. Prophylaxis can be provided with prednisone given at a dose of 50 mg at 13 hours, 7 hours, and 1 hour before the procedure. An oral antihistamine (Table 30.3) is then given 1 hour before the administration of radiocontrast material (114). The use of radiocontrast media with low osmolality can likewise reduce the risk of anaphylactoid reactions (115).

Food Allergy

Epidemiology

Food allergy affects approximately 2% of the adult population in the United States (116). Anaphylactic reactions to food requiring treatment in the Emergency Department are estimated to occur about 1,000 times a year, with a number of cases resulting in death (117). More than 90% of fatal cases of food allergy have been attributed to peanuts and tree nuts (118). A significant portion of the population is at risk, as 3 million Americans have been determined to have peanut and/or tree nut allergy. Notably, about half the members of this group have never sought medical evaluation, and only a few have epinephrine available for emergency use (119).

Relatively few foods account for the vast majority of food allergy. Whereas milk, eggs, peanuts, soy, and wheat account for 90% of food hypersensitivity in children, peanuts, fish, shellfish, and tree nuts are responsible for 85% of food-related reactions in adults. It is rare for an individual to be allergic to more than three foods (116).

Evaluation

A detailed history is important in evaluating the possibility of IgE-mediated sensitivity to food. When they occur, allergic reactions to food typically develop from a few minutes to an hour after ingestion. The absence of a close temporal relationship between exposure and the development of signs and symptoms should prompt a search for other explanations. The manifestations of allergic reactions to food can range from nausea, vomiting, and abdominal cramping to generalized urticaria and respiratory distress.

Some reported cases of anaphylactic reactions to food have been associated with factors such as exercise after a meal (120). Other case reports suggest that in highly sensitized patients, reactions can be triggered by skin contact or inhalational exposure to food particles (121).

For diagnostic purposes, *tests for food-specific IgE antibodies or food challenges* may be applicable. Although puncture skin testing and *in vitro* assays have low specificity and positive predictive values, they have excellent sensitivity and negative predictive accuracy. Only about 50% of patients with positive skin tests to food will have a reaction to *double-blind placebo-controlled food challenge*. On the other hand, negative skin tests virtually rule out IgE-mediated food sensitivity. For *in vitro* evaluation, cut-off levels of IgE that provide positive and negative predictive values of 95% and 90%, respectively, have been determined for egg, milk, peanuts, and fish (122).

Patient history regarding possible food allergy is not always reliable. Only about 40% of cases can be verified as true food-induced allergic reactions through double-blind placebo-controlled food challenges. This office-based procedure can be considered if no specific item is identified as the cause of an allergic reaction, but certain foods remain strongly suspected. It can be performed under close medical supervision by starting with minute amounts of the suspected food and stopping as soon as symptoms such as oral itching or nausea develop (123).

Management

Once a food item is identified as a possible cause of hypersensitivity reactions, it should be vigilantly eliminated from the patient's diet. Those with a history of severe allergic reaction should be prescribed epinephrine to be self-administered in case of cardiovascular or respiratory compromise due to anaphylaxis (see details in preceding section on anaphylaxis). Patients and their caregivers can obtain further support and useful updates from the Food Allergy and Anaphylaxis Network (www.foodallergy.org).

Prognosis

About one-third of adults with food allergy will lose their clinical reactivity after 1 to 2 years of allergen avoidance. However, neither skin tests nor *in vitro* tests can predict which patients would experience resolution of their food hypersensitivity (124).

Insect Venom Allergy

Evaluation

Anaphylactic reactions to insect venom account for about 50 deaths annually in the United States (125), and it is possible that additional cases are undiagnosed and unreported. Stinging insects that cause such IgE-mediated reactions include yellow jackets, hornets, wasps, honeybees, and imported fire ants. Yellow jackets dwell in the ground, whereas hornets build nests in trees and shrubs. Both can be quite aggressive and often sting with minimal provocation. Wasps build honeycomb nests in dark areas, whereas honeybees can be wild or domesticated. Imported fire ants dwell in mounds of soil mostly in the southern states, and their habitat is expanding (126).

Most insect stings typically cause localized swelling, erythema, pain, and pruritus, which are largely due to histamine, serotonin, and kinins contained in the venom. Such limited reactions are not life threatening, but potentially fatal anaphylaxis can also develop in susceptible individuals. The signs and symptoms of such serious reactions can include any combination of generalized urticaria, angioedema, and cardiovascular and/or pulmonary distress.

Localized reactions are not associated with increased risk of subsequent anaphylaxis and thus do not require any long-term intervention. Systemic allergic reactions, however, merit further evaluation and management. Skin testing and/or *in vitro* tests should be done to demonstrate the presence of IgE antibodies specific for the suspected insect venom.

Management

Adult patients with a confirmed history of systemic allergic reaction to insect venom have a 30% to 60% risk of developing anaphylaxis again in reaction to subsequent stings. Insect venom immunotherapy is thus indicated because it reduces the risk of a subsequent systemic allergic reaction to approximately 2% (127). As in any case of anaphylactic reactions, patients should carry epinephrine that can be self-administered as needed.

Prognosis

Prospective studies indicate that insect venom immunotherapy can be discontinued after 5 years of treatment. Data from follow-up evaluation over the next 5 to 10 years show that the residual risk of a systemic reaction to an insect sting is 5% to 15%. Patients who experienced a life-threatening reaction may opt to continue their treatment indefinitely (127).

Latex Allergy

The prevalence of latex hypersensitivity in the general population is less than 1%. However, certain groups have a significantly higher risk of developing this condition. For example, latex allergy is estimated to affect 24% to 60% of patients with spina bifida and genitourinary abnormalities who have undergone multiple surgeries and to affect 5% to 15% of health care workers (128). This increased risk can be attributed to a higher rate of exposure to latex gloves among these individuals.

Several proteins in the sap of the rubber tree (*Hevea brasiliensis*) have been identified as latex allergens. Exposure can occur by direct contact, parenteral administration, or inhalation of aerosolized particles. Powdered latex gloves are common sources of the latter, because latex allergens get absorbed by cornstarch powder. Individuals with latex allergy may experience similar hypersensitivity reactions to avocado, banana, chestnut, or kiwi because these foods may have cross-reactivity with latex allergens (129). IgE antibodies against latex allergens can be demonstrated by skin testing or by *in vitro* tests.

Avoidance of latex products is the only means of preventing serious allergic reactions in a sensitized individual. Primary prevention of latex allergy through the institution of latex-free environments should be encouraged. In the hospital setting, for example, only nonlatex gloves should be allowed to minimize sensitization of high-risk individuals and to avoid adverse reactions among those who are already sensitized. Affected patients should always carry epinephrine that can be self-administered in case of a life-threatening allergic reaction.

General References and Consensus Statements*

Joint Task Force on Practice Parameters. Diagnosis and management of rhinitis. Ann Allergy Asthma Immunol 1998;81:478.

Joint Task Force on Practice Parameters. **The diagnosis and management of anaphylaxis**. J Allergy Clin Immunol 1998;101:S465.

Joint Task Force on Practice Parameters. **The diagnosis and management of urticaria: a practice parameter. Part I. Acute urticaria/angioedema. Part II. Chronic urticaria/angioedema**. Ann Allergy Asthma Immunol 2000;85:521.

Joint Task Force on Practice Parameters. **Stinging insect hypersensitivity: a practice parameter**. J Allergy Clin Immunol 1999;103:963.

These Practice Parameters were developed jointly by the American Academy of Allergy, Asthma and Immunology (AAAAI), the American College of Allergy, Asthma and Immunology (ACAAI), and the Joint Council Allergy, Asthma and Immunology (JCAAI).

Specific References*

1. Hopp RJ, Bewtra AK, Watt GD, et al. Genetic analysis of allergic disease in twins. J Allergy Clin Immunol 1984;73:265.
2. Sarafino EP. Connections among parent and child atopic illnesses. Pediatr Allergy Immunol 2000;11:80.
3. Strachan DP. Family size, infection and atopy: the first decade of the "hygiene hypothesis." Thorax 2000;55:S2.
4. Kay A. Allergy and allergic diseases (First of two parts). N Engl J Med 2001;344:30.
5. Adelroth E, Rak S, Haahtela T, et al. Recombinant humanized mAb-E25, an anti-IgE mAb, in birch pollen-induced seasonal allergic rhinitis. J Allergy Clin Immunol 2000;106:253.
6. Leckie M, Brinke A, Khan J, et al. Effects of an interleukin-5 blocking monoclonal antibody on eosinophils, airway hyperresponsiveness, and the late asthmatic response. Lancet 2000;356:2144.
7. Durham S, Till S. Immunologic changes associated with allergen immunotherapy. J Allergy Clin Immunol 1998;102:157.
8. Malone DC, Lawson KA, Smith DH, et al. A cost of illness study of allergic rhinitis in the United States. J Allergy Clin Immunol 1997;99:22.
9. Meltzer EO. Quality of life in adults and children with allergic rhinitis. J Allergy Clin Immunol 2001;108:S45.
10. Blaiss MS. Cognitive, social, and economic costs of allergic rhinitis. Allergy Asthma Proc 2000;21:7.
11. Kay GG, Berman B, Mockoviak SH, et al. Initial and steady-state effects of diphenhydramine and loratadine on sedation, cognition, mood, and psychomotor performance. Arch Intern Med 1997;157:2350.
12. Skoner DP. Complications of allergic rhinitis. J Allergy Clin Immunol 2000;105:S605.
13. Ramadan HH, Fornelli R, Ortiz AO, et al. Correlation of allergy and severity of sinus disease. Am J Rhinol 1999;13:345.
14. Hisamatsu K, Ganbo T, Nakazawa T, et al. Cytotoxicity of human eosinophil granule major basic protein to human nasal sinus mucosa in vitro. J Allergy Clin Immunol 1990;86:52.
15. Alles R, Parikh A, Hawk L, et al. The prevalence of atopic disorders in children with chronic otitis media with effusion. Pediatr Allergy Immunol 2001;12:102.
16. Simons F. Allergic rhinobronchitis: the asthma-allergic rhinitis link. J Allergy Clin Immunol 1999;104:534.
17. Kapsali T, Horowitz E, Diemer F, et al. Rhinitis is ubiquitous in allergic asthmatics. J Allergy Clin Immunol 1997;S13 (abstr).
18. Gaga M, Lambrou P, Papageorgiou N, et al. Eosinophils are a feature of upper and lower airway pathology in non-atopic asthma, irrespective of the presence of rhinitis. Clin Exp Allergy 2000;30:663.
19. Grembiale R, Camporota L, Naty S, et al. Effects of specific immunotherapy in allergic rhinitis individuals with bronchial hyperresponsiveness. Am J Respir Crit Care Med 2000;162:2048.
20. Huse DM, Hartz SE, Klaus DH, et al. Does allergic rhinitis exacerbate asthma symptoms in adults? The asthma outcomes registry. Eur Respir J 1996;9:351S(abstr).
21. Braunstahl G-J, Overbeek S, Klein JA, et al. Nasal allergen provocation induces adhesion molecules expression and tissue eosinophilia in upper and lower airways. J Allergy Clin Immunol 2001;107:469.
22. Welsh P, Stricker W, Chu C, et al. Efficacy of beclomethasone nasal solution, flunisolide, and cromolyn in relieving symptoms of ragweed allergy. Mayo Clin Proc 1987;62:125.
23. Diemer FB, Sanico AM, Horowitz E, et al. Non-allergenic inhalant triggers in seasonal and perennial allergic rhinitis. J Allergy Clin Immunol 1999;103:S2 (abstr).
24. Sanico AM, Koliatsos VE, Stanisz AM, et al. Neural hyperresponsiveness and nerve growth factor in allergic rhinitis. Int Arch Allergy Immunol 1999;118:153.
25. Tovey ER, Chapman MD, Platts-Mills TA. Mite faeces are a major source of house dust allergens. Nature 1981;289:592.
26. Ehnert B, Lau-Schadendorf S, Weber A, et al. Reducing domestic exposure to dust mite allergen reduces bronchial hyperreactivity in sensitive children with asthma. J Allergy Clin Immunol 1992;90:135.
27. Tovey ER, Taylor DJ, Mitakakis TZ, et al. Effectiveness of laundry washing agents and conditions in the removal of cat and dust mite allergen from bedding dust. J Allergy Clin Immunol 2001;108:369.
28. Arlian L, Neal J, Morgan M, et al. Reducing relative humidity is a practical way to control dust mites and their allergens in homes in temperate climates. J Allergy Clin Immunol 2001;107:99.
29. Antonicelli L, Bilo MB, Pucci S, et al. Efficacy of an air-cleaning device equipped with a high efficiency particulate air filter in house dust mite respiratory allergy. Allergy 1991;46:594.
30. Huss R, Huss K, Squire E, et al. Mite allergen control with acaride fails. J Allergy Clin Immunol 1994;94:27.
31. Bartholome K, Kissler W, Baer H, et al. Where does cat allergen 1 come from? J Allergy Clin Immunol 1985;76:503.
32. Wentz PE, Swanson MC, Reed CE. Variability of cat-allergen shedding. J Allergy Clin Immunol 1990;85:94.
33. Wood R, Johnson E, Van Natta M, et al. A placebo-controlled trial of a HEPA air cleaner in the treatment of cat allergy. Am J Respir Crit Care Med 1998;158:115.
34. Avner DB, Perzanowski MS, Platts-Mills TA, et al. Evaluation of different techniques for washing cats: quantitation of allergen removed from the cat and the effect on airborne Fel d 1. J Allergy Clin Immunol 1997;100:307.
35. Wood R, Chapman M, Adkinson N, et al. The effect of cat removal on allergen content in household dust samples. J Allergy Clin Immunol 1989;83:730.
36. Perzanowski MS, Ronmark E, Nold B, et al. Relevance of allergens from cats and dogs to asthma in the northernmost province of Sweden: schools as a major site of exposure. J Allergy Clin Immunol 1999;103:1018.
37. Almqvist C, Larsson PH, Egmar AC, et al. School as a risk environment for children allergic to cats and a site for transfer of cat allergen to homes. J Allergy Clin Immunol 1999;103:1012.
38. Durham S, Walker S, Varga E, et al. Long-term clinical efficacy of grass-pollen immunotherapy. N Engl J Med 1999;341:468.

*Bold print (general references) and bold numerals (specific references) denote published controlled clinical trials, meta-analyses, or consensus-based recommendations.

39. Weiler J, Bloomfield J, Woodworth G, et al. Effects of fexofenadine, diphenhydramine, and alcohol on driving performance. A randomized, placebo-controlled trial in the Iowa driving simulator. Ann Intern Med 2000;132:354.
40. Gilmore TM, Alexander BH, Mueller BA, et al. Occupational injuries and medication use. Am J Ind Med 1996;30:234.
41. Simons FE. Non-cardiac adverse effects of antihistamines (H1-receptor antagonists). Clin Exp Allergy 1999;29:125.
42. Simons FER. H1-receptor antagonists: safety issues. Ann Allergy Asthma Immunol 1999;83:481.
43. Kernan W, Viscoli C, Brass L, et al. Phenylpropanolamine and the risk of hemorrhagic stroke. N Engl J Med 2000;343:1826.
44. Dockhorn R, Aaronson D, Bronsky E, et al. Ipratropium bromide nasal spray 0.03% and beclomethasone nasal spray alone and in combination for the treatment of rhinorrhea in perennial rhinitis. Ann Allergy Asthma Immunol 1999;82:349.
45. Lumry WR. A review of the preclinical and clinical data of newer intranasal steroids used in the treatment of allergic rhinitis. J Allergy Clin Immunol 1999;104:S150.
46. Pipkorn U, Proud D, Lichtenstein L, et al. Inhibition of mediator release in allergic rhinitis by pretreatment with topical glucocorticoids. N Engl J Med 1987;316:1506.
47. Meltzer EO, Rickard KA, Westlund RE, et al. Onset of therapeutic effect of fluticasone propionate aqueous nasal spray. Ann Allergy Asthma Immunol 2001;86:286.
48. Day J, Briscoe M, Rafeiro E, et al. Onset of action of intranasal budesonide (Rhinocort aqua) in seasonal allergic rhinitis studied in a controlled exposure model. J Allergy Clin Immunol 2000;105:489.
49. Berkowitz R, Bernstein D, LaForce C, et al. Onset of action of mometasone furoate nasal spray (NASONEX) in seasonal allergic rhinitis. Allergy 1999;54:64.
50. Jen A, Baroody F, de Tineo M, et al. As-needed use of fluticasone propionate nasal spray reduces symptoms of seasonal allergic rhinitis. J Allergy Clin Immunol 2000;105:732.
51. Allen DB. Systemic effects of intranasal steroids: an endocrinologist's perspective. J Allergy Clin Immunol 2000;106:S179.
52. Schoelzel EP, Menzel ML. Nasal sprays and perforation of the nasal septum. JAMA 1985;253:2046.
53. Pipkorn U, Pukander J, Suonpaa J, et al. Long-term safety of budesonide nasal aerosol: a 5.5-year follow-up study. Clin Allergy 1988;18:253.
54. Minshall E, Ghaffar O, Cameron L, et al. Assessment by nasal biopsy of long-term use of mometasone furoate aqueous nasal spray (Nasonex) in the treatment of perennial rhinitis. Otolaryngol Head Neck Surg 1998;118:648.
55. Baroody F, Cheng C-C, Moylan B, et al. Absence of nasal mucosal atrophy with fluticasone aqueous nasal spray. Arch Otolaryngol Head Neck Surg 2001;127:193.
56. Qvarnberg Y, Valtonen H, Laurikainen K. Intranasal beclomethasone dipropionate in the treatment of common cold. Rhinology 2001;39:9.
57. Donnelly A, Glass M, Minkwitz M, et al. The leukotriene D_4-receptor antagonist, ICI 204,219, relieves symptoms of acute seasonal allergic rhinitis. Am J Respir Crit Care Med 1995;151:1734.
58. Knapp HR. Reduced allergen-induced nasal congestion and leukotriene synthesis with an orally active 5-lipoxygenase inhibitor. N Eng J Med 1990;323:1745.
59. Miadonna A, Tedeschi A, Leggieri E, et al. Behavior and clinical relevance of histamine and leukotrienes C4 and B4 in grass pollen-induced rhinitis. Am Rev Respir Dis 1987;136:357.
60. Meltzer EO, Malmstrom K, Lu S, et al. Concomitant montelukast and loratadine as treatment for allergic rhinitis: a randomized, placebo controlled clinical trial. J Allergy Clin Immunol 2000;105:917.
61. Wilson A, Orr L, Sims E, et al. Effects of monotherapy with intra-nasal corticosteroid or combined oral histamine and leukotriene receptor antagonists in seasonal allergic rhinitis. Clin Exp Allergy 2001;31:61.
62. Reid MJ, Lockey RF, Turkeltaub PC, et al. Survey of fatalities from skin testing and immunotherapy 1985–1989. J Allergy Clin Immunol 1993;92:6.
63. Greisner WA 3rd, Settipane RJ, Settipane GA. Natural history of hay fever: a 23-year follow-up of college students. Allergy Asthma Proc 1998;19:271.
64. Bielory L. Allergic and immunologic disorders of the eye. Part II. Ocular allergy. J Allergy Clin Immunol 2000;106:1019.
65. Settipane RA, Lieberman P. Update on nonallergic rhinitis. Ann Allergy Asthma Immunol 2001;86:494.
66. Togias A. Age relationships and clinical features of nonallergic rhinitis. J Allergy Clin Immunol 1990;85:182.
67. Cianferoni A, Novembre E, Mugnaini L, et al. Clinical features of acute anaphylaxis in patients admitted to a university hospital: an 11-year retrospective review (1985-1996). Ann Allergy Asthma Immunol 2001;87:27.
68. Neugut AI, Ghatak AT, Miller RL. Anaphylaxis in the United States: an investigation into its epidemiology. Arch Intern Med 2001;161:15.
69. Pumphrey RS. Lessons for management of anaphylaxis from a study of fatal reactions. Clin Exp Allergy 2000;30:1144.
70. Kemp SF, Lockey RF, Wolf BL, et al. Anaphylaxis: a review of 266 cases. Arch Intern Med 1995;155:1749.
71. Sampson H, Mendelson L, Rosen J. Fatal and near-fatal anaphylactic reactions to food in children and adolescents. N Engl J Med 1992;327:380.
72. Yocum MW, Khan DA. Assessment of patients who have experienced anaphylaxis: a 3-year survey. Mayo Clin Proc 1994; 69:16.
73. Tharp MD, Kagey-Sobotka A, Fox CC, et al. Functional heterogeneity of human mast cells from different anatomic sites: in vitro responses to morphine sulfate. J Allergy Clin Immunol 1987;79:646.
74. Silber G, Proud D, Warner J, et al. *In vivo* release of inflammatory mediators by hyperosmolar solutions. Am Rev Respir Dis 1988;137:606.
75. Bochner B, Lichtenstein L. Anaphylaxis. N Engl J Med 1991; 324:1785.
76. Laroche D, Vergnaud MC, Sillard B, et al. Biochemical markers of anaphylactoid reactions to drugs. Comparison of plasma histamine and tryptase. Anesthesiology 1991;75:945.
77. Simons F, Roberts J, Gu X, et al. Epinephrine absorption in children with a history of anaphylaxis. J Allergy Clin Immunol 1998;101:33.
78. Korenblat P, Lundie MJ, Dankner RE, et al. A retrospective study of epinephrine administration for anaphylaxis: how many doses are needed? Allergy Asthma Proc 1999;20:383.
79. Lin RY, Curry A, Pesola GR, et al. Improved outcomes in patients with acute allergic syndromes who are treated with combined H1 and H2 antagonists. Ann Emerg Med 2000;36:462.
80. Huang SW. A survey of Epi-PEN use in patients with a history of anaphylaxis. J Allergy Clin Immunol 1998;102:525.
81. Simons FE, Gu X, Simons KJ. Outdated EpiPen and EpiPen Jr autoinjectors: past their prime? J Allergy Clin Immunol 2000; 105:1025.
82. Khan DA, Yocum MW. Clinical course of idiopathic anaphylaxis. Ann Allergy 1994;73:370.
83. Mathews K. Urticaria and angioedema. J Allergy Clin Immunol 1983;72:1.
84. Greaves M. Chronic urticaria. J Allergy Clin Immunol 2000;105: 664.
85. Cribier BJ, Santinelli F, Schmitt C, et al. Chronic urticaria is not significantly associated with hepatitis C or hepatitis G infection: a case-control study. Arch Dermatol 1999;135:1335.
86. Gala Ortiz G, Cuevas Agustin M, Erias Martinez P, et al. Chronic urticaria and *Helicobacter pylori*. Ann Allergy Asthma Immunol 2001;86:696.
87. Orfan NA, Kolski GB. Physical urticarias. Ann Allergy 1993; 71:205.
88. Weinstock LB, Kothari T, Sharma RN, et al. Recurrent abdominal pain as the sole manifestation of hereditary angioedema in multiple family members. Gastroenterology 1987;93:1116.
89. Bowen B, Hawk JJ, Sibunka S, et al. A review of the reported defects in the human C1 esterase inhibitor gene producing hereditary angioedema including four new mutations. Clin Immunol 2001;98:157.
90. Markovic SN, Inwards DJ, Frigas EA, et al. Acquired C1 esterase inhibitor deficiency. Ann Intern Med 2000;132:144.

91. Cicardi M, Agostoni A. Hereditary angioedema. N Engl J Med 1996;334:1666.
92. Nussberger J, Cugno M, Cicardi M, et al. Local bradykinin generation in hereditary angioedema. J Allergy Clin Immunol 1999;104:1321.
93. Leznoff A, Sussman GL. Syndrome of idiopathic chronic urticaria and angioedema with thyroid autoimmunity: a study of 90 patients. J Allergy Clin Immunol 1989;84:66.
94. Tong LJ, Balakrishnan G, Kochan JP, et al. Assessment of autoimmunity in patients with chronic urticaria. J Allergy Clin Immunol 1997;99:461.
95. Hide M, Francis DM, Grattan CE, et al. Autoantibodies against the high-affinity IgE receptor as a cause of histamine release in chronic urticaria. N Engl J Med 1993;328:1599.
96. Mansfield LE, Smith JA, Nelson HS. Greater inhibition of dermographia with a combination of H1 and H2 antagonists. Ann Allergy 1983;50:264.
97. Goldsobel AB, Rohr AS, Siegel SC, et al. Efficacy of doxepin in the treatment of chronic idiopathic urticaria. J Allergy Clin Immunol 1986;78:867.
98. Doeglas HM. Reactions to aspirin and food additives in patients with chronic urticaria, including the physical urticarias. Br J Dermatol 1975;93:135.
99. Cicardi M, Castelli R, Zingale LC, et al. Side effects of long-term prophylaxis with attenuated androgens in hereditary angioedema: comparison of treated and untreated patients. J Allergy Clin Immunol 1997;99:194.
100. Waytes AT, Rosen FS, Frank MM. Treatment of hereditary angioedema with a vapor-heated C1 inihibitor concentrate. N Engl J Med 1996;20:1630.
101. Kozel MM, Mekkes JR, Bossuyt PM, et al. Natural course of physical and chronic urticaria and angioedema in 220 patients. J Am Acad Dermatol 2001;45:387.
102. Gruchalla RS. Drug metabolism, danger signals, and drug-induced hypersensitivity. J Allergy Clin Immunol 2001;108:475.
103. Lazarou J, Pomeranz BH, Corey PN. Incidence of adverse drug reactions in hospitalized patients: a meta-analysis of prospective studies. JAMA 1998;279:1200.
104. Gruchalla R. Understanding drug allergies. J Allergy Clin Immunol 2000;105:S637.
105. Salkind AR, Cuddy PG, Foxworth JW. Is this patient allergic to penicillin? An evidence-based analysis of the likelihood of penicillin allergy. JAMA 2001;285:2498.
106. Adkinson NF Jr. Risk factors for drug allergy. J Allergy Clin Immunol 1984;74:567.
107. Gadde J, Spence M, Wheeler B, et al. Clinical experience with penicillin skin testing in a large inner-city STD clinic. JAMA 1993;270:2456.
108. Weiss ME, Adkinson NF. Immediate hypersensitivity reactions to penicillin and related antibiotics. Clin Allergy 1988;18:515.
109. Kelkar PS, Li JT. Cephalosporin allergy. N Engl J Med 2001;345:804.
110. Saxon A, Adelman DC, Patel A, et al. Imipenem cross-reactivity with penicillin in humans. J Allergy Clin Immunol 1988;82:213.
111. Adkinson NF Jr. Immunogenicity and cross-allergenicity of aztreonam. Am J Med 1990;88:12S.
112. Green GR, Rosenblum AH, Sweet LC. Evaluation of penicillin hypersensitivity: value of clinical history and skin testing with penicilloyl-polylysine and penicillin G. A cooperative prospective study of the penicillin study group of the American Academy of Allergy. J Allergy Clin Immunol 1977;60:339.
113. Settipane RA, Schrank PJ, Simon RA, et al. Prevalence of cross-sensitivity with acetaminophen in aspirin-sensitive asthmatic subjects. J Allergy Clin Immunol 1995;96:480.
114. Greenberger PA, Patterson R. The prevention of immediate generalized reactions to radiocontrast media in high-risk patients. J Allergy Clin Immunol 1991;87:867.
115. Barrett BJ, Parfrey PS, McDonald JR, et al. Nonionic low-osmolality versus ionic high-osmolality contrast material for intravenous use in patients perceived to be at high risk: randomized trial. Radiology 1992;183:105.
116. Sampson HA. Food allergy. Part 1. Immunopathogenesis and clinical disorders. J Allergy Clin Immunol 1999;103:717.
117. Bock SA. The incidence of severe adverse reactions to food in Colorado. J Allergy Clin Immunol 1992;90:683.
118. Bock S, Munoz-Furlong A, Sampson H. Fatalities due to anaphylactic reactions to foods. J Allergy Clin Immunol 2001;107:191.
119. Sicherer SH, Munoz-Furlong A, Burks AW, et al. Prevalence of peanut and tree nut allergy in the US determined by a random digit dial telephone survey. J Allergy Clin Immunol 1999;103:559.
120. Kidd JM 3rd, Cohen SH, Sosman AJ, et al. Food-dependent exercise-induced anaphylaxis. J Allergy Clin Immunol 1983;71:407.
121. Tan BM, Sher MR, Good RA, et al. Severe food allergies by skin contact. Ann Allergy Asthma Immunol 2001;86:583.
122. Sampson HA, Ho DG. Relationship between food-specific IgE concentrations and the risk of positive food challenges in children and adolescents. J Allergy Clin Immunol 1997;100:444.
123. Bock SA, Sampson HA, Atkins FM, et al. Double-blind, placebo-controlled food challenge (DBPCFC) as an office procedure: a manual. J Allergy Clin Immunol 1988;82:986.
124. Sampson HA. Food allergy. Part 2. Diagnosis and management. J Allergy Clin Immunol 1999;103:981.
125. The discontinuation of Hymenoptera venom immunotherapy. Report from the Committee on Insects. J Allergy Clin Immunol 1998;101:573.
126. Kemp SF, deShazo RD, Moffitt JE, et al. Expanding habitat of the imported fire ant (*Solenopsis invicta*): a public health concern. J Allergy Clin Immunol 2000;105:683.
127. Golden DB, Kagey-Sobotka A, Lichtenstein LM. Survey of patients after discontinuing venom immunotherapy. J Allergy Clin Immunol 2000;105:385.
128. Poley GE Jr, Slater JE. Latex allergy. J Allergy Clin Immunol 2000;105:1054.
129. Rodriguez M, Vega F, Garcia MT, et al. Hypersensitivity to latex, chestnut, and banana. Ann Allergy 1993;70:31.

CHAPTER 31

Approach to the Patient With Fever

PAUL G. AUWAERTER, MD

Clinicians sometimes encounter a febrile patient whose initial history and physical examination offer few clues toward achieving a diagnosis. Many patients will present with elevated temperatures, but the fever seems a secondary concern; for example, when a severe headache and meningismus focus attention on meningitis. In other circumstances, a fever with shaking chill may herald an illness soon recognized as pneumonia with the onset of a productive cough and dyspnea, or it may evolve into an apparently self-limiting viral illness. However, for isolated or persisting fevers, achieving a diagnosis often depends on medical sleuthing using a meticulous history, careful physical examination, and judicious application of diagnostic tests.

MEASUREMENT AND DEFINITIONS

Patient temperatures are reported in the United States as either centigrade (C) or Fahrenheit (F). Values may be converted according to the following:

$$°C = 5/9\,(°F - 32)$$
$$°F = (9/5)°C + 32$$

Defining normal body temperature is an imprecise science, because values obtained from modern studies rest heavily on the study method. An individual's normal oral temperature can range between 35.6 and 38.2°C (96 to 100.7°F). Normal circadian patterns cause body temperature to vary by 1°C (1.8°F), with the nadir reached typically at 6 a.m. and the peak between 4 and 6 p.m. Individual patient temperatures may differ depending on the recording instrument, because thermometers are often poorly calibrated and differ in design (mercury vs. electronic) and anatomic location of measurement (oral, axillary, rectal, tympanic).

Accurate oral readings depend on whether the probe is properly located in the sublingual pocket. Smokers may have higher than normal readings, whereas recent ingestion of a cold beverage may transiently lower oral readings. In very hot weather or after intense exercise, body temperature may rise 0.5 to 1.0°C (0.9 to 1.8°F).

The most commonly recognized "normal" body temperature of 37°C (98.6°F) is based on somewhat antiquated medical lore. Mackowiak et al. (1) described the likely 19th century origin of this criterion; it was derived from the work of a German physician, Carl Wunderlich, who obtained mostly axillary measurements in over 25,000 subjects. In his critical comparative study, Mackowiak et al. found that with modern readings in healthy men and women, the mean oral temperature was 36.8 ± 0.4° (98.2 ± 0.7°F). Rectal thermometry provides measurements with less variation, but patients and health care providers dislike this more accurate form of temperature assessment. In an effort to compare values obtained by different methods, a recent study suggested that rectal temperatures are 0.4°C (0.7°F) higher than oral and 0.8°C (1.4°F) higher than that obtained with a convenient and popular aural (tympanic membrane) device (2).

Because defining normal temperature is inexact, it is not surprising that fever terminology is also variable. Surveys of medical textbooks reveal varying proposals for defining fever that range from any temperatures greater than 37.0°C (98.6°F) to only those greater than 38.0°C (100.4°F) (3). Many clinicians define a significant fever as a temperature greater than 38.3°C (101.0°F), which is likely grounded in the classic study on fever of unknown origin (FUO) by Petersdorf and Beeson (4).

FEVER OF ABRUPT ONSET AND LIMITED DURATION

The clinician should first determine whether a fever needs to be evaluated with further investigation. Many illnesses without localizing signs in otherwise healthy individuals may be due to common viruses, such as rhinoviral infection causing the common cold. These fevers tend to be low grade, with temperatures less than 39°C (102.2°F), and do not last beyond 5 to 7 days. However, some infections that start only with fever and other nonspecific symptoms should be considered in certain situations. Table 31.1 lists selected infections that may first present in the office with fever and require additional attention.

For example, high fevers to 40°C (104°F) associated with chills, myalgia, and cough during wintertime may be due to influenza (see Chapter 33). In contrast, summertime fever in an active outdoorsman or gardener may be the first sign of a tickborne infection such as Lyme disease, ehrlichiosis, or Rocky Mountain spotted fever (see Chapter 38). Patients who use intravenous drugs or practice high-risk sex may have acute human immunodeficiency virus (HIV) infection (Chapter 39),

Table 31.1. Infections that May Present Initially with Fever Alone

Infection	Clinical Features other than Fever	Special Considerations
Anthrax (*Bacillus anthracis*)	Malaise, mild cough or chest pain; respiratory distress and mediastinitis follow	Bioterrorism agent; usually infrequent, sporadic in industrialized areas; occupational hazard of workers exposed to animals or animal products
Chickenpox (varicella)	Pruritic maculopapular rash evolves in hours to vesicles and in days to scabs	Malaise and fever precede or occur simulataneously with rash; highly contagious
Ehrlichia (*Ehrlichia chaffeensis*)	Headache, chills, myalgia; leukopenia, thrombocytopenia common	Spring, summer with tick exposure risk
German measles (rubella)	Maculopapular (occasionally confluent) rash begins on forehead and spreads to trunk and extremities	1- to 7-day prodrome of malaise, headache, mild conjunctivitis
Influenza	Headache, myalgia, chills; cough may evolve to pneumonia	Wintertime, may cause epidemics; high mortality among the chronically ill and elderly
Infectious mononucleosis (*Epstein-Barr virus*)	Pharyngitis, lymphadenopathy, splenomegaly	Atypical lymphocytes, Monospot positive 90%; differential diagnosis also includes acute HIV infection, acute viral hepatitis, rubella, acute toxoplasmosis, acute cytomegalovirus infection, adverse drug reaction
Leptospirosis (*Leptospira interrogans*)	Headache, chills, severe myalgia (calves and thighs), conjunctival suffusion, multiple organ involvement	Sudden onset of fever Acquired from contact with skin, especially if abraded, or mucous membranes of water, moist soil, or vegetation contaminated with urine of infected animals
Lyme disease (*Borrelia burgdorferi*)	Bull's eye rash classic (rash may be not noted ~20%); chills, myalgia, arthralgia, headache	Spring, summer with tick exposure risk; fever usually only with acute disease <4 wks
Malaria (*Plasmodium* species)	Headache, myalgia, back pain, abdominal pain	Any traveler with fever returning from a malarious country should be considered to have malaria until proven otherwise; rare cause of blood transfusion-related infection
Measles (rubeola)	Maculopapular rash spreading from face to neck to trunk, to feet by third day	3- to 4-day prodrome with fever, malaise, hacking cough, rhinitis, subsiding 1–2 days after onset of rash
Parvovirus (B19)	Myalgia, intense arthralgia or arthritis, lacy rash; women more afflicted than men	Exposure to daycare or school-aged children
Q fever (*Rickettsia burnetii*)	Headache, chills, anorexia, myalgias, cough, rales lasting 3 days to 2 weeks	Spread by airborne rickettsiae in dust contaminated by infected animals (cattle, sheep, goats) or by direct contact with infected animals or their tissue
Rocky Mountain spotted fever (*Rickettsia rickettsii*)	Headache, chills, myalgia; petechial rash characteristic but never present in ~10%	Spring, summer with tick exposure risk; life threatening, early treatment with doxycycline essential
Smallpox (variola major)	Malaise, headache, backache, occasional abdominal pain and vomiting; followed by maculopapular to vesicular to pustular rash beginning on face and extremities	Potential bioterrorism agent; last naturally acquired case worldwide in 1977

HIV, human immunodeficiency virus.

viral hepatitis (hepatitis B or C, see Chapter 47), or venereal diseases such as syphilis or gonorrhea (see Chapter 37) as the cause of febrile illness. Teenagers or young adults may have an isolated fever before the development of pharyngitis or lymphadenopathy associated with infectious mononucleosis (see Chapters 33 and 58). Viral exanthems may present first with fever in adolescents or adults who are not naturally immune or who were not adequately vaccinated (see Chapter 18). Recent events have made it necessary to consider also bioterrorism agents, such as anthrax and smallpox, in the evaluation of fever in certain circumstances.

In the elderly, fever generally indicates the presence of serious infection, most often caused by bacteria from urinary or respiratory sources, even when localizing symptoms are absent (5). Because significant temperature elevation may be absent in 20% to 30% of elderly patients with a serious infection, elderly patients should be considered febrile when they have an elevated body temperature of approximately 1°C (2°F) above baseline values.

DRUG FEVER

Elevation of temperature in response to a drug without the presence of rash is known as a drug fever, though it should be more properly termed "drug hypersensitivity." Although the exact incidence of drug fever is unknown, it may occur in up to 10% of hospitalized patients (6). In ambulatory patients, who are typically on fewer medications, drug fever occurs much less frequently.

Contrary to popular conceptions, drug fever usually does not cause a sustained pattern of temperature elevation. There is a variable lag time between initiation of the offending drug and onset of fever, though it most commonly occurs between the first and second weeks (7). Relative bradycardia is an important clue that may assist the physician in considering drug fever as the cause of an otherwise unexplained temperature elevation, along with a general impression that the patient is not acutely ill. Such a pulse–temperature dissociation can only be determined if a patient has a fever greater than 102°F and does not have a situation disturbing the sinoatrial node such as sick sinus syndrome or medication effect. The appropriate pulse for a given temperature is estimated by taking the last digit of the Farenheit reading and subtracting 1 and then multiplying by 10 and adding 100 (6). For example, a patient with a temperature of 104°F should have a pulse of 130 beats per minutes ($[4 - 1] \times 10 + 100$).

Patients with drug fever will often be unaware of a significant fever, and chills are uncommon. A generalized maculopapular rash may eventually arise in some patients affected by drug fever. There are no diagnostic laboratory features, although the erythrocyte sedimentation rate (ESR) may be elevated to levels exceeding 100 mm/hr, and eosinophilia may be found in a small percentage of patients. Fever induced by drugs such as barbiturates, methyldopa, phenytoin, and sulfonamides may herald the development of a serum sickness syndrome with rash, lymphadenopathy, arthritis, and nephritis. Other drugs such as procainamide, quinine, and hydralazine may cause a lupus-like syndrome with arthritis, serositis, and production of antinuclear and antihistone antibodies.

Commonly prescribed medications that are most likely to cause drug fever are listed in Table 31.2. Drugs that are not known to cause hypersensitivity reactions include aminoglycosides, digitalis preparations, and insulins.

The diagnosis of drug fever requires a high index of suspicion, because the often insidious onset may obscure the cause. Withdrawal of the suspected offending agent should result in defervescence within several days but may take weeks in drugs requiring prolonged periods of elimination (e.g., iodides, isoniazid). Conclusive evidence that a drug has caused a febrile reaction can only be proved by rechallenge, but this should not be entertained unless that medication is expected to be important for future therapy and no end-organ damage was associated with initial administration.

Table 31.2. Drugs Commonly Implicated in the Development of Fever due to Hypersensitivity

Allopurinol
Amphotericin B
Anti-thymocyte antibodies
Atropine
Azathioprine
Barbiturates
Bleomycin
Cephalosporins
Heparin
Hydralazine
Interferons
Isoniazid
Iodides (including i.v. contrast media)
Methyldopa
Penicillamine
Penicillins
Phenytoin
Procainamide
Propylthiouracil
Rifampin
Quinidine
Nonsteroidal anti-inflammatory drugs (NSAIDs)
Salicylates
Streptokinase
Sulfonamides

The most serious febrile reaction to drugs, malignant hyperthermia, occurs as an idiosyncratic response to neuroleptic medications such as haloperidol, thiothixene or phenothiazines (neurologic malignant syndrome), or certain anesthetic agents (8,9). Abrupt fever up to 41°C (105.8°F) is accompanied by altered mentation, muscular rigidity, and labile blood pressure. Few infectious processes cause temperatures elevations beyond 41°C (105.8°F), perhaps with the exception of malaria. The human body usually cannot survive fever greater than 42°C (107.6°F) (10). The differential diagnosis of extreme pyrexia otherwise includes only HIV infection, heat stroke, and central fevers due to hypothalamic injury by stroke, tumor, or infection.

FEVER OF UNKNOWN ORIGIN

Fevers of 38.3°C (101°F) or greater lasting for more than 3 weeks without a diagnosis, despite 1 week of intensive diagnostic investigation in hospital, has been the traditional definition of FUO (4,11). As a practical matter, this definition has become too restrictive because patients with FUO are less commonly hospitalized and even complex evaluations are now frequently performed on an outpatient basis. Therefore, a patient may be considered to have an FUO if temperature elevations to 38.3°C (101°F) or more persist beyond 3 weeks with negative blood culture studies and no other apparent explanation (12).

Diagnostic tests such as computed tomography (CT), magnetic resonance imaging (MRI), and serologic analyses have advanced considerably since the early published literature on FUO. Rheumatologic and infectious etiologies now comprise a smaller proportion of FUOs. Infectious causes remain the leading category, accounting for 25% to 50% of diagnoses in more recent series (13–15). Common causes of FUO (Table 31.3) account for up to half of the explanations in published series. Exhaustive lists of potential causes of FUO can be found in several reference sources (12,16).

Some recent demographic trends may be important in the evaluation of FUO. For the category of infection, classic pulmonary tuberculosis rarely leads to FUO because radiographic findings of cavitary disease suggest the proper diagnosis. *Extrapulmonary tuberculosis* such as tubercular lymphadenitis, pleural effusion, and miliary disease are the leading cause of infectious FUO in many series. These diagnoses require a high index of suspicion and confirmation by biopsy of infected tissue. Extrapulmonary tuberculosis in the

Table 31.3. Categories and Leading Diseases Causing Fever of Unknown Origin

Infections
Culture-negative endocarditis
Extrapulmonary tuberculosis
Intra-abdominal/hepatic abscess
Chronic osteomyelitis
Cytomegalovirus
Neoplasia
Lymphoma
Metastases to liver or brain
Peritoneal carcinomatosis
Renal cell carcinoma
Myelodysplastic syndrome
Rheumatologic
Temporal (giant cell) arteritis
Still disease (adult-onset, juvenile rheumatoid arthritis)
Vasculitis (polyarteritis nodosa, hypersensitivity vasculitis)
Miscellaneous
Drug fever
Granulomatous hepatitis
Sarcoidosis
Inflammatory bowel disease
Cirrhosis
Alcoholic hepatitis
Factitious fever
Habitual hyperthermia

United States is now most commonly diagnosed in foreign-born individuals who acquired the infection in their native countries (17). An individual with FUO who is a native of a country with high rates of tuberculosis (especially Mexico, the Philippines, Vietnam, India, China, Haiti, and South Korea) should be thoroughly evaluated for tuberculosis (see Chapters 34 and 41).

Because of an aging population, *malignancies* account for an increasing proportion of diagnoses in many FUO series, most significantly non-Hodgkin lymphomas (13,18). Peritoneal carcinomatosis is a particularly challenging diagnosis, because routine screening tests, including imaging studies and endoscopy, often fail to disclose the primary problem. Metastatic disease to the liver or central nervous system may cause persistent low-grade fevers. Myelodysplastic disease, historically termed preleukemia, may be responsible for fever with findings of anemia and sometimes leukopenia or thrombocytopenia.

The most common *rheumatologic* causes of FUO are diseases that lack characteristic serologic findings. Giant cell arteritis should be considered in any patient with FUO over the age of 50. Marked elevations in nonspecific inflammatory parameters such as the ESR or C-reactive protein suggest this diagnosis. The temporal arteries should be biopsied even when significant headache or visual symptoms are lacking. Still disease is another frequent cause of FUO; it is a clinical diagnosis suggested by high hectic fevers with rigors, arthralgias or arthritis, patchy and evanescent rose-colored rash, and very high serum ferritin (500 to more than 1,000 mg [mg/dl] (19).

Among *miscellaneous* causes, drug fever is a frequently overlooked consideration. Cirrhosis is an unlikely cause of FUO, although these patients with cirrhosis are prone to biliary tract infections and candidemia, which may present as isolated fever. Recurrent deep vein thromboses or chronic pulmonary emboli may occasionally cause FUO, although fevers are rarely greater than 39°C (102.2°F). Factitious fever invariably makes up a small but significant percentage of FUO. Patients presenting with factitious fever may have a medical background and have normal body temperature when it is measured under direct observation (20,21). In some series up to 20% of patients with FUO remain without a diagnosis after a thorough evaluation. However, most of these undiagnosed patients appear to have self-limited illnesses with fevers abating within 6 months (22).

Two special categories of FUO apply uniquely to the ambulatory patient. The first is FUO that lasts for more than 1 year and is not associated with laboratory abnormalities such as anemia or elevated ESR (23). The prognosis in these patients is generally excellent, and the diagnosis of *habitual hyperthermia* may be considered, especially in women who may have a slightly higher than average temperature (37.2 to 38°C, 99 to 100.5°F) but no other findings (these patients do not fit within the strict definition of FUO). The second is episodic or recurrent FUO, in which fevers occur only after weeks or months of normal temperatures. These are more often due to the miscellaneous causes of FUO (Table 31.3), but up to half of such patients remain undiagnosed (24). Patients with episodic fever who remain without diagnosis generally also have a good prognosis.

Diagnostic Approach

When a patient presents with fever, the initial evaluation should be guided by consideration of possible serious diagnoses while avoiding inappropriate or unnecessary testing for unlikely causes. Certain patients may be more thoroughly evaluated at the first visit, especially if they have an underlying chronic disorder such as HIV, active cancer, cirrhosis, organ transplantation, or splenectomy. It is important to remember that many patients with FUO are not suffering from rare and unusual diseases but rather are experiencing atypical manifestations of common illnesses (4).

For a patient who is not significantly ill and who presents with fever of less than 1 week, the office visit should focus on symptoms and signs that may guide the examiner to the most likely explanation for the illness. If no localizing symptoms are found and the patient does not appear seriously ill, then a tentative diagnosis of a viral illness is appropriate. Such patients should be reassured and advised to report if new signs or symptoms arise or if the fever persists beyond the 7 to 10 days that is consistent with self-limited viral infections.

Occasionally, a fever without localizing signs heralds an illness that should be recognized early to avoid significant morbidity and mortality. A short list of infectious considerations should include typhoid fever, malaria, ehrlichiosis, early Rocky Mountain spotted fever, or early viral hepatitis. Primary Epstein-Barr virus, cytomegalovirus, or initial HIV infections in the adult will often lack the typical features of mononucleosis-like syndromes and only present with profound malaise, fever, and liver function test abnormalities (25). Careful questioning based on recent residence or behaviors can help to determine whether these infections can be possible considerations.

If fevers persist or significant constitutional features develop (e.g., rigors, profound malaise, anorexia, weight loss, or dizziness), then the patient should be re-evaluated with consideration of whether hospitalization is appropriate. A thorough assessment of the history, including items such as residence, hobbies, travels within the last year, history of international residence, history of tuberculosis exposure, HIV risk factors, alcohol use, recently prescribed medications, and family history of febrile syndromes or autoimmune diseases, should be undertaken. The review of systems should be enumerated meticulously because even trivial symptoms may hold a clue to diagnosing the disorder.

Repeated physical examination may detect problems that are either new or slowly evolving. Areas of particular interest should include attention to all regional lymph node groups, thyroid inspection, notation of oropharyngeal ulcers or exudates, careful auscultation for cardiac murmurs, assessment of liver and spleen size, survey of all joints, examination of nail beds for splinters or clubbing, scrutiny of the skin for rash, and neurologic examination especially looking for cranial nerve abnormalities (suggesting chronic meningitis) or mononeuritis multiplex (pointing to a vasculitis). Other clues may emerge from the ocular examination, such as Roth spots on the fundus (oval retinal hemorrhages with pale centers suggesting endocarditis but only rarely seen with that illness) and scleritis, episcleritis, or uveitis (painful red eye syndromes associated with rheumatologic diseases, syphilis, tuberculosis, sarcoidosis, and inflammatory bowel disease, the diagnosis of which usually requires a slit lamp examination). Palpation of the temporal arteries may reveal cords or tenderness that suggest giant cell arteritis. In women, the pelvic examination may hold the first clue of subtle pelvic inflammatory disease or neoplasm, whereas in men the scrotal, rectal, and prostate examinations are essential to assess for an occult abscess or malignancy.

Fever Patterns

Although usually dismissed as antiquated observations, specific fever patterns can occasionally aid in suggesting the correct diagnosis and require that patients frequently obtain and log their temperatures so they can be studied (16). A stepwise daily fever elevation associated with a pulse–temperature dissociation (see Drug Fever, above) may suggest typhoid fever. Two daily fever spikes (double-quotidian fever) is a rarity but if present should suggest Still disease, a mixed malaria infection caused by more than one *Plasmodium* species, or gonococcal endocarditis. The biphasic or camelback fever pattern occurs over a 4-day interval with a steady rise and fall of temperature and may represent an infection due to dengue fever, Colorado tick fever, yellow fever, viral hemorrhagic fever, brucellosis, or leptospirosis.

Diagnostic Tests

When a patient has a significant illness or the duration of fever extends beyond 3 weeks, the laboratory may provide important direction in the investigation of fever. Minimum testing should include a complete blood count, electrolyte and liver function panels, complete urinalysis and culture, and ESR, or C-reactive protein. A chest radiograph, preferentially with posteroanterior and lateral views, should also be obtained.

At least two aerobic and anaerobic blood culture sets should be inoculated. Up to five blood culture sets may be ordered in situations in which endocarditis is a likely possibility. For example, patients with a prosthetic heart valve or those who have new cardiac murmurs or peripheral emboli may have initial blood cultures that are negative. This should prompt consideration of a valvular infection with a fastidious organism (e.g., one of the HACEK [*Haemophilus* spp., *Actinobacillus actinomycetemcomitans, Cardiobacterium hominus, Eikenella corrodens, Kingella* spp.] bacteria). If blood cultures are obtained from different sites and with at least several hours between each set, that will improve both sensitivity and specificity, the latter by helping to eliminate consideration of contaminating bacteria such as coagulase-negative staphylococci or *Propionibacterium acne*. Finally, a purified protein derivative of *Mycobacterium tuberculosis* should be placed, although the test may be negative in up to 25% of individuals with active tuberculosis.

Many additional tests can be ordered in the evaluation of an FUO, but a "shotgun" approach rarely yields useful information and may frustrate physician and patient alike while increasing costs. The efficient evaluation of this challenging condition should be guided by a comprehensive knowledge of the disorders causing this syndrome (26). A rational approach to FUO popularized by Petersdorf and Beeson (4) refers to "Sutton's Law," named after a notorious criminal of the 1930s who, when asked why he only robbed banks, replied "Why, that's where the money is." Application of this "law" to patients with FUO directs attention to an obvious abnormality that then suggests the test most likely to yield a diagnostic result, rather than proceeding with rote testing (4). In one series of patients diagnosed in a community hospital setting, 90% of patients with FUO were diagnosed by abnormalities detected either by the physical examination or by routine laboratory tests (27).

Diagnostic Imaging

CT or MRI of pertinent body areas may be helpful. Radionuclide scans are sometimes useful in the evaluation of FUO but have drawbacks. Gallium scans or indium-labeled white blood cell scans can demonstrate an abnormal area not previously considered in a patient with FUO; however, the number of false positive and false negative studies probably outweigh routine use, and ultrasonography and CT or MRI are more accurate (28–30). One exception is in the detection of an infected vascular graft or mycotic aneurysm, especially involving large vessel such as the aorta when a gallium or white blood cell scan may prove especially useful. Technetium bone scans have a role in the diagnosis of osteomyelitis but may be falsely positive, especially in areas of overlying soft tissue inflammation such as diabetic foot ulcers.

Standard transthoracic echocardiography is inadequate to rule out the presence of valvular vegetation in infectious endocarditis. Transesophageal echocardiography is superior but may fail to detect vegetations in 5% to 10% of patients with infectious endocarditis, and a repeat study should be done if clinical suspicion of the diagnosis remains high (31).

When repeated history and physical examinations and laboratory testing do not produce results, consultation may be helpful. Diagnostic consultations for FUO fall into many hands, but traditionally internists, rheumatologists, and infectious disease physicians evaluate most of these cases. If fever and a possibly associated abnormality persists, it may be advantageous, for example, to call upon a gastroenterologist or hepatologist for help with fever and transaminase evaluation or a hematologist for fever and pancytopenia. One of the most frequently overlooked strategies that may quickly lead to diagnosis is biopsy of any suspicious skin lesion or abnormal lymph node.

Bone marrow aspirate and biopsy is a generally safe procedure that may yield evidence of a disseminated granulomatous disorder and provide culture information helpful in the evaluation of fungal or mycobacterial disorders (32). Liver biopsy is an option when persisting liver function test abnormalities are not explained by noninvasive testing, although the yield of this procedure is only 5% to 17% (33). In areas of endemic fungal infection such as histoplasmosis or coccidioides, liver biopsy may still yield diagnostic information even in the absence of blood test abnormalities. Finally, exploratory laparotomy is rarely now performed because imaging technologies have greatly advanced; however, it may be occasionally required especially in disorders isolated to the peritoneum such as tuberculous peritonitis or abdominal carcinomatosis (34).

The so-called Naprosyn (naproxen) test may discriminate between fevers due to infection or malignancy (35). Fevers due to neoplasia are purportedly more responsive to the nonsteroidal anti-inflammatory agents than those caused by infection. The Naprosyn test is probably most useful in patients with a known malignancy who develop fevers of uncertain cause rather than in those with FUO new to a diagnostic evaluation.

TREATMENT

In the noncritically ill patient, reaching a diagnosis is invariably more difficult if empirical therapies obfuscate the cause of fever. Empiric trials of antibiotics have no role in the treatment of fever, unless one is certain of a diagnosis (e.g., Lyme disease manifested by erythema migrans or culture-negative endocarditis supported by echocardiographic findings). Patients with progressive illness who are suspected to have tuberculosis should have empirical therapy initiated before they become critically ill, but this should not be done with an ambulatory patient who can wait until the diagnosis of tuberculosis is certain (36).

High-dose corticosteroids should be reserved for patients with proven vasculitis or other inflammatory disorders, although lower dose steroid therapy may be helpful both diagnostically and therapeutically with cases of temporal arteritis. Occasionally, some patients with FUO have no easily definable illness but remain significantly sick with all diagnostic options exhausted. Such patients could be considered for the very careful initiation of corticosteroids to treat a putative inflammatory disorder (37).

Antipyretic Therapy

Although there is considerable evidence suggesting that fever benefits host immune defenses, especially in infectious disorders (38), physicians routinely prescribe antipyretics. There appears to be little clear benefit from treating fever with acetaminophen, aspirin, or nonsteroidal anti-inflammatory agents. Therefore, many sources suggest withholding antipyretic agents (39). Only in special situations should they be considered, such as fever in either the very young or very old at risk for febrile seizures, fever in patients unable to tolerate the increased metabolic demands because of ischemic heart disease, or in the uncommon patient who is unable to tolerate the discomfort associated with the temperature elevation (40).

Although antipyretics are perceived as benign medications, this is not always the case. Acetaminophen can be associated with hepatic or renal toxicity if higher than recommended doses (greater than 4 g/day) are taken. Patients who use ethanol or are fasting are at higher risk of hepatotoxicity from acetaminophen overdose (41). In children, aspirin has been linked to fulminant hepatitis in influenza- or varicella-related Reye syndrome, and it can increase bleeding risk and cause hepatic and renal toxicity. Corticosteroids may effectively reduce fever, but their significant side-effect profile makes them unacceptable choices for antipyresis alone.

Because fever may produce benefit, and occasionally some diagnostic insight based on its pattern, it may be best to limit the prescription of antipyretics for FUO and instead direct efforts toward the most effective antipyretic—reaching a definite diagnosis and specific therapy.

General References

Cunha BA. Fever of unknown origin. Infect Dis Clin North Am 1996;10:111.

Comprehensive discussion of the causes, diagnosis, and treatments of FUOs. This volume of Infectious Disease Clinics of North American has 13 chapters on fever and clinical illness.

Knockaert DC, Vanneste LJ, Vanneste SB, et al. Fever of unknown origin in the 1980s. An update of the diagnostic spectrum. Arch Intern Med 1992;152:51.

A relatively recent study by a group intensively studying the methods of FUO diagnosis.

Petersdorf RG, Beeson PB. Fever of unexplained origin: report of 100 cases. Medicine (Baltimore) 1961;40:1.

The classic treatise on FUO.

Simon HB. Current concepts: hyperthermia. N Engl J Med 1993;329:483.

Why fever occurs and its implications.

Specific References

1. Mackowiak PA, Wasserman SS, Levine MM. A critical appraisal of 98.6F, the upper limit of the normal body temperature, and other legacies of Carl Reinhold August Wunderlich. JAMA 1992;268:1578.
2. Rabinowitz RP, Cookson ST, Wasserman SS, et al. Effects of anatomic site, oral stimulation, and body position on estimates of body temperature. Arch Intern Med 1996;156:777.
3. Mackowiak PA. Temperature regulation and the pathogenesis of fever. In: Mandell GL, Bennett JE, Donlin R, eds. Mandell, Douglas, and Bennett's principles and practice of infectious diseases. Vol. 1. Philadelphia: Churchill Livingstone, 2000:604.
4. Petersdorf RG, Beeson PB. Fever of unexplained origin: report of 100 cases. Medicine (Baltimore) 1961;40:1.
5. Norman DC, Yoshikawa TT. Fever in the elderly. Infect Dis Clin North Am 1996;10:93.
6. Johnson DH, Cunha BA. Drug fever. Infect Dis Clin North Am 1996;10:85.
7. Mackowiak PA, LeMaistre CF. Drug fever: a critical appraisal of conventional concepts. An analysis of 51 episodes in two Dallas hospitals and 97 episodes reported in the English literature. Ann Intern Med 1987;106:728.
8. Balzan MV. The neuroleptic malignant syndrome: a logical approach to the patient with temperature and rigidity. Postgrad Med J 1998;74:72.
9. Denborough M. Malignant hyperthermia. Lancet 1998;352:1131.
10. Mackowiak PA, Boulant JA. Fever's glass ceiling. Clin Infect Dis 1996;22:525.
11. Cunha BA. Fever of unknown origin. Infect Dis Clin North Am 1996;10:111.
12. Isaac B, Kernbaum S, Burke M. Unexplained fever. Boca Raton, FL: CRC Press, 1991.
13. Larson EB, Featherstone HJ, Petersdorf RG. Fever of undetermined origin: diagnosis and follow-up of 105 cases, 1970–1980. Medicine (Baltimore) 1982;61:269.
14. Petersdorf RG. FUO: how it has changed in 20 years. Hosp Pract (Off Ed) 1985;20:84I-84M, 84P, 84T-84V passim.
15. Knockaert DC. Fever of unknown origin, a literature survey. Acta Clin Belg 1992;47:42.
16. Cunha BA. The clinical significance of fever patterns. Infect Dis Clin North Am 1996;10:33.
17. Talbot EA, Moore M, McCray E, et al. Tuberculosis among foreign-born persons in the United States, 1993–1998. JAMA 2000;284:2894.
18. Brusch JL, Weinstein L. Fever of unknown origin. Med Clin North Am 1988;72:1247.
19. Gonzalez-Hernandez T, Martin-Mola E, Fernandez-Zamorano A, et al. Serum ferritin can be useful for diagnosis in adult onset Still's disease. J Rheumatol 1989;16:412.
20. Aduan RP, Fauci AS, Dale DC, et al. Factitious fever and self-induced infection: a report of 32 cases and review of the literature. Ann Intern Med 1979;90:230.
21. Sarwari AR, Mackowiak PA. Factitious fever: a modern update. Curr Clin Top Infect Dis 1997;17:88.
22. Knockaert DC, Dujardin KS, Bobbaers HJ. Long-term follow-up of patients with undiagnosed fever of unknown origin. Arch Intern Med 1996;156:618.
23. Wolff SM, Fauci AS, Dale DC. Unusual etiologies of fever and their evaluation. Annu Rev Med 1975;26:277.
24. Knockaert DC, Vanneste LJ, Bobbaers HJ. Recurrent or episodic fever of unknown origin. Review of 45 cases and survey of the literature. Medicine (Baltimore) 1993;72:184.
25. Auwaerter PG. Infectious mononucleosis in middle age. JAMA 1999;281:454.
26. Esposito AL, Gleckman RA. A diagnostic approach to the adult with fever of unknown origin. Arch Intern Med 1979;139:575.
27. Kazanjian PH. Fever of unknown origin: review of 86 patients treated in community hospitals. Clin Infect Dis 1992;15:968.
28. Quinn MJ, Sheedy PF 2nd, Stephens DH, et al. Computed tomography of the abdomen in evaluation of patients with fever of unknown origin. Radiology 1980;136:407.
29. Knockaert DC, Vanneste LJ, Vanneste SB, et al. Fever of unknown origin in the 1980s. An update of the diagnostic spectrum. Arch Intern Med 1992;152:51.
30. Weissman AF, Fig LM, Sisson J, et al. The role of scintigraphy in the evaluation of fever of unknown origin. Am Fam Physician 1994;50:1717.
31. Ryan EW, Bolger AF. Transesophageal echocardiography (TEE) in the evaluation of infective endocarditis. Cardiol Clin 2000;18:773.
32. Volk EE, Miller ML, Kirkley BA, et al. The diagnostic usefulness of bone marrow cultures in patients with fever of unknown origin. Am J Clin Pathol 1998;110:150.
33. Holtz T, Moseley RH, Scheiman JM. Liver biopsy in fever of unknown origin. A reappraisal. J Clin Gastroenterol 1993;17:29.
34. Gleckman R. Fever of unknown origin: the value of abdominal exploration. Postgrad Med 1977;62:191.
35. Chang JC. NSAID test to distinguish between infectious and neoplastic fever in cancer patients. Postgrad Med 1988;84:71.
36. Harris HW, Mentiove S. Miliary tuberculosis. In: Schlossberg D, ed. Tuberculosis. New York: Springer-Verlag, 1994:233.
37. Suzuki A, Ohosone Y, Mita S, et al. Fever of unknown origin responding to steroid therapy. Nihon Rinsho Meneki Gakkai Kaishi 1997;20:21.
38. Roberts NJ Jr. Temperature and host defense. Microbiol Rev 1979;43:241.
39. Styrt B, Sugarman B. Antipyresis and fever. Arch Intern Med 1990;150:1589.
40. Klein NC, Cunha BA. Treatment of fever. Infect Dis Clin North Am 1996;10:211.
41. Whitcomb DC, Block GD. Association of acetaminophen hepatotoxicity with fasting and ethanol use. JAMA 1994;272:1845.

CHAPTER 32

Bacterial Infections of the Skin*

PATRICK A. MURPHY, MD

Most skin infections are trivial and can be managed at home without medical assistance. Each year, however, approximately 5% of the population develop a skin infection that requires medical attention. The severity of these infections depends on the virulence of the infecting organisms and the state of host defenses. The most common infecting organisms are *Streptococcus pyogenes* and *Staphylococcus aureus*. In otherwise healthy people, these often cause only modest morbidity and respond rapidly to appropriate treatment. They can, however, cause serious infections, especially in diabetic patients, in patients with impaired blood supply to the infected site or impaired lymphatic or venous drainage of the site, and in patients with defects in leukocytic or immunologic defense mechanisms. Serious infection is also more likely when other bacteria, or combinations of bacteria, are involved, as occurs in bites or contaminated wounds.

*Nathaniel F. Pierce, MD, contributed to earlier versions of this chapter.

SUPERFICIAL INFECTIONS CAUSED BY *S. PYOGENES* AND *S. AUREUS*

Impetigo, ecthyma, and erysipelas are superficial infections usually caused by group A hemolytic streptococci (*S. pyogenes*) and *S. aureus* (1). These infections arise from breaks in the skin that are often so minor they are unnoticed.

Impetigo

Impetigo occurs mostly among preschool children, especially in warm, humid climates or when personal hygiene is poor (2). Under these conditions, the disease is highly contagious and outbreaks may occur. Older children and adults are only occasionally affected.

Impetigo *begins as a pruritic, focal, superficial eruption of small 1- to 2-mm vesicles,* often on the face near the nares, chin, or lower extremities. There is usually no history of trauma. In several days, the vesicles change to pustules that break, become crusted, and have an erythematous base. Regional lymphadenopathy is common, but there are no constitutional symptoms. The process may spread because of scratching. Healing occurs without scarring. Impetigo may recur if personal hygiene is not improved.

Bullous impetigo is caused by strains of *S. aureus* that secrete one of the epidermolytic toxins (3). Epidemics of bullous impetigo can occur among newborns, but only sporadic cases are seen in older children, and adult cases are uncommon. The process begins as a macular erythematous rash. The characteristic thin-walled, fluid-filled, superficial bullae appear within 1 to 3 days, range from 1 cm to several centimeters in diameter, and usually involve exposed areas of the body. These bullae rupture, desquamation occurs, and healing without scarring follows in about 7 days. In its most dramatic form, this process causes the scalded skin syndrome, a disease of small children in which there is extensive superficial desquamation.

Ecthyma

Ecthyma occurs under the same conditions of poor hygiene that promote impetigo. It is characterized by 3- to 10-mm *discrete, ulcerating lesions with an adherent necrotic crust and surrounding erythema;* a small amount of pus often underlies the crust. The ulcer is sufficiently deep to cause permanent scarring. Lesions are most common on the anterior tibial surface at sites of minor trauma or insect bites. Left untreated, the lesions tend to spread distally and there may be associated lymphadenopathy; systemic symptoms, however, are lacking. Cultures of pus may yield both *S. pyogenes* and *S. aureus*. There is evidence that *S. aureus* causes a majority of the cases. Lesions with a similar appearance may result from bacteremia with *Pseudomonas aeruginosa.*

Erysipelas

Erysipelas involves progressive, often rapid spread of infection through superficial layers of skin and lymphatics. It may occur after a minor wound in normal skin but is more likely when prior injury or disease has impaired the lymphatic or venous drainage of the skin or left extensive scarring, as, for example, in a patient with chronic venous insufficiency of the lower extremities or lymphedema of the arm after radical mastectomy. Most episodes of erysipelas are caused by *S. pyogenes.* A few are caused by *S. aureus* or other agents, such as *Pasteurella multocida* or *Erysipelothrix rhusiopathiae* (see later discussion and Table 32.4), and these cannot always be distinguished clinically.

Erysipelas is characterized by a *rapidly spreading area of marked erythema with warmth, local pain, an elevated sharp margin between involved and uninvolved skin, and firm edema that gives the skin a typical "orange peel"* appearance. There may be seropurulent drainage at the inoculation site, but fluctuation and dermal necrosis are lacking. Erythema often extends centrally along superficial draining lymphatics; regional lymph nodes are often enlarged and tender. Systemic toxicity, chills, and fever are common. If it is untreated, metastatic infection may occur, and there is appreciable mortality. Facial infections are especially dangerous because of possible intracranial spread via draining lymphatics or veins. Extensive involvement of the trunk also carries an increased risk of death.

Table 32.1. Antibiotic Selection for Superficial and Pustular Skin Infections[a]

Infection	Antibiotic	Route
Superficial Infections		
Impetigo	Dicloxacillin or cephalexin	Oral
	Erythromycin	Oral
Ecthyma	As for impetigo	
Erysipelas		
Mild	Penicillin V	Oral
	Erythromycin	Oral
Severe	Penicillin G	Intravenous
Pustular Infections		
Folliculitis	None	
Furunculosis, boils	Dicloxacillin or cephalexin	Oral
	Erythromycin	Oral
Bullous impetigo	As for furunculosis	Oral
Carbuncle	As for furunculosis	Oral
	Nafcillin	Intravenous
	Vancomycin	Intravenous
Cellulitis	As for carbuncle	

[a]Dosage recommendations are in Table 32.2. Other penicillinase-resistant oral beta-lactams may also be given.

Table 32.2. Antibiotic Dosage and Schedule for Skin Infections Caused by *Streptococcus pyogenes* and *Staphylococcus aureus* in Adults

Antibiotic	Dosage
Ambulatory treatment (mild infection)	
Dicloxacillin	250 mg PO t.i.d.
Cephalexin	500 mg PO q.i.d.
Erythromycin	250–500 mg PO t.i.d.
Penicillin V	500 mg PO t.i.d.
Parenteral treatment (severe infection)	
Penicillin G	600,000–2,000,000 units IV q6h
Nafcillin or oxacillin	1–2 g IV q4–6h (dose and interval depend on severity)

Management

Bacterial cultures of the lesions of impetigo, bullous impetigo, and ecthyma usually are not helpful. Impetigo and ecthyma may reveal mixed cultures of *S. pyogenes* and *S. aureus,* or either agent alone, whereas lesions of bullous impetigo are often sterile. Blood cultures should be obtained when erysipelas is extensive or is associated with marked systemic toxicity (e.g., temperature greater than 102°F [39°C], shaking chills, severe malaise). Attempts to isolate an organism by culturing sterile saline that has been injected and withdrawn through a fine needle at the edge of the lesion have a low yield but may be helpful if usual treatment is ineffective. If there is seropurulent drainage at the site of inoculation, this should be cultured.

Antimicrobial therapy is required for all of these infections (Tables 32.1 and 32.2). To eradicate group A streptococci, antibiotic treatment should be given for 10 days, even though marked improvement may occur sooner.

Impetigo and ecthyma are treated similarly. Dicloxacillin, cephalexin, and other penicillinase-resistant beta-lactams are effective oral antimicrobials. Erythromycin is also effective where *S. aureus* are sensitive to it. Adjunctive therapy includes careful daily soaking of lesions to remove crusted debris using warm water with an iodophor (a soap that releases iodine in a nontoxic, nonstaining form, such as Betadine skin cleanser) or with a soap that contains hexachlorophene (e.g., pHisoHex). Prevention depends primarily on improved personal hygiene; the most important preventive measure is careful frequent skin cleansing with soap and water. Topical mupirocin (Bactroban) was recommended previously, but resistance develops very rapidly.

Treatment of *bullous impetigo* should be directed at penicillin-resistant staphylococci. Oral dicloxacillin and cephalexin are effective; erythromycin is an alternative where *S. aureus* are sensitive to it.

Minor episodes of *erysipelas* may be treated with oral penicillin V or erythromycin. Application of moist heat to the affected area appears to hasten clearing of the infection. Serious episodes are those with marked systemic toxicity, extensive lesions, or facial lesions and those occurring in compromised hosts (e.g., diabetics). Such patients require hospitalization and treatment with penicillin G intravenously (Tables 32.1 and 32.2). Special attention should also be paid to patients with atherosclerotic peripheral vascular disease who have infections of their lower extremities. In such patients, the affected leg should be rested and elevated; sustained pressure on any part of the leg or foot should be avoided.

Patients with preexisting damage to the veins or lymphatics of an extremity may experience repeated episodes of erysipelas that cause further damage. Patients who have numerous recurrent infections should receive continuous antibiotic prophylaxis with penicillin V (250 mg twice daily), benzathine penicillin (600,000 units intramuscularly monthly), or erythromycin (250 mg twice daily). Reduction of chronic edema by use of fitted pressure stockings or by administration of diuretics helps reduce susceptibility to this infection.

Superficial skin infections respond rapidly to appropriate therapy. Systemic toxicity and erythema associated with erysipelas usually abate within 3 or 4 days, and discrete skin lesions show marked healing within 10 days. During this period, activity should be restricted in accord with the extent of the infection. Minor lesions require no restrictions. Patients with any form of impetigo should avoid contact with infants and small children until lesions heal.

Complications

Streptococcal skin infections do not cause rheumatic fever, but they may cause *acute glomerulonephritis* if the streptococcal strain is nephritogenic. Nephritis is not prevented by antibiotic therapy. The average latency period between initial symptoms of a streptococcal skin infection and the onset of glomerulonephritis is 2 weeks. If a nephritogenic strain is known to be in the community, initial and 14-day follow-up evaluation should include a urinalysis. Most patients who develop poststreptococcal glomerulonephritis are asymptomatic, but in some, glomerulonephritis is first suggested by gross hematuria, acute hypertension, or signs of salt and water retention, such as dependent edema or congestive heart failure.

Bacteremia with metastatic infection may complicate neglected or severe episodes of erysipelas. Metastatic infection should be considered in patients with severe disease that responds poorly to treatment or if findings suggestive of distant localized infection develop. Possible metastatic infections include meningitis, endocarditis, septic arthritis, infection of preexisting pleural effusions or ascites, and solid organ abscesses (e.g., liver, spleen).

PUSTULAR INFECTIONS CAUSED BY *S. AUREUS*

These include folliculitis, furunculosis, hidradenitis suppurativa, and carbuncles. They represent increasingly severe effects of the infection of hair follicles, sebaceous glands, or sweat glands by *S. aureus,* the result being inflammation and abscess formation.

Folliculitis

Folliculitis involves minor inflammation of individual hair follicles, often with formation of small superficial pustules. There is little pain or surrounding erythema. In some people, lesions recur for months or even years. A common area of involvement is the bearded part of the face, where minor trauma from shaving may be a contributing factor.

Furunculosis

Deeper infection of follicles or cutaneous glands leads to formation of pustular furuncles. *Boils* are large furuncles. They range in diameter from about 5 mm to 2 or 3 cm and occur most commonly on hairy areas exposed to friction, trauma, or maceration (e.g., buttocks, neck, face, axillae, groin, forearms, thighs, upper back). Furunculosis may also complicate the acne of adolescence. Furuncles begin with pruritus, local tenderness, and erythema, followed by swelling and marked local pain. As pus forms in the center of the lesion, the overlying skin becomes thin, the lesion becomes elevated, pain increases, and spontaneous drainage of pus ultimately occurs, usually with prompt relief of pain and rapid healing. Furunculosis may be recurrent in some people, especially diabetics and chronic nasal carriers of *S. aureus.*

Hidradenitis Suppurativa

Hidradenitis suppurativa is a noninfectious skin disease characterized by obstruction of the ducts of apocrine sweat glands in the axilla, perineum, or groin. The process comes to light when staphylococcal infection of one or several of the obstructed glands occurs. Such episodes initially respond well to antibiotics, but because antibiotics do nothing for the primary condition, the infections recur. After several years, infection becomes chronic, with multiple scars and numerous draining abscesses and sinus tracts. By this time, the bacterial flora is usually gram negative, with *Proteus* and *Pseudomonas* commonly found.

Carbuncles

A carbuncle is a coalescent mass of deeply infected follicles or sebaceous glands with multiple interconnecting sinus tracts and cutaneous openings that drain pus ineffectively. Carbuncles usually occur in the thick skin on the back of the neck or upper back. Once formed, the lesions steadily worsen, with increasing pain, erythema, swelling, purulent drainage, and lateral enlargement; they vary in diameter from 3 to 10 cm or larger. Fever and systemic toxicity are common. Carbuncles occur with increased frequency in diabetics and may cause a major increase in the severity of diabetes. Patients may present in ketosis who are normally sustained on an oral agent or who were not previously known to be diabetic.

Management

Bacterial cultures of typical pustular lesions are usually unnecessary because virtually all are caused by *S. aureus* and most isolates prove resistant to penicillin G.

Minimal lesions, such as *folliculitis,* require little therapy. Careful, twice-daily cleansing with a mild soap, preferably one containing hexachlorophene, and avoidance of minor trauma and irritants, such as cosmetics or abrasive soaps, are usually sufficient.

Furuncles should be managed initially by gentle application of warm moist heat (as moist compresses or baths) for about 30 minutes four times a day, and by immobilizing the affected area (e.g., splinting of digits, instructing the patient to avoid pressing on the furuncle). Lesions less than 1 cm in diameter often drain spontaneously after 1 to 3 days and require no further treatment. Larger lesions, painful lesions, and lesions that do not drain spontaneously should be *drained surgically when they are fluctuant.* This can be done in the office by making a single incision into the abscess with a scalpel, after first infiltrating the incision line with 0.5% or 1.0% lidocaine for local anesthesia. Lifting the anesthetized skin with a forceps when the incision is made helps avoid pain caused by downward pressure from the scalpel. Packing with iodoform gauze for 1 or 2 days may be needed to control oozing of serosanguinous discharge after surgical drainage. Antimicrobial therapy is required only for extensive lesions such as multiple furuncles, carbuncles, or lesions associated with marked surrounding inflammation, or in diabetic patients. In such cases, oral dicloxacillin or cephalexin (Tables 32.1 and 32.2) should be given until signs of inflammation subside completely, which may take 2 weeks or longer; when antibiotics are given, indurated furuncles often resolve without becoming fluctuant.

Carbuncles require surgical drainage, which usually can be done in an outpatient facility. Patients with severe systemic toxicity, such as diabetics with carbuncles, require hospital admission and parenteral therapy with a penicillinase-resistant penicillin; vancomycin is an effective alternative for those who are allergic to penicillin.

Recurrent furunculosis may prove a frustrating problem. Management of individual episodes is as described previously, but other steps should also be taken to eliminate colonization with staphylococci. The anterior nares should be cultured. Patients whose nasal cultures contain *S. aureus* should be treated by application of mupirocin ointment to the anterior nares twice daily for 5 days. Alternatively, bacitracin ointment or gentamicin ointment may be applied three or four times daily for 14 days. During topical treatment, bacterial contamination of skin should be meticulously controlled by having the patient bathe and shampoo three times daily with a hexachlorophene soap or lotion, and by changing underclothing and bed and bath linens daily.

Recurrent furunculosis may occur in certain *disorders that impair host defenses.* Tests for diabetes mellitus should be made; if they are positive, control of blood glucose may prove beneficial (see Chapter 79). Defects in polymorphonuclear leukocyte function are a rare cause of recurrent furunculosis but should be considered in young patients who show an increased incidence or severity of infections caused by staphylococci. Gram-negative bacteria and fungi may be cultured from the furuncles of such patients. If an unusual problem, such as a leukocyte defect, is suspected, the patient should be referred to a medical center with the capability to investigate such disorders.

Hidradenitis suppurativa is a difficult problem that requires prolonged, often lifelong treatment by multiple methods. These include selective surgical drainage of abscesses; elimination of irritants such as tight clothing, antiperspirants, and shaving of the axillae; careful, frequent cleansing of skin with antiseptic agents; local application of heat; and intermittent or long-term systemic antibiotic therapy. The only curative therapy is surgical removal of all involved skin, which is easier said than done. Management of such patients is best done by physicians especially skilled in the treatment of skin disorders (see Chapter 115).

Complications

Staphylococcal skin infections may spread to other sites. This is especially true in patients with extensive inflammation and systemic toxicity, such as those with carbuncles, in whom bacteremia is common. Even an innocent-appearing furuncle can cause metastatic infection, especially in patients with a focus of increased susceptibility, such as a ventricular septal defect, an artificial heart valve, or an arthritic joint. Patients at risk for bacteremia who have such susceptible foci or whose systemic complaints (fever, focal pain) persist despite antibiotic treatment should be carefully examined for possible metastatic infection.

CELLULITIS AND WOUND INFECTIONS

Any break in the skin can become infected. This includes not only obvious trauma, such as lacerations, burns, abrasions, and animal or human bites, but also minor injuries such as scratches and insect bites. The features of the resultant infection vary widely and depend on the nature of the wound, the type of infecting organism, and the defensive responses of the infected person. In many instances, early appropriate management given on an ambulatory basis is sufficient. In others, recognition of serious infection and prompt hospitalization for vigorous medical or surgical treatment are of prime importance. Table 32.3 describes findings that require hospitalization or surgical

Table 32.3. Wound Infections: Findings that Necessitate Hospitalization or Surgical Intervention

Finding	Comment
Extensive cellulitis or erysipelas with systemic toxicity	Needs parenteral antibiotics, close observation
Diminished arterial pulse in cool, swollen, pale, infected extremity	Possible fasciitis, a surgical emergency
Cellulitis with cutaneous necrosis or subcutaneous gas	Needs parenteral antibiotics and possible surgical drainage/debridement
Closed space infection of the hand	Needs surgical drainage

Table 32.4. Causes of Life-Threatening Bacterial Cellulitis

Cause	Important Features
Gram-negative enteric bacilli, especially *Escherichia coli*	Occur in fecally contaminated wounds; gas may be present; surgical drainage required for gas or pus
Mixed anaerobic and enteric aerobic bacteria	Occur in fecally contaminated wounds; gas may be present; symptoms may progress rapidly and may include exquisite pain; surgical drainage required
Bacillus anthracis	Causes anthrax when minor wound is inoculated by spore-contaminated animal products (animal hides and hair, especially from goats); local chancre-like lesion develops, followed by systemic toxicity
Erysipelothrix rhusiopathiae	Erysipelaslike lesion with central clearing; caused by wound contamination with fish or meat products; treated with penicillin V or tetracycline
Pasturella multocida	Erysipelaslike lesion that follows a dog or cat scratch or bite; treated with penicillin V or tetracycline
Marine vibrios	Necrotizing cellulitis after minor wound is contaminated by sea water or contact with shellfish
Aeromonas hydrophila	Wound contaminated by fresh water swimming

intervention. Table 32.4 lists organisms that can cause life-threatening forms of cellulitis.

Cellulitis Caused by *S. pyogenes* and *S. aureus*

Acute cellulitis is a spreading infection of skin and subcutaneous tissues. The involved area, which enlarges steadily, is painful, tender, and intensely erythematous. Chills and fever are common, and bacteremia may occur. The lesion differs from erysipelas in that its margin is not as sharply demarcated, nor is it elevated. There may be purulent or serous drainage at the inoculation site; in severe cases, patches of involved skin may become necrotic.

The most common causes of acute cellulitis are *S. pyogenes* and *S. aureus*. Studies based on full-thickness biopsies of skin and subcutaneous fat show that more than 95% of cases are streptococcal (4). Finding gram positive cocci in drainage from the wound is presumptive evidence that they are causative. Cellulitis may progress rapidly, especially when it involves an area of chronic edema. Lower extremity infection in patients with peripheral arterial insufficiency can cause tissue necrosis and secondary infection.

Management of cellulitis should include culture of any wound drainage (as described for erysipelas) and prompt antibiotic therapy. In mild cases, treatment may be given on an ambulatory basis. The treatment should be effective for infections by penicillin-resistant staphylococci as well as penicillin-sensitive streptococci. Oral dicloxacillin or cephalexin is adequate for infections caused by either type of organism; erythromycin is a suitable alternative for patients who are allergic to penicillin (Tables 32.1 and 32.2). Local application of moist heat is a useful adjunct to antibiotic treatment; care should be taken, however, to avoid causing burns, especially in patients with impaired sensitivity to pain. Improvement is usually apparent in 3 or 4 days; during this period, patients should rest the involved area (with elevation when the cellulitis involves an extremity). Patients should be told to report promptly any worsening of the infection or of constitutional symptoms. Severe infections require hospitalization and parenteral treatment with a penicillinase-resistant beta-lactam such as nafcillin, or vancomycin. This includes patients with extensive lesions, lesions of the face, or serious toxicity.

Necrotizing Fasciitis

Most patients with an acutely swollen, painful leg have cellulitis. A very few have a much more serious infection in which the primary infectious process is in the plane of the deep fascia. The infection spreads rapidly and widely in this plane, and a whole limb may be involved in a few hours. Initially, the patient is febrile and toxic out of proportion to the visible changes in the skin, which may be minor or nonexistent. The infection causes thrombosis of small blood vessels as they cross the fascia to supply blood to the skin. The overlying skin becomes dusky blue and edematous, ultimately developing hemorrhagic bullae.

Necrotizing fasciitis is a surgical emergency; the fascia is dead over wide areas, and it must be removed back to normal bleeding tissue. Diagnosis is primarily clinical, although computed tomographic scans may show gas or edema, or both, in the plane of the deep fascia. Treatment involves long incisions with much undermining of skin edges to allow removal of necrotic material. The wounds are drained and left open to heal by secondary intention. Multiple subsequent debridements usually are necessary.

There are two distinct bacterial causes. Group A *S. pyogenes* can cause this syndrome as a single organism (5). Formerly there were epidemics of streptococcal gangrene in hospitals; presently, streptococci are the "flesh-eating bacteria" of the popular media. Streptococci do not form gas, so computed tomography may not be helpful. The other kind of necrotizing fasciitis was described by Fournier and is called Fournier's gangrene (6). It is caused by a mixed fecal flora involving several bacteria—aerobic gram negative rods and both gram positive and gram negative anaerobes. This flora typically produces abundant gas. Streptococcal fasciitis can start anywhere; Fournier's gangrene usually starts near the perineum. These cases are treated in hospital with broad-spectrum antibiotics as an adjunct to surgery; if a streptococcus is responsible, treatment can be simplified to penicillin.

Secondarily Infected Ulcers

Cutaneous ulcers are caused by a wide variety of conditions. By far the most common cause is chronic venous insufficiency, most typically associated with ulceration of the medial side of the leg, just above the ankle. Other causes of leg ulcer include any condition in which red cells aggregate and obstruct blood vessels, such as sickle cell disease and other chronic hemolytic anemias, and conditions associated with arteritis, such as rheumatoid arthritis and systemic lupus. Ulcers due to peripheral vascular disease are usually on the toes. Pressure sores are most commonly on the heels, and the ulcers of neurologic disorders overlie bony prominences such as the metatarsal heads. Management of the ulcer is generally aimed at the underlying cause and seeks to improve blood flow, reduce edema, and avoid pressure and trauma (see Chapter 95). For venous ulcers, compression stockings or bandages are the most important part of therapy.

Control of secondary infection is also important. Superficial colonization with a variety of bacteria is unavoidable and without consequence; however, infection that is deeper or laterally invasive prevents healing and may interfere with other treatments, such as skin grafting. Infection is best controlled by repeated careful cleaning and local debridement. Systemic antibiotics should be used only after all other methods have failed to control surrounding infection. The choice of antibiotic should be based on cultures of the wound or its purulent drainage. Local antibacterials are sometimes helpful. Those effective against a broad spectrum of bacterial agents include polymyxin–bacitracin–neomycin ointment, topical nitrofurazone (Furacin ointment), and the silver sulfadiazine ointment commonly used to treat burns. These should be applied three times daily until healing occurs or it is apparent that they are ineffective. Soaking with 3% acetic acid three to four times daily is helpful in controlling bacterial growth in ulcers colonized with *P. aeruginosa.*

There is good evidence that local application of fibroblast growth factors speeds healing of ulcers, but the proteins are recombinant and very expensive.

Cutaneous Diphtheria

Cutaneous ulcers and other skin lesions may become secondarily infected with *Corynebacterium diphtheriae,* causing cutaneous diphtheria. Although the cutaneous lesion may appear benign, myocarditis or neuropathy develops in approximately 3% of cases. Outbreaks have occurred in the northwest and southern parts of the United States, primarily among Native Americans or indigent urban residents (7). The presence of cutaneous diphtheria in a community should increase suspicion that skin wounds may harbor this agent. The diagnosis should be suspected when existing wounds develop a *gray-yellow or gray-brown covering membrane* and surrounding erythema. Typically, the membrane can easily be removed to reveal a clean base. Other minor skin lesions may also become infected. Typical organisms can be seen in methylene blue stains of smears from the wound and confirmed by culture on Loeffler or tellurite agar. Presumptive cases should be reported to public health officials and treated with equine diphtheria antitoxin (20,000 to 40,000 units intramuscularly or intravenously after testing for hypersensitivity to horse serum) and either erythromycin (1.5 g/day, orally) or procaine penicillin (1.2 million units/day, intramuscularly) for 7 to 10 days.

Cutaneous Anthrax

Until recently, cutaneous anthrax was a curiosity seen occasionally in agricultural areas and in factories where workers handed imported hides or wool. Now that it has been used as a bioterrorism agent, it is not clear how common it may become in the future. The cutaneous form of the disease occurs when anthrax spores become implanted under the skin, germinate, and begin to multiply. The disease is usually found on exposed skin of the hands and arms, sometimes on the face. The anthrax bacilli make two toxins: (a) an edema-forming toxin that poisons capillary endothelium and produces leaky capillaries, and (b) a lethal toxin that poisons most cells by inducing apoptosis. These two toxins account for the distinctive features of the disease. At the site of initial implantation, the skin rapidly becomes black and necrotic. The lesion is roughly circular, and diameters range from 1 to 3 cm. Although anthrax is described as causing a "malignant pustule," it is more like a vesicle, because the fluid contains bacteria but very few cells. There may be secondary vesicles around the primary one. Spreading from the primary site is an area of pronounced edema that may extend 10 cm or more from the primary lesion. There may be regional lymph node enlargement. Fever and systemic toxicity are rare except in neglected cases.

The differential diagnosis is from the vastly more common boil. Anthrax lesions are curiously painless and may itch. Big boils are very painful, as are the associated nodes. A boil may develop a black or dark red crust of coagulated blood if it has been picked at, but the anthrax lesion is black from the beginning. Edema around boils is less pronounced than that around anthrax lesions. Gram stains from boils show pus, sheets of polymorphonucleocytes, and gram positive cocci in clusters. Gram stains from anthrax vesicle fluid show big (8 μm) gram positive rods with few cells. The organisms are easily differentiated on culture, but the laboratory should be warned what it is dealing with.

Without treatment, the mortality rate of cutaneous anthrax is approximately 25%. The most suitable antibiotics for adults are quinolones (e.g., ciprofloxacin 500 mg orally twice daily) and tetracyclines (e.g., doxycycline 100 orally twice daily), given for 60 days. Penicillins, cephalosporins, and vancomycin are commonly used in children. Patients with cutaneous anthrax lesions on the head or neck or with extensive edema or signs of systemic toxicity should be hospitalized for intravenous therapy with a multidrug regimen. With treatment, the mortality rate should be well under 5%.

Bites

Bite wounds become infected with the oral, salivary, or dental flora of the biting person or animal and may cause serious local or systemic infections. Initial management before signs of infection appear is of primary importance in preventing certain infections. Appropriate prophylaxis for tetanus is required for all bite wounds (see Chapter 18).

Human bites are contaminated with a complex variety of aerobic and anaerobic oral bacteria. Without treatment, a severe necrotizing cellulitis often results. Minor lesions that break the skin should be washed thoroughly and treated with a combination of amoxicillin 875 mg and clavulanic acid (Augmentin) orally twice daily. Oral clindamycin (150 to 300 mg three times a day) is appropriate for patients who are allergic to penicillin. Antibiotics should be continued for 7 to 10 days. More severe wounds, including wounds of the hands and knuckles, require meticulous debridement and possible tendon repairs. These injuries should be referred for surgical management.

Dog bites carry the risk of local soft tissue infection with various organisms, including *P. multocida*, and raise concern about rabies. Minor abrasions, shallow punctures, and superficial lacerations require no therapy for local infection other than thorough cleansing with soap and water. Puncture wounds should be irrigated vigorously with sterile saline injected through a 20-gauge needle. More extensive or deeper bites require surgical management for debridement and, in some cases, primary closure. Amoxicillin and clavulanic acid, as described previously, should be given for bites of the hands or face. The same treatment is appropriate for patients who have signs of soft tissue infection when first seen. Patients with hand infection require surgical management and intensive antibiotic therapy.

Rabies precautions should be taken with all dog bites, including bites by domestic pets, even though the risk of rabies from domestic pets—especially when biting was provoked—is very small. The dog should be quarantined for 10 days. If the dog's owner cannot be identified, the local health department should be called to take charge of the dog. If its owner is known and can prove that the dog was vaccinated against rabies, it may be observed at its home. If it remains well, there is no risk of rabies. If the dog develops neurologic symptoms or dies, its brain should be examined immediately; prophylaxis is required if evidence of rabies is found. If the dog escapes after biting, and especially if the bite was unprovoked, rabies prophylaxis with human rabies immune globulin and human diploid cell rabies vaccine is indicated (see Chapter 18).

Bites by other domestic animals (e.g., cats) should be managed in the same way as dog bites. Cats are not routinely vaccinated against rabies and are now a greater hazard than domestic dogs. *Bites by wild animals* carry a greater risk of rabies, and rabies prophylaxis is usually required unless the animal's brain can be examined. Wild animals with the greatest risk of carrying rabies are raccoons, skunks, foxes, coyotes, and bats. The risk of rabies with rodent bites, including squirrel bites, is very small.

It is also recommended that the practitioner seek the help of the local or state health department when dealing with animal bites. Officials with knowledge of disease activity in local animal populations may be able to determine whether a particular exposure is trivial or serious and can also arrange fluorescent antibody testing and viral cultures if the animal is available. Not every animal that appears neurologically impaired has rabies; other causes of animal encephalitis are also found.

Puncture Wounds

Puncture wounds usually involve the feet or hands and may introduce infecting bacteria that cannot be removed by washing or debridement. In all instances, patients should receive appropriate prophylaxis for tetanus (see Chapter 18). *Low-risk wounds* (i.e., those not likely to be contaminated by soil or fecal material and in which the wound site is in healthy, well-vascularized tissue) need only be thoroughly washed and observed for several days for signs of developing infection. Should infection develop, any wound drainage should be cultured and treatment begun with dicloxacillin orally 250 mg three times daily or amoxicillin-clavulanate (see earlier discussion) for presumptive staphylococcal or streptococcal infection. The wound site should also be soaked in warm soapy water for 30 minutes at least four times a day.

Higher-risk wounds (i.e., those likely to be contaminated with fecal material, soil, or foreign debris and those occurring in a diabetic person or in an extremity with an inadequate blood supply) should be treated from the outset with a broad-spectrum antibiotic (in adults, ciprofloxacin 750 mg orally every 12 hours or another quinolone; in children younger than 15 years old, one of the antibiotics previously listed). The wound site should be rested and treated with warm soaks as described for low-risk wounds. The patient should promptly report any evidence of inflammation, swelling, or persisting pain. If purulent drainage develops, it should be cultured. Antibiotic management should be altered if bacteria resistant to the current treatment are isolated. If pus develops, surgical drainage usually is required.

Felon

A felon is an infection of the pulp of the distal phalanx of a finger; it usually occurs after a recognized local wound. Abscess formation and tissue necrosis are common, and bony or articular involvement may occur. If the felon is neglected or inadequately treated, severe damage, including loss of function, may occur. The most common causative agents are *S. aureus* and *S. pyogenes,* although gram negative bacilli may also be recovered. Treatment involves surgical drainage by a physician who is familiar with the procedure. Concurrent antibiotic therapy should be guided by Gram staining and culture of infected material. If Gram staining and culture are persistently negative, herpetic whitlow should be considered.

Paronychia

A paronychia is an infection, often chronic or recurrent, that involves tissue immediately adjacent to a fingernail or toenail. The affected tissue is warm, tensely swollen, erythematous, and painful. When infection is chronic, the nail may become ridged or discolored and may be lost. Paronychia occurs most often in people who bite their nails excessively or whose hands are frequently in water (e.g., dishwashers, mothers of infants). Diabetics also have an increased risk for this infection. *Candida* species appear to play an etiologic role, although a variety of bacteria usually are present. Management involves keeping hands as dry as possible (e.g., using waterproof gloves for dishwashing) and applying an anticandidal medication (e.g., nystatin cream) or a broad-spectrum antifungal agent (clotrimazole or miconazole cream) two times a day for several weeks. If localized swelling does not respond to these measures, drainage may be helpful. This can be done by sliding an 18-gauge needle, bevel down, along the nail into the involved area. Lifting the skin from the nail with the needle usually achieves drainage and relief of pain.

The major cause of paronychia of the toe (usually a great toe) is an ingrown toenail. Diagnosis and management of this problem are described in Chapter 73.

Intertriginous Infections

Approaches to diagnosis of infections involving moist intertriginous areas (toe webs, axillae, groin area) are described in Chapter 116.

General References

McDonough JJ, Stern PJ, Alexander JW. Management of animal and human bites and resulting human infections. Curr Clin Top Infect Dis 1987;3:11.

A thorough and still useful review.

Gerding DM. Foot infections in diabetic patients: role of anaerobes. Clin Infect Dis 1995;20:S283.

Important information about the microbiology of diabetic foot infections.

Specific References

1. Bisno AL, Stevens DL. Streptococcal infections of skin and soft tissues. N Engl J Med 1996;334:240.
2. Esterly NB, Nelson DB, Dunne WM Jr. Impetigo. Am J Dis Child 1991;145:125.
3. Gemmell CG. Staphylococcal scalded skin syndrome. J Med Microbiol 1995;43:318.
4. Bernard P, Bedame C, Mounier M. Streptococcal cause of erysipelas and cellulitis in adults. Arch Dermatol 1989;125:779.
5. Barker FG, Leppard BJ, Seal DV. Streptococcal necrotizing fasciitis: comparison between histological and clinical features. J Clin Pathol 1987;40:335.
6. Green RJ, Dafoe DC, Raffin TA. Necrotizing fasciitis. Chest 1996;110:219.
7. Belsey MA, Sinclair M, Roder MR, et al. *Corynebacterium diphtheriae* skin infections in Alabama and Louisiana: a factor in the epidemiology of diphtheria. N Engl J Med 1969;280:135.

CHAPTER 33

Respiratory Tract Infections*

NICHOLAS H. FIEBACH, MD
DARIUS A. RASTEGAR, MD

Respiratory tract infections are the most common acute illnesses in the United States and in the industrialized world. These infections are the most frequent causes of absences from school or work. Most upper respiratory infections (URIs) are self-diagnosed and self-treated and do not come to the attention of a physician. Lower respiratory infections (LRIs) may be minor or amenable to ambulatory treatment, but they also represent one of the leading causes of hospitalization and death in this country. The cost of respiratory tract infections in lost productivity and expenditures for treatments, including over-the-counter remedies, is estimated to be billions of dollars.

UPPER RESPIRATORY TRACT INFECTIONS

Common Cold

The common cold, or coryza, is a mild, self-limited syndrome caused usually by viral infection of the upper respiratory tract mucosa and characterized by one or more of the following symptoms: nasal discharge and obstruction, sneezing, sore throat, cough, and hoarseness.

Epidemiology and Transmission

The common cold syndrome is caused by a variety of viruses that are clinically indistinguishable from each other, yet have distinct seasonal peaks for unknown reasons. *Rhinoviruses* are the etiologic agent in 25% to 30% of colds, with seasonal peaks in early fall and middle to late spring. *Coronaviruses* account for another 10% to 15% of colds, with a seasonal peak in midwinter. *Influenza, parainfluenza, respiratory syncytial viruses, and adenovirus* are etiologic agents for another 10% to 15%, although this group more commonly causes the typical influenza syndrome (see later discussion). Bacteria associated with pharyngitis (discussed later) can also cause some common cold symptoms.

The incidence of the common cold syndrome decreases with age. On average, adults have two to four colds per year; children have six to eight (1). Because person-to-person spread of colds occurs mainly in the home and at school, schoolchildren often serve as carriers for introducing colds into a family.

Transmission of rhinovirus is most efficient by direct physical contact (2). Frequent, unconscious touching of virus-laden nasal mucosa contaminates the hands of infected individuals. Infectious material can survive on the hand for as long as 4 hours (3), during which time hand-to-hand contact with susceptible subjects transmits the virus. Self-inoculation of the nares and conjunctiva (from which the virus is passed along the lacrimal ducts to the nasal passages) then completes the transmission of the virus. Exposure to susceptible subjects across even short distances of air is an inefficient method of transmission of rhinoviruses, although aerosol transmission of particles effectively transmits some viruses (e.g., coxsackieviruses, influenza viruses, adenoviruses). Therefore, transmission of colds is probably uncommon in offices, theaters, buses, and other confined spaces if nose-to-hand-to-hand-to-nose-and-eye contact is avoided. Kissing and other exposures to oral secretions do not transmit rhinovirus efficiently.

Clinical Features

The correct diagnosis of the common cold is readily made by the patient. After an incubation period of 48 to 72 hours, the syndrome begins with mild malaise, rhinorrhea, sneezing, scratchy throat, and variable loss of taste and smell. These symptoms increase to maximal severity on the second to fourth day. Viral excretion and communicability are maximal during the period of the most severe symptoms. Fever usually is not present and rarely exceeds a 1°F (0.5°C) elevation in temperature. Cough and hoarseness may begin later, and their severity and duration are increased in cigarette smokers. Conversely, neither cigarette smoking nor exposure to cold appears to increase the attack rate of colds. Colds usually last 1 week but may persist for up to 2 weeks in 25% of cases.

Identification of the causative virus by clinical observation or readily available laboratory testing is not possible, nor is it necessary for management. The primary challenge for the physician is to identify patients with influenza, streptococcal pharyngitis, secondary bacterial sinusitis, otitis media, or more unusual URIs

*In previous editions, Frederick T. Koster, MD, and L. Randol Barker, MD, contributed to this chapter.

(see later discussion and Chapter 110), for whom antimicrobials may be beneficial. The use of sinus radiography and throat culture techniques is discussed in this chapter; pneumatic otoscopy is discussed in Chapter 110.

Treatment

Patients with typical URI syndromes can be assessed and managed appropriately by a telephone contact (4). Specific antiviral therapy for the uncomplicated common cold is not available, but symptomatic treatment is appropriate. *Systemic analgesics,* such as aspirin and acetaminophen, relieve fever, headache, and myalgias but also increase nasal secretions, possibly by decreasing the neutralizing antibody response (5). Naproxen (and presumably other *nonsteroidal anti-inflammatory drugs [NSAIDs]*) relieves the headache, myalgias, and cough without altering viral shedding or antibody response (6). *Topical analgesics* are contained in a variety of over-the-counter preparations (e.g., phenol [Chloraseptic], menthol, hexylresorcinol [Sucrets Sore Throat]) and can be recommended for amelioration of symptoms.

Bed rest is not necessary to facilitate recovery. Steam inhalation did not alleviate nasal symptoms in controlled clinical trials (7), but sipping hot chicken soup (the only soup studied) increased the clearance of nasal mucus (8). Hoarseness, caused by inflammation and edema of the vocal cords, may be relieved by voice rest (see Chapter 111). Zinc lozenges taken every 2 hours may accelerate recovery of all symptoms, but evidence from controlled trials is not conclusive; the most commonly used preparation (zinc gluconate) may also cause nausea and bad taste, and the potential for toxicity exists with prolonged use (9,10).

Nasal congestion is best relieved by *topical decongestants* (e.g., phenylephrine [NeoSynephrine], oxymetazoline [Afrin]) (11); sprays rather than drops may be more easily administered (Table 33.1) (see later discussion). Patients should be cautioned against using decongestant drops or sprays for more than 3 to 5 days to avoid the rebound effect, *rhinitis medicamentosa,* an increase in nasal congestion that occurs when decongestant medication is discontinued. Systemic effects of topical decongestants are uncommon (see Chapter 30). *Topical ipratropium* spray (0.06%) relieves rhinorrhea and sneezing but may cause blood-tinged mucus and nasal dryness (12). Nasal corticosteroids have not been shown to have a beneficial effect in the treatment of the common cold.

The effectiveness of an *oral decongestant,* pseudoephedrine (Sudafed, 30 mg over-the-counter or 60 mg by prescription; also available as Sudafed S.A., a sustained-action preparation containing 120 mg of pseudoephedrine, taken every 12 hours), has been demonstrated in some controlled trials (1,11). Pseudoephedrine did not cause blood pressure to increase in treated hypertensive patients (12). However, another over-the-counter oral decongestant, phenylpropanolamine, was banned by the U.S. Food and Drug Administration after a case-control study found that it was associated with hemorrhagic stroke in women (13).

Evidence for the effectiveness of *antihistamines* in treating the common cold has been equivocal (1,11,14). Older, sedating antihistamines (which are available over the counter; Table 33.1) may be more effective because of their anticholinergic, hence drying, effect (12). Combinations of an oral decongestant and an older antihistamine have been shown to reduce nasal symptoms and cough in controlled trials of cold treatments (11,15).

There is very limited evidence that an *expectorant* (e.g., guaifenesin, contained in many combination cold and cough remedies) is effective in URIs (11), and it is more rational and less expensive to use the individual ingredients contained in combination remedies in appropriate dosages. (See the discussion of cough suppressants in the section entitled Acute Bronchitis.)

Alternative and complementary treatments for the common cold are popular (see Chapter 5). The lack of prophylactic benefit of *vitamin C* (ascorbic acid) in preventing common colds was confirmed by a recent meta-analysis (16). There have been numerous controlled studies of vitamin C in treating the acute symptoms of the common cold. Several earlier reviews

Table 33.1. Examples of Over-the-Counter Cold Medications[a]

	Generic name	Trade name	Effectiveness	Side Effects
Antihistamines	Chlorpheniramine Diphenhydramine	Chlortrimeton; others Benadryl	Reduce sneezing, nasal mucus[b]	Drowsiness, dry mouth and nose, urinary retention
Decongestants				
Topical	Phenylephrine Oxymetazoline	NeoSynephrine; others Afrin	Reduce nasal congestion, discharge[c]	Rebound nasal congestion
Systemic	Pseudoephedrine	Sudafed; others	Decreases nasal symptoms[c]	Tachycardia, palpitations, elevated blood pressure, urinary retention
Expectorants	Guaifenesin	Robitussin; others	Marginally reduces sputum quantity[b]	None
Combinations	Antihistamine/decongestant	Many	Reduce nasal symptoms, cough[c]	Dry mouth, insomnia, nervousness, urinary retention

[a]See package labeling for dosage and schedule information.
[b]Limited or equivocal evidence from controlled trials.
[c]Evidence supported by controlled trials.

concluded that there is no significant effect (17,18), but more recent systematic reviews suggest that there may be a modest reduction in the duration and severity of symptoms with higher doses (e.g., 1 g or more daily) (16,19). However, some experts caution that such large doses may have adverse consequences in some people (20). A systematic review of the effectiveness of *Echinacea,* a plant extract, suggested that some preparations may be better than placebo in preventing or treating the common cold (21). However, there was substantial variation in the preparations investigated, and the methodologic quality of the studies was not sufficient to conclude that *Echinacea* is effective.

Antibiotics should *not* be prescribed for the uncomplicated cold. Randomized, placebo-controlled trials of treatment for uncomplicated, nonspecific URIs in adults have shown no benefit from antibiotics (22). Colored nasal discharge does not signal a bacterial infection or a complication of a cold; it simply indicates the presence in the discharge of polymorphonuclear leukocytes, which migrate into nasal secretions in response to cytokines induced by viral infection (22,23).

Patient Education

Because transmission of colds occurs chiefly by physical contact, it is reasonable to counsel patients and those around them that transmission can be minimized by hand washing, reduced finger-to-nose-and-eye contact, and reduced exposure to the cold sufferer. Clinicians should be particularly vigilant to avoid contact with the patient's secretions and should wash their hands carefully after examining the infected patient. Although clinicians with common colds may examine patients if they wash their hands and avoid sneezing on the patient, those with the flu syndrome (discussed later) should avoid patient contact.

Viral URIs may be complicated occasionally by superimposed bacterial sinusitis, otitis media, or pneumonitis. Therefore, patients should be advised to notify their health care provider of any symptoms suggesting one of these syndromes (see later discussion), each of which may require antimicrobial treatment.

Prevention. Vitamin C and *Echinacea* have not been shown, conclusively, to prevent the common cold (see previous discussion). Vaccine development is complicated by the great antigenic diversity of respiratory viruses, including more than 100 serotypes of rhinoviruses and 47 serotypes of adenoviruses.

Sinusitis

The paranasal sinuses include the frontal, ethmoid, and maxillary sinuses (Fig. 33.1). These air-filled bony cavities produce up to 2 pints of mucus every day, which normally drains into the nasopharynx. This self-cleaning occurs by movement of the mucus, propelled by cilia that line the respiratory epithelium of the sinuses, through the ostia (openings) of the sinus and the middle meatus (passageway) in the nose. The *ostiomeatal complex,* the confluence of the drainage of the frontal, ethmoid, and maxillary sinuses, is located between the middle and inferior turbinates on each side of the nasal cavity (24) (Fig. 33.2). Symptoms of nasal and sinus congestion, pain, and discharge result from inflammation of the sinuses and obstruction of the ostiomeatal complex.

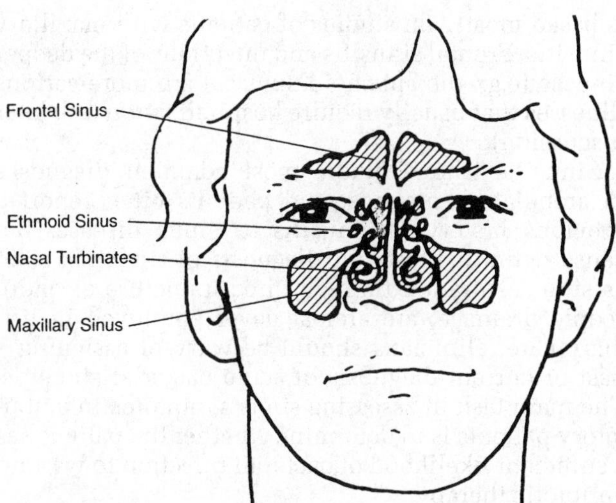

Figure 33.1. Location of the paranasal sinuses. From Williams JW, Simel DL. Does this patient have sinusitis? Diagnosing acute sinusitis by history and physical examination. JAMA 1993;270:1242, with permission.

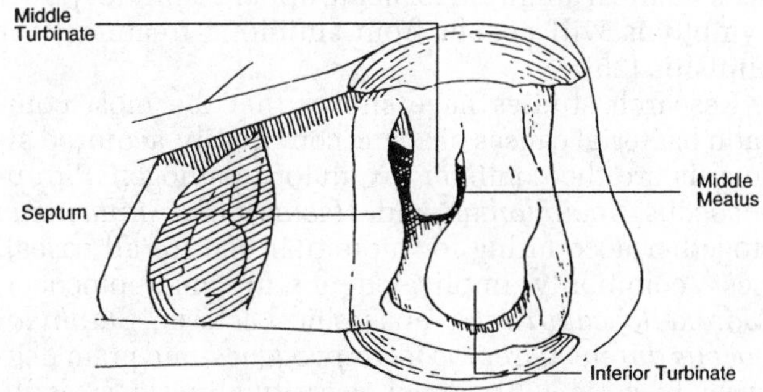

Figure 33.2. Examination of the nose (with the use of a nasal speculum). From Williams JW, Simel DL. Does this patient have sinusitis? Diagnosing acute sinusitis by history and physical examination. JAMA 1993;270:1242, with permission.

Acute bacterial sinusitis is an infection of one or more paranasal sinuses that occurs when the normal sinus drainage is impaired. Its symptoms overlap with those of nonbacterial and noninfectious causes of nasal and sinus inflammation, such as viral URIs (discussed earlier), allergic and perennial rhinitis (see Chapter 30), nasal or sinus polyps, foreign bodies, local irritation and complications from swimming and diving, immune deficiency, and anatomic abnormalities that obstruct sinus drainage. Up to 10% of cases of acute sinusitis are an extension of a dental abscess. Nursing home or homebound patients with nasogastric tubes occasionally develop sinusitis, which may manifest as a cause of persistent fever.

Most cases of sinusitis in healthy patients involve the maxillary and ethmoid sinuses, and the evidence for evaluation and treatment of sinusitis in outpatients is based mostly on studies of patients with maxillary sinusitis. Frontal sinusitis and infections of the deeper sinuses (e.g., the sphenoid sinuses) are more serious illnesses that usually require hospitalization (see later discussion).

Sinusitis is one of the most common diagnoses in ambulatory practice, and patients often report a previous history of sinusitis or sinus disease. Because definitive tests for diagnosis of sinusitis, such as sinus aspiration through direct puncture or endoscopic drainage, are almost never employed in primary care, clinicians should be wary of assigning a past or current diagnosis of acute bacterial sinusitis. The main task in assessing sinus symptoms in ambulatory patients is to determine whether the patient has a sufficient likelihood of bacterial infection to warrant antibiotic therapy.

Epidemiology

It is estimated that only 2% or less of viral URIs are complicated by the development of acute bacterial sinusitis and that fewer than 15% of patients who seek medical attention for acute upper respiratory tract symptoms will benefit from antibiotic treatment for sinusitis (25).

Research studies have shown that the most common bacterial causes of acute, community-acquired sinusitis are the common respiratory pathogens *Streptococcus pneumoniae* and *Haemophilus influenzae* (together accounting for more than half of all cases). Less commonly implicated are alpha-streptococci, *Moraxella catarrhalis,* anaerobic bacteria, *Staphylococcus aureus, Streptococcus pyogenes,* and gram negative bacteria (26). Fungi occasionally cause acute sinusitis and should be considered along with cytomegalovirus and atypical mycobacteria in immunocompromised patients.

Clinical Features and Diagnosis

Patients often seek care for suspected sinusitis because of facial pain or purulent nasal discharge. When acute bacterial sinusitis is present, the pain is caused by periosteal reaction secondary to purulent inflammation behind an obstructed ostium. The pain is dull in the early stages but becomes throbbing in later stages. Coughing, dependency, and percussion over the involved sinus may exacerbate the pain. Percussion of the teeth may be painful in maxillary sinusitis. Nontender edema of the eyelids, seen predominantly in children, may occur with uncomplicated ethmoid and maxillary sinusitis. However, the facial pain and nasal discharge associated with the viral or noninfectious causes of nasal congestion often resemble the symptoms of acute bacterial sinusitis, especially when symptoms have been present less than 1 week. Other causes of facial pain to be distinguished from sinusitis are dental abscess (see Chapter 112), migraine and cluster headache, (see Chapter 87) and trigeminal neuralgia (see Chapter 87).

Examination. The initial assessment of patients with sinus symptoms should include examination of the pharynx, nose, ears, and teeth. The nostrils may be visualized more effectively with a nasal speculum, with care taken to avoid contact with the nasal septum, which is sensitive (27). Particular attention should be directed to the area of the middle meatus, between the inferior and middle turbinates, and whether pus is present in this area (Fig. 33.2). Tapping on maxillary teeth with a probe or tongue blade may reveal tenderness, which suggests a dental abscess. Abnormal transillumination of the maxillary sinuses was found to be useful in predicting acute bacterial sinusitis in an otolaryngology practice but was only weakly predictive in a study of primary care patients (27). If it is attempted, only a concentrated halogen light source should be used; it should be placed tightly over the infraorbital rim of the patient in a completely dark room, with light transmission through the hard palate observed in the patient's open mouth. Only complete absence of light transmission, suggesting sinus opacification and infection, is helpful. Transillumination of the frontal sinuses is not useful, because they are often asymmetric in healthy patients.

Diagnostic Approach. There is no single clinical feature or easily performed diagnostic test that conclusively establishes the presence or absence of acute bacterial sinusitis. Several studies of patients with acute nasal and maxillary symptoms compared clinical findings with the results of sinus puncture and aspiration or sinus imaging studies (25). Aspiration of mucopurulent or purulent secretions, or abnormal sinus radiographs or sonograms suggestive of bacterial infection, were associated in these studies with the following clinical features: *purulent nasal discharge* reported by the patient or observed on examination; *maxillary tooth pain; facial pain or tenderness* on examination in the maxillary area; and *worsening of nasal and sinus symptoms after initial improvement* (Table 33.2). The likelihood of acute bacterial sinus infection increases with the number of these indicators present in a patient. In general, patients with purulent nasal discharge and unilateral maxillary tooth pain or facial discomfort for longer than 1 week are likely to have acute bacterial sinusitis. Patients with one or none of these findings probably do not have bacterial infection, although severe facial pain in a patient who is febrile or toxic usually warrants empiric antibiotic treatment and further evaluation. Nasopharyngeal swabs are usually contaminated with normal flora and are of no use in the evaluation.

Radiologic Examination. Diagnostic imaging of the sinuses is *not* recommended for most patients

Table 33.2. Clinical Features in Patients with Sinus Symptoms That Predict Acute Bacterial Sinusitis[a]

Symptoms Lasting 7 Days or Longer
Purulent nasal discharge (reported by the patient or observed on examination)
Maxillary tooth or facial pain or tenderness on examination
Worsening of nasal or sinus symptoms after initial improvement

[a]Patients with purulent nasal discharge *and* unilateral maxillary tooth pain or facial discomfort for 1 week or longer are likely to have acute bacterial sinusitis.

who present with acute symptoms suggesting sinusitis (24–26). Sinus radiographs demonstrating air–fluid levels or complete opacification are only 80% to 85% specific for acute bacterial sinusitis, although normal radiographs rule it out in 90% of cases (25,28). A single Waters (occipitomental) view is probably as accurate as a "sinus series" of multiple views (29). Many patients with acute nasal and sinus symptoms have intermediate findings on radiography (e.g., mucosal thickening), which are neither sensitive nor specific and which may be seen in patients with viral URIs (25). Computed tomographic (CT) scans have better sensitivity for detecting mucosal abnormalities, are able to visualize the ethmoid and frontal sinuses well, and are increasingly ordered in place of plain radiographs. However, the specificity of CT scans for diagnosing acute maxillary sinus infection may be poor; for example, a study of healthy volunteers experimentally infected with rhinovirus found that 87% had maxillary sinus abnormalities on CT scans (30). Diagnostic imaging of the sinuses is most helpful in the evaluation of unexplained headache and for patients who do not respond to therapy or who are toxic and require accurate diagnosis early.

Treatment

Randomized controlled trials of antibiotic treatment for patients with suspected acute bacterial sinusitis have provided mixed results, with several studies showing no benefit of treatment (31,32). A meta-analysis of all relevant trials concluded that antibiotic treatment was of moderate benefit (33), and a consensus panel reported that 81% of antibiotic-treated patients, compared with 66% of untreated patients, were improved at 10 to 14 days (25). This limited benefit of antibiotic treatment reflects the imprecison of diagnosis of acute bacterial sinusitis on clinical or radiographic grounds and the unavoidable inclusion in controlled studies of some patients who did not really have bacterial infections and were destined to improve regardless of treatment allocation. Recent clinical guidelines suggest that patients with mild nasal and sinus complaints should receive only symptomatic treatment, and that those with moderate or severe symptoms suggesting sinusitis (see Diagnostic Approach) should be treated with antibiotics (25). This recommendation is supported by a decision analysis which found that antibiotic treatment of patients with mild to moderate symptoms was cost-effective in reducing days sick with sinusitis (34).

Choice and Duration of Antibiotics. Amoxicillin, trimethoprim/sulfamethoxazole, amoxicillin/clavulanate, cefuroxime axetil, levofloxacin, and clarithromycin have all been proposed as first-line treatments for acute, community-acquired bacterial sinusitis (24,26) (Table 33.3). Because of concerns about more widespread antibiotic resistance among *Haemophilus* and *Streptococcus* species, some authorities recommend

Table 33.3. Oral Antibiotics Used for Ambulatory Treatment of Common Respiratory Infections

Drug (Trade Name)[a]	Available Strengths (mg)	Usual Adult Dosage and Schedule[b]	Cost[c]	Common Side Effects	Drug and Food Interactions
Penicillin V	250, 500	250–500 mg t.i.d. to q.i.d.	$	Nausea, vomiting, diarrhea, rash, vaginal candidiasis	May cause false positive clinitest for glucose, may potentiate warfarin
Amoxicillin	250, 500	250–875 mg b.i.d. to t.i.d.	$		
Amoxicillin/clavulanate (Augmentin)	250, 500, 875	250–875 mg b.i.d. to t.i.d. 500–875 mg b.i.d.	$$$		
Cefuroxime (Ceftin)	125, 250, 500	125–500 mg b.i.d.	$$$		
Cefpodoxime (Vantin)	100, 200	100–400 mg b.i.d.	$$$		
Erythromycin	250, 333, 500	250–500 mg t.i.d. to q.i.d.	$	Nausea, vomiting, abdominal pain, diarrhea	Potentiates warfarin, increases risk of lovastatin-induced rhabdomyolysis
Azithromycin (Zithromax)	250, 600	500 mg loading dose, then 250 mg q.d.	$$		
Clarithromycin (Biaxin)	500, 500SR	500 mg b.i.d., 1000 mg SR q.d.	$$$		
Doxycycline	50, 100	100 mg b.i.d.	$	Photosensitivity, nausea, vomiting, diarrhea, candidiasis	Food, milk, iron, antacids may decrease absorption
Trimethoprim (TMP)/ sulfamethoxazole (SMX)	80TMP/400SMX, (single strength), 160TMP/800SMX (double strength)	2 single-strength or 1 double-strength b.i.d.	$	Nausea, vomiting, rash, elevation of serum creatinine	Potentiates phenytoin, warfarin and sulfonylureas
Clindamycin	75, 150, 300	150–450 mg t.i.d. to q.i.d.	$$	Nausea, vomiting, diarrhea, rash, *Clostridium difficile* colitis	May potentiate neuromuscular blocking agents
Gatifloxacin (Tequin)	200, 400	200–400 mg q.d.	$$$	Nausea, vomiting, diarrhea, dizziness	Antacids inhibit absorption
Levofloxacin (Levaquin)	250, 500, 750	250–500 mg q.d.	$$$		
Moxifloxacin (Avelox)	400	400 mg q.d	$$$		

[a]No trade name is listed for drugs available in generic form.

[b]See text for recommended duration of therapy

[c]$, < $20; $$, = $20–50, $$$, > $50 for 10-day supply (5 days for azithromycin). Source: Medical Letter 2001;43:78.

initiating treatment with amoxicillin/clavulanate, cefuroxime axetil, or levofloxacin. However, a meta-analysis of clinical trials showed no advantage of cefuroxime or the newer macrolides compared to penicillin or amoxicillin (33), and a large retrospective analysis of almost 30,000 patients treated for sinusitis found that amoxicillin and trimethoprim/sulfamethoxazole were as effective as cephalosporins, fluoroquinolones, and the newer macrolides (35). In choosing an antibiotic, clinicians should consider the moderate benefits of treatment, cost, and convenience of dosing. For most patients, amoxicillin 500 mg twice daily or trimethoprim 160 mg/sulfamethoxazole 800 mg (i.e., the double-strength dosage) is an appropriate choice. For patients with severe symptoms, those who are toxic, and those in whom antibiotic-resistant bacteria may be present (e.g., frequent contact with children in day care, recent or frequent use of antibiotics, areas with a known high prevalence of antibiotic resistance), amoxicillin 500 mg/clavulanate 250 mg twice daily, cefuroxime axetil 250 mg twice daily, or levofloxacin 500 mg once daily should be prescribed.

The recommended duration of therapy for uncomplicated acute bacterial sinusitis is 10 days. Although one randomized trial compared a 3-day to a 10-day course of trimethoprim/sulfamethoxazole and found no difference in outcome at 14 days, it lacked sufficient power to detect a difference in the rates of relapse, recurrence, or serious complications (36).

Other Treatments. Although there is no conclusive evidence to support the use of adjunctive therapies for acute sinusitis (33), *improvement in sinus drainage* may be helpful. A topical decongestant, such as phenylephrine (Neo-Synephrine) 0.25% or 0.5% every 4 to 6 hours, or oxymetazoline (Afrin) 0.05% twice daily, is administered in a two-step manner: as an initial spray to decrease congestion in the membranes of the anterior nares, followed 5 to 10 minutes later by a second spray delivered deeper to the middle meatus. Use of topical decongestants should be limited to approximately 5 days to avoid rebound congestion. An oral (systemic) decongestant, such as pseudoephedrine (30 to 60 mg every 6 to 8 hours), may have a more reliable therapeutic effect in a congested nose and may be continued for the duration of symptoms (Table 33.1; see Common Cold). Evidence for the effectiveness of nasal corticosteroids in improving the symptoms of sinusitis is limited.

Pain relief is important, and codeine may be required in addition to over-the-counter analgesics and NSAIDs. Patients who plan to fly, especially in nonpressurized aircraft, should take an oral decongestant before takeoff, supplemented with topical decongestant spray every 4 hours.

Complications

Resolution of facial pain, headache, and fever is expected within several days. If no response occurs by this time, the diagnosis should be reassessed by radiography or CT scan, and referral to an otolaryngologist for antral puncture or endoscopic drainage may be advisable. For toxic patients and those with suspected frontal or ethmoid sinusitis, imaging, consultation with an otolaryngologist, and hospitalization for drainage, culture, and definitive parenteral antibiotics should be considered at initial presentation. Patients with severe facial pain benefit from early antral puncture for pain relief.

Serious complications of acute bacterial sinusitis are unusual and have been estimated to occur at a rate of only 1 in 10,000 cases (34). They constitute medical emergencies because they represent direct extension of infection to adjacent orbits, bone, blood vessels, and the central nervous system. *Nontender* periorbital edema indicates restriction of orbital venous outflow through congested ethmoid veins; it is not associated with decreased visual acuity and is appropriately managed with vigorous medical therapy. However, *tender periorbital swelling* associated with proptosis and chemosis represents orbital cellulitis and requires immediate referral to an otolaryngologist. Subsequent progression of cellulitis to subperiosteal or orbital abscess, associated with ophthalmoplegia and loss of vision, requires emergency surgical drainage. Osteomyelitis is most often a complication of frontal sinusitis. Cavernous sinus thrombosis should be suspected in the patient with signs of orbital complications plus extreme toxicity. Intracranial extension is rare but life-threatening, manifesting most commonly as meningitis. Abscesses in the brain and epidural and subdural spaces manifest more insidiously. Frontal lobe abscess may manifest as mild headache, low-grade fever, malaise, and personality change. In poorly controlled diabetics and immunocompromised hosts, invasive fungal infections of the nose and sinus can be severe and deadly; *rhinocerebral mucormycosis* may be recognized by a black eschar on the nasal turbinates.

Chronic Sinusitis

When the symptoms of acute sinusitis, especially pain and fever, subside with therapy, purulent nasal discharge may continue. Despite persistence of radiologic changes, this stage usually resolves after an additional 2 to 3 weeks of conservative management with oral decongestants.

Sinusitis is classified as *subacute* when symptoms are prolonged for 4 to 12 weeks, and *chronic* when symptoms persist longer than 12 weeks. Chronic sinusitis results from obstruction to sinus drainage and loss of the normal ciliated epithelial lining of the sinus cavity, sometimes leading to a low-grade infection by anaerobic and aerobic bacteria. Acute exacerbations may occur, caused primarily by the organisms that most commonly cause acute sinusitis (*H. influenzae* and *S. pneumoniae*). Chronic sinusitis may complicate certain systemic diseases, such as sarcoidosis, Wegener granulomatosis, immunoglobulin A deficiency, human immunodeficiency virus (HIV) infection, and allergic rhinitis with asthma. Extensive sinus disease in chronic sinusitis, indicated by bilateral occlusion of the ostiomeatal complex and severe mucosal thickening on CT scan, is associated with asthma and peripheral eosinophilia (37).

Diagnosis and Management. Persistent purulent nasal discharge and postnasal drip with associated cough, despite adequate medical therapy, are the primary features of chronic sinusitis. Facial pain and tenderness are minimal or absent. A CT scan may confirm the presence of sinus mucosal inflammation and thickening and indicate whether specific anatomic abnormalities such as polyps, mucoceles, or tumors may be involved.

Oral penicillin V or amoxicillin for 1 month is the most appropriate antimicrobial regimen; amoxicillin/clavulanate or clindamycin are alternatives (Table 33.3). Continued use of systemic decongestants, as well as a trial of *topical corticosteroids* (in dosages similar to those used for allergic rhinitis; see Chapter 30), may facilitate resolution of symptoms in chronic sinusitis (24). For patients whose symptoms do not resolve with one or more of these empiric treatments, referral to an otolaryngologist for consideration of *endoscopic or surgical drainage* is recommended.

Flu Syndrome

"Flu" is said to have been named by two Italian astrologers, who believed it was caused by the influence, or "*influenza*," of the stars. Although the term "flu-like illness" is commonly used by patients and clinicians to describe any malady thought to result from a virus, including gastroenteritis, this section describes illnesses caused by respiratory pathogens. Flu syndrome presents as the abrupt onset of malaise, myalgia, headache, and fever. Coryza and sore throat are also present. Illness is severe for 3 to 14 days, and convalescence lasts for 1 to 4 weeks. The majority of cases of flu syndrome are caused by the influenza virus during annual winter epidemics (38). Other viruses, especially parainfluenza and respiratory syncytial viruses and adenovirus, produce the same clinical syndrome and may coinfect patients with influenza (39) (Fig. 33.3).

Epidemiology

There are two genera, or types, of influenza virus that infect humans: influenza A and influenza B. Influenza A is further subtyped into strains according to variations in the surface glycoproteins, hemagglutinin (H1 through H15) and neuraminidase (N1 through N9) (40). Epidemic spread of the influenza virus is caused by the appearance in nonimmune populations of new antigenic variations of the virus. Variations of the hemagglutinin and neuraminidase antigens occur almost annually in influenza A, less often in influenza B. Major variation is called *antigenic shift* and results in pandemic spread of a new strain, almost always type A, throughout regions of the world where there is little natural immunity. The most recent pandemics occurred in the winters of 1957–1958, 1968–1969, and 1977–1978, and they varied considerably in severity. Between pandemics, minor antigenic variation, termed *antigenic drift*, occurs frequently, resulting in a new strain and epidemics during the winter almost every year. Such interpandemic spread, although less dramatic, accounts for greater cumulative morbidity and mortality because of its annual occurrence. In recent years, epidemic influenza has occurred regularly and has had a major influence on mortality and hospitalizations in this country, especially among the elderly and individuals with chronic illness. It is estimated that influenza is responsible for approximately 20,000 deaths and more than 100,000 excess hospital admissions yearly (41). Although it is often impossible clinically to distinguish infections caused by type A or type B, influenza A is responsible for greater excess mortality than type B.

Influenza virus typically circulates in the Northern Hemisphere from late November through March (Fig. 33.3). During this time there is usually a more intense peak of illness, attributable to a predominant strain, which lasts for several weeks. There may also be a second, less intense peak caused by another strain, which sometimes heralds the predominant subtype the following year (42). Influenza also occurs sporadically at other times of the year, and it may affect travelers to other parts of the world where influenza is circulating, as well as individuals exposed to persons from those areas.

Influenza virus appears to be transmitted by virus-containing small-particle aerosols dispersed by sneezing, coughing, or talking. The incubation period is 18 to 72 hours. Viral shedding persists for 5 to 10 days, but virus is present in high titer in secretions for only 48 hours after the onset of clinical illness. In the community, person-to-person transmission is rapid, with spread initially among children, then adults. In local epidemics, the incidence of cases reaches a peak in 2 to 3 weeks and persists for only 5 to 6 weeks.

Clinical Features and Diagnosis

Uncomplicated influenza, type A or B, has an abrupt onset of systemic symptoms including fever, chills, headache, myalgias, and malaise. The fever, which may rise to 106°F (41°C) in some cases, typically lasts 3 days, although it may persist for 5 to 7 days. Headache and myalgias involving the back, arms, legs, and occasionally the eyes are the predominant symptoms, persisting as long as the fever. Respiratory symptoms, such as nonproductive cough, nasal discharge, hoarseness, and sore throat, appear as systemic symptoms wane. Cough and weakness usually subside after 2 weeks but may persist longer. In the elderly, myalgias and sore throat are less common, whereas dyspnea is a more common symptom (40).

Physical findings include general toxicity, flushed face, hot skin, watery red eyes, clear nasal discharge, tender cervical lymph nodes, and occasionally localized rales in the chest. The white cell count and differential, indicated only if the patient is toxic or pneumonia is suspected, usually demonstrate mild neutropenia and relative lymphocytosis caused by absolute granulocytopenia.

Because antimicrobial therapy for influenza infections is available, it may be important to determine whether flu syndrome is caused by this specific virus. The best clinical predictors of influenza virus as the cause of flu syndrome are fever greater than 100°F

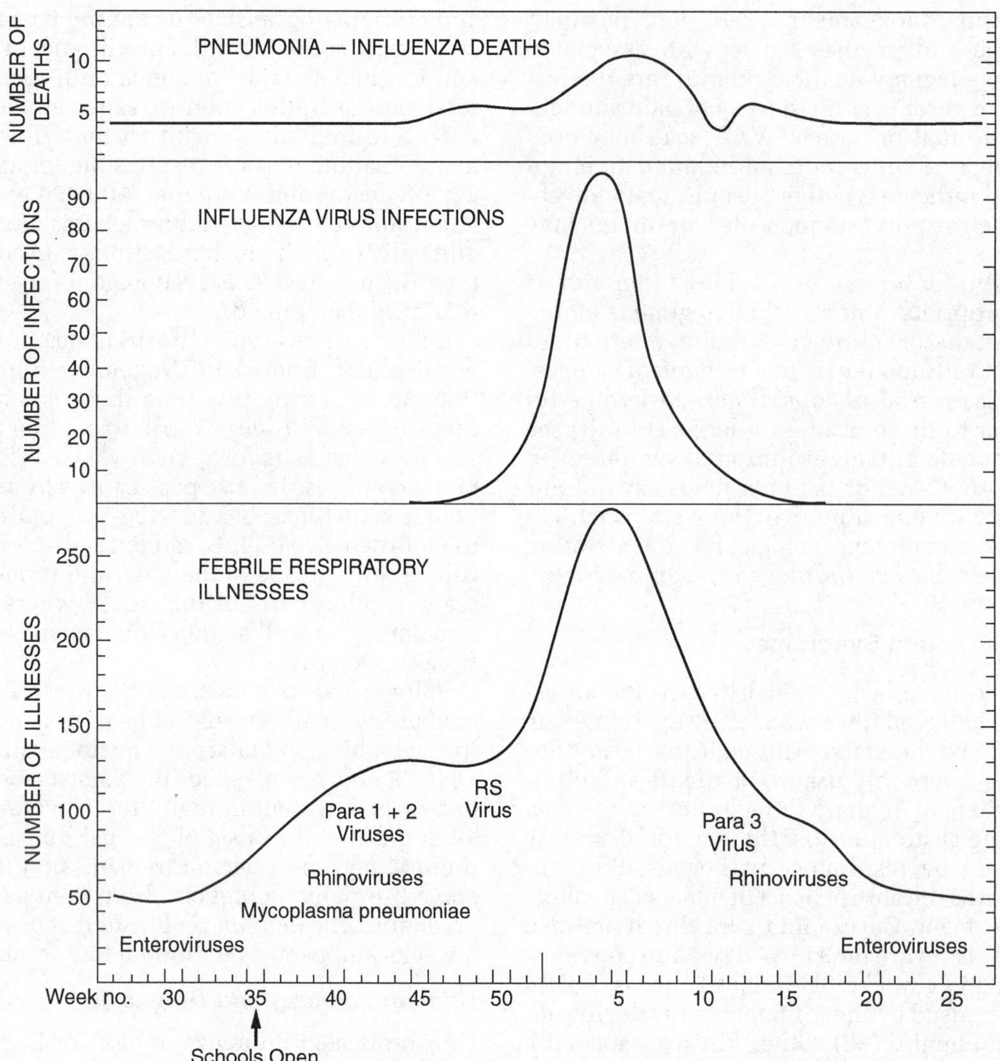

Figure 33.3. Schematic representation of the occurrence, etiology, and mortality from febrile respiratory illnesses in relation to time of year. Data are from Houston, Texas, 1975–1981. Reproduced with permission from Glezen WP. Serious morbidity and mortality associated with influenza epidemics. Epidemiol Rev 1982;4:25.

(37.8°C), cough, and abrupt onset. However, during influenza epidemics, when the prevalence of influenza infection may be 65% or higher among individuals with any respiratory symptoms, this combination is neither sensitive nor specific. Therefore, influenza should be suspected in patients who have respiratory illness during flu season (late November through March), and it should presumed to be the cause of acute respiratory illness with fever and cough when influenza is known to be circulating in the community. Clinicians can obtain information about influenza epidemics from the Centers for Disease Control and Prevention website (www.cdc.gov/ncidod/diseases/flu/weekly.htm; accessed 1/11/02) and hotline (888-232-3228) and from state and local health departments.

Diagnostic Tests. Influenza virus infection may be diagnosed by polymerase chain reaction assay, viral culture, or specific serology (comparing acute and convalescent titers). These tests, however, require specialized techniques, and the results are not available until days to weeks after a patient is evaluated. A variety of rapid test kits for point-of-care analysis are now available to clinicians (43). These tests are moderately complex and typically require multiple steps over 10 to 30 minutes. Reported sensitivity has ranged from 57% to 96% (with no clear advantage for any specific kit), but specificity is better, ranging from 88% to 100%. Therefore, a positive test reliably confirms a diagnosis of influenza infection, but a negative test does not exclude influenza or the potential benefit of specific treatment.

Treatment

Options for the specific antimicrobial treatment of influenza have expanded in recent years (41,44). In addition to *amantadine* and the related adamantane compound *rimantadine,* two neuraminidase inhibitors, *zanamivir* and *oseltamivir,* were approved for use in 1999 (Table 33.4). Amantadine and rimantadine are

Table 33.4. Antimicrobial Drugs for the Treatment of Influenza[a]

Generic name	Trade name	Active against: Type A	Active against: Type B	Dosage, route[b]	Cost[c]	Adverse effects
Amandatine	Symmetrel	Yes	No	100 mg PO b.i.d.[d,e]	$	CNS (insomnia, irritability, dizziness, decreased concentration); 10%–15% (higher in elderly); GI, 3%
Rimantadine	Flumadine	Yes	No	100 mg PO b.i.d.[d,e,f]	$$	CNS, 2%–6%; GI, 3%
Oseltamivir	Tamiflu	Yes	Yes	75 mg PO b.i.d.[e]	$$$	GI, 10%
Zanamivir	Relenza	Yes	Yes	10 mg inhaled b.i.d.	$$$	May cause bronchospasm in patients with obstructive lung disease

CNS, central nervous system; GI, gastrointestinal.
[a]See package inserts for additional information.
[b]Amantadine, rimantadine, and oseltamivir are also available as a syrup or suspension. The recommended duration of treatment for all four drugs is 5 days.
[c]In 2001, representative retail prices were: amantadine $6; rimantadine $18; oseltamivir $70; zanamivir $85.
[d]Reduce dosage in the elderly (≥ 65 years old) to 100 mg daily or less.
[e]Reduce dosage in patients with renal insufficiency (see package insert for details).
[f]Reduce dosage to 100 mg daily in patients with hepatic disease.

effective only against influenza A, whereas the newer neuraminidase inhibitors are active against both A and B strains.

All of these drugs attenuate clinical disease by reducing fever by 50% and by shortening the duration of illness by 1 or 2 days. Reductions in illness duration may be somewhat greater when influenza symptoms or fever are more severe, and there is some evidence that viral shedding (and contagion) decreases with treatment. These benefits were observed when the drug was administered within 24 to 48 hours after onset of illness, although some experts suggest treating high-risk patients who present within 3 to 4 days after symptom onset (44). Data are limited and inconclusive regarding the effectiveness of any of these drugs in treating influenza illness in high-risk patients, including the elderly (see later discussion). There is also no conclusive evidence yet that these drugs are effective in preventing serious complications of influenza (e.g., pneumonia, exacerbations of chronic diseases) (41).

Dosages, routes of administration, adverse effects, and costs of these drugs are shown in Table 33.4. Drug-resistant strains of influenza virus have been isolated from some patients treated with amantadine and rimantadine (and to a much lesser extent, oseltamivir), although no clinically significant consequences, such as subsequent outbreaks of influenza caused by resistant strains, have been observed. However, it is strongly recommended that the *duration of treatment with these drugs be limited to 5 days,* since no benefit has been shown with longer courses.

Drug treatment should be considered for patients at high risk for morbidity and mortality who develop an influenza-like illness in a community where local influenza activity has been reported. Groups at high risk include patients with chronic pulmonary, cardiovascular, metabolic, neuromuscular, or immunodeficiency diseases and patients taking immunosuppressive medications. Adults whose activities are vital to community function, including selected hospital personnel, also should be considered for drug treatment of influenza.

Choice of therapy depends on consideration of the type of influenza circulating in the community and the safety, cost, and convenience of the drugs. If influenza A is known to be circulating, rimantadine has a well-established safety profile and is not very expensive. If influenza B is also circulating, or if specific information on influenza activity is not available and the patient is very ill or is at high risk for complications, then oseltamivir or zanamivir should be considered. Zanamivir is delivered via an inhalation device which requires assembly, and elderly patients have been shown to have difficulty with its use (45).

Supportive measures are important for symptomatic relief. Bed rest and adequate fluid intake should be advised. Aspirin, 650 mg every 3 to 4 hours, or acetaminophen, 650 to 1000 mg every 4 to 6 hours (maximum 4 g daily), reduce headache, fever, and myalgia. Aspirin should be avoided in children. Sponging with tepid water is effective in lowering high fever, whereas sponging with isopropyl alcohol only increases the patient's discomfort. Relief of nasal discharge may be obtained by agents discussed previously (see Common Cold). Relief of cough with cough suppressants is discussed later (see Acute Bronchitis).

Complications

Pulmonary complications exhibit a spectrum of severity, from mild airway hyperreactivity without pulmonary infiltrates, to segmental influenza pneumonia or secondary bacterial pneumonia, to fulminant bilateral influenza pneumonia with the acute respiratory distress syndrome (ARDS). Patients should be advised that dyspnea, hemoptysis, wheezing, purulent sputum, fever persisting longer than 7 days, and, rarely, dark urine or severe muscle pain herald complications that demand prompt medical attention and sometimes hospitalization.

Airway hyperreactivity may occur after some (46), but not all, influenza infections (47) and after other viral respiratory tract infections (48). It appears to be caused by destruction of epithelial cells secondary to viral invasion and may result from heightened sensitization of afferent cholinergic irritant receptors in the respiratory mucosa. Exposure to inhaled irritants induces a vagally mediated increase in airway resistance, manifested clinically by bronchospasm, coughing, or both. Cough may also be caused by direct stimulation of cholinergic irritant receptors, because these are the receptors that mediate the cough reflex (see Chapter 59). Patients with asthma or chronic bronchitis have even greater bronchoconstrictor responses to influenza infection because of their underlying bronchial smooth muscle hyperreactivity. Airway hyperreactivity can be demonstrated for 3 to 8 weeks after infection by influenza or other viruses, and occasionally it may last for 4 to 6 months, even in patients who are not atopic.

It is likely that nonproductive cough, wheezing, and dyspnea on exertion after flu syndrome are related to airway hyperreactivity, particularly in urban areas during periods of high air pollution. Chest roentgenograms are clear. Both cough and wheezing after an otherwise uncomplicated flu-like infection may be treated with a trial of an inhaled bronchodilator (see Chapter 60) as needed and at bedtime. Patients troubled particularly by nighttime cough may obtain additional relief with 15 to 30 mg of codeine at bedtime.

During influenza epidemics, there is a twofold to threefold increase in the incidence of pneumonia (38), although influenza often is not recognized by clinicians as a primary or contributing cause in patients who are admitted to the hospital with community-acquired pneumonia (CAP) (49). The incidence of bronchitis and pneumonia associated with influenza varies with age: it is low in patients younger than 50 years of age and very high in patients older than 70 years. Mortality from pneumonia during influenza epidemics clearly increases for those with chronic pulmonary disease or congestive heart failure (50).

Primary influenza viral pneumonia is an *early* complication of influenza illness. It occurs predominantly among the elderly and patients with chronic illnesses and occasionally in healthy young adults. Within the first day or two of illness, the dry cough becomes productive and sometimes bloody, and tachypnea and dyspnea may progress rapidly to hypoxia, cyanosis, and delirium. Diffuse rales are present on examination. The chest radiograph often reveals bilateral interstitial infiltrates, but lobar consolidation may also be seen. ARDS may develop. Immediate hospitalization and intensive care are required, but the mortality rate remains high. Some patients have milder influenza pneumonia, with persistent fever, cough, dyspnea, localized rales, and normal white blood cell count, and they subsequently experience a benign course. Although there are no reported studies of antiviral drugs (Table 33.3) for the treatment of influenza pneumonia, their use is reasonable in patients in whom it is suspected.

Secondary bacterial pneumonia and bronchitis is a later complication in up to 10% of cases of influenza A, more commonly in the elderly and in patients with chronic pulmonary or cardiac disease. Pneumonitic complications of influenza B are less common but do occur (51). The presentation is typically biphasic: initial respiratory symptoms are followed by several days of clinical improvement, and then there is an exacerbation of fever with production of purulent or bloody sputum. The predominant bacterial pathogens are *S. pneumoniae, H. influenzae,* group A beta-hemolytic *Streptococcus* (GABHS) species and *S. aureus; S. aureus* has a mortality rate of approximately 50% in this setting. The diagnosis and management of pneumonia are discussed later.

Nonpulmonary complications of influenza are unusual. *Myositis,* with thigh pain and inability to walk, occurs occasionally in children and adolescents. Severe myositis with myoglobinuria and acute renal failure has been observed in adults after both influenza A and B. Guillain–Barré syndrome, encephalitis, and transverse myelitis are *neurologic complications* associated rarely with influenza infection, but no firm causal relationship has been established. *Reye syndrome* (encephalopathy and fatty liver) is a rare but severe complication of influenza, usually type B; patients present with a change in mental status and progress to coma and hepatic failure. The mean age at attack is 6 years, and the incidence has fallen markedly in recent years. The syndrome is rare in adults and, unlike the situation in children, is not associated with aspirin. With the exception of mild myositis, all of the nonpulmonary complications of influenza require hospitalization for differential diagnosis and management.

Prevention

The use of influenza vaccine and drug prophylaxis in ambulatory practice is discussed in Chapter 18.

Pharyngitis

Sore throat is among the most common symptoms seen in ambulatory medical practice. Most acute episodes of pharyngitis in adults are self-limited and of short duration, and significant complications are rare. The most important task in the evaluation of patients who complain of sore throat is to identify group A streptococcal and other bacterial infections, for which antibiotic treatment is appropriate, and to recognize less common causes of pharyngitis associated with more serious illnesses. Although many adult patients with sore throat have been treated with antibiotics in the past, it is increasingly recognized that this practice is often not appropriate.

Epidemiology

Pharyngitis in adults is caused by a variety of viral and bacterial pathogens, with no single etiology predominating (52,53). The majority of cases are caused by common viruses, most often rhinovirus, coronavirus, and adenovirus (54). Streptococcal bacteria, predominantly GABHS species, account for only 15% of cases or less. *Mycoplasma pneumoniae,* the TWAR strain of *Chlamydia pneumoniae, Arcanobacterium* (formerly *Corynebacterium*) *haemolyticum, Neisseria gonorrhoeae, H. influenzae* type b, *Corynebacterium diphtheriae, Candida* species, respiratory syncytial virus, influenza types A and B, parainfluenza, herpes simplex virus, adenovirus, and Epstein-Barr virus cause pharyngitis infrequently.

Group A Beta-hemolytic Streptococcal Pharyngitis

Clinical Features. Only 5% to 15% of episodes of acute pharyngitis in adults are caused by GABHS (55). It occurs most commonly in the winter and spring. Individuals who have regular contact with children (e.g., parents, teachers), or who have been exposed to others with diagnosed streptococcal pharyngitis, are more likely to have GABHS. The incubation period is 2 to 4 days, followed by the abrupt onset of sore throat, malaise, fever, and headache. Mild neck stiffness and gastrointestinal symptoms are sometimes present (53). All of the features of the classic syndrome, including fever, tender anterior cervical and tonsillar lymph nodes (at the angle of the jaw), and enlarged tonsils with creamy white exudate, occur in fewer than 10% of cases of streptococcal pharyngitis (56), and each of these features may occur in other types of pharyngitis. Importantly, *cough, hoarseness, and rhinorrhea are not usually present in the patient with strep throat.* The distinctive scarlatiniform rash *(scarlet fever)* is characterized by a diffuse red blush appearing on the trunk early in the disease, spreading centrifugally, blanching with pressure, and acquiring a sandpaper texture; 1 week later the skin desquamates, particularly over the palms and soles. This rash is not seen in most patients with GABHS pharyngitis. A similar rash also occurs in toxic shock syndrome and Kawasaki's syndrome and a rash associated with *A. haemolyticum* pharyngitis is localized to the trunk and does not desquamate.

Diagnosis. Because individual clinical findings are nonspecific, the diagnosis of streptococcal pharyngitis relies on clinical prediction rules, rapid antigen tests, or throat culture. Several *clinical predictions rules* for GABHS pharyngitis have been developed (53); the Centor criteria (57) are simple and straightforward, have been validated prospectively, and have emerged as a consensus tool (52,54) (Table 33.5). These criteria include: *tonsillar exudates, tender anterior cervical lymphadenopathy, history of fever* (temperature greater than 38°C [100.4°F]), and *absence of cough.* The presence of three or four of these criteria has a sensitivity of 75% and a specificity of 75% for GABHS pharyngitis, using throat culture as the reference standard. For most adults, this results in a positive predictive value of 40% to 60% when three or four criteria are present, and a negative predictive value of approximately 80% if none or only one of the criteria is present (54).

Table 33.5. Clinical Features in Patients with Sore Throat That Predict Group A Beta-hemolytic Streptococcal (GABHS) Pharyngitis[a]

Tonsillar exudate
Tender anterior cervical lymphadenopathy
History of fever *or* Temperature >38° degrees C (100.4 degrees F)
Absence of cough

[a]Patients with 3 or 4 of these features are likely to have GABHS pharyngitis; patients with 0 or 1 likely do not.

Rapid antigen tests, which use enzyme immunoassay methods to detect GABHS carbohydrate products, are commercially available for point-of-care use in ambulatory practice. Reported sensitivities and specificities vary, but on average, they are approximately 80% and 90%, respectively (54,55). For the average prevalence of GABHS in adults with sore throat (i.e., 10%), rapid antigen tests have a positive predictive value of approximately 50% and a negative predictive value of 98%. Therefore, the use of these tests in practice is no better than the clinical prediction rule in establishing the diagnosis of strep throat, but they do confirm the absence of GABHS more accurately.

Throat culture has been the gold standard for diagnosing GABHS, although a significant disadvantage is that results are not available for 24 to 48 hours. A small percentage of false negative tests may be caused by inadequate specimen collection or improper handling. False positive tests may occur if the patient is an asymptomatic carrier of GABHS and the acute pharyngitis is caused by another pathogen; this is estimated to occur in only 2% to 4% of adolescents and adults (53). Currently, many physicians prefer to send throat swabs in transport media to commercial laboratories. Inexpensive office throat culture kits are also available and have a high sensitivity (approximately 95%).

The accuracy of rapid antigen tests and throat cultures depends on *proper collection of the throat swab.* The pharynx must be viewed adequately, with elevation of the soft palate and depression of the posterior tongue (52). Use of a tongue blade and the classic "ahh" phonation by the patient may help; sometimes not having the patient stick out the tongue, or having the patient pant, is useful. The tonsillar tissue and posterior pharynx should be swabbed vigorously; adequate collection often induces a gag reflex.

Diagnostic Approach. Adult patients with sore throat should be screened for the four clinical findings (Centor criteria), as outlined previously. The clinician should also be alert to aspects of the history, symptoms, and signs that suggest other, potentially treatable or serious causes of pharyngitis (see later discussion). Patients with none or only one of the four clinical criteria should not receive further testing or antibiotic treatment, because they are unlikely to have GABHS. A consensus clinical guideline recommends (a) that patients with two or more of the criteria be tested with a rapid antigen kit and treated with antibiotics only if the result is positive; (b) that patients with two or three criteria who have positive results on the test kit, as well as all of those with four criteria, be treated with antibiotics; or (c) that testing not be used and patients with three or four criteria be treated with antibiotics (55).

Although some experts have recommended confirming negative rapid antigen tests with a throat culture, a large study found that use of the rapid test without follow-up culture was not associated with an increase in significant sequelae of GABHS (58), and consensus guidelines discourage the use of throat cultures (55). Clinicians who do not use rapid antigen tests may choose to employ throat cultures for patients with two or more of the clinical criteria, with the caveat that patients can be contacted to start or stop antibiotics when the results become known. *Symptomatic family contacts* of patients with streptococcal pharyngitis should be tested and should be treated with antibiotics if the tests or cultures are positive. Routine testing of *asymptomatic* family members is not indicated.

Rationale for Antibiotic Treatment. The benefits of treating sore throat with antibiotics, especially if GABHS can be confirmed, include prevention of acute rheumatic fever and suppurative complications and perhaps more prompt relief of symptoms and interruption of contagious spread of pharyngitis. There is a growing recognition, however, that the magnitude of the benefits of antibiotic treatment may not be as large as previously believed.

Acute rheumatic fever (59,60) is a clinical syndrome of nonsuppurative inflammatory lesions of the heart, joints, and central nervous system that follows GABHS pharyngitis. Diagnosis is based on the Jones criteria: two major criteria (carditis, polyarthritis, chorea, subcutaneous nodules, and erythema marginatum), or one major criterion and two minor criteria (fever, arthralgia, heart block, elevated acute-phase reactants including granulocytosis, erythrocyte sedimentation rate, and C-reactive protein). Evidence of recent streptococcal infection must be confirmed by either positive throat culture, streptococcal antigen test, or elevated or rising antistreptococcal antibodies. One third of acute rheumatic fever cases occur after asymptomatic streptococcal infection, but almost all cases are associated with a rise in serum antistreptolysin O (ASO). The latent period between clinical streptococcal pharyngitis and onset of acute rheumatic fever ranges from 1 to 5 weeks, with a mean of 19 days. Clinical trials have confirmed that appropriate antibiotic treatment of GABHS pharyngitis is highly effective in preventing rheumatic fever if administered within approximately 1 week after the onset of illness.

The incidence of acute rheumatic fever declined dramatically in the United States and other industrialized countries during the last century, falling to extremely low levels during the 1960s and 1970s (59). It continued to be endemic in developing countries, where it accounts for up to 40% of all cardiovascular disease. Outbreaks among school-age children and young adult military recruits in the United States in the 1980s raised fears about a resurgence of rheumatic fever, but since then its occurrence has continued to decrease to only 1 case per 1 million people per year, and the Centers for Disease Control and Prevention (CDC) dropped it as a reportable disease beginning in 1995 (61).

Because almost all of the recent, very infrequent cases of acute rheumatic fever have been in children or young adults living in close quarters, the risk in most adults after GABHS is likely to be extremely low. The reasons for the overall decline and periodic resurgence of rheumatogenic GABHS infections are not completely understood or predictable, so clinicians should be aware of emerging trends in streptococcal disease.

Suppurative complications, such as peritonsillar or retropharyngeal abscess (see later discussion), are very rare, although a quantitative review demonstrated a further reduction in their occurrence with antibiotic treatment of GABHS pharyngitis (62). However, patients with these infrequent complications often already had them at initial evaluation, or had a negative strep test initially, or were treated initially with appropriate antibiotics (55,58). Although antibiotics are often recommended for patients with GABHS pharyngitis to prevent contagion, the utility of this approach for adults in noninstitutionalized settings is not known. There is good evidence from controlled clinical trials and systematic reviews that antibiotic treatment of suspected or confirmed GABHS provides some relief of symptoms; however, therapy must be initiated within 2 to 3 days after the onset of illness, and the benefit is limited to shortening the duration of symptoms by 1 to 2 days (55,62,63).

Patients in whom GABHS is clinically suspected or confirmed by testing should be treated. In three additional groups of patients who present with sore throat, antibiotic treatment for streptococcal pharyngitis should be started and throat cultures obtained: patients with a history of rheumatic fever not currently taking prophylaxis, young patients with a strong family history of rheumatic fever, and all new cases of pharyngitis in an explosive epidemic of streptococcal disease in close populations such as groups of military personnel or students living in dormitory settings. Local health authorities should be notified promptly in this last situation.

Choice of Antibiotics. The *preferred therapy* for GABHS pharyngitis is parenteral benzathine penicillin, 1.2 million units given once intramuscularly, because it obviates nonadherence and is the only specific treatment proven in clinical trials to prevent rheumatic fever. If oral therapy is given, the recommended regimen is penicillin V, 500 mg two or three times daily for 10 days (54,55). For patients who are allergic to penicillin, erythromycin, 250 mg every 6 hours or 500 mg twice daily for 10 days, is recommended. Although a number of oral cephalosporins (10-day courses) and azithromycin (500 mg first day and 250 mg for 4 days) have clinical and bacteriologic cure rates at least as good as those of penicillin V, these extended-spectrum antibiotics should not be used as first-line treatments because of their increased costs and potentiation of antibiotic resistance (Table 33.3). Posttreatment cultures should be performed only if there is a history of rheumatic fever in the patient or in a household contact.

Symptomatic Treatment. In addition to recommending antibiotics only for patients with suspected or confirmed GABHS pharyngitis, clinicians can encourage all patients with sore throat to try antipyretics and systemic and topical analgesics (see Common

Cold) in appropriate doses, along with supportive measures such as gargling.

Other Bacterial Causes of Pharyngitis

Pharyngitis caused by *A. haemolyticum* is characterized by exudative pharyngitis, a scarlatiniform rash, fever, adenopathy, and a negative test for GABHS (54). It may be treated with erythromycin 500 mg orally twice daily for 10 days.

Gonococcal pharyngitis should be considered in patients who complain of sore throat in association with urethritis or vaginitis; it occurs alone without genital symptoms in fewer than 5% of cases and must be diagnosed by throat culture. Special culture techniques (including the use of Thayer-Martin medium, which is available in kits for office cultures, or specific swab kits with appropriate transport media) should be used to detect gonorrhea in specimens from patients practicing orogenital sex. Calcium alginate swabs should be used, because ordinary cotton swabs contain fatty acids inhibitory to gonococcal growth. Gram staining of a direct pharyngeal smear is insensitive and nonspecific. For throat cultures, *N. gonorrhoeae* must be distinguished from *Neisseria meningitidis* and *Neisseria lactamica* by carbohydrate fermentation and serology; therefore, cultures should be sent to state or regional laboratories. Patients with gonococcal infections are often coinfected with chlamydia; although coincident chlamydial pharyngitis is unusual, it is recommended that patients with gonococcal pharyngitis also be treated empirically for possible genital chlamydia infection. The recommended antibiotic regimens, based on the *1998 Guidelines for Treatment of Sexually Transmitted Diseases* (CDC), include ceftriaxone 125 mg intramuscularly in a single dose or ciprofloxacin 500 mg orally in a single dose or ofloxacin 400 mg orally in a single dose, plus azithromycin 1 g orally in a single dose or doxycycline 100 mg orally twice a day for 7 days (64). Other treatment regimens for gonococcal infections may not cure pharyngitis caused by this organism. Chapter 37 discusses sexually transmitted diseases in detail.

Diphtheria is exceedingly rare in this country. Pharyngitis and skin infections caused by *C. diphtheriae* have occurred recently only in persons from disadvantaged groups who were inadequately immunized. It should be suspected when there is a grayish membrane in the anterior nares or on the tonsils, uvula, or pharynx. Treatment must begin before bacteriologic confirmation and requires hospitalization for strict isolation, bed rest, close observation, diphtheria antitoxin, and erythromycin or penicillin for 14 days. Vaccination against diphtheria and management of exposed contacts is discussed in Chapter 18.

Throat cultures sometimes grow *other bacteria*, such as pneumococci; staphylococci; group B, C, or G streptococci; and various gram-negative enterobacteria. These species colonize the pharynx and rarely cause pharyngitis, and patients who harbor them generally should not be treated with antimicrobial agents. Some outbreaks of pharyngitis have been traced to streptococci of groups C and G, and patients with persistent sore throat and throat cultures positive for these organisms may be treated with shorter courses of the antibiotics listed for GABHS (54).

Vincent angina is an anaerobic bacterial infection of the pharynx characterized by fever, tender lymphadenitis, a large grayish-brown pseudomembrane in the pharynx, and very foul odor. It is a complication of acute necrotizing ulcerative gingivitis (see Chapter 112). Hospitalization for antimicrobial treatment with penicillin or tetracycline is the appropriate management plan.

Bacterial epiglottitis and peritonsillar abscess may present with a sore throat as the initial primary symptom but are distinguished by accompanying symptoms and signs (see later discussion).

Noteworthy Viral Causes of Pharyngitis

Infectious mononucleosis (see Chapter 58) is characterized by the clinical triad of sore throat, fever, and lymphadenopathy. It can be distinguished on clinical grounds from streptococcal infection only when hepatosplenomegaly and a maculopapular skin rash (similar to a drug eruption or rubella, typically precipitated by ampicillin) are present. Palatal petechiae may be seen in mononucleosis but may also occur with rubella or streptococcal pharyngitis. *Pharyngoconjunctival fever*, caused by several adenovirus strains, is usually accompanied by influenza-like symptoms and can be distinguished by concurrent conjunctivitis in one third of cases and a history of swimming pool exposure 1 week before onset. It has also been reported among military recruits (54). Oropharyngeal infection with *herpes simplex virus or coxsackie A virus* is distinguished by the presence of mucosal vesicles or ulcers (see Chapter 112). The vesicular enanthum in the pharynx caused by coxsackieviruses is sometimes called *herpangina*. The acute retroviral syndrome caused by *HIV infection* may manifest with fever and nonexudative pharyngitis; systemic symptoms and occasionally a rash occur also (see Chapter 39).

Chronic or Relapsing Sore Throat

Some patients describe a sore throat of several weeks' duration at their first visit. Others have either a prolonged course after an illness that began as a typical acute pharyngitis syndrome or frequent recurrence of sore throats. The conditions that can cause prolonged or recurrent pharyngitis are listed in Table 33.6. (Most are discussed in more detail elsewhere in this book, as indicated in the table.)

Chronic tonsillitis or *recurrent pharyngitis* is a clinical diagnosis made in patients with frequent sore throats (more than six in 1 year, or three or more episodes in 2 or more years), very large tonsils, and chronically enlarged, periodically tender lymph nodes. Tonsillectomy to alleviate chronic tonsillitis has been controversial in children (65); there have been no controlled trials in adults, and its indications in adults are not well established. Postoperative pain

Table 33.6. Causes of Chronic or Relapsing Sore Throat

Primary Site of Pain	Condition	See for Details
Pharynx	Chronic tonsillitis	
	Smoking (especially marijuana)	Chapters 27, 29
	Postnasal drip	Chapter 30, 59
	Infectious mononucleosis	Chapter 58
	Chronic fatigue syndrome	Chapter 58
	Agranulocytosis	
	Acute leukemia	
	Pemphigus	
Not the pharynx	Septic thyroiditis	Chapter 80
	Subacute thyroiditis	Chapter 80
	Angina (radiating to neck)	Chapter 62
	Esophageal reflux	Chapter 42
	Psychogenic	Chapter 21

and hemorrhage are the most common complications, the latter occurring in 0.5% to 2% of patients (but perhaps more often in adults) (66).

Beta-lactamase–producing organisms in the pharynx, including *S. aureus, Haemophilus* species, *Bacteroides* species, and *Branhamella catarrhalis,* can inactivate penicillin and protect mucosal streptococci; these conditions may underlie some cases of chronic tonsillitis. For recurrent pharyngitis and tonsillitis caused by group A streptococci and aerobic and anaerobic penicillin-resistant pathogens, eradication of streptococci and elimination of recurrent tonsillitis have been achieved in some patients with clindamycin, 300 mg every 8 hours, or amoxicillin/clavulanic acid (Augmentin), 500 mg every 8 hours for 7 days.

Pharyngeal Abscesses

Occasionally, after several days of symptoms of a URI, the patient develops a complicating infection of one of the closed compartments adjacent to the pharynx. The most common of these pharyngeal abscesses are *peritonsillar abscess* (also known as "quinsy") and *retropharyngeal abscess.* If one of these conditions is suspected, the patient should be referred immediately for evaluation and management by an otolaryngologist. Other conditions to consider when the patient is unable to swallow saliva because of pain are listed in Table 33.7.

Patients with *peritonsillar abscess* develop severe odynophagia; they are unable to take liquids and also may be unable to swallow their own saliva, resulting in early dehydration. The voice acquires a muffled quality, and trismus may be present. Fever, malaise, and systemic toxicity are typical. Dramatic relief may occur if the abscess drains spontaneously before the patient seeks medical attention. On physical examination, there is a swelling of the anterior tonsillar pillar at its superior pole. The involved tonsil itself may or may not be enlarged, but it is displaced medially. This condition is almost always unilateral.

The symptoms of *retropharyngeal abscess* are similar to those of peritonsillar abscess. In addition, there may be respiratory embarrassment if the process

Table 33.7. Differential Diagnosis of Severe Throat Pain, Odynophagia, and Inability to Swallow Saliva

Peritonsillar abscess	Toxic epidermal necrolysis
Retropharyngeal abscess	Stevens–Johnson syndrome
Vincent angina	Botulism
Diphtheria	Tetanus
Pharyngeal zoster	Gastroesophageal reflux
Epiglottitis	Foreign body

extends inferiorly toward the larynx. Trismus is uncommon. On examination, a swelling in the posterior oropharynx is readily seen. Lateral soft tissue radiographs of the neck may disclose expansion of the soft tissue density in the posterior pharyngeal space.

Management. Unless the airway or swallowing is compromised, needle aspiration and outpatient treatment with oral penicillin are effective (67). This can be performed by an otolaryngologist, an oral surgeon, or an experienced emergency room physician. Half of the cases of peritonsillar abscess are caused by group A *S. pyogenes.* Although some cultures grow penicillin-resistant organisms, there is no difference in cure rate between those receiving penicillin and those receiving broader-spectrum agents. The acute failure rate of needle aspiration is 6%; incision and drainage is appropriate for acute failures. Non–group A streptococcal peritonsillar abscesses recur in 10% of cases, and abscess tonsillectomy may be required for repeated recurrences (67).

Epiglottitis

Acute epiglottitis is a life-threatening but curable condition. The epiglottis serves as a valve that closes over the proximal portion of the trachea during swallowing to prevent aspiration. When the epiglottis becomes inflamed, the resultant edema causes it to curl posteriorly and inferiorly, thereby reducing the glottic aperture. Inspiration, which draws the epiglottis down, further reduces the effective airway. Epiglottitis is a rare complication of URIs. Since the introduction of the *H. influenzae* B vaccine, the incidence in children has decreased, and now the incidence in adults is higher than in children (68).

The diagnosis of epiglottitis should be suspected in patients with a sore throat, odynophagia, and muffled voice, all of short duration. Only one half of patients are febrile and show evidence of pharyngitis, and only one in three patients has cervical adenopathy. Sitting erect, complaint of dyspnea, and stridor noted on inspiration are indications of airway obstruction. Soft tissue radiographs of the neck may show edema of the epiglottis and narrowing of the aperture. The diagnosis is confirmed by indirect laryngoscopy, which reveals marked edema of the epiglottis and supraglottic tissue. This procedure must be performed only in circumstances in which emergency intubation can be carried out, because it may induce (rarely in adults) additional respiratory obstruction.

Management requires admission for observation; patients with signs of airway obstruction (as described in the previous paragraph) should be admitted to an intensive care unit, where close observation and emergency tracheotomy are possible (68). The remainder of the cases can be managed conservatively in a general ward with antibiotic treatment for the most common organisms, including *S. aureus, H. influenzae, S. pneumoniae,* and *S. pyogenes.* Use of topical or systemic corticosteroids does not prevent airway obstruction.

Telephone Assessment and Self-Care for Upper Respiratory Tract Infection

Most clinicians welcome the opportunity to assess URI symptoms initially by telephone. The telephone assessment should accomplish the following:

- Differentiate between infectious and allergic problems
- Among the patients with acute infections, distinguish those with possible bacterial infections or superinfections who should be examined to determine whether antibiotics should be prescribed
- Identify those who may have complications of a URI that require office evaluation

The following symptoms and signs should be sought: symptoms lasting longer than 3 weeks; fever lasting longer than 1 week or associated with delirium; purulent nasal discharge with sinus pain; purulent sputum, chest pain, dyspnea, or hemoptysis; ear pain or discharge; sore throat and a history of rheumatic fever; the combination of cough and fever higher than 102°F (39°C) or fever lasting longer than 4 days; hoarseness for longer than 1 month; pleuritic chest pain; marked odynophagia; and dysphagia, stridor, and difficulty in breathing.

During influenza outbreaks (late November through March), it is important to remember that the abrupt onset of fever and cough are fairly sensitive and specific for influenza infection, and that drug treatment for influenza has been shown to be effective only if started within the first 1 to 2 days of illness.

For patients not needing an office visit, simple instructions for self-care can be provided based on the measures described previously.

Increasing numbers of patients consult self-care algorithms. The book *Take Care of Yourself* by Vickery and Fries (see General References) continues to be one of the most widely distributed collections of algorithms available to the public. In an early evaluation (69), strict adherence to the algorithms for colds, influenza, cough, and sore throat would have increased the number of patient visits to a physician. Therefore, this standard set of instructions exhibited sensitivity, missing few people who needed to be examined, yet lacked specificity and led to unnecessary visits. This study pointed to the need to search for symptom complexes that better identify patients likely to be helped by a visit to a physician.

LOWER RESPIRATORY TRACT INFECTIONS

The cardinal manifestation of LRI is cough, often accompanied by auscultatory evidence of lower respiratory tract inflammation (rhonchi, rales, wheezes, signs of consolidation). Bronchitis and pneumonia are the major infectious syndromes of the lower respiratory tract in adults. A number of noninfectious conditions can also cause a cough that may be confused with a lower respiratory illness. The differential diagnosis of acute and persistent cough is summarized in Table 33.8.

Acute Bronchitis

Acute bronchitis is one of the most common clinical syndromes encountered in outpatient practice. It is defined clinically as an acute illness characterized by a cough, often accompanied by sputum production. It is differentiated from pneumonia by the absence of abnormalities on chest radiography. Bronchitis appears to be caused by inflammation of the tracheobronchial tree followed by tracheobronchial hypersensitivity that results in a cough of 1 to 3 weeks' duration. A cough that continues for longer than 3 weeks is generally referred to as a "persistent" or "chronic" cough. "Chronic bronchitis" is defined as an illness characterized by daily productive cough for at least 3 months in the absence of any other illness that may account for these symptoms (see also Chapter 60 for a discussion of chronic obstructive pulmonary disease [COPD]).

Epidemiology

Acute bronchitis in otherwise healthy adults is generally caused by viral agents, including influenza A and B, parainfluenza, respiratory syncytial virus, rhinovirus, adenovirus, and coronavirus (70). Less

Table 33.8. Conditions and Agents That Can Cause Acute or Persistent Cough

Acute (<3 wk)
Acute bronchitis/upper respiratory tract infection
  Common: influenza A and B, parainfluenza, respiratory syncytial virus, rhinovirus, adenovirus, coronavirus
  Uncommon: *Bordatella pertussis, Mycoplasma pneumoniae, Chlamydia pneumoniae*
Pneumonia
  Common: *Streptococcus pneumoniae, Hemophilus influenzae, Mycoplasma pneumoniae, Chlamydia pneumoniae,* respiratory syncytial virus
  Uncommon: *Legionella, Mycobacterium tuberculosis, Moraxella catarrhalis,* plague, varicella, tuberculosis, anthrax, hantavirus and others

Persistent (>3 wk)
Infectious
  Tuberculosis and other mycobacterium
  Fungal pneumonias: histoplasmosis, coccidioidomycosis, blastomycosis, aspergillosis
Noninfectious
  Postnasal drip
  Gastroesophageal reflux or repeated aspiration
  Asthma
  Angiotensin converting-enzyme inhibitors

commonly, acute bronchitis may be caused by bacterial agents such as *Bordetella pertussis, M. pneumoniae,* or *C. pneumoniae.* Other bacterial pathogens, such as *S. pneumoniae, H. influenzae,* or *M. catarrhalis* generally do not cause bronchitis in persons without underlying lung disease; however, they may be responsible for bacterial superinfections after an acute viral respiratory illness. Bacterial superinfection is rare in otherwise healthy adults and most commonly occurs in elderly persons and those with underlying chronic medical illness, especially chronic heart and lung disease.

Diagnosis

Patients with a cough as the predominant or only respiratory symptom may have pneumonia, bronchitis, or one of a variety of noninfectious conditions associated with persistent cough. Mucoid sputum production develops in many cases and is not helpful in distinguishing etiologic agents. Diagnostic efforts should be directed at identifying patients with pneumonia and those with noninfectious causes of cough, leaving acute bronchitis as a diagnosis of exclusion. For a primary care provider evaluating a patient with an acute illness characterized by cough, the most important question is often whether *chest radiography* is indicated for further evaluation. No single symptom, sign, or constellation of symptoms and signs can predict pneumonia reliably. However, one review suggested that the likelihood of pneumonia is diminished by the absence of signs of focal consolidation on chest examination or any of the following vital sign abnormalities: heart rate greater than 100 beats/minute, respiratory rate greater than 24 breaths/minute, oral body temperature greater than 38°C (100.4°F) (71). A chest radiograph usually is not necessary if none of these signs are present. *Gram stain* and *bacterial cultures of sputum* are not useful in the evaluation of acute bronchitis because most cases are of viral etiology and the sputum is readily contaminated by nasopharyngeal flora.

B. pertussis should be considered in adults with prolonged cough (usually defined as cough lasting longer than 2 weeks), especially if there is a history of exposure to someone with pertussis (72). Pertussis initially causes nonspecific symptoms of malaise and rhinorrhea, followed by 1 to 14 weeks of severe paroxysms of repetitive coughs terminated by an inspiratory whoop. The clinical symptoms are attenuated in previously immunized adults and children. Because of the nonspecific nature of the symptoms, 2 weeks is the duration of cough used as the threshold to initiate investigation of sporadic cases, and 1 week is used during an outbreak. Culture, using a *nasopharyngeal swab* and special medium for *Bordetella,* is the standard diagnostic assay, but it is uncommonly positive, particularly after administration of antibiotics or later in the course of illness. Direct immunofluorescent staining of organisms on a smear of nasopharyngeal secretions is useful in outbreak investigations. Diagnosis by a single positive antibody test in acute serum is increasingly used to detect sporadic cases (73).

Treatment

Antibiotics are *not* recommended for healthy adults with uncomplicated bronchitis (74). A meta-analysis of randomized controlled trials of antibiotics for bronchitis found a modest improvement in symptom duration with antibiotics (one-half day, on average) (75), but when side effects, costs, and the increasing problem of antibacterial resistance are taken into account, the risks associated with treatment appear to outweigh the potential benefits. The benefits of antibiotics for cigarette smokers appears to be the same or less than for nonsmokers (76). Sputum color is not necessarily an accurate indicator of purulence. *If pertussis is suspected,* appropriate diagnostic studies (see previous discussion) should be performed rather than using presumptive therapy with antibiotics, unless the patient is in an epidemic area. Treatment for pertussis is either erythromycin 500 mg orally four times daily or clarithromycin 500 mg orally twice daily for 7 days. Trimethoprim (160 mg)/sulfamethoxazole (800 mg) orally twice daily for 14 days is an alternative for patients who are allergic to erythromycin. Treatment options for influenza were discussed earlier in this chapter.

Treatment of cough and systemic symptoms such as fever, myalgias, malaise, and chest pain is generally symptomatic. Cough suppression may be achieved with dextromethorphan but often requires codeine sulfate, 15 to 30 mg every 4 to 6 hours, especially at bedtime (see Chapter 59). Bronchodilator treatment with a beta-agonist may help symptomatically, especially for those with evidence of bronchospasm (i.e., wheezing) on examination (70). Inhaled corticosteroids appear to be effective for patients with chronic bronchitis (77) but have not been shown to have a role in the treatment of acute bronchitis in patients without underlying lung disease. Conventional wisdom has suggested that antihistamines should be avoided to prevent inspissated secretions, although empiric data are lacking. Encouragement of good oral hydration is appropriate for all patients with respiratory tract infection.

Smokers with acute bronchitis should be strongly encouraged to stop smoking at least for the duration of the acute illness. Smokers with a history of chronic cough before their bronchitis may be more motivated to discontinue smoking permanently in the face of the acute illness. In 50% of those who discontinue smoking, the chronic cough resolves completely within 1 month. Behavioral approaches to smoking cessation are described in Chapter 27. There is no evidence that smokers who have not developed COPD will benefit from antibiotic treatment for acute bronchitis (76).

The treatment of acute exacerbations of COPD is discussed in Chapter 60.

Pneumonia

More than 3 million episodes of pneumonia occur annually in the United States, and it is responsible for more than 30 million days of disability requiring bed rest and 600,000 hospitalizations. With influenza, pneumonia ranks seventh among all diseases as a cause of death (78) and first among infectious diseases, and its mortality rate has been rising during the last two decades (79).

Definition and Distinction from Bronchitis

Pneumonia is an LRI accompanied by systemic and respiratory tract symptoms and evidence of consolidation on chest radiography. Bronchitis and pneumonia represent a continuum of LRI. Aspirated pathogens, including bacteria, fungi, and viruses, invade the bronchial epithelium and alveoli. The extent of involvement of adjacent lung parenchyma determines whether there is an infiltrate on chest radiography. Patients seen early and patients with emphysema and reduced parenchyma may fail to show any infiltrate or may show a patchy infiltrate on their chest film despite the presence of considerable inflammation. Therefore, the clinical distinction between acute bronchitis and acute pneumonia is often an arbitrary radiologic distinction. Early management and the decision for hospitalization must focus on the overall condition of the patient and the signs and symptoms of systemic toxicity and of localized pulmonary infection.

Pneumonia Syndromes and Causes

Important clues for the etiologic diagnosis of pneumonia may be obtained from knowledge of the seasonal, environmental, and occupational predilections of the various agents that cause pneumonias. Table 33.9 lists pathogens associated with different epidemiologic characteristics of patients.

Bacterial pneumonias make up the majority of all adult pneumonias, and the largest fraction of these are caused by *S. pneumoniae* (80). Pneumococcal pneumonia may occur in a previously healthy adult, or after a URI, usually with the abrupt onset of shaking chills, fever, pleuritic chest pain, and cough productive of purulent or rusty sputum. Patients with compromised pulmonary clearance of secretions (e.g., depressed consciousness, morbid obesity, abdominal surgery, chronic bronchitis, congestive heart failure, alcoholism) are predisposed to pneumococcal and other bacterial pneumonias; the onset of clinical symptoms may be more insidious in these patients.

Drug-resistant *S. pneumoniae* (DRSP) is increasingly a problem worldwide, with up to one half of isolates showing *in vitro* evidence of resistance (81). Pneumococci resistant to penicillin are often resistant to cephalosporins, macrolides, doxycycline, and trimethoprim/sulfamethoxizole as well. Characteristics of patients at higher risk for DRSP include age older than 65 years, beta-lactam therapy in the previous 3 months, alcoholism, immunosuppressive illness or medication (including corticosteroid therapy), multiple medical comorbidities, and exposure to a child in a day care center (80). The clinical significance of DRSP pneumonia is still not completely understood. There is some evidence of increased morbidity and mortality among patients infected with DRSP with high levels of resistance, but infections with intermediate resistance appear to respond well to beta-lactam treatment for pneumonia and may be of clinical significance only in the treatment of otitis media or meningitis (82).

The so-called *atypical pneumonia syndrome,* most common among patients younger than 40 years of age, is characterized by a prodrome of headache and myalgia preceding the onset of respiratory symptoms. Respiratory pathogens commonly causing "atypical pneumonia" include *M. pneumoniae, Legionella pneumophila, C. pneumoniae* (TWAR strain), a number of viruses (influenza A and B, respiratory syncytial virus, parainfluenza, adenovirus), *Chlamydia psittaci, Coxiella burnetii* (Q fever), *Coccidioides immitis,* and *Pneumocystis carinii.* Nonetheless, all of these pathogens may result in a pneumonitis that is clinically and radiographically indistinguishable from pneumococcal pneumonia (83,84); because "typical" bacterial pneumonias are also commonly preceded by a prodrome of headache, myalgias, and malaise, the designation "atypical pneumonia" is of little use in practice.

Pneumonias caused by *Mycoplasma* or *Chlamydia* often manifest with sore throat, as well as fever and

Table 33.9. Epidemiologic Characteristics Associated with Specific Community-Acquired Pneumonia Pathogens

Characteristic	Pathogens
Alcoholism	*Streptococcus pneumoniae,* anaerobes, gram-negative bacilli, tuberculosis
COPD/smoking	*S. pneumoniae, Hemophilus influenzae, Moraxella catarrhalis, Legionella*
Nursing home residency	*S. pneumoniae,* gram-negative bacilli, *H. influenzae, Staphylococcus aureus,* anaerobes, *Chlamydia pneumoniae,* tuberculosis
Poor dental hygiene	Anaerobes
Exposure to bats	*Histoplasma capsulatum*
Exposure to birds	*Chlamydia psittaci, Cryptococcus neoformans, Histoplasma capsulatum*
Exposure to rabbits	*Francisella tularensis*
Exposure to farm animals or parturient cats	*Coxiella burnetii* (Q fever)
Travel to southwest U.S.	Coccidioidomycosis
Suspected large-volume aspiration	Chemical pneumonitis, anaerobes, or obstruction
Structural lung disease (bonchiectasis, cystic fibrosis, etc.)	*Pseudomonas aeruginosa, Pseudomonas cepacia, S. aureus*
Injection drug use	*S. aureus,* anaerobes, tuberculosis, *Pneumocystis carinii*
Recent antibiotic therapy	Drug-resistant pneumococci, *Pseudomonas aeruginosa*
Endobronchial obstruction	Anaerobes

Adapted from: Niederman MS, Mandell LA, et al. Guidelines for the management of adults with community-acquired pneumonia. Am J Respir Crit Care Med 2001; 163:1730.

cough. *C. pneumoniae* may cause a biphasic illness, with severe pharyngitis and laryngitis in the first phase, followed by pneumonia (85,86).

Complications of *Mycoplasma* pneumonia include sinusitis, otitis media, myringitis (diagnostic if bullae are seen), erythema multiforme or erythema nodosum, intravascular hemolysis, meningoencephalitis, toxic psychosis, myocarditis, and pericarditis. Fulminant infection can occur irrespective of age or host status. Persistent hacking cough, lasting as long as 6 weeks despite therapy, is common and requires symptomatic relief with codeine (see Chapter 59). Relapse of the primary disease occurs in up to 10% of cases, usually 2 to 3 weeks after the initial illness, and is probably related to the fact that mycoplasma persists in bronchial epithelium for up to 14 weeks.

Pseudomonas aeruginosa is an uncommon cause of pneumonia, particularly in the outpatient setting. Risk factors for development of *P. aeruginosa* pneumonia include structural lung disease (e.g., bronchiectasis, cystic fibrosis), corticosteroid therapy, malnutrition, and recent broad-spectrum antibiotic therapy for longer than 7 days. A sputum culture that yields *P. aeruginosa* is not always indicative of true infection and may represent only colonization.

Legionnaire disease (caused by *Legionella pneumophila* and other species), in comparison with other causes of pneumonia, is more likely to be associated with headache, confusion, and diarrhea and is less likely to cause cough, expectoration, and thoracic pain (87). Laboratory abnormalities associated with Legionnaire disease include hyponatremia and elevated creatine kinase. However, that many of these symptoms, signs, and laboratory abnormalities may be seen with other typical and atypical bacterial pneumonias.

P. carinii pneumonia (PCP) should be considered if the onset of fever, cough, and dyspnea is insidious over 1 to 4 weeks and the patient is immunocompromised or has risk factors for HIV infection (see Chapter 39). The chest radiograph typically shows diffuse bilateral infiltrates but may show focal infiltrates, cysts, pneumothorax, or no abnormality (88).

Hantavirus pulmonary syndrome (HPS) is a rare pneumonitis with a high mortality rate (89), now recognized throughout the United States and western Canada. After 1 to 7 days of nonspecific viral prodrome of fever, myalgias, chills, and headache, the respiratory phase is heralded by dry cough and dyspnea, with rapid onset of pulmonary edema caused by a capillary leak syndrome. The most lethal complication is cardiogenic shock.

Influenza is an important but often overlooked cause of pneumonia during the winter flu season (48); it also contributes to occurrence of secondary bacterial pneumonias (see Flu Syndrome).

Evaluation

Physical Examination. As noted in the section on bronchitis, no specific signs or constellation of signs can confirm the diagnosis of pneumonia (71). Furthermore, the physical examination cannot reliably distinguish between bacterial and atypical pneumonia syndromes. Crepitant rales that do not clear with cough are suggestive of pneumonia of either type. Signs of consolidation (increased tactile fremitus, dullness to percussion, bronchial breath sounds, and egophony) are more common in typical bacterial pneumonia. In the early stages of pneumonia, the examination may be normal despite an infiltrate on the chest film. Alternatively, rales and rhonchi may indicate pneumonia before the appearance of an infiltrate.

Diagnostic Testing. Every patient with suspected pneumonia should have a chest radiograph to establish the diagnosis and evaluate for possible complications (80). Although chest radiography is essential for the firm diagnosis of pneumonia, a normal film does not necessarily rule out pneumonia, and radiographic patterns are not a specific indication of the cause (90). For patients with underlying heart or lung disease, measurement of oxygenation by pulse oximetry (or arterial blood gas analysis) may help to determine the need for hospitalization. Routine blood tests, including complete blood counts and serum chemistries, are of little value in determining the cause of the pneumonia but may have prognostic value and can also play a role in determining the need for hospitalization (80).

A sputum Gram stain is generally *not* recommended for the evaluation of outpatients with pneumonia (80). It can be helpful occasionally in directing initial therapy, but discordant results between Gram stain and culture in pneumococcal pneumonia, and the lack of diagnostic data for many other common respiratory pathogens including *Legionella, Mycoplasma,* and *Chlamydia*, render the Gram stain of limited utility. *Sputum cultures* likewise have limited utility in the management of ambulatory pneumonias, because sputum samples are often contaminated by oral flora and cultures are often negative if any prior antibiotic therapy has been administered (91).

Serologic testing and *cold agglutinin measurement* are usually *not* useful in the initial evaluation of patients with CAP; consensus guidelines recommend against their use to direct therapy (80). Few pathogens can be diagnosed by serologic study of the acute serum specimen; exceptions include pertussis and hantavirus infection. Rapid test kits are available for the office diagnosis of influenza, but there are limitations to their use (see Flu Syndrome). During an apparent community outbreak of a respiratory illness caused by unculturable agents, it is helpful to the public health authorities for practitioners to collect and save acute and convalescent sera for later study at reference laboratories. Guided by epidemiologic clues (Table 33.8), measurement of acute and convalescent titers for antibodies against selected infectious agents may be considered. Testing for antibodies to *M. pneumoniae,* Q fever, psittacosis, influenza, *Legionella* species, tularemia, *C. immitis,* and *Histoplasma capsulatum* is available at most state diagnostic laboratories and many commercial laboratories. The presence of serum *cold agglutinins* can be used as a rapid diagnostic test for mycoplasma pneumonia but has several drawbacks, including the requirement of delivery to the laboratory at 37°C, insensitivity, and lack of specificity.

Management

An etiologic diagnosis of pneumonia would require many different tests, and in up to 50% of cases, a specific etiology cannot be defined despite extensive diagnostic testing (92). Therefore, treatment decisions should focus on the need for hospitalization and consideration of appropriate antibiotics. The desire to avoid unnecessary hospitalizations has led to studies defining low-risk patients with CAP who can be treated as outpatients (93).

Decision about Hospitalization. A meta-analysis of pneumonia outcomes revealed multiple prognostic factors associated with increased mortality: altered mental status, male gender, absence of pleuritic chest pain, hypothermia, systolic hypotension, tachypnea, diabetes mellitus, neoplastic disease, leukopenia, and multilobar pulmonary infiltrates (94). A survey of practitioners making decisions on hospitalization for pneumonia indicated that hypoxemia, inability to maintain oral intake, and lack of patient home care support were almost universal and appropriate criteria for admission. However, practitioners usually overestimated the risk of death from pneumonia, based on examination and comorbidity, resulting in excessive use of hospitalization (95). The large *Pneumonia Patient Outcome Research Team (PORT) study,* which used data from more than 14,000 patients with CAP, established that *if the answers to all of the following three questions are "No,"* the patient is in the lowest of five risk classes (group I), with a 30-day mortality rate less than 0.4% (93):

- *Is the patient older than 50 years of age?*
- *Is one or more of the following coexisting conditions present:* neoplastic (except skin cancer), cerebrovascular, renal, or liver disease or congestive heart failure?
- *Is one or more of the following abnormalities on physical examination present:* altered mental status, pulse rate faster than 125 beats/minute, respiratory rate faster than 30 breaths/minute, systolic blood pressure lower than 90 mm Hg, temperature lower that 35°C or higher than 40°C?

If the answers to any of these three questions was "Yes," further risk assessment was determined by a point scoring system including the additional characteristics listed in Table 33.10, each of which was independently associated with increased morbidity. Patients in risk class I had a 0.1% to 0.4% risk of mortality within 30 days; class II patients (70 points or less) had a 0.6% to 0.7% risk, and class III patients (71 to 90 points) had a 0.9% to 2.8% risk. (93). Most patients in classes I and II may be safely managed as outpatients; class III patients are potential candidates for outpatient therapy or a brief inpatient observation. In contrast, patients in classes IV (91 to 130 points) and V (more than 130 points) had 30-day mortality rates of 8.2% to 9.3% and 27.0% to 31.1%, respectively, and are usually best treated in hospital settings. The PORT-derived indicators of risk can be used as general guidelines until prospective studies provide even more precise rules, but clinical judgment should supersede such rules. Complications such as concomitant meningitis or septic arthritis, hemoptysis, prior splenectomy, and need for respiratory isolation of potential tuberculosis or pneumonic plague must be considered. Moreover, a patient's social situation and personal preferences should play a role in the decision whether to hospitalize.

Table 33.10. Point Scoring System for Step 2 of the Prediction Rule for Assignment to Risk Classes II (≥70 Points), III (71–90 Points), IV, and V

Characteristic	Points Assigned[a]
Demographic factor	
Age	
Men	Age (yr)
Women	Age (yr) − 10
Nursing home resident	+10
Coexisting illness	
Neoplastic disease	+30
Liver diseae	+20
Congestive heart failure	+10
Cerebrovascular disease	+10
Renal disease	+10
Physical examination findings	
Altered mental status	+20
Respiratory rate ≥30/min	+20
Systolic blood pressure <90 mm Hg	+20
Temperature <35°C or ≥40°C	+15
Pulse ≥125/min	+10
Laboratory and radiographic findings	
Arterial pH <7.35	+30
Blood urea nitrogen ≥30 mg/dL (11 mmol/L)	+20
Sodium <130 mmol/L	+20
Glucose ≥250 mg/dL (14 mmol/L)	+10
Hematocrit <30%	+10
Partial pressure of arterial oxygen <60 mm Hg	+10
Pleural effusion	+10

[a]A total point score for a given patient is obtained by summing the patient's age in years (age minus 10 for women) and the points for each applicable characteristic.

Adapted from Fine MJ, Auble TE, Yealy DM, et al. A prediction rule to identify low-risk patients with community-acquired pneumonia. N Engl J Med 1997,336:243.

Ambulatory Management: Choice and Duration of Antimicrobial Therapy. The treatment of CAP is by necessity empiric and based on a knowledge of epidemiology and estimates of patient risk for different pathogens.

The American Thoracic Society has issued consensus guidelines for the initial treatment of immunocompetent adults with CAP (80); these guidelines are reasonable and practical but require further study to show that adherence improves outcome. The guidelines divide ambulatory patients into two groups, based on the presence or absence of cardiopulmonary disease and modifying factors that increase the risk of infection with drug-resistant pneumococcus, enteric gram-negative bacteria, or *P. aeruginosa* (Table 33.11).

For ambulatory patients with no comorbidity and no risk factors for drug-resistant *S. pneumoniae* or other modifying factors, an advanced-generation macrolide (azithromycin or clarithromycin) is recommended

Table 33.11. Modifying Factors That Increase the Risk of Infection with Specific Pneumonia Pathogens

Drug-resistant *Streptococcus pneumoniae*
- Age>65 yr
- β-Lactam therapy within the past 3 mo
- Alcoholism
- Immune-suppressive illness (including corticosteroid therapy)
- Multiple medical comorbidities[a]
- Exposure to a child in a day care center

Enteric gram-negative bacteria
- Nursing home residence
- Underlying cardiopulmonary disease
- Multiple medical comorbidities[a]
- Recent antibiotic therapy

Pseudomonas aeruginosa
- Structural lung disease (bronchiectasis, cystic fibrosis)
- Corticosteroid therapy (>10 mg of prednisone per day)
- Broad-spectrum antibiotic therapy for >7 days in the past month
- Malnutrition

[a]Includes chronic obstructive pulmonary disease, diabetes mellitus, renal insufficiency, congestive heart failure, coronary artery disease, malignancy, chronic neurologic disease, and chronic liver disease.

Adapted from: Niederman MS, Mandell LA, et al. Guidelines for the management of adults with community-acquired pneumonia. Am J Respir Crit Care Med 2001;163:1730.

Table 33.12. Outpatient Treatment of Pneumonia, Group I: Patients with No Cardiopulmonary Disease or Modifying Factors[a]

Possible Pathogens	Recommended Empiric Therapy
Streptococcus pneumoniae	Advanced-generation macrolide:
Mycoplasma pneumoniae	azithromycin or clarithromycin
Chlamydia pneumoniae	- *or* -
Hemophilus influenzae	Doxycycline[b]
Respiratory viruses	
Legionella species	
Mycobacterium tuberculosis	
Endemic fungi	
Miscellaneous	

[a]See Table 33.11 for modifying factors. Excludes patients at risk for human immunodeficiency virus infection.

[b]Because many *S. pneumoniae* isolates are resistant to tetracycline, this should only be used if the patient is allergic or intolerant of macrolides.

Adapted from Niederman MS, Mandell LA, et al. Guidelines for the management of adults with community-acquired pneumonia. Am J Respir Crit Care Med 2001;163:1730.

as first-line therapy; doxycycline is an alternative for patients who are allergic to or intolerant of the macrolides (Table 33.12). Clarithromycin and azithromycin provide coverage for pneumococcal, chlamydial, *Legionella,* and mycoplasmal infections. *Azithromycin* has the advantage of once-daily dosing. Clarithromycin, but not azithromycin, can raise blood theophylline levels, occasionally into the toxic range, and dosages of the latter drug should be monitored and adjusted.

For ambulatory patients with either cardiopulmonary illness (congestive heart failure or COPD), a risk factor for drug resistant *S. pneumoniae,* or another modifying factor, the guidelines recommend treatment with a beta-lactam *plus* a macrolide or doxycycline (Table 33.13). The beta-lactam options include oral cefpodoxime, cefuroxime, high-dose amoxicillin (1 g every 8 hours), amoxicillin/clavulanate, or parenteral ceftriaxone followed by cefpodoxime. An alternative is an antipneumococcal fluoroquinolone (gatifloxacin,

Table 33.13. Outpatient Treatment of Pneumonia, Group II: Patients with Cardiopulmonary Disease or Other Modifying Factors[a]

Possible Pathogens	Recommended Empiric Therapy
Streptococcus pneumoniae (including DRSP)	β-Lactam (oral cefpodoxime,
Mycoplasma pneumoniae	cefuroxime, high-dose amoxicillin,[b]
Chlamydia pneumoniae	amoxicillin/clavulanate, or parenteral ceftriaxone followed by cefpodoxime)
Hemophilus influenzae	*plus*
Enteric gram-negatives	Macrolide or doxycycline[c]
Respiratory viruses	-*or*-
Legionella species	Antipneumococcal floroquinolone
Moraxella catarrhalis	(gatifloxacin, levofloxacin,
Mycobacterium tuberculosis	moxifloxacin)
Endemic fungi	
Miscellaneous/mixed infections	

DRSP, drug-resistant, *S. pneumoniae.*

[a]See Table 33.11 for modifying factors. Excludes patients at risk for human immunodeficiency virus infection.

[b]One gram every eight hours.

[c]Erythromycin does not provide coverage against *H. influenzae,* so if amoxicillin is used, it should be with doxycycline or an advanced-generation macrolide (azithromycin or clarithromycin).

Adapted from Niederman MS, Mandell LA, et al. Guidelines for the management of adults with community-acquired pneumonia. Am J Respir Crit Care Med 2001;163:1730.

levofloxacin, moxifloxacin) that is active against *S. pneumoniae, M. pneumoniae, Chlamydia trachomatis, Legionella, M. catarrhalis,* and gram negative aerobes. See Table 33.3 for dosing guidelines for these drugs. Another floroquinolone, trovafloxacin, is not recommended for outpatient treatment because of reports of severe hepatotoxicity. The fluoroquinolones are generally effective against DRSP, although resistant isolates have been reported (96). Vancomycin, the ketolides, and linezolid are also active against DRSP. Many experts caution against the indiscriminate use of fluoroquinolones for outpatient treatment of pneumonia, because of concerns about the emerging resistance of pneumococci to this class of antibiotics (82).

The widespread availability of *home intravenous antibiotic services* makes it possible to avoid or shorten hospitalization yet provide the advantages of intravenous antibiotics for patients who are stable.

The duration of therapy for CAP is not precisely defined. The American Thoracic Society guidelines suggest that "typical" bacterial infections, such as pneumococcal pneumonia, should be treated for 7 to 10 days, whereas *Mycoplasma, Chlamydia,* and *Legionella* pneumonias may need longer therapy, ranging from 10 to 14 days. Because an etiologic diagnosis usually is not established in outpatients, clinicians should consider the presence of coexisting illness, the severity of illness at the onset of antibiotic therapy, and the subsequent course in determining the duration of antibiotic therapy. For most infections, a 5-day course of azithromycin is adequate therapy because of its prolonged biologic half-life.

Follow-Up. The patient should be advised to keep in close contact by telephone, maintain good hydration with oral fluids, use aspirin or acetaminophen to control fever and headache, and avoid cigarettes. A telephone contact with the patient 24 hours after the initial visit provides a check on antibiotic adherence and side effects and on the status of symptoms; also it reassures the patient that he or she has access to the physician should the condition worsen or fail to improve.

A follow-up visit to the office 3 to 4 days later will help assess response to therapy. Symptoms of pneumococcal pneumonia in the uncompromised host usually abate within 48 to 72 hours after initiation of therapy, and somewhat longer with other pathogens or compromised host defenses. If a substantial clinical response to the initial antibiotic therapy has not occurred in this time, the patient must be reevaluated. Possible reasons for clinical failure include poor adherence to the antibiotic regimen; resistance of the etiologic organism to the empiric antibiotics prescribed; unusual pathogens such as tuberculosis, viral, or fungal pneumonia; and a noninfectious cause such as pulmonary embolus or carcinoma. In any case, hospitalization usually is required to determine the cause of therapeutic failure and to provide additional treatment. Complete resolution of symptoms caused by an episode of pneumonia may not occur for 30 days or longer after diagnosis (96).

After clinical resolution of the pneumonia, a chest radiograph is recommended in 4 to 6 weeks to exclude malignancy or other persistent lung abnormalities, particularly in smokers and in patients older than 40 years of age (80). The rate of radiographic resolution depends on age and extent of pneumonic involvement; although most patients have complete clearance at 4 weeks, elderly patients and those with multilobar pneumonia or underlying lung disease can have delayed resolution (97).

Prevention of Pneumonia

Polyvalent pneumococcal and influenza vaccines are discussed in detail in Chapter 18. No special precautions need be taken to isolate the ambulatory patient with pneumonia. Household contacts of these patients need no special surveillance, with the exceptions of pneumonic disease caused by tuberculosis (see Chapter 34), tularemia, plague, or meningococci.

Pleuritis and Pleurodynia

Pneumonic infections may cause inflammation or infection of the pleura, resulting in pleuritic chest pain and the appearance of a pleural effusion. Parapneumonic effusions and empyemas are typically caused by bacterial pneumonias, but tuberculosis, atypical bacteria, viruses, fungi, and even parasites may cause pleuritis. The evaluation of pleural effusions is discussed in Chapter 59.

Pleurodynia is an uncommon acute illness usually caused by one of the coxsackieviruses. It occurs in summer and early fall. The presenting symptoms may suggest the onset of pneumonia: abrupt onset of *severe paroxysmal pain of the thorax or abdomen,* worse with cough or breathing. Other manifestations of pleurodynia include fever, headache, cough, and anorexia. The physical examination is often normal except that the patient splints to avoid pain, which is commonly felt in the lower rib cage or under the sternum. The chest radiograph is usually normal. Most patients recover within 3 days to 1 week. Rare complications are orchitis, pericarditis, and aseptic meningitis.

APPROPRIATE PRESCRIBING OF ANTIBIOTICS FOR RESPIRATORY TRACT INFECTIONS

Antibiotic prescriptions for respiratory tract infections account for 20% to 30% of all antibiotic courses for adults in this country and approximately 75% of antibiotic prescriptions written in physicians' offices (98–100). Based on data from the National Ambulatory Medical Care Surveys during the last decade, it estimated that more than 50% of adults diagnosed with URI or bronchitis, and more than 70% of adult patients visiting a health care provider for sore throat, were treated with antibiotics (99,100). A comparison of these rates with the estimated incidence in adults of acute bacterial sinusitis (15%) and GABHS pharyngitis (10%)—the principal acute URIs for which antibiotics are indicated—strongly suggests that the use of antibiotics for URIs in practice should be reduced.

The overuse of antibiotics for respiratory tract infections exposes patients to unnecessary side effects, especially allergic reactions, diarrhea, and vaginitis (Table 33.3); increases medical care costs both for individual patients and health care payors; and contributes to the increasingly serious problem of antibiotic resistance.

Antibiotic Resistance

The importance of emerging antibiotic resistance in relation to respiratory tract infections is illustrated by the increasing resistance of *S. pneumoniae* to multiple antibiotics. By the end of the 1990s, the rates of resistant strains of this key respiratory pathogen were 25% for penicillin, 29% for trimethoprim/sulfamethoxazole, 15% for cefotaxime, and 20% for macrolide antibiotics (101,102). Resistance to tetracycline was about 8%, although perhaps less for doxycycline (103). Increasing resistance also has been reported for fluoroquinolones, with rates of about 5% for older ones such as ofloxacin (104).

Although the proliferation of day care arrangements for young children and the increase in global travel also contribute to the emergence of antibiotic resistance, the frequent prescription of antibiotics for respiratory tract infections probably is a major contributor to this problem. There is evidence that individual patients who have received multiple or recent courses of antibiotics are more likely to be colonized with resistant strains of bacteria. It is also clear that rising rates of antibiotic resistance for a particular antibiotic parallel increased use of that antibiotic; efforts to decrease the use of certain antibiotics in some countries have resulted in declining rates of resistance to those antibiotics (105).

Successful Approaches to Limiting Antibiotics

Practitioners can use the following principles to limit antibiotic prescriptions for respiratory tract infections to appropriate indications:

- Specific clinical criteria offer reasonable accuracy in the selection of patients who should receive antibiotics for acute bacterial sinusitis (Table 33.2) or GABHS pharyngitis (Table 33.5).
- Nonspecific acute URI generally should not be treated with antibiotics.
- Purulent nasal secretions or productive cough by themselves do not reliably indicate the presence of an acute bacterial infection or the need for antibiotic treatment.
- Symptoms lasting longer than several days do not necessarily indicate bacterial complications or the need for antibiotics; symptoms of most viral URIs and bronchitis typically last for 1 week or longer.
- When antibiotics are indicated for acute sinusitis, GABHS pharyngitis, or pneumonia, treatment should be initiated with the recommended first-line, narrower-spectrum antibiotics; newer, broad-spectrum antibiotics usually should be considered only if there are specific reasons to suspect antibiotic resistance or more serious disease (Table 33.11).

Similar principles have been applied successfully in practice settings. A multifaceted educational intervention targeted at patients and clinicians successfully reduced antibiotic prescriptions for bronchitis from 74% to 48%, without increasing the duration of illnesses or utilization of medical services or other medications (74,106). An important component of that intervention was use of the term "chest cold" instead of "bronchitis" in referring to cough illness. This study and others emphasize the importance of providing adequate explanations to patients of the appropriate use of antibiotics.

A successful approach to patients seeking care for respiratory tract infections for whom antibiotics are not indicated should include the following:

- Determining which symptoms are most bothersome for the patient.
- Recommending or prescribing specific symptomatic treatment (see relevant sections and Table 33.1). Decongestants are often effective for nasal symptoms, systemic and topical analgesics are helpful for sore throat, and cough suppressants and sometimes inhaled bronchodilators may be useful for cough illnesses.
- Explaining to patients the natural history of many viral URIs and bronchitis, which may include the persistence of nasal symptoms or cough for 1 week or longer.
- Emphasizing to patients the personal benefits of foregoing unnecessary antibiotics (decreased exposure to adverse effects, fewer expenditures, lower risk of subsequent infection with antibiotic-resistant bacteria), as well as the importance to society of reducing antibiotic use.

Contrary to the beliefs of many clinicians, patients' expectations for antibiotics may not be insurmountable. Reduced prescribing of antibiotics is not necessarily associated with less-satisfied patients (74). Rather, patient satisfaction with encounters for respiratory complaints may have more to do with the adequacy of explanations for their illness (107). Many governmental, national, and local health care organizations are working to reduce antibiotic use for respiratory tract infections, and clinicians should increasingly be able to find support and material resources in this effort.

General References*

Snow V, Mottur-Pilson C, Gonzales R. Principles of appropriate antibiotic use for treatment of nonspecific upper respiratory tract infections in adults. Ann Intern Med 2001;134:487.

Snow V, Mottur-Pilson C, Cooper J, Hoffman JR. Principles of appropriate antibiotic use for acute pharyngitis in adults. Ann Intern Med 2001;134:506.

Snow V, Mottur-Pilson C, Hickner JM. Principles of appropriate antibiotic use for acute sinusitis in adults. Ann Intern Med 2001;134:495.

Snow V, Mottur-Pilson C, Gonzales R. Principles of appropriate antibiotic use for treatment of acute bronchitis in adults. Ann Intern Med 2001;134:518.

An important series of position papers from the American College of Physicians–American Society of Internal Medicine which provide clinical practice guidelines for the management of respiratory infections in adults.

Vickery D, Fries J. Take care of yourself: the complete illustrated guide to medical self-care. 7th ed. Cambridge: Perseus Publishing, 2000.

Simple algorithms for self-care of common medical problems, including respiratory tract infections.

Mandell GL, Douglas G, Dolin R, et al., eds. Mandell, Douglas and Bennett's Principles and Practice of Infectious Diseases. 5th ed. Philadelphia: Churchill Livingstone, 1998.

The standard textbook of infectious diseases with detailed discussions of upper and lower respiratory tract infection syndromes.

Specific References

1. Lorber B. The common cold. J Gen Intern Med 1996;11:229.
2. Gwaltney JM Jr, Moskalski PB, Hendley JO. Hand to hand transmission of rhinovirus colds. Ann Intern Med 1978;88:463.
3. Ansari SA, Springthorpe VS, Sattar JA, et al. Potential role of hands in the spread of respiratory viral infections: studies with human parainfluenza virus 3 and rhinovirus 14. J Clin Microbiol 1991;29:2115.
4. Jepson S, Holbrook JH, Hale D, et al. Management of upper respiratory tract infections by telephone. West J Med 1994; 160:529.
5. Graham NMH, Burrell CJ, Douglas RM, et al. Adverse effects of aspirin, acetaminophen, and ibuprofen on immune function, viral shedding, and clinical status in rhinovirus-infected volunteers. J Infect Dis 1990;162:1277.
6. **6.** Sperber SJ, Hendley JO, Hayden FG, et al. Effects of naproxen on experimental rhinovirus colds: a randomized, double-blind, controlled trial. Ann Intern Med 1992;117:37.
7. Forstall GJ, Macknin ML, Yen-Lieberman BR, et al. Effect of inhaling heated vapor on symptoms of the common cold. JAMA 1994;271:1109.

---

*Bold print (general references) and bold numerals (specific references) denote published controlled clinical trials, meta-analyses, or consensus-based recommendations.

8. Sakethoo K, Januszkiewicz A, Sackner MA. Effects of drinking hot water and chicken soup on nasal mucus velocity and nasal airflow resistance. Chest 1978;74:408.
9. Jackson J, Peterson C, Lesho E. A meta-analysis of zinc salts lozenges and the common cold. Arch Intern Med 1997;157: 2373.
10. Prasad A. Zinc: the biology and therapeutics of an ion. Ann Intern Med 1996;125:142.
11. Smith MBH, Feldman W. Over-the-counter cold medications: a critical review of clinical trials between 1950 and 1991. JAMA 1993;269:2258.
12. Hayden FG, Diamond L, Wood PB, et al. Effectiveness and safety of intranasal ipratropium bromide in common colds: a randomized, double-blind, placebo-controlled trial. Ann Intern Med 1996;125:89.
13. Kernan WN, Viscoli CM, Brass LM, et al. Phenylpropanolamine and the risk of hemorrhagic stroke. N Engl J Med 2000;343:126.
14. Luks D, Anderson M. Antihistamines and the common cold: a review and critique of the literature. J Gen Intern Med 1996;11:240.
15. Curley FJ, Irwin RS, Pratter MR, et al. Cough and the common cold. Am Rev Respir Dis 1988;138:305.
16. Douglas RM, Chalker EB, Treacy B. Vitamin C for preventing and treating the common cold. The Cochrane Database of Systematic Reviews 2001;4.
17. Chalmers T. Effects of ascorbic acid on the common cold: an evaluation of the evidence. Am J Med 1975;58:532.
18. Truswell AS. Ascorbic acid and the common cold [Letter]. N Engl J Med 1986;315:709.
19. Hemila H. Does vitamin C alleviate the symptoms of the common cold? A review of current evidence. Scand J Infect Dis 1994;26:1.
20. Levine M, Rumsey SC, Daruwala R, et al. Criteria and recommendations for vitamin C intake. JAMA 1999;281:1415.
21. Melchart D, Linde K, Fischer P, et al. Echinacea for preventing and treating the common cold. The Cochrane Database of Systematic Reviews 1999;4.
22. Gonzales R, Bartlett JG, Besser RE, et al. Principles of appropriate antibiotic use for treatment of nonspecific upper respiratory tract infections in adults: background. Ann Intern Med 2001;134:490.
23. Hendley JO. The host response, not the virus, causes the symptoms of the common cold [Editorial comment]. Clin Infect Dis 1998;26:847.
24. Reuler JB, Lucas LM, Kumar KL. Sinusitis: a review for generalists. West J Med 1995;163:40.
25. Hickner JM, Bartlett JG, Besser RE, et al. Principles of appropriate antibiotic use for acute rhinosinusitis in adults: background. Ann Intern Med 2001;134:498.
26. Gwaltney JM Jr. Sinusitis. In: Mandell GL, Bennett JE, Dolin R, eds. Principles and practice of infectious diseases. 5th ed. Philadelphia: Churchill Livingstone, 2000;51:676.
27. Williams JW Jr, Simel DL. Does this patient have sinusitis? Diagnosing acute sinusitis by history and physical examination. JAMA 1993;270:1242.
28. Engels EA, Terrin N, Barza M, et al. Meta-analysis of diagnostic tests for acute sinusitis. J Clin Epidemiol 2000;53:852.
29. Williams JW Jr, Roberts L Jr, Distell B, et al. Diagnosing sinusitis by x-ray: is a single Waters view adequate? J Gen Intern Med 1992;7:481.
30. Gwaltney JM Jr, Phillips CD, Miller RD, et al. Computed tomographic study of the common cold. N Engl J Med 1994;330:25.
31. Van Buchem, FL, Knottnerus JA, Schrijnemaekers VJJ, et al. Primary-care-based randomized placebo-controlled trial of antibiotic treatment in acute maxillary sinusitis. Lancet 1997;349:683.
32. Stalman W, Van Essen GA, Van Der Graaf Y, et al. The end of antibiotic treatment in adults with acute sinusitis-like complaints in general practice? A placebo-controlled double-blind randomized doxycycline trial. Br J Gen Pract 1997;47:794.
33. Williams JW Jr, Aguilar C, Makela M, et al. Antibiotics for acute maxillary sinusitis. The Cochrane Database of Systematic Reviews 2001;3.
34. Balk EM, Zucker DR, Engels EA, et al. Strategies for diagnosing and treating suspected acute bacterial sinusitis: a cost effectiveness analysis. J Gen Intern Med 2001;16:701.
35. Piccirillo JF, Mager DE, Frisse ME, et al. Impact of first-line vs. second-line antibiotics for the treatment of acute uncomplicated sinusitis. JAMA 2001;286:1849.
36. Williams JW Jr, Holleman DR, Samsa GP, et al. Randomized controlled trial of 3 vs. 10 days of trimethoprim/sulfamethoxazole for acute maxillary sinusitis. JAMA 1995;1015.
37. Newman LJ, Platts-Mills TA, Phillips CD, et al. Chronic sinusitis: relationship of computed tomographic findings to allergy, asthma, and eosinophilia. JAMA 1994;271:363.
38. Barker WH, Mullooly JP. Pneumonia and influenza deaths during epidemics: implications for prevention. Arch Intern Med 1982;142:85.
39. Gross PA, Rodstein M, LaMontagne JR, et al. Epidemiology of acute respiratory illness during an influenza outbreak in a nursing home. Arch Intern Med 1988;148:559.
40. Cox NJ, Subbarao K. Influenza. Lancet 1999;354:1277.
41. Centers for Disease Control and Prevention. Prevention and control of influenza: recommendations of the advisory committee on immunization practices. MMWR Morb Mortal Wkly Rep 2001;50(RR-4):1.
42. Glezen WP. Serious morbidity and mortality associated with influenza epidemics. Lancet 1984;4:25.
43. Rapid diagnostic tests for influenza. Med Lett Drugs Ther 1999;41:121.
44. Couch RB. Prevention and treatment of influenza. N Engl J Med 2000;343:1778.
45. Diggory P, Fernandez C, Humphrey A, et al. Comparison of elderly people's technique in using two dry powder inhalers to deliver zanamivir: randomised controlled trial. BMJ 2001;322:577.
46. Hall WJ, Douglas RG Jr. Pulmonary function during and after common respiratory infections. Annu Rev Med 1980;31:233.
47. Skoner DP, Doyle WJ, Seroky J, et al. Lower airway responses to influenza A virus in healthy allergic and non allergic subjects. Am J Respir Crit Care Med 1996;154:661.
48. Fraenkel DK, Bardin PG, Sanderson G, et al. Lower airways inflammation during rhinovirus colds in normal and in asthmatic subjects. Am J Respir Crit Care Med 1995;151:879.
49. McBean AM, Babish JD, Warren JL. The impact and cost of influenza in the elderly. Arch Intern Med 1993;153:2105.
50. Oliveira EC, Marik PE, Colice G. Influenza pneumonia: a descriptive study. Chest 2001;119:1717.
51. Baine WB, Luby JP, Martin SW. Severe Illness with influenza B. Am J Med 1980;68:181.
52. Huovinen P, Lahtonen R, Ziegler T, et al. Pharyngitis in adults: the presence and coexistence of viruses and bacterial organisms. Ann Intern Med 1989;110:612.
53. Ebell MH, Smith MA, Barry HC, et al. Does the patient have strep throat? JAMA 2000;284:2912.
54. Bisno A. Acute pharyngitis. N Engl J Med 2001;344:205.
55. Cooper RJ, Hoffman JR, Bartlett JG, et al. Principles of appropriate use for acute pharyngitis in adults: background. Ann Intern Med 2001;134:509.
56. Komaroff AL, Pass TM, Aronson MD, et al. The prediction of streptococcal pharyngitis in adults. J Gen Intern Med 1986;1:1.
57. Centor RM, Witherspoon JM, Dalton HP, et al. The diagnosis of strep throat in adults in the emergency room. Med Decis Making 1981;1:239.
58. Webb KH, Needham CA, Kurtz SR. Use of a high-sensitivity rapid strep test without culture confirmation of negative results. J Fam Pract 2000;49:34.
59. Bisno AL. Group A streptococcal infections and acute rheumatic fever. N Engl J Med 1991;325:783.
60. Stollerman GH. Rheumatic fever. Lancet 1997;349:935.
61. Centers for Disease Control and Prevention. Summary of notifiable diseases, United States. MMWR Morb Mortal Wkly Rep 1998;47(53):1.
62. Del Mar CB, Glasziou PP, Spinks AB. Antibiotics for sore throat. The Cochrane Library 2001;4.
63. Brink WR, Rammelkamp CH, Denny FW, et al. Effect of penicillin and aureomycin on the natural course of streptococcal tonsillitis and pharyngitis. Am J Med 1951;10:300.

64. Centers for Disease Control and Prevention. 1998 Guidelines for treatment of sexually transmitted disease. MMWR Morb Mortal Wkly Rep 1998;47(RR-1):1.
65. Burton MJ, Towler B, Glasziou P. Tonsillectomy versus nonsurgical treatment for chronic/recurrent acute tonsillitis. The Cochrane Library 2001;3.
66. Richardson MA. Sore throat, tonsillitis, and adenoiditis. Med Clin North Am 1999;83:75.
67. Herzon FS. Peritonsillar abscess: incidence, current management practices, and a proposal for treatment guidelines. Laryngoscope 1995;105[Suppl 74]:1.
68. Frantz TD, Rasgon BM, Quesenberry CP Jr. Acute epiglottis in adults: analysis of 129 cases. JAMA 1994;272:1358.
69. Berg AO, LoGerfo JP. Potential effect of self-care algorithms on the number of physician visits. N Engl J Med 1979;300:535.
70. Gonzales R, Sande M. Uncomplicated acute bronchitis. Ann Intern Med 2000;133:981.
71. Metlay JP, Kapoor WN, Fine MJ. Does this patient have community-acquired pneumonia? Diagnosing pneumonia by history and physical examination. JAMA 1997;278:1440.
72. Wright SW, Edwards KM, Decker MD, et al. Pertussis infection in adults with persistent cough. JAMA 1995;273:1044.
73. Nenig ME, Shinefield HR, Edwards KM, et al. Prevalence and incidence of adult pertussis in an urban population. JAMA 1996;275:1672.
74. Gonzales R, Bartlett JG, Besser RE, et al. Principles of appropriate antibiotic use for treatment of uncomplicated acute bronchitis: background. Ann Intern Med 2001;134:521.
75. Bent S, Saint S, Vittinghoff E, et al. Antibiotics in acute bronchitis: a meta-analysis. Am J Med 1999;107:62.
76. Linder JA, Sim I. Antibiotic treatment of acute bronchitis in smokers: a systematic review. J Gen Intern Med 2002;17:230.
77. Thompson AB, Muellen MB. Aerosolized beclomethasone in chronic bronchitis. Am Rev Respir Dis 1992;146:389.
78. Minio AM, Smith BL. Deaths: Preliminary data for 2000. National vital statistics reports, vol. 49, no. 12, Hyattsville, MD: National Center for Health Statistics, 2001:5.
79. Pinner RW, Teutsch SM, Simonsen L, et al. Trends in infectious disease mortality in the United States. JAMA 1996;275:189.
80. Niederman MS, Mandell LA, Anzueto A, et al. Guidelines for the management of adults with community-acquired pneumonia: diagnosis, assessment of severity, antimicrobial therapy, and prevention. Am J Respir Crit Care Med 2001;163:1730.
81. Whitney CG, Farley MM, Hadler J, et al. Increasing prevalence of multi-drug resistant *Streptococcus pneumoniae* in the United States. N Engl J Med 2000;343:1917.
82. Heffelfinger JD, Dowell SF, Jorgensen JH, et al. Management of community-acquired pneumonia in the era of pneumococcal resistance. Arch Intern Med 2000;160:1399.
83. Fang G-D, Fine M, Orloff J, et al. New and emerging etiologies for community-acquired pneumonia with implications for therapy. Medicine (Baltimore) 1990;69:307.
84. Marrie TJ, Peeling RW, Fine MJ, et al. Ambulatory patients with community-acquired pneumonia: frequency of atypical agents and clinical course. Am J Med 1996;101:508.
85. Steinhoff D, Lode H, Ruckdeschel G, et al. *Chlamydia pneumoniae* as a cause of community acquired pneumonia in hospitalized patients in Berlin. Clin Infect Dis 1996;22:958.
86. Grayston JT. Infections caused by *Chlamydia pneumoniae* strain TWAR. J Infect Dis 1992;15:757.
87. Sopena N, Sabrià-Leal, Pedor-Botet ML, et al. Comparative study of the clinical presentation of legionella pneumonia and other community-acquired pneumonias. Chest 1998;113:1195.
88. Kennedy CA, Goetz MB. Atypical roentgenographic manifestations of *Pneumocystis carinii* pneumonia. Arch Intern Med 1992;152:1390.
89. Duchin J, Koster FT, Peters CJ, et al. Hantavirus pulmonary syndrome: a new illness in the southwestern United States. N Engl J Med 1994;330:949.
90. Bartlett JG, Mundy LM. Community-acquired pneumonia. N Engl J Med 1995;333:1618.
91. Woodhead MA, Arrowsmith J, Chamberlain-Webber R, et al. The value of routine microbial investigation in community-acquired pneumonia. Respir Med 1991;85:313.
92. Ruiz M, Ewig S, Marcos MA, et al. Etiology of community-acquired pneumonia: impact of age, co-morbidity and severity. Am J Respir Crit Care Med 1999;160:397.
93. Fine MJ, Auble TE, Yealy DM, et al. A prediction rule to identify low-risk patients with community-acquired pneumonia. N Engl J Med 1997;336:243.
94. Fine MJ, Smith MA, Carson CA, et al. Prognosis and outcomes of patients with community-acquired pneumonia. JAMA 1996;275:134.
95. Fine MJ, Hough LJ, Medsger AR, et al. The hospital admission decision for patients with community-acquired pneumonia: results from the Pneumonia Patient Outcomes Research Team Cohort Study. Arch Intern Med 1997;157:36.
96. Metlay JP, Fine MJ, Schulz R, et al. Measuring symptomatic and functional recovery in patients with community-acquired pneumonia. J Gen Intern Med 1997;12:423.
97. Mittl RL Jr, Schwab RJ, Duchin JS, et al. Radiographic resolution of community-acquired pneumonia. Am J Respir Crit Care Med 1994;149:630.
98. Schwartz B, Bell DM, Hughes JM. Preventing the emergence of antimicrobial resistance: a call for action by clinicians, public health officials, and patients. JAMA 1997;278:944.
99. Gonzales R, Steiner JF, Sande MA. Antibiotic prescribing for adults with colds, upper respiratory tract infections, and bronchitis by ambulatory care physicians. JAMA 1997;278:90.
100. Linder JA, Stafford RS. Antibiotic treatment of adults with sore throat by community primary care physicians, a national survey, 1989–1999. JAMA 2001;286:1181.
101. Whitney CG, Farley MM, Hadler J, et al. Increasing prevalence of multidrug-resistant *Streptococcus pneumoniae* in the United States. N Engl J Med 2000;343:1917.
102. Hyde TB, Gay K, Stephens DS, et al. Macrolide resistance among invasive *Streptococcus pneumoniae* isolates. JAMA 2001;286:1857.
103. Ailani RK, Agastya G, Ailani RK, et al. Doxycycline is a cost-effective therapy for hospitalized patients with community-acquired pneumonia. Arch Intern Med 1999;159:266.
104. Centers for Disease Control and Prevention. Resistance of *Streptococcus pneumoniae* to fluoroquinolones—United States, 1995–1999. MMWR Morb Mortal Wkly Rep 2001;50:800.
105. Spach DH, Black D. Antibiotic resistance in community-acquired respiratory tract infections: current issues. Ann Allergy Asthma Immunol 1998;81:293.
106. Gonzales R, Steiner JF, Lum A, et al. Decreasing antibiotic use in ambulatory practice. JAMA 1999;281:1512.
107. Hamm RM, Hicks RJ, Bemben DA. Antibiotics and respiratory infections: are patients more satisfied when expectations are met? J Fam Pract 1996;43:56.

CHAPTER 34

Tuberculosis in the Ambulatory Patient

PATRICK A. MURPHY, MD

EPIDEMIOLOGY

Incidence Trends

In 1990–1992, the United States was experiencing an increase in tuberculosis incidence. The cause was the human immunodeficiency virus (HIV) epidemic, which had created a large number of susceptible hosts. In addition, the number of cases of tuberculosis (TB) caused by bacilli resistant to most or all standard antituberculosis drugs rapidly increased. These multidrug-resistant (MDR) bacilli were highly lethal for patients with HIV infection, and it was feared that they would also produce untreatable infections in the normal population. Because of these problems, there was a resurgence of interest in the disease, medical and hospital practices were changed, and there was intense follow-up of diagnosed cases by public health officers.

All this activity has paid off, and the current situation looks better (1). In 1999, there were 17,531 new cases of TB in the United States, well below the 1985 level of 22,201 and the 1992 level of 26,673. Furthermore, 43% of all the cases occurred in people who were born in other countries, and, of those, two thirds were born in Haiti, Mexico, India, China, Vietnam, or the Philippines. It seems likely that most such cases were acquired abroad and imported. The number of cases in United States natives fell 44% between 1986 and 1999, whereas the incidence in immigrants rose 53%. More than half of all immigrants with TB present within 5 years after entry into the United States. MDR TB is still virtually 100% lethal in the HIV-infected person. However, the incidence of MDR TB nationwide has decreased markedly. In 1993 there were more than 400 cases (2.5% of total) of MDR TB in persons who had never previously been treated for TB. These were presumably primary infections with a resistant organism. In 1999 there were fewer than 150 such cases (1.1%).

This improvement in the national picture can be attributed to many causes. Skin testing for TB has come back as a diagnostic procedure and is mandatory for health care workers. Patients discovered by this method are promptly given isoniazid (INH) preventive therapy. Clinical suspicion for TB by doctors has escalated, and TB is being considered as a possible cause of almost any chest illness and almost any abnormal chest radiograph. Microbiologic methods for diagnosis have improved: polymerase chain reaction (PCR) allows rapid diagnosis of TB from the sputum, and metabolic inhibition tests allow early detection of drug-resistant bacilli. Four-drug therapy for TB has virtually replaced the old two- and three-drug regimens, and therapy is commonly enforced by directly observing the patient take his or her medicines. Finally, hospitals, clinics, and prisons have refined their ventilating systems to reduce airborne transmission of TB. These changes in practice are discussed later in the chapter.

Human Immunodeficiency Virus and Tuberculosis

It is estimated that a normal adult newly infected with TB has approximately a 5% chance of developing clinical illness in the first 5 years after infection, and a total lifetime risk of approximately 10%. The other 90% of normal people infected with TB have a positive skin test but never develop clinical illness. In contrast are people who are tuberculin positive as a result of a long-standing infection and who then acquire HIV infection. Such people have an annual incidence of clinical disease of 8% to 10%, with essentially a 100% lifetime incidence (2). Even more devastating are the consequences of being HIV positive and then becoming infected with TB. Because HIV seropositivity is often unknown to or concealed by the HIV-infected person, precise estimates of annual risk in this situation are not available. However, there are enough epidemics of severe primary TB among HIV-infected people exposed to an index case of TB to make it clear that the risk must be considerably higher than the 8% to 10% noted for the situation in which TB is acquired first. The annual risk is almost certainly greater than 50% and may approach 100% (3).

There are two other reasons why HIV infection amplifies TB rates. The first is based on the intensity of exposure needed to become infected. TB is acquired by inhaling dried droplet nuclei, which typically contain one to three organisms. A normal person usually must inhale several hundred such nuclei before one of them successfully establishes a caseous focus. Most cases of TB in normal people occur after long-standing, intense exposure to an infected person living in the same house or working in daily close contact. By contrast, a person infected with HIV acquires TB after inhaling an average of less than 10 infected nuclei, meaning that HIV-infected people often acquire TB after casual contact with an infected person. The other reason why HIV infection amplifies TB rates is that the clinical disease is often severe, and many bacilli are coughed out. Each case of TB in an HIV-infected person is therefore more infectious for other people than is the average case of TB in an immunocompetent person (3).

No matter how immunosuppressed one is, one cannot develop tuberculous infection unless one is exposed to the organism. HIV infection acquired by a young male homosexual in Iowa is highly unlikely to be complicated by TB because there is little chance that he will ever be exposed to a case of pulmonary TB.

Reactivation and Primary Tuberculosis

There are now two distinct epidemiologic profiles of clinical TB. Most sporadic symptomatic cases still arise as reactivation disease in a patient who was infected many years ago and was never treated or was inadequately treated. When the patient becomes old or develops an immunosuppressive illness, the disease reactivates. Such patients are infectious for others, and TB can develop in people closely exposed to them. The response to primary tuberculous infection depends on the kind of person infected. Children are highly susceptible to TB and tend to have clinical symptoms shortly after primary infection. Primary infection in an adult usually causes no symptoms, but the newly infected person becomes tuberculin positive (4). As discussed earlier, primary TB in an HIV-infected person tends to be severe and progressive (3).

Causes

The cause of TB in an immunologically normal person residing in the United States is almost always *Mycobacterium tuberculosis.* Atypical mycobacteria, such as *Mycobacterium kansasii* and *Mycobacterium avium-intracellulare,* and certain fungi, such as *Cryptococcus neoformans* and *Histoplasma capsulatum,* may produce disease indistinguishable from TB and should be considered in the differential diagnosis. All of these diseases are more common and more severe in immunosuppressed persons. In foreign countries, bovine TB bacilli can be important.

Drug Resistance

In populations who have never been treated with antituberculosis drugs, primary resistance of tubercle bacilli to most drugs occurs at a low level (approximately 1% to 3%). Because the mechanisms of resistance are different for every drug, primary resistance to multiple drugs is uncommon. However, during the past 50 years many inner-city patients have been given antituberculosis drugs without close supervision. Such patients are likely to take drugs singly, because of real or perceived side effects from multiple drugs, and to discontinue therapy entirely after symptoms improve. Not only do the bacilli in these patients become resistant to many antituberculosis drugs, but these resistant organisms may then infect other people. In such cases, the TB is "primary" because the infected person has a new infection. Nonetheless, the tubercle bacilli may be resistant to one or more of the standard antituberculosis drugs. Even in 1965, before the HIV epidemic, children in Brooklyn who were younger than 5 years of age and had primary TB had INH-resistant organisms 15% of the time (4).

The HIV epidemic has amplified the problem of drug-resistant tubercle bacilli that already existed in large cities. It is now not uncommon for tubercle bacilli to be resistant to all three standard antituberculosis drugs: INH, rifampin (RIF), and ethambutol (EMB). Some strains have been resistant to all known antituberculosis drugs. Such MDR strains are disastrous for the HIV-infected person because the disease cannot be controlled and is rapidly fatal. MDR strains are also a major public health hazard for immunocompetent people who are exposed to intense concentrations of infectious droplet nuclei. There is no reason to believe that these organisms are any more virulent than average, and presumably a normal person infected with such strains would have a 10% lifetime risk of developing clinical disease. However, if disease developed, it could not be treated with the usual drugs.

DIAGNOSIS

History

When symptomatic, TB almost always presents with signs and symptoms of weeks' to months' duration. Almost the only time it presents as acute disease is in rare cases of acute meningitis or tuberculous pneumonia. The history should be directed toward both defining the symptom complex and determining possible exposure to known sources of disease.

Because TB has multiple presentations, chronic unexplained symptoms in any patient should be considered suspicious. Weight loss (documented over a defined period), fever (particularly in the late evenings), night sweats (to be differentiated from environmentally induced sweats), decreased appetite, and the loss of a sense of well-being are the most important nonspecific symptoms. Persistent cough (usually with sputum production), hemoptysis, and pleuritic chest pain are more specific findings suggestive of pulmonary involvement.

It is important to know whether the patient has previously had TB, has previously been skin tested for TB (and if so, when and what the results were), and when the patient has had previous chest films (and where they can be obtained).

Possibly significant history also includes any family member or close friend with known TB, any person in school or at work with known disease, and any recent history of travel to a country where TB is common.

Because extrapulmonary TB can occur in any organ (e.g., pleura, lymph nodes, endometrium, kidneys, ureters, bones and joints, skin, meninges, small intestine, peritoneum) or as a disseminated (miliary) form, chronic symptoms and signs in any organ must raise the consideration of TB.

Physical Examination

The physical examination may be entirely normal, even with obvious evidence of pulmonary disease on the chest radiograph. The following findings, when present, may be of considerable help in suggesting the diagnosis: rales localized to the upper posterior chest or auscultatory evidence of pulmonary cavitation (bronchovesicular breathing and whispered pectoriloquy), evidence of pleural effusion, supraclavicular and infraclavicular retraction, lymphadenopathy, evidence of weight loss, and fever. Although rare in the United States, large, matted, nontender cervical lymph nodes (at times with draining sinuses) are almost diagnostic of scrofula, a form of tuberculous adenitis seen primarily in children (which may also be caused by atypical mycobacteria).

Tuberculin Skin Tests

The standardized skin test (5) for evidence of tuberculous infection uses 5 units of Tween-stabilized intermediate-strength purified protein derivative (PPD), which is injected intradermally on the volar skin of the forearm. The use of control tests with "anergy panel" antigens has been abandoned. The PPD test requires intradermal injection, which is a highly skilled procedure. Tine tests and automated methods of introducing antigen into the skin such as the Heaf gun can be used in population surveys. Positive results elicited with these methods should be confirmed with the standard PPD. The PPD reaction should be read at 48 hours. A practical method for determining the diameter of the indurated area is the *ballpoint pen method:* a line is drawn from a point 1 to 2 cm away from the margin of a positive reaction; when the pen tip reaches the margin of the indurated area, definite resistance is felt; this is repeated on the opposite side, and the diameter of the indurated reaction is measured.

The diameter required for a *positive test* varies according to circumstances.

Cases in Which More Than 5 mm is Regarded As Positive:

- People with HIV infection and people receiving immunosuppressive therapy
- People with recent close contact with a case of pulmonary TB
- People with fibrotic changes on their chest radiograph suggestive of healed TB

Cases in Which More Than 10 mm is Regarded As Positive:

- In general, those with chronic illnesses known to predispose to TB and those from areas with a high incidence of TB
- People with silicosis, malnutrition (including people with gastrectomy or jejunoileal bypass), or diabetes
- Transplant recipients and people being treated with renal dialysis, corticosteroids, or cancer chemotherapy
- Children younger than 4 years of age
- Recent immigrants from high-prevalence areas
- Medical and laboratory personnel with occupational exposure
- The poor, especially injection drug users
- People from prisons, nursing homes, and other group residences

Cases in Which More Than 15 mm is Regarded As Positive:

- People who are generally healthy and not exposed to TB (testing of such persons is discouraged because most positive test results are falsely positive)

A PPD conversion requires an increase of 10 mm within 2 years for patients of any age. Note that a change from 8 to 12 mm is *not* a PPD conversion. The criteria are not foolproof and should be applied with common sense. In particular, it has been suggested that even 2 mm induration may be significant in an HIV-infected patient (6).

The tuberculin skin test is an excellent way of diagnosing recent tuberculous infection in children or young adults. Such people are rarely tuberculin positive in the absence of recently acquired tuberculous infection. The test is also useful for investigating family members or health care personnel who have had known exposure to patients with infectious TB. Because it is not specific or sensitive enough to guide a clinical decision, the tuberculin test is less useful for the evaluation of patients with nonspecific symptoms that may be caused by TB. In some populations of elderly patients, up to 50% may be tuberculin positive as a result of long-standing infection that is inactive and has nothing to do with the present illness. Fully 20% of patients who do have active clinical TB are PPD negative. When one adds in other clinical variables such as tumors, steroid therapy, radiation therapy, and organ transplantation, a negative PPD test is often uninterpretable. Also, a negative PPD test may be harmful if it is used to rule out the diagnosis of TB in a patient whose clinical state may be caused by active disease.

A person with a known positive tuberculin skin test should not have it repeated. In such patients, there is a risk of producing a very strong positive reaction characterized by tender induration, axillary adenopathy, temperature elevation, and sloughing of the epidermis after 1 week. If a patient develops this complication, it should be treated with a sterile gauze dressing impregnated with a topical steroid, such as 0.1% triamcinolone.

The Centers for Disease Control and Prevention (CDC) recommends that *previous bacille Calmette-Guérin (BCG) vaccination* be disregarded when interpreting the response to a PPD (5). The reason is that a positive PPD reaction induced by BCG tends to wane with time. There is no reliable way of determining whether a positive PPD reaction is caused by real TB or by the BCG vaccine. There is agreement that when a person is PPD tested for the first time, very pronounced reactions (greater than 20 mm) are unlikely to be a result of BCG vaccination. On the other hand, recall of PPD sensitivity induced by repetitive PPD testing in persons vaccinated with BCG is commonly seen. Necrotic tuberculin reactions are particularly common in people who were vaccinated with BCG in childhood, become health care workers, and must be PPD tested every 6 or 12 months. If the vaccination was done 20 to 30 years earlier, the first tuberculin test is commonly negative. However, with repeated testing the immunologic memory revives and the reaction becomes progressively more intense. Not only does this raise unwarranted fears of tuberculous infection, but the reactions are very painful. The CDC regulations do not cover this situation; however, it is prudent not to do more than one tuberculin test in anyone previously vaccinated with BCG.

M. tuberculosis shares antigens with related mycobacteria, so a positive skin test is not specific. However, most cross-reactions are less than 10 mm in diameter. Skin testing with specific atypical mycobacterial antigens should not be done: The antigens are not available for general use, and the results are difficult to interpret.

Persons with a remote tuberculous or atypical mycobacterial infection who have become skin-test negative may, on repeat annual skin testing, develop a positive response because the repeated exposure to antigen reinvigorates the immune response (*booster effect*) (7). Repeated testing with tuberculin skin test antigen will not induce a positive test in an uninfected person. The booster phenomenon may mimic PPD conversion in persons who are repeatedly tested, such as elderly people, in whom loss of PPD reactivity is common, and people such as hospital employees who may be skin tested frequently. The booster effect is detected by administering a second tuberculin test 2 weeks after the first test in persons who initially have a negative response. If the second response is positive, these individuals can be said to have had past infection but are not considered to have a recently acquired infection.

Current practice in hospitals is that all employees not known to be PPD positive are tested on entry. If they are PPD negative on entry and have contact with patients, they are retested annually, or more often if the hospital is in an area where TB is common.

Laboratory Evaluation

Chest Radiograph

Both posteroanterior and lateral views should be obtained. If the standard radiograph is normal but the patient has strong clinical evidence for TB, an apical lordotic view or a computed tomography scan of the chest should also be obtained. The radiologic findings typical of TB (e.g., apical scarring, hilar adenopathy with peripheral infiltrate, upper lobe cavitation, miliary infiltrate) are not specific; however, a negative chest film rules out pulmonary TB (with the rare exception of early miliary disease), making the chest film a very sensitive test.

Cultures and Smears of Sputum

Sputum for smear and culture should be obtained at least three times. A *positive sputum smear* highly suggests TB (but is not absolutely diagnostic because of the possibility of atypical infection or of contamination), and a *positive culture is diagnostic.* If sputum is difficult to obtain, one can obtain assisted sputum after the patient has inhaled hypertonic saline aerosol. This procedure is obviously dangerous to personnel and should be done only in a special room with proper precautions for infection control. If clinical features suggest infection outside the lung, smears and cultures of other body fluids such as urine and cerebrospinal fluid are appropriate.

PCR tests for *M. tuberculosis* are approved by the U.S. Food and Drug Administration for direct use on sputum. However, the tests are subject to errors due to the presence of inhibitors, and most clinical laboratories are not able to routinely offer PCR tests directly on sputum.

Cultures usually become positive within 3 or 4 weeks. Any tubercle bacillus isolated from a patient should be tested for sensitivity to standard drugs, because it may be necessary to change treatment if the organism shows resistance. The state laboratory will be glad to do this if necessary. In parts of the world with very limited funds, it may be necessary to confine drug susceptibility tests to tubercle bacilli from patients who have failed standard therapy.

Miscellaneous Laboratory Tests

In patients with active TB, the hematocrit value may be normal or low. The anemia caused by TB is normochromic and normocytic, the so-called anemia of chronic disease (see Chapter 55). The white blood cell count and differential count are usually normal; occasionally a monocytosis is seen in patients with severe disease. The urine should be tested routinely; if sterile pyuria is found, it is suggestive of renal TB and cultures should be sent for analysis.

Determinations of serum aminotransferases, alkaline phosphatase, and bilirubin may be helpful if disseminated disease or liver involvement is suspected. Also, these values provide baselines in case the patient develops hepatitis caused by antituberculosis drugs. Other procedures, such as thoracocentesis, lumbar puncture, and liver biopsy, are indicated only when specific organ involvement is suspected.

Presumptive Diagnosis

The presumptive diagnosis of active TB can be made when any of the following is found:

- A typical chest radiograph
- A positive sputum smear
- A biopsy showing caseating granulomas with or without acid-fast organisms
- A recent change (within 1 year) of the tuberculin skin test result from negative to positive, associated with other characteristic systemic symptoms or signs

The diagnosis of active TB is confirmed by a positive culture from any body fluid or biopsy specimen. All patients with a presumptive or confirmed diagnosis of TB must be reported promptly to the appropriate local health department.

Diagnosis of Tuberculosis in HIV-Infected Patients

In 1993, pulmonary TB in an HIV-positive patient was designated as an *acquired immunodeficiency syndrome (AIDS)–defining condition* (see Chapter 39). When clinical TB appears before the development of other AIDS-indicator conditions, presentation occurs in a typical fashion, with pulmonary disease predominantly in the apices and often with cavitation. Fever, sweats, cough, anorexia, and wasting are common complaints. When TB appears after AIDS is already established, many patients have progressive primary disease, with extensive lower lobe involvement, no cavitation, and hilar adenopathy (3). Extrapulmonary TB is more common in patients with AIDS and involves lymph nodes, liver, brain, meninges, bone marrow, adrenals, and the genitourinary tract. Aspiration or biopsy of the suspected site of infection should be performed for acid-fast stain and culture. If acid-fast bacilli (AFB) are found in one of these specimens, treatment for *M. tuberculosis* should be initiated while awaiting culture results, even though *M. avium-intracellulare* is more common.

MANAGEMENT AND COURSE

Treatment

When TB is diagnosed in association with systemic signs or symptoms, the patient should be treated for active disease. Patients with positive tuberculin reactions as the only manifestation of disease are more difficult to treat (see Isoniazid Treatment of Latent Tuberculosis).

Isolation

Any patient with symptomatic TB should be hospitalized at once in respiratory isolation in a negative-pressure room. Isolation must be instituted as soon as the diagnosis is made or even strongly suspected. One can never prevent a patient walking into an emergency room and exposing a doctor, two or three nurses, a clerk, a radiology technician, and other patients to the risk of TB. But an undiagnosed patient who stays on a medical ward for 2 weeks may easily expose 200 people. Isolation should be maintained until the patient is clearly noninfectious (see later discussion).

In some communities, no hospital has the required isolation rooms and MDR tubercle bacilli are uncommon or unknown. In these circumstances, a patient who has a home can be started on treatment and sent home. The logic is that everyone in the home has already been exposed. The patient is instructed not to leave the house for 2 weeks and not to allow any previously unexposed visitors for the same period. Therapy in the home should be directly observed (see later discussion), and the patient should be allowed to leave the house or have visitors only when clearly improving. It should be noted that this exception to the guidelines does not apply to patients who are homeless or are unlikely to follow directions because of alcoholism or drug addiction. It also does not apply in communities where MDR TB is common.

Drug Therapy for Tuberculosis

The imperatives of the MDR TB situation have resulted in a *standard four-drug protocol* for treatment of TB (8). There is little room for individual variation, and attempts to use nonstandard methods usually result in telephone calls from the local health department. The pressure is in favor of *rendering the patient noninfectious in the shortest possible time.* That way, fewer nurses are required to supervise the therapy.

The current standard initial regimen is as follows:

- *Isoniazid* (INH): 300 mg/day (available strengths, 100 and 300 mg)
- *Rifampin* (RIF): 600 mg/day (available strength, 600 mg)
- *Ethambutol* (EMB): 15 mg/kg per day, commonly 1,200 mg/day (available strengths, 100 and 400 mg)
- *Pyrazinamide* (PZA): 2,000 mg/day (available strength, 500 mg)

All four of these drugs are given for 2 months, and then the EMB and PZA are discontinued. INH and RIF are continued for another 4 months, making *6 months of treatment in all.* When patients are treated on a twice-weekly schedule, the daily dose of drugs is larger (Table 34.1).

After a patient's culture results become available, sensitivities should be checked. If the bacilli are susceptible to all four drugs and if directly observed therapy (discussed later) is used, more than 98% of cases of TB are permanently cured (8).

Table 34.1. Drugs for the Treatment of Mycobacterial Disease in Adults

Commonly Used Agents	Available Strengths of Oral Tablets or Capsules (mg)	Dosage: Total Once-Daily Dosage	Dosage: Twice-Weekly Dosage	Most Common Side Effects	Tests for Side Effects	Drug Interactions[a]
Isoniazid[b]	100, 300	5–10 mg/kg up to 300 mg PO or IM	15 mg/kg PO up to 900 mg	Peripheral neuritis, hepatitis, hypersensitivity	Aminotransferases (not as a routine)	Carbamazepine: increased toxicity, both drugs Disulfiram: psychosis, ataxia Phenytoin: toxicity increased
Rifampin	150, 300	10 mg/kg up to 600 mg PO	10 mg/kg up to 600 mg PO	Hepatitis, febrile reaction, purpura (rare)	Aminotransferases (not as a routine)	May reduce the effect of the following drugs due to increased hepatic metabolism: oral contraceptives, quinidine, corticosteroids, anticoagulants, disopyramide, diazepam, barbiturates, methadone, digitoxin, digoxin, oral hypoglycemics; *p*-aminosalicylic acid may interfere with absorption of rifampin
Streptomycin		15–20 mg/kg up to 1 g IM	25–30 mg/kg up to 1 g IM	Eighth nerve damage, nephrotoxicity	Vestibular function, audiograms; blood urea nitrogen and creatinine	Neuromuscular blocking agents; may be potentiated to cause prolonged paralysis
Pyrazinamide	500	15–30 mg/kg up to 2 g PO	50–70 mg/kg up to 4 g	Hyperuricemia, hepatotoxicity	Uric acid, aminotransferases	
Ethambutol	100, 400	15–25 mg/kg PO	50 mg/kg PO up to 2.5 g	Optic neuritis (reversible with discontinuation of drug; very rare at 15 mg/kg), skin rash	Red-green color discrimination and visual acuity,[c] difficult to test in a child <3 yr	

[a]Reference should be made to current literature, particularly on rifampin, because it induces hepatic microenzymes and therefore interacts with many drugs.
[b]With pyridoxine 25 mg/day for poorly nourished or pregnant patients to prevent peripheral neuropathy.
[c]Initial examination should be done at start of treatment.
Adapted from American Thoracic Society. Treatment of tuberculosis and tuberculosis infection in adults and children. Am Rev Respir Dis 134:355, 1986; and MMWR, Morb Mortal Wkly Rep 1993;42:2.

The enthusiasm for four-drug supervised therapy should not obscure the fact that this regimen is not appropriate for everyone. It is possible to cure TB with two or three drugs, but it takes longer. Patients should receive special consideration if they cannot take all of the components of the standard regimen (9).

Drug Toxicity

Patients may develop a number of toxicities from antituberculosis medications (Table 34.1).

Isoniazid. Hepatic toxicity is the most common adverse reaction; it occurs at a biochemical level in approximately 20% of patients who take the drug, and the incidence of toxicity increases with age and with excessive alcohol intake (10). Pregnant women are at increased risk for INH toxicity. Laboratory evidence of mild injury to the liver is not in itself a reason to stop the drug, however, because in most subjects the aminotransferase level returns to normal while the drug is being continued. If the patient develops jaundice or develops fever with elevated liver enzymes, the drug should be stopped. The liver injury is usually reversible and heals without further therapy. However, in some patients (elderly men and particularly those with chronic alcohol-related liver disease), the liver injury can be severe and sometimes fatal. INH liver toxicity most often occurs early in therapy, so that the first 2 to 3 months are the most critical in the detection of adverse drug reactions. Specific guidelines for monitoring for INH hepatitis are discussed later (see Prevention of Tuberculosis). Sensory peripheral neuropathy is an uncommon complication of INH therapy that occurs only in patients on an inadequate diet; it can be prevented by taking 25 mg of pyridoxine every day.

Ethambutol. The most serious side effect of EMB is *optic neuritis,* which causes decreased visual acuity and inability to distinguish the color green. This problem was seen frequently when the drug was given at a dose of 25 mg/kg. It is extremely uncommon at the current recommended daily dose of 15 mg/kg.

Rifampin. Serious allergic complications of RIF therapy, including thrombocytopenia manifested by purpura, petechiae, and hematuria; acute renal failure; and a flu-like syndrome, occur in approximately 1% of patients and necessitate cessation of therapy. There is a modest increase in hepatic toxicity that may be additive to INH toxicity, so patients taking both drugs should be supervised closely. Patients should be warned that RIF will result in an orange-red color in secretions such as urine and saliva and may irreversibly stain contact lenses. RIF accelerates the metabolism of other drugs (Table 34.1) and may necessitate an increase in the dosage of these drugs. Interaction with HIV protease inhibitors is a major problem and requires expert advice.

Special Situations

Patients with *nonpulmonary TB* can be treated with the 6-month regimen just described. Exceptions are patients with TB meningitis or bone marrow or joint infection. These patients should receive 12 months of treatment (9).

Pregnant women are difficult to treat because of the need to consider the effects of prescribed drugs on the fetus. The standard recommendation, for areas where MDR TB is uncommon, is a three-drug regimen of INH, RIF, and EMB. There is worldwide experience with this regimen, and it is generally regarded as safe. PZA is a category C drug that could be added if necessary; streptomycin (STR) is category D, and its use is discouraged. For other antituberculosis drugs, one should seek expert advice.

Patients with *renal failure* are difficult to treat because both EMB and PZA are excreted largely by the kidneys. If renal function is only moderately reduced, this situation can be dealt with by dosage reduction. However, if the patient is on hemodialysis, the calculations become a nightmare. Because the toxicity of EMB is blindness and that of PZA is severe hepatitis, errors are serious. Both INH and RIF can be given in full dosage to people with no renal function, and INH plus RIF given together for 9 months cures all forms of TB. It seems better to accept the longer treatment. If there is a real possibility of MDR TB, and a four-drug regimen is necessary, INH, RIF, PZA, and STR might be the safest. The hepatotoxicity of PZA is generally reversible, and although ototoxicity of STR is irreversible, the blood level of STR can be measured.

Patients who have HIV infection but are infected with drug-sensitive tubercle bacilli have a good prognosis for cure of their TB. It is usual to treat for 9 months rather than 6 and to be meticulous about follow-up. There is good evidence that patients with HIV as well as TB have higher relapse rates than patients with TB who are immunologically normal (11).

Drug Resistance

If the bacilli prove to be resistant to either INH or RIF, treatment should be modified to a three- or four-drug regimen in which the bacilli are susceptible to all components. Such a regimen should be continued for at least 12 months, and perhaps 18 months in a case of extensive disease. If the bacilli are resistant to both INH and RIF, the organism is by definition MDR. The patient should be referred for treatment to an expert, either at a university or at the state health department. The patient will be kept in isolation as long as bacilli are found on sputum culture. All available secondary antibiotics will be tried against the organism. A selection will be made from possibilities such as capreomycin and clofazimine. Regimens of six or seven drugs are not uncommon. If the response to the best available therapy remains poor, the addition of gamma-interferon infusions can be tried (12). If the patient is HIV infected, the outlook is probably hopeless, but there are occasional survivors (13). Details about longitudinal management of patients with drug-resistant TB are given later (see Course in Treated Patients).

Additional Therapy

The patient may have symptoms that require special management, such as high fever and toxicity for which corticosteroids may be helpful, or a pleural effusion that needs draining. The patient should be encouraged to eat an adequate diet. If the patient is eating poorly, pyridoxine (25 mg/day) should be taken with INH to prevent peripheral neuropathy. Pyridoxine should also be taken routinely by pregnant patients and by patients with other diseases that can cause peripheral neuropathy (e.g., alcoholism, diabetes, end-stage renal disease).

Course in Treated Patients

Follow-Up Schedule

Physicians in the United States are rarely expected or allowed to supervise the treatment of a patient with TB. Both death rates and recurrence rates are higher for patients treated by physicians (14), and directly observed therapy is so clearly superior for most patients that only completely reliable patients should be treated in a physician's office. Health departments will supervise therapy, test contacts and provide prophylactic INH if necessary, provide free drugs, and perform sputum cultures and radiographs as tests of cure (15). In rural areas of the United States and in other countries, the physician may have to supervise therapy for TB.

After treatment has been initiated, the patient should be seen or contacted at least once a month, chiefly to ensure drug compliance and to monitor for drug side effects. Sputum cultures should be obtained monthly for the first 3 months. At 3 months and between 6 months and 1 year, chest radiographs should be obtained. *Sputum culture should be negative after 3 months of therapy,* although occasionally nonculturable acid-fast organisms are seen on smear for longer periods. A test-of-cure culture should be done on all patients at 5 or 6 months. Because resolution of pulmonary infiltrates is often slow; the former practice of monthly chest radiography is not warranted. Chest radiographs are most helpful in excluding progression of disease and in documenting the patient's status when TB is cured.

If a patient receiving the standard four-drug therapy still has positive sputum cultures at 3 months, it is worth measuring the serum RIF level 2 hours after RIF has been given. The level should be 8 to 24 μg/mL. Occasionally a patient has a serum RIF level lower than 5 μg/mL, even as low as 1 μg/mL. If such patients are given enough RIF to get the serum RIF into the therapeutic range, the TB improves at a normal rate (16).

If the patient does not have HIV infection, has sensitive bacilli, and follows a recommended and supervised regimen for the prescribed time, then relapse is so rare (less than 1%) that postcure follow-up is not necessary. However, if the patient has HIV, the relapse rate is higher, 2% to 8%. In such cases, TB follow-up is worthwhile and can be integrated with HIV treatment (11).

Usual Response

Patients with active TB who comply with therapy have an excellent prognosis. Exceptions are patients with organisms resistant to the usual antituberculosis drugs and patients who develop adverse effects from the antituberculosis therapy. The patient should show some symptomatic improvement within 1 week after initiation of antituberculosis therapy. Improvement is usually indicated by an increased sense of well-being, an increase in appetite, and a decrease in cough, fever, and night sweats; temperature should be normal within 14 days after treatment initiation. Most patients are back to their usual state of health in 1 to 2 months.

The improvement is caused by the prompt antibacterial effects of the drugs, which lead to a decrease in the inflammatory response of the host. After 2 or 3 weeks of therapy, the patient who is improving clinically (decreased cough, absence of fever, improved appetite) can be considered *noninfectious.* If the patient is known to be infected with an MDR organism, three sputum samples must be negative on smear before the patient can be released from isolation.

Respiratory Isolation for Ambulatory Patients

Health care workers who are the first points of contact in facilities serving patients at risk for TB should be trained to ask questions to detect patients who should be isolated because of signs or symptoms suggestive of TB. Even clerks can ask questions about chronic respiratory symptoms and alert the doctor or nurse. Patients with signs or symptoms suggestive of TB should be evaluated promptly to minimize the time spent in ambulatory care areas. TB precautions should be applied while the diagnostic evaluation is being conducted.

TB precautions in the ambulatory care setting consist of placing the patient in a separate waiting area, apart from other patients and not in an open waiting area, ideally in a room meeting TB isolation requirements, and giving the patient a surgical mask and instruction to keep it on. Patients should also be given tissues and instructed to cover their mouths and noses when coughing or sneezing, if they must remove their mask to facilitate respiratory clearance.

Ventilation in ambulatory care areas serving patients at high risk for TB should be designed and maintained to reduce the risk of TB transmission. General use areas (e.g., waiting rooms) and special areas (e.g., treatment or TB isolation rooms in ambulatory areas) should be ventilated in the same manner as described for similar inpatient areas. Enhanced general ventilation or use of air disinfection techniques, such as in-room recirculation of air through high-efficiency particulate air (HEPA) filters or ultraviolet irradiation of the upper room air, may be useful. Ambulatory care settings in which patients with TB are frequently seen should have a negative-pressure room.

In general, *patients with suspected or confirmed active TB should be considered infectious* if cough is present, they are undergoing cough-inducing procedures, sputum AFB smears are positive, they are not receiving chemotherapy or have just started chemotherapy, or they have a poor clinical or bacteriologic response to chemotherapy. A person with drug-susceptible TB who is receiving adequate chemotherapy and has had a significant clinical and bacteriologic response to therapy (reduction in cough, resolution of fever, and progressively decreasing quantity of bacilli on smear) is probably no longer infectious.

Patients with active TB who need to be seen in a clinic should have appointments scheduled to avoid exposing HIV-infected or otherwise severely immunocompromised patients. This could be accomplished by setting aside certain times of the day for appointments for these patients or by having them seen in areas where immunocompromised patients are not treated.

Patients with infectious TB should have at least two negative sputum smears for AFB before being placed in indoor environments that are especially conducive to transmission (e.g., shelters for the homeless) or in settings where highly susceptible people (e.g., those with HIV infection) will be exposed (17).

Drug Resistance

The treatment of patients with drug-resistant tubercle bacilli has become common in certain U.S. cities such as New York and Miami. In other cities, drug resistance to even one antibiotic occurs less than 3% of the time, and MDR strains have rarely been observed. However, the population is so mobile that a patient who has acquired infection in one city may present for treatment in another.

Because MDR strains do not constitute the majority of strains in any city, it is customary to start treatment in all patients with a standard regimen. Exceptionally, the patient may give a clear history of exposure to a known case of MDR TB or may come from an epidemic situation where an MDR organism is known to be responsible. In these cases, the patient can be started at once on the best available regimen.

Patients infected with MDR strains may show a delayed clinical response during the first few weeks of therapy. Because the laboratory may take 8 to 10 weeks to provide sensitivity data on the original isolates, it can be difficult to detect this problem early. Newer tests based on firefly luciferase assays may permit detection of drug-resistant tubercle bacilli in as little as 8 hours, but such assays are not yet commercially available.

The cardinal rules for management of proven or suspected MDR TB are (a) never add one drug to a failing regimen (18); (b) refer the patient to the TB section of the local health department before any changes in regimen are tried; and (c) keep the patient in respiratory isolation until he or she is demonstrably cured. Control of MDR infection with chemotherapy is difficult. Treatment may require empiric regimens containing up to six drugs and lasting 18 to 36 months; at times, resectional surgery may be required (see Iseman, 1993, in General References). If a patient has MDR TB complicating HIV infection, the patient usually dies despite taking all available antituberculosis drugs.

Patient's Role in Therapy

In most of the world, TB treatment is initiated and conducted entirely in the ambulatory setting. The patient's role in the successful treatment of TB, daily self-administration of drugs for a period of 6 or 9 months and return for regular follow-up visits, is crucial. Because poor compliance accounts for most therapeutic failures in the treatment of TB, the most important function of monthly visits is the assessment, reinforcement, and documentation of compliance.

The patient should be advised about the communicable nature of TB; this is particularly important until therapy has continued for at least 2 weeks. During those first 2 weeks, patients should avoid intimate contact with others and should cough into tissue, which then should be incinerated or disposed of in closed plastic bags. After 2 weeks, most patients can be considered noncontagious, and activities can be dictated solely by their sense of well-being.

Directly Observed Therapy

Directly observed therapy (DOT) is a response to the present epidemic of uncontrolled drug-resistant TB in some U.S. cities. The preferred DOT regimen is a *four-drug, 6-month regimen.* All drugs are given twice per week, either on Monday and Thursday or on Tuesday and Friday. In general, the doses of drugs are increased over those given daily, but for each drug there is a maximum dose, which is given in Table 34.1. The patient must go to a treatment center and swallow the medication while a nurse is watching. In cities, it may be possible to have nurses take TB therapy into schools, factories, or prisons where large numbers of patients are congregated. Disabled patients can receive supervised therapy in their homes. The regimen is modified as necessary by the results of sensitivity tests on the patient's tubercle bacilli. Patients who do not keep appointments are pursued into their homes by health department personnel and, if necessary, by the police. Some states have laws that permit the incarceration of uncooperative infectious TB patients, and in extreme cases they are applied.

There is no doubt that supervised therapy is effective (15). On the other hand, this approach is an affront to human dignity, and it is not always feasible. Vast numbers of uneducated and even illiterate patients have been treated successfully by traditional methods; most societies simply do not have funds to pay for supervisors; and in rural areas, patients would have to make long journeys to be treated. The problem is that lack of compliance is difficult to predict (see Chapter 4); even such traditional indicators as alcoholism, drug addiction, and psychosis correlate significantly but poorly (19).

PREVENTION OF TUBERCULOSIS

Case Detection among Known Contacts

An integral part of initiation of care in any patient with active TB in the United States is case reporting to the local health authority and investigation of contacts. This entails tuberculin testing of all household and intimate nonhousehold contacts and retesting of nonreactors in 3 months. Reactors are examined by chest radiograph and, if free of active disease, are given chemoprophylaxis with INH (discussed later). With the exception of evaluation of family members, this type of investigation is usually difficult for a physician to carry out alone and should be done by the local city or county health department. Such departments have trained personnel who are available to visit homes and workplaces to detect cases among contacts.

Tuberculin Testing in Prevention

Ideally, the tuberculin skin test status of all people should be determined at some time in their early adult life (see earlier description of technique for skin testing). In almost all school-age children, screening for tuberculin positivity is coordinated with school health programs. In adult populations, a number of factors, such as urban residence, the presence of chronic disease, a history of residence in underdeveloped countries, and health care occupation, increase the importance of periodic tuberculin testing. This is particularly true for people for whom INH would be recommended if the PPD were positive.

Because of the increased risk of contact with unrecognized cases of TB, physicians and hospital personnel who work with populations that have an increased prevalence of TB have an increased chance of acquiring infection. Both for personal protection and because of the risk of transmitting TB to patients, these health care workers should have annual tuberculin testing and should take INH chemoprophylaxis if they convert from negative to positive.

Isoniazid Treatment of Latent Tuberculosis Infection

INH treatment for 6 to 12 months has been shown to prevent 55% to 90% of expected new cases of active TB among groups of people with latent infection who are at increased risk (17). On the basis of accumulated data, recommendations regarding whom to treat for latent TB infection and the duration of treatment have changed somewhat in recent years.

At present, INH prophylaxis (300 mg/day) is recommended for people in the following groups:

- Close contacts of active infectious cases, especially young children and HIV-infected people, regardless of PPD status
- People with recent skin test conversion (not those with booster responses)
- People with positive skin tests and an abnormal chest radiograph suggestive of old TB (i.e., apical scarring, calcified hilar lymph node)
- People with a history of old TB who have never been given antibacterial treatment
- People with positive skin tests who will be given corticosteroid or immunosuppressive therapy, who have silicosis, who have a history of a gastrectomy or jejunoileal bypass, or who have conditions such as Hodgkin's disease or HIV infection that reduce T-cell activity

In the past, patients were not given INH prophylaxis if they were older than a certain age, variously given as 35 to 55 years. The current recommendation is that persons in the groups listed, who have a TB risk that may be 30 times that of a person who is merely PPD positive, should be treated at any age. However, persons who are PPD positive and do not have any of the these risk factors should be left untreated.

Duration of Treatment. Nine months of INH therapy is recommended for patients with HIV infection or other forms of immunosuppression. It is recommended that persons younger than 18 years of age also receive 9 months of therapy. Other infected persons should receive a minimum of 6 continuous months of therapy, and preferably 9 months. For patients at especially high risk of TB whose compliance is questionable, supervised therapy may be indicated. When resources do not permit supervised daily therapy, INH may be given under supervision twice weekly at the dosage of 15 mg/kg (9).

Rifampin Plus Pyrazinamide. A 2-month regimen of RIF plus PZA has recently become popular for treatment of persons who have a positive tuberculin test but have no evidence of active TB. The idea was to give such persons prophylaxis against subsequent clinical TB in less time than the standard regimen of INH for 9 months. Unfortunately, at least 21 cases of serious liver disease with 5 deaths have been seen in such patients (20). The CDC is investigating this situation, and until the findings are reported, the regimen cannot be recommended.

Monitoring of Patients Taking INH. The guidelines recommended by the American Thoracic Society for *monitoring patients taking INH* are the following (17):

- Patients receiving preventive therapy, or responsible adults in households with children on preventive therapy, should be questioned carefully at monthly intervals for symptoms consistent with those of liver damage or other toxic effects (i.e., unexplained anorexia, nausea, or vomiting of more than 3 days' duration, fatigue or weakness of more than 3 days' duration, new and persistent paresthesias of the hands and feet) and for signs consistent with those of liver damage or other toxic effects (i.e., persistent dark urine, icterus, rash, and elevated temperature of more than 3 days' duration without explanation).
- No more than a 1-month supply of INH should be dispensed at any visit. If signs and symptoms of toxicity appear, INH should be stopped immediately and the patient should be re-evaluated. INH preventive therapy should not be prescribed if monthly monitoring cannot be accomplished. The reason for these recommendations is that an analysis of 20 fatal cases of hepatitis caused by prophylactic INH treatment showed that only 1 occurred in a patient seen every month. The great majority of the fatalities occurred in patients who were handed a year's supply of INH and never seen again (10).

Monitoring by routine laboratory tests (e.g., aminotransferases, serum bilirubin, alkaline phosphatase) is not always useful in predicting hepatic disease in INH recipients and therefore is not recommended routinely. However, in evaluating signs and symptoms such tests are mandatory. Preventive therapy should be reinstituted only if biochemical studies are normal and signs and symptoms are absent.

Because it has been recognized that monthly monitoring may fail to detect an occasional patient with severe hepatitis, monthly assessment of aminotransferase levels is recommended for patients who are in the groups at the highest risk for development of INH hepatitis: those older than 35 years of age, daily drinkers, patients concomitantly taking other potentially hepatotoxic drugs, and patients with a history of liver disease. This measurement would detect the transient aminotransferase elevation that occurs in approximately 20% of subjects taking INH; a cutoff level, such as a concentration three or five times normal, is recommended as the criterion for discontinuing INH.

General References*

Iseman MD. Treatment of multidrug-resistant tuberculosis. N Engl J Med 1993;329:784.

Practical approaches to MDR as of 1993.

Small PM, Fujiwara PI. Management of tuberculosis in the United States. N Engl J Med 2001;345:189.

The current state of the art.

Specific References

1. Center for Diseases Control and Prevention. Summary of notifiable diseases, United States, 1999. MMWR Morb Mortal Wkly Rep 2001;48:1.
2. Hopewell PC. Impact of human immune deficiency virus infection on the epidemiology, clinical features, management and control of tuberculosis. Clin Infect Dis 1992;15:540.
3. Daley CL, Small RM, Schechter GF, et al. An outbreak of tuberculosis with accelerated progression among persons infected with human immunodeficiency virus: an analysis using restriction fragment length polymorphisms. N Engl J Med 1992;326:231.
4. Reider HL, Cauther GM, Comstock GW, et al. Epidemiology of tuberculosis in the United States. Epidemiol Rev 1989;11:79.

*Bold print (general references) and bold numerals (specific references) denote published controlled clinical trials, meta-analyses, or consensus-based recommendations.

5. American Thoracic Society and Centers for Disease Control and Prevention. Targeted tuberculin testing and treatment of latent tuberculosis. Am J Respir Crit Care Med 2000;161:S221.
6. Graham NMH, Nelson KE, Solomon L, et al. Prevalence of tuberculin positivity and skin test anergy in HIV-1 seropositive and seronegative intravenous drug users. JAMA 1992;267:369.
7. Thompson NJ, Glassroth JL, Snider DE Jr, et al. The booster phenomenon in serial tuberculin testing. Am Rev Respir Dis 1979;119:587.
8. Centers for Disease Control and Prevention. Prevention and treatment of tuberculosis among patients infected with human immunodeficiency virus: principles of therapy and revised recommendations. MMWR Morb Mortal Wkly Rep 1998;47:(RR 20).
9. Small PM, Fujiwara PI. Management of tuberculosis in the United States. N Engl J Med 2001;345:189.
10. Moulding TS, Redeker AG, Kanel GC. Twenty isoniazid associated deaths in one state. Am Rev Respir Dis 1989;140:700.
11. Driver CR, Munsiff SS, Kundamel N, et al. Relapse in persons treated for drug susceptible tuberculosis in a population with high coinfection with human immunodeficiency virus in New York City. Clin Infect Dis 2001;33:1762.
12. Road I, Hacham R, Leeds N, et al. Use of adjunctive treatment with interferon gamma in an immunocompromised patient who had refractory multidrug resistant tuberculosis of the brain. Clin Infect Dis 1996;22:572.
13. Friedan TR, Sherman LF, Maw KL, et al. A multi-institutional outbreak of highly drug resistant tuberculosis. JAMA 1996;286:1229.
14. Alwood K, Keruly J, Moore-Rice K, et al. Effectiveness of supervised intermittent therapy for tuberculosis in HIV infected patients. AIDS 1994;8:1103.
15. Chaulk CP, Moore-Rice K, Rizzo R, et al. Eleven years of community-based directly observed therapy for tuberculosis. JAMA 1995;274:945.
16. Mehta JB, Shantavearape H, Byrd RP, et al. Utility of rifampin blood levels in the treatment and follow up of active pulmonary tuberculosis in patients who were slow to respond to routine directly observed therapy. Chest 2001;120:1520.
17. American Thoracic Society. Control of tuberculosis in the United States. Am Rev Respir Dis 1992;146:1623.
18. Centers for Disease Control and Prevention. National action plan to combat multidrug resistant tuberculosis. MMWR Morb Mortal Wkly Rep 1992;41:56.
19. Sumartojo E. When tuberculosis treatment fails: a social behavioral account of patient adherence. Am Rev Respir Dis 1993;147:1311.
20. Center for Disease Control and Prevention. Fatal and severe liver injuries associated with rifampin and pyrazinamide for latent tuberculous infection: revisions in American Thoracic Society and CDC recommendations. JAMA 2001;286:1445.

CHAPTER 35

Acute Gastroenteritis and Associated Conditions

RICHARD G. BENNETT, MD

Acute symptoms of gastroenteritis may follow the ingestion of a wide variety of infectious and chemical agents. Ingestion may occur because of direct person to person contact or, more commonly, via contaminated food or water. Although viral enteropathogens may spread by air transmission (1), these other routes are probably more common. With several important exceptions, the acute illnesses caused by these agents are characterized by diarrhea, with or without other gastrointestinal symptoms (nausea, vomiting, abdominal pain) or systemic symptoms and signs (anorexia, fever, malaise, orthostatic hypotension, rash, neurologic deficits).

Diarrhea is defined as an increase in the number or volume of bowel movements, which are usually fluid (see Chapter 45). The diarrhea of gastroenteritis usually begins abruptly, sometimes preceded by systemic symptoms, and the hour of onset can typically be documented by the patient. With few exceptions, the illness is self-limited and terminates within 1 to 5 days.

Tables 35.1 (infectious agents) and 35.2 (chemical agents) summarize the etiologic agents, pathophysiology, clinical and epidemiologic features, and principles of diagnosis and treatment for conditions that may occur in the United States.

Table 35.1. Characteristics of Acute Illness Caused by Ingestion of Infectious Agents

Agent	Pathogenesis	Usual Clinical Features	Frequency in USA	Usual Pattern
Bacteria				
Bacillus cereus (2)	Enterotoxin produced in food or in intestine	Vomiting if preformed toxin in food; diarrhea; rhabdomyolysis and liver failure reported	Increasing	CSO
Campylobacter jejuni (3,4)	Invasion of large and small intestine	Fever, abdominal pain, diarrhea	Common	S, CSO
Clostridium botulinum	Neurotoxin produced in food	Vomiting, diarrhea, symmetric motor paralysis, cranial nerve and respiratory paralysis, death	Uncommon	CSO
Clostridium difficile (5)	Cytotoxin and enterotoxin produced in large intestine secondary to overgrowth	Fever, abdominal pain, diarrhea (rarely bloody) in a patient currently or recently on antibiotics; relapse of up to 20%	Common in hospitalized or recently hospitalized patients	S
Clostridium perfringens	Enterotoxin released during sporulation in large intestine	Diarrhea, occasionally vomiting	Common	CSO
Escherichia coli (6)				
Enterotoxigenic	Enterotoxin produced in small intestine	Voluminous watery diarrhea without fever (traveler's diarrhea)	Common (travelers)	CSO, S
Invasive	Invasion of large intestinal mucosa	Fever, diarrhea (often bloody)	Rare	CSO, S
Adherent (7,8)	Adheres tightly to small bowel mucosa	Acute diarrhea, which may be prolonged	Unknown, probably uncommon	S
Hemorrhagic (9) (e.g., *E. coli* O157:H7)	Verotoxin or Shiga toxin produced in large bowel	Hemorrhagic colitis, may be followed by hemolytic uremic syndrome or thrombotic thrombocytopenic purpura	Common	CSO
Listeria monocytogenes (10)	Colonization	Fever, vomiting, abdominal pain, sepsis	Uncommon	CSO
Salmonella (many species)	Invasion of small and large intestine	Fever and diarrhea	Common	CSO
Salmonella typhi	Invasion of small intestine mucosa, systemic dissemination	Protracted illness: fever, malaise, headache, constipation more often than diarrhea, splenomegaly, occasionally intestinal perforation	Uncommon	S
Shigella sp.	Invasion of large intestine	Fever, diarrhea (often bloody)	Common	S
Staphylococcus aureus (11)	Enterotoxin produced in food	Vomiting dominates, diarrhea	Very common	CSO
Streptococcus group A	Invasion of upper respiratory tract	Streptococcal pharyngitis syndrome (see Chapter 33)	Uncommon (by this mode of transmission)	CSO
Vibrio cholerae (12)	Enterotoxin produced in small intestine	Voluminous watery diarrhea without fever	Rare	CSO, S
Vibrio parahaemolyticus	Probably both invasion and enterotoxin production; exact mechanism unknown	Diarrhea, abdominal cramps	Uncommon	CSO, S
Vibrio vulnificus (13)	Mechanism unknown	Fever, abdominal pain, diarrhea; septicemia, "metastatic" cutaneous lesions	Uncommon	S
Yersinia enterocolitica (14)	Invasion of small and large intestine	Fever, abdominal pain, may suggest appendicitis, diarrhea	Uncommon	CSO, S
Viruses				
Norwalk (15)	Invasion of small intestine	Vomiting and diarrhea	Common	CSO
Rotavirus (15,16)	Invasion of small intestine	Severe gastroenteritis in young children, mild in adults	Common	S
Protozoa and helminths				
Entamoeba histolytica (17)	Invasion of large intestine	Diarrhea, often chronic and bloody	Uncommon (travelers)	CSO, S
Giardia lamblia (18)	Colonization and occasional invasion of small intestine	Diarrhea, flatulence with foul-smelling stools	Uncommon (travelers)	CSO, S
Trichinella spiralis	(a) Encysted trichinae mature, mate, reproduce in small intestine; (b) larvae penetrate intestine, migrate to muscles where they cause inflammation and become encysted	Diarrhea, puffy eyes, muscle aching, fever, occasionally severe heart failure; eosinophilia typical	Uncommon	CSO, S
Cryptosporidium (19)	Colonization	Diarrhea, acute in children and healthy adults; chronic in HIV-infected patients	Common in patients with AIDS	S
Cyclospora (20)	Colonization	Diarrhea, cramping, heartburn, low-grade fever	Uncommon; more common in patients with AIDS	CSO, S

CSO, common source outbreak; S, sporadic; HIV, human immunodeficiency virus; AIDS, acquired immunodeficiency syndrome.

[a]Anal–oral transmission may occur in homosexual men.

Epidemiologic Features				
Source (Reservoir)	Transmission to Humans	Incubation Period	Diagnosis	Specific Therapy
Soil	Foodborne	2–16 h	Culture suspected food	None
Animal feces	Foodborne or waterborne[a]	24–48 h	Culture stool, blood	Erythromycin (see text)
Animal feces, soil	Foodborne (canned, low pH, anaerobic)	12–36 h	Culture food, identify toxin in food, blood, stool	Polyvalent antitoxin
Ubiquitous, especially in health care environments (spores)	Probably not necessary but may occur in hospitals[a]	2–10 days after beginning antibiotics (rarely up to 6 wk after antibiotics stopped)	Identify toxin in stool	Metronidazole or vancomycin (see text)
Human feces, animal feces, soil	Foodborne (meats)	12–24 h	Culture suspected food	None
Human feces	Foodborne	24–48 h	Culture stool, identify enterotoxin production by bacteria	None
Human feces	Foodborne (cheeses)	24–48 h	Culture stool	Same as *Shigella* (see text)
Human feces	Probably foodborne	24–48 h	Culture stool, small bowel	Antibiotics to which organism is sensitive
Animal feces	Foodborne	24–48 h	Culture stool (see text)	None
Dairy cattle	Foodborne	18 h–21 days	Stool culture; serum antilisterolysin O	Ampicillin or trimethoprim-sulfamethoxazole
Animal feces; eggs	Foodborne (many foods, see text), person-to-person[a]	12–48 h	Culture stool	Ampicillin or chloramphenicol, in selected cases only (see text)
Human feces	Person-to-person, foodborne[a]	4 days–3 wk	Culture blood, stool, antibacterial antibodies	Chloramphenicol
Human feces	Person-to-person[a]	12–48 h	Culture stool	Fluoroquinolone (see text)
Human skin, nares, mouth	Foodborne (many foods, see text)	2–8 h	Culture food, and food handlers	None
Human pharynx, skin lesions	Foodborne	1–3 days	Culture throat, food, skin lesions of food handlers	Penicillin (see Chapter 28)
Human feces	Waterborne and foodborne	12 h–5 days	Culture stools, antibacterial and antitoxin antibody	Tetracycline
Seawater	Foodborne (various types of seafood from estuary and seawater)	15–24 h	Culture stool	None
Seawater	Foodborne (various types of seafood from estuary and seawater)	24 h–2 days	Culture stool	Antibiotics for gram-negative sepsis; tetracycline
Animal feces	Foodborne, person-to-person	Probably 3–7 days	Culture stool	Doxycycline or trimethoprim-sulfamethoxazole
Human feces	Foodborne and waterborne, person-to-person (secondary cases)	1–3 days	Rise in antiviral antibody	None
Human feces	Person-to-person (secondary cases)	1–3 days	Virus antigen in stool Rise in antiviral antibody	None
Human feces	Foodborne and waterborne, person-to-person[a]	Few days to months	Examine stool for trophozoites	Metronidazole (see text)
Human feces	Waterborne, person-to-person	1–4 wk	Examine stool for trophozoites	Metronidazole (see text)
Animal muscle (swine, many wild animals)	Foodborne	2–28 days	Skin tests, antibody, muscle biopsy	Mebendazole and steroids (see text)
Fresh water; human and animal feces	Waterborne; person-to-person	?2–7 days	Examine stool for trophozoites	Evolving
Fresh water (resistant to chlorination)	Waterborne; person-to-person?; animal-to-person?	12 h–11 days	Examine stool for oocysts	Trimethoprim-sulfamethoxazole

Table 35.2. Characteristics of Acute Illness Caused by Ingestion of Chemical Agents

Agent	Pathogenesis	Clinical Features	Frequency in USA	Pattern
Seafood				
Ciguatera fish poisoning	Toxins from algae concentrated in fish, particularly predatory fish; toxins affect human cell sodium channels	Vomiting, diarrhea, paresthesias (warmth, extremities), metallic taste, blurred vision, sharp pains in extremities, respiratory paralysis	Uncommon (Florida)	CSO, S
Domoic acid (21) (amnesic shellfish poisoning)	Neuroexcitatory amino acid produced by phytoplankton and concentrated by mussels	Vomiting, cramps, headache, neurologic symptoms, anterograde amnesia, seizures, coma, death	Rare (surveillance for domoic acid in Canada)	CSO, S
Scrombroid fish poisoning	Histamine intoxication	Histamine reaction (flushing, headache, dizziness, burning of mouth and throat; urticaria, pruritus, and bronchospasm)	Uncommon (frozen and fresh fish can be affected)	CSO, S
Paralytic shellfish poisoning	Multiple neurotoxins (saxitoxins) causing motor paralysis	Paresthesias (warmth, extremities), floating sensation, dysphonia, dysphagia, weakness, and respiratory paralysis	Uncommon (surveillance for toxins in shellfish in United States)	CSO, S
Mushrooms				
Muscarine	Muscarinic cholinergic response	Colicky abdominal pain, nausea, vomiting, diarrhea, salivation, miosis, blurred vision, bradycardia, hypotension	Uncommon	CSO, S
Phalloidin (and other toxins)	Diverse cytotoxin effects, multisystemic	*Stage 1:* Nausea, abdominal pain, vomiting, bloody diarrhea, marked weakness, hypotension (shock) *Stage 2:* Clinical improvement (day 2 or 3) *Stage 3:* Severe hepatic failure, delirium, frequent fatal outcome	Uncommon	CSO, S
Miscellaneous				
Heavy metals (antimony, cadmium, copper, iron, tin, zinc)	Upper gastrointestinal irritation	Metallic taste to food, nausea, vomiting, or diarrhea	Uncommon	CSO, S
Monosodium glutamate (MSG)	Idiopathic reaction	Burning sensation in chest, neck, abdomen, extremities	Common	S

CSO, common source outbreak; S, sporadic; MSG, monosodium glutamate.

Data from Gossalin RE, Hodge HC, Smith RP, et al. Clinical toxicology of commercial products. 5th ed. Baltimore: Williams & Wilkins, 1984; and Morris JG. Natural toxins associated with fish and shellfish. In: Blaser MJ, Smith PD, Randin JI, et al. eds. Infections of the gastrointestinal tract. New York: Raven, 1995, with permission.

EPIDEMIOLOGY

Incidence and Distribution

The incidence of the conditions listed in Tables 35.1 and 35.2 varies from year to year, and the true incidence is never known because a large proportion of cases are not reported to physicians or health authorities. New national surveillance systems to establish more precise incidence rates include the Centers for Disease Control and Prevention (CDC) Emerging Infections Program Foodborne Diseases Active Surveillance Network (FoodNet, www.cdc.gov/foodnet) and the National Molecular Subtyping Network for Food-borne Disease Surveillance (PulseNet, www.cdc.gov/ncidod/dbmd/pulsenet/pulsenet.htm). Current estimates are that 76 million persons become ill, 325,000 are hospitalized, and 5,000 die each year in the United States related to eating contaminated food (22). Of 2,751 reported outbreaks investigated by the CDC between 1993 and 1997, the *cause* was established for only 878 (32%) (CDC Surveillance 3/17/00). This reflects the current limitations in diagnostic capabilities, particularly for identifying the viral pathogens thought likely to cause many outbreaks. Based on these CDC surveillance data, it is known that the greatest number of reported food-borne outbreaks are caused by *Salmonella* (357 outbreaks), followed by *Escherichia coli* (84 outbreaks), *Clostridium perfringens* (57 outbreaks), and *Shigella* (43 outbreaks). The relative numbers of outbreaks do not necessarily correlate with the number of people affected by a specific enteropathogen.

Table 35.3 summarizes for the period 1993 through 1997 the number of outbreaks, cases, and deaths resulting from the eight most commonly identified bacteria in investigations of food-borne outbreaks and the average number of cases per outbreak and overall case-fatality rates. The magnitude of disease related to enterohemorrhagic *E. coli* (i.e., strains such as *E. coli* O157:H7, which produce a potent cytotoxin known as

Epidemiologic Features				
Source	Transmission to Humans	Incubation Period	Diagnosis	Specific Therapy
Food chain of bottom-dwelling and predatory fish caught in Florida, Hawaii (red snapper, barracuda)	Foodborne	1–6 h	Clinical and epidemiologic features	Mannitol infusion, atropine for bradycardia, hypotension; symptoms may last days to months
Mussels and clams contaminated with domoic acid	Foodborne	Minutes to 48 h	Clinical and epidemiologic features	Supportive care
Bacteria acting on fish flesh (tuna, mackerel, bonito, skipjack, mahi mahi)	Foodborne ("peppery" taste of affected fish reported)	Minutes to 1 h	Clinical and epidemiologic features; elevated urine histamine level	None or antihistamines in severe cases
Toxic dinoflagellates concentrated in filter-feeding bivalves (mussels, clams, oysters, scallops)	Foodborne	<30 min	Clinical and epidemiologic features	None (lasts few hours to few days)
Amanita muscaria	Foodborne	Few minutes–few hours	Clinical and epidemiologic features	Atropine 0.1–0.5 mg s.c. or i.v.
Amanita phalloides and other *Amanita* species	Foodborne	6–15 h	Clinical and epidemiologic features	None
Containers made of alloy that includes a heavy metal	Foodborne (food prepared in, stored in, or eaten from a container from which heavy metal leached)	5 min–8 h	Clinical and epidemiologic features	None
Foods prepared with large amounts of MSG	Foodborne (Chinese restaurant foods)	3 min–2 h	Clinical and epidemiologic features	None

Table 35.3. Selected Bacterial Foodborne Outbreaks, Cases, Average Number of Cases per Outbreak, Deaths, and Case-Fatality Rate, 1993–1997

Bacteria	Outbreaks	Cases	Cases/Outbreak	Deaths	Case-Fatality Rates (per 1,000)
Bacillus cereus	14	691	49	0	0.0
Campylobacter	25	539	22	1	1.9
C. bolutlinum	13	56	4	1	18.0
C. perfringens	57	2,772	49	0	0.0
E. coli	84	3,260	39	8	2.4
Salmonella	357	32,610	91	13	0.4
Shigella	43	1,555	36	0	0.0
S. aureus	42	1,413	34	1	0.7

Data adapted from CDC Surveillance Summaries. MMWR Morb Mortal Wkly Rep 2000;SS-1:49, with permission.

verotoxin or Shiga-like toxin) has increased since the last CDC 5-year report (inclusive years 1988 through 1992), and *E. coli* went from the eighth most commonly identified cause of food-borne outbreaks to the second. Fortunately, no large outbreaks of *E. coli* have occurred in the United States since 1993 when 500 cases were reported from the western United States resulting from eating contaminated hamburger meat at fast-food restaurants (23). This improvement no doubt relates to the practice of fast-food restaurants, which now always cook hamburgers until well done. There is growing recognition that among sporadic cases of diarrhea, *E. coli* O157:H7 is the most frequently isolated bacteria from visibly bloody stool specimens (24), and many (but not all) hospital laboratories now screen such specimens for this enteropathogen (25). Although

Table 35.4. Comparison of Symptoms of Viral Versus Bacterial Gastroenteritis in Adults

	Percentage with Symptom				
	Viral Gastroenteritis		Bacterial Gastroenteritis		
Symptom	Rotavirus[a]	Norwalk Agent[b]	*Salmonella*[b]	*Shigella*[b]	*Staphylococcus aureus*
Nausea	2	85	50	45	62
Vomiting	9	84	23	39	86
Abdominal cramps	26	62	78	60	86
Diarrhea	33	44	73	100	67
Fever	5	32	49	72	10
Headache	NR	37	33	6	8

[a]From Wenman WM, Hinde D, Felthman S, et al. Rotavirus infection in adults. Results of a prospective family study. N Engl J Med 1979;301:303, with permission.
[b]From Adler JL, Zicki R. Winter vomiting disease. J Infect Dis 1969;19:668, with permission.
NR, not reported.

the most common pathogen isolated in waterborne outbreaks is *Giardia,* a large outbreak related to *Cryptosporidium* resulted in 1993 from contamination of the public water supply in Milwaukee, Wisconsin.

Outbreaks unrelated to contaminated food or water and resulting from viral enteropathogens occur most often within institutional settings (e.g., day-care centers, nursing homes, and assisted living facilities) and during the winter.

Studies of outbreaks of *viral gastroenteritis* in adults have shown that the symptoms it produces overlap with the symptoms produced by several common bacterial pathogens (Table 35.4). A viral cause is more likely when secondary cases develop in a household or institution, a pattern that suggests person to person spread rather than one-time exposure to a common food.

Sources and Modes of Transmission

The *sources and modes of transmission* of the etiologic agents causing food-borne illness are summarized in Tables 35.1 and 35.2. The features of four of the most well-recognized etiologic agents illustrate the diverse ways that food-borne disease is acquired:

1. Humans whose skin or nasal mucosa is colonized are almost always the source of *Staphylococcus aureus.* Contamination of food with small numbers of staphylococci is undoubtedly very common. Staphylococcal food poisoning occurs when contaminated foods are allowed to stand long enough for organisms to multiply and produce enterotoxin. The principal foods in which this occurs are those high in protein (ham, pork, beef, poultry, either cooked or in salads, and cream-filled cakes and pastries) and those with a high salt or sugar content (ham, salads, and custards) (11).
2. Animals are the source of the *Salmonella* serotypes that cause most human disease; only *Salmonella typhi* and *Salmonella paratyphi* are carried by humans. Transmission from animal to humans occurs chiefly by fecal contamination of equipment and personnel involved in the packaging and preparing of food, most commonly poultry and meats. Food-borne outbreaks of salmonellosis have also been recognized, particularly related to use of undercooked eggs (26). Although eggs with visible shell cracks should always be considered suspect, those with intact shells can also be infected (e.g., from a salmonella abscess in the ovary of a hen). Only hard-cooked eggs and pasteurized eggs are absolutely safe; raw egg dishes (e.g., homemade salad dressings, eggnog, ice cream) and undercooked eggs (e.g., scrambled and soft-cooked eggs) should be avoided, particularly by immunocompromised and elderly people (27).
3. *Clostridium perfringens* is a ubiquitous organism found in human and animal feces and in soil. Meats are the most frequently contaminated foods; transmission of enough organisms to produce illness occurs typically with inadequately heated or reheated meats (spores may survive at normal cooking temperatures and then germinate and multiply while foods are being held at warm temperatures or being rewarmed at temperatures that do not inhibit bacterial growth).
4. *Enterohemorrhagic E. coli* are found in the intestines of healthy livestock and can contaminate the surface of whole meat products during slaughter and processing. Most reported outbreaks have been related to *E. coli* O157:H7. Ground meats pose the highest risk because surface contamination is distributed throughout the product. The risk of illness is minimized by cooking ground red meat until it is no longer pink or until juices run clear (internal temperature 155°F). Ingestion of raw or undercooked contaminated ground meat can lead to infection that can result in bloody diarrhea and hemolytic uremic syndrome. The mortality among patients with the latter syndrome can be high. Recently, natural environmental contamination of nonmeat products (e.g., produce and apple juice) have resulted in outbreaks (28,29).

Most episodes of food-borne illness follow the *ingestion of normally safe foods that have been rendered unsafe by one or more of the following factors:* failure to refrigerate foods properly or to heat foods thoroughly, preparing foods a day or more before they are served, allowing foods to remain at warm temperatures, failure to reheat or cook foods at temperatures that kill vegetative bacteria, incorporating raw (contaminated) ingredients into foods that receive no further cooking, failure to clean and disinfect kitchen or processing plant equipment, and contamination by infected food handlers who practice poor personal hygiene. The complexity of the world's food distribution system and the difficulty in controlling food safety even at a national level are exemplified by an outbreak of salmonellosis in Finland and the United States resulting from contaminated alfalfa sprouts grown from seeds supplied by a Dutch shipper (30) and an outbreak of cyclosporiasis in North America related to raspberries from Guatemala (31).

Some food-borne illnesses are caused by the ingestion of *foods that are always unsafe* because of the presence of toxins that cannot be rendered innocuous by cooking or other means (e.g., histamine or scrombotoxin, ciguatoxin, *Amanita* toxins, paralytic shellfish toxin, mushroom toxin, and heavy metals) (32,33). A recent report of histamine poisoning associated with eating tuna burgers highlights the increasing recognition of scromboid poisoning (named for the type of fish most often associated with this illness), which is characterized by flushing, vomiting, and profuse watery diarrhea (34).

The *place* of ingestion of the etiologic agent is usually the patient's home or a restaurant and, less commonly, a social gathering or an institutional eating place.

Populations at Risk

For many of the conditions listed in Tables 35.1 and 35.2, *people are at risk at all ages,* and a single episode may not confer protective immunity against a later episode. Although most cases of acute diarrheal episodes occur in children, older adults are at increased risk from dying from gastrointestinal illnesses. Of 28,538 diarrhea-related deaths in the United States between 1979 and 1987, 78% occurred in adults 55 or more years old versus 11% in children less than 5 years old (35). A particularly high rate of diarrheal illness also occurs in people of all ages who travel to developing countries. For older adults who are commonly prescribed cardiovascular medications that can block normal physiologic responses to volume depletion, special counseling is advisable (see Chapter 41).

In the early 1980s, a wide spectrum of intestinal infections was recognized in homosexual and bisexual men and labeled the *gay bowel syndrome* (see also Chapter 98). At the time, these cases were ascribed to a combination of asymptomatic carriage of one or more enteric pathogens and unsafe sexual practices (e.g., oral–genital and genital–anal contact between subjects, exposure to multiple sexual partners). However, many of these reported cases were no doubt related to unrecognized human immunodeficiency virus (HIV) infection because this viral pathogen had not been identified at the time the term gay bowel syndrome was coined. Now, the diagnosis of HIV infection must be considered in patients with unusual diarrheal syndromes because HIV-infected patients are at increased risk for bacterial infections of the gastrointestinal tract (e.g., salmonellosis, shigellosis) and bacterial infections in general. Protracted diarrhea can herald the progression of HIV infection, and a number of enteropathogens can cause not only acute illness but also prolonged symptoms of diarrhea in patients with advanced HIV disease. *Cryptosporidium* infection, usually a benign self-limited diarrheal illness in children and healthy adults, may cause a prolonged and life-threatening illness (19). *Isospora belli,* usually not thought of as a diarrheal pathogen, may also cause diarrheal illness in these patients. Diarrheal illnesses caused by *Campylobacter jejuni,* which are usually short illnesses in normal hosts, may be prolonged in HIV-infected patients. (See Chapter 39 for additional discussion of infection in HIV-infected patients.)

PATHOGENESIS

As indicated in Tables 35.1 and 35.2, most of the etiologic agents produce symptoms caused by either inflammation of the gastrointestinal tract or physiologic events related to one or more toxins.

The common bacterial diarrheal syndromes can be separated into invasive and enterotoxigenic syndromes (Table 35.5) (8,18), and this becomes important when antibiotic treatment is considered. In *invasive disease,* the etiologic agent is found in the intestinal mucosa, and the diarrhea results from destruction of the cells of the mucosa that is often caused by the inflammation. This usually occurs in the large bowel and produces systemic symptoms (particularly fever), local symptoms (tenesmus, abdominal discomfort), and frequent small amounts of stool that contain pus cells and often blood. Shigellosis is the prototype of this syndrome. In *enterotoxigenic diarrhea,* the organisms do not invade tissue but colonize and multiply on the small bowel mucosal surface; during this process they produce enterotoxins, which act as chemical mediators and cause net secretion of fluid and electrolytes by the small bowel. Little tissue damage is produced, and inflammation of the mucosa is minimal. Symptoms consist of watery diarrhea (which may be voluminous), accompanied by minimal systemic signs, unless dehydration becomes significant. The prototypes of this syndrome are diarrheas caused by *Vibrio cholerae* and by enterotoxigenic *E. coli* (6,12).

Unfortunately, not all enteric diseases caused by bacteria fit into this simple dichotomy. Enteroadherent strains of *E. coli* have been characterized that neither invade mucosal cells nor produce enterotoxins, but they tightly adhere to the mucosal surface and produce diarrhea, presumably by interfering with normal absorptive processes. These strains produce diarrhea primarily in small children and many belong to the classic enteropathogenic serotypes (7,8). In addition, *Clostridium difficile,* a cause of antibiotic-associated

Table 35.5. Characteristics Distinguishing Invasive and Enterotoxigenic Diarrhea

Feature	Invasive Diarrhea	Enterotoxigenic Diarrhea
History	Fever, abdominal pain, tenesmus, may have blood in stool	Watery diarrhea with little or no fever or other systemic symptoms
Physical examination	Fever, abdominal tenderness; proctoscopy may be indicated	May be signs of salt and water depletion
Laboratory studies	Stool culture (may be diagnostic) Fecal leukocytes in large numbers[a] White blood cell count may be elevated	Stool culture usually negative unless special culture techniques available No or few fecal leukocytes White count usually normal, but may be elevated
Therapy	Oral fluids and electrolytes (usually only small quantities needed) Antimicrobials often indicated[b]	Oral fluids and electrolytes Bismuth subsalicylate, other symptomatic medications as needed[c] Antimicrobials not indicated
Course	Improvements in 1–2 days, particularly if appropriate antimicrobials used	Duration of 1–2 days usually; may last up to 5 days

[a]Use a drop of methylene blue stain with liquid stool
[b]See text for recommendations for specific bacterial pathogens.
[c]See text for details.

diarrhea and pseudomembranous colitis, produces two toxins: an enterotoxin (toxin A), which causes secretion of fluid into the gut lumen, and a potent cytotoxin (toxin B), which damages the gut epithelium and leads to inflammation.

PATIENT EVALUATION

Historical Information

In addition to a history of the specific symptoms, the most useful information is as follows:

- A history of *food eaten* within the past 48 hours, particularly noting any deviation from the patient's usual pattern, such as eating an unusual food (e.g., a special fish), eating at a restaurant, or attending a picnic or potluck dinner.
- A history of a *similar illness in others* (family members or members of a group who ate with the patient). This is helpful in suggesting a common source outbreak.
- The probable *incubation period.* This may be helpful in suggesting the most likely cause of a patient's illness (Tables 35.1 and 35.2). For example, the onset of symptoms immediately after ingestion always indicates chemical food poisoning, onset of symptoms within a few hours of eating strongly suggests staphylococcal food poisoning, onset within 24 to 48 hours suggests *Salmonella* infection, and onset of symptoms 1 week or more after exposure suggests a less common problem, such as *giardiasis.*
- A *history of taking antimicrobials.* Overall, no etiologic agent can be identified in approximately 80% of these patients. A history of taking clindamycin, ampicillin, or a cephalosporin currently or within the last 2 weeks, usually during hospitalization, supports the diagnosis of antibiotic-associated diarrhea caused by *C. difficile.* This agent causes syndromes that range from enterotoxigenic diarrhea to an invasive disease (see above), and rarely (0.5% of cases) it causes the syndrome of pseudomembranous colitis (36).
- A history of *neurologic symptoms* after ingestion of canned foods should always suggest botulism or one of the other sources of neurotoxins (all rare) listed in Table 35.2.
- A history revealing *risk factors for HIV infection* (see Chapter 39) and chronic diarrhea should suggest the possibility of *Cryptosporidium* (19,37), *Isospora,* or *Salmonella* infection.

Physical Examination

The physical examination is usually of minimal help in establishing a cause. Fever or significant abdominal tenderness in association with diarrhea suggests an invasive organism as the etiologic agent. Poor skin turgor and postural hypotension suggest significant salt and water deficits (uncommon in adults with diarrhea in the United States). Rare conditions in which the physical findings may be helpful are *botulism* and other neurotoxic forms of food poisoning and *trichinosis* (Tables 35.1 and 35.2).

Laboratory Studies

In most outpatients with acute gastrointestinal illness, no laboratory studies are indicated (38) unless a common source outbreak is suspected. In such cases, special cultures and tests for toxins in stools and in food, primarily for epidemiologic purposes, should be obtained.

In patients evaluated in the emergency room or in patients with a combination of diarrhea for more than 24 hours, fever, and blood in the stool or significant volume depletion, the following laboratory studies are indicated (38,39):

- *Stool culture for enterotoxigenic E. coli, Salmonella, Shigella, Campylobacter, and Yersinia.* Specifically, question whether enterotoxigenic *E. coli* is cultured routinely because not all clinical laboratories are able to identify the organism. Unfortunately, other bacteria (e.g., invasive *E. coli, Vibrio* spp.) and most viral agents cannot be identified in routine laboratory workups because of the special techniques required.

- *C. difficile tests.* Obtain either a stool cytotoxin assay (detects small amount of cytotoxin A with a sensitivity approaching 100% but takes 2 to 3 days) or stool enzyme immunoassay (sensitivity for cytotoxin A and/or B is 70% to 90%, same day) to identify enterotoxins for individuals recently hospitalized, those who are currently being treated with or have recently discontinued antibiotics, and for older residents of chronic care facilities (40).
- *Stool examination for fecal leukocytes.* The test is done by mixing a small bit of stool with methylene blue stain on a microscope slide and placing a coverslip over the mixture. After 2 or 3 minutes, the preparation is examined under the *high dry objective* for the presence of leukocytes. More than 10 leukocytes per high-powered field is indicative of an invasive pathogen.
- *A white blood cell count.* An elevated count or number of immature polymorphonuclear leukocytes supports the diagnosis of invasive diarrheal disease.

In suspected cases, the laboratory should be asked to examine the stool microscopically for *Giardia lamblia, Entamoeba histolytica,* or *Cryptosporidium* (Table 35.1). For optimal identification of trophozoites of the latter organisms, fresh stools should be examined immediately by an experienced observer. For the diagnosis of giardiasis, stools may need to be examined repeatedly. *E. histolytica* trophozoites are best identified from the mucus taken from the base of ulcerations seen at proctoscopy.

When needed to make clinical decisions, additional laboratory tests can be ordered for some conditions (Tables 35.1 and 35.2). Particularly for hospitalized patients with diarrhea and those with postantibiotic diarrhea, tests for *C. difficile* toxins must be specifically ordered because clinical laboratories typically do not culture stool for *C. difficile.* Until recently, the toxins produced by the bacterium were detected in stool specimens with tissue culture assays (requires 48 to 72 hours); enzyme immunoassays now make possible same-day results. For hospitalized patients with new diarrhea, ordering a *C. difficile* test alone is the most cost-effective approach, and stool cultures and ova and parasite examinations are usually unrevealing (41). Chapter 45 provides information about the laboratory evaluation of patients with chronic diarrhea.

MANAGEMENT

In all patients with acute diarrhea, symptomatic treatment is of primary importance. In addition, some patients may require specific therapy (i.e., antibiotics), usually indicated on the basis of the history and physical examination. Most episodes of acute diarrhea are self-limited, lasting 1 to 2 days, but occasionally symptoms last 5 to 10 days. Resolution of illness is thought to be caused by the local secretory immune response of the gastrointestinal tract.

Symptomatic Treatment

Fluid Therapy

With the exception of giardiasis, amebiasis, *C. difficile* colitis, and the more severe cases of shigellosis and salmonellosis, practically all acute diarrheal disease seen commonly in the United States can be treated with only symptomatic therapy, the mainstay of which is the replacement of fluids and electrolytes lost in the stool. Because in most patients the disease is mild and the amount of stool is small, replacement is simple. Young healthy patients should be encouraged to drink a lot of fluids, to avoid spicy foods, and otherwise to eat what they like. Foods with complex carbohydrates (e.g., cereals, rice, toast), but not foods with concentrated simple sugars (most sweet foods), may facilitate fluid reabsorption at the brush border of the intestinal mucosa and help to limit duration of diarrhea (42).

In patients who have a *very large loss of stool,* those who experience weakness and a feeling of being washed out (with or without signs of volume depletion), and older adults (who are at increased risk for hypoperfusion of vital organs with even moderate dehydration because of silent atherosclerosis), replacement should consist of fluids containing electrolytes and glucose. Oral glucose–electrolyte or carbohydrate–electrolyte replacement solutions (e.g., Pedialyte, Ceralyte) and packets containing premeasured salts and sugars that must be dissolved in water (e.g., Orlyte and Oral Rehydration Salts) are available commercially (42,43). These products have been developed primarily for treating children but are adequate for adults. Most have sodium concentrations of 50 to 75 mEq/L and substitute citrate for bicarbonate. A less complete replacement fluid can be made using constituents available at home: one pint (500 mL) water, 1/2 teaspoon table salt (NaCl), and four rounded teaspoons of table sugar (sucrose).

Because of their sugar and salt contents, *none of the following beverages is satisfactory for fluid replacement* in patients whose diarrhea is causing moderate to severe fluid loss: nondietetic soft drinks (hyperosmolar sugar solution), dietetic soft drinks (inadequate amount of simple sugars needed to facilitate intestinal fluid reabsorption), and sports drinks such as Gatorade that are designed to replace the hypotonic fluids lost with perspiration (inadequate amount of salts for replacement of intestinal fluid losses).

Patients should be instructed to replace estimated diarrheal fluid losses roughly on a 1:1 basis. Typically, 1 to 2 L should be drunk in the first 1 to 2 hours after diarrhea commences and an additional 1 to 2 L a day until symptoms resolve. Hydration is judged adequate if dilute urine is passed every 3 to 4 hours.

Patients experiencing *severe diarrhea or vomiting* that precludes easy replacement with oral replacement fluids and those who have evidence of moderate to severe salt and water depletion should receive initial intravenous fluid replacement with Ringer lactate or its equivalent. This can be accomplished in ambulatory settings, in the patient's home (see Chapter 9), or in the hospital depending on the availability of resources and the severity and duration of the patient's illness.

Other Symptomatic Measures

Several types of medications are commonly used to treat diarrhea symptomatically. *Diphenoxylate with atropine* (Lomotil) and *loperamide* (Imodium or generic, nonprescription) are agents that cause a decrease in intestinal motility and stool frequency; they may be useful to the patient at times when frequent defecation would be embarrassing. These drugs do not alter the natural course of the disease and are potentially harmful if invasive pathogens such as *Shigella* are causing the diarrhea. These medications should be avoided in frail elderly patients (particularly those recently discharged from the hospital) and those in nursing homes (in whom *C. difficile* infections are common) because toxic megacolon can be precipitated by the use of antiperistaltic drugs.

Kaolin and pectin mixtures (Kaopectate or generic, nonprescription) add to the bulk of the stool and thus the stools become less watery; actual fluid loss, however, is not affected by these agents. *Bismuth subsalicylate* (Pepto-Bismol or generic, nonprescription) has been demonstrated to decrease the volume of stools in patients with diarrhea caused by enterotoxigenic organisms and to be safe in a variety of diarrheal illnesses (44). This compound has antibacterial activity as well. It may be taken in either liquid or tablet form. The dosage is two tablets or 30 mL every half to 1 hour, as needed, up to a maximum of eight doses per 24 hours. Patients should be advised that this compound causes black stools and sometimes a blackened tongue.

In patients with *protracted vomiting,* which may occur with staphylococcal food poisoning, the antiemetic drug prochlorperazine (Compazine) may be helpful, given as a 25-mg rectal suppository two or three times daily to healthy adults and at lower dosages for the elderly.

Specific Treatment

In patients in whom *shigellosis* is strongly suspected or from whom the organism has been cultured in the stool, appropriate antibiotic treatment should be given because this will shorten the illness from 3 to 7 days to 1 to 2 days. A fluoroquinolone antibiotic (e.g., ciprofloxacin 500 mg or norfloxacin 400 mg, twice daily) for 3 days is the current drug of choice (45). An alternative therapy is trimethoprim-sulfamethoxazole, one double-strength tablet every 12 hours for 5 days (46).

If *Salmonella* is isolated from diarrheal stool, patients should not be given antibiotics unless there is evidence of systemic disease, such as high fever or other symptoms or signs of systemic infection. It has been found that routine treatment of *Salmonella* gastroenteritis with antibiotics leads to a prolongation of the carrier state in some people (47). Even without antibiotic treatment, patients may excrete *Salmonella* in the stool for several weeks to months after their acute illness has terminated. If there is systemic disease or if the patient is immunocompromised, the same antibiotics listed above for shigellosis should be prescribed, but the duration of therapy should be 3 to 7 days. Alternatively, chloramphenicol 500 mg four times a day for 3 to 7 days can be prescribed.

Patients infected with *Campylobacter* may benefit from antibiotic therapy, but controlled studies indicate primarily an effect on excretion of the organism rather than a clinical effect. Erythromycin 500 mg four times a day for 5 days seems to be the best regimen; most strains are also sensitive to similar dosages of tetracyclines, but resistance to the quinolones is now being reported (45).

In patients who develop *significant diarrhea related to antibiotics,* ideally the antibiotic should be stopped, and another substituted only if antibiotic therapy must be continued. *C. difficile* causes approximately 20% of antibiotic-associated diarrhea in hospitalized patients but is almost always responsible for severe cases of antibiotic-associated diarrhea accompanied by fever and abdominal pain (pseudomembranous colitis). The diarrhea usually begins during antibiotic treatment or within 2 weeks of stopping antibiotics; occasionally it begins weeks to months later (36). If *C. difficile* is strongly suspected, bismuth subsalicylate (see above) often helps, particularly in patients with mild to moderate diarrhea without significant systemic symptoms. Metronidazole (Flagyl), 250 mg by mouth four times a day for 10 to 14 days, shortens the illness in most patients and is indicated when severe diarrhea and other symptoms occur (e.g., low-grade fever and mild abdominal pain) (40). For the 20% of patients with relapsing infection (5) or for those with severe diarrhea and systemic manifestations of illness such as high fever, abdominal pain, or elevated blood leukocyte count indicative of pseudomembranous colitis, the much more expensive antibiotic vancomycin should be given in an oral dosage of 250 to 500 mg four times daily for 7 to 14 days (40).

Although antibiotics are definitely useful in the treatment of traveler's diarrhea, most of which is caused by enterotoxigenic *E. coli* (see Chapter 41), there is no evidence that antibiotics are useful in patients with *hemorrhagic colitis* caused by *E. coli.* In fact, accumulating evidence shows that previous exposure or empiric antibiotic treatment of diarrhea in patients who subsequently are diagnosed with *E. coli* O157:H7 infection is associated with an increased risk of hemolytic uremia syndrome (48).

Patients with *giardiasis* and *amebiasis* require appropriate antimicrobial therapy. For giardiasis, the drug of choice is metronidazole (Flagyl) 250 mg three times a day for 5 days. (Quinacrine hydrochloride, an earlier recommended treatment, is no longer available in the United States.) For moderate to severe amebic dysentery, metronidazole should be administered, 750 mg three times a day for 10 days, followed by iodoquinol (Yodoxin; previously diiodohydroxyquin), 650 mg three times a day for 3 weeks, to eradicate the cyst forms (17).

Trichinosis is treated with mebendazole 300 mg three times daily for 3 days and then 500 mg three times daily for 10 days. High dosages of prednisone (e.g., 40 to 60 mg/day) should be given simultaneously, if symptoms are pronounced, for 3 to 5 days and then tapered.

Patients with *suspected botulism* should be hospitalized in an intensive care unit immediately and should be given polyvalent antitoxin, which must be obtained through the local health department. Patients with *mushroom poisoning* caused by *Amanita muscaria* should be treated with atropine and hospitalized (Table 35.2).

Chapter 39 describes the treatable opportunistic organisms that cause diarrheal illnesses in patients with HIV infection; for one of these, cryptosporidiosis, no antibiotic therapy has been shown to be effective, but partial response with octreotide 50 mg subcutaneously every 8 hours for 48 hours has been reported.

Patient's Role in Therapy

Acute gastroenteritis, like the common cold, is often diagnosed and handled by the patient without contacting a physician. In some instances, patients contact their physician by telephone and a working diagnosis and plan of therapy can be established without an office visit. This is particularly true for healthy patients with typical symptoms of staphylococcal food poisoning. In all situations, whether the patient is examined or not, it should be stressed that care of gastroenteritis requires taking of sufficient fluids, at times supplemented by an oral electrolyte solution (see above), and by oral antibiotics if prescribed. Patients should be advised to contact their physician if diarrhea becomes worse or if they develop fever or protracted vomiting. A follow-up visit is not needed unless symptoms persist beyond 2 to 3 days or unless stool cultures have been taken and reveal that antibiotic therapy is indicated. Limitation of activity should be dictated by how the patient feels and by proximity of toilet facilities.

Course of Illness

The dehydrated patient feels almost immediate improvement when adequate oral replacement fluids are given. When the patient is given antimicrobial therapy for an invasive pathogen, diarrhea and fever should decrease notably within 24 to 36 hours.

An *atypical course* occasionally occurs after initial diagnosis and treatment. After being initially seen, any patient may develop an increase in diarrhea that could result in unanticipated significant dehydration. An increase in severity of symptoms could also occur if the patient develops antibiotic-associated enterocolitis. The occasional patient with antibiotic-resistant *Shigella* may not respond to initial therapy, indicating the need for an alternative drug. The enteric fever syndrome caused by *S. typhi* (typhoid fever), some other *Salmonella* species, and some *Yersinia* species typically begins with constipation, fever, headache, and abdominal pain, but diarrhea may develop. The progressive course and abdominal tenderness (at times suggesting acute appendicitis) are features that suggest these causes and the need for both stool and blood cultures (14). An initial episode of *ulcerative colitis* (bloody diarrhea) or an initial episode of *Crohn disease* (pain with nonbloody intermittent diarrhea that does not remit) could be misdiagnosed as shigellosis. With inflammatory bowel diseases, fluids or antibiotic therapy would not lead to resolution of symptoms.

Rarely, a patient's diarrheal symptoms may persist for more than a week. In this case, the patient should return for further evaluation, particularly repeated stool examinations, which may be necessary to confirm the diagnosis of protozoal infections.

PREVENTION

Primary Prevention

Primary prevention of the diseases discussed above can theoretically be accomplished by the following measures:

- Reducing the agent's presence in the environment;
- Increasing resistance of the host (by immunization or prophylactic antibiotics);
- Using environmental measures that block the transmission of the agent.

Regulations governing sewage treatment, water purification, and food processing, packing, and preparation provide the principal protective barriers to foodborne disease *outside the home.* Unfortunately, this is often inadequate, as evidenced by the observation that as many as 50% of poultry carcasses sold commercially in supermarkets are contaminated with *Salmonella* or *Campylobacter.* In coming years, the use of food irradiation may become more widespread, and this could drastically improve food safety (49).

In the home, almost all forms of food-borne disease can be prevented if several measures are followed routinely (Table 35.6). *Many people do not realize that*

Table 35.6. Measures to Prevent Foodborne Disease in the Home

Refrigerate all foods that are capable of supporting microbial growth (perishable foods).
Avoid keeping perishable food for long periods, even in the refrigerator.
Cook all foods at sufficiently high temperatures before serving and follow the same procedure when foods are reheated.
Avoid preparing perishable foods a day or more before they are to be served.
Avoid allowing foods to stand at warm temperatures for several hours before being served.
Avoid incorporating raw (contaminated) ingredients into foods that receive no further cooking.
Clean kitchen equipment thoroughly after it has been in contact with perishable foods.
Avoid using utensils that may contain toxic metals.
Avoid foods that are unsafe no matter how they are processed (see text).

some of the food they prepare each day is contaminated before cooking and that proper cooking and storing, not absence of contamination, is the way in which most food is rendered safe to eat. Whenever food known to be contaminated is eaten raw, the risk of food-borne disease is present. This is particularly important with respect to shellfish, which concentrate microbial organisms from the waters in which they are grown.

Despite routine testing of water by public health authorities for contamination by enteric pathogens, the number of cases of illness related to consumption of *raw seafood* continues to increase. Illnesses arise from bacteria such as *Shigella* and *Vibrio,* particularly *Vibrio vulnificus,* viruses such as hepatitis A and Norwalk, and unusual parasites in sushi (13). Some experts suggest that the risks associated with eating raw seafood are now unacceptable (50), and people at risk for gastrointestinal infections should be instructed to avoid eating uncooked seafood.

Secondary Prevention

After an outbreak of an acute enteric illness, appropriate measures should be taken to prevent additional cases. *In the household,* any foods suspected of transmitting illness should be thrown away. (In the event that an epidemiologic investigation is warranted, a sample should be submitted to the local health department.) An error in storage or cooking of the suspected food is often evident; the patient's physician should point out this error and, most important, review the standard precautions listed in Table 35.6 to prevent repeated episodes of food-borne illness. When a member of a household has an enteric infection that is transmissible from person to person (Table 35.1), this person should be instructed to wash his or her hands frequently, especially before preparing food for others. *Food-service employees* should not work until the symptoms of infectious gastroenteritis resolve. Those with shigellosis or salmonellosis should not work until two consecutive stool cultures obtained not less than 24 hours apart (and not less than 48 hours after discontinuation of antibiotics if antibiotics were given) are negative.

When *exposure outside* the home is suspected, the problem should be reported immediately to the local health department; it is the responsibility of the health department to undertake an epidemiologic investigation to protect others. Each year, investigations of 400 to 500 outbreaks of food-borne illness are reported to the CDC, and many lead to measures that interrupt potentially widespread outbreaks of diseases, some of them particularly hazardous, such as botulism.

Prophylaxis for Travelers to the Developing World

The problem of diarrheal illness and other problems related to travel are discussed in Chapter 41.

General References

Blaser MJ, Smith PD, Ravdin N, et al., eds. Infections of the gastrointestinal tract. 2nd ed. New York: Raven Press, 2002.

Comprehensive textbook.

Chin J, ed. Control of communicable diseases in man. 17th ed. Washington, DC: American Public Health Association, 2000.

A concise summary of epidemiology, management, and prevention of communicable diseases.

Centers for Disease Control and Prevention. Diagnosis and management of foodborne illnesses—a primer for physicians. MMWR Morb Mortal Wkly Rep 2001;50(RR2):1.

A useful and comprehensive review.

Centers for Disease Control and Prevention. Surveillance for waterborne-disease outbreaks—United States, 1995–1996. In: CDC Surveillance Summaries 49(SS-1), 2000.

Summarizes methods for CDC surveillance and patterns in the United States for the 1990s.

Centers for Disease Control and Prevention. Surveillance for foodborne-disease outbreaks, United States, 1993–1997. In: CDC Surveillance Summaries 49(SS-1), 2000.

Most recent summary from CDC of surveillance and patterns of foodborne disease in the United States.

Hedberg CW, Osterholm MT. Outbreaks of food-borne and waterborne viral gastroenteritis. Clin Microbiol Rev 1993;6:199.

Useful review article.

Kapikian AZ. Viral gastroenteritis. JAMA 1993;269:627.

Useful review article.

Mead PS, Slutsker L, Dietz V, et al. Food-related illness and death in the United States. Emerg Infect Dis 1999;5:607.

Useful review article.

The Medical Letter on Drugs and Therapeutics. Drugs for parasitic infections. Med Lett Drugs Ther 1998;40:1.

Periodically updated source of current recommendations for treatment.

Park SI, Giannella RA. Approach to the adult patient with acute diarrhea. Gastroenterol Clin North Am 1993;22:483.

Useful review article.

Su C, Brandt, LJ. *Escherichia coli* O157:H7 infections in humans. Ann Intern Med 1995;123:698.

Useful review article.

Specific References

1. Caul EO. Small round structural viruses: airborne transmission and hospital control. Lancet 1994;343:1240.
2. Mahler H, Pasi A, Kramer LM, et al. Fulminant liver failure in association with the emetic toxin of *Bacillus cereus.* N Engl J Med 1997;336:1142.
3. Blaser MJ, Wells JG, Feldman RA, et al. Campylobacter enteritis in the United States. Ann Intern Med 1983;98:360.
4. Skirrow MB. *Campylobacter.* Lancet 1990;336:921.
5. Fekety R, McFarland LV, Surawicz CM, et al. Recurrent *C. difficile* diarrhea: characteristics of and risk factors for patients enrolled in a prospective, randomized double-blinded trial. Clin Infect Dis 1997;24:324.
6. Levine M. *Escherichia coli* that cause diarrhea: enterotoxigenic, enteropathogenic, enteroinvasive, enterohemorrhagic, and enteroadherent. J Infect Dis 1987;155:377.
7. Clausen CR, Christie DL. Chronic diarrhea in infants caused by adherent enteropathic *Escherichia coli.* J Pediatr 1982;100:358.
8. Vial PA, Robins-Browne R, Lior H, et al. Characterization of enteroadherent-aggregative *Escherichia coli,* a putative agent of diarrheal disease. J Infect Dis 1988;158:70.
9. Su C, Brandt LJ. *Escherichia coli* O157:H7 infection in humans. Ann Intern Med 1995;123:698.
10. Dalton CB, Austin CC, Sobel J, et al. An outbreak of gastroenteritis and fever due to *Listeria monocytogenes* in milk. N Engl J Med 1997;336:100.
11. Holmberg SD, Blake FA. Staphylococcal food poisoning in the United States: new facts and old misconceptions. JAMA 1984;251:487.
12. Ouchterlony O, Holmgren J, eds. Cholera and related diarrheas. 43rd Nobel Symposium. Basel: Karger, 1980.

13. Klontz KC, Lieb S, Schreiber M, et al. Syndromes of *Vibrio vulnificus* infections: clinical and epidemiologic features in Florida cases, 1981–1987. Ann Intern Med 1988;109:318.
14. Cover TL, Aber RC. *Yersinia enterocolitica.* N Engl J Med 1989;321:16.
15. Kapikian AZ, Chanock RM. Viral gastroenteritis. In: Evans AS, ed. Viral infections of humans, 3rd ed. New York: Plenum, 1989.
16. Ho M, Glass RI, Pinsky PF, et al. Rotavirus as a cause of diarrheal morbidity and mortality in the United States. J lnfect Dis 1988;158:1112.
17. Guerrant RL. The global problem of amebiasis: current status, research needs, and opportunities for progress. Amebiasis: introduction, current status, and research questions. Rev Infect Dis 1986;8:218.
18. Stevens DP. Host-pathogen biology. Rev Infect Dis 1982;4:851.
19. Current WL, Reese NC, Ernst N, et al. Human cryptosporidiosis in immunocompetent and immunodeficient persons. N Engl J Med 1983;308:1252.
20. Soave R. *Cyclospora:* an overview. Clin Infect Dis 1997;23:429.
21. Teitelbaum JS, Zatorre RJ, Carpenter S, et al. Neurologic sequelae of domoic acid intoxication due to the ingestion of contaminated mussels. N Engl J Med 1990;322:1781.
22. Mead PS, Slutsker L, Dietz V, et al. Food-related illness and death in the United States. Emerg Infect Dis 1999;5:607.
23. Davis M, Osaki C, Gordon D, et al. Update: multistate outbreak of *Escherichia coli* O157:H7 infection from hamburgers: Western United States, 1992–1993. MMWR Morb Mortal Wkly Rep 1993;42:258.
24. Slutsker L, Ries AA. Greene KD, et al. *Escherichia coli* O157: H7 diarrhea in the United States: clinical and epidemiologic features. Ann Intern Med 1997;126:505.
25. Boyce TG, Pemberton AG, Wells JG, et al. Screening for *Escherichia coli* O157:H7—a nationwide survey of clinical laboratories. J Clin Microbiol 1995;33:3275.
26. Levine WC, Smart JF, Archer DL, et al. Foodborne disease outbreaks in nursing homes, 1975 through 1987. JAMA 1991;266:2105.
27. Mishu B, Griffin PM, Tauxe RV, et al. *Salmonella enteritidis* gastroenteritis transmitted by intact chicken eggs. Ann Intern Med 1991;115:190.
28. Armstrong GL, Hollingsworth J, Morris JG. Emerging foodborne pathogens: *Escherichia coli* O157:H7 as a model of entry of a new pathogen into the food supply of the developed world. Epidemiol Rev 1996;18:29.
29. Cody SH, Glynn MK, Farrar JA, et al. An outbreak of *Esherichia coli* O157:H7 infection from unpasteurized commercial apple juice. Ann Intern Med 1999;130:202.
30. Mahon BE, Ponka A, Hall WN, et al. An international outbreak of *Salmonella* infections caused by alfalfa sprouts grown from contaminated seeds. J Infect Dis 1997;175:876.
31. Herwaldt BL, Beach MJ, et al. The return of *Cyclospora* in 1997: another outbreak of cyclosporiasis in North America associated with imported raspberries. Ann Intern Med 1999;130:210.
32. Gosselin RE, Hodge HC, Smith RP, et al. Clinical toxicology of commercial products. 4th ed. Baltimore: Williams & Wilkins, 1976.
33. Hughes LM, Merson MR. Current concepts: fish and shellfish poisoning. N Engl J Med 1976;295:1117.
34. Becker K, Southwick K, Reardon J, et al. Histamine poisoning associated with eating tuna burgers. JAMA 2001;285:1327.
35. Lew JF, Glass RI, Gangarosa RE, et al. Diarrheal deaths in the United States, 1979 through 1987. JAMA 1991;265:3280.
36. Fekety R, Shah AB. Diagnosis and treatment of *Clostridium difficile* colitis. JAMA 1993;269:71.
37. Janoff EN, Reller LB. *Cryptosporidium* species, a protean protozoan. J Clin Microbiol 1988;25:967.
38. Canneli Y, Samore M, Shoshany O, et al. Utility of clinical symptoms versus laboratory tests for evaluation of acute gastroenteritis. Dig Dis Sci 1996;41:1749.
39. Riley LW. The epidemiologic, clinical, and microbiological features of hemorrhagic colitis. Ann Rev Microbiol 1987;41:383.
40. Mylonakis E, Ryan ET, Calderwood SB. *Clostridium difficile*-associated diarrhea: a review. Arch Intern Med 2001;161:525.
41. Siegel DL, Edelstein PH, Nachamkin I. Inappropriate testing for diarrheal diseases in the hospital. JAMA 1990;263:979.
42. Carpenter CCJ, Greenough WE, Pierce NF. Oral-rehydration therapy: the role of polymeric substrates. N Engl J Med 1988;319:1346.
43. Greenough WB, Maung UK. Oral rehydration therapy. In: Field M, ed. Current topics in gastroenterology: diarrheal diseases. New York: Elsevier, 1991:485.
44. Bierer D. Bismuth subsalicylate: its history, chemistry, and safety. Rev Infect Dis 1990;12:83.
45. Sack RB, Rahman M, Yunus M, et al. Antimicrobial resistance in organisms causing diarrheal disease. Clin Infect Dis 1997;24:S102.
46. Gotuzzo E, Oberhelman RA. Maguina C, et al. Comparison of single-dose treatment with norfloxacin and standard 5-day treatment with trimethoprim-sulfamethoxazole for acute shigellosis in adults. Antimicrob Agents Chemother 1989;33:1101.
47. Aserkoff B, Bennett N. Effect of antibiotic therapy in acute salmonellosis on the fecal excretion of *Salmonellae.* N Engl J Med 1969;281:636.
48. Wong CS, Jelacic S, Habeeb RL, et al. The risk of the hemolytic-uremic syndrome after antibiotic treatment of *Escherichia coli* O157:H7 infections. N Engl J Med 2000;342:1930.
49. Tauxe RV. Strategies for surveillance and prevention. Lancet 1998;352:10.
50. DuPont HL. Consumption of raw shellfish: is the risk now unacceptable? N Engl J Med 1986;314:707.

CHAPTER 36

Genitourinary Infections

PATRICK A. MURPHY, MD

Urinary tract infection (UTI) is one of the most common disorders seen in primary care. Most of these infections respond well to therapy, but complicated urinary infections can cause significant morbidity and mortality. This chapter provides a practical approach to the diagnosis, evaluation, management, and follow-up of ambulatory patients with UTIs. Some sexually transmitted diseases (STDs) (Chapter 37) and vulvovaginal infections (Chapter 102) may be confused with UTIs and are discussed elsewhere in this book.

GENERAL CONSIDERATIONS

Gram negative, aerobic bacteria cause 90% to 95% of UTIs in all age groups, with *Escherichia coli* accounting for approximately 80% of community-acquired infections in women and 30% to 50% of nosocomial UTIs in men and women. There are more than 100 serotypes of *E. coli,* but only 8 of these commonly cause infection. *Enterobacter, Klebsiella, Proteus* species, and *Pseudomonas* are especially important as causes of nosocomial UTIs or of infection in people with structurally abnormal urinary tracts. Gram positive bacteria cause 5% to 10% of UTIs; *Staphylococcus saprophyticus* is common in young women in the ambulatory setting (1), as is the enterococcus in nosocomial UTIs in patients of either sex. Viruses, mycobacteria, fungi, and parasites rarely cause UTIs. Fungi are most often seen in urine from patients who were recently in hospital and were or still are catheterized. Diabetes mellitus fosters fungal infection of the urine, as does failure to empty the bladder completely.

In women, the major cause of UTI is invasion of the urinary tract by bacteria that have ascended the urethra from the introitus. Women who are prone to infection have colonization of the vaginal introitus with the same serotypes of *E. coli* found in the fecal flora. Risk factors for acute UTI in women include a history of a recent UTI, increased sexual activity, use of a diaphragm and a spermicide, and failure to void after intercourse (2). There is little evidence to support the commonly held views that the direction of wiping after bowel movements or the use of oral contraceptives or tampons plays a role in the pathogenesis of UTIs in women (3).

Infection of the bladder and kidneys *in men* is unlikely unless there is a structural abnormality of the urinary tract. The much lower incidence of UTI in men has been attributed to the long male urethra, the absence of colonization by bacteria near the meatus, and an antibacterial factor—prostatic antibacterial factor—that is present in the prostatic fluid and is markedly diminished in some men who have recurrent prostatic infection. UTIs occur in some male homosexuals who have no abnormalities of the urinary tract (4) and in some men who are not circumcised (5).

The bladder has unique *intrinsic defenses* against infection. The washout of bacteria by periodic voiding is probably one important defense mechanism. The bladder mucosa also removes surface organisms, perhaps by phagocytosis, secretion of mucus, production of surface antibody, or all of these methods. This defense mechanism is severely limited if residual urine is regularly present after voiding.

Host factors play an important role in the pathogenesis of UTIs (6). UTIs occur more often and more persistently in men and women who have structural abnormalities of the urinary tract (e.g., an obstruction) or who have been catheterized or instrumented. Vesicoureteral reflux (the retrograde flow of urine from the bladder to the ureters) may be associated with ascending infection but is not necessarily causal. Infection in women occurs more often during pregnancy (4% to 6% incidence), especially in women who also have sickle cell trait (10% to 15% incidence). Diabetes mellitus does not increase the risk for development of a UTI unless there is an associated disorder of bladder emptying or the patient has been instrumented. However, once a UTI has developed in a diabetic patient, it may be more virulent.

GENERAL DIAGNOSTIC EVALUATION

The diagnosis of UTI is suggested by the history and physical examination (see later discussion) and confirmed by examination of the urine. Sometimes, radiographs and instrumentation of the urinary tract are necessary ancillary procedures.

The Patient with Irritative Symptoms—Diagnostic Approach

In young adults, UTIs are characterized by symptoms of bladder irritation such as frequency of micturition and dysuria. There may be urgency of micturition, and if a toilet is not immediately available, there may be minor leakage of urine or even complete incontinence. The urine is commonly cloudy and smells offensive. Suprapubic pressure or pain is commonly described. In a severe infection, there may be hematuria. If so, blood is evenly mixed throughout the volume of urine.

Approximately 30% of women with no fever and no symptoms other than those just described prove to have *pyelonephritis* when subjected to detailed examination (7). Clinical evidence of pyelonephritis would be temperature greater than 38.5°C, pain in the loin, chills and rigors, and evidence of frank sepsis such as tachypnea and hypotension. It is axiomatic that any woman with a UTI and a positive blood culture has pyelonephritis.

In women, usually (but not exclusively) between the ages of 15 and 50 years, *vaginal infections and STDs may mimic UTIs* (8). A pelvic examination should be performed if the history is suggestive of vulvovaginitis from candidiasis, trichomoniasis, or other infections that may account for the bladder irritative symptoms (see Chapter 37). Chlamydial or gonococcal urethritis should also be considered in sexually active women (see Chapter 37). Both of these infections are most probable in women with many sexual partners, but both are found in 2% to 4% of married women presenting for routine antenatal care (6). Chlamydial cervicitis is characterized by mucopurulent cervical discharge with endocervical edema. Gonococcal infection typically causes a purulent discharge from the cervix. Both infections are best detected by an endocervical culture, or by polymerase chain reaction (PCR) tests on urine, if available.

In children younger than 5 years of age, UTI may present in atypical ways, such as bed-wetting, fever, vomiting, or inconsolable crying. Older children generally have the same symptoms as adults. Aged people, especially if demented or psychotic, may have very few symptoms referable to the urinary tract. They commonly experience delirium, fever, urinary incontinence, or even sepsis of unknown cause. Therefore, at the extremes of life it is unwise to rely on urinary symptoms.

UTI in pregnancy, known to older obstetricians as pyelitis of pregnancy, is a highly dangerous condition (9). The diagnosis is difficult because there may be few bladder symptoms. Instead, the patient commonly has intractable vomiting in the second or third trimester, elevated blood pressure with superimposed preeclampsia or eclampsia, renal failure, sepsis, or premature labor. UTI in pregnant women usually takes the form of pyelonephritis because the ureters are dilated and atonic and ascending infection is facilitated. Most cases of frank pyelitis of pregnancy are preceded by asymptomatic bacteriuria: treatment of the bacteriuria as soon as it is discovered leads to a much lower subsequent incidence of pyelonephritis and its serious complications.

Urine Examination

The urinalysis is the most important initial study in the evaluation of the patient suspected of having a UTI, because a negative urinalysis makes a UTI unlikely and because a urinalysis may aid in the localization of an infection within the urinary tract.

Urine Collection

Collection of a *clean-catch* midstream urine specimen can be difficult, especially for women. The superiority of this procedure for reducing contamination compared with routine midstream urine collection has not been demonstrated (10). Therefore, culturing a simple midstream urine specimen voided into a sterile container should be sufficient for most outpatients of both sexes. The midstream collecting procedure may be impossible in women who are very obese or who have other disabilities. In this instance, urine must be obtained by bladder catheterization.

Catheterization of the urinary bladder is accomplished by using a no. 14 catheter inserted through the urethra into the bladder and removed when the specimen has been obtained. This requires careful preparation and cleansing of the urethra with an aseptic solution such as povidone-iodine (Betadine). Even with this precaution, a single straight catheterization has a 1% risk of inducing a new infection in ambulatory patients.

Urinalysis

If the urine specimen cannot be processed by the laboratory within 10 to 15 minutes after collection, it must be refrigerated until it reaches the laboratory.

The *uncentrifuged specimen* can be examined microscopically under a coverslip with use of the *oil immersion lens.* The finding of bacteria by this method has a 90% correlation with the subsequent culture of more than 1 million bacteria per milliliter of urine. The number of white blood cells (WBCs) in the uncentrifuged urine can be roughly quantitated microscopically *in a counting chamber by the use of the low-power lens.* In women, the finding of more than 7 WBCs/mm^3 is abnormal (although not specific for infection). The finding of 7 or fewer WBCs per cubic millimeter suggests that infection is not present. In men, the finding of any number of WBCs should be considered abnormal.

Centrifuged urine is more convenient in some ways than is uncentrifuged urine. WBC casts are more easily seen in centrifuged urine; they are important because they are positive proof of pyelonephritis. Red cells, WBCs, and bacteria are all concentrated and more easily detected. Small numbers of WBCs seen in centrifuged urine are unreliable, and pyuria should not be considered significant unless there are more than *10 WBCs per high-powered field* (HPF).

As a practical matter, microscopic examination of the urine for bacteria is difficult or impossible in most doctors' offices. Because in many cases there is little doubt about the diagnosis, it is reasonable either to treat the patient empirically (e.g., first or recurrent uncomplicated infections in women) or to use the *urine dipstick* as a rapid diagnostic aid. There may be abnormalities in tests for pH, protein, or blood, but these are nonspecific. The abnormalities specifically correlated with infection are found with the dipstick-based *nitrite test* and the *test for leukocyte esterase.* Nitrite is generated by the reductive activity of bacteria on urinary nitrate. Leukocyte esterase reflects the presence of WBCs in the urine. If both of these are positive, the specificity for UTI is greater than 90% (11,12). Not all bacteria reduce nitrate, and not all UTIs are associated with a sufficient number of WBCs in the urine to yield a positive esterase test. (For example, the sensitivity of the test is 100% for 50 WBCs/HPF or more, but it is approximately 40% for 6 to 12 WBCs/HPF.) An important cause of a false-negative nitrate test is the ingestion of large amounts of vitamin C. If the patient is symptomatic but the dipstick is negative, one should try direct demonstration of bacteriuria by microscopy or culture before deciding that infection is not present.

Urine Culture

Many women know perfectly well that they have a UTI and merely need a prescription for antibiotics with instructions to recontact the office if symptoms persist (see Management of Symptomatic Urinary Tract Infections in Women). Culture of the urine in such patients is *costly ($60 to $80) and inconvenient* and rarely affects one's decision because the patient is better before the answer is known. On the other hand, a urine culture should always be obtained before therapy in patients who have recently been hospitalized or who are seriously ill and febrile. Infections in pregnant women are so serious that urine should always be cultured. Infections in young men are sufficiently unusual that a culture should also be obtained. In other patients, clinical judgment should dictate whether a culture is done.

If a urine culture is performed, the specimen should be refrigerated during transport to the laboratory. Most patients with symptomatic UTI have at least 10^5 bacteria per milliliter of urine. However, some people develop symptoms of cystitis in the presence of 10^3 or even 10^2 organisms per milliliter of urine. If such patients are not treated, they tend to return with more severe symptoms and higher bacterial counts in the urine (13).

When urine is sent for culture, the species of bacteria isolated is also important. *Multiple species suggest contamination,* except in chronically catheterized patients or in special circumstances such as a vesicocolic fistula. Even small numbers of definite pathogens such as *E. coli* or *Klebsiella* should be regarded as suspicious. Conversely, large numbers of skin flora such as *Staphylococcus epidermidis* or diphtheroids can usually be ignored. Anaerobic bacteria virtually never cause UTI, and if they are repeatedly present, a communication with the bowel is suggested. The presence of fungi, usually *Candida,* is seldom correlated with symptoms or signs of UTI and in most cases is inconsequential.

Culture of urine specimens can be difficult in remote parts of the country. Commercially available kits allow one to dip a coated slide into fresh urine, drain it, and incubate it. Colonies develop directly on the slide, and the counts correlate well with those obtained by quantitative plate cultures (14).

Culture-Negative Urine. If the patient has symptoms of cystitis with or without pyuria but the urine does not contain visible or cultured bacteria, the most likely explanation is that the patient has urethritis, prostatitis, or vaginitis. However, adenovirus can cause symptomatic cystitis, and chemical cystitis can be caused by several chemotherapeutic agents. In patients with culture-negative pyuria, tuberculosis of the kidney, bladder stone, bladder tumor, and interstitial cystitis (discussed later) should be considered.

Localizing the Site of Infection

Several techniques may characterize a UTI as either confined to the bladder or involving the kidneys. However, in most cases it is unnecessary to try to decide whether the patient has cystitis, pyelonephritis, or prostatitis. Many patients with pyelonephritis respond to standard 3-day treatment regimens described later in this chapter.

The simplest indication that a patient has pyelonephritis or prostatitis that requires prolonged treatment is that the UTI relapses after a standard 3-day course of antibiotics that would be expected to clear a simple bladder infection. *Relapse* means that all of the infectious episodes are caused by the same organism, as defined not only by species but also by any other available characteristics such as antibiotic sensitivity or serotype. Relapsing episodes are not necessarily caused by pyelonephritis: They may be caused by persistent colonization of the introitus and multiple episodes of ascending infection. Most cases of recurrent UTI are managed by prolonged courses of antibiotics, as discussed later.

In pyelonephritis, the bacteria in the urine are usually coated with antibody. This can be detected with the use of fluorescent goat anti-human immunoglobulin. In cystitis, bacteria in the urine are generally free of antibody. This test is not absolutely reliable: Antibody-coated bacteria may be found in prostatitis, and antibody-negative bacteria may be obtained from some cases of pyelonephritis. For this reason, the test is of limited clinical value and should rarely be performed.

Other techniques are cumbersome because they require urethral or ureteral catheterization. The gold standard for localization of upper tract infection is bilateral ureteral catheterization with separate collection of the urine from each kidney. There is a less complicated bladder washout technique that detects pyelonephritis but gives no information about the side of the infection. Radiographic abnormalities such as renal cortical scars are not present in most cases of pyelonephritis. Localization of the UTI is so seldom needed in clinical practice that patients who require it should be referred to a urologist.

Imaging

Uncomplicated UTIs that respond to treatment do not require additional workup. However, some clinical situations warrant investigation for anatomic abnormalities (Table 36.1). In office practice, an intravenous pyelogram (IVP) is no longer the most appropriate way to evaluate renal anatomy. *Sonography* is quicker and less dangerous to renal function. It detects kidney size, cortical scars, stones, and hydronephrosis. If sonography is normal, IVP is unlikely to add more information (15). Sonography is particularly useful for detecting and estimating the volume of residual urine in patients who cannot empty the bladder.

Computed tomography (CT) scanning is most useful for the detection of perinephric abscess and as a prelude to operations on the kidneys. *Voiding cystourethrography* is another test that should be delegated to the urologist.

Table 36.1. Indications for Evaluating Patients Who Have Urinary Tract Infections with Ultrasonography

- Acute pyelonephritis in male patients
- Acute pyelonephritis in women with persistent high fevers or leukocytosis after 2 or 3 days of antimicrobial treatment
- Renal colic (see Chapter 51)
- Palpable bladder or renal mass
- Urea-splitting organism, usually *Proteus* spp.
- Frequently recurrent urinary tract infections in women (>3–4/yr)
- Failure to eradicate infection with appropriate therapy

MANAGEMENT OF SYMPTOMATIC URINARY TRACT INFECTIONS IN WOMEN

First Infection, Occasional Infection, or Uncomplicated Infection

Most women with UTIs experience only one or occasional uncomplicated infections. The diagnosis of a UTI can be confirmed by urinalysis and urine culture; however, as discussed earlier, a therapeutic trial is usually sufficient and is more convenient and far less costly for the patient. Although an uncomplicated infection may clear spontaneously in time, treatment with antibiotics dramatically shortens the symptomatic period and should be given. Forcing fluids, historically a common practice, is discouraged once antibiotic therapy has been initiated because it may actually dilute significantly the concentration of antimicrobial in the urine.

Antibiotic Treatment. Uncomplicated UTIs should usually be treated with an antibiotic for 3 days (Table 36.2). Three days of treatment gives the same cure rate as the traditional 7- to 10-day courses, and there is little superinfection with *Candida,* a common occurrence with the longer course. One-dose therapy was popular a number of years ago, but the cure rate is less than that attainable with 3 days of therapy.

There is a randomized controlled trial showing that UTI in presumably healthy young women can be managed effectively over the telephone (16). There is also a controlled trial showing that patients who are given antibiotics in advance can diagnose and treat their own UTIs (17).

For patients who are not pregnant, a wide range of drugs can be used. Probably the best available therapy is trimethoprim–sulfamethoxazole (TMP-SMX). This produces little in the way of allergy, kills most gram negative rods, tends to sterilize the vaginal introitus, and is inexpensive. Overall, the cure rate is 90% to 95% (18). Patients who are allergic to sulfonamides

Table 36.2. Antimicrobial Agents for Uncomplicated Urinary Tract Infections (3-Day Therapy)

Agent	Dosage and Schedule
First choice (effective and inexpensive)	
Trimethoprim-sulfamethoxazole[a] (Bactrim, Septra, generic)	1 double-strength tablet q12h
Second choice (effective)	
A Quinolone[b]	
Ciprofloxacin (Cipro)	250 or 500 mg q12h
Levoflaxacin	500 μg q12h
Norfloxacin (Noroxin)	400 mg q12h
Tetracycline[a]	500 mg q12h
Doxycycline[a]	100 mg q12h
Third choice (effective for cystitis but not for pyelonephritis)	
Nitrofurantoin (Furadantin)	50 or 100 mg q12h
Fourth choice (less effective but can be used during pregnancy)	
β-Lactams (e.g., amoxicillin, cephalexin)	250–500 mg q8h

[a] Three-day course costs less than $5.
[b] Three-day course costs $15–$20.

can be treated with a quinolone, a tetracycline, or nitrofurantoin. Because TMP-SMX has been extensively used in the last 20 years, the incidence of resistance is rising all over the country. Surveys show that resistance to TMP-SMX varies from a minimum of 7% in Pennsylvania to a maximum of 33% in Iowa (19). Resistance reported in the laboratory is not necessarily correlated with clinical failure because of the very high concentrations of antibiotics in the urine. However, at some point TMP-SMX is going to lose its effectiveness (20).

Beta-lactams such as ampicillin and cephalosporins are less effective than the four drugs mentioned earlier. However, in pregnant women there is no reasonable alternative to beta-lactams because of the risk of harm to the fetus. Therefore, a somewhat increased risk of recurrent UTI must be accepted. In the rare pregnant woman with a serious penicillin allergy, one could consider an aminoglycoside, but there is a risk of fetal deafness.

Any of the above treatments usually sterilizes the urine and produces total relief of symptoms in 24 hours or less. In very symptomatic patients, one could add the bladder analgesic *phenazopyridine* (Pyridium), 200 mg three times a day for 1 day or longer. This drug, which requires a prescription, usually alleviates annoying symptoms, especially dysuria and urgency, within hours after the first dose. The patient should be told that phenazopyridine will cause the urine to become dark orange.

If the patient remains asymptomatic after treatment, she may be regarded as cured without the need for any additional follow-up.

Points to stress to women after a UTI episode are summarized in Table 36.3. The behaviors that most often help prevent recurrent UTI are emptying the bladder after sexual intercourse and avoiding a full bladder. If a woman is using a diaphragm for contraception, a change in contraceptive method could be considered (see Chapter 100).

Table 36.3. Points to Consider in Educating Women Who Have Had an Uncomplicated Infection

Infections are often recurrent. However, the following measures may decrease the recurrence rate:

- Avoid a full bladder. This is an especially important reminder during travel.
- High fluid intake (1 L in 2–3 hr) may eradicate an infection that has just become symptomatic.
- Irritation to the urethra, as occurs with sexual intercourse, is associated with the movement of bacteria into the bladder.
- Voiding after intercourse, therefore, helps to prevent recurrent infection.
- Diaphragm use is associated with development of urinary tract infection.

Infections in the absence of structural urologic disorder are rarely, if ever, associated with the development of chronic renal failure.

Prompt recognition and treatment will help to control symptomps.

Even if recurrent infections are frequent, there is much that can be done to control symptoms.

Management of Recurrent Infection, Reinfection Type

Most women with recurrent UTIs have *reinfection* (rather than *relapse,* which is discussed below). Although the infections are symptomatic and occasionally may be associated with pyelonephritis, recurrent reinfections in women with structurally normal urinary tracts rarely, if ever, lead to chronic renal failure.

The approach to women with anatomically normal urinary tracts and the syndrome of reinfection has been vastly improved by the understanding of the pathogenesis of UTI in women. In the past, women often were treated with a variety of painful manipulations such as urethral dilation, urethral incision, transurethral resection of the bladder neck, installation of a variety of intravesical agents, and other inappropriate and ineffective maneuvers. Instead, each episode of bacterial infection should be treated as outlined previously in the section on first infections. If there are three or more recurrences in a year, the urinary tract should be evaluated for anatomic abnormalities (see earlier discussion). Patients with structural problems should be referred to the appropriate specialist (urologist or gynecologist). If the urinary tract is normal, prophylactic antimicrobials should be considered.

Prophylactic Antimicrobial Therapy

A number of studies have confirmed the efficacy of prophylaxis in reducing the frequency of UTI in women, and prophylactic therapy has dramatically improved the lives of many women with multiple UTIs. The agents that have been used are effective when given as a single small dose at bedtime. A dose taken only after sexual intercourse is also effective in patients whose recurrent UTIs are associated with sexual activity. Patient acceptance is good, and side effects are uncommon.

Many agents have been shown to be effective prophylactically, but nitrofurantoin (Furadantin), a 50-mg tablet at bedtime; TMP-SMX, 40/200 mg (half a tablet of regular strength Bactrim, Septra, or generic) at bedtime; and cephalexin (Keflex or generic), a 250-mg capsule at bedtime are used most commonly and are recommended. In some patients, the antibiotic may be effective when given on 3 days of the week. Prophylactic therapy should be continued for 6 months. If there are still frequent recurrences after the cessation of prophylaxis, prophylaxis for a longer period (e.g., 1 year) should be tried.

Estrogens

In elderly women, the vaginal cells lose glycogen, lactobacilli vanish from the vaginal flora, and the introitus becomes colonized with gram negative rods. A controlled trial demonstrated that the frequency of recurrent UTIs in elderly women can be greatly reduced (from an average incidence of 5.9 to 0.5 episodes per year) by the use of intravaginal estrogen creams (21). Treated patients used intravaginal cream containing 0.5 mg of estriol on the following schedule:

nightly for 2 weeks, then twice weekly for 8 months. Presumably, systemic estrogens would have the same effect.

CLINICAL SYNDROMES THAT MIMIC URINARY TRACT INFECTIONS IN WOMEN

There are two syndromes in women that mimic classic UTI. The urethral syndrome is common, and interstitial cystitis is rare.

Urethral Syndrome (Dysuria–Pyuria Syndrome)

The urethral syndrome is characterized by bladder irritation, frequency, urgency, and dysuria without significant (greater than 10^5) bacterial colonies per milliliter on culture. *Dysuria–pyuria syndrome* may be the better term, because *dysuria is invariable and most patients have pyuria* (more than 8 white blood cells/mm^{3}of clean uncentrifuged urine). Studies show that many women with the syndrome have bacterial infection with a low bacterial colony count (22). These infections respond to the standard therapy for uncomplicated UTI described earlier.

The urethral syndrome can also be caused by any of several sexually transmitted infections. *Chlamydia, gonorrhea, and herpes simplex* are the most common causes. Other agents such as *Mycoplasma hominis* and *Ureaplasma urealyticum* may be found, but their significance is uncertain. Any woman who has acute onset of *dysuria and has urine that is apparently sterile* may have one of these infections. The patient should have a pelvic examination to check for the signs of common STDs, and the appropriate specimens should be obtained for culture and other examinations (see Chapter 37).

If the patient has never been sexually active, or not for years, then the dysuria–pyuria syndrome is occasionally caused by a viral infection. Adenovirus is the most common cause.

Of women who have the urethral syndrome, *5% to 10% do not have a demonstrable infectious agent* even when special culture methods are used; most often these patients do not have pyuria. The cause of the syndrome in these instances is unknown. In this group, treatment with reassurance, sitz baths, and the urinary tract analgesic phenazopyridine (Pyridium), 200 mg three times a day for 5 to 10 days, will provide some relief. The patient should be informed that this medication causes the urine to appear orange. If symptoms persist, referral to a urologist is indicated for cystoscopic evaluation.

Measures to be recommended to patients with this syndrome should be identical to those outlined for UTI (Table 36.3) or, if there is vaginitis or an STD present, as outlined in Chapter 37.

Interstitial Cystitis

Interstitial cystitis is an occasionally seen disorder affecting middle-aged women that, early in its course, may be confused with the urethral syndrome. Interstitial cystitis causes symptoms of suprapubic discomfort, especially when the bladder is full, and symptoms are relieved by voiding. The patient may experience progressive loss of bladder volume and increasing urinary frequency, and eventually may have to void four to six times per hour throughout the night. The urinalysis is often normal, but hematuria may be present. The urine is sterile. This disease is difficult to diagnose. If it is suspected on the basis of the history, referral to a urologist is indicated. The urologist performs cystoscopy and often a biopsy of the bladder to establish the diagnosis (usually a normal-appearing mucosa with a very small vesical capacity is identified; tissue histology may show changes consistent with the diagnosis; mucosal hemorrhage may appear with bladder filling). Also, a cystoscopic evaluation permits the urologist to exclude other causes of the symptoms (e.g., bladder tumor). No definitive therapy has yet been developed for treatment of this condition.

Vaginitis and Cervicitis

For detailed discussion of these conditions, see Chapter 37.

SYMPTOMATIC URINARY TRACT INFECTIONS IN MEN

Bacterial Cystitis

Bacterial cystitis in men is similar in presentation to that in female patients and is diagnosed by the same method, but a urine culture should always be obtained. A UTI in a man suggests the presence of an underlying structural problem or the presence of bacterial prostatitis. In previous editions of this book, it was stated that the initial evaluation should always include a prostate examination. However, because young men who are either homosexual or uncircumcised can develop UTIs in the absence of a structural abnormality, some easing of this standard is reasonable in men from either of these groups (4,5). If a workup is initiated, sonography is preferable to IVP as a screening tool.

A small number of young boys develop UTI in the apparent absence of a structural abnormality. Most turn out to have a congenital abnormality such as urethral valves. Young men with UTIs most often have stone or hydronephrosis. Older men usually have prostatic enlargement or stones.

Bacterial cystitis in men should always be treated for a minimum of 7 to 10 days (see daily dosages and schedules for antibiotics, Table 36.2). Structural problems are so common that short courses are ineffective. Even if no structural anomaly is found, men should be carefully followed up, because many of the infections relapse. Many men with relapse-type recurrences have bacterial prostatitis; therefore, a follow-up visit 4 to 6 weeks after the initial infection should be arranged to reculture the urine and, if it is positive, to consider treatment for chronic prostatitis (discussed later).

Prostatitis

Prostatitis is classified as bacterial prostatitis (acute or chronic), nonbacterial prostatitis (prostatosis), or the much less common prostatic infections caused by a virus, a parasite, tuberculosis, a fungus, or nonspecific granulomatous changes.

Acute Bacterial Prostatitis

Acute bacterial prostatitis is characterized often by the abrupt onset of fever, chills, low back pain, and perineal pain with irritative urinary tract symptoms, although on some occasions, systemic symptoms are not pronounced. Perineal discomfort may be worsened by defecation. In addition, the patient may have initial, terminal, or occasionally total hematuria (see Chapter 49). Rectal examination usually discloses a tender, swollen, and boggy prostate. The urine and the expressed prostatic secretions contain leukocytes, and culture often grows the responsible bacterial pathogen, which most commonly is *E. coli* in older men and *Chlamydia* or *Neisseria gonorrhoeae* in younger men.

When the diagnosis is made, the patient may require hospitalization, although if systemic symptoms are minimal, ambulatory therapy is appropriate. Most antibiotics do not achieve high concentrations in prostatic fluid. The best initial choice for younger patients is *levofloxacin* (500 mg once or twice daily), which penetrates the prostate well and covers the common etiologic organisms. If quinolones cannot be used, then a number of other antibiotics may be tried. *TMP-SMX* does penetrate prostatic epithelium and is an alternative for treating *E. coli*. Penicillins and cephalosporins do not achieve effective concentrations in the prostate and are not useful. Because of the overriding effects of local antibiotic concentration, antibiotics such as *erythromycin*, which would not normally be used to treat *E. coli*, may also prove effective. Therapy with antimicrobials for acute prostatitis should be continued for 2 weeks. Dosages and schedules are listed in Table 36.2.

Bed rest and sitz baths for 20 to 30 minutes two or three times a day may provide comfort. Occasionally, prostatitis results in acute urinary retention, which requires hospitalization and urgent urologic consultation. The palpable irregularity of the prostate gland after acute infection may persist for several months. The acute infection is readily controlled, but recurrences may occur, especially in older patients.

Chronic Bacterial Prostatitis

The organisms that cause chronic bacterial prostatitis most often are gram negative bacilli, *E. coli* being the most common organism, followed by *Enterococcus, Proteus,* and *Klebsiella*. Most patients with chronic bacterial prostatitis have mild irritative symptoms (frequency, urgency, and dysuria), and occasionally there is a urethral discharge. Fever is absent. Patients may also have painless hematuria or painful ejaculation with hematospermia. On rectal examination, the prostate gland feels somewhat irregular and may be mildly tender, although the examination is often unremarkable.

Obstructive symptoms are rare. Most often the patients have intermittent symptomatic episodes that have been controlled with short courses of antibiotics. However, recurrent infection is common because of persistence of bacteria within the urinary tract. Chronic prostatitis may also be a reservoir for acute symptomatic cystitis, pyelonephritis, or epididymitis. Therefore, a prolonged course of therapy is indicated when chronic prostatitis is diagnosed clinically. If the infectious organism is sensitive, *ciprofloxacin, 250 mg twice daily for 2 weeks,* has been shown to be effective in eradicating infection in more than 60% of patients with chronic prostatitis (23).

If all efforts to eradicate infection fail, symptoms usually can be controlled with *suppressive therapy* using a low dose of *TMP-SMX,* one-half tablet of regular strength (Bactrim, Septra, or generic) nightly, indefinitely. The only way to effect a cure is by radical prostatectomy, but the morbidity of this procedure precludes its use for benign disease. Repeated prostatic massage has not been shown to be effective. Patients with refractory chronic bacterial prostatitis should be evaluated by a urologist.

Nonbacterial Prostatitis (Prostatosis)

Some patients have all of the symptoms and signs of chronic bacterial infection of the prostate, but no organism can be demonstrated. They have nonbacterial prostatitis (prostatosis), which is the most common form of prostatic inflammation. These patients have mild perineal pain and irritative symptoms on urination with *WBCs in the urine sediment, but negative urine cultures*. Culture of the secretions and urine by special techniques occasionally reveals infectious agents such as *Mycoplasma, Gardnerella vaginalis, U. urealyticum,* or *Chlamydia* species; however, the significance of these findings is unknown. Most patients with this condition cannot be cured; nevertheless, treatment with an antimicrobial such as ciprofloxacin or levofloxacin at the dosage and schedule described for acute prostatitis may control symptoms. An antispasmodic agent such as oxybutynin (Ditropan), 5 mg two to three times a day, may be tried. Therapeutic prostatic massage has not been shown to be of value.

If there is no response to therapy, the patient should be referred to a urologist to exclude conditions such as interstitial cystitis and *in situ* bladder cancer. Both conditions require cystoscopic examination for confirmation.

Prostatodynia

Patients with a syndrome called prostatodynia have symptoms suggesting prostatic inflammation but have no evidence of inflammation on physical examination, have *no WBCs in the urine or in expressed prostatic secretions, and have sterile urine cultures*. There is some evidence that the syndrome may be caused by a neurologic disorder and that muscle relaxants or alpha-sympathetic blocking agents such as phenoxybenzamine (Dibenzyline) are effective in treating it. If this syndrome is suspected, urologic consultation is suggested to confirm the diagnosis, to rule out interstitial cystitis and bladder cancer, and to initiate therapy.

Epididymitis

In young men, this infection is usually caused by sexually transmitted pathogens. Manifestations, management and course are described in Chapter 37.

The *older patient* with acute epididymitis should always have a urine culture and should be evaluated for obstruction at the bladder outlet (see Chapter 53) as soon as the acute symptoms are controlled. On rare occasions, continued pain from chronic epididymitis may occur; if it does, a urologist should be consulted, because an epididymectomy may be required.

Urethritis

Urethritis is an acute inflammation of the urethra that may be classified as gonococcal or nongonococcal. All forms of urethritis are assumed to be sexually transmitted. This topic is discussed in detail in Chapter 37.

PERSISTENT URINARY TRACT INFECTION IN MEN AND WOMEN

As noted earlier, treatment in the male or female patient of infection in a normal urinary tract with an appropriate antimicrobial should result in the sterilization of the urine within 72 hours. By this time, symptoms should have abated or at least markedly diminished. If symptoms continue, a persistent infection may be present, and the urine culture should be repeated. If the urine culture is still positive despite antibiotic therapy, further investigation is required. Modern antibiotics are so effective and the concentrations achieved in urine are so high that persistent infection is unusual.

The possibilities to be considered are that the patient is not taking the antibiotic or has taken it but vomited subsequently; the organism is totally resistant (unusual but seen with certain pseudomonads and enterococci); the patient's renal function is so poor (e.g., creatinine greater than 3 mg/dL) that little antibiotic reaches the urine; the antibiotic does not work at the current urinary pH; there is a gross structural anomaly such as a vesicocolic fistula, a leaking pyonephrosis, or a nidus of sequestered bacteria such as a staghorn calculus; or the organism is not a bacterium at all, but a fungus. Once one has decided which of the above applies, the indicated treatment is usually obvious.

RECURRENT INFECTION, RELAPSE TYPE, IN MEN AND WOMEN

Recurrent infection with the same organism is called relapse infection and implies the persistence of bacteria in tissue within the urinary tract. Relapse infection is similar to persistent infection except that in relapse the urine was shown to be sterile while the patient was taking or had completed antimicrobial therapy, whereas sterility is never demonstrated with persistent infection. Relapse occurs most often within 6 weeks after completion of a course of antimicrobial therapy. An underlying structural problem is often present in both men and women with this condition. In women, relapse is much less common than reinfection but is difficult to document because most infections are a result of *E. coli,* which has many serotypes that cannot be differentiated by routine bacteriologic laboratory techniques. Therefore, recurrent UTI caused by *E. coli* may be either relapse (same serotype) or reinfection (different serotype). On the other hand, relapse of infection with organisms other than *E. coli* may be diagnosed by routine bacteriologic culture. In women, if recurrent infection with *E. coli* occurs four times in a 12-month period or if relapse infection with other species occurs, evaluation as described previously (see Persistent Urinary Tract Infection in Men and Women) to exclude the possibility of structural abnormality is appropriate. If a structural abnormality is identified, it should be corrected if possible.

If a woman or man has a structural or functional abnormality of the urinary tract that cannot be corrected, sterilization of the urinary tract usually is not possible. In a patient who has had recurrent infections because of urine stasis caused by an atonic bladder, *intermittent straight catheterization* by the patient or a trained member of the family may help to prevent recurrent infections (see Urinary Incontinence in Chapter 54). In patients with other abnormalities, *suppressive therapy* (see regimens for prophylaxis of recurrent cystitis, discussed previously) may decrease the frequency of symptomatic exacerbations or episodes of sepsis. Relapsing infection may occur in *patients with no evidence of a structural abnormality.* In women, that usually means that the patient has chronic pyelonephritis. In men, the most common cause is chronic bacterial prostatitis. Chronic pyelonephritis is generally treated with a 6-week course of an appropriate antibiotic, on several occasions if necessary. Some patients may eventually respond to prolonged antibiotic courses of 6 months or more. These prolonged courses are generally indicated only in young patients where there is some hope of cure.

If the patient has chronic bacteriuria that cannot be eradicated, there is some evidence that the ingestion of large quantities of cranberry juice will reduce the number of symptomatic episodes (24).

INFECTION IN CATHETERIZED PATIENTS

In the ambulatory setting, one often sees patients who were catheterized while acutely ill in the hospital, developed infection, and now have bacteriuria, even though the catheter has been removed. In general, these patients should be treated based on antibiotic sensitivities, because otherwise they will probably develop symptomatic episodes of cystitis or pyelonephritis. The usual course of antibiotic is 10 days, and because recurrence is common, a cure urine culture should be done.

ACUTE PYELONEPHRITIS IN MEN AND WOMEN

Pyelonephritis is a bacterial infection of the kidney that most often results from ascending infection. It is suggested by flank pain, fever, and often, abdominal pain in addition to symptoms of bladder irritation. Bacterial infection of the kidney may also be present without any of these signs or symptoms or with only bladder irritation. The urinalysis will show changes as outlined previously, but only the presence of *WBC casts* is diagnostic of pyelonephritis.

Clinically apparent acute pyelonephritis *in men* suggests the presence of a structural problem predisposing to infection and is an indication for immediate hospitalization, parenteral antimicrobial therapy, a sonogram, and possibly other urologic investigations. If an abscess is seen or suspected, a CT scan is indicated, because abscesses usually need surgical drainage.

In women, an underlying structural problem is much less likely to be present. Therefore, the decision for hospitalization and evaluation requires careful consideration. The patient can be treated at home if she does not have complicating medical illnesses, is not severely ill, does not exhibit sepsis, is reliable, and can take antimicrobials by mouth, and if access to the physician is guaranteed should symptoms worsen. If a patient is treated at home, follow-up in 24 to 48 hours by telephone is necessary. If there has not been significant improvement during that time, the possibility of an undrained infection (caused, for example, by an obstruction or abscess) should be considered and prompt hospitalization should be arranged for parenteral antibiotics, sonography, and emergency urologic consultation.

The initial treatment for the patient treated at home can be a 10- to 14-day course of any of the antimicrobial agents listed in Table 36.2, with an appropriate adjustment based on the results of the urine culture and on sensitivity testing. Forcing fluids (once antimicrobial therapy has been started) is unnecessary and may theoretically be detrimental because the concentration of antimicrobials in the urine and in the renal tissue may be diluted. However, intake should be adequate to replace fluid losses, including the additional fluid lost by fever or by vomiting.

If the acute episode of pyelonephritis promptly resolves, follow-up in 3 to 4 weeks is appropriate. At that time, the urine culture should be sterile. If the urine is not sterile and if the organism is the same one that caused the clinical attack of pyelonephritis, the patient is a candidate for a prolonged course of antibiotic therapy (6 weeks).

ASYMPTOMATIC BACTERIURIA

Asymptomatic Bacteriuria Not Associated with Pregnancy

Asymptomatic bacteriuria is more common in women and increases in both sexes with advancing age. Among people age 20 to 50 years, bacteriuria is present in 0.5% of men and fewer than 5% of women. In contrast, 3% of men and 20% of women age 65 to 70 years have positive urine cultures. After age 80, 22% of men and 23% to 50% of women have bacteriuria (25).

In addition to advancing age, asymptomatic bacteriuria is also associated with indwelling urinary catheters, urinary incontinence, multiple medical illnesses, impairment of functional status, and impairment of mental status.

Several population studies report an unexplained increase in mortality among elderly patients with asymptomatic bacteriuria. This increase appears to be secondary to concomitant illnesses rather than a direct consequence of the bacteriuria, and treatment of the bacteria does not affect mortality (26). It is not known how often nonpregnant patients with asymptomatic bacteriuria develop symptomatic infections. Treatment with antibiotic therapy is often unsuccessful in eradicating infection and may be associated with the development of more resistant infections (27). Therefore, screening for or treatment of asymptomatic bacteriuria in nonpregnant adult women or men of any age is not recommended.

Asymptomatic Bacteriuria Associated with Pregnancy

Asymptomatic bacteriuria in pregnancy is common, affecting up to 6% of women in the first trimester. Recognition of this fact is important, because eradication of bacteriuria reduces the high incidence of symptomatic UTI that subsequently occurs during pregnancy and may increase the risk of premature birth (9). The drugs used are beta-lactams, which are known to be associated with a higher rate of recurrent infection than quinolones or TMP-SMX. Good follow-up is therefore essential.

General Reference*

Stamm WER, Hooten TM. Management of urinary tract infections in adults. N Engl J Med 1993;329:1328.

Well-referenced review article that emphasizes cost-effective strategies for treating UTIs.

Specific References

1. Latham RH, Running K, Stamm WE. Urinary tract infections in young women caused by *Staphylococcus saprophyticus.* JAMA 1893;250:3063.
2. Hooton TM, Hillier S, Johnson C, et al. *Escherichia coli* bacteriuria and contraceptive method. JAMA 1991;265:64.
3. Fihn SD. Behavioral aspects of urinary tract infection. Urology 1988;33:16.
4. Barnes RC, Daijuker R, Reddy RE, et al. Urinary tract infection in sexually active homosexual men. Lancet 1986;2:171.
5. Spach DH, Stapleton AE, Stamm WE. Lack of circumcision increases the risk of urinary tract infection in young men. JAMA 1992;267:679.
6. Sobel JD, Kaye D. Urinary tract infections. In: Mandell GL, Douglas RG, Bennett JR, eds. Principles and practice of infectious diseases. 3rd ed. New York: Churchill Livingstone, 1990.

*Bold print (general references) and bold numerals (specific references) denote published controlled clinical trials, meta-analyses, or consensus-based recommendations.

7. Fairley KF, Carson NE, Gutch RC, et al. Site of infection in acute urinary tract infection in general practice. Lancet 1971;2:615.
8. Komaroff AL. Acute dysuria in women. N Engl J Med 1984;310:368.
9. Gilstrap LC 3rd, Ramin SM. Urinary tract infections during pregnancy. Obstet Gynecol Clin North Am 2001;28:581.
10. Leisure MK, Dudley SM, Donowitz LG. Does a clean catch urine sample reduce bacterial contamination? N Engl J Med 1993;328:289.
11. James GP, Paul KL, Fuller JB. Urinary nitrite and urinary tract infection. Am J Clin Pathol 1978;70:671.
12. Pfolles M, Ringenberg B, Rames L, et al. The usefulness of screening tests for pyuria in combination with culture in the diagnosis of urinary tract infection. Diagn Microb Infect Dis 1987;6:207.
13. Stamm WE, Running K, McKwitt M, et al. Treatment of the acute urethral syndrome. N Engl J Med 1987;304:956.
14. Margileth AM, Pedreira FA, Hirschman GH, et al. Urinary tract bacterial infections. Pediatr Clin North Am 1976;23:71.
15. Filly R. Ultrasonography. In: Friedland GW, Filly R, Goris ML, et al, eds. Uroradiology: an integrated approach. New York: Churchill Livingstone, 1983.
16. Barry HC, Hickner J, Ebell MH, et al. A randomised controlled trial of telephone management of suspected urinary tract infections in women. J Fam Pract 2001;50:589.
17. Gupta K, Hooton M, Roberts PL, et al. Patient initiated treatment of recurrent urinary tract infection in women. Ann Intern Med 2001;135:S18.
18. Cue JD. Urinary tract infection and dysuria: cost conscious evaluation and antibiotic therapy. Postgrad Med 1986;80:133.
19. Karlowski JA, Jones ME, Thornsberry C, et al. Prevalence of antimicrobial resistance among urinary tract pathogens isolated from female outpatients across the US in 1999. Int J Antimicrob Agents 2001;18:121.
20. Gupta K, Hooton TM, Stamm WE. Increasing antimicrobial resistance and the management of uncomplicated community acquired urinary tract infections. Ann Intern Med 2001;135:41.
21. Raz R, Stamm WE. A controlled trial of intravaginal estriol in post-menopausal women with recurrent urinary tract infections. N Engl J Med 1993;329:753.
22. Stamm WE, Wagner KF, Ansel RL, et al. Causes of the acute urethral syndrome in women. N Engl J Med 1980;303:409.
23. Childs SJ, Goldstein EJC. Ciprofloxacin as treatment for genitourinary tract infection. J Urol 1989;141:1.
24. Avorn J, Moname M, Gurivitz JH, et al. Reduction of bacteriuria and pyuria after ingestion of cranberry juice. JAMA 1994;271:751.
25. Kaye D. Urinary tract infections in the elderly. Bull N Y Acad Med 1980;57:209.
26. Abrityn E, Mossey J, Barlin JA, et al. Does asymptomatic bacteriuria predict mortality, and does antimicrobial treatment reduce mortality in elderly ambulatory women? Ann Intern Med 1994;120:827.
27. Nicolle LE, Mayhew WJ, Bryan C. Prospective randomized comparison of therapy and no therapy for asymptomatic bacteriuria in elderly institutionalized women. Am J Med 1987;83:27.

CHAPTER 37

Sexually Transmitted Diseases

KAREN A. WENDEL, MD
JONATHAN M. ZENILMAN, MD

Sexually transmitted diseases (STDs) are common in the primary care setting. Their associated morbidity ranges from mild genitourinary pain or irritation to infertility, adverse pregnancy outcomes, facilitation of human immunodeficiency virus (HIV) transmission, and genital tract epithelial cancers. STDs are often asymptomatic. Therefore, clinicians should regularly obtain a sexual history (see Chapter 6), inquire about genitourinary symptoms, provide counseling regarding safe sexual practices (see Chapter 39), and screen persons at risk. This chapter reviews the manifestations of common STDs, their differential diagnosis, and their treatment. Vaginitis and pelvic inflammatory disease (PID) in women are discussed in Chapter 102. The STDs described in this chapter are delineated by syndrome.

GENITAL ULCER DISEASE

In the United States, genital herpes is the major cause of infectious genital ulcer disease, followed by syphilis. The prevalence of each is dependent on the patient population and geographic area, especially for syphilis, which is largely confined to urban areas and the Southeast and is the object of a national elimination campaign. Chancroid, granuloma inguinale, and lymphogranuloma venereum are rare and are usually associated with travel to endemic areas outside the United States. More than 25% of patients with genital ulceration fail to obtain a definitive diagnosis even after full microbiologic evaluation (1). The evaluation and treatment of genital ulcers is important not only for control of the primary infection but also in preventing the transmission and acquisition of HIV (2–6). Patients with genital ulcer disease should be tested for HIV infection at the time of diagnosis and 3 months after their initial presentation.

Because "classic" presentations are uncommon, pathogen-specific testing should be performed (7–9). Genital ulcers are generally attributable to sexually transmitted infections but can also be caused by local trauma and other medical conditions such as Behçet disease, Crohn disease, lichen planus, carcinoma, leishmania, fixed drug eruptions, and drug toxicities.

Treatment should be based on clinical assessment and geographic prevalence of disease (Fig. 37.1). Treatment protocols are published periodically by the Centers for Disease Control and Prevention (CDC). Often a clinician must provide empiric treatment for several possible etiologies simultaneously (1).

Herpes

Genital herpes is most often caused by sexually transmitted herpes simplex virus 2 (HSV-2), but herpes simplex virus 1 (HSV-1) now accounts for up to 30% of first-episode cases (presumably related to increased orogenital transmission). HSV-2 is almost always sexually acquired. Genital herpes is a chronic infection, and the incidence can be assessed only indirectly. Data collected from the population-based U.S. National Health and Nutritional Examination Surveys, NHANES II (1976–1980) and NHANES III (1988–1994), showed that the seroprevalence of HSV-2 infection increased by 30% between those time periods (10). In the latter period, HSV-2 prevalence was 21.9% in persons 12 years of age or older, and higher in women and African Americans. Fewer than 10% of seropositive individuals report a history of genital lesions, and up to 60% of patients with newly acquired HSV-2 infection are asymptomatic (11). With education about the manifestations of genital herpes, up to 50% of patients who previously denied symptomatic disease are able to correctly identify HSV-2 outbreaks (12).

After infection, the incubation period ranges from 2 to 20 days, with a mean of 7 to 10 days (13–15). The classic presentation of primary infection is grouped vesicular lesions 1 to 3 mm wide on an erythematous

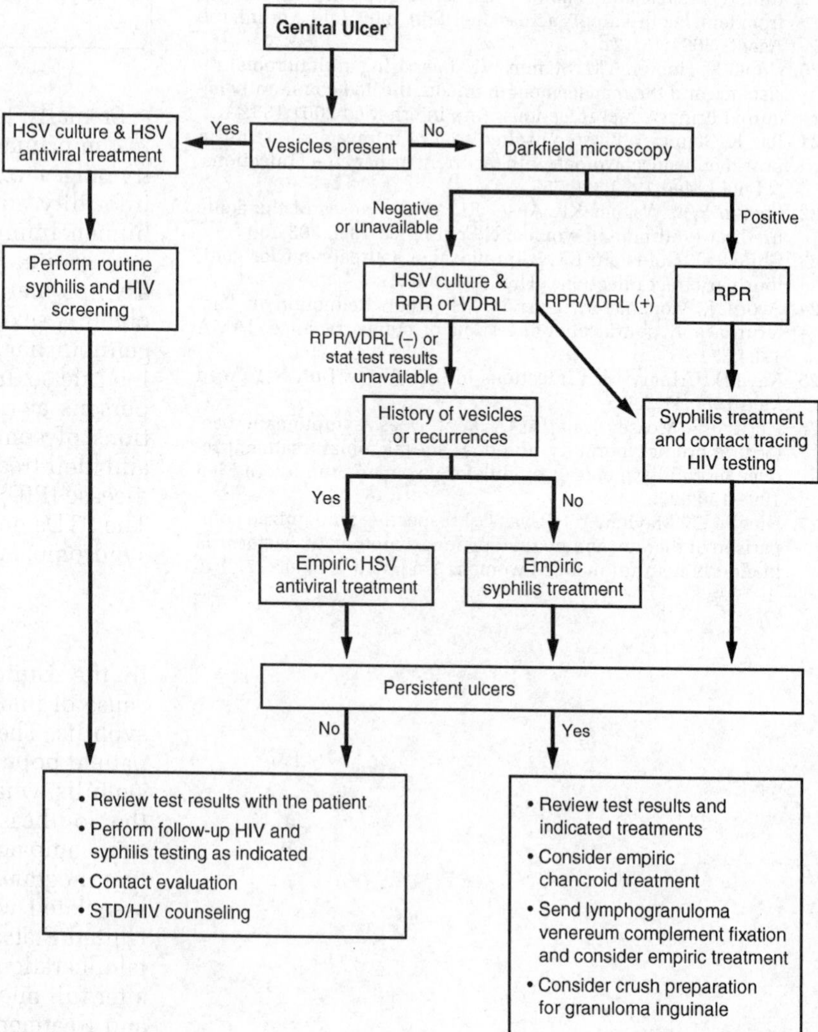

Figure 37.1. Evaluation and management of genital ulcer disease. (Important note: in outbreak settings, empiric treatment of suspected syphilis and chancroid should take priority.)

base. Without treatment, the vesicles persist for 10 to 12 days and then erode to form superficial ulcers that heal over 10 to 14 days. When symptomatic, the primary infection may have extragenital and constitutional symptoms including lymphadenopathy, fever, malaise, headache, dysuria, and hemorrhagic cervicitis.

HSV latency is established in the dorsal root ganglia of the sensory nerves innervating the infection site. The chronic phase of HSV infection is characterized by clinical recurrences and asymptomatic shedding (16,17). HSV-2 is associated with more frequent recurrences of genital lesions than is HSV-1. Higher recurrence rates are also associated with male gender and with a prolonged primary episode (younger age at acquisition) (16). Compared to the primary episode, recurrences tend to be less severe and shorter. They are often preceded by a prodrome, which can include burning, itching, or genital pain. Recurrence rates of HSV-2 vary but in a study of more than 400 people with HSV-2 infection, 38% had six or more recurrences in 1 year and 20% had ten or more (16). The highest risk of transmission is when active HSV lesions are present. Patients also shed virus when they are (2–4% of asymptomatic days), and patients are often unaware that asymptomatic shedding can transmit infection (18). On a population basis, the majority of HSV transmission occurs through asymptomatic shedding or by patients who are unaware of their infection.

Diagnosis

Except for a classic presentation, clinical diagnosis of genital herpes is difficult, and laboratory diagnostics should be used to evaluate genital lesions. Viral culture of lesion exudates is the most commonly used diagnostic test; it can also distinguish HSV-1 from HSV-2 infection, with concomitant prognostic implications. HSV culture sensitivity is highest in early disease, especially when vesicles are present. Antigen detection assays from swabs taken at the base of genital ulcers are more rapid than HSV culture and have higher sensitivity for HSV diagnosis in late-stage lesions but do not distinguish HSV-1 from HSV-2 (19). HSV DNA polymerase chain reaction (PCR) analysis of genital lesions has not been extensively studied but is a promising new diagnostic tool; it appears to have high sensitivity, but at this time is not approved by the U.S. Food and Drug Administration (FDA) (20). Papanicolaou smear and Tzanck preparations have low sensitivity.

Accurate type-specific serologic tests were not available until 1999. FDA-approved type-specific serologic assays for HSV are now available. These tests generally have sensitivities between 80% and 90% and specificities of 95% or greater (22–24). Patients seroconvert between 4 and 6 weeks after primary infection.

Use of HSV type-specific serology allows the clinician to manage difficult diagnoses and challenging counseling, such as assessing a patient with a past history of genital lesions and no diagnostic evaluation. Type-specific serologic testing can provide information regarding a patient's HSV status and thereby aids in proper counseling. Because many persons are unaware of their HSV infection, its is often difficult to determine by history whether a patient is still at risk of acquiring HSV when their sexual partner has a known history or a new diagnosis of HSV. In couples who are thought to be discordant for HSV-2 infection, type-specific serologies can clarify the true risk of acquiring new infection and can assist in counseling about sexual practices and HSV transmission.

The consequences of new HSV infection are most severe in neonates born to mothers who develop primary HSV infection during pregnancy or who have active ulcers during pregnancy. Knowing the serologic status of pregnant women and their partners would assist in counseling patients about the risks of HSV exposure in late pregnancy.

Treatment

Treatment of primary, symptomatic HSV can reduce fever and other constitutional symptoms within 48 hours (25). Skin lesions take longer to respond. Acute antiviral therapy will not cure the disease or change the subsequent natural history of recurrent disease. Treatment of recurrences can be given as episodic treatment. For patients who require episodic treatment, education regarding the symptoms of recurrences is an important part of management. These patients should have HSV antiviral medication on hand or a prescription they can readily fill when prodromal symptoms occur or lesions develop. Effective therapy for HSV recurrences requires that patients initiate treatment as early as possible—preferably within 1 day of lesion onset. Suppressive therapy can decrease the number of recurrences 70% to 80% while on therapy (1). In patients with six or more HSV recurrences in a year, suppressive antiviral treatment is effective and has been shown to significantly improve quality of life (26). The dose of antiretroviral medication needed to suppress HSV recurrences may be patient dependent, and individual titration may be necessary. Suppressive antiviral treatment also decreases asymptomatic shedding (27,28). In many patients, the frequency of HSV recurrences decreases over time. For this reason, suppressive therapy should be withdrawn periodically to re-evaluate the patient's requirements for treatment.

Antiviral therapy for HSV includes the nucleoside analogs acyclovir, famciclovir, and valacyclovir (Table 37.1). All of these agents interfere with the action of viral thymidine kinase. Famciclovir, a prodrug of penciclovir, and valacyclovir, a valine ester of acyclovir, have better absorption after oral dosing than acyclovir does. As a result, they can be taken less frequently, but they are more expensive. These drugs have little toxicity. Acyclovir has been found safe in patients using it daily for longer than 6 years (1). Topical acyclovir is not recommended for treatment of genital herpes.

In patients with HIV infection, HSV outbreaks may be more prolonged and severe, and these patients

Table 37.1. Oral Agents for Treatment of Genital Herpes

Drug	Dosage (mg)	Frequency	Duration (days)
First clinical episode			
Acyclovir	200	5 times a day	7–10
Acyclovir	400	t.i.d.	7–10
Famciclovir	250	t.i.d.	7–10
Valacyclovir	1,000	b.i.d.	7–10
Episodic therapy for recurrences			
Acyclovir	200	5 times a day	5
Acyclovir	400	t.i.d.	5
Acyclovir	800	b.i.d.	5
Famciclovir	125	b.i.d.	5
Valacyclovir	500	b.i.d.	3–5
Valacyclovir	1,000	q.d.	5
Daily suppressive therapy			
Acyclovir	400	b.i.d.	
Famciclovir	250	b.i.d.	
Valacyclovir[a]	500	q.d.	
Valacyclovir	1,000	q.d.	
Episodic therapy for recurrences in HIV-infected patients			
Acyclovir	200	5 times a day	5–10
Acyclovir	400	t.i.d.	5–10
Famciclovir	500	b.i.d.	5–10
Valacyclovir	1,000	b.i.d.	5–10
Daily suppressive therapy in HIV-infected patients			
Acyclovir	400–800	2–3 times a day	
Famciclovir	500	b.i.d.	
Valacyclovir	500	b.i.d.	

[a]Valacyclovir 500 mg q.d. may be less effective in patients with frequent recurrences (≥10 a year).

From Centers for Disease Control and Prevention. Guidelines for treatment of sexually transmitted diseases. Atlanta, GA: U.S. Department of Health and Human Services, 2002.

often require higher doses and prolonged courses of treatment for HSV. Severe episodes of HSV in immunocompromised patients, especially when HSV becomes disseminated, may necessitate hospital admission. Acyclovir-resistant HSV has been reported almost exclusively in immunosuppressed patients with prolonged exposure to the drug. Because their mechanism of action is similar, valacyclovir and famciclovir will also be ineffective. These patients require therapy with intravenous foscarnet. Patients with refractory HSV infection should have viral cultures and acyclovir drug-sensitivity testing performed at a reference center. Acyclovir-resistant HSV should be managed in consultation with an expert.

Along with antiviral therapy, counseling plays a central role in the care of patients with newly diagnosed HSV. Patients must be educated about the potential for recurrences and the availability of episodic and suppressive therapy. They should be aware that viral shedding not only occurs during the times of active lesions but also can occur during asymptomatic periods. With this in mind, they should be instructed to inform their sexual partners about their HSV status before sexual activity and to abstain from sex with uninfected partners when prodromal symptoms or active lesions are present. Patients also should be informed that the use of condoms might decrease the risk of transmission of HSV during asymptomatic periods (29). Men and women should be informed about the risks of neonatal herpes infection. Type-specific serologies for HSV may prove helpful in determining whether sexual partners are truly discordant for HSV-2 infection. Patients may obtain more HSV information by accessing informational Internet sites, including the CDC site (www.cdc.gov/nchstp/dstd/Fact_Sheets/facts_Genital_Herpes.htm; accessed 1/7/02) and the Planned Parenthood site (www.plannedparenthood.org/sti-safesex/herpes.htm; accessed 1/7/02).

Syphilis (Chancre)

For a discussion of the genital ulcers of syphilis (chancre), see the later section entitled Primary Syphilis.

Chancroid

Chancroid is caused by the gram-negative organism, *Haemophilus ducreyi.* It is relatively common in Africa, the Caribbean, and Southwest Asia but is seen infrequently in the United States. Chancroid has been seen in episodic outbreaks, especially associated with prostitution and drug use, and it is endemic in several large cities in the United States (30–32). Its incidence is likely underreported secondary to difficulties in diagnosis. In 1987 almost 5,000 cases were reported to the CDC, but in 1996 only 386 were reported (33).

The incubation period for chancroid is 4 to 7 days. Initially a papule forms; over several days, it erodes into a deep ulcer with irregular undermined borders. The ulcers are usually multiple, but they can be solitary, and they are extremely painful. Chancroid ulcers are friable and often have a purulent base. The ulcers are usually found on the coronal sulcus in circumcised men, on the prepuce in uncircumcised men, and on the labia or perineum in women (14). After 1 week, about 50% of patients develop inguinal lymphadenopathy, which is most often unilateral. Women are less likely to develop lymphadenopathy (34). Lymph nodes may become fluctuant and may rupture spontaneously. The combination of a painful ulcer and suppurative lymphadenopathy is almost pathognomonic for chancroid.

Definitive diagnosis of *H. ducreyi* requires isolation of the organism in special culture medium that is not commonly available. The sensitivity of culture is less than 80% (35). A Gram stain revealing short, wide, gram-negative rods in chains or clusters is suggestive of the diagnosis, but the sensitivity and specificity of Gram staining is generally thought to be poor (36). There is no FDA-approved PCR test for chancroid. Given these diagnostic limitations, the CDC treatment guidelines suggest that a probable diagnosis of chancroid can be based on the following criteria:

- One or more painful genital ulcers are present.
- *Treponema pallidum* is not identified on dark field examination of the ulcer exudates, and serologic

testing for syphilis is negative at least 7 days after onset of the ulcers.
- The presentation, ulcer appearance and, if present, lymphadenopathy are typical for chancroid.
- HSV culture of the ulcer exudates is negative.

The recommended treatments for chancroid include azithromycin, 1 g orally as a single dose; ceftriaxone, 250 mg intramuscularly in a single dose; ciprofloxacin, 500 mg orally twice a day for 3 days; or erythromycin base, 500 mg orally three times a day for 7 days (1). Few data are available regarding the efficacy of the short-term ceftriaxone and azithromycin regimens in HIV-infected patients. Pregnant or lactating women should avoid ciprofloxacin.

Clinical re-evaluation should be performed 3 to 7 days after initiation of therapy. Symptoms rapidly improve within 3 days after therapy begins, and clinical improvement of ulcers is usually evident in 7 days. Large ulcers may take longer than 2 weeks to heal. Healing of lymphadenopathy is slower, and large fluctuant lymph nodes may require aspiration or incision and drainage. Needle aspiration is less invasive, but patients often require re-aspiration, and for this reason incision and drainage may be preferred, because it tends to be more definitive therapy (37). Response to therapy may be slow or inadequate in uncircumcised men and in HIV-infected patients, and these patients should be monitored more closely (38–40). Overall, the cure rate with recommended therapy in HIV-negative patients is 92% or greater, and in HIV-positive patients it is 76% or greater (38–41).

Patients should be counseled to notify their recent sexual partners so that they may receive clinical evaluation and therapy if indicated. All persons who have had sexual contact with the patient within 10 days of the development of symptoms of chancroid should be treated empirically for chancroid even if no abnormalities are detected on examination. The patient should be provided HIV and syphilis testing at the time of diagnosis and instructed to return for repeat testing in 3 months (1).

Granuloma Inguinale (Donovanosis)

Granuloma inguinale is caused by the intracellular, encapsulated, short, gram-negative bacillus, *Calymmatobacterium granulomatis.* The disorder is found most commonly in tropical and subtropical areas and is rare in the United States. The incubation period is between 8 days and 12 weeks. It can manifest as large ulcerative lesions, erythematous papules with overlying granulation tissue, large papules resembling severe condyloma acuminatum, or expanding plaques of scar tissue (13). Most commonly it is a slowly progressive disorder with large, painless, friable ulcers with heaped up borders and "beefy" vascular bases. Lymphadenopathy is rare. Without treatment, granuloma inguinale is a slowly destructive process that can result in serious sequelae for the genitourinary tract. The organism is difficult to culture, and diagnosis relies on histopathology. A sample of tissue from the leading edge of an ulcer is placed between a slide and cover slip, crushed (crush preparation), and stained. The diagnosis of granuloma inguinale is made by identification of rods within cytoplasmic vacuoles of macrophages (Donovan bodies). Recommended treatments include doxycycline, 100 mg orally twice daily for at least 3 weeks, or trimethoprim–sulfamethoxazole, double-strength tablet twice daily for at least 3 weeks (1). Alternative regimens include ciprofloxacin, 750 mg twice daily for at least 3 weeks; erythromycin base, 500 mg four times a day for at least 3 weeks; or azithromycin, 1 g a week for at least 3 weeks. If lesions persist after 3 weeks of therapy has been completed, therapy should be extended until the lesions have healed completely. In patients with HIV infection, pregnant patients, and patients with slow improvement, gentamicin, 1 mg/kg intravenously every 8 hours, can be added. The benefit of empiric drug therapy for sexual contacts is not clear, but all sexual contacts within 60 days of the patient's symptom onset should be evaluated clinically.

Lymphogranuloma Venereum

Chlamydia trachomatis serovars L1, L2, and L3 are the causative organisms of lymphogranuloma venereum. The disease is rarely seen in the United States. The incubation period is between 3 and 40 days. The initial manifestation of disease is a painless papule at the site of inoculation, which erodes to form a small ulcer that heals in a few days. Patients develop painful inguinal adenopathy 7 to 30 days later, which often leads them to seek medical attention. By this time, the ulcerative lesion has usually resolved, and most patients do not recall the presence of an ulcer (13). The *groove sign* that is associated with lymphogranuloma venereum is caused by bulky lymphadenopathy that occurs on either side of the inguinal ligament but spares the area just overlying it. The major differential diagnosis is chancroid, which can produce similarly large nodes and buboes. Proctocolitis, perirectal abscesses, and rectal strictures are manifestations of lymphogranuloma venereum found in patients who engage in receptive anal intercourse (42–45). Definitive diagnosis is made by culture with serotyping of material from infected lymph nodes. However, culture is difficult, and diagnosis usually is made by clinical findings and complement fixation testing. A lymphogranuloma venereum complement fixation titer of 1:64 or greater is compatible with the diagnosis. The titer is not a useful tool for assessing severity or response to treatment and is nonspecific. Complement fixation titers can be positive in infection with non–L serovars of *C. trachomatis.* CDC guidelines recommend treatment with doxycycline, 100 mg orally twice daily for 21 days (1). Erythromycin base, 500 mg orally 4 times a day for 21 days is an alternative regimen that should be offered to pregnant or lactating women. Sexual contacts of the patient within 30 days of the development of symptoms should have clinical evaluation and urethral and cervical testing for *C. trachomatis*.

GENITAL WARTS

Genital warts are caused by infection with human papillomavirus (HPV), predominantly subtypes 6 and 11. In the United States, the prevalence of external genital warts is 1% in sexually active men and women 18 to 49 years of age (46). The prevalence of external genital warts varies by population screened and medical setting. Rates have been reported as low as 0.6% to 0.8% in health maintenance organizations and as high as 13% in STD clinics. Rates as high as 10% to 20% have been reported when both symptomatic and asymptomatic infection are assessed by sensitive HPV DNA direct-detection methods. Because many subtypes of HPV infection do not cause visible genital warts, many patients remain unaware of their infection. Risk factors for HPV infection in women include younger age, greater number of sexual partners, greater frequency of sexual intercourse, having a sex partner with genital warts, and, in some studies, failure to use condoms (46–49). In men, risk factors for genital warts include younger age, greater number of sex partners, failure to use condoms, previous STDs, and greater cigarette use (49,50). The relationship between oral contraceptive use and genital warts remains unclear (51–53). Patients with HIV or other forms of immunosuppression may be at higher risk for genital HPV infection (54,55).

HPV is a nonenveloped, double-stranded DNA virus. More than 70 HPV types have been identified, and more than 30 can infect the genital tract. HPV types 6 and 11 are the most common types causing visible genital warts, and they are rarely associated with cancers. They have been associated with laryngeal papillomatosis in infants born to women with genital warts. HPV subtypes 16, 18, 31, and 45 rarely cause visible warts and are closely associated with the development of cervical cancer and other genital cancers (56–59).

The natural history of HPV infection is variable. Genital warts may persist, enlarge, or spontaneously resolve. Spontaneous regression is more often associated with young age, and persistence is more common in immunosuppressed patients, such as those with HIV infection (60). Transmission of genital warts is primarily by sexual contact. HPV is thought to enter through minor breaks in the epithelial surface and to infect the basal cell layer (61). Given the tendency of HPV toward latent infection, the incubation period can be from months to years after acquisition.

Genital warts are most often asymptomatic, but they can be associated with pruritus, urethral or postcoital bleeding, irritation, and urethral or vaginal discharge (61). Genital warts can be located on the penis, vulva, scrotum, perineum, perianal skin, cervix, vagina, urethra, anus, or mouth. Perianal warts can occur in patients without a history of anal sex; intra-anal warts occur primarily in men and women who have had anal intercourse (62,63).

Genital warts are classified by their morphologic appearance: (a) condylomata acuminata are cauliflower-like lesions usually occurring on moist surfaces; (b) papular warts are dome-shaped lesions that are usually 1 to 4 mm in size and located on dry skin; (c) keratotic genital warts have a thickened horny surface, occur most frequently on dry skin, and are similar in appearance to common skin warts; (d) flat condylomata are subclinical lesions that are macular or slightly raised and can occur on dry or moist skin. Flat warts are generally not visible on direct examination and are most common on the cervix or on the external genitalia and perianal areas.

Diagnosis

Diagnosis of genital warts is accomplished by direct examination and can be aided by bright lighting and magnification. Anoscopy is recommended for evaluation of intra-anal warts in patients with a history of receptive anal intercourse (62). Visual inspection of the distal urethra and meatus should be performed for symptoms of terminal hematuria or abnormal urinary stream. Urethroscopy should also be considered in these cases. Because oral warts can be sexually transmitted, all patients should be questioned about oral symptoms and examined for oral warts (60). A complete examination of the genital tract should always be performed to accurately determine the extent of disease, because this may influence treatment options. The use of dilute acetic acid on areas with suspected HPV infection (acetowhite test) is not recommended because the predictive value is poor (64). HPV typing has not been shown to be of benefit in the management of genital warts.

If condylomata lata are suspected (see Secondary Syphilis), a sample for syphilis serology can be drawn and dark-field microscopy of fluid obtained from the lesions can be examined for signs of spirochetes. The clinical examination is usually diagnostic for genital warts, but biopsy should be considered when (a) the lesion is atypical; (b) the diagnosis is in doubt; (c) lesions progress during treatment; (d) there are early or frequent recurrences; (e) lesions are pigmented, indurated, ulcerated, or fixed to underlying structures; (f) individual lesions are larger than 1 cm; or (g) the patient is immunocompromised (60). Biopsy is particularly helpful when malignancy is suspected.

The differential diagnosis for genital warts is listed in Table 37.2. Bowenoid papulosis is a carcinoma *in situ* that is characterized by rough papules 2 to 4 mm in diameter with red-brown color. Buschke–Lowenstein tumor is a rare, low-grade invasive malignancy associated with HPV types 6 and 11. Bowen disease, squamous cell carcinoma, and basal cell carcinoma are other malignancies that are sometimes confused with genital warts and can be diagnosed by biopsy.

Table 37.2. Differential Diagnosis of External Anogenital Warts

Anatomic Variants	Pathologic Lesions
Skin tags	Bowenoid Papulosis
Nevi	Erythroplasia of Queyrat
Sebaceous (Tyson) glands	Bowen disease
Pearly penile papules	Condylomata lata (secondary syphilis)
Vestibular papillae	Buschke–Lowenstein tumor
	Benign tumors
	Seborrheic keratosis
	Molluscum contagiosum
	Lichen planus
	Psoriasis
	Squamous cell carcinoma

From Handsfield HH. Clinical presentation and natural course of anogenital warts. Am J Med 1997;102:16.

Treatment

Most current treatment strategies are based on destruction of the clinically visible affected tissue. The exception is imiquimod, an immune modulator, which works by enhancing the local cellular immune response. However, because infection can persist in histologically normal tissue, viral eradication and prevention of transmission to sexual partners is impossible. The goal of treatment is the alleviation of physical and psychological symptoms attributable to genital warts. The clinician must be aware and counsel the patient that side effects associated with treatment include pain, phimosis, preputial tightening, balanoposthitis, and superficial erosions or ulcerations that may facilitate the transmission of other STDs if appropriate precautions are not taken (60,62). Ablative therapy has been associated with hypopigmented and hyperpigmented scars and, rarely, hypertrophic or depressed scars (65,66). These are less likely if patients are given sufficient time to heal between treatments. Vulvadynia and other chronic pain syndromes have also been associated with ablative therapy (67). Given these risks, the possibility of spontaneous regression, and the limited benefits of treatment, patients should be aware that a decision to defer therapy and continue observation is acceptable.

Treatment can be provided by patient-applied therapy or provider-administered treatment (see later discussion). It is recommended that clinicians providing care for patients with genital warts be familiar with the use of at least one patient-applied therapy and one provider-administered therapy. If a patient has not improved significantly after three provider-administered treatments or has not had complete resolution after six treatments, the mode of treatment should be changed (1). There are insufficient data to suggest that any therapy is routinely superior to another. The choice of therapy is usually determined by wart size, wart number, anatomic site, morphology, patient preference, cost, convenience, adverse effects, risk of pregnancy, and provider experience.

Topical treatments are more effective on genital warts that are located on moist skin. In general, the first dose of patient-applied topical therapy should be applied by the clinician to demonstrate the appropriate technique of application and designate the warts to be treated. Podofilox, imiquimod, and podophyllin resin are not recommended for use during pregnancy. Surgical wart treatments are more effective than other modes of therapy in treating patients with extensive disease, oral warts, or disease on internal mucosal surfaces. Cervical warts require evaluation for squamous intraepithelial lesions and should be managed by an expert. Trichloroacetic acid (TCA) or bichloroacetic acid (BCA) and cryotherapy without use of the cryoprobe are recommended for treatment of vaginal warts. Genital warts located at the urethral meatus can be treated with cryotherapy, podophyllin resin, podofilox, or imiquimod. Recommended treatment for anal warts includes cryotherapy, TCA/BCA, and surgical methods. Surgical removal and cryotherapy are the recommended treatments for oral warts. For patients using patient-applied therapy, a follow-up visit several weeks into therapy may be useful to assess the adequacy and side effects of treatment. Risk of recurrent disease is greatest in the first 3 months after therapy.

Patient-Applied Therapy. Podofilox (Condylox) is an antimitotic agent that is the major active ingredient in podophyllin resin. Its use should be limited to a wart area of 10 cm^2 or less and a total volume of 0.5 mL/day or less (1). Podofilox 0.5% solution or gel should be applied twice daily for 3 days followed by 4 days without therapy. Treatment can be repeated for up to four cycles if needed.

Imiquimod (Aldara) is an immune stimulator. It enhances levels of interferon alpha, tumor necrosis factor, and interleukin-6 (68,69). Imiquimod 5% cream should be applied three times a week at bedtime (1). The application should be washed off with soap and water after 6 to 10 hours. In men with warts on dry skin, daily treatment may be more effective. Treatment may be continued for up to 16 weeks if needed (1).

Provider-Administered Therapy. Cryotherapy, usually with liquid nitrogen, destroys warts by cryocytolysis. It should be avoided in patients with cryoglobulinemia. The use of a cryoprobe is not recommended for the treatment of vaginal warts because of the risk of vaginal perforation and fistula formation (1). The skill and experience of the clinician in the application of cryotherapy greatly affect the efficacy and toxicity of treatment. Pain and even blistering are not uncommon. Use of topical or local anesthetics may facilitate treatment application. Cryotherapy is effective for warts on dry or moist skin. Treatments can be repeated every 1 to 2 weeks after adequate healing has occurred.

Podophyllin resin (Podofin) is an antimitotic plant compound that does not have a standardized formulation (70). It is less effective in treating warts on dry skin. Podophyllin use should be limited to a wart area of 10 cm^2 or less and a total volume of 0.5 mL per session or less (1). Podophyllin resin 10% to 25% should be applied to warts in a thin layer and allowed to dry thoroughly. Spread of the compound to normal tissues from overapplication or incomplete drying can cause significant local irritation. The patient should wash the resin off 1 to 4 hours after application. Application can be repeated weekly.

TCA (Tri-Chlor) and BCA cause chemical coagulation of proteins and thereby destroy warts. These agents work best on warts located on moist skin. TCA or BCA 80% to 90% is applied in a thin coat and allowed to dry (1). Application can be repeated weekly as needed. As with podophyllin, overapplication or incomplete drying can result in spread of the compound and damage to surrounding tissues. TCA or BCA can be neutralized with soap or sodium bicarbonate if needed.

Surgical removal by tangential scissor excision, tangential shave excision, curettage, or electrosurgery has the benefit of producing an immediate wart-free state. Surgical modes of treatment are useful for treating extensive disease but can also be used for wart areas of average size. These techniques usually require local anesthesia.

Other Treatments. Intralesional interferon has antiviral immunomodulating effects. However, this treatment requires painful intralesional injections and can be associated with systemic interferon toxicities as well as local reactions. Laser treatments are usually reserved for patients with extensive disease, genital warts refractory to other treatments, or intraurethral warts and require operator expertise.

Patients diagnosed with genital warts require counseling regarding the natural history of the disease and the associations between HPV infection and genital cancers. Patients should be aware that genital HPV infection is generally a chronic disease. It is almost always sexually transmitted, but the incubation period is long and the new appearance of genital warts does not necessarily imply a new or recent exposure. The efficacy of condoms in prevention of transmission is incomplete. Patients should be encouraged to disclose their STD history when initiating a sexual relationship with a new partner. Patients should be aware that the HPV types that are associated with cancer do not generally cause visible genital warts. HPV types associated with genital warts are unlikely to lead to malignancy. Women should be encouraged to continue regular Papanicolaou smears according to standard recommendations. Patients often perceive the diagnosis of genital warts as stigmatizing. Providing detailed information about the disease, its natural history, and treatment may ease some of the psychological distress associated with a diagnosis of a chronic STD. Counseling should also dispel misconceptions about cancer risks associated with genital warts and allow for a review of appropriate cervical cancer screening. Patients can obtain more information about genital warts and HPV infection on the Internet (www.plannedparenthood.org/sti/hpvfacts1.html; www.ama-assn.org/special/std/support/educate/stdhpv.htm; both accessed 1/7/02) or by contacting the CDC National STD Hotline, telephone number 1-800-227-8922.

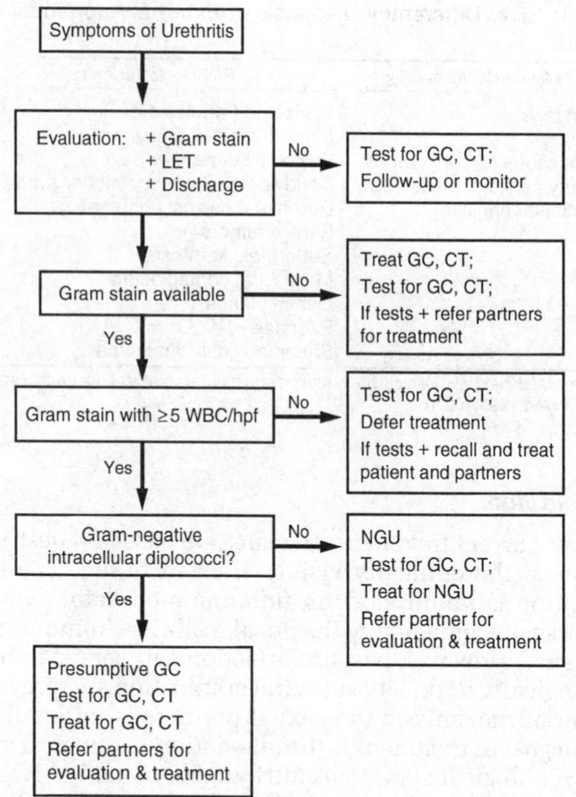

Figure 37.2. Management of symptomatic male urethritis. CT, *Chlamydia trachomatis*; GC, *Neisseria gonorrhoeae*; LET, leukocyte esterase test (urine); NGU, nongonoccocal urethritis. (Adapted from Burstein GR, Zenilman JM. Nongonococcal urethritis: a new paradigm. Clin Infect Dis 1999;28[Suppl 1]:S66.)

URETHRITIS AND CERVICITIS

Urethritis is characterized by dysuria and urethral discharge. Urethritis in men can be caused by several different pathogens, but for treatment purposes it is generally divided into two categories: gonococcal urethritis and nongonococcal urethritis (NGU). The presence of urethritis is confirmed by the clinical finding of mucopurulent discharge, Gram staining of a urethral swab with 5 or more white blood cells (WBCs) per oil immersion field, a positive leukocyte esterase test on first-void urine, or more than 10 WBCs per high-power field on microscopy of first-void urine (1). If a patient with urethral symptoms does not meet any of these criteria, he should be evaluated for gonorrhea and chlamydia but generally should not be offered empiric treatment until results of the evaluation are available. An approach to male urethritis is outlined in Fig. 37.2.

Mucopurulent cervicitis (MPC) is most commonly asymptomatic, but some women report abnormal discharge or vaginal bleeding. On examination there is mucopurulent or purulent endocervical discharge visible at the cervical os or on endocervical swab. The cervix may also be friable with easy bleeding. Women with evidence of MPC should be carefully evaluated for gonorrhea and chlamydia, but in most cases, there is no identifiable cause (1). In most women, chlamydia or gonorrhea infection is not characterized by MPC. Generally, treatment should be given only if test results confirm infection. However, in outbreak settings or in patients at high risk who are unlikely to return for test results, clinicians may consider empiric treatment for gonorrhea and/or chlamydia.

Neisseria gonorrhoeae

Gonorrhea causes an estimated 600,000 new infections each year in the United States (1). Surveillance through the CDC in 1997 demonstrated an incidence in women that peaks between the ages of 15 to 19 years and falls off rapidly after age 24 years. In men, incidence rates peak between ages 20 to 24 years and fall off significantly after age 29. Rates of gonorrhea reported to the CDC declined between 1980 and 1997. Gonorrhea is associated with younger age, non-Caucasian race, single marital status, illicit drug use, higher numbers of sexual partners, and casual or new sex partners (71–77).

N. gonorrhoeae is a gram-negative diplococcus. It is transmitted exclusively by sexual and perinatal exposure. Risk of transmission appears to be greatest from male to female during single episodes of vaginal intercourse and from female to male with multiple episodes of vaginal intercourse (78–81). Oral sex is believed to be relatively inefficient in the transmission of gonorrhea (82).

Clinical Presentation

The most common manifestations of gonorrhea infection are urethritis in men and cervicitis in women. Urethritis usually manifests 1 to 10 days after exposure and is characterized by purulent discharge and dysuria (83). A small fraction of men with gonococcal urethritis are asymptomatic (84). If left untreated, most cases of gonococcal urethritis resolve spontaneously after several weeks. Local complications of gonococcal urethritis include epididymitis, penile edema, acute prostatitis, seminal vesiculitis, and periurethral abscesses (83).

In women, the primary sites of infection are the endocervix and the urethra. Unlike men, many women do not develop overt symptoms of infection (85). When present, symptoms usually occur within 10 days and may include abnormal vaginal discharge, dysuria, or abnormal vaginal bleeding (83). Local complications of gonococcal cervicitis include infection of the Bartholin glands, salpingitis, pelvic inflammatory disease (PID) and perihepatitis (Fitz-Hugh–Curtis syndrome). Long-term complications include infertility and ectopic pregnancy.

Other than the male urethra and the cervix, gonorrhea can less commonly manifest in the anorectal area, in the oropharynx, or as disseminated gonococcal infection (DGI). Women and homosexual men may have asymptomatic anorectal gonorrheal infection or manifestations such as anal pruritus, purulent discharge, rectal bleeding, or tenesmus (86). Oropharyngeal infection is also most common in women and homosexual men and is most commonly asymptomatic (82). DGI occurs in less than 3% of all gonorrhea infections in the United States (87) and is caused by specific *N. gonorrhoeae* strains that are less likely to cause genital inflammation but more likely to cause bacteremia and disseminated disease (88). The prevalence of these strains in the United States has been decreasing. DGI is characterized by petechial or pustular skin lesions (Fig. 37.3), asymmetric arthralgia, tenosynovitis, or septic arthritis. Some patients develop septic arthritis without associated rash, arthralgias/polyarthritis, or genital disease. Less commonly, DGI is associated with osteomyelitis, endocarditis, meningitis, perihepatitis, and, in extreme cases, adult respiratory distress syndrome or the Waterhouse–Friderichsen syndrome.

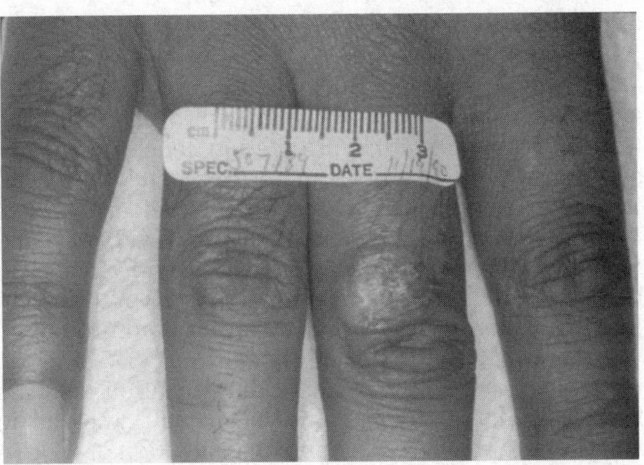

Figure 37.3. Disseminated gonococcal infection: skin lesion over the second promixal interphalangeal joint. (Photograph courtesy of Jonathan Zenilman, M.D.)

Diagnosis

The choice of diagnostic test for gonorrhea depends on the anatomic site being evaluated. In symptomatic men with urethritis, a Gram stain of urethral discharge has a sensitivity and specificity of 94% or better (89–92). Diagnosis is made by demonstration of intracellular gram-negative diplococci. To collect the male urethral sample, one hand is placed over the dorsal surface of the penis while the other attempts to move secretions forward through a stripping motion from the base of the penis to the glans. A swab is then inserted approximately 1 cm into the urethra and kept in place for approximately 30 seconds in order to absorb discharge. This sample can be used for Gram stain and gonorrhea culture. Gram staining of endocervical secretions has much lower sensitivity and therefore is not as valuable (92). When obtaining endocervical samples, the ectocervix is first cleaned with a large swab, than a small swab is inserted into the cervical os and allowed to absorb fluids for approximately 30 seconds. If STDs are of concern, samples should be obtained for gonorrhea and chlamydia testing before obtaining samples for Papanicolaou smear.

Culture is relatively inexpensive, can be performed at any site, and allows for antibiotic susceptibility testing. Nucleic acid hybridization techniques have sensitivity and specificity of approximately 85% and 98%, respectively (93). New nucleic acid amplification tests, such as ligase chain reaction (LCR) tests and PCR tests, have excellent sensitivity and specificity (approximately 95% and 99%, respectively) and allow gonorrhea testing with the use of self-administered vaginal swabs (94,95). LCR also allows for testing on urine specimens. Nucleic acid amplification tests are more expensive and have not been well assessed in rectal or oropharyngeal gonorrhea detection or in low-prevalence populations (93).

Treatment

Treatment of gonorrhea also depends on the site of infection. In general, when treating gonorrhea, it is also recommended to treat chlamydia empirically unless known rates of coinfection are low, sensitive chlamydia testing is available, and the patient is likely to return for results and treatment if needed. When choosing therapy, a clinician must consider geographic trends in antibiotic resistance. As of the year 2001, quinolone-resistant *N. gonorrhoeae* (QRNG) was common in parts of Asia and the Pacific (1). In the United States, gonorrhea antibiotic resistance and QRNG are monitored by the CDC's Gonococcal Isolate Surveillance Project (GISP). Quinolone therapy should be avoided in the treatment of infections acquired in Hawaii, the Pacific, or Asia. Quinolones are generally not recommended for pregnant women.

Recommendations for treatment of gonococcal cervicitis, urethritis, and rectal infection include single doses of cefixime, 400 mg orally; ceftriaxone, 125 mg intramuscularly; ciprofloxacin, 500 mg orally; ofloxacin, 400 mg orally; or levofloxacin, 250 mg orally (1). Other cephalosporins and quinolones may also be effective and can serve as alternative regimens when recommended regimens are unavailable. Spectinomycin, 2 g intramuscularly as a single dose, serves as an alternative regimen that is useful for patients who are intolerant of cephalosporins or quinolones, but it may not be available in some areas. Treatment of urogenital and rectal infections with the recommended regimens is effective in more than 95% of patients. Treatment of oropharyngeal infections is less effective, with reliable treatment limited to ceftriaxone 125 mg intramuscularly in a single dose or ciprofloxacin, 500 mg orally in a single dose.

Most patients with DGI require hospitalization for initial treatment. The preferred regimen is ceftriaxone, 1 g intramuscularly or intravenously daily. Other acceptable regimens include cefotaxime, 1 g, or ceftizoxime, 1 g, intravenously every 8 hours; ciprofloxacin, 400 mg, or ofloxacin, 400 mg, intravenously every 12 hours; levofloxacin, 250 mg intravenously daily; or spectinomycin, 2 g intramuscularly every 12 hours. Intravenous or intramuscular therapy should be continued for 1 to 2 days after the patient has improved clinically. Oral therapy with cefixime, 400 mg, ciprofloxacin, 500 mg, or ofloxacin, 400 mg twice daily, or with levofloxacin, 500 mg daily, should be continued until the patients has completed a 7-day course. Intravenous therapy with ceftriaxone, 1 to 2 g every 12 hours, should be extended to 10 to 14 days for evidence of meningitis or to 4 weeks for evidence of endocarditis.

According to the CDC STD treatment guidelines, all sexual contacts within 60 days of symptom onset or diagnosis of gonorrhea should be referred for medical evaluation and treatment of gonorrhea and chlamydia (1). If the patient has not been sexually active in the last 60 days, the last sexual contact should be evaluated and treated. The patient should be counseled to abstain from sexual activity until treatment is complete, symptoms have resolved, and sexual partners have been treated and are symptom free. Given the often-asymptomatic state of gonorrhea infection in women, screening of women at high risk for infection is important to control local rates of disease.

Chlamydia trachomatis

The peak incidence of chlamydia in men and women in the United States is between the ages of 15 and 29 years. Rates of chlamydia infection reported to the CDC increased between 1987 and 1997. Risk factors for chlamydia infection in women include young age, nonwhite race, low socioeconomic status, a new sex partner in the last 90 days, multiple sex partners, and failure to use condoms (96–98). Risk factors in men are less well defined but younger age, heterosexual sex, and nonwhite race are associated with infection (99–101).

Clinical Presentation

C. trachomatis is an obligate intracellular parasite (102). It exists in two different forms during its life cycle. The extracellular form is metabolically inert and is known as an elementary body. Once inside a cell, chlamydia transforms into the reticulate body, which is the metabolically active, replicative form. *C. trachomatis* infection can cause inclusion conjunctivitis, urethritis, cervicitis, epididymitis, PID, infertility, ectopic pregnancy, reactive arthritis (Reiter syndrome), proctocolitis, and perinatal infections. There is also some evidence that chlamydia infection may increase the risk of HIV acquisition (103). The effects of chlamydia infection on cervical HIV-1 viral shedding and transmission remain unclear (104,105).

Asymptomatic genital infection is common in men and women (101,106). In men, symptomatic urethritis caused by chlamydia has an incubation period between 7 and 14 days. Men may develop dysuria and penile discharge, but the discharge is usually less purulent and less abundant than that associated with gonorrhea. The discharge is clear to gray in color. Epididymitis can occur as a complication of chlamydia infection and is usually unilateral.

The majority of women with cervical or urethral chlamydia infection are asymptomatic or have only minimal symptoms (106). When symptoms are present, they may include dysuria, discharge, or abnormal bleeding. Women with PID associated with chlamydia tend to have a more subacute course (107), but they can have severe PID with associated perihepatitis. Long-term sequelae of symptomatic or asymptomatic PID include infertility and ectopic pregnancy (see Chapter 102).

Diagnosis

In men, a diagnosis of NGU can be established by obtaining a urine specimen and urethral swab (see Gonorrhea). Diagnostic criteria include 5 or more WBCs per oil immersion field on Gram stain, a positive leukocyte esterase test on first-void urine, or 10 or more WBCs per oil immersion field in first-void urine, without evidence of gram-negative diplococci on Gram stain. In women, a swab of endocervical secretions should be obtained for testing (see Gonorrhea).

The specific diagnosis of chlamydia requires culture, nucleic acid hybridization, antigen detection, or an amplification assay (PCR or LCR). Culture is the most specific test, but it can be technically and logistically difficult. In general, hybridization techniques and antigen detection have lower sensitivity than amplification tests such as PCR or LCR (94). LCR and PCR can be used on urine, self-administered swab samples, or clinician-obtained swabs (94,95). Rectal infection should be evaluated with chlamydia culture.

Treatment

Treatment for chlamydia should be given to all patients with a positive diagnostic evaluation for chlamydia. Given the high rates of gonorrhea and chlamydia coinfection in some regions, chlamydia treatment should also be considered in all patients with evidence of gonorrhea infection. The treatment regimens recommended by the CDC guidelines for uncomplicated urethritis or cervicitis include azithromycin, 1 g orally in a single dose, or doxycycline, 100 mg orally twice daily for 7 days. These two recommended treatments have equal efficacy, but azithromycin treatment has the benefit of being single-dose therapy, which may facilitate better compliance (108,109). Alternative regimens include erythromycin base, 500 mg orally four times a day for 7 days; erythromycin ethylsuccinate, 800 mg orally four times a day for 7 days; or ofloxacin, 300 mg twice a day, or levofloxacin, 500 mg orally daily, for 7 days.

Doxycycline and quinolones are contraindicated in pregnancy. Therefore, during pregnancy patients should be given erythromycin base, 500 mg orally four times a day for 7 days, or amoxicillin, 500 mg orally three times a day for 7 days. These therapies are equally efficacious, but amoxicillin has been associated with fewer gastrointestinal side effects (110). Alternative regimens in pregnant women include erythromycin base, 250 mg orally four times a day for 14 days, or erythromycin ethylsuccinate, 800 mg orally four times a day for 7 days or 400 mg orally four times a day for 14 days. Pregnant women should not be given erythromycin estolate, because it has been associated with hepatotoxicity. Azithromycin, 1 g orally as a single dose, is also an acceptable alternative in pregnant women but has not been as extensively studied. Treatment regimens for complicated chlamydia infections are provided in the sections on epididymitis (later in this chapter) and PID (see Chapter 102).

Patients being treated for chlamydia infection should be instructed to abstain from sexual activities until symptoms have resolved and 7 days have passed since their single-dose azithromycin treatment or until they have completed a 7-day course of recommended antibiotic therapy (1). All sex partners in the last 60 days should be evaluated and treated. If the patient's last sexual contact was longer than 60 days before onset of symptoms or diagnosis of chlamydia, that partner should be evaluated and treated for chlamydia. The patient should be instructed to abstain from sexual activities with any partners until they have been evaluated and completed treatment. As a result of concerns about efficacy and compliance, the CDC recommends that patients treated with erythromycin or amoxicillin be re-evaluated for chlamydia approximately 3 weeks after completion of therapy. Adolescents have high rates of reinfection after diagnosis of chlamydia, and for this reason it is also recommended to retest these patients 3 to 6 months after chlamydia treatment (111).

All sexually active women should also be screened for asymptomatic chlamydia infection. Pregnant women younger than 25 years of age with risk factors such as new or multiple sex partners should be targeted for additional chlamydia screening to prevent infection of neonates.

Nongonococcal Urethritis

Men with clinical or laboratory evidence of urethritis in the absence of gonorrhea infection are diagnosed with NGU. In the United States, 2 million cases of NGU are estimated to occur yearly (112). The etiologic agents of NGU include *C. trachomatis*, *Ureaplasma urealyticum*, *Mycoplasma genitalium*, and *Trichomonas vaginalis*. Chlamydia is the most common cause of NGU, but its prevalence in men with urethritis appears to be declining (113). In recent studies, chlamydia accounted for 15% to 41% of cases of NGU (112,114–119). The etiologic role of ureaplasma is not as well defined, but estimates of prevalence for ureaplasma are between 9% and 42% of NGU cases (112,115–119). Data connecting *M. genitalium* infection with symptomatic NGU are accumulating, and this pathogen may account for 15% to 25% of cases (114–116,120,121). *T. vaginalis* is found in 3% to 20% of men screened by urethral culture and has been clearly associated with symptoms and clinical findings of NGU (122–126). One study suggested that the prevalence of trichomonas in men may increase with age (124). In men older than 30 years of age, trichomonas and chlamydia were both identified in about 13%

of NGU cases. Rarely, HSV may be responsible for findings of NGU. Despite improved diagnostics, a significant number of NGU cases have no identifiable etiology (113,115).

Men with symptoms compatible with urethritis should be evaluated for clinical findings that confirm the diagnosis. The patient must have examination findings, urethral Gram stain results, or evidence by urine microscopy or analysis that are compatible with urethritis (see Urethritis). All such patients should be evaluated with Gram staining when available. Specific tests for gonorrhea and chlamydia should be performed as outlined previously. Testing for ureaplasma and mycoplasma is not routinely available or recommended. Trichomonas cultures of urethral swabs or centrifuged urine are recommended only for patients for whom initial therapy has failed.

Patients with clinical evidence of NGU should be treated with azithromycin, 1 g orally as a single dose, or with doxycycline, 100 mg orally twice daily for 7 days (1). Azithromycin is considerably more expensive than doxycycline, but it can be given as directly observed therapy. Failure of therapy is higher in patients with nonchlamydial NGU (113,118). Alternative regimens include erythromycin base, 500 mg orally four times a day for 7 days; erythromycin ethylsuccinate, 800 mg orally four times a day for 7 days; and either ofloxacin at 300 mg twice a day or levofloxacin at 500 mg a day for 7 days.

Patients with recurrent or persistent symptoms should be questioned about compliance with therapy and possible re-exposure. Other possible reasons for persistent symptoms are infection with tetracycline-resistant ureaplasma and infection with trichomonas (127). Culture for trichomonas infection should be performed. When re-evaluating patients with persistent symptoms, clinicians should be aware that urine PCR and LCR tests for chlamydia should not be used for re-evaluation within 3 weeks after treatment, because these tests can remain positive after therapy (128). Treatment of recurrent or persistent urethritis in patients without re-exposure or noncompliance with initial treatment should include metronidazole, 2 g orally as a single dose, with erythromycin base, 500 mg orally four times a day for 7 days, or erythromycin ethylsuccinate, 800 mg orally four times a day for 7 days (1).

Patients should be instructed to abstain from sexual activity for 7 days after initiating therapy and to refer their partners for evaluation. Unless specific testing for chlamydia is negative, all partners should be evaluated and treated for chlamydia. Partners of patients with documented trichomonas urethritis should also be referred for evaluation and treatment with metronidazole. In patients with urethritis in whom neither gonorrhea, chlamydia, nor trichomonas is identified, partner referral for evaluation is not routinely indicated.

EPIDIDYMITIS

After puberty, approximately 75% of cases of acute scrotal pain are caused by epididymitis. The most common etiologic agent depends on the age group and associated risk factors. Chlamydia and gonorrhea are the most common causes of epididymitis in sexually active men before 35 years of age (129); chlamydia is responsible for the bulk of disease (130). Men in this age group who are involved in insertive anal intercourse are also at risk for infection with enteric bacteria (131,132). Men older than 35 years and men with recent instrumentation of the urinary tract are at greatest risk for infection with enteric bacteria, although chlamydia and gonorrhea still play an important role.

Infection usually begins in the urethra or bladder and spreads to the epididymis and sometimes to the testes. The preceding urethral infection due to chlamydia and gonorrhea is asymptomatic in up to 50% of cases (132). The exposure to gonorrhea or chlamydia can occur months before symptoms develop. Patients may report preceding and concurrent dysuria and urethral discharge followed by the gradual onset of unilateral scrotal pain initially localized to the epididymis. If untreated, patients develop fever and progressive diffuse unilateral scrotal pain, edema, and erythema. A reactive hydrocele is not uncommon.

The differential diagnosis of epididymitis includes testicular torsion, torsion of the testicular appendage, testicular rupture associated with trauma, traumatic hematoma, inguinal hernia, scrotal abscess, hydrocele, varicocele, viral orchitis, testicular neoplasm, Fournier gangrene, Henoch–Schünlein purpura, renal colic, peritonitis or intraperitoneal hemorrhage with a patent processus vaginalis, and a leaking abdominal aortic aneurysm (see Chapter 97) (132). Testicular torsion and torsion of the testicular appendage are the most common alternative diagnoses (133). Expeditious diagnosis of testicular torsion is critical, because the total time of ischemia determines the viability of the testes. Therefore, when evaluating acute scrotal pain, clinicians must consider the history, risk factors, and clinical examination findings. A history of previous episodes of scrotal pain that resolved without intervention is compatible with intermittent or recurrent testicular torsion (134–136). Classically, the pain of testicular torsion is acute in onset and severe, but there is significant overlap in the clinical presentations of the common causes of acute scrotal pain. Physical findings suggestive of testicular torsion include an abnormal axis of the affected testicle, an abnormal position of the epididymis, an abnormal axis of the unaffected testicle, and abnormal elevation of the affected testicle with a palpable twist of the spermatic cord (134). Any findings on history or physical examination that are suggestive of testicular torsion should prompt emergency urologic evaluation.

Clinical findings suggestive of epididymitis were outlined by Knight and Vassy: (a) gradual onset of pain; (b) dysuria, urethral discharge, or recent genitourinary instrumentation; (c) a history of urinary tract infection, imperforate anus, neurogenic bladder, or genitourinary surgery; (d) fever of more than 101°F (38.3°C); (e) tenderness and induration at the epididymis; and (f) urinary analysis showing 10 or more WBCs or red blood cells per high-power field (134). Patients with three or more of these findings are likely to have epididymis. Evaluation of patients with epididymitis should include Gram stain and culture (or other sensitive tests) of a urethral swab for evidence of gonorrhea or chlamydia and sampling of first-void urine for leukocyte count, Gram stain, and culture (see Urethritis) (1). Patients with suspected gonorrhea or chlamydia infection should also be screened for syphilis and HIV infection.

Empiric treatment should be initiated at the time of first evaluation. Treatment in patients with a high risk of sexually transmitted epididymitis should include ceftriaxone, 250 mg intramuscularly as a single dose, with doxycycline, 100 mg orally twice daily for 10 days, or treatment with ofloxacin, 300 mg orally twice daily or levofloxacin, 500 mg orally daily for 10 days (1). In patients with epididymitis that is more likely caused by gram-negative enteric bacteria and in patients who are intolerant of cephalosporins or tetracyclines, treatment with levofloxacin (500 mg orally daily for 10 days) is recommended. Symptomatic treatment should include bed rest, scrotal elevation, and antipyretics/analgesics. Hospital admission should be considered for patients with fever, testicular abscess, toxic appearance, severe pain, immunocompromise, a history of noncompliance, or intolerance of oral intake.

Patients should have significant improvement in 3 days. Patients who fail to improve appropriately or whose symptoms do not completely resolve with treatment should be re-evaluated with consideration of the differential diagnosis outlined previously. These patients may benefit from diagnostic imaging and urosurgical evaluation. Treatment failure may indicate error in the initial diagnosis or infection with an antibiotic-resistant or atypical organism. Tuberculosis, brucellosis, Bacille Calmette-Guérin (BCG), and fungal infections are rare causes of epididymitis. If gonorrhea or chlamydia infection is suspected or proven, all of the patient's sexual partners in the last 60 days should be referred for medical evaluation and treatment. If the patient's last sexual activity was more than 60 days before diagnosis, the last partner should be referred to medical care. The patient and his sexual partners should abstain from sexual activity until symptoms have resolved and treatment has been completed.

SYPHILIS

Syphilis caused significant morbidity and mortality in the first half of the century, but after the introduction of penicillin in the 1940s, the rates of disease in the United States declined significantly (137,138). Since then, there have been epidemics at 7- to 10-year intervals. In the late 1980s, syphilis was associated with crack cocaine use and sex-for-drugs prostitution (138–140). More recently, the focus of outbreak has been in the gay community overall, and nonwhite minorities are disproportionately affected (137). Aside from the known sequelae of cardiovascular and neurologic disease and the continued morbidity from congenital syphilis, syphilis facilitates HIV transmission. The HIV epidemic, the concentration of new syphilis cases in specific geographic locations, the disproportionate impact on minority populations, and the availability of new biomedical and public health tools led the CDC to call for a new drive for syphilis elimination in 1998.

Syphilis control requires the rapid treatment of newly identified cases, aggressive contact tracing, and active screening by primary care providers. In most office settings, asymptomatic, sexually active patients should be screened for syphilis at their first visit with a nontreponemal serologic test and retested at follow-up visits if they report high-risk behaviors or have been diagnosed with another STD.

Syphilis is caused by *Treponema pallidum*. The clinical manifestations vary during the various stages of disease (Table 37.3).

Primary Syphilis

Primary syphilis is classically characterized by the development of a chancre, a painless ulcer with indurated edges and a clean base. A chancre forms 10 to 90 days (average, 21 days) after infection. Lesions begin as painless papules at the sites of sexual contact, most commonly on the genitals. Extragenital chancres are infrequent but occur primarily in the mouth (141). Approximately 30% of affected patients have multiple lesions. Chancres are frequently associated with painless regional and generalized lymphadenopathy. This painless, initial stage of disease can easily be missed, and up to 60% of patients diagnosed with syphilis have no history of ulcerative lesions (141). (See Genital Ulcer Disease for a discussion of the differential diagnosis.)

Secondary Syphilis

Approximately 50% of patients with untreated primary syphilis will develop signs of secondary syphilis. The onset of secondary syphilis usually occurs between 6 weeks and 6 months after infection. In 15% to 20% of patients, the primary chancre is still present. Secondary syphilis is a systemic disorder, the classic manifestation of which is a maculopapular, follicular, or occasionally pustular rash. The rash can be widespread and often affects the palms and soles (Fig. 37.4). Patchy alopecia may result from follicular involvement on the scalp or along the eyelids. Oral lesions known as mucous patches occur in 5% to 22% of patients and manifest as gray lesions on an erythematous base (142). Flat, waxy, wart-like lesions usually found in the moist intertriginous regions of the genital or anal areas are known as *condylomata lata*. Both mucous patches and condylomata lata are highly infectious.

Constitutional symptoms of malaise, low-grade fever, headache, and generalized lymphadenopathy are common in patients with secondary syphilis. Asymptomatic meningitis and cranial nerve palsies may also occur (141). Other, infrequent manifestations of secondary syphilis include anorexia, nausea, vomiting, jaundice, granulomatous hepatitis, proteinuria,

Table 37.3. Outline of the Clinical Stages of Syphilis

Stage	Characteristic Findings	Usual Onset after Exposure	Duration of Stage in Untreated Patients	Dark Field
Primary	Chancre—may be absent or not visible (e.g., in vagina or mouth)	10–90 days (average, 21 days)	2–6 wk	+ (Chancre, lymph nodes)
Secondary	Rash, condyloma latum, lymphadenopathy	6 wk to 6 mo	2–6 wk; recurrences in 25% over 4 yr	+ (Especially moist lesions)
Latent			May be lifelong because only ⅓ of untreated patients develop tertiary syphilis	Negative
Early	None	<1 yr after infection		
Late	None	>1 yr after infection		
Late (tertiary)				
Benign	Gumma	2–10 yr	Indolent	Negative
Cardiovascular	Aortic aneurysm Aortic insufficiency Coronary artery disease, especially of the ostia	10–30 yr	Progressive; may be fatal	Aorta may be +
Neurosyphilis		2–35 yr	Progressive; may be fatal	Brain may be +
Asymptomatic	None			
Acute syphilitic meningitis	Headache, cranial nerve lesions, papilledema	6 wk to 2 yr	Not applicable	
Meningovascular	Signs of infection depend on area involved	2–10 yr		
Paresis	Minor personality change to frank psychosis	15–35 yr		
Tabes dorsalis	Signs of posterior column degeneration	5–30 yr		

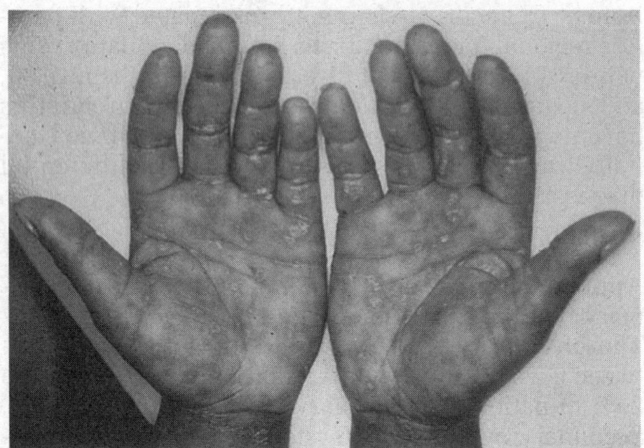

Figure 37.4. Palmar rash of secondary syphilis. (Photograph courtesy of Jonathan Zenilman, M.D.)

nephrotic syndrome, acute nephritic syndromes, gastric ulcerations or rugal hypertrophy, ocular inflammation, tinnitus, and sensorineural deafness.

Dermatologic manifestations of secondary syphilis usually resolve within 2 to 6 weeks even without treatment. One fourth of patients have a recurrence of symptoms within the first 4 years.

Latent Syphilis

Latent syphilis is the period of asymptomatic *T. pallidum* infection that begins with the resolution of secondary symptoms and ends either with treatment or with development of tertiary signs and symptoms of disease. The period is divided into two categories: *early latent* and *late latent*. The cutoff between these two categories is somewhat arbitrarily set at 1 year of infection. It is within the year of early latent syphilis that 90% of recurrences of secondary symptoms occur (143). During latent syphilis, recurrences are rare. For this reason persons with early latent syphilis also pose a higher risk of syphilis transmission.

Tertiary Syphilis

Even without appropriate treatment, only one third of patients with syphilis will develop tertiary manifestations. Since the introduction of penicillin, tertiary manifestations have become uncommon and more subtle in their presentation. There are three principal forms of tertiary syphilis: late benign (gummatous) syphilis, cardiovascular syphilis, and neurosyphilis.

Late Benign Syphilis. The classic lesion of late benign syphilis is the gumma, a granulomatous lesion that typically develops 2 to 10 years after infection. Gummas can be several centimeters in size and most commonly affect the skin (nodular or ulcerative lesions), bone, or liver. Significant morbidity and mortality can be associated with lesions in the brain or heart.

Cardiovascular Syphilis. In untreated patients, cardiovascular manifestations generally occur 5 to 30 years after initial infection. The most common manifestation is syphilitic aortitis. *T. pallidum* characteristically causes destruction of the elastic and muscular tissues of the ascending aorta, resulting in aneurysm formation, aortic ring dilatation, aortic regurgitation, and progressive heart failure. Stenosis of the coronary ostia may result in angina pectoris but is rarely associated with myocardial infarction (144).

Neurosyphilis. *T. pallidum* infection of the central nervous system (CNS) occurs at all stages of disease. Early infection may proceed to spontaneous resolution, asymptomatic meningitis, or acute aseptic meningitis. Late disease may remain asymptomatic, or patients may develop meningovascular syphilis, tabes dorsalis, or general paresis (141).

Asymptomatic neurosyphilis is defined as a reactive Venereal Disease Research Laboratory (VDRL) test for syphilis in the cerebrospinal fluid (CSF) or elevations in CSF WBC or protein concentrations in a syphilitic patient without clinical neurologic or psychiatric abnormalities. The diagnosis of asymptomatic neurosyphilis also requires that other causes of these CSF abnormalities be excluded. These abnormalities in CSF parameters are most commonly detected during secondary syphilis, and their detection in asymptomatic patients is of unclear significance. Use of penicillin in primary and secondary syphilis at doses inadequate for spirochetal eradication in the CNS has nevertheless been associated with remarkably low rates of symptomatic neurosyphilis.

Syphilitic meningitis most commonly occurs during secondary or early latent syphilis and is characterized by severe headache, meningismus, seizures, and cranial nerve involvement. Patients may develop facial palsies, sensorineural deafness, or optic nerve or primary ocular involvement (141).

Meningovascular syphilis can occur after 2 to 10 years of untreated infection. Clinical findings include headache, irritability, confusion, personality changes, emotional lability, seizures, and altered level of consciousness (145). Vasculitis of small end-arteries can produce focal findings specific to areas of involvement.

Tabes dorsalis occurs 5 to 30 years after untreated infection. Pupillomotor structures and the posterior spinal column are affected. Patients initially develop lancinating pains in their lower extremities and paresthesias. Disease progresses with the onset of sensory ataxia, loss of position and vibratory sense, areflexia, broad-based gait, incontinence, and impotence. Joint changes (Charcot joint) and neuropathic ulcers may develop. Another feature of tabes dorsalis is gastric crises with vomiting, abdominal pain, or both. Some patients also develop the classic *Argyll Robertson pupil* (small, irregular pupil that accommodates but does not react to light).

General paresis occurs in patients with untreated syphilis 15 to 35 years after infection. It is a complication of untreated syphilis that is characterized by progressive personality changes, irritability, poor judgment, memory loss, and psychotic features.

Diagnosis

There are several tools that are useful in the diagnosis and staging of syphilis. All patients diagnosed with syphilis by dark field microscopy or serologic testing should be tested for HIV infection at the time of diagnosis and, in the case of primary and secondary syphilis, at 3 months after diagnosis. Dark field microscopy and direct fluorescent antibody tests (DFA-TP) are used in early stages of syphilis to identify organisms in primary chancres and condylomata lata. Dark field microscopy is not available at all centers but is usually available at STD clinics. Patients can be referred to these centers for complete evaluation if necessary. To obtain a sample, the lesion should be lightly abraded with a gauze pad. While the lesion is squeezed, serous exudate is collected on a microscope slide or slide cover. Three microscopic samples should be evaluated immediately to avoid drying. Slides should be evaluated at 45× magnification to identify possible organisms. Any suspected organisms should be examined under oil immersion and the 100× objective. Although *T. pallidum* is a corkscrew-shaped organism with a characteristic motility, it can be difficult to differentiate from the oral spirochete, *Treponema macrodentium*. For this reason, oral lesions should not be evaluated with dark field microscopy. A negative dark field examination of a genital lesion does not rule out syphilis.

Two different types of serologic tests are available for diagnosis of syphilis and are useful during all stages of disease (Table 37.4). Nontreponemal tests include the VDRL and Rapid Plasma Reagin (RPR) tests. These tests detect nonspecific antibody to reagin, a cardiolipin–lecithin–cholesterol antigen complex. The titers of these tests usually correlate with disease activity. They cannot be used alone because of their limited sensitivity in early and late syphilis and the occurrence of false positive results. For this reason,

Table 37.4. Sensitivity and Specificity (%) of Serologic Tests for Syphilis[a] at Different Stages

	VDRL[b]		RPR[b]		FTA-ABS[b]		MHA-TP[b]	
Stage of Syphilis	Sens.	Spec.	Sens.	Spec.	Sens.	Spec.	Sens.	Spec.
Primary	80 (59–87)	98 (80–99)	86 (81–100)	98 (80–99)	98 (93–100)	98 (84–99)	82 (64–90)	99 (98–100)
Secondary	100 (99–100)	98	100 (99–100)	98	100 (99–100)	98	100 (96–100)	99
Latent	96 (73–100)	98	99	98	100 (96–100)	98	100 (96–100)	99
Tertiary (late)	71	98	73	98	96	98	94	99

[a]The consensus figures for the sensitivity and specificity are for tests done in the CDC Reference Laboratory (156) on samples derived from a well-run STD clinic. The figures in parentheses demonstrate the variability in published reports. Responsible factors include study of populations with different prevalences of syphilis and other confounding illnesses, variable performance by the laboratory, and different clinical criteria for the diagnosis of syphilis.

[b]See text for fuller discussion of these tests. MHA-TP not widely available.

a positive nontreponemal test must be followed with a specific treponemal test to confirm a diagnosis of syphilis.

Treponemal tests include the Fluorescent Treponemal Antibody Absorption (FTA-ABS) test, the Treponema Palladium particle agglutination test (TP-PA), and the microhemagglutination test for *T. pallidum* (MHA-TP or HATTS). These tests detect specific antibodies to *T. pallidum*. They have higher sensitivity and specificity than nontreponemal tests but are more difficult to perform and are more expensive. False positive results are rare but can occur in patients with autoimmune disease, viral infection, or pregnancy (146). There are also reports of false negative FTA-ABS tests in HIV-infected patients with syphilis (147). The specific treponemal tests generally should be used as confirmatory tests except in cases of suspected primary or tertiary syphilis, where the nontreponemal tests may be negative and the treponemal test may be more sensitive.

A patient is considered to have a *biologic false positive result* if the nontreponemal test is reactive and the FTA-ABS is consistently nonreactive. The titer of the nontreponemal test is usually 1:8 or less. Biologic false-positive results on nontreponemal tests are designated as acute if they are present for less than 6 months or chronic if present for longer than 6 months. Associated conditions include pneumonia, hepatitis, pregnancy, mononucleosis, measles, malaria, intravenous drug use, old age, hereditary biologic false positive status, rheumatologic disorders, chronic liver disease, and Waldenström macroglobulinemia.

The diagnosis of neurosyphilis in a patient with positive serologic tests for syphilis depends on the results of CSF analysis. Any patient with neurologic or ophthalmic signs or symptoms, evidence of tertiary aortitis or gummas, evidence of serologic treatment failure, or HIV infection and late latent syphilis should be evaluated for neurosyphilis with CSF analysis. Some experts also recommend CSF examination for patients with latent syphilis and serologic titers of 1:32 or higher. A positive CSF VDRL result is the best laboratory evidence of neurosyphilis. Although its specificity is virtually 100%, its sensitivity ranges from 10% to 89%. The CSF VDRL is less sensitive in detecting asymptomatic neurosyphilis and tabes dorsalis. However, in patients without other identifiable CNS infections, an elevated protein concentration (more than 40 mg/dL) or a WBC count greater than 5 mononuclear cells per microliter in the CSF can also indicate CNS syphilis infection. The role of the CSF FTA-ABS test in neurosyphilis diagnosis is controversial. Most researchers agree that a nonreactive CSF FTA-ABS is useful for ruling out neurosyphilis, but the significance of a reactive CSF FTA-ABS without other CSF abnormalities is unclear (148–150).

Treatment and Follow-Up

The treatment of choice for all stages of syphilis is parenteral penicillin G (benzathine, aqueous procaine, or aqueous crystalline). Combinations of benzathine penicillin and procaine penicillin or oral penicillin should not be used. The duration of treatment depends on the stage of disease. Before deciding on a treatment plan, every patient should have a thorough physical examination, including speculum examination in women, to evaluate for evidence of chancres, skin rash, ocular changes, and cardiologic or neurologic manifestations. Knowledge of a patient's HIV status is also important.

Primary and Secondary Syphilis. Primary and secondary syphilis should be treated with benzathine penicillin G, 2.4 million units intramuscularly in a single dose (1). Evidence for the efficacy of alternatives to penicillin in nonpregnant, HIV-seronegative patients is limited. Doxycycline, 100 mg orally twice a day or tetracycline, 500 mg four times a day for 14 days has been used for many years. Less is known about the efficacy of ceftriaxone, but some experts recommend 1 g/day given intramuscularly or intravenously for 8 to 10 days.

Follow-up of patients should include both physical examination and measurement of nontreponemal test titers. Follow-up should occur at 6 months and 12 months after treatment. Closer follow-up may be warranted if patients are treated with nonpenicillin regimens or if they are HIV positive. Nontreponemal test titers should decline fourfold (two dilutions) within 6 to 12 months after therapy. More than 85% of patients treated for primary or secondary syphilis eventually revert to a nonreactive nontreponemal serologic test. Approximately 10% of patients who are appropriately treated also revert to a negative FTA-ABS (151). If serologic titers have not fallen appropriately, the patient is at risk for treatment failure. Repeat HIV testing should be offered, and re-treatment should be considered if follow-up cannot be ensured. Recommended retreatment consists of three weekly intramuscular injections of benzathine penicillin G, 2.4 million units (7.2 million units total), unless CSF evaluation suggests the presence of neurosyphilis.

Latent Syphilis. Recommended treatment of early latent syphilis is benzathine penicillin G, 2.4 million units in a single dose by intramuscular injection (1). Patients who do not have documented seroconversion within the last year or clear signs of primary or secondary syphilis and who do not have a sex partner with documented primary, secondary, or early latent syphilis must be assumed to have late latent syphilis. These patients should be treated with three weekly intramuscular injections of benzathine penicillin, 2.4 million units (7.2 million units total). In nonpregnant, HIV-seronegative patients, alternatives to penicillin therapy are poorly studied. Patients with early latent syphilis may be treated with caution with the alternative regimens listed previously for primary and secondary syphilis. Patients with late latent syphilis can be treated with the alternative regimen of doxycycline, 100 mg orally twice a day, or tetracycline, 500 mg orally four times a day, for 28 days.

Clinical and serologic follow-up should be performed at 6, 12, and 24 months. Approximately 75% of patients treated for early latent syphilis and 44% of patients treated for late latent syphilis have nonreactive nontreponemal serologic tests 5 years after treatment (152). Treatment failure should be considered for patients whose titers increase fourfold, if an initial titer 1:32 or greater fails to decline at least fourfold (two dilutions) within 12 to 24 months, or if signs or symptoms of syphilis develop. These patients should have a CSF evaluation for neurosyphilis and, if negative, should be retreated for latent syphilis.

Tertiary Syphilis. Patients with gummatous or cardiovascular syphilis should be evaluated for neurosyphilis. If the CSF evaluation is normal, they should be treated with benzathine penicillin, three weekly intramuscular injections of 2.4 million units (7.2 million units total) (1). Alternatively, some experts treat patients with evidence of cardiovascular syphilis with neurosyphilis regimens. Doxycycline or tetracycline for 28 days can be considered for patients with penicillin allergy.

Patients with abnormalities on CSF examination or with evidence of ocular syphilis should be treated for neurosyphilis. Recommended treatment for neurosyphilis is aqueous crystalline penicillin G, 3 to 4 million units intravenously every 4 hours or as a continuous infusion with a daily dose of 18 to 24 million units for 10 to 14 days (1). An alternative regimen is daily intramuscular procaine penicillin, 2.4 million units, with probenecid, 500 mg orally four times a day, for 10 to 14 days. Some experts give one to three additional weekly intramuscular injections of benzathine penicillin, 2.4 million units after the intravenous treatment to achieve a total duration of therapy that is equivalent to the treatment for late latent disease. There is less clinical experience with non–penicillin-containing regimens. Ceftriaxone has been recommended by some experts when penicillin cannot be used (e.g., 2 g/day intravenously or intramuscularly for 10 to 14 days).

Response to treatment of tertiary syphilis has not been well studied. Patients with elevated CSF concentration of mononuclear cells should have repeat CSF evaluation every 6 months until the cell concentration is normal. Retreatment should be considered if the cell count has not decreased after 6 months or normalized after 2 years (1).

Pregnancy and Syphilis

In addition to the manifestations and complications already discussed, syphilis has been associated with spontaneous abortion, stillbirth, premature delivery, and perinatal death (153). Syphilis can be vertically transmitted to the neonate and results in serious systemic complications.

Pregnant patients should be treated with penicillin regimens, not with alternative regimens. Pregnant patients with penicillin allergy should be desensitized to penicillin. Some experts recommend two weekly doses of intramuscular benzathine penicillin, 2.4 million units, in pregnant women with primary, secondary, or early latent syphilis. Pregnant patients with syphilis should be managed with the assistance of an obstetrician.

HIV-Infected Patients with Syphilis

Although most HIV-infected patients can be evaluated and treated with the same diagnostic tests and treatment regimens as HIV-negative patients, clinicians should be aware of several unique considerations. Rarely, false-negative serologic test results in the setting of suggestive clinical findings for syphilis in HIV-infected patients may require biopsy of lesions for dark field examination or direct fluorescent antibody staining. HIV-infected patients with syphilis may also be at somewhat greater risk for development of neurosyphilis even at early stages of disease and may have greater rates of treatment failure with standard treatment regimens (154). Current recommendations for treatment do not differ from those for HIV-negative individuals except that all HIV-infected patients with late latent syphilis or syphilis of unknown duration should have CSF evaluation before the treatment regimen is determined (1). Recommended follow-up for HIV-infected patients is at 3, 6, 9, 12, and 24 months after therapy for primary, secondary, or early latent syphilis. Patients with late latent syphilis should be re-evaluated serologically at 6, 12, 18, and 24 months after treatment. Patients meeting previously discussed indicators for treatment failure should be reassessed with CSF evaluation and retreated.

Jarisch–Herxheimer Reaction

The Jarisch–Herxheimer reaction is an acute febrile reaction that can last for several hours and can occur within the first 24 hours of any effective treatment for syphilis. The pathogenesis is unknown, but it is thought to be related to the release of toxin by dying spirochetes. Patients often report headache, myalgias, and worsening cutaneous lesions. Antipyretics may be useful for symptomatic relief. In rare severe reactions, patients may develop transient hypotension. In pregnant women, the Jarisch–Herxheimer reaction may result in early labor or fetal distress (155). Patients with early stages of syphilis may have a greater risk of developing this reaction and should be informed about this possible side effect of treatment.

Contact Evaluation

Transmission of syphilis occurs through exposure to mucocutaneous syphilitic lesions. Therefore, primary, secondary, and early latent syphilis mark the stages of disease in which sexual partners are at risk of acquiring infection. The CDC STD treatment guidelines recommend identifying at-risk sex partners exposed to a patient within 3 months plus the duration of symptoms of primary syphilis, within 6 months plus the duration of symptoms for secondary syphilis, and within 1 year for early latent syphilis (1). Presumptive treatment should be given to all persons regardless of their serology if they have been exposed within 90 days to a case of primary, secondary, or early latent syphilis. If a person has been exposed to primary, secondary, or early latent syphilis longer than 90 days before evaluation but serologic tests are not available or follow-up is in doubt, presumptive treatment should be offered. In cases of syphilis of unknown duration, if the patient has a high titer (1:32 or more), partner notification and treatment should follow the guidelines for early syphilis. Persons with a history of exposure to a patient with latent syphilis should be managed based on the results of clinical evaluation and serologic testing.

General References

Centers for Disease Control and Prevention. 2002 Guidelines for treatment of sexually transmitted diseases. MMWR 2002 (in press).

Consensus guidelines for the management of common STDs.

Schmid GP. Approach to the patient with genital ulcer disease. Med Clin North Am 1990;74:1559.

Review of genital ulcer disease.

Wald A. New therapies and prevention strategies for genital herpes. Clin Infect Dis 1999;28[Suppl 1]:S4.

Summary of current knowledge regarding management of genital herpes

Beutner KR, Reitano MV, Richwald GA, et al. External genital warts: report of the American Medical Association Consensus Conference. AMA Expert Panel on External Genital Warts. Clin Infect Dis 1998;27:796.

Consensus statement for evaluation and management of genital warts.

Sparling PF, Handsfield HH. *Neisseria gonorrhoeae.* In: Mandell GL, Bennett JE, Dolin R, eds. Principles and practice of infectious diseases. Philadelphia: Churchill Livingstone, 2000:2242.

Infectious disease text with good summary of gonorrhea.

Jones RB, Batteiger BE. Introduction to chlamydial diseases. In: Mandell GL, Bennett JE, Dolin R, eds. Principles and practice of infectious diseases. Philadelphia: Churchill Livingstone, 2000: 1986.

Infectious disease text with good summary of chlamydia.

Burgher SW. Acute scrotal pain. Emerg Med Clin North Am 1998;16:781.

Review of the common etiologies of scrotal pain and the approach to initial diagnosis and management.

Singh AE, Romanowski B. Syphilis: review with emphasis on clinical, epidemiologic, and some biologic features. Clin Microbiol Rev 1999;12:187.

Recent review of syphilis.

Gjestland T. The Oslo Study of untreated syphilis: an epidemiologic investigation of the natural course of syphilis infection based upon a restudy of the Boeck-Bruusgaard material. Acta Derm Venereol 1955;35[Suppl. 34]:1.

Review of the natural history of syphilis.

Merritt HH. The early clinical and laboratory manifestations of syphilis of the central nervous system. N Engl J Med 1940;223:446.

Review of syphilis effects on the CNS.

Sparling PF. Diagnosis and treatment of syphilis. N Engl J Med 1971;284:642.

Classic review of syphilis.

Specific References

1. Centers for Disease Control and Prevention. 2002 Guidelines for treatment of sexually transmitted diseases. MMWR 2002 (in press).
2. Cameron DW, Simonsen JN, D'Costa LJ, et al. Female to male transmission of human immunodeficiency virus type 1: risk factors for seroconversion in men. Lancet 1989;2:403.
3. Chen CY, Ballard RC, Beck-Sague CM, et al. Human immunodeficiency virus infection and genital ulcer disease in South Africa: the herpetic connection. Sex Transm Dis 2000;27:21.
4. Greenblatt RM, Lukehart SA, Plummer FA, et al. Genital ulceration as a risk factor for human immunodeficiency virus infection. AIDS 1988;2:47.
5. Schacker T, Ryncarz AJ, Goddard J, et al. Frequent recovery of HIV-1 from genital herpes simplex virus lesions in HIV-1-infected men. JAMA 1998;280:61.
6. Stamm WE, Handsfield HH, Rompalo AM, et al. The association between genital ulcer disease and acquisition of HIV infection in homosexual men. JAMA 1988;260:1429.
7. Chapel TA, Brown WJ, Jeffres C, et al. How reliable is the morphological diagnosis of penile ulcerations? Sex Transm Dis 1977;4:150.
8. O'Farrell N, Hoosen AA, Coetzee KD, et al. Genital ulcer disease: accuracy of clinical diagnosis and strategies to improve control in Durban, South Africa. Genitourin Med 1994;70:7.
9. Zainah S, Cheong YM, Sinniah M, et al. A microbiological study of genital ulcers in Kuala Lumpur. Med J Malaysia 1991;46:274.
10. Fleming DT, McQuillan GM, Johnson RE, et al. Herpes simplex virus type 2 in the United States, 1976 to 1994. N Engl J Med 1997;337:1105.
11. Langenberg AG, Corey L, Ashley RL, et al. A prospective study of new infections with herpes simplex virus type 1 and type 2. Chiron HSV Vaccine Study Group. N Engl J Med 1999;341:1432.
12. Langenberg A, Benedetti J, Jenkins J, et al. Development of clinically recognizable genital lesions among women previously identified as having "asymptomatic" herpes simplex virus type 2 infection. Ann Intern Med 1989;110:882.
13. Rosen T, Brown TJ. Genital ulcers. Evaluation and treatment. Dermatol Clin 1998;16:673.
14. Hoffman IF, Schmitz JL. Genital ulcer disease: management in the HIV era. Postgrad Med 1995;98:67.
15. Schmid GP. Approach to the patient with genital ulcer disease. Med Clin North Am 1990;74:1559.
16. Benedetti J, Corey L, Ashley R. Recurrence rates in genital herpes after symptomatic first-episode infection. Ann Intern Med 1994;121:847.
17. Koelle DM, Benedetti J, Langenberg A, et al. Asymptomatic reactivation of herpes simplex virus in women after the first episode of genital herpes. Ann Intern Med 1992;116:433.
18. Wald A, Zeh J, Selke S, et al. Virologic characteristics of subclinical and symptomatic genital herpes infections. N Engl J Med 1995;333:770.
19. Cone RW, Swenson PD, Hobson AC, et al. Herpes simplex virus detection from genital lesions: a comparative study using antigen detection (HerpChek) and culture. J Clin Microbiol 1993;31:1774.
20. Slomka MJ, Emery L, Munday PE, et al. A comparison of PCR with virus isolation and direct antigen detection for diagnosis and typing of genital herpes. J Med Virol 1998;55:177.
21. Ashley RL, Wald A, Eagleton M. Premarket evaluation of the POCkit HSV-2 type-specific serologic test in culture-documented cases of genital herpes simplex virus type 2. Sex Transm Dis 2000;27:266.
22. Martins TB, Woolstenhulme RD, Jaskowski TD, et al. Comparison of four enzyme immunoassays with a western blot assay for the determination of type-specific antibodies to herpes simplex virus. Am J Clin Pathol 2001;115:272.
23. Whittington WL, Celum CL, Cent A, et al. Use of a glycoprotein G-based type-specific assay to detect antibodies to herpes simplex virus type 2 among persons attending sexually transmitted disease clinics. Sex Transm Dis 2001;28:99.
24. Prince HE, Ernst CE, Hogrefe WR. Evaluation of an enzyme immunoassay system for measuring herpes simplex virus (HSV) type 1-specific and HSV type 2-specific IgG antibodies. J Clin Lab Anal 2000;14:13.
25. Wald A. New therapies and prevention strategies for genital herpes. Clin Infect Dis 1999;28[Suppl 1]:S4.
26. Patel R, Tyring S, Strand A, et al. Impact of suppressive antiviral therapy on the health related quality of life of patients with recurrent genital herpes infection. Sex Transm Infect 1999;75:398.
27. Sacks SL, Shafran SD. BID Famciclovir suppression of asymptomatic genital herpes simplex virus shedding in men. Programs and abstracts of the 38th Interscience Conference on

Antibicrobial Agents and Chemotherapy, San Diego, CA, 1998.
28. Wald A, Warren T, Hu H, et al. Suppression of subclinical shedding of herpes simplex virus type 2 in the genital tract with valaciclovir. Programs and abstracts of the 38th Interscience Conference on Antimicrobial Agents and Chemotherapy, San Diego, CA, 1998.
29. Wald A, Langenberg AG, Link K, et al. Effect of condoms on reducing the transmission of herpes simplex virus type 2 from men to women. JAMA 2001;285:3100.
30. Jones C, Rosen T, Clarridge J, et al. Chancroid: results from an outbreak in Houston, Texas. South Med J 1990;83:1384.
31. Dillon SM, Cummings M, Rajagopalan S, et al. Prospective analysis of genital ulcer disease in Brooklyn, New York. Clin Infect Dis 1997;24:945.
32. DiCarlo RP, Armentor BS, Martin DH. Chancroid epidemiology in New Orleans men. J Infect Dis 1995;172:446.
33. Centers for Disease Control and Prevention. STD surveillance 1996. Atlanta: U.S. Department of Health and Human Services, Public Health Service, September 1996.
34. Plummer FA, D'Costa LJ, Nsanze H, et al. Clinical and microbiologic studies of genital ulcers in Kenyan women. Sex Transm Dis 1985;12:193.
35. Orle KA, Gates CA, Martin DH, et al. Simultaneous PCR detection of *Haemophilus ducreyi, Treponema pallidum,* and herpes simplex virus types 1 and 2 from genital ulcers. J Clin Microbiol 1996;34:49.
36. Sturm AW, Stolting GJ, Cormane RH, et al. Clinical and microbiological evaluation of 46 episodes of genital ulceration. Genitourin Med 1987;63:98.
37. Ernst AA, Marvez-Valls E, Martin DH. Incision and drainage versus aspiration of fluctuant buboes in the emergency department during an epidemic of chancroid. Sex Transm Dis 1995;22:217.
38. Ballard RC, Ye H, Matta A, et al. Treatment of chancroid with azithromycin. Int J STD AIDS 1996;7[Suppl 1]:9.
39. Kimani J, Bwayo JJ, Anzala AO, et al. Low dose erythromycin regimen for the treatment of chancroid. East Afr Med J 1995;72:645.
40. Tyndall MW, Agoki E, Plummer FA, et al. Single dose azithromycin for the treatment of chancroid: a randomized comparison with erythromycin. Sex Transm Dis 1994;21:231.
41. Malonza IM, Tyndall MW, Ndinya-Achola JO, et al. A randomized, double-blind, placebo-controlled trial of single-dose ciprofloxacin versus erythromycin for the treatment of chancroid in Nairobi, Kenya. J Infect Dis 1999;180:1886.
42. Levine JS, Smith PD, Brugge WR. Chronic proctitis in male homosexuals due to lymphogranuloma venereum. Gastroenterology 1980;79:563.
43. Mostafavi H, O'Donnell KF, Chong FK. Supralevator abscess due to chronic rectal lymphogranuloma venereum. Am J Gastroenterol 1990;85:602.
44. Papagrigoriadis S, Rennie JA. Lymphogranuloma venereum as a cause of rectal strictures. Postgrad Med J 1998;74:168.
45. Quinn TC, Goodell SE, Mkrtichian E, et al. *Chlamydia trachomatis* proctitis. N Engl J Med 1981;305:195.
46. Koutsky LA, Galloway DA, Holmes KK. Epidemiology of genital human papillomavirus infection. Epidemiol Rev 1988;10:122.
47. Meisels A. Cytologic diagnosis of human papillomavirus; influence of age and pregnancy stage. Acta Cytol 1992;36:480.
48. Syrjanen K, Vayrynen M, Castren O, et al. Sexual behaviour of women with human papillomavirus (HPV) lesions of the uterine cervix. Br J Vener Dis 1984;60:243.
49. Wen LM, Estcourt CS, Simpson JM, et al. Risk factors for the acquisition of genital warts: are condoms protective? Sex Transm Infect 1999;75:312.
50. Hippelainen M, Syrjanen S, Hippelainen M, et al. Prevalence and risk factors of genital human papillomavirus (HPV) infections in healthy males: a study on Finnish conscripts. Sex Transm Dis 1993;20:321.
51. Kataja V, Syrjanen S, Yliskoski M, et al. Risk factors associated with cervical human papillomavirus infections: a case-control study. Am J Epidemiol 1993;138:735.
52. Negrini BP, Schiffman MH, Kurman RJ, et al. Oral contraceptive use, human papillomavirus infection, and risk of early cytological abnormalities of the cervix. Cancer Res 1990;50:4670.
53. Franceschi S, Doll R, Gallwey J, et al. Genital warts and cervical neoplasia: an epidemiological study. Br J Cancer 1983;48:621.
54. Halpert R, Fruchter RG, Sedlis A, et al. Human papillomavirus and lower genital neoplasia in renal transplant patients. Obstet Gynecol 1986;68:251.
55. Matorras R, Ariceta JM, Rementeria A, et al. Human immunodeficiency virus-induced immunosuppression: a risk factor for human papillomavirus infection. Am J Obstet Gynecol 1991;164:42.
56. Durst M, Gissmann L, Ikenberg H, et al. A papillomavirus DNA from a cervical carcinoma and its prevalence in cancer biopsy samples from different geographic regions. Proc Natl Acad Sci U S A 1983;80:3812.
57. Durst M, Kleinheinz A, Hotz M, et al. The physical state of human papillomavirus type 16 DNA in benign and malignant genital tumours. J Gen Virol 1985;66:1515.
58. Gissmann L, Boshart M, Durst M, et al. Presence of human papillomavirus in genital tumors. J Invest Dermatol 1984;83[1 Suppl]:26s.
59. Koutsky LA, Holmes KK, Critchlow CW, et al. A cohort study of the risk of cervical intraepithelial neoplasia grade 2 or 3 in relation to papillomavirus infection. N Engl J Med 1992;327:1272.
60. Beutner KR, Wiley DJ, Douglas JM, et al. Genital warts and their treatment. Clin Infect Dis 1999;28[Suppl 1]:S37.
61. Handsfield HH. Clinical presentation and natural course of anogenital warts. Am J Med 1997;102:16.
62. Beutner KR, Reitano MV, Richwald GA, et al. External genital warts: report of the American Medical Association Consensus Conference. AMA Expert Panel on External Genital Warts. Clin Infect Dis 1998;27:796.
63. Carr G, William DC. Anal warts in a population of gay men in New York City. Sex Transm Dis 1977;4:56.
64. Wikstrom A, Hedblad MA, Johansson B, et al. The acetic acid test in evaluation of subclinical genital papillomavirus infection: a comparative study on penoscopy, histopathology, virology and scanning electron microscopy findings. Genitourin Med 1992;68:90.
65. Beutner KR, Conant MA, Friedman-Kien AE, et al. Patient-applied podofilox for treatment of genital warts. Lancet 1989;1:831.
66. Duus BR, Philipsen T, Christensen JD, et al. Refractory condylomata acuminata: a controlled clinical trial of carbon dioxide laser versus conventional surgical treatment. Genitourin Med 1985;61:59.
67. Reid R. The management of genital condylomas, intraepithelial neoplasia, and vulvodynia. Obstet Gynecol Clin North Am 1996;23:917.
68. Beutner KR, Spruance SL, Hougham AJ, et al. Treatment of genital warts with an immune-response modifier (imiquimod). J Am Acad Dermatol 1998;38:230.
69. Edwards L, Ferenczy A, Eron L, et al. Self-administered topical 5% imiquimod cream for external anogenital warts. HPV Study Group. Human Papilloma Virus. Arch Dermatol 1998;134:25.
70. Beutner KR, Ferenczy A. Therapeutic approaches to genital warts. Am J Med 1997;102:28.
71. Bjekic M, Vlajinac H, Sipetic S, et al. Risk factors for gonorrhoea: case-control study. Genitourin Med 1997;73:518.
72. Cooper DL, Bernstein GS, Ivler D, et al. Gonorrhea screening program in a women's hospital outpatient department: results and analysis of risk factors. J Am Vener Dis Assoc 1976;3:71.
73. Evans BA, Tasker T, MacRae KD. Risk profiles for genital infection in women. Genitourin Med 1993;69:257.
74. Gershman KA, Barrow JC. A tale of two sexually transmitted diseases: prevalences and predictors of chlamydia and gonorrhea in women attending Colorado family planning clinics. Sex Transm Dis 1996;23:481.
75. Hook EW III, Reichart CA, Upchurch DM, et al. Comparative behavioral epidemiology of gonococcal and chlamydial infections among patients attending a Baltimore, Maryland, sexually transmitted disease clinic. Am J Epidemiol 1992;136:662.

76. Mertz KJ, Finelli L, Levine WC, et al. Gonorrhea in male adolescents and young adults in Newark, New Jersey: implications of risk factors and patient preferences for prevention strategies. Sex Transm Dis 2000;27:201.
77. Upchurch DM, Brady WE, Reichart CA, et al. Behavioral contributions to acquisition of gonorrhea in patients attending an inner city sexually transmitted disease clinic. J Infect Dis 1990;161:938.
78. Holmes KK, Johnson DW, Trostle HJ. An estimate of the risk of men acquiring gonorrhea by sexual contact with infected females. Am J Epidemiol 1970;91:170.
79. Hooper RR, Reynolds GH, Jones OG, et al. Cohort study of venereal disease. I: the risk of gonorrhea transmission from infected women to men. Am J Epidemiol 1978;108:136.
80. Lin JS, Donegan SP, Heeren TC, et al. Transmission of *Chlamydia trachomatis* and *Neisseria gonorrhoeae* among men with urethritis and their female sex partners. J Infect Dis 1998;178:1707.
81. Thin RN, Williams IA, Nicol CS. Direct and delayed methods of immunofluorescent diagnosis of gonorrhoea in women. Br J Vener Dis 1971;47:27.
82. Wiesner PJ, Tronca E, Bonin P, et al. Clinical spectrum of pharyngeal gonococcal infection. N Engl J Med 1973;288:181.
83. Sparling PF, Handsfield HH. *Neisseria gonorrhoeae.* In: Mandell GL, Bennett JE, Dolin R, eds. Principles and practice of infectious diseases. Philadelphia: Churchill Livingstone, 2000:2242.
84. Handsfield HH, Lipman TO, Harnisch JP, et al. Asymptomatic gonorrhea in men: diagnosis, natural course, prevalence and significance. N Engl J Med 1974;290:117.
85. McCormack WM, Stumacher RJ, Johnson K, et al. Clinical spectrum of gonococcal infection in women. Lancet 1977;1:1182.
86. Quinn TC, Stamm WE, Goodell SE, et al. The polymicrobial origin of intestinal infections in homosexual men. N Engl J Med 1983;309:576.
87. Kerle KK, Mascola JR, Miller TA. Disseminated gonococcal infection. Am Fam Physician 1992;45:209.
88. Bohnhoff M, Morello JA, Lerner SA. Auxotypes, penicillin susceptibility, and serogroups of *Neisseria gonorrhoeae* from disseminated and uncomplicated infections. J Infect Dis 1986;154:225.
89. Janda WM, Jackson T. Evaluation of Gonodecten for the presumptive diagnosis of gonococcal urethritis in men. J Clin Microbiol 1985;21:143.
90. Juchau SV, Nackman R, Ruppart D. Comparison of Gram stain with DNA probe for detection of *Neisseria gonorrhoeae* in urethras of symptomatic males. J Clin Microbiol 1995;33:3068.
91. Luciano AA, Grubin L. Gonorrhea screening: comparison of three techniques. JAMA 1980;243:680.
92. Stamm WE, Cole B, Fennell C, et al. Antigen detection for the diagnosis of gonorrhea. J Clin Microbiol 1984;19:399.
93. Koumans EH, Johnson RE, Knapp JS, et al. Laboratory testing for *Neisseria gonorrhoeae* by recently introduced nonculture tests: a performance review with clinical and public health considerations. Clin Infect Dis 1998;27:1171.
94. Carroll KC, Aldeen WE, Morrison M, et al. Evaluation of the Abbott LCx ligase chain reaction assay for detection of *Chlamydia trachomatis* and *Neisseria gonorrhoeae* in urine and genital swab specimens from a sexually transmitted disease clinic population. J Clin Microbiol 1998;36:1630.
95. Hook EW III, Ching SF, Stephens J, et al. Diagnosis of *Neisseria gonorrhoeae* infections in women by using the ligase chain reaction on patient-obtained vaginal swabs. J Clin Microbiol 1997;35:2129.
96. Gaydos CA, Howell MR, Pare B, et al. *Chlamydia trachomatis* infections in female military recruits. N Engl J Med 1998;339:739.
97. Hughes G, Catchpole M, Rogers PA, et al. Comparison of risk factors for four sexually transmitted infections: results from a study of attenders at three genitourinary medicine clinics in England. Sex Transm Infect 2000;76:262.
98. Klausner JD, McFarland W, Bolan G, et al. Knock-knock: a population-based survey of risk behavior, health care access, and *Chlamydia trachomatis* infection among low-income women in the San Francisco Bay area. J Infect Dis 2001;183:1087.
99. Hart G. Factors associated with genital chlamydial and gonococcal infection in males. Genitourin Med 1993;69:393.
100. Magder LS, Harrison HR, Ehret JM, et al. Factors related to genital *Chlamydia trachomatis* and its diagnosis by culture in a sexually transmitted disease clinic. Am J Epidemiol 1988;128:298.
101. Stamm WE, Koutsky LA, Benedetti JK, et al. *Chlamydia trachomatis* urethral infections in men: prevalence, risk factors, and clinical manifestations. Ann Intern Med 1984;100:47.
102. Jones RB, Batteiger BE. Introduction to chlamydial diseases. In: Mandell GL, Bennett JE, Dolin R, eds. Principles and practice of infectious diseases. Philadelphia: Churchill Livingstone, 2000:1986.
103. Laga M, Manoka A, Kivuvu M, et al. Non-ulcerative sexually transmitted diseases as risk factors for HIV-1 transmission in women: results from a cohort study. AIDS 1993;7:95.
104. Ghys PD, Fransen K, Diallo MO, et al. The associations between cervicovaginal HIV shedding, sexually transmitted diseases and immunosuppression in female sex workers in Abidjan, Cote d'Ivoire. AIDS 1997;11:F85.
105. Mostad SB, Overbaugh J, DeVange DM, et al. Hormonal contraception, vitamin A deficiency, and other risk factors for shedding of HIV-1 infected cells from the cervix and vagina. Lancet 1997;350:922.
106. Cates W Jr, Wasserheit JN. Genital chlamydial infections: epidemiology and reproductive sequelae. Am J Obstet Gynecol 1991;164:1771.
107. Svensson L, Westrom L, Ripa KT, et al. Differences in some clinical and laboratory parameters in acute salpingitis related to culture and serologic findings. Am J Obstet Gynecol 1980;138:1017.
108. Martin DH, Mroczkowski TF, Dalu ZA, et al. A controlled trial of a single dose of azithromycin for the treatment of chlamydial urethritis and cervicitis: The Azithromycin for Chlamydial Infections Study Group. N Engl J Med 1992;327:921.
109. Nilsen A, Halsos A, Johansen A, et al. A double blind study of single dose azithromycin and doxycycline in the treatment of chlamydial urethritis in males. Genitourin Med 1992;68:325.
110. Brocklehurst P, Rooney G. Interventions for treating genital *Chlamydia trachomatis* infection in pregnancy. Cochrane Database Syst Rev 2000;(2):CD000054.
111. Hillis SD, Nakashima A, Marchbanks PA, et al. Risk factors for recurrent *Chlamydia trachomatis* infections in women. Am J Obstet Gynecol 1994;170:801.
112. Aral SO, Holmes KK. Social and behavioral determinants of the epidemiology of STDs: industrialized and developing countries. In: Holmes KK, Sparling PF, Mardh P-A, et al., eds. Sexually transmitted diseases. 3rd ed. New York: McGraw-Hill, 1999:39.
113. Burstein GR, Zenilman JM. Nongonococcal urethritis: a new paradigm. Clin Infect Dis 1999;28[Suppl 1]:S66.
114. Horner PJ, Gilroy CB, Thomas BJ, et al. Association of *Mycoplasma genitalium* with acute non-gonococcal urethritis. Lancet 1993;342:582.
115. Janier M, Lassau F, Casin I, et al. Male urethritis with and without discharge: a clinical and microbiological study. Sex Transm Dis 1995;22:244.
116. Jensen JS, Orsum R, Dohn B, et al. *Mycoplasma genitalium*: a cause of male urethritis? Genitourin Med 1993;69:265.
117. Romanowski B, Talbot H, Stadnyk M, et al. Minocycline compared with doxycycline in the treatment of nongonococcal urethritis and mucopurulent cervicitis. Ann Intern Med 1993;119:16.
118. Stamm WE, Hicks CB, Martin DH, et al. Azithromycin for empirical treatment of the nongonococcal urethritis syndrome in men: a randomized double-blind study. JAMA 1995;274:545.
119. McKee KT Jr, Jenkins PR, Garner R, et al. Features of urethritis in a cohort of male soldiers. Clin Infect Dis 2000;30:736.
120. Deguchi T, Komeda H, Yasuda M, et al. *Mycoplasma genitalium* in non-gonococcal urethritis. Int J STD AIDS 1995;6:144.
121. Horner P, Thomas B, Gilroy CB, et al. Role of *Mycoplasma genitalium* and *Ureaplasma urealyticum* in acute and chronic nongonococcal urethritis. Clin Infect Dis 2001;32:995.

122. Borchardt KA, al Haraci S, Maida N. Prevalence of *Trichomonas vaginalis* in a male sexually transmitted disease clinic population by interview, wet mount microscopy, and the InPouch TV test. Genitourin Med 1995;71:405.
123. Hobbs MM, Kazembe P, Reed AW, et al. *Trichomonas vaginalis* as a cause of urethritis in Malawian men. Sex Transm Dis 1999;26:381.
124. Joyner JL, Douglas JM Jr, Ragsdale S, et al. Comparative prevalence of infection with *Trichomonas vaginalis* among men attending a sexually transmitted diseases clinic [see comments]. Sex Transm Dis 2000;27:236.
125. Krieger JN, Verdon M, Siegel N, et al. Risk assessment and laboratory diagnosis of trichomoniasis in men. J Infect Dis 1992;166:1362.
126. Pillay DG, Hoosen AA, Vezi B, et al. Diagnosis of *Trichomonas vaginalis* in male urethritis. Trop Geogr Med 1994;46:44.
127. Stimson JB, Hale J, Bowie WR, et al. Tetracycline-resistant *Ureaplasma urealyticum*: a cause of persistent nongonococcal urethritis. Ann Intern Med 1981;94:192.
128. Gaydos CA, Crotchfelt KA, Howell MR, et al. Molecular amplification assays to detect chlamydial infections in urine specimens from high school female students and to monitor the persistence of chlamydial DNA after therapy. J Infect Dis 1998;177:417.
129. Berger RE, Alexander ER, Harnisch JP, et al. Etiology, manifestations and therapy of acute epididymitis: prospective study of 50 cases. J Urol 1979;121:750.
130. Grant JB, Costello CB, Sequeira PJ, et al. The role of *Chlamydia trachomatis* in epididymitis. Br J Urol 1987;60:355.
131. Berger RE, Kessler D, Holmes KK. Etiology and manifestations of epididymitis in young men: correlations with sexual orientation. J Infect Dis 1987;155:1341.
132. Burgher SW. Acute scrotal pain. Emerg Med Clin North Am 1998;16:781.
133. Lewis AG, Bukowski TP, Jarvis PD, et al. Evaluation of acute scrotum in the emergency department. J Pediatr Surg 1995;30:277.
134. Knight PJ, Vassy LE. The diagnosis and treatment of the acute scrotum in children and adolescents. Ann Surg 1984;200:664.
135. Melekos MD, Asbach HW, Markou SA. Etiology of acute scrotum in 100 boys with regard to age distribution. J Urol 1988;139:1023.
136. Stillwell TJ, Kramer SA. Intermittent testicular torsion. Pediatrics 1986;77:908.
137. St Louis ME, Wasserheit JN. Elimination of syphilis in the United States. Science 1998;281:353.
138. Nakashima AK, Rolfs RT, Flock ML, et al. Epidemiology of syphilis in the United States, 1941—1993. Sex Transm Dis 1996;23:16.
139. Gunn RA, Montes JM, Toomey KE, et al. Syphilis in San Diego County 1983–1992: crack cocaine, prostitution, and the limitations of partner notification. Sex Transm Dis 1995;22:60.
140. Rolfs RT, Goldberg M, Sharrar RG. Risk factors for syphilis: cocaine use and prostitution. Am J Public Health 1990;80:853.
141. Singh AE, Romanowski B. Syphilis: review with emphasis on clinical, epidemiologic, and some biologic features. Clin Microbiol Rev 1999;12:187.
142. Mindel A, Tovey SJ, Timmins DJ, et al. Primary and secondary syphilis, 20 years' experience. 2: Clinical features. Genitourin Med 1989;65:1.
143. Gjestland T. The Oslo Study of untreated syphilis: an epdiemiologic investigation of the natural course of syphilis infection based upon a restudy of the Boeck-Bruusgaard material. Acta Derm Venereol 1955:35[Suppl. 34]:1.
144. Burch GE, Winsor T. Syphilitic coronary stenosis, with myocardial infarction. Am. Heart J 1942:24:740.
145. Merritt HH. The early clinical and laboratory manifestations of syphilis of the central nervous system. N Engl J Med 1940;223:446.
146. Sparling PF. Diagnosis and treatment of syphilis. N Engl J Med 1971;284:642.
147. Erbelding EJ, Vlahov D, Nelson KE, et al. Syphilis serology in human immunodeficiency virus infection: evidence for false-negative fluorescent treponemal testing. J Infect Dis 1997;176:1397.
148. Dans PE, Cafferty L, Otter SE, et al. Inappropriate use of the cerebrospinal fluid Venereal Disease Research Laboratory (VDRL) test to exclude neurosyphilis. Ann Intern Med 1986;104:86.
149. Hook EW III, Marra CM. Acquired syphilis in adults. N Engl J Med 1992;326:1060.
150. Jaffe HW, Larsen SA, Peters M, et al. Tests for treponemal antibody in CSF. Arch Intern Med 1978;138:252.
151. Schroeter AL, Lucas JB, Price EV, et al. Treatment for early syphilis and reactivity of serologic tests. JAMA 1972;221:471.
152. Fiumara NJ. Serologic responses to treatment of 128 patients with late latent syphilis. Sex Transm Dis 1979;6:243.
153. Wendel GD. Gestational and congenital syphilis. Clin Perinatol 1988;15:287.
154. Berry CD, Hooton TM, Collier AC, et al. Neurologic relapse after benzathine penicillin therapy for secondary syphilis in a patient with HIV infection. N Engl J Med 1987;316:1587.
155. Myles TD, Elam G, Park-Hwang E, et al. The Jarisch-Herxheimer reaction and fetal monitoring changes in pregnant women treated for syphilis. Obstet Gynecol 1998;92:859.
156. Division of STD/HIV Prevention. Sexually transmitted disease surveillance, 1991. U.S. Department of Health and Human Services, Public Health Service. Atlanta: Centers for Disease Control and Prevention, July 1992.

CHAPTER 38

Lyme Disease and Other Tick-Borne Illnesses

JOHN A. FLYNN, MD
PAUL G. AUWAERTER, MD

Lyme disease is the most common tick-borne illness in the United States. Although it rarely causes mortality, it can have morbid complications and generates concern among patients. Other arthropod-borne illnesses such as Rocky Mountain spotted fever (RMSF) and ehrlichiosis, although less common than Lyme disease, are among the diseases requiring prompt recognition, because death can occur without proper treatment. The number of recognized tick-borne human diseases other than Lyme disease continues to expand in the United States (Table 38.1).

LYME DISEASE

Epidemiology

Since the original clinical description in 1977 of infection by the spirochete *Borrelia burgdorferi,* Lyme disease has become the most common arthropod-borne illness in the United States (1). It is endemic in more than 15 states and is responsible for a number of outbreaks in Eastern coastal areas (Fig. 38.1) (2). This spirochete was originally isolated from the *Ixodes scapularis* tick in the northeastern United States (3). Subsequently, other *Ixodes* species were found to carry this infection in California and throughout Europe and Asia. In addition to the transmitting tick vector, other animal reservoirs are involved in the tick life cycle maintaining *Borrelia* infection. In the United States, the white-footed mouse and the white-tailed deer are the preferred hosts for this very small tick, which is no larger than 2 by 3 mm in its adult form. Ticks become infected through horizontal transmission among these reservoirs. In endemic areas, up to 50% of ticks may be infected (4). Despite the high carriage rate in ticks, the probability of acquiring Lyme disease from a single tick bite is at most 3.5% in an endemic area (5). The disease incidence is greatest in the mid-spring through late fall. This correlates with periods of increased tick populations, especially biting nymphs (less than 2 mm), as well as increased outdoor activities of people in endemic areas.

Surveillance of this nationally notifiable disease has been conducted by the Centers for Disease Control and Prevention (CDC) since 1982. The following clinical care definition for this surveillance has been established and is discussed later in this chapter:

- Erythema migrans of 5 cm (2 inches) or greater, or
- At least one late manifestation of neurologic, cardiovascular, or musculoskeletal disease, and laboratory confirmation of infection with *B. burgdorferi.*

The highest number of cases in the United States are reported in the northeastern and mid-Atlantic regions. Endemic pockets also exist in northern California and in regions of Minnesota and Wisconsin. In 1999, 16,273 cases of Lyme disease were reported in 45 states and the District of Columbia, with an overall incidence rate of 6.0 per 100,000 population. Connecticut (98/100,000), Rhode Island (55/100,000), New York (24/100,000), and Pennsylvania (23/100,000) reported the highest rates that year (1). There is no gender predilection. Significant outdoor exposure (e.g., hiking, gardening) in endemic regions increases risk, although many cases have occurred without a history of much outdoor activity. In those cases for which the month of illness was identified, June (28.5%) and July (28.9%) were reported most frequently.

Clinical Manifestations and Stages

Patients may develop erythema migrans (EM) with no further symptoms even in the absence of antibiotic therapy. Others may present with one of the later manifestations of the infection without any history of EM. Lyme disease has been divided into three stages based on clinical manifestations that may occur during the infection: early localized disease, early disseminated disease, and late disease. Approximately 70% to 85% of patients with definite Lyme disease present with early localized disease. In most patients, there is no characteristic progression from one stage to the next.

Early Localized Disease

After a bite from an infected tick, an incubation period of several days to 1 month may elapse before the pathognomonic skin lesion, EM, forms at the site of the bite. Common sites include the axillae, groin, and waistline. This lesion starts as an erythematous macule or papule with an outer border and clearing center

Table 38.1. North American Tick-Borne Infections and Common Characteristics

Disease	Pathogen	Vector	Likely U.S. Geography	Clinical Hallmarks
Lyme Disease	*B. burgdorferi*	*I. scapularis* (deer tick) *I. pacificus*	Northeastern, mid-Atlantic, upper midwest, Pacific coast	Erythema migrans, facial palsy, meningitis, carditis
RMSF	*R. rickettsii*	*D. variabilis* (dog tick) *D. andersoni* (wood tick)	Southern, mid-Atlantic	Fever, headache, petechial rash
HME	*E. chaffeensis*	*A. americanum* (Lone Star tick)	New York to Texas	Fever, headache, myalgia, leukopenia, thrombocytopenia
HGE	*Anaplasma phagocytophila*	*I. scapularis* *I. pacificus*	Same as Lyme disease	Fever, headache, myalgia, leukopenia, thrombocytopenia
Relapsing fever	*B. hermsii* *B. duttonii*	*Ornithodoros species* (soft ticks)	Southwest and west	Intermittent fever, headache, petechial rash
Tularemia	*F. tularensis*	Many hard ticks	Southcentral	Ulcer, lymphadenitis,
Babesiosis	*B. microti*	*I. scapularis*	Same as Lyme disease, especially islands	Fever, anemia, malarial-like
Colorado tick fever	*Coltivirus*	*D. andersoni*	Rocky Mountains, west	Intermittent fever, headache, leukopenia

A, Amblyomma; B, Borrelia; D, Dermacentor; E, Ehrlichia; F, Francisella; HME, human monocytic ehrlichiosis; HGE, human granulocytic ehrlichiosis; *I, Ixodes; R, Rickettsia;* RMSF, Rocky Mountain Spotted Fever.

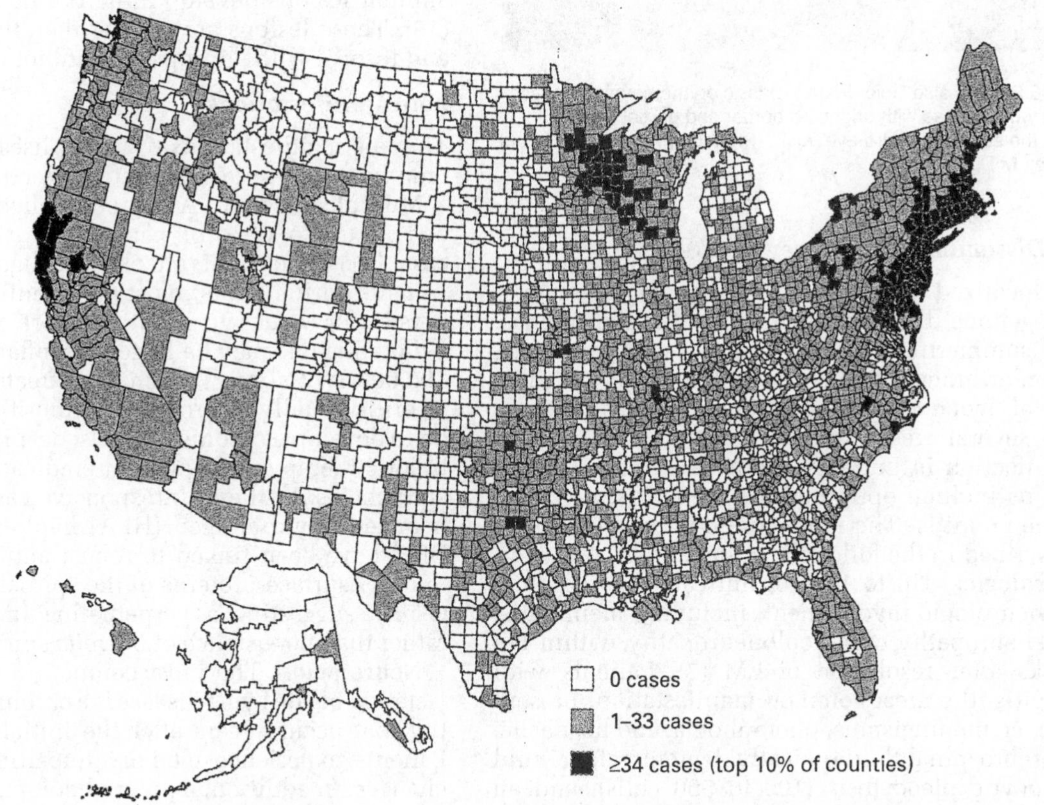

Figure 38.1. Geographic distribution of Lyme disease in the United States by county, 1982–1998. (From Orloski KA, Hayes EB, Campbell GL, et al. Surveillance for Lyme disease—United States, 1992–1998. In: CDC Surveillance Summaries, MMWR Morb Mortal Wkly Rep 2000;49(SS-3):1.)

that expands up to 15 cm in a circumferential manner over several days (Fig. 38.2; see also Color Plate). The border is sharply demarcated, warm to touch, and nontender. Only one third of patients are aware of a recent tick bite. If left untreated, EM resolves spontaneously within several weeks. If appropriate antibiotic therapy is initiated, the rash resolves in days. This rash is the single best clinical marker for this condition and occurs in up to 90% of cases (6). Most patients have some nonspecific constitutional symptoms, such as myalgia, fatigue, arthralgia, or headache. Twenty percent of patients have no manifestation other than the rash. Though often described as a "bull's-eye" rash because of central clearing, this feature is not always present, and in one study of culture-proven Lyme disease fewer than 40% of rashes had central clearing.

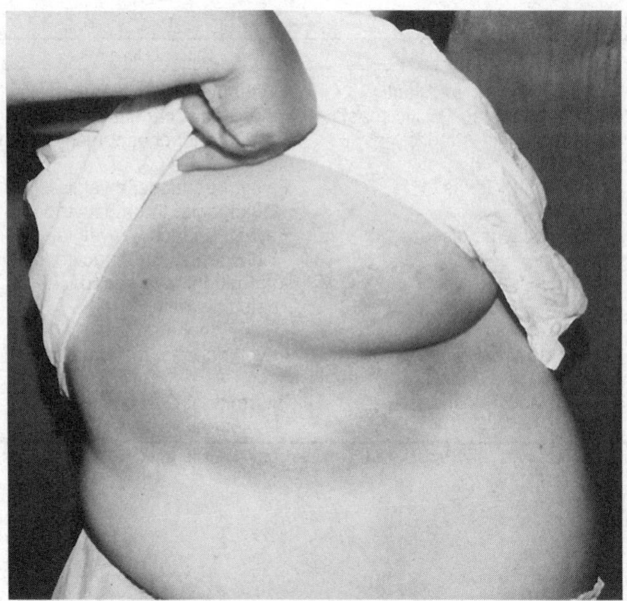

Figure 38.2. (See also Color Plate.) Classic erythema migrans rash of early Lyme disease with bright red border and partial central clearing, the so-called "bull's-eye" rash. (Photograph courtesy of Paul Auwaerter, M.D.)

Early Disseminated Disease

Early localized Lyme disease often progresses to hematogenous dissemination within the first month. During summertime, flu-like illnesses with headache, myalgia, arthralgia, and fever, without EM rash, may represent Lyme disease. End-organ effects develop within several weeks or up to 1 year after the primary infection in untreated patients. Unusual manifestations include optic neuritis, hepatitis, myositis, and pneumonitis. The more common manifestations are described in the following paragraphs.

Neurologic. Up to 15% of untreated patients develop neurologic involvement, including meningitis, cranial neuropathy, or radiculoneuropathy, within 4 to 8 weeks after resolution of EM (7). Patients with meningitis, the most common manifestation, present with fever, meningismus, photophobia, and headache. The cerebrospinal fluid typically demonstrates a mild lymphocytic pleocytosis (100 to 500 cells), and an increased protein level. A peripheral seventh nerve palsy (Bell's palsy) is the most common cranial neuropathy; it is bilateral in up to one fourth of the cases (8). Most cases resolve within 1 month regardless of treatment. Peripheral radiculoneuropathies occur less often. They may involve one or more motor or sensory nerves of the thorax or limbs in an asymmetric pattern, mimicking spinal discogenic pain or manifesting as focal weakness in the involved areas.

Cardiac. Involvement of the heart can occur in up to 10% of patients with untreated Lyme disease, typically within 3 months of developing EM. The precise incidence of Lyme carditis is unclear because the most common finding when a patient has carditis is asymptomatic first-degree atrioventricular (AV) block. Complete heart block requiring temporary pacemaker placement can may occur (9). Cardiomyopathy, pericarditis, and myocarditis have been described but appear to be rare. All cardiac involvement usually resolves within 8 weeks, and complete heart block usually recedes with antimicrobial treatment, making permanent pacemaker placement unnecessary.

Musculoskeletal. Roughly half of untreated patients develop migratory arthralgias, myalgias, tendonitis, bursitis, or bone pain. A self-limited monoarticular or oligoarticular arthritis may develop, primarily in the large joints, most often the knee. Polyarthritis is distinctly unusual. Large synovial effusions contain inflammatory fluid (5,000 to 20,000 white blood cells [WBCs] per cubic millimeter) with neutrophilic predominance.

Dermatologic. Multiple disseminated secondary annular lesions develop in half of untreated patients (10). These lesions are smaller than the initial lesion and resolve with appropriate antibiotic therapy.

Late Manifestations

The late manifestations of Lyme disease occur many months to years after the initial infection.

Musculoskeletal. A migratory oligoarthritis develops in up to 60% of patients with untreated disease (11). Recurrent attacks of oligoarthritis affect weight-bearing joints, most commonly the knee, and persist for weeks to months before resolving. Synovial effusions may be large and inflammatory (up to 100,000 WBCs/mm^3). Even in untreated patients, the arthritis usually improves. A minority of patients go on to develop a chronic arthritis, despite extensive antibiotic therapy and apparent eradication of all Lyme spirochetes. In these unresponsive cases, certain human leukocyte antigen (HLA) haplotypes (DR4 and DR2) have been linked to robust antibody responses to outer surface proteins of the spirochete (OspA and OspB), suggesting a perpetuating immune reaction rather than persistence of *Borrelia* spirochetes (12,13).

Neurologic. The most common neurologic manifestation of late Lyme disease is a chronic encephalopathy that occurs years after the initial infection (14). Patients experience memory impairment and mood changes. In addition, a polyradiculopathy with paresthesia or radicular pain of the extremities may develop with or without encephalopathy. Motor involvement is unusual. Partial improvement may occur in half of those patients who are treated with antibiotics, but the natural history tends toward a chronic progressive course. All forms of chronic neurologic Lyme disease are believed to be rare, occurring in fewer than 5% of people with untreated Lyme disease.

Dermatologic. A peculiar cutaneous affliction, *acrodermatitis chronica atrophicans,* is primarily seen in untreated patients in Europe (15). This red to blue nodular plaque develops mostly on the dorsal aspect of the hand, elbow, and extensor surface of the foot and ankle. Over time, the involved skin becomes atrophic or sclerotic. *B. burgdorferi* has been cultured from these lesions.

Diagnosis

The diagnosis of Lyme disease should be based primarily on the presence of characteristic clinical findings, exposure to an endemic area, and response to appropriate antibiotic therapy (16). The clinical presentation of EM is so distinctive that any patient presenting with this rash requires treatment for early Lyme disease. In patients with other associated findings (e.g., facial nerve palsy, complete heart block) and no history of EM, their likelihood of exposure must be considered. If it is high, serologic testing should be performed.

With the exception of tissue samples from the involved skin lesions in patients with EM, it is difficult to culture *B. burgdorferi* from any site (4). Because this technique is difficult and the skin lesion is pathognomonic, attempts at culturing skin biopsy sites are limited to research settings.

Routinely available diagnostic testing determines whether there has been an immune response to the spirochete, using an enzyme-linked immunosorbent assay (ELISA) to detect immunoglobulin M (IgM) and IgG antibodies to *B. burgdorferi.* In patients infected with Lyme disease it takes several weeks before an IgM response can be detected. This may not occur after early antibiotic use. Once positive, the IgM response can remain present for longer than a year. Although it helps to confirm exposure, it does not establish active infection. After 4 to 8 weeks, the IgG antibody response should develop in untreated patients. False positive results have been noted in a number of situations, including viral infections, rheumatoid arthritis, and other autoimmune diseases, as well as in healthy people living in endemic areas (4). In the absence of appropriate clinical and environmental findings, these laboratory studies do not have sufficient sensitivity or specificity to establish or exclude the diagnosis of Lyme disease (17).

Although criteria have been established for the interpretation of Western blot studies of Lyme disease–related antibodies, there is still difficulty with standardization and reliability of this testing (18). The CDC suggest a two-step Lyme diagnostic test strategy in which positive or equivocal ELISA studies are confirmed by Western blot testing for Lyme-specific IgM and IgG bands. These tests are available routinely. The IgM Western blot is often falsely positive and therefore should be obtained only in patients with symptoms of less than 1 month's duration. In these cases, the test is considered positive if two of three Lyme-specific bands are present. The IgG Western blot requires that at least five of ten specific bands be present. In research settings, polymerase chain reaction (PCR) has detected *B. burgdorferi* DNA in blood, synovial fluid, spinal fluid, and skin specimens (19). DNA detection with PCR continues to be fraught with technical difficulties, risk of contamination, and lack of standardization, which prevent its wide clinical use.

Treatment

Lyme disease in all stages should respond with clinical improvement to appropriate antibiotic therapy. Recognition and treatment of early Lyme disease prevents development of later manifestations. A Jarisch–Herxheimer reaction with spiking fever, rigor, and hypotension occurs in some patients within several hours after treatment. It peaks in approximately 12 hours and then resolves over 1 to 2 days, and is treated only with supportive care.

Early Manifestations

EM can be treated successfully with oral doxycycline in adults, or amoxicillin in pregnant or lactating women (Table 38.2). For people who are allergic to these medications, oral cefuroxime is an effective alternative (20). Although erythromycin has been demonstrated to be successful against EM, it is less effective in the treatment of disseminated disease. Most cases of EM resolve within days after initiation of therapy. Antibiotic therapy for 14 to 21 days is usually sufficient, although no definitive studies exist regarding the optimal duration.

Table 38.2. Antibiotic Therapy for Lyme Disease[a]

Drug	Dosage and Frequency	Duration (days)
Oral therapy for localized disease (erythema migrans)		
Doxycycline	100 mg b.i.d.	14–21
Amoxicillin	500 mg t.i.d.	14–21
-OR-		
Cefuroxime	500 mg b.i.d.	14–21
Pregnant or lactating women		
Amoxicillin	500 mg t.i.d.	14–21
Oral therapy for early disseminated disease (first-degree atrioventricular block, facial palsy, disseminated annular lesions)		
Doxycycline	100 mg b.i.d.	21–28
-OR-		
Amoxicillin	500 mg t.i.d.	21–28
Intravenous therapy for early disseminated disease (complete atrioventricular block, meningitis, neuritis)		
Ceftriaxone	2 g q.d.	14–28 (some switch to oral therapy with clinical improvement)
-OR-		
Cefotaxime	2 g q8h	
Oral therapy for late disease (arthritis)		
Doxycycline	100 mg b.i.d.	28
-OR-		
Amoxicillin	500 mg q.i.d.	28
Intravenous therapy for late disease (persistent arthritis, late neurologic disease)		
Ceftriaxone	2 g q.d.	14–28
-OR-		
Cefotaxime	2 g q8h	14–28
Penicillin G	18–24 mU IV q.d.	14–28

[a]Preferred choices are listed first, followed (after "-OR-") by alternative choices.

Patients with isolated facial palsy, minor cardiac abnormalities (e.g., first-degree AV block), or disseminated annular lesions at the time of diagnosis should be treated with a 21- to 28-day oral regimen (21). Patient with complete AV block, meningitis, or other early neuroborreliosis syndromes should receive intravenous ceftriaxone therapy for 14 to 28 days (22). Some practitioners use parenteral therapy until acute symptoms have resolved (e.g., in cases of cardiac conduction abnormalities) and then complete the course of antibiotics with oral therapy. Parenteral penicillin in equally efficacious, although ceftriaxone is used more frequently because of dosing simplicity. Patients with significant cardiac involvement may require monitoring and a temporary pacemaker.

Late Manifestations

Late manifestations of Lyme disease require longer courses of antibiotics (Table 38.2). Lyme arthritis should be treated with a 28-day course of oral antibiotics. If the patient does not respond, a 14- to 28-day course of intravenous ceftriaxone should be given (23). A small percentage of patients develop a postinfectious immune response with persistent arthritis despite extensive antibiotics. Patients with late neurologic manifestations should be treated with a 28-day course of intravenous ceftriaxone (22). Prolonged treatment with antibiotics, beyond this, is no more effective than placebo in improving persistent symptoms in patients with a history of acute Lyme disease (24). The long-term outcome for most patients with Lyme disease is favorable. One study showed no differences between patients with Lyme disease and age-matched controls without Lyme disease in difficulties with activities of daily living 1 to 11 years after diagnosis (25).

Prevention

The risk of infection with *B. burgdorferi* depends on several variables, including the prevalence of Lyme-infected ticks in the area, the number of tick bites received, and the duration that the tick is attached. If tick feeding is less than 36 to 48 hours, the risk of transmitting infection is very low. Risk increases with more extended attachment or if the tick is obviously engorged with blood. Lyme disease is not an immunizing condition. Recurrent exposure may lead to recurrent infection and clinical symptoms.

Antibiotic Prophylaxis

Several studies have examined the efficacy and cost-effectiveness of antibiotic prophylaxis after a tick bite. One report based on a decision analysis model recommended that if the risk of infection after the bite is greater than 3.6% (26), antibiotic prophylaxis should be given for anyone known to have been bitten by a tick. This threshold risk of infection, however, is higher than that observed in field studies in well-recognized endemic areas. In two placebo-controlled trials, the risk of becoming infected in an endemic area was less than 1.5% and was no greater than the risk of developing side effects from the 14 days of antibiotic treatment (5,27). An additional randomized, double-blind, placebo-controlled trial was conducted using a single 200-mg dose of doxycycline as prophylaxis within 72 hours after a tick bite. In this study, EM at the site of the tick bite developed in 0.4% of the treated group, compared with 3.2% of the placebo group. Interestingly, EM occurred only in those bitten by nymphal ticks. Adverse effects, particularly nausea, developed in 30% of the treatment group and 11% of the placebo group (28). Based on these data, some authorities recommend prophylactic therapy for early Lyme disease with a single dose of doxycycline (200 mg) if an engorged nymphal tick, acquired in an area in which *I. scapularis* is endemic, is identified on a patient (29).

Vaccination

A recently introduced vaccine (LymeRix) containing recombinant *B. burgdorferi* outer surface lipoprotein-A (L-OspA) (30,31) has been approved by the U.S. Food and Drug Administration for the prevention of Lyme disease. Vaccination requires two injections 1 month apart, with a third booster injection 1 year later. In subjects 15 to 70 years of age, vaccine efficacy was approximately 76% in the prevention of Lyme disease. To date, the frequency of adverse events has been similar in the vaccine and in the placebo group, although postmarketing surveillance continues. Chronic Lyme arthritis refractory to antibiotics has been associated with high levels of antibodies to the same Lyme antigen (OspA) that is used in the vaccine. This has raised theoretical concerns that chronic arthritis may develop in vaccinated patients after exposure to *B. burgdorferi*, but this has not occurred in practice. The decision to vaccinate patients should be individualized based on their risk of exposure. The CDC has published recommendations for the use of Lyme disease vaccine (32) (Table 38.3). This vaccination offers no protection against other tick-borne illnesses.

As of February, 2002, this product is no longer commercially available in the United States.

ROCKY MOUNTAIN SPOTTED FEVER

Mortality rates of 1% to 5% occur despite appropriate treatment of RMSF; more than 20% of untreated patients die from this most feared tick-borne illness. First described in early twentieth-century Montana and Idaho, this infection is most commonly seen east of the Mississippi River, especially in the southeastern United States. RMSF is caused by an obligate intracellular bacterium, *Rickettsia rickettsii,* that is a member of a large group of worldwide zoonotic rickettsia causing spotted fevers. The common dog tick, *Dermacentor variabilis,* transmits most cases of RMSF in the eastern United States. Transmission requires at least 6 hours of attachment to the human host. In the far western states, *Dermacentor andersoni,* the Rocky Mountain wood tick, is the main reservoir. Most cases of RMSF occur in the late spring or summer, although reports of infection during the winter come from mainly southern states. Between 500 to 1,000 cases of RMSF were reported annually during the 1990s.

Children and young adults are most commonly infected, probably because of increased outdoor exposure. Initial symptoms are often mistakenly dismissed as a routine summertime viral illness with fever, severe headache, myalgia, and arthralgia. Symptoms arise 2 to 14 days after the tick bite. The average incubation period is 7 days. Rash is the major diagnostic sign, but it tends to occur later, eventually appearing in 90% of infected patients 3 to 5 days after the initial onset of symptoms. The characteristic maculopapular rash with central petechiae typically begins on the wrists and ankles and then spreads inward toward the trunk. Involvement of the palms and soles has been considered a standard presentation of RMSF, but it does not occur in some patients. So-called "spotless" RMSF occurs in up to 10% of infected patients, especially in darker-skinned populations, necessitating a high index of diagnostic suspicion.

Once introduced to lymphatics and small blood vessels after a tick bite, *R. rickettsii* tends to invade endothelial cells, leading to a vasculitic mechanism of injury (33). Myocarditis is a leading cause of death, although pneumonitis and coma (from central nervous system vasculitis) are also common. Lumbar punctures are frequently performed for the evaluation of headache and fever. The cerebrospinal fluid is normal in most patients but shows lymphocytic or neutrophilic predominance in up to one third. Platelets are consumed at the many sites of endovascular infection, often resulting in thrombocytopenia. Elevated transaminases are noted in about half of infected patients, although clinical jaundice is seen in fewer than 10%.

The prognosis in RMSF is mainly related to the timeliness of antibiotic administration. Waiting for a characteristic rash or laboratory confirmation of infection heightens the likelihood of death. The challenge, therefore, is to recognize clinical and epidemiologic features that prompt early diagnosis. The differential diagnosis of the manifestation of RMSF includes illnesses such as measles, rubella, respiratory tract infections, gastroenteritis, disseminated meningococcal and gonococcal disease, typhoid, syphilis, other rickettsial infections, autoimmune vasculitides, thrombotic thrombocytopenic purpura, and adverse drug reactions. Although there is no uniform patient profile, consideration of this diagnosis should be prompted by a warm-weather illness in a previously healthy patient with potential tick exposure who is severely ill with fever and possible rash. Definitive diagnosis can be made by culture of *R. rickettsii* from blood, although few laboratories are equipped for this specialized undertaking (34). Skin biopsy with application of rickettsia-specific immunohistochemical antibodies may offer early diagnosis. Serologic antibody testing serves to provide only retrospective diagnosis, because sufficient antibody titers develop only during convalescence. Early clinical diagnosis remains imperative for this life-threatening infection.

Standard therapy requires administration of doxycycline (100 mg twice daily) or chloramphenicol (50 to 75 mg/kg per day), usually for 7 days. Although tetracyclines are not usually given to children because of drug staining of dental enamel, it can probably be given safely to youngsters with suspected RMSF, because a single course is unlikely to damage teeth (35).

EHRLICHIOSES

Only in the last 15 years has human infection by the genus *Ehrlichia* been known in the United States. Infection with this rickettsial agent tends to produce an illness very similar to RMSF but without rash. The Ixodidae family of ticks transmits these intracellular pathogens, usually during warm weather months. There are two different kinds of *Ehrlichia* infection, defined by whether these bacteria invade monocytes or granulocytes. A third type of erlichiosis, caused by the agent of canine ehrlichiosis, *Ehrlichia ewingii,* has also been described in humans (36).

Human Monocytic Ehrlichiosis

Human monocytotrophic ehrlichiosis (HME), first described in 1986, is an infection by *Ehrlichia chaffeensis* that occurs most commonly in the southeastern and southcentral portion of the United States, tracking the distribution of its main vector, the Lone Star tick (*Amblyomma americanum*).

Probably most patients with HME do not have symptoms or have only mild symptoms that are self-limited and do not seek medical advice. Of those patients seeking medical attention, the acuteness of illness tends to be more severe. Up to 40% of these patients require hospitalization for fever, headache, rigors, myalgia, nausea, vomiting, and abdominal pain that manifest an average of 7 days after a tick bite (37). A maculopapular rash, sometimes with petechial features, occurs in up to one third of cases. Laboratory hallmarks of HME include leukopenia and thrombocytopenia, both observed in a majority of cases, and elevations in liver transaminases. Patients who are severely ill may be admitted to the intensive care unit with an evolving picture of multiorgan system failure. Death occurs in 3% of patients, especially among the immunosuppressed.

Diagnosis may be rapidly accomplished by demonstrating characteristic morulae (mulberry-like clusters of bacteria) within monocytes or lymphocytes on examination of a peripheral blood smear. However, only about 7% of patients with HME have observable morulae. Some laboratories offer PCR detection of the organisms in blood, and this may be the most sensitive test (38). Paired acute/convalescent serologies can confirm diagnosis retrospectively. However, as with RMSF, clinical suspicion of ehrlichial infection is necessary, because delayed treatment increases the likelihood of severe infection or death.

Doxycycline (100 mg twice daily) is the treatment of choice, with mild symptoms often resolving within 24 to 48 hours after initiation. Optimal duration of therapy is uncertain, but current recommendations suggest treatment for at least 3 days after cessation of fever and clinical improvement, for a minimum course of 5 to 7 days. Severe illness can take weeks for resolution despite appropriate therapy.

Human Granulocytic Ehrlichiosis

First described in 1994, this infection of granulocytes is caused by an agent closely related to *Ehrlichia* that has recently been designated *Anaplasma phagocytophila*. This bacterium is transmitted mostly by *Ixodes persculatus*–complex ticks, therefore tracking the same distribution as Lyme disease. Much like HME, human granulocytic ehrlichiosis (HGE) probably produces subclinical disease in many cases, because populations in areas of the United States such as Wisconsin have seroprevalence rates of 15%.

Symptoms are similar to those of HME with the exception that rash is even less prevalent, affecting fewer than 10% of patients (39). Leukopenia, thrombocytopenia, and liver function abnormalities are common, although neutropenia specifically distinguishes HGE from HME (40). Severe illness can occur, including death. Morulae are identified much more commonly than in HME, with characteristic clusters identified within granulocytes in 20% to 80% of patients (41). Empiric therapy with doxycycline remains critical, because timely diagnosis cannot be achieved with available serologies, and PCR detection of blood is not widely available. The treatment regimen is identical to that for HME (described earlier).

SOUTHERN TICK-ASSOCIATED RASH ILLNESS

EM-like rashes have been described after bites of the Lone Star tick (*A. americanum*), which is not known to carry *B. burgdorferi*, the agent of Lyme disease (42). This rash has been described primarily in southern states such as the Carolinas. Southern tick-associated rash illness (STARI) appears to respond to doxycycline, and to date no chronic sequelae have been identified. A new member of the *Borrelia* species, *Borrelia lonestari*, has been identified by PCR genetic analysis as the cause of STARI but has not been cultivated from biopsy specimens to date (43).

BABESIOSIS

Babesiosis, a protozoal tick-borne infection, occurs in a similar distribution to Lyme disease because its primary vector is *I. scapularis*. New England and mid-Atlantic regions report most cases, especially coastal regions such as Cape Cod, Nantucket, Martha's Vineyard, Block Island, and Long Island. This one-celled parasite infects a wide range of animals, but the rodent strain *Babesia microti* accounts for most human cases in the United States. Two strains, WA1 and MO1, have been isolated from ill patients residing in the states of Washington, California, and Missouri (44–46).

Illness typically begins 1 to 6 weeks after a tick bite with malaise, fever, headache, myalgia, and loss of appetite. Babesia invades erythrocytes and may cause a malaria-like illness with rigors, high fevers to 40°C, hepatosplenomegaly, hemolytic anemia, and pancytopenia (47). Illness may progress to include the adult respiratory distress syndrome. Persons infected with babesia tend to be older than 50 years of age with intact spleens, but individuals at greatest risk of severe disease include immunocompromised patients and those of any age who have undergone splenectomy. Chronic infection with babesia with recrudescence of symptoms may occur more commonly than suspected after acute infection, although the exact clinical significance of this condition is unknown (48).

Diagnosis is established by examination of a peripheral blood smear and the observation of small, oval-ring forms of the parasite in 1% to 10% of erythrocytes (Fig. 38.3). This sometimes causes confusion with ring forms of falciparum malaria. Rarely, characteristic tetrad formations of babesia organisms (resembling a Maltese cross) in red blood cells easily permit confirmation. Increased antibody titers to

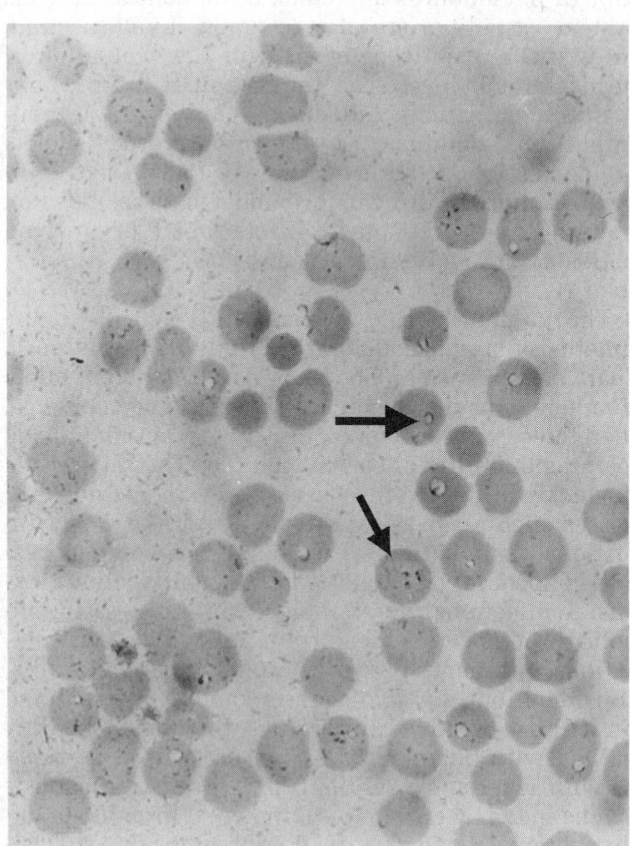

Figure 38.3. Human erythrocytes infected with *Babesia microti*. Cells display both the more commonly observed ring forms *(large arrow)* with pale central area, occasionally mistaken for malaria parasites, and the rare, pathognomonic tetrad form *(small arrow)*. (Photograph courtesy of Steve Dumler, M.D.)

B. microti (greater than 1:256) are considered diagnostic of infection, but the WA1 strain cannot be identified by standard babesia serology and requires specific antibody testing. Serology rarely offers the timely diagnosis needed for patients severely ill from babesia, but these patients usually have easily recognized levels of parasitemia on blood smear. PCR, not yet widely available, may ultimately prove to be the fastest and most reliable method for diagnosis, as with many of the tick-borne disorders. Clinical suspicion of this infection remains essential based on epidemiologic risks and presenting symptoms.

Many patients infected with babesia recover without treatment. Splenectomized patients seem to be at greatest risk of life-threatening illness with high levels of parasitemia, but severe infection may also afflict those individuals who were previously healthy. Treatment traditionally has incorporated a combination of oral clindamycin (600 mg) and quinine (650 mg) every 8 hours for 7 or more days. One recent, non-blinded trial suggested that use of both atovaquone (750 mg every 12 hours) and azithromycin (500 mg on day 1 and then 250 mg daily) for 7 days offers equal efficacy with fewer side effects (49). Patients with severe illness and profound anemia may benefit from exchange transfusion.

RELAPSING FEVER

Relapsing fever is an arthropod-borne spirochetal disease that is caused by at least 13 different species of *Borrelia* that occur in a worldwide distribution. Historically, *Borrelia recurrentis* has achieved greatest notoriety through louse-borne transmission causing vast epidemics of relapsing fever. With the single exception of endemic relapsing fever (*B. hermsii* and *B. duttonii),* tick-borne infections in North America are transmitted by hard ticks. Endemic relapsing fever is transmitted by the soft tick genus *Ornithodoros,* which are found mainly in arid environments such as the southwestern United States but extend to the northwestern and midwestern states (50).

Symptoms of relapsing fever tend to include high fever with shaking chills, headache, myalgia, arthralgia, photophobia, and lethargy. Hepatosplenomegaly, lymphadenopathy, petechial rash, neurologic abnormalities (such as facial palsy, myelitis, or radiculopathy) are present in only a minority of infected patients (51). As the name suggests, episodes of symptoms and fever alternate with an afebrile phase for 1 week or longer before returning—usually with symptoms milder than those of the initial phase. The return of fever correlates with the presence of spirochetes in the blood. Most patients average a total of two to four relapses.

Examination of the peripheral blood either by Giemsa- or Wright-stained thick and thin smears or by dark field microscopy reveals spirochetes in up to 70% of infections, although the blood rarely contains borrelia during afebrile periods. Repeated examination of blood smears may be necessary. Lyme serology tests may be falsely positive. Patients with neurologic disease may have abnormal cerebral spinal fluid.

Tetracycline (500 mg four times a day) or doxycycline (200 mg first dose, followed by 100 mg twice daily) is the preferred treatment for 10 days, although chloramphenicol (50 to 100 mg/kg per day orally or intravenously, divided every 6 hours for 10 days, and not to exceed 4 g/day) and erythromycin (500 mg four times a day) are alternatives. Neurologic disease is treated with parenteral antibiotics such as ceftriaxone (2 g intravenously every day) or penicillin G (4 mU intravenously every 4 hours) for 14 or more days. Epidemic relapsing fever can have a mortality rate of up to 40%, but endemic tick-borne disease is much milder, although death can occur. Jarisch–Herxheimer reactions have been described after initial antimicrobial therapy for relapsing fever. Because this reaction can be life-threatening, observation is urged for the first 2 hours after the start of therapy.

TULAREMIA

This infection by the gram-negative bacterium, *Francisella tularensis,* causes illness in many guises but typically involves suppurative lymph nodes with skin, eye, lung, or throat involvement. The dog tick (*D. variabilis*) and the Lone Star tick (*A. americanum*) transmit most cases in the United States, although biting flies predominate as vectors in the western states. The disease may also come from physical contact with infected animals such as rabbits, birds, beavers, squirrels, and muskrats, making hunters a group at particular risk. Despite the breadth of opportunities to acquire *F. tularensis,* this mostly rural infection has become increasingly rare since World War II for uncertain reasons. Incidence rates are now less than 0.08 per 100,000 population. In recent years, Arkansas and Missouri have reported the largest number of cases. Diagnosis is more common in the summer because of tick activity, but may occur year round.

The most common form of tularemia is ulceroglandular, accounting for 70% to 80% of reported cases (52). In this presentation, the skin tends to ulcerate and form an eschar. Regional lymph nodes that drain the ulcer may enlarge with suppuration. Other classic forms of tularemia include oculoglandular, glandular, pneumonic, oropharyngeal, and typhoidal (infection without signs of localization). Fever, chills, headache, and back pain are common with all forms.

Because of its rarity, tularemia often is not suspected, especially in its more unfamiliar forms. Cultures of blood, lymph nodes, sputum, or wounds may yield *F. tularensis* on supportive media. A clinician suspecting tularemia should alert the microbiology laboratory, because the organism, once grown, requires careful handling to prevent infection of laboratory personnel. Serologic testing for *F. tularensis* may also offer diagnostic help by demonstrating a fourfold rise in acute-to-convalescent titer, or if an acute titer higher than 1:160 is demonstrated. Streptomycin (7.5 to 10.0 mg/kg intramuscularly every 12 hours for 7 to

14 days; alternatively, 15 mg/kg intramuscularly every 12 hours for the first 3 days followed by half-dose therapy for the balance of therapy; and in the severely ill, 15 mg/kg dosing continued throughout) or gentamicin (5 mg/kg per day intravenously for 7 to 14 days) is the standard therapy. Treatment with doxycycline may result in unacceptably high rates of relapse.

TICK-BORNE VIRAL INFECTIONS

Colorado tick fever is caused by the bite of the wood tick *Dermacentor andersoni* transmitting a Coltivirus. This summertime illness is most frequently diagnosed in the Rocky Mountains and Pacific Coast regions. Perhaps fewer than 50% of individuals experience symptoms within 2 weeks after a bite by an infected tick. In symptomatic patients, a remitting fever (2-day febrile periods with a 2-day afebrile interval) that lasts for 2 weeks is common. About 20% of patients describe abdominal complaints. This viral infection is self-limited, usually necessitating only supportive care. Complicated illness is rare, although leukopenia is frequently observed. Colorado tick fever is often confused with RMSF, ehrlichiosis, or relapsing fever so prescription of doxycycline empirically is advised until the diagnosis is established. The diagnosis of Colorado tick fever may be confirmed by viral culture or viral antigen detection assays.

Tick-borne encephalitis is rare in the United States but much more common in Eurasia (53). Cases in the United States are caused by the Powassan virus, a member of the flavivirus family, transmitted by *Ixodes* ticks. Fever and headache are a frequent prodrome before evolution into encephalitic symptoms. Only supportive care is available, and chronic neurologic sequelae are common. A commercial vaccine to prevent tick-borne encephalitis is offered frequently to hikers and campers in Eastern Europe and Asia, but no recommendations exist for the United States. Only five cases have been described in this country, including four recent cases in Vermont and Maine (54).

AVOIDING TICK-BORNE ILLNESS

Despite the availability of effective antibiotics and vaccines, the best preventive measure to avoid tick-borne illnesses remains patient education about methods to limit exposure to ticks. Long pants tucked into socks should be worn when walking in woods or high grasses. Tick repellants containing 20% to 40% *N,N*-diethyl-*m*-toluamide (DEET) can decrease the risk of tick bites. In addition, individuals should carefully inspect their skin after outdoor activities to allow for rapid detection and removal of ticks.

General References*

Cunha BA, ed. Tick-borne infectious diseases: diagnosis and management. Marcel Dekker, New York, 2000.

Parola P, Raoult D. Ticks and tick-borne bacterial diseases in humans: an emerging infectious threat. Clin Infect Dis 2001;32:897.

Rahn DW, Evans J. Lyme disease. American College of Physician–American Society of Internal Medicine, Philadelphia, 1998.

A concise and comprehensive paperback text which includes 13 case studies.

CDC Lyme Disease Homepage. Available at: http://www.cdc.gov/ncidod/dvbid/lymeinfo.htm (accessed 1/7/02).

From the division of vector-borne infectious diseases of the CDC. An excellent overview of Lyme disease, appropriate for patient education with complete bibliography.

*Bold print (general references) and bold numerals (specific references) denote published controlled clinical trials, meta-analyses, or consensus-based recommendations.

Specific References

1. Centers for Disease Control and Prevention. Lyme disease—United States, 1999. MMWR Morb Mortal Wkly Rep 1999;50;181.
2. Steere AC. Lyme disease. N Engl J Med 2001;345:115.
3. Burgdorfer W, Barbour AG, Hayes SF, et al. Lyme disease: a tick-borne spirochetosis? Science 1982;216:1317.
4. Magnarelli LA, Anderson JF, Fikrig E, et al. Use of recombinant antigens of *Borrelia burgdorferi* in serologic tests for diagnosis of Lyme borreliosis. J Clin Microbiol 1996;34:237.
5. Costello CM, Steer AC, Pinkerton RE, et al. Prospective study of tick bites in an endemic area for Lyme disease. J Infect Dis 1984;150:489.
6. Gerber MA, Bell GJ, Burk GS, et al. Lyme disease in children in southwest Connecticut. N Engl J Med 1997;335:17.
7. Reik L, Steere AC, Bartenhagen NH, et al. Neurologic abnormalities of Lyme disease. Medicine (Baltimore) 1979;58:281.
8. Clark JR, Carlson RD, Sasaki CT, et al. Facial paralysis in Lyme disease. Laryngoscope 1985;95:1341.
9. McAlister HF, Klementowicz PT, Andrews C, et al. Lyme carditis: an important cause of reversible heart block. Ann Intern Med 1989;110:339.
10. Steere AC, Bartenhagen NH, Craft JE, et al. The early clinical manifestations of Lyme disease. Am J Med 1985;78:235.
11. Steere AC, Schoen RT, Taylor E. The clinical evolution of Lyme arthritis. Ann Intern Med 1987;107:725.
12. Steere AC, Dwyer E, Winchester R. Association of chronic Lyme arthritis with HLA-DR2 and HLA-DR4 alleles. N Engl J Med 1990;323:219.
13. Kalish R, Leong JM, Steere AC. Association of treatment resistant chronic Lyme arthritis with HLA-DR4 and antibody reactivity to OspA an OspB of borrelia. Infect Immun 1993;61:2774.
14. Logigian EL, Kaplan RF, Steere AC. Neurologic manifestations of Lyme disease. N Engl J Med 1990;323:1438.
15. Asbrink E, Hovmark A. Early and late cutaneous manifestations of *Ixodes*-borne borreliosis (erythema migrans borreliosis, Lyme borreliosis). Ann N Y Acad Sci 1988;539:4.
16. Steere AC, Bartenhagen NC, Craft JE, et al. The early clinical manifestations of Lyme disease. Ann Intern Med 1983;99:76.
17. Bakken LL, Case KL, Callister SM, et al. Performance of 45 laboratories participating in a proficiency testing program for Lyme disease serology. JAMA 1992;268:891.
18. Centers for Disease Control and Prevention. Recommendations for test performance and interpretation from the second national conference on serologic diagnosis of Lyme disease, 1995. MMWR Morb Mortal Wkly Rep 1995;4:590.
19. Nocton JJ, Dressler F, Rutledge BJ, et al. Detection of *Borrelia burgdorferi* DNA by polymerase chain reaction in synovial fluid from patients with Lyme arthritis. N Engl J Med 1994;330:229.
20. Nadelman RB, Luger SW, Frank E, et al. Comparison of cefuroxime axetil and doxycycline in the treatment of early Lyme disease. Ann Intern Med 1992;117:273.
21. Rahn DW, Malawista SE. Lyme disease: recommendations for diagnosis and treatment. Ann Intern Med 1991;114:472.
22. Skoldenberg B, Stiernstedt G, Karlsson M, et al. Treatment of Lyme borreliosis with emphasis on neurological disease. Ann N Y Acad Sci 1988;539:317.

23. Dattwyler RJ, Halperin JJ, Volkman DJ, et al. Treatment of late Lyme borreliosis: randomized comparison of ceftriaxone and penicillin. Lancet 1988;1:1191.

24. Klempner MS, Hu LT, Evans J, et al. Two controlled trials of antibiotic treatment in patients with persistent symptoms and a history of Lyme disease. N Engl J Med 2001;345: 85.

25. Seltzer EG, Gerber MA, Cartter ML, et al. Long-term outcomes of persons with Lyme disease. JAMA 2000;283:609.

26. Magid D, Schwartz B, Craft J, et al. Prevention of Lyme disease after tick bites: a cost effectiveness analysis. N Engl J Med 1992;34.

27. Shapiro ED, Gerber MA, Holabird NB, et al. A controlled trial of antimicrobial prophylaxis for Lyme disease after deer tick bites. N Engl J Med 1992;327:1769.

28. Nadelman RB, Nowakowski J, Fish D, et al. Prophylaxis with single-dose doxycycline for the prevention of Lyme disease after an *Ixodes scapularis* tick bite. N Engl J Med 2001;345: 79.

29. Shapiro ED. Doxycycline for tick bites–not for everyone. N Engl J Med 2001;345:133.

30. Sigal LH, Zahradnik JM, Lavin P, et al. A vaccine consisting of recombinant *Borrelia burgdorferi* outer-surface protein A to prevent Lyme disease. N Engl J Med 1998;339:216.

31. Steere AC, Sikand VK, Meurice F, et al. Vaccination against Lyme disease with recombinant *Borrelia burgdorferi* outer-surface lipoprotein A with adjuvant. N Engl J Med 1998;339: 209.

32. Centers for Disease Control and Prevention. Recommendations for the use of Lyme disease vaccine. MMWR Morb Mortal Wkly Rep 1999;48(7);1.

33. Thorner AR, Walker DH, Petri WA Jr. Rocky Mountain spotted fever. Clin Infect Dis 1998;27:1353.

34. LaScola B, Raoult D. Laboratory diagnosis of rickettsioses: current approaches to diagnosis of old and new rickettsial diseases. J Clin Microbiol 1997;35:2715.

35. American Academy of Pediatrics. Red Book: report of the Committee on Infectious Diseases. 24th ed. Elk Grove Village, IL: America Academy of Pediatrics, 1997.

36. Buller RD, Aren M, Hmeil SP, et al. *Ehrlichia ewingii*, a newly recognized agent of human ehrlichiosis. N Engl J Med 1999;341:148.

37. Fishbein DB, Dawson JE, Robinson LE. Human ehrlichiosis in the United States, 1985–1990. Ann Intern Med 1994;120: 736.

38. Comer JA, Nicholson WL, Sumner JW, et al. Diagnosis of human ehrlichiosis by PCR assay of acute phase serum. J Clin Microbiol 1999;37:31.

39. Bakken JS, Krueth J, Wilson-Dordskog C, et al. Clinical and laboratory characteristics of human granulocytic ehrlichiosis. JAMA 1996;275:199.

40. Bakken JS, Aguero-Rosenfeld ME, Tilden RL, et al. Serial measurements of hematologic counts during the active phase of human granulocytic ehrlichiosis. Clin Infect Dis 2001;32: 682.

41. Bakken JS, Dumler JS. Human granulocytic ehrlichiosis. Clin Infect Dis 2000;31:554.

42. Shapiro ED, Gerber MA. Lyme Disease. Clin Infect Dis 2000;31:533.

43. James AM, Liveris D, Wormser GP, et al. *Borrelia lonestari* infection after a bite by an *Amblyomma americanum* tick. J Infect Dis 2001;183:1810.

44. Quick RE, Herwaldt BL, Thomford JW, et al. Babesiosis in Washington state: a new species of *Babesia*. Ann Intern Med 1993;119:284.

45. Persing DH, Herwaldt BL, Glaser C, et al. Infection with a *Babesia*-like organism in northern California. N Engl J Med 1995;332:172.

46. Herwaldt B, Persing DH, Precigout EA, et al. A fatal case of babesiosis in Missouri: identification of another piroplasm that infects humans. Ann Intern Med 1996;126:172.

47. Gelfand JA, Callahan MV. Babesiosis. Curr Clin Top Infect Dis 1998;18:201.

48. Krause PJ, Spielman A, Telford SR III, et al. Persistent parasitemia after acute babesiosis. N Engl J Med 1998;339:160.

49. Krause PJ, Lepore T, Sikand VK, et al. Atovaquone and azithromycin for the treatment of babesiosis. N Engl J Med 2000;343:1454.

50. Dworkin MS, Anderson DE Jr, Schwan G, et al. Tick-borne relapsing fever in northwestern United States and southwestern Canada. Clin Infect Dis 1998;26:122.

51. Horton JM, Blaser MJ. The spectrum of relapsing fever in the Rocky Mountains. Arch Intern Med 1985;145:871.

52. Evans ME, Gregory DW, Schaffner W, et al. Tularemia: a 30 year experience with 88 cases. Medicine (Baltimore) 1985;64: 251.

53. Centers for Disease Control and Prevention. Arboviral disease—United States, 1994. MMWR Morb Mortal Wkly Rep 1995;44:641.

54. Centers for Disease Control and Prevention. Outbreak of Powassan encephalitis—Maine and Vermont, 1999–2001. MMWR Morb Mortal Wkly Rep 2001;50:761.

CHAPTER 39

Human Immunodeficiency Virus Infection*

DARIUS A. RASTEGAR, MD
MICHAEL I. FINGERHOOD, MD

In the two decades since the onset of the human immunodeficiency virus (HIV) epidemic, the prognosis for patients in the United States has greatly improved (1). Highly active antiretroviral treatment (HAART) and prophylaxis for opportunistic infections have significantly lowered the mortality from acquired immunodeficiency syndrome (AIDS) and have improved the lives of many. These changes have made the care of HIV-infected patient more rewarding yet more complex.

The role of primary care practitioners in caring for HIV-infected individuals is controversial. Some studies have found poorer patient survival and lower adherence with guidelines among physicians who care for small numbers of patients (generally five or less). However, less is known about how the care provided by more experienced generalists compares with specialists. Most would agree that ongoing experience with the care of HIV-infected patients is important and that a physician with only a few HIV-infected patients should consider referring these patients to an expert.

Primary care practitioners certainly do play an important role in identifying those who are infected and counseling those at risk of becoming infected. The goal of this chapter is to review these matters and to provide the generalist with an overview of the issues involved in the ambulatory care of HIV-infected patients. This chapter cannot cover all the details of antiretroviral therapy and HIV-related complications; other resources for obtaining more extensive and up to date information are listed under General References.

GENERAL CONSIDERATIONS

Causes

HIV is a member of the *lentivirus subfamily of human retroviruses* and was found to be the etiologic

*Janet Horn, MD, and Lori Fantry, MD, MPH, contributed to this chapter in previous editions.

agent of AIDS in 1983. These viruses code for an enzyme known as reverse transcriptase, which permits transcription of viral RNA into proviral DNA and subsequent integration into the host's cellular genome, leading to a persistent and latent infection. The retroviruses are associated with diseases of long incubation period, involvement with the hematopoietic and central nervous systems, and immune suppression. Other related human retroviruses include HIV-2 and the human T-cell lymphotropic viruses (HTLV-I, and HTLV-II). HIV-2, found primarily in West Africa, has also been associated with AIDS but has a more prolonged incubation period (2). HTLV-1 has been associated with tropical spastic paraparesis and T-cell leukemia/lymphoma, and HTLV-II has not yet been associated definitively with any human disease (3).

Epidemiology

The Centers for Disease Control and Prevention (CDC) estimates that 800,000 to 900,000 Americans are infected with HIV (4). Worldwide, over 36 million adults are HIV infected. As of the end of 2000, 774,467 cases of AIDS in the United States had been reported to the CDC and 322,865 persons were known to be living with AIDS (5).

Most HIV infection occurs in adults who belong to the major risk groups for HIV infection: men who have sex with men, injection drug users, heterosexual partners of infected persons, and infants of infected women. Rarely are the risk factors for acquisition of HIV infection unknown. As of the end of 2000, 46% of AIDS cases reported to the CDC were in men who have sex with men, 25% were injection drug users, and 11% in persons who had heterosexual exposure to the virus. However, among newly diagnosed cases of HIV infection reported to the CDC from July 1999 to June 2000, 28% were in men who had sex with men, 10% among injection drug users, and 18% from heterosexual contact (6). This suggests that in the United States, like much of the rest of the world, HIV infection is increasingly being transmitted by heterosexual contact.

Transmission and Prevention of Transmission

Primary care practitioners play an important role in counseling patients at risk of acquiring HIV. However, doing so requires actually evaluating a patient's risk of infection; practitioners frequently do not do this because it involves questions about an individual's sexual practices and drug use—topics that physicians (and patients) are often uncomfortable discussing (7). Primary care practitioners should ask all their patients about their sexual practices, as well as drug and alcohol use, in an open and nonjudgmental fashion and educate them about the risks they may be taking.

HIV-1 occurs in highest concentrations in blood and semen. It also occurs in lower concentrations in cervical and vaginal secretions, saliva, tears, breast milk, and amniotic fluid. HIV transmission is most commonly through blood and semen, but vaginal secretions and breast milk also have been implicated in the transmission process.

Sexual Transmission

HIV infection can be transmitted during sexual intercourse between men and between men and women. The risk of transmission varies depending on a number of factors, including the type of sexual practice, the HIV viral RNA level of the infected person, and likely other factors (yet to be determined) in the immune system of the uninfected person.

The following patterns, practices, and situations carry the greatest risk of infection:

- Unprotected receptive anal intercourse, especially if the mucosal lining has been torn, which may happen with penile insertion itself but is more likely to happen with such sexual practices as fisting. The estimated per-episode risk with anal receptive intercourse is 0.8% to 3.2%.
- Unprotected vaginal intercourse—the estimated per-episode risk is 0.05% to 0.15%. A study of HIV-discordant (one HIV infected, the other not) heterosexual couples in Uganda reported a 0.11% per-episode risk, and there was no difference in transmission rates from females to males or vice versa (8).
- Unprotected vaginal or rectal intercourse when either partner has genital ulceration (e.g., due to primary syphilis, chancroid, or genital herpes). Genital ulcers can act as conduits for infected blood from or for infected semen, blood, or vaginal secretions into the person with the ulcer.

The *prevention of sexual transmission of HIV* requires that sexually active people choose sexual practices that eliminate the high-risk situations listed above, as well as other lower risk practices, including oral–genital contact. In the care of every patient who is sexually active and in public education messages, the fundamentals of safe, possibly safe, and definitely unsafe sex should be clearly communicated (Table 39.1). Specific instructions for the most effective use of condoms (Table 39.2) are particularly important. Postexposure prophylaxis with antiretroviral medication after sexual contact with someone who is infected (similar to postoccupational exposure prophylaxis; see Occupational Exposure, below) may be considered in certain situations (9).

The risk of sexual transmission also varies depending on the serum level of HIV RNA ("viral load") in the infected person. In a study of 415 discordant heterosexual couples in Uganda, researchers reported an average transmission rate of approximately 12 per 100 person-years. However, there were no instances of transmission when the infected partner's HIV RNA level was below 1,500 (10).

Transmission Through Transfusion of Blood and Blood Products

HIV can be transmitted only by whole blood, blood cellular components, plasma, and clotting factors. No

Table 39.1. Safe Sex Guidelines

Safe sex practices
Massage
Hugging
Mutual masturbation
Social kissing (dry)
Body-to-body rubbing
Voyeurism, exhibitionism, fantasy
Possibly safe sex practices
French kissing (wet)
Anal intercourse with condom[a]
Vaginal intercourse with condom[a]
Limiting the number of partners with whom one has sex
Unsafe sex practices
Semen, vaginal fluid, menstrual blood, or urine in mouth or in contact with the skin where there is an open cut or sore
Anal intercourse without condom[a]
Vaginal intercourse without condom[a]
Rimming (oral–anal contact)
Fisting (possible percutaneous inoculation with blood from trauma caused by inserting fist into anus)
Having sex when either partner has an open genital sore

[a]See instructions for condom users in Table 39.2.

Table 39.2. Instructions for Condom Users

Use a condom every time you have intercourse.
Always put the condom on the penis before intercourse begins.
Put the condom on when the penis is erect.
Do not pull the condom tightly against the tip of the penis. Leave a small empty space—about 1 or 2 cm—at the end of the condom to hold semen. Some condoms have a nipple tip that will hold semen.
Unroll the condom all the way to the bottom of the penis.
If the condom breaks during intercourse, withdraw the penis immediately and put on a new condom.
After ejaculation withdraw the penis while it is still erect. Hold onto the rim of the condom as you withdraw so that the condom does not slip off.
Use a new condom each time you have intercourse. Throw used condoms away.
If a lubricant is desired, use water-based lubricants such as contraceptive jelly. Lubricants made with petroleum jelly may damage condoms. Do not use saliva because it may contain virus.
Store condoms in a cool dry place if possible.
Condoms that are sticky or brittle or otherwise damaged should not be used.

Adapted from Population Reports XIV, No. 3, 1986.

other blood products (e.g., immune globulin preparations, albumin, plasma protein fraction, hepatitis B vaccine) have been implicated.

The risk of acquiring HIV through a blood transfusion is now infinitesimally small. The estimated risk of HIV infection is 1:153,000 per unit of blood transfused (11). This low risk has been achieved by blood donor education programs (to eliminate donors who belong to high-risk groups), uniform blood product screening since April 1985, HIV-inactivating treatment of clotting factor concentrates, the use of autologous blood transfusions for elective surgery, and efforts to avoid all nonessential transfusions.

Needle Transmission

Sharing of needles by injection drug users accounts for a large proportion of patients with AIDS in the United States. HIV-infected patients in this group pose a threat to both needle partners and sexual partners. In developing countries, this mode of transmission may also occur because of reuse of improperly cleaned needles and syringes for the injections of medicines.

Definitive interruption of transmission by injection drug use requires that the user discontinue the practice as part of a recovery program (see Chapter 29). The interruption of transmission by those who continue injection drug use requires that they avoid needle sharing. Therefore, drug treatment can serve the dual purpose of treating addiction and preventing HIV transmission. Syringe and needle exchange programs have been shown to decrease needle sharing and to decrease spread of HIV infection. Some have advocated that physicians prescribe clean needles to injection drug users who would otherwise not have access to them to prevent transmission of HIV and other bloodborne diseases. It is unknown whether cleaning needles with bleach before reuse is effective in preventing infection. Protective behaviors have been difficult to promote in this subset of people who engage in a variety of high-risk behaviors.

Perinatal Transmission

Although several modes may account for perinatal transmission from an HIV-infected woman to her infant, most infants acquire their infection at or near the time of delivery because of inoculation or ingestion of maternal blood. Intrauterine transmission by cord blood is less common. Transmission can also occur postnatally through breast-feeding. It is estimated that 7% to 39% of infants born to HIV-infected mothers become infected, with the highest rates occurring in infants born to mothers with high viral loads, late-stage disease, early fetal membrane rupture, and placental inflammation.

Prevention of perinatal transmission requires primary prevention through safer sex practices and secondary prevention through HIV testing and subsequent counseling of HIV-infected women about the risks of pregnancy. Antiretroviral therapy with zidovudine or nevirapine has been shown to reduce transmission of HIV to the fetus, and dual antiretroviral therapy (with zidovudine and lamivudine) is more effective than monotherapy. However, the current standard of care in the United States is to treat pregnant women who have an HIV RNA level over 1,000 copies/mL with a three-drug regimen with the goal of lowering the HIV RNA level to an undetectable level. It has been shown that transmission to the infant is rare if the HIV RNA level is below 500 copies/mL at the time of delivery. In addition, elective cesarean section appears to reduce the risk of transmission but is probably only of benefit if the mother does not receive or respond to antiretroviral treatment (i.e., has an HIV RNA over 1,000 copies/mL) (12).

Casual Contact and the Risk of Human Immunodeficiency Virus Transmission

Casual transmission of HIV does not occur. Thus, household contacts of HIV-infected patients who are not sexual partners are not at risk during ordinary circumstances. Although the virus has been isolated in urine and saliva, there have been no documented cases of transmission through kissing or through exposure to urine, stool, or saliva. However, it is generally recommended that the same precautions taken to prevent transmission of hepatitis B in the household setting should be observed by HIV-infected people (see Chapter 47).

Occupational Exposure

The possibility of transmission of HIV to health care workers and caretakers in the patient's household has been of concern since the identification of HIV as the cause of AIDS. The cumulative results of several studies of health care workers have shown that health care workers are at an extremely low but finite risk of occupational infection with the virus. The predominant occupational risk for infection is through accidental needlestick exposure. Most cases of HIV transmission by needlestick exposure have occurred via a large-bore needle. Accidental infection is preventable by conscientious use of *universal precautions* (Table 39.3). "Universal" refers to the fact that these precautions should be followed in the direct care and in the handling of the body fluids of *all* patients (not just those known to be HIV infected).

If a health care worker has a percutaneous injury (needlestick or cut) or contact of mucous membrane (eye or mouth) or nonintact skin with blood, tissues, or other body fluids, the source patient should be assessed clinically and, if consent is obtained, that patient should be tested for HIV infection. As soon as possible after exposure, the exposed worker should be counseled and, if consent is obtained, tested for HIV infection. If the source patient is HIV negative and has no clinical indicators of or risk factors for HIV infection, no further follow-up of the exposed worker is necessary. The U.S. Public Health Service recommends postexposure prophylaxis for occupational exposures to HIV in certain situations depending on type of exposure and exposure source (13). General guidelines for postexposure prophylaxis use for percutaneous injuries and mucous membrane and nonintact skin exposures are given in Tables 39.4 and 39.5, respectively. Postexposure prophylaxis should be initiated within 1 to 2 hours after exposure. The optimal duration of therapy is unknown, but 4 weeks is suggested. Most health care institutions have postexposure protocols and resources for their employees; the National Clinicians' Postexposure Prophylaxis Hotline run by staff at the University of California-San Francisco and San Francisco General Hospital is another resource for obtaining advice regarding

Table 39.3. Health Care Workers' Universal Precautions that Should Be Used in the Care of *All* Patients

Wear gloves for touching blood and body fluids, mucous membranes, or nonintact skin of the patient.
Wash hands immediately before and after patient care.
Wear gown, mask, and goggles if aerosolization or splattering of blood or body fluids is likely.
Handle sharp instruments with great care and discard them immediately in containers designed for this purpose. Used venipuncture needles MUST NOT be recapped.
Clean blood spills promptly with disinfectant such as 1:10 dilution of bleach.
Refrain from direct patient care if you have exudative skin lesions.

Table 39.4. Recommended HIV Postexposure Prophylaxis for Percutaneous Injuries

	Infection status of source				
Exposure Type	HIV Positive Class 1[a]	HIV Positive Class 2[a]	Source of Unknown HIV Status[b]	Unknown Source[c]	HIV Negative
Less severe[d]	Recommend basic 2-drug PEP	Recommend expanded 3-drug PEP	Generally, no PEP warranted; however, consider basic 2-drug PEP[e] for source with HIV risk factors[f]	Generally, no PEP warranted; however, consider basic 2-drug PEP[e] in settings where exposure to HIV-infected persons is likely	No PEP warranted
More severe[g]	Recommend expanded 3-drug PEP	Recommend expanded 3-drug PEP	Generally, no PEP warranted; however, consider basic 2-drug PEP[e] for source with HIV risk factors[f]	Generally, no PEP warranted; however, consider basic 2-drug PEP[e] in settings where exposure to HIV-infected persons is likely	No PEP warranted

[a]HIV positive, class 1—asymptomatic HIV infection or known low viral load (e.g., <1,500 RNA copies/mL). HIV positive, class 2—symptomatic HIV infection, AIDS, acute seroconversion, or known high viral load. If drug resistance is a concern, obtain expert consultation. Initiation of postexposure prophylaxis (PEP) should not be delayed pending expert consultation, and because expert consultation alone cannot substitute for face-to-face counseling, resources should be available to provide immediate evaluation and follow-up care for all exposures.

[b]Source of unknown HIV status (e.g., deceased source person with no samples available for HIV testing).

[c]Unknown source (e.g., a needle from a sharps disposal container).

[d]Less severe (e.g., solid needle and superficial injury).

[e]The designation "consider PEP" indicates that PEP is optional and should be based on an individualized decision between the exposed person and the treating clinician.

[f]If PEP is offered and taken and the source is later determined to be HIV negative, PEP should be discontinued.

[g]More severe (e.g., large-bore hollow needle, deep puncture, visible blood on device, or needle used in patient's artery or vein).

HIV, human immunodeficiency virus; AIDS, acquired immunodeficiency syndrome.

Source: Centers for Disease Control and Prevention. Updated U.S. Public Health Service guidelines for the management of occupational exposures to HBV, HCV, and HIV and recommendations for postexposure prophylaxis. MMWR Morb Mortal Wkly Rep 2001;50(no. RR-11):1, with permission.

Table 39.5. Recommended HIV Postexposure Prophylaxis for Mucous Membrane Exposures and Nonintact Skin[a] Exposures

	Infection status of source				
Exposure Type	HIV Positive Class 1[b]	HIV Positive Class 2[b]	Source of Unknown HIV Status[c]	Unknown Source[d]	HIV Negative
Small volume[e]	Consider basic 2-drug PEP[f]	Recommend basic 2-drug PEP	Generally, no PEP warranted; however, consider basic 2-drug PEP[f] for source with HIV risk factors[g]	Generally, no PEP warranted; however, consider basic 2-drug PEP[f] in settings where exposure to HIV-infected persons is likely	No PEP warranted
Large volume[h]	Recommend basic 2-drug PEP	Recommend expanded 3-drug PEP	Generally, no PEP warranted; however, consider basic 2-drug PEP[f] for source with HIV risk factors[g]	Generally, no PEP warranted; however, consider basic 2-drug PEP[f] in settings where exposure to HIV-infected persons is likely	No PEP warranted

[a]For skin exposures, follow-up is indicated only if there is evidence of compromised skin integrity (e.g., dermatitis, abrasion, or open wound).

[b]HIV Positive, Class 1—asymptomatic HIV infection or known low viral load (e.g., <1,500 RNA copies/mL). HIV Positive, Class 2—symptomatic HIV infection, AIDS, acute seroconversion, or known high viral load. If drug resistance is a concern, obtain expert consultation. Initiation of postexposure prophylaxis (PEP) should not be delayed pending expert consultation, and because expert consultation alone cannot substitute for face-to-face counseling, resources should be available to provide immediate evaluation and follow-up care for all exposures.

[c]Source of unknown HIV status (e.g., deceased source person with no samples available for HIV testing).

[d]Unknown source (e.g., splash from inappropriately disposed blood).

[e]Small volume (i.e., a few drops).

[f]The designation "consider PEP" indicates that PEP is optional and should be based on an individualized decision between the exposed person and the treating clinician.

[g]If PEP is offered and taken and the source is later determined to be HIV negative, PEP should be discontinued.

[h]Large volume (i.e., major blood splash).

HIV, human immunodeficiency virus; AIDS, acquired immunodeficiency syndrome.

Source: Centers for Disease Control and Prevention. Updated U.S. Public Health Service guidelines for the management of occupational exposures to HBV, HCV, and HIV and recommendations for postexposure prophylaxis. MMWR Morb Mortal Wkly Rep 2001;50(no. RR-11):1, with permission.

postexposure prophylaxis (phone: 888-448-4911; internet: www.ucsf.edu/hivcntr).

SEROLOGIC DIAGNOSIS AND COUNSELING

Indications for Serologic Testing

Primary care practitioners are the front line of identifying patients infected with HIV and at risk of acquiring the infection. HIV testing and counseling are indicated both to prevent further transmission of disease and to allow people already infected to be identified so that they can seek appropriate medical care. This is especially important now that we have potent drugs to halt the progression of HIV and prevent infection in newborns.

According to the CDC, voluntary testing should be performed in all patients who have sexually transmitted diseases, are current or former injection drug users, are hemophiliacs, have active tuberculosis (TB), have received blood transfusions or blood products between 1978 and 1985, are prostitutes, are from developing countries with high rates of HIV infection, have regular sexual partners with risk factors or known to be HIV infected, have signs or symptoms suggestive of HIV infection, consider themselves at risk for HIV infection or request testing, or are exposed to blood or other at-risk body fluids (including health care workers who perform invasive procedures); all pregnant women should also have voluntary testing performed. There is a growing list of conditions associated with HIV infection that should also provoke consideration of HIV testing; some of these are listed in Table 39.6.

Pretest and Posttest Counseling

The most important aspect of HIV testing is pretest and posttest counseling. Because of the ominous meaning of HIV infection, it is important to ensure privacy and to allow sufficient time to respond to the patient's feelings and questions. Many settings require the patient's written informed consent as part of pretest counseling. Recommended points of discussion during counseling are shown in Table 39.7. Information about behaviors associated with the risk of acquiring HIV infection is important in both stages of counseling. Details have also been published regarding counseling of patients infected with HTLV-I and HTLV-II (3).

Information about available printed materials useful in posttest counseling and about regional programs for HIV-infected patients can be obtained by contacting the National AIDS Information Clearing House (P.O. Box 6003, Rockville, MD 20850; telephone 800-458-5231).

Serologic Tests

Antibody to HIV usually appears 6 to 12 weeks after infection but may take as long as 6 months to appear. However, the body's immune response to HIV does not lead to elimination of the virus from host tissues. As described above, a persistent carrier (and persistent

Table 39.6. Factors that Should Trigger Consideration of Testing for Human Immunodeficiency Virus

Historical factors
Alcohol or drug use/detoxification
Psychiatric hospitalization
Homelessness
Unsafe sexual practices
Multiple partners
Men who have sex with men
Sex with prostitutes
Clinical factors
Any sexually transmitted disease, including
Herpes
Gonorrhea
Trichomonas
Syphilis
Hepatitis B
Pelvic inflammatory disease
Genital condyloma
Abnormal Pap smear
Other infections, including
Tuberculosis
Pneumonia
Recurrent vaginal candidiasis
Herpes zoster
Hepatitis C
Skin conditions
Psoriasis
Seborrhea
Molluscum contagiosa
Other conditions
Unexplained weight loss
Bell palsy/other neuropathies
Generalized lymphadenopathy/unexplained focal adenopathy
Lymphoma
Mononucleosis syndrome
Pulmonary hypertension
Congestive heart failure (unexplained)
Renal failure
Idiopathic thrombocytopenic purpura (ITP)
Thrombotic thrombocytopenic purpura (TTP)

Table 39.7. HIV Pretest and Posttest Counseling: Points for Discussion

Pretest counseling
Meaning of positive test
Positive test means HIV infection
Positive test does *not* mean AIDS[a]
Positive test means patient is an HIV carrier
Confidentiality of test results and medical information
Availability of anonymous and confidential counseling and testing sites
Potential adverse psychosocial consequences if information becomes known, e.g., possible adverse effects on employment, housing, insurance status
Sources of additional AIDS/HIV-related information[b]
Means for reducing risk of HIV transmission or exposure (depends on patient's current or likely high-risk behaviors)
"Safe sex" practices (see Tables 39.1 and 39.2)
Sterilization of intravenous drug equipment
Treatment for drug addiction
Discontinuation of sharing intravenous needles
Posttest counseling
Interpretation of HIV antibody test results
Information about long-term chances of developing symptoms
Planning for medical follow-up
Referral to psychosocial support services
Reinforcement of recommendations for prevention of HIV transmission/exposure
Discussion of notification of sexual partners or needle-sharing partners
Reproductive issues in women

[a]Most people with a positive test will develop AIDS. Length of time from infection to development of AIDS is variable but averages 10 years.

[b]A single source for information is the National AIDS Information Clearing House. P.O. Box 6003, Rockville, MD 20850 (800-458-5231).

HIV, human immunodeficiency virus; AIDS, acquired immunodeficiency syndrome.

seropositive) state follows infection with this type of virus. The diagnosis of HIV infection is based on detection of *anti-HIV antibodies* by the enzyme-linked immunosorbent assay (ELISA), confirmed by the more specific Western blot (WB) method. In the WB method, several individual HIV proteins are transferred onto nitrocellulose paper and reacted against the patient's serum and known positive and negative sera; HIV antibody is detected by an anti-human immunoglobulin antibody coated with an enzyme that, in the presence of substrate, produces a colored band. A positive WB test (the presence two of three colored bands representing p24, gp41, and gp120 or gp160) indicates that the patient has been infected with HIV (14).

ELISA tests are reported as positive or negative. WB tests are reported as positive, negative, or indeterminate. The routine processing of a specimen that is positive on initial ELISA testing always includes rerun of the ELISA, to confirm the result, followed by the WB test. The currently used ELISA tests have a sensitivity greater than 99% and a specificity of 99.5%. False positive ELISA tests (ELISA positive, WB negative) may occur when nonspecific serologic reactions are present in patients who have other types of immunologic abnormalities or who have had multiple transfusions or multiple pregnancies. False positives generally occur in patients from groups at low risk of acquiring HIV infection. False negative ELISA results may occur in recently infected patients who have not made an antibody response.

Patients whose WB tests are reported as indeterminate are those whose sera yield only one of the necessary positive color bands. In most cases, the person is not infected with HIV, especially if the person is at low risk. However, this result may signify that a person is in the process of primary infection and will eventually convert to WB positive. For this reason, the patient should be tested again; if the result remains indeterminate, testing should be repeated in 3 to 6 months. If the WB pattern remains indeterminate for 6 months—in the absence of any known risk factors or clinical findings to suggest HIV infection—the test may be considered negative. Patients who have risk factors or findings compatible with HIV-induced disease should have continued evaluation.

The Food and Drug Administration also has licensed *home HIV test kits.* These systems require the purchaser to pierce his or her skin with the lancet supplied in the kit, place a few drops of blood on a filter paper test card, and then send the sample to a central laboratory. Routine testing with ELISA and, if necessary, WB is then performed. The Food and Drug Administration has also approved an oral specimen collection device, which consists of a pad placed between the gum and cheek for 2 minutes and then sent to a laboratory in a vial. Sensitivity and specificity for both systems are reported to be comparable with routine testing on serum. Counseling is provided over the telephone.

HIV RNA level ("viral load") should not be used for screening purposes, except when acute HIV infection is suspected. The sensitivity and specificity of this test for diagnosing chronic infection is poorer than the ELISA and WB tests; some chronically infected patients have undetectable viral loads, and false positive viral loads can also occur (15).

PATHOGENESIS AND NATURAL HISTORY

Pathogenesis of Disease in Human Immunodeficiency Virus-Infected Patients

HIV causes illness by impairing important components of the patient's immune system, making the patient susceptible to a wide variety of infections. This virus also causes illness by its direct effect on other body systems, especially the nervous system (15).

HIV preferentially infects human *T lymphocytes of the helper/inducer subset* (also called *CD4 cells*), resulting in both quantitative and qualitative defects in helper cell function. Because helper T lymphocytes are crucial in cell-mediated immunity, HIV infection impairs this type of immunity, making the patient susceptible to a number of opportunistic infections. Uninfected people usually have more than 800 CD4 cells/mm^3 of blood, whereas HIV-infected patients with opportunistic infections usually have less than 200 CD4 cells/mm^3. Thus, monitoring the CD4 cell count has become useful for predicting the degree of suppression of a patient's cell-mediated immunity, guiding the differential diagnosis of new symptoms, and deciding when to initiate antiretroviral treatment and prophylaxis for opportunistic infection (see below).

Other abnormalities of immune function are also found in HIV-infected people. HIV can infect and impair the function of macrophages and monocytes and CD4 lymphocytes. HIV infection may also result in B-lymphocyte activation and nonspecific hypergammaglobulinemia, which may impair the *de novo* antibody response to some antigens; this may place the patient at increased risk for infection with encapsulated bacteria. In addition, some studies suggest that HIV infection may cause derangements in polymorphonuclear neutrophil phagocytosis and intracellular killing.

Although most of the illnesses in patients with HIV infection are caused by impaired resistance to infection, a number of clinical manifestations are direct consequences of HIV infection or the immune response to HIV infection. There is good evidence that the virus plays an etiologic role in some neurologic syndromes. The virus may directly affect the nervous system both centrally and peripherally, causing HIV meningitis, dementia, and peripheral neuropathy. In addition, the virus, or in some cases the immune response to the virus, causes disease in the gastrointestinal tract, heart, lungs, and possibly the kidneys.

Natural History and Prognosis in Human Immunodeficiency Virus Infection

The mean length of time from seroconversion to symptomatic AIDS in untreated patients is 10 years. The time from infection to symptoms, however, varies considerably from person to person and probably reflects variations in individuals' immune systems and the infectivity of different strains of the virus. Expanded use of antiretroviral therapy, prophylaxis against opportunistic infections, and treatment of AIDS-associated conditions result in delayed progression and longer life expectancies for HIV-infected people. An overview of the natural history of HIV infection, based on CD4 counts and viral load, is shown in Fig. 39.1. Because the virus may remain clinically silent with no demonstrable signs of immunodeficiency or symptoms for many years, asymptomatic patients play a major role in transmitting the virus.

Primary Human Immunodeficiency Virus Infection

Primary HIV infection ("acute retroviral syndrome") is usually symptomatic in the form of a mild to severe flu-like illness. The most common signs and symptoms are fever, malaise, myalgia, and rash (Table 39.8). The syndrome is nonspecific and cannot be differentiated from other acute viral illnesses on the basis of signs or symptoms alone. Patients often do not seek medical attention and even when they do, primary HIV infection is often not recognized. There is a wide range of less common presentations of primary HIV infection that have been reported; some are listed in Table 39.8.

The incubation period (time from exposure to onset of illness) for the acute syndrome may range from 5 days to 3 months, usually 2 to 4 weeks. During the period of initial infection, blood virus levels are high, HIV is widely disseminated, and there is a transient decrease in circulating CD4 cells. There is an immune response to HIV between 1 week and 3 months after infection, and antibodies are detectable 6 to 24 weeks after the initial exposure. The early immune response is associated with a dramatic decrease in viremia, but viral replication is never completely curtailed, particularly in lymphoid tissue.

Because of the nonspecific nature of the illness, primary care practitioners need to maintain a high index of suspicion to identify patients with primary HIV infection. The diagnosis can be made by measuring HIV RNA level (viral load) or HIV p24 antigen; an elevated viral load (usually over 100,000 copies/mL) or detectable p24 antigen, in the presence of a negative HIV ELISA, establishes the diagnosis. Viral load is a more sensitive test (100%) than the p24 antigen (89%) but is less specific (97% vs. 100% for p24 antigen); however, specificity for viral load rises to 100% if a cutoff of 10,000 copies/mL is used (15). Recognizing primary HIV infection is important because it can help prevent further transmission and gives the opportunity to test for transmission of resistant virus (see section on resistance testing).

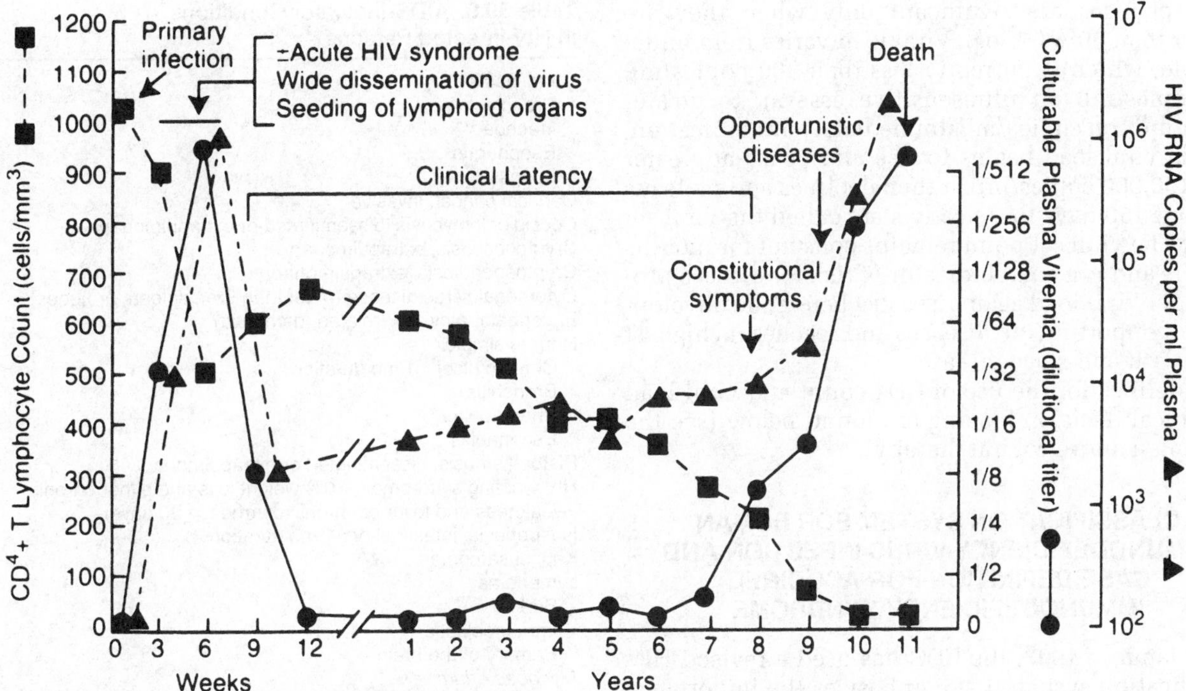

Figure 39.1. Natural history of HIV infection, based on CD4 counts and viral load. (From Fauci AS, Pantaleo G, Stanley S, et al. Immunopathogenic mechanisms of HIV infection. Ann Intern Med 1996;124:654, with permission.)

Table 39.8. Manifestations of Primary Human Immunodeficiency Virus Infection

Common signs and symptoms
Fever
Malaise
Myalgia/arthralgia
Rash
Headache
Sore throat
Night sweats
Lymphadenopathy
Less common signs and symptoms
Oral ulcers
Oral candidiasis (thrush)
Weight loss
Nausea/vomiting
Hepatosplenomegaly
Thrombocytopenia
Leukopenia
Transaminitis
Other reported manifestations
Clinical hepatitis
Acute pneumonitis
Vascultitis
Nephrotic syndrome/acute renal failure
Rhabdomyolysis
Neuropathy (including radiculopathy, Guillain-Barré syndrome, Bell palsy)
Aseptic meningitis/meningoencephalitis
Aplastic anemia
Opportunistic infections (esophageal candidiasis, pneumocystis pneumonia, etc.)

Prognostic Indicators

The marker of disease progression that is most familiar to clinicians and has served the test of time is the *CD4 lymphocyte count.* The absolute number and percentage of CD4 lymphocytes gives the clinician an indication of the degree of immunosuppression and hence can be used to determine what types of associated conditions the patient is susceptible to and give an estimate of life expectancy. The absolute number of CD4 cells is subject to more variability than the percentage because of normal biologic fluctuations in total lymphocyte counts. Within a year of seroconversion, CD4 cell counts usually drop 200 to 300/mm^3 from the normal range of 800 to 1200. This decline is followed by an increase to near baseline and then a slow decline of less than 100 cells per year (Fig. 39.1). People with CD4 cell counts greater than 500 are usually asymptomatic and have virtually no risk of developing an AIDS-indicator condition, except for TB, cervical cancer, recurrent bacterial pneumonias, or superficial Kaposi sarcoma (KS), within 18 months. In contrast, those with CD4 cell counts of 100 or less are often symptomatic and have a 60% chance of developing an AIDS-indicator disease (excluding TB, cervical cancer, and recurrent bacterial pneumonias) within 18 months.

A second prognostic indicator of disease progression is *HIV viral load* (measured as circulating HIV RNA). Among patients with equivalent CD4 lymphocyte counts, patients with higher viral loads on average have a more rapid a fall in CD4 counts and clinical disease progression (17). Viral loads are an important way to monitor the effectiveness of antiretroviral therapy; a change in viral load usually occurs before a change in CD4 lymphocyte count, so changes in therapy can be made sooner if viral load is used. Nevertheless, changes in viral load should be interpreted with caution because there is wide intrapatient variation and serial changes are significant only when they are greater than 50% (.3 log). Viral load varies from undetectable, which is currently less than 400 copies/mL (50 copies/mL on ultrasensitive assays), to greater than 1 million copies/mL. Immediately after infection, plasma viral load begins to rise and peaks at greater than 100,000 copies/mL. It then declines and plateaus in about 150 days to a steady state called the viral set point. The viral set point remains constant for months to years and is a good indicator of risk for disease progression. Viral load again rises just before the development of opportunistic diseases and reaches its highest value with end-stage disease.

Guidelines for the use of CD4 count and viral load in clinical decision-making are found below (see the section on antiretroviral therapy).

CLASSIFICATION SYSTEM FOR HUMAN IMMUNODEFICIENCY VIRUS INFECTION AND CASE DEFINITION FOR ACQUIRED IMMUNODEFICIENCY SYNDROME

Since January 1993, the CDC has used a revised HIV classification system that emphasizes the importance of the CD4 (T lymphocyte) count. This replaced the previous classification system published by the CDC in 1986, based exclusively on clinical disease criteria. Patients are now classified according to three categories of CD4 cell counts:

1. More than 500/mm^3;
2. 200 to 499/mm^3;
3. Less than 200/mm^3.

They are also classified according to three clinical categories:

A. Asymptomatic, acute HIV, or persistent generalized lymphadenopathy;
B. Symptomatic, not A or C conditions;
C. AIDS-indicator conditions.

Once a person meets criteria for symptomatic HIV or AIDS, that person remains in the same category or advances to a more advanced stage despite interventions that may eliminate symptoms or increase CD4 cell counts. Patients in categories 3 or C meet the case definition of AIDS.

Symptomatic disease in category B includes any condition attributable to immunodeficiency from HIV infection or complicated by HIV infection (except those in categories A and C). Examples of these conditions include bacillary angiomatosis; oropharyngeal candidiasis; vulvovaginal candidiasis that is persistent, frequent, or poorly responsive to therapy; cervical dysplasia (moderate or severe) or cervical carcinoma *in situ*; constitutional symptoms such as fever (38.5°C or higher) or diarrhea lasting more than 1 month; oral hairy leukoplakia; herpes zoster of more than one dermatome or recurring at least once; idiopathic thrombocytopenic purpura; listeriosis; pelvic inflammatory disease; and peripheral neuropathy.

Table 39.9. AIDS-Indicator Conditions in HIV-infected Persons

Candidiasis
Bronchi
Trachea
Esophagus
Lungs
Cervical cancer, invasive
Coccidioidomycosis, disseminated or extrapulmonary
Cryptococcosis, extrapulmonary
Cryptosporidiosis, extrapulmonary
Cytomegalovirus disease (other than liver, spleen, or nodes)
Encephalopathy, HIV related (dementia)
Herpes simplex
Chronic ulcer >1 mo duration
Bronchitis
Pneumonitis
Esophagitis
Histoplasmosis, disseminated or extrapulmonary
HIV wasting syndrome (>10% weight loss and either chronic weakness and fever or chronic diarrhea, ≥30 days)
Isosporiasis, intestinal of >1 mo duration
Kaposi sarcoma
Lymphoma
Burkitt
Immunoblastic
Primary of the brain
Mycobacterium
M. avium complex, disseminated or extrapulmonary
M. kansasii, disseminated or extrapulmonary
M. tuberculosis, pulmonary or extrapulmonary
Other species, disseminated or extrapulmonary
P. carinii pneumonia
Pneumonia, two or more episodes within a year
Progressive multifocal leukoencephalopathy
Salmonella septicemia, recurrent
Toxoplasmosis, brain

HIV, human immunodeficiency virus; AIDS, acquired immunodeficiency syndrome.

Adapted from Centers for Disease Control and Prevention. 1993. Revised classification system for HIV infection and expanded surveillance case definition for AIDS among adolescents and adults. MMWR Morb Mortal Wkly Rep 1992; 41 (No. BR-17), with permission.

The CDC has also expanded the list of *AIDS-indicator conditions* (Table 39.9). In addition to the 23 clinical conditions originally used to define AIDS, pulmonary TB, recurrent pneumonia (at least two episodes per year), and invasive cervical cancer are now AIDS-indicator diseases.

INITIAL EVALUATION AND TREATMENT OF THE HUMAN IMMUNODEFICIENCY VIRUS-INFECTED PATIENT

Baseline History, Physical Examination, and Laboratory Studies

The apparently asymptomatic patient with HIV infection requires an initial evaluation and ongoing psychosocial support and medical assessment. This section describes important manifestations to be sought in initial and subsequent evaluations of HIV-positive patients and prophylactic guidelines, as established by the U.S. Public Health Service in collaboration with the Infectious Diseases Society of America (18). Descriptions of symptomatic manifestations are found under Symptomatic Human Immunodeficiency Virus-Infected Patient, below.

In addition to the HIV-oriented review of systems summarized in Table 39.10, seropositive patients should be asked about a history of sexually transmitted diseases, TB, or a positive purified protein derivative (PPD) test; exposure to or history of hepatitis B; immunosuppressive therapy (e.g., an asthmatic patient who intermittently requires corticosteroids); and previous immunizations, including pneumococcal and hepatitis B vaccines. Important information to obtain in the social history includes current sexual practices (type and number of sexual partners), types of contraception used, and past or present injection drug use.

The *baseline physical examination* should include all organ systems, with special emphasis on the oral cavity, skin, lymph nodes, and, in women, the reproductive system. Physical manifestations in these organ systems are particularly important because diseases may be found that are potentially treatable (i.e., seborrheic dermatitis) or that carry prognostic significance (i.e., oral candidiasis).

The *baseline laboratory evaluation* should establish a database that will be useful for identifying already present abnormalities and for comparison when abnormalities are identified at a later time in the care of the patient. This database should include a complete blood count (including a differential and platelet count), hepatitis B surface antigen and antibody, syphilis serology, *Toxoplasma* antibody, HIV viral load, and CD4 lymphocyte count. Baseline serologic tests for antibody to cytomegalovirus (CMV) are not generally useful because of the high prevalence of positive tests in the normal population. Unless the patient has a history of a positive PPD skin test or TB, the patient should have a PPD. A chest radiograph should be performed in all patients who have a positive PPD (5 mm or more induration) or have respiratory symptoms or a history of respiratory disease. Table 39.9 gives suggested guidelines for periodic monitoring.

Many patients who complain of no symptoms at baseline will have one or more abnormalities found on physical examination or laboratory evaluation, most commonly generalized lymphadenopathy (see definition below), reduced CD4 count, elevated HIV viral load, or mild suppression of the elements of the bone marrow (19). If a history of constitutional symptoms (weight loss, fevers, night sweats) is elicited, this should be evaluated further, as discussed in the next section. Findings in the oral cavity that may not cause symptoms but suggest some degree of immunodeficiency include oral hairy leukoplakia or early *Candida* infection (see descriptions below). A finding of an isolated low platelet count may be indicative of immune thrombocytopenic purpura. Laboratory abnormalities (e.g., hypochromic anemia) should be evaluated in the same manner as in a non–HIV-infected patient.

Table 39.10. HIV-oriented Review of Symptoms

General: Weight loss, fever, night sweats
Skin: New rashes, pigmented lesions, itching
Lymphoid system: Asymmetric or rapidly growing lymph nodes.
HEENT: Change in vision, unusual headaches, congestion or running nose, oral lesions
Respiratory: Cough, shortness of breath, decrease in exercise tolerance
Gastrointestinal: Pain or difficulty in swallowing, nausea or vomiting, diarrhea, painful defecation
Neuropsychiatric: Difficulty thinking, depression, change in personality, numbness or tingling, muscle weakness, loss of sensation

HIV, human immunodeficiency virus.

Health Maintenance: Monitoring Schedules, Immunizations, and Opportunistic Infection Prophylaxis

Table 39.11 outlines the recommended monitoring schedule for HIV-infected patients according to CD4 cell count. Table 39.17 and this section address immunizations and opportunistic infection prophylaxis to prevent first episodes of preventable diseases. Later sections address the treatment of opportunistic infections (see Symptomatic Human Immunodeficiency Virus-Infected Patient) and the schedule for viral load monitoring and the initiation and long-term use of antiretroviral drugs (Antiretroviral Treatment).

Prevention of First Episodes of Opportunistic Infections

Preventive care for HIV-infected patients should include various vaccinations (Table 39.12). Pneumococcal pneumonia is the leading cause of bacterial pneumonia in HIV-infected patients; *pneumococcal vaccine* is recommended for all HIV-infected patients. It should be given early in the course of HIV infection or, if given in later stage disease, after the patient has

Table 39.11. Health Maintenance in the HIV-infected Patient: Monitoring Timing and Frequency Based on CD4 count

CD4 Count (per mm^3)	>500	200–499	100–200	<100
CD4 cell count	3–6 mo[a]	3 mo	3 mo	3 mo
HIV viral load	3–6 mo[a]	3 mo	3 mo	3 mo
Syphilis serology	12 mo	12 mo	12 mo	12 mo
Hepatitis B serology	Once	Once	Once	Once
Tuberculosis screening[b]	12 mo	12 mo	12 mo	12 mo
Pap smear	6–12 mo	6–12 mo	6–12 mo	6–12 mo
Ophthalmologic exam (CMV)	No	No	No	6 mo

[a]A patient on antiretroviral therapy should be monitored every 3 months; a longer interval may be sufficient if not on therapy, especially if the viral load is relatively low.
[b]When positive, do not repeat.
HIV, human immunodeficiency virus; CMV, cytomegalovirus.

Table 39.12. Health Maintenance in HIV-infected Individuals: Immunizations and Antimicrobial Prophylaxis to Prevent First Episodes of Opportunistic Disease in Adults

Pathogen	Indication	First Choice	Alternative
Category I: Strongly Recommended as Standard of Care			
Pneumocystis carinii	CD4 count <200 or oropharyngeal candidiasis	TMP/SMZ, 1 SS; or DS q.d	Dapsone 50 mg BID or 100 mg q.d.; or Aerosolized pentamidine; 9 mo or Atovaquone 1500 mg q.d.
Mycobacterium tuberculosis Isoniazid-sensitive	PPD reaction ≥5 mm or prior positive PPD without treatment or contact with active TB case	Isoniazid 300 mg + pyridoxine 50 mg q.d. × 9 mo; or Isoniazid 900 mg + pyridoxine 100 mg b.i.w. × 9 mo; or Rifampin 600 mg + pyrazinamide[a] 20 mg/kg q.d. × 2 mo	Rifabutin 300 mg + pyrazinamide 20 mg/kg q.d. × 2 mo; or Rifampin 600 mg q.d. × 4 mo.
M. tuberculosis Isoniazid-resistant	Same as above, with high probability of exposure to isoniazid-resistant tuberculosis	Rifampin 600 mg + pyrazinamide[a] 20 mg/kg q.d. × 2 mo[a]	Rifabutin 300 mg + pyrazinamide[a] 20 mg/kg q.d. × 2 mo; or Rifampin 600 mg q.d. × 4 mo.; or Rifabutin 300 mg q.d. × 4 mo.
M. tuberculosis multidrug-resistant	Same as above, with high probability of exposure to multidrug-resistant tuberculosis	Consult public health authorities.	None
Toxoplasma gondii	IgG antibody to *Toxoplasma* and CD4 count <100	TMP/SMZ, 1 DS q.d.	TMP-SMZ, 1 SS q.d.; or Dapsone 50 mg q.d. + pyrimethamine 50 mg q.w. + leukovorin 25 mg q.w.; or Atavoquone 1500 mg q.d. ± pyrimethamine 25 mg q.d. + leukovorin 10 mg q.d.
Mycobacterium avium complex	CD4 count <50	Azithromycin 1200 mg q.w.; or Clarithromycin 500 mg b.i.d.	Rifabutin 300 mg q.d.; or Azithromycin 1200 mg q.w. + rifabutin 300 mg q.d.
Varicella zoster virus (VZV)	Significant exposure to chickenpox or shingles for patients who have no history of either condition or, if available, negative antibody to VZV	Varicella zoster immune globulin (VZIG), 5 vials (1.25 mL each) im administered ≤96 h after exposure, ideally within 48 h	None
Category 2: Generally recommended			
Streptococcus pneumoniae	All patients	Pneumococcal vaccine	None
Hepatitis B	All susceptible (anti-HBc-negative) patients	Hepatitis B vaccine (3 doses)	None
Influenza A	All patients (annually, before influenza season)	Influenza vaccine	Rimantadine 100 mg b.i.d.; or Amantadine 100 mg b.i.d.

All medications are p.o. unless otherwise noted.

[a]Use with caution; severe cases of hepatotoxicity reported with this combination (see text).

HIV, human immunodeficiency virus.

Source: 1999 USPHS/IDSA guidelines of the prevention of opportunistic infections in persons infected with HIV. MMWR Morb Mortal Wkly Rep 1999;48:40–59.

responded to antiretroviral therapy. The evidence for the efficacy of the pneumococcal vaccine is mixed: A randomized controlled trial in Uganda unexpectedly showed a trend toward increased pneumococcal disease among vaccine recipients (20), whereas an analysis of a U.S. database of HIV-infected patients suggested a benefit for those with CD4 counts over 500 (21). The *influenza vaccine* has been shown to be effective and safe in HIV-infected adults (22).

Hepatitis B vaccine should be given in hepatitis B surface antigen and antibody-negative patients who have continued risk factors for hepatitis B because of the increased risk for chronic hepatitis in HIV-infected patients. Although data on the efficacy of *other killed or inactivated vaccines* is not available, it is still recommended that routine vaccines such as tetanus are given to HIV-infected patients.

Live attenuated vaccines such as polio, typhoid, and yellow fever should not be given. Measles vaccine, however, has been shown to be safe in HIV-infected children and can be given according to the recommendations for HIV-negative people. For details regarding dosages and schedules of immunizations, see Chapter 18.

Antimicrobial Prophylaxis

Table 39.12 delineates recommendations for antimicrobial prophylaxis for infections caused by *Pneumocystis carinii*, *Mycobacterium avium*, and *Toxoplasma gondii*. These indications for prophylaxis are guided largely by CD4 counts and not symptomatic infection. Recommended prophylaxis regimens for other opportunistic infections, initiated *after episodes of symptomatic infection*, are found below (Symptomatic Human Immunodeficiency Virus-Infected Patient).

Pneumocystis carinii pneumonia (PCP) prophylaxis should be initiated when the CD4 cell count is less than 200 or if the patient already has had PCP or has oral candidiasis (18). Doses and regimens for the oral agents effective for prophylaxis are shown in Table 39.12. Oral trimethoprim-sulfamethoxazole

(TMP-SMZ) is the preferred agent because it has been shown to be most efficacious and it also has the added benefit of being inexpensive (less than $50 for a year of treatment).

The most common side effects with TMP-SMZ prophylaxis, in descending order of frequency, include rash, pruritus, nausea and vomiting, fever, anemia, neutropenia, and elevated liver function tests. These side effects often occur within the first month of starting therapy, but some, especially cutaneous reactions and fever, may occur even years after initiation of therapy. These side effects occasionally necessitate discontinuation of therapy. Often, however, TMP-SMZ can be reintroduced, especially when given in gradually increasing doses using the liquid formulation.

If life-threatening reactions occur, such as Stevens-Johnson syndrome, or if the patient is unwilling to restart TMP-SMZ because of prior side effects, dapsone, aerosolized pentamidine, or atovaquone can be substituted. The major toxicities of dapsone are rash and cytopenias. The side effects of aerosolized pentamidine (300 mg every 4 weeks administered over 20 to 25 minutes with a jet nebulizer) include cough and bronchospasm, most often seen in smokers or in patients with pre-existing asthma. Pretreatment with a metered-dose bronchodilator often prevents this problem. In addition, because of the risk of aerosolization of a mycobacterial infection not previously suspected, use of aerosolized pentamidine should be used only in specially designated areas and in patients proven not to have active TB. Atovaquone is another oral alternative to TMP-SMZ but is much more expensive than the other prophylactic agents (~$10,000 a year). Side effects of atovaquone include rash and diarrhea.

All HIV-infected patients with *positive tuberculin tests* (defined as 5 mm or more of induration), regardless of age, should be treated prophylactically with isoniazid 300 mg for at least 9 months or rifampin and pyrazinamide for 2 months (18). The rifampin and pyrazinamide combination has been associated with cases of severe hepatotoxicity and even death; it should be used with caution, especially for patients receiving other hepatotoxic drugs and those with a history of alcoholism or chronic liver disease. Furthermore, it is recommended that liver enzymes be checked at baseline and after 2, 4, and 6 weeks of treatment (18a). If the patient is known to have been exposed to a strain that is resistant to isoniazid but sensitive to rifampin, rifampin should be used as preventive therapy (see details in Chapter 34).

Patients with antibodies to *T. gondii* and CD4 cell counts less than 100 cells/mm^3 should be given TMP-SMZ (one double-strength dose per day) for prophylaxis (18). Dapsone and pyrimethamine are acceptable alternatives if TMP-SMZ is not tolerated. Folinic acid is also given, with the regimen at 25 mg/wk to prevent bone marrow toxicity associated with pyrimethamine.

Prophylaxis is recommended against *M. avium* complex (MAC) when CD4 cell counts are less than 50 cells/mm^3 and has been shown to reduce the risk of disseminated infection and overall mortality (23). Effective regimens include azithromycin 1200 mg once a week, clarithromycin 500 mg twice daily, or rifabutin 300 mg daily. Azithromycin and clarithromycin are more efficacious than rifabutin, and azithromycin has the added advantage of once weekly dosing.

Oral ganciclovir has been shown to prevent *CMV retinitis* in patients with low CD4 cell counts (24), but because of toxicity and difficulty defining which patients are at risk, CMV prophylaxis is not routinely recommended (18). Ophthalmologic screening every 6 months for CMV retinitis is recommended for patients with CD4 cell counts less than 75 cells/mm^3.

Fluconazole has been shown to reduce the risk of invasive fungal infections (esophageal candidiasis and cryptococcosis) for patients with advanced AIDS (CD4 counts < 50/mL) but does not reduce overall mortality (25). For this reason, and because of concerns about the development of drug resistance, the routine use of fluconazole as prophylactic agent is not recommended (18).

Since the advent of new antiretroviral agents that can raise CD4 cell counts for prolonged periods (see below), there has been increasing evidence that primary (and in some cases secondary) prophylaxis can be discontinued once the CD4 cell count rises above the value used as the threshold for initiation. Discontinuation of primary prophylaxis for *P. carinii*, *T. gondii*, and MAC has been shown to be safe when patients have a sustained increase in CD4 counts above the prophylaxis threshold.

Coexisting Medical Problems

HIV-positive patients are as likely as HIV-negative patients to have common acute or chronic diseases. The two groups should be approached in the same way in addressing these problems and in addressing indicated preventive care (see Chapter 14).

Many HIV-infected patients describe minor problems, such as fatigue, night sweats, mild chronic diarrhea, pruritus, and low-grade temperature elevation, for which specific infectious causes cannot be identified. Many of these problems may be manifestations of chronic HIV infection. In addition, for some patients, a focus on somatic concerns is the way in which they present their mental distress (see Chapter 21 for a detailed discussion of somatization). When an identifiable opportunistic infection has been excluded (see below) and there is no evidence of a conventional infection, simple palliative measures should be recommended. Patients should be encouraged to discuss their mental distress at the same time that they are queried and advised about physical symptoms.

Psychosocial and Ethical Aspects

Dealing with the psychosocial issues accompanying the diagnosis of asymptomatic HIV infection is often more difficult than the medical management. Patients who have learned they have a fatal disease that may have been acquired sexually and is stigmatizing for a variety of reasons usually feel extremely isolated and despondent. Because patients' emotional responses

Table 39.13. Indications for the Initiation of Antiretroviral Therapy in the Chronically HIV-1–Infected Patient

Clinical Category	CD4 Cell Count	Plasma HIV RNA	Recommendation
Symptomatic (AIDS, severe symptoms)	Any value	Any value	Treat
Asymptomatic, AIDS	$CD4^+$T cells <200/mm^3	Any value	Treat
Asymptomatic	$CD4^+$ T cells >200/mm^3 but <350/mm^3	Any value	Treatment should generally be offered, though controversy exists.
Asymptomatic	$CD4^+$T cells >350/mm^3	>30,000 (bDNA) or >55,000 (RT-PCR)	Some experts would recommend initiating therapy, recognizing that the 3-yr risk of developing AIDS in untreated patients is >30%. In the absence of very high levels of plasma HIV RNA, some would defer therapy and monitor the $CD4^+$ T-cell count and level of plasma HIV RNA more frequently. Clinical outcomes data after initiating therapy are lacking.
Asymptomatic	$CD4^+$T cells >350/mm^3	<30,000 (bDNA) or <55,000 (RT-PCR)	Many experts would defer therapy and observe, recognizing that the 3-yr risk of developing AIDS in untreated patients is <15%.

HIV, human immunodeficiency virus; AIDS, acquired immunodeficiency virus; RT-PCR, reverse transcriptase polymerase chain reaction.
Source: Guidelines for the use of antiretroviral agents in HIV-1 infected adults and adolescents. February 4, 2002. www.hivatis.org.

may impair the ability to process information, it is important to check their comprehension of the facts, to be prepared to reiterate points covered in the posttest counseling session (Table 39.7), and to respond to the feelings and questions that these points will evoke. The patient must understand how the virus is and is not transmitted, the usual course of the disease, and available therapeutic interventions.

The HIV-infected patient has an intense need for hope and support. In addition to ensuring the patient of one's ongoing support and using counseling techniques that are helpful for a patient in crisis (see Chapter 20), it is appropriate to offer psychologic or psychiatric consultation after the diagnosis of HIV positivity. Among the possible psychosocial consequences of this diagnosis are the uncovering of homosexuality in men whose gay orientation has been confidential; the threatened loss of family, social, and occupational relationships; an increase in the release of irresponsible promiscuity in antisocial people; and an increased risk of suicide. These problems particularly require expert counseling.

HIV-positive patients should be assured of confidentiality about their condition but at the same time should be instructed to inform others who may have been infected by them. Although asymptomatic HIV infection is not reportable in most jurisdictions, the patient's physician may have a responsibility to inform others who may be infected if the patient will not do so. This raises the difficult conflict between the patient's right to confidentiality and the rights of other people to protect their health. Laws governing physicians' actions and obligations and ethical aspects of caring for an HIV-infected patient are discussed further in a later section (Public Health and Legal Responsibilities of the Physician).

Table 39.14. Strategies to Improve Adherence

- Inform patient, anticipate, and treat side effects.
- Avoid adverse drug interactions.
- If possible, reduce dose frequency and number of pills.
- Negotiate a treatment plan, which the patient understands and to which he/she commits.
- Take time, multiple encounters to educate, and explain goals of therapy and need for adherence.
- Establish readiness to take medication *before* first prescription is written.
- Recruit family and friends to support the treatment plan.
- Develop concrete plan for specific regimen, relation to meals, daily schedule, side effects.
- Provide written schedule and pictures of medications, daily or weekly pill boxes, alarm clocks, pagers, other mechanical aids to adherence.
- Develop adherence support groups or add adherence issues to regular agenda of support groups.
- Develop linkages with local community-based organizations around adherence with educational sessions and practical strategies.

Source: Guidelines for the use of antiretroviral agents in HIV-1 infected adults and adolescents. February 4, 2002. www.hivatis.org.

ANTIRETROVIRAL TREATMENT

Multiple clinical trials have shown that HAART dramatically increases CD4 counts, decreases viral load, delays clinical progression, and prolongs life. However, the duration of the efficacious effect and the optimal stage for initiation of therapy are unknown. Development of resistance and long-term side effects of antiretrovirals are concerns in patients on HAART. The long-term side effects include dyslipidemia (dysmorphic changes and hyperlipidemia), hyperglycemia, peripheral neuropathy, and avascular necrosis. As a result, debate exists over whether to delay initiation of antiretroviral therapy. Consensus recommendations for antiretroviral treatment were extensively revised in 2001 and are shown in Table 39.13. Most importantly, patients must be willing and able to comply with HAART with the recognition that a very high level of compliance with medication regimen is necessary to prevent viral resistance and treatment failure. Strategies for optimizing adherence are outlined in Table 39.14. Treatment recommendations released in 2001 and summarized in Table 39.15 include treatment with at least three agents, usually two nucleoside reverse transcriptase inhibitors (NRTI) and a nonnucleoside reverse transcriptase inhibitors (NNRTI) or protease inhibitor (26). Up to date recommendations are available from the U.S. government (website: www.hivatis.org).

Table 39.15. Recommended Antiretroviral Agents for Initial Treatment of Established HIV Infection

	Column A	Column B
Strongly recommended	Efavirenz Indinavir Nelfinavir Ritonavir + Indinavir Ritonavir + Lopinavir[a] Ritonavir + Saquinavir (SGC[b] or HGC[b])	Stavudine + Didanosine Stavudine + Lamivudine Zidovudine + Didanosine Zidovudine + Lamivudine
Recommended as alternatives	Abacavir Amprenavir Delavirdine Nelfinavir + Saquinavir-SGC Nevirapine Ritonavir Saquinavir-SGC	Didanosine + Lamivudine Zidovudine + Zalcitabine
No recommendation: insufficient data[c]	Hydroxyurea in combination with antiretroviral drugs Ritonavir + Amprenavir Ritonavir + Nelfinavir Tenofavir	
Not recommended: should not be offered	All monotherapies, whether from Column A or B[d] Saquinavir-HGC[e]	Stavudine + Zidovudine Zalcitabine + Didanosine Zalcitabine + Lamivudine Zalcitabine + Stavudine

Antiretroviral drug regimens are comprised of one choice each from columns A and B.
Drugs are listed in alphabetical, not priority, order.
[a]Coformulated as Kaletra.
[b]Saquinavir-SGC, soft-gel capsule (Fortovase); Saquinavir-HGC, hard-gel capsule (Invirase).
[c]This category includes drugs or combinations for which information is too limited to allow a recommendation for or against use.
[d]Zidovudine monotherapy may be considered for prophylactic use in pregnant women with low viral load and high CD4+ T-cell counts to prevent perinatal transmission.
[e]Use of saquinavir-HGC (Invirase) is not recommended, except in combination with ritonavir.
HIV, human immunodeficiency virus.
Source: Guidelines for the use of antiretroviral agents in HIV-1–infected adults and adolescents. February 4, 2002. www.hivatis.org.

Baseline viral loads and CD4 counts give the most useful information about prognosis without treatment. The CD4 count has increasingly been viewed as the guide for deciding on when to initiate HAART. The viral load is the best guide for monitoring the effectiveness of therapy and deciding when to change antiretroviral therapy. Once HAART is initiated, achieving an undetectable viral load should be the goal. In clinical trials, this is achieved in excess of 80% of patients after 1 year of therapy, whereas in most clinical settings it is achieved in only 40% to 60% of patients.

Recently, several developments have appreciably altered the approach to antiretroviral therapy and monitoring its efficacy: recent debate over the benefits and risks of early versus delayed initiation of HAART (Table 39.16), the recognition of long-term toxicity of HAART, and the use of resistance testing to guide therapy (particularly changes in therapy).

Antiretroviral Drugs

There are currently three classes of antiretroviral drugs available: NRTIs, the NNRTIs, which have the same mechanism of action as the NRTIs but a different structure, and the protease inhibitors, which act at a different locus in the process of viral replication than NRTIs or NNRTIs. Table 39.17 summarizes practical information about available antiretroviral drugs.

The development of agents that act at different loci in the viral replication cycle has led to the application of principles used with other infectious agents to prevent resistance and promote eradication, such as the principles applied in the treatment of TB. The hallmark of these principles is the use of several agents simultaneously.

Table 39.16. Risks and Benefits of Delayed Initiation of Therapy and of Early Therapy in the Asymptomatic HIV-infected Patient

Risks and benefits of delayed initiation of therapy
- Benefits of delayed therapy
  - Avoid negative effects on quality of life (i.e., inconvenience)
  - Avoid drug-related adverse events
  - Delay in development of drug resistance
  - Preserve maximum number of available and future drug options when HIV disease risk is highest
- Risks of delayed therapy
  - Possible risk of irreversible immune system depletion
  - Possible greater difficulty in suppressing viral replication
  - Possible increased risk of HIV transmission

Risks and benefits of early therapy
- Benefits of early therapy
  - Control of viral replication easier to achieve and maintain
  - Delay or prevention of immune system compromise
  - Lower risk of resistance with complete viral suppression
  - Possible decreased risk of HIV transmission
- Risks of early therapy
  - Drug-related reduction in quality of life
  - Greater cumulative drug-related adverse events
  - Earlier development of drug resistance, if viral suppression is suboptimal
  - Limitation of future antiretroviral treatment options

HIV, human immunodeficiency virus.
Source: Guidelines for the use of antiretroviral agents in HIV-1 infected adults and adolescents. February 4, 2002. www.hivatis.org.

Table 39.17. Characteristics of Antiretroviral Drugs

Nucleoside Analogues							
Generic Name	Zidovudine (AZT)	Didanosine (ddI)	Zalcitabine (ddC)	Stavudine (d4T)	Lamivudine (3TC)	Tenofovir	Abacavir (ABC)
Trade Name	Retrovir	Videx	Hivid	Zerit	Epivir	Viread	Ziagen
Form	100- and 300-mg tablets	25-, 50-, 100-, 150-, and 200-mg chew tablets, 125-, 200-, 250-, and 400-mg (enteric-coated) capsule	0.375- and 0.75-mg tabs	15-, 20-, 30-, and 40-mg capsules; 1 mg/mL oral solution	150-mg tablets 10 mg/mL oral solution	300-mg tablets	300-mg tablets
Dosing Recommendations	300-mg b.i.d. or 200 mg t.i.d.; with 3TC as Combivir 1 tablet b.i.d.; with 3TC and abacavir as Trizivir 1 tablet b.i.d.	>60 kg: 400 EC capsule qD, or 200 mg chew tabs 2 qD, or 100 mg tabs 2 b.i.d. <60 kg: 250 EC capsule qD, or 125 mg tabs 2 qD.	0.75 mg t.i.d.	>60 kg: 40 mg b.i.d. <60 kg: 30 mg b.i.d.	150 mg b.i.d.; with AZT as Combivir (1 tablet b.i.d.); with AZT and abacavir as Trizivir (1 b.i.d.)	300 mg p.o. qD	300 mg b.i.d.; with AZT and 3TC as Trizivir 1 b.i.d.
Major Toxicity	Bone marrow suppression: anemia, neutropenia; nausea, vomiting, headache, insomnia, asthenia; lactic acidosis (rare).	Pancreatitis; peripheral neuropathy; nausea, diarrhea; lactic acidosis (rare).	Peripheral neuropathy; stomatitis; pancreatitis; lactic acidosis (rare).	Peripheral neuropathy; lactic acidosis (rare).	Lactic acidosis (rare).	Nausea, vomiting, diarrhea Lactic acidosis (?)	Hypersensitivity (2%–5%) with fever, nausea, vomiting, anorexia, cough, dyspnea, malaise and morbilliform rash. May be life-threatening especially with rechallenge. Lactic acidosis (rare).

Non-Nucleoside Reverse Transcriptase Inhibitors (NNRTIs)			
Generic Name	Nevirapine	Delavirdine	Efavirenz
Trade Name	Viramune	Rescriptor	Sustiva
Form	200-mg tablets	100-mg and 200-mg tablets	50-, 100-, and 200-mg capsules
Dosing Recommendations	200 mg p.o. qD × 14 days, then 200 mg p.o. b.i.d.	400 mg p.o. t.i.d.	600 mg p.o. qD at hs
Major Toxicity	Rash—may require hospitalization; rare cases of Stevens-Johnson syndrome; hepatitis	Rash; headaches; increased aminotransferase levels	Dizziness; sleep disorder; bad dreams, confusion, amnesia, agitation, hallucinations, poor concentration—usually resolyes after 2 weeks; take hs; rash, rare reports of Stevens-Johnson syndrome. Avoid in pregnancy.

Protease Inhibitors						
Indinavir	Ritonavir	Saquinavir		Nelfinavir	Amprenavir	Lopinavir & Ritonavir
Crixivan 200-, 333-, and 400-mg capsules	Norvir 100-mg capsules; 600 mg/7.5 mL p.o.-solution	Invirase 200-mg capsules (hard gel caps)	Fortovase 200-mg capsules (soft gel caps)	Viracept 250-mg tablets; 50 mg/g oral powder	Agenerase 50- and 150-mg capsules 15 mg/mL	Kaletra 133.3 mg lopinavir + 33.3 mg ritonavir capsules; 80 mg lopinavir + 70 mg ritonavir per mL oral solution
Usual Dose						
800 mg q 8h 800 mg q 12 h with ritonavir Separate with ddI dose by 1 h	600 mg b.i.d.; 400 mg b.i.d. with fortavase; 100–200 b.i.d. with indinavir. Separate with ddI dose by 2 h	800 mg t.i.d. (not recommended); 400 mg b.i.d. with ritonavir	1,200 mg t.i.d.; 400 mg b.i.d. with ritonavir	1,250 mg b.i.d.; 750 mg t.i.d.	1200 mg b.i.d.	400 mg lopinavir + 100 mg ritonavir (3 capsules) b.i.d.
Side Effects						
GI intolerance; nephrolithiasis or nephrotoxicity; headache; asthenia; dizziness; rash; metallic taste; ITP, alopecia; increased indirect bilirubinemia (inconsequential); fat redistribution; hyperglycemia; hyperlipidemia	GI intolerance; parasthesias; taste perversion; triglycerides increase; aminotransferase increase, CPK increase, and uric acid increase; pancreatitis; fat redistribution; hyperglycemia; hyperlipidemia	GI intolerance; headache; transaminase increase; fat redistribution; hyperglycemia; hyperlipidemia	GI intolerance; headache; transaminase increase; hypoglycemia; fat redistribution; hyperglycemia; hyperlipidemia	Diarrhea; fat redistribution; hyperglycemia; hyperlipidemia	GI intolerance; rash (usually at 1–10 weeks), Stevens-Johnson syndrome; parasthesias; increase in aminotransferases; fat redistribution; hyperglycemia; hyperlipidemia	GI intolerance; asthenia; increased aminotransferases; fat redistribution; hyperglycemia; hyperlipidemia

Because so many agents are available currently, there are many ongoing trials to determine which particularcombinations are most efficacious for lowering the viral load. With several agents being used simultaneously, there is a high likelihood of side effects and drug–drug interactions. Because of the exceedingly rapid pace at which these new drugs and the related clinical trial data are being released, primary care providers should consult sources of timely updates (see General References) or consult an expert when making decisions regarding antiretroviral therapy.

Overall Strategies in Antiretroviral Treatment

The viral load and CD4 count are both used to monitor the patient's response to therapy; however, the viral load is the guide for deciding on changes in antiretroviral therapy. Changes in CD4 count lag behind changes in viral load. Because patient compliance in taking HAART is crucial to avoid resistance, both verbal and written patient instructions about dosages and intervals are essential.

When HAART is initiated or changed, the viral load should be monitored 2 to 4 weeks later and then at 3-month intervals to assess continued efficacy. A .5 to 1.0 log decrease in viral load (e.g., from the hundreds of thousands to tens of thousands) should be achieved after 2 to 4 weeks of therapy. Patient compliance should be reviewed whenever there is a failure in suppressing viral load to an undetectable level. A transient increase in viral load, which resolves after about 1 month, may follow vaccine administration or an intercurrent acute illness.

When the viral load fails to suppress or rebounds to a detectable level, resistance to one or more drugs is likely. Compliance should be reviewed with development of strategies to improve adherence. Resistance testing should be performed to assess which of the antiretrovirals has lost effectiveness because of viral mutations (27) (see next section).

Drug Resistance

It is now understood that loss of the antiviral response to HAART (as indicated by increased viral load and decreased CD4 count) is usually caused by the virus' ability to mutate. The best way to prevent development of resistance is to maximally suppress viral replication and to sustain this; the only other way is not to expose the patient to antiretroviral medications in the first place (particularly if the patient is not ready for the commitment that HAART requires). When resistance develops to some of the antiretroviral agents, it may also develop simultaneously to a similar drug that has never been used. Thus, knowledge of the cross-resistance patterns of various antiretroviral agents is important in changing therapy.

Resistance mutations are random events, and the chance that a particular mutation will appear rises with the level of viral replication. The development of resistance is directly related to a patient's compliance in taking the prescribed dosage at the appropriate time. Taking antiretrovirals at a reduced dosage results in drug levels at which selection for drug-resistant variants can occur. Furthermore, taking only one or two antiretrovirals increases the chance that the virus may become resistant to one or both. Resistance testing is most useful in two situations: for patients on HAART who are failing therapy (i.e., viral load is detectable) to guide decisions regarding therapy changes and for patients with primary HIV infection ("acute retroviral syndrome") to detect transmission of resistant virus (28). Resistance testing only gives reliable information about drugs a patient is currently taking; a patient may have virus with resistance mutations to other drugs (particularly if they have been exposed to them previously), but these may not be detected in the absence of the selective pressure of taking that drug.

Genotypic resistance testing is now easily available through many major laboratories. The test is costly (~U.S.$300 to 500), but this expense is negligible when compared with the cost of continuing ineffective antiretroviral medications. The viral load usually has to be above 1,000 copies/mL for the test to be performed, and the results are generally reported as a series of mutations identified by a letter-number-letter sequence (e.g., M184V). The number is the codon where the mutation has been detected, the first letter is the wild-type amino acid at that codon, and the last letter is the amino acid that has been substituted for it (i.e., M184V is a replacement of methionine with valine at the 184 codon). Interpretation of genotypic resistance testing is complex because some isolated mutations confer high-level resistance to a medication, whereas in other cases multiple mutations or specific combinations of mutations are needed for resistance to develop. Updated databases of resistance mutations are available through a number of Internet sites, including the one maintained by the International AIDS Society-USA (www.iausa.org). Results of resistance testing must be considered in conjunction with knowledge of what antiretrovirals the patient has taken in the past. If noncompliance is contributing to resistance, a new HAART regimen should not be prescribed until obstacles to compliance are addressed and resolved.

SYMPTOMATIC HUMAN IMMUNODEFICIENCY VIRUS-INFECTED PATIENT

General Principles

The most important aspect of the primary care of the symptomatic HIV-infected patient is building rapport and trust with the patient. Many newly diagnosed HIV-positive patients are young and have been previously healthy; symptoms and illness are often new to them. They may either overreact to each symptom or deny symptoms entirely. Good rapport with patients is thus essential for having them disclose information and for distinguishing the significance of new symptoms.

The CD4 lymphocyte count is the most useful marker for making treatment decisions in the care of HIV-infected patients. Importantly, it serves as a guide for generating a differential diagnosis for symptoms. When a patient's CD4 count is greater than 500 cells/mm^3, new symptoms are most likely to be due to non–HIV-associated conditions. When a patient's CD4 count is between 200 and 500, new symptoms should lead to a careful search for a possible HIV-related illness. Finally, when a patient's CD4 count is less than 200, new symptoms are more likely to be due to an opportunistic infection.

Human Immunodeficiency Virus Complications

The four most common AIDS-indicator conditions are PCP, disseminated MAC, esophageal candidiasis, and the HIV wasting syndrome. With widespread use of prophylaxis, the first two conditions have become less common. Most complications of HIV can be diagnosed and treated in ambulatory settings with only severely ill patients requiring hospitalization. This section briefly addresses the approach to the most common HIV-related complications; more information is available in the resources listed in General References at the end of this chapter.

Constitutional Manifestations and Lymphadenopathy

Fatigue is probably the most common symptom described by HIV-infected people. Causes of fatigue include high levels of HIV virus in the blood, anemia, testosterone deficiency, medication side effect, and depression. The first three causes may be diagnosed by blood test. In the case of high levels of virus in the blood, HAART may ameliorate symptoms of fatigue. Anemia may be treated with once weekly injections of erythropoietin, and testosterone deficiency may be treated with testosterone replacement by patch or injection. Fatigue related to medications often improves after the first few weeks of therapy but may warrant a change in medication. Treatment of depression is outlined in Chapter 24.

Fevers, night sweats, or weight loss may be the presenting manifestations of an opportunistic infection or a malignancy or they may be due to HIV infection itself. When one or more of these symptoms are present, a careful evaluation for a treatable problem is mandatory. Some constitutional symptoms (e.g., fever or diarrhea lasting longer than 1 month) categorize the patient as having symptomatic HIV infection. The laboratory evaluation of fever, chills, or night sweats should include a complete blood count with differential, liver function tests, chest radiograph, urinalysis, serum cryptococcal antigen test if CD4 count is near or below 200, blood cultures, and sputum cultures if sputum is available. If the history, physical examination, and these screening laboratory data do not reveal an explanation for fever, a more extensive workup should be performed. Considerations should be given to obtaining blood cultures for MAC if the CD4 count is less than 100 and to looking for an occult infection using computed tomography (CT) of the chest and/or abdomen. A drug-related fever should also be considered, with sulfa drugs a common offender. Disseminated MAC infection typically causes weight loss and spiking fevers in the absence of arthralgias. This species of mycobacterium is not communicable.

Lymphadenopathy may represent reaction to HIV, infection with another agent, or a malignancy. Generalized lymphadenopathy (defined as nodes 1 cm or greater in diameter in two or more noncontiguous extrainguinal sites) may persist during the first 6 months after diagnosis of HIV. Nodes most often enlarged are anterior and posterior cervical, axillary, submental, and femoral nodes; preauricular and epitrochlear nodes are rarely enlarged. Patients with generalized lymphadenopathy often have one or more other abnormalities in the history, physical examination, or laboratory evaluation, but no single abnormality coexists predictably with adenopathy. Lymphadenopathy per se has not been found to be predictive of the patient's future course.

If a patient's lymphadenopathy is most pronounced in the inguinal region, with or without an active genital lesion or a history of a lesion, sexually transmitted diseases such as chancroid or lymphogranuloma venereum should be considered. If lymphadenopathy is localized in one area, progressively enlarging, associated with constitutional symptoms, or of a different texture (very firm or irregular), biopsy should be considered to exclude malignancy, especially non-Hodgkin lymphoma.

Respiratory Tract Manifestations

HIV-infected patients with a high CD4 count, presenting with cough, most often have a simple bronchitis. If the chest radiograph of an HIV-infected patient shows a lobar infiltrate, sputum should be obtained and processed for a Gram stain and routine culture. Mycobacterial and fungal stains and culture should also be considered. With the widespread use of PCP prophylaxis and HAART, *Streptococcus pneumoniae* (pneumococcus) has become the most common cause of pneumonia in HIV-infected individuals. Treatment of lobar pneumonia should be based on guidelines for empiric treatment of pneumonia, described in Chapter 33, unless or until a specific pathogen is identified.

Pneumocystis carinii *Pneumonia*

Before widespread use of PCP prophylaxis, many HIV-infected patients experienced at least one episode of PCP in the course of their disease. Compared with other pneumonias, the symptoms of PCP are usually less acute in onset and sputum is usually scant and thin. Common complaints include fever, night sweats, dyspnea, and nonproductive cough. Dyspnea is most often the predominant or sole symptom. The duration of respiratory symptoms is usually 1 to 3 weeks, although the systemic symptoms may have been present for several months. Because many of these patients have been previously healthy, their clinical presentation may be subtle. For example, it is common for a patient with PCP to have had no more than a mild dry cough and a modest decrease in exercise tolerance. Thrush may be present or may have occurred in the past as an indicator of immunosuppression. The physical examination is often nonspecific. Fever, tachycardia, and tachypnea may be present and, if so, indicate more severe disease. Auscultation of the chest is often unremarkable, and the chest radiograph may be normal in up to 15% of cases.

HIV-infected patients with only a history of respiratory symptoms should undergo a stepwise laboratory evaluation that is designed to diagnose or rule out PCP and other pulmonary infections. Ambulatory pulse oximetry performed in the office provides objective evidence for whether oxygen desaturation is responsible for symptoms of dyspnea. Chest x-ray should be performed if pneumonia is clinically suspected. In patients with abnormal chest radiographs, the pattern of infiltrates is helpful in determining the next step. A lobar infiltrate on radiograph and a history of acute onset of symptoms is most consistent with a community-acquired pneumonia, either typical (e.g., pneumococcal) or atypical (e.g., mycoplasmal). A lobar infiltrate in the presence of subacute or chronic symptoms is more consistent with mycobacterial or fungal disease. A diffuse interstitial pattern is the most common presenting pattern on a chest radiograph in patients with PCP.

In the presence of pneumonia or hypoxia, an attempt should be made to make a specific diagnosis by inducing the production of sputum. *P. carinii* is diagnosed by microscopic examination of sputum, either by silver stain or direct fluorescent antibody. Examination of induced sputum for *P. carinii* has a sensitivity of approximately 80% in selected patients, although its negative predictive value is low. Therefore, if a specific diagnosis is not made on induced sputum, the patient should undergo fiberoptic bronchoscopy with bronchoalveolar lavage. Sputum can also be stained and cultured for mycobacteria, fungi, and viruses.

Patients who are not hypoxic can be safely treated in the ambulatory setting using oral medications. There are several options for ambulatory treatment: the first-line agent for the treatment of PCP is TMP-SMX (15 mg/kg/day of TMP + 75 mg/kg/day of SMX in three to four divided doses for 21 days). The typical adult dose is two double-strength tablets three times a day. If the patient is allergic to or unable to tolerate TMP-SMX, dapsone with TMP (15 mg/kg/day of TMP + 100 mg/day of dapsone for 21 days) or atovaquone (750-mg suspension orally twice a day with meals for 21 days) may be used. Symptomatic improvement usually occurs within 24 to 48 hours, but it may be slower in some patients. The chest radiograph may take several weeks to revert to normal. Patients should not be considered to have failed treatment until at least 5 to 7 days of therapy without improvement have elapsed. At this time, discontinuation of the initial therapy and substitution of an alternative drug is warranted. Of patients with first episodes of PCP, over 90% recover. Higher mortality rates are seen in patients who develop severe hypoxemia. Secondary prevention for PCP should be instituted after the acute episode.

Tuberculosis

Mycobacterial infections are well-recognized complications of immunosuppression. The incidence of *M. tuberculosis*, which is highly communicable, is increasing in patients with AIDS, and TB may be the presenting illness in some HIV-infected patients. To reflect this, the 1993 CDC case definition for AIDS added pulmonary TB as an AIDS-indicator condition (Table 39.9). Chapter 34 discusses the approach to prophylaxis and treatment of TB in HIV-infected patients, including patients infected with multidrug-resistant strains of *M. tuberculosis*.

Neurologic Manifestations

The nervous system is often involved in patients with HIV infection. More than 10% of patients with AIDS have an initial AIDS-indicator neurologic disease (Table 39.9). Involvement of the nervous system may be categorized as disease secondary to HIV infection itself, disease secondary to opportunistic pathogens or neoplasms, and disease related to medication toxicity. Manifestations may be caused by diseases of the central nervous system (CNS) or the peripheral nervous system.

Peripheral Neuropathy

Peripheral neuropathies occur at all stages of HIV infection. When caused directly by HIV, symptoms usually present as a distal symmetric sensory neuropathy. Bell palsy and varicella zoster are two infectious causes of peripheral neuropathy that may occur at even high CD4 counts. Neuropathy also commonly occurs as a toxic side effect of several of the antiretroviral medications, most notably stavudine and didanosine—again, usually a distal sensory neuropathy. Neuropathy due to these medications may resolve with discontinuation of the medication but often persist even after discontinuation. Symptoms of peripheral neuropathy may be controlled with tricyclic antidepressants or some of the antiseizure medicines, including gabapentin and lamotrigine (see Chapter 92). When symptoms are related to medication toxicity, treatment often requires a change in HAART regimen.

Global Central Nervous System Disorders Caused by Human Immunodeficiency Virus

In later stages of HIV infection, many patients develop the AIDS dementia complex, a disorder characterized by cognitive, motor, and behavioral dysfunction. Dementia is the most common CNS complication of

AIDS and is included in the CDC case definition of AIDS (Table 39.9). Diagnostic features include positive HIV serology, history of cognitive/behavioral changes (especially impaired concentration and attention, apathy, and memory loss), and associated neurologic findings including hyperreflexia, hypertonia, signs of myelopathy (spastic paraparesis or ataxia), and frontal release signs (29). In early stages of HIV infection of the CNS, the mental status and neurologic examinations can be completely normal. Cerebrospinal fluid (CSF) findings are nonspecific: normal or slightly elevated protein concentration, normal glucose concentration, and a slight mononuclear pleocytosis. CT or magnetic resonance imaging of the brain may show cerebral atrophy with changes in white matter.

Before making a working diagnosis of AIDS dementia, it is important to exclude metabolic or toxic encephalopathies, opportunistic infections, neoplasms, and neurosyphilis. The Mini-Mental Status Examination is helpful for identifying cognitive abnormalities in a brief office interview (see Chapter 26, Table 26.1). In a patient whose Mini-Mental Examination is normal, neuropsychologic testing may be useful in assessing suspected early AIDS dementia and in following the course of the disease. This may be especially important in assessing patients whose work requires a high level of cognitive function. Characteristic abnormalities include difficulty with complex sequencing, impairment of fine and rapid motor movements, and slowed verbal fluency. In rare instances, brain biopsy may be indicated to exclude other metabolic, neoplastic, or infectious causes. In patients with high viral loads, cognitive function may improve after initiation of HAART.

Opportunistic Central Nervous System Infections

The clinical presentation of opportunistic CNS infections may be subtle. Headache and fever are the most common presenting symptoms of CNS infections, although fever may not be present. Focal neurologic findings and meningismus are found in fewer than half of patients with CNS infection. Therefore, a high index of suspicion must be maintained in any HIV-positive patient with a low CD4 count with new onset of severe headache, a change in a usual headache pattern, or persistent headache. Because sinusitis may present with fever and a headache and is common in HIV-infected patients, this diagnosis should be considered as well.

Opportunistic infections of the CNS generally occur in HIV-infected patients with CD4 counts below 200. *Cryptococcus neoformans* is the most common pathogen causing meningitis in AIDS patients; this meningitis usually presents as a nonfulminant process. Focal CNS disease is most often caused by *T. gondii*, although primary CNS lymphoma, tuberculoma, or cryptococcoma may present in the same way. Progressive multifocal leukoencephalopathy may also present as a focal CNS disease. This is a progressive demyelinating disorder caused by reactivation of a papovavirus in immunosuppressed patients, including those with AIDS. It presents as a subacute disease, progressing over several weeks, with focal neurologic deficits without alteration of consciousness until its terminal stages.

Because the physical examination usually is not diagnostic, a thorough laboratory evaluation is important in any patient with new neurologic symptoms. The evaluation should begin with magnetic resonance imaging or contrast-enhanced CT of the head to exclude mass lesions. The presence of a ring-enhancing lesion is characteristic for toxoplasmosis, although lymphoma and other causes cannot be excluded. Because toxoplasmosis is the most common cause of such a lesion and because definitive diagnosis requires a brain biopsy, it is reasonable to begin empirical treatment for toxoplasmosis (usually with oral pyrimethamine, folinic acid, and sulfadiazine) on the basis of the CT. If after 10 to 14 days of therapy the patient has not clinically improved or the CT shows no improvement, further diagnostic measures should be considered.

Unless the CT shows a mass lesion that might lead to herniation, lumbar puncture should also be performed in evaluating new CNS symptoms. CSF should be evaluated for opening pressure, cell count, protein and glucose concentrations (with a simultaneous serum glucose), Gram stain, India ink preparation, culture for bacteria, mycobacterial and fungal stains and cultures, cryptococcal antigen, and a serologic test for syphilis. Cryptococcal meningitis may be present even with few or no cells in the CSF; in most cases, cryptococcal antigen is present in both the CSF and the serum. A working diagnosis of neurosyphilis should be considered in the presence of a positive serum VDRL, CSF pleocytosis, and negative cultures and stains for other organisms, even if the CSF VDRL is negative. Once opportunistic infections and neoplasms are excluded, especially in a patient in whom mental status changes are pronounced, the AIDS dementia complex should be the working diagnosis.

Psychiatric Manifestations

Psychiatric disorders may predate the acquisition of HIV infection in some patients, and treatment of patients with a pre-existing psychiatric illness and HIV infection may be extremely challenging. Virtually all HIV-infected patients go through a stressful experience upon learning that they are infected. In the months to years that follow diagnosis of HIV infection, patients may require supportive counseling and the assistance of professional social workers and social service agencies to deal with psychosocial problems. Over the course of their illness, many patients develop symptoms of depression (30). Apathy and mental slowing are often prominent in the presentation of major depression in HIV-infected patients, and paranoid thoughts or other symptoms of functional psychosis may accompany symptoms that suggest delirium or cognitive impairment.

For major depression, which is more common in HIV-infected persons than in the general population, antidepressant treatment is usually effective. The usual dosages of all antidepressants are appropriate for patients in the early stages of HIV infection. The dosages should be lower than the usual recommended dosages in patients who are in the late stages, and these patients seem to be more sensitive to all of the effects of antidepressants. (See Chapter 24 for practical information about antidepressants.) Psychostimulant drugs (e.g., methylphenidate) may be particularly helpful in alleviating the apathy in depressed HIV-infected patients.

For patients who develop psychotic symptoms, the high-potency neuroleptic haloperidol is recommended because it has few anticholinergic side effects. Psychotic symptoms in HIV-infected patients respond to low dosages of haloperidol (e.g., 1 to 5 mg one to three times a day). Details regarding the use of neuroleptic drugs are found in Chapter 25.

Oral Cavity and Gastrointestinal Manifestations

The oral and gastrointestinal manifestations of HIV infection may be caused by opportunistic pathogens or, in the case of some patients with diarrhea, by nonopportunistic pathogens.

Oral Lesions

Oral lesions are common in HIV-positive patients and are often the first symptoms of immunodeficiency. The most common oral problem is thrush, or candidiasis, which occurs most typically as a whitish coating of the oral mucosa or tongue (see Chapter 112, Fig. 112.6). Five percent to 10% of patients develop thrush within the first 6 months of known HIV infection, and it occurs in half of patients at some point in their disease. Other manifestations of oral *Candida* infection are angular cheilosis and erythema without coating. Mycostatin liquid (500,000 units swish and swallow five times a day) or clotrimazole troches (10 mg five times a day) usually control symptoms of thrush. Symptoms usually resolve within 10 to 14 days of treatment; if they fail, systemic therapy with fluconazole 100 mg daily for 10–14 days should be used.

Other oral manifestations of HIV infections include oral hairy leukoplakia, KS, mass lesions secondary to neoplasms and opportunistic infections, aphthous ulcers, and periodontal disease. Oral hairy leukoplakia presents as symptomless hypopigmented shaggy lesions, histologically showing hyperparakeratosis of the mucosa, on the lateral aspects of the tongue. It may be confused with thrush, from which it may be distinguished by scraping the lesion and examining the scrapings microscopically after application of potassium hydroxide (see technique, Chapter 117). The absence of typical fungal forms generally excludes thrush. A distinct HIV gingivitis that may lead to severe periodontitis and occasionally acute necrotizing gingivitis may occur despite good oral hygiene. Management of periodontal disease may include topical treatment (e.g., chlorhexidine) or systemic antibiotics. Management of these problems requires coordination of care with a dentist. Oral KS appears as bluish, black, flat lesions, usually on the hard palate. Biopsy of suspicious lesions establishes the diagnosis.

Esophagitis

Esophagitis should be considered when the patient complains of odynophagia, dysphagia, or retrosternal chest pain. The most common cause of esophagitis in HIV-infected patients is *Candida albicans*; most patients have oral thrush concomitant with or preceding esophagitis. Candida infection distal to the oral cavity constitutes an AIDS-indicator condition. Esophagitis may also be caused by herpes simplex virus or CMV. Less commonly, aphthous ulcers, KS, primary lymphoma, and esophageal squamous cell carcinoma may be the cause of esophageal symptoms. In a patient with odynophagia, empiric treatment for candida esophagitis with oral fluconazole is indicated (200 mg orally the first day, followed by 100 mg/day). If symptoms do not improve within 7 to 10 days of treatment, the patient should be further evaluated with endoscopy.

Gastric and Hepatobiliary Diseases

The stomach is the most common gastrointestinal location for visceral KS; lesions are commonly found by endoscopy. Most patients already have cutaneous KS. Gastric lymphomas may also be found. Acalculous cholecystitis occurs occasionally in HIV-infected patients. Sonography shows sludge in the gallbladder with edema of the gallbladder wall.

Parenchymal hepatic disease is common in HIV-infected patients, most often related to coinfection with hepatitis C. Commonly, elevated concentrations of serum alkaline phosphatase and serum aminotransferases are present. Hepatitis C is often more fulminant in the setting of coinfection with HIV (31). In patients with a good prognosis related to HIV, treatment with alpha-interferon and ribavirin for hepatitis C should be considered (see treatment of hepatitis C in Chapter 47). MAC is the most common opportunistic liver pathogen in patients with advanced HIV (CD4 <50). In MAC-related hepatitis, alkaline phosphatase levels are usually elevated out of proportion to other liver enzymes, and the diagnosis can be rapidly established by liver biopsy.

Diarrhea

Diarrhea occurs in many patients during the course of HIV infection (32). Additionally, many of the antiretroviral medications, especially the protease inhibitor nelfinavir, can cause symptomatic diarrhea. Large-volume diarrhea, often with associated crampy abdominal pain and weight loss, is commonly caused by both opportunistic and conventional enteric pathogens. *G. lamblia,* salmonella, shigella, and *Campylobacter* are possible causes of diarrhea in otherwise healthy patients with HIV. Pathogenic mostly in patients with low CD4 counts, *I. belli,* microsporidia, and cryptosporidium usually cause large-volume watery diarrhea in the absence of fever. CMV and MAC cause diarrhea in individuals with very low CD4 counts. Both are associated with fever, but patients with CMV colitis generally have more abdominal pain and bloody diarrhea compared with patients with MAC who usually have nonbloody diarrhea. Multiple stool specimens for culture and microscopic examination for ova and parasites are necessary to diagnose each of these entities. Some entities, such as CMV and MAC, require more invasive procedures such as small or large bowel biopsy for diagnosis. When careful evaluation does not yield a cause (about one-third of the time), diarrhea can be ascribed to HIV infection itself. Aggressive fluid resuscitation and the use of rice-based cereal are essential to prevent dehydration and wasting in patients, many of whom are already underweight. Chapter 35 contains details regarding the diagnosis and management of gastroenteritis caused by conventional pathogens.

In patients who practice receptive anal intercourse, perianal herpetic ulcerations may account for proctalgia and tenesmus, as may a number of other sexually transmitted infections (e.g., syphilis, gonorrhea, and chlamydia).

Human Immunodeficiency Virus Wasting Syndrome

The diagnosis of HIV wasting is made in patients with the combination of pronounced weight loss (10% or more from baseline) and either chronic diarrhea or chronic weakness and fever in the absence of other opportunistic infection or malignancy (33). Optimal use of antiretroviral drugs and of therapy for lesions of the oral cavity and esophagus, in conjunction with good nutrition, is essential. Men should be evaluated for testosterone deficiency and treated with androgen replacement if abnormality is found (see Chapter 85). Consideration of underlying depression should also be made.

Cutaneous Manifestations

Seborrheic dermatitis and psoriasis are the most commons cutaneous problems seen in HIV-infected patients. Diagnosis and management of these two conditions are described in Chapter 116.

KS, which occurs mostly in homosexual men with HIV, is an AIDS-defining complication of HIV. KS presents as painless violaceous papules, usually .5 to 2 cm in diameter, often multiple, occurring most commonly on the face, on the extremities, and in the oral cavity. The lesions are bluish in light-skinned patients and may appear nearly black in dark-skinned patients. KS requires a biopsy for definitive diagnosis. KS may also involve the lungs, oral cavity, and the gastrointestinal tract. The treatment of KS varies from the use of liquid nitrogen for skin lesions to the use of systemic chemotherapy for visceral involvement (34).

A number of the invasive opportunistic infections of HIV-infected patients, such as cryptococcosis, atypical mycobacterial infection, and histoplasmosis, may present with cutaneous lesions that are rather insignificant in appearance. In the presence of symptoms of systemic disease, one should be highly suspicious and consider biopsy of new skin lesions.

Mucocutaneous herpes simplex virus infection, described in Chapter 117, is another syndrome often seen in HIV-infected patients and if persistent for more than a month is also an AIDS-indicator condition. Shingles, or reactivation of latent varicella-zoster infection, is also common in HIV-infected patients and may involve multiple dermatomes. Diagnosis is based on a cytologic examination of the vesicle fluid (the Tzanck smear), viral cultures, or polymerase chain reaction (see details in Chapter 117). The mucocutaneous erosions caused by these viruses also predispose the patient to local and disseminated bacterial superinfection. Diagnosis and treatment for herpes virus infections are summarized in Chapter 117.

Other Organ Systems

Other organ systems are involved in HIV-infected patients, although not as often as those mentioned above.

Ophthalmologic

The predominant ophthalmologic disease is CMV retinitis, which may be completely asymptomatic but if left untreated progresses to blindness. The incidence of CMV retinitis has declined dramatically with the advent of HAART over the past 5 years (35). Routine funduscopic examination is crucial, especially in patients with CMV disease in the past and in patients with CD4 counts less than 100. Diagnosis is confirmed by an ophthalmologist because the lesions, which are hemorrhagic and exudative, are specific for this entity.

Hematologic

Anemia occurs commonly in the late stages of HIV infection. It may be related to HIV infection itself or, less commonly, may be secondary to involvement of the bone marrow by one of the opportunistic infections, such as TB, MAC, or histoplasmosis. Anemia may also be secondary to adverse effects of medications, especially zidovudine and sulfa drugs. Anemia should be investigated as outlined in Chapter 55. Patients with advanced HIV and symptomatic anemia with low erythropoietin levels can be treated with erythropoietin injections. Thrombocytopenia may occur at any stage of HIV. It is usually immune based, related to the HIV virus itself, and generally responds to treatment with antiretroviral therapy; alternatively, corticosteroids and splenectomy can also be effective. Leukopenia occurs as a direct result of the HIV virus and can be exacerbated by medications. Treatment of leukopenia should be based on attempting to decrease the HIV viral load with HAART. Granulocyte colony-stimulating factor can be given if the absolute neutrophil count falls below 500 cells/mm^3.

Renal

Both reversible and irreversible renal abnormalities are encountered in patients with HIV infection. Although some of these abnormalities may be caused by

HIV infection, many result from identifiable causes, especially drug toxicity. HIV-related nephropathy reveals focal sclerosing glomerulonephritis on biopsy. Some patients do respond to therapy with corticosteroids (36).

Cardiac

The diagnostic approach to cardiac disease in HIV-infected patients should also focus on identifiable causes other than HIV infection. A distinct HIV cardiomyopathy has been described. In such cases, HIV RNA has been isolated directly from myocytes. Coxsackie B virus, CMV, and toxoplasmosis are infectious causes of HIV-related cardiomyopathy (37). Additionally, atherosclerotic heart disease is likely to be seen more often in HIV patients related to hyperlipidemia induced by many HAART regimens; it is recommended that patients started on HAART have baseline and follow-up lipid panels checked. HIV-infected patients with hyperlipidemia are generally treated in the same way that uninfected patients are (see Chapter 82).

Gynecologic

With the increase in the numbers of HIV-infected women, involvement of the reproductive tract has been recognized. Women with HIV infection often have chronic vulvovaginal candidiasis or herpes, poorly responsive to therapy, as the first manifestation of underlying immunodeficiency. Immunosuppressed women may also be at more risk for the progression to malignancy of cervical papillomavirus infection. HIV-positive women should have an initial Pap smear, followed by a repeat in 6 months. If both are normal, follow-up Pap smear should be repeated every 12 months. All HIV-positive women with abnormal Pap smears should have colposcopy performed.

PROBLEMS UNIQUE TO SPECIFIC PATIENT POPULATIONS

Injection Drug Users

Injection drug users have difficult medical and social problems, even in the absence of HIV disease. Hospital admission for complications related to drug use, including endocarditis, thrombophlebitis, and cellulitis, is common. Thus, when an injection drug user is infected with HIV, the care becomes even more challenging.

Many individuals with substance abuse can be compliant with complicated HAART regimens. However, because the patient's best chance of durable success is with their initial HAART regimen, poor compliance can be disastrous in the long run. Compliance with office visits is a useful predictor for likely compliance with HAART. Therefore, initiation of HAART in patients with substance abuse should generally be delayed until individuals show up for at least two consecutive office visits.

If a patient continues to use drugs and miss office visits, referral to a methadone program might be beneficial. It is important to note that drug interactions occur between several antiretrovirals, most notably the NNRTIs, and methadone that results in increased clearance of methadone. Patients on methadone and started on an NNRTI usually need their methadone dose raised. Additionally, one of the NNRTIs, efavirenz, may give a false positive result for marijuana on a urine drug screen. Treatment of substance abuse is described in Chapter 29.

Women

Most women infected with HIV in the United States are injection drug users or are sexual partners with men who have a history of injection drug use. Many women in the latter group may not know their partner has put them at risk and do not find out about their HIV diagnosis until they are pregnant or symptomatic. Barrier contraception (condom use by the partner) is of paramount importance to prevent not only pregnancy but also transmission of HIV (for details, see Sexual Transmission, above). Antiretroviral therapy during pregnancy reduces the risk of transmission of HIV to the fetus and thus should be prescribed to pregnant HIV-infected women (see Perinatal Transmission, above) (12). Efavirenz (teratogenic) and the combination of stavudine and didanosine (lactic acidosis) should be avoided during pregnancy.

SPECIAL CONSIDERATIONS

Social and Economic Issues

Patients with AIDS are faced not only with coping with a fatal disease, which is sexually transmissible, but also with the social stigma attached to the disease. These patients must confront the need to inform their sexual partners (for the partners' own protection), the risk of losing close friends, and isolation from their family. They must also face the risk of employment, housing, or insurance discrimination. Women must face the effect of this disease on their childbearing future, as well as the effect on children they are already rearing. In addition to the medical complications of AIDS, common social and economic problems, the patient's provider must repeatedly present unpleasant facts to the patient and help the patient come to terms with them.

The patient's financial stress may be ameliorated somewhat by the fact that AIDS (and some HIV-related illnesses that do not meet diagnostic criteria for AIDS) qualifies a patient for Social Security disability. This means that the patient receives Social Security income immediately but must wait 24 months before receiving Medicare health insurance. A patient who meets the needs criteria for Supplemental Security Income can obtain health insurance through Medicaid immediately (see Chapter 9 for further information). In 2001, the 1-year retail cost of an average HAART regimen was $12,000, giving an idea of the size of the health care cost of AIDS, even for the ambulatory patient.

A newer and rather unusual problem that has arisen since the advent of HAART is patients having unexpected restored health after years of considering themselves to be terminally ill. This has raised many psychologic and practical issues, including making plans for a future never expected, returning to work after being on disability, and the guilt of surviving when so many early in the epidemic did not.

In addressing the social aspects of the patient's disease, the patient's right to privacy and confidentiality should be ensured at the outset, and patients should be asked to specify the people to whom they plan to disclose the nature of their illness. Many AIDS patients require counseling to cope with these decisions and the many changes in their lives caused by their disease. In addition to provider input, the supportive counseling of a social worker or nurse educator and help from community-based support groups should be enlisted.

Death and Dying

Because AIDS is in many a fatal disease, dealing with the issues of death and dying is extremely important. It is probably not appropriate to begin such discussions when a patient first learns of the HIV diagnosis other than to answer questions about the prognosis frankly. It should be emphasized that HIV infection has a long latency period. Hope is extremely powerful in maintaining the patient's psychological and physical well-being.

The more appropriate time to explore the issues of death and dying is when the patient develops signs and symptoms related to progressive disease. Open discussions should be initiated about financial planning and about advance directives regarding resuscitation and other aspects of care when one may not be competent. These discussions should take place early in the course of AIDS while the patient is still fully competent. Issues of death, dying, and bereavement are discussed in further detail in Chapter 13, and Chapter 12 describes legal considerations in specifying and documenting advance directives.

Public Health and Legal Responsibilities of the Physician

No disease in recent times has emphasized to a greater extent the confrontation between the defense of individual privacy and the protection of public health. Clearly, this remains a major challenge to health care professionals dealing with HIV infection. The physician's primary responsibility is to the patient. The unique trust inherent in the physician–patient relationship allows the physician to guide the patient to protect those who may be at risk because of sexual contact. The physician has the responsibility of emphasizing to the patient, on multiple occasions if necessary, the importance of informing sexual or needle-sharing partners. Guidelines governing the physician's responsibility when the patient refuses to inform others are included in many state laws, and advice regarding these guidelines should be sought from public health authorities in one's state. Many states now have confidential programs for sexual partner notification.

Physicians are required by law to report all newly diagnosed cases of AIDS, using confidential morbidity report forms. In addition, some states now require reporting of most symptomatic HIV-associated diseases.

Information and Support for Household Members

People who live with or care for HIV-infected patients at home have special needs. Most importantly, they need clear information about the transmission of HIV infection, about both the safety of nonintimate contact with the patient and the risks and precautions related to intimate contact. Household caretakers should be advised to follow the universal precautions recommended to health care workers for the care of all patients (Table 39.3).

People close to patients with HIV infection and AIDS invariably have a variety of intense emotional reactions and must also confront distressing social implications of the patient's illness. Thus, taking the time to share information and respond to questions from patients' caretakers is a critical part of caring for patients with HIV and AIDS.

General References*

American Medical Association website: www.ama-assn.org/special/hiv.
Offers updates on HIV care and links to other useful sites.

Bartlett JG, Gallant JE. Medical management of HIV infection. Baltimore: Johns Hopkins University, Department of Infectious Diseases, 2001.
Practical manual, especially regarding details about medications and evaluation of complications, updated every year. To order, call 800-787-1254. Interim updates at www.hopkins-aids.edu.

Bartlett JG, Finkbeiner AK. The guide to living with HIV infection, 4th ed. Baltimore: Johns Hopkins University Press, 1998.
An invaluable practical resource for caretakers and family members.

Cotton DJ, ed. AIDS clinical care. Massachusetts Medical Society, Waltham.
Excellent monthly review of issues related to HIV care, including a feature topic, case history, and review of recent journal articles. Can also be accessed online at www.accnewsletter.org. (subscription required to view full text).

Johns Hopkins AIDS Service website: www.hopkins-aids.edu.
Offers updates on latest developments, access to a web version of John Bartlett's handbook, and answers to questions submitted by patients and providers.

Practice guidelines. For federally approved treatment guidelines and information, the HIV/AIDS Treatment Information Service may be called: 800-448-0440 (TDD/Deaf access, 800-243-7012) Monday through Friday, 9 a.m. to 7 p.m. EST, fax 301-738-6616, P.O. Box 6303, Rockville, MD 20849-6303, or accessed by the internet at www.hivatis.org.

Specific References

1. Lee LM, Karon JM, Selik R, et al. Survival after AIDS diagnosis in adolescents and adults during the treatment era, United States, 1984–1997. JAMA 2001;285:1308.
2. Markowitz DM. Infection with the human immunodeficiency virus type 2. Ann Intern Med 1993;118:211.

*Bold print (general references) and bold numerals (specific references) denote published controlled clinical trials, meta-analyses, or consensus-based recommendations.

3. Centers for Disease Control and Prevention and USPHS Working Group. Guidelines for counseling persons infected with human T-lymphotrophic virus type I (HTLV-1) and type II (HTLV-2). Ann Intern Med 1993;118:448.
4. Centers for Disease Control and Prevention. World AIDS Day—December 1, 2000. MMWR Morb Mortal Wkly Rep 2000;49:1061.
5. Centers for Disease Control and Prevention. HIV and AIDS—United States, 1981–2000. MMWR Morb Mortal Wkly Rep 2001;50:430.
6. Centers for Disease Control and Prevention. HIV/AIDS surveillance report. www.cdc.gov 2000;12.
7. Epstein RM, Morse DS, Frankel RM, et al. Awkward moments in patient-physician communication about HIV risk. Ann Intern Med 1998;128:435.
8. Gray RH, Wawer MJ, Brookmeyer R, et al. Probability of HIV-1 transmission per coital act in monogamous, heterosexual, HIV-1 discordant couples in Rakai, Uganda. Lancet 2001;357:1149.
9. Lurie P, Miller S, Hecht F, et al. Postexposure prophylaxis after nonoccupational HIV exposure. JAMA 1998;280:1769.
10. Quinn TC, Mawer MJ, Sewankambo N, et al. Viral load and heterosexual transmission of human immunodeficiency virus type 1. N Engl J Med 2000;342:921.
11. Cummings PD, Wallace EL, Schorr JB. Exposure of patients to human immunodeficiency virus through the transfusion of blood components that test antibody-negative. N Engl J Med 1989;321:941.
12. Perinatal HIV Guidelines Working Group. Public health service task force recommendations for the use of antiretroviral drugs in pregnant HIV-1 infected women for maternal health and interventions to reduce perinatal HIV-1 transmission in the United States. www.hivatis.org January 24, 2001.
13. Centers for Disease Control and Prevention. Updated U.S. Public Health Service guidelines of the management of occupational exposures to HBV, HCV, and HIV and recommendations for postexposure prophylaxis. MMWR Morb Mortal Wkly Rep 2001;50:1.
14. Centers for Disease Control and Prevention. Interpretation and use of the Western blot assay for serodiagnosis of human immunodeficiency virus type I infections. JAMA 1989;262:3395.
15. Daar ES, Little S, Pitt J, et al. Diagnosis of primary HIV-1 infection. Ann Intern Med 2001;134:25.
16. Panteleo G, Graziosi C, Fauci AS. The immunopathogenesis of human immunodeficiency virus infection. N Engl J Med 1993;328:327.
17. Saksela K, Stevens CE, Rubinstein P, et al. HIV-1 messenger RNA in peripheral blood mononuclear cells as an early marker for risk of progression to AIDS. Ann Intern Med 1995;123:641.
18. Centers for Disease Control and Prevention. United Sates Public Health Service/Infectious Disease Society of America guidelines for prevention of opportunistic infections in persons infected with HIV. MMWR Morb Mortal Wkly Rep 1999;48:40.
18a. American Thoracic Sociey/Centers for Disease Control and Prevention. Update: Fatal and severe liver injuries associated with rifampin and pyrazinamide for latent tuberculosis infection and revisions in American Thoracic Society/CDC recommendations—United States, 2001. Am J Repir Crit Care Med 2001;164:1319.
19. Moss AR, Bachetti P. Natural history of HIV infection. AIDS 1989;39:55.
20. French N, Nakiyingi J, Carpenter LM, et al. 23-Valent pneumococcal polysaccharide vaccine in HIV-1-infected Ugandan adults: double-blind, randomised and placebo controlled trial. Lancet 2000;355:2106.
21. Dworkin MS, Ward JW, Hanson DL, et al. Pneumococcal disease among human immunodeficiency virus-infected persons: incidence, risk factors, and impact of vaccination. Clin Infect Dis 2001;32:794.
22. Tasker SA, Treanor JJ, Paxton WB, et al. Efficacy of influenza vaccination in HIV-infected persons: a randomized double-blind, placebo controlled trial. Ann Intern Med 1999;131:430.
23. Pierce M, Crampton S, Henry D, et al. A randomized trial of clarithromycin as prophylaxis against disseminated MAC infection in patients with advanced acquired immunodeficiency syndrome. N Engl J Med 1996;335:384.
24. Spector SA, McKInley GF, Lalezari JP, et al. Oral ganciclovir for the prevention of cytomegalovirus disease in persons with AIDS. N Engl J Med 1996;334:1491.
25. Powderly WG, Finklestein DM, Feinberg J, et al. A randomized trial comparing fluconazole with clotrimazole troches for prevention of fungal infections in patients with advanced human immunodeficiency virus infection. N Engl J Med 1995;332:700.
26. United States Department of Health and Human Services. Guidelines for the use of antiretroviral agents in HIV-infected adults and adolescents. February 2002. Published at www.hivatis.org.
27. Weinstein MC, Goldie SJ, Losina E, et al. Use of genotypic resistance testing to guide HIV therapy: clinical impact and cost-effectiveness. Ann Intern Med 2001;134:440.
28. Hirsch MS, Brun-Vezinet F, D'Aquila RT, et al. Antiretroviral drug resistance testing in adult HIV-1 infection: recommendations of an International AIDS Society-USA panel. JAMA 2000;283:2417.
29. McArthur JC, Sacktor N, Selnes O. Human immunodeficiency virus-associated dementia. Semin Neurol 1999;19:129.
30. Boyle BA, Goldenberg D. Current issues in antiretroviral and psychiatric therapy for HIV-infected patients. AIDS Reader 2000;10:508.
31. Soriano V, Garcia-Samaniego J, Rodriguez-Rosado R, et al. Hepatitis C and HIV infection: biological, clinical, and therapeutic implications. J Hepatol 1999;31[Suppl 1]:119.
32. Kartalija M, Sande MA. Diarrhea and AIDS in the era of highly active antiretroviral therapy. Clin Infect Dis 1999;28:701.
33. Nemechek PM, Polsky B, Gottlieb MS. Treatment guidelines for HIV-associated wasting. Mayo Clin Proc 2000;75:386.
34. Dezube BJ. Acquired immunodeficiency syndrome-related Kaposi's sarcoma: clinical features, staging, and treatment. Semin Oncol 2000;27:424.
35. Whitcup SM. Cytomegalovirus retinitis in the era of highly active antiretroviral therapy. JAMA 2000;283:653.
36. Winston JA, Burns GC, Klotman PE. Treatment of HIV-associated nephropathy. Semin Nephrol 2000;20:293.
37. Rerkpattanapipat P, Wongpraparut N, Jacobs LE, et al. Cardiac manifestations of acquired immunodeficiency syndrome. Arch Intern Med 2000;160:602.

C H A P T E R 40

Ambulatory Care for Selected Infections Including Osteomyelitis, Lung Abscess, and Endocarditis

JOHN G. BARTLETT, MD

Usually, the three types of infections reviewed in detail in this chapter are managed initially with intravenous antibiotics administered in the hospital. Patients with these infections are often seen first in an office setting, and the long courses of antibiotics used to treat them are then completed after discharge from the hospital. These infections involve diverse bacteria and different anatomic sites but share a propensity for relapse caused by persistent bacteria at the infected site. This explains the requirement for prolonged courses of antimicrobial treatment. Antibiotics may be administered by two different routes out of hospital: the oral route, to complete a course initiated parenterally during hospitalization, and the intravenous route, using the same regimen provided for inpatients and administered by home health agencies (see Gilbert, et al., in General References) (see Chapter 9).

EXPANDING ROLE OF ORAL ANTIBIOTICS

In the past, there was reluctance to prescribe oral antibiotics to be taken at home for most serious infections; however, this approach is gaining acceptance because of a number of studies indicating efficacy (1–5). The advantages of home use of oral agents are patient convenience, the notable reduction in cost, and a reduction in nosocomial infections. These and other considerations are summarized in Table 40.1. Average charges for hospital care that includes intravenous antibiotics are about $1,000/day, whereas for intravenous antibiotics given at home the average charge is $300 to $400/day and for oral agents the cost is $1 to $6/day. The issue of patient convenience is obvious. With regard to nosocomial infections, the cost in terms of morbidity, mortality, and hospital charge is substantial. In 1992, it was estimated that nosocomial infections accounted for 19,000 deaths (0.9% of hospitalized patients) and were a contributing factor in the deaths of 58,000 patients (2.7%). The extension in-hospital stay averaged 4 days for those with nosocomial infections, at an average cost of $2,100 (6). Of particular concern in recent years has been nosocomial acquisition of tuberculosis (especially the multiply resistant strains); *Clostridium difficile*–associated colitis, which is now recognized largely as a nosocomial complication; and Legionnaires disease. Hospitals also remain the major source of problem pathogens such as *Pseudomonas aeruginosa,* multiply resistant gram-negative bacilli, methicillin-resistant *Staphylococcus aureus,* and vancomycin-resistant *Enterococcus.*

Some types of infectious diseases have traditionally been treated with parenteral antibiotics but may sometimes be treated with oral agents: *P. aeruginosa* urinary tract infections (including bacterial prostatitis), pulmonary infections in patients with cystic fibrosis, some forms of osteomyelitis, tricuspid valve endocarditis caused by *S. aureus* in intravenous drug abusers, fever in the patient with neutropenia (see Chapter 10), some cases of pyelonephritis, most cases of pneumonia (see Chapter 33), and selected fungal infections that traditionally have required amphotericin B.

Newer Antimicrobial Agents

Much of the progress in this area has resulted from the development of oral antimicrobial agents in four classes that have an expanded spectrum of activity: cephalosporins, fluoroquinolones, beta-lactam–beta-lactamase inhibitor combinations, and the triazole antifungal agents. Among the *cephalosporins* and *carbecephams,* the agents with an expanded spectrum of activity for oral administration include cefaclor, cefuroxime axetil, cefprozil, cefpodoxime, loracarbef, and cefixime. All of these agents are active against most strains of Enterobacteriaceae; activity against major gram-positive cocci is variable, and none of these agents is active against *P. aeruginosa,* enterococci, or methicillin-resistant *S. aureus.* In general,

Table 40.1. Advantages and Disadvantages of Home Treatment with Oral Antimicrobial Agents

Advantages
Cost reduction
Patient convenience
Reduced nosocomial infections
Demonstrated efficacy
Disadvantages
Bioavailability
Need for supportive care or monitoring
Compliance
Possible legal liability
Selected infections that require parenteral agents
Serious side effects that require immediate care

these drugs are advocated for respiratory tract infections, skin and soft tissue infections, and urinary tract infections. The *fluoroquinolones* include norfloxacin, ciprofloxacin, ofloxacin, gatifloxacin, moxifloxacin, and levofloxacin. There are slight differences among these agents in bioavailability, spectrum of activity, pharmacology, and side effects. In general, ciprofloxacin is favored for infections involving *P. aeruginosa*; levofloxacin gatifloxacin, and moxifloxacin are preferred for infections in which *Streptococcus pneumoniae* is an established or suspected pathogen. *S. aureus* strains are developing resistance to the fluoroquinolones, and resistance to one implies resistance to the entire group. The only available oral *beta-lactam–beta-lactamase inhibitor* is amoxicillin plus clavulanate (Augmentin), which has the spectrum of amoxicillin plus organisms that are penicillin resistant because of beta-lactamase production: *S. aureus,* many gram negative bacilli, *Haemophilus influenzae,* and many anaerobes.

For oral treatment of serious anaerobic infections, either of two older drugs, metronidazole and clindamycin, is usually an option.

Newer Antifungal Agents

The triazoles include ketoconazole, fluconazole, and itraconazole. These drugs are now supplanting amphotericin B for many fungal infections. All three are effective against most strains of *Candida albicans* and may be used for mucocutaneous candidiasis, but their use for parenchymal and systemic *Candida* infections is limited. Fluconazole has established efficacy for cryptococcosis. Itraconazole now appears to be the preferred agent for most cases of histoplasmosis, blastomycosis, and paracoccidioidomycosis and for many cases of coccidioidomycosis and aspergillosis.

RISKS AND BURDENS OF HOME TREATMENT

The use of oral agents in the home setting for infections traditionally treated with intravenous antibiotics in the hospital is not without some risks and burdens. Supportive care requiring some hospital resources for very sick patients is an example. Although monitoring of drug levels is rarely an issue with oral agents, compliance is always a concern, and physicians have been notoriously unable to predict which patients will take their medications (see Chapter 4). In many communities, this issue is now addressed for tuberculosis by direct observation of pill taking, although here the circumstances are somewhat different because antituberculosis drugs can be given twice weekly and the need is justified on the basis of public health concerns. Certain pathogens are difficult or impossible to treat with currently available oral agents. These include the fluoroquinolone-resistant strains of *P. aeruginosa,* many infections involving methicillin-resistant *S. aureus,* and cytomegalovirus. An additional concern about outpatient management is the fact that patients are not under direct observation, so emergency care is not immediately available for serious side effects. The major example is immunoglobulin E–mediated hypersensitivity caused by beta-lactam agents, which occurs with a frequency of about 1:2,500 to 1:25,000 courses of penicillin G. Finally, there may be concern about legal liability when the use of oral antibiotics is not considered the standard of care, even if efficacy and safety seem well established. Because many third-party payers now mandate home care for stable patients who require long-term antibiotics, the latter concern is unlikely to deter expanded home treatment.

OSTEOMYELITIS

Definition

Osteomyelitis is an infection of bone. There are *four major categories:* osteomyelitis due to hematogenous spread of infection, osteomyelitis secondary to a contiguous focus of infection, infection of prosthetic joints, and osteomyelitis associated with vascular insufficiency. These four categories differ in terms of patient age, bones involved, predisposing conditions, usual bacterial pathogens, and presentation (Table 40.2). Osteomyelitis is also classified as *acute or chronic:* acute osteomyelitis indicates newly recognized bone infection, whereas chronic osteomyelitis indicates prior infection or clinical symptoms exceeding 10 days (3).

Clinical Presentation and Bacteriology

Hematogenous

Hematogenous osteomyelitis is classically described as a disease of *children,* usually younger than 16 years of age, which is usually caused by *S. aureus* (3). The tendency for this infection to occur during active growth reflects the enhanced susceptibility of the vascular network of the metaphysis, especially of the femur or tibia. About one third of the patients have a history of preceding nonpenetrating trauma in the area that is subsequently involved. The infection begins in the metaphyseal sinusoidal veins; it is contained by the epiphyseal growth plate and tends to spread laterally, with perforation of the cortex and lifting of the loose periosteum.

Hematogenous osteomyelitis of the long bones in *adults* is rare, different in presentation, and

Table 40.2. Types of Osteomyelitis

	Hematogenous	Secondary to Contiguous Infection	Complications of Vascular Insufficiency
Approximate proportion of all cases (%)	20	50	30
Most common age groups	1–16 yr, >50 yr	Any age	>50 yr
Bones involved	Long bones (children) Vertebrae (adults)	Hip, femur, tibia, digits	Feet
Predisposing causes	Trauma Bacteremia	Surgery Soft tissue infection	Diabetes mellitus Vascular insufficiency
Usual bacteria	*Staphylococcus aureus* Gram negative bacilli	Often polymicrobial: Gram negative bacilli, *S. aureus*	Usually polymicrobial: gram negative bacilli, anaerobes, streptococci, *S. aureus*
Presentation			
Initial episode	Fever, local pain swelling, tenderness, limited movement	Fever, local pain swelling, tenderness, limited movement	Ulceration drainage ± pain
Recurrent episode	Sinus drainage ± pain	Sinus drainage ± pain	Drainage ± pain

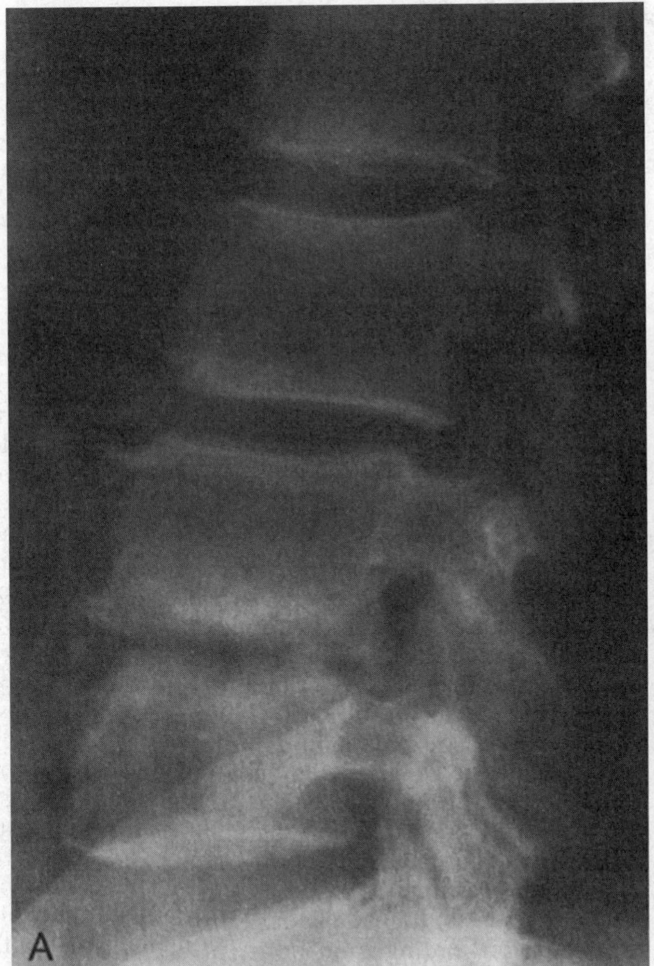

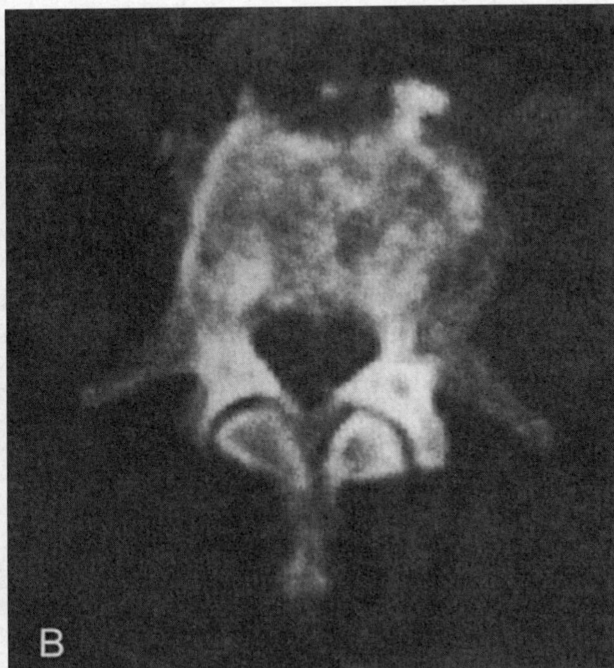

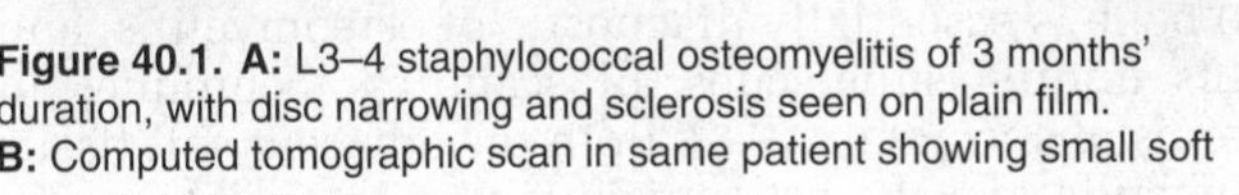

Figure 40.1. A: L3–4 staphylococcal osteomyelitis of 3 months' duration, with disc narrowing and sclerosis seen on plain film. **B:** Computed tomographic scan in same patient showing small soft tissue abscess and minimal bone destruction. Note hazy bone outline (From Post MJD, ed. Computed tomography of the spine. Baltimore: Williams & Wilkins, 1984:740.)

bacteriologically distinct. In these patients, the growth cartilage has been resorbed so that the subarticular space is more vulnerable, and the periosteum is firmly attached so that subperiosteal abscess formation is uncommon. The most common form of hematogenous osteomyelitis in adults involves the vertebrae (Fig. 40.1), and the most common pathogens are gram-negative bacilli and *S. aureus*. The initial site of infection is the richly vascularized bone adjacent to cartilage; there is subsequent involvement of adjacent bone plates and of the intervertebral disc. The infection may extend longitudinally to involve adjacent vertebrae, anteriorly to produce a paraspinal abscess, or posteriorly to form an epidural abscess.

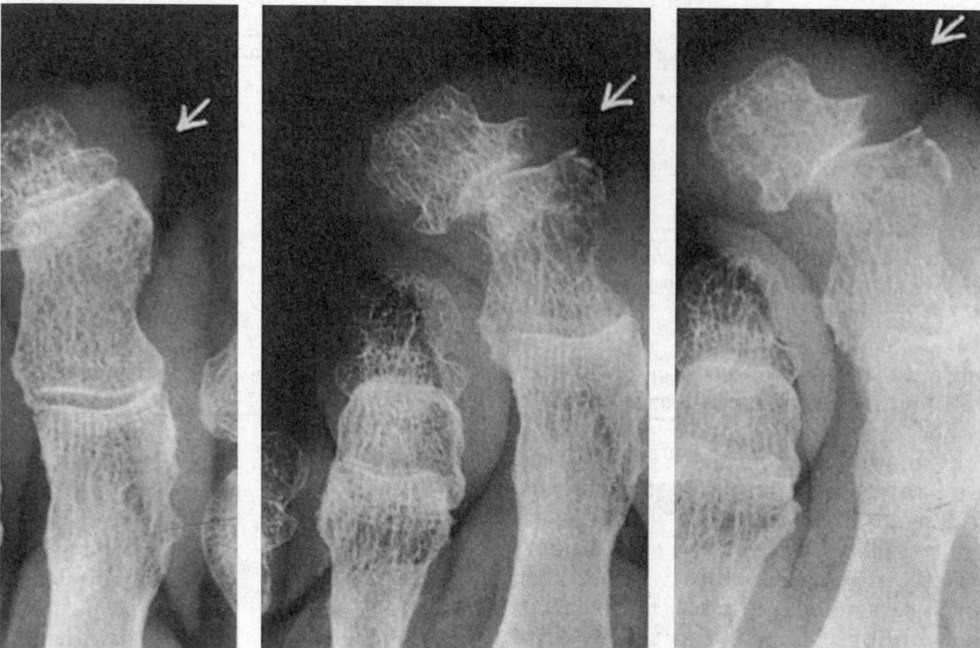

Figure 40.2. Arrows indicate, from left to right, infected soft corn, sinus tract, and osteomyelitis in the distal interphalangeal joint. As destruction increases, the joint becomes dislocated. (From Gamble FO, Yale I. Clinical foot roentgenology. Baltimore: Williams & Wilkins, 1966.)

Patients with acute hematogenous osteomyelitis usually present with precipitous onset of pain, swelling, chills, and fever. With vertebral osteomyelitis, there is fever with back pain, stiffness, and often point tenderness over the infected vertebra. Many patients have a more subacute presentation, with vague symptoms of 1 to 2 months' duration before presentation and few constitutional complaints. One well-described variant is the Brodie abscess (also called a cold abscess): subacute staphylococcal osteomyelitis located in the metaphysis of a long bone, which manifests with local pain and fever. Patients with recurrent or chronic osteomyelitis often simply note increased or persistent drainage and pain after an episode involving the same anatomic location.

Contiguous Infection

Osteomyelitis secondary to a contiguous focus of infection accounts for at least half of all cases. The most common precipitating factor is previous surgery, usually involving the lower extremities, such as open reduction of fractures of the femur or tibia. Next in frequency is a soft tissue infection involving the digits of the hands or feet. These infections usually become apparent within 1 month after the precipitating event, although many patients have chronic or recurrent infections that occur intermittently for years or decades.

Prosthetic Joint Infections

Infections that complicate prosthetic joints are classified as acute (within 12 weeks after surgery) or chronic (within 3 to 24 months after surgery) (3). Later infections may result from transient bacteremia in a fashion analogous to the pathogenesis of endocarditis, with the joint serving as a susceptible nidus. The presentation of an infected prosthesis is a painful, unstable joint, often with little or no fever and nonspecific radiographic findings. The diagnosis is best established with semiquantitative culture of an aspirate from the joint space or bone–cement interface. *Staphylococcus epidermidis* accounts for 75% of cases; next in frequency are *S. aureus,* streptococci, *Peptococcus magnus,* enteric gram-negative bacilli, and *Candida* spp.

Vascular Insufficiency

Osteomyelitis associated with vascular insufficiency is most common in patients with diabetes mellitus or severe atherosclerosis (7,8). The most common sites of infection are the toes and small bones of the feet, usually with overlying soft tissue infections (Fig. 40.2). These infections are often detected on routine radiographs performed to evaluate the chronic draining sinuses or skin ulcers that are so common in the patients at risk. Probing that demonstrates extension of ulcers to bone is essentially diagnostic of osteomyelitis, and this finding supersedes all scanning techniques in terms of specificity (7,8). Both the adjacent soft tissue infection and the osteomyelitis usually involve *polymicrobial flora* that may include anaerobic bacteria, coliforms, pseudomonads, streptococci, and *S. aureus.*

Laboratory Evaluation

Diagnostic studies include radiographs, radionuclide studies, computed tomography (CT), or magnetic resonance imaging (MRI) to demonstrate typical bone changes and cultures to identify the etiologic organism.

The earliest changes on plain radiographs are lytic lesions; other findings may include soft tissue swelling, periosteal reaction, cortical irregularity, demineralization, and sequestrum formation. However, typical changes are not visible on plain films until 30% to 50% of the bone has been resorbed, and this usually requires 10 to 14 days. In a patient with a normal plain film but clinical findings suggesting osteomyelitis, a technetium bone scan or an indium In 111 leukocyte scan can be helpful. Both of these tests are sensitive in early osteomyelitis (70% to 90%), but they lack specificity (50% to 75%) (3,9,10). The bone scan uses technetium Tc 99 as a marker bound to diphosphonate which concentrates in bone because of incorporation at sites of osteoblastic activity. Abnormal studies may occur when there is increased blood flow associated with soft tissue infections or with osteoblastic activity caused by other processes, such as degenerative joint disease. If a three-phase technetium scan (immediate, showing flow; 15-minute, showing blood pooling; and 4-hour showing bone imaging) is used, soft tissue infections give positive images in the first two phases but only bony infection gives positive images in all three phases. Most authorities regard ^{99}Tc scanning as the preferred scintigraphic method (9,11). CT and MRI are also useful in showing osteomyelitis. CT scans are particularly helpful for guiding needle biopsy or percutaneous aspirations. MRI is particularly sensitive and may show osteomyelitis before changes are evident by scintigraphy (3). Prosthetic material that is ferromagnetic is a contraindication to MRI, but most materials now used in orthopedic surgery do not interfere.

Because antimicrobial treatment, often prolonged, is the mainstay of management, accurate bacteriologic data are helpful for making the diagnosis and planning treatment. The list of possible organisms is long, and sensitivity patterns for these organisms show considerable variation, making empiric selection of antimicrobials hazardous. These considerations may justify an aggressive attempt to identify the responsible organism. Conclusive bacteriologic studies require isolation of the pathogen from bone or blood cultures.

Under ideal circumstances, an orthopedist should perform a *needle aspiration* over the involved bone, either blindly or, preferably, under CT guidance (12). If subperiosteal pus is obtained, surgical drainage is mandatory. If no pus is obtained, the needle is inserted into bone to obtain a specimen. The diagnostic yield with a needle aspirate of bone is approximately 60%, and for a surgical biopsy it is approximately 90% (3). Cultures from draining sinus tracts tend to show poor correlation with cultures obtained directly from bone (13). Needle aspirate specimens should be submitted for Gram stain and for culture of aerobic and anaerobic bacteria. Care must be exercised in the interpretation of culture results, even of bone aspirates, because these are often contaminated, especially if the specimen is obtained by traversing soft tissue infections (14). Organisms recovered in low concentrations, especially those growing only in the broth culture, must be viewed with skepticism. Common skin contaminants include *S. epidermidis,* diphtheroids, and *Propionibacterium.* These organisms tend to cause osteomyelitis only in the presence of prosthetic devices. Gram staining of exudate or tissue aspirate should verify the culture results and represents an important correlate in determining the etiologic organism. The semiquantitative results of cultures are an important and often overlooked component of interpreting culture results, especially when the organisms detected are common contaminants.

Treatment

General Principles

Immobilization was commonly advocated for the treatment of osteomyelitis in the preantibiotic era. However, it appears to be less important at present, and most authorities conclude that strict immobilization is unnecessary.

Antimicrobial Treatment: Acute Osteomyelitis. For newly diagnosed or acute osteomyelitis, the standard recommendation has been a 3- to 6-week course of parenteral antibiotics (14–16). This recommendation is based on several studies noting that patients often developed recurrent or chronic disease when treatment lasted less than 21 days. The standard regimen for acute staphylococcal osteomyelitis in adults is a penicillinase-resistant penicillin such as nafcillin, given intravenously at a dosage of 1.5 to 2 g every 6 hours. Alternative parenteral regimens are cefazolin (1.0 to 1.5 g every 8 hours), vancomycin (1 g every 12 hours), or clindamycin (600 mg every 8 hours) (3). In stable patients, these regimens can be initiated in the hospital and completed at home.

To decrease cost, length of hospitalization, and patient discomfort, a *modified regimen,* consisting of a short course of parenteral antibiotics followed by a prolonged course of oral agents, has been developed (3). The intravenous antibiotic is given for at least 3 days, or until the patient is afebrile, or for an arbitrarily defined period such as 1 to 2 weeks. An alternative oral agent selected by *in vitro* sensitivity tests is then taken by mouth, usually at home, to complete a total 3- to 6-week course, usually 4 weeks. The drugs recommended for oral administration are clindamycin (300 mg every 6 hours), an oral antistaphylococcal penicillin such as dicloxacillin or cephalexin (500 mg every 6 hours), or a fluoroquinolone. It should be noted that the importance of bactericidal activity and the relative merits of drugs for bone penetration as factors in drug selection are debated issues that remain unresolved.

Antimicrobial Treatment: Chronic Osteomyelitis. Therapeutic guidelines are less precise for chronic osteomyelitis. Because necrotic bone may serve as a nidus for sequestered bacteria, surgical excision of dead tissue and adequate debridement are often essential components of treatment. Antibiotic selection should be based on bacteriologic diagnosis using deep aspirates or, preferably, cultures obtained from bone. The daily dosage, route of administration, and duration of treatment are somewhat arbitrary, but most authorities recommend prolonged courses. The initial treatment may consist of parenteral antibiotics for 1 to 3 months in the hospital or in the home, followed by oral agents for several months (16). An alternative approach is the use, from the outset of treatment, of oral agents to which the patient's infecting organism is sensitive, for extended periods, such as 6 months or longer (3). Fluoroquinolones such as ofloxacin or ciprofloxacin, alone or in combination with clindamycin or metronidazole, have established efficacy for osteomyelitis with a mixed anaerobic–coliform flora (3). Oral cephalosporins may also be used for infections involving gram negative bacilli; metronidazole by mouth is preferred for oral treatment of deep infections involving anaerobes, although clindamycin and amoxicillin–clavulanate (Augmentin) are probably effective as well. Various authors have used a variety of dosages of these antibiotics. Guidelines should be sought in published reports or the most current editions of manuals on the use of antibiotics for specific infections.

Late Complications

The major complication of osteomyelitis is recurrence that may happen months, years, or decades after the initial event. The patient should be warned of this potential complication. The clinical features of recurrences are fever, draining sinuses, local pain, increased sedimentation rate, and the typical changes noted on radiographs or scans, as summarized previously. Chronic osteomyelitis may be complicated by secondary amyloidosis, although it has become extremely rare since the advent of antibiotics. Another complication is epidermoid carcinoma arising in a draining sinus of osteomyelitis, which occurs in 0.2% to 1.5% of cases, with a mean delay of 34 years (17).

Patients with orthopedic devices such as prosthetic joints are at risk for infection after transient bacteremia. However, unlike the situation with endocarditis, there are no guidelines from authoritative sources to direct preventive treatment. It is reasonable to administer prophylactic antibiotics for those procedures that are considered a risk by the American Heart Association for patients susceptible to endocarditis (see Table 93.13 in Chapter 93). However, the major pathogens for infected orthopedic devices are *S. aureus, S. epidermidis,* and to a lesser extent, *Streptococcus* spp., whereas endocarditis prophylaxis is directed primarily against *Streptococcus.* For the former organisms, some recommend prophylaxis with an oral cephalosporin or clindamycin: one dose taken 1 hour before dental work in patients with periodontal disease or potential dental infection and two subsequent doses (18). However, the American Academy of Oral Medicine has deferred issuing a formal standard for antibiotic prophylaxis in patients with orthopedic prostheses.

LUNG ABSCESS

Definition

The term *lung abscess* refers to pulmonary suppuration with parenchymal necrosis caused by bacterial infection. The lesions are traditionally classified on the basis of clinical and bacteriologic observations. Lung abscesses are considered *acute or chronic* depending on the duration of symptoms at the time of initial presentation, with the usual dividing line being 4 to 6 weeks. Clinically, lung abscesses are often grouped as *putrid* lung abscess, in reference to the foul odor of sputum that is regarded as diagnostic of anaerobic infection, or *nonspecific* lung abscess, indicating that aerobic sputum cultures have not grown out a pathogen. Anaerobic bacteria are the presumed pathogens in these latter cases also. Lung abscesses may also be classified clinically as primary or secondary, depending on predisposing conditions. *Primary* lung abscesses are those that occur in patients who are prone to aspiration or in previously healthy patients. *Secondary* abscesses are complications of a local lesion such as a pulmonary malignancy or of a systemic disease that compromises immunologic defenses. Approximately 80% of lung abscesses are primary; 60% are putrid, and 40% are nonspecific (probably mostly anaerobic) (19). Patients with lung abscess often present in the ambulatory care setting because of the chronicity of these infections. Most patients are hospitalized for diagnostic studies and initial treatment with intravenous antibiotics. The hospital course is usually followed by prolonged courses of antibiotics and follow-up chest radiographs.

Clinical Presentation and Bacteriology

Many bacteria are potential pulmonary pathogens, but few organisms are likely to cause parenchymal necrosis. The most common pathogens are anaerobic bacteria that make up the normal flora of the gingival crevice and are aspirated during periods of altered consciousness. The usual pathogens in such cases are *Prevotella* spp., *Bacteroides* spp., anaerobic streptococci, and *Fusobacterium nucleatum* (19). The most common aerobic bacteria that cause suppurative pulmonary infections are *S. aureus* and *Klebsiella pneumoniae;* less common causal pathogens are *Streptococcus pyogenes, S. pneumoniae, H. influenzae, P. aeruginosa, Legionella, Nocardia,* and enteric gram-negative bacilli other than *K. pneumoniae.* It is important to exclude other etiologic agents, such as mycobacteria and fungi, that may cause chronic abscesses requiring an entirely different antimicrobial regimen. Tuberculosis should be suspected in any patient with a lung abscess, especially in patients with a cough that has lasted for 1 month to 1 year, nonputrid sputum, and typical clinical features of night sweats and weight loss.

Patients with anaerobic lung abscesses usually have indolent complaints that last for weeks or even months. Common symptoms include fever, malaise, cough, and sputum production. Pleuritic pain and hemoptysis are common and may persuade a chronically ill patient to seek medical attention. Chills are occasionally noted, but true rigors are rare. The common observation of anemia and weight loss reflects the chronicity of many of these infections. The sputum is usually purulent, and putrid odor is noted in approximately 60% of bacteriologically confirmed anaerobic lung abscesses. The usual sites of involvement are the anatomic segments of the lung where aspiration is most likely to occur by gravitational flow in the recumbent position. These are the superior segments of the lower lobes and the posterior segments of the upper lobes. Less common abscess sites are the basilar segments of the lower lobes, which are dependent in the upright or semiupright position.

Lung abscesses caused by aerobic bacteria are usually found in specific clinical settings. Staphylococcal pulmonary infections with abscess formation are particularly common in young children and in adults with influenza or hospital-acquired pneumonia.

Klebsiella is often suspected as a cause of lung abscess in alcoholic patients, but even in these patients anaerobic organisms are far more common. The immunologically compromised patient may have pulmonary suppuration caused by a variety of bacterial and nonbacterial organisms, but anaerobes appear to be distinctly unusual in this population.

Laboratory Examination

The initial evaluations in patients with symptoms of lung abscess are those recommended for patients with suspected pulmonary infections in general. These include a chest radiograph, a complete blood count, blood cultures, and an examination of expectorated sputum. Gram staining of respiratory secretions typically shows a mixed or polymicrobial flora. The lung abscess usually is readily apparent with the chest radiograph (Fig. 40.3), although other causes of a pulmonary cavity must be considered in the differential diagnosis. Alternative considerations include a cavitating neoplasm, cavitating pulmonary infarction, tuberculosis, fungal infection, an infected pulmonary cyst or bulla, and a loculated empyema (i.e., pleural space infection) with an air–fluid level caused by a bronchopleural fistula, gas-producing organisms, or Wegener granulomatosis.

When a cavitary lesion appears to be caused by bacterial infection, there is controversy about the approach to identifying the likely pathogen. Sputum should be examined using Gram stain and Ziehl–Nielson stain to determine from the outset whether an anaerobic pathogen or *Mycobacterium tuberculosis* is the likely cause of the abscess.

Expectorated sputum is easily obtained from most patients, and standard cultures usually show a predominance of an aerobic organism when it is the etiologic pathogen. The problem with these specimens is that they are inappropriate for anaerobic culture, and the results with aerobic cultures are often misleading because of contamination by bacteria that reside in the upper airway.

Bronchoscopy is generally not useful for microbiologic studies except for mycobacterial and nonbacterial pathogens; an exception is specimens that are obtained with a specialized double catheter and are cultured quantitatively for aerobes and anaerobes.

Antimicrobial Treatment

Antimicrobials are the mainstay of treatment for lung abscess (Table 40.3). The best-studied regimens are those for anaerobic lung abscesses, because these account for most cases. Nevertheless, there is considerable controversy regarding the selection of agents and the duration of treatment.

Anaerobic Infections

With regard to drug selection, the initial antimicrobial agent recommended by most authorities is *clindamycin,* which is active against most anaerobic bacteria. In approximately 25% of patients, anaerobic organisms resistant to penicillin are present, and almost all of these organisms are highly sensitive to clindamycin. Not surprisingly, comparative trials showed that clindamycin was superior to penicillin in terms of primary response rate and duration of fever after the institution of treatment (20), two factors that may allow earlier hospital discharge. The initial treatment is usually given parenterally (600 mg intravenously every 8 hours) until the patient is afebrile and there is subjective improvement. This usually requires 3 to 7 days but may require considerably longer in patients with very large lung abscesses, those with prolonged symptoms before treatment, and those with pleural complications (primary empyema). The major alternative antibiotics are amoxicillin–clavulanate (875 mg orally twice daily) or penicillin (10 million units intravenously daily) plus metronidazole (500 to 750 mg twice daily).

Aerobic Infections

Guidelines for antimicrobial selection are less precise for lung abscesses involving other organisms. In these cases, the antibiotic is selected on the basis of *in vitro* sensitivity tests. Abscesses involving *S. aureus* or gram-negative bacilli are regarded as more serious infections, and intravenous antibiotics should be given for a more prolonged period; in selected stable patients, the intravenous regimen can be completed at home.

Duration of Treatment

Rigorous studies to determine the optimal duration of antimicrobial treatment for lung abscesses have not been done. The duration of treatment is arbitrary, but most authorities recommend at least 6 weeks or longer depending on results of serial radiographs. Antibiotics

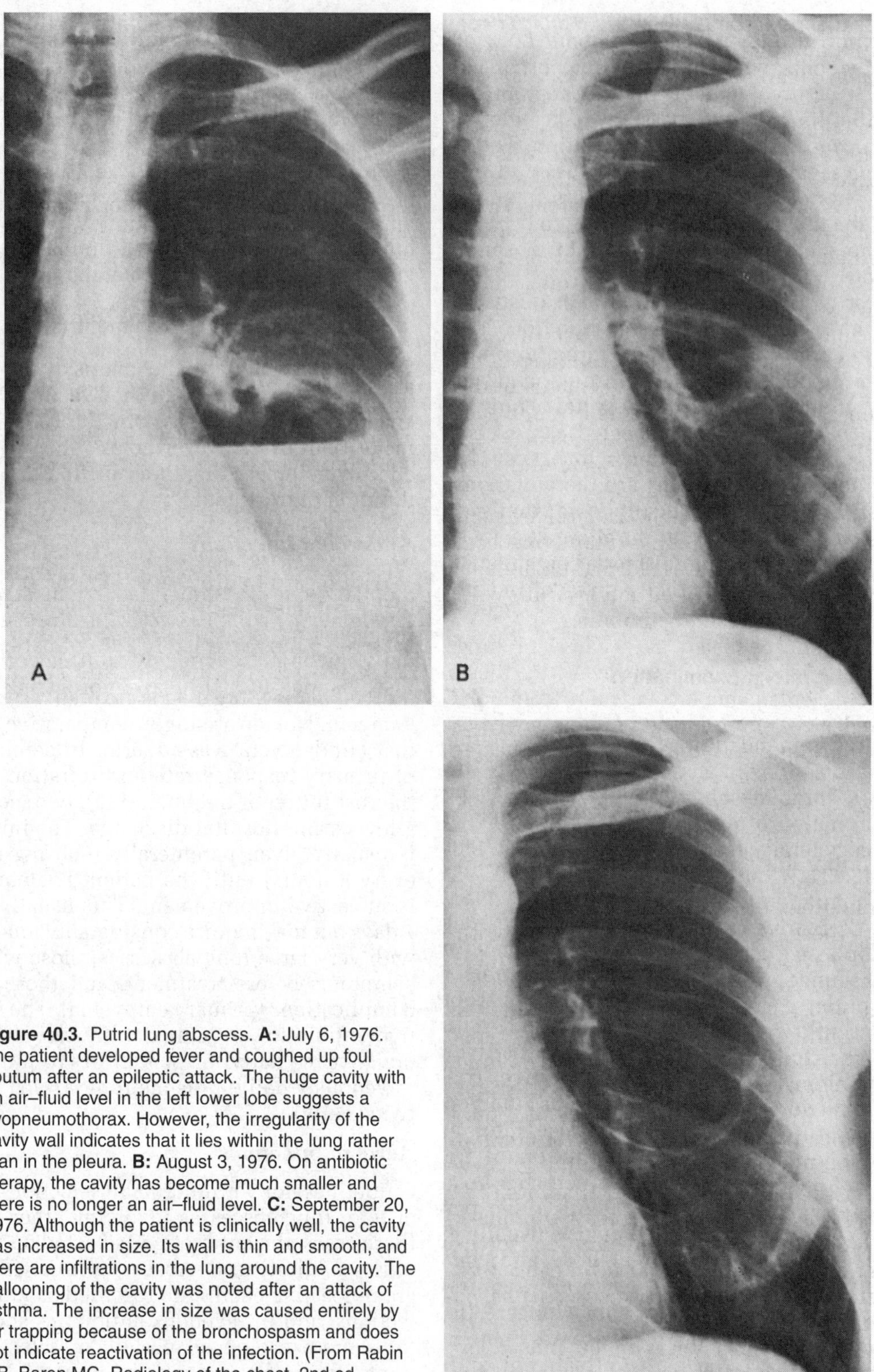

Figure 40.3. Putrid lung abscess. **A:** July 6, 1976. The patient developed fever and coughed up foul sputum after an epileptic attack. The huge cavity with an air–fluid level in the left lower lobe suggests a pyopneumothorax. However, the irregularity of the cavity wall indicates that it lies within the lung rather than in the pleura. **B:** August 3, 1976. On antibiotic therapy, the cavity has become much smaller and there is no longer an air–fluid level. **C:** September 20, 1976. Although the patient is clinically well, the cavity has increased in size. Its wall is thin and smooth, and there are infiltrations in the lung around the cavity. The ballooning of the cavity was noted after an attack of asthma. The increase in size was caused entirely by air trapping because of the bronchospasm and does not indicate reactivation of the infection. (From Rabin CB, Baron MG. Radiology of the chest. 2nd ed. Baltimore: Williams & Wilkins, 1980:340.)

are given until the chest radiograph either is clear or shows only a small stable residual lesion (Fig. 40.3). These recommendations are based on experiences in which patients have had relapses despite treatment for at least 1 month; in these patients, the infiltrate was still resolving when drugs were discontinued, and the patients were subsequently readmitted for recurrent abscesses in the same pulmonary segment. The usual oral regimen with clindamycin is 300 mg four times daily.

Table 40.3. Antimicrobial Regimens for Primary Lung Abscess

Intravenous[a]	Oral[a]	Comments
Aqueous penicillin G 5–10 million units/d	Penicillin G or V 500–750 mg q.i.d. or Amoxicillin 500 mg q.i.d. or	Regarded as standard *Advantages:* Inexpensive and well tolerated *Disadvantages:* Approximately 20% fail to respond and additional patients have delayed response
	Amoxicillin–clavulanate 875 mg b.i.d.[b]	*Advantage:* Coverage for organisms that produce β-lactamase *Disadvantage:* Expensive
	or	
Clindamycin 600 mg every 6–8 hr	Clindamycin 300 mg q.i.d.	*Advantage:* Opitmal response rates *Disadvantages:* Expensive; side effects include diarrhea in 10% to 20% of patients and occasional patients with pseudomembranous colitis

[a]Intravenous treatment until patient is afebrile and clinically improved; oral treatment is given either to complete an arbitrary total course of 3 to 6 weeks of treatment or until chest radiographs show clearance or a small, stable residual lesion.
[b]Both strengths listed are for amoxicillin; both contain 125 mg of clavulanate.

Regardless of the total duration of treatment, adequate follow-up is necessary to ensure resolution with serial radiographs. These should be obtained at 2- to 3-week intervals, or earlier if there is clinical deterioration. Most patients with lung abscess treated with antibiotics improve clinically before there is demonstrable improvement in the chest radiograph; cavities gradually close, but 20% to 30% persist beyond 6 weeks, and the roentgenographic criteria for cure as defined previously may require several months (21).

Inadequate Response to Treatment

Failure to show progressive improvement, especially if accompanied by clinical symptoms, necessitates a change in medical therapy, bronchoscopy (to rule out obstruction), or, on rare occasions, surgery. The major indications for surgery are an abscess that is totally refractory to antibiotic treatment, life-threatening or persistent hemorrhage, and abscesses occurring in association with an obstructed bronchus (22).

ENDOCARDITIS

Definition and Epidemiology

Endocarditis, an infection involving the heart valves, usually is caused by bacteria but occasionally by other microbes such as *Rickettsia* or fungi. There is a spectrum of clinical findings, but patients with the subacute form of the disease may have symptoms that are notably vague and nonspecific. The principal criteria for making the diagnosis are documented fever, heart murmur, and positive blood cultures. A unique feature of the disease is that most patients have continuous bacteremia, so that blood cultures are positive in 95% of patients, regardless of the temporal relationship between blood samplings and temperature profile.

The annual incidence of acquired *native valve endocarditis* in the United States is 1.7 to 6.2 per 100,000 population. The incidence is much higher among injection drug users: 150 to 2,000 per 100,000. Mitral valve prolapse (MVP) is the most common structural abnormality predisposing to endocarditis: the annual incidence in patients with MVP is approximately 100 per 100,000. *Prosthetic valve endocarditis* may account for up to 25% of cases in developed countries. The incidence of endocarditis after prosthetic valve insertion is approximately 1% in the first 12 months and 2% to 3% at 60 months. (23)

All patients with endocarditis should be hospitalized for a complete diagnostic evaluation, supportive care, and initiation of treatment with antibiotics, given intravenously. This discussion addresses the management of these patients in the ambulatory care setting after hospital discharge.

Treatment

Antimicrobial Treatment Out of Hospital

Antibiotics are selected for patients with endocarditis according to *in vitro* sensitivity tests, with emphasis on bactericidal activity. Most patients are treated with specific regimens according to guidelines from authoritative sources. The standard of treatment has traditionally been 4 to 6 weeks of intravenous antibiotic therapy. Many authorities now endorse a 2-week regimen of penicillin and streptomycin for infections caused by penicillin-sensitive strains of *Streptococcus viridans* and *Streptococcus bovis* (24), and most recommend prolonged courses for patients with prosthetic valve endocarditis (25). If intravenous antibiotics are planned for several weeks, part of the parenteral course can be administered at home to expedite hospital discharge.

Abbreviated courses of intravenous or oral antibiotics have been suggested for staphylococcal tricuspid valve endocarditis occurring as a complication of intravenous drug abuse (1,26). The advantages of this plan are that it is substantially less expensive, it reduces the problem of venous access, and it appears to be highly effective. The *oral regimen* studied most extensively is ciprofloxacin (750 mg twice daily) plus rifampin (300 mg twice daily), but *S. aureus* is showing escalating rates of resistance to all fluoroquinolones, so use should be restricted to cases showing good bactericidal activity *in vitro*. Alternatively, treatment may begin with intravenous agents such as nafcillin (2 g every 4 hours) with or without gentamycin (1 mg/kg every 8 hours) for 2 weeks, followed by oral administration of ciprofloxacin or cephalexin (500 mg every 6 hours) (27,28). The duration of treatment should be 4 weeks.

Patients with *prosthetic valve endocarditis* have infections that have proved particularly difficult to cure without intervening surgery. Nevertheless, intravenous antibiotics are given with the aim of avoiding reoperation; this is a realistic goal with antibiotic-sensitive organisms. The most common pathogen in these cases is *S. epidermidis,* which is treated for at least 6 weeks with intravenous drugs selected on the basis of *in vitro* sensitivity tests. The usual regimen is a penicillinase-resistant penicillin (nafcillin or oxacillin, 2 g every 4 hours) or vancomycin (30 mg/kg daily) for at least 6 weeks combined with gentamycin (1 mg/kg every 8 hours) for the first 2 weeks (24). For methicillin-resistant strains, the regimen is vancomycin and rifampin (300 mg orally every 12 hours) for at least 6 weeks and gentamycin for 2 weeks. Many authorities recommend prolonged courses of oral antibiotics after the initial intravenous regimen, such as dicloxacillin or cephalexin in a divided dose of 2 g/day. Because these patients are often stable, it is reasonable to complete a course of dicloxacillin or cephalexin combined with rifampin, 600 to 900 mg/day, out of hospital. This oral regimen is continued for arbitrarily defined periods that range from several weeks to 6 months or longer (25). Because *rifampin reduces the effect of warfarin,* which is part of the medical regimen of patients with prosthetic valves, patients taking rifampin typically need an increase in their warfarin dosage.

Long-Term Follow-Up and Prognosis

Patients with endocarditis treated medically or surgically should be monitored carefully after discontinuation of antibiotics. Major *complications* during this recovery phase include congestive heart failure, relapse, mycotic aneurysms, and recurrences involving new organisms.

Blood cultures are commonly recommended after discontinuation of antibiotic treatment, usually 2 to 3 days later. Patients who have had an inadequate course of therapy usually relapse within this time frame. Relapse after the recommended course of therapy is least common with viridans streptococci (about 2%); it is more common with most other pathogens (23). Patients most likely to relapse are those with prosthetic valve endocarditis and/or endocarditis involving organisms resistant to antibiotics. The presence of positive blood cultures without a clearly identifiable portal of entry in the recovery phase is presumptive evidence of relapse. The usual recommendation is another course of antibiotics or surgery for a refractory infection. The choice between these two approaches is made on the basis of the extent of the initial treatment course, underlying valve disease, and the *in vitro* sensitivity of the organism, with particular attention to bactericidal activity. The patient should also be warned of the possibility of relapse and should be instructed to monitor temperature, especially in the evening, when elevations are most likely to be noted.

Cardiac function should be monitored carefully during and after antibiotic treatment for endocarditis. Valve replacement is a rather common practice during active infection, especially in the 6% to 20% of patients who satisfy certain, often somewhat arbitrary criteria. It should be noted, however, that the mortality rate of surgery performed during active infection is substantially higher than that of surgery performed on an elective basis. When possible, valve replacement should be conducted 6 weeks or longer after antibiotics have been discontinued. The major indication is congestive heart failure that proves difficult to control with medical management.

Mycotic aneurysms may become apparent at any time during the course of endocarditis, but most become clinically apparent several months or even years after treatment. These lesions usually occur at arterial bifurcations and have been reported in up to 15% of cases. The vessels most often involved are intracranial; next in frequency are chest and abdominal arteries. The diagnostic evaluation usually consists of CT, when the central nervous system is involved, or arteriography for lesions suspected there or in other locations. Surgical correction is almost always indicated.

Anticoagulation is usually avoided during active endocarditis because of the danger of bleeding from unrecognized aneurysms or from embolic infarctions. However, in patients who are receiving anticoagulants for prosthetic valves, anticoagulation should be continued in the absence of a bleeding complication.

It must be remembered that any patient with endocarditis is at risk for another infection. These patients should be warned about this potential complication with any endoscopic, surgical, or dental procedures. It is good practice to supply all patients who are at risk for endocarditis with the wallet-sized card provided by the American Heart Association that contains recommendations for *antibiotic prophylaxis* to be used with various procedures (see Table 93.13 in Chapter 93). This serves the dual role of emphasizing the importance of prophylaxis to the patient and ensuring that specific guidelines will be available to health professionals who may be performing procedures on the patient that can cause bacteremia.

General References*

Gilbert DN, Dworkin RJ, Raber SR, Leggett JE. Outpatient parenteral antimicrobial-drug therapy. N Engl J Med 1997;12:829.

Detailed review of available infusion systems and of medical information related to parenteral administration of antibiotics to outpatients.

*Bold print (general references) and bold numerals (specific references) denote published controlled clinical trials, meta-analyses, or consensus-based recommendations.

Osteomyelitis

Lew DP, Waldvogel FA. Osteomyelitis. N Engl J Med 1997;336:999.
Thorough, well-referenced reviews, updated periodically.

Lung Abscess

Bartlett JG. Anaerobic bacterial infections of the lung and pleural space. Clin Infect Dis 1993;16:S248.

Gopalakrishna KV, Lerner PI. Primary lung abscess. Cleve Clin Q 1975;42:3.

Perlman LV, Lerner E, D'sops N. Classification and analysis of 97 cases of lung abscess. Am Rev Respir Dis 1969;99:390.

Endocarditis

Mylonakis E, Calderwood SB. Infective endocarditis in adults. N Engl J Med 2001;345:1318.
Excellent review.

Specific References

1. Dworkin RJ, Sande MA, Lee BL, et al. Treatment of right-sided *Staphylococcus aureus* endocarditis in intravenous drug users with ciprofloxacin and rifampin. Lancet 1989;2:1071.
2. Gentry LO, Rodriguez-Gomez G. Ofloxacin versus parenteral therapy for chronic osteomyelitis. Antimicrob Agents Chemother 1991;35:538.
3. Lew DP, Waldvogel FA. Osteomyelitis. N Engl J Med 1997;336:999.
4. Malik IA, Abbas Z, Karim M. Randomized comparison of oral ofloxacin alone with combination of parenteral antibiotics in neutropenic febrile patients. Lancet 1992;339:1092.
5. Nelson JD. A critical review of the role of oral antibiotics in the management of hematogenous osteomyelitis. In: Remington RS, Swartz MN, eds. Clinical topics in infectious diseases, vol 4. New York: McGraw-Hill, 1996:64.
6. Black J, Hunt TL, Godley PJ, et al. Oral antimicrobial therapy for adults with osteomyelitis or septic arthritis. J Infect Dis 1987;155:968.
7. Centers for Disease Control and Prevention. Public focus: surveillance, prevention and control of nosocomial infections. MMWR Morb Mortal Wkly Rep 1992;41:783.
8. Eneroth M, Larsson J, Apelquist J. Deep foot infections in patients with diabetes and foot ulcer. J Diabetes Comp 1999;13:254.
9. Grayson ML, Gibbons GW, Balogy K, et al. Probing to bone in infected pedal ulcers: a clinical sign of underlying osteomyelitis in diabetic patient. JAMA 1995;273:721.
10. Littenberg B, Mushlin AL. Technetium bone scanning in the diagnosis of osteomyelitis: a meta-analysis of test performance. J Gen Intern Med 1992;7:158.
11. Kothan NA, Pelchoritz DJ, Meyer JS. Imaging of musculoskeletal infections. Radiol Clin N Amer 2001;39:653.
12. Tumeh SS, Tohmeh AG. Nuclear medicine techniques in septic arthritis and osteomyelitis. Rheum Dis Clin North Am 1991;17:559.
13. Howard CB, Einhorn M, Dagan R, et al. Fine-needle bone biopsy to diagnose osteomyelitis. J Bone Joint Surg Br 1994;76:311.
14. Sugarman B, Hawes S, Musher DM, et al. Osteomyelitis beneath pressure sores. Arch Intern Med 1983;143:683.
15. Mackowiak POA, Jones SR, Smith JW. Diagnostic value of sinus-tract cultures in chronic osteomyelitis. JAMA 1978;239:2772.
16. Levinson ME, Mangura CT, Lorber B, et al. Clindamycin compared with penicillin for the treatment of anaerobic lung abscess. Ann Intern Med 1983;98:466.
17. Bell S. Further observations on the value of oral penicillins in chronic staphylococcal osteomyelitis. Med J Aust 1976;2:591.
18. Norden C, Nelson JD, Mader JT, et al. Evaluation of new anti-infective drugs for the treatment of infections of prosthetic hip joints: Infectious Diseases Society of America and the Food and Drug Administration. Clin Infect Dis 1992;15[Suppl 2]:S177.
19. Wagner DK, Collier BC, Rytel MW. Long-term intravenous antibiotic therapy in chronic osteomyelitis. Arch Intern Med 1985;145:1073.
20. West WF, Kelly P, Martin WJ. Chronic osteomyelitis. I: Factors affecting the results of treatment in 186 patients. JAMA 1970;213:1837.
21. Bartlett JG. Anaerobic bacterial infections of the lung. Chest 1987;91:901.
22. Norden CW. Antibiotic prophylaxis in orthopedic surgery. Rev Infect Dis 1991;13:S842.
23. Delahaye F, Hoen B, McFadden E, et al. Treatment and prevention of endocarditis. Expert Opin Pharmacother 2002;3:131.
24. Mader JT, Norden C, Nelson JD, et al. Evaluation of new anti-infective drugs for the treatment of osteomyelitis in adults: Infectious Diseases Society of American and the Food and Drug Administration. Clin Infect Dis 1992;15[Suppl 1]:S155.
25. Landay MJ, Christensen EE, Bynum LJ, et al. Anaerobic pleural and pulmonary infection. AJR Am J Roentgenol 1980;134:233.
26. Hagan JL, Hardy JD. Lung abscess revisited: a survey of 184 cases. Am Surg 1983;197:755.
27. Bisno AL, Dismukes WE, Durak DT, et al. Antimicrobial treatment of infective endocarditis due to viridans streptococci, enterococci, and staphylococci. JAMA 1989;261:1471.
28. Chambers HF, Miller RT, Newman MD. Right-sided *Staphylococcus aureus* endocarditis in intravenous drug abusers: two-week combination therapy. Ann Intern Med 1988;109:619.

CHAPTER 41

International Medicine: Care of the Traveler and of the Immigrant Patient

STEPHEN D. SEARS, MD, MPH
NATHANIEL W. JAMES IV, MD

CARE OF THE TRAVELER

International travel is increasing in popularity. Americans are visiting exotic locales and trekking to increasingly remote regions of the world. It is now estimated that 25 to 40 million Americans travel by air to foreign countries each year. Many others take boats, cruises, or cars to Canada and Mexico. Of these millions, it is estimated that 4 to 8 million journey to developing areas of the world where they encounter infectious diseases that are uncommon in developed countries. Malaria, schistosomiasis, yellow fever, polio, typhoid fever, and amebiasis are just a few of the diseases that are more prevalent in tropical developing countries. Many travelers make little or no provision for the prevention of illness while traveling. This is unfortunate because the overall attack rate for several infectious diseases is much higher in international travelers than it is in comparable populations that remain at home (1). This fact is well illustrated by the results of a study of Swiss travelers that found that three-fourths had at least one symptom of infectious illness while traveling; of the 16,500 travelers surveyed in this study, more than 30% had at least one episode of a diarrheal illness. In a follow-up study, not only were travelers found to have illnesses while traveling, but almost one-third became ill within a month of returning home. Another study of 2,000 travelers returning to the United Kingdom found that 43% became ill during or shortly after their journeys (2). In another review, 75% of travelers did not take sufficient basic precautions against infection (3).

These studies offer a small glimpse into the medical problems of travelers. Even so, there is no reliable measurement of the amount or severity of disease encountered by the traveler. Only a portion of the most dramatic cases of illness in travelers, such as malaria, Lassa fever, or African trypanosomiasis, are usually reported to public health authorities. For instance, recent outbreaks of leptospirosis (4) and coccidiomycosis (5) only came to light well after the travel-related exposures. At present, there is no mechanism for obtaining accurate surveillance data on the occurrence of illness in American travelers, nor are there data on significant risk factors for acquiring infectious diseases. This lack of data hampers scientific investigation of interventional strategies in travelers. Even so, significant progress has been made in the prevention of malaria, traveler's diarrhea, and diseases for which immunizations exist.

To prevent unnecessary illness, it is imperative that travelers undertake appropriate *pretrip health planning.* When approached by a person about to embark upon an international journey, it is important for the clinician to ascertain several key aspects of the proposed trip. *Where are you going? Where will you stay? What is the purpose of your trip? Where will you be eating? In restaurants or in private homes? Is sex with other travelers or local residents likely?* With this information, one can categorize the types and magnitude of risk. A businessperson staying for a short time in a first-class hotel in a large city in a developing country has different risks than does a college student who will be living in villages in several developing countries. Most travelers fit somewhere between these two extremes, and a travel consultation must be individualized to fit the traveler's lifestyle, itinerary, medical history, use of medications, allergies, and previous immunizations.

There are several *sources for current recommendations.* Immunizations, malaria prevention, food and water safety, diarrhea, schistosomiasis, and a number of general health hazards are topics that should be discussed with the traveler. Two useful resources that are updated yearly provide practical information on these issues: *Health Information for International Travel,* published by the U.S. Public Health Service (available from the Centers for Disease Control and Prevention, Atlanta, GA 30333) and *Vaccination Certificate Requirements for International Travel and Health Advice to Travelers,* published by the World Health Organization (available from WHO Publication Center, 49

Sheridan Ave., Albany, NY 12210). Other valuable resources include the International Association for Medical Assistance to Travelers (IAMAT, 417 Center St., Lewistown, NY 14092), which provides information on tropical diseases and a list of English-speaking physicians overseas, and the Centers for Disease Control and Prevention (CDC) Traveler's Information Hotline (404-332-4559; will fax current information on all regions).

In addition, *travel medicine websites* have proliferated. At least 65 websites cover a variety of topics, including consumer advice, professional societies, outbreak updates, traveling with chronic illnesses, epidemiology of infectious diseases, and consumer products. For a partial listing, see Table 41.1.

Immunizations

Vaccines are now available against a number of the major viral and bacterial diseases encountered in developing areas. For patients traveling to these areas, it is necessary to administer travel-specific vaccines and to update primary vaccines (Table 41.2). Immunizations can be broadly separated into those that are legally required and those that are recommended. *Legally required vaccinations* are public health measures that certain countries demand before entry, to benefit the country as a whole, whereas *recommended immunizations* are designed to benefit only the patient. No vaccines are legally required to enter or return to the United States. However, many countries have strict entry requirements, and travelers who arrive without proper vaccination certificates may be denied entry, quarantined, or possibly vaccinated at the point of entry. Therefore, it is important to determine what vaccines are required before beginning a journey.

Currently, the only legally required vaccination is for yellow fever, and each country has its own requirements. In the past, smallpox and cholera vaccinations

Table 41.1. Travel-related Websites

	Website
Authoritative travel medicine recommendations	
CDC Yellow Book	www.CDC.gov/travel/yellowbk99.pdf
CDC and Prevention Travel Information	www.cdc.gov/travel/travel
Health Canada Online	www.hc-sc.gc.ca
Pan American Health Organization	www.paho.org
Databases for travel medicine practitioners	
American Society of Travel Medicine and Hygiene	www.astmh.org
The Medical Letter	www.medicalletter.com
Shoreland's Travel Health Online	www.tripprep.com
Consumer websites	
Medical Advisory Services for Travelers Abroad	www.masta.org
International Society of Travel Medicine	www.istm.org
Travax Pre Travel Advice	www.shoreland.com
Medical assistance for overseas travelers	
International Association for Medical Assistance To Travelers	www.iamat.org or www.sentex.ntNIAMAT
International Federation of Red Cross and Red Crescent Societies	www.ifrc.org
U.S. State Department	www.state.gov
World Health Organization	www.who.int

CDC, Centers for Disease Control and Prevention.

Table 41.2. Vaccines and Immune Globulin for International Travel

Vaccine/Immune Globulin	Patient Age	Route	Dose	Booster	Comments
Yellow fever	>9 mo	s.c.	0.5 mL	0.5 mL q10yr	May be required.
Cholera	6 mo–4 yr	s.c. or i.m.	0.2 mL	0.2 mL q6mo	May be required.
	5–10 yr		0.3 mL	0.3 mL q6mo	Limited efficacy.
	>10 yr		0.5 mL	0.5 mL q6mo	
Typhoid parenteral	<10 yr	s.c.	0.25 mL	0.25 mL q3yr	Local reactions common.
	>10 yr		0.50 mL	0.5 mL q3yr	
Typhoid oral (TY21a)	>1 yr	Oral	1 dose q.o.d. × 4	Repeat series q5yr	Keep refrigerated, avoid antibiotics.
Typhoid parenteral (ViCPS)	≥2 yr	i.m.	0.5 mL	2 yr	Well tolerated.
Poliomyelitis					
OPV	All ages	Oral	3 doses	1 dose pretravel	IPV is preferable for adults.
IPV	All ages	s.c.	3 doses	1 dose q10yr	
Japanese encephalitis	<3 yr	s.c.	0.5 mL	1 dose at 1 and 4 yr	Delayed allergic reactions.
	>3 yr		1.0 mL		
Hepatitis A					
Havrix	2–17 yr	i.m.	0.5 mL × 2	6–12 mo then 10 yr	Consider screening for anti-HAV in frequent travelers.
	>17 yr	i.m.	1 mL × 2	6–12 mo then 10 yr	
Vaqta	2–17 yr	i.m.	0.5 mL × 2	6–12 mo then 10 yr	
	>17 yr	i.m.	1 mL × 2	6–12 mo then 10 yr	
Immune globulin (short term <3 mo)	<23 kg	i.m.	0.5 mL	—	Immune globulin is used for prophylaxis of hepatitis A; consider screening for anti-HAV in frequent travelers.
	23–45 kg		1.0 mL	—	
	>45 kg		2.0 mL	—	
Tetanus-diphtheria	>7 yr	i.m.	3 doses	1 dose q10yr	Always use combined vaccine.
Meningitis A, C, Y, W135	>2 yr	i.m.	0.5 mL	Unclear	For specific areas of travel.
Rabies	All ages	i.m.	1.0 mL (3 doses)	1 dose q2yr	Still requires postexposure treatment.
		i.d.	0.1 mL (3 doses)	1 dose q2yr	i.d. only approved for HDCV.
Hepatitis B	All ages	i.m.	1.0 mL (3 doses)	Unclear	Protection lasts 5–7 yr.

OPV, oral polio vaccine; IPV, inactivated polio vaccine; HDCV, human diploid cell vaccine.

were required by many countries, but in 1980, the World Health Organization declared the global eradication of smallpox, and on January 1, 1982, smallpox was deleted from the list of diseases subject to regulation. Although cholera vaccination is not endorsed by the World Health Organization for entry into any country, some local authorities may still require proof of cholera vaccination, especially if the traveler is arriving from endemic areas.

Yellow Fever

Yellow fever, once almost controlled, has made a dramatic resurgence (6). Although generally rare in travelers, two yellow fever deaths in Americans visiting the Amazon Basin were recently reported (7). Yellow fever vaccine, containing a live attenuated strain of the yellow fever virus, is one of the most important and effective vaccines. It is required by some countries before travelers are allowed entrance, particularly when areas to be visited are endemic for yellow fever and when travelers have recently left a country endemic for yellow fever. If yellow fever exists in the country of destination, the traveler should be vaccinated regardless of the regulations of the country (Figs. 41.1 and 41.2). The vaccine is nontoxic and induces long-lasting immunity. Although the yellow fever vaccine is quite safe, there have been recent reports of rare adverse effects. Therefore, the vaccine should only be

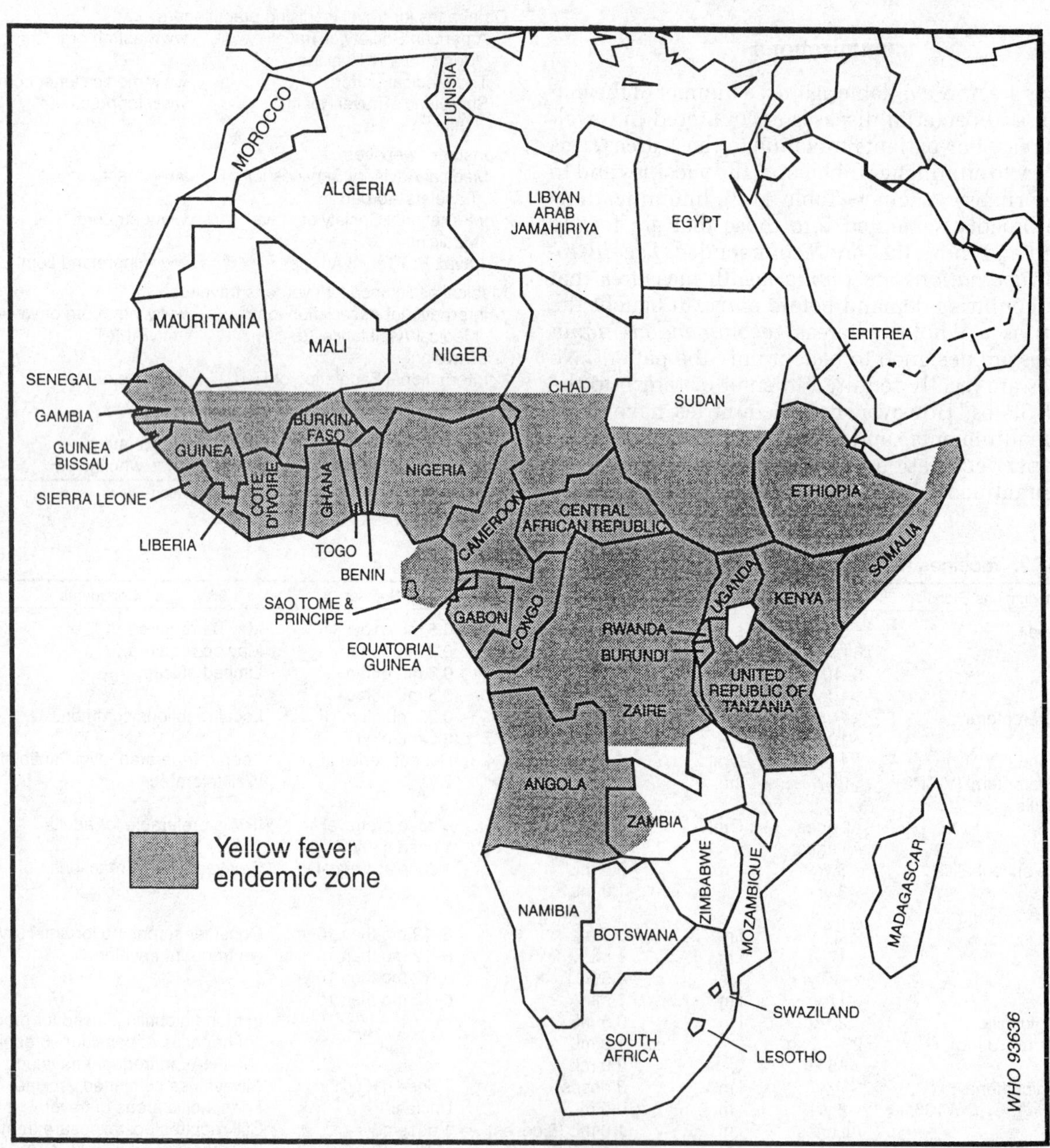

Figure 41.1. Yellow fever endemic zone in Africa. (From Centers for Disease Control and Prevention. Health Information for International Travel, 1999–2000, DHHS, Atlanta, GA, with permission.)

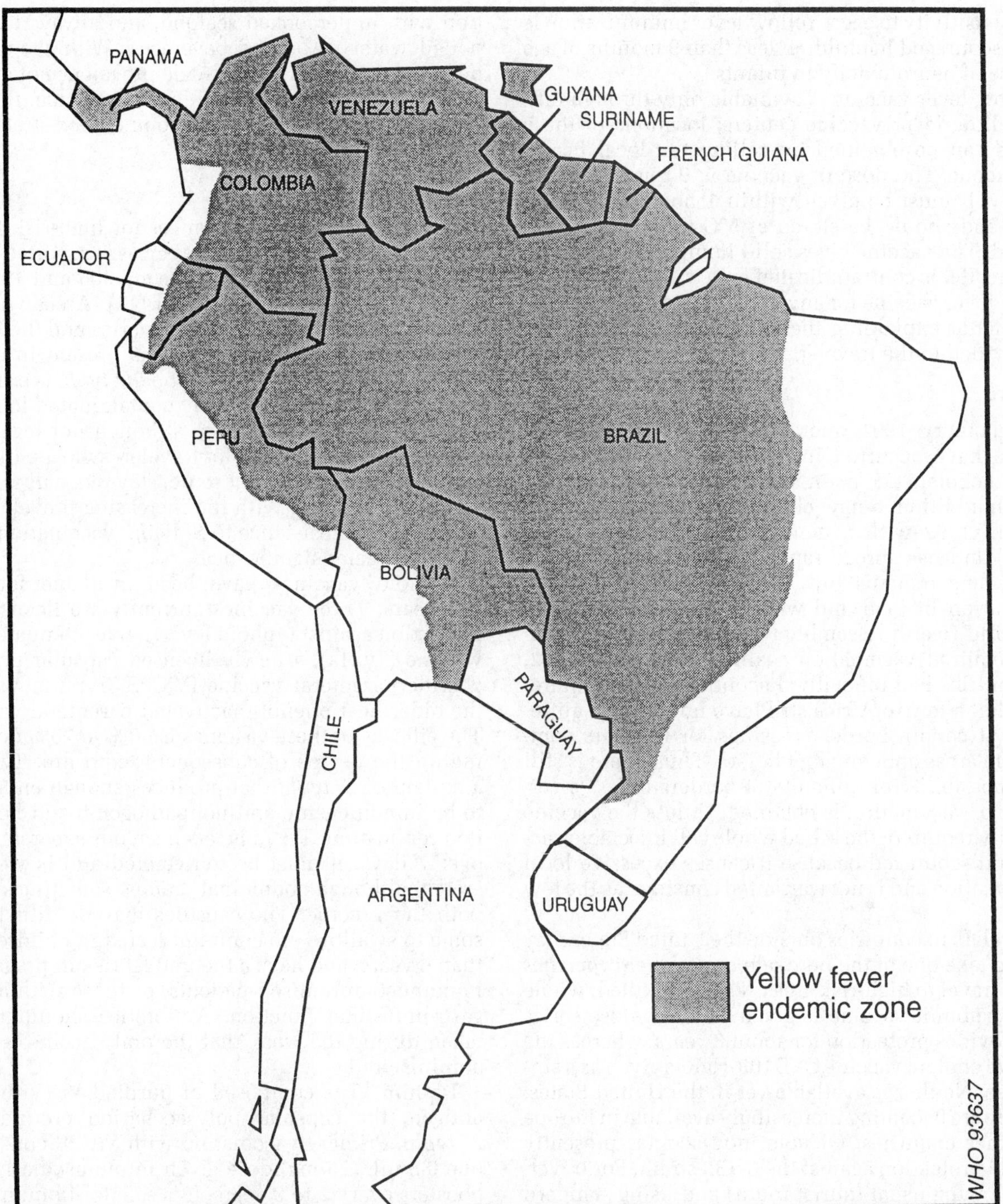

Figure 41.2. Yellow fever endemic zone in the Americas. (From Centers for Disease Control and Prevention. Health Information for International Travel, 1999–2000, DHHS, Atlanta, GA, with permission.)

given to travelers who will be at risk for yellow fever. Mild reactions occur in 1% to 5% of patients. These include mild headache, myalgia, low-grade fever, or other minor symptoms 5 to 10 days after inoculation.

Because yellow fever vaccine is a live attenuated virus, it could pose a risk to pregnant women, although teratogenicity has not been encountered. Pregnant women who must travel to areas endemic for yellow fever should be vaccinated. It is presumed that the unknown but small risk to the fetus is less than the risk to the mother. If at all possible, the trip should be postponed until after delivery. The vaccine is contraindicated in immunocompromised patients, including patients with acquired immunodeficiency syndrome with CD4 counts below 200. Because the vaccine strain is grown in chick embryo culture, it should not be given to travelers with known hypersensitivity to eggs. Yellow fever immunization is also discouraged in children less than 9 months of age because of neurotoxicity in infants.

Yellow fever vaccine is available only through official yellow fever vaccine centers; locations of these centers can be obtained by calling the local health department. The dose of vaccine is 0.5 mL subcutaneously. It must be given within 1 hour of reconstitution and should be stored at 5°C until it is reconstituted. The vaccine gives solid immunity for at least 10 years. If it is contraindicated for a traveler to receive yellow fever vaccine for any of the above reasons, a detailed letter explaining the contraindications should be provided to the traveler.

Cholera

Since January 1991, more than a million cases of cholera have occurred in South and Central America, and cholera occurs in nearly all developing countries. In addition, a new cholera epidemic erupted in India in 1992 with a non-01 vibrio cholerae strain (0-139) and has spread rapidly (8). Even so, the risk to travelers remains low, especially for those who use caution in food and water acquisition. In 1973, the World Health Assembly recommended discontinuing required vaccination against cholera. By 1992, all countries had officially discontinued this requirement, but a few in Africa still have unofficial requirements at certain border crossings for travelers coming from areas endemic for cholera. Thus, there is still some possibility of difficulty at borders unless a certificate of vaccination is obtained. Unless the vaccine is legally required, the killed whole cell injectable vaccine is discouraged because it causes excessive local inflammation and is not warranted considering the low risk.

Travelers in countries outside the United States may wish to take one of the new safe *oral cholera vaccines* if they travel to high-risk areas. The oral, killed, whole cell, B subunit vaccine is given as a two-dose series and provides protection for about 3 years, whereas the oral live cholera vaccine CVD103-HgR is given as a single dose. Neither is available yet in the United States, but they are becoming increasingly available in Europe and other countries. Of note, no vaccines presently provide protection against the 0-139 strain. For travelers following usual tourist routes and using standard precautions in countries endemic for cholera, the estimated attack rate is less than 1 per 100,000 returning travelers, but recent studies in Japanese travelers suggest that the rate of cholera infection may be much higher than previously assumed (9). Furthermore, the estimated rates are likely to be significantly underestimated because many cholera episodes may be not be distinguished from other episodes of traveler's diarrhea, and being treated overseas, they may not be reported to the CDC. Nonetheless, rather than recommend immunization routinely, clinicians should emphatically instruct travelers to areas endemic for cholera not to eat uncooked vegetables, to use caution with undercooked seafood, and always to drink boiled water or bottled beverages. With the continued increases in the worldwide prevalence of cholera coupled with reported antibiotic resistance, the new oral vaccines may become a recommended strategy for travelers in the future (10).

Typhoid Fever

Typhoid fever remains a danger for high-risk travelers; more than 70% of the 2,445 cases reported to the CDC in the United States between 1985 and 1994 occurred after international travel (11). Areas with the greatest risk are parts of South America and the Indian subcontinent, although the risk is present in almost all developing countries. *Salmonella typhi* is transmitted by the ingestion of fecally contaminated food and water. Typhoid vaccination, although not legally required, is recommended for travelers who are likely to stray off the usual tourist route, stay in small villages, and eat local food. With the increasing prevalence of antimicrobial resistance to *S. typhi,* vaccination takes on even greater significance.

Typhoid vaccines have been available for over 100 years. Three vaccines currently are licensed for protection against typhoid fever: a live attenuated oral vaccine (Ty21a), a newly licensed capsular polysaccharide parenteral vaccine (ViCPS, Typhim Vi), and the older heat-phenol-inactivated parenteral vaccine. The efficacy of these vaccines is 60% to 70% depending on the degree of subsequent exposure. Ty21a is a mutant of *S. typhi* that produces enough endotoxin to be immunogenic and nonpathogenic and has limited replication. Ty21a is taken as four separate doses over 7 days; it must be refrigerated and is well tolerated, although abdominal cramps sometimes occur with the vaccine. The capsules may be difficult for some to swallow, are contraindicated in children less than 6 years, and have a theoretical risk in pregnancy, immunocompromised patients, or those with altered gastrointestinal function. Antibiotics should not be taken during the week that the oral vaccine is being administered.

Typhim Vi is composed of purified Vi (Virulence) antigen, the capsular polysaccharide produced by *S. typhi.* Primary vaccination with ViCPS consists of one 0.5-mL (25-mg) dose given intramuscularly with boosters every 2 to 3 years. It is safe for immunocompromised travelers, is well tolerated, and is not affected by concurrent antibiotics. The vaccine is not recommended for children under 2 years of age because of poor immunogenicity at this age. The heat-phenol-inactivated parenteral vaccine should always be used without the paratyphoid component. The parenteral vaccine often causes pain at the injection site, fever, headache, and malaise for 1 to 3 days. If the traveler has never been vaccinated, the primary sequence is two inoculations 1 month apart (see Table 41.2 for dosages). The parenteral inactivated vaccine causes significantly more adverse events and is not more effective than either ViCPS or Ty21a. The two modern vaccines are vastly improved in regards to adverse effects compared with the whole-cell parenteral vaccine. Therefore, either oral Ty21a or ViCPS is generally preferred.

Polio

Paralytic poliomyelitis had been eradicated from the Americas (12), but recently there were reports of a cluster of polio cases in the Dominican Republic. In developing countries outside the Americas polio rates are falling, but travelers should still be protected. Travelers who have previously completed a primary series with either the Sabin (oral, live) or Salk (parental, inactivated) vaccine should have a booster dose if they have not previously received a booster as an adult. A history of at least three doses of oral polio vaccine (OPV, Sabin) or four doses of inactivated polio vaccine (IPV, Salk) with IPV boosters each 5 years until age 18 is evidence of adequate primary immunization. Such fully immunized people need only one dose of polio vaccine before traveling to high-risk areas. If a traveler is only partially immunized, the primary series should be completed.

Adults who require a primary series should receive IPV. Recently, a new IPV of enhanced potency has been released (eIPV). IPV is preferred in adults because the risk of OPV-associated paralysis is somewhat higher in adults than in children. If children are not already vaccinated, they should receive a primary series. New guidelines for primary polio immunization with eIPV rather than OPV have just been released. If an unimmunized adult traveler does not have time to complete a primary IPV series before departure, a single dose of OPV may offer reasonable protection. On return, primary immunization with IPV should be completed. Live (OPV) vaccine should not be given routinely to women known to be pregnant, although teratogenicity has not been shown. If the risk of polio is significant and the pregnant woman is unimmunized, primary vaccination with IPV would be prudent. Because OPV is a live virus, immunocompromised patients and their families should not receive OPV; instead they should be immunized with IPV. Table 41.2 summarizes information regarding dosages for polio vaccines.

Tetanus and Diphtheria

Tetanus occurs worldwide but is slightly more common in the tropics. Many adults may not be protected against tetanus (13), so it is important to keep tetanus immunization up to date in travelers. Boosters must be given every 10 years regardless of age. Travelers, if they injure themselves, are less likely to seek medical help, so adequate pretravel immunization becomes more important. Diphtheria is endemic in many developing countries and is currently epidemic in the countries of the former Soviet Union. Most cases occur in unimmunized or partially immunized people. Therefore, routine immunization with tetanus-diphtheria rather than with tetanus toxoid alone should be given. For primary immunization, patients older than 7 years should receive three doses of tetanus-diphtheria. (Before age 7, the primary immunizing agent is the diphtheria-pertussis-tetanus combination.) The first doses are 1 to 2 months apart and the third 6 to 12 months later. Local reactions may occur within 12 to 48 hours after vaccination. Severe local reactions can occur in adults if the booster is given within a short time of the previous vaccine. The only contraindication to tetanus-diphtheria is a history of hypersensitivity reactions after immunization.

Varicella

A live attenuated vaccine against varicella virus (chickenpox) was released in the mid-1990s. Varicella occurs worldwide, is highly contagious, and can be severe in adults. The primary series in childhood is a single dose of vaccine, and in those older than 12 years, it is two doses given 1 month apart. Long-term travelers should be immune; if immune status is not known, serologic testing may be indicated. The vaccine is contraindicated in pregnant women and those with compromised immunity.

Hepatitis A

Hepatitis A (HA) continues to be an important risk for travelers to many areas of the developing world and is the most common vaccine-preventable disease of travelers. Although the risk is less for people who travel on ordinary tourist routes and stay for short periods, it may be considerable for those who bypass the tourist routes and stay for extended periods. HA illness may be asymptomatic but can also be severe, with jaundice and significant morbidity. Protection against HA is strongly recommended for international travelers to developing areas (14). Although immune globulin provides passive protection against HA for a few months and is safe and effective, HA vaccine (active immunization) is generally preferred for most travelers. Two vaccines are licensed, Havrix (SKF) and Vaqta (Merck), and both prevent approximately 90% of expected HA infections. A new combination vaccine for HA and hepatitis B (HB) is also available (see below). Travelers to HA-endemic areas should ideally receive the first dose of vaccine at least 1 month before travel. Recent evidence suggests that vaccine is protective even when given immediately before a trip, although protective antibodies may not be measurable. Immune globulin is less expensive and is still a reasonable choice for travelers making only one trip who need limited (up to 3 months) HA protection. For travelers leaving immediately, administering both immune globulin and HA vaccine is both safe and effective.

The recommended schedules for both Havrix and Vaqta include a primary immunization for all patients and a booster in 6 to 12 months for patients 2 to 18 years of age. A booster for travelers over 18 ensures optimal long-term protection. The dosage of immune globulin may be based on weight, but for adults injection of 2 mL for stays of less than 3 months is adequate in practice. HA vaccines are well tolerated and adverse events are rare. The only side effect of immune globulin is muscle soreness at the injection site. Immune globulins for intramuscular injection prepared in the United States carry no risk of transmission of human immunodeficiency virus (HIV) or other infectious agents, but those produced in developing countries should not be used. Pregnancy is not a contraindication to immune globulin. Screening for anti-HA virus in frequent travelers should also be considered.

Hepatitis B

HB vaccination is now recommended for all infants and adolescents. Although the risk of (HB) is generally low for the routine traveler, this may be an opportunity to provide this important vaccine. Health care workers who are likely to have contact with blood or secretions from patients in areas endemic for HB should receive the HB vaccine. Travelers who will live for more than 6 months in countries with a high prevalence of HB antigenemia should also be strongly considered for vaccination. The prevalence of HB virus carriers is 5% to 15% in sub-Saharan Africa and Southeast Asia, including China and Indonesia, and 1% to 5% in North Africa, South Central Asia, and Southern Europe. Because HB can be transmitted through sexual contact, travelers should be counseled appropriately when going to endemic areas. Vaccination or HB immune globulin prophylaxis may be appropriate for people who are likely to have sexual contacts. Primary adult vaccination consists of three intramuscular doses of 1 mL of vaccine. The first two doses are given 1 month apart, and the third dose should be given 6 months later. This is often difficult in travelers, and accelerated vaccine schedules have been defined and may be useful for travelers with high exposure risks (see additional details in Chapter 18). A combination vaccine (Twinrx, GlaxoSmithKline) may be given to travelers who need to be protected against HA and HB, as long as there is time to provide two doses (1 month apart) before departure. It is not approved for children.

Rabies

Rabies remains uncontrolled in many areas of the developing world, but the risk to short-term travelers is low. Rabies transmission occurs when the rabies virus is introduced into open cuts or wounds, usually through the bite of an infected animal, so counseling on avoidance of animal bites and avoiding street dogs is essential. *Pre-exposure rabies prophylaxis,* which consists of three inoculations of human diploid cell killed virus vaccine (HDCV), purified chick embryo cell vaccine (PCEC) or rabies vaccine adsorbed (RVA) (1 mL intramuscularly on days 0, 7, and 21 or 28) is appropriate for long-term travelers who will live in endemic areas. People who anticipate animal exposure, such as veterinarians, animal handlers, and laboratory workers, should be vaccinated and should also receive a booster dose of vaccine (1 mL) every 2 years. Children are especially at risk because of the increased likelihood of contact with stray dogs. The new vaccines (HDCV, PCEC, and RVA) are more immunogenic and cause fewer reactions than the old duck embryo vaccine. Occasional local reactions and rare systemic reactions such as headaches, myalgias, and dizziness may occur. Vaccine from animal brain tissue is still being used in some developing countries, so if travelers require rabies vaccine, they should be sure to obtain the HDCV, PCEC, or RVA.

The HDCV may also be administered to travelers by the intradermal route (0.1 mL on days 0, 7, and 21 or 28) if the three-dose series is completed 30 days or more before departure. The PCEC and RVA should not be administered intradermally. If there is not sufficient time before departure, one of the intramuscular rabies vaccine should be used. Intradermal rabies vaccine is as immunogenic as intramuscular vaccine, but because the dose is one-tenth of the intramuscular dose, it is less costly. The HDCV should not be administered by the intradermal route when chloroquine or mefloquine, which may interfere with the immune response to the HDCV, is being used.

Pregnancy is not a contraindication to pre-exposure prophylaxis. If the previously vaccinated traveler is exposed to rabies, he or she should still seek medical help for *postexposure immunization* (see Chapter 18). Any animal bite should be thoroughly cleansed with soap and water to help reduce the risk of rabies.

Tuberculosis

Tuberculosis (TB) continues to be a worldwide health problem, but the risk to the short-term traveler is small. *Mycobacterium tuberculosis* is primarily a respiratory pathogen contracted by inhaling droplet nuclei, but unpasteurized milk products can also spread the disease. Travelers who will be spending extended periods in TB endemic areas should have a tuberculin skin test before departure. Bacillus Calmette-Guérin (BCG) vaccine use is controversial, and most U.S. experts do not recommend it. Periodic skin tests in long-term travelers are recommended to detect subclinical infections.

Measles, Mumps, Rubella, and Influenza

In most developing and developed countries other than the United States, measles, mumps, and rubella remain uncontrolled. Therefore, children should receive routine immunizations against these diseases before travel. Adolescents and adults who have neither had these diseases nor been immunized against them are at risk of becoming infected while traveling. People born after 1957 should have a booster dose of vaccine if they have not already received it. Rubella vaccine is indicated for females of child-bearing age without serologic evidence of prior rubella infection (see Chapter 18).

Certain travelers may benefit from pretrip vaccination with influenza and pneumococcal vaccine. Influenza causes morbidity and mortality throughout the world and poses a risk to unvaccinated travelers. Influenza vaccination should be considered for high-risk travelers who did not receive influenza vaccine the previous fall if they are traveling to the tropics (where influenza occurs throughout the year), traveling in large tourist groups (which may include persons from areas of the world where influenza viruses are circulating), or traveling to the Southern Hemisphere during April through September. Increasing penicillin resistance in pneumococci throughout the world is also of concern, and pneumococcal vaccine should be given to patients at increased risk. Chapter 18 contains details regarding risk groups, dosages, and schedules for these vaccines.

Japanese Encephalitis

Japanese encephalitis is a mosquito-borne viral encephalitis that occurs in epidemics in much of Asia, including China, and endemically in the tropical areas of Southeast Asia. The risk to short-term travelers and those who confine their travel to urban centers is low. People at greatest risk are those living for prolonged periods in endemic or epidemic areas (Fig. 41.3). A vaccine to protect against Japanese encephalitis is now available in the United States. The vaccine (JE-VAX, Japanese encephalitis vaccine, inactivated; distributed by Connaught Laboratories) should be considered for patients planning long-term residence in endemic areas and for travelers visiting rural farming areas or sleeping in unscreened rooms in endemic or epidemic areas. It is especially recommended for people staying more than 1 month in an endemic country. Japanese encephalitis vaccine is associated with a 10% to 20% rate of side effects, including fever, headache, myalgias, and malaise. Serious allergic reactions have also been documented, which may be delayed up to 1 week after immunization. Even so, the vaccine is immunogenic, efficacious, and safe and has been used to vaccinate millions of people. Vaccinees should be observed for 30 minutes after immunization and should be warned about the possibility of delayed allergic reaction. The primary series consists of three subcutaneous injections at weekly intervals, with boosters at 1 and 4 years, and the initial series should be completed at least 3 weeks before departure.

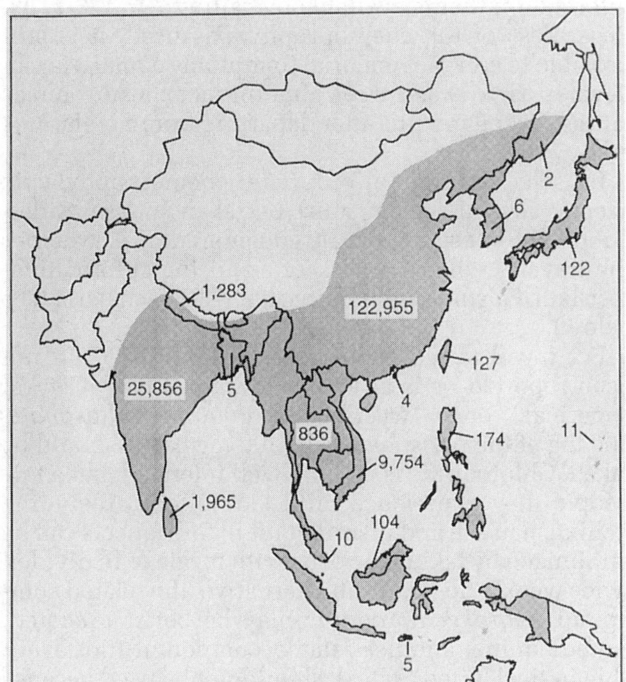

Figure 41.3. Reported Japanese encephalitis cases by endemic countries and regions of Southeast Asia where viral transmission is proven or suspected, 1986–1990. (From Tsai TF. Japanese encephalitis vaccines. In: Plotkin SA, Mortimer E, eds. Vaccines, 2nd ed. Philadelphia: W.B. Saunders, 1994, with permission.)

Meningococcal Meningitis

Meningococcal meningitis occurs throughout the developing world, often in devastating epidemics. Although cases in American travelers are rare, vaccine may be indicated for persons going to countries with high rates of infection. Areas where pretravel immunization has been recommended in the past include Northern India, Nepal, and Kenya. Risk is seasonal in the meningitis belt of Sahel (sub-Saharan Africa), including the dry inland regions of west African countries. Vaccine is required for entry into Saudi Arabia for pilgrims traveling to Mecca for the Hajj. Although meningococcal meningitis epidemics have occurred in Latin America, the prevalent type has been B, a serotype not covered by the vaccine. The vaccine available for use in the United States is the A, C, Y W-135 Quadrivalent vaccine (Menomune, Connaught). The dose of vaccine is 0.5 mL given subcutaneously, with boosters recommended between 3 and 5 years.

Miscellaneous Vaccines: Typhus, Plague, Lyme, Anthrax, and Tick-borne Encephalitis

Typhus vaccine is no longer available, and the disease poses little risk except for those working with louse-infected refugees. Anecdotal cases of typhus have been reported in travelers to remote areas and empiric treatment with doxycycline is effective and curative.

Plague exists in certain rural areas in Africa, Asia, and North and South America. Vaccination is not recommended for most travelers, but if the traveler will have direct contact with wild rodents in plague-enzootic areas, vaccination may be considered. Local and systemic reactions after plague vaccine are common. Instead of vaccination, travelers considered to be at high risk for plague due to unavoidable exposures in epidemic areas should consider short-term antibiotic prophylaxis with tetracycline (500 mg twice daily) or doxycycline (100 mg daily). Trimethoprim-sulfamethoxazole can be substituted in children.

Lyme disease is found in temperate regions of Europe, Asia, and the United States and is generally not transmitted in the tropics (see Chapter 38). A safe and effective vaccine has been licensed, but because of genospecies diversity of the infectious agent, *Borrelia burgdorferi*, the vaccine is not likely to be efficacious outside North America. Avoiding tick habitats, using repellants, and checking daily for ticks is the recommended strategy to avoid exposure.

Tick-borne encephalitis (spring–summer encephalitis) is a viral infection of the central nervous system occurring in western and central Europe, including the countries of the former Soviet Union. Transmission is from infected ticks, but infection can be acquired by consuming unpasteurized dairy products. Effective vaccines are available in Europe but are not licensed in the United States. Available data do not support their use in travelers.

Anthrax vaccine is produced from a culture filtrate of *Bacillus anthracis* and has been licensed since 1970. Its use is controversial and is confined to military personnel.

Timing of Vaccines

Many travelers see a physician just before their departure. In this situation, all active immunizations can be given concurrently. The simultaneous administration of injectable cholera and yellow fever vaccine may rarely be associated with lower than expected antibody levels to both vaccines. The clinical relevance of this is unknown because injectable cholera vaccine is almost never given. Simultaneous administration of multiple vaccines produces good antibody responses to all the antigens. However, when it is possible, multiple vaccinations should be spread out over time, and all should be completed by 1 week before arrival in a developing country to decrease the likelihood of reactions and to ensure that adequate antibody levels have been attained (15). When vaccines are administered concurrently, they should be given with separate syringes at different body sites. Killed vaccines can be given at the same time as immune globulin. With certain live attenuated vaccines (especially measles, mumps, rubella), passively acquired antibody may interfere with replication of the vaccine virus and poses the possibility of decreasing the efficacy of the vaccine. Therefore, if possible, live virus vaccines should be given at least 14 days before the administration of immune globulin and probably 3 months after administration. Immune globulin does not interfere with yellow fever or OPV, both of which are live.

Malaria Prophylaxis

Malaria is a potentially fatal parasitic disease caused by infection of red blood cells with *Plasmodium* species. It is usually transmitted by *Anopheles mosquitoes* but can be acquired from transfused blood and intravenous drug use. Malaria tends to be more severe in "immunologically virgin" travelers than in residents of endemic areas. The disease is characterized by high fevers, chills, sweats, myalgias, and headache with no obvious focal signs or symptoms of infection. Malaria exists worldwide. The risk of contracting malaria varies from country to country and from season to season depending on local conditions such as rainfall, altitude, and mosquito density. Because malaria is almost totally preventable in travelers, there should be no deaths in travelers caused by malaria. Each year, however, American travelers still die because of inadequate protection against malaria. Prevention of malaria requires minimizing mosquito contact and taking appropriate prophylactic medicine (16).

To avoid mosquito exposure, travelers should sleep in screened rooms and under mosquito nets. Anopheles mosquitoes feed predominantly from dusk to dawn. Therefore, travelers who must be out during this time should try to cover the body with clothing and use insect repellent on exposed areas. Long-sleeved shirts, long-legged trousers, and occasionally a face net should be worn if at all possible. Mosquito repellent containing *N,N*-diethylmetatoluamide (DEET, 20% to 40%) should be applied to exposed skin. Use of 100% DEET is not recommended and can be toxic for children. Outdoor nighttime activity should be avoided whenever possible. Permethrin, a repellant and insecticide of low toxicity, can be applied to bed nets, clothing, and tents. Permethrin has been shown to decrease clinical malaria cases in African children when applied to bedding. It is available in most pharmacies and sporting goods stores (17).

Even with appropriate mosquito protection, travelers may get bitten by malarious mosquitoes. It is therefore necessary to take an appropriate *chemoprophylactic* drug (Table 41.3) when traveling to a malarious area. Malaria chemoprophylaxis should preferably begin 1 to 2 weeks before travel and should continue for 4 weeks after leaving the malarious areas. Before deciding on a chemoprophylactic regimen, it is important to obtain recent information regarding country-specific malaria risk. The CDC maintains up to date information that is available by calling 707-488-7788. Regardless of the chemoprophylaxis used, it is still possible to contract malaria. Symptoms of malaria can develop as early as 1 week after initial exposure and as late as several months after departure from a malarious area.

In selecting the appropriate chemoprophylactic agents, several factors must be taken into consideration. The most important consideration is whether the traveler will be at risk of acquiring chloroquine-resistant *Plasmodium falciparum* (CRPF) malaria (see below).

For travel to malarious areas where CRPF has not been reported or is at a very low level (e.g., Central America), once weekly *chloroquine phosphate,* 500 mg of the phosphate salt (300 mg base), should be taken. Chloroquine is usually well tolerated, but a few people may experience mild side effects, including itching, nausea, and disorientation. Side effects can be minimized by taking the drug with meals or in divided twice weekly doses. As an alternative, the related compound *hydroxychloroquine* may be better tolerated. Amodiaquine, another related compound (not available in the United States), should not be used because of associated hepatotoxicity and bone marrow depression. When chloroquine is used for prolonged periods at high dosages, as in the therapy of rheumatoid arthritis, it may be associated with a severe retinopathy. This serious side effect is extremely rare when chloroquine

Table 41.3. Drugs Used in the Prophylaxis of Malaria[a]

Drugs	Adult Dosage	Pediatric Dosage
Chloroquine phosphate (Aralen)	500 mg salt orally, once/wk	5 mg/kg base (8.3 mg/kg salt) orally, once/wk, up to a maximal dose of 300 mg base
Hydroxychloroquine sulfate (Plaquenil)	400 mg salt orally, once/wk	5 mg/kg base (6.5 mg/kg salt) orally, once/wk, up to a maximal adult dose of 310 mg base
Mefloquine	228 mg base (250 mg salt) orally, once/wk	15–19 kg: ¼ tablet/wk 20–30 kg: ½ tablet/wk 31–45 kg: ¾ tablet/wk >45 kg: 1 tablet/wk
Doxycycline	100 mg orally, once/day	>8 yr of age: 2 mg/kg of body weight orally/day, up to adult dose of 100 mg/day
Atovoquine/Proguanil (Malarone)	250 mg/100 mg daily, 1–2 days, before and for 7 days after entering malaria area	10–20 kg: ¼ tablet 21–30 kg: ½ tablet 31–45 kg: ¾ tablet
Proguanil (not available in United States)	200 mg orally, once/day in combination with weekly chloroquine	<2 yr: 500 mg/day 2–6 yr: 100 mg/day 7–10 yr: 150 mg/day >10 yr: 200 mg/day
Primaquine	15 mg base (26.3 mg salt) daily, once/day for 14 days	0.3 mg/kg base (0.5 mg/kg salt) orally once/day for 14 days
For presumptive therapy: pyrimethamine-sulfadoxine (Fansidar)	3 tablets (75 mg pyrimethamine and 1500 mg sulfadoxine orally as a single dose)	5–10 kg: ½ tablet 11–20 kg: 1 tablet 21–30 kg: 1.5 tablets 31–45 kg: 2 tablets >45 kg: 3 tablets

[a]See text for indications according to geographic region and *Plasmodium* species.

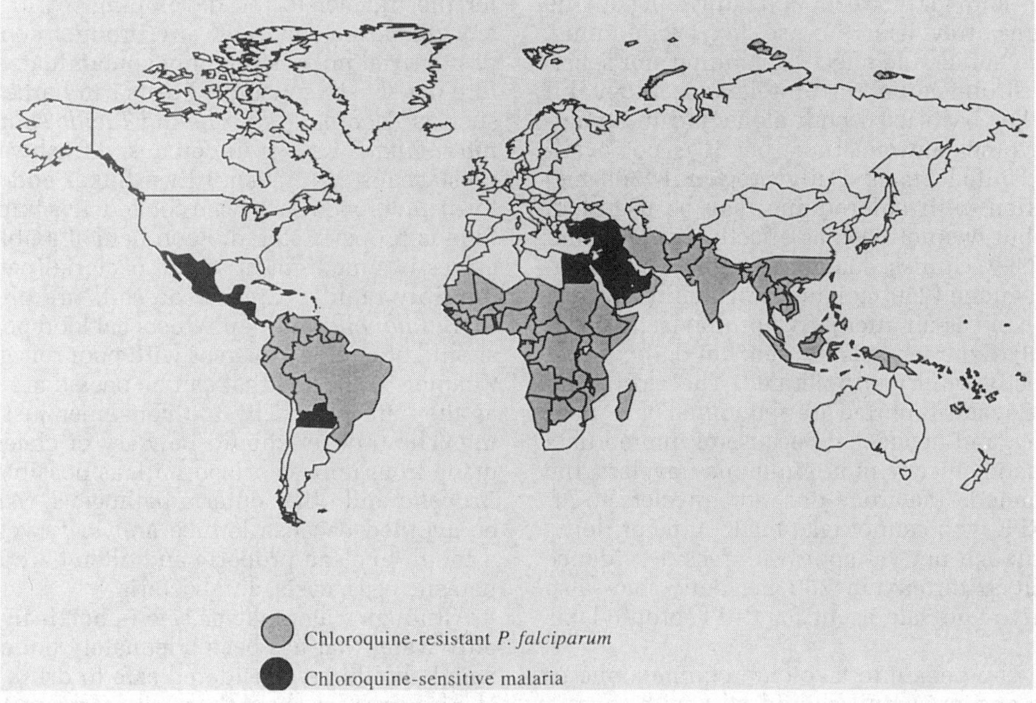

Figure 41.4. Distribution of malaria and chloroquine-resistant *Plasmodium falciparum*, 1997. (From Centers for Disease Control and Prevention. Health Information for International Travel, 1999–2000, DHHS, Atlanta, GA, with permission.)

is used at the low dosages for malaria chemoprophylaxis. The risk of retinopathy appears to increase after a cumulative dosage of 100 g of base, and periodic retinal examinations should be considered in travelers who have taken this much chloroquine. Chloroquine is safe in pregnant and lactating women and should be recommended to pregnant women traveling to malaria endemic zones.

Most malaria endemic areas now have strains of *P. falciparum* that are resistant to chloroquine, and travelers to these areas (Fig. 41.4) are at risk of contracting chloroquine-resistant malaria if chloroquine alone is used for chemoprophylaxis. For these areas, once a week *mefloquine* (250 mg) is recommended. In two areas, eastern Thailand and rural Cambodia, mefloquine resistance has been reported. Minor side effects reported with mefloquine include dizziness, insomnia, vivid dreaming including nightmares, and gastrointestinal disturbances that tend to be transient and self-limited. It has been associated rarely with serious adverse reactions such as psychoses and convulsions at higher doses than used for prophylaxis. Mefloquine has occasionally been associated with asymptomatic bradycardia and a prolonged QT interval and should be used with caution, if at all, by travelers who take beta-blockers, quinidine, calcium channel blockers, or other cardiac drugs that alter conduction. Mefloquine should also be used with caution, if at all, in travelers with a seizure disorder or underlying psychosis. Mefloquine is safe in the second and third trimesters of pregnancy. There is insufficient information regarding its safety in the first trimester. Mefloquine prophylaxis should begin 1 week before travel to malarious areas, and it should be continued weekly for 4 weeks after leaving such areas.

There are a number of *alternative chemoprophylactic regimens for CRPF.* For travelers who are unable to take mefloquine or those traveling to areas where mefloquine resistance has been reported, daily doxycycline is an acceptable regimen. Prophylaxis with doxycycline (100 mg) should begin 1 to 2 days before, during, and for 4 weeks after traveling to the malarious area. Travelers who use doxycycline must be alert to potential side effects, including sun sensitivity and gastrointestinal tract intolerance. Proguanil (Paludrine) has been used both alone and in combination with other antimalarials, but it is not available in the United States. Daily proguanil (200 mg) in combination with chloroquine may be useful in East Africa but has not been as effective in Thailand and Papua New Guinea. Malarone, a fixed combination of atovaquone (250 mg) and proguanil (100 mg), is now available as an alternative prophylactic agent for CRPF (18). Experience is limited, but daily dosing appears effective and well tolerated. The most common adverse events reported are abdominal pain, nausea, vomiting, and headache. Because of limited data on prophylactic efficacy in nonimmune travelers, the CDC recommends Malarone only for travelers to areas with CRPF who cannot take mefloquine or doxycycline. Although not yet approved, recent evidence suggests that azithromycin 250 mg daily may also be an effective and safe agent for CRPF prophylaxis (19).

Travelers who decide to take chloroquine alone or chloroquine and proguanil should take with them a treatment supply (three tablets) of pyrimethamine-sulfadoxine (Fansidar). These travelers are at risk of acquiring CRPF and should be advised to take the Fansidar promptly if they have a febrile illness and cannot obtain medical care (Table 41.3). Mefloquine should not be used for self-treatment because of the likelihood of dosage-dependent side effects.

Routine malaria prophylaxis with chloroquine or mefloquine does not prevent delayed attacks of malaria from *Plasmodium vivax* or *Plasmodium ovale* because these species have an extraerythrocytic chronic liver phase not eradicated by these two agents. *Primaquine* is an 8-aminoquinolone drug that is effective against the chronic liver forms of vivax and ovale malaria. For travelers with minimal mosquito exposure and short stays in endemic areas, primaquine is not routinely indicated. However, primaquine prophylaxis should be considered in travelers who have had extended stays in areas endemic for either *P. vivax* or *P. ovale* malaria and who have had significant mosquito exposure. Primaquine, 15 mg of base daily for 14 days, is usually given during the last 2 weeks of chloroquine chemoprophylaxis. Primaquine can cause hemolysis in people with glucose 6-phosphate deficiency and has several other potential side effects, such as headache, nausea, vomiting, and gastrointestinal distress. Before treatment with this drug, the patient's glucose 6-phosphate deficiency status should be determined.

Food and Water

The traveler should learn the mantra for food and water safety: "boil it, cook it, peel it, or forget it." Food and water are the most common vehicles for the introduction of infectious agents into the body. It is best for the traveler to the developing world to consider any *uncooked* food and any product containing unpasteurized milk as possibly contaminated and therefore not safe to consume. Meats can harbor pathogens such as *Trichinella spiralis* and *Taenia solium* and *Taenia saginata.* Raw or undercooked freshwater fish and crustaceans can transmit liver flukes and tapeworms. Even after foods have been cooked, it is imperative that food is properly stored. Food held at ambient temperatures is a medium in which bacterial pathogens can multiply rapidly. Creamy desserts are often vehicles for *Salmonella* and staphylococcal food poisoning and should be avoided in areas with poor refrigeration (see Chapter 35). Fruits that can be peeled are safe as long as they are peeled by the consumer just before eating. The traveler should be wary of cheese products made from unpasteurized milk as possible sources of *Brucella* and other enteric pathogens. Salads should be avoided because lettuce and leafy vegetables are difficult to clean properly and often harbor infectious parasite eggs, cysts, and bacteria.

Although water may be safe in hotels in large cities, only water that has been adequately boiled or chlorinated should be considered safe to drink. If the traveler is uncertain about the purity of the water, it should be boiled. Routine chlorination may not kill all parasites. In areas where purified water is not available or where hygiene and sanitation are poor, travelers are advised to drink only the following beverages: those that use boiled water, such as hot tea or coffee; canned or bottled carbonated beverages, including carbonated bottled water and soft drinks; and beer or wine.

Boiling is by far the most reliable method of making water safe to drink. If the water contains sediment or floating matter, it should be strained with a cloth before boiling or chemical treatment. The water should be boiled vigorously for at least 10 minutes to kill cysts, viruses, and bacteria and then allowed to cool to room temperature. If boiling is not possible, water can be *chemically disinfected* with tincture of iodine or tetraglycine hydroperiodide tablets. The purification tablets can be purchased from a pharmacy or a sporting goods store. The traveler should follow the manufacturer's instructions. If the water is cloudy, the number of tablets should be doubled. If the water is extremely cold, it should be allowed to warm up before the tablets are added. Tincture of iodine should be used as follows. Per quart or liter of water, for clean water, use 5 drops and let sit 30 minutes. For cloudy or cold water, use 10 drops and let sit several hours.

Water may also be adequately purified by the use of small portable *water filters* that are available in sporting goods stores. These remove all water-borne parasitic and bacterial agents and some remove viruses. The water can be consumed immediately after treatment.

It should be remembered that where water may be contaminated, ice (as well as containers for drinking) should also be considered contaminated. If at all possible, boiled or bottled water should be used for making ice, rinsing drinking vessels, and brushing teeth. If boiled or bottled water is unavailable, the hot water tap can be used as a last resort. Although many infectious agents do not grow at these temperatures, hot tap water is by no means completely safe.

Diarrhea

Diarrhea is the most common illness among travelers to developing countries, occurring in 30% to 60%, and it affects the enjoyment of the trip for many people. Most cases do not pose a serious health threat; however, some episodes are severe and may lead to dehydration. Cases occur when fecally contaminated food or water is ingested, so the precautions mentioned above for food and water should be followed. Even with good personal hygiene and avoidance of suspect food and water, the attack rate for traveler's diarrhea remains high. Approximately 70% of episodes are caused by bacterial agents, with more than 50% caused by enterotoxigenic *Escherichia coli*. Less common etiologies include protozoa and viruses, but no organism is found in 10% to 40% of cases (Table 41.4). Because the causative agents can be assumed to be bacterial three-fourths of the time, several strategies to prevent bacterial diarrhea or to treat it early have been studied (20).

Table 41.4. Common Causes of Traveler's Diarrhea[a]

Bacteria (50%–70%)	Protozoa (0%–20%)	Viruses (0%–20%)
Escherichia coli	*Giardia*	Rotavirus
Campylobacter	*Entamoeba*	Calcivirus
Salmonella	*Cryptosporidia*	Enterovirus
Shigella	*Cyclospora*	

[a]No organism found (10%–40%).

Prophylaxis

A consensus conference on traveler's diarrhea held at the National Institutes of Health recommended against the routine use of prophylactic antimicrobials (21). The potential risk of adverse reactions to the prophylactic agent was thought to outweigh the benefits. Although routine prophylaxis was not thought to be appropriate, it was also concluded that some travelers may wish to consult with their physician and may elect to use prophylactic antimicrobial agents for travel under special circumstances, once the risks and benefits are clearly understood. The antimicrobials that have been used in this way include ciprofloxacin (250 or 500 mg/day), norfloxacin (400 mg/day), ofloxacin 300 mg/day, doxycycline (100 mg/day with meals), and trimethoprim-sulfamethoxazole (one double-strength tablet daily), continued for 2 days after departure from a developing country. If prophylaxis is used, it should be limited to less than 3 weeks, and the quinolones listed are preferred in most cases because of the excellent coverage for the enteric pathogens, with consequent high efficacy rates (prevents more than 95% of expected illness) and low rate of adverse reactions. If doxycycline is being used for another indication (e.g., malaria prophylaxis or acne), additional antidiarrheal prophylaxis is not needed; because of possible photosensitivity, people taking doxycycline should wear hats and garments that prevent sun exposure.

Pepto-Bismol, a nonprescription product containing bismuth subsalicylate, can also prevent approximately 65% of diarrhea episodes; the dosage is two tablets four times a day with meals. Pepto-Bismol turns the tongue and stools black, and it may cause tinnitus.

Examples of travelers who would benefit from prophylaxis are those with pre-existing medical conditions (e.g., cardiovascular disease) that would place the person at great risk if diarrhea and even mild dehydration develop. Prophylaxis is also sometimes appropriate for people who will be at high risk for a very limited time (e.g., volunteers in a refugee camp for less than 3 weeks).

Treatment

Most cases of diarrhea are self-limited and may require only rest and replacement of fluids and salts. This can best be accomplished with oral rehydration solution (ORS; e.g., CeraLyte, Cera Products, Inc., Columbia, MD), but certain home-available fluids (e.g., juices, soups) can also be used. Especially when diarrhea is severe, ORS should be used because it contains a complete formulation to replace the needed electrolytes in the appropriate concentrations. The traveler should drink a volume of ORS to approximate the volume of diarrhea losses, although an exact balance of intake and output is not necessary. If no commercial ORS is available, a similar solution can be made by adding one-half teaspoon salt, one-half teaspoon baking soda, and 4 tablespoons sugar to 1 pint (500 mL) water. (If baking soda is not available, 1 teaspoon salt should be used.) The electrolyte concentrations of fluids for sweat replacement (e.g., Gatorade) are not equivalent to ORS. Any ORS remaining after 24 hours should be discarded because there is a chance of bacterial contamination.

Early antimicrobial treatment with ciprofloxacin (250 or 500 mg twice daily), levofloxacin (500 mg daily), norfloxacin (400 mg twice daily), doxycycline (100 twice daily), or trimethoprim-sulfamethoxazole (one double-strength tablet twice daily) will shorten the episode caused by susceptible strains of bacteria. Generally, the drug should be started soon after diarrhea begins and continued for 3 days, although a single dose of ciprofloxacin (500 mg) or levofloxacin (500 mg) has been shown to be effective (22). Recently, campylobacter resistant to quinolones has been increasing in prevalence. Preliminary studies suggest that azithromycin 500 mg daily may be effective therapy for this organism and for travelers diarrhea in general. If the illness is thought to be *shigellosis* on the basis of signs and symptoms (blood in the stool, fever, and severe cramps), one of the quinolones for 5 days is the regimen of first choice; the second choice would be trimethoprim-sulfamethoxazole for 5 days. Most shigellae are resistant to tetracyclines and sulfa, however.

Antimotility drugs such as diphenoxylate/atropine (Lomotil) and loperamide (Imodium) may provide temporary relief when diarrhea is especially inconvenient, such as during a long bus trip or other emergent situations. There continues to be concern that dysentery can be prolonged if antimotility drugs are used, and these agents should be used with care (if at all) with fever or dysentery because of potential clinical deterioration with an invasive bacterial pathogen. They have been used together with antimicrobial agents such as the quinolones to provide more rapid relief than might occur with the antimicrobial alone; however, the improvement is marginal. If loperamide (no prescription needed), which does not cause atropine-like side effects, is used, the dose is two 2-mg tablets after each voluminous watery stool.

Bismuth subsalicylate (Pepto-Bismol) is also helpful, although large amounts are needed to significantly reduce diarrhea. The dosage is 30 mL liquid (or two tablets) every half hour to 1 hour, up to eight doses in 24 hours. Precautions with this drug include complications caused by the salicylates it contains and by the fact that it binds tetracyclines. Kaopectate, Enterovioform, and Streptotriad are not efficacious and should not be used.

The choices among the modalities described above should be based on the patient's symptoms. Fluid replacement should be encouraged for any episode of diarrhea and is all that is necessary in mild cases. For diarrhea of moderate severity (two to three unformed stools per day, no fever, no symptoms of frank dysentery, i.e., severe crampy pain or bloody stools), nonspecific symptomatic therapy may be all that is needed. Either bismuth subsalicylate or loperamide is useful. Antimicrobial agents should be used only for moderately severe to severe illness (more than four unformed stools per day, mild fever, dysentery). Some travel experts advocate taking antimicrobial agents at the first sign of diarrhea to minimize the length of the illness episode. Balancing adverse drug effects with symptomatic relief is the goal.

For diarrhea that is very severe, is associated with repeated vomiting, or does not improve after several days, the traveler should be advised to consult a physician rather than attempt self-treatment. A doctor should also be consulted if there is blood in the stool; if there is a fever higher than 101°F, especially if accompanied by shaking chills; or if antimicrobial therapy does not provide rapid improvement.

Finally, in preparation for possible diarrhea, the traveler should be reminded that *toilet tissue* is difficult to find in many developing countries and that it is prudent to take a supply. Additional information regarding the pathogenesis, epidemiology, and treatment of diarrheal illnesses is contained in Chapter 35.

Schistosomiasis

Schistosomiasis is one of the world's major public health problems. Three predominant species exist (*Schistosoma mansoni, S. japonicum,* and *S. haematobium*) and are found worldwide (Figs. 41.5 through 41.7). Although few travelers are aware of schistosomiasis, it is a common disease in much of the developing world (23). After infection, the disease may lie dormant until it causes problems later in life. People contract schistosomiasis by wading or swimming in fresh or estuary water that harbors the snail vector of this trematode parasite. The cercariae (larval stage) can penetrate the skin and pass into the bloodstream without causing any symptoms at the time. Symptoms that may occur with schistosomiasis depend on the stage of the infection. Sometimes, there may be a rash at the site where the cercariae invaded, but this is uncommon. About 4 or 5 weeks after infection, an episode of fever, cough, and general malaise may occur. Still later (6 months to several years), more severe complications may occur, usually related to liver or urinary tract disease.

In recent years, severe cases of schistosomiasis have occurred in Americans after river rafting in Ethiopia and after swimming in fresh water in Kenya. Although treatment has improved with the advent of praziquantel, it is better to advise travelers to avoid fresh water contact in endemic areas and thereby prevent disease acquisition. For a returning traveler who has been exposed to fresh water in a schistosome-endemic area, screening tests, including a complete blood count and specific serology, may be useful. This is particularly important in a patient with unexplained systemic symptoms. Eosinophilia in the peripheral blood may be present during the initial stages of the parasitic infection, although it is not a constant finding in late chronic infections. Positive serology indicates likely exposure, especially in the nonimmune traveler. If serology is positive, a further laboratory evaluation

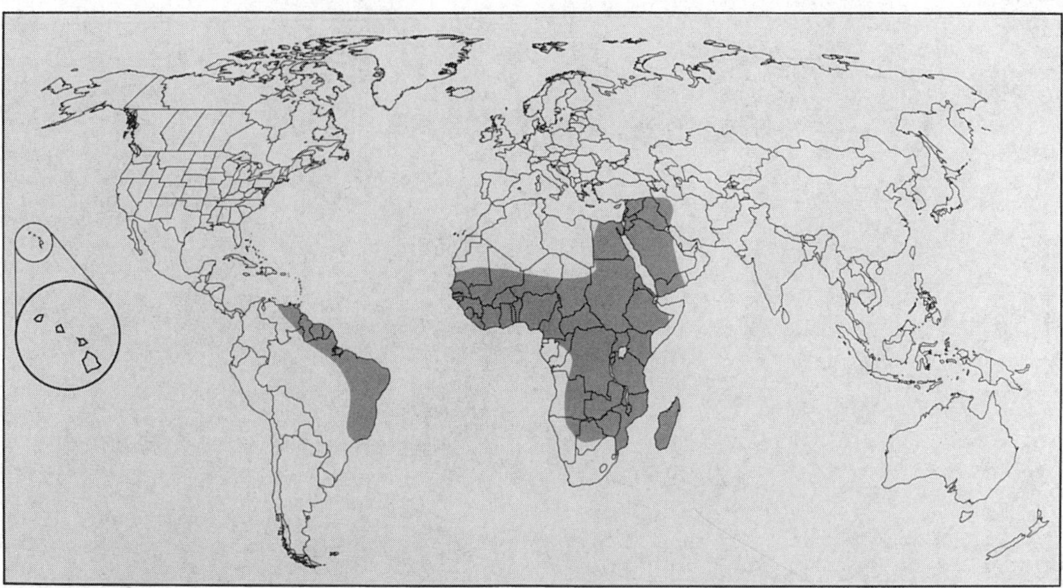

Figure 41.5. Geographic distribution of *Schistosoma mansoni.* (From Guerrant RL, Walker DH, Weller PH. Tropical infectious diseases: principles, pathogens, and practice. New York: Churchill Livingstone, 1999, with permission.)

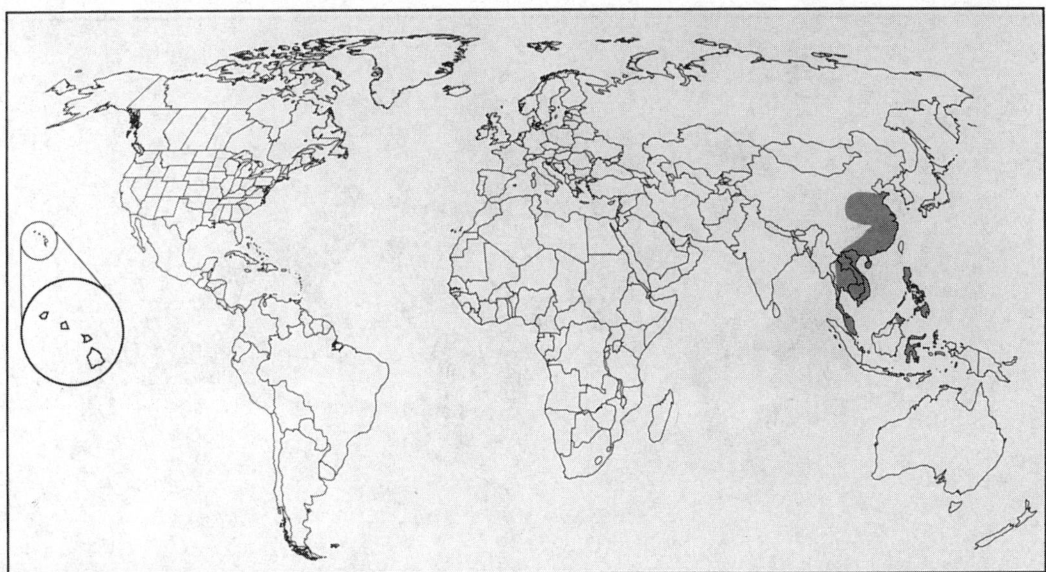

Figure 41.6. Geographic distribution of *Schistosoma japonicum.* (From Guerrant RL, Walker DH, Weller PH. Tropical infectious diseases: principles, pathogens, and practice. New York: Churchill Livingstone, 1999, with permission.)

including urinalysis and stool examination for ova should be undertaken, recognizing that the acute syndrome described above may occur before there is detectable egg excretion. Proven or strongly suspected acute schistosomal infection requires treatment with *praziquantel* (Biltricide), which is effective in early schistosomal infection. This drug is supplied in 600-mg tablets, scored so that they can be broken into four 150-mg units. Treatment is accomplished in 1 day by giving a single dose of 40 mg/kg for *S. mansoni* or *S. haematobium* and three doses (20 mg/kg each) 4 to 6 hours apart for *S. japonicum.*

Dengue

In recent years the incidence of dengue fever has increased dramatically in most of the countries in the Caribbean (Fig. 41.8). Dengue fever is a mosquito-borne viral illness transmitted by *Aedes aegypti* mosquitoes. It also occurs in parts of tropical Asia, Africa, and the Pacific. Dengue fever is characterized by sudden onset of high fevers, severe frontal headaches, joint and muscle pains, and a general feeling of malaise. In addition, many patients have nausea, vomiting, and a maculopapular rash that typically

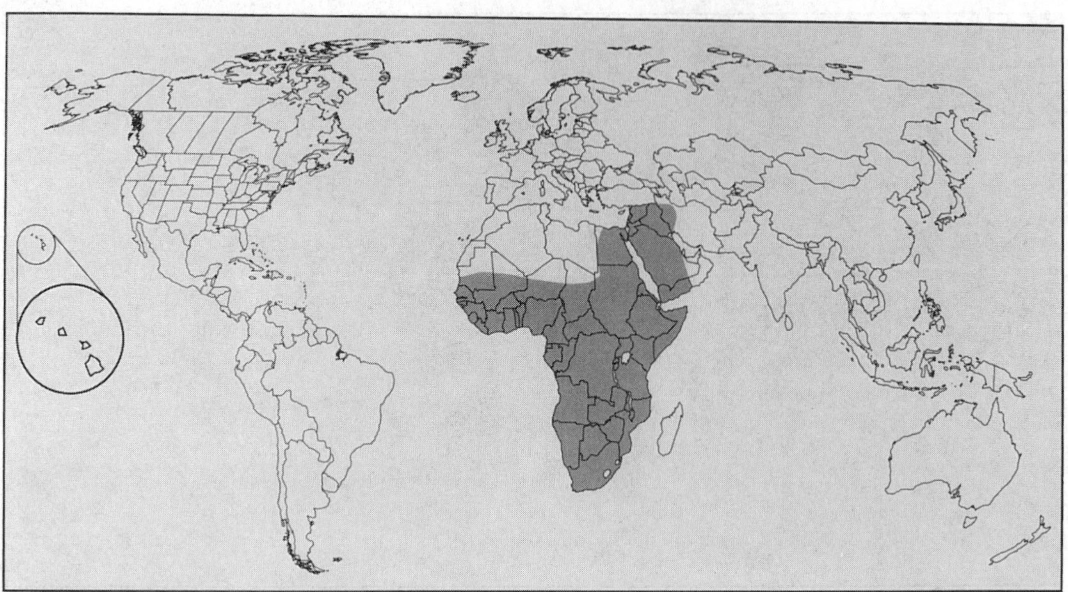

Figure 41.7. Geographic distribution of *Schistosoma haematobium.* (From Guerrant RL, Walker DH, Weller PH. Tropical infectious diseases: principles, pathogens, and practice. New York: Churchill Livingstone, 1999, with permission.)

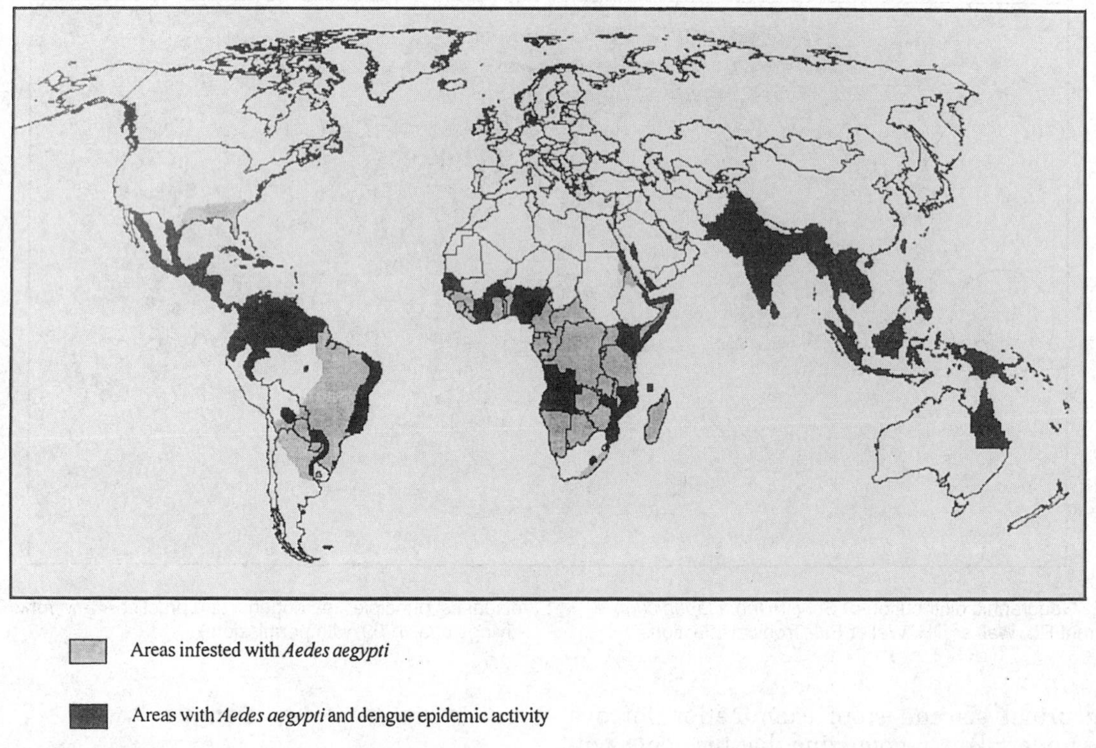

Figure 41.8. World distribution of dengue, 1996. (From Centers for Disease Control and Prevention. Health Information for International Travel, 1999–2000, DHHS, Atlanta, GA, with permission.)

appears 3 to 5 days after the onset of fever. The rash may spread from the trunk to the arms, legs, and face and generally is benign and self-limited, although prolonged convalescence is often seen. Most dengue is subclinical or nonspecific in presentation, but it may also present as a severe and fatal hemorrhagic disease, called dengue hemorrhagic fever. Currently, there is no specific treatment for dengue and vaccines are not available. Travelers to areas where dengue is endemic therefore need to take precautions to avoid mosquito bites (see Malaria Prophylaxis, above). Unlike the *Anopheles* mosquito (malaria vector), which is a nocturnal biter, the *Aedes* mosquitoes (dengue) are out and feeding during the day. In addition, *Aedes*

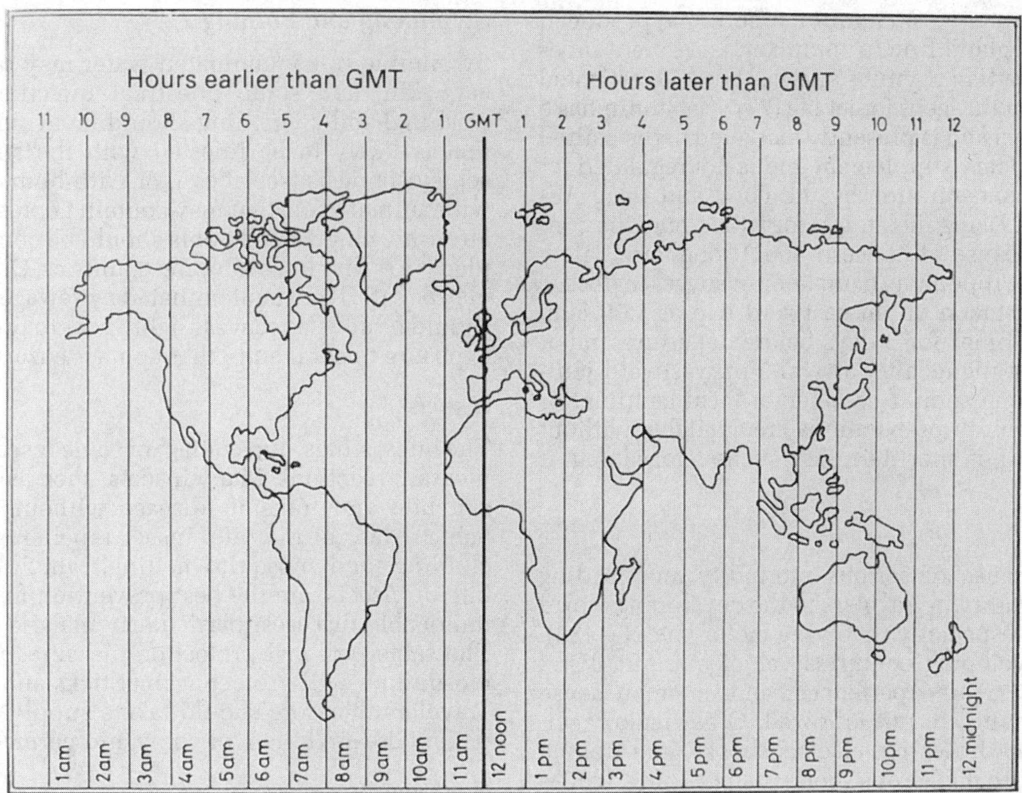

Figure 41.9. Time zones (jet lag typically occurs when five or more zones are crossed). *GMT,* Greenwich meridian time. (From Walker E, Williams G, Raeside F, et al. ABC of health travel, 4th ed. London: BMJ Publishing Group, 1997, with permission.)

are well adapted to an urban environment, breeding in trees, cans, and wells near human dwellings. Because increasing numbers of travelers have become ill with dengue, precautions to avoid mosquito exposure need to be rigorously followed when endemic areas are visited (24).

Miscellaneous Health Concerns

Human Immunodeficiency Virus-infected Traveler

Infection with HIV should not preclude travel. However, health risks for the HIV-infected traveler require special considerations (25). The efficacy of vaccination, the risks of live virus vaccines, the risk of acquiring enteric infections, and the late expression of latent infections such as TB, malaria, and fungal diseases require careful pretrip counseling (for details on HIV infection, see Chapter 39). HIV-infected travelers can receive the usual vaccines if the CD4 count is above 200, but live vaccines should not be given if the count is lower.

Air Travel and Jet Lag

Recent studies suggest an increased risk of venous thromboses in air travelers. Prevention by stretching and walking during flights should be encouraged. Cabin pressure is generally maintained at altitudes of approximately 8,000 feet, which lowers the PaO_2 to between 60 and 70 mm Hg in healthy travelers. Individuals with chronic lung disease may need supplemental oxygen. Those with recent myocardial infarction or significant underlying cardiovascular compromise should generally avoid travel unless absolutely necessary (26).

Jet lag seems to be nearly universal for travelers traversing several time zones (Fig. 41.9), although some seem to be more affected than others. Traveling eastward is associated with increased jet lag compared with traveling west. More than simple travel fatigue, jet lag occurs when the body's physiologic clock has not yet adjusted to the new time zone. Symptoms include sleepiness during the daytime, lying awake and hungry at night, and often a feeling that one's thinking processes are not quite normal. Several days to a week are usually needed to recover completely from jet lag.

Although time is the only cure, a *few suggestions* seem to help. Patients should be advised to avoid overeating and excess alcohol ingestion during air travel and to keep a light snack handy for middle of the night hunger. Before a long trip, travelers can adjust by going to bed 1 hour earlier or later for each time zone crossed. Also, they should be advised to try to schedule a day of rest after passing six or more time zones before proceeding with their business or vacation. Travelers should be encouraged to adjust to local times for eating and sleeping as soon as possible after arrival. Taking a mild sleeping medication before bed for 2 or 3 days may also help to get back on schedule (see also Chapter 7). *Melatonin,* a hormone produced in the pineal gland from tryptophan, is a potent modulator of circadian rhythms and has been investigated as a prophylactic agent for jet lag (27). Melatonin has a hypnotic effect and is presently marketed in the United States as a dietary supplement and is not regulated for purity and concentration by the Food and Drug Administration. Using melatonin for jet lag remains controversial because of concern about long-term safety and efficacy. Proponents of melatonin suggest a dosage of 3 to 5 mg taken on an eastward trip at 3:00 a.m. "destination time" for 3 days before departure and at bedtime for 4 nights after arrival. For westward journeys, 3 to 5 mg should be taken at local bedtime for 4 days. Melatonin preparations are available without prescription. For short-term use such as for jet lag, it appears safe.

Accidents

The major cause of serious morbidity and leading cause of mortality in travelers to the developing world is accidents, especially involving motor vehicles (28). In many developing countries vehicles are in disrepair, drivers are inexperienced, and common sense rules for driving are not followed. Other major accidents include drowning, electric shocks, and trauma associated with dangerous sports (hang gliding, whitewater rafting). Injury prevention strategies should be part of routine travel advice (29). Defensive driving is a must. In developing areas, roads are generally not as well built as in developed areas, road hazards are common, and often animals sleep in the roads at night. Compounding the problems of accidental trauma is the usual lack of a developed emergency medicine infrastructure. Many countries have no formal emergency transport system, and hospital supplies are often lacking. Blood is often not available or not carefully screened, and quality control is not available. For serious trauma, it is often best to arrange transport to a medical facility in or operated by a developed nation.

Injectable Medications and Blood Transfusions

Travelers should be advised to avoid, if possible, receiving any injectable medication or blood transfusions when traveling in the developing world. Both HB and HIV can be readily transmitted by this route because needles and syringes may not always be sterilized properly. In addition, blood in most developing countries is not routinely screened for HIV (and may also not be screened for HB).

Motion Sickness

Travelers with a history of motion or sea sickness can attempt to avoid these symptoms by taking one of the antihistamines useful for this problem or ginger root derivatives. There are a number of medications available for symptom control, but in a recent study of whale watchers in the North Sea, meclizine, cyclizine, dimenhydrinate, and ginger root (given as candy or in a 250-mg tablet) were found to have equivalent efficacy (30). Further details are found in Chapter 89.

Swimming and Bathing

Swimming in contaminated water may result in eye, ear, skin, and some intestinal infections. Wading, washing, and swimming should be avoided in water that is likely to be infested with the snail hosts of schistosomiasis (see above) or with human sewage or with animal urine that may contain *Leptospira.* Generally, only chlorinated pools should be considered safe places to swim in developing countries. Ocean beaches may be safe, if not contaminated by sewage, but bathers should be advised to wear light shoes to protect against exposure to coral and other contact hazards.

Insects

The bites, stings, and contact of some insects cause unpleasant reactions. Many insects, such as mosquitoes, can bite and transmit disease without the traveler being aware of the bite. Insect repellents, protective clothing, and mosquito netting, which prevent the bite of insects, are the best prevention for some communicable diseases, particularly malaria (see above). The same personal protection measures used against mosquitoes will protect against ticks and biting flies. Travelers therefore should take a supply of insect repellent cream, lotion, or spray and permethrin.

Sunburn

Sunburn is a particular hazard in tropical and high-glare environments. Sunshades, sunscreens (see Chapter 118), broad-brimmed hats, and protective clothing are important preventive measures. Many sunscreen lotions must be reapplied after bathing or heavy perspiration. For maximal protection, travelers should apply all sunscreen products before going outside. A small percentage of people who take the tetracycline antibiotics (including doxycycline) may develop an exaggerated burn after exposure to the sun; this may be important if this antibiotic is being taken daily for diarrhea or malaria prevention.

High Altitude

High altitudes can be a problem for people with preexisting heart or lung disease, and portable oxygen may be advisable for these situations. Rapid exposure to altitudes more than 8,000 feet above sea level can cause serious medical problems. The incidence and severity of mountain sickness are related to the altitude, rate of ascent, and prior acclimatization. Initial symptoms include dizziness, headache, extreme fatigue, chilliness, nausea, and vomiting. More severe symptoms may also occur, most commonly difficulty in concentrating, extreme shortness of breath, and more severe headache. In most people, symptoms are mild and clear within 24 to 48 hours. If symptoms persist or are severe, a return to lower altitude may be required. Administration of oxygen generally relieves acute symptoms. Preventive measures include adequate rest before travel, avoidance of alcohol and tobacco, and decreased physical activity at high altitude.

The carbonic anhydrase inhibitor acetazolamide (Diamox) has been shown to reduce the time needed for acclimatization to high altitudes. It is prescribed at a dosage of 250 mg three times a day beginning 1 day before ascent and continued for 2 to 3 days after ascent. Dexamethasone is also effective in minimizing altitude sickness. In a recent report, both acetazolamide and dexamethasone (2 mg four times a day or 4 mg twice daily) were effective and reasonably well tolerated, although depression after dexamethasone withdrawal has been observed. Nifedipine may prevent high altitude pulmonary edema but has not been shown clearly to prevent or treat altitude sickness (31). Although acetazolamide is considered the drug of choice for the prevention of high altitude sickness, the definitive treatment consists of moving to a lower altitude as soon as possible. Acetazolamide should not be used by sulfa-allergic people.

Snakes and Scorpions

Poisonous snakes live in many developing countries, although most travelers will never see them unless they visit a zoo. If travelers will be walking through brush or jungle or will be walking at night, they should wear good-quality leather boots that cover the ankle. Not all snake bites are poisonous and not all poisonous snake bites are fatal, but immediate treatment by a physician is essential. If possible, the traveler should bring the snake for identification.

Scorpion bites are painful but seldom dangerous, except possibly to infants. Exposure to bites can be avoided by sleeping under mosquito netting and shaking clothing and shoes before putting them on.

Contact with marine life in tropical seas can be associated with minor discomfort such as sea bathers' eruption or may be more serious with exposure to jelly fish toxins, bites of sea snails, or lion fish. Most marine hazards are avoided by using good judgment and common sense while swimming, snorkeling, and diving.

Medicines

If travelers are taking prescribed medications, they should obtain an adequate supply before leaving and keep all medications in their luggage. Many medications are sold without prescription overseas. However, the traveler should be cautious about purchasing these medicines. Although medicines made by recognized pharmaceutical companies are generally of high quality, the quality of other medicines may not be guaranteed. The traveler should be advised not to self-medicate, because many medicines have serious side effects.

Pregnant Women and Children

Some medications used commonly in travelers should not be given to pregnant women, in particular doxycycline (impairs tooth development in the infant) and Fansidar (see Malaria Prophylaxis, above) (32). Travel late in pregnancy may precipitate labor. In fact, many airlines do not allow air travel during the final month. Women prone to vaginal yeast infections, especially if antibiotics are taken, may want to take antifungal agents.

Immunizations recommended for children are, in general, the same as those recommended for adults (Table 41.2), except that yellow fever vaccine is not usually required under 1 year of age (33). Routine infant vaccinations are even more important for children traveling to developing countries because diphtheria, whooping cough, polio, and measles are common. The dosages of medicines have to be adjusted for children. This is especially important for malaria medications. Because children may be restless on long airline trips, some parents are tempted to sedate their children. This is discouraged, however, because children may react adversely to sedatives.

Sexually Transmitted Diseases

Engaging in casual sex may be more common in travelers than previously recognized (34). The risk of contracting sexually transmitted diseases is high in some parts of the world. Very importantly, HIV infection has become a global health problem. In addition to the risk of HIV infection, sexually transmitted pathogens such as penicillinase-producing *Neisseria gonorrhoeae* are becoming increasingly common. Likewise, less common pathogens such as chancroid and lymphogranuloma venereum and HB are more common in certain areas. To reduce the risk of sexually transmitted infections, travelers need to be discriminating in sexual relations and avoid multiple partners, anonymous partners, prostitutes, and people who have had multiple sexual partners. If a traveler chooses to have sexual relations, condoms should always be used during intercourse.

Miscellaneous Infections

Many people experience a *traveler's cold* during a trip. These are thought to be caused by infection with respiratory viruses to which the traveler has no immunity. Travelers should bring their favorite cold remedy and an extra box of tissues with them. Erythromycin is sometimes used for travel-related respiratory infection, but its efficacy is unknown. *Fungal infections,* especially jock itch (tinea cruris) and athlete's foot (tinea pedis), may also be more common, especially in hot humid environments. Travelers should wear clean dry socks, or sandals when possible, and use antifungal powders and ointments as needed.

In recent years, *American cutaneous leishmaniasis* has also occurred sporadically in people who have visited the area endemic for this disease (southern Texas to northern Argentina, chiefly Mexico and Central America). The etiologic agents are protozoa of the *Leishmania* species, which are inoculated by female sandflies that inhabit forested lowlands. The skin lesion of American cutaneous leishmaniasis evolves over weeks to months from a papule to a nodule to an ulcer with raised indurated borders that eventually heals with a scar. Diagnosis requires identification of organisms in skin scrapings or biopsied tissue.

Using insect repellent and wearing long sleeves and trousers are usually effective in preventing sandfly bites.

Long-Term Travelers

Recommendations for long-term travelers are generally the same regarding food and water, immunizations, and malaria prophylaxis. However, the need for certain interventions may increase. For example, the reasons for immunizing short-term travelers against HB, typhoid, rabies, meningitis, or Japanese encephalitis may not be compelling, but the benefit for a long-term traveler will be greater because the duration of time at risk is greater. Hence, the need for complete immunizations for endemic diseases of the area should be stressed. With recommendations for universal HB protection for infants, the importance of this vaccine for young travelers living overseas should be stressed. Furthermore, travelers may be willing to avoid fresh garden salads for short times, but long-term residents may choose to grow their own garden or find safe vegetables.

The commonly used antimalarials (chloroquine, mefloquine, and Paludrine) can all be used safely for several years if indicated; therefore, long duration of stay is not a contraindication for these drugs, although the cost of long-term usage must be discussed when choosing an antimalarial.

If the traveler hires people to work in the house, these employees should be screened medically before starting work. The examination should include a chest radiograph to rule out active TB and stool analysis to rule out fecal parasites and *S. typhi*.

Medical Emergencies

Becoming ill overseas can be frightening and challenging. If the traveler becomes seriously ill or injured while traveling, the U.S. consulate can provide advice on where to go for help. In addition, the International Association for Medical Assistance to Travelers publishes a book listing English-speaking physicians (call 716-754-4883). Also, local Rotary or Lions Clubs can be helpful.

International Traveler's Health Kit

The following is a suggested first aid and health kit that represents the minimal necessary equipment for the traveler to the developing world (items can be obtained from various travel catalogs and suppliers):

- International Immunization Card with documentation of vaccines received
- Appropriate medication for malaria prophylaxis
- Mosquito repellent
- Water purification tablets, tincture of iodine, or water filters
- Oral rehydration salt packets (available in the United States from CERA Products, Columbia, MD, 410-997-2334, and Jianas Brothers, Kansas City, MO, 816-421-2880).
- Antimicrobial medication for treatment or prevention of diarrhea as arranged with the traveler's physician
- Imodium or Lomotil, if indicated
- Sunscreen
- Adhesive bandages (for blisters)
- A spare pair of glasses or at least the lens prescription
- Any prescription medication the traveler takes regularly
- Legible copies of prescriptions for medications
- The traveler's favorite cold remedy
- Fever thermometer
- Aspirin or acetaminophen (paracetamol in most other countries)
- Astringent or antiseptic
- Antifungal powder
- Toilet paper

Post-Travel Screening

Most people who acquire viral, bacterial, or parasitic infections in developing countries become ill within 6 weeks after returning, but certain infectious diseases, such as malaria and schistosomiasis, may not manifest themselves until later. The traveler should be advised to seek medical help for any unexplained symptoms during the 12 months after the end of a trip. When an unexplained late illness occurs, it is necessary to identify all of the developing countries that the traveler visited to know which infectious disease risks he or she encountered.

For travelers who stay for long periods in the developing world, it is prudent to provide routine screening on arrival home. This should include a complete blood count with differential, liver function tests, TB skin test, stool examination for occult blood, urinalysis, and stool examination for ova and parasites. If these tests all are normal, the traveler has probably not acquired a serious unrecognized infectious disease, but post-trip surveillance for another 6 months is still warranted.

IMMIGRANT PATIENTS

Legal immigration to the United States during the last 25 years has reached levels not seen since the early 1900s. Approximately 750,000 new legal immigrants arrive each year. This new wave of immigration is fueled in part by recent conflicts and human rights abuses. Legal immigrants include refugees, those aliens admitted with special status for humanitarian reasons via resettlement programs, and nonrefugees who arrive without resettlement assistance.

Refugees comprise less than 20% of the total legal immigration to the United States and receive limited cash assistance and services through local resettlement programs. These local refugee resettlement programs are nongovernmental organizations working in cooperation with state refugee coordinators who help to distribute federal and state money at the local community level for the initial resettlement of refugees. Refugees, if able, are expected to work and can apply for *permanent resident alien cards* after 1 year. After 5 years, permanent resident aliens over the age of 18 can petition for U.S. citizenship, and children who have resident alien cards automatically become citizens if either parent obtains citizenship.

Three other groups of immigrants include nonrefugee legal aliens, international adoptees, and undocumented aliens, which often includes migrant workers. Nonrefugee legal aliens comprise the bulk of U.S. immigration. These individuals are expected to be financially self-sufficient and may include family members rejoining previously admitted refugees. In recent years, couples and individuals seeking to build or expand families have increasingly turned to international adoptions. Undocumented aliens have captured much attention in recent years and have special health care needs because they are often uninsured and are afraid of being exposed to authorities. The health care of many migrant workers, including immigrants, is complicated by the potential for discontinuity of medical services as they follow employment opportunities, often farm related, throughout the United States (35). Given these different categories of immigrants dispersed throughout the United States, it is especially important for primary care practitioners to have knowledge of the health care needs of these populations.

Issues of Culture

One of the challenges of providing immigrant health care is understanding culture-bound health beliefs, practices, and treatments. Immigrants often lack an understanding of basic physiology or the principles of infectious diseases and may explain illness on the basis of a bad wind that has entered the body, possession by a spirit or demon, or an imbalance of opposing forces such as hot and cold or yin and yang (36). Practices that appear to have no purpose in the treatment of a specific malady may be encountered, including ritual scarring, uvulectomy, "female circumcision," and male circumcision. Other culture-bound health treatments include coining, cupping, pinching, massage, ceremonies to exorcise an evil spirit, consumption of herbal teas or alcohol, or inhalation of herbal steams (Fig. 41.10). White tape impregnated with an aromatic substance may be applied to the temple to relieve headaches or to the back or joints to relieve pain. Traditional Cambodian women believe it is important to have a fire built under the bed and to remain on the bed consuming hot spicy food for weeks after the delivery of a new baby. Failure to do this may result in the perception that healing will never be complete and future complaints of pelvic pain, backaches, other complications may ensue, requiring expensive medical evaluations.

Often, local healers are consulted (37). There may be little trust in the Western-trained practitioner, who resorts to obtaining a detailed history, physical examination, and often laboratory data and x-rays before issuing a prescription. Phlebotomy or x-ray imaging may even be perceived as injurious. Instead, the refugee or immigrant patient may prefer to approach a family member, elder, monk, shaman, or other traditional healer, believing these healers possess insight that Western-trained practitioners lack (38).

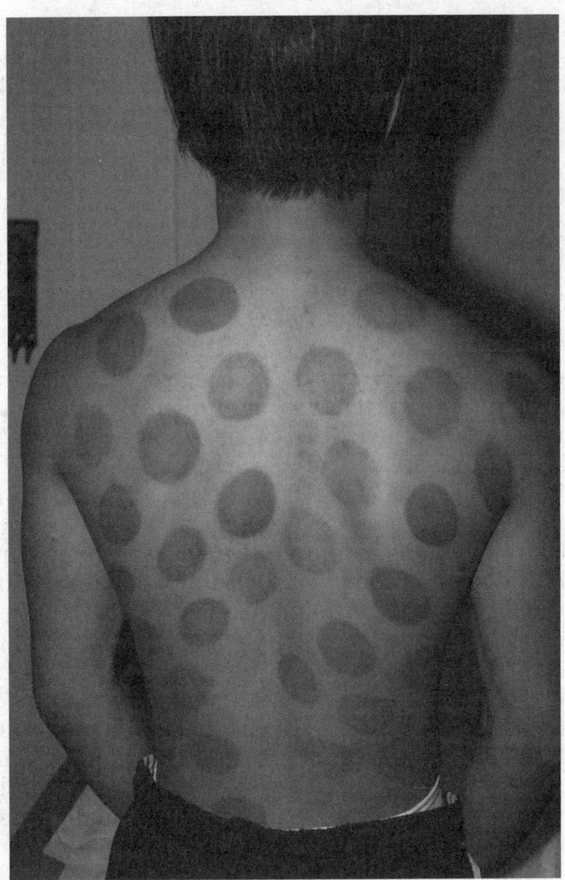

Figure 41.10. Cupping. Cambodian refugee adolescent with fever, sore throat, and tonsillar exudate. (Portland, Maine 1997. Courtesy of Maine Medical Center Audiovisual Department.)

The concept of cancer screening or regular preventive health or dental care visits is often not highly evolved, if at all. Preventive health care may take the form of a tattoo or wearing of amulets. The risks from exposure to tobacco smoke, alcohol, and environmental substances, such as lead in homes or mercury in freshly caught fish, may be poorly understood or unknown.

The traditional doctor–patient relationship may not be effective or understood in different cultures. For instance, a Muslim woman will likely not allow an examination by a male practitioner except in an emergency and may even feel uncomfortable being in the same room with him unless her father, husband, or brother accompanies her. Some holidays may have direct medical relevance as well, most notably the Muslim holy month of Ramadan, during which able-bodied adults must fast from sun up to sun down. Some individuals interpret this to include medications. In Asian cultures, it is disrespectful to pat the head of a child as a gesture of kindness or to sit slouched or with the bottom of the foot exposed. The Asian patient who does not make eye contact may be adhering to traditional norms of respect, although this can be misinterpreted as disinterest or passivity. An Asian patient may also tend to agree with or defer to the health care professional because to do otherwise may be considered discourteous. Contrary to Western belief that bad news should be communicated directly to an individual by laying out the facts, some cultural groups believe that bad news must be conveyed through a trusted family member or friend, an approach that may stand in conflict with our concern for patient confidentiality.

Practitioners and support staff should be careful to record names and birth dates as accurately as possible. Many Southeast Asian cultures invert the name after arriving in the United States so that Nguyen Van Thong in Vietnam becomes Thong Van Nguyen in the United States, because Nguyen is really the family name and Thong is the given name. Some cultures may use the same name for the family name and given name as in Mohamed Mohamed. Dates of birth are usually recorded in Day-Month-Year format overseas. These dates can easily be misinterpreted in the United States so that, for example, 12-05-1981 on overseas documents or as written by the patient translates incorrectly to December 5, 1981 and correctly to May 12, 1981. Vietnamese children are considered to be age 1 at birth and their age increments increase on the lunar New Year. As simple and inconsequential as these issues may seem, they can lead to many problems, including patient registration errors, Medicaid reimbursement denials, and child growth chart and immunization record errors.

Interpreters

Language differences pose the greatest potential barrier to the health care of the refugee and immigrant patient (39). Hospitals and medical practices that accept federal health care reimbursement are required to provide interpreters. There are no standards that define interpreter qualifications or when an interpreter is needed. In many large cities, trained medical interpreters are readily available, but this may not be the case in smaller communities. As a rule, children should not be used for medical interpreting. Telephone language line services have become a popular substitute and may be superior in situations requiring a high degree of confidentiality. These services have up to 140 different languages available. Use of high quality speakerphones or telephones with dual handsets optimize use of these services. Available telephone interpreter services include *LanguageLine Services* (http://www.languageline.com), *Pacific Interpreters* (http//www.pacificinterpreters.com), and *CyraCom International* (http://www.cyracom.net), among others. Many informed consent documents are not available in the appropriate language. If available they may be too complex or the patient may be illiterate. Fortunately, vaccine information statements are now becoming available in different languages on the Internet at http://www.immuneize.org/vis/index.htm.

Overseas Medical Examination

All refugees and overseas applicants for U.S. immigrant visas must undergo medical examinations before embarking for the United States. The standards for this screening are established by the CDC, National Center for Infectious Diseases, Division of Quarantine and published at the website for this organization (http://www.cdc.gov/ncidod/dq/index.htm). "Panel physicians" designated by the U.S. Department of State administer the examination. Documentation is on U.S. Department of State form OF-157. A supplement to form OF-157 is used to document immunizations. The overseas medical examination seeks to identify physical or mental health problems of public health significance. Health problems are designated as class A conditions, those that may potentially preclude U.S. immigration, and class B conditions, which are of sufficient public health concern that they be brought to the attention of consular authorities. Emphasis is placed on TB, HIV, syphilis, and other sexually transmitted disease screening for patients age 15 or over. TB is screened by chest x-ray. Those with suspected or confirmed active pulmonary TB or positive tests for syphilis should be fully treated before being allowed to travel to the United States. HIV disease does not automatically preclude U.S. immigration.

Entering the United States

Quarantine officials located at U.S. ports of entry review the overseas medical examination and directly notify state public health officials of the need to conduct medical follow-up for conditions of public health significance on a case by case basis. Refugees often have had disrupted medical care due to conflict, dislocation, deprivation, and life in refugee camps, and they are considered to be at greater risk for TB than nonrefugee immigrants. Consequently, state public health officials are notified of all new refugee arrivals for purposes of follow-up tuberculin skin testing. When a refugee relocates within the United States, the public health system may lose contact with the patient and fail to complete follow-up TB screening. TB screening and other follow-up health recommendations for refugees are issued by the U.S. Office of Refugee Resettlement in consultation with the CDC.

Initial Health Screening Examination in the United States

There are no standard guidelines for health care follow-up of refugees and immigrants beyond those that cover specific diseases and conditions of public health significance. Even so, all refugees and immigrants should undergo complete and thorough health screening shortly after U.S. arrival and establish a relationship with a primary care practitioner. Because of language and cultural barriers, medical data gathering may depend disproportionately on the physical examination and laboratory studies. Refugees are more likely than nonrefugee immigrants to have undiagnosed or inadequately managed health problems. Some of these problems may present for the first time in adults, whereas ordinarily they would have been diagnosed and managed by pediatricians in the United States. Disorders of growth and development, genetic disorders, and rheumatic and other valvular heart disease are a few examples. Children often are seen first in primary care clinics because they require school physicals and immunizations and are often eligible for Medicaid.

Existing Medical Records

The initial health screening examination should begin with a review of any overseas medical documents. The patient should have a copy of the OF-157 and supplement and may have other overseas medical records. Any accessible records that have been generated as a consequence of public health intervention after U.S. arrival should also be reviewed. This might include tuberculin skin test results, additional chest x-rays, TB clinic records, immunization records, or other health records.

Medical History

A complete medical history should be obtained using an interpreter if necessary. The names of medications that are currently being used and that have been brought from overseas should be recorded. Software programs like MICROMEDEX are helpful in being able to rapidly identify some overseas medications. Additional helpful information includes migration history and information on accompanying family members and those left behind. Refugees may have suffered war-related physical trauma, emotional trauma, or torture. A patient's languages and dialects, both written and spoken, should be documented. Literacy, years of education, and work experience may be predictors of ability to adapt and acculturate in the United States. It should be determined if a woman or couple of childbearing age is familiar with birth control options, and family planning desires should be addressed.

Physical Examination

The physical examination should be as complete as possible and may require a same-sex practitioner. It should include height, weight, hearing, and vision assessment. The pelvic examination should include cervical cancer, gonorrhea, and chlamydia screening. This is particularly true for refugee girls and women who may be victims of rape as a war crime or in refugee camps and may be unable to verbalize these atrocities. Scars or deformities acquired as a consequence of battle, land mine, torture, or other injury should be documented.

Screening Laboratory Tests

The decision to obtain screening laboratory and other studies should follow generally accepted guidelines for age- and sex-matched patients. Additional screening tests to consider in refugees and immigrants include a complete blood count and differential, varicella antibody, HB surface antigen (HBsAg), HB surface antibody, rapid plasma reagin, HIV antibody, and stool test for ova and parasites.

Special Refugee and Immigrant Health Considerations

Certain medical problems are more prevalent among refugee and immigrant patients than other patients in a typical U.S. medical practice. The initial health screening examination and subsequent follow-up care should to focus on these specific areas.

Tuberculosis

The overseas medical examination should reduce the likelihood that a patient with active pulmonary TB will enter the United States. Nevertheless, refugees and immigrants occasionally slip through with active pulmonary or extrapulmonary disease. Far more common are refugees who have had a negative chest x-ray during the overseas medical examination but have a positive purified protein derivative (PPD) skin test upon arrival in the United States. These patients are usually asymptomatic, are not infectious, and do not pose an immediate public health risk. They should undergo an additional chest x-ray, history, and physical examination. If determined to have latent TB infection, they should receive preventive therapy according to established guidelines. Directly observed therapy is preferred. This prophylactic therapy is intended to interrupt the risk of developing reactivation of pulmonary TB. Prior receipt of BCG vaccine should be ignored when considering preventive therapy because of a positive PPD. Prior BCG vaccination is known to cause a positive PPD skin test for variable periods of time after immunization. However, a positive PPD skin test cannot reliably be attributed to the vaccine. If patients are found to have active pulmonary or extrapulmonary disease, immediate appropriate therapy and reporting to public health authorities is necessary (see Chapter 34). Other mycobacterial diseases, including leprosy, may occur with greater prevalence in refugees and immigrants.

Hepatitis B

HB is more prevalent in developing countries than in the United States. Sixty percent of Southeast Asian patients may have one or more serologic marker for HB, and in parts of Southeast Asia, HB carrier prevalence approaches 15%. For this reason, serologic screening for HBsAg is important to identify carriers and should be done even for the rare patient who has received HB immunization overseas. The high prevalence of HB surface antibody may also make routine screening for this marker more cost effective than blanket immunization. Refugee and immigrant patients who lack both markers should be considered for immunization.

HBsAg carrier patients require careful counseling. They may easily misunderstand the implications of this finding or even confuse a discussion about HB virus infection for HIV disease. Diagnosis of this disorder may stigmatize the patient in ways that are poorly understood by the practitioner. These patients should also undergo additional initial screening to stratify them with regard to risk for hepatocellular carcinoma or progression of their disease. This may include HB E antigen and antibody, hepatitis C antibody, hepatitis delta antigen and antibody, and alanine aminotransferase. Either HA IgG antibody testing or HA vaccine should be considered. There is no good data regarding the age, frequency, or method of screening for hepatocellular carcinoma. Periodic screening with alfafetoprotein and ultrasound has been suggested.

Anemia

Anemia is commonplace in refugee patients. Reversible causes include general nutritional factors and iron deficiency. Iron deficiency is usually a consequence of a chronic excess loss of dietary iron due to menses, hookworm disease, schistosomiasis, or other cause of persistent blood loss. The most common nonreversible cause of anemia in Southeast Asian refugees is beta-thalassemia, hemoglobin E, or a combination of the two conditions. Eosinophilia is another commonly encountered hematologic condition in refugees and immigrants and is frequently associated with one or more helminthic infections.

Screening for these conditions begins with a complete blood count and differential and, if indicated, iron studies, followed by hemoglobin electrophoresis and stool and urine testing for ova and parasites. Patients of reproductive age identified as having one or more of the hemoglobinopathies may be considered for genetic counseling.

Parasites

Parasites, often in association with eosinophilia, are commonly encountered in refugee and immigrant patients from tropical or subtropical countries. Screening or empiric treatment for parasites should be considered for these patients. Empiric treatment with albendazole, 200 mg twice a day for 5 days, has been suggested as a cost-effective approach to common parasite management in adults (40). The standard practice of ordering three stool samples for ova and parasites may need to be reconsidered. Although this approach is typically used to achieve adequate sensitivity, often the first sample in a refugee or immigrant patient returns positive for one or more pathogens. Initially identified parasites can be treated first and additional testing ordered as necessary to assess for cure and detect additional parasites. Limited English proficiency or misinterpretation of instructions can lead to misuse of stool sample kits, especially if each individual in a large family receives three at a time. In addition, stool sample kits for ova and parasites are expensive and typically contain polyvinyl alcohol and formalin preservatives, both of which are toxic if ingested. Stool testing for ova and parasites has a good chance of detecting parasites with an intestinal or biliary phase of the life cycle but will likely miss blood and tissue parasites. Thick and thin smears for malaria should be considered in any refugee or immigrant patient in whom chronic malaria is suspected or in an acute febrile illness.

Syphilis

Although a test for syphilis is mandatory for refugees and immigrants age 15 or over and is included as part of the routine overseas medical examination, additional testing detects cases missed during the overseas medical examination or acquired since the examination was administered. A positive test for syphilis in a patient who previously tested negative may prompt further investigation for possible HIV disease, other sexually transmitted diseases, and screening of children who may not have been previously tested.

Immunization Delay

Immunizations should be updated at the time of the overseas medical examination but may be mid-series or never started depending on when the examination was performed, the availability of immunization products, or time factors. Delayed immunizations need to be updated. Adults and children may be behind on routine childhood vaccines. Careful documentation of immunization should be provided to the refugee and immigrant patient because proof of immunization will be required when application is made for adjustment of citizenship status with the U.S. Immigration and Naturalization Service. It can be very difficult to obtain an accurate history of prior varicella infection. Given the difficulty of storing this vaccine and the need for two doses of vaccine over the age of 13, it may be cost effective to routinely perform varicella serologic testing for all new refugee and immigrant patients.

Delayed Growth and Development

Delayed growth and development are often a source of concern to health care professionals. There are no readily available, standardized, country-specific growth charts for children from the variety of different countries represented by recent refugees and immigrants. Poverty, nutrition, parasitosis, sanitation, and availability of medical care impact growth and development. In many developing or war-torn regions, these factors are quite variable from region to region and from time to time. Standardized growth charts for children from these regions, if they do exist, may not account for these variables, and U.S. health professionals may find these charts more difficult to interpret than charts that are routinely used in the United States. Growth and development can be plotted on standardized U.S. growth curves, expecting some delays for certain children. Many Southeast Asian refugee children fall at or below the fifth percentile for height and weight upon arrival in the United States and move up on the curve with time. Failure to advance along the growth curve should prompt appropriate evaluation for possible failure to thrive. Although rare, specific nutritional deficiencies resulting in such conditions as scurvy and rickets should always be considered in refugees coming out of very harsh conditions (41).

Other Health Problems

Hypertension, diabetes, gout, malignancy, and many other health problems may be detected on routine screening of refugees and immigrants. In some cases, a prior diagnosis may have been established and the patient may have been treated. They may arrive in the United States on a dwindling supply of medications that usually must be changed to incorporate more readily available drugs. Alternatively, they may have had inadequate, sporadic, or no treatment at all for these health problems. Dental problems are very common (42). Appropriate follow-up, workup, and referral to specialists and dentists must be coordinated.

Post-Traumatic Stress Disorder and Depression

Refugees are both victims and survivors. They are displaced from their homeland because of a reasonable fear of persecution. Many have been directly or tangentially involved in fighting, imprisonment, rape, execution of family members, torture, ethnic cleansing, or other atrocities. Often refugees from the same country share strikingly similar histories with regard to the events that led up to their ultimate escape and resettlement. Some have lived for years in refugee camps. Children have been born and raised in these camps and may never have known a normal existence. Other refugees have been luckier, having fled encroaching fighting to live with relatives or on their own in a neighboring country (43). The psychological impact of these experiences can vary greatly from mild to severe disability. Patients may present with sleep disturbance or other somatic complaints. As the patient becomes established, patterns of interrupted employment, lack of interest in the children, or complete withdrawal may emerge. There may be evidence of depressed mood and blunted affect by examination.

There is a common refugee experience that is characterized by loss, grief, dislocation, migration, adaptation, and acculturation within the country of final asylum. Adaptation can be understood as the modifications undertaken by immigrants, within the new surroundings, to maintain life and culture as close as possible to what it used to be. Acculturation is the process of taking on the new culture and may be at odds with adaptive responses.

One striking example is the rapid acculturation of refugee and immigrant youth when compared with their parents. Western values that tolerate freedom of expression and the chance to date and move about for teens and young adults often clash with traditional family values, compounding some of the usual complexities of parent–adolescent interaction. Furthermore, refugee and immigrant adolescents who have been in the United States for more than a few years typically have learned English more quickly than their parents and have ceased native language development. In what would seem to be an inversion of normal life, parents often must depend on their children to be their spokespersons in all family and personal matters.

Additional factors, including lack of community, inadequate job skills, gender role reversal, academic problems, poverty stricken surroundings, and hopelessness, can contribute to the propensity that refugees, in particular, will suffer from posttraumatic stress disorder and depression.

Physical Trauma

Physical trauma as a consequence of fighting, land mines, and torture is encountered in refugee patients, including children. These injuries may impact the ability to work or attend school. Awareness, documentation of the extent of these injuries, and prompt attention to rehabilitation is important to maximize functional ability.

Anticipatory Guidance

Refugee and immigrant patients should be helped to begin to take an active role in preventive health care. Additional visits to establish primary health care and annual examinations to achieve better compliance with preventive health measures may be needed. Often refugee and immigrant patients must return at 2 and 6 months after the initial examination to complete immunization series. These are opportunities to see how they are adjusting and to reinforce use of smoke detectors, child safety seats, and seat belts. Other important issues include housing safety (fire escape or other egress in the event of a fire), smoking, passive smoke exposure, the need for cancer screening examinations such as mammography, family planning, and sexually transmitted disease prevention. Concerns about their children can also be reviewed, including school adjustment, fighting, guns, gang involvement, substance abuse, early sexual activity, and use of the Internet.

General References

Advice For Travelers. Med Lett 1999;41:39.

Up to date summary.

Barnett ED, Chen R. Children and international travel: immunizations. Pediatric Infect Dis J 1995;14:982.

A good review of the issues unique to the pediatric traveler.

Dupont HL, Steffen R. Textbook of travel medicine and health. Ontario: BC Decker, 1997.

Comprehensive textbook of travel medicine. Also on compact disc.

Freedman DO, ed. Infectious Disease Clinics of North America, Travel Medicine, Vol. 12, No 2, July 1998, W.B. Saunders Company.

A compendium of travel-related topics.

Guerrant RL, Walker DH, Weller PF. Tropical infectious diseases: principles, pathogens, and practice. Philadelphia: Churchill Livingstone, 1999.

Authoritative textbook of tropical medicine.

Health Information for International Travel. Center for Disease Control and Prevention. DHHS, Atlanta, GA.

The Yellow Book; practical and comprehensive manual updated yearly.

Health Information for International Travel. Supplement to Morbidity and Mortality Weekly Report, DHHS Publication No. (CDC) 92-8280, Atlanta, Centers for Disease Control and Prevention.

A practical manual, updated yearly, available free of charge.

Joe JR, Malach RS, Willis W, et al. Developing cross-cultural competence: a guide for working with young children and their families. Baltimore: Paul H. Brookes Publishing Co., 1995.

A review of the cultural issues of immigration.

Jong EC, ed. The medical clinics of North America. Travel Medicine 1999;83(4).

Good review of travel medicine.

Jong EC, McMillan R. The travel and tropical medicine manual, 2nd ed. Philadelphia: W.B. Saunders, 1995.

A relevant manual written for the clinician that contains a list of travel clinics.

Keystone JS, Kozarsky PE, Freedman DO. Internet and computer-based resources for travel medicine pactitioners. Clin Infect Dis 2001;32:757.

A complete listing of online resources.

Knirsch CA. Travel medicine and health issues for families traveling with children. Adv Pedaitr Infect 1999;14:163.

A good summary of issues for families traveling with children.

Mathews DS, Pust RE, Cordes DH, et al. Prevention and treatment of travel-related illness. Am Fam Physician 1991;44:1343.

Practical information.

Patterson JE, Patterson TF, Bia FJ, et al. Assuring safe travel for today's elderly. Geriatrics 1989;44:44.

Good review of age-related health risks.

Rose SR. International travel health guide, 11th ed. North Hampton, MA: Travel Medicine, 2000.

Complete travelers' health book, updated annually.

Ryan ET, Kain KC. Health advice and immunizations for travelers. N Engl J Med 2000;342:1716.

An up to date summary.

Schroeder D. Staying healthy in Asia, Africa, and Latin America, 5th ed. Stanford, CA: Avalon Travel Publishing, 2000.

A handbook that contains the nuts and bolts of health maintenance for traveling in the developing regions of the world.

Walker PF, Jaranson J. Refugee and immigrant health care. Med Clin North Am 1999;83:1103.

Good concise review.

Specific References

1. Cossar JN, Reid D, Fallon RJ, et al. A cumulative review of studies on travelers, their experience of illness and the implications of these findings. J Infect 1990;21:27.
2. Reid D, Dewar RD, Fallon RJ, et al. Infection and travel: the experience of package tourists and other travelers. J Infect 1990;2:65.
3. Packham CJ. A survey of notified travel-associated infections: implications for travel health advice. JL Pub Hill Med 1995; 17:217.
4. Outbreak of Leptospirosis among white water rafters, Costa Rica. MMWR Morb Mortal Wkly Rep 1997;46:577.
5. Coccidiomycosis in travelers returning from Mexico—Pennsylvania, 2000. MMWR Morb Mortal Wkly Rep 2000;49: 1004.
6. Robertson SE, Hull BP, Tomori O, et al. A decade of reemergence. JAMA 1996;276:1157.
7. Fatal yellow fever in a traveler returning from Venezuela. MMWR Morb Mortal Wkly Rep 1999;49:33.
8. Mahon BE, Mitz ED, Greene, KD, et al. Reflection of global changes in cholera epidemiology. JAMA 1996;276:307.
9. Wittlinger F, Steffen R, Watanabe H, et al. Risk of cholera among Western and Japanese travelers. J Travel Med 1995;2:154.
10. Sanchez JL, Taylor DN. Cholera. Lancet 1997;349:1825.
11. Mermin JH, Townes JM, Gerber M, et al. Typhoid fever in the United States, 1985–1994. Arch Intern Med 1998;158:663.
12. Eradication of paralytic poliomyelitis in the Americas. MMWR Morb Mortal Wkly Rep 1992;41:681.
13. Hilton E, Singer C, Kozarsky P, et al. Status of immunity to tetanus, measles, mumps, rubella, and polio among U.S. travelers. Ann Intern Med 1991;115:32.
14. Lemon SM, Thomas DL. Vaccines to prevent viral hepatitis. N Engl J Med 1997;336:196.
15. Falvo C, Horowitz H. Adverse reactions associated with simultaneous administration of multiple vaccines to travelers. J Gen Intern Med 1994;9:255.
16. Juckett G. Malaria prevention in travelers. Am Fam Phys 2000;59:2523.
17. Lobel HO, Kozansky PE. Update on prevention of malaria in travelers. JAMA 1997;278:1767.
18. Shanks GO, Gordon DM, Klotz FW, et al. Efficacy and safety of atovaquone/proguanil as suppressive prophylaxis for plasmodium falciparum malaria. Clin Infect Dis 1998;27:494.
19. Taylor WRJ, Richie TL, Fryauff DJ, et al. Malaria prophylaxis using azithromycin: a double-blind, placebo-controlled trial in Irian Jaya, Indonesia. Clin Infect Dis 1999;28:74.
20. Ericsson DC. Traveler's diarrhea: epidemiology, prevention, and self-treatment. Infect Dis Clin North Am 1998;12:285.
21. Consensus Conference. Travelers diarrhea. JAMA 1985;253: 2700.
22. Adachi JA, Ostrosky-Zeichner L, DuPont HL, et al. Empirical antimicrobial therapy for traveler's diarrhea. Clin Infect Dis 2000;31:1079.
23. Jelinek T, Nothdurft H, Loscher T. Schistosomiasis in travelers and expatriates. J Travel Med 1996;3:160.
24. Jelinek T. Dengue fever in international travelers. Clin Infect Dis 2000;31:144.
25. Karp CL, Neva FA. Tropical infectious diseases in human immune deficiency virus-infected patient. Clin Infect Dis 1999;28:947.
26. Bettes TN, McKenas DK. Medical advice for commercial air travelers. Am Fam Phys 1999;60:801.
27. Petrie K, Dawson AG, Thompson L, et al. A double-blind trial of melatonin as a treatment for jet lag in international cabin crew. Biol Psych 1993;33:526.
28. Hargarten SW, Barker TD, Guptill K, et al. Overseas fatalities of United States citizen travelers: an analysis of deaths related to international travel. Ann Emerg Med 1991;20:622.
29. Bratton RL. Advising patients about international travel: what they can do to protect their health and safety. Postgrad Med 1999;106:57.
30. Schmid R, Schick T, Steffen R, et al. Comparison of seven commonly used agents for prophylaxis of sea sickness. J Travel Med 1994;1:203.
31. Dumont L, Mardiroscoff C, Tramer M. Efficacy and harm of pharmacological prevention of acute mountain sickness, quantitative systematic review. Brit Med J 2000;321:267.
32. Samual BU, Barry M. The pregnant traveler. Infect Dis Clin North Am 1998;12:325.
33. Sood SK. Immunization for children traveling abroad. Pediatr Clin North Am 2000;47:435.
34. Matteeli A, Carosi G. Sexually transmitted diseases in travelers. Clin Infect Dis 2001;32:1063.
35. Mobed K, Gold EB, Schenker MB. Occupational health problems among migrant and seasonal farm workers. West J Med 1991;157:367.
36. Kleinman A, Eisenburg L, Good B. Culture, illness, and cure. Ann Intern Med 1978;88:251.
37. Aronson L. Traditional Cambodian health beliefs and practices. Rhode Island Med J 1987;70:73.
38. Kraut AM. Healers and strangers. JAMA 1990;263:1807.
39. Haffner L. Translation is not enough interpreting in a medical setting. West J Med 1992;157:255.
40. Muenning P, Pallin D, Sell RL, et al. The cost effectiveness of strategies for the treatment of intestinal parasites in immigrants. N Engl J Med 1999;340:773.
41. Yip R, Scanion K, Towbridge F. Improving growth status of Asian refugee children in the United States. JAMA 1992;267:937.
42. Hayes EB, Talbot SB, Matheson ES, et al. Health status of pediatric refugees in Portland, Maine. Arch Pediatr Adolesc Med 1998;152:564.
43. Shepherd J, Faust S. Refugee health care and the problem of suffering. Bioethics Forum 1993;9:307.

SECTION 5

Gastrointestinal Problems

CHAPTER 42

Disorders of the Esophagus: Dysphagia, Noncardiac Chest Pain, and Gastroesophageal Reflux

PHILIP O. KATZ, MD

PHYSIOLOGY OF SWALLOWING

Normal swallowing requires the coordination of the skeletal muscles of the pharynx, the cricopharyngeus muscle (the upper esophageal sphincter), and the proximal third of the esophagus, with the smooth muscle of the distal body of the esophagus and the lower esophageal sphincter (LES). Thus, the initiation of swallowing is voluntary, but involuntary processes subsequently propel the swallowed bolus through the esophagus into the stomach. The following sequence of events occurs during normal swallowing: relaxation of the upper esophageal sphincter to permit entry of the bolus into the esophagus, closure of the sphincter to prevent esophageal or pharyngeal regurgitation and aspiration, propulsion of the bolus distally by esophageal peristalsis, relaxation of the LES to allow easy entrance of the bolus into the stomach, and prompt closure of the LES to prevent reflux of gastric contents.

DYSPHAGIA

Dysphagia, difficulty in swallowing, may result from a disturbance of any of the anatomic structures or of the physiologic events involved in normal swallowing. It is an extremely specific symptom and should never be dismissed as an emotional problem or symptom of globus hystericus (discussed later in this chapter). The patient often says that food sticks in his or her chest, often pinpointing the precise area. Occasionally, dysphagia may be accompanied by pain on swallowing, *odynophagia,* but the two symptoms are distinct and may occur independently. Two types of dysphagia exist: oropharyngeal dysphagia (the inability to initiate the act of swallowing) and esophageal dysphagia (difficulty in transporting material down the esophagus).

Clinical Evaluation

History

Because of the complexity of the swallowing mechanism, the causes of dysphagia are varied. Certain aspects of the history are helpful in elucidating the underlying disorder. Difficulty in swallowing solids strongly suggests an anatomic obstruction such as carcinoma, stricture, or esophageal ring, whereas difficulty in swallowing solids and liquids suggests a motility disturbance such as achalasia, scleroderma, or diffuse esophageal spasm (DES).

The history may also be useful in identifying the region of abnormal function as either oropharyngeal or esophageal. Symptoms suggestive of *oropharyngeal dysphagia* include difficulty in initiating a swallow, regurgitation of liquid through the nose, aspiration with swallowing, and an inability to propel a bolus of food into the esophagus. Patients with *esophageal dysphagia* complain of retrosternal fullness after swallowing and of the feeling that food is stuck at a certain point in the esophagus, often relieved by regurgitation. Esophageal dysphagia is most commonly caused by structural abnormalities (ring, stricture, or tumor) but may be caused by reflux esophagitis or a primary motility disorder. Several common causes of dysphagia are listed in Table 42.1.

Mild weight loss may be described by patients with any type of chronic dysphagia, the result of a voluntary decrease in intake of food that often accompanies their symptoms. More severe weight loss with anorexia suggests carcinoma or achalasia.

Special Studies

To delineate the cause of dysphagia, one or more of the following procedures should be used: radiologic studies, esophagoscopy, and esophageal motility studies. The workup can establish a diagnosis in 95% of cases. Consultation with a gastroenterologist is recommended for most patients with dysphagia, both for evaluation of the clinical problem and for the performance of esophagoscopy and motility studies.

Radiology. The initial study in most patients with dysphagia is usually a *barium swallow,* a procedure that can identify motility disturbances and anatomic deformities. It is typically ordered by the primary caregiver. A barium swallow is the easiest procedure for the patient to tolerate (it takes only 15 to 20 minutes and is associated with essentially no discomfort). As with all radiologic studies, the radiologist should be told which disorders are most suspected. Without this communication, the radiologist may perform a routine barium swallow looking only for carcinoma, stricture, or reflux. Special techniques must be applied to identify esophageal rings and diverticula. Careful fluoroscopic control is required to evaluate motility. In addition, to observe the rapid activity of pharyngeal contractions and to detect abnormal esophageal contractions, the barium swallow should be recorded on videotape or cine film if oropharyngeal dysphagia is suspected. A marshmallow should be added if esophageal dysphagia is suspected. This will help localize the site of the obstruction. A double contrast study (carbon dioxide pellets are added to the barium meal to distend the esophagus) should be performed to identify mucosal abnormalities associated with gastroesophageal reflux. In this way, barium studies often can detect both organic and functional abnormalities that have led to dysphagia. However, a negative study does not exclude either anatomic (e.g., reflux esophagitis, small ulcers, or early cancer) or motor disorders of the esophagus, and a positive study seldom permits a specific diagnosis to be made; therefore, a barium swallow is almost always followed by endoscopy or esophageal manometry. In fact, there is a debate among gastroenterologists about the need for a barium swallow; many clinicians are comfortable in doing endoscopy initially, unless a high obstruction is suspected.

Endoscopy. *Esophagoscopy* is an essential part of the evaluation of dysphagia. Because the barium swallow may miss some lesions, endoscopy should be performed in all patients with persistent dysphagia, particularly in those with persistent difficulty in swallowing solid food. Esophagoscopy is complementary to the radiographic examination. The procedure is well tolerated and can be performed on an ambulatory basis even in the elderly. When a lesion is detected by radiography, endoscopy provides the most direct approach to establish the nature of the lesion, whether inflammatory or neoplastic. Biopsies and brushings for cytologic evaluation can be obtained under visual guidance. Furthermore, the instrument may disrupt esophageal webs or rings that are causing the dysphagia and thus may be both a diagnostic and a therapeutic tool. Inability to pass the endoscope through the esophagus into the stomach confirms an anatomic cause of the dysphagia and rules out a primary motor disturbance (e.g., achalasia). The patient's experience with upper gastrointestinal endoscopy is described in Chapter 45.

Recording of Esophageal Motility. *Esophageal manometry* is the best procedure for the evaluation of esophageal motor function (Table 42.2). This study measures the strength, function, and coordination of

Table 42.1. Types of Dysphagia

Symptoms	Causes
	Oropharyngeal
Nasal regurgitation, cough, aspiration with swallowing, difficulty initiating swallow	Central nervous system: cerebrovascular accident, Parkinson disease, brainstem tumors Muscle: Myasthenia, polymyositis, thyroid disease, systemic lupus erythematosus Structural: Web, Zenker diverticulum, extrinsic compression
	Esophageal
Dysphagia for solids	Carcinoma, stricture (continuous) Ring, diverticulum, esophagitis (intermittent)
Dysphagia for solids and liquids	Motility disorder, severe narrowing from tumor, stricture, esophagitis

Table 42.2. Esophageal Motility Disorders

Disorder	Manometry: Esophageal Body	Manometry: Lower Esophageal Sphincter	Primary Symptoms
Primary			
Achalasia	Absent peristalsis, low amplitude	High pressure, normal, incomplete relaxation (may be normal early in the disease)	Dysphagia, regurgitation, chest pain
Diffuse esophageal spasm	Simultaneous contractions mixed with normal peristalsis	Normal pressure, 1/3 with incomplete relaxation	Chest pain, dysphagia
Nutcracker esophagus	High amplitude, normal peristalsis	Normal pressure	Chest pain
Hypertensive LES	Normal amplitude	High pressure, normal relaxation	Chest pain
Ineffective esophageal motility	Nontransmitted, low amplitude (<30 mm Hg) in >20% of swallows with some normal peristalsis	Normal pressure	Dysphagia, chest pain, often seen in reflux disease
Secondary			
Reflux esophagitis	Ineffective motility	Low pressure may be seen	Heartburn, dysphagia
Scleroderma	Aperistalsis (smooth muscle), low amplitude	Low to absent pressure	Regurgitation, heartburn
Polymyositis	Proximal muscle disorder (low amplitude, disordered peristalsis)	Normal pressure	Regurgitation, oropharyngeal dysphagia

LES, lower esophageal sphincter.

the upper esophageal sphincter and LES and the body of the esophagus in response to a swallow. The procedure is well tolerated, takes only about 30 minutes, and involves the passage of a narrow catheter through the nose or the mouth into the stomach. Recordings are made of the amplitude and coordination of contractions within the pharynx and esophagus. Various motility abnormalities can be diagnosed by use of this technique. Esophageal manometry should be performed in all patients for whom a structural cause for the dysphagia cannot be found.

Specific Causes of Dysphagia

Carcinoma of the Esophagus

Cancer of the esophagus should always be suspected as the cause of dysphagia in patients over the age of 40. The incidence of esophageal adenocarcinoma is rising faster than that of any other malignancy in white men in the United States and has superseded squamous cell cancer of the esophagus as the most common esophageal cancer. Adenocarcinoma of the gastric cardia is also rising in incidence (1). Overall, esophageal cancer is still relatively rare—approximately 12,000 cases per year in the United States. African-American men are still more likely to develop squamous cell esophageal cancer than are white men or are women. The predisposing factor for adenocarcinoma is Barrett esophagus, a replacement of the normal squamous cells of the gastroesophageal junction by columnar cells. Predisposing factors for squamous cell carcinoma include cigarette smoking, heavy alcohol use, lye strictures, and achalasia.

Squamous cell cancer is most common in the middle to distal third of the esophagus. Adenocarcinoma occurs primarily in the distal third of the esophagus. Carcinoma of the cardia of the stomach may extend into the lower esophagus and obstruct the esophageal lumen.

Diagnosis. The diagnosis of esophageal cancer is generally made only after symptoms have developed, by which time the lesion is already advanced, with involvement of regional lymph nodes. In patients with predisposing conditions, such as Barrett mucosa, earlier detection of the cancer may be achieved by regular endoscopic surveillance every 2 to 3 years with biopsy and cytologic brushings of the entire esophagus. Most patients present with dysphagia for solid food for several months that progresses to dysphagia for solids and liquids, usually with progressive weight loss. Odynophagia (pain on swallowing) may accompany the dysphagia. Occult blood loss is common but hematemesis is unusual.

The diagnostic workup in all patients includes a barium swallow and upper endoscopy. If the radiograph is negative, the endoscopic examination may still reveal mucosal lesions. When the tumor is already defined by radiograph, endoscopy is necessary to establish a histologic diagnosis, which is important in deciding whether surgery or radiation therapy is indicated. Multiple biopsies and directed brush cytologies obtained via the endoscope provide a positive tissue diagnosis in more than 95% of cases of esophageal cancer. However, radiologic evaluation remains important because it provides useful information about the degree of esophageal obstruction, the length of the tumor, and the appearance of the fundus of the stomach. With the combined use of these two techniques, cancer of the esophagus can be differentiated from other esophageal lesions, such as peptic stricture of the esophagus, achalasia, severe esophagitis, and esophageal varices.

After the diagnosis is confirmed, a computed tomography of the chest and abdomen should be considered to evaluate the possibility of extraesophageal extension, but it is most useful to rule out hepatic metastases. Endoscopic ultrasound is being used with increased frequency for staging. It is now the most sensitive and specific method for staging this disease and should be considered in all preoperative evaluations (2). Regardless of the staging procedure, more than 50% of patients who present with dysphagia and have tumor apparently confined to the esophagus have extensive incurable disease at operation (3).

Therapy. Therapy for esophageal cancer is generally *surgery* or *radiation.* The choice between these two forms of therapy depends on the cell type and the location of the neoplasm. Adenocarcinoma is less radiosensitive, usually occurs in the distal third of the esophagus, and therefore is better suited for a surgical approach. Squamous cell carcinoma is radiosensitive, and numerous studies suggest that radiation of lesions in the distal and middle thirds of the esophagus is as effective as is surgery (see Chapter 10 for a discussion of radiotherapy in the treatment of cancer). Surgical resection is more extensive and less well tolerated in patients with more proximal tumors. The combination of radiotherapy and resection has been reported to improve survival, but more experience with this approach is needed. Whatever the therapy, the prognosis is poor: 75% of patients die within 1 year of diagnosis and 90% die by 5 years (3). Patients with adenocarcinoma detected during regular screening of Barrett mucosa have a better prognosis, with reported survival rates as high as 80% (3). Chemotherapy has met with some recent success in patients with unresectable adenocarcinoma and should be considered also as a means of downstaging patients before surgery. Some advocate preoperative chemotherapy even in patients with resectable cancer.

Palliation (maintenance of an open esophagus so that the patient can swallow food and saliva) should be the major aim of therapy if the tumor is not resectable. Dilation of the lumen with mercury-weighted rubber dilators, guidewire-assisted polyvinyl dilators, or various balloon dilators may all achieve successful palliation. Treatment with thermal coagulating dilators or laser therapy occasionally may be helpful. Esophageal prostheses have been used in palliation, particularly with tracheoesophageal fistulas. Chemotherapy or surgical palliation should also be considered in selected cases. Unfortunately, no well-designed clinical trials that compare different modalities have been done, so the choice of palliation must be individualized after consultation with a surgeon, an oncologist, and a gastroenterologist.

Achalasia

Achalasia is characterized by the complete absence of esophageal peristalsis and failure of LES relaxation. The condition occurs in all age groups, with a peak incidence in the fourth and fifth decades. The incidence of this disorder is approximately 1 in 100,000 population per year. Men and women are equally susceptible to the disease. Patients present most commonly with progressive dysphagia for both solids and liquids and, often, with regurgitation of ingested material. Pulmonary symptoms such as nocturnal coughing and even aspiration pneumonia may be the initial mode of presentation. Occasionally, substernal chest pain is associated with the dysphagia.

Pathogenesis. The pathogenesis of achalasia is unknown. Several studies have described abnormalities in the myenteric ganglion cells in the distal esophagus (LES zone), in the body of the esophagus, and in the vagal nucleus and its peripheral fibers. However, these findings have not been consistent. Pharmacologic studies have further supported the concept of denervation of the esophagus. There is an exaggerated response of the LES and the body of the esophagus to cholinergic stimulation and to the hormone gastrin, consistent with the concept of denervation hypersensitivity. The cause of the neuropathic injury is unknown.

Diagnosis. The routine chest radiograph often suggests the diagnosis. The normal gastric air bubble is absent, and an air–fluid level in the dilated esophagus is sometimes seen behind the heart. With a very dilated and tortuous esophagus, the mediastinum appears widened. The typical features on barium esophagogram (Fig. 42.1) include smooth tapered narrowing of the distal end of the esophagus that fails to open properly, retention of barium and secretions in the more proximal esophagus, and absence of peristalsis. The distal narrowing is often described as a bird beak or pen quill deformity. The patient must be examined while upright to demonstrate the height of the retained barium-filled column.

Esophageal manometry demonstrates three distinct abnormalities in patients with achalasia: absence of peristalsis of the smooth muscle of the esophagus, failure of the LES to relax after a swallow, and elevated LES pressure. If possible, manometry should be done in every patient suspected of having the disease to confirm the diagnosis. In achalasia, the basal LES pressure usually is elevated, at times to very high levels, and the degree of relaxation is incomplete. Thus, there is a constant high-pressure zone that impedes the passage of the esophageal contents. Peristalsis is also absent, further impairing the propulsion of the bolus distally. Manometry may demonstrate high-amplitude, simultaneous, repetitive contractions that are not peristaltic. These patients are classified by some as having vigorous achalasia and often have severe chest pain (4).

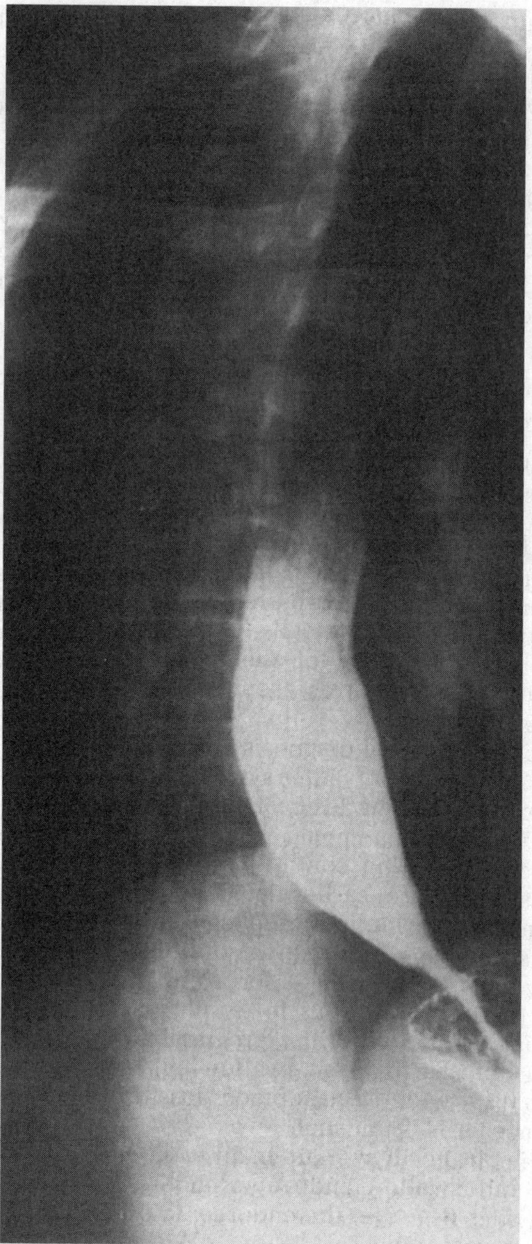

Figure 42.1. Barium swallow in a patient with achalasia. The esophagus is dilated and the tapered distal segment never opens normally. Under fluoroscopy, no peristalsis is seen, but simultaneous contractions are noted.

Patients who present early in the course of disease with mild symptoms and minimal esophageal dilation may, at manometry, appear to have normal LES relaxation (because of a manometric artifact) and normal sphincter pressure and yet have true achalasia. In such cases, technetium-labeled food studies with the patient in the upright position should be performed to confirm delayed emptying and the abnormal LES (5).

Differential Diagnosis. Achalasia must be differentiated from other disorders that lead to obstruction of the passage of food into the stomach. *Esophageal strictures,* both peptic and neoplastic, and *carcinomas at the esophagogastric junction* may result in symptoms and even in a radiographic and manometric picture similar to that of achalasia (6). Thus, all such patients should be evaluated with endoscopy. Failure to pass the endoscope into the stomach indicates an anatomic obstruction. *Scleroderma,* with its associated esophageal motility disturbance, may result in dysphagia with diminished peristalsis seen on the radiograph. If stricture has not occurred, the patient will demonstrate a wide-open sphincter through which barium passes easily. By the time patients with esophageal scleroderma develop stricture and dilation of the esophagus that may mimic achalasia, they usually have other obvious stigmata of scleroderma (particularly tight skin of the face and hands or Raynaud phenomenon). Furthermore, on esophageal manometry the LES pressure in scleroderma is low rather than high, as it is in achalasia, but, as in achalasia, the disorder of motility is confined to the smooth muscle portion (distal two-thirds) of the esophagus, with a normally functioning proximal segment. In patients from South America, *Chagas disease* may result in a megaesophagus and present with manometric patterns identical to that of achalasia. Patients with *idiopathic intestinal pseudo-obstruction* have a manometric pattern similar to that of achalasia; esophageal manometry may be used to help confirm the diagnosis.

Therapy. Two types of definitive therapy exist for achalasia: pneumatic dilation and surgery. Both forms of therapy are aimed at reducing the pressure gradient between the esophagus and the stomach, thus decreasing the severity of the dysphagia. The aperistalsis and impaired sphincter relaxation persist after therapy. *Pneumatic dilation,* an outpatient procedure, is performed by a trained gastroenterologist. The esophagus is aspirated completely before the dilation. After premedication with analgesics and sedatives, a balloon dilator is passed into the stomach. Under fluoroscopic guidance, the balloon portion is positioned across the LES. It is then inflated for 10 to 30 seconds, causing a forceful disruption of the LES muscle. The dilator is then removed and can be expected to be blood streaked. The patient usually experiences chest pain during the procedure. The major risk of the procedure is esophageal perforation, which occurs in up to 5% of dilations. Satisfactory results (long-term improvement in dysphagia, weight gain, and decrease in retention of barium) can be expected in approximately 85% of cases. In successful cases, there is immediate relief of symptoms. The patient is observed for 4 to 6 hours and discharged. Dilation can be repeated if symptoms of dysphagia recur or worsen, but most patients have only minimal symptoms for many years after therapy. Repeat esophageal manometry is not necessary if symptoms have been relieved.

Surgical therapy involves a transection of the circular muscle of the LES zone to the level of the mucosa, the Heller myotomy. This surgical approach provides results similar to those after pneumatic dilation, with a success rate of 80% to 85%. The procedure may cause significant reflux esophagitis in 10% to 25% of patients. As a result of this complication, some advocate combining a fundoplication with the myotomy. Until recently, the procedure required a thoracotomy, but it can now be performed by either a laparoscopic or thoracoscopic approach. These minimally invasive techniques have made myotomy a better tolerated procedure with shorter hospitalizations, but because pneumatic dilation can be performed on outpatients, it is usually the procedure of choice. Surgery is reserved for failure of repeated dilations to provide symptomatic relief, esophageal perforation secondary to pneumatic dilation, inability to perform dilation because of the shape of the esophagus or the presence of a large epiphrenic diverticulum, and inability to exclude carcinoma.

Medical therapy with nitrates, calcium channel blockers (Table 42.3), and even mercury bougienage

Table 42.3. Therapy for Esophageal Motility Abnormalities Associated with Chest Pain

Treatment Modality	Dose	Mode of Administration	Major Complications
Reassurance			
Nitrates[a]			
Nitroglycerin	0.4 mg SL	Usually before meals and PRN	Headache
Isosorbide	10–30 mg p.o.	30 min before meals	
Anticholinergics			
Dicyclomine (Bentyl)	10–20 mg	4 times a day	Dry mouth, blurred vision
Sedatives/antidepressants			
Diazepam (Valium)	2–5 mg	4 times a day	Drowsiness
Trazodone (Desyrel)	50–100 mg	4 times a day	Drowsiness, impotence
Imipramine (Tofranil)	50 mg	At bedtime	Drowsiness
Calcium channel blockers[a]			
Nifedipine (Procardia)	10–30 mg	4 times a day	Dizziness, nausea, dyspepsia
Diltiazem (Cardizem)	90 mg	4 times a day	Headache, edema, nausea
Smooth muscle relaxants[a]			
Hydralazine[a]	20–50 mg	3 times a day	Headache, lupuslike syndrome
Static dilation	50 French	Repeat as needed	None
Pneumatic dilation[b]			Perforation (3%–5%)
Esophagomyotomy[c]			Gastroesophageal reflux (20%)

[a]Orthostatic hypotension is a common complication of this class of drugs.

[b]May be indicated if dysphagia is a prominent symptom.

[c]Rarely indicated (intractability).

may offer transient improvement in some patients. Pharmacologic therapy should be reserved for patients in whom pneumatic dilation or myotomy is contraindicated or for patients with very mild disease.

Botulinum toxin, injected into the LES via endoscopy, has been studied as a treatment of achalasia (7). A decrease in LES pressure and improved esophageal emptying are seen immediately after injection. An initial success rate of 70% to 80% has been reported after the first injection, with most patients relapsing (and requiring repeat treatment) in 6 months to 1 year. This procedure can be performed by a trained endoscopist and has no more risk than esophagoscopy alone. The therapy should be considered for patients in whom surgery has high risk and in whom the risk of perforation with pneumatic dilation is also high, but not as a long-term treatment option.

Complications. Many studies suggest that patients with achalasia are at increased risk of esophageal cancer. The incidence of this complication ranges from 6% to 29% in various series (6). Cancer in patients with achalasia should not be confused with cancer of the esophagogastric junction presenting with an achalasia-like picture. The cancer that develops in patients with primary achalasia usually occurs many years after the diagnosis of achalasia has been established, is of the squamous cell type, and generally occurs in the midportion of the esophagus. There is no evidence that successful therapy of achalasia prevents the development of cancer. Thus, patients with achalasia are sometimes considered for periodic endoscopy with esophageal cytology every 3 to 5 years after diagnosis, although no definitive studies have been done to support this recommendation.

Diffuse Esophageal Spasm

Clinical Presentation. Symptomatic DES (8) is a disorder characterized by intermittent nonperistaltic (simultaneous) esophageal contractions that result in dysphagia and substernal chest pain. The disorder is seen equally in both sexes and at all ages (although it appears to be rare in children). The dysphagia is intermittent and is experienced for both solids and liquids. The pain is also intermittent and may be provoked by certain foods, particularly hot and cold beverages. At other times, the pain occurs spontaneously and may even awaken the patient at night. The pain is highly variable in quality and is sometimes described as knife-like or as dull and crushing; it may radiate to the neck, back, or arms. It may be brief or last for hours. Because of its location, radiation, and crushing quality, it is often confused with the pain of ischemic heart disease. When no cardiac disease is found, many of these patients are incorrectly believed to have a psychogenic disturbance.

Diagnosis. The procedures for the diagnosis of this condition include radiographic studies and esophageal manometry. A carefully performed *barium swallow,* or *videoesophagogram,* may demonstrate nonperistaltic, spontaneous, and simultaneous contractions (tertiary waves) of the body of the esophagus. However, these abnormal contractions are often encountered during routine barium swallow and by themselves do not make a diagnosis of esophageal spasm without the appropriate clinical history. Furthermore, because DES is an intermittent condition, the barium swallow may be normal or too insensitive to detect the motility disturbance. Because the barium study is not specific, it should be done only on patients with dysphagia. Patients with suspected DES should have *esophageal motility studies* to confirm the diagnosis, even if they have had a barium swallow. Provocative agents (e.g., edrophonium) can be used during the motility studies to identify more clearly patients who experience chest pain of esophageal origin (described later in this chapter) (9).

Therapy. Therapy for DES and other motility disorders that cause chest pain is discussed in greater detail later in this chapter and is listed in Table 42.3.

Other Primary Motility Disorders

In addition to achalasia and DES, three distinct primary motility abnormalities of the esophagus have been described that are associated rarely with dysphagia. The *nutcracker esophagus* and the *hypertensive LES* (excessively high LES pressures with normal esophageal peristalsis) are two abnormalities associated primarily with chest pain and, rarely, with dysphagia; they are discussed later in this chapter. Some patients with dysphagia referred for esophageal motility testing demonstrate contractions in the distal esophagus with amplitude of smooth muscle contraction below 30 mm Hg in more than 30% of swallows. This is called *ineffective esophageal motility* because contractions of this low amplitude are incapable of effective propagation of a bolus. This abnormality is seen commonly with gastroesophageal reflux, and rarely it may be seen with dysphagia alone.

Secondary Motility Disorders

Chronic reflux esophagitis (discussed later) may cause scarring of the distal esophagus, which can result in decreased force of esophageal contractions and/or ineffective esophageal motility, either of which can lead to dysphagia. There is ample evidence that acute acid reflux does not induce esophageal spasm, but chronic reflux may cause symptoms and motility abnormalities that are radiographically similar. Treatment is aggressive antireflux therapy. Improvement in dysphagia and contraction abnormalities is variable, but the pain of chronic reflux usually diminishes with treatment.

Abnormalities of esophageal contractions associated with dysphagia may be seen in patients with hyperthyroidism or hypothyroidism, amyloidosis, and myotonic dystrophy. Diabetes mellitus has been associated with multiple radiographic and manometric abnormalities, but patients are seldom symptomatic. Collagen vascular disease, particularly scleroderma, may affect the esophagus as well. Chronic idiopathic intestinal pseudo-obstruction may produce manometric abnormalities indistinguishable from those of achalasia. Many authorities have used esophageal manometry to help make this diagnosis. Use of the term *presbyesophagus* should be abandoned. Aging itself does not produce significant alteration of esophageal motility.

Scleroderma of the Esophagus

The esophagus is involved in up to 80% of patients with scleroderma. At times the esophageal symptoms are the presenting complaints that lead to the diagnosis. Indeed, the esophagus may demonstrate the characteristic abnormalities even before skin changes occur. The main symptoms of esophageal scleroderma are heartburn and dysphagia. The cause for these symptoms can be readily appreciated by examining the changes in esophageal motility. In esophageal scleroderma, the LES pressure is very low, resulting in free gastroesophageal reflux. In addition, the peristaltic waves initially are of reduced amplitude, progressing later to complete aperistalsis in the smooth muscle portion of the esophagus, sparing the skeletal muscle portion. Because peristalsis is impaired, the refluxed acid remains in the esophagus for an abnormally long time, perhaps accounting for the common development of an esophageal stricture in this disorder. Thus, the dysphagia may be caused by the primary motor abnormality or may signify the development of a peptic stricture.

The pathogenesis of scleroderma is unknown. In the esophagus, the disorder is not simply secondary to replacement of muscle fibers with collagen because the motility dysfunction can be demonstrated in the absence of histopathologic changes. It has been suggested that there is a neural defect in the esophagus rather than a primary myogenic disorder (10).

Scleroderma is a chronically progressive disease for which no specific treatment exists. Therapy of esophageal manifestations is directed at symptomatic relief and prevention of strictures.

Patients with scleroderma, whether they have dysphagia or heartburn, should be referred to a gastroenterologist for evaluation of esophageal motility and to rule out reflux esophagitis and stricture formation. If reflux is present, the patient should be treated with intensive antireflux therapy (Table 42.4) to try to prevent stricture formation. Strictures should be dilated by bougienage, followed by long-term medical therapy with proton pump inhibitors. In general, patients with scleroderma require a high dosage of an H_2 antagonist or a proton pump inhibitor (Table 42.4) for treatment of esophagitis. Antireflux surgery should be avoided because the motility disorder may lead to significant dysphagia after fundoplication.

Esophageal Webs and Rings

Dysphagia for solid foods may be caused by esophageal webs or rings. An *esophageal web* is a mucosal structure that protrudes into the lumen, most commonly in the proximal esophagus. The association of iron deficiency anemia with a proximal esophageal web constitutes the *Plummer-Vinson syndrome*. *Esophageal rings* are located in the distal esophagus and may be either mucosal or muscular; rings can be demonstrated in up to 10% of the population but rarely cause symptoms.

The ring that occurs just above the gastroesophageal junction is called *Schatzki ring*. The origin of these lesions is unclear, but they are probably acquired. They are often found in asymptomatic individuals. There is some evidence that gastroesophageal reflux is associated with the development of Schatzki ring.

Symptoms arise when the ring narrows the esophageal lumen to less than 13 mm in diameter and are rare if the lumen is more than 20 mm in diameter. A typical presenting symptom of a patient with an esophageal ring is intermittent dysphagia for solid foods. The patient may point to the area of the ring. At times a bolus of food may become impacted; the patient then regurgitates and then may be able to resume eating without further difficulty. The intermittency of the dysphagia, the chronicity of the condition, and the difficulty in making the diagnosis unless specifically suspected often result in misdiagnosis and inappropriate therapy.

The diagnosis of esophageal ring is best made by barium swallow with a barium-coated marshmallow. The lower esophageal ring is best detected when the lower segment of the esophagus is distended, as it is during a Valsalva maneuver. Endoscopy is sometimes helpful to differentiate rings from annular strictures secondary to either reflux esophagitis or carcinoma. Cervical webs are often missed on conventional radiography but may be detected with cine studies. The webs usually are detected on the anterior surface of the esophagus, and lateral and oblique films are needed to demonstrate these lesions. Endoscopy often fails to visualize cervical webs and may disrupt the lesion during blind passage of the instrument into the esophagus. The endoscope may reveal an esophageal ring during air sufflation of the distal esophagus.

If the webs are associated with iron deficiency, treatment of the anemia causes rapid regression of the web. Otherwise, therapy involves mechanical disruption of the ring or web as well as reassurance, along with the recommendation to chew food well and slowly. Bougienage with a large-caliber dilator often disrupts the lower esophageal ring with complete relief of the dysphagia. The procedure causes transient discomfort but much less pain than does pneumatic dilation. It is ordinarily done by a gastroenterologist. Rarely, symptoms may persist after bougienage, and pneumatic dilation or even surgery may be necessary.

Globus Sensation

Globus sensation is a diagnosis often incorrectly made in patients with dysphagia who have no demonstrable organic disease. However, this condition does not produce dysphagia and should not be used to explain away the symptom of dysphagia. Patients with globus describe the sensation of a lump in the throat, but they

Table 42.4. Treatment of Gastroesophageal Reflux

Intervention	Specific Change	Mechanism of Improvement
Lifestyle changes		
Elevate head of bed (6- to 8-inch blocks)		Decreased acid contact time
Avoid drugs that decrease LES pressure	Theophylline, nitrates, calcium channel blockers, benzodiazepines	Avoids decrease of lower sphincter pressure
Avoid irritants	Citrus, coffee	Avoids direct mucosal damage
Stop smoking		Removes inhibition of H2 blockers, increases lower sphincter pressure
Avoid eating before sleep	3 h	Avoids gastric distension
Antacids	As needed	Decreases gastric acid
Alginic acid (Gaviscon)	As needed	Barrier protectant
H_2 antagonists (OTC)	As needed	Decreases gastric acid
Pharmacologic therapy		
H_2 antagonists[a]		
Cimetidine (Tagamet)	400 mg b.i.d. (nonerosive symptomatic disease) 800 mg b.i.d. (erosive esophagitis)	Decreases acid secretion
Ranitidine (Zantac)	150 mg b.i.d. (nonerosive symptomatic disease) 150 mg q.i.d. (erosive esophagitis)	
Famotidine (Pepcid)	20 mg b.i.d. (nonerosive symptomatic disease) 40 mg b.i.d. (erosive esophagitis)	
Nizatidine (Axid)	150 mg b.i.d. (all forms of reflux disease)	
Metoclopramide (Reglan)	5–10 mg q.i.d.	Metoclopramide increases LES pressure, increases esophageal clearance, and accelerates gastric emptying
Sucralfate (Carafate)	1 g q.i.d.	Mucosal protection (not FDA approved for treatment of reflux)
Proton pump inhibition		
Lansoprazole (Prevacid)	30 mg/day (am) 15 mg/day (am) maintenance	
Omeprazole (Prilosec)	20 mg/day (am)	Decreases acid secretion
Rabeprazole (Aciphex)	20 mg/day (am)	Decreases acid secretion
Pantoprazole (Protonix)	40 mg/day (am)	
Esomeprazole (Nexium)	40 mg/day (am) acute 20 mg/day(am) acute, maintenance	
Surgery	Nissen fundoplication	Creates intra-abdominal esophagus and augments antireflux barrier
	Belsey Mark IV repair	
	Hill procedure	
Endoscopic treatment	Suturing device	Mechanism unknown
	Radiofrequency energy to sphincter	Barrier tightening, decreased sphincter relaxation?

[a]Nocturnal H_2 antagonists are insufficient antireflux therapy.

do not actually have difficulty swallowing. At times, these symptoms may be more pronounced with eating. However, when specifically questioned, patients deny dysphagia or food sticking or being held up in this region and they state that the symptom is present even when they are not eating. The pathogenesis of this condition is unknown, but hypertonicity of the upper esophageal sphincter, as a primary disorder or as a consequence of esophageal reflux, has been suggested. Gastroesophageal reflux should be ruled out (see below) before a psychologic disturbance (see Chapter 21) is diagnosed. Reassurance and an explanation of the problem form the basis for treatment. Mild sedation may be helpful. The significance of this disorder is mainly its differentiation from other conditions that produce true dysphagia.

ESOPHAGEAL CHEST PAIN

Chest pain is a common and difficult diagnostic challenge. It is now well accepted that esophageal disease can be implicated as a cause of recurrent chest pain. The prevalence of esophageal chest pain is unknown. However, 10% to 30% of first cardiac catheterizations done to evaluate chest pain are normal. At least 50% of patients with normal coronary catheterizations have identifiable esophageal abnormalities; 50% of patients with normal coronary arteries continue to be disabled by chest pain, despite being told that they do not have heart disease (11). These patients often continue to receive antianginal medications, continue to have approximately two physician visits a year for chest pain, and are hospitalized about once a year for continuing evaluation, at significant cost (11).

Etiology and Pathogenesis

Esophageal chest pain has been attributed to stimulation of esophageal chemoreceptors by acid reflux or of mechanoreceptors by smooth muscle spasm or esophageal distension. Cold or hot liquids may cause severe chest pain, suggesting an alteration in temperature receptors in the esophagus. Transient myoischemia may be a cause of pain in patients with spastic motility disorders. Such patients have an increased frequency of psychiatric disorders and have personality profiles similar to those of patients with the irritable bowel syndrome (see Chapter 44), suggesting that chronic stress may play a role in the pathogenesis of chest pain. Panic disorder has been diagnosed in up to one-third of patients with chest pain and normal coronary angiograms (12).

Two major abnormalities have been associated with esophageal chest pain: esophageal motility disorders and gastroesophageal reflux disease (GERD). Studies using ambulatory pH monitoring have demonstrated gastroesophageal reflux in approximately 45% of patients with unexplained chest pain. The typical symptom of gastroesophageal reflux—heartburn—is seen in about half of patients with GERD-related chest pain. Approximately 30% of patients with esophageal chest pain have a demonstrable motility disorder, and of this group, the most common disorder is the *nutcracker esophagus* (hypertensive esophagus, supersqueezer). This manometric abnormality is characterized by normal peristaltic contractions in the distal esophagus with contraction amplitude greater than 2 standard deviations above normal (less than 180 mm Hg) associated with chest pain (Table 42.2). Many of these patients have prolonged duration of contractions as well. *DES* (see above) is the motility disorder usually considered the principal cause of esophageal chest pain; however, studies have found it to be uncommon, representing less than 10% of esophageal motility abnormalities in patients with noncardiac chest pain (13). Other disorders, such as an *isolated elevated LES pressure* (hypertensive LES) and *achalasia,* are rarely associated with noncardiac chest pain. A large number of patients (approximately 35%) have contraction abnormalities that do not fit into one of the four categories defined here. These patients have been historically grouped under the general category of *nonspecific esophageal motility disorders;* however, these patients have had their motility abnormalities re-evaluated and are now classified as having ineffective esophageal motility. This abnormality is defined as low amplitude esophageal contractions (<30 mm Hg) in more than 20% of swallows (see Table 42.2) (14).

Evaluation requires consultation with a gastroenterologist. Few patients have spontaneous chest pain during stationary esophageal motility testing (even if esophageal motility is abnormal), but chest pain is often reproduced when the esophagus is stimulated with intravenous edrophonium (Tensilon). This cholinergic agonist reproduces chest pain accompanied by high-amplitude esophageal contractions in 20% to 30% of patients with chest pain and normal coronary arteries (11). Edrophonium does not cause narrowing of the coronary arteries nor does it cause chest pain in normal subjects or in patients with irritable bowel syndrome. A positive test indicates that the chest pain is of esophageal origin.

Diagnosis

Unfortunately, the history is not reliable in differentiating esophageal from cardiac pain or in differentiating the various esophageal causes of chest pain. Location, exertional onset, and radiation do not distinguish the two entities. Heartburn, dysphagia, or odynophagia suggests an esophageal etiology, but overlap does exist. Pain lasting longer than 1 hour or pain that awakens the patient from sleep is more likely to be esophageal but is occasionally seen with cardiac disease. Therapeutic trials with antacids or nitrates do not distinguish between the two diseases. Intraesophageal acid perfusion can cause pain and ST-T wave changes indistinguishable from that due to coronary artery disease, so cardiac disease must be ruled out before the esophagus can be implicated. A musculoskeletal etiology should be sought by careful examination of the chest wall and the costochondral joints. Peptic ulcer disease should be excluded by history, and if biliary tract disease is suspected, it should be excluded by ultrasound. Endoscopy is normal in 80% to 90% of cases and should not be done routinely (15). If heartburn is present, consideration should be given to a short (3- to 4-week) therapeutic trial of antireflux therapy. If this trial is unsuccessful, the patient should be referred, if possible, to a gastroenterologist who has equipment to perform 24-hour ambulatory esophageal pH monitoring. With this latter method, the frequency of reflux can be assessed, episodes of pain can be correlated with episodes of reflux, and esophageal pH can be monitored during exercise. If this study is negative, esophageal manometry with provocative testing with edrophonium should be performed. Using this systematic approach, an esophageal etiology can be established in more than 60% of patients with noncardiac chest pain.

Treatment

If gastroesophageal reflux is diagnosed, treatment should proceed as outlined later in this chapter, although most patients require higher dosages of proton pump inhibitors for pain relief. Treatment of patients who have only positive provocative tests is more difficult and controversial (Table 42.3). Once cardiac disease has been ruled out, reassurance should be given to all patients, specifically indicating that the esophagus, and not the heart, is the cause of their pain. Many experience a decrease in pain with this single intervention. Patients with spastic disorders or with nutcracker esophagus may respond to a nitrate or a calcium channel blocker. Hydralazine may be tried in patients with symptomatic esophageal spasm if nitrates or calcium blockers are not successful. Trazodone HCl (Desyrel), an antidepressant, has been used successfully to relieve chest pain in these patients and is particularly useful in patients with other symptoms suggestive of depression. Imipramine (50 mg at bedtime) also has been shown to lower the frequency of esophageal chest pain (16). This dosage, lower than that used to treat depression, is suspected to have a visceral analgesic effect on smooth muscle. Tranquilizers and anticholinergics have been used successfully in some patients. Patients with symptoms unresponsive to these measures may respond to biofeedback or to other psychologic interventions. Rarely surgery with a long esophageal myotomy is required in patients with severe pain in whom pharmacologic therapy has failed. Many patients with esophageal chest pain, whatever the cause, continue to have intermittent symptoms despite therapeutic intervention.

GASTROESOPHAGEAL REFLUX

GERD is common in the United States. Approximately 10% of Americans experience daily heartburn and up to 33% have symptoms monthly. Most patients complain of burning substernal pain that radiates upward, often aggravated by meals and by lying down and relieved by sitting up. Approximately 10% of people have chest pain that is similar to that of angina pectoris as the sole manifestation of reflux. An unknown number of people have hoarseness, cough, or wheezing as manifestations of GERD (17). In most cases the diagnosis and treatment of GERD can be managed successfully by the primary care provider; however, 10% to 15% of patients develop complications and require referral to a gastroenterologist.

Etiology and Pathogenesis

The etiology of GERD is unknown. Several defects contribute to the development and progression of the disease. By far the most significant is an abnormality of the antireflux barrier: the LES. Two major abnormalities of the LES are associated with an increased frequency of reflux: *a low basal LES pressure* and *transient LES relaxation* unassociated with a swallow. The latter abnormality is the most common cause of an episode of reflux. Abnormal esophageal epithelial resistance (increased permeability to hydrogen ions), abnormalities of gastric emptying, gastric distension, and the nature of the gastric refluxate (acid, pepsin, and bile) all contribute to the development of GERD.

Diagnosis

Several diagnostic tests are readily available to establish the clinical diagnosis. No single test provides complete information about the cause and consequences of reflux, so careful selection among the available modalities is required. In patients with mild heartburn, a therapeutic trial of what has been termed phase I therapy, including antacids or H_2 receptor antagonists in over the counter doses, may be an effective diagnostic approach. Studies have evaluated the utility of high dose proton pump inhibitors (the equivalent of 40 to 60 mg omeprazole daily for 1 to 2 weeks) to determine if symptoms are relieved (18). If successful, no further workup may be needed. Patients with dysphagia and chest pain should be considered for early study to determine the cause of their symptoms. If the diagnosis of reflux disease is established, treatment can proceed as outlined below. Also, patients with symptoms for more than 10 years, especially if they are 50 years or older, should have early endoscopy because of their higher prevalence of Barrett esophagus (see below).

A *barium swallow* is the simplest, least expensive procedure to perform in the evaluation of symptomatic GERD, but it is normal 40% to 60% of the time and should therefore be used primarily in the evaluation of patients with suspected reflux who also have dysphagia (see above). Several other points are important in interpreting a barium study. Hiatal hernia is present in 40% to 60% of the general population. Mild free reflux may be seen in 30% of normal individuals. These findings, together or alone, should not be used to make a diagnosis of reflux disease. The presence of mucosal irregularities, stricture, or esophageal ulcer suggests a high likelihood (85% to 95%) that GERD is present.

Endoscopy (esophagoscopy) is the best study for the diagnosis and evaluation of reflux esophagitis or of other complications of GERD such as stricture or Barrett epithelium. If esophagitis is present at endoscopy, the diagnosis of GERD is established with 95% certainty, and no further workup is required. If a stricture is encountered, it should be biopsied to rule out carcinoma (dilation may be done at the same sitting in some patients). If Barrett mucosa is observed, biopsies can be taken to confirm the diagnosis and to rule out dysplasia or *in situ* carcinoma.

The diagnosis of GERD is established in most patients by the combination of history, response to therapy, and endoscopy. If the diagnosis is still in doubt or the patient presents with an atypical symptom, 24-hour *ambulatory pH monitoring* should be performed. (Endoscopy may be normal in 40% of patients in whom reflux is subsequently verified by prolonged intraesophageal pH monitoring.) The test is performed by placing a 2-mm flexible antimony probe transnasally 5 cm above the LES. The probe is connected to a recording box similar to an ambulatory electrodiagraphic monitor and worn about the waist. The patient can then be observed at home eating a normal diet. Ambulatory monitoring is extremely useful in patients with noncardiac chest pain, in patients with chronic pulmonary or otolaryngologic symptoms suggestive of reflux, or in patients with typical symptoms when a diagnosis is elusive. Probes may be placed at multiple levels in the esophagus to evaluate patients with atypical symptoms. All patients who are being considered for surgery should have pH monitoring to confirm the diagnosis before the operation. The study is extremely reproducible and is currently the most sensitive and specific diagnostic test for the presence of abnormal acid reflux.

A suggested approach to the diagnosis of GERD is outlined in Fig. 42.2.

Treatment

Treatment has traditionally been divided into phases (Table 42.4), implying that each is a distinct step to be followed in all patients. At present it is accepted

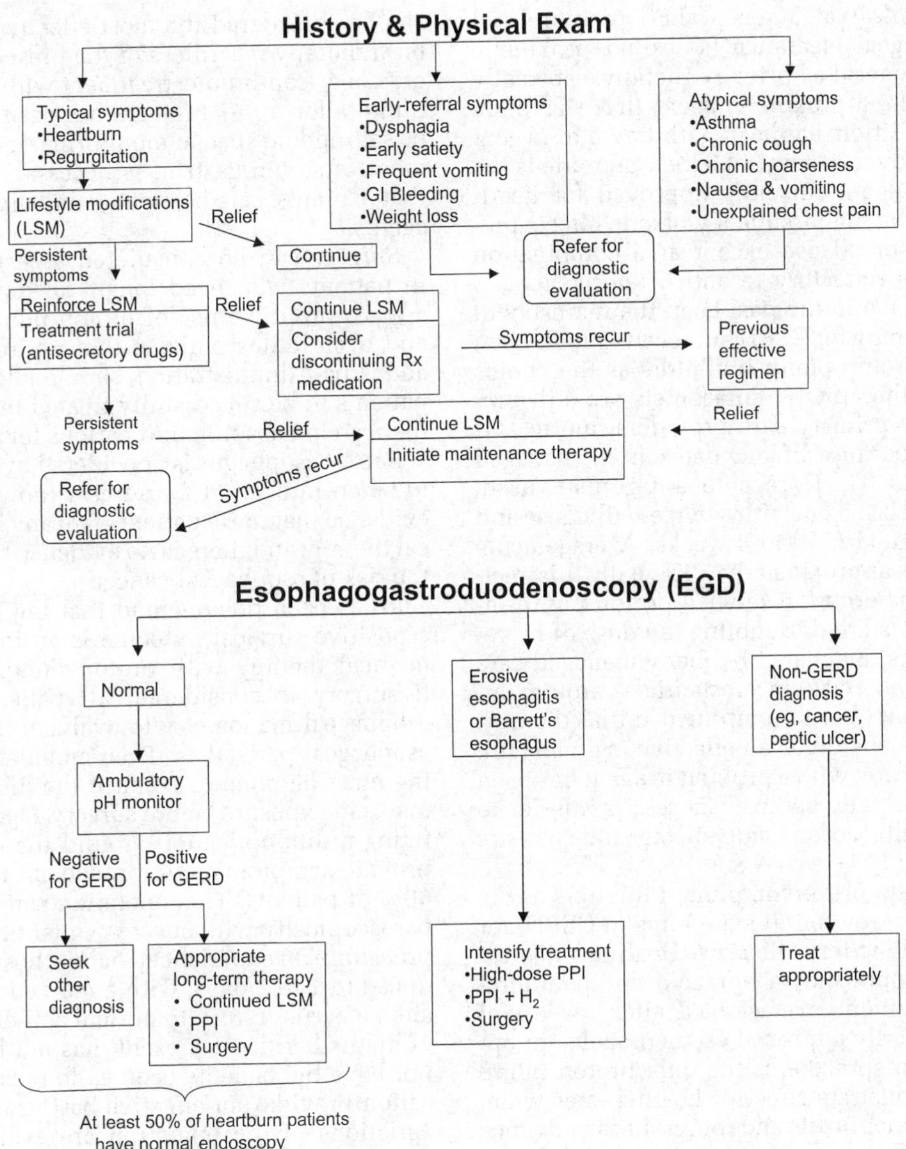

Figure 42.2. Approach to patients with gastroesophageal reflux.

that therapy should be individualized using a combination of lifestyle modifications (historically *phase I therapy*) and pharmacologic or surgical interventions The overall goals of treatment are the complete relief of symptoms to improve the quality of life of the patient, the healing of erosive esophagitis if present, and the prevention of symptomatic relapse or complications.

Lifestyle modifications include elevating the head of the bed on 6- to 8-inch blocks or using a wedge designed to be placed in the bed under the shoulders and upper back. The patient should avoid sleeping on more pillows because this might actually increase abdominal pressure and contribute to more reflux. Certain foods (e.g., coffee, citrus juice, and spices) are direct esophageal irritants and should be avoided. The patient should be instructed not to lie down after a meal because this promotes greater reflux. Avoidance of food 3 hours before going to bed has also been shown to decrease episodes of reflux. Drugs that decrease LES pressure (e.g., calcium channel blockers, nitrates, sedatives, and theophylline) should be avoided. Antacids and over the counter H_2 antagonists can be considered adjuncts to lifestyle modifications and should be used as needed to relieve daytime symptoms. The current practice of using proton pump inhibitors as first-line therapy has relegated lifestyle modifications to a minor role in many guidelines, though the American College of Gastroenterology guidelines recommend that such modifications are part of any treatment program for GERD. Few would use behavioral modification as the only therapy for established GERD.

Pharmacologic therapy is aimed at decreasing gastric acid secretion (H_2 antagonists or proton pump inhibitors). Agents that augment LES pressure and improve esophageal clearance (so-called prokinetic agents) are rarely used as primary therapy, especially because cisapride, a prokinetic agent that was often used for this condition, has been withdrawn from general use due to adverse events. Metoclopramide is the only prokinetic agent currently approved for heartburn; however, the high frequency of side effects precludes its widespread use except as a combination agent in patients refractory to antisecretory therapy. H_2 antagonists have in the past been the mainstay of antisecretory therapy for GERD but recently have been supplanted by proton pump inhibitors as the choice even for initial therapy. H_2 antagonists are still prescribed by many primary care providers due to low initial costs or because of mandates from managed care organizations. If an H_2 receptor antagonist is used, treatment should be begun with a twice-daily dose and should be continued for 6 to 8 weeks. Average acute healing rates are approximately 50% with this regimen. If symptoms do not resolve, a proton pump inhibitor should be started. Doubling the dose of H_2 receptor antagonists, mandated by many managed care algorithms, does not result in substantial symptom improvement compared with continued initial therapy, so should not be considered an effective regimen (19). Combination therapy with a prokinetic agent has been abandoned, principally because success is inferior to proton pump inhibitors and side effects (and cost) are greater.

Current data support proton pump inhibitors as the most effective therapy for all symptoms of GERD, for both acute and long-term therapy. Healing rates for omeprazole, lansoprazole, rabeprazole, and pantoprazole are equivalent and average 85% after 8 weeks of therapy. The recently approved esomeprazole, an optical isomer of omeprazole, is the only proton pump inhibitor to demonstrate superior healing rates when compared with omeprazole and represents an advance in antisecretory therapy (20). Proton pump inhibitors should be considered in all patients as potential first-line agents for treatment.

Long-Term Treatment

GERD is a chronic disease. Symptomatic and endoscopic relapse of esophagitis is seen in up to 80% of patients initially treated successfully. Therefore, most patients require some form of long-term therapy (21,22), which must be individualized. H_2 receptor antagonists at full dosage are approved for maintenance treatment but are effective in maintaining symptomatic and endoscopic remission in fewer than 50% of patients. The proton pump inhibitors give the best symptomatic relief, and all five are effective agents in maintaining symptom relief and remission of esophagitis (approximately 85% of patients, on daily therapy) (22). It is now clear that it may be as difficult to maintain symptomatic remission in patients with nonerosive GERD as it is to treat patients with erosive esophagitis or Barrett esophagus so proton pump inhibitors can be considered the most effective agents for long-term therapy regardless of the presence or absence of erosions. Continuous treatment with proton pump inhibitors for up to 11 years has been demonstrated to be safe and no special monitoring, including measurement of serum gastrin, is necessary (23). It is likely that patients can be treated indefinitely with these agents.

Surgery can be considered as a treatment option in patients who need long-term daily medical therapy. Appropriate use of proton pump inhibitor therapy, even in doses higher than approved by the Food and Drug Administration, should allow essentially all patients to be successfully treated medically; as such there are no absolute indications for surgery.

Barrett esophagus is considered by some authorities to be an indication for surgery; however, there is no evidence that these patients fare any better with medical therapy and there is no evidence that surgery alters the risk of esophageal cancer.

It has been documented that the best predictor of a positive surgical outcome is an initial response to medical therapy with proton pump inhibitors (24). If surgery is considered, all patients should have esophageal manometry to evaluate LES pressure and esophageal peristalsis. Then ambulatory pH monitoring must be done to confirm the diagnosis of abnormal acid exposure before surgery. Operations incorporating a fundoplication around the distal esophagus provide symptomatic improvement in approximately 90% of patients. This operation can now be done laparoscopically with success equal to that of the open procedure. In experienced hands, hospitalization is reduced to 1 to 2 days, with a marked decrease in pain and an earlier return to normal activity. Simple repair of hiatus hernia, if present, has not been as effective nor have the benefits been as long lasting. Fundoplication provides an effective barrier to reflux. Several variations of the operation are available, and local surgical expertise generally dictates the specific operation that is performed. Complications include dysphagia, which may require esophageal dilatation, and the gas-bloat syndrome from inability to belch. Recent data indicate that over half of the patients treated with antireflux surgery have returned to using medication 10 years or more after the operation, a reminder that this intervention may not be permanent (25). The clinician should also be reminded that there is a learning curve for this operation, estimated at 20 to 30 procedures. Care in selecting an experienced surgeon is critical. Antireflux surgery for patients with scleroderma should be avoided at all costs, because it may markedly exacerbate dysphagia. Vagotomy is not indicated in the treatment of GERD.

The Food and Drug Administration has approved two endoscopic therapies for GERD: radiofrequency ablation of the LES region and an endoscopic sewing device. Each has been evaluated in only a small number of patients in uncontrolled single studies. Further evaluation is needed to determine the role of these procedures in GERD.

Complications

The complications of reflux include hemorrhage, ulcerations, stricture formation, and development of Barrett mucosa. Esophagitis is the cause of 5% to 10% of all cases of upper gastrointestinal hemorrhage. Peptic ulcers and strictures must be differentiated from malignancy and from ingestion of caustic substances. The presence of a midesophageal ulcer or stricture should raise the suspicion of Barrett mucosa (columnar-type mucosa that replaces the squamous mucosa of the tubular esophagus). This type of mucosa has characteristic staining features that differentiate it from normal gastric tissue. This metaplastic intestinal type of epithelium is a premalignant condition. Patients with Barrett mucosa should therefore undergo regular endoscopic surveillance (every 2 to 3 years) for the development of cancer.

HIATUS HERNIA

Herniation of a part of the stomach through the diaphragm through the normal esophageal hiatus into the thorax is called a hiatus hernia. The defect is common, but the precise prevalence is very much influenced by the zeal of the radiologist during the performance of an upper gastrointestinal series. Estimates of prevalence therefore range from 30% to 60% overall. The defect is twice as common in women as in men and is extremely common in elderly people, affecting perhaps 70% to 80% of the population who are older than age 60. Many clinicians still erroneously correlate hiatus hernia with reflux esophagitis, but certainly a hernia may exist without producing symptomatic reflux and reflux may occur without hernia. If a patient has clear-cut reflux esophagitis, the treatment should not be influenced by the presence of a hiatus hernia. If a patient who does not have reflux is inadvertently discovered to have a hiatus hernia, no treatment is indicated. (In the past, needless surgery was done to reduce a hiatus hernia in patients whose symptoms were not clearly attributable to the defect.) A large hiatus hernia (>5 cm) may predispose to more serious reflux and itself cause symptoms of chest pain or dysphagia.

A *paraesophageal hernia,* the hernia of part of the stomach through the diaphragm adjacent to the gastroesophageal junction, is potentially dangerous because about one-third of the time the hernia incarcerates and produces acute obstruction, which is a surgical emergency.

General References*

DeVault KR, Castell DO. **Updated guidelines for the diagnosis and treatment of gastroesophageal reflux disease.** Am J Gastroenterol 1999;94:1434.

The guidelines of the American College of Gastroenterology. This guideline statement has been endorsed by the other major GI societies.

Katz PO. Treatment of gastroesophageal reflux disease: use of algorithms to aid in management. Am J Gasteroenterol 1999; 94[Suppl]:3.

A general overview of treatment.

Katz PO, Castell DO. Approach to the patient with unexplained chest pain. Am J Gastroenterol 2000;95[Suppl]:4.

A review of the current management of this problem.

Sampliner RE. Practice Parameters Committee of the American College of Gastroenterology. **Practice guidelines on the diagnosis, surveillance, and therapy of Barrett's esophagus.** Am J Gastroenterol 1998;93:1028.

Guidelines for management of Barrett esophagus.

Specific References

1. Devesa SS, Blot WJ, Fraumeni JF Jr. Changing patterns in the incidence of esophageal and gastric carcinoma in the United States. Cancer 1998;83:2049.
2. McLoughlin RF, Cooperberg PL, Mathieson JR, et al. High resolution endoluminal ultrasonography in the staging of esophageal carcinoma. J Ultrasound Med 1995;14:725.
3. Fleischer DE, Haddad NG. Neoplasms of the esophagus. In: Castell DO, ed. The esophagus, 3rd edition. Philadelphia: Lippincott, Williams & Wilkins, 1999:235.
4. Bondi JL, Goodwin DH, Garrett JM. Vigorous achalasia: its clinical interpretation and significance. Am J Gastroenterol 1972;58:145.
5. Katz PO, Richter JE, Cowan R, et al. Apparent complete lower esophageal sphincter relaxation in achalasia. Gastroenterology 1986;90:978.
6. Meijssen MAC, Tilanus HW, van Blankenstein M, et al. Achalasia complicated by oesophageal squamous cell carcinoma. A prospective study in 195 patients. Gut 1992;33: 155.
7. Pasricha PJ, Rai R, Ravich WJ, et al. Botulinum toxin for achalasia: long-term outcome and predictors of response. Gastroenterology 1996;110:1410.
8. Richter JE, Castell DO. Diffuse esophageal spasm: a reappraisal. Ann Intern Med 1984;100:242.
9. Katz PO, Dalton CB, Richter JE, et al. Esophageal testing of patients with non-cardiac chest pain or dysphagia. Results of three years experience with 1161 patients. Ann Intern Med 1987;106:593.
10. Cohen S, Fisher R, Lipshutz W, et al. The pathogenesis of esophageal dysfunction in scleroderma and Raynaud's disease. J Clin Invest 1972;51:2663.
11. Katz PO. Approach to the patient with non cardiac chest pain. Semin Gastroenterol Dis 2001;12:38.
12. Katon W, Hall ML, Russo J. Chest pain: relationship of psychiatric illness to coronary arteriographic results. Am J Med 1988;84:1.
13. Dalton CB, Castell DO, Hewson EG, et al. Diffuse esophageal spasm. A rare motility disorder not characterized by high-amplitude contractions. Dig Dis Sci 1991;36:1025.
14. Leite LP, Johnston BT, Barrett J, et al. Ineffective esophageal motility: the primary finding in patients with nonspecific esophageal motility disorder. Dig Dis Sci 1997;42:1859.
15. Cherian P, Smith LF, Bardhan KD, et al. Esophageal tests in the evaluation of non-cardiac chest pain. Dis Esoph 1995;8: 129.
16. Cannon RO, Quyyumi AA, Mincemoyer R, et al. Imipramine in patients with chest pain despite normal coronary angiograms. N Engl J Med 1994;330:1411.
17. Locke GR, Talley NJ, Fett SL, et al. Prevalence and clinical spectrum of gastroesophageal reflux: a population-based study in Olmsted County, Minnesota. Gastroenterology 1997;112: 1448.
18. Fass R, Fennerty MB, Ofman JJ, et al. The clinical and economic value of a short course of omeprazole in patients with noncardiac chest pain. Gastroenterology 1998;115:42.
19. **19.** Kahrilas PJ, Fennerty MB, Joelsson B. High- versus standard-dose ranitidine for control of heartburn in poorly responsive

*Bold print (general references) and bold numerals (specific references) denote clinical trials, meta-analyses, or consensus-based recommendations.

acid reflux disease: a prospective, controlled trial. Am J Gastroenterol 1999;94:92.
20. Kahrilas PJ, Falk GW, Johnson DA, et al. Esomeprazole improves healing and symptom resolution as compared with omeprazole in reflux oesophagitis patients: a randomized controlled trial. Aliment Pharmacol Ther 2000;14:1249.
21. Howden CS, Castell DO, Cohen S, et al. The rationale for continuous maintenance treatment of reflux esophagitis. Arch Intern Med 1995;155:1465.
22. Vigneri S, Termini R, Leandro G, et al. A comparison of five maintenance therapies for reflux esophagitis. N Engl J Med 1995;333:1106.
23. Klinkenberg-Knol EC, Festen HPM, Jansen JBMJ, et al. Long-term treatment with omeprazole for refractory reflux esophagitis. Ann Intern Med 1994;121:161.
24. So JB, Zeitels SM, Rattner DW. Outcomes of atypical symptoms attributed to gastroesophageal reflux treated by laparoscopic fundoplication. Surgery 1998;124:28.
25. Spechler S, Lee E, Ahnen D, et al. Long-term outcome of medical and surgical therapies for gastroesophageal reflux disease: follow-up of a randomized controlled trial. JAMA 2001;285:2331.

CHAPTER 43

Peptic Ulcer Disease

PHILIP O. KATZ, MD

EPIDEMIOLOGY AND NATURAL HISTORY

Peptic ulcer disease is still a common problem, even though the incidence of duodenal ulcers has decreased over the last 40 years (1) and hospital admissions for uncomplicated duodenal ulcer have essentially disappeared. The incidence of gastric ulceration has not changed over this time (1) nor has the incidence of complications, such as bleeding, perforation, obstruction, and penetration, of peptic ulcers in general (2). The economic impact of ulceration is over 5 billion dollars a year in the United States (3).

Until relatively recently, duodenal ulcer was twice as common and gastric ulcer slightly more common in men than in women, but currently the prevalence of both is approximately the same in men and women (2). Also, the incidence of duodenal ulcer has fallen markedly in younger age groups, so that the prevalence and incidence of duodenal and gastric ulcers are now higher in older compared with younger age groups (4).

Ulcers are usually less than 1 cm in diameter, although giant ulcers (larger than 2.5 cm) occasionally occur. Duodenal ulcers are almost always located in the duodenal bulb or immediately postbulbar, within 3 cm of the pyloric duodenal junction. Ulcers distal to the duodenal bulb should raise the suspicion of the Zollinger-Ellison syndrome (discussed later in this chapter) or Crohn disease of the duodenum. Gastric ulcers are most commonly located on the lesser curvature, at the junction of the body and antrum of the stomach. There is no risk of cancer in a duodenal ulcer, but 1% to 3% of gastric ulcers not attributable to nonsteroidal anti-inflammatory drugs (NSAIDs) are malignant.

Untreated duodenal ulcer disease can be chronic. Estimates are that 50% to 90% of patients have a recurrence, often asymptomatic, within 1 year of diagnosis if curative therapy is not given (5). The rate of recurrences peaks over 5 years and then decreases over 10 to 20 years (6,7). The recurrence rate of gastric ulcers has not been studied as extensively but appears to be lower (5). Both duodenal and gastric ulcers tend to recur in the same place as the index ulcer. Long-term studies suggest that bleeding or perforation occurs at a rate of 1% to 3% a year, with a lifetime incidence of approximately 20% (8), if the ulcer is not adequately treated. Recurrent hemorrhage occurs in approximately 50% of patients who have had a prior bleed. The complication rate may be reduced by maintenance therapy (9) and can be eliminated if the bacterium *Helicobacter pylori* is eradicated (see below). The major risk of death from ulcer disease is on the first presentation (10).

PATHOPHYSIOLOGY

Duodenal Ulcer

Duodenal ulcer disease has always been viewed as the result of an imbalance between the normal duodenal defense mechanisms and the amount of acid delivered to the duodenum from the stomach. Multiple abnormalities have been identified that result in this imbalance: increased parietal cell mass, increased capacity of parietal cells to secrete acid, increased vagal drive to secrete acid, defective inhibition of gastrin release and of gastric secretion after gastric acidification or after a meal (these first four abnormalities result in a considerably increased acid production compared with normal), abnormally rapid gastric emptying, and altered duodenal defense mechanisms, including bicarbonate secretion, mucus production, vascular integrity, and endogenous prostaglandin production. It is now clear that these imbalances are caused by hypersecretory states, ingestion of NSAIDs, and, most importantly, by *H. pylori* infection.

Gastric Ulcer

The pathogenesis of gastric ulceration is unclear. It is generally believed that the basic defect in gastric ulcer formation is the disruption of the gastric mucosal barrier. This barrier can be broken by such irritants as bile, alcohol, and aspirin. These experimental observations help explain the epidemiologic data associating alcohol with acute gastritis and aspirin with gastric ulcers and erosions. Furthermore, in patients with gastric ulcers, radiologic and manometric studies have suggested an increased duodenal gastric reflux. This reflux of bile across an incompetent pyloric sphincter results in the disruption of the mucosal barrier. Once the barrier is broken, hydrogen ion may diffuse back into the gastric cells, leading to ulceration via local histamine release, vasodilation, and tissue damage. Thus, according to this concept, gastric ulcer formation requires injury to the gastric mucosal barrier and the presence of some, but not necessarily an excessive amount of, acid. *H. pylori* infection has been associated with gastric ulcer disease in most patients, and the presence of gastritis may make the mucosa more susceptible to injury.

RISK FACTORS

Helicobacter pylori

It is now well accepted that *H. pylori* infection is the most common and important risk factor for duodenal ulcer. The risk of gastric ulcer is probably multifactorial, although many gastric ulcers are associated with *H. pylori* and the decreased recurrence of gastric ulcer after eradication of infection suggests that *H. pylori* is a risk factor.

H. pylori is a gram-negative spiral organism found exclusively in gastric epithelium. It may be seen in the duodenal bulb in regions where there is gastric metaplasia. In the United States, the organism is found in 10% of healthy people under 30 years of age and in approximately 60% of healthy people over age 60 (11). The rate of infection varies by country and by region of the United States and is higher in lower socioeconomic areas and in developing countries (11). The organism is probably spread by person to person contact.

H. pylori is the etiologic agent for chronic nonerosive antral gastritis (see below), is present in the stomach in 70% of patients with a peptic ulcer, and is the most common cause of that disease (12). It is estimated that 15% to 20% of infected patients will develop an ulcer in their lifetime. Other diseases associated with *H. pylori* infection are the rare B-cell mucosa-associated lymphoid tissue (MALT) lymphoma and gastric adenocarcinoma.

Eradication of the organism appears to result in accelerated duodenal ulcer healing (13) and significantly decreased ulcer recurrence 1 and 2 years after treatment (13,14). The rate of reinfection is unknown but appears to be less than 1% up to 5 years after treatment. Eradication of *H. pylori* also reduces recurrent bleeding in patients who have bled.

NON-*HELICOBACTER PYLORI* ULCERS

It is becoming clear that 20% to 30% of gastroduodenal ulcers may be *H. pylori* negative (15,16). Most of these are NSAID related (see above), some probably due to surreptitious use. False negative *H. pylori* screening tests may, in part, account for these findings; the availability of more than one reliable test for *H. pylori* should improve the practitioner's ability to detect the organism (see below). Prior use of antibiotics, particularly macrolides, or proton pump inhibitors (PPIs) within 6 weeks of *H. pylori* testing also may result in false negative tests. The bacterium *Helicobacter heilimannii* (formerly *Gastrospirillum hominus*) is a urease producing gram negative organism found to infect gastric mucosa and has been reported in some patients with *H. pylori*-negative ulcers who have not taken NSAIDs (17).

Nonsteroidal Anti-inflammatory Drugs

There is good evidence that all *NSAIDs* can cause gastric and duodenal ulcers. The greatest risk of NSAID-induced gastric or duodenal toxicity appears to be in people over 60 years of age (18), in patients with a history of a gastrointestinal "event" (peptic ulcer or hemorrhage), in patients who are taking corticosteroids or anticoagulant drugs concurrently, and in patients taking a dose of an NSAID that is two or more times the usual prescribed dose (19). Prospective and retrospective studies have concluded that chronic use of corticosteroids by patients who are not taking NSAIDs does not increase the risk of peptic ulcer disease or its complications (20). The COX-2 specific NSAIDs (celecoxib and rofecoxib) are associated with a significantly lower risk of gastric ulceration and major complications, including gastrointestinal bleeding, compared with traditional nonselective NSAIDs (21,22). These NSAIDs should be strongly considered in patients who require anti-inflammatory drugs, especially those at risk for complications from this class of agents.

Other Factors

Genetic factors were once thought to play an important role in the development of peptic ulcers, but since the recognition of the major risk factors—*H. pylori* and NSAIDs—for peptic ulcer disease, the role of inheritance appears to be minimal (23).

The role of *stress* in the pathogenesis of peptic ulcer disease seems clinically evident but has been difficult to quantitate. In fact, in a case–control study, the number of stressors in the lives of patients with duodenal ulcer was no greater than in control subjects (24).

Cigarette smoking has been repeatedly demonstrated to be associated with an increased frequency of duodenal ulcer disease, with frequencies ranging between 33% and 100% above those found among nonsmokers (25,26). Cigarette smoking may increase the frequency of recurrence if *Helicobacter* is not eradicated (27). There is no epidemiologic evidence that alcohol is ulcerogenic, although it is a known cause of acute gastritis. Coffee, although not ulcerogenic, may exacerbate symptoms of peptic disease.

Certain disease states have been associated with an increased risk of peptic ulcer disease. Evidence of such associations must be carefully evaluated in light of the relatively high prevalence of ulcer disease in the general population and the frequent use of ulcerogenic drugs. However, there is good evidence linking peptic ulcer disease with chronic obstructive pulmonary disease, alcoholic cirrhosis, and chronic renal failure (28–30).

Conditions that lead to increased gastric acid secretion also predispose to ulcer disease. The Zollinger-Ellison syndrome, or gastrinoma (discussed later in this chapter), is the best example of such a condition. Extensive small bowel resection may also lead to hyperplasia of antral gastrin-containing cells and result in ulcer disease. Retained antrum after gastric surgery (rarely seen today) is another example of a situation in which uninhibited acid production is associated with recurrent ulcerations.

Many drugs other than NSAIDs are reputed to be ulcerogenic, although the evidence is not well established for most of them. Aspirin is one drug that causes gastric and duodenal ulcers. Experimentally, aspirin disrupts the gastric mucosa both physiologically and anatomically, leading to ulcer formation. The risk of gastric ulcer increases sixfold when patients use more than three aspirins a day (31). Aspirin use also increases the risk of bleeding from peptic lesions (see Chapter 56). Enteric-coated or buffered aspirin has no advantage over regular aspirin with respect to these untoward effects. Alcohol used concomitantly with aspirin increases the risk for ulcer bleeding.

DIAGNOSIS

History

The most common symptom of peptic ulcer disease is epigastric distress—vague discomfort or a feeling of gnawing hunger—usually in the midline. If actual pain occurs, it is typically aching or burning.

Classically, the distress of duodenal ulcer occurs 1 to 3 hours after a meal and may awaken the patient from sleep, usually between 1 and 2 a.m.; it is relieved within minutes by food, antacids, or vomiting. Pain is minimal before breakfast. In patients with gastric ulcers, the history is more variable. In some, a similar distress–food–relief pattern exists, whereas in others there is no relationship with food. Occasionally, the distress is actually exacerbated by food.

Other less common symptoms of ulcer disease include nausea, vomiting, and dyspepsia. However, in some patients with ulcers, one or more of these symptoms may occur in the absence of typical ulcer pain. Weight loss occurs in up to 50% of patients with a benign gastric ulcer and is therefore not a helpful feature in distinguishing a benign from a malignant ulcer. Patients with duodenal ulcer often gain weight because they eat more in an attempt to control their pain.

The history may also suggest certain complications. Pyloric obstruction presents first with early satiety and then with persistent vomiting, often of undigested food. A change in the quality of the pain or radiation of the pain to the back or shoulder suggests penetration of the ulcer. A history of melena suggests bleeding.

Occasionally, one of these complications is the first clinical manifestation of peptic ulceration.

Physical Examination

The physical examination may provide supportive, although nonspecific, information. Localized epigastric tenderness is common. The presence of a succussion splash 4 hours or more postprandially is evidence of gastric outlet obstruction. Rectal examination should be included in the initial physical examination to obtain a stool specimen for testing for occult blood.

Radiologic Studies

Confirmation of the presence of peptic ulcer disease has in the past been made by use of barium studies or endoscopy, but endoscopy is now used almost exclusively because it is more accurate and because endoscopy allows biopsy of the mucosa for *H. pylori*. *Currently, there should be few if any indications to use barium radiographs to make the diagnosis of peptic ulcer disease.*

Endoscopy

Endoscopy is the diagnostic procedure of choice in the diagnosis of peptic ulcers. Experienced endoscopists are able to diagnose up to 95% of gastroduodenal ulcers (the ulcer ultimately has been proved by a second endoscopy or by surgery) (32). Guidelines for when to perform endoscopy in a patient with suspected peptic ulcer disease can only be suggested. In patients with typical symptoms of duodenal ulcer, a diagnosis can be strongly suggested, but not confirmed, by response to a therapeutic trial of medical therapy. Patients with persistent abdominal pain refractory to medical treatment or with recurrent symptoms after "curative" therapy should undergo endoscopy. Other indications for endoscopy include suspected outlet obstruction, active or suspected gastrointestinal bleeding, the need to evaluate equivocal or indeterminate findings on upper gastrointestinal series, if performed, and the need to confirm the presence or absence of *H. pylori*. No follow-up endoscopic evaluation of an uncomplicated duodenal ulcer is required because the risk for malignancy is nil.

All gastric ulcers should be biopsied to be certain they are benign. If, therefore, despite current guidelines, a gastric ulcer has been diagnosed by radiograph, endoscopy should be done, even if the ulcer looks benign, so that it can be biopsied (33). The ulcers should then be followed until they have healed, as confirmed by endoscopy. For a review of patient experience during endoscopy, see Chapter 45.

Gastric Analysis

Gastric secretory studies have enhanced the understanding of the pathophysiology of ulcer disease but have very little clinical usefulness. Although many patients with duodenal ulcer disease can be shown to hypersecrete acid, more than half of such patients actually have normal levels of acid production. Furthermore, the presence of hypersecretion does not predict the development of ulcer disease in an individual patient. Dyspepsia with a negative radiograph is not an indication for gastric analysis.

In patients with gastric ulcers, gastric analysis is not helpful. No reliable criteria exist to differentiate benign from malignant gastric ulcers.

The main indications for gastric analysis are for preoperative evaluation of patients with suspected Zollinger-Ellison syndrome (see below) or in postgastrectomy patients with recurrent ulcer disease. However, gastric analysis is not useful as an indicator of the type of surgery needed; more acid production does not necessarily require more gastric resection (34).

Serum Gastrin Measurements

Measurements of the level of gastrin in the blood are readily available and are useful in the evaluation of patients with suspected hypersecretory conditions. The fasting basal serum gastrin level is usually normal (less than 150 pg/mL) in patients with duodenal and gastric ulcer disease but is elevated, often to very high levels (usually 1,000 pg/mL or more), in patients with the Zollinger-Ellison syndrome (see below). In patients with frequently recurrent ulcers and in patients refractory to conventional therapy—features suggestive of the syndrome—two or three fasting serum gastrin determinations should be made to rule out this condition because the levels may fluctuate.

Diagnosis of *Helicobacter pylori*

Several diagnostic tests are available for the detection of *H. pylori* infection (35–37) (Table 43.1). *The gold standard is histologic testing* (38), using at least two biopsies obtained endoscopically from different parts of the antrum to ensure that the infection is not missed. This method has a sensitivity and specificity of 85% to 100%. It is time consuming, requires analysis by an experienced pathologist, and is expensive. *H. pylori* is identified in the mucosa with the use of hematoxylin and eosin, Warthin-Starry, or Giemsa stains. The sensitivity for cultures (essentially done for research only) is 50% to 95%, but the specificity approaches 100%.

For patients undergoing endoscopy, one of the most cost-effective tests is the rapid *urease (CLO) test*. In this commercially available test, the biopsy is placed in a gel-containing urea, phenol red, and a bacteriostatic agent. *H. pylori* causes a color change from yellow to red if the test is positive. This test is approximately 95% sensitive and 95% specific.

Several noninvasive tests are available for use in ambulatory patients (39). One of these is a fingerstick serologic test for the detection of immunoglobulin G (IgG) antibody. The method is approximately 90% sensitive and specific. A decline in IgG concentration correlates well with eradication of *H. pylori* 12 to 24 months after treatment (36).

Table 43.1. Diagnostic Tests for *Helicobacter pylori*

Method	Specimen	Cautions	Sensitivity (%)	Specificity (%)	Comments
		For Patients Who Do Not Require Endoscopy			
Serology test (in office)	Serum or whole blood	Lipidemia	90–95	90	Performed in 5–20 min; detects IgG (elevated in patients with *H. pylori*).
Multiwell ELISA (in laboratory)	Serum	Recent antibiotics make interpretation of a single sample difficult; 1%–5% of patients do not produce detectable antibody	90–95	90	Decrease in paired antibody titers can be assessed. Patients with rapid antibody decrease are cured. Persistent antibody after therapy is common and may slowly decrease (12–18 mo), which may represent cure or continued infection.
Urea breath test	Breath sample	Antibiotics and PPIs can cause false-negative results; should be done 4 weeks or more after last antibacterial therapy; not affected by H_2-receptor antagonists	95	95	Urease of *H. pylori* generates labeled CO_2 from breakdown of ingested urea. Breath sample taken 20–40 min after fasting. Patient ingests isotope in liquid (^{13}C) or capsule (^{14}C).
		For Patients Undergoing Endoscopy and Biopsy			
Rapid Urease test	1–2 mucosal biopsies	Same as for breath test: do not take samples from ulcers or lesions	90	98	Simple biopsy test: Urease of *H. pylori* generates ammonia and causes pH change. One-step test, no reagents, result in 1–24 hr. Least expensive method of endoscopic diagnosis.
Histology	2 mucosal biopsies	Still regarded by many as the gold standard for *H. pylori* detection	95	98	Simple and very accurate: Specimen can be reexamined in equivocal cases. Provides a permanent record. Special stains occasionally necessary to detect organism.
Culture of biopsy	1–2 mucosal biopsies	3–6 days on moist, brain–heart blood agar in Campy pac or 10% CO_2, 37°C	80	100	Provides antibiotic sensitivity information (if necessary).

ELISA, enzyme-linked immunosorbent assay; PPI, proton pump inhibitors.

The *urea breath test* is another noninvasive test. It entails giving the patient ^{13}C-labeled urea by mouth and then measuring the patient's breath for the labeled bicarbonate, which is generated when *H. pylori* splits the urea. This test is 96% sensitive and 98% specific. The ^{13}C test is read by a mass spectrometer, so the expired air must be sent out of the office for reading. This is a reliable noninvasive test for evaluation of eradication of the organism (35).

Summary

If endoscopy is planned, a rapid urease test is the diagnostic procedure of choice for *H. pylori.* If a patient with a duodenal (or gastric) ulcer has a negative rapid urease test, a serologic test should be performed to rule out a false negative result. This is more cost effective (and accurate) than histologic examination or culture (37,40). Follow-up, if necessary, should include the urea breath test. If endoscopy is not necessary, diagnosis can be made by serology unless there is a history of prior *H. pylori* infection.

MEDICAL THERAPY

The treatment of peptic ulcer disease involves two issues: healing of the ulcer and prevention of its recurrence. Both can be accomplished with successful eradication of *H. pylori,* if present. Acute treatment also includes relief of pain with pharmacologic agents. Rarely, a patient is refractory to medical treatment or has complications and requires surgery.

Nonpharmacologic Therapy

There is no evidence that dietary modification affects either the symptoms or the course of peptic ulcer disease. Frequent feedings, bland diets, increased milk consumption, and decreased consumption of spices and fruit juices have never been demonstrated to affect healing. Although alcohol and caffeine increase acid secretion, no evidence exists that discontinuing either of these substances enhances healing, and it is reasonable to allow patients to continue to consume them in moderation. Dietary restrictions should be limited to substances that cause symptoms; otherwise, patients should be allowed to eat as they wish.

The most important nonpharmacologic intervention is to discontinue cigarette smoking (see Chapter 27) (25,27). Cigarette smoking both increases the risk and delays the healing of duodenal ulcers. Impaired healing of duodenal ulcers in smokers compared with nonsmokers has been repeatedly demonstrated in controlled trials with H_2 antagonists. The impact of smoking is more dramatic when recurrence of ulcers is examined. Nonsmokers who are not prescribed maintenance therapy and do not have *H. pylori* eradicated have a yearly recurrence rate of approximately 20% (equal to smokers treated with maintenance therapy) compared with a recurrence rate of approximately 70% in nontreated smokers in whom the organism is not eradicated (27). Smoking may predispose patients to perforation and bleeding. The effect of smoking on gastric ulceration appears to be similar to that on duodenal ulceration, although it has not been studied as extensively. If *H. pylori* is eradicated, duodenal ulcers do not appear to recur even if smoking is continued. Nevertheless, it seems prudent to recommend smoking cessation in these patients.

Aspirin and other NSAIDs are well-known risk factors for gastric erosions and ulcers. There is a trend toward an increased risk of duodenal ulcers and erosions as well. All such agents should be discontinued, if possible, when a patient has a peptic ulcer.

Pharmacologic Therapy

Duodenal Ulcer

Patients with a proven diagnosis of duodenal (or gastric) ulcer associated with *H. pylori* infection should receive treatment aimed at eradication of *H. pylori* and appropriate pharmacologic therapy to decrease duodenal ulcer pain. Appropriate treatment results in healing of 85% to 95% of duodenal ulcers and reduction of duodenal ulcer recurrence to less than 1% per year. There are several important treatment principles: Therapy with a single antibiotic is not effective, no single regimen has proven effective for all patients, and substitution of an antibiotic of the same class for a recommended antibiotic (e.g., ampicillin for amoxicillin or doxycycline for tetracycline) results in a dramatic decrease in healing rates. Each regimen discussed in this section should be evaluated based on efficacy, antimicrobial resistance, side effects, compliance, cost, and previous treatment.

Several regimens have received Food and Drug Administration (FDA) approval (41) (Table 43.2). Dual therapy and non–PPI-based regimens, though FDA approved, are no longer considered to be as effective as PPI-based triple therapy:

1. Triple therapy with bismuth subsalicylate (two tablets four times a day), metronidazole (250 mg four times a day), and tetracycline (500 mg four times a day) taken for 14 days, prepared as a blister pack for each day's dosage. More than 60% of the doses must be completed to ensure optimal eradication rates. Side effects have been variable with this regimen, ranging from 10% to 30%, and may be reduced by the addition of a PPI. A single daily dose of a PPI will increase compliance, which is the key to a successful regimen. Patients who are intolerant of tetracycline can be given amoxicillin (500 mg four times a day) in its place.
2. The regimen that is favored, especially by gastroenterologists, is called *PPI-based triple therapy.* Several regimens have been approved by the FDA, and eradication rates of up to 95% have been reported with 7 to 14 days of treatment with a PPI twice a day, amoxicillin (1,000 mg twice a day), and clarithromycin (500 mg twice a day). To ensure an optimal response, treatment for at least 10 days appears important. Metronidazole (500 mg twice daily) may be substituted for amoxicillin, usually with similar healing rates, but lower healing rates may be seen in parts of the country where metronidazole resistance is high. Current estimates are that metronidazole resistance rates are approximately 15% and clarithromycin resistance rates are approximately 7%. Amoxicillin and tetracycline resistance is uncommon. The newest PPI, esomeprazole, can be used once a day (40 mg). All currently available PPIs can be used to treat *H. pylori* though pantoprazole regimens have not been approved by the FDA. It is likely that no further treatment beyond 14 days is required for treatment of duodenal ulcer when a PPI-based triple therapy is used.

It is hoped that future treatment will be simpler and equally effective.

If *H. pylori* is successfully eradicated, maintenance therapy should not be needed. If symptoms recur after seemingly successful treatment, the patient should be tested for the presence of the organism (urea breath test or repeat endoscopy, depending on availability and cost). If *H. pylori* is present, it is probably not

Table 43.2. Therapeutic Options for Eradication of *H. pylori*

Regimen	Drugs	Dosage	Duration
Dual therapy	Omeprazole	40 mg q.d.	2 wk
	Clarithromycin	500 mg t.i.d.	
	or		
	RBC	400 mg b.i.d.	4 wk
	Clarithromycin	500 mg t.i.d.	2 wk
Bismuth-based triple therapy	Bismuth subsalicylate	2 tablets q.i.d.	2 wk
	Metronidazole	250 mg q.i.d.	
	Tetracycline or	500 mg q.i.d.	
	amoxicillin	500 mg q.i.d.	
PPI-based triple therapy	Metronidazole or	500 mg b.i.d.	10–14 days
	amoxicillin	1000 mg b.i.d.	
	PPI[a]		
	Amoxicillin	1000 mg b.i.d.	10–14 days
PPI[a] plus two antibiotics	Clarithromycin	500 mg b.i.d.	
Quadruple therapy	Bismuth-based triple therapy plus PPI[a]	Triple therapy plus PPI[a]	14 days

[a]See Table 43.3.

RBC, ranitidine and bismuth citrate; PPI, proton pump inhibitor.

Table 43.3. Drugs Approved for the Treatment of Peptic Ulcer Disease

Drug	Available Strength	OTC	Generic	Initial Dose	Principal Side Effects[a]
H_2 receptor blockers					
Cimetidine (Tagamet)	100, 200, 300, 400, 800 mg	+	+	400 mg b.i.d. or 800 mg at bedtime	Gynecomastia, confusion, impotence, blood dyscrasia, drug interaction
Ranitidine (Zantac)	75, 150, 300 mg	+	+	150 b.i.d. or 300 mg at bedtime	Gynecomastia, impotence, hepatitis (rare)
Famotidine (Pepcid)	10, 20, 40 mg	+	–	20 mg b.i.d. or 40 mg at bedtime	Headache, decreased libido, depression, mild increase in aminotransferase
Nizatidine (Axid)	75, 150, 300 mg	+	–	150 mg b.i.d. or 300 mg at bedtime	Sweating, urticaria (<1%), somnolence, elevated liver enzymes
Proton pump inhibitors[b]					
Omeprazole (Prilosec)	10, 20, 40 mg	–	–	20 mg/day (DU) 40 mg/day (GU)	Headache, dizziness, rash, diarrhea, abdominal pain
Lansoprazole (Prevacid)[c]	15, 30 mg	–	–	30 mg/day	Diarrhea, abdominal pain
Rabeprazole (Aciphex)[c]	20 mg	–	–	20 mg/day	Headache
Pantoprazole (Protonix)[c]	40 mg	–	–	40 mg/day	Chest pain, headache, diarrhea
Esomeprazole (Nexium)[c]	20, 40 mg	–	–	20–40 mg/day	Headache, diarrhea, nausea, abdominal pain
Sulcrafate (Carafate)	1 g	–	–	1 g q.i.d. or 2 g q.i.d.	Constipation

[a]1%–10% of patients.

[b]For eradication of *H. pylori* infection, all PPIs are given b.i.d. (i.e., twice the initial dose listed in the table) for 10–14 days except esomeprazole, 40 mg, which is given once a day.

[c]Not approved by FDA for treatment of gastric ulcer.

OTC, over the counter.

reinfection but incomplete treatment, and another course of treatment should be prescribed. If *H. pylori* is not found, evaluation for another cause of symptoms should be pursued.

There are other therapeutic options. Though the combination of PPIs with antibiotics is the preferred method of treatment of *H. pylori*-associated ulcers, antisecretory agents such as antacids and H_2 receptor antagonists are effective in relief of symptoms and may still be used in selected patients with intolerance to PPIs or with *H. pylori*-negative ulcers. The currently available drugs used in the treatment of peptic ulcer disease are listed in Table 43.3.

Antacids are rapidly acting and are effective in transient relief of acute symptoms. In fact, a large selection of antacids is available, either calcium carbonate, aluminum, or magnesium based. Though their acid neutralizing capacity varies, most standard antacids raise intragastric pH to close to 6 for about 1 hour. This neutralizing effect is similar to that of a meal. Because of the short duration of action, large doses (on the order of 200 to 400 mEq/day) are needed for ulcer healing. This requires six to seven doses per day, which can be difficult for patients to comply with and is associated with diarrhea with magnesium-containing antacids and perhaps constipation with aluminum-based products. Healing rates of approximately 75% have been shown to occur in patients with duodenal ulcers after 4 weeks of treatment (42).

Histamine receptor antagonists were the mainstay of therapy before the development of the current *H. pylori* directed regimens to treat peptic ulcer disease. Four H_2 receptor antagonists are available for use: cimetidine, ranitidine, famotidine, and nizatidine (Table 43.3). The former two are available as generic compounds, and all are available in over the counter dosage formulations. They are used to treat ulcers in full dose given twice daily or as a nocturnal dose. When used in FDA-approved dosing schedules, H_2 receptor antagonists reduce acid production by 30% to 50%, keep intragastric pH above 3 (the critical value for ulcer healing) for 8 to 12 hours, and effectively heal more than 80% of peptic ulcers after 6 to 8 weeks of therapy (43). Side effects are infrequent (rare abdominal discomfort, nausea, and vomiting). Cimetidine appears to have the greatest potential for interaction with drugs that effect the cytochrome P450 system such as diazepam, phenytoin, warfarin, and theophylline, and therefore is less useful than the others. When H_2 blockers are used as primary therapy, recurrence is common so long-term maintenance therapy with one-half the standard dose of drug is usually needed (44).

Sucralfate forms a protective coating on the mucosa of the stomach and duodenum. It is as effective as H_2 blockers in the healing of duodenal ulcers (and probably in the healing of gastric ulcers, also) but has the disadvantage of requiring multiple dosing (Table 43.3). It has been largely replaced by PPIs as initial and maintenance therapy for peptic ulcer disease.

In the case of *H. pylori*-negative duodenal ulcer (probably caused by NSAIDs), traditional treatment with H_2-receptor antagonists or PPIs in recommended doses should be given. Maintenance therapy should be considered only if severe gastrointestinal bleeding was associated with a duodenal ulcer. This can be accomplished with one-half the daily dose of whatever drug was given for acute healing.

Gastric Ulcer

In general, the same drugs available to treat duodenal ulcers are effective in the treatment of gastric ulcer (Table 43.3). If *H. pylori* is present (and it should be sought), it should be eradicated (Table 43.2), regardless of whether NSAIDs are thought to be implicated.

Healing must be documented by endoscopy. No dietary restriction affects healing, and hospitalization (in the absence of complications) is unnecessary. NSAIDs, including aspirin, should be discontinued, if possible.

Smoking cessation should be strongly recommended. Maintenance therapy is necessary if the ulcer was due to *H. pylori*, until the infection is eradicated.

The prevention and treatment of gastropathy, associated with NSAIDs, are discussed in Chapter 77.

SURGICAL THERAPY

Surgery is effective therapy for the relief of ulcer symptoms and for the prevention of ulcer recurrence. With current medical therapy, surgery is almost never necessary except in emergencies: perforation, uncontrolled hemorrhage, gastric outlet obstruction, and, rarely, intractability.

Because today most operations are performed on an emergency basis, the type of surgery is generally decided upon in the operating room after the surgeon has evaluated the gastroduodenal area.

Duodenal Ulcer

Three major operations are currently used for duodenal ulcer: *vagotomy with pyloroplasty, vagotomy with antrectomy,* and *parietal cell (or highly selective) vagotomy.* The first two procedures involve a selective vagotomy (gastric vagal fibers only) plus a drainage procedure to facilitate gastric emptying postoperatively. The third procedure involves cutting vagal fibers to the body (acid-secreting cells) of the stomach, preserving antral innervation, and eliminating the need for a drainage procedure. Vagotomy with pyloroplasty has the lowest mortality, shortest operation time, and a recurrence rate of 6% to 8%. Vagotomy with antrectomy is technically more difficult and may predispose patients to more postoperative morbidity (because an anastomosis to the remaining stomach is required) but has the lowest recurrence rate (less than 2%) (45). Postoperative complications (Table 43.4) are significantly more common with either procedure than with parietal cell vagotomy. A parietal cell vagotomy has a recurrence rate of 10% at 10 years (45), approximately four to five times that of vagotomy with antrectomy. Long-term complications (of dumping syndrome and diarrhea) are less than 60% those of vagotomy with antrectomy. In the hands of experienced surgeons, a parietal cell vagotomy is the operation of choice. The higher recurrence rate (which can be managed medically in 80%) is an acceptable trade-off for the decreased complication rate.

Gastric Ulcer

For gastric ulcers, the type of surgery is less certain because understanding of the condition is less clear. In contrast to duodenal ulcer disease, a vagotomy may not be indicated in all patients with a gastric ulcer who undergo surgery. However, in patients who have evidence of concomitant duodenal ulcer disease (approximately 10% to 40% of patients with gastric ulcers) and in patients who have pyloric ulcers, which generally behave as duodenal ulcers, a vagotomy is clearly indicated. If the ulcer is within the antrum, an antrectomy or hemigastrectomy that includes the ulcer is often the preferred operation. When the ulcer cannot be included in the gastric resection, a full-thickness biopsy of the ulcer should be taken for frozen section to rule out malignancy. The recurrence rate for gastric ulcers after these types of operation is very low (1% to 2%).

After antrectomy or hemigastrectomy, the stomach may be anastomosed to the duodenum (Billroth I anastomosis) or to the jejunum (Billroth II). The type of anastomosis is determined by the surgeon based on the degree of duodenal deformity and on technical considerations.

Postgastrectomy Syndromes

Many problems develop after gastrectomy (Table 43.4). In 10% of patients, postgastrectomy complications are severe. Many of these conditions result from the altered physiology created by the surgery.

ZOLLINGER-ELLISON SYNDROME

The Zollinger-Ellison syndrome dramatically represents the relationship between gastrin, acid secretion, and ulcer formation. The syndrome results from a *non–beta islet cell tumor* of the pancreas that autonomously secretes gastrin and is therefore called a *gastrinoma.* In most cases multiple tumors are present, most commonly found in the head of the pancreas. These tumors vary considerably in size from several millimeters, often undetectable at surgery, to huge masses that may even be palpable through the abdominal wall. Approximately two-thirds of gastrinomas are malignant in their biologic behavior and histologic appearance; they can metastasize and can be a cause of death, although generally they are slow growing.

With the introduction of readily available measurement of gastrin, the appreciation of the clinical features of Zollinger-Ellison syndrome has changed. The original description of the syndrome focused on the virulent nature of the ulcer diathesis and on the atypical location for the ulcers. It is now recognized, however, that 75% of ulcers in patients with Zollinger-Ellison syndrome occur in the duodenal bulb and appear as routine single duodenal ulcers. However, the finding of postbulbar and jejunal ulcerations should alert the clinician to the possibility of the syndrome. More than one-fourth of patients undergo ulcer surgery before the diagnosis of the syndrome, which is usually made only when anastomotic ulcers develop. Diarrhea is another common symptom, occurring in more than one-third of patients, and may precede the formation of ulcers by several years; however, 7% of patients have diarrhea and never develop an ulcer. (The diarrhea is caused principally by the increased secretion of gastric acid, which, when it enters the duodenum, lowers the pH of the normally alkaline duodenal fluid and thereby interferes with absorption of water and electrolytes.)

Diagnosis

The diagnosis of Zollinger-Ellison syndrome should be considered under the following conditions: Failure

Table 43.4. Postgastrectomy Syndromes

Syndrome	Clinical Features	Pathophysiology	Diagnosis and Treatment
Early			
Stomal dysfunction	Vomiting, gastric retention	Edema, inflammation, hypokalemia	Electrolyte repletion, time, no suction
Duodenal stump dehiscence	Pain, fever, signs of abscess, sepsis, death	Billroth II anastomosis: tension and poor closure, adjacent pancreatitis, excessive inflammation in area of surgery	Reoperation
Afferent loop syndrome	Pain, vomiting bile without food, may occur acutely or chronically	Billroth II anastomosis: afferent loop too long, kinked, twisted, herniated etc.; loop fills, then empties	Reoperation
Vagotomy complications			
Transient dysphagia	Dysphagia	Lower esophageal sphincter dysfunction	Usually transient, disappears in 1–2 wk
Diarrhea	Diarrhea transient or slight, 20–40% of patients; troublesome, 5%; occurs mainly with selective vagotomy and drainage procedure	Most common after truncal vagotomy; appears to be related to increased output of dihydroxy bile salts, the cause of which is uncertain	Cholestyramine, Amphojel
Late or persistent			
Dumping syndrome	Early phase: with or shortly after meals—nausea, abdominal fullness or pain, cramping, palpations, dizziness, sweating	Distension of gastric pouch and upper jejunum from rapid emptying; peripheral intravascular volume depletion from rapid entry of fluid into jejunum due to osmotic changes in jejunum; vasomotor symptoms related to release of vasoactive substances into circulation, such as serotonin and bradykinin	Small frequent meals, high protein, low carbohydrate, small volume of liquids only
	Late phase: symptoms of hypoglycemia	Early hyperglycemia → insulin production → late hypoglycemia	
Gastric cancer	Increased incidence of 3%–5% in gastric stump 15–20 yr after surgery	Possibly related to chronic gastritis developing after gastrectomy	Endoscopy for diagnosis, surgical resection
Diarrhea	Chronic diarrhea	Rapid gastric emptying, lactose intolerance unmasked by vagotomy, malabsorption, Z-E syndrome, bile acid output increased, bacterial overgrowth	Lactose-free diet; if no response, malabsorption workup (Chapter 45)
Stomal or recurrent ulcer	Recurrent ulcer symptoms; hemorrhage in approximately 50%	Hyperacidity caused by inadequate resection, incomplete vagotomy, retained antrum, unrecognized Z-E syndrome (gastrinoma)	Endoscopy; H_2 antagonists, (successful in 80%), reoperation
Anemia	Iron deficiency	Chronic blood loss; impaired iron absorption	Repletion of deficient nutrient
	Nutritional anemia	Defective vitamin B_{12} absorption because of decreased intrinsic factor production (resection and gastritis); possible blind loop bacterial overgrowth; folate deficiency	
Osteomalacia	Bone pain	Diminished calcium intake, poor vitamin D absorption; duodenal bypass	

Z-E, Zollinger-Ellison.

of medical therapy, giant ulcer, multiple ulcers, postbulbar or jejunal ulcers, anastomotic ulcer, ulcer disease in association with diarrhea (but not diarrhea secondary to drugs), and radiographic or secretory evidence of gastric hypersecretion.

The diagnosis of Zollinger-Ellison syndrome is usually based on the fasting serum gastrin concentration, normally less than 150 pg/mL. Elevations greater than 1,000 pg/mL in association with the typical clinical picture are nearly diagnostic of a gastrinoma. However, in patients with mild elevations of the serum gastrin concentration (between 150 and 300 pg/mL) and in postoperative patients, differentiation between Zollinger-Ellison syndrome and other causes for hypergastrinemia is important. Consultation with a gastroenterologist is advisable. Other conditions that may lead to hypergastrinemia include retained antrum, G-cell hyperplasia, postvagotomy plus pyloroplasty, small portion of the population with routine duodenal ulcer disease, and pernicious anemia. Also, H_2 receptor blockers cause a slight increase in the serum gastrin concentration, so these drugs should be stopped 12 hours before blood is drawn for the measurement. PPIs may cause elevation of serum gastrin for weeks to months after being stopped.

Differentiation of these disorders from the Zollinger-Ellison syndrome requires the use of provocative tests, the secretin and calcium infusion tests, generally performed by a gastroenterologist. The *secretin test* is preferred because it is more reliable and is safer. In both tests, the response of the serum gastrin level to the infusion of a stimulating substance is monitored. In the secretin test, the serum gastrin level rises, usually within the first half hour after the injection of secretin in patients with Zollinger-Ellison syndrome, whereas in all other disorders the gastrin level falls or is unchanged.

In the *calcium infusion test,* serum gastrin determinations are made immediately before and then repeatedly for 4 hours after the intravenous administration of calcium. In all conditions, the gastrin level increases. However, in the Zollinger-Ellison syndrome, the response is exaggerated with a rise more than 50% over basal levels.

Gastric analysis may provide further supportive data. Marked hypersecretion is found in both the basal state and after pentagastrin stimulation. Because the stomach is being influenced by an autonomous tumor, further stimulation with exogenous pentagastrin provides little additional stimulation to secretion. Thus, the basal acid output to maximal acid output ratio is 0.6 or greater in this syndrome. However, there is considerable overlap with normal values, so the gastric secretory data alone cannot be used to make the diagnosis.

Various attempts have been made to localize the gastrinoma in the hope that excision of an isolated tumor would be curative. Unfortunately, such efforts have been unsuccessful because multiple tumors are often present, small lesions are undetectable by surgical inspection of the pancreas, and these tumors often have metastasized by the time surgical exploration is performed (34). The use of selective pancreatic venography with measurements of gastrin levels from each venous site may provide an improved method to localize the gastrinoma.

Therapy

Because the tumor mass is rarely localized and therefore rarely curable by local resection, therapy is directed at the end organ. Total gastrectomy historically has been the procedure of choice. Although little evidence exists to suggest that gastrectomy alters the biologic behavior of the gastrinoma, it does prevent the consequences of the hypersecretion of acid. In the past, patients died from this condition most often because of the virulent nature of the ulcer diathesis, including frequent recurrences, diarrhea, and even malabsorption, as well as multiple operations. Complete removal of the end organ prevents these complications. In some patients a parietal cell vagotomy may be an alternative to gastrectomy.

In recent years it has become clear that medical therapy is successful in controlling the ulcer disease and the diarrhea and that surgery is most often unnecessary. The PPIs (Table 43.3) are also extremely successful in controlling acid secretion in these patients, although high doses are often required. Long-term treatment with these agents is approved and is safe.

NONULCER DYSPEPSIA

Dyspepsia is a symptom of persistent epigastric discomfort, occasionally related to meals and sometimes associated with nausea, belching, or bloating. It is estimated to be present in 7% of the U.S. population, most of whom rarely seek medical treatment. When patients with dyspepsia are evaluated with endoscopy, only 20% to 25% have demonstrable peptic ulcer disease or gastric cancer. Nonulcer dyspepsia presents a diagnostic and therapeutic dilemma.

If large groups of patients with nonulcer dyspepsia are evaluated, four major diseases are found to be associated: irritable bowel syndrome, cholelithiasis, gastroesophageal reflux, and chronic pancreatic disease. In irritable bowel syndrome (see Chapter 44) the dyspepsia is associated with diffuse abdominal pain and altered bowel habits. Patients with gastroesophageal reflux disease have associated heartburn (see Chapter 42). Chronic pancreatic disease is less common but is usually associated with more severe pain and steatorrhea. The most difficult diagnostic dilemma, because of the high prevalence of gallstones in the general population, is distinguishing patients with symptomatic gallstones from patients with dyspepsia and asymptomatic (incidental) gallstones (see Chapter 96). It is now well established that patients with dyspepsia do not respond to cholecystectomy unless they have had an identifiable attack of acute cholecystitis or a history of biliary colic. The absence of either should suggest that gallstones are not the cause of dyspepsia.

Patients without one of these identifiable conditions are said to have *essential dyspepsia.* The etiology of this condition is unknown. A small subset of patients has been described with delayed gastric emptying of solids; however, correlation of improvement of symptoms with treatment has been poor. Approximately 50% of patients have *H. pylori* gastritis (see previous discussion). Again, symptomatic response to treatment for this infection has been inconsistent. It is clear that patients with essential dyspepsia do not have increased basal acid secretion nor has a definite association with stress been documented.

The patient with essential dyspepsia can be difficult to manage. The yield of diagnostic procedures is low and, particularly with cholelithiasis, may be confusing. Response to empiric therapy with H_2 blockers or PPIs has been disappointing and may be misleading and lead to inappropriate long-term therapy.

Until more controlled trials are available, patients younger than 40 years with a short history and no evidence of organic disease by physical examination and appropriate laboratory tests should be treated with reassurance, some modification of their diet, and avoidance of caffeine, alcohol, and tobacco. Drugs with a low incidence of side effects—such as H_2 blockers or PPIs—may be used, if necessary, in short courses of 3 to 4 weeks (Table 43.3). If no response occurs in 4 weeks and no evidence of reflux disease or irritable bowel syndrome is present, endoscopy should be performed. If endoscopy is negative, the other diagnoses should be pursued. Patients over age 50 are candidates for early investigation (within 1 to 2 weeks), particularly if symptoms are severe and have occurred for the first time. In this group the diagnostic yield for endoscopy is 60% (46). Patients who are not responsive to these measures are often treated for *H. pylori* infection (see above) if these organisms are demonstrated on gastric biopsy; however, data from placebo controlled trials suggest that treatment of *H. pylori* does not result in long-term relief of essential or nonulcer dyspepsia (47) An individualized approach is necessary using a combination of antisecretory agents, reassurance, and supportive care. The long-term prognosis is good with or without treatment in patients in whom endoscopy is negative.

GASTRITIS

Gastritis—inflammation of the stomach mucosa—is a nonspecific diagnosis that is made by endoscopic biopsy. It may be variably associated with dyspepsia, although a cause and effect relationship has not been documented. Several types of gastritis are seen in clinical practice.

Acute erosive, or *hemorrhagic, gastritis* is seen most commonly in seriously ill hospitalized patients; in patients taking NSAIDs, including aspirin; after heavy alcohol ingestion; and rarely in patients prescribed potassium chloride or iron supplements. Symptoms are variable but usually include nausea or vomiting and gastrointestinal bleeding that requires hospitalization.

Nonerosive or *chronic antral gastritis* is a histologic entity commonly seen in the general population, particularly the elderly. It is now well accepted that this condition is caused by *H. pylori* infection. However, it is unclear whether the histologic (or endoscopic) entity of gastritis is associated with symptomatic disease. There has been no demonstrated correlation between eradication of *H. pylori,* histologic resolution of gastritis, and relief of dyspepsia, bloating, abdominal pain, gas, and so on. In practice, patients with these syndromes should be treated as having nonulcer dyspepsia. Symptomatic treatment of patients with nonerosive gastritis is the same as it is for patients with nonulcer dyspepsia.

General References

Feldman M, Scharschmidt F, Sleisenger MH, eds. Sleisenger and Fordtran's gastrointestinal and liver disease: pathophysiology, diagnosis, management, 6th ed. Philadelphia: W.B. Saunders, 1997.
The standard text.

Specific References*

1. Munnangi S, Sonnenberg A. Time trends of physician visits and treatment patterns of peptic ulcer disease in the United States. Arch Intern Med 1997;157:1489.
2. Kurata JH. Epidemiology: peptic ulcer risk factors. Semin Gastrointest Dis. 1993;4:2.
3. Sonnenberg A, Everhart JE. Health impact of peptic ulcer in the US. Am J Gastroenterol 1997;92:614.

*Bold print (general references) and bold numerals (specific references) denote published controlled clinical trials, meta-analyses, or consensus-based recommendations.

4. Sonnenberg A. Temporal trends and geographic variations of peptic ulcer disease. Aliment Pharmacol Ther 1995;9[Suppl2]:3.
5. The ACG Committee on FDA-Related Matters. Current status of maintenance therapy in peptic ulcer disease. Am J Gastroenterol 1988;83:607.
6. Fry J. Peptic ulcer disease: a profile. Br Med J 1964;2:809.
7. Greibe J, Bugge P, Gjorup T, et al. Long-term prognosis of duodenal ulcer: follow-up study and survey of doctors' estimates. Br Med J 1977;2:1572.
8. Penston JG, Wormsley KG. Review articles: maintenance treatment with H_2 receptor antagonists for peptic-ulcer disease. Aliment Pharmacol Ther 1997;6:3.
9. Bardhan KD, Hinchliffe RFC, Bose K. Low dose maintenance treatment with cimetidine in duodenal ulcer: intermediate term results. Postgrad Med J 1986;62:347.
10. Bonnevie O. Survival in peptic ulcer. Gastroenterology 1978; 75:1055.
11. Pounder RE, Ng D. The prevalence of *Helicobacter pylori* infection in different countries. Aliment Pharmacol Ther 1995;9[Suppl 2]:33.
12. National Institutes of Health. *Helicobacter pylori* in peptic ulcer disease. JAMA 1994;272:65.
13. Graham DY, Lew GM, Evans DG, et al. Effect of triple therapy (antibiotics plus bismuth) on duodenal ulcer healing. A randomized controlled trial. Ann Intern Med 1991;115:266.
14. Hentschel E, Brandstatter G, Dragosics B, et al. Effect of ranitidine and amoxicillin plus metronidazole on the eradication of *Helicobacter pylori* and the recurrence of duodenal ulcer. N Engl J Med 1993;328:308.
15. Laine L, Hopkins RJ, Girardi LS. Has the impact of *Helicobacter pylori* therapy on ulcer recurrence in the US been overstated? A meta-analysis of rigorously designed trials. Am J Gastroenterol 1998;93:1409.
16. Gisbert JP, Blanco M, Mateos JM, et al. *H. pylori* negative duodenal ulcer. Prevalence and causes in 774 patients. Dig Dis Sci 1999;44:2295.
17. Goddard AF, Logan RP, Atherton JC, et al Healing of duodenal ulcer after eradication of *Helicobacter heilmannii.* Lancet 1997;349:1815.
18. Fries JF, Miller SR, Spitz PW, et al. Toward an epidemiology of gastropathy associated with nonsteroidal antiinflammatory drug use. Gastroenterology 1989;96:647.
19. Lanza FL. A guideline for the treatment and prevention of NSAID-induced ulcers. Am J Gastroenterol 1998;93:2037.
20. Conn HO, Poynard T. Corticosteroid therapy does not induce peptic ulcer. J Intern Med 1994;236:619.
21. Langman MJ, Jensen DM, Watson DJ, et al. Adverse upper gastrointestinal effects of rofecoxib compared with NSAIDs. JAMA 1999;282:1929.
22. Silverstein FE, Faich G, Goldstein JL, et al. Gastrointestinal toxicity with celecoxib vs nonsteroidal anti-inflammatory drugs for osteoarthritis and rheumatoid arthritis: the CLASS study: A randomized controlled trial. JAMA 2000;284:1247.
23. Del Valle J, Cohen H, Laine L, et al. Acid peptic disorders in Textbook of Gastroenterology. Vol 1. Philadelphia: Lippincott, Williams & Wilkins, 1999:1370.
24. Piper DW, McIntosh JH, Ariotti DE, et al. Life events and chronic duodenal ulcer: a case control study. Gut 1981;22:1011.
25. McCarthy DM. Smoking and ulcers: time to quit [Editorial]. N Engl J Med 1984;311:726.
26. Kurata JH, Nogawa AW. Meta-analysis of risk factors for peptic ulcer. Nonsteroidal anti-inflammatory drugs, *Helicobacter pylori*, and smoking. J Clin Gastroenterol 1997;24:2.
27. Sontag S, Graham DY, Belsito A, et al. Cimetidine, cigarette smoking, and recurrence of duodenal ulcer. N Engl J Med 1984;311:689.
28. Stemmermann GN, Marcus EB, Buist AS, et al. Relative impact of smoking and reduced pulmonary function in peptic ulcer risk. A prospective study of Japanese men in Hawaii. Gastroenterology 1989;96:1419.
29. Kirk AP, Dooley JS, Hunt RH. Peptic ulceration in patients with chronic liver disease. Dig Dis Sci 1980;25:756.
30. Kang JY, Wu AY, Sutherland IH, et al. Prevalence of peptic ulcer in patients undergoing maintenance dialysis. Dig Dis Sci 1988;33:774.

31. Aspirin Myocardial Infarction Study Research Group. A randomized, controlled trial of aspirin in persons recovered from myocardial infarction. JAMA 1980;243:661.
32. Dooley CP, Larson AW, Stace NH, et al. Double contrast barium meal and upper gastrointestinal endoscopy. A comparative study. Ann Intern Med 1984;101:538.
33. Committee on Endoscopic Utilization. Appropriate use of gastrointestinal endoscopy. Manchester, MA: American Society for Gastrointestinal Endoscopy, June 6, 1986.
34. McCarthy D. The place of surgery in the Zollinger-Ellison syndrome. N Engl J Med 1980;302:1344.
35. Cutler AF, Havstad S, Ma CK, et al. Accuracy of invasive and noninvasive tests to diagnose *Helicobacter pylori* infection. Gastroenterology 1995;109:136.
36. Cutler AF, Prasad VM. Long-term follow-up of *Helicobacter pylori* serology after successful eradication. Am J Gastroenterol 1996;91:85.
37. Fallone CA, Mitchell A, Paterson WG. Determination of the test performance of less costly methods of *Helicobacter pylori* infection. Clin Invest Med 1995;18:177.
38. Faigel DO, Furth EE, Childs M, et al. Histological predictors of active *Helicobacter pylori* infection. Dig Dis Sci 1996;41:937.
39. Graham DY, Evans DJ, Peacock J, et al. Comparison of rapid serological tests (FlexSure HP and QuickVue) with conventional ELISA for detection of *Helicobacter pylori* infection. Am J Gastroenterol 1996;91:942.
40. Greenberg PD, Koch J, Cello JP. Clinical utility and cost effectiveness of *Helicobacter pylori* testing for patients with duodenal and gastric ulcers. Am J Gastroenterol 1996;91:228.
41. Walsh JH, Peterson WL. The treatment of *Helicobacter pylori* infection in the management of peptic ulcer disease. N Engl J Med 1995;334:984.
42. Peterson WL, Sturdevant RAL, Frankl HD, et al. Healing of duodenal ulcer with an antacid regimen. N Engl J Med 1977;297:341.
43. Lanzon-Miller S, Pounder RE, Hamilton MR, et al. Twenty four hour intragastric acidity and plasma gastrin concentration before and during treatment with either ranitidine or omeprazole. Aliment Pharmacol Therap 1987;1:239.
44. Van Deventer GM, Elashoff JD, Reedy TJ, et al. A randomized study of maintenance therapy with ranitidine to prevent recurrence of duodenal ulcer. N Engl J Med 1989;320:113.
45. Jordan PH Jr, Thornby J. Should it be parietal cell vagotomy or selective vagotomy–antrectomy for treatment of duodenal ulcer? A progress report. Ann Surg 1987;205:572.
46. Talley NJ, Phillips SF. Nonulcer dyspepsia: potential causes and pathophysiology. Ann Intern Med 1988;108:865.
47. Talley NJ, Hunt RH, What role does *Helicobacter pylori* play in dyspepsia and nonulcer dyspepsia? Arguments for and against *H. pylori* being associated with dyspeptic symptoms. Gastroenterology 1997;113[Suppl 6]:567.

CHAPTER 44

Irritable Bowel Syndrome

BRIAN E. LACY, PhD, MD

OVERVIEW

Irritable bowel syndrome (IBS) is one of the most common medical conditions diagnosed in primary care practice today. It is characterized by chronic abdominal pain and a change in the frequency or character of bowel movements, without a clear-cut cause. In the Western world, IBS accounts for nearly 12% of visits to primary caregivers and approximately 28% of all referrals to gastroenterologists (1). For many patients, IBS is a chronic problem that greatly affects all aspects of daily life. Fortunately, research over the last several decades has led to a significant advance in our understanding of the pathophysiology of the disorder. This has enabled the medical profession to move forward from a model that primarily involved observing and describing the symptoms of IBS to a true biopsychosocial model that comprehends all aspects of the disease.

DEFINITION

Over the years, IBS has been given a number of different labels, including nervous colitis, spastic colitis, mucus colitis, unstable colon, and irritable colon. These labels should all be discarded because they are both imprecise and inaccurate. In addition, these misleading terms are often quite stressful to the patient because they may be confused with other disorders, such as ulcerative colitis.

The term "irritable bowel syndrome" may lead many patients and clinicians to believe that the disorder is just a vague amalgamation of complaints. However, IBS is actually a fairly specific constellation of findings (described below). At times the intestinal tract does seem "irritable" due to underlying abnormalities in gastrointestinal motility and to alterations in visceral sensitivity. For these reasons IBS remains an appropriate and inclusive term.

IBS is currently defined on the basis of criteria established by a panel of international experts in Rome in 1998 (2). The Rome criteria define IBS as a chronic disorder of abdominal pain or discomfort present for at least 12 weeks (which need not be consecutive) over the previous 12 months, with at least two of the following three features: abdominal pain relieved with defecation, pain associated with a change in stool frequency, or pain associated with a change in stool consistency. Recently, some clinicians have altered the temporal criteria of the definition to make it more applicable to daily patient care. Thus, abdominal pain present for a substantial period of time over the last 3 months would also qualify as IBS if it were relieved with defecation and associated with either a change in stool frequency or stool consistency. This may help minimize recall bias that is inherent in asking the patient to remember symptoms over the previous 12-month period.

PREVALENCE AND EPIDEMIOLOGY

IBS is a disorder found worldwide, with a prevalence in the United States of 15% to 20% (1). IBS may present in all age groups, including children. Most patients begin to develop their typical symptoms in the late teenage years or early 20s, although the problem may not be diagnosed for many years. Peak prevalence occurs in the third and fourth decades of life, and the prevalence decreases in the sixth and seventh decades of life. Although IBS can be diagnosed at any age, a new diagnosis of IBS should be made cautiously in patients more than 60 years of age, because other diseases (colon cancer, diverticulitis) may have similar presenting symptoms. It is important to note that for most patients IBS is a chronic disorder. Once diagnosed, most patients still are symptomatic to some degree 5 years later (3), although 25% to 30% no longer meet the diagnostic criteria (1).

There appears to be a similar prevalence of IBS between whites and African Americans (4). The prevalence is somewhat lower in Hispanics (1). In general, women are nearly three times more likely to be diagnosed with IBS than are men (1). The underlying reasons for the female preponderance are unknown.

PATHOGENESIS

Overview

IBS was once thought to represent a nervous disorder of the gut, hence the terms "nervous colitis" or "spastic colitis." However, our concept of IBS has changed considerably over the last 50 years. To label IBS a "colitis" is inappropriate because the disorder affects multiple parts of the gastrointestinal tract. It is now believed that IBS is a complex disorder in which a number of physiologic processes are involved. These include abnormalities in intestinal motility, alterations in visceral sensory function, and changes in central nervous system processing of sensory information. The realization that the gut and the brain are intimately connected now plays a central role in the theory of the pathogenesis of IBS.

Altered Gut Motility

Although a number of different patterns of abnormal intestinal motility have been described in patients with IBS, no one pattern is pathognomonic of the disorder. In general, the signs and symptoms of IBS, and the alterations in gastrointestinal motility that underlie them, appear to be related predominantly to an exaggeration of normal patterns of intestinal motility.

Enhanced Visceral Sensitivity

Abdominal pain is a critical part of the definition of IBS. A number of studies have demonstrated that patients with IBS have an increased sensitivity to pain within the gastrointestinal tract (5-7). Many of these studies have used balloon distention of the gastrointestinal tract to measure this heightened sensitivity. During these studies a balloon is placed in the intestinal tract (rectum, sigmoid colon, ileum) and is gradually inflated. Patients with IBS perceive balloon distention at much lower levels of inflation and also describe the distention as more painful than do patients without IBS. This increased sensitivity to pain is not a generalized phenomenon, however, because patients with IBS do not have lower thresholds for somatic pain, when measured by the cold water immersion test. These experiments demonstrate that patients with IBS are very sensitive to stimuli within the gut and suggest that they may interpret normal intestinal function as painful in many circumstances.

Central Nervous System Influences

It has been suggested that patients with IBS may process sensory information from the intestinal tract differently than do patients without IBS (1). In addition, other stimulation, such as stress, anxiety, or depression, may modulate sensory processing and influence the perception of pain. These findings have significant implications, especially in regard to the treatment of IBS. Therapy focused only on the intestinal tract may not be nearly as successful as a multisystem approach.

Other Factors

Clinicians and patients commonly question whether there are unique events that produce IBS or increase the likelihood of developing IBS later in life. Two studies demonstrated that an infectious gastroenteritis may increase the likelihood of developing IBS later in life (8,9). Many patients recall the persistence of bloating, abdominal pain, and altered bowel habits after an acute infectious illness (i.e., traveler's diarrhea). The precise mechanism is unknown, but several explanations have been offered (9). An infectious process may injure the enteric nervous system, the intrinsic nerve supply responsible for coordinating peristaltic activity within the gastrointestinal tract. Another possibility involves immune hypersensitivity, where recurrent exposure to an otherwise benign substance might induce inflammation and possibly intestinal dysmotility. Also, some experts believe an infectious agent could induce a cycle of chronic mucosal inflammation, eventually leading to altered gut motility. However, biopsies of colonic mucosa in patients with documented IBS are not different from specimens from control subjects, which argues against the hypothesis that mucosal inflammation plays a significant role in the development of the disease.

Many published reports suggest that previous physical or sexual abuse plays a role in the development of IBS. Several studies have shown a higher prevalence of physical or sexual abuse in patients (primarily women) with IBS than in control groups (10). Clearly, a history of abuse is an important factor to consider in patients with functional bowel disorders, and this issue should be considered during the initial evaluation. Other psychological stressors may play a role as well and should be explored in the evaluation of patients with IBS (1).

HEALTH CARE BEHAVIOR AND ECONOMIC COSTS OF IRRITABLE BOWEL SYNDROME

The costs of diagnosing and treating patients with IBS are staggering. More than three million clinician visits occur each year for the primary reason of IBS. A study in 1995 revealed that the annual cost of IBS-related health care (physician visits, diagnostic tests) in the United States was more than eight billion dollars (11). That does not include associated indirect costs, such as lost productivity, lost wages, over the counter medications, and copayments for health care, which may be as much as three times as high.

In addition to being a costly disease to diagnose and treat, IBS also has a significant impact both in the workplace and at school (11). IBS is now second only to the common cold as the reason for days missed from work and school. Overall, patients with IBS miss three times as many work days as those without IBS (12). Chronic ill health from IBS may also affect the workplace in a variety of other ways. These patients may miss important meetings, cancel business-related travel, or may even be denied, or have to forgo, promotions at work.

The health care behavior of patients with IBS deserves special attention. Although 15% to 20% of U.S. adults fulfill the criteria for IBS, not all of those with symptoms seek professional medical evaluation. In fact, only 25% to 33% of those who meet the criteria for IBS seek medical care (13). Most patients with IBS do not seek medical advice for a variety of reasons, including the presence of less severe symptoms, the fear of being diagnosed with a severe life-threatening disorder (i.e., cancer), financial reasons, or the embarrassment of discussing their symptoms. In the United States, patients who do seek health care are more likely to be women. This pattern is fairly constant throughout the world. Patients who do seek a caregiver for the treatment of IBS are also likely to have seen more than one caregiver for their problem. In addition, patients who seek advice for IBS are nearly three times more likely to see clinicians for other non-IBS related symptoms as well (14). Patients with IBS who visit health care providers are more likely to have comorbid pathologic illness (anxiety, depression, somatization, or panic disorder) than are patients who do not seek medical attention.

DIAGNOSIS

One important aspect related to the diagnosis and treatment of patients with IBS is that unnecessary diagnostic tests and procedures are often performed. These tests may be simple and safe (repeated blood work or abdominal ultrasounds), they may be invasive (flexible sigmoidoscopy or colonoscopy), or they may be expensive (repeated computed tomographies of the abdomen or pelvis). Furthermore, several studies have shown that patients with IBS are three times more likely to undergo unnecessary surgery, such as appendectomy, hysterectomy, or exploratory laparotomy, than are patients without IBS (15–17). Numerous office visits, tests, procedures, and unnecessary surgery all lead to a significant increase in yearly health care costs for patients with IBS. Studies have demonstrated that the yearly increased health care costs for patients with IBS are greater than for patients without IBS, with an average yearly escalation in cost of $1,000 to $1,500 (18,19).

Most patients with IBS are diagnosed after having symptoms for months to years. The average time between the onset of symptoms and the diagnosis of IBS is just over 3 years (20).

The diagnosis of IBS does not need to be a difficult, prohibitively expensive experience for either patient or caregiver. After a careful interview, physical examination, and a few simple tests, the diagnosis should be made, often at the first office visit. IBS should not be a diagnosis of exclusion nor should the patient be told or led to believe that "it is all in your head." One important question to consider at the initial interview is why is the patient coming to you now? An understanding of the timing of the office visit and of the circumstances that prompted it is critical in terms of how the history is taken, what additional parts of the physical examination might need to be performed, and how the treatment plan should be initiated.

History

The two most common presenting complaints are those of *abdominal pain* and *altered bowel habits.* Which of these two components is emphasized depends on which is the more disturbing to the patient. This, in turn, is determined by the intensity of each symptom, by the patient's reaction to it, and by the disruptive effects of the symptom on the patient's function and activities. For example, some patients are less bothered by abdominal pain, which can be hidden from others, but are perturbed by urgent diarrhea, which interferes with their job or social functions. The pattern of symptoms varies considerably from person to person but remains fairly consistent for a given individual, with changes for an individual occurring predominantly in intensity or frequency of occurrence. Typically, symptoms are intermittent, with symptom-free periods lasting days, weeks, or, rarely, months. However, an occasional patient will have daily symptoms without remission.

The presence of abdominal pain is required for the diagnosis (see Rome criteria, above) of IBS. The pain is not a single acute episode but rather is chronic in nature. It should be temporally related to defecation in some way; pain related to urination, menstruation, or exertion suggests an alternative diagnosis. Abdominal pain must be present for at least 12 weeks out of the preceding 12 months, although this time does not need to be consecutive. Alternatively, some clinicians question their patients about whether they have had pain for a significant amount of time (>25%) over the preceding 3 months. The quality of pain varies among patients, although for most patients the character of the pain remains fairly stable over time. Some patients describe the pain as crampy in nature, whereas others describe it as sharp or burning. The location of the pain may vary from person to person but remains fairly consistent for the same person over time. The pain is more commonly present on the left side of the abdomen than on the right and is most common in the left lower quadrant. Some patients complain of pain in the suprapubic area or describe a deep-seated pelvic pain that localizes toward the rectum. Some patients describe pain that radiates into their lower back, akin to "labor pains," and uncommonly the pain radiates down into their legs. The pain is often difficult to localize for the patient and usually does not occur in a well-circumscribed area. When asked to localize their pain, many patients cover a broad area of their abdomen with their hand opened up. Others describe a belt-like, or band-like, distribution that originates in the left lower quadrant and extends across the midline. The timing of the pain is usually unpredictable, which is one of the most frustrating aspects of this disorder. Quite often, the onset of pain does not appear to correlate with any single known precipitating stressful event; instead, periods of illness may correlate with general periods of stress over many years. It is important to try to identify life experiences or interpersonal relationships that constitute stress for a particular patient and then incorporate this information into the treatment plan. For example, tests at school may provoke increased symptoms in students, and stressful presentations or situations (business meetings, trials, family emergencies) may also produce increased symptoms. It is not uncommon for a patient to complain of debilitating daily abdominal pain, but to have no pain, with undisturbed sleep, at night. However, patients with IBS often suffer from sleep disturbances, and the interruption of sleep is occasionally accompanied by abdominal pain. Also, patients with IBS often relate that they sleep well but that their typical pain begins immediately upon awakening.

Based on the results of large survey studies, a normal pattern of defecation ranges from three bowel movements per week to three per day. Patients with IBS have altered patterns of defecation, and, as with pain, these altered patterns, though variable from person to person, are fairly consistent for a given individual, changing only in periodicity and intensity. Patients with IBS are usually considered to have one of three patterns of altered defecation: constipation predominant, diarrhea predominant, or alternating constipation and diarrhea. For patients who are prone to diarrhea, many find that the first stool in the morning is of normal consistency. However, subsequent bowel movements become increasingly loose and are associated with significant urgency, abdominal cramps, and flatulence. The urgency and cramps are temporarily relieved by the passage of stool but quickly return and precipitate yet another bowel movement. As bowel evacuation ends, stools are primarily liquid or mostly mucus, and some patients are left feeling drained. Many patients with IBS are concerned about variations in the size and character of the stool, because they believe these variations represent an anatomic problem within the colon, such as cancer. Formed stools may be compressed and of narrow pencil-sized diameter because of the molding effect of rectosigmoid spasm. In other instances spasm of the colon results in prolonged transit of stool, which produces dehydrated, rocky hard, pellet-like stool, called scybala. Mucus may cover the stools or may be passed alone. Stools may be mistakenly referred to as "diarrhea" when they consist of frequently passed small quantities of soft fragments that are narrow in caliber. Explosive defecation may result from evacuation of gas along with the stool. Fecal incontinence (usually slight staining of the undergarments), which occurs in about 20% of patients with IBS, may result from the repetitive reflex relaxations that occur in association with repetitive spastic distal colonic contractions.

Patients with IBS often describe increased stool frequency in the postprandial period. In addition, many patients also describe increased fecal urgency and more severe lower abdominal cramps and spasms during this same time period. This reflects a heightened gastrocolic reflex, which normally occurs 30 to 45 minutes after a medium to large-sized meal.

Bloating and gaseous abdominal distention are common complaints of patients with IBS as are complaints of belching, burping, and bloating. However, studies have demonstrated that patients with IBS who have such complaints do not have more intestinal gas than do normal subjects (21). Instead, they have a decreased tolerance to distention from normal amounts of gas, which may be related to hypermotility of their intestinal tract and to a lowered threshold for distention-inducing spasm. Some patients have persistent complaints of severe cramps, pain, and distention in either the left upper quadrant or the right upper quadrant. Symptoms are usually abated by the passage of flatus, often assisted by patients placing themselves in a knee–chest position. These conditions, although uncommon, are referred to as the *splenic flexure syndrome* or the *hepatic flexure syndrome*, respectively. Gas, because it tends to rise, usually forms pockets under the splenic flexure, which is the highest portion of the colon in the upright position. Concomitant rectosigmoid spasm may also prevent the normal release of this gas and thus further exacerbate symptoms.

Patients with IBS also commonly complain of indigestion, heartburn, epigastric pain, and mild nausea. Heartburn, or gastroesophageal reflux disease, is extremely common in the United States, affecting more than 40% of adult Americans (see Chapter 42). Thus, it is not surprising that some patients with IBS also suffer from gastroesophageal reflux disease. However, many of the other complaints, generally categorized as dyspeptic symptoms, often reflect the same abnormal pathophysiologic processes that occur in the colon and small intestine in patients with IBS. Overall, it is estimated that 40% to 50% of patients with IBS have dyspeptic symptoms. This overlap of symptoms reinforces the point that IBS is an appropriate term for this disorder, because it does encompass problems and complaints referable to the entire gastrointestinal tract.

As mentioned previously, a history of abuse (physical, mental, or emotional) is often seen in patients with functional bowel disorders. This issue should be raised at some point in the evaluation process. The timing of this discussion depends on both the patient and the practitioner. Many practitioners like to raise this issue at the time of the first visit, whereas others feel more comfortable once a relationship with the patient is established after several visits. It is critical, however, that when the issue is raised, it is done in an appropriate setting and with an appropriate amount of time available.

Although the symptoms described above are commonly seen in patients with IBS, they are nonspecific and can also be present in other disorders (see Differential Diagnosis, below). However, there are some important signs or "red flags" that need to be immediately considered because they usually indicate the presence of another disease process. Weight loss is not associated with IBS per se and warrants a more thorough investigation. As previously noted, up to 50% of patients who seek medical advice for symptoms of IBS have some associated psychological disorder, such as depression or anxiety. It is thus not uncommon to have a patient with both IBS and depression who loses weight, but the weight loss is due to the depression and not due to IBS. Anemia, heme-occult positive stool, and gastrointestinal bleeding are not directly associated with IBS. Any evidence of bleeding or anemia warrants thorough investigation. Constitutional symptoms such as fatigue, myalgias, arthralgias, fevers, chills, and night sweats may rarely be seen in patients with IBS, although they are more commonly due to another disorder. Attention should be paid to the family history and specific questions about the presence of inflammatory bowel disease, celiac disease, and any type of gastrointestinal malignancy should be asked. Finally, patients with IBS usually have one pattern of altered bowel habits. A sudden change in this pattern, from chronic diarrhea to constipation, for example, warrants investigation.

Physical Examination

A thorough physical examination should be performed at the time of initial evaluation. This ensures the patient that complaints are being taken seriously, even if the symptoms are classic for IBS and have been present for many years. A thorough examination is also necessary to exclude other disorders

The physical examination is generally normal. The patient may, however, appear anxious or distressed during the interview and examination. Vital signs, including weight, should be taken and recorded. Examination of the lower abdomen may reveal some tenderness or firmness, especially in the left lower quadrant over the sigmoid colon. Stool is often present in the sigmoid colon, both in patients with and without IBS, and can usually be palpated. Patients with IBS often have spasms in the sigmoid colon, which may account for the tenderness. Signs of rebound and guarding should not be present; they warrant looking for an alternative diagnosis. The caregiver should also look for evidence of masses in the abdomen, check for abdominal bruits, and listen for a succussion splash, which can be seen in patients with gastroparesis, and attempt to palpate the liver and spleen.

A digital rectal examination should be performed in all patients. The presence of an anal fissure may explain a history of rectal bleeding, especially in patients with constipation and straining. The presence of a fistula or significant perianal disease raises the possibility of Crohn disease. Patients with IBS often have some tenderness in the rectum, due to visceral hypersensitivity, rectal spasms, and muscular contractions. However, significant tenderness, evidence of a mass, or the presence of blood in the rectum warrants further investigation

Laboratory Tests

In patients with IBS the goals of testing are to establish the diagnosis as early as possible, to look for coexisting/alternative diagnoses, and to avoid performing unnecessary tests. A limited number of easily performed tests, coupled with a thorough history and physical examination, can readily diagnose the disorder in most patients. If the patient has predominant symptoms of diarrhea, then stool samples should be sent for routine culture and examination for ova and parasites, *Clostridism difficile* cytotoxin, and fecal leukocytes. Routine laboratory tests that should be performed include a complete blood count and erythrocyte sedimentation rate or C-reactive protein. These tests should all be normal in patients with IBS. An elevated sedimentation rate, a low hemoglobin concentration, or the presence of fecal leukocytes is incompatible with a primary or sole diagnosis of IBS and needs to be investigated.

In some patients, a more thorough initial evaluation is warranted. In patients with urgency, tenesmus, and discomfort in the left lower quadrant, flexible sigmoidoscopy is recommended to rule out ulcerative colitis, infectious proctitis, or cancer. A more thorough evaluation may also be appropriate for patients with a strong family history of inflammatory bowel disease or colorectal cancer or with abnormal findings on physical examination or laboratory tests. These patients may require more invasive tests such as colonoscopy, upper endoscopy, a full small bowel follow-through, or a computed tomography of the abdomen and pelvis.

Differential Diagnosis

When a patient with IBS is first evaluated in the office, with complaints of abdominal pain and altered bowel habits, the differential diagnosis seems incredibly broad (Table 44.1). However, as the interview progresses and the chronicity of symptoms becomes more apparent and after the physical examination is performed and is essentially normal, the differential diagnosis narrows considerably.

Table 44.1. Differential Diagnosis of Irritable Bowel Syndrome

- Inflammatory bowel disease
  - Crohn disease
  - Ulcerative colitis
- Nonspecific colitis
  - Collagenous colitis
  - Lymphocytic colitis
- Malabsorption
  - Celiac disease
  - Tropical sprue
  - Pancreatic insufficiency
  - Bacterial overgrowth
  - Lymphoma
  - Amyloidosis
- Lactose intolerance
- Food sensitivities
- Food allergies
- Urogynecologic sources of pain
  - Ovarian cysts
  - Endometriosis
  - Interstitial cystitis
  - Uterine fibroids
  - Pelvic inflammatory disease
- Other disorders
  - Viral gastroenteritis
  - Diabetic diarrhea
  - Intestinal ischemia
  - Malignancy
  - Eosinophilic enteritis
  - Mastocytosis
  - HIV enteropathy
  - Whipple disease

Many adult Americans develop some intolerance to lactose after the age of 30. If not recognized, continued ingestion of milk or milk products can lead to abdominal bloating, distention, and loose frequent stools, especially in the postprandial period. If the patient is placed on a lactose-free diet and all symptoms disappear, then the diagnosis is that of lactose intolerance (see Chapter 45). However, for most patients with IBS, a lactose-free diet in and of itself will not eliminate all symptoms. Some patients have both IBS and lactose intolerance, and symptoms of bloating, gas, and more frequent stools may improve with cessation of lactose intake. However, complaints of abdominal pain, rectal spasms and cramps, and fecal urgency persist. Treatment for these symptoms of IBS is discussed below.

One critical issue for many patients is differentiating IBS from inflammatory bowel disease, especially if they have previously been diagnosed with nervous colitis or spastic colitis. The absence of anemia and a normal erythrocyte sedimentation rate is reassuring, as is a normal physical examination (absence of perianal disease and no evidence of extraintestinal manifestations of IBD). Sigmoidoscopy or colonoscopy are not indicated for such patients.

Many patients are also quite concerned that their symptoms represent an underlying malignancy. Of course, no one test can eliminate the possibility that a malignancy exists, especially in a very early stage. However, the patient should be reassured that with a normal physical examination, normal initial testing (complete blood count, erythrocyte sedimentation rate, heme-occult tests), and the absence of a family history of a gastrointestinal malignancy, it is unlikely that more rigorous invasive testing will uncover a malignancy. This reassurance, coupled with routine follow-up examinations to look for new findings or changes in symptoms, weight, or blood count, is both safe and effective.

TREATMENT

General Principles

Because the underlying etiology of IBS is unknown, treatment focuses on the relief of symptoms. Successful management of IBS requires that the practitioner is interested in both the patient and the underlying disorder, that both patient and practitioner have a clear understanding of the current state of knowledge of IBS, and, above all, that both parties recognize the chronic nature of the disorder. This latter point implies acceptance of a prolonged cooperative therapeutic endeavor between patient and caregiver.

Treatment begins with the first interview and physical examination, which should be designed to establish a relationship of mutual interest and confidence and which should be thorough enough to demonstrate to the patient that the caregiver has taken the complaints seriously. Attention to the details of all contributing factors, including diet, emotions, professional and interpersonal relationships, and the patient's fears and concerns, provides ample evidence to the patient that these are important factors that must be addressed in the overall treatment plan. The worst mistake that a practitioner can make is to downplay the symptoms on the grounds that they exist only in the patient's mind.

It is important to take the time to explain to the patient the present understanding of the pathophysiology of IBS and the factors that influence it. This helps to emphasize to the patient that the disorder is chronic in nature, although it can usually be managed successfully through cooperation between patient and caregiver. The demonstrated ability of the caregiver to predict the course of the disorder promotes confidence on the patient's behalf. Furthermore, if patients know what to anticipate and understand that treatment can be expected to ameliorate rather than eliminate the disorder, they are better prepared to face recurrent episodes or flares, which otherwise can be frustrating, disappointing, and even frightening. Labeling and understanding the disorder can be reassuring to patients and may provide them with the patience required to wait for gradual improvement. At the same time, the positive implications of the diagnosis should be underscored, emphasizing that IBS, although chronic in nature, does not lead to cancer or colitis and does not alter life expectancy.

Diet

Even when the patient keeps a meticulous daily log relating onset of symptoms to food intake, it is often difficult to make direct associations with any degree of specificity or certainty. Patients often convince themselves that they are allergic to every type of food and suddenly find themselves only taking in water and small amounts of rice or crackers, which may still produce symptoms. It is best to explain to individuals who have postprandial distress that, although some foods may be bothersome, it is usually the act of eating that aggravates or precipitates the symptoms rather than the individual food itself. It is important to stress to these patients that they are not truly allergic to food. Some patients find that they react badly to certain types of foods, such as carbonated beverages, caffeine, fatty or greasy foods, alcohol, high-fructose beverages, sorbitol, or certain spices, although there are no convincing data that these foods as a group are more likely to produce problems than other foods. Patients may wish to abstain from these foods for a period and note whether symptoms recur on at least two occasions when each substance is reintroduced. Any food that is definitely associated with precipitation of symptoms should obviously be avoided, although one should be careful not to create a dietary cripple.

Some patients with constipation-predominant IBS derive benefit from a diet that includes a large amount of bran. This can be administered as two tablespoons of miller's unprocessed bran three times a day and can usually be purchased in a health food store. Bran has been shown to increase the size of stool and the frequency of its passage. Initially, bran may produce an increase in flatulence, and patients should be warned of this effect. However, most patients find that this side effect is short lived. The dosage should be titrated for each patient, weighing the beneficial effects against the annoying side effects, although maximum beneficial effects are usually achieved if the patient can consume 30 g/day.

Pharmacotherapy: General Principles

IBS is characterized by complaints of abdominal pain, bloating, and either constipation or diarrhea. Given the complex pathophysiology of IBS and the complicated interplay between the gut, the enteric nervous system, and the brain, it is really not surprising that no single agent has ameliorated the symptoms of IBS. Because all symptoms cannot be resolved with the use of only one medication, treatment needs to be individualized for each patient and should be aimed at the predominant symptom. As an example, at the first visit the patient may wish to focus on the treatment of constipation, whereas at later visits, after some progress has been made in treating constipation, the treatment of pain may become a priority. Because IBS is a chronic waxing and waning disease and because no drug has been shown to be persistently beneficial, although medications are often required, they should be prescribed sparingly and discontinued as soon as possible.

Constipation

Initial treatment should involve life-style modifications, changes in diet, and use of fiber supplements (see Chapter 46). Patients should be counseled to increase fluid intake to a minimum of 64 ounces per day, take in foods with natural fiber (bran cereals, pears, peaches, stewed prunes, plums), and to try to defecate at the same time each day. Many patients find that a daily morning regimen of fiber cereal, stewed prunes or prune juice, and then strong coffee or tea is all that is required. Attempting to defecate 30 to 45 minutes after breakfast may encourage a bowel movement, because this is the time when the gastrocolic reflex is present and most active.

Fiber supplements (methylcellulose, psyllium, polycarbophil, coarse bran, or ispaghula husk; Table 44.2) are all available over the counter or at health food stores. All these products act as hydrophilic agents to bind water and prevent excess dehydration of the stools in patients who are constipated. In patients with significant diarrhea, these agents can also act to bind excess water and increase the bulk of the stool. Although widely used in the treatment of IBS for nearly 30 years, controlled trials have not consistently demonstrated a therapeutic effect (22,23). Also, up to 20% of patients develop significant bloating and abdominal distention with these agents, which often

Table 44.2. Medications Used in the Treatment of Irritable Bowel Syndrome

Constipation	
Fiber products	Methylcellulose (Citrucel) Psyllium (Metamucil) Polycarbophil (Equalactin) Coarse bran or ispaghula husk
Misoprostol	
Erythromycin	
Colchicine	
Osmotic agents	Lactulose Go-lytely Miralax
5HT-4 agonists	Tegaserod (awaiting FDA approval)
Diphenoxylate-atropine	Lomotil
Loperamide	Imodium
Resin binding agents	Cholestyramine
Opioids	DTO - deodorized tincture of opium
Bloating	
Antispasmodic agents	Dicyclomine (Bentyl) Clidinium (Librax) Levsin (Hyoscyamine)
Antiflatulents	Simethicone (Mylicon) Charcoal Enzyme replacements
Abdominal pain	
Antispasmodics	See above
Tricyclic antidepressants	Amitriptyline Nortriptyline Desipramine
Anticholinergic agents	
SSRIs	Fluoxetine, luvoxamine, paroxetine, sertraline
Non-narcotic agents	Acetaminophen Tramadol (Ultram) Gabapentin (Neurontin) Carbomazepine (Tegretol)

requires stopping therapy. Nevertheless, given their ease of use, their availability, and their proven safety, these agents are still considered first-line therapy. Patients will often use over the counter laxatives such as milk of magnesia or magnesium citrate, which may be effective if constipation is not severe.

When dietary supplements and over the counter medications fail, one of a number of prescription medications may be tried. *Lactulose* is a nonabsorbable sugar that can be titrated from a dose of one tablespoon per day to up to three tablespoons three times a day, if necessary. Common side effects include bloating and abdominal cramps. Some patients respond well to the use of *polyethylene glycol* solutions, either in the form commonly used before colonoscopy (Go-lytely or Nu-lytely) or in a powdered form that can be titrated over time (Miralax). *Misoprostol*, a prostaglandin agent commonly used to protect the stomach from nonsteroidal agents, may produce loose stools or diarrhea in 10% to 15% of patients. A trial is usually initiated at 100 μg twice a day and then titrated upward to a maximum of 200 μg four a day. The most common side effect is abdominal cramps. *Liquid erythromycin* (EES suspension, 200 mg/5 mL), although not commonly used, can be very effective in some patients with constipation. Patients are usually begun on a lower dose (50 mg four times a day) and then titrated up to 250 mg three or four times a day. Side effects include abdominal cramps, mild nausea, and the possibility of developing oral candidiasis or vaginal yeast infections. However, many patients are quite concerned about the long-term use of antibiotics and prefer to avoid this therapy. *Colchicine* (0.6 mg tablets) can be an effective agent because it stimulates rectosigmoid peristaltic activity. One or two tablets in the morning, 30 to 45 minutes before scheduled bathroom time, can be very beneficial in some patients. A new medication, *tegaserod* (Zelnorm), is currently under review by the FDA and has shown promising results during testing; it acts differently than the nonselective agents described above, because it selectively binds to serotonin receptors in the gut that are directly involved in initiating the peristaltic reflex. Preliminary results have shown that this medication reduces complaints of constipation, increases orocecal transit time, and improves symptoms of bloating and abdominal pain in up to two-thirds of women with constipation-predominant IBS (24). Time and experience will tell whether this new class of drug will be able to provide significant relief of symptoms for this difficult problem.

Diarrhea

Patients with complaints of loose poorly formed stools may benefit from low dose fiber products, as described above, to help absorb excess water and provide more bulk for the stools. Some patients find that the use of these agents in wafer form (i.e., Metamucil wafer), especially at night, is most beneficial, because these agents avoid the addition of even more fluids to the diet. Significant diarrhea may respond to *loperamide* (Imodium), one to two tablets every 6 to 8 hours if necessary; its efficacy has been established in a controlled trial (25). Loperamide decreases intestinal transit, thereby allowing more fluid to be absorbed. It also increases external anal sphincter tone and may decrease incontinence and soiling in some patients. Care should be taken to discontinue medication as soon as the diarrhea is controlled to avoid inducing constipation, especially in patients who are prone to having alternating constipation and diarrhea. Loperamide is preferable to diphenoxylate-atropine (Lomotil), a commonly used opiate, because of its longer duration of action and its relative lack of extraintestinal effects. Patients who have strongly diarrhea-predominant IBS and who do not respond to the medications mentioned above may benefit from *tincture of opium* (deodorized tincture of opium). Patients can start with one or two drops each morning in a small amount of water or juice and slowly increase the dose as necessary. Refractory cases may also respond to *cholestyramine*, 9 g once or twice a day, which binds bile acids that may play a role in causing diarrhea in patients with IBS.

Abdominal Pain

The underlying cause of abdominal pain in patients with IBS is thought to be due to both heightened visceral sensitivity and abnormal contractions within the intestinal tract. As such, therapy for pain over the last two decades has focused on the use of antispasmodic agents to blunt or minimize smooth muscle contractions within the gut. Although there are ample theoretical grounds for prescribing *antispasmodic medications*, clinical experience with them has been disappointing. Most studies that have looked at these medications have been poorly designed, poorly controlled, and have not shown significant benefits above placebo. Nevertheless, some patients improve with antispasmodic drugs, particularly those whose symptoms are induced by meals and those who complain of tenesmus. When used for those whose symptoms are related to meals, anticholinergics should be prescribed 30 to 45 minutes before meals so that the major benefit of the drug will be available at the time of anticipated symptoms. Patients with tenesmus should take the drug on a regular basis, timing the dose so that it is given as close as possible to 1 hour before anticipated symptoms. There is no evidence that one anticholinergic drug is better than another, but it seems logical to use drugs that have the highest ratio of antispasmodic to antisecretory effect, so that a large dose can be administered to suppress smooth muscle spasm without producing undesirable side effects such as dry mouth. *Mebeverine*, a spasmolytic agent with little or no antisecretory effect, is available in most countries outside of the United States and is prescribed in doses of 100 to 200 mg four times a day (one-half hour before meals if symptoms are meal related). In the United States, *dicyclomine hydrochloride* (Bentyl) is given in dosages of 10 to 20 mg three or four times a day, as tolerated. The major side effects are tachycardia and orthostatic hypotension. Thus, baseline and follow-up recordings of pulse rate and blood pressure with the patient seated and standing are very important. Dicyclomine should be prescribed in very small quantities to elderly people who are susceptible to orthostatic changes. Tolerance usually does not develop, but a change to a different anticholinergic may be helpful if benefit decreases. A therapeutic trial should be carried out for at least 3 weeks to test the efficacy of the drug.

Analgesic medications should be avoided if possible and when used should be prescribed in the lowest dose possible. Aspirin and acetaminophen, although generally safe, usually are not beneficial. Narcotics should not be prescribed because IBS is a chronic disorder and long-term use of narcotics leads to tolerance and addiction and can interfere with other forms of management (cognitive therapy, behavior modification). Several tricyclic antidepressants (amitriptyline, nortriptyline, desipramine) have been well studied in patients with IBS and shown to be effective. Treatment should begin with a low dose, usually 10 to 25 mg each night, and should be advanced slowly. Effective doses for relief of chronic abdominal pain are generally much less (one-fourth to one-third the usual dose) than those required for depression. Unfortunately, these agents do have side effects, most of which are related to their anticholinergic properties. These side effects can limit their therapeutic potential and include dry mouth, dry eyes, sedation, weight gain, cardiac arrhythmias, and hypotension. A new class of antidepressants, the *selective serotonin reuptake inhibitors* show promise in the treatment of IBS patients with chronic abdominal pain. Although more expensive than tricyclic antidepressants, they have fewer side effects, are generally safer, and are well tolerated. Although data are now emerging that selective serotonin reuptake inhibitors may be beneficial for relief of chronic abdominal pain, these data are limited at present only to case reports and small abstracts, and there are no large well-controlled studies yet to confirm these initial views.

Bloating

This is one of the most difficult gastrointestinal complaints to treat. Most medications designed to alleviate gaseous distention have proved to be disappointing. However, *simethicone* (Mylicon), two to four tablets with meals, or *activated charcoal*, four tablets with meals and at bedtime, can be prescribed as a therapeutic trial. *Enzyme replacements* (Phazyme, Pancrease, Viokase) provide some benefit in a limited number of patients, but the overall results have been disappointing. Some patients respond well to the use of antispasmodics, described above.

Psychological Management

Psychological management begins with the recognition of depression (see Chapter 24), anxiety (see Chapter 22), panic disorder (see Chapter 22), or a somatization disorder (see Chapter 21). Symptoms of IBS often are anxiety provoking and sometimes are perpetuated by social reinforcement (secondary gain). Psychological evaluation and management usually can be effectively performed by the interested practitioner without the need for psychiatric referral. IBS itself is not an indication for psychiatric consultation. Referral should be reserved for patients who would need expert psychotherapy whether or not they have IBS.

Psychological management is dictated by answers to the following questions: Is there evidence of anxiety, and are the symptoms aggravated by stress? If so, what are the specific stressors? Is the patient depressed? Does gratification from illness behavior reinforce the illness? What misconceptions does the patient have about IBS? Treatment usually requires a multifocal approach, including making the patient aware of the problem, using counseling sessions, cognitive behavioral therapy, stress management, and the use of medications to treat the associated, or underlying, anxiety, depression, or somatization disorder. It is now demonstrated that this multifocal approach can be very successful (26).

Alternative Medicines

Many patients resort to natural remedies (e.g., peppermint oil) and herbal medications after traditional medications have failed to provide relief. In these cases, the clinician should ask the patient to bring in the medications or the labels to ensure that the patient is not ingesting harmful substances.

PROGNOSIS

For most patients with IBS, the disease is a chronic disorder during which the patient may have relatively symptom-free periods intermixed with exacerbations of pain, bloating, or diarrhea. Longitudinal studies have shown that more than 75% of patients initially diagnosed with IBS retain that diagnosis 5 years after the initial diagnosis was made (27,28). It is unclear whether the 25% of patients who do not retain the diagnosis of IBS at 5 years have had spontaneous resolution of their symptoms or whether these patients were treated successfully with complete resolution of their symptoms. Most studies follow patients who have been referred to specialists for their care and thus may report patients with more severe symptoms. This referral pattern of more severe patients may account for the chronic nature of the disorder seen in many studies. No data suggest that the diagnosis of IBS increases the likelihood of developing cancer or increases the likelihood of developing some other disease.

ACKNOWLEDGMENT

Special thanks to Dr. Marvin M. Schuster, now retired, for his many tireless years of teaching, research, and patient care in the field of irritable bowel syndrome.

General References*

Akehurst R, Kaltenthaler E. **Treatment of irritable bowel syndrome: a review of randomised controlled trials.** Gut 2001;48:272.

Drossman DA, Whitehead, WE, Camilleri M. **Irritable bowel syndrome: a technical review for practice guideline development.** Gastroenterology 1997;112:2120.

Klein KB. **Controlled treatment trials in the irritable bowel syndrome.** Gastroenterology 1988;95:232.

Jailwala J, Imperiale TF, Kroenke K. **Pharmacologic treatment of the irritable bowel syndrome: a systematic review of randomized, controlled trials.** Ann Intern Med 2000;133:136.

Thompson WG, Longstreth GF, Drossman DA, et al. Functional bowel disorders and functional abdominal pain. Gut 1999;45[Suppl II]:43.

Specific References

1. Drossman DA, Whitehead, WE, Camilleri M. Irritable bowel syndrome: a technical review for practice guideline development. Gastroenterology 1997;112:2120.

2. Hammer J, Talley NJ. Diagnostic criteria for the irritable bowel syndrome. Am J Med 1999;107(SA):55.

3. Kay L, Jorgensen T, Jensen KH. The epidemiology of irritable bowel syndrome in a random population: prevalence, incidence, natural history and risk factors. J Intern Med 1994; 236:23.

4. Taub E, Cuevas JL, Cook EW, et al. Irritable bowel syndrome defined by factor analysis: gender and race comparisons. Dig Dis Sci 1995;40:2647.

5. Accarino A, Azpiroz F, Malagelada JR. Selected dysfunction of mechanosensitive intestinal afferents in irritable bowel syndrome. Gastroenterology 1995;108:636.

6. Mayer EA, Gebhart GF. Basic and clinical aspects of visceral hyperalgesia. Gastroenterology 1994;107:271.

7. Mayer EA, Raybould HE. Role of visceral afferent mechanisms in functional bowel disorders. Gastroenterology 1990;99: 1688.

8. Gwee KA, Graham JC, McKendrick MW, et al. Psychometric scores and the persistence of irritable bowel after infectious diarrhoea. Lancet 1996;347:150.

9. Gwee KA, Leong YL, Graham C, et al. The role of psychological and biological factors in postinfective gut dysfunction. Gut 1999;44:400.

10. Drossman DA, Laserman J, Nachman G, et al. Sexual and physical abuse in women with functional and organic gastrointestinal disorders. Ann Intern Med 1990;113:828.

11. Whitehead WE, Burnett CK, Cook ED, et al. Impact of irritable bowel syndrome on quality of life. Dig Dis Sci 1996;41:2248.

12. Drossman DA, Li Z, Andruzzi E. U.S. householder survey of functional gastrointestinal disorders. Prevalence, sociodemography, and health impact. Dig Dis Sci 1993;38:1569.

13. Talley AJ, Gabriel SE, Harmsen WS, et al. Medical costs in community subjects with irritable bowel syndrome. Gastroenterology 1995;109:1736.

14. Talley NJ, Zinsmeister AR, Van Dyke C, et al. Epidemiology of colonic symptoms and the irritable bowel syndrome. Gastroenterology 1991;101:927.

15. Burns DG. The risk of abdominal surgery in irritable bowel syndrome. South Afr Med J 1986;70:91.

16. Doshi M, Heaton KW. Irritable bowel syndrome in patients discharged from surgical wards with non-specific abdominal pain. Br J Surg 1994;81:1216.

17. Fielding JF. Surgery and the irritable bowel syndrome: the singer as well as the song. J Irish Med 1983;76:33.

18. Levy RL, Stang P, VonKorff M, et al. The comparative cost of IBS in an HMO. Gastroenterology 2000;118:A398.

19. Eisen GM, Weinfurt KP, Hurley J, et al. The economic burden of irritable bowel syndrome in a managed care organization. Am J Gastroenterol 2000;95:A748.

20. IBS national survey study, July 1998; data on file, Glaxo-Welcome.

21. Maxton DG, Martin DF, Whorwell PJ, et al. Abdominal distention in female patients with irritable bowel syndrome: exploration of possible mechanisms. Gut 1991;32:662.

22. Cook IJ, Irvine EJ, Campbell D, et al. Effect of dietary fiber on symptoms and rectosigmoid motility in patients with irritable bowel syndrome. Gastroenterology 1990;98:66.

23. Lucey MR, Clark ML, Lowndes J, et al. Is bran efficacious in irritable bowel syndrome. A double-blind, placebo-controlled crossover study. Gut 1987;28:221.

24. Prather CM, Camilleri M, Zinsmeister AR, et al. Tegaserod accelerates orocecal transit in patients with constipation-predominant irritable bowel syndrome. Gastroenterology 2000;118:463.

25. Conn PA, Read NW, Holsworty CD, et al. Role of loperamide and placebo in management of irritable bowel syndrome. Dig Dis Sci 1984;29:239.

26. Drossman DA, Thompson WG. The irritable bowel syndrome: review and a graduated multicomponent treatment approach. Ann Intern Med 1992;116:1009.

27. Svendsen JH, Munck LK, Andersen JR. Irritable bowel syndrome: prognosis and diagnostic safety. A 5-year follow-up study. Scan J Gastroenterol 1985;20:415.

28. Owens DM, Nelson DK, Talley NJ. The irritable bowel syndrome: long term prognosis and the patient-physician interaction. Ann Intern Med 1995;122:107.

*Bold print (general references) and bold numerals (specific references) denote published controlled clinical trials, meta-analyses, or consensus-based recommendations.

C H A P T E R 45

Selected Gastrointestinal Problems I: Bleeding, Diarrhea, Abdominal Pain

LAWRENCE J. CHESKIN, MD
BRIAN E. LACY, M.D, PhD

GASTROINTESTINAL BLEEDING

The presence of blood in the stool or in the upper gastrointestinal (GI) tract is always a significant finding that requires thorough investigation. GI bleeding may manifest as occult blood, melena (black stool) or intermittent hematochezia (overtly bloody stool), or hematemesis. Massive hemorrhage, whatever the source, requires immediate hospitalization and often emergency diagnostic procedures. Otherwise, the evaluation of GI bleeding can often be performed in an ambulatory setting. Table 45.1 shows the common conditions associated with GI bleeding.

Tests for Detection of Blood in Stool

In normal subjects, the hemoglobin concentration of the stool is less than 2 mg hemoglobin per gram of stool, as measured by tagged red cell assay. The most commonly used test for fecal occult blood is the *modified guaiac slide test (Hemoccult)*. This test depends on the peroxidase activity of hemoglobin and reflects the concentration of hemoglobin in the stool. In mass screening programs, 1% to 16% of subjects have positive test results. Of these, 2% to 17% prove to have cancer (2% to 14% early stage cancer) (1) and 9% to 36% have adenomatous polyps. The rest have other causes of bleeding (e.g., gastritis, peptic ulcer) or no detectable source. The test is more specific than it is sensitive; one study predicted that testing stool for occult blood in asymptomatic people older than 45 years of age as the primary screening method would fail to detect half of the cases of colorectal cancer (2). Because colonic cancers and polyps may bleed intermittently, sensitivity is improved when multiple stool specimens are evaluated. Left-sided lesions are detected more often than right-sided ones. Among asymptomatic patients with a positive slide test who have carcinoma, more than 80% have early lesions limited to the bowel. Therefore, a positive test for occult blood in the stool requires further investigation and may favorably influence the patient's prognosis.

Laxatives increase the numbers of both true positive and false positive results of the Hemoccult test (probably by an irritant effect on the normal colonic mucosa and on colonic lesions such as cancer). For this reason, some screening programs recommend a high-bulk diet for several days before the stool is tested in the hope of maximizing the discovery of occult lesions. False negative results are more likely in patients taking large doses of vitamin C. Positive tests without clinical significance may result variably from hemoglobin or from peroxidase-rich foods (rare red meat and uncooked vegetables such as broccoli, turnips, and cauliflower), and from iron compounds. Salicylates and other nonsteroidal anti-inflammatory agents (NSAIDs) can cause occult GI bleeding, either because of a direct irritant effect on the stomach or duodenum or because of unmasking of an underlying lesion. Rehydration of the fecal material also increases the false positive rate and is not recommended.

The optimal number and the timing of collection of stool samples have not been determined. The object is to detect bleeding from lesions that are known to bleed sporadically. To enhance compliance, convenience for the patient is also important. The usual recommendation is to obtain two different samples from three different stools over 3 days every year in patients older than 40 years of age (see Chapter 14) (1). Patients should avoid raw red meat, large doses of vitamin C or aspirin, and NSAIDs for 3 days before and during the period of testing. The stool slides can be stored up to 6 days if necessary without a decrease in the sensitivity of the test.

Evaluation of Patients with Gastrointestinal Bleeding

Choosing Appropriate Tests

The history and physical examination direct the sequence of the various tests used to investigate GI bleeding. The patient's age, medical history, and social history; the nature of associated symptoms; and the severity of bleeding are all important factors. For

Table 45.1. Common Causes of Gastrointestinal Bleeding

Occult Bleeding
Gastritis, especially caused by nonsteroidal anti-inflammatory agents or ethanol
Peptic ulcer disease
Colonic polyps
Colonic cancer
Gastric cancer
Esophagitis

Melena
Peptic ulcer disease
Hemorrhagic gastritis
Gastric cancer

Hematochezia
Diverticulosis
Angiodysplasia
Rectal outlet disorders (hemorrhoids, cryptitis, fissures)
Inflammatory bowel disease
Colonic polyps
Colonic cancer

Hematemesis
Peptic ulcer disease
Esophageal varices
Mallory–Weiss tear
Hemorrhagic gastritis
Gastric cancer

example, patients with peptic symptoms or with risk factors such as use of NSAIDs (see Chapter 43) require an initial evaluation of their esophagus, stomach, and duodenum, whereas patients with a change in bowel habits require an initial evaluation of their colon and rectum. In general, patients younger than 50 years of age are less likely to have a colonic lesion than are older patients. Peptic disease and benign rectal lesions are more evenly distributed among adults of all ages.

In asymptomatic patients with occult fecal blood and in patients with hematochezia but no other symptoms, the lower bowel should generally be investigated first. In patients with hematemesis or melena but no other symptoms, the upper GI tract should be investigated first. A reasonable approach to the evaluation of lower and upper GI bleeding is described in the next two sections.

Lower Gastrointestinal Tract

For patients presenting with hematochezia, flexible proctosigmoidoscopy is usually the first test done to evaluate the lower bowel. If inconclusive, it should be followed by an *air-contrast barium enema* or a *colonoscopy.* Barium enema is slightly less costly than *flexible sigmoidoscopy;* and colonoscopy is approximately four times as costly (six times, if performed with polypectomy). In patients older than 40 years of age, colonoscopy should be performed as the initial test.

The finding of hemorrhoids, polyps, or even a rectal cancer on flexible sigmoidoscopy does not obviate the need to examine the rest of the colon. However, in patients younger than 40 years of age, if the pattern of bleeding is consistent with rectal disease (see Chapter 98) and a rectal lesion is seen during proctosigmoidoscopy, colonoscopy is not always necessary. Also, diverticulosis (see Chapter 46), found on barium enema, should not be considered the cause of intermittent mild hematochezia until colonoscopy has failed to provide another explanation.

For patients with occult fecal blood and no localizing symptoms, a colonoscopy or a flexible sigmoidoscopy plus a barium enema is the minimum recommended workup (1).

Proctosigmoidoscopy. Anorectal lesions are poorly visualized by barium enema. Cryptitis, bleeding hemorrhoids, fissures, and proctitis can be seen only by rigid or flexible proctoscopy. Even rectal polyps and cancer are much better revealed by proctoscopy than by a barium enema. The preparation of the patient for this procedure and the patient's experience during the procedure are described below.

Flexible sigmoidoscopy is used to evaluate the rectum and descending colon. It is better tolerated and identifies more proximal lesions than does rigid proctosigmoidoscopy. It is most useful in screening asymptomatic patients for colorectal adenoma or carcinoma (3). It is not recommended for evaluating patients with GI bleeding because colonoscopy is still required to exclude more proximal colonic lesions.

Barium Enema. The barium enema is a valuable test in the detection of colonic lesions. Even in patients with suspected anorectal disease, a colonoscopy or barium enema is indicated to rule out other lesions, particularly in those patients who are at high risk for polyps and cancer. The barium enema may also detect diverticula, inflammatory bowel disease, strictures, extraluminal masses, or intramural filling defects from endometriosis or metastatic tumor.

The double-contrast (air-contrast) barium technique is preferred in the search for a colonic source of bleeding. This technique has the advantage over the conventional single-contrast barium enema in that it provides much better detail of the mucosa. Early changes of inflammatory bowel disease can also be detected by this technique, although with a lesser sensitivity than colonoscopy. However, because of the risk of perforation, the double-contrast barium enema should not be performed in patients with a suspected obstructing lesion or acute diverticulitis.

Patient Experience. The patient's colon must be cleaned before the study can be performed satisfactorily. A reasonable regimen is the ingestion of 2 to 3 L of liquids and a low-residue diet (see Chapter 46) the day before the examination and administration of a laxative, such as 2 to 4 tablespoons of milk of magnesia that night; on the morning of the examination, a sodium phosphate (Fleet) enema is self-administered. This preparation is effective in approximately 90% of patients. Patients who are chronically constipated may need 2 days of preparation. The preparation often causes cramping and urgency, but it is important to the examination and should be encouraged.

The patient should be told that the barium will be introduced into the rectum through a lubricated plastic enema tip while the patient lies on his or her left side on a hard table. Often a balloon is then inflated around the tip to seal the rectal ampulla. The patient is then told to lie supine while the barium is allowed to flow in, intermittently, under fluoroscopic observation. Often, the patient experiences cramping during this process. After the colon is filled, several films are taken, with the patient in various positions. The barium is then evacuated. The films are developed and an additional film is taken after evacuation. The entire procedure takes 45 to 60 minutes.

The air-contrast barium enema differs from the standard technique in that a smaller amount of very dense barium is introduced, followed by insufflation of air. All patients experience cramping during this procedure (usually more than is experienced during the standard barium enema), and atropine may be given to inhibit cramping. The patient is flatulent for several hours after the procedure.

Colonoscopy. Colonoscopy is indicated in patients with GI bleeding of suspected colonic origin, either as the initial test or as a follow-up examination when proctosigmoidoscopy and barium enema have not provided an unequivocal diagnosis. Most gastroenterologists perform colonoscopy instead of a barium enema plus flexible sigmoidoscopy because of its higher positive predictive value in the evaluation of rectal bleeding (4). Also, in patients with polyps, colonoscopy provides a way to remove the polyps without major surgery. An experienced endoscopist can reach the cecum in more than 95% of cases (5). The complications from the procedure are mainly perforation and hemorrhage; the overall complication rate for diagnostic colonoscopy is 0.3% to 0.4%, with a mortality rate of 0.02% (6). If polypectomy is performed, the morbidity rate increases to 1% to 2%, but the mortality rate remains the same.

The sensitivity of colonoscopy in experienced hands is much higher than that of even an air-contrast barium enema (see previous discussion): Only 2% of polyps are not diagnosed. In a study of anemic patients with occult bleeding, colonoscopy revealed polyps (greater than 5 mm in diameter) or cancer in 15% of patients with negative barium enema examinations; of patients with rectal bleeding, 34% had a significant lesion (including 11% with cancer) when the barium enema was reported as negative or simply as showing diverticulosis (7).

Patient Experience. Preparation for colonoscopy usually includes a liquid diet for 2 or 3 days and laxatives and enemas (prescribed by the consulting gastroenterologist). An alternative preparation is to drink 4 L of a nonabsorbed isosmolar salt solution the night before the procedure (Golytely or Colyte). Elderly patients may have difficulty ingesting this amount of fluid, in which case the standard laxative preparation (see Barium Enema) may be preferable. Just before the procedure, the patient is sedated intravenously (usually with meperidine plus diazepam or midazolam). During the procedure, the patient may experience discomfort when the bowel is distended with air for inspection and as the colonoscope is maneuvered through the bowel lumen. There is no additional discomfort when a biopsy or polypectomy is performed. The duration of the procedure is variable, depending on the tortuosity of the colon, the presence of disease, and the skill of the endoscopist, but the average is 30 to 60 minutes. Someone must be available to accompany the patient home after the procedure because of possible lingering sedation. For patients who are at high risk of endocarditis (see Chapter 65), antibiotic prophylaxis must be given before and after the procedure (see Chapter 93).

Upper Gastrointestinal Tract

The sequence of tests performed in evaluating the upper GI tract depends on the severity of the bleeding and the suspected diagnosis. *Upper endoscopy,* or *esophagogastroduodenoscopy (EGD),* has become the procedure of choice for most patients with upper GI bleeding. An *upper GI series* is sometimes done first in patients with suspected peptic disease or carcinoma when the bleeding is chronic or occult. On the other hand, if an inflammatory process is suspected (esophagitis or gastritis), endoscopy should be done because contrast radiography is less sensitive in detecting mucosal lesions that are not severe. Also, in patients with acute bleeding, *endoscopy* is indicated because actively bleeding lesions can often be treated at the time of the procedure, by endoscopic sclerotherapy in the case of bleeding esophageal varices or by electrocautery in the case of bleeding ulcers or angiodysplasias. If an upper GI series has been performed first and is negative or reveals a gastric ulcer (Chapter 43) or a tumor, upper endoscopy should be the next routine procedure. The upper GI series and upper endoscopy have approximately the same cost. If the upper and lower GI tracts have been evaluated in a patient with GI bleeding and the studies have been negative, a *small bowel series* should be considered to investigate the possibility of Crohn disease and other disorders that affect mainly the small intestine.

Radiologic Studies. The *upper GI series* is helpful in the detection of mass lesions in the esophagus and stomach and in identifying gastric and duodenal ulcerations, although it does not allow mucosal biopsy for *Helicobacter pylori.* It is well tolerated and inexpensive. The patient's experience during the performance of an upper GI series is described in Chapter 43.

The conventional *small bowel series* is very poor at detecting small lesions of the intestine (e.g., cancer, leiomyoma). Disorders such as Crohn disease or lymphoma are more likely to be revealed by radiography (although a definitive diagnosis can be made only by biopsy). These sources of bleeding are uncommon and should be suspected only when the more common conditions (peptic ulcer disease, colonic polyps) have been excluded. The patient should be warned that the small bowel series requires spending 1 to 5 hours in the radiology department, during which time films are taken every 30 minutes.

Endoscopy. Upper endoscopy is the most widely used means of investigating GI blood loss. This technique not only is more sensitive than radiography but also provides a direct means of obtaining specimens for histologic examination. Because of its greater sensitivity, endoscopy is indicated even if barium studies have been negative in the evaluation of a suspected upper GI source of bleeding.

Patient Experience. Upper endoscopy is an outpatient procedure that usually takes less than 15 minutes. The patient fasts overnight before the procedure. Just before the procedure, the patient is sedated with intravenous medication (meperidine plus diazepam or midazolam) and the throat is anesthetized with a topical anesthetic. Some gagging is common during passage of the endoscope into the esophagus. Under direct vision, mucosal biopsies and cytologic brushings can be obtained from suspicious lesions for histologic confirmation. Biopsies are completely painless. Complications include perforation and bleeding but are extremely uncommon. Newer, smaller-caliber endoscopes have greatly improved patient tolerance of the procedure. After the procedure, because of the sedation, someone must be available to drive the patient home. The patient typically has a sore throat for several hours.

Occult and Obscure Gastrointestinal Bleeding

Occult bleeding is defined as chronic slow bleeding occurring from the GI tract, manifesting either as iron deficiency anemia or a positive fecal occult blood test. Evaluation of occult bleeding should always start with a lower GI examination, preferably with a colonoscopy, especially in individuals older than 40 years of age, unless the history is strongly suggestive of an upper GI lesion. If the colonoscopy is negative, proceeding to an upper endoscopy is reasonable.

Obscure bleeding is defined as persistent GI bleeding, occult or overt, for which no source is identified by upper and lower endoscopy. Arteriovenous malformations, peptic ulcer disease, erosions in larger hiatal hernias, and NSAID use are some of the causes of obscure bleeding. Obscure bleeding does not necessarily correspond to small-volume bleeding: It can range from occult to massive bleeding. Evaluation of obscure bleeding should start with a repeat endoscopy from both directions. If these are again unrevealing, evaluation of the entire duodenum and proximal jejunum with a push enteroscopy is cost-effective and should be the next step. (Push enteroscopy is performed by passing from above a colonoscope as far as possible beyond the duodenum [8,9]). A duodenal or small bowel biopsy should be obtained for celiac disease during upper endoscopy, especially in young Caucasian patients with a history of diarrhea and persistent iron deficiency anemia. Barium studies may be helpful in patients with a negative endoscopic examination. For small bowel lesions, enteroclysis (the introduction through a catheter of contrast medium into the small bowel) is significantly more sensitive than standard barium small bowel follow-through and should be the next test if the expertise is available. A radioisotope-labeled red blood cell scan (the so-called "bleeding scan") and mesenteric angiography should be considered in cases of overt bleeding that remain undiagnosed. Bleeding scans and angiography are helpful only when the rate of bleeding exceeds 0.1 to 0.4 mL/min and 0.5 mL/min, respectively, at the time of the study (10,11). Even in the absence of active bleeding, however, angiography may sometimes be helpful if characteristic vascular patterns of a Dieulafoy lesion (a dilated submucosal blood vessel that has eroded through the overlying mucosa), tumor, or vascular malformation are seen. Exploratory laparotomy with intraoperative enteroscopy is sometimes necessary in patients who require repeated tranfusions due to recurrent bleeding and in whom the source of bleeding remains unidentified despite extensive evaluation as described previously. All patients with persistent bleeding should be evaluated for a disorder of hemostasis (e.g., von Willebrand disease) if an anatomic cause of bleeding has not been identified (see Chapter 56).

Selected Lesions That Bleed

The most common cause of upper GI bleeding—peptic disease—is discussed in Chapter 43. Common causes of lower GI bleeding include benign anorectal disorders (Chapter 98), inflammatory bowel disease (discussed later in this chapter), and diverticulosis (Chapter 46).

Colonic Polyps

Colonic polyps or colonic cancer should be suspected in any patient older than 40 years of age who has GI bleeding or a change in bowel habits. Bleeding may be occult or may occur as intermittent hematochezia. The patient is often totally asymptomatic but may complain of a change in bowel habits, abdominal pain, or passage of mucus through the rectum. It is believed that all cancers of the colon (except those associated with ulcerative colitis, discussed later) arise from these benign epithelial tumors, although only a small percentage of premalignant polyps grow into invasive cancers. It has been estimated that it takes a minimum of 7 years for an early polyp to become an invasive cancer. Therefore, the removal of polyps before they become malignant has the potential to prevent the occurrence of colonic cancer in predisposed individuals. Although polyps are most common in the rectosigmoid region, they may be found anywhere in the colon. The detection of a polyp on proctoscopy or barium enema is an indication for referral to a gastroenterologist.

The risk of polyps' becoming malignant is related to their histologic type and size. *Hyperplastic polyps* make up 10% to 30% of all colorectal polyps. They tend to be small (less than 0.5 cm in diameter) and to be located in the distal colon or rectum, and they probably have no malignant potential. *Villous and tubular adenomas* make up almost two thirds of all colorectal polyps, are found in 25% of people by age 50 years (and in 50% by age 80), and carry a definite risk of malignant transformation that increases as they increase in size (12). The risk that a villous adenoma larger than 2 cm in diameter is cancerous is greater than 50% (Table 45.2) (13). Fortunately, if the cancer remains confined to the mucosa of the polyp *(carcinoma in situ),* colonoscopic polypectomy is curative. Once the cancer has infiltrated the stalk of the polyp,

Table 45.2. Polyps: Relationship of Size, Histologic Type, and Risk of Carcinoma

	% That Are Cancerous		
Histologic Type	<1 cm	1–2 cm	>2 cm
Tubular adenoma	1.0	10.2	34.7
Intermediate type	3.9	7.4	45.8
Villous adenoma	9.5	10.3	52.9

From Muto T, Bussey HJ, Morson BC. The evolution of cancer of the colon and rectum. Cancer 1975;36:2251.

surgery is indicated. Because the cancerous change in the polyp may be focal, single biopsies of a polyp are not sufficient to exclude the presence of a malignancy; instead, the entire polyp must be excised.

Once an adenomatous polyp has been detected, surveillance for additional polyps is indicated. In 30% of patients more than one polyp is present at the time of initial investigation, and the risk of recurrence rises with the number and size of polyps that are initially discovered (14). Subsequent development of new polyps occurs in at least 10% of patients. The patient should continue to be tested yearly for occult blood in the stool. The finding of a single positive test is an indication for a repeat evaluation. Even when the stools are negative for blood, periodic evaluation of the colon is still recommended. Colonoscopy should be repeated in 3 years. If a follow-up examination reveals no further polyps, the screening interval may be increased to once every 5 years.

Multiple polyposis syndromes are rare inherited abnormalities that are significant for their malignant potential. *Familial polyposis, Gardner syndrome,* and *Turcot syndrome* all are associated with multiple adenomatous polyps of the colon and therefore carry a high risk for development of carcinoma. Gardner syndrome includes osteomas and soft tissue tumors, and Turcot syndrome includes tumors of the central nervous system. Familial polyposis and Gardner syndrome are inherited as autosomal dominant defects, while Turcot syndrome in an autosomal recessive manner. The diagnosis of a polyposis syndrome is usually made when the patient is in his or her twenties, with cancer developing in virtually all patients by some 20 years later. There is considerable controversy about the therapy for these conditions. Colonic resection is indicated, but its extent and timing are not uniformly agreed on. Ideally, when rectal polyps are present, a proctocolectomy should be performed to eliminate the risk of cancer. However, because the patients are generally asymptomatic and young, the prospect of an ileostomy (see Chapter 46) is often overwhelming to them. Newer operations involving ileorectal pull-through procedures are now available, and results are encouraging (see Chapter 46). Cyclooxygenase-2 (COX-2) inhibitors (e.g., celecoxib), have been demonstrated to reduce the number of polyps in patients with familial polyposis syndromes (15). Whether these agents are of use also in patients with sporadic adenomatous polyps and whether they reduce the risk of malignant transformation remain to be seen. Consultation with a gastroenterologist and a GI surgeon is recommended as soon as the diagnosis is made.

Colonic polyposis syndromes should be distinguished from conditions associated with juvenile polyps or hamartomas that are of low malignant potential. The *Peutz–Jeghers syndrome* consists of multiple hamartomas, predominantly of the small intestine, associated with buccal and cutaneous pigmentation. Although the malignant potential of the hamartomas is low, duodenal and ovarian carcinomas have been reported in 2% to 5% of patients. Rarely, juvenile polyps may occur throughout the GI tract. In the absence of associated extracolonic manifestations, this syndrome is called *generalized juvenile polyposis*; when accompanied by alopecia, nail bed changes, hyperpigmentation, and malabsorption, it is called the *Cronkhite–Canada* syndrome.

Colorectal Cancer

Epidemiology and Etiology. Cancers of the colon and rectum account for 14% of all cancers and are the second leading cause of cancer death overall in the United States. Overall, there is approximately a 5% lifetime chance of developing a colorectal cancer.

Colorectal cancer occurs with increasing frequency in older age groups, with two thirds occurring in people older than 65 years of age. Geographic differences in the mortality rate from this neoplasm suggest an etiologic role for dietary and environmental factors. In particular, a high-fat, low-fiber diet appears to be associated with an increased risk of colorectal cancer. For unclear reasons, the proportion of cancers in the right side of the colon has increased in recent years, with a commensurate drop in the proportion of rectosigmoid lesions (16). Currently, about half of colorectal cancers are within reach of the flexible sigmoidoscope. The remaining half are proximal to the splenic flexure and accessible only with a colonoscope. The three main predisposing conditions for colorectal cancer are colonic polyps, familial polyposis (see previous discussion), and ulcerative colitis (discussed later). The presence of these conditions dictates the need for a strict colonoscopic surveillance program and, at times, even prophylactic surgery to prevent the development of cancer. (See below for the risk of cancer in ulcerative colitis.) Although it is accepted that a family history of colorectal cancer predisposes a person to polyps and colorectal cancer, there is some evidence that the risk does not rise significantly above that of the general population unless more than one first-degree relative has had colorectal cancer (17).

Screening Tests. Because of the high incidence of colon cancer and its precursor, the colonic polyp, screening tests should be performed routinely in all patients older than 50 years old. Patients at high risk should be screened at an earlier age (Table 45.3). A number of large, randomized trials showed that annual or biennial fecal occult blood testing decreases the 8- to 15-year cumulative mortality from colorectal cancer by 16% to 33%, compared with no screening (18–21). Hemoccult cards are convenient for the patient because they can be mailed to the practitioner's office without a significant loss in sensitivity. For asymptomatic patients, it is recommended that such

Table 45.3. Colon Cancer Screening

Risk Category	Recommendation
Average risk	Begin at age 50 yr with annual fecal occult blood testing *plus one of the following:* Flexible sigmoidoscopy every 5 yr, *or* Flexible sigmoidoscopy + double-contrast barium enema every 5–10 yr *or,* Colonoscopy every 10 yr (arguably the best screening method).
Second- or third-degree relative with colorectal cancer	Same as for average risk.
First-degree relative with colon cancer or adenomatous polyps diagnosed before age 60 yr	Same as for average risk but begin at age 40 yr.
Two or more first-degree relatives with colon cancer, or one first-degree relative with colon cancer or adenomatous polyps diagnosed before age 60 yr	Colonoscopy every 5 yr beginning at age 40 yr or 10 yr younger than the earliest diagnosis in family.
Hereditary Nonpolyposis Colon Cancer (HNPCC), defined as three relatives with colon cancer, two of them being first-degree relatives of the third, at least two generations affected, and one with colon cancer diagnosed before age 50 yr	Colonoscopy every 1–2 yr, beginning at age 20–25 yr or 10 yr younger than the earliest colon cancer diagnosis in the family, whichever comes first.
Familial Adenomatous Polyposis	Flexible sigmoidoscopy annually, beginning at age 10–12 yr

Modified from: Burt RW (2000) and Byers et al. (1997); See general references.

screenings be combined with a yearly rectal examination and with flexible sigmoidoscopy every 5 years (22).

A retrospective case-control study of patients 45 years of age and older who had been monitored for 17 years revealed that screening sigmoidoscopy reduced deaths from colon cancer by almost 60% (3). However, because of the insensitivity of the test for fecal occult blood (see earlier discussion) and because flexible sigmoidoscopy is limited to the descending colon, a substantial number of cancers may be missed (24% in a recent study [23]). It is reasonable, therefore, to consider whether colonoscopy at age 50 years, repeated (if normal) every 10 years, might not be the best screening test for colon cancer (24). Admittedly, a randomized, prospective study is needed to answer the question definitively.

Diagnosis

History. The chromosomal changes that accompany the progression of normal colonic mucosa to adenoma and then to carcinoma have been elucidated (25). There may soon be a means to detect people who are at increased risk for development of colorectal cancer so that surveillance can be focused on them. Currently, most patients with adenocarcinoma of the colon are diagnosed only after symptoms have developed. Fewer than one third are asymptomatic at the time of diagnosis (26), yet it is in this group that the highest chance for cure exists. The major presenting symptoms (26,27) are abdominal pain (25% to 75%) and a change in bowel habits (20% to 50%), either constipation or diarrhea. Abdominal pain is least common among patients with cancer of the rectum, where even large lesions can be accommodated without producing symptoms. Gross blood in the stool is another common complaint, occurring in 75% of patients with rectal cancer and 30% to 40% of patients with colonic cancer above the rectum. This hematochezia, however, is often mistakenly attributed to hemorrhoids. Presentation with anemia or with weight loss is also common.

Physical Examination. The findings on physical examination vary according to the location and extent of the lesion. The primary tumor may be palpable as an abdominal mass, particularly in cancer of the right colon, where lesions can remain asymptomatic for long periods. Metastatic disease may be suggested by the presence of a large, hard, nodular liver; ascites; or peripheral adenopathy or by the palpation of a mass in the cul-de-sac on rectal examination. Signs of anemia may be present, particularly in lesions of the cecum and ascending colon, which can bleed covertly for months or even years before the diagnosis is made. Most patients have a positive test result for occult blood sometime during their course of illness.

Barium Enema. The diagnosis of colon cancer is sometimes made by barium enema. Findings may include a polypoid mass, stenosis (either as a stricture or with an "apple-core" appearance), distortion of the mucosa, and localized rigidity of the bowel wall. At times, distortion or fixation of adjacent structures may be seen. The development of a gastrocolic fistula, best seen on barium enema, is also suggestive of a primary colonic neoplasm.

It has traditionally been said that the accuracy of the barium enema for the diagnosis of colon cancer is excellent, except at opposite ends of the large bowel. The cecum is often difficult to evaluate because of the inability to cleanse the region completely or, at times, to distinguish a prominent ileocecal valve or sphincter from a mass. The rectum is also difficult to visualize optimally, because often it is obscured by the balloon through which the barium is administered. Therefore, proctoscopy or flexible sigmoidoscopy is usually recommended in addition to a barium enema for patients with suspected colorectal carcinoma (7).

Endoscopy. The role of endoscopy in the diagnosis of colorectal cancer continues to increase. Some polypoid lesions, even if large or sessile, can be removed via the colonoscope, avoiding surgery in many cases.

In addition, colonoscopy has an important role in the identification of other colonic lesions. The prevalence of coexistent polyps in patients with colon cancer is high, ranging from 10% to 30%. These residual polyps may develop later into carcinomas, accounting for the incidence (5% to 10%) of a second colon cancer in patients with cancer of the colon who have been monitored for up to 25 years (13). In addition, synchronous colon carcinomas occur in 3% to 5% of patients. Therefore, colonoscopy is helpful in ensuring that the rest of the colon is free of neoplastic lesions. Optimally, colonoscopy should be performed preoperatively; otherwise, it should be done within the first year postoperatively. In a very large survey, the sensitivity of colonoscopy for the detection of colorectal carcinoma was 95%, whereas that of barium enema was 83% (7). There is also a significant miss rate for colonoscopy: For precursor polyps, colonoscopy failed to detect 27% of lesions 0.5 cm or smaller and 6% of lesions 1 cm or larger (28).

Carcinoembryonic Antigen. Carcinoembryonic antigen (CEA) is a normal fetal antigen found in the blood of many patients with colorectal carcinoma (from 30% of patients with local disease to 83% of patients with metastatic disease). It is also commonly found in higher than normal titers in the blood of patients with other malignancies, in cigarette smokers, and with a variety of benign conditions, including peptic ulcer, pancreatitis, diverticulitis, and inflammatory bowel disease. Therefore, the CEA titer is not a useful screening test for the presence of colorectal cancer.

Although its efficacy and cost-effectiveness for this purpose have been questioned (29), the assay may be helpful in the postoperative treatment of patients who have increased blood CEA levels at the time of diagnosis. Persistently elevated CEA concentrations postoperatively suggest metastatic disease; falling levels that then rise on follow-up evaluation suggest reemergence of the malignancy, usually at a remote site.

Therapy. Surgery is the most effective therapy for most cases of colon carcinoma. Inoperable tumors (including metastatic tumors) respond 20% to 40% of the time to 5-fluorouracil (5-FU) combined with leucovorin, preferably prescribed by or with the advice of an oncologist. However, there is no clear effect of such therapy on survival. (5-FU is usually well tolerated but occasionally mucositis, with severe diarrhea, occurs.) Operable tumors at an advanced stage (stage C or D; Table 45.4) should be treated with the same drugs, and in such cases, there is some survival benefit (30). It is not yet clear whether patients with stage B cancer profit from adjuvant therapy (31).

Anal cancers should be treated, if possible, in specialized centers with radiation and chemotherapy and then, if possible, should be surgically removed.

Preoperative Evaluation. Before surgery, most patients should undergo evaluation for metastatic disease. Liver function tests should be performed routinely, as well as computed tomography (CT) or ultrasound study of the liver. In patients with bowel obstruction or bleeding, surgery may still be needed as palliation, despite the presence of liver metastases. In patients who are asymptomatic from their bowel lesions, the presence of multiple hepatic metastases should deter surgical intervention (single hepatic metastases are often resectable). However, abnormal liver function tests alone should not be considered absolute evidence of metastatic disease, nor should normal test results be considered to exclude hepatic metastases. A histologic diagnosis should be made, if possible. Needle liver biopsy is a simple way to obtain tissue and may be guided by ultrasound or CT. A preoperative CEA concentration should also be determined as a baseline.

Table 45.4. Colon Carcinoma

	Staging and 5-Year Survival Rate	
Classification[a]	Microscopic Findings	% Survival
A	Disease limited to mucosa	95
B	Tumor extends to serosa	60–70
C	Tumor extends to serosa and nodes involved	<40
D	Distant metastases	<5

[a]Modification of the Dukes classification.

For patients requiring an ostomy, preoperative evaluation by an enterostomal therapist is helpful, not only to discuss with the patient problems and concerns about the ostomy, but also to mark the proper location of the ostomy preoperatively (see Chapter 46).

Prognosis. The prognosis of colorectal carcinoma is based on several variables. The major variable is the extent of the tumor, in terms of its invasion through the bowel wall and its lymph node involvement (Table 45.4). Vessel invasion and the degree of differentiation of the tumor histologically also affect survival. The pathologist's interpretation of the resected specimen is much more meaningful than the surgeon's estimation of curability.

Follow-Up Care. Most patients undergoing resection for colorectal cancer do well in the early postoperative period. Diarrhea may be present early, but it is usually transient and easily controlled with antidiarrheal medication. The patient with a colostomy needs continued follow-up care by the surgeon and the enterostomal therapist to ensure proper functioning and handling of the ostomy (see later discussion).

The long-term follow-up is aimed at detection of recurrence or spread of the cancer and at continued surveillance for new colonic lesions. Most commonly, metastases occur in adjacent nodes, with eventual spread to the liver. Physical examinations, liver function tests, and CEA determinations usually are done every 2 to 6 months for 3 to 5 years. Abdominal CT scans must be obtained to assess a confirmed rise in CEA levels or liver function tests, but whether long-term outcome is improved is unclear, despite earlier detection of recurrent tumor.

To evaluate for synchronous colonic lesions, colonoscopy should be performed within the first 6 to 12 months postoperatively, if it has not already been done preoperatively. If no lesions are found, colonoscopy should be repeated 3 years later. The interval may then be increased to once every 5 years if no recurrence or adenomatous polyps are detected. Yearly evaluation for occult fecal blood loss should also be performed, with three to six Hemoccult cards. If any of these are positive, colonoscopy should be repeated.

Arteriovenous Malformations of the Colon

Arteriovenous malformations of the colon are a common source of GI bleeding (32,33), most often in the elderly and in patients with chronic renal failure. A variety of terms have been used to describe these abnormalities, including *angiodysplasia, hemangioma,* and *vascular ectasia.* The etiology of the disorder is unknown. Although the lesions may occur throughout the GI tract, they appear most commonly in the mucosa of the cecum and ascending colon, where multiple lesions are often found, ranging in size from 1 mm to more than 1 cm. An association of angiodysplasia of the colon with aortic stenosis has been observed repeatedly (32).

The prevalence of angiodysplasias and the frequency with which they cause bleeding are uncertain. With increasing use of endoscopy and selective angiography, the disorder is being recognized more often. In one study of patients older than 60 years of age without a history of GI bleeding, submucosal vascular ectasia was detected in 53% and mucosal lesions in 27% (32). Angiodysplasias may be the most common cause of bleeding from the right colon, and they and diverticula are the most common causes of major lower intestinal bleeding in the elderly (33).

These lesions, when they bleed, often produce hematochezia. The bleeding is sometimes brisk and may be massive, but occult blood loss may also occur and seems to be an increasingly common presentation of this disorder (34). Bleeding often stops spontaneously, but it commonly recurs. The lesions cannot be detected by barium enema, are not recognizable from the serosal surface by the surgeon, and are often overlooked by the pathologist. The diagnosis is best made by selective arteriography (by which a malformation can be visualized even when the bleeding has stopped) or by colonoscopy. However, as with diverticula, the mere presence of angiodysplasias does not incriminate them as the source of bleeding, and other potential sources should be sought. Endoscopic therapy with a heater probe, injection sclerotherapy, argon plasma coagulation, or laser ablation of discrete mucosal lesions can be performed by an experienced gastroenterologist. Lesions that are resistant to endoscopic therapy and continue to bleed should be treated by surgical resection of the involved segment of colon. However, angiodysplasias may be present diffusely throughout the intestinal tract and therefore not amenable to endoscopic or surgical therapy. Intra-arterial vasopressin or embolization at angiography may be helpful for actively bleeding lesions of the small and/or large bowel. Medical therapy with a combination of mestranol, 0.05 mg, and norethindrone, 1 mg, may be helpful in preventing rebleeding and decreasing transfusion requirements in patients with diffuse intestinal angiodysplasias (35). Combination therapy is associated with significant adverse effects in both men (gynecomastia, testicular atrophy) and women (vaginal bleeding), and bleeding may recur once the therapy is stopped. Nonetheless, medical therapy may be extremely helpful in selected patients.

Clinicians should be aware of this disorder, especially in elderly patients with GI bleeding in whom the initial evaluation is unrevealing, but the diagnosis is made only after consultation with a gastroenterologist or radiologist.

DIARRHEA

Diarrhea is a troublesome problem that almost everyone has experienced. In infants and children, diarrhea can rapidly lead to death if untreated. The frail elderly also are at increased risk, when they become volume depleted, for strokes or other major ischemic events. In most adult cases, the diarrheal illness begins abruptly, lasts only a day or two, and resolves without serious sequelae (see Chapter 35). Only occasionally does the illness continue for longer than 1 week or do symptoms recur after the initial attack. The task facing the clinician is to identify the few patients with a significant underlying disorder who may require a specific therapeutic approach.

Definition

Patients complaining of diarrhea usually have an increase in the frequency and fluid volume of the bowel movement. Stool weight is the best objective measurement of diarrhea, with mean weights in the United States ranging normally between 100 and 200 g/day. In the patient with chronic diarrhea, objective documentation of daily fecal output is sometimes necessary (see later discussion). Most patients with significant diarrhea produce more than 200 g of stool per day. A subset of patients with diarrhea present with the frequent passage of small volumes of liquid stool. Patients with inflammatory conditions or space-occupying lesions of the rectum may present in this fashion. Patients with the irritable bowel syndrome have stool volumes either within or slightly above the normal range. Patients with secretory forms of diarrhea or small-bowel disorders with malabsorption often pass very large volumes of stool, in the range of 500 to 1000 g/day or more.

Pathophysiology

There are four basic mechanisms of diarrhea: osmotic load within the intestine, which results in retention of water within the lumen; excessive secretion of electrolytes and water into the intestinal lumen; exudation of protein and fluid from the intestinal mucosa; and altered intestinal motility resulting in rapid transit through the colon.

Osmotic diarrhea occurs when poorly absorbed material retains fluid within the intestinal lumen. This mechanism operates in patients with malabsorption or with lactose intolerance, in which undigested sugars accumulate within the intestinal lumen and exert a considerable osmotic load. Magnesium-containing laxatives and some magnesium-containing antacids (e.g., Maalox) probably produce diarrhea through a similar mechanism.

Secretory diarrhea occurs when the intestinal mucosa secretes increased amounts of water and electrolytes under the stimulation of a variety of substances. Cholera is the prototype, but a number of other enterotoxin-producing organisms (e.g., enterotoxigenic *Escherichia coli*) produce diarrhea in the same way (see Chapter 35). Other substances that induce secretory diarrhea include bile acids and long-chain fatty acids (e.g., after ileal resection, in Crohn disease, with a malabsorption syndrome), certain GI hormones, and anthraquinone laxatives. Many of these stimulating agents have been shown to increase intracellular cyclic adenosine monophosphate (cAMP) and to inhibit sodium potassium adenosine triphosphatase (ATPase). The increase in cAMP leads to increased secretion.

Exudative diarrhea results from the outpouring of protein, blood, or mucus from an inflamed or ulcerated mucosa. Ulcerative colitis, Crohn disease, invasive infections (see Chapter 35), and infiltrative disorders such as Whipple disease or lymphoma are examples of this mechanism.

Motility disorders may lead to diarrhea, although the exact correlation between the abnormal motility and the diarrhea is not completely understood. The irritable bowel syndrome (see Chapter 44) is generally believed to be a motor disorder that causes abdominal pain and altered bowel habits, with diarrhea predominating in many patients. Diabetes mellitus may also lead to diarrhea caused by neurogenic dysfunction. Other conditions, such as scleroderma, can lead to stasis of the bowel with resultant bacterial overgrowth, steatorrhea, and diarrhea.

It is not always possible to identify one particular mechanism to account for diarrhea in a given patient; sometimes more than one mechanism is operative. However, an appreciation of pathophysiology enables the clinician to understand the clinical features of a diarrheal illness better and to select appropriate therapy.

Evaluation of Acute Diarrhea

Acute diarrhea caused by infectious agents or by ingested toxins is discussed in greater detail in Chapter 35. Most patients who present to the clinician with a sudden onset of diarrhea have a benign, self-limited illness. These patients do not require extensive evaluation and can simply be reassured. However, a small percentage of such patients have a significant underlying illness for which specific therapy is needed.

If diarrhea persists for longer than 72 hours or if there is gross blood in the stool, an evaluation is indicated. In any case, the patient should always be evaluated before medicine is prescribed, because in certain situations even nonspecific antidiarrheal therapy may be harmful. In particular, it has been shown that opiate-containing antidiarrheal drugs such as diphenoxylate (Lomotil) or loperamide (Imodium) can prolong the course of acute infectious diarrhea by hindering the natural mechanisms that clear the body of the organism (36) and can potentiate the development of the hemolytic-uremic syndrome in patients infected with *E. coli* O157:H7 (37).

History

The history reveals whether the illness is acute or chronic and also provides clues to the underlying cause. The sudden onset of loose, watery stool is most commonly caused by an infectious process, and much less often by ingestion of drugs or poisons. Infectious diarrhea is likely to affect more than one person. Often, no specific bacterial agent is identified and the syndrome is assumed to be a viral gastroenteritis. Bacteria can cause diarrhea by a direct effect on the bowel or by elaboration of a toxin that produces intestinal dysfunction. Toxin-induced diarrhea, often associated with vomiting, begins within 6 hours after ingestion of contaminated food, whereas bacteria-induced diarrhea does not begin for 12 to 24 hours. Examples of toxin-induced diarrhea are enterotoxigenic *E. coli* infection and staphylococcal, clostridial, and *Bacillus cereus* food poisoning. Bloody diarrhea should never be ascribed to viral or toxin-mediated diarrhea; it is more likely to be caused by bacterial infection *(Shigella, Campylobacter, Yersinia, Salmonella,* enterohemorrhagic and enteroinvasive *E. coli*), ulcerative colitis, diverticulosis, ischemic bowel disease, or radiation colitis. Information about recent travel (see Chapter 41) should include not only trips out of the country but also camping or fishing trips within the United States. *Giardia,* for example, may be carried by beavers, which contaminate water supplies and cause both epidemic outbreaks and individual cases of acute diarrhea among campers and hikers. Recent use of drugs is a common cause of new-onset diarrhea (Table 45.5) that may not be readily recognized by the clinician or the patient. Magnesium-containing antacids, broad-spectrum antimicrobials, hydralazine, and quinidine are commonly used drugs that can lead to diarrhea (see later discussion). A history of recent antibiotic therapy, multiple affected friends or family members, associated symptoms such as abdominal or rectal pain, tenesmus, or a history of anal intercourse may provide clues to the etiology of diarrhea.

A number of intestinal infections are seen more commonly in immunocompromised individuals (e.g.,

Table 45.5. Common Drugs That May Induce Diarrhea

Antimicrobials[a]
Clindamycin
Ampicillin
Cephalosporins
Antacids
Magnesium-containing
Antihypertensive Agents
Hydralazine
Propranolol
Cardiovascular Agents
Digitalis
Quinidine
Antimetabolites
Colchicine
Alcohol
Nutritional Supplements
Hyperosmolar solutions (enteral feedings)
Potent Diuretics
Furosemide
Bumetanide

[a]All antimicrobials can induce diarrhea.

those with human immunodeficiency virus [HIV] infection, lymphoma, or immunosuppressive therapy after organ transplantation). Appropriate questions should be asked to identify patients who are at risk for HIV infection (see Chapter 39). Patients with CD4-positive T lymphocyte counts lower than 50/mm^3 or viral burdens greater than 70,000 copies/mL are at particular risk for acquiring infections. In addition to being more susceptible to conventional bacterial and parasitic infections, immunocompromised individuals are at risk for diarrhea from unusual organisms such as *Microsporidium, Cyclospora, Isospora belli, Cryptosporidium, Mycobacterium avium-intracellulare, Cytomegalovirus, Herpes simplex,* and *Candida.*

Physical Examination

The physical examination in acute diarrhea is generally unremarkable. The patient's state of hydration should be estimated because it is an important measure of the severity of the diarrhea and of the need for hospitalization. Some inflammatory and infectious diarrheas are associated with intermittent fever. Abdominal examination usually reveals no more than mild diffuse tenderness. The bowel sounds usually are active or hyperactive. Rectal examination is essential because diarrhea may be the initial manifestation of obstructing rectal carcinoma; furthermore, in the geriatric population, fecal impactions may result in overflow diarrhea, and constipating agents may be mistakenly recommended.

Stool Examination

If diarrhea has continued for longer than 3 to 4 days, the stool should be examined for the presence of blood, leukocytes, and enteric pathogens. Blood in the stool suggests mucosal disruption and is not a feature of osmotic, secretory, or motor diarrhea. Inflammatory conditions such as ulcerative colitis and pseudomembranous colitis (see Chapter 35), as well as *Shigella* and invasive strains of *E. coli,* often cause bloody diarrhea.

Fecal leukocytes are best seen by microscopic examination of the liquid portion of the stool after staining with methylene blue or Gram stain (see Chapter 35, where the technique is described). The recently developed latex agglutination test for the neutrophil product lactoferrin is more sensitive and more specific and can be performed rapidly (38). Fecal leukocytes are not seen in infectious processes that do not invade the mucosa such as viral enteritis, in toxin-mediated diarrhea such as cholera, or in infection with noninvasive *E. coli* (see Chapter 35). *Salmonella, Shigella, Amoeba,* and *Campylobacter,* which are invasive organisms, typically lead to exudation of fecal leukocytes, as does chronic inflammatory bowel disease. In these conditions, in which the mucosal barrier is broken, the course of the diarrheal illness is unpredictable and may even become life-threatening. The absence of fecal leukocytes or blood, even in a single specimen, is therefore reassuring, and in these cases the disease is usually transient.

Stool cultures for bacterial pathogens should be obtained in all patients who have fecal leukocytes. Specific isolation techniques are needed to diagnose *Yersinia* and *Campylobacter,* common causes of acute diarrhea, and should be requested. Acute infectious diarrhea secondary to infection by *Salmonella* or *Shigella* or other invasive organisms is impossible to differentiate from acute inflammatory bowel disease, especially without a stool culture. In the absence of fecal leukocytes, stool cultures are generally negative and are not routinely recommended. Gram staining of the stool for bacteria is not helpful except in cases of suspected staphylococcal enterocolitis or gonococcal proctitis.

Examination of the stool for parasites such as *Entamoeba histolytica* and *Giardia lamblia* is important if diarrhea persists for more than a few days, even in the absence of a history of travel, because the organism can be passed by contact with a carrier. Microscopic examination of the inflammatory exudate of a patient with acute amebic colitis almost always demonstrates motile trophozoites, but only if the slide is prewarmed (e.g., over a light bulb) and then examined immediately. Also, contamination with urine or feces should be avoided. Slides sent to a laboratory for processing are unlikely to reveal amebae. Rectal biopsy may identify the organisms in the exudate. Serologic tests for amebae can be useful but do not distinguish recent from distant infection. Measurement of acute and convalescent titers is more specific for recent infection but gives the diagnosis only in retrospect. *Giardia* can be detected on examination of fresh stool in only about half of affected patients. Duodenal aspiration or biopsy is more sensitive in diagnosing giardiasis. A recently introduced enzyme-linked immunosorbent assay (ELISA) test for giardia antigen in stool has a sensitivity of 96% and a specificity of 100% (39). This test becomes negative after eradication of the infection and probably will replace all other tests for diagnosing *Giardia* infection. If there is a history of recent antibiotic use, three stool specimens should be evaluated for *Clostridium difficile* toxin. Several new rapid tests for *C. difficile* toxins A and B have high sensitivities and specificities (40).

Endoscopy

Flexible sigmoidoscopy is important in patients who have acute diarrhea associated with fecal leukocytes or bloody diarrhea if the cause is not obvious. The examination should be performed without a prior enema, because enemas may alter the appearance of the mucosa and reduce the chance of detecting intestinal pathogens such as amebae. The marginal diagnostic return in examining the entire colon is quite small, so flexible sigmoidoscopy is preferable to colonoscopy in this situation.

Many acute diarrheal illnesses produce a similar abnormal but nonspecific mucosal appearance on sigmoidoscopy. However, certain findings suggest specific diseases. In viral enteritis, giardiasis, toxin-mediated diarrhea, drug-induced diarrhea, and other conditions not accompanied by fecal leukocytes or blood loss, the sigmoidoscopy is normal. In *ulcerative colitis,* the rectal mucosa is involved in at least 95% of cases, and the mucosa is uniformly abnormal with bleeding and a granular, friable appearance. *Crohn disease* uncommonly affects the rectum, but it is often apparent in the sigmoid or more proximal portions of the colon. It may appear as discrete aphthoid ulcers or patches of grossly abnormal mucosa with normal intervening tissue. *Amebiasis* occasionally produces flask-shaped ulcers that may be single or multiple, with normal intervening mucosa; more often, however, it produces a pattern very similar to that of ulcerative colitis. In *shigellosis,* multiple small, superficial ulcers may be seen, but the appearance may also be indistinguishable from that of ulcerative colitis. *Pseudomembranous colitis* is identified by the presence of numerous raised yellow plaques covering an inflamed mucosa. Occasionally a carcinoma or large villous adenoma may be detected by sigmoidoscopy. Sigmoidoscopy also provides an opportune time to obtain samples of stool and exudate for culture and microscopic examination. The patient's experience with sigmoidoscopy is described in Chapter 46.

Radiographic Studies

Radiography is of limited use in the evaluation of acute diarrhea and may, in fact, be confusing. In patients with suspected inflammatory bowel disease or ischemic colitis, plain films of the abdomen may demonstrate an irregular appearance of the bowel wall secondary to mucosal edema, often described as "thumbprinting." In the gravely ill patient with fulminant colitis, the radiograph may confirm the presence of toxic megacolon. In most cases of acute diarrhea, a plain film is not needed. Barium studies during the acute phase of the diarrhea are likewise not needed and in certain conditions may even be hazardous, as in patients with severe colitis or ischemic bowel disease. A small bowel series in acute viral enteritis may be frighteningly abnormal, resembling sprue, and yet may rapidly return to normal after resolution of the acute illness.

Evaluation of Chronic Diarrhea

The approach to patients with either acute diarrhea that lasts longer than 3 to 4 days or chronic diarrhea (lasting longer than 4 weeks) is very much the same. Although the clinician may be reassured by knowing that the majority of such patients do not have a serious progressive or disabling disease, the patient requires a specific diagnosis and effective therapy. The differential diagnosis is so varied, and the available tests are so numerous, that the diagnostic workup of chronic diarrhea poses a difficult problem. The following discussion provides a practical approach to this problem.

History

The history is often helpful in differentiating organic from functional diarrhea (e.g., irritable bowel syndrome; see Chapter 44). If organic diarrhea is suspected, it is important to determine whether the pathogenic mechanism is osmotic, secretory, motor, or exudative (see earlier discussion). Patients should be asked to describe the characteristics of the stools, whether they are too frequent, loose, excessive in volume, malodorous, floating, or associated with fever, blood, mucus, tenesmus, bloating, or excessive flatus.

In patients with so-called *functional diarrhea,* the history of diarrhea often dates back many months or years, although occasionally it can be traced to a specific acute diarrheal illness. Despite the chronicity, no sequelae, such as weight loss, anemia, or hypoalbuminemia, have occurred. The patient typically complains of several watery, at times explosive bowel movements early in the morning, and then no subsequent movements the rest of the day. Nocturnal bowel movements are rare. The total stool output is usually small—often less than 200 g/day and rarely, if ever, more than 500 g/day. Mucus often is present. There is no blood in the stool unless secondary conditions (e.g., anal fissures) have developed. Postprandial pain is a feature of irritable bowel syndrome (see Chapter 44) but is absent in many patients. The condition often waxes and wanes in severity, and stress often exacerbates the symptoms.

The most common cause of chronic secretory diarrhea is *laxative abuse.* It should be suspected in apparently healthy patients with large-volume diarrhea, especially if they have *melanosis coli* (spotty or diffuse brownish mucosal pigmentation) on sigmoidoscopic examination. Although such patients may have emotional problems with which the clinician must deal (see Chapter 21), often the abuse simply reflects a misconception about the frequency of normal bowel movements and an attempt to adhere to that standard.

In patients with organic disease, the history may indicate the part of the intestinal tract that is involved. The passage of a large volume of frothy, malodorous stool without blood suggests small-bowel diarrhea, often secondary to malabsorption. The frequent passage of small volumes of poorly formed, bloody stools suggests inflammatory, exudative disorders of the colon such as ulcerative colitis. The presence of recognizable fat droplets (oil) suggests malabsorption, often secondary to pancreatic insufficiency. (Floating stools and undigested food in the stools are not always helpful observations because they may be seen in both organic and functional diarrheal states.) The association of diarrhea with the ingestion of certain dietary products (milk, fruit, hyperosmolar solutions, sorbitol-containing gum or candy) may not be recognized by the patient unless he or she is specifically asked. A detailed drug history is also important, because many drugs can cause diarrhea (Table 45.5; see later discussion).

Other symptoms may help the physician to arrive at a specific diagnosis. *Arthritis* and *arthralgias* may suggest the presence of one of several uncommon bowel diseases, such as inflammatory bowel disease or

Whipple disease; conversely, diarrhea may be an important feature of Reiter syndrome (see Chapter 78). *Weight loss,* in the absence of anorexia, should suggest malabsorption, hyperthyroidism, or a malignant tumor. *Abdominal pain* may reflect the irritable bowel syndrome (see Chapter 44), in which case it is generally in the left lower quadrant or the suprapubic region; or a disease of the small bowel (e.g., Crohn disease), in which case it is often periumbilical or in the right lower quadrant; or a gastrinoma (Zollinger–Ellison syndrome), in which case peptic ulcers are responsible for upper abdominal pain.

A history of previous GI or biliary surgery, intravenous drug abuse, or anal intercourse, or a family history of inflammatory bowel disease or celiac sprue, may sometimes provide clues to the etiology of diarrhea. Some patients may report fecal incontinence as diarrhea; incontinence is rarely reported voluntarily and should be specifically inquired about.

Physical Examination

The physical examination may reveal additional information about the cause of the diarrhea. Patients with malabsorption may have evidence of weight loss, peripheral neuropathy (secondary to vitamin B deficiency), and carpopedal spasm (secondary to hypocalcemia). Erythema nodosum and pyoderma gangrenosum are seen in some cases of inflammatory bowel disease. Hyperpigmentation is a feature of both Whipple disease and Addison disease. Diabetic diarrhea is often associated with other evidence of autonomic dysfunction, such as postural hypotension. Nondeforming arthritis is a feature of Whipple disease and of inflammatory bowel disease. Hepatosplenomegaly and lymphadenopathy suggest lymphoma or Whipple disease. The abdominal examination may reveal an arterial bruit or an aortic aneurysm, which suggests ischemic bowel disease. A rectal examination may disclose perianal disease (e.g., abscesses or fistulas secondary to Crohn disease), a rectal tumor, or a fecal impaction.

Endoscopy

Flexible sigmoidoscopy, done primarily if an infectious etiology is suspected or if disease is thought to be limited to the rectosigmoid region (e.g., ulcerative proctitis), may be performed during the initial visit without a prior cleansing enema. Examination and biopsy of the rectosigmoid mucosa may suggest specific etiologies (ulcerative colitis, Crohn disease, amebiasis, pseudomembranous colitis, Whipple disease, or amyloidosis). Even a grossly normal-appearing mucosa is worth biopsying, because collagenous colitis or microscopic colitis, for example, may be present in patients with chronic watery diarrhea. The finding of melanosis coli in a patient complaining of diarrhea indicates laxative abuse. At the time of sigmoidoscopy, stool specimens are obtained for microscopic evaluation and culture. Gonococcal proctitis appears similar to ulcerative proctitis (discussed later) and requires direct plating on a warm special culture medium (Thayer–Martin) with prompt incubation. Routine stool cultures should be taken as well. The stool should be examined for leukocytes, blood, fat (Sudan stain), and parasites (see Chapter 35).

Colonoscopy, which does require bowel preparation, may be a preferable procedure, especially in patients 40 years of age or older, an age when the incidence of colon cancer begins to rise. In approximately one third of patients with chronic diarrhea, a histologic diagnosis is made after colonoscopy and biopsy (41).

After this initial evaluation, the cause of the chronic diarrhea in most patients is either evident or strongly suspected. It is usually possible to distinguish functional from organic diarrhea, to detect evidence of inflammatory or infiltrative disease, to suspect the presence of malabsorption, to characterize the diarrhea as small bowel or large bowel, and even to suggest the underlying pathophysiology. Further evaluation is then dictated by the results of this initial workup.

Laboratory Studies

Laboratory studies should be selected to support the clinical impression, but they rarely are able to make or exclude a specific diagnosis. In general, the possibility of blood loss (stool Hemoccult and hematocrit value), malnutrition (serum albumin concentration), and fluid-electrolyte imbalance are assessed.

Radiologic Studies

A plain film of the abdomen may reveal pancreatic calcifications (indicative of chronic pancreatitis), a dilated small bowel, or an abnormal bowel contour (as in inflammatory bowel disease or lymphoma).

In the patient older than 40 years of age who has chronic or recurrent diarrhea, a *colonoscopy* is preferred by the majority of gastrointerologists during the initial evaluation. In younger patients, colonoscopy is unlikely to be useful unless a specific disorder is suspected. The presence of blood in the stool, at any age, is a clear indication for a colonoscopy or barium enema, regardless of the presence of hemorrhoids or fissures. Neoplastic and inflammatory conditions may be diagnosed in this way, and ulcerative colitis and Crohn disease of the colon can be differentiated in most cases. When inflammatory bowel disease is suspected, if a barium enema is done, an attempt should be made to reflux contrast material into the terminal ileum to rule out Crohn disease of the ileum.

The timing of the barium enema is important. Barium interferes with the collection of stool for measurement of volume and fat and with the detection of parasites. A barium enema should be delayed for 1 week after a rectal biopsy to avoid colonic perforation. The patient's experience with the barium enema is discussed earlier.

A *small bowel series* (see above for a discussion of the patient's experience with this procedure) is helpful in distinguishing mucosal disease (celiac sprue), inflammatory conditions (Crohn disease), and infiltrative processes (Whipple disease or amyloidosis). In addition, a small bowel series is indicated in postsurgical patients to clarify the anatomy (e.g., blind loop, fistula) and to detect localized areas of dilation and stasis.

Other Studies

A *quantitative 72-hour stool collection,* although regarded as unpleasant by both the patient and laboratory personnel, is a very informative test. It should be used early in the evaluation of patients in whom the initial routine workup does not suggest a diagnosis. The test can be performed in the ambulatory setting by having the patient collect all stool in a preweighed container supplied by the clinical laboratory. The test should be performed before barium studies or other invasive tests are done. A log of daily food intake and bowel activity is kept, and all nonessential medications are avoided. The normal stool weight is less than 200 g/day (or volume less than 200 mL/day). Most patients with irritable bowel syndrome or other functional forms of chronic diarrhea have stool weights and volumes within this range. A stool volume of more than 1000 mL/day suggests a secretory diarrhea or malabsorption.

Fecal fat should also be measured during this collection. Normally less than 9% of ingested fat is secreted in the stool per day (4 to 7 g on an average American diet containing 60 to 100 g of fat). Fecal fat excretion of more than 14 g/day is considered steatorrhea. It is important to remember that severe diarrhea by itself can cause fat malabsorption with fecal fat values between 7 and 14 g/day. Although it is less reliable, a qualitative test for stool fat by Sudan stain can be useful as a rapid screening test for steatorrhea. The presence of steatorrhea dictates a different approach to the remainder of the workup (see later discussion). In the absence of excessive fat excretion or evidence of an exudative process (e.g., inflammatory bowel disease), high-volume diarrhea suggests a secretory process.

The *osmotic gap* of the stool can help differentiate secretory from osmotic diarrhea (42). The osmotic gap can be calculated as $290 - 2\,([Na^+] + [K^+])$. The concentration of Na^+ and K^+ in homogenized stool water can be directly measured. The sum of the concentrations of these ions is multiplied by 2 to account for unmeasured anions. The final product is then subtracted from 290 because studies have shown that in the distal intestine, the stool osmolality equilibrates with the osmolality of plasma. In pure osmotic diarrhea, the stool osmotic gap is greater than 125. In pure secretory diarrhea, the osmotic gap is less than 50. In mixed osmotic and secretory diarrhea, the osmotic gap may be between 50 and 125. A fecal pH of less than 5.3 is suggestive of carbohydrate malabsorption. However, fecal pH is higher if there is associated malabsorption of fat and protein.

Urine and stool specimens should be sent for spectrophotometry or thin-layer chromatography to detect anthraquinones, bisacodyl, or phenolphthalein in patients with suspected laxative abuse.

In patients with suspected secretory diarrhea, further evaluation usually requires hospitalization and consultation with a gastroenterologist. In secretory diarrhea, having the patient ingest nothing by mouth for 48 hours does not alter the volume of diarrhea, whereas in osmotic diarrhea the stool volume significantly decreases. If laxative abuse is ruled out, a secretagogue-secreting tumor can be investigated by measuring serum gastrin (Zollinger–Ellison syndrome) or serum vasoactive intestinal peptide.

Evaluation of Malabsorption

When the quantitative or qualitative fecal fat determination indicates steatorrhea, the evaluation of the diarrhea should be focused on the cause of malabsorption. Malabsorption can result from small-intestinal disease, pancreatic disease, hepatobiliary disease, or gastric disease. A series of diagnostic studies is used initially to define the organ involved and then to diagnose the specific disease. Consultation with a gastroenterologist is generally recommended to help perform and analyze these various tests.

The *D-xylose* test measures the absorptive capacity of the proximal small bowel and is useful in distinguishing malabsorption from maldigestion (pancreatic enzyme deficiency). D-Xylose does not require the pancreatic stage of digestion to be absorbed by an intact small-intestinal mucosa. After absorption it enters the blood and is excreted in the urine. The test is performed in the same manner as an oral glucose tolerance test and can be performed in the ambulatory setting by most clinical laboratories. A 25-g oral dose of xylose is given, and the patient's urine is collected over the next 5 hours. The test is considered positive if urinary excretion of D-xylose is less than 5 g in 5 hours or the plasma concentration is less than 20 mg/dL one hour after ingestion of D-xylose. A blood sample is collected 1 hour after ingestion. In disorders of the intestinal mucosa (e.g., celiac disease, Whipple disease), xylose is poorly absorbed and low levels are found in the serum and urine. Uncommonly, massive bacterial overgrowth may also produce an abnormal D-xylose test that reverts to normal with antibiotic treatment. Because an abnormal xylose test suggests mucosal disease, a *small-bowel biopsy* should be performed next. Dehydration, renal insufficiency, third spacing of fluid, vomiting, and hypothyroidism may spuriously decrease urine (but not serum) levels of D-xylose.

If the D-xylose test is normal, maldigestion, usually caused by *pancreatic insufficiency,* is the most likely cause of steatorrhea. In chronic pancreatitis, pancreatic calcifications may be seen on an abdominal plain film, and diabetes mellitus is sometimes present. Pancreatic insufficiency can be confirmed by measuring pancreatic secretions or by measuring intraluminal contents after a test meal. These tests involve intubation of the duodenum, with collection of intraluminal contents. Other methods do not require intubation but simply entail urine collection; for example, the *bentiromide test* uses a nonabsorbable synthetic peptide (500 mg of bentiromide) that is cleaved by the pancreatic enzyme chymotrypsin to release para-aminobenzoic acid, which is then absorbed and measured when it is excreted in the urine. Urinary excretion of less than 85 mg of para-aminobenzoic acid in 6 hours is considered positive. This test has a sensitivity of 85% and specificity of 95% (43). Measurement of *fecal concentrations of the pancreatic enzymes chymotrypsin and elastase* also have a high sensitivity and specificity for pancreatic insufficiency, and they are much easier to perform than the bentiromide test (44). Often, however, if a presumptive diagnosis of pancreatic insufficiency is made, the patient is treated empirically with pancreatic enzymes (e.g., Viokase, three to six tablets with meals, or Pancrease, two to three tablets with meals). If the diagnosis is correct, symptoms are moderately improved but not entirely eliminated. Diagnostic and therapeutic decisions should be made in consultation with a gastroenterologist.

Endoscopic biopsy of the small intestine is often useful in the detection of various disorders that can cause malabsorption or diarrhea, or both. Disorders that may be diagnosed by small-bowel biopsy include sprue, Whipple disease, intestinal lymphoma, amyloidosis, lymphangiectasia, and eosinophilic gastroenteritis. Giardiasis can also be diagnosed by examination of the intestinal mucosa and the intestinal mucus or fluid.

Disorders of the terminal ileum (Crohn disease, ileal resection) may also lead to diarrhea and malabsorption. Evaluation may include a *Schilling II test* or a *bile salt breath test.* The Schilling II test measures vitamin B_{12} absorption, which is abnormal in disorders of the terminal ileum, the site of B_{12} absorption. Absorption is impaired despite the presence of intrinsic factor (see Chapter 55) or the administration of antibiotics.

Similarly, the *bile salt breath test* measures bile acid absorption, which is also abnormal in disorders of the terminal ileum, the site of bile salt absorption. The patient is given orally a radiolabeled (^{14}C) bile salt. In the presence of terminal ileal disease, the bile salt is malabsorbed and excess acid reaches the colon, where bacteria deconjugate it and release $^{14}CO_2$, which diffuses across the colon and is excreted in the breath. Therefore, in ileal disease, the level of $^{14}CO_2$ in the patient's expired air is abnormally high. The same abnormality can be seen when there is bacterial overgrowth in the small bowel, so that the bile acid is deconjugated and metabolized there instead of in the colon. Bile acid malabsorption caused by bacterial overgrowth is reversed when the patient is given antibiotics. Both the Schilling test and the bile salt breath test are performed by nuclear medicine specialists.

Specific Causes of Chronic Diarrhea

Lactose Intolerance

Lactose is by far the most commonly malabsorbed carbohydrate. Lactose intolerance results from a deficiency or total absence of the enzyme lactase in the brush border of the intestinal mucosa, which causes maldigestion and therefore malabsorption of lactose. The unabsorbed carbohydrate exerts an osmotic effect that draws water into the intestinal lumen. In the colon, the lactose is metabolized by bacteria to organic acid, CO_2, and hydrogen. The acid contributes to the diarrhea by both an osmotic effect and an irritant effect on the colonic mucosa. The unabsorbed carbohydrate, if present in sufficient quantities (the critical amount varies widely), may cause diarrhea, gaseousness, bloating, and abdominal cramps.

Lactose intolerance may be present either as an inherited condition, "lactase nonpersistence" after childhood, or one that is acquired because of damage to the intestinal epithelium (e.g., infectious enteritis, sprue). Even in patients with a genetic disorder, the onset of the disease is unpredictable and may not occur until adult life. The secondary cases are usually, but not always, reversible if the underlying disease is successfully treated. The severity of the clinical symptoms is highly variable.

In some patients even small amounts of lactose produce severe symptoms, but in others large quantities may be consumed with no or only minimal symptoms. Isolated lactase deficiency is most common in African Americans (70% to 100% prevalence) and in Asians (more than 90%) but may also be found in 12% of the white population in the United States (45). The condition is more pronounced in certain clinical settings: when superimposed on another diarrheal disorder, most commonly irritable bowel syndrome; after gastric surgery, which permits rapid delivery of lactose to the small bowel; and when a patient consumes extra amounts of milk as part of (misguided) therapy for ulcer disease.

The diagnosis of lactose intolerance is suggested by the history and the response to a lactose-free diet. However, almost one third of patients with symptomatic lactose intolerance may not have made the correlation between dietary intake and the resulting symptoms, because a wide variety of foods contain lactose, ranging from bread to instant coffee.

Ordinarily, a 3-week trial of a diet that is free of milk and milk products is a satisfactory therapeutic trial to test the diagnosis of lactose intolerance. Other tests are indicated only in equivocal cases or when the patient's nutritional status would be compromised by eliminating milk products unnecessarily.

Specific tests for the diagnosis of *lactose intolerance* include the *lactose tolerance test* and the *hydrogen breath test.* The lactose tolerance test measures changes in the concentration of serum glucose at 1 and 2 hours after ingestion of 50 g of lactose. A rise in glucose of 20 mg/100 mL above the fasting level is normal. The test has approximately a 30% false positive rate, and its validity depends on a variety of factors besides simply the presence of the lactase enzyme. The hydrogen breath test is easier to perform and is more accurate. Unabsorbed lactose is fermented by colonic bacteria, and the resultant hydrogen is absorbed and expired in the breath. In normal subjects, after a 25 g lactose load, there is only a trace amount of hydrogen in the expired air, whereas in lactase-deficient patients substantial levels are recorded. An increase in breath hydrogen of 20 ppm above baseline within 4 hours is considered positive. This test is widely available; it is usually performed by a nuclear medicine specialist or in a gastroenterology laboratory, and it requires 2 to 4 hours of the patient's time.

Fecal Impaction

Although it is the result of chronic constipation, fecal impaction (46) commonly causes diarrhea. The adults most at risk for impaction are elderly sedentary people, often those who are bedridden. The feces are usually impacted in the rectum or in the rectosigmoid region but occasionally may extend high up into the colon (rarely, even to the cecum). The leaking of colonic fluid around the impaction, which results in the passage of frequent, small-volume, watery bowel movements, accounts for the diarrhea. Other symptoms are common but are usually nonspecific: a sense of fullness in the rectum, vague lower abdominal pain, nausea, and headache. On physical examination, the firm stool is palpable in the left lower quadrant of the abdomen, which is best examined bimanually (a finger of one hand in the rectum and the other hand on the abdomen). The impaction is best removed manually if it is low enough, or through the sigmoidoscope if it is not. Repeated enemas (e.g., a Fleet enema) may be helpful once some of the very hard stool is removed. Complications of impaction include recurrent urinary tract infection (because of compression of the ureters, more common in women), urinary incontinence, intestinal obstruction, perforation of the colon, and local ulceration (stercoral ulcer). Prevention of fecal impaction is an important goal in the sedentary elderly population and is best done by increasing dietary fiber, adding a bulk laxative if necessary, and urging that at least 2 quarts of liquid be ingested each day, in addition to that consumed in the course of meals. Patients should also be sure to respond promptly to the urge to defecate.

Ulcerative Colitis

Ulcerative colitis is a chronic inflammatory disorder of the colonic and rectal mucosa; its cause is unknown. It is recommended that patients with this condition be monitored by their primary care provider in consultation with a gastroenterologist. The disorder may affect patients of any age, with a peak incidence in the third decade and a second peak in the seventh decade.

The clinical picture of ulcerative colitis is highly variable (Table 45.6). The disorder may be limited to the rectum (ulcerative proctitis) or may involve the entire colon. Symptoms may range from occasional rectal bleeding, even without diarrhea, to profuse purulent and bloody diarrhea. The severity of the initial presentation and the extent of disease at the time of the initial attack have been shown to be useful predictors of the eventual course of the disease (47). Most patients (approximately 60%) have mild disease, that is, fewer than four bowel movements a day without fever, weight loss, or hypoalbuminemia. The vast majority of these patients have colitis limited to the rectosigmoid region or descending colon. Approximately 10% to 15% of patients with ulcerative colitis develop severe pancolitis with accompanying deterioration in their general health. Another 25% have moderate disease with more troublesome diarrhea, often containing blood, accompanied by crampy lower abdominal pain. Patients with moderate or severe disease may also have systemic symptoms of fever, fatigue, and weight loss. The clinical course is characterized by periodic exacerbations that generally respond well to adjustments in medical therapy. The smallest group of patients with ulcerative colitis consists of those with severe disease. This group includes the 1% of patients who present initially with fulminant colitis. In patients with severe colitis, symptoms may suddenly worsen, with profuse diarrhea, rectal bleeding, and high fevers. Plain films of the abdomen may demonstrate a dilated bowel (toxic megacolon). Mortality is high in this group of patients.

Table 45.6. Severity of Ulcerative Colitis

Severity	Description
Mild	<4 bowel movements daily with no blood or only small amount of blood No systemic signs of toxicity ESR <30 mm/hr
Moderate	>4 bowel movements daily Systemic signs and symptoms including low-grade fever, fatigue, and weight loss
Severe	≥6 bowel movements daily with blood Signs of systemic toxicity including high fever, tachycardia, anemia ESR >30 mm/hr

ESR, erythrocyte sedimentation rate.

Because there is no specific test for, or histopathology of, ulcerative colitis, the diagnosis depends on the constellation of symptoms, the appropriate endoscopic and histologic appearance of the colonic mucosa, the exclusion of other inflammatory conditions, and the natural history of the disorder. Patients with acute presentations, depending on the circumstances, must be differentiated from patients with infectious diarrheas caused by *Salmonella, Shigella,* or *Campylobacter* (see Chapter 35); amebiasis; Crohn disease (Table 45.7); and ischemic colitis. (Patients with *ischemic colitis* present with acute abdominal pain and the passage of bloody stool; this is a disease of middle-aged or older people who usually have evidence of generalized atherosclerosis.)

Treatment. *Medical therapy* for ulcerative colitis is determined by the severity of the attack and the extent of disease, and it should be individualized. (The use of antidiarrheal drugs in patients with chronic diarrhea is discussed later in this chapter.) Mild attacks may respond to sulfasalazine (Azulfidine, 4 to 6 g/day) or to 5-aminosalicylic acid (ASA) agents (mesalamine, 2 to 4.8 g/day, or olsalazine, 1.5 to 3.0 g/day), whereas moderate or severe attacks require treatment with oral or intravenous steroids (equivalent to prednisone 40 to 60 mg/day). Steroids are very useful for acute exacerbations, especially in patients with severe disease or toxic symptoms, but they are not helpful in preventing relapses. Conversely,

Table 45.7. Differentiating Features of Crohn Disease and Ulcerative Colitis

Feature	Crohn Disease	Ulcerative Colitis
Symptoms	Pain and diarrhea are the prominent symptoms; bleeding is uncommon	Bloody diarrhea with tenesmus and lower abdominal cramps
Distribution	Can occur anywhere in the gastrointestinal tract from mouth to anus	Usually limited to the colon
Endoscopic features	Skip lesions with normal intervening mucosa, deep serpiginous ulcers, rectal sparing, anal skin tags, and perianal fistulas	Continuous involvement; mucosa appears granular, ulcerated, and friable; rectum is involved with variable proximal extension
Microscopic features	Transmural inflammation, submucosal fibrosis, focal granulomas, discrete mucosal ulcers	Mucosal inflammation, crypt distortion, crypt abscesses, lymphoid aggregates
Radiology	Terminal ileal involvement and narrowing (string sign), ileal strictures, fistulas; colonic haustrations remain normal	Rectal involvement, ground-glass appearance of mucosa, flattening of haustral markings (lead pipe sign)
Complications	Fistulas, ileal obstruction, abscesses	Toxic megacolon, bleeding, cancer

sulfasalazine is of limited value in the treatment of acute attacks but has been shown to reduce the frequency of exacerbations and may allow reduction of the dosage of steroids. Topical mesalamine or corticosteroids in the form of enemas or suppositories may be sufficient therapy for mild to moderate distal colitis. Patients with severe disease who do not improve after 7 to 10 days of high-dose steroid therapy may require either intravenous cyclosporine, 4 mg/kg per day, or surgery. A minority of patients with ulcerative colitis become steroid dependent and need 6-mercaptopurine (6-MP) or azathioprine for 3 to 4 months before steroids can be successfully tapered, followed by long-term therapy with these agents. For the maintenance of remission in ulcerative colitis, oral mesalamine or sulfasalazine is recommended. Chronic treatment with oral corticosteroids has not been shown to prevent recurrences and is not recommended. Azathioprine or 6-MP, 1.5 to 2.5 mg/kg day, may be used in patients who are steroid dependent or refractory to corticosteroids or 5-ASA agents, preferably in consultation with a gastroenterologist.

It has been discovered that nicotine alleviates symptoms in patients with ulcerative colitis (48), but whether it should be recommended treatment remains to be clarified.

Surgery in ulcerative colitis is curative, and patients should be counseled early in their course about the role of surgery in the treatment of this disorder. Patients should be informed about the indications for surgery and the types of operations that are available. Early attention to this issue enables the patient to accept an operation more readily if it is needed. Surgery for ulcerative colitis involves a proctocolectomy with an ileostomy to which a stomal appliance is attached to ensure continence (see Chapter 46. Construction of a continent ileostomy (Kock pouch) avoids the need for a stomal appliance, but the procedure is technically difficult and often requires revision. Another alternative is construction of an internal pouch from a loop of small bowel anastomosed to the anus (Park's procedure). These last two procedures are most successful in motivated young patients who are undergoing elective colectomy.

Cancer of the Colon. The risk of colorectal cancer is increased 5 to 10 times in patients with ulcerative colitis (49). The major risk factors are duration of disease (risk increases significantly after 8 to 10 years of disease), extent of colonic involvement (pancolitis carries the highest risk, whereas the risk in patients with ulcerative proctitis is similar to that of the general population), and age at onset of disease (patients younger than 25 years of age at the time of onset have the highest risk, independent of the extent of disease). The cancer may be found anywhere in the colon, although most commonly it is within the rectum or rectosigmoid. It may be multicentric and does not arise in adenomatous polyps. It is important that the patient know about the risk of cancer because it may influence a decision to undergo colectomy. After they have had the disease for 8 to 10 years, high-risk patients should have yearly evaluations of the colon by colonoscopy. Because dysplastic changes of the colonic mucosa have been identified as precancerous and have been shown to correlate closely with the development of cancer elsewhere in the colon, serial colonic and rectal biopsies should be obtained during this yearly colonoscopy in high-risk patients.

Crohn Disease

Crohn disease, or *regional enteritis,* is a chronic inflammatory condition of unknown cause involving all layers of the intestine, as opposed to just the mucosa (as in ulcerative colitis; see Table 45.7). The condition most commonly affects the terminal ileum, but any area from the esophagus to the anus can be involved. The onset of the disease most commonly occurs in adolescence or young adulthood. The incidence of Crohn disease has been rising in recent years, particularly Crohn disease of the colon.

Presentation. Crohn disease may be localized initially to the small bowel, involve small bowel and colon, or be confined to the colon only. The inflammatory process often remains confined to the initial site of involvement unless surgery is performed. Recurrence is the rule after surgery, and the condition may then involve additional segments of bowel. Spontaneous progression of the disease tends to occur in a proximal (orad) direction. As the inflammatory process persists, the bowel wall becomes thickened and stenotic, leading to bowel obstruction. Fistula formation is characteristic and may involve any contiguous structure. As a result, abscess formation and infection can complicate the clinical course. Diarrhea, abdominal pain, and weight loss are the most common symptoms. Unlike ulcerative colitis, rectal bleeding is not a prominent feature unless the colon is the major site of involvement.

The *differential diagnosis* includes disorders of both the small and the large bowel. Occasionally the patient presents with fever and acute right lower quadrant pain resembling acute appendicitis. When there is terminal ileal involvement, Crohn disease must be distinguished from lymphoma and tuberculosis. Colonic involvement may suggest ulcerative colitis, ischemic colitis, or carcinoma. Involvement of the distal small bowel and the right colon, the presence of characteristic skip areas, stricturing of the bowel, perianal disease, and fistula formation are helpful diagnostic features that suggest Crohn disease.

Treatment. *Medical therapy* for Crohn disease is similar to that for ulcerative colitis, depending heavily on corticosteroids and 5-ASA preparations or sulfasalazine. For mild to moderate active Crohn disease, 5-ASA agents or sulfasalazine (see earlier discussion for dosing schedule) should be used as first-line agents. Metronidazole (1–2 gm per day) or ciprofloxacin (1g/day) is as effective as mesalamine or sulfasalazine and may be used in patients who are allergic or intolerant to them or in combination with the first-line agents. Long-term metronidazole therapy is, however, associated with development of peripheral neuropathy in some individuals. Patients with severe disease usually require a course of prednisone, 40 to 60 mg/day until the symptoms resolve, followed by a slow taper. A monoclonal antibody to tumor necrosis factor alpha (Infliximab), given in a single intravenous dose of 5 mg/kg, may be used as adjunctive therapy in individuals not responding to steroids. Patients with severe or fulminant disease require aggressive treatment, which often includes hospitalization, parenteral hyperalimentation, and either intravenous cyclosporine or oral tacrolimus. Surgery may become necessary if response to medical therapy is not optimal. As in ulcerative colitis, steroids are not effective in preventing relapses and should not be used for maintenance of remission. After the control of acute disease, mesalamine, sulfasalazine, metronidazole, ciprofloxacin, 6-MP, or azathioprine may be used for maintenance therapy. Infliximab is effective in closing fistulas in one third or more of the patients (50). However, some patients require periodic infusions every 8 to 12 weeks to prevent recurrence. Although they are not as effective, antibiotics, 6-MP, and azathioprine may also be useful in the treatment of fistulizing Crohn disease.

Because of the complexity of the disease, management should be accomplished by, or in consultation with, a gastroenterologist.

Surgery is sometimes necessary in Crohn disease for resection of fibrotic obstructing lesions, drainage of abscesses, and resection of complicated fistulas. Occasionally the disease is refractory to medical therapy and the diseased bowel must be resected. It must be recognized that surgery is not intended to be curative, so removal of normal bowel to achieve wide, disease-free margins is not indicated. In the rare patient whose disease is extensive and unresponsive to medical and surgical intervention or in whom a short-bowel syndrome has developed secondary to the disease and to repeated surgery, long-term home parenteral hyperalimentation can be beneficial to provide good nutritional support and ameliorate symptoms.

Course. Despite its chronicity and tendency for recurrence, Crohn disease takes a highly variable course. Prolonged asymptomatic periods occur, even after years of disease activity and multiple operations. There is a poor correlation between clinical severity and the radiologic appearance of the disease, so follow-up radiographs are not indicated unless there is a suspicion of a new development in the disease (e.g., a fistula). The risk of colorectal carcinoma is elevated significantly only in Crohn disease involving the colon, and even then probably not to the same degree as in ulcerative colitis. Mortality from the disease is low, but morbidity is high. Because the natural history is so variable, the clinician should approach the patient with Crohn disease in a positive and hopeful fashion, yet be aware of the potential for significant morbidity. All patients should be monitored in close consultation with a gastroenterologist.

Drug-Induced Diarrhea

A variety of commonly used medications can cause diarrhea (Table 45.5). The diarrhea may be a direct result of the pharmacologic activity of the drug (e.g., magnesium-containing antacids, colchicine), or the mechanism for the induction of diarrhea may be unknown (e.g., hydralazine, propranolol). The diarrhea may also signify drug toxicity (e.g., digitalis). Certain drugs have repeatedly been associated with diarrhea (antibiotics, antacids, quinidine, digitalis, and alcohol), whereas in other cases (hydralazine, propranolol), the relationship is rare and not well defined.

Diarrhea associated with antibiotics may range from a mild increase in the frequency and volume of stools to a toxic, life-threatening condition. Diarrhea may develop during the course of antibiotic therapy, or after parenteral or oral use, but it may also occur up to months after discontinuation of the drugs. The antibiotics most commonly associated with diarrhea are ampicillin, tetracycline, clindamycin, and the cephalosporins.

In the more severe forms of antibiotic-associated diarrhea, the diarrhea is bloody and is accompanied by abdominal cramps and fever. Endoscopy may reveal pseudomembranes, which appear as raised yellowish plaques on edematous, friable mucosa. Histologically, these pseudomembranes are collections of fibrin, mucin, and leukocytes. Proliferation of *C. difficile* and the elaboration of its toxin cause pseudomembranous colitis. This organism accounts for the vast majority of cases of pseudomembranous colitis and for 20% to 30% of antibiotic-associated diarrhea in general. The toxin elaborated by *C. difficile* can be assayed in stool. The organism can also be cultured, but it is difficult to grow. Because culture is less sensitive than the toxin titer and does not correlate as well with symptoms, it is not recommended.

Therapy involves discontinuation of the antibiotics and, in cases of pseudomembranous colitis, administration of metronidazole (Flagyl), 500 mg four times a day for 7 days (see Chapter 35). This antimicrobial agent is effective against clostridial organisms, and the response is fairly rapid. Relapses after discontinuation of metronidazole are not uncommon. In such cases, a second course should be administered. Vancomycin may be prescribed (125 to 500 mg orally four times a day for 7 days) for cases repeatedly resistant or relapsing after metronidazole. Oral cholestyramine has also been used effectively to bind the toxin. Antidiarrheal medications are contraindicated because they may actually prolong the duration of the disease. It is probably unnecessary to treat patients who are found to have *C. difficile* toxin–positive stools, as is common in nursing homes, unless there are accompanying symptoms or an outbreak is in progress. Symptomatic patients can be treated with bismuth subsalicylate (Pepto-Bismol), 30 mL or 2 tablets every 4 hours, while results of the assay for the toxin are awaited.

Postsurgical Diarrhea

A variety of surgical procedures may result in diarrhea. Predictably, *extensive small-bowel resections* (e.g., for mesenteric vascular occlusions) result in severe diarrhea and steatorrhea (short-bowel syndrome). Management of such cases requires careful attention to nutritional factors and often use of narcotics for control of the diarrhea. Long-term home hyperalimentation has allowed patients to overcome the severe malabsorption that would accompany massive small-bowel resection.

Resection of the ileum is less well tolerated than resection of the jejunum, because the ileum serves as the only site for absorption of bile acids. When the ileal resection is limited (less than 100 cm), the total bile acid pool remains sufficient to prevent significant steatorrhea. However, there is still an excessive loading of bile acids into the colon, where they stimulate mucosal secretion and result in diarrhea. Therapy for this form of diarrhea is aimed at binding the fecal bile acids with an agent such as cholestyramine. The dosage is 4 g given before meals and at bedtime. When ileal resection is more extensive (more than 100 cm), the total bile acid pool becomes diminished below the critical level needed for proper digestion and absorption of fat, and steatorrhea develops. The use of cholestyramine in this situation further depletes the bile acid pool and worsens the steatorrhea and diarrhea. Therefore, dietary fat should be supplied in the form of medium-chain triglycerides, which do not require bile acids for absorption. Commercial preparations are available (e.g., Portagen), and consultation with a nutritionist as well as a gastroenterologist is recommended.

Diarrhea may also occur after *gastric surgery* with vagotomy. At times the vagotomy causes diarrhea by altering intestinal motility and, for unclear reasons, by increasing the concentration of fecal bile acids. Therapy with cholestyramine has been successful in this postvagotomy syndrome. Gastric surgery may also unmask latent lactase deficiency or, rarely, latent celiac disease. The blind loop syndrome with resultant bacterial overgrowth, dumping syndrome, inadvertent gastroileal anastomosis, and gastrocolic fistula are all complications that can result in diarrhea in patients who have undergone gastrectomy (see Chapter 43).

Diarrhea occurs rarely after routine cholecystectomy, in association with an increased concentration of fecal bile acids. Therapy with cholestyramine is effective. Subtotal colectomy, with an ileal-rectal anastomosis (e.g., for multiple polyposis), often results in diarrhea that is usually easily controlled by antidiarrheal medication and diminishes with time. Segmental colonic resection usually does not result in diarrhea because of the large functional reserve of the normal colon.

Symptomatic Antidiarrheal Therapy

Diarrhea is merely a symptom, and therapy, if possible, should be directed at the primary underlying process. However, a wide variety of agents are available for symptomatic control of diarrhea. The efficacy of these agents is highly variable, and the mechanism of action of many is poorly understood. Symptomatic treatment should be avoided in patients with acute infectious diarrhea (except at minimal dosages to prevent marked discomfort), because early suppression of bowel movements in these conditions prolongs the diarrhea.

Hydrophilic bulk-forming agents, such as psyllium (Metamucil, Konsyl), have been shown to improve the consistency of ileostomy and colostomy effluent (see earlier discussion). These agents, which paradoxically are also used in treating constipation, are particularly useful in patients with irritable bowel syndrome (Chapter 44).

Another group of antidiarrheal medications consists of those classified as *absorbents,* on the premise that these agents absorb factors within the intestinal lumen that cause diarrhea. Medications of this group include kaolin and pectin (Kaopectate), bismuth salts (Pepto-Bismol), aluminum hydroxide (Amphojel), and cholestyramine (Questran). Most are available over the counter, but their value is not well established. However, Pepto-Bismol has been shown to be effective in controlling the symptoms of traveler's diarrhea (see Chapter 35). Cholestyramine is effective in treating bile acid–induced diarrhea, as occurs in patients after ileal resection, vagotomy, or cholecystectomy. This drug also may bind other compounds, such as digoxin and warfarin, and thereby decrease their absorption.

Opioid derivatives are probably the most effective antidiarrheal medications. Opiate drugs delay the transit of intraluminal contents through the small and large intestines. A central effect is also likely. In patients with extensive small-bowel resection, codeine may be the only effective form of therapy. The synthetic agents diphenoxylate–atropine (Lomotil) and loperamide (Imodium) are also effective and are generally well tolerated. The atropine in Lomotil contributes little to its antidiarrheal effect and may cause significant toxicity. Imodium has the theoretical advantages of a more favorable ratio of GI effects to central nervous system effects and a longer duration of action. An over-the-counter formulation is now available. Imodium has the practical disadvantage of being expensive. The development of megacolon, prolongation of symptoms, and worsening of pseudomembranous colitis have all been linked to the injudicious use of these agents in patients with bacterial diarrhea. The potential risk for abuse is theoretically less for Imodium.

Another group of drugs that is under investigation is classified as *antisecretory.* Some of these drugs inhibit the synthesis of prostaglandins, which increase intestinal secretion by stimulating adenylate cyclase activity within intestinal cells. (Adenylate cyclase is the enzyme that catalyzes the formation of cAMP, the concentration of which influences certain transport systems in cell membranes.) Other drugs of this class inhibit adenylate cyclase directly. For example, indomethacin inhibits prostaglandin synthesis and has been shown experimentally to inhibit the effect of enterotoxin. Propranolol, an inhibitor of adenylate cyclase, suppresses bile acid–induced fluid accumulation in intestinal loops. Certain diuretics (e.g., ethacrynic acid) that act on electrolyte transport have also been shown to be effective enterotoxin antagonists. Endorphin-like peptides are also under study as antidiarrheal agents. Investigation into their mechanism of action may lead to the development of new effective forms of therapy against diarrhea. A somatostatin analog (octreotide) is available for the treatment of GI endocrine tumors (e.g., vasoactive intestinal peptide–secreting tumor, gastrinoma, carcinoid). It is not recommended for use in other forms of diarrhea.

Because there are few data to allow an objective comparison of the various antidiarrheal medications, the choice of drug must be based on efficacy, safety, and cost. For acute, self-limited illnesses, drugs such as Kaopectate and bismuth salts are often tried by patients, even before a health care provider is consulted. For such patients, diphenoxylate–atropine (Lomotil) or loperamide (Imodium) is highly effective. Patients should be instructed to use medication after a diarrheal movement and not to exceed 8 tablets/day. Loperamide may provide longer diarrhea-free intervals with fewer side effects (51). Oral rehydration therapy (see Chapters 35 and 41) is important, especially with voluminous diarrhea in the frail elderly and in children. Both glucose-based and rice-based electrolyte solutions are available for rehydration. Commercial rehydration solutions designed for athletes (e.g., Gatorade) have inadequate concentrations of electrolytes and therefore are not satisfactory in the treatment of diarrhea.

For patients with chronic diarrhea, the choice of medication is based on the severity and cause of the diarrhea. In patients with the diarrhea-predominant form of the irritable bowel syndrome (Chapter 44), hydrophilic agents may be useful. The dosage should be titrated to the desired bowel habits, with dosages ranging from 1 teaspoon to 2 tablespoons per day mixed in 8 ounces of juice or water per dose. In patients with diarrhea from other causes, diphenoxylate–atropine or loperamide should be tried. These medications can be given in divided doses throughout the day. Diarrhea can also be prevented by taking one or two tablets before engaging in an event associated with diarrhea (e.g., meals, examinations).

In more severe cases of diarrhea, narcotics are necessary. Tincture of opium is convenient because it can easily be titrated (by the drop) to control diarrhea at the lowest possible dosage. A recommended starting dosage is six drops every 4 to 6 hours, to be adjusted by one or two drops per dose depending on the patient's response. Codeine, at a dose of 15 to 30 mg, may also be used with the same dosage schedule.

ABDOMINAL PAIN

Abdominal pain is one of the most common presenting complaints of ambulatory patients. Many patients complain of having chronic pain that is constant or recurrent, and in this population it is important to consider functional as well as organic causes for the symptom. Acute abdominal pain (onset within 24 hours before the patient seeks help) almost always reflects an organic process. In any case, whether chronic or acute, abdominal pain resulting from an organic cause is more often a symptom of GI disease than of non-GI disease.

The caregiver's response to the patient with abdominal pain is influenced by the rapidity of onset, apparent severity, location, and accompanying signs and symptoms (e.g., fever, GI bleeding, diarrhea) that may suggest a specific process. Although there is no information about the relative frequency of the various causes of abdominal pain, experience suggests that, most often, *acute pain* is self limited (abates within hours) and the pain is usually attributed (without proof) to viral gastroenteritis or dietary indiscretion. *Chronic pain,* if associated with an organic process, is most often caused by peptic, gallbladder, or diverticular disease, chronic relapsing pancreatitis (primarily in alcoholics), or carcinoma (most commonly pancreatic or colonic). The symptoms and signs that accompany these processes are discussed in a general way in this chapter and more specifically in the chapters devoted to these conditions. Chronic pain that is not associated with a demonstrable organic process is most often caused by the irritable bowel syndrome (see Chapter 44).

The significance of pain is determined by two major factors: the characteristics of the pain and the characteristics of the patient. The significance of pain to the patient depends on its severity and frequency, the degree to which it interferes with daily life or sleep patterns, and its meaning (both implied and symbolic). Even severe pain can be tolerated for brief periods if it appears infrequently, whereas less severe pain may be less tolerable if it interrupts important activities or disturbs sleep. Pain that has no anticipated end is generally less well tolerated than pain that, even though intense, has a predictable span. The threshold of pain tolerance varies considerably from one individual to another, because of both neurologic and psychological factors. When pain suggests to the patient a serious underlying disorder, such as cancer, this concern itself may decrease tolerance for the pain. Also, pain that is primarily organic may be reinforced by the secondary psychosocial gains it provides.

Elderly patients with abdominal pain require special attention (52). Even serious underlying conditions may be manifested by minimal subjective complaints and objective signs. For example, the diagnoses of appendicitis and of ruptured appendix are easily missed because pain may not be severe and fever and leukocytosis may be minimal or absent. Therefore, careful follow-up of abdominal pain in the elderly warrants repeated abdominal and rectal examinations and serial determinations of body temperature and laboratory tests (e.g., white blood cell and differential counts).

Management of any type of pain can be significantly improved by consideration of certain general principles. For example, reassurance that pain can be relieved by medication or surgery can significantly raise the threshold of tolerance. On the other hand, the existence of severe pain sensitizes patients to additional, less intense pain (e.g., lumbar puncture, venipuncture), and the patient's overreaction to the second pain should not be taken to imply that the primary pain is psychogenic. Another common misconception is that alleviation of pain by placebo implies psychogenic origin; in fact, organic pain may be more readily relieved by placebo than psychogenic pain is. A post hoc rationalization that accounts for this phenomenon views the patient with organic pain as a person who wants desperately to get rid of the pain, whereas the person with psychogenic pain may be unwilling to give it up because of secondary gain.

Types of Abdominal Pain

A few general concepts concerning abdominal pain are reviewed here because understanding them can be helpful in making a diagnosis. Pain involving the digestive system can be visceral, parietal, referred, neurogenic, or psychogenic. Pain caused by metabolic disease is ordinarily visceral or neurogenic.

Visceral Pain

Visceral pain can result from spasm or stretching of the muscle wall of a hollow viscus, from distention of the capsule of a solid organ such as the liver, or from inflammation and ischemia of a visceral structure. Tenderness associated with visceral pain (sometimes including rebound tenderness) is often felt directly over the part of the digestive system that is involved, although small bowel tenderness is usually not well localized (except for the terminal ileum). Abdominal viscera are insensitive to cutting, tearing, crushing, and burning.

Parietal Pain

The parietal peritoneum, mesentery, and posterior peritoneal covering are sensitive to forces similar to those that affect the viscera, but the omentum and anterior abdominal wall are less sensitive. Parietal tenderness is more localized than visceral tenderness, and rebound tenderness is experienced over the involved area. Parietal pain that is the result of generalized inflammation (peritonitis) encompasses a large area of the peritoneum. A rigid abdomen, associated with pain, usually means that the inflammation is severe.

Referred Pain

Both visceral and parietal pain may be referred to a remote site along shared nerve pathways (dermatomes). Gallbladder pain, for example, typically radiates to the infrascapular area, and right diaphragmatic pain to the right shoulder. Esophageal pain can be confused with the pain of myocardial ischemia because the sites to which the pain radiates may be identical (e.g., the neck and left arm). The more severe the visceral pain, the more likely it is to be referred to the back, as with esophageal spasm or cholecystitis. The skin overlying the dermatome to which the pain is referred may be hypersensitive. Deep palpation of the primary site of the painful organ may intensify the pain, not only locally but also at its referred site. However, the reverse is not true: Deep palpation over the referred site does not usually enhance pain over the primary site.

Abdominal Pain Caused by Metabolic Disease

Metabolic disease may produce intestinal pain by a direct effect on the alimentary tract (e.g., when intestinal spasm is induced by porphyria, lead poisoning, or familial Mediterranean fever). In hereditary angioneurotic edema, C1 esterase deficiency may produce intestinal swelling, which can cause pain as a result of partial obstruction or intestinal spasm. On the other hand, metabolic disorders may secondarily produce GI pain; for example, hyperparathyroidism can produce a painful peptic ulcer or pancreatitis. Hyperlipidemia also can cause pancreatitis, but it can be associated with abdominal pain in the absence of pancreatic disease.

Neurogenic Pain

Neurogenic abdominal pain (causalgia) is experienced by the patient as a burning sensation along the route of distribution of the nerve and is sometimes associated with hyperesthesia. Usually the spinal root is involved by herpes zoster, carcinoma, or arthritis, but peripheral neuropathies caused by operative trauma or diabetes mellitus may also produce neurogenic abdominal pain. There is no relationship of neurogenic pain to digestive function (e.g., eating, defecating).

Psychogenic Pain

Psychogenic pain may represent a conversion reaction that results in the perception of pain when no organic dysfunction exists, or it may result from psychophysiologic reactions characterized by pathologic or physiologic responses to psychological stress (see Chapter 21). For example, emotional stress can lead to painful intestinal spasm in patients with irritable bowel syndrome (Chapter 44). This spasm is a measurable physiologic event. Similarly, stress may lead to peptic symptoms as a result of gastric hypersecretion, which also can be quantitated. Pain or tenderness that represents a conversion reaction (emotions converted into somatic complaints) may disappear during periods of distraction. Such pain may be inconsistent and incompatible with known neuroanatomy and neurophysiology.

Historical Clues to Diagnosis

Although the successful diagnosis of conditions that manifest with abdominal pain depends on meticulous pursuit of leads that are provided by the history and physical examination, familiarity with standard questions and examination techniques assists in ensuring completeness. A history of previous episodes of pain, medications taken (e.g., NSAIDs, warfarin), and the existence of a chronic disease (e.g., diabetes mellitus, diverticulosis) is important. Questions relating to local features include the nature and quality of the pain; its location, radiation, intensity, timing, duration, and course; and the factors that precipitate, aggravate, and alleviate it. Associated symptoms and signs include tenderness, fever and chills, anorexia, nausea and vomiting, diarrhea and constipation, obstruction, borborygmus, rectal bleeding, passing of mucus, jaundice, and genitourinary symptoms. Although aggravation of pain by emotional tension is seen with functional disorders such as irritable bowel syndrome, the pain of many organic disorders can also be accentuated by emotional stress.

Rapidity of Onset of Pain

The temporal development of abdominal pain is an important factor that guides the physician in evaluation. In particular, pain that develops abruptly or within minutes and becomes rapidly severe is ominous (Table 45.8).

In addition, situations in which a silent period follows the initial symptoms are notoriously deceptive problems. For example, a perforated viscus or an intestinal infarction may be characterized by resolution of the intense initial pain hours after perforation or infarction first occurs and by a recurrence of pain several hours later when peritonitis and volume depletion are well established.

Almost always, therefore, if the patient complains of an abrupt onset of severe abdominal pain on the day that he or she visits the clinician, even if the pain has resolved and the abdominal examination is unrevealing, a complete blood count, urinalysis, chest radiograph, plain and upright films of the abdomen, and close surveillance over several hours are imperative.

When the onset of pain is more gradual, many more causes are possible, and considerable judgment is necessary in determining the urgency and direction of the evaluation. The caregiver must be guided by the patient's history, the nature and location of the pain, and the examination. In all cases, follow-up examination is warranted. Newly experienced abdominal pain, even if it is believed to be innocuous, should never be dismissed without follow-up (at least by telephone) within a few days so that any important new symptoms are not missed. It is best for the clinician to initiate this follow-up because it obviates the need for the patient to decide whether a change in symptoms is important enough to trouble the practitioner.

Table 45.8. Causes of Acute Abdominal Pain According to Rapidity of Onset

Intestinal Causes	Extraintestinal Causes
Abrupt Onset (Instantaneous)	
Perforated ulcer	Ruptured aneurysm or aortic dissection
Ruptured abscess or hematoma	Ruptured ectopic pregnancy
Intestinal infarct	Pneumothorax
Ruptured esophagus	Myocardial infarct
	Pulmonary infarct
Rapid Onset (Minutes)	
Perforated viscus	Ureteral colic
Strangulated viscus	Renal colic
Volvulus	Ectopic pregnancy
Pancreatitis	Splenic infarct
Biliary colic	
Mesenteric infarct	
Diverticulitis	
Penetrating peptic ulcer	
High intestinal obstruction	
Appendicitis (gradual onset more common)	
Gradual Onset (Hours)	
Appendicitis	Cystitis
Strangulated hernia	Pyelitis
Low small intestinal obstruction	Salpingitis
Cholecystitis	Prostatitis
Pancreatitis	Threatened abortion
Gastritis	Urinary retention
Peptic ulcer	Pneumonitis
Colonic diverticulitis	
Meckel diverticulitis	
Crohn disease	
Ulcerative colitis	
Mesenteric lymphadenitis	
Abscess	
Intestinal infarct	
Mesenteric cyst	

Adapted from Ridge JA, Way LW. Abdominal pain. in: Sleisenger MH, Fordtran JS, eds. Gastrointestinal disease, 5th ed. Philadelphia: WB Saunders, 1993;156.

Nature and Location of Pain

Esophageal pain is usually described as pressing, constricting, or burning (Tables 45.9 and 45.10). It is usually located in the substernal area and, when severe, radiates through to the back. The location of the pain is a good clue to the location of the underlying disease. Although pain from the lower esophageal region may be referred higher, lesions high in the esophagus do not refer to the lower part of the esophagus (see also Chapter 42).

Gastric pain is usually experienced in the subxiphoid area or the left upper quadrant. Although

Table 45.9. Nature and Location of Gastrointestinal Pain

Organ involved	Nature of Pain	Location of Pain
Esophagus	Burning, constricting	Upper lesions: high substernal Lower lesions: low sternal or referred upward Severe: back
Stomach	Gnawing discomfort, sensation of hunger	Epigastric Left upper quadrant
Duodenum	Gnawing discomfort, sensation of hunger	Epigastric
Small intestine	Aching, cramping, bloating, sharp	Diffuse Periumbilical Terminal ileum: right lower quadrant
Colon	Aching, cramping, bloating, sharp	Lower abdomen Sigmoid: left lower quadrant Rectum: midline and sacrum
Pancreas	Excruciating, constant	Upper abdomen radiating to back
Gallbladder	Severe, later dull ache	Right upper quadrant Radiates to right scapula or interscapular area
Liver	Ache, occasionally sharp	Right lower rib cage Right upper quadrant if liver is enlarged

gastritis is perceived as a true pain (often burning or cramping in quality), the distress caused by both duodenal and gastric ulceration is experienced as a gnawing discomfort or as a hunger sensation rather than as pain. The discomfort caused by peptic ulcer is often precipitated by fasting and is relieved by eating. The pain of peptic ulcer usually awakens the patient between 1 and 3 a.m. In contrast, pain of gastritis may be aggravated by eating or relieved only momentarily and then subsequently intensified over 10 to 15 minutes. A change from ulcer distress to a burning, boring, or knife-like pain (especially when there is radiation through to the back) is an indication of penetration. Pain that is precipitated by meals also suggests gastric outlet obstruction (often caused by pyloric channel ulcer) or high intestinal obstruction (see also Chapter 43).

Duodenal pain is felt also in the epigastric area or slightly to the right of it, and it may radiate through to the back. When an ulcer is perforated, the pain appears abruptly in the epigastric region and later settles into the right lower quadrant as gastric contents are spilled into the right gutter.

Small-intestinal pain is generally diffuse and poorly localized. It is experienced in the periumbilical area and, when severe, radiates through to the back. Pain deriving from the terminal ileum may be localized to the right lower quadrant. Uncommonly, it may radiate down the leg. Small intestinal pain is generally crampy, sharp, or aching. *Bloating, distention,* and *dull ache* are terms that often are associated with prolonged mechanical obstruction or reflex ileus, whereas more acute forms may be manifested by sharp, steady pain. Associated fever and chills suggest inflammatory bowel disease.

Colonic pain is better localized, often to the lower abdomen. *Sigmoid pain* is felt in the left lower quadrant, and *rectal pain* is often described by the patient as being located over the rectum, usually in the midline. Gas pocketed in the splenic flexure of the colon (seen most commonly in patients with the irritable bowel syndrome) produces left upper quadrant or left chest pain that may be confused with the pain of myocardial ischemia. Temporary relief is obtained by passing gas (see also Chapter 44). Colonic pain generally is crampy or of an aching quality unless perforation occurs, and then it is often severe and constant. Associated fever and chills suggest diverticulitis, diverticular abscess, or ulcerative colitis.

Pancreatic pain is excruciating and constant and usually located in the upper abdomen with radiation through to the back, but it may be felt in almost any area of the abdomen. Chronic pancreatic pain (caused by inflammation, pseudocyst, or carcinoma) is similar in nature and location to acute pancreatic pain but may be less severe. Pancreatitis is almost invariably associated with vomiting. If vomiting is not present, other diagnoses (e.g., pancreatic carcinoma) should be considered.

Appendicitis often begins as diffuse abdominal pain that intensifies over hours as it settles in the right lower quadrant. The pain of appendicitis is often aggravated by extension of the right leg.

Gallbladder pain generally begins in the right upper quadrant or epigastrium and radiates to the interscapular area or to the right infrascapular area. It is excruciatingly severe, may be aggravated by deep inspiration, and is replaced by a dull, aching sensation that persists for hours after the severe pain subsides. Tenderness can often be elicited by deep palpation under the rib in the area of the gallbladder, especially during deep inspiration. Gallbladder pain often appears several hours after a heavy meal. Associated fever and chills suggest ascending cholangitis (see also Chapter 96).

Hepatic pain localizes over the liver, and a tender liver can be demonstrated by palpation of its edge during deep inspiration or by fist percussion over the lower right rib cage anteriorly (or over the right upper quadrant if the liver is enlarged).

Genitourinary pain (e.g., renal colic) is discussed in Chapters 36 and 51.

Physical Examination

The patient's general appearance provides clues about the severity, the duration, and often the cause of the underlying condition. The cold, sweat, and pallor of shock along with the marble skin (superficial vessels seen over blanched skin) indicating vasoconstriction are signs of significant hemorrhage. Tachycardia and perspiration are seen in both shock and sepsis, but the skin in shock is cold and clammy, whereas in sepsis it is warm and moist. Signs of sepsis suggest bacterial enteritis, inflammatory bowel disease, intra-abdominal abscess, cholangitis, pancreatitis, peritonitis, or pyelonephritis.

Table 45.10. Differential Diagnosis of Abdominal Pain Caused by Gastrointestinal Disorders

A. Character, Location, Production or Relief

Disorder	Character	Location	Produced or Relieved by
Peptic ulcer	Gnawing hunger discomfort, occasionally burning, gastric (within minutes after meals); duodenal (usually several hours after meals)	Subxiphoid, may radiate to back	Produced by empty stomach, relieved by food, antacids, or H_2-receptor blockers
Penetrating ulcer	Severe, boring, constant pain	Subxiphoid radiating to back	May awaken patient in early morning hours, may be relieved by antacids or H_2-receptor blockers
Perforated ulcer	Abrupt, severe pain followed within 6 hr by deceptive refractory period with diminishing of pain	Initially epigastric, then right lower quadrant (right gutter)	Initial pain spontaneous, peritonitis aggravated by movement
Small bowel obstruction	Crampy severe pain with partial obstruction, constant pain develops with complete obstruction or strangulation	Generalized periumbilical or localized over strangulation	Relieved by intubation decompression
Large bowel obstruction	Crampy pain initially, constant pain with subsequent distention or strangulation, onset less sudden than upper intestinal obstruction	May be localized or generalized	Occasionally relieved by intubation decompression
Intestinal infarct	Severe, excruciating, abrupt onset	Generalized	Relieved only by surgery
Intussusception	Sudden onset severe crampy pain	Periumbilical	Temporary relief may occur with emesis
Appendicitis	Initially colic then continuous with varying intensity	Initial colic in periumbilical area, subsequently continuous in right lower quadrant, occasional perineal radiation	Aggravated by extension of right leg
Pancreatitis	Severe, constant pain	Epigastric, radiation to back or lower abdomen	Often initiated by alcoholic binge or eating after binge, by common duct obstruction, penetrating ulcer, or blunt trauma
Cholecystitis	Constant, severe pain preceding nausea and vomiting; subsidence of pain followed by aching	Right upper quadrant radiating to infrascapular region	Precipitated by heavy meal and aggravated by deep inspiration
Biliary colic	Crampy, severe pain	Epigastric, radiating to right upper quadrant and subscapular region	Precipitated by heavy meal within 1–3 hr
Diverticulitis	Crampy or continuous pain	Left lower quadrant, may radiate to back	Relieved by anticholinergics and antibiotics
Crohn disease	Crampy with partial obstruction and continuous pain with inflammatory mass	Periumbilical or right lower quadrant, may radiate to back	May be precipitated by milk, relieved by defecation or intubation decompression
Ulcerative colitis	Crampy pain usually, may be constant with toxic dilation	Often left lower quadrant or any area of colon, generalized with toxic megacolon or perforation	Precipitated by emotional stress or infection; toxic magacolon by opiates or enemas; relieved temporarily by defecation

B. Abnormal Physical Findings, Associated Signs, and Laboratory Features

Disorder	Abnormal Physical Findings	Associated Signs and Symptoms	Laboratory Features
Peptic ulcer	Subxiphoid tenderness	Nausea, vomiting, retrosternal burning; weight gain with duodenal ulcer; weight stable or loss with gastric ulcer	Endoscopic or radiographic demonstration of ulcer, possible occult blood in stool or melena, and iron deficiency anemia
Penetrating ulcer	Marked subxiphoid tenderness	Writhing, clutching abdomen	Amylase may be elevated
Perforated ulcer	Initially rigid with rebound, during refractory stage tenderness disappears to return later, absence of liver dullness with intraperitoneal air	Patient lies rigidly still, pale, perspiring; emesis may be present	Upright film shows free air under diaphragm; leukocytosis
Small bowel obstruction	Borborygmus, high-pitched sound with rushes initially; later quiet abdomen; tenderness may be mild or rebound tenderness may be present	Emesis (may be feculent with lower obstruction), obstipation, may be weak with shocklike appearance	Plain film of abdomen showing air–fluid levels may show stepladder pattern
Large bowel obstruction	Initially hyperperistalsis with high-pitched rushes, subsequently distention and decrease in bowel signs	Nausea but less vomiting than with high obstruction, obstipation, or marked constipation	Large bowel distention with air–fluid levels and no air demonstrated distal to obstruction
Intestinal infarct	Quiet bowel sounds, tenderness present but not commensurate with pain, later rebound tenderness	Shock, bloody diarrhea, melena, vomiting; history of intestinal angina	Leukocytosis, hemoconcentration; bloody fluid on paracentesis; plain film of abdomen may reveal normal gas pattern or no gas pattern due to fluid-filled loops

Table 45.10—*continued.* Differential Diagnosis of Abdominal Pain Caused by Gastrointestinal Disorders

B. Abnormal Physical Findings, Associated Signs, and Laboratory Features

Disorder	Abnormal Physical Findings	Associated Signs and Symptoms	Laboratory Features
Intussusception	Tender mass in abdomen, high-pitched peristaltic rushes	Initially normal stool after onset, then blood, mucus, and constipation; vomiting is late; fever after strangulation	Barium enema demonstrates coiled spring appearance of invagination; with ileocecal intussusception, small bowel loop is in colon
Appendicitis	Localized rebound tenderness, hyperesthesia over area	Initially diarrhea, then constipation; nausea and vomiting may be present; fever, tachycardia; rectal tenderness in right perirectal area	Leukocytosis
Pancreatitis	Marked epigastric tenderness, guarding and upper abdominal distention; the pain of chronic pancreatic disease may be less pronounced	Emesis almost invariable, fever, with hemorrhagic pancreatitis purple color in flank or periumbilical region; emesis is less common in patients with chronic pancreatic disease	Marked leukocytosis, hyperamylasemia; serum calcium depression on days 2 to 4, toxic psychosis on days 2 to 4; radiograph may show calcification, localized ileus, or colon cutoff sign; upper gastrointestinal series demonstrates pancreatic enlargement and spicules in C loop of duodenum; may have left pleural effusion
Cholecystitis	Tenderness over gallbladder area, especially on deep inspiration; Murphy sign may be positive	More common in obese women ≥40 yr or older after pregnancy; high incidence among some American Indian populations	Leukocytosis; plain film may show calcified stone; stones seen on ultrasonography; TcHIDA nonvisualized; cholanglograms may show radiopaque stones
Biliary colic	As for cholecystitis	As for cholecystitis; jaundice may be present	Radiopaque stones may be seen on plain film; stones seen on ultrasonography; intravenous cholangiogram may show dilated duct; bilirubin, alkaline phosphatase increase; may have hyperamylasemia
Diverticulitis	Guarding and tenderness in left lower quadrant	Constipation, fever, tachycardia; rectal tenderness on left; may have urinary frequency or dysuria from pericolonic involvement	Leukocytosis, barium enema shows diverticula but may not visualize during acute episode, may show partial obstruction
Crohn disease	Tender mass in right lower quadrant, borborygmus	Nausea, vomiting, diarrhea, fever; may have perirectal fistula; tender mass in right rectal area, occasional clubbing	Anemia, elevated sedimentation rate; small bowel series shows cobblestone appearance or string sign
Ulcerative colitis	Tender over involved area, distended especially over transverse colon with toxic megacolon	Frequent passing of small amounts of bloody liquid stool; tenesmus with rectal involvement; fever, tachycardia, arthralgia, erythema nodosa; proctoscopy reveals bleeding and friability	Anemia; elevated sedimentation rate; barium enema demonstrates ulcerations, shortening, effacement of colon

Modified from Handbook of Differential Diagnosis, vol 2, part 1: The abdomen. Nutley, NJ: Rocom Press, 1974.

The position assumed by the patient may be characteristic of a particular disorder. A position of truncal flexure often typifies patients with pancreatitis, whereas patients with gallbladder colic tend to pace or writhe about and appear restless in their unsuccessful attempt to find a comfortable position. This is in sharp contrast to the immobile position assumed by patients with peritonitis, who attempt to avoid even the slightest jarring movement.

Inspection of the abdomen is facilitated by using incident lighting to visualize abdominal asymmetry and to outline masses and pulsations. In thin patients with partial obstruction, peristaltic intestinal movement may be seen through the abdominal wall, and churning peristalsis may coincide with reports of crampy abdominal pain. Flank discoloration *(Gray–Turner sign)* or periumbilical discoloration *(Cullen sign)* results from retroperitoneal or intraperitoneal hemorrhage dissecting into the subcutaneous tissues and may indicate hemorrhagic pancreatitis. A strangulated hernia may protrude visibly from ventral defects, from the inguinal area, or into the scrotum, where peristaltic contractions may occasionally be appreciated. Patients with subphrenic abscess or gallbladder disease may have inspiratory pain that results in splinting and avoidance of deep inspiration.

Auscultation should always be performed before palpation so that abdominal sounds may be evaluated before they are altered by palpation. At times borborygmus is audible without the stethoscope. Specifically, one should search for hyperperistaltic or hypoperistaltic sounds, for the high tinkles of obstruction, and for bruits suggesting vascular distortion from aneurysms, atherosclerosis, compression of blood vessels, or invasion of blood vessels (e.g., invasion of the splenic artery in advanced pancreatic carcinoma).

Although a silent abdomen implies reflex ileus, bowel sounds may also be quiet or significantly diminished late in the course of mechanical obstruction. Whenever obstruction (especially gastric outlet obstruction) is considered, an attempt should be made to elicit a succussion splash. This is done by placing the stethoscope over the area (e.g., the stomach) and shaking the patient gently but abruptly. A sloshing sound indicates the presence of air and fluid. This finding in the stomach 3 hours or more after eating or drinking indicates delayed gastric emptying or, rarely, marked hypersecretion.

Gentle percussion should precede palpation and is an excellent means for detecting rebound tenderness, masses, and tympany (either generalized or localized) over an area of ileus or obstruction. Because air rises to the area between the liver and the abdominal wall, absence of liver dullness with the patient in a recumbent position is an important finding indicating the presence of free air in the abdominal cavity.

Before *palpation,* it is wise to ask the patient to point to the site of maximum pain. Gentle palpation should at first avoid that site to minimize the chances that muscle guarding will interfere with the examination. The patient should be lying perfectly supine with knees flexed to facilitate relaxation of abdominal muscles. Guarding may be localized over specific lesions (often inflammatory), or there may be marked rigidity if pain is severe, as in perforation or penetration. Subxiphoid tenderness suggests an active ulcer. Tenderness over the liver, especially when the liver edge is brought down against the examining finger by deep inspiration, suggests inflammation in this organ. With gallbladder disease, tenderness is localized to the region of the gallbladder, and with cystic or common duct obstruction, a distended viscus can sometimes be felt as well. Right lower quadrant tenderness is found with appendicitis or with Crohn disease involving the ileum or the ileocecal area. A left lower quadrant tender sigmoid cord is felt most commonly with irritable bowel syndrome but can also indicate diverticular disease. A distinct tender mass in the right lower quadrant suggests inflammation (usually Crohn disease) extending beyond the bowel; a similar finding in the left lower quadrant suggests diverticulitis. Board-like rigidity indicates an intra-abdominal catastrophe such as perforation or infarction. Pulsatile masses should be differentiated from laterally expansile masses because the former can represent a mass overlying an artery, whereas the latter implies aneurysmal dilation. When localized perforation has occurred, rebound tenderness may be localized over the area. Hyperesthesia may exist over the segmental distribution of the spinal nerve that innervates the particular area of the viscus. This finding is detected by gently rubbing the fingers over the skin of the involved dermatome.

Rectal examination can be extremely helpful in localizing areas of tenderness as well as in palpating masses through the rectum. Periappendiceal abscesses can sometimes be identified in this manner, as can a perforated diverticulum. On digital examination the finger should complete a circle that includes the entire perirectal area.

Genital and pelvic examination, like the rectal examination, should be performed in all patients with abdominal pain because it can detect hernias as well as genitourinary and other pelvic problems.

If analgesic drugs have been administered, it is useful to reexamine the patient after pain has been relieved to identify masses or localized tenderness that may have been obscured by guarding and rigidity.

Laboratory Tests

A complete blood count, urinalysis, and test for occult blood in the stool are required in every person with serious acute abdominal pain, as are a chest radiograph and plain and upright films of the abdomen. Other laboratory tests should be ordered as indicated by the specific findings.

A low hematocrit value or hemoglobin concentration can call attention to intraperitoneal or retroperitoneal bleeding, whereas hemoconcentration raises consideration of mesenteric vascular occlusion. A high leukocyte count and a high erythrocyte sedimentation rate suggest inflammation or infection. Blood in the urine points to kidney disease as a possible source of pain.

The presence of occult blood in the stool reinforces concern about the GI tract as a source of painful symptoms; it may be an early sign of vascular ischemia or intussusception or a sign of more common lesions such as peptic ulcer, polyp, or inflammatory bowel disease.

Radiology

Plain and upright films of the abdomen are helpful in delineating gas patterns, which may demonstrate displacement of intestine by intra-abdominal masses or may show localized loops of ileus, as with *pancreatitis* or *pyelonephritis.* Air is distributed more widely in the small bowel in *reflex ileus* and in *intestinal obstruction.* In the latter, the typical stepladder pattern is often encountered, with slight separation of the loops caused by edema of the wall of the small bowel; an upright film demonstrates air–fluid levels in the dilated loops. Absence of air distal to a specific point suggests *obstruction* at that point. *Volvulus* can be diagnosed on the plain film, which demonstrates a sausage-shaped air-filled or air- and fluid-filled viscus coming to an apex. In gastric volvulus, the greater curvature is seen above the lesser curve, and a double air–fluid level is a classic finding, one level being in the lesser curvature of the fundus and the other in the antrum (because of the inverted U-shaped stomach under these conditions). Free air under the diaphragm on the upright film indicates a *perforated viscus* unless the patient has had recent surgery (at which time air was introduced) or has *pneumatosis cystoides intestinalis,* in which case a large amount of air may appear

Table 45.11. Ultrasound, Computed Tomographic (CT) Scanning, and Magnetic Resonance Imaging (MRI): Comparison of the Technique and the Patient Experience

Characteristic	Ultrasound	CT	MRI
Basis of tissue attenuation	Tissue elasticity, acoustic impedance	Electron density; linear attenuation coefficient	Nuclear resonance
Radiation dose or toxic effect	None known at diagnostic energy levels	8–10 R (skin exposure)	None known
Morphologic detail	Good	Excellent	Excellent
Contrast medium useful	No	Iodinated intravascular and oral agents; diatrizoate meglumine (Gastrografin)	No (in abdomen)
Time for examination	½–1 hr	½–1 hr	1 hr
Operator skill	Substantial	Minimal	Minimal
Ease of interpretation	Complex, many artifacts	Straightforward	Moderately straightforward
Preparation	Nothing by mouth after midnight (for pelvis, three glasses of water 1 hr before study and do not void)	Evacuate barium from recent gastrointestinal studies (or wait 1 wk)	None
Cooperation	Lie still, supine, be able to hold breath	Lie still, supine, be able to hold breath	Lie still, supine, breathe quietly

Adapted from Ferrucci JT Jr. Body ultrasonography [first of two parts]. N Engl J Med 1979;300:538.

subdiaphragmatically from ruptured pseudocysts. The important clue to pneumatosis cystoides intestinalis is the presence of free air in the absence of signs or symptoms of perforation or peritonitis. Radiopaque gallbladder or kidney stones or pancreatic calcification seen on plain films may help corroborate a suspected diagnosis or point attention toward one of these organs.

Contrast studies have been largely replaced by endoscopic procedures in the evaluation of patients with abdominal pain. Endoscopy is both more sensitive and more specific than contrast radiology of the bowel, although it is considerably more expensive. An *upper GI series* (see Chapter 43) is useful if extrinsic compression on the stomach or duodenum or partial gastric outlet obstruction is suspected at endoscopy. *Barium enema* (see earlier discussion in this chapter) can be useful in demonstrating a low site of obstruction and reducing an intussusception. A barium enema should always be preceded by digital examination of the rectum and by proctoscopy to be certain that the rectum is normal (e.g., that there is no rectal carcinoma). When pain is thought to result from gallbladder disease (see Chapter 96) and opaque stones are not visible on plain abdominal films, ultrasonography is an excellent means of demonstrating stones in the gallbladder, although it is not reliable in detecting ductal stones. An *oral cholecystogram* may demonstrate radiolucent stones; if the gallbladder is not visualized with reinforced dosage, a diseased gallbladder is likely. A *TcHIDA or PipHIDA radioisotopic study* may demonstrate obstruction of the common or cystic duct. This technique requires injection of isotope and serial views for 1 hour. (A sonogram is usually performed beforehand to localize the gallbladder.)

Ultrasonography is also useful in showing pancreatic edema or pseudocysts, evaluating a suspected abdominal aortic aneurysm, and evaluating a patient who is difficult to examine for an intra-abdominal mass; this technique has the advantage of avoiding irradiation. Sonography is often unsatisfactory in obese patients and in those with metal abdominal sutures because adipose tissue and metal reflect sound.

Computed tomography (CT) is a sensitive means of demonstrating masses, infarcted tissue, and cysts, but it is expensive and exposes the patient to radiation.

Magnetic resonance imaging (MRI) is not used as an initial imaging study of the abdomen but is used selectively to define mass lesions, especially in the liver, kidneys, or adrenal glands, and vascular abnormalities, such as hemangiomata and renal or hepatic vein thrombosis. It is considerably more expensive than a CT scan. HASTE MRI, a newer technique (53,54), can demonstrate viscera without movement artifact. It is also effective in showing flowing fluids and therefore can demonstrate partial or complete vascular occlusion.

Table 45.11 compares the ultrasound, CT, and MRI techniques and the patient experience during the performance of these procedures.

Selective mesenteric angiography should be performed in patients with suspected mesenteric vascular ischemia (particularly in elderly patients with postprandial abdominal pain) or mesenteric vascular occlusion (e.g., women taking contraceptive medication). This is particularly helpful in older patients, because normal arteriographic findings rule out mesenteric vascular disease; on the other hand, occlusion of even two of the three major aortic branches (celiac, superior mesenteric, and inferior mesenteric arteries) can occur without symptoms of mesenteric vascular disease. It may be prudent to hospitalize the patient for this procedure. The patient experience is similar to that described for renal arteriography (see Chapter 67).

Endoscopy

Upper GI endoscopy (esophagoscopy, gastroscopy, duodenoscopy) requires referral to a gastroenterologist. It should be considered the ambulatory procedure of choice to diagnose upper GI disease and to obtain a biopsy for diagnosis (e.g., when cancer is suspected). Endoscopy should be performed promptly when abdominal pain is associated with upper GI bleeding (see earlier discussion), but these patients should be hospitalized. The patient's experience during the procedure has already been described.

Proctoscopy should be performed in any patient with abdominal pain and rectal bleeding or a change in bowel habits and in any patient in whom inflammatory bowel disease (proctitis, ulcerative colitis, Crohn disease) is suspected. Moreover, anal lesions such as hemorrhoids and fissures are best demonstrated by proctoscopy. The procedure routinely should precede roentgenographic examination of the lower bowel, because the barium enema does not visualize the lower rectum.

For *proctosigmoidoscopy,* whether prior preparation is appropriate depends on the suspected pathology. If *proctosigmoidoscopy* is performed to detect or biopsy a mass lesion, a laxative is used the day before and a cleansing enema is given on the morning of the procedure. On the other hand, mucosal lesions (e.g., inflammatory bowel disease) are best demonstrated without preparation (other than a natural bowel movement the morning of the procedure). Most enema preparations tend to produce some mucosal edema that may obscure mucosal lesions. Proctosigmoidoscopy is not painful, but an uncomfortable sensation is produced by the distension of the rectosigmoid region by the instrument used and by air.

Fiberoptic sigmoidoscopy can usually be performed if a laxative is administered the day before and an enema is given on the morning of the procedure. Many general physicians have been trained to perform this procedure, but in the absence of such training, referral to a gastroenterologist is appropriate. The patient's experience during the procedure has already been described.

Colonoscopy, like upper endoscopy, requires referral to a gastroenterologist. It should be considered in patients with abdominal pain who have occult rectal bleeding, in those with suspected diffuse colonic inflammatory disease (ulcerative colitis, Crohn disease) or suspected ischemic colitis, and in patients with polypoid lesions on barium enema who require biopsy or, often, resection of the lesion. Colonoscopy cannot be performed within a day or two after a barium radiograph of the lower or upper GI tract. The patient's experience during the procedure has already been described.

In addition to concerns about facts relating to endoscopy, many patients have specific apprehensions and misconceptions that can be managed appropriately only if the patient is encouraged to express them. The most common questions concern the indication for the procedure, its anticipated benefits, and technical details about the procedure itself, including prior preparation, side effects, and risks. Much of the patient's anxiety can be allayed if the referring practitioner can answer these questions appropriately. The clinician may find it helpful to emphasize that the fiberoptic instruments can be passed with little discomfort and that photographs can be taken for detailed study, as well as brushings for cytology and biopsy for histology.

Treatment

The treatment of patients with abdominal pain depends on the severity of the pain, its rapidity of onset, and the nature of the underlying condition, if known. Severe pain with an abrupt or rapid onset often reflects a GI disorder that will require surgical intervention (Table 45.8). Hospitalization and consultation with a surgeon should be requested immediately in almost all such cases. Less severe pain (pain that does not prevent the patient from ambulating, talking normally, thinking coherently, and so on) should not be treated aggressively with analgesic drugs until an attempt has been made to establish a diagnosis, because the pain often abates spontaneously within minutes or hours and does not recur. In such circumstances, no further evaluation is indicated. If the pain recurs or persists and the cause is not obvious, the screening tests described in this chapter should be performed. If these tests do not provide a diagnosis, referral to a gastroenterologist is indicated.

As a general rule, analgesic drugs may be prescribed to patients with persistent pain, but opiates should be avoided if possible, because they can aggravate the underlying condition. (For example, morphine may aggravate pancreatitis by producing duodenal and ampullary spasm, thus enhancing pancreatic duct obstruction, and opiates or anticholinergics may produce toxic megacolon in patients with active ulcerative colitis.) Furthermore, there is a risk of narcotic addiction in any patient whose pain is likely to be of prolonged duration.

ACKNOWLEDGMENT

We are grateful to Dr. Hemant Pande for his valuable contribution in writing this chapter.

General References*

Gastrointestinal Bleeding

American College of Physicians. **Suggested technique for fecal occult blood testing and interpretation in colorectal cancer screening.** Ann Intern Med 1997;126:808.

Barkin JS, Ross BS. Medical therapy for chronic gastrointestinal bleeding of obscure origin. Am J Gastroenterol 1998;93:1250.

Burt RW. Colon cancer screening. Gastroenterology 2000;119:837.

Byers T, Levin B, Rothenberger D, et al. American Cancer Society guidelines for screening and surveillance for early detection of colorectal polyps and cancer; update 1997. American Cancer Society Detection and Treatment Advisory Group on Colorectal Cancer. CA Cancer J Clin 1997;47:154.

Fleisher M, Winawer SJ, Zauber AG, et al. Accuracy of fecal occult blood test interpretation. National Polyp Study Work Group. Ann Intern Med 1991;114:875.

Kim YI. AGA technical review: impact of dietary fiber on colon cancer occurrence. Gastroenterology 2000;118:1235.

Potter GD, Sellin JH. Lower gastrointestinal bleeding. Gastroenterol Clin North Am 1988;17:341.

Ransohoff DF, Lang CA. Sigmoidoscopic screening in the 1990s. JAMA 1993;269:1278.

*Bold print (general references) and bold numerals (specific references) denote published controlled clinical trials, meta-analyses, or consensus-based recommendations.

Ransohoff DF, Lang CA. Screening for colorectal cancer with the fecal occult blood test: a background paper. Ann Intern Med 1997;126:811.

The supporting data for the ACP position (see American College of Physicians, 1997).

Winawer SJ, Fletcher RH, Miller L, et al. **Colorectal cancer screening: clinical guidelines and rationale.** Gastroenterology 1997;112:594.

Consensus guidelines endorsed by the American Gastroenterological Association, the American Cancer Society, the American College of Gastroenterology, the American Society for Gastrointestinal Endoscopy, and others.

Winawer SJ, Zauber AG, Ho M, et al. Prevention of colorectal cancer by colonoscopic polypectomy. The National Polyp Study Workgroup. N Engl J Med 1993;329:1977.

Zuckerman GR, Prakash C, Askin MP, et al. **AGA technical review on the evaluation and management of occult and obscure gastrointestinal bleeding.** Gastroenterology 2000;118:201.

Diarrhea

Aranda-Michel J, Giannella RA. Acute diarrhea: a practical review. Am J Med 1999;106:670.

Cranston D, McWhinnie D, Collin J. Dietary fibre and gastrointestinal disease. Br J Surg 1988;75:508.

Fine KD, Schiller LR. **AGA technical review on the evaluation and management of chronic diarrhea.** Gastroenterology 1999;116:1464.

Mylonakis E, Ryan ET, Calderwood SB. *Clostridium difficile*–associated diarrhea: a review. Arch Intern Med 2001;161:525.

Sawer MK, Gehlbach SH. Bacterial disease of the colon. Prim Care 1988;15:125.

Simon D. Pharmacotherapy of gastrointestinal tract infections in patients with AIDS. Pract Gastroenterol 1993;17(3):9.

Abdominal Pain

Ferrucci JT Jr. Body ultrasonography [first of two parts]. N Engl J Med 1979;300:538.

Good review of the clinical uses of sonography, with useful comparison of computed tomographic scanning.

Glasgow RE, Mulvihill SJ. Abdominal pain, including the acute abdomen. In: Feldman M, Scharschmidt BF, Sleisenger HH, eds. Sleisenger and Fordtran's gastrointestinal and liver disease. 6th ed., vol. 1. Philadelphia: WB Saunders, 1997:80.

Handbook of differential diagnosis. Vol. 2, part I: the abdomen. Nutley, NJ: Rocom Press, 1974.

Excellent illustrations by M. F. Netter and good tables.

Nathan L, Huddleston JH. Acute abdominal pain in pregnancy. Obstet Gynecol Clin North Am 1995;33:55.

Pearigen PD. Unusual causes of abdominal pain. Emerg Med Clin North Am 1996;14:593.

Specific References

1. American College of Physicians. Suggested technique for fecal occult blood testing and interpretation in colorectal cancer screening. Ann Intern Med 1997;126:808.
2. Allison JE, Feldman R, Tekawa IS. Hemoccult screening in detecting colorectal neoplasm: sensitivity, specificity, and predictive value. Long term follow-up in a large group practice setting. Ann Intern Med 1990;112:328.
3. Selby J-V, Friedman GD, Quesenberry CP Jr, et al. A case-control study of screening sigmoidoscopy and mortality from colorectal cancer. N Engl J Med 1992;326:653.
4. Irvine EJ, O'Connor J, Frost RA, et al. Prospective comparison of double contrast barium enema plus flexible sigmoidoscopy v. colonoscopy in rectal bleeding. Gut 1988;29:1188.
5. Waye JD, Bashkoff E. Total colonoscopy: is it always possible? Gastrointest Endosc 1991;37:152.
6. Kavic SM, Basson MD. Complications of endoscopy. Am J Surg 2001;181;319.
7. Rex DK, Rahmani EY, Haseman JH, et al. Relative sensitivity of colonoscopy and barium enema for detection of colorectal cancer in clinical practice. Gastroenterology 1997;112:17.
8. Foutch PG, Sawyer R, Sanowski RA. Push-enteroscopy for diagnosis of patients with gastrointestinal bleeding of obscure origin. Gastrointest Endosc 1990;36:337.
9. Zaman A, Katon RM. Push enteroscopy for obscure gastrointestinal bleeding yields a high incidence of proximal lesions within reach of a standard endoscope. Gastrointest Endosc 1998;47; 372.
10. Dusold R. Burke K, Carpentier W, Dyck WP. The accuracy of technetium-99m-labeled red cell scintigraphy in localizing gastrointestinal bleeding. Am J Gastroenterol 1994;98:345.
11. Zuckerman DA, Bocchini TP, Birnbaum EH. Massive hemorrhage in the lower gastrointestinal tract in adults: diagnostic imaging and intervention. AJR Am J Roentgenol 1993;161:703.
12. O'Brien MJ, Winawer SJ, Zauber AG, et al. The National Polyp Study: patient and polyp characteristics associated with high-grade dysplasia in colorectal adenomas. Gastroenterology 1990;98:371.
13. Muto T, Bussey HJ, Morson BC. The evolution of cancer of the colon and rectum. Cancer 1975;36:2251.
14. Bond JH. Polyp guideline: diagnosis, treatment, and surveillance for patients with colorectal polyps. Practice Parameters Committee of the American College of Gastroenterology. Am J Gastroenterol 2000;95:3053.
15. Steinbach G, Lynch PM, Phillips RKS, et al. The effect of celecoxib, a cyclooxygenase-2-inhibitor, in familial adenomatous polyposis. N Engl J Med 2000;342:1946.
16. Devesa SS, Chow WH. Variation in colorectal cancer incidence in the United States by subsite of origin. Cancer 1993;71:3819.
17. Grossman S, Milos ML. Colonoscopic screening of persons with suspected risk factors for colon cancer. I: family history. Gastroenterology 1988;94:395.
18. Hardcastle JD, Chamberlain JO, Robinson MH, et al. Randomized controlled trial of fecal occult-blood screening for colorectal cancer. Lancet 1996;348:1472.
19. Kewenter J, Brevinge H, Engaras B, et al. Results of screening, rescreening, and follow-up in a prospective, randomized study for detection of colorectal cancer by fecal occult blood testing: results for 68,308 subjects. Scand J Gastroenterol 1994;29:468.
20. Kronborg O, Fenger C, Olsen J, et al. Randomized study of screening for colorectal cancer with faecal-occult-blood test. Lancet 1996;348:1467.
21. Mandel JS, Bond JH, Church TR, et al. Reducing mortality from colorectal cancer by screening for fecal occult blood. N Engl J Med 1993;328:1365.
22. Rex DK, Johnson DA, Lieberman DA, et al. Colorectal cancer prevention 2000: recommendations of the American College of Gastroenterology. Am J Gastroenterol 2000;95:868.
23. Lieberman DA, Weiss DG, for the Veterans Affairs Cooperative Study Group. One-time screening for colorectal cancer with combined fecal occult-blood testing and examination of the distal colon. N Engl J Med 2001;345:555.
24. Detsky AS. Screening for colon cancer: can we afford colonoscopy? [Editorial]. N Engl J Med 2001;345:607.
25. Kinzler KW, Nilber TMC, Vogelstein B, et al. Identification of a gene located at chromosome 5q21 that is mutated in colorectal cancers. Science 1991;251:1366.
26. Speights VO, Johnson MW, Stoltenberg PH, et al. Colorectal cancer: current trends in initial clinical manifestations. South Med J 1991;84:575.
27. Steinberg SM, Barkin JS, Kaplan RS, et al. Prognostic indicators of colon tumors: the Gastrointestinal Tumor Study Group experience. Cancer 1986;57:1866.
28. Rex DK, Cutler CS, Lemmel GT, et al. Colonoscopic miss rates of adenomas determined by back-to-back colonoscopies. Gastroenterology 1997;112:24.
29. Moertel CG, Fleming TR, Macdonald JS, et al. An evaluation of the CEA test for monitoring patients with resected colon cancer. JAMA 1993;270:943.
30. Macdonald JS, Astrow AB. Adjuvant therapy of colon cancer. Semin Oncol 2001;28:30.
31. Buyse M, Piedbois P. Should Dukes' B patients receive adjuvant therapy? A statistical perspective. Semin Oncol 2001;28;20.
32. Boley SJ, Sammartano R, Adams A, et al. Nature and etiology of vascular ectasias of the colon. Gastroenterology 1977;72:650.

33. Cheung PS, Wong SK, Boey J, et al. Frank rectal bleeding: a prospective study of causes in patients over the age of 40. Postgrad Med J 1988;64:364.
34. Coppell MS, Gupta A. Changing epidemiology of GI angiodysplasia with increasing recognition of clinically milder cases. Am J Gastroenterol 1992;87:201.
35. Barkin JS, Ross BS. Medical therapy for chronic gastrointestinal bleeding of obscure origin. Am J Gastroenterol 1998;93:1250.
36. Dupont HL, Hornick RB. Adverse effects of Lomotil therapy in shigellosis. JAMA 1973;226:1525.
37. Cimolai N, Carter JE, Morrison BJ, et al. Risk factors for the progression of *Escherichia coli* O157:H7 enteritis to hemolytic-uremic syndrome. J Pediatr 1990;116:589.
38. Fine KD, Ogunji F, George J, et al. Utility of a rapid fecal latex agglutination test detecting the neutrophil protein, lactoferrin, for diagnosing inflammatory causes of chronic diarrhea. Am J Gastroenterol 1998;93:1300.
39. Garcia LS, Shimizu RY. Evaluation of nine immunoassay kits (enzyme immunoassay and direct fluorescence) for detection of *Giardia lamblia* and *Cryptosporidium parvum* in human fecal specimens. J Clin Microbiol 1997;35:1526.
40. Vanpoucke H, De Baere T, Claeys G, et al. Evaluation of six commercial assays for rapid detection of *Clostridium difficile* toxin and/or antigen in stool specimens. Clin Microbiol Infect 2001;7:55.
41. Shah RJ, Fenoglio-Preiser C, Bleau BL, et al. Usefulness of colonoscopy with biopsy in the evaluation of patients with chronic diarrhea. Am J Gastroenterol 2001;96:1091.
42. Eherer AJ, Fordtran JS. Fecal osmotic gap and pH in experimental diarrhea of various causes. Gastroenterology 1992;103:545.
43. Lang C, Gyr K, Stalder GA, et al. Assessment of exocrine pancreatic function by oral administration of *N*-benzoyl-L-tyrosyl-*p*-aminobenzoic acid (Bentiromide): 5 years' clinical experience. Br J Surg 1981;68:771.
44. Carroccio A, Verghi F, Santini B, et al. Diagnostic accuracy of fecal elastase 1 assay in patients with pancreatic maldigestion or intestinal malabsorption: a collaborative study of the Italian Society of Pediatric Gastroenterology and Hepatology. Dig Dis Sci 2001;46:1335.
45. Scrimshaw NS, Murray EB. The acceptability of milk and milk products in populations with a high prevalence of lactose intolerance. Am J Clin Nutr 1988;48:1079.
46. Tramonte SM, Brand MB, Mulrow CD, et al. The treatment of chronic constipation in adults. J Gen Intern Med 1997;12:15.
47. Edwards FC, Truelove SC. The course and prognosis of ulcerative colitis. Part III: complications. Gut 1964;5:7.
48. Pullan RD, Rhodes J, Garresh S, et al. Transdermal nicotine for active ulcerative colitis. N Engl J Med 1994;330:811.
49. Lennard-Jones JE, Morson BC, Ritchie JK, et al. Cancer surveillance in ulcerative colitis. Lancet 1983;2:149.
50. Panaccione R, Canadian Consensus Group on the use of infliximab in Crohn's disease. Infliximab for the treatment of Crohn's disease: review and indication for clinical use in Canada. Can J Gastroenterol 2001;15:371.
51. Palmer KR, Corbett CL, Holdsworth CD. Double blind cross-over study comparing loperamide, codeine, and diphenoxylate in the treatment of chronic diarrhea. Gastroenterology 1980;79:1272.
52. Sanson TG, O'Keefe KP. Evaluation of abdominal pain in the elderly. Emerg Med Clin North Am 1996;14:615.
53. Beall DP, Regan F. MRI of bowel obstruction using HASTE sequence. J Comput Assist Tomogr 1996;20:823.
54. Regan F, Fradin J, Khazan R, et al. Choledocholithiasis: evaluation with MR cholangiography. AJR Am J Roentgenol 1996;168:1441.

CHAPTER 46

Selected Gastrointestinal Problems II: Constipation, Diverticular Disease, Ostomy Care

LAWRENCE J. CHESKIN, MD

CONSTIPATION

Definition

Constipation is often defined as the infrequent, difficult passage of stool. However, it may mean different things to different people: that the stools are too infrequent, too difficult to expel, too hard, or too small, or that there is a sensation of incomplete evacuation. Of these, frequency of bowel movements is the most readily measured parameter. Several studies have identified a wide variation in the frequency of bowel movements among normal subjects of both sexes and of all ages, ranging from three per day to three per week (1). Therefore, someone who has fewer than three bowel movements per week is constipated, by definition. On the other hand, a change in frequency of movements, for example, from two per day to three per week, may also signify constipation. However, it is probably not necessary to do a workup or to treat people merely because they report fewer than three bowel movements per week. Even one movement per week is acceptable if it does not represent a recent change in bowel frequency and is not associated with symptoms such as pain on defecation or bloating. Constipation is among the most prevalent gastrointestinal (GI) complaints, accounting for more than 2.5 million physician visits in the United States annually and more than half a billion dollars in sales of laxatives (2). The prevalence of constipation increases with age, and it is more common in women and in lower socioeconomic groups (2,3).

Almost always, constipation is caused by a delay in transit within the colon or by a pelvic outlet delay (4) (see also Chapter 44). A wide variety of conditions can affect colonic transit (Table 46.1). There may be structural abnormalities that obstruct the passage of intraluminal contents, or there may be conditions that alter colonic motility. Evaluation of patients with constipation must therefore include consideration of a wide variety of possible etiologies. Although it is difficult to be precise about the relative frequencies of the various causes, chronic constipation (months or longer) is most commonly the result of a motility disorder (as in sedentary people eating a low-fiber diet or in patients with the irritable bowel syndrome), the use of constipating drugs, local anorectal problems (fissures, hemorrhoids, tumors), or pelvic outlet delay.

Table 46.1. Causes of Constipation

Idiopathic Causes (Possible Mechanisms)
Dietary factors: low residue
Motility disturbances: colonic inertia or spasm (irritable bowel syndrome)
Sedentary living

Structural Abnormalities
Anorectal disorders: fissures, thrombosed hemorrhoids, rectocele
Strictures
Tumors

Endocrine/Metabolic Causes
Hypercalcemia
Hypokalemia
Hypothyroidism
Diabetes mellitus
Uremia
Pregnancy

Neurogenic Causes
Cerebrovascular events
Hirschsprung disease
Parkinson disease
Multiple sclerosis
Spinal cord tumors
Trauma

Smooth Muscle/Connective Tissue Disorders
Amyloidosis
Scleroderma

Drugs
Antacids: aluminum- and calcium-containing compounds
Anticholinergics
Antidepressants
Calcium channel blockers (especially veropamil)
Cholestyramine
Narcotics
Sympathomimetics: pseudoephedrine

Psychogenic Causes (Especially Depression)

Evaluation

History

The history provides the most useful information about the etiology of constipation. It may reveal a gross misconception about normal bowel habits or a neurotic preoccupation with bowel function. Reassurance that there is a broad range of normal bowel frequency may be all that is needed in many cases of self-defined constipation. It is important to determine the onset and duration of constipation and whether it represents a recent change in frequency of bowel movement. Associated symptoms such as straining, abdominal pain, bloating, and distention may shed light on the severity of symptoms. A detailed dietary history should be obtained, and the amount of dietary fiber intake should be estimated. Patients should be questioned regarding symptoms that may suggest a systemic process (e.g., hypothyroidism, hyperparathyroidism, scleroderma), a neurologic disorder (e.g., cerebrovascular disease, Parkinson disease), or intake of drugs (e.g., anticholinergics, calcium channel blockers, opiates, antidepressants), which are known to impair colonic motility. Most systemic and neurologic diseases are almost certain to affect organs outside the GI tract so that, in addition to constipation, patients have symptoms that reflect extraintestinal dysfunction. On the other hand, even local processes (e.g., strictures, tumors) often produce other GI symptoms in addition to constipation, such as abdominal pain or rectal bleeding. Therefore, rectal bleeding should always be thoroughly evaluated (see later discussion), even though in constipated patients it often is caused by perianal disease (e.g., fissures, hemorrhoids). Abdominal pain with constipation is also a prominent feature of the irritable bowel syndrome (see Chapter 44). Most patients with idiopathic diet-related or drug-induced constipation are otherwise asymptomatic, although a complaint of a bloated sensation is common if constipation is prolonged. A history of the type, frequency, and duration of laxative use may highlight a dependence on laxatives or may even suggest a psychological disorder if the laxative use is inappropriate.

Physical Examination

The physical examination should be focused on the identification of underlying causes of constipation. The general examination is rarely helpful unless an enlarged thyroid or abdominal mass is detected. Rectal examination is often helpful because it can identify fissures and hemorrhoids as well as anal stenosis or stricture secondary to surgery or inflammation. The anal sphincter is normally closed. A gaping anal opening or asymmetry of the anal opening may indicate a neurologic disorder (spinal cord trauma, peripheral neuropathy) that impairs sphincteric function. After inspection, a careful digital examination should be performed to evaluate the strength of the anal sphincters, the presence of masses, the consistency of the stool, and the presence of any painful or tender areas. The patient should be asked to strain and the amount of perineal descent should be noted. In general there should be 2 to 3 cm of perineal descent with straining. In patients with pelvic floor disorders, there may be no descent or paradoxic perineal ascent. The stool should also be tested for occult blood.

Laboratory Tests

Before any endoscopic evaluation, basic laboratory testing is sometimes helpful. Serum creatinine, urea nitrogen and electrolytes, especially Na^+, K^+, and Mg^{2+}, should be checked. Thyroid function tests should be performed if hypothyroidism is suspected.

Endoscopy

Most gastroenterologists believe that endoscopy should be performed routinely for newly constipated patients in whom the cause is not obvious. There is, however, no firm evidence on which to base this recommendation (5). Patients age 50 years and older should have colonoscopy because of their increased risk of colon cancer. Even a good air-contrast barium enema is not a substitute for endoscopy, because subtle mucosal abnormalities cannot be detected and because the most distal 15 to 20 cm of the colon are difficult to evaluate radiographically. Anoscopy also may be needed to search properly for hemorrhoids or fissures (see Chapter 98).

In patients younger than 50 years of age, flexible sigmoidoscopy is probably a reasonable substitute for colonoscopy unless there has been evidence of other worrisome symptoms such as GI bleeding or weight loss.

Flexible sigmoidoscopy can be performed in the practitioner's office with the patient in the knee–chest position on a routine examining table or in the left lateral position. Sigmoidoscopy should be performed to the highest level possible, with limitations imposed by the patient's tolerance of the procedure, the presence of stool, and the length of the instrument (a flexible sigmoidoscope is usually 60 cm in length and can often be passed to the splenic flexure). The patient's experience during flexible sigmoidoscopy and colonoscopy is described in Chapter 45.

Inflamed *hemorrhoids* and *fissures* found during anoscopy or flexible sigmoidoscopy may be secondary to constipation, but they may also cause pain on defecation and thereby promote constipation. These lesions are also common causes of bleeding in the chronically constipated patient. A spotty or diffuse brown pigmentation of the mucosa, known as *melanosis coli,* is indicative of *chronic laxative abuse,* particularly of the anthraquinone family (e.g., cascara, senna, aloe). A mass lesion, such as a *carcinoma* or *polyp,* may also be identified by flexible sigmoidoscopy or colonoscopy.

A *rectal biopsy* may diagnose amyloidosis, ulcerative colitis, or Crohn disease, and a deeper, suction biopsy of a rectal valve may diagnose Hirschsprung disease. Biopsies of the rectal mucosa can be taken safely below the peritoneal reflection (approximately 12 cm proximal to the anus in men, 8 cm in women). Punch biopsies can be performed by any clinician who has had appropriate training and experience. Suction biopsies should be performed only by a surgeon or gastroenterologist. Rectal biopsy should be painless unless a tender, inflamed lesion is biopsied; if it is done properly, the risks of bleeding and perforation, the major complications, are low.

Radiographic Studies

Radiographic examination is helpful primarily in the detection of obstructing lesions. The plain film of the abdomen may occasionally diagnose an obstructing carcinoma before endoscopy has been done. The presence of a megacolon or a volvulus, of either the sigmoid colon or the cecum, also may be easily diagnosed by a plain film. Some practitioners obtain a barium enema after flexible sigmoidoscopy in all patients with new-onset constipation, rather than simply performing a colonoscopy. As stated earlier, colonoscopy is probably the preferable procedure, although the two approaches have not been prospectively compared. Obstructing neoplasms and strictures can be identified by barium studies, although more subtle mucosal lesions may be missed. The radiologist also may comment on the motility of the colon, particularly if there is significant spasm or if haustral markings are absent, as is seen in patients who use laxatives habitually and in those who have an atonic megacolon.

Other Studies

Colonic motility tests and *transit studies* are additional procedures that may provide insight into the pathophysiology of constipation. These studies are generally available only in specialized centers. They should be performed for the few patients who are severely impaired by constipation and who are refractory to conventional therapy.

Colonic motility studies are performed by placing catheters to monitor intracolonic pressures in the rectal and sigmoid regions. The study can identify various patterns of colonic activity in patients with constipation (6). In some, high-amplitude phasic contractions are seen spontaneously, as well as in response to stimulation. This type of segmental activity is sometimes associated with pain and is believed to cause constipation by impeding the distal flow of luminal contents. In other patients, an atonic pattern is found, characterized by a decreased response to stimulation and a loss of resistance to distention.

Colonic transit time can be measured by plotting the expulsion of radiopaque markers (Sitzmarks, commercially available) after daily ingestion of a capsule containing 24 markers. Once a steady state is reached, the number of markers entering the GI tract must equal the number being excreted, and the transit time in hours is equal to the number of markers still in the colon on plain film (7). Moreover, the distribution of these markers may have a relationship to the underlying motility disturbance. The retention of markers only in the rectum suggests a failure of expulsion, whereas retention throughout the colon suggests generalized colonic inertia.

Defecography is the study of the process of defecation (8). It can provide useful information when anatomic abnormality of the anorectal region is suspected as the cause of constipation. In this test, the patient evacuates thick barium under fluoroscopic monitoring while sitting on a special commode. Defecography can also be performed scintigraphically. Anomalies such as intussusception and rectocele can be revealed by this technique. However, patients may find the test embarrassing, impairing the validity of the results.

Anorectal manometry is helpful in excluding Hirschsprung disease if it demonstrates a normal rectoanal inhibitory reflex. It may also provide useful information regarding pelvic floor function (6).

Treatment

The treatment for constipation should, if possible, be based on correction of the underlying abnormality; for example, a systemic disease that can be treated (e.g., hypothyroidism) or a constipating drug that can be stopped. The use of laxatives as a reflex response to complaints of constipation should be discouraged. Successful therapy must include discussion with the patient about the broad limits of normal bowel function and the patient's own concepts of normal bowel activity.

Bowel Retraining

Bowel retraining is an important initial aspect of therapy for patients whose constipation does not have an identifiable and remediable cause. The patient should be encouraged to have a regular daily routine with time set aside for having a bowel movement, preferably within 5 to 10 minutes after a meal, to take advantage of the strong stimulus of the gastrocolic reflex. This behavior modification program allows the patient to become more aware of and responsive to the normal urges to defecate. Patients should be advised always to respond to such urges. In severely constipated patients, a bowel retraining program may be initiated, with enemas or suppositories used to enhance bowel activity at the desired time. For enemas, lukewarm tap water should be used, because all other solutions may be irritating if used repetitively. The enema should also be done soon after eating a meal to take advantage of the gastrocolic reflex. For suppositories, bisacodyl (Dulcolax) should be used, again just after eating; however, these suppositories should not be used for more than a few days, because they may eventually be irritating. Glycerin suppositories are commonly used but are not very effective.

Diet

Dietary fiber has long been considered an important factor in bowel function but there is as yet no evidence that this is so (5). However, patients with constipation do often respond to an increase in fiber in their diet, and there is evidence that oroanal transit times are decreased when intake of dietary fiber is increased (9).

Table 46.2. Fiber Content of Various Foods

Type of Food	Dietary Fiber per Average Serving (g)
Vegetables	
Beans (navy, lima, kidney, baked)	8.5–10.0
Beans (string)	2.0
Broccoli	3.2
Brussels sprouts	2.3
Cabbage	2.0
Carrots	2.0
Celery	1.0
Corn	2.6
Corn on the cob	5.9
Lettuce	1.0
Potato (baked with skin)	3.0
Potato (french fried)	1.6
Peas (canned)	6.0
Rice	0.8
Fruit	
Apple with peel	2.0
Apple juice	0.0
Banana	1.5
Grapefruit (fresh)	0.6
Orange	2.0
Peach	2.0
Raspberries	4.6
Strawberries	1.6
Bread	
Whole wheat	1.3
White, rye, French	0.7
Cereal	
All-Bran (100%)	8.4
Corn flakes	2.6
Wheaties	2.6
Other Foods	
Meats: chicken, liver, fish, lamb	0.0
Cheese, milk, yogurt	0.0

As an initial step in treatment, therefore, the patient should be advised to follow a diet rich in fiber. As listed in Table 46.2, a variety of foods are high in fiber. As a practical matter, it may be reasonable to add a commercial fiber preparation to a high-fiber diet. Maintaining an adequate intake of fluids (1.5 to 2 L/day), although particularly difficult for some older patients with constipation, is also helpful (10).

Laxatives

Despite numerous warnings, laxatives are still popular in the treatment of constipation. The presence of 700 or more commercially available laxatives and enema preparations attests to the widespread use of these agents. The mechanism of action for most laxatives is poorly understood, and the potential for toxicity is often underestimated (Table 46.3). Few data are available for comparison among the various laxatives, and the decision to use a particular laxative often is determined by individual preference rather than by objective evidence of efficacy or safety.

There are a number of different mechanisms by which a laxative effect may be achieved. *Bulk-forming agents* are natural or synthetic polysaccharides or cellulose derivatives that exert their laxative effect

Table 46.3. Laxatives

Classification and Active Ingredient	Examples	Dosage	Average Onset of Action	Potential Adverse Effects
Bulk				
Psyllium seed	Konsyl	1 tsp to 2 tbsp/day	12–24 hr or longer	Increased gas and bloating sensation; bowel obstruction if stricture is present
	Effer-Syllium			
	Perdiem (with senna)			
Plus dextrose	Metamucil			
Bran		4 + tbsp/day		
Calcium polycarbophil	FiberCon	4–8 tablets/day		
Emollient (Softeners)				
Docusate sodium	Colace, Peri-Colace (with cassanthranol)	1–3 caps/day	24–48 hr	
	Surfak			
Stimulant				
Phenolphthalein	Ex-Lax	1–2 tablets (100–200 mg)	6–8 hr	Dermatitis; electrolyte Imbalance, melanosis coli
Bisacodyl	Dulcolax	2–3 tabs (10–15 mg)	6–12 hr	
Senna	Senokot, Perdiem (with psyllium)	1–4 tsp or 2–4 tabs	6–12 hr	
Cascara (casanthranol)	Peri-Colace (with dioctyl sodium)	1–2 tabs	8–12 hr	
Carbon dioxide	Ceo-two suppositories	1–2	10–30 min	
Osmotic				
Ricinoleic acid	Castor oil	1–2 tsp		Electrolyte Imbalance
Lactulose[a]	Cephulac, Chronulac	1–2 tbsp/day	24–48 hr	Excessive gas production
Magnesium salts	Milk of Magnesia, magnesium citrate	2–4 tbsp	3–6 hr or less	Hypermagnesemia, hypocalcemia, hyperphosphatemia in chronic renal failure
Sodium salts	Phospho-Soda	2 tbsp in 1/2 glass of water	2–6 hr	
	Fleet enema (sodium phosphate)	120 mL	2–5 min	Dehydration; hypocalcemia; hyperphosphatemia in chronic renal failure

[a]Requires a prescription.

primarily by absorbing water and increasing fecal mass. Psyllium seed and bran are examples of such laxatives. In addition to their hydrophilic properties, these agents are metabolized by colonic bacteria, resulting in accumulation of osmotically active metabolites. These laxatives are effective in increasing the frequency and in softening the consistency of stool. There have been isolated reports of obstruction secondary to use of hydrophilic agents in patients with esophageal or small-bowel strictures. In most cases, however, this type of laxative is highly effective and the potential for adverse effects appears to be low. However, in patients with an atonic form of constipation, particularly with megacolon, these agents are often ineffective and produce an uncomfortable sensation of bloating and gaseousness at high dosages. Bloating is common in all patients when they begin to take bulk agents, but it is usually transient and can be minimized by increasing the dosage gradually over a period of weeks. A meta-analysis found that laxatives and fiber increased the frequency of bowel movements by a mean of 1.4 times per week (11). Fiber and bulk laxatives also reduced constipation-related abdominal pain.

Docusate sodium (Colace) is often labeled as a *stool softener* or a wetting agent. It works by lowering surface tension, allowing water to enter the stool more easily. It is generally well tolerated.

The *saline laxatives* are magnesium or sodium salts (e.g., milk of magnesia, sodium phosphate) which are poorly absorbed and therefore act as hyperosmolar solutions. They may also stimulate the release of cholecystokinin, a hormone that stimulates colonic motility. Complications include hypermagnesemia in patients with renal failure and hypocalcemia from phosphate overdoses.

Stimulant laxatives, such as anthraquinone derivatives (senna, aloe, cascara) and diphenylmethane compounds (phenolphthalein, bisacodyl), exert their effects primarily by altering electrolyte transport by the intestinal mucosa and thereby increasing intestinal motor activity. The effect of these agents is claimed to be more specific on the colon. Phenolphthalein, an ingredient found in many over-the-counter preparations, has been associated with severe allergic dermatitis and the Stevens–Johnson syndrome. The chronic use of the anthraquinone derivatives has been reported to induce damage to the myenteric plexus and therefore may eventually impair bowel motility. Agents such as these that affect electrolyte transport may result in significant hypokalemia, factitious diarrhea, protein-losing enteropathy, and salt overload. Although these agents are undoubtedly effective, their chronic use may lead to significant side effects, and they should be avoided when possible.

Castor oil, previously thought to be a stimulant laxative, is now understood to exert its cathartic effect by alteration of intestinal fluid and electrolyte secretion. Ricinoleic acid, the active ingredient of castor oil, has effects on the small and large intestine similar to those of bile acids: It inhibits absorption of sodium and glucose and stimulates fluid and electrolyte secretion by increasing cellular cyclic adenosine monophosphate (cAMP) and by inhibiting sodium–potassium adenosine triphosphatase (ATPase). This increase in intraluminal fluid content may then secondarily affect intestinal motility. Its use is not recommended because of the potential for fluid–electrolyte disturbances.

Lactulose (Cephulac or Chronulac syrup) is a semisynthetic disaccharide that is not metabolized by intestinal enzymes. As a result, water and electrolytes are retained within the intestinal lumen by the osmotic effect of this undigested sugar. In addition, this agent is converted by colonic bacteria to organic acids, which may further alter electrolyte transport or affect colonic motility, or both. Lactulose is commonly used in patients with hepatic encephalopathy (see Chapter 47). It has also been shown to be an effective laxative in patients with chronic constipation. There is little information on the relative merits of lactulose and bulk laxatives except that lactulose is expensive and requires 24 to 48 hours to achieve its effect.

Surgery

Surgery is rarely necessary in the treatment of constipated patients. However, it is required for resection of an obstructing lesion, and myectomy may be needed for treatment of Hirschsprung disease. Various procedures have been recommended for patients with megacolon with recurrent volvulus, ranging from simple tacking down of the loose mesentery to resection of bowel. Finally, in severe cases of intractable constipation, extensive surgery has been advocated, varying from resection of redundant sigmoid loops to subtotal colectomy with ileal proctostomy. The exact role and precise indication for this type of surgery remain to be more clearly defined, but there is evidence that subtotal colectomy is effective and well tolerated in patients with severe atonic constipation (12).

Summary of Recommendations

Therapy for constipation should always be directed first at identifying and treating any underlying disorder (Table 46.1). If the constipation is drug induced, the drug should be discontinued (if possible) or an alternative that is less constipating should be substituted. Otherwise, fiber and fluids should be added to the diet, and, if necessary, a bulk laxative should be prescribed. When constipation is idiopathic, caused by an irreversible underlying disorder (e.g., diabetes mellitus), or secondary to a necessary drug, dietary changes and some form of laxative therapy may be necessary.

In practically all patients with constipation, a high-fiber diet or a bulk laxative is helpful. The amount of dietary fiber or bulk laxative that is needed varies from patient to patient and must be determined individually. Because the only significant side effect from this form of therapy is excessive gas and a bloated sensation, the dosage can be gradually increased until either the constipation is resolved or the side effects become too uncomfortable. For most patients, this form of therapy is successful and appears to be very safe on a chronic, defined (i.e., not as-needed) basis. No other laxatives are needed.

However, in patients with partial bowel obstruction (as recognized on radiography) and in those with an atonic form of constipation (e.g., institutional megacolon), the high fiber–bulk laxative approach usually is not effective. A patient with constipation caused by partial obstruction usually must be treated surgically. A patient with an atonic colon may need a stimulant laxative. Senna compounds, bisacodyl (either as a tablet or as a suppository), or enemas are most effective in such cases. Combinations of a stimulant laxative with a bulk agent (e.g., Perdiem) or with a softener (e.g., Peri-Colace) are reasonable and effective forms of therapy. Bulk agents alone in such cases simply distend the already distended bowel further without improving bowel function.

Special consideration must be given to the bedridden or chair-bound patient. In such patients, use of laxatives may result in incontinence because the patient may not be able to recognize or respond quickly enough to the sudden urge to defecate. In these circumstances, bulk agents are useful to keep the stool soft (Table 46.3), but suppositories or enemas should also be used (simple tap water enemas are usually sufficient), with the patient already positioned on the commode. In this fashion, the embarrassment and soilage of fecal incontinence can be avoided and fecal impactions can be prevented. Enemas or suppositories may be used regularly (daily to every third day) to prevent fecal impactions and overflow diarrhea and incontinence.

A pamphlet for patients, entitled, *What Is Constipation?,* is sponsored by the National Institute of Arthritis, Diabetes, Digestive and Kidney Diseases. (This pamphlet may be ordered [and then duplicated] from Clearinghouse, 1555 Wilson Boulevard, Suite 600, Rosslyn, VA 22209-2461.)

DIVERTICULAR DISEASE OF THE COLON

Definitions

The terminology for conditions subsumed under the phrase *diverticular disease* is widely misunderstood. The phrase refers to a variety of clinical states that may differ in etiology and prognosis. The nomenclature of diverticular disease of the colon is listed in Table 46.4. As can be seen from this classification, *diverticulosis* is simply the presence of colonic diverticula, without presuming that there are accompanying signs and symptoms. *Symptomatic diverticular disease* is diverticulosis associated with pain or altered bowel habits in the absence of evidence of diverticular inflammation. *Diverticulitis* is inflammation of one or more diverticula, generally implying perforation of

Table 46.4. Nomenclature of Diverticular Disease of the Colon

Diverticulosis (presence of multiple diverticula)
Asymptomatic
Symptomatic (pain, altered bowel habits)
Complicated by hemorrhage
Diverticulitis (necrotizing inflammation in one or more diverticula)
With microperforation (local inflammation)
With macroperforation, manifested by abscess, fistula, peritonitis, obstruction, or hemorrhage
Prediverticular state: muscular thickening and shortening of colonic wall without recognizable diverticula

a diverticulum, and it is almost always symptomatic. The *prediverticular state* is characterized by some of the radiographic, pathologic, and often clinical features of diverticulosis without the formation of diverticula. The distinctions among these entities are more than semantic, because the pathophysiology and natural history of each is probably different.

Epidemiology and Pathogenesis

The prevalence of diverticular disease in Western countries is strongly correlated with age: Approximately 20% of men and women older than 40 years of age, 50% of those older than 60 years, and as many as 66% over age 85 have diverticulosis of the colon (13). These figures reflect a striking rise in the frequency of the condition over the last 70 years (in the early 20th century, only 5% of people over 60 years old were affected), coincident with the advent of milling, which removes two thirds of the fiber content of flour. In addition, it is known that vegetarians have a much lower prevalence of diverticular disease than nonvegetarians. In a prospective study of almost 48,000 men, a low-fiber diet increased the risk of development of diverticular disease by two- to threefold over a 4-year period (14). This evidence led to the hypothesis that a low-fiber diet increases intraluminal pressure and that the increased pressure leads to herniation of the mucosa through weakened or porous parts of the colonic muscle. In support of this hypothesis is the demonstration in some cases of diverticular disease of higher resting pressures in the colon and of exaggerated contractile activity in response to meals and cholinergic stimulation (3). Therefore, both a low-fiber diet and disordered colonic motility have been implicated in the pathogenesis of diverticulosis.

Another aspect in the pathogenesis of this condition is the weakness in the colonic wall through which the mucosa herniates to form the diverticulum. The site of herniation occurs at areas of least resistance, most often at points of penetration of intramural vessels through the circular muscle layer. The association of colonic diverticula with scleroderma and with Marfan and Ehlers–Danlos syndromes suggests that loss of muscle mass or defects in collagen may be important factors. Changes in collagen synthesis are known to occur with aging and may explain the increased prevalence of diverticular disease in elderly people. Therefore, the formation of diverticula may also involve a degenerative process of the colonic muscle with a change in tensile strength of the wall of the colon.

Asymptomatic Diverticulosis

A substantial majority of patients with diverticulosis detected on barium enema are entirely asymptomatic. The diverticula may be localized to the sigmoid colon or may involve the entire colon diffusely. The sigmoid colon is almost always involved (95% of the time), and sigmoid diverticula account for 75% of all colonic diverticula (13). It is believed that this predilection is explained by the narrow caliber of the sigmoid colon, which results in higher intraluminal pressures and hence a greater risk of herniation. The more distal the position in the colon, the higher the prevalence of diverticula. However, rectal diverticula rarely occur.

The natural history of diverticulosis is variable. A large majority of patients never present clinically, either because their diverticulosis is asymptomatic or because the symptoms are not severe enough to cause them to seek medical attention. Symptomatic diverticular disease manifests either as painful diverticular disease (75%) or as diverticulitis or hemorrhage (25%) (15). In most cases, diverticula precede the onset of symptoms by several years. In a minority of cases, however, typical symptoms precede anatomic disease (the prediverticular state).

Although a diet high in fiber may be beneficial in preventing the development of diverticula, there is little evidence that therapy for asymptomatic diverticulosis is of any value in preventing or even delaying the occurrence of symptomatic diverticular disease or of such complications as diverticulitis or hemorrhage. Maintenance of regular bowel habits without the use of laxatives is probably the best advice for patients who are asymptomatic. It is also prudent to alert patients to the manifestations of symptomatic diverticular disease and to urge them to seek medical care promptly should such symptoms develop.

Painful Diverticular Disease

Diagnosis

Diverticular disease may at times become symptomatic. When the predominant symptoms are abdominal pain and an alteration in bowel habits, the cause is usually painful diverticular disease. The hallmark of this disease is abdominal pain without evidence of an inflammatory process. The pain may be colicky or steady, is generally in the left lower quadrant, and is usually made worse by meals (presumably because of gastrocolic reflex) and at least partially relieved by having a bowel movement or by passing flatus. Bowel habits, usually during the painful episodes, often become irregular, with development of constipation, diarrhea, or both in an alternating fashion. Constipation is more common than the other alterations in bowel habits. These attacks are usually episodic rather than continuous. Symptoms may also include nausea, heartburn, and flatulence.

Physical examination may reveal tenderness, at times significant, in the left lower quadrant of the abdomen. A tender sigmoid loop, which feels like a sausage, may be palpable, but there is no other palpable mass and the entire abdominal examination is often unremarkable. The stool should be negative for occult blood, but rectal bleeding may be found because of coincidental rectal outlet disorders such as fissures or hemorrhoids. The presence of fever, leukocytosis, or peritoneal signs points toward the more serious diagnosis of diverticulitis.

Proctosigmoidoscopy, if performed during an attack, shows a normal colonic mucosa. However, considerable pain and spasm may be caused by the procedure.

Colonoscopy or *barium enema* (see Chapter 45) is important both for diagnosing diverticulosis and for excluding other reasons for the symptoms. Spasm may be a feature of diverticular disease, but fistulas or a mass suggests diverticulitis, carcinoma, or Crohn disease. Particularly in elderly patients, in whom the prevalence of diverticulosis is so high, it is important not to assume that the patient's symptoms have been explained once diverticula are found; carcinoma, for example, may be the real cause.

Therapy

The therapy for symptomatic diverticular disease is based on the assumption that a low-fiber diet and increased colonic pressure are important pathogenetic factors. Diets high in fiber (Table 46.2) are prescribed and have been shown to be effective in improving bowel transit and relieving symptoms (16). Commercial preparations of hydrophilic colloids made from vegetable fiber are available and convenient, but they are more expensive than dietary sources (Table 46.3). Patients should be instructed about high-fiber diets and, if necessary, should be given fiber supplements at a dosage of 4 to 10 g (1 tablespoon one to three times a day in a glass of water or juice). Artificial fiber products in tablet form are also available (e.g., Fiberall, FiberCon).

In addition to dietary maneuvers, anticholinergic drugs or antispasmodic drugs may be helpful for the relief of abdominal pain. Although these agents are not of proven value for this condition, some patients do respond. Dicyclomine (Bentyl), at a dosage of 10 to 20 mg before meals and at bedtime, or hyoscyamine (e.g., Levsin, also available in sustained-release and sublingual formulations) 0.125 to 0.375 mg every 4 hours as needed may be helpful. Other, more potent anticholinergics may produce adverse side effects and may aggravate the constipation.

The patient should be told that the course of the disease is unpredictable and that attacks will probably be experienced at irregular intervals (months to years) for the rest of his or her life. There is no benefit in continuing to take medication for the condition between attacks, but maintenance of a high-fiber diet is prudent.

Diverticulitis

Diverticulitis results from perforation of one or more diverticula, usually in the sigmoid colon. Perforation may result from persistently high colonic pressures, from abrasion by a fecalith, or from an inflammatory process that weakens the wall of the diverticulum. Usually the perforation is initially microscopic and is well confined by the omentum and the mesentery, but it may be grossly evident with free perforation (macroperforation), generalized peritonitis, abscess formation, and fistulization. Diverticulitis increases in incidence with age and with duration of the underlying diverticulosis, and it is more common in patients who have many diverticula. Fistulas may form to the bladder (colovesicular fistula is most common), vagina (especially after hysterectomy), small bowel, or skin (17). *Diverticulitis is the most common complication of diverticulosis.* The long-term risk for development of diverticulitis among patients with diverticulosis is 10% to 25% (13), but it is probably much lower in patients with asymptomatic diverticulosis.

Diagnosis

The cardinal symptoms of acute diverticulitis are abdominal pain and fever. In classic cases, the pain is severe, abrupt in onset, and persistent, worsening with time and localizing to the left lower quadrant. The pain is often accompanied by anorexia, nausea, and vomiting. Altered bowel habits, especially constipation, are common. Urinary tract symptoms and purulent vaginal discharge may occur because of fistula formation or because of inflammation of contiguous structures.

Abdominal tenderness and fever are found on physical examination. Localized peritonitis may be indicated by marked direct and rebound tenderness over the involved area, usually most pronounced in the left lower quadrant. The abdomen is often distended and tympanitic to percussion and the bowel sounds diminished. A mass may be felt at the site of inflammation in the left lower quadrant or on pelvic or rectal examination. Rectal bleeding occurs in approximately 25% of patients and is usually occult.

Leukocytosis is almost always present. Pyuria and/or hematuria may be found when there is involvement of the bladder or ureter.

The presentation of acute diverticulitis may be muted in the elderly patient. A high degree of suspicion is required in this population, because there may be no fever, no leukocytosis, and minimal abdominal pain.

The *differential diagnosis* includes painful diverticular disease, carcinoma of the colon, and inflammatory or ischemic bowel disease. The presence of peritonitis, fever, and leukocytosis rules out simple symptomatic diverticular disease. The other conditions are distinguished from diverticulitis by their clinical course and by barium enema or endoscopy.

The *diagnosis* of acute diverticulitis is made largely on clinical grounds, but some tests may be useful in confirming the clinical impression. Plain abdominal radiographs (flat and upright or decubitus views) may show signs of ileus and the location of the inflammatory mass, or they may show air in the bladder in some cases of colovesical fistula. Plain films are also important in detecting free air caused by perforation, a surgical emergency. A limited flexible sigmoidoscopy is indicated in many cases when the diagnosis is in doubt, both to rule out other processes in the left colon and to see whether there are indeed diverticula in the sigmoid colon. Once their presence is verified, the procedure is terminated to avoid worsening or causing free perforation. Weeks later, after successful medical therapy, it is safe to complete the examination of the rest of the colon by colonoscopy. This is not so much to make the diagnosis of diverticulitis as to exclude other conditions, such as carcinoma or Crohn disease. Abdominal computed tomography (CT) can be very helpful in visualizing diverticular abscesses in the pericolonic tissues, and it has largely supplanted other radiographic and endoscopic modalities as an adjunct to the clinical diagnosis of diverticulitis (18).

Therapy

Most patients with diverticulitis should be hospitalized, placed on bowel and bed rest, and given analgesics, intravenous hydration, and antimicrobial drugs (such as clindamycin and gentamicin, or cefotetan to treat both aerobic and anaerobic infection). Selected patients, particularly younger patients who are otherwise healthy and who have only mild tenderness and low-grade fever, may be treated on an ambulatory basis with oral broad-spectrum antibiotics (e.g., trimethoprim–sulfamethoxazole, double-strength twice daily, plus metronidazole, 500 mg every 6 hours for 10 days to 2 weeks).

Although more than 75% of patients respond to conservative medical management, it is wise to obtain surgical consultation early in the hospital course to facilitate operative intervention should it prove necessary. The patient's condition usually improves markedly in 3 to 10 days if medical therapy is successful. For patients who respond to conservative management, a recurrence rate of 20% to 25%, mostly in the first 5 years, can be expected (19).

Failure to resolve the acute inflammatory process, recurrent attacks of diverticulitis, and obstructive stricture formation are indications for surgical intervention. It seems reasonable that patients be placed on a high-fiber diet after recovery from an acute episode of diverticulitis.

Diverticular Bleeding

Diverticular disease is the most common cause of gross lower GI bleeding in adults, followed closely by bleeding from angiodysplasias (20). Both diverticulosis and angiodysplasias are common in the older population, and both are commonly found in the proximal colon. Diverticular bleeds, in contrast to diverticulitis, occur in the right colon in two thirds of cases (even though diverticula are much more common in the left colon) (21). The average age of patients with diverticular bleeding is approximately 70 years (22). Bleeding is the presenting manifestation of diverticular disease in approximately 16% of patients (23,24). The exact cause of diverticular bleeding is uncertain. Diverticulitis is rarely, if ever, associated with gross bleeding. There is no evidence that dietary therapy reduces the risk of hemorrhage. Most instances of bleeding occur in patients who are otherwise asymptomatic.

Massive hemorrhage is a common mode of presentation for diverticular bleeding, although in many cases the bleeding is occult and chronic. Massive lower GI bleeding in a patient known to have diverticula is not necessarily diverticular in origin: In 30% of cases, colonoscopy detects a second lesion (e.g., cancer or angiodysplasia) (21). Occult bleeding also should be ascribed to diverticulosis only after other causes have been excluded by a thorough evaluation (see Chapter 45).

Patients with diverticular hemorrhage require hospitalization for hemodynamic stabilization, diagnosis, and therapy. Approximately 70% of patients stop bleeding spontaneously. In the subset of patients who continue to bleed, angiography is the initial procedure of choice, especially if the bleeding is very brisk. During angiography, transcatheter embolization (with autologous blood clot, Gelfoam, or another agent) can be attempted and is sometimes very effective in patients who are poor surgical candidates. Angiography results usually are negative when the bleeding is slow and intermittent, and in such patients a radionucleotide bleeding scan, and a colonoscopy after a standard bowel preparation, should be considered. Emergency surgery is indicated when the bleeding is persistent. It involves a segmental colectomy when the bleeding site has been identified but colonoscopic interventions have failed, or subtotal colectomy with ileorectal anastomosis when the bleeding site in the colon has not been identified. The recurrence rate after the first episode of diverticular bleeding is 20% to 25%; it is approximately 50% after the second episode and increases with each subsequent episode of bleeding (25). Patients with two or more episodes of significant diverticular bleed should be considered for elective surgical resection (26).

CARE OF PATIENTS WITH COLOSTOMY OR ILEOSTOMY

Ostomies are openings of a portion of the GI tract—usually the ileum or the colon—that have been surgically diverted to the abdominal wall. It is estimated that there are more than 1 million *ostomates* (the preferred term for people with ostomies) in North America. The amount of time devoted in medical school curricula and postgraduate training to the care of ostomies is not commensurate with these numbers, and few health care providers have the necessary background to be appropriately helpful to the ostomate. This is particularly unfortunate in light of the fact that the partial or total colectomy that results in an ileostomy or colostomy often cures the underlying condition, leaving a healthy patient who is capable of normal function, assuming that he or she receives appropriate preoperative preparation and postoperative ostomy care.

Ninety percent of *ileostomies* are performed for ulcerative colitis. Less often, they are done for other conditions, such as Crohn disease of the colon or familial polyposis. Most of the patients are young, 75% or more being between 20 and 45 years of age.

In contrast, *colostomies* are usually performed for cancer of the rectum or, less often, for diverticulitis or for neurologic impairment or gunshot wounds that have led to incontinence. Both children and young adults with congenital disorders (e.g., imperforate anus) may have colostomies, but 80% of patients who have colostomy surgery are over the age of 50 years.

Appropriate management of the stoma begins before surgery and continues for a short period after successful surgery and for a longer period when old problems persist or new ones arise.

Preoperative Care

Ostomy management should begin as soon as ostomy surgery is seriously considered. For preparation of the patient to be most effective, family members should be included, because the approach is best tailored to meet the needs of the patient and the family. Preparation should include a brief description of the surgery, emphasizing the benefits to be derived, and of the stoma, stressing the fact that the stoma itself need not interfere with any aspect of future life except for vigorous body contact sports. Emphasis is placed on the fact that modern developments in appliances permit normal functioning and that there is no way that anyone will be able to tell that the clothed patient has an ostomy. After these introductory comments, the patient and family should be given an opportunity to voice their concerns and to ask questions, both during this first discussion and later, after the initial shock has worn off.

Many resources are available during the preoperative stage: the informed practitioner or surgeon, specially trained stoma nurses or enterostomal therapists (most of whom are nurses who have had specialized training at one of the schools of enterostomal therapy), and members of the visiting committee of the local chapter of the United Ostomy Association. The latter are usually trained lay ostomates who are specifically selected whenever possible to match the patient in age and sex (and often in socioeconomic status), so that the patient can identify readily with the visitor. The benefits to be derived from the visiting team cannot be overemphasized; even the most comforting professionals cannot be as reassuring to the patient as some kindred soul who has undergone similar surgery, has adjusted to it, and is leading a healthy, productive, and joyful life.

Pamphlets available through the local chapters of ostomy organizations can promote the patient's acceptance of the procedure, provide an optimistic projection for the future, and educate the patient in the use of ostomy appliances and colostomy irrigation. In addition, videotapes on preoperative preparation are available; they are particularly useful when viewed by the patient after the first discussion of the topic, because they not only depict healthy ostomates who discuss their initial and subsequent adjustment but also provide basic anatomic facts and information concerning appliances. Such knowledge allays fears and misconceptions and provides the basis for logical questions.

What to Tell the Patient about Conventional Ileostomy

Conventional ileostomies require that the patient continuously wear a pouch, which is applied to the body with the use of a skin barrier (a wafer-like adhesive) to provide a watertight seal. In this manner the intestinal contents (a better term than *stool* or *waste material*) discharge into the pouch, which can be emptied into the toilet simply by unclipping the end of the pouch four or five times a day. The contents are liquid and usually odorless. The pouch is flat and cannot be detected through the clothing or even in a bathing suit. The seal is tight enough so that the ostomate can swim, dive, dance, and participate in sports such as skiing or baseball. Modern materials are so effective that the pouch can be worn for a week at a time without being removed.

What to Tell the Patient about a Kock or Internal Pouch

The Kock or internal pouch (sometimes called "continent ileostomy") consists of several loops of small intestine sutured to each other and opened so that they form a reservoir pouch (artificial rectum) within the abdomen. This reservoir is connected to the abdominal wall with a short segment of ileum and opens much as a conventional ileostomy does, except that it can be placed much lower on the abdomen because it will not require an external pouch if it performs well. Between the pouch and the short ileal conduit, a nipple valve is constructed by inverting the ileum into the pouch in such a manner that it prevents leakage and therefore provides continence. To evacuate the contents of the pouch, the patient inserts a Silastic catheter into it through the ileostomy and the nipple valve. The ileal contents then drain through the catheter into the toilet bowl. Although frequent drainage is necessary initially, eventually most patients drain three or four times a day. Because it does not require an external appliance, the stoma can be placed near the groin, permitting the wearing of brief attire, such as a bikini.

This type of surgery is not recommended for patients who have Crohn disease involving the ileum. Moreover, one third of the operations are initially unsuccessful in providing total continence and therefore require revision, and in some instances more than one revision. These factors must be taken into consideration when deciding the appropriate form of surgery for the patient, especially when patients with conventional ileostomies ask about the advisability of converting their conventional, well-functioning ileostomy to the continent ileostomy. This operation also is not appropriate for people who have neurologic disorders that impair manual dexterity and interfere with insertion of the Silastic catheter. For these reasons, the Kock procedure has been largely replaced by the endorectal pull-through operation.

What to Tell the Patient about Sphincter-Saving Operations

The operation that has largely replaced the Kock pouch as a continent procedure is the *endorectal pull-through with ileal pouch.* Like the Kock procedure, the endorectal pull-through involves the construction of a reservoir pouch formed by suturing several adjacent loops of small bowel to each other and opening up the contiguous walls to form a reservoir. The distal (efferent) limb is then brought through the rectal stump, which has been denuded of its mucosa, and the distal ileum is sutured to the distal rectal wall from inside. The denuded rectum then adheres to the serosal surface of the efferent ileal limb. Thus, the anal sphincters are spared and nerve damage from anterior dissection is avoided. This approach can be used when rectal involvement from ulcerative colitis is not so severe that it prevents lifting the mucosa off the submucosal surface and removing it. Generally this procedure is contraindicated in Crohn disease because of the risk of local inflammation around the intestinal surface and anastomosis and because of the danger of fistula formation. When successful, this sphincter-forming surgery can preserve continence. The construction of an adequate reservoir and the appropriate placement of the efferent limb are technically difficult. Therefore, this procedure should be performed only by surgeons who have had substantial experience with the operation.

The *ileoanal anastomosis,* an increasingly popular procedure, differs from the endorectal pull-through in that, in the former procedure, the ileal pouch is attached directly to the anus.

What to Tell the Patient about Colostomy

There are basically four different types of colostomies: the *dry colostomy,* the *wet colostomy,* the *loop colostomy,* and the *continent colostomy* using a magnetic cap. Most permanent colostomies are dry sigmoid colostomies, which result from rectal resection, usually for cancer of the rectum. Because only the rectum has been removed, the usual stool consistency is not altered. This is an important feature because it means that patients who have frequent and erratic bowel habits, as in the irritable bowel syndrome, will continue to have these bowel habits and therefore will have unpredictable evacuation. They will probably have to wear an appliance. Patients who have more regular bowel habits can often develop controlled evacuations by use of irrigation (enemas) that they initially administer for proper control, daily at first and later, in most instances, every 2 days. Some colostomates simply wear a small adhesive bandage or gauze pad, although most prefer to wear a small appliance (stoma cap) to protect against incontinence during those few days a year when they develop the same episodes of diarrhea that affect the general population. Patients who have irritable bowel syndrome (see Chapter 44) or more frequent bowel movements when they are stressed will continue to have similar symptoms after surgery and therefore may not achieve continence during intervals between irrigations.

The wet colostomy refers to loose stool that occurs when a colostomy is situated proximal to the splenic flexure. This type of colostomy usually is performed as a temporary bypass and is generally less desirable because evacuations are more frequent and cannot be controlled by irrigation, and because the contents are malodorous because of colonic bacterial action. A permanent ileostomy is generally preferable to a permanent wet colostomy. The wet colostomy requires an appliance large enough to contain the colonic evacuations.

Loop colostomies and double-barrel colostomies are performed as (usually temporary) diverting procedures in the proximal colon. The loop is brought over a glass or plastic rod, and the resultant irregular oblong shape may make fitting a watertight appliance difficult.

Informed consent for colostomy requires that the patient be made aware of possible postoperative impotence. If impotence does occur, psychological adjustment to it is improved with preoperative counseling. Impotence is uncommon among ileostomates, but some degree of sexual impairment occurs in 80% of colostomates, 50% of whom are totally impotent after surgery. This occurs because of the wide resection that is necessary for rectal cancer surgery, the major indication for a colostomy, as well as the advanced age of the typical colostomate compared with the ileostomate. Patients may be reassured that sexual counseling is available if problems arise and that many couples find alternative satisfactory means of sexual gratification. It is appropriate to offer men the possibility of penile prostheses or intracavernosal or transurethral delivery of a vasodilating drug to produce potency (see Chapter 6). These concerns are less significant for the female ostomate, who does not experience impaired performance, although impaired gratification may still be an important factor.

Postoperative Management

Only late postoperative problems are discussed here, because the early problems will be managed in the hospital. Four major categories of problems are psychological adjustment, sexual adjustment, appliance management, and local and physiologic problems. Again, all can be minimized by appropriate preoperative preparation and counseling of the patient and the patient's family by an informed health care provider working with the appropriate members of the health care team.

Psychological Adjustment

A concerted effort should be made postoperatively by the medical team, the family, and particularly the spouse to restore self-esteem and foster independence. During the early postoperative months, men tend to depend on their wives for nursing care, but women seem to prefer help from other women (daughters, mothers, sisters) rather than from husbands. This is explained by the fact that wives express more concern about being physically unacceptable to the husband than vice versa. Attendance at meetings of local ostomy chapters is a good way to prepare the family during the postoperative period. Formal psychotherapy may be needed if depression is severe, if suicidal inclinations appear prominent, or if behavior is bizarre.

Sexual Adjustment

If debilitating illnesses, such as inflammatory bowel disease, have led to decreased libido and impaired sexual function, ileostomy may lead to improved postoperative sexual function and more satisfactory sexual relations. This is less often true when colostomies, performed with proctectomy and radical pelvic dissection, lead to neurologic impairment of potency. Even in these circumstances, psychological factors may play a major role.

In general, impaired sexual relationships may result from neurologic impairment, depression with loss of libido, inhibitions caused by a sense of humiliation and embarrassment, or, in some unfortunate instances, rejection by the spouse. An awareness of these possibilities will prepare the practitioner to assist with preventive or corrective measures. Frank discussions with the male patient may, in some instances, indicate the advisability of urologic referral for treatment of impotence (see Chapter 6).

Appliance Management

Modern improvements have impressively decreased the number of problems that are directly attributable to the appliance.

Skin Problems. Skin breakdown, a problem that used to plague 50% of ileostomates, is now uncommon because of effective skin barriers that have replaced the old cement adhesives. Hypersensitivity to adhesives or to the pouch can be diagnosed when the contour of skin reaction conforms to that of the adhesive or the pouch. If hypersensitivity is suspected, a patch test using the arm or trunk distant from the stoma may confirm the suspicion. Skin problems are more common among ileostomates than colostomates, because ileostomy effluent contains digestive enzymes. Skin that has been excoriated by ileal leakage should be treated with a cortisone spray, such as Kenalog, and an antifungal powder, such as Mycostatin, neither of which interferes with adherence of the appliance. Patients with more serious skin problems should be referred to gastroenterologists and to enterostomal therapists experienced with ostomy care. Skin complications of proximal colostomies may be similar to those of ileostomies.

Odor. Odor problems are more commonly encountered by colostomates than ileostomates because of putrefactive bacteria present in the colon. Some bacterial colonization of the ileum takes place after colectomy, but odor problems occur only occasionally in 50% of ileostomates and more often in about a third. Sudden increase in gas and odor may signify partial intestinal obstruction. Dietary factors such as oils, fat-soluble vitamins, eggs, and onions may be associated with offensive odors and may be diagnosed by a careful dietary history or by use of an elimination diet. Odors may also be caused by malabsorption resulting from small-bowel disease or resection. A number of deodorants are available that can be placed into the pouch (Nilodor, Banish, and aspirin), and oral bismuth subgallate also may be helpful.

Leakage. Under ordinary circumstances, leakage is rarely seen with new appliances, but it may become a problem if pregnancy or postoperative weight gain (e.g., in a patient previously emaciated from inflammatory bowel disease) changes body contour, requiring refitting of the appliance. The stoma may shrink during the first 6 to 8 weeks after surgery, and good follow-up care is vital for at least the first postoperative year. Minimal bleeding at the stoma may occur occasionally and is no cause for alarm. A soft, wet cloth should be used to clean the stoma, because dry materials can stick to the surface and cause bleeding. Skin excoriation can occur as a result of perspiration under the pouch, particularly in hot weather. This can be prevented by wearing a cover over the pouch and powdering the skin liberally.

Equipment Update

Stoma nurses and enterostomal therapists are usually familiar with state-of-the-art supplies and equipment. Such products include the following:

- Durahesive flexible wafer (Sur-Fit Natura) allows removal and replacement of the pouch without disturbing the skin barrier, helps avoid discomfort and skin irritation, and allows easy repositioning for supine bedside drainage without removal of the pouch.
- Stomahesive paste and Stomahesive protective powder can be used to fill in skin irregularities around the stoma.
- The Guardian two-piece system has a drainable pouch with replaceable filters.
- First Choice drainable pouch with convex barrier is a one-piece unit that provides excellent skin protection for flush, recessed, or retracted stomas.
- Ile-Sorb absorbent gel packets placed in the pouch transform diarrheal water into a gel, which keeps the contents of the pouch away from the stoma.
- Closed-pouch styles and closed minipouches are interchangeable with the two-piece units for patients who have colostomies.

- Stoma caps provide a convenient stomal covering for discharge that is controlled by irrigation. The caps contain a carbon cloth filter to absorb the odorous components of flatus.

Local and Physiologic Complications

Ileostomates are much more likely to experience complications of this type than are colostomates, and most of these complications appear within the first year after surgery. Obstruction caused by volvulus, herniation, or adhesions is the most common problem; prolapse, retraction, and fistula formation are seen less often. These problems usually require consultation with a surgeon or gastroenterologist and often need surgical correction. Crampy abdominal pains, abdominal distention, vomiting, and excessive diarrheal discharge suggest the presence of obstruction. Gastroenteritis may mimic some of these symptoms, but it persists only for several days.

Because of the absence of normal colonic absorptive function, ileostomates may be susceptible to dehydration or electrolyte imbalance (particularly salt depletion), especially in hot weather because of sweating and increased incidence of infectious diarrhea. For this reason, ileostomates should be encouraged to increase water and salt intake during the summer unless there are medical contraindications. Antidiarrheal agents such as deodorized tincture of opium, Lomotil, or Imodium may be needed during these periods and also should be available during travel to countries where traveler's diarrhea may be a problem (see Chapter 41).

With these minimal precautions, neither ileostomy nor colostomy imposes any dietary restrictions, except that ileostomates should avoid excessive quantities of peanuts or fibrous foods such as bean sprouts (Table 46.2), which have been reported to be associated with obstruction. Taken in moderation, however, these foods usually present no problem.

Effects of Small-Bowel Resection or Colectomy on Handling of Medications

For the most part colectomy does not influence drug absorption, because most drugs are absorbed in the small bowel. A major exception is sulfasalazine (Azulfidine), one of the drugs most commonly used for inflammatory bowel disease. The inactive form of this drug is broken down by colonic bacteria into an active constituent that is reabsorbed into the bloodstream and secreted in connective tissue of the gut. Colectomy obviously can seriously impair this process. On the other hand, because sulfasalazine is most effective for colonic involvement in inflammatory bowel disease, it is not often required after colectomy.

When resection of parts of the small bowel is performed for the treatment of inflammatory bowel disease, the patient is left with decreased absorptive surface and often intestinal hurry. This rapid transit may lead to poor absorption of medications and foodstuffs. Particularly, enteric and sustained-release preparations should be avoided under these circumstances. Patients with short-bowel syndrome are especially prone to have problems and may benefit from medications prescribed in liquid rather than tablet form because liquid is more rapidly absorbed.

Residual inflammatory disease and bacterial overgrowth in the terminal ileum of ostomy patients may result in poor absorption of vitamin B_{12} and the need for vitamin B_{12} replacement.

Colostomy Irrigation

Although a few colostomates (with distal colostomy) find that they can have controlled bowel movements by careful dietary manipulations, the vast majority use irrigation to control evacuation. This simply involves the instillation of 1 L of warm tap water through the colostomy. The replacement of the old irrigating catheter with the blunt cone (which is placed against the stoma to prevent backflow) has virtually eliminated the problems of perforation. Although tepid water is preferred to avoid cramping, some patients find cold water more effective. It is normal for patients to have an initial evacuation followed within one-half hour by further excretion; for this reason, the patient should be advised to continue wearing the irrigation sleeve (long pouch) with the end closed for one-half hour after irrigation. Cramps experienced during the irrigation may be caused by rapid instillation of water, from air distention of the bowel resulting from failure to expel the air from the irrigating tip, or from obstruction. Constipation and diarrhea should be handled in the same way as in patients who have intact colons (see earlier discussion in this chapter and in Chapter 45), relying on dietary manipulations as much as possible (prunes and bran for constipation, hard cheeses and rice for diarrhea).

ACKNOWLEDGMENT

We are grateful to Dr. Hemant Pande for his valuable contribution in revising this chapter.

General References*

Constipation

Cranston D, McWhinnie D, Collin J. Dietary fibre and gastrointestinal disease. Br J Surg 1988;75:508.

A review of the relationship of fiber to constipation, diverticular disease, and colorectal cancer.

Locke GR III, Pemberton JH, Phillips SF. **AGA technical review on constipation.** Gastroenterology 2000;119:1766.

Wald A. Constipation. Med Clin North Am 2000;84:1231.

Diverticular Disease

Camilleri M, Lee JS, Viramontes B, et al. Insights into the pathophysiology and mechanisms of constipation, irritable bowel syndrome, and diverticulosis in older people. J Am Geriatr Soc 2000;48: 1142.

*Bold print (general references) and bold numerals (specific references) denote published controlled clinical trials, meta-analyses, or consensus-based recommendations.

Deckmann RC, Cheskin LJ. Diverticular disease in the elderly. J Am Geriatr Soc 1993;40:986.
A general review with emphasis on presentation in the elderly.
Schroetz DJ Jr. Uncomplicated diverticulitis: indications for surgery and surgical management. Surg Clin North Am 1993;73:965.

Colostomy or Ileostomy

Beart RW Jr. Sphincter saving operations for chronic ulcerative colitis. Adv Surg 1990;23:195.
Camilleri M, Lee JS, Viramontes B, et al. Insights into the pathophysiology and mechanisms of constipation, irritable bowel syndrome, and diverticulosis in older people. J Am Geriatr Soc 2000;48:1142.
Deckmann RC, Cheskin LJ. Diverticular disease in the elderly. J Am Geriatr Soc 1993;40:986.
A general review with emphasis on presentation in the elderly.
Mullen BD, McGinn KA. The ostomy book: living comfortably with colostomies, ileostomies and urostomies. Boulder: Bull Publishing, 1992.
Schroetz DJ Jr. Uncomplicated diverticulitis: indications for surgery and surgical management. Surg Clin North Am 1993;73:965.
Schuster MM, Bengel JR. Ileostomy and colostomy management. In: Spittell J Jr, ed. Clinical medicine, vol. 10. New York: Harper & Row, 1982:1.
White CA, Hunt JC. Psychological factors in postoperative adjustment to stoma surgery. Ann R Coll Surg Engl 1997;79:3.

Specific References

1. Connell AM, Hilton C, Irvine G, et al. Variation of bowel habit in two population samples. BMJ 1965;2:1095.
2. Sonnenberg A, Koch TR. Physician visits in the United States for constipation: 1958–1986. Digest Dis Sci 1989;34:606.
3. Loche GR III. The epidemiology of functional gastrointestinal disorders in North America. Gastroenterol Clin North Am 1996;25:1.
4. Nyam DC, Pemberton JH, Ilstrup DM, et al. Long-term results of surgery for chronic constipation. Dis Colon Rectum 1997;40:273.
5. Locke GR III, Pemberton JH, Phillips SF. AGA technical review on constipation. Gastroenterology 2000;119:1766.
6. Wald A. Colonic and anorectal motility testing in clinical practice. Am J Gastroenterol 1994;89:2109.
7. Metcalf AM, Phillips SF, Zinsmeister AR, et al. Simplified assessment of segmental colonic transit. Gastroenterology 1987;92:40.
8. Wald A, Caruana BJ, Freimanis MG, et al. Contributions of evacuation proctography and anorectal manometry to evaluation of adults with constipation and defecatory difficulty. Dig Dis Sci 1990;35:481.
9. Voderholzer WA, Schatke W, Muhldorfer BE, et al. Clinical response to dietary fiber treatment of chronic constipation. Am J Gastroenterol 1997;92:95.
10. Anti M, Pignataro G, Armuzzi A, et al. Water supplementation enhances the effect of high-fiber diet on stool frequency and laxative consumption in adults with functional constipation. Hepatogastroenterology 1998;45:727.
11. Tramonte SM, Brand MB, Mulrow CD, et al. The treatment of chronic constipation in adults. J Gen Intern Med 1997;12:15.
12. Nyam DC, Pemberton JH, Ilstrup DM, et al. Long-term results of surgery for chronic constipation. Dis Colon Rectum 1997;40:273.
13. Parks TG. Natural history of diverticular disease of the colon. Clin Gastroenterol 1975;4:53.
14. Aldoori WH, Giovannucci EL, Rimm EB, et al. A prospective study of diet and the risk of symptomatic diverticular disease in men. Am J Clin Nutr 1994;60:757.
15. Hughes LE. Postmortem survey of diverticular disease of the colon: I. Diverticulosis and diverticulitis. Gut 1969;10:336.
16. Hyland JM, Taylor I. Does a high fibre diet prevent the complications of diverticular disease? Br J Surg 1980;67:77.
17. Woods RJ, Lavery IC, Fazio VW, et al. Internal fistulas in diverticular disease. Dis Colon Rectum 1988;31:591.
18. Welch CE. Computerized tomography scans for all patients with diverticulitis. Am J Surg 1988;155:366.
19. Larson DM, Masters SS, Spiro HM. Medical and surgical therapy in diverticular disease: a comparative study. Gastroenterology 1976;71:734.
20. Levien DH, Mazier WP, Surrell JA, et al. Safe resection for diverticular disease of the colon. Dis Colon Rectum 1989;32:30.
21. Tedesco F, Waye J, Raskin J, et al. Colonoscopic evaluation of rectal bleeding: a study of 304 patients. Ann Intern Med 1978;89:907.
22. Deckmann RC, Cheskin LJ. Diverticular disease in the elderly. J Am Geriatr Soc 1993;40:986.
23. McGuire HH, Haynes BW. Massive hemorrhage from diverticulosis of the colon: guidelines for therapy based on bleeding patterns observed in fifty cases. Ann Surg 1972;175:847.
24. Ramanath HK, Hinshaw JR. Management and mismanagement of bleeding colonic diverticula. Arch Surg 1971;103:311.
25. McGuire HH Jr. Bleeding colonic diverticula: a reappraisal of natural history and management. Ann Surg 1994;220:653.
26. The Standards Task Force, American Society of Colon and Rectal Surgeons. Practice parameters for sigmoid diverticulitis. Surg Laparos Endosc Percutan Tech 2000;10:142.

CHAPTER 47

Diseases of the Liver

ESTEBAN MEZEY, MD

HEPATITIS

Hepatitis is an inflammatory condition that may be localized in the liver or may be part of a generalized systemic process. Acute hepatitis is usually a self-limited disease. The principal causes of acute hepatitis are viruses, drugs, and alcohol. Chronic hepatitis is unresolved hepatitis that has persisted for longer than 6 months. Cirrhosis is often the principal consequence of chronic hepatitis.

Acute Hepatitis

Viral Hepatitis

Viral hepatitis is a systemic infection whose principal manifestations are hepatic. The four types of viral hepatitis that are well-defined, separate entities are

Table 47.1. Comparison of Selected Characteristics of Various Types of Viral Hepatitis

Characteristic	Type A	Type B	Type C	Type E
Hepatitis A antibody	Appearance of or increase in titer	Absent or no change in titer	Absent or no change in titer	Absent or no change in titer
Hepatitis B surface antigen	Absent	Present in early stage of illness	Absent	Absent
Hepatitis C antibody	Absent	Absent	Appears 10–20 wk after infection	Absent
Incubation period	15–50 d	50–160 d	15–160 d	35–40 d
Route of infection	Oral and parenteral	Usually parenteral, also oral or sexual	Usually parenteral, also oral or sexual	Oral
Age preference	Children	Any age	Any age	15–40 yr
Seasonal incidence	Autumn–winter, epidemic outbreaks	All year	All year	Epidemic outbreaks
Severity	Usually mild	Often severe	Often mild	Mild, severe in pregnancy
Mortality	0.1%	0.1%–1.0%	0.1%	0.5% (20% in pregnancy)
Prophylactic value of gammaglobulin	Good	Good with hyperimmune hepatitis B globulin	Unclear	Unclear
Hepatitis vaccine	90%–100% efficacy	90% efficacy		

designated type A, B, C, and E. Delta hepatitis (hepatitis D virus) is infection by a defective virus-like particle that is dependent on persisting or concomitant infection with type B virus.

The characteristic features of types A, B, C, and E hepatitis are shown in Table 47.1. Type A hepatitis, previously known as infectious hepatitis, is more common than the other types. It is usually transmitted by the fecal-oral route and has a particularly high incidence wherever people come in close contact under poor hygienic conditions. A number of epidemics have been described after fecal contamination of the water or food supply. Ingestion of contaminated shellfish has been associated with both sporadic cases and epidemics.

Type B hepatitis, previously called serum hepatitis, is usually transmitted by the parenteral route from blood, blood products, or contaminated needles. It is also commonly transmitted by sexual contact and from the mother to the fetus. Delta hepatitis is transmitted by the same routes as type B hepatitis (1). Its incubation period ranges from 3 to 13 weeks. Infection with the delta agent may become manifest as a biphasic pattern of hepatitis when there is simultaneous infection with hepatitis B virus, or as a clinical exacerbation of hepatitis in patients who are carriers of hepatitis B virus with or without chronic liver disease. Delta hepatitis has been implicated in cases of fulminant hepatitis and in worsening of chronic liver disease with more rapid progression to cirrhosis. However, the incidence of delta hepatitis is unknown.

Hepatitis C virus accounts for most cases of hepatitis acquired by blood transfusion, although it is now more commonly transmitted by other routes. In the West, 4% of cases of hepatitis C are acquired by blood transfusion, 38% by parenteral use of illicit drugs, 10% by sexual or household exposure to people who have had hepatitis or multiple partners, 2% by occupational exposure to infected blood, and 1% by dialysis (2). The source of infection in approximately 45% of cases is unknown; a large proportion of these patients are in a low socioeconomic level. Skin tattoos are also a risk factor. Ear piercing in men and intranasal cocaine use have been found to be more common in blood donors infected with hepatitis C virus than in noninfected donors (3).

Hepatitis E virus is a common cause of hepatitis epidemics in developing countries, but it can also occur sporadically in developed countries. The virus is transmitted by the fecal-oral route, usually by ingestion of contaminated water. It is associated with a high mortality rate in pregnant women (4).

Hepatitis G virus is a single-stranded RNA virus that has a genomic sequence similar to hepatitis C virus. It is present in 1.8% of healthy blood donors and often is found in the blood of patients with hepatitis C infection. In a few cases hepatitis G is the only virus identified in patients with hepatitis, and in most of these cases the hepatitis is mild. However, definitive proof is lacking to implicate hepatitis G virus as a causative agent of hepatitis.

Clinical Presentation. The symptoms of the various types of hepatitis are similar. However, in contrast to the other types of viral hepatitis, acute viral hepatitis C is usually a mild illness that is very likely to persist and develop into chronic hepatitis if left untreated. Most cases of hepatitis are anicteric; patients have a few nonspecific symptoms, such as fatigue and nausea, and the disease is often misdiagnosed as a flu-like illness. The correct diagnosis, if suspected, is made by demonstrating bilirubin in the urine and an increase in the level of serum aminotransferases. In icteric disease, the symptoms that usually precede jaundice are anorexia, fatigue, abdominal discomfort, and nausea. Erythematous skin rashes, urticaria, arthralgias, and low-grade fever may also appear. These initial symptoms are followed within 10 days by the appearance of dark urine, often pruritus, and jaundice. It is at this stage that most patients seek medical attention. On physical examination, a tender, palpable liver is found in approximately 70% of the patients. Posterior cervical lymphadenopathy and splenomegaly may also be present. Jaundice usually increases in intensity during the first few days and then begins to decrease, disappearing completely by 2 to 8 weeks after onset.

Laboratory Features. A mild degree of transient anemia, granulocytopenia, lymphocytosis with the appearance of atypical lymphocytes, and mild hemolytic anemia, with an increase in the reticulocyte count, are commonly found in patients with viral hepatitis. Both the direct (conjugated) and the total fraction of serum bilirubin rise; the height reached by the total bilirubin is an indication of the severity of the disease. However, total serum bilirubin concentrations higher than 30 mg/dL are almost invariably caused by complicating hemolysis. The serum aminotransferases usually rise before the onset of detectable jaundice, may reach levels as high as several thousand units, and may remain elevated for several weeks. The height reached by the aminotransferases in the serum provides only a rough estimate of the degree of hepatocellular injury and is of no prognostic value. However, a rapid fall in aminotransferases from a high peak to normal in less than 1 week may be an indication of fulminant hepatitis with massive necrosis and collapse of liver parenchyma. The serum alkaline phosphatase usually rises in the early, cholestatic phase of hepatitis, remains elevated throughout the illness, and is often the last serum enzyme to return to normal levels after clinical recovery. The concentration of serum albumin is normal in acute hepatitis. Serum gammaglobulins often are transiently elevated. The prothrombin time is usually normal and, if prolonged, is usually responsive to the administration of vitamin K. Prolongation of the prothrombin time with no response to vitamin K administration suggests severe hepatitis; if the prolongation increases, it is indicative of fulminant hepatitis. Vitamin K, 10 to 15 mg, is usually given by the subcutaneous route; when it is given intravenously, the rate of administration should be no faster than 1 mg/minute to avoid an anaphylactoid response.

Imaging Studies. Imaging of the liver by either ultrasonography or computed tomography (CT) scanning is not useful in the diagnosis or management of acute viral hepatitis. However, ultrasonography is useful to confirm a decrease in liver size in hospitalized patients with severe necrosis and fulminant hepatitis in whom the liver cannot be palpated.

Immunologic Features. A marked advance in the diagnosis of hepatitis occurred with the discovery in 1964 of an antigenic substance in the blood that was later documented to be associated only with type B hepatitis. This antigen, initially named Australian antigen because it was first detected in the serum of an Australian aborigine, is now designated hepatitis B surface antigen (HBsAg). In 1973, the hepatitis A antigen was discovered, and the determination of serum antibodies to this antigen began to be used for the identification of type A hepatitis. Delta virus, which is associated with HBsAg, was discovered in 1977. In 1989, an antibody to hepatitis C was developed as a diagnostic test for the identification of parenterally transmitted non-A, non-B hepatitis (5). The hepatitis C RNA test became available soon thereafter. Antibodies to hepatitis E virus (anti-HEV) are used to detect hepatitis E infection. A hepatitis E RNA test is also available for clinical studies.

In acute type A hepatitis, fecal excretion of hepatitis A antigen (HA Ag) can be demonstrated a few days before the increase in serum aminotransferases, rises to a peak during maximal serum aminotransferase elevation, and then falls as jaundice appears. Antibody to hepatitis A (anti-HA, predominantly immunoglobulin M [IgM]) appears in the serum as HA Ag, disappears from the stool, and rises rapidly to high levels. Afterward, antibody titers (predominantly IgG) remain detectable for at least 10 years, indicative of immunity against reinfection. Because hepatitis A infection is very common, many healthy people have detectable anti-HA in the serum. The prevalence of positive anti-HA is approximately 30% in the United States and as high as 90% in certain areas of Latin America and Asia (6). Hence, identification of an acute episode of hepatitis as type A requires a high titer of anti-HA of the IgM class or the appearance of or a rise in anti-HA titer in the serum collected during the convalescent stage compared with the acute stage of hepatitis.

The hepatitis B virus by electron microscopy appears as a double-shelled, 42-nm spherical particle, originally called the Dane particle. The outer shell of this particle is HBsAg, and the inner core contains an antigen that has been designated the hepatitis B core antigen (HBcAg). The inner core also contains double-stranded DNA and DNA polymerase activity. In acute type B viral hepatitis, HBsAg first appears in the blood 1 to 2 weeks before and usually disappears by 2 to 3 months after the onset of clinical symptoms (Fig. 47.1). Antibody to hepatitis B core antigen (anti-HBc) appears in the serum at the onset of clinical symptoms, reaches a peak soon after the maximal level of serum aminotransferase is reached, and then falls gradually, becoming undetectable 1 to 2 years after the infection. Antibody to the hepatitis B surface antigen (anti-HBs) usually appears during the convalescence, when HBsAg is no longer detectable, and then persists for many years. The presence of HBsAg or IgM anti-HBc during the acute illness is evidence that the hepatitis is caused by the hepatitis B virus (7). Persistence of HBsAg in the serum beyond 3 months after the infection suggests that the patient has become a chronic carrier of the hepatitis B virus (8). The presence of high titers of anti-HBc but absent anti-HBs is usually found in association with HBsAg in the carrier state. The presence of anti-HBs indicates that the patient has had a prior infection with type B hepatitis and now is immune to reinfection. In 1972 a new antigen called e antigen was discovered in HBsAg-positive sera. The e antigen (HBeAg), although associated only with type B hepatitis, is immunologically distinct from HBsAg and HBcAg. HBeAg appears transiently in the serum during the early phase of acute type B hepatitis. In chronic carriers of HBsAg, the presence of HBeAg is a marker of active virus replication and correlates with infectivity of the carrier (9). Some studies suggest that the presence of HBeAg in the chronic carrier

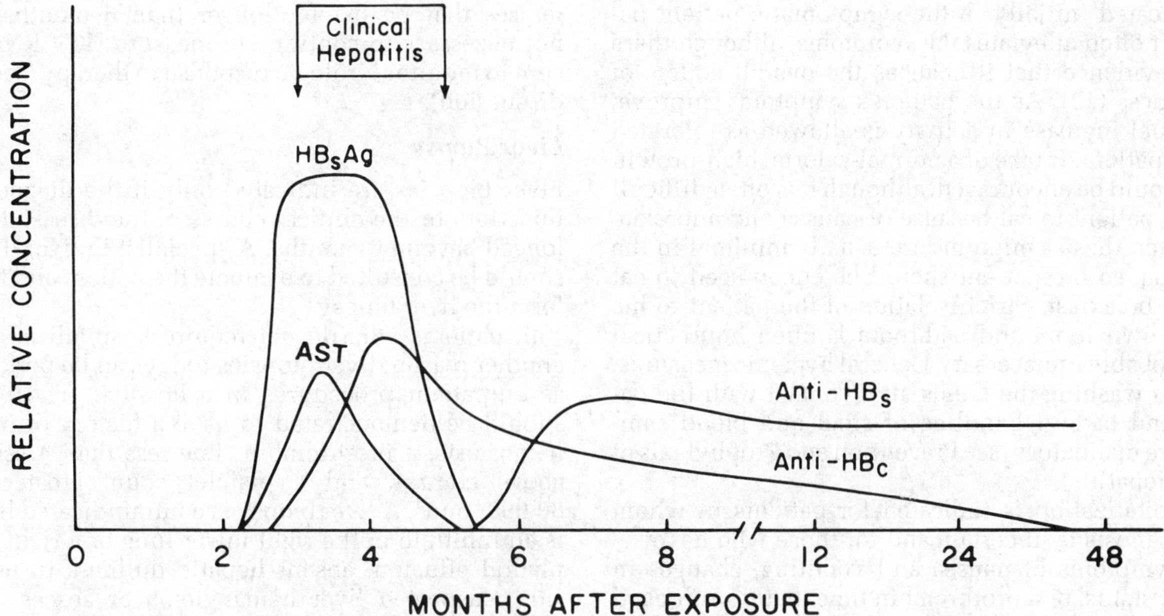

Figure 47.1. Pattern of appearance of hepatitis B surface antigen (HbsAg) and antibodies to hepatitis surface antigen (anti-HBs) and to hepatitis B core antigen (anti-HBc) in acute hepatitis B infection. AST, aspartate aminotransferase. (From Mezey, E. Specific liver diseases. In Halsted JH, Halsted CH, eds. The laboratory in clinical medicine. 2nd ed. Philadelphia: WB Saunders, 1981.)

is an indicator of progression of acute hepatitis B to chronic hepatitis or cirrhosis. Hepatitis B DNA (HBV DNA) is also used to detect the hepatitis B virus and to obtain information on viral load.

Hepatitis delta virus (HDV) is a defective virus-like particle that is composed of a small RNA genome surrounded by delta antigen (HDAg) and a coat of HBsAg. Acute hepatitis delta infection (1) is associated with a brief rise in delta antigen (HDAg) that lasts approximately 10 days and is followed by the appearance of delta antibody (anti-HD). Initially the antibody is of IgM type, lasting 10 to 20 days; this is followed by the appearance of IgG anti-HD. A characteristic of hepatitis delta infection is a lowering of HBsAg titers; probably hepatitis D virus requires hepatitis B virus for its replication.

Hepatitis C is caused by a single-stranded RNA virus. There are at least five major genotypes of the hepatitis C virus, which have different geographic distributions and influences on the clinical course of the disease and its response to therapy (10). Hepatitis C virus RNA (HCV RNA) is detectable within 10 days after infection and persists during the development of acute and chronic hepatitis. Anti-HC becomes detectable 12 to 15 weeks after infection. In most cases, it persists in the blood regardless of the outcome of the disease (11).

Hepatitis E is caused by a 27- to 34-nm, nonenveloped, RNA single-stranded, polyadenylated virus. Acute hepatitis E (HEV) infection is associated with rises of IgM and IgG anti-HEV antibodies. IgM anti-HEV is found in more than 90% of patients 1 week to 2 months after the onset of the illness. IgG anti-HEV appears after the IgM antibody response, and its titer rises after the acute illness, remaining detectable for 1 to 4.5 years. HEV infection in the serum and stool can be detected by reverse transcriptase-polymerase chain reaction (RT-PCR) measurement of HEV RNA (4).

At present, the practical usefulness of the immunologic markers for hepatitis is as follows. Hepatitis A infection is confirmed by the demonstration of a rise in anti-HA titer in the serum collected during convalescence as compared with the acute stage of hepatitis, or preferably, during the acute illness, by the presence of anti-HA of the IgM class. Infection with hepatitis B is usually confirmed by the presence of HBsAg, but if the antigen is absent and it is clinically indicated, the diagnosis can be confirmed by demonstrating IgM anti-HBc. The determination of anti-HBs is useful to find out whether a person is immune to hepatitis B or whether that person is a candidate for prophylaxis (see Prevention and Prophylaxis of Viral Hepatitis). HBV DNA is useful in monitoring the virologic response of chronic hepatitis B to treatment. Acute hepatitis C infection is diagnosed by the detection of hepatitis C RNA, whereas chronic hepatitis C is diagnosed by detection of hepatitis C RNA or by anti-HC 6 months or longer after the onset of illness. The false-positive detection of anti-HC is less than 10% and occurs principally in chronic autoimmune hepatitis (see later discussion). Hepatitis D, as a cause of fulminant hepatitis or recurrent type B hepatitis, is diagnosed by the presence of HDAg or IgM anti-HD. Hepatitis E is diagnosed by showing initially the presence of IgM anti-HEV in the serum, or later in the course of the infection the appearance of IgG anti-HEV.

Management

Acute viral hepatitis usually resolves completely in 1 to 3 months. There is no specific therapy. Bed rest is indicated initially in the symptomatic patient because it often alleviates the symptoms, although there is no evidence that it changes the overall course of the illness (12). As the patient's symptoms improve, a gradual increase in activity is allowed as tolerated by the patient. Intake of a normal-calorie, high-protein diet should be encouraged, although it is often difficult for the patient to eat because of nausea and anorexia. However, these symptoms are usually minimal in the morning, so the patient should be encouraged to eat a large breakfast. Strict isolation of the patient to his or her own room and bathroom is often impractical and probably unnecessary. General hygienic measures, such as washing the hands after contact with the patient and careful handling of stool and blood samples, are mandatory (see Prevention and Prophylaxis of Viral Hepatitis).

Hospitalization is indicated for patients in whom the diagnosis is uncertain and for those who have severe symptoms of nausea and vomiting, changes in mental status, or a prothrombin time that is prolonged more than 4 seconds above the control value. Patients with very high levels of serum bilirubin (greater than 30 mg/dL), who most likely have severe hemolysis complicating their hepatitis, should be hospitalized. By contrast, the magnitude of elevation of serum amino-transferase by itself, is not an indication for hospitalization. In addition, it is advisable to admit to the hospital patients who do not have somebody at home who can observe and help them.

Nausea can be controlled with oral diphenhydramine, 25 mg three times a day, or by prochlorperazine, 10 mg two to four times a day, without danger of central nervous system depression. Acetaminophen, 500 mg four times a day, can be safely given for abdominal discomfort (the risk of hepatotoxicity occurs at much higher dosages). No sedatives should be given, because they may precipitate hepatic encephalopathy. Corticosteroids are of no value in the treatment of acute viral hepatitis.

Patients should be monitored at intervals varying from 1 to 3 weeks and should not be discharged from ambulatory care until all symptoms have disappeared and all laboratory tests have returned to normal. Patients are advised not to ingest alcoholic beverages until 1 month after all laboratory tests have returned to normal.

Patients with hepatitis who are asymptomatic can return to light work despite abnormal liver tests such as hyperbilirubinemia and elevations of the serum aminotransferases and alkaline phosphatase. Patients in whom the elevation of serum bilirubin is high enough to cause jaundice can also return to work but may need a note of their condition to their employer to avoid concern on the part of coworkers.

In patients with hepatitis B, HBsAg should be measured after 6 months. If HBsAg is still detectable at that time, a hepatologist should be consulted for further management. In patients with hepatitis C, chronicity is defined as elevations of serum aminotransferases that persist for longer than 6 months. It is not necessary to continue to measure HCV RNA, except to monitor virologic response to therapy (see later discussion).

Liver Biopsy

Liver biopsies are indicated only if the diagnosis is uncertain or the clinical course of the disease is prolonged beyond 6 months. A specialist in liver disease should be consulted to evaluate the patient and to perform the liver biopsy.

In patients who do not require hospitalization for another reason, liver biopsies today can be performed as outpatient procedures in a hospital. The patient should be demonstrated to have a history of normal hemostasis, a prothrombin time less than 4 seconds above control, and a platelet count greater than 80,000/ mm^3. A liver biopsy is contraindicated if there is an infiltrate in the right lower lung or a right-sided pleural effusion, absent hepatic dullness to percussion, suspected liver hemangioma or abscess, massive ascites, extrahepatic obstruction, or severe anemia (hemoglobin less than 10 g/dL).

Patient Experience. After application of local anesthesia, the liver biopsy is performed by the intercostal right subcutaneous route using suction with a needle 1.6 mm in diameter. It entails minimal risk when done by a skilled operator. The most common complication is pleuritic pain lasting a few hours after the biopsy, which is noted in approximately 5% of the cases. The most serious complications are bleeding and bile peritonitis, which occur in fewer than 1% of cases. The risk of mortality from liver biopsy is 0.2%. After the procedure, patients are observed for approximately 4 hours and then, if no complications have occurred, are sent home accompanied by a friend or relative.

Prognosis

Most patients with acute viral hepatitis recover from their illness without any sequelae. The mortality rate from all types of hepatitis is less than 0.1%. The principal cause of death is the development of fulminant hepatitis, which is more common in type B hepatitis. Fulminant hepatitis usually overcomes the patient within 10 days after the onset of the symptoms of hepatitis. Older patients and patients with other medical illnesses, such as diabetes mellitus, are more likely to have a prolonged course and a higher mortality rate. Type E hepatitis, transmitted by the fecal-oral route, results in a high mortality rate in pregnant women. Indications of a poor prognosis are changes in mental status, a nonpalpable liver that is also small on hepatic scan, a liver that decreases rapidly in size, or a prothrombin time that is prolonged more than 4 seconds above normal.

Chronic hepatitis occurs in approximately 85% of untreated patients with hepatitis C, and 15% to 20% of those patients eventually develop cirrhosis. Chronic hepatitis occurs in 3% to 5% of patients with type B hepatitis, of whom 6% to 20% develop cirrhosis within 5 years. Chronic hepatitis and cirrhosis do not occur after type A or type E hepatitis. These complications should be suspected in patients with hepatitis B or who continue to have clinical and laboratory evidence of liver disease 6 months after the onset of acute hepatitis (13). Most patients clear the HBsAg from their serum within 3 months of the onset of the illness. Approximately 10% of patients with type B hepatitis become chronic carriers of HBsAg. Chronic carriers of HBsAg with abnormal levels of serum aminotransferases should be evaluated for the development of chronic active hepatitis by liver biopsy. An increased incidence of hepatocellular carcinoma has been found in carriers of HBsAg or hepatitis C RNA.

Differential Diagnosis

A number of other viruses have been reported to cause hepatitis. *Cytomegalic inclusion infection,* usually clinically inapparent in the adult, can present with manifestations of hepatitis in patients being administered immunosuppressive therapy, in those who have diseases characterized by immunosuppression (see Chapter 39), or after blood transfusions in healthy subjects. The diagnosis can be made promptly, if necessary, by examination of biopsy specimens for intranuclear inclusions and detection of the virus in tissue with specific antibodies. Alternatively, the diagnosis can be made by detection of cytomegalovirus (CMV) antigenemia or by culture of the urine. *Mononucleosis* (caused by the Epstein-Barr virus, EBV) is often associated with hepatocellular dysfunction with mild transient jaundice in 5% to 10% of patients. It is diagnosed by the presence in the serum of a heterophil antibody that is not absorbed by guinea pig kidney or by a positive mononucleosis spot test. Demonstration of IgM EBV antibodies specific for Epstein-Barr virus confirms the diagnosis (see Chapter 58).

Hepatitis caused by *leptospirosis* should be suspected in patients who have been in close contact with rodents or with food, water, soil, or other material contaminated with the urine of rodents; the diagnosis is established by recovery of *Leptospira* in culture of the blood or by a rise in antibodies in the course of the disease. *Drug-induced hepatitis* (see later discussion) manifests with clinical features that are indistinguishable from those of viral hepatitis, and a history of drug intake is a most important clue in suspecting the diagnosis. *Alcoholic hepatitis* (discussed later) usually develops after recent heavy alcohol ingestion; the serum aminotransferases are rarely elevated more than 10 times above normal, and the elevation is primarily in the serum aspartate aminotransferase (AST). In patients with marked cholestasis—as evidenced by persistent elevation of the bilirubin, high serum alkaline phosphatase, and pruritus in association with persistently dark urine and light stools—the diagnosis of *extrahepatic biliary obstruction* should be entertained. An abnormal sonogram may provide a clue to extrahepatic obstruction if the biliary ducts are found to be dilated, and the patient should then be referred to a specialist in liver diseases for further evaluation.

Prevention and Prophylaxis of Viral Hepatitis

General hygienic measures, such as washing the hands after contact with the patient, are the most effective means of preventing the spread of hepatitis from the patient to others. The patient's dishes and eating utensils can be shared by other people only if they have been cleaned and heated to more than 120°F for 15 to 20 minutes in a dishwasher after the patient has used them. Assignment of the patient to a separate bathroom is ideal but often impractical. The viruses can be present in feces, blood, and other body fluids of the patient; any of these materials should be handled with care. Because the virus appears in the stool during the prodromal period of hepatitis, the precautions mentioned should be taken routinely in environments where there is a high risk of development of hepatitis, such as in institutions for the mentally retarded.

The screening of blood for HBsAg and anti-hepatitis C before transfusion has markedly decreased the risk of posttransfusion infection by hepatitis B and hepatitis C viruses to 1 in 63,000 and 1 in 100,000 units transfused, respectively (14). Other sources of type B and type C hepatitis that can easily be controlled are contaminated needles, pins used to test sensation, and dental and surgical instruments. All used needles or pins should be discarded in specially labeled bottles containing 40% formalin, which is known to inactivate the hepatitis viruses. The preferred method for cleaning surgical and dental instruments is by heat sterilization. The risk that most health care workers who are HBsAg positive pose to their patients is minimal if high standards of hygiene are maintained. The exceptions are dentists and surgeons (15), who often develop cuts on their hands while operating. Dentists are urged to wear gloves regardless of whether they are HBsAg positive, to protect themselves and their patients. Patients who have had hepatitis B or hepatitis C and have recovered (clinically and serologically) may be infectious for many years and therefore should not be allowed to donate blood. Spouses of patients with hepatitis B should receive hepatitis B vaccine. Unvaccinated sexual partners of patients who have recovered from hepatitis B may be at risk. Sexual partners of patients with chronic hepatitis C who are in monogamous relationships have less than a 2% risk of infection. Food handlers with hepatitis A infection should not return to their work with food until 4 months after the onset of symptoms, because hepatitis A virus can be detected in the stool for that long.

Standard immune serum globulin (ISG) is known to prevent the clinical manifestations of hepatitis A in 80% to 90% of persons when administered within 2 weeks after exposure. However, it does not prevent subclinical infection. The recommended dosage of standard ISG is 0.02 mL/kg. Hepatitis A vaccine is indicated for close personal contacts of patients with known hepatitis A, inmates of institutions during an epidemic of hepatitis A, and travelers to areas where hepatitis is endemic. It is not indicated for casual acquaintances or coworkers of the patient or for people who are known to have anti-HA antibody in their serum. To obtain immediate and long-term protection in people recently exposed to hepatitis A, the vaccine is combined with the administration of ISG. The hepatitis A vaccine results in the development of protective anti-HA antibody 2 weeks after its administration, a protection that lasts approximately 6 months, at which time a booster dose is given to extend the protection for up to 10 years. The vaccination (Havrix or Vaqta) is given as an injection of 0.5 mL to children and adolescents aged 2 to 17 years and as a 1-mL injection to adults (16).

The role of standard ISG in the prevention of type B hepatitis is uncertain. *Hepatitis B immune globulin* (containing a high titer of anti-HBs) prevents approximately 75% of cases of type B hepatitis (if given immediately after exposure) in people who have been stuck with needles contaminated by HBsAg-positive patients, in sexual partners of HBsAg-positive patients, in newborns of HBsAg-positive mothers, and in staff personnel of dialysis units (17). It is not indicated for casual or work contacts of patients with type B hepatitis or for patients who have been demonstrated to have anti-HBs. Testing for anti-HBs should be done routinely before administration of hepatitis B immune globulin, provided that the results of the tests can be obtained within 1 week after exposure to the virus.

Chapter 18 contains details regarding indications, dosages, and schedules for primary prevention of hepatitis B with *hepatitis B vaccine,* postexposure prophylaxis for adults and newborn infants exposed to people who have active hepatitis B or are known HBsAg carriers, and postexposure prophylaxis for adults exposed to people whose HBsAg status is unknown.

There have been insufficient studies to know whether the incidence of posttransfusion hepatitis C or hepatitis E is decreased by the administration of standard ISG. No vaccines are currently available for the prevention of hepatitis C or hepatitis E.

Drug-Induced Hepatitis

The liver is the principal organ concerned with drug metabolism; hence, it is not surprising that it is also a principal target for drug toxicity. Every drug has the potential for producing hepatocellular damage. Drug-induced hepatitis results from either direct hepatotoxicity or an idiosyncratic reaction (host hypersensitivity). Hepatotoxic reactions caused by direct toxins such as carbon tetrachloride and inorganic phosphorus are dose dependent and reproducible with a brief interval after exposure to the drug. Idiosyncratic reactions are the more common response to drugs. Characteristically, they are not dose dependent, occur in only a small number of people who are exposed, and are preceded by a sensitizing period of 1 to 4 weeks of exposure or a history of exposure. Drug reactions may be cholestatic, may simulate viral hepatitis, or may combine features of both processes.

Cholestatic Reactions. Cholestasis is caused by a direct dose-related effect of the administration of anabolic steroids and oral contraceptives. Cholestasis occurs in 1% to 2% of patients receiving anabolic steroids but less often after the ingestion of oral contraceptive drugs. Jaundice and pruritus are prominent symptoms. The elevated serum bilirubin is composed principally of the direct conjugated fraction. Serum alkaline phosphatase and cholesterol are elevated, whereas serum aminotransferases are normal or only slightly elevated. Cholestasis disappears soon after withdrawal of the offending drug.

A much larger number of drugs cause cholestasis through *hypersensitivity.* Examples are phenothiazine derivatives such as chlorpromazine, antibiotics such as erythromycin, antithyroid drugs such as propylthiouracil and methimazole, hypoglycemic agents such as tolbutamide and chlorpropamide, immunosuppressant drugs such as azathioprine, and cytotoxic drugs such as chlorambucil. Common clinical features of these drug reactions are fever, right upper quadrant abdominal pain, pruritus, skin rash, and eosinophilia. Serum aminotransferases are moderately elevated (less than 10 times normal). The clinical and laboratory abnormalities usually subside between 2 and 4 weeks after discontinuation of the drug, although on occasion cholestasis persists for months to years. Severe pruritus is treated with cholestyramine (Questran) given in a dosage of 4 g three times a day before meals. Relief of pruritus is obtained in 4 to 7 days after starting this medication. Patients with cholestasis should be hospitalized whenever the jaundice persists unchanged or increases 2 to 4 weeks after discontinuation of the drug, to investigate the possibility of other causes of cholestasis (see Chapter 96).

Hepatocellular Reactions. Most agents that produce direct hepatocellular damage are toxins rather than drugs. Acetaminophen, however, is a drug that produces hepatic necrosis in all people if ingested in a large dose (greater than 10 g), usually in a suicide attempt. Alcoholics and patients taking drugs such as phenobarbital, which are inducers of microsomal enzymes, are at risk for development of hepatic necrosis after the ingestion of lower doses of acetaminophen. Shortly after ingestion the patient develops nausea and vomiting, but evidence of hepatocellular damage often does not become apparent until 48 hours later, when serum aminotransferases rise and the prothrombin time becomes prolonged. The patient's condition then deteriorates; jaundice appears and central nervous system depression may occur. The mortality rate of patients who took an overdose of acetaminophen was found to be 3.5% in one large study (18). Therefore, patients who are known or suspected to have ingested toxic amounts of acetaminophen should be hospitalized for support and treatment (ordinarily with *N*-acetylcysteine).

There has been a marked increase in the use of *herbal medications* in the Western world in recent years (19). Some of these products, the ingredients of which are often poorly defined, are hepatotoxic. A history of taking herbal medicines should be sought in any patient with unexplained liver disease.

Idiosyncratic hepatocellular reactions have been reported after the administration of a number of drugs, the most common of which are isoniazid, alpha-methyldopa, nitrofurantoin, ketoconazole, sulfonamides, terbinafine (Lamisil), 3-hydroxy-3-methyglultaryl coenzyme A (HMG-CoA) reductase inhibitors (statins), troglitazone, phenylbutazone, and halothane. Asymptomatic increases in serum aminotransferases, which subside despite continued administration of the drug, have been reported in 5% to 10% of patients taking isoniazid or alpha-methyldopa 1 dopa. Because of the often transient nature of the serum aminotransferase elevations, there is no need to monitor these tests in asymptomatic patients. However, the development of symptoms of fatigue and anorexia or of nausea and general malaise is an indication for the determination of serum aminotransferase concentrations; if aminotransferase activity is increased, the drug should be discontinued immediately, because this often heralds the onset of severe hepatocellular damage. In some cases rifampin, an occasional cause of hepatotoxicity itself, potentiates the hepatotoxic effects of isoniazid. The incidence of acute hepatitis in patients taking these latter two drugs is 0.1% to 0.3%. Women and older patients are more likely to be affected. The onset of the reaction is between 1 and 10 weeks after the start of therapy. The symptoms, laboratory tests, and findings on liver biopsy are indistinguishable from those of viral hepatitis (see earlier discussion), so serologic tests to rule out viral hepatitis are often obtained. The hepatitis usually resolves within a few weeks after the drug is discontinued. However, a mortality rate as high as 12% has been reported for severe hepatitis caused by isoniazid. Moreover, chronic active liver disease can develop if the drug responsible for the hepatitis is continued. Administration of corticosteroids is not indicated in drug-induced hepatitis.

Alcoholic Hepatitis. This condition is seen most often after prolonged heavy alcohol intake. Women are more susceptible to alcoholic liver disease than men are, and it usually does not develop in men who drink less than 40 g of ethanol per day or in women who drink less than 20 g per day (equivalent to 4 and 2 ounces [120 and 60 mL] of 86 proof whiskey, respectively). Many of the presenting clinical characteristics of patients with alcoholic hepatitis (e.g., anorexia, significant fatigue, jaundice, tender hepatomegaly) are indistinguishable from those of viral hepatitis. However, patients with alcoholic hepatitis are more likely to have fever and leukocytosis. The elevation of the serum aminotransferases is rarely 10 times above normal, and often there is a prolongation of the prothrombin time. The elevation of AST is characteristically greater than that of alanine aminotransferase (ALT). Patients with alcoholic hepatitis and jaundice should be admitted to the hospital and have a definite diagnosis established by liver biopsy, if not contraindicated by abnormal hemostatic function. Liver biopsy differentiates alcoholic hepatitis from drug-induced hepatitis and viral hepatitis and gives an indication of any underlying chronic liver disease. The illness is often more severe than in patients with viral hepatitis, and decompensation with hepatic encephalopathy and death can occur. Approximately one third of patients with alcoholic hepatitis have been shown to progress to cirrhosis, often within 6 months (20). However, if patients can abstain from further drinking of alcohol (see Chapter 28), approximately one third recover completely, both clinically and histologically, usually within 1 month.

Chronic Hepatitis

Chronic hepatitis is inflammation of the liver detected by abnormal liver tests or abnormal liver histology that has persisted for longer than 6 months. The spectrum of chronic hepatitis varies from a benign, reversible process to an unrelenting process that often progresses to cirrhosis. Liver biopsy is essential both for the diagnosis and to establish the severity of the disease and the need for treatment. The liver histology is graded semiquantitatively according to the degree of necrosis and inflammation (minimal, mild, moderate, or severe activity) and staged for the amount of fibrosis and the presence of cirrhosis (21).

The principal causes of chronic hepatitis are infection with a hepatitis virus (type B or C), autoimmune disease (formerly called lupoid hepatitis), and drugs such as isoniazid, alpha-methyldopa, and nitrofurantoin. In addition, patients with Wilson disease, alpha-1-antitrypsin deficiency, or primary biliary cirrhosis may present with clinical and histologic features of chronic hepatitis.

The onset of chronic hepatitis is usually insidious. The patient may be asymptomatic, with liver disease detected by aminotransferase elevations on routine testing, or there may be symptoms of general malaise, fatigue, abdominal discomfort, anorexia, and jaundice. In about one third of the patients, the disease evolves from a clinically overt episode of acute hepatitis. Physical examination in patients with chronic hepatitis often reveals hepatomegaly and sometimes, when the disease is more advanced, splenomegaly, spider angiomas, palmar erythema, and gynecomastia. Elevations of serum aminotransferases may be the only laboratory abnormality, but elevations of bilirubin and globulins are also common. Decreases in serum albumin and prolongation of the prothrombin time reflect loss of hepatocellular function and a poor prognosis. Older male patients are more likely to have HBsAg in the serum and to present with an acute onset of illness. Patients with chronic hepatitis caused by hepatitis C virus may have arthralgias, vasculitis, palpable purpura, and peripheral neuropathy caused by type II cryoglobulinemia. Often these patients have false-negative test results for anti-hepatitis C and undetectable hepatitis C RNA because these factors are concentrated in the cryoprecipitates (22).

Patients with *autoimmune hepatitis* are more likely to be women and to present with acne, amenorrhea, arthralgia and arthritis, pleurisy, or intermittent fever (23). In addition, they may have associated thyroiditis, Sjögren syndrome, ulcerative colitis, glomerulonephritis, or hemolytic anemia. Laboratory tests on these patients show evidence of immunologic hyperactivity: Serum gammaglobulin is often markedly elevated, and there is elevation in the titers of antinuclear antibodies and smooth muscle antibodies. A small subgroup of patients with chronic autoimmune hepatitis have normal titers of antinuclear antibodies but elevated liver–kidney microsomal (anti-LKM) antibodies. In addition, antimitochondrial antibodies are found in 15% of these patients.

The diagnosis of *Wilson disease* (which affects approximately 1 in 1 million people) should be considered in all patients, particularly those younger than 25 years of age, who have clinical and laboratory features of otherwise unexplained chronic hepatitis (24). Wilson disease is discussed in more detail in the section on cirrhosis. The diagnosis of chronic hepatitis caused by *alpha-1-antitrypsin deficiency* (which affects 1 in 1,000 people) is suggested by the finding of an absent or low alpha-1-globulin on serum protein electrophoresis (25). The diagnosis is established by demonstrating a low value of alpha-1-antitrypsin in the serum by quantitative measurement and by protease inhibitor (Pi) typing (25). The common allele is PiM; liver disease occurs in approximately 20% of people who are homozygous for the allele PiZ. Liver biopsy reveals periodic acid–Schiff (PAS)–positive cytoplasmic inclusions that are resistant to diastase in both homozygous and heterozygous patients for the allele PiZ. There is no known medical therapy for this deficiency, which is transmitted by codominant inheritance. The diagnostic characteristics of *primary biliary cirrhosis* are discussed later in the section on cirrhosis. The diagnosis of *drug-induced chronic hepatitis* (see Drug-Induced Hepatitis) depends on a careful history and the demonstration of improvement of the patient after discontinuation of drugs that are known to produce this illness. In most cases, chronic active hepatitis caused by drugs reverts to normal after discontinuation of the offending drug.

The clinical course of patients with chronic active hepatitis is variable. Patients can be asymptomatic for a long time, have periods of intermittent worsening and remission, or have a progressive course to cirrhosis and death if untreated. Delta hepatitis is associated with clinical exacerbation of chronic hepatitis B and more rapid progression to cirrhosis (1).

Therapy. *Corticosteroids* are beneficial for symptomatic patients with chronic autoimmune hepatitis. Clinical, biochemical, and histologic improvement and even remission have been observed, and mortality rates have been reduced after therapy with corticosteroids (23). Prednisone or prednisolone, 40 to 60 mg, is given initially to suppress the activity of the disease and then is tapered slowly, usually over 1 to 3 months, to a maintenance dosage of 10 to 20 mg. Symptomatic improvement followed by a fall in serum aminotransferases occurs during the first few weeks. Treatment with corticosteroids is decreased to the smallest dosage possible to maintain normal or minimally increased values of the serum aminotransferases. Discontinuation of the corticosteroid therapy often results in a relapse. *Azathioprine* at an initial dosage of 100 mg/day in combination with prednisone is often effective in maintaining a remission (23). Asymptomatic patients with chronic hepatitis are usually treated only if they have persistent elevations of serum aminotransferases, histologic evidence of at least a mild grade of activity, and evidence of early fibrosis. Administration of corticosteroids to patients with chronic viral hepatitis is contraindicated because it appears to favor replication of hepatitis viruses, resulting in a higher morbidity and mortality (26).

Interferon-alfa-2b therapy is effective in eliminating evidence of viral replication (HBeAg) and in normalizing serum aminotransferase in more than one third of patients with type B hepatitis who are treated (27). Higher dosages and prolonged administration of interferon-alfa result in improvement in 15% to 25% of patients with chronic delta hepatitis (13). *Lamivudine,* a nucleoside analog, in an oral dose of 100 mg/day, results in a decrease in HBV DNA to undetectable levels in 95% of patients after 6 months of treatment, and in a normalization of ALT levels in 52% at 6 months and 70% at 1 year (28). These effects are associated with improvement in liver histology in 75% of patients. After 6 to 8 months of therapy, however, viral mutants that are resistant to the therapy begin to appear; in these cases after discontinuation of the therapy the HBV DNA and ALT return to pretreatment levels as the virus returns to the wild type. Approximately 30% of patients receiving lamivudine for 1 year who experienced a loss of HBeAg remained in remission for 6 months after the therapy (29).

Interferon-alfa-2b therapy (3 million units subcutaneously three times a week) *in combination with oral ribavirin* (1,000 to 1,200 mg orally) given for 48 weeks reduces hepatitis C RNA to undetectable levels and normalizes serum aminotransferases in half of patients with type C hepatitis, but the relapse rate within 6 months after completion of therapy is approximately 50% (29). Hence, the rate of sustained virologic and biochemical response is only 20% to 30%. The response is as high as 65% when the hepatitis C genotype is 2 or 3, as opposed to genotypes 1 and 4. Preliminary studies indicate that *pegylated interferon-alfa-2b,* which requires only one weekly injection and results in more sustained blood levels of interferon, combined with ribavirin, results in a higher virologic and biochemical response. Decisions about the use of interferon, lamivudine, and ribavirin should be made in consultation with a hepatologist.

No specific therapy exists for type E hepatitis.

UNEXPLAINED ELEVATIONS OF LIVER ENZYMES IN THE SERUM

Elevations of serum aminotransferases and alkaline phosphatase are occasionally found in normal subjects or in patients without suspected liver disease. In such a situation the abnormality should first be confirmed by repeat testing. Next, it is important to remember that elevated serum aminotransferases and alkaline phosphatase do not necessarily originate from the liver. For example, elevated serum aminotransferases can be caused by injury to the heart and striated muscle; if the source of the serum aminotransferases is muscle, the more specific creatine kinase will also be elevated. Elevation of serum gammaglutamyl transpeptidase (GGTP) is useful to confirm the hepatic origin of elevated serum aminotransferases, because, unlike the latter enzymes, it does not originate from damaged muscle. Elevation of GGPT alone, however, should not be used as an indication of liver damage, because GGPT is a microsomal enzyme and elevations may occur as a result of ingestion of drugs that are microsomal enzyme inducers, such as phenytoin (Dilantin), phenobarbital, and ethanol. An isolated increase of serum alkaline phosphatase can originate from liver or bone. The hepatic origin of alkaline phosphatase can be confirmed by demonstration of an elevated 5′-nucleotidase value; unlike alkaline phosphatase, this enzyme is present only in the liver and in the epithelium of the bile ducts. By contrast, an elevated serum alkaline phosphatase accompanied by a normal serum 5′-nucleotidase value is almost invariably caused by bone disease; a common cause of such an occurrence is a paget disease of bone. Any persistent elevation of serum aminotransferases for longer than 6 months that remains unexplained is an indication for liver biopsy to rule out chronic hepatitis. A persistent elevation of serum alkaline phosphatase in the absence of an elevated serum bilirubin can occur in patients with fatty liver, which is common in diabetic and obese patients, or it can be the result of space-occupying lesions, such as granulomas or metastatic carcinoma. A CT scan with contrast of the liver is recommended in these cases to rule out metastatic carcinoma, but a liver biopsy is indicated only if the CT scan shows a space-occupying lesion or if there is clinical suspicion of diseases such as tuberculosis or sarcoidosis that may result in hepatic granulomas.

ALCOHOLIC FATTY LIVER

Alcoholic fatty liver results from alterations of lipid metabolism caused by alcohol and therefore occurs in all persons who ingest alcohol in excessive amounts. It is manifested mainly by a feeling of abdominal fullness caused by hepatomegaly and mild elevation of the serum aminotransferases (rarely more than twice normal). On occasion, marked fatty infiltration is associated with symptoms of malaise, weakness, anorexia, tender hepatomegaly, and even jaundice. These symptomatic patients require further evaluation, occasionally including liver biopsy, to distinguish fatty liver from alcoholic hepatitis and cirrhosis. The treatment of fatty liver consists of abstinence from alcohol. With abstinence, the abnormal accumulation of fat disappears within 4 to 6 weeks. As the patient's condition improves, the liver decreases in size and becomes nontender. Serum bilirubin and aminotransferase values promptly return to normal. Recurrent episodes of symptomatic fatty liver are common after heavy alcohol ingestion, but there is no evidence that this lesion itself leads to cirrhosis.

NONALCOHOLIC STEATOHEPATITIS

Nonalcoholic steatohepatitis is a chronic disease of unknown origin characterized by fatty infiltration and hepatocellular damage with inflammation in patients who lack a history of significant alcohol ingestion. (30). It is a very common cause of elevated serum aminotransferase concentrations. It is more common in women. Obesity and type 2 diabetes are found in 80% and in 50% to 75% of patients, respectively (30,31). Most of the patients are asymptomatic and liver disease is discovered by finding elevated serum aminotransferases. The principal symptoms, when present, are fatigue and right upper abdominal discomfort. Hepatomegaly is a finding in 90% of the patients, but splenomegaly is rare. The serum ALT level is usually higher than the serum AST, which helps in differentiating nonalcoholic from alcoholic steatohepatitis. The serum ferritin and transferrin saturation values are often elevated, but few of these patients are homozygous for the hemochromatosis (HFE) gene. If the diagnosis is in doubt, it can be confirmed by ultrasonography. Liver biopsy is indicated in symptomatic patients with serum aminotransferase elevations of more than 6 months' duration. Patients with evidence of moderate to severe fibrosis on liver biopsy have at least a 5% risk of progressing to cirrhosis. Weight reduction by intake of a calorie-restricted, low-fat diet often results in a decrease in fatty infiltration, improvement of symptoms, a decrease in liver size, a fall in serum triglycerides, and sometimes a fall in serum aminotransferase concentrations.

CIRRHOSIS

Cirrhosis is a chronic diffuse liver disease characterized by widespread hepatic fibrosis and nodule formation. The fibrosis is the result of extensive destruction of liver cells, and the nodularity represents regeneration. For clinical purposes, cirrhosis can be classified into the following major categories: alcoholic, viral (hepatitis B and C), cardiac, and biliary cirrhosis; Wilson disease; hemochromatosis; and schistosomiasis. The onset of cirrhosis is usually insidious and is associated with nonspecific symptoms such as fatigue, anorexia, weight loss, nausea, and abdominal discomfort. As the disease progresses, signs of hepatocellular failure become prominent: jaundice, edema, ascites, electrolyte abnormalities, bleeding tendencies, spider angiomas, palmar erythema, gynecomastia, impotence, and loss of axillary and pubic hair. Hepatomegaly and portal hypertension resulting in splenomegaly and a venous collateral circulation are common. The most severe complications of cirrhosis are hepatic encephalopathy, bleeding from esophageal and/or gastric varices, infection (e.g., spontaneous bacterial peritonitis), and hepatorenal syndrome. Patients with alcoholic cirrhosis often have recurring episodes of hepatocellular failure, precipitated by superimposed alcoholic hepatitis and fatty infiltration induced by alcohol ingestion. Clinical improvement often occurs after abstinence from alcohol and after bed rest and optimal nutrition. Rapid deterioration of patients with cirrhosis should raise the suspicion of a complicating hepatocellular carcinoma. Common laboratory findings in patients with cirrhosis include anemia, a normal or slightly decreased leukocyte count, and moderate thrombocytopenia. The most common abnormal liver tests are hyperbilirubinemia, a depressed serum albumin, elevated serum globulins, and a prolonged prothrombin time.

Differential Diagnosis

The diagnostic characteristics of some of the other types of cirrhosis are as follows.

Cardiac Cirrhosis. Cardiac cirrhosis develops only after prolonged and severe cardiac failure, usually caused by valvular disease, particularly in patients with tricuspid incompetence or constrictive pericarditis. Jaundice, hepatomegaly, and ascites are prominent features, but the diagnosis can be established with certainty only by liver biopsy. Treatment of cardiac failure—for example, treatment of constrictive pericarditis by pericardiectomy—results in improvement of liver function.

Primary Biliary Cirrhosis. Primary biliary cirrhosis (32) is a chronic disease of unknown cause that is characterized by progressive intrahepatic cholestasis and is most often seen in middle-aged women. The principal manifestations are jaundice with pruritus, hepatomegaly, hypercholesterolemia with the formation of xanthoma and xanthelasma, and steatorrhea caused by the decreased delivery of bile acids to the intestine. Antimitochondrial antibodies are found in 95% of these patients, and their presence is virtually diagnostic. Liver biopsy in the early stages reveals injury to the septal and large intralobular bile ducts with surrounding accumulation of inflammatory plasma cells and lymphocytes and with granuloma formation. In the end stages of the disease, cirrhosis develops that is almost indistinguishable from other causes of nonalcoholic cirrhosis. Treatment with ursodeoxycholic acid has been found to reduce serum bilirubin and aminotransferases, delay clinical progression of the disease, and increase survival without liver transplantation (33).

Primary Sclerosing Cholangitis. Primary sclerosing cholangitis (PSC) is a chronic cholestatic disease of unknown etiology caused by inflammation and obstruction of the bile ducts. It has a prevalence of 1 to 7 cases per 100,000 population and is more common in men. There is strong association between PSC and inflammatory bowel disease, both ulcerative colitis and Crohn disease, with a prevalence greater than 50% in most studies (34). The patients may initially be asymptomatic and present with laboratory values indicating cholestasis, such as elevations of serum bilirubin and alkaline phosphatase, or they may be symptomatic and present with abdominal pain, pruritus, jaundice, or fever. Hepatomegaly is common. Perinuclear antineutrophilic cytoplasmic (pANCA) antibodies are found in approximately 80% of patients, but this test is not very specific. Low-titer antimitochondrial antibodies are present in about 5% of patients. Dilated bile ducts may be seen by sonography, but visualization of the bile ducts by endoscopic retrograde cholangiopancreatography (ERCP) is essential to establish the diagnosis. It usually demonstrates multiple strictures and beading of the intrahepatic and extrahepatic biliary tree. Liver biopsy typically shows portal and periportal inflammation and fibrosis, initially often concentric around bile ductules. The disease often progresses to cirrhosis. The most serious complications of PSC are cholangiocarcinoma in 7% to 15% of patients and cancer of the colon in those patients with associated inflammatory bowel disease. There is no proven medical therapy for PSC. Major dominant bile duct obstructions, resulting often in bacterial cholangitis, are treated with ballooning, stenting of the bile ducts, and antibiotics. The development of permanent jaundice is an indication for liver transplantation (see later discussion).

Wilson Disease. Wilson disease is a rare disorder of copper metabolism that is inherited as an autosomal recessive disorder (24). Its symptoms result from hepatic and neurologic dysfunction. In children the principal symptoms are caused by liver involvement, whereas in adults neurologic symptoms tend to predominate. The diagnosis should be suspected in all children or young adults who develop cirrhosis, because treatment with copper-chelating agents can arrest the disease and alleviate all symptoms. A characteristic finding that is virtually diagnostic is the presence of Kayser–Fleischer rings, which are greenish-brown rings found on the posterior surface and in the periphery of the cornea. Because these rings cannot often be seen by the naked eye, it is important to refer all suspected patients to an ophthalmologist for slit-lamp examination of the cornea. Serum ceruloplasmin, the copper-binding protein, is reduced in most, but not all, cases. Histologic examination of a liver biopsy is not diagnostic. However, quantitative determination of copper with a finding of more than 250 μg per gram of dry liver weight or the urinary excretion of more than 50 μg copper in 24 hours is diagnostic. Hospitalization is not required for treatment of Wilson disease with D-penicillamine, a chelating agent with considerable toxicity that is best administered by a hepatologist.

Hemochromatosis. Hemochromatosis is an inherited disorder of iron metabolism that results in excessive body iron; it is characterized principally by cirrhosis, diabetes mellitus, and grayish pigmentation of the skin. Other symptoms are cardiac failure and arrhythmias, peripheral neuritis, arthritis, and testicular atrophy. The iron overload appears to be caused by an increased absorption of dietary iron, and the mode of inheritance is autosomal recessive. The hemochromatosis (HFE) gene has been identified. The primary mutation in the gene is C282Y (substitution of cysteine by tyrosine). Another mutation is H63D (substitution of histidine by aspartate). The homozygous C282Y/C282Y mutation is responsible for 61% to 92% of the cases of hemochromatosis around the world. Compound heterozygotes (C282Y/H63D) have a fourfold increased risk of hemochromatosis, compared with the general population. Homozygous genotype H63D/H63D is not associated with increased iron deposition (35). The disease usually appears in people older than 40 years of age, and it develops earlier in men, probably because of the menstrual loss of iron in women. The diagnosis is made by demonstrating a high serum iron concentration (greater than 150 μg/dL), a high saturation of iron-binding protein (greater than 50%), and increased serum ferritin, usually in a patient with a positive family history (36). The finding of the genotype C282Y/C282Y confirms the diagnosis of hemochromatosis. Therapy consists of removal of excess iron by repeated phlebotomy (1 to 2 units weekly) with the goal of achieving a serum ferritin concentration between 25 and 50 ng/mL.

Schistosomiasis. Hepatic schistosomiasis may occur in people from tropical areas who have been infected by schistosome cercariae while swimming or walking in infested water. The liver disease is caused by the deposition of ova of *Schistosoma mansoni* in the portal areas, with the development of an inflammatory reaction, often with granuloma formation and periportal fibrosis. Jaundice is uncommon in these patients at presentation. The most common laboratory abnormalities are increases in serum alkaline phosphatase and mild elevations of serum bilirubin and aminotransferases. The diagnosis of active infection is made by demonstrating motile *Schistosoma* ova on fresh examination of rectal biopsy, and the diagnosis of liver involvement is made by showing the presence of ova capsules on liver biopsy.

Management

The treatment of uncomplicated cirrhosis consists of voluntary restriction of activity if the patient has weakness and fatigue, a diet that is high in protein but low in salt, and abstinence from alcohol (see Chapter 28). This regimen almost invariably results in improvement of hepatocellular function in patients with alcoholic cirrhosis and occasionally in patients with nonalcoholic cirrhosis. Tranquilizers and sedatives should be avoided. Infection and gastrointestinal bleeding, which in addition to alcohol ingestion are common precipitating factors of decompensation, should be sought and treated. Vitamin K, 15 mg subcutaneously, may improve prolongation of the prothrombin time. Multivitamins and folic acid, 1 mg/day, may be given if the patient's dietary intake appears to be inadequate or if there is evidence of vitamin deficiencies. Potassium deficiency is common and may contribute to the precipitation of hepatic encephalopathy, but its extent is difficult to assess because serum potassium concentration is a poor reflection of the total body potassium. However, when the serum potassium concentration falls below 3.5 mEq/L, the deficit often can be replaced by giving 30 mL of 10% potassium chloride orally two or three times a day, if tolerated or K-Dur tablets, 20 mEq, two or three times daily.

Fluid retention is treated with sodium restriction (500 mg of sodium chloride per day) and diuretics. The induced diuresis should be slow and should result in a loss of no more than 2.27 kg (5 lb) of weight per week because of the danger of precipitating electrolyte depletion and hypokalemia. Diuresis can be initiated by spironolactone, 100 mg a day, and the dosage can be increased gradually to 200 mg/day to obtain a diuresis. A loop diuretic (e.g., furosemide) is added to the regimen gradually if diuresis is inadequate. The dosage of the diuretics is decreased or their use is discontinued if the patient develops hyponatremia or impaired renal function. Patients with ascites that is unresponsive to sodium restriction and high dosages of diuretics should be referred to a hepatologist for management by either therapeutic paracentesis or transjugular intrahepatic portasystemic stent-shunt (TIPS). The development of acute hepatic encephalopathy manifested by asterixis or changes in mental status is an indication that the patient should be hospitalized for evaluation and treatment. Acute and chronic gastrointestinal bleeding is also an indication for hospitalization.

Lactulose is the principal therapy for hepatic encephalopathy. Lactulose is a nonabsorbable synthetic disaccharide that reduces blood ammonia and improves encephalopathy in more than 80% of patients when administered in dosages of 20 to 30 g (30 to 45 mL) three to four times a day. Lactulose usually is effective only when it also increases the frequency of bowel movements. Other than producing mild abdominal cramps and flatulence, lactulose is devoid of side effects. The mechanism of its action is not well defined, but its effectiveness is related to its ability to trap nitrogen in the stool and decrease ammonia production. Some of the decrease in ammonia production may be caused by a decrease in contact time of the stool with colonic bacteria. Patients with cirrhosis should be prescribed a normal protein diet of 50 to 70 g/day, which is sufficient to maintain an anabolic state. Higher amounts of protein are of no benefit and can result in the development of encephalopathy. If encephalopathy develops while the patient is on a normal protein diet, it is initially controlled with lactulose therapy with minimal or no reduction of the intake of protein. However, oral protein may need to be restricted if the encephalopathy is not controlled by lactulose. If adequate protein intake can not be achieved because of worsening hepatic encephalopathy, then oral or enteral formulas of casein hydrolysates (Ensure) are indicated. The administration of adequate protein, which results in a positive nitrogen balance, decreases muscle wasting and improves serum albumin and hepatic encephalopathy. (20) A change from animal protein to a vegetable protein diet may also improve hepatic encephalopathy. The exact mechanism whereby vegetable protein is better tolerated is unknown. However, vegetable protein contains smaller amounts of ammonia, methionine, and aromatic acids, and it also results in alterations of small intestinal and colonic bacterial flora so that the excretion of fecal nitrogen is increased (37). The beneficial effects of a vegetable protein diet and lactulose on hepatic encephalopathy are additive. Patients with decompensated cirrhosis who are not responding to therapy should be considered for liver transplantation and should be referred to a hepatologist for evaluation.

Transplantation

Liver transplantation has become an important option for some patients with end-stage liver disease. In general, patients should be referred to a transplantation center for consideration of liver transplantation if they have fulminant hepatitis or if they have developed cirrhosis with impaired hepatic synthetic function, hyperbilirubinemia, ascites, and/or encephalopathy. Results in patients who do undergo transplantation are excellent compared with patients who do not. For example, in patients with hepatitis C and end-stage liver disease, the 5-year survival rate is approximately 70%, compared with less than 50% in untransplanted patients with comparable disease (38)—this, despite the almost universal recurrence of hepatitis C in the allograft (39). Results in patients with other causes of cirrhosis are comparable.

General References*

Alter MJ, Mast EE. The epidemiology of viral hepatitis in the United States. Gastroenterol Clin North Am 1994;23:437.

Update on the epidemiology of all forms of viral hepatitis.

Di Bisceglie AM, Carithers RL Jr, Gores GJ. Hepatocellular carcinoma. Hepatology 1998;28:1161.

Progress report on epidemiology, pathogenesis, diagnosis, and treatment.

Lauer GM, Walker, BD. Hepatitis C virus infection. N Engl J Med 2001;345:41.

Maddrey WC, Schiff ER, Sorrell MF. Transplantation of the liver. 3rd ed. Hagerstown, MD: Lippincott Williams & Wilkins, 2000.

Mezey E. Fatty liver. In Schiff ER, Sorrell MF, Maddrey WC, eds. Schiff's diseases of the liver. 8th ed. Philadelphia: JB Lippincott, 1999:1185.

Discusses various causes, clinical presentation, and management of fatty liver.

Zakim D, Boyer TD. Hepatology: a textbook of liver disease. 4th ed. Philadelphia: WB Saunders, 2002.

A comprehensive textbook of liver disease.

Zimmerman HJ. Hepatotoxicity: the adverse effects of drugs and other chemicals on the liver. 2nd ed. Philadelphia: Lippincott Williams & Wilkins, 1999.

A comprehensive source of information on drug hepatotoxicity.

Specific References

1. Rizzetto M, Verme G, Gerin JL, et al. Hepatitis delta virus disease. Prog Liver Dis 1986;8:417.
2. Alter MJ. Epidemiology of hepatitis C in the West. Semin Liver Dis 1995;15:5.
3. Conry-Cantinela C, VanRaden M, Gibble J, et al. Routes of infection, viremia, and liver disease in blood donors found to have hepatitis C infection. N Engl J Med 1996;334:1691.
4. Krawczynski K, Aggarwal R, Kamili S. Hepatitis E. Infect Dis Clin North Am 2000;14:669.
5. Kuo G, Choo Q-L, Alter HJ, et al. An assay for circulating antibodies to a major etiologic virus of human non-A, non-B hepatitis. Science 1989;244:362.
6. Szmuness W, Dienstag JC, Purcell RH, et al. Distribution of antibody to hepatitis A antigen in urban adult populations. N Engl J Med 1976;295:755.
7. Krugman S, Overby LR, Mushahwar IK, et al. Viral hepatitis, type B: studies on natural history and prevention re-examined. N Engl J Med 1979;300:101.
8. Sampliner RE, Hamilton FA, Iseri OA, et al. The liver histology and frequency of clearance of the hepatitis B surface antigen (HBsAg) in chronic carriers. Am J Med Sci 1979;277:17.
9. Grady GF and the U.S. National Heart and Lung Institute Collaborative Study Group. Relation of e antigen to infectivity of HBsAg-positive inoculations among medical personnel. Lancet 1976;2:492.
10. Bukh J, Miller RH, Purcell RH. Genetic heterogeneity of hepatitis C virus: quasispecies and genotypes. Semin Liver Dis 1995;15:41.
11. Alter MJ, Margolis HS, Krawczynski K, et al. The natural history of community-acquired hepatitis C in the United States: The Sentinel Counties non-A, non-B Hepatitis Study Team. N Engl J Med 1992;327:1899.
12. Repsher LH, Freebern RK. Effects of early and vigorous exercise on recovery from infectious hepatitis. N Engl J Med 1969;281:1393.
13. Hoofnagle JH, DiBisceglie AM. The treatment of chronic viral hepatitis. N Engl J Med 1997;336:347.
14. Schreiber GB, Busch MP, Kleinman SH, et al. The risk of transfusion-transmitted viral infections: The Retrovirus Epidemiology Donor Study. N Engl J Med 1996;334:1685.
15. The Incident Investigation Teams and others. Transmission of hepatitis B to patients from four infected surgeons without hepatitis B antigen. N Engl J Med 1997;336:178.
16. Lemon SM, Thomas DL. Vaccines to prevent viral hepatitis. N Engl J Med 1997;336:196.
17. Seeff LB, Koff RS. Passive and active immunoprophylaxis of hepatitis B. Gastroenterology 1984;86:958.
18. Black M. Acetaminophen hepatotoxicity. Annu Rev Med 1984;35:577.
19. Chitturi S. Herbal hepatotoxicity: an expanding but poorly defined problem. J Gastorenterol Hepatol 2000;15:1093.
20. Mezey E. Treatment of alcoholic liver disease. Semin Liver Dis 1993;13:210.
21. Desmet VJ, Gerber M, Hoofnagle JH, et al. Classification of chronic hepatitis: diagnosis, grading, and staging. Hepatology 1994;19:1513.
22. Agnello V, Chung RT, Kaplan LM. A role for hepatitis C virus in type II cryoglobulinemia. N Engl J Med 1992;327:1490.
23. Obermayer-Straub P, Strassburg CP, Manns MP. Autoimmune hepatitis. J Hepatol 2000;32[Suppl 1]:181.
24. Sternlieb I, Scheinberg IH. Chronic hepatitis as a first manifestation of Wilson's disease. Ann Intern Med 1972;76:59.
25. Fagerhol MK, Laurell CB. The polymorphism of prealbumins and α_1-antitrypsin in human sera. Clin Chim Acta 1967;16:199.
26. Lam KC, Lai CL, Trepo C, et al. Deleterious effect of prednisolone in HBsAg-positive chronic active hepatitis. N Engl J Med 1981;304:380.
27. Hoofnagle JH, Shafritz DA, Popper H. Chronic type B hepatitis and the healthy HBsAg carrier state. Hepatology 1987;7:758.
28. Dienstag JL, Schiff ER, Wright TL, et al. Lamivudine as initial treatment for chronic hepatitis B in the United States. N Eng J Med 1999;341:1256.
29. Lin OS, Keeffe EB. Current treatment strategies for chronic hepatitis B and C. Annu Rev Med 2001;52:29.

*Bold print (general references) and bold numerals (specific references) denote published controlled clinical trials, meta-analyses, or consensus-based recommendations.

30. James OF, Day CP. Non-alcoholic steatohepatitis (NASH): a disease of emerging identity and importance. J Hepatol 1998; 29:495.
31. Sheth SG, Gordon FD, Chopra S. Nonalcoholic steatohepatitis. Ann Intern Med 19997;126:137.
32. O'Donohue J, Williams R. Primary biliary cirrhosis. QJM 1996; 89:5.
33. Poupon, RE, Bonnand AM, Chretien Y, et al. Ten-year survival in ursodeoxycholic acid-treated patients with primary biliary cirrhosis: The UDCA-PBC Study Group. Hepatology 1999;29: 1668.
34. Angulo P, Lindor KD. Primary sclerosing cholangitis. Hepatology 1999;30:325.
35. Bacon BR, Olynyk JK. Brunt EM, et al. HFE gene genotype in patients with hemochromatosis and other liver diseases. Ann Intern Med 1999;130:953.
36. Bassett ML, Halliday JW, Ferris RA, et al. Diagnosis of hemochromatosis in young subjects: predictive accuracy of biochemical screening tests. Gastroenterology 1984;87:628.
37. Greenberger NJ, Carley J, Schenker S, et al. Effect of vegetable and animal protein diets in chronic hepatic encephalopathy. Am J Dig Dis 1977;22:845.
38. Fattovich G, Guistina G, Degos F, et al. Morbidity and mortality in compensated cirrhosis type C: a retrospective follow-up study of 384 patients. Gastroenterology 1997;112:463.
39. Gane EJ, Portmann BC, Naoumov NV. Long-term outcome of hepatitis C infection after liver transplantation. N Engl J Med 1996;334:815.

SECTION

6

Renal and Urologic Problems

CHAPTER 48

Proteinuria

EDWARD S. KRAUS, MD

Normally less than 150 mg of protein per 24 hours is present in urine, although values may be as high as 300 mg/24 hours in adolescents. Sixty percent of this urinary protein is plasma protein (two thirds of it is albumin) that has been filtered by glomeruli and only partially reabsorbed by renal tubules. The remaining 40% is synthesized and secreted into the urine by the renal tubules and by the more distal portions of the urogenital tract.

Increased urinary protein excretion (proteinuria) may be caused by renal disease, either glomerular dysfunction that allows more protein to be filtered or changes in the renal tubules resulting in decreased reabsorption of filtered proteins. Alternatively, increased urinary protein excretion may reflect increased metabolic generation of protein. Proteinuria is often encountered in the general population, not selected for any health risks (2% to 5% prevalence). In most instances, proteinuria is simply an abnormal laboratory finding in an asymptomatic patient with no significant impact on present or future health. Approximately 1% of those who have proteinuria when screened have renal or systemic disease with significant physiologic sequelae (1). Currently, screening for proteinuria is not recommended for the general population (2), but it should be performed in selected groups at risk for renal disease (see Office Assessment of Patients with Proteinuria). This chapter discusses the methods of detection of protein in the urine and describes an approach to the evaluation and treatment of patients with proteinuria.

METHODS FOR DETECTING PROTEINURIA

Office screening for proteinuria is easily accomplished by several accessible and inexpensive semiquantitative methods described in detail in this chapter. Most methods are sensitive (dipstick detects 20 to 30 mg of albumin per deciliter; sulfosalicylic acid and heat and acetic acid detect 5 to 10 mg of protein per deciliter), so positive results may be obtained when testing concentrated urine even though 24-hour urinary protein excretion is normal. With all of these methods, false-positive and false-negative results may occur (Table 48.1).

Dipstick

A dipstick is the most practical and easiest test for semiquantitation of urinary proteins. When moistened with urine, the stick becomes yellow if protein is absent. As protein concentration increases, interference with the dye–buffer combination results in an increasingly green color. Although it is simple and inexpensive, the technique has several limitations. Because the color reaction is pH dependent, false-positive reactions may be observed if the urine is alkaline (pH greater than 7.5). This error can be avoided by adding a drop of strong acid (e.g., 1 N HCl) before testing to ensure that the pH in the urine is less than 7.0. Also, the dipstick method is sensitive primarily to albumin; globulins or parts of globulins (e.g., heavy or light chains, Bence Jones protein) may be missed. Because of these limitations, an alternative method of screening for proteinuria should be available in the practitioner's office. Either of the methods described in this section is satisfactory.

Sulfosalicylic Acid

Another easy and inexpensive semiquantitative test for proteinuria is protein precipitation with a 3% to 10% solution of sulfosalicylic acid (SSA). SSA is available from some pharmacies or from hospital laboratories. SSA is used most often to detect globulins or light chains, because the dipstick is insensitive to these proteins. However, false-positive test results occur if the urine is already turbid. In this situation the urine must be filtered before it is tested. False-positive results also occur when the test is done within 3 days after administration of iodinated radiographic contrast medium or certain drugs (Table 48.1). In addition, the SSA test detects proteins of prostatic and vaginal origin. These contaminants can be avoided by not palpating the prostate before collecting urine from men and by obtaining a clean voided urine specimen from women, which should show no or only a few vaginal cells microscopically.

Heat and Acetic Acid

The heat and acetic acid method is more time-consuming and is recommended as a second method

Table 48.1. Urinary Constituents that Alter the Results of Protein Screening Tests

Urinary Constituent	Dipstick	Sulfosalicyclic Acid	Heat and Acetic Acid
Radiographic contrast media	No effect	False positive	False positive
Drugs and drug metabolites[a]	No effect	False positive	False positive
Bence Jones protein	False negative	No effect	False negative[b]
Highly alkaline urine	False positive	False negative	False negative
Urine turbidity	No effect	False positive	False positive
Vaginal or prostatic secretion	No effect	False positive	False positive

[a]Tolbutamide, tolmetin, chlorpromazine, sulfisoxazole, and high dosages of cephalosporins and penicillin.

[b]Precipitated protein may disappear rapidly and be missed with continued heating.

Modified from Bradley M, Schumann GB, Ward PCJ. Examination of urine. In: Henry JB, ed. Todd–Sanford–Davidsohn clinical diagnosis and management by laboratory methods. 16th ed. Philadelphia: WB Saunders, 1979.

of urine protein testing only if SSA is not available. Glacial acetic acid may be purchased at a photography store and must be diluted for accurate results. The diluted solution, 1 volume of glacial acetic acid to 2 volumes of water, may be stored and used as necessary. The test is performed by heating the top of a test tube containing approximately 10 mL of urine. After the top of the urine begins to boil rapidly, three or four drops of the diluted acetic acid is added. Reheating to boiling causes a white precipitate to form if protein (either globulin or albumin) is present in the urine specimen. False-positive results occur if the specimen is contaminated with prostatic or vaginal secretions and in the presence of certain drugs or radiographic contrast media (Table 48.1). Furthermore, the rapid boiling can mask the visualization of a transient precipitation of Bence Jones protein.

OFFICE ASSESSMENT OF PATIENTS WITH PROTEINURIA

Patients may present for evaluation of proteinuria that has been discovered during evaluation for school, military service, employment, or insurance. If these patients are otherwise healthy, a screening test for proteinuria should be repeated two or three times in the office before further workup is performed. Transient nonrecurrent mild proteinuria may be seen in association with changes in systemic hemodynamics caused by the stress of fever, exercise, exposure to cold, or decompensated congestive heart failure and therefore may not reflect a progressive renal disease.

Historically, chronic proteinuria should be suspected if the patient acknowledges reports of abnormal urinalysis performed as part of previous screening examinations. Patients also may be aware of prior renal or urologic problems but may not associate them with proteinuria. Therefore, a detailed urologic history should be obtained, including history of infection or stones, prior radiologic evaluations, and family history of renal insufficiency. Because drugs such as gold, penicillamine, captopril, and nonsteroidal anti-inflammatory agents can cause proteinuria, medications should be reviewed thoroughly. Proteinuria may represent only one facet of a systemic illness suggested by dermatologic, rheumatologic, infectious, and cardiovascular review of systems. The date of onset of edema, nocturia, or hypertension may help determine the duration of a disease associated with proteinuria. Occasionally, the patient may have noticed foaming of the urine on voiding if proteinuria has been massive.

Physical examination should be reviewed for the presence of signs that may be associated with the cause of renal disease (e.g., diabetic retinopathy; abdominal masses suggestive of polycystic kidneys; rashes, murmurs, or arthropathy indicative of systemic illness), or that may result from renal disease (e.g., edema), or both (e.g., hypertension).

If screening examinations reveal proteinuria, further laboratory evaluation should include several studies. First, a microscopic urinalysis should be performed. The presence of other abnormalities (e.g., hematuria, casts, inflammatory cells) suggests specific patterns of renal disease of which proteinuria may be just a part. Second, serum creatinine concentration or creatinine clearance should be measured to identify whether renal filtration function is impaired (see Chapter 52). Third, proteinuria should be quantitated by either examination of a 24-hour urine sample or determination of the protein/creatinine ratio in a single voided sample. This helps classify the disorder (see next section) and assists in the development of the differential diagnosis.

24-Hour Urine Collection for Protein

A clean container without preservatives, usually a gallon jug, is given to the patient with instructions about the collection process. The 24-hour collection is best done on a day when the patient will be using a single toilet, and it is helpful for the patient to place a note on the toilet on the day of collection, as a reminder to collect all required specimens. On the day of collection, the first voided morning specimen is discarded, and then all urine voided during the next 24 hours, including the next morning's first voided specimen, is collected in the container. Once the urine is collected, it is not critical when protein determination is done. If there is excessive delay, however, bacterial growth can falsely raise protein concentrations. Therefore, it is advisable to refrigerate the urine specimen until it is brought to the laboratory, if it is not brought in on the day the collection is completed. Alternatively, if refrigeration is not possible, 1 to 2 g of boric acid should be added to the container. Other preservatives (e.g., strong acids, thymol) must be avoided because they interfere with the protein assay.

Quantitation of urine protein is a precise measurement in a well-controlled laboratory, and any value greater than 200 mg/day is considered abnormal. Proteinuria is classified as nonnephrotic if the excretion is between 200 and 3,500 mg in 24 hours, and as nephrotic (definitely indicative of glomerular disease) if the excretion is greater than 3,500 mg in 24 hours, regardless of the presence or absence of other manifestations of the nephrotic syndrome (e.g., low serum albumin, edema, high serum cholesterol). The simultaneous measurement of urinary creatinine is helpful as an index of the adequacy of collection. Most patients who are of average body mass produce between 800 and 1,500 mg of creatinine per day (21 to 26 mg/kg per day in adult men, 16 to 22 mg/kg per day in adult women).

Protein/Creatinine Ratio

An excellent correlation exists between 24-hour urinary protein excretion and the protein/creatinine concentration ratio (milligrams per deciliter of protein divided by milligrams per deciliter of creatinine), as determined in a random sample of urine obtained during normal daytime activity (3). A ratio greater than 0.2 is considered abnormal. A ratio greater than 3.5 represents nephrotic-range proteinuria. The ratio may overestimate 24-hour urinary protein excretion in certain circumstances, most notably when urine is collected after strenuous exercise, from patients with diabetes mellitus, or from patients whose daily urinary creatinine excretion is considerably less than 1 g (e.g., frail adults). Conversely, determination of this ratio from a first morning urine specimen may underestimate daily urinary protein losses (see Orthostatic Proteinuria). The urinary protein/creatinine ratio is especially useful if a 24-hour collection is difficult to obtain or if there is doubt about the completeness of the sample.

NONNEPHROTIC PROTEINURIA

A variety of primary renal and systemic diseases may be associated with nonnephrotic range proteinuria. Also, most, if not all, patients with nephrotic-range proteinuria may at some time have had non–nephrotic-range protein excretion. Evaluation is best defined by considering patients who have normal physical examinations and laboratory profiles (i.e., isolated proteinuria) separately from those patients with other stigmata of disease, such as active urinary sediment or hypertension (nonisolated proteinuria).

Isolated Proteinuria in Apparently Healthy Patients

If the initial evaluation is negative except for the presence of isolated proteinuria, the proteinuria may be further classified as persistent (25% to 30% of patients) or intermittent (70% to 75% of patients) (4). The practitioner can determine which pattern is present by obtaining five or six specimens for semiquantitative analysis over several months. Also, the 24-hour urine protein excretion is almost always less than 1 g in patients with isolated proteinuria. If the total protein excretion is greater than 2 g/24 hours, the chance of significant occult kidney disease is high, and further investigation for nonisolated proteinuria should be considered.

Intermittent Proteinuria

A study of patients with intermittent isolated proteinuria screened by dipstick (protein in fewer than 80% of specimens) revealed definite abnormalities by light microscopy in the renal tissue of approximately 60% of patients; the remainder had normal or almost normal biopsy findings (5). The significance of these findings is unclear, however, in light of another study that retrospectively analyzed the prognostic significance of proteinuria in male college students and found no excess mortality 37 to 45 years later. Morbidity was not studied (6). The Framingham study reported that overall mortality and cardiovascular mortality rates in men were slightly but significantly increased (approximately threefold) in association with proteinuria, in some cases intermittent (7). Analysis of data from the Multiple Risk Factor Intervention Trial (MRFIT) more recently demonstrated that proteinuria is associated with higher all-cause and cardiovascular mortality rates among men with other risk factors for coronary heart disease (i.e., hypertension, elevated serum cholesterol, and cigarette smoking) (8).

In any case, patients who are found to have asymptomatic intermittent proteinuria and who have no evidence of systemic or renal disease can be given an optimistic prognosis. It is unnecessary to perform a kidney biopsy in these patients, but it would be prudent to monitor them yearly with measurement of urine protein excretion, a urinalysis, and determination of serum creatinine. Should deterioration in renal function, significant increase in protein excretion, or new abnormalities occur, reassessment and possibly a renal biopsy would become necessary.

Persistent Proteinuria

Patients with protein in more than 80% of urine specimens screened by dipstick are defined as having persistent proteinuria. The disorder may be further classified by evaluating the effect of posture. *Orthostatic persistent proteinuria* is present when the patient is in the upright position only. *Constant persistent proteinuria* is not influenced by the position of the patient.

Orthostatic Proteinuria. A simple method of determining the presence of this phenomenon is to have the patient collect two urine specimens. The patient rests quietly for 2 hours and then voids just before retiring in the evening to ensure an empty bladder on assuming the recumbent posture. The patient then does not get out of bed for 8 hours. On arising, he or she voids completely into a container labeled *recumbent urine (Specimen 1)*. The patient then stays up but is not vigorously active and collects all subsequent urine over the next 8 hours. This specimen is labeled *ambulatory urine (Specimen 2)*. The protein concentrations in the two urine specimens are compared. This protocol may be simplified if the patient does not drink during the night. In the morning after overnight fluid deprivation, two or more urine specimens are collected consecutively. The first specimen is marked *recumbent* and should be collected immediately on arising. The patient should then resume normal intake of fluid. The second specimen, collected after the patient has been up, active, and ambulating normally for 8 hours, is labeled *ambulatory*. A semiquantitative test (dipstick or SSA) and a measurement of urine concentration to confirm antidiuresis are performed on each sample (4). In patients with orthostatic proteinuria, the recumbent protein excretion is negligible but proteinuria is found when the patient assumes the upright posture.

A renal biopsy is not necessary in the evaluation of a patient with oz thostatic prosteinuria; however, when biopsies have been done as part of a research protocol, minor abnormalities have been defined in approximately one half of the patients, and the others have had a biopsy that appeared normal on light microscopy (studies using electron or immunofluorescent microscopy have not been done) (4). However, it would be prudent to monitor the patient by measuring urinary protein excretion and serum creatinine on a yearly basis even after the proteinuria has cleared.

If orthostatic persistent proteinuria is documented, the prognosis seems to be excellent. Military recruits with this problem have been monitored for 20 years; none developed renal failure, and approximately 80% were no longer proteinuric (9). Not all patients who were free of protein in the urine at 10-year follow-up remained protein free after 20 years, but none showed significant deterioration in renal function. A 35 year follow-up of these same patients did suggest that some developed a decline of renal function greater then expected for normal aging (10).

Constant Proteinuria. In most patients with constant proteinuria, diverse morphologic changes are identified in kidney biopsy specimens. Few long-term studies of these patients have been made, but the course is likely to be indolent. Renal failure develops very rarely, although most patients develop abnormal urine sediment and 50% develop hypertension (11). It is not necessary to perform a renal biopsy if there are no other findings, but yearly re-evaluation is appropriate and should include blood pressure measurement, urinalysis, and determination of 24-hour protein excretion and serum creatinine and creatinine clearance. If proteinuria exceeds 2 g/day, additional evaluation including a sonogram or intravenous pyelogram and collagen vascular screens may be appropriate.

Nonisolated Proteinuria

If an abnormality related to proteinuria is discovered during initial evaluation (e.g., hypertension, hematuria, casts in the urine, renal failure), further investigation may be necessary. The direction and extent of the investigation depend on the nature of the abnormality. Renal biopsy may be indicated, especially if hematuria, red blood cell casts, mild renal failure, or evidence of systemic disease (e.g., systemic lupus erythematosus [SLE]) is present. Table 48.2 lists some additional investigations that may be indicated to evaluate abnormalities associated with proteinuria. A telephone consultation with a nephrologist may be helpful in determining the need for further evaluation.

Table 48.2. Selected Investigations That May Be Appropriate in the Diagnosis of Proteinuria That Is Not Isolated or Is Nephrotic

Antineutrophil cytoplasmic antibody (ANCA) if vasculitis is suspected
Antinuclear antibody if systemic lupus erythematosus is suspected
Antistreptolysin (ASO) titer if there is a possibility of poststreptococcal glomerulonephritis
Complement (C3, C4) if glomerulonephritis is suspected
Complete blood count to provide a baseline evaluation for subsequent use and to provide a clue to a systemic illness (e.g., leukemia)
Erythrocyte sedimentation rate or C-reactive protein if collagen vascular disease is suspected
Fasting blood sugar to consider the possibility of diabetes mellitus
Hepatitis B surface antigen, hepatitis C antibodies by second- or third-generation enzyme-linked immunosorbent assay (ELISA), if hepatitis-associated vasculitis may be present
Radiologic evaluation: Ultrasound, computed tomography, magnetic resonance imaging or on occasion intravenous pyelogram or voiding cystourethrogram to provide evidence for structural renal disease
Rapid plasma reagin (RPR) with history or risk factors for sexually transmitted disease
Serum albumin if nephrotic range proteinuria is present
Serum electrolytes (Na^+, K^+, Cl^-, HCO_3^-, Ca^{2+}, PO_4^{2-}) to provide a screen for abnormalities subsequent to renal disease
Serum and urine protein electrophoresis and immunofixation electrophoresis if multiple myeloma is suspected
Uric acid to screen for urate-related renal disease
Urine culture if pyuria is present
Radiograph of chest to provide evidence for systemic disease (e.g., sarcoidosis)

Microalbuminuria

Among diabetic patients, small increases in urinary albumin excretion (below the detectability limits for usual laboratory screening methods) have been associated with an increased likelihood (up to nine times greater incidence) of development of diabetic nephropathy, retinopathy, and cardiovascular complications, even in patients who are normotensive (12). Several clinical studies have now demonstrated that the use of angiotensin-converting enzyme (ACE) inhibitors (13–17) slows the rate of development of these complications (see Chapter 69). Other investigators (18–19) have demonstrated the renoprotective effect of ACE inhibitors for patients with nondiabetic nephropathy and macroalbuminuria (both nonnephrotic and nephrotic).

Clinical practice recommendations (see American Diabetes Association, 2001, in General References) have been published encouraging that both patients with insulin-dependent diabetes for at least 5 years and all non–insulin-dependent diabetic patients be screened annually for the presence of microalbuminuria. Although semiquantitative dipstick assays exist for the detection of microalbuminuria, quantitative assays performed by a laboratory are still preferred. Microalbuminuria is defined by excretion of 30 to 300 mg albumin in a timed 24-hour urine collection or an albumin/creatinine ratio greater than or equal to 30 μg/mg in a spot urine sample. An abnormal result should be rechecked two or three times over several months.

If microalbuminuria is found repeatedly and does not improve with tighter glycemic control, ACE inhibitor therapy should be considered. (The use of angiotensin receptor blockers for this purpose is currently under investigation.) Stabilization or a fall of up to 30% to 50% in urinary albumin excretion over the ensuing 3 to 6 months indicates response to this intervention. Patients should be monitored for a rise in serum creatinine or the development of hyperkalemia during the first few weeks after initiation of ACE inhibitor therapy and with each dose increase. Serum creatinine often increases slightly as a result of ACE inhibitor therapy (usually to less than 15% to 20% above the patient's baseline concentration) and then reaches a plateau. If serum creatinine increases to a more significant extent, the drug usually should be discontinued or the dose decreased to one that was previously well-tolerated.

NEPHROTIC PROTEINURIA

If a 24-hour protein quantitation reveals more than 3.5 g of protein or if the protein/creatinine ratio is greater than 3.5, nephrotic-range proteinuria is established by definition and is indicative of glomerular disease. Once nephrotic-range proteinuria has been identified, consultation with a nephrologist (if not already obtained) is appropriate to help decide the extent of the workup and to provide suggestions for treatment. There are many causes of nephrotic syndrome, but few conditions are seen with significant frequency in general medical practice (Table 48.3). Clinical and laboratory assessments for systemic illness should be performed first in an effort to establish the etiology of the nephrotic syndrome (e.g., detection of Bence Jones proteinuria, collagen vascular screens for SLE). Table 48.2 lists some of the laboratory evaluations that may be helpful in determining the cause of renal disease. If nephrotic-range proteinuria develops in a patient who has been diabetic for longer than 10 years, the renal lesion is almost always diabetic glomerulosclerosis, particularly if the patient also has diabetic microaneurysms in the retina. In this setting, a renal biopsy usually is unnecessary. On the other hand, a biopsy usually is necessary to diagnose a specific primary renal disease if a diagnosis cannot be made by other tests (e.g., detection of Bence Jones proteinuria, rectal biopsy for amyloid), or it may be needed to guide therapy or to help determine prognosis (e.g., SLE).

Table 48.3. Causes of Nephrotic Syndrome in Adults[a]

- Most common
  - Diabetes mellitus
  - Idiopathic membranous glomerulopathy
  - Idiopathic lipoid nephrosis (including minimal change disease, mesangial proliferative glomerulonephritis, focal segmental glomerulosclerosis)
- Less common
  - Proliferative glomerulonephritis (crescentic glomerulonephritis)
  - Membranoproliferative glomerulonephritis
  - Collagen vascular disease
  - Amyloidosis

[a]An extensive list of potential causes of nephrotic syndrome can be found in Falk RJ, Jennette JC, Nachman PH. Primary glomerular disease. In: Brenner BM, ed., Brenner and Rector's the kidney. 6th ed. Philadelphia: WB Saunders, 2000:1267.

Renal Biopsy

Patient Experience. In general, in patients without renal failure and normal hemostasis, percutaneous biopsy is performed under local anesthesia with computed tomographic or sonographic guidance. This technique permits the nephrologist to sample the lower portion of the kidney, avoiding the hilar vessels and the renal collecting system. With percutaneous biopsy, the patient usually experiences minimal discomfort and is able to be out of bed in 6 to 12 hours.

The biopsy core is approximately 1 mm in diameter and 10 to 20 mm in length. Usually two such tissue cores are obtained. The risk associated with percutaneous renal biopsy is small if it is performed by an experienced physician.

Microscopic hematuria after the procedure is almost inevitable, and usually there is a small hematoma at the biopsy site on the surface of the kidney. However, it usually is of no clinical consequence. Gross hematuria occurs in 5% to 10% of patients, but less than 5% of this group require a transfusion to replace blood loss. Fewer than 1 in 1,000 patients require nephrectomy because of continued massive bleeding, and death from biopsy is rare. A renal arteriovenous fistula may develop after biopsy, but it usually closes spontaneously. Rarely, this complication may require treatment if bleeding continues or if hypertension develops (see Stiles et al., 2000, in General References). Even more rarely, there may be perforation of another viscus.

When percutaneous biopsy is not feasible (e.g., obesity, ectopic location, small size of kidney), open transjugular or laparoscopic biopsy can be obtained; some surgeons perform this procedure under local anesthesia in selected patients (see Stiles et al., 2000, in General References).

Regardless of the technique of obtaining the biopsy, the evaluation of tissue by a pathologist experienced in preparation and interpretation of renal biopsy material includes light, immunofluorescent, and electron microscopy.

The practitioner who has referred to a nephrologist a patient for whom a renal biopsy has been performed should expect communication of the following: the probable diagnosis, based on all aspects of the microscopic assessment; whether specific therapy for the condition is indicated; and what prognostic judgment can be made.

TREATMENT OF PATIENTS WITH PROTEINURIA

Patient care is directed at diagnosis, education, surveillance, and treatment of any underlying disease (renal biopsy findings may help target specific interventions). If proteinuria is believed to be caused by a drug, the agent should be discontinued. Proteinuria from drugs may take several months to resolve, and occasionally it is permanent. In addition, judicious use of ACE inhibitors has been associated with a decrease in proteinuria and perhaps stabilization of renal function and improvement of protein and lipid metabolism (13–20). As discussed earlier, when ACE inhibitors are used there should be surveillance for hyperkalemia and acute renal failure.

If either edema or hypoalbuminemia is present, special therapy may be indicated. In the absence of renal failure, albumin synthesis is either increased or normal in patients with the nephrotic syndrome. Until recently, treatment included provision of a high-protein diet (2 to 3 g of protein per kilogram of dry weight, that is, estimated or actual weight before edema developed). Currently, mild to moderate protein restriction rather than protein supplementation is advised, because it is believed that high protein intake may lead to progressive renal dysfunction by producing hyperfiltration (21). ACE inhibitor therapy (and possibly angiotensin receptor blockers) may also ameliorate these findings. Appropriate standards for protein intake and pharmacologic intervention in this setting remain controversial and are a subject of intense research.

In the presence of edema, salt restriction to a tolerable level, such as a no-added-salt diet (approximately 2 to 3 g/day of sodium; see Chapter 67) is appropriate. If the edema is more severe and is unresponsive to sodium chloride restriction, cautious use of a loop diuretic (furosemide, torsemide, or bumetanide) may be necessary. No attempt should be made to rid the patient entirely of edema, which could risk contraction of the circulating volume, with serious consequences. Potassium-sparing diuretics (spironolactone, triamterene, or amiloride) may be added if renal failure is absent. Metolazone or thiazides may be added if loop diuretics have not been entirely adequate. Monitoring of serum potassium is important for selection and adjustment of the diuretic regimen, especially if ACE inhibitors are used in this setting. In many instances, the patient can establish the correct diuretic dosage schedule by keeping a diary of weights and drug intake. If acceptable control is still not achieved, consultation with a nephrologist is appropriate.

Numerous extrarenal complications are associated with nephrotic syndrome. These include alterations in cellular immunity leading to increased infections, hyperlipidemia, and changes in calcium and bone metabolism. Nephrotic syndrome can be associated with a hypercoagulable state with thrombosis of the renal veins as well as other vessels. Clues to the development of this complication include pulmonary embolism, sudden deterioration in renal function, significant increase in the level of proteinuria, back or flank pain, and the development of hematuria. Suspicion of this complication requires hospitalization of the patient for urgent evaluation. Patients with nephrotic syndrome should be counseled about risk factors for deep venous thrombosis, such as long periods of immobilization. This is especially true for patients with membranous glomerulonephritis, although renal vein thrombosis has been reported in all types of glomerulonephritis.

Prediction of the course and selection of specific therapy in patients with nephrotic-range proteinuria depend on the pathologic pattern that is identified in the biopsy. Patients with nephrotic-range proteinuria need regularly scheduled office visits at 1- to 4-month intervals. Usually this follow-up is done by the primary care provider and the patient sees the nephrologist only once a year. The office visit provides an opportunity to review the patient's symptoms and to perform a limited physical examination (which, at a minimum, should include weight, volume assessment, and blood pressure) as well as to evaluate the 24-hour urine protein excretion or a protein/creatinine ratio, the renal function (creatinine or creatinine clearance), and the serum electrolytes if diuretics are being used. Less often, an assessment of the serum albumin may be necessary.

General References*

Ibrahim HN, Rosenberg ME, Hostetter TH. Proteinuria. In: Seldin DW, Giebisch G, eds. The kidney: physiology and pathophysiology. 3rd ed. Philadelphia: Lippincott Williams & Wilkins, 2000:2269.

Excellent summary of the physiologic basis, evaluation, and treatment of proteinuria.

Keane WF. Proteinuria: its clinical importance and role in progressive renal disease. Am J Kidney Dis 2000;35[Suppl 1]:S97.

Overall review of the association of microalbuminuria and cardiovascular disease, of proteinuria and the progression of renal disease, and recent studies evaluating the effect of pharmacologic interventions that reduce proteinuria on renal outcomes.

Stiles KP, Yuan CM, Chung EM, et al. Renal biopsy in high-risk patients with medical diseases of the kidney. Am J Kidney Dis 2000; 36:419.

Review of conventional and alternative methods for biopsy of the kidney with discussion of contraindications and complications.

Standards of medical care for patients with diabetes mellitus. American Diabetes Association. Diabetes Care 2001;24[Suppl 1]: S33.

Consensus statement enumerating evidence-based clinical practice guidelines for evaluation and management of proteinuria.

Specific References

1. Iseki K, Iseki C, Ikemiya Y, et al. Risk of developing end-stage renal disease in a cohort of mass screening. Kidney Int 1996;49:800.
2. Woolhandler S, Pels RJ, Bor DH, et al. Dipstick urinalysis screening of asymptomatic adults for urinary tract disorders. I: Hematuria and proteinuria. JAMA 1989;262:121.
3. Ginsberg JM, Chang BS, Matarese RA, et al. Use of single voided urine samples to estimate quantitative proteinuria. N Engl J Med 1983;309:1543.

*Bold print (general references) and bold numerals (specific references) denote published controlled clinical trials, meta-analyses, or consensus-based recommendations.

4. Robinson RR. Isolated proteinuria in asymptomatic patients. Kidney Int 1980;18:395.
5. Muth RG. Asymptomatic mild intermittent proteinuria: a percutaneous renal biopsy study. Arch Intern Med 1965;115:569.
6. Levitt JI. The prognostic significance of proteinuria in young college students. Ann Intern Med 1967;66:685.
7. Kannel WB, Stampfer MJ, Castelli WP, et al. The prognostic significance of proteinuria: the Framingham study. Am Heart J 1984;108:1347.
8. Grimm RH, Svendsen KH, Kasiske B, et al. Proteinuria is a risk factor for mortality over 10 years of follow-up. MRFIT Research Group, Multiple Risk Factor Intervention Trial. Kidney Int 1997;63[Suppl]:S10.
9. Springberg PD, Garrett LE, Thompson AL Jr, et al. Fixed reproducible orthostatic proteinuria: results of a 20-year follow-up study. Ann Intern Med 1982;97:516.
10. Martin-Arevalo DL, Yee J, Pugh J, et al. Fixed and reproducible orthostatic proteinuria: a 35-yr follow-up study. J Am Soc Nephrol 1996;7:1323(abst).
11. King SE. Diastolic hypertension and chronic proteinuria. Am J Cardiol 1962;9:669.
12. Nelson RG, Knowler WC, Pettitt DJ, et al. Assessment of risk of overt nephropathy in diabetic patients from albumin excretion in untimed urine samples. Arch Intern Med 1991;151:1761.
13. Lewis EJ, Hunsicker LG, Bain RP, et al. The effect of angiotensin-converting enzyme inhibition on diabetic nephropathy. N Engl J Med 1993;329:1456.
14. Mathiesen ER, Hommel E, Giese J, et al. Efficacy of captopril in postponing nephropathy in normotensive insulin dependent diabetic patients with microalbuminuria. BMJ 1991;303:81.
15. Ravid M, Savin H, Jutrin I, et al. Long-term stabilizing effect of angiotensin-converting enzyme inhibition on plasma creatinine and on proteinuria in normotensive type II diabetic patients. Ann Intern Med 1994;118:577.
16. Sano T, Kawamura T, Matsumae H, et al. Effects of long-term enalapril treatment on persistent micro-albuminuria in well-controlled hypertensive and normotensive NIDDM patients. Diabetes Care 1994;17:420.
17. Heart Outcomes Prevention Evaluation Study Investigators. Effects of ramipril on cardiovascular and microvascular outcomes in people with diabetes mellitus: results of the HOPE study and MICRO-HOPE substudy. Lancet 2000;45:601.
18. The GISEN Group (Gruppo Italiano di Studi Epidemiologici in Nefrologia). Randomised placebo-controlled trial of effect of ramipril on decline in glomerular filtration rate and risk of terminal renal failure in proteinuric, non-diabetic nephropathy. Lancet 1997;349:1857.
19. Ruggenenti P, Perna A, Gherardi G, et al. Renoprotective properties of ACE-inhibition in non-diabetic nephropathies with non-nephrotic proteinuria. Lancet 1999;354:359.
20. Praga M, Hernandez E, Montoyo C, et al. Long-term beneficial effects of angiotensin-converting enzyme inhibition in patients with nephrotic proteinuria. Am J Kidney Dis 1992;20:240.
21. Brenner BM, Lawler EV, Mackenzie HS. The hyperfiltration theory: a paradigm shift in nephrology. Kidney Int 1996;49:1774.

CHAPTER 49

Hematuria

DAVID A. SPECTOR, MD

Normal individuals excrete up to 2 million red blood cells (RBCs) into the urine daily; this is equivalent to one to three RBCs per high-power microscopic field (HPF) with standard urinalysis techniques. The finding of greater numbers of RBCs in the urine constitutes abnormal hematuria, although the exact level separating normal from abnormal is arbitrary. Benzidine- or orthotolidine-impregnated, hemoglobin-sensitive dipsticks, widely used as screening tests for hemoglobinuria (usually caused by lysis of RBCs in the urine and therefore an indication of hematuria), are less sensitive than microscopy but are usually positive in urine that contains three RBCs per HPF. The rate at which RBCs lyse depends on the concentration of the urine in which they are found and the duration of time they are exposed. Usually some lysis occurs within a few minutes, especially when the urine is dilute. There are certain limits to the use of hemoglobin-sensitive dipsticks (Table 49.1).

Microscopic hematuria may or may not indicate serious genitourinary tract disease (1,2). The symptoms, signs, and laboratory findings associated with hematuria and the clinical setting in which it occurs help considerably in predicting the seriousness of the finding. For example, gross hematuria or hematuria associated with proteinuria or pyuria is highly predictive of a significant disease. Conversely, asymptomatic microhematuria in a young adult has little predictive value.

PSEUDOHEMATURIA

A large number of substances can impart a color to urine that may be mistaken for hematuria (3). *Exogenous sources* of some of these substances are listed in Table 49.2. *Endogenous substances* capable

Table 49.1. Limits of Dipstick Method for Detection of Blood in the Urine

Reasons for a Positive Test
Hematuria greater than approximately 5–10 RBCs/HPF
Hematuria with lysis of RBCs
  From hypotonic urine (specific gravity <1.008)
  From highly alkaline urine (pH >6.5)
Hemoglobinuria from intravascular hemolysis
Myoglobinuria from muscle injury
False positive reactions
  From hypochlorite (bleach) contamination of container
  From peroxidase (from heavy growth of bacteria)

Reasons for a False Negative Test
Vitamin C: Ingestion of large amounts of vitamin C (>200 mg/d) results in diminished oxidation potential of the test material. The dipstick test may miss trace quantities of blood, although usually there is a quantitative decrease in the estimate of blood (such as 3+ to 2+). (This is of concern only if RBCs are observed but the dipstick test is negative.)
Formaldehyde: Ingestion of bacterial suppressant agents (such as Mandelamine or Hiprex) that produce formaldehyde in acid urine or contamination of the container with formaldehyde diminish the oxidizing potential of the reagent strips. This results in a quantitative estimate error or, if hematuria is minimal, false negative result.

HPF, high-power field; RBCs, red blood cells.

Table 49.2. Exogenous Substances That May Cause Pseudohematuria[a]

Type	Examples
Medications	
Analgesics	Phenacetin, phenazopyridine (e.g., Pyridium)
Antimicrobials	Nitrofurantoin, rifampin, sulfonamides
Antimalarials	Chloroquine, primaquine
Laxatives	Anthraquinones: cascara, senna, danthron (e.g., Modane or Dorbane)
Anticancer agents	Doxorubicin, daunorubicin
Others	Deferoxamine (an iron-chelating agent), levodopa, phenothiazines, methyldopa (rare)
Vegetable Dyes	
Anthocyanins: beets, blackberries	
Paprika	
Rhubarb	
Fuscin (a reddish dye used in topical agents)	
Others	
Antiseptics	Mercurochrome, phenols, cresols, povidone-iodine (Betadine)
Urate crystals (in acid urine)	

[a]Some of these agents cause hemoglobinuria.

of producing a reddish hue include porphyrins, myoglobin, and hemoglobin. Myoglobin and hemoglobin also cause positive reactions in tests for RBCs. Therefore, when the urine dipstick is positive and the microscopy is negative for RBCs, myoglobinuria or hemoglobinuria should be suspected. Both are serious findings and warrant further evaluation. Myoglobinuria indicates substantial muscle disease or injury, and hemoglobinuria indicates significant hematuria (with lysis of RBCs) or hemolysis. However, the dipstick reaction will be falsely positive in the presence of oxidizing substances (e.g., if there is heavy hypochlorite (bleach, chlorine) or peroxidase (from bacteria) contamination of the urine specimen or its container). A false-negative dipstick test may also occur when formaldehyde (e.g., present as a breakdown product of methenine) or large amounts of vitamin C are in the urine, because both substances decrease the sensitivity of the test reagent.

INNOCENT HEMATURIA

Microscopic hematuria often is identified after a genitourinary tract examination such as a pelvic or prostate examination, cystoscopy or bladder catheterization, or biopsy of prostate, bladder, or kidney. Occasionally, gross hematuria may be seen in this setting. Gross or microscopic hematuria is also sometimes present after vigorous exercise such as swimming, lacrosse, boxing, football, or running. This finding is most common in long-distance runners, and in one study, 18% of athletes were found to have hematuria after the completion of a marathon (4). Hematuria in all such settings subsides in 24 to 48 hours. It does not signify underlying genitourinary disease if it resolves quickly and does not recur spontaneously. In exercisers (especially runners), proteinuria or cast formation sometimes accompanies the hematuria, and the red cells have been found to be dysmorphic, suggesting that the bleeding site is the glomerulus.

HEMATURIA WITH PYURIA

If a patient is found to have hematuria associated with pyuria (with or without irritative symptoms such as frequency, urgency, or dysuria), an infectious cause is most likely and bacterial cultures of the urine should be obtained. If a specific organism is identified, appropriate antimicrobial therapy should be given (see Chapter 36). After treatment, the patient should be monitored carefully (including urinalysis) for 4 to 6 weeks to ensure that the hematuria has been eradicated and does not recur. If irritative symptoms suggesting infection have been present and the routine culture is sterile, a *sexually transmitted disease* (especially *Chlamydia* infection or gonorrhea), a viral infection, or tuberculosis (now a rare cause of hematuria) should be suspected. *Chlamydia trachomatis* infection (see Chapters 36 and 102), especially may be manifested by hematuria and pyuria with minimal irritative symptoms. When a sexually transmitted infection is suspected but cannot be proved, a therapeutic trial of an antimicrobial drug may be given (see Chapters 36 and 102). *Viral cystitis* is a fairly common infection of young women. It has a short-lived natural course (2 to 3 days), and it is nonrecurrent. Suspicion of *tuberculosis of the urinary tract* requires several weeks to confirm by culture. (An acid-fast stain of a voided specimen of urine is not a reliable indicator because of the regular presence of acid-fast material from smegma bacilli. These bacilli would be eliminated by obtaining a catheterized urine specimen but most experts suggest simply waiting for the culture results in the typical patient in whom tuberculosis is a consideration.) Rarely, one may encounter a patient who is from an area endemic for schistosomiasis, and in this situation, the presence of hematuria should raise a question of this infection. Because noninfectious disorders of the bladder (including malignancies) may also present with irritative symptoms (see Chapter 53), one should ensure that those symptoms have abated after treatment, especially in patients older than 50 years of age, and it is probably prudent to confirm that the patient's urinalysis is normal 4 to 6 weeks after completion of treatment for this infection.

HEMATURIA WITH PROTEINURIA, RED BLOOD CELL CASTS, OR DYSMORPHIC RED BLOOD CELLS

Hematuria associated with proteinuria reflects either glomerulonephritis or interstitial nephritis. When proteinuria is greater than 2 g in 24 hours or RBC casts are present, the diagnosis is probably glomerulonephritis (see Chapter 48). The morphologic appearance on microscopy of the RBCs may help differentiate glomerular from nonglomerular bleeding (5). This observation takes advantage of the deformation of the cytoplasmic content of RBCs after their passage into the Bowman space. If more than 80% of at least 100 (counted) RBCs appear dysmorphic (abnormal size, shape, and cytoplasmic staining) by Wright stain (or phase contrast microscopy, if available) of the urinary sediment, glomerular bleeding is very likely. In particular, acanthocytes (ringform RBCs with vesicle-shaped protrusions), when present, almost always indicate glomerular disease (6). If glomerulonephritis is suspected, estimation of the glomerular filtration rate and quantitative 24-hour urine protein excretion are indicated. Also, a thorough evaluation for a possible cause should be conducted. Chapter 48 suggests an approach. Although any form of glomerulonephritis may be present, immunoglobulin A nephropathy (Berger disease) (7), Alport syndrome (hereditary nephritis, often associated with deafness), and thin basement membrane disease are especially likely in situations in which the hematuria has been an incidental finding. Each of these diseases is characterized by recurrent episodes of microscopic or gross hematuria, variable or no proteinuria, and a variable course. A nephrologist should be consulted when these or other forms of glomerulonephritis are suspected. Often the nephrologist will perform a renal biopsy (see Chapter 48) to establish the diagnosis, estimate the prognosis, and determine treatment.

ASYMPTOMATIC ISOLATED MICROHEMATURIA

The prevalence of isolated microscopic hematuria depends on the stringency of the diagnostic criteria (e.g., number of RBCs per HPF, number of "positive" tests required) and the population studied. For example, in each of five studies of young adults, less then 1% of the study population had asymptomatic hematuria (8). In contrast, in multiple studies of high-risk older men, 13% to 21% of the population had asymptomatic hematuria (9).

Causes of Asymptomatic Hematuria

Most series describing the causes of microscopic hematuria come from the urology-oriented literature and emphasize diagnoses likely to be made by cystoscopic and radiographic evaluation (Table 49.3).

In all series, no specific diagnosis was made for many patients, in part because patient evaluations were usually incomplete. For example, most series did not include a renal biopsy, which may have revealed glomerular or interstitial disease (10,11). The importance of this omission was borne out by one study in which 51 of 65 adult patients with hematuria with minimal or no proteinuria and a negative urologic workup had a specific diagnosis established only after the performance of a renal biopsy (10).

Table 49.3. Distribution (%) of Selected Urologic Findings in Asymptomatic Patients with Microhematuria

Finding	Mariani et al. (13) (694 pts., HMO Urology Referrals[a])	Golin and Howard (17) (246 pts., Urology Referral)	Khadra et al. (18) (982 pts., Hematuria Clinic[b])	Mohr et al. (19) (781 pts., Rochester MN Population[c])	Bard (1) (177 Women, Urology Referral)	Messing et al. (20) (192 Men>50 Yr Screened for Hematuria)
Neoplasia	8.5	9.3	5.4	1.0	0	8.3
Other disorders						
Renal calculi	3.4	0	4.0	3.3	1.6	8.9
Ureteral calculi	0.6	1.0	0	0.9	0.6	
Nephritis/renal insufficiency	1.2	2.0	9.4	14.4	0	1.0
Benign prostatic hypertrophy	16.5	8.0	—[f]	37.7	—	47.4
Urinary tract infection	4.3	2.0	13.0	0.5	—[d]	2.6
Urethrotrigonitis/prostatitis	37.7	18.0	—[f]	1.8	32.6	—
Any finding[e]	88.3	47.6	31.8	62.5	63.0	84.9

[a]Original series of 1,000 patients included 309 patients with gross hematuria.
[b]Original series of 1,930 patients included 948 with gross hematuria.
[c]Complete urologic workup not performed on all patients.
[d]Women with urinary tract infection excluded from study.
[e]Includes those listed above in addition to other findings that may or may not have been related to the hematuria. These include hydronephrosis, renal cysts, polycystic kidney disease, vesicoureteral reflux, interstitial and radiation cystitis, diverticula, ureteropelvic junction obstruction, ureterocele, cystocele, neurogenic bladder, atrophic vagina, scarred kidney, cystitis cystica, polyps, papillary necrosis, calcified renal mass, and trabeculated bladder. Some patients in all series had more than one disorder.
[f]Unable to determine from data.

In addition, most series did not include quantitation of 24-hour urine calcium and uric acid. Hypercalciuria (more than 300 mg/24 hours) or hyperuricosuria (more than 750 mg/24 hours in women; more than 800 mg/24 hours in men) has been shown to cause hematuria (presumably as a result of irritation of the tubules by microcrystals), and thiazide therapy (which reduces calciuria) or allopurinol stops the bleeding in these circumstances (12).

In general, neoplasia is more commonly reported in series comprising older individuals or patients referred to urologists; conversely, neoplasia is rarely found in population-based series of young patients. Renal biopsy, when performed, often reveals a glomerular cause of hematuria in younger patients in whom the workup is otherwise unrevealing, and it also may reveal glomerular lesions in up to 40% of cases, even in elderly patients (11). As in patients with combined hematuria and proteinuria, the most likely biopsy findings in patients with asymptomatic hematuria are immunoglobulin A nephritis, followed by Alport disease and thin basement membrane disease (11).

EVALUATION OF PATIENTS WITH HEMATURIA

Pseudohematuria and drug-induced hematuria (Table 49.4) should be ruled out. The evaluation then depends on associated symptoms, on whether the bleeding is gross or microscopic, and on the results of the complete urinalysis (discussed earlier). Localization of the site of the bleeding in the genitourinary tract is the first priority. The associated symptoms and the history of temporal events often provide diagnostic clues. For example, colicky flank pain suggests that the hematuria is emanating from the ureter, whereas dysuria and urinary frequency suggest that the bleeding is from the bladder. All patients should be asked about the temporal relationship of the hematuria to exercise, to ingestion of medications or food, and to trauma. The urinalysis is helpful also if findings suggest glomerular disease or infection (see earlier discussion). In some studies, the seriousness of the underlying lesion was proportional to the number of RBCs per HPF, and patients with gross hematuria were especially at risk for serious or life-threatening illness (13).

Table 49.4. Examples of Drugs Causing Hematuria

Antimicrobials
Penicillin analogs[a]
Cephalosporin analogs[a]
Sulfa analogs[a]
Polymycin[a]
Rifampin[a]

Analgesics and Anti-Inflammatory Agents
Aspirin[b]
Aminosalicylic acid[b]
Nonsteroidal anti-inflammatory agents[a]

Diuretics
Furosemide[a]
Ethacrynic acid[a]
Thiazides[a]

Anticoagulants
Warfarin (Coumadin)[c]

Other
Cyclophosphamide[d]
Ifosfamide (Isex, an antineoplastic agent)[d]
Danazol[d]

[a]Infrequent bleeding caused by interstitial nephritis, usually occurring within days to weeks of taking drugs; usually reversible.

[b]Infrequent bleeding caused by medullary/papillary necrosis, usually following many months or years of combination analgesic preparations; partially reversible.

[c]An underlying cause of hematuria is often found and a workup should be considered (Cuttino JT Jr, Clark RL, Feaster SH, Zwicke DL. The evaluation of gross hematuria in anticoagulated patients: efficacy of i.v. urography and cystoscopy. AJR Am J Roentgenol 1987;149:527.)

[d]Bleeding caused by hemorrhagic cystitis in 10%–20% of patients; dose-related and usually reversible.

A focused history and physical examination should be performed to seek clues to illnesses with which hematuria is associated (e.g., a nodular prostate suggestive of prostate cancer, cutaneous or other abnormalities suggestive of a collagen vascular disease). When the history and physical examination, together with selected laboratory procedures (e.g., urine culture) and treatment (e.g., antimicrobial agents), do not support a working diagnosis, certain laboratory data should be obtained. This evaluation should include a complete blood count, an estimate of glomerular function (e.g., serum creatinine), a sickle cell preparation (in the appropriate host), a 24-hour urine specimen for determination of calcium and uric acid concentrations (see earlier discussion), and an intravenous pyelogram with tomography (if the creatinine concentration is not significantly elevated and the patient has no history of dye allergy). In patients with a suspected bleeding disorder, a platelet count and measurement of the prothrombin, partial thromboplastin, and bleeding times should be done. Even if an underlying bleeding diathesis is identified, the search for a pathologic process in the genitourinary tract should continue, because one is usually identified (see Chapter 56). In patients older than 40 to 50 years of age, two or three fresh morning urine specimens should be evaluated by a cytology laboratory for the presence of tumor cells. The sensitivity of cytology in this setting is 30% when an upper tract tumor is present and 50% to 90% when a bladder tumor is present (with higher rates of detection for higher grades of cancer). However, because cystoscopy (discussed later) is the diagnostic procedure of choice when bladder cancer is suspected, many urologists suggest that cytology not be done until after cystoscopy has been performed, and then only when that procedure is negative for cancer but the clinician remains suspicious of the presence of a urinary tract neoplasia. In recent years a number of methods of detecting voided protein tumor markers (e.g., BTA, NMP22, Lewis x Antigen, CD44V) have been promoted for use in evaluating recurrence of bladder tumors (9). Although the use of voided tumor markers in the evaluation of patients with hematuria is promising, the available data are insufficient currently to warrant their routine use for that purpose.

Nevertheless, if neoplasia is a consideration (patient older than 40 to 50 years of age or younger but with a risk factor for bladder cancer), a urologist should be consulted and the patient should undergo cystoscopy (see Chapter 53) (14). Risk factors for bladder cancer include a heavy occupational exposure (e.g., to aromatic amines, dyes, benzidine, paint ingredients [see Chapter 8]); prolonged daily use of analgesics (phenacetin, acetaminophen, and aspirin combinations have been reported to be associated with genitourinary cancer); heavy smoking; and a history of pelvic irradiation or use of cyclophosphamide. If neoplasia is a strong consideration, the urologist might also suggest evaluation of the patient by sonography, computed tomographic (CT) scanning, magnetic resonance imaging, or renal angiography.

If neoplasia is not strongly considered and persistent hematuria is present or recurrent, the patient should be referred to a nephrologist for consideration of renal biopsy (see Chapter 48).

If no etiologic basis for microscopic hematuria is initially found, follow-up evaluations should be performed. Although in some patients microhematuria is transient and benign, in others with persistent hematuria, genitourinary neoplasms or calculi are discovered 1 to 3 years after the onset of hematuria (15,16).

Gross Hematuria

If gross hematuria is present, the evaluation should proceed initially in the same manner as for microscopic hematuria, but there are several caveats. Blood clots in the urine suggest that bleeding is from the bladder. Clots may occasionally result from upper urinary tract bleeding, although in that situation ureteral colic is likely to occur. It should be remembered that plasma protein may be lost into the urine (and then be detected by qualitative or quantitative testing) in large quantities yet not reflect a glomerular disease. However, the concentration of urinary protein rarely exceeds 1 g/day when it occurs as a result of blood in the urine alone. The *three-glass test* is sometimes useful in determining the site of gross bleeding. This test is performed by having the patient void into containers in a sequence: The initial 10 mL of urine represents the urethral specimen, the *middle portion* of urine voided is nondiagnostic of a specific location, and blood in the *terminal portion* (the last few drops of urine) suggests that the site is likely to be the prostate, bladder neck, or proximal urethra. Blood present in all three specimens is not specific for the site of origin. The finding of blood in one of three specimens may correlate with clinical symptoms, but this relationship is not reliable.

In patients with persistent gross hematuria, a urologist should always be consulted promptly, because the most opportune time to identify the site is when the bleeding is active.

The surveillance of a patient found to have gross hematuria depends on the cause (Table 49.5). If no cause is found, close surveillance (every 6 months for several years) is indicated, because some of these patients have a serious underlying disorder, such as a tumor or glomerulonephritis. This surveillance should include reviewing the history, performing a physical examination, obtaining a urinalysis and determining the urea nitrogen and creatinine concentrations, and, in situations in which a tumor is considered, obtaining a urine specimen for cytologic examination and referring the patient to a urologist for a cystoscopic examination.

Table 49.5. Diagnosis Established in Patients with Gross Hematuria

Diagnosis	Percentage
Nondiagnostic	52.5
Renal cancer	0.9
Urothelial cancer	0.1
Bladder cancer	19.3
Prostate cancer	0.6
Stone disease	3.2
Urinary tract infection	13.0
Nephrologic disease	10.3
	(100.0)

Adapted from Khadra MH, Pickard RS, Charlton M, et al. A prospective analysis of 1,930 patients with hematuria to evaluate current diagnostic practice. J Urol 2000;163:524–527; and represents 948 patients with gross hematuria from an original series of 1,930 patients who were referred to a hematuria clinic with either gross or microscopic findings.

HEMATOSPERMIA

The presence of blood in the ejaculate of men is an alarming but usually innocuous symptom. This problem occurs most often in men older than 40 years of age, and most often the episodes recur over several weeks or months. If hematospermia occurs in an otherwise asymptomatic man who has a normal physical examination (including rectal examination of the prostate and seminal vesicles) and a normal urinalysis, the patient should be reassured that it is innocuous and that no further workup is necessary. If there is any abnormality, further evaluation for benign prostatic hypertrophy or cancer of the prostate, seminal vesicles, bladder, or urethra should be considered and a urologist should be consulted.

General References*

Abarbanel J, Benet AE, Lask D, et al. Sports hematuria. J Urol 1990;143:887.

Buntix F, Wauters H. **The diagnostic value of microscopic hematuria in diagnosing urological cancer: a meta-analysis.** Fam Pract 1997;14:63.

Leary FJ, Aguilo JJ. Clinical significance of hematospermia. Mayo Clin Proc 1974;49:815.

Sutton JM. Evaluation of hematuria in adults. JAMA 1990;263:2475.

Grossfeld GD, Carroll PR. Evaluation of asymptomatic microscopic hematuria. Urol Clin North Am 1998;25:661.

Specific References

1. Bard RH. The significance of asymptomatic microhematuria in women and its economic implications. Arch Intern Med 1988;148:2629.

*Bold print (general references) and bold numerals (specific references) denote published controlled clinical trials, meta-analyses, or consensus-based recommendations.

2. Mohr DN, Offord KP, Melton LJ III. Isolated asymptomatic microhematuria: a cross-sectional analysis of test-positive and test-negative patients. J Gen Intern Med 1987;2:318.
3. Young DS, Pestaner LC, Gibberman V. Effects of drugs on clinical laboratory tests. Clin Chem 1975;21:1D.
4. Siegel AJ, Hennikens CH, Solomon HS, et al. Exercise-related hematuria: findings in a group of marathon runners. JAMA 1987;241:391.
5. Chang BS. Red cell morphology as a diagnostic aid in hematuria. JAMA 1984;252:1747.
6. Kohler H, Wandel E, Brunck B. Acanthocyturia: a characteristic marker for glomerular bleeding. Kidney Int 1991;40:115.
7. D'Amico G. Clinical features and natural history in adults with IgA nephropathy. Am J Kidney Dis 1988;12:353.
8. Woolhandler S, Pels RJ, Bor DH, et al. Dipstick urinalysis screening of asymptomatic adults for urinary tract disorders. JAMA 1989;262:1214.
9. Grossfeld GD, Litwin MS, Wolf JS Jr, et al. Evaluation of asymptomatic microscopic hematuria in adults: the American Urological Association best practice policy. Part I: definition, detection, prevalence, and etiology. Part II: patient evaluation, cytology, voided markers, imaging, cystoscopy, nephrology evaluation, and follow-up. Urology 2001;57:599.
10. Copley JB, Hasbargen JA. Idiopathic hematuria: a prospective evaluation. Arch Intern Med 1987;147:434.
11. Topham PS, Harper SJ, Furness PN, et al. Glomerular disease as a cause of isolated microscopic hematuria. QJM 1994;87:329.
12. Andres A, Praga M, Bello I, et al. Hematuria due to hypercalciuria and hyperuricosuria in adult patients. Kidney Int 1989;36:96.
13. Mariani AJ, Mariani MC, Macchioni C, et al. The significance of adult hematuria: 1000 hematuria evaluations including a risk–benefit and cost-effectiveness analysis. J Urol 1989; 141:350.
14. Carter WC III, Rous SN. Gross hematuria in 110 adult urologic hospital patients. Urology 1981;18:342.
15. Murakami S, Igarashi T, Hara S, et al. Strategies for asymptomatic microscopic hematuria: a prospective study of 1,034 patients. J Urol 1990;144:99.
16. Nieuwhof C, Doorenbos C, Grave W, et al. A prospective study of the natural history of idiopathic non proteinuric hematuria. Kidney Int 1996;49:222.
17. Golin AL, Howard RS. Asymptomatic microscopic hematuria. J Urol 1980;124:389.
18. Khadra MH, Pickard RS, Charlton M, et al. A prospective analysis of 1,930 patients with hematuria to evaluate current diagnostic practice. J Urol 2000;163:524.
19. Mohr DN, Offord KP, Owen RA, et al. Asymptomatic microhematuria and urologic disease: a population based study. JAMA 1986;256:224.
20. Messing EM, Young TB, Hunt VB, et al. Home screening for hematuria: results of a multi-clinic study. J Urol 1992;148: 289.

CHAPTER 50

Hypokalemia*

JOHN E. ANDERSON, MD

Hypokalemia—serum potassium concentration less than 3.5 mEq/L—occurs in fewer than 1% of normal, healthy people. It is, however, common in ambulatory practice, and is often the consequence of drug therapy or disease. Although it is often thought to be trivial and is sometimes ignored, hypokalemia may be important in disorders such as hypertension, cardiovascular disease, and cerebrovascular disease. When severe, it can be life-threatening, but even mild hypokalemia may also predispose to death. Loss of potassium through the gastrointestinal tract or the kidneys accounts for most cases of hypokalemia seen in ambulatory practice, with less common causes occasionally encountered. The physiology of potassium homeostasis, the clinical consequences of potassium depletion, an approach to the differential diagnosis, and the management of hypokalemia are reviewed in this chapter.

PHYSIOLOGIC BACKGROUND

The serum potassium concentration depends on the total body potassium content and the distribution

*Kevin A. Rossiter, MD, contributed to this chapter in the last edition.

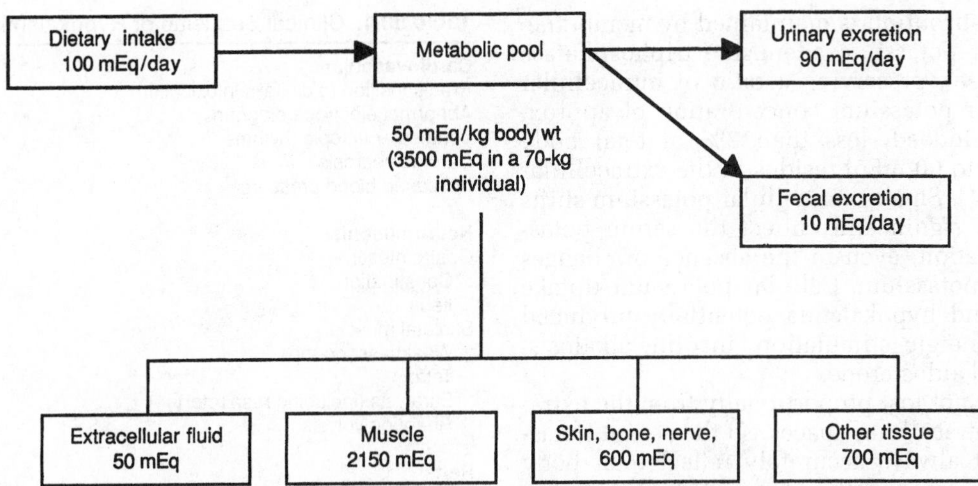

Figure 50.1. Balance of potassium. (Adapted from Kliger AS, Hayslett JP. Disorders of potassium. In: Brenner BM, Stein JH, eds. Acid-base and potassium homeostasis. New York: Churchill Livingstone, 1978.)

of potassium between the intracellular and extracellular spaces. Total body potassium, normally about 50 mEq/kg, is determined by the external balance between the intake and excretion of potassium. In health, excretion matches intake and total body potassium remains essentially constant (Fig. 50.1). The internal balance or distribution of potassium between the intracellular and extracellular spaces may vary even in the absence of changes in the external balance of potassium (1).

External Potassium Balance

The average intake of potassium is approximately 1 mEq/kg body weight per day. Normally about 90% is absorbed and excreted in the urine, and the remainder is eliminated in the stool (Fig. 50.1). With illness, however, gastrointestinal tract losses can be substantially greater. Diarrhea can cause acute losses of large amounts of potassium in stool, and progressive chronic renal failure results in substantially increased potassium elimination by the colon. This adaptation preserves normal serum potassium until renal failure is very severe. Only trivial amounts of potassium are lost through the skin (less than 5 mEq/day) unless sweating becomes profuse. The rate of urinary potassium excretion is adjusted in proportion to intake, the kidney being the major regulator of potassium balance. Potassium is freely filtered by the glomerulus and is almost completely reabsorbed in the proximal parts of the nephron, so urinary potassium excretion is largely a function of distal tubular secretion. The rate of potassium secretion (and excretion) (Fig. 50.2) is affected by dietary potassium intake, the serum potassium concentration, the luminal flow rate, distal sodium and chloride delivery, distal transepithelial voltage, acid–base balance, the plasma aldosterone concentration, and antidiuretic hormone concentration. Any factor that increases the urinary flow rate, distal sodium delivery, or aldosterone secretion; or decreases distal

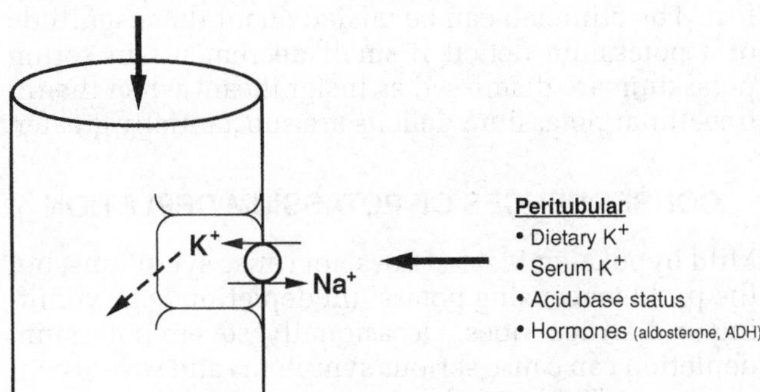

Figure 50.2. Factors influencing potassium secretion by the distal tubule. ADH, antidiuretic hormone. (Modified from Giebisch G. Physiology of potassium metabolism. In: Whelton A, Walker WG, eds. Potassium in cardiovascular and renal medicine. New York: Marcel Dekker, 1986.)

chloride delivery; or causes metabolic alkalosis will stimulate potassium secretion and predispose to the development of potassium depletion. Urinary potassium excretion can be reduced to a minimum of 5 to 25 mEq/day. Although dietary deficiency of potassium may exacerbate other causes of hypokalemia (e.g., diuretic-induced), hypokalemia caused by diet alone is rare in otherwise normal patients unless intake is severely limited for prolonged periods. Therefore, when hypokalemia is encountered, there is almost always some significant factor or disease that must be investigated.

Internal Potassium Balance

Almost all of the body potassium is located intracellularly, with only the smallest portion in the extracellular space. This distribution is maintained by membrane-bound sodium–potassium adenosine triphosphatase (Na^+-K^+-ATPase), preserving a ratio of intracellular to extracellular potassium concentration of approximately 30:1. Indeed, less than 2% of total body potassium (50 to 60 mEq) resides in the extracellular space (Fig. 50.1). Small transcellular potassium shifts can, therefore, significantly affect the serum potassium concentration, even in the absence of changes in total body potassium. Cellular potassium uptake is increased and hypokalemia potentially produced by beta-2-adrenergic stimulation, insulin, alkalosis, anabolism, and aldosterone.

Potassium is not lost proportionally from the extracellular and intracellular spaces, so the serum potassium does not always accurately reflect total body stores. Nevertheless, in the absence of major alterations in internal potassium balance, there is a roughly linear inverse relationship between the decrement in the serum potassium concentration and the magnitude of the potassium deficit: The serum potassium falls approximately 0.3 mEq/L for each 100 mEq of potassium depletion. This relationship is valid for deficits up to approximately 500 mEq. With larger deficits, the serum potassium falls less for every 100 mEq of potassium lost. The clinician can be misled about the magnitude of a potassium deficit if small decrements in serum potassium are dismissed as insignificant when the intracellular potassium deficits are substantially greater.

CONSEQUENCES OF POTASSIUM DEPLETION

Mild hypokalemia itself does not cause symptoms, but the problem causing potassium depletion (e.g., vomiting or diarrhea) does. Occasionally, severe potassium depletion can cause serious symptoms and severe consequences (Table 50.1).

Table 50.1. Clinical Sequelae of Hypokalemia

Cardiovascular
Predisposition to digitalis intoxication
Abnormal electrocardiogram
Ventricular ectopic rhythms
Cardiac necrosis
Increased blood pressure

Neuromuscular
Gastrointestinal
  Constipation
  Ileus
Skeletal muscle
  Weakness, cramps
  Tetany
  Paralysis (including respiratory)
  Rhabdomyolysis

Renal
Decreased renal blood flow
Decreased glomerular filtration rate
Renal hypertrophy
Pathologic alterations (interstitial nephritis)
Predisposition to urinary tract infection

Fluid and Electrolyte
Polyuria and polydipsia
  Renal concentrating defect
  Stimulation of thirst center
  ADH release (?)
Increased renal ammonia production
  Predisposition to hepatic coma
  Altered urinary acidification
Renal chloride wasting
Metabolic alkalosis
Sodium retention
Hyponatremia (with or without concomitant diuretic)

Endocrine
Decrease in aldosterone
Increase in renin
Altered prostaglandin metabolism
Decrease in insulin secretion (carbohydrate intolerance)

ADH, antidiuretic hormone.

Modified from Tannen RL. Potassium disorders. In: Kokko J Fluids and electrolytes. Philadelphia: WB Saunders, 1986.

Effect on Cardiovascular and Neuromuscular Systems

Of greatest concern is the effect of hypokalemia on the *heart.* Severe potassium depletion may rarely be a cause of myocardial necrosis, but less severe changes in potassium balance can clearly affect cardiac conduction and rhythm. When hypokalemia is present, characteristic pathologic electrocardiographic changes may be seen (Fig. 50.3). Hypokalemia has also long been known to predispose patients to digitalis intoxication, manifested by a variety of rhythm disturbances. Whether mild to moderate hypokalemia *per se* can cause dangerous ventricular arrhythmias is controversial (2), but it is clear that hypokalemia can cause serious arrhythmias in patients with underlying heart disease (3).

Both *smooth and skeletal muscle function* can be altered by potassium depletion. Severe hypokalemia can cause gastrointestinal tract dysmotility, resulting in ileus. Proximal muscle weakness can progress to paralysis. The respiratory muscles may be involved, resulting in respiratory failure. Hypokalemia may also predispose to rhabdomyolysis, at least in part by interfering with exercise-induced vasodilation. On the other hand, postural hypotension and a decrease in systemic vascular resistance have been reported in potassium-depleted patients. Rarely, tetany may be seen even in the absence of changes in pH or serum calcium.

Effect on Blood Pressure

Although hypokalemia is often considered a complication of therapy for hypertension, increasing evidence implicates a role for potassium in the pathophysiology and evolution of hypertension and other cardiovascular and cerebrovascular diseases. Populations that consume a low-potassium diet have been found to have a high prevalence of hypertension and cardiovascular disease (4,5). Large studies also show that a person's blood pressure is partly potassium dependent (6,7). The risk of hypertension has been found to increase

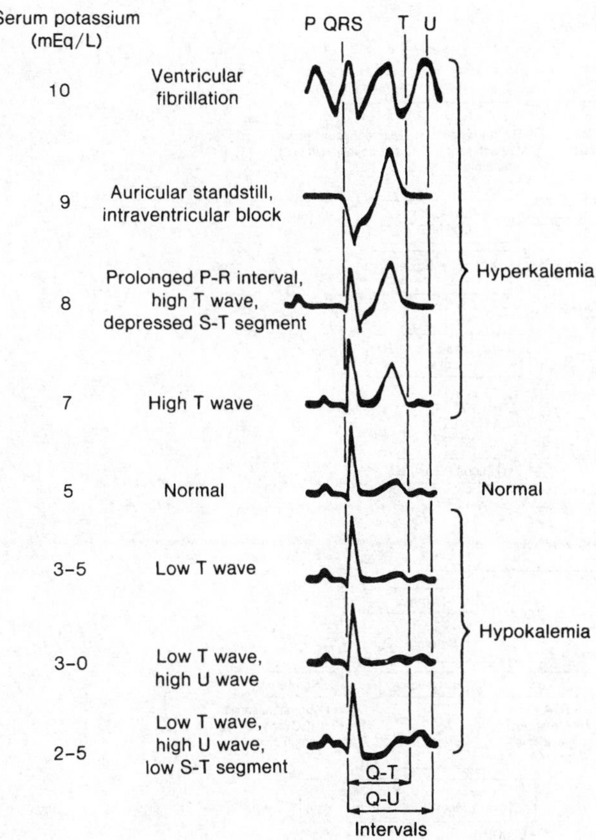

Figure 50.3. Electrocardiogram in assessment of potassium. (Adapted from Burch GE, Winsor T. A primer of electrocardiography. 6th ed. Philadelphia: Lea & Febiger, 1972:128.)

as the amount of potassium consumed in the diet decreases, independent of the sodium intake (8). The mechanisms for the effect of potassium on blood pressure are unclear, but these observations suggest that simple interventions may lower a patient's likelihood of developing hypertension (9–11). Studies show that supplementation of the diet with 48 to 120 mEq/day can lower blood pressure (12,13). The correction of hypokalemia by dietary means or pharmacologic supplementation can enhance the treatment of hypertension with minimal risk and expense (14). The effect of increased dietary potassium may be greater than the effect of similar amounts of potassium chloride supplementation, perhaps because dietary potassium may be associated with citrate rather than chloride anions. In addition, beyond its effect on hypertension, potassium supplementation has been shown to reduce the risk of cerebrovascular disease and stroke (15).

Effect on the Kidney

The most characteristic alteration in renal function is an impaired ability to concentrate the urine. The defect is generally mild, and the polyuria sometimes seen may be caused in large part by direct stimulation of thirst. Prolonged severe potassium depletion can produce reversible reductions in the glomerular filtration rate and renal blood flow. Rarely, acute renal injury can occur. Progressive chronic renal failure can develop, with chronic tubulointerstitial disease as the pathologic finding.

Effect on the Endocrine System

Hypokalemia inhibits the synthesis of aldosterone, increases plasma renin activity, and decreases insulin secretion as well as insulin action. The latter effect may worsen a patient's control of diabetes mellitus. Renal ammonia production, directly stimulated by hypokalemia, may precipitate or aggravate hepatic encephalopathy in patients with severe liver failure.

DIFFERENTIAL DIAGNOSIS AND MANAGEMENT

Typically, the most common causes of hypokalemia (diuretic use, vomiting, diarrhea) can be determined from the history. For less obvious cases, the approach described in Figure 50.4 is recommended (16).

Deficient Potassium Intake

Potassium is widely distributed in many foods, especially fruits, raw vegetables, fish, beef, and pork (Table 50.2). Therefore, inadequate potassium intake is an unusual cause of hypokalemia except in some high-risk situations (dietary fads, pica, alcoholism, cachexia). Insufficient dietary potassium intake during anabolic states as cells take up potassium, as when malnourished patients are fed and with treatment for megaloblastic anemia (17), may lead to hypokalemia. In such patients, the urinary potassium excretion is less than 10 to 20 mEq/day while they are hypokalemic unless there is a compounding problem. Dietary deficiency of potassium, particularly in the elderly, may also exacerbate diuretic-induced hypokalemia.

Transient Disorders of Internal Potassium Balance

Beta-2-adrenergic agonists lower the serum potassium concentration by stimulating cellular potassium uptake. A reduction in serum potassium is commonly seen when beta-2-adrenergic agonists (administered by any route) are used in the treatment of asthma or premature labor. Although the decrease in serum potassium is usually mild, significant hypokalemia can occur. This usually resolves within hours after the drug is discontinued. Similarly, *high levels of endogenous catecholamines* released during stress may explain transient reductions in serum potassium (which resolve with or without potassium supplementation) that are sometimes seen during acute illness, delirium tremens, and acute myocardial infarction (17,18).

Metabolic and respiratory alkalosis are associated with small shifts of potassium from the extracellular to the intracellular space. This may sensitize the patient to digitalis, even in the absence of total body potassium depletion.

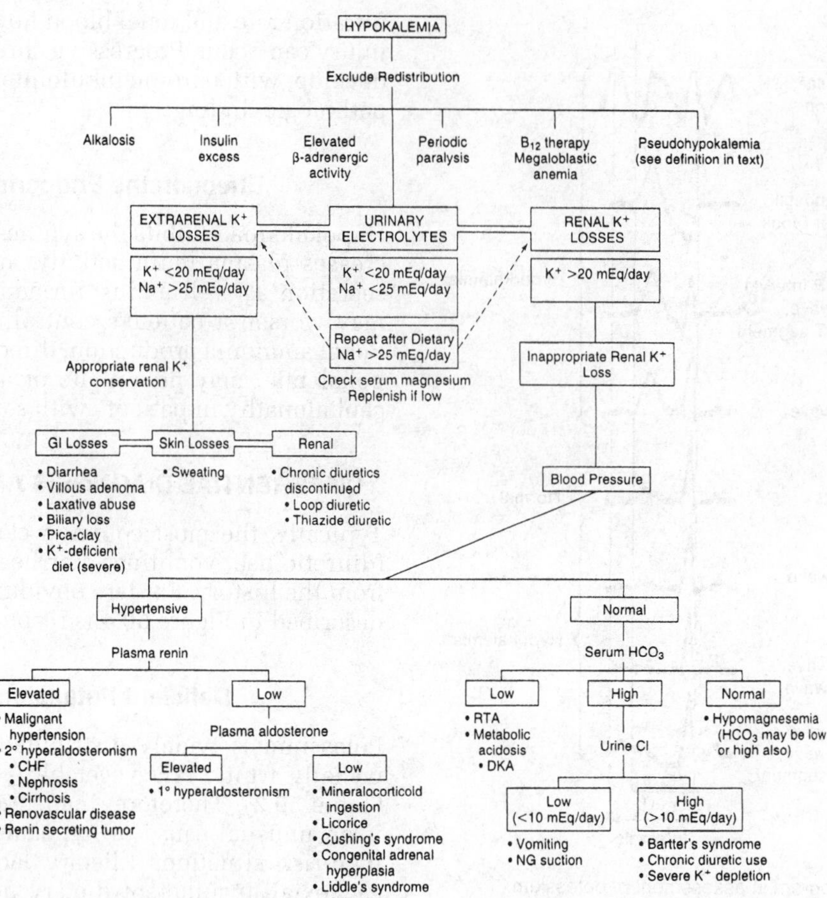

Figure 50.4. Diagnostic approach to hypokalemia. RTA, renal tubular acidosis; DKA, diabetic keloacidosis; NG, nasogastric; CHF, congestive heart failure. (Modified from Narins RG, Jones ER, Stom MC, et al. Diagnostic strategies in disorders of fluid, electrolyte and acid-base homeostasis. Am J Med 1982;72:496.)

Insulin stimulates cellular potassium uptake in liver and skeletal muscle, independent of its effects on glucose transport. This dose-dependent action forms the basis for use of insulin in the treatment of severe hyperkalemia. When insulin is used to correct hyperglycemia and the initial serum potassium is normal, hypokalemia may ensue.

Hypokalemic periodic paralysis is a rare familial disorder characterized by spontaneous episodes of paralysis that may be precipitated by a variety of stimuli, including insulin, glucose, and a high-carbohydrate meal. A similar syndrome may also be seen in hyperthyroidism, especially in Asian men. Although a profound fall in the serum potassium is regularly demonstrated during paralysis, urinary potassium excretion decreases dramatically, signifying an intracellular shift of potassium. In the thyrotoxic form, beta-blocking agents may be effective in preventing attacks.

Vitamin B_{12}, when administered in the therapy of megaloblastic anemia, can cause large intracellular shifts of potassium as metabolic activity is increased in hematopoietic cells. Provision of adequate quantities of potassium and careful monitoring prevent this complication.

Finally, other rare causes of transient hypokalemia have been reported. *Pseudohypokalemia* can result when metabolically active cells incorporate potassium after a specimen of blood has been drawn and left at room temperature. This may occur in leukemia. Hypothermia can lower plasma potassium to 3.0 mEq/L or less because of potassium uptake into cells. Rare cases of barium salt poisoning caused by contamination of table salt have been reported; hypokalemia in this setting results from blockade of potassium channels and inhibition of potassium egress from cells.

External Losses of Potassium

If there is no reason to suspect an extracellular to intracellular shift of potassium, the patient is likely to be potassium depleted. In this case, the next step is to determine where the potassium was lost—via a renal or an extrarenal route. This often can be accomplished by measuring the urinary potassium concentration. If renal potassium excretion is high (greater than 20 mEq/L on a spot urine specimen or greater than 20 mEq in a 24-hour collection) despite hypokalemia, excessive renal potassium losses are, at least in part, responsible for potassium depletion. On the other hand, a renal potassium excretion that is appropriately low suggests an extrarenal loss of potassium, with appropriate renal conservation.

Table 50.2. Some Common Potassium-Rich Foods

Food Source	Average Portion	Potassium (mEq)
Vegetables		
Artichoke	1 large	22.0
Beans		
Cooked dried	1/2 cup	10.7
Lima	5/8 cup	10.8
Brussels sprouts	7 medium	7
Corn	1 ear	5.0
Potato		
White	1 boiled	7.3
Sweet	1 boiled	7.7
Tomato		
Fresh	1 medium	9.4
Canned	1/2 cup	5.6
Squash, winter	1/2 cup boiled	11.9
Meats		
Hamburger	1 patty	9.8
Rib roast	2 slices	11.2
Fish, haddock	1 medium fillet	8.0
Clams	4 large	6.0
Oysters	6 medium	3.1
Fruits		
Apple	1 medium	2.8
Applesauce	1/3 cup	1.7
Apricots	3 medium	7.2
Avocado	1/2 pitted	15.5
Banana	1 6-inch	9.5
Cantaloupe	1/4 medium	6.4
Dates	10 pitted	16.6
Fruit cocktail	1/2 cup	4.3
Grapefruit	1/2 medium	3.5
Melon	1/4 small	6.4
Orange	1 small	7.7
Peach	1 medium	5.2
Pear	1 medium	6.7
Plum	2 medium	7.7
Prunes, dried	10 medium	17.8
Raisins	1 tablespoon	2.0
Strawberries	10 large	4.2
Watermelon	1 slice	15.4
Juice		
Grapefruit	1 cup	10.4
Orange	1 cup	12.4
Pineapple	1 cup	9.2
Prune	1 cup	15.0
Tomato	1 cup	13.7
Vegetable	1 cup	14.1
Nuts		
Peanuts, roasted	1 tablespoon	2.0
Peanut butter	2 tablespoon	2.0
Mixed nuts	3.5 oz	2.0
Milk		
Buttermilk	9 oz	8.0
Skim milk	8 oz	8.5
Whole milk	8 oz	9.0

GASTROINTESTINAL LOSSES RESULTING IN POTASSIUM DEFICIENCY

Diarrhea

Potassium and bicarbonate are normally present in the stool in high concentrations. When diarrhea is significant, hypokalemia may result. This often is associated with a non–anion gap hyperchloremic metabolic acidosis (caused by the loss of bicarbonate). Occasionally, hypokalemia may be a clue to the presence of a villous adenoma of the colon or surreptitious laxative abuse. Diarrheal states in general are often associated with clinical contraction of the extracellular fluid volume, detected on physical examination by weight loss, low jugular venous pressure, poor skin turgor, tachycardia, and orthostatic hypotension. Urinary potassium excretion should be low when potassium deficiency results from intestinal losses, because, in this setting, the kidney conserves potassium maximally. However, this is true only when the volume status of the patient is maintained. If diarrhea is severe and volume contraction develops, secondary hyperaldosteronism occurs as a protective strategy to preserve salt balance. Potassium losses are accelerated in the urine paradoxically.

Loss of Gastric Fluid

Hypokalemia is well known to accompany vomiting or gastric drainage, yet gastric fluid contains only small amounts of potassium (approximately 5 to 10 mEq/L). The major route of potassium loss in this setting is the urine. The loss of gastric chloride induces metabolic alkalosis, chloride deficiency, extracellular volume depletion, and secondary hyperaldosteronism. The increased filtered load and increased distal delivery of bicarbonate, decreased distal delivery of chloride, and high levels of aldosterone all act together to stimulate secretion of potassium. The urine has a high concentration of potassium but a very low concentration of chloride. Under these circumstances, correction of potassium depletion and of metabolic alkalosis requires provision of adequate amounts of chloride, potassium, and sodium. Potassium administered with anions other than chloride is not retained but is excreted in the urine (19).

RENAL LOSSES RESULTING IN POTASSIUM DEFICIENCY

Diuretics

Diuretics that act proximally to potassium secretory sites accelerate potassium excretion by increasing the amount of sodium and water delivered to the distal nephron while simultaneously stimulating the release of aldosterone. Loop diuretics (furosemide, bumetanide, torsemide) and thiazide diuretics act in this way. The serum potassium concentration usually reaches a nadir within 7 days after beginning therapy (20). The degree of potassium depletion depends on the concurrent sodium intake. Some diuretics cause more severe hypokalemia than others (20): At standard doses, thiazide and thiazide-like diuretics induce an average fall in the serum potassium concentration of 0.6 mEq/L. Furosemide causes less potassium depletion, with an average fall in potassium concentration of only 0.3 mEq/L. The use of multiple kaliuretic diuretics acting at different nephron sites (e.g., furosemide and thiazide) is likely to cause significant hypokalemia (21).

Urinary potassium levels lower than 3.0 mEq/L suggest one of two situations: *excessive sodium intake* that increases the amount of sodium and water delivered to the distal nephron, which in turn accelerates potassium secretion, or *an unrecognized potassium-wasting state* such as primary or secondary hyperaldosteronism (22). Both should be considered if significant hypokalemia develops after the introduction of potassium-wasting diuretics, particularly if the potassium level before treatment was low.

Monitoring Potassium in Patients Receiving Diuretics

Before administration of diuretics, the serum potassium (as well as the concentrations of other electrolytes, blood urea nitrogen, and serum creatinine) should be measured. If the value is initially normal, serum potassium should be measured approximately 1 and 4 weeks after initiation of, or an increase in, the dosage of a diuretic. Most patients who develop hypokalemia will have done so within the first week. Subsequently, semiannual assessment is probably adequate in nonedematous, stable, well-nourished patients unless other indications arise. Edematous patients have major underlying diseases, and those with heart failure are often treated with digitalis, so the risk of serious consequences of hypokalemia is greater. Monitoring should be more frequent in these patients.

Prevention and Treatment of Diuretic-Induced Hypokalemia

Whether mild diuretic-induced hypokalemia is dangerous remains controversial. When a diuretic is indicated, one should use simple measures that minimize the risk of hypokalemia. These include using the lowest effective dosage of a diuretic agent and prescribing a moderate restriction of dietary salt (75 to 100 mEq sodium per day or 2 to 2.5 g sodium or 4 to 6 g sodium chloride). Increased dietary potassium intake should also be suggested (Table 50.2), because it is easy for a patient to accomplish, is cost-effective, and may be associated with other benefits such as lower blood pressure and decreased risk of stroke, hypertension, and other cerebrovascular diseases (see earlier discussion).

Even with preventive measures, approximately 30% of diuretic-treated patients become hypokalemic in the range of 3.0 to 3.5 mEq/L (17). If the diuretic must be continued and normalization of the serum potassium must be restored, especially for patients with indications for potassium maintenance therapy listed in Table 50.3 (22), the decision must be made whether to use potassium supplements or potassium-sparing diuretics. Because hydrogen is lost along with potassium, diuretic-induced hypokalemia is usually associated with metabolic alkalosis. Replacement must be with *potassium chloride* (Table 50.4), not potassium with poorly absorbed anions, because the latter increase the electronegativity of tubules and thus further increase potassium loss (19). Salt substitutes are composed mostly of potassium chloride (approximately 50 to 65 mEq/teaspoon) and are a cheap and effective alternative. However, diuretic-induced hypokalemia may seem to be refractory even to large doses of potassium chloride because the renal clearance of potassium remains high during continued diuretic therapy (23). In one study, potassium chloride at dosages up to 96 mEq/day normalized the serum potassium in only 8 of 16 hypertensive patients with diuretic-induced hypokalemia (23).

Table 50.3. Indications for Potassium Maintenance Therapy

Digitalis therapy
Predisposition to hepatic coma
Serum potassium concentration <3.0 mEq/L
Development of glucose intolerance
Underlying cardiac disease
Symptoms attributable to hypokalemia

With permission from Tannen RL. Diuretic induced hypokalemia. Kidney Int 1985; 28:988.

Table 50.4. Commonly Available Potassium Chloride Supplements

Product	Amount (mEq)
Extended-release tablets	
Micro-K Extentabs, Slow K, Klor-Con 8	8
K-Dur, K-Norm, K-Tab, Ten-K, Micro-K 10 Extentabs, Klor-Con 10	10
K-Dur	20
Powders for solution (flavored)[a]	
K-Lor (also 15 mEq), Kato, Klor-Con Klor-Con 125 (25 mEq)	20/packet
Suspension (no taste)	
Micro-K LS	20/packet
Efflorescent granules or tablets (flavored)[a]	
Klorvess, Klor-Con/EF (25 mEq)	20
Solutions (flavored)[a]	
Klorvess 10%, Rum-K 15%	20–30/15 mL

[a]Taste is generally improved by chilling.

Potassium-sparing diuretics (including spironolactone, triamterene, and amiloride) offer several advantages, such as reducing urinary potassium losses, minimizing the development of metabolic alkalosis by reducing acid excretion (spironolactone), and limiting renal magnesium wasting. In one study, conversion from hydrochlorothiazide (with or without potassium supplements) to hydrochlorothiazide plus amiloride or hydrochlorothiazide plus triamterene without potassium supplements increased the serum potassium by approximately 0.5 to 0.7 mEq/L and brought it into the mid-normal range (24).

The *major risk* of attempts to raise the serum potassium is overshoot hyperkalemia. To avoid this, all patients beginning therapy with potassium supplements or potassium-sparing agents should be assessed for risk factors for hyperkalemia. These include renal insufficiency (obvious elevations of serum creatinine greater than 1.2 mg/dL), diabetes mellitus, age 75 years or older, and the ingestion of other agents known to interfere with potassium homeostasis (e.g., angiotensin-converting enzyme inhibitors, nonsteroidal anti-inflammatory drugs, cyclosporine, heparin). Therefore, all patients who are beginning therapy to raise their serum potassium level should have their serum potassium measured after 1 and 4 weeks and then at least every 6 to 12 months, if not more often as indicated. If a hypokalemic patient is found to have renal insufficiency or other risk factors for hyperkalemia, potassium supplements and potassium-sparing diuretics are generally contraindicated.

Assessment of 24-hour urinary potassium excretion along with the serum potassium helps in predicting how best to supplement (or restrict) potassium intake. For example, if the patient is taking 40 mEq of potassium supplementation a day, has a 24-hour urinary excretion of 80 mEq potassium, and has a plasma potassium concentration of 3.0 mEq/L, then more supplements (dietary or pharmacologic) are indicated. Even in the patient with normal renal function, potassium supplements and potassium-sparing diuretics generally should not be given together or along with other drugs that interfere with potassium homeostasis.

Excessive Urinary Potassium Losses (Renal Potassium Wasting)

The differential diagnosis in the setting of renal potassium wasting is complex, but it can be simplified by assessing the acid–base status and the blood pressure of the patient (Fig. 50.4) (16).

Hypokalemia Accompanied by Hypertension

If hypokalemia secondary to renal potassium wasting is accompanied by an elevated blood pressure, renin (angiotensin) or mineralocorticoid (or glucocorticoid) excess is suggested. Several causes must be considered (Table 50.5). The evaluation of such a patient is complex (25,26). Although certain basic diagnoses may be made in an office, referral to a center experienced in the evaluation of these syndromes may still be necessary.

Unless the cause is readily apparent (e.g., a patient with essential hypertension treated with diuretics), one should beware of surreptitious diuretic abuse (see later discussion). The first step in the evaluation of renal potassium wasting in a hypertensive patient is the determination of plasma renin activity (Fig. 50.4, p. 678). An elevated renin concentration suggests primary renin excess, as may be caused by renovascular, accelerated, malignant hypertension, or rarely a renin-producing tumor. On the other hand, if the renin concentration is low, the plasma renin activity should be remeasured along with the plasma aldosterone level. If both levels are low, the presence of excessive amounts of endogenous or exogenous steroids, other than aldosterone, is likely: Certain types of licorice, chewing tobacco, carbenoxolone, and steroid-containing nasal sprays are rare exogenous causes of this syndrome. Finally, if the renin level is low but the simultaneous aldosterone level is high, primary aldosteronism is strongly suggested. The sensitivity and specificity of this screening test may be increased by determining the aldosterone/renin ratio 2 hours after administration of 25 mg of captopril. In primary aldosteronism, the ratio remains high, but it is suppressed in patients with essential hypertension (27,28).

Most patients with primary aldosteronism are asymptomatic. Clinical manifestations, when present, in addition to hypertension, are related to potassium depletion and occur only when such depletion is severe. These include weakness, paralysis, tetany, arrhythmias, polyuria, and polydipsia. Edema is less common than would be expected because of adaptive factors that diminish sodium retention. Patients with primary aldosteronism usually have hypokalemia, but as many as 25% have serum potassium levels higher than 3.5 mEq/L. However, many of these patients manifest hypokalemia if challenged with potassium-wasting diuretics or with large intakes of sodium chloride (200 mmol/day, approximately 4 to 5 g of sodium or 10 to 12 g sodium chloride). Both of these interventions result in increased delivery of sodium and water to the distal nephron, where, under the influence of excessive aldosterone, sodium is reabsorbed and potassium and hydrogen ions are secreted. Hypokalemia and metabolic alkalosis ensue. Indeed, the development of severe hypokalemia after the initiation of thiazide therapy is sometimes a clue to a hypermineralocorticoid state. On the other hand, a serum potassium level greater than 4.0 mEq/L in a patient on a high-sodium diet (documented by a 24-hour urinary sodium excretion of approximately 200 mEq/day) virtually excludes the diagnosis (29).

When the combination of hypokalemia, suppressed plasma renin activity, and elevated aldosterone concentration make the diagnosis of primary hyperaldosteronism likely, localization procedures such as computed tomography or magnetic resonance imaging should be undertaken by the consultant to distinguish adenomas from bilateral adrenal hyperplasia. The treatment of adenomas has primarily been surgical, and excision has often led to the cure of hypertension and hypokalemia. If bilateral hyperplasia is found, surgery is not indicated because it is seldom

Table 50.5. Causes of Hypertension with Associated Renal Potassium Wasting

Hyperreninemic Forms
Renovascular
Renin tumor
Malignant or accelerated essential hypertension

Hyporeninemic Steroid-Dependent Forms
Mineralocorticoid
- Exogenous
  - Licorice, desoxycorticosterone, fludrocortisone, chewing tobacco, carbenoxolone
- Endogenous
  - Adrenal adenoma
  - Adrenal glomerulose hyperplasia
  - Enzyme deficiency: 17-OHase; 11-OHase
  - Liddle syndrome

Glucocorticoid
- Endogenous
  - Cushing syndrome, pituitary, ectopic ACTH, adrenal cortical
- Exogenous

With permission from Narins RG, Jones ER, Stom MC, et al. Diagnostic strategies in disorders of fluid, electrolyte and acid-base homeostasis. Am J Med 1982; 72:496.

curative. A trial of spironolactone is useful in almost all patients. Large doses (up to 400 mg daily) are sometimes necessary and the full effects may not be seen for several weeks. Failure of spironolactone to normalize the blood pressure while normalizing hypokalemia strongly suggests that, regardless of the presence or absence of an adenoma to explain the aldosterone excess, surgery would probably not resolve the hypertension. Although spironolactone has been the mainstay of medical therapy for primary aldosteronism, amiloride (up to 40 mg/day) is also effective and may be the drug of choice for patients who are intolerant of spironolactone (29).

Normotensive Renal Potassium Wasting

If renal potassium wasting is discovered in a normotensive patient, the acid–base status should be evaluated (Fig. 50.4, p. 678). If metabolic acidosis is present, renal tubular acidosis or diabetic ketoacidosis is suggested (although the latter is usually apparent by findings other than renal potassium wasting). If metabolic alkalosis is present, measurement of urinary chloride provides an important clue to the underlying process. If the urinary chloride concentration is low, the likely cause is upper gastrointestinal fluid loss. If the urinary chloride is high, the cause may be the coincident use of diuretics during the time of the sampling, but other causes are possible, such as Bartter syndrome (see later discussion). Diuretic abuse and self-induced vomiting are common concealed causes of hypokalemia and metabolic alkalosis.

Urinary electrolyte evaluation with respect to diuretics is often frustrating. The half-life of the various diuretics must be considered. Most loop diuretics, with the exception of torsemide, have fairly short half-lives despite the common perception that they are long acting. Therefore, excess urine chloride may be seen during the period of active or recent drug use with apparently paradoxical low urine chloride after the drug has left the urine.

Magnesium depletion and potassium depletion often go hand in hand, and magnesium depletion can cause renal potassium wasting. Hypomagnesemia is a common finding in up to 40% of hypokalemic patients. Although the mechanism is incompletely understood, enhanced aldosterone secretion is believed to play a role. Hypomagnesemia (of any cause) can produce hypokalemia as a result of fecal as well as urinary losses. Therefore, serum magnesium should be measured during the evaluation of any patient with refractory hypokalemia.

Bartter and Gitelman Syndromes

Bartter syndrome manifests with hypokalemic metabolic alkalosis, excessive urinary potassium losses, and normal blood pressure, without edema. Plasma renin activity and aldosterone levels are significantly elevated. This syndrome appears to result from an inherited defect resulting in abnormally low sodium chloride reabsorption by the thick ascending limb of the loop of Henle combined with high aldosterone levels stimulated by volume depletion. This presentation is mimicked by diuretic abuse and surreptitious vomiting, from which Bartter syndrome must be differentiated. A urine screening test for surreptitious use of diuretics should be done. Also urinary chloride is elevated in Bartter syndrome and decreased in surreptitious vomiting, both of which may result in hypokalemic metabolic alkalosis. Hypokalemia is usually refractory to potassium supplementation but may be ameliorated by administration of prostaglandin synthesis inhibitors such as nonsteroidal anti-inflammatory drugs or amiloride 5 to 10 mg/day (24).

Gitelman syndrome also causes hypokalemic metabolic alkalosis, excessive urinary potassium losses, and normal blood pressure, without edema but is distinguished by hypomagnesemia and hypocalcuria. A defect in the thiazide-sensitive sodium chloride transporter causes patients with this condition to act as if they were exposed to thiazide diuretics (30).

General References*

Gennari FJ. Hypokalemia. N Engl J Med 1998;339:451.

Greenberg A, et al. Primer on kidney diseases, 2nd Edition. New York: Academic Press, 1998.

Rose BD, Post TW. Clinical physiology of acid-base and electrolyte disorders. 5th ed. New York: McGraw-Hill, 2001.

Weiner ID, Wingo CS. Hypokalemia: consequences, causes, and correction. J Am Soc Nephrology 1997;8:1179.

Specific References

1. Sterns RH, Cox M, Feig PU. Internal potassium balance and the control of the plasma potassium concentration. Medicine (Baltimore) 1981;60:339.
2. Siegel D, Hulley SD, Black DM. Diuretics, serum and intracellular electrolyte levels, and arrhythmias in hypertensive men. JAMA 1992;267:1083.
3. Kuller LH, Hulley SB, Cohne JD, et al. Unexpected effects of treating hypertension in men with electrocardiographic abnormalities: a critical analysis. Circulation 1986;73:114.
4. Langford HG. Dietary potassium and hypertension: epidemiological data. Ann Intern Med 1983;98[Suppl]:770.
5. Linas SL. The role of potassium in the pathogenesis and treatment of hypertension. Kidney Int 1991;39:771.
6. INTERSALT Research Group. INTERSALT: an international cooperative study on electrolytes and blood pressure. BMJ 1988;297:319.
7. McCarron DA, Morris CD, Henry HJ, et al. Blood pressure and nutrient intake in the United States. Science 1984;224:1392.
8. Frisancho AR, Leonard WR, Bollettino LA. Blood pressure in blacks and whites and its relationship to dietary sodium and potassium intake. J Chronic Dis 1984;37:515.
9. Appel LJ, Moore TJ, Obarzanek E, et al. A clinical trial of the effects of dietary patterns on blood pressure. DASH Collaborative Research Group. N Engl J Med 1997;336:1117.
10. Brancati FL, Appel LJ, Seidler AJ, et al. Effect of potassium supplementation on blood pressure in African Americans on a low-potassium diet: a randomized, double-blind, placebo-controlled trial. Arch Intern Med 1996;156:61.
11. Siani A, Strazzullo P, Giacco A, et al. Increasing the dietary potassium intake reduces the need for antihypertensive medication. Ann Intern Med 1991;115:753.
12. Siani A, Strazzullo P, Russo L, et al. Controlled trial of long term oral potassium supplements in patients with mild hypertension. BMJ 1987;294:1453.

*Bold print (general references) and bold numerals (specific references) denote published controlled clinical trials, meta-analyses, or consensus-based recommendations.

13. Svetkey LP, Yarger WE, Feussner JR, et al. **Double-blind, placebo-controlled trial of potassium chloride in the treatment of mild hypertension.** Hypertension 1987;9:444.
14. Whelton PK, Jiang H, Cutler JA, et al. Effects of oral potassium on blood pressure: metaanalysis of randomized controlled clinical trials. JAMA 1997;277:1624.
15. Khaw KT, Barrett-Connor E. Dietary potassium in stroke-associated mortality: a 12-year prospective population study. N Engl J Med 1987;316:235.
16. Narins RG, Jones ER, Stom MC, et al. Diagnostic strategies in disorders of fluid, electrolyte and acid–base homeostasis. Am J Med 1982;72:496.
17. Sterns RH, Spital A. Disorders of internal potassium balance. Semin Nephrol 1987;7:399.
18. Morgan DB, Young RM. Acute transient hypokalemia: new interpretation of a common event. Lancet 1982;2:751.
19. Kassirer JP, Berkman PM, Lawrenz DR, et al. The critical role of chloride in the correction of hypokalemic alkalosis in man. Am J Med 1965;38:172.
20. Morgan DB, Davidson C. Hypokalemia and diuretics: an analysis of publications. BMJ 1980;280:905.
21. Nader PC, Thompson JR, Alpern RJ. Complications of diuretic use. Semin Nephrol 1988;8:365.
22. Tannen RL. Diuretic-induced hypokalemia. Kidney Int 1985; 28:988.
23. Papademetriou V, Burris J, Kukich S, et al. Effectiveness of potassium chloride or triamterene in thiazide hypokalemia. Arch Intern Med 1985;145:1986.
24. Ridgeway NA, Ginn DR, Alley K. Outpatient conversion of treatment to potassium-sparing diuretics. Am J Med 1986;80:785.
25. Gordon RD. Mineralocorticoid hypertension. Lancet 1994;344: 240.
26. Stewart PM. Mineralocorticoid hypertension. Lancet 1999;353: 1341.
27. Laragh JH, Brenner BM. Hypertension: pathophysiology, diagnosis, and management. New York: Raven Press, 1990.
28. Lyons DF, Kem DC, Brown RD, et al. Single dose captopril as a diagnostic test for primary aldosteronism. J Clin Endocrinol Metab 1988;57:892.
29. Young WF Jr., Klee GG. Primary aldosteronism: diagnostic evaluation. Endocrinol Metab Clin North Am 1988;17:367.
30. Simon DB, Nelson-Williams C, Bia MJ. Gitelman's variant of Bartter's syndrome, inherited hypokalemic alkalosis, is caused by mutations in the thaizide-sensitive Na-Cl cotransporter. Nat Genet 1996;12:24.

CHAPTER 51

Urinary Stones

DAVID A. SPECTOR, MD

Urinary stones are common in the United States. Although urologic intervention or nephrologic consultation may occasionally be required, most patients with stones can be evaluated, treated, and monitored by the primary care provider. This chapter reviews the various manifestations of stone disease, the types of urinary stones, the evaluation of patients with stones, the acute and chronic treatment of patients with urinary stones, and when to obtain consultation for these patients.

PRESENTATION OF URINARY STONE DISEASE

Patients with urinary stone disease may present with acute colic, persistent or recurrent urinary tract infection, isolated hematuria, no symptoms but a stone discovered incidentally on a radiograph taken for other purposes, or a prior history of stones.

Acute Colic

Presentation

Most patients with urinary stones at some time have an acute episode of colic. The stone, if obstructing, causes ureteral spasm, resulting in intermittent pain, which is often severe. The location of the pain depends on the location of the stone in the ureter, but it is most often felt in the flank; then, as the stone moves distally, pain radiates in a characteristic pattern around the groin and into the testicles in men or into the labia majora in women. Nausea, vomiting, and other gastrointestinal symptoms that often suggest a primary gastrointestinal problem may be associated with pain. Examination reveals an uncomfortable, restless patient. There may be costovertebral tenderness as well as deep tenderness in the abdomen. More importantly, no signs of peritoneal irritation (guarding, rebound, rigidity) are present. Fever is not present unless infection has developed in the obstructed urinary tract.

Urinalysis demonstrates microscopic (or gross) hematuria in 91% of cases (1). The presence of pyuria is important because chronic bacterial infection may be associated with the development of urinary stones; however, pyuria may be absent even if infection is present in the situation of complete urethral obstruction.

Diagnosis and Management

The aims of management of colic should be relief of discomfort, surveillance for infection, and determination of whether the stones will pass spontaneously or will require surgical removal. The *abdominal radiograph* (kidneys, ureters, and bladder, or KUB) is useful in monitoring the site and progression of the stone. Approximately 90% of renal stones are radiodense and can be seen on a good-quality KUB radiographs. The size and position of the stone help determine the likely course of the episode of colic and the urgency of intervention. In general, stones that are smaller than 5 mm pass spontaneously, those between 5 and 10 mm have a 50% chance of passing spontaneously, and those larger than 10 mm usually require surgical removal. The common sites where stones become lodged are in the renal calyx, in the ureteropelvic junction, in the ureter at the pelvic brim where the ureter begins to pass over the iliac vessels, in the lower third of the ureter, and at the ureterovesical junction. If there is doubt about whether calcification seen on plain film is within the urinary tract, an oblique view may help. It is also important to review old abdominal films taken for any reason to see whether a stone was present previously.

An *intravenous pyelogram* (IVP) or (unenhanced) helical CT of the abdomen should also be obtained as soon as possible in the patient with colic because it helps establish the diagnosis, especially in patients with radiolucent stones, and it provides certain important information that aids in management. For decades, IVP was the standard test for patients with renal colic, but unenhanced helical CT has become the imaging technique of choice for the examination of patients with suspected renal calculi (2). Although it is more expensive, helical CT is faster and requires no contrast dye exposure. On the other hand, IVP gives more information regarding anatomic urinary tract abnormalities, which might predispose to stone formation (e.g., medullary sponge kidney, diverticula). Rarely, a urologist might need to be consulted for consideration of either an *antegrade pyelogram* (i.e., via a catheter passed percutaneously into the renal pelvis) or a *retrograde pyelogram*. These methods are safe for patients with a history of allergy to IVP dye.

Occasionally a patient with a history strongly suggestive of renal colic may have another cause for the pain. A dissection of the aorta, acute back strain or lumbar disc disease, the passage of blood clots in the ureters (as in sickle cell disease or renal infarct), and, rarely, malingering should be considered. A malingerer is often difficult to identify at first, and such patients may give a classic history of acute renal colic while relating a history of allergy to IVP dye. Often these patients have blood (obtained from a fingerstick or oral injury) in the urine specimen they give for analysis. (For further information on malingering, see Chapter 21.)

Several factors help in the decision whether to hospitalize a patient with renal colic, to obtain urgent urologic consultation, or to treat the patient at home. First, the patient with nausea and vomiting cannot be ensured of an adequate fluid intake or adequate oral analgesia and should be admitted to a hospital. Second, fever suggests infection proximal to an obstructing stone, and urgent urologic consultation should be obtained. Third, if the CT scan or IVP reveals a nonfunctioning kidney (completely obstructed ureter), a partially obstructed ureter from a solitary kidney, or urine extravasation, urgent urologic consultation should be obtained. Fourth, if the stone is larger than 10 mm, spontaneous passage is very unlikely and urologic consultation should be obtained. Of all stones that become symptomatic, 80% are ureteral, and 85% to 90% of these pass spontaneously. Therefore, only 10% to 15% of ureteral stones require interventional treatment (3).

Most patients can be treated at home. Forced hydration of 2 to 3 L of fluid every 24 hours is necessary to maintain a good urinary flow and to help in moving the stone. When the patient is voiding, all of the urine voided during the period of intermittent colic should be collected and strained through an old stocking, a fine knit screen, or a filter paper so that the passed stone may be saved and analyzed. Some patients may not realize that a passed "stone" may resemble gravel more than a pebble.

It is important to prescribe oral analgesic medication, such as oxycodone (generic, 5 mg, 1 to 3 tablets) or Tylox, which contains oxycodone and acetaminophen (1 to 3 capsules), every 3 to 4 hours, to control the discomfort. Phenothiazine (e.g., Phenergan, 25 mg) given with the narcotic provides additional relief by controlling any associated nausea. Some prostaglandin synthesis inhibitors such as indomethacin (Indocin or generic, 50 mg three to four times per day), ketorolac

(Toradol, 10 mg every 4 to 6 hours orally; or 30 mg intravenously or intramuscularly every 6 hours), or diclofenac (Voltaren, 50 mg orally two to three times daily) may provide effective analgesia in renal colic (4). This effect may result from reductions in renal pelvic pressure caused by a decreased glomerular filtration rate and from a reduction of ureteral edema. These or other nonsteroidal anti-inflammatory drugs may be tried in combination with traditional analgesics if symptoms of colic are prolonged (with appropriate cautions for adverse effects, especially in the elderly).

The patient should be hospitalized if fever, uncontrolled pain, or vomiting develops. If symptoms of colic are intermittent and well controlled at home, the patient should be monitored with a weekly radiograph of the abdomen to determine the progression of the stone. If by 6 weeks the stone has not passed, it is unlikely that spontaneous passage will occur, and urologic consultation should be obtained. For occupational or social reasons, some patients want to consider earlier surgical removal and therefore ask their physicians to request urologic consultation sooner.

Stones that pass from the ureter into the bladder usually pass with ease through the urethra. In the event of a bladder outlet obstruction, a stone may be retained in the bladder *(bladder stone),* where it may grow and in time become an infection stone (see Struvite Stones).

Patient Requiring Urologic Referral. When a patient is referred to a urologist for *stone removal,* there are several options. During endoscopy, lower ureteral stones may be removed with the use of a grasping forceps that is inserted through a cystoscope or ureteroscope or pulverized by ultrasonic, electrohydraulic, or laser lithotripsy. These procedures are similar to cystoscopic examination but require general or spinal anesthesia and hospitalization (see Chapter 53 for discussion of these endoscopes). These procedures have a success rate greater than 95% and a low rate of complications. Until the early 1980s, stones located more proximally required removal by open ureterolithotomy, open pyelolithotomy, or, in the case of a staghorn calculus, nephrolithotomy. However, two new techniques, *percutaneous nephrostolithotomy* (PCNL) and *extracorporeal shock wave lithotripsy* (ESWL), have supplanted traditional open stone removal operations. Both techniques give results similar to operative stone removal but are associated with less convalescence time and less morbidity.

PCNL requires that the patient be sedated and an IVP be performed to localize the kidney and the stone. Under fluoroscopy, a percutaneous nephrostomy tube is placed near the posterior axillary line. Subsequently, the tract is dilated and various nephroscopes, buckets, and forceps are used to extract the calculi. For struvite calculi (also called triple phosphate or "infection" stones; see later discussion), *hemiacidrin (Renacidin) irrigation* is sometimes useful to dissolve residual stones. Antegrade radiographs are performed to confirm stone removal and ureteral patency. Successful removal occurs with more than 95% of renal stones and 88% of ureteral stones. On the other hand, PCNL is associated with a significant incidence of complications, including hemorrhage (5% to 12%), arteriovenous fistulae (0.6%), perforation/extravasation (5% to 26%), and fever or sepsis (3% to 11%) (5). Typically, a 2- to 3-day hospitalization is needed for a patient to undergo PCNL.

The number of centers providing ESWL has multiplied rapidly in recent years. ESWL sometimes requires that the patient have anesthesia (usually spinal), but most often it is performed with only intravenous sedation, after which the stone is located by ultrasound or fluoroscopically. A shock wave, generated by an electrode similar to a spark plug, is focused by the lithotripter for a precise impact on the stone (Fig. 51.1). When the shock wave encounters calculus material that has different acoustic properties from surrounding tissue, a tensile force is produced that shatters that material. This treatment takes an average of 30 to 45 minutes. ESWL usually is done in outpatient settings. After ESWL, fragments of stone usually pass in the urine for a few days and cause mild colic. Retreatment is needed in a few patients, and macroscopic hematuria occurs transiently in most.

The selection of treatment modalities for a given patient depends in part on the characteristics of the stone being treated and in part on local resources and expertise. Where all modalities are available, ESWL used alone is the treatment of choice in 70% of patients. Patients who are suitable for treatment with ESWL are those who have single or multiple renal stones less than 20 mm in diameter, some patients with smaller staghorn stones (those in which the pelvis is not dilated), and some with stones located in the upper third of the ureter. Larger calculi, most staghorn calculi, and calculi composed of cystine (see later discussion) are usually treated by percutaneous nephrolithotomy in combination with ESWL, or by open operation alone.

Results of ESWL are excellent. For patients with stones less than 10 mm in size that are located in the kidney or ureter, 90% become stone free or are left with small, asymptomatic residual fragments. Convalescence from ESWL requires several days. Most patients experience some flank discomfort from the trauma to the kidney. This discomfort often requires use of analgesics for a few days. Immediate complications of ESWL are uncommon, but renal or perirenal tissue injury has been demonstrated in experimental studies and suggested by MRI and tissue enzyme release in up to 85% of patients. Between 1% and 8% of patients develop new hypertension or experience exacerbation of pre-existing hypertension within 3 years after ESWL treatment (6,7). The frequency of this complication may depend on the type of lithotripter.

Other Patterns of Stone Presentation

Urinary stones usually produce symptoms that suggest acute colic, at least at some time in their course.

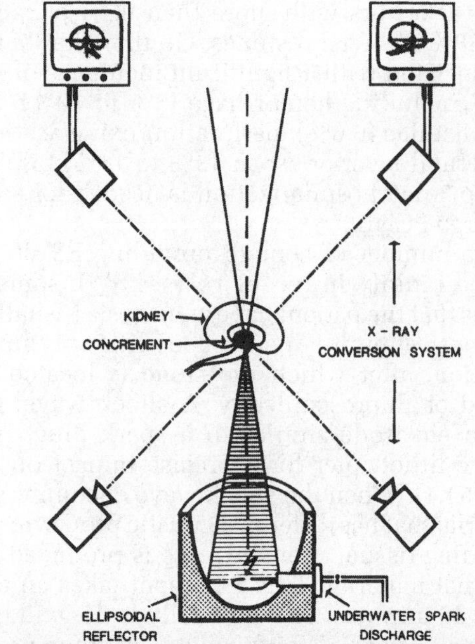

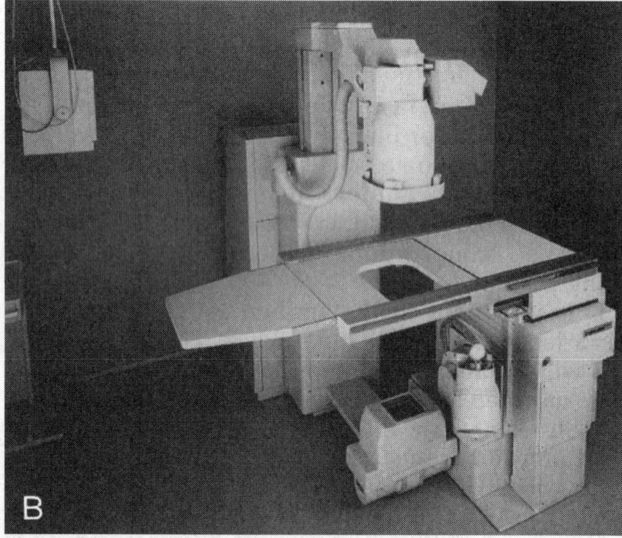

Figure 51.1. A: Schematic drawing of the technical arrangement of a modern lithotripter. (From Chaussey C, Schmidt E, Jocham D. Non-surgical treatment of renal calculi with shock waves. In Roth RA, Finlayson BF, eds. *Clinical management of urolithiasis.* Baltimore: Williams & Wilkins, 1993.) **B:** Photograph of a modern lithotripter. (Courtesy of Domier Medical Systems, Inc, Kennesaw, GA.)

When stones are discovered in patients who do not have colic, these patients require the same evaluation and management as do patients who have passed a stone associated with colic (see Diagnostic Workup for Patients with Urinary Stone Disease).

TYPES OF STONES AND THEIR CAUSES

There are four main types of urinary calculi: calcium oxalate or phosphate, uric acid, struvite–triple phosphate (magnesium ammonium phosphate), and cystine. Calcium stones are by far the most common. Table 51.1 shows the classification of stone-forming patients by the type of stone passed.

It is important to be familiar with the metabolic disorders these patients may have. This understanding is helpful in planning a diagnostic evaluation and specific therapy (see later sections in this chapter). This is particularly true in the evaluation of the patient with the most common stone type, calcium.

Calcium Stones

Table 51.2 shows the metabolic and clinical disorders in calcium stone formers. This table shows that in almost 80% of patients who have had a calcium stone, a specific disorder can be identified as the cause. In addition to the common disorders shown in the table, other metabolic disorders, such as hypocitraturia, may

Table 51.1. Classification of Stone-Forming Patients by Type of Stone Passed

Type of Stone	Coe Series (1,431 Patients)	Other Series Combined (1,870 Patients)
Calcium oxalate (with or without phosphate)	69[a]	63.2[a]
Calcium phosphate	2	7.4
Calcium and uric acid	10	
Uric acid	2	5.4
Cystine	1	2.5
Struvite	7	21.5
Unknown	10	

[a]All values expressed as percentages of patients in each category.

From Coe FL. Nephrolithiasis: pathogenesis and treatment. Chicago: Year Book Medical Publishers, 1988.

Table 51.2. Metabolic and Clinical Disorders in 989 Calcium Oxalate Stone Formers

Disorders	No. of Patients (%) Men	Women
Systemic Disease		
Primary hyperparathyroidism[a]	26 (4)	24 (10)
Sarcoid	6 (1)	1 (1)
Cushing syndrome	5 (1)	1 (0.4)
Paget disease	1 (0.1)	4 (2)
Renal tubular acidosis, type I	7 (1)	4 (2)
Enteric hyperoxaluria[b]	39 (5)	13 (5)
No Systemic Disease		
Idiopathic (hereditary) hypercalciuria	213 (29)	121 (49)
Hyperuricosuria	126 (17)	9 (4)
Both disorders	120 (16)	22 (9)
No metabolic disorders[c]	186 (26)	52 (11)
Total	**729**	**249**

[a]Seventeen additional patients had primary hyperparathyroidism: either their stones were admixed with uric acid, struvite, or cystine; they had stones with no calcium; or their stone type was unknown.

[b]Includes primary hyperoxaluria (three patients) and hyperoxaluria as a consequence of intestinal bypass for obesity.

[c]Urinary citrate data not available; hypocitraturia has been found alone or in combination with other disorders in 19% of hypercalciurias.

From Coe FL. Nephrolithiasis: pathogenesis and treatment. Chicago: Year Book Medical Publishers, 1988.

promote urinary calcium salt precipitation. Hypocitraturia is present as the sole metabolic abnormality in 10% (8) and as one of two or three abnormalities in 19% (9) of calcium stone formers. Urine pH, which affects the prevalence of many types of stones (see Urinanalysis), has little influence on the formation of calcium oxalate stones, but calcium phosphate stones are promoted with a pH greater than 6. The approach to these disorders is discussed later in this chapter.

Uric Acid Stones

Uric acid stones are caused by the high insolubility of undissociated uric acid (its pK of 5.7 means that 50% of uric acid is undissociated at pH 5.7 and 90% is undissociated at pH 4.7). Three factors are associated with uric acid stone formation: hyperuricosuria, highly acid urine, and low urinary volume. The lifetime incidence of uric acid stones in the general population is very low (Table 51.3). On the other hand, uric acid stones are very prevalent in patients who have gout, asymptomatic hyperuricemia, and hyperuricosuria, and probably in patients with a history of gout and no hyperuricemia. Many patients have passed uric acid stones long before a gouty attack has occurred. It is known that many patients with gout produce an abnormally high fraction of their daily acid load as titratable acid rather than as ammonium and therefore have an unusually low average urinary pH. Furthermore, patients with chronic diarrhea and those with excessive fluid loss from the skin may have highly concentrated urine, which predisposes them to the formation of uric acid calculi. Patients who have myeloproliferative disease and those with solid tumors that are undergoing lysis may have excessive uric acid excretion, which may be associated with uric acid stones and tubular plugs of urate. Patients with gout also have more calcium stones than people in the general population (10). The association may result from crystallization of uric acid, which then forms a nidus for calcium deposition.

Table 51.3. Prevalence of Urate Stones in Various Populations

Population	Lifetime Incidence (%)
General population	0.01
Patients with gout	22
Hyperuricosuria in primary gout[a] (mg/24 hr)	
<300	11
300–699	21
700–1100	35
>1100	50
Hyperuricemia in men[b] (mg/dL)	
7–8	12.7
8–9	22
>9	40

[a]Adapted from Yu T-F, Gutman AB. Uric acid nephrolithiasis in gout. Ann Intern Med 1967;67:1133.

[b]Adapted from Hall AP, Barry PE, Dawber TR, McNamara PM. Epidemiology of gout and hyperuricemia. Am J Med 1967;42:27.

Table 51.4. Urinary Cystine Excretion

Subjects	Excretion (mg/d)
Normal individuals	<100
Heterozygotes for cystinuria	150–300
Homozygotes for cystinuria	>600

Struvite Stones (Infection Stones)

It is generally believed that infection stones form primarily as a consequence of the hydrolysis of urea and the production of ammonium by the bacterial enzyme urease. The production of ammonia leads to a highly alkaline urine, which promotes the precipitation of magnesium, ammonium, and phosphate. These are the components of the infection-induced or struvite stone. Most urea-splitting organisms are *Proteus* species; however, *Pseudomonas, Klebsiella, Staphylococcus,* and some *Escherichia coli* strains are capable of producing urease. Struvite stones do not form *de novo* but almost always are a complication of another primary stone disease in which infection has become superimposed, and they are especially likely to grow into staghorn calculi (large stones that cannot pass the ureteropelvic junction and that form a cast of all or a portion of the pelvicaliceal system).

Cystine Stones

Cystine stones are rare and usually are seen in young patients, because the onset is usually in childhood. The stone forms because of crystallization of cystine when the urine is supersaturated with this substance, which occurs when there is an inherited defect in renal tubular resorption of filtered cystine. This is a particularly virulent form of stone disease and may be associated with staghorn calculi. In addition to cystinuria, there is usually urinary loss of other basic amino acids, including ornithine, lysine, and arginine. The disorder is an inherited autosomal recessive trait, although some heterozygous patients have excess cystine excretion, as is shown in Table 51.4. Cystine is much less soluble in acid urine than it is in alkaline urine; therefore, cystine stones generally form when urine is acid and cystine excretion is greater than 400 mg/24 hours.

NATURAL HISTORY OF URINARY STONE DISEASE

Urinary calculus disease is a chronic illness. Once a stone has formed there is a tendency for recurrence, and management should be tailored to the stone activity, the type of stone, and any associated metabolic abnormality.

Stone activity—the number of stones formed and the change in size of existing stones—is an important, although at times difficult, determination. It requires a yearly review of stones passed and removed,

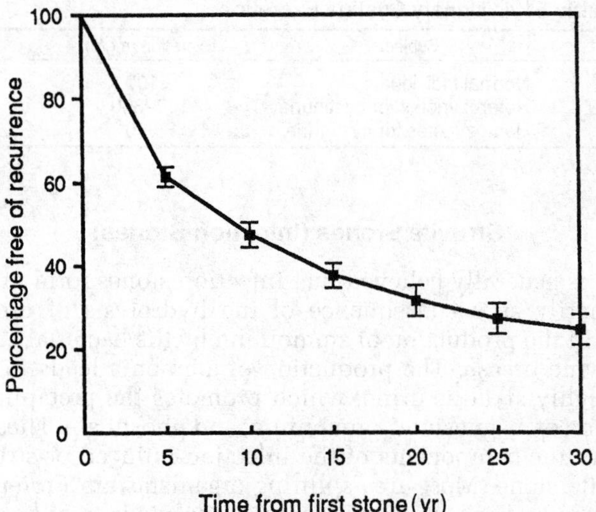

Figure 51.2. Life-table calculation of the time course of recurrence after a first renal stone in 515 patients. (Reproduced with permission from Sutherland JW, Parks JH, Coe FL. Recurrence after a single renal stone in a community practice. *Miner Electrolyte Metab* 1985;11:267)

as well as an evaluation by abdominal radiography of the increase in size of known stones or the appearance of new stones. The activity of urinary calculi depends on a number of factors: stone type, associated metabolic abnormality, treatment received (both specific and nonspecific), and age. Therefore, precise rates of recurrence cannot be given with accuracy.

Nevertheless, two studies have provided useful and corroborative information regarding the recurrence rate after passage of a first urinary stone. In one retrospective study of 515 patients who were monitored after a single (first) stone and given no medications to prevent a recurrence, there was a 50% recurrence rate at approximately 9 years and about 75% recurrence by 25 years (11). These data are presented as a graph in Fig. 51.2. Another study of patients who passed their first calcium stone showed a recurrence in half of the patients by 5 years and in two-thirds by 9 years (12).

Therefore, it is suggested that evaluation for associated metabolic abnormalities be undertaken in every patient who has formed a new stone, because recurrence is likely, the basic assessment is noninvasive and inexpensive, and a workup may uncover an especially virulent or an important systemic disease or metabolic defect responsible for stone formation.

DIAGNOSTIC WORKUP FOR PATIENTS WITH URINARY STONE DISEASE

Evaluation of patients with stone disease can be accomplished entirely in an ambulatory setting. This evaluation depends on a directed history and physical examination, stone analysis if available, and certain laboratory measurements. The extent of the evaluation of patients passing a first stone is somewhat controversial. Some suggest an abbreviated evaluation, because not all patients have recurrent stones and because all treatment modalities have potential side effects; others, citing the likelihood of eventual recurrence, fully evaluate patients after the first stone passage (see Coe et al., 1992, in General References). The approach outlined in this section is a reasonable and commonly used method for evaluation of patients who have had a urinary calculus (13).

History

A directed medical history is important in determining the activity of stone disease as well as in providing clues to the nature of the stone. The number of passed stones, the frequency of attacks of colic or hematuria, and any history of infection should be obtained. Previous abdominal radiographs and, most importantly, chemical analysis of prior stones should be obtained, if possible. The *family history* may provide a clue to cystine stones, uric acid stones (gout), and many calcium stones (e.g., those associated with idiopathic hypercalciuria). The *dietary history* may reveal excessive intake of sodium, animal protein, purine, or oxalate (see Types of Stones and Their Causes). High-protein meat diets are associated with production of metabolic acids (which leech bone and cause hypercalciuria), increased urine excretion of urate, and decreased excretion of urinary citrate, all of which may predispose to the development of stone disease. The approximate daily *fluid intake* is also an important part of the history. Some people ingest as little as 500 to 700 mL/day and therefore have concentrated urine most of the day. The *medication history* is important. For example, aspirin at high dosages (more than 5 g/day) and probenecid are associated with increased uric acid excretion and may cause a predisposition to uric acid calculi. On the other hand, use of the xanthene oxidase inhibitor allopurinol has led to development of xanthene stones. Use of calcium-containing antacids (e.g., Titralac, Tempo, Tums) as well as vitamins A and D and loop diuretics (e.g., furosemide) may be associated with hypercalciuria and calcium stone formation. Acetazolamide (Diamox) may be associated with development of chronically alkaline urine and a higher incidence of calculi made of calcium phosphate. Vitamin C at high dosages can cause hyperoxaluria. Triamterene (contained in Dyazide) and its metabolites (14), as well as acyclovir and indinavir (15), have been found as a nidus in urinary calculi (or as the only constituent). Moreover, certain medications have been shown to decrease calcium excretion (e.g., thiazides) or uric acid excretion (e.g., allopurinol), whereas loop diuretics promote hypercalciuria and interfere with results of testing in a patient who is being evaluated for renal stone disease. The *occupational history* is important because environmental temperature (and therefore fluid losses) and accessibility to fluids are factors that influence stone formation by promoting decreased output of highly concentrated urine.

Physical Examination

Physical examination (when there is no colic) occasionally gives clues to specific problems. For example, band keratopathy (stippled calcification of the perimeter of the cornea, which may require a slit-lamp for visualization) may be seen in hyperparathyroidism, or there may be signs of sarcoidosis, hyperthyroidism, inflammatory bowel disease, neoplasia, or gouty arthritis. Most often, however, the examination is normal.

Urinalysis

The urinalysis provides a simple assessment that may give specific direction to the determination of the cause of the urinary calculus. It is important that the urinalysis be complete, including the determination of pH. The pH is usually acid in patients with a uric acid or a cystine stone and is invariably alkaline in patients with struvite stones. Also, the pH may suggest the presence of renal tubular acidosis: Because the first voided morning urine is usually acid, a urine pH greater than 6.0 in such a specimen suggests the possibility of renal tubular acidosis. The microscopic analysis may show hematuria (although this is often absent in the intercritical period), crystals, or evidence of infection. Crystals of cystine have the appearance of a benzene ring and are highly suggestive of cystinuria. Other crystals are more variable and are not diagnostic but may give a clue to the stone composition in patients with lithiasis (see Coe et al., 1992, in General References for photographs of typical examples).

Stone Analysis

If a stone is available, it should be analyzed to determine its composition, because the stone type determines the approach to evaluation and treatment. Stones can be analyzed inexpensively at commercial laboratories and may be mailed without preservative for this purpose.

Laboratory Assessment

A laboratory analysis is important even for patients in whom a stone is available for analysis (Table 51.5). This evaluation is necessary because it is increasingly recognized that many patients have more than one metabolic disorder that predisposes them to stone formation. For example, struvite stones often start as some other primary stone type, most often calcium; patients with a calcium oxalate stone may have hypercalciuria, hyperuricosuria, or hypocitraturia. Patients usually comply with the testing necessary for proper evaluation of a metabolic disorder if they understand the ease with which it can be accomplished, the substantial rate of recurrent calculi, and the effectiveness of specific therapy for metabolic problems (see Preventive Treatment of Urinary Calculus Disease). Furthermore, the 24-hour urine volume and sodium content provide objective guides as to when the most basic interventions, such as increasing fluid intake (if urinary volume is low) or decreasing salt intake (if sodium excretion is high), are useful (see General Measures).

Table 51.5. Laboratory Assessment of Patients with Urinary Calculi[a]

Measurement
24-Hour urinary volume
24-Hour urinary calcium[b]
24-Hour urinary uric acid[c]
24-Hour urinary creatinine
24-Hour urinary oxalate
24-Hour urinary citrate
24-Hour urinary sodium
Urinalysis
Urine cystine screen (cyanide–nitroprusside test)
Urine culture (if pyuria)
Urine pH (taken on first voided morning specimen collected under mineral oil)
Serum calcium
Serum phosphorus
Serum uric acid
Serum chloride
Serum bicarbonate
Serum creatinine
Serum urea nitrogen

[a] During evaluation patients should follow their usual diet and life habits.

[b] The 24-hour urine container should contain 15 mL concentrated HCl (with warning to avoid contact).

[c] The 24-hour urine container should contain a few crystals of thymol to retard bacterial overgrowth.

Laboratory assessment of patients who have formed urinary calculi is simple and noninvasive and can be performed easily in the office. It is important that this initial evaluation be accomplished *without modifying the patient's diet or habits* so that an underlying process associated with urinary calculus disease is not masked. The reasons for obtaining most of the studies listed in Table 51.5 are self-evident. Urinary creatinine is measured to monitor the completeness of collections (normally about 1 gm of creatinine is excreted 1 day, more if muscular and less if wasted) and to estimate the glomerular filtration rate. Urinary sodium (reflecting dietary intake) is measured because increased urinary sodium excretion promotes hypercalciuria. Serum calcium should be repeated at least once, and ionized calcium should be determined if possible, because the latter is a more accurate index of hypercalcemia. Urinary citrate should be measured in patients with calcium stones. Citrate combines with calcium to form a soluble complex, thus reducing the availability of calcium for crystallization with oxalate or phosphate, and it also directly inhibits crystallization of these substances.

Several commercially prepared 24-hour urine kits have become available (from Urocor Inc., Oklahoma City, Oklahoma, or Mission Pharmacal Co., San Antonio, Texas) that allow for measurement of all urinary constituents listed in Table 51.5 (including pH and cystine) from a single 24-hour urine sample. The kit, including jugs for urine, is mailed directly to the

Table 51.6. Situations in Which Hyperoxaluria May Be Expected

Hereditary overproduction (usually virulent stone disease with frequent recurrences and nephrocalcinosis, often occurring before age 12 yr)
Methoxyflurane anesthesia (immediately after)
Ethylene glycol ingestion (immediately after)
Chronic inflammatory bowel disease affecting the ileum, ileal resection, or small bowel bypass
Cellulose phosphate ingestion (during entire period of ingestion)
Oxalate gluttony (tea, spinach, rhubarb)

Table 51.7. Causes of Hypercalciuria that May Not Be Associated with Hypercalcemia

Idiopathic hypercalciuria
Administration of loop diuretics (furosemide, ethacrynic acid, or bumetanide)
Excessive salt ingestion
Exogenous adrenal corticosteroids
Cushing syndrome
Paget disease of bone
Immobilization
Progressive bone disease
Malignant tumors
Hyperthyroidism
Sarcoidosis
Renal tubular acidosis
Other causes of metabolic acidosis
Medullary sponge kidney
Severe phosphate deprivation

patient, who returns a sample alliquot of the 24-hour urine to the company for analysis.

An *IVP*, if not done previously as part of the evaluation of an episode of acute colic, could be done as part of the search for underlying structural disease (e.g., anatomic abnormality of the lower urinary tract, medullary sponge kidney).

In addition to the laboratory assessment outlined in Table 51.5, *parathyroid hormone* should be measured if hypercalcemia (see Chapter 81) or hypophosphatemia is present, or if stone analysis indicates that the stone is made up of calcium phosphate. Finally, urinary oxalate should be measured when hyperoxaluria is suspected (Table 51.6). It is not done routinely because hyperoxaluria is uncommon and the analysis cannot be done reliably by all laboratories.

Hypercalciuria

Although calcium excretion varies somewhat with intake of calcium and of protein, generally the upper limits of calcium excretion for patients eating a normal diet are 250 mg/24 hours for women and 300 mg/24 hours for men. Patients with *hypercalciuria without hypercalcemia* deserve special attention because they are seen commonly and because of the variable pathogenesis of their stones. Table 51.7 lists the causes of hypercalciuria that may not be associated with hypercalcemia.

Most patients have idiopathic hypercalciuria from either a *renal leak* (renal hypercalciuria, 5% of stone formers) or *excessive gastrointestinal absorption* of calcium (absorptive hypercalciuria). In the latter instance, which is far more common, there is excess gastrointestinal absorption (and then excretion) of calcium after the ingestion of calcium. The differentiation of renal from absorptive hypercalciuria requires the use of an *oral calcium tolerance test* (16), which is not routinely recommended in a general medical office practice but should be performed by a nephrologist or urologist specializing in stone disease. However, it is important to be aware that some patients with absorptive hypercalciuria may have normal calcium excretion if they inadvertently restrict their calcium intake on the day of the urine collection. Therefore, it is advantageous to ensure that the patient continues his or her usual diet for a few days before and during the metabolic evaluation.

PREVENTIVE TREATMENT OF URINARY CALCULUS DISEASE

General Measures

Patients who have formed even a single stone should be educated about the nature of urinary calculi, their natural history, the importance of regular surveillance, and the effectiveness of therapy. Eliminating dietary excesses or deficiencies will probably help control calcium stone formation in many patients, although controlled studies providing proof of efficacy of dietary interventions are not available (17). Increasing fluid intake has long been a mainstay of treatment of all types of urinary calculi. In a randomized, prospective study of nearly 200 patients, increasing fluid intake to achieve a urine volume of greater than 2 L reduced recurrence of calculi by more than 50% during 5 years of follow-up (18).

The decision to use specific therapy (especially pharmacologic therapy) must be made on an individual basis. The rate of stone recurrence for a large population of patients may not apply to an individual patient. It is prudent to use only general and dietetic therapeutic measures if the patient has passed only a single stone and has no evidence of urinary stones on radiography. However, for recurrent stone formers and patients with radiographic evidence of stones, more specific measures should be used (see later discussion).

Diet

Diet can play a role in most conditions in which stones form. Because obtaining a detailed diet history is often impractical in the office, it is usually helpful to have a dietitian or nutritionist evaluate the patient, both to determine dietary excesses or deficiencies and to begin to plan dietary therapy, depending on the results of the evaluation for metabolic abnormalities. Specific dietary restrictions are discussed under the various stone types.

Fluid Intake

A low urine volume, reflecting low fluid intake, is common in many stone formers. Regardless of the type of stone that has been formed, patients should maintain a high intake of fluids to ensure a urinary output of 2 to 4 L/day. This high urinary output prevents supersaturation, and the high flow rate may wash out small crystalline formations before they produce any obstructive or irritative symptoms.

Patients who have had several urinary stones are likely to continue to do so. Such patients should be prescribed a high fluid intake throughout the day and night (19). This can be accomplished by having the patient drink 2 to 4 L through the day and then take one or two glasses of water before retiring. This should result in a nocturnal diuresis necessitating voiding 3 to 4 hours later, at which time a further ingestion of one or two glasses of water will continue the diuresis until morning. Older patients may not require the intake of fluid before retiring to bed since there is an age related change in solute diuresis resulting in natural nocturia in the elderly. Although this method is annoying to the patient, once the habit is formed it is a small nuisance compared with subsequent stone formation. Continuing to encourage patients is critical to the success of the treatment program.

Avoidance of Dehydration

Patients should be counseled to avoid dehydration, and the resulting concentrated urine, when participating in sports or during travel or work.

Specific Therapy for Calcium Stone Formers

Calcium is present in most urinary calculi, and hypercalciuria is the most common disorder uncovered during the evaluation of patients with urinary calculus disease. In addition to the general measures described earlier in this chapter, there are several specific therapies.

Dietary Measures

Because dietary calcium restriction usually results in a fall in urinary calcium excretion, it has been advocated for patients with calcium stones and hypercalciuria. However, no controlled studies have confirmed the efficacy of this measure. In fact, in two large epidemiologic analyses, dietary calcium was found to be *inversely* related to the risk of developing renal calculi, with a 46% reduction of risk in men and a 35% reduction of risk in women who ingested dietary calcium in the highest versus the lowest quintile (20,21). Furthermore, in a randomized trial, men receiving a normal calcium diet (with restricted salt and animal protein) had less chance of recurrent stones than men on a low calcium diet (21a). Although the mechanism whereby higher dietary calcium might protect against stones is uncertain, it is known that greater calcium binding of gut oxalate results in decreased oxalate absorption and reduced urinary oxalate excretion. Therefore, apart from the probable increase in urinary stones, dietary calcium restriction may actually cause significant additional effects, such as reduced bone mineral density and negative calcium balance. Therefore, dietary calcium restriction is no longer recommended as a general policy in treating calcium stones. On the other hand, supplemental calcium (e.g., calcium carbonate tablets) has been shown to be a risk factor for renal calculi and should be avoided in patients with renal stones (20,21).

A number of authorities suggest limiting animal protein intake to 1 g/kg daily in patients with renal calculi. In addition to increasing calcium excretion, dietary animal protein intake increases excretion of uric acid and lowers urinary citrate excretion (probably because of acid production consequent to animal protein catabolism). These latter two changes predispose to formation of calcium stones. A direct relationship has been demonstrated between animal protein intake and calcium stone formation (20,21). A randomized trial in men who experienced recurrent urinary calculi in association with hypercalcinuria showed a significant reduction in stone recurrence over 5 years in those who restricted animal protein (529 mg/day) and salt intake compared with those on a low calcium diet (21a).

Similar circumstantial data suggest that high dietary potassium intake and the prevention of hypokalemia may independently reduce the risk of calcium stones. Potassium bicarbonate, but not sodium bicarbonate, reduces calcium excretion (22), and potassium deprivation increases calcium excretion (23). Furthermore, a higher dietary potassium intake was associated with a 50% reduction in the risk of calcium stones (20). It seems sensible, then, to avoid hypokalemia and, when alkali (citrate) is indicated, to provide it as the potassium salt (see Potassium Citrate). Finally, because dietary sodium chloride enhances calciuria, all patients with calcium stones should have modest restriction of dietary salt.

Thiazide Diuretics

Thiazide administration has been shown to result in a fall in urinary calcium excretion by as much as 50% to 60% within a day or two. Thiazides are an ideal theoretical choice (if hypokalemia is avoided) in the treatment of renal hypercalciuria, but thiazides also seem to be effective in absorptive hypercalciurias and even in patients with calcium stones associated with normal calcium excretion. Many studies attest to a 60% to 90% efficacy of a thiazide in reducing the frequency of calcium stones in all types of stone formers. Although there are serious methodologic concerns about some of these studies (24), two prospective trials demonstrate at least a 50% reduction in stone recurrence in patients taking thiazide (25,26), and most experts consider thiazide the drug of choice in hypercalciurics. However, because of their tendency to raise serum calcium, thiazides should be avoided in patients who are already hypercalcemic (e.g., those with hyperparathyroidism or sarcoidosis).

Any thiazide diuretic may be used, but trichlormethiazide (2 to 4 mg) or hydrochlorothiazide (25 to 50 mg) twice daily, or chlorthalidone (25 to 50 mg) once daily are most commonly prescribed. However, the exact dosage of thiazide to be used for the prevention of urinary calculi is uncertain. The incidence of side effects was almost 35% in one early study (27) in which a 50-mg dose of hydrochlorothiazide was given twice a day, the regimen that usually resulted in maximal hypocalciuria. Most side effects were seen soon after initiation of the drug. Intolerance of thiazides can be limited to less than 10% of patients by increasing the dosage gradually and reducing it if side effects develop. Although thiazides increase the plasma uric acid concentration (see Chapter 76), this is not detrimental to patients with urate stones. Chapter 50 provides a discussion of management of the hypokalemic complications of thiazides. If a potassium-sparing diuretic is used, amiloride, 5 to 10 mg daily, is the drug of choice. A preparation containing amiloride and hydrochlorothiazide (e.g., Moduretic) may be used. Triamterene should not be given because of the association of this agent with the formation of urinary calculi (see earlier discussion in History). The best choice for prevention or treatment of thiazide-induced hypokalemia is the addition of oral potassium citrate (see next section). This provides both potassium and base. The latter increases urinary citrate, which is reduced as a consequence of thiazide therapy (28). Citrate therapy has also been useful in hypercalciuric patients who continue to form stones despite thiazide therapy, presumably by increasing urinary citrate concentration (see next section) (29).

Potassium Citrate

Potassium citrate (e.g., Polycitra-K, Urocit-K) is useful in many metabolic conditions associated with renal stones. It is prescribed at a dosage of 0.5 to 2 mEq/kg per day in two to four doses daily. Potassium citrate is available as Polycitra-K solution (2 mEq potassium per milliliter) or crystal packets (30 mEq potassium per packet) to be mixed in water or juice, and as Urocit-K tablets (5 or 10 mEq potassium per tablet). Its usefulness results from the alkalinizing effect on the urine (for calcium stones associated with renal tubular acidosis, hyperuricosuria, and diarrheal syndromes, and for uric acid and cystine stones); an increase in urinary citrate, a natural inhibitor of stone formation (for calcium stones associated with hypocitraturia); and a mild reduction in calciuria. In a placebo-controlled prospective, randomized trial, 30 to 60 mEq potassium citrate daily reduced stone events by 90% compared with placebo and to pretreatment rates in hypocitraturic calcium stone formers (30).

The goals of treatment are to provide enough base to increase urinary pH to 6.0 and 7.0 and to restore normal urinary citrate excretion (more than 320 mg/day and as close as possible to the normal mean of 640 mg/day). A 24-hour urinary citrate excretion or urinary pH measurement should be obtained to determine the adequacy of the initial dosage. Once an acceptable level is achieved, it should be confirmed every 6 to 12 months.

Orthophosphate (Inorganic Phosphate)

The administration of inorganic phosphate (e.g., K-Phos) has been shown to reduce urinary calcium and the formation of calcium stones, in part by complexing gut calcium and thereby decreasing absorption, and in part by increasing urine inhibitors of stone formation. Although some trials suggest that orthophosphate reduces renal calculi (31), others do not, and no controlled trial is available. Because of the large doses required and the high incidence of gastrointestinal side effects, this therapy is discouraged for patients without consultation from a nephrologist.

Cellulose Phosphate

Taken with meals, this ion-exchange resin (Calcibind) binds calcium so that it is not absorbed. Early studies suggested that this agent might be useful in hyperabsorptive hypercalciuria, but the only controlled trial did not show efficacy (24). Because the incidence of significant side effects, including osteoporosis, may be high, cellulose phosphate is not recommended without consultation with a nephrologist.

Patients with Calcium or Uric Acid Stones Who Are Found to Have Hyperuricosuria

Patients with calcium stones who have hyperuricosuria and those who have mixed calcium and uric acid stones should be treated as if they had pure uric acid stones.

If purine gluttony is present, hyperuricosuria can be modified by dietary restriction of purine-rich foods, such as liver, kidney, and fish roe. However, dietary excess is not often the problem, and other means are necessary.

Uric acid stone formation can be significantly modified by *increasing the urinary pH.* Increasing the pH of the urine from 4.5 to 5.5 or 6.5 increases uric acid dissociation from 15% to 40% and 80%, respectively. Alkalinization can be accomplished by the administration of sodium bicarbonate several times a day. However, because sodium bicarbonate often causes gastrointestinal discomfort and gas, citrate salts (e.g., Polycitra-K solution, which contains 2 mEq of base per milliliter, as previously discussed) are more palatable and therefore preferable. Most patients require 10 mL three times a day, but the dosage should be adjusted as necessary based on the results of regular urine pH testing. The metabolism of citrate results in the generation of bicarbonate. During the initial week of treatment and periodically thereafter, the patient should be taught to measure the urinary pH several times a day using simple pH strips to ensure proper alkalinization (urine pH greater than 6.5).

Should these agents not be effective in controlling recurrence of uric acid stones, if the urine pH cannot be kept above 6.5, or if uric acid excretion is greater than 650 mg/day, *allopurinol* (which decreases uric acid production) may be used and effectively reduces stone recurrence. Allopurinol (Zyloprim, available in 100- and 300-mg tablets) should be initiated at a dosage of 100 mg once a day and raised to a level that controls uric acid excretion (to less than 500 or 600 mg/day); doses greater than 300 mg are divided in two daily doses. Complications from allopurinol are usually minor (minor skin rash, drug fever, precipitation of an acute gouty attack), but the drug can have serious side effects and should be discontinued when a skin rash or fever occurs, because fatal systemic vasculitis has been reported. The use of allopurinol is especially important as a preventive measure in patients who have excess uric acid excretion because of a myeloproliferative disease or in anticipation of tumor lysis during treatment of neoplastic disease.

Hyperoxaluria

In patients with hyperoxaluria, the aim is lower oxalate excretion (normal excretion is less than 45 mg/day). Treatment depends to some extent on the cause of hyperoxaluria. Reduction of foods with high oxalate content (spinach, rhubarb, chard, nuts, cocoa, and chocolate) helps in many cases of mild hyperoxalemia. The most common setting of severe hyperoxaluria and oxalate stones is in patients with malabsorption, especially in cases of ileal resection. In such circumstances, gut calcium, which ordinarily precipitates with oxalate, binds instead to fats, allowing oxalate to be readily absorbed. Treatment in such circumstances may be complicated and might include reducing dietary oxalate and fat, supplementing calcium and magnesium, prescribing cholestyramine resin to bind oxalate, administering potassium citrate, and recommending high fluid intake. Nephrology consultation for help in managing this complex problem is appropriate.

Cystinuria

Stone formers with cystinuria generally have virulent disease and are best treated in consultation with a nephrologist. Usually it is necessary to increase urine output to 3 L/day and to raise urinary pH in a manner similar to that used in patients with uric acid stones (see Uric Acid Stones). If stone activity continues, one may use D-penicillamine, tiopronin (which has fewer side effects), or the angiotensin-converting enzyme inhibitor captopril, all of which form complexes with cystine and prevent its precipitation.

Struvite or Infection Stones

Infection stones are particularly virulent. Untreated patients with infected staghorn calculi often develop sepsis and require urgent nephrectomy. Among 177 consecutive patients with staghorn calculi, renal-related death occurred in 67% of those patients who refused treatment, in 3% of those who were treated without clearance of stone fragments, and in none of those who had complete clearance of fragments (32). In view of this morbidity and mortality and with the recent advance in techniques for controlling infection stones, early urologic referral for surgical intervention is imperative. The goal of surgery in such patients is to remove the stone totally, as suggested by an American Urologic Association consensus panel (33). This may be accomplished by a variety of approaches, including PCNL, ESWL, combinations of PCNL and ESWL, and open surgery, as discussed earlier. There are inherent advantages and disadvantages to each technique, and ultimately the choice for a given patient must depend on a number of considerations, including the size and location of the stone or stones and the preference of the surgeon. The mortality rate for these procedures in experienced hands is less than 1%.

In addition to the surgical treatment of infection stone disease, medical therapy is an important adjunct. Associated metabolic abnormalities should be sought and treated. Specific antimicrobial therapy is necessary in conjunction with surgery, and, where stones cannot be removed surgically, suppressive therapy with antimicrobials may decrease for a period the incidence of septicemia. The use of oral agents that prevent infecting bacteria from splitting urea (urease inhibitors) has been shown to decrease recurrence of some struvite stones by preventing the formation of highly alkaline urine caused by the ammonium produced by urea-splitting organisms. Acetohydroxamic acid (Lithostat) may be used as an adjunct to antimicrobial therapy and surgery in patients with struvite stones. Acetohydroxamic acid, 250 mg, three to four times a day or a total dosage of 10 to 15 mg/kg per day (but never more than 1.5 g/day) should be used only when the patient is infected with urea-splitting organisms, as evidenced by a high urinary pH. Because of its teratogenic effects, it is contraindicated in women who are pregnant. Also it is not effective in the presence of moderate renal failure (i.e., creatinine 2.5 mg/dL or higher, or creatinine clearance 20 mL/minute or less). Side effects occur in almost 30% of patients and some are serious, such as thrombophlebitis and hemolysis. Experience with the drug is still limited, and consultation with a urologist is appropriate before prescribing it.

Urinary Calculi In Patients Without An Identifiable Metabolic Disorder

Approximately 10% to 15% of stone formers are found after evaluation not to have an identified metabolic disorder and may respond to general measures and to treatment with thiazides and/or potassium citrate, as outlined previously (34).

General References*

Coe FL, Favus MJ, Pak CYC, et al. Kidney stones: medical and surgical management. Philadelphia: Lippincott-Raven, 1996.

A multi-authored textbook that covers all aspects of stone disease.

Coe FL, Parks JH, Asplin JR. The pathogenesis and treatment of kidney stones. N Engl J Med 1992;327:1141.

This review covers medical aspects of urinary stone disease and provides an extensive documentation of the literature.

Pearle MS. Prevention of nephrolithiasis. Curr Opin Nephrol Hypertens 2001;10:203.

An up-to-date review of dietary and medical interventions for renal calculi.

*Bold print (general references) and bold numerals (specific references) denote published controlled clinical trials, meta-analyses, or consensus-based recommendations.

Segura JW, Preminger GM, Assimos DG, et al. **Ureteral stones clinical guidelines panel summary report on the management of ureteral calculi.** J Urol 1997;158:1915.

Evidence-based guidelines for the urologic management of ureteral stones.

Specific References

1. Li J, Kennedy D, Levine M, et al. Absent hematuria and expensive computerized tomography: case characteristics of emergency urolithiasis. J Urol 2001;165:782.
2. Smith RC, Varanelli M. Diagnosis and management of acute ureterolithiasis: CT is truth. AJR Am J Roentgenol 2000; 175:3.
3. Chaussy CG, Fuchs GJ. Current state and future developments of noninvasive treatment of human urinary stones with extracorporeal shock wave lithotripsy. J Urol 1989;141:782.
4. **4.** Labrecque M, Dostaler LP, Rousselle R, et al. Efficacy of nonsteroidal anti-inflammatory drugs in the treatment of acute renal colic: a meta-analysis. Arch Intern Med 1994;154:1381.
5. Lingeman JE. Lithotripsy and surgery. Semin Nephrol 1996;16: 487.
6. Lingeman JE, Woods J, Toth PD, et al. The role of lithotripsy and its side effects. J Urol 1989;141:793.
7. Yokoyama M, Shoji F, Yanagizawa R, et al. Blood pressure changes following extracorporeal shock wave lithotripsy for urolithiasis. J Urol 1992;147:553.
8. Preminger GM. The metabolic evaluation of patients with recurrent nephrolithiasis: a review of comprehensive and simplified approaches. J Urol 1989;141:760.
9. Wilson DM. Clinical and laboratory approaches for evaluation of nephrolithiasis. J Urol 1989;141:780.
10. Yu T-F, Gutman AB. Uric acid nephrolithiasis in gout: predisposing factors. Ann Intern Med 1967;67:1133.
11. Sutherland JW, Parks JH, Coe FL. Recurrence after a single renal stone in a community practice. Miner Electrolyte Metab 1985; 11:267.
12. Blacklock NJ. The pattern of urolithiasis in the Royal Navy. In: Hodgkinson A, Nordin BE, eds. Renal stone symposium. London: Churchill 1969:33.
13. Rivers K, Shetty S, Menon M. When and how to evaluate a patient with nephrolithiasis. Urol Clin North Am 2000;27:203.
14. Ettinger B, Oldroyd NO, Surgel F. Triamterene nephrolithiasis. JAMA 1980;244:2443.
15. Kopp JB, Miller KD, Mican JAM, et al. Crystalluria and urinary tract abnormalities associated with indinavir. Ann Intern Med 1997;127:119.
16. Pak CYV, Kaplan RA, Bone H, et al. A simple test for the diagnosis of absorptive, resorptive and renal hypercalciurias. N Engl J Med 1975;292:497.
17. Parivar F, Low RK, Stoller ML. The influence of diet on urinary stone disease. J Urol 1996;155:432.
18. **18.** Borghi L, Meschi T, Amato F, et al. Urinary volume, water and recurrences in idiopathic calcium nephrolithiasis: a 5-year randomized prospective study. J Urol 1996;155:839.
19. Pak CY, Sakhaee K, Crowther C, et al. Evidence justifying a high fluid intake in treatment of nephrolithiasis. Ann Intern Med 1980;93:36.
20. Curhan GC, Willett WC, Rimm ER, et al. A prospective study of dietary calcium and other nutrients and the risk of symptomatic kidney stones. N Engl J Med 1993;328:833.
21. Curhan GC, Willett WC, Speizer FE, et al. Comparison of dietary calcium with supplemental calcium and other nutrients as factors affecting the risk for kidney stones in women. Ann Intern Med 1997;126:497.

21a. Borghi L, Schianchi T, Meschi T, et al. Comparison of two diets for the prevention of recurrent stones in idiopathic hypercalciuria. N Engl J Med 2002;346:77.

22. Lemann J Jr, Gray RW, Pleuss JA. Potassium bicarbonate, but not sodium bicarbonate, reduces urinary calcium excretion and improves calcium balance in healthy men. Kidney Int 1989;35:688.
23. Lemann J Jr, Pleuss JA, Gray RW, et al. Potassium administration reduces and potassium deprivation increases urinary calcium excretion in healthy adults. Kidney Int 1991;39:973.
24. Churchill DN. Medical treatment to prevent recurrent calcium urolithiasis: a guide to critical appraisal. Miner Electrolyte Metab 1987;13:294.
25. Ettinger B, Citron JT, Livermore B, et al. Chlorthalidone reduces calcium oxalate calculus recurrence but magnesium hydroxide does not. J Urol 1988;139:679.
26. Laerum E, Larsen S. Thiazide prophylaxis of urolithiasis: a double-blind study in general practice. Acta Med Scand 1984; 215:383.
27. Yendt ER. Medical management of calcium stones. In: Roth RA, Finlayson B, eds. Stones: clinical management of urolithiasis. Baltimore: Williams & Wilkins, 1983:187.
28. Nicor MJ, Peterson R, Sakhaee K, et al. Use of potassium citrate as potassium supplement during thiazide therapy of calcium nephrolithiasis. J Urol 1984;131:430.
29. Pak CYC, Peterson R, Sakhaee K, et al. Correction of hypocitraturia and prevention of stone formation by combined thiazide and potassium citrate therapy in thiazide-unresponsive hypercalciuric nephrolithiasis. Am J Med 1985;79:284.
30. **30.** Barcelo P, Wuhl O, Servitge E, et al. Randomized double-blind study of potassium citrate in idiopathic hypocitraturia calcium nephrolithiasis. J Urol 1993;150:1761.
31. Thomas WC Jr. Use of phosphates in patients with calcareous renal calculi. Kidney Int 1978;13:390.
32. Teichman JM, Long RD, Hulbert JC. Long-term renal fate and prognosis after staghorn calculus management. J Urol 1995;153:1403.
33. **33.** Segura JW, Preminger GM, Assimos DG, et al. Nephrolithiasis Clinical Guidelines Panel summary report on the management of staghorn calculi. The American Urological Association Nephrolithiasis Clinical Guidelines Panel. J Urol 1994;151:1648.
34. Coe FL. Treated and untreated recurrent calcium nephrolithiasis in patients with idiopathic hypercalciuria, hyperuricosuria, or no metabolic disorder. Ann Intern Med 1977;87:404.

CHAPTER 52

Chronic Renal Insufficiency

GARY R. BRIEFEL, MD

Renal insufficiency, either presenting as a primary renal event or complicating another illness, is a common clinical problem. Data derived from the Third National Health and Nutrition Examination Survey indicate that there are almost 11 million people in the United States who have a serum creatinine concentration greater than 1.5 mg/dL (1). The understanding of the reasons why patients who have renal insufficiency progress to renal failure has increased, and the ability to modify the natural history has improved. Because patients with beginning stages of renal insufficiency are often discovered by the primary care provider, it is important to be familiar with the initial phases of evaluation and management. It has also been recognized that the predialysis management of patients who develop end-stage renal disease has an impact on subsequent morbidity. Therefore, coordination between the primary care provider and the nephrologist is important.

The healthy kidney performs a wide variety of functions that contribute to the maintenance of the internal environment of the body. In addition to its role in maintaining the balance of water and electrolytes, the kidney has important endocrine and metabolic functions. It produces hormones responsible for normal bone formation (1,25-dihydroxyvitamin D_3), red blood cell production (erythropoietin), and blood pressure control (renin, prostaglandins). The kidney is responsible for degrading a number of polypeptide hormones, including parathyroid hormone (PTH), insulin, gastrin, and prolactin. Also, the kidney serves as a major excretory route for many toxic metabolic wastes and a wide variety of drugs or their breakdown products.

In parallel with the progressive destruction of renal mass that occurs with many chronic kidney diseases, patients pass through a sequence of clinical stages before reaching *end-stage renal disease* (ESRD), the point when dialysis is required. The divisions between these stages are somewhat arbitrary and may vary among patients; nevertheless, these distinctions are useful in predicting the kinds of abnormalities that are to be expected for any given degree of renal dysfunction. Frequent reference to the glomerular filtration rate (GFR) throughout this chapter should not be interpreted to mean that the precise value of this measurement must be known to manage the patient. Before ESRD, the blood urea nitrogen (BUN) and serum creatinine concentrations are often within the normal range, despite a 50% to 60% fall of the GFR to as low as 50 mL/minute. Signs and symptoms, if present during this stage, are usually attributable to the underlying disease (e.g., diabetes mellitus, hypertension). As renal function declines further (GFR, 20 to 50 mL/minute), the BUN and serum creatinine levels become noticeably increased and some metabolic abnormalities appear (e.g., metabolic acidosis, carbohydrate intolerance, and reduced synthesis of 1,25-dihydroxyvitamin D_3). Also at this point, the kidney's ability to respond to acute changes in body fluid and electrolyte composition is reduced. In this stage of renal insufficiency, although the BUN and serum creatinine concentrations are increased (azotemia), symptoms attributable to the retention of nitrogenous wastes are absent. However, the patient may begin to experience symptoms related to anemia (fatigue), loss of urine-concentrating ability (polyuria), or volume expansion (dyspnea or edema).

When the GFR falls below 20 mL/minute (serum creatinine concentration usually greater than 5 mg/dL), the patient enters the stage of renal failure. This stage is associated with a further reduction in the ability of the kidney to maintain homeostasis and is characterized by multiple biochemical abnormalities (e.g., hypocalcemia, hyperphosphatemia, metabolic acidosis) and fluid overload. The term *uremia* is used to describe the entire set of signs, symptoms, and metabolic disturbances that occur in advanced kidney failure (GFR less than 10 mL/minute, serum creatinine concentration usually greater than 8 mg/dL) and that may affect virtually all organ systems. Examples of uremic manifestations include nausea, vomiting, and anorexia (gastrointestinal tract); lassitude, reversal of the sleep–wake cycle (nervous system); heart failure, hypertension (cardiovascular system); pruritus (skin); and infertility (endocrine system).

EPIDEMIOLOGY OF CHRONIC RENAL INSUFFICIENCY

There is excellent information on the epidemiology of patients who require renal replacement therapy (dialysis or renal transplantation) and enter the ESRD Program (the Medicare-funded program that provides coverage for virtually all patients in the United States who need dialysis). These data are collected and analyzed by the federally funded United States Renal Disease System (USRDS) (2). At the end of 1999, more than 320,000 patients were being treated for ESRD under the Medicare program in the United States with either dialysis or kidney transplantation. Since 1972, the year Medicare coverage was extended to patients with chronic renal failure who needed dialysis, the incidence of end-stage renal failure in patients who enter dialysis and transplant programs has increased from 71 million per year to more than 311 million per year in 1999. In actual numbers, 87,000 new patients entered the ESRD Program in 1998, and this figure has been increasing yearly by almost 5%. The incidence and prevalence of ESRD is projected to increase further over the next 10 years (Fig. 52.1) in concert with the aging of the population. Medicare expenditures for the ESRD Program in 1999 were $12.7 billion, and total costs reached $17.9 billion (Fig. 52.2).

The incidence of ESRD requiring dialysis has been noted to be 30% to 40% higher in men than in women and to peak between the ages of 65 and 74 years. The rate has also been estimated to be three to four times greater in nonwhites than in whites, because of either higher prevalence of hypertension or a greater end-organ sensitivity to the effect of hypertension in nonwhites. The reported distribution of dialysis patients entering the ESRD Program by primary renal diagnosis is diabetic nephropathy, 39.5%; hypertensive/large vessel disease, 25.2%; glomerulonephritis, 9.1%; secondary glomerulonephritis/vasculitis, 2.2%; interstitial nephritis, 3.8%; cystic/hereditary/congenital kidney disease, 2.8%; neoplasms/tumors, 1.7%; miscellaneous/unknown, 15.7% (Table 52.1) (2). Patients with renal disease related to acquired immunodeficiency syndrome (AIDS) remain a small fraction of the total, with an incidence rate of 1.4 new patients per million population.

CLASSIFICATION

Kidney diseases are often classified according to whether they produce acute or chronic renal failure. *Acute renal failure* (ARF) is defined as a deterioration of glomerular filtration that occurs over days or weeks, whereas the course of *chronic renal failure* often runs from months to years. Many diseases that cause ARF are reversible, and recovery is often complete (e.g., aminoglycoside nephrotoxicity). ARF is not commonly encountered in the ambulatory setting,

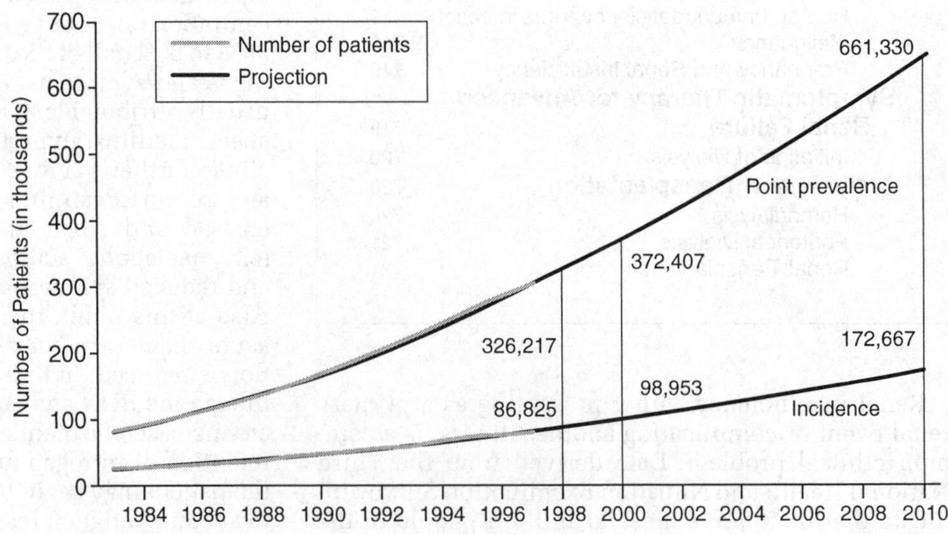

Figure 52.1. The past, current and projected incidence and prevalence of end-stage renal disease. (Modified from U.S. Renal Data System: USRDS 2000 annual data report.)

Table 52.1. Primary Renal Disease Demographics for Dialysis Patients Entering the End-Stage Renal Disease (ESRD) Program (1994–1998)

Dialysis	No. Patients	% of Total	Median Age (yr)	Age (%)			Gender (%)		Race/Ethnicity (%)				
				<20	20–64	>64	Male	Female	White	Black	Native American	Asian	Hispanic
All ESRD	382,490	100.0	63	100	100	100	100	100	100	100	100	100	100
Diabetes	150,978	39.5	64	1.6	40.9	39.0	35.3	44.1	39.8	37.9	62.4	42.2	58.8
Glomerulonephritis (GN)	34,997	9.1	57	30.5	10.2	7.4	10.4	7.7	9.9	7.2	7.9	14.8	9.1
Secondary GN/ vasculitis	8,490	2.2	47	9.8	3.0	1.2	1.4	3.2	2.2	2.3	2.1	2.2	2.4
Interstitial nephritis/ pyelonephritis	14,429	3.8	66	6.7	3.2	4.3	4.0	3.5	4.7	2.1	2.0	3.2	2.7
Hypertensive/large vessel disease	96,268	25.2	70	5.1	17.0	34.5	26.9	23.3	23.7	30.4	11.5	21.8	16.2
Cystic/hereditary/ congenital	10,801	2.8	52	24.9	3.4	1.6	3.0	2.6	3.6	1.4	1.5	2.1	2.6
Neoplasms/tumors	6,498	1.7	69	0.6	1.2	2.3	2.0	1.4	2.1	1.1	1.0	0.8	1.0
Miscellaneous conditions	12,299	3.2	56	4.5	3.7	2.6	3.9	2.4	3.0	4.1	1.4	1.1	2.0
Biology uncertain	13,712	3.6	68	7.0	2.8	4.4	3.9	3.2	4.0	2.8	2.4	4.1	3.5
Missing	34,018	8.9	51	9.2	14.6	2.7	9.2	8.6	6.9	10.7	8.0	7.7	1.8

Modified from US Renal Data System, USRDS 2000 Annual Data Report.

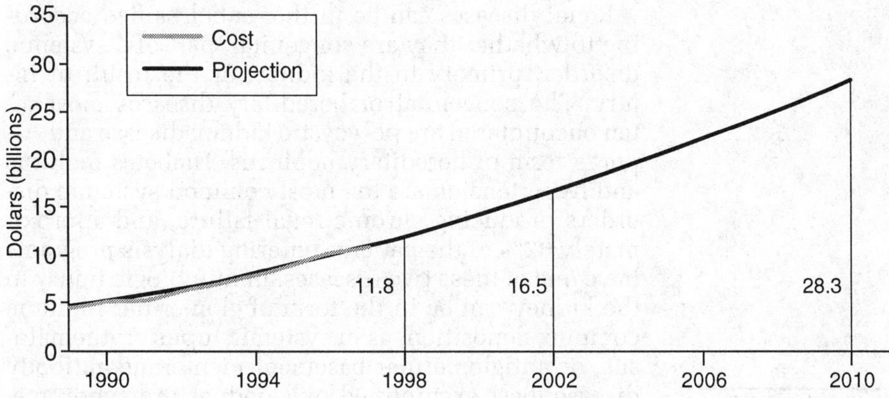

Figure 52.2. Estimated Medicare costs for the End-Stage Renal Disease Program. (Modified from U.S. Renal Data System: USRDS 2000 annual data report.)

but it may be seen with obstruction, drug nephrotoxicity (e.g., angiotensin-converting enzyme [ACE] inhibitors), or rapidly progressive glomerulonephritis. Recovery from diseases that produce chronic renal failure is less common. Some illnesses that produce ARF may not be entirely reversible and can progress to ESRD (e.g., Goodpasture syndrome, acute cortical necrosis). Conversely, some chronic forms of renal disease can improve spontaneously or with therapy and may never progress to the point of necessitating dialysis treatments (e.g., membranous glomerulopathy, the nephropathy of systemic lupus erythematosus).

The causes of kidney failure may be further subdivided into those with prerenal, renal, or postrenal components. *Prerenal azotemia* is caused by factors that produce a decrease in renal perfusion. Diminished perfusion may result from anatomic lesions such as might occur with renal artery stenosis, but more commonly it is related to decreased cardiac output (heart failure), vasodilation (septic shock), or volume depletion (vomiting, diarrhea, or excessive diuretic use). Prerenal azotemia caused by volume depletion, for example, may often be superimposed on existing chronic renal failure from other causes. *Postrenal azotemia* is caused by obstructing lesions that occur distal to the kidney parenchyma, involving the renal pelvis, ureters, bladder, or urethra. Common examples of such lesions are prostatic enlargement, nephrolithiasis, and retroperitoneal cancers.

Most diseases that cause chronic renal failure directly involve the kidney parenchyma and are classified according to the anatomic region that is primarily affected (Table 52.2). *Glomerular lesions* can be caused by proliferation of endothelial or mesangial cells (e.g., postinfectious glomerulonephritis), thickening of the basement membrane (e.g., membranous glomerulopathy, diabetic nephropathy), glomerulosclerosis (e.g., focal sclerosis), or combinations of the three (e.g., membranoproliferative glomerulonephritis). Any of the diseases that cause glomerular lesions, if sustained, can lead to chronic glomerulonephritis. Clinically, glomerular diseases are often associated with hypertension, edema, renal insufficiency, hematuria, and proteinuria.

Table 52.2. Classification of Kidney Diseases that May Result in Chronic Renal Failure

Prerenal diseases
Renal artery stenosis S
Hepatorenal syndrome S
Renal parenchymal diseases
Glomerular diseases
Membranous glomerulonephritis (GN) I
Membranoproliferative GN I
Focal glomerulosclerosis I
HIV nephropathy S
Rapidly progressive GN I
Goodpasture syndrome I, S
Lupus nephritis I, S
Immunoglobulin A nephropathy I
Alport syndrome (hereditary nephritis) H, S
Diabetic glomerulosclerosis M, S
Tubulointerstitial diseases
Drug-induced interstitial nephritis N[a]
Chronic pyelonephritis with reflux
Analgesic nephropathy N
Radiation nephritis N
Polycystic kidney disease H, S
Sickle cell nephropathy S
Heavy metal nephropathy N
Gouty nephropathy M, S
Medullary cystic disease H
Vascular diseases
Thrombotic thrombocytopenic purpura S
Hemolytic-uremic syndrome S
Scleroderma kidney S
Hypertensive nephropathy S
Vasculitis I, S
Wegener granulomatosis I, S
Miscellaneous
Myeloma kidney N, S
Amyloidosis S
Fibrillary glomerulopathy I
Postrenal diseases
Nephrolithiases
Bilateral ureteral obstruction
Bladder outlet obstruction

H, Hereditary; I, immunologically mediated; M, metabolic; N, nephrotoxic; S, part of a systemic disorder.

[a]See Table 52.4.

Diseases that affect primarily the tubulointerstitial areas of the kidney are characterized morphologically by interstitial inflammation, fibrosis, and tubular atrophy. In the past, these lesions were often equated with bacterial infections of the kidney (pyelonephritis), but today most are caused by toxins (e.g., analgesics, heavy metals), metabolic derangements (e.g., hyperuricemia, hypercalcemia), or immunologic disorders (e.g., methicillin-induced interstitial nephritis). The glomeruli are only secondarily involved in the tubulointerstitial diseases. *Polycystic and medullary cystic kidney diseases* are a subgroup of the tubulointerstitial nephropathies and are characterized histologically by the presence of a multitude of thin-walled cysts derived from tubular epithelium. Patients with interstitial forms of kidney disease are not usually hypertensive or edematous, and they often produce large volumes of urine with high sodium content. Typically, nonnephrotic-range proteinuria (i.e., less than 3 g/day), sterile pyuria, and hyperchloremic metabolic acidosis are present.

Lesions of the renal vessels may be located in the main renal arteries (e.g., atherosclerosis, fibromuscular dysplasia), in medium-sized arteries or arterioles (e.g., polyarteritis nodosa, scleroderma, atheroembolic disease), or in the renal veins (e.g., renal vein thrombosis). Renal insufficiency is a result of reduction in blood flow to the glomeruli. Involvement of the renal vessels is often part of a systemic illness that also affects vessels in other areas of the body. The clinical features of the renal vasculitides are very similar to those of glomerulonephritis except that nephrotic-range proteinuria (by definition more than 3 g/day) is uncommon.

A number of renal diseases can variably affect one or more of the kidney's anatomic regions. For instance, renal involvement in *multiple myeloma* may take the form of a diffuse thickening of the glomerular basement membrane (light-chain nephropathy), or more often it causes a tubulointerstitial nephropathy. *Systemic lupus erythematosus* is another example of a disease that can produce either glomerular or tubulointerstitial damage.

Renal diseases can be further subclassified according to whether they are congenital, part of a systemic disorder, primary to the kidney, or the result of injury. The congenital or hereditary diseases most often encountered are polycystic kidney disease and Alport's form of hereditary nephritis. Diabetes mellitus and hypertension are the most common systemic disorders producing chronic renal failure, and approximately 62% of the patients entering dialysis programs have one of these two diseases. Immunologic injury to the kidney can be in the form of glomerular immune complex deposition, as in systemic lupus erythematosus, or antiglomerular basement membrane antibody disease, best exemplified by Goodpasture syndrome. Most immunologically mediated diseases affect predominantly the vessels or glomeruli, but they can also damage the tubulointerstitial areas, as is seen in drug-induced interstitial nephritis (e.g., methicillin). Drugs (e.g., aspirin) and toxins (e.g., heavy metals) most often produce damage to the interstitium. Metabolic disorders (e.g., diabetes mellitus, oxalosis) can result in damage to any region of the kidney.

PATHOPHYSIOLOGY OF UREMIA

The course of many chronic kidney diseases is characterized by the progressive loss of functioning nephrons. The kidney undergoes a number of adaptive changes that allow most patients with chronic renal failure to have few signs or symptoms until approximately 80% of the original number of nephrons has been lost.

Once a certain level of renal impairment has been reached, further deterioration seems to be inevitable, even when the original insult is transient and other causes of additional damage have been excluded. The mechanism that has been postulated to explain the progressive nature of renal disease is related to the adaptive response to injury (3). According to this

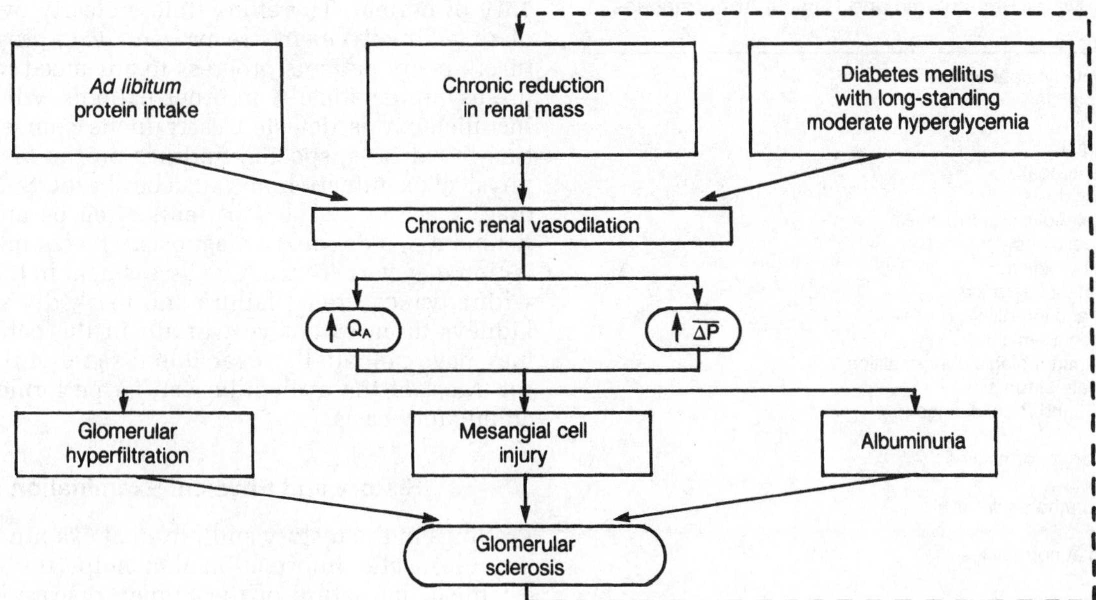

Figure 52.3. Proposed sequence of events whereby a chronic reduction in kidney mass and the consequent increase in glomerular pressures and flows lead to progressive renal damage. Q_A, Blood flow; ΔP, transcapillary hydraulic pressure. (Redrawn from Brenner BM, Meyer TW, Hostetter TH. Dietary protein intake and the progressive nature of kidney disease: the role of hemodynamically mediated glomerular injury in the pathogenesis of progressive glomerular sclerosis, aging, renal ablation, and intrinsic renal disease. N Engl J Med 1982;307:652.)

hypothesis, after a reduction in nephron mass, renal vasodilation occurs and leads to hyperperfusion of the remaining glomeruli. These changes are considered to be adaptive because they result in increased GFRs. However, experiments have shown that this state of *glomerular hypertension,* if sustained, can in itself be harmful (Fig. 52.3). Glomeruli of nephrons exposed to prolonged hyperperfusion begin to leak protein, become sclerotic, and eventually are destroyed. Current theories implicate toxicity from the filtered proteins, perhaps mediated by release of cytokines or other inflammatory products, as an important mechanism of renal parenchymal damage. As more and more nephrons are lost, the stimulus for hyperperfusion of the residual nephrons is increased and the process becomes self-perpetuating. There is evidence that many diseases that produce limited kidney damage (e.g., patchy cortical necrosis, analgesic nephropathy, radiation nephritis) may progress to ESRD by this mechanism.

The ability of the impaired kidney to maintain the concentrations of individual components of the body's fluids within normal limits is variable. The concentrations of substances that are simply filtered and neither secreted nor resorbed by the tubule, such as urea, begin to rise early in the course of renal impairment (GFR 50% of normal). In contrast, the serum concentration of phosphorus, which is under the influence of PTH, is kept within the normal range until more than approximately 80% of renal function is lost. This is because in renal failure, increased PTH activity progressively reduces the amount of phosphorus resorbed by the tubule (normally 80% of filtered phosphorus is resorbed), in parallel with the reduction in renal mass. Once the GFR falls below about 20% of normal, this mechanism can no longer keep pace, and the serum phosphorus level begins to rise. Other solutes, such as sodium and potassium, are even better regulated, and their concentrations are maintained within the normal range until the GFR is less than 5 mL/minute.

Eventually the reserve capacity of the kidney is overwhelmed and a number of signs, symptoms, and metabolic abnormalities appear that are characteristic of uremia (Table 52.3). Uremia is a complex syndrome that results from the failure of the kidney to fulfill its excretory, endocrine, and metabolic functions. In the patient with ESRD, virtually every organ system is affected to some degree. The mechanisms for only some of the abnormalities that appear in uremia are well understood. Efforts to explain the metabolic consequences of renal failure by the retention of toxic wastes are only partially satisfying. Because urea is easily measured, it is the putative toxin that has been most thoroughly examined. Other nitrogenous waste products (e.g., ammonia, guanidinosuccinic acid), middle molecules (polypeptides of intermediate molecular weight), and a variety of organic and inorganic compounds have been implicated in the pathogenesis of uremia. Each of these toxins, individually or together, potentially could interfere with a specific cellular metabolic function and give rise to a manifestation of uremia.

Not all manifestations of uremia can be attributed to the retention of metabolic waste products. Many well-described endocrine and metabolic derangements are of equal significance in the pathogenesis of uremia.

Table 52.3. Major Physiologic and Clinical Abnormalities of Uremia

Fluid and electrolyte abnormalities
- Volume expansion
- Hyperkalemia
- Hypocalcemia
- Hyperphosphatemia
- Metabolic acidosis

Endocrine-metabolic abnormalities
- Vitamin D deficiency
- Hyperparathyroidism
- Carbohydrate intolerance
- Impotence and infertility
- Hypertriglyceridemia

Hematologic-immunologic abnormalities
- Impaired platelet function
- Abnormal T- and B-cell function
- Anemia

Cardiovascular abnormalities
- Hypertension
- Accelerated atherosclerosis
- Pericarditis

Dermatologic abnormalities
- Pruritus
- Increased pigmentation
- Acne

Gastrointestinal abnormalities
- Nausea and vomiting
- Anorexia
- Pancreatitis

Neuromuscular abnormalities
- Peripheral neuropathy
- Seizures
- Coma
- Asterixis
- Myoclonus

A deficiency of certain hormones results when the failing kidney is no longer able to produce them in adequate quantities (e.g., erythropoietin, 1,25-dihydroxyvitamin D_3). Other hormones normally degraded or metabolized by the kidney may be present in excess (e.g., PTH, insulin, prolactin). Alternatively, the damaged kidney may elaborate an excess of hormone (e.g., renin). Hormone levels or activity may also be altered as a consequence of abnormal protein binding (e.g., thyroid hormone), peripheral resistance (e.g., insulin, PTH), or loss of feedback control (e.g., luteinizing hormone).

DIAGNOSIS OF CHRONIC RENAL INSUFFICIENCY

Presentation

Kidney disease can most easily be recognized when it is associated with clearly defined clinical symptoms such as urinary tract obstruction or laboratory findings such as proteinuria or hematuria. The recognition of one of these abnormalities is helpful in focusing the ensuing diagnostic evaluation. Often, the presence of renal disease is discovered during the evaluation of a systemic disease of which renal dysfunction is only a part (e.g., diabetes mellitus, hypertension).

Because of the remarkable reserve and adaptive capabilities of the kidney, symptoms of uremia do not appear until glomerular filtration is reduced to 10% to 15% of normal. Therefore, unless clearly overt signs of renal involvement are present (e.g., gross hematuria), many patients progress to advanced renal failure asymptomatically. In other patients, whose renal insufficiency is detected early in its course by routine blood tests, specific findings on the history and physical examination may also be absent. Special laboratory testing in these patients often permits establishment of a definitive diagnosis. The complete evaluation may vary from a brief assessment in the patient with advanced renal failure and markedly shrunken kidneys to an extensive workup in the patient who may have potentially reversible disease of recent onset. Most of the evaluation can be performed on an ambulatory basis.

History and Physical Examination

Findings in the history and physical examination can provide useful information that helps the clinician establish the nature of the kidney disease, estimate its duration, and determine its effect on the patient. One of the major goals in evaluating the patient with recently identified renal failure is to distinguish patients with primary, acquired kidney disease from those whose renal failure is caused by familial, congenital, or systemic illness.

The family history should be reviewed for the presence of polycystic kidney disease, Alport syndrome, medullary sponge kidney, hypertension, diabetes mellitus, or renal failure. The presence of a hereditary form of renal disease in the family should help establish the etiology of the patient's kidney problem. Next, the patient's medical history should be reviewed carefully, with a particular emphasis on discovering the presence of a systemic illness that can cause renal failure (e.g., hypertension, diabetes mellitus, collagen vascular disorders). Patients with AIDS can develop a nephropathy that manifests with nephrotic syndrome and often progresses to renal failure (4). In the absence of symptoms related to a systemic illness, the patient should be questioned about symptoms associated with abnormalities of the urinary tract. Dysuria, frequency, renal colic, hesitancy, or urinary incontinence points to an abnormality of the lower urinary tract as the cause of the patient's renal dysfunction.

In addition to the symptoms that may prove useful in establishing a diagnosis, several symptoms (e.g., nausea, vomiting, fatigue, nocturia, itching, restless leg) are nonspecific. These "uremic" symptoms are present in most patients with advanced renal failure.

Because symptoms of renal failure often do not appear until late in the course, it is sometimes difficult to pinpoint the time of onset of the disease. Important clues can occasionally be found when records of past physical examinations performed for work, insurance, or military purposes are reviewed.

Because certain drugs can cause renal dysfunction (e.g., heroin, analgesics, nonsteroidal anti-inflammatory drugs [NSAIDs], aminoglycosides) or aggravate pre-existing renal insufficiency (e.g., diuretics)

Table 52.4. Some Commonly Used Drugs that May Adversely Affect Renal Function

Antibiotics
Aminoglycosides (ATN)
Penicillins (IN)
Tetracyclines (increased azotemia and acidosis)
Analgesics
Aspirin (PN and reduction in RBF)
Phenacetin (PN and IN)
Nonsteroidal analgesics (IN, nephrotic syndrome, and reduced RBF)
Diuretics
Thiazides (volume depletion and IN)
Loop agents (volume depletion and IN)
Miscellaneous
Radiocontrast materials (ATN)
Methysergide (retroperitoneal fibrosis causing obstructive uropathy)
Penicillamine (NS)
Gold (NS)
Acyclovir, indinavir, methotrexate (crystal induced ARF)
Mitomycin C (TTP-HUS)
H_2-receptor antagonists (interfere with secretion of creatinine and produce false elevations of the serum creatinine concentration)
ACE inhibitors (precipitate renal failure in patients with renovascular disease)

ATN, Acute tubular necrosis; IN, interstitial nephritis; NS, nephrotic syndrome; PN, papillary necrosis; RBF, renal blood flow.

(Table 52.4), there should be a complete inventory of past and current drug use.

The physical examination should be focused on a search for signs of systemic illnesses and for genitourinary structural abnormalities. These might include high blood pressure, hypertensive or diabetic retinopathy, vascular bruits, vasculitic skin rashes (palpable purpura), gouty tophi, or ocular abnormalities (e.g., band keratopathy of hypercalcemia). Enlarged kidneys on palpation may be found in patients with polycystic disease or hydronephrosis. A pelvic or rectal examination should be performed to evaluate causes of lower urinary tract obstruction, such as prostatic or cervical cancer. If obstruction or flaccid neurogenic bladder is suspected, the bladder should be catheterized or evaluated by sonography after the patient voids to measure residual volume (see Chapter 54). A residual volume that is larger than 200 to 300 mL should raise concern for bladder outlet obstruction (see Chapter 53) or neuropathic bladder (most commonly seen in diabetic patients). Signs of heart failure, pericarditis, or neuropathy are most often related to the stage of renal failure and are not helpful in establishing the cause.

Laboratory Investigation

Laboratory testing of patients with chronic renal insufficiency establishes the severity and the origin of the kidney disease and determines the presence of complicating abnormalities.

Diagnostically, the *urinalysis* can often provide important information. Red blood cells (RBCs), particularly when associated with RBC casts, are most indicative of a glomerular or vascular lesion. In the presence of isolated hematuria, the presence of dysmorphic RBCs in the urinalysis can suggest an upper urinary tract source. Leukocytes, with or without casts, are found in the interstitial nephropathies. Hyaline or granular casts are not indicative of a specific pathologic process.

The *urine dipstick* is only a rough guide to the amount of proteinuria (see Chapter 48). Most dipsticks are designed to detect only albumin and may therefore miss the presence of other proteins, such as light-chain proteins. The dipstick measures only the concentration of protein, so the reading must be interpreted in conjunction with the urine specific gravity. The finding of 1+ proteinuria on two consecutive tests taken 3 months apart is considered abnormal and requires further evaluation (5). Patients who are high risk for the development of kidney disease (e.g., diabetics, hypertensives, African Americans) should be checked for microalbuminuria (urine albumin excretion between 30 and 300 mg/day) by means of specific urinary dipsticks for albumin or by antibody techniques. The finding of microalbuminuria in these populations is associated with an increased risk of renal and cardiovascular events and demands further evaluation and treatment (5). When quantification of proteinuria is desired, a 24-hour urine specimen should be obtained; it can also be used to calculate the creatinine clearance (see later discussion). Alternatively, the protein/creatinine ratio may be determined in a specimen of urine as described in Chapter 48. The finding of nephrotic-range proteinuria (excretion of more than 3 g/day or a spot urine protein/creatinine ratio greater than 3) usually indicates a glomerular lesion, whereas lesser amounts are seen in some glomerular or vascular disorders and in most interstitial forms of nephritis. In patients older than 40 years of age with unexplained renal insufficiency, regardless of the amount of urinary protein detected by dipstick, a serum and urine electrophoresis should be obtained to exclude the possibility of multiple myeloma.

Selected tests should be ordered when an *immunologically mediated disease* is suspected, such as in a patient with vasculitis or an unexplained nephritic picture (RBC casts, nephrotic proteinuria). For example, measurement of the serum complement levels (C3 and C4) and screening for the presence of antistreptococcal antibodies, antinuclear antibodies, rheumatoid factor, and cryoglobulins may be of value when collagen vascular disease or poststreptococcal glomerulonephritis is suspected. Measurement of antineutrophil cytoplasmic antibodies (ANCAs) is useful in diagnosing cases of systemic vasculitis, including Wegener granulomatosis and polyarteritis nodosa. Hepatitis B surface antigen (see Chapter 47) can be demonstrated in the blood of some patients with membranous glomerulopathy and in those with some forms of vasculitic renal disease. Hepatitis C infections are associated with mixed cryoglobulinemia and membranoproliferative glomerulonephritis. Hepatitis B and C antigens and antibodies should also be assayed in any patient being referred for dialysis or transplantation, because precautions to prevent the spread of hepatitis

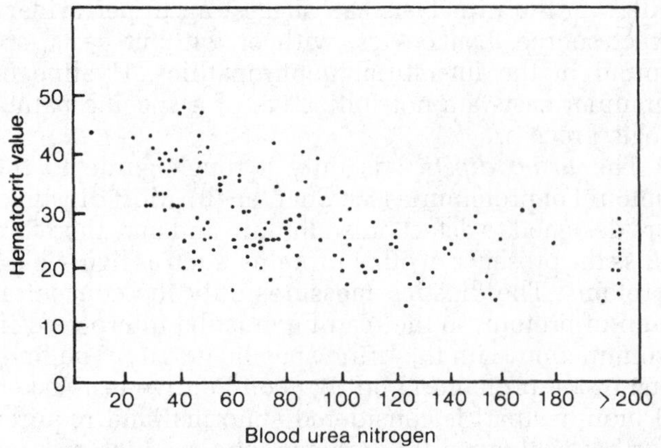

Figure 52.4. Relationship of blood urea nitrogen concentration to the hematocrit value in patients with chronic renal failure. (From Erslev AJ. Erythrocyte function of the kidney. In: Wesson LG, ed. Physiology of the human kidney. New York: Grune & Stratton, 1969:521.)

must be taken if the patient is a potential carrier. A test for human immunodeficiency virus (HIV) antibodies (see Chapter 39) should be performed in patients with nephrotic syndrome or renal failure who are at risk for HIV infection. In general, a nephrologist should be consulted to help guide this workup.

The *severity of anemia* (see Chapter 55) roughly parallels the BUN concentration, as shown in Fig. 52.4. The absence of anemia in patients with renal insufficiency should suggest either recent onset, the presence of polycystic kidney disease, or hydronephrosis. Both polycystic kidney disease and hydronephrosis can be associated with normal or elevated hematocrit values. The peripheral blood smear should be examined carefully for abnormalities associated with diseases that can produce renal failure. Rouleaux formation may be present in multiple myeloma, and leukopenia may be associated with collagen vascular diseases. A microangiopathic hemolytic anemia may be seen in patients with thrombotic thrombocytopenic purpura, the hemolytic-uremic syndrome, postpartum renal failure, accelerated hypertension, or scleroderma.

Measurements of the concentrations of blood glucose, serum electrolytes (Na, K, Cl, HCO_3, Ca, PO_4), and uric acid are helpful in patient monitoring. Hypercalcemia may suggest a tumor or hyperparathyroidism. The uric acid concentration is usually increased in patients with renal insufficiency, but a level greater than 12 mg/dL may indicate the presence of primary hyperuricemia or a myeloproliferative disorder.

Some *measure of overall kidney function* is needed to determine the degree of impairment, monitor the progression of disease, assess the effects of therapy, and adjust the dosage of drugs that are excreted by the kidney. The GFR is the standard means of expressing the level of renal function. In clinical practice, the GFR may be estimated from the serum creatinine concentration, from the endogenous CrCl, or from formulas that incorporate the patient's serum creatinine level, age, and weight.

The normal GFR is approximately 100 to 140 mL/minute in men and 85 to 115 mL/minute in women. A gradual deterioration of GFR with age occurs, even in the absence of overt renal disease, in 70% of individuals (6,7). The following equation may be used for estimating the expected creatinine clearance in healthy men.

$$\text{GFR} = 133 - 0.64 \times \text{Age}$$

where the GFR is expressed in milliliters per minute and the age in years. The clearance for women 50 years of age or older is approximately 5 to 10 mL/minute less than for men. At age 70, for example, an individual without renal disease may have lost 30% of his or her previous GFR.

The serum creatinine concentration is a better indicator of renal function than is the level of BUN, because the latter is affected by such nonrenal factors as volume status, diet, intestinal bleeding, liver function, and protein catabolism. The general relationship between serum creatinine concentration and GFR is shown in Fig. 52.5. When trying to determine the extent of renal impairment, it is important to remember that the serum creatinine concentration for any given level of GFR varies among individuals, because the relationship between the two values is significantly influenced by nonrenal factors such as the patient's muscle mass and age. Creatinine is produced by muscle, and its production rate directly parallels the muscle mass. The amount of creatinine produced per day also falls with age. As can be seen in Fig. 52.5, a small or elderly patient may have a doubling of the serum creatinine concentration, from 0.8 to 1.6 mg/dL, and still be within the "normal" range. Also, a young, muscular patient who produces 1.5 g of creatinine per day will have a GFR of 30 mL/minute when his or her serum creatinine concentration is 5 mg/dL, whereas

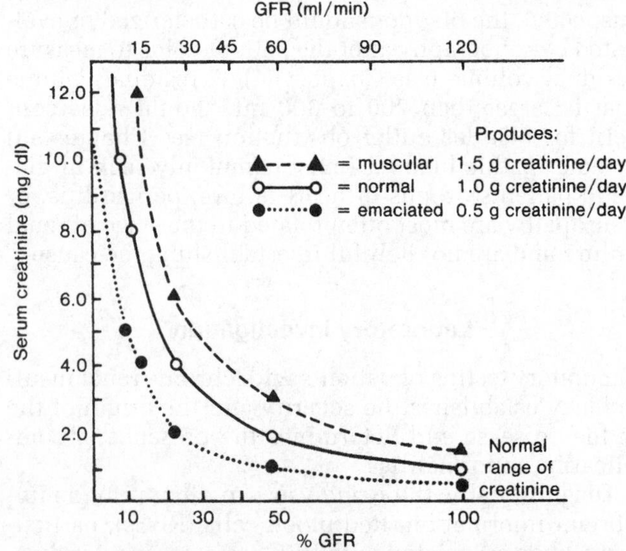

Figure 52.5. Relationship of the serum creatinine concentration to glomerular filtration rate in patients with different muscle mass.

an elderly, frail patient who produces only 0.5 g of creatinine per day will have a creatinine clearance of only 10 mL/minute at the same serum creatinine concentration. Therefore, although an elevated serum creatinine value almost always reflects abnormal renal function, a creatinine concentration in the "normal" range does not mean that GFR is normal, particularly if there is other evidence for the presence of renal disease. Once the factors affecting the level of serum creatinine concentration are understood, the physician should have a clinically useful measure of overall renal function.

Because of the difficulties in estimating the level of renal function from the serum creatinine concentration alone, alternative methods for estimating the GFR are available. These methods are generally used to adjust dosages of drugs that are excreted by the kidney or to assess renal function in elderly or small patients.

The endogenous creatinine clearance is a reasonable approximation of GFR in patients with normal or modestly reduced function but overestimates the GFR in those with advanced renal failure. The formula used for calculating clearance is

$$\text{Creatinine clearance} = UV/P \div 1{,}440$$

where U is the urine creatinine in milligrams per deciliter, V is the urine volume in milliliters in 24 hours, P is the plasma creatinine concentration in milligrams per deciliter, and 1,440 is the number of minutes in 24 hours. The result is expressed in milliliters per minute. A correction can be made for body surface area, but in adults this is not needed for usual clinical purposes. A 24-hour urine collection is used to determine daily creatinine production (i.e., $U \times V$). To confirm the adequacy of this collection, the expected daily creatinine production may be estimated by multiplying body weight by $[28 - (0.2 \times \text{Age})]$ for men and $[23.8 - (0.17 \times \text{Age})]$ for women. For example, the expected daily creatinine production in a 50-year-old man weighing 70 kg would be $70 \times [28 - (0.2 \times 50)] = 1{,}260$ mg.

In collecting the 24-hour urine, the patient should be instructed to choose a convenient time to begin the collection—usually upon rising in the morning. At this time the patient voids and discards the urine but collects all subsequent urine until the same time the following day, when the patient again voids and adds that specimen to the collection. The blood sample for measurement of creatinine is usually obtained at the end of the collection period, but it may be drawn at any time during the collection. The estimation of GFR by measurement of creatinine clearance is often inaccurate, mainly because of collection errors. Although radionuclide measurements of GFR that do not require urine collection are available, there is rarely a need for such accuracy in office practice, and these tests are reserved largely for research purposes.

An alternative to calculating the creatinine clearance that avoids the difficulties entailed in collecting urine samples and can be performed in the office is based on a formula that takes into account the patient's body weight (in kilograms) and age:

$$\text{GFR} = [(140 - \text{Age}) \times \text{Weight}] \div [72 \times \text{Serum creatinine concentration}]$$

(The GFR value obtained should be multiplied by 0.85 in the case of a small woman.) It should be recognized that the value of GFR determined by the preceding formula or by measurement of the creatinine clearance may vary significantly from the more accurate determination of GFR by inulin clearance. For clinical purposes, however, these differences are generally considered insignificant.

When monitoring the course of kidney disease, it should be recalled that the serum creatinine concentration increases in a nonlinear fashion as renal function declines (Fig. 52.5). In the early stages of renal insufficiency, when the GFR falls by 50%, the absolute increase in the serum creatinine concentration is small. Therefore, most of the loss of functioning nephrons occurs at levels of serum creatinine that would be considered only modestly increased. Once the GFR is reduced to 20% to 30% of normal, the curve expressing the relationship between serum creatinine and GFR rises steeply. The absolute changes in serum creatinine concentration that occur when ESRD is present are therefore less significant, in relation to losses of GFR, than those seen in early renal insufficiency.

Alternative methods of *monitoring the progression of renal disease* have been devised to overcome the limitations of using the serum creatinine concentration alone and because sequential measurements of creatinine clearance are often impractical or improperly done. A plot of the reciprocal of the serum creatinine concentration [$1/S_{cr}$] versus time (Fig. 52.6) produces a function that parallels the rate of decline in GFR. In many, but not all, patients, the plot is linear, with the slope reflecting the rate of progression and the horizontal axis intercept the estimated time of end-stage renal failure. It has been suggested that the slope is constant for an individual and that any deviation reflects the effects of therapy or the presence of a superimposed process. There are limitations to this method for monitoring renal function. Comparisons of [$1/S_{cr}$] versus GFR measured with radioisotope techniques have disclosed discordances in up to 45% of cases (8). For example, the slope of $[\text{Cr}]^{-1}$ may overestimate or underestimate the rate of change of GFR using the radioisotope techniques. In some cases, the slope of the [$1/S_{cr}$] remains stable while true GFR declines, or vice versa. These discrepancies are caused in part by changes in creatinine metabolism that occur in patients with renal failure. Therefore, mathematical formulations may be useful, but they must be interpreted only in conjunction with the remainder of the clinical and laboratory information. It is also important to understand that changes in GFR (reflected by an increasing serum creatinine concentration or a falling creatinine clearance) are not necessarily related to permanent changes in intrinsic kidney

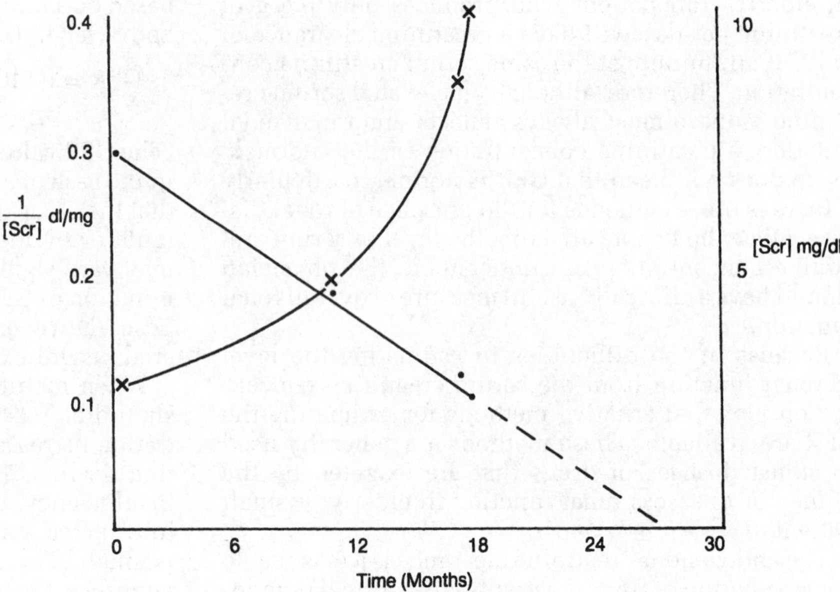

Figure 52.6. Relationship between the serum creatinine concentration ([Scr], *line with* x *marks*) and the reciprocal of serum creatinine concentration (1/[Scr], *solid line*) over time in a patient during an 18-month period. The linear relation suggests that nephrons are being lost at a constant rate. This kind of plot can also be used to monitor the course of renal failure. By extending the line derived from observed data, it is possible to make a rough estimate *(dashed line)* of when dialysis will be necessary.

function and may be caused by other factors (see Treating Reversible Causes of Deterioration in Renal Function).

Renal Imaging Techniques

Anatomic and functional evaluation of the kidney can be obtained through a variety of tests, not all of which need be performed on any individual patient. Renal imaging techniques in chronic renal failure should be used to establish renal size, detect remediable lesions, and determine etiology.

Renal sonography is a reliable means of estimating kidney size and usually detects the presence of significant hydronephrosis. Because of the risk of radiocontrast dye toxicity in patients with renal impairment (discussed later), the sonogram should be used in place of the intravenous pyelogram (IVP) as the initial imaging technique in most instances. Median kidney length as measured by sonography is 11.2 cm on the left and 10.9 cm on the right. Renal size is slightly less in women than in men and decreases with age in both sexes (9). An abdominal radiograph including kidneys, ureters, and bladder (KUB), with tomograms if necessary, is the simplest and least expensive test for estimating renal size but does not detect the presence of hydronephrosis. Normal kidney length as measured by radiography is approximately 12 to 13 cm, or roughly the same as three to four lumbar vertebrae and discs. The kidneys appear longer when measured by radiography because of a projection effect. Small kidneys by either technique usually indicate advanced chronic renal disease. However, normal or large kidneys may be seen in chronic renal failure (e.g., diabetes mellitus, amyloidosis).

Hydronephrosis caused by obstruction should be ruled out in every patient with chronic renal insufficiency. If the screening sonogram reveals the presence of hydronephrosis, a urologist should be consulted. Subsequent evaluation of the obstructed kidney by the urologist may include an IVP, a retrograde pyelogram, a computed tomographic (CT) scan, magnetic resonance imaging (MRI), or a sonographically guided percutaneous antegrade pyelogram. These evaluations are selected to localize the precise site of the obstruction and to identify its nature. The choice of the procedure depends on the preference of the urologist or radiologist. However, an added advantage of the antegrade pyelogram technique is that it allows simultaneous placement of a percutaneous nephrostomy tube for drainage. Occasional cases of nondilated hydronephrosis occur, so further evaluation is indicated, even when the sonogram is normal, if the suspicion of obstruction is high (e.g., a patient with a history of renal colic or intra-abdominal malignancy). HASTE MRI can be used to distinguish between acute and chronic obstruction (10).

In the past, *the IVP* was the most useful radiographic test in determining the cause of renal failure in diseases that produce gross anatomic abnormalities such as chronic pyelonephritis, nephrolithiasis, or obstruction from papillary necrosis. Although the cysts in patients with polycystic kidney disease are detected by IVP, renal ultrasound or spiral CT (see next paragraph) are better screening techniques. The IVP is not useful in patients with parenchymal disorders that are not associated with gross anatomic defects. The IVP is of value only when the creatinine concentration is relatively low (e.g., less than 2.0 to 2.5 g/dL). When it is used in patients with renal insufficiency, IVP-associated dehydration may injure the kidney and can be avoided (see later discussion).

CT scans, particularly the high-speed spiral CT scan, have proved useful for the evaluation of renal stones, renal masses, and cysts, and for visualizing the renal vessels. *Nuclear medicine imaging techniques,* useful in the evaluation of patients with hypertension caused

Table 52.5. Clinical Presentations of Atheromatous Renal Disease

Acute renal failure following reduction in blood pressure (particularly with ACE inhibitors)
Progressive azotemia in a patient with known renovascular disease
Azotemia associated with new-onset hypertension or a change in severity of hypertension
Unexplained azotemia in an elderly patient with peripheral vascular disease
Progressive renal failure with evidence of cholesterol embolization

Adapted from Jacobson HR. Ischemic renal disease: an overlooked entity? Kidney Int 1988;34:729.

by unilateral renal artery stenosis, have been found to be less reliable in detecting bilateral renovascular disease (RVD). Bilateral atheromatous RVD (Table 52.5), an often overlooked cause of renal failure (11), is more difficult to diagnose with radionuclide studies because the standard renal scan relies on asymmetric blood flow as a diagnostic criterion. When blood flow to both kidneys is reduced, it is difficult to distinguish bilateral renal artery stenosis from parenchymal disease. Captopril renography, which depends on captopril-induced hemodynamic alterations (and is helpful in diagnosing unilateral renal artery stenosis in the absence of significant renal failure), may be of value and should be tried in patients with renal insufficiency and suspected bilateral RVD, but it often is not diagnostic (12). Doppler or duplex sonography has been used as a screening tool for diagnosing bilateral renal artery stenosis, but these modalities do not provide anatomic detail and are operator dependent. An arteriogram should be obtained if the index of suspicion is high and a therapeutic decision (e.g., balloon dilation) would be made based on the results. Gadolinium-enhanced magnetic resonance imaging has become another less invasive means of assessing the renal arteries in high-risk patients with suspected renal artery stenosis. It avoids the use of potentially nephrotoxic radiographic dyes and the use of intra-arterial catheters. Carbon dioxide angiography provides good definition without the use of traditional dyes. Intravenous digital subtraction angiography has been suggested as a lower-risk method of imaging the renal arteries, because the risks of dye-induced ARF or atheroembolic disease appear to be reduced, probably because of the lesser amount of dye given and the use of smaller catheters. Finally, high-speed spiral CT scans produce excellent images of the renal arteries and veins. Given the complex decisions encountered when evaluating patients with suspected ischemic renal artery disease, a vascular surgeon, a radiologist, or a nephrologist should be consulted before the arteriogram is ordered. The most difficult decisions arise in patients with probable diabetic nephropathy, who often have significant peripheral vascular disease. The decision to perform angiography is usually based on the clinical judgment that the course deviates from what is usually seen in diabetics, or when the vascular component seems prominent (severe hypertension, claudication, bruits).

The incidence of *radiocontrast-induced ARF* seems highest in patients with renal insufficiency (serum creatinine concentration greater than 2 mg/dL), diabetic patients, and the elderly. Although incidence rates as high as 50% in these groups have been reported, most of these cases are clinically insignificant and reversible. More recent reviews of ARF in high-risk patients have found lower rates (9% to 16%), and it has been suggested that a greater awareness of the role of preprocedure and postprocedure hydration is proving to be of benefit (13). The use of low-osmotic radiocontrast agents (sodium meglumine ioxaglate, iohexol) appears to reduce, but does not eliminate, the occurrence of postangiography ARF in patients with pre-existing renal insufficiency (14). The use of the antioxidant acetylcysteine (600 mg orally 2×/d the day before and the day of the study) in combination with intravenous saline has been shown to reduce the frequency of renal function deterioration after the administration of nonionic, low-osmolality radiocontrast agents in patients with renal insufficiency (15). The benefits of giving mannitol infusions or other pretreatments prophylactically are still unsettled. In summary, the presence of renal insufficiency should not be considered an absolute contraindication to the performance of intravascular dye studies, particularly when the needed information cannot be obtained by alternative means. Because the decline in renal function after use of radiocontrast materials appears to be particularly preventable by avoiding volume depletion, patients should be instructed to maintain salt intake (6 to 8 g/day) and fluid intake (1 to 2 L/day) both before and after the examination. Low-osmotic radiocontrast agents should be used for patients who have pre-existing renal insufficiency.

Renal Biopsy

Once the baseline data have been accumulated, a nephrologist should be consulted to help interpret the information and to decide whether a renal biopsy is indicated. Early consultation with a nephrologist (if the serum creatinine concentration is greater than 1.5 mg/dL or other signs of significant renal disease are present) is advisable. A complete record of past laboratory investigations, a recent urinalysis, and a recent renal ultrasound test should be provided for patients who are being referred for evaluation of chronic renal insufficiency. If the diagnosis remains unknown despite all available information, a renal biopsy provides histologic information and, for many disease entities, is the most specific diagnostic test available. The biopsy should be considered when the diagnosis is uncertain, to estimate prognosis, to help demonstrate renal involvement of a systemic illness, and to help make therapeutic decisions. Most renal biopsies can be performed percutaneously with the use of local anesthesia. Although overnight observation in the hospital is still common, many nephrologists perform renal biopsies in ambulatory surgery settings with 6 to 8 hours of postprocedure monitoring (see Chapter 48). If the kidneys are very small or renal failure is advanced, a biopsy is usually not done.

MONITORING THE PATIENT WITH RENAL INSUFFICIENCY

The interval between visits is determined by the stage of renal insufficiency, the rate of progression, and the presence of complicating disorders. Early in the course, patients should have office visits scheduled every 4 to 6 months for monitoring of their symptoms, signs (e.g., weight, blood pressure, edema), and laboratory data (e.g., serum creatinine concentration, BUN, electrolytes, complete blood count, urinalysis, and possibly creatinine clearance). As renal failure progresses, visits must be spaced more closely, usually at 1-month intervals until dialysis becomes necessary. Drug dosages of prescription, over-the-counter, and herbal medications should be reviewed at each visit and adjusted according to the degree of renal dysfunction (see Drug Use in Renal Insufficiency).

COURSE AND PROGNOSIS

The underlying renal disease largely determines prognosis. Many renal diseases have characteristic rates of progression. For example, patients with polycystic kidney disease typically have very indolent courses and some never progress to ESRD. More aggressive courses, with advanced renal failure developing within months to a year, are more likely to occur in patients with diseases such as rapidly progressive glomerulonephritis, systemic sclerosis, or malignant hypertension. However, most renal diseases fall into an intermediate group, with ESRD developing within 1 to 5 years after the initial diagnosis.

Therapy

Goals

The goals of therapy fall into four major categories. The first is to treat the underlying renal disease, if possible (e.g., corticosteroids or chlorambucil for membranous nephropathy). The second is to slow the progression of renal deterioration by modifying the known or suspected factors that aggravate the primary process (e.g., treatment of hypertension, hyperglycemia, glomerular hyperperfusion) and avoiding factors that may aggravate existing renal failure (e.g., NSAIDs). The third goal is to treat the specific complications of renal disease (e.g., acidosis) as they occur, and to prevent the long-term complications of uremia before they can become fully established (e.g., secondary hyperparathyroidism). Finally, the patient should be referred to a dialysis and transplantation center well before the need for renal replacement therapy (see Dialysis and Transplantation).

Specific Treatments

Once a diagnosis is established, a nephrologist should be consulted, if not already accomplished, to determine whether effective therapy is available for the patient's renal disease. In general, the earlier in the course a treatment is started, the more likely it is to be successful in halting or reversing the disease. When the patient's renal disease is advanced or the effectiveness of the treatment is not well established, it is often advisable to forgo potentially toxic therapies, because the hazards often outweigh the benefits.

Many immunologically mediated renal diseases (e.g., membranous nephropathy, Wegener disease, Goodpasture syndrome, lupus nephritis) may respond to treatment with corticosteroids, cytotoxic agents, or plasmapheresis. For others (e.g., immunoglobulin A nephropathy), there is no proven effective therapy. Patients with immunologically mediated renal disease who require therapy should be under the care of a rheumatologist or nephrologist.

When the renal disease is associated with a metabolic disorder such as occurs in diabetes mellitus, it is critical to treat the underlying abnormality (e.g., hyperglycemia). Treatment directed at metabolic control may slow the course of renal deterioration but is not likely to result in significant reversal of established disease.

When a drug (e.g., methicillin, indomethacin) or other toxic substance (e.g., a heavy metal) is identified as the cause of renal failure, the offending agent should be withheld or avoided. A trial of corticosteroids may be given to patients with drug-induced interstitial nephritis, but this treatment is still controversial and the decision should be made in conjunction with a nephrologist.

Vascular lesions in the kidney caused by malignant hypertension may resolve slowly, but usually only partially, with control of blood pressure. In some patients this correlates with significant improvement in the GFR. Patients with renal failure secondary to bilateral RVD may have significant improvement in their renal function after successful angioplasty or bypass surgery, particularly if intervention occurs before renal insufficiency becomes too far advanced (serum creatinine less than about 4 mg/dL).

Obstructing lesions of the urinary tract may require surgical excision (e.g., benign prostatic hypertrophy) or urinary diversion (e.g., retroperitoneal fibrosis) to preserve or improve renal function. Other cases can be managed more conservatively (e.g., intermittent straight catheterization of the bladder) if the lesion is not amenable to surgical therapy (e.g., flaccid neurogenic bladder).

Nonspecific Treatments

There are important treatment options that can reduce the rate of renal deterioration by as much as one half, even when no specific therapies can be directed at the primary renal disorder. The first involves the use of a *protein-restricted diet* to retard the progression of renal disease in order to delay or even obviate dialysis (16–18). The GFR in healthy animals and humans varies directly with protein intake. Dietary protein restriction has been shown in animal experiments, using various models of partial renal injury, to reduce the degree of compensatory hypertrophy and hyperperfusion (see Pathophysiology of Uremia) and to forestall

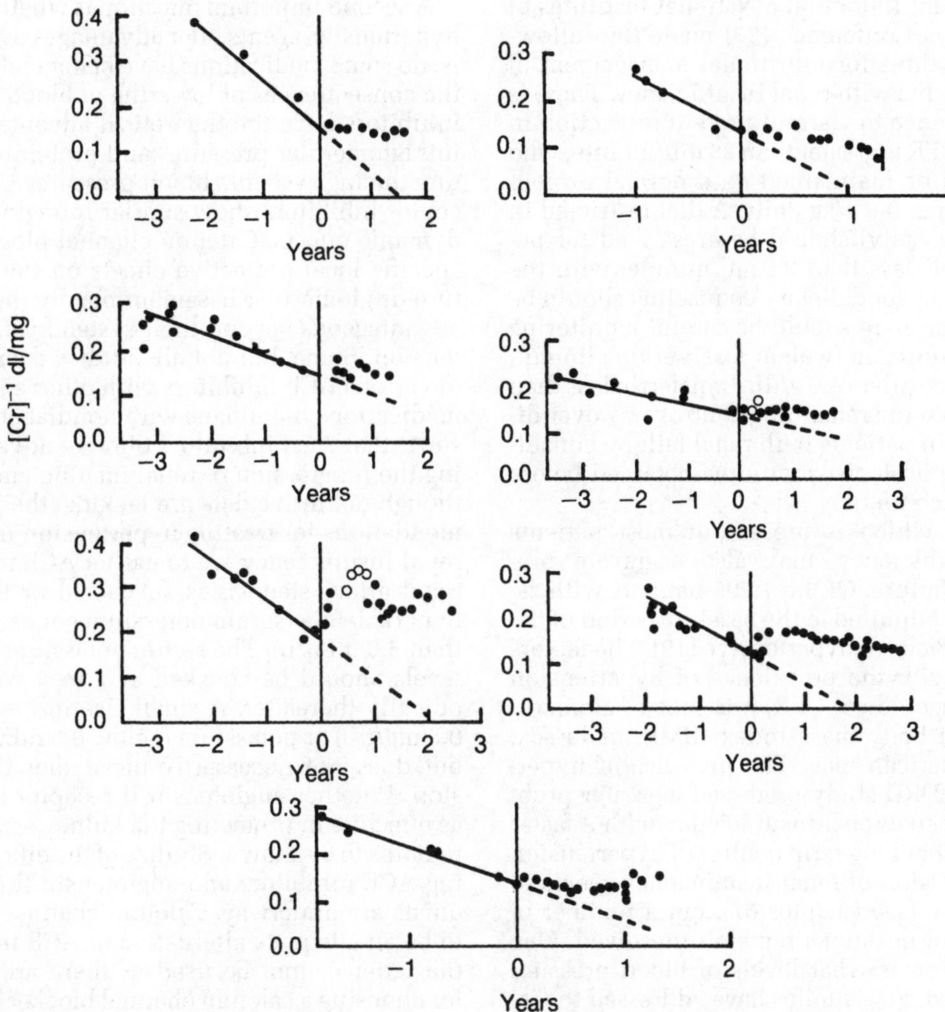

Figure 52.7. Data showing how the rate of progression of renal failure in seven different patients, as determined by a plot of the reciprocal of the serum creatinine concentration over time, was affected by the institution at time 0 of a low-phosphorus, low-protein diet. A decrease in the slope reflects stabilization of renal function. The dashed line indicates the projected course. (Data redrawn from Mitch WM, Walser M, Steinman TI, et al. Effect of a keto acid–amino acid supplement to a restricted diet on the progression of chronic renal failure. N Engl J Med 1984;311:623.)

the development of glomerular sclerosis, proteinuria, and progressive renal failure. Dietary treatments have been extensively studied in humans as well (Fig. 52.7). The other intervention that has been shown to protect the kidney is treatment of the hypertension that is commonly found in renal diseases of all types. Most of the studies that investigated diet therapy and control of blood pressure divided the patient populations into those with and without diabetes. Therefore, the following discussion pertains to non-diabetic patients. See also the section on diabetes mellitus.

Despite several small studies that seemed to confirm the benefits of dietary protein restriction in humans, questions remained about its value in the treatment of chronic renal failure. Some, but not all, of these questions were resolved by the Modification of Diet in Renal Disease (MDRD) Study (18). Patients with varying degrees of renal insufficiency (GFR, 25 to 55 mL/minute) were randomly assigned into a usual blood pressure group (mean arterial pressure [MAP], 107 mm Hg) or a low blood pressure group (MAP, 92 mm Hg). ACE inhibitors were used in a significant proportion of both groups. On the basis of an intention-to-treat analysis, despite the achievement of dietary and blood pressure goals, there were no significant differences between the interventions in rate of decline of GFR (as measured by radioisotope techniques), time until dialysis was required, or mortality. Although the mean protein intake between the groups was different, there was considerable variation and overlap among individual patients. When the data from the group with advanced renal failure were reanalyzed, correlating actual achieved dietary protein intake with GFR (controlling for other factors known to influence the rate of decline in GFR), it was concluded that, within the range 0.5 to 1.0 g/kg daily protein intake, a lower intake was associated with a slower rate of decline in GFR (19).

Based on current literature, a National Institutes of Health Consensus Conference (20) made the following recommendations for nutritional management of nondiabetic patients with renal insufficiency. There is insufficient evidence to warrant protein restriction in patients whose GFR is greater than 25 mL/minute, who therefore should be maintained on a normal protein intake of more than 0.8 g/kg daily. A diet restricted in protein (0.6 g/kg daily) should be prescribed for patients with a GFR less than 25 mL/minute, with the understanding that good dietary counseling should be available and that there should be careful monitoring for signs of malnutrition (weight loss, serum albumin concentration lower than 4.0 g/dL, transferrin less than 200 mg/dL). Given the remaining controversy over dietary restriction in patients with renal failure, consultation with a nephrologist should be obtained before embarking on such therapy.

Hypertension, which is present in most patients with renal insufficiency, may also aggravate preexisting kidney failure. Of the 1,795 patients with renal insufficiency admitted to the baseline period of the MDRD study, 83% were hypertensive (19). The factors that correlated with the prevalence of hypertension included older age, lower GFR, presence of glomerular disease, high body mass index (BMI), male sex, and African American race. The presence of hypertension in the MDRD study predicted a greater probability of progressive renal insufficiency with a faster rate of decline. That long-term control of hypertension slows the progression of renal insufficiency seems to be beyond debate (see Chapter 67), but a number of important clinical questions remain unresolved. One important question is what levels of blood pressure should be targeted. Few studies have addressed the issue of whether renal function is better preserved by lowering blood pressure to less than the usual target of 140/90 mm Hg. In addition to varying the protein intake, patients in the MDRD study were randomly assigned to receive usual or aggressive antihypertension therapies. Patients in the aggressively treated group (MAP target, 92 mm Hg) whose GFRs were between 25 and 55 mL/minute had a more rapid decline in renal function during the first 4 months than those in the usual care group (MAP target, 107 mm Hg) but a more gradual decline thereafter. It was postulated that the initial rapid decline was hemodynamically mediated and did not reflect actual kidney damage. The beneficial effect of aggressive blood pressure control was greatest in patients with proteinuria (greater than 1 g/day). These findings led to the recommendation that the target blood pressure should be 130/80 to 130/85 mm Hg for patients with chronic renal insufficiency without proteinuria, but blood pressure in patients with renal insufficiency associated with proteinuria of greater than 1 g/day should be lowered to levels near 125/75 mm Hg. Currently, the recommendations for treating hypertension in African Americans, who seem to be more susceptible to the damaging effects of high blood pressure, are not different from those for other populations.

A second important question is whether certain antihypertensive agents offer advantages over others—that is, do some medications have beneficial effects beyond the consequences of lowering of blood pressure? ACE inhibitors have the theoretical advantage of reducing intraglomerular pressures and proteinuria in addition to reducing systemic blood pressures. Angiotensin receptor inhibitors show similar intraglomerular hemodynamic effects. Calcium channel blockers may have specific local protective effects on the renal vasculature or glomerular basement membrane that could be advantageous beyond their systemic effects on hypertension. Some, but not all, studies comparing the use of various ACE inhibitors with other antihypertensive medications in humans with nondiabetic renal failure show that ACE inhibitors offer an advantage in slowing the progression of renal insufficiency (21–23). Although definitive data are lacking, the general recommendations for treating hypertension in patients with renal insufficiency are to use an ACE inhibitor unless renal artery stenosis is suspected or the patient has hyperkalemia (serum potassium concentration greater than 5.0 mEq/L). The serum potassium and creatinine levels should be checked at 1 to 2 weeks and periodically thereafter. A small rise in creatinine (below 0.5 mg/dL) or potassium (below 0.5 mEq/L) may occur but does not necessarily mean that therapy should stop. Whether angiotensin II receptor antagonists are as effective in protecting the kidney as ACE inhibitors remains to be shown. Studies of the efficacy of combining ACE inhibitors and angiotensin II receptor antagonists are underway. Calcium channel blockers seem to be an adequate alternative to ACE inhibitors when the latter cannot be used or there are other reasons for choosing a calcium channel blocker. Whether there are differences between the types of calcium channel blockers in terms of renal protective effect is still unclear. The presence of proteinuria is an independent risk factor for the progression of renal insufficiency. Higher rates of protein excretion are associated with more rapid declines in renal function. Reducing protein excretion with ACE inhibitors or angiotensin receptor antagonists can attenuate the losses.

Therapy directed at correcting volume overload in patients with mild to moderate renal insufficiency is similar to that for patients with normal renal function and hypertension. A salt-restricted diet (e.g., 2 g/day) may be attempted as a first step. Loop diuretics such as furosemide, bumetanide, or torsemide can be added if salt restriction is insufficient or if nondiuretic drugs (e.g., hydralazine, captopril) lead to secondary salt retention. Thiazides are generally avoided in patients with GFRs lower than 30 mL/minute because they often lose their diuretic effect. Except in rare circumstances, and only then with careful monitoring, potassium-sparing diuretics (spironolactone, triamterene, amiloride) should not be used in patients with significant renal impairment because of the increased risk of hyperkalemia. In patients who have refractory edema or advanced renal failure with severe salt retention, it may be necessary to use large daily doses of diuretic (furosemide up to 400 mg, bumetanide up to 10 mg, or torsemide up to 200 mg) or to use a combination of loop diuretic and thiazide (e.g., metolazone 2.5 to 5 mg) (24). Patients need to have their body weight and blood chemistries closely monitored when using combination diuretic therapy, because some patients experience exaggerated responses.

There is often a fine line between effective blood pressure control and hypotension when potent diuretics and antihypertensives are being used; therefore, careful monitoring of blood pressure (both supine and upright) and of serum creatinine concentration is necessary. With the use of potent drugs such as minoxidil (see Chapter 67), bilateral nephrectomy (which results in the requirement for dialysis) for the treatment of refractory cases of hypertension can usually be avoided.

Left ventricular hypertrophy is present in more than 60% of patients starting dialysis, and cardiovascular disease is the leading cause of death in patients with ESRD (25). Long-term control of hypertension, starting in the predialysis period, is important in reducing the risk of left ventricular hypertrophy and atherosclerosis in patients receiving dialysis treatment.

Treating Reversible Causes of Deterioration of Renal Function

Before any change in serum creatinine concentration is attributed to natural progression of the underlying renal disease, several alternative possibilities should be considered (Table 52.6).

Extracellular volume depletion is probably the most common cause for a fall in GFR. It may be related to an intercurrent illness associated with anorexia, fever, gastrointestinal losses of sodium and water, excessive salt restriction, or diuretic use. The usual clinical signs of volume depletion (low jugular venous pressure, orthostatic hypotension, tachycardia, decreased skin turgor, and weight loss) may be absent. Weight loss between office visits is usually the most important diagnostic clue to the presence of volume depletion. The urinary sodium concentration or urine osmolality, usually helpful in establishing the diagnosis of volume depletion in oliguric patients, is of little value in the patient with chronic renal failure because concentrating and salt-conserving abilities in these patients are often impaired.

Patients with decompensated congestive heart failure may also have superimposed prerenal azotemia.

Table 52.6. Causes of Renal Functional Deterioration

Volume depletion (salt and water depletion)
Congestive heart failure
Drug nephrotoxicity
Ureteral or urethral obstruction
Orthostatic hypotension
Microcrystal deposition (e.g., acute severe hyperuricemia)
Hyperphosphatemia–hypercalcemia
Hypertension
Radiocontrast materials (oral and parenteral)
Glomerular hyperperfusion

Optimal treatment of heart failure may improve renal function in these patients (see Chapter 66).

Drugs given for treatment of various other disorders can be related to worsening of renal function (Table 52.4). A careful review of both prescribed and over-the-counter medications is therefore necessary when assessing unexpected changes in kidney function. Of the drugs prescribed in the ambulatory setting, diuretics and NSAIDs are probably the most common offenders. Diuretics can aggravate pre-existing renal failure by inducing intravascular volume depletion and, less commonly, by producing an interstitial nephritis. Careful monitoring of the blood pressure, weight, BUN, and serum creatinine concentration helps detect early signs of prerenal azotemia in patients receiving diuretics. Withholding diuretic therapy for several days usually allows intravascular volume and GFR to return to baseline values.

Use of NSAIDs can result in a deterioration in kidney function, either by causing a reversible redistribution of renal blood flow or by producing an interstitial nephritis. NSAIDs are most likely to reduce GFR in patients with prerenal states (e.g., volume depletion, congestive heart failure, nephrosis). At this time it cannot be said that one nonsteroidal compound is safer to use in the patient with renal insufficiency than another. It is therefore best to avoid them altogether once the GFR is less than 50 mL/minute.

There are numerous reports of reversible renal dysfunction when ACE inhibitors were administered to patients with bilateral renovascular disease or renal artery stenosis of a solitary kidney. The former group should be considered for further diagnostic evaluation of their vascular disease.

Obstruction, because of its reversibility, should always be considered in patients with a fall in the GFR. This is particularly true in elderly men who are predisposed to prostatic hypertrophy and in diabetic patients who may have autonomic neuropathy affecting bladder emptying. Drugs that reduce bladder tone (e.g., antidepressants, antispasmodics, antiparkinsonian drugs with anticholinergic properties) should always be considered as causes of urinary retention. If obstruction is a possibility, the postvoid residual volume should be measured (see Chapter 53).

Microcrystal deposition in the kidney has been suggested as a cause of progressive deterioration in patients with azotemia. Serum uric acid concentrations are often elevated in patients with renal insufficiency. However, there is no evidence that reducing the serum uric acid concentration will prevent further deterioration when the original kidney disease was not caused by tophaceous gout. Allopurinol therefore is not used unless it is needed to control symptomatic gout.

Dietary Management

The major goals of dietary management in the patient with chronic renal insufficiency are to optimize intravascular volume, correct electrolyte abnormalities, relieve uremic symptoms, and prevent or slow

Table 52.7. Dietary Management of Renal Failure[a]

Therapy	Goals
Salt: 4–6 g/d	Maintain intravascular volume
Fluid: 1–3 L/d	Avoid dehydration
Potassium: If [K] >5.5 mEq/L, restrict intake to 2–2.4 g/d	Prevent hyperkalemia
Protein: Restrict intake to 0.55–0.6 g/kg per day (50% rich in essential amino acids)	Relieve uremic symptoms Retard progression of renal failure
Calories: 35–45 kcal/kg per day	Maintain nutrition
Calcium: 1–1.5 g/d	Maintain [Ca] = 9–10 mg/dL
Vitamins: multivitamin + folate	Replace vitamins lacking in protein-restricted diet
Phosphorus: Restrict intake to 800 mg/d	Prevent secondary hyperparathyroidism

[a]A dietician should be consulted to teach the patient how to achieve these intakes.

the progression of kidney disease (Table 52.7). The dietary and general treatment of nephrotic syndrome, occasionally a component of chronic renal failure, is discussed in Chapter 48.

The *volume of the intravascular space* is directly related to salt balance, which is in turn regulated by the kidney. As renal function declines, the ability of the kidney to maintain salt balance in response to changes in sodium intake becomes limited, especially when the changes occur abruptly. The intravascular volume may be depleted if the intake of salt is reduced (e.g., excessive salt restriction, anorexia) or if there are losses of salt (e.g., vomiting, diarrhea, diuretics). A reduction in intravascular volume can lead to a further increase in the BUN and to serum creatinine concentrations above the baseline values (prerenal azotemia). Conversely, the intravascular volume will increase if the intake of salt is suddenly augmented (dietary indiscretion), and the patient can develop hypertension, edema, or heart failure.

Most patients with chronic renal insufficiency maintain sodium balance on a salt intake of 4 to 6 g/day. Patients with congestive heart failure or hypertension may need further limitation of salt intake (2 g/day of salt), whereas the rare patient with severe salt-wasting nephropathy may require salt supplements to prevent volume depletion. Most of these latter patients have some form of interstitial renal disease.

Salt intake should be adjusted to maintain intravascular volume at the level that maximizes the GFR for any given degree of renal failure. Assessment of the state of the intravascular volume can be aided by obtaining serial body weights (rapid changes in weight are usually caused by fluid gains or losses), performing a physical examination (e.g., orthostatic change of pulse and blood pressure, jugular venous pressure, skin turgor, edema), and measuring changes in the BUN and serum creatinine concentrations (increases in the level of BUN are proportionately greater than those of the serum creatinine concentration in states of volume depletion). It is often useful to establish an "ideal weight." This is the weight at which the patient has optimal renal function without overt signs of volume overload. For some patients (e.g., those with congestive heart failure or nephrotic syndrome), a small amount of edema is acceptable because worsening of azotemia may develop when further diuresis is attempted. Whenever there is a significant change in the GFR, the intravascular volume and the ideal weight should be re-evaluated.

When the GFR falls as a result of volume depletion, it is necessary to restore the intravascular volume. This can be accomplished either by adding salt to the diet or by prescribing sodium chloride (600 mg four times a day) or sodium bicarbonate tablets (600 mg four times a day) until the patient's weight and GFR return to baseline values. If oral replacement is not practical (e.g., because of persistent vomiting), the patient should be given intravenous therapy, usually in the hospital.

If volume overload develops or persists despite salt restriction, diuretics can be used to increase salt excretion (Table 52.8). Because the thiazide diuretics, with the exception of metolazone (Zaroxolyn), lose their effectiveness when the GFR falls below 30 mL/minute, it is often necessary to use a loop diuretic, such as furosemide (Lasix), torsemide (Demadex), or bumetanide (Bumex). Another loop diuretic, ethacrynic acid (Edecrin), has been associated with an unacceptable level of ototoxicity and should not be used in patients with renal insufficiency. The potassium-sparing diuretics spironolactone (Aldactone), triamterene (Dyrenium), and amiloride (Midamor; also in Moduretic) are also best avoided without consultation from a nephrologist when there is significant renal failure because of the risk of inducing serious hyperkalemia.

Potassium restriction is usually unnecessary until the late stages of renal failure (GFR less than 15 mL/minute), except in the small number of patients with the syndrome of hyporeninemic hypoaldosteronism (see next paragraph), but careful monitoring of serum potassium levels is indicated nonetheless. If hyperkalemia develops, potassium restriction to between 2 and 2.4 g/day (40 to 50 mEq/day) is necessary. A dietitian should be consulted to help plan a potassium-restricted diet. Foods with high potassium content include dairy products, many greens, beans, potatoes, tomatoes, bananas, dates, prunes, raisins, and citrus fruits. Patients who are on sodium-restricted diets must also be informed that many salt substitutes are unacceptable because they are often composed of potassium salts.

The association of hyperkalemia and hyperchloremic metabolic acidosis in patients with mild to moderate renal insufficiency (GFR greater than 25 mL/minute) should lead one to consider the presence of the hyporenin hypoaldosterone syndrome (26). This syndrome occurs most often in azotemic patients with hypertension, diabetes mellitus, or interstitial nephritis. This disorder probably has many causes, but it is caused in part by a suppression of the renin–aldosterone axis. The diagnosis is usually made on clinical grounds, after excluding other reasons for hyperkalemia (e.g., high potassium intake, drugs that reduce renal excretion of potassium), but it can be

Table 52.8. Diuretics in Renal Failure

Drug	Available Strengths (mg)	Dosage (mg/d)	Route of Excretion	Comments
Thiazides (Hydrochlorothiazide)	25, 50	12.5–50	Renal	May induce volume depletion and hyperuricemia. Loses effectiveness if GFR <30 mL/min but may be used in combination with loop diuretics in advanced renal failure.
Metolazone (Zaroxolyn)	2.5, 5, 10	5–20	Renal	May induce volume depletion and hyperuricemia. Effective when GFR >10 mL/min.
Furosemide (Lasix)	20, 40, 80	20–400	Renal	May induce volume depletion and hyperuricemia. Effective when GFR >5 mL/min. May produce ototoxicity and rarely interstitial nephritis. May increase nephrotoxicity of antibiotics.
Bumetanide (Bumex)	0.5, 1, 2	1–10	Renal	May induce volume depletion and hyperuricemia. Side effects include ototoxicity and muscle pains and may also increase the risk of antibiotic nephrotoxicity.
Torsemide (Demadex)	5, 10, 20, 100	5–100	Hepatic/renal	Longer half-life than other loop diuretics.
Ethacrynic acid (Edecrin)	—	Avoid	Hepatic	Usually avoided in renal failure because the risk of ototoxicity is significantly higher than with furosemide or bumetanide.
Spironolactone (Aldactone)	—	Avoid	Hepatic	Avoid when GFR <50 mL/min due to the risk of inducing serious hyperkalemia.
Triamterene (Dyrenium)	—	Avoid	Renal	Same as above
Amiloride (Midamor)	—	Avoid	Renal	Same as spironolactone

GFR, glomerular filtration rate.

more firmly established by the demonstration of a low plasma renin concentration that fails to rise after stimulation with furosemide (Lasix, 40 mg orally) and upright posture for 2 hours. The patient should also have no evidence of glucocorticoid deficiency (random cortisol concentration, 15 to 25 mg/mL; see Chapter 81). Because, in the absence of aldosterone, potassium excretion by the kidney depends on an adequate urine flow rate (1.5 to 2 L/day), patients with this syndrome are at risk for development of severe hyperkalemia during periods of salt restriction or volume depletion. Normotensive patients may be treated with a mineralocorticoid (fluorohydrocortisone [Florinef], 0.1-mg tablets, ½ to 1 tablet/day). Alternatively, if hypertension is present or develops after administration of the mineralocorticoid, the patient may be treated with a combination of furosemide (Lasix, 40 to 80 mg twice a day) plus sodium bicarbonate (600 mg four times a day). The furosemide is used to promote a good urine flow rate, whereas the sodium bicarbonate helps prevent salt depletion and also is of use in correcting the associated metabolic acidosis. The goal of therapy is to keep the serum potassium concentration within the normal range. Because therapy is often complicated, these cases are best managed with the help of a nephrologist or endocrinologist.

Although diluting and concentrating abilities are impaired in renal failure, most patients can ingest 1 to 3 L of fluid daily without developing hyponatremia. If hyponatremia occurs, fluids should be limited to less than 1.5 L/day to prevent water intoxication.

Protein-restricted diets, in addition to their use in reducing the rate of decline in kidney function, are indicated for patients with advanced renal failure (GFR less than 20 mL/minute) who develop nausea, vomiting, or other symptoms attributable to uremia. Because many end products of protein metabolism have been implicated in the causation of the uremic syndrome, therapy consists of reducing protein intake to approximately 0.6 g/kg of body weight per day (approximately 40 g of protein per day in a 70-kg patient). Normal protein intake in the United States exceeds 70 g/day. Half of the protein intake should be in the form of meats, fish, eggs, or milk, because these foods are rich in essential amino acids. For the patient consuming a protein-restricted diet to maintain adequate nutritional balance, total caloric intake must be adjusted to provide 35 to 45 kcal/kg per day. This can be accomplished by increasing the intake of fats and carbohydrates.

Because protein-restricted diets are often deficient in vitamins, calcium, and phosphorus, patients should receive a daily vitamin supplement and 1 to 1.5 g of elemental calcium per day (a single 600-mg calcium carbonate tablet provides 250 mg of elemental calcium). The reduction in dietary phosphorus is desirable (see later discussion), so phosphorus supplements are not given.

Considering the complexity of such diets and the need for individualization of salt, mineral, protein, and potassium intake, consultation with a dietitian or a nephrologist proficient in prescribing renal diets is suggested. Constant encouragement and supervision of dietary therapy are needed. The success of dietary treatment often depends on the involvement of family members as well as an enthusiastic dietitian.

Calcium and Phosphorus

Renal osteodystrophy is a general term that encompasses osteitis fibrosa, osteomalacia, and a variety of other bone lesions that occur in patients with kidney failure. The pathophysiologic factors that lead to osteodystrophy originate in the early stages of renal failure, although clinical manifestations generally do not develop until the patient is on dialysis.

The pathophysiology of renal osteodystrophy is complex but can be briefly summarized as follows: PTH hypersecretion occurs in response to an absolute or relative deficiency of the active form of vitamin D (see later discussion). The relative deficiency of vitamin D, in turn, leads to diminished calcium absorption, skeletal resistance to the effects of PTH, and resetting of the setpoint of PTH secretion in response to calcium.

The increased rate of PTH secretion is successful at keeping serum calcium and phosphorus levels within the normal range until the GFR is less than 30 mL/minute. In more advanced renal failure, hypocalcemia and hyperphosphatemia develop. Hyperphosphatemia further blunts the calcemic response to PTH and diminishes vitamin D secretion. The most important consequence of prolonged secondary hyperparathyroidism is the development of bone disease (osteitis fibrosa cystica).

Osteomalacia, in renal insufficiency, is caused partly by the failure of the diseased kidney to convert 25-hydroxyvitamin D_3 to its more active form, 1,25-dihydroxyvitamin D_3. The active form of vitamin D is necessary for normal bone mineralization. Serum levels of vitamin D can be in the normal range in patients with renal failure, but with GFRs greater than 30 mL/minute such levels may still represent a relative deficiency of the vitamin, because increased levels of vitamin D would be expected in response to the low calcium concentration in renal failure. Absolute deficiencies of vitamin D are found once the GFR falls below 30 mL/minute. Abnormal collagen synthesis, titration of bone buffers, and accumulation of aluminum in the bone matrix have also been implicated in the pathogenesis of osteomalacia.

Patients with renal insufficiency should have periodic measurements of calcium, phosphorus, magnesium, and alkaline phosphatase. Determination of PTH levels, when necessary, should be by an assay that measures the intact or amino-terminal hormone. Bone radiographs or biopsies are not routinely obtained in patients not yet receiving dialysis, unless the patient has symptomatic bone disease.

The clinical features of deranged calcium and phosphorus metabolism, including bone pain, fractures, and proximal myopathy, are not often seen until after the patient is on dialysis. However, it is generally acknowledged that preventing parathyroid hyperplasia is easier than reversing it once it is established. Therefore, therapy to correct these abnormalities should begin during the early stages of renal failure (Table 52.9).

Based on a knowledge of calcium, phosphorus, and vitamin D alterations in early renal insufficiency, it is possible to outline a plan of therapy directed at reducing the incidence and severity of osteodystrophy in late renal insufficiency. The goals of therapy are to limit the rise in PTH secretion that usually accompanies renal failure and to prevent the development of osteomalacia. These goals can be achieved by maintaining a positive calcium balance, providing vitamin D, and reducing phosphorus intake.

Table 52.9. Steps in the Management of Calcium and Phosphorus Balance in Patients with Renal Failure

Therapy	Goals
A. GFR 50–30 mL/min	
Calcium supplements (1–1.5 g/d)	Maintain serum calcium concentration at 9–10 mg/dL
Vitamin D (Rocaltrol 0.25–0.5 μg/d, available in 0.25-μg tablets, Hectoral 5-μg three times a week)	Maintain serum calcium concentration at 9–10 mg/dL
GFR <30 mL/min	
B. Restrict phosphorus intake (800 mg/d)	Maintain serum phosphorus concentration at 4.0–6.0 mg/dL
Phosphorus–binding antacids (calcium carbonates or sevalemer [RenaGel] taken with meals)	Maintain serum phosphorus concentration at 4.0–6.0 mg/dL

GFR, glomerular filtration rate.

Because calcium absorption is diminished in patients with renal insufficiency, the first step in treatment is to ensure an adequate intake of calcium. This is particularly important for patients on protein-restricted diets, which often contain only 300 to 400 mg of calcium per day (normal calcium intake is 800 to 1,000 mg/day). Supplements in the form of calcium carbonate (generic), 600 mg four times per day, provide 1,000 mg of elemental calcium per day. Calcium lactate (generic, 300 mg, in two tablets four times a day) may be substituted if the carbonate is not tolerated because of constipation or bloating.

It was shown in a prospective, controlled trial that low dosages of orally administered vitamin D (Rocaltrol) given to patients with GFRs between 60 and 20 mL/minute can reverse some of the biochemical and histologic evidence of osteodystrophy (27). If, after consultation with a nephrologist, it is decided to treat early, initially the lowest dosage of the vitamin D preparation should be selected, and the dosage should be raised every 4 weeks until the serum calcium is in the upper range of normal. It appears, from experience, that most patients with renal insufficiency cannot tolerate a Rocaltrol dosage greater than 0.5 μg/day without developing hypercalcemia. Hypercalcemia may be associated with increases in the serum creatinine concentration, which should be reversible once the dosage of vitamin D is reduced and calcium levels return to the normal range. Because of the frequency of hypercalcemia and its potential effects on renal function, it is crucial that serum calcium levels be monitored weekly after a change in dosage, until the serum calcium concentration stabilizes, and monthly thereafter. There does not appear to be any value to monitoring the levels of vitamin D metabolites during therapy. In general, one expects to see a fall in the levels of alkaline phosphatase and PTH. Suppression of PTH to "normal" levels with vitamin D therapy leads to a syndrome of adynamic bone disease in dialysis patients who manifest a resistance to PTH. The precise degree to which PTH should be suppressed in pre-ESRD patients is uncertain, but values lower than 200 pg/mL should be avoided (28).

Vitamin D therapy should not be initiated when serum calcium or phosphorus levels are greater than 10.5 and 6 mg/dL, respectively, because of the possibility of inducing metastatic calcification or renal dysfunction. If the serum phosphorus concentration is elevated, as is common in patients whose GFR is less than 30 mL/minute, it is necessary to first reduce the level of phosphorus to normal before starting vitamin D therapy.

The serum phosphorus concentration may rise after institution of vitamin D therapy because both calcium and phosphorus absorption are increased. If dietary phosphate restriction (approximately 800 mg/day) is not sufficient to maintain serum phosphorus levels within the normal range, phosphate binders must be used (see later discussion).

The form of vitamin D used is important, because preparations (e.g., vitamin D_2, vitamin D_3) that require final activation by the kidney have proved to be ineffective at the usual dosages. The most commonly used vitamin D preparation that does not require renal activation is 1,25-dihydroxyvitamin D_3(Rocaltrol). When given orally, Rocaltrol (0.25 to 1.0 μg/day) is effective in improving calcium absorption and raising serum calcium levels in azotemic patients.

Restriction of *dietary phosphorus* to approximately 800 mg/day (normal intake is 1 to 1.8 g/day) should be initiated when the serum phosphorus level first becomes elevated. This degree of phosphorus restriction can be achieved by restricting the intake of protein to 60 g/day (foods such as eggs, meat, and fish contain 15 mg of phosphorus per gram of protein, and dairy products 20 to 30 mg/g). Despite restriction of phosphorus intake, the serum phosphorus level often becomes elevated when the GFR falls below 30 mL/minute. At this juncture it is necessary to start treatment with phosphate binders. Calcium-containing compounds such as calcium carbonate and calcium acetate, which bind phosphate in the intestine and thereby reduce phosphate absorption, have supplanted the use of oral antacids containing aluminum hydroxide (AlternaGEL or Amphojel) or aluminum carbonate (Basaljel). This is based on the demonstration that aluminum from the antacids is absorbed and can accumulate in the brain and bones of patients with renal failure. This aluminum accumulation has been implicated in the pathogenesis of the dialysis dementia syndrome (myoclonus, seizures, and dementia), anemia (see Chapter 55), and a particular form of osteomalacia (characterized by the appearance of aluminum in the mineralization front of bone studied histochemically) that develop in some patients with ESRD. Nephrologists now recommend the addition of aluminum-containing compounds only in refractory cases of hyperphosphatemia. Other medications (Table 52.10) should not be given simultaneously with phosphate binders because their absorption may be increased or decreased. Furthermore, calcium citrate and aluminum-containing binders should not be given simultaneously, because citrate increases the absorption of aluminum. The initial dosage of antacid should be 1 or 2 tablets or capsules given with meals; the dosage should be increased (at 2-week intervals) until the serum phosphorus concentration is reduced to between 4 and 6 mg/dL. Serum phosphorus levels should be monitored every 1 to 2 months to avoid the syndrome of phosphate depletion (low serum phosphorus), which may result in muscle weakness, osteomalacia, and fractures. Many patients report constipation with calcium salts and object to the number of pills.

Table 52.10. Drugs Whose Bioavailability Is Altered by Phosphate Binders

Decreased
Digoxin
Oral anticoagulants
Tetracycline
Anticholinergics
Aspirin
Chlorpromazine
Increased
Penicillin
Pseudoephedrine

A serious concern has been raised about the use of calcium-containing phosphate binders in patients with renal failure. A study in which young dialysis patients were screened with electron-beam CT scans revealed significant cardiac calcification (which in the general population is associated with atherosclerosis) in 14 of 16 subjects who were between 20 and 30 years of age. One correlate of cardiac calcification was higher calcium intake (29). A new option for binding phosphate is to use a non–calcium-containing, nonabsorbable resin called sevelamer hydrochloride (RenaGel). The starting dose should be two to three 403-mg capsules taken three times per day with meals and titrated to normalize the phosphorus level. Sevelamer hydrochloride also lowers total and low-density lipoprotein cholesterol concentrations. This product is as effective as calcium carbonate, but it is considerably more expensive and some patients complain of gastric bloating.

Acidosis

A mild hyperchloremic (normal anion gap) metabolic acidosis develops commonly in patients with early renal insufficiency (Fig. 52.8). This occurs because the decrease in production of ammonia by the failing kidney results in inability of the kidney to excrete metabolically produced acids (sulfates and phosphates). The hypochloremic (with an abnormal anion gap) acidosis that is commonly associated with renal failure usually does not appear until the GFR has fallen below 20 mL/minute.

Chronic metabolic acidosis contributes to the long-term complications of patients who have renal failure by decreasing bone mineralization and suppressing protein synthesis. The goal of treating the acidosis is to maintain a serum bicarbonate level greater than 20 mEq/L. If protein restriction (see Dietary Management), which reduces the exogenous acid load, is

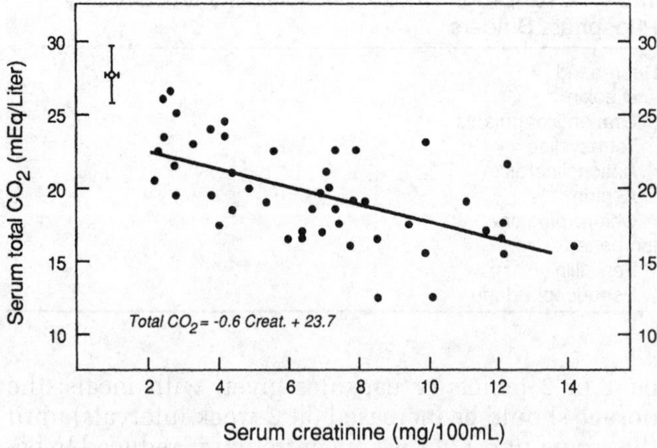

Figure 52.8. Relationship between serum bicarbonate and serum creatinine concentrations in patients with chronic renal insufficiency. (From Widmer B, et al. The influence of graded degrees of chronic renal failure. Arch Intern Med 1979;139:1099.)

insufficient to restore buffering capacity, base in the form of sodium citrate liquid (1 mL liquid = 1 mEq bicarbonate) can be given. Dosages of 30 to 60 mEq/day of base, given in divided doses, are generally sufficient to maintain acid–base balance. Sodium bicarbonate (600 mg = 14 mEq base) can also be used, but it is less well tolerated than citrate because of gastrointestinal complaints such as belching and bloating. Finally, $CaCO_3$, given as a calcium supplement and phosphate binder, may also be effective in correcting the acidosis.

Anemia

A normochromic, normocytic anemia develops in patients with chronic renal failure, and its severity is proportional to the degree of renal insufficiency (Fig. 52.4). Up to 45% of patients with a serum creatinine concentration of 2 mg/dL are anemic (30). The anemia of renal failure results mainly from decreased erythropoietin production. Other causes of anemia (e.g., iron deficiency) must also be considered.

All patients should be prescribed a multivitamin regimen that includes folate to replace the vitamins lacking in the restrictive diets. Blood transfusion, when necessary, should not be withheld for fear of sensitizing a potential transplant recipient. Patients who have received multiple blood transfusions have higher rates of retention of functioning transplanted kidneys than do those who have not received transfusions. Iron deficiency is almost universal in patients on hemodialysis, but it may also occur in the predialysis patient, particularly if multiple blood samples have been taken or if there is bleeding. Iron deficiency is best diagnosed in patients with chronic renal failure by measuring the level of serum ferritin. The serum iron and iron-binding capacity are often low in patients with renal failure, but a transferrin saturation less than 15% should suggest the possibility of iron deficiency. The values of serum ferritin that are associated with normal iron stores are higher in patients with renal failure than in those without kidney disease. Therefore, the laboratory should be consulted to interpret serum ferritin levels properly in the uremic patient. The treatment of iron deficiency is the same in azotemic patients as in any other patient (see Chapter 55).

Patients whose hemoglobin levels fall below 11 g/dL or who have symptoms related to anemia should be treated with recombinant human erythropoietin (Epogen, Procrit) given at dosages of 80 to 120 units/kg subcutaneously, two to three times per week (31,32) or darbepoetin alfa (Aranesp) 0.45 mcg/kg SC weekly or 0.75 mcg/kg SC every other week. The higher dosages are associated with a more rapid response but can result in more difficulty controlling blood pressure. Therefore, unless there is some urgency to correct the anemia, starting at the lower dosages is recommended. Most patients become asymptomatic when the hemoglobin level is between 11 and 12 g/dL. Even patients who are not iron deficient but are taking erythropoietin should be given ferrous sulfate 300 mg and 1 mg of folic acid daily because iron and vitamin stores can be depleted rapidly. In some patients, blood pressure may become more difficult to control with this treatment, and it is therefore recommended that blood pressure measurements be taken on a weekly basis until the hematocrit level stabilizes (usually 6 to 8 weeks). Despite evidence that correction of anemia improves quality of life and may reduce long-term cardiovascular complications, only a minority of uremic patients are treated with erythropoietin before starting dialysis treatment. The reasons for suboptimal use of erythropoietin in the predialysis population are not known, but they may be related to unfamiliarity with treatment issues or difficulties in obtaining reimbursement. For the treatment to be reimbursable, Medicare rules require that the injections be given in the office or clinic. Many patients complain that there are many obstacles (i.e., large prepayments) to obtaining private insurance coverage for erythropoietin, given its expense.

DRUG USE IN RENAL INSUFFICIENCY

The incidence of adverse drug effects is increased in patients with renal failure, a fact that is attributable largely to the alterations in pharmacokinetics that occur as renal function declines. Adverse drug effects in these patients can be divided into those that are caused by abnormal drug metabolism (e.g., increased incidence of digitalis toxicity) and those that are caused by an effect on renal function that is part of the anticipated pharmacologic action of the drug (e.g., reduction in GFR with diuretics or NSAIDs) (33). In renal failure, drug bioavailability, volume of distribution, and protein binding may be abnormal; however, the most significant derangement is the prolongation of half-life of many drugs or their metabolites. Therefore, it is necessary to have a basic understanding of how a drug's administration should be modified when renal failure is present.

Because even over-the-counter preparations (e.g., aspirin, ibuprofen, magnesium-containing antacids) have the potential for causing toxicity, patients should be reminded to telephone their primary care provider before using nonprescription drugs. Whenever possible, drugs that require no modification of dosage or that do not affect kidney function adversely should be substituted for those with a greater potential for inducing toxicity. The avoidance of drugs with marginal efficacy will help reduce the frequency of adverse effects.

A complete review of drug usage in renal failure may be found in *Drug Prescribing in Renal Failure,* published by the American College of Physicians (34). Guidelines are provided in this section for the drugs most commonly prescribed in ambulatory practice (Tables 52.11 and 52.12).

Before initiating therapy with a drug that requires dosage modification in renal failure, it is necessary to have an accurate estimation of GFR. Predicting the GFR from the serum creatinine level alone is not recommended; rather, one should either measure the creatinine clearance directly or use one of the formulas for estimating GFR (see earlier discussion and equations).

Depending on what modifications are required for a particular drug, an appropriate loading and maintenance dosage can be chosen. A loading dose must be given whenever rapid achievement of therapeutic drug levels is desired. Maintenance dosages are adjusted either by lengthening the interval between administrations or by reducing the size of each dose. The use of nomograms or tables does not guarantee that adverse drug effects will not occur. The monitoring of serum drug levels is often helpful, particularly when using drugs with low toxic/therapeutic ratios. Finally, the list of drugs should be reviewed periodically and the patient questioned specifically about side effects.

Table 52.11. Some Commonly Used Drugs that Should Be Avoided in Patients with Renal Failure (GFR <30 mL/min)

Antimicrobials
- Cephaloridine (Loridine)
- Tetracyclines
- Nitrofurantoin (Macrodantin)
- Nalidixic acid (NegGram)
- Analgesics
- Aspirin
- NSAIDs (e.g., Motrin, Naphosyn)
- Meperidine (Demerol)

Diuretics
- Potassium-sparing diuretics (Aldactone, Moduretic, Dyrenium)
- Ethacrynic acid (Edecrin)
- Thiazides (e.g., Diuril)

Antacids
- Magnesium-containing antacids (e.g., Maalox, Mylanta)

Hypoglycemic drugs
- Acetohexamide (Dymelor)
- Chlorpropamide (Diabinese)
- Metformin (Glucophage)

Drugs used in the treatment of gout
- Phenylbutazone (Butazolidin)
- Sulfinpyrazone (Anturane)
- Probenecid (Benemid)

GFR, glomerular filtration rate.

Table 52.12. Some Commonly Used Drugs that Require Dosage Reduction in Renal Failure (GFR <50 mL/min)

Cardiovascular drugs
- Digoxin (Lanoxin)
- Nadolol (Corgard)
- Atenolol (Tenormin)
- Procainamide (Pronestyl)
- Disopyramide (Norpace)

Antihypertensive drugs
- Captopril (Capoten)
- Clonidine (Catapres)

H_2-Receptor antagonists
- Cimetidine (Tagamet)
- Ranitidine (Zantac)

Hypoglycemic drugs
- Insulin
- Acetohexamide
- Chlorpropamide

Drugs used in the treatment of gout
- Allopurinol (Zyloprim)

Antibiotics
- Most penicillins
- Some cephalosporins
- Quinolones
- Many antiviral agents

Antimicrobials

When renal impairment is not advanced (i.e., GFR greater than 50 mL/minute), no change is necessary for most commonly used antimicrobials in the dosages used in ambulatory practice; this includes penicillins, cephalosporins, erythromycin, metronidazole, chloramphenicol, and quinolones. However, the administration of tetracyclines, with the exception of doxycycline, is discouraged in the patient with impaired renal function, because these drugs tend to increase the urea nitrogen concentration and other nitrogen end products and could increase symptoms of uremia. With a GFR of less than 50 mL/minute, many antibiotics require dosage modification and it is therefore important to check the pharmacokinetics of the drug.

When treating urinary tract infections in patients with GFRs lower than 50 mL/minute, urinary antiseptic drugs such as nitrofurantoin (Macrodantin) or nalidixic acid (NegGram) should not be used, because they are ineffective and there is an increased risk of systemic toxicity associated with the retention of metabolites. Antimicrobials such as ampicillin, fluoroquinolones, and the cephalosporins, which are secreted by the renal tubular cells, achieve a high urine concentration even when the GFR is very low; they are effective in the treatment of urinary tract infections in patients with advanced renal failure. Trimethoprim–sulfamethoxazole is also effective in patients with impaired renal function. The dosage of ciprofloxacin or levofloxacin should be reduced by 50% when the GFR falls below 30 mL/minute.

Antiviral agents, including acyclovir, ganciclovir, amantadine, lamivudine, and zidovudine (AZT), all require dosage modification when GFR falls below 50 mL/minute.

Analgesics

The dosages of acetaminophen, codeine, oxycodone (Tylox), morphine, and pentazocine (Talwin) require no modification in renal failure. Furthermore, none of these drugs adversely affects kidney function in patients with chronic renal insufficiency. There is some epidemiologic evidence that the regular, heavy use of acetaminophen is associated with an increased risk of renal damage. The use of meperidine (Demerol) for more than two to three doses is hazardous because of the accumulation of its metabolites, which may induce seizures.

The use of NSAIDs, including aspirin, is generally not recommended in patients with renal insufficiency because they predictably result in a 25% to 50% decrease in GFR (35). The effects of NSAIDs on GFR result from changes in renal blood flow consequent to inhibition of renal prostaglandin synthesis and are greatest in patients who have diminished effective circulatory volume (patient taking diuretics and those with congestive heart failure). The reduction in GFR is generally reversible once the NSAID is discontinued, but the return to baseline may take up to 1 month. It is unclear whether the reduction in GFR associated with NSAIDs results in any permanent harm to the kidney.

There are several possible approaches to the patient with renal insufficiency for whom it is believed important to use an NSAID. Sulindac (Clinoril) appears not to affect renal prostaglandin synthesis to the same extent as the other NSAIDs, and it is generally considered to produce lesser effects on GFR in patients with mild renal insufficiency (36). The nonacetylated salicylates are only weak inhibitors of prostaglandin synthesis and theoretically should not affect renal function. Currently, however, there are no data on the safety of nonacetylated salicylates in patients with renal insufficiency. When NSAIDs are given to patients with renal failure, it is necessary to monitor kidney function carefully. It is probably prudent to discontinue use of these drugs if more than a minimal change in renal function is seen.

Patients with renal insufficiency are predisposed to development of salt retention, hyponatremia, and hyperkalemia when given NSAIDs. Hyperkalemia is more common when NSAIDs are given in conjunction with potassium-sparing diuretics or ACE inhibitors. Finally, there have been numerous case reports of patients with previously normal renal function who developed ARF with nephrotic syndrome, as an idiosyncratic reaction, after having been given NSAIDs. When examined by biopsy, these patients usually are found to have an interstitial form of nephritis.

Psychoactive Drugs

For the patient with renal failure, no alteration in dosage is necessary for the benzodiazepines (e.g., Valium, Ativan), neuroleptics (e.g., Haldol, Thorazine), or tricyclic antidepressants (e.g., Pamelor), because all are metabolized chiefly by the liver. Although antipsychotic drugs such as clozapine (Clozaril) and olanzapine (Zyprexa) do not require dose adjustments in patients with renal insufficiency, resperidone (Risperdal) dosages do have to be reduced. The metabolism of serotonin reuptake inhibitors such as fluoxetine (Prozac) and sertraline (Zoloft) is unclear. The phenothiazines and tricyclics must be used with caution because they have significant anticholinergic properties and, accordingly, may cause urinary retention. All psychoactive drugs are capable of causing excessive sedation in patients with advanced renal failure. Lithium, which is renally excreted, should be used with great caution once the GFR falls below 50 mL/minute. Levels must be monitored frequently (see Chapter 24).

Antacids, H_2-Receptor Antagonists, and Proton Pump Inhibitors

Many commonly prescribed or over-the-counter antacids contain magnesium compounds as a major constituent, and magnesium toxicity may occur when the GFR is less than 30 mL/minute. Therefore, patients should be instructed to use antacids that are based on aluminum (as opposed to magnesium). Because, with prolonged ingestion, significant amounts of aluminum are absorbed and accumulate in the tissues of patients with renal failure, these drugs should be prescribed only for periods of less than 1 month. Sucralfate, although containing aluminum, may be used because the compound is minimally absorbed compared with other aluminum-containing compounds.

The dosage of the H_2-receptor antagonists cimetidine, ranitidine, and famotidine must be reduced by 50% as the creatinine clearance falls below 30 mL/minute. All can cause an increase in serum creatinine levels, probably because of inhibition of the tubular secretion of creatinine.

No significant dosage alterations are required for the proton pump inhibitors such as omeprazole, lansoprazole, rabeprazole, and pantoprazole.

Cardiovascular Drugs

Both loading and maintenance dosages of digoxin must be reduced once the GFR is diminished to less than 50 mL/minute—the loading dosage by 75% and the maintenance dosage by 50%. Despite the use of nomograms (37) and the monitoring of drug levels, digoxin toxicity remains a problem in the uremic patient. Therefore, whenever feasible, other treatments for heart failure should be tried before resorting to digoxin.

A large variety of beta-blocking agents are now available, and each has slightly different pharmacologic or pharmacokinetic properties. The most important consideration in patients with renal failure is the route of excretion. The dosages of propranolol (Inderal), metoprolol (Lopressor), labetalol (Normodyne), carvedilol

(Coreg), and penbutolol (Levatol), all of which are metabolized by the liver, are unchanged even in advanced renal failure. Atenolol (Tenormin), nadolol (Corgard), pindolol (Visken), carteolol (Cartrol), timolol (Blocadren), and the metabolites of acebutolol (Sectral) are excreted largely by the kidney and require dosage reduction. All beta-blocking agents should be used with caution in patients with impaired renal function, because they may reduce cardiac output and thereby aggravate azotemia.

The dosage interval should be increased twofold to fourfold to avoid toxicity when giving procainamide (Pronestyl) or disopyramide (Norpace) to patients with renal failure. Monitoring of blood levels of the drug and, in the case of procainamide, its active metabolite (*N*-acetylprocainamide) is important in guiding therapy. Once the GFR falls below 10 mL/minute, the dosages of flecainide, encainide, and tocainide should be halved. Quinidine and amiodarone do not require dosage modification, even in advanced renal failure.

The use of antihypertensive drugs in patients with renal failure is discussed in Chapter 67.

Hypoglycemic Agents

The half-life of insulin is prolonged in renal failure, so attention to dosage is required in the diabetic patient with developing renal insufficiency to avoid hypoglycemia. The oral hypoglycemic agents acetohexamide and chlorpropamide have active metabolites that accumulate in renal failure and may produce prolonged hypoglycemia. Therefore, patients with type 2 diabetes who are taking oral hypoglycemic agents should switch to shorter-acting agents such as tolbutamide (Orinase), glipizide (Glucotrol), or glyburide (Micronase, Diabeta) once their GFR falls below 50 mL/minute.

Rosiglitazone (Avandia) and pioglitazone (Actors) requires no dosage adjustment in patients with renal failure. On the other hand, the use of metformin (Glucophage) is discouraged in the presence of even modest degrees of renal insufficiency, because the incidence of lactic acidosis increases as GFR declines.

Anticonvulsants

The dosage of phenytoin (Dilantin) is essentially unchanged in renal failure because an increased volume of distribution and a shortened half-life are offset by reduced protein binding. Because the unbound fraction of phenytoin is increased, its therapeutic and toxic effects occur at lower measured total serum levels in patients with renal failure than they do in patients without renal insufficiency (Fig. 52.9). Similarly, the dose of valproate is unchanged in patients with renal insufficiency, but levels of free valproate may be increased. Gabapentin (Neurontin) dosages require modification as renal failure progresses. Carbamazepine (Tegretol) dosing is unchanged with renal insufficiency.

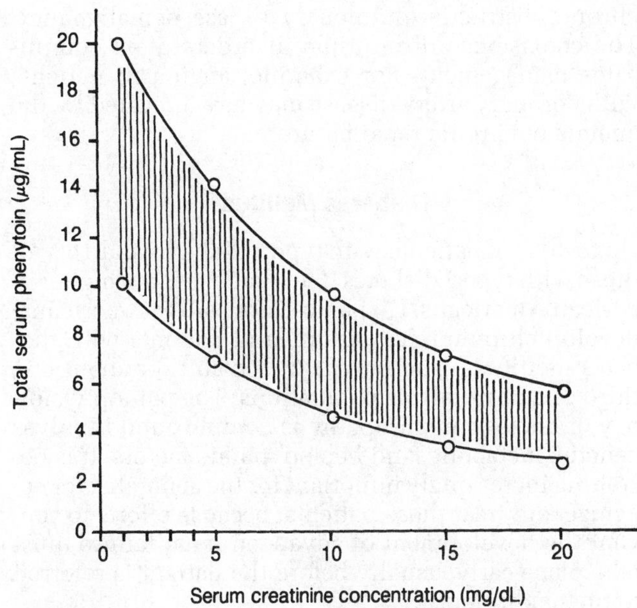

Figure 52.9. Range of total serum phenytoin concentrations that provide therapeutic levels of free drug in patients with varying degrees of renal failure. (Redrawn from Reidenberg NM, Affirme M. Influence of disease on binding of drugs to plasma proteins. Ann N Y Acad Sci 1973;226:115.)

Drugs Used in the Treatment of Gout

Colchicine may be used for the prophylactic treatment of symptomatic gout in usual dosages (0.6 to 1.2 mg/day). The incidence of colchicine myopathy appears to be increased in patients with kidney impairment, and when it is prescribed the patient should be monitored closely for this complication by measuring of creatinine phosphokinase concentration and muscle strength. The dosage of allopurinol must be reduced to 200 mg/day in patients with GFRs lower than 50 mL/minute and to 100 mg/day when the GFR is less than 30 mL/minute. The uricosuric agents probenecid (Benemid) and sulfinpyrazone (Anturane) are ineffective when the GFR falls below 50 mL/minute and should therefore not be used. Indomethacin (Indocin) is almost entirely metabolized by the liver, so it does not accumulate even in advanced renal failure. However, patients who receive indomethacin for the treatment of acute gout must have their BUN and serum creatinine concentrations monitored carefully, because indomethacin can cause a transient worsening of renal function.

CHRONIC RENAL INSUFFICIENCY AND COEXISTING DISORDERS

Nonrenal diseases often occur in patients with uremia. In some patients, such as those with systemic lupus erythematosus or diabetes mellitus, the renal disease is part of a generalized illness that affects many other organ systems. Other patients may have diseases unrelated to the kidneys, such as coronary artery disease, chronic obstructive pulmonary disease, or malignancy. The coexistence of multiple disorders often complicates management. For example, angina in patients with coronary artery disease may be aggravated by the anemia of chronic renal failure.

Diabetes Mellitus

Up to 40% of patients with type 1 diabetes and 10% of those with type 2 diabetes (the incidences are higher in African Americans, Hispanics, and Native Americans) develop chronic renal failure, and patients with diabetes mellitus (usually type 2) account for about one third of many dialysis populations. The pathophysiology of diabetic nephropathy is complex and involves genetic, metabolic, and hemodynamic factors. It is becoming increasingly important for the generalist to recognize and treat these patients, because efforts to prevent the development of advanced renal failure must take place early, usually before the patient is referred to the nephrologist.

Proteinuria (greater than 300 mg/day), as detected by a urine dipstick, is the earliest clinical manifestation of diabetic nephropathy; it is seen 10 to 15 years after the onset of type 1 diabetes mellitus and sooner in patients with type 2. By this time, pathologic changes of diabetic glomerulosclerosis are well established. More subtle degrees of proteinuria, so-called microalbuminuria (30 to 300 mg/24 hours), predicts the development of diabetic nephropathy and identifies a subpopulation of patients who need more aggressive therapy, including tight glucose and blood pressure control. Without specific interventions, a high proportion of patients (50%) with type 1 disease who have microalbuminuria develop renal insufficiency. The predictive value of microalbuminuria in type 2 diabetes is weaker (20% to 40%).

The Council on Diabetes Mellitus of the National Kidney Foundation has published guidelines for the screening and treatment of diabetic patients with microalbuminuria (38). Screening for microalbuminuria should be performed annually for all diabetics between the ages of 12 and 70 years. Although timed urine collections are more accurate and preferable, measurement of a morning spot urine for albumin and creatinine, using a specific assay to detect microalbuminuria, is a more practical alternative. Microalbuminuria is present if the albumin excretion rate is between 30 and 300 mg/24 hours or the albumin/creatinine ratio is between 30 and 300 mg/g on two occasions in a 3-month period. Urine protein may be falsely elevated if the patient is performing strenuous exercise, has a febrile illness, has a urinary tract infection, or is in heart failure. Studies have shown that treatments (usually involving the use of ACE inhibitors or angiotensin-receptor blockers) that reduce proteinuria have significant renoprotective effects in patients with or without hypertension (39,40).

Short-term studies of patients with early diabetes showed that tight glycemic control can reverse some of the abnormalities, such as hyperfiltration, that are thought to be important in the development of diabetic nephropathy. The Diabetes Control and Complications Trial (DCCT) (41) showed that the development of microalbuminuria could be forestalled and that the amount of established albuminuria could be reduced when intensive therapy with multiple-dose insulin or an insulin pump was coupled with frequent glucose monitoring in patients with type 1 diabetes. There is no evidence for a threshold effect of glycemic control below which the risk of developing microbalbuminuria is forestalled; therefore, lowering the blood glucose level as much as possible is recommended (42). Although similar data are lacking for populations of patients with early type 2 diabetes, the results of the STENO study (43), which included a group that received intensive therapy aimed at controlling glucose, blood pressure, and dyslipidemia, suggested that it makes sense to attempt better glucose control in these patients as well.

The prevention of progressive renal insufficiency should be the major goal in treating patients with early diabetic nephropathy. Hypertension is often present in diabetic patients, particularly if they have evidence of nephropathy. A number of studies in both type 1 and type 2 diabetes have demonstrated that the speed of renal deterioration is correlated with the degree of hypertension and that reducing the blood pressure to normal levels slows the rate. Animal studies and short-term human studies suggest that ACE inhibitors and nondihydropyridine calcium channel blockers provide additional protective effects beyond those afforded by the lowering of blood pressure. These impressions have been confirmed in large-scale, randomized studies (44). Most nephrologists would now recommend the use of an ACE inhibitor as first-line antihypertensive therapy in diabetic patients with nephropathy. Although hyperkalemia and renal insufficiency (in patients with bilateral renal artery stenosis) are uncommon complications of ACE inhibitor therapy, the serum potassium and creatinine levels should be checked approximately 1 week after starting treatment. A decrease in GFR, reflected in a small but measurable increase in serum creatinine level, is expected and should not be a reason for discontinuing the ACE inhibitor (45). Two clinical trials have demonstrated that the angiotensin-receptor blockers, irbesartan and losartan, can reduce proteinuria and slow the progression of renal insufficiency in hypertensive, nephropathic patients with type 2 diabetes (46,47). In at least one study, the nondihydropyridine calcium channel blockers verapamil and diltiazem were as effective as lisinopril in reducing protein excretion and the rate of decline in GFR in patients with type 2 diabetes mellitus, renal insufficiency, and proteinuria (48). Regardless of which antihypertensive agent is used, it is important to maintain good control of the blood pressure (130/85 mm Hg or lower).

The renoprotective effect of ACE inhibitors appears to extend to normotensive patients with type 1 diabetes and probably also to those with type 2 (49–52). The HOPE trial (53) demonstrated the value of using ramipril to reduce cardiovascular events in diabetic patients who were considered to be at high risk, including those with microalbuminuria. Therefore, the consensus recommendation is to treat all diabetic patients who have microalbuminuria or macroalbuminuria, regardless of blood pressure, with ACE inhibitors or angiotensin-receptor blockers unless contraindicated.

As in nondiabetic patients, the value of a low-protein diet in retarding the progression of renal damage in diabetic populations remains controversial. If such therapy is attempted, it is important to refer the patient to a dietitian who is familiar with the prescription of the diets and who will work with the patient over time to help with compliance.

Renal disease may reduce the requirement for insulin, an effect related at least in part to decreased hormone degradation in the renal tubules as nephrons are progressively lost. Some oral hypoglycemic agents, notably chlorpropamide and acetohexamide, also have prolonged half-lives in uremic patients. As a consequence of these pharmacologic abnormalities, the first overt manifestation of renal disease in some diabetic patients is the occurrence of hypoglycemia. Therefore, the dosage of insulin or oral hypoglycemic drugs should be assessed regularly in patients with renal impairment.

Diabetes *per se* is not a contraindication to dialysis or transplantation, although the course of diabetic patients is more complicated than that of patients with isolated renal failure. The form of therapy best suited for those patients with ESRD is uncertain. Hemodialysis, peritoneal dialysis, and transplantation have their proponents. Diabetic patients should be reminded that dialysis and transplantation are supportive therapies for renal dysfunction and will not improve their diabetes (see Dialysis and Transplantation). The microvasculopathy that destroys the kidney also affects the retinal and peripheral vessels. Because blindness and peripheral vascular disease are important causes of morbidity and mortality in the dialysis and transplantation population, it is critical for these patients to have appropriate attention to their eyes (see Chapter 79) and feet (see Chapter 73).

Heart Disease

Patients with congestive heart failure or angina often require more frequent monitoring as renal function declines. Diuretics may lose their effectiveness, or as anemia worsens patients with ischemic heart disease may become more symptomatic. In this situation transfusions are necessary if there has been an inadequate response to antianginal therapy, although erythropoietin may be useful in improving the anemia.

Patients with renal failure have been noted to have an accelerated rate of atherogenesis. This may be explained by the presence of hypertension, glucose intolerance, hyperhomocysteinemia, hypertriglyceridemia, and reduced levels of high-density lipoproteins in this group of patients.

Human Immunodeficiency Virus Infection

A *chronic,* progressive nephropathy characterized by proteinuria and renal failure can be seen in patients with AIDS. Most of these patients have a history of intravenous drug abuse, but AIDS nephropathy has also been found in patients with other HIV exposures. The prognosis of these patients is grim, and many die from infections, complications, or inanition before they reach the point of needing dialysis. Small studies have reported a beneficial effect of steroids alone or in combination with highly active antiretroviral therapy (HAART) on the course of HIV nephropathy (54,55), but treatment remains frustrating. The early experience with dialysis in AIDS patients was poor (56); more recent reports suggest a more optimistic prognosis, particularly for asymptomatic patients and those treated with HAART (57,58). The experience is best for patients who are HIV positive but have unrelated renal failure.

Malignancy

Renal failure resulting from hypercalcemia, sepsis, or drug nephrotoxicity is not an uncommon occurrence in patients who are dying with a malignancy. In many of these patients it would be inappropriate to prolong their lives by initiating dialysis. However, patients with multiple myeloma or other neoplasms who may have a long survival time might benefit from dialysis. Dialysis in patients with neoplastic diseases should be recommended only after careful discussion with the patient, the family, an oncologist, and a nephrologist.

Pregnancy and Renal Insufficiency

The presence of even mild renal insufficiency has important ramifications for the health of the mother and baby. The frequency of hypertensive complications is increased and proteinuria is exacerbated in women with renal disease who become pregnant. Aside from the increased incidence of hypertension, women who have antepartum serum creatinine levels of 1.4 mg/dL or less do not generally experience a worsening of renal function during the pregnancy. The renal outcome for women with initial serum creatinine levels greater than 1.4 mg/dL is not as good; almost half experience a decline in renal function during pregnancy, a decline that persists in many (59). Prematurity and low birth weight are much more common in babies born to women with renal insufficiency, but fetal survival is greater than 90% in most series when women get appropriate prenatal attention and high-quality neonatal intensive care is available.

SYMPTOMATIC THERAPY FOR ADVANCED RENAL FAILURE

Patients with advanced renal failure (GFR less than 10 mL/minute) invariably develop a variety of uremic symptoms. Gastrointestinal disturbances such as nausea, anorexia, and vomiting are common. Treatment involves further restriction of protein (see Dietary Management) or use of antiemetics (e.g., prochlorperazine [Compazine]). Itching is often a bothersome problem of unknown etiology. Reduction of serum phosphorus to normal levels and the use of skin lubricants (see Chapter 116) and antihistamines (e.g., diphenhydramine [Benadryl], 25 to 50 mg four times/day) are all worth 1- to 3-week trial periods. Ultraviolet light therapy may also be helpful, but this requires consultation with a dermatologist who performs this type of therapy. Fatigue, heart failure, and angina may be caused by worsening anemia or volume overload and should respond to erythropoietin or diuretics. Neuromuscular symptoms, such as myoclonus, restless legs, and disturbed sleep, are signs of advanced uremia and should serve as warnings that more severe abnormalities (e.g., seizures, coma) may soon develop.

Although the patient and physician should try to minimize the symptoms of uremia with conservative therapy including protein-restricted diets, there is a point when this effort becomes counterproductive and dialysis should be started.

Initiation of Dialysis

There are no absolute laboratory criteria defining the time at which dialysis should be initiated, but most patients in whom dialysis is started have serum creatinine concentrations of approximately 8 to 10 mg/dL. Many nephrologists believe that diabetics develop uremic symptoms at lower levels of BUN and creatinine concentrations than do nondiabetics. Delay in starting dialysis can lead to the development of severe peripheral neuropathy, malnutrition, or pericarditis from which complete recovery might not be possible. A low serum albumin (less than 4.0 g/dL), reflecting malnutrition, has been shown to be a strong predictor for increased mortality in both dialysis and predialysis populations. As patients become uremic, there is a tendency for them to spontaneously decrease their food intake, which predisposes these patients to malnutrition. Most nephrologists would consider any sign of malnutrition, such as weight loss or low serum albumin (not attributable to other causes), to be an indication for starting dialysis (60). A National Kidney Foundation consensus group recommended that dialysis be started when the creatinine clearance falls below that provided by peritoneal dialysis on a weekly basis (i.e., 9 to 14 mL/minute), particularly if there is evidence of malnutrition or signs of uremia (61).

The importance of timely referral to a nephrologist for dialysis planning cannot be overemphasized. Late referral, defined as less than 3 months before the actual initiation of dialysis, has been associated with poorer metabolic control, lower likelihood of being treated with erythropoietin for anemia, greater chance of starting hemodialysis with a temporary catheter, starting dialysis as an inpatient, and having higher medical care costs and higher mortality rates (62,63). If the patient is not already under the care of a nephrologist, referral for dialysis planning should take place when the serum creatinine concentration is 4 mg/dL or the creatinine clearance is less than 30 mL/minute. In some instances the primary care provider may question whether referral for dialysis treatments is appropriate. This question most often arises in very old patients, those with severe heart disease, significant cognitive impairment, malignancies, or otherwise short life expectancies. Several sets of guidelines have been developed to help assist in these difficult decisions (64,65).

DIALYSIS AND TRANSPLANTATION

In 1998, more than 200,000 patients were being maintained on dialysis in the United States. Most facilities provide hemodialysis, peritoneal dialysis, and transplantation (or referral to a transplantation center) for patients with ESRD (Table 52.13). Either form of dialysis therapy can be performed at a center or at the patient's home. Some patients choose dialysis as a permanent form of treatment, whereas others undergo dialysis temporarily until they receive a kidney transplant. Although dialysis does not correct all of the metabolic abnormalities of chronic renal failure, it has enabled thousands of patients to lead productive lives. The nephrologist often serves as primary care provider for patients who do not have one. For those patients who do, it is important for the nephrologist and the generalist to coordinate care carefully.

Hemodialysis

The hemodialysis procedure involves circulating the patient's blood through a machine that corrects electrolyte abnormalities and can remove excess fluid and toxic metabolic wastes. In the case of slowly progressive renal failure, provisions for dialysis should be made months in advance of need. The goal of dialysis therapy is to maintain health at a level consistent with a normal lifestyle. Therefore, it is not advisable to wait for signs and symptoms of far-advanced uremia (e.g., pericarditis, seizures, coma, bleeding) to appear before initiating dialysis. The patient should be referred to a nephrologist associated with a dialysis center when the creatinine clearance approaches 30 mL/minute. In this way the patient can be familiarized with the

Table 52.13. Treatments for End-Stage Renal Failure

Hemodialysis
Home
Hospital based
Satellite or self-care (e.g., those not situated in a hospital)
Peritoneal dialysis
Continuous ambulatory peritoneal dialysis
Continuous cyclic peritoneal dialysis
Intermittent peritoneal dialysis
Renal transplantation
Living donor transplant
Living unrelated donor transplant
Cadaveric transplant

various forms of therapy offered at that facility and become acquainted with the staff.

Before starting dialysis, it is necessary to provide vascular access to allow for the repeated venipunctures required for this form of therapy. It is important that the access be placed well before the patient needs dialysis treatments; otherwise, it is necessary to use temporary access techniques (central vein or femoral vein cannulation), which are associated with both short-term problems (pneumothorax, infection) and long-term complications (subclavian vein stenosis or thrombosis). The preferred access is the arteriovenous fistula, which is usually created at the wrist of the nondominant arm. The creation of a fistula can be performed, in most instances, under local anesthesia and often in an outpatient surgical unit. Because a 2- to 3-month maturation period is often necessary before the fistula can be used, arrangements for the creation of the fistula should be made early, and always before the GFR falls to less than 10 to 15 mL/minute. If the patient's vessels are inadequate to support the creation of an arteriovenous fistula, an alternative would be to insert a synthetic (Dacron, Gore-Tex) graft under the skin of the forearm. In most cases the synthetic graft can be used within 3 weeks after placement. The most common complications after placement of a fistula or graft are clotting and infection.

Hemodialysis is performed in most centers three times a week, and each session lasts 3 to 4 hours. Except for needle insertion, the procedure is not painful, but some patients do experience muscle cramps, headaches, or nausea during or just after dialysis. Hospital-based dialysis should be reserved for patients who require intensive monitoring. Home dialysis is encouraged for patients with good home situations who have willing and able partners. Home dialysis patients have the advantage of more flexible schedules and a greater sense of control than do hospital-based patients; for these reasons, they have a greater chance of maintaining their previous lifestyle. The remainder of the patients can be treated at outpatient dialysis centers. Small, uncontrolled studies suggest that short daily or slow nocturnal hemodialysis offers better metabolic control and sense of well-being, compared with traditional intermittent hemodialysis.

As a group, hemodialysis patients have an 80% survival rate for the first year; by 5 years, the survival rate falls to approximately 55%. The development of long-term complications of chronic renal failure, including progressive neuropathy, osteodystrophy, cardiovascular disease, and an array of endocrine disturbances, reflects the fact that dialysis does not correct all of the metabolic disturbances of uremia.

Peritoneal Dialysis

Peritoneal dialysis procedures involve the instillation of dialysis fluid through a catheter into the abdominal cavity. Fluid and toxic solutes are transferred across the mesenteric capillary bed into the dialysis fluid, which is then removed through the catheter. Improvements in the techniques of peritoneal dialysis have increased its popularity among patients. In the past, peritoneal dialysis required 12 to 16 hours of being connected to an automatic cycling machine, two to three times a week (*intermittent peritoneal dialysis*). Even then, its simplicity and freedom from hemodynamic complications made this form of therapy attractive, particularly to the elderly and to those with heart disease. Today, *continuous ambulatory peritoneal dialysis* (CAPD) has almost completely replaced the older, machine-based therapy. In this technique, the patient constantly carries 2 to 3 L of dialysis solution in the abdomen (66). The fluid is exchanged four times a day, every day. However, because fluid movement is determined by gravity and no machine is necessary, the patient is able to perform dialysis at home, at work, or virtually anywhere. This degree of freedom is one of the most attractive aspects of CAPD. Its other attributes, at least theoretically, are that it provides greater removal of higher–molecular-weight substances than hemodialysis does and that the continuous nature of the dialysis eliminates the large swings in concentration of electrolytes and creatinine that occur with the more intermittent forms of therapy. Also, the abdominal catheter for CAPD can be placed at the time of the first dialysis and does not require a maturation period. The major difficulty associated with peritoneal dialysis is the development of peritonitis. The incidence in the typical patient is about one infection every 12 to 24 months, but these infections usually respond to antimicrobial therapy and continued peritoneal dialysis, and often treatment of peritonitis does not require hospitalization. However, the peritoneal dialysis catheter may need periodic replacement.

Continuous cyclic peritoneal dialysis (CCPD) is a variant of peritoneal dialysis in which the patient is connected to an automated cycling device that performs the exchanges while the patient is sleeping, further reducing the impact of dialysis on the patient's daytime schedule.

Comparative survival statistics between hemodialysis and peritoneal dialysis are difficult to interpret because of significant population selection biases. Whether hemodialysis or peritoneal dialysis is used depends on the center to which the patient is referred and patient preference. At most dialysis facilities, the patient has a choice and may change dialysis modes if the outcome of one is unsatisfactory.

Renal Transplantation

Of all available therapies, successful renal transplantation provides for the most complete correction of the uremic syndrome. Innovations in antirejection therapy, such as use of the potent immunosuppressant drugs cyclosporine, tacrolimus, sirolimus, mycophenolate mofetil, and monoclonal antibodies (OKT3), have improved the rate of graft survival.

The success of renal transplantation depends on the antigenic similarity between donor and recipient.

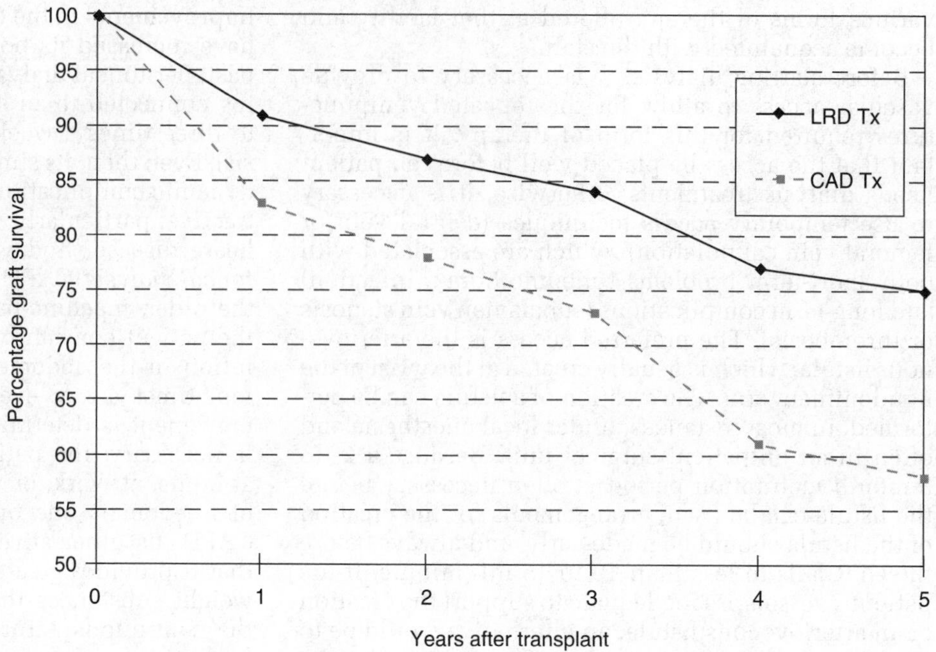

Figure 52.10. Two-year kidney graft survival according to donor source in patients treated with cyclosporine. (Modified from Agodoa LYC, Held PJ, Port FK, eds. U.S. Renal Data System: USRDS 1996 annual data report. Bethesda, MD: National Institute of Diabetes and Digestive and Kidney Diseases, 1996.)

Except in the case of identical twins (in which rejection does not occur), the best results are found with living related donor, human leukocyte antigen (HLA)–identical transplants. In this instance, kidney survival is greater than 90% at 2 years. More commonly performed are HLA-matched sibling-to-sibling or parent-to-child organ transplantations, with a success rate of 92% at 1 year and 87% at 2 years (Fig. 52.10). Patient survival for non–HLA-identical living related donor transplants is greater than 90% at both 1 year and 2 years. Most patients (more than 75%) do not have the possibility of a living related donor and must await a cadaveric transplant, which, despite the best tissue typing, has a significantly lower success rate of 83% at 1 year and 77% at 2 years. Patient survival rates for cadaveric transplants are 90% at 1 year and 88% at 2 years. Comparison of survival statistics between cadaveric transplants and dialysis patients is complicated because of selection bias. Transplant recipients tend to be younger, have better myocardial function, and have fewer coexisting illnesses than their dialysis counterparts. If these factors are taken into account, no significant difference in survival rate can be found between patients receiving cadaveric kidney transplants and those being treated by dialysis.

Patients with uncomplicated renal transplantation usually require a 4- to 7-day hospitalization. The use of laparoscopic donor nephrectomy has reduced the convalescence of donors and increased the frequency of living related and living unrelated donor transplants (67). After transplantation (except with identical twins), the patient requires lifelong immunosuppression, usually with a combination of cyclosporine (Sandimmune) or tacrolimus (Prograf); prednisone; and azathioprine (Imuran), sirolimus (Rapamune), or mycophenolate mofetil (CellCept). The patient must understand that there is always the risk of rejection and the possibility of graft failure, with a return to dialysis. Although there is no doubt that a successfully functioning transplant restores health better than any other therapy, patients on immunosuppressive therapy have considerable risks from corticosteroid use and immunosuppression, including obesity, diabetes, cataracts, osteoporosis, serious infections, and malignancies.

The primary care provider can be of great value in advising which forms of therapy might coincide best with the patient's expectations. Often, patients have a better understanding of their choices if they visit a dialysis or transplantation unit and talk with patients or staff. The decision to suggest renal transplantation is most clear-cut in adolescents or young adults who wish to pursue an active, vigorous life, have a job, and have intact sexual functions. This is particularly so if a well-matched living donor is available. Elderly patients and those with extensive multisystem disease may not be able to tolerate the rigors of transplantation. For others, a period of dialysis and assessment of the patient's adjustment to this therapy often helps in determining whether to continue dialysis or consider transplantation. Often, the patient who adjusts well to dialysis can be fully rehabilitated and can maintain a job as efficiently as the patient with a successful renal transplantation. At present it appears that quality of life is the most important criterion determining which form of therapy is selected, because survival appears to be similar in patients undergoing either cadaveric transplantation or dialysis.

The personal financial impact of chronic renal failure and the cost of hemodialysis and transplantation, which initially were prohibitively expensive, have been minimized for patients and their families by extension of the Medicare program to patients younger than 65 years of age with ESRD. Nevertheless, patients often have to leave their jobs because of chronic illness or because of the time requirements of therapy.

Despite advances in dialysis and transplantation in recent years, the best hope for patients with chronic renal disease lies in prevention and appropriate therapy in the early stages of renal insufficiency. These objectives must be accomplished by the patient's primary care physician.

General References*

Bakris BL, Williams M, Dworkin L, et al. **Preserving renal failure in adults with hypertension and diabetes: a consensus approach.** Am J Kidney Dis 2000;36:646.

Consensus recommendations for the treatment of hypertension, renal insufficiency, and proteinuria based on review of relevant literature.

Brenner BM, Rector FC, eds. The kidney. 5th ed. Philadelphia: WB Saunders, 1996.

Useful general nephrology text.

Felsefeld AJ. Considerations for the treatment of secondary hyperparathyroidism in renal failure. J Am Soc Nephrol 1997;8:993.

Review of pathophysiology and treatment of renal bone disease.

Materson BJ, Preston RA. Prevention of diabetic nephropathy. Hosp Pract 1997;32:129.

Current review on the effects of intensive therapy on the outcome of long-term complications of type 1 diabetes.

Pereira BJG. Optimization of pre-ESRD care: the key to improved dialysis outcomes. Kidney Int 2000;57:351.

A review of the issues relating to the management of patients with chronic renal insufficiency.

Remuzzi G, Ruggenenti P, Benigni A. Understanding the nature of renal disease progression. Kidney Int 1997;51:2.

Latest theories explaining the mechanisms that lead to progressive renal failure.

Uribarri J. Acidosis in chronic renal insufficiency. Semin Dial 2000;13:232.

Review of the causes, clinical consequences, and treatment of uremic acidosis.

Specific References

1. Jones C, McQuillan G, Kusek J, et al. Serum creatinine levels in the US population: Third National Health and Nutrition Examination Survey. Am J Kid Dis 1998;32:992.
2. U. S. Renal Data System: 2001 Annual Data Report. National Institute of Diabetes and Digestive and Kidney Disease. Bethesda, MD: U. S. Department of Health and Human Services, 2001.
3. Brenner BM, Meyer TW, Hostetter TH. Dietary protein intake and the progressive nature of kidney disease: the role of hemodynamically mediated glomerular injury in the pathogenesis of progressive glomerular sclerosis, aging, renal ablation, and intrinsic renal disease. N Engl J Med 1982;307:652.
4. Rao TKS, Friedman EA, Nicastri AD. The types of renal disease in the acquired immunodeficiency syndrome. N Engl J Med 1987;316:1062.
5. **5.** Keane WF, Eknoyan G. Proteinuria, albuminuria, risk, assessment, detection, elimination (PARADE): a position paper of the National Kidney Foundation. Am J Kidney Dis 1999;33: 1004.
6. Lindeman RD, Tobin J, Shock NW. Longitudinal studies on the rate of decline in renal function with age. J Am Geriatr Soc 1985;33:278.
7. Rowe JW, Andres R, Tobin JD, et al. Age-adjusted standards for creatinine clearance. Ann Intern Med 1976;84:567.
8. Walser M, Drew DH, LaFrance ND. Reciprocal creatinine slopes often give erroneous estimates of progression of chronic renal failure. Kidney Int 1989;36(S27):S-81.
9. Emanian SA, Nielsen BN, Pederson JF, et al. Kidney dimensions at sonography: correlation with age, sex, and habitus in 665 adult volunteers. AJR Am J Roentgenol 1993;160:83.
10. Regan F, Petronis J, Bohlman M, et al. Perirenal MR high signal: a new and sensitive indicator of acute ureteric obstruction. Clin Radiol 1997;52:445.
11. Greco BA, Breyer JA. Atherosclerotic ischemic renal disease. Am J Kidney Dis 1997;29:167.
12. Geyskes GG, Dei HY, Puylaert CB, et al. Renovascular hypertension identified by captopril-induced changes in the renogram. Hypertension 1987;9:451.
13. **13.** Parfrey PS, Griffitch SM, Steinman TI, et al. Contrast material-induced renal failure in patients with diabetes mellitus, renal insufficiency or both: a prospective controlled study. N Engl J Med 1989;320:1.
14. Lautin EM, Freeman NJ, Schoenfeld AH, et al. Radiocontrast-associated renal dysfunction: a comparison of lower-osmolaity and conventional high-osmolality contrast media. AJR Am J Roentgenol 1991;157:59.
15. Tepel M, van der Giet M, Schwartzfeld C, et al. Prevention of radiographic-contrast-agent–induced reductions in renal function by acetylcysteine. N Engl J Med 2000;343:180.
16. Bergstrom J. Discovery and rediscovery of low protein diets. Clin Nephrol 1984;21:29.
17. Maschio G, Oldrizzi L, Tessitore N, et al. Effects of dietary protein and phosphorus restriction on the progression of early renal failure. Kidney Int 1982;22:371.
18. Klahr S, Levey AS, Beck GH, et al. The effects of dietary protein restriction and blood-pressure control on the progression of chronic renal disease. N Engl J Med 1994;330:877.
19. Levey AS, Adler S, Caggiula AW, et al. Effects of dietary protein restriction on the progression of advanced renal disease in the Modification of Diet in Renal Disease Study. Am J Kidney Dis 1996;27:652.
20. **20.** Striker G. Report on a workshop to develop management recommendations for the prevention of progression in chronic renal disease. J Am Soc Nephrol 1995;5:1537.
21. **21.** Hannedouche T, Landais P, Goldfarb B, et al. Randomized controlled trial of enalapril and beta blockers in non-diabetic chronic renal failure. Br Med J 1994;309:833.
22. Maschio M, Alberti D, Janin G, et al. Effect of angiotensin converting enzyme inhibitor benazepril in the progression of renal insufficiency. N Engl J Med 1996;334:939.
23. Zuccelli P, Zuccla A, Borghi M, et al. Long-term comparison between captopril and nifedipine in the progression of renal insufficiency. Kidney Int 1992;42:452.
24. Rose BJ. Diuretics. Kidney Int 1991;29:336.
25. Levin A, Singer J, Thompson CR, et al. Prevalent left ventricular hypertrophy in the redialysis population: identifying opportunities for intervention. Am J Kidney Dis 1996;27:347.
26. Phelps KR, Lieberman RL, Oh MS, et al. Pathophysiology of the syndrome of hyporeninemic hypoaldosteronism. Metabolism 1980;29:186.
27. **27.** Barker LRI, Louise Abrams SM, Roe C, et al. 1,25(OH)2 D3 administration in moderate renal failure: a prospective double blind trial. Kidney Int 1989;35:661.
28. Torres A, Lorenzo V, Hernandez D, et al. Bone disease in predialysis, and CAPD patients: evidence of a better bone response to PTH. Kidney Int 1995;47:1434.
29. Goodman WG, Goldin J, Kuizon BD, et al. Coronary-artery calcification in young adults with end-stage renal disease who are undergoing dialysis. N Engl J Med 1987;316:73.
30. Kazmi WH, Annamaria TK, Khan S, et al. Anemia: an early complication of chronic renal insufficiency. Am J Kidney Dis 2001;38:803.
31. Eschbach JW, Egrie JC, Dowing MR, et al. Correction of the anemia of end-stage renal disease with recombinant human erythropoietin: results of a combined phase I and II clinical trial. N Engl J Med 1987;316:73.

*Bold print (general references) and bold numerals (specific references) denote published controlled clinical trials, meta-analyses, or consensus-based recommendations.

32. Lim VS, DeGowin RL, Zavala D, et al. Recombinant human erythropoietin treatment in pre-dialysis patients: a double-blind placebo controlled trial. Ann Intern Med 1989;110:108.
33. Bennett WM, Plamp C, Porter GA. Drug related syndromes in clinical nephrology. Ann Intern Med 1977;87:582.
34. Aronoff GR, Bennett WM, Berns JS, et al. Drug prescribing in renal failure. Dosing guidelines for adults. 4th ed. Philadelphia, PA: American College of Physicians, 1999.
35. Clive DM, Stoff JS. Renal syndromes associated with nonsteroidal anti-inflammatory drugs. N Engl J Med 1984:310:563.
36. Eriksson L, Stufelt G, Thysell H, et al. Effects of sulindac and naproxen on prostaglandin secretion in patients with impaired renal function and rheumatoid arthritis. Am J Med 1990;89:313.
37. Aronson JK. Clinical pharmacokinetics of cardiac glycosides in patients with renal dysfunction. Clin Pharmacokinet 1983;8:155.
38. Bennett PH, Haffner S, Kasiske BL, et al. Screening and management of microalbuminuria in patient with diabetes mellitus: recommendations to the Scientific Advisory Board of the National Kidney Foundation from an ad hoc committee of the Council on Diabetes Mellitus of the National Kidney Foundation. Am J Kidney Dis 1995;25:107.
39. Parving HH, Lehnert H, Brochnew-Mortensen, et al. The effect of irbesartan on the development of diabetic nephropathy in patient with type 2 diabetes. N Engl J Med 2001;345:870.
40. Ravid M, Lang R, Rachmani R, et al. Long-term renoprotective effect of angiotensin-converting enzyme inhibition in non-insulin-dependent diabetes mellitus: a 7-year-follow-up study. Arch Intern Med 1996;156:286.
41. The Diabetes Control and Complications Research Group. The effect of intensive treatment of diabetes of the development and progression of long-term complication in insulin-dependent diabetes mellitus. N Engl J Med 2001;329:997.
42. Chaturvedi N, Bandinello S, Mangili R, et al. Microalbuminuria in type 1 diabetes: rates, risk factors and glycemic threshold. Kidney Int 2001;60:219.
43. Gaede P, Vedel P, Parving HH, et al. Intensified multifactorial intervention in patients with type 2 diabetes mellitus and microalbuminuria: the STENO type 2 randomized study. Lancet 1999;353:617.
44. Lewis EJ, Hunsicker LG, Bain RP, et al. The effect of angiotensin-converting enzyme inhibition on diabetic nephropathy. N Engl J Med 1993;239:1456.
45. Bakris GL, Weir MR. ACE inhibitor-associated elevations in serum creatinine: is this a cause for concern? Arch Intern Med 2001;160:685.
46. Lewis EJ, Hunsicker LG, Clarke WR, et al. Renoprotective effect of the angiotensin receptor antagonist irbesartan in patients with nephropathy due to type 2 diabetes. N Engl J Med 2001;345:851.
47. Brenner BM, Cooper ME, de Zeeuw D, et al. Effects of losartan on renal and cardiovascular outcomes in patients with nephropathy due to type 2 diabetes. N Engl J Med 2001;345:851.
48. Bakris GL, Copley JB, Vicknair N, et al. Calcium channel blockers versus other antihypertensive therapies on progression of type 2 diabetes and nephropathy. Kidney Int 1996;50:1641.
49. Ravid M, Savin H, Jutrin I, et al. Long-term stabilizing effect of angiotensin-converting enzyme inhibition on plasma creatinine and on proteinuria in normotensive type 2 diabetic patients. Ann Intern Med 1993;118:577.
50. Laffel LM, McGill JB, Gans DJ, et al. The beneficial effect of angiotensin-converting enzyme inhibitional with captopril in diabetic nephropathy in normotensive type 1 patients with microalbuminuria. Am J Med 1995;99:497.
51. Jerums J, Allen TJ, Campbell DJ, et al. Long-term comparison between perindopril and nifedipine in normotensive patients with type 1 diabetes and microalbuminuria. Am J Kidney Dis 2001;7:890.
52. Parving H, Hommel E, Jensen BR, et al. Long-term comparison between perindopril and nifedipine in normotensive patient with type 1 diabetic patients. Kidney Int 2001;60:228.
53. Effects of an angiotensin-converting-enzyme inhibitor, ramipril, on cardiovascular events in high-risk patients. N Engl J Med 2000;342:145.
54. Smith MC, Austen JL, Carey JT, et al. Prednisone improves renal function and proteinuria in human immunodeficiency virus-associated nephropathy. Am H Med 1996;101:41.
55. Nacarrete JE, Pastan SO. Effect of highly active antiretroviral treatment and prednisone in biopsy-proven HIV-associated nephropathy [Abstract]. J Am Soc Nephrol 2000;11:93A.
56. Rao TKS, Friedman EA, Nicastri AD. The types of renal disease in the acquired immunodeficiency syndrome. N Engl J Med 1996;101:41.
57. Ifudu O, Mayers JD, Mathew JJ, et al. Uremia therapy with end-stage renal disease and human immunodeficiency virus infection: has the outcome changed in the 1990s? Am J Kidney Dis 1997;29:549.
58. Ahuja TS, Borucki M, Grady J. Highly active antiretroviral therapy improves survival of HIV-infected hemodialysis patients. Am J Kidney Dis 2000;36:574.
59. Jones DC, Hayslett JP. Outcome of pregnancy in women with moderate or severe renal insufficiency. N Engl J Med 1996;335:226.
60. Hakim RM, Lazarus JM. Initiation of dialysis. J Am Soc Nephrol 1995;6:1319.
61. NKF-DOQI Clinical Practice Guidelines for Peritoneal Dialysis Adequacy: guidelines 1 and 2. Am J Kidney Dis 2001;37(S1):S70.
62. Ratcliffe PJ, Phillips RE, Oliver DO. Late referral for maintenance dialysis. Br Med J (Clin Res Ed) 1984;288:441.
63. Ifudu O, Dawood M, Homel P, et al. Excess morbidity in patients starting uremia therapy without prior care by a nephrologist. Am J Kidney Dis 1996;28:841.
64. Renal Physicians Association and American Society of Nephrology. Clinical practice guidelines on shared decision making in the appropriate initiation and withdrawal from dialysis. Rockville, MD: Renal Physicians Association, 2000.
65. Mendelssohn DC, Barrett BJ, Brownscombe LM, et al. Elevated levels of serum creatinine: recommendations for management and referral. CMAJ 1999;161:414.
66. Levey AS, Harrington JT. Continuous peritoneal dialysis for chronic renal failure. Medicine (Baltimore) 1982;61:330.
67. Cadeddu JA, Ratner L, Kavoussi LR. Laparoscopic donor nephrectomy. Semin Laparosc Surg 2000;7:195.

CHAPTER 53

Bladder Outlet Obstruction

RAY E. STUTZMAN, MD

The bladder, bladder outlet, prostate, and urethra may be affected by a wide variety of conditions that result in symptoms of urinary obstruction or bladder irritability. These lower urinary tract symptoms are common, especially in older men.

Benign prostatic hyperplasia (BPH) is the most common cause of bladder outlet obstruction in men older than 50 years of age. Autopsy studies show that 50% to 60% of men older than 50 years have significant enlargement of the prostate caused by BPH, and the prevalence increases with age. A number of other conditions also cause lower urinary tract symptoms in the male, including urethral stricture, carcinoma of the prostate, neurogenic bladder, bladder calculus, prostatitis, bladder neck contracture, urethritis, chronic cystitis, interstitial cystitis, and carcinoma of the bladder. Functional obstruction, seen in both women and men, may result from chronic bladder distention, debilitating disease, psychogenic retention, or medications.

HISTORY

Bladder outlet obstruction secondary to BPH is characterized by symptoms of urinary hesitancy, diminished force and caliber of the stream, and postvoid dribbling. The symptoms of urinary frequency, urgency, and nocturia result from a diminished functional bladder capacity, bladder muscle hypertrophy, and often bladder instability. The bladder hypertrophy results in increased intravesical pressure during voiding, thereby providing compensation for the obstruction. In time, however, the bladder decompensates, and this may lead to residual urine, infection, hematuria, hydronephrosis, and renal failure.

Patients with *urethral stricture* usually have a history of urethral trauma, instrumentation (most commonly an indwelling Foley catheter), or urethritis and, in association with symptoms of bladder outlet obstruction, may notice a split stream. *Carcinoma of the prostate* can manifest with obstructive symptoms, which often are of shorter duration than those seen in patients with BPH, in whom symptoms of outlet obstruction usually progress over several years. Recent onset of back or bone pain, anorexia, or weight loss suggests malignancy. *Neurogenic bladder* should be suspected if other symptoms of neurologic disease are present, if disorders of bowel or sexual function coexist with bladder outlet obstruction, or if a systemic disease that causes neurologic bladder dysfunction (e.g., diabetes mellitus, spinal cord injury) exists.

A review of current and recently used medications (Table 53.1) is mandatory in the evaluation of the patient with symptoms of bladder outlet obstruction. Anticholinergic agents, antispasmodics, antiparkinsonian drugs, and many antidepressant drugs depress bladder muscle contractility; sympathomimetic agents (e.g., ephedrine and other decongestants found in over-the-counter cold remedies), beta-blocking agents, and levodopa increase bladder outlet resistance. Diuresis (from a diuretic, glucosuria, or a large, brisk fluid intake) may overstretch a partially decompensated detrusor muscle and cause acute urinary retention.

It is important to distinguish *outlet obstructive bladder symptoms* (hesitancy, decreased stream, postvoid dribbling) from *irritative bladder symptoms* (frequency, urgency, nocturia). Although anatomic or functional obstruction may produce either type of symptoms, irritative symptoms are seen with cystitis, prostatitis, bladder stones, and bladder carcinoma. Finally, the differentiation of polyuria from urinary frequency and nocturia from enuresis (involuntary bedwetting) can be made by appropriate questioning.

The American Urological Association (AUA) Measurement Committee has developed a *symptom assessment tool* (Table 53.2; see pg. 727) for patients with prostatism. This prostate symptom score is based on the answers to seven questions concerning urinary symptoms. Each question allows the patient to choose one of five answers scaled to indicate increasing severity of the particular symptom. The answers are assigned points from 0 to 5. The total score can therefore range from 0 to 35 (asymptomatic to very symptomatic). There is an additional single question to assess the quality of life. The answer to this question ranges from "delighted" to "terrible," or 0 to 6. The International Consensus Committee (ICC), under the patronage of the World Health Organization (WHO), has agreed to use the symptom index for BPH. The ICC

Table 53.1. Selected Pharmacologic Agents with Known Influence on Bladder Function

Drugs that Increase Bladder Tone and Contractility
Bethanecol (Urecholine)

Drugs that Decrease Bladder Contractility
Anticholinergic drugs (e.g., Pro-Banthine, Donnatal, Ditropan)
Antihistamines
Calcium antagonists (verapamil, nifedipine, diltiazem)
Prostaglandin inhibitors (e.g., ibuprofen)
Tricyclic antidepressants (e.g., imipramine, nortriptyline)
β_2-Adrenergic antagonists (e.g., terbutoline)

Drugs that Increase Bladder Outlet Resistance
Adrenergic agonists (e.g., ephedrine, Sudafed)
Antiparkinsonian drugs (e.g., levodopa, Sinemet)
β-Adrenergic antagonists (e.g., propranolol)
Estrogens

Drugs that Decrease Outlet Resistance
Antispasticity drugs (e.g., diazepam, Baclofen)
α-Adrenergic antagonists (e.g., doxazosin, prazosin, phenoxybenzamine, terazosin)

Drugs that Increase Urinary Volume
Diuretics

strongly recommends that all physicians who counsel patients with symptoms of prostatism use these measures not only during the initial interview but also during and after treatment in order to monitor response.

PHYSICAL EXAMINATION

The physical examination of the patient with lower urinary tract symptoms should be carefully focused, with special emphasis on the urinary tract.

The *abdominal examination* may reveal several findings: a distended bladder from retention, renal tenderness (infection or hydronephrosis) or a renal mass (hydronephrosis, neoplasm, or cystic disease), and inguinal hernia from straining at urination when outlet obstruction is present. In the male patient, the *examination of the penis* may reveal phimosis or urethral meatal stenosis that could cause partial obstruction. The examination of the epididymides may show evidence of acute or chronic infection, which may be a complication of bladder outlet obstruction and concomitant prostatitis. A brief *neurologic examination,* particularly of the anal sphincter tone, genital and perineal sensation, and motor, sensory, and reflex activity of the lower extremities, may disclose abnormalities that suggest a neurogenic bladder as the cause of the patient's symptoms.

A careful *rectal examination* of the prostate is important in evaluating the patient with suspected BPH or prostatic carcinoma. Although there are certain limits, rectal palpation permits examination of the lateral lobes of the prostate and the posterior lobe, adjacent to the apex. The anterior lobe cannot be felt, and rarely is the median lobe palpable unless it is markedly enlarged. BPH most commonly involves the lateral and median lobes; moreover, the size of the prostate gland as estimated by rectal examination is not directly related to the degree of urinary obstruction.

The most important information obtained from the rectal examination is the *consistency of the prostate gland.* The patient may be examined when he is in the lateral decubitus, knee–chest, or standing–bending position. The patient should void as fully as possible before the examination, because a full bladder can distort the size of the prostate. The patient should be told that he may feel the urge to void when the prostate is examined. To prevent anal sphincter spasm, appropriate time should be taken to explain the procedure to the patient. Using ample lubricant, one should dilate the anal sphincter slowly and gently by gradually inserting the finger through the anus and asking the patient to bear down slightly. This examination permits the determination of shape, size, and consistency of the prostate; the presence of tenderness; any other rectal masses; and the adequacy of anal sphincter tone.

The normal prostate is palpable 2 to 5 cm from the anal verge through the anterior rectal wall. The examining finger can normally reach over the top (base) of the prostate, as well as over each lateral border. A median sulcus is appreciated in the midline. The palpable prostate can be compared in size, configuration, and consistency with the tip of the nose.

BPH often results not only in obliteration of the median sulcus but also in a failure of the examining finger to reach the base of the gland. The consistency of the gland in BPH is smooth and rubbery, similar to the thenar eminence of the hand. The gland is not tender unless prostatitis is present. BPH may be characterized by symmetric or asymmetric enlargement and can be nodular. The clinical differentiation between carcinoma and asymmetric or nodular BPH usually is based on the degree of induration or hardness of the gland.

Classically, prostatic carcinoma is characterized by a rock-hard nodule or mass involving one or both posterior lobes. The zygomatic arch of the face has a similar consistency to that of prostatic carcinoma. However, not all hard nodules are found on biopsy to be cancer, nor are all cancerous nodules hard. Granulomatous prostatitis, prostatic calculi, spheroids of BPH, or nodularity resulting from transurethral resection of the prostate (TURP) may manifest as prostatic nodules and induration. Only 30% to 40% of prostatic nodules biopsied as suspicious for carcinoma are positive on histologic examination.

If prostatic carcinoma is suspected, it is important to determine the extent of the local lesion—single nodule, diffuse involvement, or extension outside the capsule—and to refer the patient to a urologist.

PRELIMINARY LABORATORY ASSESSMENT

If the patient is thought to have bladder outlet obstruction caused by BPH, the need and urgency for urologic consultation must be determined. A urinalysis and a determination of the urinary flow rate (see later

Table 53.2. International Prostate Symptom Score (I-PSS)[a]

	Not at All	Less Than 1 Time in 5	Less Than Half the Time	About Half the Time	More Than Half the Time	Almost Always	Your Score
Incomplete emptying: Over the past month, how often have you had a sensation of not emptying your bladder completely after you finished urinating?	0	1	2	3	4	5	____
Frequency: Over the past month, how often have you had to urinate again less than 2 hours after you finished urinating?	0	1	2	3	4	5	____
Intermittency: Over the past month, how often have you found you stopped and started again several times when you urinated?	0	1	2	3	4	5	____
Urgency: Over the past month, how often have you found it difficult to postpone urination?	0	1	2	3	4	5	____
Weak stream: Over the past month, how often have you had a weak urinary stream?	0	1	2	3	4	5	____
Straining: Over the past month, how often have you had to push or strain to begin urination?	0	1	2	3	4	5	____
	None	1 time	2 times	3 times	4 times	5 or more times	
Nocturia: Over the past month how many times did you most typically get up to urinate from the time you went to bed at night until the time you got up in the morning?	0	1	2	3	4	5	____
						Total I-PSS Score =	____

Quality of Life

	Delighted	Pleased	Mostly Satisfied	Mixed (About Equally Satisfied and Dissatisfied)	Mostly Dissatisfied	Unhappy	Terrible
If you were to spend the rest of your life with your urinary condition just the way it is now, how would you feel about that?	0	1	2	3	4	5	6

[a]From International Consensus Committee under patronage of the World Health Organization. Handy cards containing this information are currently available at no cost from Merck and Co., Inc., telephone 215-652-7300.

discussion), a urine culture (if pyuria is present), and measurement of serum creatinine or, sometimes, measurement of the postvoid residual volume (see later discussion) provide the data to aid in making this decision. A measurement of serum *prostate-specific antigen* (PSA) should be obtained in the evaluation of patients with suspected carcinoma.

Prostate-Specific Antigen and Screening for Prostate Cancer

PSA is an enzyme synthesized only by prostatic epithelial cells. The ejaculate contains a high concentration of PSA, which is responsible for the liquefaction of the seminal coagulum. However, PSA is not specific for prostate carcinoma. Elevated serum PSA concentrations may be found in prostate carcinoma, glandular hyperplasia associated with BPH, acute bacterial prostatitis, prostate abscess, prostatic infarction, and manipulation of the prostate (e.g., cystourethroscopy, needle biopsy of the prostate, TURP). Ejaculation within 48 hours can elevate the PSA. Digital rectal examination and transrectal ultrasound (TRUS) do not appear to alter significantly the level of serum PSA. In 70% of men, PSA is less that 2 ng/mL. It is estimated that 40% to 50% of men with prostate carcinoma have a PSA greater than 10 ng/mL, whereas fewer than 5% of patients with BPH have such a high concentration. When the clinician elects to screen for asymptomatic prostate cancer in a man, the serum PSA determination is not adequate but should be used in conjunction with a digital rectal examination.

There remains controversy concerning the routine screening of men for asymptomatic prostate cancer. A popular position is the recommendation that all men between the ages of 50 and 75 years who also have at least a 10-year life expectancy should have a yearly PSA and digital rectal examination. It has been suggested from a simulation model that screens beginning earlier (at age 40 years) and occurring only biennially (instead of annually) may be more effective and less resource intensive than annual screening (1). On the other hand, there is no evidence yet that early detection of asymptomatic prostatic cancers has changed survival, although it may lead to significant mental and physical morbidity (e.g., anxiety, morbidity related to surgery or radiation). Therefore, screening for prostate cancer remains controversial. Accordingly, one should always discuss the risks and benefits of an evaluation aimed at the early detection of prostate cancer with patients who might be considered candidates for screening. Ongoing studies on the course of prostate cancer may ultimately guide clinicians concerning this consideration.

Men who have a family history of prostate cancer are at increased risk, and many of these men on explanation of the pros and cons of screening elect to be screened yearly, starting at age 40 years. African Americans also have an increased risk of developing prostate cancer and usually elect to be screened when fully informed about the pros and cons of screening. In both of these instances, the patient should understand the implications and subsequent diagnostic and therapeutic considerations of finding a biopsy positive for cancer.

PSA density (PSAD), a quotient of serum PSA and prostate volume determined by ultrasonography performed by a urologist or ultrasonographer, is used by some specialists to distinguish BPH from prostate cancer in a patient with a history or physical examination that raises concern about cancer. More specialists suggest that the rate of change in PSA levels over time (PSA velocity), rather than the PSAD, may be a sensitive and specific early clinical marker for the development of prostate cancer (2). A serial increase in 1 year of 0.75 ng or more over baseline is strongly suggestive of prostatic carcinoma despite normal digital rectal examinations. An increase in volume of the prostate in BPH occurs more slowly, so PSA does not rise rapidly in that condition. If a significant increase in PSA levels occurs, TRUS and prostate biopsy (both done by the consulting urologist or ultrasonographer) should be considered. PSA exists in both a bound and a free form. Patients with prostate cancer often have less free (unbound) PSA, usually less than 10%, whereas patients with BPH usually have more than 25% free PSA. The value of determining the PSA serum-to-urinary ratio in patients with suspected BPH or cancer of the prostate is under investigation (3); it is not currently recommended in routine practice.

Patient Experience. Needle biopsy of the prostate is usually done in a urologist's office or in an ultrasound suite. Prostate biopsy currently is most commonly done in conjunction with TRUS (see later discussion). No anesthesia or sedation is required, and the patient can eat and drink normally on the day of the procedure. Aspirin and other nonsteroidal anti-inflammatory agents (except for COX-2 inhibitors) should be stopped for 1 week, and anticoagulants should be stopped until the anticoagulant effect has gone, to avoid an increased risk of bleeding. A prophylactic antimicrobial (usually a fluoroquinolone) is given on the evening before and the morning of the procedure. The procedure usually takes 20 to 30 minutes, and the patient feels no more discomfort than with a typical rectal examination. The ultrasound probe, which is slightly larger than the index finger, is introduced into the rectum, allowing the prostate gland to be visualized. Usually a total of 10 to 12 needle core specimens are obtained from suspicious as well as normal areas. The biopsy apparatus has a spring-loaded gun mechanism, and the operator informs the patient that a loud noise will be heard when it is fired. The patient usually remains under surveillance for 30 to 60 minutes to be sure that the procedure was accomplished without incident. Most men notice a slight amount of blood in their urine or stool for a day or two. Bloody semen may be experienced for several ejaculations. The patient should be informed that these findings are common and of no concern unless they persist.

Most important, serum PSA concentration is the most reliable marker for response to treatment in prostate carcinoma. Serum PSA values should be negligible within 3 to 4 weeks after a radical prostatectomy. The failure of this to occur is an indication of residual disease. Elevated PSA concentrations also drop after primary radiation therapy, but they never reach zero. Regardless of the treatment, a subsequent rising PSA level means progression of the disease.

UROLOGIC INVESTIGATION

Urodynamic Assessment

Urodynamic evaluation of the urinary tract includes urinary flow rate (uroflowmetry) and cystometry. *Uroflowmetry* can be done by the generalist because it is easy to perform, is noninvasive, and may provide valuable information about the degree of obstruction and thereby guide the initiation of treatment. *Urinary flow rate* may be assessed by measuring the volume of urine voided during a 5-second period. Normal males have 5-second volumes exceeding 75 mL, whereas men with urinary obstruction have flows of less than 50 mL in 5 seconds. *Cystometry,* which includes pressure flow measurements, is performed by a urologist and is indicated for patients with clinical suspicion of voiding dysfunction unrelated to bladder outlet obstruction. This situation primarily involves patients with urgency, frequency, or a suggestion of a neurologic disorder. Cystometry involves simple bladder catheterization with manometric measurements as sterile fluid is infused. There is no evidence that routine cystometry and pressure flow measurements are of value in the management of urinary outlet obstruction secondary to BPH.

If the patient has hematuria, recurrent or persistent urinary tract infection, or renal failure and the diagnosis of BPH is likely, the patient is usually a candidate for surgery, and referral to a urologist is appropriate

Table 53.3. Indications for Surgery in Patients with Benign Prostatic Hypertrophy

Intractable symptoms not satisfactorily controlled by medical therapy
Urinary retention
Frequently recurrent or persistent urinary tract infection
Recurrent gross bleeding
Unacceptably high postvoid residual urine (e.g., >400–500 mL) not controlled with medical therapy
Bladder calculi
Evidence of obstruction affecting the ureters or kidneys

(Table 53.3). If there is no indication for surgery, then no further evaluation is necessary at this juncture, and medical therapy may be considered if symptoms are bothersome to the patient.

NONSURGICAL TREATMENT OF BLADDER OUTLET OBSTRUCTION

Nonsurgical therapy for BPH currently relies on two different pharmacologic approaches:

- Eliminating the dynamic component of the bladder outlet obstruction through the use of alpha-adrenergic antagonists (e.g., terazosin, doxazosin, tamsulosin)
- Producing a state of androgen deprivation with luteinizing hormone–releasing hormone (LHRH) antagonists, antiandrogens, or 5α-reductase inhibitors (e.g., finasteride)

Bethanechol (Urecholine), a cholinergic agent commonly prescribed in the past for an adynamic bladder without outlet obstruction, is rarely used today because of the cardiovascular and gastrointestinal side effects and the availability and ease of intermittent catheterization.

The rationale for use of alpha-antagonists in BPH is based on the fact that smooth muscle makes up a significant component of the human prostate, and their precise physiologic effects are increasingly understood (4). In fact, the prostate is composed primarily of glandular epithelium, smooth muscle, and connective tissue. Several alpha-blockers have been used, including doxazosin, terazosin, and other selective long-acting alpha-1-adrenergic blockers, such as tamsulosin. The typical dosage of terazosin (e.g., Hytrin, available in 1-, 2-, 5-, and 10-mg tablets) is 1 to 10 mg/day in one or two daily doses. The blood pressure must be monitored, and the drug should be started at a dosage of 1 mg at bedtime (to minimize the hypotensive effect) and increased in 3 to 7 days if no response has occurred. Doxazosin (e.g., Cardura, available in 1-, 2-, 4-, and 8-mg tablets) is taken as 1 to 8 mg/day in a single dose. If the patient is taking other antihypertensive agents, closer monitoring of the blood pressure is needed. Generally, dosage adjustment can be made weekly. Tamsulosin (Flomax) has a single daily dose of 0.4 mg and has no significant effect on blood pressure. Alpha-blockers are probably best avoided in patients who initially have low blood pressure. In selected patients with minimal to moderate outlet symptoms, the results of treatment with alpha-blockers have been excellent, with a measured increase in urinary flow rate, decrease in some of the irritative voiding symptoms, and minimal side effects. Alpha-blockers are effective in both larger and smaller glands.

Hormonal therapy (androgen deprivation), including castration, has long been known to decrease the size of the prostate when BPH is present. However, the side effects of either medical or surgical castration precluded such therapy except in elderly symptomatic patients who were considered to be at too high a risk for surgical intervention or for the administration of an anesthetic. The development of a 5α-reductase inhibitor, *finasteride* (Proscar), has significantly altered the management options for patients with BPH. Finasteride produces a profound fall in serum and intraprostatic dihydrotestosterone (DHT) levels without lowering testosterone levels. It possesses no androgenic, antiandrogenic, or steroid hormone–related properties. In approximately 30% of patients it causes a 30% reduction in prostate volume over 6 months. Long-term administration of finasteride has not been associated with clinically significant adverse effects, and there have been no significant changes in other hormone parameters. Patients who take finasteride have a drop of approximately 50% from their pretreatment PSA level. The dosage of finasteride (Proscar) is 5 mg orally every day in a single dose. It must be given for at least 6 months for the trial to be considered adequate. If the patient stops finasteride, the prostate size will return to pretreatment levels and the bladder outlet obstructive symptoms will recur. If the patient does benefit from finasteride, the drug should be continued indefinitely. The administration of finasteride does not preclude surgical treatment (see later discussion) if the patient alters his decision to take the drug for any reason or fails to respond to the medication after 6 months. Finasteride is most effective in glands that are larger on examination, usually considered to be larger than 40 g by urologists (5); glands that are very large (more than 70 g) are usually so large that the examiner cannot reach the base (upper portion) with the examining finger, assuming the bladder is not distended.

Finasteride, terazosin, or both were compared by Lepor et al. with placebo in men with BPH (6). Terazosin was effective in this study, but finasteride was not, and the combination was no more effective than terazosin alone. However, in an accompanying editorial, Walsh pointed out that BPH is a heterogenous disorder and that the Lepor study did not control for prostate gland size, as was done in the earlier finasteride study (7). Walsh suggested, as indicated previously, that finasteride should be used only when the gland is large, whereas alpha-antagonists can be used with both large and small glands. Currently and commonly, as an end result of the Lepor study (7), the combination of finasteride and alpha-agonists is used (see later discussion).

Estrogens are thought to play a considerable causative or permissive role in BPH; estrogen deprivation, therefore, may represent a useful treatment in patients with this condition. Aromatase inhibitors have attracted attention for use in the treatment of several estrogen-dependent clinical disorders. These agents are under investigation and cannot be recommended yet.

Saw palmetto (*Serenoa repens*), an herbal extract from the berry of the saw palmetto tree and now readily available over the counter, is gaining popularity as a treatment for symptoms of prostatism. The medication is very popular in Europe. It seems to be more effective than a placebo, although the mechanism of action is not known (8). It has no effect on PSA levels. Other herbal agents, such as beta-sitosterol plant extract (9) and rye grass pollen extract (10), are under investigation.

In summary, most patients with mild or moderate symptoms of bladder outlet obstruction should be reassured and can be followed by watchful waiting. If they do have significant bothersome symptoms, a trial of saw palmetto may be tried and is generally well tolerated. If after 6 months the symptoms remain bothersome, therapy with alpha-blockers may be substituted. If the prostate is large, finasteride can be added if an adequate response is not achieved with alpha-blockers alone. There is no evidence that saw palmetto combined with either of these agents adds benefit. In the special situation of a patient who has partial urinary retention after an operative procedure (discussed later) or from medication, an alpha-blocker is appropriate to give him a trial at voiding without a catheter or surgery. (Also, these patients can use intermittent self-catheterization for up to 4 to 6 weeks to see whether they are able to return to their prior voiding pattern—see later discussion.)

For patients requiring invasive procedures because symptoms are intolerable despite a trial of medical treatment or because of another indication for surgery (Table 53.3), the most accepted method still is a TURP. However, some urologists prefer newer modalities, such as transurethral vaporization of the prostate, transurethral needle ablation of the prostate, or transurethral microwave hyperthermia, and one must be superficially familiar with such procedures (discussed later).

When surgery is a consideration and a patient is referred to a urologist, several further assessments often are made before a surgical procedure is performed.

FURTHER EVALUATION OF BLADDER OUTLET OBSTRUCTION

Imaging

Intravenous urography once was used routinely in the evaluation of men with bladder outlet obstructive symptoms, but because it is invasive and has some side effects, this is no longer true. It now is limited, for the most part, to evaluation of the patient with hematuria (see Chapter 49). If an intravenous urogram is believed to be necessary, one should determine that the serum creatinine concentration is less than 1.8 mg/dL. If the patient gives a history of a previous reaction, even if mild or moderate in severity, there is approximately a 35% chance of a recurrent reaction. However, nonionic contrast agents may be used with a much lower risk. A decision to perform a study in this instance must be made on an individual basis and in consultation with a radiologist and urologist.

Ultrasonography of the urinary tract, a simple, noninvasive technique, appears to provide more useful information and is used more commonly. It is the procedure of first choice to evaluate the upper urinary tract for the presence of hydronephrosis, stones, renal masses, and anomalies. Ultrasonography is useful to quantitate the postvoid residual urine, identify bladder calculi, and estimate the size of the prostate.

Transrectal ultrasonography (TRUS), because it can clearly visualize the prostate, is in common use. This procedure is useful when evaluating a patient with an abnormal prostate on rectal examination or an elevated PSA. It is usually initiated by a urologist and usually is done in combination with a prostate biopsy. The size of the prostate gland can be calculated and abnormal areas within the gland can be delineated; cancer, for example, is usually hypoechoic. If cancer is suspected or known, TRUS assists in staging (i.e., extensive local disease or invasion of the seminal vesicles). TRUS is used for localization during needle biopsy of the prostate. The patient experience with this procedure was described previously.

A *renal scan* may be used to evaluate renal blood flow or delayed excretion suggestive of obstruction.

A *retrograde ureteropyelogram,* done in conjunction with cystoscopy by a urologist, provides visualization of the ureters, renal pelvis, and calyces. The contrast medium used during this procedure is rarely absorbed and can be used safely in patients with contrast media allergy (e.g., from an intravenous pyelogram).

If the history suggests a urethral stricture (see later discussion), a *retrograde urethrogram* may be performed. This procedure requires instillation of contrast material into the urethra with appropriate radiographs. Anesthesia is not needed during this procedure, and only minimal discomfort is experienced during injection into the urethra.

Instrumentation

One gains considerable information in the evaluation of a patient with symptoms of bladder outlet obstruction by performing several invasive procedures. Because these procedures may be associated with the development of infection, they should not be done casually.

Bladder Catheterization for Postvoid Volume

Insertion of a urethral catheter immediately after a patient has voided allows measurement of the amount of residual urine (more than 100 mL is abnormal) and helps determine whether there is a urethral stricture. There is a risk of urosepsis if infection is present; also, hematuria or urinary retention may result from the instrumentation. Now ultrasound has virtually replaced catheterization in the determination of the postvoid residual volume. *Ultrasound* of the lower abdomen and pelvis accurately estimates postvoid residual urine without an invasive procedure such as catheterization. Simple to use, accurate, portable ultrasound units are available and are useful for any clinician. If a neurogenic bladder is suspected, the patient should be referred to a urologist for a consultation and the performance of a formal cystometrogram and possibly a cystourethroscopy.

Cystometrogram

A cystometrogram is easily performed by a urologist, or, in the case of bedside cystometry (see Chapter 54), by a generalist experienced in this technique, in the office. The procedure is similar to a catheterization for residual urine. After the catheter is placed, a sterile solution is used to fill the bladder; the detrusor response to the increasing volume is recorded and classified, and the various pressure-flow relationships are demonstrated.

Cystourethroscopy

Cystourethroscopy, performed by a urologist usually in the office suite or outpatient unit, is a procedure that permits visualization of the entire urethra, the prostate, and the bladder.

Patient Experience. For cystourethroscopy using topical anesthesia without premedication, a lighted rigid or flexible instrument, typically 6 mm in diameter, is used. The patient often perceives a feeling of suprapubic pressure as the bladder is being filled with the irrigating fluid, but the degree of discomfort is usually slight. The examination takes just a few minutes. However, if a retrograde ureteropyelogram is performed, another 15 minutes may be required. After cystoscopy, patients often experience dysuria. The patient should be advised about this possibility and informed that it may be relieved by voiding while sitting in a bathtub filled with warm water or by taking phenazopyridine (Pyridium), 100–200 mg three times a day for 1 or 2 days. Hematuria after cystoscopy is also common and may persist for 2 or 3 days. The patient should be informed of this possibility, reassured that it is not uncommon, and advised to force fluids (2 to 3 L/day). Infection in the urinary tract occurs only rarely after cystoscopy. Occasionally, acute urinary retention results from edema of the prostate subsequent to instrumentation. If this complication occurs, insertion of an indwelling catheter is necessary. An uncommon long-term complication of cystoscopy is urethral stricture (discussed later). The use of smaller instruments and new, flexible cystoscopes has decreased the incidence of this complication.

The urologist learns a great deal from the cystoscopic examination. The entire urethra is seen. The size of the prostate, the degree of occlusion, trabeculation in the bladder, the presence of a bladder stone, and diverticula are all directly visualized. This information is most important in helping the urologist determine the need for and the type of surgery.

SURGICAL TREATMENT OF BLADDER OUTLET OBSTRUCTION

Benign Prostatic Hyperplasia

For more than 50 years, the traditional operative approaches for BPH have been TURP and open prostatectomy. Questions have been raised about the morbidity and mortality of these procedures (11). Several simpler and less invasive surgical therapies have been developed or are being investigated. These newer surgical options are discussed in this section.

As an alternative to any treatment, particularly with acute or chronic urinary retention, the patient may remain on long-term indwelling catheterization or have clean intermittent catheterization. Suprapubic cystostomy, used extensively in the past, is rarely needed today because of the improvement in urethral catheters and the widespread use of intermittent catheterization. Occasionally, suprapubic catheterization is used acutely, and in this situation the fistula heals quickly after the catheter is removed, provided that any outlet obstruction has been removed. Long-term catheterization of any sort is associated with recurrent urinary tract infections and urosepsis; therefore, other options (medical, described earlier, or surgical, described in this section) for treating a patient with bladder outlet obstruction should always be considered first.

Surgical Management of Benign Prostatic Hyperplasia

Transurethral Resection of the Prostate. TURP is the most commonly used procedure in the surgical treatment of BPH. It requires hospitalization for 1 to 2 days, although occasionally it is done as an outpatient procedure; general or spinal anesthesia is used. TURP is also the most effective procedure for BPH, with improvement in about 85% of men undergoing this surgery.

Complications have been minimized by the use of smaller, more efficient instruments; by improved lighting; and by isotonic irrigating fluids. Nevertheless, bleeding, infection, and plasma hypoosmolality (from absorption of irrigation fluid) may occur. Long-term complications occur in fewer than 5% to 15% of operations and include urethral stricture, bladder neck contracture, and incontinence (12). An emerging problem with TURP is related to its increasingly infrequent use and the subsequent fall in experience in its performance, particularly among younger urologists.

A common consequence of TURP is *retrograde ejaculation,* a situation characterized by the ejaculation of semen into the bladder rather than externally through the urethra. This phenomenon occurs because the bladder neck is opened as part of the TURP and cannot subsequently contract, as is necessary to produce antegrade ejaculation. Retrograde ejaculation results in sterility but does not usually affect orgasm. This consequence should be discussed with sexually active patients and their partners before prostatectomy. TURP should not produce organic erectile impotence; however, psychogenic impotence may follow TURP or other genitourinary surgery. The management of psychogenic impotence is described in Chapter 6.

Most patients can resume normal physical and sexual activity in approximately 4 weeks after TURP. However, complete healing of the prostatic fossa usually takes 2 to 3 months, and during this period, a urinalysis may reveal white and red blood cells.

Open Prostatectomy. Open prostatectomy requires a slightly longer hospitalization and recovery period. This approach is used when, in addition to having a large prostate, the patient has a bladder condition that can be repaired at the same time (e.g., bladder diverticulum, bladder stone). Organic erectile impotence occurs in approximately 5% to 15% of men undergoing this surgery, and the percentage may be higher when the perineal approach is used. If this complication occurs, an evaluation should be performed before the impotence is attributed to the surgery and presumed to be irreversible. Urinary incontinence occurs in about 3% to 5% of men undergoing open prostatectomy. As with TURP, complications with open prostatectomy are related to the experience of the surgeon.

It is important for a patient undergoing any form of prostatectomy for BPH to understand that the entire prostate gland is not removed. Because of the presence of residual prostate tissue, these patients have a risk equal to that of the general population of ultimately developing prostatic carcinoma. The decision regarding prostate cancer screening is, therefore, unaffected by this procedure (see earlier discussion). Because residual prostatic tissue remains, recurrent symptoms or complications from prostatic hypertrophy may develop later. The frequency of recurrence depends primarily on the extent of the initial surgery and is highly variable.

Transurethral Incision of the Prostate and Bladder Neck. Transurethral incision of the prostate (TUIP) is gaining increasing favor and is replacing TURP in selected cases (13). The indication for incision of the prostate is the same as for TURP, except that it may be used in younger men and in patients whose prostate gland seems to be of almost normal size on rectal examination, usually considered to be less than 30 g by urologists. Incision is performed primarily through the muscle of the bladder neck and through the prostate adenoma to the level of the verumontanum. Usually two incisions are made. In comparing TUIP with TURP, there are fewer complications with TUIP, and the postoperative flow rates and relief of symptoms are comparable with either procedure. There are no significant differences in subjective prostate-related symptoms or uroflowmetry between the two procedures. However, there is a higher incidence of bladder neck contracture after TURP. Besides being associated with lower complication rates, including retrograde ejaculation, than TURP, TUIP requires a shorter operative period and postoperative stay and decreased postoperative morbidity. Some urologists perform TUIP using only local anesthesia. The only major disadvantage of TUIP is the potential for missing major localized prostate cancer; for this reason, some urologists advocate either a biopsy of the prostate or at least one loop incision (similar to that done in TURP) for tissue at the time of the TUIP.

Other Procedures to Relieve Bladder Neck Obstruction. *Balloon dilation* of the prostatic urethra was used in the past but is no longer recommended and is not effective in the long term.

A permanently implanted *urethral stent,* made of various materials ranging from stainless steel to a biodegradable substance, has been used with varying results. The placement of a urethral stent is limited primarily to high-risk patients who have urinary retention and are poor operative risks. The advantages of the stent are that there is no significant intraoperative or postoperative hemorrhage and no need for an indwelling urethral catheter, the procedure can usually be done under local anesthesia, and the patient most often does not require hospitalization. Stent dislodgement, urinary infection, and stone formation on the stent have been reported. In selected cases, it is considered as an alternative to a chronic indwelling catheter or intermittent clean catheterization.

Transurethral microwave hyperthermia (TUMT) is an outpatient procedure now approved by the U.S. Food and Drug Administration that seems to improve the patient's symptoms objectively and subjectively without causing significant tissue damage. The temperature of the prostate is raised to approximately 45° to 55°C. Findings after hyperthermia of the prostate show that there is a definite improvement, on the order of 50%, in the obstructive symptoms. This procedure is well tolerated, with only a few transient and usually mild adverse effects. Histologic analysis of material obtained after hyperthermia shows significant tissue reaction and evidence of widespread cell death of prostate tissue. On the other hand, TRUS measurement of the size of the gland has failed to demonstrate any overall reduction in the volume of the prostate during follow-up.

Laser Treatment of the Prostate. The use of lasers may be an alternative to TURP (14). The laser is in direct contact with the prostatic urethra, resulting in incision and vaporization of prostatic tissue. Studies of laser prostatectomy suggest that acute or delayed complications typical of TURP are seen. Laser prostatectomy may be performed as an outpatient procedure, with benefits similar to those of TURP, transurethral vaporization of the prostate (TVP), and transurethral needle ablation (TUNA).

Transurethral Vaporization of the Prostate. TVP provides results comparable to those of TURP (15). A more powerful electrical current in the resectoscope loop results in vaporization of tissue with minimal bleeding. There is also a wedge loop that can provide vaporization as well as removal of prostatic tissue.

This results in less bleeding, shorter catheterization, and a shorter hospital stay. Some of these procedures are done on an outpatient basis, with removal of the catheter within 24 to 48 hours. Another advantage of TVP is that most of the equipment necessary for this procedure is available in most operating rooms and hospitals; expensive equipment, as is required for laser therapy, is not needed.

Transurethral Needle Ablation. TUNA is a technique involving the insertion of a needle transurethrally into the prostate, causing tissue necrosis by radio frequency. This procedure can be done on an outpatient basis under local anesthesia, usually with an indwelling catheter for 1 to 2 days and low morbidity (16).

Urethral Stricture

A urethral stricture may be treated with urethral dilation, transurethral incision of the stricture, or open urethral surgery. The method selected depends on the length and location of the stricture, the patient's overall health, and the urologist's experience.

PROSTATIC CARCINOMA

Prostatic carcinoma is the most commonly diagnosed cancer among American men and the second most common cause of cancer death in men. Prostate cancer will develop in approximately 9% of white and 11% of black men in the United States in their lifetime. A newborn U.S. male child has approximately a 3% to 4% chance of dying from prostate cancer. Family history and race are definite risk factors for the development of carcinoma of the prostate. Men with prostatic cancer may present with bladder outlet obstruction, although cancer is a far less common cause with this presentation than is BPH. The most common physical findings leading to the diagnosis of adenocarcinoma of the prostate are a prostatic nodule or induration discovered on rectal examination of the prostate and an elevated PSA. Either finding should lead to a urologic consultation and biopsy of the prostate. Approximately 30% to 40% of prostatic nodules or induration in the prostate are adenocarcinomas. The prevalence of unsuspected or incidental carcinoma of the prostate found at biopsy or TURP ranges from 4% in the fourth decade to 80% in the ninth decade of life. The prevalence at autopsy may be higher because many cancers begin in the outer periphery of the prostate gland and are missed by incomplete TURP or by random biopsy.

The management of prostatic carcinoma is somewhat controversial. The presenting PSA, the clinical stage of the disease, and the Gleason score must all be considered.

Gleason Scoring System

The tissue obtained by biopsy (see previous discussion) is described by use of the *Gleason Scoring System* for adenocarcinoma of the prostate. This system divides the cancer into five histologic grades, with Gleason pattern 1 being well differentiated and Gleason pattern 5 being poorly differentiated carcinoma. The cancer patterns are scored based on the predominant histologic grade seen at two sites. The most differentiated cancers (and those with the best prognosis) would be scored as grade 1 + 1, or a Gleason score of 2. The most poorly differentiated cancers would be scored as grade 5 + 5, or a Gleason score of 10. Prostate tumors are multifocal within the prostate in more than 80% of cases. Prostatic intraepithelial neoplasia (PIN) may be reported on biopsy. PIN is an architecturally benign prostatic acinus or duct lined by cytologically atypical cells. It is now well recognized that high-grade PIN is a premalignant lesion for prostate cancer. When high-grade PIN is found on needle biopsy, the chance of detecting carcinoma on subsequent biopsies is 30% to 50%. All of this information assists the urologist in planning the management options.

Staging

The stage of the disease is established clinically by digital rectal examination, PSA level, and, in selected cases, a bone scan. The TNM (tumor, nodes, metastasis) classification is most commonly used, but the Whitmore–Jewett staging system is familiar and is used by many (17) (Table 53.4). Table 53.5 compares these two systems. TRUS may be helpful in the assessment of local disease and in estimating the volume of neoplasm. This is usually done in conjunction with biopsy of the prostate (see earlier discussion). Magnetic resonance imaging or computed tomography scanning usually is not indicated. Significant in TNM classification is T1c, a tumor identified by needle biopsy performed because of an elevated PSA but with a normal rectal examination. Regional lymph node metastases are assessed by the N designation in the TNM system and by the D_1 designation in the Whitmore–Jewett classification. Distant metastases are identified by the M designation in the TNM and by the D_2 designation in the Whitmore–Jewett classification.

If the neoplasm is limited to the prostate (i.e., no evidence of local spread or metastatic disease) and the patient is younger than 75 years of age, has an anticipated survival of 10 or more years, and has no

Table 53.4. Whitmore–Jewett Staging of Prostatic Carcinoma

Stage	Description
A	Clinically undetectable; found on pathologic examination after prostatectomy
A1	Focal and well differentiated
A2	Diffuse (>5%) or poorly differentiated
B	Limited to prostate on rectal examination
B1	Solitary nodule; <1.5 cm; one lobe
B2	One whole lobe or both lobes
C	Locally extending outside of prostatic capsule or into seminal vesicles
D	Metastatic disease
D1	Pelvic lymph-node metastases
D2	Distant metastases, usually bone

Table 53.5. TNM Classification and Whitmore–Jewett Staging System

TNM	Description	Whitmore-Jewett	Description
T1a	Nonpalpable, with 5% or less of resected tissue with cancer (TURP or open prostatectomy)	A1	Same as TNM
T1b	Nonpalpable, with greater than 5% of resected tissue with cancer (TURP or open prostatectomy)	A2	Same as TNM
T1c	Nonpalpable, but serum PSA is elevated	0[a]	Same as TNM
T2a	Palpable, half of 1 lobe or less	B1N	Palpable nodule, less than 1 lobe
T2b	Palpable, greater than half of 1 lobe but not both lobes	B1	Palpable, less than 1 lobe
T2c	Palpable, involves both lobes	B2	Palpable, 1 entire lobe or more
T3a	Palpable, unilateral capsular penetration	C1	Palpable, outside capsule, not into seminal vesicles
T3b	Palpable, bilateral extracapsular extension	C2	Same as TNM
T3c	Palpable, invasion of seminal vesicles	C3	Same as TNM
T4	Tumor is fixed or invades adjacent structures (i.e., bladder neck, sphincter, rectum, pelvic wall)	C4	Same as TNM
N	Regional lymph node metastases	D1	Same as TNM
M	Distant metastases (i.e., bone)	D2	

PSA, prostate-specific antigen; TURP, transurethral resection of the prostate.

[a]Not defined in original Whitmore–Jewett classification.

Modified from Partin AW, Yoo S, Carter HB, et al. The use of prostate-specific antigen, clinical stage and Gleason score to predict pathological stage in men with localized prostate cancer. J Urol 1993;150:110.

contraindicating medical diseases, he is a candidate for a curative treatment. Radiation therapy and radical prostatectomy are primary considerations. Radical prostatectomy appears to provide slightly less morbidity and longer survival. In the hands of a urologist experienced in this type of surgery, the complications usually are minimal and fewer than 2% of patients develop total incontinence, although many experience minor episodes of incontinence that persist for 6 to 12 months or longer after the surgery. A modification of the traditional radical prostatectomy permits the removal of all cancerous tissue yet attempts to spare the pelvic nerves that control erection; there is preservation of preexisting potency in up to 70% of younger patients who undergo such a procedure at the hands of a urologist who is experienced in it.

Stage A (T1, N0 M0) prostatic carcinoma is disease unsuspected on rectal examination of the prostate. It may discovered at the time of prostatectomy, usually TURP, for obstructive symptoms thought to be secondary to BPH. If carcinoma is reported, the percentage or volume of neoplasm compared with the total amount of tissue removed and the histologic grade of the neoplasm should be noted. This information aids in the management and determination of prognosis. Stage A is further subdivided into stage A1 (T1a) disease, well-differentiated carcinoma in less than 5% of resected tissue. All other incidentally discovered carcinomas are stage A2 (T1b) and are considered potentially more aggressive. The urologist initiates a metastatic evaluation with a nuclear bone scan. PSA should be measured if not already done, always before treatment and, because it is of great value in monitoring the progress of a patient, after treatment.

If there is no evidence of local or distant metastatic disease, the management in stage T1a disease is controversial. In a younger patient (before age 65 years) with T1a disease who is at higher risk for recurrence because of his expected longevity, radical prostatectomy is recommended. For the older patient (after approximately 65 years), observation is often recommended. The patient with T1b disease is at considerable risk for development of metastases, and radical prostatectomy or radiation is recommended.

The management of stage T1c, biopsy done because of an elevated PSA, is also controversial. Management options include watchful waiting, radical prostatectomy, and radiation therapy. The age of the patient, the grade of the tumor, and the estimated volume of the cancer (e.g., number of positive biopsy cores) must be considered in recommending management.

Stage B (T2, N0 M0) carcinoma is defined as disease limited to the prostate gland that is detected clinically either as a nodule or as diffuse hardness with no extension or fixation. If the neoplasm is limited to the prostate and the patient is younger than 75 years of age, has an anticipated 10-year survival, and has no contraindicating medical diseases, he is a candidate for curative radical prostatectomy or definitive radiation therapy.

Stage C (T3 and T4, N0 M0), local extensive prostatic cancer, is usually treated by definitive radiotherapy, with or without adjuvant hormonal therapy. The decision to treat a patient who has prostate cancer with radiotherapy also requires a risk–benefit discussion by the urologist, oncologist, or radiotherapist. Although radiotherapy is usually well tolerated, there is some risk for the subsequent development of symptomatic chronic proctitis, typically manifested by bleeding and tenesmus, impotence, and chronic cystitis usually associated with bleeding. The prevalence of these complications is variable and depends in part on the dosage of radiotherapy and the size of the delivery port. The age and general health of the patient are major considerations in determining management options. If significant bladder outlet obstruction is present, the patient may also need a TURP; this combination of treatments results in an increased risk of urinary incontinence.

The obturator and iliac nodes are usually the first sites of metastases, and these structures are positive in up to 50% of patients with prostatic cancer. Current imaging techniques, including computed tomography and magnetic resonance imaging, are not reliable in detecting early lymph node metastases and are not routinely indicated in the preoperative evaluation of a patient with prostate cancer. A PSA level greater than 20 μg is suggestive of nodal metastases, but such a level does not preclude surgical or radiation therapy.

Metastatic, or stage D (M+), prostatic cancer is managed by hormonal therapy (i.e., androgen deprivation) via surgery (castration) or drugs. Studies show that hormonal therapy initiated at the time of diagnosis does not prolong survival but may delay the onset of symptomatic metastases, compared with hormonal therapy initiated only in response to symptoms (e.g., bone pain). Diethylstilbestrol (3 mg/day) and orchiectomy give similar results, producing an 85% to 90% partial symptomatic response rate in previously untreated patients. The duration of response averages 18 months, although occasionally prolonged remissions occur. There is no advantage to combining orchiectomy and estrogen therapy. In general, estrogen therapy, which causes salt and water retention, should be avoided in patients who also have an edema-forming illness (e.g., congestive heart failure, chronic liver disease, nephrotic syndrome) not controlled by diuretics. Because of these side effects, diethylstilbestrol is no longer commonly used. LHRH analogs (leuprolide, goserelin) are just as effective as surgical castration. These analogs, in combination with potent antiandrogens (flutamide, bicalutamide), provide total androgen blockage. However, data do not indicate that the total androgen blockage provides long-term survival any better than either chemical or surgical castration alone. However, an antiandrogen (e.g., flutamide—see earlier discussion) is recommended for the first 3 to 6 weeks in patients initially starting on LHRH agonists, because these drugs initially cause a rise in the testosterone, which then drops after approximately 3 to 4 weeks.

One should be aware of the effects of androgen ablation by either chemical or surgical castration. Patients after several years may experience osteopenia and osteoporosis, anemia, loss of libido, hot flashes (as experienced in some women after menopause), and some loss of well-being and masculine prowess.

No new treatment has been offered for metastatic prostate cancer since androgen ablative therapy was introduced more than 60 years ago. A number of investigational trials have used cytotoxic chemotherapy in all stages of prostatic carcinoma, but no method is as effective as androgen deprivation. Cytotoxic chemotherapy also is only partially effective in patients who fail hormonal therapy or who have extensive metastatic disease. Tumor necrosis factor and suramin are used by some but without overwhelming benefit. Gene therapy, antiangiogenesis drugs, vaccines, and cell death promoters are under current investigation.

Much of the controversy in the diagnosis and treatment of prostatic cancer results from the inability to assess accurately the influence of prostatic cancer on longevity (18,19). Many patients with low-grade and low-stage disease should be treated by watchful waiting, particularly those older than 75 years of age. A more aggressive approach should be taken in younger patients (30 to 60 years). It is estimated that a significant number of young patients with prostate cancer have a genetic basis for their disease, so their family members should be screened and monitored closely (see earlier discussion). It is currently typical to offer aggressive treatment, primarily radical prostatectomy, to younger men with prostate cancer in the belief that they have a more virulent form of the disease. Radiation therapy is recommended primarily for patients approximately 70 years of age or older with locally confined disease and for younger patients with T3 disease (stage C) who are not considered surgical candidates because of comorbidities.

Table 53.6. Survival of Men with Appropriately Managed Prostatic Carcinoma Using Both the Whitmore–Jewett and the TNM Systems

Stages	% Men Surviving with Prostate Cancer at Various Stages Who Receive Treatment		
	5 yr	10 yr	15 yr
A1 T1		Normal life expectancy	
A2	50–80	40–70	15–35
B T2	50–90	40–70	15–40
C T3	15–70	5–60	0–30
D M+	5–30	3–10	0–3

Controversy remains regarding the use of adjuvant hormonal therapy in the treatment of prostate cancer. For patients who are surgical candidates, there are no data to support the use of hormonal therapy before surgery. In selected patients, especially those with T3 disease (stage C), radiation therapy plus hormonal therapy should be considered.

Cryotherapy, or freezing of the prostate, is still experimental and is not recommended currently in the primary treatment of prostate cancer.

A diet with excessive fat or low selenium or both is considered to be a risk factor in the development of prostate cancer. Because of fact, alteration of the diet with supplements of lycopene (cooked tomatoes), broccoli, and similar vegetables and/or supplemental vitamin E may benefit longevity once cancer has been diagnosed. Larger studies are needed, however, before one becomes more prescriptive.

Because prostatic cancer occurs in older men who often have coexisting diseases that influence longevity and because the natural history of the disease is quite variable, there is great range in survival among men with prostate cancer. The current best estimates for survival with various stages of prostatic cancer with the treatments discussed here are listed in Table 53.6.

URINARY INCONTINENCE

Urinary incontinence is a common problem of the elderly and of younger women. It may be a manifestation of urinary outlet obstruction. The evaluation and management of patients with urinary incontinence is described in Chapter 54.

General References*

Barry MJ. Prostate-specific antigen testing for early diagnosis of prostate cancer. N Engl J Med 2001;344:1373.

A review of the controversies of PSA testing starting with a typical clinical vignette.

Kirby R, Fitzpatrick J, Kirby M, et al. Shared care for prostatic disease, ed 2. Oxford, UK: ISIS Medical Media Ltd., 2000.

A clear review with case studies of the common problems of the prostate.

Chapple CR, McConnell JD, Tubaro A, eds. Benign prostatic hypertrophy: current therapy. London: Martin Dunitz Ltd, 2000.

A good review of medical and surgical treatments of benign prostatic hypertrophy.

Naz RK, ed. Prostate: basic and clinical aspects. New York: CRS Press, 1997.

A complete and well referenced monograph covering benign prostatic hypertrophy and prostate cancer.

Blasko JC, Lange PH. Prostate cancer: the therapeutic challenge of locally advanced disease. N Engl J Med 1997;337:340.

A thorough review.

Oesterling JE. Benign prostate hyperplasia: medical and minimally invasive treatment options. N Engl J Med 1995;332:99.

A thorough review of therapeutic possibilities in managing men with symptomatic BPH.

The Finasteride Study Group. **The effect of finasteride in men with benign prostatic hyperplasia.** N Engl J Med 1992;327:1185.

The initial and now classic study.

Walsh PC. Benign prostate hyperplasia. In: Walsh PC, Retik AB, Stamey TA, et al., eds. Campbell's urology. 7th ed. Philadelphia: WB Saunders, 1998.

Cuellar DC, Kyprianou N. Future concepts in the medical therapy of benign prostatic hyperplasia. Curr Opin Urol 2001;11:27.

A thoughtful review of the use of drugs and herbal agents n this condition.

Holtgrewe HL. Surgical management of benign prostatic hyperplasia in 2001: a pause for thought. J Urol 2001;166:177.

A reflective essay.

Specific References

1. Ross KS, Carter HB, Pearson JD, et al. Comparative efficiency of prostate-specific antigen screening strategies for prostate cancer detection. JAMA 2000;284:1399.
2. Carter HB, Pearson JD, Metter EJ, et al. Longitudinal evaluation of prostate-specific antigen levels in men with and without prostate disease. JAMA 1992;267:2215.
3. Hillebrand M, Bastian M, Steiner M, et al. Serum to urinary prostate-specific antigen ratios in patients with benign prostate hyperplasia and prostate cancer. Anticancer Res 2000;20(6D):4995.
4. Michelotti GA, Price DT, Schwinn DA. Alpha 1-adrenergic receptor regulation: basic science and clinical implications. Pharmacol Ther 2000;88:281.
5. Boyle P, Gould AL, Roehrborn CG. Prostate volume predicts outcome of treatment of benign prostate hyperplasia with finasteride: meta-analysis of randomized clinical trials. Urology 1996;48:398.
6. Lepor H, Willingford WO, Barry MJ, et al. The efficacy of terazosin, finasteride, or both in benign prostatic hyperplasia. Vetrans Affairs Cooperative Studies Benign Prostatic Hyperplasia Study Group. N Engl J Med 1996;335:533.
7. Walsh P. Treatment of benign prostate hyperplasia. N Engl J Med 1996;335:586.
8. Gerber GS. Saw palmetto for the treatment of men with lower urinary tract symptoms. J Urol 2000;163:1408.
9. Wilt TJ, MacDonald R, Ishani A. beta-sitosterol for the treatment of benign prostatic hyperplasia systematic review. BJU Int 1999;83:976.
10. MacDonald R, Ishani A, Rutks I, et al. A systematic review of Cernilton for the treatment of benign prostatic hyperplasia. BJU Int 2000;85:836.
11. Roos NP, Wennberg JE, Malenka DJ, et al. Mortality and reoperation after open and transurethral resection of the prostate for benign prostatic hyperplasia. N Engl J Med 1989;320:1120.
12. Mebust WK, Holtgrewe HL, Cockett ATK, et al. Transurethral prostatectomy: immediate and postoperative complications: a cooperative study of 13 participating institutions evaluating 3885 patients. J Urol 1989;141:243.
13. Jepsen JV, Bruskewitz RC. Recent developments in the surgical management of benign prostatic hyperplasia. Urology 1998;51:23.
14. Gerber GS. Lasers in the treatment of benign prostatic hyperplasia. Urology 1995;45:193.
15. Fraundorfer MR, Gilling PJ, Kennett KM, et al. Holmium laser resection of the prostate is more cost effective than transurethral resection of the prostate: results of a randomized prospective study. Urology 2001;57:454.
16. Kahn SA, Alphonse P, Tewari A, et al. An open study on the efficacy and safety of transurethral needle ablation of the prostate in treating symptomatic benign prostatic hyperplasia: the University of Florida experience. J Urol 1998;160:1707.
17. Garnick MB, Fair WR. Prostate cancer: emerging concepts. Ann Intern Med 1996;125:118.
18. Adolfsson J, Carstensen J. Natural course of clinically localized prostate adenocarcinoma in men less than 70 years old. J Urol 1991;146:96.
19. Wason J, Fleming C, Bruskewitz R, et al, for The Prostate Patient Outcome Research Team. The treatment of localized prostate cancer: what are we doing, what should we know, and what should we be doing? Semin Urol 1993;11:23.

*Bold print (general references) and bold numerals (specific references) denote published controlled clinical trials, meta-analyses, or consensus-based recommendations.

CHAPTER 54

Urinary Incontinence

THOMAS E. FINUCANE, MD
E. JAMES WRIGHT, MD

Urinary incontinence (UI) is defined in a variety of ways. *Dorland's Medical Dictionary* refers to "constant or frequent involuntary passage of urine" due to failure of voluntary sphincter control. A more functional definition is "the involuntary passage of urine that causes problems for the patient or caregivers," acknowledging that the definition of incontinence depends in part on social context. The wide variability in estimates of prevalence is due in part to differences in definition. Among adults, these estimates tend to increase with increasing age and with increasing disability. Involuntary loss of small amounts of urine is surprisingly common in perfectly healthy young women. A majority of elderly persons in nursing homes are incontinent.

Perhaps more importantly, estimating the effectiveness of treatments depends on the definitions of effectiveness that are used. Storage and voiding depend on an intricate interplay of voluntary and involuntary factors, and intervention often leads to small improvements in frequency or volume of spillage with a greater or lesser improvement in health. Another factor that makes evaluation of treatments difficult is the natural history of the disease, which is chronic, fluctuating, and often progressive. Distinguishing treatment effect from natural variability can be difficult. Finally, psychological factors are central in the evaluation and treatment of UI; the problem is not simply one of urodynamics.

PATHOPHYSIOLOGY

Urine flows when intravesical pressure exceeds pressure in the urethra. Innervation of the bladder is complex, but two important generalizations help in managing the various types of UI. The first generalization concerns the effects of upper motor neuron (UMN) and lower motor neuron (LMN) disease on bladder function. UMN lesions, such as stroke, cord injury or multiple sclerosis, tend to cause loss of inhibition of reflexes, as they do with skeletal muscle, and therefore lead to hyperreflexia and spasticity. In contrast, LMN lesions, such as diabetic neuropathy, interrupt the reflex arc and tend to cause flaccidity. (The term "neurogenic bladder", referring either to spastic detrusor contractions with UMN disease or a flaccid bladder with LMN disease, is ambiguous and should be avoided.)

The second generalization concerns autonomic innervation and can be remembered with the simple mnemonic that *Sympathetics favor Storage*. Alpha-adrenergic agents tend to increase urethral pressure and relax the detrusor, whereas adrenergic blockers have the opposite effect. Cholinergic agonists tend to relax the sphincter, and anticholinergics to increase its pressure. Remembering this balance, the yin and yang of urine, allows ready understanding of drug therapy and unintended drug side effects.

CLINICAL SYNDROMES

Stress Incontinence

The diagnosis of stress incontinence is made when rises in intra-abdominal pressure and thus intravesical pressure, as with sneezing, laughing, coughing, lifting, or just rising from a chair, cause urine to leak. Although a variety of abnormalities, or combinations of abnormalities, can cause stress incontinence, the final common pathway is that pressure in the urethral sphincter is so low that the rise in intra-abdominal pressure can overcome it, causing leak of urine. Usually only small volumes of urine are lost in this clinical form of UI.

Urge Incontinence

Patients with urge incontinence have, as the name suggests, a sudden irresistible urge to void. If the length of warning is shorter than the time required to get to a toilet, incontinence results. Usually large volumes of urine are lost. Involuntary detrusor contractions are the cause. These are common in neurologically normal persons, where the term "detrusor instability" is often used; in patients with UMN lesions, "detrusor hyperreflexia" is favored. The terms *uninhibited, spastic, hyperactive, overactive,* and *unstable bladder* also refer generally to this situation, and the use of these terms has confused the literature in this field. Local irritation, as with stone, infection, or tumor, can cause or worsen urge incontinence, presumably by increasing afferent traffic in the reflex arc. In many cases urge incontinence is idiopathic (1).

Overflow Incontinence

Patients with severe bladder distention can leak either small or large amounts of urine. Distention may occur because intravesical pressure is low, because intraurethral pressure is high, or both. High intraurethral pressure in men is most commonly caused by prostatic enlargement, but most men with obstruction are not incontinent (see Chapter 53). In women, the most common cause of high intraurethral pressure is prior surgery. The most common cause of low intravesical pressure in both sexes is diabetic neuropathy.

Functional Incontinence

Some patients lack mobility, or motive, or opportunity to get to a toilet in time. Cognitive, emotional, pharmacologic, and environmental factors all contribute to a patient's developing functional incontinence. Usually large volumes of urine are lost in this clinical form of UI.

Mixed Incontinence

In many patients, a combination of factors contributes to incontinence. These patients may present with a mixed picture, most commonly urge and stress incontinence. A relatively common problem is the incontinence pattern of stress-induced urge. In this situation, increases in abdominal pressure (and thus bladder pressure) induce an uninhibited bladder contraction and a sense of urgency followed by loss of urine, usually in large quantities. Detrusor hyperactivity with impaired contractility (DHIC) has been reported as a common syndrome in frail elderly patients, and it appears mostly to be a problem among nursing home residents. Mild urge incontinence coupled with the inability to transfer independently (functional incontinence) in frail and impaired elders, especially those in nursing homes, is another common recognizable presentation.

Recent-Onset Incontinence

In a previously continent patient, the recent onset of incontinence is an important problem for the clinician to recognize and address. Recent-onset incontinence may be transient and reversible. In a patient who is otherwise stable, medication, urinary tract infection, and stool impaction are problems important to consider and treat if present. New UI can also be an early sign of delirium or depression, and these conditions are also important to consider and treat if present. UI for the patient is often extremely devastating. It is often thought in an older person to be the beginning of infirmity and dependency. One must address this concern thoughtfully and effectively to help the patient fully.

EVALUATION

History

The history especially is the cornerstone of evaluation, beginning with a commonsense evaluation for easily reversible problems (see earlier discussion). Young, ambulatory patients seen in the office most often have stress incontinence, whereas elderly persons who are frail, and especially nursing home residents, are more likely to have urge or mixed incontinence. Table 54.1 lists several specific areas that should be covered in the history. In cognitively intact patients, a clear history of urge or stress incontinence (or both) may be enough information to initiate a trial of therapy. Obstructive symptoms are predictive of overflow incontinence in elderly men, but most men with prostatic obstruction are not incontinent.

A bladder record or voiding diary can at times be helpful in getting a clear picture of voiding pattern. Such a record can easily be made by asking the patient to record the times of voiding and of accidents and describe the accidents in terms of the circumstances (e.g., rushing to the toilet [typical of urge] or coughing [typical of stress], and whether the lost volume is large [typical of urge] or small [typical of stress]). For patients with cognitive impairment who cannot abstract and summarize their experience with voiding, the record (in this instance usually completed by a caregiver) can provide valuable information in planning a behavioral intervention. Cognitively intact patients can usually provide enough history to help guide therapy, but at times a bladder record is useful for them as well. Indeed, such a record may serve as the document of the pretreatment period to which the effect of treatment can be compared. Patients who are unwilling to complete such records are often poorly

Table 54.1. Specific Areas to Cover in the History when Evaluating Patients with Urinary Incontinence

- Specific symptoms
  - Acute/chronic/recurrent
  - Daily pattern (consider voiding diary; see text)
  - Stress or urge pattern
  - Precipitants
  - Polyuria
- Obstructive symptoms
  - Hesitancy
  - Decreased stream
  - Dribbling
- Irritative symptoms
  - Dysuria
  - Frequency
- Previous treatment
- Pelvic surgery or radiation
- Medications
  - Adrenergic or cholinergic modulators (see text)
  - Narcotics
  - CNS-active drugs
  - Calcium channel blockers
- Neurology
  - Known relevant neurologic problems
  - Change in sexual or bowel function
- Environmental
  - What does it take to toilet?

committed to sustaining a treatment program for their problem.

Medication history deserves special emphasis. First, sympathomimetic and anticholinergic drugs should be suspected as a cause of UI if problems develop with emptying the bladder (as predicted by the mnemonic "Sympathetics favor Storage"). An elderly man who presents with urinary retention, for example, should be queried carefully about recent consumption of antihistamine-decongestant cold remedies or other new medications. Narcotics and calcium channel blockers also cause urinary retention. In patients with limited cognitive reserve, any drug that interferes with executive function (decisions and interpretative reasoning) can make the situation worse. Finally, rapid-acting diuretics can cause incontinence, but two points should be borne in mind. First, once in a steady state, diuretics do not by themselves increase the total amount of urine a patient produces each day. Second, thiazide diuretics, especially when used at low doses for hypertension, actually have almost no diuretic effect. (How they lower blood pressure is uncertain, but the effect is almost certainly *not* due to intravascular volume contraction.)

Physical Examination

The examination should be focused on identifying neuropsychiatric disease and impaired mobility. Marked extracellular fluid volume overload may be an important contributor, especially to nocturnal incontinence. A palpable bladder after an attempt to void is a significant but infrequent finding suggesting overflow incontinence. Fecal impaction is important to evaluate, especially if the UI is recent in onset or has worsened.

Signs of serious UMN or LMN disease are usually present if that disease is responsible for incontinence. If perineal sensation or anal sphincter tone is abnormal, more detailed neurologic evaluation is indicated. In particular, if a patient has new-onset UI, and there are signs of lower lumbar or sacral nerve dysfunction, then the cauda equina syndrome must be considered (see Chapter 86).

Prostate size on rectal examination is neither sensitive nor specific for diagnosis of outlet obstruction. Similarly, pelvic organ prolapse in elderly women has limited diagnostic value in defining the cause or type of incontinence.

Further Testing

The Agency for Healthcare Research and Quality recommends that all incontinent patients have a determination of post-void residual volume (PVR), either by catheterization or preferably by ultrasound, done just after voiding, as well as a urinalysis (2). For healthy ambulatory patients who give a clear history of chronic, stable UI of the stress, urge, or mixed type and who have a normal PVR, no further testing is indicated. If the PVR is high, then the problem is more complicated than simply low pressures in the urethra (leading to stress incontinence) or uninhibited bladder contractions (leading to urge incontinence). Furthermore, the risk of hydronephrosis or recurrent urinary tract infection is increased. Additional evaluation may be necessary to explain the elevated PVR. Authors vary in their definition of an "abnormal" PVR, and there is no absolute value that can be invoked independent of the clinical picture. Further, PVR is by no means constant from measurement to measurement.

If, after this initial evaluation, diagnosis is uncertain to the extent that a treatment plan cannot be clearly initiated, additional evaluation may be useful. This situation most commonly occurs in elderly male diabetic patients who have symptoms of overflow incontinence. Failure to empty completely might result from high intraurethral pressure due to prostate disease, from low intravesical pressure due to autonomic neuropathy, or from a combination of the two conditions. Cystometry (described later) can help the practitioner make this distinction. Further diagnostic testing may also be useful in patients whose symptoms remain unacceptable after conservative management and who are willing to consider surgery. Further investigation may of course be indicated if the initial evaluation discovers unexpected, incidental abnormalities, such as hematuria, a prostate nodule, unexplained pyuria, or urinary retention.

Cystometry

In bedside cystometry, a catheter is placed and the bladder is filled. The volume at which the urge to void is first felt, the volume at which the urge is uncontrollable, and any involuntary contractions can all be measured. With laboratory-performed multichannel cystometrogram, intra-abdominal pressure is measured with either a rectal or a vaginal probe, allowing true detrusor pressure to be calculated from the measured intravesical pressure. The value of a multichannel cystometrogram is uncertain in a typical generalist practice, but it is most likely to be useful with uncooperative patients who cannot relax and with those for whom surgery is contemplated.

Urethrocystoscopy. This procedure is not required in the evaluation of a patient for isolated incontinence. However, it may be part of the evaluation of suspected tumor, stone, foreign body, or recurrent infection if these problems are considered to be associated with the patient's incontinence.

Imaging Tests. Other than determination of PVR by ultrasound, imaging of the upper and lower urinary tract is not part of the evaluation of isolated incontinence. As with urethrocystoscopy, imaging may be needed to evaluate other problems, such as impaired renal function, possible tumor or stone, or hematuria or pyuria found on urinalysis.

TREATMENT

In general, treatment of stress incontinence emphasizes strategies to decrease sudden increases in abdominal pressure while increasing pressure in the urethral sphincter, and treatment of urge incontinence focuses on both keeping bladder volumes low and anticipating the need to toilet. In many cases incontinence is mixed in origin, and both approaches should be taken. The effectiveness of the various interventions in UI is measured in a variety of ways, and direct comparisons are not always possible. Many of the reported trials are done with very few subjects and may not have power to detect differences. Further, all of the medications touted as effective in treating patients with UI can have serious side effects.

General Principles

Several principles apply generally to the treatment of adult patients with UI:

- First and foremost, a careful review of medications used by the patient should be done. Those that might be associated with incontinence should be stopped, if possible, as a therapeutic trial.
- Mixed urge and stress incontinence is common, and combining treatments for each condition is often more effective than single treatment.
- Incontinent patients should be instructed to void at regular, relatively short intervals, because urge and stress incontinence may both be reduced when bladder volume is kept small. A schedule may be suggested to cognitively intact patients, and scheduled toileting (i.e., by the clock) can help patients who are unable to toilet independently.
- Patients, particularly those with overflow or urge incontinence, should be counseled not to hurry when they have to void. A leisurely stance for men, double voiding (voiding a second time a few minutes after the initial try), and Credé maneuvers (pressure applied suprapubically while attempting to void) may improve emptying. It is unknown why cold temperature or the sound of running water tend to encourage emptying, but they may be tried.
- Nocturnal incontinence may result from a change with aging in the diurnal variability of antidiuretic hormone (ADH) production (see Chapter 81), with a concomitant nocturnal increase in urine production, and may have less to do with mobilization of edema or with drinking fluids in the evening.
- An incontinent patient who does not have any other symptoms of urinary tract infection is unlikely to improve as a result of antibiotic treatment to sterilize the urine. Patients with cognitive impairment or loss of bladder sensation may not be able to report symptoms of a UTI, and it is possible that treatment with antimicrobials (see Chapter 36) might help in some cases when "asymptomatic" bacteriuria is found. However a study of nursing home patients showed that eradication of incidental bacteriuria had no effect on incontinence (3).
- Despite its long record of use in the treatment of UI in women, current opinion suggests that there is no rigorous evidence to show that estrogen (plus progesterone when appropriate) is effective treatment (4–7). Nevertheless, many still hold the opinion that estrogens could be tried for isolated UI in one very special circumstance: They may be tried for a period of 1 month with appropriate precautions in women with atrophic vaginitis (see Chapter 106) when incontinence is part of the presentation of this problem.
- Data about the use and benefit of the various types of absorbent products now widely used are very limited. Disposable products may lead to fewer problems with skin breakdown than nondisposable products. In many cases, the balance of cost (which can be significant) and convenience is determinative.
- There is some evidence that a structured intervention with patient education, counseling, and frequent interaction with providers may be an important part of any treatment effect. Some communities have multidisciplinary continence clinics that can be considered. Patient-focused educational materials are quite helpful, and several are recommended (see General References).

Urge or Mixed Incontinence

Several behavioral modification treatments are commonly used in this situation. *Bladder training* (also called bladder retraining) is probably effective for cognitively intact patients, but it requires an intensive effort, including education, encouragement, and positive reinforcement (8). Patients are taught to recognize the sense of precipitate voiding and to postpone the urge, using distraction or relaxation techniques. The goal simply is to void on a schedule rather than in response to the urge to urinate. If the patient is unsuccessful in delaying the urge to void, the schedule may be redone, shortening the interval until the next scheduled void; or, the patient may simply stay on the same schedule and learn to ignore the interpolated voiding urges.

Habit training, which is distinct from bladder training, can be done when the patient has an identifiable pattern of voiding (for example, when incontinence occurs after an avoidable stimulus, such as consumption of an iced drink). Bladder records are especially useful in this regard. The patient is toileted in anticipation of situations where incontinence would be expected. Patients are best selected for habit training when they are generally not able to learn to achieve bladder continence, as they would in bladder training. Habit training is usually most suitable for patients living at home with a caregiver.

The following techniques are suggested for bladder training:

- Begin the patient on an every-2-hour toileting schedule for 3 days. For example, have the patient void on arising at 6 a.m., and then at 8 a.m., 10 a.m., 12 noon, 2 p.m., 4 p.m., and so on.
- After 2 days, review the bladder records. Note timing of episodes of incontinence and of toiletings when patient does not void.
- Alter the schedule accordingly. For instance, if the patient does not void at 10 a.m. but is wet by noon,

Table 54.2. Drug Treatment for Urinary Incontinence

	Drug Name	Dose and Frequency			Comments
		Initial	Usual	Max	
Urge incontinence	Oxybutinin	2.5 mg b.i.d.	5 mg t.i.d.	5 mg q.i.d.	Dry mouth, constipation, other anticholinergic effects, glaucoma
	Tolterodine	1 mg q.i.d.	1 mg b.i.d.	2 mg b.i.d.	Less toxic, less effective, expensive
	Oxybutinin extended release	5 mg q.d.	10 mg q.d.	30 mg q.d.	Same as oxybutinin regular release
Alternatives with limited efficacy data	Imipramine[b]	10 mg h.s.	25 mg b.i.d.	25 mg t.i.d.	Anticholinergic effects, especially dry mouth
	Propantheline	7.5 mg q.d.	7.5 mg t.i.d.	15 mg q4h	Anticholinergic effects, especially constipation
	Dicyclomine[a]	10 mg q.d.	10 mg q.d.	40 mg t.i.d.	Anticholinergic effects, especially constipation
Stress incontinence (limited data available)	Pseudophedrine[a]	15 mg q.d.	15 mg b.i.d.	30 mg t.i.d.	Can worsen hypertension, heart disease
	Imipramine[b]	10 mg h.s.	25 mg b.i.d.	25 mg t.i.d.	Anticholinergic effects, especially dry mouth

[a]Off-label use
[b]Off-label use. Labeled for enuresis.

eliminate the 10 a.m. session and toilet the patient at 11 a.m.

- After each modification, or when incontinence worsens, keep 3 days of bladder records and confirm appropriateness of schedule.

Prompted voiding, yet another behavior modification modality, is effective in reducing episodes of incontinence with patients who are cognitively impaired and unable to toilet independently. The protocol comprises monitoring for wetness, when wetness is identified prompting the patient to void, and then providing positive reinforcement after voiding. This treatment is typically used in nursing homes and assisted living homes.

Oxybutynin and *tolterodine* are antimuscarinic drugs that are effective in the treatment of urge incontinence (Table 54.2). The latter is newer and thought to be less toxic, but it is more expensive than the former. *Propantheline* and *imipramine* may be effective, but the evidence is limited and these drugs have serious side effects, especially in the elderly. They should be used with caution and in low doses in this population. These agents probably also act through both antimuscarinic and adrenergic properties. Dry mouth is a common side effect of all these drugs, and many other anticholinergic side effects can also ensue. It is implausible to imagine that the anticholinergic effects of these systemic drugs are confined to the urethral sphincter and detrusor. *Flavoxate,* an agent formerly highly touted in the treatment of UI, is ineffective.

Stress Incontinence

Pelvic floor muscle exercises (PFME) are more effective in treating stress incontinence in adult women than is sham treatment or no treatment. A majority of women report significant benefit (9). The mechanism by which these exercises lead to improvement is uncertain. They may be effective for men following radical prostatectomy (10). PFME are often combined with or compared to biofeedback, vaginal cones (a form of weight-lifting), or electrical stimulation of the pelvic floor. The data are variable, but, of these treatments, biofeedback seems to offer the best results. Many elderly women do not persist with PFME, although one study of women with a mean age of 50 years found that 5 years later most were still doing the exercises at least weekly and were doing well (11).

Generally, PFME should be tried by women with stress and/or urge incontinence, because these exercises are relatively simple, without harm, and often very effective. A patient may get a good sense of these exercises from reading the lay literature (see General References). If the patient appears motivated but has not achieved success by doing the exercises suggested, the patient may benefit from referral to a multidisciplinary continence clinic.

The following techniques are suggested for pelvic floor muscle exercises:

- First, identify the pelvic muscles. This can be done by starting and stopping the flow of urine. The same muscle groups are used when trying to inhibit the passage of flatus. Place a hand on the anterior abdomen to be sure these muscles are relaxed. (It is common to tighten them inadvertently when learning these exercises).
- Second, learn to control these muscles. One should be able to void about a teaspoon of urine at a time.
- Third, train these muscles. At first, hold each contraction for about 3 seconds. Before arising in the morning, do this five times. Gradually add "exercise sessions" during the day, until 15 repetitions of 3 seconds each are performed three times a day.
- Fourth, the clinician should encourage the continued use of these exercises.

Bladder training (discussed earlier for urge or mixed incontinence) has been reported to be useful in women with stress incontinence (12).

Drug treatment of stress incontinence is based on limited evidence. The drug with the best evidence of efficacy, phenylpropanolamine, is now off the market because of concerns about toxicity. Other alpha-adrenergic agonists have similarly limited evidence of effectiveness and also have substantial risk, especially in frail patients with cardiovascular disease. Very limited data may justify a trial of oxybutynin or tolterodine in relatively well patients who are troubled by their symptoms and who do not respond to behavioral interventions. Side effects from these drugs are also common, and the patient must be monitored carefully.

Surgical Treatment

Surgical therapy for incontinence continues to evolve for both men and women. More than 100 procedures for incontinence have been described. Most have been abandoned; a few are performed with acceptable levels of satisfaction and risk. The search continues for a least invasive, effective procedure that corrects or compensates for the variety of dysfunctions that cause incontinence.

There are few well designed, randomized trials, and the lack of standardization in measuring outcomes makes comparisons difficult. However, procedures used by urologists and gynecologists have been variably successful, and none can be clearly shown to be a "gold standard." The generalist considering referral of a patient for surgery should consider the impact of the incontinence, the expectations for outcome, the tolerance for risk, the existing comorbidities, local surgical expertise, and preference. Patients should usually have a trial of medical and behavioral therapy before referral is considered.

All procedures designed to correct incontinence in women carry potential risk for injury to the bladder, urethra, ureters, and bowel. Procedures that attempt to suspend or support portions of the urethra and anterior vaginal wall can cause urinary retention, and urgency or worsened prolapse of other pelvic organs are also risks of surgery. Because of anatomic proximity and shared innervation, changes in bowel and sexual function may also be affected by incontinence surgery. Table 54.3 summarizes some of the currently used surgical procedures.

Table 54.3. Some Current Surgical Procedures Used to Treat Urinary Incontinence

Procedure	Indication	Hospitalization	"Cure" rate (%)	Special complications	Comment
Retropubic colposuspension	Stress in women	2–4 days	Up to 85 at 10 yr	Voiding dysfunction 20%, usually transient (3 wk to 3 mo)	Restricted activity of 4–8 wk is typical
Laproscopic colposuspension	Stress in women	1–2 days	30–80	Same as above but less	
Pubovaginal or suburethral slings (includes tension-free vaginal type)	Stress in women	1–2 days	80–85 at 3–7 yr 60–70 if preoperative symptoms included urgency	Retention up to 7%; frequency/urgency 10%–12%	
Urethral bulking agents: collagen	Stress in women and men	Outpatient	50–60 after an average of two injections improve but only 15–30 are cured	Transient (1–3 days) retention; embolization and material migration in men, minimal in women; must be tested for allergy to collagen used	Typically requires two or more injections at 4–6 wk; typically used when more invasive surgery cannot be done; treatment usually lasts 2–4 yr and can be repeated
Artificial urinary sphincter	Stress in women		Limited use	Infection, erosion, mechanical failure	Occasionally used in women with difficult-to-manage recurrent incontinence and a rigid (pipestem) urethra
Artificial urinary sphincter	Stress in men	1 day	90–95	Infection, malfunction, erosion of cuff in 2%–7%	Uses a Silastic reservoir, cuff and in-line pump; patient mechanically pumps fluid from cuff to reservoir to void so requires dexterity and adequate recognition of the need to void; often used if incontinence has resulted from prostate surgery
Sacral neuromodulation	Urge	Outpatient local anesthesia for temporary or permanent placement is required	About 80% of patients achieve 50% or greater reduction in incontinent episodes		Low-level pulsed electrical stimulation to appropriate sacral nerves; requires at first an external stimulator for 2–7 days of adjustment; this temporarily stimulator is replaced permanently if effective; permanent implantation requires surgical implantation and the battery lasts 5–7 yr
Bladder augmentation	Urge		Improves urge incontinence in about 70%	Goal is to increase bladder capacity and weaken contractions; a patch of intestine is added to bladder or a mucosal diverticular is created; up to 75% of patients require subsequent intermittent catheterization	

From references 13–21.

General References*

Blaivas JG, Romanzi LJ, Heritz DM. Urinary incontinence: pathophysiology, evaluation, treatment overview and nonsurgical management. In: Walsh PC, Retik AB, Vaughan ED, et al., eds. Campbell's urology. 7th ed. Philadelphia: WB Saunders Co, 1997.

Resnick NM, Yolla SV. Geriatric incontinence and voiding dysfunction. In: Walsh PC, Retik AB, Vaughan ED, et al., eds. Campbell's urology. 7th ed. Philadelphia: WB Saunders, 1997.

Both chapters are well referenced and encyclopedic with many photographs and graphs.

Ham RJ, Lekan-Rutledge DA. Ham RJ, Sloane PD, eds. Incontinence in primary care geriatrics. 3rd ed. St Louis: Mosby, 1997.

A case-based review.

Cardozo L, Stoskin D, Kirby M. Urinary incontinence in primary care. Oxford, UK: ISIS Medical Media, 2000.

A terse, practical, short monograph.

Clinical practice guideline no. 2. Urinary incontinence in adults: acute and chronic management. Aging Health Care Policy and Research, Publication No. 96-0682. Rockville, MD: U.S. Department of Health and Human Resources, Public Health Service, 1996.

A useful publication, but some of the information is now dated.

Burgio RL, Pearce KL, Lucco AJ. Staying dry: a practical guide to bladder control. Baltimore: Johns Hopkins University Press, 1989.

A very valuable guide for patients.

Specific References

1. Drake MJ, Mills IW, Gillespie JI. Model of peripheral autonomous modules and a myovesical plexus in normal and overactive bladder function. Lancet 2001;358:401.
2. Agency for Healthcare Research and Quality. Clinical Practice Guidelines Archive. Available at: http://www.ahrq.gov/clinic/cpgarchv.htm (accessed 1/7/02).
3. Ouslander JG, Schapira M, Schnelle JF, et al. Does eradicating bacteriuria affect the severity of chronic urinary incontinence in nursing home residents? Ann Intern Med 1995;122:749.
4. Grady D, Brown JS, Vittinghoff E, et al., for the HERS Research Group. Postmenopausal hormones and incontinence: the Heart and Estrogen/Progestin Replacement Study. Obstet Gynecol 2001;97:116.
5. Fantl JA, Cardozo LD, Ekberg J, et al. Estrogen therapy in the management of urinary incontinence in post-menopausal women: a meta-analysis. Obstet Gynecol 1994;83:12.
6. Jackson S, Shepherd A. Brookes S, et al. The effect of estrogen supplementation on post-menopausal urinary stress incontinence: a double-blind placebo controlled trial. Br J Obstet Gynaecol 1999;106:711.
7. Ouslander JG, Greendale GA, Uman G, et al. Effects of oral estrogen and progestin on the lower urinary tract among female nursing home residents. J Am Geriat Soc. 2001;49:803.
8. Hirsch C. Review: inconclusive evidence suggests that bladder training improves urge incontinence. ACP Jour Club 1999;67.
9. Hay-Smith EJC, Bo K, Berghmans LCM, et al. Pelvic floor muscle training for urinary incontinence in women. Cochrane Database of Systemic Reviews, Issue 1, 2001.
10. Van Kampen M, De Weerdt W, Van Poppel H, et al. Effect of pelvic-floor re-education on duration and degree of incontinence after radical prostatectomy: a randomized controlled trial. Lancet 2000;355:98.
11. Bo K, Talseth T. Long-term effect of pelvic floor muscle exercise 5 years after cessation of organized training. Obstet Gynecol 1996;87:261.
12. Wyman JF, Fantl JA, McClish DK, et al. Quality of life following bladder training in older women with urinary incontinence. International Urogynecology Journal Pelvic Floor Dysfunction 1997;8:223.
13. Colombo M, Millani R, Vitobello P, et al. Randomized comparison of Burch colposuspension versus anterior colporrhaphy in women with stress urinary incontinence and anterior vaginal wall prolapse. Br J Obstet Gynecol 2000;107:544.
14. Leach GE, Bmochowski RR, Appell RA, et al. Female stress urinary incontinence clinical guidelines panel summary report on surgical management of female stress urinary incontinence. J Urol 1997;158:875.
15. Burton G. A three year prospective randomized urodynamic study comparing open and laparoscopic colposuspension. Neurourol Urodyn 1997;16:353.
16. Sand PK, Winkler H, Blackhurst DW, et al. A prospective randomized study comparing modified Burch retropubic urethropexy and suburethral sling for treatment of genuine stress incontinence with low-pressure urethra. Am J Obstet Gynecol 2000;182:30.
17. Ulmsten U, Falconer C, Johnson P, et al. A multicenter study of tension-free vaginal tape (TVT) for surgical treatment of stress urinary incontinence. Int Urogynecol J 1998;210:9.
18. Groutz A, Blaivas JG, Kesler SS, et al. Outcome results of transurethral collagen injection for female stress incontinence: assessment by urinary incontinence score. J Urol 2000;164:2006.
19. Klutke JJ, Subir C, Andriole G, et al. Long-term results after antegrade collagen injection for stress urinary incontinence following radical retropubic prostatectomy. Urology 1999;53:974.
20. Bosch JL, Groen J. Sacral nerve neuromodulation in the treatment of patients with refractory motor urge incontinence: long-term results of a prospective longitudinal study. J Urol 2000;163:1219.
21. Leng WW, Blalock HJ, Frederksson WH, et al. Enterocystoplasty or detrusor myectomy? Comparison of indications and outcomes for bladder augmentation. J Urol 1999;161:758.

*Bold print (general references) and bold numerals (specific references) denote published controlled clinical trials, meta-analyses, or consensus-based recommendations.

SECTION 7

Hematologic Problems

CHAPTER 55

Anemia

LARRY WATERBURY, MD

GENERAL CONSIDERATIONS

Anemia, a reduction of the proportion of red blood cells or of hemoglobin in the blood, is a condition, like hypoxia or jaundice, that always reflects a primary underlying disease. Although sometimes symptoms (e.g., shortness of breath on exertion) or signs (e.g., pallor) are associated with anemia, the diagnosis of the condition depends essentially on one or more laboratory measurements, such as the hematocrit value (Hct) or the hemoglobin concentration (Hb). In general, anemia is defined in a man as an Hct of less than 42% or an Hb of less than 14 g/100 mL and in a woman as an Hct less than 37% or Hb less than 12 g/100 mL. When anemia is diagnosed, other measurements (see Approach to Evaluation of Anemia) are important in establishing the cause of the process and selecting appropriate therapy.

Most routine complete blood counts (CBCs) obtained in clinical practice in the United States are determined by automated counting methods (Table 55.1). The CBC usually reports the Hb, Hct, red blood cell count (RBC), white blood cell count (WBC), mean corpuscular volume (MCV), mean corpuscular hemoglobin (MCH), and mean corpuscular hemoglobin concentration (MCHC). One commonly used automated system (Coulter) measures the Hb, RBC, and MCV, and from these variables calculates the Hct, MCH, and MCHC. With the use of the automated counters, the indices (MCH, MCHC, MCV), especially the MCV, are precise, accurate measurements that can be used in approaching the diagnostic workup of anemia. The calculated Hct is slightly lower than that obtained by centrifugation (i.e., packed cells trap plasma, distorting the ratio of red cells to plasma). The red cell distribution width (RDW) calculated by most automated systems is a measure of variation in size. It is often increased in many anemias (e.g., moderate to severe iron deficiency, megaloblastic anemias, many hemolytic anemias, anemias associated with reticulocytosis).

APPROACH TO EVALUATION OF ANEMIA

The routine database that should be obtained on every anemic patient includes the Hct, Hb, MCV, MCHC, and reticulocyte count (Table 55.2). A smear of the peripheral blood should be examined. On the basis of all of these data and a complete history and physical examination, the physician can progress a long way toward an etiologic diagnosis of the anemia. Three questions should be asked:

1. *What is the MCV?* With the use of the automated counters, the MCV is a direct measurement of red cell size. The normal range varies among individual laboratories, but it is approximately 82 to 98 fL. Actually, it is helpful to use a broader normal range, 80 to 100 fL, to classify the anemia as microcytic (MCV less than 80 fL), normocytic (MCV 80 to 100 fL), or macrocytic (MCV greater than 100 fL). Microcytic and macrocytic anemias have very limited differential diagnoses, so by simply noting the MCV the diagnostic approach can easily be focused when the anemia is microcytic or macrocytic.
2. *What is the basic mechanism of the anemia?* There are only three ways patients become anemic: decreased effective production of red blood cells, bleeding, or hemolysis. The most helpful laboratory measurement in defining the mechanism of anemia is the reticulocyte count. This count is used to assess the appropriateness of the response of the bone marrow to anemia. The normal reticulocyte count is approximately 1%, representing the 1% of new cells that are released into the circulation from the bone marrow daily (the ordinary red cell life span being approximately 100 days). Under the stimulus of erythropoietin, in the anemic patient, the bone

Table 55.1. Representative Normal Values (Coulter S)

Laboratory Measurements	Men	Women
Hemoglobin, g/dL of blood	14–18	12–16
Hematocrit value, %	42–54	37–47
MCV, fL	82–98	82–98
MCH, pg	27–32	27–32
MCHC, g/dL of red blood cells	31.5–36	31.5–36

MCV, mean corpuscular volume; MCH, mean corpuscular hemoglobin; MCHC, mean corpuscular hemoglobin concentration.

Table 55.2. Routine Database for Anemic Patients

Hematocrit value
Hemoglobin concentration
Mean corpuscular volume
Mean corpuscular hemoglobin concentration
Reticulocytic count (and calculation of reticulocytic index)
Evaluation of a peripheral blood smear

Table 55.3. Reticulocyte Index

$$\text{Reticulocyte index} = \text{Reticulocyte count} \times \frac{\text{Patient Hct}}{\text{Normal Hct}}$$

Example: reticulocyte count 6%, hematocrit 15%

$$\text{Reticulocyte index} = 6\% \times \frac{15\%}{45\%} = 2\%$$

marrow should be able to triple acutely its output of new cells; if anemia is chronic and severe, the bone marrow may be able to increase its output of cells to eight to ten times normal. This increased bone marrow activity is reflected in an appropriately elevated reticulocyte count. The reticulocyte count must be adjusted for the level of anemia to obtain a value known as the *reticulocyte index* (Table 55.3), a more accurate reflection of erythropoiesis. In patients with bleeding or hemolysis, the reticulocyte index should be at least 3%. In patients with anemia caused by decreased production of red blood cells, the reticulocyte index is less than 3%, and often it is less than 1.5%.

In addition to the reticulocyte index, serial Hct measurements over a few days or weeks may provide clues to the mechanism of the anemia. Total shutdown of production in the marrow in the absence of bleeding or hemolysis results in a fall in the Hct of only 3 or 4 percentage points per week. If the value has fallen more rapidly, bleeding or hemolysis must have taken place. Anemia with an appropriate reticulocyte response in the absence of bleeding usually means hemolysis.

3. *Does the patient have another problem that is commonly associated with anemia?* Table 55.4 lists anemias commonly associated with various clinical characteristics and diseases. For this purpose, race and sex are also taken into consideration. Women are iron deficient more often than are men, and African American patients are more likely than whites to have hemoglobinopathies or glucose-6-phosphate dehydrogenase (G6PD) deficiency.

In summary, the initial database should enable the physician to classify the anemia on the basis of the

Table 55.4. Anemias Associated with Various Clinical Settings

Female
Iron deficiency

African Americans
G6PD deficiency, hemoglobinopathies, thalassemia

Mediterranean Origin
G6PD deficiency, thalassemia

Far East Origin
Hemoglobinopathies, thalassemia

Viral Infections
Immune hemolysis
Decreased production

Bacterial Infection
Anemia of inflammation
Microangiopathic hemolysis
Oxidative hemolysis (G6PD deficiency)
Other hemolytic mechanisms

Malignancy
Iron deficiency caused by bleeding from a colon cancer
Microangiopathic hemolysis
Immune hemolysis
Decreased production

Alcoholic Liver Disease
Bleeding
Hypersplenism
Folate deficiency
Decreased production
Sideroblastic anemia
Iron deficiency
Hemolysis

Hyperthyroidism or Hypothyroidism
Decreased production
Pernicious anemia
Iron deficiency

Renal Failure
Decreased production
Hemolysis
Bleeding

Aortic Valve Replacement
Microangiopathic hemolysis

Malignant Hypertension
Microangiopathic hemolysis

Rheumatoid Syndromes
Anemia of inflammation
Iron deficiency
Immune hemolysis

Collagen Vascular Disease
Immune hemolysis
Anemia of inflammation

Drugs
α-Methyldopa: Immune hemolysis
Quinine/quinidine: Immune hemolysis
Penicillin: Immune hemolysis (rare)
Chloramphenicol: Dose-related marrow depression; idiosyncratic aplastic anemia
Gold: Aplastic anemia
Antituberculosis drugs: Sideroblastic anemia
Phenytoin: Megaloblastic anemia (folate); pure red cell aplasia
Sulfa/sulfones: G6PD hemolysis
Methotrexate: Megaloblastosis
Amphotericin, cis-platinum, zidovudine: Production defect

G6PD, glucose-6-phosphate dehydrogenase.

MCV, categorize the basic mechanism of the anemia, and consider possible causes based on the patient's problem list. This initial assessment should then suggest the appropriate further diagnostic workup.

ANEMIA WITH A LOW MEAN CORPUSCULAR VOLUME

Table 55.5 lists the anemias commonly associated with a low MCV. For the most part, the diagnosis rests between iron deficiency anemia and thalassemia. Occasionally the anemia of chronic inflammation or, even more rarely, that of sideroblastic anemia is microcytic; more often, they are normocytic or, in the case of sideroblastic anemia, macrocytic.

Iron Deficiency Anemia

Although dietary iron deficiency does occur in the infant and during the rapid growth phase of adolescence, in the United States iron deficiency usually occurs only as a result of bleeding. Iron deficiency from menstruation and from pregnancy is extremely common in women; however, iron deficiency in a man or in a postmenopausal woman should be considered to be caused by gastrointestinal bleeding until proven otherwise.

Diagnosis

The history and physical examination may yield information that suggests the presence of iron deficiency (1). Such information includes a history of multiple pregnancies in a woman; strange dietary habits such as the eating of ice, starch, or clay (pica); any history of gastrointestinal bleeding; and physical findings of a sore tongue, brittle and ridged fingernails, spoon nails, or cheilosis. The physical findings are seen only in patients with long-standing and severe iron deficiency.

Most of the body's iron is incorporated in hemoglobin, but approximately one third of it is stored in reticuloendothelial sites, primarily in the spleen, liver, and bone marrow. In patients with slow continued bleeding, the reticuloendothelial iron stores supply iron to the bone marrow until the stores are depleted. It is at this point that iron deficiency anemia begins to develop. In iron deficiency, cell size (MCV) correlates with the degree of anemia, so very mild iron deficiency anemia may be associated with normal-sized cells (see Mild Iron Deficiency) (2). The MCV progressively decreases as the anemia becomes more severe, but the MCHC usually remains normal until the Hct falls to less than 30%. As the anemia becomes more marked, the red cells also become progressively more distorted (poikilocytosis). Table 55.6 illustrates the relationship between the Hct, the MCV, and the degree of red cell distortion (poikilocytosis) seen in iron deficiency anemia of varying degrees of severity.

Often the diagnosis of iron deficiency is obvious after the initial history, physical examination, and standard laboratory evaluation. If not, a number of other tests may be useful. One of the most useful is a baseline MCV measurement, because iron deficiency is an acquired microcytic anemia and in thalassemia microcytosis is lifelong. The *reticulocyte index* is inappropriately low for the degree of anemia. The *serum iron concentration* (SI) is low, but it is usually low also in patients with acute or chronic inflammation or malignancy. Furthermore, an acute infectious process such as pneumococcal pneumonia causes an immediate drop in the SI, even though the patient is not iron deficient. Classically, the *total iron-binding capacity* (TIBC) is elevated. It is a measure of serum transferrin, the iron transport protein that supplies bone marrow red blood cell precursors with iron. However, many iron-deficient patients have a normal TIBC, and the TIBC may be low in cases of chronic inflammation or malignancy regardless of whether iron deficiency is present. In iron deficiency, cell receptors (marrow red cells) for transferrin increase and result in an increase in circulating *transferrin receptor* levels, which can be measured. This test can be helpful in distinguishing iron deficiency from the anemia of chronic disease (3), but the sensitivity and specificity are relatively low (4), nor is the test universally available. In fact, none of these tests is completely reliable in the diagnosis of iron deficiency, especially in patients with comorbidities.

Table 55.5. Causes of Anemia with Low Mean Corpuscular Volume

Iron deficiency
Thalassemia
Anemia of chronic inflammation (occasionally)
Sideroblastic anemia (congenital, rare)
Some hemoglobinopathies (e.g., HbE)
Aluminum toxicity

Table 55.6. Representative Database at Various Stages in the Slow Development of Severe Iron Deficiency Anemia[a]

Hct (%)	42	42	35	27	19
MCV (82–98 fL)	92	88	82	75	68
MCHC (32–36 g/dL)	33	33	33	31	29
SI (65–175 μg/dL)	70	60	35	20	20
TIBC (250–375 μg/dL)	300	300	300	400	450
Serum ferritin (10–200 μg/mL)	60	30	5	3	1
Peripheral smear	Normal	Normal	Normal	1+ poikilocytosis 1+ hypochromia	4+ poikilocytosis 4+ hypochromia
Bone marrow iron stores	Present	Absent	Absent	Absent	Absent

Hct, Hematocrit value; MCV, mean corpuscular volume; MCHC, mean corpuscular hemoglobin concentration; SI, serum iron; TIBC, total iron-binding capacity.

[a]Numbers in parentheses are the range of normal values.

Table 55.7. Inappropriately Normal or Elevated Serum Ferritin Levels

Acute liver disease
Cirrhosis
Hodgkin disease
Acute leukemias
Solid tumors (occasionally)
Fever
Acute inflammation
Renal dialysis patients
After taking oral iron for 2–3 wk or after recent treatment with parenteral iron

Measurement of serum ferritin is the most useful noninvasive test in the assessment of body iron stores (5). Ferritin is a water-soluble complex of iron and a binding protein, apoferritin. The serum ferritin concentration reflects the status of the reticuloendothelial stores and, in general, is a more specific test than the SI and TIBC in the diagnosis of iron deficiency. A low serum ferritin concentration almost always reflects iron deficiency. A very high serum ferritin concentration usually signifies iron overload, as in the patient who has received multiple transfusions. However, in many situations (e.g., inflammatory disease, chronic renal failure), the serum ferritin may be spuriously normal or even elevated in the presence of iron deficiency anemia (Table 55.7). In these situations it may be difficult to make a definitive diagnosis of iron deficiency without a bone marrow iron stain. Response to a therapeutic trial of iron may allow a presumptive diagnosis of iron deficiency. In general, it is inappropriate to subject people to an expensive and uncomfortable evaluation of their gastrointestinal tract without persuasive proof of iron deficiency; on rare occasions, such proof may require a bone marrow iron stain. The *bone marrow iron stain* is the most definitive way to prove a diagnosis of iron deficiency because iron stores are depleted when iron deficiency anemia is present and are normal or elevated in patients with microcytic anemia from other causes.

Treatment

After institution of oral iron therapy, the reticulocyte response is maximal at about 7 to 10 days. The Hct begins to rise after approximately 1 week, and in the uncomplicated case, a normal Hct is reached in a few weeks. However, it takes many months of therapy for patients to replete their iron stores (the status of which can be evaluated, by repeat measurement of serum ferritin, after iron therapy is concluded). Iron absorption is variable and unpredictable. Even under optimal conditions, only a fraction of ingested iron is absorbed. In the menstruating woman with iron deficiency anemia, treatment for 1 year or longer may be necessary. Iron deficiency is common in menstruating women, especially in those with heavy menstrual periods and a history of multiple pregnancies. Some may require perpetual iron therapy to maintain a normal Hct. Standard treatment with oral iron consists of 1 tablet of iron (e.g., ferrous sulfate, 300 mg, which contains 60 mg of elemental iron) three times daily on an empty stomach (1 hour before meals). It is difficult for patients to take the noontime dose, and it is reasonable to omit it. There are numerous preparations of iron other than ferrous sulfate, but there is usually no justification for recommending any of them unless a reduction in the dosage of elemental iron is required (see Side Effects). Generally, time-release capsules and enteric-coated preparations are to be avoided. They are costly and absorption is variable. Oral iron should be taken between meals, separate from H_2 blockers, antacids, and proton pump inhibitors. Preparations containing iron, including ferrous sulfate, can be obtained without prescription.

Side Effects

Approximately 15% of patients have gastrointestinal side effects from oral iron—most commonly constipation, but nausea, abdominal cramping, and diarrhea are also seen. If such side effects develop, the practitioner may elect to administer iron only once a day or may instruct the patient to take iron with meals instead of on an empty stomach (but not with tea or antacids). Taking iron with food decreases iron absorption by approximately 50%, but absorption is still sufficient to replenish the body's iron if treatment is continued long enough. If symptoms still continue after these alterations in dosage and schedule, it may be helpful to decrease the individual dosage of oral iron. If the dosage is decreased to less than 40 mg of elemental iron, symptoms often abate. This can be done by using pediatric liquid preparations, which usually are well tolerated.

If these adjustments in the dosage and schedule of oral iron administration are made, parenteral iron is rarely indicated. However, parenteral therapy is indicated in patients with small or large bowel inflammation, rapid gastrointestinal transit, or malabsorption, or if the patient has severe iron deficiency and noncompliance has been repetitively proven. Iron dextran has been the most commonly used form of parenteral iron, but ferric gluconate in sucrose appears to be a safer preparation (6); it is now used preferentially in patients undergoing renal dialysis and may be prescribed to other patients as well. Parenteral iron is usually given in small doses intramuscularly or intravenously. If the intravenous route is chosen, the infusion must be given slowly. Guidelines for the dosage of parenteral iron are provided in the *Physicians' Desk Reference* but may be calculated grossly from the patient's age and Hb value (Table 55.8). A test dose is administered 1 hour before the first therapeutic dose to ensure that the patient is not allergic to the preparation. Injections may be given daily until the calculated required dosage has been administered. Large doses of intravenous iron, appropriately diluted and given over several hours, are not approved by the U.S. Food and Drug Administration (FDA) but are generally safe when supervised by experienced clinicians. Side effects from parenteral iron include pain and rash at the

Table 55.8. Representative Total Body Iron Deficits (mg) at Various Body Weights and Hemoglobin Concentrations

	Iron Deficit at Various Hemoglobin Levels			
Patient Weight (lb)	4 g/dL	6 g/dL	8 g/dL	10 g/dL
100	2250	1750	1400	1000
120	2650	2100	1650	1150
140	3050	2500	1950	1350
160	3550	2850	2200	1550
180	3950	3200	2500	1750

Table 55.9. Globin Chain Composition of Normal Adult Hemoglobins

Type	Composition	Percentage of Total in Normal Adults
Hgb A	$\alpha_2\beta_2$	97
Hgb A_2	$\alpha_2\delta_2$	2
Hgb F	$\alpha_2\gamma_2$	1

injection site, arthralgias, staining of the skin, fever, and rare anaphylactoid reactions.

Thalassemia

In the normal adult, three types of hemoglobins are present in mature red cells: A, the major component, and two minor components, A_2 and F (fetal). Each hemoglobin molecule consists of four heme groups and four globin chains; the globin chains in each molecule are of two different types. All three hemoglobins have two α-globin chains but differ in their second set of globin chains (β, γ, or δ) (Table 55.9).

Thalassemia is an inherited defect in globin chain production. Anemia is caused by a combination of decreased hemoglobin production and, usually, mild hemolysis. β-Thalassemia is seen in the United States primarily in African American patients, patients from Southeast Asia, and patients of Mediterranean (Greek or Italian) origin. The genetics of α-thalassemia are complicated, and the disorder appears to have a wider racial distribution than does β-thalassemia, but it is especially common in African Americans (7). Most patients are heterozygous and are clinically asymptomatic but may have microcytosis. The diagnosis is important, because the entity is often confused with iron deficiency anemia, resulting in lifelong repetitive workups for gastrointestinal bleeding and inappropriate treatment with iron. Microcytosis in African American patients is more likely to be caused by α-thalassemia than by iron deficiency.

Diagnosis

Table 55.10 lists the typical database for the patient with heterozygous α- or β-thalassemia. The combination of a low MCV and only a very mild anemia should alert the practitioner to the diagnosis, because in iron deficiency the degree of microcytosis parallels the severity of the anemia (Table 55.6).

In the forms of β-thalassemia most commonly seen in the United States, there is a decreased production of β chains with a compensatory increase in the production of δ chains, resulting in a decreased production of hemoglobin A and an increased production of hemoglobin A_2. This increase can be assessed by electrophoresis of the hemoglobin and is a definitive diagnostic test for β-thalassemia. Less commonly in this country, increases in hemoglobin F may be seen in patients with β-thalassemia.

Table 55.10. Heterozygous Thalassemia: Typical Database

Data Value	Typical Value
Hematocrit value	37%
MCV	69 fL
MCH	20 pg
MCHC	32 g/dL
Reticulocyte count	2.5%
Red blood cell morphology	Microcytosis, poikilocytosis, stippling
Ferritin	Normal or increased

MCV, mean corpuscular volume; MCH, mean corpuscular hemoglobin; MCHC, mean corpuscular hemoglobin concentration.

The α-thalassemias are more difficult to diagnose because a decreased production of α chains affects the relative concentrations of all of the normal adult hemoglobins. A definitive diagnosis of one of the α-thalassemia syndromes may be difficult and may require family studies or techniques available primarily in research laboratories. However, the diagnosis of presumptive α-thalassemia in the setting of an appropriate database (hematologic values consistent with the diagnosis in the absence of iron deficiency and of β-thalassemia) is reasonable even in the absence of laboratory confirmation.

Patient Education

It is important to explain to patients with heterozygous thalassemia that the clinical features of their condition mimic those of iron deficiency. The patient should be put on guard against repetitive diagnostic workups for iron deficiency. The clinician should emphasize the benign nature of the illness and that the anemia, being mild, usually does not cause any symptoms. The patient should be cautioned against taking oral iron, because thalassemic patients actually have an increase in iron stores. Genetic counseling is important; a couple, both heterozygous for β-thalassemia, has a 25% chance of having a child with homozygous β-thalassemia. Furthermore, the genes for thalassemia and those for hemoglobin S and C are alleles. Hemoglobin S–β-thalassemia is a clinically significant disease.

Miscellaneous

The anemia of chronic disease and the anemia of malignancy may be associated with a low MCV (although the MCV is usually normal). These entities are discussed later in this chapter (see Anemias with Normal Mean Corpuscular Volume and an Inappropriately Low Reticulocyte Index). Sideroblastic anemias (characterized by increased iron stores and ringed sideroblasts in the bone marrow) are occasionally microcytic, and some hemoglobinopathies are associated with a low MCV (hemoglobin E). The former conditions are best treated in consultation with a hematologist; the latter are seen primarily in Southeast Asians. Aluminum toxicity, now seen infrequently in dialyzed patients with chronic renal failure, sometimes causes a further reduction in red cell mass, with microcytosis (8).

ANEMIA WITH A HIGH MEAN CORPUSCULAR VOLUME

An MCV greater than 100 fL is abnormal, and an attempt should be made to explain the abnormality. Table 55.11 lists conditions associated with an increased MCV (9). For the most part, the diseases associated with an elevated MCV are liver disease, the megaloblastic anemias (including drug-induced megaloblastosis), and the refractory anemias with hypercellular bone marrows (myelodysplastic syndromes). Occasionally an elevated MCV measured by the automatic counter is spurious, caused by red cell antibodies (cold agglutinins). Because young red blood cells are large, patients with a marked reticulocytosis may have an increased MCV.

Liver Disease

Chronic hepatocellular and obstructive liver disease results in cholesterol loading in the lipid portion of the red cell membrane so that the cell increases in size. The MCV is often elevated but is usually not greater than 115 fL (Table 55.12). On smears, cells appear to be round and centrally targeted, without significant variation in shape. This morphologic abnormality is not a cause of anemia. However, patients with liver disease often have other reasons to be anemic (bleeding, hemolysis, folic acid deficiency). The severe alcoholic often has an increased MCV even in the absence of overt liver disease or marked megaloblastosis (10). Presumably the elevated MCV results from periodic episodes of alcoholic liver disease, folic acid deficiency, or both. Because of poor diet, the alcoholic often becomes folic acid depleted. In addition, alcohol interferes with folic acid metabolism.

Table 55.11. Differential Diagnosis of Mean Corpuscular Volume Greater Than 100 fL

Spurious
Reticulocytosis (marked)
Liver disease
Alcoholism
Myelodysplastic syndromes
Myelophthisis
Drugs
Megaloblastic anemias
Normal variant

Megaloblastic Anemia

A megaloblast is a larger than normal hematopoietic precursor with a nucleus that contains characteristic granular chromatin, the result of abnormal DNA synthesis (11). Table 55.13 lists the various etiologies of megaloblastic anemia related to deficiency of vitamin B_{12} (cobalamin) or folic acid (essential cofactors in DNA synthesis). The body's stores of B_{12} are such that a diet without this vitamin (one in which animal protein is completely excluded) would not result in megaloblastosis due to B_{12} deficiency for several years; therefore, dietary B_{12} deficiency is extremely rare. By far the most common cause of B_{12} deficiency is pernicious anemia, an acquired autoimmune defect of the gastric mucosa resulting in deficient formation of intrinsic factor, which binds ingested B_{12} and allows its absorption in the terminal ileum. Patients with pernicious anemia are usually elderly and often complain of sore mouth, indigestion, and constipation or diarrhea. Neurologic problems, including peripheral neuropathy, dorsal column dysfunction (loss of vibratory and position sense in the lower extremities), and changes in affect are common. If the deficiency is not corrected, lateral column dysfunction (weakness and spasticity)

Table 55.12. Laboratory Features in Three Conditions Associated with an Elevated MCV

Feature	Liver Disease	Megaloblastic Anemia	Myelodysplastic Syndrome
Mean corpuscular volume	Usually <115 fL	Often >115 fL	Usually <115 fL
White blood cell count (WBCs)	Variable	Often decreased	Often decreased
Platelet count	Variable	Often decreased	Often decreased
Red blood cell (RBC) morphology	Target cells, no poikilocytosis	Marked anisocytosis and poikilocytosis, macro-ovalocytes	Marked anisocytosis and poikilocytosis, may mimic megaloblastic anemia
Nucleated RBCs	Not common	Common	Common
WBC morphology	Normal	Hypersegmented nuclei of neutrophils	May have abnormal mononuclear cells, no nuclear hypersegmentation of neutrophils
Platelet morphology	Normal	Normal	May be large and degranulated
RBC folate	Depends on diet	Decreased in folate deficiency, normal or slightly decreased in B_{12} deficiency	Normal or elevated
Serum B_{12}	Normal	Decreased in B_{12} deficiency, may be slightly decreased in folate deficiency	Normal or elevated

Table 55.13. Causes of Megaloblastosis Due to Vitamin B_{12} or Folic Acid Deficiency

Vitamin B_{12}
Pernicious anemia (acquired or congenital)
Gastrectomy
Ileal resection
Crohn disease and tropical sprue
Fish tapeworm infestation
Blind loop syndrome
Nutritional deficiency (vegan diet, rare)
Familial selective malabsorption (Imerslund-Grasbeck disease)

Folic Acid
Dietary (old age, alcoholism, chronic disease)
Malabsorption (sprue)
Hemodialysis
Severe exfoliative skin disease (e.g., psoriasis)
Drugs
- Interference with absorption or use (phenytoin, alcohol)
- Dihydrofolate reductase inhibitors (methotrexate, trimethoprim)

Increased requirements
- Pregnancy
- Infancy
- Hemolysis (e.g., sickle cell anemia)

also occurs. The anemia develops so slowly that patients often have very low Hcts and yet remarkably good cardiovascular compensation for their anemia. Such patients usually have an expanded total blood volume and are prone to develop heart failure if given transfusions. B_{12} deficiency from other causes (Table 55.13) is less common. Patients who have had total gastrectomy or ileal resection or who have ileal disease (Crohn disease, tropical sprue) are likely to develop B_{12} deficiency and should receive prophylactic vitamin B_{12}. B_{12} deficiency after partial gastrectomy is less common. There is evidence that B_{12} malabsorption may occur and lead to neuropsychiatric sequelae secondary to vitamin B_{12} deficiency, despite normal hematologic values and normal Schilling tests (discussed later in this chapter). In such cases, vitamin B_{12} levels are usually low, although often not as low as in pernicious anemia. Diagnosis may require more sensitive (and more expensive) tests of B_{12} metabolism, such as measurement of serum or urine methylmalonic acid and serum homocysteine (12). The mechanism of B_{12} deficiency in such patients is unclear, although it may be caused, at least in some patients, by an inability to absorb food-bound B_{12} even though they secrete normal amounts of intrinsic factor (13). If such problems are suspected, the patient should be referred to a hematologist or a neurologist for further evaluation. A therapeutic trial of vitamin B_{12} is often recommended.

In contrast to vitamin B_{12}, the body's stores of folic acid are depleted rapidly when patients eat a diet deficient in folate. (The main sources of folate in the diet are leafy vegetables, fruits, nuts, and liver.) Therefore, folic acid deficiency is most often dietary. For example, pregnant women have an increased need for folate and without prenatal supplementation may develop folate deficiency, as may patients whose dietary intake is severely restricted because of chronic disease or multiple surgical procedures. Intestinal malabsorption for any reason is also a common cause of folate deficiency. Finally, a number of drugs may be associated with folate deficiency: Phenytoin (Dilantin) interferes with folate absorption, alcohol interferes with folate utilization, and methotrexate and trimethoprim–sulfamethoxazole (Bactrim, Septra) interfere with folate metabolism. Also, some chemotherapeutic agents (e.g., hydroxyurea, cytosine arabinoside, methotrexate, azathioprine) that are used in the treatment of cancer, or to induce immunosuppression in patients with a variety of disorders, cause megaloblastosis by inhibiting DNA synthesis.

Diagnosis

The morphology of the peripheral blood and bone marrow is the same in patients with folic acid and in those with vitamin B_{12} deficiencies (11). With a severe megaloblastic anemia, the MCV often is significantly increased. An MCV greater than 120 fL is almost always caused by a megaloblastic anemia. The red cells in the peripheral blood are characterized by marked variation in size and shape. The common cell is a macro-ovalocyte (large egg-shaped cell). One may also see Howell–Jolly bodies (nuclear fragments), Pappenheimer bodies (iron granules), and nucleated red blood cells. The nuclei of the neutrophils are often hypersegmented, and commonly there is a neutropenia and thrombocytopenia. The bone marrow is typically markedly cellular, revealing characteristic megaloblastic changes of all cell lines. The bone marrow iron stain usually reveals increased numbers of iron-containing nucleated red blood cells (sideroblasts).

Folic Acid and Vitamin B_{12} Assay. Classically, in vitamin B_{12} deficiency the serum B_{12} level is quite low (less than 100 pg/mL) and the serum folate level is high. Spuriously normal B_{12} levels may occasionally be seen in B_{12} deficiency (see earlier discussion), and spuriously low levels may be seen without B_{12} deficiency in some patients with folic acid deficiency (Table 55.14). The serum folate assay has little clinical usefulness in the workup of megaloblastic anemia

Table 55.14. Vitamin B_{12} and Folate Concentrations

Serum B_{12} Concentration
Spuriously low in some patients with folate deficiency
Spuriously low in some pregnant patients
May be spuriously low in patients taking large daily doses of vitamin C
May be low in strict vegetarians
May be elevated for weeks after one injection of B_{12}
Increased in myeloproliferative syndromes

RBC Folate Concentration
Reflects chronic folate deficiency
Falsely low in some patients with B_{12} deficiency
Falsely high in patients with reticulocytosis

Serum Folate Concentration
A measure of recent dietary intake of folate
May be low, normal, or elevated in B_{12} deficiency

secondary to folic acid deficiency. The red cell folate concentration does reflect chronic folate deficiency, although it may be falsely low in some patients with vitamin B_{12} deficiency (Table 55.14).

Schilling Test. The Schilling test is a measure of B_{12} absorption and requires the measurement of total radioactivity excreted during a 24-hour period after ingestion of radioactive vitamin B_{12}. This test is useful primarily in cases in which the data are confusing and for patients already treated with vitamin B_{12}, in whom the serum levels are no longer helpful. The Schilling test requires a cooperative patient who can collect a 24-hour urine sample. The test includes the following steps: After voiding, the patient takes 0.5 μCi of cobalt-labeled vitamin B_{12} (^{60}Co or ^{57}Co cyanocobalamin) by mouth. A 24-hour urine collection is initiated; at 2 hours, 1 mg of B_{12} is given by injection (the flushing dose) and the percentage of the radioactive B_{12} excreted in 24 hours is determined. Normally 7% or more of the dose is excreted in 24 hours. Incomplete collection results in a spuriously low Schilling test and a false diagnosis of B_{12} malabsorption. In addition, if there is severe megaloblastic anemia, there are changes in the gastrointestinal mucosa that affect B_{12} absorption. For example, the Schilling test may be abnormal in patients with folic acid deficiency, because of the effect of folate deficiency on the intestinal mucosa, until the megaloblastic process has been treated for a week or two (Table 55.15).

Table 55.16 outlines a stepwise approach to the use of the laboratory in differentiating between folic acid and vitamin B_{12} deficiency in a patient with a megaloblastic anemia.

After a diagnosis of vitamin B_{12} deficiency is established and treatment is initiated (see later discussion), there is no need for periodic determination of serum vitamin B_{12}.

Other Laboratory Features. Megaloblastic anemias are essentially hemolytic in that there is marked destruction of abnormally formed cells within the marrow (ineffective erythropoiesis), which often results in indirect hyperbilirubinemia and an elevated concentration of serum lactate dehydrogenase. The serum iron concentration is usually elevated, and the reticulocyte index is inappropriately low.

Gastric achlorhydria is present in pernicious anemia, and antibodies to gastric mucosal cells and to intrinsic factor are often present, as are other autoantibodies, especially antithyroid and antiadrenal antibodies. The most useful of these findings is the assay of anti–intrinsic factor antibody in serum, which is reasonably specific for pernicious anemia and is present in approximately 70% of cases. Anti–intrinsic factor antibody assay may be helpful in the occasional patient with megaloblastic anemia of uncertain etiology. There is an increased prevalence of thyroid disease (hypothyroidism, hyperthyroidism, and euthyroid goiter) in patients with pernicious anemia.

Table 55.15. Causes, Other Than Pernicious Anemia, of a Positive Schilling Test

Incomplete urine collection
Renal failure
Some patients with megaloblastic anemia before treatment
Gastric antibodies to intrinsic factor
Defective intrinsic factor
Drugs (alcohol, colchicine, cholestyramine)
Pancreatic insufficiency
Partial gastrectomy

Treatment

The usual treatment for B_{12} deficiency is monthly intramuscular administration of 1,000 μg of vitamin B_{12} for the rest of the patient's life. Many physicians treat patients daily while they are in the hospital, particularly if they have neurologic signs; however, there is little evidence that this practice is more efficacious than simply starting maintenance monthly injections. There is evidence that B_{12} deficiency secondary to pernicious anemia can be treated successfully with daily oral vitamin B_{12}, 2 mg a day (14). Tablets of vitamin B_{12} are available over the counter in dosages of up to 1 mg.

Folic acid, 1 to 5 mg daily, is adequate treatment for patients with folic acid deficiency. Treatment should be given at least until a normal Hct is reached and should be continued if the patient is not eating an adequate diet or if the underlying cause persists (e.g., malabsorption). Patients with a chronic hemolytic state, such as children with sickle cell anemia, patients on hemodialysis (folic acid is dialyzable), and pregnant patients, should receive prophylactic treatment.

With appropriate treatment of megaloblastic anemia, there is a rapid reticulocytosis, which reaches a peak at approximately 7 to 10 days; the Hct begins to rise in approximately 1 week, and in uncomplicated cases, it rises at a rate of 4 to 5 percentage points per week. The leukopenia and thrombocytopenia respond dramatically, and leukocyte and platelet counts may return to normal in a day or two. There is a variable response of the neurologic complications of vitamin B_{12} deficiency. Megaloblastic madness usually abates dramatically. Dorsal column problems and peripheral neuropathies usually improve, but more slowly. Lateral spinal tract signs are usually refractory to treatment.

Table 55.16. Differentiating Between Folate and B_{12} Megaloblastosis

Etiology by History	RBC Folate	Serum B_{12}	Interpretation	Further Testing
Suggests folate	↓	Normal or ↑	Folate deficiency	None
Suggests folate	↓	Slightly ↓	Folate deficiency	Recheck B_{12} after folate treatment for 1 week
Suggests B_{12}	Normal or ↑	↓	B_{12} deficiency	None
Suggests B_{12}	↓	↓	B_{12} deficiency	May confirm with Schilling test
All other combinations → Schilling test				

Myelodysplastic Syndromes

These syndromes are acquired disorders of bone marrow stem cells that usually are seen in elderly patients and that at presentation may mimic a megaloblastic anemia (15). However, the morphologic features of the bone marrow, and usually the peripheral smear, are different (Table 55.12). White blood cell and platelet morphology may be abnormal, the serum vitamin B_{12} and folic acid levels are high, and the patients do not respond to folic acid or vitamin B_{12} therapy. In the bone marrow, ringed sideroblasts (red cell precursors containing granules of iron that form a ring around the nuclei) are common, as are "megaloblastoid changes." Approximately 25% of patients develop acute nonlymphocytic leukemia, usually within 1 year but sometimes only after several years.

ANEMIAS WITH NORMAL MEAN CORPUSCULAR VOLUME AND APPROPRIATE RETICULOCYTE INDEX (HEMOLYSIS AND BLEEDING)

Anemias caused by bleeding and hemolysis are associated with an appropriate bone marrow response manifested by an appropriate reticulocyte index (Table 55.3). The MCV is usually normal; however, if the reticulocyte count is high, the MCV may be slightly elevated. The diagnosis of hemolysis is suggested by an anemia with a reticulocyte index of at least 3% in the absence of overt bleeding. Bleeding is far more common than hemolysis, and bleeding in certain body sites (e.g., retroperitoneal bleeding in patients taking anticoagulants, bleeding into the site of a hip fracture) may be associated with a marked drop in Hct and a high reticulocyte count without external evidence of blood loss. Furthermore, the correction of anemias that are caused by decreased bone marrow production may also yield a database that mimics hemolysis, as in patients with an appropriate reticulocyte response after being treated with iron, folic acid, or vitamin B_{12}, or after alcohol withdrawal.

Approach to Hemolysis

It is appropriate to attempt to prove that hemolysis is occurring before obtaining diagnostic tests in a search for specific etiologies. The diagnostic approach to hemolysis varies depending on whether the hemolysis is primarily intravascular or extravascular.

Intravascular Hemolysis

Table 55.17 lists hemolytic mechanisms associated with intravascular destruction of red blood cells. Almost all of them require that the patient be hospitalized, and, if possible, diagnostic testing and treatment should be planned in consultation with a hematologist. In intravascular hemolysis, red cell lysis occurs within the vascular space, resulting in hemoglobinemia. The plasma becomes visibly red or brown (methemoglobinemia) at a low concentration of hemoglobin (approximately 30 mg/100 mL). Free hemoglobin initially binds to haptoglobin (a binding protein produced in the liver). Once haptoglobin is saturated, free hemoglobin passes through the glomerulus and hemoglobinuria occurs. Some of the hemoglobin in the renal tubules is absorbed by the renal tubular cells, which slough into the urine several days later and stain positively for iron (urine hemosiderin). The latter test, therefore, is helpful in documenting the presence of intravascular hemolysis several days after it has occurred. Table 55.18 suggests an appropriate database when hemolysis is suspected in the clinical states associated with intravascular hemolysis.

Table 55.17. Clinical States Associated with Intravascular Hemolysis

Acute hemolytic transfusion reactions
Severe and extensive burns
Physical trauma (e.g., march hemoglobinuria)
Severe microangiopathic hemolysis (e.g., aortic valve prosthesis, TTP)
G6PD deficiency
Paroxysmal nocturnal hemoglobinuria

G6PD, glucose-6-phosphate dehydrogenase; TTP, thrombotic thrombocytopenic purpura.

Table 55.18. Appropriate Database when Intravascular Hemolysis Is Suspected

Observation of the color of the serum/plasma
Observation of the color of the urine
Measurement of free plasma hemoglobin
Heme pigment test of the urine if there are no red cells in the urine sediment
Measurement of serum haptoglobin
Iron stain of urine sediment for hemosiderin several days after a presumed hemolytic event

Extravascular Hemolysis

Most hemolysis occurs extravascularly within cells of the reticuloendothelial system. A diagnosis of extravascular hemolysis is more difficult to prove than that of intravascular hemolysis. There is no hemoglobinemia, hemoglobinuria, or hemosiderinuria. Haptoglobin is only partially saturated because there is only a slight leakage of free hemoglobin into the circulation. There may be indirect hyperbilirubinemia, but this is an insensitive sign of hemolysis. There is an increase in fecal and urine urobilinogen, but this is difficult to quantitate. Other tests of hemolysis, such as red cell survival, are difficult, and the results are not known for several days. The clinician often must be satisfied with only a presumptive diagnosis of extravascular hemolysis. Therefore, if extravascular hemolysis is suspected, it may be appropriate to obtain tests diagnostic of specific disease states based on a knowledge of the patient's other problems and on the baseline database (Table 55.19).

Information from the Peripheral Smear

In hemolytic states the peripheral smear often reveals only evidence of the response of the bone marrow to hemolysis (large polychromatophilic or finely stippled red cells). It is a common misconception that one

Table 55.19. Most Common Causes of Extravascular Hemolysis

Autoimmune hemolysis
Delayed hemolytic transfusion reactions
Hemoglobinopathies
Hereditary spherocytic and nonspherocytic anemias
Hypersplenism
Hemolysis with liver disease

always sees fragmented red cells on smear; they are seen only in microangiopathic hemolytic anemias. However, the smear may give further clues about the specific cause of the hemolysis, as indicated below.

Spherocytes. Spherocytes are seen in small numbers in many hemolytic states. When present in large numbers, they suggest either hereditary spherocytosis, autoimmune hemolysis, or one of the hemoglobin C hemoglobinopathies.

Elliptocytes. In large numbers, these cells suggest a diagnosis of hereditary elliptocytosis.

Fragmented Cells (Schistocytes). Sharply pointed, fragmented cells (helmet cells, spiculated cells, triangle cells) are seen in microangiopathic states (see later discussion).

Spiculated Cells. Sometimes spiculated cells are seen in patients with severe liver disease and hemolysis (usually in a terminal stage of liver disease). Spiculated cells are also one type of schistocyte found in the blood of patients with microangiopathic hemolysis.

Bite Cells (Blister Cells). Bite cells are sometimes seen in patients with oxidative hemolysis (e.g., G6PD deficiency). In bite cells, all of the hemoglobin appears to be pushed to one side of the cell.

Poikilocytosis and the Hemoglobinopathies. In patients with sickle cell disease and in the various other sickle cell syndromes, the peripheral smear is often diagnostic (see later discussion).

Hemolysis with a Positive Coombs Test

Once hemolysis is suspected, the diagnostic testing should be guided by the patient's problem list (16,17). Because of the relatively common occurrence of immune hemolysis and the important therapeutic implications of such a diagnosis, it is desirable to obtain a Coombs test at this stage in the workup.

Positive Direct Coombs Test

The direct Coombs test is done by mixing the patient's cells with Coombs antiserum containing antibody to immunoglobulin G (IgG) and to complement. If the test is positive, the physician should first ascertain from the laboratory personnel that the positive result is attributable to antibody and/or complement on the red cell surface. If this is the case, it is important to determine whether the antibody is an alloantibody or an autoantibody.

Alloantibodies are antibodies induced by prior transfusion or, in a woman, by placental transfer of fetal red cells. The antibodies are directed against specific minor red cell antigens, and it is important to identify them in case future transfusions are necessary. Ordinarily the antibody is present primarily in the patient's plasma and is identified by an antibody screen (indirect Coombs test). However, a direct Coombs test would also be positive because of the presence of alloantibodies if the patient had been recently transfused with cells that were still circulating and sensitized by the antibody.

Table 55.20. Comparison of Alloantibody and Autoantibody

Test	Alloantibody	Autoantibody
Direct Coombs' test	Often negative; may be positive if sensitized foreign red cells are still circulating	Positive
Indirect Coombs' test	Positive	Positive or negative
Antibody screen (panel)	Specificity is seen	Panagglutination, no specificity seen

Table 55.21. Autoimmune Hemolysis Caused by a Warm Antibody: Differential Diagnosis

Idiopathic
Secondary
- Infection (particularly viral)
- Drugs
  - α-Methyldopa
  - Penicillin
  - Quinine/quinidine
- Collagen vascular disease (systemic lupus erythematosus)
- Lymphoproliferative disorders
- Miscellaneous (e.g., thyroid disease, malignancy)

In a patient with hemolysis, if there has not been a recent transfusion, a positive direct Coombs test usually implies the presence of an autoantibody. In this situation the antibody may be present in the serum as well as on the surface of the red cells. Table 55.20 describes the differences between alloantibodies and autoantibodies. Autoantibodies are classified as either warm antibodies or cold antibodies. Warm antibodies are usually IgG and cannot be identified by direct agglutination of red cells; a Coombs test is required to detect them. Cold antibodies are usually IgM, cause direct agglutination of red cells in the cold, and result in a positive Coombs test because of fixation of complement to the red cell.

Hemolysis Caused by Warm Antibodies

Table 55.21 lists the conditions commonly associated with autoimmune hemolysis resulting from a warm antibody. Patients may develop such antibodies secondary to the use of certain drugs or to any of a number of conditions, including infections (particularly viral), collagen vascular disease (systemic lupus erythematosus [SLE]), lymphoproliferative diseases, and other malignancies. The classic example of a drug that induces a positive Coombs test is alpha-methyldopa (Aldomet) (18).

Autoimmune hemolysis is a relatively infrequent condition; sometimes it precedes the development of SLE or lymphoma. Patients usually have anemia, which may be severe. On physical examination, the spleen is slightly enlarged in 50% of patients, and mild jaundice and fever are not uncommon. The peripheral smear shows marked polychromatophilia, spherocytosis, and often, but not always, an elevated reticulocyte index. Autoimmune hemolysis that is temporary, such as that caused by drug administration or a viral infection, usually requires no treatment (although if a drug is implicated, it should be discontinued). The process gradually remits over 2 to 3 weeks. Patients with chronic primary autoimmune hemolysis should be referred to a hematologist, who usually prescribes corticosteroids, which are usually effective if first given at a reasonably high dosage and slowly tapered as the anemia improves. Occasionally, splenectomy is required for refractory cases. In patients with secondary chronic autoimmune hemolysis, treatment of the underlying disease is the most important therapy. Autoimmune hemolysis may sometimes present as a fulminant life-threatening anemia, sometimes associated with reticulocytopenia. In such cases patients should be hospitalized immediately and transfused despite the incompatible cross-match.

Cold Agglutinin Hemolysis

The most common etiology of autoimmune hemolysis caused by a cold antibody is a viral illness or *Mycoplasma* pneumonia (19). Severe hemolysis is rare. Chronic idiopathic cold agglutinin hemolysis or cold agglutinin hemolysis secondary to a lymphoproliferative disease is often more refractory to treatment with steroids and splenectomy than is the case with warm antibody hemolysis. Transfusion therapy may be a problem in such cases, because the antibody is a panagglutinin and reacts with all blood types; therefore, a compatible cross-match may be impossible to obtain. Ordinarily, the IgM antibody in cold agglutinin hemolysis is not significantly hemolytic, and transfusions with warmed washed red cells may be attempted when absolutely necessary (20).

Hemolysis with Fragmented Red Cells on Peripheral Smear

Table 55.22 lists the conditions associated with hemolysis and the presence of fragmented red cells on peripheral smear. The peripheral blood contains sharply pointed poikilocytes (schistocytes). Such cells are characteristic and are clearly differentiated from abnormally shaped red cells seen in other conditions (21). The hemolysis may be severe and in such cases is usually intravascular, resulting in hemoglobinemia, hemoglobinuria, haptoglobin saturation, and subsequently, hemosiderinuria (see earlier discussion). Red cell fragmentation may occur after insertion of a prosthetic, usually an aortic, valve. Rarely this may be associated with clinically significant hemolysis. More often, red cell fragmentation is caused by arteriolar lesions (e.g., fibrin, inflammation) that cause damage to the cells as they pass through the damaged vessel. When fragmented red blood cells are accompanied by thrombocytopenia, one should consider the possibility of disseminated intravascular coagulation (see Chapter 56) or of thrombotic thrombocytopenic purpura. This latter syndrome is often accompanied by fever and neurologic deficits, which characteristically fluctuate. If this condition is suspected, the patient should be hospitalized immediately and treated in consultation with a hematologist. The hemolytic-uremic syndrome is a related (perhaps identical) syndrome, more common in children, that is characterized by the prominence of renal failure over other organ dysfunction.

Table 55.22. Hemolysis with Fragmented Red Cells on Peripheral Smear: Differential Diagnosis

Aortic value prosthesis
Arteritis (e.g., malignant hypertension, polyarteritis)
Disseminated intravascular coagulation
Thrombotic thrombocytopenic purpura
Hemolytic-uremic syndrome
Malignancy
Giant hemangiomas
Renal transplant rejection
Eclampsia
Metastatic cancer (gastric)
Some chemotherapy

Hemolysis with Enlarged Spleen (Hypersplenism)

Not all large spleens cause cytopenias, and the degree of cytopenia does not necessarily correlate with the size of the spleen (22). Thrombocytopenia and leukopenia are more common than is anemia. Splenomegaly, from almost any cause, may result in hypersplenism, but the syndrome is seen most often in patients who have chronic liver disease and congestive splenomegaly. Splenomegaly is sometimes seen in patients with hemolysis from other mechanisms, such as autoimmune hemolysis or hereditary spherocytosis. Rarely, splenectomy is necessary because of severe cytopenias resulting from hypersplenism. Occasionally patients with Felty syndrome (see Chapter 77) are benefited by splenectomy, as are some patients with chronic leukemia or lymphoma.

Glucose-6-Phosphate Dehydrogenase Deficiency

G6PD deficiency (23) is seen primarily in African American patients in the United States. Inheritance is sex linked. Ten percent of African American males are affected (hemizygotes), as are 20% of African American females (heterozygotes). In these patients, hemolysis caused by G6PD deficiency is an acute intravascular hemolytic event usually precipitated by infection or an oxidant drug. Drugs known to precipitate hemolysis include sulfonamides, nitrofurantoin, and primaquine. Caucasian-type G6PD deficiency is seen primarily in patients from Mediterranean countries and usually is more severe than the African type, sometimes causing chronic, persisting, partially compensated hemolysis.

Diagnosis after a hemolytic event may be difficult, especially in the female heterozygote. Screening tests for G6PD deficiency may give a normal result at this time, and even the affected hemizygote African American male may have a normal screening test for several weeks after hemolysis (young cells contain more G6PD activity). Occasionally a characteristic cell (bite cell) is seen in the peripheral blood during a hemolytic event.

Although the frequency of the genetic defect is high, the incidence of severe hemolysis with provocation (infection, drugs) is low. Ordinarily, routine screening before treatment with a known oxidant drug (e.g., sulfonamide) is not recommended. Affected patients should be given a list of drugs to avoid (23).

Sickle Cell Disorders

Approximately 8% of the African American population in the United States carry the sickle cell gene (24). The gene is also present to much less an extent in Greeks, Italians, Arabians, and people from India. Hemoglobin S results from a mutation in the β-globin chain in hemoglobin that, when oxygen tension is reduced, causes the formation of rigid polymers that distort the shape of the red blood cell and increase its rigidity, leading to tissue ischemia and infarction. A number of common inherited disorders involving hemoglobin S are listed in this section.

Sickle Cell Trait

Most people who are heterozygous for hemoglobin S (sickle cell trait) are completely well and are not anemic. The peripheral smear appears normal, although sickling is seen if the blood is deoxygenated. Hemoglobin electrophoresis reveals approximately 40% hemoglobin S and 60% hemoglobin A; hemoglobins A_2 and F are present in normal concentration.

Most patients with sickle trait lead a normal life. However, rare clinical events attributable to the presence of sickle cell hemoglobin do occur. For example, splenic infarction at high altitudes (above 10,000 feet) has been reported. (Oxygen pressures in commercial aircraft are high enough that people with sickle cell trait may fly safely.) Occasionally, infarctions occur in more vital organs during vigorous exercise. All people with sickle cell trait have renal tubular dysfunction resulting in hyposthenuria; on occasion, severe hematuria may occur from hypertonicity in the renal medulla, resulting in sickling and leading to ischemia and tubular infarction. People with sickle cell trait have a higher incidence of renal infections, especially during pregnancy.

It is important to identify patients with sickle cell trait so that they may be given genetic counseling. A couple, both heterozygous for hemoglobin S, should be informed that they have a 25% chance of having a child with sickle cell anemia.

Sickle Cell Anemia (Hemoglobin SS)

Sickle cell anemia exists in approximately 0.15% of the African American population (24–26). The disease is usually severe, resulting in significant morbidity as well as shortened life expectancy. However survival has improved considerably in the last 30 years. Mean survival in SS disease is about 45 years, and it is about 64 years in persons with hemoglobin SC disease (27). One of the most disturbing clinical features of the illness is the occurrence of painful vaso-occlusive episodes: recurrent episodes of severe pain, usually in the limbs and the abdomen, caused by sickling-induced ischemia. Patients have a lifelong, often severe anemia, with Hct values that range from the mid-teens to the high twenties. The primary mechanism of the anemia is extravascular hemolysis. There is a chronic reticulocytosis and a chronic indirect hyperbilirubinemia. The patients usually have a leukocytosis, the white cell count rising occasionally as high as 30,000 to 40,000 cells/mL during a painful crisis. A mild thrombocytosis is also common. The peripheral smear shows markedly distorted red cells, including characteristically sickled cells. On electrophoresis, only hemoglobin S with a variable amount of hemoglobin F (no hemoglobin A) is detected.

The multiple and repetitive episodes of organ ischemia caused by sickling result in a host of abnormalities. The bones characteristically appear abnormal on radiography, revealing old infarctions that mimic the changes of osteomyelitis. The medullary spaces are usually widened by the marked compensatory expansion of bone marrow. The spine often takes on a distorted appearance, and aseptic necrosis of the femoral head (and, rarely, of the humeral head) is common, sometimes requiring joint replacement. Puberty is often delayed. Splenomegaly usually disappears by 8 years of age because of repeated infarctions of the spleen. An adult with sickle cell anemia is essentially autosplenectomized. This lack of splenic function contributes to the propensity for infections, related especially to a decreased ability to resist pneumococcal infections. Gallstones (pigment stones) are common, and sicklers do develop cholecystitis, which may be extremely difficult to differentiate clinically from a syndrome of intrahepatic cholestasis secondary to sickling in the hepatic sinusoids. There is some hazard to surgery, but patients with recurrent abdominal pain consistent with cholecystitis, who have gallstones, should probably have elective cholecystectomy (see Chapter 96). Pregnancy in women with SS disease is complicated by an increased risk of pyelonephritis, pulmonary infarction, antepartum hemorrhage, prematurity, and fetal death. With time, patients develop cardiomegaly and chronic myocardial disease related to repetitive microinfarctions of the heart. Murmurs are common and may suggest rheumatic or congenital heart disease. Patients with sickle cell anemia develop venous thromboses and pulmonary embolism. They also develop thromboses *in situ* in the lungs, followed, after many years, by chronic scarring and fibrosis. Pulmonary thrombosis/embolism may lead to pulmonary hypertension and heart failure. Cerebral vascular accidents are common, including infarction and intracerebral and subarachnoid hemorrhage. Seizures are common as well. Up to 75% of patients with sickle cell anemia develop leg ulcerations that may be chronic and extremely difficult to heal. Patients with sickle cell anemia are prone to serious retinopathy, which rarely may lead to blindness because of plugging of small retinal capillaries and subsequent neovascularization. It is important for these patients to be examined yearly by an ophthalmologist, because some of the problems can be prevented by photocoagulation of abnormal new retinal vessels (28).

Hemoglobin SC Disease

The genes that code for hemoglobin S and hemoglobin C are alleles. The C hemoglobin mutation is common in African Americans (approximately 2% prevalence), and patients doubly heterozygous for S and C constitute approximately 0.15% of that population. The syndrome is similar to that of SS disease but is usually somewhat more mild. In contrast to sickle cell anemia, the spleen is palpable in 50% of adult patients.

Hemoglobin S–β-Thalassemia

Patients doubly heterozygous for hemoglobin S and β-thalassemia trait have a syndrome similar to sickle cell anemia but usually more mild. Characteristically the MCV is low. The spleen may be palpable, and hemoglobin electrophoresis reveals 70% to 80% hemoglobin S and smaller amounts of hemoglobin A and F (the reverse of the pattern in sickle cell trait).

Treatment

Vaso-Occclusive Episodes. Painful vaso-occlusive episodes are often severe and may last for a few hours to several days and occasionally for several weeks. They may be associated with high fever and neutrophilia, which makes it difficult but important to differentiate crises from infection. No specific therapy exists. When pain is persistent, hospitalization is indicated. It is important to treat patients in painful crisis aggressively. Relatively large doses of intravenous narcotics are frequently needed. Routine, rather than as-needed (prn) orders, are appropriate in the hospital. Patients with sickle cell disease metabolize narcotics rapidly, and doses need to be repeated every 2 hours. Patient-controlled analgesia has been found to be useful (29). Although narcotic abuse can occur, sickle cell pain, like pain due to cancer, should be treated based on the patient's description and tolerance of the pain. The data suggest that prompt, aggressive treatment of pain decreases hospitalizations and emergency room visits (30).

Infection. As mentioned, patients with sickle cell anemia are prone to infections, especially with the pneumococcus. Patients with sickle cell anemia should receive pneumococcal vaccine (see Chapter 18) and should be encouraged to seek medical help at the first evidence of infection or fever.

Hemolytic and Aplastic Crises. In adults, acceleration of hemolysis is unusual. If the Hct drops significantly below baseline, it is probably because of decreased marrow production, associated with infection. Hemolytic episodes are much more common in children. If they occur, hospitalization and transfusion are often necessary. Patients with chronic severe hemolysis have an increased requirement for folic acid, and folic acid deficiency may occur, resulting in reticulocytopenia and more severe anemia. Therefore, daily folic acid therapy (1 mg) is reasonable for all patients with sickle cell anemia.

Thromboembolization. When patients with sickle cell disease develop deep vein thrombosis or pulmonary embolism, they should be treated with anticoagulants, as would any patient with such problems (see Chapter 57). However, venography should be avoided because of the danger of development of leg ulcers in any patient with SS hemoglobin whose lower extremities are traumatized. It is often difficult to distinguish pulmonary thrombotic/embolic problems from pneumonia. The *acute chest syndrome,* an episode characterized by chest pain, shortness of breath, and cough—often with fever and a pulmonary infiltrate—is common in patients with sickle cell anemia and usually warrants hospitalization to evaluate the diagnostic possibilities and institute appropriate treatment. When it is associated with significant hypoxia the syndrome can be fatal, and patients may benefit from exchange transfusion. There is evidence that the use of incentive spirometry during pain crises may decrease pulmonary complications in sickle cell disease.

Leg Ulcers. Leg ulcers are often large and are particularly refractory to treatment. Skin grafting is frequently only temporarily helpful. It is important to keep the ulcers clean, to elevate the legs frequently, and to use surgical stockings and elastic wraps (see Chapter 95).

Hematuria. Patients with sickle cell trait, sickle cell anemia, SC disease, or sickle cell thalassemia are all prone to bouts of severe hematuria related to sickling and to medullary ischemia precipitated by the hypertonicity of the renal medulla. Bleeding can occur for days or even weeks. Maintenance of a high urine flow is important to prevent clots from causing obstruction. Usually the hematuria stops spontaneously.

Priapism. Priapism is common in SS and SC disease and often results in permanent impotence once it has resolved. If urologic intervention is to be attempted, it must be done within a few hours of the onset of the priapism. It is often only temporarily helpful. Once impotence has occurred, penile protheses are often helpful (see Chapter 6).

Preventive Treatment with Hydroxyurea. A large controlled study demonstrated that treatment with hydroxyurea does decrease the incidence of painful crises in some patients with sickle cell anemia (31). The mechanism may be partly (but not completely) caused by increased intracellular levels of hemoglobin F. The benefit is modest in most patients, and a therapeutic trial requires close monitoring by a hematologist. The long-term side effects of hydroxyurea must be weighed carefully before a patient is prescribed this therapy (31). There is a growing experience with stem cell transplantation in children with sickle cell syndromes (32).

Recommendations for Preventive Care

Patients with sickle cell disorders have a lifelong chronic illness and require frequent and recurrent use of the health care system. The patient needs one general practitioner who is familiar with his or her case. The availability of emergency care 24 hours a day is also exceedingly important.

Infection. There should be rapid evaluation of fever, chills, or other signs of infection. The patient should be immunized with the pneumococcal, influenza, and *Haemophilus influenzae* type B vaccines (see Chapter 18). Because heart murmurs and cardiomegaly are common, it is often difficult to know whether a patient with sickle cell anemia has valvular heart disease. If any doubt exists, it is reasonable to prescribe prophylactic antibiotics before dental procedures (see Chapter 93).

Folic Acid. It is generally recommended that patients receive 1 mg of folic acid daily.

Ophthamologic Examination. Patients should see an ophthalmologist yearly.

Transfusions. In general, transfusions should be avoided because of the dangers of iron overload, sensitization to minor red cell antigens, infection, and other hazards of transfusion. Exchange transfusion (supervised by a hematologist) may help interrupt a prolonged pain crisis and is indicated in severe, life-threatening acute chest syndrome (discussed earlier), and hypertransfusion is useful in preventing recurrent neurologic vascular events. Alloimmunization occurs much more frequently in patients with sickle cell disease than in other patients with anemia because of minor red cell antigen incompatibilities in racially mismatched blood (33). This can be minimized by routinely doing extended crossmatches using blood matched for the predominant offending antigens (Duffy, Kidd, Kell, E, C).

The question of prophylactic transfusion for patients with sickle cell disease who are undergoing surgery with a general anesthetic has been long debated. A large multicenter study suggested there is no benefit to aggressive exchange transfusion over simple preoperative transfusion to hemoglobin levels of about 10 g/dL (34).

Hydroxyurea. Patients with frequent, severe, life-altering, painful vaso-occlusive episodes should be referred to a hematologist for consideration for therapy with hydroxyurea.

ANEMIAS WITH NORMAL MEAN CORPUSCULAR VOLUME AND AN INAPPROPRIATELY LOW RETICULOCYTE INDEX

Mild normocytic anemias without appropriate reticulocyte responses are among the most common problems seen in clinical practice. Before considering possible etiologies and embarking on a diagnostic workup, it is important to be sure that the Hct/Hb is reproducibly low. Moreover, the normal values for the testing laboratory should be known. For example, in some laboratories an Hct of 35% in a woman is normal. One should also consider the variation in normal values related to age, sex, pregnancy, and other factors. Finally, one should be sure that volume overload is not the cause. Volume shifts may result in swings in Hct of 6 or 8 percentage points. Table 55.23 lists the differential diagnosis of a normocytic anemia with an inappropriately low reticulocyte count.

Table 55.23. Anemia with a Normal Mean Corpuscular Volume and Low Reticulocyte Index: Differential Diagnosis

Renal failure
Anemia of chronic disease (inflammatory disease and malignancy)
Anemia of hypoendocrine states (hypothyroidism, etc.)
Mild (early) iron deficiency
Combined iron deficiency and megaloblastic anemia
Drug-induced marrow depression
Primary bone marrow disorders
Bone marrow infiltration (myelophthisis)
Bleeding or hemolysis plus one of the above

Primary Bone Marrow Disorders

A minority of patients in this category of anemia (i.e., normal MCV, low reticulocyte index) have primary bone marrow disorders and need referral to a hematologist/oncologist. They require bone marrow aspiration or biopsy, and it is helpful to talk with them about the procedure before their referral visit.

Patient Experience. The procedure sounds more frightening than the experience. Patients should be told that the procedure is usually done in the specialist's office and usually takes only 15 to 30 minutes. The patient lies on the side or abdomen. The usual site is the posterior superior iliac spine. A local anesthetic is used to deaden pain receptors in the dermis and the periosteum. The aspirate or biopsy needles are small in diameter, and the procedure when done by an experienced clinician is minimally uncomfortable. Very anxious patients can be given an oral or parenteral analgesic or a mild sedative for anxiety, or both, before the procedure if they bring someone with them to drive them home. A Band-Aid is all that is used after the procedure, and acetaminophen is all that is needed for postprocedure discomfort.

Anemia of Renal Failure

Patients with uremia are anemic primarily because of decreased production of erythropoietin (35). The red cell morphology on smear is usually normal, but occasionally spiculated cells (burr cells) may be seen. Some patients have a microangiopathic peripheral smear. There may be a mild thrombocytopenia, and the nuclei of the neutrophils may be hypersegmented even in the absence of folic acid deficiency. The Hct depends on the degree of renal failure (see Fig. 52.4 in Chapter 52). Significant anemia is unusual if the creatinine concentration is less than 2 mg/100 mL. The Hct values that are seen in patients with renal failure who are undergoing dialysis are extremely variable (from the low teens, requiring transfusion, up to the mid-thirties). Recombinant human erythropoietin is helpful for the treatment of anemia of renal failure. Responses can be dramatic, and although the preparation is expensive, side effects are few (e.g., hypertension in some patients) (36). Erythropoietin levels are not reliable in predicting response to erythropoietin injections in patients with mild renal insufficiency. Patients in renal failure may also be anemic because of iron deficiency (secondary to blood loss) or because of folate deficiency (because folic acid is dialyzable). Some patients with glomerulonephritis or arteritis have a microangiopathic hemolytic anemia.

Anemia of Chronic Disease

Any chronic inflammatory disease (e.g., rheumatoid arthritis) or malignant disease can cause mild to moderate anemia, unrelated to blood loss or hemolysis (37–39). (If the Hct is less than 25%, another explanation should be sought). It is important to note that other chronic illnesses are not associated with this kind of anemia. Red cell morphology is usually normal, but sometimes the MCV is less than 80 fL, requiring differentiation of the process from other causes of a microcytic anemia (see earlier discussion). The serum iron concentration and the total iron-binding capacity are low; the percentage of saturation may be just as low as it is in iron deficiency (less than 10%). The serum ferritin is normal or elevated, and bone marrow iron stores are normal or increased. Treatment with erythropoietin can sometimes be helpful in certain patients (e.g., those with cancer, HIV infection, rheumatoid arthritis) who have severe, symptomatic anemia if the serum erythropoietin level is less than 500 IU/mL (and especially if it is less than 100 IU/mL) (40–42).

In addition to chronic infections, acute infection or inflammation causes a decrease in serum iron, reticulocytopenia, and a decrease in bone marrow red cell production. If present for 1 week or longer, an acute inflammatory process may result in a fall in the Hct of several percentage points.

Mild Early Iron Deficiency

Although severe iron deficiency results in microcytic anemia (discussed earlier), in the early stages mild iron deficiency may result in anemia with a normal peripheral smear and a normal MCV. Diagnosis can usually be made by measurement of serum ferritin or by a bone marrow iron stain. In addition, a patient with severe iron deficiency, when it accompanies a macrocytic anemia such as a megaloblastic anemia (e.g., an alcoholic patient with iron deficiency and folic acid deficiency) may have a severe anemia that is normocytic. The reticulocyte count is inappropriately low until (in the alcoholic patient) alcohol is withdrawn and iron and folate are administered.

Anemia in the Elderly

Old age *per se* is not an explanation for a significant normocytic anemia (43). The Hct in healthy patients in their seventies is only slightly lower than the normal adult range (Table 55.1). However, it is in elderly patients that frustrating, mild, unexplained, normocytic anemias occur. In such patients the following possible explanations should be considered: fluid overload, blood loss from phlebotomy if the patient has been hospitalized recently, and any recent inflammatory disease (viral or bacterial infection, inflammatory joint problem) that may depress bone marrow production and, if present for several days, may result in a drop in Hct. If none of these explanations seems appropriate and there is no reason to suspect an underlying problem, it is reasonable simply to monitor the Hct without further diagnostic workup. If it is known that the onset of the anemia is recent (e.g., if there is a record of a normal Hct finding 3 months previously), other efforts should be made to explain it. For example, the possibility of occult gastrointestinal bleeding with early iron deficiency or the anemia of chronic disease or malignancy should be entertained. There is evidence that unexplained anemias are more common in elderly poor persons with inadequate access to health care and that in the very old anemia is associated with an increased mortality risk (44).

General References*

Charache S, Johnson CS, eds. Sickle cell disease. Hematol Clin North Am 1996;10:1221.

Hoffman R, Benz EJ, Shattil SJ, et al., eds. Hematology: Basic Principles and Practice. 3rd ed. New York: Churchill Livingstone, 2000.

Waterbury L. Hematology. 4th ed. Baltimore, MD: Williams & Wilkins, 1996.

Specific References

1. Cook JD. Clinical evaluation of iron deficiency. Semin Hematol 1982;19:6.
2. England JM, Ward S, Down MC. Microcytosis, anisocytosis and the red cell indices in iron deficiency. Br J Haematol 1976;34:589.
3. Suominen P, Punnonen K, Rajamaki A, et al. Serum transferrin receptor and transferrin receptor-ferritin index identify healthy subjects with subclinical iron deficits. Blood 1998;92:2934.
4. Junca J, Fernandez-Aviles F, Oriol A, et al. The usefulness of serum transferring receptor in detecting iron deficiency in the anemia of chronic disorders. Haematologica 1998;83:676.
5. Halliday JW, Powell LW. Serum ferritin and isoferritins in clinical medicine. Prog Hematol 1979;11:229.
6. Faich G, Strobos J. Sodium ferric gluconate complex in sucrose: safer intravenous iron therapy than iron dextrans. Am J Kidney Dis 1999;33:464.
7. Pierce HI, Kurachi S, Sofroniadou K, et al. Frequencies of thalassemia in American blacks. Blood 1977;49:981.
8. Kaiser L, Schwartz KA. Aluminum induced anemia. Am J Kidney Dis 1985;5:348.
9. Davidson RJL, Hamilton PJ. High mean red cell volume: its incidence and significance in routine hematology. J Clin Pathol 1978;31:493.
10. Colman N, Herbert J. Hematologic complications of alcoholism: overview. Semin Hematol 1980;17:164.
11. Lindenbaum J. Status of laboratory testing in the diagnosis of megaloblastic anemia. Blood 1983;61:624.

---

*Bold print (general references) and bold numerals (specific references) denote published controlled clinical trials, meta-analyses, or consensus-based recommendations.

12. Lindenbaum J, Healton EB, Savage DG, et al. Neuropsychiatric disorders caused by cobalamin deficiency in the absence of anemia or macrocytosis. N Engl J Med 1988;318:1720.
13. Carmel R, Sinow RM, Siegel ME, et al. Food cobalamin malabsorption occurs frequently in patients with unexplained low serum cobalamin levels. Arch Intern Med 1988;148:1715.
14. Kuzminski AM, De Giacco EJ, Allen RH, et al. Effective treatment of cobalamin deficiency with oral cobalamin. Blood 1998;92:1191.
15. Ganser A, Haelyer D. Clinical course of myelodysplastic syndromes. Hematol Oncol Clin North Am 1992;6:607.
16. Collins PW, Newland AC. Treatment modalities of autoimmune blood disorders. Semin Hematol 1992;29:64.
17. Pirofsky G. Clinical aspects of autoimmune hemolytic anemia. Semin Hematol 1976;13:251.
18. Salama A, Mueller-Eckhardt C. Immune-mediated blood cell dyscrasias related to drugs. Semin Hematol 1992;29:54.
19. Jacobson LB, Longstreth GF, Edgington TS. Clinical and immunologic features of transient cold agglutinin hemolytic anemia. Am J Med 1973;54:514.
20. Jefferies LC. Transfusion therapy in autoimmune hemolytic anemias. Hematol Clin North Am 1994;8:1087.
21. Brain MC. Microangiopathic hemolytic anemia. N Engl J Med 1969;281:833.
22. Dameshek W. Hypersplenism. Bull N Y Acad Med 1955;31: 113.
23. Beutler E. Glucose-6-phosphate dehydrogenase deficiency. N Engl J Med 1991;324:169.
24. Abramson H, Bertles JF, Wethers DL, eds. Sickle cell disease. St Louis: Mosby, 1973.
25. Charache S. Treatment of sickle cell anemia. Annu Rev Med 1981;32:195.
26. Vichinsky EP. Comprehensive care in sickle cell disease: its impact on morbidity and mortality. Semin Hematol 1991;28: 220.
27. Platt OS, Brambilla DJ, Rosse WF, et al. Mortality in sickle cell disease: life expectancy and risk factors for early death. N Engl J Med 1994;330:1639.
28. King W, Nadel AJ. Ophthalmologic complications in hemoglobinopathies. Hematol Oncol Clin North Am 1991;5:535.
29. McPherson E, Perlin E, Finke H, et al. Patient-controlled analgesia in patients with sickle cell vaso-occlusive crisis. Am J Med Sci 1990;299:10.
30. Brookoff D, Polomano RA. Treating sickle cell pain. Ann Intern Med 1992;116:364.
31. Charache S, Barton FB, Moore RD. Hydroxyurea and sickle cell anemia: clinical utility of a myelosuppressive "switching" agent. The Multicenter Study of Hydroxyurea in Sickle Cell Anemia. Medicine (Baltimore) 1996;75:300.
32. Walters MC, Storb R, Patience M, et al. Impact of bone marrow transplantation for symptomatic sickle cell disease: an interim report. Blood 2000;95:1918.
33. Vichinsky EP, Earles A, Johnson RA, et al. Alloimmunization in sickle cell anemia and transfusion of racially unmatched blood. N Engl J Med 1990;322:1617.
34. Vichinsky EP, Haberkern CM, Neumayr L, et al. A comparison of conservative and aggressive transfusion regimens in the perioperative management of sickle cell disease: the Preoperative Transfusion in Sickle Cell Disease Study Group. N Engl J Med 1995;333:206.
35. Erslev AJ. Management of anemia of chronic renal failure. Clin Nephrol 1974;2:174.
36. Eschbach JW, Eqrie JC, Downing MR, et al. Correction of the anemia of end-stage renal disease with recombinant human erythropoietin: results of a combined phase I and II clinical trial. N Engl J Med 1987;316:73.
37. Cartwright GE. The anemia of chronic disorders. Semin Hematol 1966;3:351.
38. Cash JM, Sears DA. The anemia of chronic disease: spectrum of associated diseases in a series of unselected hospitalized patients. Am J Med 1989;87:638.
39. Means R, Krantz SB. Progress in understanding the pathogenesis of the anemia of chronic disease. Blood 1992;80:1639.
40. Henry DH, Beall GN, Benson CFA, et al. Recombinant human erythropoietin in the treatment of anemia associated with human immunodeficiency virus (HIV) infection and zidovudine therapy. Ann Intern Med 1992;117:739.
41. Ludwig H, Fritz E, Leitgeb C, et al. Prediction of response to erythropoietin treatment in chronic anemia of cancer. Blood 1994;84:1056.
42. Pincus T, Olsen NJ, Russell I, et al. Multicenter study of recombinant human erythropoietin in correction of anemia in rheumatoid arthritis. Am J Med 1990;89:161.
43. Lipschitz DA, Udupa KB, Milton KY, et al. Effects of age on hematopoiesis in man. Blood 1984;63:502.
44. Izaks GJ, Westendorp RG, Knook DL. The definition of anemia in older persons. JAMA 1999;281:1714.

CHAPTER 56

Disorders of Hemostasis

LARRY WATERBURY, MD
PHILIP D. ZIEVE, MD

In a healthy person a number of different processes interact to ensure that blood is maintained in a fluid state until the integrity of a blood vessel wall is compromised; at that point, a plug is rapidly formed to prevent exsanguination. Three major systems are involved in this regard: the vasculature itself, the blood platelets, and the coagulation system.

EVALUATION OF PATIENTS

The history is the most important aid in determining whether a patient has a hemorrhagic diathesis (1). Patients with congenital disorders of hemostasis or acquired disorders of long standing almost certainly have had unexpectedly excessive bleeding in response to minor trauma or to surgery. The clinician should ask

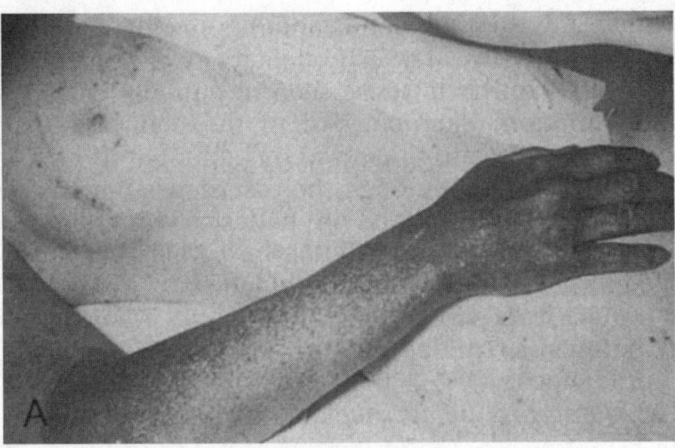

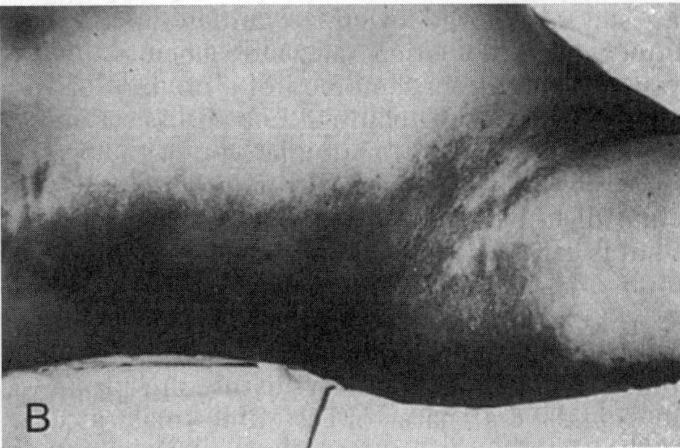

Figure 56.1. Bleeding caused by thrombocytopenia compared with bleeding caused by abnormal coagulation. **A:** Immune thrombocytopenic purpura with typical petechial lesion. **B:** Hemophilia A with extensive purpuric bleeding. (From Zieve PD, Levin J. Disorders of hemostasis. Philadelphia: W.B. Saunders, 1976, with permission.)

Table 56.1. Laboratory Evaluation of Hemostatic Function

System	Screening Tests	Specific Tests
Blood vessels	None	Depends on suspected underlying disorder (see text)
Platelets		
Quantitative	Scanning of a stained smear of the peripheral blood	Platelet count
Qualitative	Bleeding time	Platelet aggregation
Coagulation	Partial thromboplastin time, prothrombin time, thrombin time	Factor assays

specifically whether the patient has required transfusion after an operative procedure or a seemingly minor trauma.

Bleeding caused by injury to the vasculature is overwhelmingly more common than bleeding caused by defective hemostasis. Therefore, patients with gastrointestinal or genitourinary hemorrhage, for example, are more likely to have a lesion (e.g., a peptic ulcer, carcinoma, diverticulum, or tumor of the kidney or of the bladder) that has bled than a disorder of hemostasis. Similarly, nosebleeds, bleeding gums, or excessive menstrual flow probably reflect local (usually benign) problems. Furthermore, even if patients have hemostatic dysfunction, they are likely to bleed from local lesions, the propensity to bleed of which has been accentuated by the hemostatic abnormality.

Specific disorders of hemostasis may be suspected strongly on the basis of the patient's history and because of characteristic findings on physical examination (Fig. 56.1; see below), but in almost all instances, laboratory tests are required before a specific diagnosis can be made. Screening tests, procedures that are extremely sensitive to alterations in hemostasis, are ordinarily relied on first in a patient with a suspected hemorrhagic diathesis (Table 56.1). If any of these tests are abnormal or if it is strongly suspected that a disorder of hemostasis exists, even if the tests are not abnormal, more specific tests are indicated; these are best performed in consultation with a hematologist.

DISORDERS OF BLOOD VESSELS

Vascular disease is diagnosed uncommonly as a cause of a hemorrhagic diathesis, in part because, except for trauma, disorders of the vasculature that result in untoward bleeding are rare (2), and in part because there is no reliable screening test to detect generalized vascular dysfunction. The primary hemorrhagic manifestation of vascular disease is purpura, a confluent purplish discoloration of the skin caused by extravasation of blood from cutaneous and subcutaneous blood vessels. Although patients with an abnormal vasculature may occasionally experience bleeding from large blood vessels, most commonly they bleed into the skin or mucous membranes. Because purpura is a common response to minor trauma, it cannot in itself be taken as evidence of an underlying hemorrhagic diathesis.

Cutaneous Lesions

Unexplained bruises, especially on the lower extremities, are common and usually are not associated with an underlying disease process. A history of easy bruising therefore is unlikely, in itself, to lead to a diagnosis of a disorder of hemostasis. Similarly, *senile purpura,* which occurs characteristically on the dorsum of the hand and the extensor surfaces of the forearms, does not represent a generalized hemorrhagic diathesis but results from the loss of connective tissue support to intracutaneous blood vessels, which then are easily traumatized and bleed within the substance of the skin. Identical lesions are seen sometimes in patients with Cushing syndrome or in patients who have received corticosteroid therapy.

Allergic purpura (3,4) is a hypersensitivity reaction to an antigenic stimulus that usually cannot be identified (although sometimes a drug or an infection can be incriminated as a provocative agent). Characteristically, patients develop a symmetric petechial rash, which is most prominent on the extremities. The lesions are slightly raised, distinguishing them from the petechiae of thrombocytopenia. No hemostatic dysfunction is associated with this condition; the cutaneous manifestations of the disorder are part of a widespread small-vessel vasculitis, the manifestations of which also may include arthralgias (sometimes with evidence of joint effusions), fever, malaise, abdominal pain, gastrointestinal bleeding, and renal disease caused by a focal glomerulonephritis that occasionally may progress to chronic renal failure. There is no specific treatment for this condition; although if the patient is taking a drug that is suspected to be a sensitizing agent, it should be discontinued. In fact, because the offending agent is often not readily identified, the administration of all drugs that are not absolutely essential to care should be discontinued. Most patients recover spontaneously within 3 or 4 weeks, but sometimes signs and symptoms of the disease continue or recur for up to a year. Patients should be reassured while they are symptomatic that unless they have evidence of progressive renal disease, they will ultimately recover.

Autoerythrocyte sensitization (5) is a disorder, predominantly of women, characterized by apparently spontaneous painful ecchymoses, usually on the lower extremities and anterior trunk. The disorder is named as it is because of a belief at one time that it arose as the result of a hypersensitivity response to the patients' red cells or red cell stroma, and in fact the lesions can sometimes be produced by injection of autologous red cells into the skin of these patients. It has become apparent, however, that virtually all patients with the disorder are severely psychoneurotic and, in some instances, frankly psychotic; many people believe now that the lesions are self-inflicted.

Cryoglobulinemia (6) as a primary abnormality or as a special feature of an underlying disease such as dysproteinemia (see Dysproteinemia later in this chapter), lymphoma, or collagen vascular disease may also cause purpuric bleeding, especially on the lower extremities. The cryoglobulins may be isolated monoclonal proteins or may be immune complexes of monoclonal IgG or IgM and polyclonal IgG or of mixed polyclonal immunoglobulins. There is often an associated glomerulonephritis and, in the patient with immune complex formation, sometimes evidence of hepatitis B or hepatitis C infection.

The diagnosis of cryoglobulinemia may be made by placing a sample of the patient's serum in a refrigerator overnight and then inspecting the serum to see whether a white gel or precipitate has formed that disappears when the specimen is warmed. The blood for this test should be drawn in a warm syringe and then allowed to clot and retract in a 37°C water bath. Primary cryoglobulinemia is poorly responsive to treatment; secondary cryoglobulinemia may respond to treatment of the underlying disease.

Patients with other vasculitides sometimes also present with petechia-like lesions and systemic disease (e.g., renal or pulmonary disease) typically much more severe than it is in patients with allergic purpura. These conditions are sometimes associated with antineutrophilic cytoplasmic antibodies. Such patients are best managed in consultation with a rheumatologist.

Mucocutaneous Lesions

Some patients with vascular disease are prone to bleeding from the oral, nasal, or gastrointestinal mucosa, as well as from the skin. Such patients may present to their providers not only with cutaneous hemorrhage but with bleeding gums, epistaxis, hematemesis, or melena.

Amyloidosis

Mucocutaneous bleeding may be a symptom of amyloidosis because of the deposition of amyloid within the walls of blood vessels (7). Periorbital bleeding and bleeding in skin folds are especially common. The skin in the areas of hemorrhage sometimes appears thickened because of palpable amyloid deposits within it. Patients suspected of having this disorder should have biopsies with appropriate staining and serum and urine electrophoresis in an attempt to make a specific diagnosis.

Dysproteinemia

Myeloma or macroglobulinemia may be associated with untoward bleeding, either because of increased viscosity of the blood or because the coating of blood vessels and platelets with the abnormal protein interferes with normal hemostatic function (8). Abnormal coagulation is also common in patients with these disorders. Patients suspected of having dysproteinemia should have samples of their serum and urine examined by electrophoresis in an attempt to demonstrate a monoclonal protein. If the diagnosis of dysproteinemia seems likely on the basis of this test and the clinical presentation, consultation with a hematologist or oncologist is appropriate.

Vitamin C Deficiency

There are three situations in which symptomatic vitamin C deficiency (scurvy) might be seen in this country: in chronic alcoholics, food faddists, and chronically ill or debilitated patients (9). Because humans, unlike most animals, are unable to synthesize vitamin C, they depend on exogenous sources such as fruits or leafy vegetables. People who cannot or will not eat an adequate diet of foods that contain the vitamin are subject to the manifestations of scurvy. The signs and symptoms of scurvy are attributable largely to the formation of defective connective tissue, because of the human body's absolute dependence on vitamin C for the synthesis of normal collagen. Mucocutaneous bleeding is common in patients with vitamin C deficiency who characteristically have large ecchymoses on their extremities, bleeding gums, and, very suggestive of this disorder, perifollicular hemorrhages that appear commonly on the lower extremities and anterior trunk. Sometimes patients with vitamin C deficiency develop hemarthroses similar to those seen in patients with severe coagulation disorders. All manifestations of scurvy are readily reversed by administration of vitamin C, so that although the disorder is uncommon it should be considered in patients with compatible signs and symptoms. Vitamin C deficiency can be confirmed by assay of the blood, but this is usually unnecessary because if the diagnosis is suspected, a therapeutic trial of vitamin C (250 mg once a day) is innocuous.

Hereditary Hemorrhagic Telangiectasia

Hereditary hemorrhagic telangiectasia is an inherited abnormality of blood vessels (an autosomal dominant condition) in which there is dilation of abnormally thin-walled venules and capillaries (10). The dilations result in characteristic telangiectases, which are small, flat, red, or purple lesions that blanch on pressure. They occur throughout the body but can be seen externally most commonly on the lips, tongue, hand, and mucous membranes of the nose. Lesions of larger blood vessels also occur in this disease, most commonly pulmonary arteriovenous fistulas, which develop in up to one-third of patients and may cause high-output heart failure. Vascular malformations of the liver or the brain also may occur. The mucocutaneous lesions may bleed excessively when traumatized. Recurrent epistaxis is the most common symptom of patients with the disorder, but the most troublesome problem is recurrent gastrointestinal bleeding, which is difficult to manage. Accessible lesions can ordinarily be treated by local compression. No pharmacologic agent will alter the course of the condition, but symptoms are variable; many patients experience little difficulty during the course of their life.

DISORDERS OF PLATELETS

Platelets provide a cellular defense against the loss of blood from traumatized vessels, especially where blood flow is relatively rapid, as it is on the arterial side of the circulation and in the left heart. Platelets are particularly effective in sealing leaks from small arterioles and capillaries; when platelets are abnormal, either quantitatively or qualitatively, these vessels bleed most prominently. The platelet plug is initiated by contact of platelets with subendothelial collagen, which is exposed by injury to the vascular intima. The absorption of a protein, von Willebrand factor (see below), to specific receptor sites on the platelet surface is important in the mediation of this process. Thereafter, aggregating agents such as thrombin and adenosine diphosphate cause the accretion of platelets at that site, eventually forming an adhesive plug that within minutes prevents the further flow of blood. Eventually, the plug is replaced by fibrin laid down by the activation of the coagulation mechanism, which occurs simultaneously with the initiation of platelet plug formation.

Thrombocytopenia is one of the most common acquired disorders of hemostasis. The normal platelet count is between 150,000 and 400,000/mm^3, but the platelet count ordinarily must be reduced to below 50,000/mm^3 before untoward bleeding is observed, and even then bleeding usually does not occur unless the patient is traumatized. So-called spontaneous bleeding is unlikely unless the platelet count is reduced below 20,000/mm^3. There is a general impression that there is a higher risk of bleeding when thrombocytopenia is secondary to decreased bone marrow production rather than to decreased survival of platelets. For example, patients with immune thrombocytopenia may not have significant bleeding even with platelet counts as low as 5,000/mm^3. At any given platelet count, the risk of bleeding varies with the cause of thrombocytopenia.

The characteristic lesion of thrombocytopenia is the petechia, a small purpuric hemorrhage occurring on the skin or mucous membranes, especially at sites of elevated capillary pressure, such as the lower extremities, the forearm after inflation of a blood pressure cuff, or the face after prolonged crying or coughing. In fact, if capillary pressure is raised high enough or if capillaries are damaged after sunburn, for example, petechiae may be seen in otherwise normal people. Although cutaneous bleeding may be the first clue to the diagnosis of thrombocytopenia, morbidity from the disorder is more likely to result from gastrointestinal or genitourinary hemorrhage. As previously mentioned, if bleeding from these sites occurs, the patient should be examined at an appropriate time to determine whether an organic lesion, such as a carcinoma of the colon or of the kidney, has bled in association with defective hemostasis. The most feared complication of thrombocytopenia is intracerebral bleeding that, although it occurs infrequently, is still one of the major causes of death in patients with the disorder.

Evaluation of the Thrombocytopenic Patient

The best screening test for the evaluation of the numbers of platelets in the blood is observation of a stained smear of the peripheral blood. With relatively little experience it is easy to determine whether the platelet count is unusually low or high. In un-anticoagulated blood (e.g., from a fingerstick), at least one clump of platelets should be seen, on the average, in every oil immersion field. In anticoagulated blood, one platelet should be seen for every 10 to 20 red cells. If a quantitative abnormality is suspected, a precise platelet count can be obtained. The bleeding time is not useful as a screening test for detecting quantitative abnormalities of platelets or for predicting which patients are likely to bleed excessively when traumatized (11). However, despite its limitations, the bleeding time is still used commonly to evaluate qualitative abnormalities of platelet function, described later in this chapter.

Patients with an immune thrombocytopenia (see below) characteristically have increased amounts of gamma globulin adsorbed to their platelets. Tests to detect these proteins are widely available but have proved to be nonspecific and therefore of little value in establishing a precise diagnosis.

In ambulatory practice, many patients are encountered with mild thrombocytopenia, the precise pathophysiology of which is not clear. Many patients are found to have thrombocytopenia during the course of routine hematologic studies performed to obtain baseline data or as part of an evaluation of an apparently unrelated condition. The first task for the clinician is to rule out spurious thrombocytopenia secondary to marked platelet clumping affecting the accuracy of the automated platelet count. This artifact is usually secondary to antibodies to the anticoagulant used to obtain blood for a complete blood count. When spurious thrombocytopenia is suspected, blood should be collected using another anticoagulant (usually citrate) and the platelet count should be repeated. The technician should inspect a smear from anticoagulated blood for increased clumping. Once spurious thrombocytopenia has been ruled out, if the platelet count is more than 50,000/mm^3 in such circumstances and the history, physical examination, and other hematologic evaluations do not suggest an underlying disease that urgently requires diagnosis and treatment, it is probably justifiable simply to follow the patient with serial platelet counts performed monthly until it is determined how stable the counts are.

Symptomatic thrombocytopenia caused by decreased production of platelets is usually observed in conjunction with processes such as aplastic anemia, leukemia, myelodysplasia, disseminated tuberculosis, or metastatic carcinoma that affect other hematologic cell lines. In contrast, severe thrombocytopenia caused by increased destruction of platelets does not necessarily indicate the presence of a disease process that is affecting parts or systems of the body other than the blood platelets or their precursors. To be reasonably certain about the pathophysiology of thrombocytopenia, however, it is sometimes necessary to perform an aspiration of the bone marrow and to evaluate the numbers of megakaryocytes and the appearance of the other blood-cell precursors. Patients who have thrombocytopenia because of diseases involving the bone marrow, except in cases of megaloblastic anemia, have reduced numbers of megakaryocytes. If the thrombocytopenia is severe, it is likely that abnormalities of production of, or qualitative changes in, other cell lines also will be noted. On the other hand, if the patient is thrombocytopenic because of increased destruction of platelets, the numbers of megakaryocytes will be increased and the marrow will otherwise appear normal (although increased erythroid activity might be seen in those patients who are bleeding). It has been proposed (12,13) that bone marrow aspiration need not be done routinely in patients with isolated thrombocytopenia (thought to be immune mediated). In any case, patients with severe thrombocytopenia (<30,000/mm^3) require consultation with a hematologist.

Decreased Production of Platelets

Decreased production of platelets is a common mechanism for thrombocytopenia in ambulatory patients (Table 56.2). Apparent suppression of thrombopoiesis is often associated with viral infections such as upper respiratory infections, infectious mononucleosis, and childhood exanthems. In most cases, bone marrow aspirates show megakaryocytes in normal or reduced numbers, although they sometimes appear morphologically abnormal. At other times, increased numbers of megakaryocytes are seen, suggestive of a destructive process (perhaps immunologic) to which the marrow has responded with increased production of platelets. In general, patients with benign *viral infections* are not likely to have severe thrombocytopenia and so are not at major risk of bleeding. The process ordinarily dissipates as the infection resolves.

Table 56.2. Etiology of Thrombocytopenia by Mechanism

Decreased production
Primary bone marrow disorders (leukemia, myelodysplasia, aplastic anemia, myeloma)
Replacement (by metastatic cancer, etc.)
Infection
Drugs
Ineffective myelopoiesis
Megaloblastic anemia
Decreased survival/increased sequestion
Immune thrombocytopenia
Thrombotic thrombocytopenic purpura/hemolytic-uremic syndrome
Disseminated intravascular coagulation
Large spleen syndrome

Certain drugs predictably produce thrombocytopenia by affecting thrombopoiesis. Among these, cytotoxic agents are unlikely to be administered by the general practitioner. Although thiazide diuretics have been reported to produce mild to moderate thrombocytopenia commonly, a clear-cut cause and effect relationship has not been demonstrated. In the reported studies, platelet counts have fallen several weeks after the beginning of therapy, sometimes associated with morphologically abnormal megakaryocytes. Rarely, however, thiazides have been clearly implicated in immunologically induced destructive thrombocytopenia (see Increased Destruction of Platelets, below). Thiazide diuretics also are a common cause of allergic purpura (see above), but patients with this condition have normal platelet counts.

A large number of drugs have been implicated, on occasion, in the production of thrombocytopenia by the suppression of thrombopoiesis. Therefore, if patients are symptomatic from thrombocytopenia or have counts below 50,000/mm^3 and the cause of thrombocytopenia is unknown, it would be reasonable to discontinue administration of all drugs that are not considered absolutely essential.

Management

Clearly, if the cause of the decreased platelet production can be removed (e.g., discontinuing administration of an offending drug), that should be done. If there is no evidence of mucous membrane or internal bleeding, treatment of the thrombocytopenia itself usually is unnecessary. Patients with severe bleeding should receive platelet transfusions when thrombocytopenia is due to decreased platelet production and counts are less than 50,000/mm^3. Some patients with chronic diseases of the bone marrow, such as myelodysplasia or aplastic anemia, may require periodic platelet

Table 56.3. Immune Thrombocytopenia

Primary (ITP, autoimmune thrombocytopenia)
Secondary immune thrombocytopenia
Acute
Viral infections
Drugs (e.g., quinine, quinidine, sulfa, heparin)
Posttransfusion purpura
Chronic
Collagen vascular disorders (e.g., lupus, scleroderma)
Lymphoproliferative disorders (chronic lymphocytic leukemia, lymphoma, macroglobulinemia, Hodgkin disease)
Other autoimmune disorders (e.g., Hashimoto thyroiditis, Graves disease, sarcoidosis, biliary cirrhosis)

ITP, idiopathic thrombocytopenic purpura.

transfusions. Such patients should be followed by a hematologist or an oncologist as well as by a primary caregiver.

Increased Destruction of Platelets

In ambulatory practice probably the most common cause of thrombocytopenia is thrombocytopenia secondary to an immune mechanism (Table 56.3). Patients with *autoimmune thrombocytopenia* (12–14) characteristically present with petechiae. Physical examination reveals no other evidence of disease; in particular, the spleen usually is not palpable. It is helpful to look at platelet morphology on a peripheral blood smear. Typically, platelets are large and sometimes elongated in severe destructive thrombocytopenia as opposed to the small platelets seen when the thrombocytopenia is due to decreased production. The smear should be made with blood from a fingerstick because anticoagulants cause platelets to swell. Bone marrow aspirates appear normal except for increased numbers of megakaryocytes. An acute disease, often preceded by an otherwise benign viral infection, is seen more commonly in children and, by definition, lasts less than 6 months. The chronic illness (often still called idiopathic thrombocytopenic purpura) lasts longer than 6 months and is seen more often in women than men (ratio of 3 or 4 to 1). It sometimes is associated with an underlying lymphoproliferative disorder or a collagen vascular disease, especially systemic lupus erythematosus and, more rarely, autoimmune hemolytic anemia. There is an increased incidence of immune thrombocytopenia in association with human immunodeficiency virus (HIV) infection (15) (see Chapter 39). Autoimmune thrombocytopenia has been shown to be caused by an antibody adsorbed to the surface of circulating platelets that results in their premature destruction by the reticuloendothelial system. It has been demonstrated that the disorder is characterized by ineffective production of platelets as well (16).

Many drugs (17) have been associated with thrombocytopenia on an immunologic basis. Heparin is the drug most commonly implicated (see Chapter 57). Many other drugs (e.g., quinine, quinidine, and sulfa) have been implicated rarely. Also, several cases have been reported in which heroin addicts have thrombocytopenia of an immune type, apparently produced by heroin (or an adulterant used with it). If a patient presents to the practitioner with severe thrombocytopenia caused by increased destruction of circulating platelets, it is important to ask what drugs the patient is taking and to consider stopping them if there is any question that the drugs are involved in the process.

It is not unusual for *alcoholics* to develop thrombocytopenia, usually to a moderate degree, after a binge. Alcohol appears to damage platelet membranes, causing their premature destruction, and to inhibit compensatory increase in platelet production by marrow megakaryocytes. Once the binge is over, the platelet count returns to normal (or transiently higher than normal) in 4 to 5 days. Alcoholics of long standing who have developed cirrhosis of the liver and portal hypertension may have chronic thrombocytopenia because of increased sequestration of platelets in their spleens.

Management

An American Society of Hematology Practice Guidelines Panel has made recommendations about the treatment of autoimmune thrombocytopenia (12,13). The panel found no experimental evidence on which recommendations could be based, so they resorted to achieving a consensus among experts. The recommendations that follow are not precisely those of the panel but are consistent with its views. If the platelet count is less than 20,000/mm^3, treatment should be instituted immediately with the equivalent of 60 to 100 mg (1 mg/kg of body weight) of prednisone, even if the patient is asymptomatic or has only a few petechiae. Patients with mucous membrane or internal bleeding should be hospitalized; patients with severe internal bleeding should receive intravenous gamma globulin (which corrects immune thrombocytopenia more rapidly than do corticosteroids) in the hospital as well. Such bleeding will usually not occur if the platelet count is over 30,000/mm^3. In general, the risk of major bleeding appears greater in elderly patients (18,19).

Most patients with platelet counts of 20,000 to 30,000/mm^3 or less because of chronic immune thrombocytopenia ultimately require splenectomy. Treatment of immune thrombocytopenia in patients with HIV infection is the same as it is for patients who do not have HIV infection, but in the former group zidovudine, 1 g/day, also has been shown to be effective (20,21).

Although approximately 70% of patients respond within days to corticosteroids with a rise in platelet count sufficient to maintain adequate hemostasis, most relapse as the dosage is tapered. (A reasonable schedule is to reduce the dosage by 10 mg/day each week to half the initial dosage and then by 5 mg/day each week.) If patients do not respond to corticosteroids initially, if mucous membrane or internal bleeding recurs, or if the platelet count falls below 30,000/mm^3 as the dosage of corticosteroids is tapered, splenectomy is indicated. Adequate platelet counts (greater than 50,000/mm^3) are maintained in approximately 80% of splenectomized patients.

Increased Sequestration of Platelets

Patients with large spleens often have thrombocytopenia because of redistribution of platelets within a larger splenic pool, most commonly because of congestive splenomegaly associated with portal hypertension. Splenectomy reverses thrombocytopenia but is rarely indicated, because usually the thrombocytopenia is not severe and splenectomy should be considered only if there is a clear-cut hemorrhagic diathesis and if the underlying disease responsible for the enlarged spleen permits an operation to be performed.

Increased Use of Platelets

Patients with disseminated intravascular coagulation characteristically have thrombocytopenia, almost always in association with multiple defects in coagulation. Such patients often present acutely ill because of the underlying disease that has incited the hemostatic disorder. For example, in patients with various complications of pregnancy, with disseminated carcinoma, or in some patients with septicemia, hemostatic mechanisms have been activated because of exposure of the circulating blood to thromboplastic material. The hemorrhagic diathesis is manifest most commonly by widespread bruising, petechiae, and mucous membrane bleeding, occasionally, but not often, associated with evidence of venous or arterial thrombosis. In addition to thrombocytopenia, patients have disordered coagulation, which can be identified by measuring the prothrombin time, the partial thromboplastin time, and the concentration of fibrinogen in the plasma, and by the demonstration of increased titers of fibrinogen and fibrin degradation products in the plasma or serum. These products are formed by the lysis of fibrinogen and fibrin by plasmin, the major proteolytic enzyme of the blood. Patients who are strongly suspected of having disseminated intravascular coagulation or in whom the diagnosis has been made should be hospitalized for further treatment and to identify and treat the underlying disease.

Qualitative Disorders of Platelets

A number of inherited abnormalities of platelets have been identified that result in impaired hemostasis even though platelet counts are often within normal limits. In general, the hemorrhagic diathesis associated with these conditions is milder than it is in patients with severe thrombocytopenia. Practitioners are unlikely to see these patients, but if patients have unexplained bleeding, such as purpura, epistaxis, or menorrhagia, with apparently normal coagulation and normal or slightly reduced platelet counts, it is reasonable to perform a bleeding time (see below), which is often abnormal in patients with qualitatively abnormal platelets. Similar abnormalities may be acquired in patients with various disease states (22), most commonly uremia; in fact, patients with chronic renal failure who have a tendency to bleed often improve after hemodialysis.

Perhaps the most common acquired qualitative disorder of blood platelets occurs after the ingestion of aspirin, which often prolongs the bleeding time and irreversibly interferes with platelet aggregation and the release of certain intracellular platelet constituents. Although untoward bleeding is unusual in patients who have taken aspirin, the drug may intensify a preexisting tendency to bleed. Other nonsteroidal anti-inflammatory drugs also may impair platelet function, but, compared with aspirin, the effect is even less predictable and is more quickly reversible when the drug is stopped.

Patient Experience. The bleeding time should be performed using a commercially available, spring-loaded, disposable device (Simplate) that makes a small incision in the forearm. The examiner should puncture the skin with the disposable lancet. A blood pressure cuff should be inflated to 40 mm Hg above the elbow during the test. The time between the instant the puncture is made and the point at which blood from the wound can no longer be adsorbed onto a piece of filter paper is the bleeding time (normally 2 to 9 minutes). The patient should be warned of the very transient sharp pain that will be experienced when the wound is made and of the small scar, usually inapparent, that may form when the wound heals.

Thrombocytosis

Platelet counts above 400,000 mm^3, unless associated with a myeloproliferative disorder such as polycythemia vera, myeloid metaplasia, or chronic granulocytic leukemia, are not in themselves associated with an increased risk of morbidity from excessive bleeding or clotting. However, they may signify the presence of an underlying disease that requires attention. If thrombocytosis exists, the most common causes are *inflammatory disease* and *solid tumor malignancies.* Other causes include the post splenectomy state, acute bleeding, inflammatory bowel disease, and severe chronic iron deficiency. In secondary thrombocytosis, the platelet count is usually (but not always) less than $1,000,000/mm^3$.

Patients with chronic myeloproliferative disorders (polycythemia vera, primary myelofibrosis, essential thrombocythemia), if they have thrombocytosis, usually have large distorted platelets on smear and other hematologic abnormalities typical of the particular disease. Many of those patients also have splenomegaly. The platelet counts may be over $1,000,000/mm^3$. The treatment of thrombocytosis associated with chronic myeloproliferative disease should be planned in consultation with a hematologist.

COAGULATION DISORDERS

The generation of a solid fibrin clot from circulating soluble fibrinogen is the body's major defense against the loss of blood from the vasculature, especially from blood vessels larger than the capillary, arteriole, and venule. Coagulation is initiated by the exposure of proteins to thromboplastic substances (tissue factor) when blood vessels are injured. Thereafter, a series of enzymatic reactions occurs that results in the conversion of fibrinogen by the proteolytic enzyme thrombin to fibrin. The best screening tests to detect abnormalities of clotting are the activated partial thromboplastin time (aPTT) and the prothrombin time (PT). The aPTT and the PT measure different phases of the early parts of the coagulation process, but both measure the later phase of the process—the conversion of prothrombin to thrombin and the subsequent conversion of fibrinogen to fibrin.

There are enzymatic mechanisms that oppose coagulation and prevent unwarranted widespread clotting of the blood when a blood vessel is injured. A number of cases have been reported of patients with an increased tendency to thrombosis and low levels of activity of one of the various protease inhibitors that normally circulate in the blood and regulate coagulation (see Chapter 57). *The fibrinolytic system* generates the proteolytic enzyme plasmin, which adsorbs to the clots and results in their ultimate dissolution. Fibrinolytic therapy is commonly used in the treatment of various thrombotic diseases (e.g., acute myocardial infarction), but such therapy requires hospitalization.

Patients who have a deficiency of one or more of the coagulation proteins are more likely to have extensive soft tissue bleeding or major hemorrhage in response to trauma than are patients with disorders of the vasculature or of blood platelets (petechiae, discussed earlier in this chapter, are never a sign of abnormal coagulation). Hereditary disorders of coagulation are rare. They are ordinarily readily diagnosed because of the history of life-long bleeding and, in the case of hemophilia, because of a history of characteristic hemorrhage into joints and soft tissues. Patients who have a severe hemorrhagic diathesis because of a hereditary abnormality of clotting almost always have markedly low levels of the deficient coagulation protein. Therefore, screening tests such as the aPTT are almost always abnormal and provide clues to the presence of the disorder. It is unlikely that the practitioner will encounter such patients because most of them are diagnosed in childhood and are treated by hematologists thereafter. However, if such a patient is encountered who is suspected of having a hereditary disorder of coagulation but who has not previously been diagnosed, referral to an appropriate center would be warranted.

von Willebrand disease (23,24) is an inherited abnormality of hemostasis (autosomal dominant) in which there is a reduction in the concentration or structure of a protein, the von Willebrand factor, which ordinarily binds to platelets and mediates their adhesion to subendothelial collagen in the course of platelet plug formation (see above). Normally, von Willebrand factor forms a complex with antihemophilic globulin (factor VIII:C), the protein that is deficient in the blood of patients with classic hemophilia, so that patients with von Willebrand disease often have reduced levels of factor VIII. The qualitative disorder of platelets is reflected in a prolonged bleeding time and decreased platelet adhesiveness. The platelets of these patients characteristically do not aggregate *in vitro*, as normal platelets do, when exposed to the obsolete antibiotic ristocetin. The course of the disease and the extent of the laboratory abnormalities vary from one patient to another, but in general the hemorrhagic diathesis is milder than it is in hemophilia A. Patients bleed most commonly from their gastrointestinal tract; it is not unusual that symptoms of the disease are not apparent until the patient is an adult. The bleeding time and aPTT are useful screening tests. The diagnosis and treatment of patients with von Willebrand disease require the ongoing participation of a hematologist.

Table 56.4. Advice To Give Patients with a Disorder of Hemostasis

Take only medicine prescribed by your caregiver. Do not take aspirin or cold remedies.
Take acetaminophen (e.g., Tylenol) instead of aspirin.
Avoid unnecessary trauma.
Wear an identification bracelet identifying your bleeding disorder.
Call your care giver
If you experience any abnormal bleeding.
Before you visit your dentist.
If you are hospitalized for any reason.

Acquired disorders of coagulation are more common than are congenital ones. By their nature they are more likely to be associated with multiple defects in hemostasis, such as those seen in patients with disseminated intravascular coagulation (discussed earlier in this chapter) or in patients taking anticoagulant drugs (see Chapter 57). The diagnosis and management of these problems are discussed in those sections.

Rarely, an isolated clotting factor deficiency is acquired, often in association with a lymphoproliferative or collagen vascular disease. Such a deficiency may or may not be revealed by a hemorrhagic diathesis but is almost always associated with an abnormal aPTT or an abnormal PT. Patients with unexplained long aPTTs or PTs should be referred to a hematologist for evaluation.

ADVICE TO PATIENTS WHO HAVE A DISORDER OF HEMOSTASIS

Table 56.4 lists some rules to give patients who have hemostatic dysfunction (see Chapter 57, Table 57.4). It is also important that the patient know the name of his or her disease and its clinical manifestations.

General References

Colman RW, Hirsh J, Marder VJ, et al., eds. Hemostasis and thrombosis: basic principles and clinical practice, 4th ed. Philadelphia: Lippincott Williams & Wilkins, 2000.

An authoritative exhaustively referenced text.

Jennette JC, Falk RJ. Small-vessel vasculitis. N Engl J Med 1997;337: 1512.

Ratnoff OD, Forbes CD, eds. Disorders of hemostasis. New York: Grune & Stratton, 1996.

A well-edited review.

Specific References

1. Collier BS, Schneiderman P. Clinical evaluation of hemorrhagic disorders: the bleeding history and differential diagnosis of purpura. In: Hoffman R, Benz EJ Jr, Shattil SJ, et al., eds. Hematology.

Basic principles and practice, 3rd ed. New York: Churchill Livingstone, 2000:1252.
2. Bick RL. Vascular disorders associated with thrombohemorrhagic phenomena. Semin Thromb Hemost 1979;5:167.
3. Calabrese LH, Duna GF. Drug-induced vasculitis. Curr Opin Rheumatol 1996;8:34.
4. Blanco R, Martinez-Taboada VM, Rodriguez-Valverde V, et al. Cutaneous vasculitis in children and adults: associated diseases and etiologic factors in 303 patients. Medicine 1998;77:403.
5. Ratnoff OD. The psychogenic purpuras: a review of autoerythrocyte sensitization, autosensitization to DNA, "hysterical" and factitial bleeding, and the religious stigmata. Semin Hematol 1980;17:192.
6. Monti G, Galli M, Invernizzi F, et al. Cryoglobulinaemias: a multi-centre study of the early clinical and laboratory manifestations of primary and secondary disease. QJM 1995;88:115.
7. Kyle RA, Greipp RR. Amyloidosis (AL): clinical and laboratory features in 229 cases. Mayo Clin Proc 1983;58:665.
8. Perkins HA, MacKenzie MR, Fudenberg HH. Hemostatic defects in dysproteinemias. Blood 1970;35:695.
9. Reuler JB, Broudy VC, Cooney TG. Adult scurvy. JAMA 1985; 253:805
10. Peery WH. Clinical spectrum of hereditary hemorrhagic telangiectases (Osler-Weber-Rendu disease). Am J Med 1987;82:989.
11. Rodgers RPC, Levin J. A critical reappraisal of the bleeding time. Semin Thromb Hemost 1990;16:1.
12. George JN, Woolf SH, Raskob GE, et al. Idiopathic thrombocytopenic purpura: a practice guideline developed by explicit methods for the American Society of Hematology. Blood 1996;88:3.
13. The American Society of Hematology ITP Practice Guideline Panel. Diagnosis and treatment of idiopathic thrombocytopenic purpura: recommendations of the American Society of Hematology. Ann Intern Med 1997;126:319.
14. George JN, el-Harake MA, Raskob GE. Chronic idiopathic thrombocytopenic purpura. N Engl J Med 1994;331:1207.
15. Morris L, Distenfeld A, Amorosi E, et al. Autoimmune thrombocytopenic purpura in homosexual men. Ann Intern Med 1982;96:714.
16. Gernsheimer T, Stratton J, Ballem PJ, et al. Mechanisms of response to treatment in autoimmune thrombocytopenic purpura. N Engl J Med 1989;320:974.
17. Aster RH. Drug-induced immune thrombocytopenia: an overview of pathogenesis. Semin Hematol 1999;36[1 Suppl 1]:2.
18. Guthrie TH Jr, Brannan DP, Prisant LM. Idiopathic thrombocytopenic purpura in the older adult patient. Am J Med Sci 1988;296:17.
19. Cortelazzo S, Finazzi M, Buelli M, et al. High risk of severe bleeding in aged patients with chronic idiopathic thrombocytopenic purpura. Blood 1991;77:31.
20. Walsh C, Krigel R, Lennette E, et al. Thrombocytopenia in homosexual patients. Prognosis, response to therapy, and prevalence of antibody to the retrovirus associated with acquired immune deficiency syndrome. Ann Intern Med 1985;103:542.
21. Landonio G, Cinque P, Nosari A, et al. Comparison of two dose regimens of zidovudine in an open, randomized, multicentre study for severe HIV-related thrombocytopenia. AIDS 1993;7:209.
22. George JN, Shattil SJ. The clinical importance of acquired abnormalities of platelet function. N Engl J Med 1991;324:27.
23. Ruggeri ZM, Zimmerman TS. von Willebrand factor and von Willebrand disease. Blood 1987;70:895.
24. Sadler JE. A revised classification of von Willebrand disease. For the Subcommittee on von Willebrand Factor of the Scientific and Standardization Committee of the International Society on Thrombosis and Haemostasis. Thromb Haemost 1994;71:520.

C H A P T E R 57

Thromboembolic Disease

LARRY WATERBURY, MD
PHILIP D. ZIEVE, MD

Patients with acute vascular occlusions, whether venous or arterial, may require hospitalization for initial diagnosis and treatment. However, now with the availability of low molecular weight heparin, some patients can be diagnosed and treated on an ambulatory basis by their primary caregivers. More and more the care of the patient with thromboembolic disease is the responsibility of the generalist.

VENOUS THROMBOEMBOLISM

Risk Factors

Most patients who present to the clinician with venous occlusion have formed clots in the veins of the lower extremities. The primary pathologic process is stasis of blood (e.g., as might be seen in people who are chronically ill, obese, or for other reasons lead sedentary lives or who have sustained trauma to their lower limbs). *Upper extremity deep vein thrombosis* (DVT) in ambulatory patients is uncommon but in general is associated with many of the same risk factors and complications as is lower extremity thrombosis and warrants the same diagnostic and therapeutic considerations (1). Indwelling venous catheters and overuse of the extremity are particularly associated with upper extremity venous thrombosis.

There is an association between the use of *oral contraceptive agents* and venous thromboembolism. The risk is increased three- to sixfold, even with the relatively low dose estrogen preparations now in use (2).

The risk exists only during the time the contraceptive is being used but does not increase with duration of use (3). The risk of thromboembolic disease in patients receiving postmenopausal hormonal replacement is much smaller.

Occasionally, an underlying *malignancy,* not always apparent, is associated with venous (or arterial) thromboembolic disease (1,4–6). Also occasionally, an *inherited deficiency of a naturally occurring anticoagulant* (e.g., *protein C,* an inhibitor of activated coagulation factors V and VIII; *protein S,* a cofactor in reactions that involve protein C; or *antithrombin III,* an inhibitor of thrombin and of several other activated coagulation factors) is implicated in the genesis of recurrent thrombosis (7). *Resistance to activated protein C* is the most common inherited abnormality in patients with DVT; the condition is due to a mutation in the factor V molecule, so-called *factor V Leiden* (7). Five percent of the U.S. white population are heterozygotes for factor V Leiden (significantly less common in African, Asian, Hispanic, and Native Americans) (8). Two percent of the population are heterozygotes for the *prothrombin gene mutation (G20210A mutation).* Both conditions are associated with less of a thrombotic risk than deficiencies of protein C, protein S, or antithrombin III but significantly increase the risk of thrombosis when other acquired or inherited risk factors are present as well. Also, rarely, an inherited or acquired abnormality of fibrinogen (a *dysfibrinogenemia*), revealed usually by a prolonged thrombin time (see Chapter 56) or of fibrinolysis, may be associated with thromboembolic disease.

Antibodies to phospholipid or, more precisely, to protein–phospholipid complexes, may potentiate venous and arterial thromboses (9). Some of these antibodies are identified by their ability to prolong various phospholipid-dependent coagulation tests (e.g., the recalcified plasma clotting time, the Russell viper venom time, and the activated partial thromboplastin time [aPTT]). These antibodies are identified by mixing studies in which they prolong the clotting tests of normal plasma. Such antibodies were first recognized in patients with systemic lupus erythematosus (SLE) and are sometimes called *lupus anticoagulants.* Other antiphospholipid antibodies directed against cardiolipin may be detected as well. Concordance is limited between lupus anticoagulants and anticardiolipin antibodies. Antiphospholipid antibodies are present in about one-third of patients with SLE, often in patients with other diseases of connective tissue, and uncommonly in the rest of the population (principally older people). The inhibition of coagulation test is an *in vitro* phenomenon. *In vivo* the antibodies are associated with venous and arterial thrombosis. The incidence of thrombotic events is highest in patients with SLE (in whom immune thrombocytopenia is also frequently present). In other people the risk is not well defined, but in one large retrospective study the risk was five times that in a control group, when the antibody titers were high (10). Currently, it seems prudent to test for antiphospholipid antibodies in all patients with SLE who have a thrombotic event or who are contemplating pregnancy (these antibodies are associated with an increased incidence of spontaneous abortion) and in other patients who experience thrombotic events without associated risk factors. The antibodies characteristically persist for months, or sometimes years, and may recur. When patients with antiphospholipid antibodies develop venous or arterial thromboses, they should be anticoagulated (see below). Patients with antiphospholipid antibodies and a history of prior spontaneous abortion may be treated during pregnancy with heparin (coumarin anticoagulants cause fetal abnormalities; see below) followed by 4 to 6 weeks of a coumarin or heparin after delivery, when the risk of thrombosis is highest.

Hyperhomocystinemia, a risk factor for arterial thrombosis, appears to predispose patients to venous thrombosis as well. In one study, 10% of patients with DVT had elevated plasma levels of homocysteine (11).

Patients without apparent risk factors who experience recurrent thromboses or patients who have a positive family history who experience one thromboembolic event should be evaluated for an inherited or acquired abnormality of coagulation, preferably in consultation with a hematologist. Assays of coagulation factors or of their inhibitors should be done by an experienced laboratory at least 2 months after an acute event and after anticoagulation has been discontinued for at least 10 days. However, anticoagulants do not affect the measurement of phospholipid antibody titers, factor V Leiden, the prothrombin gene mutation, and homocysteine levels.

Presentation and Evaluation

Superficial thrombophlebitis is readily recognized as inflammation of a visible tender, often palpably thrombosed, vein. There is no risk of embolism from such clots, unless the deep veins are also involved. In one study, superficial thrombophlebitis was much more likely to be associated with DVT if the superficial veins were not varicose (12) (see Chapter 95). Otherwise, treatment does not require administration of anticoagulant drugs (see below) and is confined to nonsteroidal anti-inflammatory drugs, elevation of the extremity, local moist heat, and, if there is concomitant infection, antibiotics. However, many believe that patients with phlebitis of the entire superficial saphenous vein to the groin should be anticoagulated. If DVT is suspected in a patient with superficial phlebitis, ultrasonography (see below) should be performed.

Signs and symptoms of pulmonary embolism (see Chapter 59) may be the sole manifestation of venous thrombosis in the deep veins of the lower extremities. More commonly, patients present with swelling, pain, and tenderness of the affected extremity, although swelling alone may be the presenting symptom. In any case, the prevention of pulmonary embolism is the primary reason why diagnosis and treatment of venous thrombosis are urgent. On the basis of history and physical examination alone, however, it is difficult to distinguish DVT from other processes. In one large series more than two-thirds of patients suspected clinically of having a DVT were found to have other etiologies (13). Therefore, patients suspected of having thrombosis of the deep veins or of having had pulmonary embolism must undergo specific diagnostic studies so that appropriate therapy for venous thromboembolism may be instituted. The test of reference is *contrast venography*. If characteristic filling defects are seen in radiographs of the veins after injection of contrast material, the diagnosis is established. However, because of the relative difficulty, discomfort, and occasional side effects of the procedure, noninvasive tests have largely replaced venography in the diagnosis of DVT.

Patient Experience. Contrast venography is performed after injection of the contrast medium into a dorsal vein of the foot. The patient should be warned that the procedure sometimes is associated with unpleasant burning or cramping in the lower extremity while the dye is being injected (especially in patients with phlebitis). Venography itself may cause thrombosis; the incidence of superficial vein thrombosis and DVT, proved by repeated venography, is approximately 2% (14,15).

One of two noninvasive tests is commonly used in the diagnosis of DVT: *impedance plethysmography* (IPG) (16–18) and *Doppler ultrasonography* (19). Both depend on the skill of the technician who performs the test, and the sensitivity and specificity of the tests should be established by every vascular laboratory. Both tests are more sensitive in detecting thrombosis in deep veins of the thigh but are insensitive in detecting thrombosis in deep veins of the calf. However, calf vein thrombi are unlikely to embolize unless they first propagate into the thigh (20,21). Because of limitations in the specificity of IPG (e.g., false positive tests are common in patients with right-sided heart failure or with conditions that cause external venous compression), ultrasonography is the test that is almost always used in the United States. The sensitivity of IPG has been questioned as well (22). Doppler ultrasonography (19) (so-called duplex ultrasonography) combines ultrasonography with Doppler technology to provide visualization of the venous channels and a measurement of the flow of blood through them. During the performance of the test, an external probe is applied to the thigh and the failure of the vein underlying the probe to collapse is a sensitive and specific sign of thrombosis.

A model has been developed to establish the pretest probability of DVT and to estimate the predictive value of these noninvasive tests (23) (Table 57.1). By use of the pretest probability, a sensible diagnostic and therapeutic approach to patients with suspected DVT has been suggested (Table 57.2). Even though the approach cannot be considered definitive until larger scale prospective studies have been done, it does provide some direction on the basis of objective data rather than on unsubstantiated clinical impression, as has often been the case in the past. On the basis of the model, patients with low pretest probability and normal ultrasonography (nearly half the study group) can be considered not to have a DVT.

Table 57.1. A Model for Predicting Pretest Probability for Deep Vein Thrombosis (DVT)

Major points
- Active cancer (including treatment within previous 6 mo)
- Recent immobility for more than 3 days, whatever the cause (e.g., bed rest, paralysis, plaster cast)
- Major surgery within 4 wk
- Tenderness along the distribution of the deep venous system
- Measurable swelling of the thigh and calf
- Calf swelling alone >3 cm on symptomless side (measured 10 cm below tibial tuberosity)
- At least two first-degree relatives with a history of DVT

Minor points
- Recent trauma (within 60 days) to the symptomatic leg
- Pitting edema (symptomatic leg only)
- Dilated superficial veins (nonvaricose, in symptomatic leg only)
- Hospitalization within 6 mo
- Erythema of symptomatic leg

Probability of DVT
- High
  - ≥3 major points and no alternative diagnosis
  - ≥2 major points, ≥2 minor points, and no alternative diagnosis
- Low
  - 1 major point, ≥2 minor points, and an alternative diagnosis
  - 1 major point, ≥1 minor point, and no alternative diagnosis
  - 0 major points, ≥3 minor points, and an alternative diagnosis
  - 0 major points, ≥2 minor points, and no alternative diagnosis
- Moderate
  - All other combinations

Modified from Wells PS, Hirsh J, Anderson DR, et al. Accuracy of clinical assessment of deep-vein thrombosis. Lancet 1995;345:1326, with permission.

Table 57.2. Predictive Value of Ultrasonography (US)

Pretest Probability	Normal	Abnormal
Low	DVT ruled out	Venography (treat for DVT if abnormal)
Moderate	Repeat US in 1 wk (treat for DVT if abnormal)	Treat for DVT
High	Venography (treat for DVT if abnormal)	Treat for DVT

DVT, deep vein thrombosis.

Modified from Wells PS, Hirsh J, Anderson DR, et al. Accuracy of clinical assessment of deep-vein thrombosis. Lancet 1995;345:1326, with permission.

There are also some *newer tests*. Some centers now use *magnetic resonance venography* in the diagnosis of DVT. It is a relatively expensive technique but has sensitivity and specificity in excess of 95% (24). *Thromboscintigraphy*, by use of ^{99M}Tc-apcitide, a labeled peptide that binds to the glycoprotein IIb/IIIa receptors of platelets, is now approved for diagnosis of DVT as well; its sensitivity and specificity, compared with contrast venography, are greater than 70% (25).

Patients with *calf vein thrombosis* alone do not need to be given anticoagulant drugs (see below); they can be treated in the same way as are patients with superficial thrombophlebitis. If ultrasonography (or IPG) is unavailable, however, patients with venographically demonstrable calf vein thrombosis should be anticoagulated because there is no easy way, on follow-up, to detect propagation of the clot.

Patient Experience. Doppler ultrasonography takes about 10 minutes to perform and is painless; the patient lies quietly while transducers are placed on the thigh. During the test, a probe is applied with gentle pressure over the vein being evaluated. Optimally, the patient needs to lie prone.

If patients have signs and symptoms of *pulmonary embolism* (see Chapter 59), the first diagnostic procedure should be a *ventilation/perfusion scan of their lungs.* If the scan is negative or is read as low probability and the patient has signs and symptoms of venous occlusion of the lower extremities, further diagnostic studies should be done (see above) to establish that diagnosis. Many centers use *spiral computed tomography* as a substitute for ventilation/perfusion scans of the lungs (see Chapter 59), but the sensitivity and specificity of the test in the diagnosis of pulmonary embolism are not yet well established (26). Because of the relatively poor specificity of ventilation/perfusion scans in diagnosing pulmonary embolism, there is evidence that the use of noninvasive testing for lower extremity thrombosis can be helpful in making decisions about further testing and treatment (27,28).

D-Dimer

D-dimer is a degradation product of cross-linked fibrin. Most patients with thromboembolism have elevated plasma D-dimer levels. Specificity of the test is low because levels are frequently increased in patients after surgery, with malignancy, with central lines, and so forth. However, the assay does have negative predictive value when combined with an estimate of pretest probability. In patients with low risk, a negative D-dimer assay essentially rules out venous thromboembolism. However, in populations at high risk for DVT (e.g., cancer patients, patients seen in the emergency room), the negative predictive value is less than 80% (29). Also, there is as yet no standardized assay for measurement of the product.

Treatment

The most important therapy for patients with DVT in the lower extremities is anticoagulation, instituted to prevent extension of the clot. The larger the clot, the more likely it is to break off and become an embolus. Anticoagulation is usually instituted in the hospital with heparin, which is administered 4 to 5 days along with warfarin. The advent of low molecular weight heparin, however, does provide an option now for patients to be treated at home (see below).

Warfarin

Warfarin is the coumarin commonly used in the anticoagulation of ambulatory patients. Coumadin is the brand name product that is commonly prescribed; other products, including generic products, are reliable but are not interchangeable because of variation in bioavailability. Ordinarily, patients who have been hospitalized for diagnosis and initial treatment of venous thromboembolic disease are given warfarin while heparin is being administered so that by the time heparin is discontinued, the full effect of the coumarin has become established. Coumarins interfere with the synthesis of vitamin K-dependent clotting factors (factors II, VII, IX, and X) by the liver. Their effect is not fully realized until they have been given for approximately 5 days. The administration of warfarin usually is initiated in dosages of 5 mg/day (1-, 2-, 2.5-, 4-, 5-, 7.5-, and 10-mg tablets are available) and then adjusted, depending on the therapeutic response, which is monitored by use of the prothrombin time.

There is an internationally accepted uniform system for reporting the prothrombin time (30). The system dictates that all results are related to those obtained by use of a standardized thromboplastin, the critical reagent used in the performance of the test. The relationship is expressed as an *International Normalized Ratio (INR),* and laboratories doing prothrombin times should report their results in terms of the INR. (The INR is the ratio of the patient's prothrombin time to the normal standard prothrombin time of the testing laboratory, raised by an exponent, the International Sensitivity Index [ISI], supplied by the manufacturer of the thromboplastin.) Because there is still some question about the reliability of the ISI provided by a given manufacturer, however, it is best, if possible, to have sequential prothrombin times done by the same laboratory or, if a different laboratory is to be used, to have prothrombin times done on the same plasma by both laboratories to establish the appropriate standards of comparison.

In most circumstances, the goal of anticoagulant therapy with warfarin is to maintain the INR between 2.0 and 3.0 because it is within this range that a reasonable therapeutic effect is achieved and the risk of untoward bleeding is relatively small. The ratio of the patient's prothrombin time to that of the control will vary, depending on the ISI of the thromboplastin that is used. These recommendations result in significantly lower prothrombin times than have been thought appropriate in the past. During the first several weeks of administration of warfarin, the prothrombin time should be measured at least every few days until it is determined that the proper dosage schedule has been achieved. Thereafter it is appropriate to measure the anticoagulant response every 2 to 4 weeks, depending on the stability of the anticoagulant response (see also Factors Affecting Response, below). At the same time it is prudent to examine the patient's urine and stool for occult blood and to assess the hematocrit value or hemoglobin concentration.

During the course of anticoagulation with coumarin compounds, patients should be instructed to avoid predictable trauma such as might be expected from playing contact sports or from working in an environment associated with a high risk of injury. Intramuscular injections should not be given to the anticoagulated patient; subcutaneous injections, done properly, are safe. Venipunctures are also safe, but the wound should be compressed for 10 to 15 minutes after

Table 57.3. Some Factors That May Affect a Patient's Response to Warfarin

Enhanced Response	Reduced Response
Vitamin K deficiency	Barbiturates
Liver disease	Carbamazepine (Tegretol)
Drugs	Chlordiazepoxide (Librium)
Anabolic steroids	Cholestyramine
Amiodarone	Griseofulvin
Cimetidine[a]	Nafcillin
Clofibrate	Rifampin
Cotrimoxazole (e.g., Bactrim)	Sucralfate
Erythromycin	Spironolactone
Isoniazid	Foods[b]
Metronidazole (Flagyl)	Avocado
Miconazole	Fish
Phenylbutazone	Broccoli
Piroxicam (Feldene)	Spinach
Propranolol	Cabbage
Sulfinpyrazone	Kale
	Cauliflower

[a]The effect of other H_2 blockers is uncertain.
[b]Rich in vitamin K.

the needle is withdrawn. Arterial punctures are contraindicated as outpatient procedures, for which prolonged compression and observation of the puncture site are impractical.

Factors Affecting Response. Ordinarily, patients taking a given dose of warfarin maintain a consistent hypoprothrombinemic response, once a steady state is reached. However, a number of factors might alter the patient's responsiveness to warfarin after a period of stability (Table 57.3). Sometimes, the amount of vitamin K ingested in the patient's diet might be altered drastically, increasing the potency of warfarin if less vitamin K is ingested and decreasing it if considerably more is ingested. Significantly decreased ingestion of vitamin K is almost always associated with a markedly decreased intake of food (e.g., in patients who are anorexic because of illness or who have instituted severe dietary restrictions in an attempt to lose weight). The effect of reduction in intake of vitamin K is most pronounced in those patients who are concomitantly receiving antibiotics, which inhibit the synthesis of vitamin K by normal flora of the intestinal tract. Because the vitamin K–dependent clotting factors are synthesized in the liver and because coumarins are metabolized by the liver, patients who develop intercurrent hepatic illness (e.g., hepatitis) should be watched carefully for enhanced effective anticoagulation. In such a circumstance, it would be wise to measure prothrombin times more frequently but it would not be necessary to discontinue warfarin unless bleeding ensued or the prothrombin time became significantly prolonged over the baseline therapeutic control.

One of the major problems in dealing with a patient taking coumarin anticoagulants is the possibility of *drug interaction*. A number of pharmacologic agents potentiate the anticoagulant effect of coumarins, and a few inhibit it. (Table 57.3 lists the drugs for which good supporting evidence is available; other possible interactions for which the evidence is less strong are listed on p. 233S in reference 31.) One should be cautious, however, when initiating any new forms of therapy or discontinuing old ones in a patient who is receiving coumarin anticoagulants. Prothrombin times should be checked more frequently for several weeks to ensure that the pharmacologic response to coumarin has not been altered. In general, the likelihood of a potentiated response is much higher than that of an inhibitory one, so there is greater risk of an increased susceptibility to bleeding than of an inhibition of anticoagulation. One should also be careful about the use of drugs such as aspirin that have an effect on hemostasis that might be enhanced by warfarin or that may produce bleeding by injuring the gastric mucosa. Other nonsteroidal anti-inflammatory drugs (see Chapter 77) also have at least a potential for compromising hemostasis and should be used cautiously.

Complications. By far the major complication experienced by patients taking coumarin anticoagulants is hemorrhage (32,33). In general, the risk of hemorrhage is increased by the intensity of treatment and by the presence of comorbid conditions (e.g., hepatic or renal disease) (32,34). The risk appears greatest within the first month of initiation of treatment. Elderly patients, who are likely to be more ill, to have a greater propensity to fall, to have lesions that are prone to bleed, and to be taking multiple medications, are probably at greater risk. Minor episodes (e.g., small bruises and bleeding gums after brushing of the teeth) are relatively common but ordinarily do not require a change in the dose schedule of the anticoagulant. Occult rectal bleeding, minor bleeding from hemorrhoids, microscopic hematuria, and menorrhagia are encountered in less than 10% of patients. When bleeding of this kind is observed, every attempt must be made to establish the site of bleeding by the use of appropriate diagnostic studies (35). If prothrombin times have been maintained within the therapeutic range, the rapidity and extent of bleeding will dictate whether the anticoagulant drug should be discontinued, at least temporarily. Major genitourinary or gastrointestinal bleeding sufficient to lower the hematocrit value or hemoglobin concentration or bleeding of any degree in the central nervous system dictates prompt discontinuation of the anticoagulant and immediate hospitalization for further diagnosis and treatment. It is prudent to administer 25 mg of vitamin K 1 (AquaMEPHYTON) intravenously at a rate no greater than 5 mg/min while arranging for hospitalization. (The prothrombin time will begin to shorten in 4 to 6 hours and, in most patients, will be in a safe range in 12 to 24 hours.) Bleeding is often associated with an independent organic process (e.g., a peptic ulcer, a carcinoma of the colon, or a genitourinary abnormality); bleeding of this kind is likely to occur even when the prothrombin time is in the therapeutic range (36).

There is a major risk in the use of coumarin compounds in *pregnant patients* (37,38). Major hemorrhagic complications occur in the fetus as well as teratogenic effects unrelated to the anticoagulant action. Therefore it is recommended that pregnancy is avoided in women who are being treated with coumarin drugs because a normal infant can be expected only about two-thirds of the time. The risk of

Table 57.4. Advice To Be Given to Patients Taking a Coumarin Anticoagulant

Take only medicines prescribed by your doctor. Do not take mineral oil, laxatives, aspirin (or any product such as a cold remedy that contains aspirin), or any other proprietary anti-inflammatory agents or any multivitamin preparation that contains vitamin K. You may take acetaminophen (e.g., Tylenol) instead of aspirin for pain.
Take your coumarin at the same time each day.
Avoid wide variation in the kinds and amounts of food you eat, especially fish, broccoli, spinach, cabbage, kale, or cauliflower.
Do not drink more than one or two glasses of beer or wine or the equivalent of more than 1 ounce (1 "shot") of whiskey a day.
Avoid any activity that might expose you unnecessarily to trauma—for example, contact sports.
Call your doctor immediately
- If you experience any abnormal bleeding.
- Before you visit the dentist.
- Before seeing any other physician.
- If you cannot keep your scheduled appointment.
- Before leaving on a trip.
- If you are hospitalized, for any reason, without your doctor knowing about it.

heparin in pregnancy is less clear-cut; an increased incidence of fetal wastage has been reported (37) but also has been disputed. In any case, if anticoagulation is necessary, heparin is clearly safer than coumarins (see below) (38,39). Advice for management of patients who are taking a coumarin compound and who are to undergo a surgical procedure is provided in Chapter 93.

Rarely, patients given a coumarin anticoagulant will develop *hemorrhagic infarcts* in their skin (often in women's breasts) within 10 days, with eventual sloughing of necrotic tissue. This complication is much more likely in people with protein C or protein S deficiency (see above). Under such circumstances, the drug ordinarily is stopped immediately (although it is unclear whether it is necessary to do so).

Table 57.4 provides useful information for patients at the onset of anticoagulation or at the time that the patient is discharged from the hospital. Selection of patients who can follow these rules will diminish considerably the incidence of hemorrhagic complications in patients taking anticoagulant drugs (see also Chapter 56, Table 56.5).

Heparin

Unfractionated heparin is not commonly prescribed to outpatients. If, however, because of unacceptable side effects unrelated to its anticoagulant activity a coumarin could not be used, subcutaneous heparin has sometimes been required after hospitalization. It has typically been administered every 12 hours in doses designed to maintain the aPTT at 1.5 to 2 times control 6 hours after administration (40). Once a dosage regimen is established by this technique (usually in the range of 15,000 to 17,500 units twice a day), it probably is unnecessary to measure the aPTT again unless the patient develops bleeding or recurrent thrombosis. It has been demonstrated that prevention of recurrent thromboembolism is comparable with that achieved by the use of warfarin (40). So-called low-dose heparin (5,000 units two to three times a day) is inadequate treatment for patients with established thrombosis (41).

Low Molecular Weight Heparin And Heparinoids. In recent years, a number of *low molecular weight heparins* that appear to have significant advantages over conventional unfractionated heparin have been developed. The new preparations have greater bioavailability, a more predictable dose response, and a longer half-life than the standard product (42). There is also a lesser risk of drug associated thrombocytopenia (see below). These differences permit the administration of a fixed dose of heparin subcutaneously once or twice a day and eliminate the need to monitor the patient's aPTT. A number of clinical trials (43–45) and meta-analyses (46,47) have concluded that the efficacy and safety of low molecular weight heparin are at least as good as that of unfractionated heparin. Several studies have demonstrated the safety of treatment in the outpatient setting, but strict adherence to one of the outpatient protocols is required (48). Currently, two low molecular weight heparins are licensed for the treatment of venous thromboembolism in the United States: enoxaparin and tinzaparin. Dalteparin and danaparoid (a heparinoid; see below) are currently approved for prophylaxis only. If low molecular weight heparin is used, it is still appropriate to start warfarin concurrently, unless there is a contraindication to its use (see above).

Danaparoid (Orgaran) is a mixture of low molecular weight sulfated glycosaminoglycans from which the heparin has been removed. Its effects on coagulation are similar, but slightly different, than those of heparin. Sufficiently large trials comparing danaparoid with low molecular weight heparin have not yet been reported to assess relative risks and benefits precisely.

Heparin-induced Thrombocytopenia. Unfractionated heparin causes a fall in the platelet count in up to 10% to 20% of patients to whom it is administered (49). Most of these patients have so-called *heparin-induced thrombocytopenia*, type I, a benign process of no clinical significance that typically develops within 1 to 2 days and often spontaneously abates, despite the continued administration of heparin. Counts will fall within the normal range or mild thrombocytopenia may develop. Up to 3% of patients, however, develop antibody-mediated thrombocytopenia, also known as *heparin-induced thrombocytopenia, type II (HIT-II)*. HIT-II occurs within 4 to 10 days and is due to the emergence of antibody against a complex of heparins and platelet factor 4. Platelet counts are ordinarily not as low as those seen in other immune thrombocytopenias and average 60,000 m/L. The risk of HIT-II is much less with the use of low molecular weight heparin or heparinoids (45). There is a 30% risk of recurrent HIT-II if heparin is given again within the ensuing 3 months, in which case counts typically fall within hours (50). After 3 months (by which time antibodies usually have disappeared), the risk of recurrence, after re-exposure, is uncertain.

Up to 50% of patients with HIT-II develop venous and/or arterial thrombosis, perhaps as a result of platelet activation. Venous thromboemboli are four times as common as arterial; either may develop for up to a month after the onset of the illness.

The *diagnosis* of HIT-II is made clinically on the basis of the time course and degree of thrombocytopenia after administration of heparin and the associated thromboembolic complications, if present. The diagnosis can be confirmed by assay of the HIT-II antibody, but that is not often readily available.

Treatment of HIT-II demands immediate cessation of unfractionated heparin. Patients with very low platelet counts (<20,000 m/L) or with thrombotic complications should be hospitalized. Heparinoids (danaparoid, see above) can be substituted for heparin (5% cross-reactivity), but low molecular weight heparins have considerably more cross-reactivity and should not be used (49). Other drugs—lepirudin (51), a recombinant hirudin, or argatroban (52), a direct inhibitor of thrombin—are alternative choices.

Prevention of HIT-II is best done by using unfractionated heparin sparingly; by simultaneous administration of warfarin, as above, and discontinuation of heparin within 5 days; or by preferential use of low molecular weight heparins or heparinoids.

Other Complications. Prolonged use of unfractionated heparin (4 months or more) in dosages exceeding 10,000 units/day has been reported to cause *osteoporosis;* spontaneous spinal and rib fractures have been observed. The risk of this complication developing is unknown, nor is it known whether low molecular weight heparin ever causes osteoporosis. Until more data are accumulated, treatment with heparin for longer than 3 months is at least relatively contraindicated.

Both standard heparin (especially the bovine preparation) and low molecular weight heparin also commonly cause *reversible elevation* of *aminotransferase activity,* without other evidence of hepatic dysfunction (53). No pathologic correlation with this reaction has been identified, so if it occurs, heparin may continue to be administered.

Finally, both standard and low molecular weight heparin predictably suppress aldosterone production and induce hyperkalemia in 7% to 8% of treated patients (54). The risk is especially great in patients prone to hyperkalemia for other reasons (e.g., diabetes mellitus, chronic renal disease); in such patients, potassium levels should be measured every 3 to 4 days.

Thrombolytic Therapy. The use of thrombolytic therapy in DVT remains controversial. The rate and percent lysis is higher than with anticoagulation alone, and this may result in a lower incidence of the postphlebitic syndrome, although this has not been proven in well-controlled studies. The best candidates are young patients with large proximal DVTs with significant swelling and pain. It is very important to obtain informed consent because many patients are not willing to accept an increased bleeding risk to prevent the postphlebitic syndrome (55). Patients must be hospitalized before thrombolytics can be administered.

Interruption of the Inferior Vena Cava. It is appropriate to place a vena caval filter in patients with DVT and an absolute contraindication to anticoagulation or in a patient who experiences a pulmonary embolism while appropriately anticoagulated. It also may be reasonable in the patient with very poor pulmonary vascular reserve (e.g., after a large pulmonary embolism) who could not tolerate even a small recurrent pulmonary embolism. It is clear that caval interruption is only a temporary preventive measure with no difference in mortality at 2 years. There is, however, an increased incidence of recurrent DVT compared with that of patients who have been anticoagulated (56).

Aspirin

A meta-analysis has concluded that aspirin is of some use in reducing the incidence of DVT and, especially, pulmonary emboli in immobilized patients (57,58). There is no justification for prescribing aspirin as a treatment of venous thrombosis.

Course

It has been standard practice for many years to continue anticoagulation for at least 3 months in patients with DVT (59). It is likely that patients who have developed DVT in response to a transient risk (e.g., surgery, trauma) may not need anticoagulation for longer than 4 to 6 weeks (60,61). However, a randomized prospective study suggests that patients without apparent risks should be treated for 6 months after a first episode of venous thromboembolism (62). Some patients with persistent risk (e.g., cancer, recurrent thromboembolic disease, or abnormalities of hemostasis that predispose them to thrombosis; see above) should be treated indefinitely (60,63).

Patients should be advised to avoid prolonged sitting or standing in one position, elevate their legs for two to three periods of 30 minutes each day, and wear elastic stockings to promote venous return. Although the effectiveness of these maneuvers has not been established, there is little or no risk associated with any of them, and they may be of some value.

When a decision is made to discontinue anticoagulation therapy, it may be terminated abruptly without fear of an increased risk of early recurrence of venous thrombosis; the so-called rebound phenomenon has never been demonstrated.

Recurrent DVT is difficult to diagnose (64); it is not a common problem in appropriately managed patients (see above). Many patients who have had a documented acute DVT develop recurrent pain and swelling of the same extremity without evidence of recurrent thrombosis. Even contrast venography may be equivocal in such patients because of persistent occlusion of a vein by a previous clot. In such circumstances, Doppler ultrasonography is probably the most reliable test, if it (or IPG) has been demonstrated to have become normal after treatment of an acute thrombotic event; normalization occurs in 70% of patients by 3 months and in 90% by 9 months (16). If ultrasonography (or IPG) has not become normal and if a contrast venogram is not interpretable or if recurrent thrombosis has been definitively diagnosed, anticoagulation for a year is probably reasonable. Most experts recommend anticoagulation for at least a year after a second DVT and longer if there are ongoing risk factors.

Postphlebitic Syndrome

Some patients, after repeated attacks of thrombosis of the veins of the lower extremities, develop chronic changes in those veins with loss of competence of the valves and hemorrhage of small tributary veins, leading to chronic edema and discoloration of the legs and ankles (65). Sometimes painful stasis ulcers that make it difficult for the patient to move about also develop. The treatment of this postphlebitic syndrome is the promotion of venous return from the lower extremities by the use of support stockings during the day and by elevation of the lower extremities for several hours each day. In those patients who have developed ulcers, bed rest with persistent elevation of the extremity above the level of the heart is recommended and, if necessary, administration of appropriate antibiotics. On such a regimen, the ulcers usually heal, although they may recur if the patients are not careful to continue to follow prescribed conservative therapy (see Chapter 95). Signs and symptoms of chronic venous insufficiency are often manifest in patients with no history or evidence of DVT (66).

When to Hospitalize a Patient with a Deep Vein Thrombosis

Patients should be hospitalized for diagnosis and treatment of DVT if studies are not otherwise readily available, if there is evidence of a serious associated disease (e.g., malignancy, heart failure), if there is a suspicion of pulmonary embolism, or if low molecular weight heparin is not an option as initial therapy (see above).

ARTERIAL THROMBOEMBOLISM

Unlike clots that form in the venous circulation, arterial thrombosis (see also Chapters 64, 91, and 94) is primarily initiated by platelet plug formation, begun by the adherence of ambient platelets to altered surfaces in arterial vessels and complicated frequently by a breaking off this plug, which then embolizes to obstruct more distal vessels (see also Chapters 62, 91, and 94). The major risk factor, by far, is *atherosclerosis*, but rarely underlying *malignancy*, an *antiphospholipid antibody*, or *hyperhomocystinemia* may be associated with an increased propensity to arterial thrombosis (see above). Symptoms and signs of thromboembolism appear more abruptly than those of venous occlusion and commonly are associated with necrosis of tissue that had been fed by the now obstructed vessel. Heparin and coumarin anticoagulants, both experimentally and clinically, are of little use in preventing the formation of such clots or in preventing their propagation. (There is, however, compelling evidence that warfarin anticoagulation decreases considerably the risk of arterial emboli in patients with chronic atrial fibrillation; see Chapter 64. Warfarin is also prescribed commonly for patients with dilated cardiomyopathy; see Chapter 66.) There is a great deal of interest, therefore, in the use of drugs that interfere with platelet plug formation and that might be useful in the prophylaxis of arterial thromboembolism.

Class I Antiplatelet Agents: Aspirin

Aspirin interferes with platelet function and therefore inhibits platelet plug formation. It interferes with the formation of a potent aggregating and vasoconstricting substance, thromboxane A_2, formed in platelets by the metabolism of prostaglandins. Aspirin inhibits the rate-limiting enzyme in this reaction, cyclooxygenase; as a result, the aggregation of platelets by collagen or connective tissue is inhibited and the release of substances, which themselves stimulate platelet aggregation, is impaired.

Aspirin inhibits not only prostaglandin synthesis in platelets but also the formation by vascular endothelium of prostacyclin, a potent inhibitor of platelet aggregation. Although there is no precise information on the proper dosage of aspirin to be administered to achieve an optimal effect (presumably at the point where there is maximum inhibition of thromboxane A_2 synthesis and minimum inhibition of prostacyclin synthesis) (67), there is no evidence that aspirin at any dosage is thrombogenic.

Unless aspirin is administered to patients with an underlying hemostatic disorder (including the administration of an anticoagulant drug; see above), a hemorrhagic diathesis is unusual. However, aspirin does have a toxic effect on the mucosa of the gastrointestinal tract that may result in bleeding or may increase the likelihood of hemorrhage from pre-existent peptic ulcerations (68).

A number of studies have been performed to assess the efficacy of aspirin for *secondary prevention* of thromboembolic events in patients with a history of cardiovascular and cerebrovascular disease. A meta-analysis (a statistical evaluation of the sum of all published interpretable trials) of 70,000 patients with a history of arterial vascular disease or of a condition that predisposes patients to vascular disease reported that allocation to antiplatelet treatment (essentially aspirin) reduced overall vascular events by approximately 25% and reduced death from vascular events by 18% (57). There was no significant difference between patients with cardiovascular disease and those with cerebrovascular disease and no significant difference in effect between 75 and 325 mg/day of aspirin. A study of 333 men with stable angina, a subset of the large Physicians' Health Study, reported that 325 mg of aspirin every other day did not affect the frequency of chest pain but did reduce risk of a first myocardial infarction by 87% during the 5 years of the study (69).

It is reasonable to recommend aspirin, 75 to 325 mg/day, to patients with transient ischemic attacks, unstable angina, stable angina, myocardial infarction, thrombotic stroke, or peripheral arterial disease (70,71). There is little risk of major hemorrhagic side effects at these dosages (325 mg/day, in fact, increases the risk only slightly) (68,72).

It has become a routine in most centers to administer aspirin (325 mg/day) indefinitely to patients who have undergone coronary artery bypass surgery. Aspirin is also used in a wide variety of patients in whom maintenance of vascular patency is important (e.g., after angioplasty or after a procedure to establish vascular access for hemodialysis) (57,73).

There have also been three studies of aspirin in the *primary prevention* of atherosclerotic disease (given prophylactically to apparently healthy people) (74–76). The combined studies showed a one-third reduction in the number of nonfatal myocardial infarctions (77) but no reduction in overall mortality from vascular disease. A later expanded meta-analysis of studies of 30,000 healthy people who were at apparently low risk of atherosclerotic disease showed minimal benefit of antiplatelet therapy (again, primarily aspirin) in protecting against vascular events, including death from vascular disease (57). There is therefore no compelling reason to prescribe aspirin as a prophylactic agent to such people.

Class II Antiplatelet Agents: Dipyridamole

Dipyridamole inhibits the breakdown of cyclic AMP, leading to an inhibition of platelet activation. The U.S. Food and Drug Administration has approved the combination of aspirin plus extended release dipyridamole (combined tablet, Aggrenox, 25 mg/200 mg twice a day) in patients with a previous history of stroke or transient ischemic attack, but there is no evidence that dipyridamole, alone or in combination, is effective.

Class III Antiplatelet Agents: Ticlopidine, Clopidogrel

Ticlopidine (Ticlid) and clopidogrel (Plavix) inhibit the aggregation of platelets by adenosine diphosphate. A multicenter study showed ticlopidine to be approximately 20% more effective than aspirin in preventing death from any cause and in preventing fatal and nonfatal major strokes in a population of men and women who had recently experienced transient ischemic attacks or minor strokes (78). It has also been shown to be beneficial in patients with coronary artery disease (57). However, the incidence of side effects, especially diarrhea, was considerably greater than with aspirin, and severe reversible neutropenia occurred in approximately 1% of patients. Rare cases of thrombotic thrombocytopenic purpura have also been reported (79). The recommended dosage is 250 mg twice a day, resulting in a cost more than 100 times that of aspirin. If prescribed, the manufacturer recommends the patient's white blood cell count and differential count should be measured every 2 weeks for 3 months.

Clopidogrel (75 mg/day) was compared with aspirin (325mg/day) in the CAPRIE trial in patients with a recent myocardial infarction, ischemic stroke, or peripheral vascular disease; it had a significant but modest increase in risk reduction over aspirin with comparable side effects (80). Because it does not cause neutropenia and is associated less often with thrombotic thrombocytopenic purpura than is ticlopidine (81), clopidogrel has essentially become the class III antiplatelet agent of choice. However, because of its cost, it should be prescribed primarily for suitable patients who cannot take aspirin.

Class IV Antiplatelet Agents: Inhibitors of Glycoprotein IIb/IIIa Platelet Receptors (Abciximab, Eptifibatide, Tirofiban)

Multiple studies are ongoing to evaluate the role of this newer class of platelet inhibitors in various arterial ischemia syndromes, but none of the drugs is suitable for use in ambulatory patients.

General References*

American College of Chest Physicians Conference on Antithrombotic Therapy. Chest 1995;108:225S.

Bauer, KA. The thrombophilias: Well-defined risk factors with uncertain therapeutic implications. Ann Intern Med 2001;135:367.

Ginsberg JS. Management of venous thromboembolism. N Engl J Med 1996;335:1816.

A consensus on the use of antithrombotic therapy using evidence-based criteria.

Tapson YF, Carroll BA, Davidson BL, et al. The diagnostic approach to acute venous thromboembolism. Clinical practice guideline. American Thoracic Society. Am J Respir Crit Care Med 1999;160:1043.

Thomas DP, Roberts HR. Hypercoagulability in venous and arterial thrombosis. Ann Intern Med 1997;126:638.

Concise review of the subject.

Specific References

1. Prandoni P, Polistena P, Bernardi E, et al. Upper extremity deep vein thrombosis. Risk factors, diagnosis, and complications. Arch Intern Med 1997;157:57.
2. Vandenbroucke JP, Rosing J, Bloemenkamp KW, et al. Oral contraceptives and the risk of venous thrombosis. N Engl J Med 2001;344:1527.
3. Vessey M, Mant D, Smith A, et al. Oral contraceptives and venous thromboembolism: findings in a large prospective study. BMJ 1986;292:526.
4. Goldberg RJ, Serreff M, Gore JM, et al. Occult malignant neoplasm in patients with deep venous thrombosis. Arch Intern Med 1987;147:251.
5. Prandoni P, Lensing AWA, Buller HR. Deep-vein thrombosis and the incidence of subsequent symptomatic cancer. N Engl J Med 1991;327:1128.
6. Sack GH, Levin J, Bell WR. Trousseau's syndrome and other manifestations of chronic disseminated coagulopathy in patients with neoplasms: clinical, pathophysiologic, and therapeutic features. Medicine (Baltimore) 1977;56:1.
7. Selegsohn U, Lubetsky A. Genetic susceptibility to venous thrombosis. N Engl J Med 2001;344:1222.
8. Ridker PM, Miletich JP, Hennekens CH, et al. Ethnic distribution of factor V Leiden in 4047 men and women. Implications for venous thromboembolism screening. JAMA 1997;277:1305.
9. Love PE, Santoro SA. Antiphospholipid antibodies: anticardiolipin and the lupus anticoagulant in systemic lupus erythematosus (SLE) and in non-SLE disorders. Prevalence and clinical significance. Ann Intern Med 1990;112:682.

*Bold print (general references) and bold numerals (specific references) denote published controlled clinical trials, meta-analyses, or consensus-based recommendations.

10. Ginsberg KS, Liang MH, Newcomer L, et al. Anticardiolipin antibodies and the risk for ischemic stroke and venous thrombosis. Ann Intern Med 1992;117:997.
11. den Heijer M, Koster T, Blom HJ, et al. Hyperhomocysteinemia as a risk factor for deep-vein thrombosis. N Engl J Med 1996;334:759.
12. Bergquist D, Jaroszewski H. Deep vein thrombosis in patients with superficial thrombophlebitis of the leg. BMJ 1986;292:658.
13. Birdwell NL, Raskob GE, Whitsett TL, et al. The clinical validity of normal compression ultrasonography in outpatients suspected of having deep venous thrombosis. Ann Intern Med 1998;128:1.
14. Bettmann MA, Robbins A, Braun SD, et al. Contrast venography of the leg: diagnostic efficacy, tolerance, and complication rates with ionic and nonionic contrast media. Radiology 1987;165:113.
15. Lensing AWA, Prandoni P, Buller HR, et al. Lower extremity venography with Iohexol: results and complications. Radiology 1990;177:503.
16. Huisman MV, Buller HR, ten Cate JW, et al. Utility of impedance plethysmography in the diagnosis of recurrent deep-vein thrombosis. Arch Intern Med 1988;148:681.
17. Huisman MV, Buller HR, ten Cate JW, et al. Management of clinically suspected acute venous thrombosis in outpatients with serial impedance plethysmography in a community hospital setting. Arch Intern Med 1989;149:511.
18. Hull RD, Hirsh J, Carter CJ, et al. Diagnostic efficacy of impedance plethysmography for clinically suspected deep-vein thrombosis. Ann Intern Med 1985;102:21.
19. White RH, McGahan JP, Daschbach MM, et al. Diagnosis of deep-vein thrombosis using duplex ultrasound. Ann Intern Med 1989;111:297.
20. Moser KM, LeMoine JR. Is embolic risk conditioned by location of deep venous thrombosis? Ann Intern Med 1981;94:439.
21. Philbrick JT, Becker DM. Calf deep venous thrombosis. A wolf in sheep's clothing. Arch Intern Med 1988;148:2131.
22. Anderson DR, Lensing AWA, Wells PS, et al. Limitations of impedance plethysmography in the diagnosis of clinically suspected deep-vein thrombosis. Ann Intern Med 1993; 118:25.
23. Wells PS, Hirsh J, Anderson DR, et al. Accuracy of clinical assessment of deep-vein thrombosis. Lancet 1995;345:1326.
24. Evans AJ, Sostman HD, Witty LA, et al. Detection of deep venous thrombosis: prospective comparison of MR imaging and sonography. J Magn Reson Imag 1996;6:44.
25. Taillefer R. Radiolabeled peptides in the detection of deep venous thrombosis. Semin Nucl Med 2001;31:102.
26. Rathbun SW, Raskob GE, Whitsett TL. Sensitivity and specificity of helical computed tomography in the diagnosis of pulmonary embolism: a systematic review. Ann Intern Med 2000;132: 227.
27. Stein PD, Hull RD, Pineo G. Strategy that includes serial noninvasive leg tests for diagnosis of thromboembolic disease in patients with suspected acute pulmonary embolism based on data from PIOPED. Arch Intern Med 1995;155:2101.
28. Wells PS, Ginsberg JS, Anderson DR, et al. Use of a clinical model for safe management of patients with suspected pulmonary embolism. Ann Intern Med 1998;129:997.
29. Bounameaux H, de Moerloose P, Perrier A, et al. Plasma measurement of D-dimer as diagnostic aid in suspected venous thromboembolism: an overview. Thromb Haemost 1994;71:1.
30. Koepke JA, Triplett DA. Standardization of the prothrombin time—finally. Arch Pathol Lab Med 1985;109:800.
31. Hirsh J, Dalen JE, Deykin D. Oral anticoagulants. Mechanism of action, clinical effectiveness, and optimal therapeutic range. Chest 1995;108:231S.
32. Landefeld CS, Beyth RJ. Anticoagulant-related bleeding: clinical epidemiology, prediction, and prevention. Am J Med 1993;95:315.
33. Levine MN, Raskob G, Landefeld S, et al. Hemorrhagic complications of anticoagulant treatment. Chest 1995;108:276S.
34. Fihn SD, McDonell M, Martin D, et al. Risk factors for complications of chronic anticoagulation. A multicenter study. Ann Intern Med 1993;118:511.
35. Jaffin BW, Bliss CM, Lamont JT. Significance of occult gastrointestinal bleeding during anticoagulation therapy. Am J Med 1987;83:269.
36. Culclasure TF, Bray VJ, Hasbargen JA. The significance of hematuria in the anticoagulated patient. Arch Intern Med 1994;154:649.
37. Hall JG, Pauli RM, Wilson KM. Maternal and fetal sequelae of anticoagulation during pregnancy. Am J Med 1980;68:122.
38. Letsky EA, de Swiet M. Thromboembolism in pregnancy and its management. Br J Haematol 1984;57:543.
39. Ginsberg JS, Hirsh J, Turner DC, et al. Risk to the fetus of anticoagulant therapy during pregnancy. Thromb Haemost 1989;61:197.
40. Hull R, Delmore T, Carter C, et al. Adjusted subcutaneous heparin versus warfarin sodium in the long-term treatment of venous thrombosis. N Engl J Med 1982;306:189.
41. Hull R, Delmore T, Genton E, et al. Warfarin sodium versus low-dose heparin in the long term treatment of venous thrombosis. N Engl J Med 1979;301:855.
42. Hirsh J, Levine MN. Low molecular weight heparin. Blood 1992;79:1.
43. Hull RD, Raskob GE, Rosenbloom D, et al. Treatment of proximal vein thrombosis with subcutaneous low-molecular-weight heparin vs intravenous heparin. Arch Intern Med 1997;157: 289.
44. Koopman MM, Prandoni P, Piovella F, et al. Treatment of venous thrombosis with intravenous unfractionated heparin administered in the hospital as compared with subcutaneous low-molecular-weight heparin administered at home. N Engl J Med 1996;334:682.
45. Levine M, Gent M, Hirsh J. A comparison of low-molecular-weight heparin administered primarily at home with unfractionated heparin administered in the hospital for proximal deep-vein thrombosis. N Engl J Med 1996;334:677.
46. Lensing AWA, Prins MH, Davidson BL, et al. Treatment of deep venous thrombosis with low-molecular weight heparins. A meta-analysis. Arch Intern Med 1995;155:601.
47. Siragusa S, Cosmi B, Piovella F, et al. Low-molecular-weight heparins and unfractionated heparin in the treatment of patients with acute venous thromboembolism: results of a meta-analysis. Am J Med 1996;100:269.
48. Boccaion H, Elias A, Chale JJ, et al. Clinical outcome and cost of hospital vs home treatment of proximal deep vein thrombosis with a low-molecular-weight heparin: the Vascular Midi-Pyrenees study. Arch Intern Med 2000;160:1769.
49. Warkentin TE, Chong BH, Greinacher A. Heparin-induced thrombocytopenia: towards consensus. Thromb Haemost 199;879:1.
50. Warkentin TE, Kelton JG. Temporal aspects of heparin-induced thrombocytopenia. N Engl J Med 2001;344:1286.
51. Demasi R, Bode AP, Knupp C, et al. Heparin-induced thrombocytopenia Am Surg 1994;60:26.
52. Lewis BE, Wallis DE, Berkowitz SE, et al. Argatroban anticoagulant therapy in patients with heparin-induced thrombocytopenia. Circulation 2001;103:1838.
53. Dukes GE, Sanders SW, Russo J, et al. Transaminase elevations in patients receiving bovine or porcine heparin. Ann Intern Med 1984;100:646.
54. Oster JR, Singer I, Fishman LM. Heparin-induced aldosterone suppression in hyperkalemia. Am J Med 1995;98:575.
55. O'Meara JJ, McNutt RA, Evans AT, et al. A decision analysis of streptokinase plus heparin as compared with heparin alone for deep-vein thrombosis. N Engl J Med 1994;330:1864.
56. Decousus H, Leizorocicz A, Parent F, et al. A clinical trial of vena caval filters in the prevention of pulmonary embolism in patients with proximal deep-vein thrombosis. Prevention du Risque d'Embolie Pulmonaire par Interruption Cave Study Group. N Engl J Med 1998;338:409.
57. Antiplatelet Trialists' Collaboration. Collaborative overview of randomized trials of antiplatelet therapy. I. Prevention of death, myocardial infarction, and stroke by prolonged antiplatelet therapy in various categories of patients. BMJ 1994;308:81.
58. Antiplatelet Trialists' Collaboration. Collaborative overview of randomized trials of antiplatelet therapy. III. Reduction in

venous thrombosis and pulmonary embolism by antiplatelet prophylaxis among surgical and medical patients. BMJ 1994; 308:235.
59. Coon WW, Willis PW III. Recurrence of venous thromboembolism. Surgery 1973;73:823.
60. Duiguid DL. Oral anticoagulant therapy for venous thromboembolism. N Engl J Med 1997;336:433.
61. Petitti DB, Strom BL, Melmon KL. Duration of warfarin anticoagulant therapy and the probabilities of recurrent thromboembolism and hemorrhage. Am J Med 1986;81:255.
62. Schulman S, Rhedin A-S, Lindmarker P, et al. A comparison of six weeks with six months of oral anticoagulant therapy after a first episode of venous thromboembolism. N Engl J Med 1995;332:1661.
63. Schulman S, Granqvist S, Holmström M, et al. The duration of oral anticoagulant therapy after a second episode of venous thromboembolism. N Engl J Med 1997;336:393.
64. Leclerc JR, Jay RM, Hull RD, et al. Recurrent leg symptoms following deep vein thrombosis. A diagnostic challenge. Arch Intern Med 1985;145:1867.
65. Beyth RJ, Cohen AM, Landefeld S. Long-term outcomes of deep-vein thrombosis. Arch Intern Med 1995;155:1031.
66. Editorial. Post-thrombotic venous disorders. Lancet 1985;1:1488.
67. FitzGerald GA, Oates JA, Hawiger J, et al. Endogenous biosynthesis of prostacyclin and thromboxane and platelet function during chronic administration of aspirin in man. J Clin Invest 1983;71:676.
68. Roderick PJ, Wilkes HC, Meade TW. The gastrointestinal toxicity of aspirin: an overview of randomized controlled trials. Br J Clin Pharmacol 1993;35:219.
69. Ridker PM, Manson JE, Gaziano JM, et al. Low-dose aspirin therapy for chronic stable angina. A randomized placebo-controlled clinical trial. Ann Intern Med 1991;114:835.
70. Hennekens CH, Buring JE, Sandercock P, et al. Aspirin and other antiplatelet agents in the secondary and primary prevention of cardiovascular disease. Circulation 1989;80:749.
71. Willard JE, Lange RA, Hillis LD. The use of aspirin in ischemic heart disease. N Engl J Med 1992;327:175.
72. Hirsh J, Dalen JE, Fuster V, et al. Aspirin and other platelet-active drugs. The relationship among dose, effectiveness, and side effects. Chest 1995;108:247S.
73. Antiplatelet Trialists' Collaboration. Collaborative overview of randomized trials of antiplatelet therapy. II. Maintenance of vascular graft or arterial patency by antiplatelet therapy. BMJ 1994;308:159.
74. Manson JE, Stampfer MJ, Coldity GA, et al. A prospective study of aspirin use and primary prevention of cardiovascular disease in women. JAMA 1991;266:521.
75. Peto R, Gray R, Collins R. Randomized trial of prophylactic daily aspirin in British male doctors. BMJ 1988;296:313.
76. The Steering Committee of the Physicians' Health Study Research Group. Final report on the aspirin component of the ongoing physicians' health study. N Engl J Med 1989;321:129.
77. Hennekens CH, Peto R, Hutchison GB, et al. An overview of the British and American aspirin studies [Letter]. N Engl J Med 1988;318:923.
78. Hass WK, Easton JD, Adams HP Jr, et al. A randomized trial comparing ticlopidine hydrochloride with aspirin for the prevention of stroke in high risk patients. N Engl J Med 1989;321:501.
79. Bennett CL, Weinberg PD, Rozenberg-Ben-Dror K, et al. Thrombotic thrombocytopenic purpura associated with ticlopidine: a review of 60 cases. Ann Intern Med 1998;128:541.
80. CAPRIE Steering Committee. A randomized, blinded, trial of clopidogrel versus aspirin in patients at risk for ischaemic events (CAPRIE). Lancet 1996;348:1329.
81. Bennett CL, Connors JM, Carwile JM, et al. Thrombotic thrombocytopenic purpura associated with clopidogrel. N Engl J Med 2000;342:1773.

CHAPTER 58

Selected Disorders of Lymph Nodes and Lymphocytes

LARRY WATERBURY, MD
PHILIP D. ZIEVE, MD

INFECTIOUS MONONUCLEOSIS

Infectious mononucleosis is one of several infections that are caused by herpes viruses. Others include cytomegalovirus (CMV) infections, herpes simplex infections (see Chapters 102 and 117), and varicella-zoster infections (see Chapter 117).

Epidemiology and Pathogenesis

The Epstein-Barr virus (EBV) is the cause of infectious mononucleosis (1,2), an acute febrile illness that, in the United States, affects primarily teenagers and young adults (the age group between 15 and 25 years). Infection with the virus is extremely common; for example, more than 50% of college students of both sexes have antibodies to it, and each year 12% of college students who do not have antibodies to EBV develop them (most of them in the course of clinical mononucleosis) (3). Because of the ubiquity of exposure early in life, infectious mononucleosis is rare in people over the age of 35 and when it does occur may present atypically (see below). The virus seems to be spread by oral contact, first infecting B lymphocytes in the oral pharynx that subsequently generate a T-cell response that results in atypical lymphocytosis in the peripheral blood.

Table 58.1. Signs and Symptoms of Infectious Mononucleosis

Common Symptoms	Percent	Common Signs	Percent	Less Common Signs and Symptoms	Percent
Malaise	100	Adenopathy	100	Jaundice	10
Sore throat	85	Fever	90	Arthralgia	5
Warmth, chilliness	70	Pharyngitis	85	Skin rash	5
Anorexia	70	Splenomegaly	60	Diarrhea	5
Headache	50	Bradycardia	40	Photophobia	5
Cough	40	Periorbital edema	25		
Myalgia	25	Palatal enanthem	25		

Signs and Symptoms

Clinical illness usually begins after a 1- to 2-month incubation period. Classically, patients have pharyngitis, lymphadenopathy, splenomegaly, and marked atypical lymphocytosis. Table 58.1 lists the relative frequency of the characteristic signs and symptoms associated with the illness. Pharyngitis occasionally can be extremely severe and is often accompanied by an exudate, which may be foul smelling. Rarely, it may be so severe that it leads to respiratory obstruction. Of the few patients who do not have pharyngitis (especially children), most simply have a nonspecific febrile illness associated with malaise. Other patients have mild jaundice and a syndrome that mimics infectious hepatitis. Posterior cervical adenopathy is characteristic of almost all patients, and there is often generalized lymph node enlargement as well; approximately 60% have an enlarged spleen. Some patients may experience a protracted course with nonspecific symptoms, slight to moderately tender lymphadenopathy, and splenomegaly that persist for weeks. Most patients are significantly improved by the end of 3 weeks.

Patients usually present to the practitioner at the end of the first week with a nonspecific illness characterized by malaise and perhaps by anorexia, mild headache, and fever (up to 104°F). Adenopathy, splenomegaly, and pharyngitis usually appear at about this time and slowly resolve over the following weeks. However, as noted below, the classic laboratory features of the disease may not be present until the second or third week of the clinical illness. Patients over 40 years of age tend to have more prolonged fever and less adenopathy than do young adults (4,5).

Laboratory Features

The hematocrit value is usually normal, although occasionally mild hemolysis and rarely a severe autoimmune hemolytic anemia are seen. The peripheral white cell count is usually elevated, reaching its height during the second and third weeks of the clinical illness. Early in the course there may be a severe absolute neutropenia, and occasionally the absolute neutrophil count is less than 500/μL. The differential count of the white cells is characterized by an absolute lymphocytosis with large numbers (more than 10% of the total white cell population) of atypical lymphocytes (large lobulated or indented nuclei and vacuolated or bluish cytoplasm). The platelet count is normal to slightly decreased in most patients; severe thrombocytopenia may occur rarely. Slight increases in the activity of hepatic enzymes are common but never reach the height seen in viral hepatitis; however, older patients tend to have more marked hepatic dysfunction, and in this group jaundice is common (4).

Table 58.2. Serologic Evidence of Epstein-Barr Virus (EBV) Infection

IgM antibody to viral capsid antigen (IgM anti-VCA). Appears early in primary infection and disappears within 3 to 6 mo.

IgG antibody to viral capsid antigen (IgG anti-VCA). Appears slightly later than IgM anti-VCA and remains detectable for life.

Antibodies to the early antigen (EA) complex of EBV of the diffuse (D) type (anti-D). Anti-D antibodies appear early in primary infection and disappear by 2 to 3 mo. A significant number of patients do not develop these antibodies.

Antibodies to EB nuclear antigen (anti-EBNA). Anti-EBNA appears 6–12 wk after symptoms and is detectable for life.

Serologic Features

Diagnosis is based on the presence of typical clinical features and characteristic serologic tests. A number of different EBV antibodies have been identified (6). They are summarized in Table 58.2. *Immunoglobulin M antibody to viral capsid antigen* (IgM anti-VCA) appears within 1 to 6 weeks after onset of infection and disappears within 3 to 6 months; a rising titer during the first few weeks of clinical illness is the most useful, and generally the most easily available serologic, evidence of recent primary infection. *Antibodies to the early antigen complex of EBV of the diffuse (D) type* (known as anti-D antibodies) also appear early in primary infection and disappear by 2 to 3 months, but anti-D antibody testing is much less available than IgM anti-VCA testing. *Heterophil antibodies (nonspecific antibodies secondary to the immune response to EBV)* are elevated in most patients, peaking in weeks 2 to 5 of clinical illness, and present in low titer for up to a year.

Differential absorption studies are needed to identify the presence of those heterophil antibodies that are specific for infectious mononucleosis (the antibodies are absorbed by bovine red cells but not by guinea pig kidney). A number of rapid diagnostic tests are commercially available. Some use horse red cells in a latex agglutination assay (the "Monospot" test), and others use enzyme-linked immunosorbent assays. In general, the kits are quite sensitive and specific and are the tests of choice for diagnosis (7). Most patients do not require EBV antibody testing. In patients with classic symptoms of infectious mononucleosis, a positive rapid test is sufficient serologic confirmation for the diagnosis for clinical purposes. Some 5% to 10% of patients with clinical infectious mononucleosis and serologic evidence of recent primary EBV infection are heterophil antibody negative (7). Another 5% to 10% of patients with clinical features of infectious mononucleosis, also heterophile negative, have another illness (e.g., CMV infection, toxoplasmosis) (8).

Complications

Severe complications of infectious mononucleosis are rare but do occur. They include neurologic problems (encephalitis, meningitis, peripheral neuropathy, Guillain-Barré syndrome), bacterial superinfection, and splenic rupture (9). The latter has accounted for occasional deaths, especially because the diagnosis is easily missed. The diagnosis should be suspected if there is a recent history of sudden, brief, sharp, abdominal pain. Occasional deaths have been seen also with severe pharyngitis and airway obstruction. All these complications are even more rare when the mononucleosis syndrome is caused by an infectious agent other than the EBV (see below). The pharyngitis in infectious mononucleosis may closely resemble that of exudative streptococcal pharyngitis, and all patients should have throat cultures to rule out bacterial infection.

Treatment

No specific treatment exists for infectious mononucleosis, and all that is usually necessary is patient education and supportive care. There is no evidence that prolonged bed rest is helpful. It is reasonable for patients to avoid strenuous activities until they feel strong enough to participate. Contact sports should be avoided if the spleen is tender or significantly enlarged. Because splenomegaly may persist for months, however, it seems unreasonable to avoid such sports until the spleen is no longer palpable. Although contacts do occasionally develop infectious mononucleosis, there is no evidence that the disease is highly infectious and patients should not be rigidly restricted from interpersonal contacts (3). (Although the patient continues to shed the virus for up to 18 months after onset of the illness [10], close personal exposure during this period only occasionally results in transmission of the disease.)

Surgery may be needed for splenic rupture, although some cases have been handled with just transfusion support (9). Corticosteroids are usually reserved for patients with severe pharyngitis or impending airway obstruction (11) and other rare life-threatening complications of the illness. Controlled studies have not proven steroids or steroids plus acyclovir to be clinically useful (12,13).

Other Causes of the Mononucleosis Syndrome

Cytomegalovirus Infection

Although CMV infections may cause devastating clinical illness in the newborn (*in utero*) and in the immunocompromised host, infection in the noncompromised adult causes a clinical syndrome essentially indistinguishable from infectious mononucleosis except that exudative pharyngitis is unusual in CMV infection. Unlike exposure to EBV, which has occurred in most adults in the United States by age 25, primary CMV infections usually occur at an older age, making CMV mononucleosis the most common cause of the mononucleosis syndrome in patients over 30 years of age. Up to 50% of people over the age of 40 have antibodies to CMV, although most do not have a history of infection. Diagnosis can be made by finding an increased titer of serum IgM antibody to CMV.

Toxoplasmosis

Acute toxoplasmosis, although usually asymptomatic in people with normal immune responses, may cause a syndrome that resembles infectious mononucleosis, but pharyngitis does not occur and splenomegaly and lymphadenopathy are usually not as prominent. Also, patients usually do not develop hepatitis or the hematologic manifestations of EBV infections. Diagnosis usually depends on a constellation of serologic findings indicative of recent primary infection (a positive Sabin-Feldman dye test, the presence of anti-IgM antibodies by an indirect fluorescent antibody test, or the demonstration of rising titers of IgG antibodies by indirect fluorescent antibody).

Other Infections

Other conditions, besides mononucleosis, CMV, and toxoplasmosis, can cause the mononucleosis syndrome (8): Viral hepatitis (see Chapter 47), acute human immunodeficiency virus infection (Chapter 39), and human herpesvirus 6 infection. Sometimes an etiologic agent cannot be identified even after extensive serologic testing. Table 58.3 suggests a stepwise plan for the serologic evaluation of patients with the mononucleosis syndrome. Seronegative patients need further evaluation only if symptoms persist for more than a week or two or if symptoms intensify or if worrisome adenopathy persists (see The Undiagnosed Patient with Lymphadenopathy, below).

CHRONIC FATIGUE SYNDROME

Since 1985, there has been an epidemic in the United States, predominantly in young women, of an illness characterized universally by debilitating fatigue and by a host of other symptoms (sore throat, tender lymph nodes, myalgia, joint pain, headaches, malaise, impaired memory or concentration), many of them suggestive of EBV infection. Initially, people who complained of these symptoms were thought to have chronic mononucleosis because of the demonstration of antibodies to EBV in their blood. It soon became evident, however, that antibody titers to a number of viruses (retroviruses, CMV, human herpesvirus type 6, Coxsackie B virus, measles) were elevated in the blood of these patients, casting doubt on the role of EBV as an etiologic agent of the illness. Extensive

Table 58.3. Stepwise Serologic Testing in the Diagnosis of the Cause of the Mononucleosis Syndrome

1. Typical clinical features with a positive heterophil slide test. This essentially establishes a diagnosis of infectious mononucleosis, usually caused by EBV. *Recommendation:* No further testing is needed.
2. Typical clinical features with a negative heterophil slide test at the time the patient first presents to the physician. *Recommendation:* Draw acute serum samples (save frozen in two containers) for pertinent serologic testing for EBV (IgM VCA and IgG EBNA antibodies), toxoplasmosis, CMV, HIV. Repeat heterophil slide test during the third week of clinical illness. If positive, no further testing is necessary. If negative, repeat EBV serology (at least 2 wk after acute sample) and send with one of the acute serologic samples for EBV IgM anti-VCA testing and IgG EBNA antibodies. If the EBV serologies are diagnostic of recent infection, no further testing is necessary.
3. Typical clinical features, negative slide test at week 3 of clinical illness, and negative EBV serology (negative IgM anti-VCA and negative or positive IgG EBNA). *Recommendation:* Draw convalescent sera for testing for toxoplasmosis, CMV, and send with acute sera for appropriate serologic testing. Consider HIV infection in patients at risk.
4. Typical or atypical clinical features with negative serologies for all of the above. Consider other causes (e.g., leukemia, lymphoproliferative disease, granulomatous disease, collagen vascular disease). *Recommendation:* Consider lymph node biopsy and other tests (e.g., bone marrow aspiration and biopsy).

EBV, Estein-Barr virus; VCA, viral capsid antigen; EBNA, Epstein-Barr nuclear antigen; CMV, cytomegalovirus; HIV, human immunodeficiency virus.

seroepidemiologic study by the Centers for Disease Control and Prevention has revealed no consistent association with any infectious agent (14). Therefore, the illness was renamed the chronic fatigue syndrome, and criteria were formulated for its diagnosis (15). It has become obvious that the prevalence of psychiatric illness (e.g., depression, somatoform disorder, anxiety) is increased considerably in patients with the syndrome, so that it is tempting to believe that all the symptoms reflect underlying psychopathology. Studies have failed to identify differences between control subjects and cases in a host of tests of immunologic function (16). Affected patients are likely to remain symptomatic indefinitely; they need the understanding and support of their families and their caregiver and specific attention to psychiatric problems when they are manifest (see Chapters 21, 22, and 24). The likelihood of patients returning to totally normal function is low (17). Poor prognostic features include older age, more chronic illness, the presence of comorbid psychiatric disease, and a persistent belief by the patient that the illness has a physical cause (18). Psychiatric intervention, especially cognitive therapy, may be helpful (19,20).

CHRONIC LYMPHOCYTIC LEUKEMIA

Clinical Features

Chronic lymphocytic leukemia (CLL) is the most common type of leukemia in the United States. It is primarily a disease of older men (21) in that two-thirds of patients are 60 or older and two to three times as many men are afflicted as are women. A mild tendency for the disease to segregate in families suggests that genetic factors may play a role in its acquisition (22).

Many patients are asymptomatic when diagnosed (see below), but complaints of malaise and increased fatigability are common. Ultimately, most patients develop generalized lymphadenopathy and splenomegaly.

A persistent absolute lymphocytosis (greater than 10,000/μL for 3 months or longer) is the hallmark of the disease; lymphocyte counts as high as 200,000 to 300,000/μL may be seen occasionally. Other tests (bone marrow aspiration, lymph node biopsy) are ordinarily not necessary to establish the diagnosis.

As the disease progresses, hypogammaglobulinemia, anemia, granulocytopenia, and thrombocytopenia may develop. Autoimmune disorders (autoimmune hemolytic anemia and thrombocytopenia and pure red cell aplasia) develop in 10% to 15% of patients.

Treatment and Course

The survival of patients with CLL correlates best with the stage of their disease at diagnosis (23,24). For example, asymptomatic patients with only an absolute lymphocytosis (about 25% of the patients) have an essentially normal life expectancy. Patients with lymphadenopathy alone have a median survival of 6 to 8 years (about 50% of patients), and patients with significant anemia or thrombocytopenia (about 25% of patients) have a median survival of 2 to 3 years.

There is no good evidence that treatment influences survival, but it can be helpful in decreasing the severity of signs and symptoms in the later stages of the disease. Thus, stable asymptomatic patients with or without lymphadenopathy or splenomegaly do not require treatment. On the other hand, patients with marked constitutional symptoms (weight loss, severe malaise) or with symptomatic anemia or thrombocytopenia should be treated. For years standard treatment of CLL included alkylating agents (e.g., chlorambucil) and prednisone. Recent studies suggest that treatment of CLL with the purine analogue fludarabine results in a higher rate of remission (especially complete remission) and in more prolonged remissions than does treatment with alkylating agents (although without an improved survival) (25). Aggressive treatment (including bone marrow and stem cell transplant) of early stage disease in younger patients with CLL is undergoing active investigation. Patients with autoimmune hemolysis and thrombocytopenia require more aggressive treatment with corticosteroids, and splenectomy is sometimes necessary in severely anemic or thrombocytopenic patients who are unresponsive to corticosteroids. A hematologist or medical oncologist should be consulted at the time of diagnosis of CLL and should be involved in the care of patients who require treatment.

Differential Diagnosis

A number of neoplastic conditions other than CLL may be associated with a chronic lymphocytosis:

macroglobulinemia, B- and T-cell lymphomas, hairy cell leukemia, prolymphocytic leukemia, and adult T-cell leukemia. The morphology of the cells, evaluation of peripheral lymphocyte surface markers by flow cytometry, or other manifestations of the disease usually lead to the correct diagnosis. These conditions should be managed in close consultation with an oncologist.

A syndrome has been recognized (26), most often in older people, characterized by a clonal proliferation of large granular T lymphocytes (up to 10,000/mm^3) and, usually, chronic neutropenia. Anemia (rarely, red cell aplasia) and thrombocytopenia are uncommon. Lymphocytic infiltration of the bone marrow and spleen (with splenomegaly) is characteristic; lymph node involvement is rare. Some patients have coexistent seropositive rheumatoid arthritis; most patients, with or without arthritis, have serologic abnormalities (e.g., in addition to increased titers of rheumatoid factor, antinuclear antibodies, polyclonal hypergammaglobulinemia, and circulating immune complexes). The major morbidity from the disease is caused by recurrent bacterial infections; otherwise, most patients require no treatment and their mortality rate is low.

THE UNDIAGNOSED PATIENT WITH LYMPHADENOPATHY: WHEN TO RECOMMEND LYMPH NODE BIOPSY

Lymphadenopathy is a common physical finding that is associated with multiple disease processes (27). The decision about when to biopsy an enlarged lymph node is difficult (28). The problem arises most often in younger patients. Older patients with localized lymphadenopathy unexplained by infection or inflammation should be assumed to have cancer until proven otherwise, and the biopsy decision, therefore, is usually an easy one. However, lymphadenopathy in children and in young adults is usually caused by inflammation, and biopsy is usually not diagnostic. The clinician is often concerned in such circumstances about the possible harm from a delay in the diagnosis of a malignancy (Hodgkin disease or non-Hodgkin lymphoma most commonly) or a granulomatous condition (e.g., tuberculosis, sarcoid) for which specific treatment is indicated. However, harm can result from unnecessary biopsy. For the patient, there is both psychologic and physical discomfort from the procedure, and most important, there can be uncertainty about the interpretation of the biopsy of a reactive node. The histology of reactive nodes, especially those encountered in the mononucleosis syndrome, can be difficult to interpret. Reed-Sternberg cells (ordinarily pathognomonic of Hodgkin disease) can be seen in the nodes of patients with infectious mononucleosis, and reactive nodes can sometimes look like and be interpreted as diagnostic of Hodgkin disease or of non-Hodgkin lymphoma. Because of these problems, biopsy of a lymph node should be avoided in a patient with the mononucleosis syndrome if possible.

Table 58.4. When to Recommend Lymph Node Biopsy in the Teenager and Young Adult

Features against early biopsy
- Mononucleosis syndrome, especially when proven serologically.
  - Ear–nose–throat symptoms (earache, sore throat, coryza tonsillar, or dental infection).
  - Lymph nodes less than 2 cm in diameter.
  - Normal chest radiograph, especially when associated with one of the above.

Features for early biopsy
- Systemic illness with atypical features of the mononucleosis syndrome and without serologic proof of a cause of the mononucleosis syndrome (see Table 58.3).
- Lymph nodes greater than 2 cm in diameter and an abnormal chest radiograph, absence of ear–nose–throat symptoms, or no proof of a typical mononucleosis syndrome.
- Localized supraclavicular lymphadenopathy. This may be seen in the mononucleosis syndrome but in its absence is suggestive of mediastinal (right supraclavicular) or abdominal (left supraclavicular) granulomatous or neoplastic disease.

If a specific diagnosis cannot be made on the basis of clinical features and serologic studies, few criteria can be relied on to decide whether a biopsy is indicated. However, one helpful retrospective study reported that in the age range of 9 to 25 years, three variables were important in determining whether a lymph node biopsy might be diagnostic of an illness requiring specific treatment (29): the size of the node to be tested by biopsy, the presence or absence of ear–nose–throat symptoms, and the presence or absence of an abnormality on chest radiograph. Nodes greater than 2 cm in diameter were more likely to contain important histologic information than were smaller nodes. An abnormal chest radiograph (adenopathy, infiltrate) in a patient with peripheral adenopathy correlated with useful biopsy information. Patients with cervical lymphadenopathy but without any ear– nose–throat symptoms were more likely to have a diagnostic lymph node biopsy. A recent study developed a prediction rule that, if validated, may be useful in deciding which patients with adenopathy should be biopsied (30). Table 58.4 summarizes some of the features that can be used, especially in the young patient, to help determine the advisability and timing of a lymph node biopsy.

General References*

Rai KR, Patel DV. Chronic lymphocytic leukemia. In: Hoffman R, Benz EJ, Shattil SJ, et al., eds. Hematology: basic principles and practice, 3rd ed. New York: Churchill Livingstone, 2000:1350.

Sullivan JL. Infectious mononucleosis and other Epstein-Barr virus-associated diseases. In: Hoffman R, Benz EJ, Shattil SJ, et al., eds. Hematology: basic principles and practice, 3rd ed. New York: Churchill Livingstone, 2000:812.

Specific References

1. Evans AS, Niederman JC, McCollum RW. Seroepidemiologic studies of infectious mononucleosis with EB virus. N Engl J Med 1968;279:1121.

*Bold print (general references) and bold numerals (specific references) denote published controlled clinical trials, meta-analyses, or consensus-based recommendations.

2. Strauss SE, Cohen JI, Tosato G, et al. Epstein-Barr virus infections: biology, pathogenesis, and management. Ann Intern Med 1993;118:45.
3. Sawyer RN, Evans AS, Niederman JC, et al. Prospective studies of a group of Yale University freshmen. I. Occurrence of infectious mononucleosis. J Infect Dis 1971;123:263.
4. Horwitz CA, Henle W, Henle G, et al. Infectious mononucleosis in patients aged 40 to 72 years: report of 27 cases, including 3 without heterophil-antibody responses. Medicine (Baltimore) 1983;62:256.
5. Auwaerter PG. Infectious mononucleosis in middle age. JAMA 1999;281:454.
6. Evans AS, Niederman JC, Cenabre LC, et al. A prospective evaluation of heterophile and Epstein-Barr versus specific IgM antibody tests in clinical and subclinical infectious mononucleosis: specificity and sensitivity of the tests and persistence of antibody. J Infect Dis 1975;132:546.
7. Linderholm M, Borman J, Juto P, et al. A comparative evaluation of nine kits for rapid diagnosis of infectious mononucleosis and Epstein-Barr virus-specific serology. J Clin Microbiol 1994;32:259.
8. Evans AS. Infectious mononucleosis and related syndromes. Am J Med Sci 1978;276:325.
9. Asgari MM, Begos DG. Spontaneous splenic rupture in infectious mononucleosis: a review. Yale J Biol Med 1997;70:175.
10. Miller G, Niederman JC, Andrews LL. Prolonged oropharyngeal excretion of Epstein-Barr virus after infectious mononucleosis. N Engl J Med 1973;288:229.
11. McGowan JE Jr, Chesney PJ, Grossley KB, et al. Guidelines for the use of systemic glucocorticoids in the management of selected infections. Working Group on Steroid Use, Antimicrobial Agents Committee, Infectious Disease Society of America. J Infect Dis 1992;165:1.
12. Tynell E, Aurelius E, Brandell A, et al. Acyclovir and prednisolone treatment of acute infectious mononucleosis: a multicenter, double-blind, placebo-controlled study. J Infect Dis 1996;174:324.
13. Torre D, Tambini R. Acyclovir for treatment of infectious mononucleosis: a meta-analysis. Scand J Infect Dis 1999;31: 543.
14. Mawle AC, Nisenbaum R, Dobbins JG, et al. Seroepidemiology of chronic fatigue syndrome: a case-control study. Clin Infect Dis 1995;21:1386.
15. Fukuda K, Straus SE, Hickie I. The chronic fatigue syndrome: a comprehensive approach to its definition and study. Ann Intern Med 1994;121:953.
16. Mawle AC, Nisenbaum R, Dobbins JG, et al. Immune responses associated with chronic fatigue syndrome: a case-control study. J Infect Dis 1997;175:136.
17. Bombardier CH, Buchwald D. Outcome and prognosis of patients with chronic fatigue vs chronic fatigue syndrome. Arch Intern Med 1995;155:2105.
18. Joyce J, Hotopf M, Wessely S. The prognosis of chronic fatigue and chronic fatigue syndrome: a systematic review. Q J Med 1997;90:223.
19. Deale A, Chalder T, Marks I, et al. Cognitive behavior therapy for chronic fatigue syndrome: a randomized controlled trial. Am J Psych 1997;154:408.
20. Sharpe M, Hawkins K, Simkin S, et al. Cognitive behaviour therapy for the chronic fatigue syndrome: a randomized controlled trial. BMJ 1996;312:22.
21. Skinnider LF, Tan L, Schmidt J, et al. Chronic lymphocytic leukemia. A review of 745 cases and assessment of clinical staging. Cancer (Philadelphia) 1982;50:2951.
22. Conley CL, Misiti J, Laster AJ. Genetic factors predisposing to chronic lymphocytic leukemia. Medicine (Baltimore) 1980;59:323.
23. Rai KR, Han T. Prognostic factors and clinical staging in chronic lymphocytic leukemia. Hematol Oncol Clin North Am 1990;4:447.
24. Rozman C, Montserrat E. Chronic lymphocytic leukemia. N Engl J Med 1995;333:1052.
25. Rai KR, Peterson BL, Appelbaum FR, et al. Fludarabine compared with chlorambucil as primary therapy for chronic lymphocytic leukemia. N Engl J Med 2000;343:1750.
26. Loughran TP, Starkebaum G. Large granular lymphocyte leukemia. Report of 38 cases and review of the literature. Medicine (Baltimore) 1987;66:397.
27. Libman H. Generalized lymphadenopathy. J Gen Intern Med 1987;2:48.
28. Greenfield S, Jordan MC. The clinical investigation of lymphadenopathy in primary care practice. JAMA 1978;240:1388.
29. Slap GB, Brooks SJ, Schwartz JS. When to perform biopsies of enlarged peripheral lymph nodes in young patients. JAMA 1984;252:1321.
30. Vassilakopoulos TP, Pangalis GA. Application of a prediction rule to select which patients presenting with lymphadenopathy should undergo a lymph node biopsy. Medicine 2000;79:338.

SECTION

8

Pulmonary Problems

CHAPTER 59

Common Pulmonary Problems: Cough, Hemoptysis, Dyspnea, Chest Pain, and Abnormal Chest X-Ray*

IRINA PETRACHE, MD
STEVE N. GEORAS, MD

Patients who develop acute respiratory problems usually present with symptoms that result in the rapid diagnosis and treatment of the underlying disorder. On the other hand, chronic diseases of the lung that cause slowly progressive symptoms may go undetected unless incidentally discovered as part of a general medical evaluation. This chapter discusses common pulmonary problems with which the general practitioner is often confronted: cough, hemoptysis, dyspnea, noncardiac chest pain, and the abnormal chest x-ray.

COUGH

Cough is an important defense mechanism that clears the airways of both secretions and inhaled particles (1). Although it is often associated with other respiratory symptoms, cough may be the symptom that prompts a patient to seek medical advice, especially if it is associated with complications (e.g., fear of serious disease, exhaustion, insomnia, life-style change, pain, hoarseness, or urinary incontinence). A cough is composed of three phases: a deep inspiration, closure of the glottis accompanied by a rapid increase in intrathoracic pressure, and a final opening of the glottis with an explosive release of pressure.

Mucosal neural receptors that initiate a *cough reflex* are located throughout the nasopharynx, ears, larynx, trachea, and bronchi down to the level of the terminal bronchioles. They are rapidly adapting receptors with thin myelinated nerve fibers and show varied sensitivities to different stimuli. Stimulation of these receptors in the nasopharynx may also cause sneezing. In contrast, stimulation of laryngeal receptors may initiate cardiovascular, bronchoconstrictor, and laryngoconstrictor reflexes, whereas stimulation of tracheal and bronchial receptors may also cause bronchospasm and airway mucus secretion. After activation of the receptors, impulses are conducted along afferent pathways in the ninth and tenth cranial nerves to the cough center located diffusely in the medulla. The reflex is complete through efferent pathways that cause forceful contraction of the diaphragm and other expiratory muscles. Although many different stimuli activate these receptors, all initiate cough by some form of mechanical or chemical irritation. Additional factors, such as acute inflammation of the airways, may disrupt the bronchial mucosa, increase its permeability, and expose the receptors. The accompanying increases in respiratory secretions will lead to cough. Environmental pollutants, such as cigarette smoke, can directly stimulate the receptors without necessarily provoking an inflammatory reaction. Finally, although stimulation of irritant receptors may cause reflex bronchoconstriction, the bronchospasm itself, through reflex pathways, induces cough.

Acute Cough Syndromes

Table 59.1 shows the causes of cough. Generally, acute coughs are self-limited (less than 3 weeks) and are caused by viral *upper respiratory tract infections* (2). In contrast, cough that is triggered by mild bronchospasm may persist for weeks to months after a viral upper respiratory tract infection (see below). Usually, viral infections, atypical pneumonias, and *Pneumocystis carinii* pneumonia are associated with nonproductive coughs, and bacterial infections are associated with significant sputum production. Younger patients tend to have a more productive cough associated with *pneumonia,* whereas older individuals, especially those with chronic obstructive pulmonary disease (COPD), may retain secretions because of impaired ability to clear them. When a productive cough follows a typical viral syndrome, it may signal the development of a superimposed bacterial bronchitis or pneumonia. High concentrations of air pollutants, such as

*Philip L. Smith, E. James Britt, and Peter B. Terry contributed to this chapter in previous editions.

Table 59.1. Causes of Cough

Causes	Examples
Common causes	
Acute	
Inflammation	Tracheitis, bronchitis, pneumonia
Irritation	Environmental pollutants
Bronchospasm	Infection
Chronic	
Inflammation	Bronchitis, pollution, cigarettes, bronchiectasis, aspirated foreign body, chronic pneumonia (tuberculous and nontuberculous mycobacterial infection, *Pneumocystis* pneumonia in AIDS)
Irritation	Cigarettes, cancer, postnasal drip
Bronchospasm	Asthma, heart failure
Less common causes	
Drug induced	Angiotensin-converting enzyme inhibitor, beta-blockers (oral or ophthalmic), inhaled medication
Irritation	Esophageal reflux, chronic aspiration, auditory canal stimulation (cerumen, hair), aortic aneurysm
Inflammation	Sarcoid, alveolitis, bronchiolitis obliterans organizing pneumonia (BOOP)

AIDS, acquired immunodeficiency syndrome.

insoluble gases (e.g., ozone, SO_3, or NO_2), which are not irritating to the upper airway, can cause either a dry or a productive cough secondary to chemical irritation.

Chronic Cough Syndromes

A persistent cough (generally lasting more than 3 weeks) is often more bothersome than the acute cough syndrome described above. The most common cause of chronic coughing is *cigarette smoking* (2). The so-called smokers' cough, a manifestation of *chronic bronchitis,* is generally described as hacking, worse in the morning, and productive or dry, as sputum is often ignored by cigarette smokers. The number of cigarettes smoked bears little relationship to the development of cough. Perhaps because they inhale more deeply, smokers of marijuana may complain of a persistent cough after smoking only one to two cigarettes daily. Patients with central *bronchogenic and mediastinal tumors* often present with cough, whereas patients with metastatic tumors or peripheral lung cancers that arise outside the airways or beyond irritant receptors seldom do. In nonsmokers, the most common cause of chronic cough is *postnasal drip,* resulting from chronic sinusitis or allergic rhinitis (1,2). The postnasal drip syndrome is also the single most common cause of cough for which patients seek medical attention (1). It is important to recognize that *bronchospasm* in smokers, as well as nonsmokers, can be associated with a chronic dry cough. Cough may be the only manifestation of mild *asthma* (cough variant asthma) and need not be associated with dyspnea, wheezing, or changes in baseline pulmonary function (3).

Gastroesophageal reflux disease (GERD) may present with only minimal gastrointestinal symptoms and a significant nagging cough and, occasionally, hoarseness (see Chapter 42). A nocturnal cough that is precipitated or increased by lying flat makes this diagnosis more likely, but cough due to congestive heart failure is also often initiated by the patient lying down. A dry hacking cough associated with dyspnea is common in patients in *heart failure* (see Chapter 66). Similarly, cough may precede the complaint of dyspnea in patients with pulmonary emboli or bronchiolitis obliterans organizing pneumonia (a patchy pneumonia, probably immunologic, often idiopathic, that often responds to treatment with corticosteroids). *Bronchiectasis and chronic pulmonary infections,* such as tuberculosis or nontuberculous mycobacterial pneumonia in immunocompetent patients, and *Pneumocystis carinii* pneumonia in patients with acquired immunodeficiency syndrome (AIDS), commonly cause coughing. A chronic nonproductive cough occurs in up to 10% of patients taking an *angiotensin-converting enzyme inhibitor* and remits shortly (within 4 weeks) after the drug is discontinued. Because angiotensin-converting enzyme inhibitors are the treatment of choice for many conditions (e.g., congestive heart failure), it may be worth trying to "treat through" the cough in some patients. A recent study found that the thromboxane antagonist picotamide was highly effective at relieving angiotensin-converting enzyme–induced cough (4); however, this drug is currently not available in the United States. Other pharmacologic approaches can be used, including cromolyn sodium (e.g., via metered-dose inhalers, two puffs four times a day), baclofen (5 mg three times a day for 1 week, 10 mg three times a day for 3 weeks), low-dose theophylline, or sulindac. However, these regimens have not been studied in controlled settings or with large numbers of patients (5). The incidence of cough is negligible with angiotensin II receptor antagonists; thus a trial of these agents may also be reasonable.

There are numerous less common causes of chronic cough. A chronic cough may be caused by a process that stimulates the neural receptors in the pleura and pericardium. Even *impacted cerumen* in the external auditory canal can elicit a chronic cough. If the history and physical examination are unrevealing, it is often tempting to attribute chronic cough to a psychogenic cause; however, this is a rare cause of coughing, most often reported in children (1).

Evaluation

The acute and chronic cough syndromes are evaluated in similar ways. Usually, a history and physical examination yield a presumptive diagnosis. Information should be obtained about the development, duration, character, and precipitants of the cough; environmental or occupational exposure; smoking history; and any history of asthma or COPD. A history of constant swallowing or of throat clearing is associated with postnasal drip, even though the patient may deny many other symptoms associated with sinusitis.

Although the physical examination seldom provides a specific diagnosis, it may provide important clues. Careful examination of the ears, nose, throat, and lungs may yield relevant clues to a diagnosis. Cobblestoning in the posterior oropharynx represents lymphoid hyperplasia and is commonly seen in patients with chronic sinusitis. Examination of the chest may reveal rhonchi caused by the loose secretions that result from acute or chronic infection. A localized wheeze suggests a bronchogenic tumor, whereas wheezing at end-expiration suggests active bronchospasm. Finally, the physical examination allows the quality and severity of the cough to be observed. A harsh cough associated with loose secretions is characteristic of tracheobronchitis resulting from viral upper respiratory tract infection. When little or no coughing occurs in the course of the visit, the patient should be asked to cough to determine whether the cough is productive or is associated with wheezing. This is also useful because some patients refuse to admit to expectoration of sputum and often unconsciously swallow their secretions.

If a diagnosis is not obvious after a history and physical examination, a chest x-ray is indicated. It may reveal a tumor, a pneumonia, or another chronic inflammatory process involving the lung parenchyma. The x-ray also may demonstrate atelectasis associated with a bronchogenic tumor or an aspirated foreign body or bilateral hilar adenopathy suggesting sarcoidosis. Three diagnoses account for almost 100% of chronic coughs in nonsmokers with normal chest x-rays: postnasal drip, asthma, and GERD (1). In patients with a normal x-ray, spirometry can be used to look for obstructive airways disease. However, a normal spirogram does not necessarily exclude the diagnosis (see Chapter 60). When the chest x-ray is normal, bronchoscopy seldom provides additional useful information (2). Although a proximal bronchogenic tumor can be hidden on a chest x-ray by the mediastinal shadows, patients with these tumors often have associated hemoptysis (see below). If the history, physical examination, chest x-ray, and spirogram are unrevealing and if the patient's cough persists after stopping new medicines, including angiotensin-converting enzyme inhibitors and beta-blockers (including eye drops) (6), referral to a subspecialist may be appropriate. Additional tests would include methacholine challenge (asthma), high-resolution chest computed tomography (CT) (bronchiectasis, interstitial lung disease), sinus x-ray or CT (chronic sinusitis), 24-hour pH probe (GERD), and, rarely, bronchoscopy (endobronchial tumor or aspirated foreign body) or cardiac evaluation (heart failure). Irwin et al. (2) developed a useful algorithm for evaluating chronic cough (Fig. 59.1).

Therapy

Specific therapy of the various acute inflammatory and irritating processes likely to cause coughing is discussed in detail in individual chapters dealing with these topics.

In general, viral tracheobronchitis requires only symptomatic therapy because coughing usually subsides spontaneously in 2 to 4 weeks. Patients with persistent coughing and a history or physical examination compatible with bronchospasm may benefit from bronchodilators. Treatment should begin with an inhaled beta-2-sympathomimetic agonist. A detailed therapeutic approach to the pharmacologic treatment of bronchospasm is presented in Chapter 60.

Cessation of cigarette smoking and avoidance of a polluted environment may be the most important aspects of the therapy of both acute and chronic cough. It is often difficult to convey to a smoker that smoking as few as one or two cigarettes a day causes airway irritation and inflammation. Ipratropium bromide may improve cough and decrease sputum production in patients with chronic bronchitis (see Chapter 60) (1).

Removal of impacted cerumen in the auditory canal provides immediate relief (see Chapter 110). The treatment of postnasal drip and GERD are discussed in Chapters 33 and 42, respectively. In most patients, cough will improve within 1 week of initiation of therapy for postnasal drip, but it may take months to resolve in the case of GERD, even with optimal therapy (2). Approximately one-fourth of patients with chronic cough referred for subspecialty evaluation had more than one cause (2). Thus, if specific therapy does not eliminate the cause, additional testing and treatment should be pursued.

After specific therapy has been initiated, the use of *antitussives* should be considered. Despite the enormous demands made for antitussives, there are few situations in which these preparations are absolutely necessary. Moreover, the expectoration of sputum is a major goal in the therapy of patients with chronic obstructive airway disease. Therefore, when antitussives are needed in patients with productive coughs, it is usually better to attempt cough reduction (not total suppression), primarily to allow patients to sleep and to avoid posttussive syncope, stress incontinence, or straining of the chest wall or abdominal muscles. In the United States, several hundred cough and decongestant preparations, usually sold as combination products, are available. Many of these preparations combine so-called expectorants with antitussives and should be avoided because, insofar as they have an effect, they work at cross purposes. In prospective double-blind studies of patients with cough associated with the common cold, the combination of dexbrompheniramine, an antihistamine (contained, for example, in Cheracol and Drixoral), and pseudoephedrine, a vasoconstrictor (6 mg/120 mg twice a day, orally for 1 week), reduced symptoms compared with placebo (7), as did naproxen (500 mg loading dose, then 200 to 500 mg three times a day orally for 5 days) (8). Another randomized study of 97 patients with cough secondary to upper respiratory tract infections found no difference between guaifenesin alone versus guaifenesin plus codeine or guaifenesin plus dextromethorphan in reducing coughing (9).

Antitussives act on the cough reflex either by anesthetizing the peripheral irritant receptors or by increasing the threshold of the cough center. The two most effective nonnarcotic antitussives are *dextromethorphan* and *benzonatate,* although the latter has not been rigorously studied in a placebo controlled randomized

Table 59.2. Nonnarcotic Antitussives

Drug	Brand Name	Usual Dose	Site of Action	Comment
Dextromethorphan	Many preparations	15–30 mg four times a day	Central	Considered most effective central agent
Benzonatate	Tessalon	100–200 mg four times a day	Peripheral	Considered most effective peripheral agent

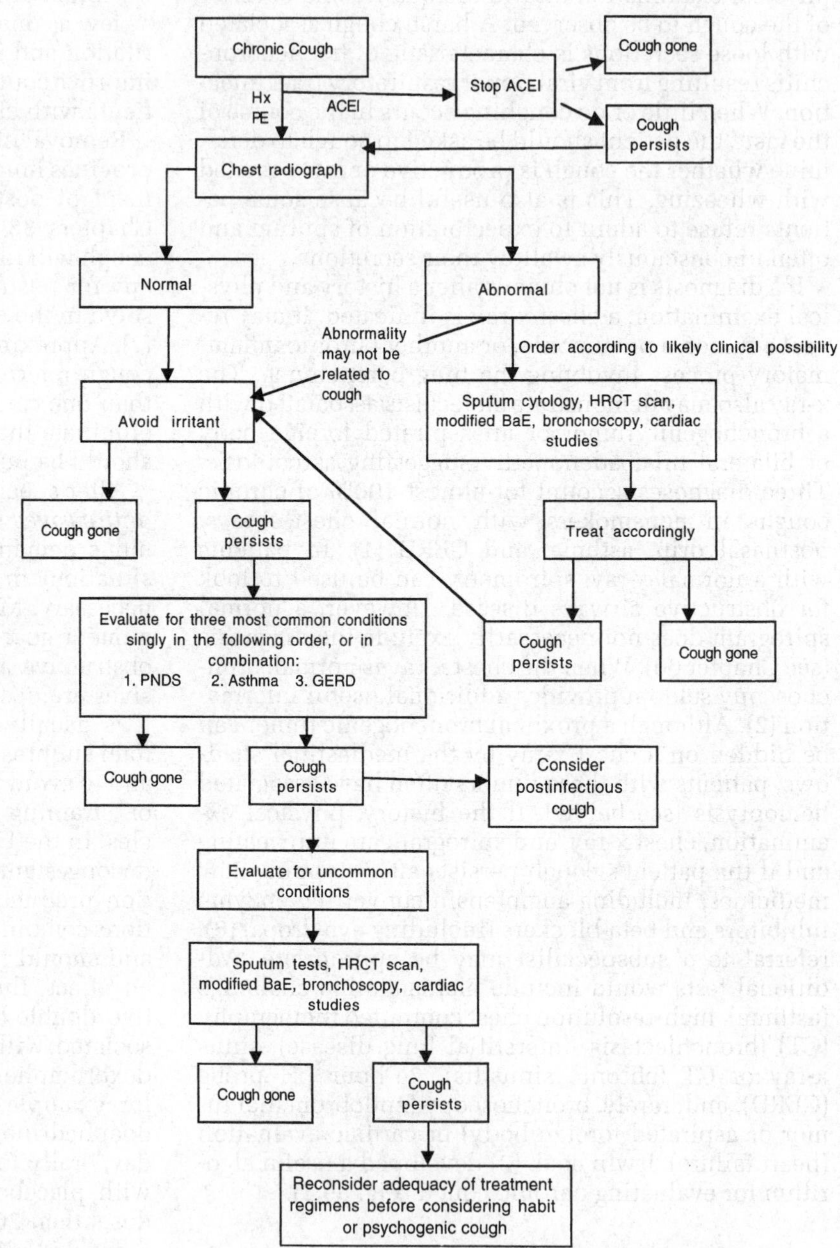

Figure 59.1. Guidelines for evaluating chronic cough in immunocompetent adults. *ACEI*, angiotensin-converting enzyme inhibitor; *BaE*, barium esophagography; *GERD*, gastroesophageal reflux disease; *HRCT*, high-resolution computed tomography; *Hx*, history; *PE*, physical examination; *PNDS*, postnasal drip syndrome. (From Irwin RS, Boulet LP, Cloutier MM, et al. Managing cough as a defense mechanism and as a symptom. A consensus panel report of the American College of Chest Physicians. Chest 1998;114:133S, with permission.)

trial (Table 59.2). Dextromethorphan is chemically derived from the opiates; however, it is classified as nonnarcotic because at prescribed dosages it has no sedative or analgesic effects and therefore has little potential for abuse. It is available over the counter in a variety of preparations (e.g., Dimetane DX). Dextromethorphan suppresses cough centrally. Occasionally, the drug causes nausea, dizziness, or vertigo, and overdosage of more than 200 mg may lead to central nervous system (CNS) depression. Benzonatate is a peripherally acting anesthetic similar to tetracaine. Rarely, it causes headaches, dizziness, and nausea or gastrointestinal upset. The drug should not be chewed or sucked because this will result in an unpleasant taste and prolonged oral pharyngeal anesthesia. Overdosage has been associated with CNS stimulation and tremors, which may lead to seizures followed by profound CNS depression. It is reasonable to treat patients initially with dextromethorphan and, if intolerable cough persists, to substitute benzonatate.

If nonnarcotic antitussives are ineffective, *codeine* can be tried. Many clinicians prescribe codeine preferentially to patients with persistent cough because it is a more potent cough suppressant than the nonnarcotic agents. Codeine is effective in dosages of 15 to 30 mg administered every 3 to 6 hours. The common side effects—nausea, vomiting, constipation, dry mouth, and sedation—are usually not experienced at these lower dosages.

HEMOPTYSIS

Hemoptysis is defined as the expectoration of blood from below the vocal cords. It can range from flecks of blood in sputum to the coughing of large amounts (more than 1 L) of blood. Distinguishing between hemoptysis and hematemesis can occasionally be difficult. Blood from the lungs is usually bright red and frothy, has an alkaline pH, and is usually mixed with sputum containing macrophages and white blood cells. Often, patients with hemoptysis complain of a tickling or irritation in their chest. On the other hand, hematemesis is characterized by blood that is darker brown, has an acid pH, and is mixed with food particles. Sometimes blood from a lesion in the sinuses or in the upper airway will be aspirated and later expectorated, making it appear that the bleeding occurred in the lower respiratory tract. A careful history and physical examination must be performed to avoid inappropriate evaluation or treatment. The patient should be instructed to collect and save the bloody sputum so that the hemoptysis can be quantified. Nevertheless, a history of hemoptysis should not be ignored if a patient cannot produce a specimen on command because the symptoms can be intermittent. The various pulmonary causes of hemoptysis are summarized in Table 59.3.

In the typical ambulatory practice, *chronic bronchitis* is by far the most common cause of blood streaking of the sputum, followed by *lung cancer* 10% to 20% of the time. The likelihood of a particular diagnosis depends on the patient population (e.g., smokers vs. nonsmokers) (10). *Bronchiectasis* in the industrial world is less common today because of mass screening for tuberculosis, childhood vaccinations for measles and whooping cough, and antibiotic treatment of serious respiratory infections. *Active cavitary tuberculosis* is also a less common cause of hemoptysis than it once was, but residual upper lobe bronchiectasis, the result of old tuberculosis infection, is still seen. *Bronchogenic carcinoma* (see Chapter 61) presents with hemoptysis at two stages: Blood-streaked sputum may be a brief manifestation of a small irritative mucosal lesion. This symptom may resolve only to be replaced later by major hemoptysis from a large endobronchial tumor that is friable or necrotic or is eroding central vessels. Usually blood from a *necrotizing pneumonia* or a *lung abscess* is mixed with pus, and the sputum

Table 59.3. Pulmonary Causes of Hemoptysis

Causes	Examples
Common	
Inflammation	Bronchitis, bronchiectasis (including cystic fibrosis), tuberculosis, pneumonia, lung abscess
Neoplasm	Lung cancer
Less common	
Inflammation	Goodpasture syndrome, idiopathic pulmonary hemosiderosis, Wegener granulomatosis, SLE, systemic necrotizing vasculitis
Infection	Parasitic, pre-existing cavitary disease with mycetoma (old Tb or fibrocystic sarcoidosis), broncholithiasis
Neoplasm	Bronchial carcinoid, endobronchial metastasis
Vascular disease	Pulmonary embolus with infarction, arteriovenous malformation, aortic aneurysm, mitral stenosis, tricuspid endocarditis, pulmonary hypertension
Iatrogenic cause	Bronchoscopy, transthoracic lung biopsy, transtracheal oxygen catheter, transtracheal suctioning, pulmonary artery catheterization, airway stenting
Drugs	Anticoagulation, aspirin, thrombolytics, crack cocaine, solvents, penicillamine
Chest trauma	
Foreign body	

SLE, systemic lupus erythematosus; Tb, tuberculosis.

appears red-brown or red-green. Hemoptysis from *pulmonary emboli,* a manifestation of pulmonary infarction, is rare, due to the lung's dual blood supply, unless patients have significant heart or lung disease (11). Even with the advent of fiberoptic bronchoscopy, the cause of hemoptysis remains undiagnosed 8% to 15% of the time (12,13). The 5-year survival rate for patients with cryptogenic hemoptysis (hemoptysis with normal chest x-ray and a negative bronchoscopy) is very good (85% to 95%) (12).

Less common causes of hemoptysis are also listed in Table 59.3, but this ranking reflects to some extent the location of a practice. For example, mycetomas and parasitic infections that cause hemoptysis are much more common in areas of the country where those problems are endemic. Hemoptysis is common in *bronchial carcinoids* by virtue of their endobronchial location and marked vascularity. Hemoptysis caused by *pulmonary metastasis* from a solid tumor is rare. Its presence raises the possibility of endobronchial metastases, which are most common in patients with breast, colon, and kidney cancer and those with malignant melanoma. Patients with *mitral stenosis* and pulmonary vascular congestion are prone to hemoptysis with any source of lung irritation. Although certainly less common today, this valvular abnormality is often silent and the history of rheumatic fever forgotten. Patients taking the *anticoagulants* warfarin or heparin may develop hemoptysis, especially if there is an associated inflammation of the airways. Occasionally, *blunt chest trauma* produces hemoptysis in an otherwise healthy individual. Very rarely, hemoptysis is due to intrathoracic endometriosis, in which case it occurs at the time of menstruation.

Evaluation

The diagnostic evaluation of hemoptysis is aimed at determining the cause, localizing the site, and quantifying the amount of bleeding. The history and physical examination are directed at uncovering clues to the causes outlined in Table 59.3. An attempt should be made to quantitate the amount of hemoptysis by history and by collection of expectorated blood. Massive hemoptysis, generally defined as greater than a few hundred milliliters of blood during a 24-hour period, represents a medical emergency, and survival of the patient depends on rapid diagnosis and treatment (14).

During the physical examination, extrathoracic sources of bleeding from the nasal passages, sinuses, and pharynx should be sought. Physical findings may be helpful. Digital clubbing may be seen in non–small cell lung cancer, lung abscess, or bronchiectasis. Scattered ecchymoses, multiple petechiae, or gastrointestinal bleeding suggests a defect in hemostasis, and telangiectasia of the skin, lips, or buccal mucosa is consistent with hereditary hemorrhagic telangiectasis (or Osler-Weber-Rendu syndrome). Ulceration and crusting of the nasal septum may represent upper airway involvement of Wegener granulomatosis. The significance of unilateral wheezing or crackles must be interpreted with caution because these sounds may be produced by aspirated blood or secretions rather than by endobronchial tumor.

A chest x-ray is essential because acute inflammatory diseases, such as active tuberculosis, pneumonia, and lung abscess, will produce obvious radiographic abnormalities. Typically, lung cancers associated with hemoptysis are centrally located squamous cell carcinomas, and approximately half are cavitary. However, localization of the bleeding source is often precluded by bilateral aspiration of blood or by the presence of bilateral pulmonary disease. Patients with bronchitis often have normal chest x-rays, and the findings on plain film of focal bronchiectasis may be nonspecific. If the bronchiectasis is a result of old tuberculosis, however, apical scarring may suggest the diagnosis; otherwise, there may be increased or crowded lung markings, thickened dilated bronchi, multiple cystic cavities (1 to 3 mm in diameter), or infiltrates due to recurrent infection. The chest CT is more sensitive than the chest x-ray in detecting bronchiectasis and is generally sufficient to make the diagnosis (15). Differentiating bronchitis from bronchiectasis by history and chest x-ray is sometimes difficult. This distinction may not be critical, however, because the acute medical management of bronchitis and bronchiectasis in patients with hemoptysis is the same.

When the chest x-ray is normal or nonlocalizing, endobronchial malignancy is the principal diagnosis to exclude, although bronchitis is the most likely diagnosis. Individuals under 40 years old, including smokers, with hemoptysis that has lasted less than 1 week are unlikely to have cancer. In such patients, observation is a reasonable initial approach (16).

Persistent or recurrent hemoptysis mandates a thorough evaluation that includes bronchoscopy. Patients with normal chest x-rays who are at increased risk for lung cancer (over 40 years old, greater than 20-pack-year cigarette smoker) should undergo bronchoscopy. Still, only about 5% of these patients will have lung cancer discovered at bronchoscopy (see Chapter 61) (16,17). Sputum cytology may provide the diagnosis in as many as half of these patients, but bronchoscopy is generally still required to locate the site of malignancy (lung vs. upper aerodigestive tract) and to plan for therapy. In the evaluation of recurrent or persistent hemoptysis, most clinicians view bronchoscopy and chest CT as complementary, the CT being helpful in guiding the bronchoscopy and/or angiography to the regions of highest yield (15,18).

Therapy

Blood irritates the tracheobronchial tree and triggers constant coughing, which by itself is traumatic. Mild cough suppression may help (see above), but the patient must be able to expectorate blood as it accumulates. Specific treatment depends on the underlying cause of hemoptysis. Chronic bronchitis, with intercurrent hemoptysis, is usually treated on an ambulatory basis with antimicrobial drugs (see Chapter 60) for 10 to 14 days; in such circumstances blood streaking of the sputum usually stops in 2 to 3 days.

No clinical criteria or radiographic signs predict massive hemoptysis, and the quantity of hemoptysis does not necessarily indicate the seriousness of the patient's underlying disease. Thus, given the tendency for rebleeding and the often unpredictable clinical course, a low threshold for hospitalization is warranted. If there is massive hemoptysis, consideration should be given to early bronchoscopy and/or interventional angiography with bronchial artery embolization (14,19).

DYSPNEA

Breathing is an unconscious act that usually occurs effortlessly, yet even normal people become aware of their breathing during deep sighs or during moderate to severe exercise. Dyspnea, the abnormal uncomfortable sensation of breathlessness, is difficult to define because patients often cannot accurately perceive or quantitate the feeling. Similar to an individual's threshold for the recognition of pain, the complaint of dyspnea depends on both the individual's limit for discomfort and the specific circumstances that provoke shortness of breath. Thus, dyspnea must be defined in terms of what is abnormal for a particular individual in the context of his or her level of fitness and of the amount of activity that is associated with breathlessness. Some patients become dyspneic with relatively small measurable alterations in ventilation, whereas others (e.g., patients who are hyperventilating with Kussmaul breathing) may not complain of dyspnea. Fortunately, a reasonable correlation exists between the degree of dyspnea and objective measurements of physiologic dysfunction.

Often, the actual complaint of dyspnea may not be expressed as such, and it may vary depending on the type of precipitating illness and on whether it developed abruptly or over a longer period. Thus, asthmatic patients may complain of tightness in the chest and acute shortness of breath, whereas patients with acute pulmonary embolism (PE) may state that their breath has suddenly "been taken away," and they cannot get enough air even though they ventilate easily. A sensation of air hunger or suffocating is typical for congestive heart failure. In contrast, patients with emphysema or neuromuscular diseases may note an increased effort or work of breathing and may modify their life-styles and dismiss the sensation of breathlessness as part of their advancing age.

Normal Ventilation

No single mechanism is responsible for dyspnea. Because dyspnea is the result of a variety of diverse influences acting alone or together, a brief discussion of the control of ventilation may help the practitioner understand the complexity of dyspnea and the reason why this sensation often does not immediately respond to correction of obvious physiologic abnormalities. Normally, ventilation is coupled to the individual's metabolic demands as reflected in the oxygen consumption and carbon dioxide elimination necessary to meet a given level of activity. These needs are sensed by peripheral (carotid and aortic bodies) and central (medullary) chemical chemoreceptors that respond to the O_2, CO_2, and pH of blood and cerebrospinal fluid. The acute stimulation of these receptors provokes changes in minute ventilation. In addition, the control and regulation of the rate and pattern of breathing are influenced by the reflex effects of activation of neural receptors that lie in the lung parenchyma, airways, blood vessels, respiratory muscles, and chest wall. For example, receptors in the chest wall and diaphragm will respond to increased stiffness (decreased compliance) in the lung that occurs with fluid accumulation or with interstitial fibrosis. In addition, interstitial edema may activate C fibers located in the alveolar interstitium and may cause reflex dyspnea in patients with pulmonary edema. Other receptors located in the airway epithelium cause rapid shallow breathing, coughing, and bronchospasm when irritating substances are inhaled. Finally, the CNS alone can cause large alterations in breathing that lead to hyperventilation in association with anxiety attacks (see Chapter 22). This discussion should help in understanding, for example, why the correction of arterial hypoxemia alone in a patient with an asthmatic attack usually does not relieve the sensation of breathlessness. In this situation, dyspnea results from the complex interaction of both chemical and neural stimuli to breathe, coupled with an individual's response to these signals. Therefore, correction of only one of these problems is not sufficient to abolish dyspnea. A detailed consensus panel report on the pathophysiology and management of dyspnea has been published (20).

Evaluation

The causes of dyspnea are diverse and include essentially all diseases that result in significant functional impairment of either the respiratory system (gas exchange and pulmonary mechanics) or the cardiovascular system (circulatory and cardiac function) and any hematologic abnormality that impairs oxygen delivery. Table 59.4 summarizes the general disease categories likely to cause abnormal breathlessness.

In ambulatory practice, the major causes of dyspnea are obstructive airway disease and atherosclerotic and hypertensive heart disease, either alone or in combination. The prevalence of symptomatic lung disease in a specific geographic region or socioeconomic group is further modified by the prevalence of cigarette use, urban pollution, and occupational exposure to inhaled

Table 59.4. Causes of Dyspnea

	Acute	Chronic
Common		
Pulmonary		
Obstructive airway disease	Asthma, bronchitis	Asthma, COPD
Restrictive lung disease	Pneumothorax	Diffuse interstitial lung disease, pleural effusion
Inflammatory	Pneumonia	
Vascular	Pulmonary embolism	
Cardiac	CHF (angina equivalent)	CHF (cardiomyopathy)
Other	Psychogenic	Chronic anemia, obesity
Less Common		
Pulmonary		
Upper airway obstruction	Epiglottitis, foreign body aspiration	Goiter
Restrictive lung disease		Diaphragm paralysis, neuromuscular disease, kyphoscoliosis, pulmonary metastases (lymphangitic)
Vascular		Pulmonary hypertension (thromboembolic, idiopathic), hepatopulmonary syndrome (cirrhosis)
Cardiac		CHF (pericardial disease)
Other	CO intoxication, acute blood loss or hemolysis, thyroid disease	

CHF, congestive heart failure; CO, carbon monoxide; COPD, chronic obstructive pulmonary disease.

toxic substances. The clinical circumstances and sequence of events in which dyspnea occurs will aid in its evaluation.

One of the first steps in evaluating a patient who complains of dyspnea is deciding whether the symptoms reflect an acute or a chronic event because the more serious causes of dyspnea tend to present abruptly. In general, dyspnea of sudden onset is easier to evaluate, but the workup must proceed quickly to determine whether the patient should be admitted to the hospital for more intensive evaluation and therapy. On the other hand, the evaluation of chronic dyspnea can usually be accomplished more slowly in an ambulatory setting.

Acute Dyspnea

The history, physical examination, and chest x-ray form the focal point of the evaluation of a patient with acute dyspnea. In a young patient, the medical history and physical examination alone often suggest the presumptive diagnosis. When necessary, additional distinction of primary cardiac from pulmonary disorders will be aided by the chest x-ray, spirogram, and electrocardiogram.

Acute tracheobronchitis should be considered in the middle-aged smoker with cough, dyspnea, and purulent sputum in association with a clear chest x-ray. When wheezing and rhonchi are present, the term *asthmatic bronchitis* is often used. *Spontaneous pneumothorax* (see below) presents with sudden sharp chest pain and dyspnea. A small but significant pneumothorax on chest x-ray can easily be missed, and diagnostic accuracy will be improved with an expiratory film. Previously undiagnosed *interstitial lung disease, bullous lung disease,* and *cystic fibrosis* may also present with spontaneous *pneumothoraces.* In these cases, the chest film should demonstrate characteristic abnormalities.

Acute dyspnea in association with fever, cough, and purulent sputum with localized infiltrates suggests *pneumonia,* usually bacterial (see Chapter 33). Diffuse infiltrates and nonproductive cough suggest atypical pneumonia (see Chapter 33).

The patient with acute dyspnea and known *heart failure* has usual cardiac symptoms and signs, including paroxysmal nocturnal dyspnea, crackles, cardiomegaly, and a symmetric interstitial pattern with or without pleural effusions (see Chapter 66). *Psychogenic dyspnea,* or the hyperventilation syndrome, has a rapid onset and is usually found in conjunction with anxiety disorders (see Chapter 22). This syndrome should be considered in young patients in whom dyspnea is unrelated to exertion and is associated with somatic complaints and excessive fearfulness (21).

Less common but important causes of acute dyspnea include acute *foreign body aspiration,* usually evident from the history of aspiration and a physical examination that demonstrates decreased breath sounds over the part of the lung supplied by the occluded bronchus. During the heating season or in certain industrial settings, *carbon monoxide intoxication* should be considered as a cause of headaches and dyspnea. Diagnosis requires a high degree of suspicion and awareness of the problem. Confirmation requires measurement of carboxyhemoglobin with a co-oximeter. The partial pressure of oxygen measured in the arterial blood gas sample will remain normal.

Pulmonary Embolism

PE is a major life-threatening cause of acute dyspnea, but the diagnosis can be difficult. Its evaluation requires a systematic approach with a logical sequence of diagnostic testing. Approximately 75% of patients presenting with suspected deep vein thrombosis (DVT) or PE do not have these conditions (22).

The incidence of PE is high in patients with chronic obstructive lung disease or congestive heart failure and in those with risk factors for venous thromboembolism (e.g., cancer, prolonged immobilization, or a strong family history of DVT; see Chapter 57) (22,23). In general, the risk of venous thromboembolism and PE is higher in men. In a prospective study of older women (>60 years of age), obesity, heavy cigarette smoking, and high blood pressure were significant risk factors for PE (24). In younger women, the use of oral contraceptives substantially increases the risk of PE (see Chapter 57) (23). The physical examination is usually not helpful in the diagnosis, especially because many of the patients have underlying respiratory and cardiovascular diseases that may themselves produce abnormal physical findings: tachycardia, tachypnea, distended neck veins, and an accentuated second pulmonic heart sound.

Most laboratory tests are not useful in the diagnosis of PE. Chest x-rays are often abnormal, but the findings are nonspecific (localized infiltrates or oligemia, atelectasis, an elevated hemidiaphragm, or a pleural effusion). The arterial blood gas tensions are also often abnormal (reduced $Pa{O_2}$ and $Pa{CO_2}$) but are not helpful diagnostically, in part because of considerable variation and in part because of the high prevalence of cardiopulmonary diseases that alters both the $Pa{O_2}$ and $Pa{CO_2}$.

The most widely used procedure in the screening of patients for PE is a ventilation/perfusion (V/Q) scan of the lungs. Whether the patient is hospitalized before having the scan depends on the severity of the presentation.

Patient Experience. Little discomfort is associated with a lung scan. The patient should be instructed that he or she will inhale a mixture of oxygen and xenon for 3 to 4 minutes, followed by a venous injection of radioactive-labeled technetium. Several different projections are then recorded on a scanner while the patient is lying on a table.

The V/Q scan is a highly sensitive test, but it can be nonspecific depending on the configuration, location, and number of perfusion defects seen. There are well-established criteria for interpreting the results of V/Q scans. In general, the greater the perfusion defects without corresponding ventilation defects, the "higher probability" the scan. If the V/Q scan is normal, the diagnosis of an acute PE is excluded. Conversely, a high probability scan is associated with an 85% to 90% chance of PE. Unfortunately, only 10% to 15% of patients with suspected PE will have a high probability scan, and less than 5% will be normal (25). Most patients will have an intermediate probability (or nondiagnostic) V/Q scan and require further testing to confirm or exclude the diagnosis. It is worth remembering that a "low probability" scan does not exclude the diagnosis of PE. In particular, if there is a high clinical suspicion, up to 40% of patients with low probability V/Q scans will have documented PE on pulmonary angiography (25).

In patients with nondiagnostic V/Q scans, abnormal compression ultrasonography (or impedance plethysmography) may detect a proximal DVT and confirm the need for anticoagulation (26). Approximately 10% of these patients will have a DVT detected by initial testing and should be hospitalized for initiation of anticoagulant therapy (see Chapter 57). Because ultrasonography does not detect calf vein thromboses, some patients with an initially negative test are at risk for propagating a thrombus and having a PE. This occurs 2% to 15% of the time, depending on risk factors for DVT. If there is adequate cardiopulmonary reserve, serial noninvasive testing (e.g., at days 5 and 10) is a reasonable strategy. Alternatively, if clinical suspicion for PE is high or there is limited cardiorespiratory reserve, pulmonary angiography may be warranted.

Spiral CTs are being increasingly used to test for PE noninvasively (27,28). In a spiral CT, the x-ray tube rotates continuously in the same direction while the patient moves through the scanner without stopping. By injecting a carefully timed bolus of contrast medium, images can be obtained in a single breath hold that allow visualization of the main, lobar, and segmental pulmonary arteries in most patients. Newer scanners with faster acquisition times and higher resolution are entering the market. The diagnosis of a PE is usually obvious as a low-density filling defect within the vessel lumen. The advantages of a spiral CT include its relatively quick acquisition time (although this is usually an issue in the unstable patient and not in the ambulatory setting) and its ability to diagnose abnormalities within the lung parenchyma and mediastinum. In several studies, unsuspected abnormalities (e.g., pneumothorax, cancer) were found in 10% to 30% of subjects undergoing spiral CT to "rule out PE" (28). If, due to underlying lung disease, the V/Q scan is difficult to interpret, the spiral CT may be especially helpful.

There are several disadvantages of a spiral CT. First, there is a lack of widely agreed upon standards for diagnosing PE by spiral CT, and a highly trained interpreter with a knowledge of bronchovascular anatomy (and its variants) is essential. This is in contrast to V/Q scans, the interpretation of which was validated prospectively in large and well-designed studies (e.g., PIOPED, 25). Second, it is clear that spiral CT will miss PEs in the subsegmental vessels. The exact incidence and significance of subsegmental PEs are both unknown and controversial. Some argue that subsegmental emboli may be clinically insignificant and that anticoagulation can be withheld in this setting if there is no other evidence of DVT (e.g., negative compression ultrasonography). However, experience in this regard is limited, and long-term studies with large numbers of patients will be needed. Diagnostic algorithms incorporating spiral CT into the PE workup have been proposed (28), and practitioners are encouraged to become familiar with the expertise at their institution.

The resolution of PE varies and can occur as early as 1 to 2 weeks in patients who have had small emboli. With larger emboli and in patients with underlying cardiopulmonary disease, there may be angiographic evidence of emboli that persists for 2 or 3 months (29). If chest pain occurs after discharge, a subsequent lung scan, chest CT (and perhaps, depending on the results, angiography) is necessary to determine whether embolization has recurred.

Evaluation of Chronic or Progressive Dyspnea

In contrast to acute dyspnea, chronic dyspnea is usually more difficult to diagnose and often requires more extensive diagnostic procedures; therefore, the evaluation should proceed in a logical sequence to avoid expensive and invasive laboratory testing. Because shortness of breath is appropriate to certain levels of activity depending on the fitness of the individual, the clinician must decide whether the patient's symptoms are abnormal and over what period they have developed. Many patients with chronic cardiopulmonary disease or chronic anemia adapt to the insidious onset of dyspnea by subconsciously changing daily habits and avoiding physical activity. The degree of dyspnea should be determined by comparing the patient's abilities to perform work with an appropriate peer group and with his or her baseline performance. Thus, the complaint of dyspnea in a 35 year old who normally runs 5 miles and now becomes short of breath after running only 2 miles should not be ignored.

The most useful initial test is the chest x-ray, which is often abnormal and therefore directs subsequent evaluation. Patients with *COPD* associated with emphysema have hyperinflation, decreased lung markings, and often evidence of bullous formation (see Chapter 60). Large *pleural effusions, lung cancer,* or *heart disease* associated with dyspnea results in obvious changes in the chest roentgenogram with evidence of fluid occupying at least half of one hemithorax, large mass lesions, or cardiomegaly, respectively. *Interstitial lung disease* that has led to fibrosis is revealed by chest x-ray, although the precise cause often requires intensive investigation (see below). *Unilateral hemidiaphragm paralysis* results in obvious asymmetry in lung expansion. Patients with this condition often describe orthopnea secondary to difficulty with diaphragmatic excursion in the recumbent position.

Patients with dyspnea and a normal or nonspecific chest x-ray represent a challenging group to diagnose. An approach to the evaluation of these patients is

Table 59.5. Workup of Chronic Dyspnea when the Initial Workup (e.g., Chest X-Ray, Spirometry) is Unrevealing

Disease Suspected	Test
Pulmonary	
Obstructive airway disease	Home peak flow monitoring, bronchoprovocation
Interstitial lung disease	Helium lung volumes, diffusing capacity, high-resolution chest CT
Respiratory muscle weakness	Helium lung volumes, diffusing capacity, inspiratory/expiratory pressures
Pulmonary hypertension (thromboembolic, idiopathic)	V/Q scan, echocardiography, pulmonary angiography
Unclear	Helium lung volumes, diffusing capacity
Cardiac	
Coronary artery disease	ECG/MUGA: rest ± exercise
Cardiomyopathy	Echocardiogram
Other	
Thyroid disease	Thyroid function tests
Anemia	Hemoglobin concentration or hematocrit value
Mixed cardiac/respiratory disease	Cardiopulmonary exercise testing
Deconditioning	Cardiopulmonary exercise testing
Anxiety/hyperventilation	Cardiopulmonary exercise testing

CT, computed tomography; V/Q, ventilation/perfusion ___; ECG, electrocardiogram; MUGA, multiple gated acquisition scan.

shown in Table 59.5. Most of these patients have obstructive lung disease. A spirogram is useful to screen for occult lung disease because a normal spirogram nearly excludes significant parenchymal disease. Although patients with exercise-induced asthma may have a normal spirogram during symptom-free periods, more commonly there is evidence of slight reduction in the baseline forced expiratory volume as a percentage of forced vital capacity. Home peak flow monitoring may confirm the diagnosis in these patients. Additional specialized procedures that aid in the diagnosis of exercise-induced asthma are discussed in Chapter 60. One study reported 72 patients referred for evaluation of chronic dyspnea not diagnosed by history, physical examination, chest x-ray, or spirometry. The two most common diagnoses were asthma/reactive airway diseases (approximately 17%) and hyperventilation syndrome (approximately 20%), but there was a wide spectrum of underlying diseases in the remaining cases. Notably, 20% of patients remained undiagnosed despite extensive evaluation (30).

In general, *obesity* is not associated with dyspnea unless body weight is markedly increased (50% to 100% or more or 100 pounds or more over ideal weight). *Primary pulmonary hypertension* may be associated with subtle dilation of the pulmonary arteries on chest x-ray and is most commonly seen in young asthenic women. *Upper airway obstruction* due to *goiter*, for example, often is not apparent on a routine posteroanterior and lateral chest x-ray. Anemia does not usually cause dyspnea unless it has developed acutely (blood loss or hemolysis) or unless it is relatively severe (e.g., hematocrit values of 20% or less). Some patients with advanced *hepatic cirrhosis* complain of severe dyspnea, especially worse when upright ("platypnea"). These patients experience excess shunting of blood through abnormal vascular channels in the lung (the *hepatopulmonary syndrome*) (31).

In patients in whom the diagnosis is uncertain, laboratory testing should include a hemoglobin determination or hematocrit value to determine whether the patient has severe anemia or erythrocytosis, and thyroid function studies if there are symptoms of thyroid dysfunction (e.g., unexplained weight gain, fatigue).

Complete pulmonary function tests should be performed. In addition to baseline spirometry (see Chapter 60), other pulmonary function tests include the measurement of *total lung capacity* and *functional residual capacity,* which quantitate the degree of hyperinflation or restriction. Categorization of a disorder as obstructive or restrictive will direct the clinician to a narrowed list of causes. *The diffusing capacity* measures the amount of alveolar capillary surface area available for gas exchange. Thus, the diffusing capacity is reduced in patients with PE and other vascular occlusive diseases and in patients with emphysema. In contrast, an elevated diffusing capacity is found in conditions that elevate the pulmonary blood volume—for example, erythrocytosis, early congestive heart failure, or obesity. Measurement of inspiratory and expiratory pressures helps characterize neuromuscular problems. *Flow-volume loops* help identify upper airway sources of obstruction. The experience of the patient during the performance of these tests is described in Chapter 60.

Cardiovascular testing should be performed. The use of specialized noninvasive cardiovascular evaluation, including *echocardiograms* and *nuclear scanning* to assess right and left ventricular function or the presence of valvular heart disease is discussed in Chapters 65 and 66.

If a patient is dyspneic on exertion and baseline testing of cardiopulmonary function, as described above, is normal or only mildly abnormal, *exercise testing* should be considered. In general, two types of exercise tests are available. The first is a standard *cardiac stress test,* during which the patient is exercised and observed for the development of chest pain and for electrocardiographic or radionuclide ischemic changes (see Chapter 62). The second type of exercise testing is a *cardiopulmonary stress test* in which cardiac function, pulmonary gas exchange, ventilation, and physical fitness are quantitated at specific work loads. The two types of tests are similar, but the patient should be told that the cardiopulmonary test requires continuous exercise while breathing into a mouthpiece, and measurement of oxygenation is made either by an oximeter or by means of an indwelling arterial line. Such complicated cardiopulmonary stress testing is justified and useful to determine whether dyspnea is due to cardiac disease; pulmonary disease, including exercise-induced asthma or occult pulmonary vascular disease; deconditioning; or combinations of the above. This type of testing is particularly useful in evaluating patients for disability compensation because static pulmonary function and noninvasive cardiac testing may not accurately predict the functional state of a given patient during actual working conditions. The referring clinician can usually determine presumptively the most likely cause for dyspnea and can make the appropriate referral for the specific exercise test. In large hospital centers with combined cardiopulmonary laboratories, simultaneous consultation and exercise testing by cardiologists and pulmonologists may be available. Stress testing can also be useful in deciding whether or not the patient needs supplemental oxygen (see Chapter 60).

This approach to the evaluation of dyspnea will almost always answer the questions necessary for diagnosis of the underlying condition and for establishment of a therapeutic regimen.

Therapy

Treatment of dyspnea is primarily aimed at therapy of the underlying cardiac, pulmonary, neuromuscular, or hematologic disorders that cause abnormal breathlessness. In certain patients with underlying irreversible lung disease, specific measures that improve respiratory muscle function may alleviate symptomatic dyspnea. Training programs that increase both muscle strength and endurance are available in selected pulmonary rehabilitation centers and have resulted in decreased shortness of breath in some patients. Because anxiety and depression are commonly associated with the development of chronic cardiopulmonary disorders associated with dyspnea, appropriate anxiolytics or antidepressants may be useful (see Chapter 22). In patients with pulmonary disease, buspirone (20 to 30 mg/day) may be an effective anxiolytic and does not impair respiratory drive. Selective serotonin reuptake inhibitors may be particularly useful in patients with panic attacks (21). In patients with terminal lung diseases (e.g., cancer, COPD, interstitial pulmonary fibrosis), the primary caregiver should make plans to deal with progressive dyspnea and end of life care. Having a discussion early on (and not in the setting of an acute decompensation) can by itself be quite reassuring. Low-dose narcotics (e.g., morphine sulfate) can be extremely useful as a palliative therapy for terminally ill dyspneic patients. Some subjects obtain marked relief from nebulized morphine, which may act via bronchial opioid receptors. The optimal dosing of nebulized morphine is unknown (typically started at 20 mg morphine sulfate in 5 mL normal saline) and requires further study.

NONCARDIAC CHEST PAIN

Chest pain is a particularly frightening symptom because of the widespread knowledge and concern about heart disease; however, nonspecific musculoskeletal pain is more common than angina, especially in younger patients (less than 40 years old). Most patients with chest pain can be evaluated and treated in an ambulatory setting; a few patients require referral to a specialist. The common noncardiac cause of chest pain is discussed in this section, which should be read in conjunction with Chapter 62.

Afferent neural impulses responsible for thoracic pain are carried by the sympathetic chain, vagus, and phrenic nerves. Visceral structures, which include the lung, diaphragm, heart, and esophagus, all lie within the thoracic cage and have overlapping innervation. Chest pain arising from these different organs often has similar referral patterns; thus, irritation of the diaphragmatic pleura, diaphragm, or pericardium from either thoracic or abdominal disease causes chest pain that radiates to the shoulder. In addition, patients may have difficulty localizing pain from the deeper anatomic structures within the chest, whereas diseases involving the superficial structures, muscles, and ribs are more easily localized. Because there is no sensory innervation of the lung parenchyma, alveolar or interstitial disease does not cause chest pain unless the pulmonary vasculature, bronchi, or pleura are involved. Studies have found that enhanced visceral (esophageal) pain perception underlies many cases of unexplained angina-like chest pain (32). Table 59.6 lists causes of chest pain.

Musculoskeletal pain is common in young individuals who increase their exercise abruptly (including patients who acutely hyperventilate as part of an anxiety state; see Chapter 22). A history of unusual exertion with increased breathing plus tenderness of intercostal muscles usually suffices to make this diagnosis.

Pain caused by *tracheitis* or *tracheobronchitis* is a distinctive substernal burning sensation that is precipitated by coughing and is most often associated with viral respiratory infections. This is in contrast to the sharp, stabbing, pleuritic chest pain experienced with pneumonia. The latter is clearly localized to the chest wall and arises from stretching the inflamed parietal pleura during breathing or coughing. *Pleurodynia* (or epidemic myalgia), characterized by fever, headache, and sudden onset of intense lower thoracic pleuritic pain, is usually due to Coxsackie B viruses.

Other causes of chest pain include *costochondritis* (Tietze syndrome), which is an anterior localized pain

Table 59.6. Causes of Chest Pain

Causes	Examples
Common	
Chest wall	Nonspecific musculoskeletal, costochondritis, Tietze syndrome
Cardiac	Angina
Pulmonary	Tracheitis, pleurodynia, pneumonia
Gastrointestinal	Esophageal reflux/spasm
Neurologic	Cervical spine disease (radicular)
Less common	
Chest wall	Herpes zoster, thoracic outlet syndrome, fractured rib, tumor
Cardiac	Aortic dissection, pericarditis
Pulmonary	Pneumothorax, pulmonary hypertension, pulmonary infarction
Gastrointestinal	Peptic ulcer disease, abdominal infection/peritonitis

associated with tenderness over one or more costochondral junctions; *herpes zoster,* which commonly causes unilateral aching or itching, limited to one dermatome, which may precede by several days the eruption of vesicles; *rib fracture or bone metastases,* which are more chronic and pleuritic in nature; and *cervical spine disease* with referred pain to the chest (see Chapter 70). Acute stabbing chest pain can occur with a *spontaneous pneumothorax,* which occurs primarily in young men or in older patients with obstructive pulmonary disease. Often, a small (less than 20%) pneumothorax is not accompanied by significant dyspnea in otherwise healthy individuals. Pleuritic chest pain that follows the abrupt onset of dyspnea should raise the suspicion of a PE. The pain associated with *pulmonary hypertension* is heavy and aching and often similar to that of cardiac ischemia (see Chapter 62). *Gastrointestinal disorders,* such as GERD or gastric or duodenal ulcer, are usually distinguished from cardiopulmonary chest pain by their association with eating and by their relief by antacids (see Chapters 42 and 43).

Evaluation

Many common causes of noncardiac chest pain can be diagnosed by a thorough history and physical examination. Because discrete anatomic structures must be involved to cause noncardiac chest pain, the physical examination is more useful in the diagnosis of noncardiac chest pain than in the diagnosis of dyspnea and hemoptysis. Inspection of the chest wall may reveal the characteristic unilateral eruption of herpes zoster along a dermatome. Light palpation over the chest wall elicits pain and crepitus from fractured ribs. Mild pressure over the costochondral junctions anteriorly reproduces the pain of Tietze syndrome. (In general, cardiac pain is not worsened by pressure over the chest wall.) In pneumonia or pulmonary infarction, a distinct friction rub can be heard directly over the specific area of chest pain. With pericardial involvement, a friction rub that varies with respiration or with the cardiac cycle is usually present. A thorough abdominal examination is important because diseases involving the abdominal visceral organs can cause referred chest pain that is indistinguishable from that produced by involvement of the thoracic structures. Often, laboratory studies and a chest x-ray will not be necessary for the diagnosis of these common causes of chest pain.

Therapy

The treatment of chest pain requires therapy of the underlying disease process, as well as analgesic drugs for the pain itself. Tracheal irritation is limited to the duration of the viral illness but can be treated by cough suppression and bronchodilators (see Cough, above). Tietze syndrome is treated with standard anti-inflammatory agents and heat. Although the pain of herpes zoster is often severe, it may be controlled with mild narcotics such as codeine, 30 to 60 mg every 4 to 6 hours. The chest pain experienced in pulmonary hypertension often does not respond to treatment with nonnarcotic analgesics, and narcotics may be required if the hypertension does not improve with treatment.

Pleuritic pain in patients with pneumonia or PE responds to specific therapy of the inflammatory process. Nevertheless, narcotics may be needed to reduce splinting of the chest wall and thereby to prevent atelectasis. Codeine (60 mg every 4 hours) is usually adequate therapy.

ABNORMAL CHEST X-RAY

A chest x-ray must always be compared with prior films because an abnormality that has been stable in size for more than 2 years is almost certainly benign and may not require further evaluation. Also, depending on the appearance of the abnormality and the patient's age, the most appropriate plan may be observation with serial chest x-ray.

Specific Patterns Indicative of an Abnormal Chest X-Ray

This section reviews common abnormalities that indicate the presence of pulmonary disease that requires further evaluation.

Air Bronchogram

Normally, bronchi beyond the mainstem division cannot be seen; however, when the alveoli surrounding a bronchus are devoid of air because of consolidation, or less commonly, collapse, an air bronchogram (Fig. 59.2) can be seen. The presence of an air bronchogram indicates an alveolar filling process and is most commonly seen in pneumonia and pulmonary

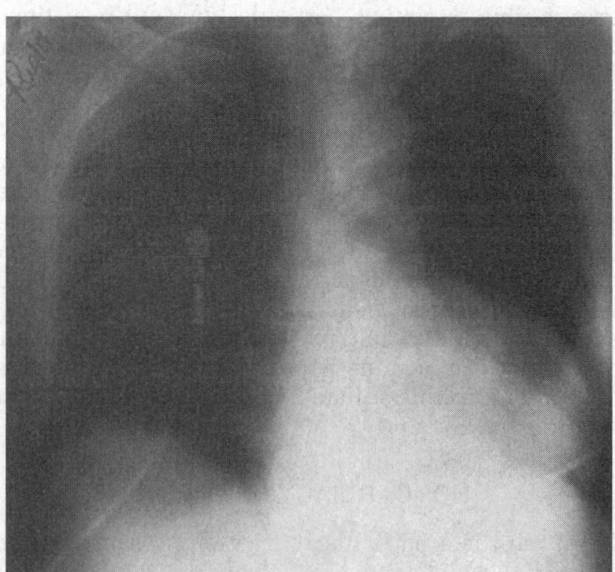

Figure 59.2. Air bronchogram. The patient had fever and sputum production; the initial x-ray demonstrates a branching air bronchogram seen behind the heart on the left, which is consistent with a lower lobe infiltrate.

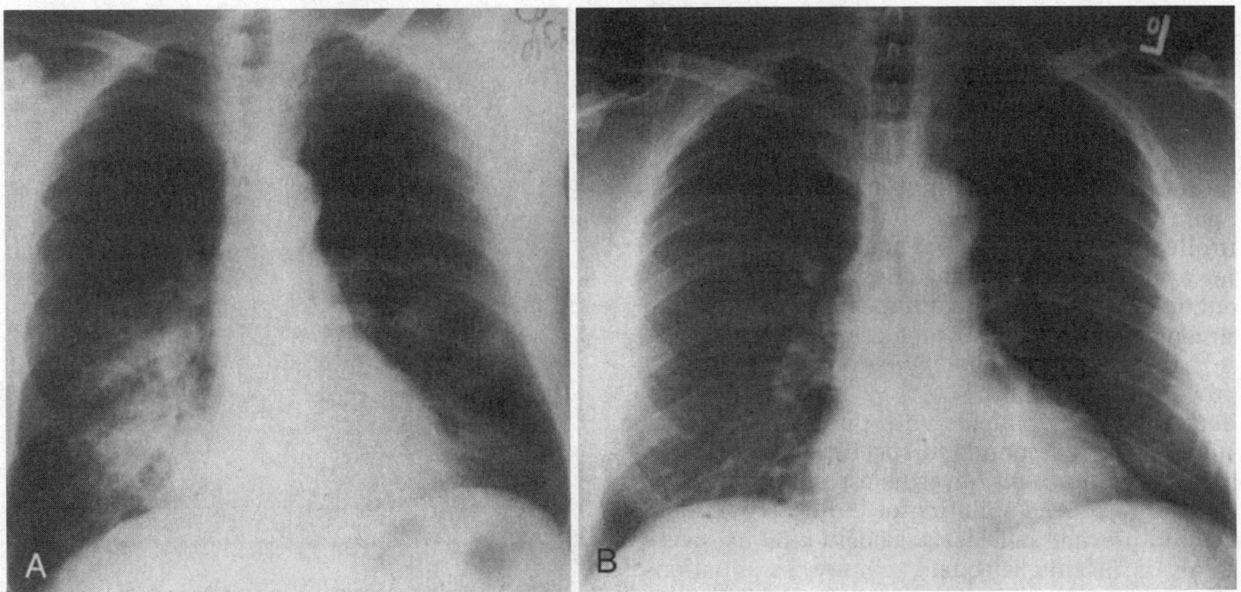

Figure 59.3. Silhouette sign. A middle lobe infiltrate obscures the border of the heart **(A)**. A previous x-ray is shown for comparison **(B)**.

edema (cardiogenic and noncardiogenic). However, an air bronchogram is not present in every consolidated lung because bronchi may fill with secretions or exudate. Therefore its absence is less significant than its presence.

Silhouette Sign

The obliteration on a chest x-ray of the margin of a normally opaque structure in the chest by an abnormal pulmonary density is called the silhouette sign. If the clinician has knowledge of thoracic anatomy and of spatial relations, the silhouette sign can be used to localize abnormalities within the lung parenchyma. Edges of organs that are in contact with parenchymal infiltrates will be obliterated because the normal air interface is eliminated. On the other hand, intrathoracic lesions that are not anatomically contiguous will not interfere with the outlines of nearby structures. For example, obliteration of the right or left cardiac borders, which are anterior, localizes an abnormality to the right middle lobe or the lingular segment of the left upper lobe respectively (Fig. 59.3). In contrast, an infiltrate that overlaps but does not obliterate the cardiac border is posterior and represents a lower lobe lesion. Lower lobe abnormalities obliterate diaphragmatic borders and on the lateral chest x-ray are seen as an increased density over the vertebrae (spine sign). Obliteration of the left border of the aortic knob, a posterior structure, occurs with lesions in the apical posterior segment of the left upper lobe, whereas obliteration of the ascending aorta, an anterior structure, occurs with lesions in the anterior segment of the right upper lobe.

Collapse

The collapse (Fig. 59.4) or diminution in volume of the whole lung, a lobe, or a segment of one of the lobes can be an important clue to the presence of asymptomatic pulmonary disease, such as bronchogenic carcinoma, or it may be the cause of a symptom, such as dyspnea in an asthmatic patient with mucous plugging. The primary mechanisms that cause pulmonary collapse are *bronchial obstruction* from either an intrinsic bronchial mass or an extrinsic or intrinsic stenosis of the bronchus, *compression of the lung* from a large pleural effusion or from a pneumothorax, *peripheral bronchial plugging* with subsequent pulmonary collapse, and *contraction of the lung* secondary to chronic inflammatory disease. The signs of collapse are related to anatomic landmarks within the lung and are manifested by displacement of the fissure in the lung, loss of aeration within the pulmonary parenchyma, and crowding of the vascular and bronchial lung markings. Other signs that suggest collapse reflect the secondary effects of loss of lung volume such as elevation of the diaphragm, shift of the mediastinal structures toward the collapsed area, diminution of the size of a hemithorax, compensatory hyperinflation, hilar displacement, and tracheal deviation. These latter signs are much more difficult to interpret in patients with underlying lung disease, in whom many of these signs may exist in the absence of collapse.

Septal Markings

Normally, lung markings reflect vascular patterns within the pulmonary parenchyma and are rarely due to the bronchi or the lymphatics. Three types of linear shadows represent septal markings within the lung: *Kerley A lines,* thin nonbranching lines several inches long radiating from the hilum that appear to cross blood vessels; *Kerley B lines* (Fig. 59.5), up to 1 inch in length, found at the lateral lung bases, on the posteroanterior film or in the retrosternal clear space on the lateral film, radiating from the pleura; and *Kerley*

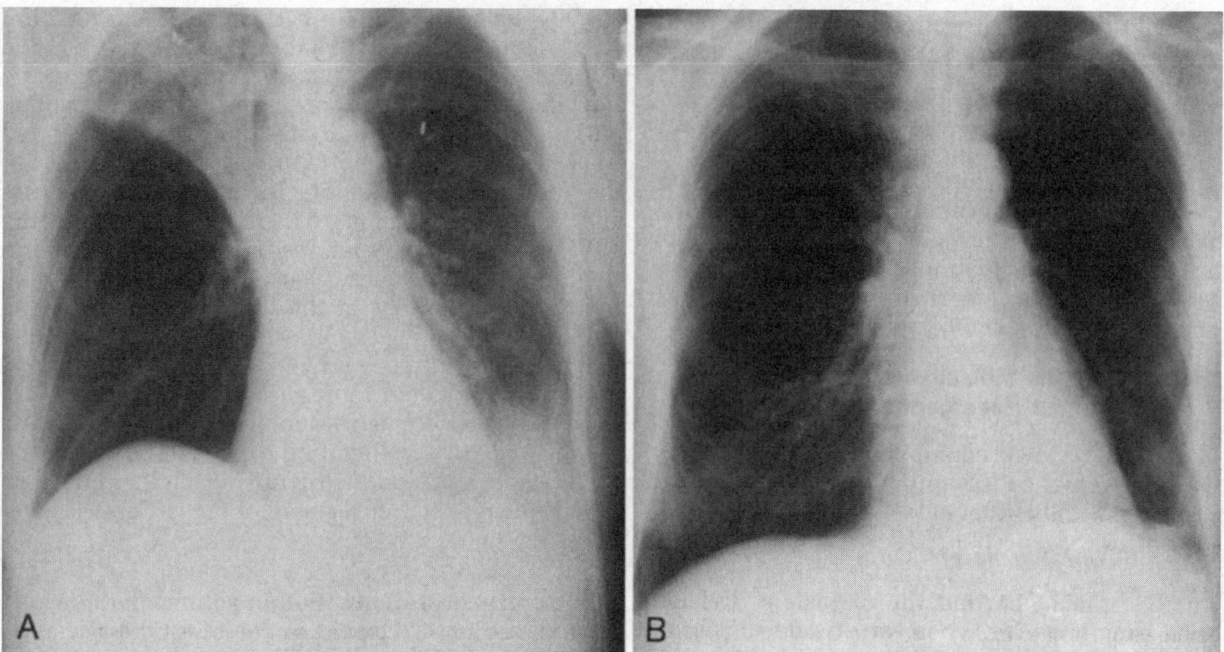

Figure 59.4. Collapse. This demonstrates collapse of the right upper lobe and partial collapse of the left lower lobe in a patient complaining of cough and increased sputum **(A).** The middle lobe fissure is displaced upward, and there is blunting of the left hemidiaphragm.

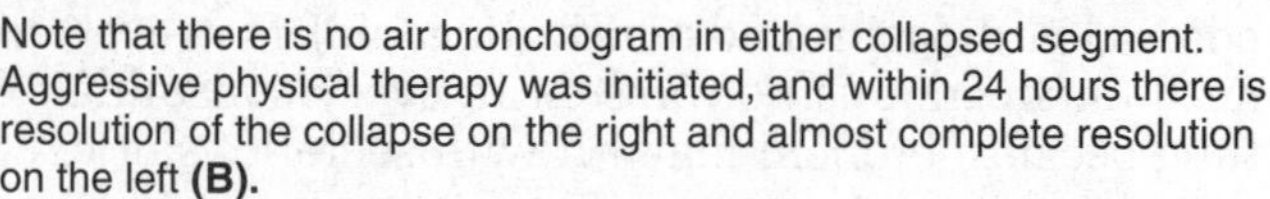

Note that there is no air bronchogram in either collapsed segment. Aggressive physical therapy was initiated, and within 24 hours there is resolution of the collapse on the right and almost complete resolution on the left **(B).**

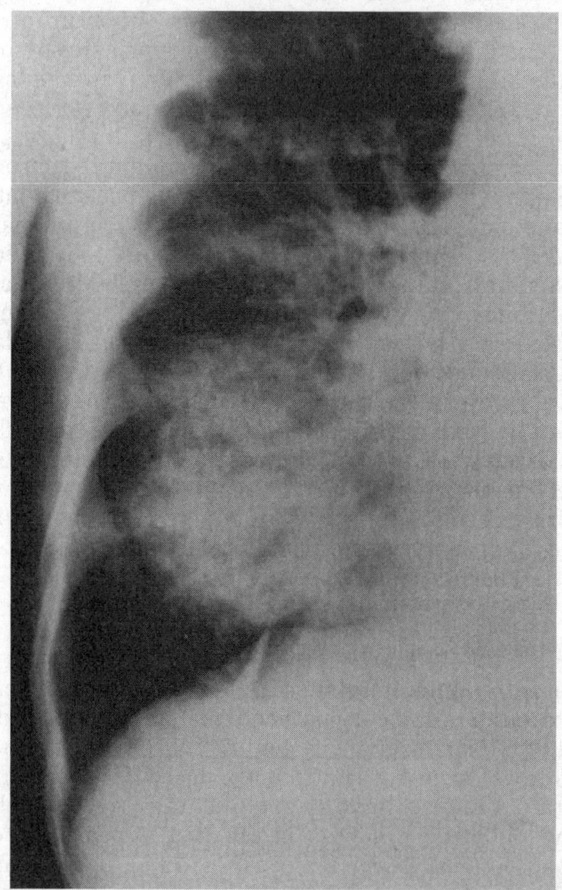

Figure 59.5. Kerley B lines. A close view of the right lower lung in a patient with congestive heart failure demonstrates horizontal linear lines that run to the edge of the lung.

C lines, fine interlacing structures throughout the lung parenchyma that produce a spider-web appearance. The fine linear or reticular pattern represented by Kerley's lines are specific for interstitial lung disease. The most common cause of these lines is interstitial edema caused by congestive heart failure.

Common Problems in Patients with Abnormal Chest X-Rays

In this section, three general categories are discussed in which the chest x-ray provides the basis for diagnosis and further evaluation. A general approach is outlined, including the initial evaluation that should be completed by the clinician before referral to a pulmonary specialist or a thoracic surgeon. Often, this diagnostic evaluation can be completed in an ambulatory setting.

Infiltrates

Infiltrates represent alveolar or interstitial lung disease and seldom show borders except at pleural surfaces. They may be radiographically separated into diffuse and focal infiltrates. *Diffuse* implies bilateral generalized involvement, if not of the entire lungs, then at least most of both lung fields. *Focal* implies discrete lesions that may or may not be bilateral but that have intervening normal lung tissue between the localized lesions.

Alveolar. *Alveolar infiltrates* (Fig. 59.6A) can be recognized by their fluffy margins, their coalescence into rosette formations, their occasional butterfly configuration involving hilar and central lung

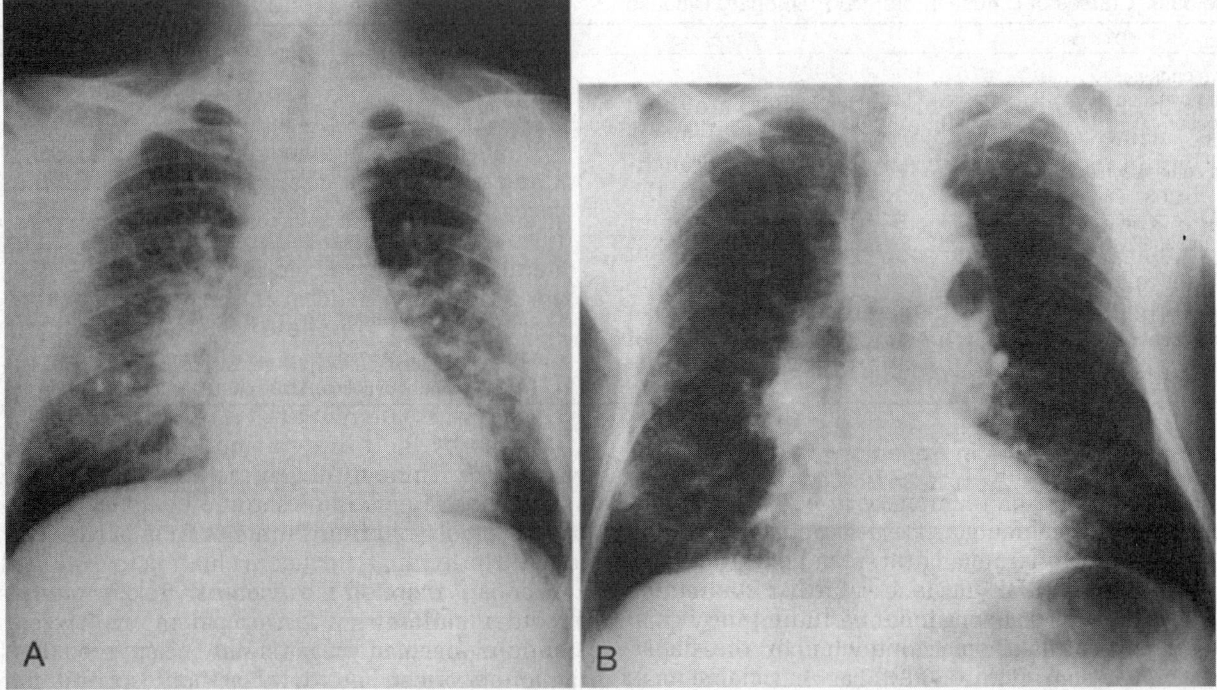

Figure 59.6. A: Alveolar patterns. This patient has progressive dyspnea after inhaling fumes from an automobile accident. Compared with B, little air is visible in the infiltrate because fluid is filling the alveoli. **B:** Interstitial pattern. This demonstrates bilateral interstitial infiltrates in a patient with progressive dyspnea and with fibrosis on biopsy. Compared with A, there is a lacy reticular appearance with accentuation of the air spaces by the fibrosis.

zones, and the presence of air bronchograms or air alveolograms.

Although there are numerous causes of diffuse interstitial pulmonary disease, there are few causes of diffuse alveolar lung disease. Therefore, the distinction between an alveolar and an interstitial process is important. Unfortunately, it is not always possible to distinguish between the two entities, and there may be a combination of both. Moreover, a disorder that begins as an interstitial process can often merge into an alveolar process, such as interstitial edema in early congestive heart failure progressing to florid pulmonary edema.

The causes of *diffuse alveolar pulmonary disease* of the lung are shown in Table 59.7. The three most common causes are *infection, edema,* and *hemorrhage,* and they are characterized by rapid progression and regression. In contrast, diffuse interstitial disease develops more slowly. Therefore, the time course for the development of pulmonary symptoms and roentgenographic abnormalities is an important aspect in the differential diagnosis of diffuse lung disease.

Interstitial. An *interstitial pattern* may be primarily linear (reticular) or may consist of multiple, discrete, noncoalescent, round nodules, 1 to 5 mm in diameter (Fig. 59.6B). Although there can be a summation effect, these small nodular densities retain a distinct identity in comparison with the larger fluffier infiltrates characteristic of alveolar disease. In certain disease processes, such as tuberculosis, histoplasmosis, or healed viral pneumonia, these nodules may calcify and thus appear more dense. *Honeycombing* is

Table 59.7. Causes of Diffuse Alveolar Pulmonary Disease

Disorder	Common	Uncommon
Infection (pus)	Pneumonia	
Edema (fluid)	Cardiac and noncardiac pulmonary edema	
Hemorrhage (blood)		Anticoagulation, trauma, hemoptysis, Goodpasture syndrome, idiopathic pulmonary hemosiderosis
Cells		Bronchoalveolar cell cancer, lymphoma, sarcoidosis, eosinophilic granuloma, pulmonary eosinophilic disorders
Foreign material		Lipoid pneumonia
Protein		Alveolar proteinosis

seen in advanced interstitial lung disease and represents end-stage irreversible scarring with thickened or dilated airways. It can be identified on a chest x-ray as round or oval irregular air spaces that have a reasonably uniform diameter of 1 to 10 mm and are arranged in web-like bunches, thus giving the impression of a honeycomb. Honeycombing is seen in a variety of fibrosing lung diseases, including idiopathic pulmonary fibrosis, sarcoidosis, asbestosis, chronic hypersensitivity pneumonitis, and eosinophilic granuloma. Bilateral interstitial infiltrates in the lower lung fields are a commonly seen radiographic pattern. The most common diagnoses with this pattern are bronchiectasis, chronic aspiration, collagen vascular diseases, asbestosis, sarcoidosis, or idiopathic pulmonary

Table 59.8. Causes of Diffuse Interstitial Pulmonary Disease

Disorder	Common	Uncommon
Known causes		
Cardiovascular	Early heart failure	
Infection	Atypical and viral pneumonia, *Pneumocystis* infection	Miliary tuberculosis, fungal pneumonia
Collagen vascular disease		Scleroderma, rheumatoid arthritis, systemic lupus erythematosus
Occupational (*Pneumoconiosis*)		Asbestosis, silicosis, coal miner's pneumoconiosis
Hypersensitivity and drug reactions		Hypersensitivity pneumonitis, nitrofurantoin, amiodarone, cytotoxic drugs
Physical agents		Radiation
Neoplastic		Lymphoma, lymphangitic spread of tumor
Unknown causes		
	Sarcoidosis	Idiopathic pulmonary fibrosis, eosinophilic granuloma, lymphocytic interstitial pneumonitis

fibrosis. Localized interstitial processes often represent residues of prior pulmonary infections. If new, they may represent acute processes such as mycoplasma pneumonia or lymphangitic spread of carcinoma.

Although interstitial lung disease can be idiopathic, this is a diagnosis of exclusion, and the primary goal in the evaluation is to determine whether a treatable disease is present (Table 59.8). The initial medical history, physical examination, and laboratory testing should be oriented toward evaluating the patient for the presence of sarcoidosis, pulmonary involvement associated with collagen vascular disease, granulomatous lung infection (mycobacterium, fungus), or pneumoconiosis secondary to occupational exposure (see Chapter 8). Additional testing often includes complete pulmonary function testing (spirometry, lung volumes, diffusing capacity, room air arterial blood gas measurement), formal cardiopulmonary exercise testing, chest CT, and fiberoptic bronchoscopy with lavage and transbronchial lung biopsy. The transbronchial lung biopsy is often useful in diagnosing and guiding therapy in patients with sarcoidosis, lymphangitic spread of tumor, infectious disease, collagen vascular pulmonary diseases, and idiopathic pulmonary fibrosis. If the tissue obtained with transbronchial biopsy is inadequate for diagnosis, consultation with a thoracic surgeon for a surgical lung biopsy (video assisted thoracoscopy or open lung biopsy) may be indicated.

Slowly Resolving or Recurrent Infiltrates. *Endobronchial tumor* must be considered in patients who have a slowly resolving pneumonia. Most patients with community-acquired pneumonia respond rapidly to antibiotic therapy, and their chest x-ray will return to baseline over 2 to 4 weeks (see Chapter 33). In one study, radiographic resolution of pneumonia was inversely related to age and was delayed in smokers, patients with multilobar infiltrates, and in hospitalized patients (33). Patients with chronic obstructive lung disease (see Chapter 60) who have difficulty mobilizing their bronchial secretions and patients with superimposed congestive heart failure or with necrotizing or multilobar pneumonia may have pulmonary infiltrates that persist for 4 to 5 months. If a patient shows symptomatic improvement and slow but progressive roentgenographic clearing, observation is warranted. If roentgenographic abnormalities persist and the patient fails to show clinical improvement or if the pulmonary infiltrate is found in an asymptomatic individual, further evaluation to exclude lung cancer is warranted (see Chapter 61). In contrast to an older patient, a younger patient with recurrent sinopulmonary infections should be suspected of having an abnormal host defense such as cystic fibrosis or an immunoglobulin deficiency state, which may escape detection until adolescence or early adulthood. In addition, an undiagnosed immunodeficiency such as AIDS should be considered if a patient with a presumed community acquired pneumonia fails to respond to appropriate antibiotics (see Chapter 39).

Older patients with *recurrent pneumonias* should also be evaluated for the possibility of lung cancer. In evaluating patients with recurrent pneumonia, it is essential to review previous chest x-rays to document the anatomic location and the characteristics of the recurrent pulmonary infiltrate. In general, if a pneumonia recurs in multiple lobes or in pulmonary segments that are unrelated anatomically, bronchogenic carcinoma is unlikely. For example, a recurrent pneumonia that initially involves the right upper lobe and subsequently the right lower lobe is unlikely to be the result of a single endobronchial tumor. In addition to the anatomic location, the time during which recurrent pneumonias have occurred should be considered. If the interval is more than 2 years, malignancy is unlikely.

Apical. Often, roentgenographic patterns that range from increased pulmonary markings or minor scarring to cystic or cavitary disease in the upper lobes will be interpreted by a radiologist as showing old granulomatous disease or active tuberculous infection. The evaluation of these patients includes questioning about previous tuberculous lung disease (including the type and duration of antituberculous therapy) and an assessment of the reactivity of the tuberculin skin test. Comparison with prior chest x-rays is useful because the activity of an infiltrate cannot be determined from an isolated chest x-ray. If old chest x-rays demonstrate that no change has occurred, further evaluation may be unnecessary. The evaluation and treatment of patients with tuberculosis are discussed in Chapter 34.

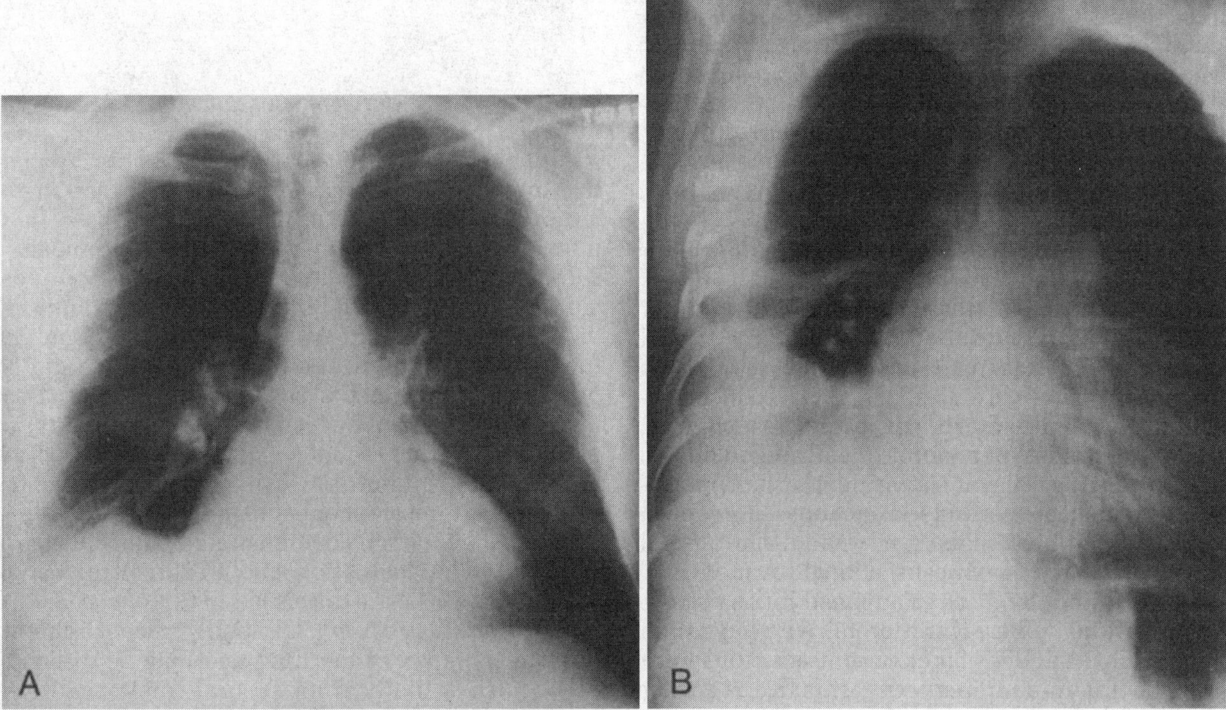

Figure 59.7. Subpulmonic effusion. The diaphragm appears to be elevated on the right **(A).** This represents subpulmonic fluid; when the patient is placed in the right lateral decubitus position **(B),** fluid layers on the right and tracks in the minor fissure and along the apex and the diaphragm.

Superior sulcus tumors, usually squamous cell carcinomas, arise in the extreme apex of the lung and may be difficult to distinguish from pleural thickening or old granulomatous disease. Later in the disease course, x-rays may reveal erosion of adjacent ribs or vertebrae by the tumor (see Chapter 61).

Pleural Effusion

Small amounts of free fluid within the pleural space will obliterate the costophrenic or costocardiac angles. Because the density of pleural fluid is greater than the density of the lung, a subpulmonic collection will laterally displace the crest of the diaphragm (Fig. 59.7A). An increased density between the stomach gas bubble and pulmonary tissue may also indicate the presence of fluid within the pleural space. The diagnosis of a large pleural effusion is not difficult because fluid within the pleural space on an upright chest x-ray will form a concave density across the chest cavity; decubitus x-rays will demonstrate free flowing pleural fluid in the dependent hemithorax (Fig. 59.7B). If the patient is recumbent, the pleural fluid will layer over the entire hemithorax, causing the lung to appear opaque.

In general, when pleural effusion is seen on a chest x-ray, a sample should be obtained for analysis. The obvious exception is a patient who develops acute pulmonary edema associated with a rapidly developing pleural effusion that resolves with therapy for congestive heart failure (see Chapter 66). The causes of pleural effusion are listed in Table 59.9. A diagnostic thoracentesis to determine the cause of the effusion can generally be done when the thickness of the fluid between the inner border of the rib and lung is more than 1 cm on a lateral decubitus x-ray. The fluid should be sent for white blood cell and differential count, total protein concentration, lactate dehydrogenase (LDH) concentration, glucose concentration,

Table 59.9. Causes of Pleural Effusion

Effusion	Common	Uncommon
Transudate	CHF Cirrhosis, nephrosis	Pericardial disease Myxedema, peritoneal dialysis
Exudate		
Malignancy	Metastatic disease (solid tumors)	Lymphoma, mesothelioma
Infection	Bacterial (parapneumonia and empyema), tuberculosis	Atypical pneumonias, fungal, viral, parasites (amebiasis, paragonimiasis)
Trauma	Hemothorax	Chylothorax
Gastrointestinal		Pancreatitis, esophageal rupture, subphrenic abscess
Collagen vascular disease		Systemic lupus erythematosus, rheumatoid arthritis
Miscellaneous	Postcoronary artery bypass surgery	Pulmonary infarction, benign asbestos effusion, drug hypersensitivity, postmyocardial infarction syndrome, uremia, trapped lung, lymphatic abnormalities

CHF, congestive heart failure.

Gram stain, cultures (aerobic and anaerobic bacteria, mycobacterium, fungus), pH (if there is a parapneumonic effusion), and cytopathology (if malignancy is suspected). Most pleural effusions are clear and straw colored, and deviations from this norm may be diagnostically helpful. For example, a bloody effusion suggests tumor and, less commonly, PE with infarction, tuberculosis, or trauma; a lime-green effusion suggests tuberculosis; a white milky effusion suggests a chylous exudate; and a viscous fluid with feculent odor strongly suggests an anaerobic empyema.

It is important to classify pleural effusion as either transudative or exudative (34,35). *Transudates* caused by increased hydrostatic pressure or decreased plasma oncotic pressure have low protein and LDH concentration and are generally due to congestive heart failure, cirrhosis with ascites, or nephrotic syndrome. They do not require further diagnostic evaluation, and treatment is directed at the underlying cause. *Exudates,* due to increased protein permeability of the pleural blood vessels, are generally caused by inflammation or tumor infiltration. Exudates are defined by one of the following criteria: pleural fluid protein concentration that is greater than 50% of the concentration of serum protein, pleural fluid LDH concentration that is greater than 60% of the concentration of serum LDH, or pleural fluid LDH concentration that is greater than 67% of the upper limit of normal serum LDH (34). Pleural effusions with protein concentrations greater than 3 g/100 mL are nearly always exudates. If the pleural fluid is defined as exudative but the clinical picture is more consistent with a transudate, the serum–pleural fluid albumin gradient should be measured. If this is greater than 1.2 g/dL, the effusion is probably transudative (35). A cell count and pleural fluid cytologic study should be performed because the presence of polymorphonuclear leukocytes in pleural fluid suggests acute inflammation and infection, whereas more than 50% lymphocytes suggests tuberculosis or malignancy. The presence of more than 5% pleural mesothelial cells makes the diagnosis of tuberculosis unlikely. Low pleural fluid glucose concentration (less than 50 mg/dL) occurs in infections (parapneumonic, tuberculosis), rheumatoid arthritis, and occasionally malignancy. Pleural fluid pH determination is important not only in the differential diagnosis (an acidic pH is seen with infection, malignancy, severe inflammation, esophageal rupture) but also in the management of parapneumonic pleural effusions. In this setting, a pH below 7.20 signals the possibility of a complicated parapneumonic effusion, which would require a more aggressive approach (36). If a pleural effusion is bloody or appears infected, the patient should be hospitalized for further diagnostic studies and therapy (e.g., chest tube drainage, pleural biopsy).

Pneumothorax

There are three major types of pneumothorax: spontaneous, iatrogenic, and traumatic. Of these, the general practitioner is most commonly faced with a spontaneous pneumothorax either in a young healthy individual or in an older patient with underlying pulmonary disease. In the former, a subpleural apical bleb ruptures into the pleural space, causing varying amounts of air to collect. Patients with spontaneous pneumothoraces tend to be tall, thin, young, male smokers (37). These patients generally are at rest when they first experience symptoms. In the older patient, emphysema with concomitant bullous disease is commonly associated with a pneumothorax (Fig. 59.8). The abrupt onset of pleuritic chest pain or dyspnea is characteristic. Pneumothoraces are diagnosed by demonstrating a visceral pleural line on the chest x-ray.

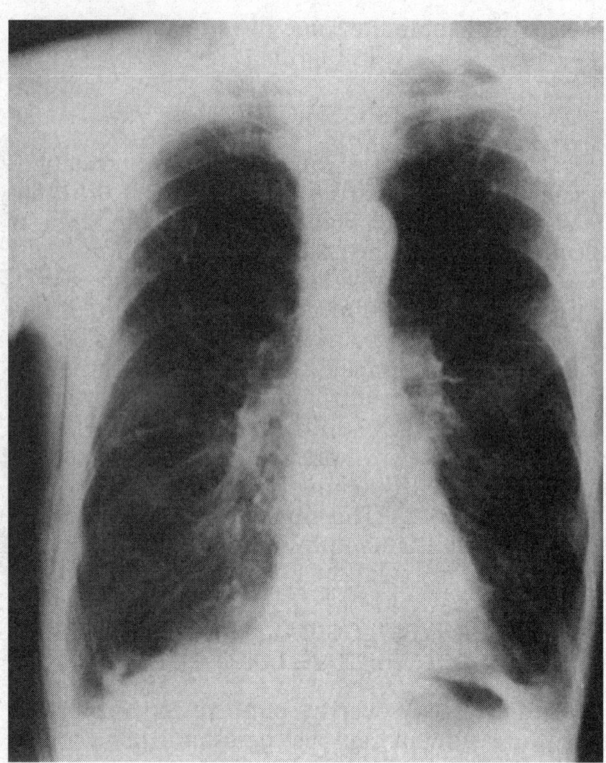

Figure 59.8. Pneumothorax. If the x-ray is not carefully examined, the pneumothorax in the right lower lung can easily be missed. Note the widespread bullae throughout the lung.

After the diagnosis of pneumothorax is made, the patient may need observation (ambulatory or inpatient) or insertion of a chest tube. For patients with a pneumothorax greater than 15% of the volume of the hemithorax, needle or catheter aspiration (e.g., using a thoracentesis kit) can obviate the need for hospitalization. This should only be performed by experienced personnel, because of the risk of visceral pleural laceration. In general, patients with underlying lung disease should be hospitalized and may require a chest tube because of their limited pulmonary reserve. On the other hand, a healthy patient with a small pneumothorax (less than 15%) who is not in distress may remain at home and may be followed by serial chest x-rays. The rate of reabsorption is slow; assuming approximately 1.25% of the volume is reabsorbed per day (37), a 15% pneumothorax will take approximately 12 days to reabsorb spontaneously. Supplemental oxygen can enhance the rate of reabsorption by decreasing alveolar nitrogen content and thus increasing the transpulmonary nitrogen gradient.

Solitary Nodule

A solitary nodule is a radiologic finding that always requires evaluation. A detailed discussion of the problem is to be found in Chapter 61.

General References*

George RB, Light RW, Matthay MA, et al. Chest medicine. Essentials of pulmonary and critical care medicine, 3rd ed. Baltimore: Williams & Wilkins, 1995.

Concise complete general textbook of pulmonary medicine.

Irwin RS, Boulet LP, Cloutier MM, et al. **Managing cough as a defense mechanism and as a symptom.** A consensus panel report of the American College of Chest Physicians. Chest 1998;114:133S.

A thorough review by leaders in the field.

Reed JC. Chest radiology. Plain film patterns and differential diagnoses, 4th ed. St. Louis: Mosby-Year Book, 1997.

A thorough textbook that gives a discussion and comprehensive differential diagnosis of common radiographic patterns of chest disease.

Tapson VF, Fulkerson WJ, Saltzman HA. Venous thromboembolism. Clin Chest Med 1995;16:229.

Up to date monograph on epidemiology, pathophysiology, diagnosis, and treatment.

Wasserman K, ed. Principles of exercise testing & interpretation: including pathophysiology and clinical applications, 3rd ed. Philadelphia: Lippincott Williams & Wilkins, 1999.

A standard and up to date reference on exercise testing.

Specific References

1. Irwin RS, Madison JM. The diagnosis and treatment of cough. N Engl J Med 2000;343:1715.
2. Irwin RS, Curley FJ, French CL. Chronic cough: the spectrum and frequency of causes, key components of the diagnostic evaluation, and outcome of specific therapy. Am Rev Respir Dis 1990;141:640.
3. Corrao WM, Braman SS, Irwin RS. Chronic cough as the sole presenting manifestation of bronchial asthma. N Engl J Med 1979;300:633.
4. Malini PL, Strocchi E, Zanardi M, et al. Thromboxane antagonism and cough induced by angiotensin-converting-enzyme inhibitor. Lancet 1997;350:15.
5. Luque CA, Vazquez Ortiz M. Treatment of ACE inhibitor-induced cough. Pharmacotherapy 1999;19:804.
6. Diggory P, Heyworth P, Chau G, et al. A. Unsuspected bronchospasm in association with topical timolol—a common problem in elderly people: can we easily identify those affected and do cardioselective agents lead to improvement? Age Ageing 1994;23:17.
7. Curley FJ, Irwin RS, Pratter MR, et al. Cough and the common cold. Am Rev Respir Dis 1988;138:305.
8. Sperber SJ, Hendley JO, Hayden FG, et al. Effects of naproxen on experimental rhinovirus colds. A randomized, double-blind, controlled trial. Ann Intern Med 1992;117:37.
9. Croughan-Minihane MS, Petitti DB, Rodnick JE, et al. Clinical trial examining the effectiveness of three cough syrups. J Am Board Fam Pract 1993;6:109.
10. Johnston H, Reisz G. Changing spectrum of hemoptysis. Underlying causes in 148 patients undergoing diagnostic flexible fiberoptic bronchoscopy. Arch Intern Med 1989;149:1666.

*Bold print (general references) and bold numerals (specific references) denote published controlled clinical trials, meta-analyses, or consensus-based recommendations.

11. Moser KM. Pulmonary embolism. In: Murray JF, Nadel JA, eds. Respiratory medicine, 2nd ed. Philadelphia: W.B. Saunders, 1994.
12. Adelman M, Haponik EF, Bleecker ER, et al. Cryptogenic hemoptysis. Clinical features, bronchoscopic findings, and natural history in 67 patients. Ann Intern Med 1985;102:829.
13. Hirshberg B, Biran I, Glazer M, et al. Hemoptysis: etiology, evaluation and outcome in a tertiary referral hospital. Chest 1997;112:440.
14. Cahill BC, Ingbar DH. Massive hemoptysis: assessment and management. Clin Chest Med 1994;15:147.
15. Tasker AD, Flower CD. Imaging the airways. Hemoptysis, bronchiectasis, and small airways disease. Clin Chest Med 1999;20:761.
16. O'Neil KM, Lazarus AA. Hemoptysis. Indications for bronchoscopy. Arch Intern Med 1991;151:171.
17. Poe RH, Israel RH, Marin MG, et al. Utility of fiberoptic bronchoscopy in patients with hemoptysis and a nonlocalizing chest roentgenogram. Chest 1988;93:70.
18. McGuinness G, Beacher JR, Harkin TJ, et al. Hemoptysis: prospective high-resolution CT/bronchoscopic correlation. Chest 1994;105:1155.
19. Mal H, Rullon I, Mellot F, et al. Immediate and long-term results of bronchial artery embolization for life-threatening hemoptysis. Chest 1999;115:996.
20. American Thoracic Society. Dyspnea. Mechanisms, assessment, and management: a consensus statement. Am J Respir Crit Care Med 1999;159:321.
21. Smoller JW, Pollack MH, Otto MW, et al. Panic anxiety, dyspnea, and respiratory disease. Am J Respir Crit Care Med 1996;154:6.
22. Ginsberg JS. Management of venous thromboembolism. N Engl J Med 1996;335:1816.
23. Goldhaber SZ. Pulmonary embolism. N Engl J Med 1998;339:93.
24. Goldhaber SZ, Grodstein F, Stampfer MJ, et al. A prospective study of risk factors for pulmonary embolism in women. JAMA 1997;277:642.
25. The PIOPED Investigators. Value of the ventilation/perfusion scan in acute pulmonary embolism. Results of the prospective investigation of pulmonary embolism diagnosis (PIOPED). JAMA 1990;263:2753.
26. Hull RD, Raskoh G, Ginsberg JS, et al. A noninvasive strategy for the treatment of patients with suspected pulmonary embolism. Arch Intern Med 1994;154:289.
27. Gefter W, Hatabu H, Holland GA, et al. Pulmonary thromboembolism: recent developments in diagnosis with CT and MR imaging. Radiology 1995;197:561.
28. Lipchik RJ, Goodman LR. Spiral computed tomography in the evaluation of pulmonary embolism. Clin Chest Med 1999;20:731.
29. Dalen JE, Banas JS Jr, Brooks HL, et al. Resolution rate of acute pulmonary embolism in man. N Engl J Med 1969;280:1194.
30. DePaso WJ, Winterbauer RH, Lusk JA, et al. Chronic dyspnea unexplained by history, physical examination, chest roentgenogram, and spirometry: analysis of a seven-year experience. Chest 1991;100:1293.
31. Lange P, Stoller J. The hepatopulmonary syndrome. Ann Intern Med 1995;122:521.
32. Goyal RK. Changing focus on unexplained esophageal chest pain. Ann Intern Med 1996;124:1008.
33. Mittl RL Jr, Schwab RJ, Duchin JS, et al. Radiographic resolution of community-acquired pneumonia. Am J Respir Crit Care Med 1994;149:630.
34. Light RW, MacGregor I, Luchsinger PC, et al. Pleural effusions: the diagnostic separation of transudates and exudates. Ann Intern Med 1972;77:507.
35. Light RW. Diagnostic principles in pleural disease. Eur Respir J 1997;10:476.
36. Light RW, Rodriguez RM. Management of parapneumonic effusions. Clin Chest Med 1998;19:373.
37. Light RW. Management of spontaneous pneumothorax. Am Rev Respir Dis 1993;148:245.

CHAPTER 60

Obstructive Airways Diseases: Asthma and Chronic Obstructive Pulmonary Disease

ROBERT A. WISE, MD
MARK C. LIU, MD

Obstructive lung diseases are the most common chronic pulmonary diseases encountered in ambulatory practice. *Asthma, chronic bronchitis, and emphysema are the most common of these disorders.* Less common conditions that lead to chronic obstructive lung disease include bronchiectasis, chronic forms of bronchiolitis, and cystic fibrosis. These disorders have different clinical presentations, causes, and prognoses, but all share the same physiologic abnormality—chronic airflow limitation.

EPIDEMIOLOGY

Obstructive airways diseases are increasing in prevalence and severity throughout the world. Over the past two decades, the prevalence of obstructive lung diseases in the United States increased by about 40%. It is estimated that 16 to 30 million Americans have been diagnosed with chronic obstructive pulmonary disease (COPD) or asthma. More than 100,000 deaths are attributed to chronic bronchitis and emphysema, the fourth leading cause of death, with increasing death rates mainly in women and minorities; 5,000 deaths are caused by asthma, disproportionately in inner-city minorities, but without overall increase in the past decade (1). The direct health care costs for chronic bronchitis, emphysema, and asthma are about $14 billion. Between 1979 and 1998, the age-adjusted mortality from chronic obstructive lung disease increased 42%, which is particularly notable because the all-cause death rate in the United States fell by 18% during this period (2,3).

PATHOPHYSIOLOGIC ABNORMALITIES IN OBSTRUCTIVE LUNG DISEASE

The diagnosis, severity, clinical course, and response to treatment can best be established by objective tests of lung function. How these disorders lead to chronic airflow limitation and how this limitation is measured in the ambulatory patient are discussed below.

Forced Expiratory Spirometry

Obstructive lung diseases cause the lung to empty slowly during a forced expiratory maneuver. Normal people can forcefully expel all of the air that can leave their lungs (the vital capacity) within 4 to 6 seconds. People with established obstructive lung disease may continue to expire during a forced expiratory maneuver for 10 to 20 seconds or more.

Forced Expiratory Vital Capacity and Forced Expiratory Volume in 1 Second

The forced expiratory vital capacity (FVC) test is used to diagnose and follow the course of obstructive lung diseases. The test is performed by having the patient blow forcefully into a device that records the volume of air leaving the lungs as a function of time. The record of the maneuver is called a *spirogram*, and the test itself is called *forced expiratory spirometry*. Devices that record the spirogram may either measure flow directly (a pneumotachometer) and calculate volume electronically or measure volume directly (a spirometer). Many such devices are commercially available and are accurate and reliable, but it is important to ascertain that the devices meet established standards that are promulgated for either screening or diagnostic purposes (4,5). More common than inaccurate equipment is the inability of the technician to elicit maximum effort from the test subject. A good spirometry technician must be both enthusiastic and demanding. Although diagnostic spirometers require daily calibration, office spirometers do not (5). Anyone caring for patients with obstructive lung diseases should have ready access to spirometry. General indications for spirometry are listed in Table 60.1.

Table 60.1. Indications for Spirometry

Establish diagnosis of obstructive lung disease.
Establish prognosis of obstructive lung disease.
Evaluate acute bronchodilator response.
Evaluate response to treatment.
Measure physiologic impairment for disability rating.
Evaluate thoracic and nonthoracic surgical risk.

Table 60.2. Criteria for Good Spirometry Session

At least three technically acceptable maneuvers.
Rapid start of expiration.
Continuous effort without hesitation or coughing.
Prolonged effort until plateau (at least 6 sec).
At least two reproducible maneuvers.
FEV_1 and FVC within 5% or 200 mL of highest value.

FEV_1, 1-second forced expiratory volume; FVC, forced vital capacity.

The *forced expiratory maneuver* is performed by having the patient take a maximal inspiration and then forcefully blow all of the air into the spirometer. A technically satisfactory maneuver is one that has a rapid onset, has a smooth contour without hesitation or coughing, and is prolonged until airflow ceases, with a minimum duration of 6 seconds. The test is repeated until three technically satisfactory maneuvers are obtained, two of which give reproducible measurements. Reproducible measurements are defined as being within 5% of each other or within 200 mL, whichever is greater (Table 60.2).

Many measures can be derived from the forced expiratory spirogram, but the most useful are the total amount of air leaving the lung, the FVC; the amount of air leaving the lung in the first second, the FEV_1; and the percentage of total air that leaves the lung in the first second, the FEV_1/FVC ratio or FEV_1%. The volume measures are expressed as absolute values adjusted to reflect the volume of gas at body temperature with 100% humidity. The FEV_1 and FVC are compared with predicted values based on age, gender, race, and height from a healthy reference population, usually as a percent of predicted (6). Airflow limitation is present when the FEV_1/FVC ratio is reduced below the value found in 95% of healthy nonsmokers (Table 60.3), although many people use an operational definition of an FEV_1/FVC ratio less than 0.70. The severity of airflow obstruction is determined by the reduction in FEV_1. Because diseases of airflow limitation also cause increased trapping of gas in the lung at the end of a forced expiration, FVC commonly is reduced as well. This should not, however, be confused with disorders that are associated with small lungs, the *restrictive lung diseases* (see Chapter 59). Despite the low FVC, the maximum gas volume of the lung—the *total lung capacity* (see below)—is usually increased in patients with obstructive disease. Typically, restrictive lung diseases cause an increase in FEV_1/FVC ratio in combination with a reduced FVC (Table 60.4 and Fig. 60.1).

The degree to which airflow limitation can be reversed rapidly is measured by performing spirometry

Table 60.3. Predicted Normal and Lower Limits of Normal FEV_1/FVC Ratio for 68" Tall Person

	Men		Women	
Age (yr)	Predicted (%)	Lower Limit Normal (%)	Predicted (%)	Lower Limit Normal (%)
20	85.0	76.7	86.7	77.6
30	83.5	75.2	84.1	75.1
40	82.0	73.7	81.6	72.6
50	80.4	72.2	79.1	70.0
60	78.9	70.6	76.6	67.5
70	77.4	69.1	74.1	65.0
80	75.9	67.6	71.5	62.5

FEV_1, 1-second forced expiratory volume; FVC, forced vital capacity.

Adapted from Crapo RO, Morris AH, Gardner RM. Reference spirometric values using techniques and equipment that meet ATS recommendations. Am Rev Respir Dis 1981;123:659, with permission.

Table 60.4. Interpretation of Spirometry

Ventilatory Defect	FEV_1	FVC	FEV_1/FVC
Obstructive	Decreased	Normal or decreased	Decreased
Restrictive	Decreased	Decreased	Normal or increased

FEV_1, 1-second forced expiratory volume; FVC, forced vital capacity.

before and after treatment with an inhaled bronchodilator. A positive response of either FEV_1 or FVC to bronchodilators is defined as greater than a 12% increase above baseline and an increment of at least 200 mL. Although this test is helpful in determining the potential for improvement when there is a rapid response to inhaled bronchodilators, many patients without a rapid response show improvement after several weeks or months of treatment with bronchodilators or anti-inflammatory agents.

Patient Experience. Forced expiratory spirometry can be safely and accurately performed in people with normal lung function and in those with advanced lung disease, even those who are critically ill. After a nose clip is attached, the patient inspires deeply and then forcefully expires for about 6 seconds. Because of the high pleural pressures, patients occasionally experience light-headedness during the maneuver. This can be minimized by having the patient sit during the test. Some patients experience soreness of the chest wall or abdomen for a day or two after the test, although analgesics are rarely needed.

Flow-Volume Loops

Forced expiratory airflow is high during the initial part of expiration and gradually falls to zero throughout the maneuver. The forced expiratory maneuver can be plotted as flow in relation to volume. If this is also done during a forced inspiration, the resultant display is called a flow-volume loop. Flow-volume loops can be readily calculated and displayed with small computers attached to flow or volume measuring devices. The flow-volume loop does not give information about the presence of obstructive airway

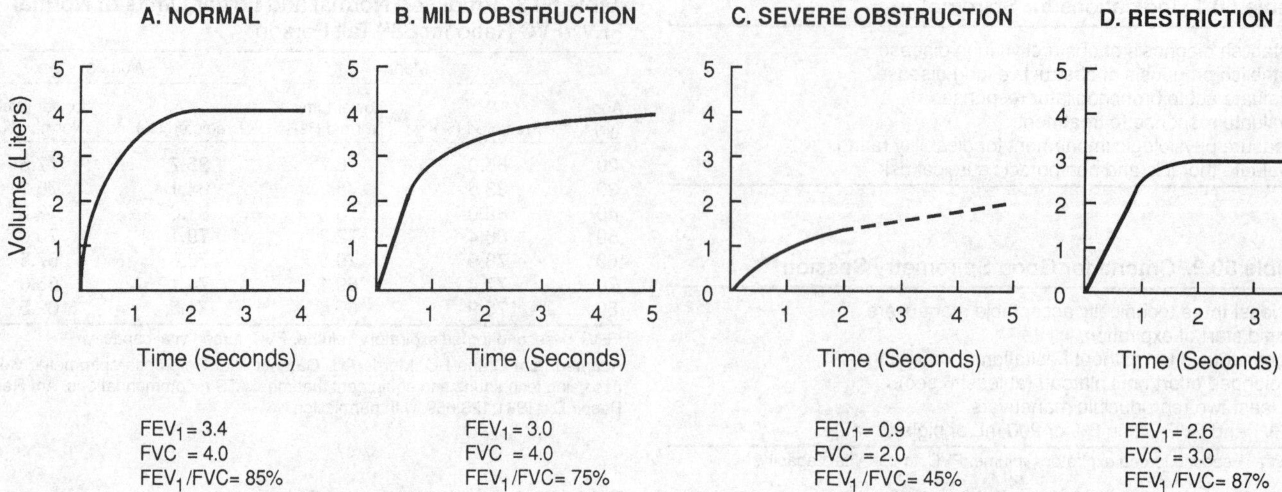

Figure 60.1. Spirographic tracings of forced expiration. Exhaled volume is plotted against time. The forced vital capacity (*FVC*) is represented by the total volume expired. One-second forced expiratory volume (*FEV_1*) is the volume of air expired during the first second. **A:** Normal spirogram. **B:** Spirogram from a patient with mild obstructive airways disease. **C:** Spirogram from a patient with severe obstructive defect. If the spirogram were incorrectly terminated after 2 seconds, the FVC would be artificially reduced (see text). When it is performed correctly (*dotted lines*), it is obvious that there is airway obstruction and that there is no restrictive disease. **D:** Spirogram showing restrictive pulmonary disease (FEV_1/FVC is normal but FVC is reduced).

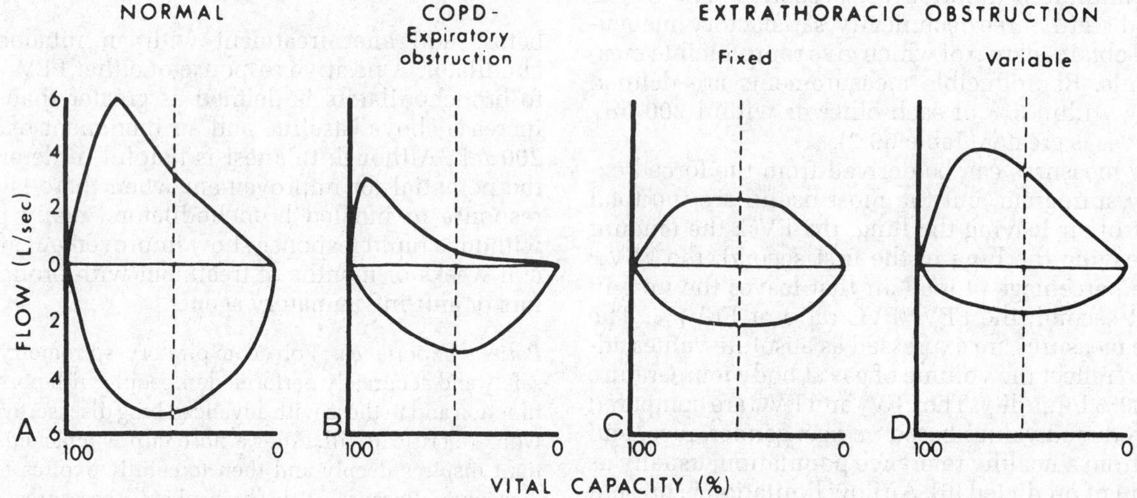

Figure 60.2. Flow-volume curves (loops) of maximal forced expiration (*top*) and maximal inspiration (*bottom*). Expiratory and inspiratory flow is plotted against lung volume expressed as a percentage of vital capacity. The *dotted line* can be used to compare flow rates at 50% of the vital capacity, where inspiratory flow rates normally exceed expiratory flow rates. **A:** Normal flow-volume curves. **B:** Flow-volume curves illustrating expiratory airflow obstruction showing decreased flow rates at all points in lung volume throughout maximal expiration. **C:** Fixed extrathoracic airway obstruction (cancer or stenosis of the larynx) produces a pattern where there is a decrease and flattening of both inspiratory and expiratory flow-volume curves. Inspiratory flow rate at 50% of the vital capacity is equal to similar expiratory flow rate. **D:** Variable extrathoracic obstruction (vocal cord paralysis) produces a pattern where there is a decrease and flattening of maximal inspiratory flow-volume curves. Inspiratory flow rates at 50% of the vital capacity are less than similar expiratory flow. (Modified from Hyatt RE, Black LF. The flow-volume curve: a current perspective. Am Rev Respir Dis 1973;107:191, with permission.)

disease that is not present in the traditional volume-time tracing of the spirogram and does not allow the easy hand measurement of the FEV_1 that can be done with volume-time tracings. The flow-volume loop is useful to detect upper airway disorders that affect the early portions of the forced expiration or that impede forced inspiration. Such disorders include laryngeal tumors, tracheal stenosis, or vocal cord paralysis (7) (Fig. 60.2). Because these disorders of the upper airway may mimic the dyspnea and wheezing of obstructive lung diseases and because they are potentially curable, the flow-volume loop can provide important information when the diagnosis is uncertain.

Other Lung Function Tests

Ordinarily, tests of lung function other than spirometry are not feasible to implement in the clinic or office setting and require referral to a pulmonary function laboratory. They are mainly helpful in the initial diagnostic evaluation of patients with lung disease.

Measurement of lung volume by *helium dilution, nitrogen washout, or body plethysmography* are helpful tests to establish the diagnosis of obstructive lung disease. The total lung capacity is usually increased (hyperinflation), as is the residual volume (air trapping) in both emphysema and acute asthma. In contrast, restrictive disorders such as sarcoidosis, asbestosis, or interstitial pulmonary fibrosis cause reduction in lung volume. Because helium dilution and nitrogen washout measure lung volume only in units of lung that are well ventilated, they tend to underestimate the true lung volume in people with emphysematous bullae or acute asthma with air trapping. Body plethysmography, which measures compressible gas volume in the chest, is more accurate in these conditions but because of the expense and technical difficulty of this measurement is often unavailable. In most circumstances, the dilution or washout methods provide sufficient accuracy to distinguish obstructive lung diseases from restrictive lung diseases.

Patient Experience (Lung Volume Measurements). With the helium dilution and nitrogen washout methods, the patient quietly breathes either a mixture of helium and oxygen or pure oxygen for 5 to 7 minutes. Because these tests require complete collections of expired gas, the patient must be able to form a tight seal around a mouthpiece. After the resident gas in the lung is measured (functional residual capacity), the patient performs two or three slow vital capacity maneuvers for calculation of the subdivisions of lung volume.

With the body plethysmography method, the patient sits in a tightly sealed box, about the size of a small closet, and breathes through a mouthpiece. At intervals, the technician closes a shutter on the mouthpiece and instructs the subject to perform a panting maneuver against the closed mouthpiece. The test is safe and painless, although a rare individual finds the box too confining. After the resident compressible gas in the lung is measured (thoracic gas volume), the patient performs several slow vital capacity maneuvers.

Measurement of the *carbon monoxide diffusing capacity (DCO)* by the single-breath method measures the effective area of the alveolar-capillary membrane available for gas transfer. Because of the destruction of alveolar septa, the DCO is reduced in emphysema. The magnitude of reduction in DCO is correlated with the physiologic severity of emphysema, as well as the amount of emphysema found in high-resolution computed tomographies of the chest (8,9).

Because the DCO is also reduced in diseases that affect the interstitium of the lung (e.g., pulmonary fibrosis and sarcoidosis) and diseases that affect the pulmonary blood vessels (e.g., pulmonary emboli and pulmonary arterial hypertension), a reduction in DCO must be interpreted in the context of other lung function tests and clinical findings. Because the DCO is often elevated in asthma and is decreased in emphysema, it helps determine the degree of reversibility of lung function that can be expected. When the diffusing capacity is below 50% to 60% of the predicted value, about half of the individuals with obstructive lung disease have oxygen desaturation with exercise and may benefit from supplemental oxygen (10). When the DCO exceeds 60% of predicted, oxygen desaturation with exercise is uncommon.

Patient Experience (Diffusing Capacity). The patient takes in a full vital capacity breath of gas containing a small concentration of carbon monoxide and holds his or her breath for 10 seconds. The maneuver is conducted two or three times to obtain reproducible measurements. The amount of carbon monoxide taken up does not cause appreciable increases in carboxyhemoglobin, and the test can be safely performed in patients who are anemic or who have coronary artery disease.

The expired alveolar air is analyzed to determine the rate of uptake of carbon monoxide. The test requires a 10-second breath-hold and about 1 L of vital capacity to collect an accurate sample of alveolar gas. Therefore, those who are unable to hold their breath because of dyspnea or coordination or who have less than 1 L of vital capacity often cannot perform this test.

Mechanisms of Airflow Limitation

Because the common finding of obstructive airways diseases is a reduction in forced expiratory airflow, it is important to understand the mechanism by which this reduction occurs. During forceful expiration, the pleural pressure rises around both the alveoli and the conducting airways. The pressure in the alveoli is slightly higher than the pleural pressure because the lung has elastic properties that tend to compress the alveolar gas, similar to an inflated latex balloon. This pressure difference between the alveoli and the pleural space is called the *elastic recoil pressure* and is equal to the distending pressure that prevents collapse of the alveolus. During expiration, the pressure near the alveoli is close to alveolar pressure but falls along the length of the airways because of the airway resistance. As pleural pressure is increased, the expiratory flow increases and the pressure drop along the airway becomes greater. When the pressure in the airway falls below a critical level with respect to the surrounding pleural pressure, the condition of flow limitation occurs. Under the condition of flow limitation, further increases in pleural pressure do not increase airflow. The precise mechanism by which flow limitation occurs is not fully understood, but it has been hypothesized that there is development of a narrowing at a site in the airway that acts like a nozzle or a fluttering of the airway that creates turbulence.

Although it is not understood exactly what occurs at the site of flow limitation in the airway, the general pathophysiologic processes that lead to reduced flows during forced expiration are understood (Table 60.5). Everyone has flow limitation during a forced expiration, but people with obstructive airways disease demonstrate flow limitation with less

Table 60.5. Mechanisms of Airflow Limitation

Mechanism	Disease	Anatomic Correlate
Decreased elastic recoil	Emphysema	Destruction of alveolar septa
Increased airway resistance	Chronic bronchitis	Peribronchial fibrosis, mucous gland hyperplasia
Increased airway collapsibility	Asthma	Smooth muscle hyperplasia, submucosal inflammation, mucous plugging of small airways

effort and at lower airflow. The three lung abnormalities that reduce flow during forced expiration are decreased lung recoil pressure, increased resistance of the airways, and increased tendency of airways to collapse. Decreased lung recoil pressure causes a lower distending pressure between the airway and the surrounding pleural pressure, thereby promoting the tendency of the airways to narrow. Increased resistance of the airways, particularly in the periphery of the lung, causes increased pressure drops along the airways during expiration, promoting the tendency of the airways to narrow. Increased airway collapsibility caused by bronchial smooth muscle constriction, inflammatory products encroaching upon the airway lumen, or decreased tethering of the airway by the alveolar septa also causes airways to collapse more easily.

In general, one can attribute the airflow limitation in *emphysema* to the decreased elastic recoil of the lung, the airflow limitation in *chronic bronchitis* to the increased peripheral airway resistance, and the airflow limitation in asthma to the increased tendency of airways to collapse. Although all these disorders are classified as *obstructive lung diseases,* it must be emphasized that physical obstruction of the airways is not the only mechanism causing reduced forced expiratory flow.

ASTHMA

Definition

Asthma is a disorder characterized symptomatically by cough, chest tightness, shortness of breath, and wheezing associated with limitation of airflow (see above). The symptoms may be acute and episodic or may wax and wane over long periods. One or more of the symptoms may be dominant, but usually all are present. The airflow obstruction is variable and may return to the normal range between exacerbations. Between episodes, most asthmatics are symptom free, but they are susceptible to attacks of wheezing, cough, and chest tightness when exposed to various "triggers." Common triggers for asthma attacks are shown in Table 60.6. Nearly all asthmatics have inflammation of the airways and bronchial hyperreactivity (11).

About 1 in 20 residents of the United States has asthma, and it is even more common in other developed countries. About half of the asthmatics in the United States have onset of the disease during childhood. In the prepubertal age group, the disease is more common in males, whereas the reverse is true for adults. About half of the children with asthma will have spontaneous resolution of their disease by young adulthood, though it may recur in the third or fourth decades. After age 30, asthma prevalence increases with advancing age.

Table 60.6. Common Triggers for Asthma

Exercise	Viral respiratory infections
Cold Air	Strong odors/irritants
Seasonal aeroallergens	Cigarette smoke
Ragweed pollen	Perfume
Tree pollen	Detergents
Grass pollen	Air pollutants
Indoor aeroallergens	
Dust mite feces	
Cockroach trailings	
Warm-blooded animals (e.g. cats, mice, dogs)	
Mold spores	

Allergy to common aeroallergens is present in most childhood asthmatics, and chronic allergic exposure is considered to be a potential underlying cause in the development of childhood asthma and an exacerbating trigger. In the older population, specific allergies are not as tightly linked to the presence of asthma, although those with allergies are more likely to have asthma than those without allergies (12).

Pathophysiology

Airways Reactivity

In asthmatics, bronchospasm can be induced by either allergic, irritant, or physicochemical stimuli. This increased tendency to have bronchospasm is synonymously called bronchial reactivity, airways reactivity, bronchial hyperreactivity, or bronchial hyperresponsiveness. This characteristic is defined by exaggerated declines in lung function after inhalation challenge with nonspecific bronchoconstrictor agents such as methacholine or histamine, with physical agents such as cold dry air ventilation or exercise-induced hyperpnea, or with specific allergenic agents such as inhaled antigens.

Virtually all asthmatics with active disease display airways reactivity, and the degree of reactivity correlates roughly with the severity of asthma. About one in eight individuals without clinical asthma also shows laboratory evidence of airways reactivity. Most smokers with mild chronic obstructive lung disease without clinical evidence of asthma have airways reactivity (13). Therefore, laboratory evidence of airways reactivity is not by itself diagnostic of asthma. However, testing for airways reactivity is useful when a negative result can rule out the diagnosis of asthma: the person with chronic persistent cough (see Chapter 59), episodic unexplained dyspnea (see Chapter 59), or occupationally associated respiratory symptoms. Although the testing procedure for airway reactivity is not complex, it is not performed on a regular basis except in specialty clinics and therefore usually requires referral to a pulmonary function laboratory.

Patient Experience (Airway Reactivity Testing). The testing procedure is safe if the baseline level of lung function is no more than moderately impaired (FEV_1 >60% predicted). Before the test, the patient should not use oral theophylline for 48 hours, short-acting inhaled bronchodilators for 8 hours, or long-acting inhaled bronchodilators for 24 hours. Oral or inhaled corticosteroids or other anti-inflammatory drugs may be continued. The patient breathes increasing concentrations of methacholine, either through repeated vital capacity breaths or through quiet tidal breathing. After each concentration, spirometry is performed. When the FEV_1 falls by 20% or more or the highest concentration is reached, the test is terminated and the bronchoconstriction is reversed with an inhaled bronchodilator. When conducted in a supervised setting, the test is safe, although some people with reactive airways experience coughing or chest tightness (14).

Specific airway inhalation challenge with antigen is rarely necessary for clinical purposes unless it is absolutely necessary to document whether a specific agent exacerbates asthma, such as a work-related exposure where employment decisions must be made. However, the response to specific antigen challenge does give insight into the pathogenesis of chronic asthma. After inhalation of an antigen of sufficient dose, acute bronchoconstriction lasts for 20 to 60 minutes, the early-phase reaction. Untreated, this early bronchospasm resolves within 1 to 2 hours, although it may be reversed with inhaled bronchodilators. Approximately 4 to 24 hours later, however, bronchospasm recurs in less than half of allergic people. It is generally thought that the *early-phase reaction* is due to bronchial smooth muscle constriction but that the *late-phase* reaction is the consequence of inflammatory cell recruitment with consequent airway mucosal edema and bronchoconstriction.

Exercise-induced bronchospasm is present in nearly all asthmatics if challenged sufficiently. After cessation of vigorous exercise, normal individuals show a small amount of bronchodilation. In contrast, susceptible asthmatics develop bronchoconstriction 5 to 20 minutes after stopping exercise. Similar responses can be elicited by breathing cold dry air. Postulated causes for exercise-induced bronchoconstriction include increases in the osmolality of the airway fluid lining layer because of drying of the airways causing release of inflammatory mediators, direct response of the airways to cooling during exercise hyperpnea, or vascular engorgement of the bronchial mucosa (15,16). Exercise-induced bronchospasm can be effectively prevented by pretreatment with either an inhaled beta-2-adrenergic agonist, a leukotriene inhibitor, or a mast-cell stabilizer such as cromolyn (see below).

Patient Experience (Exercise Bronchoprovocation). The patient should avoid bronchodilators in the same fashion as for methacholine challenge testing and should also avoid leukotriene antagonists and mast-cell stabilizing agents such as cromolyn or nedocromil for 24 hours. The patient exercises on a bicycle ergometer or treadmill to tolerance. After stopping exercise, spirometry is performed several times for the next 30 minutes. If bronchospasm occurs, it is reversed with an inhaled bronchodilator (14).

Airway Inflammation and Remodeling

The mechanisms that cause nonspecific airways reactivity are not entirely understood; however, it is now recognized that airway inflammation is linked to the presence of airways reactivity. Even mild asymptomatic asthmatics show submucosal infiltration with neutrophils, eosinophils, monocytes, T lymphocytes, and mast cells; edema; vascular engorgement; subepithelial collagen and fibronectin deposition; and epithelial desquamation. Patients with more long-standing asthma show hyperplasia of smooth muscle, goblet cell metaplasia, and mucous gland hypertrophy. It is thought that the chronic changes in airway morphology contribute to the nonreversible changes in lung function found in long-standing asthmatics (17).

Numerous theories explaining how airway inflammation leads to airways reactivity and remodeling have been advanced. It is likely that asthma is the common expression of several mechanisms or that one mechanism is predominant in some situations but not others. Whatever the mechanism, there is strong evidence that treatment of the underlying airway inflammation can reduce airways reactivity and improve asthma symptoms (18). There is no evidence, however, that anti-inflammatory treatment can prevent remodeling of the airways and improve long-term lung function (19).

Pathophysiology of the Acute Asthmatic Attack

The acute asthmatic attack may occur suddenly as a consequence of exposure to an allergic or irritant substance, producing severe bronchospasm in an individual with previously well-controlled asthma and normal lung function. More commonly, the attack occurs after many days of progressive reductions in lung function, increasing lability of lung function, progressive exertional dyspnea and cough, nocturnal awakening and increasing requirements for symptomatic use of inhaled bronchodilators (20).

During the acute attack, bronchospasm, mucosal edema, and mucous plugging lead to narrowing and closure of small peripheral airways. This causes an increase in resistance to inspiratory and expiratory airflow and, more important, trapping of air. The patient must breathe at high lung volume to keep the airways open. The consequences of this hyperinflation are increased work of breathing, impaired mechanical advantage of the shortened respiratory muscles and of the flattened diaphragm, pulmonary hypertension, and markedly negative inspiratory swings in pleural pressure to initiate airflow. If the attack is severe or prolonged, respiratory muscle fatigue can occur with consequent hypoventilation, carbon dioxide retention, hypoxemia, respiratory failure, and death (21). Arterial blood gas tensions in nonsevere asthma attacks usually show hypocapnia from hyperventilation. A normal arterial carbon dioxide tension may indicate either resolution of the attack or impending respiratory failure and must therefore be correlated with other clinical features (22). Ventilation-perfusion mismatch accounts for the hypoxemia that accompanies an asthma attack; however, treatment with beta-adrenergic bronchodilators usually worsens ventilation-perfusion matching, causing transient worsening hypoxemia as the asthma attack improves. Resolution of the attack is often preceded by the expectoration of copious secretions with small mucous plugs. As the attack resolves, dyspnea and chest tightness disappear before wheezing resolves, whereas abnormalities of lung function can persist for many days or weeks (23).

Clinical Presentations

Clinical presentations of asthma differ with regard to chronicity and to inciting factors. There is broad overlap between these categories of asthma, and they should not necessarily be considered to have differing underlying mechanisms.

Extrinsic or allergic asthma is a condition in which the worsening of the asthma can be clearly associated with exposure to a specific allergen (Table 60.6). In more than 80% of cases, allergic asthma is associated with allergic rhinitis. The most common perennial allergens associated with worsening of asthma include molds (particularly Alternaria), house dust mite feces, cockroach trailings, cat secretions, and mouse feces (24,25). The most common seasonal allergens include ragweed (autumn), tree pollen (spring), and grass pollens (summer). Diagnosis of a specific allergen triggering asthma requires a history of worsening asthma after exposure, improvement of the asthma when the allergen is removed, and positive wheal and flare reaction to the offending agent on allergy skin testing. Clear association of asthma with a specific allergen is important because control of the environmental exposure or specific immunotherapy can be time consuming, expensive, or impractical. When an aeroallergen is clearly associated with asthma symptoms, immunotherapy with weekly allergy injections may lead to mild, although transient, improvement in the disease (26). In most cases, however, asthma is adequately treated in the absence of immunotherapy (27).

Intrinsic or nonallergic asthma is a condition in which there is no clear association with specific allergen exposure. This form of asthma is more common in adults than in children and typically causes perennial symptoms. Acute episodes may be triggered by viral illnesses, but often no specific provocative stimulus can be found. In about half of the cases, the asthma persists or worsens throughout life, leading to incompletely reversible abnormalities of pulmonary function. When this is associated with chronic cough and sputum production, it is often called *chronic asthmatic bronchitis* and may be difficult to distinguish from smoking-related chronic obstructive lung disease. The cause of this form of asthma is unclear. Many patients show some traits of allergic tendencies with elevation of serum IgE levels and eosinophilic airway inflammation, but allergy skin testing is usually negative. In some cases, it appears that the onset of the disease followed a severe lower respiratory tract viral infection, whereas in others it may be associated with long-term exposure to specific allergens or respiratory irritants (17,28).

Occupational asthma (see Chapter 8) is a condition in which a specific occupational exposure leads to cough, wheezing, and chest tightness. If exposure to the offending antigen persists, a chronic asthmatic condition with sensitivity to nonspecific agents may occur. If exposure to the sensitizing agent is stopped soon enough, symptoms and nonspecific airway reactivity often resolve, although it may take up to 2 years. Because the prognosis for remission is better in those who cease exposure early, the caregiver needs to diagnose occupational asthma early and to initiate steps to avoid continued exposure (29). Common substances that may cause occupational asthma are shown in Table 60.7.

Reactive airways dysfunction syndrome is a disorder that follows an intense short-term exposure to a toxic nonallergenic substance such as sulfuric acid, nitric acid, chlorine, or hydrochloric acid fumes. After the exposure—often the result of an industrial accident

Table 60.7. Occupational Exposures Causing Asthma

Agent	Specific Examples	Occupation
Birds	Pigeons, chickens	Pigeon breeders, poultry workers
Chemicals	Hexachlorophene, formalin, ethylene diamine, metabisulfite	Hospital workers, photographers, food preparation workers, water purification workers
Crustaceans	Crabs, shrimp	Food processing workers
Drugs	Antibiotics, sulfa derivatives	Workers in pharmaceutical industry, agricultural feed mixing
Enzymes	*Bacillus subtilis,* trypsin, papain	Detergent handlers, pharmaceutical industry workers
Epoxy resins	Anhydride compounds	Workers in manufacturing, auto body repair
Laboratory animals	Rats, mice, rabbits, guinea pigs	Laboratory workers, veterinarians
Metals	Platinum, nickel, chromium, cobalt, vanadium	Workers in metal plating, leather tanning, hard metal industry
Plants	Grain dust, flour	Grain handlers, bakers, millers
Plastics and rubber	TDI (toluene di-isocyanate), DDI (diphenylmethane di-isocyanate), Azodicarbonamide	Polyurethane plastic, paint, varnish, and rubber workers
Soldering fluxes	Colophony, aminoethylethanolamine	Electronics, aluminum fabrication workers
Vegetable products	Gum acacia	Printing workers
Wood dust	Cedar, redwood	Carpenters, construction workers, woodmill workers

Adapted from Chan-Yeung M. Occupational asthma. Chest 1990;98:148S, with permission.

or fire—and resolution of the resultant acute lung injury, the individual is left with chronic airways reactivity to nonspecific physicochemical agents such as tobacco smoke or cold air. The disorder may resolve after several months but often leads to chronic airways reactivity (30).

Exercise-induced bronchospasm is present in most asthmatics, although some children and young adults may experience asthma only after exercise. Although this syndrome may be confused with exertional dyspnea or angina, careful questioning will reveal that the dyspnea occurs after a 5- to 20-minute symptom-free interval after the cessation of exercise. Exercise-induced bronchospasm is thought to be caused by the airway cooling and drying, leading to hyperosmolar fluids lining the airways and to the release of bronchoconstrictor and vasodilator mediators (16). For this reason, exercise-induced bronchospasm is often worse in cold dry environments, whereas a warm humid environment like an indoor swimming pool is often well tolerated. The symptoms can be prevented by inhalation of a beta-agonist bronchodilator or sodium cromolyn (see below) about 20 minutes before exercise.

Triad asthma (Sampter syndrome) is a syndrome of nasal polyps, asthma, and aspirin sensitivity. One of three asthmatics with nasal polyps has aspirin sensitivity, in comparison with 1 in 15 asthmatics without nasal polyps. These individuals often have severe chronic asthma and occasionally experience systemic anaphylactic reactions to aspirin or aspirin-like compounds, including nonsteroidal anti-inflammatory drugs (NSAIDS) (31). Even asthmatics who are aware that they are sensitive to aspirin (10% of asthmatics) may be inadvertently using compounded drugs that contain aspirin (see Chapter 30 for a list of common medicines that contain aspirin). The mechanism by which this occurs is thought to involve blockade of cyclooxygenase-derived prostaglandins and the induction of lipoxygenase-derived leukotrienes from inflammatory cells. Surgical removal of the nasal polyps may make the asthma better, but the polyps often recur and require long-term topical or systemic corticosteroid treatment. If aspirin is required for treatment of another condition, rapid desensitization can be performed, but daily maintenance doses of aspirin are required to sustain the effect. Aspirin-sensitive asthma is an indication for the use of leukotriene antagonists or inhibitors such as montelukast, zafirlukast, or zileuton, because increased leukotriene production is a prominent feature of this syndrome. Specific cyclooxygenase-2 inhibitors appear to be well-tolerated by patients with aspirin sensitivity, likely due to the lack of effect on the constitutive form of cyclooxygenase (32).

Cough-variant asthma is a condition in which wheezing, dyspnea, and chest tightness are minimal symptoms, but chronic cough is the major complaint. Approximately 30% of patients with chronic persistent cough of more than 8 weeks duration have airways reactivity and respond to treatment with bronchodilators or corticosteroids (33,34).

Allergic bronchopulmonary aspergillosis (ABPA) is an uncommon form of asthma that is difficult to treat and can lead to chronic respiratory failure. The disorder is caused by local allergic reaction to noninvasive *Aspergillus* or to other fungal species colonizing the airway. *Aspergillus fumigatus*, a ubiquitous saprophyte, is the most common organism, but other fungi can cause the same syndrome. The chronic inflammatory condition leads to dilation and bronchiectasis of the central airways, recurrent mucous plugging and segmental atelectasis, and eventually fibrotic destruction of lung parenchyma. Criteria for the diagnosis of ABPA include recurrent atelectasis and pulmonary infiltrates; radiographic evidence of proximal bronchiectasis or mucoid impactions, blood, and sputum eosinophilia; immediate skin test reactivity to *Aspergillus*; serum precipitins to *Aspergillus*; elevated serum IgE; and specific IgG and IgE antibodies to *Aspergillus* by radioallergosorbent tests or enzyme-linked immunosorbent assay testing (see below) (35).

The usual treatment consists of systemic corticosteroids with starting dosages of 0.5 to 1.0 mg/kg per day of prednisone or its equivalent. At least 6 months of therapy are usually required, but many patients are never able to tolerate permanent steroid cessation. Inhaled or systemic antifungal therapy is not helpful in eradicating the offending agent, although there is evidence that long-term treatment with oral agents such as itraconazole may be beneficial in reducing the steroid dose (36,37). Early diagnosis and treatment are necessary to prevent the progressive bronchiectasis and lung fibrosis that can occur. The effectiveness of therapy is monitored with serum IgE levels and chest x-rays. Because ABPA is found in approximately 10% of patients with cystic fibrosis, the clinician should consider screening for cystic fibrosis by measurements of sweat chloride concentrations or by genetic analysis in patients with ABPA.

Refractory asthma is defined as dyspnea, wheezing, and frequent exacerbations despite maximum therapy with bronchodilators and inhaled and systemic corticosteroids (38). When symptoms are intractable, the possibility should be considered that a condition that mimics asthma (see below) is present. Other circumstances that may contribute to intractable asthma include an occult persistent exposure to an allergen or irritant at home or at work, use of beta-blockers either systemically or as eye drops, use of aspirin or related drugs, exposure to dietary chemicals such as sulfites, hypothyroidism or hyperthyroidism, gastroesophageal reflux, sinusitis, bronchopulmonary aspergillosis, and mucocutaneous fungal infection. However, the most likely cause of refractory asthma is nonadherence to prescribed treatment, a behavior that is often underestimated (39).

Catastrophic asthma occurs in individuals who experience rapid deterioration of asthma with fatal or near-fatal consequences. In most cases this occurs in people with severe underlying disease, but it can occur without such a history. The severity of the attack is often not recognized by the patient or by caregivers, and the ability to predict such events is poor. About one-third of fatal asthma attacks are preceded by recurrent hospitalizations, but only 1 of 20 are preceded by previous near-fatal attacks. The prognosis of patients who have had a near-fatal attack of asthma is poor, with 10% dying within 1 year (40).

Wheezing that is not due to asthma may be confused by the patient or the clinician with asthma, often as an intractable case. Such conditions include congestive heart failure, mitral stenosis, cystic fibrosis, immotile cilia syndrome, immunoglobulin deficiency, laryngeal tumors, vocal cord paralysis, laryngospasm, airway foreign body, hypereosinophilic syndromes, endobronchial sarcoidosis, bronchiolitis obliterans, Churg-Strauss vasculitis, multiple pulmonary emboli, reaction to angiotensin-converting enzyme inhibitors, and, in underdeveloped countries, pertussis and diphtheria (38,41). A common disorder mimicking severe episodic asthma is *vocal cord dysfunction syndrome* where inspiration is accompanied by paradoxical closure of the vocal cords (42). Careful examination may allow differentiation of upper airway conditions from asthma. Upper airway obstructions cause monophonic (i.e., single pitch) inspiratory or inspiratory–expiratory high-pitched sounds (stridor) heard loudest over the central airways. In contrast, asthmatic wheezing causes polyphonic expiratory sounds that are heard loudest over the chest. When there is a question of upper airway obstruction, laryngoscopy and flow-volume loops should be obtained, particularly during a symptomatic episode.

Evaluation of Chronic Asthma

Medical History and Clinical Interview

A thorough medical history is essential for establishing the diagnosis of asthma and for guiding treatment. The following factors should be evaluated: duration, frequency, and severity of attacks; seasonal variation of disease; specific trigger factors; occupational and recreational exposures; home conditions; other allergic conditions; and medication use and adherence.

Asthmatics describe their episodic shortness of breath differently than do patients with other forms of lung disease or heart failure. Asthmatics use terms such as *chest tightness* and *wheeziness* rather than *air hunger*, *suffocation*, or *rapid breathing*. Asthmatics often say the site of obstruction is in their neck. They report more difficulty with inspiration than expiration in contrast to patients with emphysema, who cannot distinguish inspiratory from expiratory distress (43,44).

Asthma should not be considered well controlled if there is more than occasional requirement for symptomatic use of inhaled bronchodilators or if there is nocturnal awakening with symptoms. The presence of nocturnal symptoms is such a characteristic feature of asthma that the absence of this history should stimulate the investigation of other causes of episodic wheezing and chest tightness. Although pollen seasons and common aeroallergens vary geographically, asthma that is worse in the early fall suggests ragweed allergy; worse in the summer, grass pollen allergy; and worse in the spring, tree pollen allergy. Specific asthma triggers (Table 60.6) should be elicited. Because the symptoms of asthma may follow an allergic exposure by 2 to 24 hours, elicitation of such exposures requires careful questioning or the maintenance of a prospective asthma diary recording exposures, symptoms, and peak flow. Occupational exposures may be obvious (Table 60.7) but can also occur from operations in an adjacent work space or via ventilation systems. Strong evidence of an occupational trigger exposure is the absence of symptoms on weekends and during vacations. Occasionally, it is necessary to have a worksite inspection performed by an expert in occupational medicine (see Chapter 8).

In cases in which it is unclear whether the home exposure is important, the patient should be questioned about whether the asthma worsened upon moving to a new home and whether it improves during periods away from home. Perennial allergen and irritant exposures at home contribute to the chronic airway inflammation that causes asthma, particularly in children. House dust mites feed on desquamated human skin and produce allergenic feces that are easily respirable. Dust mites thrive in a humid warm environment, particularly in feather pillows, comforters, carpets, upholstered furniture, and mattresses. Cockroaches and their excreta are highly allergenic. Pets, particularly cats and dogs, secrete antigen in their saliva that may persist in the home environment many years after the pets are no longer present. Frequent vacuuming, while useful in eliminating home allergens, also disperses antigen into the air for several hours. Smokers in the home also disperse irritant sidestream smoke that worsens asthma. Humidifiers or other causes of high ambient humidity promote the growth of molds and of dust mites. Some exposures may be difficult to uncover. Urea-formaldehyde foam insulation can cause low-level irritant exposure that is a potential aggravator of asthma. Newly varnished floors or furniture can give off isocyanate fumes that worsen asthma (45). Toluene di-isocyanate exposure can trigger severe asthma in those who use polyurethane paint or varnish, heavy mold exposure occurs in those who engage in water sports or boating; and seminal fluid allergy can rarely occur in those who have coitus (46–48).

Knowledge of associated allergic conditions is helpful. Histories of allergic rhinitis, eczema, and urticaria can assist in determining specific asthma triggers and would support more specific therapies directed toward those allergens. Chronic allergic or infectious sinusitis can exacerbate asthma, and symptoms of sinus pain or drainage should be elicited (49).

Gastroesophageal reflux may trigger nocturnal asthma either through reflex distension and irritation of the esophagus or through aspiration of gastric contents into the larynx and lower airways (50,51). *Tartrazine* (yellow dye no. 5) is found in yellow or orange foods, particularly powdered orange juice substitutes. Although tartrazine was once thought to be a common cause of asthma in aspirin-sensitive individuals, it is now considered that true tartrazine sensitivity is exceedingly rare (52). *Sulfites*, present in dried fruits, wines, processed potatoes, seafood, and salad greens, can cause acute asthma attacks. The mechanism is thought to be from production of sulfur dioxide. Although some patients attribute asthma symptoms to ingestion of *monosodium glutamate*, found in Asian cooking or snack foods, it is rare that this trigger can be verified objectively (53). It should not be assumed that asthmatics do not smoke *cigarettes*. In some urban populations, as many as 40% of asthmatics are cigarette smokers. Air pollution, particularly respirable particulates, ozone, SO_2, and NO_2, have been implicated as an exacerbating factor in asthma during atmospheric inversions in the summer (54–56).

Only approximately 50% of asthmatics adhere to their prescribed drug regimen, often without admitting this to the caregiver. Adherence worsens as the drug program becomes more complex, and there is less adherence with drugs that prevent but do not relieve symptoms (57). It is important to elicit in a friendly and supportive manner whether the patient is actually following the prescribed program. This can be aided by questions such as "How often do you have difficulty taking your medications on a routine basis?" or "What problems have you had in taking your medicines?" Barriers to adherence (see Chapter 4) include failure to accept or understand the benefit and purpose of medication and environmental controls, the high cost of drugs and supplies, frequent dosing of multiple drugs, side effects of treatment, and disorganized stressful living conditions. These elements need to be explored and modified when possible.

Physical Examination

The physical examination of the patient with asthma should be directed toward confirming the diagnosis, estimating the severity of disease, evaluating related conditions, and ruling out other disorders that mimic asthma.

During an *acute asthmatic attack*, the patient appears frightened and fatigued. The respiratory pattern is deep and slow with a prolonged expiratory phase but may progress to rapid shallow breathing with expiratory grunting that heralds the onset of respiratory failure. Speech is telegraphic or absent. Coughing is ineffective. The chest appears hyperinflated, with reduced tidal expansion compared with the strong respiratory efforts. The sternomastoid muscles are contracted with each inspiration during severe episodes. Hyperinflation of the lungs causes the lower lateral ribcage to move inward with each inspiratory contraction of the flattened diaphragm rather than outward as normally occurs. Tachycardia is present, with weakening of the pulse during inspiration. An inspiratory fall in systolic blood pressure (*pulsus paradoxus*) of more than 15 mm Hg is present in severe attacks but may disappear with the onset of respiratory failure (58,59). The chest has diffuse polyphonic expiratory wheezes but in the most severe attacks may be silent. Inspiratory wheezing suggests the presence of upper airway obstruction, whereas localized or monophonic wheezing suggests mechanical bronchial obstruction from tumor or foreign body. Absent breath sounds in one hemithorax with wheezing in the other should raise the possibility of *pneumothorax*—a potentially lethal complication.

In chronic asymptomatic asthma, the examination of the chest may be entirely normal. The presence of mild airflow obstruction can be determined by listening for wheezes during a forced expiration. However, this finding is neither sensitive nor specific for asthma. Associated allergic rhinitis causes the nasal mucosa to be pale and edematous. Nasal polyps appear as tan-gray mucoid lesions that obstruct the nasal aperture.

Examination should be directed at disorders that may mimic asthma. Listening over the neck during forced inspiration or with the arm extended over the head can bring out inspiratory stridor with upper airway obstruction. Findings of congestive heart failure such as chest crackles, cardiomegaly, or mitral murmurs should be carefully evaluated. High-pitched monophonic localized inspiratory squeaks suggest the presence of bronchiolitis.

Laboratory Testing

Spirometry (see above) should be performed in all asthmatics in the asymptomatic phase and periodically during the course of therapy to establish a baseline severity and to monitor therapy. Persistent abnormalities of pulmonary function, which form the basis for recurrent attacks of asthma, are present in the asymptomatic phase. The chest x-ray is usually normal in asymptomatic asthma but shows hyperinflation during acute attacks. ABPA (p. 815) shows characteristic central bronchiectasis and signs of mucoid impaction. During severe acute asthma attacks, pneumothorax or pneumonia may require specific treatment. Peripheral blood eosinophilia is common in asthma, particularly if the patient has not been exposed to corticosteroids. Microscopic examination of unstained sputum can distinguish eosinophils from neutrophils when there is purulence, guiding the need for corticosteroids versus antibiotics (60). In severe corticosteroid-treated asthma, however, neutrophils may predominate, even in the absence of bacterial infection (61). Other features characteristic of asthmatic sputum are *Charcot-Leyden crystals*, which are spear-shaped crystals derived from eosinophil granules; *Curschmann spirals*, which are mucous casts of small airways; and *Creola bodies*, which are clumps of desquamated ciliated epithelial cells.

Skin testing for specific allergens is helpful to diagnose specific allergies, particularly when environmental control procedures are costly or difficult, such as changing occupations or residences or eliminating a beloved pet. However, positive allergy skin tests do not indicate allergy to a particular substance as the cause of asthma unless there is a compatible history. *Radioallergosorbent tests (RASTs)* measure allergen-specific IgE in the blood and may be substituted for

Table 60.8. Components of Asthma Treatment

Monitor symptoms and lung function.
Control adverse environmental exposures.
Educate patient and family.
Administer drug therapy.

skin testing. *Total serum IgE* is elevated in asthma but is useful mainly for diagnosis and monitoring of ABPA (see p. 815). *Methacholine challenge* is helpful when the diagnosis of asthma is uncertain. A normal methacholine challenge in a symptomatic person virtually eliminates the diagnosis of active asthma. *Flow-volume loops* and *nasopharyngoscopy* are useful tests to determine whether vocal cord dysfunction is mimicking asthma (42).

Treatment

The goal of the treatment of asthma is to keep the patient symptom free day and night, with full activity levels, normal lung function, absent side effects, and satisfaction with the process of care. For most patients who can adhere to a comprehensive asthma management plan, this is a realistically attainable goal.

Treatment in the ambulatory setting has four major components: monitoring of symptoms and lung function, control of environmental triggers, education of the patient and family, and drug therapy (Table 60.8).

Home Monitoring of Lung Function

Monitoring lung function with objective tests is important in asthmatics who have to use symptomatic bronchodilator treatments more than twice per week or who have experienced severe attacks. Inexpensive peak flow monitors are commercially available. Recording peak flow gives an indication of maximal lung function, can forecast the worsening of asthma before severe symptoms develop, allows objective identification of harmful environmental or occupational exposures, and facilitates telephone contact between the patient and medical caregivers. A practical regimen is to record the peak flow daily in the morning. If it is less than 80% of the patient's personal best level, additional recordings during the day are warranted. The determination of a patient's personal best level can be obtained during a 2- or 3-week period of intensive asthma treatment and should be periodically updated. Asthma diaries are helpful in recording patterns of peak flow variation, symptoms, and use of symptomatic bronchodilators (Fig. 60.3).

Control of Environmental Triggers and Complicating Conditions

Environmental controls for asthma include the identification and removal of nonspecific irritants and the reduction of exposure to specific allergens. *Smoking cessation* is essential and may require repeated strong personalized messages, referral to smoking cessation group programs, and drug therapy (see Chapter 27). Household members should also be discouraged from smoking in the house.

Gastroesophageal reflux may worsen asthma, although it is controversial whether treatment is indicated in the absence of reflux symptoms. Small frequent feedings; elevation of the bed; and antacids, histamine-2 receptor blockers, or proton pump blockers may be prescribed (see Chapter 42). *Allergic or infectious sinusitis* should be aggressively treated with antibiotics, intranasal steroids, or surgical procedures (62).

Common specific perennial *allergen sources* include house dust mite, cockroaches, molds, and pets. *House dust mites* can be controlled by maintaining low humidity, removing carpeting and stuffed furniture from the bedroom, and covering mattresses and pillows with impermeable covers. Asthmatics should avoid vacuuming or entering a freshly vacuumed area for 1 to 2 hours or should wear a protective face mask. High efficiency vacuum cleaners are available but are of unproven value. Bedding should be washed weekly in hot water (above 130°F) to eliminate dust mites. *Fur-bearing animals* shed allergenic saliva and urine, and should be eliminated from the household if they exacerbate asthma. If the patient or family is unwilling to part with the pet, other partially effective measures include washing the pet frequently, excluding the pet from the asthmatic's bedroom, and blocking forced hot air vents in the asthmatic's bedroom (63). *Cockroach infestation* is a particularly important cause of asthma in inner cities and can be controlled with insecticides, although repeated treatment is required. The preferred methods of cockroach control are boric acid powder, poison baits, and traps (64). *Insecticide sprays*, particularly cholinesterase inhibitors, can cause severe asthma exacerbations by themselves. *Molds* can be controlled in the home by the use of dehumidifiers and by providing adequate ventilation in the kitchen and bathroom. Mouse antigens are ubiquitous in the inner city. They have an uncertain relationship to asthma, but elimination of mice is a prudent measure (65). Indoor air cleaning devices using high-efficiency filters or electrostatic filters can diminish suspended particles of tobacco smoke and mold spores, but they have not been found to improve asthma symptoms in controlled studies (66). Therefore, they are not recommended for routine use and do not substitute for other methods of environmental control. Room or house humidifiers should be avoided because they can increase concentrations of mold spores and house dust mites.

During specific pollen allergy seasons or high air pollution days, asthmatics should stay indoors at midday when the pollen concentration and air quality are worst. Outdoor exercise during high air pollution periods should be avoided because high levels of ventilation increase the damaging effect of air pollutants. Closing doors and windows and using a recirculating air conditioner minimize indoor pollen and air pollution exposure.

Exposure to occupational allergens should be controlled by ventilation changes in the workplace. If

ASTHMA SYMPTOM AND PEAK FLOW DIARY

__My predicted peak flow
__My personal best peak flow
__My Green (OK) Zone (80-100% of personal best)
__My Yellow (Caution) Zone (50-80% of personal best)
__My Red (Danger) Zone (below 50% of personal best)

Date	a.m.	p.m.	a.m.	p.m.	a.m.	p.m.	a.m.	p.m.	a.m.	p.m.	a.m.	p.m.	a.m.	p.m.
Peak flow reading														
No asthma symptoms														
Mild asthma symptoms														
Moderate asthma symptoms														
Serious asthma symptoms														
Medicine used to stop														
Urgent visit to the doctor														

1. Take your peak flow reading every morning (a.m.) when you wake up and every night (p.m.) at bedtime. Try to take your peak flow readings at the same time each day. If you take an inhaled beta$_2$-agonist medicine, take your peak flow reading *before* taking that medicine. Write down the highest reading of three tries in the box that says peak flow reading.
2. Look at the box in the upper left of this sheet to see whether your number is in the green, yellow, or red zone.
3. In the space below the date and time, put an "X" in the box that matches the symptoms you have when you record your peak flow reading.
4. Look at your asthma control plan for what to do when your number is in one of the zones and you have asthma symptoms.
5. Put an "X" in the box beside "medicine use" if you took *extra* asthma medicine to stop your symptoms.
6. If you made any visit to your doctor's office, emergency room, or hospital for treatment of an asthma episode, put an "X" in the box marked "urgent visit." Tell your doctor if you went to the emergency room or hospital.

No symptoms = No symptoms (wheeze, cough, chest tightness, or shortness of breath) even with normal physical activity.
Mild symptoms = Symptoms during physical activity, but not at rest. It does not keep you from sleeping or being active.
Moderate symptoms = Symptoms while at rest; symptoms may keep you from sleeping or being active.
Serious symptoms = Serious symptoms at rest (wheeze may be absent); symptoms cause problems walking or talking; muscles in neck or between ribs are pulled in when breathing.

Figure 60.3. Asthma symptom and peak flow diary.

not possible, personal respiratory protection or even job reassignment is required to control exposures. Sources of nonspecific respiratory irritants should be avoided. These include unvented gas, kerosene, or wood burning stoves and heaters. In highly sensitive individuals, aerosol sprays and perfumed cosmetics may worsen asthma and should be eliminated.

Drugs that worsen asthma such as aspirin and other NSAIDS and beta-adrenergic blockers should be avoided or should be monitored closely if no alternatives are possible. Many patent medications for upper respiratory infections, sinusitis, gastroenteritis, musculoskeletal pain, or menstrual pain contain aspirin, which can worsen asthma in susceptible individuals, and the use of such drugs should be avoided. Beta-adrenergic blockers may inadvertently be used as eye drops for treatment of glaucoma, with the potential for severe asthma exacerbation.

Although not based on experimental evidence, annual influenza vaccination is recommended for asthmatics of all ages because the infection can precipitate severe and prolonged exacerbations of asthma (67). In some individuals, there is concern that influenza vaccine may worsen asthma, but overall the risk is small (68,69).

Education of the Asthmatic

Education of the patient is an important obligation of the caregiver (70). Excellent materials are available on the Internet from volunteer and government agencies to assist in this process (71–73). The specific aims of the education should be to recognize the signs and symptoms of asthma, to use the peak flow meter correctly, to take medication properly, to establish and follow treatment plans for exacerbations, to avoid and control asthma triggers, and to make appropriate use of urgent medical care. Important specific topics are listed in Table 60.9.

Asthmatic patients need to be instructed in the proper use of *metered-dose inhalers (MDIs)* used to deliver inhaled medications. Patients should be observed using their inhaler during office visits, and proper technique should be repeatedly taught because some studies have shown that 40% of asthmatics do not use their inhalers properly. Proper technique is described in Table 60.10. For patients who cannot perform this maneuver properly despite training and practice, the effectiveness of the MDI can be enhanced by use of a spacer or reservoir device. Some drugs are available in single- or multiple-dose dry powder inhalers or breath-triggered MDIs. These devices are breath activated and are effective for people with poor coordination; however, they require good inspiratory flows to work properly. In the uncommon cases where use of an MDI is not effective, small electrically powered nebulizers can deliver bronchodilators. However, use of nebulizers is limited by their lack of portability, their expense, and the need for meticulous cleaning and preparation of solutions. Rinsing the mouth after inhalation of drugs effectively reduces local oropharyngeal side effects and minimizes systemic absorption.

Table 60.9. Components of Asthma Education

Description of asthma
What asthma medicines do
Community resources for asthma patients and their families
Correct use of metered-dose inhaler and nebulizer
How to use a peak flow meter
How to record an asthma diary
Warning signs of asthma attacks
Asthma trigger control plan
Steps to manage an asthma attack
School, work, and exercise activity plans

Table 60.10. Proper Use of Metered-Dose Inhaler (MDI)

Action	Reason for Action
Shake MDI gently.	Disperses drug evenly with vehicle. Check that canister is full.
Hold the MDI two fingerbreadths from the widely opened mouth.	The larger droplets will rain out in the air rather than impact in the mouth. This prevents mouth and throat irritation with some vehicles and thrush with inhaled corticosteroids.
Breathe normally and pause at quiet end-expiration.	Inhaling from a low lung volume allows greater peripheral penetration of the drug.
Actuate the MDI at the onset of inspiration and slowly inhale over 4–6 s.	Slow inspiratory flow rates enhance deposition of particles in the peripheral airways and reduce turbulence and impaction in the upper airway.
Hold the breath for 5–10 s at total lung capacity.	Small respirable particles will be allowed to settle in the smaller airways during the breath-hold.
Exhale slowly.	Slow expiration reduces exhalation of drug from the lung.

Adapted from Newhouse MT, Dolovitch MB. Control of asthma by aerosols. N Engl J Med 1986;315:870, with permission.

Table 60.11. Self-Management of Acute Exacerbations

Monitor peak flow and symptoms.
Use inhaled beta-adrenergic agonist every 20 min for three doses, then every 3–4 h for 6–12 h as needed.
Contact provider or visit emergency department if there is incomplete response to initial treatment and peak flow is 50%–70% of baseline.
Go to emergency department if poor response to initial therapy or if peak flow is <50% of baseline, or if patient is so breathless that he or she cannot speak in complete sentences.

Each asthmatic should have a well-understood action plan for treatment of exacerbations and should also understand signs of worsening asthma and what action should be taken. Such a plan should be based on the patient's history of severity of exacerbations, access to health care, and reliability. A typical action plan is shown in Table 60.11.

Drug Treatment for Asthma

Drugs should be used in the treatment of asthma in a stepped approach to normalize activity levels and lung function and to minimize exacerbations (Table 60.12). Once control of asthma is achieved, the program can be slowly tapered to maintain the lowest necessary drug dosage. It is important to distinguish between drugs that are used for short-term relief of symptoms and drugs that are used for long-term control of the underlying disease. Failure of the patient to understand this distinction often leads to underuse of anti-inflammatory agents and to overreliance on inhaled short-acting bronchodilators, with consequent failure to meet the goals of asthma care.

Table 60.12. Stepwise Approach to Asthma Care

	Symptoms	Lung Function	Quick Relief Drugs	Long-term Control Drugs
Step 1: Mild intermittent	Symptoms less than twice weekly	FEV_1 or PEFR 80% or greater of predicted	Short-acting inhaled beta-agonists	None needed
	Brief exacerbations		Use of beta-agonist more than twice weekly may indicate need to start control treatment	
	Nocturnal symptoms less than two times per month			
Step 2: Mild persistent	Symptoms more than twice weekly but not daily	FEV_1 or PEFR 80% or greater of predicted	Short-acting inhaled beta-agonists	Low-dose inhaled corticosteroid, or cromolyn, or nedocromil, or sustained-release theophylline
	Limitation of activity during exacerbations		Use of beta-agonist more than once daily may indicate need to increase control treatment	
	Nocturnal symptoms more than two times per month			
Step 3: Moderate persistent	Daily symptoms	FEV_1 or PEFR 60%–80% predicted	Short-acting inhaled beta-agonists	Medium-dose inhaled corticosteroid, or additional controller (e.g., salmeterol, formoterol, theophylline, or leukotriene inhibitor)
	Daily use of short-acting bronchodilator		Use of beta-agonist more than once daily may indicate need to increase control treatment	
	Nocturnal symptoms more than once weekly			
Step 4: Severe persistent	Continual symptoms	FEV_1 or PEFR 60% predicted or less	Short-acting inhaled beta-agonists	High-dose inhaled corticosteroid and long-acting bronchodilator (e.g., salmeterol, formoterol, theophylline, or leukotriene inhibitor) or oral corticosteroid as needed to treat and prevent exacerbations
	Limited physical activity		Use of beta-agonist more than once daily may indicate need to increase control treatment	
	Frequent exacerbations Frequent nocturnal symptoms			

Principles of stepwise care of asthma

Gain control of asthma as quickly as possible, then decrease treatment to the least medication necessary to maintain control.

A short course of oral corticosteroids may be needed at any step to gain control of asthma or treat exacerbations.

Review treatment at 1- to 6-mo intervals for possible stepwise reduction in treatment.

If control is not maintained, review patient inhaler technique, adherence, and control of environmental irritants, allergens, or adverse drug response (e.g., aspirin, beta-blockers).

FEV, one-second forced expiratory volume; PEFR, peak expiratory flow rate.

Adapted from National Heart, Lung, and Blood Institute. Expert Panel Report II: Guidelines for the Diagnosis and Management of Asthma (see General References, Consensus Statements and Guidelines for Management of Asthma and COPD).

Table 60.13. Beta-Sympathomimetic Agonists

Generic Name	Trade Name	β_2 Selectivity	Onset of Action (min)	Inhalation Peak Effect (min)	Duration of Effect (h)	Dosage Form
Metaproterenol	Alupent	$\beta_2 >>> \beta_1$	1–5	30–60	2–5	Metered-dose inhaler, 650 μg/puff Nebulized solution, 5%, or premixed 0.4%–0.6% ampules
Terbutaline	Brethine	$\beta_2 >>> \beta_1$	1–5	—	2–5	Oral tablets 2.5 or 5.0 mg Injection, 1 mg/mL
Pirbaterol	Maxair	$\beta_2 >>> \beta_1$	5	30–60	4–5	Metered-dose inhaler, 200 μg/puff
Albuterol	Proventil Ventolin Volmax Xopenex[a]	$\beta_2 >>>> \beta_1$	5–15	60–90	3–6	Metered-dose inhaler, 90 μg/puff Nebulized solution 0.5% or premixed 0.083% ampules Oral tablets 4.0–8.0 mg
Salmeterol	Serevent	$\beta_2 >>>>> \beta_1$	10–20	180	12	Metered-dose inhaler, 25 μg/puff Dry-powder inhaler, 50 μg/dose
Formoterol	Foradil	$\beta_2 >>>>> \beta_1$	2–10	120	12	Dry-powder inhaler, 12 μg/dose

[a]Isomeric form of albuterol.

Inhaled short-acting selective beta-2-agonists should be prescribed for patients with mild asthma. Use should be confined to the minimum number of inhalations needed to control symptoms. Table 60.13 lists several selective beta-2-agonists available in MDIs. The choice of which beta-2-agonist to use should be made initially on the basis of the symptomatic relief of the patient and on cost because little else distinguishes most of the agents available by prescription in the United States. Nonprescription inhalers should be avoided because many contain epinephrine, which has potentially serious cardiovascular side effects aside from its alpha- and beta-1-adrenergic properties. Because selective beta agonists are so effective in relieving symptoms of bronchospasm, but without treating the underlying airway inflammation, they have the potential for permitting patients to increase exposure to harmful agents and to delay more definitive treatment. There does not seem to be any harmful or beneficial effect of the regular use of short-acting bronchodilators compared with symptomatic use (74). Therefore, it is reasonable to use them only to control symptoms.

Long-acting selective beta agonists may lead to the development of tolerance to their protective effect against nonspecific bronchial challenge, whereas the acute bronchodilating effects of the drugs are unchanged (75). The typical MDI contains 200 to 300 inhalations and therefore should last about 3 to 4 weeks or longer. More frequent use of bronchodilator MDIs usually indicates the need for more intensive anti-inflammatory therapy. In general, however, modern selective beta agonists are safe and effective drugs, and they should not be withheld from the symptomatic asthmatic. The most common side effects are tremor and cardiac arrhythmias. An often neglected side effect of chronic use of beta agonists is hypokalemia (apparently caused by an intracellular shift of potassium), which can be corrected with supplemental potassium (see Chapter 50). Long-acting beta agonists such as salmeterol (Serevent) or formoterol (Foradil) that have a slower onset and longer duration of action are used for long-term control of symptoms but should be avoided for acute relief of symptoms because that may lead to excessive adrenergic stimulation. Therefore, drugs in this class should be prescribed in conjunction with a shorter acting agent to be used for acute relief of symptoms. Monotherapy with a long-acting beta agonist, although effective for treatment of exercise-induced bronchospasm, is not as effective as inhaled corticosteroids for control of persistent symptoms (76–78).

If bronchodilators are used to treat asthma symptoms more than twice weekly (excluding prophylactic use for exercise), an inhaled anti-inflammatory agent should usually be prescribed. *Inhaled nonsteroidal antiallergy drugs* include cromolyn (Intal-2 metered sprays four times a day) and nedocromil (Tilade-2 metered sprays two to four times a day). These agents have few side effects but have limited efficacy for control of asthma. These agents are, however, effective for prevention of exercise-induced bronchospasm. Their use is limited, however, by the lack of availability of the high-concentration preparations that have been shown to be most effective, the recommended frequency of dosing, and the high cost of these drugs. In patients with mild persistent disease, it is an acceptable alternative to prescribe a long-acting bronchodilator, such as inhaled salmeterol or formoterol, or oral long-acting theophylline. In mild persistent asthma, particularly those who exhibit aspirin sensitivity, leukotriene inhibitors and antagonists are effective (79–82). Some patients, however, show little or no response to leukotriene inhibitors, which may reflect genetic polymorphisms of the enzymes that produce leukotrienes (83).

Inhaled corticosteroids are important anti-inflammatory agents and have become the mainstay of treatment for patients with persistent asthma symptoms. They reduce airway inflammation and airway reactivity (84). Most of the side effects are caused by local effects such as oral candidiasis and dysphonia, which can be avoided by use of a spacer/reservoir device or by rinsing the mouth with water after each

Table 60.14. Approximate Comparative Daily Dosages for Inhaled Corticosteroids in Adults

Drug	Low Dose	Medium Dose	High Dose
Beclomethasone	168–504 μg	504–840 μg	>840 μg
40–42 μg/puff	4–12 puffs	12–20 puffs	>20 puffs
80–84 μg/puff	2–6 puffs	6–10 puffs	>10 puffs
Budesonide turbuhaler	200–400 μg	400–600 μg	>600 μg
200 μg/dose	1–2 inhalations	2–3 inhalations	>3 inhalations
Flunisolide	500–1,000 μg	1,000–2,000 μg	>2,000 μg
250 μg/puff	2–4 puffs	4–8 puffs	>8 puffs
Fluticasone	88–264 μg	264–660 μg	>660 μg
44–50 μg/puff	2–6 puffs		
100–110 μg/puff		2–6 puffs	>6 puffs
220–250 μg/puff			>3 puffs
Triamcinolone	400–1,000 μg	1,000–2,000 μg	>2,000 μg
100 μg/puff	4–10 puffs	10–20 puffs	>20 puffs

Adapted from National Heart, Lung, and Blood Institute. Expert Panel Report II: Guidelines for the Diagnosis and Management of Asthma (see General References, Consensus Statements and Guidelines for Management of Asthma and COPD).

use. Although biochemical evidence of chemical adrenal suppression and increased bone metabolism is found with high-dose inhalation (more than 1,200 μg/day) of these agents, clinically noteworthy systemic toxicity is rarely observed. However, reports of increased prevalence of glaucoma in older people receiving large doses of inhaled steroids and transiently decreased growth in children receiving moderate doses of inhaled steroids emphasize the importance of using the smallest effective dose (85,86). Inhaled corticosteroids available in the United States include beclomethasone, budesonide, flunisolide, fluticasone, and triamcinolone. All are approximately equivalent in efficacy and side effects, although some have more convenient dosages and delivery devices. The drug is usually started at a dosage that is adequate to control asthma symptoms and is decreased to the lowest effective dosage (87). The effect of a change in dosage of inhaled corticosteroids may take 3 to 4 weeks to ascertain. Table 60.14 shows the equivalence of available formulations of inhaled corticosteroids.

If inhaled corticosteroids do not control symptoms and optimize lung function, consideration should be given to adding a second long-acting drug, such as an oral or inhaled long-acting beta agonist, a leukotriene inhibitor, or a long-acting oral theophylline preparation, to control asthma (88–92). Long-acting agents are particularly helpful when symptoms occur at night. A long-acting *theophylline* preparation may be given at a dosage of 400 to 1,200 mg/day in one or two daily doses. Theophylline should be started at a low dosage that is increased at weekly or longer intervals with monitoring of symptoms. It is not clear that monitoring of blood levels is necessary in the absence of side effects. Theophylline is a mild bronchodilator and also has a modest anti-inflammatory effect (93,94). Side effects of theophylline include anorexia, nausea, gastroesophageal reflux, anxiety, and palpitations. Serious toxic effects at serum levels above 20 μg/mL include seizures and atrial and ventricular tachyarrhythmias. Because theophylline is metabolized by the liver, there are interactions with numerous other drugs. Erythromycin, ciprofloxacin and other quinolones, and cimetidine decrease theophylline metabolism and elevate serum levels. Cigarette smoking and hyperthyroidism are associated with increased metabolism and decreased theophylline levels. Congestive heart failure and hepatic insufficiency require a reduction in dosage.

An oral long-acting beta agonist, albuterol (2- to 4-mg tablets), may be given twice daily. Maximal doses of oral beta-adrenergic agonists are often limited by tremor and a sensation of nervousness and therefore should be titrated upward starting at one-half to one-fourth the maximum recommended dose. Tolerance to this side effect occurs over several weeks, whereas the bronchodilator action is retained. The availability of *inhaled long-acting beta agonists* such as salmeterol and formoterol has eliminated the use of oral agents except in circumstances where cost, adherence, or patient preference dictate their use.

Antileukotriene drugs, leukotriene receptor antagonists (zafirlukast-Accolate, 20 mg twice a day; montelukast-Singulair 10 mg once daily), and 5-lipoxygenase inhibitors (zileuton-Zyflo, 600 mg four times a day) are useful in some asthmatics (82). Antileukotriene drugs are best reserved for the patient with mild or moderate asthma, for the patient with aspirin sensitivity, for the athlete who suffers from exercise-induced asthma, and for the patient who is unwilling or unable to use adequate doses of inhaled steroids. The leukotriene receptor blockers have the theoretical disadvantage compared with lipoxygenase inhibitors that they do not inhibit all classes of bronchoconstrictor leukotrienes. In practice, however, they appear to be equivalent agents, and the receptor antagonists have the practical advantages that they require less frequent dosing and do not require monitoring of hepatic function to detect the occasional hepatic dysfunction that occurs with zileuton. Rarely, patients treated with leukotriene antagonists develop a syndrome similar to Churg-Strauss vasculitis (95). Some patients do not respond to these agents, and treatment should be abandoned if there is no apparent benefit.

Inhaled anticholinergic drugs (e.g., ipratropium bromide) are safe and effective bronchodilators in asthma, and they add some marginal benefit when added to beta-2-adrenergic agonists, particularly during an acute exacerbation (96).

When these measures are ineffective in controlling asthma or when previously stable asthma is punctuated by an exacerbation, *oral corticosteroids* should be used. These may be prescribed as a 5- to 14-day course starting at 30 to 60 mg/day of prednisone or equivalent prednisolone and either stopping abruptly or tapering gradually. In more severe cases, tapering of the steroids may take several months or require chronic treatment with daily or every other day prednisone. In dosages above 20 mg/day for long periods, serious complications, including diabetes mellitus, posterior subcapsular cataracts, osteoporosis with compression fractures, and hypothalamic–pituitary–adrenal axis suppression, are common. Because of the serious side effects of chronic steroid use, vigorous efforts should be made to optimize adherence with environmental controls and maximum inhalational drug therapy in these patients. Other disorders that mimic asthma should be investigated. If long-term steroids are necessary, tuberculin skin testing should be considered, although the benefit of isoniazid prophylaxis compared with monitoring with chest x-rays in this setting is controversial (97). In those receiving long-term corticosteroid therapy, particularly postmenopausal women, prophylaxis of corticosteroid-induced osteoporosis with vitamin D and calcium supplements or bisphosphonates is recommended (see Chapter 103).

For asthmatic patients who cannot taper steroids, several options may be considered, although none is well established at present. These include methotrexate, cyclosporine, troleandomycin, oral gold salts, hydroxychloroquine, dapsone, inhaled lidocaine, and intravenous immunoglobulin infusions (98–100). Monoclonal antibodies to IgE may be forthcoming, although initial clinical results show marginal benefit (101). If gastroesophageal reflux and associated asthma exacerbations can be documented by esophageal pH probe recording and medical treatment is not helpful, surgical treatment of the reflux should be considered (102) (see Chapter 42). Initiation of these treatments should be undertaken by someone familiar with the treatment of steroid-dependent asthmatics because many such patients will have other diagnoses or can be successfully tapered with consistent comprehensive asthma care.

Emergency Treatment of the Acute Asthma Attack

When asthma fails to respond to home management (Table 60.12), the patient should be instructed to receive emergency treatment in a hospital emergency department or a similarly equipped facility. Both patients and clinicians should understand that untreated severe asthma can be fatal and should recognize the individual at risk (103) (Table 60.15). Treatment should be initiated with nebulized treatments of selective beta-adrenergic agonists given as three treatments in the first 60 to 90 minutes (Table 60.16). MDI administration of four to eight inhalations using a reservoir device is as effective as nebulizer therapy and may be used when a nebulizer is not readily available (104).

Table 60.15. Risk Factors for Fatal Asthma

Risk factor
Previous episode of mechanical ventilation for asthma
Hospitalization for asthma in previous year
Steroid-dependent asthma
Nonadherence to medical treatment
Overuse of inhaled beta-adrenergic agonists
Recent steroid taper or abrupt withdrawal
Lack of objective measures of asthma severity
Psychiatric disorder
Inner-city residence, poverty

Table 60.16. Dosages of Inhaled Beta-Adrenergic Agonists in Acute Asthma Exacerbations in Adults

Drug	Dose (Nebulized in 3–5 mL Sterile Saline Solution)
Albuterol	2.5 mg (0.5 mL of 0.5% solution)
Metaproterenol	15 mg (0.3 mL of 5% solution)
Isoetharine	5 mg (0.5 mL of 1% solution)

Supplemental oxygen should be given to patients who are hypoxemic or to those in whom arterial oxygen saturation is unknown. Because bronchodilators initially can worsen ventilation-perfusion matching, oxygen saturation may fall during the early phases of treatment even as lung function is improving. Peak flow measurement or spirometry should be performed on admission and after each nebulizer treatment to determine response. Arterial blood gases should be checked in patients who appear severely ill to determine whether hypercapnia is present and whether mechanical ventilation might be required. A chest x-ray should be performed in patients in whom the possibility of pneumonia, pulmonary edema, or pneumothorax is suspected. Serum theophylline levels should be measured in patients taking theophylline to guide possible therapy with this drug. Serum electrolytes may reveal hypokalemia from excess beta agonist use.

If the initial treatment is unsuccessful, one should initiate systemic corticosteroids at a dosage of 60 to 125 mg prednisolone intravenously every 6 hours (105). Hourly treatments with nebulized bronchodilators should be continued and the response measured. If there is no response to nebulized bronchodilators over the first 2 to 3 hours, subcutaneous epinephrine 0.2 to 0.4 mg or terbutaline 0.25 mg may be administered (106). In patients with peak flow less than 50% of baseline, intravenous theophylline may be beneficial in improving lung function and preventing hospital admission, starting with an infusion of 0.6 mg/kg lean body weight (107,108). The infusion rate should be 0.3 mg/kg for patients with hepatic disease or for those taking drugs that diminish aminophylline metabolism. In patients not previously taking theophylline, a loading dose of 5 to 6 mg/kg should be given. In those who have been taking theophylline, the dosage should be guided by serum levels, with no more than a 3 mg/kg loading dose. Intravenous fluids should be given for dehydration, but excessive administration of intravenous fluids may worsen the asthma by promoting airway mucosal edema.

After the initial treatment, if the patient shows peak flow or FEV_1 less than 25% of baseline, develops altered sensorium, has an arterial oxygen tension less than 60 mm Hg on supplemental oxygen, or has arterial carbon dioxide tension greater than 40 mm Hg, he or she should be transferred to an intensive care facility for further treatment, monitoring, and possible mechanical ventilation. In some circumstances, noninvasive positive pressure ventilation may prevent the need for intubation (109).

In most circumstances, the response to the first 4 hours of therapy should determine whether the patient needs to be admitted to the hospital. Considerations that favor hospitalization include peak flow less than 40% of baseline, continued severe symptoms, a recent history of failed emergency treatment, a history of respiratory failure, and inadequate home support or access to medications.

Management of the Pregnant Asthmatic

Pregnancy has an unpredictable effect on asthma—about one-third of patients experience no change in symptoms, one-third improve, and one-third get worse. Poorly controlled asthma may pose an increased risk of prematurity, intrauterine growth retardation, and perinatal morbidity. Prolonged or severe asthmatic attacks with hypoxemia or acid-base disturbances pose risks to the fetus, which has borderline oxygenation. Thus, prompt and aggressive management of acute asthmatic episodes should take precedence over concerns that the medications used to manage asthma may pose theoretical risks to the fetus.

In pregnant women, during an acute asthmatic attack initial treatment should include supplemental oxygen to maintain an oxygen saturation of greater than 95% to prevent fetal hypoxemia. Epinephrine should be avoided if possible because of its tendency to reduce placental blood flow. Fetal monitoring should also be instituted in all but mild asthma attacks.

In general, management of pregnant and nonpregnant asthmatics is the same. Control of symptoms should be attempted with minimal use of medications, but no special attempt to discontinue medications is indicated.

Beta-2-adrenergic agents and theophylline are smooth muscle relaxants and may therefore inhibit uterine contractions during labor. They have been used for decades and are generally safe for the fetus. Epinephrine causes vasoconstriction because of its alpha-adrenergic properties and may diminish placental and fetal blood flow. The most commonly used systemic corticosteroids, prednisone and prednisolone, cross the placenta poorly, so steroid production by the fetus is unaffected. Adrenal steroid suppression in the mother, however, may require administration of supplemental corticosteroids during the stresses of labor and delivery. Long-term use of oral steroids in other conditions has been associated with lower birth weight infants, so it is prudent to maximize inhaled forms of therapy before instituting long-term oral steroids. The benefits of inhaled steroids and cromolyn outweigh any potential risk to the pregnant asthmatic or her fetus. As a general rule, it is prudent to rely on drugs that have a long record of safe experience in pregnant asthmatics (see General References, Management of Asthma During Pregnancy).

Course and Prognosis

Asthma that begins at an early age generally improves, and rates of prolonged remission have been reported from 30% to 70%. The severity of asthma correlates with the remission rate, so children with mild disease are likely to remit, whereas those with severe disease often continue to be symptomatic. Some childhood asthmatics experience a remission but then have a recurrence of asthma in adulthood. Such patients tend to develop disease that is persistent and severe.

Patients who first develop asthma as adults have more rapid decline of lung function with aging, which may lead to irreversible airway obstruction (110). Additional risk factors such as cigarette smoking, environmental exposures, and infection may influence the progression of asthma to COPD (see below).

Death from asthma or one of its complications is uncommon, with overall death rates in the United States of about 1.5 per 100,000 population. Considering disease prevalence (approximately 12 to 17 million asthmatics in the United States), this is a low mortality rate. However, asthma mortality increased 31% between 1980 and 1990, with the greatest burden of death sustained by inner-city African-American males. Since 1988, the U.S. death rate from asthma has tended to stabilize or decrease in association with the wider use of inhaled corticosteroids (1). Similar trends have been documented in other countries as well (111).

CHRONIC OBSTRUCTIVE PULMONARY DISEASE

Definition

Many attempts to define COPD have been made, leading to some confusion about terminology. The American Thoracic Society definition follows: Chronic obstructive pulmonary disease (COPD) is a disorder characterized by abnormal tests of expiratory flow that do not change markedly over periods of several months' observation. The qualification is intended to distinguish COPD from asthma. The airflow obstruction may be structural or functional. Specific causes of airflow obstruction such as localized disease of the upper airways, bronchiectasis, and cystic fibrosis are excluded. Bronchial hyperreactivity may be present with COPD as measured by an improvement in airflow following the inhalation of beta-adrenergic agents or worsening after inhalation of methacholine or histamine (112). COPD may further be subclassified into emphysema and chronic bronchitis.

Emphysema is defined by morphologic criteria as abnormal dilation of the terminal airspaces of the lung with destruction of alveolar septa in the absence of interstitial fibrosis (113). Whereas a formal diagnosis of emphysema requires gross anatomic inspection of the lung, a clinical diagnosis can be reasonably based on a compatible history, physical examination, pulmonary function tests, and radiographic studies. *Panacinar emphysema* is a condition in which all of the airspaces in an acinus are equally dilated. Typically, the bases of the lung are more involved than the apices. This is the usual finding in alpha-1-antitrypsin deficiency and in some elderly nonsmoking individuals. *Centroacinar emphysema* describes the condition in which the respiratory bronchiole at the proximal end of the acinus is more dilated than other portions of the acinus. Commonly, the apices of the lung are more involved in this disorder, which occurs predominantly in cigarette smokers. Peripheral airways disease is commonly associated with centroacinar emphysema, manifested by inflammation, fibrosis, and tortuosity of the terminal and respiratory bronchioles. The physiologic abnormality is the consequence of both the emphysema and the small airway narrowing and fibrosis.

Chronic bronchitis is a condition of chronic cough and sputum production that excludes other specific disorders such as bronchiectasis, tuberculosis, or cystic fibrosis. The formal epidemiologic definition of this disorder is the presence of cough and sputum production for the majority of days of the week for at least 3 months of the year for at least 2 years in a row. However, nearly everyone with chronic bronchitis has cough and sputum production on a perennial basis. Chronic bronchitis is common in cigarette smokers and is often incorrectly perceived by the patient to be a normal smoker's cough. The morbid anatomy of chronic bronchitis shows hyperplasia and hypertrophy of the mucous glands of the large central airways with central mucous plugging, variable degrees of smooth muscle hyperplasia, and airway wall thickening and inflammation (114,115). Chronic bronchitis can occur in the absence of major physiologic abnormalities, and the extent that it contributes to mortality and morbidity in COPD is controversial. In patients with advanced COPD, mortality is best predicted by the postbronchodilator FEV_1, with little additional information provided by other clinical factors (116). Some epidemiologic studies of people with less severe disease have shown some excess mortality associated with a productive cough, but the magnitude is not large (117). Approximately 30% of those with abnormal lung function report a productive cough, and the magnitude of the physiologic abnormality is worse in those who report more severe cough and sputum production. COPD patients with chronic cough and phlegm are more prone to exacerbations of COPD than those without. Some smokers with chronic bronchitis can develop severe airflow limitation without emphysema. These individuals are best classified as having *chronic obstructive bronchitis* or, when there is prominent reversible airflow obstruction, *chronic asthmatic bronchitis*.

Natural History

COPD is a chronic disease that has its origins in early adulthood, or possibly even childhood, but does not produce symptoms or impairment of activity until it is far advanced, usually in late middle age or in the elderly. The normal aging process causes slowly progressive degeneration of lung function after young adulthood, so a normal person loses approximately 20% of vital capacity and approximately 25% of FEV_1 between the ages of 25 and 75. The average decline in FEV_1 is about 30 mL/yr, with some acceleration after the age of 65. These changes are the result of loss of elastic recoil in the lung from the degradation of elastin fibers, similar to the changes that occur in the skin that cause wrinkles. In most cigarette smokers, the rate of decline of FEV_1 is normal or only moderately increased. In susceptible smokers, however, there is an accelerated degeneration of lung function, 80 to 150 mL/yr loss of FEV_1 (118,119). Over the course of several decades, this leads to progressive breathlessness and, if unchecked, to disability, respiratory failure, and death. It has been suggested that children who have serious respiratory ailments or exposure to respiratory toxins such as passive cigarette smoke will be at increased risk for development of COPD because of impaired lung function as young adults and consequently less reserve capacity (Fig. 60.4).

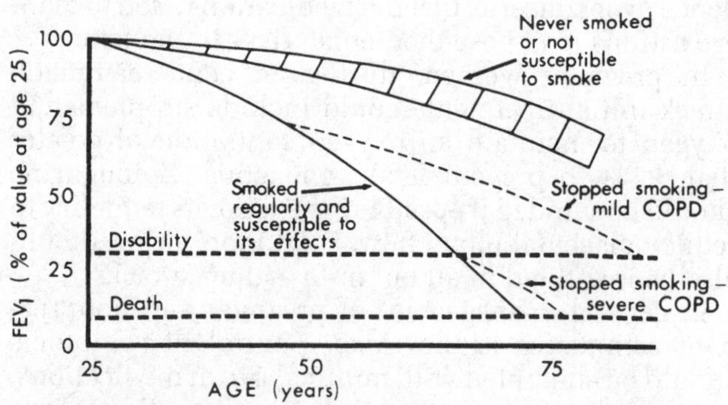

Figure 60.4. Effect of risk factors from smoking on the loss of lung function (forced expiratory volume in 1 second [FEV_1]). The *upper curves* are derived from subjects who do not smoke or are not susceptible to the effects of smoking. They lose lung function gradually throughout adult life (15–30 mL/yr). *Lower curves* show accelerated loss of lung function in subjects who are susceptible to the effects of cigarette smoke. At age 65 there is respiratory disability because FEV_1 has decreased to 25% to 30% of predicted (1–1.2 L), and further functional deterioration will eventually cause death because of complications of respiratory insufficiency. If that subject stops smoking, life may be prolonged but a respiratory death may still eventually result. If intervention is initiated earlier in life (40–50 yr) when there is mild chronic obstructive pulmonary disease, accelerated loss of lung function is reversible and a respiratory death may be avoided. Although this figure illustrates theoretical loss of FEV_1 for an adult cigarette smoker, susceptible smokers will lose lung function at different rates, thereby becoming disabled at different ages. (Modified from Fletcher C, Peto R. The natural history of chronic airflow obstruction. BMJ 1977;1:1645, with permission.)

Because of the reserve capacity of the lungs, the early stages of COPD do not cause any limitation of activity. When the FEV_1 reaches approximately 50% of predicted, there is ventilatory limitation of exercise capacity, but this is often ignored or attributed to deconditioning; heavy exercise is progressively curtailed. Respiratory infections may cause severe and prolonged symptoms in this phase of the disease, prompting the patient to seek medical care. When the FEV_1 reaches approximately 30% to 35% of predicted (about 1.2 L in a man and 1.0 L in a woman), symptoms prevent normal execution of daily living and work activities, and about half of the afflicted individuals stop working. With continued decline in the FEV_1, chronic hypoxemia, hypercapnia, and cor pulmonale develop. Viral infections, mucous plugging, or respiratory irritants—including exposure to air pollutants—can precipitate episodes of acute respiratory failure, leading to hospitalization, mechanical ventilation, or death. More than half of the patients with COPD compatible with emphysema die within 10 years after initial diagnosis, whereas approximately 15% of those with chronic asthmatic bronchitis die in the first decade after diagnosis (120). The prognosis for the COPD patients has not improved over the last 35 years.

Cigarette smoking is a major risk factor for development of COPD. Both observational studies and clinical trials have shown that cessation of smoking earlier in the course of disease can slow the rate of degeneration of lung function to the normal or near-normal range (121,122).

Pathogenesis

It is impossible to predict which individuals are susceptible to COPD. However, several risk factors have been identified that increase an individual's risk for developing COPD (123,124) (Table 60.17). Among these risk factors, *cigarette smoking* is the most prominent and potentially the most amenable to change. The mechanism by which cigarette smoking leads to COPD is thought to be mediated by pro-inflammatory components of cigarette smoke such as the hydrocarbon compound *acrolein*. Fourfold to fivefold increases in the numbers of activated neutrophils are present in the terminal air spaces and the peribronchial regions in smokers. These cells produce elastase that can destroy the elastin elements in the alveolar walls and induces emphysema in animal models. Normally, the small amount of neutrophil elastase is inactivated by antiproteases present in serum and lung liquid lining layer, alpha-1-antitrypsin being present in the largest quantities.

Table 60.17. Risk Factors for Developing COPD

Established risk factors
Cigarette smoking
Age
Male sex
Reduced lung function
Accelerated decline in lung function
Occupational dust exposure
Alpha-1-antitrypsin deficiency (Pi-ZZ phenotype)
Probable and possible risk factors
Air pollution
Childhood respiratory infections
Allergic diathesis
Airways reactivity
Low socioeconomic status
Poor nutrition
ABO blood type
ABH nonsecretor status
Family members with COPD

COPD, chronic obstructive pulmonary disease.

Adapted from Burrows B. Airways obstructive diseases: pathogenetic mechanisms and natural histories of the disorders. Med Clin North Am 1990;74:547; and from Higgins M. Risk factors associated with chronic obstructive lung disease. Ann NY Acad Sci 1991;624:7, with permission.

There is increasing evidence that proteases secreted by alveolar macrophages and alveolar lining cells, including the cathepsins and matrix metalloproteinases play a pathobiologic role in development of emphysema (125–128). These enzymes degrade a range of matrix proteins and inactivate the antiproteases that protect the lung from enzymatic destruction. Animals exposed to high levels of cigarette smoke are protected from emphysema if they are genetically unable to produce matrix metalloelastase. Animals that overexpress matrix metallocollagenase are highly susceptible to development of emphysema, and this enzyme has been found in increased quantities in smokers who develop emphysema (129). Thus, although we are not certain which enzymes are critical to the development of pulmonary emphysema, it seems likely that the balance between free protease activity within the alveolus and alveolar duct and local antiprotease activity determines the rate of destruction of the lung parenchyma. Mechanical factors may also play a role, because emphysema patients who undergo lung volume reduction surgery have accelerated decline in pulmonary function after the surgery, which causes increased stress on the lung parenchyma.

Alpha-1-antitrypsin deficiency is an uncommon genetic disorder (found in about 1 in 2,500 whites of European descent) in which the circulating levels of antiproteases are less than 10% of normal. Normal alpha-1-antitrypsin activity is produced by the allele Pi-M (protease inhibitor M), for which approximately 90% of the population are homozygous. Pi-S is an allele with intermediate antiprotease activity, and Pi-Z is an allele with marked reduction in antiprotease activity. More than 75 minor alleles of the Pi gene have been identified, although most are rare and are uncommonly associated with disease. Individuals who are homozygous for the Pi-Z phenotype are at the greatest risk for developing premature emphysema. Such individuals account for approximately 1% to 2% of cases of emphysema. The Pi-Z phenotype is the result of a single DNA base substitution causing an amino acid substitution that prevents secretion of the material from liver cells (130). Serum levels are less than 15% of normal, despite hepatic intracellular accumulation of the enzyme inhibitor. In addition, the Pi-Z inhibitor has a slower reaction rate in neutralizing proteases, so what is secreted is less effective. Most studies have shown little increased risk for emphysema in people with intermediate levels of alpha-1-antitrypsin—the Pi-MS, Pi-MZ, and Pi-SZ phenotypes—suggesting a threshold level of antiprotease activity for development of premature emphysema in deficient patients. Although affected people present for medical care with severe emphysema in the third and fourth decades, many people with alpha-1-antitrypsin deficiency have normal or only mildly abnormal lung function if they do not smoke (131).

Other *genetic factors* may play a role in susceptibility to COPD, but they are poorly understood at present. Recent evidence has linked polymorphisms of epoxide hydrolase, involved in detoxification of oxidative species, and tumor necrosis factor-alpha with susceptibility to COPD (132–134).

Occupational exposure to a number of mineral and organic dusts has been implicated in the development of COPD (135). In most of these circumstances, however, the offending agents are additive or synergistic with the effects of cigarette smoking, and it is rare to find occupationally related symptomatic COPD in the absence of cigarette smoking. The mechanism is presumed to be the result of nonspecific irritation or activation of alveolar macrophages, enhancing lower respiratory inflammation. Although far-advanced silicosis and asbestosis may be associated with airflow obstruction, the predominant lesion in these disorders is fibrosis with localized compensatory emphysema and honeycombing, leading to restrictive ventilatory defects. Occupational exposure to sensitizing agents found in grain, wood, cotton dust, and polyurethane compounds not only may cause asthma but may also lead to fixed airflow obstruction with chronic asthmatic bronchitis if the exposure is prolonged.

Nonspecific airway reactivity occurs in approximately 70% of people with COPD, even those with mild abnormalities and minimal symptoms, and is more common in women than in men (136). However, the interpretation of this finding is controversial. One school of thought, the so-called Dutch hypothesis, holds that this is a constitutional state that predisposes the individual to develop accelerated degeneration of pulmonary function when exposed to cigarette smoke or to other environmental agents (137). The alternative viewpoint is that airways reactivity is a marker for inflammatory or geometric changes that have already occurred and therefore is the result of the disease process, not the cause.

The magnitude of airway reactivity correlates with the rate of decline of lung function (138,139) and with markers of inflammation. Whereas inflammatory mediators or airway wall thickening may contribute to increased tendency for airways to narrow, it is also possible that destruction of alveolar septal attachments and thickening of airway walls, which are the result of smoking-induced inflammation and early emphysema, lead to the increased tendency of the airways to constrict (140). This hypothesis is supported by the finding that airway reactivity is inversely correlated with baseline lung function in smokers (13), does not disappear with smoking cessation, and is induced in animals with emphysema caused by proteolytic enzymes (141).

Abnormal lung function, particularly the FEV_1/FVC ratio during early adulthood, is a predictor of accelerated degeneration in lung function, a phenomenon known as *the horse-race effect* (142). People with lower lung function have already experienced some increased decline in lung function. Even individuals within the normal range of lung function who show lower spirometric indices have increased mortality from lung disease and other causes.

Aging is normally associated with changes in lung function, including reduction in vital capacity and FEV_1 and increases in residual volume and functional residual capacity. Physiologically, all these changes can be attributed to a reduction in the elastic recoil of the lung that accompanies the aging process. The mechanism for these changes is unknown but is presumed to be the cumulative effect of endogenous and exogenous factors that degrade the elastin in the lung and the balance of processes that repair or prevent this damage. Emphysema of the panacinar type, which is similar to that occurring with alpha-1-antitrypsin deficiency, is found in some elderly nonsmoking individuals, particularly women. Development of emphysema in smokers may reflect either the additive effects of toxic exposure that accelerate the normal aging of the lung or interference with the processes that inhibit such degeneration. Most of the increased mortality from COPD over the last two decades has been confined to individuals over the age of 65, raising the possibility that the disease is being unmasked as mortality from heart disease, stroke, and infectious diseases is declining (143).

COPD is more common among the poor and poorly educated. Although cigarette smoking is more common in lower socioeconomic groups, the indigent have worse lung function even when adjusted for smoking status. Race is not thought to be a component; some evidence suggests that African Americans are less susceptible to COPD than whites (144). Factors that may contribute include crowded living conditions with exposure to frequent viral respiratory infections, indoor air pollutants from heating or cooking devices in poorly ventilated homes, poor nutrition, exposure to passive cigarette smoke, inadequate access to medical care for childhood respiratory infections, or increased exposure to respiratory irritants and toxins in the workplace (see Chapter 8). Although COPD mortality rates are highest in white men, women and African Americans have shown disproportionate increases in COPD mortality over the past decade, likely reflecting changing smoking patterns over the past 30 years (143).

The evidence that high levels of *air pollution* are important in the genesis of COPD is suggestive but not definitive (145). In animal models, high levels of NO_2 and ozone can induce emphysema independently and can potentiate protease-induced emphysema, suggesting that oxidant air pollutants inhibit lung protective mechanisms. There is more convincing evidence that acid aerosols, ozone, and fine particulates contribute to COPD exacerbations, hospitalizations, and death (146–150).

Whereas allergic tendencies are strongly associated with the presence of asthma and symptoms of cough and wheeze in nonsmokers, the effect of atopy on respiratory symptoms and on decline in lung function in smokers is less clear. In part, this may be because of the tendency of adolescents and young adults with highly reactive airways to avoid cigarette smoking. Some evidence suggests that allergies or nonspecific elevation of serum IgE levels contribute to the development of fixed airway obstruction in smokers (138).

Evaluation of the Patient With Chronic Obstructive Pulmonary Disease

History

COPD must be considered a diagnostic possibility in all individuals who smoke, even in the absence of respiratory symptoms. The caregiver should inquire about smoking habits in every patient encounter. Specific questioning about the age at onset, average number of packs per day, and number and duration of quit attempts should be elicited. Often, patients report being nonsmokers to the caregiver when they have only recently quit smoking. Other respiratory symptoms such as cough, phlegm, and exertional dyspnea should be quantified. Morning sputum production is often erroneously considered to be normal by smokers. Shortness of breath can be detected by asking whether the individual has trouble keeping up with peers doing routine activities such as walking, sports, or work activities. More advanced dyspnea is roughly quantified by distance walked or flights of stairs walked before stopping. Sleep disturbances are a common and often overlooked symptom of COPD and may impair quality of life more than exertional dyspnea.

Physical Examination

Although historical and physical findings of COPD may confirm the diagnosis when they are present, they are usually apparent with advanced disease (see below for spirometric guidelines). The absence of these findings is not sensitive enough to exclude the diagnosis in the person at risk (Table 60.18) (151,152).

In advanced COPD, general physical findings include those caused by hyperinflation: increase in resting chest anteroposterior diameter, elevation of the clavicles, widening of the xiphocostal angle, and increase in the intercostal spaces. The distance between the larynx and the sternal notch is reduced to less than 4 cm (152). With inspiration there is diminished movement of the ribcage and increased movement of the abdominal wall. The patient has hypertrophied and well-defined abdominal and sternomastoid muscles but diminished muscle mass in the thighs and legs. The characteristic seated posture is leaning forward with both hands on the knees to fix the shoulders, permitting more effective use of the accessory cervical

Table 60.18. Sensitivity and Specificity of History and Physical Findings for Diagnosis of Moderate COPD

Historical Items			
Historical Finding	Cutoff	Sensitivity (%)	Specificity (%)
Age	≥75 yr	13	99
Previous diagnosis of COPD	Yes vs. no	80	74
Smoking history	≥70 pack-yr	40	95
Dyspnea severity (5-point scale)	≥4	60	75
Phlegm	2 oz or more in a.m. when present	20	95
Theophylline use	Yes vs. no	60	71
Steroid use	Yes vs. no	40	87
Inhaler use	Yes vs. no	27	94
Home oxygen	Yes vs. no	20	96
Physical Examination Items			
Physical Finding	Cutoff	Sensitivity (%)	Specificity (%)
Initial impression[a]	Yes vs. no	25	95
Diaphragm excursion	<2 cm TLC vs. RV	12	98
Chest percussion	Increased resonance	32	94
Cardiac dullness	Decreased area	16	99
Blow out a match	≤10 cm	53	88
Wheeze	Yes vs. no	9	100
Reduced breath sounds	Yes vs. no	65	96
Forced expiratory time	>10 sec	12	99
Cardiac point of maximum impulse	Abdominal	27	98
Final overall opinion	Yes vs. no	51	93

[a]Based on general inspection.

COPD, chronic obstructive pulmonary disease; TLC, total lung capacity; RV, residual volume.

Adapted from Badgett RG, Tanaka DJ, Hunt DK, et al. Can moderate chronic obstructive pulmonary disease be diagnosed by historical and physical findings alone? Am J Med 1993;94:188, with permission.

muscles. This may lead to hyperkeratosis of the anterior thighs. Pursed-lip breathing and prolonged time of expiration are spontaneously adopted to diminish the energy expenditure of breathing. The fingers often show tobacco staining. Clubbing of the nails is rare and suggests the presence of bronchiectasis or bronchogenic carcinoma. Chest percussion shows increased resonance and low diaphragms that move poorly with full inspiration and expiration. Auscultation shows diminished transmission of breath sounds over areas of emphysema and is the most reliable physical finding indicative of chronic airflow limitation. Early inspiratory crackles indicate opening of closed airways and are common in COPD, whereas late and pan-inspiratory crackles are more common with interstitial lung diseases (153). Wheezing may be elicited in most COPD patients by forced expiration, but the presence of wheezing during quiet breathing is more common with reversible bronchospasm.

In far-advanced disease with *cor pulmonale,* elevated right atrial pressures cause neck vein distension, peripheral edema, and hepatomegaly. The pulmonary hypertension and distension of the right ventricle cause a pronounced cardiac impulse in the epigastrium and along the left sternal border. Tricuspid regurgitation from dilation of the right ventricle and pulmonary hypertension causes a systolic murmur over the epigastrium and along the left sternal border that increases with inspiration. In contrast to other forms of pulmonary hypertension, a ventricular heave and increased intensity of the second heart sound are not usually appreciated because of the interposed emphysematous lung.

Additional Studies

The ability to blow out a paper match from more than 10 cm away with an open mouth is a rudimentary lung function test that is helpful when abnormal, but it is not sensitive. Another simple bedside lung function test is to measure the forced expiratory time with a stethoscope over the trachea during a FVC maneuver. However, it is not sensitive enough in practice to screen for airflow limitation (154).

The *chest x-ray* is abnormal only in advanced disease and so is not a good diagnostic screening test. Signs of COPD include hyperinflation with flattening of the diaphragm, increased retrosternal airspace on the lateral view, narrow cardiac silhouette, paucity and tapering of peripheral blood vessels, and bullae (155). In some smokers with COPD, particularly those with bronchitis symptoms, there may be small rounded opacities or increased linear markings that represent thickened airway walls.

High-resolution computed tomography of the chest is becoming the standard for evaluation of emphysema in the absence of an anatomic diagnosis (156). In practice, however, this study is rarely necessary because less expensive tests of lung function—spirometry and the diffusing capacity—are usually adequate to distinguish asthma from emphysema and to follow the course of the disease and the response to treatment.

Spirometry (see above) should be performed initially for diagnosis and assessment of severity. It is not clear whether spirometry should be performed for COPD screening in asymptomatic smokers, because the sole effective means of halting disease progression, smoking cessation, should be universally promoted regardless of lung function. After initial diagnosis of COPD, however, spirometry should be repeated to monitor progression of the disease and response to treatment, particularly when there is a change in the patient's health status (157). As a general rule, FEV_1 measurements greater than 80% predicted indicate mild obstruction, 30% to 80% predicted indicate moderate obstruction, and less than 30% predicted indicate severe obstruction. Peak flow monitoring, useful in asthma, may be misleading in COPD, because the peak flow can be well maintained despite worsening disease.

Sensitive tests, such as the *single-breath nitrogen washout test,* measure the function of the small airways. Such tests are abnormal in most smokers and do not predict who will develop symptomatic COPD. Therefore, they are not routinely recommended. In smokers, forced expiratory spirometry is effective in screening for COPD. With serial measures of spirometry, it is possible to identify individuals who are demonstrating accelerated declines in lung function before symptoms intervene. Of spirometric indices, a FEV_1/FVC ratio below 70% predicts future decline in lung function (142).

Bronchodilator testing can reveal reversible bronchospasm, and the postbronchodilator measure of FEV_1 is the best overall predictor of life expectancy in COPD. Failure to respond rapidly to a single dose of an inhaled bronchodilator does not indicate that lung function will not improve with more long-term treatment. About one in five patients who does not demonstrate a rapid bronchodilator response will show improvement in lung function after several weeks of treatment with bronchodilators or corticosteroids (158). Abnormal methacholine reactivity is common in COPD but does not usually provide sufficient information to warrant its routine use.

The *carbon monoxide diffusing capacity test* (see above) is helpful in distinguishing emphysema from asthma. Cigarette smokers without emphysema have mild reductions in diffusing capacity because of the accumulation of carbon monoxide in the blood, which is only partially reversible with smoking cessation. A diffusing capacity below 70% of the predicted value is present with emphysema but may also be found with interstitial fibrosis and pulmonary vascular diseases. In chronic asthmatic bronchitis, the diffusing capacity tends to be preserved (159).

Measurements of lung volume (see above) help distinguish obstructive lung diseases from restrictive lung diseases. They are particularly helpful during the initial assessment or when it is unclear whether an interstitial process is present such as that caused by occupational exposure to silica or asbestos. Measurements of airway resistance and lung compliance are often abnormal in COPD but do not add useful clinical information in most circumstances.

Exercise testing is indicated in individuals who demonstrate reduction in diffusing capacity below 50% to 60% of predicted and who are not hypoxemic at rest, if supplemental oxygen is being considered for improving exercise capacity. Exercise testing should be performed in a monitored facility. Measurement of oxygen saturation with a pulse oximeter usually suffices to determine whether oxygen should be prescribed. More complex and invasive exercise testing with measurement of arterial blood gas tensions, oxygen consumption, and ventilation are used for evaluation for disability (see Chapter 9) or if the cause for dyspnea is unclear.

Hypoxemia occurs in COPD as a consequence of ventilation-perfusion mismatching. In those with advanced disease, particularly obese individuals, hypoventilation and hypercapnia also promote hypoxemia. With exercise, particularly at higher altitude, hypoxemia can worsen because of impairment of diffusion of oxygen across the alveolar-capillary membrane. Measurement of arterial oxygen saturation should be done for patients who have moderately advanced disease, with FEV_1 below about 1.5 L, because this group is at risk to have chronic hypoxemia and to develop cor pulmonale. At higher altitudes, hypoxemia develops with less severe pulmonary involvement, and oxygen tensions should be measured more liberally. When the FEV_1 falls below 1.0 L, chronic hypercapnia becomes more common, often in the patients with the least dyspnea.

Other blood tests are indicated only as needed for the general care of the patient. An elevated hematocrit value is uncommon in COPD in comparison with similar levels of hypoxemia at altitude, but when it does occur, it should alert the clinician to the possible presence of chronic hypoxemia (160). Hypokalemia and hypomagnesemia are common as a consequence of beta-adrenergic agonists in conjunction with diuretics and, if severe, may contribute to respiratory muscle failure (161).

Screening evaluation for *severe alpha-1-antitrypsin deficiency* can be done with serum protein electrophoresis to see if there is a marked decrease in the alpha-1-globulin level. Genotyping or measurements of protease inhibitor levels are more specific and can detect intermediate deficiencies. Screening should be reserved for situations when there is a family history suggesting alpha-1-antitrypsin deficiency or when the patient has severe COPD at a relatively young age.

Cystic fibrosis may present in adulthood with chronic cough and phlegm associated with chronic airflow limitation. It should be suspected if there is radiographic evidence of bronchiectasis, a family history of cystic fibrosis or severe chronic childhood lung disease, if the patient has ABPA (p. 815), or if sputum cultures persistently grow mucoid colonies of *Pseudomonas*. Elevations of chloride in sweat iontophoresis samples confirm the diagnosis, but genetic testing is now widely available to test for polymorphisms of the *CFTR* gene.

The *electrocardiogram* in COPD shows a vertical or indeterminate heart axis and low voltage. Enlarged P waves, right axis deviation, or right ventricular hypertrophy is present with cor pulmonale. Echocardiography can confirm right ventricular dilation and tricuspid valve insufficiency. *Doppler studies* of tricuspid retrograde flow can be used to estimate pulmonary artery pressures, but these may be inaccurate with severe lung hyperinflation. Transesophageal echocardiography (see Chapter 65) gives better views, but the more invasive nature of the procedure limits its application. In most circumstances echocardiography should be reserved for patients in whom there is a question of associated left ventricular dysfunction or of valve disease.

Sputum examination by Gram stain or wet preparation during exacerbations can help determine whether there is a predominance of neutrophils or eosinophils, guiding the choice between corticosteroids and antibiotics. The presence of green phlegm, a marker for neutrophil myeloperoxidase, is a sensitive finding for the presence of a high bacterial load in sputum (162). Culture of the sputum is unnecessary unless pneumonia is present or unusual or resistant organisms are suspected. The role of lower respiratory tract bacterial infections in causing COPD exacerbations is unclear, but common pathogens such *as Streptococcus pneumoniae*, *Haemophilus influenzae*, or *Moraxella (Branhamella) catarrhalis* can be found in the lower airways in about half of COPD flares (163).

Management

The components of care in COPD consist of education about the disease, prevention of disease progression, treatment of complications, drug treatment to maximize lung function, and rehabilitation to optimize activity levels.

Education is important so that the patient can develop an understanding of what COPD is, how it is caused, and what possible courses the disorder may take. The patient should be given realistic expectations about the long-term progressive but variable course of the disease, tempered by the understanding that temporary worsening symptoms are preventable and treatable. The patient should try to achieve maximum social and physical functioning and to make use of whatever family, social, and medical support is available. Simple measures such as the availability of special parking areas for the disabled, wheelchairs and motorized carts in shopping malls and airports, portable oxygen, and oxygen supplementation during air travel are not always known by patients with advanced COPD, who may unnecessarily confine themselves to home and become socially isolated. Local volunteer health associations commonly sponsor groups in which these issues are discussed, and they often provide instructional materials via the internet (American Lung Association http://www.lungusa.org,

National Heart Lung and Blood Institute http://www.nhlbi.nih.gov/health/public/lung/index.htm). Patients and their families should understand that the dyspnea that occurs with exertion is not harmful to the lung and that with appropriate pacing of activities, a certain level of dyspnea is actually desirable to achieve and maintain physical conditioning. Inquiries about sexual functioning should not be avoided. Education of the patient's bed partner about proper techniques and the use of prophylactic bronchodilators and oxygen can establish more normal sexual functioning, even with severe disease. Advance directives regarding intensive or long-term medical care should be discussed with patients and their families, and the clinician should encourage this communication. Both clinician and patient should understand that episodes of acute respiratory failure in COPD that require mechanical ventilation are often successfully treated, but that the long-term survival is poor, although unpredictable, in those who have incapacitating dyspnea, cor pulmonale, or poor nutrition (164–166).

Prevention of disease progression and complications is one of the most important goals of treatment. By the time most patients present with advanced disease, they have discontinued smoking, although a sizable minority have not. Many with mild or moderate disease continue to smoke, unaware of their illness and the potential for arresting its progression by smoking cessation. The practical approaches to smoking cessation are discussed in Chapter 27. In the patient with lung disease, the clinician should deliver a strong personalized smoking cessation message that emphasizes the definite and progressive nature of the disease, the likelihood of early disability with continued smoking, and the potential for arresting the disease when smoking is stopped. Referral to a smoking group program and use of bupropion and nicotine replacement therapy improve smoking cessation rates.

Exposure to respiratory irritants should be avoided in the workplace and the home, and if the disease is complicated by allergy or overlaps with allergic asthma, environmental control measures should be instituted. Smoking of marijuana and cocaine may cause airway irritation, and although there is little evidence that they contribute to airway reactivity or to development of COPD, their use should be discouraged.

Pneumococcal vaccination (see Chapter 18) is recommended, although the evidence of its particular efficacy in COPD is lacking (167,168). *Influenza vaccination annually* (see Chapter 18) or amantadine/rimantadine prophylaxis for unimmunized individuals during an influenza epidemic can prevent or attenuate this potentially fatal infection. During influenza epidemics, the use of neuraminidase inhibitors such as zanamivir and oseltamivir can minimize the severity of infection if taken within 48 hours of onset of the illness (169,170).

Patients with alpha-1-antitrypsin deficiency are candidates for intravenous replacement therapy with protease inhibitors, although the long-term benefits of this treatment are somewhat disappointing, particularly in those with mild impairment and those with severe impairment (171–173).

Treatment of Complications

Tracheobronchial infections are common in COPD, heralded by a change in the quantity, viscosity, or color of sputum. Although many infections are initiated by viruses, bacterial contamination or superinfection of the lower respiratory tract is common. Broad-spectrum and inexpensive antibiotics such as tetracycline, erythromycin, amoxicillin, or trimethoprim- sulfamethoxazole can shorten the duration of these symptoms if there are symptoms suggestive of infection (174). When the patient is intolerant of first-line antibiotics or when there is a evidence of resistant organisms, cephalosporin, amoxicillin-clavulanate, macrolide, or quinolone antibiotics should be prescribed (175). Antibiotics generally should be given only in exacerbations where there is the triad of cough, dyspnea, and change in sputum color or quantity. The oral route of administration is preferred if tolerated by the patient.

Chronic hypoxemia causes pulmonary hypertension and cor pulmonale, a condition associated with poor survival if untreated. Oxygen therapy prolongs survival and improves physical and psychologic functioning in hypoxemic patients with COPD (176,177). When indicated (Table 60.19), oxygen can be administered with a nasal cannula. Oxygen concentrators, compressed oxygen tanks, and liquid oxygen storage reservoirs are all suitable for home use (178). Portable liquid oxygen systems and small compressed oxygen tanks with reservoir devices or demand valves allow mobility out of the home and should be used whenever possible. Oxygen should be prescribed at the lowest level necessary to maintain an arterial oxygen saturation at or above 90%, usually 1 to 4 L/min. Supplemental oxygen must be used for at least 18 h/day to have a significant impact on survival. The patient should understand that oxygen is used to prevent cardiac complications and not just to relieve dyspnea. Transtracheal oxygen catheters are used for the occasional patient who requires high oxygen concentrations or who cannot tolerate a nasal cannula (179).

If desaturation occurs with exercise, increased flows of oxygen during activity can improve exercise tolerance and enhance the ability to engage in an exercise conditioning program. *Nocturnal hypoxemia* in COPD is common and often unsuspected. The need to screen for nocturnal oxygen desaturation and the benefit of treatment in terms of survival is not known.

Table 60.19. Indications for Continuous Oxygen Therapy

Arterial oxygen tension $\leq$ 55 mm Hg or sat $O_2 \leq$ 88% while in usual state of health
Arterial oxygen tension $\leq$ 60 mm Hg or sat $O_2 \leq$ 89% with evidence of chronic hypoxemia such as erythrocytosis, ankle edema, venous engorgement, electrocardiographic p-pulmonale, or psychologic impairment

Preliminary evidence suggests that nocturnal oxygen prevents progression of pulmonary hypertension in COPD patients with nocturnal desaturation (180–182). Nonetheless, it is prudent to test for nocturnal hypoxemia (in a sleep center or a hospital) in individuals who have erythrocytosis, unexplained peripheral edema without waking abnormalities of blood gases, or daytime hypersomnolence.

When *pulmonary hypertension* and *cor pulmonale* are present, treatment consists of continuous oxygen to overcome hypoxemia and diuretics to control peripheral edema. Digitalis is not useful unless there is concomitant left ventricular disease or atrial tachyarrhythmias. Calcium channel blockers can vasodilate the pulmonary circulation, but they often worsen hypoxemia and their benefit is not established. Almitrine, a respiratory stimulant not available in the United States, improves arterial oxygen tension through improved ventilation-perfusion matching but does not reduce pulmonary artery pressure (183,184). Phlebotomy increases exercise capacity when the hematocrit exceeds 55%, but persistent erythrocytosis suggests inadequate oxygen supplementation or another cause (185).

Supraventricular tachyarrhythmias are common in patients with COPD, as a consequence of right atrial enlargement, increased endogenous adrenergic tone, hypoxemia, and drug treatment, particularly theophylline. Treatment is similar to that in patients who do not have pulmonary disease (see Chapter 64). However, the presence of COPD should not prevent evaluation for treatable causes of arrhythmias such as pulmonary embolism, hyperthyroidism, or valvular heart disease, which may be more difficult to diagnose in these patients.

Control of *mucus hypersecretion* with the use of expectorants and with physical means such as high frequency chest wall oscillation is not of proven benefit in improving lung function, although symptoms are sometimes improved (186).

Hypercapnia may actually be an adaptive response to obstructive lung disease by decreasing the work of breathing, preventing respiratory muscle fatigue, and allowing a diminished sensation of dyspnea. Respiratory stimulants may therefore be detrimental over long periods. Bronchospasm (see below), obesity (see Chapter 83), and sleep apnea (see Chapter 7) are reversible conditions that can contribute to hypercapnia and therefore should be treated. Narcotics and sedatives with potential for respiratory depression should be avoided.

Malnutrition is present in 50% of patients with advanced COPD, usually when the FEV_1 is less than 35% of predicted. This is the consequence of increased metabolic demands, insufficient caloric intake, and possibly elaboration of cachexia-producing cytokines such as tumor necrosis factor-alpha. Body weight less than 90% of ideal is associated with increased mortality and decreased exercise capacity in patients with otherwise similar lung function (187). Although clinical trials of nutritional supplementation have been disappointing, it is prudent to monitor body weight in COPD patients and prescribe caloric supplementation as needed because those patients who do gain weight show improved survival (188).

Drug Therapy to Maximize Functional Status

Bronchodilators and anti-inflammatory agents are used in COPD to reverse bronchospasm and to prevent bronchoconstriction in response to provocative agents. Small amounts of bronchoconstriction and air trapping can cause marked deterioration in symptoms, and conversely, small amounts of bronchodilation can cause considerable improvement in functional capacity. Inhaled corticosteroids do not alter the progression of COPD but do tend to reduce exacerbations. They should be reserved for patients who have an asthmatic component to their disease or those who have frequent exacerbations (189–192).

Stepped drug treatment should use the minimum number of agents and the least frequent dosing schedule possible, starting with the agents having the greatest benefit and least toxicity. The recommended stepped treatment approach is to initiate treatment with anticholinergic bronchodilators or a short-acting beta-adrenergic agent. If both are required, a combination inhaler of ipratropium and albuterol is available (Combivent). Long-acting agents such as inhaled salmeterol or oral theophylline can be added to the initial therapy. In individuals who have frequent exacerbations, inhaled corticosteroids or a combination inhaler of inhaled corticosteroids and long-acting bronchodilator may be added (157). Chronic use of systemic corticosteroids should be reserved for individuals with very frequent or life-threatening exacerbations who cannot tolerate their discontinuation. Response to treatment is judged by symptomatic improvement and by spirometry.

Ipratropium bromide (Atrovent) is an inhaled anticholinergic drug that causes 4 to 8 hours of bronchodilation through inhibition of vagal stimulation of the airways. It appears to be particularly effective in patients with chronic asthmatic bronchitis and does not lead to tolerance. Although it is usually more expensive than beta agonists, it is the usual choice for first-line therapy. The dosage is started at two MDI inhalations three times daily and can be increased to six inhalations four times daily. Systemic side effects are uncommon, even with relatively high doses (193). Local side effects include mouth irritation and cough, which can be diminished by good inhaler technique or by use of a spacer. Although ipratropium provides sustained benefit in patients with moderate disease, it does not inhibit progression of the disease if smoking is continued (121). Tiotropium (Spiriva), not yet approved in the United States, is a promising anticholinergic bronchodilator which has the benefit of once-daily dosing (194,195).

Beta-adrenergic agonists are used at dosages comparable with those used in asthma (see above). Although there is concern that self-medication with these agents is overused in asthmatics, the dosages used in COPD are often less than are needed to achieve adequate bronchodilation (196). The dosages of inhaled selective beta agonists should be increased before oral agents are prescribed so that tremor and hypokalemia are minimized. Long-acting inhaled beta agonists such as salmeterol (Serevent) or formoterol (Foradil) are useful because of the long duration of action and documented benefit on quality of life (197,198). Combination inhaler therapy with a beta agonist and an anticholinergic provides better bronchodilation than either agent alone and the simplified treatment regimen may aid compliance (199,200). Spacer devices, breath-actuated MDIs, and dry-powder inhalers of beta-adrenergic agonists are useful for those who cannot coordinate the use of conventional MDIs (see above).

Theophylline is best taken in a long-acting preparation once or twice daily. Although it is possible to monitor blood levels, there is only a rough correlation between side effects and serum levels. If typical side effects such as nausea, vomiting, tremor, or tachyarrhythmias occur, the dose should be adjusted irrespective of serum levels. The use of theophylline in COPD has diminished in recent years because of the availability of long-acting inhaled agents, but it is still an effective and inexpensive second-line drug (201). As with asthma, this drug is most useful for the prevention of nocturnal symptoms. Although the bronchodilating effects of theophylline are moderate compared with inhaled drugs, it has other pharmacologic actions that improve the well-being of the COPD patient, including improvement in diaphragm function, prevention of respiratory muscle fatigue, increased ventilatory drive, potentiation of catecholamine function, prevention of microvascular permeability, increased mucociliary clearance, prevention of late-phase antigen responses, inhibition of mast cell histamine release, and suppression of leukocyte activation (202). Clinical trials showing improvement in functional status beyond that gained from the effects of bronchodilation are consistent with improvement in respiratory muscle function (203,204). New drugs that are more specific inhibitors of phosphodiesterase-4 have not yet been approved in the United States but hold the promise of similar efficacy with less toxicity.

Oral corticosteroids are effective for treatment of COPD exacerbations (205,206). Among chronic symptomatic patients, some 10% to 20% show substantial short-term improvement, defined as 25% or greater increase in FEV_1. In general, the patients studied have had far-advanced disease and have not differed from other COPD patients except in their steroid response (207). Some have suggested that long-term low-dose oral steroids may slow the progression of the disease, but the evidence is not strong in comparison to the well-defined side effects of such treatment. Most patients with COPD who are on chronic corticosteroids can safely taper the dose at the equivalent of 5 mg of prednisone per week and exclusively reserve their use for exacerbations (208).

Inhaled corticosteroids have a limited role in the treatment of COPD. It is now established that inhaled corticosteroids do not alter the progression of COPD in those who continue to smoke. They may be useful in patients who have an overlap between asthma and COPD or who have frequent exacerbations. Inhaled corticosteroids can reduce the frequency of exacerbations and improve airways reactivity (189,191). Although often recommended, it is difficult to determine if an individual patient will respond to inhaled steroids based on a trial of oral corticosteroids.

Treatment of Chronic Obstructive Pulmonary Disease Exacerbations

COPD exacerbations (209,210) are characterized by worsening dyspnea, cough, and increased sputum production. On average, patients with COPD have three exacerbations per year, but there is wide variation. Only half of these come to the attention of caregivers. Precipitating events include respiratory and nonrespiratory infections, exposure to respiratory irritants and air pollution, or comorbid conditions such as heart failure, pulmonary embolism, myocardial ischemia, or pneumothorax. The management of these exacerbations depends on their severity. Patients with severe acute onset of dyspnea; evidence of hypoxemia such as mental confusion, cyanosis, or desaturation; new onset of chest pain, edema, or arrhythmias; and those with important comorbidities or inadequate social support should be referred for hospitalization. Arterial blood gas studies and chest radiographs are useful for evaluating the etiology and severity of acutely ill patients, but spirometry adds little to the clinical decision-making process. Increasing the frequency and intensity of inhaled short-acting bronchodilators for several days is effective in most cases. A hand-held inhaler and spacer is usually adequate, but a nebulizer may be needed for those who cannot coordinate well. Patients who have increasing dyspnea accompanied by a change in the quantity or color of phlegm should be prescribed an antibiotic. A brief course of corticosteroids, equivalent to 30 to 40 mg of prednisone for 7 to 14 days, will shorten the duration of symptoms.

Pulmonary Rehabilitation

Lacking the capacity to restore damaged lung parenchyma, efforts should be made to optimize activity levels through rehabilitation programs. The content of such programs varies widely but includes some or all of the following elements: education about COPD and its treatment, nutritional counseling, psychological support, pacing and energy conservation training for daily activities, aerobic exercise conditioning, and upper extremity strength training. Generally, these programs have demonstrated improved exercise endurance and sense of well-being without changes in lung function. The benefit of some components of these programs are better documented than others (211). If a coordinated rehabilitation program is not accessible, many of these elements can be provided individually to ambulatory patients. For example, a regular daily walk for 15 to 30 minutes at a pace that induces mild to moderate dyspnea can be safely prescribed for most patients with COPD. Instructional materials and support groups for patients and families are widely available through volunteer agencies and the internet.

Surgery

Surgical resection of bullae is rarely indicated for treatment of COPD. An individual with a single large bulla that occupies more than one-third of the hemithorax with preserved carbon monoxide diffusing capacity is likely to do best after bullectomy (212). Unilateral or bilateral lung transplantation is indicated in some patients with advanced emphysema, usually in individuals below age 60 when the FEV_1 is below 25% predicted or if severe pulmonary hypertension is present (213). The goal of lung transplantation is to improve quality of life, but it is not clear that survival is improved (214,215). Lung transplantation is limited by availability of donor organs and accessibility to transplant centers. Lung volume reduction surgery is a promising procedure, where lung tissue is removed surgically, leads to increased elasticity of the remaining lung and may improve the contour and function of the diaphragm. The operative mortality from the procedure ranges from 4% to 10%; the duration of benefit is about 2 to 4 years in those who survive (216,217). Selection criteria for this operation are not well defined; however, the benefits are greatest in those with the most severe emphysema in the upper regions of the lung. Until controlled studies are available to define patient selection and efficacy, lung volume reduction surgery should be approached as a procedure with limited application (218). The perioperative management of patients with COPD is discussed in Chapter 93.

Prognosis (See Also Natural History, Above)

In general, the prognosis of patients with chronic airways obstruction can be estimated from the FEV_1. One study showed that in moderate obstruction, when FEV_1 was greater than 1.25 L, the 5-year survival of patients was only slightly decreased from that of matched controls. If FEV_1 was between 0.75 and 1.25 L, 5-year survival decreased to approximately 66% of expected, and if less than 0.75 L, to 33% of expected (120). Cardiac disease, resting tachycardia, hypercapnia, and hypoxemia pose additional risks to survival, whereas a significant response to bronchodilator therapy (greater than 10% improvement in FEV_1) is associated with improved survival. Serial tests of lung function help identify patients with excessive rates of decline.

General References*

Asthma

Barnes PJ, ed. Asthma. 2nd ed. Philadelphia: Lippincott-Raven, 1997.
A comprehensive treatise on asthma.

Busse WW, Holgate ST. Asthma and rhinitis. 2nd ed. Malden, MA: Blackwell Science, 2000.
An authoritative text on asthma pathophysiology and the scientific basis of treatment.

Busse WW, Lemanske RF, Jr. Advances in immunology: asthma. N Engl J Med 2001;344:350.

Szefler SJ, Leung DYM, eds. Severe asthma: pathogenesis and clinical management. Vol. 86 in series Lung biology in health and disease, edited by Claude Lenfant. New York: Marcel Dekker, 1996.
Excellent reference for treatment of steroid-dependent asthma. Good treatment of drug adherence issues.

Chronic Obstructive Pulmonary Disease

Barnes PJ. Chronic obstructive pulmonary disease. N Engl J Med 2000;343:269.
An excellent review of pathobiology of COPD.

Cherniack NS, ed. Chronic obstructive pulmonary disease. Philadelphia: W.B. Saunders, 1991.
A multiauthored text with authoritative reviews of all aspects of chronic obstructive pulmonary disease.

Ferguson GT. **Recommendations for the management of COPD.** Chest 2000;117:23S.
A summary and comparison of treatment guidelines for COPD.

Senior RM, Anthonisen NR. Chronic obstructive pulmonary disease (COPD) Am J Respir Crit Care Med 1998;157:139S.
Brief authoritative review of clinical and pathobiological aspects of COPD.

Consensus Statements and Guidelines for Management of Asthma and COPD

Agency for Healthcare Research and Quality. **A clinical practice guideline for treating tobacco use and dependence: a US Public Health Service report.** JAMA 2000;283:3244.

American College of Obstetricians and Gynecologists (ACOG) and The American College of Allergy, Asthma and Immunology (ACAAI). The use of newer asthma and allergy medications during pregnancy. Ann Allergy Asthma Immunol 2000;84:475.

American Thoracic Society. **Standards for the diagnosis and care of patients with chronic obstructive pulmonary disease.** Am J Respir Crit Care Med 1995;152:S77.

American Thoracic Society. Pulmonary rehabilitation—1999. Am J Respir Crit Care Med 1999;159:1666.

Bach PB, Brown C, Gelfand SE, et al. **Management of acute exacerbations of chronic obstructive pulmonary disease: a summary and appraisal of published evidence.** Ann Intern Med 2001;134:600.

COPD Guidelines Group of the Standards of Care Committee of the British Thoracic Society. **BTS guidelines for the management of chronic obstructive pulmonary disease.** Thorax 1997;52:S1.

Joint Task Force on Practice Parameters. **Practice parameters for the diagnosis and treatment of asthma.** Joint Task Force on Practice Parameters, representing the American Academy of Allergy Asthma and Immunology, the American College of Allergy, Asthma and Immunology, and the Joint Council of Allergy, Asthma and Immunology. J Allergy Clin Immunol 1995;96(5 Pt 2):707 (1998 update at http://www.jcaai.org/Param/Asthma.htm).

National Asthma Education and Prevention Program Expert Panel Report II. **Guidelines for the diagnosis and management of asthma.** HHS publication 97-451. Bethesda, MD: The National Heart, Lung and Blood Institute, 1997, 1999. (http://www.nhlbi.nih.gov/guidelines/asthma/asthgdln.htm).

National Asthma Education and Prevention Program Working Group. **Considerations for Diagnosing and Managing Asthma in the Elderly.** NIH publication 96-3662. Bethesda MD: The National Heart, Lung and Blood Institute, 1996. (http://www.nhlbi.nih.gov/guidelines/asthma/asthgdln.htm).

National Asthma Education Program Working Group. **Management of asthma during pregnancy.** NIH publication 93-3279A. Bethesda, MD: The National Heart, Lung and Blood Institute, 1992. (http://www.nhlbi.nih.gov/guidelines/asthma/asthgdln.htm).

Pauwels RA, Buist AS, Calverley PM, et al. **Global strategy for the diagnosis, management, and prevention of chronic obstructive pulmonary disease.** NHLBI/WHO Global Initiative for Chronic Obstructive Lung Disease (GOLD) Workshop summary. Am J Respir Crit Care Med 2001;163:1256.

Siafakas NM, Vermeire P, Pride NB, et al. Optimal assessment and management of chronic obstructive pulmonary disease (COPD).

*Bold print (general references) and bold numerals (specific references) denote published controlled clinical trials, meta-analyses, or consensus-based recommendations.

The European Respiratory Society Task Force. Eur Respir J 1995;8:1398.

Snow V, Lascher S, Mottur-Pilson C. **Evidence base for management of acute exacerbations of chronic obstructive pulmonary disease.** Ann Intern Med 2001;134:595.

Specific References

1. Sly RM. Decreases in asthma mortality in the United States. Ann Allergy Asthma Immunol 2000;85:121.
2. National Heart, Lung, and Blood Institute. Morbidity & Mortality 2000: chartbook on cardiovascular, lung, and blood diseases. Bethesda, MD: U.S. Department of Health and Human Services, Public Health Service, National Institutes of Health, 2000. Available from URL: http://www.nhlbi.nih.gov/resources/docs/00chtbk.pdf.
3. American Lung Association. Available from URL: http://www.lungusa.org/data/.
4. American Thoracic Society. Standardization of Spirometry, 1994 Update. Am J Respir Crit Care Med 1995;152:1107.
5. Ferguson GT, Enright PL, Buist AS, et al. Office spirometry for lung health assessment in adults: a consensus statement from the National Lung Health Education Program. Chest 2000;117:1146.
6. American Thoracic Society. Lung function testing: selection of reference values and interpretative strategies. Am Rev Respir Dis 1991;144:1202.
7. Hyatt RE, Black LF. The flow-volume curve: a current perspective. Am Rev Respir Dis 1973;107:191.
8. Morrison, NJ, Abboud, RT, Ramadan, F, et al. Comparison of single breath carbon monoxide diffusing capacity and pressure-volume curves in detecting emphysema. Am Rev Respir Dis 1989;139:1179.
9. Gelb AF, Schein M, Kuei J, et al. Limited contribution of emphysema in advanced chronic obstructive pulmonary disease. Am Rev Respir Dis 1993;147:1157.
10. Owens GR, Rogers RM, Pennock BE, et al. The diffusing capacity as a predictor of arterial oxygen desaturation during exercise in patients with chronic obstructive pulmonary disease. N Engl J Med 1984;310:1218.
11. Busse WW, Lemanske RF. Advances in immunology: asthma. N Engl J Med 2001;344:350.
12. Burrows B, Martinez FD, Halonen M, et al. Association of asthma with serum IgE levels and skin-test reactivity to allergens. N Engl J Med 1989;320:271.
13. Tashkin DP, Altose MD, Bleecker ER, et al. The lung health study: airway responsiveness to inhaled methacholine in smokers with mild to moderate airflow limitation. Am Rev Respir Dis 1992;145:301.
14. American Thoracic Society. Guidelines for methacholine and exercise challenge testing—1999. Am J Respir Crit Care Med 2000;161:309.
15. O'Byrne PM. Leukotriene bronchoconstriction induced by allergen and exercise. Am J Respir Crit Care Med 2000;161:S68.
16. Gilbert IA, McFadden ER Jr. Airway cooling and rewarming. The second reaction sequence in exercise-induced asthma. J Clin Invest 1992;90:699.
17. Bousquet J, Jeffery PK, Busse WW, et al. Asthma: from bronchoconstriction to airways inflammation and remodeling Am J Respir Crit Care Med 2000;161:1720.
18. Barnes PJ. Inhaled glucocorticoids for asthma. N Engl J Med 1995;332:868.
19. CAMP Research Group. Long-term effects of budesonide or nedocromil in children with asthma. The Childhood Asthma Management Program Research Group. N Engl J Med 2000;343:1054.
20. McFadden ER Jr. Exertional dyspnea and cough as preludes to acute attacks of bronchial asthma. N Engl J Med 1975;292:555.
21. Molfino NA, Nannini LJ, Martelli AN, et al. Respiratory arrest in near-fatal asthma. N Engl J Med 1991;324:285.
22. McFadden ER Jr, Lyons HA. Arterial blood gas tensions in asthma. N Engl J Med 1968;278:1027.
23. McFadden ER Jr, Kiser R, DeGroot WJ. Acute bronchial asthma: relations between clinical and physiologic manifestations. N Engl J Med 1973;288:221.
24. Eggleston PA, Arruda LK. Ecology and elimination of cockroaches and allergens in the home. J Allergy Clin Immunol 2001;107[3 Suppl]:S422.
25. Weiss ST, Horner A, Shapiro G, et al. The prevalence of environmental exposure to perceived asthma triggers in children with mild-to-moderate asthma: data from the Childhood Asthma Management Program (CAMP). J Allergy Clin Immunol 2001;107:634.
26. Creticos PS, Reed CE, Norman PS, et al. Ragweed immunotherapy in adult asthma. N Engl J Med 1996;334:501.
27. Adkinson NF Jr, Eggleston PA, Eney D, et al. A controlled trial of immunotherapy for asthma in allergic children. N Engl J Med 1997;336:324.
28. Sporik R, Holgate ST, Platts-Mills TA, et al. Exposure to house-dust mite allergen (Der p I) and the development of asthma in childhood. A prospective study. N Engl J Med 1990;323:502.
29. Venables KM, Chan-Yeung M. Occupational asthma. Lancet 1997;349:1465.
30. Alberts WM, do Pico GA. Reactive airways dysfunction syndrome. Chest 1996;109:1618.
31. Szczeklik A. Aspirin-induced asthma: pathogenesis and clinical presentation. Allergy Proc 1992;13:163.
32. Stevenson DD, Simon RA. Lack of cross-reactivity between rofecoxib and aspirin in aspirin-sensitive patients with asthma. J Allergy Clin Immunol 2001;108:47.
33. Irwin RS, Madison JM. The diagnosis and treatment of cough. N Engl J Med 2000;343:1715.
34. Johnson D, Osborn LM. Cough variant asthma: a review of the clinical literature. J Asthma 1991;28:85.
35. Kauffman HF, Tomee JF, van der Werf TS, et al. Review of fungus-induced asthmatic reactions. Am J Respir Crit Care Med 1995;151:2109.
36. Wark P, Wilson AW, Gibson PG. Azoles for allergic bronchopulmonary aspergillosis (Cochrane review). Cochrane Database Syst Rev 2000;3:CD001108.
37. Stevens DA, Schwartz HJ, Lee JY, et al. A randomized trial of itraconazole in allergic bronchopulmonary aspergillosis. N Engl J Med 2000;342:756.
38. Luskin AT. Recalcitrant asthma: an allergist's approach. Allergy Proc 1990;11:281.
39. Rand CS, Mellins RB, Malveaux F, et al. The role of patient adherence in fatal asthma. In: Sheffer A, ed. Fatal asthma. New York: Marcel Dekker, 1998:429.
40. McFadden ER Jr, Warren EL. Observations on asthma mortality. Ann Intern Med 1997;127:142.
41. Byrd RP Jr, Krishnaswamy G, Roy TM. Difficult-to-manage asthma. How to pinpoint the exacerbating factors. Postgrad Med 2000;108:37.
42. Newman KB, Mason UG 3rd, Schmaling KB. Clinical features of vocal cord dysfunction. Am J Respir Crit Care Med 1995;152:1382.
43. Mahler DA, Harver A, Lentine T, et al. Descriptors of breathlessness in cardiorespiratory diseases. Am J Respir Crit Care Med 1996;154:1357.
44. Govindaraj M. What is the cause of dyspnea in asthma and emphysema? Ann Allergy 1987;59:63.
45. Sporik R, Squillace SP, Ingram JM, et al. Mite, cat, and cockroach exposure, allergen sensitization, and asthma in children: a case-control study of three schools. Thorax 1999;54:675.
46. Fabbri LM, Picotti G, Mapp CE. Late asthmatic reactions, airway inflammation and chronic asthma in TDI sensitized subjects. Eur Respir J 1991;13:136s.
47. Shah A, Sircar M. Postcoital asthma and rhinitis. Chest 1991;100:1039.
48. Holden TE, Sherline DM. Bestiality, with sensitization and anaphylactic reaction. Obstet Gynecol 1973;42:138.
49. Muller BA. Sinusitis and its relationship to asthma. Can treating one airway disease ameliorate another? Postgrad Med 2000;108:55.
50. Gibson PG, Henry RL, Coughlan JL. Gastro-oesophageal reflux treatment for asthma in adults and children. Cochrane Database Syst Rev 2000;2:CD001496.

51. Alexander JA, Hunt LW, Patel AM. Prevalence, pathophysiology, and treatment of patients with asthma and gastroesophageal reflux disease. Mayo Clin Proc 2000;75:1055.
52. Virchow C, Szczeklik A, Bianco S, et al. Intolerance to tartrazine in aspirin-induced asthma: results of a multicenter study. Respiration 1988;53:20.
53. Woessner KM, Simon RA, Stevenson DD. Monosodium glutamate sensitivity in asthma. J Allergy Clin Immunol 1999; 104:305.
54. Koenig JQ. Air pollution and asthma. J Allergy Clin Immunol 1999;104:717.
55. Friedman MS, Powell KE, Hutwagner L, et al. Impact of changes in transportation and commuting behaviors during the 1996 Summer Olympic Games in Atlanta on air quality and childhood asthma. JAMA 2001;285:897.
56. Abbey DE, Petersen F, Mills PK, et al. Long-term ambient concentrations of total suspended particulates, ozone, and sulfur dioxide and respiratory symptoms in a nonsmoking population. Arch Environ Health 1992;48:33.
57. Rand CS, Wise RA. Adherence with asthma therapy in the management of asthma. In: Szefler SJ, Leung DYM, eds. Lung biology in health and disease. Vol. 86. Severe asthma: pathogenesis and clinical management. New York: Marcel Dekker, 1995:435.
58. Shim C, Williams MH Jr. Pulsus paradoxus in asthma. Lancet 1973;1:530.
59. McFadden ER Jr, Kiser R, DeGroot WJ. Acute bronchial asthma: relations between clinical and physiologic manifestations. N Engl J Med 1973;288:221.
60. Epstein RL. Constituents of sputum; a simple method. Ann Intern Med 1972;77:259.
61. Wenzel SE, Szefler SJ, Leung DY, et al. Bronchoscopic evaluation of severe asthma. Persistent inflammation associated with high dose glucocorticoids. Am J Respir Crit Care Med 1997;156:737.
62. de Benedictis FM, Bush A. Rhinosinusitis and asthma: epiphenomenon or causal association? Chest 1999;115:550.
63. de Blay F, Chapman MD, Platts-Mills TA, et al. Airborne cat allergen (Fel d I). Environmental control with the cat in situ. Am Rev Respir Dis 1991;143:1334.
64. Gergen PJ, Mortimer KM, Eggleston PA, et al. Results of the National Cooperative Inner-City Asthma Study (NCICAS) environmental intervention to reduce cockroach allergen exposure in inner-city homes. J Allergy Clin Immunol 1999;103:501.
65. Phipatanakul W, Eggleston PA, Wright EC, et al. Mouse allergen. I. The prevalence of mouse allergen in inner-city homes. The National Cooperative Inner-City Asthma Study. J Allergy Clin Immunol 2000;106:1070.
66. Wood RA, Johnson EF, Van Natta ML, et al. A placebo-controlled trial of a HEPA air cleaner in the treatment of cat allergy. Am J Respir Crit Care Med 1998;158:115.
67. Cates CJ, Jefferson TO, Bara AI, et al. Vaccines for preventing influenza in people with asthma (Cochrane review). Cochrane Database Syst Rev 2000;4:CD000364.
68. Nicholson KG, Nguyen-Van-Tam JS, Ahmed AH, et al. Randomised placebo-controlled crossover trial on effect of inactivated influenza vaccine on pulmonary function in asthma. Lancet 1998;351:326.
69. Kramarz P, Destefano F, Gargiullo PM, et al. Does influenza vaccination prevent asthma exacerbations in children? J Pediatr 2001;138:306.
70. Liu C, Feekery C. Can asthma education improve clinical outcomes? An evaluation of a pediatric asthma education program. J Asthma 2001;38:269.
71. See URL: http://www.nhlbi.nih.gov/health/index.htm.
72. See URL: http://www.lungusa.org/asthma/.
73. See URL: http://www.vh.org/Providers/ClinGuide/AsthmaIM/Default.html.
74. Drazen JM, Israel E, Boushey HA, et al. Comparison of regularly scheduled with as-needed use of albuterol in mild asthma. N Engl J Med 1996;335:841.
75. Cheung D, Timmers MC, Zwinderman AH, et al. Long-term effects of a long-acting beta 2-adrenoceptor agonist, salmeterol, on airway hyperresponsiveness in patients with mild asthma. N Engl J Med 1992;327:1198.
76. Simons FE, the Canadian Beclomethasone Dipropionate-Salmeterol Xinafoate Study Group. A comparison of beclomethasone, salmeterol, and placebo in children with asthma. N Engl J Med 1997;337:1659.
77. Lemanske Jr RF, Sorkness CA, Mauger EA, et al. Inhaled corticosteroid reduction and elimination in patients with persistent asthma receiving salmeterol—a randomized controlled trial. JAMA 2001;285:2594.
78. Lazarus SC, Boushey HA, Fahy JV, et al. Long-acting $\beta 2$-agonist monotherapy vs continued therapy with inhaled corticosteroids in patients with persistent asthma: a randomized controlled trial. JAMA 2001;285:2583.
79. Edelman JM, Turpin JA, Bronsky EA, et al. Oral montelukast compared with inhaled salmeterol to prevent exercise-induced bronchoconstriction. A randomized, double-blind trial. Ann Intern Med 2000;132:97.
80. Malmstrom K, Rodriguez-Gomez G, Guerra J, et al. Oral montelukast, inhaled beclomethasone, and placebo for chronic asthma. A randomized, controlled trial. Montelukast/Beclomethasone Study Group. Ann Intern Med 1999;130:487.
81. Leff JA, Busse WW, Pearlman D, et al. Montelukast, a leukotriene-receptor antagonist, for the treatment of mild asthma and exercise-induced bronchoconstriction. N Engl J Med 1998;339:147.
82. Drazen JM, Israel E, O'Byrne PM. Drug therapy: treatment of asthma with drugs modifying the leukotriene pathway. N Engl J Med 1999;340:197.
83. Silverman ES, Drazen JM. Genetic variations in the 5-lipoxygenase core promoter. description and functional implications. Am J Respir Crit Care Med 2000;161:77S.
84. Juniper EF, Kline PA, Vanzieleghem MA, et al. Effect of long-term treatment with an inhaled corticosteroid (budesonide) on airway hyperresponsiveness and clinical asthma in nonsteroid-dependent asthmatics. Am Rev Respir Dis 1990;142:832.
85. Lipworth BJ. Systemic adverse effects of inhaled corticosteroid therapy: a systematic review and meta-analysis. Arch Intern Med 1999;159:941.
86. Childhood Asthma Management Program (CAMP) Research Group. Long-term effects of budesonide or nedocromil in children with asthma. N Engl J Med 2000;343:1054.
87. Barnes PJ. Inhaled glucocorticoids for asthma. N Engl J Med 1995;332:868.
88. Evans DJ, Taylor DA, Zetterstrom O, et al. A comparison of low-dose inhaled budesonide plus theophylline and high-dose inhaled budesonide for moderate asthma. N Engl J Med 1997;337:1412.
89. Greening AP, Ind PW, Northfield M, et al. Added salmeterol versus higher-dose corticosteroid in asthma patients with symptoms on existing inhaled corticosteroid. Allen & Hanburys Limited UK Study Group. Lancet 1994;344:219.
90. Laviolette M, Malmstrom K, Lu S, et al. Montelukast added to inhaled beclomethasone in treatment of asthma. Montelukast/Beclomethasone Additivity Group. Am J Respir Crit Care Med 1999;160:1862.
91. Lofdahl CG, Reiss TF, Leff JA, et al. Randomised, placebo controlled trial of effect of a leukotriene receptor antagonist, montelukast, on tapering inhaled corticosteroids in asthmatic patients. BMJ 1999;319:87.
92. Pauwels RA, Lofdahl CG, Postma DS, et al. for the Formoterol and Corticosteroids Establishing Therapy (FACET) International Study Group. Effect of inhaled formoterol and budesonide on exacerbations of asthma. N Engl J Med 1997;337:1405.
93. Kidney J, Dominguez M, Taylor PM, et al. Immunomodulation by theophylline in asthma. Demonstration by withdrawal of therapy. Am J Respir Crit Care Med 1995;151:1907.
94. Weinberger M, Hendeles L. Theophylline in asthma. N Engl J Med 1996;334:1380.
95. Wechsler ME, Garpestad E, Flier SR, et al. Pulmonary infiltrates, eosinophilia, and cardiomyopathy following corticosteroid withdrawal in patients with asthma receiving zafirlukast. JAMA 1998;279:455.
96. Stoodley RG, Aaron SD, Dales RE. The role of ipratropium bromide in the emergency management of acute asthma

exacerbation: a meta-analysis of randomized clinical trials. Ann Emerg Med 1999;34:8.
97. Schatz M, Patterson R, Kloner R, et al. The prevalence of tuberculosis and positive tuberculin skin tests in a steroid-treated asthmatic population. Ann Intern Med 1976;84:261.
98. Dykewicz MS. Newer and alternative non-steroidal treatments for asthmatic inflammation. Allergy Asthma Proc 2001;22:11.
99. Davies H, Olson L, Gibson P. Methotrexate as a steroid sparing agent for asthma in adults. Cochrane Database Syst Rev 2000;2:CD000391.
100. Aaron SD, Dales RE, Pham B. Management of steroid-dependent asthma with methotrexate: a meta-analysis of randomized clinical trials. Respir Med 1998;92:1059.
101. Milgrom H, Fick RB Jr, Su JQ, et al. Treatment of allergic asthma with monoclonal anti-IgE antibody. N Engl J Med 1999;341:1966.
102. Larrain A, Carrasco E, Galleguillos F, et al. Medical and surgical treatment of nonallergic asthma associated with gastroesophageal reflux. Chest 1991;99:1330.
103. Strunk RC. Identification of the fatality-prone subject with asthma. J Allergy Clin Immunol 1989;83:477.
104. Idris AH, McDermott MF, Raucci JC, et al. Emergency department treatment of severe asthma. Metered-dose inhaler plus holding chamber is equivalent in effectiveness to nebulizer. Chest 1993;103:665.
105. Littenberg B, Gluck EH. A controlled trial of methylprednisolone in the emergency treatment of acute asthma. N Engl J Med 1986;314:150.
106. Appel D, Karpel JP, Sherman M. Epinephrine improves expiratory flow rates in patients with asthma who do not respond to inhaled metaproterenol sulfate. J Allergy Clin Immunol 1989;84:90.
107. Wrenn K, Slovis CM, Murphy F, et al. Aminophylline therapy for acute bronchospastic disease in the emergency room. Ann Intern Med 1991;115:241.
108. Rossing TH, Fanta CH, Goldstein DH, et al. Emergency therapy of asthma: comparison of the acute effects of parenteral and inhaled sympathomimetics and infused aminophylline. Am Rev Respir Dis 1980;122:365.
109. Thys F, Roeseler J, Delaere S, et al. Two-level non-invasive positive pressure ventilation in the initial treatment of acute respiratory failure in an emergency department. Eur J Emerg Med 1999;6:207.
110. Lange P, Parner J, Vestbo J, et al. A 15-year follow-up study of ventilatory function in adults with asthma. N Engl J Med 1998;339:1194.
111. Goldman M, Rachmiel M, Gendler L, et al. Decrease in asthma mortality rate in Israel from 1991–1995: is it related to increased use of inhaled corticosteroids? J Allergy Clin Immunol 2000;105:71.
112. American Thoracic Society. Standards for the diagnosis and care of patients with chronic obstructive pulmonary disease (COPD) and asthma. Am Rev Respir Dis 1987;136:225.
113. National Heart, Lung, and Blood Institute, Division of Lung Diseases. Workshop report: the definition of emphysema. Am Rev Respir Dis 1985;132:182.
114. Jeffery PK. Morphology of the airway wall in asthma and in chronic obstructive pulmonary disease. Am Rev Respir Dis 1991;143:1152.
115. Jeffery PK. Structural and inflammatory changes in COPD: a comparison with asthma. Thorax 1998;53:129.
116. Anthonisen NR, Wright EC, Hodgkin JE, IPPB Trial Group. Prognosis in obstructive pulmonary disease. Am Rev Respir Dis 1986;133:14.
117. Peto R, Speizer FE, Cochrane AL, et al. The relevance in adults of air-flow obstruction, but not of mucus hypersecretion, to mortality from chronic lung disease: results from 20 years of prospective observation. Am Rev Respir Dis 1983;128:491.
118. Fletcher C, Peto R. The natural history of chronic airflow obstruction. BMJ 1977;1:1645.
119. U.S. Surgeon General. The health consequences of smoking: chronic obstructive lung disease. DHHS Publication No. 84–50205. Washington, DC: U.S. Government Printing Office, 1984.
120. Burrows B, Bloom JW, Trayer GA, et al. The course and prognosis of different forms of chronic airways obstruction in a sample from the general population. N Engl J Med 1987;317:1309.
121. Anthonisen NR, Connett JE, Kiley JP, et al. Effects of smoking intervention and the use of an inhaled anticholinergic bronchodilator on the rate of decline of FEV1. The Lung Health Study. JAMA 1994;272:1497.
122. Scanlon PD, Connett JE, Waller LA, et al. Smoking cessation and lung function in mild-to-moderate chronic obstructive pulmonary disease. The Lung Health Study. Am J Respir Crit Care Med 2000;161:381.
123. Viegi G, Scognamiglio A, Baldacci S, et al. Epidemiology of chronic obstructive pulmonary disease (COPD). Respiration 2001;68:4.
124. Higgins M. Risk factors associated with chronic obstructive lung disease. Ann N Y Acad Sci 1991;624:7.
125. Chapman HA Jr, Munger JS, Shi GP. The role of thiol proteases in tissue injury and remodeling. Am J Respir Crit Care Med 1994;150(Pt 2):S155.
126. Zheng T, Zhu Z, Wang Z, et al. Inducible targeting of IL-13 to the adult lung causes matrix metalloproteinase- and cathepsin-dependent emphysema. J Clin Invest 2000;106:1081.
127. Imai K, Dalal SS, Chen ES, et al. Human collagenase (matrix metalloproteinase-1) expression in the lungs of patients with emphysema. Am J Respir Crit Care Med 2001;163:786.
128. Hautamaki RD, Kobayashi DK, Senior R, et al. Requirement for macrophage elastase for cigarette smoke-induced emphysema in mice. Science 1997;277:2002.
129. Finlay GA, O'Driscoll L, Russell KJ, et al. Matrix metalloproteinase expression and production by alveolar macrophages in emphysema. Am J Respir Crit Care Med 1997;156:240.
130. Crystal RG, Brantly ML, Hubbard RC, et al. The alpha-1-antitrypsin gene and its mutations: clinical consequences and strategies for therapy. Chest 1989;95:196.
131. Silverman EK, Province MA, Rao DC, et al. A family study of the variability of pulmonary function in α_1-antitrypsin deficiency: quantitative phenotypes. Am Rev Respir Dis 1990;142:1015.
132. Sandford AJ, Chagani T, Weir TD, et al. Susceptibility genes for rapid decline of lung function in the lung health study. Am J Respir Crit Care Med 2001;163:469.
133. Sakao S, Tatsumi K, Igari H, et al. Association of tumor necrosis factor alpha gene promoter polymorphism with the presence of chronic obstructive pulmonary disease. Am J Respir Crit Care Med 2001;163:420.
134. Higham MA, Pride NB, Alikhan A, et al. Tumour necrosis factor-alpha gene promoter polymorphism in chronic obstructive pulmonary disease. Eur Respir J 2000;15:281.
135. Garshick E, Schenker MB, Dosman JA. Occupationally induced airways obstruction. Med Clin North Am 1996;80:851.
136. Kanner RE, Connett JE, Altose MD, et al. Gender difference in airway hyperresponsiveness in smokers with mild COPD. The Lung Health Study. Am J Respir Crit Care Med 1994;150:956.
137. Sluiter HJ, Keoter GH, de Monchy JG, et al. The Dutch hypothesis (chronic non-specific lung disease) revisited. Eur Respir J 1991;4:479.
138. O'Connor GT, Sparrow D, Weiss ST. The role of allergy and nonspecific airway hyperresponsiveness in the pathogenesis of chronic obstructive pulmonary disease. State of the art review. Am Rev Respir Dis 1989;140:225.
139. Tashkin DP, Altose MD, Connett JE, et al. Methacholine reactivity predicts changes in lung function over time in smokers with early chronic obstructive pulmonary disease. Am J Respir Crit Care Med 1996;153:1802.
140. Drazen JM, Hirschman C, Macklem PT, et al. Mechanics of bronchoconstriction influenced by inflammation. In: Holgate ST, ed. The role of inflammatory processes in airway hyperresponsiveness. Boston: Blackwell, 1989.
141. Bellofiore S, Eidelman DH, Macklem PT, et al. Effects of elastase-induced emphysema on airway responsiveness to methacholine in rats. J Appl Physiol 1989;66:606.
142. Burrows B, Knudson RJ, Camilli AE, et al. The horse-racing effect and predicting decline in forced expiratory volume in one second from screening spirometry. Am Rev Respir Dis 1987;135:788.

143. Wise RA. Changing smoking patterns and mortality from chronic obstructive pulmonary disease. Prev Med 1997;26:418.
144. Viegi G, Scognamiglio A, Baldacci S, et al. Epidemiology of chronic obstructive pulmonary disease (COPD). Respiration 2001;68:4.
145. Hodgkin JE, Abbey DE, Euler GL, et al. COPD prevalence in nonsmokers in high and low photochemical air pollution areas. Chest 1984;86:830.
146. American Thoracic Society. Health effects of outdoor air pollution. Am J Respir Crit Care Med 1996;153:3.
147. Bates DV, Sizto R. The Ontario Air Pollution Study: identification of the causative agent. Environ Health Perspect 1989;79:69.
148. Schwartz J. Is there harvesting in the association of airborne particles with daily deaths and hospital admissions? Epidemiology 2001;12:55.
149. MacNee W, Donaldson K. Exacerbations of COPD: environmental mechanisms. Chest 2000;117:390S.
150. Samet JM, Dominici F, Curriero FC, et al. Fine particulate air pollution and mortality in 20 U.S. cities, 1987–1994. N Engl J Med 2000;343:1742.
151. Badgett RG, Tanaka DJ, Hunt DK, et al. Can moderate chronic obstructive pulmonary disease be diagnosed by historical and physical findings alone? Am J Med 1993;94:188.
152. Straus SE, McAlister FA, Sackett DL, et al. The accuracy of patient history, wheezing, and laryngeal measurements in diagnosing obstructive airway disease. CARE-COAD1 Group: Clinical Assessment of the Reliability of the Examination-Chronic Obstructive Airways Disease. JAMA 2000;283:1853.
153. Piirila P, Sovijarvi AR, Kaisla T, et al. Crackles in patients with fibrosing alveolitis, bronchiectasis, COPD, and heart failure. Chest 1991;99:1076.
154. Schapira RM, Schapira MM, Funahashi A, et al. The value of the forced expiratory time in the physical diagnosis of obstructive airways disease. JAMA 1993;270:731.
155. Sanders C. The radiographic diagnosis of emphysema. Radiol Clin North Am 1991;30:1019.
156. Coxson HO, Rogers RM, Whittall KP, et al. A quantification of the lung surface area in emphysema using computed tomography. Am J Respir Crit Care Med 1999;159:851.
157. Pauwels RA, Buist AS, Calverley PM, et al. Global strategy for the diagnosis, management, and prevention of chronic obstructive pulmonary disease. NHLBI/WHO Global Initiative for Chronic Obstructive Lung Disease (GOLD) Workshop summary. Am J Respir Crit Care Med 2001;163:1256.
158. Eaton ML, Green BA, Church MS, et al. Efficacy of theophylline in irreversible airflow obstruction. Ann Intern Med 1980;92:758.
159. Knudson RJ, Kaltenborn WT, Burrows B. Single breath carbon monoxide transfer factor in different forms of chronic airflow obstruction in a general population sample. Thorax 1990;45:514.
160. Oren R, Beeri M, Hubert A, et al. Effect of theophylline on erythrocytosis in chronic obstructive pulmonary disease. Arch Intern Med 1997;14:1474.
161. Lipworth BJ, McDevitt DG, Struthers AD. Prior treatment with diuretic augments the hypokalemic and electrocardiographic effects of inhaled albuterol. Am J Med 1989;86:653.
162. Stockley RA, O'Brien C, Pye A, et al. Relationship of sputum color to nature and outpatient management of acute exacerbations of COPD. Chest 2000;117:1638.
163. Sethi S, Murphy TF. Bacterial infection in chronic obstructive pulmonary disease in 2000: a state-of-the-art review. Clin Microbiol Rev 2001;14:336.
164. Menzies R, Gibbons W, Goldberg P. Determinants of weaning and survival among patients with COPD who require mechanical ventilation for acute respiratory failure. Chest 1989;95:398.
165. Martin TR, Lewis SW, Albert RK. The prognosis of patients with chronic obstructive pulmonary disease after hospitalization for acute respiratory failure. Chest 1982;82:310.
166. Rieves RD, Bass D, Carter RR, et al. Severe COPD and acute respiratory failure. Correlates for survival at the time of tracheal intubation. Chest 1993;104:854.
167. Simberkoff MS, Cross AP, Al-Ibrahim M, et al. Efficacy of pneumococcal vaccine in high-risk patients. Results of a Veterans Administration Cooperative Study. N Engl J Med 1986;315:1318.
168. Williams JH Jr, Moser KM. Pneumococcal vaccine and patients with chronic lung disease. Ann Intern Med 1986;104:106.
169. Nichol KL, Margolis KL, Wuorenma J, et al. The efficacy and cost effectiveness of vaccination against influenza among elderly persons living in the community. N Engl J Med 1994;331:778.
170. Bridges CB, Fukuda K, Cox NJ, et al. Prevention and control of influenza. Recommendations of the Advisory Committee on Immunization Practices (ACIP). MMWR Morb Mortal Wkly Rep 2001;50:1.
171. Alkins SA, O'Malley P. Should health-care systems pay for replacement therapy in patients with alpha(1)-antitrypsin deficiency? A critical review and cost-effectiveness analysis. Chest 2000;117:875.
172. The Alpha-1-Antitrypsin Deficiency Registry Study Group. Survival and FEV_1 decline in individuals with severe deficiency of 1-antitrypsin. Am J Respir Crit Care Med 1998;158:49.
173. Seersholm N, Wencker M, Banik N, et al. Does alpha1-antitrypsin augmentation therapy slow the annual decline in FEV_1 in patients with severe hereditary alpha1-antitrypsin deficiency? Eur Respir J 1997;10:2260.
174. Anthonisen NR, Manfreda J, Warren CWP, et al. Antibiotic therapy in exacerbations of chronic obstructive pulmonary disease. Ann Intern Med 1987;106:196.
175. Snow V, Lascher S, Mottur-Pilson C. Evidence base for management of acute exacerbations of chronic obstructive pulmonary disease. Ann Intern Med 2001;134:595.
176. Medical Research Council Working Party. Long term domiciliary oxygen therapy in chronic hypoxic cor pulmonale complicating chronic bronchitis and emphysema: report of the Medical Research Council Working Party. Lancet 1981;1:681.
177. Nocturnal Oxygen Therapy Trial Group. Continuous or nocturnal oxygen therapy in hypoxemic chronic obstructive lung disease: a clinical trial. Ann Intern Med 1980;93:391.
178. O'Donohue WJ Jr. Home oxygen therapy. Med Clin North Am 1996;80:611.
179. Tarpy SP, Celli BR. Long-term oxygen therapy. N Engl J Med 1995;333:710.
180. Fletcher EC, Donner CF, Midgren B, et al. Survival in COPD patients with a daytime PaO_2 greater than 60 mm Hg with and without nocturnal oxyhemoglobin desaturation. Chest 1992;101:649.
181. Fletcher EC, Luckett RA, Goodnight-White S, et al. A double-blind trial of nocturnal supplemental oxygen for sleep desaturation in patients with chronic obstructive pulmonary disease and a daytime PaO_2 above 60 mm Hg. Am Rev Respir Dis 1992;145:1070.
182. Chaouat A, Weitzenblum E, Kessler R, et al. A randomized trial of nocturnal oxygen therapy in chronic obstructive pulmonary disease patients. Eur Respir J 1999;14:1002.
183. Weitzenblum E, Schrijen F, Apprill M, et al. One year treatment with almitrine improves hypoxaemia but does not increase pulmonary artery pressure in COPD patients. Eur Respir J 1991;4:1215.
184. Winkelmann BR, Kullmer TH, Kneissl DG, et al. Low-dose almitrine bismesylate in the treatment of hypoxemia due to chronic obstructive pulmonary disease. Chest 1994;105:1383.
185. Chetty KG, Light RW, Stansbury DW, et al. Exercise performance of polycythemic chronic obstructive pulmonary disease patients. Effect of phlebotomies. Chest 1990;98:1073.
186. Poole PJ, Black PN. Mucolytic agents for chronic bronchitis or chronic obstructive pulmonary disease. Cochrane Database Syst Rev 2000;CD001287.
187. Wilson DO, Rogers RM, Wright EC, et al. Body weight in chronic obstructive pulmonary disease. Am Rev Respir Dis 1989;139:1435.
188. Ferreira IM, Brooks D, Lacasse Y, et al. Nutritional intervention in COPD: a systematic overview. Chest 2001;119:353.
189. Lung Health Study Research Group. Effect of inhaled triamcinolone on the decline in pulmonary function in chronic obstructive pulmonary disease. N Engl J Med 2000;343:1902.

190. Vestbo J, Sorensen T, Lange P, et al. Long-term effect of inhaled budesonide in mild and moderate chronic obstructive pulmonary disease: a randomised controlled trial. Lancet 1999;353:1819.
191. Pauwels RA, Lofdahl C-G, Laitinen LA, et al. Long-term treatment with inhaled budesonide in persons with mild chronic obstructive pulmonary disease who continue smoking. N Engl J Med 1999;340:1948.
192. Burge PS, Calverley PMA, Jones PW, et al. Randomised, double blind, placebo controlled study of fluticasone propionate in patients with moderate to severe chronic obstructive pulmonary disease: the ISOLDE trial. BMJ 2000;320:1297.
193. Gross NJ, Petty TL, Friedman M, et al. Dose response to ipratropium as a nebulized solution in patients with chronic obstructive pulmonary disease. A three-center study. Am Rev Respir Dis 1989;139:1188.
194. Casaburi R, Briggs DD Jr, Donohue JF, et al. The spirometric efficacy of once-daily dosing with tiotropium in stable COPD: a 13-week multicenter trial. Chest 2000;118:1294.
195. van Noord JA, Bantje TA, Eland ME, et al. A randomised controlled comparison of tiotropium and ipratropium in the treatment of chronic obstructive pulmonary disease. Thorax 2000;55:289.
196. Ferguson GT, Cherniack RM. Current concepts: management of chronic obstructive pulmonary disease. N Engl J Med 1993;328:1017.
197. Rennard SI, Anderson W, ZuWallack R, et al. Use of a long-acting inhaled β2-adrenergic agonist, salmeterol xinafoate, in patients with chronic obstructive pulmonary disease. Am J Respir Crit Care Med 2001;163:1087.
198. D'Urzo AD, De Salvo MC, Ramirez-Rivera A, et al. In patients with COPD, treatment with a combination of formoterol and ipratropium is more effective than a combination of salbutamol and ipratropium : a 3-week, randomized, double-blind, within-patient, multicenter study. Chest 2001;119:1347.
199. Combivent Inhalation Solution Study Group. Routine nebulized ipratropium and albuterol together are better than either alone in COPD. Chest 1997;112:1514.
200. Friedman M, Serby CW, Menjoge SS, et al. Pharmacoeconomic evaluation of a combination of ipratropium plus albuterol compared with ipratropium alone and albuterol alone in COPD. Chest 1999;115:635.
201. Lam A, Newhouse MT. Management of asthma and chronic airflow limitation. Are methylxanthines obsolete? Chest 1990;98:44.
202. Pauwels RA. New aspects of the therapeutic potential of theophylline in asthma. J Allergy Clin Immunol 1989;83(2 Pt 2):548.
203. Murciano D, Auclair MH, Pariente R, et al. A randomized, controlled trial of theophylline in patients with severe chronic obstructive pulmonary disease. N Engl J Med 1989;320:1521.
204. Wrenn K, Slovis CM, Murphy F, et al. Aminophylline therapy for acute bronchospastic disease in the emergency room. Ann Intern Med 1991;115:241.
205. Niewoehner DE, Erbland ML, Deupree RH, et al. Effect of systemic glucocorticoids on exacerbations of chronic obstructive pulmonary disease. N Engl J Med 1999;340:1941.
206. Thompson WH, Nielson CP, Carvalho P, et al. Controlled trial of oral prednisone in outpatients with acute COPD exacerbation. Am J Respir Crit Care Med 1996;154:407.
207. Mendella LA, Manfreda J, Warren CPW, et al. Steroid response in stable chronic obstructive pulmonary disease. Ann Intern Med 1982;96:17.
208. Rice KL, Rubins JB, Lebahn F, et al. Withdrawal of chronic systemic corticosteroids in patients with COPD: a randomized trial. Am J Respir Crit Care Med 2000;162:174.
209. Bach PB, Brown C, Gelfand SE, et al. Management of acute exacerbations of chronic obstructive pulmonary disease: a summary and appraisal of published evidence. Ann Intern Med 2001;134:600.
210. Pauwels RA, Buist AS, Calverley PM, et al. Global strategy for the diagnosis, management, and prevention of chronic obstructive pulmonary disease. NHLBI/WHO Global Initiative for Chronic Obstructive Lung Disease (GOLD) Workshop summary. Am J Respir Crit Care Med 2001;163:1256.
211. American College of Chest Physicians and American Association of Cardiovascular and Pulmonary Rehabilitation. Pulmonary rehabilitation: joint ACCP/AACVPR evidence-based guidelines. Chest 1997;112:1363.
212. Nickoladze GD. Functional results of surgery for bullous emphysema. Chest 1992;101:119.
213. The American Society for Transplant Physicians (ASTP)/American Thoracic Society (ATS)/European Respiratory Society (ERS)/International Society for Heart and Lung Transplantation (ISHLT). International guidelines for the selection of lung transplant candidates. Am J Respir Crit Care Med 1998;158:335.
214. Trulock EP 3rd. Lung Transplantation for COPD. Chest 1998; 113[4 Suppl]:269S.
215. Hosenpud JD, Bennett LE, Keck BM, et al. Effect of diagnosis on survival benefit of lung transplantation for end-stage lung disease. Lancet 1998;351:24.
216. Gelb AF, McKenna RJ Jr, Brenner M, et al. Lung function 4 years after lung volume reduction surgery for emphysema. Chest 1999;116:1608.
217. Flaherty KR, Kazerooni EA, Curtis JL, et al. Short-term and long-term outcomes after bilateral lung volume reduction surgery: prediction by quantitative CT. Chest 2001;119: 1337.
218. Fessler HE, Wise RA. Lung volume reduction surgery: is less really more? Am J Respir Crit Care Med 1999;159:1031.

CHAPTER 61

Lung Cancer

LINDA F. BARR, MD

Lung cancer is the leading cause of visceral cancer and of cancer-related death in the United States. In 1999 there were an estimated 171,600 new cases of lung cancer and 158,900 deaths from the disease. For each lung cancer patient, there is an average of 14.7 years of life lost prematurely (1). Because of its close association with tobacco smoke, lung cancer is generally a preventable tumor. However, the diagnosis usually occurs late in the course of the disease after metastasis has occurred and determined the outcome. Recent advances in the management of lung cancer have been due to the addition of, and improvement in, chemotherapy for the treatment of non–small cell lung cancer (NSCLC). New radiologic methods offer the promise of improved lung cancer detection to better direct therapy in an effort to enhance survival.

EPIDEMIOLOGY

Tobacco

Eighty percent to 90% of lung cancers are caused by tobacco smoke, most importantly from cigarettes, but also from pipes and cigars. The increasing death rate from lung cancer in the past 50 years lags 20 years behind a parallel rise in cigarette smoking. Ominously, although the prevalence of current cigarette use has declined over more than 30 years, it has significantly increased among high school students in the United States from 27.5% in 1991 to 36.4% in 1997. Further, cigar smoking has increased by 50% among all age groups (2). The lifetime lung cancer mortality for the general population is approximately 10% for moderate smokers, 20% for heavy smokers, and 1% for nonsmokers (3), a compelling statistic because 47 million Americans smoke. For smokers, the most important determinant of lung cancer risk is the duration of cigarette smoking, and the number of cigarettes smoked per day has a multiplicative effect (4). The risk of lung cancer increases approximately with the fourth power of the number of years of smoking and the square of the number of cigarettes smoked daily (5). Because of the duration effect, individuals who start smoking before the age of 15 years are four times more likely to develop lung cancer than those who begin after the age of 25 years (4). Further, the exposure to smoke from others' cigarettes ("passive smoking") leads to an increased risk of lung cancer (6). The risk of lung cancer declines after 5 years from cessation of smoking and continues to decrease with duration of time from quitting; for former heavy smokers, some risk remains.

The amount of tar in each cigarette does not correlate with cancer risk. This is because smokers of low tar and low nicotine increase the depth and length of their cigarette inhalation to get their required dose of nicotine (7).

Occupational Exposure

Other exposures that increase the risk for lung cancer and examples of relevant occupations are listed in Table 61.1 (8). It is especially important to identify people with asbestos exposure. Not only do asbestos-exposed individuals have an increased incidence of mesothelioma, they also have a sixfold greater risk of developing lung cancer than the general population. Those exposed people who smoke are 60 times more likely to develop bronchogenic carcinoma than are nonsmoking nonexposed people (9).

Radon

The risk of radon as a pulmonary carcinogen has received a great deal of public attention. Radon is a naturally produced radioactive gas that is found

Table 61.1. Occupational Agents Associated with Lung Cancer

Agent	Occupational Examples
Arsenic	Copper smelting, pesticide manufacturing, manufacture of "pressure-treated" wood
Asbestos	*Historically:* production, shipfitters; *Currently:* maintenance and construction workers exposed to asbestos insulation, mechanics exposed to asbestos brake linings.
Beryllium	Mining, refining, manufacture of ceramics, electronic and aerospace equipment.
Bis(chloromethyl)ether	Production, construction.
Cadmium	Electroplating, manufacture of plastics and alloys, pigments, battery electrodes
Chromium, hexavalent	Manufacturing of pigments, stainless steel, plating.
Mustard gas	Production, warfare
Nickel	Manufacturing of stainless steel, nonferrous alloys, batteries, and electroplating.
Polycyclic aromatic compounds	Aluminum production, coal gasification, coke production, soot, and iron and steel founding
Radon	Mining
Vinyl chloride	Production of polyvinyl chloride
Probably carcinogens	
Acrylonitrile	Manufacture of acrylic fiber for textiles, pipes
Diesel exhaust	Mining, trucking, construction
Formaldehyde	Manufacture, biology
Silica	Mining, masonry, concrete, pottery

Based on classifications of the International Agency for Research on Cancer and the National Institute of Occupational Safety and Health.

universally in the soil and air. The contribution of radon exposure to excess lung cancer in uranium and other underground miners (including those who mine iron, zinc, tin, and fluorspar) is well established. Of unproven but theoretical concern is the lung cancer risk due to exposure to radon from contaminated soil beneath some homes. By extrapolation from miners' data, it is estimated that such exposure may be responsible for a relative risk of 1.14 (95% confidence interval = 1.0 to 1.3) at 150 Bq/m^3 (the standard measure of radiation exposure) and may account for 6,000 to 36,000 lung cancer deaths each year in the United States. There may be a greater than additive risk for cigarette smoking and home radon exposure (10). Because of uncertainty in the risk estimates, it has been suggested that homes should be tested for radon using commercially available tests and corrective measures taken when the exposure rate approaches 150 Bq/m^3. Whether such measures are effective in reducing the risk of lung cancer is unknown.

Other Risk Factors

It is important to consider other groups with increased risk of bronchogenic carcinoma. First, those with *previous lung cancers* or with other tobacco-associated cancers are at a markedly increased risk of developing a second cancer of the respiratory or upper digestive tract (discussed later). Second, some studies suggest that *genetic predisposition* may influence the risk of lung cancer. Stratified case-control studies controlled for cigarette smoking have determined that lung cancer patients have an odds ratio of 1.7 to 5.3 for having a first-order relative with lung cancer (11,12). This increased risk may be due to an inadequacy of DNA repair capacity: Studies of the repair of bleomycin- and benzo[a]pyrene diol-epoxide–induced chromatid damage (the latter is a carcinogenic derivative of tobacco smoke) show significant differences in the DNA repair ability of lymphocytes derived from lung cancer patients and those from age- and ethnicity-matched control subjects (13). Alternately, genetic differences in lung cancer risk may reflect differences in the functioning of enzymes in the metabolic pathways of carcinogens.

Third, the presence of *chronic lung disease* may increase lung cancer risk. This has been described both for chronic obstructive pulmonary disease (14) and for interstitial disease (15). Fourth, human immunodeficiency virus infection is associated with a relative risk of lung cancer of 6.5 compared with the general population. As with acquired immunodeficiency syndrome-defining malignancies, lung cancer is more aggressive and manifests a worsened prognosis in the human immunodeficiency virus-positive patient (16).

SCREENING

The diagnosis of lung cancer is generally made in the last quarter of the tumor's life cycle, usually after metastases have occurred and essentially have determined the outcome (17). This observation underlies the dismal survival of patients with the disease: For all stages combined, 5-year survival for patients with NSCLC is 14% and for those with small cell lung cancer (SCLC) is 6%, with no significant change over the past two decades. However, 50% of patients with disease discovered at a localized stage survive (18). Thus, there is much interest in detecting lung cancers at an earlier curable stage. As with other adult solid tumors, lung cancers have a long preclinical phase characterized by accumulating genetic changes over a decade or more. This may reflect the relationship between tumor size and doubling time. A tumor of 1 mm has already undergone 20 doublings and one of 1 cm, 30 doublings. Over the extrapolated range of tumor doubling times, this implies a lifespan of 5 to 10 years with continued genetic damage, angiogenesis, and metastasis occurring along the way (19). Earlier large randomized studies at multiple centers showed that screening cigarette smokers with yearly chest x-rays and sputum cytology improved the detection of cancer and the survival (time from detection to death) but did not lead to a significant reduction in mortality (20). It is controversial whether this paradox is due to lead time bias (the time of diagnosis moved forward, but the date of death unaffected) or overdiagnosis (some of the tumors never would have progressed to clinical disease) (21) or whether the tumors were not detected at an early enough point in their development to have altered outcome.

The same debates surround the development of low-energy chest computed tomography (CT) as a screening tool for lung cancer (22). This technique is more sensitive than chest x-ray and detects nodules below 1 cm.

Using low-energy chest CT, the Early Lung Cancer Action Project found noncalcified nodules in 23% of screened symptom-free volunteers who were 60 years or older and had at least a 10-pack-year cigarette smoking history with no prior cancer. Only 20% of these nodules were identified on chest x-ray. These nodules were managed similarly to those in the protocol described for solitary pulmonary nodules (SPNs; see below). Twelve percent of these nodules were malignant, of which 85% were stage I, and all were NSCLCs (23). The incidence of malignant nodules in these asymptomatic smokers in this CT study was 7%, similar to the 6.4% incidence of unsuspected malignant nodules found in the lung specimens of patients undergoing lung volume reduction surgery (24). Current studies will determine whether low-energy CT screening improves the mortality for these patients with lung cancer.

In addition to improving radiologic methods for lung cancer detection, ongoing research has focused on developing lung cancer biomarkers. Candidate abnormalities found in cigarette smokers include mutations in *ras* and *p53* genes and DNA sequence loss at three loci: 3p14 (the location of the *FHIT* tumor suppression gene), 9p21 (the location of the *p16* tumor suppressor gene), and 17p13 (the location of the *p53* tumor suppressor gene). Differences between lung cancer patients and control subjects have also been found for the functional status of members of the family of enzymes responsible for carcinogen activation and degradation and the ability of patients' lymphocytes to repair the genetic damage induced by the cigarette carcinogen benzo[a]pyrene (13,25). Measurement of these markers is not yet clinically useful.

In summary, screening patients at risk for lung cancer has not yet been determined to affect mortality and therefore cannot be currently recommended.

HISTOLOGY

Lung cancer is classified broadly into two major groups—*NSCLC* and *SCLC*—both of which are associated with cigarette smoking. The distribution of these cancers is 80% and 20%, respectively. In the NSCLC category, approximately 36% of patients have *squamous cell carcinomas,* 45% have *adenocarcinomas,* 9% have *large cell carcinomas,* 2% to 4% have *bronchioalveolar carcinomas,* and 1% to 2% have *carcinoids.* There is significant heterogeneity in the histology: 45% of patients with NSCLC have mixed NSCLC phenotypes, 10% to 20% of NSCLC tumors have SCLC-like neuroendocrine features, and 9% of SCLC have regions of NSCLC tumor cells (26). This heterogeneity supports the hypothesis that all pulmonary cancers arise from a single pluripotent stem cell that has the capacity to differentiate into the major bronchoalveolar mucosal cell types, including neuroendocrine, glandular, and epithelial.

The past 15 to 20 years have seen a significant shift in NSCLC subtypes from a majority squamous cell to a majority adenocarcinoma, occurring in North America but not Europe. This has been attributed to the use of "low tar" cigarettes in the United States and Canada, which lead to a deeper inhalation pattern that allows the peripheral lung (where adenocarcinomas generally arise) greater carcinogen exposure. A contributor may be the increased proportion of women with lung cancer, a population that is more prone to adenocarcinomas (27,28).

The incidence of bronchioloalveolar carcinoma has doubled over the past 20 years, and in one study, this tumor constituted 15% of all lung cancers (29). The reason for this increase is unclear. Patients with this cancer tend to be younger, are more likely to be female, and are less likely to be smokers than are those with other lung cancers. The treatment of bronchioloalveolar carcinoma is similar to that of other non–small cell carcinomas. However, this tumor has a greater propensity to spread locally compared with other NSCLC phenotypes, and repeated surgical excisions may be necessary (30).

Malignant mesothelioma is a pleural tumor strongly associated with asbestos exposure. This tumor usually presents with a pleural effusion. The diagnostic yield of thoracentesis for mesothelioma is less than 40%, improved only by 10% by repeat thoracentesis and pleural needle biopsy. Thus, thoracoscopic-guided biopsy or open lung biopsy may be required for this diagnosis. The differentiation of mesothelioma from adenocarcinoma is an occasional problem and may necessitate electron microscopy or staining for immunohistochemical markers. The treatment of mesothelioma entails debulking surgery, with either intracavitary or external radiation; chemotherapy is sometimes given. The prognosis is poor (31).

HISTORY

The symptoms of lung cancer may be categorized as those caused by the mass effect of the tumor in the airway, those caused by impingement of the tumor on extrapulmonary mediastinal structures, those of paraneoplastic syndromes, and those of distant metastases.

Pulmonary Symptoms

Ninety percent of patients with lung cancer have symptoms at the time of diagnosis, and most of these symptoms are respiratory. The respiratory manifestations include cough, dyspnea, chest pain, hemoptysis, and symptoms related to postobstructive pneumonia. Cough occurs in almost all patients during the course of lung cancer. *Cough* and sputum production are nonspecific symptoms in smokers, but the appearance of a chronic cough, with or without expectoration, or the change in cough pattern in an older smoker should raise a suspicion of lung cancer.

Hemoptysis (generally blood-streaked sputum) is the initial manifestation of cancer in many patients. If there is no other explanation that can be diagnosed by history, physical examination, and a routine chest x-ray, the issue for patients with mild hemoptysis is whether to proceed with a bronchoscopic investigation into the cause. Factors that favor bronchoscopy are patient age greater than 40 years, an abnormal chest x-ray, a history of hemoptysis of more than 1 week, a history of tobacco smoking, a chronic cough, or the presence of anemia or weight loss. Lung cancer is found at bronchoscopy in one-third of patients with hemoptysis and one or more of these risk factors (32). Whether bronchoscopy is indicated in the absence of these risk factors is unclear. With rare exceptions, a negative bronchoscopy is reliable for excluding cancer in patients with hemoptysis and negative radiologic studies (33).

Chest pain is reported by approximately half of patients with lung cancer on presentation, usually as an intermittent dull ache on the side of the tumor. The cause of this pain is unclear, and if the tumor appears otherwise resectable, this symptom should not preclude surgery. A more severe pain may indicate metastatic disease to the parietal pleura or to a bone and may necessitate a bone scan or a positron emission tomography (PET scan). Shoulder pain, sometimes mistaken for arthritis, may be caused by a *Pancoast* (superior sulcus) tumor (see below) or may be caused by a tumor involving the diaphragm.

Dyspnea in a patient with lung cancer may be caused directly by the primary tumor or may be due to factors indirectly related to the tumor, those due to treatment of the cancer, and those due to other concurrent medical disease. Primary tumor related etiologies include tumor obstruction of airway with postobstructive atelectasis or pneumonia, pleural effusion, lymphangitic carcinomatosis, or pericardial tumor involvement. Dyspnea indirectly related to the cancer may be due to pulmonary embolism, an electrolyte or hormonal disorder due to a paraneoplastic syndrome, or due to inanition. Radiation may result in pneumonitis. Chemotherapeutic agents may cause anemia or other toxicities that may contribute to this symptom. Finally, because cigarettes are a common risk factor for other medical conditions, patients with lung cancer may have pre-existing lung disease, usually chronic obstructive lung disease or cardiac disease.

Extrapulmonary Thoracic Symptoms

Extrapulmonary symptoms caused by intrathoracic extrapulmonary extension include superior vena cava syndrome, Pancoast tumor syndrome, Horner syndrome, dysphagia, hoarseness, and cardiac disease. Patients with such symptoms should be rapidly evaluated for definitive diagnosis and treatment.

The superior vena cava syndrome consists of edema and rubor of the upper trunk and face, sometimes with syncope. It is caused by obstruction of the superior vena cava by involvement of the mediastinum with tumor. The chest x-ray usually shows a right upper lobe mass, a widened mediastinum, and, in 25% of cases, a right pleural effusion.

The Pancoast syndrome is caused by a tumor that is located at the pulmonary apex and that involves adjacent structures such as the chest wall, lymphatics, ribs, vertebrae, vessels, and nerves. The tumor may cause shoulder pain, arm pain, and paresthesia, usually in the ulnar distribution, indicating encroachment of the brachial plexus.

Horner syndrome is due to tumor invasion of the lower cervical or upper thoracic sympathetic trunk and consists of miosis, ptosis, enophthalmos, facial flushing, and anhidrosis on the affected side.

Hoarseness may be caused by involvement of the trachea with tumor or by vocal cord paralysis caused by entrapment of the recurrent laryngeal nerve, usually on the left, by a mediastinal mass. This symptom should be evaluated with a flow-volume loop (done in a pulmonary function laboratory) or by laryngoscopy. Based on these studies, a CT may be indicated to evaluate the upper airway, mediastinum, and pulmonary parenchyma.

Wheezing, although usually caused by small airways obstruction, may also be produced by upper airway or bronchial obstruction by an intrinsic or extrinsic mass. Therefore, upper airway involvement should be ruled out in all wheezing patients by auscultation over the neck. The presence of stridor or of monophonic wheezing that localizes to the neck should be emergently evaluated with flow-volume loops and/or laryngoscopy.

Mediastinal tumors or enlarged lymph nodes can cause dysphagia by extrinsically impinging on the esophagus. Finally, lung cancers can invade the pericardium and produce tamponade.

Extrathoracic Symptoms

Anorexia, cachexia, weight loss, and fever are common in patients with lung cancer, particularly as the disease advances. Extrathoracic metastatic disease is found at autopsy in most patients with NSCLC and in almost all patients with SCLC. Metastases may be seen in any organ. Common metastatic sites for lung cancer include the pleura, bone, brain, liver, and adrenal glands. In addition, SCLC frequently invades the bone marrow, leading to hematologic abnormalities.

Paraneoplastic Syndromes

Paraneoplastic syndromes are common in patients with lung cancer. It is important to recognize that the symptoms of the paraneoplastic syndrome may precede the other symptoms of lung cancer; manifestations of these syndromes may mimic metastatic disease and mislead treatment decisions; and these symptoms generally improve with successful treatment of the underlying malignancy.

Endocrine syndromes may be seen in 10% to 15% of patients. The most common is *hypercalcemia*, secondary to a parathyroid hormone-related protein, with an N-terminus homologous with that of normal parathyroid hormone so that it binds to the parathyroid hormone receptor. This syndrome is usually caused by a NSCLC. The syndromes of *inappropriate antidiuretic hormone release* and of *ectopic adrenocorticotropic hormone secretion* are less common and more likely to be seen in patients with SCLC. Increased levels of these ectopic hormones can be found in the blood of many more patients with SCLC than in the few percent that manifest these syndromes. The syndrome of inappropriate antidiuretic hormone release is associated with hyponatremia and is treated with fluid restriction. The ectopic adrenocorticotropic hormone syndrome is characterized by mild hypertension, hyperglycemia, hypokalemia, alkalosis, and occasional hyperpigmentation but generally without the other manifestations of Cushing syndrome.

Clubbing and hypertrophic pulmonary osteoarthropathy are common in, although not limited to, patients with lung cancer. Clubbing is seen in one-third of patients with lung cancer. Hypertrophic pulmonary osteoarthropathy with pain, swelling and tenderness, and positive bone scan of affected bones may be seen in as many as 10% of these patients, and lung cancer is the underlying cause in more than 80% of adult cases of this osteoarthropathy.

Neurologic paraneoplastic processes are rare but dramatic and may be the presenting symptoms of SCLC (34). In the *Eaton-Lambert syndrome*, proximal muscle weakness and paresthesias may mimic myasthenia gravis from which it can be distinguished by electromyography. The diagnosis of other neurologic paraneoplastic syndromes, including peripheral neuropathies, subacute cerebellar degeneration, cortical degeneration, polymyositis, and intestinal dysmotility, may be facilitated by the measurement of type I antineuronal nuclear antibody (ANNA-1/Hu-1) (34).

Hematologic abnormalities may occur in patients with lung cancer and mesotheliomas. An increased tendency to clot may be manifest either as typical or atypical (*Trousseau syndrome*) venous or arterial thromboembolic disease (see Chapter 57). Anemia and reactive thrombocytosis are common.

PHYSICAL EXAMINATION

The purpose of a careful physical examination in patients with lung cancer is to determine the presence of metastatic disease, to evaluate the patient's candidacy for therapy, and to assess the patient's functional capacity, which is a major contributor to prognosis. Constitutional findings are important: Weight loss may be evidence of advanced disease. Attention must be paid to areas of pain or tenderness, which may indicate boney metastasis. The examination should also include an evaluation of lymph nodes in the anterior and posterior cervical, supraclavicular, and axillary regions; suspicious lymph nodes are those greater than 1 cm in diameter, are hard in consistency, or are fixed. Hoarseness or the signs of superior vena cava syndrome or of Horner syndrome should be noted. The pulmonary examination may reveal evidence of chronic lung disease and local wheezing or bronchial breath sounds from bronchial obstruction or basilar dullness from a pleural effusion. D'Espene sign, the inappropriate transmission of whispered pectoriloquy below the level of the T2 vertebral body, suggests mediastinal involvement with tumor. The cardiac examination, including evaluation of jugular veins, is important in preoperative assessment and also for determination of malignant pericardial effusion. The presence of hepatomegaly (liver span more than 13 cm) may suggest hepatic metastases. The extremities may demonstrate clubbing, edema, or cyanosis. A careful neurologic examination is important for evidence of brain metastases.

DIAGNOSTIC PROCEDURES

Chest X-Ray

A review of old chest x-rays can demonstrate the rapidity of disease onset and may aid in prognostication. A mass with a doubling time of less than 2 weeks or greater than 450 days is unlikely to be malignant. (For a more extensive discussion of radiologic characteristics helpful in differentiating benign from malignant pulmonary lesions, see Solitary Pulmonary Nodule, below.)

Certain chest x-ray patterns are suggestive of particular types of lung cancer. Squamous cell and small cell carcinomas tend to be centrally located, and adenocarcinomas and large cell carcinomas tend to arise peripherally. Centrally located tumors are more likely to present with symptoms of obstruction: atelectasis, pneumonia, and dyspnea. SCLC may demonstrate only hilar adenopathy with no visible primary tumor on the initial chest x-ray. Squamous cell carcinoma is the most likely bronchogenic carcinoma to cavitate, although even this tumor cavitates uncommonly.

Bronchioloalveolar cell carcinoma also usually presents peripherally and tends to be multifocal. This cancer has a variety of radiologic manifestations and may appear as a single mass or as multiple nodules, or it may imitate a pneumonia. Malignant mesothelioma is associated with a pleural effusion, and the underlying pleural surface is thickened and lumpy.

Computed Tomography and Magnetic Resonance Imaging of the Chest

A CT of the chest is routine in the evaluation of patients with suspected lung cancer to determine the anatomic extent of the tumor and to guide diagnostic and therapeutic procedures (reviewed in Ref. 35). CT may demonstrate additional lesions that are unseen on chest x-ray. Further, CT may aid in characterizing the size, shape, and composition of these lesions. For example, CT is better than the chest x-ray in determining calcification of a solitary pulmonary nodule; a densely calcified nodule is more likely to be benign. Also CT may demonstrate fat in a nodule, highly suggestive of a hamartoma. In addition, the presence and size of mediastinal or hilar lymph nodes can be evaluated by CT. Nodes greater than 1 cm in diameter have a 60% chance of representing metastatic disease (36), and if a surgical cure is contemplated, sampling by transbronchial needle aspiration (TBNA), mediastinoscopy, or mediastinotomy is required (see below). Finally, extending CT cuts down through the upper abdomen may demonstrate hepatic or adrenal metastases, although these radiographic findings will require biopsy if therapy would be influenced by the histology of these lesions. CT is neither sensitive nor specific in detecting the invasion of chest wall or mediastinal structures. Magnetic resonance imaging (MRI) is not as informative as CT for evaluating pulmonary parenchymal disease, nor is it helpful for evaluating mediastinal nodes. MRI is superior to CT in specific cases—for example, for the evaluation of the possibility of chest wall or vascular invasion by tumor and for the examination of superior sulcus tumors.

Positron Emission Tomography

PET, using the glucose analogue fluorodeoxyglucose, is a new imaging technique that may have a role in the evaluation of patients with SPNs and in the staging of lung cancer (see Staging, below). Fluorodeoxyglucose is taken up more avidly by more metabolically active cells and is not metabolized. Cancer tissue is enhanced by this method, whereas normal tissue is not. There are false positives: Inflammatory lesions can also light up. Further, some tumors are falsely identified as benign by this study (see Solitary Pulmonary Nodules, below).

Sputum Cytology

The frequency of diagnosis of lung cancer from cytology submitted from spontaneously expectorated sputum depends on the cell type and the location of the tumor (37). Squamous cell tumors shed cells into the airways, and cytologies are positive approximately 80% of the time. However, patients with a peripheral adenocarcinoma have positive cytologies less than 5% of the time. Patients should be instructed to produce a forceful cough. Three early morning specimens should be collected in a tightly fitting container, and if they cannot be submitted to the laboratory within 2 to 3 hours of collection, a fixative should be added and the specimens can be pooled and submitted together. Saccomanno solution, which contains alcohol and Carbowax, is one of the best fixatives. More than three samples does not increase the likelihood of a positive diagnosis of cancer. If the patient is not producing sputum, induction by the inhalation of an aerosolized solution of saline can be helpful. The patient inhales normal saline or a balanced salt solution (Hanks' BSS) that is aerosolized by an ultrasonic nebulizer (DeVilbiss 3583). In general, sputum induction is not a routine office procedure and should be done by experienced personnel. In addition to the sputum collected immediately after induction, good material is produced on the following morning. The addition of chest vibration or percussion does not improve the yield from sputum cytology. In cases in which there is obstruction of the bronchus as evidenced by the physical examination or the chest x-ray, it is reasonable to start collecting sputum after therapy, including antibiotics and perhaps bronchodilators, which may reestablish airway patency and allow sputum to be produced.

Bronchoscopy

Bronchoscopy is useful for both the diagnosis and staging of bronchogenic carcinoma (38). Bronchoscopy is important to search for a second synchronous malignancy and to evaluate vocal cord function. A fixed vocal cord suggests involvement of the recurrent laryngeal nerve in the mediastinum. Furthermore, the bronchoscope visualizes the proximal extent of the tumor, which is helpful in planning surgery (tracheal "sleeve" resections allow resection of tumors close to the carina). Multiple diagnostic procedures may be done through the bronchoscope: Transbronchial biopsy using forceps, brushing for cytology, and bronchoalveolar lavage. In addition, transbronchial needle aspiration (TBNA) allows sampling of hilar, subcarinal, and other mediastinal lymph nodes. Fiberoptic bronchoscopy is an outpatient procedure and can be done comfortably using mild sedation (e.g., midazolam or propofol), a short-acting narcotic (fentanyl), a drying agent (usually atropine or glycopyrrolate), and topical lidocaine. Occasional circumstances dictate preoperative endotracheal intubation or the use of a rigid bronchoscope, which are done with general anesthesia.

The diagnostic yield of bronchoscopy is 60% to 80% for tumors greater than 2 cm in diameter and 20% to 40% for those less than 2 cm and is higher for visualized masses in the central airways. Necrotic tumors, submucosal carcinomas, and large tumors that displace feeding bronchi may be more of a diagnostic challenge and may require more than one bronchoscopic procedure to obtain diagnostic material. Many peripheral tumors are accessible by bronchoscope using fluoroscopically guided needles, brushes, and biopsy forceps. However, masses that are smaller than 2 cm or in the outer third of the lung are usually better approached by percutaneous transthoracic needle aspiration (PTNA).

Although generally a safe and well-tolerated procedure, potential complications of bronchoscopy include pulmonary hemorrhage, pneumothorax, laryngospasm or bronchospasm, and transient cardiac arrhythmias. Patients with primary or secondary coagulation disorders, thrombocytopenia, uremia, pulmonary hypertension, or the superior vena cava syndrome are at an increased risk for bleeding. Pneumothorax complicates approximately 5% of transbronchial forceps biopsies and less than 1% of TBNA aspiration procedures, although only half of these patients require a chest tube. Transient atrial and ventricular arrhythmias occur in approximately 5% of elderly patients and may be related to transient hypoxemia or the induction of the vagal response by passage of the bronchoscope through the upper airway. However, death is rare and almost always is associated with a transbronchial biopsy that has caused significant bleeding (39).

Patients may have a low-grade fever after bronchoscopy, but the occurrence of pneumonia is low. Although the incidence of bacteremia during bronchoscopy is less than 2%, some advocate prophylactic antibiotics for patients at risk for bacterial endocarditis (39).

The interval between a myocardial infarction and safe performance of fiberoptic bronchoscopy is unknown and must be established on an individual basis, balancing the goals of the procedure and the therapeutic implication of the results.

Patient Experience. Bronchoscopy may be performed on an ambulatory basis by a pulmonologist or a thoracic surgeon. The patient is told to fast (including liquids) for 12 hours before bronchoscopy (although generally medicines may be taken with a sip of water) and not to eat for approximately 2 hours after its completion when the effects of topical anesthesia wear off. The only discomfort the patient will experience is coughing caused by irritation of the trachea and main bronchi, which is treated with topical lidocaine. There is usually no pain associated with this procedure. Although there may be a low-grade fever (less than 100.5°F oral) or blood-streaked hemoptysis during the first 24 hours after bronchoscopy, the patient should call the pulmonologist or go to the Emergency Room for higher fever, hemoptysis of greater than this volume, chest pain or severe shoulder pain (which may indicate a pneumothorax), or exacerbation of shortness of breath.

In the unusual situation in which sputum cytology demonstrates malignancy but the chest x-ray and chest CT do not localize a suspicious area ("occult carcinoma"), a long bronchoscopic procedure is undertaken under general anesthesia, in which a meticulous upper airway evaluation is followed by sequential sampling of each pulmonary segment. Positive findings mandate a confirmatory procedure in which repeat sampling is done of subsegments corresponding to the positive material. The yield of this procedure is 13% to 35%, and up to 15% of these patients have multicentric carcinomas. New metachronous primary lung cancer develops in these patients at the rate of 5% per year. Almost all these patients are heavy smokers and have increased surgical morbidity and mortality; thus, lung-sparing surgery or photodynamic therapies may be indicated (40).

Percutaneous Transthoracic Needle Aspiration

CT-directed PTNA of the lung is most useful when a mass or a nodule is located peripherally near the pleura or in the apex of the lung. It is especially helpful in the diagnosis of metastatic carcinoma because these tumors arise outside of the airway and are difficult to diagnose by bronchoscopy, particularly when they are less than 2 cm in size. It may also be preferred when infection is in the differential diagnosis because the interpretation of the significance of an infectious agent obtained by bronchoscopy is complicated by the passage of the scope through the nonsterile nasopharynx or oropharynx. PTNA is performed by either a radiologist or pulmonologist with fluoroscopic or CT guidance. The technique and experience of the operator and of the cytopathologist are of paramount importance in the success of the procedure, and the yield is increased with a repeat procedure. However, the false negative rate for any fluoroscopically guided procedure is significant. Thus, nondiagnostic or nonspecific findings require follow-up, the nature of which is determined by the adequacy of the sample and the clinical scenario. PTNA is an outpatient procedure, done with local anesthetic, and requires a cooperative patient (41).

Contraindications to the procedure include large blebs or blood vessels that are in the direct path of the needle; a patient with an uncontrollable cough, in which case general anesthesia may be necessary; and contralateral pneumonectomy, in which case the production of a pneumothorax would be devastating. In addition, patients with pulmonary hypertension have an increased risk of bleeding.

Patient Experience. Patients may receive intravenous sedation and local anesthetic. The patient will feel a mild pressure with the introduction of the needle. Otherwise, there is no significant pain. Potential complications include a 5% risk of bleeding (usually of minimal amount) and a 10% to 15% risk of pneumothorax (one-half of these require chest tube insertion). Most patients can resume normal activity within 24 hours.

Mediastinoscopy, Mediastinotomy, and Thoracoscopy

Mediastinoscopy and mediastinotomy are indicated when enlarged mediastinal lymph nodes or masses cannot be adequately sampled by less invasive techniques (TBNA or PTNA; see above). Lymph nodes accessible to cervical mediastinoscopy are those in the pretracheal area from the thoracic inlet to 1 cm beyond the carina bilaterally. Those anterior to the aortic arch and in the aortic-pulmonary window are not accessible to the cervical mediastinoscope and require anterior mediastinotomy. Potential complications include wound infection, injury to major vascular structures, and recurrent laryngeal nerve paralysis (42). These procedures are done by thoracic surgeons and require general anesthesia and hospitalization.

A biopsy done through a thoracoscope may be better tolerated than one done during a limited thoracotomy, and thoracoscopy may also be helpful, in selected cases, in the removal of peripheral lung masses (43) and in diagnosing the cause of pleural effusions. A medical thoracoscopy can be done under general anesthesia or in the sedated patient with local anesthetic. The visceral and parietal pleuras are examined with either a rigid or fiberoptic endoscope inserted through a chest tube.

A video-assisted thoracic surgical procedure usually requires general anesthesia. The procedure involves

Table 61.2. Staging of Non–Small Cell Lung Cancer: TNM Definitions

Primary tumor (T)	
TX	Primary tumor cannot be assessed or tumor proven by presence of malignant cells in sputum or bronchial washings but not visualized by imaging on bronchoscopy
TO	No evidence of primary tumor
Tis	Carcinoma *in situ*
T1	Tumor 3 cm or less in greatest dimension, surrounded by lung or visceral pleura, without bronchoscopic evidence of invasion more proximal than lobar bronchus (i.e., not in main bronchus)[a]
T2	Tumor with any of the following features of size or extent: More than 3 cm in greatest dimension Involves main bronchus, 2 cm or more distal to the carina Invades the visceral pleura Associated with atelectasis or obstructive pneumonitis that extends to the hilar region but does not involve the entire lung
T3	Tumor of any size that directly invades any of the following: chest wall (including superior sulcus tumors), diaphragm, mediastinal pleura, or pericardium; tumor in the main bronchus less than 2 cm distal to the carina but without involvement of the carina; or associated atelectasis or obstructive pneumonitis
T4	Tumor of any size that invades any of the following: mediastinum, heart, great vessels, trachea, esophagus, vertebral body, or carina; or tumor with a malignant pleural effusion[b] or pericardial effusion, or satellite nodule(s) within the primary bearing lobe
Lymph node (N)	
NX	Regional lymph nodes cannot be assessed
NO	No regional lymph node metastasis
N1	Metastasis in ipsilateral peribronchial or ipsilateral hilar lymph nodes, including direct extension
N2	Metastasis in ipsilateral mediastinal or subcarinal lymph node(s)
N3	Metastasis in contralateral mediastinal, contralateral hilar, ipsilateral or contralateral scalene, or supraclavicular lymph node(s)
Distant metastasis (M)	
MX	Presence of distant metastasis cannot be assessed
MO	No distant metastasis
M1	Distant metastasis[c]

[a]The uncommon superficial tumor or any size with its invasive component limited to the bronchial wall, which may extend proximal to the main bronchus, is also classified as T1.

[b]Most pleural effusions associated with lung cancer are caused by tumor. However, there are a few patients in whom multiple cytologic examinations or pleural fluid are negative for cancer. In these cases, the fluid is nonbloody and is not an exudate. When these elements and clinical judgment dictate that the effusion is not related to tumor, the effusion should be excluded as a staging element and the patient should be staged T1, T2, T3. Pericardial effusion is classified according to the same rules.

[c]Tumor nodule(s) in the ipsilateral lung nonprimary tumor-bearing lobe are classified as M1.

From Mountain CF. Revisions in the international system for staging lung cancer. Chest 1997;111:1710, with permission.

inducing a controlled pneumothorax and single lung ventilation, followed by the insertion of the instruments through additional incision(s). The patient generally has 2 to 3 days of hospital observation with a chest tube in place after thoracoscopy. The incidence of complications is similar to that of the closed procedures (44).

STAGING

The staging of the patient with lung cancer has two goals: to determine the anatomic extent of the tumor and to determine the physiologic capacity of the patient to undergo therapy.

Non–Small Cell Lung Cancer

For NSCLC, the anatomic extent of the tumor is defined by the TNM classification system, where T is the tumor size, N is the nodal involvement, and M is the distant metastasis. The TNM categories are then grouped into four stages with therapeutic and prognostic implications (Tables 61.2, 61.3, and 61.4).

Mediastinal nodal involvement may be assessed by chest CT, with sampling of lymph nodes larger than 1 cm in transverse diameter, by bronchoscopy (TBNA aspiration), or by mediastinoscopy or surgery. Recent studies indicate that PET may be complementary to CT for this examination (45,46). PETs have superior

Table 61.3. Staging of Non–Small Cell Lung Cancer—New International Revised Stage Grouping

Stage 0	Tis
Stage IA	T1, NO, MO
Stage IB	T2, NO, MO
Stage IIA	T1, N1, MO
Stage IIB	T2, N1, MO
	T3, NO, MO
Stage IIIA	T1-3, N2, MO
	T3, N1, MO
Stage IIIB	T4, Any N, MO
	Any T, N3, MO
Stage IV	Any T, Any N, M1

From Mountain CF. Revisions in the international system for staging lung cancer. Chest 1997;111:1710, with permission.

Table 61.4. Five-year Survival of Non–Small Cell Lung Cancer by Stage at Presentation

Stage	TNM	Frequency (%)	5-Yr Survival (%)
IA	T1NOMO	~10	67
IB	T2NOMO		57
IIA	T1NIMO		34
IIB	T2NIMO	~13	24
	T3NOMO		22
IIIA	T1-3N2MO	~22	13
	T3N1MO		9
IIIB	T4anNMO	~22	7
	T1-4N3MO		3
IV	T1-4N0-3M1	~32	1

From Bunn PA Jr, Mault J, Kelly K. Adjuvant and neoadjuvant chemotherapy for non-small cell lung cancer: a time for reassessment? Chest 2000;117:119S, with permission.

sensitivity to CTs for the detection of lymph node activity; however, PETs cannot adequately distinguish between intrapulmonary lymph nodes and those in the mediastinum nor between hyperplastic and neoplastic disease, thus mandating sampling of positive areas.

The major sites of NSCLC metastases are brain, bones, liver, and adrenal glands. The extent of routine pretreatment evaluation of these sites has been controversial. However, two large meta-analyses have demonstrated that the negative predictive value of a good clinical evaluation for metastatic disease is more than 97% (47,48). This has led the American Thoracic Society/European Respiratory Society to recommend the NSCLC staging evaluation in Table 61.5 (49). These recommendations may need to be modified for the individual patient. For example, constitutional signs or symptoms of advanced disease or evidence of borderline operability by physiologic criteria may necessitate a more aggressive staging evaluation.

Recent studies suggest that whole body PET may have a place in the preoperative staging of patients with potentially resectable NSCLC. PET has good sensitivity and specificity for the detection of distant metastases (45,46). In one prospective study of 102 patients, PET resulted in a change in tumor stage in 62 (45). However, because there is a 17% false positive rate for distant metastases, these areas need to be sampled. In addition, PET has poor specificity for the brain. Finally, there are as yet no data on whether the staging information from PET improves survival.

Both patients with NSCLC and those with SCLC should have their performance status evaluated. The performance status determines both the ability to undergo therapy and is a major contributor to the prognosis (50). Common scales for this measurement are the ECOG and Karnofsky scales, which measure the patient's physiologic status due both to the cancer and to concurrent medical problems (Table 61.6).

Table 61.5. Pretreatment Evaluation of Patients with Lung Cancer

Part A: Recommended tests for all patients
- Complete blood count
- Electrolytes, calcium, alkaline phosphatase, albumin, AST, ALT, T bili, creatinine
- Chest roentgenogram
- CT of chest through the adrenals[a]
- Pathologic confirmation of malignancy[b]

Part B: Recommended tests for selected but not all patients

Test	Indication
CT of liver with contrast or liver ultrasound	Elevated liver function tests; abnormal non–contrast-enhanced CT of liver or abnormal clinical evaluation
CT of brain with contrast or MRI brain	CNS symptoms or abnormal clinical evaluation
Radionuclide bone scan	Elevated alkaline phosphatase (bony fraction), elevated calcium, bone pain, or abnormal clinical evaluation
Pulmonary function tests	If lung resection or thoracic radiotherapy planned
Arterial blood gases	Patients with borderline resectability due to limited cardiopulmonary status
Quantitative radionuclide perfusion lung scan or exercise testing to evaluate maximum oxygen consumption	Patients with borderline resectability due to limited cardiopulmonary status

[a]May not be necessary if patient has obvious M1 disease on chest x-ray or physical exam.

[b]While optimal in most cases, tissue diagnosis may not be necessary in some cases where the lesion is enlarging and/or the patient will undergo surgical resection regardless of the outcome of a biopsy.

CT, computed tomography; AST, aspartate aminotransferase; ALT; alanine aminotransferase; CNS, central nervous system; MRI, magnetic resonance imaging; T bili, total bilirubin.

Modified from American Thoracic Society/European Respiratory Society. Pretreatment evaluation of non-small-cell lung cancer. Am J Respir Crit Care Med 1997;156:320, with permission.

Table 61.6. Performance Status Scales

Karnofsky Performance Scale[a]	
Point	Description
100	Normal: no complaints; no evidence of disease
90	Able to perform normal activity; minor signs/symptoms of disease
80	Normal activity with effort; some signs/symptoms of disease
70	Cares for self, unable to perform normal activity or do active work
60	Requires occasional assistance but is able to care for most personal needs
50	Requires considerable assistance and frequent medical care
40	Disabled; requires special care and assistance
30	Severely disabled; hospitalization indicated; death not imminent
20	Very sick; hospitalization and active supportive treatment are necessary
10	Moribund; fatal processes progressing rapidly
0	Dead
ECOG Performance Status Scale[b]	
Grade	Criteria
0	Fully active, able to carry on all predisease activities without restriction (Karnofsky 90–100)
1	Restricted in physically strenuous activity but ambulatory and able to carry out work of a light or sedentary nature, for example, light housework or office work (Karnofsky 70–80)
2	Ambulatory and capable of all self-care but unable to carry out any work activities. Up and about ≥50% of waking hours (Karnofsky 50–60)
3	Capable of only limited self-care, confined to bed or chair ≥50% of waking hours (Karnofsky 30–40)
4	Completely disabled, cannot carry on any self-care, totally confined to bed or chair (Karnofsky 10–20)

[a]From Vaporiciyan AA, Nesbitt JC, Lee JS, et al. Neoplasms of the thorax: cancer of the lung. In: Bast RC, Kufe DW, Pollock RE, et al., eds. Cancer medicine, 5th ed. Hamilton, Ontario: BC Decker Inc., 2000, with permission.

[b]From American Society of Clinical Oncology. Clinical practice guidelines for the treatment of unresectable non-small-cell lung cancer. J Clin Oncol 1997;15:3002, with permission.

Small Cell Lung Cancer

SCLC is classified by a two-stage system. In *limited stage disease,* the cancer is confined to the hemithorax and the regional lymph nodes (including mediastinal, ipsilateral hilar, and supraclavicular nodes), which essentially delineate the extent of disease that can be contained within a tolerable radiation port. *Extensive stage disease* is that which lies outside these boundaries. SCLC is a more aggressive tumor than NSCLC and metastasizes early and widely. Therefore, the staging on presentation is more extensive than with NSCLC. The staging of SCLC patients generally entails the same recommendations as in part A of Table 61.5, as well as additional studies. Because 38% of these patients have bone involvement at presentation, a bone scan is indicated. One-fourth of patients have liver metastases; because liver function tests are not sensitive for metastases, a CT through the liver is necessary. Because the central nervous system is involved in one-half of the patients with SCLC and does not cause symptoms in 10%, a head CT is indicated. A bone marrow aspirate and biopsy may be required if no other metastatic sites are found. The performance status needs to be evaluated, as for NSCLC (see above).

TREATMENT

Non–Small Cell Lung Cancer

The most important prognostic criterion for NSCLC is the TNM classification because it defines resectable, and thus most of the potentially curable, disease. Surgery is the standard treatment for those without clinical evidence of mediastinal or metastatic disease and is an option for selected patients with tumor involvement of the mediastinum or chest wall. Chemotherapy and radiotherapy improve survival of some stages.

Stages I, II, and IIIA

Surgical resection results in a 5-year survival of 70% and 50% for patients with clinical stage I and stage II NSCLC, respectively, and is appropriate for selected patients with stage IIIA disease for whom 5-year survival is 15% by presurgical staging (although better for those defined by surgical staging). These results indicate significant mortality even in patients with disease that appears to be local at presentation. Postoperative radiation therapy alone, although improving local control, has had little effect on survival for these patients. However, adjuvant or neoadjuvant (preoperative) platinum-based chemotherapy (e.g., cisplatin or carboplatin), generally in combination with other chemotherapeutic agents and external radiation, has been shown to improve survival for stage IIIA disease. It is controversial whether this regimen improves survival for stages I and II disease (51). However, these protocols may improve symptoms, and survival may be changed by newer therapies currently being studied (52).

Stage IIIB and IV

The 5-year survival for patients with stage IIIB disease is 5% and for stage IV disease is rare. Median survival times with best available therapies are 6 to 10 months. For these patients, performance status is the key to determining further therapy. For stage IIIB patients, chemotherapy with a platinum-based regimen and definitive local radiation therapy is indicated for patients with good performance status. This should be started soon after diagnosis, because a delay in therapy may negate the survival benefit. For stage IV patients, chemotherapy is appropriate for patients with good performance status; local radiotherapy should be used for palliation (53). However, for the subgroup of patients with solitary brain metastases and otherwise resectable lung cancer (stage I or II), there may be a role for combined thoracotomy and craniotomy, in conjunction with chemotherapy (54).

Surgical Considerations

Patients with NSCLC tumors that appear anatomically localized after staging evaluation are considered surgical candidates if the risks of the thoracotomy, and of the removal of functional lung tissue, are considered medically reasonable. The prediction of residual lung function after resection is based on pulmonary function studies. If radiologic studies show an irregular distribution of underlying lung disease, a nuclear perfusion study may be needed to determine the contribution of the proposed lung resection to the total lung function; the predicted postoperative forced expiratory volume in 1 second (FEV_1) is calculated from this fraction. All patients should be evaluated as potential candidates for both pneumonectomy and lobectomy in case operative findings dictate that the former will be necessary for cure. A pneumonectomy is feasible if the preoperative FEV_1 is 2 L or more or 80% of predicted, if the maximum voluntary ventilation is 50% or more of predicted, or if the maximal oxygen consumption on exercise testing is more than 20 mL/kg/min. Alternatively, a lobectomy or pneumonectomy is feasible if the predicted postoperative FEV_1 is 0.8 L or more or 40% of predicted. For borderline cases, or when the degree of dyspnea or disability is greater than the FEV_1 would predict, a DLCO of 40% or more of predicted or a change of oxygen saturation of 2% or less with exercise suggests that a patient is operable. Many surgeons also rely on the patient's exertional tolerance: Good tolerance as demonstrated by the ability to walk a flight of stairs or by excellent baseline activity level predicts adequate functional reserve to tolerate pulmonary resection. Patients who do not meet these criteria or those who have hypoxemia or hypercarbia on baseline arterial blood gas have a high risk for respiratory complications after thoracotomy. Additional considerations such as cardiovascular status, other comorbid disease, and the informed patient's wishes need to be considered in the surgical decision (55).

Possible postoperative pulmonary complications of patients undergoing thoracotomy include the need for prolonged mechanical ventilatory support or the development of bronchospasm, atelectasis, bronchitis or pneumonia, or prolonged chest tube air leak. Several preoperative measures decrease the risk for these complications in patients with chronic obstructive lung disease. These include the sustained cessation of smoking, use of inhaled bronchodilators and inhaled steroids (for asthmatics), treatment of pulmonary infection with antibiotics, and treatment of increased secretions with measures such as chest physiotherapy, postural drainage, and/or flutter valve. Finally, all patients need to be taught how to use the incentive spirometer.

Thoracotomy results in a temporary decrease in vital capacity of 30% (in part due to pain and atelectasis) and increased upper airway bacterial load. Thus, important postoperative measures include using adequate but not excessive pain control and encouraging the patient to cough frequently and to use the incentive spirometer. Both cancer and chronic obstructive lung disease are independent risk factors for deep venous thrombosis and pulmonary embolism. Therefore, as with all surgical patients, early ambulation, lower extremity sequential compression devices, and, when surgically feasible, low-dose unfractionated or low molecular weight heparin are important preventative measures. Normal activities can be resumed within several weeks of surgery, depending on the pulmonary reserve.

Radiotherapy

Definitive radiotherapy is not as effective a therapy as surgery, but it offers a potential for cure or for prolonged survival when surgery is not an option. Although compromised lung function may limit the ability to deliver radiation, definitive external radiotherapy may cure 15% to 20% of patients with stage I and II disease who have contraindications to surgery (56). As discussed earlier, radiotherapy has a role in stage IIIA, IIIB, and IV disease and, possibly as part of a multimodal approach, in stage I and II disease.

The complications of external radiation include pneumonitis, pulmonary fibrosis, and dysphagia from transient esophagitis. The rate of these complications depends on the time and dosage of radiation delivery and the volume of normal tissue exposed. However, complication rates have fallen in recent years as techniques have improved. Minimizing pulmonary risk in a patient with underlying lung disease requires individualization of radiation protocols by the radiation oncologist, taking into account the extent of the pulmonary disease and the anatomy of the tumor.

Palliative Therapies

For patients who are not candidates for other therapies, local symptom palliation may be accomplished by palliative external beam radiation therapy. Palliative radiotherapy is delivered over shorter intervals and in lower dosages than those used for definitive therapy, and it relieves hemoptysis, superior vena cava syndrome, and dyspnea in 60% to 80% of patients. However, it is rare for vocal cord paralysis to respond. Although less than 20% of NSCLC patients with atelectasis respond to radiotherapy, 57% of those with SCLC (see below) re-expand collapsed lobes or lungs (57).

Laser therapy, brachytherapy, and the bronchoscopic placement of prosthetic stents are other options for the symptomatic relief of major airway obstruction (40). These procedures may require hospitalization and need to be performed by physicians familiar with their use. The neodynium-yttrium aluminum garnet laser is useful for debulking endobronchial obstructing lesions. Symptomatic relief is immediate and dramatic but may last 1 to 3 months in two-thirds of patients because of tumor regrowth. Thus repeated procedures may be required, with increasing procedure-related mortality.

Endoscopically placed brachytherapy with iridium-192 is used to reduce either endobronchial or extraluminal compressing masses. This therapy relieves symptoms more rapidly than external radiation, although not as rapidly as laser therapy, and has a longer duration of response with fewer complications compared with laser. Brachytherapy also does not cause the regional pneumonitis that limits the use of external radiation. The risks of endobronchial brachytherapy and laser therapy are bronchial perforation and hemorrhage with asphyxiation. In addition, local edema with critical airway occlusion can complicate laser therapy, and fistulas may form after brachytherapy.

Brachytherapy can also be delivered intraoperatively by permanent implantation of iodine-125 or palladium-103 seeds. Chest wall lesions may be treated with temporary iridium-192 seeds. This type of brachytherapy is particularly helpful for superior sulcus tumors. The roles of laser or brachytherapy as definitive therapies for bronchogenic carcinoma remain to be defined (58).

Role of Consultants

Given the above therapeutic considerations, patients with NSCLC should be considered for referral to specialists based on tumor stage and on the patient's functional and medical status. Tumors of stages I, II, and IIIA are potentially resectable, and patients in these categories should be referred for surgical evaluation, depending on comorbid medical conditions and pulmonary function, as outlined above. Patients in these stages who are not surgical candidates should be referred to a radiation oncologist for possible external radiation therapy.

Patients with NSCLC of tumor stages II and III and those with stage IV tumors who have good physiologic function should also be referred to a medical oncologist for evaluation for chemotherapy. The role of combined chemotherapy and radiation therapy for subgroups is being defined, and the medical oncologist may involve a radiation oncologist in the treatment protocol. Patients with bone pain, pulmonary symptoms due to airway obstruction, and brain metastases should be referred to a radiation oncologist for palliative therapy. As noted above, some patients with solitary brain metastases and stage I or II NSCLC may be candidates for neurosurgical intervention (51,53).

Hospice care (see Chapter 13) is a consideration for patients with stage IV tumors and significant comorbid conditions and for those with poor performance status or who have failed repeated therapies.

Small Cell Lung Cancer

Almost all patients with SCLC have either clinically evident or subclinical metastases at presentation. Except for the rare isolated SCLC, surgery is generally not an option, and the mainstay of treatment is chemotherapy. Therefore, all these patients should be

Table 61.7. Influence of Therapy on Survival of Patients with Small Cell Lung Cancer

Era	Survival: Limited Disease	Survival: Extensive Disease
Prechemotherapy		
Supportive care (median)	3 mo	1.5 mo
Surgery (5 yr)	<1%	
Radiotherapy (5 yr)	1%–3%	
Chemotherapy		
Single agent (median)[a]	6 mo	4 mo
Combination		
Median	10–14 mo	7–11 mo
5 yr	2%–8%	0–1%
Combination with chest irradiation		
Median	12–16 mo	7–11 mo
5 yr	6%–12%	0–1%

[a]Some recent results suggest that longer median survival may be possible in selected patients.

From Ihde DC. Chemotherapy of lung cancer. N Engl J Med 1992;327:1434, with permission.

referred to a medical oncologist; this consultant will usually involve a radiation oncologist. Chemotherapy (in conjunction with radiotherapy for patients with limited disease) increases survival for most patients with extensive and limited disease and has the potential for cure of a few patients with limited disease. Combination chemotherapy results in initial response rates of 65% to 90%, including 10% to 40% complete responses, depending on the stage. Unfortunately, relapse is the rule, and salvage chemotherapy is significantly less efficacious (59). The standard chemotherapeutic protocol uses a combination of two to four agents given every 3 to 4 weeks for six to eight courses. The current common regimen uses cyclophosphamide, daunorubicin, and vincristine. Cisplatin and etoposide may also be given. Some protocols add cranial irradiation. The major toxicity of the chemotherapeutic agents used for SCLC is nausea and vomiting, myelosuppression, alopecia, neurotoxicity, and cardiomyopathy (see Chapter 10 for other common adverse effects of chemotherapy). Table 61.7 shows the influence of combination chemotherapy on the survival of patients with SCLC. These survival statistics have not changed appreciably over the past 15 years, although newer agents seem promising. Chemotherapy for lung cancer may be given to ambulatory patients and is administered by an oncologist.

The patient's quality of life is as important as survival, and newer protocols track this outcome. For those with dyspnea, treatment involves addressing the underlying cause(s). In addition, for the appropriate patient, narcotics need to be considered for palliation.

FOLLOW-UP OF PATIENTS SURVIVING LUNG CANCER

Lung cancer is most likely to recur within the first 5 years, although 9% of patients with resected stage I disease may have recurrences more than 5 years after treatment. One-third of these first reappearances are local. Although lung cancers can metastasize anywhere, the most common sites are regional lymph nodes, brain, lung, liver, and bone (60).

Patients who have had a lung cancer have a significant risk of a second primary cancer. In one large study of patients with resected stage I NSCLC, one-third had second synchronous or metachronous cancers discovered over 10 years of follow-up, of which one-third were second primary lung cancers (60). Chemotherapy increases the incidence of leukemia and of myelodysplastic syndromes. Cranial irradiation may produce central nervous system toxicity, and symptoms may not appear for several years.

Follow-up at least every 3 to 4 months for the first few years after resection of a lung cancer, and at least yearly thereafter, is advised to detect metastases or local recurrence and second primary malignancies. Patients with lung cancers may be a group for which serial low-energy CT and/or PET may be useful screening maneuvers, although this has not been studied. Close attention to standard recommendations for early detection of extrapulmonary cancers, such as yearly history and physical examination, monitoring for occult fecal blood, and routine mammography, are advisable. Symptoms of bone pain may be assessed with bone scans and x-rays. Neurologic signs or symptoms may be evaluated by head CT or MRI (gadolinium enhances the sensitivity). Chest symptoms can be evaluated with x-ray, CT, and/or bronchoscopy. Abdominal CT is more sensitive than liver function studies for the evaluation of patients with signs or symptoms of hepatic metastases.

CHEMOPROPHYLAXIS

In addition to encouraging patients to stop smoking, there has been much interest in the concept of chemoprophylaxis to both inhibit and reverse pulmonary carcinogenesis. Pulmonary carcinogenesis is believed to involve the progressive accumulation of genetic lesions and pathologic dysplasia. There likely is a "field defect" involving the interaction of genetic predisposition with environmental triggers. Patients who have had a previous carcinoma are at high risk for developing a second primary tumor.

Potential chemoprophylactic agents include vitamins: the retinoids, the carotenoids, alpha-tocopherol, and a potential detoxifying (antioxidant) agent, *N*-acetylcysteine. To date, the results of large primary prevention trials of at-risk populations have been discouraging. Indeed, both the CARET study, which tested the combination of beta-carotene and retinyl palmitate against placebo for 18,314 men and women (including 14,254 cigarette smokers), and the ATBC trial which examined the effects of beta-carotene, with or without alpha-tocopherol, in 29,133 cigarette-smoking men found that beta-carotene significantly increased the risk of lung cancer (reviewed in ref. 28). The EUROSCAN trial found no tumor-free or survival advantage of supplemental retinyl palmitate and/or *N*-acetylcysteine for 2,592 patients with head and neck or lung cancers (61).

PLEURAL EFFUSIONS

Patients with bronchogenic carcinoma and pleural effusion usually have dyspnea and cough, although one-fourth are asymptomatic. In contrast, most patients with malignant mesothelioma and effusion have chest pain that is usually dull and nonpleuritic. In one-third of patients with carcinomatous pleurisy, the effusions are bilateral, and three-fourths of patients have moderate to large pleural effusions. Indeed, the absence of a mediastinal shift in the setting of a large effusion is highly suggestive of a tumor either fixing the mediastinum, obstructing a main bronchus, or simulating an effusion in the pleural space.

There are two categories of pleural effusion in the setting of lung cancer: carcinomatous involvement of the pleura (malignant effusion) and paramalignant effusion in which the pleura is not involved with tumor. Malignant effusions are usually exudative, are serosanguinous or bloody, and may have a lymphocytosis, a low pH, and a low glucose concentration (see Chapter 59). Elevated amylase (salivary isotype) in a patient without an esophageal rupture may be seen in pleural effusions with adenocarcinoma, and elevated hyaluronic acid may be seen in those associated with malignant mesothelioma. The paramalignant effusion may be either exudative or transudative and may be due to mediastinal or peripheral carcinoma obstructing lymph drainage, central venous obstruction due to tumor, or secondary to postobstructive pneumonia or atelectasis. Becuase patients who smoke and are older are at increased risk of coronary artery disease, congestive heart failure needs to be considered in the differential diagnosis of a transudative effusion in this group of patients.

The patient with a malignant effusion is not surgically curable, and most patients die within 6 months of diagnosis. However, those with paramalignant effusions may be candidates for surgery, generally as part of a combined modality therapy. Thus, the cause of pleural effusion needs to be established in patients with otherwise curable bronchogenic carcinoma, as well as for those with nonresectable carcinoma to help direct palliative therapy.

Thoracentesis, with cytologic evaluation of fluid, provides diagnoses in more than two-thirds of cases of malignant effusions, with the yield improved by repeating the procedure, as well as by blind pleural biopsy. Potential complications of these procedures include pneumothorax (5% to 10%), bleeding (approximately 1%), and parietal pleural seeding (1% to 2%). Unfortunately, for 10% to 20% of patients with malignant effusions, these studies are nondiagnostic. Both thoracentesis and pleural biopsy are routinely done in an ambulatory setting, the latter only by pulmonologists or thoracic surgeons.

Thoracoscopy (discussed earlier) is a more sensitive examination for pleural disease in the patient with suspected malignant effusion. Thoracoscopically directed pleural biopsy correctly identifies malignancy in 95% of affected patients (62). More studies are needed to validate the promise of PET for differentiating malignant from benign pleural effusions (63).

Patient Experience. For thoracentesis and pleural biopsy, patients are administered a local anesthetic before the insertion of a needle into the pleural space. The patient feels the injection of lidocaine, which stings for a few seconds until the onset of anesthesia. Lung re-expansion usually causes some coughing and may be associated with a chest sensation that some patients find uncomfortable or even painful. Pneumothorax, which may be either due to needle trauma of the lung or to the sucking in of air into an emptied pleural space in the setting of a noncompliant lung, may be associated with increased shortness of breath or chest of shoulder pain on the affected side. However, pneumothorax may be asymptomatic, so a postthoracentesis chest x-ray is mandatory for all patients. The pneumothorax may be followed in an outpatient with serial chest x-rays or may require chest tube placement, depending on the clinical scenario.

For diagnostic medical thoracoscopy, a short-acting sedative (e.g., midazolam or propofol) and a short-acting opiate (fentanyl) are injected intravenously. Then a small incision is made under local anesthesia and an endoscope is passed into the pleural space. Patients feel pressure during the performance of the procedure. For video-assisted thoracic surgery, patients require general anesthesia.

Both thoracentesis and thoracoscopic evaluation of the pleura take approximately 30 minutes to perform.

The treatment of pleural effusions in the setting of lung cancer depends on the cause. Systemic chemotherapy is the main option for patients with malignant effusions due to SCLC and is one option for patients with unresectable NSCLC. Otherwise, various palliative procedures may be tried.

Those patients with effusions secondary to mediastinal lymphatic obstruction may be candidates for external radiotherapy. Effusions secondary to postobstructive processes may be amenable to external radiotherapy or to laser therapy, brachytherapy, or placement of a prosthetic stent, all procedures directed at reestablishing bronchial patency.

Large malignant effusions, which usually recur after they are drained, may be treated with repeated thoracentesis. However, the most common approach to the malignant effusion is pleurodesis. In general, the optimal candidate for this procedure is one who has already demonstrated symptom relief with thoracentesis and has a prognosis of greater than a few months. Patients with bulky pleural disease or central bronchial obstruction are less likely to respond to pleurodesis because the lung needs to re-expand and the pleural surfaces to appose in order to seal. Pleurodesis is helpful in three-fourhts of selected patients. Surgical pleural abrasion or pleurectomy has a higher morbidity and mortality than closed pleurodesis but may be useful for certain patients (62).

Patient Experience. For pleurodesis, the pleural space is drained as completely as possible with a chest tube in the hospital, and a sclerosing agent (talc, doxycycline, or bleomycin) is instilled into the pleural space. The patient generally requires narcotics while the chest tube is in. The chest tube is clamped, and the patient is told to move sequentially in different positions over the subsequent several hours. Doxycycline pleurodesis may be painful, and simultaneous lidocaine instillation and/or narcotics are usually given. Talc pleurodesis may produce fever, with onset at 4 to 12 hours that may last for 72 hours. The sclerosing agent may need to be reinstilled after a few days if the first treatment is ineffective. Pleurodesis generally requires hospitalization, but for some patients with unloculated effusions, a pig-tail catheter can be inserted on an ambulatory basis for the delivery of the sclerosing agent.

SOLITARY PULMONARY NODULE

An SPN is defined as a single focal spherical density in the pulmonary parenchyma that is not associated with any other parenchymal process or with adenopathy. Its diameter is variously designated in the medical literature as up to 3 to 4 cm. One-half of these lesions are malignant, either primary pulmonary cancers or metastases from an extrapulmonary source. Surgical resection is possible in 80% of those with an SPN, and the 5-year survival rate is 40%. These figures are significantly better than those for lung cancer as a group. The nonmalignant lesions are due to a diverse group of processes, including the residua of prior granulomatous diseases (e.g., tuberculosis or fungal infection), hamartomas, bronchial adenomas, organizing pneumonia, pulmonary infarcts, and arteriovenous malformations (64). The management of the SPN for an individual patient is based on a risk–benefit analysis, including the probability that the nodule is malignant, the risks of the contemplated diagnostic and therapeutic procedures, the accuracy of biopsy techniques, the risk that a delay in therapy will affect outcome, and, finally, the informed patient's preference.

There are four possible strategies for managing a patient with an SPN. The first is to do no further follow-up. The second is to refer the patient for an immediate invasive study for diagnosis. The third is to refer the patient for immediate surgical excision. The fourth is to observe the SPN carefully over time ("watchful waiting") for any signs that would move the patient to one of the other management strategies. The course of action for any individual patient is determined by the answers to four questions and may be aided by PET.

Question 1: Is the visualized lesion really an SPN? It has been estimated that 10% to 20% of lesions interpreted as possible SPNs on the initial chest x-ray are not actual SPNs (65). In these cases, what appeared to be a pulmonary nodule may actually be an extraparenchymal process (e.g., bone, vascular, or chest wall lesion), or alternatively, the pulmonary nodule may not be a solitary process (i.e., additional disease is present). Other radiologic studies, including a review of old films and CTs, may be helpful.

Question 2: What is the age and stability of the nodule? Comparing the current studies with prior x-rays is needed to answer this question. The doubling time for a pulmonary malignancy ranges from 20 to 400 days. Thus, the lack of growth of an SPN for several years is sufficient evidence of benign disease.

Question 3: What are the characteristics of the patient that increase the risk for malignancy? The establishment of smoking status (or other toxic exposure as outlined in Table 61.1) is one cornerstone of this investigation. The second is the patient's age: The prevalence of malignancy in SPNs is 1% in patients less than 35 years old but increases rapidly with years above this age (66). Furthermore, the history of a prior malignancy mandates a more aggressive approach because in 80% of these patients, the SPN will prove to be either a primary or metastatic malignancy (67). It is important that an SPN in a patient with a known extrapulmonary primary tumor is biopsied because these nodules are more likely to be a new primary tumor of the lung than to be a metastasis (68).

Question 4: What are the risk characteristics of the nodule? The most important risk characteristic of an SPN is its growth rate, as previously discussed. Second, although calcification may be seen in malignant disease, certain patterns of calcification favor a benign diagnosis. A dense central nidus and a diffuse or laminated pattern of calcification are reliable signs of healed granuloma. A popcorn pattern of calcification suggests a hamartoma. However, an eccentric nidus of calcification is uninformative and may be due to a cancer engulfing a prior calcified lesion. CT densitometry is more sensitive than chest x-ray for demonstrating calcification (69).

Other characteristics are also important to examine. A nodule of greater than 3 cm in diameter is likely malignant. Further, an irregular lesion with poorly defined or spiculated borders has a high likelihood of malignancy.

To answer these questions, the workup of the SPN includes first obtaining the necessary films to verify the presence of an SPN, examining all prior x-rays, and, finally, obtaining a chest CT to confirm the presence of disease, demonstrate associated disease, examine the characteristics of the nodule (including size, shape, and the presence of calcification, fat, fluid, and vessels), and evaluate the diagnostic approach.

Two of these management strategy groups should fall out immediately from this initial appraisal. For one group of patients, the benign nature of the process may be assured after some or all of these steps; these patients will not require further evaluation. Patients who have a high risk of malignancy based on the above criteria should undergo a staging evaluation (as per above discussion) and should be referred for surgery if appropriate. For the patient who does not fall into one of these two groups, the decision as to whether to refer the patient for an immediate biopsy or whether to adopt a watchful waiting approach may be aided by the findings from a PET. Prospective studies show a sensitivity of PETs for all SPNs is 90% to 92% and specificity is 83% to 90%. The sensitivity of PET decreases to 80% for nodules less than 1.5 cm, and carcinoids, bronchoalveolar carcinomas, and a few adenocarcinomas may be missed (70,71). Thus follow-up of negative scans (the watchful waiting strategy) is mandatory. A positive PET would favor the immediate biopsy strategy.

The diagnostic techniques for obtaining a biopsy of an SPN include fluoroscopically directed PTNA; fluoroscopically directed transbronchial biopsy or TBNA, done through a fiberoptic bronchoscope; thoracoscopic biopsy; or thoracotomy. These procedures have been discussed earlier. The diagnostic yield of PTNA is 70% to 90% and of transbronchial biopsy is 30% to 70% (64,72). Nonneoplastic causes of peripheral nodules (especially certain infections) may be diagnosed by transbronchial biopsy or PTNA. However, the specter of false negative results mandates that nonspecific findings are followed by either another procedure or by watchful waiting. The choice of the initial diagnostic technique and of the follow-up management is best determined by a pulmonologist in consultation with the patient.

Based on the discussion above, the watchful waiting strategy would be appropriate management, for example, for a patient less than 35 years old with no risk factors and with a small well-defined nodule that is negative on PET, a patient with a nodule of less than 2.5 cm that has been unchanged in size for 2 years by prior chest x-rays, a patient with few risks who has had negative diagnostic studies, or a patient for whom the risk of the diagnostic and therapeutic procedures outweigh the risks of watchful waiting. Given the range of tumor doubling times, it is unlikely that the delay inherent in this strategy would result in a significant decrease in survival for the patient with a pulmonary nodule that is malignant (66). A scheme for monitoring serial x-rays might be to obtain repeat films every 3 to 4 months for 1 year, then every 6 months for 1 year, and then to repeat at yearly intervals thereafter. The total number of years to follow a nodule depends on the suspicion of malignancy based on the above criteria. For patients for whom the level of suspicion is low, serial studies for 2 years are adequate. For the patient for whom the level of suspicion for malignancy is high, a 5-year follow-up is necessary to encompass the unusually slow-growing carcinoma (usually an adenocarcinoma).

General References

Feld R, Ginsberg RJ, Payne DG, et al. Lung. In: Abeloff MD, Armitage JO, Lichter AS, et al., eds. Clinical oncology, 2nd ed. Philadelphia: Churchill Livingstone, 2000:1398.

Vaporiciyan AA, Nesbitt JC, Lee JS, et al. Cancer of the lung. In: Bast RC, Kufe DW, Pollock RE, et al., eds. Cancer medicine, 5th ed. London: BC Decker, 2000:1227.

Specific References*

1. Smith RA, Glynn TJ. Epidemiology of lung cancer. Radiol Clin North Am 2000;38:453.
2. Wingo PA, Ries LA, Giovino GA, et al. Annual report to the nation on the status of cancer 1973–1996, with a special section on lung cancer and tobacco smoking. J Natl Cancer Inst 1999;91:675.
3. Peto R. Influence of dose and duration of smoking on lung cancer rates. IARC Sci Publ 1986;74:23.
4. American Thoracic Society. Cigarette smoking and health. Am J Respir Crit Care Med 1996;153:861.
5. Doll R, Peto R. Cigarette smoking and bronchial carcinoma: dose and time relationships among regular smokers and life-long nonsmokers. J Epidemiol Community Health 1978;32:303.
6. Zhong L, Goldberg MS, Parent ME, et al. Exposure to environmental tobacco smoke and the risk of lung cancer: a meta-analysis. Lung Cancer 2000;27:3.
7. National Cancer Institute. The FTC cigarette test method for determining tar, nicotine, and carbon monoxide yields of U.S. cigarettes. Report of the NCI expert committee. Smoking and Tobacco Control Monograph No. 7. Bethesda, MD: U.S. Department of Health and Human Services, Public Health Service, National Institutes of Health, National Cancer Institute; NIH Publ. No. 9-4028, 1996.
8. Steenland K, Loomis D, Shy C, et al. Review of occupational lung carcinogens. Am J Ind Med 1996;29:474.
9. Selikoff IJ, Hammond EC. Asbestos and smoking. JAMA 1979;242:458.
10. Lubin JH, Boice JD, Lung cancer risk from residential radon: meta-analysis of eight epidemiologic studies. J Natl Cancer Inst 1997;89:49.
11. Shaw GL, Falk RT, Pickle LW, et al. Lung cancer risk associated with cancer in relatives. J Clin Epidemiol 1991;44:429.
12. Saraceno J, Spivack SD. Strategies for early detection of lung cancer. Clin Pulm Med 1999;6:66.
13. Amos CI, Xu W, Spitz MR. Is there a genetic basis for lung cancer susceptibility? Recent Results Cancer Res 1999;151:3.
14. Tockman MS, Anthonisen NR, Wright EC, et al. Airways obstruction and the risk for lung cancer. Ann Intern Med 1987;106:512.
15. Hubbard R, Venn A, Lewis S, et al. Lung cancer and cryptogenic fibrosing alveolitis: a population-based cohort study. Am J Respir Crit Care Med 2000;161:5.
16. Katariya K, Thurer RJ. Malignancies associated with the immunocompromised state. Chest Surg Clin North Am 1999;9:63.
17. Weiss W, Seidman H, Boucot KR. The Philadelphia Pulmonary Neoplasm Research Project: symptoms in occult lung cancer. Chest 1978;73:57.
18. Fry WA, Menck HR, Winchester DP. The National Cancer Data Base report on lung cancer. Cancer 1996;77:1947.
19. Rom WN, Hay TC, Lee TC, et al. Molecular and genetic aspects of lung cancer. Am J Respir Crit Care Med 2000;161:1355.
20. Frost JK, Ball WC Jr, Levin ML, et al. Early lung cancer detection: results of the initial (prevalence) radiologic and cytologic screening in the Johns Hopkins study. Am Rev Respir Dis 1984;130:549.
21. Parkin DM, Moss SM. Lung cancer screening: Improved survival but no reduction in deaths—the role of "overdiagnosis." Cancer 2000;89:2369.
22. Patz EF Jr, Goodman PC, Bepler G. Screening for lung cancer. N Engl J Med 2000;343:1627.
23. Henschke CI, McCauley DI, Yankelevitz DF, et al. Early Lung Cancer Action Project: overall design and findings from baseline screening. Lancet 1999;354:99.

*Bold print (general references) and bold numerals (specific references) denote published controlled clinical trials, meta-analyses, or consensus-based recommendations.

24. Hazelrigg SR, Boley TM, Weber D, et al. Incidence of lung nodules found in patients undergoing lung volume reduction. Ann Thorac Surg 1997;64:303.
25. Goodman GE. Prevention of lung cancer. Crit Rev Oncol Hematol 2000;33:187.
26. Vaporiciyan AA, Nesbitt JC, Lee JS, et al. Neoplasms of the thorax: cancer of the lung. In: Bast RC, Kufe DW, Pollock RE, et al., eds. Cancer medicine, 5th ed. Hamilton, Ontario: BC Decker, 2000:1227.
27. Thun MJ, Lally CA, Flannery JT, et al. Cigarette smoking and change in the histopathology of lung cancer. J Natl Cancer Inst 1997;89:1580.
28. Franceschi S, Bidoli E. The epidemiology of lung cancer. Ann Oncol 1999;10[Suppl 5]:S3.
29. Auerbach O, Garfinckel L. The changing pattern of lung carcinoma. Cancer 1991;68:1973.
30. Barkley JE, Green MR. Bronchioloalveolar carcinoma [Review]. J Clin Oncol 1996;14:3277.
31. Chahinian AP, Pass HI. Malignant mesothelioma. In: Bast RC, Kufe DW, Pollock RE, et al., eds. Cancer medicine, 5th ed. Hamilton, Ontario: BC Decker, 2000.
32. Snider GL. When not to use the bronchoscope for hemoptysis [Editorial]. Chest 1979;76:1.
33. Adelman M, Haponik EF, Bleecker ER, et al. Cryptogenic hemoptysis: clinical features, bronchoscopic findings, and natural history of 67 patients. Ann Intern Med 1985;102:829.
34. Patel AM, Davila DG, Peters SG. Paraneoplastic syndromes associated with lung cancer. Mayo Clin Proc 1993;68:278.
35. Shaham D, Guralnik L. The solitary pulmonary nodule: radiologic considerations. Semin Ultrasound CT MR 2000;21:97.
36. McLoud TC, Bourgouin PM, Greenberg RW, et al. Bronchogenic carcinoma: analysis of staging in the mediastinum with CT by correlative node mapping and sampling. Radiology 1992;182:319.
37. Mehta AC, Marty JJ, Lee FYW. Sputum cytology. Clin Chest Med 1993;14:69.
38. Arroliga AC, Matthay RA. The role of bronchoscopy in lung cancer. Clin Chest Med 1993;14:87.
39. Haponik EF, Kvale P, Wang KP. Bronchoscopy and related procedures. In: Fishman AP, ed. Pulmonary disease and disorders, 2nd ed. New York: McGraw-Hill, 1988:437.
40. Cortese DA, Edell ES. Role of phototherapy, laser therapy, brachytherapy, and prosthetic stents in the management of lung cancer. Clin Chest Med 1993;14:149.
41. Khouri NF, Stitik FP, Erozan YS, et al. Transthoracic needle aspiration biopsy of benign and malignant lung lesions. AJR Am J Roentgenol 1985;144:281.
42. McElvein RB. Procedures in the evaluation of chest disease. Clin Chest Med 1992;13:1.
43. Miller DL, Allen MS, Deschamps C, et al. Video-assisted thoracic surgical procedure: management of a solitary pulmonary nodule. Mayo Clin Proc 1992;64:462.
44. Boutin C, Viallat JR, Cargnino P, et al. Thoracoscopy in malignant pleural effusions. Am Rev Respir Dis 1981;124:588.
45. Pieterman, RM, van Putten JW, Meuzelaar JJ, et al. Preoperative staging of non-small-cell lung cancer with positron-emission tomography. N Engl J Med 2000;343:254.
46. Dwamena BA, Sonnad SS, Angobaldo JO, et al. Metastases from non-small cell lung cancer: mediastinal staging in the 1990s—Meta-analytic comparison of PET and CT. Radiology 1999;213:530.
47. Silvestri GA, Littenberg B, Colice GL. The clinical evaluation for detecting metastatic lung cancer: a meta-analysis. Am J Respir Crit Care Med 1995;152:225.
48. Hillers TK, Sauve MD, Guyatt GH. Analysis of published studies on the detection of extrathoracic metastases in patients presumed to have operable non-small cell lung cancer. Thorax 1994;49:14.
49. American Thoracic Society/European Respiratory Society. Pretreatment evaluation of non-small-cell lung cancer. Am J Respir Crit Care Med 1997;156:320.
50. Stanley KE. Prognostic factors for survival in patients with inoperable lung cancer. J Natl Cancer Inst 1980;65:25.
51. Reif MS, Socinski MA, Rivera MP. Evidence-based medicine in the treatment of non-small-cell lung cancer. Clin Chest Med 2000;21:107.
52. Wagner H. Postoperative adjuvant therapy for patients with resected non-small cell lung cancer: still controversial after all these years. Chest 2000;117:110S.
53. American Society of Clinical Oncology. Clinical practice guidelines for the treatment of unresectable non-small-cell lung cancer. J Clin Oncol 1997;15:2996.
54. Kelly K, Bunn PA. Is it time to reevaluate our approach to the treatment of brain metastases in patients with non-small cell lung cancer. Lung Cancer 1998;20:85.
55. Dunn WF, Scanlon PD. Preoperative pulmonary function testing for patients with lung cancer. Mayo Clin Proc 1993;68:371.
56. Dosoretz DE, Galimarini MS, Rubenstein JH, et al. Local control in medically inoperable lung cancer: an analysis of its importance in outcome and factors determining the probability of tumor eradication. Int J Radiat Oncol Biol Phys 1993;27:507.
57. Slawson R, Scott R. Radiation therapy in bronchogenic carcinoma. Radiology 1979;132:175.
58. Hilaris BS, Mastoras DA. Contemporary brachytherapy approaches in non-small-cell lung cancer. J Surg Oncol 1998;69:258.
59. Bunn PA, Carney DN. Overview of chemotherapy for small cell lung cancer. Semin Oncol 1997;24[Suppl 7]:S69.
60. Martini N, Bains MS, Burt ME, et al. Incidence of local recurrence and second primary tumors in resected stage I lung cancer. J Thorac Cardiovasc Surg 1995;109:120.
61. Van Zandwijk N, Dalesio O, Pastorino U, et al, for the European Organization for Research and Treatment of Cancer Head and Neck and Lung Cancer Cooperative Groups. EUROSCAN, a randomized trial of vitamin A and N-acetylcysteine in patients with head and neck cancer or lung cancer. J Natl Cancer Inst 2000;92:977.
62. American Thoracic Society. Management of malignant pleural effusions. Am J Respir Crit Care Med 2000;162:1987.
63. Erasmus JJ, McAdams HP, Rossi SE, et al. FDG PET of pleural effusions in patients with non-small cell lung cancer. AJR Am J Roentgenol 2000;175:245.
64. Lillington GA, Caskey CI. Evaluation and management of solitary and multiple pulmonary nodules. Clin Chest Med 1993;14:111.
65. Khouri NF, Meziane MA, Zerhouni EA, et al. The solitary pulmonary nodule. Assessment, diagnosis and management. Chest 1987;91:128.
66. Cummings SR, Lillington GA, Richard RJ, et al. Managing solitary pulmonary nodules. The choice of strategy is a "close call." Am Rev Respir Dis 1986;134:453.
67. Neifeld JP, Michaelis LL, Doppman JL. Suspected pulmonary metastases: correlation of chest x-ray, whole lung tomography, and operative findings. Cancer 1977;39:383.
68. Cahan WG. Multiple primary cancers of the lung, esophagus and other sites. Cancer 1977;40:1954.
69. Siegelman SS, Zerhouni EA, Leo FP, et al. CT of the solitary pulmonary nodule. AJR Am J Roentgenol 1980;135:1.
70. Lowe VJ, Fletcher JW, Gobar L, et al. Prospective investigation of positron emission tomography in lung nodules. J Clin Oncol 1998;16:1075.
71. Prauer HW, Weber WA, Romer W, et al. Controlled prospective study of positron emission tomography using the glucose analogue [18f]fluorodeoxyglucose in the evaluation of pulmonary nodules. Br J Surg 1998;85:1506.
72. Cortese DA. Solitary pulmonary nodule: observe, operate or what [Editorial]? Chest 1982;81:662.

SECTION 9

Cardiovascular Problems

CHAPTER 62

Coronary Artery Disease

MARK D. KELEMEN, MD, MSc
NISHA CHANDRA STROBOS, MD

Chest pain is one of the most common complaints of patients in an ambulatory practice. The major early objective in the diagnosis of such patients is the separation of noncardiac from cardiac pain. Chapters 42 and 59 describes the various causes of noncardiac chest pain. This chapter describes the pathogenesis of coronary artery disease (CAD) and its most common clinical symptom, angina pectoris. Chapter 63 describes the posthospital medical care and rehabilitation of patients who have had a myocardial infarction.

CAD caused by atherosclerosis is one of the most common ailments in the Western world, and it remains the leading nontraumatic cause of disability and death in the United States. Increased public awareness and health education have dropped CAD mortality by more than 20% in the last 25 years. However, CAD is still the leading cause of death among American men and women (1). Patients with chest pain often seek medical attention. It is essential that health care providers know how to respond to such patients in order to make appropriate diagnostic and therapeutic decisions. In the approach to the patient with chest pain, a detailed history and physical examination must not be replaced by sophisticated procedures but should allow the clinician to select the most appropriate diagnostic tests.

PATHOGENESIS

The endothelium plays an integral role in the defense against atherosclerosis and in modulating vascular tone and preventing thrombosis in blood vessels. These endothelial functions are affected by the presence of CAD risk factors, even before atherosclerosis is evident. In the earliest stages, circulating monocytes adhere to endothelial cells (via adhesion molecules) and migrate into the intima of the blood vessel, where they ingest oxidatively-modified low-density lipoprotein (LDL) and get trapped as foam cells. Collections of foam cells, known as fatty streaks, have been found in early childhood. Foam cells die, leading to the development of a lipid core, and smooth muscle cells are signaled to migrate from the media, destroying the internal elastic lamina of the vessel in the process. Calcification of the plaque occurs early and may be able to be visualized noninvasively by electron beam computed tomography (EBCT, see later discussion). The arterial wall begins to thicken and remodel. We now know from intravascular ultrasound studies that encroachment of plaque into the lumen of a coronary artery is a late process and reflects advanced disease (arterial cross-sectional area is reduced by 40% before a lesion is visible as "significant" CAD at catheterization).

The progression of atherosclerosis is accelerated by three processes: endothelial dysfunction, inflammation, and thrombosis. The advanced lesion is characterized by a core of lipid and necrotic tissue surrounded by a fibrous cap. This cap contains collagen, and its characteristics are closely related to the risk of plaque rupture, which is the major cause of acute coronary syndromes. Specifically, the thinner the cap, the more likely it is that rupture will occur. Shear stress at the edge or "shoulder" region of a plaque, inflammation at the endothelial surface of the cap, or internal degradation of the cap by enzymes known as metalloproteinases also are important determinants of the likelihood of plaque rupture. A ruptured plaque leads very quickly to thrombus formation. Complete occlusion of a coronary vessel by thrombus on a ruptured plaque typically causes an acute transmural myocardial infarction (MI) characterized by ST elevation on the electrocardiogram (ECG). Nonocclusive thrombus can cause unstable angina or an MI, without ST elevation. Nonocclusive thrombus may not cause symptoms, but instead may change plaque geometry and lead to rapid plaque growth. Transmural and nontransmural MIs are treated very differently (2,3). Studies have shown that an acute MI may be more likely to occur in an area that was previously not severely narrowed (i.e., less than 50% luminal reduction by angiography) than in an area that was more severely narrowed (i.e., more than 70% reduction) (4,5). It is true, however, that atherosclerotic narrowing of a coronary artery by 70% or greater is more likely than a less severe narrowing to cause exertional angina. The discordance between plaque severity and the development of acute MI indicates that coronary disease is not simply a mechanical problem.

Most patients with classic angina by history have fixed atherosclerotic lesions of 70% or more in at least one major coronary artery. Angina is caused by a mismatch between myocardial oxygen supply and demand. Supply is affected by coronary perfusion pressure and coronary vascular resistance. Flow is autoregulated over a wide variety of perfusion pressures, and therefore most of the changes in flow are due to changes in resistance (i.e., vasodilation). However, the coronary bed beyond a significant flow-limiting stenosis is already maximally vasodilated, so that small increases in demand (e.g., increased heart rate and blood pressure during exercise) may result in myocardial ischemia. Demand is related to heart rate, systolic blood pressure, and wall tension. Wall tension is determined by ventricular pressure, cavity size, and wall thickness. Exercise and emotional stress have potent effects on these variables and, not coincidentally, are the common triggers for ischemic chest pain.

RISK FACTORS

Both genetic and environmental risk factors influence the development of atherosclerotic heart disease. The recognition of risk factors is especially important because many of these conditions can be modified to prevent disease. Landmark epidemiologic surveys such as the Framingham Heart Study have helped to define levels of risk for the individual risk factors. Treatment guidelines have recently been revised to include the important interactions between individual risk factors and age. Risk calculators (CAD event risk over 10 years) are available on the Internet at http://www.intmed.mcw.edu/clincalc/heartrisk.html (accessed 1/7/02). The 27th Bethesda Conference was designed to bring attention to specific patients at high risk for the development of CAD events (6). This work has been incorporated into the National Cholesterol Education Program (NCEP) Expert Panel on Detection, Evaluation and Treatment of High Blood Cholesterol in Adults (Adult Treatment Panel III or ATP-III) (see Chapter 82) (7). The concepts of "risk" and "risk factor" are important in understanding and using the guidelines. The Bethesda Conference outlined four categories of risk based on observational studies and efficacy studies (clinical trials). These risk factors are summarized in Table 62.1.

Table 62.1. Risk Factors for Cardiovascular Disease (CVD)

Category 1 (Factors for Which Interventions Have Been Proved to Lower CVD Risk)
Cigarette smoking
Elevated low-density lipoprotein (LDL) cholesterol
High fat/cholesterol diet
Hypertension
Left ventricular hypertrophy
Thrombogenic factors (as affected by aspirin)
Category 2 (Factors for Which Interventions are Likely to Lower CVD Risk)
Diabetes mellitus
Physical inactivity
Low levels of high-density lipoprotein (HDL) cholesterol[a]
Triglycerides
Small, dense LDL particle size
Obesity
Postmenopausal status (women)
Category 3 (Factors Associated with Increased CVD Risk That, if Modified, Might Lower Risk)
Psychosocial factors
Elevated Lipoprotein (a)
Elevated Homocysteine
Oxidative stress
No alcohol consumption
Category 4 (Factors Associated with Increased Risk That Cannot be Modified)
Age
Male gender
Low socioeconomic status
Family history of early-onset CVD

[a]May now be considered a Category 1 risk factor; see text. Adapted from Pasternak RC, Grundy SM, Levy D, et al. 27th Bethesda Conference: matching the intensity of risk factor management with the hazard for coronary disease events. Task Force 3. Spectrum of risk factors for coronary heart disease. J Am Coll Cardiol 1996;27:978.

Category I risk factors are those for which interventions have been proven to reduce the risk of CAD events. They include smoking, elevated LDL cholesterol, diet high in saturated fat, hypertension, left ventricular hypertrophy, and "thrombogenic factors," which are unnamed but have the potential of being reduced by aspirin.

Category II risk factors are those for which interventions are likely to lower CAD risk. They include diabetes mellitus, physical inactivity, low levels of high-density lipoprotein (HDL) cholesterol, increased levels of triglycerides, obesity, and postmenopausal estrogen deficiency. Since the publication of these findings, diabetes has been reclassified as a CAD "risk equivalent" based on data suggesting that diabetic patients without known CAD have survival rates similar to those of nondiabetic patients who have experienced an MI. The ATP-III guidelines focus attention on the so-called "metabolic syndrome," which incorporates abdominal obesity, atherogenic dyslipidemia (elevated triglycerides, small LDL particles, low HDL cholesterol), elevated blood pressure, insulin resistance (with or without glucose intolerance), and prothrombotic and proinflammatory states. Patients with this syndrome are now appropriately targeted for intensive lipid modification. Low HDL cholesterol, with the publication of the Veterans Affairs High Density Lipoprotein Intervention Trial (VA-HIT) (8), may now be considered a category I risk factor, because intervention to raise HDL cholesterol (i.e., with gemfibrozil) in this trial reduced the incidence of cardiovascular events (9). Although postmenopausal status correctly identifies a cardiac risk factor; there has been no evidence to date that hormone replacement therapy reduces cardiac risk (10). At this time, the American Heart Association does not recommend hormone replacement therapy *for the express purpose* of reducing CAD risk.

Category III risk factors are those associated with increased CAD risk that may, if modified, lower risk. These include the so-called "putative" or "emerging" risk factors such as depression, elevated lipoprotein (a) levels, and hyperhomocysteinemia. This list should probably be expanded to include inflammatory markers (elevated white blood cell count, high-sensitivity C-reactive protein, and soluble adhesion molecules, and evidence of *Chlamydia* infection), thrombotic risk factors (plasminogen activator inhibitor-1), and sleep apnea. Coronary calcification as measured by EBCT (11) can correctly be considered a category III risk factor for now, but it may need to be reclassified (like diabetes mellitus) as a CAD risk equivalent because it functionally measures the subclinical coronary artery plaque burden. Moderate alcohol intake (1 to 3 drinks per day) may reduce CAD risk (see p. 868).

Category IV risk factors are those that are associated with increased risk but cannot be modified. They include age, male gender, low socioeconomic status, and family history of early-onset CAD. Positive family history has been defined as CAD in a male first-degree relative younger than 55 years of age or in a female first-degree relative younger than 65 years of age. These factors are usually taken into consideration with the available risk scoring systems.

DIAGNOSIS

History

Character and Location of Ischemic Pain

The discomfort of myocardial ischemia may be described in a variety of ways; because many individuals do not describe it as a pain, it is often more effective to ask the patient to describe any discomfort. Some describe it as squeezing, crushing, burning, or smothering, whereas others describe a shortness of breath or simply a feeling of heaviness. Some patients may hold their clenched fist in the middle of the chest to describe the discomfort. A sharp pain is unlikely to be of cardiac origin, but the patient should be asked to characterize it further. To some people, "sharp" may mean severe rather than knife-like or piercing.

Angina, as classically described, begins and ends gradually, usually over 2 to 5 minutes, and is usually steady in character, although it can occasionally wax and wane. If ischemic pain continues for longer than 20 minutes, MI is more likely. The discomfort is midline and substernal; it often radiates to the shoulder, arm, hand, or fingers, usually to the left. Radiation down the inside of the arm into the fingers supplied by the ulnar nerve is classic. Pain may also radiate into the neck, the lower jaw, or the interscapular region. Occasionally, a patient has pain only in a referred location and experiences no chest discomfort at all. Sometimes, the discomfort suggests another condition to the patient and he or she consults a primary care provider for "heartburn" or a dentist for jaw pain ascribed to a toothache. The pain of myocardial ischemia is diffuse and cannot easily be localized. Rarely is the patient able to point with one finger to the location; when pain can be localized in this way, it is likely to be noncardiac in origin. The elderly, especially the frail elderly, are more likely to experience atypical pain (or dyspnea instead of pain) with respect to character and location.

The Canadian Cardiovascular Society Classification (CCS) System (12) was designed to provide a simple way of grading anginal symptoms. *Class I angina* occurs with strenuous, rapid, or prolonged exertion but not with ordinary physical activity. Patients with *class II angina* experience slight limitation of ordinary activity. Class II angina occurs on walking or climbing stairs rapidly; walking uphill; walking or climbing stairs after a meal, in cold, or in wind; or under emotional stress. *Class III angina* produces marked limitations of ordinary physical activity. Angina occurs on walking one or two blocks on level terrain or climbing one flight of stairs under normal conditions and at a normal pace. With *class IV angina*, the most severe type, the patient is unable to carry on any physical activity without discomfort; anginal symptoms may be present at rest. A higher CCS class is associated with more extensive CAD and a higher risk of CAD events.

Precipitating Factors

The single most important diagnostic feature of the discomfort of myocardial ischemia is its predictable relationship to exertion, emotional stress, or other situations that may either increase myocardial oxygen demand or reduce supply. The cause of atypical pain, pain in an unusual location or of an unusual character, may be clarified by this relationship. Pain that is experienced at rest, if it is caused by ischemia, suggests unstable angina or MI.

Anxiety and mental stress are important and often overlooked provoking factors in many patients. Myocardial oxygen demand may be increased by anxiety to an extent and duration greater than that produced by exercise, resulting in prolonged pain. Angina is more likely to occur during cold or windy weather because of increased peripheral vascular resistance and, consequently, increased myocardial work. Sexual intercourse may also trigger episodes of angina owing to increased myocardial oxygen demand. Sometimes ischemic discomfort follows a heavy meal, perhaps because of the shunting of blood to abdominal viscera and increased sympathetic tone. Nocturnal angina may be a manifestation of left ventricular failure due to an increase in left ventricular end-diastolic pressure resulting from the augmentation in venous return that occurs when the patient is supine. Similarly, patients who describe breathlessness and chest pain with exertion may have angina as a consequence of left ventricular failure.

Relief of Ischemic Pain

Because angina is caused by a discrepancy between oxygen supply and demand, relief of pain is achieved by increasing coronary blood flow or decreasing oxygen demand. Most people must stop or at least slow the activity responsible for precipitating the pain before it is relieved. Angina is also typically relieved by sublingual nitroglycerin. The practitioner and the patient both need to know that the relief of chest pain by nitroglycerin is not specific for myocardial ischemia. For example, the pain of esophageal spasm is commonly relieved by nitroglycerin. A placebo effect may relieve chest discomfort from other causes as well.

Physical Examination

The physical findings in patients with CAD are nonspecific. The examination should be done with particular attention to uncovering circumstantial evidence that would support the diagnosis of CAD: high blood pressure, evidence of abnormal lipid metabolism such as tendon xanthomas or xanthelasma, funduscopic changes reflecting long-standing hypertension or diabetes mellitus, or evidence of peripheral vascular disease. A complete cardiovascular examination should include measurement of the blood pressure in both arms and auscultation of the carotid and femoral arteries and the abdominal aorta. Special attention should be paid to excluding significant valvular disease, especially aortic stenosis, because severe aortic stenosis can itself cause angina pectoris. If suspected, aortic stenosis should be confirmed by echocardiography (see Chapter 65).

Electrocardiogram

A 12-lead ECG should be obtained as soon as possible in a patient with suspected CAD, although in many cases it is completely normal. The most reliable ECG sign of chronic ischemic heart disease is a pathologic Q wave, recorded by the leads of the ECG that are measuring electrical activity of a part of the myocardium that has been previously infarcted (Fig. 62.1A). The differential diagnosis of Q waves on an ECG includes prior MI, healed myocarditis, an infiltrative myocardial disorder such as amyloidosis or sarcoidosis, and the Wolff–Parkinson–White syndrome (usually with characteristic findings of preexcitation, see Chapter 64). Nonspecific ST-T wave changes, abnormalities of conduction (except for left bundle branch block, discussed later), and arrhythmias do not help establish the diagnosis of myocardial ischemia. However, ST-segment depression with a flat or downsloping ST segment is indicative of subendocardial ischemia (Fig. 62.1B). It is seldom present in the resting ECG of patients with ischemic heart disease unless they are experiencing angina at the time the tracing is being recorded. On the other hand, transient ischemic changes are seen commonly when a patient with CAD is exercised to a point at which chest pain develops. Such ECG changes, appearing with exercise or pain and resolving with rest or with the resolution of pain, are usually an indication of myocardial ischemia. Therefore, the necessity of repeating the ECG at rest or after the chest pain has resolved cannot be overemphasized. ST-segment elevation during chest pain (Fig. 62.1C) suggests MI or variant angina (discussed later). T-wave inversion in an ECG taken at rest is a nonspecific finding but can occur after infarction or as a specific transient finding in a patient experiencing angina. Therefore, ECG changes noted during episodes of chest pain not only can confirm the diagnosis of

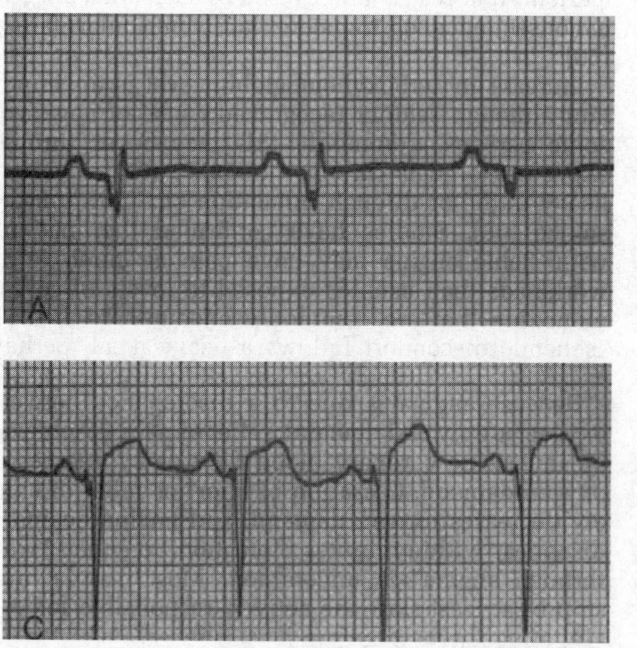

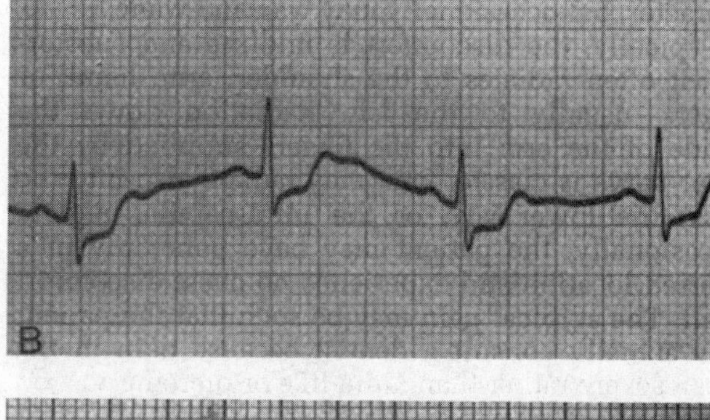

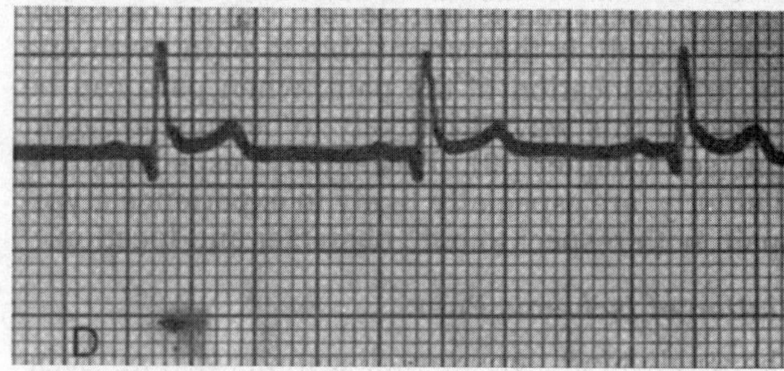

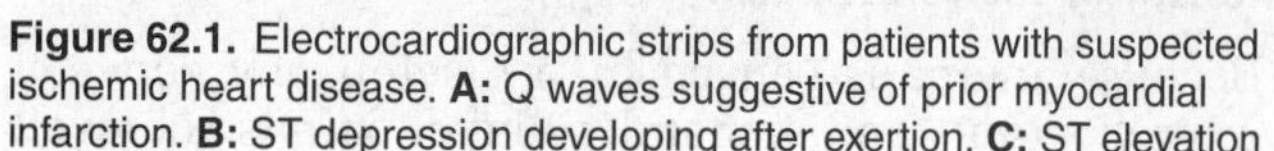

Figure 62.1. Electrocardiographic strips from patients with suspected ischemic heart disease. **A:** Q waves suggestive of prior myocardial infarction. **B:** ST depression developing after exertion. **C:** ST elevation during coronary artery spasm (variant angina). **D:** Early repolarization (a normal variant).

myocardial ischemia but also may indicate the extent and location of the ischemic myocardium. As a general rule, the more widespread the changes on the ECG, the more myocardium is involved. ST-segment elevation in the absence of chest pain is common in the resting ECG of healthy young adults and is caused by rapid or "early" repolarization of the ventricle. This pattern (Fig. 62.1D) is usually noted in the mid-left chest leads (V_2 through V_4) but may be more widespread. ST-segment elevation from pericarditis is diffuse and can be associated with PR-segment depression.

The presence of ST-T abnormalities in an otherwise healthy person is a nonspecific finding and should not be considered confirmation of CAD. There is a high association of left bundle branch block (LBBB) with organic heart disease (see Chapter 64), especially CAD. Right bundle branch block (RBBB), on the other hand, is seen commonly in the absence of other cardiac abnormalities.

Stress Testing

Exercise Electrocardiography

The exercise stress test not only is a means of establishing the diagnosis of myocardial ischemia but also can be used to assess the efficacy of antianginal therapy, to identify patients who are likely to have more severe CAD and a large area of myocardium at risk, and to assess serially the degree of conditioning or exercise capacity in patients of all age groups. The American College of Cardiology (ACC)/American Heart Association (AHA) exercise testing guidelines (13) outline the recommendations for the use of exercise testing in establishing the diagnosis of CAD, in assessing risk and prognosis in patients with symptoms or a prior history of CAD, and the use of exercise testing after MI. The usefulness of exercise testing in establishing the diagnosis of CAD is based in part on the likelihood that the patient has this condition (i.e. the "pretest probability" of CAD). This can be determined by the patient's age, gender, and symptoms. For example, exercise testing would not be expected to add much to establishing a diagnosis of CAD in an older patient with typical angina (who has a high pretest probability of CAD) or in a young, asymptomatic individual (who has a low pretest probability of CAD). The usefulness of stress testing in these situations would be limited, respectively, by false-negative and false-positive findings. The ACC/AHA guidelines (13) recommend exercise testing to diagnose CAD in adult patients with an intermediate pretest probability of CAD based on gender, age, and symptoms. For patients with known CAD, the guidelines recommend stress testing for those with a significant change in clinical status. Patients with unstable angina, decompensated heart failure, severe aortic stenosis, or uncontrolled hypertension should not be referred for stress testing because of an unacceptably high risk of provoking a cardiac event with exercise.

The rationale of exercise stress testing is that as the work performed by the patient increases, cardiac work is increased. This increase in work results in an increase in myocardial oxygen utilization, which demands an increase in coronary blood flow. If narrowed or obstructed coronary arteries prevent the required increase in coronary blood flow, myocardial ischemia may occur and be manifested as chest pain or ECG changes (14).

The simplest and least expensive exercise stress test is the graded, symptom-limited exercise treadmill test. This requires the patient to be monitored with a 12-lead ECG while walking on a treadmill at workloads that can be progressively increased by increasing the speed and inclination of the device. A stationary bicycle ergometer (with hand pedals) may be substituted for a treadmill, permitting the patient to exercise with his or her arms instead of legs. Although it is not commonly used, this method of stress testing permits a patient to exercise who may otherwise be unable to do so because of lower extremity claudication, arthritis, or amputation. It may also be useful in the evaluation of patients who have chest pain predominantly or exclusively with work that involves the arms and shoulders.

A simple algorithm can be used to decide the type of stress test to recommend (Fig. 62.2). First, the patient's ability to exercise should be assessed. If the patient can walk up a flight of stairs carrying laundry or groceries, for example, a treadmill exercise protocol can generally be chosen to allow the patient to achieve a level of cardiac work that permits meaningful information to be obtained from the test. If the patient cannot perform this task, or one that is comparable, a pharmacologic stress test with cardiac imaging (discussed later) should generally be recommended. The patient's baseline ECG should be reviewed to determine whether baseline ST-segment abnormalities exist that might lower the predictive value of exercise-induced changes. False-positive stress tests are often encountered in patients taking medications such as digoxin or amiodarone, in women, and in patients with left ventricular hypertrophy or mitral valve prolapse (15). In such patients and in those with baseline ST-segment abnormalities, intraventricular conduction defects (i.e., LBBB or RBBB), or other conduction system disorders (e.g., Wolff–Parkinson–White syndrome), the sensitivity of the exercise stress test can be enhanced by concurrent radioisotopic or echocardiographic imaging (see later discussion). The choice

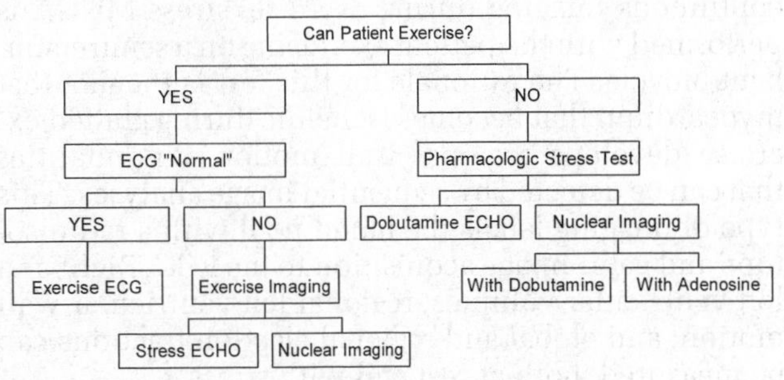

Figure 62.2. An algorithm for determining the appropriate stress test. See text for a description of the procedures.

between radioisotopic or echocardiographic imaging depends largely on the expertise of local laboratories.

Radioisotope Imaging

Radioisotope imaging can enhance the specificity of stress testing by evaluating myocardial function or flow (16). Radioisotope imaging can be used in conjunction with either treadmill exercise testing or pharmacologic stress testing, using either dobutamine to increase cardiac work or adenosine or dipyridamole to alter coronary blood flow (see later discussion). Commonly used imaging modalities include radioisotope imaging with thallium 201– and/or technetium 99–based agents (e.g., ^{99m}Tc-sestamibi). The usefulness of ^{201}Tl as a perfusion tracer is based on its ability to function as an analog of ionic potassium. It is very efficiently extracted by healthy myocardial cells, and uptake is proportional to regional perfusion and myocardial viability. ^{99m}Tc-sestamibi has a shorter half-life (6 hours) than does ^{201}Tl (73 hours), allowing a larger tracer dose to be administered. This and its higher emission energy make it an excellent agent for cardiac imaging. ^{99m}Tc-sestamibi is particularly useful in obese patients and in patients with large breasts (because of possible attenuation of the radioisotopic images in the area of the anterior myocardium).

Both ^{201}Tl and ^{99m}Tc-sestamibi can be used to assess regional myocardial blood flow, either by planar imaging or by single-photon emission computed tomography (SPECT). Imaging usually occurs at two separate times: the stress scan, obtained very shortly after the patient has exercised or received a pharmacologic agent, and the rest scan, obtained either before or several hours after stress. The radioisotope is injected intravenously at the time of peak exercise (or at the time of peak infusion during a pharmacologic stress test), and scintigraphic images are obtained shortly thereafter, depicting regional myocardial perfusion at the time of peak stress. The rest scan is typically obtained several hours later and shows redistribution of the isotope. Ischemia is indicated by the filling in of a cold spot defined on the stress images (i.e., normalization or "redistribution" of a radioisotopic defect), and infarction is indicated by a persisting cold spot or one with only partial redistribution.

Radioisotope imaging with stress gated blood pool scans (multiple gated acquisition, or MUGA) can also be used to assess myocardial ischemia. To allow for continuous imaging during exercise, stress MUGA is performed with the patient exercising on a semirecumbent bicycle. The rationale for this test is the fact that myocardium that becomes ischemic during graded exercise develops regional wall motion abnormalities that can be detected by sequential image analyses. This type of imaging labels the blood pool with a radioisotope and gates image acquisition to the ECG. Right and left ventricular volumes, regional left ventricular wall motion, and global and regional ejection fractions can be measured, both at rest and with stress.

The cost of stress testing with radioisotope scanning is usually several times that of a standard exercise test.

Stress Echocardiography

Two-dimensional echocardiography can be used instead of radioisotope scanning to detect areas of regional myocardial dysfunction (as evidenced by a wall motion abnormality) with exercise or pharmacologic stress (17,18). Typically, baseline images are first obtained at rest to determine the adequacy of the echocardiographic images. If these images are technically inadequate (e.g., because of obesity or severe obstructive lung disease), then radioisotope images are preferable. If the rest images are technically adequate, the patient undergoes treadmill exercise stress and then images are reacquired immediately, using special software to allow for direct comparison of pre-exercise and postexercise images. If pharmacologic stress testing with dobutamine (see next section) is employed, the dose of dobutamine is increased in a stepwise fashion, and echocardiographic images are typically obtained each time the dose is increased. The safety of dobutamine stress echocardiography is comparable to that of a routine exercise stress test (17,19,20). The sensitivity, specificity, and cost of the test are similar to those of radioisotopic stress testing. Stress echocardiography may be preferred in some cases, because some information is provided that is not obtained with radioisotopic scanning (e.g., the presence of pericardial effusion, ventricular hypertrophy, or valve abnormality); it also avoids exposure to radioactivity.

Pharmacologic Stress Testing

Patients who are unable to exercise because of physical limitations can be evaluated after intravenous administration of dipyridamole, adenosine, or dobutamine in conjunction with an imaging modality. Dipyridamole and adenosine dilate all coronary vessels and generally increase flow to all areas of the heart. Enhanced dilation of normal coronary arteries, compared to that which occurs in significantly narrowed vessels, augments differences in flow that usually are not apparent at rest. These agents are suitable for use with radioisotopic imaging modalities that may readily demonstrate this flow heterogeneity. Because they affect flow, but not heart rate or contractility, they are used only in conjunction with radioisotopic imaging but generally not with echocardiography. After administration of dipyridamole or adenosine followed by either ^{201}Tl or ^{99m}Tc-sestamibi (i.e., the stress image), myocardium supplied by a narrowed coronary artery typically demonstrates a perfusion defect that "fills in" during the rest image. Because of its ultrashort duration of action, adenosine is preferred to dipyridamole for this test.

Dobutamine is a beta-1 agonist that at high dosages (20 to 40 μg/kg per minute intravenously) increases myocardial contractility and heart rate in a manner and extent similar to exercise. Heart rate may not be affected to the same extent as contractility, and atropine is often administered intravenously to increase the heart rate to the maximal predicted heart rate for age. Dobutamine may be used in conjunction with either echocardiography or radioisotopic imaging for the diagnosis of CAD.

Mild side effects (nausea, flushing, headaches) are common with dipyridamole, adenosine, and dobutamine. Dipyridamole and adenosine (but not dobutamine) can produce severe bronchospasm and therefore must be used with great caution in patients so predisposed. Adenosine can also cause transient heart block. Because dobutamine increases atrioventricular conduction, it should not be used in patients with atrial flutter and should be used carefully in patients with atrial fibrillation.

Implications of an Abnormal Stress Test

If treadmill exercise stress testing is performed, factors affecting prognosis include the degree of ST-segment depression, how rapidly ST-segment depression develops during exercise, and how long it persists in recovery. In addition, an ischemic ECG response that is accompanied by hypotension generally implies a large amount of myocardium at risk. The best studies of stress test responses and prognosis are for radioisotopic imaging. The number, size, and location of abnormalities on stress myocardial perfusion studies reflect the location and extent of functionally significant coronary stenoses (21). Both radioisotopic and echocardiographic imaging can detect left ventricular dilation with stress, a finding that suggests global, severe ischemia. Lung uptake of a radioisotopic tracer indicates stress-induced left ventricular dysfunction and suggests multivessel CAD. Many studies have shown that high-risk abnormal stress tests are associated with an increased risk of cardiac events. On the other hand, normal radioisotopic or echocardiographic stress tests are associated with a benign prognosis. In a review of 16 studies involving almost 4,000 patients over 2 years, a negative perfusion scan was associated with a 0.9% rate of cardiac death per year, similar to that of the general population (22).

Ambulatory Electrocardiography

The ambulatory ECG (Holter monitor) may also be useful in detecting myocardial ischemia. However, it is not a good tool for screening patients to make the diagnosis of CAD. In patients with CAD who are symptomatic during ambulatory ECG monitoring, ST-segment elevation or depression can be observed during episodes of pain and at other times as well (silent ischemia; see later discussion). In patients with silent ischemia, the ambulatory ECG is particularly useful in quantitating the degree and frequency of ischemia and in assessing the efficacy of therapy.

Electron Beam Computed Tomography

Studies in the 1970s demonstrated that coronary calcification (detected by cardiac fluoroscopy) was useful in identifying patients with angiographically significant CAD (23). EBCT is a highly sensitive technique for detecting coronary artery calcium and may be useful to diagnose CAD noninvasively (11). ECG gating allows data acquisition within one or two breathholds, making it a fast test with limited radiation exposure. The images obtained by this technique allow the determination of a calcium score, which is an index of calcium deposition in multiple arterial segments and is a good approximation for overall plaque burden in the coronary tree. High calcium scores are associated with increased risk for MI (24). The test offers improved discrimination over conventional risk factors in the identification of people with CAD (25). The negative predictive value of EBCT is high (26). The cost implications and the appropriate populations in whom the test is most likely to be useful have not yet been defined.

Cardiac Catheterization and Coronary Arteriography

Coronary arteriography is defined as radiographic visualization of the coronary vessels after the injection of radioopaque contrast medium (27). This technique provides direct information about the presence of CAD and defines the distribution and severity of obstructive coronary lesions. The images obtained are stored as either 35-mm cine film or as a digital recording. Percutaneous or cutdown techniques of the femoral or brachial arteries allow insertion of sheaths for the introduction of selective catheters for the right and left coronary ostia, saphenous bypass grafts, or internal mammary arteries. Arteriography is performed as part of cardiac catheterization, which may also include left ventriculography and hemodynamic assessment. Because coronary anatomy varies, nomenclature can also vary. Fig. 62.3 shows diagrammatically the coronary arteries and their branches as they appear on coronary arteriography. There are three major coronary arteries: the left anterior descending, the left circumflex, and the right coronary artery. The coronary tree can be divided into 29 segments, but the extent of disease is usually defined as one-vessel, two-vessel, three-vessel, or left main disease, with significant disease taken to mean the presence of a 50% or greater reduction in diameter (some operators and texts use 70% or greater).

The 1999 ACC/AHA Guidelines for Coronary Angiography (27) outline the indications and contraindications for the procedure. The guidelines recommend arteriography for those with CCS class III or IV angina on medical treatment (marked limitations of ordinary physical activity due to angina or angina at rest, discussed earlier) and those with high-risk criteria on noninvasive testing regardless of angina severity. It may also be reasonable to consider coronary arteriography for patients with angina that has improved with medical treatment but remains present, those whose noninvasive testing results demonstrate progressively worsening abnormalities, those who cannot tolerate medical therapy, those with angina who cannot be adequately risk stratified because of disability or illness, and those whose occupation involves the safety of others (e.g., pilots, bus drivers) and who have abnormal, but not high-risk, stress test results.

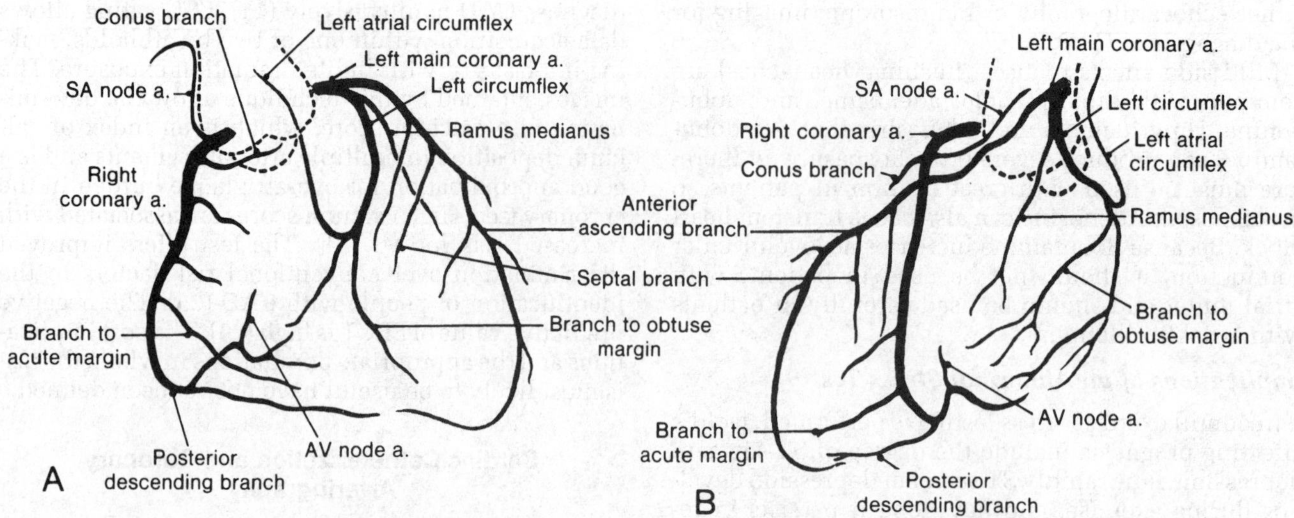

Figure 62.3. Anatomic representation of the coronary arteries. These vessels are represented as they would be seen on the angiogram. No attempt to convey the third dimension has been made. Careful study of the changes in position of the various branches with rotation of the heart is essential to intelligent interpretation of arteriograms. **A:** Anteroposterior. **B:** Lateral. (From Abrams HL, Adams DF. The coronary arteriogram: structural and functional aspects [First of two parts]. N Engl J Med 1969;281:1276.)

Inherent in the recommendation for coronary arteriography is the assumption that the patient is a potential candidate for coronary revascularization. If the patient's general medical condition or other medical problems preclude revascularization, or if the patient refuses to consider revascularization regardless of catheterization results, arteriography is ill advised.

Indications for percutaneous coronary intervention (including angioplasty and stenting) (28) and coronary artery bypass surgery (29) are reviewed in separate ACC/AHA guidelines and are discussed later in this chapter.

Patient Experience. The patient may undergo cardiac catheterization as part of an evaluation during a hospitalization, but the test itself does not require the patient to be admitted to the hospital. The procedure is not painful, and the patient remains awake throughout the study. Approximately 1 hour before the procedure, the patient is given a sedative, usually diazepam (Valium), 5 to 10 mg orally. After the patient is brought to the catheterization laboratory, either the area of the brachial artery or the femoral artery is prepared for sterile procedure. The site of introduction of the catheter is usually chosen based on the preference of the operator but also is guided by the presence and extent of peripheral vascular disease. Typically, a catheter is introduced percutaneously through a wire that is threaded through an introducer needle, but if vascular access is difficult, a larger incision may be necessary to directly visualize the artery. Under fluoroscopic guidance, the catheter is threaded to the coronary sinuses and the orifices of the right and left coronary arteries are injected sequentially with contrast medium. The patient is asked to hold his or her breath during the few seconds of the injection. In addition to this part of the test, which visualizes the coronary arteries, additional studies are performed to measure ventricular pressures and to assess left ventricular contraction during injection of dye directly into the left ventricular cavity. During ventriculography, focal wall motion abnormalities, ventricular aneurysms, and valvular lesions such as mitral regurgitation can be assessed in addition to the measurement of overall left ventricular function and ejection fraction. At the end of the procedure, the catheter is withdrawn and pressure is applied to the arteriotomy site to achieve hemostasis. If a larger incision was necessary, it is sutured.

During the procedure, the patient may feel slightly woozy from the sedation. There is usually no pain except for the moment when the needle is initially introduced, and there is some pressure as the catheter is held in place. There may be a sensation of hot flushing when the dye is injected, particularly when the larger bolus of dye is injected into the left ventricle during ventriculography.

Risks and Relative Contraindications

The major complications of coronary arteriography are MI, stroke, and death. These risks are related to the experience of the laboratory performing the study and the type of patient undergoing the test. Risks tend to be lower in young, otherwise healthy patients and higher in older patients with poor left ventricular function, particularly those with associated peripheral vascular disease and those who are clinically unstable (e.g., patients with cardiogenic shock, recent acute MI, or decompensated heart failure) at the time of the procedure. In a survey of almost 60,000 patients, mortality from angiography was 0.11%; MI occurred in 0.05%, and stroke in 0.07%; vascular access complications were more common (0.43%) (30).

There are no absolute contraindications to coronary arteriography. Relative contraindications include renal failure, active gastrointestinal bleeding, acute stroke, severe anemia, coagulopathy, unexplained fever or active untreated infection, severe uncontrolled hypertension, allergic reaction to angiographic contrast agents, and decompensated congestive heart failure. Renal insufficiency has been the most well studied complication: it occurs in up to 5% of patients without preexisting renal dysfunction and in 10% to 40% of patients with baseline renal insufficiency. More than 75% of patients who develop renal insufficiency recover normal renal function, although 10% of these patients may require dialysis. Pretreatment with intravenous hydration (0.45% saline) and limiting the amount of intravenous contrast material used are the most effective means to avoid renal dysfunction. The major predictors of contrast allergy are prior contrast allergy (risk of subsequent reaction, 50%), iodine allergy, and shellfish allergy. These conditions should be discussed with a patient before referral for angiography. The use of nonionic contrast medium, pretreatment with corticosteroids, and treatment with antihistamines may reduce allergic complications.

TREATMENT OF ANGINA PECTORIS

General Therapeutic Considerations

In evaluating and treating patients with angina, it is of paramount importance to identify and treat underlying contributing factors and to modify cardiac risk factors that promote CAD progression if possible.

Hypertension is often present in patients with angina. There is a linear relationship between left ventricular work and myocardial oxygen demand. Left ventricular systolic pressure increases in response to an increase in peripheral vascular resistance. Both systolic and diastolic hypertension can increase myocardial oxygen demand. An attempt should always be made to reduce resting blood pressure to normal in patients with chronic hypertension, including those with isolated systolic hypertension. This can be of crucial importance in reducing the frequency and severity of angina pectoris in the hypertensive patient. Beta-blockers and calcium channel blockers (see Chapter 67) are excellent choices in such patients because they have other antianginal properties as well. Agents such as hydralazine and minoxidil, which cause a reflex tachycardia, are less desirable.

It is important to achieve a maximal level of pulmonary compensation in patients with *angina and coexisting lung disease* (see Chapter 60). Chronic hypoxemia and acidosis and the increased work of breathing in patients with pulmonary disease increase myocardial oxygen demand or decrease myocardial oxygen delivery, or both. Beta-selective bronchodilators are less likely to accelerate the heart rate and are often useful in such patients. Unfortunately, the treatment of angina in patients with severe lung disease is often limited by a real, or perceived, need to avoid the use of beta-blockers (see later discussion).

Abstinence from tobacco products is essential, because nicotine in tobacco can cause coronary vasoconstriction. Techniques that are used to achieve this goal are described in Chapter 27. Similarly, passive tobacco smoke should be avoided.

The possibility of *hyperthyroidism* (see Chapter 80) in patients with angina should never be overlooked, particularly in older patients or in those with increasing angina. Often, particularly in the older patient, other obvious signs of hyperthyroidism are not present. For example, hyperthyroidism may be manifested only by an increased frequency or severity of angina, an increase in heart rate in people with atrial fibrillation, or increasing heart failure.

Anemia is also important to consider in patients with angina, particularly if the hemoglobin concentration falls to less than 7 g/dL, when cardiac output must increase to maintain adequate peripheral oxygen delivery at rest. Obviously, this problem is exacerbated in those patients with concomitant chronic lung disease and hypoxemia.

Heart failure (see Chapter 66) in patients with angina should always be optimally treated. The real possibility that heart failure is producing angina at rest (see later discussion) or nocturnal angina should be considered. Diuretics, vasodilators, and beta-blockers may be useful in patients with rest or nocturnal angina and may reduce the frequency and severity of angina. The calcium channel blocker, amlodipine, may also be useful in this setting, because it has little negative inotropic effect, reduces preload and afterload, helps decrease left ventricular end-diastolic pressure, and lowers peripheral vascular resistance.

Lipids and Diet

It is believed that most of the recent decline in mortality from heart disease is related to primary and secondary risk factor reductions (31). These observations are supported by the West of Scotland Coronary Prevention Study, which demonstrated a significant mortality reduction with treatment of hyperlipidemia in asymptomatic people, the greatest benefit occurring in patients with other risk factors for CAD (32). The value of secondary prevention was also established by the Scandinavian Simvastatin Survival Study (33) and the Cholesterol and Recurrent Events (CARE) trial (34), each of which demonstrated a significant reduction in mortality when LDL levels were lowered to approximately 100 to 120 mg/dL. Other trials also have clearly demonstrated coronary artery lesion regression with vigorous, sustained normalization of elevated cholesterol to an LDL cholesterol level of less than 100 mg/dL (35). The NCEP guidelines (7) indicate that the goal LDL cholesterol level is less than 100 mg/dL in patients with angina or known CAD. In addition to discussing recommendations for lipid-lowering drug therapy, the guidelines also recommend a multifaceted lifestyle approach to reduce risk. This approach calls for reducing the intake of saturated fats to less than 7% of total calories and reducing dietary cholesterol to less than 200 mg/day. Achieving an ideal body weight and increasing physical activity are also advised. This subject is discussed in more detail in Chapter 82. There is also benefit to treating patients with low values of HDL cholesterol. The use of gemfibrozil to raise HDL cholesterol levels was shown to reduce the risk of major cardiovascular events in patients with CAD (9).

Alcohol

Alcohol is an acute pressor agent and may be responsible for as many as 10% of all cases of hypertension (36). However, moderate drinking (1 to 3 drinks per day) is accompanied by an increase in HDL cholesterol (37). The extent to which the increase in blood pressure associated with heavy drinking mitigates the beneficial effect on HDL remains to be determined. In an editorial, Victor and Hansen commented, "In the absence of alcohol related illness, therefore, a drink or two a day still seems safe and advisable from a cardiovascular standpoint" (38).

Antioxidants

Although antioxidants may be important in inhibiting atherosclerosis, clinical trials of antioxidant therapy have not demonstrated conclusive long-term benefit. In the Heart Outcomes Prevention Evaluation (HOPE) study, for example, approximately 9,500 patients at high risk for cardiovascular events were randomly assigned to therapy with either 400 IU of vitamin E or placebo for an average of 4.5 years. There was no apparent effect of treatment with vitamin E on cardiovascular outcomes in this study (39).

Fish Oil

Epidemiologic studies in the early 1990s suggested that eating fish conferred protection against CAD. However, in 1995, after studying 44,895 male health professionals, Ascherio et al. reported no beneficial effect of increasing fish intake from 1 to 2 servings per week to 5 to 6 per week (40).

Postmenopausal Hormone Replacement Therapy

Several studies have shown that the acute administration of estrogen can cause coronary vasodilatation and reverse endothelial dysfunction in postmenopausal women with CAD. In addition, several observational studies have shown that postmenopausal women with CAD who take hormone replacement therapy (HRT) have a decreased risk of recurrent cardiovascular events compared with women who do not (41,42). Based on these data, two randomized, placebo-controlled studies evaluated the role of HRT in postmenopausal women with chronic stable CAD. The Heart and Estrogen/Progestin Replacement Study (HERS) (43) showed that HRT did not result in a reduced risk of cardiovascular death or nonfatal MI, and the Estrogen Replacement and Atherosclerosis Study (ERAS) (44) failed to show an effect of HRT on the angiographic progression of atherosclerotic heart disease. There is also evidence that postmenopausal HRT increases the risk of venous thromboembolic disease (43,45) and gallbladder disease (43) in women with CAD. Therefore, routinely recommending HRT to postmenopausal women for the purposes of reducing cardiovascular morbidity or mortality is not advised at this time.

Physical Conditioning

Physical conditioning can also improve the exercise tolerance and psychological well being of patients with stable angina. Most large communities have developed supervised exercise programs for patients with CAD. The benefits of physical conditioning and exercise programs for patients with heart disease are described in detail in Chapter 63. The AHA recently published guidelines for exercise in various patient groups that are available on their website (www.aha.org; accessed 1/7/02). Patients with angina should be counseled to avoid physical activities that are known to provoke their symptoms. Health care providers should specifically discuss the safety of sexual intercourse, a subject that people are often reluctant to broach (see Chapter 63). The level of sexual activity or participation in any stressful physical activity that is appropriate ideally should be based on the results of an exercise stress test. The energy requirements for a broad range of activities are summarized in Chapter 63 (Table 63.5).

Medical Treatment

The basic objective in treating patients with angina pectoris is not only to relieve or prevent symptoms but also to prevent disease progression. The former goal may be achieved by medical therapy that improves the relationship between myocardial oxygen demand and supply. The latter goal may be accomplished by preventing platelet aggregation and by decreasing the growth of atherosclerotic plaque and the risk of plaque rupture. The major advance in the medical management of angina has been the demonstration that long-acting antiplatelet and antithrombotic agents and vigorous lipid-lowering therapy can improve outcomes in selected patients with CAD. Angina that occurs with exercise is usually caused by an increase in myocardial oxygen demand that cannot be met because of fixed arterial obstruction. A decrease in or cessation of the work that produced the angina usually results in a prompt reduction in myocardial oxygen demand. Therefore, rest or a decrease in the level of activity may relieve angina in 1 to 2 minutes. If anxiety is a contributing or provoking factor, it may take longer for myocardial work to decrease and the episode of angina may be prolonged. Table 62.2 lists practical information about the drugs used most often in the treatment of angina.

Nitrates

Traditionally, nitroglycerin and related compounds have been an inexpensive mainstay of treatment of patients with angina pectoris. Initially these agents were thought to increase coronary blood flow by producing coronary artery dilation. Although nitrates may

Table 62.2. Selected Drugs Used in the Treatment of Angina[a]

Class	Brand Name[d]	Available Strengths	Usual Starting Dosage	Usual Maximum Dosage	Onset	Duration
Nitrates						
Nitroglycerin (sublingual)[b]	Nitrostat and others	0.15-, 0.30-, 0.40-, 0.60-mg tablets	1 tablet (0.4 mg) at time of, or in anticipation of, pain	2–3 tablets at time of pain over 15 min	30 sec	3–5 min
Topical						
Ointment	Nitro-Bid, Nitrol	2% ointment	½ inch every 4–6 hr as needed	4–5 inches q3–4 hr	30–60 min	3–6 hr
Patch[c]	Transderm Nitro, Nitro-Dur, and Nitrodisc	2.5-, 5-, 10-, 15-mg/24 hr rated release (0.1, 0.2, etc., mg/hr)	5 mg	2–3 patches that deliver 15 mg/24 hr	30 min	24 hr
Long-Acting						
Isosorbide[b] dinitrate	Isordil, Sorbitrate, and others	5-, 10-, 20-mg tablets, oral; 40-mg tablets or capsules, oral	10 mg b.i.d. or t.i.d.	60–80 mg b.i.d. or t.i.d.	15–30 min	4–6 hr
Isosorbide mononitrate	Ismo	20 mg	20 mg b.i.d. given 7 hr apart	40 mg b.i.d. given 7 hr apart	60 min	5 hr after 2nd dose
β-Adrenergic Blockers[b]						
Propranolol[b]	Inderal	10-, 20-, 40-, 80-mg tablets, oral	10–20 mg t.i.d. or q.i.d.	320 mg/day in divided doses	1–1.5 hr	4–6 hr
Nadolol	Corgard	40-, 80-, 120-mg tablets, oral	40 mg q.d.	240 mg	1–2 hr	24 hr
Atenolol	Tenormin	50-, 100-mg tablets, oral	50 mg q.d.	100–150 mg	1–2 hr	24 hr
Metoprolol	Lopressor	50, 100 mg or 100 mg XL	100 mg in two divided doses; in older persons, 25 mg b.i.d.	200 mg b.i.d.	1–2 hr	24 hr
Calcium Channel Blockers						
Nifedipine	Procardia	10-mg capsule	10 mg t.i.d. or q.i.d.	40 mg q6 hr	20–30 min	8 hr
Nifedipine, extended release	Procardia XL Adalat CC	30, 60, 90 mg	30 mg q.d. (for converting pts from t.i.d. to XL, add up mg dose, e.g., 30 mg t.i.d. = 90 mg XL	90 mg q.d.	1–2 hr	>24 hr
Verapamil	Calan, Isoptin	80-, 120-mg tablets	80 mg t.i.d. or q.i.d.	120 mg q.i.d.	30–45 min	6–8 hr
Verapamil SR	Isoptin SR Calan SR	120, 180, 240 mg	120–180 mg q.d.	240 mg b.i.d.	1–2 hr	24 hr
Diltiazem	Cardizem	30-, 60-, 90-, 120-mg tablets	30 mg q.i.d.	60 mg q6 hr	30–45 min	6–8 hr
Diltiazem CD	Cardizem CD	120, 180, 240, 300, 360 mg	180–240 mg q.d.	360 mg q.d.	1–2 hr	24 hr
Nicardipine	Cardene	20-, 30-mg capsules	20 mg t.i.d.	40 mg t.i.d.	30–120 min	8 hr
Amlodipine	Norvasc	2.5, 5, 10 mg	5 mg q.d., increase dosage after 3–5 days, small or elderly pts start 2.5 mg q.d.	10 mg q.d.	Several hours	24 hr

[a]Other drugs, other dosages of the drugs listed, and combinations of different drugs are marketed. The drugs and dosages shown are the ones most often used.

[b]Generic available.

[c]The brand name of these preparations is followed by a number (5, 10, 15, 20). It is important to know whether that number refers to milligrams per 24 hours (Transderm-Nitro or Nitrodisc) or to square centimeters of the patch (Nitro-Dur). Nitro-Dur contains 4 mg/cm of patch, reported now as release per hour.

[d]Other brands may be available.

increase coronary blood flow in patients with spasm or may increase collateral flow to obstructed vessels, evidence suggests strongly that the mechanism of action of nitrates in most patients is not an increase in blood flow but a decrease in myocardial oxygen demand and peripheral vascular resistance. These compounds produce dilation of the venous circulation, which reduces venous return and decreases ventricular volume. The decrease in ventricular volume improves the efficiency of the heart and decreases wall tension. These effects ultimately reduce myocardial oxygen demand. Nitrates also produce arterial dilation to a lesser degree, and thereby reduce the resistance to ventricular ejection. This effect further decreases myocardial oxygen demand by reducing left ventricular work. Therefore, the beneficial antianginal effect of nitrates is caused primarily by peripheral vasodilation.

Sublingual nitroglycerin is still the drug of choice for the relief and prevention of discrete episodes of angina pectoris in most patients. The initial dose should be small (0.4 mg) to minimize unpleasant side effects (flushing, headache, light-headedness) in patients in whom higher dosages may be unnecessary. Patients should be taught that it is important that their pain be relieved as soon as possible, and they should be instructed to take nitroglycerin whenever such symptoms appear. Use of nitroglycerin in this way may do more than simply prevent ischemic pain. Angina often produces anxiety, which may increase heart rate and blood pressure and thereby increase myocardial oxygen demand. This may lead to a vicious cycle in which ischemia may be worsened and the severity and duration of angina increased. If pain is not relieved by 2 to 3 tablets of nitroglycerin (the patient should wait for at least 5 minutes between doses), or if the need for nitroglycerin increases suddenly and dramatically, the patient should be instructed to call his or her health care provider or go to an emergency facility immediately because of the danger of impending MI. Because nitroglycerin may lose potency on storage, patients should be advised not to keep tablets longer than 3 to 4 months after opening the bottle. If the use of nitroglycerin does not result in the relief of angina and the usual side effects are not experienced, the problem may be caused by outdated medicine that has lost its potency rather than by a change in cardiac status. Prophylactic use of nitroglycerin is of particular value in patients who have angina in response to specific and reproducible stress despite other therapies. For example, the patient who develops angina after walking from a car to a place of work can be instructed to take nitroglycerin after the car is parked, wait a few minutes, and then walk to work, thereby preventing pain altogether. The use of prophylactic nitroglycerin before sexual intercourse may also prevent angina and may alleviate the anxiety that is naturally associated with sexual activity when angina is anticipated.

It is important to teach the patient to use sublingual nitroglycerin correctly. The patient should cease the activity that has caused angina, take sublingual nitroglycerin, and sit down to avoid the possible untoward effects of hypotension (increased in the standing position). The most common side effects of nitroglycerin therapy are flushing and headache; both may diminish with increasing usage of the drug. A nitroglycerin lingual spray has been developed that is designed to deliver 0.4 mg of nitroglycerin sublingually with each compression of the nebulizer. Some patients find this preparation more acceptable and more reliable than the tablet.

Long-acting nitrates. As shown in Table 62.2, long-acting nitrates are available in a variety of preparations. Careful studies confirm the clinical efficacy of both nitroglycerin ointment and isosorbide tablets (46,47). In selecting among available oral preparations, the major considerations should be efficacy, convenience, and cost. Using these criteria, *long-acting isosorbide* is probably the best choice for ambulatory patients. A *nitrate patch* for once-a-day use also is available. It provides controlled release of 0.2, 0.4, or 0.6 mg/hour of nitroglycerin through a semipermeable membrane applied to the skin by means of an adhesive tape. The patch delivers a standardized dose, but constant serum levels of nitrate predispose to the development of tolerance and the patch should therefore be removed for a period of the day (e.g., at night) (48).

The side effects of all long-acting nitrates are similar to those produced by sublingual nitrates. Some patients are unable to take long-acting nitrates because of persistent headache, but for most this is not a problem. Nitrates can also produce orthostatic hypotension and occasionally syncope.

Sildenafil (Viagra) is a drug used for the treatment of erectile dysfunction. The drug inhibits cyclic guanosine monophosphate (cGMP)–specific phosphodiesterase type 5, allowing cGMP to accumulate in the corpus cavernosum of the penis. Because nitrates increase levels of cGMP and sildenafil inhibits its breakdown, the combination of sildenafil and nitrates may result in severe hypotension. Therefore, as discussed in Chapter 63, sildenafil should not be used by men who are taking nitrates of any kind.

Beta-Blocking Agents

A number of beta-blockers are currently available in the United States. These agents vary in their cardioselectivity, in their metabolism, and, to some degree, in their side effects (see later discussion and Chapters 64 and 67).

In many respects, beta-blockade is an ideal approach to the treatment of angina. It decreases heart rate, myocardial contractility, and, in many patients, systemic blood pressure. These effects alone or in combination significantly reduce myocardial oxygen consumption and thereby attenuate the frequency or severity of angina in most patients.

An added benefit for patients with ischemic heart disease is that beta-blockade often effectively prevents arrhythmias (see Chapter 64). It may decrease or eliminate premature ventricular contractions (PVCs), and the ventricular rate in patients with atrial fibrillation may also be decreased. Furthermore, when

PVCs are frequent, the number of hemodynamically effective ventricular contractions is diminished, which decreases coronary as well as peripheral perfusion. In patients who are in atrial fibrillation, decreasing the ventricular response improves left ventricular dynamics by decreasing heart rate, increasing diastolic filling period, and decreasing myocardial oxygen consumption.

The dosage of a beta-blocker can be rapidly increased over hours or days until the desired effect is obtained. The heart rate is a useful guide to treatment; sinus bradycardia at a resting rate of 50 and 60 beats/minute is a reasonable goal. However, the ideal dosage is one that not only results in mild sinus bradycardia at rest but also blocks an increase in heart rate with exercise. The dosage necessary to produce this effect and that necessary to relieve angina pectoris may vary considerably.

Although beta-blockers are an important part of the management of congestive heart failure (CHF) (see Chapter 66), the acute effect of these drugs is to decrease myocardial contractility, and they should not be used in patients with decompensated CHF.

Extreme caution must be exercised when using any beta-blocker in a patient with second- or third-degree block (see Chapter 64), because life-threatening bradycardia can be precipitated in such patients.

The nonselective beta-blockers (propranolol, nadolol, pindolol, timolol, carvedilol) are contraindicated in patients with intrinsic asthma. A history of allergic asthma or bronchospasm during pulmonary infections should therefore be sought in all patients for whom beta-blockers are being considered. Furthermore, patients with chronic obstructive lung disease may develop increased bronchospasm from beta-blockers even if they have no history of allergic or intrinsic asthma; in such patients, a selective beta-blocker with minimal beta-2-blocking effects should be used. Metoprolol and atenolol are both cardioselective and can often be used safely in such patients and in patients with peripheral arterial disease, particularly Raynaud disease, in whom nonselective beta-blockers may exacerbate symptoms. However, even these agents have beta-2-blocking effects at moderate and high dosages and should be used cautiously in these situations.

Although impotence occurs in 1% or less of the susceptible population, it is a major reason for discontinuing the drug in young and middle-age men. This side effect can sometimes be overcome by prescribing a beta-blocker with poor lipid solubility and therefore less penetration of the nervous system (e.g., atenolol instead of propranolol). Atenolol may also be less likely to cause depression or to alter sleep patterns, occasional reported side effects of other beta-blockers.

Calcium Channel Blockers

Calcium channel blockers reduce the influx of calcium into the slow channels of the myocardium and smooth muscle (see Chapter 64) and thereby cause several important hemodynamic effects—dilation of coronary arteries, prevention of coronary vasospasm, and production of systemic vasodilation—that effectively reduce preload and afterload. They have been shown to be effective in the treatment of both stable and unstable angina and are also effective antihypertensive agents. A number of calcium channel blockers are currently available (Table 62.2). Although many are effective in the treatment of hypertension (see Chapter 67), only a few are currently approved for use in patients with angina: nifedipine, nicardipine, amlodipine, verapamil, diltiazem, and bepridil. A meta-analysis suggested that the use of short-acting calcium blockers, when used to treat hypertension, is associated with adverse outcomes (49). More recently, another meta-analysis compared patients treated with diuretics, beta-blockers, angiotensin-converting-enzyme (ACE) inhibitors, or clonidine to those treated with intermediate-acting or long-acting calcium channel blockers and showed that those treated with calcium antagonists had a higher risk of MI, congestive heart failure, and major cardiovascular events (50). Although calcium channel blockers are effective in treating patients with angina, it seems reasonable to consider other therapies first and to use calcium antagonists only if other antianginal medications do not relieve symptoms.

Nifedipine is a potent coronary and systemic vasodilator and may be used for angina and for the treatment of hypertension. The common side effects of nifedipine are dizziness, flushing, headache, nausea, diarrhea, and, because of systemic vasodilation, peripheral edema. The major adverse effect is significant hypotension, which, in association with a reflex tachycardia, can actually intensify myocardial ischemia in a few patients. All side effects can usually be controlled by a reduction in dosage of the drug. Nifedipine and other calcium channel blockers should be used cautiously in patients taking digoxin, because excretion of digoxin may be inhibited and digitalis toxicity may be induced. At higher dosages in patients with reduced left ventricular function, negative inotropy may be observed with nifedipine.

Nicardipine is structurally similar to nifedipine but is less likely to cause hypotension or left ventricular dysfunction. It may be useful in patients with angina and borderline blood pressure.

Amlodipine also has been shown to be an effective antianginal and antihypertensive agent. Its safety in patients with significant left ventricular dysfunction (51) makes it a particularly attractive anti-ischemic agent in patients with angina and reduced left ventricular ejection fraction. Added advantages are its once-a-day dosing and the infrequent incidence of side effects. It has few if any effects on the atrioventricular (AV) node. Reflex tachycardia after administration is also unusual.

Verapamil is often prescribed for the treatment of hypertension or arrhythmia but is also an effective antianginal agent. However, it has a more potent negative inotropic effect than other calcium channel blockers and significantly retards AV conduction. Therefore it should not be used in patients with compromised left ventricular function or in those with sinus bradycardia, sick sinus syndrome, or AV block (see Chapter 64). In these situations, amlodipine or nicardipine are safer choices. Verapamil may be particularly beneficial in the patient with a supraventricular arrhythmia who also has angina.

Diltiazem also significantly retards AV conduction, but it has less of a negative inotropic effect than does verapamil and, in contrast to nifedipine, is unlikely to cause hypotension or other side effects (e.g., flushing, headache, edema). It is available as a twice-a-day or a once-a-day preparation.

Bepridil, although approved for treatment of patients with stable angina, is not often used because of the risk of QT-interval prolongation and torsades de pointes.

Caution must be exercised when treating older patients with calcium blockers, especially if used in conjunction with a beta-blocker or other agents that slow AV conduction (e.g., digitalis) or if used in patients with pre-existing conduction system disease. In such patients, significant heart block and bradycardia can be precipitated but usually resolve after stopping administration of the calcium blocker or after the administration of calcium intravenously. This effect, most commonly seen with verapamil and diltiazem, may occur with other calcium blockers, but not with amlodipine.

Anticoagulants and Antiplatelet Drugs

Aspirin (81 to 325 mg) remains the cheapest agent to reduce platelet aggregation. The AHA/ACC guidelines on the management of chronic stable angina recommend daily aspirin, in the absence of contraindications, for all patients with this condition (52). If aspirin is absolutely contraindicated, clopidogrel (75 mg), an inhibitor of adenosine 5′-diphosphate (ADP)–induced platelet aggregation, may be used. It is generally preferable to ticlopidine, a drug with a similar mechanism of action, because ticlopidine has a slow onset of action and is more often associated with the development of neutropenia and, occasionally, thrombotic thrombocytopenic purpura in some patients. Despite their occasional use, there are no data to support the use of anticoagulants or dipyridamole in patients with angina.

Angiotensin-Converting Enzyme Inhibitors

ACE inhibitors reduce morbidity and mortality in patients with CHF (see Chapter 66) and should be part of the treatment regimen of patients with CHF and angina. The recent HOPE trial (53) demonstrated that the ACE inhibitor ramipril reduced mortality and the risk of MI and stroke in patients with vascular disease or diabetes plus one other cardiovascular risk factor who were not known to have left ventricular dysfunction or CHF. Although the routine use of ACE inhibitors cannot be recommended for all patients with CAD, it should certainly be considered, particularly if there is coexistent hypertension or diabetes mellitus.

Initiating and Adjusting Long-Acting Drugs for Angina

The choice of an antianginal regimen should be made after evaluation of the patient's age, angina frequency, lifestyle, and possible mechanism of angina. In addition, the patient's financial resources should be considered, because many drugs, although effective, are expensive and not available as generic substitutes. In patients with stable angina, either a nitrate preparation or a beta-blocker may be started initially (Table 62.2). A calcium channel blocker may be prescribed to patients who have variable chest pain, in whom coronary artery spasm (see Variant Angina) may be playing a role, and to those intolerant of beta-blockers. If the patient does not improve, the dosage may be increased weekly until a response is achieved. If the type of treatment selected initially fails to help at a maximally tolerated dosage, another agent can be added or substituted. Because nitrates and beta-blockers decrease myocardial oxygen demand by different mechanisms, concomitant use of the two types of therapy is reasonable. If it is necessary to stop beta-blocker therapy, it should be tapered over several days to avoid the risk of precipitating angina, which may occur when a beta-blocker is abruptly discontinued.

Patients who fail to improve after maximal medical management for angina pectoris are often considered for coronary arteriography and possible revascularization. It is therefore important to make certain that maximally-tolerated doses of medications are used before considering medical therapy unsuccessful. In general, maximal medical therapy for angina consists of a beta-blocker, a long-acting nitrate, and a calcium channel blocker in doses that either achieve the desired effect or cannot be increased because of the development of side effects. In addition, all patients with angina should take daily aspirin (or clopidogrel if aspirin is absolutely contraindicated).

Percutaneous Transluminal Coronary Angioplasty

Percutaneous transluminal coronary angioplasty (PTCA) is an important option for the treatment of CAD that cannot be controlled by medical therapy. This technique has the ability to restore nearly normal coronary flow in diseased native coronary arteries, without the cost and morbidity of bypass surgery. It involves the compression of a critical coronary lesion against the wall of the affected coronary artery by means of an inflatable balloon mounted on a special catheter. Patients are identified as candidates for PTCA after cardiac catheterization has clearly delineated coronary anatomy and after it has been determined that bypass surgery would otherwise be indicated. PTCA was initially used to treat patients with single-vessel, proximal, discrete, noncalcific coronary lesions. However, in skilled hands, PTCA is also an appropriate treatment for multivessel CAD. Although there are no absolute contraindications to the procedure, patients with arterial dissection or eccentric and long stenotic lesions are poor candidates and have a higher risk of complications and restenosis with PTCA. These patients are best treated with surgery.

Patients who are appropriate candidates for PTCA undergo the procedure either immediately after cardiac catheterization or at a later time, depending on the clinical situation and the needs of the particular patient. The techniques used for PTCA are similar to those employed for cardiac catheterization and coronary arteriography, described earlier in this chapter. The major difference is that instead of the simple injection of contrast dye for diagnostic purposes, PTCA involves the use of a preshaped guiding catheter through which a balloon catheter (with the balloon deflated) is inserted. Under fluoroscopic guidance, the balloon is postioned midway across the lesion to be dilated. The balloon is then inflated with increasing pressures until there is no more indentation of the balloon and dye injections through the guiding catheter show normal flow and a sufficiently patent coronary artery.

The major limitations of balloon angioplasty are abrupt vessel closure and restenosis. The usual restenosis rate after PTCA is 30%, but the rate can be as high as 40% to 50%. Restenosis most commonly occurs within the first 6 months and can be successfully treated by a second PTCA. A lack of symptoms after 6 to 8 months usually indicates a favorable long-term prognosis. The use of *intracoronary stents* has reduced the rates of both abrupt vessel closure and restenosis (54,55). Intracoronary stents are typically stainless steel cylindrical structures and are often self-expanding. They are available in a variety of lengths and sizes. Stents are usually delivered and deployed on balloon catheters using the guiding catheters and guidewires described previously. Although stents are usually deployed after balloon dilation, followed by a second high-pressure dilation after stent placement, direct stenting without predilation is also feasible.

Barring complications, the patient's experience during PTCA (with or without intracoronary stent placement) and the time required for the procedure are the same as for coronary angiography (see previous discussion). The only exception is that many patients experience chest pain during inflation of the balloon in the coronary artery. The incidence of major side effects (including coronary artery dissection, MI, and sudden death) is related to the skill and experience of the operator and can be as low as 1% to 4%. Overall, the procedure is successful 80% to 90% of the time. Patients can usually be discharged the day after the procedure and often can return to work 1 week later. After successful angioplasty and stent placement, patients are prescribed aspirin indefinitely and clopidogrel or ticlopidine for 4 to 6 weeks. Patients taking ticlopidine can develop leukopenia, so blood counts should be checked at 2-week intervals.

Surgical Management

Coronary artery bypass graft (CABG) surgery is one of the most common surgical procedures performed in this country today. It is generally accepted that patients with incapacitating angina pectoris who have good left ventricular function and who have failed maximal medical therapy should be considered candidates for coronary arteriography and subsequent surgery. Early studies demonstrated that CABG surgery prolongs survival compared with medical therapy in patients with stable angina who have 50% or greater stenosis of the left main coronary artery (56) or who have triple-vessel CAD and a left ventricular ejection fraction between 35% and 50% (57). Long-term follow-up indicates that, in patients with normal left ventricular function, surgery does not result in a survival benefit compared to medical therapy, even in patients with left main or triple-vessel CAD (58,59).

CABG surgery usually involves the use of saphenous vein bypass grafts and implantation of an internal mammary artery into the native coronary artery circulation or the placement of radial artery conduits as bypass grafts. Some surgeons also use radial or gastric arterial conduits in patients undergoing repeat surgical procedures. The technique used is often based on the surgeon's preference and experience.

The procedure is usually performed through a median sternotomy using cardiopulmonary bypass and cardioplegic arrest. Newer, minimally invasive techniques use a limited thoracotomy incision and are associated with less postoperative pain, a shorter stay in the intensive care unit, earlier discharge from the hospital, and a more rapid recuperation. Bypass procedures can be performed on the beating heart, thereby avoiding some of the complications of traditional cardiopulmonary bypass surgeries. Some centers have little, if any, experience with these newer techniques, and they are not available in every community. These operations may also be technically more challenging and, understandably, there is a shortage of long-term outcome data compared with conventional bypass techniques.

CABG surgery results in complete (or nearly complete) relief of angina pectoris initially in approximately 60% of properly selected patients; another 20% have a significant decrease in angina (60). There is a demonstrable increase in exercise tolerance after surgery in approximately 60% to 80% of such patients.

Patients with good left ventricular function have a 1% to 2% mortality rate from surgery, and fewer than 4% of patients develop evidence of MI during the perioperative period. Perioperative MI is more likely to occur in older patients and in patients with severe disease distal to a proximal obstruction. Another major complication of bypass surgery is stroke, which may be caused by cerebral hypoperfusion or arterial embolization, or both. The risk of perioperative stroke varies from less than 1% to about 6% depending on the patient's risk factors (61,62); it is highest in patients older than 70 years of age and in those with preexisting cerebrovascular disease or a previous stroke (63–65). Patients with significant atherosclerosis of the proximal or ascending aorta or of the carotid or intracranial cerebral arteries are also at increased risk.

Neuropsychiatric complications of CABG include problems with memory and other cognitive functions. The prevalence of these disturbances varies from about 10% to 80% soon after surgery, depending on the manner in which neurocognitive function is assessed (66,67). In general, neuropsychiatric disturbances resolve slowly over several months.

Historically, up to 30% of patients have developed recurrent angina within 5 years after bypass surgery. The diagnosis of recurrent angina should be confirmed by exercise stress testing. The initial treatment is the same as it is for patients who have not had bypass surgery: beta-blockers, nitrates, or calcium channel blockers. Patients who prove to be unresponsive to medical treatment should undergo coronary arteriography in an effort to delineate new lesions that could be amenable to percutaneous angioplasty or repeat CABG. In an attempt to prevent formation of such lesions, it is now common practice to administer aspirin to patients after bypass surgery (see Chapter 57) and to treat hyperlipidemia aggressively (see Chapter 82).

The *postpericardiotomy syndrome* may develop after bypass surgery, usually within 2 to 4 weeks (but sometimes as early as a few days or as late as 6 months after the operation). The syndrome is characterized by fever, fatigue, pleuritic chest pain, and often pleural and pericardial effusions. Laboratory examination shows leukocytosis and an elevated erythrocyte sedimentation rate. Large effusions may require drainage, but most patients respond to diuretics and a nonsteroidal anti-inflammatory agent (e.g., indomethacin, 25 to 50 mg three times a day for 1 to 2 weeks). Patients who are refractory to such treatment usually respond to prednisone, initially 60 mg a day for 2 to 3 days, with tapering of the dosage over 7 to 10 days. Constrictive pericarditis is a late rare complication of the postpericardiotomy syndrome; when it occurs, pericardial stripping is often necessary.

Atrial fibrillation is common after CABG surgery, occurring in 30% to 40% of patients (and in more than 50% in those older than 75 years of age). The arrhythmia often resolves spontaneously without specific therapy, but it may be persistent and may require anticoagulation, cardioversion, or both. The incidence of postoperative atrial fibrillation may be reduced by the prophylactic use of beta-blockers or amiodarone (68,69).

Dysesthesia, swelling, and itching are common in the leg from which the vein was harvested and can persist for several months. The swelling usually responds to the use of support hose or elevation of the legs periodically during the day. If the itching is severe and there is no evidence of local infection, topical corticosteroid ointments are often effective.

CABG surgery has been shown to prolong life in several patient subsets (see earlier discussion). In addition, 60% of patients who either were working just before bypass surgery or discontinued work because of cardiac symptoms return to work after surgery. Early ambulation is advisable, and the role of cardiac rehabilitation, as early as 6 to 8 weeks postoperatively, cannot be overemphasized (see detailed discussion in Chapter 63).

Patient Experience. Most patients are discharged within 5 to 7 days after CABG if the operation and postoperative recuperation have been uncomplicated. Usually, the patient is transferred from an intensive care unit to an intermediate care unit within 24 hours; early and aggressive mobilization is standard. After discharge, a structured, self-directed exercise program is commonly used. It is recommended that patients not operate a motor vehicle for 6 to 8 weeks after surgery.

Other Therapies

Although conventional medical therapy and improved revascularization techniques result in improvement in angina for most patients, there are still some who fail to improve despite these therapies. Others cannot be treated with certain classes of medications or cannot tolerate maximal doses as a result of side effects. In addition, some patients, particularly those with diffuse and/or distal coronary disease, are not appropriate candidates for either PTCA or CABG. If conventional treatments cannot be employed or fail to relieve symptoms, alternative therapies should be considered.

Enhanced external counterpulsation (EECP) should be considered in patients with class III or IV angina who remain symptomatic despite maximally-tolerated medical therapy and who are not believed to be candidates for either PTCA or CABG. EECP is available only in practices with specialized equipment. It involves the use of inflatable pneumatic cuffs that are wrapped around the patient's lower legs and thighs and are sequentially inflated and deflated (using compressed air) in relation to the cardiac cycle. The use of high pressure (300 mm Hg) allows blood to be pumped back to the heart during early diastole in an attempt to increase coronary blood flow and possibly to promote the development of collateral coronary circulation. The patient undergoes therapy for 1 hour each day, 5 days each week in the office setting, usually for a total of 7 weeks. EECP appears to decrease the number of episodes of angina and to improve exercise tolerance (70). It is reimbursed by many insurance companies and by Medicare.

Chelation therapy is designed to "leach" calcium out of atherosclerotic plaque by the repeated intravenous administration of ethylenediamine tetra-acetic acid (EDTA). Although many patients with refractory angina undergo, or are interested in, this form of treatment, a review of published clinical studies of chelation therapy indicates that it is of no clinical benefit (71). Because chelation therapy may produce a number of serious adverse effects, it is not recommended for the treatment of patients with angina.

Many new techniques are being studied in an attempt to improve coronary blood flow in patients with refractory angina who are not candidates for conventional revascularization procedures. These include transmyocardial laser revascularization, therapeutic angiogenesis (gene therapy to stimulate blood vessel growth in the heart), and percutaneous *in situ* coronary venous arterialization (percutaneous catheter-based coronary bypass). The percutaneous coronary bypass procedure is a new, experimental approach that uses a catheter and a self-expanding connector to create a fistula between a critically narrowed coronary artery and an adjacent coronary vein (72). Whether these experimental techniques become part of the treatment regimen for patients with angina will depend on the results of ongoing trials.

UNSTABLE ANGINA

Unstable angina is a term used to describe pain caused by cardiac ischemia that is becoming more intense, is occurring more frequently (often provoked by diminishing effort, perhaps even at rest), and is relieved less readily by nitroglycerin. The syndrome has also been called "crescendo angina" and "preinfarction angina." Sometimes unstable angina develops in a patient with previously stable, reasonably controlled angina; at other times, it develops in a patient with recent onset of ischemic symptoms. During the episode, the ECG shows ST-segment elevation or depression or T-wave inversion, which reverts to normal when the pain has abated. Because of the increased risks of MI and sudden death and because of the need for aggressive medical therapy, patients with unstable angina should be hospitalized. Although some cases of unstable angina can be managed successfully with aspirin, heparin, beta-blockers, and other antianginal therapy alone (which may include calcium channel blockers or nitroglycerin, as discussed previously), some patients may benefit from more aggressive antiplatelet therapy (e.g., an intravenous glycoprotein IIb/IIIa inhibitor) or from early coronary arteriography and revascularization. Consultation with a cardiologist should be considered when evaluating patients with unstable angina to identify the subset of patients who are at highest risk and to decide on the optimal therapeutic strategy for each patient.

VARIANT ANGINA

Variant angina (Prinzmetal angina) is, in a sense, unstable in that it occurs usually at rest; however, unlike typical angina, it does not occur on exertion or in response to emotional stress. Attacks of pain are experienced often at the same time each day; often, they awaken the patient early in the morning. During the attacks, there is ST-segment elevation that reverts to baseline when the attack is over; in about one third of the patients there are also transient AV blocks or arrhythmias (including ventricular tachycardia or fibrillation). Unlike unstable angina, pain is usually promptly relieved by sublingual nitroglycerin.

Coronary artery spasm often plays a major role in the pathogenesis of variant angina. Two groups of patients have been identified. By far the larger group (85% of patients) have fixed, often proximal obstruction of a major coronary artery; angina in this group often is associated with spasm of the artery near the site of obstruction. The variant syndrome in this group of patients commonly occurs after months or years of stable typical angina pectoris or after an MI.

The smaller group with variant angina (15% of patients) have normal coronary arteries but have spasm of one of the arteries, which reduces blood supply to the myocardium, resulting in ischemic pain. These patients are usually younger and are predominantly women. There is usually no history of typical angina or MI in these patients, and there is rarely a history of a systemic arteritis syndrome. The ST-segment elevation observed during the anginal attack is a manifestation of coronary artery spasm. It can often be confirmed by arteriography. It is important to perform arteriography in such patients, because those with normal coronary arteries are obviously not candidates for CABG or PTCA and most respond favorably to treatment with calcium channel blockers, the drugs of choice in such patients. If used without calcium channel blockers, beta-blockers may potentiate coronary artery spasm because of unopposed alpha-adrenergic vasoconstriction.

Angina and MI, probably caused by coronary vasospasm, have also been reported in otherwise healthy patients who use *cocaine*. Coronary vasospasm usually occurs acutely after ingestion or inhalation of cocaine, but it can also be observed up to an hour after use as a result of vasoactive byproducts of cocaine metabolism. Prolonged episodes of angina in such patients usually respond well to treatment with calcium channel blockers because concurrent hypertension is common.

ANGINA WITH NORMAL CORONARY ARTERIES

There are some individuals who have chest pain that is characteristic of angina but are found to have normal coronary arteries on arteriography. Many different possible causes have been described, including coronary vasospasm (see previous discussion), abnormal coronary vasodilator reserve (caused by either easily-identifiable cardiac disease, such as aortic stenosis or hypertrophic cardiomyopathy, or by disease of small coronary vessels that are not visualized on arteriography), narrowing of a major coronary artery not demonstrated by the conventional views obtained during routine arteriography (i.e., a false-negative study), or noncardiac chest pain (especially esophageal disease; see Chapter 42). The prognosis of these patients is generally favorable, with survival being comparable to that of age- and sex-matched controls (73), but chest pain is often recurrent and may result in frequent visits to emergency departments or to the practitioner's office.

SILENT ISCHEMIA

Many episodes of myocardial ischemia are painless. Such "silent ischemia" may be detected either during exercise treadmill testing or by continuous ECG monitoring. Asymptomatic ischemic ST-segment changes on ECG monitoring are common in patients with CAD and have been correlated with transient abnormalities in myocardial perfusion and function.

Many ambulatory patients with stable angina experience asymptomatic episodes of ischemia that often occur at low heart rates during activities of everyday life, without an apparent significant increase in myocardial oxygen demand; such episodes may even be precipitated by mental stress. Studies in patients with unstable angina or in patients in the early postinfarction phase have identified silent ischemia to be a powerful predictor of poor outcome (74,75). Patients with unstable angina who also have silent ischemia have a significantly greater frequency of bypass surgery, angioplasty, or recurrent symptomatic angina than patients without silent ischemia (75). The presence of silent ischemia within the first 3 days after an MI has also been shown to be associated with a greater frequency of recurrent ischemic events. Although several studies have identified silent ischemia to be a poor prognostic factor for patients with CAD, it is unknown whether treatment of such patients in an attempt to eliminate these episodes improves prognosis.

CORONARY ARTERY DISEASE IN WOMEN

A large body of data suggests that women with CAD have outcomes that are worse than those of men with comparable disease (15,76). CAD is the leading cause of death in women in the United States. The diagnosis of CAD in women is harder to establish because symptoms are often atypical and false-positive stress tests are more common. Hence, clinicians must be alert to atypical presentations in women and, if noninvasive testing is warranted, stress testing with radioisotopic or echocardiographic imaging should be considered. The treatment of angina in women is the same as that previously described.

PROGNOSIS

The mortality rate of patients with angina depends on a number of factors, including age, the extent and severity of CAD, left ventricular function, and medical comorbidity. The prognosis for older patients, those with diabetes mellitus, and women (see previous section) is worse than for others with angina.

In general, a 2-year mortality rate of approximately 1.3% has been reported (77). In contrast, the crude first-year mortality rate remains between 10% and 30% for patients with unstable angina (see previous discussion), 8% to 10% for patients surviving 30 days after MI, and 5% to 10% for those with stable angina of 2.5 years' duration (78–81).

Stress testing (see earlier discussion) helps assess prognosis in patients with angina. Patients with angina who have positive exercise stress tests have an annual incidence of subsequent cardiac events and mortality that is higher than that of patients who have negative stress tests (82). The prognosis of patients is worse when ST-segment depression occurs early in exercise, is downsloping, and persists long after termination of exercise. If cardiac catheterization and/or an assessment of left ventricular function have been obtained, these data can also help determine prognosis in patients with angina. The two most important determinants of mortality in patients with CAD are the location and extent of coronary artery occlusion and the left ventricular ejection fraction (83). Data from the Coronary Artery Surgery Study (CASS) registry of more than 14,000 patients indicate that the annual mortality rate is 2% for patients with one-vessel disease, 4% for two-vessel disease, 8% for three-vessel disease (84), and 27% to 37% for left main disease (56). For patients with left ventricular dysfunction, even if not severe (i.e., left ventricular ejection fraction 35% to 50%), these figures are considerably worse (57).

General References*

Gersh BJ, Braunwald E, Bonow RO. Chronic coronary artery disease. In: Braunwald E, Zipes DP, Libby P, ed. Heart disease: a textbook of cardiovascular medicine. 6th ed. Philadelphia: WB Saunders, 2001:1272.

A complete discussion of the diagnosis and management of angina pectoris.

Specific References

1. American Heart Association. 2001 Heart and stroke statistical update. Dallas, Texas: American Heart Association, 2000.
2. Ryan TJ, Antman EM, Brooks NH, et al. 1999 Update: ACC/AHA guidelines for the management of patients with acute myocardial infarction. A report of the American College of Cardiology/American Heart Association Task Force on Practice Guidelines (Committee on Management of Acute Myocardial Infarction). J Am Coll Cardiol 1999;34:890.
3. Braunwald E, Antman EM, Beasley JW, et al. ACC/AHA guidelines for the management of patients with unstable angina and non–ST-segment elevation myocardial infarction: a report of the American College of Cardiology/American Heart Association Task Force on Practice Guidelines (Committee on the Management of Patients With Unstable Angina). J Am Coll Cardiol 2000;36:970.
4. Little WC, Constantinescu M, Applegate RJ, et al. Can coronary angiography predict the site of a subsequent myocardial infarction in patients with mild-to-moderate coronary artery disease? Circulation 1988;78:1157.
5. Ambrose JA, Tannenbaum MA, Alexopoulos D, et al. Angiographic progression of coronary artery disease and the development of myocardial infarction. J Am Coll Cardiol 1988;12:56.
6. 27th Bethesda Conference: matching the intensity of risk factor management with the hazard for coronary disease events. J Am Coll Cardiol 1996;27:957.
7. Expert Panel on Detection, Evaluation, and Treatment of High Blood Cholesterol in Adults. Executive summary of the Third Report of the National Cholesterol Education Program (NCEP) Expert Panel on Detection, Evaluation, and Treatment of High Blood Cholesterol in Adults (Adult Treatment Panel III). JAMA 2001;285:2486.
8. Boden WE. High-density lipoprotein cholesterol as an independent risk factor in cardiovascular disease: assessing the data from Framingham to the Veterans Affairs High-Density Lipoprotein Intervention Trial. Am J Cardiol 2000;86:19L.
9. Rubins HB, Robins SJ, Collins D, et al. Gemfibrozil for the secondary prevention of coronary heart disease in men with low

*Bold print (general references) and bold numerals (specific references) denote published controlled clinical trials, meta-analyses, or consensus-based recommendations.

levels of high-density lipoprotein cholesterol. N Engl J Med 1999;341:410.

10. Hulley S, Grady D, Bush T, et al. Randomized trial of estrogen plus progestin for secondary prevention of coronary heart disease in postmenopausal women: Heart and Estrogen/Progestin Replacement Study (HERS) Research Group. JAMA 1998;280:605.

11. O'Rourke RA, Brundage BH, Froelicher VF, et al. American College of Cardiology/American Heart Association Expert Consensus Document on electron-beam computed tomography for the diagnosis and prognosis of coronary artery disease. J Am Coll Cardiol 2000;36:326.

12. Campeau L. Grading of angina pectoris. Circulation 1976;54:522(letter).

13. Gibbons RJ, Balady GJ, Beasley JW, et al. ACC/AHA guidelines for exercise testing: executive summary. A report of the American College of Cardiology/American Heart Association Task Force on Practice Guidelines (Committee on Exercise Testing). Circulation 1997;96:345.

14. Detrano R, Gianrossi R, Mulvihill D, et al. Exercise-induced ST segment depression in the diagnosis of multivessel coronary disease: a meta analysis. J Am Coll Cardiol 1989;14:1501.

15. Wenger NK. Coronary heart disease in women: clinical syndromes, prognosis, and diagnostic testing. Cardiovasc Clin 1989;19:173.

16. Beller GA, Gibson RS. Sensitivity, specificity, and prognostic significance of noninvasive testing for occult or known coronary disease. Prog Cardiovasc Dis 1987;29:241.

17. Dagianti A, Penco M, Agati L, et al. Stress echocardiography: comparison of exercise, dipyridamole and dobutamine in detecting and predicting the extent of coronary artery disease. J Am Coll Cardiol 1995;26:18.

18. Ryan T, Vasey CG, Presti CF, et al. Exercise echocardiography: detection of coronary artery disease in patients with normal left ventricular wall motion at rest. J Am Coll Cardiol 1988;11:993.

19. Mertes H, Saivada SG, Ryan T, et al. Symptoms, effects, and complications associated with dobutamine stress echocardiography: experience in 1118 patients. Circulation 1993;88:15.

20. Secknus MA, Marwick TH. Evolution of dobutamine echocardiography protocol and indications: safety and side effects in 3,011 studies over 5 years. J Am Coll Cardiol 1997;29:1234.

21. Ritchie JL, Bateman TM, Bonow RO, et al. Guidelines for clinical use of cardiac radionuclide imaging. Report of the American College of Cardiology/American Heart Association Task Force on Assessment of Diagnostic and Therapeutic Cardiovascular Procedures (Committee on Radionuclide Imaging), developed in collaboration with the American Society of Nuclear Cardiology. J Am Coll Cardiol 1995:25:521.

22. Brown KA. Prognostic value of thallium-201 myocardial perfusion imaging: a diagnostic tool comes of age. Circulation 1991;83:363.

23. Bartel AG, Chen JTT, Peter RH, et al. The significance of coronary calcification detected by fluoroscopy: a report of 360 patients. Circulation 1974;49:1247.

24. Raggi P, Callister TQ, Cooil B, et al. Identification of patients at increased risk of first unheralded acute myocardial infarction by electron-beam computed tomography. Circulation 2000;101:850.

25. Guerci AD, Arad Y, Agatston A. Predictive value of EBCT scanning. Circulation 1998;97:2583.

26. Budhoff MJ, Georgiou D, Brody A, et al. Ultrafast computed tomography as a diagnostic modality in the detection of coronary artery disease: a multicenter study. Circulation 1996;93:898.

27. Scanlon PJ, Faxon DP, Audet AM, et al. ACC/AHA guidelines for coronary angiography. A report of the American College of Cardiology/American Heart Association Task Force on practice guidelines (Committee on Coronary Angiography). Developed in collaboration with the Society for Cardiac Angiography and Interventions. J Am Coll Cardiol 1999;33:1756.

28. Smith SC Jr, Dove JT, Jacobs AK, et al. ACC/AHA guidelines of percutaneous coronary interventions (revision of the 1993 PTCA guidelines)—executive summary. A report of the American College of Cardiology/American Heart Association Task Force on Practice Guidelines (Committee to Revise the 1993 Guidelines for Percutaneous Transluminal Coronary Angioplasty). J Am Coll Cardiol 2001;37:2215.

29. Eagle KA, Guyton RA, Davidoff R, et al. ACC/AHA guidelines for coronary artery bypass graft surgery: executive summary and recommendations. A report of the American College of Cardiology/American Heart Association Task Force on Practice Guidelines (Committee to Revise the 1991 Guidelines for Coronary Artery Bypass Graft Surgery). Circulation 1999;100:1464.

30. Noto TJ Jr, Johnson LW, Krone R, et al. Cardiac catheterization 1990: a report of the Registry of the Society for Cardiac Angiography and Interventions (SCA&I). Cathet Cardiovasc Diagn 1991;24:75.

31. Hunink MGM, Goldman L, Tosteson ANA, et al. The recent decline in mortality from coronary heart disease, 1980–1990. The effect of secular trends in risk factors and treatment. JAMA 1997;277:535.

32. Shepherd J, Cobbe SM, Ford I, et al. Prevention of coronary heart disease with pravastatin in men with hypercholesterolemia. West of Scotland Coronary Prevention Study Group. N Engl J Med 1995;333:1301.

33. Scandinavian Simvastatin Survival Study Group. Baseline serum cholesterol and treatment effect in the Scandinavian Simvastatin Survival Study (4S). Lancet 1995;345:1274.

34. Sacks FM, Pfeffer MA, Moye LA, et al. The effect of pravastatin on coronary events after myocardial infarction in patients with average cholesterol levels. Cholesterol and Recurrent Events Trial Investigators. N Engl J Med 1996;335:1001.

35. Brown G, Albers JJ, Fisher LD, et al. Regression of coronary artery disease as a result of intensive lipid lowering therapy in men with high level of apolipoprotein B. N Engl J Med 1990;323:1289.

36. Randin D, Vollenweider P, Tappy L, et al. Suppression of alcohol-induced hypertension by dexamethasone. N Engl J Med 1995;332:1733.

37. Langer RD, Criqui MH, Reed DM. Lipoproteins and blood pressure as biological pathways for effect of moderate alcohol consumption on coronary heart disease. Circulation 1992;85:910.

38. Victor RG, Hansen J. Alcohol and blood pressure: a drink a day. N Engl J Med 1995;332:1782.

39. Yusuf S, Dagenais G, Pogue J, et al. Vitamin E supplementation and cardiovascular events in high-risk patients. The Heart Outcomes Prevention Evaluation Study Investigators. N Engl J Med 2000;342:154.

40. Ascherio A, Rimm EB, Stampfer MJ, et al. Dietary intake of marine n-3 fatty acids, fish intake, and the risk of coronary disease among men. N Engl J Med 1995;332:977.

41. Grady D, Rubin SM, Petitti DB, et al. Hormone therapy to prevent disease and prolong life in postmenopausal women. Ann Intern Med 1992;117:1016.

42. Sullivan JM, Vander-Zwaag R, Hughes JP, et al. Estrogen replacement and coronary artery disease: effect on survival in postmenopausal women. Arch Intern Med 1990;150:2557.

43. Hulley S, Grady D, Bush T, et al. Randomized trial of estrogen plus progestin for secondary prevention of coronary heart disease in postmenopausal women. Heart and Estrogen/Progestin Replacement Study (HERS) Research Group. JAMA 1998;280:605.

44. Herrington DM, Reboussin DM, Brosnihan KB, et al. Effects of estrogen replacement on the progression of coronary-artery atherosclerosis. N Engl J Med 2000;343:522.

45. Grady D, Wenger NK, Herrington D, et al. Postmenopausal hormone therapy increases risk for venous thromboembolic disease. The Heart and Estrogen/Progestin Replacement Study. Ann Intern Med 2000;132:689.

46. Danahy DT, Aronow WS. Hemodynamics and antianginal effects of high-dose oral isosorbide dinitrate after chronic use. Circulation 1977;56:205.

47. Thadani U, Fung HL, Darke AC, et al. Oral isosorbide dinitrate in angina pectoris: comparison of duration of action and dose–response relation during acute and sustained therapy. Am J Cardiol 1982;49:411.

48. Elkayam U. Tolerance to organic nitrates: evidence, mechanisms, clinical relevance, and strategies for prevention. Ann Intern Med 1991;114:667.

49. Psaty BM, Smith NL, Siscovick DS, et al. Health outcomes associated with antihypertensive therapies used as first-line agents: a systematic review and meta-analysis. JAMA 1997;277:739.

50. Pahor M, Psaty BM, Alderman MH, et al. Health outcomes associated with calcium antagonists compared with other first-line antihypertensive therapies: a meta-analysis of randomised controlled trials. Lancet 2000;356:1949.

51. Packer M, O'Connor CM, Ghali JK, et al. Effect of amlodipine on morbidity and mortality in severe chronic heart failure. N Engl J Med 1996;335:1107.

52. Gibbons RJ, Chatterjee K, Daley J, et al. ACC/AHA/ACP-ASIM guidelines for the management of patients with chronic stable angina: executive summary and recommendations. A Report of the American College of Cardiology/American Heart Association Task Force on Practice Guidelines (Committee on Management of Patients with Chronic Stable Angina). Circulation 1999;99:2829.

53. Yusuf S, Sleight P, Pogue J, et al. Effects of an angiotensin-converting-enzyme inhibitor, ramipril, on cardiovascular events in high-risk patients. The Heart Outcomes Prevention Evaluation Study Investigators. N Engl J Med 2000;342:145.

54. Fischman, DL, Leon, MB, Baim, DS, et al. A randomized comparison of coronary stent placement and balloon angioplasty in the treatment of coronary artery disease. N Engl J Med 1994;331:496.

55. Serruys PW, de Jaegere P, Kiemeneij F, et al. A comparison of balloon expandable stent implantation with balloon angioplasty in patients with coronary artery disease. N Engl J Med 1994;331:489.

56. Chaitman BR, Fisher LD, Bourassa MG, et al. Effect of coronary bypass surgery on survival patterns in subsets of patients with left main coronary artery disease. Report of the Collaborative Study in Coronary Artery Surgery (CASS). Am J Cardiol 1981;48:765.

57. Passamani E, Davis KB, Gillespie MJ, et al. A randomized trial of coronary artery bypass surgery: survival of patients with a low ejection fraction. N Engl J Med 1985;312:1665.

58. Caracciolo EA, Davis KB, Sopko G, et al. Comparison of surgical and medical group survival in patients with left main coronary artery disease: long-term CASS experience. Circulation 1995;91:2325.

59. Caracciolo EA, Davis KB, Sopko G, et al. Comparison of surgical and medical group survival in patients with left main equivalent coronary artery disease: long-term CASS experience. Circulation 1995;91:2335.

60. Hultgren HN, Peduzzi P, Detre K, et al. The 5 year effect of bypass surgery on relief of angina and exercise performance. Circulation 1985;72[Suppl 5]:79.

61. Puskas JD, Winston AD, Wright CE, et al. Stroke after coronary artery operation: incidence, correlates, outcome, and cost. Ann Thorac Surg 2000;69:1053.

62. Roach GW, Kanchuger M, Mangano CM, et al. Adverse cerebral outcomes after coronary bypass surgery. Multicenter Study of Perioperative Ischemia Research Group and the Ischemia Research and Education Foundation Investigators. N Engl J Med 1996;335:1857.

63. McKhann, GM, Goldsborough, MA, Borowics, LM, et al. Predictors of stroke risk in coronary artery bypass patients. Ann Thorac Surg 1997;63:516.

64. Yoon BW, Bae HJ, Kang DW, et al. Intracranial cerebral artery disease as a risk factor for central nervous system complications of coronary artery bypass graft surgery. Stroke 2001;32:94.

65. van der Linden, Hadjinikolaou L, Bergman P, et al. Postoperative stroke in cardiac surgery is related to the location and extent of atherosclerotic disease in the ascending aorta. J Am Coll Cardiol 2001;38:131.

66. van Dijk D, Keizer AM, Diephuis JC, et al. Neurocognitive dysfunction after coronary artery bypass surgery: a systematic review. J Thorac Cardiovasc Surg 2000;120:632.

67. Newman, MF, Kirchner, JL, Phillips-Bute, B, et al. Longitudinal assessment of neurocognitive function after coronary-artery bypass surgery. N Engl J Med 2001;344:395.

68. Daoud EG, Strickberger A, Man KC, et al. Preoperative amiodarone as prophylaxis against atrial fibrillation after heart surgery. N Engl J Med 1997;337:1785.

69. Guarnieri T, Nolan S, Gottlieb SO, et al. Intravenous amiodarone for the prevention of atrial fibrillation after open heart surgery. The Amiodarone Reduction in Coronary Heart (ARCH) trial. J Am Coll Cardiol 1999;34:343.

70. Arora RR, Chou TM, Jain D, et al. The multicenter study of enhanced external counterpulsation (MUST- EECP): effect of EECP on exercise-induced myocardial ischemia and anginal episodes. J Am Coll Cardiol 1999;33:1833.

71. Ernst E. Chelation therapy for coronary heart disease: an overview of all clinical investigations. Am Heart J 2000;140: 139.

72. Oesterle SN, Reifart N, Hauptmann E, et al. Percutaneous in situ coronary venous arterialization: report of the first human catheter-based coronary artery bypass. Circulation 2001;103:2539.

73. Proudfit WL, Bruschke AVG, Sones FM. Clinical course of patients with normal or slightly or moderately abnormal coronary arteriograms: 10 year follow-up of 571 patients. Circulation 1980;62:712.

74. Gottlieb SO, Gottlieb SH, Achuff SC, et al. Silent ischemia on Holter monitoring predicts mortality in high-risk postinfarction patients. JAMA 1988;259:1030.

75. Gottlieb SO, Weisfeldt ML, Ouyang P, et al. Silent ischemia as a marker for early unfavorable outcomes in patients with unstable angina. N Engl J Med 1986;314:1214.

76. Chandra NC, Ziegelstein RC, Rogers WJ, et al. Observations of the treatment of women in the United States with myocardial infarction: a report from the National Registry of Myocardial Infarction—I. Arch Intern Med 1998;158:981.

77. Thompson SG, Kienast J, Pyke SDM, et al. Hemostatic factors and the risk of myocardial infarction or sudden death in patients with angina pectoris. N Engl J Med 1995;332:635.

78. Anderson HV, Cannon CP, Stone PH, et al. One-year results of the thrombolysis in myocardial infarction (TIMI) IIIB clinical trial: a randomized comparison of tissue-type plasminogen activator versus placebo and early invasive versus early conservative strategies in unstable angina and non-Q wave myocardial infarction. J Am Coll Cardiol 1995;26:1643.

79. Califf RM, White HD, Van de Werf F, et al. One-year results from the Global Utilization of Streptokinase and TPA for Occluded Coronary Arteries (GUSTO-I) Trial. Circulation 1996;94:1233.

80. GUSTO Investigators. An international randomized trial comparing four thrombolytic strategies for acute myocardial infarction. N Engl J Med 1993;329:673.

81. Hennekens CH, Buring JE, Sandercock P, et al. Aspirin and other antiplatelet agents in the secondary and primary prevention of cardiovascular disease. Circulation 1989;80:749.

82. Ellstad MH, Wan MKC. Predictive implications of stress testing: follow-up of 2700 subjects after maximum treadmill stress testing. Circulation 1975;51:363.

83. Califf RM, Mark DB, Harrell FE, et al. Importance of clinical measures of ischemia in the prognosis of patients with documented coronary artery disease. J Am Coll Cardiol 1988;11:20.

84. Mock MB, Ringqvist I, Fisher LD, et al. Survival of medically treated patients in the Coronary Artery Surgery Study (CASS) registry. Circulation 1982;66:562.

CHAPTER 63

Postmyocardial Infarction Care and Cardiac Rehabilitation

KERRY J. STEWART, EDD
ROY C. ZIEGELSTEIN, MD

EPIDEMIOLOGY OF MYOCARDIAL INFARCTION

Overview

Cardiovascular diseases remain the major cause of mortality in the United States, accounting for approximately 950,000 deaths annually. These conditions as a whole are responsible for about 41% of all deaths in this country (1). About half of these deaths are caused by myocardial infarction (MI). Although the overall death rate after MI has decreased, the rate of hospitalizations for MI has been stable or has slightly increased over the last decade. The greater number of patients surviving an MI has increased the number of individuals who may be considered for cardiac rehabilitation and secondary prevention (2). In both older and younger patients, mortality after MI could be reduced still further with more consistent use of interventions known to benefit patients after MI, which is the focus of this chapter (3).

Patients who survive an acute MI are far more likely to suffer recurring illness or death from coronary artery disease (CAD). There are approximately 7.3 million people alive today with a history of heart attack in the United States (1). Two of every three survivors of MIs do not make a complete recovery but still have a good long-term prognosis. The longitudinal care of the patient who has survived an MI is usually the responsibility of the patient's primary care provider.

Demographic Subgroups

Five percent of MIs occur in patients younger than 40 years of age, and 45% of people who have MIs are under age 65. Strikingly, approximately 85% of deaths from MI occur in patients over age 65 (4).

It is estimated that in the United States, 1 man in 5 will have an MI before age 60 and that 1 in 10 to 15 men in this age group will die prematurely of atherosclerotic heart disease. These risks are two to three times lower in age-matched women under the age of 65; they are only slightly lower in women over age 65 (4). Death rates from CAD are highest among African-American men and women. Whereas the mortality from cardiovascular disease has declined for men over the last two decades, it has increased for women during this period (1).

Data from the Cardiovascular Health Study show that the *prevalence of MI* in older men (i.e., the history of having had MI) ranges from 18% for ages 65 to 69 to 30% for ages 80 to 84 (4). The prevalence of MI in women ranges from 9.5% for ages 65 to 69 to 17.9% for ages 85 and greater. These findings appear to be related to the higher incidence and prevalence of CAD throughout the adult years in men.

For *patients hospitalized with an acute MI,* women, particularly African-American women, have higher case mortality than men both during hospitalization and in the 48 months after discharge (5). The higher mortality in women admitted for acute MI has been found in all age groups irrespective of type of treatment (6).

PROGNOSIS OF PATIENTS DISCHARGED FROM CORONARY CARE UNITS

Survivors of Myocardial Infarction

Mortality

Over the last two decades, the in-hospital mortality rate for patients with Q-wave MI has decreased, whereas that of non–Q-wave MI has remained the same. The overall in-hospital mortality for acute MI is now 10% to 15% (7). Although the in-hospital mortality rate is higher for patients with Q-wave MI, there is a higher long-term mortality for those with non–Q-wave MI. The overall first-year mortality for hospital survivors of an MI is approximately 10% to 15% (7,8). Most of the deaths in the first year occur during the 3 months after discharge, and they occur chiefly in patients with one or more of the high-risk characteristics listed in Table 63.1.

The *classification of acute MI developed by Killip* according to the presence and severity of congestive heart failure (CHF) on admission to the hospital is one of the most useful prognostic indices. Class I patients have no evidence of CHF on admission, class II patients have mild CHF, class III patients present with pulmonary edema, and class IV patients have cardiogenic shock. Figure 63.1 shows the strikingly different survival rates among patients in these four classes (9). Recently, there has been improvement in survival rates in each of the Killip classes, but the classification remains a valid index of morbidity and mortality after MI.

The clinical factors predictive of an increased mortality after hospital discharge are listed in Table 63.1. Patients with the greatest risk of mortality during the first year after an MI have one or more of the following: a previous MI; development of early (within 10 days) post-MI angina accompanied by transient ST-segment or T-wave changes; an ejection fraction of 40% or less; late hospital phase (predischarge) complex ven-

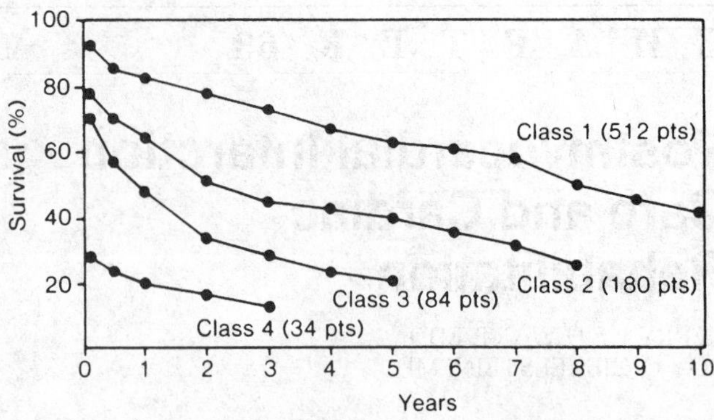

Figure 63.1. Survival after acute myocardial infarction based on Killip classification (810 patients admitted to the Duke Medical Center Coronary Care Unit from 1967 to 1978). (From Rosati RA, Harris PJ. Acute myocardial infarction. In: Fries J, Ehrlich GE, eds. Prognosis: contemporary outcomes of disease. Bowie, MD: Charles Press, 1981:275, with permission.)

tricular arrhythmia; proximal left main, left anterior descending, or three-vessel CAD; a positive stress test at low workload within a few weeks after MI; presence of ischemic ST changes on resting electrocardiogram (ECG) taken 1 month or longer after MI; and low heart rate variability (the amount of heart rate fluctuation around the mean heart rate) (10). The GISSI-2 study also clearly showed that the significantly increased risk of in-hospital mortality with older age persists after discharge (11). Left ventricular (LV) aneurysm developing within 2 days of the acute MI also brings a high risk of death during the first year, independent of LV function (12). In addition to these cardiac complications, post-MI depression is strongly associated with post-MI mortality, even after controlling for other known predictors of survival (13).

In patients who are *clinically stable 1 to 6 months after hospitalization* for an acute MI or unstable angina, the presence of ischemic ST-segment depression on the resting ECG is the strongest predictor of morbidity and mortality over the ensuing 3 years. Posthospitalization stress testing is predictive of future coronary events in stable patients only when ischemia (1 mm or greater ST-segment depression on exercise ECG) or a reversible perfusion defect (on thallium exercise test) is present at a low workload (5 metabolic equivalents [METs] or less) or when there is evidence of exercise-induced LV dysfunction (LV cavity dilation and/or increased thallium uptake by the lung during exercise) (14). Each of these high-risk subsets has made up less than 3% of study populations.

Table 63.1. Characteristics Associated with Increased Mortality After Discharge of Patients Who Have Had an MI

Admission characteristics
- History of a previous MI
- CHF (chest x-ray or Killip classification)
- History of hypertension
- Extent of LV ischemia (radionuclide scintigraphy, cardiac enzymes)

Characteristics at discharge
- Early (within 10 days) post-MI angina, with transient ST–T changes[a]
- LV ejection fraction $<40\%$ (radionuclide ventriculography, arteriography)
- Complex ventricular arrhythmia[b] (Holter monitor)
- Left main proximal, left anterior descending, or three-vessel CAD (arteriography)
- Positive limited early post-MI ECG stress test (within 2–3 weeks after MI)
- Ventricular aneurysm developing in acute stage of MI

Characteristics after discharge
- ECG abnormalities, especially ischemic ST-segment depression, $\geq$1 month after MI
- Decreased heart rate variability
- Cigarette smoking
- Depression

[a]Mortality risk highest when ECG shows ischemia at a distance (i.e., transient ischemic ST changes in myocardial location that is different from the location of the patient's MI).

[b]Multifocal premature ventricular contractions (PVCs), runs of two or more sequential ectopic ventricular beats, or PVCs with R on T pattern.

MI, myocardial infarction; CHF, congestive heart failure; LV, left ventricular; ECG, electrocardiogram; CAD, coronary artery disease.

Morbidity

Postinfarction angina occurs during the year after an MI in many patients (15). In patients who are free of angina or other cardiac symptoms in the hospital, a predischarge exercise stress test may be performed safely. Patients who can exercise to 5 to 6 METs or to 70% to 80% of the age-predicted maximal heart rate without an abnormal ECG or blood pressure response have a low 1-year mortality (16). Exercise testing increases the ability to predict whether a patient will develop angina. Angina during the years after an MI occurs in almost 90% of patients with positive stress tests but in only about one in three patients with a negative stress test (15). Patients with a post-MI symptom limited stress test showing early ischemic ST-segment changes (1 mm or more exercise-induced ST-segment depression) or limited work capacity (5 METs or less) have two or more times the risk of recurrent MI and of death over the ensuing year (17). As described below (see Risk Stratification Before Hospital Discharge), patients with abnormal predischarge stress tests are often catheterized to decide on the advisability of revascularization.

Postinfarction medical complications other than angina include CHF, life-threatening arrhythmias and sudden death, intracavity thrombi with stroke and systemic emboli, and post-MI syndrome (Dressler syndrome).

The *psychologic and social sequelae* during the year after an MI depend on both the severity of the patient's MI and the patient's premorbid psychosocial situation (see below for a more detailed discussion of this topic).

Patients With Unstable Angina

Unstable angina is defined as pain caused by cardiac ischemia that is occurring more frequently, is being provoked by less effort, is occurring at rest, or is being relieved less readily by nitroglycerin. Other characteristics are described in Chapter 62.

Patients discharged from the cardiac care unit with the diagnosis of unstable angina have 1-year morbidity and mortality rates similar to those of patients discharged with the diagnosis of a completed MI (18). Studies show that the resting ECG and the response to exercise stress testing are especially helpful in predicting future events in patients who are clinically stable after admission for unstable angina (14). The lack of ischemic ST-segment changes during exercise testing helps to identify patients at lower risk (19).

In an individual patient with unstable angina, a more precise prognosis can be given by defining the coronary anatomy by *cardiac catheterization and coronary angiography.* In studies of patients with unstable angina, coronary angiography has shown that left main CAD is more common in patients discharged with the diagnosis of unstable angina than in those discharged with the diagnosis of a completed MI (15% vs. 5%, respectively). Another 10% have diffuse CAD, 10% have normal coronary arteries and are presumed to have coronary artery spasm or small vessel disease as the cause of their chest pain, and the remaining 65% are equally divided among single, double, and triple coronary vessel disease (20). This information is clinically important because of the demonstrated superiority of surgical over medical treatment of left main CAD. The prognoses associated with each of the above patterns and the management of unstable angina are described in Chapter 62.

Survivors of Cardiac Arrest Who Have Not Had a Myocardial Infarction

The first-year mortality rate of survivors of out-of-hospital cardiac arrest who have not had an MI is approximately three times the mortality rate of survivors of out-of-hospital cardiac arrest who subsequently are shown to have completed an MI. In a study of more than 200 survivors of out-of-hospital cardiac arrest followed for over 4 years, the rate of recurrence of ventricular fibrillation or sudden death in patients without an acute MI was 31%, compared with 5% for out-of-hospital survivors of cardiac arrest who subsequently evolved ECG changes of acute MI. The median time to recurrent circulatory arrest was 20 weeks. More than 70% of the episodes of ventricular fibrillation were unexpected or occurred during sleep or during the usual activities of daily living (21).

Because the survivors of ventricular fibrillation not associated with an MI have a high risk of sudden death they require aggressive and highly individualized treatment. The multiplicity of recent advances in electrophysiology, antiarrhythmics, automatic implantable defibrillators, and the many innovative surgical approaches to medically intractable, but symptomatic, ventricular dysrhythmias dictate prompt referral of such high-risk patients to a consulting cardiologist. This topic is discussed in more detail in Chapter 64.

RISK STRATIFICATION BEFORE HOSPITAL DISCHARGE

In 1997, the American College of Physicians published the recommendations for in-hospital risk stratification of MI patients, summarized in Figs. 63.2 and 63.3 (see General References). This three-phase scheme delineates decision-making that is supported by outcome data from clinical trials. It was published to guide the care of MI patients before they are discharged from the hospital. It draws on a mix of *baseline characteristics and findings from continuous reevaluation of the patient.* Depending on clinical findings, a patient may have undergone thrombolysis, revascularization, or neither in the acute and nonacute phase of risk stratification. In the *predischarge evaluation*, patients at intermediate or low risk (60% to 70% of MI patients) should have assessment of their LV function and noninvasive stress testing. Often, those patients can be discharged after stays as short as 4 to 5 days. The postdischarge prognosis of MI patients and their appropriate management depends on the predischarge evaluation, postdischarge reevaluations, and the rehabilitation and medical approaches described in this chapter.

REHABILITATION AND MANAGEMENT AFTER MYOCARDIAL INFARCTION

Most patients discharged after MI can expect to return to most of their usual activities within a few weeks

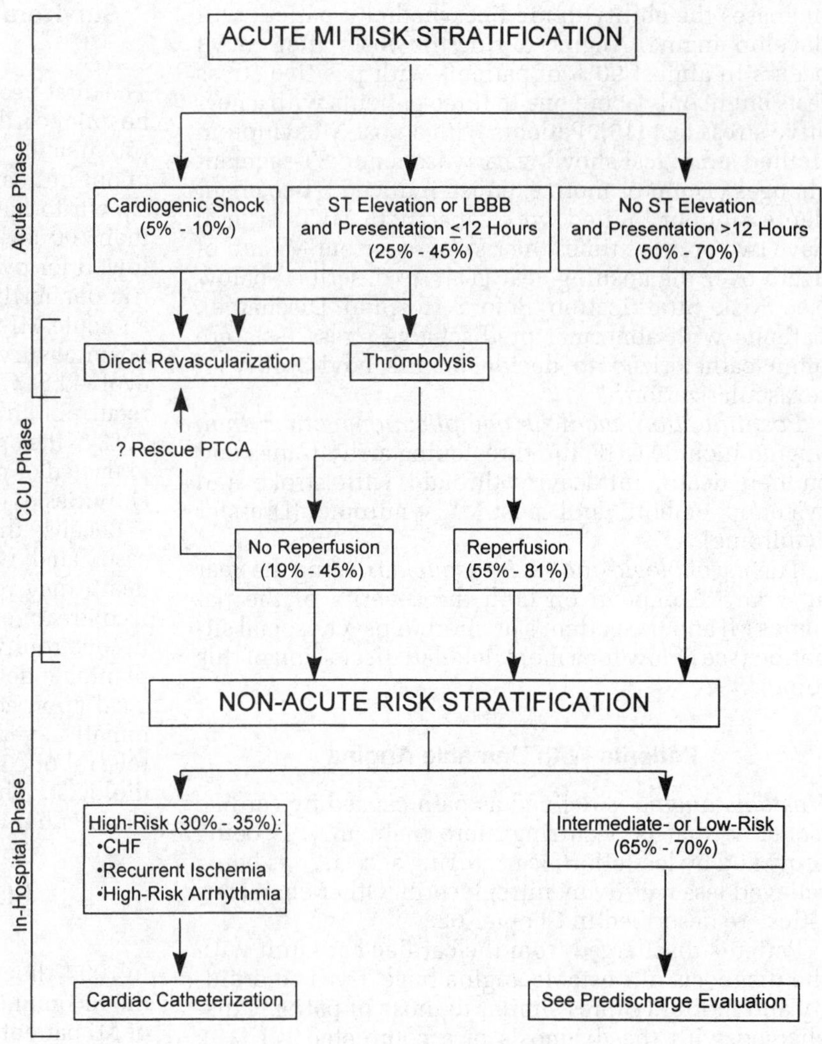

Figure 63.2. Flow diagram of risk stratification after myocardial infarction. *CCU,* coronary care unit; *CHF,* congestive heart failure; *LBBB,* left bundle branch block; *MI,* myocardial infarction; *PTCA,* percutaneous transluminal coronary angioplasty; *ST,* ST segment. (From Clinical Guidelines Part I and II. Guidelines for risk stratification after myocardial infarction [American College of Physicians]. Ann Intern Med 1997;126:556, with permission.)

to months. For a smaller number of patients, complications of their MI make this outcome impossible. In either situation, an organized plan for care should be followed (Table 63.2). This plan should include the education of the patient and the patient's family. Because of shorter hospital stays, much of the patient education previously included in inpatient cardiac rehabilitation is now conducted in outpatient programs.

Patient Education

Most hospitals initiate education about MI when the patient is clinically stable. The educational program is often the responsibility of a cardiac rehabilitation professional. Patient education should cover the nature of coronary heart disease, cardiac symptoms, cardiac drugs, modification of major risk factors (smoking, hypertension, hyperlipidemia, obesity, and inactivity) and guidelines for resumption of physical activities (including sexual activity) and return to work. It should be emphasized that MI is a manifestation of a disease process that has been going on for many years. Many patients attribute their MI to what they were doing at the moment it actually occurred. Patients must understand that the MI would very likely have occurred regardless of what they were doing that particular day and that the likelihood of a recurrence may best be diminished by following prescribed medical therapy and making lifestyle changes.

Individualized information should be provided in a *predischarge conference* at which the patient and the patient's family members are encouraged to ask questions. The conference should include review of any adverse prognostic features identified before discharge (Table 63.1); the medications prescribed at discharge; discussion of specific plans for cardiac rehabilitation, diet, and smoking modification; a chance for ventilation about emotional stress-laden issues; and realistic appraisal of expectations of return to work or usual levels of physical activity. Because of the high frequency of postinfarction angina, it is especially important to describe this symptom to patients who have never had it and to point out to all patients that it may occur with the increased activity recommended for the coming

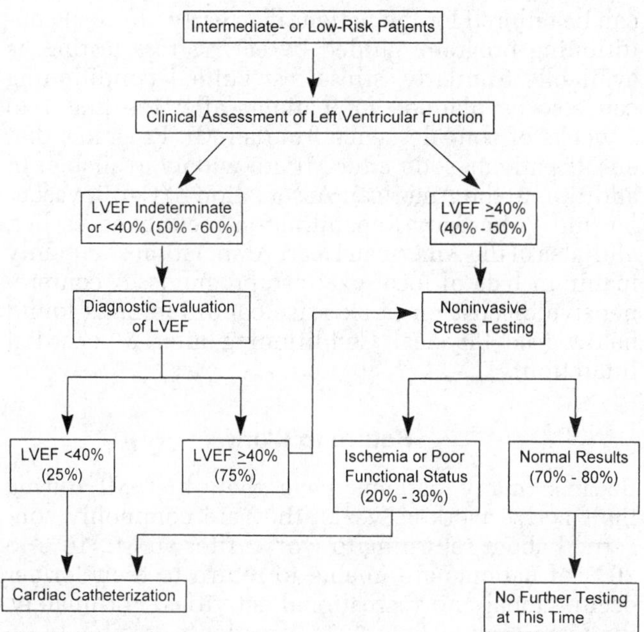

Figure 63.3. Flow diagram for predischarge risk stratification after myocardial infarction. *LVEF,* left ventricular ejection fraction. (From Clinical Guidelines Parts I and II. Guidelines for risk stratification after myocardial infarction [American College of Physicians]. Ann Intern Med 1997;126:556, with permission.)

Table 63.2. Plan of Care for MI Survivors After Hospital Discharge

Patient education (objectives for all patients)[a]
- Understands disease process (damage to the heart that heals in a few months, leaves a scar)
- Understands likely prognosis
- Understands and follows progressive activity schedule[b]
- Understands approximate timetable for return to work[b]
- Understands importance of controlling major risk factors (smoking, hypercholesterolemia, hypertension) and takes action to control them
- Knows how to recognize principal cardiac symptoms (angina, tachycardia, heart failure, hypotension) and understands how to use sublingual nitroglycerin
- Participates in group classes after discharge[c]
- Gets answers to questions specific to his or her lifestyle

Medical management
- Review in-hospital course for prognosis characteristics (see Table 63.1) and for medications prescribed at discharge
- Assess and reinforce above patient education
- Check periodically for complications of infarction (see Table 63.6)
- Check for behavior–psychiatric complications
- Check ECG 2–3 months after discharge
- Beta-blocker, ACE inhibitor, and aspirin treatment[d]
- Referral for physical conditioning[d]

[a]Essential to include the patient's spouse in all aspects of education.
[b]Serial exercise stress tests may be used to plan progressive activity (see text).
[c]If programs are available in the community.
[d]See text for details.
MI, myocardial infarction; ACE, angiotensive converting enzyme.

weeks. Every patient should be given sublingual nitroglycerin, and the correct use of this drug should be reviewed.

Because patients may not retain the information they hear in the hospital, it is important to provide this information in writing and to assess and reinforce patient understanding of it after discharge. The patient education booklet *After a Heart Attack* (single copies available without charge from local chapters of the American Heart Association) gives a useful general account of the disease process, prognosis, coronary risk factors, and rehabilitation process.

Many hospitals have developed *group classes for MI survivors and their spouses.* Typically, patients and their spouses are invited to participate in a number of weekly meetings during the first or second month after discharge. Sessions are usually led by a cardiac rehabilitation professional such as a nurse, social worker, clinical exercise physiologist, or cardiologist, with the objective of having participants raise questions about the recovery period to provide mutual support by sharing experiences with each other. Additional resources available in many communities are patient-run heart clubs and supervised physical conditioning programs (see Physical Conditioning after Myocardial Infarction, below). The American Association of Cardiovascular and Pulmonary Rehabilitation (401 North Michigan Avenue, Chicago, IL 60611-4267; 312-321-5146; http://www.aacvpr.org) publishes a national directory of cardiac rehabilitation programs and is a good source of professional and patient materials, including *Guidelines for Cardiac Rehabilitation* (see General References). There are also several nationally distributed newsletters for patients with CAD (e.g., *The Heartline,* Coronary Clubs, Inc., 9500 Euclid Ave., Cleveland, OH 44195; telephone 216-444-3690). In recent years, the *WorldWide Web* has offered a wealth of patient information dealing with heart disease prevention and rehabilitation. Some examples include the sites of the Johns Hopkins Bayview Medical Center (http://www.jhbmc.jhu.edu/cardiology/cardiology.html) and of the American Heart Association (http://www.amhrt.org). Patients can also be directed to support groups such as The Mended Hearts (http://www.mendedhearts.org). Many of these sites provide links to other sources of patient information, support, and online newsletters.

Postdischarge Appointments

In general, each patient who has had an MI should be encouraged to contact his or her primary care provider or cardiologist at least once during the first week at home to discuss any questions that arise, and an office visit should be scheduled within 2 to 3 weeks. Before this visit, it is important to review the patient's hospital summary to determine whether adverse prognostic features were present (Table 63.1) and to identify the medications prescribed at discharge. The visit should be divided between an assessment of the patient's progress in rehabilitation (physical activity level, diet and smoking modifications, emotional status, understanding of the overall plan of care, expectation about return to work) and an assessment of the patient's medical status (manifestations of ischemia and heart failure, blood pressure status, and review of current medications). Two or more additional office visits, similar to the first visit, should be scheduled during the 3 months after an MI, and the patient should be encouraged to telephone at any time about symptoms or questions.

Risk Stratification at 3 to 6 Weeks

About 3 to 6 weeks after MI, a *maximal exercise stress test* should be considered, because this can provide helpful therapeutic and prognostic information regarding the patient's disease. Table 63.3 summarizes the criteria and recommendations of the American College of Physicians, based on stratification into low-risk and moderate-risk findings in this stress test. The stress test is also used to assess functional capacity, to guide the return to work, and to provide goals (e.g., target heart rate, MET level) for an exercise prescription. About 3 months after hospital discharge, an ECG should be obtained; this should be used as the patient's new baseline tracing.

Activity Schedule

Table 63.4 contains a practical summary (for use by the patient) of symptom recognition and a schedule of progressive physical activities for the first 2 months after MI. Table 63.5 lists a broad array of activities corresponding to the recommended energy levels during and after the recuperation period. Resumption of activities with different energy requirements should be gradual; in particular, the duration of certain activities should be brief at first, with gradual increase, according to how the patient feels. The schedule in Table 63.4 can be given to most patients. A more aggressive plan can be tailored for the patient if an early physical conditioning program, guided by early stress testing, is available. Similarly, stress test guided conditioning can also be planned for patients after the first 1 to 2 weeks of convalescence from an MI. Programs that enroll patients soon after MI are widely available. In addition to the American Association of Cardiovascular and Pulmonary Rehabilitation mentioned earlier, affiliates of the American Heart Association commonly maintain lists of local exercise programs. A comprehensive discussion of exercise conditioning is found below (see Physical Conditioning after Myocardial Infarction).

Table 63.3. Recommendations According to Stress Test Risk Stratification 3 to 6 Weeks After MI

Low-risk patients

These patients have a peak workload of 5 METs[a] or more in the absence of exercise-induced angina pectoris or ST-segment depression.

Recommendations: Further diagnostic testing is unlikely to identify patients at an even lower risk and is therefore not indicated. The effect, if any, of medical or surgical therapy on the prognosis of these patients is difficult to demonstrate because of their very low risk. Treatment should emphasize the reduction of risk factors, especially the control of hypertension, cessation of smoking, modification of diet, and exercise training.

Moderate-risk patients

These patients have a peak workload of less than 5 METs, a peak systolic pressure of less than 110 mm Hg, or severe myocardial ischemia, defined as angina or ischemic ST-segment depression of 2 mm or more appearing at a heart rate of 130 to 140 bpm or less.

Indication for coronary arteriography: In patients at moderate risk, coronary arteriography is indicated.

[a]MET (metabolic equivalent) is the energy requirement for a certain level of activity. One MET is the energy requirement at rest. See METs for common activities in Table 63.5.

bpm, beats per minute; MI, myocardial infarction.

From American College of Physicians. Evaluation of patients after recent acute myocardial infarction (position paper). Ann Intern Med 1989;110:485, with permission.

Return to Work

Because many patients have their first MI during their active working years, they are commonly concerned about returning to work. After an MI, 10% to 20% of patients are unable to return to their former occupational and recreational activities. Fortunately, the remaining 80% to 90% of patients are able to do so within 2 to 6 months. In fact, 88% of those younger than age 65 are able to return to their usual work after an MI (1). Patients who do not return to work within 6 months of MI are unlikely ever to return to work (22), and this is often caused by psychological and not physical factors (see Psychological Problems, below). Telling the patient, soon after discharge, to expect to return to work is important in preventing disability caused by psychological factors. Obviously, the type of work is also an important consideration. Patients whose occupations involve mental stress and hectic schedules should be advised to return to work on a part-time basis at first, leaving plenty of time for rest and relaxation. For patients whose work involves significant physical exertion, the timing of return to work can be based on the information in Tables 63.4 and 63.5 and guided by the results of exercise stress testing and monitored responses during a supervised rehabilitation program. From Table 63.5, it is evident that most occupations require an energy level of 6 METs or less. Occupational activities classified as heavy work, such as digging ditches, require energy expenditure of 7 METs or more. Certain activities may produce an increased workload on the heart because of psychological stress (e.g., driving a vehicle) or because they entail significant resistive exercise (e.g., carpentry, plumbing, shoveling, operating pneumatic tools, or carrying objects heavier than 30 pounds).

Patients with MIs complicated by poorly controlled angina, CHF, or arrhythmias should be evaluated in conjunction with a consulting cardiologist (see Medical Complications, below) before a plan for returning to work and other activities is recommended. Some of these patients qualify for *permanent medical disability* (see Chapter 9) or for job retraining through vocational rehabilitation. The *fundamental difference between impairment and disability* caused by CAD was underscored in the report of the 1989 Bethesda Conference on Insurability and Employability of the Patient with Ischemic Heart Disease (23). Impairment is

Table 63.4. Activity Schedule and Symptom Recognition for Patients Convalescing from MI[a]

General points

All activities, including sitting and lying down, require energy. The amount of energy required to perform a specific activity is expressed as METs. One MET is your resting energy requirement. As activities become more strenuous, the amount of energy required (METs) also increases, as does the workload imposed on your heart.

The schedule recommended in this program is based on the number of METs needed for various activities. Some specific recommendations are given for each of the first 3 months after your return to home. Table 63.5 gives the energy requirements for a wide variety of additional activities. If the table omits your favorite activities, ask your doctor about them.

Warnings: Generally the following activities impose an added strain on your heart and should be avoided, especially during the first 3 months after a heart attack:

- Taking very hot or cold showers or baths
- Holding your breath while exercising, lifting, or straining
- Working in a bent or stooped position or with arms held above your head
- Doing work that requires continuous tensing of your muscles
- Working or exercising during very hot, cold, humid, or windy weather (in bad weather, plan your regular exercise at a nearby shopping mall)
- Working or exercising during the first hour after a meal or after consuming alcohol
- Consuming excessive amounts of alcohol (e.g., more than 1–2 ounces of whiskey, 2–3 beers, 1–2 glasses of wine per day)
- Walking or exercising on a hill or an inclined surface
- Engaging in any activity that creates emotional stress or worry for you

Recommended activity schedule[b]

First month (1–3 METs)

From discharge to 1 week

Regular exercise: Walk 5 min at a leisurely pace once a day on a level surface.

Some specific advice: This week, primarily get used to being at home. Occupy yourself with sit-down activities such as watching television, playing cards, sewing, painting, or sketching. Avoid lifting objects heavier than 5 lb or doing activities that require reaching above your head. You may go up and down the stairs. However, take your time and limit the number of times you need to climb them. Do all of the things you were doing in the hospital. Get up and get dressed each day. You may be surprised at how tired and weak you feel. This is natural. Be sure to take rest periods when you need them, particularly after meals and before you exercise or climb the stairs.

Week 2

Regular exercise: Walk 5 min at a leisurely pace twice a day.

Some specific advice: Continue all of your previous activities and add others, such as taking rides in the car (however, no driving yet), cooking a meal, washing clothes in a machine (have someone else remove them), making your bed, attending a relaxing movie, going out to dinner, going shopping with your family (let others lift things from the shelves to the basket and carry the groceries), shooting pool, playing shuffleboard, throwing a softball underhand, playing a piano or organ.

Weeks 3 and 4

Regular exercise: Advance gradually to walking 10 min at a leisurely pace twice a day.

Some specific advice: Continue your previous activities and others, such as going to religious services, sweeping floors, polishing furniture, driving the car (beginning with short drives, avoiding heavy traffic).

Second month (3–5 METs)

Regular physical exercise: Progressively increase leisurely walking from 15 min once a day at a slightly faster pace to 30 min once or twice a day.

Some specific advice: Table 63.5 lists the approximate energy requirements of each activity. You may gradually increase your activities by adding additional activities and spending more time at them; consult Table 63.5 for activities requiring 5 METs or less (or more).

Recognizing heart symptoms

Your heart will give you warning signs if it is not ready for increased activity. Here are some guidelines to use:

Pulse: Locate your pulse and count the number of times it beats for 15 sec and multiply that number by 4. This is your heart rate for 1 min. Take your pulse before you begin your walk or any new activity and at the end of the activity. Contact your health care provider before resuming exercise if:

- There is an increase of 20 heartbeats or more per minute in postexercise pulse over pre-exercise pulse
- Your heart rate exceeds 120/min[c]
- You detect abnormal heart action: pulse becoming irregular, fluttering or jumping in chest or throat, very slow pulse rate, sudden burst of rapid heartbeats

Chest pain: Contact your health care provider before resuming exercise if you experience pain or pressure in the chest, arm, or throat precipitated by exercise or following exercise. Remember to take your nitroglycerin and rest if you do experience pain.

Dizziness: Contact your health care provider before resuming exercise if you become dizzy, light-headed, or faint during exercise.

Breathing difficulty: Contact your health care provider before resuming exercise if you become short of breath during or after a new exercise, or if you awaken from sleep short of breath.

[a]Information in Table 63.5 should be given to patients who receive the instructions in this table.
[b]Pace of these activities may be scaled up or down by results of early post-MI stress test when available.
[c]These figures may be markedly modified by results of early stress test or medication.
MI, myocardial infarction.

a medically defined disorder and is an important component of disability, but it is just one of several factors that determine the overall ability of a person to perform meaningful work. Additional factors that affect disability include other medical disorders, age, sex, education, training, and psychosocial support. The main points in the report state that most MI patients can return to work; prognosis can be estimated by clinical examination and noninvasive studies that evaluate LV function (echocardiogram), myocardial jeopardy (thallium stress test), and electrical instability (Holter monitor); cardiac catheterization is not routinely required; special assessment may be needed for jobs requiring sudden or sustained high effort or heat exposure (e.g., firefighters) or for those in whom sudden disability may endanger others (e.g., airline pilots); a trial period of progressively increasing part-time work may be necessary for smooth transition from total disability

Table 63.5. Energy Requirements of Certain Activities

Activity Level	Self-Care or Home	Occupational	Recreational	Physical Conditioning
Very light (≤3 METs)	Washing, shaving, dressing Desk work, writing, washing dishes Driving car[a]	Sitting (clerical, assembling) Standing (store clerk, bartender) Driving truck[a] Crane operator[a]	Shuffleboard Horseshoes Bait casting Billiards Archery[a] Golf (cart)	Walking (level, at 2 mph) Stationary bike (very low resistance) Very light calisthenics
Light to moderate (3–5 METs)	Cleaning windows Raking leaves Weeding Power lawn mowing Waxing floors (slowly) Painting Carrying objects 15–30 lb[b]	Stocking shelves (light objects)[b] Light welding Light carpentry[b] Machine assembly Auto repair Paper hanging[b]	Dancing Golf (walking) Sailing Horseback riding Volleyball Tennis (doubles) Sexual intercourse[a] (see details in the text)	Walking (3–4 mph) Level bicycling (6–8 mph) Light calisthenics
Moderate (5–7 METs)	Easy digging in garden Level hand lawn mowing Climbing stairs (slowly) Carrying objects 30–60 lb[b]	Carpentry (exterior home building)[b] Shoveling dirt[b] Pneumatic tools[b]	Badminton (competitive) Tennis (singles) Snow skiing (downhill) Light backpacking Basketball Football Skating (ice and roller) Horseback riding (gallop)	Swimming (breast stroke)
Heavy (7–9 METs)	Sawing wood[b] Heavy shoveling[b] Climbing stairs (moderate speed) Carrying objects 60–90 lb[b]	Tending furnace[b] Digging ditches[b] Pick and shovel[b]	Canoeing[b] Mountain climbing[b] Fencing Paddleball Touch football	Jogging (5 mph) Swimming (crawl stroke) Rowing machine Heavy calisthenics Bicycling (12 mph)
Very heavy (9 METs)	Carrying loads upstairs[b] Carrying objects 90 lb or more Climbing stairs (quickly) Shoveling heavy snow[b] Shoveling for 10 min (16 lb)	Lumberjack[b] Heavy laborer[b]	Handball Squash Ski touring over hills[b] Vigorous basketball	Running (6 mph) Bicycling (≥13 mph or steep hill) Rope jumping

[a]May cause added psychologic stress that will increase work of the heart.

[b]May produce disproportionate myocardial demands because of use of arms or isometric exercise. See further discussion regarding isometric (resistive) exercise in physical conditioning section of this chapter.

From Haskell WL. Design and implementation of cardiac conditioning programs. In: Hellerstein HK, ed. Rehabilitation of the coronary patient. New York: John Wiley & Sons, 1978:203, with permission.

to full-time work; and maximal functional capacity should be evaluated as soon as the clinical status is stable usually 3 to 5 weeks after uncomplicated MI, 7 weeks after coronary bypass surgery, and 1 week after coronary angioplasty in patients who have not had an MI.

Although cardiac rehabilitation, including education, counseling, and behavioral intervention, has many benefits, it has not been shown to alter the rates of return to work. This was the conclusion of the 1995 *Cardiac Rehabilitation Guidelines* of the Agency for Health Care Policy and Research (see General References). The expert panel reported that although education and counseling may improve a patient's potential for return to work, many other factors play a role in return to work, including willingness of the employer to rehire the patient, the patient's level of job satisfaction, economic incentives, and perceived stress of the job.

Sexual Activity

It is safe for patients who are symptom free during usual activities of daily living to resume sexual intercourse within 4 to 6 weeks of their MI. Available data suggest that the energy requirement approximates 3 METs during foreplay and afterplay and 5 METs at climax (24). These are equivalent to the oxygen demands of a brisk walk around the block or climbing one flight of stairs. In a study of patients after MI, coitus accounted for less than 1% of sudden deaths. These usually occurred during extramarital affairs in which the men were considerably older than their companions and often were inebriated at the time of intercourse (25).

The Myocardial Infarction Onset Study (26) also provides information about the risk of sexual activity in patients with cardiac disease and is of particular benefit to those counseling individuals about sexual activity after an MI. Although this study confirmed that sexual activity can trigger MI, the risk appears to be small and transient. Importantly, the relative risk of triggering an MI in individuals with a history of angina or previous MI is not greater than it is in those without prior cardiac disease.

This same study also indicated that regular exercise appears to reduce, and possibly to eliminate, the small increased risk of MI associated with sexual activity. Thus, health care providers who counsel patients after an MI can reassure them that the risk of triggering an MI during sexual activity is particularly low for those who exercise regularly. When counseling patients about resumption of sexual activity, one should *give specific advice* and encourage questions. The pamphlet *Sex and Heart Disease,* available from the American Heart Association (http://americanheart.org/Heart_and_Stroke_A_Z_Guide/sex.html), is a helpful adjunct to counseling. Frequency of sexual intercourse can be similar to the frequency before the patient's MI. Sexual foreplay without completion of intercourse can be recommended to patients who wish to resume sex cautiously. In general, sexual activity can be resumed in the position that was most gratifying before the MI; however, patients should avoid positions in which they support their weight on their arms because this requires sustained isometric type of work (see Physical Conditioning after Myocardial Infarction, below) and may put extra stress on the heart. Sexual activity should be engaged in when both partners are relaxed. It is best to abstain from intercourse for 2 or 3 hours after eating a large meal because eating increases the work of the heart.

Inability to return to a previous pattern of sexual activity may be caused by angina (precipitated by intercourse), new medications, or psychological stress associated with the recent MI. If an otherwise stable patient develops angina during intercourse, sublingual nitroglycerin can be taken just before sexual activity.

Erectile dysfunction may be particularly common in men with CAD because the two conditions share common risk factors. For this reason, practitioners may be asked about the use of sildenafil (Viagra) by patients recovering from an MI. Sildenafil inhibits cyclic guanosine monophosphate (cGMP)-specific phosphodiesterase type 5, thereby inhibiting the breakdown of cGMP and allowing it to accumulate in the corpus cavernosum of the penis. A recent study in men with severe coronary stenosis showed that oral sildenafil did not produce any adverse cardiovascular effects, even in coronary flow (27). Although caution should be used when prescribing sildenafil to patients with CAD, particularly if the individual is not regularly physically active, it may be appropriate in the absence of low blood pressure or aortic stenosis. It must be emphasized, however, that sildenafil should not be used by men who are taking medicines that contain organic nitrates of any kind, including nitroglycerin. Because nitrates cause an increase in cGMP and sildenafil inhibits its breakdown, the combination of sildenafil and any nitrate may result in dramatic, and potentially dangerous, reductions in arterial blood pressure. The evaluation and management of drug-induced and psychological sexual dysfunction, both of which may occur after MI, are discussed in Chapter 6.

Psychological Problems

It is normal for patients to experience *symptoms of anxiety and depression* during the first few weeks after discharge from the hospital. Some of these symptoms are caused by misconceptions about the nature and prognosis of MI and may respond to simple reassurance and clarification. Most patients do well when encouraged to express their concerns and reassured that their response is normal. A small supply of a minor tranquilizer (see Chapter 22) or a short-acting hypnotic (see Chapter 7) can be prescribed if needed. As noted earlier (see Patient Education), participation in group classes and group exercise programs can also help patients adjust to changes in their lives after MI.

Another common psychological complication of MI is an *inappropriate fear of physical activity of any kind* (i.e., the so-called cardiac cripple or ergophobic). Early participation in supervised physical activity, including the treadmill test, and exercise conditioning have been shown to enhance the patient's self-confidence and ability to perform physical tasks (28). Having the spouse observe the early treadmill test establishes confidence in the spouse that his or her partner is not a cardiac cripple. In some medical centers, spouses are offered an opportunity to walk on the treadmill as well. This serves to establish a reference point for estimating ability to engage in activity. Engaging in a wide range of activities in the months after an MI is important because self-confidence is task specific (28,29). Most cardiac exercise programs (see below) emphasize activities using the legs, such as walking and jogging. Although this increases self-confidence in tasks requiring leg work, it does little for arm self-confidence. To increase arm self-confidence, patients must practice arm exercises as well (29,30). This is especially important for patients who plan to return to work that requires upper body and arm efforts. The use of resistance training in cardiac rehabilitation also helps to increase self-confidence.

Another common problem is *denial of illness persisting beyond the first few days in the hospital.* The behavior associated with persistent denial may create substantial risks. This is especially true of patients who are extremely competitive and are used to controlling most of the circumstances of their lives (31). They are typically determined to return to work as soon as possible and will refuse cardiac rehabilitation on the basis that they can do it better on their own. This behavior arouses anxiety, fear, and concern in the spouse and family and may lead to significant marital conflict. An open discussion with patient and spouse, with each acknowledging the other's concerns, can often lead to resolution of these conflicts and more appropriate behavior from each partner.

At times it is useful to teach patients to use *various forms of feedback* to guide their activities. Specifically, patients are taught to use a target heart rate based on an exercise stress test; to observe themselves and how they feel, with the basic instruction to rest if fatigue or any cardiac symptoms occur during exercise; to call their primary care provider or cardiologist if symptoms persist after using nitroglycerin; and to view the spouse as a source of feedback. In most cases, the spouse's observation of how the patient looks is remarkably accurate. If a wife says her husband looks tired or does not look right, she is probably right (and vice versa). By having the patient agree to consider these comments as well meaning, the patient will usually comply with the spouse's advice. Thereafter, the number of reminding behaviors from the spouse is reduced progressively, and the rehabilitation process can proceed with greater enthusiasm from both partners. With more difficult patients or when there is pre-existing marital strife, the consultation of a psychiatrist or psychologist may be helpful in managing adjustment problems.

Some patients have *severe psychological and behavioral problems after MI* that may interfere with their rehabilitation. The most common problem is *persistent depression,* which may have characteristics of a major or minor depressive illness or may present as an adjustment disorder characterized by anxiety, depression, somatization, or a mixture of these responses (32). The diagnosis and management of these problems are discussed in Chapters 21, 22, and 24.

About 40% of patients have either minor or major depression soon after an MI (32). *Major depression* occurs in 15% to 20% of patients and is associated with a three- to fourfold increased cardiovascular mortality at 6 months (13). Individuals with major depression soon after an MI are likely to remain depressed for at least several months and possibly longer (32). Thus, the practitioner who views depression as an expected reaction that is likely to improve and not likely to influence recovery may be missing an opportunity to improve the patient's quality of life and health. Because major depression typically does not resolve spontaneously, the patient who leaves the hospital depressed may continue to experience mood disturbance at the very time when participation in risk-reducing behaviors is critical. Patients with depression after an MI are less likely to adhere to recommended behavior and lifestyle changes intended to reduce the risk of subsequent cardiac events (33).

These findings highlight the importance of recognizing symptoms of depression and offering patients appropriate treatment, which should include a program of cardiac rehabilitation (34). A study in which depressive symptoms were present in 20% of patients after a major coronary event showed that symptoms resolved in two-thirds of these patients after a program of cardiac rehabilitation (35). Unfortunately, patients with depression are more difficult to recruit and retain in these programs than are individuals without depression (36,37). When depression is identified in a patient recovering from an MI, the practitioner should encourage the individual to socialize and to increase interactions with friends and family. Depression resolves more rapidly after an MI when patients have good social support (38). Social support may even buffer the adverse effects of depression on prognosis. The 1-year cardiac mortality of depressed patients with the lowest levels of perceived social support has been observed to be more than five times that of depressed patients with the highest levels of perceived social support (38).

Several small studies report that the selective serotonin reuptake inhibitors (SSRIs) are safe and effective in patients with ischemic heart disease, some of whom had recently sustained an MI (39–41). In light of these studies and the general absence of significant cardiovascular side effects of the SSRIs, antidepressants in this class are preferable to tricyclic antidepressants (TCAs) in patients with depression after an MI who require antidepressant therapy. TCAs may increase resting heart rate, produce orthostatic hypotension, and adversely affect intracardiac conduction and, possibly, the susceptibility to ventricular arrhythmias (42). In a study that compared the effects of the SSRI paroxetine to those of the TCA nortriptyline in patients with ischemic heart disease and major depression, patients treated with the TCA experienced significantly more adverse cardiac events than those treated with paroxetine (40). The results of larger trials investigating the benefit of psychosocial interventions and antidepressant drug treatment in patients who are recovering from an MI should be available in the next few years to help guide the therapy of these high-risk individuals. The treatment of depression is described in detail in Chapter 24.

Studies show that the basic components of *coronary-prone behavior* (type A behavior) are time urgency and free-floating hostility. Long working hours, sustained drive, reasonable competitiveness, and enthusiasm do not appear to constitute coronary-prone behavior. In some patients, the basic components of type A behavior can be modified. Such modification has been associated with significant decrease in morbidity and mortality (43).

Medical Therapy

Overview

There is evidence that beta-blockers and aspirin reduce the risk of morbidity and mortality after MI. For certain subgroups of patients, long-term treatment with angiotensin-converting enzyme (ACE) inhibitors also improves prognosis. Despite the widespread use of calcium channel blockers after MI, there is no evidence that treated patients benefit. The evidence for current recommendations regarding each of these classes of drugs is thoroughly reviewed by Hennekens et al. (see General References).

Beta-Adrenoreceptor Blockers

Beta-blocker therapy is recommended for patients who have had an MI. Treatment should begin during the initial hospitalization and should be continued indefinitely. The benefits of beta-blocker therapy are modest in low-risk patients (i.e., younger patients without a prior MI or those who have not had an anterior MI or who do not now have complex ventricular ectopy or significant LV dysfunction) (44), but it is generally recommended that unless a clear contraindication exists, even low-risk patients should receive beta-blockers indefinitely. When there are contraindications to beta-blockers, they should not be used. When initiated early in the course of an infarction (within 6 hours), beta-blockers may limit or reduce infarct size. Later in the postinfarct time period, the mechanism for a reduction in mortality is the prevention of reinfarction and the antiarrhythmic property of beta-blockers. The *overall magnitude of benefit* from the use of beta-blockers seems to be about a one-third reduction in first-year mortality (from approximately 6% to 4% when all randomized patients are considered) and about the same magnitude of reduction in reinfarction during the first post-MI year; these benefits may extend beyond 1 year in some subgroups. *Contraindications* to the use of beta-blockers include asthma, bradycardia, and insulin-treated diabetes mellitus. Although CHF is commonly considered a contraindication to the use of beta-blockers, an improvement in survival and reduction in expected coronary events have been found even with a history of CHF, as long as the CHF is clinically compensated when beta-blocker therapy is initiated (45). The *recommended dosage* of a beta-blocker is the amount required to produce attenuation of heart rate and blood pressure response to exercise without producing side effects. The characteristics of the available beta-blocking drugs are summarized in Chapter 67.

The issue of *duration of beta-blocker therapy* is of great practical relevance in the clinical management of post-MI patients because of the their potential side effects (e.g., depression, easy fatigability, and cold extremities). The benefits of the long-term use of beta-blockers are still debated (46). Several long-term studies examining their benefit postinfarction support a duration for their use of 2 to 3 years after an acute MI. After this time, the survival benefits are less certain. It is reasonable to conclude that if a patient is tolerating the therapy without the described side effects, beta-blocker use should be continued indefinitely.

Antiplatelet Therapy

Daily aspirin is recommended for all patients who have had an MI. Although the efficacy of other types of antiplatelet therapy is less well established, clopidogrel or ticlopidine may be substituted for aspirin if true aspirin allergy is present. If the risk is acceptable, warfarin anticoagulation is also a reasonable alternative for secondary prevention of MI in patients unable to take aspirin or for those with atrial fibrillation, LV thrombus, or extensive wall motion abnormality. Multiple randomized trials of antiplatelet therapy for secondary prevention of vascular disease show that prolonged treatment with aspirin has no effect on nonvascular mortality but reduces vascular *mortality* by approximately 15% and nonfatal vascular *events* (stroke or MI) by approximately 30% in patients with pre-existing cardiac or cerebral vascular diseases (47). Post-MI benefits are similar to those in patients after stroke and transient ischemic attack. *In absolute terms,* the benefits of antiplatelet therapy accrued to about 40 per 1,000 treated patients during the first month of treatment after an acute MI and to about 40 per 1,000 patients with a history of MI who were treated for 3 years. There is no difference in the degree of protection afforded by aspirin alone at a dosage of 325 mg/day and that afforded by higher aspirin dosages or other antiplatelet agents. Aspirin, 100 mg/day, has also been shown to improve coronary artery bypass graft patency at 4 months (90% of grafts patent vs. 68% in the placebo group) (48) and to decrease significantly the frequency of restenosis after percutaneous transluminal coronary angioplasty (49) and thrombolysis (50). For additional details regarding antiplatelet agents, see Chapter 57.

Angiotensin-converting Enzyme Inhibitors

All patients who have had an MI and whose LV ejection fraction is less than 40% should receive an ACE inhibitor in the absence of specific contraindications (see MI management guidelines in General References). Although the benefit of ACE inhibitors may be less in those with normal or mildly reduced LV function, even these patients should be considered for treatment with ACE inhibitors, in addition to aspirin and beta-blockers. The purpose for the use of these agents after an MI is to prevent LV remodeling and recurrent ischemic events.

In *chronic ischemic congestive cardiomyopathy,* the long-term use of ACE inhibitors is associated with significant improvement in morbidity and mortality irrespective of severity and symptoms of failure. A large placebo-controlled study showed that patients with recent MI and LV dysfunction (ejection fraction of 40% or less by radionuclide ventriculography) who were randomized to captopril experienced a modest reduction in cardiovascular and overall mortality, progression to severe heart failure, and recurrent MI during 3 years of treatment (51). Another large study showed that asymptomatic patients with LV ejection fraction of 35% or less who were randomized to enalapril also experienced a reduction in mortality or progression to heart failure during 3 years of treatment (52). The benefits accrued chiefly to patients with the lowest ejection fractions. In asymptomatic patients with reduced ejection fractions, ACE inhibitors should be started at low dosages (e.g., enalapril 2.5 mg/day; captopril 6.25 mg three times daily) with gradual increases (e.g., enalapril up to 10 mg/day; captopril up to 25 or 50 mg three times daily) guided by blood pressure response and renal function. Characteristics of ACE inhibitors are summarized in Chapter 67.

Calcium Channel Blockers

Calcium channel blockers are not recommended for secondary prevention after an MI. Because calcium channel blockers have not been demonstrated to significantly improve mortality in MI survivors, they should only be used in patients with symptomatic ischemia or hypertension that is not controlled despite treatment with beta-blockers and other agents known to improve survival after an MI. Calcium channel blockers may also be appropriate for patients with good LV function who have specific contraindications to beta-blockers or tolerate them poorly.

Smoking, Hyperlipidemia, Hypertension, and Exercise

Smoking

All patients who smoke after an MI should be counseled to stop. Post-MI morbidity and mortality are significantly reduced in patients who discontinue smoking. Smokers who have survived an MI are usually motivated to stop; practical ways to assist them, including the prescription of nicotine substitution products, are described in Chapter 27.

Lipid-lowering Diet and Drugs

A low saturated fat and low cholesterol diet (the American Heart Association Step II diet) should be recommended to all patients after an MI. Patients whose low density lipoprotein (LDL) cholesterol is greater than 125 mg/dL despite diet should receive lipid-lowering drug therapy in an attempt to lower the LDL cholesterol below 100 mg/dL. Patients who have a normal total cholesterol but whose high density lipoprotein (HDL) cholesterol is less than 35 mg/dL should have an exercise program recommended in an attempt to raise HDL cholesterol. Drug therapy (e.g., with niacin or gemfibrozi) may be considered for this purpose as well. Studies show that lipid-lowering drug therapy improves the prognosis of MI survivors (53–55). In the large Scandinavian Simvastatin Survival Study (4S) of secondary prevention, men and women 35 to 70 years, with cholesterol in the range 213 to 309 mg/dL despite an 8-week trial of diet, were randomized to simvastatin 20 to 40 mg daily or placebo (53). Simvastatin subjects had the following *6-year absolute benefits* when compared with placebo subjects: survival, 91.3% versus 87.6%; one or more CAD events, 19% versus 28%; and risk of undergoing myocardial revascularization procedures, 11.3% versus 17.2%. The mean changes in total cholesterol, LDL cholesterol, and HDL cholesterol in the treatment group were −25%, −35%, and +8%, respectively. In 1994, an expert panel of the National Cholesterol Education Program recommended treatment to attain a target LDL level of 100 mg/dL post-MI (see General References). The 4S study and the more recent pravastatin trial in post-MI patients with total cholesterol levels below 240 mg/dL and LDL levels 115 to 174 mg/dL both provide indirect support for the 1994 recommendation (53,55). The third report of the National Cholesterol Education Program (see General References), issued in May 2001, updated the recommendations for the clinical management of high blood cholesterol. This report retains the recommendation to attain a target LDL level of 100 mg/dL post-MI. If the baseline LDL cholesterol is greater than 130 mg/dL, intensive life-style therapy and maximal control of other risk factors (i.e., obesity, hypertension) should be started. However, for most patients, an LDL-lowering drug will be required to achieve the target LDL along with life-style change. The new recommendations also suggest drug therapy as an option if the LDL is between 100 and 129 mg/dL.

As pointed out in the American College of Physicians risk stratification report (see General References), lipid levels measured within 24 to 48 hours of an MI are accurate and can guide post-MI secondary prevention decisions. Detailed information regarding cholesterol and atherosclerotic disease is found in Chapter 82.

Exercise

The role of formal exercise programs in rehabilitation after MI is described in detail below (see Physical Conditioning after Myocardial Infarction).

Medical Complications

Table 63.6 lists the principal medical complications of MI, the procedures that may be useful in diagnosing or evaluating them, and potential therapies. As noted above (see Risk Stratification before Hospital Discharge), complications identified early are addressed very aggressively before or shortly after

Table 63.6. Medical Complications of MI

Complications	Diagnostic Procedures for Selected Patients[a]	Management Approaches
Angina or other evidence of reversible ischemia	ECG stress testing, radionuclide stress testing, Holter monitor for silent ischemia, coronary arteriography	Standard antianginal therapy (see Chapter 62), coronary artery bypass or PTCA for selected patients, physical conditioning
CHF	Radionuclide ventriculography or echocardiography (reduced ejection fraction, segmental dysfunction, rupture, ventricular aneurysm)	Afterload reduction, diuretics, inotropics, ?beta-blockers, ?anticoagulants (see Chapter 66 for treatment of heart failure); surgery in a few selected patients
Arrhythmias	Holter monitor; ECG stress testing, electrophysiologic study in selected patients	Beta-blockers, other antiarrhythmics (see Chapter 64); surgery or implanted defibrillator in selected patients
Post-MI syndrome (Dressler)	Echocardiography (pericardial effusion)	Aspirin or other anti-inflammatory agents (see text)
Systemic emboli	Echocardiography (intracardiac thrombus)	Anticoagulant therapy (see Chapter 57); surgery in selected patients

[a]Should be coordinated and interpreted by consulting cardiologist.

MI, myocardial infarction; ECG, electrocardiogram; CHF, congestive heart failure; PTCA, percutaneous transluminal coronary angioplasty.

discharge. In general, the use of sophisticated and costly procedures to evaluate the complications listed in Table 63.6 should be coordinated by a consulting cardiologist.

Postinfarction Angina

As pointed out in the discussion of prognosis above, angina is common in survivors of MI. The evaluation and medical management of angina are described in detail in Chapter 62. Because protection of the heart from transient ischemia may be especially important during recovery from an MI, it is advisable to prescribe beta-blockers in most patients (see above) and to undertake aggressive evaluation and management of patients who develop angina within the first 3 months after MI. Because of the poor prognosis associated with angina that occurs very early after an MI, patients with this problem after hospital discharge should be referred to a cardiologist for consideration of coronary catheterization and possible coronary revascularization.

Postinfarction Symptomatic Congestive Heart Failure

Postinfarction symptomatic CHF usually develops before discharge from the hospital. Currently, most patients have their LV ejection fraction measured as part of their evaluation before discharge, so that those at increased risk of developing symptomatic CHF after discharge are known. As noted above, it has been shown that ACE inhibitors delay deterioration in functional capacity and improve survival in patients with CHF after MI (51). The use of ACE inhibitors and other agents for CHF is described in detail in Chapter 66. Selected patients with persistent CHF may have segmental or global LV dysfunction or mitral regurgitation that may improve after cardiac surgery and may benefit from referral to a cardiologist.

Postinfarction Arrhythmias

A substantial proportion of MI survivors have *complex ventricular arrhythmias* (see criteria in Table 63.1) on 24-hour ambulatory ECG monitoring after the first week of hospitalization. Controlled trials do not show that the suppression of ventricular ectopy with drug therapy improves mortality. Routine testing to determine whether ventricular arrhythmia is present after an MI is therefore not recommended. The Cardiac Arrhythmia Suppression Trial revealed that the use of type I antiarrhythmic agents (encainide and flecainide) in such patients was associated with about three times the sudden death rate of that with the use of placebo (56). In addition, the use of antiarrhythmic agents in the posthospital treatment of patients with the *combination of complex ventricular arrhythmias and low ejection fractions* documented at the end of their stay in the hospital remains controversial. Early trials using type I drugs did not establish efficacy; however, recently reported trials using the type III drug amiodarone suggest a significant reduction in arrhythmias and arrhythmia-related deaths in this high-risk subset of patients (57,58). Studies evaluating the benefits of implantable defibrillators in specific high-risk populations have supported prior beliefs that defibrillators prolong life when compared with antiarrhythmic drugs (59,60). Details regarding all options for the management of symptomatic arrhythmias are discussed in detail in Chapter 64.

Postmyocardial Infarction (Dressler) Syndrome

It is estimated that 3% to 4% of patients develop this complication, usually within 1 to 8 weeks after an MI. The syndrome is characterized by the pain of pericarditis (substernal pain relieved by leaning forward and increased with inspiration), presence of a friction rub, a pericardial effusion (which can best be demonstrated by echocardiography), malaise, fever, leukocytosis, and often a unilateral or bilateral pleural effusion. The principal considerations in the differential diagnosis are pulmonary embolism and recurrence or extension of the recent MI.

A patient with suspected Dressler syndrome should be considered for hospitalization. A possible recurrent MI should be addressed by monitoring, serial ECGs, and measurement of cardiac enzymes. Evaluation for pulmonary embolization requires a ventilation-perfusion lung scan or pulmonary angiography. If these tests do not show an explanation for the patient's symptoms, the clinical diagnosis of Dressler syndrome can be made with reasonable assurance. Echocardiographic evidence of a pericardial effusion and an elevated erythrocyte sedimentation rate may also be present.

Dressler syndrome usually responds to salicylates or indomethacin; in patients who do not respond to these drugs, prednisone gives prompt relief of symptoms. However, the use of steroids within 4 weeks of an MI may alter postinfarction healing and may increase the risk of myocardial rupture. The use of steroids should therefore be limited to patients who are more than 4 weeks postinfarction. Once the diagnosis is secure and symptoms are controlled, the patient can be discharged. The anti-inflammatory drug chosen in the hospital should be administered for a few weeks after discharge. Patients who have recurrent symptoms when anti-inflammatory treatment is discontinued should resume treatment for another month or longer.

Arterial Embolization

Arterial embolization occurs after hospitalization in 5% to 10% of MI survivors. The emboli seem to originate from mural thrombi that are typically seen in the LV apex adjacent to akinetic or dyskinetic wall segments. Approximately 30% to 40% of hearts with akinetic or dyskinetic LV apices show mural thrombi on the echocardiogram. Because of these facts, anticoagulation (see Chapter 57) in patients with mural thrombi is generally recommended, although the impact and appropriate duration of anticoagulation have not been assessed in a prospective trial. However, most cardiologists anticoagulate MI survivors who have mural thrombi for 3 to 6 months. In patients with LV systolic dysfunction, warfarin use is associated with improved survival and reduced morbidity (61). Patients with atrial fibrillation or a history of embolic events should also be considered for systemic anticoagulation with warfarin.

Referral for Cardiology Consultation

Selected MI survivors may benefit from coronary angioplasty or cardiac surgery by having their symptoms reduced or their prognosis improved. Patients in the following groups should be referred promptly to a cardiologist to ensure optimal medical therapy and to obtain an opinion about the advisability and the timing of invasive procedures:

- Patients with *uncontrolled angina* refractory to medical therapy, with a markedly positive exercise stress test at low workload or with evidence of LV dysfunction during exercise (e.g., increased lung uptake of thallium during exercise);
- Patients with a *ventricular aneurysm*;
- Patients with *CHF refractory to medical therapy* (ACE inhibitors, digitalis, and diuretics);
- Patients with *structural complications* such as ventricular septal defect (suggested by holosystolic murmur and thrill at the left sternal border), papillary muscle rupture (suggested by refractory CHF and holosystolic apical murmur), segmental akinesis, or ventricular aneurysm;
- Patients with *electrical instability* (e.g., symptomatic bradycardia, high-grade atrioventricular blocks, ventricular tachycardia, or other arrhythmias).

Home Care for Acute Myocardial Infarction

A 1971 controlled trial in Great Britain showed that for patients with uncomplicated acute MIs the outcome is similar whether the patient is cared for in the home or in an intensive care unit (62). Because hospital care is the norm for an acute MI in the United States, it is unlikely that home care will gain significant acceptance. However, management at home may be appropriate for an occasional patient who has a stable acute MI and objects to hospitalization, who is demented and would predictably become very disoriented and agitated in a cardiac care unit, or who consults a health care provider several days after the onset of symptoms of infarction. The scheme for rehabilitation after MI described in this chapter can be adapted to these situations.

MANAGEMENT OF UNSTABLE ANGINA AFTER DISCHARGE FROM HOSPITAL

Of patients admitted to a hospital with unstable angina but without MI, 15% to 30% continue to have pain despite vigorous medical management. Patients in this group have an estimated 25% 1-year mortality rate. Therefore, most are evaluated and referred for coronary angioplasty or coronary artery bypass surgery. These interventions relieve or eliminate symptoms in most cases and improve survival for those with left main CAD, three-vessel disease, and two-vessel disease with LV dysfunction.

To date, the rehabilitation of the medically managed patient with unstable angina has not been studied as systematically as the rehabilitation of the patient after MI. These patients should receive education similar to that recommended for patients after MI regarding the nature of CAD, the recognition of symptoms, and the control of risk factors (see above). Because these patients do not have an ischemic injury that may take 2 or more months to heal, they often return to their usual activities more rapidly than patients who have had an MI. This is true particularly if their angina is well controlled and a stress test shows good effort tolerance (9 METs or more) and minimal or no changes caused by ischemia or LV dysfunction. Additional information regarding the management of unstable angina is found in Chapter 62.

PHYSICAL CONDITIONING AFTER MYOCARDIAL INFARCTION

Regular exercise, with the goal of attaining the physiologic adaptation known as the *conditioning effect,* is safe and beneficial for almost all patients after MI, just as it is for healthy people and patients with most chronic diseases. The basic principles of exercise training are applicable to people with and without heart disease. *Low-intensity exercise* that does not produce a conditioning effect may be associated with health benefits (see Chapter 16). Cardiac rehabilitation programs are excellent resources to which patients can be referred for a supervised exercise program. Contemporary programs are also experienced in addressing the individualized exercise and learning needs of each patient in the rehabilitation setting.

Cardiovascular principles related to exercise are described in considerable detail in Chapter 16; important principles regarding the musculoskeletal system are described in Chapter 68. A brief summary of these principles are provided here.

The body adapts to the kind and amount of physical demands placed on it. The response is *specific,* with the greatest changes observed only in those parts of the body on which demands are placed. For exercise to improve fitness, it must *overload* the muscles or organ system involved in the exercise. To overload is to exercise at a greater intensity than the intensity to which one is accustomed. *Threshold of training* is the amount of exercise that must be done to produce fitness improvements. Because the effects of exercise are specific to the type of activity engaged, an optimal exercise program should include a variety of activities designed to improve each of the major components of fitness. These are cardiovascular endurance, muscle strength, muscle endurance, and flexibility.

The principal hemodynamic adaptation to cardiovascular or aerobic exercise in patients with heart disease takes place in the peripheral vascular and muscular systems. Trained muscles can extract more oxygen from a given blood flow, and there is a better distribution of the cardiac output. Heart rate and blood pressure are lower at rest and at a given submaximal workload. As a result, the patient can do more work with less cardiac effort (i.e., less myocardial oxygen demand). This is extremely beneficial to cardiac patients who have limited blood supply through the coronary arteries. Angina may occur at the same threshold, that is, the same double product (heart rate × systolic blood pressure), but this threshold is reached at a higher level of body work or MET level. METs are used to rate the energy requirement of different physical activities, as indicated by the amount of oxygen extracted during those activities. One MET is 3.5 mL O_2/kg body weight per minute and is equivalent to oxygen requirement at rest; 2 METs are twice the resting requirements, and so on. (See Table 63.5 for the METs required for a broad range of activities.) In patients with CAD, the increase in angina-free exercise capacity achieved with regular exercise is similar to that achieved with medications such as beta-blockers and nitrates. In healthy people who practice aerobic exercise, there are also changes in the heart itself, including increase in diastolic volume, increase in ejection fraction at rest and to a greater extent during exercise, and enhancement of contractility. Few studies show any of this central effect in cardiac patients. However, there is evidence that cardiac patients may achieve central changes if they train hard and long enough (63). Improvement in coronary collateral circulation or myocardial perfusion has been shown in patients who participate in regular physical exercise and adhere to a low-fat diet (64). However, the independent effect of exercise on CAD progression is not yet known.

In recent years, there is also increased recognition of the importance of resistive training for individuals with and without cardiovascular disease. The American Heart Association issued a Scientific Advisory on "Resistance Exercise in Individuals With and Without Cardiovascular Disease" (see General References). This advisory, which has been endorsed by the American College of Sports Medicine, notes that after careful screening and risk stratification, and when appropriately prescribed, resistance training is an effective method for improving muscular strength and endurance, preventing and managing a variety of chronic medical conditions, modifying cardiac risk factors, and enhancing psychosocial well-being. Examples of resistance training are weight lifting, push-ups, sit-ups, isometrics, and hand grips. Most activities requiring lifting and straining, such as weight training, have a large static component. In such activities there is increased peripheral vascular resistance, with subsequent increase in blood pressure but little increase in heart rate or cardiac output. Such exercises do not bring about enhancement in oxygen extraction, so they are generally not aerobic. There are inadequate data to suggest that brief episodes of moderate resistive exercise are dangerous. In fact, studies show that cardiac patients who were required to carry or lift weights or to perform isometric exercise after MI had fewer ischemic electrocardiographic changes and arrhythmias during resistive exercise than during aerobic exercises (65). Gradual involvement in resistive training may therefore be beneficial and desirable, especially for patients whose jobs require static efforts.

Cardiac Rehabilitation

Participation in a formal cardiac rehabilitation program should be recommended to all patients after an MI. These programs reduce cardiovascular mortality and the risk of subsequent cardiac events, improve symptoms and exercise tolerance, improve blood lipids, increase the likelihood of smoking cessation, improve quality of life and psychosocial outcomes, and promote compliance. *Cardiac Rehabilitation Clinical Practice Guidelines* (see General References) from the Agency for Health Care Policy and Research defined the scientific basis for recommendations for multifactorial cardiac rehabilitation services that include medical evaluation, prescribed exercise, cardiac risk factor modification, and education, counseling, and behavioral interventions. Provision of these services is physician directed and is typically implemented by a team of health care professionals that may include nurses, clinical exercise physiologists, and physical therapists. Unfortunately, despite the scientific evidence demonstrating the benefits of cardiac rehabilitation, the report points out that only 11% to 20% of the several millions of patients with coronary heart disease participate in cardiac rehabilitation programs.

Benefits of Conditioning

Cardiac patients who exercise regularly and have become conditioned show better control of angina and enhancement of physical working capacity. Because of the peripheral cardiovascular adaptations described earlier, angina pectoris occurs at higher exercise levels. This increased anginal threshold allows the patient to do more work, and at any given level of work the patient feels more comfortable because the work represents a lower percentage of a now higher maximal capacity. Similar benefits for patients with LV dysfunction and chronic heart failure have also been demonstrated (66,67). *Rating of perceived exertion* (RPE) is a scale that measures how hard any given level of work feels (Table 63.7). The RPE is administered during exercise testing. The patient is asked to rate the work at each stage of the test. After conditioning, the RPE is lower at any given stage and is associated with a lower heart rate and blood pressure (68). RPE is also a useful

Table 63.7. Rate of Perceived Exertion (RPE) Scale

6
7 Very, very light
8
9 Very light
10
11 Fairly light
12
13 Somewhat hard
14
15 Hard
16
17 Very hard
18
19 Very, very hard
20

From Borg G. Subjective effort in relation to physical performance and working capacity. In: Pick HL, ed. Psychology: from research to practice. New York: Plenum, 1978:333, with permission.

way to prescribe exercise. This approach focuses on how the patient actually feels and correlates closely with the target heart rate and desired MET level. For most cardiac patients, a prescription at 13 to 14 ("somewhat hard" to "hard") on the RPE scale is both safe and effective for cardiovascular conditioning.

The *effect of exercise training on longevity in patients after MI* has been established. Meta-analysis of the combined results of 10 randomized clinical trials demonstrates a 25% reduction in cardiovascular mortality, although not in nonfatal reinfarction for patients in rehabilitation programs (69). Benefits of exercise conditioning on the psychometric profile are not firmly established (see Greenland and Chu in General References).

Risks of Conditioning

With proper selection, supervision, monitoring, and precautions, physical conditioning for cardiac patients has proved to be remarkably safe. Cumulative data from more than 1.5 million person-hours of exercise, done predominantly 3 months after MI, show that the risks of ventricular fibrillation, acute MI, and death are 1 in 10,000 to 1 in 32,000, 1 in 253,000, and 1 in 100,000 to 1 in 212,000 person-hours of exercise, respectively (70). There is no comparable large series on exercise conditioning earlier than 3 months after MI. In the authors' experience with exercise programs beginning an average of 10 days after hospital discharge, there have been few serious complications during exercise over a 20-year period. These patients exercise three times a week, for an average of 6 to 8 weeks, at a conditioning heart rate of approximately 80% of what they safely achieved on a post-MI stress test, performed before starting the exercise program.

Cardiovascular Medications and Conditioning

Many patients who enroll in exercise programs are taking one or more medications. Many of these medications alter the cardiovascular response to exercise. Patients enrolled in a conditioning program should always be stress tested (see below) while taking their regular medications, and the effects of their drugs must be considered in interpreting test results. For example, beta-blockers attenuate the heart rate response to exercise. Thus, heart rate is not useful as an end point for stress testing or as a parameter for the patient to monitor during exercise conditioning. In a patient on a beta-blocker, symptoms, ECG changes, fatigue, and RPE (Table 63.7) are used as end points during stress testing. These parameters are also useful for establishing the exercise prescription in patients on certain medications. Table 63.8 summarizes the *effects of a number of commonly prescribed cardiac drugs on the hemodynamic response to exercise.*

Patients taking a variety of drugs have been evaluated and have participated safely in physical conditioning programs. There is some controversy regarding the effect of beta-blockers on the response to training. It has been suggested that beta-blockers may attenuate the beneficial effects of training. A clinical trial (71) to establish whether a beta-blocker (propranolol) or a calcium channel blocker (diltiazem) limits exercise capacity and training effect showed that neither drug interfered with muscle strength. After starting propranolol, maximal aerobic capacity was reduced by 20%, whereas a 20% increase in aerobic capacity from this reduced level occurred with training while subjects continued to use the drug. Thus, although a training effect can be achieved while using a beta-blocker, its use may limit the full benefit of exercise training as measured by maximal aerobic capacity. On the other hand, for patients who are limited by ischemia, the use of a beta-blocker may allow the patient to achieve workloads that may not otherwise be attained without anti-ischemic medication.

Referral for Conditioning

The decision to refer a patient for physical conditioning after MI depends on the patient's clinical status,

Table 63.8. Effect of Various Classes of Medications on Hemodynamic Status During Exercise

Drug	Peak Heart Rate	Peak Systolic Blood Pressure
Antihypertensives		
ACE inhibitors	=	↓
Hydralazine	↑	↓
Minoxidil	↑	↓
Clonidine	↓	↓
Methyldopa	↓	↓
Prazosin	↑	↓
Nitrates	↑	↓
Antiarrhythmics	=	↓
Beta-blockers	↓	↓
Digitalis[a]	=	↑
Calcium blockers		
Nifedipine	↑	↓
Diltiazem	=	↓
Verapamil	↓	↓

[a]Patients with congestive heart failure.

↓, decreased; ↑, increased; =, no discernible effect; ACE, angiotensin-converting enzyme.

Modified from Powles ACP. The effect of drugs on the cardiovascular response to exercise. Med Sci Sports Exerc 1981;13:252, with permission.

motivation, and the availability of well-supervised and staffed programs designed for such patients. Whereas participation is often limited by third-party insurance reimbursement, a key factor in increasing compliance to cardiac rehabilitation is a specific instruction from the health care provider to the patient to participate in such a program. Medically supervised programs, offering ECG monitoring and the immediate availability of emergency care, often accept patients within 1 to 2 weeks of hospital discharge. If such a program is not available, cautious guidelines such as those shown in Table 63.4 are appropriate. After 2 months, when no supervised program is available, patients with uncomplicated MI can be advised to increase their exercise levels gradually, using the results of a stress test to establish target heart rates or RPE.

Before beginning a conditioning program, the patient should have an ECG stress test (see Chapter 62 for a description of the patient's experience), the results of which are used in planning the exercise program. In general, the conditioning target heart rate is 70% to 85% of the maximal heart rate safely achieved on the stress test.

Contraindications

A patient should not be enrolled in or should discontinue a conditioning program if the following problems are present: poorly controlled angina, severe dyspnea at low workloads, moderate to severe uncontrolled hypertension at rest (diastolic above 110 mm Hg), complex arrhythmias (Table 63.1), atrial fibrillation with a rapid ventricular response, second- or third-degree heart block, significant valvular or congenital heart disease, significant orthopedic or pulmonary limitations, chronic alcoholism, or recent acute physical or mental illness.

Exercise Programs

Exercise sessions should be supervised by personnel trained in exercise physiology and cardiopulmonary resuscitation, with immediate availability of monitoring and resuscitative equipment. Programs that accept patients soon after MI should have equipment for continuous ECG monitoring. Sessions are usually held *three times a week on nonconsecutive days.* The total duration of an average session is about 45 minutes. The pattern for a workout is illustrated in Fig. 63.4. During the stimulus phase, the patient exercises at an intensity that elicits a heart rate or RPE (see above) that falls within the prescribed target zone. Figure 63.5 shows recommendations for exercise intensity based on heart rate response during an exercise stress test. Exercising near the 70% level, for 20 to 30 minutes, promotes fitness, and beginners should be instructed to maintain intensity near this level. Experienced exercisers can advance to the 85% level if a more intense workout is desired. The stimulus, or period at the target heart rate, is preceded by 5 to 10 minutes of warmup and is followed by 5 to 10 minutes of cool-down (Fig. 63.4). Warmup and cool-down should include

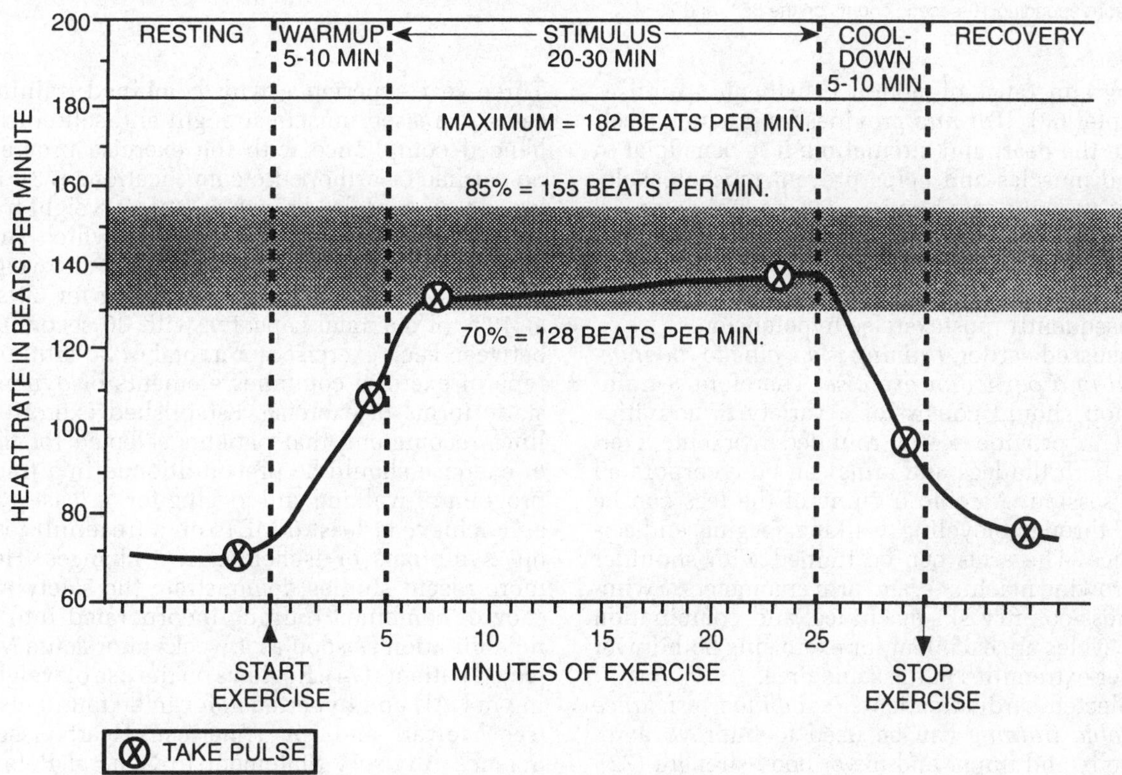

Figure 63.4. The exercise training program.

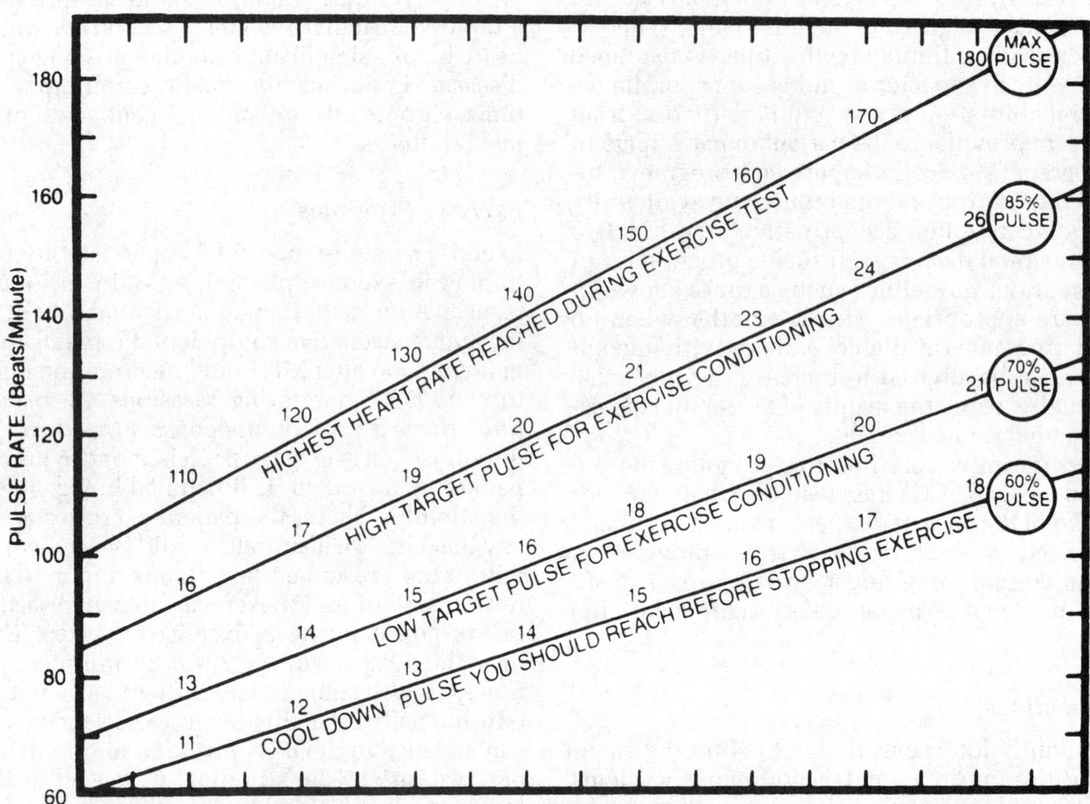

Figure 63.5. Target pulse rates for 10-second counts that should be measured the first 10 seconds after exercise. (To convert the count to beats per minute, multiply by 6.) To determine a patient's target pulse rate range, identify the highest rate safely achieved during the most recent exercise test on the top line (maximum pulse line) and then locate the corresponding 10-second counts on the 85% and 70% lines directly below. These two values represent the limits of target rate range for exercise conditioning. (From Haskell WL. Design and implementation of cardiac conditioning programs. In: Wenger NK, Hellerstein HK, eds. Rehabilitation of the coronary patient. New York: Wiley, 1978:209, with permission.)

stretching and range-of-motion calisthenic exercises (see Chapter 68). *Warmup* provides for gradual acceleration of the heart and circulation; it is beneficial to joints and muscles and helps prevent musculoskeletal injuries. *Cool-down* provides for gradual deceleration of the cardiovascular system and prevents pooling of blood in the muscles when exercise stops abruptly. Pooling can lead to a precipitous drop in venous return and, consequently, postexercise hypotension.

As discussed earlier, *training is specific to the muscles used in a particular exercise.* Therefore, a training session should consist of a variety of activities designed to provide a well-rounded workout. Exercises for both the legs and arms can be incorporated into the session. Aerobic training of the legs can be achieved through bicycling, walking, jogging, and aerobic dance. The arms can be trained with shoulder wheels, rowing machines, and arm ergometers. Swimming, cross-country ski machines, and combination arm–leg cycles are excellent for exercising both lower and upper extremities at the same time.

For selected cardiac patients, *combined resistance and aerobic training* can be used to improve aerobic capacity and upper and lower body strength (72). Three-year experience with combined training indicates increased muscle strength and self-efficacy, enhanced compliance with the exercise program, and no cardiac or orthopedic complications (73). In combined training (also known as circuit weight training), the patient uses machines, each of which stresses a different muscle group, and moves from weight machine to weight machine, performing for 30 seconds at 40% of maximal capacity, with 30 seconds of rest between each exercise, for a total of 20 minutes. This type of exercise combines elements of dynamic and static forms of exercise. Established exercise guidelines recommend that patients selected for this type of exercise should be preconditioned in a traditional program of walking and jogging for at least 3 months and achieve at least 6 METs on a treadmill test without symptoms or ischemic ECG changes. However, more recent studies demonstrate the safety and efficacy of combined training incorporated into cardiac rehabilitation as soon as 4 weeks after acute MI in selected patients (74). Reviews on the use of weight training in CAD and hypertension can be found elsewhere (see Stewart and the American Heart Association Science Advisory Statement in General References).

Alternatives to weight machines, particularly for patients at high risk or for those who are markedly deconditioned or who are participating very soon after MI, are rubber band devices, pulley weights, wrist weights, and light dumbbells.

Termination of Supervised Training

Criteria for terminating supervised exercise training and transfer to nonsupervised maintenance programs are not clearly established. ECG monitoring for 6 to 8 weeks, and longer, during early exercise programs is generally recommended. Clinical stability and functional capacity above 7 to 8 METs (Table 63.5) are generally accepted exit criteria.

After a few months of supervised exercise, repeated stress testing is useful for measuring the change in physical working capacity and for adjusting more accurately the optimal exercise training intensity.

Long-Term Maintenance of Physical Conditioning

Long-term compliance with formal exercise programs is often poor. It is necessary to exercise regularly at the proper intensity, frequency, and duration if physical fitness is to be maintained. Measurable deterioration in the conditioning effect occurs after missing only a few weeks. The time required to retrieve lost ground seems to be directly related to the length of time without exercise and the degree of physical fitness achieved before cessation of exercise. Exercise must become a part of a person's weekly routine, not something that is done only sporadically or only during the recovery from MI.

General References*

1996 Surgeon General's report on physical activity and health (S/N 017-023-00196-5). U.S. Department of Health and Human Services, Centers for Disease Control and Prevention, National Center for Chronic Disease Prevention and Health Promotion, The President's Council on Physical Fitness and Sports.

Significant reviews and summaries promoting the benefits of life-style changes.

American Association of Cardiovascular and Pulmonary Rehabilitation. Guidelines for cardiac rehabilitation programs, 3rd ed. Champaign, IL: Human Kinetics, 1999.

Provides criteria for patient selection and exercise training.

American College of Physicians Guidelines for risk stratification after myocardial infarction. Ann Intern Med 1997;126:556.

Expert Panel on Detection, Evaluation, and Treatment of High Blood Cholesterol in Adults. **National Cholesterol in Education Program: second report of the Expert Panel on Detection, Evaluation, and Treatment of High Blood Cholesterol in Adults (Adult Treatment Panel II).** Circulation 1994;89:1329.

Expert Panel on Detection, Evaluation, and Treatment of High Blood Cholesterol in Adults. **National Cholesterol in Education Program: second report of the Expert Panel on Detection, Evaluation, and Treatment of High Blood Cholesterol in Adults (Adult Treatment Panel III).** NIH Publication No. 01-3670, May 2001. (http://www.nhlbi.nih.gov/guidelines/cholesterol/atp3xsum.pdf)

Detailed review of evidence plus explicit guidelines for controlling lipid levels in patients with and without CAD.

Greenland P, Chu JS. Efficacy of cardiac rehabilitation services with emphasis on patients after myocardial infarction. Ann Intern Med 1988;109:650.

Review paper.

Hennekens CH, Albert CM, Goldfried SL, et al. Adjunctive drug therapy of acute myocardial infarction: evidence from clinical trials. N Engl J Med 1996;335:1660.

Critical review of all clinical trials of the use of ACE inhibitors, nitrates, calcium channel blockers, antiarrhythmic agents, and magnesium in patients with MI.

Peterson DM. Exercise and physical activity in the adult population: a general internist's perspective. J Gen Intern Med 1993;8:149.

Review of benefits and risks of physical activity. Contains specific instructions for patients for whom the primary physician recommends exercise.

Peterson ED, Shaw LS, Califf RM. Risk stratification after myocardial infarction. Ann Intern Med 1997;126:561.

Physical activity and cardiovascular health. NIH Consensus Statement 13(3):1–33, Dec. 18–20, 1995.

Expert panel reviews data suggesting physical activity as a major focus for prevention.

Physical activity and public health: a recommendation from the Centers for Disease Control and Prevention and the American College of Sports Medicine. JAMA 1995;273:4.

Summary statements by organizations heading effort to promote increasing physical activity as a means of prevention.

Pollock ML, Franklin BA, Balady GJ, et al. AHA Science Advisory. Resistance exercise in individuals with and without cardiovascular disease: benefits, rationale, safety, and prescription: an advisory from the Committee on Exercise, Rehabilitation, and Prevention, Council on Clinical Cardiology, American Heart Association; Position paper endorsed by the American College of Sports Medicine. Circulation 2000;101:828.

Provides a review of the literature and recommendations for patient selection and resistance training prescription.

Ryan TJ, Antman EM, Brooks NH, et al. **1999 update: ACC/AHA guidelines for the management of patients with acute myocardial infarction. A report of the American College of Cardiology/American Heart Association Task Force on Practice Guidelines (Committee on Management of Acute Myocardial Infarction).** J Am Coll Cardiol 1999;34:890.

Guidelines based on critical assessment of 280 published articles. Excellent explanation of the evidence base for rational and cost-effective predischarge care of MI patients.

Stewart KJ, Franklin BA, Squires RW. Resistance training in patients with coronary artery disease. In: Graves J, Franklin B, eds. Resistance training for health and rehabilitation. Champaign, IL: Human Kinetics, 2001.

Review article on resistance training.

Wenger NK, Froelicher ES, Smith LK, et al. **Cardiac rehabilitation clinical guideline no. 17.** Rockville, MD: U.S. Department of Health and Human Services, Public Health Service, Agency for Health Care Policy and Research and National Heart, Lung, and Blood Institute. AHCPR Pub. No. 96-0673, October 1995.

Written by leaders in the field of cardiac rehabilitation and based on critical review of published research.

Books for Lay People On Exercise And Conditioning

American College of Sports Medicine. ACSM fitness book. Champaign, IL: Human Kinetics, 1992.

Iknoian T. Fitness walking. Champaign, IL: Human Kinetics, 1995.

Sharkey BJ. Fitness and health, 4th ed. Champaign, IL: Human Kinetics, 1997.

Specific References

1. American Heart Association. 2001 heart and stroke statistical update. Dallas, TX: American Heart Association, 2000.
2. Rosamond WD, Chambless LE, Folsom AR, et al. Trends in the incidence of myocardial infarction and in mortality due to

*Bold print (general references) and bold numerals (specific references) denote published controlled clinical trials, meta-analyses, or consensus-based recommendations.

coronary heart disease, 1987 to 1994. N Engl J Med 1998;339: 861.
3. Ellerbeck EF, Jencks SF, Radford MJ, et al. Quality of care for Medicare patients with acute myocardial infarction: a four-state pilot study from the cooperative cardiovascular project. JAMA 1995;273:1509.
4. Heart and Stroke Facts. 1997 statistical supplement. Dallas: American Heart Association, 1997.
5. Tofler GH, Stone PH, Muller JC, et al. Effect of gender and race in prognosis after MI: adverse prognosis for women, particularly black women. J Am Coll Cardiol 1987;9:473.
6. Chandra NC, Ziegelstein RC, Rogers WJ, et al. Observations of the treatment of women in the United States with myocardial infarction: a report from the National Registry of Myocardial Infarction. I. Arch Intern Med 1998;158:981.
7. Furman MI, Dauerman HL, Goldberg RJ, et al. Twenty-two year (1975 to 1997) trends in the incidence, in-hospital and long-term case fatality rates from initial Q-wave and non-Q-wave myocardial infarction: a multi-hospital, community-wide perspective. J Am Coll Cardiol 2001;37:1571.
8. McGovern PG, Pankow JS, Shahar E, et al. Recent trends in acute coronary heart disease—mortality, morbidity, medical care, and risk factors. The Minnesota Heart Survey Investigators. N Engl J Med 1996;334:884.
9. Rosati RA, Harris PJ. Acute myocardial infarction. In: Fries JF, Ehrlich GE, eds. Prognosis: contemporary outcomes of disease. Bowie, MD: Charles Press, 1981.
10. van Ravenswaaij CMA, Kollee LAA, Hopman JCW, et al. Heart rate variability. Ann Intern Med 1993;118:436.
11. Maggioni AP, Maseri A, Fresco C, et al. Age-related increase in mortality among patients with first myocardial infarctions treated with thrombolysis. The Investigators of the Gruppo Italiano per lo Studio della Sopravvivenza nell'Infarto Miocardico (GISSI-2). N Engl J Med 1993;329:1442.
12. Meizlish JL, Berger HJ, Plankey M, et al. Functional left ventricular aneurysm after acute myocardial infarction. N Engl J Med 1984;16:1001.
13. Frasure-Smith N, Lesperance F, Talajic M. Depression following myocardial infarction. Impact on 6-month survival. JAMA 1993;270:1819.
14. Moss AJ, Goldstein RE, Hall J, et al. Detection and significance of myocardial ischemia in stable patients after recovery from acute event. JAMA 1993;269:2379.
15. Waters DD, Theroux P, Halphen C, et al. Clinical predictors of angina following myocardial infarction. Am J Med 1979;66:991.
16. Mark D, Froelicher V. Exercise treadmill testing and ambulatory monitoring. In: Califf R, Mark D, Wagner G, eds. Acute coronary care. St. Louis: CV Mosby, 1995:767.
17. Theroux P, Marpole DGF, Bourassa MG. Exercise stress testing in the postmyocardial infarction patient. Am J Cardiol 1983;52:664.
18. Anderson HV, Cannon CP, Stone PH, et al. One-year results of the Thrombolysis in Myocardial Infarction (TIMI) IIIB clinical trial. A randomized comparison of tissue-type plasminogen activator versus placebo and early invasive versus early conservative strategies in unstable angina and non-Q wave myocardial infarction. J Am Coll Cardiol 1995;26:1643.
19. U.S. Department of Health and Human Services, Public Service Agency for Health Care Policy and Research, National Heart, Lung and Blood Institute. Clinical practice guideline. Unstable angina: diagnosis and management. AHCPR Publication No. 94-0602, No. 10, March 1994.
20. Plotnick GD. Approach to the management of unstable angina. Am Heart J 1979;98:243.
21. Schaffer WA, Cobb LA. Recurrent ventricular fibrillation and modes of death in survivors of out-of-hospital ventricular fibrillation. N Engl J Med 1975;293:259.
22. Russell RO Jr, Abi-Mansour P, Wenger NK, et al. Return to work after coronary artery bypass surgery and percutaneous transluminal angioplasty: issues and potential solutions. Cardiology 1986;73:306.
23. DeBusk RF. Report of the twentieth Bethesda Conference. Insurability and employability of the patient with ischemic heart disease. 38th Annual Scientific Session. Anaheim, CA: American College of Cardiology, March 1989.
24. Hellerstein HK, Friedman EH. Sexual activity in the post-coronary patient. Arch Intern Med 1970;125:987.
25. Ueno M. The so-called coitus death. Jpn J Legal Med 1963; 17:330.
26. Muller JE, Mittleman A, Maclure M, et al. Triggering myocardial infarction by sexual activity. Low absolute risk and prevention by regular physical exertion. Determinants of Myocardial Infarction Onset Study Investigators. JAMA 1996;275:1405.
27. Herrmann HC, Chang G, Klugherz BD, et al. Hemodynamic effects of sildenafil in men with severe coronary artery disease. N Engl J Med 2000;342:1622.
28. Ewart CK, Taylor CB, Reese LB, et al. Effects of early postmyocardial infarction exercise testing on self-perception and subsequent physical activity. Am J Cardiol 1983;51:1076.
29. Ewart CK, Stewart KJ, Kelemen MH, et al. Self-efficacy mediates strength gains during circuit weight training in men with coronary artery disease. Med Sci Sports Exerc 1986;18:531.
30. Gillilan RE, Chopra AK, Kelemen MH, et al. Prediction of compliance to target heart rate during walk-job exercise in cardiac patients by a self-efficacy scale. Med Sci Sports Exerc 1984;16:115.
31. Baile WF, Engel BT. A behavioral strategy for promoting treatment compliance following myocardial infarction. Psychosom Med 1978;40:412.
32. Schleifer SJ, Macari-Hinson MM, Coyle DA, et al. The nature and course of depression following myocardial infarction. Arch Intern Med 1989;149:1785.
33. Ziegelstein RC, Fauerbach JA, Stevens SS, et al. Patients with depression are less likely to follow recommendations to reduce cardiac risk during recovery from a myocardial infarction. Arch Intern Med 2000;160:1818.
34. Duryee R. The efficacy of inpatient education after myocardial infarction. Heart Lung 1992;21:217.
35. Milani RV, Lavie CJ, Cassidy MM. Effects of cardiac rehabilitation and exercise training programs on depression in patients after major coronary events. Am Heart J 1996;132:726.
36. Guiry E, Conroy RM, Hickey N, et al. Psychological response to an acute coronary event and its effect on subsequent rehabilitation and lifestyle change. Clin Cardiol 1987;10: 256.
37. Blumenthal JA, Williams RS, Wallace AG, et al. Physiological and psychological variables predict compliance to prescribed exercise therapy in patients recovering from myocardial infarction. Psychosomatic Med 1982;44:519.
38. Frasure-Smith N, Lespèrance F, Gravel G, et al. Social support, depression, and mortality during the first year after myocardial infarction. Circulation 2000;101:1919.
39. Shapiro PA, Lesperance F, Frasure-Smith N, et al. An open-label preliminary trial of sertraline for treatment of major depression after acute myocardial infarction (the SADHAT Trial). Sertraline Anti-Depressant Heart Attack Trial. Am Heart J 1999;137: 1100.
40. Roose SP, Laghrissi-Thode F, Kennedy JS, et al. Comparison of paroxetine and nortriptyline in depressed patients with ischemic heart disease. JAMA 1998;279:287.
41. Strik JJ, Honig A, Lousberg R, et al. Efficacy and safety of fluoxetine in the treatment of patients with major depression after first myocardial infarction: findings from a double-blind, placebo-controlled trial. Psychosom Med 2000;62: 783.
42. Roose SP, Glassman AH. Cardiovascular effects of tricyclic antidepressants in depressed patients with and without heart disease. J Clin Psychiatry 1989;50[Suppl]:1.
43. Friedman M. Diagnosis and treatment of type A behavior as a medical disorder. Prim Cardiol 1989;15:68.
44. Furberg CD, Friedwald WT, Eberlein KA. Proceedings of the workshop on the implications of recent beta-blocker trials for postmyocardial infarction patients. Circulation 1983; 67:1.
45. Chadda K, Goldstein S, Byington R, et al. Effect of propranolol after acute myocardial infarction. Circulation 1986;73:503.

46. Viscoli CM, Horowitz RI, Singer BH. Beta blockers after myocardial infarction: influence of first year clinical course on long-term effectiveness. Ann Intern Med 1993;118:99.
47. Antiplatelet Trialists' Collaboration. Collaborative overview of randomized trials of antiplatelet therapy. I. Prevention of death, myocardial infarction, and stroke by prolonged antiplatelet therapy in various categories of patients. BMJ 1994;308:81.
48. Lorenz RL, Schacky CV, Weber M, et al. Improved aorto-coronary bypass patency by low-dose aspirin (100 mg daily): effects on platelet aggregation and thromboxane formation. Lancet 1984;1:1261.
49. Thornton MA, Greventzig AR, Hollman J, et al. Coumadin and aspirin in prevention of recurrence after transluminal coronary angioplasty: a randomized study. Circulation 1984;69:72.
50. ISIS-2. Randomised trial of intravenous streptokinase, oral aspirin, both or neither among 17,187 cases of suspected acute myocardial infarction. Lancet 1988;2:349.
51. Pfeffer M, Braunwald E, Moye L, et al. Effect of captopril on mortality and morbidity in patients with left ventricular dysfunction after myocardial infarction. N Engl J Med 1992;327:669.
52. SOLVD Investigators. Effects of enalapril on mortality and development of heart failure in asymptomatic patients with reduced left ventricular ejection fractions. N Engl J Med 1992;32:685.
53. Randomised trial of cholesterol lowering in 4444 patients with coronary heart disease: the Scandinavian Simvastatin Survival Study (4S). Lancet 1994;344:1383.
54. Rossouw JE, Lewis B, Rifkind BM. The value of lowering cholesterol after myocardial infarction. N Engl J Med 1990;323:1112.
55. Sacks FM, Pfeffer MA, Moye LA, et al. The effect of pravastatin on coronary events after myocardial infarction in patients with average cholesterol level. N Engl J Med 1996;335:1001.
56. Echt DS, Liebson PR, Mitchell LB, et al. Mortality and morbidity in patients receiving encainide, flecainide, or placebo: the Cardiac Arrhythmia Suppression Trial. N Engl J Med 1991;324:781.
57. European Myocardial Infarct Amiodarone Trial Investigators. Randomised trial of effect of amiodarone on mortality in patients with left-ventricular dysfunction after recent myocardial infarction. Lancet 1997;349:667.
58. Canadian Amiodarone Myocardial Infarction Arrhythmia Trial Investigators. Randomised trial of outcome after myocardial infarction in patients with frequent or repetitive ventricular premature depolarisations. Lancet 1997;349:675.
59. Moss AJ, Hall WJ, Cannom DS, et al. Improved survival with an implanted defibrillator in patients with coronary disease at high risk for ventricular arrhythmias. N Engl J Med 1996;335:1933.
60. The Antiarrhythmic versus Implantable Defibrillator (AVID) Investigators. A comparison of antiarrhythmic-drug therapy with implantable defibrillator in patients resuscitated form near-fatal ventricular arrhythmias. N Engl J Med 1997;337:1576.
61. Al-Khadra AS, Salem DN, Rand WM, et al. Warfarin anticoagulation and survival: a cohort analysis from the Studies of Left Ventricular Dysfunction. J Am Coll Cardiol 1998;31:749.
62. Mather HG, Pearson NG, Read KLQ, et al. Acute myocardial infarction: home and hospital treatment. BMJ 1971;1:334.
63. Ehsani AA, Heath GH, Hagberg JM, et al. Effects of 12 months of intense exercise training on ischemic ST-depression in patients with coronary artery disease. Circulation 1981;64:1116.
64. Schuler G, Hambrecht R, Schlierf G, et al. Regular exercise and low fat diet: effects on progression of coronary artery disease. Circulation 1992;86:1.
65. Taylor JL, Copeland RB, Cousin AL, et al. The effect of isometric exercise on the graded exercise test in patients with stable angina. J Cardiopulm Rehab 1981;1:450.
66. Coats AJS, Adampoulos S, Meyer TC, et al. Effects of physical training in chronic heart failure. Lancet 1990;335:63.
67. Sullivan MJ, Higgambotham MB, Cobb FR. Exercise training in patients with severe left ventricular dysfunction: hemodynamics and metabolic effects. Circulation 1988;78:506.
68. Gutmann MC, Squires RW, Pollack ML, et al. Perceived exertion–heart rate relationship during exercise testing and training in cardiac patients. J Cardiovasc Rehab 1981;1:52.
69. Oldridge NB, Guyatt GH, Fischer ME, et al. Cardiac rehabilitation after myocardial infarction: combined experience of randomized clinical trials. JAMA 1988;260:945.
70. Council on Scientific Affairs, American Medical Association. Physician-supervised exercise programs in rehabilitation of patients with coronary heart disease. JAMA 1981;245:1463.
71. Stewart KJ, Effron MB, Vaeni SA, et al. Effects of diltiazem or propranolol during exercise training of hypertensive men. Med Sci Sports Exerc 1990;22:171.
72. Kelemen MH, Stewart KJ, Gillilan RE, et al. Circuit weight training in cardiac patients. J Am Coll Cardiol 1986;7:38.
73. Stewart KJ, Mason M, Kelemen MH. Three year participation in circuit weight training improves muscular strength and self-efficacy in cardiac patients. J Cardiopulm Rehab 1988;8:292.
74. Stewart, KJ, McFarland LD, Weinhofer JJ, et al. Safety and efficacy of weight training soon after acute myocardial Infarction. J Cardiopulm Rehabil 1998;18:37.

CHAPTER 64

Arrhythmias and Other Abnormalities of Cardiac Conduction

SHELDON H. GOTTLIEB, MD
HUGH CALKINS, MD

Contraction of the heart is normally the result of a well-orchestrated electromechanical system. The orderly function of the system is maintained by the domination of the heart rate by a single pulse generator known as the pacemaker, by the relatively fast and uniform conduction of the electrical signal via specialized conduction pathways, and by the relatively long and uniform duration of the electrical signal relative to its velocity of conduction through these pathways, which ensures uniform electrical excitation and contraction of the heart. An arrhythmia is any disturbance in the normal sequence of impulse generation and conduction in the heart.

Arrhythmias may occur in the absence of heart disease, they may be symptoms of severe disease, or may themselves cause disease. Their significance and the need for treatment must be evaluated in the context of the clinical situation in which they occur. A precise etiologic diagnosis and an understanding of the pharmacology of the medications used are necessary to treat arrhythmias effectively.

PHYSIOLOGY OF IMPULSE GENERATION AND CONDUCTION

Action Potential

Muscle contraction is stimulated by an electrical impulse, the action potential. In skeletal muscle, the action potential lasts several milliseconds, and the electrical activity is essentially dissipated before the beginning of contraction. In cardiac muscle, however, the action potential lasts several hundred milliseconds, almost as long as the contraction itself (Fig. 64.1). In this way, the action potential not only stimulates contraction of the heart but also determines the duration and intensity of contraction. Furthermore, as long as the action potential is maintained, the heart cannot be stimulated to contract again.

The action potential is generated by depolarization and repolarization of the muscle cell (Fig. 64.2). In the resting state, the intracellular concentration of potassium is high and that of sodium is low compared with the extracellular fluid. These gradients are maintained by metabolic activity within the cell membrane. The resting membrane potential is strongly negative (i.e., there is an electrochemical gradient across the membrane so that the inside of the membrane is negatively charged compared with the outside of the membrane). If an electrical stimulus is applied, the membrane becomes very permeable to sodium ions, which rapidly leak into the cell (phase 0). The membrane is thus depolarized (loses its negative charge) and, in fact, is transiently positively charged (overshoot). Repolarization occurs relatively slowly as chloride (phase 1), calcium ions (phase 2), and then potassium ions (phase 3) move back into the cell and thereby restore the resting potential (phase 4) (Fig. 64.2) (1).

Relationship to the Electrocardiogram

In the heart, the phases of rapid depolarization and overshoot correspond to the QRS complex of the electrocardiogram (ECG); phase 2 corresponds to the ST segment, and phase 3 to the T wave (Fig. 64.2). During phase 2 the membrane is absolutely, and in phase 3 it is relatively, refractory to propagation of another electrical impulse.

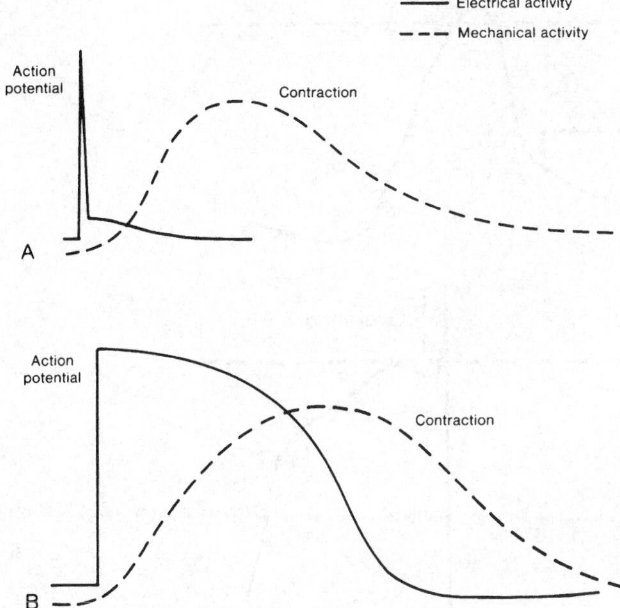

Figure 64.1. Comparison between relative time scales of electrical *(continuous curve)* and mechanical *(interrupted curve)* activity in **(A)** skeletal and **(B)** cardiac muscle. (From Noble D. The initiation of the heart beat. Oxford, England: Clarendon Press, 1975, with permission.)

Fast and Slow Currents

In most cardiac tissue, excitation is propagated by the rapidly depolarizing sodium current so that the impulses are conducted rapidly. However, in the sinoatrial node and the proximal part of the atrioventricular (AV) node, excitation is propagated by a slowly depolarizing current generated by the influx of calcium ions into the cell. Also, in diseased cardiac muscle, the sodium current may be inhibited and depolarization may occur entirely via the slow calcium current; therefore, the action potential may be conducted very slowly. This difference in conduction velocity between cells depolarized by the sodium versus the calcium current has important implications in the generation and treatment of arrhythmias (see later discussion).

Pacemaker Generation

In most cardiac cells, an action potential is not generated until an electrical stimulus is applied. In pacemaker cells, slow spontaneous depolarization occurs until a threshold is reached, whereupon phase 0 rapidly ensues (Fig. 64.2); this process is called *automaticity.* In the absence of heart block, the heart rate is controlled by the pacemaker cells that depolarize most rapidly, because then the action potential is conducted rapidly throughout the heart and initiates rapid depolarization of other cells, even if they already have begun spontaneous slow depolarization. Automaticity is affected by the rate of slow spontaneous depolarization and the threshold potential. Automaticity is enhanced by increased sympathetic tone, decreased vagal tone, increased catecholamine concentration in the blood, thyroid hormone, and digitalis. It is suppressed by decreased sympathetic tone, increased vagal tone, decreased thyroid hormone concentration, and various drugs (e.g., those used in the treatment of arrhythmias). Antiarrhythmic drugs may also increase automaticity under some conditions; this phenomenon, known as proarrhythmogenesis, is discussed later.

Impulse Generation and Conduction

Sinoatrial Node

The sinoatrial (SA) node is composed of pacemaker cells and is located at the junction of the right atrium and the superior vena cava (Fig. 64.3). The cells of the SA node spontaneously depolarize more rapidly than any other cells within the heart and thereby control the heart rate.

Atrioventricular Node

The AV node is the part of the specialized conduction system that carries the electrical impulse from the atrium to the ventricle. The AV node lies at the junction of the right atrium and the interventricular septum, just above the tricuspid valve. Conduction through the AV node, which is mediated by calcium channels, is unique in that it is relatively slow; as a result, there is a 100- to 200-msec delay between activation of the atria and ventricles. This delay is important because it ensures that ventricular contraction occurs after atrial contraction is complete, which maximizes filling of the ventricle with blood. Another unique property of the AV node is that conduction is decremental. This means that as more impulses arrive at the AV node, fewer get through, and those that do conduct through the AV node travel at a slower rate. The property of decremental conduction allows the AV node to serve as a protective gate that does not respond to extremely rapid impulses generated in the atria, thereby protecting the ventricles from rapid stimulation (e.g., during atrial fibrillation). The AV node also has intrinsic pacemaker activity, similar to that of the sinus node but slower (usually at a rate of 40 to 60 beats/minute). Because of the slower rate, the AV node may function as a subsidiary pacemaker if the SA node fails.

Bundle of His

When the action potential leaves the AV node, it enters the specialized conducting fibers known as the bundle of His. The main bundle of His divides into three branches: the right bundle branch, which runs along the right ventricular surface of the septum, the anterior superior branch, which runs along the left ventricular surface of the septum, and the posterior inferior branch, which runs along the posterior wall of the left ventricle. The action potential is conducted through the bundle branches and into the myocardium by a widespread network of smaller fibers known as Purkinje fibers.

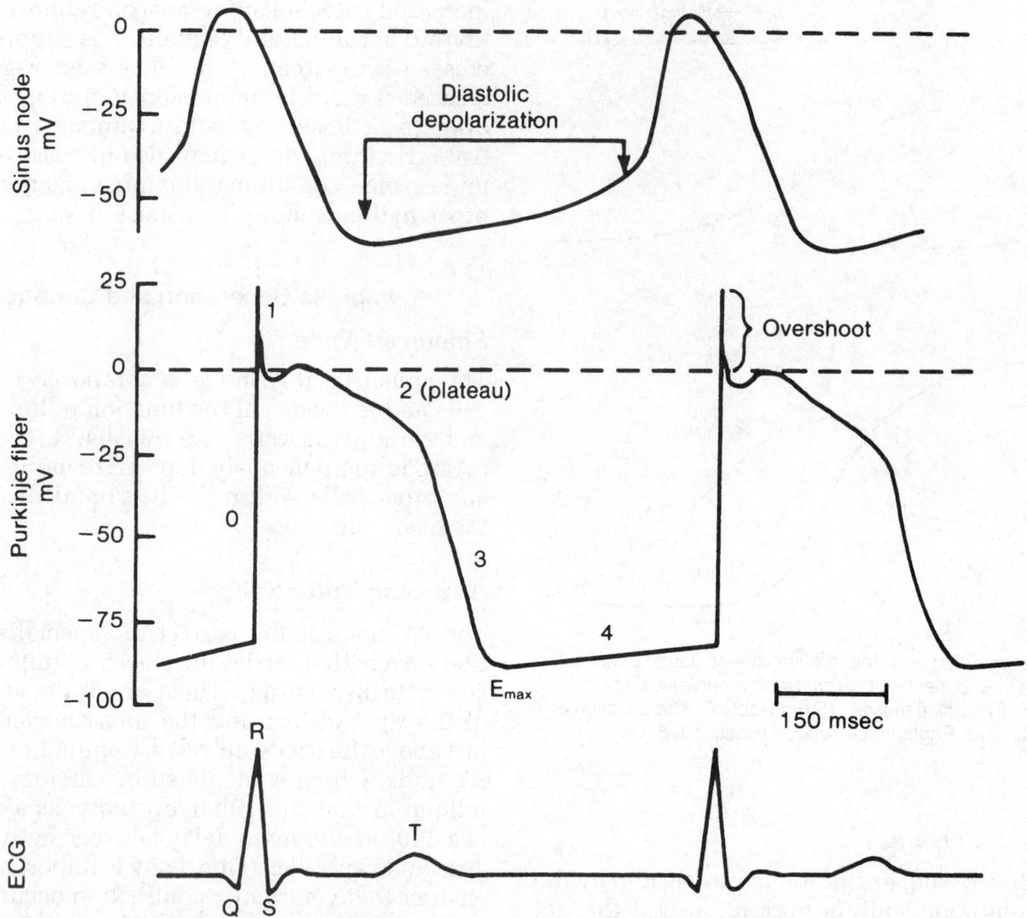

Figure 64.2. Transmembrane potentials from the sinus node and a Purkinje fiber. Note the spontaneous diastolic depolarization in the upper panel, characteristic of pacemaker fibers. The numbers in the middle panel are explained in the text. The lower panel shows the correlation of the time sequence of changes in the action potential with the surface electrocardiogram. Alterations in depolarization are reflected in changes in the QRS duration of the surface record; those in repolarization are associated with alterations in the Q–T interval. (From Singh BN, Collett JT, Chew CYC. New perspectives in the pharmacologic therapy of cardiac arrhythmias. Prog Cardiovasc Dis 1980;22:243.)

MECHANISM OF CARDIAC ARRHYTHMIAS

There are three basic causes of disturbance in the rhythm of the heart: suppression or enhancement of initiation or propagation of the action potential, reentry of the action potential into a pathway through which it has already passed, and triggered activity (1). More than one of these mechanisms may be operative in producing a particular arrhythmia (e.g., ectopic supraventricular tachycardia in a patient with sinus node dysfunction).

Suppression or Enhancement of Initiation or Propagation of Action Potential

A disease process that interferes with pacemaker activity within the SA node or with the movement of the electrical impulse through the normal conduction pathways of the heart results in abnormal slowing of the heart rate (bradyarrhythmia) and/or in one of the various forms of heart block.

Enhanced automaticity of a part of the cardiac conduction system may result in the initiation of an impulse more rapidly than is normally generated by the SA node. If that happens episodically, occasional premature contractions occur, the nature of which depends on the location of the ectopic pacemaker. On the other hand, if there is rapid sustained firing of the ectopic focus, a tachyarrhythmia ensues.

Reentry

Most clinically significant arrhythmias result from reentry (Fig. 64.4). Reentrant arrhythmias occur in the setting of two anatomically or functionally distinct conduction pathways, unidirectional conduction block in one of the pathways, and slowed conduction. When these three conditions are fulfilled, the electrical impulse may travel down one limb of the reentrant circuit and return via the second limb of the circuit, resulting in a "short circuit" or "circus" arrhythmia. Less commonly, arrhythmias result from

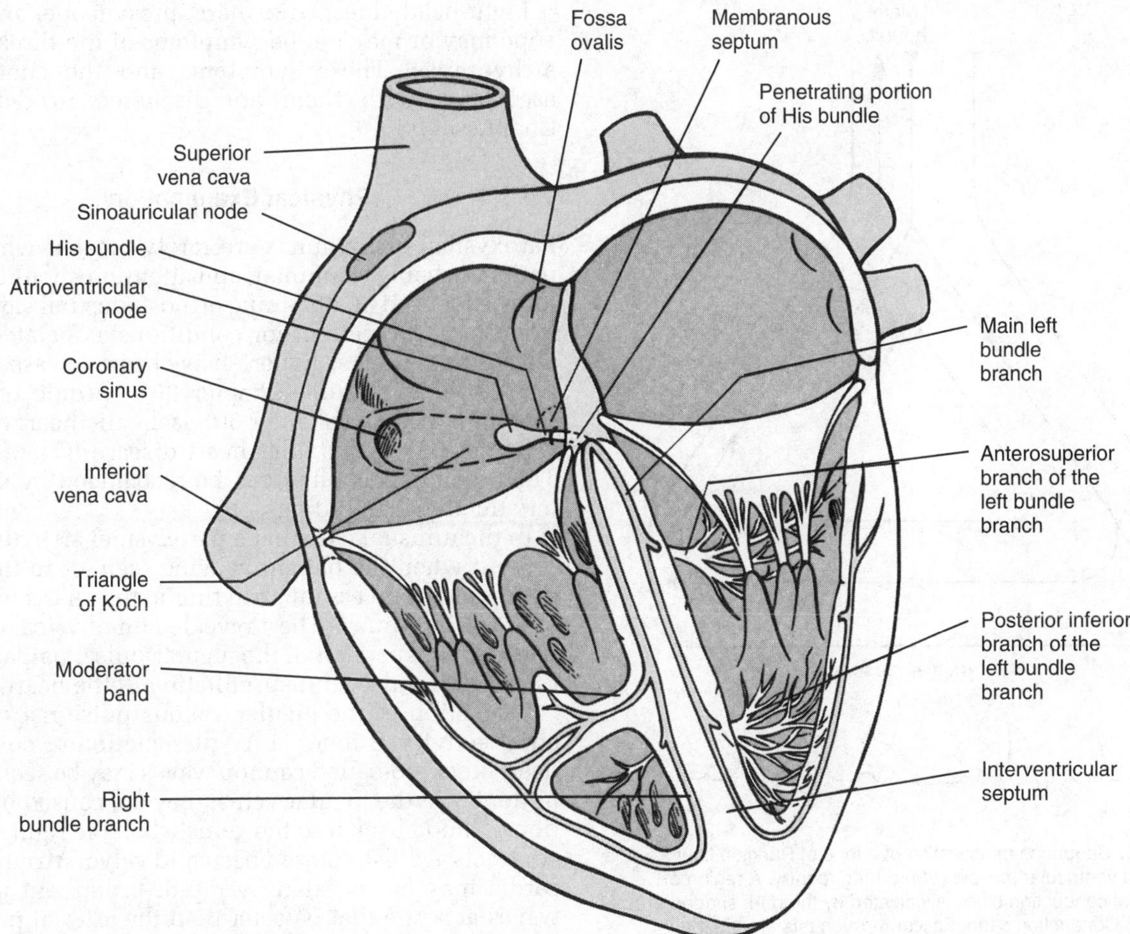

Figure 64.3. Anatomy of impulse generation. (From Willerson JT, ed. Treatment of heart diseases. London: Gower Medical Publishers, 1992. By permission of Mosby International.)

anatomic abnormalities such as an accessory AV connection, as in the case of the Wolff–Parkinson–White (WPW) syndrome.

Triggered Activity

Triggered arrhythmias are less common; they result from afterdepolarizations that follow an action potential and that reach threshold for triggering additional impulses (2). Examples of triggered arrhythmias include torsades de pointes, multifocal atrial tachycardia, and atrial tachycardia resulting from digitalis toxicity (see later discussion).

DIAGNOSIS OF ARRHYTHMIAS: GENERAL CONSIDERATIONS

History

Arrhythmias may or may not cause symptoms. Symptoms are caused by an appreciation of the irregular rhythm (palpitations) (3,4) or by a reduction in cardiac output (light-headedness, dizziness, presyncope, syncope, dyspnea, diaphoresis, chest pain, anxiety).

When taking a history from a patient with a suspected arrhythmia, it is important to define the onset, regularity, and duration of symptoms and whether any factors seem to trigger symptoms (e.g., drinking coffee, smoking, exercise, emotional stress, taking or forgetting to take medications).

It is important to determine whether there is a history or symptoms of an underlying disease that may be associated with arrhythmia (e.g., hypertension, heart failure, ischemic or valvular heart disease, thyrotoxicosis), because the prognosis and recommended treatment depend to a large extent on the nature and severity of underlying heart disease. Patients should be asked about a family history of arrhythmias or sudden death; the taking of stimulant drugs either illicitly (see Chapter 29) or as an attempt to lose weight (see Chapter 83); and about the taking of prescription drugs that can cause arrhythmias (digitalis, theophylline, diuretics, beta-blockers, alpha-agonists, tricyclic antidepressants, and antihypertensives).

Palpitations are heartbeats that are sensed, usually because the beats are fast or irregular. However, they do not necessarily imply a significant arrhythmia, and they may represent only sinus tachycardia in an

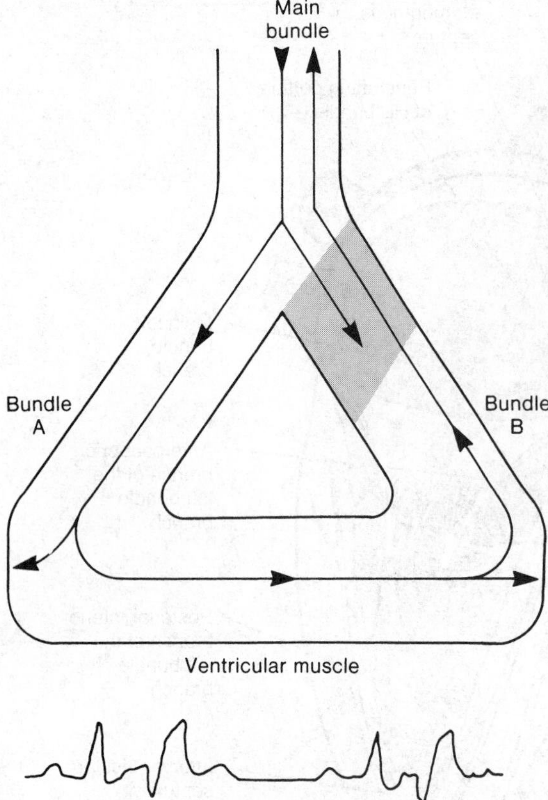

Figure 64.4. Sequence of activation of a loop of Purkinje fiber bundles and ventricular muscle (VM) during reentry. A region of unidirectional conduction block is indicated by the dark shaded area in branch B. Conduction cannot occur through this area in the antegrade direction (from B to VM), but only in the retrograde direction (from VM to B). Slow conduction is present in the loop. The bottom of the figure shows a possible electrocardiographic pattern that may result from this type of reentry. (From Wit AL, Rosen MR, Hoffman BF. Electrophysiology and pharmacology of cardiac arrhythmias. II: Relationship of normal and abnormal electrical activity of cardiac fibers to the genesis of arrhythmias. B: Re-entry, Section I. Am Heart J 1974;88:664.)

otherwise healthy person, especially if the patient is prone to somatization and hypochondriasis (3). In contrast, patients with paroxysmal supraventricular arrhythmias may be misdiagnosed as having a panic disorder (see Chapter 22) (5). Clinical descriptors of palpitations that are predictive of an arrhythmia include "heart fluttering," "heart stopping," and "irregular heartbeat" (1,3). Palpitations are often localized to the area of the apex beat, but paroxysmal supraventricular tachycardias (PSVTs) are commonly sensed in the side of the neck or under the upper sternum. Some people seem to sense the compensatory pause (see later discussion) after an extra heartbeat, but some may sense the extra beat itself. Often the contraction after an extra beat is more powerful than a normal beat (so-called postextrasystolic potentiation), and this stronger beat may be the one that is sensed. Supraventricular beats are more commonly sensed as palpitations than are ventricular beats; in fact, prognostically significant runs of ventricular tachycardia may be asymptomatic.

Light-headedness, dizziness, presyncope, and syncope may or may not be symptoms of life-threatening arrhythmias. These symptoms and the conditions associated with them are discussed in detail in Chapter 89.

Physical Examination

Paroxysmal arrhythmias are rarely present when the patient is being examined, and attention should therefore be focused on obtaining orthostatic vital signs and examining the patient for conditions associated with arrhythmia, such as hypertensive heart disease (Chapter 67), heart failure (Chapter 66), chronic obstructive lung disease (Chapter 60), ischemic heart disease (Chapter 62), or valvular heart disease (Chapter 65). These conditions often can be recognized by characteristic physical findings.

In the unusual case that a paroxysmal arrhythmia is present when the patient is being seen, or in the case of chronic or incessant arrhythmia, the characteristics of the arrhythmia are best revealed on physical examination by inspection of the jugular pulse, palpation of the arterial pulse, and auscultation of the heart.

Inspection of the jugular venous pulse may reveal atrial activity. If there is AV dissociation or complete heart block, so-called cannon waves may be seen intermittently in the jugular veins; they are caused by ejection of blood back into the veins when the right atrium contracts against a closed tricuspid valve. Atrial tachycardia may be revealed by rapid, prominent jugular waves at a rate that is faster than the arterial pulse or heart sounds.

Auscultation of the heart also establishes the ventricular rate and rhythm and the intensity of the first heart sound (S_1), the most useful heart sound in the evaluation of arrhythmia. For example, variation in the intensity of S_1 during a regular tachycardia suggests AV dissociation; variation during a regular bradycardia suggests second- or third-degree heart block. The intensity of S_1 is also a function of the P–R interval. A loud S_1 suggests a short P–R interval; a soft S_1 suggests a long P–R interval, caused, for example, by digitalis toxicity or electrolyte abnormalities (for other cardiac conditions affecting the intensity of S_1; see Chapter 65).

Use of the Electrocardiogram

It is essential to obtain an ECG when evaluating a patient who is having or is suspected of having had an arrhythmia. Without it, with few exceptions, a specific diagnosis is impossible (6). Often, ambulatory (Holter) monitoring, an event monitor (loop recorder) (7), or an exercise ECG is indicated to detect a sporadic arrhythmia or an arrhythmia that is induced by stress (8). Even less commonly, a complex arrhythmia cannot be diagnosed accurately by standard ECG, and an intracavitary electrophysiologic study must be obtained by catheterization in order to make a precise diagnosis. Upright tilt table testing may be necessary to differentiate presyncope or syncope caused by an arrhythmia from neurocardiogenic syncope (also called vasodepressor or vasovagal syncope). The use of this test is discussed in Chapter 89.

Surface Resting Electrocardiogram

A number of features of the standard ECG must be assessed.

Atrial Activity. Atrial activity is best assessed in leads 2, 3, aVF, and V_1. The presence of P waves must be identified. If P waves are present, their configuration and their relationship to the QRS complexes must be established. Normally the P–R interval is between 0.12 and 0.20 seconds (each 1-mm segment on the ECG is equal to 0.04 second), and each QRS complex is preceded by a P wave whose vector is such that the P wave is upright in leads 2, 3, and aVF. If P waves are not present, other evidence of atrial activity (fibrillation or flutter waves) should be sought.

Ventricular Activity. The duration of the QRS complexes (normally less than 0.10 second) should be measured and the regularity of ventricular activity assessed. A basically regular rhythm may be interrupted by so-called premature beats—QRS complexes that appear before the next regular beat is expected. If premature beats are present, it should be noted whether they have a fixed relationship to the preceding normal beat and whether their configuration is the same as that of the regularly occurring complexes.

Ambulatory Electrocardiogram

The ambulatory (Holter) ECG records on magnetic tape the electrical activity of the heart, usually for a 24- to 48-hour period (9). The recording device is small and does not interfere with any of the patient's activities (except bathing and swimming). The technique is useful in the following circumstances:

- Assessing whether suspicious symptoms (e.g., palpitation, light-headedness, dizziness, syncope) in a patient with a normal resting ECG are caused by an episodic arrhythmia
- Assessing whether episodic, but potentially life-threatening, arrhythmias are occurring in a patient with known heart disease (e.g., ischemic heart disease, congestive heart failure)
- Assessing the efficacy of antiarrhythmic therapy or the function of a cardiac pacemaker
- Assessing whether there is episodic evidence of overt or silent ischemia

A minority of episodic arrhythmias are detected during 24 hours of Holter monitoring (10). If symptoms are infrequent, it may be necessary to record the ambulatory ECG for 48 to 72 hours or to use an event monitor (see later discussion). The patient should be asked to keep a record of symptoms while being monitored, to determine whether those symptoms are attributable to arrhythmia. Patients should be instructed to record symptoms associated with their palpitations, including dizziness, nausea, shortness of breath, chest discomfort, or arm pain (10).

If symptoms are infrequent, an *event monitor,* also known as a *cardiac event recorder* or *external loop recorder,* may be useful in making a diagnosis of an arrhythmia (7). These pager-sized devices are worn clipped to the patient's belt or dress during all daily activities. The patient wears two chest electrodes that are attached to the monitor by snap-on leads. The patient may easily remove the monitor and leads to shower or bathe, and fresh electrodes are easily applied by the patient. Event monitors record a 30- to 60-second "loop" of the patient's cardiac electrical activity on a computer chip. If the patient experiences symptoms, he or she may activate the device by pushing a button; this saves the loop of beats in the device memory. The recorded ECG is then transmitted via an audiotelephonic interface to a central monitor, where the rhythm strip is printed out and sent to the referring clinician. The recording technician will contact the referring clinician directly if potentially dangerous arrhythmias are detected. The devices are usually worn for 30 days, or until an event is recorded. If events are extremely infrequent, an *insertable loop recorder* may be advised. These devices, similar in size and shape to a permanent pacemaker, are implanted under the skin in the upper chest. The patient does not need to be hospitalized for the procedure, and the device may remain in place for more than a year; these devices are easily explanted. They are activated with the use of a magnetic wand, and the transmission procedure is similar to that used for a standard event monitor. Studies show that event monitors, when used for the diagnosis of intermittent palpitations, are more likely than Holter monitors to record diagnostic arrhythmias and do so at a lower cost (10). The cost of Holter monitoring and event monitoring is approximately five to ten times that of a standard ECG.

Exercise Electrocardiogram

Exercise ECG is described in detail in Chapter 62. It is a useful test in the evaluation of patients who have symptoms suggestive of an arrhythmia during or after exercise and, in those with premature ventricular contractions, to determine whether they become more or less frequent during or after exercise (see Ventricular Premature Beats) (11). It may also be helpful in assessing the adequacy of rate control in patients with atrial fibrillation.

GENERAL PRINCIPLES IN MANAGEMENT OF ARRHYTHMIAS

Once it has been established that a patient has a particular arrhythmia, the practitioner must decide whether treatment is necessary. A general principle is that treatment should be limited to symptomatic patients with prognostically significant arrhythmias (12) and that antiarrhythmic medications should be avoided whenever possible (13). It must also be determined whether the arrhythmia is secondary to a noncardiac process (e.g., hypoxia, electrolyte imbalance, fever, drug toxicity) or a cardiac process (e.g., heart failure, ischemia, pericarditis, digitalis intoxication), the correction of which will restore a normal cardiac rhythm.

If specific therapy is indicated, an appropriate regimen must be selected: one or more of the antiarrhythmic drugs, electrical conversion of the arrhythmia, a cardiac pacemaker or antitachycardia device, catheter or surgical ablation of the arrhythmia focus, or a combination of these regimens. It must be determined whether the potential benefits of the proposed antiarrhythmic therapy outweigh the risk of proarrhythmia (see later discussion) and whether the cost, side effects, and inconvenience of the therapy are justified.

An important and often difficult issue to determine is whether hospitalization is required for the initiation of therapy.

A consensus exists that antiarrhythmic therapy should be initiated in the hospital for patients with hemodynamically unstable arrhythmias, such as sustained ventricular tachycardia, or for initiation of antiarrhythmic agents (other than amiodarone) in patients with significantly compromised cardiac function as evidenced by a left ventricular ejection fraction (EF) lower than 40%. Antiarrhythmic therapy can be initiated on an ambulatory basis in patients with functionally normal hearts in the absence of a hemodynamically compromising arrhythmia. Although there is some debate, many cardiologists believe that, in the absence of a hemodynamically compromising arrhythmia, even patients with an EF lower than 40% can have amiodarone initiated as an outpatient (14).

Some antiarrhythmic drugs prolong the Q–T interval and may induce torsades de pointes (polymorphic ventricular tachycardia; see later discussion), particularly when therapy is first started (see www.torsades.org for a list of these drugs). Two such drugs are sotalol and dofetilide, and patients generally need to be monitored as inpatients when beginning therapy with these agents. Given this risk, a cardiologist should be consulted whenever these two drugs are begun. Consultation with a cardiologist may also be helpful in deciding which patients beginning therapy with other antiarrhythmic drugs, such as procainamide, quinidine, disopyramide, and flecainide, require hospitalization for continuous ECG monitoring.

Pharmacology of Antiarrhythmic Drugs

Antiarrhythmic drugs are grouped commonly into four classes (1,15). Class I drugs, whose prototype is quinidine (16), interfere with the fast inward sodium current. Class II drugs, whose prototype is propranolol, affect sympathetically mediated excitability. Class III drugs, such as sotalol or amiodarone (17), prolong the duration of the action potential by decreasing the late inward (phase 3) potassium current. Class IV drugs, whose prototype is verapamil, block calcium-mediated slow channel currents in the myocardium (18).

Digitalis and adenosine do not fit into this classification scheme. Strictly speaking, digitalis is not an antiarrhythmic drug in that it does not have a direct effect on membrane function. It acts indirectly as an antiarrhythmic agent by increasing vagal activity, thereby increasing the refractory period of the specialized conduction tissue of the atria and slowing the velocity of the action potential through the AV node. Digitalis also increases the frequency of fibrillatory waves in atrial fibrillation, thereby presenting more impulses to the AV node, making the node refractory to conduction (this process is called *concealed conduction*). General considerations in the use of digitalis, including dosages, choice of a preparation, and recognition and treatment of toxicity are discussed in Chapter 66. The pharmacology and use of adenosine are discussed below.

Table 64.1 shows some of the characteristics of the orally administered antiarrhythmic drugs that can be used to treat an ambulatory patient.

Most antiarrhythmic drugs have a low toxic/therapeutic ratio, and some are exceedingly toxic (Table 64.2). In addition to direct toxic effects, antiarrhythmic drugs often have complex interactions with commonly used drugs such as digoxin, warfarin, and certain antihistamines and antibiotics (see Torsades de Pointes), and may paradoxically induce arrhythmias and increase the incidence of sudden cardiac death, a clinical scenario called *proarrhythmia*. Proarrhythmic effects can include virtually any arrhythmia but often are seen as an increase in the frequency of premature ventricular contractions (PVCs) or a sudden onset of ventricular tachycardia, torsades de pointes, or ventricular fibrillation. Although in the past it was believed that proarrhythmic effects of drugs are usually seen within several days after an antiarrhythmic drug is started or the dosage is changed, the results of the Cardiac Arrhythmia Suppression Trial (CAST) make it clear that these effects of drugs may be delayed (19). In general, the proarrhythmic effects of antiarrhythmic drugs are usually seen in patients with severe heart disease, as evidenced by an EF of less than 40% (20,21).

The risk of antiarrhythmic drug treatment has been highlighted by several clinical trials and reviews based on meta-analyses. An almost fourfold increase in mortality was demonstrated in patients with myocardial dysfunction and nonsustained ventricular tachycardia after a myocardial infarction (MI) when they were treated with either flecainide or encainide (19). Also, a significant increase in post-MI mortality has been shown in patients treated with any class I antiarrhythmic agent (22). A meta-analysis of patients with atrial fibrillation treated with quinidine showed an increased mortality (23), and an analysis of antiarrhythmic drug use in the Stroke Prevention in Atrial Fibrillation Trial reported an almost fivefold increased risk of cardiac death among patients with heart failure who were receiving an antiarrhythmic drug (24).

Class I Drugs

All class I drugs block the sodium channel (see earlier discussion), but the effect on the duration of the action potential and on repolarization varies depending on the kinetics of the blockage. This fact has practical

Table 64.1. Characteristics of Antiarrhythmic Drugs

Drug	Common Brand Name	Effects on ECG	Half-Life (hr)	Time to Steady State (days)	Available Strength (mg)	Usual Oral Dosage	Maximal Daily Dosage (mg)	Therapeutic Plasma Level
Class IA								
Quinidine	Generic	Prolongs QRS, Q–T, and (±) P–R	6	1–2	200 (sulfate), 342 (gluconate)	200–600 mg q6–8h	1800 (s); 2400 (g)	3–7 μg/mL
Procainamide	Pronestyl	Prolongs QRS, Q–T, and (±) P–R	3–4	1	250, 500, 750 (sustained release)	500–1,000 mg q3–4h or q6h (sustained release)	4,000	3–8 μg/mL[a]
Disopyramide	Norpace	Prolongs QRS, Q–T, and (±) P–R	6–9	1–2	100, 150	150 mg q.i.d.	1,200	2–4 μg/mL
Class IB								
Mexiletine	Mexitil	Shortens Q–T	10–12	2–3	150, 200, 250	200–300 mg q8h	1,200	0.5–2 μg/mL
Class IC								
Flecainide	Tambocor	Prolongs P–R, QRS, Q–T, bradycardia	12–27	2–3	100	200 mg q.d.	600	0.2–1.0 μg/mL
Propafenone	Rythmol	Prolongs P–R, QRS, but not Q–T	2–10 (90% of patients), 10–32 (10% of patients)	Depends on genetically determined metabolic rate	150, 300	450–900 mg in three divided doses	900	0.2–1.5 μg/mL
Class II (see Table 64.3)								
Class III								
Amiodarone	Cordarone	Prolongs P–R, QRS	53	8 days after loading dose	200	100–600 mg q.d.	800	Not useful
Sotalol	Betapace	Slows HR, prolongs QTc; no effect on QRS	12	3–4	80, 160	80–160 b.i.d. to t.i.d.	480–640[b]	Not useful
Dofetilide[c]	Tikosyn	Prolongs QT; no effect on other conduction parameters	10	NA	0.125 mg, 0.25 mg, 0.5 mg	0.125–0.5 mg b.i.d.[d] (4–8 μg/kg IV bolus)	0.5 mg b.i.d.	Not useful
Ibutilide	Corvert	Prolongs QT	6	NA	0.1 mg/mL solution (10 mL) for injection	NA (1 mg IV over 10 min if $\geq$ 60 kg; 0.1 mg/kg if $<$ 60 kg)	NA	Not useful
Class IV								
Verapamil	Calan, Isoptin	Prolongs P–R	4.5–12	1–2	40, 80, 120, 180, 240 (sustained release)	80–120 mg q8h or 120–360 mg sustained release q.d.	480	125–400 ng/mL
Diltiazem	Cardizem	Prolongs P–R	3.5	1	30, 60, 90, 120 or 180, 240, 300 CD	30–120 mg t.i.d. to q.i.d. daily or 120–480 mg CD q.d.	480	Not useful

s, Sulfate; g, gluconate; CD, continuous delivery; ECG, electrocardiogram; NA, not applicable.

[a] It may also be important to measure, especially in patients in cardiac or renal failure, the level of the active metabolite of procainamide, *N*-acetylprocainamide (NAPA—therapeutic level 6–20 μg/mL).

[b] Elimination is mainly in the urine. Dosages should be lowered in patients with renal insufficiency.

[c] Drug is available only to prescribers who have received dosing and treatment education and have passed a certifying examination (see Tikosyn.com).

[d] Dose decreased for renal insufficiency or if QT $>$ 500 msec or $>$ 15% baseline.

Table 64.2. Adverse Effects of Antiarrhythmic Drugs

Drug	Cardiac		Noncardiac	
	Common	Uncommon	Common	Uncommon
Class IA				
Quinidine	Decreased digoxin excretion; may precipitate digitoxicity	Ventricular arrhythmias, myocardial depression, hypotension	Nausea, diarrhea, tinnitus, vertigo, rash, fever, warfarin interaction (↑ INR)	Hepatic dysfunction, thrombocytopenia, hemolytic anemia
Procainamide	None	Myocardial depression	Nausea, vomiting	Agranulocytosis, lupus-like syndrome
Disopyramide	Myocardial depression; should be used with caution in patients with severe or poorly compensated congestive heart failure	Severe hypotension in absence of known heart disease	Anticholinergic effects, especially urinary retention, dry mouth, blurred vision, constipation, aggravation of narrow-angle glaucoma	Acute psychoses, cholestasis
Class IB				
Mexiletine	None	Increased frequency of ventricular arrhythmias	Nausea, vomiting, indigestion, dizziness, tremor	Sleep disturbances, fatigue
Class IC				
Flecainide	Increased frequency of ventricular arrhythmias, myocardial depression; use with caution in patients with ejection fraction <40%	New supraventricular arrhythmias, congestive heart failure	Dizziness, visual disturbances, dyspnea, nausea, tremor	Constipation, edema, abdominal pain
Propafenone	Conduction delay	? Congestive heart failure	Unusual taste, constipation	Nausea, blurred vision, dizziness
Class II				
Propranolol[a]	Bradycardia, myocardial depression	Anginal syndrome may worsen if drug suddenly discontinued	Fatigue, nausea, vomiting, depression, impotence, potentiates bronchospasm in patients with asthma	Peripheral vascular insufficiency, hyperglycemia, alopecia
Class III				
Amiodarone	Bradycardia, increased heart block, increased digoxin concentration	Ventricular arrhythmias	Nausea, corneal microcrystallization, thyroid function abnormalities, decreased pulmonary diffusing capacity, abnormalities in liver function tests, tremor, ataxia, peripheral neuropathy, warfarin interaction (↑ INR)	Blue tint of exposed skin, pulmonary fibrosis
Sotalol	Bradycardia, fatigue, increased QTc	Torsade de pointes in 3%–5%	Dyspnea	
Dofetilide	Prolongs QT interval, torsades de pointes, ventricular tachycardia, chest pain	—	Dizziness, headache, insomnia, nausea, diarrhea, dyspnea, respiratory infection, rash	Confusion, parasthesias, and paralysis
Ibutilide	Prolongs QT interval; torsades de pointes, heart block, hypotension, ventricular arrhythmia	—	Headache, nausea	—
Class IV				
Verapamil	Bradycardia, prolongation of P–R interval, peripheral edema, increased digoxin level	Precipitation of congestive heart failure or pulmonary edema, severe hypotension, heart block	Dizziness, headache, constipation, nausea	Confusion, sleep disorders
Diltiazem	Bradycardia, prolongation of P–R interval	Heart block, increased digoxin level	Dizziness, headache, constipation	Rash, itching

INR, International normalized ratio.

[a]Other β-blocking agents have the same adverse effects, although bronchospasm and peripheral vascular insufficiency may be less likely with use of cardioselective β-blockers (see Table 64.3).

application in the choice of drugs for treatment of specific arrhythmias and in the use of a combination of drugs (e.g., mexiletine plus quinidine) (1), although it would be advisable to combine these drugs only after consultation with a cardiologist.

Class I drugs have been subdivided into three classes: IA, IB, and IC (Table 64.1).

Class IA Drugs. Class IA drugs prolong the duration of the action potential (Fig. 64.1) and so prolong the QRS and Q–T interval and the effective refractory period. These drugs include quinidine, procainamide, and disopyramide.

Quinidine. In addition to its direct effects on the heart, quinidine blocks parasympathetic stimulation by the vagus nerve and may enhance AV conduction (and the ventricular rate) in some patients. For this reason, patients with supraventricular tachyarrhythmias should generally be treated with a drug to slow AV nodal conduction (e.g., digitalis, a beta-blocker) before they are given quinidine. Quinidine also is a moderately potent inhibitor of alpha-adrenergic activity and may cause orthostatic hypotension (16).

Several preparations of quinidine are available; quinidine sulfate is the recommended preparation on the basis of cost, but quinidine gluconate may have fewer gastrointestinal side effects. A sustained-release preparation containing gluconate (Quinaglute Dura Tabs) may be preferred in some patients because it can be given every 8 to 12 hours.

Table 64.1 shows the time necessary to reach a steady state after administration of usual dosages of quinidine. If a faster effect is desired, loading doses may be given (e.g., 300 mg every 3 hours for three doses); in this circumstance hospitalization is advisable, both to monitor the effect of the drug and because the arrhythmia presumably is more dangerous.

Although quinidine has been used to treat a large variety of supraventricular and ventricular arrhythmias, it is rarely used to treat arrhythmias today because of the fear of proarrhythmia (particularly in patients with structural heart disease), the availability of other effective and safer antiarrhythmic drugs, and the development of gastrointestinal side effects in a large proportion of patients taking the drug. The indications for quinidine should be regularly and critically reviewed (16).

There are a number of possible *toxic effects* of quinidine. The most common are gastrointestinal (especially diarrhea) and occur often within hours after the drug is administered. Cinchonism (tinnitus, headache, visual disturbances) should not be seen if blood levels are checked periodically and if the dosage is appropriately adjusted. Hypersensitivity reactions (e.g., rash, arthralgias, immune thrombocytopenia, hemolytic anemia) occur occasionally.

Cardiac toxicity is usually dose related, often signaled by a prolongation of the Q–T interval; Q–T prolongation of 50% or more beyond baseline is an indication for reduction of the dosage of quinidine. Serious toxicity is manifested by a high degree of AV block, ventricular tachycardia, torsades de pointes (see later discussion), or ventricular fibrillation—all emergency situations that may require cardiorespiratory support and warrant immediate hospitalization. Occasionally, patients taking quinidine die suddenly, sometimes with low plasma levels of the drug. Patients with prolonged Q–T intervals before institution of therapy with quinidine may be more prone to sudden death and therefore should not be given the drug. Greater care is warranted in women taking quinidine, because quinidine causes greater Q–T prolongation in women than in men at equivalent serum concentrations (25). Patients receiving quinidine (or other drugs that prolong the Q-T interval, such as procainamide or sotalol) should be checked by ECG periodically (e.g., every 6 months) to monitor the Q–T interval. Those patients whose Q–T interval exceeds 450 msec, or whose Q–T increases consistently over time, should be referred to a cardiologist to re-evaluate the need for the particular drug or to consider either a reduction in dose or discontinuation of the drug.

Quinidine may have *interactions with other drugs.* Because patients prescribed quinidine are commonly treated with digitalis as well, it is especially important to recognize that digoxin levels may increase significantly in patients given quinidine. Quinidine decreases the excretion of digoxin by the kidneys, so it is important to monitor serum digoxin concentrations when quinidine is first prescribed and to alter the dosage of digoxin to prevent digitalis intoxication.

Quinidine is an alpha-adrenergic blocker and, if it is prescribed with vasodilators (e.g., nitrates, nifedipine, hydralazine, prazosin, angiotensin-converting enzyme inhibitors) or with potent diuretics (e.g., furosemide), it can cause symptomatic (especially postural) hypotension.

Drugs that are metabolized by hepatic microsomal enzymes may alter the pharmacokinetics of quinidine, and, conversely, quinidine may alter the kinetics of one of these drugs. For example, phenytoin may accelerate the metabolism of quinidine, shortening its effect, and quinidine may inhibit the metabolism of warfarin, prolonging its effect.

Most importantly, the patient and clinician must both be aware of the need to avoid other drugs that prolong the Q–T interval. Drugs that prolong the Q–T interval and/or induce torsades de pointes are listed on a convenient website at *www.torsades.org* (accessed 1/7/02).

Procainamide. The suppressive effects of procainamide on the electrical activity of the heart are the same as those of quinidine, but, unlike quinidine, procainamide has little effect on vagal or alpha-adrenergic activity.

Like quinidine, procainamide may be used to treat many supraventricular arrhythmias. Its use today is limited because of concerns about proarrhythmia, the availability of other effective and safer antiarrhythmic drugs, and the very high proportion of patients who develop a lupus-like syndrome (discussed later) after being treated with procainamide on a long-term basis.

The *noncardiac toxicity* of procainamide is different from that of quinidine. Gastrointestinal symptoms occur less often, and, when they do, nausea and vomiting are more common than diarrhea. Fever (often with shaking chills) or granulocytopenia occurs occasionally.

Within 3 months, 50% of people taking procainamide develop antinuclear antibodies (ANAs), and 90% do so within 12 months (26). Twenty percent to 30% of patients with ANAs develop a lupus-like syndrome characterized by serositis (pleuritis, pericarditis, synovitis), fever, hepatomegaly, and a positive lupus erythematosus preparation. Unlike classic systemic lupus erythematosus, vasculitis is not a manifestation of drug-induced lupus, so that renal disease, for example, does not occur. Most important, the syndrome abates, usually within days, when the drug is discontinued (ANAs may persist for months). The major threat of the syndrome is hemorrhagic pericarditis, and one must watch for signs and symptoms of pericardial tamponade. For these reasons, procainamide is not recommended for long-term use.

Disopyramide. Disopyramide has direct membrane effects very much like those of quinidine and, like quinidine, blocks parasympathetic activity. It is licensed for the treatment of specific ventricular arrhythmias: unifocal or multifocal PVCs and ventricular tachycardia. Like quinidine and procainamide, disopyramide is rarely used in ambulatory practice for treatment of patients with supraventricular or ventricular arrhythmias. Perhaps the most common use of disopyramide today is in the treatment of patients with vasodepressor syncope (see Chapter 89). The effectiveness of disopyramide in the treatment of this common condition is caused by its vagolytic and negative inotropic effects.

The noncardiac toxicity of disopyramide is caused mainly by its anticholinergic effects, which include dry mouth, blurred vision, urinary hesitancy, and constipation. For these reasons, disopyramide is in general not advised for elderly patients. Nausea, vomiting, and diarrhea are less common than after administration of quinidine or procainamide. The cardiac toxicity of the drug is, in part, similar to that of quinidine in that it can prolong the Q–T interval and produce torsades de pointes (see later discussion). Disopyramide may also cause or intensify heart failure or cause profound hypotension in patients who have compromised left ventricular function; it should not be administered to such patients.

Class IB Drugs. Class IB drugs shorten repolarization and the Q–T interval and have little effect on the duration of the QRS complex. This class includes phenytoin and mexiletine. Class IB drugs are generally not effective for supraventricular arrhythmias.

Phenytoin. Phenytoin decreases automaticity and the duration of the action potential in the Purkinje fibers of the myocardium. Its use is limited in the treatment of arrhythmias. Phenytoin toxicity is discussed in detail in Chapter 88.

Mexiletine. Mexiletine has electrophysiologic effects similar to those of lidocaine. Adverse effects include nausea, tremulousness, dizziness, and anxiety. It may be useful in combination with a class IA or class III drug (see later discussion), but consultation with a cardiologist is advised before it is prescribed.

Class IC Drugs. Class IC drugs slow conduction and widen the QRS complex but cause only small changes in refractoriness or the Q–T interval. The class IC drugs currently available, flecainide and propafenone, are both highly effective against serious ventricular arrhythmias and may be particularly useful in the treatment of supraventricular arrhythmias, especially atrial fibrillation. Because flecainide has been shown to be associated with a high incidence of sudden death (more than three times that among patients treated with placebo) when used in patients with ventricular dysfunction after MI (19), it should generally not be used in patients with ischemic heart disease, particularly if the EF is less than 40%. Common noncardiac side effects are nausea and epigastric pain. These are controlled largely by dosing with meals to reduce peak drug levels. Class IC drugs should be used with great caution in patients with atrial flutter, because their anticholinergic effects may increase AV conduction and result in 1:1 conduction of atrial flutter at a heart rate of 250 to 300 beats/minute. These drugs should be used only in consultation with a cardiologist.

Class II Drugs (Sympathetic Blocking Agents)

These drugs block the effects of catecholamines (which may potentiate the development of arrhythmias) and slow conduction in the atria, AV node, and myocardium.

Beta-blockers are used to slow the ventricular response in patients with atrial tachyarrhythmia; occasionally, in the process, they convert paroxysmal atrial tachycardia, atrial flutter, or atrial fibrillation to normal sinus rhythm. In addition, ventricular arrhythmias initiated by exercise or ischemia (see Chapter 62) or associated with the congenital long Q–T syndrome (see later discussion in this chapter) may be prevented by the use of these drugs. Low dosages of a beta-blocker (e.g., sustained-release metoprolol) may be effective in controlling heart rate in patients with atrial fibrillation or in maintaining normal sinus rhythm in patients who have been cardioverted (see later discussion). Beta-blockers are the only antiarrhythmic medications that have been convincingly shown to reduce the incidence of sudden death after MI (22). Their use in this regard is discussed in detail in Chapter 63.

A range of *side effects* are associated with the use of beta-blockers. Although they are useful in the management of chronic heart failure (see Chapter 66), beta-blockers can precipitate heart failure if their dose is not appropriately titrated in patients with poor ventricular function. They are also contraindicated in patients with bronchial asthma. Gastrointestinal side effects (primarily nausea and diarrhea) occur occasionally. Most beta-blockers occasionally cause hair thinning; this effect appears to be reversible when the dosage is reduced or the drug is discontinued.

The properties of the currently available beta-blocking agents are listed in Table 64.3. Propranolol

Table 64.3. Characteristics of Currently Available β-Blockers

	Acebutolol (Sectral)	Labetalol (Normodyne Trandate)	Atenolol (Tenormin)	Metoprolol (Lopressor)	Nadolol (Corgard)	Pindolol (Visken)	Propranolol (inderal)	Timolol (Blocadren)	Carvedilol (Coreg)[a]
β-Blocking plasma levels	0.2–2.0 μg/mL	0.7–3.0 μg/mL	200–500 ng/mL	50–100 ng/mL	50–100 ng/mL	50–100 ng/mL	50–100 ng/mL	5–10 ng/mL	—
Half-life (hr)	3–4	5–6	6–9	3–4[b]	14–24	3–4	3.5–6[b]	4	7–10
Active metabolites	Yes	No	No	No	No	No	Yes	No	No
Predominant route of elimination	HM	HM	RE (mostly unchanged)	HM	RE	RE (40% unchanged) and HM	HM	RE (20% unchanged) and HM	HM (50% higher plasma levels in elderly and in chronic renal failure)
β_1-Blockade potency ratio (propranolol = 1.0)	0.3	0.3	1.0	1.0	1.0	6.0	1.0	6.0	0
Relative β_1 selectivity	+	0	+	+	0	0	0	0	0
Available strengths (mg)	200, 400	100, 200, 300	50, 100	50, 100; or 25, 50, 100, 200 XL	40, 80, 120, 160	5, 10	10, 20, 40, 60, 80; and 60, 80, 120, 180 mg long-acting	10	3.125, 6.25, 12.5, 25.0
Usual maintenance dosage	200–600 mg b.i.d.	100–600 mg b.i.d.	50–100 mg q.d.	50–100 mg b.i.d. or 50–200 mg XL q.d.	40–50 mg q.d.	5–20 mg t.i.d.	40–80 mg q.i.d. or 120–160 mg long-acting once a day	20 mg b.i.d.	25 b.i.d.

HM, hepatic metabolism; RE, Renal excretion.

[a]Has significant α-blocking activity; orthostasis is commonly experienced.

[b]Long-acting preparation also available.

Modified from Frishman WH. Beta-adrenoceptor antagonists: new drugs and new indications. N Engl J Med 1981;305:550.

crosses the blood–brain barrier and may cause such side effects as depression and sleep disturbance, although the evidence supporting an association between the use of beta-blockers and depression is not strong (27). Atenolol and metoprolol are long acting, do not cross the blood–brain barrier, and are cardioselective. The dose of atenolol may need to be carefully titrated in patients with renal insufficiency, because it is largely cleared by renal excretion. The main advantage of the longer-acting agents or sustained-release preparations is the likelihood of better compliance.

Class III (Potassium Current Blockers)

Amiodarone. Amiodarone is a potent drug that effectively suppresses both supraventricular and ventricular arrhythmias (17). Especially at high dosages (more than 300 mg/day), it is associated with a number of troublesome side effects, including photosensitivity, corneal microdeposits, hypothyroidism or hyperthyroidism, pulmonary interstitial fibrosis, hepatotoxicity, and a variety of neurologic complaints. However, the use of the drug is not associated with a high risk of proarrhythmia, and amiodarone is the only antiarrhythmic agent that has not been shown in clinical trials to be associated with an increased risk of cardiac death. Each 200-mg tablet of amiodarone contains 75 mg of iodine; the likelihood of thyroid dysfunction is therefore high when the drug is taken chronically (28).

Amiodarone also interacts with many other drugs and, for example, may potentiate the toxic effects of digoxin and of beta-blocking agents. It also interferes with the metabolism of warfarin and may markedly prolong the prothrombin time (17). Because of these problems, the risks and benefits of amiodarone must be considered on a patient-by-patient basis. Today amiodarone is one of the most commonly used drugs to treat atrial fibrillation (see later discussion). Amiodarone is also frequently used in the treatment of patients with sustained ventricular arrhythmias. A cardiologist familiar with the drug should be closely involved in the patient's care. Because of a long mean half-life (almost 2 months), the effects may persist for weeks after the drug is discontinued.

Meta-analyses of the use of amiodarone in high-risk patients after MI (29) show a modest mortality benefit: the number needed to treat to avoid one additional death is 71. Post-MI patients whose left ventricular EF is less than 40% or who have frequent ventricular arrhythmias (nonsustained ventricular tachycardia or more than 10 PVCs per minute) should be seen in consultation with a cardiologist to decide on the most appropriate therapy.

Sotalol. Sotalol is a racemic mixture of both a class II agent (i.e., a beta-blocker, L-sotalol) and a class III agent (D-sotalol) (30). The indications for its use are the same as for amiodarone, and it has fewer extracardiac side effects. However, because serious ventricular arrhythmias are seen in 3% to 5% of patients, it should be used with caution in patients with impaired ventricular function and should not be initiated on an ambulatory basis if the patient has underlying structural heart disease.

Sotalol, which previously carried an indication only for ventricular arrhythmias, has recently been repackaged with extended patent protection as Betapace-AF and marketed specifically for control of atrial fibrillation in patients with or without structural heart disease. Because of the risk of torsades de pointes (see later discussion), however, a patient beginning sotalol must be monitored as an inpatient for at least several days.

Other Agents. Dofetilide and ibutilide are class III agents that have been approved relatively recently for the treatment of arrhythmias. *Dofetilide* is approved by the U.S. Food and Drug Administration for the treatment of atrial arrhythmias. It is used in ambulatory practice for the maintenance of sinus rhythm in patients who have been converted from atrial fibrillation. *Ibutilide* is useful either to acutely convert atrial fibrillation by itself or to facilitate electrical cardioversion of atrial fibrillation. Because there is no oral form of the drug, it has no role in ambulatory practice.

Class IV Drugs (Calcium Channel Blockers)

Calcium channel blockers are effective and useful drugs for controlling supraventricular arrhythmias. Conduction through the AV node is dependent on calcium-mediated currents. By blocking these currents, calcium channel blockers may control the ventricular response in atrial fibrillation and may convert to sinus rhythm supraventricular arrhythmias that depend on conduction through the AV node. Verapamil may be useful in an ambulatory setting for the conversion of paroxysmal AV node reentry tachycardia (AVNRT) (discussed later) to sinus rhythm. Doses of 80 to 120 mg orally may be used safely in patients known to have AVNRT; conversion to sinus rhythm usually occurs in 30 to 60 minutes. Alternatively, a dose of 5 to 10 mg intravenously may convert AVNRT in minutes. If the drug is not effective, referral to a hospital emergency room should be considered. Oral verapamil at dosages of 240 to 360 mg/day may be used for prophylaxis against supraventricular arrhythmias. Verapamil may also be used at dosages of 240 to 360 mg/day for control of heart rate in patients with atrial fibrillation. Diltiazem at dosages of 120 to 300 mg/day may also be effective. The dihydropyridine calcium channel blockers, such as nifedipine and amlodipine, are not useful for control of atrial arrhythmias, nor are calcium channel blockers in general effective for control of ventricular arrhythmias.

Calcium channel blockers such as verapamil and diltiazem, which may be useful in AVNRT, can cause a dangerous acceleration of the heart rate in patients with the WPW syndrome by increasing conduction in the accessory pathway. If supraventricular tachycardia degenerates to atrial fibrillation in patients with the WPW syndrome who are treated with a calcium channel blocker, the ventricular rate may suddenly accelerate to more than 300 beats/minute. For this reason, calcium channel blockers should not be used in patients with a known accessory pathway.

Verapamil is metabolized by the liver and should be used with caution in patients with impaired hepatic function. Both verapamil and diltiazem are available in extended-release formulations that can be taken once daily. Except perhaps for initial dosage titration, the once-daily formulations are preferred over the short-acting forms. Occasionally, elderly patients are very sensitive to diltiazem and require only 30 mg three times daily.

The most common *side effects* of calcium channel blockers are headache, light-headedness, dizziness, hypotension, peripheral edema, and constipation. Both verapamil and diltiazem interfere with renal clearance of digoxin and may precipitate digitalis intoxication. All calcium channel blockers are myocardial depressants, and both verapamil and diltiazem may suppress the SA node, decrease heart rate, and prolong the P–R interval. Verapamil should be used with caution in patients with left ventricular dilation and EF of 40% or less, although diltiazem may be used with caution in such patients. There is concern that the use of short-acting calcium channel blockers (i.e., nifedipine, verapamil, diltiazem) may be associated with an increased risk of cardiovascular morbidity and mortality, but an increased risk does not appear to be present in patients using long-acting calcium channel blockers (31).

Pacemaker Therapy

Implantable electrical pulse generators (pacemakers) are the treatment of choice for patients with symptomatic bradyarrhythmias and heart block (32,33). The decision to implant a pacemaker and the type of unit to use must be determined in consultation with a cardiologist. In general, patients in atrial fibrillation who require a pacemaker (see later discussion) require ventricular demand pacemakers. Most patients in sinus rhythm are best served by a multiprogrammable AV sequential unit. The modest increases in cost and complexity of the AV sequential units appear to be more than offset by the improved long-term physiologic response of patients. Pacemaker generators are less than 0.5 cm thick and may function for up to 10 years. Pacemaker leads are easily implantable via a percutaneous transvenous technique and rarely become dislodged, even during vigorous activity. Symptoms are relieved in most patients who are symptomatic because of bradyarrhythmias and conduction block (see later discussion).

Patient Experience. The units are implanted subcutaneously under local anesthesia in the pectoral area, and the pacemaker lead is inserted via the cephalic vein or directly with the use of a special introducer into the axillary or subclavian vein and lodged in the apex of the right ventricle or in the right atrial appendage. The procedure takes about 1.5 hours; the patient experiences some discomfort when the anesthetic is injected and, often, an unpleasant sensation when the tissues are manipulated to create a pocket for the pacemaker unit.

After the procedure, patients, depending on their age and condition, are discharged from the hospital late on the same day, or on the next day. Patients with sedentary jobs may return to work within 1 week after pacemaker insertion, but patients with more active jobs should be kept off work for up to 6 weeks to allow the wound to heal completely. After that, there is little or no discomfort; the unit feels like part of the chest wall, and there are no restrictions on the patient's activity. Microwave ovens do not interfere with pacemaker functions, but cellular phones may do so if they are held directly over the pacemaker (34). Magnetic resonance scanning is absolutely contraindicated in patients with permanent pacemakers.

Patients with implanted pacemakers require systematic, long-term follow-up. The frequency of follow-up depends on the original indication for the pacemaker. Patients who require constant pacing must be seen more often (approximately every 3 months) than patients who require episodic pacing (approximately every 4 to 6 months). At these visits the function of the pacemaker must be assessed with a 12-lead ECG and a computerized pacemaker analyzer, which measures pacemaker data including battery voltage and lead resistance.

The pacemaker and its registration number should be entered into the patient's record, and the patient should keep the registration card for the pacemaker on his or her person in the event of malfunction of the instrument or an emergency intercurrent problem.

Cardioversion

The electrical conversion of atrial tachyarrhythmias is done by the application of a short burst of direct current to the chest wall. The shock is synchronized with the QRS complex of the ECG to avoid applying it during the vulnerable period of the cardiac cycle, when ventricular tachycardia or fibrillation might be induced.

Cardioversion is a more reliable technique for the conversion of tachyarrhythmias than is the administration of antiarrhythmic drugs. It may be required on an emergency basis if a patient has developed severe heart failure, hypotension, or ischemia as a result of an arrhythmia. Otherwise, the procedure should be planned with the cardiologist, who will attempt the conversion.

There are a number of considerations in deciding whether elective cardioversion is appropriate for a patient with atrial fibrillation (35) (see later discussion).

The most cost-effective strategy, in terms of quality-adjusted life years, is to attempt cardioversion before initiation of antiarrhythmic therapy. Typically, patients are anticoagulated for at least 3 weeks before elective cardioversion and for 4 weeks afterward. However, clinical trials have shown that if transesophageal echocardiography (TEE) does not reveal an atrial thrombus, cardioversion may be done without anticoagulation beforehand (36). (The need for anticoagulation for at least 4 weeks after cardioversion, however, is not obviated.) If atrial fibrillation recurs soon after cardioversion, an antiarrhythmic agent can be started and cardioversion can be repeated (37).

Patient Experience. Cardioversion is done by a cardiologist in a hospital, either with an anesthesiologist or with a nurse experienced in administering conscious sedation, and with resuscitation equipment available. The patient is sedated, usually with intravenous midazolam given to effect. Normally the patient cannot recall afterward the details of the procedure. For atrial fibrillation, cardioversion is attempted at 200 watt-seconds; if that is unsuccessful, the energy level is increased and other shocks are administered until there is conversion or until a level of 360 watt-seconds is reached. If an initial attempt using anteroposterior patch placement fails, another attempt at cardioversion can be undertaken using an apex–base paddle position. If this is unsuccessful, cardioversion can be repeated either with a defibrillator capable of delivering a biphasic waveform or by delivering the shock through an intracardiac electrode (referred to as internal cardioversion). Administration of ibutilide (38,39), a relatively new class III antiarrhythmic agent, immediately before cardioversion can also lower the amount of energy required for cardioversion. With the recent availability of biphasic waveforms, this approach is rarely required. Complications, embolism or a new arrhythmia, are unusual. After cardioversion, the patient is observed for several hours while rhythm is monitored and then discharged if the rhythm is stable.

When to Refer a Patient for an Invasive Electrophysiologic Study

Several categories of patients should be referred for electrophysiologic study; most of these patients will already be under the care of a cardiologist. They include patients with a sustained wide complex tachycardia and those who have survived an episode of sudden cardiac death; patients with nonsustained ventricular tachycardia (particularly in the setting of a prior MI) who are thought to be at increased risk of sudden cardiac death; patients with syncope of unknown origin in the setting of structural heart disease; and patients who are considered to be candidates for a curative catheter ablation procedure for treatment of any of a large variety of supraventricular arrhythmias (including WPW syndrome, PSVT (p. 904), atrial flutter, and atrial tachycardia) and also some types of ventricular arrhythmias (i.e., idiopathic ventricular tachycardia). Although empiric antiarrhythmic drug treatment is appropriate for many patients with PSVT and other types of supraventricular arrhythmias, many patients either fail or are intolerant of such therapy, and others prefer an attempt at radiofrequency catheter ablation to taking drugs the rest of their lives (40).

Patient Experience. The patient's experience during electrophysiologic study is similar in some respects to that during cardiac catheterization (see Chapter 62) in that the patient must lie flat on a table in a cardiac catheterization laboratory. Catheters usually are advanced, under fluoroscopy, through the femoral vein rather than through the artery, as is done during coronary angiography. The procedure takes longer than does coronary catheterization; the average diagnostic procedure takes about 1 to 2 hours, whereas a radiofrequency catheter ablation procedure can take up to 4 or 5 hours. In a typical diagnostic procedure, intracardiac electrical activity is recorded and the heart is stimulated (either pharmacologically or electrically through a catheter) in an attempt to determine how easily an arrhythmia may be induced. If a significant arrhythmia is induced and does not resolve spontaneously, antiarrhythmic drugs or electrical cardioversion is used to restore the patient's intrinsic rhythm. The risks of a diagnostic electrophysiologic procedure are slight. The risks associated with catheter ablation vary based on the target arrhythmia. There is a small risk that a permanent pacemaker will be required, because of the induction of complete heart block during an ablation procedure, in no more than 1% of patients (40). The risk of major morbidity (e.g., stroke, MI, significant valve damage) or mortality is approximately 0.1%. Patients are usually treated with aspirin for several weeks after an ablation procedure to reduce the risk of embolization.

SPECIFIC ARRHYTHMIAS

Sinus Tachycardia

Definition and Causes

In adults, the normal sinus rate is 60 to 100 beats/minute. Sinus tachycardia, a sinus rhythm at a rate greater than 100 beats/minute, is usually a physiologic rhythm in that the rate is ordinarily appropriate to the physiologic state of the patient, a state that requires an increased cardiac output to meet increased metabolic demands. The maximal sinus heart rate that can be attained varies with age but usually does not exceed 140 beats/minute unless demands are excessive (e.g., vigorous exercise). The common factors that stimulate an increase in the rate of sinus rhythm, other than exercise, are fever (an increase of approximately 10 beats/minute for each Fahrenheit degree rise in body temperature), emotional stress, intravascular volume depletion, heart failure, hypoxia, and a variety of drugs that affect the autonomic nervous system, including caffeine, aminophylline, amphetamine, alcohol, antidepressants, phenothiazines, and calcium channel blockers of the dihydropyridine class (e.g., nifedipine).

Physical Findings

A regular rapid pulse and heart rate are detected, although there may be a slight variation in rate, called sinus arrhythmia. S_1 is normal, and the jugular pulsations are normal.

Electrocardiogram

A P wave precedes each QRS complex; the P–R interval is normal for the rate (0.16 to 0.17 sec at rates faster than 130/minute), and the P-wave vector is normal (upright P waves in II, III, and aVF).

Treatment

In most cases, persistent sinus tachycardia need not be treated; it is the underlying condition that requires therapy. Digitalis, especially, should not be used to treat a patient with sinus tachycardia unless there is associated heart failure.

In the occasional patient with an unexplained sinus tachycardia for whom a thorough evaluation fails to reveal an underlying cause, and in whom tachycardia is symptomatic, the use of small dosages of a beta-blocker may be justified. Low-dose beta-blockers may also be helpful in treating the anxiety and tachycardia associated with anticipated stressful situations.

Sinus Bradycardia

Definition and Causes

Sinus bradycardia is a heart rate slower than 60 beats/minute (41). Impulse generation in the sinus node is often slow in aerobically well-conditioned people (e.g., long-distance runners, heavy laborers) because of high vagal tone. In fact, trained athletes may have asymptomatic sinus bradycardia with resting heart rates as low as 40 beats/minute. Inappropriately low sinus rates are also commonly caused by increased vagal tone, as is seen in association with pain, vomiting, or vasovagal syncope. A hypersensitive carotid sinus, more common in elderly people, may result in marked bradycardia when the sinus is compressed by a tight collar or by the patient's tensing his or her neck. Parasympathomimetic drugs such as neostigmine, tranquilizers, phenothiazines, digitalis, and sympatholytic drugs such as methyldopa, clonidine, and all beta-blockers also may produce sinus bradycardia. Vagally induced bradycardia may be severe and result in asystole (and loss of consciousness) when the stimulus is marked or prolonged or occurs in a hypoxic patient.

Physical Findings

A regular slow pulse and heart rate are detected. S_1 is normal, and the jugular pulsations are normal.

Electrocardiogram

A P wave precedes each QRS complex; the P–R interval is normal for the rate (up to 0.20 to 0.21 sec), and the P-wave vector is normal (upright P waves in II, III, and aVF).

Treatment

Asymptomatic sinus bradycardia discovered as an incidental finding does not require treatment. If there are no ECG signs of conduction block and structural heart disease is not present, resting heart rates as low as 40 beats/minute may be well tolerated. However, patients who present with symptoms of light-headedness or syncope and are found to have sinus bradycardia may have underlying sinus node disease or may be subject to paroxysms of tachycardia and bradycardia, the so-called sick sinus syndrome (see next section). Patients with sinus bradycardia and symptoms should be evaluated with an ambulatory ECG to determine whether they have this condition. In any case, patients with symptomatic sinus bradycardia, not caused by a drug, are best treated with permanent pacemaker implantation.

Sick Sinus Syndrome

Definition and Causes

The term *sick sinus syndrome* refers to a heterogeneous group of arrhythmias involving defective impulse generation by the sinus node or abnormal impulse conduction in the atria and AV node (42). The syndrome is characterized by periods of inappropriate sinus bradycardia (often severe, with rates between 25 and 40 beats/minute), which may precede or follow supraventricular tachyarrhythmias, and by varying degrees of sinoatrial block, sometimes including sinus arrest. The rubrics *bradycardia–tachycardia syndrome* and *tachycardia–bradycardia syndrome* are sometimes used, depending, respectively, on whether bradycardia precedes or follows a tachyarrhythmia.

The sick sinus syndrome is caused by degenerative fibrotic changes within the sinus node. It is often associated with similar abnormalities in other parts of the cardiac conduction system that result in varying degrees of atrioventricular and intraventricular block. These pathologic changes are much more common in patients older than 60 years of age. Although their precise cause is unknown, they are often associated with hypertensive or ischemic heart disease.

Symptoms and Signs

Many patients are asymptomatic. When symptoms do occur, they are produced either by spontaneous sinus arrest or by the tachyarrhythmia itself (palpitations). If there is coexistent left ventricular dysfunction or coronary artery disease, symptoms of heart failure or ischemia may occur due to reduced cardiac output or increased cardiac demand.

The physical examination is often normal unless the patient is examined during an episode of bradyarrhythmia or tachyarrhythmia, in which case the findings depend on the type of arrhythmia that is present (see later discussion). Sometimes light carotid sinus massage produces symptomatic bradyarrhythmia in a patient with sick sinus syndrome who is in normal sinus rhythm.

Electrocardiogram

The ECG may be normal or may simply reveal sinus bradycardia. Often, there are varying degrees of sinoatrial block, characterized by varying P–P intervals on the ECG. Sometimes sinus arrest occurs, manifested by absent P waves and associated, usually, with a junctional escape rhythm. Some patients have atrial fibrillation with a slow ventricular response, reflecting a concomitant AV conduction abnormality (see earlier discussion). The ECG changes of the various atrial tachyarrhythmias are described later in the discussions of these entities.

If there is a history of unexplained syncope or palpitations and the resting ECG is normal, ambulatory ECG monitoring is indicated (see Diagnosis of Arrhythmias).

Treatment and Course

The treatment of choice for patients with the sick sinus syndrome who are symptomatic from bradyarrhythmias is permanent pacemaker implantation (see Pacemaker Therapy). Otherwise, symptoms are often progressive. Patients with minor symptoms (e.g., light-headedness, dizziness) often find that they feel significantly better after pacemaker therapy.

Tachyarrhythmias associated with the syndrome generally are not prevented by electrical pacing. However, pacing does allow the use of drugs such as digitalis, calcium channel blockers, amiodarone, and beta-blockers that depress the sinus node and increase the likelihood of sinus arrest or asystole. It is reasonable, after a pacemaker is implanted, to administer metoprolol 25 mg twice a day, and to increase the dosage to 50 mg or 100 mg twice a day in an attempt to prevent tachyarrhythmias. If the beta-blocker is not effective, diltiazem or verapamil may be administered in low doses as well, unless the patient has a depressed EF. If tachyarrhythmias continue, consideration should be given, in conjunction with the consulting cardiologist, to the use of another antiarrhythmic drug (see previous discussion).

Patients with sick sinus syndrome have an incidence, unaffected by pacemaker therapy, of arterial embolization of approximately 10% per year, caused by associated paroxysmal atrial arrhythmias. If tachyarrhythmias are not well controlled, these patients should be anticoagulated with warfarin. The sick sinus syndrome is not itself associated with increased mortality. Life expectancy in these patients is a function of the patient's age and comorbid conditions (42). Patients with chronic atrial fibrillation or supraventricular tachycardia as a manifestation of sick sinus syndrome should be treated with warfarin (discussed later) or with aspirin if the patient cannot or will not take warfarin. Warfarin may be started approximately 2 to 3 days after a permanent pacemaker is implanted.

Premature Atrial and Junctional Contractions

Definition and Causes

Premature atrial contractions (PACs) and premature junctional contractions (PJCs) are commonly seen in patients who are otherwise well. They often are induced by the same stimuli that produce sinus tachycardia, especially caffeine or nicotine. However, in patients with congestive heart failure or chronic pulmonary disease, PACs or PJCs may progress to atrial fibrillation or flutter.

Symptoms and Signs

Usually patients are unaware of PACs or PJCs. Occasionally they note the PAC or PJC as a palpitation; the clinician, on listening to the heart or palpating the arterial pulse, is aware of a slight irregularity in the cardiac rhythm.

Electrocardiogram

PACs are reflected in the ECG by a premature, morphologically abnormal P wave followed by a premature, morphologically normal QRS complex. Often these impulses are not conducted (Fig. 64.5), in which case, if the P wave is buried in the preceding T wave, a false diagnosis of sinus arrest may be made. At other times the premature impulse may be aberrantly conducted, the result of relative refractoriness of one of the bundle branches (usually a right bundle branch pattern is seen after the premature atrial beat).

PJCs are reflected in the ECG by a retrograde P wave (negatively deflected in leads II, III, and aVF) that may follow, be hidden in, or precede a morphologically normal but premature QRS complex.

Treatment

Patients with PACs or PJCs who are otherwise well do not require treatment. Rarely, it may be necessary to prescribe a beta-blocker, or another antiarrhythmic agent such as sotalol or amiodarone, to reduce the frequency of PACs in patients who have annoyingly frequent palpitations. In patients who have underlying cardiac or pulmonary disease with associated systolic dysfunction, digitalization may prevent the progression of PACs to atrial fibrillation (43). Quinidine or

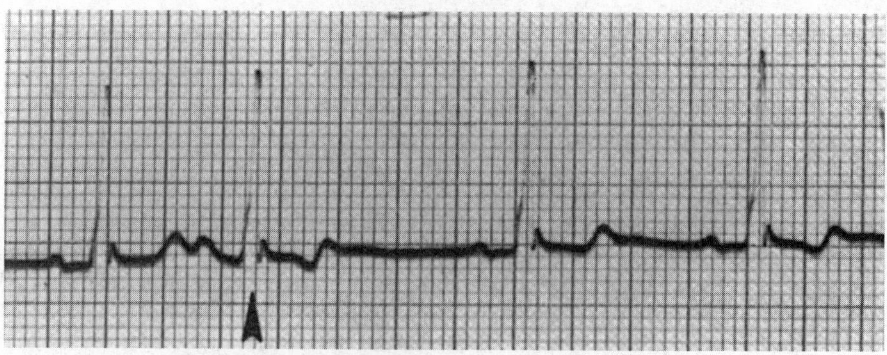

Figure 64.5. A premature atrial contraction *(arrowhead)*. Note the normal configuration of the premature QRS complex.

procainamide is also effective in the control of PACs, but the risk associated with the use of these drugs usually is not warranted (see earlier discussion).

Paroxysmal Supraventricular Tachycardia

Definition and Causes

The term *paroxysmal supraventricular tachycardia* (PSVT) refers to a group of supraventricular arrhythmias that start and terminate abruptly and generally result from reentry (44). The most common cause of PSVT is atrioventricular nodal re-entrant tachycardia (*AVNRT*), which accounts for two thirds of all cases of PSVT (45). AVNRT occurs in the setting of two functionally distinct conduction pathways in the region of the AV node (called the fast and slow pathways). The second most common cause of PSVT is an accessory pathway–mediated tachycardia called *orthodromic AV reciprocating tachycardia.* This type of tachycardia, accounting for approximately one third of all cases of PSVT, results when the electrical impulse travels from the atria to the ventricles via the AV node and returns to the atria via an accessory pathway that connects the atrium and ventricle. The third, and least common cause of PSVT, accounting for fewer than 5% of all cases, is a *reentrant or triggered atrial tachycardia* that is confined to the atrium.

The heart rate during episodes of PSVT may vary from 130 to 240 beats/minute. In general, PSVT involving an accessory pathway tends to be more rapid and PSVT caused by an atrial tachycardia tends to be slower. However, because of a tremendous amount of overlap, the rate of the tachycardia usually is not helpful in establishing a diagnosis.

Nonparoxysmal atrial tachycardia with block (caused by gradually accelerated automaticity of an ectopic atrial focus) as a manifestation of digitalis toxicity is now rarely seen. If nonparoxysmal atrial tachycardia occurs in association with an AV conduction abnormality (commonly 2:1 block) and the patient is taking digitalis, the drug should be withheld and the serum potassium concentration should be measured. If the patient is hypokalemic, potassium repletion is in order; usually this can be accomplished by administration of oral potassium salts (i.e., 20 mEq three times a day; see Chapter 50). Patients with refractory arrhythmias with block caused by digitalis toxicity should be hospitalized for more aggressive treatment.

Symptoms and Signs

PSVT can usually be suspected or diagnosed based on a careful history. The most important features of PSVT are its abrupt onset and termination and its sustained rapid and regular rate. Patients may also complain of dyspnea, diaphoresis, light-headedness, presyncope, or chest pain. Often the patient is able to terminate the arrhythmia abruptly by performing actions that increase vagal stimulation of the heart, such as a Valsalva maneuver, coughing, or placing a cold wet towel over the face (diving reflex). Often, polyuria is experienced for as long as the arrhythmia lasts; this may be due to atrial dilatation and to release of atrial natriuretic peptide (46).

Attacks often occur spontaneously but may be precipitated by physical or emotional stress, caffeine, or nicotine. They may be as short as a few seconds and as long as several weeks. The frequency of the attacks is also variable: Some people have attacks every day, some only a few times during their entire lives.

On examination, a rapid, regular arterial pulse and heart rate are noted, often faster than that measured in patients with sinus tachycardia and usually not associated with the same stimuli. When the atria and ventricles contract simultaneously, cannon waves are seen in the jugular veins.

Electrocardiogram

PSVT is characterized by a rapid, regular heart rate. There is a fixed relationship of the P wave to the QRS complex. If the impulse is generated in the AV node (as in AVNRT), the P wave may be buried in the QRS complex, but the process can be identified by the normal appearance of the QRS complex and the regularity of the rate. When the P wave is visible, it may follow the QRS complex (in some nodal reentry rhythms and most accessory pathway reentry rhythms). It may also precede the QRS complex and may appear morphologically normal (atrial reentry or ectopic rhythm), in which case the diagnosis can be made (by ECG) only if the rate is high enough to make sinus tachycardia unlikely. The P wave also may be hidden in the T wave, but again the regularity of the rate and the usually normal duration of the QRS complex establish the diagnosis (6,45).

If the ECG obtained from a patient with PSVT demonstrates various degrees of AV block (Fig. 64.6), the most likely cause of the arrhythmia is an atrial tachycardia. The presence of an accessory pathway–mediated tachycardia can be completely eliminated, and the possibility of AVNRT is most unlikely.

Treatment and Course

Therapy for PSVT always starts with attempts to increase vagal tone. As mentioned earlier, the patient often has learned to do this. If the arrhythmia persists despite the patient's efforts, carotid sinus massage should be applied. This must be done after auscultation of the carotid arteries to ensure that there are no bruits; if there are, carotid sinus massage is contraindicated. The carotid sinus is at the point of maximal impulse of the carotid artery in the neck. The right sinus should be massaged first for up to 20 seconds; if that has no effect, the left sinus should be massaged. The two sinuses should never be massaged simultaneously. During massage, the patient's ECG should be monitored continuously, and resuscitation equipment should be available.

If carotid sinus massage fails, pharmacologic therapy is indicated. This is best done in an emergency room or a similar facility and always with continuous

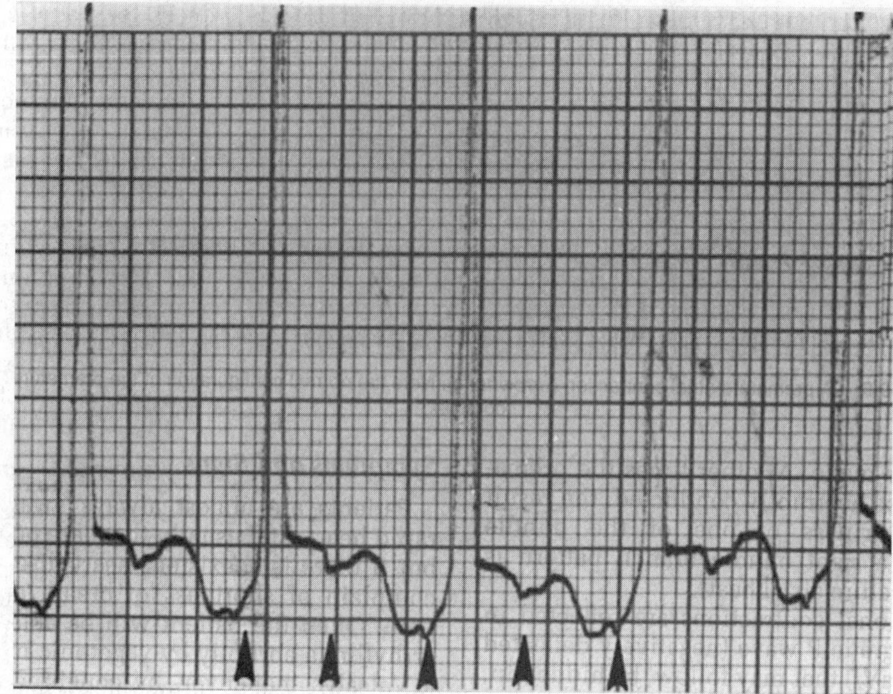

Figure 64.6. Supraventricular tachycardia with 2:1 AV block; the arrowheads point to consecutive P waves.

ECG monitoring. The drug of choice is adenosine (which slows conduction through the AV node), 6 to 18 mg, because the effect of the drug is dissipated in only 10 to 15 seconds after intravenous administration; it usually converts the arrhythmia to normal sinus rhythm within 5 to 10 seconds. It is critical that adenosine be administered as a bolus into a rapidly flowing intravenous line. This is best accomplished by using a stopcock and immediately flushing the line with 10 mL of saline after injection of the adenosine. If PSVT persists after administration of adenosine, electrical cardioversion should be considered. Administration of intravenous adenosine should be performed only in a setting where emergency defibrillation can be performed. Alternatives to adenosine include verapamil (80 to 120 mg orally or 5 to 10 mg intravenously), diltiazem (60 to 120 mg orally) (discussed earlier), or propranolol (40 to 80 mg orally or 1 to 4 mg intravenously). As noted previously, calcium channel blockers may increase conduction in the accessory pathway in patients with WPW syndrome. Calcium channel blockers therefore should not be used to treat PSVT in patients who are known to have an accessory pathway, in order to avoid dangerous acceleration of the ventricular rate if PSVT degenerates to atrial fibrillation.

PSVT can be prevented or the number of episodes reduced with the use of a large variety of antiarrhythmic agents. If an initial episode of PSVT terminates spontaneously and is associated with mild symptoms, it would be reasonable to instruct the patient about techniques to terminate the arrhythmia and to delay initiation of antiarrhythmic therapy. On the other hand, if the patient has had multiple episodes of tachycardia, has required emergency room evaluation for termination of tachycardia, or has symptoms of hemodynamic compromise, chronic antiarrhythmic therapy or radiofrequency catheter ablation is indicated.

Digoxin may be used to treat PSVT and is perhaps the most convenient, best tolerated, least expensive, but least effective medication for this purpose. Beta-blockers and calcium channel blockers are somewhat more effective, are more expensive, and, when once-a-day dosing is used, are equally convenient. On the other end of the spectrum are class 1C antiarrhythmic agents such as propafenone and flecainide, which are effective but even more expensive and less convenient. Although amiodarone can be used to treat patients with PSVT, this drug is rarely prescribed because of the benign nature of this arrhythmia, the potential for serious side effects of the drug (see earlier discussion), and the alternative of radiofrequency catheter ablation.

Over the past 10 years, radiofrequency catheter ablation (described earlier) has emerged from an experimental technique to become first- or second-line therapy for the treatment of patients with PSVT (47). Success rates exceed 95%, complications are rare (less than 1%), and the procedure is well tolerated. For this reason, patients with PSVT should be informed about the existence of a curative catheter-based procedure that can be considered as an alternative to lifelong antiarrhythmic therapy or that can be used if antiarrhythmic therapy fails. Electrophysiologic testing and radiofrequency catheter ablation should be recommended as first-line therapy if PSVT occurs in the setting of WPW syndrome (see later discussion). Because of the potentially life-threatening nature of WPW syndrome, these patients should be referred for

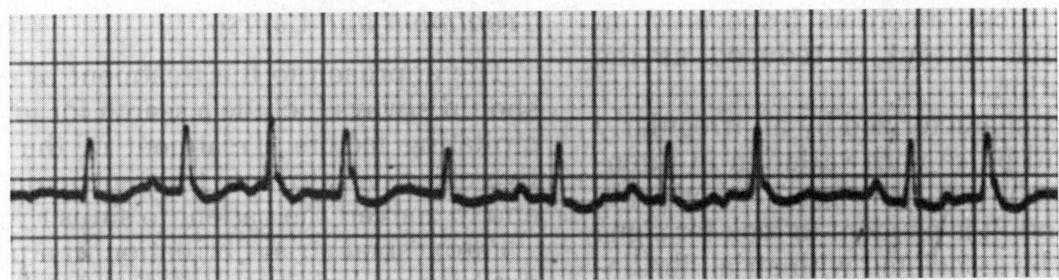

Figure 64.7. Multifocal atrial tachycardia. Note the variation in the morphology of the P waves and the duration of the P–R intervals.

electrophysiologic testing and radiofrequency catheter ablation (40). Similarly, if a patient with PSVT has symptoms of severe hemodynamic compromise (i.e., syncope), electrophysiologic testing and radiofrequency catheter ablation should be considered early in management.

Although PSVT is generally a benign arrhythmia, it rarely disappears without treatment. Once a patient has had one episode of PSVT, other episodes will probably occur. In most patients the frequency of episodes of PSVT increases over time. In contrast to this generally benign course, the prognosis of patients with PSVT who have WPW syndrome, severe structural heart disease, or symptoms of hemodynamic compromise is not as favorable. For this reason, more aggressive approaches to treatment are used early in these settings.

Multifocal Atrial Tachycardia

Multifocal atrial tachycardia is a chaotic supraventricular arrhythmia characterized on ECG by varying morphology of the P waves, varying P–R intervals, and a rapid heart rate, usually 100 to 200 beats/minute; QRS morphology is normal, and every QRS complex is preceded by a P wave (Fig. 64.7) (48). The arrhythmia usually is seen in patients with serious underlying disease, especially decompensated chronic obstructive pulmonary disease, and is better treated by, for example, improving ventilatory function than by attempting directly to suppress the rhythm. Digitalis does not alter this arrhythmia (which is usually well tolerated) and therefore should not be administered. Either verapamil or diltiazem may be used to control the heart rate in patients with multifocal atrial tachycardia. Oral dosages of 40 to 80 mg three to four times a day of verapamil or 30 to 60 mg three to four times a day of diltiazem should be tried. If they are effective, a sustained-release preparation of verapamil or diltiazem at the same total daily dosage may be used.

Atrial Fibrillation

Definition and Causes

Atrial fibrillation is defined electrophysiologically as the generation of multiple reentry wave fronts by the atria. It is usually triggered by a premature atrial contraction (PAC) (see earlier discussion) that triggers the development of these wave fronts and results in an atrial rate in excess of 300 beats/minute. These impulses enter the AV node randomly. Because of the unique conduction properties of the AV node, including slow conduction and decremental conduction, only a small proportion of the impulses are conducted to the ventricle. This results in a much slower (100 to 180 beats/minute) and irregularly irregular ventricular rate.

The prevalence of atrial fibrillation increases with age and with the development of structural heart disease (49). When atrial fibrillation occurs in the absence of any evidence of structural heart disease in patients younger than 50 years of age, it is called *lone atrial fibrillation*. In some patients, factors that trigger episodes of atrial fibrillation can be identified (e.g., physical or emotional stress, alcohol, nicotine, caffeine). The major noncardiac illness associated with atrial fibrillation is hyperthyroidism; in the presence of a fast ventricular response refractory to drugs given to slow the ventricular rate atrial fibrillation may be the first clue to the diagnosis (50).

Hypertensive and rheumatic heart disease (especially if it involves the mitral valve) also predisposes to the development of atrial fibrillation, but almost every kind of myocardial disorder has been associated with it. In addition, the tachyarrhythmic component of the sick sinus syndrome (see earlier discussion) may be atrial fibrillation.

Symptoms and Signs

Atrial fibrillation can be asymptomatic. The most common symptoms of atrial fibrillation are palpitations and fatigue. If the ventricular response is fast, patients often complain of feeling disoriented, lightheaded, weak, or faint as well, especially if they are elderly. Because atrial contraction normally provides approximately 20% of the total cardiac output, patients with incipient heart failure, ischemic heart disease, or valvular heart disease may develop symptoms and signs of those disorders (especially on exertion) when cardiac output is reduced as the result of atrial fibrillation.

Atrial fibrillation is characterized by an irregularly irregular heartbeat and pulse, with variation in intensity of the sounds (including murmurs) on both auscultation and palpation. It is prudent to look for signs of diseases known to be associated with atrial fibrillation (coronary heart disease, heart failure, hypertension, mitral stenosis or regurgitation, and hyperthyroidism),

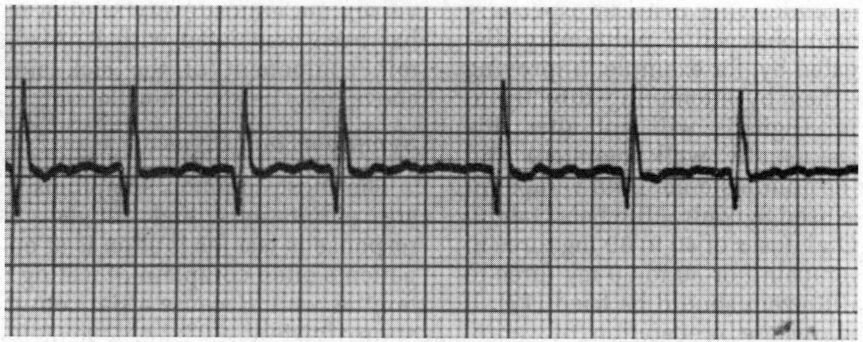

Figure 64.8. Atrial fibrillation. The ventricular rate is 90 to 100 beats/minute, indicative (because digitalis had not been administered) of an associated disorder of atrioventricular conduction.

especially because those signs may be subtle or may be altered by the arrhythmia.

Electrocardiogram

The ECG shows rapid irregular fibrillatory atrial activity at rates of 300 to 500/minute; no P waves are present. The ventricular rhythm is irregularly irregular, at rates that at onset are usually 150 to 200/minute, unless there is coexistent disease in the AV node or the patient is taking a medication that slows AV conduction, in which case slower rates are likely (Fig. 64.8).

The QRS complex is usually morphologically normal. Occasionally there is aberrant conduction of an impulse in the ventricles, after a beat that has been preceded by a long pause. The aberrant beat usually has a right bundle branch block (RBBB) configuration. This so-called Ashman phenomenon is caused by prolonged refractoriness of (usually) the right bundle branch after the long pause. These aberrant beats must be distinguished from ventricular premature beats. Apart from their typical relationship to a preceding long R–R interval, aberrant beats are often triphasic (RSR′) in lead V_1, and their initial vector is the same as that of the normally conducted beats; neither of these features is characteristic of ventricular premature beats.

Other Studies

In addition to an ECG and chest x-ray, all patients presenting for the first time with atrial fibrillation should have thyroid function studies and a two-dimensional echocardiogram. Unusual causes of atrial fibrillation, such as atrial myxoma or chronic pericardial effusion, may require echocardiography for diagnosis.

Treatment and Course

The approach to the treatment of atrial fibrillation should always include a search for underlying or precipitating factors. Treatment of the arrhythmia has two objectives: to slow the ventricular rate if it is fast and to convert the rhythm to sinus rhythm if possible.

Paroxysmal atrial fibrillation in a patient who does not have underlying heart disease often reverts to normal sinus rhythm once precipitating factors (e.g., fever, stress, alcohol, nicotine) are controlled or removed. Specific treatment is indicated in the following circumstances: a rapid ventricular response associated with symptoms (e.g., extreme fatigue, syncope, angina, shortness of breath); the presence of known underlying structural severe heart disease (e.g., aortic stenosis, severe mitral stenosis, ischemic heart disease, chronic congestive failure), because such patients are unlikely to revert to normal sinus rhythm spontaneously; and persistent atrial fibrillation, especially if the resting ventricular rate is greater than 110 beats/minute or if the rate after moderate exercise (e.g., climbing a flight of stairs) is greater than 150 beats/minute.

Symptomatic patients and patients with underlying structural heart disease usually require admission to the hospital immediately after onset of the arrhythmia for cardioversion (see previous discussion) or for pharmacotherapy. Elective cardioversion of atrial fibrillation should be considered if the arrhythmia has been present for less than 6 months and significant atrial enlargement (i.e., greater than approximately 5 cm) is not present. Successful cardioversion and maintenance of sinus rhythm are unlikely if atrial fibrillation has been present for longer than 6 months or if marked atrial enlargement is noted on echocardiography. Although a comparison of rate control and cardioversion strategies failed to show that those randomly assigned to cardioversion achieved greater symptomatic improvement or improved quality of life (35), cardioversion is still recommended to many patients in whom maintenance of sinus rhythm is believed to be likely, to patients in whom rate control in atrial fibrillation may be difficult to achieve, or in an effort to avoid chronic anticoagulation. If electrical cardioversion is recommended, the patient should be anticoagulated for at least 3 weeks and then considered for elective cardioversion unless a TEE-guided approach is employed (see earlier discussion). In general, cardioversion restores normal sinus rhythm in most patients, but the relapse rate is high—50% in 1 year and 90% in 3 years—unless an underlying disorder can be identified and corrected or the atrial fibrillation has been of short duration.

Following a second episode of sustained atrial fibrillation, antiarrhythmic therapy is often used, after a repeat successful cardioversion, in an attempt to maintain sinus rhythm. Because no study has demonstrated that treatment of patients who have atrial fibrillation with antiarrhythmic therapy prolongs survival or reduces the incidence of strokes, the main indication for antiarrhythmic therapy should be the reduction of symptoms.

The selection of an appropriate antiarrhythmic agent for maintaining normal sinus rhythm depends to a large degree on whether structural heart disease is present. For patients with no structural heart disease, almost any antiarrhythmic agent is safe. Class IC antiarrhythmic agents such as flecainide or propafenone or the class III antiarrhythmic agent sotalol are often used as first-line antiarrhythmic therapy in this setting. If these are ineffective, low-dose amiodarone can be considered. In contrast, the risk of proarrhythmia is high among patients with impaired ventricular function. Perhaps the most effective and safest antiarrhythmic agent in this setting is low-dose amiodarone (100 to 200 mg/day). It should be recognized that atrial fibrillation is a difficult arrhythmia to treat and that even with the most effective antiarrhythmic agents, sinus rhythm can be maintained during long-term follow-up in fewer than 50% of patients.

If antiarrhythmic therapy fails or is poorly tolerated, the goal of treatment should be to achieve adequate rate control and effective long-term anticoagulation (51). When rate control is attempted, the goal should be to achieve a resting ventricular rate between 70 and 100 beats/minute and a rate after modest exercise of less than 150 beats/minute. Digoxin slows the ventricular response in acute atrial fibrillation, but it does not enhance conversion to sinus rhythm and has limited use in controlling heart rate in chronic atrial fibrillation (52). When it is used in an acute situation, 0.75 to 1.0 mg digoxin should be given by mouth, followed by 0.125 to 0.25 mg/day.

In contrast to digoxin, calcium channel blockers such as verapamil (120 to 240 mg/day, sustained release), diltiazem (120 to 240 mg/day, sustained release), or small dosages of a beta-blocker (e.g., atenolol 25 to 50 mg/day, metoprolol 25 mg twice a day, propranolol 10 to 20 mg four times a day) effectively control heart rate during exercise and are preferred to digoxin (see General Principles in Management of Arrhythmias). Once effectiveness is demonstrated, those drugs may be taken once daily in a sustained-release form at the same total daily dosage.

In patients with chronic atrial fibrillation and a rapid ventricular rate in whom pharmacologic approaches to heart rate control are ineffective or result in intolerable side effects, electrophysiologic modification or ablation of the AV node and permanent pacemaker implantation should be performed (53).

Radiofrequency catheter ablation is emerging as an alternative treatment strategy for selected patients with *paroxysmal* atrial fibrillation that is refractory to pharmacologic therapy (53). Evidence suggests that paroxysmal atrial fibrillation is commonly triggered by rapid bursts of tachycardia arising from muscle sleeves that extend from the left atrium into the pulmonary veins. Radiofrequency catheter ablation, targeting these pulmonary vein sleeves, may cure atrial fibrillation in up to 70% of such patients (54,55). The role of radiofrequency catheter ablation in the management of patients with persistent or chronic atrial fibrillation (other than ablation of the AV junction) has not been established.

A slow ventricular response to atrial fibrillation in untreated patients suggests an associated disorder of AV conduction. Such patients do not require specific therapy for the arrhythmia (other than anticoagulation) unless they are hemodynamically compromised (i.e., in refractory heart failure) and their heart rate is slower than 60 to 70 beats/minute, in which case implantation of a pacemaker may be indicated.

Anticoagulation. Patients with chronic atrial fibrillation are at increased risk of arterial embolization. For example, the Framingham study reported that, over a 24-year period, patients with chronic atrial fibrillation with and without rheumatic heart disease had, respectively, a 17-fold and a 5-fold increase in the incidence of stroke (56). Overall, the incidence of arterial embolization in untreated patients with chronic atrial fibrillation is approximately 10% a year (51). In general, patients should be anticoagulated with warfarin for at least 3 weeks before, and at least 4 weeks after, elective cardioversion (see earlier discussion). An alternative approach is to refer the patient for TEE and, if no intracardiac clots are demonstrated, to perform cardioversion without preliminary anticoagulation but followed by at least 4 weeks of warfarin therapy (36). Prospective randomized trials support the use of anticoagulants in patients with chronic atrial fibrillation if there are no contraindications (57). Anticoagulation with warfarin to obtain an international normalized ratio (INR) of 2.0 to 3.0 is recommended for all patients with atrial fibrillation who are older than 65 years of age or who have other risk factors for stroke such as hypertension, diabetes, or a prior transient ischemic episode or stroke. In patients who cannot or will not take warfarin, some studies support the use of aspirin, 325 mg/day, particularly in young patients with no risks for embolism (58,59).

Apart from the morbidity and mortality associated with atrial embolization, the prognosis of patients with atrial fibrillation depends on the nature and extent of underlying heart disease.

Atrial Flutter

Definition and Causes

Atrial flutter is a reentrant arrhythmia that is confined to the right atrium and results in an atrial rate of about 300 beats/minute. Usually there is a 2:1 AV conduction block so that the ventricular response is about 150 beats/minute, and in contrast to atrial fibrillation, both atrial and ventricular responses are regular. Atrial flutter is almost always seen in patients who have underlying disease—ischemic heart disease, rheumatic heart disease, congestive cardiomyopathy, atrial septal defect, mitral valve disease, chronic obstructive pulmonary disease, or thyrotoxicosis—the same diseases often associated with atrial fibrillation. In contrast to atrial fibrillation, however, atrial flutter is rarely seen in patients who are otherwise healthy.

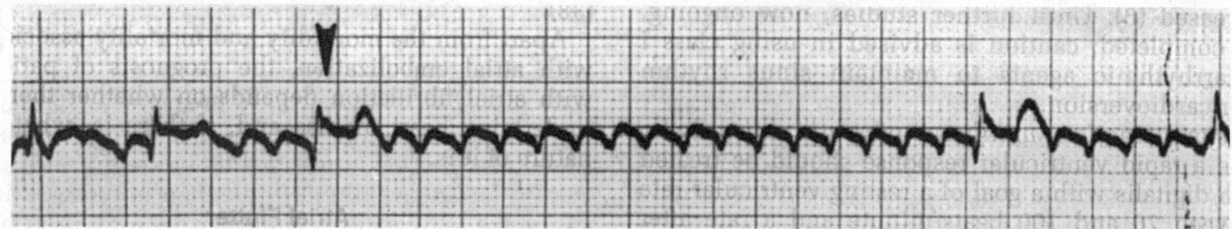

Figure 64.9. Atrial flutter. The flutter waves are clearly revealed after carotid sinus massage *(arrowhead)*.

Symptoms and Signs

Patients are usually aware of a rapid heart rate; whether other symptoms develop depends on the severity and nature of the underlying heart disease.

A regular, rapid heart rate and atrial pulse are detected. Sometimes the flutter waves are visible in the jugular pulse. An S_4 is occasionally audible (in contrast to atrial fibrillation).

Electrocardiogram

In atrial flutter, the ECG commonly shows rapid, regular sawtooth flutter waves at about 300 beats/minute (Fig. 64.9); P waves are absent. The ventricular response is regular, usually at about 150 beats/minute, and the QRS complex is ordinarily morphologically normal. If the AV node is diseased or the patient is taking a medication that slows AV conduction, higher degrees of AV block may be seen, usually a multiple of 2 (e.g., 4:1, 8:1). Aberrant conduction (see Atrial Fibrillation) is unusual.

If the diagnosis is unclear, carotid sinus massage may help distinguish atrial flutter from other paroxymal supraventricular tachyarrhythmias. It usually causes an abrupt temporary slowing of the rate; flutter waves, which may have been difficult to detect at a higher rate, are visible in the ECG, most commonly in leads II, III, aVF, and V_1 (Fig. 64.9). Diagnostic workup is the same as for atrial fibrillation.

Treatment and Course

Atrial flutter is often a chronic and very refractory arrhythmia that is difficult to treat with medical therapy. The initial goal of therapy should be to slow the ventricular response, but, in contrast to the situation with atrial fibrillation, it is often difficult to lower the ventricular rate with drugs.

If there is no contraindication, electrical cardioversion (see previous discussion) is the treatment of choice if atrial flutter persists, even if there is a high degree of AV block. Most patients can be converted to normal sinus rhythm, usually after application of a much lower energy shock than is necessary to convert atrial fibrillation. If atrial flutter recurs after cardioversion, antiarrhythmic therapy or radiofrequency catheter ablation should be considered.

Considerations regarding pharmacologic therapy for atrial flutter are the same as for atrial fibrillation (see previous discussion). Perhaps the only difference is that atrial flutter is even less likely to respond to antiarrhythmic therapy. Patients who have recurrent symptomatic atrial flutter despite pharmacologic treatment should be considered for an electrophysiologic study with possible radiofrequency catheter ablation of the reentry circuit. Radiofrequency catheter ablation of atrial flutter can be accomplished successfully in more than 95% of patients and with a very low incidence of complications (60,61). Radiofrequency catheter ablation has been demonstrated to be more effective than antiarrhythmic therapy for treatment of atrial flutter (61).

Ventricular Premature Beats

Definition and Causes

Ventricular premature beats (VPBs) or premature ventricular contractions (PVCs) are impulses generated in the ventricles, usually as the result of reentry of an impulse conducted down from the atria through the AV node, but sometimes as the result of the firing of an ectopic (parasystolic) focus.

Occasional VPBs occur in many healthy people sporadically during their lives, more often in older people. However, often VPBs are associated with underlying organic heart disease (e.g., hypertensive heart disease, ischemic heart disease, cardiomyopathy, mitral valve prolapse). The frequency of VPBs may be increased in people both with and without heart disease by caffeine, alcohol, sympathomimetic drugs, tricyclic antidepressants, phenothiazines, hypokalemia, hypomagnesemia, hypoxia, or emotional stress. VPBs are a common manifestation of digitalis intoxication. Exercise usually abolishes VPBs in people without structural heart disease; conversely, an increase in the number of VPBs after exertion is highly suggestive of structural heart disease.

Symptoms and Signs

Patients may be unaware that they have had a VPB, but often they experience a palpitation, sensing either the premature beat itself or the more forceful normal beat that follows it after a compensatory pause.

Electrocardiogram

The ECG shows a premature ventricular response with a morphologically abnormal, often bizarre, wide QRS complex (62). No P wave precedes a VPB, but by retrograde conduction a P wave sometimes follows it. The ST segment and the T wave have an opposite vector

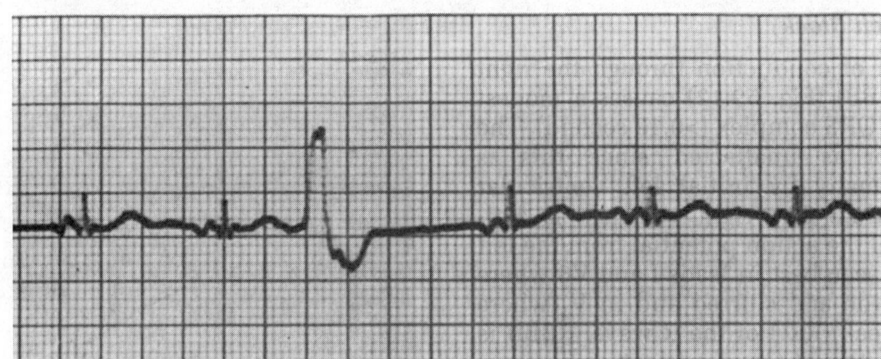

Figure 64.10. Premature ventricular beat. Note that the R–R interval between the two normal beats separated by the PVB is the same as that between two normal beats separated by another normal beat.

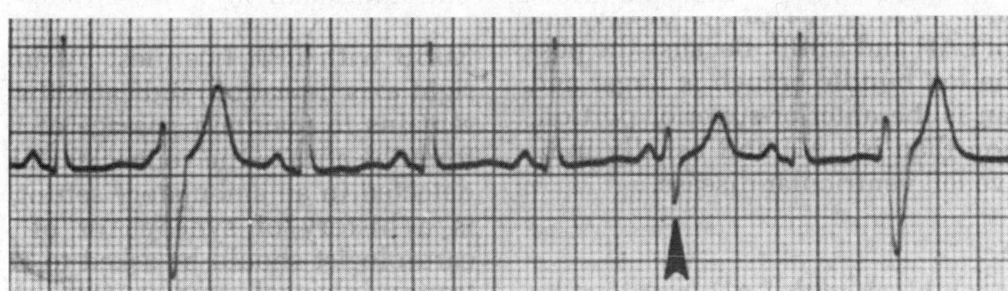

Figure 64.11. Premature ventricular beats caused by the firing of an ectopic focus. The arrowhead points to a fusion beat.

from the QRS complex. Typically, a VPB is followed by a compensatory pause; that is, the R–R interval between two normal beats separated by a VPB is the same as that between two normal beats separated by another normal beat if the patient is in normal sinus rhythm (Fig. 64.10). This occurs because retrograde conduction of the premature beat to the AV node blocks the succeeding sinus beat.

When VPBs are caused by reentry, they have a fixed temporal (coupled) relationship to the preceding normal beats. When they are caused by the firing of an ectopic (parasystolic) focus, they have no fixed relationship to the preceding normal beats but do have a regular pattern (i.e., the ectopic intervals are constant or are multiples of a constant). Ectopic beats may occasionally fuse with normal beats, producing a complex that is intermediate between the two (Fig. 64.11).

Treatment and Course

VPBs in patients with otherwise normal hearts are not harmful. However, there is an increased incidence of sudden death and MI in patients with VPBs who have underlying ischemic heart disease (11). It has not been demonstrated that suppression of VPBs in these latter patients alters their course (13). Because all antiarrhythmic agents have potentially serious side effects (Table 64.2), the practitioner must consider for each patient the relative risks of treating versus not treating VPBs. The following generalizations may be useful:

- Apparently healthy young people with asymptomatic ventricular premature beats probably do not need treatment (63).
- Apparently healthy young people with VPBs causing symptomatic palpitations also do not need pharmacologic treatment. If symptoms interfere with normal lifestyle despite reassurance, a trial of a low-dose beta-blocker, such as metoprolol extended release 25 to 50 mg/day, may abolish VPBs and relieve symptoms. Beta-blockers should be discontinued after several weeks; often VPBs do not recur and no further treatment is necessary.
- Patients with significant structural heart disease (evidenced by an EF of less than 40%) and symptomatic ventricular arrhythmias, especially symptomatic multifocal premature ventricular beats with a frequency of greater than ten per hour or runs of ventricular tachycardia, have an increased risk of sudden death. The treatment of these patients remains highly controversial, and they should be referred to a cardiologist for consideration of electrophysiologic testing or empiric treatment with a class III antiarrhythmic agent. The Multicenter Automatic Defibrillator Implantation Trial (MADIT) demonstrated that placement of an implantable defibrillator improves survival among patients with a prior MI and an EF of less than 35% who have inducible sustained ventricular tachycardia during electrophysiologic testing that is not suppressed with intravenous procainamide (64,65). Sustained ventricular tachycardia is usually defined as ventricular tachycardia that lasts longer than 30 seconds or requires termination because of hemodynamic compromise, whereas nonsustained ventricular tachycardia terminates spontaneously within 30 seconds. The Multicenter Unsustained Tachycardia Trial (MUSST) confirmed these findings and demonstrated that placement of an implantable defibrillator improves survival among patients with a prior MI and an EF of less than 40% who have inducible sustained ventricular tachycardia during electrophysiologic testing (66). Based on the results of this study, it is now recommended that patients with nonsustained

ventricular tachycardia, in the setting of an *ischemic cardiomyopathy,* undergo electrophysiologic testing and that an implantable defibrillator be implanted in those patients with inducible ventricular tachycardia. The optimal approach to management of nonsustained ventricular tachycardia in the setting of a *nonischemic cardiomyopathy* is unknown and is currently under investigation.

- When ventricular arrhythmias occur in the setting of congestive heart failure, an attempt should be made to achieve a maximal state of cardiac compensation before antiarrhythmic therapy is instituted. Hemodynamic compensation may decrease or eliminate VPBs so that specific antiarrhythmic therapy is not needed. Disopyramide and flecainide are myocardial depressants and are specifically contraindicated in patients whose hearts are enlarged and hypocontractile. Furthermore, patients in severe chronic heart failure, many of whom are taking diuretics, are more likely to experience problems such as hypokalemia, hypomagnesemia, alkalosis, hypoxemia, and digitalis toxicity, thus increasing the risk of serious side effects from antiarrhythmic agents (67). Such patients are best treated in consultation with a cardiologist.
- Patients with structural heart disease who have a sustained ventricular arrhythmia (sustained monomorphic ventricular tachycardia or ventricular fibrillation) are best managed based on the results of electrophysiologic testing. Implantable defibrillators are the treatment of choice in this patient population (68). This approach requires hospitalization and consultation with a cardiologist. Radiofrequency catheter ablation in this patient population is generally used as adjunctive therapy in patients who have undergone placement of an implantable defibrillator and are experiencing frequent shocks due to recurrent slow sustained monomorphic ventricular tachycardia (69).
- Sustained ventricular tachycardia that occurs in the absence of structural heart disease (referred to as idiopathic ventricular tachycardia) is generally associated with a benign prognosis. Treatment is indicated for relief of symptoms. This type of ventricular tachycardia usually responds to treatment with most types of antiarrhythmic agents including beta-blockers, calcium channel blockers, and class 1C antiarrhythmic agents. Radiofrequency catheter ablation, which has success rates greater than 90% and a low incidence of complications, is another commonly employed treatment option in this patient population (70).
- Primary care providers occasionally assume the care of patients who are taking antiarrhythmic agents because of a history of symptomatic ventricular arrhythmias caused by structural heart disease. Consultation with a cardiologist is advisable before stopping the therapy.
- The possibility that a patient may experience a proarrhythmic effect from an antiarrhythmic agent must always be kept in mind (see earlier discussion).

Preexcitation Syndrome

Definition and Causes

The atria and ventricles are electrically isolated from each other by the AV groove, and the electrical signal from the atrium is conducted to the ventricle via the AV node and conducting system. If the AV groove is short-circuited by muscle fibers, if muscle fibers from the atria enter the His bundle below the AV node, or if muscle fibers from the His bundle bypass the bundle branches, a variable portion of the right or left ventricle is depolarized early. These short-circuiting fibers are known as accessory atrioventricular, nodoventricular, and fasciculoventricular pathways—the atriofascicular bypass tract and the intranodal bypass tract, depending on their location (Fig. 64.12).

The classic example of preexcitation is the *WPW syndrome.* This syndrome is characterized electrocardiographically by a short P–R interval followed by a wide QRS complex, which is a fusion beat between the ventricular myocardium that is preexcited and that which is excited via normal conduction pathways (Fig. 64.13). The portion of the complex caused by preexcitation is called the delta wave because of its resemblance to the Greek capital letter Δ. If the accessory bundle connects the atria with the left ventricle, the ECG pattern resembles right bundle branch block (type A WPW). On the other hand, if the connection is with the right ventricle, the pattern resembles left bundle branch block (type B WPW); the negative delta wave in lead II in this situation may be taken for a Q wave, and the mistaken diagnosis of remote MI may be made.

If the atrial fibers insert into the bundle of His and short-circuit the AV node, the P–R interval is short but no delta wave is seen, because below the AV node conduction occurs along the usual pathways. This syndrome is known as the *Lown–Ganong–Levine (LGL) syndrome.* A number of other variants of preexcitation syndrome have been described but are much rarer than these two more common disorders (71).

The ECG manifestations of preexcitation may vary from time to time within a given patient because, if conduction occurs through the normal anatomic pathways rather than through accessory fibers, no preexcitation is seen on the ECG. If preexcitation is facilitated because of disease in the AV node or because of drugs that suppress conduction through the AV node (e.g., digitalis, calcium channel blockers, beta-blockers), abnormalities on the ECG are seen.

Supraventricular arrhythmias are found in 13% to 60% of patients with preexcitation. PSVT is most commonly observed, but atrial fibrillation and flutter also occur (72). Accessory pathways can conduct anterograde (from the atrium to the ventricle), retrograde (from the ventricle to the atrium), or both. The morphology of the QRS complex during the tachyarrhythmia depends on the direction in which the reentrant tachycardia occurs. If reentry occurs with anterograde conduction through the AV conducting system and retrograde conduction through an accessory pathway, then the ventricles are depolarized through the normal

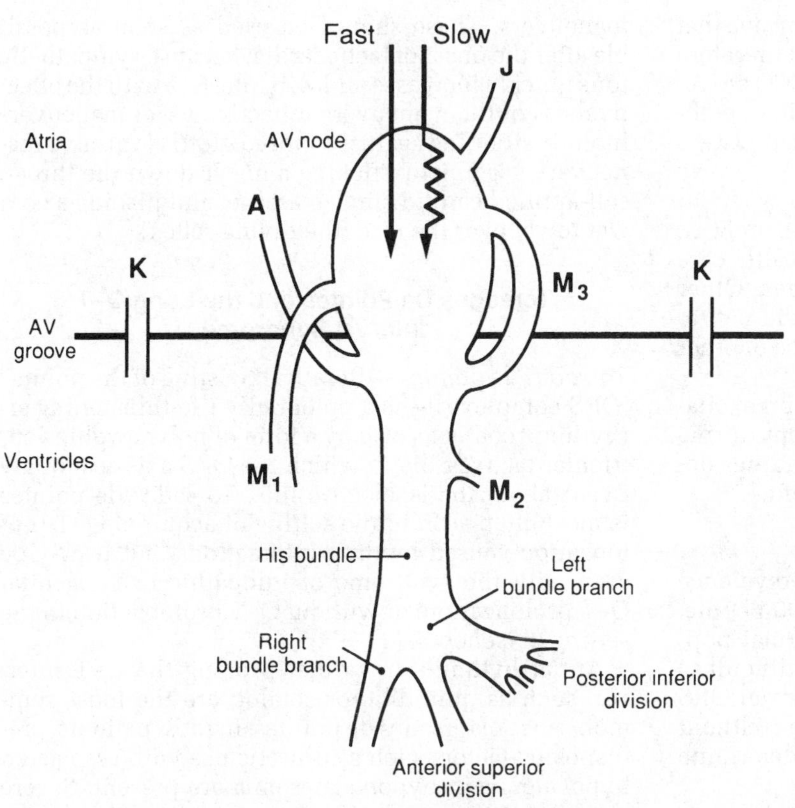

Figure 64.12. Schematic diagram of possible accessory conduction pathways (old eponymic nomenclature in parentheses.) A, Atriofascicular (atrio-Hisian) bundles; K, accessory atrioventricular (Kent) bundles; J, intranodal bypass (James) tracts; M (Mahaim) fibers—M1, accessory nodoventricular; M2, accessory fasciculoventricular; M3, nodofascicular fibers. Dual atrioventricular node pathways are represented by the fast and slow symbols. (Adapted from Wellens HJJ, Brugada P, Penn OC. The management of preexcitation syndromes. JAMA 1987;257:2325.)

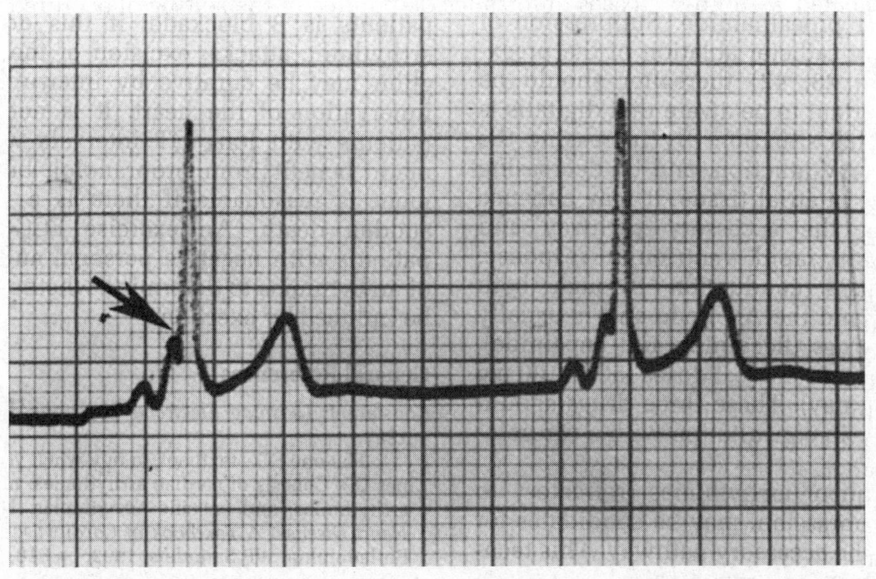

Figure 64.13. The Wolff–Parkinson–White syndrome. Note delta wave.

AV conduction system and the QRS duration during the tachyarrhythmia may be normal (i.e. no delta wave is seen during tachycardia). This type of tachycardia, known as *orthodromic atrioventricular reentrant tachycardia (AVNRT),* is by far the most common supraventricular tachycardia in patients with the WPW syndrome. In a small percentage of patients with the WPW syndrome and AVNRT, the circuit is established in the opposite direction, with depolarization of the ventricle over the accessory pathway. In this circumstance, known as *antidromic AVNRT,* the QRS complex is wide and the arrhythmia can easily be confused with ventricular tachycardia.

It should be noted that the term *preexcitation* refers to evidence of an anterograde-conducting accessory pathway on the ECG. *WPW syndrome* refers to a specific syndrome of supraventricular tachycardia in the setting of preexcitation on the ECG. A patient who has evidence of preexcitation on the ECG but no supraventricular tachycardia is properly described as having *asymptomatic preexcitation.* Accessory pathways that conduct only in the retrograde direction and therefore are not associated with a delta wave on the ECG are referred to as *concealed accessory pathways;* these pathways cannot be identified by a routine 12-lead ECG.

Symptoms and Signs

Preexcitation may be an incidental finding on an ECG, or it may come to the attention of the health care provider because of symptoms of palpitations. Other symptoms of tachyarrhythmia depend on the nature of the arrhythmia and the presence or absence of other structural heart disease.

There are no physical findings caused by preexcitation other than occasionally a loud S_1, except during periods of tachyarrhythmia, and then the findings depend on the type of arrhythmia that is present.

Prevalence

Preexcitation syndromes are not rare. The prevalence of preexcitation is between 1 and 3 per 1,000 people, or approximately 0.15% to 0.3% of the normal population (72). Accurate prevalence rates are difficult to obtain, because short P–R intervals with normal QRS durations are commonly seen in people without arrhythmias, so no studies are done to determine whether a bypass tract exists.

Preexcitation syndromes occasionally may be associated with certain forms of congenital heart disease. Preexcitation of the WPW type is associated with Ebstein anomaly of the tricuspid valve, corrected transposition of the great vessels, and hypertrophic cardiomyopathies (71).

Treatment and Course

The presence of preexcitation in an asymptomatic patient is associated with an annual risk of sudden cardiac death of approximately 0.1%. Because this is not markedly greater than the risk of sudden cardiac death in the general population and because treatment is associated with some risk, current guidelines recommend that asymptomatic patients who have evidence of preexcitation on their ECG not be treated (73). Exceptions to this rule are competitive athletes and people in high-risk occupations (e.g., bus drivers, pilots). In these settings it is reasonable to consider performing an electrophysiologic study to determine whether the accessory pathway has the capacity to conduct rapidly (which increases the risk of sudden cardiac death fivefold) and whether a sustained arrhythmia can be induced. In these settings, radiofrequency catheter ablation is often performed. All patients with evidence of preexcitation on their ECG should be instructed to contact their health care provider if symptoms subsequently develop. Because of the increased risk of sudden cardiac death among symptomatic patients with preexcitation (WPW syndrome), electrophysiologic testing with radiofrequency catheter ablation is now recommended as first-line therapy.

Patients with occasional symptoms can often be taught to break the arrhythmia with the use of vagal maneuvers. These should be tried as soon as possible after the onset of tachycardia, because sympathetic tone quickly increases and will interfere with the effectiveness of the maneuvers. Effective vagal maneuvers include straining against a closed glottis (Valsalva maneuver), gagging by sticking a finger down the throat, self-applied carotid sinus massage, and placing a cold wet towel over the face (the diving reflex).

Torsades De Pointes and the Long Q–T Interval Syndrome

Torsades de pointes—literally, "twisting of the points" (QRS complexes)—is a potentially life-threatening arrhythmia characterized by a form of polymorphic ventricular tachycardia in which the QRS axis seemingly twists about the isoelectric line. Torsades de pointes is most often seen in the setting of acquired Q–T prolongation caused by drug interactions, but it may be seen with the syndrome of idiopathic or congenital Q–T prolongation, or without Q–T prolongation in the setting of ischemia (2).

Antiarrhythmic drugs that prolong the Q–T interval, such as quinidine or sotalol, are the most common cause of torsades de pointes. In most patients, predisposing factors such as diuretic use with associated hypokalemia or hypomagnesemia are present. Severe bradycardia is another important predisposing factor, as is female gender, which is associated with 70% of cases of torsades de pointes in the setting of acquired Q–T prolongation (74). Besides antiarrhythmic drugs, a variety of other drugs may cause Q–T prolongation and have been associated with torsades de pointes. These include antidepressants; antihistamines of the H_1-blocking type (astemizole and terfenadine); and some antibiotics, particularly erythromycin (75). Although the incidence of torsades de pointes in patients taking these drugs is rare, they should be used with caution in women; in patients who are taking several of these drugs in combination, especially in the setting of hypokalemia (76) or hypomagnesemia (77); and in patients with the long Q–T syndrome.

In contrast to acquired Q–T prolongation, idiopathic or congenital long Q–T syndrome is a relatively rare congenital disorder in which delayed repolarization is expressed as a long Q–T interval (longer than 0.45 second when corrected for heart rate) (78). In some families, the inheritance is autosomal recessive and is associated with nerve deafness; in others, the inheritance is autosomal dominant and hearing is normal. Diagnostic criteria, using a point scale, have been published (79). The long Q–T interval predisposes to torsades de pointes, which often causes syncope and may cause sudden death, especially in the setting of acute stress (78). The Q–T interval should be measured routinely in the ECG of patients who complain of syncope for which there is no explanation.

The most effective treatment of symptomatic patients with the *congenital* long Q–T syndrome is beta-blocker therapy, in contrast to *acquired* Q–T prolongation in which bradycardia may provoke torsades de pointes. If beta-blocker therapy does not suppress arrhythmic attacks, excision of the left stellate ganglion, interrupting sympathetic innervation of the heart, may be curative. Appropriate treatment reduces the long-term mortality rate from 50% to less than 5%. It is not known whether patients with long Q–T intervals who are asymptomatic benefit from antiadrenergic therapy, but certainly treatment is reasonable if there is a family history of sudden death. An exercise ECG is indicated for patients with negative personal and family histories of arrhythmias to determine whether arrhythmias can be induced by exertion.

Arrhythmias in Pregnancy

Clinically significant arrhythmias occur rarely during pregnancy, but the awareness of ventricular ectopy and ventricular tachycardia is increased (80). The most common arrhythmia, other than isolated premature atrial beats and premature ventricular beats, is PSVT (see pg. 917) caused by AV node reentry, a common arrhythmia (see previous discussion). Occasionally, nonsustained ventricular tachycardia is detected as an incidental finding in an otherwise asymptomatic patient. Antiarrhythmic treatment options are limited in pregnancy—fluoroscopy, which is necessary for radiofrequency catheter ablation, is contraindicated, and antiarrhythmic drug options are limited. Beta-blockers, especially atenolol, have been reported to be safe during pregnancy, and quinidine and procainamide have been used as well (80). Submaximal exercise stress testing has been shown to be safe up to 25 weeks' gestation (81); ventricular arrhythmias that suppress with exercise are thought to have a benign prognosis (82). Patients with symptomatic arrhythmias should be referred to a cardiologist for evaluation.

HEART BLOCK

Heart block, a delay or failure of conduction of the cardiac impulse, is categorized electrocardiographically.

Right Bundle Branch Block

RBBB, a delay or block of conduction through the right bundle branch (Fig. 64.14), causes a modest prolongation of the QRS complex (longer than 0.12 second). The initial QRS vector is unaffected because it is accounted for normally by initial left ventricular (septal) depolarization. The right ventricle is activated by a spread of the action potential from the left ventricle, which is seen best in leads I and V_6, where the S waves are wide and slurred, and in V_1, where there is a double peak (RR′) of the R wave. RBBB is sometimes seen on the ECG of patients who have otherwise normal hearts. More often it is associated with an underlying congenital or acquired disorder, such as atrial septal defect and hypertensive or ischemic heart disease. Patients with newly acquired RBBB have an increased risk of cardiovascular morbidity and death from cardiovascular disease (83).

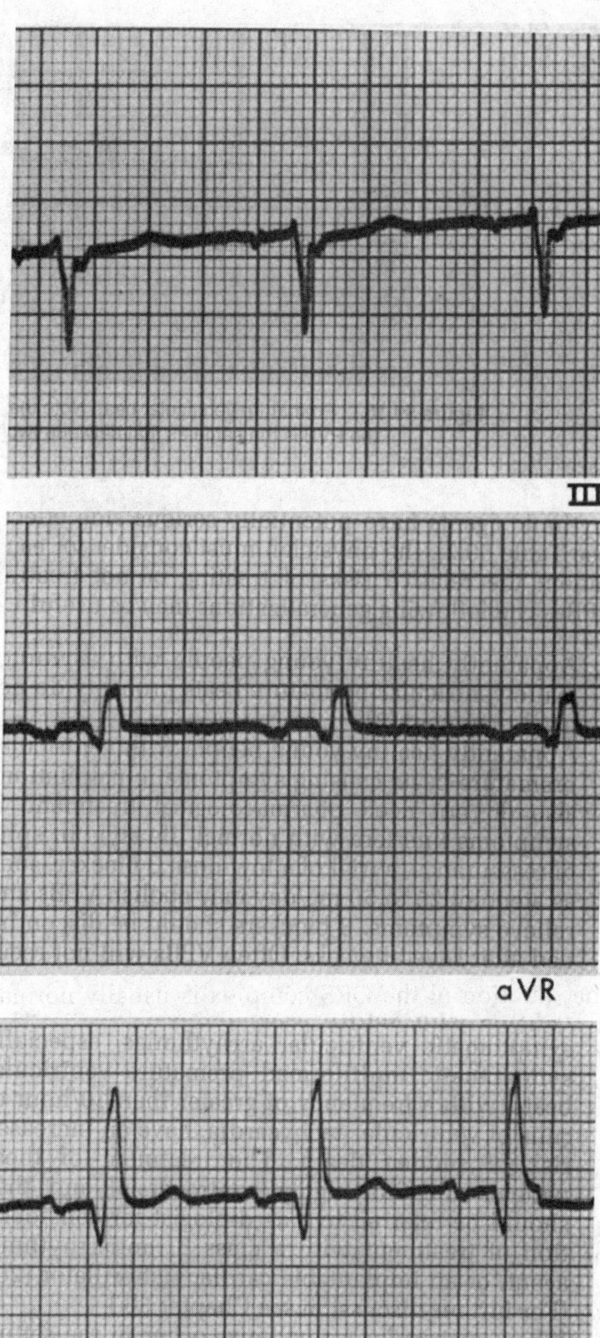

Figure 64.14. Right bundle branch block and left anterior hemiblock (bifascicular block).

Left Bundle Branch Block

LBBB, a delay or block of conduction through the left bundle branch (Fig. 64.15), causes a marked prolongation of the QRS complex (0.14 to 0.16 second). The entire sequence of ventricular depolarization is affected so that the QRS complex is widened and the QRS axis is directed to the left and posteriorly. Abnormal repolarization is reflected in the T wave, which

Figure 64.15. Left bundle branch block.

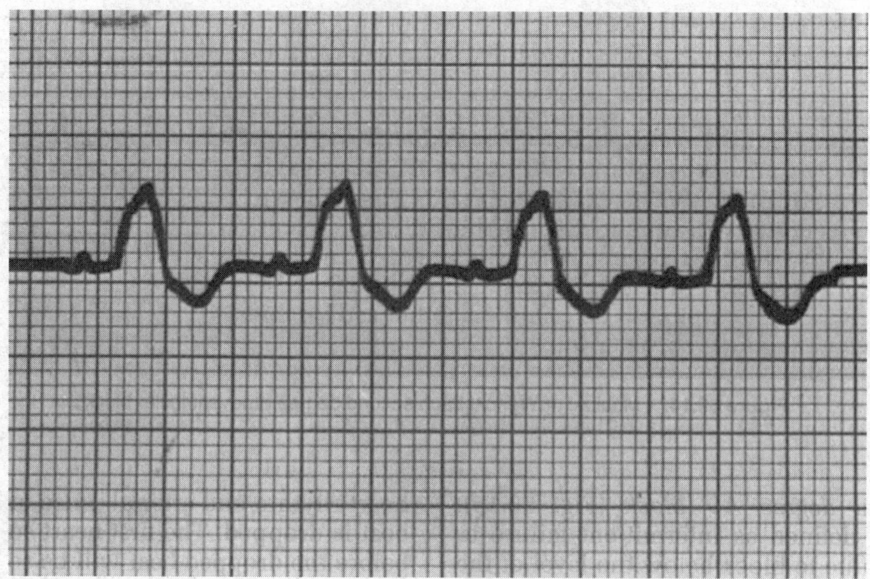

is always in the direction opposite that of the QRS complex.

LBBB almost always signifies heart disease, usually ischemic heart disease or cardiomyopathy (84).

Hemiblocks

Left Anterior Hemiblock. If there is delay or block of the cardiac impulse in the anterosuperior portion of the left bundle branch (Fig. 64.3), the corresponding wall of the left ventricle is activated late, resulting in marked left-axis deviation on the ECG (Fig. 64.14). The duration of the QRS complex is usually normal or slightly prolonged (longer than 0.10 second). The causes of left anterior hemiblock (LAH) are the same as those of LBBB. LAH is occasionally seen in patients with no discernible heart disease. Whatever the cause, LAH is not in itself a poor prognostic sign and, at least in an ambulatory setting, requires no specific therapy.

Left Posterior Hemiblock. If there is delay or block of the cardiac impulse in the posterior portion of the left bundle branch (Fig. 64.3), activation of the posterior wall of the left ventricle is delayed. The ECG pattern of left posterior hemiblock (LPH) is characterized by marked right-axis deviation (more than +110 degrees). The causes of LPH are the same as those of LAH and LBBB. Because the posterior portion of the left bundle branch is larger and better perfused than the anterosuperior portion, LPH is less common than LAH and usually indicates more extensive left ventricular disease (85).

Bifascicular Block

RBBB with LAH (manifested by an RBBB pattern and left-axis deviation; Fig. 64.14) or RBBB with LPH (manifested by an RBBB pattern and right-axis deviation) indicates that only one pathway remains to maintain passage of the cardiac impulse from the atria to the ventricles. If bifascicular block is detected in an ambulatory setting, especially if there is a history of syncope or light-headedness, a cardiologist should be asked to advise whether electrophysiologic studies (see Diagnosis of Arrhythmias) or pacemaker implantation is indicated. The risk that unselected patients with bifascicular block will develop complete heart block is 2% to 4% per year (86).There is conflicting evidence, however, about the course of patients with bifascicular block: some report no increased morbidity, and others report a considerably shortened survival time. Although there is no consensus about how to deal with the problem, the prognosis seems to be related to the extent of the underlying disease.

First-Degree Heart Block

Definition and Causes. The P–R interval normally varies with heart rate but should not exceed 0.20 second in people in normal sinus rhythm. First-degree AV block is defined as a prolonged P–R interval. The block may be caused by a prolongation of conduction in any of the structures between the SA node and the bundle of His (Fig. 64.3). Most commonly, when the QRS duration is normal, a long P–R interval is caused by a delay in conduction in the AV node. When first-degree block coincides with LBBB, it is likely that there is a delay in conduction in the His bundle. A prolonged P–R interval with RBBB may be caused by a block in the AV node or in the bundle of His.

A prolongation of the P–R interval is usually caused by degenerative, ischemic, or inflammatory changes in the AV conduction systems. It is commonly seen in older people without other evidence of heart disease, in patients who have had an inferior wall MI, or in association with myocarditis (including acute rheumatic fever). Drugs such as digitalis, which affect vagal activity, and sympatholytic drugs also may produce first-degree AV block.

Symptoms and Signs. First-degree AV block in itself does not produce symptoms or abnormal physical findings except that S_1 is reduced in intensity.

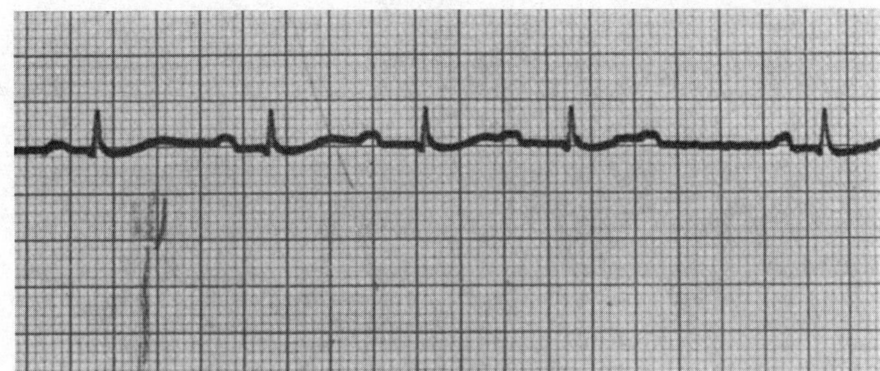

Figure 64.16. Mobitz-I or Wenckebach second-degree atrioventricular block.

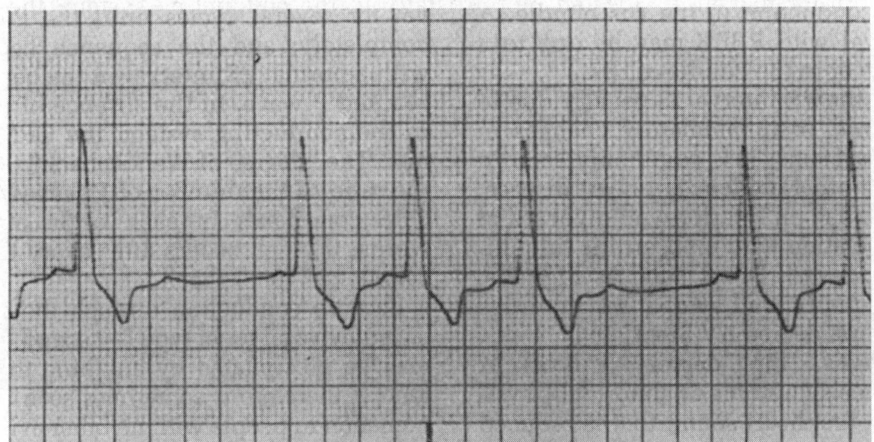

Figure 64.17. Mobitz-II second-degree atrioventricular block.

Treatment and Course. Patients with first-degree AV block who are asymptomatic and who have no other evidence of heart disease need not be treated. If patients with first-degree block complain of lightheadedness or dizziness, an ambulatory ECG or event monitor should be obtained (see Use of the Electrocardiogram), because some of these patients can have episodic higher degrees of block.

Second-Degree AV Block

Definition and Causes. Second-degree AV block is present when some, but not all, P waves are followed by QRS complexes. Second-degree AV block is caused by conduction delay or block either in the AV node or in the conduction system below the AV node, most commonly resulting from ischemic heart disease, cardiomyopathy, or drug toxicity (e.g., calcium channel blockers). The site of the block has important therapeutic implications.

Mobitz-I or Wenckebach Second-Degree AV Block. Second-degree AV block within the AV node results in the Wenckebach phenomenon. It is characterized by progressive lengthening of the P–R interval with shortening of the R–R interval for several cycles until the P wave is blocked completely (87) (Fig. 64.16); then the sequence begins again, often with a normal P–R interval in the beat that follows the blocked P wave. In the absence of disease elsewhere in the conducting system, the QRS complex is normal. The degree of Wenckebach block is characterized by the ratio of the number of P waves to the number of QRS complexes in each cycle of block. In other words, if block occurs after every third P wave, it is called 3:2 Wenckebach.

Because conduction through the AV node is influenced by vagal tone, type I second-degree AV block may be precipitated by anything that increases vagal tone. It therefore is sometimes seen as a transient phenomenon in people with no other evidence of heart disease. Otherwise, it is produced by the same processes that are associated with first-degree AV block.

Mobitz-II Second-Degree AV Block. Mobitz-II block is defined as intermittent failure to conduct a P wave caused by block below the level of the AV node (Fig. 64.17). The P–R interval of the conducted beat before a blocked P wave is usually normal. The block may be intermittent, or it may occur in a fixed 2:1 or 3:1 ratio. Coexistent bundle branch block is commonly seen. Progression to higher degrees of block or to asystole may occur rapidly.

Vagal influences have little effect on conduction below the AV node, so changes in vagal tone do not influence Mobitz-II block. However, the block may be precipitated by medications such as beta-blockers, which decrease conduction through the bundle of His. The common causes of Mobitz-II block are degenerative or ischemic changes in the His–Purkinje system.

Figure 64.18. Third-degree heart block.

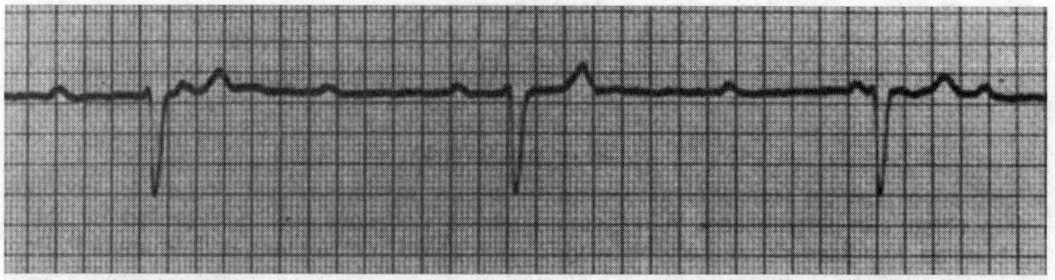

Symptoms and Signs

Mobitz-I Second-Degree AV Block. Patients are often asymptomatic but if vagal tone is increased (e.g., by digitalis or a beta-blocker or central sympatholytics such as clonidine), profound bradycardia may ensue, sometimes with rates lower than 30 beats/minute. Such patients may complain of light-headedness, syncope, or extreme fatigue.

Physical findings are subtle; irregularity of the heart rhythm and arterial pulse may be noted when a beat is dropped. The S_1 of the last beat before the dropped beat is softer than that of the first beat after the pause (because of the variation in P–R interval; see Chapter 65).

Mobitz-II Second-Degree AV Block. Symptoms and physical findings are similar to those of patients with Mobitz-I block except that they are not influenced by changes in vagal activity and the intensity of S_1 is constant.

Treatment and Course

Mobitz-I First-Degree AV Block. Asymptomatic patients need not be treated, because the risk of rapid progression of the block and of asystole is slight. Symptomatic patients usually have pronounced bradycardia. If so, medications that may be increasing the block should be discontinued. If such medications are essential to the patient's management, a cardiac pacemaker should be implanted (see Pacemaker Therapy).

Mobitz-II Second-Degree AV Block. Because of the high risk of rapid progression of the block and of asystole, all patients, even if asymptomatic, should be treated with a permanent cardiac pacemaker unless a reversible cause is identified and treated.

Patients with a history of light-headedness or dizziness who have new bundle branch block should be suspected of having had Mobitz-II block. This suspicion often can be confirmed with the use of an ambulatory ECG or event monitor (see Use of the Electrocardiogram). An intracardiac ECG (discussed earlier), if necessary, may also show prolonged conduction through the His bundle.

Third-Degree (Complete) Heart Block

Definition and Causes. Complete heart block occurs when there is total failure of conduction of impulses from the atria through the AV junction to the bundle of His (or, more rarely, if all three fascicles below the His bundle are diseased). The life of the patient then depends on the escape of a ventricular pacemaker. A rhythm generated in the upper portion of the His bundle may have a QRS configuration nearly identical to that of normally conducted impulses and has a rate between 40 and 60 beats/minute (Fig. 64.18). It is more likely to be a stable rhythm than is a rhythm generated by a lower pacemaker. If the pacemaker is located more distally in the conducting system, the ventricular rate decreases, the QRS morphology becomes wider and more bizarre, and the risk of asystole increases. In children or young adults, complete heart block may occur because of congenital defects in development of the AV cushion or of the conduction system itself; in such cases, escape rhythms are usually generated high in the bundle of His. In older people, complete heart block is most commonly caused by degenerative and fibrotic changes in the conduction system. It is also seen sometimes in association with infiltrative disease of the myocardium (e.g., sarcoid, amyloid), inflammatory processes (e.g., rheumatoid arthritis), and myocardial infections (e.g., bacterial endocarditis with valve ring abscess) or ischemic heart disease. Occasionally digitalis toxicity may produce complete heart block, as may excessive dosages of beta-blockers, amiodarone, or calcium channel blockers.

Complete heart block is a subcategory of *AV dissociation,* a situation in which the atria and ventricles are depolarized independently. In instances of AV dissociation other than complete heart block, the ventricles may be paced independently because of enhancement of the rate of discharge of a latent ventricular pacemaker (e.g., ventricular tachycardia) or because of marked slowing of the rate of discharge of the ordinarily dominant atrial pacemaker. In these instances, the ventricular rate is usually greater than the atrial rate and is also usually greater than in patients with complete heart block.

Symptoms and Signs. A major symptom of complete heart block is sudden loss of consciousness (a Stokes–Adams attack), the result of asystole or tachyarrhythmia (ventricular tachycardia or fibrillation). The asystole is caused by failure of the ventricular pacemaker; the tachyarrhythmia is caused by escape of another focus when the idioventricular rate falls too low (a variant of the bradycardia–tachycardia syndrome; see Sick Sinus Syndrome). If the heart begins to pump effectively again within seconds, as it usually does, the patient promptly regains consciousness and is alert and oriented. If perfusion of vital organs is delayed, seizure-like activity (ordinarily not generalized) and even death may ensue. Patients who are unconscious for more than a few minutes may not become fully alert for hours.

Complete heart block in patients with underlying myocardial disease can cause symptoms of heart failure (see Chapter 66), primarily because of further reduction in cardiac output as the result of bradycardia.

Physical findings of heart block are all attributable to the dissociation between atrial and ventricular contraction: Variation in the intensity of S_1, variation in systolic blood pressure, variation in the intensity of heart murmurs and of S_3 and S_4, and the appearance of cannon waves in the jugular pulse. The heart rate, of course, is slow.

Treatment and Course. The treatment of complete heart block is permanent pacemaker implantation unless a reversible cause is identified and treated. Even patients with a potentially reversible cause of complete heart block usually require hospitalization for temporary transvenous pacemaker therapy until normal rhythm is restored. The life expectancy of treated patients with complete heart block who have no other evidence of cardiac or systemic disease is excellent and approaches that of their age-matched cohort. Patients with complete heart block caused by coronary disease have a prognosis that is determined by the extent of their underlying coronary artery disease and their myocardial function.

General References*

Constant J. Learning electrocardiography. Boston: Little, Brown, 1997.
The one ECG textbook to buy when you are buying only one.

Podrid PJ, Kowey PR, eds. Cardiac arrhythmia: mechanisms, diagnosis and management. Baltimore: Williams & Wilkins, 1995.
A well-edited and clinically very useful and accessible textbook.

Specific References

1. Task Force of the Working Group on Arrhythmias of the European Society of Cardiology. The Sicilian gambit: a new approach to the classification of antiarrhythmic drugs based on their actions on arrhythmogenic mechanisms. Circulation 1991;84:1831.
2. Tan HL, Hou CJ, Lauer MR, et al. Electrophysiologic mechanisms of the long QT interval syndromes and torsades de pointes. Ann Intern Med 1995;122:701.
3. Barsky AJ. Palpitations, arrhythmias, and awareness of cardiac activity. Ann Intern Med 2001;134:832.
4. Zimetbaum P, Josephson ME. Evaluation of patients with palpitations. N Engl J Med 1998;338:1369.
5. Lessmeier TJ, Gamperling D, Johnson-Liddon V, et al. Unrecognized paroxysmal supraventricular tachycardia: potential for misdiagnosis as panic disorder. Arch Intern Med 1997;157:537.
6. Zipes DP. Clinical application of the electrocardiogram. J Am Coll Cardiol 2000;36:1746.
7. Zimetbaum PJ, Josephson ME. The evolving role of ambulatory arrhythmia monitoring in general clinical practice. Ann Intern Med 1999;130:848.
8. Calkins H. Premature ventricular depolarizations during exercise. N Engl J Med 2000;343:879.
9. Crawford MH, Bernstein SJ, Deedwania PC, et al. ACC/AHA guidelines for ambulatory electrocardiography: executive summary and recommendations: A Report of the American College of Cardiology/American Heart Association Task Force on Practice Guidelines (Committee to Revise the Guidelines for Ambulatory Electrocardiography). Developed in Collaboration With the North American Society for Pacing and Electrophysiology. Circulation 1999;100:886.
10. Kinlay S, Leitch JW, Neil A, et al. Cardiac event recorders yield more diagnoses and are more cost-effective than 48-hour Holter monitoring in patients with palpitations: a controlled clinical trial. Ann Intern Med 1996;124:16.
11. Jouven X, Zureik M, Desnos M, et al. Long-term outcome in asymptomatic men with exercise-induced premature ventricular depolarizations. N Engl J Med 2000;343:826.
12. Cannom DS, Prystowsky EN. Management of ventricular arrhythmias: detection, drugs, and devices. JAMA 1999;281:172.
13. Zipes DP, Wellens HJJ. What have we learned about cardiac arrhythmias? Circulation 2000;102:IV-52.
14. Goldschlager N, Epstein AE, Naccarelli G, et al. Practical guidelines for clinicians who treat patients with amiodarone. Practice Guidelines Subcommittee, North American Society of Pacing and Electrophysiology. Arch Intern Med 2000;160:1741.
15. Vaughan Williams EM. Significance of classifying antiarrhythmic actions since the cardiac arrhythmia suppression trial. J Clin Pharmacol 1991;31:123.
16. Grace AA, Camm AJ. Quinidine. N Engl J Med 1998;338:35.
17. Connolly SJ. Evidence-based analysis of amiodarone efficacy and safety. Circulation 1999;100:2025.
18. Abernethy DR, Schwartz JB. Calcium-antagonist drugs. N Engl J Med 1999;341:1447.
19. Echt DS, Liebson PR, Mitchell LB, et al. Mortality and morbidity in patients receiving encainide, flecainide, or placebo. The Cardiac Arrhythmia Suppression Trial. N Engl J Med 1991;324:781.
20. Horowitz LN. Proarrhythmia: taking the bad with the good. N Engl J Med 1988;319:304.
21. Pratt CM, Eaton T, Francis M, et al. The inverse relationship between baseline left ventricular ejection fraction and outcome of antiarrhythmic therapy: a dangerous imbalance in the risk-benefit ratio. Am Heart J 1989;118:433.
22. Teo KK, Yusuf S, Furberg CD. Effects of prophylactic antiarrhythmic drug therapy in acute myocardial infarction: an overview of results from randomized controlled trials. JAMA 1993;270:1589.
23. Coplen SE, Antman EM, Berlin JA, et al. Efficacy and safety of quinidine therapy for maintenance of sinus rhythm after cardioversion: a meta-analysis of randomized control trials. Circulation 1990;82:1106.
24. Flaker GC, Blackshear JL, McBride R, et al. Antiarrhythmic drug therapy and cardiac mortality in atrial fibrillation. The Stroke Prevention in Atrial Fibrillation Investigators. J Am Coll Cardiol 1992;20:527.
25. Benton RE, Sale M, Flockhart DA, et al. Greater quinidine-induced QTc interval prolongation in women. Clin Pharmacol Ther 2000;67:413.
26. Blomgren SE, Condemi JJ, Bignall MC, et al. Antinuclear antibody induced by procainamide: a prospective study. N Engl J Med 1969; 281:64.
27. Ried LD, McFarland BH, Johnson RE, et al. Beta-blockers and depression: the more the murkier? Ann Pharmacother 1998;32:699.
28. Newman CM, Price A, Davies DW, et al. Amiodarone and the thyroid: a practical guide to the management of thyroid dysfunction induced by amiodarone therapy. Heart 1998;79:121.
29. Amiodarone Trials Meta-Analysis Investigators. Effect of prophylactic amiodarone on mortality after acute myocardial infarction and in congestive heart failure: meta-analysis of individual data from 6500 patients in randomised trials. Lancet 1997;350:1417.
30. Hohnloser SH, Woosley RL. Sotalol. N Engl J Med 1994;331:31.
31. Alderman MH, Cohen H, Roque R, et al. Effect of long-acting and short-acting calcium antagonists on cardiovascular outcomes in hypertensive patients. Lancet 1997;349:594.
32. Gregoratos G, Cheitlin MD, Conill A, et al. ACC/AHA guidelines for implantation of cardiac pacemakers and antiarrhythmia devices: a report of the American College of Cardiology/American Heart Association Task Force on Practice Guidelines (Committee on Pacemaker Implantation). J Am Coll Cardiol 1998;31:1175.
33. Bryce M, Spielman SR, Greenspan AM, et al. Evolving indications for permanent pacemakers. Ann Intern Med 2001;134:1130.
34. Hayes DL, Wang PJ, Reynolds DW, et al. Interference with

*Bold print (general references) and bold numerals (specific references) denote published controlled clinical trials, meta-analyses, or consensus-based recommendations.

cardiac pacemakers by cellular telephones. N Engl J Med 1997;336:1473.

35. Hohnloser SH, Kuck KH, Lilienthal J. Rhythm or rate control in atrial fibrillation—Pharmacological Intervention in Atrial Fibrillation (PIAF): a randomised trial. Lancet 2000;356:1789.

36. Klein AL, Grimm RA, Murray RD, et al. Use of transesophageal echocardiography to guide cardioversion in patients with atrial fibrillation. N Engl J Med 2001;344:1411.

37. Catherwood E, Fitzpatrick WD, Greenberg ML, et al. Cost-effectiveness of cardioversion and antiarrhythmic therapy in nonvalvular atrial fibrillation. Ann Intern Med 1999;130:625.

38. Volgman AS, Carberry PA, Stambler B, et al. Conversion efficacy and safety of intravenous ibutilide compared with intravenous procainamide in patients with atrial flutter or fibrillation. J Am Coll Cardiol 1998;31:1414.

39. Oral H, Souza JJ, Michaud GF, et al. Facilitating transthoracic cardioversion of atrial fibrillation with ibutilide pretreatment. N Engl J Med 1999;340:1849.

40. Calkins H, Yong P, Miller JM, et al. Catheter ablation of accessory pathways, atrioventricular nodal reentrant tachycardia, and the atrioventricular junction: final results of a prospective, multicenter clinical trial. Circulation 1999;99:262.

41. Mangrum JM, DiMarco JP. The evaluation and management of bradycardia. N Engl J Med 2000;342:703.

42. Andersen HR, Nielsen JC, Thomsen PE, et al. Long-term follow-up of patients from a randomised trial of atrial versus ventricular pacing for sick-sinus syndrome. Lancet 1997;350:1210.

43. Levy S, Breithardt G, Campbell RW, et al. Atrial fibrillation: current knowledge and recommendations for management. Working Group on Arrhythmias of the European Society of Cardiology. Eur Heart J 1998;19:1294.

44. Ganz LI, Friedman PL. Supraventricular tachycardia. N Engl J Med 1995;332:162.

45. Kalbfleisch SJ, el Atassi R, Calkins H, et al. Differentiation of paroxysmal narrow QRS complex tachycardias using the 12-lead electrocardiogram. J Am Coll Cardiol 1993;21:85.

46. Levin ER, Gardner DG, Samson WK. Natriuretic peptides. N Engl J Med 1998;339:321.

47. Cheng CH, Sanders GD, Hlatky MA, et al. Cost-effectiveness of radiofrequency ablation for supraventricular tachycardia. Ann Intern Med 2000;133:864.

48. Kastor JA. Multifocal atrial tachycardia. N Engl J Med 1990;322:1713.

49. Allessie MA, Boyden PA, Camm AJ, et al. Pathophysiology and prevention of atrial fibrillation. Circulation 2001;103:769.

50. Klein I, Ojamaa K. Thyroid hormone and the cardiovascular system. N Engl J Med 2001;344:501.

51. Falk RH. Atrial fibrillation. N Engl J Med 2001;344:1067.

52. Falk RH, Knowlton AA, Bernard SA, et al. Digoxin for converting recent-onset atrial fibrillation to sinus rhythm: a randomized, double-blinded trial. Ann Intern Med 1987;106:503.

53. Scheinman MM, Morady F. Nonpharmacological approaches to atrial fibrillation. Circulation 2001;103:2120.

54. Jais P, Haissaguerre M, Shah DC, et al. A focal source of atrial fibrillation treated by discrete radiofrequency ablation. Circulation 1997;95:572.

55. Haissaguerre M, Jais P, Shah DC, et al. Spontaneous initiation of atrial fibrillation by ectopic beats originating in the pulmonary veins. N Engl J Med 1998;339:659.

56. Wolf PA, Kannel WB, McGee DL, et al. Duration of atrial fibrillation and imminence of stroke: the Framingham study. Stroke 1983;14:664.

57. Matchar DB, McCrory DC, Barnett HJ, et al. Medical treatment for stroke prevention. Ann Intern Med 1994;121:41.

58. Albers GW. Choice of antithrombotic therapy for stroke prevention in atrial fibrillation: warfarin, aspirin, or both? Arch Intern Med 1998;158:1487.

59. Albers GW, Dalen JE, Laupacis A, et al. Antithrombotic therapy in atrial fibrillation. Chest 2001;119:194S.

60. Natale A, Newby KH, Pisano E, et al. Prospective randomized comparison of antiarrhythmic therapy versus first-line radiofrequency ablation in patients with atrial flutter. J Am Coll Cardiol 2000;35:1898.

61. Nabar A, Rodriguez LM, Timmermans C, et al. Effect of right atrial isthmus ablation on the occurrence of atrial fibrillation: observations in four patient groups having type I atrial flutter with or without associated atrial fibrillation. Circulation 1999;99:1441.

62. Brugada P, Brugada J, Mont L, et al. A new approach to the differential diagnosis of a regular tachycardia with a wide QRS complex. Circulation 1991;83:1649.

63. Bikkina M, Larson MG, Levy D. Prognostic implications of asymptomatic ventricular arrhythmias: the Framingham Heart Study. Ann Intern Med 1992;117:990.

64. Moss AJ, Hall WJ, Cannom DS, et al. Improved survival with an implanted defibrillator in patients with coronary disease at high risk for ventricular arrhythmia. Multicenter Automatic Defibrillator Implantation Trial Investigators. N Engl J Med 1996;335:1933.

65. Moss AJ. Implantable cardioverter defibrillator therapy: the sickest patients benefit the most. Circulation 2000;101:1638.

66. Buxton AE, Lee KL, DiCarlo L, et al. Electrophysiologic testing to identify patients with coronary artery disease who are at risk for sudden death. Multicenter Unsustained Tachycardia Trial Investigators. N Engl J Med 2000;342:1937.

67. Cooper HA, Dries DL, Davis CE, et al. Diuretics and risk of arrhythmic death in patients with left ventricular dysfunction. Circulation 1999;100:1311.

68. Kastor JA. Michel Mirowski and the automatic implantable defibrillator. Am J Cardiol 1989;63:1121.

69. Morady F. Radio-frequency ablation as treatment for cardiac arrhythmias. N Engl J Med 1999;340:534.

70. Coggins DL, Lee RJ, Sweeney J, et al. Radiofrequency catheter ablation as a cure for idiopathic tachycardia of both left and right ventricular origin. J Am Coll Cardiol 1994;23:1333.

71. Gollob MH, Green MS, Tang AS, et al. Identification of a gene responsible for familial Wolff-Parkinson-White syndrome. N Engl J Med 2001;344:1823.

72. Al Khatib SM, Pritchett EL. Clinical features of Wolff-Parkinson-White syndrome. Am Heart J 1999;138:403.

73. Calkins H, Langberg J, Sousa J, et al. Radiofrequency catheter ablation of accessory atrioventricular connections in 250 patients: abbreviated therapeutic approach to Wolff-Parkinson-White syndrome. Circulation 1992;85:1337.

74. Makkar RR, Fromm BS, Steinman RT, et al. Female gender as a risk factor for torsades de pointes associated with cardiovascular drugs. JAMA 1993;270:2590.

75. Drici MD, Knollmann BC, Wang WX, et al. Cardiac actions of erythromycin: influence of female sex. JAMA 1998;280:1774.

76. Gennari FJ. Hypokalemia. N Engl J Med 1998;339:451.

77. Weisinger JR, Bellorin-Font E. Magnesium and phosphorus. Lancet 1998;352:391.

78. Towbin JA. New revelations about the long-QT syndrome. N Engl J Med 1995;333:384.

79. Schwartz PJ, Moss AJ, Vincent GM, et al. Diagnostic criteria for the long QT syndrome: an update. Circulation 1993;88:782.

80. Page RL. Treatment of arrhythmias during pregnancy. Am Heart J 1995;130:871.

81. Carpenter MW, Sady SP, Hoegsberg B, et al. Fetal heart rate response to maternal exertion. JAMA 1988;259:3006.

82. Sami M, Kraemer H, Harrison DC, et al. A new method for evaluating antiarrhythmic drug efficacy. Circulation 1980;62:1172.

83. Schneider JF, Thomas HE, Kreger BE, et al. Newly acquired right bundle-branch block: the Framingham Study. Ann Intern Med 1980;92:37.

84. Schneider JF, Thomas HE Jr, Kreger BE, et al. Newly acquired left bundle-branch block: the Framingham study. Ann Intern Med 1979; 90:303.

85. Kulbertus HE, Demoulin JC. The left hemiblocks: significance, prognosis and treatment. Schweiz Med Wochenschr 1982;112:1579.

86. Dhingra RC, Wyndham C, Amat-y-Leon F, et al. Incidence and site of atrioventricular block in patients with chronic bifascicular block. Circulation 1979;59:238.

87. Upshaw CB Jr, Silverman ME. The Wenckebach phenomenon: a salute and comment on the centennial of its original description. Ann Intern Med 1999;130:58.

CHAPTER 65

Common Cardiac Disorders Revealed by Auscultation of the Heart

EDWARD P. SHAPIRO, MD

During the past two decades, significant changes have occurred in techniques for diagnosis of, and strategies for, intervention in valvular heart disease. For a detailed review and discussion of controversial aspects, the reader is referred to the American College of Cardiology/American Heart Association Guidelines for the Management of Patients with Valvular Disease, published in its full form (1) or executive summary (2). These valuable aides can be accessed on the Web at www.acc.org and www.americanheart.org, respectively.

HEART SOUNDS

First Heart Sound (S_1)

The first heart sound is a high-frequency sound produced by closure of the atrioventricular (AV) valves, that is, M_1 (mitral valve closure) followed by T_1 (tricuspid valve closure). Mitral valve closure is louder than tricuspid valve closure.

Abnormally wide splitting of the first heart sound is produced by delays in closure of the tricuspid valve, as in patients with right bundle branch block, ventricular ectopic beats, idioventricular rhythm, or left ventricular (LV) pacing. In mitral stenosis, mitral valve closure may be so delayed that tricuspid valve closure may actually precede mitral valve closure.

Increased intensity of the first heart sound is associated with a rapid increase in ventricular pressure, which occurs when the ventricles are presented with an increased volume (e.g., ventricular septal defect and atrial septal defect) or with a wide-open AV valve at the end of diastole, which occurs when there is shortening of the AV filling time (e.g., atrial tachycardia and conditions associated with a short P-R interval) and when AV filling time is prolonged (e.g., mitral stenosis).

Reduced intensity of the first heart sound may indicate an immobile valve (e.g., severe mitral regurgitation or stenosis) or a long P-R interval.

Second Heart Sound (S_2)

The second heart sound is produced by closure of the semilunar valves, that is, A_2 (aortic valve closure) followed by P_2 (pulmonic valve closure). Normal splitting of the second heart sound occurs at the height of inspiration, when the splitting may be as wide as 0.10 seconds and is caused by the increase in stroke volume in the right heart with the increase in venous return with inspiration. The two components of the second heart sound are normally synchronous and virtually single during expiration.

Abnormally wide splitting of S_2 without change in expiration is characteristic of an atrial septal defect or anomalous pulmonary venous return. S_2 is widely split but variable in patients with right bundle branch block or pulmonic stenosis. In the presence of severe aortic stenosis, A_2 is delayed beyond P_2, resulting in wide splitting during expiration with no splitting during inspiration (reversed or paradoxical splitting). Paradoxical splitting of the second heart sound also occurs in the presence of a left bundle branch block, severe hypertension, or severe LV failure.

Increased intensities of A_2 and P_2 are features of aortic and pulmonary hypertension, respectively. Decreased intensities of A_2 or P_2 are features of an immobile or severely thickened aortic or pulmonic valve.

Gallops

The identification of a gallop sound affords valuable information about diagnosis, prognosis, and treatment. Gallops are diastolic sounds and appear to be related to the two periods of filling of the ventricles: the rapid filling phase (the S_3, or ventricular diastolic gallop) and the presystolic filling phase related to atrial systole (S_4, or atrial gallop).

The *atrial gallop sound*, or S_4, is a low-frequency presystolic sound and is found in patients with primary myocardial disease, coronary artery disease, systemic or pulmonary hypertension, or severe aortic or pulmonic stenosis. The atrial gallop indicates severity of the underlying disorder, and as the patient's condition improves, the sound may become fainter or disappear. With ventricular hypertrophy, an S_4 is a fixed finding of no prognostic significance. An atrial gallop is commonly heard in people above the age of 65, even in the absence of heart disease or hypertension (see Doppler Echocardiography, below).

The *ventricular gallop sound,* or S_3, is a low-frequency sound (see Chapter 66). It occurs with the same timing as the normal physiologic third sound, approximately 0.14 to 0.16 seconds after the second heart sound. The third sound is a normal finding in children, pregnant women, and in young adults up to the age of 30 (see discussion of Doppler Echocardiography, below). An S_3 gallop otherwise is a feature of severe cardiac decompensation, whatever the underlying cause (e.g., hypertension, coronary artery disease, rheumatic heart disease), and indicates a poor prognosis.

Ejection Sounds (Clicks)

Ejection sounds are produced at the time of ejection of blood from the left ventricle into the aorta or from the right ventricle into the pulmonary artery. The sound may originate in a thickened valve or dilated great vessel. The *aortic ejection sound* is located in the area of aortic auscultation—namely, from the second right intercostal space in a straight line to the cardiac apex—and occurs 0.05 seconds after M_1. It is a high-frequency sound, often called a click. In the presence of systemic hypertension, the aortic ejection sound is an indication of severity. It disappears as hypertension improves. Aortic ejection clicks may also be heard in patients with aortic stenosis, aneurysm of the ascending aorta, and aortic insufficiency.

Pulmonic ejection sounds (or clicks) are often localized to the second left intercostal space and may increase in intensity with expiration. They occur immediately after M_1. Pulmonic clicks are a feature of valvular pulmonic stenosis and of pulmonary hypertension.

A *midsystolic clicking sound,* with or without a late systolic murmur, may indicate mitral valve prolapse (see below).

Opening Snaps

An opening snap occurs because of a stenotic, but still mobile, mitral or tricuspid valve. The mitral opening snap is best heard between the pulmonic area and the cardiac apex. It occurs 0.04 to 0.12 seconds after S_2 in early diastole. It is heard in patients with a thickened mitral valve. The earlier the snap, the more severe the stenosis. The tricuspid opening snap is best heard at the lower left or right sternal border and occurs immediately after S_2 in early diastole.

Murmurs

Evaluation of a heart murmur is one of the most common tasks that confronts a practitioner conducting a physical examination. Virtually all normal people have a systolic murmur at some time in their lives. On the other hand, a murmur may be a sign of serious underlying cardiac or noncardiac disease. It is important to distinguish innocent murmurs from those that reflect an underlying disorder and to appropriately select the tests that will lead to the precise diagnosis and proper management.

General Characteristics of Murmurs

A murmur is a series of audible vibrations produced by turbulence in the circulation. These vibrations can be characterized by intensity, pitch, shape, quality, and timing in the cardiac cycle; precordial location of maximal intensity; and radiation.

The *intensity or loudness* of a murmur is, by convention, graded on a scale of 1 to 6. A grade 1 murmur is audible only after concentrated auscultation. A grade 2 murmur is faint but readily audible. A grade 3 murmur is prominent but not loud. Grade 4 murmurs are loud and are often, but not always, associated with a palpable thrill. A grade 5 murmur is very loud and can be heard with only the edge of the stethoscope touching the chest wall. A grade 6 murmur is heard with the stethoscope held 1 cm above, but not actually touching, the chest wall.

The *pitch of a murmur* refers to the frequency of the sound, from high to low. High-frequency murmurs usually reflect high velocity or high pressure.

The *shape of a murmur* refers to the change in intensity throughout the duration of the sound, for example, crescendo (increasing in intensity), decrescendo (decreasing in intensity), or constant.

The *quality of a murmur* refers to the nature of the sound: harsh, blowing, musical, cooing, rumbling, and so forth. Although these terms are not precise, they are useful in identifying various benign and significant conditions, as described below.

The *timing of a murmur* is particularly important in establishing the cause of the sound—first, whether the murmur is systolic, diastolic, or continuous and, second, whether it is heard in early, middle, or late systole or diastole. Murmurs that last throughout systole are called holosystolic. Late diastolic murmurs are sometimes called presystolic.

The *location of a murmur* refers to the site on the chest wall where the sound is loudest. The direction of radiation refers to the other sites where the murmur, although less intense, can still be heard; those sites may be outside the chest (e.g., the back or neck). Aortic murmurs may be heard anywhere in a straight line from the second right interspace to the apex. Pulmonic murmurs are heard best at the second left intercostal space; tricuspid murmurs, at the lower left sternal border; and mitral murmurs, at the cardiac apex radiating into the axilla.

There are two kinds of systolic murmurs: ejection and regurgitant murmurs. The ejection systolic murmur may be an innocent flow murmur or it may reflect organic heart disease. The regurgitant murmur may be caused by dilation of the annulus of the valve in an otherwise normal heart or may represent organic heart disease.

The *ejection murmur* is a crescendo/decrescendo (or diamond-shaped) murmur caused by the turbulence of blood flowing through either the aortic or the pulmonic valve. The murmur is most commonly midsystolic and ends before the second or closing sound (S_2) of the valve from which the murmur was generated; that is, aortic ejection murmurs end before A_2 and pulmonic ejection murmurs end before P_2. The loudness of the murmur depends in part on the pressure gradient across the valve and in part on other factors, such as thickness of the chest and the cardiac output; the shape depends on the acceleration and deceleration of blood flow across the valve as systole proceeds. When diastole is prolonged—for example, by a premature ventricular contraction—ejection murmurs become louder because of the passage of a large volume of blood through the valve. In general, the greater the cardiac output, the louder the murmur. Increases in cardiac output caused by hypermetabolic states, such as anemia, fever, or thyrotoxicosis, increase the loudness of the murmur. Decreases in cardiac output, as in congestive heart failure, decrease the loudness of the murmur.

Regurgitant murmurs are murmurs produced by backward flow of blood from a high-pressure chamber to a compartment of lower pressure. Intensity may be constant, as in mitral regurgitation, tricuspid regurgitation, or ventricular septal defect, or may be decrescendo, as in aortic and pulmonary regurgitation.

A number of maneuvers can be performed to alter the intensity of a systolic murmur and to help determine its origin. For example, the Valsalva maneuver reduces intrathoracic venous return and softens the murmur of aortic stenosis while intensifying that of hypertrophic cardiomyopathy (HCM). Squatting, which increases venous return, has the opposite effect. Isometric handgrip, which increases blood pressure and therefore reduces forward flow, softens the murmur of aortic stenosis and intensifies that of mitral regurgitation.

Innocent Murmurs

Innocent murmurs are a series of vibrations that are produced in the absence of significant abnormalities of cardiac anatomy or function (Table 65.1). Innocent murmurs can usually be distinguished from significant murmurs by the absence of other physical, radiologic, or electrocardiographic evidence of disease. Also, innocent murmurs are usually in early systole or midsystole, are grade 1 or 2 in intensity, and vary with respiration and position. Occasionally, echocardiography (see below) is done to clarify the cause of a murmur, but more elaborate studies, such as stress tests, radionuclide studies, and cardiac catheterization, are used only after it has been decided that a murmur is not innocent and that a more precise diagnosis is necessary.

Table 65.1. Benign or Innocent Systolic Murmurs

Vibratory ejection systolic murmur
Continuous murmur of venous hum
Pulmonic ejection systolic murmur
Aortic ejection systolic murmur
Murmur associated with pregancy

The most common innocent *systolic murmur of childhood* and young adulthood that is clearly recognizable as benign based on the characteristics of the murmur alone is the musical or vibratory midsystolic murmur (best heard at the lower left sternal border) caused by the vibration of the leaflets of the pulmonary valve.

The *venous hum* is a continuous murmur, loudest in the neck, caused by altered flow through the jugular veins. It can be eliminated by turning the patient's head, compressing the internal jugular vein on the side where the murmur is heard, or placing the patient in the supine position.

The *pulmonic ejection systolic murmur* is a systolic crescendo/decrescendo murmur generated by the flow of blood through the pulmonary valve. It is loudest in the left second intercostal space or at the midleft sternal border.

Similarly, the *aortic ejection systolic murmur* is an early systolic murmur generated by the flow of blood through the aortic valve. It is loudest in the right second intercostal space or at the apex of the heart. This innocent or flow murmur, caused by sclerosis of the aorta or the aortic valve, is the most common benign systolic murmur in middle-aged or elderly patients and may have a cooing quality. An echocardiogram may be necessary to rule out LV hypertrophy and aortic stenosis.

Benign flow murmurs are commonly heard in *pregnant women*. Because of the normally increased stroke volume at 28 to 30 weeks' gestation, diastolic filling sounds and systolic ejection murmurs of turbulent flow are common. In pregnant women also, an S_3 may be prominent enough to be confused with the middiastolic murmur of mitral stenosis. The S_3 of pregnancy may be distinguished from the murmur of mitral stenosis, however, by the absence of an opening snap and by the accompanying hyperdynamic apical movement. An echocardiogram is indicated occasionally in some patients to make a precise diagnosis.

In a pregnant woman it is critical to compare the femoral and brachial pulses and the blood pressures in the presence of a heart murmur because coarctation of the aorta may present with a soft heart murmur and, if left undiagnosed, may rarely result in aortic dissection or rupture.

Clinical Applications of Echocardiography

Echocardiography is a valuable adjunct to the clinical assessment in patients suspected of having cardiovascular disease (3). This technique uses high-frequency pulsed sound waves to record echoes of cardiac structures as they move within a beam of sound directed into the chest.

To record a *transthoracic M-mode ECG*, an ultrasound transducer is placed at one point on the chest wall and rocked to inscribe an arc that encompasses several areas of the heart sequentially. The transducer serves as a source of the sound beam and a receiver of the echoes. A *transthoracic two-dimensional (2D) echocardiogram* is recorded using a pulse transducer that is automatically directed across an arc, providing a simultaneous view of the cardiac structures, which is recorded on videotape. Both modes are usually combined and reported together. These procedures do not cause discomfort, but the patient ideally must be able to lie flat for approximately 20 minutes for performance of the test.

Echocardiography allows visualization of all four cardiac valves, the aortic root, both atria, the right ventricle, the left ventricle including all individual wall segments (Fig. 65.1), and the pericardium. The size and function of these structures are analyzed and patterns of specific diseases may be recognized.

2D echocardiography is particularly helpful in assessing LV function in patients with ischemic heart disease, in whom regional structure and function are most important. It should be understood that echo assessment of overall or regional LV function is usually semiquantitative. Wall motion is usually categorized as normal or as mildly, moderately, or severely depressed. If an ejection fraction is reported, this often represents a visual estimate by the echocardiographer. Small differences reported in serial studies of the same patient, therefore, may not represent an important change unless the studies have been compared side by side by the same observer. Some laboratories use software that allows more quantitative reporting, but the value of this has not yet been adequately established. The noninvasive nature of the test and its ease of performance make 2D echocardiography extremely useful for assessing patients with cardiac decompensation or suspected organic heart disease.

The 2D echocardiogram is diagnostic in cases of pericardial effusion, HCM, congestive cardiomyopathy, mitral valve stenosis or prolapse, aortic regurgitation, intracardiac masses, and Ebstein anomaly of the tricuspid valve. The technique is helpful in ischemic heart disease with regional wall motion abnormalities; aortic stenosis; infectious endocarditis; cardiac tamponade; atrial septal defect; other forms of congenital heart disease, such as ventricular septal defect, tetralogy of Fallot, and bicuspid aortic valve; and any other structural abnormality of the heart.

Doppler echocardiography is an extremely useful tool for the detection and quantification of the severity

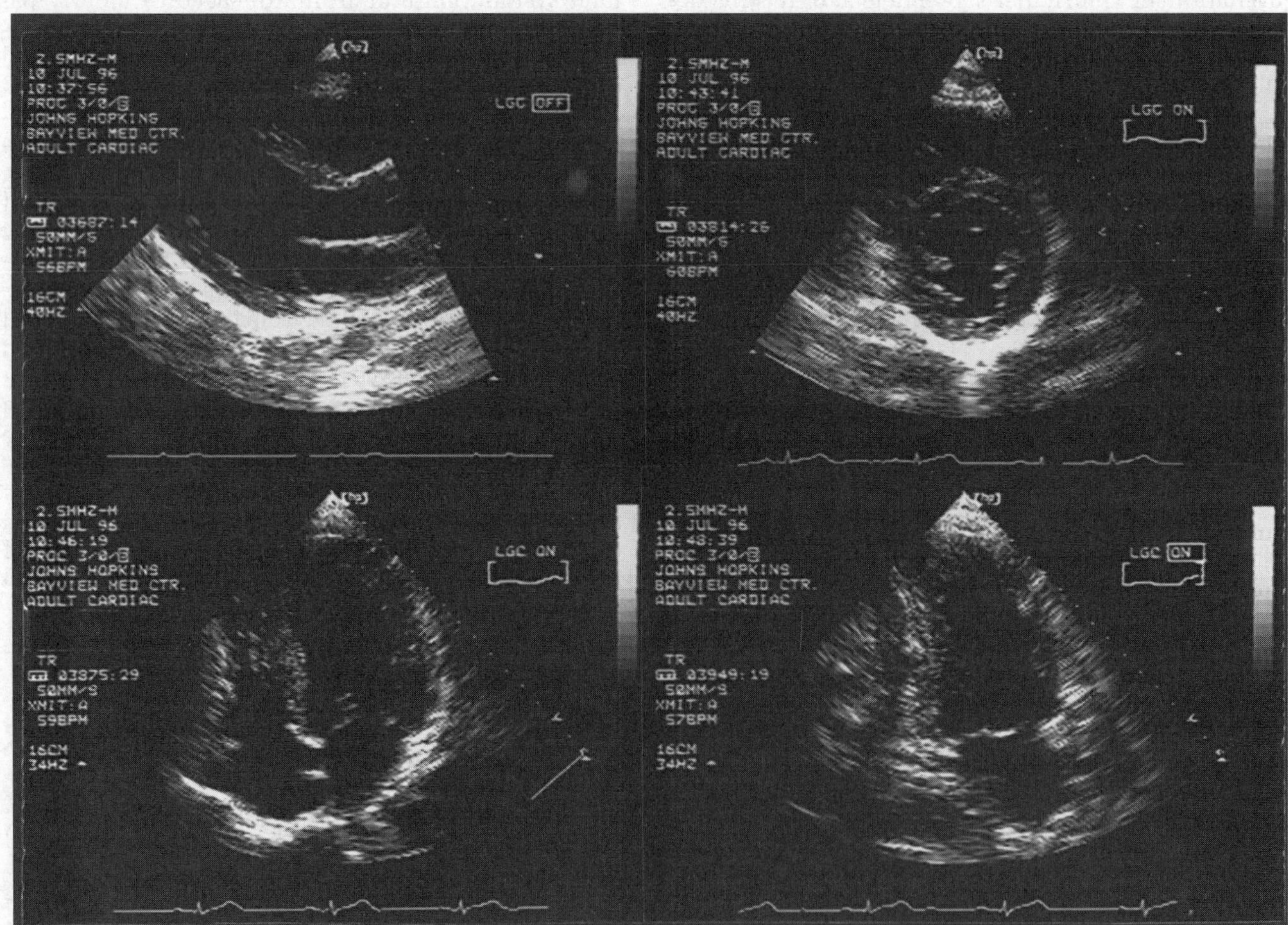

Figure 65.1. The four basic views of the two-dimensional echocardiogram. Tomographic slices obtained from different vantage points and angles reveal valvular structure and all left ventricular walls. **Upper left:** Parasternal long axis view demonstrating septum and posterior wall. **Upper right:** Parasternal short axis view displaying a "breadloaf" slice of the left ventricle. **Lower left:** Apical four-chamber view revealing septum, apex, and lateral wall. **Lower right:** Apical two-chamber view, revealing inferior wall, apex, and lateral wall.

of valvular heart disease. High-frequency sound is directed at a column of moving red blood cells, and the reflected sound is analyzed for changes in frequency, which indicate the direction and velocity of flow. Flow velocity information is color coded and superimposed on the 2D echocardiographic image, providing visual representation of blood flow through the heart and great vessels.

In valvular stenosis, a high-velocity jet of blood is detected distal to the stenosis; the higher the transvalvular gradient, the higher the velocity of the jet. The pressure gradient across a valve and the area of the aortic (4) and mitral (4,5) valves can also be calculated, providing precise quantification of the severity of aortic and mitral stenosis.

Valvular regurgitation can be detected by reverse flow and its severity estimated, usually by measuring the extent to which the regurgitant jet is detectable in the chamber proximal to the leaking valve. For example, mitral regurgitation is considered severe on a color Doppler study if the regurgitant jet occupies more than 40% of the area of the left atrium during systole (6). A small degree of regurgitation of the tricuspid valve is usually seen in normal subjects and does not represent disease. The presence of tricuspid regurgitation allows the estimation of right ventricular systolic pressure, which is equal to the pulmonary artery systolic pressure in the absence of pulmonic valvular disease. This is useful in the detection and follow-up of patients with pulmonary hypertension of any cause. Small amounts of mitral and pulmonic regurgitation are usually seen in normal people and are not a cause for concern if the echocardiographer comments that the extent is "mild." Small amounts of aortic regurgitation are also frequently seen and are considered normal if their extent is graded as "trivial."

Doppler echocardiography is often used to detect *diastolic dysfunction*, a frequent contributor to the development of congestive heart failure, especially in the elderly (see Chapter 66). The normal diastolic flow pattern consists of two phases: passive filling during early diastole (termed the E wave), which is aided by elastic recoil of the ventricle, and filling during late diastole (termed the A wave) due to atrial contraction. In young normal people, the left ventricle is pliable and elastic recoil during diastole is vigorous, resulting in brisk early filling, hence a large E wave. Very little filling then remains to be accomplished during late diastole, hence a small A wave. The ratio of early to late filling (the E/A ratio) therefore is high, typically about 1.5 to 2.0 in normal people in their thirties or forties. However, the left ventricle loses its pliability in patients with LV hypertrophy, other forms of chronic heart disease, and even during the process of normal aging. Early diastolic elastic recoil then becomes ineffective in aiding filling, and the E wave becomes small. To compensate, a substantial proportion of filling must occur during late diastole, and the A wave enlarges. The E/A ratio is thus reduced, and when it falls below 1, "grade I diastolic dysfunction" is said to be present. This pattern is also called "abnormal relaxation." Grade I diastolic dysfunction is a normal finding in people older than age 65.

However, the E/A ratio is an imperfect index of diastolic function because the velocity of early LV filling depends on several factors in addition to LV relaxation. For instance, a high left atrial pressure, which occurs in congestive heart failure, causes a high AV pressure gradient, which accelerates early filling irrespective of LV stiffness, resulting in a large E wave and a high E/A ratio. This pattern is called pseudonormalization of the E/A ratio, or "grade II diastolic dysfunction." Distinguishing pseudo-normal from normal may require ancillary Doppler procedures such as repeating the recording during a Valsalva maneuver or measuring flow through the pulmonary vein, but the presence of grade II diastolic dysfunction should be considered in the elderly and in people with LV hypertrophy, in whom there is likely to be grade I dysfunction at baseline. Common causes of grade II diastolic dysfunction include systolic dysfunction, valvular heart disease, fluid overload, and episodes of ischemia. When grade II diastolic dysfunction occurs in the absence of those conditions, "diastolic heart failure" is considered to be present. This latter phenomenon is commonly seen in the elderly in the presence of LV hypertrophy or severe hypertension.

When the E/A ratio exceeds 2.0, "grade III diastolic dysfunction" or a "restrictive pattern" is said to be present. This occurs in restrictive cardiomyopathy and constrictive pericarditis, but also in all conditions that cause grade II diastolic dysfunction, when they are severe.

Several conditions may produce the pattern of grade II or III diastolic dysfunction in the absence of congestive heart failure. For example, in significant mitral regurgitation that is well compensated, the left atrial pressure in *early* diastole may be elevated due to the large "v" wave, increasing the E/A ratio, but the *mean* diastolic pressure may not be high enough to cause pulmonary congestion. Also, in patients who have recently converted from atrial fibrillation to sinus rhythm, a transient atrial myopathy is often present, resulting in a small "A" wave and a high E/A ratio (7).

In patients in whom a large E wave is present, an S_3 is often audible. These include normal people less than 30, elderly patients with congestive heart failure, and patients with constrictive cardiomyopathy, in whom the early diastolic sound is called a pericardial knock. In patients in whom a large A wave is present, an S_4 is usually audible. These include normal elderly people and patients with LV hypertrophy due to hypertension or aortic stenosis.

A common limitation of standard transthoracic echocardiography is that ultrasound penetrates lung and bone poorly, and the available acoustic window is limited in many patients, resulting in poor-quality studies. The technique of *transesophageal echocardiography* (TEE) has extended the diagnostic utility of echocardiography by allowing high-quality studies, with markedly increased resolution, in all patients (8). Additional structures can be assessed, including the venae cavae, coronary sinus, pulmonary veins, atrial septum, atrial appendages, pulmonary artery, and ascending and descending aorta. Valve leaflets are seen with great clarity. Resolution is adequate to detect atheroma on the walls of the aorta. The method transforms a noninvasive imaging modality into a semi-invasive one; the procedure is similar to esophagoscopy and is often performed in a hospital's endoscopy unit, often on an outpatient basis. The patient is asked to fast for 6 to 8 hours and is treated with a pharyngeal topical anesthetic and intravenous sedation. The patient is then assisted in swallowing a small (i.e., 1-cm diameter) echo transducer mounted on a gastroscope-like tube. Visualization of the cardiac structures from the esophagus and stomach is usually accomplished in about 20 minutes. The examination may include the intravenous injection of agitated saline, which creates ultrasonic contrast via tiny bubbles, to assess for right-to-left shunting. Complications of TEE are rare and include inability to intubate the esophagus successfully (1.9%), pulmonary difficulties such as bronchospasm (0.07%), cardiac arrhythmias (0.08%), and bleeding (0.02%) (9). Esophageal perforation is extremely rare.

The indications for TEE are evolving. The method allows visualization of almost the entire aorta and is sensitive (97.7%) and specific (76.9%) in the diagnosis of aortic dissection (10). The method is much better than transthoracic echo for visualizing cardiac sources of embolus, such as thrombus in the left atrium or left atrial appendage, sluggish blood flow in the left atrium, atrial septal aneurysm, patent foramen ovale, and complex aortic atheroma, sometimes with attached thrombus. Therefore, it is often ordered in patients with cryptogenic strokes (i.e., strokes in patients without evidence of atheroma in the carotid or vertebral systems). This is the method of choice for assessing the function of prosthetic mitral valves and for visualizing vegetations or intracardiac abscesses caused by endocarditis. TEE is sometimes indicated when transthoracic echo quality is poor and information about cardiac structure or function is deemed crucial.

SELECTED DISORDERS ASSOCIATED WITH ABNORMAL HEART SOUNDS

Aortic Stenosis

Stenosis of the aortic valve obstructs the flow of blood into the aorta and therefore raises the LV pressure above the aortic pressure. The pressure gradient across the valve is related to the severity of the stenosis. The elevated pressure results in a concentric hypertrophy of the left ventricle. Symptoms develop when the left ventricle can no longer compensate for the pressure load; the heart fails and the cardiac output declines.

Aortic stenosis may occur at any one of several levels. The most common obstruction (75% of patients) is at the aortic valve, although patients with subvalvular and supravalvular aortic stenosis may have symptoms and signs of severity similar to those of valvular disease. It is particularly important to differentiate fixed aortic outflow obstruction from idiopathic hypertrophic disease, in which the obstruction is dynamic in nature (Table 65.2; see below).

Causes and Epidemiology

In patients below the age of 30, aortic stenosis is most likely to be caused by a congenitally stenotic unicuspid valve. Between the ages of 30 and 65, a bicuspid aortic valve, which has become calcified and gradually more rigid over the years, is the most common cause of aortic stenosis. Rheumatic valvular disease accounts for less than 25% of cases of isolated aortic stenosis in patients between the ages of 30 and 70 years. Over the age of 65, degeneration and sclerosis of the valve account for most cases of aortic stenosis. With the decline of rheumatic fever and the aging of the population, degenerative (calcific) aortic stenosis in the elderly has become the most common form of the disease that is encountered. Except in the elderly, in whom the prevalence is the same in both sexes, isolated aortic stenosis is three to four times more common in men.

Table 65.2. Comparison of Valvular Aortic Stenosis and Hypertrophic Cardiomyopathy

	Valvular Aortic Stenosis	Hypertrophic Cardiomyopathy
Symptoms	Dyspnea, angina, syncope, or near-syncope.	Dyspnea, angina, syncope, or near-syncope.
Signs	Systolic ejection murmur loudest at aortic area or at apex; louder if patient squats.	Systolic ejection murmur loudest at left lower sternal border; louder if patient stands or performs a Valsalva maneuver.
	A_2 may not be audible.	A_2 is usually audible.
	S_4 is common.	S_4 is very common.
	Ejection sounds are common.	Ejection sounds are uncommon.
	Carotid upstroke is delayed.	Carotid upstroke is brisk.
Electrocardiogram	LVH and strain pattern.	LVH and strain pattern; Q waves in inferior and lateral leads are common.
Chest radiograph	LVH is a late sign.	LVH may occur but unpredictably.
	Aortic valve is always calcified (may be seen only on fluoroscopy).	Aortic valve is not calcified.
	Ascending aorta may be dilated.	Ascending aorta is not dilated.
Echocardiogram	Characteristic echos of valvular calcification and valvular stenosis.	Disproportionate septal hypertrophy and systolic anterior displacement of mitral valve may be present.

LVH, left ventricular hypertrophy.

Natural History and Symptoms

Patients with aortic stenosis are usually asymptomatic until late in the course of their disease. Mild to moderate obstruction does not greatly compromise LV function, and even patients with severe stenosis may compensate for years before they develop symptoms. Mortality is minimal during the asymptomatic phase of the disease. However, after the development of symptoms there is a precipitous decline in survival and if the lesion is not corrected, the average patient dies in about 4 years.

The earliest symptoms are easy fatigability and excessive dyspnea after unusual exercise. Syncope or near-syncope with effort (see Chapter 89), angina (see Chapter 62), and dyspnea on usual exercise (see Chapter 66) are indicative of severe valvular obstruction. Patients with heart failure do not survive as long (2 years) as do patients with syncope (3 years) or angina (5 years). Sudden death occurs in approximately 15% of symptomatic patients.

Physical Findings

Patients with aortic stenosis usually have a loud (grade 3 to 4) systolic ejection murmur. The maximal intensity of the murmur is at the second right intercostal space or at the cardiac apex. At the apex the murmur often has a musical cooing quality. There is often a thrill in the suprasternal notch or the second right intercostal space. However, the loudness of the murmur may not correlate with the severity of stenosis. Also, if cardiac output is reduced, as in congestive heart failure, or if the diameter of the chest is increased, the intensity of the murmur may be less than it otherwise would be. A late peak to the murmur suggests severe obstruction, but this may be difficult to appreciate with a stethoscope, and absence of the late peak does not mean that obstruction is not severe. Augmentation of the murmur when the patient suddenly squats and diminution of the murmur when the patient stands or performs a Valsalva maneuver are characteristic of aortic stenosis.

The systolic murmur, although it may not be loud, is an invariable sign of aortic stenosis; other cardiac sounds depend on the nature of the stenotic lesion. An early systolic ejection click is commonly heard when the valve is still mobile. The second aortic sound (A_2) is often not audible when the valve is so rigid that S_2 has only one component (P_2). Paradoxical splitting of the second heart sound, in the absence of left bundle branch block, is a sign of severity. A small pulse pressure (less than 30 mm Hg) also indicates severe obstruction (in elderly people, the pulse pressure may be normal despite severe stenosis). A slowly rising pulse—best assessed by palpation of a carotid artery—is characteristic. Under the age of 40, an S_4 is another sign of severe obstruction; over the age of 40, S_4 is common because of the high prevalence of hypertensive and ischemic heart disease and does not correlate with severity of stenosis.

Based on a review of available evidence of the precision and accuracy of the clinical examination for abnormal systolic murmurs, the likelihood of aortic stenosis is increased by the presence of effort syncope, slowly rising carotid pulse, mid or late systolic peak of murmur, soft or absent S_2, apical to carotid delay, or brachioradial delay (11). The regurgitant early diastolic murmur of aortic insufficiency is heard in 30% to 40% of patients with aortic valve stenosis.

Laboratory Evaluation

An ECG, a chest x-ray, and an echocardiogram should be obtained routinely in a patient suspected of having aortic stenosis.

Electrocardiogram. The ECG is usually normal until stenosis becomes severe, at which point LV hypertrophy (Table 65.3 and Fig. 65.2) and nonspecific ST depression and T-wave inversion are common, but not invariable. In older patients particularly, an abnormal ECG cannot be relied on to reflect severity because there are often other reasons why it might be abnormal.

Chest X-Ray. Calcification of the aortic valve is always present in patients with aortic stenosis who are older than 40, but often fluoroscopy is necessary to reveal it. Poststenotic dilation of the ascending aorta is also commonly seen. The heart size and configuration are usually normal until the disease is far advanced.

Echocardiogram. Echocardiography reveals immobile and usually calcified aortic valve leaflets. An increase in ventricular wall thickness on echocardiography implies severe obstruction if there is no other cause for hypertrophy. Doppler echocardiography (see above) can provide an estimate of the transaortic gradient and the aortic valve area. The valve area is

Table 65.3. Principal Electrocardiographic Features of Left Ventricular Hypertrophy

Electrocardiographic Criteria	Point System for Diagnosis[a]
Negative components of P in $V_1 \geq 1$ mm and $\geq .04$ sec	3 points
QRS	
Largest limb lead R or S ≥ 20 mm or largest chest lead S before transition or R after transition ≥ 30 mm	3 points
OR	
Largest S before transition plus largest R after transition = 45 mm;	
Frontal plane axis ≥ -30 degrees	2 points
Duration in extremity lead ≥ 0.09 sec	1 point
Intrinsicoid deflection ≥ 0.05 sec	1 point
ST–T	
In general, opposite QRS:	
Without digitalis	3 points
With digitalis	1 point

[a]Interpretation of point score: 6 points, left ventricular hypertrophy; 5 points, probable left ventricular hypertrophy; 4 points, possible left ventricular hypertrophy. If only voltage criteria are met, ECG may be designated as borderline, and left ventricular hypertrophy is suggested only by voltage and should be excluded by other clinical means.

Modified from Horan LG, Flowers NC. Electrocardiography and vectorcardiography. In: Braunwald E, ed. Heart disease: a textbook of cardiovascular medicine. Philadelphia: WB Saunders, 1980;229, with permission.

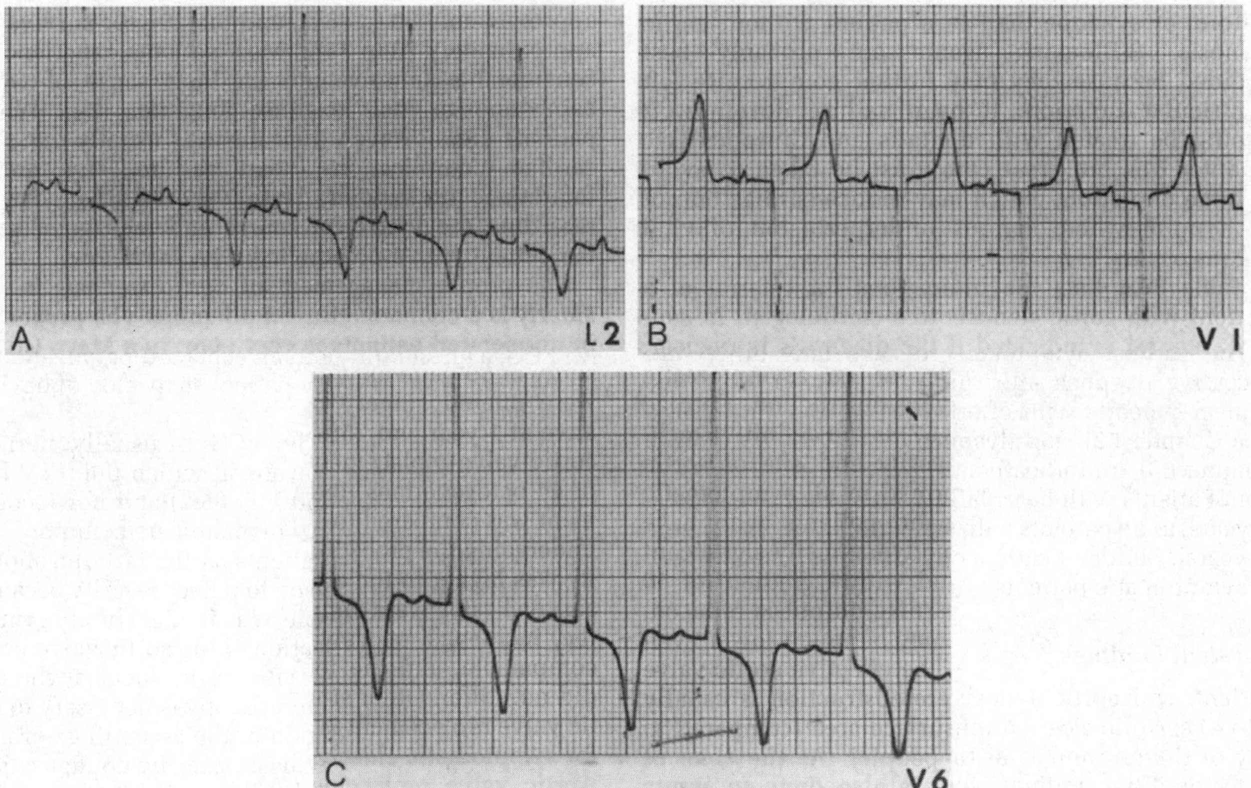

Figure 65.2. Electrocardiogram of a patient with left ventricular hypertrophy (Table 65.3).

generally considered a better measure of severity of aortic stenosis than the gradient because the gradient may be deceptively low in the presence of reduced cardiac output caused by LV dysfunction, even with severe stenosis (see below). Doppler echocardiography is helpful in distinguishing aortic stenosis from aortic valve sclerosis, in which no gradient is present.

Management

Asymptomatic patients with mild or moderate disease should be reassessed every 12 months so that signs of progressive disease can be detected promptly. Reassessment should include interval history, pertinent physical examination, ECG, chest x-ray, and echocardiogram. The asymptomatic patient with severe aortic stenosis presents a management dilemma. Although sudden death is extremely rare in asymptomatic patients (<1% per year), symptoms may appear suddenly and progress rapidly to sudden death (as early as 3 months after symptoms appear). Seventy percent of asymptomatic patients progress to symptoms within 3 years. Although these factors suggest that prophylactic valve replacement might be indicated in asymptomatic patients with severe disease, this must be weighed against the operative mortality (3% to 12%), the risk of prosthetic valve complications (1% to 2% per year), and the fact that many patients would be operated on needlessly (12). Patients with severe asymptomatic aortic stenosis therefore should be referred to a cardiologist. However, many cardiologists recommend that asymptomatic patients be followed extremely closely without prophylactic surgery. These issues should be discussed with the patient. It is accepted practice to perform aortic valve replacement in asymptomatic patients with severe (or sometimes moderate) aortic stenosis who require other open heart procedures, such as coronary artery bypass grafting.

Patients should be cautioned to avoid undue exertion because acute heart failure, arrhythmia, and sudden death are more likely under such circumstances. The risk of subacute bacterial endocarditis is increased in patients with aortic stenosis and is unrelated to the severity of the stenosis (the risk is unchanged after aortic valve surgery; see below). Therefore, antibiotic prophylaxis (see Chapter 93) is necessary before dental and surgical procedures.

Atrial arrhythmias are uncommon; if they occur, they must be treated aggressively (see Chapter 64) because they are more likely to cause angina, heart failure, or syncope than in a patient without aortic stenosis. Beta-blockers should be best avoided in patients with severe aortic stenosis, because they may compromise LV function. If heart failure develops, it should be treated with digitalis and diuretics (see Chapter 66), but great care must be taken to avoid volume depletion, which may reduce cardiac output to a point where serious underperfusion of vital organs occurs.

Table 65.4 lists the indications for referral of a patient with aortic stenosis to a cardiologist. In general, referral is indicated if the diagnosis is unclear, the

Table 65.4. Indications for Referral of Patients with Aortic Stenosis

If there is a question about the diagnosis or severity
If the patient is symptomatic
If the asymptomatic patient has signs of severe obstruction
Physical signs
Small pulse pressure (<30 mm Hg)
Late peak of systolic murmur
Diminished A_2
Paradoxical splitting of A_2
Electrocardiogram
Left ventricular hypertrophy
ST depression and T-wave inversion
Chest x-ray
Left ventricular hypertrophy
Echocardiogram
Concentric left ventricular hypertrophy
Doppler-calculated gradient greater than 50 mm Hg or valve area less than 0.75 cm^2

patient is symptomatic, or an asymptomatic patient has evidence of severe obstruction. Cardiac catheterization (see Chapter 62) is the definitive technique for assessing the severity and site of aortic stenosis. It should be performed in all symptomatic patients. Hemodynamically significant stenosis is usually associated with a gradient of 50 mm Hg or greater (unless cardiac output is reduced, in which case the gradient may be much lower even if there is severe stenosis). The effective aortic valve orifice in patients with severe obstruction is usually less than 0.4 or 0.5 cm^2 per m^2 of body surface area (compared to 1.6 to 2.6 cm^2 per m^2 in normal people). Many laboratories report absolute, rather than normalized, valve areas. At some centers, aortic stenosis is considered severe if the valve area is less than 0.75 cm^2. At others, valve areas of less than 1.0 cm^2 are considered severe, 1.0 to 1.5 cm^2 considered moderate, and more than 1.5 cm^2 considered mild. At the time of catheterization, angiography is also done to assess LV function, the patency of the coronary arteries, and the degree, if any, of aortic and mitral regurgitation.

The cardiologist is likely to recommend replacement of the stenotic aortic valve with a prosthesis in all symptomatic patients and in asymptomatic patients with signs of severe obstruction who are found to have LV dysfunction or other high risk features.

Operative mortality in patients without LV failure is 5% to 10%; in patients with LV failure it is 10% to 25%. The patient's postoperative health and long-term survival depend on a number of factors (including age, general health, and LV function), but overall, the 5-year survival is approximately 80% to 85% and the 10-year survival is approximately 70% to 75%. Most patients experience a considerable improvement in their sense of well-being and exercise tolerance. If death does occur, it is usually due to a cardiac complication (heart failure, myocardial infarction, or sudden death). (For further details regarding the long-term course and management of the patient with a prosthetic valve, see below.)

The proper management of *aortic stenosis in the elderly* is a common clinical challenge. The prognosis in unoperated patients is very poor; in a Mayo Clinic study of 50 patients with a mean age of 77 years who were offered surgery but refused, only 57% were alive at 1 year and 25% at 3 years (13). In a study of aortic valve replacement in the elderly (14), a group of 44 octogenarians undergoing aortic valve replacement was compared with a group of 83 younger patients undergoing the procedure. Although the early mortality was higher in the elderly (14% vs. 4%), 2-year survival rates were similar (73% vs. 90%, an insignificant difference), the incidence of valve-related complications was comparable, and the total duration of hospital stay did not differ. Other studies confirm that aortic valve replacement is the most appropriate therapy for symptomatic elderly patients with aortic stenosis. Aortic valve replacement should not be withheld because of age itself, although intercurrent illness, common in the elderly, may complicate decision making.

Percutaneous balloon valvuloplasty is a technique in which one or more balloons are placed across a stenotic aortic valve and are then inflated in an attempt to reduce the severity of stenosis. This method has achieved excellent results in children with congenital aortic stenosis. In adults, it has been applied mainly to elderly patients or to those who are poor surgical candidates for other reasons. Although the transaortic gradient is usually reduced and initial clinical improvement is achieved, overall results have not been encouraging because high rates of death (24%) and recurrences of severe symptoms of aortic stenosis (47%) have been reported within 6 months of the procedure. Long-term survival after the procedure is dismal and resembles the natural history of untreated aortic stenosis (15). At present, aortic valvuloplasty for adults has been abandoned at most centers and should be considered only in extraordinary circumstances, for example, for a severely symptomatic and hemodynamically compromised patient who requires urgent management of aortic stenosis as a "bridge" to aortic valve replacement.

Hypertrophic Cardiomyopathy

HCM is a disease of cardiac muscle characterized by severe myocardial hypertrophy, in the absence of conditions that cause secondary hypertrophy of the heart muscle, such as hypertension and aortic stenosis. The left ventricle is hypercontractile and during systole ejects essentially all of its blood, leaving a "clenched fist" with very high wall stress. HCM has been called by a variety of names, including asymmetric septal hypertrophy (because of predominant hypertrophy in the septal region) and idiopathic hypertrophic subaortic stenosis (because of the common presence of a dynamic outflow tract gradient). However, some patients with HCM do not have asymmetric septal hypertrophy and may have either concentric hypertrophy or only apical hypertrophy of the left ventricle. In addition, not all patients with HCM have evidence of a dynamic outflow tract gradient. In contrast to the microscopic appearance of secondary LV hypertrophy, in which the fibers are enlarged but are properly oriented, the myofibrils in HCM are characterized by myofibrillary disarray.

Causes and Epidemiology

The prevalence of HCM in young adults is thought to be about 2 per 1,000 (16) but is higher in the elderly. The disease occurs as a familial inherited disease in about 60% of cases and as a sporadic disease, without affected first-degree relatives, in the remainder. Men and women are equally likely to be affected. In the familial form, the mode of inheritance is autosomal dominant in about 75% of pedigrees. A variety of mutations has been identified in patients with HCM, including in the beta-myosin heavy chain gene (chromosome 14), the cardiac troponin T gene (chromosome 1), and the alpha-tropomyosin gene (chromosome 15). All these genes code for sarcomeric proteins. The presence of these mutant components perturbs overall contractile function, and cardiac hypertrophy develops as a compensatory response.

Natural History and Symptoms

As echocardiography has become more widely used for the evaluation of patients with heart murmurs, it has become clear that most patients with HCM are asymptomatic or have only mild symptoms. Unless there is a family history of sudden death, the prognosis in this group is excellent; one study (17) of 25 patients showed neither death nor progression of disease over a 4.4-year follow-up period.

The most common symptom of patients with HCM is dyspnea, but patients also often complain of angina (with or without evidence of occlusive coronary artery disease) and syncope or near-syncope. These symptoms are much more likely to be induced by exertion than to occur spontaneously.

Once marked symptoms develop, some patients become rapidly worse, with progressive heart failure, angina, or arrhythmias. The most troublesome feature of the illness is its propensity to cause sudden death. The incidence of sudden death is approximately 3% to 4% per year in symptomatic patients with HCM, but some families have a particularly high incidence, depending on the specific mutation in the pedigree. For example, survival is poor in cardiac troponin T mutations but near normal in alpha-tropomyosin mutations (18).

Physical Findings

Clinical and laboratory features that distinguish aortic stenosis from HCM are listed in Table 65.2. The characteristic signs of the disease are a sustained LV apical impulse, a loud S_4, and a harsh systolic ejection murmur, loudest at the left lower border of the sternum and often accompanied by a thrill. The location of the murmur helps to distinguish the condition from valvular aortic stenosis. Other distinguishing features are as follows: The second heart sound (A_2) is usually audible, a diastolic murmur is rare, the pulse pressure is normal, ejection sounds are uncommon, and, most important, the upstroke of the carotid pulse is brisk. In addition, the murmur of HCM is augmented when the patient stands or performs a Valsalva maneuver and is diminished when the patient squats—the opposite of the findings in patients with aortic stenosis. The murmur often diminishes rapidly during the release phase of the Valsalva maneuver.

Laboratory Evaluation

An ECG, chest x-ray, and echocardiogram should be obtained routinely in patients suspected of having HCM. Genetic testing to identify the specific mutation should be considered (see below).

Electrocardiogram. The ECG is abnormal in most patients and is always abnormal in patients with obstruction. Typically, there is evidence of LV hypertrophy (Fig. 65.2 and Table 65.3), and there is nonspecific ST depression and T-wave inversion. Q waves are often seen in the inferior and lateral leads, reflecting septal hypertrophy.

Chest X-Ray. The left ventricle is sometimes enlarged, but unpredictably so. In contrast to aortic valvular stenosis, the aortic valve is not calcified and the ascending aorta is not dilated.

Echocardiogram. Echocardiography is diagnostic; it usually demonstrates a thickened ventricular septum, hypertrophied out of proportion to the posterior wall of the left ventricle, although concentric or apical hypertrophy is sometimes present. Cavity obliteration, or near cavity obliteration, usually occurs during systole. The mitral valve apparatus moves anteriorly during systole (systolic anterior motion), where it may contribute to obstruction of the outflow tract. Also, the aortic leaflets may close suddenly in early systole and reopen as systole continues. (These abnormalities of the aortic valve may be present only after the patient is administered amyl nitrite.)

Management

The goal of therapy is to reduce the hypercontractile state of the left ventricle. Currently this is best done by means of the calcium channel blocker verapamil (80 to 120 mg four times a day or a sustained-release preparation once a day) unless the patient has signs or symptoms of heart failure. Alternatively, a beta-blocker may be prescribed (e.g., metoprolol, 25 to 100 mg twice daily, or an equivalent sustained-release preparation). Angina, especially, is often relieved by treatment, but dyspnea also may be decreased as a result of a slower heart rate and of more time for the ventricle to fill. Although it is not clear that the risk of sudden death is reduced by therapy, most patients are symptomatically improved or at least stabilized by treatment. Disopyramide, a type 1A antiarrhythmic agent (see Chapter 64) with negative inotropic properties, has also been used successfully in patients with HCM, but possible proarrhythmic effects of the drug, due to prolongation of the Q-T interval, have not been well studied in this population.

Drugs that increase ventricular contractility or decrease ventricular volume (digitalis, vasodilators, beta-adrenergic stimulants, and diuretics) are best avoided if possible. Patients, even if asymptomatic, should avoid undue exertion (e.g., running).

There is an increased risk of endocarditis in patients with HCM, and these patients should therefore receive antibiotic prophylaxis before dental and surgical procedures (see Chapter 93).

Many patients with HCM eventually become refractory to beta-blockers or verapamil or develop intolerable side effects from those medications. Two new therapies have potential and are currently being studied. First, dual-chamber cardiac pacing, even in the absence of bradyarrhythmias, may result in a reduction in the symptoms of angina, dyspnea, and presyncope over 6 to 12 weeks. Some (19,20), but not all (21,22), studies have shown that objective measures of disease, such as exercise treadmill time and outflow tract gradient, also improve with this therapy. Second, studies suggest that alcohol ablation of a portion of the septum (injected during catheterization) causes a localized infarction with widening of the outflow tract and reduced gradient (23). Long-term trials have not yet been completed. The use of these techniques on a nonexperimental basis is still controversial. Patients with HCM who show progression of symptoms or intolerance of medical treatment should be referred to a cardiologist for consideration of these alternative treatments.

Surgical removal of a portion of the hypertrophied septum (septal myectomy) should be considered in severely symptomatic patients should other forms of therapy fail. Such a decision should be made in consultation with a cardiologist and a cardiac surgeon. Improved surgical techniques have reduced the perioperative mortality of this procedure to less than 5% (although it may be significantly higher in the elderly); symptoms are usually relieved (24) and long-term mortality is improved.

An implantable cardiac defibrillator may be placed in patients who have survived sudden death, have family members who have died suddenly, have high-risk mutations on genetic testing, or have been observed to have life-threatening ventricular arrhythmias.

Screening of relatives by echocardiography may detect other family members with the syndrome. In that case, referral to a center that can perform genetic testing to identify the specific mutation and offer genetic counseling should be considered.

Atrial Septal Defect

Atrial septal defect of the ostium secundum type (in the midportion of the septum) is one of the most common congenital cardiac diseases diagnosed in adults. It causes, until late in the course (see below), a left-to-right atrial shunt with a volume overload of the right ventricle and overperfusion of the lungs.

Causes and Epidemiology

The defect is more common in females; the reported female/male ratio ranges from 1.5 to 3.5:1. Occasionally the defect is associated with other cardiac abnormalities, including mitral valve prolapse and HCM.

Natural History and Symptoms

Patients with atrial septal defect are usually asymptomatic until their third or fourth decade. Thereafter, symptoms almost always develop (usually dyspnea on exertion, fatigue, and palpitations), the result of heart failure and supraventricular arrhythmias. Less commonly, symptoms of pulmonary embolism (see Chapter 59) or paradoxical embolism (e.g., a stroke) occur. Virtually all patients are symptomatic by age 60. In fact, three-fourths of untreated patients are dead by age 50 and 90% by age 60. Increased pulmonary blood flow eventually produces pulmonary vascular disease and, consequently, pulmonary hypertension in approximately 15% of patients (25). When this happens, the left-to-right shunt first decreases and then reverses; at that point, cyanosis develops. Coexistent atherosclerotic or hypertensive cardiovascular disease may complicate the course of older patients with atrial septal defect and may make diagnosis and treatment more difficult.

Physical Findings

Atrial septal defect usually causes a wide fixed splitting of the second heart sound due to late closure of the pulmonic valve as a result of increased flow into the right atrium and right ventricle. A soft blowing systolic pulmonic ejection murmur and a low to medium frequency mid-diastolic flow murmur across the tricuspid valve are common. The precordium may be hyperdynamic with a palpable S_3. If pulmonary hypertension has developed (see below), clubbing and cyanosis may be observed, and P_2 is accentuated. Signs of right ventricular failure (edema, distended neck veins, hepatomegaly) are common late in the disease.

Laboratory Evaluation

An ECG, a chest x-ray, and an echocardiogram should be obtained routinely in a patient suspected of having an atrial septal defect.

Electrocardiogram. The ECG displays an incomplete right bundle branch block or rSR′ in lead V_1 90% to 95% of the time. If the defect is of the secundum type, a vertical frontal plane axis or right axis deviation is usually present. The presence of frank right ventricular hypertrophy suggests that pulmonary hypertension has developed. Ostium primum atrial septal defect, a less common form of atrial septal defect that occurs as part of the spectrum of endocardial cushion defect, is distinguished by the presence of left axis deviation. Atrial fibrillation occurs commonly in symptomatic patients; atrial flutter and paroxysmal atrial tachycardia occur less often.

Chest X-Ray. The chest x-ray in this disease is almost always abnormal and shows increased pulmonary vascularity with a prominent main pulmonary artery and increased heart size (Fig. 65.3). The right pulmonary artery is usually more prominent than the left because of differential flow.

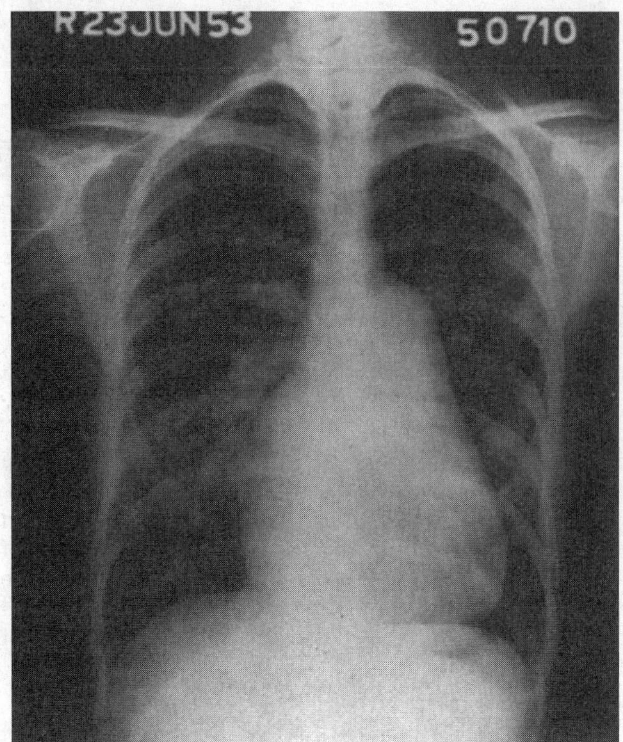

Figure 65.3. Chest x-ray of a patient with atrial septal defect.

Echocardiogram. The echocardiogram demonstrates right ventricular enlargement and paradoxical motion of the ventricular septum with respect to the posterior wall of the left ventricle. These findings are also seen with other lesions that cause volume overload of the right ventricle, such as tricuspid and pulmonic regurgitation, and partial anomalous pulmonary venous return. Flow across the atrial septum can often be visualized by using color Doppler echocardiography. Contrast echocardiography, in which agitated saline is injected intravenously and is visualized echocardiographically as bubbles, usually can detect the presence of some right-to-left shunting across the atrial septum, even if the direction of the shunt is predominantly left-to-right.

Management

Patients suspected of having an atrial septal defect should be referred to a cardiologist for definitive diagnosis. The cardiologist usually performs TEE and, if the patient is over 40 years old, cardiac catheterization (see Chapter 62 for a description of the patient experience). All patients, even if they are asymptomatic, should have their defect repaired if pulmonary blood flow is more than 1.5 times systemic blood flow. The operative mortality is less than 2%, although some degree of persistent right ventricular or LV dysfunction is common in adults. If severe pulmonary hypertension has developed (pulmonary pressure equal to or greater than the systemic pressure), corrective surgery is generally contraindicated, but patients with lesser degrees of pulmonary hypertension may still benefit from repair of the defect. Survival after corrective surgery is influenced by the age of the patient and the degree of persistent cardiac dysfunction. Patients with otherwise normal hearts have normal survival rates after successful repair of the atrial defect and usually can resume normal activity. Endocarditis prophylaxis is unnecessary for patients with isolated atrial septal defect (see Chapter 93).

Mitral Regurgitation

Mitral regurgitation may develop because of an abnormality of any part of the mitral valve apparatus: the valve leaflets, the chordae tendineae, the papillary muscles, or the annulus. Such abnormalities may result in either acute or chronic signs and symptoms, depending on the nature of the lesion.

An incompetent mitral valve allows regurgitation into the left atrium of blood from the left ventricle. The reduced load on the ventricle reduces the tension in the ventricular muscle and allows it to use more energy in contraction. Therefore, in patients with chronic mitral regurgitation, cardiac output remains normal for years until, because of age or intercurrent disease, the ventricle can no longer compensate and heart failure ensues. In patients with acute mitral regurgitation, ventricular compensation is inadequate and heart failure develops abruptly.

Chronic Mitral Regurgitation

Causes and Epidemiology. Chronic mitral incompetence in adults may occur in association with a variety of disorders. Rheumatic fever is the cause of only 5% to 15% of cases. Otherwise, chronic mitral regurgitation is most often caused by papillary muscle necrosis (the result of ischemic heart disease), an inherited (e.g., Marfan syndrome or mitral prolapse; see below) or an acquired disorder of connective tissue, idiopathic calcification of the valve (primarily a disorder of the elderly), endocarditis, left ventricular dilatation, or congenital maldevelopment of the mitral apparatus.

Natural History and Symptoms. The left ventricle characteristically adapts to the increased preload of mitral regurgitation by adding new sarcomeres in series, which returns preload toward normal. The chamber becomes larger and more compliant and fully compensates for the volume overload by increasing the end-diastolic volume and stroke volume. Patients may therefore remain asymptomatic for many years, even for their entire lives, if the regurgitation is not severe (26). Characteristically, when symptoms do develop, they appear gradually over years as LV dysfunction slowly develops, and the ability to compensate for the loss of more than half of the stroke volume back into the left atrium is lost. Dyspnea and fatigue are the usual symptoms of LV failure. Supraventricular arrhythmias, especially atrial fibrillation, are likely to develop if left atrial enlargement becomes marked, compromising somewhat the ability of the heart to compensate. Acute pulmonary edema occasionally occurs but is uncommon. Sometimes severe pulmonary hypertension develops without much enlargement of the left atrium. Early surgical correction of the lesion in patients with pulmonary hypertension and signs of right ventricular hypertrophy is important.

In a series of symptomatic patients with mitral regurgitation, 80% treated medically survived 5 years and 60% survived 10 years (27). Moderately to severely symptomatic patients do less well; in one report 46% of patients with chronic rheumatic mitral insufficiency survived 5 years (28).

Physical Findings. A high-pitched holosystolic murmur, loudest at the apex, is characteristic of chronic mitral regurgitation (patients with mild regurgitation may have only a late systolic murmur). The holosystolic murmur is constant in intensity and radiates always to the axilla and sometimes to the back and the base of the heart. It is best heard when the patient is in the left lateral decubitus position. The murmur is diminished when the patient stands or performs a Valsalva maneuver and is intensified when the patient squats. If regurgitation is severe, the precordium is usually hyperdynamic and there is an S_3 gallop. S_1 is soft. If pulmonary hypertension has developed, an S_4 gallop, a loud P_2, and a right ventricular heave may be appreciated. Signs of right ventricular failure—edema, hepatomegaly, distended neck veins, hepatojugular reflux—may also be seen late in the course of this disease.

Laboratory Evaluation. An ECG, a chest x-ray, and an echocardiogram should be obtained routinely if a patient is suspected of having mitral regurgitation.

Electrocardiogram. The ECG shows evidence of left atrial enlargement (Fig. 65.4 and Table 65.5) and, if present, of atrial fibrillation. The pattern of LV hypertrophy (Fig. 65.2 and Table 65.3) is often seen as well, primarily in patients with severe disease. A pattern of right ventricular hypertrophy (Table 65.6), indicating pulmonary hypertension is less common and, when seen, is cause for great concern.

Chest X-Ray. LV and left atrial enlargement are common. On a posteroanterior film, elevation of the left bronchus and prominence of the left atrial appendage are the earliest signs of left atrial enlargement; a double density is seen posteriorly when the left atrium is grossly enlarged (Fig. 65.5).

Echocardiogram. Echocardiography demonstrates left atrial and LV enlargement and hyperdynamic motion of the left ventricle, especially the septum. 2D echocardiography can usually define the etiology of the valvular disease (i.e., rheumatic, prolapsing, ischemic). Color Doppler echocardiography (see above) is sensitive in detecting mitral regurgitation and can estimate its severity.

Table 65.5. Principal Electrocardiographic Features of Left Atrial Enlargement

P wave	
Axis	+45 degrees to −30 degrees
Amplitude (II, III, aVF) duration	>0.11 sec (broad)
Component (V_1)	
Early	Positive but inside normal
Late	Negative, ≥0.04 area units[a]

Modified from Horan LG, Flowers NC. Electrocardiography and vectorcardiography. In: Braunwald E, ed. Heart disease: a textbook of cardiovascular medicine. Philadelphia: WB Saunders, 1980;226, with permission.

[a]Area units = mm-sec. One small block on standard ECG paper = 0.04 mm-sec.

Table 65.6. Electrocardiographic Criteria of Right Ventricular Hypertrophy in Adults without Conduction Defects Known *Not* to Have Infarction

Sign	Points[a]
Ratio reversal (R/S V_5:R/S V_1 ≤0.4)	5
qR in V_1	5
R/S ratio in V_1>1	4
S in V_1 <2 mm	4
R in V_1 + S in V_5 or V_6 >10.5 mm	4
Right -axis deviation >100 degrees	4
S in V_5 or V_6 ≥7 mm and each ≥2 mm	3
R/S in V_5 or V_6 ≤1	3
R in V_1 ≥7 mm	3
S_1, S_2, and S_3 each ≥1 mm	2
S_1 and Q_3 each ≥1 mm	2
R′ in V_1 earlier than 0.08 sec and ≥2 mm	2
R peak in V_1 or V_2 between 0.04 and 0.07 sec	1
S in V_5 or V_6 >2 mm but <7 mm	1
Reduction in V lead R/S ratio between V_1 and V_4	1
R in V_5 or V_6 <5 mm	1

Modified from Horan LG, Flowers NC. Electrocardiography and vectorcardiography. In: Braunwald E, ed. Heart disease: a textbook of cardiovascular medicine. Philadelphia: WB Saunders, 1980;226, with permission.

[a]Interpretation of point score: 10 points, right ventricular hypertrophy; 7 to 9 points, probable right ventricular hypertrophy or hemodynamic overload; 5 to 6 points, possible right ventricular hypertrophy or hemodynamic overload. These criteria do not take into account serial ECG comparisons. Such additional data may alter the interpreter's impression of the likelihood of fixed enlargement or dynamic overload.

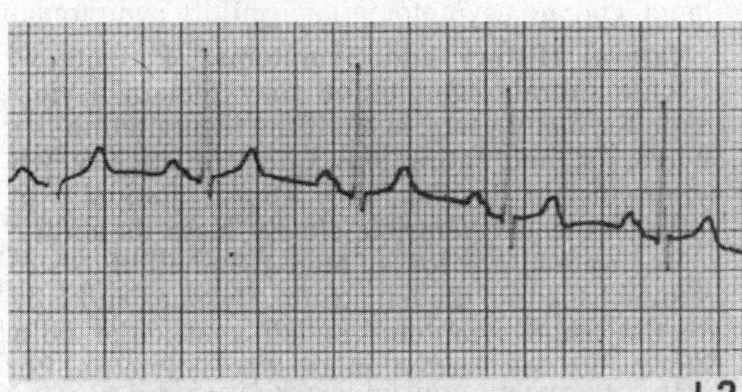

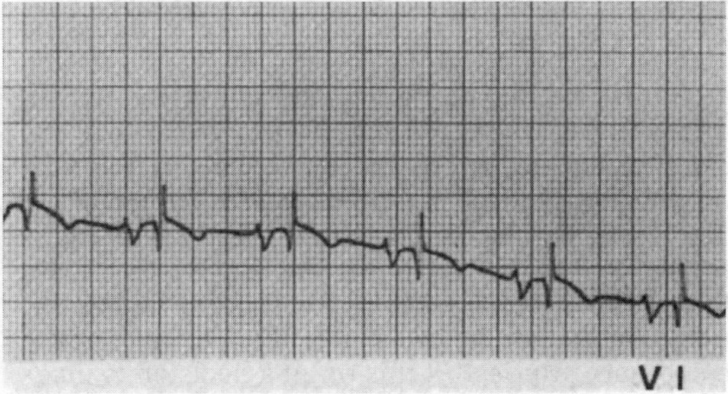

Figure 65.4. Electrocardiogram of a patient with left atrial enlargement (Table 65.5).

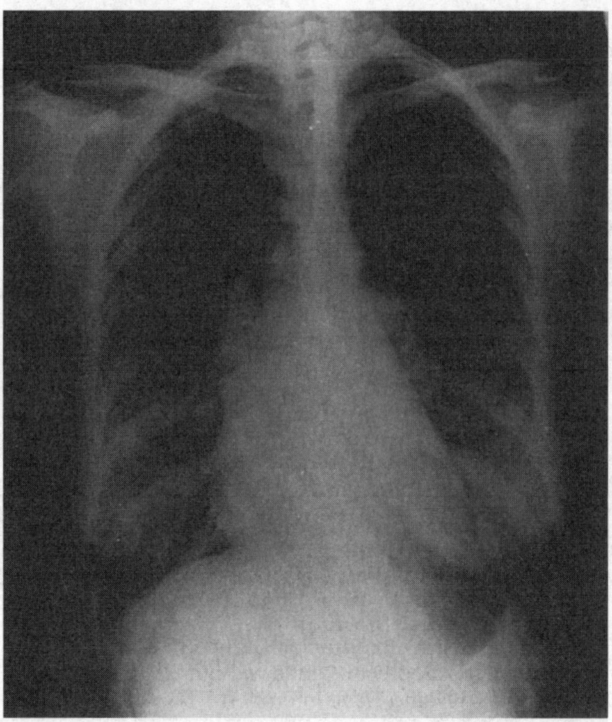

Figure 65.5. Chest x-ray of a patient with left atrial enlargement. Note the straight left heart border and the calcification of the wall of the left atrium.

Management. Patients who have mild disease (graded by the clinical examination and Doppler echocardiography) can be managed medically (see below). Antibiotic prophylaxis against bacterial endocarditis should be administered before all dental and surgical procedures (see Chapter 93). If atrial fibrillation is present, restoration of sinus rhythm should be attempted to reduce the risk of embolism and slow progression of atrial enlargement, unless the left atrium is greatly enlarged or mitral regurgitation has been present for years. (A detailed discussion of the treatment of atrial fibrillation is in Chapter 64.) However, the development of atrial fibrillation may represent a marker of severe or progressive disease, the management of which is discussed below. Likewise, the new onset of heart failure may signal either worsening of mitral regurgitation or the development of secondary LV dysfunction and may constitute an indication for surgical intervention.

The management of moderate and severe mitral regurgitation depends on the severity of symptoms and on LV function. In patients who are symptomatic with fatigue, congestive heart failure, or arrhythmias, mitral valve replacement or repair may be indicated and referral to a cardiologist should be made (Table 65.7). It is likely that cardiac catheterization and angiography (see Chapter 62) will be done to confirm the diagnosis, establish the severity of the lesion, and evaluate the function of the left ventricle and, often, the patency of the coronary arteries. At this point a decision is made about the value of operative repair of the lesion. Unless the patient has severe noncardiac disease or LV function is so severely reduced that the patient would not tolerate an operation, replacement or repair of the defective valve is very likely to be recommended. The operative mortality is largely dependent on preoperative ejection fraction but averages about 2% to 5%.

Table 65.7. Indications for Referral of Patients with Mitral Regurgitation

Dyspnea or fatigue
Development of supraventricular arrhythmia, particularly atrial fibrillation
An asymptomatic patient with moderate or severe disease, especially if there is progressive cardiac enlargement or an ejection fraction less than 60%
Uncertainty about the diagnosis
Acute mitral regurgitation
Patients with mitral valve prolapse who have symptomatic arrhythmias; chronic, moderate, or severe mitral regurgitation; infectious endocarditis; or transient ischemic attacks

Because mitral regurgitation is often well tolerated for years or even decades, many patients are asymptomatic. However, the long-standing chronic volume overload often results in a gradual deterioration in LV function, which greatly increases the risk and reduces the benefit of mitral valve repair or replacement when it eventually becomes necessary. Progressive LV dysfunction may be difficult to detect using the usual means of assessment of wall motion (echocardiography and gated blood pool scanning) because regurgitation into the low-pressure left atrium reduces the afterload of the left ventricle during ejection and results in exaggerated wall motion and falsely optimistic estimates of contractility. Many patients develop irreversible LV dysfunction before they report symptoms, even if the ejection fraction has remained within normal limits. In patients with severe mitral regurgitation caused by flail leaflet, this insidious ventricular dysfunction results in a high annual mortality rate (4.1%) even if symptoms are minimal or absent and early surgery is associated with an improved prognosis (29). In this group, at the end of a follow-up period of 10 years, 90% of patients have either undergone surgical treatment or died. These observations, coupled with recent success in mitral valve repair procedures (see below), which avoid saddling the patient with the burdens of a prosthetic valve, suggest that surgery should be performed earlier in the course of the disease than had previously been recommended, even in patients who are asymptomatic or mildly symptomatic. The diagnosis of moderate or severe mitral regurgitation is therefore an indication for referral of the patient to a cardiologist. The recommendation may be to follow patients with ejection fractions above 60% (measured by annual echocardiograms or gated blood pool scans), looking for an increase in end-diastolic or end-systolic dimension or a reduction in wall motion. However, in patients with ejection fractions near the low end of normal (55% to 60%) or below or end-systolic dimension of greater than or equal to 4.5 cm, early surgery will probably be advised (30).

Afterload reduction by use of an arteriolar vasodilator may be particularly useful in this condition; by lowering peripheral resistance, ejection of blood into the aorta, rather than back into the left atrium, is favored. Intravenous vasodilator therapy can result in dramatic hemodynamic improvement in hospitalized patients with congestive heart failure caused by mitral regurgitation. Based on that observation, it seems reasonable to use oral vasodilators in patients with mitral regurgitation who are not yet ready for surgery. If a beneficial hemodynamic effect could be sustained, it might be possible to delay the development of LV dysfunction or symptoms and postpone the need for surgery. Although this approach is often taken in asymptomatic patients, the efficacy of long-term vasodilator therapy in this regard has not been well studied, and recommendations based on randomized trials cannot be made. However, the use of vasodilators in patients with congestive heart failure caused by mitral regurgitation is well established.

The health and survival of patients who have undergone successful valve replacement depend on a number of factors (also see below). Advanced age, the presence of concomitant mitral stenosis, reduced LV function (ejection fraction under 50%), and severity of symptoms preoperatively (New York Heart Association class III or IV; see Chapter 66) are adverse factors that reduce long-term postoperative survival. In general, patients with mitral regurgitation on the basis of ischemic heart disease do less well than patients with rheumatic heart disease. Nevertheless, even patients with one or more adverse risk factors live longer, on the average, with a prosthetic valve than they would without one, and most patients are able to be more active than they were before surgery. The overall 10-year survival for patients who have undergone successful mitral surgery is approximately 70%. Postoperatively, anticoagulation with warfarin is used routinely to prevent thromboembolic complications in patients with mechanical prosthetic valves (see Chapter 57).

Surgical reconstruction of the incompetent mitral valve has been shown to be an excellent alternative to mitral valve replacement, particularly for valves leaking because of myxomatous degeneration (see Mitral Valve Prolapse, below). Repair is most likely to be feasible if the etiology of the mitral regurgitation is flail posterior leaflet. Repaired valves usually maintain their competency (92%), seem not to be susceptible to infectious endocarditis, and do not require chronic anticoagulation (1). Valve repair results in better operative mortality, long-term survival, and postoperative ejection fraction than does valve replacement (31). The decision about whether to recommend valve repair or replacement depends on the availability of a surgeon who is skilled at this procedure and is usually made in consultation with the cardiologist and the cardiac surgeon.

Acute Mitral Regurgitation

Causes and Epidemiology. Acute mitral incompetence is most often caused by rupture of the chordae tendineae, the cords that connect the valve cusps to the papillary muscles of the left ventricle. Most of the time the cause of the rupture is myxomatous degeneration of the valve (see Mitral Valve Prolapse, below), although occasionally acute mitral regurgitation is caused by papillary muscle rupture or dysfunction (complications of myocardial infarction) or by perforation of a mitral cusp as the result of bacterial endocarditis. The disorder is primarily encountered in middle-aged and elderly patients.

Natural History and Symptoms. Because the left atrium is suddenly presented with a volume load to which it cannot rapidly accommodate, acute pulmonary edema is much more common in patients with acute, compared with chronic, mitral regurgitation.

Physical Findings. A harsh holosystolic murmur of constant intensity, loudest at the apex, is characteristic; if a posterior cord has ruptured, the murmur may radiate to the base of the heart and may mimic the murmur of aortic stenosis. Sometimes an early systolic or midsystolic, or even a crescendo/decrescendo, murmur is heard. An S_3 gallop is almost always heard, and an S_4 gallop is common. Unlike the situation in patients with chronic mitral regurgitation, S_1 is normal or even loud. Signs of left-sided heart failure (rales) and right-sided failure (edema, distended neck veins) are also common.

Laboratory Findings

Chest X-Ray. The chest x-ray shows marked pulmonary congestion. The left atrium and the left ventricle are minimally enlarged.

Echocardiogram. Chamber enlargement is usually not seen, but increased systolic motion of the valve is common. If the chordae have ruptured, the flailing chordae or marked prolapse of the leaflets into the left atrium may be visualized by 2D echocardiography. Doppler echocardiography allows detection of the lesion, but Doppler criteria for estimating the severity of acute mitral regurgitation are not yet established.

Management. Patients suspected of having acute mitral regurgitation should be hospitalized immediately for diagnosis, treatment of acute heart failure, and consideration for early operative repair.

Mitral Valve Prolapse

Causes and Epidemiology

Systolic prolapse of a leaflet of the mitral valve into the left atrium has proved to be a common phenomenon. Women are more likely to be affected than are men, although reported sex ratios vary considerably. The exact nature of this abnormality is not entirely clear, but in most cases, the condition appears to be inherited (autosomal dominant), with reduced penetrance in men and children. Histologic study of prolapsing valves removed at operation shows myxomatous degeneration, a proliferation of the spongiosa layer of mucopolysaccharides into the fibrosa layer of collagen, resulting in a weakness in the supporting structure of the valve. This abnormality is also seen in a number of known disorders of connective tissue, including Marfan syndrome and Ehlers-Danlos syndrome. However, echocardiographic prolapse is also often reported in patients with documented coronary artery disease, hypertrophic cardiomyopathy and atrial septal defect, and these cases may represent secondary prolapse in which the valve is normal but changes in ventricular geometry cause prolapsing of the leaflets. In these secondary cases, the click and associated symptoms (see below) usually are not present.

Natural History and Symptoms

Most patients are asymptomatic, and the condition is identified during a routine physical examination. Less often, patients complain of palpitations, chest pain, or dyspnea. The palpitations reflect arrhythmias (see below) or, more commonly, just an awareness of sinus tachycardia. The chest pain is often vague and inconstant and, rather than constituting a true part of the mitral valve prolapse syndrome, may represent ascertainment bias (32). That is, patients with nonspecific complaints may be found to have mitral valve prolapse coincidentally, and an incorrect association is made (33). Similarly, dyspnea in the absence of significant mitral regurgitation may be unrelated to the syndrome (34).

In most patients the syndrome is benign. However, in approximately 15% of patients significant mitral regurgitation occurs, and patients may complain of dyspnea caused by LV failure. Approximately 3% to 4% of patients require mitral valve surgery during a follow-up period of about 8 years (35).

Some studies have suggested that patients with mitral valve prolapse are at risk for embolic strokes (36), but others have ascribed this finding to ascertainment bias (34). The risk of infective endocarditis in patients with mitral valve prolapse is approximately five times that of the general population. This risk is highest in patients with mitral regurgitation or thickened mitral leaflets.

The most feared complication of mitral valve prolapse, sudden death, is extremely rare. The risk is higher in patients with a family history of sudden death or in patients with a prolonged Q-T interval on their ECG (see below).

The hemodynamic and infectious complications appear to be more common in men than in women and in patients who have mitral regurgitation at the time of presentation. The echocardiographic findings of thickening and redundancy of the mitral leaflet also identify patients with mitral valve prolapse who are at higher risk (37). These findings allow targeting of prophylactic antibiotic therapy and frequent follow-up of specific groups.

Physical Findings

The characteristic finding in patients with mitral prolapse is a midsystolic click, best heard at the lower left sternal border, caused by sudden tensing of the prolapsed valve. It occurs later than the systolic ejection sound heard commonly in association with systemic hypertension (see above). Very often the click is followed immediately by a crescendo late systolic murmur that continues until A_2.

The physical findings may vary from time to time in any given patient and may also vary with the position of the patient. Standing generally augments the click and makes it occur earlier in systole, because afterload is reduced and the ventricle becomes smaller with respect to the mitral valve, increasing the prolapse. Squatting and isometric handgrip increase afterload and have the opposite effect. In those rare instances in which chronic mitral regurgitation has developed, the typical physical findings—including the holosystolic murmur—of this condition will be encountered (see above).

The mitral valve prolapse syndrome is commonly associated with skeletal abnormalities, such as scoliosis and pectus excavatum, suggesting that valve prolapse may be only one component of a generalized disease of connective tissue.

Laboratory Findings

Electrocardiogram. The ECG is usually normal, especially in asymptomatic patients. Symptomatic patients may show nonspecific ST-T wave changes, usually in the inferior leads, and sometimes prolongation of the Q-T interval. A variety of arrhythmias may occur in patients with mitral valve prolapse. The most common are premature ventricular contractions and paroxysmal supraventricular tachycardia.

Echocardiogram. The echocardiogram usually is diagnostic in this condition. It shows late systolic or holosystolic prolapse of one or both leaflets of the mitral valve. Sometimes, however, the echocardiogram shows no abnormalities despite the typical cardiac findings. These patients probably have minor degrees of prolapse. Mitral regurgitation, if present, can be detected by Doppler echocardiography (see above).

Management

Asymptomatic patients need no treatment but should be reassessed by interval history, physical examination, and echocardiogram every few years. Care should be taken to ensure that the diagnosis does not produce unwarranted anxiety. Patients who have a systolic murmur or echocardiographic evidence of thickening or redundancy of the mitral leaflet should receive prophylaxis against bacterial endocarditis before dental or surgical procedures (see Chapter 93). Other patients probably do not need prophylaxis.

Patients with palpitations should have ambulatory electrocardiographic monitoring or event monitoring to determine the severity of their arrhythmia, and therapy should be prescribed on the basis of the type of arrhythmia that is present (see Chapter 64). A beta-blocking agent is often a drug of choice in the treatment of these patients and also in those with mitral prolapse who complain of chest pain or who have persistent palpitations caused by sinus tachycardia (e.g., long-acting propranolol, usual dosage 40 to 120 mg/day, or atenolol 25 to 50 mg/day). The mechanism of action of the drug in the relief of pain is unknown but may be explained by the fact that many untreated patients have been shown to have increased blood levels of norepinephrine and to have increased sympathetic tone.

Patients with symptomatic mitral regurgitation should be treated as described above. Referral to a cardiologist is recommended at any time patients become symptomatic from arrhythmia (other than sinus tachycardia), chronic mitral regurgitation, or thromboembolism.

A pamphlet published by the American Heart Association, titled "Mitral Valve Prolapse," provides a clear explanation of the syndrome to patients and may help allay the anxiety that many patients with mitral valve prolapse feel regarding their risk of complications. The booklet is available through local American Heart Association offices. Information is also available through the American Heart Association website at http://www.americanheart.org.

Mitral Stenosis

Stenosis of the mitral valve obstructs the flow of blood out of the left atrium and therefore raises the left atrial pressure above the LV diastolic pressure. The pressure gradient across the valve and the area of the valve orifice are measures of the severity of the stenosis. Because of the increase in left atrial pressure, there is an increase in pressure in the pulmonary blood vessels and a tendency to develop atrial fibrillation. The pulmonary congestion and atrial fibrillation account for most of the symptoms of the disease.

Causes and Epidemiology

By far the most common cause of mitral stenosis in adults is rheumatic fever (although a history of rheumatic fever can be elicited in only 50% of patients with pure mitral stenosis). Pure mitral stenosis occurs in 40% of all patients with rheumatic heart disease. The rest of the time there is associated mitral regurgitation, aortic valve disease, and, uncommonly, tricuspid valve disease. Two-thirds of patients with rheumatic mitral stenosis are women.

Natural History and Symptoms

On average, there is a latent period of nearly 20 years between an attack of acute rheumatic fever and the development of symptomatic mitral stenosis (38). Thus, symptoms usually do not develop before the fourth decade. The severity of symptoms is quite variable. In fact, some people are never symptomatic, some are mildly symptomatic indefinitely, and some develop progressively severe cardiopulmonary decompensation. Of the patients with progressive disease, it has been estimated that an average of 7 years elapses between the onset of symptoms and the development of total disability (class IV cardiac status; see Chapter 66). In one series the 5-year survival from that point in patients treated medically was only 15% (39).

Pulmonary congestion causes many of the symptoms of mitral stenosis: dyspnea, orthopnea, and paroxysmal nocturnal dyspnea. If left atrial pressure rises acutely because of a sudden stress, frank pulmonary edema may occur. Hemoptysis caused by rupture of small bronchial veins or by pulmonary edema is not unusual.

As the disease progresses, pulmonary hypertension develops followed by symptoms of right heart failure: edema, distended neck veins, a tender liver, and ascites. At this point, the flow of blood into the left heart is limited and the pulmonary arterioles hypertrophy, diminishing the risk of pulmonary edema. Low cardiac output is responsible for the fatigue that is a common complaint of patients at this stage.

Atrial fibrillation (see Chapter 64) complicates the course of 40% to 50% of patients with mitral stenosis. The 20% reduction in blood flow across the mitral valve by the subsequent loss of left atrial contraction may intensify symptoms of heart failure and fatigue.

At some time in their course, 20% of patients with mitral stenosis experience symptomatic thromboembolism, most often to the brain; 80% of these patients are in atrial fibrillation.

Physical Findings

A mid-diastolic rumbling murmur with presystolic accentuation is characteristic of mitral stenosis. It is best heard at, and is often limited to, the cardiac apex. To hear it, it may be necessary to turn the patient to the left lateral position and to have him or her expire fully. Sometimes the patient must be exercised before the murmur is audible. The murmur is best heard with the bell of the stethoscope pressed lightly against the chest. A loud first heart sound and opening snap (see above) usually accompany the murmur when the valve is mobile. Late in the course, signs of pulmonary hypertension (a loud P_2 and a right ventricular heave) and of right heart failure may be found.

Laboratory Findings

Electrocardiogram. The ECG shows left atrial enlargement (Fig. 65.4 and Table 65.5) in 90% of patients who are in sinus rhythm. With the development of pulmonary hypertension, signs of right ventricular hypertrophy appear (Table 65.6).

Chest X-Ray. Left atrial enlargement (see above and Fig. 65.5) is seen in virtually all patients with symptomatic mitral stenosis, but the size of the left atrium does not correlate with the severity of stenosis. Late in the course right ventricular and right atrial hypertrophy are seen as well. Symptomatic patients are also likely to show radiologic signs of pulmonary congestion, the severity of which determines the findings that are seen (see Chapter 66). Calcification of the mitral valve is not unusual in patients with long-standing mitral stenosis, but it is better visualized by fluoroscopy or echocardiography than by a plain x-ray.

Echocardiogram. Mitral stenosis can be easily diagnosed by echocardiography. Mitral valve thickening can be seen; there is reduced excursion of the anterior leaflet of the valve and abnormal anterior motion of the posterior leaflet during diastole (it normally moves posteriorly). The severity of the stenosis can be accurately assessed by 2D and Doppler echocardiography (see above).

Management

Asymptomatic patients in normal sinus rhythm need no treatment except prophylaxis for bacterial endocarditis when they are to undergo dental or surgical procedures (see Chapter 93) and warfarin in some cases (see below). Newly diagnosed adult patients with mitral stenosis do not ordinarily require prophylaxis for beta-hemolytic streptococcal infection unless they have had an attack of rheumatic fever within the last 5 to 10 years or are in a population where beta-hemolytic streptococcal infection is more prevalent (e.g., military personnel or hospital workers). Patients who have received prophylaxis throughout childhood should continue to receive it indefinitely. When prophylaxis is necessary, the best regimen is 1 to 2 million units of benzathine penicillin G intramuscularly once a month.

Asymptomatic patients who develop atrial fibrillation, however, should be considered for balloon valvuloplasty because atrial fibrillation has its own long-term sequelae that should be avoided if possible (40). Valvuloplasty should also be considered in asymptomatic patients with moderate or severe mitral stenosis who are planning pregnancy because symptoms are likely to occur in late pregnancy and pulmonary edema may occur during labor.

Mildly symptomatic patients should be treated with diuretics and sodium restriction (see Chapter 66 for a detailed discussion of the treatment of heart failure). Because it does not affect the hemodynamic abnormality, digitalis is not useful in this situation unless rapid atrial fibrillation or flutter develops. Although the use of beta-blockers has been advocated in patients with mitral stenosis in normal sinus rhythm (to reduce heart rate and prolong the diastolic filling period), randomized studies have not demonstrated a clinical benefit (41).

Warfarin anticoagulants should be administered to patients with mild mitral stenosis who have had one or more episodes of systemic or pulmonary thromboembolism (see Chapter 57), who are in atrial fibrillation, or who have echocardiographic evidence of left atrial enlargement. All patients with moderate or severe mitral stenosis should be treated with anticoagulants.

The poor prognosis of symptomatic medically treated patients with severe or progressive disease (see Natural History and Symptoms, above) dictates that such patients should be offered a mechanical procedure to improve transmitral flow, either percutaneous balloon valvuloplasty or valve surgery. Percutaneous valvuloplasty can be achieved using a balloon catheter passed through the venous system and then across the atrial septum to the mitral valve. This procedure is generally effective in patients who have low LV end-diastolic pressures, who do not have New York Heart Association class IV symptoms, and in whom the echocardiogram shows good mitral valve mobility and minimal valvular or subvalvular thickening and calcification. It is contraindicated in patients who have moderate-to-severe mitral regurgitation or a left atrial thrombus by TEE (1). In a prospective randomized trial comparing percutaneous valvuloplasty with open surgical commissurotomy in suitable patients, after the procedure the size of the mitral valve orifice and functional class were better in the percutaneous group than in the surgical group (40). Of the patients who underwent percutaneous valvuloplasty, 72% were asymptomatic after 3 years, compared with 57% of the surgically treated patients. The better hemodynamic results, lower costs, and elimination of need for thoracotomy suggest that balloon valvuloplasty should be considered for all suitable patients. The procedure is well tolerated and effective even in elderly frail patients. From the patient's perspective, the procedure is similar to a catheterization. Patients sometimes feel faint during balloon inflation. An overnight hospitalization is required.

In patients requiring mechanical release of mitral valve obstruction who are not suitable for percutaneous valvuloplasty, the preferred surgical procedure depends on the anatomy of the valve at the time of operation. If possible, a mitral commissurotomy is performed. The operative mortality of this procedure is low (1% to 3%) and the results are excellent for a number of years. However, after commissurotomy, 10% of patients within 5 years and 60% within 10 years require reoperation because of restenosis or because of the development of symptomatic mitral regurgitation or symptomatic aortic stenosis. If a prosthetic valve is implanted, the operative mortality is 3% to 10%; the course of patients who survive surgery depends on a number of factors (see below) but certainly is better than that of symptomatic patients treated medically. Table 65.8 lists the reasons to refer patients with mitral stenosis to a cardiologist.

Aortic Regurgitation

An incompetent aortic valve allows regurgitation into the left ventricle of blood ejected into the aorta. To compensate for the increased volume load, the left ventricle dilates and hypertrophies, so the effective stroke volume may be normal for a long time. Eventually, however, the left ventricle cannot maintain the workload, and clinical signs and symptoms of heart failure ensue.

Table 65.8. Indications for Referral of Patients with Mitral Stenosis

Asymptomatic or symptomatic patients who develop atrial fibrillation or show evidence of pulmonary hypertension
Dyspnea or recurrent attacks of pulmonary edema
Symptomatic disease of the aortic or tricuspid valve
Women, whether symptomatic or not, who wish to become or who are pregnant
Patients with chronic obstructive lung disease
Patients with angina pectoris

Modified from Brandenburg RO, Fuster V, Giuliani ER. Valvular heart disease. When should the patient be referred? Pract Cardiol 1979;5:50, with permission.

Causes and Epidemiology

Aortic regurgitation may be caused by disease of the aortic valve cusps or dilation of the aortic root. Rheumatic fever now accounts for less than 15% of cases of chronic aortic valvular incompetence (42), many fewer cases than it did 20 to 30 years ago. Congenital aortic valvular incompetence caused by a bicuspid valve accounts for 12% of cases. Bacterial endocarditis is the most common cause of acute aortic valvular incompetence. Traumatic rupture of a cusp of the aortic valve is uncommon.

Chronic aortic regurgitation is caused by dilation of the aortic root in 12% of cases, most commonly idiopathic. Rare causes include rheumatoid arthritis, ankylosing spondylitis, Reiter syndrome, congenital disorders of connective tissue (Marfan syndrome, Ehlers-Danlos syndrome, and osteogenesis imperfecta), and syphilitic aortitis. Acute aortic regurgitation caused by dilation of the aortic root is most commonly caused by aortic dissection, usually associated with medial necrosis of the aorta. Dissection is associated with systemic hypertension in approximately 50% of cases; occasionally a primary disorder of connective tissue, such as Marfan syndrome, can be incriminated. Aortic regurgitation in general is more common in men than women, but there are specific exceptions (e.g., rheumatoid arthritis).

Natural History and Symptoms

In chronic aortic regurgitation, volume overload is usually tolerated for years or decades because of adaptive dilation and hypertrophy that maintains cardiac performance in or near the normal range. Patients may therefore remain asymptomatic for up to 20 years or have only mild dyspnea on exertion. However, the chronically overloaded heart eventually develops irreversible structural and functional damage, often during the asymptomatic period (43). When symptoms do develop (progressively more severe dyspnea, orthopnea, paroxysmal nocturnal dyspnea, and less often, angina), they reflect an ominous deterioration in the condition.

Patients with acute aortic regurgitation develop fulminant pulmonary edema because of the inability of the left ventricle to compensate for the sudden volume load and for the abrupt rise in LV end-diastolic pressure. Marked dyspnea and weakness may be experienced virtually overnight and in most cases within 2 or 3 months. Other symptoms depend on the underlying cause: fever, for example, if it is endocarditis; severe pain in the chest, if it is due to aortic dissection.

Physical Findings

Patients with chronic aortic regurgitation have a characteristic high-frequency early diastolic decrescendo murmur, best heard at the aortic area and at the left sternal border. The duration (but not the intensity) of the murmur correlates with the severity of the lesion, so the murmur is holodiastolic in patients with severe chronic aortic regurgitation. Often there is an accompanying harsh systolic ejection murmur as well, heard at the base of the heart. Severe aortic regurgitation may also cause a loud apical diastolic murmur (the Austin Flint murmur), simulating the murmur of mitral stenosis. Unlike the situation in true mitral stenosis, however, S_1 in patients with aortic regurgitation is sometimes soft, the result of premature closure of the mitral valve, and there is no opening snap. If aortic regurgitation is moderate or severe, the pulse pressure is ordinarily wide, reflecting peripheral vasodilation. The combination of an increased systolic pressure and a reduced diastolic pressure (sometimes as low as 30 mm Hg) produces characteristic changes in the peripheral pulse (e.g., water-hammer pulse, pistol-shot sounds heard over the femoral artery) and a typical bobbing of the head with each heart beat.

Patients with acute aortic regurgitation often show signs of left- and right-sided heart failure. The regurgitant diastolic murmur is lower pitched and shorter than it is in patients with chronic aortic incompetence; S_1 is often absent and S_3, uncommon with chronic regurgitation, is usually present. The pulse pressure is normal, the result of intense peripheral vasoconstriction.

Laboratory Findings

Electrocardiogram. The ECG also reflects the severity and duration of aortic regurgitation. Patients with chronic disease show the ECG pattern of LV hypertrophy (Fig. 65.2 and Table 65.3), whereas patients with acute disease do not (although they commonly do show nonspecific ST-T wave changes).

Chest X-Ray. The size of the heart in patients with aortic regurgitation depends on the duration and severity of the disease. Patients with chronic severe disease have very large left ventricles, but patients with acute regurgitation may have no cardiac enlargement at all.

Echocardiogram. Echocardiography with Doppler is useful in confirming the diagnosis and assessing LV function and the degree of hypertrophy. Premature mitral valve closure is helpful in confirming very severe aortic regurgitation. The severity of aortic regurgitation can also be estimated by Doppler echocardiography using a number of described criteria.

Management

Asymptomatic patients with mild aortic regurgitation need not be treated but should be assessed once or twice a year by interval history, physical examination, and chest x-ray. Yearly ECGs and echocardiograms should also be obtained. Prophylaxis for bacterial endocarditis is indicated when patients are to undergo dental or surgical procedures (see Chapter 93).

Vasodilating drugs acutely reduce the regurgitant volume and have long been known to be useful in improving hemodynamics in the short term. Randomized clinical trials demonstrate that long-term treatment with hydralazine (44), nifedipine (45), or enalapril

(46) reduces end-diastolic and end-systolic volumes and increases ejection fraction in asymptomatic or minimally symptomatic patients with moderate or severe aortic regurgitation. A reduction in the extent of hypertrophy can also be demonstrated. Angiotensin-converting enzymes seem to be the most potent in this regard (46), probably because suppression of the renin–angiotensin system inhibits the development of detrimental hypertrophy. These data suggest that vasodilator therapy has the potential to delay the need for valve replacement and should be prescribed in patients with moderate or severe aortic regurgitation even if they are asymptomatic. Patients should then be assessed once or twice a year by interval history, physical examination, and chest x-ray. Yearly ECGs and echocardiograms should also be obtained. If evidence of worsening LV dilation, hypertrophy, or LV function is detected, valve repair or replacement should be considered.

Table 65.9 lists the reasons to refer patients with aortic regurgitation to a cardiologist. In general, referral is indicated in patients with chronic disease to consider whether to recommend aortic valve replacement for symptomatic patients and for asymptomatic patients with physical findings of severe disease (widened pulse pressure, holodiastolic murmur, increasing LV enlargement, decreasing ejection fraction) (47). All patients with suspected acute aortic regurgitation should be seen by a cardiologist as soon as possible. The cardiologist is likely to perform cardiac catheterization (see Chapter 62) to assess the severity of the lesion, the presence of other valvular disease or coronary artery disease, and the function of the left ventricle. Patients with marked LV diastolic and systolic enlargement and ejection fractions of less than 50% are at high risk of requiring aortic valve replacement for symptoms of deteriorating LV function within 3 years (43).

When patients with chronic aortic regurgitation develop symptoms of congestive heart failure, 50% are dead within 2 years (48). Thus, valve replacement is warranted in all symptomatic patients, preferably before severe LV dysfunction develops. The operative mortality is 3% to 10%, but of the patients who survive surgery, 77% live 10 years or more (49) and their quality of life is usually significantly improved (see below). Symptoms of congestive heart failure are responsive to diuretics, digitalis, and vasodilators.

Table 65.9. Indications for Referral of Patients with Aortic Regurgitation

Uncertainty about the diagnosis
Symptomatic chronic aortic incompetence (dyspnea, fatigue, angina)
Acute aortic incompetence
Asymptomatic patients with evidence of severe chronic aortic incompetence: widened pulse pressure, holodiastolic murmur, left ventricular hypertrophy, progressive cardiac enlargement, falling ejection fraction, or echocardiographic end-systolic valvular dimension greater than 4.5 cm

Modified from Brandenburg RO, Fuster V, Giuliani ER. Valvular heart disease. When should the patient be referred? Pract Cardiol 1979;5:50, with permission.

The Patient With a Prosthetic Valve

Although patients usually demonstrate clear improvement in symptoms and prognosis after valve replacement, they should not be considered cured. Despite refinements in design, no valve currently available is free of potential serious complications, which, because they may occur many years after surgery, dictate careful long-term follow-up of all patients who have prosthetic valves.

Many varieties of mechanical valves and tissue (bioprosthetic) valves have been developed. The most commonly used mechanical valves are the Starr-Edwards ball-in-cage series, the Bjork-Shiley tilting disk valve, and the St. Jude valve, which has two semicircular tilting leaflets. The most common tissue valves are the Hancock and Carpentier-Edwards valves, which are constructed of porcine aortic valve leaflets that have been fixed in glutaraldehyde, and various valves constructed from bovine pericardium. The mechanical prosthetic valves are extremely durable but are thrombogenic (see below), and patients who receive them require long-term anticoagulation with warfarin. Bioprosthetic valves are less thrombogenic (1) but are also less durable, often requiring late valve replacement because of structural degeneration (see below).

Potential Complications

Thromboembolic phenomena are perhaps the most common life-threatening complications of prosthetic valves and may present as sudden stroke, myocardial infarction, or peripheral arterial occlusion. Alternatively, thrombus may accumulate around the valve ring and prevent proper valve motion, resulting in gradual or sudden obstruction of flow and the development of severe congestive heart failure. Thromboembolic events have been more common with prosthetic valves in the mitral than in the aortic position. Despite treatment with full anticoagulation, the incidence of thromboembolic complications with most mechanical valves is approximately 1% to 2% per year (50). The incidence is lower with the St. Jude valve. Perivalvular leakage resulting in regurgitation occasionally develops in the postoperative period and may require reoperation.

Prosthetic valve endocarditis develops in 2% to 3% of patients and may present as a febrile illness, a new murmur of valvular regurgitation or stenosis, hemodynamic deterioration, or embolization. Because the infection is at the site of a foreign body, the prognosis for recovery with standard antibiotic therapy is worse than in native valve endocarditis. Recurrence after one trial of medical therapy is generally an indication for replacement of the valve. Prognosis is worse in infections that develop within 60 days of surgery (72% mortality), in which contamination may have occurred at operation, than in those that develop later (45% mortality), when transient bacteremia may be the source of infection.

Late valvular degeneration is a significant problem after tissue valve implantation. Histologic studies reveal fibrin deposition, tears in the leaflets, and calcification that commonly results in some degree of valvular stenosis or regurgitation 5 to 15 years after operation. In some cases in which clinical deterioration occurs, reoperation is required. In a multicenter trial (51), the 11-year probability of reoperation for structural failure of bioprosthetic valves was 15% for those in the aortic position and 36% for those in the mitral position. The process of structural degeneration is greatly accelerated in children but also occurs commonly in young adults (younger than age 35).

Bleeding complications are more common with the mechanical valves, which always require full anticoagulation. In the multicenter trial mentioned above (51), the 11-year probability of bleeding complications was 42% with mechanical valves and 26% with bioprosthetic valves. However, these figures may not reflect the current risk of bleeding because in the 1970s, when most patients were recruited into that study, the recommended prothrombin time ratio was 2 to 2.5 times control. Current recommendations are for less vigorous anticoagulation. Because the prothrombin time varies from laboratory to laboratory, the standard is expressed as the International Normalized Ratio (INR) (see Chapter 57). The current recommendation is that the INR is maintained at 2.5 to 3.5 (see below). In patients at high risk of a thromboembolic event, aspirin may be added to the regimen.

Physical and Laboratory Findings

Auscultatory findings after valve replacement are variable. In general, the ball-in-cage valves produce loud opening and closing clicks. In the aortic position, therefore, there is a prominent systolic ejection click, and S_2 is loud and metallic. In the mitral position, S_1 is loud and there is a prominent systolic opening click after S_2, which is similar in timing to the opening snap of mitral stenosis. With the Bjork-Shiley and St. Jude valves, the closing sounds are loud but the opening sounds are variable. Porcine valves are the most physiologic, and as in a native valve, the closing sounds are audible but opening sounds are rare. All valves in either position produce systolic ejection murmurs. Diastolic flow murmurs are common with the Bjork-Shiley valve in the mitral position.

It is important to document the baseline physical examination repeatedly so that the significance of any changes that occur in association with new symptoms can be assessed. The most reliable sign of prosthetic valve dysfunction is the loss or muffling of the opening and closing clicks. New regurgitant murmurs may occur. Congestive heart failure may develop.

The 2D echocardiogram may show abnormal, delayed, or intermittent leaflet motion. Doppler echocardiography (see above) is particularly helpful in accurately detecting and quantifying new valve gradients and regurgitation. Tissue valves are often well visualized and can be assessed by echocardiography. However, mechanical valves are not well seen by transthoracic echocardiography, and TEE is usually required to assess valve anatomy if there is clinical suspicion or Doppler evidence of impaired prosthetic valve function. Fluoroscopy is usually very helpful if restriction of mechanical leaflet motion is being investigated.

Management

Management of the patient with a prosthetic valve should begin before the valve is implanted; the selection of the proper type of valve for the individual patient is crucial. A tissue valve is most appropriate for the patient who is likely to be noncompliant with anticoagulation or who is at high risk for bleeding complications. These individuals include alcoholics; patients with psychiatric problems, unexplained syncope, or previous gastrointestinal bleeds; patients whose occupations put them at high risk of injury; and elderly patients. Women of child-bearing age who desire future pregnancies should receive pulmonary autografts (Ross procedure) or tissue valves (see below), but in the latter case they should be made aware that valve replacement may have to be repeated in 8 to 10 years. Young men or women who do not anticipate pregnancy and who will tolerate anticoagulation are better off with the more durable mechanical valves so that reoperation is not necessary. These decisions are usually made by the cardiac surgeon after discussing the options with the patient, but it is important that the practitioner communicate his or her opinions to the surgeon well in advance.

All patients with mechanical valves in the aortic or mitral position must be fully anticoagulated with warfarin indefinitely (see Chapter 57). For aortic prostheses, the INR should be maintained between 2.0 and 3.0 (target INR of 2.5) for bileaflet valves (i.e, St. Jude valves) and tilting disk valves (i.e., Medtronic Hall valves), provided the patient is in sinus rhythm and does not have left atrial enlargement. The target INR should be 3.0 (range 2.5 to 3.5) for patients with a St. Jude or Medtronic Hall aortic valve who are in atrial fibrillation, who have another disk valve (i.e., a Bjork-Shiley valve) in the aortic position, and for all patients with a mitral prosthetic valve (52). An alternative recommendation for patients at higher risk is a target INR of 2.5 (range 2.0 to 3.0) in combination with aspirin, 80 to 100 mg a day. For patients with a caged ball (Starr-Edwards) valve or for patients considered at high risk of systemic embolism (e.g., patients with atrial thrombi), a target INR of 3.0 (range 2.5 to 3.5) is recommended in combination with aspirin, 80 to 100 mg/day (52). The incidence of thromboembolism is 9% annually without anticoagulation and 1% to 2% with warfarin. If an elective surgical procedure is planned, the modification of warfarin therapy should be individualized. In most patients, warfarin may be safely discontinued 3 days before surgery and resumed afterward (see details in Chapter 93). However, temporary substitution of intravenous heparin should be considered if there has been a recent thromboembolus, a Bjork-Shiley valve is present, or if one (for mitral valves) or three (for aortic valves) of the following risk factors are present: atrial fibrillation, LV dysfunction, previous thromboembolism, hypercoagulable condition, and mechanical prosthesis (52). Antiplatelet agents (see Chapter 57) are not adequate to prevent thromboembolic complications, which occur at an annual rate of 7.5% with aspirin treatment (50). The low molecular weight heparins have not been adequately studied for this purpose; there are numerous cases of both successes and failures with this approach in the medical literature. The routine addition of low dose (80 to 100 mg) aspirin to warfarin has been advocated for patients with the following risk factors for thromboembolism: prior embolization, vascular disease, or hypercoagulable state. This maneuver reduces the risk of thromboembolism but increases the incidence of bleeding complications.

Patients with tissue valves in the aortic position should be anticoagulated for 3 months after operation only, so that endothelialization of the valve may occur. Warfarin should then be discontinued unless risk factors for thromboembolism are present. In that case, warfarin should be continued with a target INR of 2 to 3. There is controversy over whether tissue valves in the mitral position require long-term anticoagulation. Most cardiologists would discontinue warfarin after 3 months and then use aspirin only, unless risk factors for thromboembolism were present. In that case, warfarin should be continued with a target INR of 2.5 to 3.5. Strict antibiotic prophylaxis against endocarditis is indicated. Table 93.13 lists regimens recommended by the American Heart Association before and after various procedures.

Prosthetic valve dysfunction is an indication for referral to a cardiologist, who will usually recommend TEE and cardiac catheterization. See Table 65.10 for reasons to refer a patient with a prosthetic valve to a cardiologist.

Pregnancy in a Patient With a Prosthetic Valve

Pregnancy poses a serious problem in patients with mechanical prosthetic valves. The ingestion of warfarin during pregnancy results in a definite increase in the incidence of fetal death and birth defects (see Chapter 57). The spontaneous abortion rate is approximately 30%, probably because warfarin crosses the placenta and predisposes the fetus to intrauterine hemorrhage. Between 8% and 16% of the liveborn infants have various birth defects, most commonly nasal hypoplasia with stippled epiphysis (a specific warfarin embryopathy), as well as optic atrophy, microcephaly, and mental retardation.

Table 65.10. Indications for Referral of Patients with Prosthetic Valves

Progressive symptoms of congestive heart failure
Progressive cardiac enlargement
Changes in prosthetic heart sounds
Pregnancy or the desire to become pregnant
Embolization
Endocarditis

On the other hand, the risk of thromboembolism is greater during pregnancy, and discontinuation of anticoagulation greatly increases the danger of systemic embolism. In one study (53), systemic embolism was seen in 31% of such patients despite antiplatelet therapy. Most of the patients had Starr-Edwards valves.

There is no consensus regarding the management of early pregnancy when a mechanical prosthetic valve is in place. Some authors recommend substituting full-dose heparin, which does not cross the placenta, for warfarin during the first trimester of pregnancy. However, such therapy requires prolonged hospitalization, and the incidence of fetal death appears to be high with this regimen as well (see Chapter 57). The safety and efficacy of low molecular weight heparin in this situation have not been established. The proper management of anticoagulation at the end of pregnancy is more clearly defined. If warfarin has been given, it should be replaced by heparin 2 weeks before delivery is expected. Heparin can then be stopped at the onset of labor to prevent peripartum hemorrhage. Aspirin is not effective in preventing thromboembolism in these patients.

Most clinicians strongly counsel patients with mechanical prosthetic valves to avoid pregnancy. Patients with valves should be well aware of the risks if pregnancy is contemplated. Pregnancy or the desire to become pregnant is an indication for referral to both a cardiologist and an obstetrician specializing in high-risk patients.

Pregnancy for the patient with a tissue (bioprosthetic) valve is much safer because anticoagulation can be avoided. Antiplatelet agents have a role here.

The best approach to these problems is to avoid valve replacement in women in whom future pregnancy is likely; if possible, mitral stenosis should be managed medically, with percutaneous valvuloplasty, or with surgical commissurotomy and mitral regurgitation with medical therapy or valve repair. If valve replacement is necessary in such a patient, the surgeon should be strongly urged to use a bioprosthesis rather than a mechanical valve, and the patient should be aware that eventual reoperation will probably be necessary. For the aortic valve, the pulmonary autograft (Ross procedure) provides good long-term results without the need for anticoagulation. In this procedure, the pulmonary valve is autotransplanted into the aortic position and is replaced with a cadaveric homograft.

General References*

Bonow RO, Carabello B, DeLeon, AC, et al. **ACC/AHA guidelines for the management of patients with valvular heart disease.** J Am Coll Cardiol 1998;32:1486.

A consensus statement covering all aspects of valvular disease.

*Bold print (general references) and bold numerals (specific references) denote published controlled clinical trials, meta-analyses, or consensus-based recommendations.

Braunwald E, Zipes D, Libby P, eds. Heart disease: a textbook of cardiovascular medicine. 6th ed. Philadelphia: W.B. Saunders, 2001.
Encyclopedic review of cardiac physical examination, heart sounds, and cardiac graphic techniques.
Constant J. Bedside cardiology. Boston: Little, Brown, 1976.
The best teaching text for understanding the physiological basis of heart sounds and how to hear and describe them.

Specific References

1. Bonow RO, Carabello B, DeLeon, AC, et al. ACC/AHA guidelines for the management of patients with valvular heart disease. J Am Coll Cardiol 1998;32:1486.
2. Bonow RO, Carabello B, DeLeon, AC, et al. ACC/AHA guidelines for the management of patients with valvular heart disease. Circulation 1998;98:1949.
3. Feigenbaum H. Echocardiography. 5th ed. Philadelphia: Lea & Febiger, 1994.
4. Hatle L, Angelsen B. Doppler ultrasound in cardiology, physical principles and clinical applications. Philadelphia: Lea & Febiger, 1985.
5. Faletra F, Pezzano A Jr, Fusco R, et al. Measurement of mitral valve area in mitral stenosis: four echocardiographic methods compared with direct measurement of anatomic orifices. J Am Coll Cardiol 1996;28:1190.
6. Helmcke F, Nanda NC, Hsiung MC, et al. Color Doppler assessment of mitral regurgitation with orthogonal planes. Circulation 1987;75:175.
7. Shapiro EP, Effron MB, Lima S, et al. Transient atrial dysfunction after conversion of chronic atrial fibrillation to normal sinus rhythm. Am J Cardiol 1988;62:1202.
8. Daniel WG, Mugge A. Transesophageal echocardiography. N Engl J Med 1995;332:1268.
9. Daniel WG, Erbel R, Kasper W, et al. Safety of transesophageal echocardiography. Circulation 1991;83:817.
10. Nienaber CA, von Kodolitsch Y, Nicolas V, et al. The diagnosis of thoracic aortic dissection by noninvasive imaging procedures. N Engl J Med 1993;328:1.
11. Etchells E, Bell C, Robb K. Does this patient have an abnormal systolic murmur? JAMA 1997;277:564.
12. Carabello BA. Indications for valve surgery in asymptomatic patients with aortic and mitral stenosis. Chest 1995;108:1678.
13. O'Keefe JH Jr, Vlietstra RE, Bailey KR, et al. Natural history of candidates for balloon aortic valvuloplasty. Mayo Clin Proc 1987;62:986.
14. Olsson MA, Granstrom L, Lindblom D, et al. Aortic valve replacement in octogenarians with aortic stenosis: a case-control study. J Am Coll Cardiol 1993;7:1512.
15. Lieberman EB, Bashore TM, Hermiller JB, et al. Balloon aortic valvuloplasty in adults: failure of procedure to improve long-term survival. J Am Coll Cardiol 1995;26:1522.
16. Maron BJ, Gardin JM, Flack JM, et al. Prevalence of hypertrophic cardiomyopathy in a general population of young adults. Echocardiographic analysis of 4111 subjects in the CARDIA Study. Coronary Artery Risk Development in (Young) Adults. Circulation 1995;92:785.
17. Spirito P, Chiarella F, Carratino L, et al. Clinical course and prognosis of hypertrophic cardiomyopathy in an outpatient population. N Engl J Med 1989;320:749.
18. Watkins H, McKenna WJ, Thierfelder L, et al. Mutations in the genes for cardiac troponin T and alpha-tropomyosin in hypertrophic cardiomyopathy. N Engl J Med 1995;332:1058.
19. Fananapazir L, Cannon RO, Tripodi D, et al. Impact of dual-chamber permanent pacing in patients with obstructive hypertrophic cardiomyopathy with symptoms refractory to verapamil and beta-adrenergic blocker therapy. Circulation 1992;85:2149, 1992.
20. Kappenberger LJ, Linde C, Jeanrenaud X, et al. Clinical progress after randomized on/off pacemaker treatment for hypertrophic obstructive cardiomyopathy. Europace 1999;1:77.
21. Maron BJ. Appraisal of dual-chamber pacing therapy in hypertrophic cardiomyopathy: too soon for a rush to judgment? J Am Coll Cardiol 1996;27:431.
22. Maron BJ, Nishimura RA, McKenna WJ, et al. Assessment of permanent dual chamber pacing as a treatment for drug-refractory symptomatic patients with obstructive hypertrophic cardiomyopathy: A randomized, double-blind crossover study. Circulation 1999;99:2927.
23. Spencer WH. Alcohol septal ablation in hypertrophic obstructive cardiomyopathy: the need for a registry. Circulation 1999;102:600.
24. ten Berg JM, Suttorp MJ, Knaepen PJ, et al. Hypertrophic obstructive cardiomyopathy. Initial results and long-term follow-up after Morrow septal myectomy. Circulation 1994;90:1781.
25. Craig RJ, Selzer A. Natural history and prognosis of atrial septal defect. Circulation 1968;37:805.
26. Gaasch WH, John RM, Aurigemma GP. Managing asymptomatic patients with chronic mitral regurgitation. Chest 1995;108:842.
27. Rapaport E. Natural history of aortic and mitral valve disease. Am J Cardiol 1981;35:221.
28. Munoz S, Gallardo J, Diaz-Gorrin JR, et al. Influence of surgery on the natural history of rheumatic mitral and aortic valve disease. Am J Cardiol 1975;35:234.
29. Ling LH, Enriquez-Sarano M, Seward JB, et al. Clinical outcome of mitral regurgitation due to flail leaflet. N Engl J Med 1996;335:1417.
30. Ross J Jr. The timing of surgery for severe mitral regurgitation. N Engl J Med 1996;335:1456.
31. Enriquez-Sarano M, Schaff HV, Orszulak TA, et al. Valve repair improves the outcome of surgery for mitral regurgitation. A multivariate analysis. Circulation 1995;91:1022.
32. Devereux RB, Kramer-Fox R, Brown WT, et al. Relation between clinical features of the mitral prolapse syndrome and echocardiographically documented mitral valve prolapse. J Am Coll Cardiol 1986;8:763.
33. Quill TE, Lipkin M, Greenland P. The medicalization of normal variants: the case of mitral valve prolapse. J Gen Intern Med 1988;3:267.
34. Freed LA, Levy D, Levine RA, et al. Prevalence and clinical outcome of mitral valve prolapse. N Engl J Med 1999;341:1.
35. Zuppiroli A, Rinaldi M, Kramer-Fox R, et al. Natural history of mitral valve prolapse. Am J Cardiol 1995;75:1028.
36. Barnett JHM, Boughner DR, Taylor DW, et al. Further evidence relating mitral valve prolapse to cerebral ischemic events. N Engl J Med 1980;302:139.
37. Marks AR, Choong CY, Sanfilippo AJ, et al. Identification of high-risk and low-risk subgroups of patients with mitral-valve prolapse. N Engl J Med 1989;320:1031.
38. Selzer A, Cohn K. Natural history of mitral stenosis: a review. Circulation 1972;45:878.
39. Oleson KH. The natural history of 271 patients with mitral stenosis under medical treatment. Br Heart J 1962;24:349.
40. Reyes VP, Raju BS, Wynne J, et al. Percutaneous balloon valvuloplasty compared with open surgical commissurotomy for mitral stenosis. N Engl J Med 1994;331:961.
41. Stoll BC, Ashcom TL, Johns JP, et al. Effects of atenolol on rest and exercise hemodynamics in patients with mitral stenosis. Am J Cardiol 1995;75:482.
42. Haydar HS, He GW, Hovaguimian H, et al. Valve repair for aortic insufficiency: surgical classification and techniques. Eur J Cardiothorac Surg 1997;11:266.
43. Siemienczuk D, Greenberg B, Morris C, et al. Chronic aortic insufficiency: factors associated with progression to aortic valve replacement. Ann Intern Med 1989;110:587.
44. Greenberg B, Massie B, Bristow JD, et al. Long-term vasodilator therapy of chronic aortic insufficiency. A randomized double-blinded, placebo-controlled clinical trial. Circulation 1988;78:92.
45. Scognamiglio R, Fasoli G, Ponchia A, et al. Long-term nifedipine unloading therapy in asymptomatic patients with chronic severe aortic regurgitation. J Am Coll Cardiol 1990;16:424.
46. Lin M, Chiang HT, Lin SL, et al. Vasodilator therapy in chronic asymptomatic aortic regurgitation: enalapril versus hydralazine therapy. J Am Coll Cardiol 1994;24:1046.
47. Brandenburg RO, Fuster V, Giuliani ER. Valvular heart disease. When should the patient be referred? Pract Cardiol 1979;5:50.

48. Massell BF, Ameccua FJ, Czohiczer G. Prognosis of patients with pure or predominant aortic regurgitation in the absence of surgery. Circulation 1966;34[Suppl 2]:164.
49. Corti R, Binggeli C, Turina M, et al. Predictors of long-term survival after valve replacement for chronic aortic regurgitation; is M-mode echocardiography sufficient? Eur Heart J 2001;22:808.
50. Cannegieter SC, Rosendaal FR, Briet E. Thromboembolic and bleeding complications in patients with mechanical heart valve prostheses. Circulation 1994;89:635.
51. Hammermeister KE, Sethi GK, Henderson WG, et al. A comparison of outcomes in men 11 years after heart-valve replacement with a mechanical valve or bioprosthesis. N Engl J Med 1993;328:18.
52. Stein PD, Albert JS, Bussey HI, et al. Antithrombotic therapy in patients with mechanical and biological prosthetic heart valves. Chest 2001;119[1 Suppl]:220S.
53. Salazar E, Zajarias A, Gutierrez N, et al. The problems of cardiac valve prostheses, anticoagulants and pregnancy. Circulation 1984;70[Suppl 1]:169.

CHAPTER 66

Heart Failure

SHELDON H. GOTTLIEB, MD
ROY C. ZIEGELSTEIN, MD

DEFINITION

The amount of blood that the heart pumps per minute (the cardiac output) is normally precisely adjusted to meet the metabolic needs of the body. The cardiac output may increase twofold or threefold as a person goes from rest to exercise. An increase in cardiac output may occur within the space of one heartbeat by a decrease in vagal tone, which causes an increase in heart rate. After several seconds of exercise, sympathetic tone increases, which causes a further increase in cardiac output by increasing the heart rate and the amount of blood pumped per heartbeat (the stroke volume). Neural regulation of the peripheral circulation shunts blood flow away from the kidneys and redistributes it to the working muscle groups. The increased cardiac output soon brings about an increase in the amount of blood returning to the right side of the heart (the venous return); this leads to a further increase in cardiac output in response to the increased filling pressure and increased stretch in the heart muscle (the Frank-Starling principle).

If the heart, working at a normal filling pressure, is unable to pump enough blood to maintain tissue perfusion pressure and thereby to meet the metabolic needs of the body, compensatory neural and hormonal mechanisms that cause remodeling of the heart are brought into play. These adjustments may acutely or gradually cause symptoms and signs recognized as the syndrome of *heart failure.*

Most heart failure patients are either *presymptomatic* or *undiagnosed* (1). *Acute heart failure,* manifest usually by pulmonary edema (recognized by the abrupt onset of extreme breathlessness and evidence of alveolar edema by physical and radiologic examination), warrants immediate hospitalization for diagnosis of the underlying or precipitating cause and for treatment. Patients with *advanced heart failure,* who are severely symptomatic at rest, despite compliance with an evidence-based heart failure regimen (see below), require urgent consultation with a cardiologist. All other patients with heart failure have *chronic heart failure,* which can usually be managed in an ambulatory setting.

EPIDEMIOLOGY

About 4,700,000 Americans alive today have heart failure (2). The prevalence of heart failure increases greatly in patients over 60 years old (Fig. 66.1). The incidence of heart failure is approximately 0.3 per 1,000 per year under age 45, remains constant at approximately 3 per 1,000 per year in the middle-age groups, and increases to 10 per 1,000 in patients over the age of 65 (3). The incidence among men is slightly higher than among women in the 45- to 84-year-old range but is higher among women in the 85- to 94-year-old range (4).

There are currently almost 1 million hospital discharges for heart failure in the United States each year (438,000 men and 540,000 women) (2). Between 1973 and 1995, the annual hospitalization rates for congestive heart failure (CHF) among patients over age 65 more than tripled, from approximately 60 per 10,000 people to more than 200 per 10,000. Between 1980 through 1988, mortality from heart failure rose, but

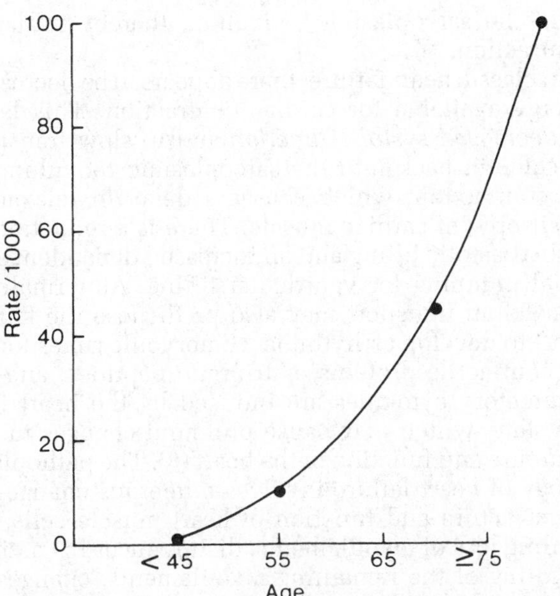

Figure 66.1. The prevalence of heart failure reported from physicians' offices as a function of patient age. Note the marked increase in the sixth and seventh decades. Between 10% and 20% of patients older than age 60 followed regularly by a physician have a history of heart failure. This percentage is likely to increase as preventive measures after myocardial infarction become more effective and because patients are more likely to be discharged alive from hospital after admission with a diagnosis of heart failure. (From McKee P, Castelli W, McNamara P, et al. The natural history of congestive heart failure: the Framingham study. N Engl J Med 1971;285:1441, with permission.)

there was a decline between 1988 and 1995. This decrease in mortality probably reflects in part improved treatment because the percentage of hospitalized CHF patients who died fell from 11.3% in 1981 to 6.1% in 1993 associated with a decrease in the average length of stay and an increase in costs and in the use of cardiac procedures and costs (5).

PHYSIOLOGY

The Heart as a Pump

Length–Tension Relationship: Frank-Starling Principle and Preload

As heart muscle is stretched, it develops increased tension. The relationship of length to tension defines the *compliance* of heart muscle; the inverse of compliance is *stiffness.* If the ventricle is distended with blood, pressure develops within the cavity. A higher pressure is needed to distend the ventricle to a given volume in a less compliant (i.e., stiffer) ventricle. The pressure needed to stretch the ventricle to a given end-diastolic volume is called the *preload,* clinically measured as the *left ventricular end-diastolic pressure* (LVEDP). The relationship between the volume of the ventricle just before contraction and the force developed during contraction defines the Frank-Starling principle (6,7). If the LVEDP is plotted against stroke work (the stroke volume times the mean blood pressure), a ventricular function curve is defined (Fig. 66.2). It can be seen from this relationship that the normal ventricle is compliant: It develops an adequate amount of force during contraction with a low preload. However, as the ventricle fails, it requires a higher preload to increase its stroke work (Fig. 66.2).

Afterload

Afterload is the dynamic resistance against which the heart contracts. It determines the degree of stress within the myocardium. Systolic blood pressure closely approximates and is clinically the most useful indicator of afterload. Afterload determines the ease or speed of ventricular contraction; hence, the stroke volume and ejection fraction (the portion of the ventricular volume that is ejected with each beat) is a function of afterload.

Contractility and Inotropic State

The relationship of preload (LVEDP) to stroke work (stroke volume × mean blood pressure) defines the functional state of cardiac muscle (see above). The relative position of the curve defines the inotropic state of the muscle. For example, infusing the heart with an inotropic substance such as digitalis causes the ventricular function curve to shift to the left, i.e., to perform a higher stroke work at a given preload, assuming that afterload is kept constant. In other words, the contractility of the heart is increased.

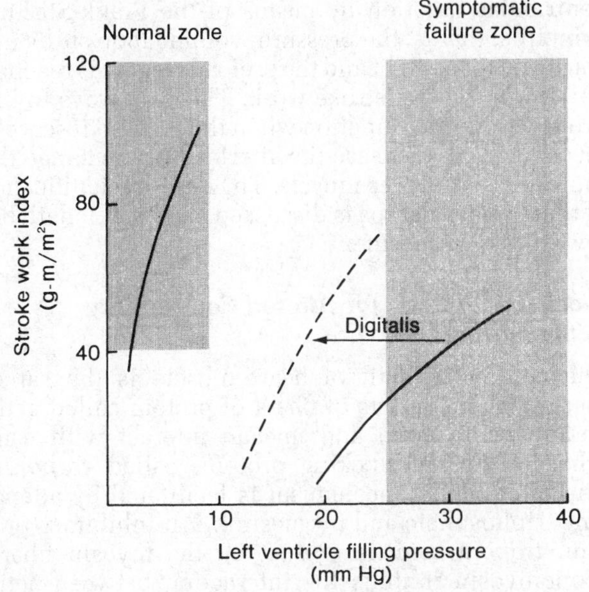

Figure 66.2. "Ventricular function curves" show the relationship between left ventricular filling pressures and stroke work. The position of the curve defines the inotropic state of the heart. Note that for a given curve (i.e., a given inotropic state), the function of the heart, or the amount of work the heart is capable of performing, varies with the left ventricular filling pressure. (Adapted from Weisfeldt ML. Congestive heart failure: pathophysiology and the evaluation of ventricular function. In: Harvey AM, Johns RJ, McKusick VA, et al., eds. The principles and practice of medicine. New York: Appleton-Century-Crofts, 1984, with permission.)

Relationship Between Preload, Afterload, and Inotropic State (Contractility)

If the end-diastolic pressure–volume relationship (curve) is kept constant, an increase in afterload or a decrease in inotropic state causes a decrease in the volume of the pressure–volume loop (i.e., a depression in ventricular function) as measured clinically by the ejection fraction or stroke volume. Thus, if afterload (end-systolic blood pressure) increases, ventricular function measured by the pressure volume loop or by the ejection fraction (normally 50% to 75%) decreases. A compensatory response is for the LVEDP, or preload, to increase, which restores the ventricular function (pressure–volume loop) to baseline. A further increase in afterload leads to a further depression in ventricular function, which again may be restored by an increased preload (i.e., by increasing LVEDP). The *preload reserve* is the LVEDP above which the pulmonary capillary oncotic pressure is exceeded; fluid then passes into the alveoli, and pulmonary congestion, with symptoms of cough and dyspnea, occurs. Any increase in afterload that occurs when the preload reserve is reached causes a decrease in ventricular function and a worsening in symptoms of congestion. The preload reserve varies with the compliance of the ventricle as measured by the position of the LV pressure–volume relationship. If heart muscle is made stiffer or less compliant by a chronic disease process such as hypertension or aortic stenosis or by an acute process such as ischemia or increased heart rate, a higher filling pressure is necessary to set the level of ventricular function by means of the Frank-Starling principle, that is, the pressure–volume loop shifts upward and to the right and the preload reserve is reached at a lower level of stroke work. The only ways to improve ventricular function when the preload reserve is reached are to decrease the afterload or to change the inotropic state of the muscle. The clinical significance of these relationships is discussed at greater length below under Management.

Biochemical Basis for Altered Contractility in the Failing Heart

The contractile unit of heart muscle is the sarcomere, which consists of fibers of protein called actin and myosin. *Actin* and *myosin* interact with each other by an interlocking protein, called *troponin.* The interlocking mechanism is facilitated by adenosine triphosphate and magnesium. An inhibitory protein, *tropomyosin,* is present on the myosin fibers. Tropomyosin inhibits the interaction between actin and myosin and allows the muscle to relax. Calcium inhibits the tropomyosin complex, frees the interlocking troponin, and allows actin and myosin to interact and to develop tension. Calcium is therefore necessary for myocardial contraction to take place. Large amounts of calcium are stored within the heart in the *sarcoplasmic reticulum.* Excitation–contraction coupling takes place in heart muscle when an action potential causes a release of calcium from the sarcoplasmic reticulum, thereby initiating contraction.

In classic heart failure, there appears to be decreased energy available for cardiac contraction. This leads to *decreased systolic function* and to slow transport of calcium back into the sarcoplasmic reticulum after contraction, which causes a delay in relaxation (lusitropy) of cardiac muscle. There is a reduction in early diastolic filling and an increased dependence on atrial pumping for ventricular filling. Abnormalities in calcium transport may also predispose the failing heart to develop arrhythmias. Embryonic genes for fetal contractile proteins, natriuretic peptides, and inflammatory cytokines are induced by the heart failure state, which may cause profound changes in the structure and function of the heart (8). The pathophysiology of heart failure involves numerous changes in the structure and function of heart muscle cells, including loss of myofilaments, disturbances in calcium handling of the remaining myofilaments, changes in receptor density, and alterations in signal transduction. One of the fundamental processes underlying this condition is the progressive loss of cardiac muscle cells, leading to structural changes in the heart and to an increase in collagen synthesis. It appears that this progressive loss is the result of cell death, either by *necrosis* (an unregulated process that most likely cannot be interrupted), *apoptosis* (a highly regulated process that can theoretically be prevented by specific and early intervention), or both (9). Indeed, it has been surmised that the beneficial effect of some drugs used to treat heart failure may involve the inhibition of apoptosis.

In 30% to 50% of patients with the clinical syndrome of heart failure, systolic function as judged by the ejection fraction is normal but diastolic function (relaxation) is impaired. This leads to inadequate LV filling. Any compensatory increase in heart rate shortens diastole disproportionately more than systole, which leads to a further reduction in both LV filling and the time available for calcium uptake; therefore, both systolic function and diastolic compliance worsen (10).

Compensatory Mechanisms

Heart Rate

The neural and hormonal responses to heart failure lead to an increase in heart rate in an attempt to maintain cardiac output. This may lead to rapid deterioration in systolic and diastolic function because of the disproportionate shortening of diastole relative to systole as heart rate increases (see above). The difference between the maximum heart rate during exercise and the resting heart rate (the heart rate reserve) is decreased and the normal vagally mediated resting R-R interval variability is markedly blunted in heart failure. The degree of blunting is highly correlated with plasma norepinephrine levels, which may be very high in advanced heart failure (11).

Hypertrophy and Dilation

Left ventricular hypertrophy (LVH) and dilation may allow compensation of the failing heart to be maintained for many years. The stress in the wall of the heart varies with the radius of the ventricular cavity. If the heart is subjected to a *volume load,* it dilates to accommodate the load and to increase its ability to eject the load (the Frank-Starling principle; see above). However, ventricular dilation causes an increase in ventricular wall stress, which stimulates ventricular hypertrophy. Eventually, the heart becomes both dilated and hypertrophied, and the ratio of wall thickness to cavity size returns to normal, which normalizes wall stress. Therefore, a state of compensated ventricular dilation is achieved. The response to a *pressure overload* is different. An increase in wall stress in the absence of volume overload leads to cellular hypertrophy; wall stress per unit area returns to normal, but the cavity size is unchanged.

Activation of the Neurohormonal System

The neurohormonal activation triggered by the inability of the failing heart to maintain an effective arterial blood pressure and tissue perfusion is a major cause of the syndrome of heart failure (12). Neurohormonal activation leads to an increase in peripheral vascular resistance, a redistribution of cardiac output (maintaining flow to the heart and brain and reducing it to the kidneys, skin, splanchnic organs, and skeletal muscle), and to the retention of salt and water. In less severe heart failure, when the resting cardiac output is normal, redistribution occurs only during exercise. In severe heart failure, when the resting cardiac output is significantly decreased, redistribution occurs at rest. The decrease in blood flow is functionally most important in the kidneys. Decreased renal blood flow causes a release of renin from the juxtaglomerular apparatus, which leads to increased plasma angiotensin activity. *Angiotensin* is a potent vasoconstrictor and acts both directly on smooth muscle and indirectly by increasing norepinephrine release from vascular nerve endings. Norepinephrine and angiotensin may directly damage myocardial cells. Prolonged increased plasma norepinephrine levels lead to a decreased density of beta-1-adrenergic receptors on cardiac myocytes and thereby may decrease the normal myocardial response to sympathetic stimulation. The increase in angiotensin activity leads to an increase in aldosterone production, which causes an increase in sodium resorption from the distal nephron, thereby increasing plasma volume.

Increased aldosterone levels also contribute to hypokalemia and hypomagnesemia that may make the failing heart more susceptible to ventricular arrhythmias. Aldosterone also appears to stimulate myocardial fibrosis, which in turn may play a role in hypertrophy and dilatation of the ventricle (13). The renal resorption of sodium is also facilitated by an increased filtration fraction at a given glomerular filtration rate, which causes increased sodium reabsorption in the proximal nephron. Paradoxically, hyponatremia may result from increased thirst and consumption of free water, triggered by increased levels of circulating renin, angiotensin, aldosterone, and antidiuretic hormone and by a decreased renal responsiveness to atrial natriuretic peptide (14). The effect of angiotensin on thirst and on sodium appetite is striking (15). The importance of these compensatory responses to neurohormonal activation in the management of patients with heart failure is discussed below.

DIAGNOSIS

Causes of Heart Failure

When the diagnosis of heart failure is made, it is essential to determine the most likely etiology because the treatment and prognosis of heart failure vary greatly depending on its cause. Heart failure is caused by one of three basic mechanisms: an increased workload to which the heart cannot accommodate, a disorder of the myocardium so that it is unable to accommodate normal workloads, or a restriction of ventricular filling so that an adequate stroke volume cannot be achieved. Table 66.1 lists selected examples of these conditions. In the United States, the most common condition associated with heart failure is hypertension, followed closely by ischemic heart disease (16).

The most common precipitating causes of acute heart failure are noncompliance with medication or diet in a patient with previously compensated heart failure, acute myocardial ischemia or infarction, poorly controlled hypertension, arrhythmia, valvular disease, and pneumonia. In patients for whom the precipitating cause is not obvious, it is important to

Table 66.1. Causes of Heart Failure

- Increased workload to which the heart cannot accommodate
  - High-output states
    - Hyperthyroidism[a]
    - Anemia[a]
    - Systemic arteriovenous fistulas[a]
    - Certain dermatologic disorders (e.g., psoriasis, erythroderma)[a]
  - Valvular regurgitation or left-to-right shunts[a]
  - Increased impedance to injection
    - Systemic hypertension[a]
    - Pulmonary hypertension
    - Pulmonic or aortic stenosis[a]
- Disorders of myocardium so that the heart is unable to accommodate normal workloads
  - Cardiomyopathies (viral, familial, drug induced [cytotoxic chemotherapy, chronic use of amphetamines, cocaine])
  - Myocardial infarction
  - Restriction of ventricular filling
  - Pericardial constriction or effusion[a]
  - Atrial myxoma[a]
  - Mitral and tricuspid valvular stenosis[a]
  - Increased ventricular stiffness
    - Infiltrative myocardial disease (e.g., amyloid, hemochromatosis)
    - Ventricular hypertrophy
    - Hypertrophic cardiomyopathy

[a]Indicates causes of heart failure that are potentially treatable by specific therapy.

Adapted from Weisfeldt ML. Congestive heart failure: pathophysiology and the evaluation of ventricular function. In: Harvey AM, Johns RJ, McKusick VA, et al, eds. The principles and practice of medicine. New York: Appleton-Century-Crofts, 1984:185, with permission.

consider arrhythmia (see Chapter 64), covert ischemia (see Chapter 62), and pulmonary embolism (see Chapter 59). In addition, it is important to inquire about psychosocial stress, which may lead to increased energy demands and is often associated with increased salt and water intake.

Right- and Left-sided Heart Failure

Heart failure was historically classified as *right sided* (e.g., as evidenced by jugular venous congestion, hepatic enlargement, ascites, or peripheral edema; see below) or *left sided* (as evidenced by signs and symptoms of pulmonary congestion; see below) depending on which chamber or chambers was compromised. Although this diagnostic scheme is occasionally encountered in clinical discourse and is enshrined in the International Classification of Diseases, 9th revision (ICD-9) diagnostic codes, it is now primarily of historical interest.

Functional Classification

The amount of physical activity that a patient can perform without symptoms of heart failure determines functional class. Several classification schemes that are useful in categorizing patients in this regard are presented in Tables 66.2 and 66.3. Correctable disease may be present despite severe symptoms, so the functional classification provides useful prognostic information only within selected subsets of patients. Functional class is best determined by questioning the patient regarding performance during well-defined daily activities. For example, a patient may be asked about his or her tolerance for walking a specified number of flights of stairs, walking a specific distance, or carrying a specific load. The patient should also be questioned regarding which customary interpersonal, household, or work activities have had to be modified (see Chapter 63 for metabolic requirements of daily activities). Several quality of life measures have been developed specifically for heart failure; these measures may be useful in evaluating the patient's impairment and response to treatment (17).

History

No symptoms, signs, or laboratory tests are pathognomonic of heart failure. The significance of symptoms and signs compatible with heart failure must be inferred based on the patient's overall condition and the stage at which the patient appears to be in the natural history of his or her disease. Clinical criteria for the diagnosis of heart failure are listed in Table 66.4.

The most common symptoms of heart failure are dyspnea and fatigue. *Dyspnea* in heart failure is a symptom of increased LVEDP with pulmonary venous and capillary congestion. Increased pulmonary congestion decreases lung compliance and vital capacity. The work of breathing increases and breathing becomes rapid, shallow, and forced. *Fatigue,* caused by low cardiac output, is often described as a general sense of weakness or "lack of ambition." Some patients may complain of fatigue rather than dyspnea. Fatigue may be a symptom of low cardiac output with hypotension caused by overaggressive diuresis, especially when there is concomitant use of converting enzyme inhibitors and beta-blockers. A complaint of dyspnea or fatigue may be difficult to interpret because effort intolerance may bear little or no relationship to objective measures of circulatory, ventilatory, or metabolic dysfunction during exercise; factors other than the degree of hemodynamic dysfunction may be important. These include musculoskeletal status, muscle deconditioning, arthritis, body composition, obesity, motivation, comorbid depression, and tolerance of discomfort.

Table 66.2. Assessment of Functional Capacity

New York Heart Association Classification[a]	Severity of Symptoms[b]	Max. Oxygen Uptake (mL/min/kg)[b]	Goldman's Specific Activity Scale (METs)[c,d]
I Patients with cardiac disease but without resulting limitations of physical activity. Ordinary physical activity does not cause undue fatigue, palpitations, dyspnea, or anginal pain.	None to mild	>20	10
II Patients with cardiac disease resulting in slight limitation of physical activity. They are comfortable at rest. Ordinary physical activity results in fatigue, palpitations, dyspnea, or angina pain.	Mild to moderate	16–20	5–6
III Patients with cardiac disease that results in marked limitation of physical activity and causes fatigue, palpitations, dyspnea, or anginal pain.	Moderate to severe	10–16	3.6–4.2
IV Patients with cardiac disease that results in inability to carry on any physical activity without discomfort. Symptoms of cardiac insufficiency or of the anginal syndrome may be present even at rest. If any physical activity is undertaken, discomfort is increased.	Severe	<10	2–2.3

[a]The Criteria Committee of the New York Association, Inc. Diseases of the heart and blood vessels, nomenclature and criteria for diagnosis, 6th ed. Boston: Little, Brown, 1964.

[b]Adapted from Weber KT, Janiski JS. Cardiopulmonary exercise testing. Philadelphia: W.B. Saunders, 1986.

[c]Adapted from Goldman L, Hashimoto B, Cook EF, et al. Comparative reproducibility and validity of systems for assessing cardiovascular functional class: advantages of new specific activity scale. Circulation 1981;64:1227.

[d]METs, Metabolic equivalents of activity.

Table 66.3. Goldman's Specific Activity Scale[a]

	Any Yes	No
1. Can you walk down a flight of steps without stopping? (4.5–5.2 METs[b])	Go to no. 2	Go to no. 4
2. Can you carry anything up a flight of eight steps without stopping (5–5.5 METs) or can you a. Have sexual intercourse without stopping (5–5.5 METs) b. Garden, rake, weed (5.6 METs) c. Roller skate, dance foxtrot (5–6 METs) d. Walk at a 4 miles/hr rate on level ground (5–6 METs)	Go to no. 3	Class III
3. Can you carry at least 24 pounds up eight steps (10 METs) or can you a. Carry objects that are at least 80 pounds (8 METs) b. Do outdoor work—shovel snow, spade soil (7 METs) c. Do recreational activities such as skiing, basketball, touch football, squash, handball (7–10 METs) d. Jog/walk 5 miles/hr (9 METs)	Class I	Class II
4. Can you shower without stopping (3.6–4.2 METs) or can you a. Strip and make bed (3.9–5 METs) b. Mop floors (4.2 METs) c. Hang washed clothes (4.4 METs) d. Clean windows (3.7 METs) e. Walk 2.5 miles/hr (3–3.5 METs) f. Bowl (3–4.4 METs) g. Play golf (walk and carry clubs) (4.5 METs) h. Push power lawn mower (4 METs)	Class III	Go to no. 5
5. Can you dress without stopping because of symptoms? (2–2.3 METs)	Class III	Class IV

[a]See legend to Table 66.2.

[b]METs, Metabolic equivalents of activity.

Table 66.4. Diagnostic Criteria for Heart Failure. Criteria 1 and 2 should be fulfilled in all cases

1. Symptoms and/or signs of heart failure (at rest or during exercise[a])
   Dyspnea on ordinary exertion
   Paroxysmal nocturnal dyspnea
   Orthopnea
   Nocturnal cough
   History of acute pulmonary edema
   S_3 gallop
   Crackles at the lung bases
   Jugular venous distension
   Hepatojugular reflux
   Bilateral ankle edema
2. Objective evidence of cardiac dysfunction (at rest)
   Evidence of LV dysfunction (both systolic and diastolic) by imaging techniques
   An abnormal ECG with evidence of LV enlargement or scar
   Cardiothoracic ratio >0.5
   Elevated brain natriuretic peptide (BNP)[b] levels
3. Response to treatment directed toward heart failure (in cases where diagnosis is in doubt)

[a]Note that patients who are functional class I (see text) would have objective evidence of cardiac dysfunction, a history of symptoms and signs compatible with heart failure, and be receiving treatment for heart failure in order to fulfill the criteria for the diagnosis of heart failure.

[b]Note that the role of brain natriuretic peptide (BNP) in the diagnosis and management of heart failure in ambulatory practice is in evolution. BNP, because of its high negative predictive value, may be very useful in ruling out heart failure or in following its clinical course (see text).

LV, left ventricular; ECG, electrocardiogram.

Adapted from Task Force on Heart Failure of the European Society of Cardiology. Guidelines for the diagnosis of heart failure. Eur Heart J 1995;16:741, with permission.

Orthopnea is dyspnea in the recumbent position. It is often experienced by patients with heart failure, although it may also be a symptom of patients with obstructive lung disease or obesity. Blood normally pools in the lower extremities when a person is upright. When a person lies down, there is an increase in venous return to the heart; in a patient with heart failure, this may result in an increase in LVEDP that is significant enough to cause pulmonary venous congestion. The severity of orthopnea is often assessed by the number of pillows the patient must use to be able to breathe comfortably in the recumbent position.

Patients with heart failure often have a *nonproductive cough,* especially when in the recumbent position; at times this is the patient's premonitory symptom of decompensated heart failure and may precede the development of dyspnea by several days. The cough is caused by pulmonary venous congestion and usually improves with diuresis.

Paroxysmal nocturnal dyspnea (PND) is characteristic of poorly compensated heart failure; it typically occurs several hours after falling asleep and is relieved by sitting up in bed or by getting out of bed and sitting in a chair. Because PND often is associated with wheezing, it must be distinguished from the nocturnal shortness of breath sometimes experienced by people with obstructive lung disease (see Chapter 60). Periodic, or Cheyne-Stokes, breathing is a symptom of severe heart failure with low cardiac output; during the hyperpneic phase this respiratory pattern may be confused with PND and should be distinguished from obstructive sleep apnea (see Chapter 7).

A history of *edema* or weight gain (from retention of salt and water) is often elicited from patients with heart failure. Many also give a history of having taken digitalis, diuretics, or an angiotensin-converting enzyme (ACE) inhibitor in the past for a "heart problem." *Chest pain* caused by myocardial ischemia is common in patients with heart failure (see Chapter 62). Decompensated heart failure caused by salt and water overload may cause ischemic chest pain due to LV dilation with increased LV oxygen demands. Heart failure caused by systolic or diastolic dysfunction (see below) may rapidly decompensate because of ischemia, especially if there is associated paroxysmal mitral regurgitation caused by acute papillary muscle dysfunction. This may happen in association with exercise in patients with stable ischemic heart disease or may occur paroxysmally and at rest in patients with unstable ischemic heart disease (see Chapter 62). The symptomatic response to nitroglycerin does not by itself differentiate between dyspnea caused by ischemia with acute LV dysfunction and dyspnea caused by chronic heart failure; sublingual nitroglycerin may relieve symptoms of congestion caused by either condition (see below).

Nocturia, a common symptom of heart failure, often occurs early in the illness. It is caused by the redistribution in cardiac output that occurs in the recumbent position, restoring in part blood flow to the kidney that, in the upright position, has been diverted to other organs. The circadian pattern of atrial natriuretic peptide release may also be disturbed (see above).

Decreased cardiac output by itself, or in association with disturbed sleep patterns caused by orthopnea, PND, and Cheyne-Stokes respirations or with concomitant cerebrovascular disease, may lead to *impairment in mental function,* ranging from mild confusion to overt psychosis. However, the most common neuropsychiatric complaints are mild chronic anxiety and depression; these may be the presenting complaints, especially in elderly patients with previously undiagnosed heart failure (18).

Symptoms of *gastrointestinal congestion* may be seen in patients with chronic poorly compensated heart failure. Chronically increased right heart pressure may cause passive congestion of the liver, with swelling and discomfort in the right upper quadrant of the abdomen. Chronic constipation is also a common complaint and may be due to medication, inactivity, and lack of fiber in the diet.

Physical Findings

The physical findings in heart failure depend on its cause, the degree to which neurohormonal compensatory mechanisms are invoked (see above), the degree to which cardiac remodeling has progressed, and whether the heart failure is uncompensated or compensated.

Uncompensated Heart Failure

In chronic uncompensated or poorly compensated heart failure, there are signs of an attempt at pulmonary and cardiac compensation (increased respiratory and heart rate), signs of cardiac remodeling (increased heart size), and signs of increased renin, angiotensin, and aldosterone activity (vascular redistribution and evidence of cardiac, pulmonary, and peripheral congestion). Congestion is manifest by a ventricular gallop sound (S_3), pulmonary crackles, jugular venous distension, hepatojugular reflux, and peripheral pitting edema.

Increased heart size may be recognized by inspection, palpation, and percussion of the precordium. The precordium should be palpated with the patient in the supine and the left lateral position. The location, quality, and size of the point of maximal impulse (PMI) should be noted. The PMI of a dilated and enlarged heart is displaced laterally and caudally and is heaving and diffuse. The PMI of a concentrically enlarged heart is not displaced but may be thrusting or sustained.

Sinus tachycardia, defined as a resting heart rate in an adult of greater than 100 beats/min, is a sensitive but nonspecific sign of heart failure; it is a compensatory mechanism to increase cardiac output (see below). In patients with poorly compensated heart failure, a relative tachycardia of 85 to 95 beats/min may be seen. The tachycardia shortens diastolic filling time and may lead to further deterioration in function (see above).

The second pulmonic sound (P_2) is often accentuated in patients in LV failure because of increased pulmonary artery pressure. *Paradoxical splitting of the second heart sound,* an indication of prolonged LV ejection time, may be heard in patients with chronic heart failure and is often associated with a left bundle branch block.

The *ventricular or S_3 gallop sound* is the most specific sign of heart failure (19). The sound is heard shortly after the second heart sound (S_2) and is caused by sudden restriction of filling in a noncompliant left ventricle. It is usually heard using the bell of the stethoscope directly over the PMI and may be audible only when the patient is in the left lateral position. The sound is low pitched and often may be sensed by the cadence of the heart sounds rather than specifically heard. The cadence closely approximates the word *Kentucky* (pronounced kyn-TUC-ky). The middle syllable is accentuated to represent the loud second heart sound caused by increased pulmonary artery pressure in patients in heart failure. The timing of the last syllable closely approximates the timing of the third heart sound, when the word is repeated at a rate of 85 to 100 times a minute.

Crackles (formally called rales) are high-pitched sounds (similar to the sound of a clump of hair rubbed between the fingers) produced by the sudden filling with air of fluid-filled alveoli. They are a sign of moderately to severely decompensated left heart failure.

Neck vein distension and hepatojugular reflux are insensitive but specific findings of heart failure (20). In chronic heart failure, right ventricular filling pressure usually increases as the LVEDP increases. With time, the right ventricle becomes less compliant; as heart size increases, the pericardium may also restrain the heart and thereby limit filling.

Neck vein distension is assessed while the patient is semirecumbent, with a small pillow supporting the neck and the head turned slightly away from the examiner. Ideally, the internal rather than the external jugular vein is inspected because the latter contains valves and may not reflect accurately the right heart pressure. Internal jugular venous distension is seen as a broad-based fullness in the anterior cervical triangle. An arbitrary reference point may be chosen (e.g., the sternal angle; this approximates in many the level of the right atrium), and the column of blood above this point may be measured without regard for the angle of elevation of the thorax. The value of this observation is that accurate serial assessments are possible, permitting the examiner to confirm worsening failure (increasing jugular venous pressure) or to recognize a too vigorous diuretic response (abnormally low jugular venous pressure).

Hepatojugular reflux is assessed by having the patient lie supine and semirecumbent at 45 degrees. The patient is asked to breathe normally and is warned that the examiner will apply pressure over the right upper quadrant of the abdomen. Patients so warned comply and do not hold their breath or perform the Valsalva maneuver, which distends the jugular vein and makes the sign impossible to elicit. The pressure on the vena cava causes right ventricular end-diastolic pressure and right atrial pressure to rise and to remain elevated; this is seen as jugular venous distension.

Peripheral pitting edema is a common but not specific sign of heart failure. It occurs in the dependent portions of the body, which in ambulatory patients means the feet and lower legs. Edema in heart failure is caused by increased resorption of salt and water by the kidney. An increase in weight may precede pitting edema as an early objective manifestation of decompensated heart failure. Patients should be encouraged to weigh themselves daily or at least three times a week, and they should record the values and bring the weight record with them at each visit.

It is worth noting that calcium channel blockers (see below) are a common cause of pitting edema, so if a patient is taking one of these drugs, peripheral edema is not necessarily caused by heart failure. Unilateral pitting edema is also commonly seen in the vein-harvest leg after coronary artery bypass surgery.

Because of low cardiac output and vascular redistribution, patients' extremities may be cool and their nail beds may be cyanotic. Delayed capillary filling in the skin of the abdomen may be apparent when the examiner's hand is removed after assessing hepatojugular reflux. In patients with decompensated heart failure, hepatic congestion may produce jaundice, hepatomegaly, and abdominal pain that mimic acute hepatitis.

Compensated Heart Failure

In contrast to the findings in patients with acute or chronic uncompensated heart failure, there may be few or no specific physical findings in patients with compensated heart failure at rest other than signs of increased heart size. A presystolic gallop or fourth heart sound (S_4) can be heard in most patients with longstanding high blood pressure or ischemic heart disease who are in normal sinus rhythm. The fourth heart sound is thought to be caused by atrial contraction into a stiff ventricle (see also below). A soft systolic murmur, approximately grade 1 to 2/6, is commonly heard at the PMI or along the left sternal border in patients with chronic compensated heart failure. This murmur usually represents a minor degree of mitral or tricuspid insufficiency. A soft first heart sound may be due to a prolonged P-R interval. This may suggest digitalis toxicity or may be due to beta-blockers, amiodarone, or a combination of these drugs.

Laboratory Diagnosis

Brain Natriuretic Peptide

A rapid assay for brain natriuretic peptide (BNP) has recently been developed and may be a useful new tool for the diagnosis of CHF. BNP is produced by the ventricles in response to stress (e.g., elevated pressure, neurohormonal stimulation). Although not yet widely available, it may prove to be diagnostically most useful because of its high negative predictive value. In other words, a low level of BNP virtually rules out heart failure (21). The Food and Drug Administration recently approved a point-of-care BNP assay that provides results within about 15 minutes. A moderately increased level of BNP is suggestive but not diagnostic by itself. High levels of BNP are diagnostic of heart failure, but in practice, such patients are highly likely to have typical symptoms and signs of heart failure on physical examination, chest x-ray, and electrocardiogram (ECG). BNP may be very useful in guiding treatment. In one study in which treatment was guided either by BNP levels or by clinical signs and symptoms alone, the number of significant cardiac events in the "BNP group" was reduced by nearly 50% compared with the control group (22). BNP may therefore become one of the most useful tools in the diagnosis and management of heart failure in ambulatory practice.

Chest X-Ray

The chest x-ray is an important diagnostic procedure for the evaluation of suspected heart failure. The radiologic signs of heart failure are cardiac enlargement and pulmonary congestion.

A number of factors influence heart size on the chest x-ray, including body build, the depth of inspiration when the film is taken, and the chambers that are enlarged. Nevertheless, determination of the ratio of the transverse diameter of the heart to the greatest diameter of the chest, the cardiothoracic ratio, is a reliable and valid measurement of heart size and should be part of the database of every patient who is thought to have or to have had heart failure. The normal cardiothoracic ratio is less than 0.5. The pulmonary vasculature should be examined and signs of vascular redistribution, caused by pulmonary venous hypertension, and of enlarged hilar vessels, caused by acute or chronic pulmonary hypertension, should be noted.

Normally, the lower lobes of the lungs are better perfused than the upper lobes. The earliest radiologic sign of pulmonary congestion is reduction of blood flow to the lower lobes caused by compression of vessels by extravascular fluid that has gravitated to the lung bases. In early heart failure, there is simply an equalization of the size of the vessels to the upper and lower lobes; as congestion increases, the vessels to the upper lobes become more prominent, the so-called cephalization of flow. More severe failure is manifest by signs of interstitial edema and ultimately by alveolar edema and a transudative pleural effusion (see Chapter 59).

Electrocardiogram

No changes in the ECG are diagnostic of heart failure. However, the ECG may reflect an underlying disease (e.g., LVH caused by hypertension; Q waves or ST-T wave changes caused by infarction) or the presence of an unstable rhythm (e.g., atrial fibrillation with rapid ventricular response) that has caused heart failure. Changes reflecting chamber enlargement or hypertrophy (especially LVH or left atrial enlargement), conduction system disease (especially first-degree atrioventricular block and bundle branch block), or an abnormal rhythm (especially sinus tachycardia, atrial fibrillation, or ventricular ectopy) are common. *A normal ECG is rarely seen in patients with chronic LV dysfunction.* Because of this, it has been proposed that the ECG should be used as a triage tool, which could reduce by 50% the number of echocardiograms ordered for the evaluation of suspected heart failure (23).

Patients with hypertrophy of the heart may show only minor nonspecific ST-T wave changes. Grossly abnormal changes are commonly seen in the ECG of patients who have both dilation and hypertrophy of the left ventricle. The most common manifestations of LVH are *left axis deviation, increased QRS voltage and QRS duration, and ST-T wave changes.* Although there are numerous ECG criteria for LVH, a clinically useful criterion is the index of Lewis: net positivity in lead 1 plus net negativity in lead 3 equals 2.0 mV or more (see also Chapter 65). Also, an R wave greater than 11 mm in aVL is highly specific for LVH.

Conduction abnormalities are common in patients in heart failure, especially left bundle branch block. Left bundle branch block may be an early sign of congestive cardiomyopathy, especially when it occurs in young patients. It is nearly always a sign of organic heart disease.

Left atrial enlargement is diagnosed by the presence of a negative P wave with an area of greater than 1 mm^2 in lead V_1. It commonly is seen in the ECG of a patient with acute heart failure and may disappear as the patient is treated and the volume of the heart decreases.

Right ventricular hypertrophy is most reliably diagnosed in adults by a shift of the QRS axis toward the right greater than 90 degrees in combination with altered precordial R-wave progression (see also Chapter 65).

Certain ECG changes suggest a decreased ejection fraction, especially in patients with heart failure caused by ischemic heart disease. These include Q waves in leads 1, aVL, and V_1 through V_4 with persistently upward coving of the ST segments in the precordial leads (seen in patients with extensive anterior wall infarctions with aneurysms) and deep Q waves in both inferior and precordial leads with QRS duration greater than 0.1 second (suggesting ischemic cardiomyopathy) (23). *Low QRS voltage* (less than 10 mm in precordial leads and less than 5 mm in limb leads) is commonly caused by pericardial effusion, hypothyroidism, or infiltrative disease of the heart (e.g., amyloid), but also may be seen in patients with severe emphysema or marked obesity.

Echocardiography

The two-dimensional echocardiogram with Doppler is a reliable technique for determining ventricular size and thickness, the presence of valvular and structural abnormalities, the evaluation of systolic and diastolic function, and the presence or absence of pericardial effusion. If not previously performed, a two-dimensional echocardiogram should be obtained in all patients with a clinical diagnosis of heart failure to assess LV function. This is particularly important because heart failure due to LV systolic dysfunction may be difficult to distinguish from heart failure with normal LV function (i.e., diastolic dysfunction) by history and physical examination alone (see below). Echocardiography should be considered for patients with suspected valvular or pericardial disease or for patients in whom the cause of heart failure is unclear. In the primary care setting, echocardiography is unlikely to be useful in the evaluation of patients with suspected heart failure in patients with a normal ECG and a chest x-ray showing a cardiothoracic ratio below 0.5 (23). (The use of echocardiography in the diagnosis of valvular heart disease is discussed more fully in Chapter 65.)

Two-dimensional echocardiography with color-flow Doppler is useful in estimating the ejection fraction and detecting valvular stenosis or regurgitation. Pulmonary artery pressures may be estimated accurately but only in patients who have tricuspid regurgitation; this includes most patients with heart failure. Two-dimensional echocardiography with pulsed Doppler evaluation of mitral valve flow velocity is also useful in differentiating between systolic and diastolic dysfunction (24).

Radionuclide Angiography

Radionuclide angiography (gated blood pool scan or multigated acquisition study) is a technique for visualizing the cardiac chambers throughout the cardiac cycle. The major advantages of this technique over echocardiography are that good images may be obtained even in patients who are obese or who have severe chronic lung disease, and the ejection fraction may be determined precisely.

Radionuclide angiography is an effective tool to evaluate LV wall motion abnormalities, including ventricular aneurysm, and to evaluate LV function and diastolic compliance. The general practitioner does not ordinarily consider radionuclide angiography without the advice of a cardiologist. In most institutions, echocardiography has largely replaced radionuclide angiography as a diagnostic tool because it provides much more information regarding systolic and diastolic function, without radiation.

Cardiac Catheterization and Myocardial Biopsy

Cardiac catheterization (see Chapter 62) should be considered in any patient in chronic heart failure in whom an etiologic and anatomic diagnosis has not been made by noninvasive techniques. The sudden onset of heart failure with cardiomegaly in a previously healthy patient is an indication for immediate referral to a cardiologist. Cardiac catheterization may be the only way to diagnose pericardial disease. Myocardial biopsy may be useful in young patients suspected of having a cardiomyopathy who have the sudden onset of heart failure of uncertain cause. Approximately one-third of patients with chronic dilated cardiomyopathy are found, by cardiac catheterization, to have significant coronary disease (25). The procedure should be considered in all patients who have dilated cardiomyopathy of uncertain origin, especially in diabetic patients, who may have severe coronary heart disease with no symptoms of chest pain.

Exercise Testing

It is often difficult to determine the functional status of patients with heart failure, and functional limitation is often overestimated or underestimated. Studies show that the most precise determination of functional classification is given by exercise testing with assessment of oxygen consumption (26). The protocol used should be one in which the level of exercise is increased in small increments. The test should be obtained in consultation with a cardiologist or a pulmonologist and only if functional classification cannot be satisfactorily determined by clinical means. The 6-minute walk test, in which the distance that the patient is able to walk in 6 minutes is measured, correlates well with function assessed by measurement of oxygen consumption and also with prognosis. It is a useful, inexpensive tool for the assessment of functional status, and changes in performance can be tracked over time (27). A carefully taken history is also useful and inexpensive (see above).

Systolic Versus Diastolic Dysfunction

The clinical signs and symptoms of heart failure may result from systolic or diastolic dysfunction of the myocardium (see above). It is important to determine whether one or both of these mechanisms are operative to prescribe appropriate treatment.

In patients with heart failure caused by *systolic dysfunction,* the heart is dilated, often hypertrophied, and the inotropic state of the heart is impaired relative to the afterload so that the ejection fraction, and often the blood pressure, is decreased. A reduced ejection fraction, detected by echocardiography or gated blood pool scan, and an S_4 on auscultation may be the only signs of compensated systolic dysfunction. In uncompensated systolic dysfunction, resting tachycardia is usually present and an S_3 may also be heard. The heart is usually enlarged on chest x-ray, and Q waves, QRS widening, or left bundle branch block may be present on the ECG.

In patients with signs and symptoms of heart failure caused by *diastolic dysfunction,* the ventricle is less compliant (i.e., stiffer) and early diastolic passive filling of the left ventricle is decreased. Therefore, immediately before atrial systole, the atrium has a greater than normal volume and pressure and by the Frank-Starling principle the force of atrial contraction is increased. Clinically, this may be detected by a palpable presystolic apical filling wave or heard as a loud S_4. On pulsed Doppler echocardiography, diastolic dysfunction may be diagnosed by the increased velocity of the atrial component of diastolic filling relative to the peak velocity of the early diastolic rapid filling phase (see Chapter 65 for a more detailed discussion of this topic) (24).

The diagnosis of diastolic dysfunction is more difficult to make clinically than is that of systolic dysfunction. The diagnosis should be suspected in patients with evidence of increased filling pressure (jugular venous distension and pulmonary redistribution of blood flow) and concomitant elevation of blood pressure.

MANAGEMENT

The goal of therapy is not merely to control symptoms but to treat specifically the underlying causes of heart failure if possible (Table 66.1). If the underlying disease cannot be effectively treated (Fig. 66.3), an attempt should be made to increase the capacity of the heart to do work or to decrease the amount of work that the heart has to do. Table 66.5 shows the various measures that can be used to accomplish these goals in ambulatory patients. These measures are discussed in detail below.

General Principles

Lifestyle and Nonpharmacologic Therapies

It is not always possible to improve the function of the failing heart, but it usually is possible to decrease the metabolic needs of the body by encouraging a patient to stop smoking (see Chapter 27), to avoid emotional stress, and to get an adequate amount of rest (Table 66.6). A thorough understanding of the patient's home and work environment and the relationship of the patient to his or her supporting family members and caregivers is important. When possible, the recommended treatment regimen should be discussed with the patient and the patient's family.

The ambulatory patient should be encouraged to exercise (see Chapter 63) but to take care to avoid exertion to the point of causing further symptomatic cardiac decompensation. Sometimes this simply means performing the same activities more slowly.

There is a decreased stimulus to renin, angiotensin, and aldosterone production during supine rest, and even severely disabled patients may be able to lead socially useful and satisfying lives if they rest in the afternoon and in the early evening or before social or business engagements. Strict bed rest, which causes muscle weakness and deconditioning, should be strongly discouraged. The best advice may be for patients with chronic stable heart failure to participate in an exercise training regimen, in which the exercise is supervised at levels shown to be beneficial in controlled trials (28,29).

It is important that the temperature and humidity of the patient's home and work environment are controlled. Patients should be encouraged to have air conditioners for the summer months to reduce the extra demand placed on the heart by hot humid weather.

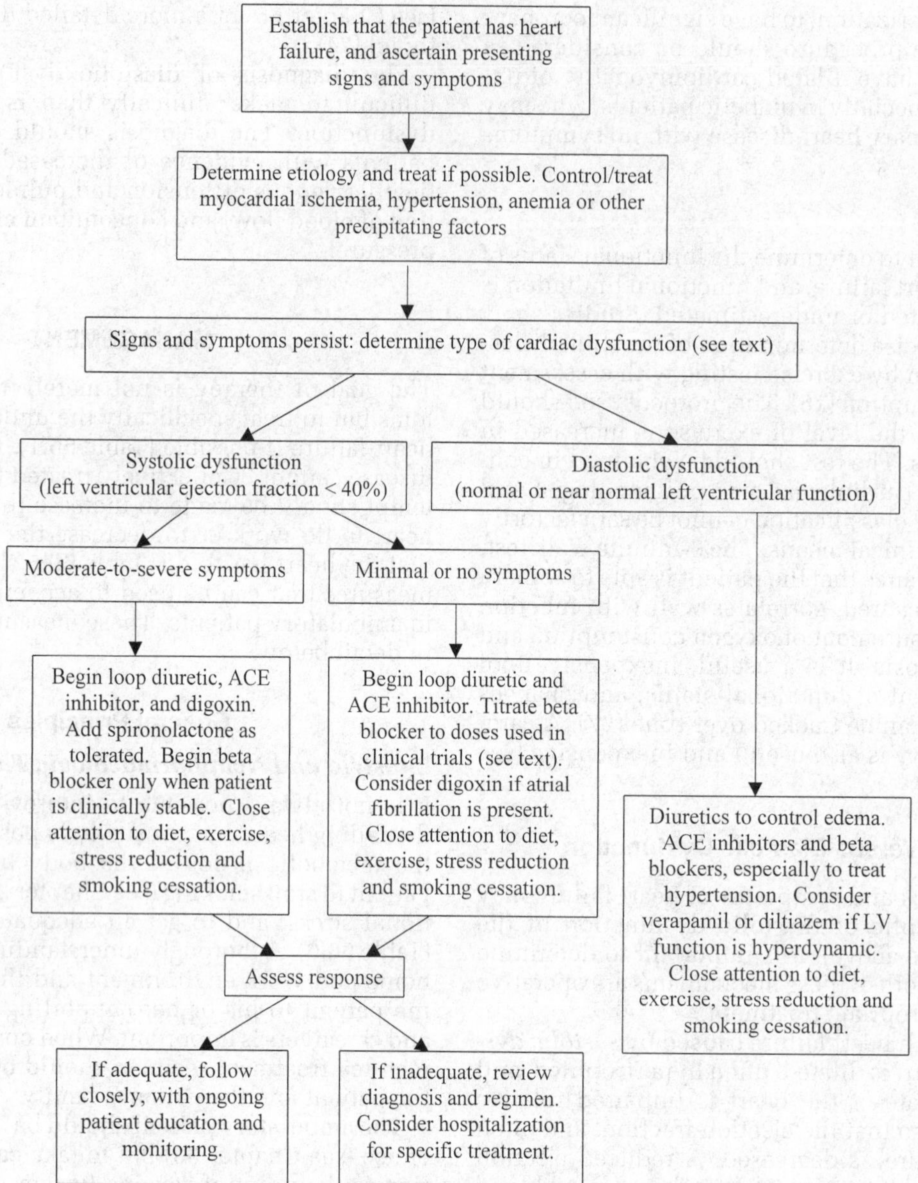
Establish that the patient has heart failure, and ascertain presenting signs and symptoms
Determine etiology and treat if possible. Control/treat myocardial ischemia, hypertension, anemia or other precipitating factors
Signs and symptoms persist: determine type of cardiac dysfunction (see text)
Systolic dysfunction (left ventricular ejection fraction < 40%)
Diastolic dysfunction (normal or near normal left ventricular function)
Moderate-to-severe symptoms
Minimal or no symptoms
Begin loop diuretic, ACE inhibitor, and digoxin. Add spironolactone as tolerated. Begin beta blocker only when patient is clinically stable. Close attention to diet, exercise, stress reduction and smoking cessation.
Begin loop diuretic and ACE inhibitor. Titrate beta blocker to doses used in clinical trials (see text). Consider digoxin if atrial fibrillation is present. Close attention to diet, exercise, stress reduction and smoking cessation.
Diuretics to control edema. ACE inhibitors and beta blockers, especially to treat hypertension. Consider verapamil or diltiazem if LV function is hyperdynamic. Close attention to diet, exercise, stress reduction and smoking cessation.
Assess response
If adequate, follow closely, with ongoing patient education and monitoring.
If inadequate, review diagnosis and regimen. Consider hospitalization for specific treatment.

Figure 66.3. Algorithm for treatment of heart failure.

Table 66.5. Measures Used in Ambulatory Treatment of Heart Failure

Increasing capacity of heart to do work
Appropriate drug regimen (see text)
Control of atrial fibrillation and other arrhythmias (see Chapter 64)
Pacemaker (see text)
Decreasing amount of work that heart has to do
Appropriate drug regimen (see text)
Compliance with medication and diet
Adequate rest
Control of other medical illness (e.g. anemia, diabetes, hypertension)
Home oxygen
Exercise training in selected patients

Diet

There is surprisingly little experimental evidence that a severely salt-restricted diet is of long-term benefit in controlling heart failure in patients who respond well to moderate dosages of diuretics. We are not aware of any published randomized clinical trials of low salt diet in heart failure in the modern era. It is commonly observed, however, that sudden increases in salt intake may precipitate acute pulmonary edema in patients who have moderately well-compensated chronic heart failure. Holiday seasons are particularly dangerous in this regard, probably also because of the increased activity and emotional stress. The various types of salty food that the patient is likely to eat should be anticipated, based on the patient's cultural background. Examples of frequently eaten salty food include breakfast meats such as sausage, bacon, and scrapple; deli meats including "low-salt" ham; salt pork or fatback in cooking vegetables; and many foods prepared by traditional ethnic cooks. Many patients attempt to substitute condiments in place of salt and

Table 66.6. Suggested Topics for Patient, Family, and Caregiver Education and Counseling

General counseling
- Explanation of heart failure and the reason for symptoms
- Cause or probable cause of heart failure
- Expected symptoms
- Symptoms of worsening heart failure
- What to do if symptoms worsen—how to obtain help in an emergency
- Self-monitoring with daily weights
- Explanation of treatment/care plan
- Clarification of patient's responsibilities for self-management
- Importance of cessation of tobacco use
- Role of family members or other caregivers in the treatment/care plan
- Availability and value of qualified local support group
- Importance of obtaining vaccinations against influenza and pneumococcal disease

Prognosis
- Life expectancy
- Advance directives
- Advice for family members in the event of sudden death

Activity recommendations
- Recreation, leisure, and work activity
- Exercise
- Sex, sexual difficulties, and coping strategies

Dietary recommendations
- Sodium restriction
- Avoidance of excessive fluid intake
- Fluid restriction (if required)
- Alcohol restriction (complete abstinence if heart failure is due to alcohol)

Medications
- Effects of medications on quality of life and survival
- Dosing
- Likely side effects and what to do if they occur
- Coping mechanisms for complicated medical regimens
- Availability of lower cost medications or financial assistance
- Importance of compliance with the treatment/care plan

are not aware that ketchup, hot sauce, soy sauce, and other sauces have high sodium concentrations. Homebound patients may eat prepared foods such as frozen pancakes and waffles or frozen convenience dinners, or they may have fast food brought to their home by family and neighbors; most patients are unaware that the sodium content of these foods is often higher than Atlantic Ocean seawater (1 g sodium/100 g seawater) (30). A no-added-salt diet, which contains approximately 2 to 3 g of sodium, suffices for most patients in compensated heart failure. Patients with poorly compensated heart failure may require a diet that contains 500 mg to 1 g of sodium, along with a restriction of volume intake to 1.5 L or less. The caregiver must take the time to give specific concrete advice about diet and nutrition.

A high-soluble-fiber diet may help avoid constipation and straining (see Chapter 46). Referral to a dietitian may be essential for patients with frequent episodes of cardiac decompensation caused by noncompliance with advice about salt and fluid restriction. Guidelines for planning these diets and a list of foods to be avoided by patients being treated for heart failure are given in Chapter 67.

Patients with heart failure may wish to know whether they can continue to drink alcoholic beverages. More than 2 ounces of alcohol a day may increase blood pressure and may impair cardiac function. In any patient with a cardiomyopathy apparently related to prolonged heavy alcohol use, total abstinence from alcohol is essential. A recently published large prospective cohort study, however, suggests that moderate alcohol consumption (approximately 1 oz/day) may decrease the risk of development of heart failure in older persons. This effect may be due to the association of moderate alcohol consumption with lower risk of development of coronary artery disease and type 2 diabetes. Moderate alcohol consumption may also decrease blood pressure (31).

Drugs that Promote Positive Sodium Balance

A number of commonly used drugs can promote a positive sodium balance: Renal sodium retention may be caused by corticosteroids and estrogens, for example. Nonsteroidal anti-inflammatory drugs (NSAIDs) other than aspirin are strongly associated with the development of heart failure; one study showed an odds ratio of 10.5 for the development of heart failure among patients with known heart disease who took NSAIDs (32). It is important to note that the effects of cyclooxygenase-2 inhibitors (e.g., celecoxib or rofecoxib) on kidney function may be similar to those of the nonselective NSAIDs (33). Some antacid preparations contain a significant amount of sodium. Patients with heart failure should not receive these drugs, or if the drugs are necessary, the patients should be monitored closely for symptoms of increased heart failure or electrolyte disturbance. There is no convincing evidence that aspirin has a deleterious effect on patients with heart failure; indeed, its use appears to be associated with lower mortality, especially in patients with coronary disease and heart failure (34). Unless there is a definite history of aspirin allergy or a history of aspirin-induced gastrointestinal or intracerebral bleeding, it seems advisable for patients with heart failure who are not taking warfarin to take daily aspirin, especially if they have associated coronary disease.

Drugs that May Directly or Indirectly Impair Left Ventricular Function

Calcium channel blockers depress LV function and should be avoided in patients with systolic dysfunction. Second-generation drugs (felodipine and amlodipine; see below) may be an exception, but they should be considered only if the patient's blood pressure remains poorly controlled despite the careful titration to appropriate doses of ACE inhibitors, beta-blockers, and diuretics. The antiarrhythmic agents disopyramide and flecainide should not be used in patients with systolic dysfunction.

Drug Therapy

The goal of drug therapy for heart failure is to relieve symptoms, improve function, and prolong life. Clinical trials demonstrate that it is possible to achieve these goals in most patients with chronic heart failure, although in clinical practice appropriate drugs are often not titrated to doses shown to achieve these goals in randomized controlled trials (35).

There may be important differences in the therapeutic approach to patients whose heart failure is caused by systolic dysfunction (dilated left ventricle with decreased ejection fraction) as opposed to patients whose heart failure is caused primarily by diastolic dysfunction (hypertrophied stiff heart with a normal or increased ejection fraction) (see above). Although many patients, especially older patients with chronic hypertension, have heart failure due to diastolic dysfunction, there are at present no clinical trials to guide therapy for this condition.

Diuretic Drugs

Diuretic drugs are used when it is impossible to treat the underlying cause of heart failure or when signs and symptoms of congestion persist despite treatment of the underlying condition. Although diuretic drugs have not been shown to prolong life (with the exception of spironolactone in certain patients with heart failure; see below), they relieve symptoms and improve function in most patients with heart failure. Diuretics reduce symptoms of circulatory congestion by increasing sodium and water excretion.

The goal of diuretic therapy is to reach and maintain the patient's "dry weight." Physiologically, this is the weight at which signs of peripheral congestion are substantially relieved and the LV filling pressure remains near the preload reserve (i.e., function is optimized via the Frank-Starling principle). Clinically, this is the weight at which peripheral edema is no more than a trace, jugular venous distension is absent, hepatojugular reflux, if present, is no more than a few centimeters above the clavicle with the patient reclining at 45 degrees supine, the blood urea nitrogen and creatinine determinations are at, or slightly above, baseline, and there are no symptomatic orthostatic blood pressure changes. After diuresis to the dry weight, the decrease in ventricular wall stress (i.e., afterload) and the improvement in ventricular contraction brought about by a decrease in heart size and peripheral vascular resistance often lead to a prompt improvement in ventricular function and, in hypertensive patients, a reduction in blood pressure.

There are three classes of diuretics in common use: thiazides (e.g., hydrochlorothiazide) and thiazide-like agents (e.g., metolazone, chlorthalidone), the so-called loop diuretics (e.g., furosemide, bumetanide, and torsemide), and the potassium-sparing diuretics (spironolactone, triamterene, and amiloride) (Table 66.7).

The *thiazides* and the *thiazide-like diuretics* act on the early portion of the distal convoluted tubule of the nephron; they cause a moderate increase in the excretion of sodium and chloride. Potassium and hydrogen losses are accentuated because of the increased delivery of solute to the terminal portion of the distal tubule, where potassium secretion occurs and is modulated by aldosterone. Thiazide-like agents such as metolazone act on both the proximal and distal convoluted tubules of the nephron and may be particularly effective in patients with very low renal blood flow.

The *loop diuretics* inhibit tubular resorption of chloride and sodium in the ascending limb of the loop of Henle. These diuretics are potent and result in a substantial increase in the excretion of sodium, chloride, and water. Like thiazides, the loop diuretics increase the delivery of solute to the more distal portion of the nephron, where potassium and hydrogen secretion is accentuated.

Potassium-sparing diuretics act on the terminal portion of the distal convoluted tubule, where only a small proportion of sodium is reabsorbed; by themselves they are only weak diuretics. However, they may be especially useful in combination with a thiazide or loop diuretic in preventing hypokalemia or when a patient becomes refractory to the more potent diuretics. The effect of thiazides and loop diuretics may be dampened by the resorption of sodium in the terminal portion of the distal convoluted tubule because they act proximal to the portion of the distal nephron where aldosterone influences sodium resorption. *Spironolactone*

Table 66.7. Characteristics of Selected Diuretic Drugs

Generic Name	Brand Name	Available Preparations	Usual Daily Dosage (mg/day)	Frequency of Dosing (per day)	Onset of Effect	Peak Effect	Duration
Hydrochlorothiazide	Generic	25-, 50-, 200-mg tablet	25–100	1–2	2 h	4 h	12 hr or more
Chlorthalidone	Generic, Hygroton	50-, 100-mg tablet	50–100	1	2 h	6 h	24 h
Metolazone	Zaroxolyn	2.5-, 5-, 10-mg tablet	2.5–10	1	1 h	2 h	12–14 h
Indapamide	Lozol	2.5-mg tablet	2.5–5.0	1	1 h	2 h	28 h
Furosemide	Lasix	20-, 40-, 80-mg tablet	20–160	1–2	1 h	1–2 h	6 h
Ethacrynic acid	Edecrin	50-mg tablet	50–100	1–2	30 min	2 h	6–8 h
Bumetanide	Bumex	0.5-, 1-mg tablet	0.5–2	1–2	30 min to 1 h	1–2 h	4 h
Torsemide	Demadex	20-, 40-mg tablet	20–40	1	30 min to 1 h	3 h	12 h
Triamterene	Dyrenium	100-mg capsule	100–300	1–2	2 h	6–8 h	12–16 h
Spironolactone	Aldactone	25-mg tablet	50–400	1–2	Gradual onset	2–3 days after initiation of therapy	2–3 days after cessation of therapy
Amiloride	Midamor	5-mg tablet	5–10	1	2 h	6–10 h	24 h

is structurally similar to aldosterone and competitively inhibits aldosterone binding to cellular receptors. *Triamterene* and *amiloride* block sodium resorption and potassium excretion but do not compete with aldosterone or even depend on its presence to be effective. These diuretics may cause life-threatening increases in the serum potassium level. Patients should usually not receive potassium supplementation while taking them. Also, patients with renal failure or patients taking an ACE inhibitor are at increased risk for developing hyperkalemia if given these diuretics. Serum potassium must be monitored carefully when these agents are used.

Use of Diuretic Drugs. When used in the treatment of heart failure, diuretics should always be prescribed with another agent (e.g., an ACE inhibitor or a beta-blocker). In patients with normal renal function, therapy should start with the lowest effective dosage of a thiazide compound (Table 66.7). Generic hydrochlorothiazide is the drug of choice. Many patients with mild heart failure may effectively control symptoms by use of the drug every other day or three times a week, along with use of an ACE inhibitor and beta-blocker. Patients with progressive disease, associated with worsening renal perfusion and albuminuria, should not be treated with a thiazide diuretic, which may decrease renal perfusion. In these cases, a loop diuretic—furosemide, bumetanide, torsemide—should be prescribed (Table 66.7) (ethacrynic acid is no longer widely used). These drugs are often effective in low oral dosages. Furosemide and bumetanide are available in generic forms and torsemide will soon also be available in generic formulation. Bumetanide and torsemide are less ototoxic than furosemide and their bioavailability orally is higher than that of furosemide. However, furosemide is still the most popular of these drugs, in part because of cost. Furosemide should be started at a dosage of 20 mg/day and increased as necessary for control of symptoms. Although a single dose of furosemide or bumetanide is commonly administered each day, these drugs are short acting (half-life of 1 to 1.5 hours), and patients with moderate to severe heart failure may require a second dose given in the late afternoon to effect a negative sodium balance. Torsemide has a longer half-life and may be effective given once daily, even in patients with moderately severe heart failure.

Dosages of furosemide higher than 160 to 240 mg/day are rarely required and may cause ototoxicity. Patients who require such large doses of diuretic for control of congestive symptoms should probably be referred to a cardiologist for evaluation. It may be necessary in these cases to substitute bumetanide or torsemide for furosemide or to add a thiazide diuretic in modest dosages (12.5 to 25 mg of hydrochlorothiazide or 2.5 to 5 mg of metolazone). Combination with a thiazide diuretic may markedly potentiate the effect of loop diuretics, leading to a rapid mobilization of fluid, and thereby allow these patients to be treated in an ambulatory setting and without the use of intravenous diuretics. Careful monitoring of electrolyte levels is essential (see below). A potassium sparing diuretic may be appropriate in certain circumstances. In particular, spironolactone should be considered in patients with severe heart failure due to systolic dysfunction because it has been shown to reduce morbidity and mortality in these patients (36). The diuretic dosage should be reduced when the dry weight is achieved and the patient should be weighed daily and should keep a written record of the weights to review with the care provider

Side Effects of Diuretics

Hypokalemia. The thiazide and loop diuretics have marked kaliuretic effects, and especially in edematous patients, hypokalemia is a common complication of the use of diuretic therapy. Hypokalemia may lead to fatigue, muscle cramps, and depression and often precipitates arrhythmias or digitalis toxicity. A high sodium diet predisposes to hypokalemia in patients taking loop diuretics because of aldosterone-mediated sodium–potassium exchange in the distal tubule. Patients with persistent hypokalemia should be encouraged to adhere to a very low sodium diet. The justification for sodium restriction must be explained to the patient in concrete terms. If hypokalemia persists despite a low sodium diet and treatment with an ACE inhibitor, a potassium-sparing diuretic such as triamterene or spironolactone should be used in preference to potassium salts. Potassium supplementation should be discontinued before the administration of a potassium-sparing diuretic and the patient's electrolyte concentration must be monitored carefully when these medications are started, when the dosage is adjusted, or when there is a change in the severity of the heart failure. Patients with diabetes and renal disease, who commonly have some degree of hypoaldosteronism and hyperkalemia (type 4 renal tubular acidosis), may be very sensitive to the potassium-sparing effects of these drugs. The serum potassium should be measured again 3 days to 1 week later; the goal is to maintain serum potassium concentration in the high normal range. The usual dosage of triamterene is 50 to 100 mg one to three times a day and of spironolactone, 12.5 to 100 mg once or twice daily. The higher dose ranges must be used with caution, especially in diabetics, as noted above. The indications for and use of potassium salts in patients taking diuretics are fully discussed in Chapter 50.

Hyponatremia. The loop diuretics and the thiazides may occasionally be associated with hyponatremia by impairing free water clearance, so caution is especially appropriate in patients who tend to consume large quantities of fluid. These diuretics also may be associated with hyponatremia when the extracellular volume has become contracted (a potent stimulus to the release of antidiuretic hormone) and fluid intake has not been restricted. Usually, the hyponatremia may be corrected by restricting water intake to less than 1 L/day. Finally, the thiazides may be associated rarely with hyponatremia in euvolemic patients who also are severely potassium depleted. This situation clinically resembles the syndrome of inappropriate secretion of antidiuretic hormone, although the exact mechanism of the complication is not fully known. The drug must be withdrawn until hyponatremia is corrected.

Contraction of the Extracellular Volume. Diuretics exert their therapeutic effect by causing a net loss of sodium, chloride, and water. If the response is excessive, depletion of the extracellular fluid compartment (the maintenance of which depends on sodium and chloride) occurs. This may have catastrophic consequences such as postural hypotension, sometimes with loss of consciousness, precipitation of ischemia caused by changes in cerebral, coronary, or renal blood flow or precipitation of hyperosmolar coma in diabetics. These complications are especially common when loop diuretics are used but may occur after the use of thiazides or combination diuretics, especially in patients also taking an ACE inhibitor. The patient should be monitored carefully, therefore, for evidence of excessive contraction of extracellular volume by daily self-assessment of weight and the presence or absence of edema and frequent assessment by the caregiver of the degree of fullness of the neck veins and of orthostatic changes in the blood pressure and pulse and of glucose levels in diabetics.

Acid-Base Disturbance. By their different actions on the nephron, diuretics have an effect on acid-base balance. The thiazides and the loop diuretics are often associated with the generation and maintenance of a metabolic alkalosis. This usually requires no therapy. To correct the alkalosis, the associated volume and potassium deficiency would have to be corrected. If the volume were replenished, the effect of the diuretic would be negated. Therefore, usually only potassium-sparing diuretics or potassium chloride supplements are given (see Chapter 50). If the alkalosis is thought to be detrimental, for example, in patients with respiratory failure, the diuretic should be discontinued or the dosage reduced.

Potassium-sparing diuretics may be associated with diminished hydrogen ion excretion and therefore with a mild metabolic acidosis. This is usually of no consequence and requires no treatment.

Hyperuricemia. Thiazides and loop diuretics commonly elevate the concentration of serum urate by blocking urate secretion by the proximal renal tubules or enhancing resorption through contraction of extracellular volume. However, symptomatic gout is not usual, nor is the elevation of uric acid likely to cause renal injury or stone formation. Therefore, unless gout does occur, routine measurement of uric acid and treatment are unnecessary. The treatment of diuretic-induced gout is discussed in Chapter 76; in general it is the same as it is for primary gout and does not require discontinuation of the diuretic. If NSAIDs are used in treatment, the patient should be monitored closely for volume overload and for changes in renal function. Consultation with a rheumatologist may be advisable if gout is severe or recurrent in a patient with heart failure.

Hyperglycemia. Thiazides and, less commonly, loop diuretics may cause glucose intolerance. Hypoglycemic therapy may be required (or changed, in diabetic patients already receiving a hypoglycemic agent) if the diuretic is to be continued (see Chapter 79).

Lipid Abnormalities. Thiazides may increase triglyceride concentrations in the blood. In patients with lipid abnormalities, a loop diuretic at low dosages (10 to 20 mg) may be preferable to a thiazide.

Other Effects. Thiazides are occasionally associated with a hypersensitivity-induced small vessel vasculitis (see Chapter 56), thrombocytopenia (see Chapter 56), and hypercalcemia (see Chapter 81) and may be associated with impotence. Furosemide at high dosages has been associated with the development of interstitial nephritis and renal failure, especially in patients with marked proteinuria. Spironolactone, which structurally is related to estrogen, may cause gynecomastia and may reduce libido in men or cause impotence; these side effects usually resolve within a few weeks of discontinuing the drug. Even when diuretics have substantially relieved the signs and symptoms of CHF, other medications are usually necessary to optimize function and prolong life.

Digitalis

Digitalis may help restore cardiac compensation by increasing the inotropic state, or contractility, of cardiac muscle, thereby increasing the ejection fraction at a given preload and afterload, as described above. It appears to act by increasing the delivery of calcium to the contractile apparatus of the heart. Digoxin is the only positive inotropic agent that has been convincingly shown both to improve function and quality of life and not to increase mortality in patients with symptomatic heart failure (37). Because digoxin is indicated only for patients with heart failure caused by systolic dysfunction, it is ordinarily used in patients treated also with a diuretic and an ACE inhibitor (see below).

Indications for Use of Digitalis Drugs. Digitalis reduces symptoms of heart failure and decreases the hospitalization rate for heart failure (37). It improves ventricular performance by moderating the heart rate of patients in atrial fibrillation or atrial flutter and by improving contractility in patients with heart failure due to systolic dysfunction. However, the degree to which digitalis preparations increase ventricular contractility is modest and the toxic-to-therapeutic ratio is small. Furthermore, the indiscriminate use of digitalis as a first-line medication for control of heart failure has led to its use in many patients in whom heart failure is not caused primarily by a decrease in the inotropic state of myocardial muscle. Such patients include those whose heart failure is caused by systemic hypertension, those with diastolic dysfunction or restriction to LV filling, and those in whom symptoms of fatigue are caused by a decreased cardiac output induced by excessive diuresis. In a classic definitive study, overall mortality was not higher with digitalis than with placebo (37), and digitalis was most beneficial in patients who were most symptomatic and had marked LV dysfunction.

Recommendations for Use of Digitalis Compounds. Digitalis glycosides should be prescribed only for patients with symptomatic CHF caused by systolic dysfunction (LV ejection fraction 40% or lower, cardiothoracic ratio 0.5 or higher). It is also a useful drug for certain types of arrhythmias (see Chapter 64).

The Glaxo-Burroughs-Wellcome preparation of digoxin, Lanoxin, has a bioavailability of approximately 75% and an intermediate duration of action (half-life of 36 to 48 hours). Digitalis elixir in capsules, Lanoxicaps (50-, 100-, and 200-μg capsules), has a bioavailability of nearly 100% and is useful when careful titration of the dosage is important, as in small elderly patients. Digitalization is best accomplished in an ambulatory patient by daily administration of the drug at the maintenance dosage (see below). Within four or five half-lives of the drug (approximately 7 days), full digitalization is ordinarily achieved.

The effect of digitalis on the patient's condition should be monitored and reassessed periodically. If there is no objective decrease in heart size or improvement in exercise capacity after a 1- or 2-month trial of digitalis therapy, the drug should probably be discontinued. Digitalis should be used cautiously in older patients and in any patient known to have impaired renal function. There is no evidence that elderly patients are intrinsically more sensitive to digitalis compounds, but they have a smaller body mass, often have impaired renal excretion of the drug, and have higher serum levels for a given oral dosage of the drug.

The average dosage of digoxin in patients with normal renal function is 250 μg/day (200 μg/day of Lanoxicap). Lower doses should be prescribed in patients with known impairments of renal function.

Digitalis may interact with other medications, and because of its low therapeutic ratio, the possibility of an interaction should be considered when any medication is added to the regimen of a patient already taking digoxin. The administration of quinidine causes a decreased renal excretion of digoxin, which may lead to digitalis toxicity; similar effects have been seen when digitalis is prescribed along with either of the calcium channel blockers verapamil or diltiazem (but not with nifedipine). The antiarrhythmic agent amiodarone may increase bioavailability of digoxin; the dosage of digoxin must be reduced and levels monitored when these drugs are used concomitantly. The use of thiazides and loop diuretics may lead to digitalis toxicity either because of increased retention of digoxin secondary to decreased renal blood flow or because of increased sensitivity to digitalis as the result of hypokalemia or hypomagnesemia. Cholestyramine and some antacids impair digoxin absorption and may result in a subtherapeutic effect.

Recognition and Treatment of Digitalis Toxicity. Digitalis toxicity commonly is caused by administration of too much digitalis, overdiuresis (often with associated hypokalemia and/or hypomagnesemia), intercurrent development of renal insufficiency, or administration of drugs that interact with digitalis to increase its plasma concentration. Digitalis toxicity is especially common in older patients in an ambulatory practice. In one large trial, 2% of the digitalized patients required hospitalization for suspected digitalis toxicity (37).

The manifestations of digitalis toxicity may be difficult to recognize in older patients and in patients whose normal baseline level of function is not familiar to the practitioner. They include changes in the cardiovascular system, gastrointestinal tract, and central nervous system. The most common cardiac manifestations of digitalis toxicity are progressive slowing and regularization of the heart rate (i.e., development of a nodal rhythm) of patients in atrial fibrillation and frequent premature ventricular contractions. Digitalis toxicity should be suspected in any patient who is taking digitalis and has premature ventricular contractions or in any patient in atrial fibrillation whose heart rate falls below 60 and becomes regular. Because digitalis both increases automaticity and decreases conduction through the AV node, paroxysmal atrial tachycardia with block may be seen. The peripheral pulse in paroxysmal atrial tachycardia with block is usually 100 to 120 beats/min (see Chapter 64). Cardiac toxicity may occur in the absence of other signs or symptoms of digitalis overdose.

Gastrointestinal side effects are common manifestations of digitalis intoxication. They include anorexia, mild nausea, and occasionally vomiting and diarrhea.

Digitalis may cause changes in the sensorium ranging from mild confusional states to frank delirium and psychosis. In an older patient it may be difficult to determine, without stopping the drug, whether these symptoms are caused by primary cerebral disease or digitalis excess. Digitalis is structurally related to estrogen and may cause gynecomastia, decreased libido, or impotence in men.

The diagnosis of digitalis toxicity is based on clinical and laboratory findings. If symptoms compatible with digitalis toxicity are present, especially in elderly patients, the drug should be stopped immediately. The patient should be reassessed in approximately 3 to 5 days. If symptoms have abated, a presumptive diagnosis of digitalis intoxication is warranted.

Although digoxin levels should not be checked routinely, it is appropriate to do so in cases of suspected toxicity. An adequately digitalized patient has a serum digoxin concentration of approximately 0.8 to 1.2 ng/mL; most toxic patients have concentrations above 1.8 ng/mL. However, if a patient has symptoms compatible with digitalis toxicity and his or her serum digoxin level is within the normal range, toxicity has not been ruled out because at therapeutic digoxin levels, hypokalemic patients may develop digitalis toxicity. Most patients with digitoxicity can be treated by temporary withdrawal of the medication and reinstitution of it at a lower dosage. Often, diuretic therapy must also be modified or potassium or magnesium supplements administered. However, patients with symptomatic arrhythmias are best hospitalized for a few days so that they can be monitored closely.

It is appropriate for all patients taking digitalis, and certainly for those who develop toxicity, to have the indications for digitalis therapy carefully reviewed to be sure that the patient clearly has systolic dysfunction or requires the drug for control of atrial arrhythmias (see Chapter 64).

Beta-Blockers

Activation of the neurohormonal system in heart failure leads to a chronic increase in sympathetic stimulation of the heart. This is facilitated by the resetting of aortic and cardiac baroreceptors that lose their inhibitory effectiveness. Chronic sympathetic stimulation of the heart leads to the down-regulation of beta-1-adrenergic receptors and may directly damage cardiac myocytes, thereby leading to further deterioration of myocardial function in CHF. A series of clinical trials shows convincingly that beta-blockers improve LV function, quality of life, and survival in patients with heart failure (38–40). Certainly all patients with moderate and stable heart failure due to LV systolic dysfunction should receive beta-blockers unless there is a specific and definite contraindication to this therapy. The recently reported preliminary results of the COPERNICUS study suggest that the beta-blocker carvedilol improves morbidity and mortality even in patients with more severe heart failure due to LV dysfunction (40). The usual protocol is to begin with low doses of either the beta-1-selective inhibitor metoprolol or of carvedilol, an alpha-1- and nonselective beta receptor inhibitor. Doses are then titrated upward in an attempt to achieve doses similar to those used in the Metoprolol CR/XL Randomized Intervention Trial in Heart Failure (38) (approximately 150 mg of the long-acting microencapsulated Toprol-XL) or in the U.S. Carvedilol Heart Failure Trials Program (39) (approximately 25 mg twice daily of carvedilol). In practice, titration of beta-blockers to the doses used in clinical trials may be limited by bradycardia or by symptomatic hypotension, particularly in older patients and in those receiving ACE inhibitors concomitantly. It is also important to note that beta-blocker therapy should not be initiated if the patient has signs of decompensated heart failure.

Importance of Hypertension Control in Patients in Heart Failure

Hypertension increases ventricular wall stress, and therefore the afterload on the heart, and reduces the cardiac output, especially as the heart begins to fail. It also triggers vascular remodeling (8,16). It is essential, therefore, that hypertension is controlled in patients in heart failure. This subject is discussed in detail in Chapter 67.

Vasodilators

Physiologic Rationale for Vasodilator Therapy. The signs and symptoms of heart failure are caused by the compensatory responses triggered by the inability of the heart, at a normal filling pressure, to maintain tissue perfusion (see above). Neurohumoral compensatory mechanisms result in an increase in LV preload and afterload. In the setting of LV dysfunction, these compensatory mechanisms lead to a further deterioration of cardiac function. The judicious use of vasodilator agents may optimize cardiac function, prevent further deterioration of LV function, improve the patient's functional state, and prolong the life of patients in chronic heart failure. Drugs that are predominantly *venodilators,* such as nitroglycerin preparations, primarily cause a decrease in preload, thereby relieving symptoms of vascular congestion. Venodilators are most useful in patients with severe heart failure in whom preload reserve is exceeded during exercise, which leads to an increase in LVEDP and to pulmonary vascular congestion. This also may occur at rest in association with ischemia in patients with ischemic heart disease or in association with progression of disease in patients with cardiomyopathy or valvular heart disease. Venodilators should not be used in patients with heart failure caused by restriction to ventricular filling (e.g., hypertrophic cardiomyopathy) or in patients with aortic stenosis in whom a reduction in preload may lead to a marked decrease in cardiac output. *Arteriolar vasodilators* increase cardiac output primarily by decreasing afterload (i.e., decreasing ventricular wall stress during contraction), thereby allowing the myocardium to contract more efficiently. These medications are most effective in patients with severe peripheral and central congestion who have signs of peripheral hypoperfusion, such as cool hands and acrocyanosis. It is important to note that arteriolar vasodilators increase cardiac output only if preload remains near the preload reserve. With afterload reduction, the left ventricle unloads more efficiently and volume shifts from the thorax to the abdomen and the peripheral venous circulation, thereby lowering preload. However, if preload drops significantly, cardiac output cannot be maintained, and the blood pressure falls. Thus, in an ambulatory setting, vasodilators must be used with caution and often with a concomitant adjustment of diuretic dosage.

Nitrates. Nitroglycerin in various formulations is an effective venodilator at the low end of the dosage range and a mixed venodilator and arteriolar dilator at higher dosages. The practitioner should be familiar with the use of nitrates in several forms (see Chapter 62): short-acting sublingual nitrates, long-acting nitrates taken orally, and nitroglycerin dermal patches. *Sublingual nitroglycerin* is generally used in a dosage of 0.4 mg. The medication is sensitive to body heat, light, and moisture and must be kept in a sealed dark glass or metal container. Patients should be encouraged to purchase new sublingual nitroglycerin every 6 months to ensure that the medication is active. Sublingual nitroglycerin may be used liberally to control symptoms of pulmonary congestion during normal physical activity such as walking up stairs, shopping, and so forth. Small bottles of 25 tablets may be prescribed and should be kept in strategic locations in the patient's home, car, and workplace. An effective *long-acting medication* is isosorbide dinitrate (generic, Isordil, Sorbitrate) in dosages of 5 to 20 mg orally, two to three times a day. If symptoms have not improved within a few days, the dosage should be increased. Dosages as high as 40 to 60 mg orally, three times a day, may be used safely depending on the patient's blood pressure response. Before and after each increase in the dosage, the patient should be checked for orthostatic hypotension. If there is a drop of more than 15 to 20 mm Hg systolic blood pressure 3 minutes after rising from the supine to the standing position, the dosage should be decreased slightly. *Nitroglycerin dermal patches* give sustained high blood levels of nitrate. Tolerance to the effect of sustained levels of nitroglycerin develops after 7 to 10 days of continuous use of nitroglycerin patches, and patients should be advised to remove the patch at bedtime and reapply a fresh patch upon awakening. The usual dosage is a 0.2- to 0.6-mg/h patch, applied in the morning and removed at bedtime. The patient should not be concerned about having the patch in contact with water during bathing or swimming; if it does fall off, however, a new one should be applied.

The most common side effects of nitrate therapy are headache and nausea. Skin irritation is occasionally seen with the use of dermal patches. Headache can usually be controlled by aspirin or acetaminophen, and it usually abates after several days of nitrate therapy. Gastrointestinal side effects of long-acting oral nitrates can occasionally be eliminated by switching to a different preparation of long-acting nitroglycerin or switching to nitroglycerin patches. Rubbing alcohol should be used to remove nitroglycerin dermal patches. If skin irritation develops, a different brand of patch should be tried.

Angiotensin-converting Enzyme Inhibitors. As discussed, the syndrome of heart failure is caused in large part by the stimulation of the renin–angiotensin–aldosterone system by the kidney (Fig. 66.4). ACE inhibitors block the conversion of angiotensin I to angiotensin II, a potent vasoconstrictor and a regulator of renin and aldosterone production. They cause a marked decrease in angiotensin II levels approximately 30 minutes to 2 hours after administration. ACE inhibitors also inhibit the degradation of bradykinin, a potent vasodilator. ACE inhibitors are thus effective vasodilators; they also block aldosterone-mediated salt and water retention.

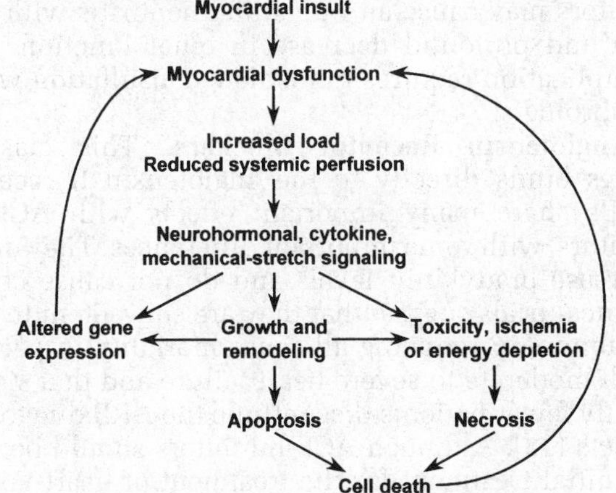

Figure 66.4. Interaction between myocardial injury, activation of the renin–angiotensin system, altered gene expression, and ventricular remodeling, which leads to myocardial dysfunction. (From Braunwald E, Bristow MR. Congestive heart failure: fifty years of progress. Circulation 2000;102:IV-14, with permission.)

ACE inhibitors appear to be the most effective vasodilators currently available for the treatment of heart failure. They retain their effectiveness after long-term use and have been shown to decrease the rate of progression of LV dysfunction and to decrease the rate of hospital admission in patients with heart failure (41). ACE inhibitors are first-line agents for treatment of heart failure caused by systolic dysfunction. All such patients should be prescribed an ACE inhibitor, unless a significant contraindication to its use, such as a history of allergic reactions to the drug or significant renal failure, is present. ACE inhibitors are also recommended to prevent or delay the development of symptomatic heart failure in patients with asymptomatic LV systolic dysfunction (42).

The currently available ACE inhibitors for use in CHF and their dosage ranges are shown in Table 66.8. Captopril is most useful for initiating ACE inhibitor therapy because of its short half-life, rapid onset of action (approximately 30 minutes), and wide dosage range. In patients with obvious signs of circulatory congestion, a dose of 12.5 mg of captopril should be given and the blood pressure checked in 1 hour. The usual effective dosage of captopril for heart failure is 12.5 to 50 mg three times a day. Patients who are hyponatremic or at their dry weight, or who are known to have significant renal vascular disease, should be started at 6.25 mg (one-half of a 12.5-mg cross-scored tablet) and their diuretic dosage should be decreased (because the danger of symptomatic hypotension is greater in such situations). Patients who are stable and have mild heart failure may respond well to enalapril 2.5 to 20 mg twice a day or lisinopril 5 to 40 mg/day in one dose. Both of these are prodrugs and their onset of action is approximately 2 to 4 hours. Symptomatic improvement is usually seen in several days, with maximal benefit after 3 months, although further improvement is often seen with longer treatment.

Because ACE inhibitors block the effect of aldosterone, potassium-sparing diuretics or supplementation may need to be decreased and potassium levels and renal function should be monitored 3 to 7 days after initiation of therapy, again at 2 to 4 weeks and periodically thereafter. ACE inhibitors also block angiotensin-mediated vasoconstriction, which may maintain renal perfusion pressure in patients with renal insufficiency. If serum creatinine or the potassium level rises after the initiation of ACE inhibitor therapy, diuretic dosages should be halved; the ACE inhibitor dose may need to be reduced and titrated upward more gradually. Consultation with a cardiologist or nephrologist may be helpful in this situation. Some studies suggest that aspirin, especially at high dosages, may

Table 66.8. Vasodilators Useful in Treating Heart Failure

Type of Drug	Drug	Available Tablet Strength	Usual Dosage
Organic nitrate			
	Isosorbide dinitrate (Isordil)	10, 20, 40 mg	10–40 mg b.i.d. or t.i.d.
	Nitroglycerin dermal patches[a]	0.1, 0.2, 0.4, and 0.6 mg/h	0.2–0.6 mg/h
Arteriolar vasodilator			
	Hydralazine (Apresoline)	10, 25, 50, 100 mg	25–75 mg q.i.d.
Calcium channel blockers			
	Nifedipine (Procardia)	30, 60, 90 mg sustained release	30–90 mg q.d.
	Felodipine (Plendil)	5, 10 mg	2.5–10 mg q.d.
	Amlodipine (Norvasc)	2.5, 5, 10 mg	5–10 mg q.d.
	Diltiazem (Cardizem)[b]	120, 180, 240, 300, 360 mg sustained release	120–360 mg q.d.
	Verapamil (Calan, Isoptin)[b]	120, 180, 240, 300, 360 mg sustained release	120–360 mg q.d.
Angiotensin-converting enzyme (ACE) inhibitors			
	Captopril (Capoten)	12.5, 25, 50, 100 mg	6.25–50 mg t.i.d.
	Enalapril (Vasotec)	2.5, 5, 10, 20 mg	2.5–20 mg b.i.d.
	Lisinopril (Zestril, Prinivil)	2.5, 5, 10, 20, 30, 40 mg	5–40 mg q.d.
	Benazepril (Lotensin)	5, 10, 20, 40 mg	10–40 mg q.d.
	Quinapril (Accupril)	5, 10, 20, 40 mg	5–20 mg b.i.d.
	Trandolapril (Mavik)	1, 2, 4 mg	1–4 mg q.d.
	Fosinopril (Monopril)	10, 20, 40 mg	5–40 mg q.d.
	Ramipril (Altace)	1.25, 2.5, 5, 10 mg	2.5–5 mg b.i.d.
Angiotensin receptor blockers (ARBs)[c]			
	Losartan (Cozaar)	25, 50, 100 mg	25–100 mg q.d.
	Valsartan (Diovan)	80, 160 mg	80–320 mg q.d.
	Irbesartan (Avapro)	75, 100, 300 mg	100–300 mg q.d.
	Candesartan (Atacand)	4, 8, 16, 32 mg	2–32 mg q.d.

[a]To avoid development of tolerance, an 8- to 12-h period without topical nitrates should be scheduled daily. Usually, this means applying nitroglycerin patches upon awakening and removing them at bedtime.

[b]Should be used only in patients with heart failure caused by diastolic dysfunction or when ischemia is a major reason for left ventricular decompensation. Short-acting preparations are not recommended, and available tablet strengths refer only to sustained-release preparations.

[c]None of the angiotensin receptor blockers has been approved for use in heart failure at this time. Their use should be limited to patients who do not tolerate ACE inhibitors (see text).

interfere with the vasodilating effects of ACE inhibitors (34); this effect does not seem to be clinically important at the usual dosages of aspirin used in patients with concomitant coronary heart disease and heart failure. It seems prudent, however, to use the lowest effective dosage of aspirin in these patients.

Side Effects. The most common side effect of ACE inhibitors is cough. A persistent, nonproductive, hacking cough is seen in 2% to 10% of patients treated with these drugs, although a less bothersome cough may be noted in many patients. This rate may be as high as 44% in Asian populations and tends to be more frequent in women (42). Decreasing the dosage or switching to a different converting enzyme inhibitor is only occasionally helpful. The cough is thought to be caused by the stimulation by bradykinin (the levels of which are increased by these drugs) of vagal afferents that trigger the cough reflex. Patients who have had significant symptomatic relief of heart failure after ACE inhibitor therapy may wish to try continuing the drug at a lower dosage or to learn to live with the cough. Often, the drug must be discontinued, in which case therapy with an angiotensin receptor blocker (ARB), should be considered (see below). If medication cost is paramount, hydralazine and long-acting nitrates may be tried. Because cough may itself be a symptom of heart failure (see above) or of a number of other conditions (see Chapter 59), the practitioner should be as certain as possible that the drug has caused the cough before discontinuing it.

Other side effects related to ACE inhibitors are uncommon. The ones most often seen are skin rash in patients taking captopril and angioedema in patients taking long-acting inhibitors (enalapril, lisinopril). These side effects warrant stopping the drug. Taste alteration and neutropenia are rarely seen. Rarely, ACE inhibitors may cause an interstitial nephritis with sudden and profound decrease in renal function. This complication requires immediate consultation with a nephrologist.

Angiotensin Receptor Blockers. This class of drugs binds directly to the angiotensin II receptor. ARBs share many important effects with ACE inhibitors, with some important differences. They do not increase bradykinin levels and do not cause cough. Clinical trials suggest that they are equipotent to ACE inhibitors in reducing all-cause mortality in patients with moderate to severe heart failure and that significantly fewer patients discontinue the ARB due to side effects (43). Although ACE inhibitors should be used as initial treatment for the treatment of heart failure, ARBs are a reasonable alternative when ACE inhibitors are contraindicated or are not tolerated because of cough. Several ARBs are currently available that may be given once a day (Table 66.8). The same cautions apply as for ACE inhibitors with regard to dosing.

Hydralazine. Hydralazine is an effective direct arteriolar vasodilator. In properly selected patients and when used in effective dosages, hydralazine may increase the cardiac output as much as twofold. This improved cardiac output may persist chronically in patients who respond initially. The combination of hydralazine and long-acting nitroglycerin has been shown to prolong survival in patients with severe heart failure treated concomitantly with diuretics and digitalis (44). Because the benefit of ACE inhibitors (see above) is greater than that of hydralazine and isosorbide, this combination should only be used when patients cannot tolerate ACE inhibitors or ARBs.

Calcium Channel Blockers. These drugs interfere with contractility of smooth muscle by blocking the entry of calcium into muscle cells, resulting in vasodilation, especially of the arterioles. All the currently available calcium channel blockers also depress myocardial contractility, although with calcium channel blockers of the *nifedipine* class, afterload reduction caused by vasodilation may offset the direct cardiac depressant effects and cardiac output may be maintained or may increase. In such patients afterload reduction is predominant, but these drugs should still be used with great caution in patients with severe LV dysfunction (ejection fraction 30% or less) and only if blood pressure is not controlled using ACE inhibitors and beta-blockers. The second-generation drugs *felodipine* and *amlodipine* may be effective in some patients with cardiomyopathy (45) because of their vasodilatory properties.

Verapamil is an arteriolar vasodilator that has a significant negative effect on cardiac contraction and relaxation. It may be particularly useful, at dosages of 120 to 360 mg/day (in sustained-release preparations), in patients with heart failure caused by diastolic dysfunction, but because of its negative inotropic effect, it should not be used in patients who have a congestive cardiomyopathy or an ejection fraction less than 45%. *Diltiazem,* in sustained-release dosages of 120 to 360 mg/day, may also be used for treatment of angina or hypertension in patients with heart failure caused by diastolic dysfunction. Common side effects of calcium channel blockers include headache, hypotension, nausea, constipation, and pedal edema (not caused by volume overload). Short-acting calcium channel blockers have been associated with increased mortality in patients in heart failure and their use should be avoided.

Summary of General Recommendations for Use of Afterload Reduction Therapy in an Ambulatory Setting. Unless specifically contraindicated, all patients with LV systolic dysfunction should be treated with an ACE inhibitor for the treatment and/or prevention of heart failure. If ACE inhibitors are contraindicated because of rash or angioedema or are poorly tolerated because of cough, an ARB may be substituted. If neither an ACE inhibitor nor an ARB is tolerated (e.g., because of renal failure), the combination of hydralazine and isosorbide is appropriate. Although no mortality benefit has been demonstrated in patients receiving calcium channel blockers, amlodipine or felodipine may be used in patients with persistently elevated blood pressure despite the use of an ACE inhibitor, an ARB, and/or a beta-blocker.

The patient's weight should be measured daily; signs of circulatory congestion (dependent edema, jugular venous distension and hepatojugular reflux, liver enlargement) should be assessed each time the physician sees the patient.

Symptomatic postural hypotension is a common complication of vasodilator therapy in patients in whom diuresis has been excessive. If this happens, the dosage of diuretic, not that of the vasodilator, should be reduced.

Compliance Issues

A major cause of mortality and morbidity in patients with heart failure is poor compliance with prescribed regimens. The average heart failure patient takes three to seven medications, and patients with other common comorbidities may be taking many more (46–48). Not surprisingly, patients often do not appropriately take the medications they are prescribed. Both over- and underdosing of medications occur, particularly as regimens become more complicated. Poor compliance with medications is a particular problem in those with depression, a common comorbidity in patients with heart failure. Patients with depression are three times as likely to be noncompliant with medical treatment regimens as are patients without depression (49).

Suggestions for enhancing compliance with medical treatment regimens in heart failure patients are as follows:

1. Patients should carry a list of their medications with them at all times.
2. They should bring both the list and all their medications, in the dispensed bottles, with them each time they visit their health care provider.
3. An "ABCD" arrangement of medicines is an easy-to-remember way to review medications and ensure that guideline recommendations are being followed:
   - **A.** Is the patient receiving an **A**CE inhibitor or an ARB and has it been titrated to a maximally tolerated dose?
   - **B.** Is the patient receiving a **b**eta-blocker and has it been titrated to a maximally tolerated dose?
   - **C.** If the patient is taking a **c**alcium channel blocker, can it be titrated downward or eliminated?
   - **D.** If the patient is receiving **d**igoxin, are there signs of digitalis toxicity or do any of the medications potentially interact with digoxin? If the patient is receiving a **d**iuretic, is the volume status optimal?

Home Oxygen Therapy

Patients with severe end-stage heart failure and arterial oxygen desaturation at rest caused by low cardiac output or concomitant pulmonary disease may feel more comfortable, especially while sleeping, with the use of low-flow nasal oxygen. The most efficient way to supply oxygen for therapy at home is by means of an oxygen generator, which is usually rented. The presence of oxygen desaturation should be documented (most easily done by use of a pulse oximeter) before oxygen is prescribed.

Anticoagulation Therapy

Patients with chronic severe CHF are at increased risk for pulmonary and peripheral emboli. Studies show an incidence of peripheral arterial embolization in these patients that ranges from 2% to 5% per year (50). A patient with a markedly dilated LV cavity or a patient with an LV aneurysm, especially if in atrial fibrillation, should be considered for treatment with warfarin anticoagulants (see Chapter 57). There have not been any controlled trials of anticoagulation in patients with heart failure. After adjusting for differences in baseline characteristics, warfarin use was associated with improved survival and reduced morbidity in patients with LV systolic dysfunction among patients enrolled in the Studies of Left Ventricular Dysfunction (51). Of note, warfarin use was not assigned in a randomized controlled fashion, and data on compliance with therapy, the intensity of anticoagulation, and complications of therapy were not reported. Warfarin therapy may be hazardous in patients with severe heart failure who may have wide swings in prothrombin time caused by hepatic dysfunction and multiple drug interactions. In such circumstances, the prothrombin time should be checked more frequently, perhaps every few weeks, or within 2 to 4 days after a medication known to interact with warfarin has been introduced or the dosage of warfarin or an interacting medication is changed.

Control of Arrhythmias in Heart Failure and Atrio-Biventricular Pacing

One of the cardinal features of CHF is a tendency to develop arrhythmias. Between 30% and 50% of patients with chronic heart failure die suddenly, presumably of ventricular tachyarrhythmias, although some studies show bradyarrhythmias to be as likely a cause of death. Holter monitoring is seldom useful in evaluating patients without symptomatic arrhythmias. Patients with symptomatic arrhythmias should be referred to a cardiologist for evaluation.

Amiodarone may be useful in some patients with heart failure and arrhythmias (see Chapter 64). Although amiodarone is effective in reducing the incidence of several arrhythmias, additional studies are still needed to determine which patients with heart failure should be treated with amiodarone. Some studies suggest that treatment with amiodarone reduced arrhythmic deaths in patients with heart failure who were considered to be at high risk of death from arrhythmia (52). In these studies, amiodarone was used at a dose of 200 to 400 mg once a day. Amiodarone interacts with digitalis and may precipitate digitalis toxicity; it also markedly potentiates the effect of warfarin anticoagulants.

It is expected that the implantable defibrillator will supplant the use of antiarrhythmic agents in patients with heart failure who are considered to be at high risk of sudden death from arrhythmia based on symptoms or significant ventricular ectopy. Consultation with a cardiologist is recommended for all such patients.

Permanent transvenous atrio-biventricular pacing (leads pacing the atrium and both ventricles) has recently been examined as a treatment for patients with heart failure who have LV systolic dysfunction, are in sinus rhythm, and have a significant intraventricular conduction delay (53). The rationale for this therapy is that the conduction delay may adversely affect LV systolic function by producing asynchronous ventricular contraction. A recent study in a small number of patients with moderate-to-severe heart failure showed that this form of pacing improved exercise tolerance and quality of life and decreased the need for hospitalizations (54). It is not yet clear which patients should be referred for this therapy. Ongoing studies should clarify the type of patient who is most likely to benefit from atrio-biventricular pacing.

Operative Correction of Problems Causing Heart Failure

The most commonly encountered surgically correctable problems in patients with chronic congestive failure include ischemic heart disease with revascularizable lesions or with resectable ventricular aneurysm, valvular heart disease, and atrial septal defect. Any patient who is in heart failure caused by a surgically correctable cause of myocardial dysfunction should be considered for operative correction, and consultation with a cardiologist should be obtained. Patients whose heart failure is secondary to reversible LV dysfunction may not be easily distinguished by history, physical examination, and echocardiography from those with irreversible ventricular impairment. Noninvasive stress testing may be helpful to detect ischemia or to assess myocardial viability in patients who are candidates for revascularization. Referral to a cardiologist may help select the appropriate noninvasive test or to determine which patients are appropriate for cardiac catheterization and coronary angiography.

Heart transplants should be considered for patients in severe refractory heart failure. The procedure is being performed in specialized centers throughout the United States. There are a number of contraindications to transplantation, including age of 70 or greater; irreversible severe renal, hepatic, or pulmonary disease; severe peripheral or cerebral vascular disease; insulin-requiring diabetes mellitus; and psychiatric impairment, so the proportion of eligible patients with heart failure is small. Even so, because of the scarcity of donated cadaver organs, the wait for an available compatible heart can be many months, during which time the patient may succumb to his or her disease.

Community Health Services

Many community health services are available to help the caregiver deal with the patient and the patient deal with the illness.

Home Visits

In two situations, home visits by the patient's health care provider or a visiting nurse should be considered in the management of a patient in heart failure: when the patient has repeatedly returned to the office or has been readmitted to the hospital with heart failure caused by dietary neglect or by failure to use medications correctly (see below) and when the homebound patient's symptoms are so severe (New York Heart Association class IV, Table 66.2) that he or she is unable to come for an office visit without becoming exhausted.

Information Booklets

The American Heart Association has useful free booklets that describe low salt diets and the management of CHF for the patient and family. These booklets may be obtained from local chapters of the American Heart Association. The American Heart Association website also has excellent information for patients with heart failure at http://www.americanheart.org/chf/working/index.htm. Extensive information, which is quite pertinent and useful, is also available on numerous other WorldWide Web sites.

Exercise Programs

Graduated regular exercise may improve exercise tolerance and increase daily activities and general well-being in some patients with heart failure, even in patients with severe LV dysfunction caused by ischemic heart disease. The improvement in function is thought to be caused by improved efficiency of the skeletal muscles; there is no evidence that myocardial function can be improved by exercise. Patients may also develop a sense of increased confidence in their ability to function.

Patients with class I to III CHF may be trained to exercise to 60% of their maximal heart rate for 20 minutes a day, 3 days a week. Exercise may be contraindicated entirely in patients who are in uncompensated left heart failure or whose heart failure is caused by valvular heart disease. Isometric exercise should be prescribed with caution in patients in heart failure because of the extra afterload this form of exercise imposes on the heart. Well-supervised circuit weight training may be safe. Muscle toning exercises using 1-kg hand weights are safe and may safely be used to help maintain function in all but the most frail patients with heart failure.

PROGNOSIS

The prognosis in heart failure is related clinically to the LV ejection fraction, the functional status of the patient, the initial response to treatment, the patient's compliance with the treatment regimen, the patient's age and comorbidities, and the cause of the heart failure. Physiologically, prognosis is related most importantly to LVEDP and to the degree of neurohumoral activation and LV remodeling. Most patients in chronic CHF die suddenly, presumably from ventricular arrhythmia (55). Other common causes of death are progressive heart failure and cerebral and peripheral embolization (50). In the Framingham study, which included heart failure from all causes, the probability of dying within 5 years of onset of heart failure was 62% for men and 42% for women (4,55). The median survival after the onset of heart failure was 1.7 years in men and 3.2 years in women (55). The cause of heart failure in most of these patients was hypertension or ischemic heart disease. Heart failure complicating uncorrected aortic stenosis is a particularly ominous sign, and most of these patients die within 3 years (see Chapter 65) unless aortic valve surgery is performed.

In general, prognosis is related to the patient's functional class (Table 66.2). Patients in functional class I have an annual mortality of approximately 10%. Patients in functional class IV have an annual mortality of nearly 50% (55). It is important that the practitioner not give a prognosis to the patient and family until the optimal level of response to therapy has been achieved. It has been observed that the median survival in advanced heart failure is similar to that of patients with metastatic breast cancer. Hence, it is appropriate to discuss advance directives and living wills with the patient early in the course of treatment.

Over the 40-year period from 1948 to 1988 (before the widespread use of ACE inhibitors and beta-blockers), there was no improvement in survival for patients with heart failure (55). However, in recent years the treatment of CHF in the ambulatory setting has evolved rapidly, and the outlook for these patients, although guarded, is no longer as grim (5).

Hospital Readmission

Patients discharged from the hospital with the diagnosis of heart failure have a high readmission rate. Factors associated with hospitalization include poor compliance with medications, inadequate treatment of associated hypertension and ischemic heart disease, and underuse of ACE inhibitors (56). Comprehensive outpatient programs, which include intensive education of the patient and family, social service support, titration of medications, and close follow-up, have demonstrated reductions in hospitalization rates of up to 87%, associated with clinically significant decreases in sodium intake from 3,400 to 2,100 mg/day and increases in the daily dosages of ACE inhibitors (57,58).

Patients treated successfully for heart failure should be advised to pay attention even to subtle signs and symptoms that may precede overt decompensation. Mild dyspnea or a slight change in weight should not be ignored because they may be followed, not by a gradual escalation in the severity of the condition, but by severe and seemingly abrupt deterioration that requires readmission to the hospital. Decreasing the likelihood of hospital readmission requires (a) patient education about the importance of sodium restriction and careful monitoring of weight, (b) the titration of medications to doses shown in clinical trials to be effective, (c) patient compliance with the medical treatment regimen, (d) decreasing the incidence of potentially preventable disease (e.g., influenza or pneumonia), (e) meticulous management of other medical illness (e.g., diabetes and hypertension), (f) constant monitoring of symptoms, and (g) timely reporting of increases in weight or development of symptoms to the patient's health care provider.

PREVENTION OF HEART FAILURE

It has been shown in asymptomatic patients that the development of symptomatic heart failure may be predicted by the finding of cardiac enlargement on echocardiography (41). The prognosis of these patients may be improved by treatment with ACE inhibitors, which may delay the development of overt heart failure in patients with LV dysfunction (41,59).

Although preventing or delaying the development of symptoms in individuals with existent LV dysfunction is important and feasible, the major impact on heart failure prevention will result from a reduction in the prevalence of hypertension, diabetes mellitus, hyperlipidemia, and cigarette smoking and the adoption of a healthier diet and regular exercise programs by a greater proportion of the population. Much time and effort has gone into identifying the medicines and interventions that will improve and prolong the lives of those with heart failure. The focus now needs to shift to making certain that patients get those medicines and, more importantly, trying to make sure that a greater number of our population will never need them.

General References*

Cohn JN. The management of chronic heart failure. N Engl J Med 1996;335:490.

Authoritative concise review.

Gomberg-Maitland M, Baran DA, Fuster V. Treatment of congestive heart failure: guidelines for the primary care physician and the heart failure specialist. Arch Intern Med 2001;161:342.

An excellent review of heart failure management.

Specific References

1. Haas GJ. Management of asymptomatic left ventricular dysfunction. Cleve Clin J Med 2001;68:249.
2. American Heart Association. 2001 heart and stroke statistical update. Dallas, TX: American Heart Association, 2000.
3. Centers for Disease Control and Prevention. Changes in mortality from heart failure–United States, 1980–1995. JAMA 1998;280:874.
4. Kannel WB. Vital epidemiologic clues in heart failure. J Clin Epidemiol 2000;53:229.
5. Polanczyk CA, Rohde LE, Dec GW, et al. Ten-year trends in hospital care for congestive heart failure: improved outcomes and increased use of resources. Arch Intern Med 2000;160:325.
6. Lakatta EG. Starling's law of the heart is explained by an intimate interaction of muscle length and myofilament calcium activation. J Am Coll Cardiol 1987;10:1157.
7. Katz AM, Lorell BH. Regulation of cardiac contraction and relaxation. Circulation 2000;102:IV69.
8. Hunter JJ, Chien KR. Signaling pathways for cardiac hypertrophy and failure. N Engl J Med 1999;341:1276.
9. Kang PM, Izumo S. Apoptosis and heart failure: a critical review of the literature. Circ Res 2000;86:1107.
10. Litwin SE, Grossman W. Diastolic dysfunction as a cause of heart failure. J Am Coll Cardiol 1993;22:49A.
11. Porter TR, Eckberg DL, Fritsch JM, et al. Autonomic pathophysiology in heart failure patients. Sympathetic-cholinergic interrelations. J Clin Invest 1990;85:1362.
12. Schrier RW, Abraham WT. Hormones and hemodynamics in heart failure. N Engl J Med 1999;341:577.
13. Brilla CG. Aldosterone and myocardial fibrosis in heart failure. Herz 2000;25:299.
14. Michell AR. Effective blood volume: an effective concept or a modern myth. Perspect Biol Med 1996;39:471.
15. Fitzsimons JT. Angiotensin, thirst, and sodium appetite. Physiol Rev 1998;78:583.
16. Levy D, Larson MG, Vasan RS, et al. The progression from hypertension to congestive heart failure. JAMA 1996;275:1557.
17. Green CP, Porter CB, Bresnahan DR, et al. Development and evaluation of the Kansas City Cardiomyopathy Questionnaire: a new health status measure for heart failure. J Am Coll Cardiol 2000;35:1245.
18. Vaccarino V, Kasl SV, Abramson J, et al. Depressive symptoms and risk of functional decline and death in patients with heart failure. J Am Coll Cardiol 2001;38:199.
19. Harlan WR, Oberman A, Grimm R, et al. Chronic congestive heart failure in coronary artery disease: clinical criteria. Ann Intern Med 1977;86:133.
20. Butman SM, Ewy GA, Standen JR, et al. Bedside cardiovascular examination in patients with severe chronic heart failure: importance of rest or inducible jugular venous distension. J Am Coll Cardiol 1993;22:968.
21. Maisel AS, Koon J, Krishnaswamy P, et al. Utility of B-natriuretic peptide as a rapid, point-of-care test for screening patients undergoing echocardiography to determine left ventricular dysfunction. Am Heart J 2001;141:367.
22. Troughton RW, Frampton CM, Yandle TG, et al. Treatment of heart failure guided by plasma amino terminal brain natriuretic peptide (N-BNP) concentrations. Lancet 2000;355:1126.
23. Davie AP, Francis CM, Love MP, et al. Value of the electrocardiogram in identifying heart failure due to left ventricular systolic dysfunction. BMJ 1996;312:222.
24. Nishimura RA, Tajik AJ. Evaluation of diastolic filling of left ventricle in health and disease: Doppler echocardiography is the clinician's Rosetta Stone. J Am Coll Cardiol 1997;30:8.
25. Hare JM, Walford GD, Hruban RH, et al. Ischemic cardiomyopathy: endomyocardial biopsy and ventriculographic evaluation of patients with congestive heart failure, dilated cardiomyopathy and coronary artery disease. J Am Coll Cardiol 1992;20:1318.
26. Jennings GL, Esler MD. Circulatory regulation at rest and exercise and the functional assessment of patients with congestive heart failure. Circulation 1990;81:II5.
27. Bittner V, Weiner DH, Yusuf S, et al. Prediction of mortality and morbidity with a 6-minute walk test in patients with left ventricular dysfunction. SOLVD Investigators. JAMA 1993;270:1702.
28. Coats AJ. Exercise training for heart failure: coming of age. Circulation 1999;99:1138.

*Bold print (general references) and bold numerals (specific references) denote published controlled clinical trials, meta-analyses, or consensus-based recommendations.

29. Keteyian SJ. How hard should we exercise the failing human heart? J Cardiopulm Rehabil 2001;21:164.
30. MacGregor GA, de Wardener HE. Salt, diet and health: Neptune's poisoned chalice: the origins of high blood pressure. Cambridge: Cambridge University Press, 1998.
31. Abramson JL, Williams SA, Krumholz HM, et al. Moderate alcohol consumption and risk of heart failure among older persons. JAMA 2001;285:1971.
32. Page J, Henry D. Consumption of NSAIDs and the development of congestive heart failure in elderly patients: an underrecognized public health problem. Arch Intern Med 2000;160:777.
33. Swan SK, Rudy DW, Lasseter KC, et al. Effect of cyclooxygenase-2 inhibition on renal function in elderly persons receiving a low-salt diet. A randomized, controlled trial. Ann Intern Med 2000;133:1.
34. Krumholz HM, Chen YT, Radford MJ. Aspirin and the treatment of heart failure in the elderly. Arch Intern Med 2001;161:577.
35. Cleland JG, Swedberg K, Poole-Wilson PA. Successes and failures of current treatment of heart failure. Lancet 1998;352 [Suppl 1]:SI19.
36. Pitt B, Zannad F, Remme WJ, et al. The effect of spironolactone on morbidity and mortality in patients with severe heart failure. Randomized Aldactone Evaluation Study Investigators. N Engl J Med 1999;341:709.
37. The Digitalis Investigation Group. The effect of digoxin on mortality and morbidity in patients with heart failure. N Engl J Med 1997;336:525.
38. Effect of metoprolol CR/XL in chronic heart failure: Metoprolol CR/XL Randomised Intervention Trial in Congestive Heart Failure (MERIT-HF). Lancet 1999;353:2001.
39. Packer M, Bristow MR, Cohn JN, et al. The effect of carvedilol on morbidity and mortality in patients with chronic heart failure. U.S. Carvedilol Heart Failure Study Group. N Engl J Med 1996;334:1349.
40. Tendera M, Ochala A. Overview of the results of recent betablocker trials. Curr Opin Cardiol 2001;16:180.
41. Vasan RS, Larson MG, Benjamin EJ, et al. Left ventricular dilatation and the risk of congestive heart failure in people without myocardial infarction. N Engl J Med 1997;336:1350.
42. Brown NJ, Vaughan DE. Angiotensin-converting enzyme inhibitors. Circulation 1998;97:1411.
43. Pitt B, Poole-Wilson PA, Segal R, et al. Effect of losartan compared with captopril on mortality in patients with symptomatic heart failure: randomised trial—the Losartan Heart Failure Survival Study ELITE II. Lancet 2000;355:1582.
44. Cohn JN, Archibald DG, Ziesche S, et al. Effect of vasodilator therapy on mortality in chronic congestive heart failure. Results of a Veterans Administration Cooperative Study. N Engl J Med 1986;314:1547.
45. Packer M, O'Connor CM, Ghali JK, et al. Effect of amlodipine on morbidity and mortality in severe chronic heart failure. N Engl J Med 1996;335:1107.
46. Miller NH, Hill M, Kottke T, et al. The multilevel compliance challenge: recommendations for a call to action. A statement for healthcare professionals. Circulation 1997;95:1085.
47. Monane M, Bohn RL, Gurwitz JH, et al. Noncompliance with congestive heart failure therapy in the elderly. Arch Intern Med 1994;154:433.
48. Bennett SJ, Milgrom LB, Champion V, et al. Beliefs about medication and dietary compliance in people with heart failure: an instrument development study. Heart Lung 1997;26:273.
49. DiMatteo MR, Lepper HS, Croghan TW. Depression is a risk factor for noncompliance with medical treatment: meta-analysis of the effects of anxiety and depression on patient adherence. Arch Intern Med 2000;160:2101.
50. Dries DL, Rosenberg YD, Waclawiw MA, et al. Ejection fraction and risk of thromboembolic events in patients with systolic dysfunction and sinus rhythm: evidence for gender differences in the studies of left ventricular dysfunction trials. J Am Coll Cardiol 1997;29:1074.
51. Al Khadra AS, Salem DN, Rand WM, et al. Warfarin anticoagulation and survival: a cohort analysis from the Studies of Left Ventricular Dysfunction. J Am Coll Cardiol 1998;31:749.
52. Connolly SJ. Evidence-based analysis of amiodarone efficacy and safety. Circulation 1999;100:2025.
53. Varma C, Camm AJ. Pacing for heart failure. Lancet 2001;357:1277.
54. Cazeau S, Leclercq C, Lavergne T, et al. Effects of multisite biventricular pacing in patients with heart failure and intraventricular conduction delay. N Engl J Med 2001;344:873.
55. Ho KK, Anderson KM, Kannel WB, et al. Survival after the onset of congestive heart failure in Framingham Heart Study subjects. Circulation 1993;88:107.
56. Chin MH, Goldman L. Factors contributing to the hospitalization of patients with congestive heart failure. Am J Public Health 1997;87:643.
57. Rich MW, Beckham V, Wittenberg C, et al. A multidisciplinary intervention to prevent the readmission of elderly patients with congestive heart failure. N Engl J Med 1995;333:1190.
58. West JA, Miller NH, Parker KM, et al. A comprehensive management system for heart failure improves clinical outcomes and reduces medical resource utilization. Am J Cardiol 1997;79:58.
59. Garg R, Yusuf S. Overview of randomized trials of angiotensin-converting enzyme inhibitors on mortality and morbidity in patients with heart failure. Collaborative Group on ACE Inhibitor Trials. JAMA 1995;273:1450.

CHAPTER 67

Hypertension

L. RANDOL BARKER, MD, ScD

High blood pressure (HBP), or hypertension, is the most common problem addressed at office visits to internists and general practitioners (see Table 1.3). The ambulatory management of this condition is a longitudinal process requiring skill in enlisting the patient's cooperation and in selecting, monitoring, and adjusting treatment. Hypertension has been studied extensively by epidemiologists and clinicians. The recommended care of patients with hypertension is based on findings from numerous clinical and epidemiologic studies.

EPIDEMIOLOGY

Incidence and Prevalence

Incidence

It has been estimated that 1.8 million adults in the United States develop hypertension each year (1).

Prevalence

As shown in data from the most recent National Health and Nutritional Examination Survey (NHANES) (Table 67.1), the prevalence of hypertension increases with age in all gender and race/ethnic subgroups. In this survey, hypertension was defined as a mean systolic blood pressure (SBP) on a single occasion of 140 mm Hg or greater, a mean diastolic blood pressure (DBP) of 90 mm Hg or greater, or current treatment for hypertension with prescribed medication. Because it has been shown that some survey subjects are normotensive at repeat visits (2), the figures from NHANES overstate somewhat the prevalence of sustained hypertension.

Isolated systolic hypertension is seen mainly in the elderly. The prevalence of isolated systolic hypertension is approximately 6% in persons 60 to 69 years of age and approximately 18% in persons age 80 years and older (3).

Of those individuals with hypertension, approximately 75% have stage 1 hypertension, which is defined as an SBP of 140 to 159 mm Hg or a DBP of 90 to 99 mm Hg (see Clinical Classification). Therefore, in a typical practice, decisions must be made most often for patients with stage 1 hypertension.

Table 67.1. Prevalence of High Blood Pressure[a] by Age and Race/Ethnicity for Men and Women, U.S. Population 18 Years of Age and Older

Age (yr)	African American[b]	White[c]	Mexican American
Men			
18–29	6.8	4.4	2.8
30–39	20.9	12.8	9.3
40–49	36.8	23.4	22.4
50–59	55.9	41.8	36.0
60–69	63.6	51.3	53.8
70–79	68.0	60.3	52.1
80 and older	62.4[d]	60.3	70.5[d]
Women			
18–29	2.0[d]	0.6[d]	1.0[d]
30–39	11.3	4.6c	6.2
40–49	30.5	12.7	10.6
50–59	47.9	36.8	33.5
60–69	77.8	50.9	59.3
70–79	72.6	66.9	67.0
80 and older	80.5[d]	74.3	71.0[d]

[a]Systolic blood pressure ≥140 mm Hg or diastolic blood pressure ≥90 mm Hg or taking antihypertension medication.

[b]Excludes Hispanic blacks.

[c]Excludes Hispanic whites.

[d]Estimate is based on sample size not meeting minimum requirement of NHANES III design, or relative standard error is greater than 30%.

From Burt VL, Whelton P, Roccella EJ, et al. Prevalence of hypertension in the US adult population: results from the Third National Health and Nutrition Examination Survey, 1988–1991. Hypertension 1995;23:305.

Secular Trends

Two secular trends in the United States probably reflect the beneficial impact of widespread attention to hypertension and other cardiovascular risk factors in the past three decades (4):

- The prevalence of hypertension in adults has decreased. This may reflect lifestyle changes that are known to prevent blood pressure (BP) increase (see Primary Prevention).
- The age-adjusted mortality rates from the two major consequences of hypertension have decreased. Between 1972 and 1990, stroke mortality decreased by almost 60%, and coronary heart disease mortality decreased by approximately 50%.

Other recent trends are a cause for concern (4):

- There has been an increase in the age-adjusted incidence of stroke and end-stage renal disease and the prevalence of congestive heart failure (CHF)—three problems for which hypertension is commonly an antecedent risk factor.
- Level of awareness of HBP, proportion being treated, and proportion with controlled HBP decreased modestly in the most recent national survey (Table 67.2), according to data from the third NHANES. In that survey, the majority of those with uncontrolled HBP (most frequently a modest elevation in SBP) were persons who have access to medical care (5). Persons older than 65 years of age accounted for the largest absolute number of subjects with uncontrolled HBP. Mexican Americans had the lowest rate of controlled HBP (15%).

Table 67.2. Trends in the Awareness, Treatment, and Control of High Blood Pressure in Adults: United States, 1976–1994[a]

	NHANES II (1976–1980)	NHANES III (Phase 1) 1988–1991	NHANES III (Phase 2) 1991–1994
Awareness (%)	51.0	73.0	68.4
Treated (%)	31.0	55.0	53.6
Controlled[b] (%)	10.0	29.0	27.4

[a]Adults age 18 to 74 years with systolic blood pressure (BP) ≥140 mm Hg or diastolic BP ≥90 mm Hg or taking antihypertensive medication.

[b]Systolic BP <140 mm Hg and diastolic BP <90 mm Hg.

From Burt VL, Whelton P, Roccella EJ, et al. Prevalence of hypertension in the US adult population: results from the Third National Health and Nutrition Examination Survey, 1988–1991. Hypertension 1995;23:305.

PRIMARY PREVENTION

Many subgroups in the population have an increased risk for development of sustained hypertension, including people who are overweight or sedentary, have high-normal BPs, consume excessive amounts of salt or alcohol, are African American, or have a family history of hypertension. Clinical trials have shown that weight reduction, regular exercise (aerobic and low intensity), reduced salt or alcohol intake, and a diet rich in vegetables and fruits but low in animal fat can prevent the development of hypertension and reduce BP (6–8). Other lifestyle changes that have been evaluated in clinical trials have been found to have inconsistent or unproved efficacy in the prevention or treatment of hypertension. These include stress reduction and increased intake of potassium, fish oil, magnesium, and dietary fiber (7).

The widespread adoption of measures known to help prevent hypertension and of other measures known to protect cardiovascular health (e.g., not smoking) would reduce significantly the cardiovascular morbidity in the population. In addition to public health approaches, physicians can help by recommending these measures to all patients and especially to those who have a family history of hypertension or have high-normal BPs (see later discussion). A later section of this chapter describes practical details regarding nonpharmacologic measures for controlling or preventing hypertension.

RISKS AND RISK REDUCTION

Risks Attending Untreated Hypertension

Risk Related to Blood Pressure

For the patient and the physician, the single most important concept in approaching hypertension is that high BP increases the risk of symptomatic cardiovascular disease (stroke, coronary artery disease, CHF, renal insufficiency) during the patient's entire life. This concept was elucidated best by the longitudinal observations on subjects in the Framingham study, which used 140/90 mm Hg as the threshold BP for hypertension (9). A number of other longitudinal studies corroborated the major findings of this study (10). A recent reanalysis of the Framingham data showed that subjects entering the study with high-normal BP (SBP, 130 to 139 mm Hg; DBP, 85 to 89 mm Hg) had increased risk of cardiovascular disease (11). In addition, analysis of data from multiple longitudinal studies indicated that incremental increases in SBP and in pulse pressure are the most powerful predictors of cardiovascular events in the population of older patients with hypertension (12).

In summary, longitudinal studies have established the following overall facts about blood pressure and the risk of cardiovascular disease:

- Risks increase progressively with both SBP and DBP at all BP levels. In the elderly, SBP and pulse pressure especially affect risk.
- The annual risk of major cardiovascular events is higher for older patients at all BP levels.
- At all ages and BPs, the annual incidence of events is somewhat higher for men than for women.

Coexisting Cardiovascular Risk Factors

One or more other treatable risk factors are present in many subjects with hypertension. These risk factors may affect a patient's prognosis far more than hypertension does. This is illustrated by the fact that two hypothetical patients with the following risk-factor profiles have similar long-term cardiovascular risks:

Age	Cigarettes per Day	Total Cholesterol	Diastolic Blood Pressure
50	0	180mg/day	125 mm Hg
50	30	220mg/dL	95 mm Hg

Baseline Target Organ Damage

In addition to BP level, age, gender, and other risk factors, *coexisting cardiovascular abnormalities* (target organ damage) increase the size of the risk. This is illustrated in Table 67.3, which summarizes findings in subgroups of placebo-treated subjects from the Veterans Administration Therapeutic Trial.

Table 67.3. Placebo-Treated Subjects, Veterans Administration Trial: Impact of Blood Pressure and Cardiovascular Abnormalities on Attack Rate

Risk Factor at Entry[a] and Diastolic Blood Pressure (mm Hg)	No. Patients	Attack Rate[b]
Without abnormality		
90–104	36	0.145
109–114	51	0.173
With abnormality		
90–104	48	0.352
105–114	50	0.426

[a]Cardiovascular and renal abnormalities, defined as follows: Presence of any of the following: grade 2 or greater hypertensive retinopathy, cardiomegaly on chest radiograph, left ventricular hypertrophy on electrocardiogram, evidence of renal damage, myocardial infarction, congestive heart failure, cerebrovascular accident.

[b]Rate observed during 3 years.

Adapted from Veterans Administration Cooperative Study Group on Antihypertensive Agents. Effects of treatment on morbidity in hypertension. III: Influence of age, diastolic pressure, and prior cardiovascular disease; further analysis of side effects. Circulation 1972;45:991.

Risk Reduction by Treatment of Hypertension

A number of placebo-controlled clinical trials completed between 1970 and 1985 demonstrated that pharmacologic treatment reduces risks in *middle-age adults with diastolic hypertension* (13). Table 67.4 summarizes for each of the major trials (14–18) the principal characteristics and percent reduction in expected morbidity and mortality. Six placebo-controlled clinical trials reported between 1985 and 1997 (19–24) showed convincingly that pharmacologic treatment also reduces morbidity and mortality in *older persons with HBP, including those with isolated systolic hypertension.* The principal characteristics and results of these trials are summarized in Table 67.5.

Meta-analysis of data current to 1999 from all placebo-controlled trials and head-to-head comparisons of antihypertensive drugs from four classes—thiazide diuretics, beta-blockers, angiotensin-converting enzyme (ACE) inhibitors, and calcium antagonists—showed that the overall benefits of BP control are similar for drugs from each of these classes (25). One class (calcium antagonists) was associated with an increased risk of coronary heart disease and a greater reduction in stroke risk, both findings of borderline significance. Additional meta-analyses by the same consortium (Blood Pressure Lowering Trialists Collaboration) will be undertaken in 2003 to include the added data expected from a number of ongoing clinical trials (see World Health Organization, 1990, in General References). The questions being addressed in ongoing trials include: (a) Are angiotensin II–receptor blockers (ARBs) as effective as or more effective than existing antihypertensive drugs? (b) Does drug treatment benefit hypertensive patients older than 80 years of age (HYVET trial)? (c) Does concurrent drug treatment of mild-to-moderate hypercholesterolemia add to the benefit conferred by antihypertensive drugs (ALLHAT trial)? In 2002, large single RCTs showed that the ARB losartin performed better than atenolol in preventing cardiovascular morbidity and mortality in both nondiabetic and diabetic patients with essential HBP and left ventricular hypertrophy (25a,25b).

Relative Risk Reduction

Aggregate analysis of clinical trial results has shown that *in the first few years of treatment,* there is a 42% reduction in expected stroke incidence and fatality (95% confidence interval [CI], 33% to 50%) and a 14% reduction in coronary heart disease incidence and fatality (95% CI, 4% to 22%) (13). Additional analyses of clinical trial results have shown that treatment of HBP reduces the expected incidence of CHF by more than 50% (26) and that the largest impact on incident CHF is in older patients with isolated systolic hypertension and evidence of a previous myocardial infarction (MI) (27). Treatment also prevents the onset or worsening of renal insufficiency, although population-based data suggest that among African Americans control of

Table 67.4. Clinical Trials in Adults with Diastolic Hypertension

	VA (Mild)	VA (Severe)	Australian[a]	Oslo	MRC
No. of patients	380	143	3,427	785	17,354
Average age, yr	51	51	50	45	51 (male) 53 (female)
% Female	0	0	37	0	48
Range of DBP at entry (mm Hg)	90–104	115–129	95–109	90–109	90–109
Principal medications	TZ, R, H	TZ, R, H	TZ or BB M C	TZ or BB M	TZ or BB M or BB TZ or C
Approximate % reduction in cardiovascular morbidity and mortality	35	75	30	25	19

VA, Veterans Administration; DBP, diastolic blood pressure; MRC, Medical Research Council (British); TZ, thiazide diuretic; R, reserpine; H, hydralazine; BB, beta-blocker; M, methyldopa; C, clonidine.

[a]Control group in this study got no treatment (all other control groups got placebo).

Table 67.5. Clinical Trials in Older People with Hypertension

	EWPHE	Coope and Warrender	STOP-Hypertension	MRC	SHEP	SYST-EUR
No. of patients	840	884	1,627	4,396	4,736	4,695
Average age (range), yr	72 (60–97)	69 (60–79)	75 (70–84)	70 (65–74)	72 (60–80 or more)	70
% Female	70	70	63	58	57	66
Mean BP at entry (mm Hg)	182/101	197/100	195/102	185/91	170/77	174/87
Principal medications	TZ TZ/TRIAM M	AT TZ M	TZ/AMIL AT, METOP PIND	TZ/AMIL AT	CTHAL AT	NITREND ENAL TZ
Approximate % reduction in cardiovascular morbidity and mortality	29	24	40	17	32	31

EWPHE, European Working Party on High Blood Pressure in the Elderly; STOP-Hypertension, Swedish Trial in Old Patients with Hypertension; MRC, Medical Research Council (British); SHEP, Systolic Hypertension in the Elderly Program; SYST-EUR, Systolic Hypertension in Europe; BP, blood pressure; TZ, thiazide; TRIAM, triamterene; M, methyldopa; AT, atenolol; CTHAL, chlorthiadone; AMIL, amiloride; METOP, metoprolol; NITREND, nitrendipine; PIND, pindolol; ENAL, enalapril.

HBP may not protect renal function as effectively as in Caucasians (1).

Gender. Meta-analysis of data from seven clinical trials that included both men and women showed that the relative risk reduction attributable to treatment was *similar for both genders* (28).

Absolute Risk and Risk Reduction

As noted previously, the absolute risk of cardiovascular disease is much higher among patients with hypertension who are elderly and those with target organ damage or multiple risk factors. Figure 67.1 shows the combined impact of these patient characteristics on absolute risk. The absolute benefit of treatment is also much higher when patients with these characteristics are treated. Bearing in mind the approximate one-third reduction in morbidity and mortality that was found in the trials summarized in Tables 67.4 and 67.5 and using the information summarized in Fig. 67.1, it can be seen that the absolute benefits of treatment differ greatly for groups of patients with similar BPs. For example:

In a 70-year-old man with three major risk factors and a BP of 160/90 mm Hg, the 10-year risk of a major cardiovascular event is approximately 45%. A one-third reduction in risk would mean that about 15 of an expected 45 events would be prevented in a group of 100 such patients treated for 10 years. Stated another way, the *number needed to treat* for 10 years to prevent one event would be 6 or 7.

In a 40-year-old man with a BP of 160/90 mm Hg and no major risk factors, the 10-year risk of a major cardiovascular event is approximately 10%. A one-third reduction in risk would mean that about 3 of an expected 10 events would be prevented in a group of 100 such patients treated for 10 years. In this instance, the *number needed to treat* for 10 years to prevent one event would be about 33.

It is likely that the findings from randomized controlled trials underestimate the potential benefits of BP lowering, for a number of reasons:

- They use intention-to-treat assignment to analyze results.
- Cross-over between treatment groups occurs (no treatment to active treatment or active treatment to discontinuation of treatment).
- The average duration of treatment is 3 to 5 years, so benefits accruing over longer treatment intervals are not detected.

Gender. Absolute risk reduction differs by type of cardiovascular event in men and women (28). In women, the major benefit is reduction in stroke. This benefit is especially pronounced in African American women, a finding that is partly explained by the greater absolute risk of stroke in these women (29). In men, treatment prevents as many coronary disease events as cerebrovascular events. This difference is thought to reflect the greater absolute risk of coronary events in untreated men.

Nonpharmacologic Measures

In clinical trials, nonpharmacologic measures (weight reduction, salt restriction, physical exercise, and a

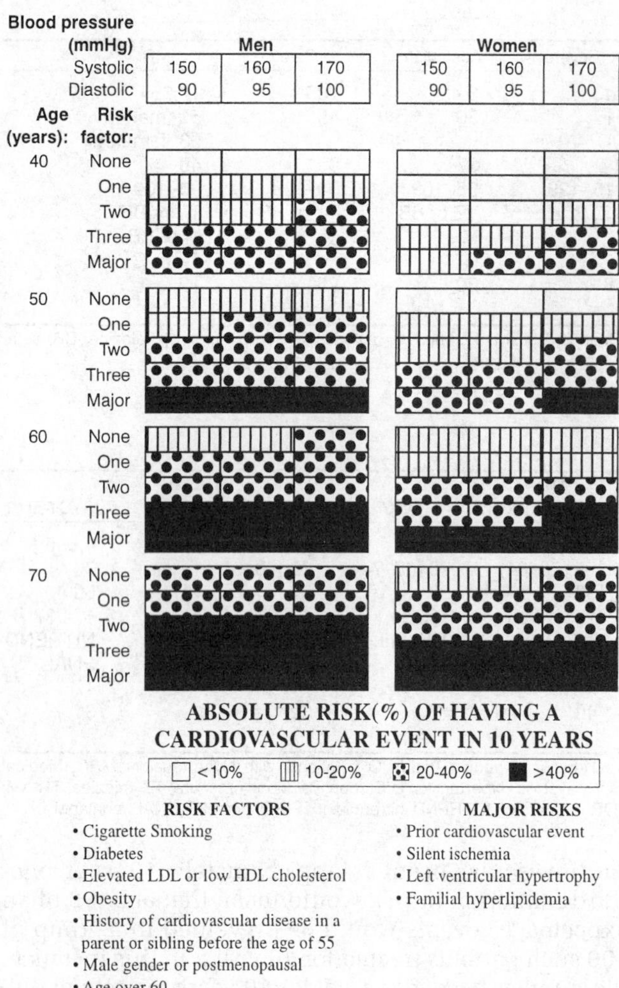

Figure 67.1. Matrix developed to help in decisions regarding the active treatment of hypertension. (Shading patterns shown in box represent absolute risks during 10 years.) (From Jackson R, Barham P, Bills J, et al. Management of raised blood pressure in New Zealand: a discussion document. BMJ 1993;307:107.)

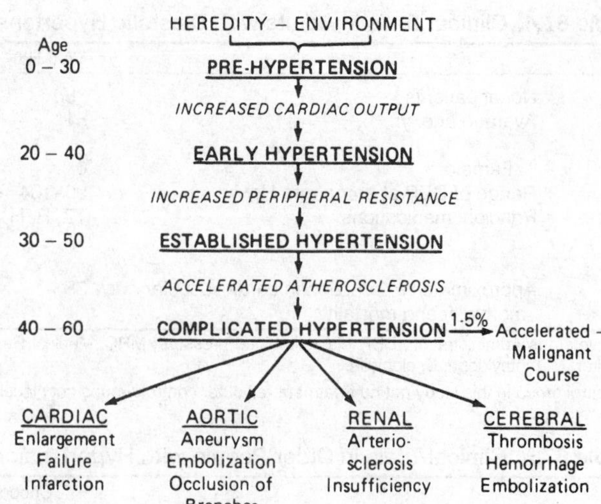

Figure 67.2. A representation of the natural history of untreated essential hypertension. (From Kaplan N. Clinical hypertension. 6th ed. Baltimore: Williams & Wilkins, 1994;110.)

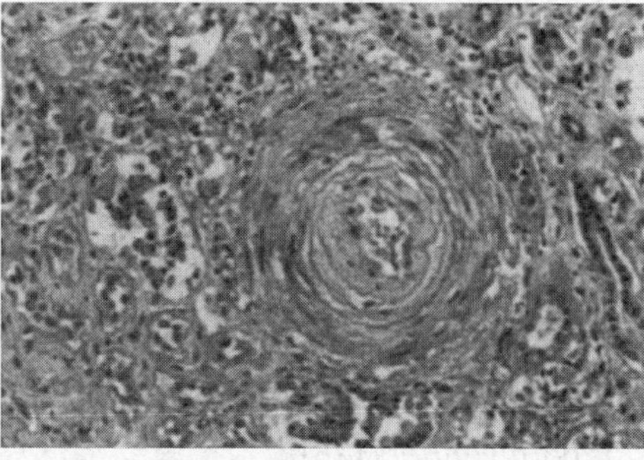

Figure 67.3. Hyperplastic arteriosclerosis in renal tissue from a patient with essential hypertension.

high-vegetable, low-fat diet) have been shown to reduce BP in hypertensive subjects (4). Although these trials were not designed to detect the impact of nonpharmacologic measures on cardiovascular morbidity and mortality, it is likely that they are efficacious (8,30).

PATHOPHYSIOLOGY AND NATURAL HISTORY OF ESSENTIAL HYPERTENSION

It is estimated that 95% to 99% of hypertensives do not have an identifiable cause for their hypertension. Their problem has been designated *essential hypertension,* a condition whose antecedents are probably a mix of genetic and environmental factors (4). Several abnormal physiologic characteristics have been demonstrated in essential hypertension; these provide a conceptual basis for understanding the clinical consequences of hypertension and the mechanisms of action of antihypertensive drugs.

As indicated in Fig. 67.2, the patient with established essential hypertension has an increase in peripheral arterial resistance; this is hypothesized to be the final consequence of either or both of two mechanisms: Inappropriate renal retention of salt and water or increased endogenous pressor activity. Serial studies on small numbers of subjects have suggested that a stage of increased cardiac output may precede the stage of increased peripheral resistance (31). This earlier stage may be manifested in some young hypertensives as a high resting heart rate. In general, however, the evaluation of the individual patient with essential hypertension does not yield much information about the dominant mechanism contributing to that patient's HBP.

The major complications of untreated HBP are named in Fig. 67.2. These complications can be seen as the clinical manifestations of two pathophysiologic processes that are operating during many silent years of increased peripheral resistance: *Trauma to the vessels in the arterial circulation,* leading to accelerated atherosclerosis in large vessels and to obliterative changes (Fig. 67.3) or thinning and rupture in small vessels, and *increase in the work load of the heart,* leading to CHF or angina pectoris.

MEASURING THE BLOOD PRESSURE

Standard Practices

A number of factors can affect the level of the BP that is measured by a sphygmomanometer (32). To ensure the validity of the measured BP and to ensure that comparable information is obtained in repeated observations, the following standard practices should be followed at each visit (4,33,34):

1. *Ensure that the patient has not smoked, chewed or snuffed tobacco, eaten a meal, or ingested caffeine or alcohol within 30 minutes* before measurement. Nicotine and caffeine cause a transient rise in BP, and eating can cause a transient decrease in BP, especially in elderly persons.
2. *Select cuff of appropriate size.* The width of the rubber bladder in the cuff should be 40% to 50% of the upper arm circumference. The ratio of bladder length to width is 2:1 in most adult cuffs, meaning that a bladder that encircles approximately 80% of the arm will have the right width. When bladder dimensions are too small for the patient's arm, the measured BP obtained may be higher than the actual BP (Fig. 67.4). Overestimation of the BP because of small cuff size can be minimized by using large adult cuffs (bladder dimensions about 30 × 15 cm) for all adult patients.
3. *Apply the cuff to the subject's arm* so that the lower margin is 2.5 cm above the antecubital space and the middle of the inflatable bladder is aligned with the brachial artery pulse.
4. *Have the patient sit with back supported in a chair for a few minutes. Measure the BP with the arm passively supported across the chest or resting on a table* so that the stethoscope head is placed over the brachial artery pulse at the level of the heart (about the level of the junction of the fourth intercostal space with the lower left sternal border). Sitting unsupported or actively holding one's arm across the chest can cause the SBP and DBP to increase by 5 to 10 mm Hg. Standing (in the untreated patient) may cause an increase and recumbency a decrease in the BP.
5. *In a new patient, measure the pressure in each arm.* If a difference between arms is noted and confirmed on repeated measurement, take all subsequent BPs in the arm with the higher pressure. The most common cause of arm-to-arm difference, which occurs in some patients with atherosclerotic disease, is partial occlusion of blood flow proximal to the brachial artery.
6. *Record the first Korotkoff sound (KS) for SBP.* The cuff pressure should be high enough to obliterate the radial pulse; by ensuring that this occurs, one avoids reading a falsely low SBP resulting from the *silent auscultatory gap* that occasionally occurs between the first and second Korotkoff sounds.
7. *Deflate the cuff slowly (about 2 mm Hg/second).* This prevents underestimation of the SBP and overestimation of the DBP. Both may occur with too rapid deflation, especially in a patient with a relatively slow resting heart rate. Underestimation of SBP may occur if the patient has an auscultatory gap.
8. *Record the fifth Korotkoff sound (disappearance) for DBP.*
9. *Wait 30 seconds* before repeating measurement in the same arm to permit the return of the blood that has transiently filled the veins distal to the inflated cuff.
10. *Use the average of two readings* in the same arm to designate the patient's BP. If the two measurements of SBP or DBP differ by more than 5 mm Hg, repeat measurements until a stable level is reached.
11. *To detect orthostatic hypotension before initiating antihypertension treatment, and after starting or increasing therapy with antihypertensive drugs,* record the BP with the patient standing for at least 1 minute. In treated patients, consider also measuring the BP after a standard exercise (e.g., ten steps on a footstool or walking a fixed distance), because the orthostatic effect of drugs is often more pronounced after exercise.
12. *Record BP, pulse rate, position, arm, and cuff size* (if a large cuff is used), thereby ensuring that these conditions will be duplicated when BPs are measured at subsequent visits.

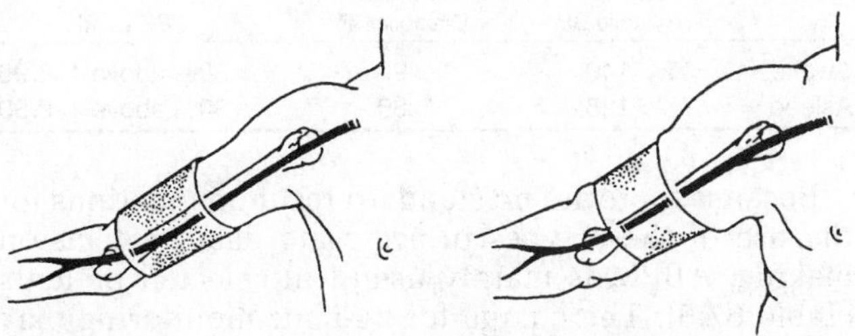

Figure 67.4. On the right, bladder width is small for arm, and full cuff pressure is never applied to artery. An erroneously high pressure results. On the left, bladder width is adequate for arm, and full cuff pressure is applied to brachial artery. (Reproduced with permission from the American Heart Association.)

Special Situations

Atrial Fibrillation. In patients with atrial fibrillation, whose beat-to-beat stroke volume and BP differ because of varying intervals between ventricular beats, record the average of several SBP and DBP values.

Pseudohypertension. When the wall of the brachial artery is rigid from calcification, the cuff pressure needed to compress the artery may greatly exceed the intra-arterial pressure, and a very high cuff pressure may be assumed, incorrectly, to be the actual BP. This condition, which has been called *pseudohypertension,* can be tentatively diagnosed by the finding that the (presumably calcified) radial artery does not collapse when the pulse is obliterated during cuff inflation; there is substantial intraobserver and interobserver variability in the interpretation of this maneuver (35). Definitive diagnosis of pseudohypertension requires arterial catheterization to directly measure the BP, which is then compared with the cuff pressure. It is important to consider pseudohypertension in the evaluation of patients—usually older patients with widespread atherosclerosis—who describe hypotensive symptoms despite apparently normal or high cuff pressures. A practical approach to management when pseudohypertension is suspected is described later (see Orthostatic Symptoms).

White-Coat Hypertension and White-Coat Effect. Among patients with stage 1 hypertension in the physician's office (see Clinical Classification), 20% or more have normal average daytime BPs if measured at home (36). This pattern is referred to as *white-coat hypertension*. Many patients with apparent white-coat hypertension have normal BPs when the measurement is repeated after the patient has rested quietly in the office. The *white-coat effect* refers to an average office-measured BP that is higher than the average daytime BP. Up to 40% of patients have a white-coat effect of 20/10 mm Hg or more (37). This effect is largest in patients with stage 2 or 3 HBP. Although cohort studies have indicated that patients with white-coat hypertension do not have excess cardiovascular risks, cross-sectional studies have found increased risk of left ventricular hypertrophy (LVH) in such patients (38), and there is evidence that some develop sustained HBP (i.e., elevated home *and* office pressures) (37). Management decisions for patients who demonstrate these patterns are discussed later in this chapter (see Treatment: General Considerations).

Self-Measurement and Ambulatory Blood Pressure Monitoring

Self-measurement by the patient or someone else and ambulatory blood pressure monitoring (ABPM) are two ways in which the snapshot type of information obtained at office visits can be expanded. Critical assessment of experience with these two methods yields the following conclusions (4,37,39):

- Neither method was used to classify the subjects in the observational studies and clinical trials, described earlier, that are the basis for current treatment guidelines. Therefore neither method is recommended for routine assessment and management of patients.
- The findings from cross-sectional and prospective studies have shown that target organ disease (e.g., LVH) and long-term risks correlate better with BPs from ABPM than with office BPs.
- Both self-measurement and automated ABPM can be helpful when office BPs do not seem to be sufficient for making clinical decisions (Table 67.6) or when patients wish to be more involved in monitoring the status of their BP.
- On the basis of findings from multiple studies, and using a cutoff point of two standard deviations above the mean BP in patients with normal pressure or untreated HBP, it has been recommended that home readings of 135/85 mm Hg or more should be considered hypertensive (4,37).

Table 67.6. Situations in Which Self-Measurement Devices or Automated Noninvasive Ambulatory Blood Pressure Monitoring Devices May Be Useful for Clinical Decisions

"Office" or "white-coat" hypertension: blood pressure repeatedly elevated in office setting but repeatedly normal out of office
Evaluation of apparent drug resistance
Evaluation of nocturnal blood pressure changes
Episodic hypertension
Hypotensive symptoms associated with antihypertensive medications or autonomic dysfunction
Carotid sinus syncope and pacemaker syndromes[a]

[a]Along with electrocardiographic monitoring.

From The Sixth Report of the Joint National Committee on Prevention, Detection, Evaluation, and Treatment of High Blood Pressure. Arch Intern Med 1997;157:2413.

- Self-measurement has a specificity of 85% for identifying white-coat hypertension.
- A large proportion of patients do not adhere to correct technique for self-measurement, and/or they obtain BPs that differ from simultaneous BPs by ABPM.

Home measurement devices. Many devices are available, ranging from inexpensive ($20 to $30) simple units that require auscultation with a stethoscope to more expensive ($50 to $150) electronic units that display the BP digitally. These devices are reviewed periodically to help consumers select among them. *Finger monitors* are not accurate and should not be recommended (40). When a patient decides to measure BPs at home, it is essential to confirm at periodic office visits that the patient's technique is satisfactory and that similar pressures are obtained with the home monitoring device and the office unit.

ABPM devices. These are portable devices that measure cuff pressures frequently over a 24-hour period. Patients are instructed to hold the arm still during automatic cuff inflation and to keep a diary and report dizziness, headache, or other symptoms of interest. Reports display average daytime, nighttime, and 24-hour pressures; frequencies and temporal distribution of selected pressures; and the *BP load* (e.g., percentage of waking pressures higher than 140/90 mm Hg or sleeping pressures higher than 120/80 mm Hg). The American Society of Hypertension has selected as abnormal an overall average 24-hour SBP greater than 135 mm Hg and a DBP greater than 85 mm Hg and has selected the following as *"probable abnormal" awake or asleep BPs* (39):

	Average Systolic BP	Average Diastolic BP	BP Load
Awake	>140	>90	>30% above 140/90
Asleep	>125	>80	>30% above 120/80

Because there are no standard recommendations for the use of these types of aggregate data in decision making, ABPM is mainly useful in selected patients (Table 67.6). The charge for 24-hour monitoring may range from $150 to $450.

One clinical trial comparing treatment decisions based on average office BPs to decisions based on average BPs measured by ABPM concluded that the latter decisions led to less intensive BP treatment and a better sense of well-being but did not reduce the overall cost of treatment (41).

Blood Pressure Variability

There are a number of psychological, biologic, and pharmacologic causes of BP variability. These factors should be considered when deciding what the measured BP means in an individual patient, in addition to following the standard approach to measuring the BP (described earlier).

Normal Patterns. In a 24-hour period, the average person's resting BP fluctuates (SBP, 20 to 40 mm Hg; DBP, 10 to 20 mm Hg) (37). The lowest BPs occur during sleep. These ranges occur in patients with normal BP and in hypertensive patients who are or are not taking antihypertensive drugs. During ordinary activities such as walking, talking on the telephone, attending a meeting, dressing, eating, and working at a desk, slight increases in both the SBP (5 to 20 mm Hg) and the DBP (5 to 10 mm Hg) may occur in untreated subjects. During and after vigorous exercise, the SBP may rise as much as 60 mm Hg and there may be a modest decrease in the DBP.

Common causes of transient or short-term high BP are white-coat hypertension (described earlier); mental stress, both intellectual and psychological; self-medication with excessive amounts of nonprescription sympathomimetic decongestants; nicotine, caffeine, or alcohol use shortly before BP measurement; and alcohol or sedative–hypnotic withdrawal.

Common causes of transient or short-term decrease in a patient's BP are volume contraction during an illness that causes fluid losses or reduced intake; bed rest for several days; hospitalization with or without strict bed rest; and the postprandial state in elderly persons.

EVALUATION OF THE HYPERTENSIVE PATIENT

Clinical Classification

In its sixth report (JNC-6), issued in 1997, the Joint National Committee on Detection and Evaluation of High Blood Pressure revised the national standards for clinical classification of adult patients with high BP (4). The JNC-6 classification, which is also used by the World Health Organization/International Society of Hypertension (WHO/ISH) in its 1999 Guidelines (42), is shown in Table 67.7. It differs in two ways from the classification published in 1993:

1. A new clinical category has been added: optimal BP (i.e., SBP, 120 mm Hg or less and DBP, 80 mm Hg or less).
2. There are now three instead of four stages (or "grades" in the WHO/ISH Guidelines), according to BP level. Old stage 4 (SBP, 210 mm Hg or greater; DBP, 120 mm Hg or greater) has been eliminated because of the infrequency of stage 4 disease.

The JNC and WHO/ISH recommendations for treatment of patients with stage 1, 2, or 3 HBP are based on the burden of coexisting risk factors and target organ disease (Fig. 67.1). These recommendations are discussed later (see Treatment of Hypertension).

Table 67.7. Classification of Blood Pressure for Adults Age 18 Years and Older[a]

Category	Systolic (mm Hg)		Diastolic (mm Hg)
Optimal[b]	<120	and	<80
Normal	<130	and	<85
High-normal	130–139	or	85–89
Hypertension[c]			
Stage 1	140–159	or	90–99
Stage 2	160–179	or	100–109
Stage 3	≥180	or	≥110

[a]Not taking antihypertensive drugs and not acutely ill. When systolic blood pressure (SBP) and diastolic blood pressure (DBP) fall into different categories, the higher category should be selected to classify the individual's blood pressure status. Isolated systolic hypertension is defined as SBP ≥140 mm Hg and DBP <90 mm Hg and staged appropriately (e.g., 170/82 mm Hg is defined as stage 2 isolated systolic hypertension). In addition to classifying stages of hypertension on the basis of average blood pressure levels, clinicians should specify presence or absence of target organ disease and additional risk factors. This specificity is important for risk classification and treatment (see Table 67.10).

[b]Optimal blood pressure with respect to cardiovascular risk is <120/80 mm Hg. However, unusually low readings should be evaluated for clinical significance.

[c]Based on the average of two or more readings taken at each of two or more visits after an initial screening.

From The Sixth Report of the Joint National Committee on Prevention, Detection, Evaluation, and Treatment of High Blood Pressure. Arch Intern Med 1997;157:2413.

The classification of patients should be addressed using values obtained by standard methods for BP measurement (detailed earlier) on two or more occasions after the initial detection of HBP. This approach is important because being labeled hypertensive can result in increased sick days, increased life insurance premiums, or employment restrictions for the patient (43). A variable characteristic such as BP will regress with repeated measurements to the person's usual level, which may be normal in some subjects whose initial BP is high. Two research findings underline the latter point: First, a sizable proportion of people who are found to be hypertensive at an initial screening visit do not have HBP at follow-up visits (2); and second, SBP and DBP predictably decrease when daily measurements are made over several weeks (44).

Clinical Presentation

There are several ways in which patients with high BP present to physicians.

History of Hypertension

On their initial visit, many patients state that they have hypertension. For some of these patients, recorded BPs from other sources are available. Some are taking antihypertensive drugs, presumably for sustained hypertension. Based on this information, on BP recordings made at the initial and follow-up visits, and on clinical and laboratory data regarding target organs, the patient's hypertension can usually be classified with confidence.

High Initial Blood Pressure

In practice, patients found to have an elevated SBP or DBP should have their BP remeasured within the following time intervals: 1 year for high-normal BP (SBP,

130 to 139 mm Hg or DBP, 85 to 89 mm Hg); 2 months for stage 1 (SBP, 140 to 159 mm Hg, or DBP, 90 to 99 mm Hg); 1 month for stage 2 (SBP, 160 to 179 mm Hg, or DBP, 100 to 109 mm Hg); and 1 week for stage 3 (SBP, 180 mm Hg or greater, or DBP, 110 mm Hg or greater) (4). Even very high initial BPs, especially when they are measured in emergency departments, may represent transient elevations.

Patients with transient high BPs or with high-normal BPs are at increased risk for development of sustained hypertension. They should be informed about this, and they should be advised to avoid excess salt and to follow other practices that reduce the likelihood of developing hypertension (see Primary Prevention).

Options for evaluating patients with *suspected white-coat hypertension* were described previously (see Ambulatory Monitoring and Home Measurement).

Chronic Hypertension

Hypertension is chronic if the average SBP is greater than 140 mm Hg or the average DBP is greater than 90 mm Hg at multiple office visits. At a patient's first visit, there may be evidence of chronic hypertension (e.g., a pre-existing electrocardiogram [ECG] that shows LVH, fundal hemorrhages or exudates found on physical examination). Eye ground findings indicative of arteriolosclerosis (grade 1, narrowing of arteriolar lumen; grade 2, arteriovenous crossing changes) are less specific indicators of chronic hypertension and should not be substituted for BP measurements on multiple occasions. Most patients with chronic hypertension are in JNC stage 1 or 2 (Table 67.7) when they first present to the physician.

The prognosis for untreated chronic hypertension and the benefits of treatment were summarized earlier (see Risks and Risk Reduction).

Accelerated Hypertension

Hypertension is accelerated when there is clinical evidence of severe arteriolosclerosis, meaning either *grade 3 or 4 hypertensive retinopathy* (grade 3, hemorrhages or fresh exudates; grade 4, papilledema) or *renal insufficiency* for which there is no apparent cause except the hypertension. Before they develop evidence of accelerated hypertension, most of these patients have had very high BPs (i.e., JNC stage 3) for several years.

The prognosis in *untreated accelerated hypertension* is poor: approximately 95% of these patients die from cardiac, renal, or central nervous system complications within 5 years after initial presentation. Control of BP and use of dialysis (for those with end-stage renal disease) have dramatically improved the prognosis in these individuals.

Hypertensive Emergency

A hypertensive emergency exists when elevation of the BP will predictably contribute to a catastrophic outcome within hours or days. Patients with one of two types of hypertensive emergency—hypertensive encephalopathy and dissecting aneurysm of the thoracic aorta—may present initially in an office setting. If either of these diagnoses is suspected, the patient should be transported immediately to a hospital emergency department for evaluation and treatment.

Hypertensive encephalopathy is the result of cerebral edema that develops gradually over 24 hours or longer in a patient with severe hypertension. In such a patient, global cerebral symptoms, such as headache, confusion, and irritability, have usually been present and progressive for hours or days. Papilledema may be present. Hypertensive encephalopathy should not be diagnosed until intracerebral mass or hemorrhage, which may also manifest with hypertension, has been excluded by computed tomographic (CT) scanning. Diffuse or focal white matter edema in the supratentorial compartment is usually be seen on the scan (45).

Thoracic aortic dissection results from an expanding hematoma in the wall of the aorta. The patient with acute dissection usually has a history of known hypertension and presents with a story of sudden anterior chest pain or tearing pain in the back. Two noninvasive imaging modalities—CT and magnetic resonance imaging—are very sensitive and specific diagnostic tests for dissection. By definition, a *proximal dissection* involves the aorta between the aortic root and the left subclavian artery (palpated pulse intensity and BP levels may be decreased in either arm; there may be a murmur of aortic regurgitation) and a *distal dissection* involves only that part of the aorta distal to the left subclavian artery.

The prognosis in encephalopathy or aortic dissection—if diagnosed before irreversible damage has occurred—depends on prompt hospitalization for antihypertension treatment and, for some patients with dissection, surgery. Despite the overwhelming threat to life without treatment, good outcomes can be achieved with appropriate intervention.

Hypertensive Urgency

The term *hypertensive urgency* is often used to categorize patients with severe hypertension (e.g., SBP, 210 mm Hg or more, or DBP, 120 mm Hg or more) who may have evidence of target organ disease but are asymptomatic. Some authors advocate lowering of the BP within a few hours, using doses of oral medications with prompt onset of action. There is no evidence for benefit—and there is some evidence for harm (e.g., stroke, MI)—in asymptomatic patients whose BP is treated hourly until the BP is lowered (37). As discussed later (see Treatment of Hypertension), with currently available drugs it is usually possible, and more appropriate, to control severe hypertension within a few days.

Baseline Evaluation: Overview

The baseline evaluation of patients with sustained hypertension has five objectives:

1. To assess the status of *target organs* affected by hypertension

2. To identify clues to the presence of *secondary hypertension*
3. To guide the selection of *initial treatment*
4. To establish the *pretreatment status* of the patient's electrolytes, renal function, and other characteristics that may be affected by antihypertensive drugs
5. To detect the presence of additional *cardiovascular risk factors*

Table 67.8 lists by source the information that is recommended to accomplish these five objectives at baseline. These recommendations match the consensus recommendations of the 1997 JNC report (4).

Target Organ Status

At baseline evaluation, most patients with sustained hypertension, including those with accelerated hypertension, have no symptoms attributable to their hypertension. In the past, it was thought that headache, tinnitus, epistaxis, and dizziness were common symptoms of hypertension, but community-based studies have demonstrated that these symptoms are not more prevalent in hypertensive than in normotensive subjects (46).

The major morbidity of HBP is the result of cardiac, cerebral, and renal disease. Baseline information about the target organs affected by HBP often helps in making decisions about follow-up care (see Recommendations Regarding Initial Treatment).

Heart

A history of symptoms caused by CHF or by coronary artery disease is occasionally obtained at the baseline evaluation. Auscultation of the heart commonly

Table 67.8. Recommended Baseline Evaluation of the Patient with Sustained Hypertension

	Reason for Obtaining Information				
Information	End-organ Status	Clues to Presence of Secondary Hypertension	Selection of Treatment	Factors Modified by Treatment	Additional Cardiovascular Risk Factors
Interview, old records					
Age and race		X	X		
Blood pressure levels		X	X	X	
Hypertension treatment, results, side effects		X	X		
Family history		X	X		X
Congestive heart failure	X		X		
Angina	X		X		
Transient ischemic attack or cerebrovascular accident	X				
Renal disease	X	X	X		
Comprehension of hypertension			X	X	
Diet (Na, K, fats)		X	X	X	X
Exercise habits			X		X
Current medications[a]		X	X	X	X
Alcohol use		X	X		
Tobacco use					X
Current life stresses		X	X		X
Coexisting conditions[b]		X	X		
Periodic sympathetic symptoms		X			
Physical examination					
Weight		X	X	X	
Blood pressure (right, left, resting, standing)		X	X	X	
Heart rate and rhythm		X	X	X	
Eye grounds	X		X		
Peripheral pulses	X	X	X		
Heart	X				
Lungs			X		
Abdomen (mass, bruit)		X			
Neurologic	X				
Laboratory findings					
Complete blood count				X	
Calcium level		X		X	
Creatinine level	X	X	X	X	
Potassium level		X	X	X	
Sodium level			X		
Fasting glucose level			X	X	
Cholesterol (total, high-density lipoprotein) level[c]				X	X
Uric acid level			X	X	
Urinalysis		X		X	
Electrocardiogram	X		X		

[a]identify medications that can cause hypertension or counteract antihypertensive drugs (e.g., oral contraceptives, tricyclic antidepressants, sympathomimetic decongestants, appetite suppressants, corticosteroids, nonsteroidal anti-inflammatory drugs, cyclosporine, erythropoietin, monoamine oxidase inhibitors, venlafaxine).

[b]See Table 67.16.

[c]2001 Recommendations of the National Cholesterol Education Program: obtain a fasting lipid profile beginning at age 20 years and every 5 years thereafter (see Chapter 82).

reveals accentuation of the aortic second sound and a systolic ejection murmur. Infrequent auscultatory findings include a systolic ejection sound at the base of the heart, paradoxical splitting of the second heart sound, or a short, high-pitched diastolic murmur at the base. Evidence of LVH may be found at baseline evaluation, either on physical examination (left ventricular heave or fourth heart sound) or on the ECG. Evidence of left-atrial abnormality is the earliest change on the ECG, reflecting atrial contraction against a left ventricle with decreased compliance during diastole. The ECG criteria for LVH are summarized elsewhere (see Table 65.3 in Chapter 65). The sensitivity of the ECG for detecting LVH is less than 50%, using the echocardiogram as the gold standard. The concentric hypertrophy typical of hypertension causes only a modest increase in the left ventricle silhouette on the chest radiograph, and the plain film of the chest is the least sensitive test for identifying changes from LVH.

Because of its cost, an *echocardiogram* to check for LVH should be considered only in situations where it may affect a treatment decision—such as a patient with stage 1 HBP, no other cardiovascular risk factors, and physical examination findings suggesting significant HBP (discussed earlier); or a patient with refractory stage 2 or 3 HBP, no other end-organ signs of HBP, and evidence suggesting that there is white-coat hypertension (see earlier discussion).

The *functional abnormalities associated with LVH* have been studied extensively. In some asymptomatic patients, the ejection fraction (measured by echocardiogram) is normal during rest but shows a subnormal increase during exercise. In hypertensive patients with symptoms of left ventricular failure, echocardiographic studies have revealed that some have global left ventricular dysfunction; some have functional subaortic stenosis; some have a hyperkinetic left ventricle with a normal or high ejection fraction and diminished relaxation during diastole; and some in the latter group (usually older patients) have cavity obliteration during diastole (47). Because appropriate drug therapy for patients in these groups differs in important ways (see later sections), it is recommended that hypertensive patients with signs and symptoms of heart failure should have an echocardiogram to ensure that the drugs selected for them are likely to improve rather than worsen the heart failure.

Most symptoms of *coronary artery disease* in hypertensive patients are related to occlusive disease of the coronary arteries. Some hypertensive patients who describe exertional angina and who have normal coronary arteriograms may have ischemia caused by increased resistance of the microvasculature of the myocardium (48).

Kidney

Simple tests of kidney status (urinalysis and serum creatinine concentration) are normal in the majority of hypertensive patients at baseline. In patients with a high baseline BP, the finding of an elevated creatinine concentration, proteinuria (sometimes more than 1 g/24 hours), or microscopic hematuria may signify accelerated hypertension. In such patients, other forms of renal or urologic disease should be excluded before these findings are attributed to hypertension. *Microalbuminuria* (albumin/creatinine ratio greater than 30 mg/g in a spot urine sample) may occur, especially in patients with stage 2 or 3 HBP. Its prognostic significance in patients without diabetes is unknown, and checking for it is not recommended as part of the baseline evaluation (49).

Central Nervous System

A history of stroke or transient ischemic attacks, an asymptomatic carotid bruit, or neurologic findings of a remote stroke may be present at baseline evaluation, but most patients do have evidence of cerebrovascular disease when they are first evaluated.

Eye

Ophthalmic symptoms attributable to HBP (decreased acuity from retinal hemorrhages or retinal detachment) are uncommon. However, examination of the retina has been emphasized in the evaluation of hypertensive patients because it offers direct inspection of blood vessels affected by hypertension. Most patients with chronic hypertension have evidence of arteriolosclerosis (grade 1 or 2 hypertensive retinopathy), but these findings have little practical value because they are not specific for hypertension, and there is significant interobserver and intraobserver variability in detecting them. Grade 3 retinopathy (hemorrhages or exudates) should be sought in patients with stage 3 HBP (Table 67.7); these changes are specific for accelerated hypertension.

Evaluation for Secondary Hypertension

Information obtained at the baseline evaluation or during follow-up identifies those patients who may have hypertension secondary to a reversible cause. Because surgically curable causes of HBP are uncommon, only highly selected patients should undergo the costly evaluations needed to diagnose these problems (4).

Chronic Alcoholism

In some individuals, *heavy, chronic alcohol use* causes sustained hypertension. For patients found to have both HBP and alcoholism at the baseline evaluation, BP control should be attempted initially through detoxification and treatment of the alcoholism (see Chapter 28). The BP becomes normal in those with alcohol-induced hypertension within about 1 week after discontinuation of alcohol.

Concurrent Use of a Medication that Can Cause High Blood Pressure

This cause of HBP should be considered in any patient concurrently who is using one of the medications that occasionally cause BP elevation (see list in footnote to Table 67.8). Although there is a detectable increase in the BP in most women who take *oral contraceptives,* the BP usually remains within the normal range with preparations that contain less than 50 μg of estrogen, the amount contained in currently prescribed products (see Chapter 100 for practical considerations related to oral contraceptives). *Estrogen* in the doses used for postmenopausal hormone replacement therapy, about one-sixth of the amount in oral contraceptives, usually does not cause the BP to rise. In one longitudinal study, women receiving hormone replacement therapy actually had less aging-related increase in SBP than these not receiving it (50). Because estrogen may occasionally cause hypertension, women who take it should have their BP monitored. *Cydosporine* commonly causes HBP related to generalized arterial vasoconstriction. It responds well to calcium antagonists.

To confirm that a medication is the cause of a patient's hypertension, there should be evidence that the patient had a normal BP before use of the medication, and the patient's BP should become normal within a few weeks after discontinuation of the medication (if this can be done safely).

Renovascular Hypertension

It is estimated that 0.5% or fewer of all hypertensive patients have renovascular hypertension (RVH), which is hypertension caused by unilateral stenosis of the main or of a segmental renal artery (51). In patients younger than 40 years of age, the cause is usually fibromuscular hyperplasia of the renal artery. In older patients, atherosclerosis of the renal artery is the usual cause. There is probably no racial or sexual predominance in the population of patients with RVH (52). Smoking is more common in all groups of patients with RVH (53).

A number of clinical findings increase the probability that a patient with HBP has RVH:

- The presence of a unilateral abdominal bruit radiating to the flank. The sensitivity of this finding is about 40% (54)
- Well-documented recent (span of 1 or 2 years) change from normal BP to stage 2 or 3 hypertension (Table 67.7)
- Onset of HBP before the age of 20 or after the age of 50 years
- Evidence of accelerated hypertension (i.e., grade 3 or 4 hypertensive retinopathy or renal insufficiency caused by hypertension) in any patient
- Unexplained renal failure, especially with a normal urinary sediment
- Recurrent episodes of flash pulmonary edema in a patient with chronic HBP
- Hypertension that is refractory to maximal tolerated doses of multiple antihypertensive drugs
- Unexplained refractoriness to previously effective drugs
- Doubling of the patient's serum creatinine concentration after initiation of an ACE inhibitor (suggests bilateral renal artery stenosis)

If a patient has one or more of these findings and is a candidate for surgery, the following choices can be presented:

1. *Use medication to control the hypertension*, including drugs not previously tried in those patients whose hypertension seems refractory to maximal doses of multiple drugs. This choice is supported by the findings that RVH usually responds to medical therapy and that most patients with renal artery stenosis caused by atherosclerosis (which the most common cause of RVH) either show no change after revascularization or need to resume drug treatment within 1 year or longer after surgery (51,55). Because control of systemic HBP will not prevent progressive renal failure caused by bilateral renal artery stenosis (ischemic nephropathy), patients whose renal function worsens despite control of HBP should be considered for evaluation and possible revascularization (55).
2. *Undergo evaluation for renal artery stenosis.* Before undergoing tests, the patient should declare an interest in accepting revascularization (balloon angioplasty or surgery) if testing shows renal artery stenosis. Also the patient should understand that if renal artery stenosis is found, the only way to establish whether renovascular HBP is present is to await the BP response to revascularization.

There are two generally accepted *criteria for confirmed RVH* (51):

- Durable postrevascularization cure (BP of 140/90 mm Hg or less, off medicine) or significant improvement (SBP or DBP reduced by at least 15% without a change in medication), *or*
- Much less medication needed to maintain a normal BP

Screening Tests. The major noninvasive screening tests for RVH currently available comprise one functional test (captopril scintirenography) and three imaging techniques (duplex ultrasonography, magnetic resonance angiography [MRA], and CT angiography). The sensitivity and specificity of these tests has been the focus of many studies in which they have been compared to contrast arteriography as the gold standard. The performance characteristics vary widely because of differences in the criteria set for an abnormal test. Published ranges are as follows (56):

	Sensitivity	Specificity
Captopril scintirenography	57–94%	71–98%
Duplex ultrasonography	17–100%	67–98%
MRA, nonenhanced	33–100%	65–96%
MRA gadolinium-enhanced	88–100%	75–100%
CT angiography (CTA)	94–100%	95–99%

According to a meta-analysis of all published studies of these screening tests, CT angiography and gadolinium-enhanced MRA performed significantly better than the other three tests (56). Smaller numbers of patients have been studied with these newer imaging techniques, so their role has yet to be definitively established. In selecting a screening test for RVH, the

Table 67.9. Clinical Index of Suspicion (Pretest Probability) for Renovascular Hypertension

Moderate Suspicion (5%–15%)
Very severe diastolic hypertension (≥120 mm Hg) at baseline
Change over 1 to 2 years from normal blood pressure to severe diastolic hypertension (≥110 mm Hg) in patients <20 or >50 years old
Hypertension refractory to pharmacologic treatment
Episodic flash pulmonary edema
High Suspicion (≥25%)
Severe diastolic hypertension (≥110 mm Hg) with either progressive renal insufficiency or grade 3 or 4 hypertensive retinopathy plus resistance to aggressive pharmacologic treatment
Severe diastolic hypertension (≥110 mm Hg) with incidentally detected asymmetry of kidney size

Adapted from Mann SG, Pickering TG. Detection of renovascular hypertension: state of the art—1992. Ann Intern Med 1992;117:845.

following additional considerations may be helpful:

- Screening is most likely to be of value when it is undertaken in patients with a moderately high (5% to 15%) or very high (25% or greater) pretest probability of RVH, on the basis of clinical features (Table 67.9).
- Renal artery duplex ultrasonography is highly operator dependent, and visualization is difficult in overweight patients.
- Captopril scintirenography may be less useful in patients with moderate renal insufficiency and in elderly patients, in whom atherosclerotic renal artery stenosis does not usually cause renin-dependent HBP (55).
- MRA is safe in patients with renal insufficiency, and gadolinium enhancement increases the ability of MRA to detect stenotic lesions in segmental renal arteries.
- CT angiography may be less accurate in patients with a creatinine concentration greater than 1.7 mg/dL (57).

Patient Experience. In *captopril scintirenography,* the patient receives an injection of tracer material and undergoes scintigraphic scanning twice: Before and after receiving a standard dose of captopril. The two-stage procedure takes about 3 hours. If the patient is currently taking an ACE inhibitor or an ARB, it should be withheld on the day of the test. Other current antihypertensive medications may be continued. The test measures quantitative and qualitative changes in renal flow or filtration to detect asymmetry between the two kidneys. The test depends on the influence of captopril on the renal handling of radioactive tracers. In a kidney with significant renal artery stenosis, there is angiotensin II–mediated constriction of the postglomerular arterioles; captopril reduces or eliminates this construction, thus lowering the glomerular filtration rate and leading to a change in the renal handling of tracer materials. There may be a compensatory increase in glomerular filtration rate in the contralateral kidney, which magnifies the difference in handling of ratiotracers.

The patient experience for the noninvasive imaging tests—*MRA, CT angiography, and duplex ultrasonography*—is similar to that described for neurologic evaluations in Chapter 86.

Anatomic Diagnosis. For the patient in whom screening is positive for probable RVH—and for some patients in whom the clinical suspicion of RVH is quite high (i.e., 25% or higher pretest probability; Table 67.9)—the patient should be referred for renal arteriography. Noninvasive study with intravenous digital subtraction angiography usually does not provide adequate detail to make a decision for intervention.

If arteriography shows unilateral renal artery stenosis and the patient has fibromuscular hyperplasia, percutaneous transluminal renal angioplasty (PTRA) is the revascularization treatment of choice. The cure rate is approximately 60% (55). Neither PTRA nor surgery has produced very satisfactory long-term results if renal artery stenosis caused by atherosclerosis is present; the cure rate approximately 30% in these patients (55). The use of a stent after PTRA may improve long-term results.

Patient Experience: Renal Arteriography. The patient experience is similar to that described for cerebral arteriography in Chapter 86. For both studies, femoral artery catheterization is used, and, when a small catheter is used, the patient does not need hospital admission.

Kidney Disease

Kidney disease should be suspected as a possible cause of HBP in patients with a history of hematuria, stones, or recurrent pyelonephritis; in patients in whom large kidneys (e.g., from obstruction or polycystic disease) or a large bladder (after voiding) is palpated; and in patients for whom the urinalysis suggests acute or chronic glomerulonephritis (i.e., proteinuria and/or many casts, especially red cell casts). If obstructive uropathy is suspected, a sonogram should be obtained. In patients with established chronic renal failure and small kidneys, it is usually impossible to determine whether the hypertension or the renal disease was the initial problem.

Mineralocorticoid Hypertension

The most common cause of mineralocorticoid hypertension (58) is hyperaldosteronism, and the most common clue to this cause is a baseline potassium level significantly below normal for which there is no explanation such as diuretic use or gastrointestinal fluid loss. Hypertensive patients with this finding should be asked about excessive consumption of licorice, which contains glycyrrhetinic acid, a moiety with mineralocorticoidlike activity; there are case reports of hypertension that abated when the patient discontinued consuming large amounts of licorice. The ambulatory evaluation of a patient with suspected primary hyperaldosteronism is discussed in detail in Chapter 50.

Pheochromocytoma

Clues to the presence of pheochromocytoma (59,60) are a history of a hypermetabolic state (which may resemble hyperthyroidism) or of paroxysms of symptoms caused by increased sympathetic nervous system activity (tachycardia, palpitations, diaphoresis), with associated severe headaches. The absence of such symptom clusters virtually excludes the presence of pheochromocytoma. Paroxysms last from minutes to several hours, but usually less than 1 hour. In approximately 75% of patients with pheochromocytoma, paroxysms occur at least once a week; the remaining patients either experience multiple attacks on most days or experience an attack only once every few months. These symptoms are especially important when there is no evidence for more common causes for them, such as hyperthyroidism (see Chapter 80), reactive hypoglycemia (see Chapter 81), migraine or cluster headaches (see Chapter 87), or panic attacks and other anxiety disorders (see Chapter 22).

Paroxysmal and persistent hypertension are equally common in patients with pheochromocytoma. Orthostatic hypotension, with or without symptoms, is present in some patients, presumably because of vasodilation caused by predominant beta-2 sympathetic activity.

Additional findings that increase the prior probability of pheochromocytoma are a marked change in BP or heart rate in response to minor injury, parturition, or general anesthesia; a neurocutaneous syndrome (von Recklinghausen disease or von Hippel–Lindau syndrome); a blood relative with a pheochromocytoma; and type II multiple endocrine neoplasia (medullary carcinoma of the thyroid or parathyroid adenoma, or both, with symptoms suggesting pheochromocytoma).

Screening Tests. Because pheochromocytoma is uncommon, the best practice is to screen only those patients in whom clinical suspicion is high and to refer for consultation or more costly diagnostic evaluation only those patients with positive screening tests. Measurement of 24-hour urinary excretion of one or more of the three markers for increased pressor synthesis (catecholamines, metanephrines, and vanillylmandelic acid) is a screening test that has satisfactory performance characteristics. When used in a patient with an estimated 5% pretest probability of having a pheochromocytoma (e.g., a hypertensive patient with unexplained paroxysms of headache, tachycardia, and/or diaphoresis), excess excretion of any of the three markers would increase to 35% to 45% the probability (positive predictive value) that the patient has pheochromocytoma; and normal results would increase from 95% to approximately 99% the probability (negative predictive value) that the patient does not have pheochromocytoma (61). An alternative test, measurement of the plasma level of normetanephrine or metanephrine, may have better performance characteristics but is not yet available for routine screening (60).

Screening Procedures. For the 24-hour urine tests, the patient is given a plastic container that contains a fixed amount of a strong acid and is instructed to collect a 24-hour specimen. The same specimen can be used to screen for catecholamines, metanephrines, and vanillylmandelic acid. With modern assay techniques, no foodstuffs and only a small number of drugs interfere with test results: Measured *catecholamines* may be increased by methyldopa, labetalol, rapid withdrawal of clonidine, ethanol, tetracycline, erythromycin, L-dopa, theophylline, hypoglycemia, isoproterenol, and prochlorperazine; measured *metanephrines* may be increased by monoamine oxidase inhibitors, labetalol, ethanol, clonidine withdrawal, and occasionally methyldopa; measured *vanillylmandelic acid* may be decreased by monoamine oxidase inhibitors and clofibrate and may be increased by nalidixic acid, levodopa, labetalol, and clonidine withdrawal. In patients who have normal BPs between paroxysms of hypertension, the urine specimen should be taken when the patient is hypertensive. In a patient with especially concerning symptoms whose marker excretion is normal, it is reasonable to repeat the test one or more times.

Diagnostic Tests. Patients with positive screening tests should undergo definitive diagnostic testing to localize the presumed tumor. This process has been improved by the availability of radioisotope scanning using labeled iodobenzylguanidine, followed by CT scanning or magnetic resonance imaging of the site that takes up this substance. Almost all pheochromocytomas are located in the adrenal glands; 1% to 3% may be located in the posterior mediastinum. Of these tumors, 90% can be totally removed at surgery. Up to 10% are found to be malignant at surgery.

Sleep Apnea

Sustained hypertension occurs in some patients with obstructive sleep apnea. From small numbers of reports, it appears that the hypertension abates in response to treatment with continuous positive airway pressure (62) (see Chapter 7).

Coarctation of the Aorta

Clues to the presence of this condition are hypertension in a relatively young patient (most are recognized in the pediatric age group); decreased BP in the lower extremities, suggested by diminished or absent femoral pulses and corroborated by auscultation over the popliteal artery, using a large cuff; and evidence of collateral arterial circulation either on inspection of the trunk or on the plain chest radiograph, which may also show poststenotic dilation of the aorta. In a minority of patients, the coarctation occurs proximal to the left subclavian artery, and the BP is high only in the right arm. To confirm the presence of a coarctation, the patient must undergo aortography.

Status of Factors Modified by Treatment of Hypertension

Table 67.8 lists factors that should be addressed or documented at baseline because they may be modified as part of the treatment plan or as a consequence of treatment. These include information obtained from the history (patient's understanding of hypertension, usual diet, alcohol consumption, current medications), from the physical examination (weight, BP, heart rate and rhythm, edema), and from laboratory tests (creatinine, electrolytes, fasting glucose, complete blood count, uric acid, cholesterol, and urinalysis).

Status of Other Cardiovascular Risk Factors

Coexisting cardiovascular risk factors are common in patients with hypertension. They greatly affect a patient's long-term probability of morbidity and mortality (Fig. 67.1). Therefore, the baseline evaluation of a hypertensive patient should include checking for other risk factors, and these factors should be considered in planning the overall management. These factors include gender, family history of premature cardiovascular disease, tobacco use (see Chapter 27), high-cholesterol or high-salt diet, hypercholesterolemia (see Chapter 82), sedentary living (see Chapter 16), stressful lifestyle, obesity (see Chapter 83), and diabetes mellitus (see Chapter 79).

TREATMENT OF HYPERTENSION

General Considerations

Goals of Treatment

When sustained hypertension has been confirmed, the goal of treatment is to reduce the patient's risk of future cardiovascular disease by restoring the BP to normal and controlling other risk factors. Normal BP is defined as office SBP and DBP values lower than 140 and 90 mm Hg, respectively, or home SBP and DBP values lower than 135 and 85 mm Hg (4,42). *For diabetic patients and for patients with CHF or chronic renal failure,* a BP lower than 130/85 mm Hg is now recommended (4,42). For patients in whom goal BPs cannot be attained, partial BP control confers some benefit (63).

Timetable. In patients who choose a nonpharmacologic regimen (discussed later), a trial of this approach for 6 to 12 months is usually needed to evaluate its impact on the BP. When drug treatment is selected, a goal of satisfactory BP control without significant drug side effects can usually be achieved within 1 to 3 months.

White-Coat Hypertension and White-Coat Effect. There are not adequate data to define BP goals or treatment recommendations for patients with these patterns of BP elevation (see Measuring the Blood Pressure). At least one large study showed similar 4-year rates of cardiovascular morbidity in patients with high office BPs (stages 1 to 3) who did or did not manifest a "white-coat" effect (lower, often still high, daytime BPs) and were treated on the basis of their office BPs (64). As noted previously, the current consensus is that home BPs of 135/85 mm Hg or greater should be considered elevated, meaning that the goal BP for these and other patients' home BPs should be less than these levels (4).

Intensity of Blood Pressure Lowering. Because of the suggestion that an on-treatment DBP lower than 85 mm Hg may increase risk (a "J-curve" effect), particularly in patients with pre-existing coronary artery disease (65), some authorities recommended in the early 1990s that the DBP should not be reduced below 85 mm Hg. However, no J-curve pattern was reported in the Systolic Hypertension in the Elderly Program (SHEP), in which the average on-treatment DBP was 68 mm Hg (22). A subsequent clinical trial (Hypertension Optimal Treatment, HOT), which was designed to compare the effects of on-treatment DBPs of 90 mm Hg or less, 85 mm Hg or less, and 80 mm Hg or less, did not find evidence of a J-curve effect (66). In this trial, diabetic patients randomly assigned to the most aggressive BP lowering measures had a lower incidence of cardiovascular events than those treated less aggressively. This result was not found for nondiabetic trial participants.

Initiating Treatment According to Risk Stratification

Beginning with its 1997 report (4), the JNC has recommended an overall treatment strategy that considers BP goals, risk stratification, and selection of drugs according to the findings of randomized controlled trials. This strategy is summarized in Figs. 67.5 and 67.6 and in Table 67.10. The WHO/ISH guidelines recommend a similar overall approach (42).

Special considerations for the treatment of hypertension in *adolescents, elderly persons, and pregnant women* are discussed in later sections of this chapter.

For stage 2 or stage 3 HBP (sustained DBP of 100 mm Hg or more), initial treatment with antihypertensive drugs is recommended for all patients.

Table 67.10. Risk Stratification and Initial Treatment[a]

Blood Pressure Stages (mm Hg)	Risk Group A (No Risk Factors[b] and No TOD/CCD)[c]	Risk Group B (At Least One Risk Factor, Not Including Diabetes, and No TOD/CCD)	Risk Group C (TOD/CCD or Diabetes, With or Without Other Risk Factors)
High-normal (130–139/85–89)	Lifestyle modification	Lifestyle modification	Drug therapy
Stage 1 (140–159/90–99)	Lifestyle modification (up to 12 mo)[d]	Lifestyle modification (up to 6 mo)[d]	Drug therapy
Stages 2 and 3 (≥160/≥100)	Drug therapy	Drug therapy	Drug therapy

TOD, target organ disease; CCD, clinical cardiovascular disease (see Table 67.11).

[a]Lifestyle modification should be adjunctive therapy for all patients recommended for pharmacologic therapy.

[b]Major risk factors (see Fig. 67.1).

[c]For example, a patient with diabetes and a blood pressure of 142/94 mm Hg plus left ventricular hypertrophy should be classified as having stage 1 hypertension with target organ disease (left ventricular hypertrophy) and with another major risk factor (diabetes). This patient would be categorized as stage I, risk group C, and recommended for immediate initiation of pharmacologic treatment.

[d]For patients with multiple risk factors, consider drugs as initial therapy plus lifestyle modifications.

From The Sixth Report of the Joint National Committee on Prevention, Detection, Evaluation, and Treatment of High Blood Pressure. Arch Intern Med 1997;157:2413.

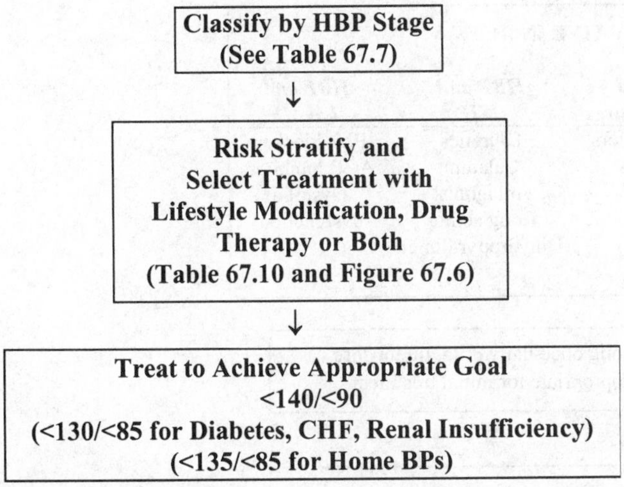

Classify by HBP Stage (See Table 67.7)

↓

Risk Stratify and Select Treatment with Lifestyle Modification, Drug Therapy or Both (Table 67.10 and Figure 67.6)

↓

Treat to Achieve Appropriate Goal <140/<90 (<130/<85 for Diabetes, CHF, Renal Insufficiency) (<135/<85 for Home BPs)

Figure 67.5. Overall treatment strategy. (Adapted from The Sixth Report of the Joint National Committee on Prevention, Detection, Evaluation, and Treatment of High Blood Pressure. Arch Intern Med 1997;157:2413, and 1999 World Health Organization/International Society of Hypertension Guidelines Subcommittee. WHO/ISH guidelines for the management of hypertension. J Hypertens 1999;17:151.)

For stage 1 HBP (sustained SBP 140 to 159 mm Hg or DBP 90 to 99 mm Hg), an individualized approach to initial treatment is recommended. Figure 67.1 shows the graded impact of BP level, other risk factors, target organ damage, and clinical cardiovascular disease on the 10-year prognosis in these patients. Initial treatment with antihypertensive drugs is recommended for all stage 1 patients in risk group C (Table 67.10)—that is, those who have diabetes, target organ damage (Table 67.11), or a history of clinical cardiovascular disease. The presence at baseline of *multiple other cardiovascular risk factors* (smoking, hypercholesterolemia, age older than 60 years, male gender, postmenopausal status, strong family history of cardiovascular morbidity) also favors initial drug treatment. For patients with stage 1 HBP who do not have these associated characteristics, it is reasonable to try nonpharmacologic treatment for up to 1 year (risk group A—no risk factors) or for 6 months (risk group B—one risk factor, not including diabetes), especially in those patients who voice a strong preference to try this approach.

Nonpharmacologic Treatment (Lifestyle Modification)

A number of nonpharmacologic modalities that require a change in lifestyle can either prevent the development of HBP (see Primary Prevention) or lower BP. Among patients who are taking antihypertensive drugs, these measures may enable motivated patients to decrease or discontinue drugs and maintain control of their HBP (see Step-Down Therapy).

Although there have been no clinical trials to determine the impact of any these measures on clinical cardiovascular disease, there is evidence that nonpharmacologic control of HBP may be as effective as pharmacologic control in preventing LVH (67). Those individual measures for which there is convincing evidence for effectiveness in lowering BP include following: a healthy diet, reducing weight, reducing daily intake of salt, increasing physical exercise, and limiting alcohol intake (4). Maintenance of lifestyle modification, and its benefits, requires ongoing motivation of the patient (see Chapter 4). For motivated patients with stage 1 HBP and few or no associated risk factors, one or more lifestyle modifications can be tried as primary treatment (Table 67.10). Additionally, these for all subgroups (gender, age, race) measures should be recommended, when pertinent, to all patients who are beginning treatment with antihypertensive drugs.

Healthy Diet

A diet that is rich in fruits and vegetables and low in saturated and total fat (the DASH diet) has been shown to reduce BP independently of exercise, salt reduction, and weight reduction (6). The effect on BP occur within 8 weeks. Long-term impact probably persists in those who adhere to the diet. Because this diet reduces other risk factors, it should be recommended to motivated patients in conjunction with other nonpharmacologic measures. Recently it was shown that for all subgroups (gender, age, race) salt reduction is additive to the DASH diet's effect on BP (68).

Weight Reduction (4,37)

In overweight persons, a decrease in BP may occur after only modest weight loss (e.g., about 10 pounds) (4,37). Practical approaches to weight reduction are described in Chapter 83.

Salt Restriction

Limitation of daily sodium intake to 100 mmol (about 2 g) of elemental sodium, which is equivalent to 4 to 6 g of salt, should be recommended to all patients with hypertension (69). The impact of salt reduction occurs over a period of weeks. If BP decreases to and remains at normal levels, salt limitation should be maintained as definitive therapy.

Tables 67.12 and 67.13, which can be copied for distribution to patients, summarize what patients need to know to follow a low-salt diet. When giving this information to a patient, it is important to point out that approximately 75% of one's daily intake of salt usually comes in processed foods (see "What Not to Eat" column in Table 67.13) and that there are many ways to make food tasty without adding salt (see "Add New Flavors to Your Food" in Table 67.12).

Salt use and diuretics. As discussed later, when a patient continues to ingest a large amount of salt while taking diuretics, potassium wasting is increased. Therefore salt restriction may both prevent excessive potassium loss and facilitate BP reduction in patients taking diuretics.

Physical Exercise

Moderate-intensity exercise (e.g., gardening, walking, cycling), *lifestyle exercise* accumulated during the day

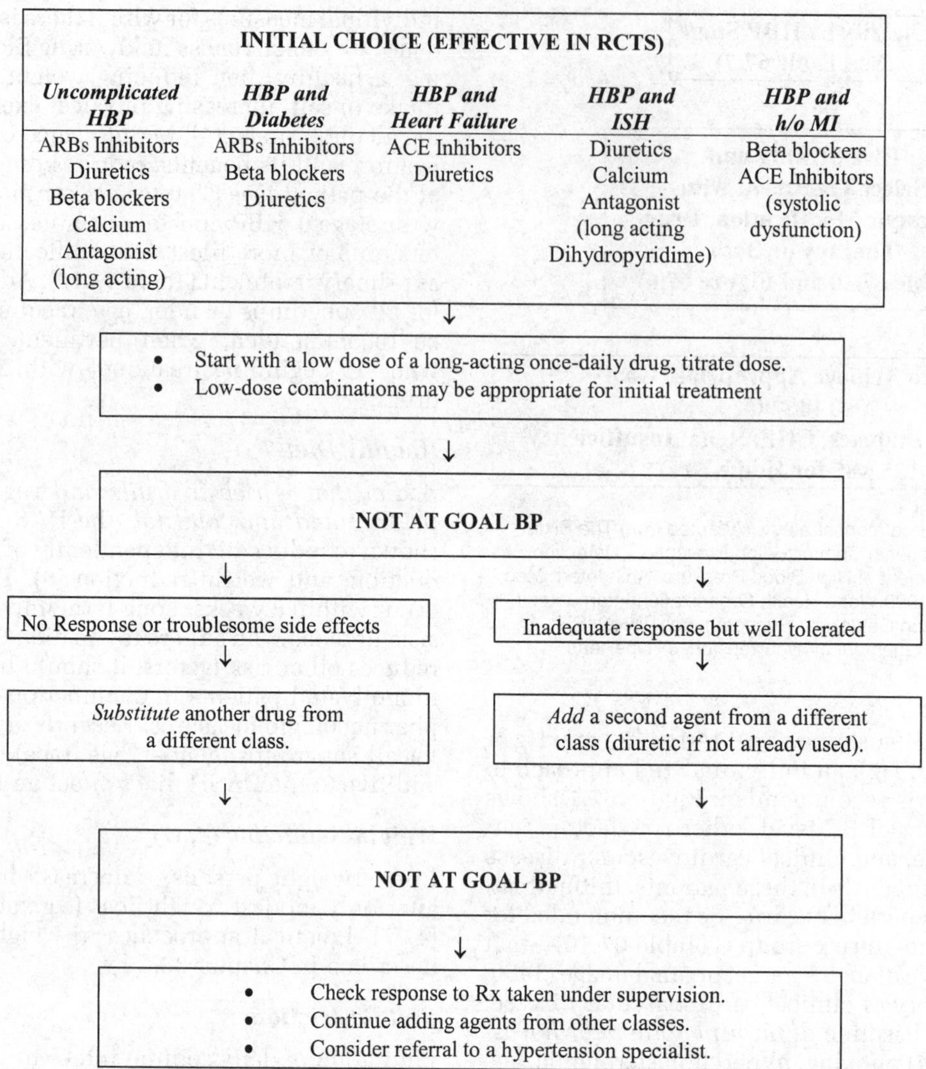

Figure 67.6. Guidelines for selecting and adjusting antihypertensive drug therapy. (Adapted from The Sixth Report of the Joint National Committee on Prevention, Detection, Evaluation, and Treatment of High Blood Pressure. Arch Intern Med 1997;157:2413, and 1999 World Health Organization/International Society of Hypertension Guidelines Subcommittee. WHO/ISH guidelines for the management of hypertension. J Hypertens 1999;17:151.)

Table 67.11. Manifestations of Target Organ Disease or Clinical Cardiovascular Disease

Organ System	Manifestations
Cardiac	Clinical, ECG, or radiologic evidence of coronary artery disease; LVH or "strain" by ECG or LVH by echocardiography; left ventricular dysfunction or cardiac failure
Cerebrovascular	Transient ischemic attack or stroke
Peripheral vascular	Absence of one or more major pulses in extremities (except for dorsalis pedis) with or without intermittent claudication; aneurysm
Renal	Serum creatinine $\geq$130 μmol/L (1.5 mg/dL); proteinuria (1+ or greater); microalbuminuria
Retinopathy	Hemorrhages or exudates, with or without papilledema

ECG, electrocardiographic; LVH, left ventricular hypertrophy.

From The Fifth Report of the Joint National Committee on Detection, Evaluation, and Treatment of High Blood Pressure (JNC V). Arch Intern Med 1993;153:154.

(e.g., using stairs instead of elevators, walking to work), and the *high-intensity exercise* needed to attain cardiac conditioning have BP-lowering effects (4,37). The decrease in cardiovascular mortality that is associated with exercise may be partly related to its impact on BP. Chapter 16 provides details regarding the health benefits and practical aspects of physical exercise.

Physical Activities While Taking Antihypertensive Drugs. Most patients want to be informed about the implications of hypertension and antihypertensive drug therapy for ordinary physical activity. Subjects with untreated hypertension have the same patterns of BP fluctuation during exercise as normotensive subjects, only at higher pressures: With vigorous exercise, the SBP rises (as much as 60 mm Hg) while the DBP may rise or fall slightly. Similar patterns are usually found in patients treated with antihypertensive drugs. The effects of a number of antihypertensives and other cardiovascular drugs on BP during exercise are

Table 67.12. Information for Patients Who Are Advised to Follow a 2-g Sodium Diet

Americans eat about 20 times more sodium than they need, most of which comes from salt, Which is one source of sodium.

Sodium is:

found naturally in foods, even those that do not taste salty.

added to food by manufacturers in food processing.

added in cooking in the form of salt, baking powder, baking soda, or seasonings such as monosodium glutamate (MSG).

added as salt to food at the table.

☐ In the body, sodium acts like a sponge to hold water in the body tissues. Sometimes the body cannot get rid of enough of the sodium. High blood pressure may result. If not controlled, high blood pressure leads to stroke, kidney failure, and heart disease.

☐ Using no salt in cooking or at the table and eliminating highly salted food cuts down the sodium level of the food you eat to about 2000 mg day.

Add New Flavors to Your Food!

☐ Herbs and spices can give new zest to your unsalted cooking.

☐ A little herb goes a long way. If you are making your own substitution without the benefit of a recipe, try ¼ teaspoon of dried herb or spice to:

a recipe for 4 servings,

a pound of meat, poultry, fish, or vegetable or 2 cups of sauce.

If you are using red pepper or garlic powder start with only ⅛ teaspoon. Taste and add a little more depending on your preference.

☐ If you use fresh herbs use four times the amount of dried herb. Instead of ¼ teaspoon of dried herb use 1 full teaspoon of fresh herb.

☐ Add dried herbs to soups and stews during the last hour of cooking.

☐ Use whole spices in slow-cooking dishes and add them at the beginning of the cooking period.

☐ When using ground spices, add them 15 minutes before the end of the cooking period. If adding them to uncooked dishes, add them several hours before serving. As a start, try one or a combination of the following popular herbs:

Basil	Rosemary
Celery seed	Sage
Marjoram	Savory
Mint	Thyme

Beware of Hidden Sodium!

Processed Foods

Salt is added to many packaged, convenience, "fast," and canned foods. Examples are packaged dinners (e.g., macaroni and cheese), packaged coatings and "helpers," combination dinners (e.g., frozen meals and casserole dishes), canned soups, dried soups, canned vegetables, and frozen vegetables with sauces.

"Fast Foods"

Generally, meals served at "fast food" places are high in sodium. A typical meal of a hamburger, french fries, and a vanilla shake can total more than 1000 mg of sodium—more than half of your total daily allowance. Remember pizza, hot dogs, burgers, fried chicken, fried fish, omelettes, and tacos served at fast food places are usually high in sodium. Just one whole dill pickle contains 1900 mg of sodium, almost the total allowed in this diet.

Read labels carefully. Foods that list salt or sodium as ingredients should be avoided. Compare different brands of the same product. It is unnecessary to purchase special dietetic foods. Many dietetic foods contain sodium or salt, so read the labels carefully.

Additives

☐ Sodium may be added to food as a preservative; for quick cooking; to soften or loosen skins of fruits and vegetables; to cure meats, fish, sausage; to stop growth of molds. Additives that contain sodium include:

Monosodium glutamate (MSG)
Baking soda
Disodium phosphate
Sodium alginate
Sodium benzoate
Sodium hydroxide
Sodium nitrate
Sodium propionate
Sodium sulfite

Some Tips on Eating Out!

☐ Select restaurants that offer *à la carte* service.

☐ For breakfast, order from the allowed cereals. Poached or boiled eggs with toast may be ordered at most restaurants.

☐ For lunch, try fruit or tossed salads; roast beef, sliced chicken, or turkey breast sandwich; and fruit for dessert.

☐ At dinner, try fruit (fresh, canned, or frozen), fruit juice, or fruit cup as an appetizer.

☐ If you select broiled meats, fresh fish, or chicken, you may request that no salt or other condiments like garlic salt or onion salt be added before or after broiling.

☐ Inside cuts of roast beef, lamb, pork, veal, chicken, and turkey have less sodium than outside cuts. Trim off the edges that would have been salted. Ask that it be served without gravy or sauce.

☐ In ordering rice, ask if it has been cooked in salted water. Some restaurants cook rice without salt. Rice pilaf is usually prepared with salt.

☐ You can count on baked potato. For toppings use butter, margarine, or sour cream.

☐ If in doubt about cooked vegetables, order sliced tomatoes or a salad such as tossed salad, lettuce wedge, or fruit salad. Try lemon or oil and vinegar for the dressing. Ask the waiter to leave off the croutons!

☐ Help yourself to the bread basket, but avoid salted breadsticks and crackers with salted tops.

☐ For dessert select fruit, sherbet, ice cream, or plain yogurt.

☐ Most airlines provide "special meals." A low-sodium meal may be ordered at no extra cost when you make your flight reservation.

☐ Fast food menu items (except for the salad bar where you can select low-sodium items) have usually been salted. If food can be prepared to order, request that no salted seasonings be added.

To Sum it Up

☐ Using less salt is advisable for almost everyone, even children, so let the whole family join in.

☐ Avoid shaking salt on your food. Substitute a blend of herbs for your salt shaker.

☐ Cook without salt. Try leaving it out of recipes.

☐ Experiment with new flavors by using herbs and spices. Fine restaurants rely on herbs, spices, and the natural flavor of food, not salt, for good taste.

☐ Avoid fast foods and other processed foods high in sodium.

☐ Read the labels of foods and medicines to find "hidden" sodium. Look for the symbol: Na; look for the words: salt, sodium, soda, brine.

☐ Become familiar with foods that are high in sodium.

☐ Low-sodium salt, such as "Lite Salt," is a combination of sodium and potassium. Do not be misled that it is free of sodium. It has about half the sodium content of regular salt.

Use of low-sodium salt and salt substitutes can be dangerous because of the very high potassium content. It is essential that you ask your doctor if you may use them. Also ask how much you may use each day.

Modified from "Health Is In—Salt Is Out," courtesy of The Maryland High Blood Pressure Coordinating Council.

Table 67.13. Food List for Patients Who Are Advised to Follow a 2-g Sodium Diet (Shows What *to* Eat and What *Not* to Eat)[a]

	What to Eat	What Not to Eat
Vegetables	**Fresh and Most Frozen Vegetables** Artichoke Asparagus Avocado Bamboo shoots Bean sprouts Beets Broccoli Brussels sprouts Cabbage Carrots Cauliflower Celery Chicory Collards Corn Cucumber Dried beans Dried peas Eggplant Endive Escarole Green beans Kale Kohlrabi Leeks Lettuce Lima beans Mixed vegetables Mushrooms Mustard greens Okra Onion Parsley Parsnips Peas Peppers Potato, sweet or white Pumpkin Radishes Rutabaga Scallions Soybeans Spinach Squash—summer, acorn, winter Tomato Tomato juice, low sodium Turnip V-8 juice, low sodium Water chestnuts Watercress Wax beans Yams *Note:* Low-sodium canned vegetables may be used.	Canned vegetables Canned tomato juice Canned vegetable juice Frozen peas Frozen lima beans Frozen vegetables with seasoned sauce Olives Pickled vegetables Pickles Sauerkraut Seaweed
Protein Foods	**Lean Fresh Meat** Beef Lamb Liver Pork Veal	Bacon Canned meats Corned beef Dried chipped beef Ham, cured or "low salt" Hotdogs Luncheon meats Salt pork Sausage Scrapple Smoked meats Salted or pickled meats Meat extenders and "helpers" TV and frozen meat dinners "Fast food" meats
	Breads Cracked wheat French Hamburger roll Hot dog roll Italian Raisin Rye Vienna White, enriched Whole wheat **Crackers** Matzoh Melba toast Rusk Rye Krisp Zwieback **Cereals** Barley Cream of wheat, regular Cornmeal Granola Grits, regular Oatmeal, regular Petijohns Popcorn, unsalted Puffed Rice Puffed Wheat Ralston Rice Shredded Wheat Special K Tapioca Wheatena **Pastas, Cooked Without Salt** Macaroni Noodles Spaghetti	Danish pastries Muffins Pancakes Pizza Spoonbread Stuffing mix Sweet rolls Waffles **Crackers/Snack Foods** Crackers with salted tops Pretzels Soda crackers Consider crackers, chips, pretzels to be high in sodium unless labeled as "unsalted" **Cereals** Dry cereals, except those listed under "What to Eat" Instant grits Instant hot cereals Salted popcorn **Pastas** Chow mein noodles Prepackaged meals, such as macaroni, noodle, or spaghetti dinners
Fruits	**Fresh, Frozen, Canned, or Dried Fruit** Apple Apple juice Applesauce Apricots Banana Berries Cantaloupe Cherries Cranberries Dates Figs Grapefruit Grapefruit juice Lemon Nectarine Orange Orange juice Peach Pear Pineapple Pineapple juice Plums Prunes Prune juice Raisins Raspberries Rhubarb	Dried fruits that contain sodium preservative

Category	Allowed	Avoid
Fresh Fish	Bass, Bluefish, Carp, Cod, Flounder, Haddock, Hake, Halibut, Ocean perch, Pike, Pollack, Pompano, Porgy, Red snapper, Rockfish, Salmon, Shad, Sole, Swordfish, Trout, Tuna, Whitefish	Anchovy, Canned fish, Commercially frozen fish, "Fast food" fish, Herring, Salted fish, Sardines, Smoked or pickled fish, TV and frozen fish dinners
Fresh Shellfish	Crab, Lobster, Oysters[b], Shrimp	Crabs, prepared with salty seasoning, Mussels, Scallops
Peanut Butter		
Dried Beans, Cooked Without Salt, Salt pork, or Ham		Canned beans
Leen Fresh Poultry	Capon, Chicken, Cornish hen, Duck, Goose, Turkey	Canned chicken, Canned turkey, Commercial fried chicken, TV dinners, Turkey roll, Frozen turkey or chicken casseroles/pies, Frozen omelet, Frozen souffle, Frozen quiche
Beverages	Alcoholic beverages, in moderation; Club soda; Cocoa; Coffee—ground, instant, decaffeinated; Soft drinks; Sugar-free beverages, in moderation; Tea—loose, teabags, instant; Tonic water; Wine	
Breads, Crackers	**Breads**: Cinnamon, Corn and molasses; **Crackers**: Any crackers with unsalted tops	**Breads**: Biscuits, Cornbread, Croutons, packaged
(Fruits, continued)	Grapes, Grape juice, Honeydew, Strawberries, Tangerine, Watermelon	
Desserts	Custard, homemade; Fruit; Fruit cake; Fruit cobbler; Gelatin desserts, all flavors; Ice cream; Ice milk; Lady fingers; Sherbert; Sponge cake, homemade; Yogurt, plain	Commercially prepared cake, cookies, pies; Donuts; Pudding mixes; Sweet rolls
Seasonings	Garlic, fresh or powdered; Herbs and spices; Horseradish, fresh or prepared; Lemon, juice and peel; Onion, fresh, powdered, or flaked; Pepper; Tabasco sauce; Vanilla extract; Vinegar; Wine; Worcestershire sauce (used sparingly)	Barbeque sauce; Catsup; Celery salt; Chili sauce; Cooking wine (has salt added); Garlic salt; Lemon pepper seasoning; Meat tenderizers; Monosodium glutamate (MSG); Onion salt; Pickle relish; Prepared mustard; Salt, seasoned or plain; Sea salt; Soy sauce; Steak sauce
Dairy Products	Skim milk; Dry milk; Evaporated milk; Yogurt, plain; Brie; Cheddar; Colby; Cottage; Gruyere; Monterey Jack; Mozzarella; Muenster; Natural Swiss; Neufchatel; Port du Salut; Ricotta; Cheese labeled "low sodium" or "unsalted"	Buttermilk (commercial); Condensed milk; "Fast food" shakes; Bule; Camembert; Cheezola; Edam; Feta; Gouda; Limburger; Parmesan; Processed cheese, American and Swiss; Processed foods; Processed spreads; Provolone; Roquefort; Romano; Slim Line cheese; Tilsit

[a]Useful conversions: 100 mg of sodium = 4.35 mEq of sodium; 100 mg of sodium = 250 mg of salt; 1 teaspoon of salt = 6 g of sodium.

[b]If from saltwater bed, rinse saltwater out with fresh water.

Adapted from "Health Is In—Salt Is Out," courtesy of The Maryland High Blood Pressure Coordinating Council.

summarized in Table 63.XX in Chapter 63. In general, it is reasonable to inform patients that their hypertension does not make them different and to reassure them that they can engage in all of their usual activities after beginning treatment for hypertension.

Moderation or Discontinuation of Alcohol Intake

For persons who are social drinkers, drinking up to 2 ounces/day (e.g., 2 cans of beer, 2 glasses of wine, 2 one-jigger drinks) may reduce cardiovascular risk (4,37). In patients with alcoholism, abstinence may be efficacious as the only treatment or as adjunctive treatment for coexisting hypertension. Approaches useful in the detection and treatment of alcoholism are described in Chapter 28.

Dietary Potassium

Consuming a diet with substantial potassium content may facilitate the BP-lowering effects of weight reduction, salt restriction, or antihypertensive drugs (70). Increased potassium intake usually occurs as a consequence of changing to a low-sodium diet, which tends to contain more potassium-rich natural foods (e.g., fresh fruits and vegetables) in place of processed food. Because potassium deficiency may cause the BP to increase, maintenance of a normal serum potassium concentration (3.5 mEq/L or higher) probably facilitates the BP-lowering effect of diuretics.

Cognitive and Behavioral Techniques

Cognitive and behavioral techniques include biofeedback, stress management, meditation, and muscle relaxation techniques. Critical assessment of clinical trials of these techniques does not support the efficacy of any of them as a primary method for decreasing BP (4). Motivated patients may wish to use one of these techniques as an adjunct to another primary treatment strategy. Muscle relaxation techniques useful for stress reduction are described in Chapter 22.

Other Substances and Nutrients

Adequate intake of *calcium and magnesium* or supplemental *garlic* may promote BP reduction, but there is no evidence that increased amounts of either of these nutrients should be recommended (37). Although *fish oils* may lower BP, they are associated with adverse effects that counterbalance the small benefit. *Caffeine and nicotine* may transiently raise BP, but their elimination does not lower BP. The amount of nicotine in nicotine substitution products used in smoking cessation aids described in Chapter 27 does not usually raise BP (71).

Pharmacologic Treatment: General Recommendations

To date, objective methods for selecting the most appropriate antihypertensive drug for an individual patient have not been developed. Therefore drug treatment for most patients should be initiated and adjusted using the strategies outlined in the algorithms in Figs. 67.5 and 67.6, adapted from the guidelines published by the JNC (4) and WHO/ISH (42). The recommendations in Fig. 67.6 for initial choice of antihypertensive drugs are based on clinical trials demonstrating that active drug treatment decreases morbidity and mortality. One or more large placebo-controlled trials have demonstrated this for each of five classes of drugs: diuretics, beta blockers, ACE inhibitors, and calcium antagonists and ARBs (25,25a,25b). The evidence from individual trials of drugs in the first four classes was pooled in two sets of meta-analyses published in 2000. The first set (25), which supported the efficacy of all four classes of drugs, used data from both placebo-controlled trials and head-to-head comparison of drugs. The second set (72), which included only head-to-head comparisons, found evidence that patients assigned to long-acting calcium antagonists had higher risks of coronary artery disease than those assigned to the other three classes. Additional meta-analyses, which will include trials of drugs from these four classes and from the newest class, the ARBs, will be conducted in 2003, at which time data will be available from a large number of trials in progress (73).

Figure 67.6 lists four conditions for which there is clinical trial evidence that drugs from specific classes may be especially effective: Diabetes, heart failure, isolated systolic hypertension, and history of MI. These conditions and other factors that may guide drug selection are discussed later (see Individualizing Drug Selection).

The impact of most antihypertensive drugs on BP occurs within 1 to 7 days. For patients with stage 1 or stage 2 HBP, it is reasonable to evaluate the response to medications within 1 month. Patients with stage 3 hypertension (e.g., SBP, 180 mm Hg or more, or DBP, 110 mm Hg or more) should be evaluated frequently until there is evidence that the BP is responding to the drugs or dosages prescribed.

PHARMACOLOGIC TREATMENT: SPECIFIC CONSIDERATIONS

This section summarizes recommendations regarding monotherapy and combination therapy with currently available antihypertensive drugs; information about available products, dosages, and common side effects (Tables 67.14 and 67.17); and selected indications and contraindications according to patient characteristics, coexisting conditions (Table 67.15), and common drug–drug interactions (Table 67.16).

Classes of Antihypertensive Drugs

Antihypertensive drugs belong to one of the following classes listed in Table 67.14: diuretics, adrenergic inhibitors, calcium antagonists, ACE inhibitors or ARBs, and direct vasodilators.

Because drugs from each class of antihypertensive agents are available in preparations that are effective for 24 hours or longer, it is prudent to attempt to control a patient's BP with a *once-a-day medication schedule.*

Many proprietary antihypertensive drugs are substantially more expensive than *generic preparations.*

Generic preparations are available for each class of drug except the newest class, the ARBs (Table 67.14).

Monotherapy

Monotherapy with drugs from each class, with the exception of vasodilators, can be chosen initially. The vasodilators hydralazine and minoxidil usually require cotreatment with an adrenergic inhibitor to prevent reflex tachycardia. In systematic studies, it has been shown that 50% or more of patients respond to low-dose monotherapy alone (74,75). Increasing the dosage of the initial drug, substituting another drug, or adding a drug or drugs from another class are strategies that make it possible to achieve the goal BP (Fig. 67.5) in most patients who do not respond to or do not tolerate the initial regimen (Fig. 67.6).

Initial monotherapy with a low dosage of a diuretic (e.g., 12.5 to 25 mg of hydrochlorothiazide daily), a beta-blocker (e.g., 25 to 50 mg of atenolol daily) is appropriate for many patients (37). The rationale for this recommendation is that drugs from one of these two classes have been the principal drugs in placebo-controlled trials demonstrating that treatment decreases mortality and major morbidity. In a smaller number of clinical trials, ACE inhibitors and long-acting calcium antagonists have seemed to be as effective as diuretics and beta-blockers (25), although there is suggestive evidence that calcium antagonists either show no benefit in, or may harm, subsets of patients at high risk for MI (72).

Because of the increased incidence of heart failure in patients taking the alpha-blocker doxazosin in a head-to-head comparison of drugs from the major classes, alpha-blockers should not be selected for initial monotherapy (76). Alpha-blockers may be appropriate in treating selectively patients who would be candidates for alpha-blocker treatment of symptoms from benign prostate hypertrophy (see Chapter 53).

Drug Combinations

The principal advantage of combining agents is successful BP control—often with relatively low dosages of drugs from different classes—in patients whose BP is not controlled with monotherapy. This advantage has been demonstrated in a number of studies, including one that randomly allocated nonresponding patients to two-drug combinations of drugs from each of the following classes: diuretic (hydrochlorothiazide), beta-blocker (atenolol), ACE inhibitor (captopril), alpha-blocker (prazosin), calcium antagonist (diltiazem-SR), and central-acting alpha-agonist (clonidine) (77). In the HOT trial of more aggressive BP lowering, combination therapy was necessary in about 70% of subjects to achieve DBPs lower than 90 mm Hg (66).

Fixed-Dose Combination Tablets

Drugs from two or more classes of antihypertensive agents (usually a low-dose thiazide diuretic plus a nondiuretic) are available in a number of fixed-dose combinations. The appropriate combination tablets may provide additional convenience at no additional cost.

Drug Combinations with Beneficial or Risky Synergies

Two antihypertensive drug combinations have been shown to have beneficial synergistic effects:

- An *ACE inhibitor* added to a *thiazide or loop diuretic:* May prevent diuretic-induced hypokalemia
- An *adrenergic inhibitor* (beta-blocker or central-acting alpha-agonist) plus a *vasodilator* (hydralazine or minoxidil): the former prevents reflex tachycardia induced by the latter, enabling the patient to take these potent vasodilations.

Certain two-drug combinations may have potentially harmful synergistic effects:

- An *ACE inhibitor* combined with a *potassium-sparing diuretic* and/or potassium supplements: May cause hyperkalemia.
- A *beta-blocker* plus a *nondihydropyradine calcium antagonist*: May cause heart block.

Adding a Diuretic

The addition of a diuretic has been shown to enhance the antihypertensive effect of all nondiuretic drugs. Therefore, in a patient who does not achieve control with one of the nondiuretic drugs, the *addition of a low dosage of a thiazide diuretic* should be considered. Higher doses of a thiazide, a more potent loop diuretic, or a potassium-sparing diuretic may be needed in some patients who have edema due to sodium retention. An especially potent regimen—the combination of a loop diuretic (e.g., furosemide) with a low dosage of a diuretic active at the distal convoluted tubule (e.g., a thiazide or metolazone)—may occasionally be needed to control volume overload in a patient whose hypertension is related to this (78).

Demographic Characteristics

In general, *African American subjects* respond less often than whites to ACE inhibitor and beta-blocker monotherapy and more often to monotherapy with diuretics; calcium antagonists and alpha-blockers are also effective as monotherapy. In a large proportion of *older patients* with diastolic or isolated systolic hypertension, low-dose diuretic monotherapy is effective; long-acting nondihydropyridine calcium antagonists have also been shown to be effective in controlling the BP in older patients (4,42). *Gender* has not been correlated with selected advantages or disadvantages of any classes of antihypertensive drugs. Because the potent vasodilator minoxidil causes marked hirsutism, it is not an acceptable medication for women. Additional considerations in managing hypertension in *adolescents, older patients*, and *pregnant patients* are discussed in later sections of this chapter.

Table 67.14. Oral Antihypertensive Drugs[a]

Drug Classes and Drugs	Trade Name	Usual Dose Range in Total mg/day (Frequency per Day)	Available Strengths (mg)	Selected Side Effects and Comments[b]
Diuretics (Partial List)				
Thiazide and thiazide-like diuretics				Biochemical abnormalities: ↓ potassium, ↓ sodium, ↑ uric acid Sexual dysfunction: ↑ calcium, ↓ magnesium, ↑ cholesterol, ↑ glucose, short term ↑ cholesterol Rare: blood dyscrasias, photosensitivity, pancreatitis, hyponatremia
Chlorthalidone (G)	Hygroton	12.5–50 (1)	25, 50	
Hydrochlorothiazide (G)	Hydrodiuril, Microzide, Esidrix	12.5–50 (1)	12.5, 25, 50	
Indapamide (G)	Lozol	1.25–5 (1)	2.5	(Less or no hypercholesterolemia)
Metolazone	Mykrox	0.5–1.0 (1)	0.5	
	Zaroxolyn	2.5–10 (1)	2.5, 5	
Loop Diuretics				
Bumetanide (G)	Bumex	0.5–4 (2–3)	0.5, 1	(Short duration of action, no hypercalcemia)
Ethacrynic acid	Edecrin	25–100 (2–3)	50	(Only nonsulfonamide diuretic, ototoxicity)
Furosemide (G)	Lasix	40–240 (2–3)	20, 40, 80	(Short duration of action, no hypercalcemia)
Torsemide	Demadex	5–100 (1–2)	5, 10, 20, 100	(Long duration of action)
Potassium-Sparing Agents				Hyperkalemia
Amiloride (G)	Midamor	5–10 (1)	5	
Spironolactone (G)	Aldactone	25–100 (1)	25, 50, 100	(Gynecomastia)
Triamterene (G)	Dyrenium	25–100 (1)	50, 100	
Adrenergic Inhibitors				
Peripheral-Acting Agents				
Guanadrel	Hylorel	10–75 (2)	10, 25	(Postural hypotension, diarrhea)
Guanethidine	Ismelin	10–150 (1)	10, 25	(Postural hypotension, diarrhea)
Reserpine (G)[c]	Serpasil	0.05–0.25 (1)	0.1, 0.25	(Nasal congestion, sedation, depression, activation of peptic ulcer)
Centrally Acting				Sedation, dry mouth, bradycardia, withdrawal hypertension
Clonidine (G)[d]	Catapres	0.2–1.2 (2–3)	0.1, 0.2	(More withdrawal)
Guanabenz (G)	Wytensin	8–32 (2)	4, 8	
Guanfacine (G)	Tenex	1–3 (1)	1, 2	(Less withdrawal)
Methyldopa (G)	Aldomet	500–3000 (2)	250, 500	(Hepatic and "autoimmune" disorders)
α-Blockers				Postural hypotension
Doxazosin (G)	Cardura	1–16 (1)	1, 2, 4, 8	
Prazosin (G)	Minipress	2–30 (2–3)	1, 2, 5	
Terazosin (G)	Hytrin	1–20 (1)	1, 2, 5, 10	
β-Blockers				Bronchospasm, bradycardia, heart failure, may mask insulin-induced hypoglycemia Less serious: impaired peripheral circulation, insomnia, fatigue, decreased exercise tolerance, ↓ high-density lipoprotein cholesterol, hypertriglyceridemia (except agents with intrinsic sympathomimetic activity)
Acebutolol (G)[e, f]	Sectral	200–800 (1)	200, 400	
Atenolol (G)[e]	Tenormin	25–100 (1–2)	25, 50, 100	
Betaxolol (G)[e]	Kerlone	5–20 (1)	10, 20	
Bisoprolol (G)[e]	Zebeta	2.5–10 (1)	5, 10	
Carteolol[e]	Cartrol	2.5–10 (1)	2.5, 5	
Metoprolol (G)[e]	Lopressor	50–300 (2)	50, 100	
	Toprol-XL	50–300 (1)	50, 100, 200	
Propranolol (G)	Inderal	40–480 (2)	10, 20, 40, 60, 80	
Timolol (G)	Blocadren	20–60 (2)	5, 10, 20	

Combined α- and β-Blockers				Postural hypotension, bronchospasm
Carvedilol	Coreg	12.5–50 (2)	3.125, 6.25, 12.5, 25	
Labetalol (G)	Normodyne, Trandate	200–1,200 (2)	100, 200, 300	
Direct Vasodilators				Headaches, fluid retention, tachycardia
Hydralazine (G)	Apresoline	50–300 (2)	10, 25, 50, 100	(Lupus syndrome, sensory neuropathy)
Minoxidil (G)	Loniten	15–100 (1)	2.5, 10	(Hirsutism)
Calcium Antagonists				
Nondihydropyridines				Conduction defects, worsening of systolic dysfunction, gingival hyperplasia ankle edema
Diltiazem (G)	Cardizem SR	120–360 (2)	60, 80, 120	(Nausea, headache, lupus-like rash)
	Cardizem CD,	120–360 (1)	120, 180, 240, 300	
	Dilacor XR, Tiazac			
Verapamil (G)	Isoptin, Calan	40, 80, 120 (3)		
	Isoptin SR, Calan SR	90–480 (2)	120, 180, 240	(Constipation)
	Verelan, Covera HS	120–480 (1)	120, 180, 240, 360	
Dihydropyridines				Ankle edema, flushing, headache, gingival hypertrophy
Amlodipine	Norvasc	2.5–10 (1)	2.5, 5, 10	
Felodipine	Plendil	2.5–20 (1)	5, 10	
Isradipine	DynaCirc	5–20 (2)	2.5, 5	
	DynaCirc CR	5–20 (1)	5, 10	
Nicardipine (G)	Cardene SR	60–90 (2)	20, 30	
Nifedipine (G)	Procardia XL, Adalat CC	30–120 (1)	30, 60, 90	
Nisoldipine	Sular	20–60 (1)	10, 20, 30, 40	
Angiotensin-Converting Enzyme (ACE) Inhibitors				Common: cough Rare: angioedema, hyperkalemia, rash, loss of taste, leucopenia, hepatotoxicity, pancreatitis, acute renal failure with bilateral renal artery stenosis, ↑ fetal loss if given in second or third trimester
Benazepril	Lotensin	5–40 (1–2)	5, 10, 20, 40	
Captopril (G)	Capoten	25–150 (2–3)	12.5, 25, 50, 100	
Enalapril (G)	Vasotec	50–40 (1–2)	2.5, 5, 10, 20	
Fosinopril	Monopril	10–40 (1–2)	10, 20	
Lisinopril	Prinivil, Zestril	5–40 (1)	5, 10, 20, 40	
Moexipril	Univasc	7.5–15 (2)	7.5, 15	
Perindopril	Aceon	4–8 (1–2)	2, 4, 8	
Quinapril	Accupril	5–80 (1–2)	5, 10, 20, 40	
Ramipril	Altace	1.25–20 (1–2)	1.25, 2.5, 5, 10	
Trandolapril	Mavik	1–4 (1)	1, 2, 4	
Angiotensin II Receptor Blockers				Similar to ACE Inhibitors but do not cause cough and rarely cause , angioedema, loss of taste, or hepatotoxicity
Candesartan	Atacand	8–32 (1)	4, 8, 16, 32	
Eprosartan	Teveten	400–800 (1–2)	400, 800	
Irbesartan	Avapro	150–300 (1)	150, 300	
Losartan	Cozaar	25–100 (1–2)	25, 50	
Perindopril	Aceon	4–8 (1–2)	2, 4, 8	
Telmisartan	Micardis	40–80 (1)	40, 80	
Valsartan	Diovan	80–320 (1)	80, 160	

G, generic available.

[a]These dosages may vary from those listed in the *Physicians' Desk Reference,* which may be consulted for additional information. The listing of side effects is not all-inclusive, and clinicians are urged to refer to the package insert for a more detailed listing.

[b]Parentheses indicate individual drug effect; all others are class effects.

[c]Also acts centrally.

[d]Also available as transdermal therapeutic system (Catapres TTS) in patches that deliver .1 to .3 mg daily for 7 days.

[e]Cardioselective.

[f]Has intrinsic sympathomimetic activity.

Adapted from the Sixth Report of the Joint National Committee on Prevention, Detection, Evaluation, and Treatment of High Blood Pressure. Arch Intern Med 1997;157:2413.

Table 67.15. Guidelines for Selecting Drug Treatment of Hypertension

Class of Drug	Compelling Indications	Possible Indications	Compelling Contraindications	Possible Contraindications
Diuretics	Diabetes Heart failure Elderly patients Systolic hypertension		Frequent: Gout	Sexually active males
β-Blockers	Angina After myocardial infarct Diabetes Tachyarrhythmias Migraine	Heart failure Pregnancy	Asthma and COPD Heart block[a]	Athletes and physically active patients Peripheral vascular disease
ACE inhibitors	Heart failure Diabetes Left ventricular dysfunction After myocardial infarct Nondiabetic renal disease		Pregnancy Hyperkalaemia Bilateral renal artery stenosis	
Calcium antagonists	Angina Elderly patients Systolic hypertension	Peripheral vascular disease	Heart block[b]	Congestive heart failure[c]
α-Blockers	Prostatic hypertrophy	Glucose intolerance Dyslipidaemia		Orthostatic hypotension
Angiotensin II antagonists	ACE inhibitor cough	Heart failure	Pregnancy Bilateral renal artery stenosis Hyperkalaemia	

ACE, angiotensin-converting enzyme; COPD chronic obstructive pulmonary disease.

[a]Grade. 2 or 3 atrioventricular block.

[b]Grade 2 or 3 atrioventricular block (contraindication for verapamil or diltiazem).

[c]Verapamil or diltiazem.

Adapted from 1999 World Health Organization/International Society of Hypertension Guidelines Subcommittee, WHO/ISH guidelines for the management of hypertension, J Hypertens 1999;17:151.

Miscellaneous Coexisting Medical Conditions

Coexisting medical conditions may influence the selection of antihypertensive drugs. Figure 67.6 and Table 67.15 list for each class of drugs *compelling indications,* meaning that there is evidence for drug-specific benefits from randomized controlled trials. Table 67.15 also lists for each class of antihypertensives coexisting conditions that constitute possible indications, compelling contraindications, and possible contraindications.

Nondiabetic Renal Disease

Based on meta-analysis of trials that compared multiple drugs, it appears that ACE inhibitors may have a selective renoprotective effect independent of their BP-lowering effect in patients with nondiabetic renal disease (79). On the other hand, BP reduction with drugs from all classes has delayed the progression of chronic renal failure. The level of 130/85 mm Hg, or lower, was associated with optimal renoprotection. This finding was especially true in patients with 1 g/day or more of proteinuria, including African Americans, a group at high risk for development of end-stage renal disease (52). In one study, an even lower on-treatment BP–approximately 125/75 mm Hg—was found to provide optimal renoprotection in African American patients (80). In summary, any antihypertensive drug or drug combination that controls the BP to 130/85 mm Hg or less is appropriate for patients with renal disease.

Diabetes Mellitus

HBP is up to twice as common in diabetic patients than in matched nondiabetic individuals, and there is an association between type 2 diabetes, hypertension, and the insulin resistant state known as "syndrome X" (hyperinsulinemia, dyslipidemia, and obesity) (81). Nonpharmacologic lifestyle changes that decrease insulin resistance (weight reduction and increased exercise) may theoretically be especially important in treating this subset of hypertensive patients.

The recommended on-treatment goal of 130/85 mm Hg or less for diabetic patients (4,42) was supported by the findings of the HOT Trial, which, like the United Kingdom Prospective Diabetes Study (UKPDS) trials, showed that more aggressive antihypertensive drug treatment reduces both microvascular (nephropathy, retinopathy) and macrovascular complications of type 2 diabetes (66,82,83). Two nondiuretic classes of antihypertensive drugs were shown to be equally efficacious in the UKPDS: ACE inhibitors (captopril) and beta-blockers (atenolol). Two drug comparison trials showed significantly lower cardiovascular event rates among diabetic patients taking ACE inhibitors versus dihydropyridine calcium antagonists (84,85). Although calcium antagonists were used in HOT, the findings from these two trials suggest that other classes may be more beneficial. In this regard, it is important to recognize that *cotreatment with diuretics* has been fundamental to BP control in major trials that have shown benefits in diabetic patients with HBP (83–86).

In patients with *type 1 diabetes with nephropathy* (urine albumin, 30 mg/day or more), ACE inhibitors should be used, because they have been shown to reduce proteinuria and delay loss of renal function even in nonhypertensive diabetic patients (87). In type 2 diabetes with nephropathy and HBP, ARBs have been studied extensively (88). ARBs confer renoprotection, and there is evidence that the addition of an ACE inhibitor may enhance this effect. The impact of ARBs on overall cardiovascular morbidity and mortality has not yet been established.

A potential unique role for ACE inhibitors in type 2 diabetic patients was found in the MICRO-HOPE trial. In this placebo-controlled trial, addition of the ACE inhibitor ramipril at a fixed dose (10 mg) to patients' current regimens reduced microvascular and macrovascular end points in diabetic patients (89). The benefit of treatment was at least partly independent of BP lowering, suggesting that ramipril and other ACE inhibitors may have a unique vascular protective effect in diabetes.

Pretreatment and posttreatment *standing BPs* should always be measured in diabetic patients. When orthostasis is found, presumably caused by neuropathy, the standing pressure should be monitored and included in treatment decisions.

Left Ventricular Hypertrophy

The finding of LVH on either a baseline ECG or an echocardiogram is a powerful independent predictor of cardiovascular morbidity (90). LVH may regress when BP is reduced by weight reduction, by salt restriction, or by antihypertensive drugs from all classes except direct vasodilators (91). To date, no class of antihypertensive drug has been shown to have a unique advantage in reducing LVH, although a meta-analysis of several small studies suggested an advantage for ACE inhibitors (92). In addition, it is not known whether reversal of LVH offers health benefits beyond those associated with BP reduction (90).

In the subset of patients with the combination of LVH on ECG, symptoms of heart failure, and echocardiographic evidence for *diastolic dysfunction*, a calcium channel blocker or a beta-blocker may provide symptomatic relief as the result of a modest decrease in contractility (47). In the short term, these drugs do not appear to decrease the late-diastolic stiffness that is present in these patients (93). Over a longer period (3 years), diastolic function does improve in association with regression of LVH in patients treated with ACE inhibitors (94).

Cost of Antihypertensive Drugs

Brand name drugs, especially newer drugs, typically cost the patient more than $1 per dose. Even generic drug prices fluctuate according to what manufacturers choose to charge. This may explain why studies have shown that up to 35% of Americans with hypertension report that they have difficulty affording their prescribed medications (95).

The least expensive generic regimens ($10 to $40 per month) are monotherapy with a generic thiazide diuretic, beta-blocker (atenolol or propranolol), short-acting alpha-blocker (prazosin), ACE inhibitor (captopril), short-acting nondihydropyridine (verapamil), or reserpine. Because the recommended starting dose of hydrochlorthiazide (12.5 mg) is available only in a relatively expensive capsule form, it is cheaper to use half-tablets of inexpensive 25-mg tablets.

When combination therapy is needed, a *combination product* may be less expensive than the component drugs purchased separately.

Drug–Drug Interactions

Table 67.16 provides drug interaction information that may be important in selecting and monitoring both antihypertensive agents and other drugs. This information is not exhaustive. Today, pharmacists usually can provide prompt responses to queries about drug interactions.

Drug Side Effects

The most common side effects for each class or subclass of antihypertensive drugs are listed in Table 67.14.

Modification of the regimen may be needed if drugs control the hypertension but cause troublesome side effects. After any drug has been initiated, the patient should be encouraged to discuss any drug-associated disturbances, such as reduced mental alertness, mood change, or impairment in physical exercise or sexual activity. From 5% to 20% of enrollees discontinue therapy in the trials of most antihypertensive drugs because of such side effects, and many notice minor side effects as long as they are taking antihypertensive drugs. Even taking a placebo for hypertension is associated commonly with side effects. For many side effects, the frequency is similar in active-drug and placebo patients. Table 67.17 summarizes the frequency of some of the side effects that were systematically enumerated in patients taking a prototypic drug from each of the principal classes or a placebo.

The data in Table 67.17 are from one large clinical trial. Evidence-based review of the literature (37) and practical experience lead to the following conclusions regarding a number of important symptomatic side effects:

- *Cough* is common (up to 30%) in patients taking *ACE inhibitors*; it begins and remits shortly after starting or stopping (or reducing) the drug. ARBs can be substituted.
- *Angioedema* may occur, rarely, more than 1 month after initiation of *ACE inhibitor* or ARB use and recurs when an ACE inhibitor is inadvertently readministered. It can be life-threatening if it affects the upper airway.

Table 67.16. Selected Drug Interactions with Antihypertension Therapy

Class of Agent	Increase Efficacy	Decrease Efficacy	Effect on Other Drugs
Diuretics	Diuretics that act at different sites in the nephron (e.g., furosemide + thiazides)	Resin-binding agents NSAIDs Steroids	Diuretics raise serum lithium levels. Potassium-sparing agents may exacerbate hyperkalemia due to ACE inhibitors.
β-Blockers	Cimetidine (hepatically metabolized β-blockers) Quinidine (hepatically metabolized β-blockers) Food (hepatically metabolized β-blockers)	NSAIDs Withdrawal of clonidine Agents that induce hepatic enzymes, including rifampin and phenobarbital	Propranolol induces hepatic enzymes to increase clearance of drugs with similar metabolic pathways. β-Blockers may mask and prolong insulin-induced hypoglycemia. Heart block may occur with nondihydropyridine calcium antagonist. Sympathomimetics cause unopposed α-adrenoceptor–mediated vasoconstriction. β-Blockers increase angina-inducing potential of cocaine.
ACE inhibitors	Chlorpromazine or clozapine	NSAIDs Antacids Food decreases absorption (moexipril)	ACE inhibitors may raise serum lithium levels. ACE inhibitors may exacerbate hyperkalemic effect of potassium-sparing diuretics.
Calcium antagonists	Grapefruit juice (some dihydropyridines) Cimetidine or ranitidine (hepatically metabolized calcium antagonists)	Agents that induce hepatic enzymes, including rifampin, phenytoin, and phenobarbital	Cyclosporine levels increase[a] with diltiazem, verapamil, mibefradil, or nicardipine (but not felodipine, isradipine, or nifedipine). Nondihydropyridines increase levels of other drugs metabolized by the same hepatic enzyme system, including carbamazepine, digoxin, quinidine, sulfonylureas, and theophylline. Verapamil may lower serum lithium levels.
α-Blockers			Prazosin may decrease clearance of verapamil.
Centrally acting α_2-agonists and peripheral neuronal blockers		Tricyclic antidepressants (and probably phenothiazines) Monoamine oxidase inhibitors Sympathomimetics or phenothiazines antagonize guanethidine or guanadrel Iron salts may reduce methyldopa absorption	Methyldopa may increase serum lithium levels. Severity of clonidine withdrawal may be increased by β-blockers. Many agents used in anesthesiology are potentiated by clonidine.

ACE, angiotensin converting enzyme; NSAIDs, nonsteroidal anti-inflammatory drugs.

[a]This is a clinically and economically beneficial drug–drug interaction because it both retards progression of accelerated atherosclerosis in heart transplant recipients and reduces the required daily dosage of cyclosporine.

From The Sixth Report of the Joint National Committee on Prevention, Detection, Evaluation, and Treatment of High Blood Pressure. Arch Intern Med 1997;157:2413. See Physicians' Desk Reference and Frishman WH, Sonnenblick EH. Cardiovascular pharmacotherapeutics. New York: McGraw-Hill, 1997.

- Because they are *teratogenic,* ACE inhibitors, ARBs, and beta blockers contraindicated during pregnancy.
- *Ankle swelling* is common (up to 25%) in patients taking *calcium antagonists* and can be a reason for reducing the dose or replacing this class of drug. Edema is often present (as part of total-body volume expansion) in patients who require the potent vasodilator *minoxidil.* Loop diuretic treatment, not discontinuation of minoxidil, is appropriate for these patients.
- *Impotence* is common (up to 20%) in men taking *diuretics* and should be addressed before and during treatment.
- *Incontinence* is increased in patients with baseline detrusor instability taking *diuretics* and constitutes a reason not to initiate diuretic treatment.
- *Frequent gouty arthritis* may occur after initiation of *diuretic* treatment and constitutes a reason to select an alternative treatment.
- *Peripheral vascular disease* has not been shown to worsen on *beta-blocker* treatment. Beta-blocker treatment is reasonable in patients with peripheral vascular disease, especially those with coexisting coronary artery disease.
- *Depression* is not increased in patients taking *beta-blockers.* Patients taking *reserpine* above the recommended maximum daily dose (0.25 mg) may develop reversible depression at any time during long-term treatment. Reserpine should not be initiated in patients with concurrent or past depression.
- *Hirsuitism* predictably occurs, and is pronounced, in patients taking *minoxidil.* For this reason, women do not tolerate this drug.
- *A lupus-like syndrome* is occasionally caused by *hydralazine.* It has the following features in most affected subjects: it occurs after 6 months or more of exposure to 200 mg/day or more, begins as new arthritis or arthralgia, rarely affects the kidneys, stimulates the production of antinuclear antibodies, and remits entirely within a few months after discontinuation of hydralazine (rarely, a patient has persistent rheumatologic symptoms or

Table 67.17. TOMHS Participants Attending the 12-Month Visit Who Reported a Worsening or New Condition Through the 12-Month Visit ($N = 96$)

	Antihypertensive Agent					
Condition	Acebutolol	Amlodipine Maleate	Chlorthalidone	Doxazosin Mesylate	Enalapril Maleate	Placebo
Tiredness or fatigue	45 (36.3)	36 (30.8)	43 (34.7)	38 (31.1)	33 (26.8)	72 (33.8)
Weakness	21 (16.9)	18 (15.3)	20 (16.3)	15 (12.3)	17 (13.8)	38 (17.8)
Trouble falling asleep	21 (16.8)	14 (11.9)	22 (17.7)	19 (15.8)	22 (17.9)	43 (20.2)
Nightmares	12 (9.6)	10 (8.5)	8 (6.5)	10 (8.2)	2 (1.6)	18 (8.5)
Nervousness	12 (9.7)	17 (14.4)	14 (11.3)	18 (14.8)	18 (14.6)	43 (20.2)
Feeling depressed	23 (18.4)	21 (17.8)	19 (15.4)	20 (16.4)	24 (19.5)	41 (19.2)
Decreased frequency of sex	22 (17.7)	23 (19.5)	24 (19.5)	16 (13.2)	27 (22.0)	27 (12.7)
Decreased interest in sex	14 (11.3)	16 (13.6)	19 (15.4)	14 (11.6)	20 (16.3)	24 (11.3)
Drowsiness or sleepiness	30 (24.2)	31 (26.3)	37 (29.8)	29 (24.0)	33 (26.8)	47 (22.1)
Faintness, dizziness	23 (18.4)	22 (18.6)	24 (19.4)	28 (23.0)	28 (22.8)	44 (20.7)
Light-headedness when standing up	21 (16.8)	19 (16.1)	23 (18.5)	35 (28.7)[a]	36 (29.3)[a]	8 (3.8)
Headaches	27 (22.1)	27 (22.9)	26 (21.7)	38 (31.4)	31 (25.2)	72 (34.3)
Numbness or tingling	23 (18.4)	28 (23.9)	24 (19.4)	29 (24.0)	19 (15.4)	34 (16.0)
Stuffy nose	42 (33.9)	38 (32.5)	34 (27.4)	48 (40.0)	57 (46.3)	77 (36.3)
Dry mouth	23 (18.4)	22 (18.6)	26 (21.0)	24 (19.7)	27 (22.0)	41 (19.2)
Rash	13 (10.4)	14 (11.9)	22 (17.7)	22 (18.2)	29 (23.8)	39 (18.3)
Cough	29 (23.2)	34 (28.8)	28 (22.6)	32 (26.2)	35 (28.7)	48 (22.6)
Swelling of feet, ankles	14 (11.2)	16 (13.6)	11 (8.9)	13 (10.7)	14 (11.4)	31 (14.6)
Nausea or vomiting	9 (7.2)	10 (8.5)	16 (13.1)	12 (9.8)	10 (8.1)	33 (15.5)
Muscle pain or cramps	31 (24.8)	35 (29.9)	31 (25.6)	34 (27.9)	31 (25.2)	69 (32.7)
Increased urination	41 (32.8)	35 (29.7)	37 (30.1)	43 (35.2)	45 (36.6)	63 (29.6)

TOMHS, Treatment of Mild Hypertension Study.

[a] $p < .01$ for comparison with placebo group.

From Treatment of Mild Hypertension Research Group. A randomized, placebo-controlled trial of a nutritional-hygienic regimen along with various drug monotherapies. Arch intern Med 1991;151:1413.

antinuclear antibodies long after discontinuation of hydralazine).

- *Peripheral sensory neuropathy* may also be caused by *hydralazine.* It manifests as paresthesias and numbness and responds to pyridoxine, 50 mg/day, or to discontinuation of the hydralazine.
- *Orthostatic exaggeration of the BP-lowering effect* can occur with *any antihypertensive drug.* Therefore, patients should be asked about orthostatic symptoms and should have a standing BP measured to check for asymptomatic orthostasis after every change in the regimen. For those with an orthostatic fall in SBP of more than 15 mm Hg, a standing BP should also be measured after exercise (e.g., 10 steps on a footstool or walking a fixed distance) because exercise can exacerbate drug-induced orthostatic hypotension. For patients who report that they have orthostatic symptoms shortly after taking their daily medication, the standing BP should be measured when symptoms are present—either at home by the patient or in the office—because profound but transient orthostatic hypotension can occur in some patients (see Problems in the Course ofTreatment).

In many clinical trials, *quality-of-life indices* have been used to measure the impact of antihypertensive drugs on patients' energy levels, mental health, physical abilities, and social functioning. In one study, patients taking each of the major classes of drugs or placebo reported modest improvement in most of these measures 4 years after starting treatment (96).

Impact on Serum Lipid Concentrations. Although thiazide diuretics at low dosages can cause a short-term increase in total cholesterol and beta-blockers may decrease high-density lipoprotein cholesterol and increase triglycerides (97), these unfavorable effects did not persist in a 4-year study of monotherapy that compared a low-dose thiazide diuretic, a beta-blocker, an ACE inhibitor, a nondihydropyridine calcium antagonist, and a long-acting alpha-blocker (98). The JNC consensus recommendations indicate that any lipid abnormality should be addressed according to current recommendations (see Chapter 82) and that antihypertensive drugs, including low-dose diuretics, should be used according to the scheme in Fig. 67.6 (4).

Step-Down Therapy

Patients who are taking one or more antihypertensive drugs may want to take measures that enable them to reduce or discontinue drug treatment. Based on the results of a clinical trial in middle-aged adults, about one third of patients who have reduced weight and restricted salt can maintain control of their HBP without previously administered antihypertensive drugs (99). Similarly, about one third of older patients receiving monotherapy for HBP were able to maintain normal BP when drugs were discontinued after 3 months of lifestyle change (salt restriction and/or weight reduction) (100).

Promoting Adherence to Pharmacologic Treatment

Adherence to treatment as a generic feature of ambulatory care is discussed in detail in Chapter 4. Because poor adherence is common in patients with hypertension, the problem has been studied extensively. Nonjudgmental statements such as the following have been shown to be effective in eliciting accurate information from patients for whom antihypertensive drugs are prescribed: "People often have difficulty taking their medicines for one reason or another and we are interested in finding out any problems that occur so that we can understand them better." After this statement, patients are asked whether they ever miss tablets and are encouraged to discuss any problems they are having with taking medicine.

Certain strategies have been shown to improve adherence to antihypertension treatment. Several of these should be used routinely. More intensive strategies should be used for those patients who appear to be especially noncompliant (see Chapter 4).

Strategies recommended for all patients include the following:

- Ensure that the patient knows several critical facts about hypertension: that it increases the risk of disabling illness (stroke, heart disease, kidney failure) or premature death; that it is usually asymptomatic when initially detected; that treatment reduces the risk of illness or premature death by at least one third; and that treatment is continuous for life. This information is covered well in patient information pamphlets available from the American Heart Association. One of these pamphlets should be offered to each patient as an adjunct to a verbal summary of this information, and the patient's comprehension of the fundamentals of hypertension should be ascertained periodically. (For further information on techniques for effective patient education, see Chapter 4.)
- Prescribe drugs that can be taken once per day (Table 67.14).
- Have patients state how they are taking their medication at each visit, including what they have taken "today" and, for drugs with a duration of action shorter than 12 hours, when the last dose was taken. Patients taking multiple drugs should be encouraged to bring their bottles of medicine to every visit.
- Ensure that supervision is provided frequently enough. During the first year of treatment, this should probably be at least every 3 months, at scheduled visits.
- Ensure that the practice is planned to maximize convenience for the patient, meaning that waiting time is brief, telephone access to the practice is easy, requests for appointment changes are accommodated, and prescription renewals are easy to obtain.

For patients who admit poor compliance, the reason should be explored and addressed (see practical approaches for detecting and addressing noncompliance in Chapter 4).

For patients with uncontrolled hypertension in whom poor compliance is suspected but not admitted, the following strategies have been shown to help:

- Have the adult with whom the patient has the most contact (usually the spouse) become an active participant in promoting adherence. This other adult should know the treatment regimen and should be asked to provide specific reinforcement for medication taking.
- Have the patient or another person take BP measurements at home and bring the record to office visits. The home measuring technique should be observed periodically, using the equipment that is used at home.
- Observe the patient's BP response for several hours after the prescribed medication is taken under supervision in the office (101).
- Have the patient participate in group meetings with other hypertensive patients, coordinated by someone skilled in promoting group support mechanisms.

PROBLEMS IN THE COURSE OF TREATMENT

Four problems that occur during the long-term treatment of many patients with hypertension are the need for adjustment of the antihypertension regimen, instability in BP control, orthostatic symptoms, and intercurrent illness.

Medication Adjustment

Within 3 months after initiation of pharmacologic treatment, most patients should have satisfactory BP control without significant medication side effects. In the ensuing months and years, minor or major changes in the medical regimen will be needed for some patients. Each medication change brings the possibility for medication error. Therefore, whenever a medication adjustment is contemplated, the reason should be well established. Whenever medication adjustments affect one or more of the medications that the patient is already taking, it is important to write down the new instructions for the patient.

Instability in Blood Pressure Control

General Approach

Most patients in whom satisfactory control has been achieved will have at some follow-up visits either uncontrolled HBP or, less often, overcontrolled HBP. At those visits, one can usually identify the probable cause and design a plan to restore satisfactory control. In assessing loss of BP control for which the cause is unclear, it is always useful to *check the BP in both arms* (to rule out pseudocontrol in an arm that may have a stenotic artery proximal to the brachial artery) and to *review the information recorded at the most recent visit when the BP was controlled and ask, "What is different today?"* The differential diagnosis of instability in BP control is summarized in Table 67.18, divided into common and uncommon causes. Before revising a patient's regimen, a prompt follow-up visit should usually be scheduled to determine whether the loss of control is persistent.

Home monitoring of the BP, either by the patient or by someone else, can be useful in assessing apparent

Table 67.18. Differential Diagnosis of Instability in Blood Pressure Control

Common Causes	Uncommon Causes
Noncompliance	Concurrent medications[a]
Increased salt consumption	Tolerance
Weight gain	Sleep apnea
Psychological stress	Refractory hypertension
Increased use of or withdrawal from ethanol	
Intercurrent illness[b]	

[a]See footnote to Table 67.8 and Table 67.16.
[b]See text.

loss of response to antihypertensive drugs. If this strategy is used, the patient should obtain and document the following information: BP, arm, position, heart rate, time since last dose of each medication. The currently marketed home monitoring devices range from inexpensive devices that require skill in auscultation to more expensive electronic devices that give digital readouts. If one plans to rely on data from home monitoring, it is advisable to have the patient (or family member) bring the device to the office periodically to check technique and accuracy.

Noncompliance

Noncompliance, or overcompliance, can often be identified by nonjudgmental inquiry, as described earlier (see Promoting Adherence) and in Chapter 4. Patients who have deliberately discontinued medications will often explain their reasons.

Some patients simply omit their medications on the day of the visit. On the other hand, some take their medications consistently but incorrectly. Because the cause may be an error in dispensing of medication, patients who report that they are complying should be asked to telephone the office and read the information on their medication bottles or to bring their medication bottles to the next visit.

If patients with uncontrolled BPs report taking their medication correctly, this can be further evaluated by having them take their medicine under supervision in the office and then measuring the BP response for several hours (101).

Changes in Salt Consumption or Weight Gain

Increase in salt consumption may lead to a positive sodium balance, which can blunt the effects of antihypertensive drugs. Because of increased thirst, this problem is not uncommon in the summer months. The converse situation—negative sodium balance from inadequate replacement of sweat—may cause an overresponse to antihypertensive drugs. Increased salt consumption should be suspected whenever loss of BP control is associated with a weight gain of 2 to 3 lb (1 kg) or more, with or without edema. A brief review of the patient's current diet often helps support this hypothesis. Management consists of having the patient resume moderate sodium restriction or substituting more potent diuretic treatment. Temporary use of furosemide (e.g., 20 to 40 mg daily for a few days) to eliminate excess sodium is often useful in this situation. For patients in whom sodium overload is a recurrent problem, furosemide in dosages adjusted by the patient to maintain a stable weight is effective.

If the patient's weight gain is associated with increased caloric intake, reduced caloric intake, leading to weight reduction, may restore the response to antihypertensive medications (see Chapter 83).

Psychological Stress

In a patient who is adhering faithfully to treatment, intercurrent psychological stress may explain the failure to respond as usual to antihypertensive drugs. The cause is probably an increase in sympathetic nervous system activity accompanying psychological stress.

Stress may be associated only with visits to a physician's office (see Special Situations: White-Coat Hypertension and White-Coat Effect), especially if the patient is being seen by a new physician, and the rise in BP may be strictly transient. This problem can be minimized by ensuring that the patient is at ease before the BP is measured and by *repeating the measurement later in the visit* if the initial pressure is high. If stress is suspected as the reason for elevated office BPs, home BP measurements may provide better information for judging the effectiveness of treatment and may spare patients from inappropriate increases in antihypertensive drugs and the associated side effects.

Psychological stress may also be caused by a serious job- or family-related crisis. Brief inquiry may reveal additional stress-related symptoms, such as headache, dyspepsia, sleeplessness, and irritability. In such patients, management consists of supportive counseling (see Chapter 20) and, if deemed appropriate, short-term prescription of an anxiolytic medication (see Chapter 22).

Excess Alcohol or Withdrawal from Alcohol

Because hypertension can occur as a manifestation of excessive alcohol intake or of alcohol withdrawal, it is important to check for alcohol abuse in a patient who has previously had controlled hypertension (see Chapter 28). Unstable BP control caused by alcohol withdrawal is probably most common in patients whose medical appointments occur after a weekend.

Concurrent Medications

A number of prescribed and over-the-counter (OTC) medications may attenuate the response to some or most antihypertensive drugs (Table 67.16, footnote to Table 67.8). Some drugs can potentiate the response to antihypertensive medications (Table 67.16). Antagonism of antihypertensive agents has been assessed for two common classes of drugs, both available in OTC and prescription formulations: (a) *decongestants* containing sympathomimetics, which may raise the BP but do not impair the response to antihypertensives when the recommended OTC dosage is taken (102); and (b) *nonsteroidal anti-inflammatory drugs,* some of which have been shown to raise BP or to interfere with the response to antihypertensives, or both (103,104).

Sleep Apnea

Sleep apnea can cause HBP or explain instability in response to antihypertension treatment in some patients. This has two implications for patient care: inquire about symptoms of sleep apnea in nonresponding patients (see Chapter 7) and consider effective treatment of sleep apnea as the explanation when a patient's HBP is easier to control after the patient's sleep problem has been identified and treated (105).

Hypertension that Becomes Refractory to Treatment

Rarely, a patient's BP becomes refractory to previously effective drugs and none of the other causes is identified. In such patients, two questions must be answered:

1. *Is the hypertension really refractory to a previously effective regimen?* This question can be answered best by direct observation of medication taking and measurement of the BP response for 2 to 5 hours in the office (101). Although there is little published information on the subject, confirmed loss of response can be caused either by tolerance to an antihypertensive drug or by progression of the physiologic factors that underlie the patient's HBP. Increased doses of the current regimen or change to another is indicated when this explanation is hypothesized.
2. *If refractoriness is confirmed, what is the reason?* This question is especially important for the occasional patient whose refractory hypertension is confirmed and who does not respond to other antihypertensive drugs. This situation is unusual (106) and suggests that one of the causes of secondary hypertension may be present, especially new renovascular hypertension (see Secondary Hypertension).

Resistant Hypertension

Occasionally, a newly-diagnosed patient fails to respond to a variety of antihypertensive drugs at high dosages (106). Apparently resistant hypertension can be assessed by direct observation of response to drugs during several hours in the office (101). Regimens that may be particularly effective in controlling resistant hypertension, each of which can be given in forms that allow once-a-day dosing, are the following:

- A vasodilator (minoxidil or hydralazine) with a beta-blocker and a diuretic. A loop diuretic is often required to control the fluid retention that minoxidil typically induces. Because of predictable hirsutism, minoxidil should not be considered for most women.
- An ACE inhibitor in conjunction with a calcium channel blocker and a diuretic or in combination with a minoxidil–beta-blocker–diuretic regimen.
- High-dose furosemide in conjunction with two potent nondiuretic drugs.
- A high-dose long-acting alpha-blocker plus a diuretic.

If no regimen controls the BP in a patient with resistant hypertension, evaluation for a surgically treatable cause of hypertension, especially RVH, is indicated (see previous discussion).

Orthostatic Symptoms

Many patients taking antihypertensive drugs describe brief orthostatic dizziness or faintness, particularly when they first stand up in the morning. Usually, either sitting for a few minutes before standing or a modest reduction in drug dose alleviates the problem.

At times, a patient who has satisfactory BPs at office visits describes pronounced orthostatic symptoms lasting 1 hour or longer after taking medicine. In this situation, it is important to reduce or discontinue the medication promptly. If such a patient has severe hypertension when not taking medicine, it is helpful to evaluate objectively the orthostatic symptoms before reducing medications (Fig. 67.7).

Occasionally a patient—usually an older person—describes orthostatic symptoms related to medications at a time when the standing BP is measured as normal or high. In patients with known atherosclerosis (e.g., carotid bruits), this may be caused by *positional cerebral ischemia* (107). In such patients, the problem may also be pseudohypertension, a measurement artifact caused by a difficult-to-compress calcified brachial artery (see Measuring the Blood Pressure). For practical purposes, when either positional cerebral ischemia or pseudohypertension is suspected, a trial of less (or no) antihypertensive drugs is appropriate; if the patient's symptoms improve, it is reasonable to withhold antihypertensive drugs or to prescribe doses that do not cause the symptoms.

Intercurrent Illness

During long-term treatment, most hypertensive patients develop acute or chronic conditions that require adjustment of their antihypertensive drugs. For patients with selected chronic conditions, one or more antihypertensive drugs may be advantageous or inappropriate, as summarized in Table 67.15. Several common intercurrent problems require extra caution with any antihypertensive drug regimen.

Acute Illness

All patients with hypertension have intercurrent acute illnesses. The following factors, which *increase a person's sensitivity to antihypertensive drugs,* may accompany some of those intercurrent illnesses:

- Reduced intake of food, including salt
- Bed rest: In previously healthy individuals, bed rest for longer than a few days produces a modest reduction in recumbent BPs and may cause a marked reduction in standing BP.

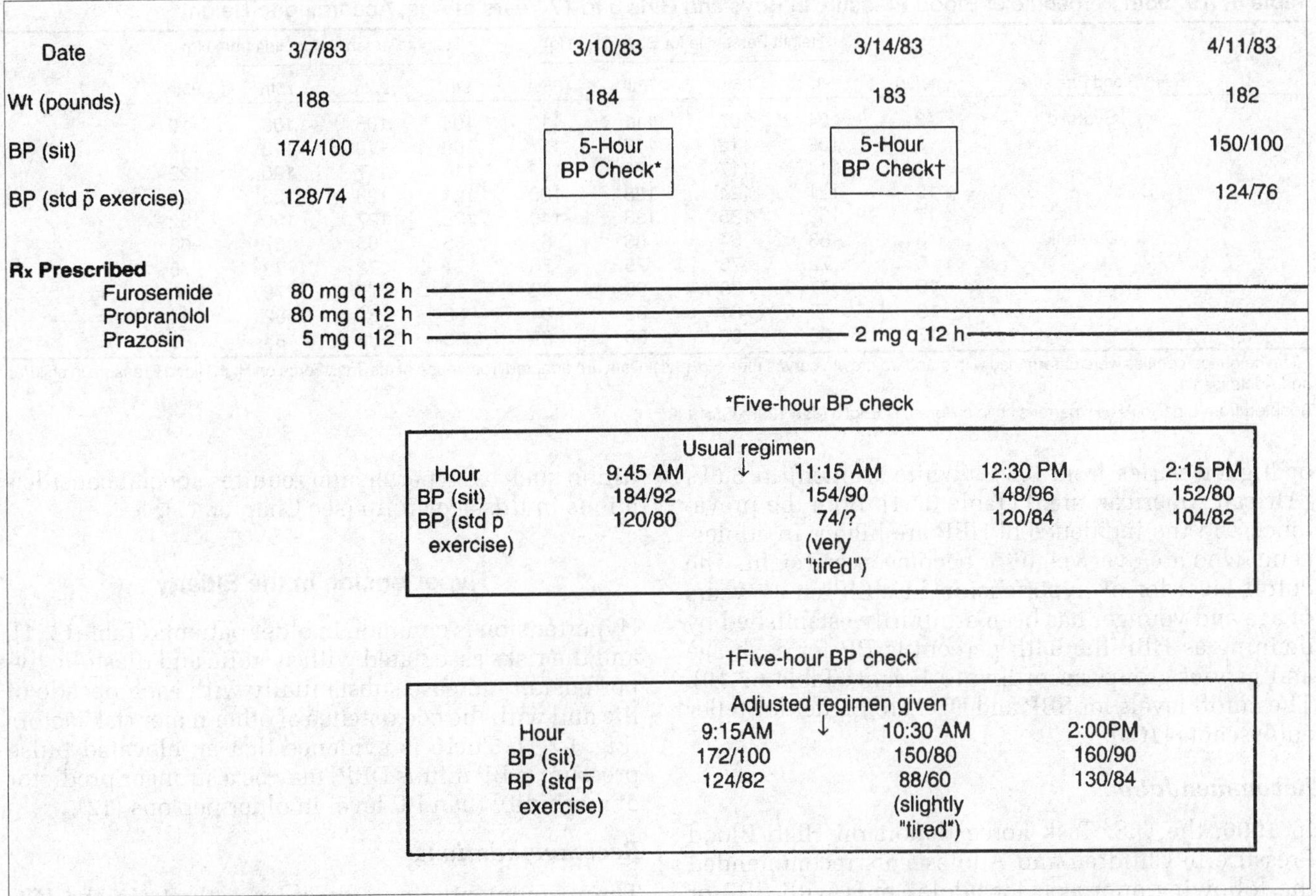

Date
3/7/83
3/10/83
3/14/83
4/11/83
Wt (pounds)
188
184
183
182
BP (sit)
174/100
5-Hour BP Check*
5-Hour BP Check†
150/100
BP (std p̄ exercise)
128/74
124/76
Rx Prescribed
Furosemide
80 mg q 12 h
Propranolol
80 mg q 12 h
Prazosin
5 mg q 12 h
2 mg q 12 h
*Five-hour BP check
Usual regimen
Hour
BP (sit)
BP (std p̄ exercise)
9:45 AM
184/92
120/80
11:15 AM
154/90
74/?
(very "tired")
12:30 PM
148/96
120/84
2:15 PM
152/80
104/82
†Five-hour BP check
Adjusted regimen given
Hour
BP (sit)
BP (std p̄ exercise)
9:15AM
172/100
124/82
10:30 AM
150/80
88/60
(slightly "tired")
2:00PM
160/90
130/84

Figure 67.7. Office evaluation of a 54-year-old woman who had severe hypertension at baseline (230/140 mm Hg) and who complained of transient "tiredness" after taking her medicine each day. The tiredness was not present when she came for routine afternoon visits. Office evaluation confirmed that the tiredness was caused by orthostatic hypotension that occurred for 1 to 2 hours after her morning dose of prazosin. (From Barker LR. Five-hour blood pressure check to assess hypertension not responding to conventional therapy. Md Med J 1986;35:94.)

- Volume loss caused by vomiting, diarrhea, or hyperglycemia
- Vasodilation caused by febrile illness

If lower BPs are documented or if the patient describes orthostatic symptoms, short-term decrease or withholding of antihypertensive drugs will protect the patient from the additional morbidity of hypotension or electrolyte depletion (e.g., in a patient taking diuretics). The patient's usual antihypertensive regimen should be resumed gradually as the BP returns to hypertensive levels. In some situations (e.g., after major surgery), the previous regimen may not be needed for 1 month or longer.

New Stroke or Myocardial Infarction

In patients who remain hypertensive after a transient ischemic attack or completed stroke, one large placebo-controlled study of antihypertensive treatment (ACE inhibitor plus diuretics) showed a significant reduction in the occurrence of second strokes and other cardiovascular events (108).

The hypertensive patient who has had a recent myocardial infarction (MI) may have a normal BP or less severe hypertension during convalescence. Because this fall in BP may be transient, the BP should be evaluated at least monthly in the first 3 to 4 months after discharge.

Preplanned Surgery

Antihypertensive therapy in relation to preplanned surgery is addressed in Chapter 93.

HYPERTENSION IN SELECTED SUBGROUPS

Hypertension in Adolescents

Epidemiology

There are no longitudinal or clinical trial data relating BP level or treatment of HBP to health outcomes in adolescents and children.

In young adults (age 18 to 29 years), the crude prevalence of hypertension, defined as 140/90 mm Hg

Table 67.19. 95th Percentile of Blood Pressure in Boys and Girls 3 to 17 Years of Age, According to Height[a]

		Height Percentile for Boys (mm Hg)				Height Percentile for Girls (mm Hg)			
Blood Pressure	Age (yr)	5th	25th	75th	95th	5th	25th	75th	95th
Systolic	3	104	107	111	113	104	105	108	110
	6	109	112	115	117	108	110	112	114
	10	114	117	121	123	116	117	120	122
	13	121	124	128	130	121	123	126	128
	17	132	135	138	140	126	127	130	132
Diastolic	3	63	64	66	67	65	65	67	68
	6	72	73	75	76	71	72	73	75
	10	77	79	80	82	77	77	79	80
	13	79	81	83	84	80	81	82	84
	17	85	86	88	89	83	83	85	86

[a] The height percentiles were determined with standard growth curves (see Fig.11.1). Data are adapted from those of the Task Force on High Blood Pressure in children and Adolescents.

Adapted from Sinaiko AR. Hypertension in children. N Engl J Med 1996;335:1968.

or higher, varies from 0.6% (white women) to 6.8% (African American men) (Table 67.1). Both the prevalence and the incidence of HBP are higher in adolescents who are overweight or become overweight. The cutoff level for of hypertension in children 17 years of age and younger has been arbitrarily established by defining as HBP the 95th percentile BP for each age and gender group, according to height (Table 67.19). The cutoff levels for SBP and DBP are higher for taller adolescents (109).

Recommendations

In 1996, the U.S. Task Force Report on High Blood Pressure in Children and Adolescents recommended the following approach for adolescents with SBP or DBP levels approaching or above the 95th percentile (Table 67.19) (110):

- Measure BPs on at least three separate occasions before classifying the BP.
- Advise weight reduction, if needed.
- Advise avoidance of markedly elevated salt intake.
- Encourage physical activity.
- Encourage discontinuation of smoking cigarettes (nonsmokers should be discouraged from starting the habit).
- Examine for other risk factors (e.g., serum lipids, glucose).

For patients whose BPs remain above the 95th percentile despite nonpharmacologic measures, pharmacologic treatment is recommended. The goal is a BP below the 95th percentile for the patient's age and height. The baseline evaluation and the principles for selecting individual antihypertensive drugs for adolescents are essentially the same as for adults. However, because of their teratogenic effects, ACE inhibitors and ARBs should not be used in pregnant or sexually active teenage girls.

Adolescents who do not respond to treatment or who have "red flags" for secondary hypertension should be evaluated for treatable causes of their HBP (see Evaluation for Secondary Hypertension).

Because of the psychological and social stresses associated with adolescence, the care of a chronic condition such as hypertension requires special considerations in this age group (see Chapter 11).

Hypertension in the Elderly

Hypertension is common in older patients (Table 67.1), and the risks associated with systolic and diastolic hypertension increase substantially with each decade of life and with the coexistence of other major risk factors (Fig. 67.1). There is evidence that an elevated pulse pressure (SBP minus DBP) may be a stronger predictor of morbidity than BP level in older persons (12).

Recommendations

The recommendations for older patients in the JNC and WHO/ISH reports (4,42) are based on the findings from the six clinical trials summarized in Table 67.5 (17–24). The most recent, the Syst-Eur trial for patients with isolated systolic hypertension, showed that nitrendipine, a long-acting dihydropyridine calcium antagonist, had an effect similar in magnitude to that of regimens used in earlier trials (23). The principal JNC recommendations for older patients are the following:

- For older persons with sustained DBPs of 90 mm Hg or greater, reduction of the pressure to less than 90 mm Hg is recommended.
- For older persons with a SBP greater than 140 mm Hg, reduction of the pressure to less than 140 mm Hg is now recommended; an interim goal of 160 mm Hg or less is regarded as appropriate in patients with very high pretreatment SBPs.
- A trial for up to 1 year of nonpharmacologic measures before drugs are prescribed is regarded as appropriate initial treatment for older patients with stage 1 hypertension (Table 67.7), particularly those without target organ disease.

Several general points about the published clinical trials in older patients are helpful in making decisions for individual patients:

- *Stage 1 hypertension* (SBP, 140 to 159 mm Hg; DBP, 90 to 100 mm Hg): Although the JNC now recommends BP reduction in older persons with stage 1 HBP, this recommendation is made recognizing that (a) the clinical trials enrolled and showed benefits for patients with stage 2, not stage 1, HBP and (b) on-treatment BPs were not as low as those currently recommended.

- *Demographic features:* The clinical trial populations consisted of healthy men and women whose mean ages ranged from 69 to 75 years. Women, whose hypertension-related morbidity and mortality are similar to those of men after age 60, were heavily represented. Notably, African American subjects were not included in three U.S. trials and were underrepresented in the fourth (SHEP). For healthy patients older than 80 years of age, the impact of HBP treatment is being investigated in a large placebo-controlled trial, HYVET, which will compare active treatment with a diuretic or a calcium antagonist (73).
- *Antihypertensive medications:* Low-dose diuretic treatment was used as first-line treatment in five of the six trials summarized in Table 67.5, and in at least one trial (British Medical Research Council) benefit accrued to the diuretic-treated subjects but not to subjects treated with a beta-blocker (atenolol) (21).
- *Morbidity and mortality:* Treatment reduced morbidity and mortality in subjects with either isolated systolic hypertension or the combination of systolic and diastolic hypertension. The absolute benefit was substantial. During 5 years, stroke, MI, or cardiovascular death was prevented in 50 to 150 of 1,000 subjects.

Caveats Regarding Drug Treatment

Several special characteristics of older persons should be considered in deciding how to treat their hypertension.

Orthostatic hypotension unrelated to drugs is fairly common in elderly patients (111). The explanation may be an increase in sedentary activity or blunting of autonomic reflexes. Therefore, it is important to obtain baseline and follow-up standing BPs (including standing after walking) in older patients taking antihypertensive drugs.

Both *pseudohypertension* and *white-coat hypertension* (see Measuring the Blood Pressure) may be more prevalent in older persons, especially those who describe orthostatic symptoms despite apparent high pressures at office visits and in those who have no target organ disease.

Other characteristics of older subjects that increase the risks associated with antihypertensive drugs include the following:

- Salt and fluid intake may vary significantly from week to week.
- Concomitant large-vessel atherosclerosis (kidneys, brain, heart) may increase the risk of ischemic damage resulting from drug-induced hypotension.
- Errors in taking medication may be increased.
- Drug excretion rates are generally reduced as a function of aging.

These and other characteristics that are important in the care of older persons are discussed in Chapter 12. *Three precautions* minimize the risks of antihypertensive drugs in older patients: using the lowest recommended dosage and increasing the dosage slowly, keeping the drug schedule simple, and decreasing or discontinuing drugs if there are signs or symptoms of significant orthostatic hypotension or other annoying side effects.

Hypertension in Pregnancy

This section addresses BP and HBP assessment and management in women who are pregnant or lactating (112). For *nonpregnant women,* longitudinal studies have delineated the risks of HBP, and clinical trials have demonstrated the benefits of treatment (Tables 67.4 and 67.5). The negligible impact on BP of oral contraceptives and estrogen replacement in most women was addressed in an earlier section (see Evaluation for Secondary Hypertension).

Normally, the SBP does not change during pregnancy but the DBP *falls by about 10 mm Hg during the first and second trimesters,* then reverts to the prepregnancy level in the third trimester. The maximal fall occurs between the 13th and 20th weeks. It is probably caused by the general vasodilation that accompanies pregnancy. An increase in renin and aldosterone levels also occurs in normal pregnancy.

Hypertension (SBP, 140 mm Hg or higher, or DBP, 90 mm Hg or higher) is present or develops in 6% to 8% of pregnancies in the United States.

Based on previous records or history from the patient, it should be possible at the first prepartum visit to decide for most women whether they are usually normotensive or have chronic hypertension. This decision is helpful in managing the following *four categories of hypertension* that have been defined by the National High Blood Pressure Education Program Working Group on High Blood Pressure in Pregnancy (112):

- Chronic hypertension
- Preeclampsia–eclampsia
- Preeclampsia superimposed on chronic hypertension
- Gestational hypertension

This recently-recommended classification differs from that issued previously by naming gestational hypertension as a distinct category.

Chronic Hypertension in Pregnancy

Chronic hypertension is defined as an SBP of 140 mm Hg or greater or a DBP of 90 mm Hg or greater diagnosed before pregnancy or appearing before the 20th week of pregnancy. It is more common in pregnant women who are in their thirties because the prevalence of hypertension increases with age (Table 67.1).

There are two important questions to consider in patients with chronic hypertension:

1. *Should a woman with chronic hypertension avoid pregnancy?* In the woman with uncomplicated stage 1 or stage 2 HBP (Table 67.7), there is only a small increase in the risk to the mother or to the infant. However, in women with stage 3 HBP or evidence of target organ disease (cardiomegaly, renal impairment, or eye ground changes of accelerated hypertension), infant mortality is greatly increased; these women should be advised to avoid pregnancy.
2. *How should chronic hypertension be treated during pregnancy?* On the basis of critical assessment of the literature, which contains no high-quality clinical trials, the following approaches are supported (37):
   a. A patient who becomes pregnant while taking a nondiuretic antihypertensive medication should substitute methyldopa (labetalol or hydralazine if methyldopa is not tolerated) for her usual medication and should continue treatment unless she becomes hypotensive during the pregnancy.
   b. A patient who becomes pregnant while taking a diuretic for hypertension can continue this treatment. In these patients, it is important to confirm that chronic hypertension was documented before drug treatment was initiated.
   c. For patients with chronic hypertension who are not already taking antihypertensives, treatment for the hypertension should be considered. The evidence favors treatment for women with longstanding stage 2 HBP or already-present target organ disease. Untreated women with uncomplicated stage 1 HBP have pregnancy outcomes similar to those of normotensive women.
   d. Methyldopa can be recommended, based on the finding of improved fetal survival in a single controlled trial of methyldopa treatment (without diuretics) for women with chronic hypertension and on the fact that methyldopa, hydralazine, labetalol have been found to be safe during pregnancy.
   e. ACE inhibitors and ARBs should be avoided, because fetal abnormalities have been reported with these classes of drug.
   f. The long-term effects of calcium antagonists on the fetus are unknown.

Preeclampsia–Eclampsia

Preeclampsia is a pregnancy-induced syndrome in which the clinical data must be carefully considered before making the diagnosis, in particular to distinguish it from pre-existing chronic hypertension and gestational hypertension. A number of factors increase the risk of developing preeclampsia (Table 67.20). Untreated preeclampsia is associated with a high incidence of fetal mortality and with maternal morbidity, especially the convulsive syndrome known as eclampsia. The major pathophysiologic derangement in preeclampsia is placental hypoperfusion caused by abnormal implantation of the trophoblast; this state leads to endothelial damage, which initiates the release of compounds that cause generalized vasospasm, reduced plasma volume and cardiac output, decreased glomerular filtration rate, and compromised perfusion of the placenta, kidneys, liver, and brain (113).

Table 67.20. Risk Factors for Preeclampsia

Primigravida
Familial history of preeclampsia/eclampsia
Diabetes mellitus
Multiple gestation
Extremes of age
Pre-existing hypertensive vascular or renal disease
Hydatidiform mole
Fetal hydrops, but not isoimmunization *per se*
Previous history of preeclampsia/eclampsia

Diagnosis. The criteria for the diagnosis of preeclampsia are as follows:

1. *Development of new hypertension after the 20th week of pregnancy.* SBP of 140 mm Hg or DBP of 90 mm Hg is the recommended cutoff value for hypertension in this instance; however, close observation is recommended for women who remain normotensive but show either SBP increases of 30 mm Hg or more or DBP increases of 15 mm Hg or more from early values (average of values before 20 weeks' gestation), especially if these BP increases are accompanied by proteinuria or a uric acid concentration of 6 mg/dL or higher. If previous BP is unknown, readings of SBP 140 mm Hg or higher or DBP 90 mm Hg or higher after 20 weeks' gestation are considered sufficiently elevated to satisfy the BP criterion for preeclampsia.
2. *The development of new proteinuria,* in the absence of urinary tract infection, during the last trimester (two clean-catch specimens obtained at least 4 hours apart that reveal 1+ proteinuria by dipstick or more than 300 mg of protein in a 24-hour specimen).

In the absence of proteinuria, preeclampsia is highly suspected when increased BP appears accompanied by headache, blurred vision, and abdominal pain, or by abnormal laboratory test results, specifically low platelet counts and abnormal liver enzyme values.

The development of new, *generalized edema* during the last trimester is another manifestation of preeclampsia. *Dependent edema* alone is not a predictor of preeclampsia; it is seen in approximately one third of pregnant women whose BP remains normal.

Eclampsia is defined as the occurrence in a woman with preeclampsia of seizures that cannot be attributed to other causes.

Treatment. Most preeclampsia develops late in the third trimester, when the fetus is mature and delivery, the definitive treatment, can be planned promptly. The usual predelivery management for preeclampsia, under the supervision of the patient's obstetrician, is hospital admission, modified bed rest, frequent monitoring of maternal BP and fetal status, and antihypertensive drugs. Clinical trials have not shown clear benefits from any of these measures (114).

Preeclampsia resolves within 6 weeks after delivery. Approximately 25% of primigravidas with preeclampsia develop it during a future pregnancy. However, epidemiologic studies have shown that women with a history of preeclampsia do not have an increased risk for development of chronic hypertension (115).

Prevention. No measures have been shown convincingly to prevent preeclampsia. Salt restriction and aspirin, previously thought to be efficacious, have been no better than placebo in large clinical trials. This is also true for calcium supplementation, although it may decrease the risk of one component of preeclampsia, hypertension.

Preeclampsia Superimposed on Clinical Hypertension

There is ample evidence that preeclampsia may occur in women who have chronic hypertension. The diagnosis of superimposed preeclampsia is highly likely with the following findings:

1. In women with hypertension and no proteinuria early in pregnancy (less than 20 weeks' gestation), new-onset proteinuria, defined as the urinary excretion of 300 mg or more protein in a 24-hour specimen, is present.
2. In women with hypertension and proteinuria before 20 weeks' gestation, in whom any of the following is seen:
   a. Sudden increase in proteinuria
   b. Sudden increase in blood pressure in a woman whose hypertension was previously well controlled
   c. Thrombocytopenia (platelet count less than 100,000 cells/mm^3)
   d. Increase in alanine aminotransferase or aspartate aminotransferase to abnormal levels.

Gestational Hypertension

Gestational hypertension is defined as the development of new HBP after the 20th week of pregnancy without proteinuria. In some, it may be an early manifestation of preeclampsia; in others, previously unrecognized chronic HBP. The final determination that a woman does not have the preeclampsia syndrome can be made only after delivery. Without treatment, the outcome of pregnancy in women with this form of HBP is usually good.

Management of Hypertension During Lactation

Because breast-feeding is practiced widely, some women who need antihypertensive drugs seek advice regarding breast-feeding (116). Most drugs appear in breast milk, but the calculated dose consumed by the suckling infant ranges from 0.001% to 5% of the standard therapeutic dose tolerated by infants without toxicity. Based on what is known of antihypertensive drugs, the following drugs, if needed, are regarded as compatible with lactation: atenolol, propranolol, methyldopa, captopril, and hydrochlorothiazide.

General References*

The sixth report of the Joint National Committee on Detection, Evaluation, and Treatment of High Blood Pressure. Arch Intern Med 1997;157:2413.

1999 World Health Organization/International Society of Hypertension Guidelines Subcommittee.**WHO/ISH guidelines for the management of hypertension.** J Hypertens 1999;17:151.

These two well-referenced consensus papers concur almost entirely.

World Health Organization/International Society of Hypertension Blood Pressure Lowering Treatment Trialists' Collaboration. **Protocol for prospective collaborative overviews of major randomized trials of blood-pressure-lowering treatments.** J Hypertens 1990;16:127.

Describes meta-analyses that should provide reliable data about the effects of newer classes of BP-lowering drugs. In total, 36 clinical trials eligible for inclusion in this project have been identified. The first round of analyses, has been published (**25**). The second round of analyses will be conducted in 2003.

Loggie JMN. Pediatric and adolescent hypertension. Boston: Blackwell Scientific, 1992.

Definitive text on hypertension in adolescents.

Mulrow CD (ed.) **Evidence-based hypertension.** London: BMJ Publishing Co., 2001.

Answers to most practical questions about the diagnosis and treatment of HBP, using referenced sources that are rated according to the quality of research design.

Specific References

1. Perneger TV, Klag MJ, Whelton PK. Projections of hypertension-related renal disease in middle-aged residents of the United States. JAMA 1993;269:1272.
2. Carey RM, Reid RA, Ayers CR, et al. The Charlottesville blood-pressure survey: value of repeated blood-pressure measurements. JAMA 1976;236:847.
3. Borhani NO, Applegate WB, Cutler JA, et al. Systolic Hypertension in the Elderly Program (SHEP): baseline characteristics of the randomized sample. I: Rationale and design. Hypertension 1991;17[Suppl II]:2.
4. The Sixth Report of the Joint National Committee on Prevention, Detection, Evaluation, and Treatment of High Blood Pressure. Arch Intern Med 1997;157:2413.
5. Hyman DJ, Pavlik VN. Characteristics of patients with uncontrolled hypertension in the United States. N Engl J Med 2001;345:479.
6. Appel LJ, Moore TJ, Obarzanek E, et al. for the DASH Collaborative Research Group. A clinical trial of the effects of dietary patterns on blood pressure. N Engl J Med 1997;336:1117.
7. National High Blood Pressure Education Program Working Group. Report on primary prevention of hypertension. Arch Intern Med 1993;153:186.
8. Trials of Hypertension Prevention Collaborative Research Group. The effects of nonpharmacologic interventions on blood pressure of persons with high normal levels. Results of Trials of Hypertension Prevention, phase 1. JAMA 1992;267:1213.
9. Kannel WB, Sorlie P. Hypertension in Framingham. In: Paul O, ed. Epidemiology and control of hypertension. Miami: Symposia Specialists, 1975.
10. MacMahon S, Peto R, Cutler J, et al. Blood pressure, stroke, and coronary heart disease: part 1. Prolonged differences in blood pressure: prospective observational studies corrected for the regression dilution bias. Lancet 1990;335:765.

---

*Bold print (general references) and bold numerals (specific references) denote published controlled clinical trials, meta-analyses, or consensus-based recommendations.

11. Vasan RS, Larson MG, Leip EP, et al. Impact of high-normal blood pressure on the risk of cardiovascular disease. N Engl J Med 2001;345:1291.
12. Blacher J, Staessen JA, Girerd X, et al. Pulse pressure not mean pressure determines cardiovascular risk in older hypertensive patients. Arch Intern Med 2000;160:1085.
13. Collins R, Peto R, MacMahon S, et al. Blood pressure, stroke, and coronary heart disease: part 2. Short-term reductions in blood pressure: overview of randomized drug trials in their epidemiological context. Lancet 1990;335:827.
14. The Australian therapeutic trial in mild hypertension. Lancet 1980;1:1261.
15. Helgeland A. Treatment of mild hypertension: a five-year controlled drug trial. The Oslo study. Am J Med 1980;69:725.
16. Medical Research Council Working Party. MRC trial of treatment of mild hypertension: principal results. Br Med J 1985;291:97.
17. Veterans Administration Cooperative Study Group on Antihypertensive Agents. Effects of treatment on morbidity in hypertension: results in patients with diastolic blood pressures averaging 115 through 129 mm Hg. JAMA 1967;202:116.
18. Veterans Administration Cooperative Study Group on Antihypertensive Agents. Effects of treatment on morbidity in hypertension: results in patients with diastolic blood pressures averaging 90 through 114 mm Hg. JAMA 1970;212:1143.
19. Amery A, Birkenheager W, Brixko P, et al. Mortality and morbidity results from the European Working Party on High Blood Pressure in the Elderly trial. Lancet 1985;1:1349.
20. Coope J, Warrender TS. Randomized trial of treatment of hypertension in elderly patients in primary care. Br Med J 1986;293:1145.
21. MRC Working Party. Medical Research Council trial of treatment of hypertension in older adults: principal results. Br Med J 1992;304:405.
22. SHEP Cooperative Research Group. Prevention of stroke by antihypertensive drug treatment in older persons with isolated systolic hypertension. JAMA 1991;265:3255.
23. Staessen JA, Fagard R, Thijs L, et al., for the Systolic Hypertension—Europe (Syst-Eur) Trial Investigators. Morbidity and mortality in the placebo-controlled European Trial on Isolated Systolic Hypertension in the Elderly. Lancet 1997;350:757.
24. Swedish Trial in Old Patients with Hypertension (STOP-Hypertension). Morbidity and mortality in the Swedish Trial in Old Patients with Hypertension. Lancet 1991;338:1281.
25. Blood Pressure Lowering Treatment Trialists' Collaboration. Effects of ACE inhibitors, calcium antagonists, and other blood-pressure-lowering drugs: results of prospectively designed overviews of randomized trials. Lancet 2000;355:1955.
25a. Dahlof B, Devereux RB, Kjeldsen SE, et al. Cardiovascular morbidity and mortality in the Losartan Intervention for Endpoint reduction in hypertension study (LIFE): a randomised trial against atenolol. Lancet 2002;359:995.
25b. Lindholm LH, Ibsen H, Dahlof B, et al. Cardiovascular morbidity and mortality in patients with diabetes in the Losartan Intervention For Endpoint reduction in hypertension study (LIFE): a randomised trial against atenolol. Lancet 2002;359:1004.
26. Moser M, Hebert PR. Prevention of disease progression, left ventricular hypertrophy and congestive heart failure in hypertension treatment trials. J Am Coll Cardiol 1996;27:1214.
27. Kostis JB, Davis BR, Cutler J, et al. Prevention of heart failure by antihypertensive drug treatment in older persons with isolated systolic hypertension. JAMA 1997;278:212.
28. Gueyffier F, Boutitie F, Boissel JP, et al. Effect of antihypertensive drug treatment on cardiovascular outcomes in women and men: a meta-analysis of individual patient data from randomized, controlled trials. Ann Intern Med 1997;126:761.
29. Quan A, Kerlikowske K, Gueyffier F, et al. Efficacy of treating hypertension in women. J Gen Intern Med 1999;14:718.
30. Trials of Hypertension Prevention Collaborative Research Group. Effects of weight loss and sodium reduction intervention on blood pressure and hypertension incidence in overweight people with high-normal blood pressure: Trials of Hypertension Prevention, Phase II. Arch Intern Med 1997;157:657.
31. Birkenhager WH, Krauss XH, Schalekamp MADH, et al. Consecutive haemodynamic patterns in essential hypertension. Lancet 1972;1:560.
32. Baker RH, Ende J. Confounders of auscultatory blood pressure measurement. J Gen Intern Med 1995;10:223.
33. Perloff D, Grim C, Flack J, et al., for the Writing Group. Human blood pressure determination by sphygmomanometry. Circulation 1993;8:2460.
34. Prisant LM, Alpert BS, Robbins CS, et al. American National Standard for nonautomated sphygmomanometers: summary report. Am J Hypertens 1995;8:210.
35. Tsapatsaris NP, Napolitana GT, Rothchild J. Osler's maneuver in an outpatient setting. Arch Intern Med 1991;151:2209.
36. Pickering TG, James GD, Boddie C, et al. How common is white coat hypertension? JAMA 1988;259:225.
37. Mulrow CD (ed.) Evidence-based hypertension. London: BMJ Publishing Co., 2001.
38. Grandi AM, Broggi R, Colombo S, et al. Left ventricular changes in isolated office hypertension: a blood pressure-matched comparison with normotension and sustained hypertension. Arch Intern Med 2001;161:2677.
39. Pickering T. Recommendations for the use of home (self) and ambulatory blood pressure monitoring. American Society of Hypertension Ad-Hoc Panel. Am J Hypertens 1996;9:1.
40. Nesselroad JM, Flacco VA, Phillips DM, et al. Accuracy of automated finger blood pressure devices. Fam Med 1996;28:189.
41. Staessen JA, Byttebier G, Buntinx F, et al. Antihypertensive treatment based on conventional or ambulatory blood pressure measurement. A randomized controlled trial. Ambulatory Blood Pressure Monitoring and Treatment of Hypertension Investigators. JAMA 1997;278:1065.
42. 1999 World Health Organization/International Society of Hypertension Guidelines Subcommittee. WHO/ISH guidelines for the management of hypertension. J Hypertens 1999;17:151.
43. Haynes RB, Sackett DL, Taylor DW, et al. Increased absenteeism from work after detection and labeling of hypertensive patients. N Engl J Med 1978;299:741.
44. Engel BT, Gaarder KR, Glasgow MS. Behavioral treatment of high blood pressure. I: Analyses of intra- and interdaily variations of blood pressure during a one-month, baseline period. Psychosom Med 1981;43:255.
45. Weingarten KL, Zimmerman RD, Pinto RS, et al. Computed tomographic changes of hypertensive encephalopathy. AJNR Am J Neuroradiol 1985;6:395.
46. Weiss NS. Relation of high blood pressure to headache, epistaxis, and selected other symptoms: the United States Health Examination Survey of Adults. N Engl J Med 1972;287:631.
47. Shepherd RFJ, Zachariah PK, Shub C. Hypertension and left ventricular diastolic function. Mayo Clin Proc 1989;64:1521.
48. Brush JE Jr, Cannon RO III, Schenke WH, et al. Angina due to coronary microvascular disease in hypertensive patients without left ventricular hypertrophy. N Engl J Med 1988;319:1302.
49. Rosa TT, Palatini P. Clinical value of microalbuminuria in hypertension. J Hypertens 2000;18:645.
50. Scuteri A, Bos AJG, Brant LJ, et al. Hormone replacement therapy and longitudinal changes in blood pressure in postmenopausal women. Ann Intern Med 2001;135:229.
51. Detection, evaluation, and treatment of renovascular hypertension. Working Group on Renovascular Hypertension. Arch Intern Med 1987;147:820.
52. National High Blood Pressure Education Program Working Group. 1995 Update of the working group reports on chronic renal failure and renovascular hypertension. Hypertension 1997;29:744.
53. Nicholson JP, Alderman MH, Pickering TG, et al. Cigarette smoking and renovascular hypertension. Lancet 1983;1:765.
54. Turnbull JM. Is listening for abdominal bruits useful in the evaluation of hypertension? JAMA 1995;274:1299.
55. Safian RD, Textor SC. Renal-artery stenosis. N Engl J Med 2001;344:431.

56. Vasbinder GBC, Nelemans PJ, Kessels AGH, et al. Diagnostic tests for renal artery stenosis in patients suspected of having renovascular hypertension: a meta-analysis. Ann Intern Med 2001;135:401.
57. Olbricht CJ, Paul K, Prokop M, et al. Minimally invasive diagnosis of renal artery stenosis by spiral computer tomography angiography. Kidney Int 1995;48:1332.
58. Stewart PM. Mineralocorticoid hypertension. Lancet 1999;353:1341.
59. Manger WM, Gifford RW Jr. Pheochromocytoma: current diagnosis and management. Cleve Clin J Med 1993;60:365.
60. Pacak K (Moderator), NIH Conference. Recent advances in genetics, diagnosis, localization, and treatment of pheochromocytoma. Ann Intern Med 2001;134:315.
61. Young MJ, Dmuchowski C, Wallis JW, et al. Biochemical tests for pheochromocytoma: strategies in hypertensive patients. J Gen Intern Med 1989;4:273.
62. Zwillich CW. Is untreated sleep apnea a contributing factor for chronic hypertension? JAMA 2000;283:1880.
63. Taguchi J, Freis ED. Partial reduction of blood pressure and prevention of complications in hypertension. N Engl J Med 1974;291:329.
64. Verdecchia P, Schillaci G, Borgioni C, et al. Prognostic significance of the white coat effect. Hypertension 1997;29:1218.
65. Farnett L, Mulrow CD, Linn WD, et al. The J-curve phenomenon and the treatment of hypertension: is there a point beyond which pressure reduction is dangerous? JAMA 1991;265:266.
66. Hansson L, Zanchetti A, Carruthers SG, et al. Effects of intensive blood-pressure lowering and low-dose aspirin in patients with hypertension: principal results of the Hypertension Optimal Treatment (HOT) randomized trial. HOT Study Group. Lancet 1998;351:1755.
67. Stamler R, Grimm RH Jr, Dyer AR, et al. Cardiac status after four years in a trial of nutritional therapy for high blood pressure. Arch Intern Med 1989;149:661.
68. Vollmer WM, Sacks FM, Ard, J, Appel LJ, et al. Effects of diet and sodium intake on blood pressure: subgroup analysis of the DASH-Sodium Trial. Ann Intern Med 2001;135:1019–1028.
69. Midgley JP, Matthew AG, Greenwood CMT, et al. Effect of reduced dietary sodium on blood pressure: a meta-analysis of randomized controlled trials. JAMA 1996;275:1590.
70. Whelton PK, He J, Cutler JA, et al. Effects of oral potassium on blood pressure: meta-analysis of randomized controlled clinical trials. JAMA 1997;277:1624.
71. Khoury Z, Comans P, Keren A, et al. Effects of transdermal nicotine patches on ambulatory ECG monitoring findings: a double-blind study in healthy smokers. Cardiovasc Drugs Ther 1996;10:179.
72. Pahor M, Psaty BM, Alderman MH, et al. Health outcomes associated with calcium antagonists compared with other first-line antihypertensive therapies: a meta-analysis of randomized controlled trials. Lancet 2000;356:2949.
73. World Health Organization/International Society of Hypertension Blood Pressure Lowering Treatment Trialists' Collaboration. Protocol for prospective collaborative overviews of major randomized trials of blood-pressure lowering treatments. J Hypertens 1998;16:127.
74. Materson BJ, Reda DJ, Cushman WC, et al. Single-drug therapy for hypertension in men. N Engl J Med 1993;326:914.
75. Treatment of Mild Hypertension (TOMH) Research Group. A randomized, placebo-controlled trial of a nutritional-hygienic regimen along with various drug monotherapies. Arch Intern Med 1991;151:1413.
76. ALLHAT Collaborative Research Group. Major cardiovascular events in hypertensive patients randomized to doxazosin vs chlorthalidone: the antihypertensive and lipid-lowering treatment to prevent heart attack trial (ALLHAT). JAMA 2000;283:1967.
77. Materson BJ, Reda DJ, Cushman WC, et al. Results of combination anti-hypertensive therapy after failure of each of the components. J Human Hypertens 1995;9:791.
78. Ellison DH. The physiologic basis of diuretic synergism: its role in treating diuretic resistance. Ann Intern Med 1991;114:886.
79. Giatras I, Lau J, Levey AS. Effect of angiotensin-converting enzyme inhibitors on the progression of nondiabetic renal disease: a meta-analysis of randomized trials. Angiotensin-Converting Enzyme Inhibitor and Progressive Renal Disease Study Group. Ann Intern Med 1997;127:337.
80. Lazarus JM, Bourgoignie JJ, Buckalew VM, et al. Achievement and safety of a low blood pressure goal in chronic renal failure. The Modification of Diet in Renal Disease Study Group. Hypertension 1997;29:641.
81. Reaven GM, Lithell H, Landsberg L. Hypertension and associated metabolic abnormalities: the role of insulin resistance and the sympathoadrenal system. N Engl J Med 1996;334:374.
82. UK Prospective Diabetes Study Group. Efficacy of atenolol and captopril in reducing risk of macrovascular and microvascluar complications in type 2 diabetes: UKPDS 39. BMJ 1998;317:713.
83. UK Prospective Diabetes Study Group. Tight blood pressure control and risk of macrovascular and microvascular complications in type 2 diabetes: UKPDS 38. BMJ 1998;317:703.
84. Tatti P, Pahor M, Byington RP, et al. Outcome results of the fosinopril versus amlodpine cardiovascular events randomized trial (FAXCET) in patient with hypertension and NIDDM. Diabetes Care 1998;21:597.
85. Estacio RO, Jeffers BW, Hiatt WR, et al. The effect of nisoldipine as compared to enalapril on cardiovascular outcomes in patients with non-insulin-dependent diabetes and hypertension. N Engl J Med 1998;338:645.
86. Kaplan NM. Management of hypertension in patients with Type 2 diabetes mellitus: guidelines based on current evidence. Ann Intern Med 2001;135:1079–1083.
87. The ACE Inhibitors in Diabetic Nephropathy Trialist Group. Should all patients with type 1 diabetes mellitus and microalbuminuria receive angiotensin-converting enzyme inhibitors? Ann Intern Med 2001;134:370.
88. Hostetter TH. Prevention of end-stage renal disease due to type 2 diabetes. N Engl J Med 2001;345:910.
89. Heart Outcomes Prevention Evaluation (HOPE) Study Investigators. Effects of ramipril on cardiovascular and microvascular outcomes in people with diabetes mellitus: results of the HOPE study and MICRO-HOPE substudy. Lancet 2000;355:253–259.
90. Devereaux RB. Regression of left ventricular hypertrophy: how and why? JAMA 1996;275:1517.
91. Schmieder RE, Martus P, Klingbeil A. Reversal of left ventricular hypertrophy in essential hypertension: a meta-analysis of randomized double-blind studies. JAMA 1996;275:1507.
92. Schmieder RE, Martus P, Klingbeil A. Reversal of left ventricular hypertrophy in essential hypertension: a meta-analysis of randomized double-blind studies. JAMA 1996;275:1507.
93. Kass DA, Wolff MR, Ting CT, et al. Diastolic compliance of hypertrophied ventricle is not acutely altered by pharmacologic agents influencing active processes. Ann Intern Med 1993;119:466.
94. Franz IW, Tonnesmann U, Muller JF. Time course of complete normalization of left ventricular hypertrophy during long-term antihypertensive therapy with angiotensin converting enzyme inhibitors. Am J Hypertens 1998;11:631.
95. Magarian GJ. Reserpine: a relic from the past or a neglected drug of the present for achieving cost containment in treating hypertension? J Gen Intern Med 1991;6:561.
96. Grimm RH Jr, Grandits GA, Cutler JA, et al., for the TOMHS Research Group. Relationships of quality-of-life measures to long-term lifestyle and drug treatment in the treatment of mild hypertension study. Arch Intern Med 1997;157:638.
97. Kasiske BL, Ma JZ, Kalil RS, et al. Effects of antihypertensive therapy on serum lipids. Ann Intern Med 1995;122:133.
98. Grimm RH Jr, Flack JM, Grandits GA, et al. Long-term effects on plasma lipids of diet and drugs to treat hypertension. JAMA 1996;275:1549.
99. Stamler R, Stamler J, Grimm R, et al. Nutritional therapy for high blood pressure: final report of a four-year randomized controlled trial—the Hypertension Control Program. JAMA 1987;257:1484.
100. Whelton PK, Appel LJ, Espeland MA, et al. Sodium restriction and weight loss in the treatment of hypertension in

older persons: a randomized controlled trial of nonpharmacologic interventions in the elderly (TONE). JAMA 1998;279: 839.

101. Barker LR. Five-hour blood pressure check to assess hypertension not responding to conventional therapy. Md Med J 1986;35:94.
102. Kroenke K, Omori DM, Simmons JO, et al. The safety of phenylpropanolamine in patients with stable hypertension. Ann Intern Med 1989;111:1043.
103. Johnson AG, Nguyen TV, Day RO. Do nonsteroidal anti-inflammatory drugs affect blood pressure? A meta-analysis. Ann Intern Med 1994;121:289.
104. Radack K, Deck C. Do nonsteroidal anti-inflammatory drugs interfere with blood pressure control in hypertensive patients? J Gen Intern Med 1987;2:108.
105. Becker JM, Brandenburg U, Penzel T, et al. Blood pressure and sleep apnea: results of long-term nasal continuous positive airway pressure therapy. Cardiology 1991;79:84.
106. Alderman MH, Budner N, Cohen H, et al. Prevalence of drug resistant hypertension. Hypertension 1988;11:ii.
107. Meyer JS, Leiderman H, Denny-Brown D. Electroencephalographic study of insufficiency of the basilar and carotid arteries in man. Neurology 1956;6:455.
108. aPROGRESS Collaborative Group. Randomized trial of a peridopril-based blood-pressure-lowering regimen among 6105 individuals with previous stroke or transient ischaemic attack. Lancet 2001;358:1033.
109. Sinaiko AR. Hypertension in children. N Engl J Med 1996;335:1968.
110. Update on the 1987 Task Force Report on high blood pressure in children and adolescents: a working group report from the National High Blood Pressure Education Program. Pediatrics 1996;98:649.
111. Caird FI, Andrews GR, Kennedy RD. Effect of posture on blood pressure in the elderly. Br Heart J 1973:35:527.
112. Report of the National High Blood Pressure Education Program Working Group on High Blood Pressure in Pregnancy. Am J Obstet Gynecol 2000;183:S1.
113. Zuspan FP, Samuels P. Preventing eclampsia. N Engl J Med 1993;329:1265.
114. Sibai BM. Treatment of hypertension in pregnant women. N Engl J Med 1996;335:257.
115. Chesley LC, Annitto JE, Cosgrove RA. The remote prognosis of eclamptic women: sixth periodic report. Obstetrics 1976;124:446.
116. Newton ER. Lactation and its disorders. In: Mitchell GW Jr, Bassett LW, eds. The Female Breast and Its Disorders. Baltimore: Williams and Wilkins, 1990.

SECTION 10

Musculoskeletal Problems

C H A P T E R 68

Approach to Musculoskeletal Injuries

RONALD P. BYANK, MD
ALI MOSHIRFAR, MD
SIMON C. MEARS, MD, PhD
JAMES F. WENZ, MD

Sports and physically demanding recreational activities have become increasingly popular in modern life for all age groups. As a result of this increased level of participation, patients frequently present to generalists seeking professional advice and treatment for orthopedic problems. Most of the injuries associated with exercise also may occur in nonexercising people who suffer injury caused by falls, missteps, overactivity, or minor motor vehicle accidents. Evaluation and management are similar for exercising and nonexercising patients with these injuries.

This chapter provides a systematic approach to the evaluation of a patient with musculoskeletal complaints and common sports medicine issues such as sprains, strains, and tendinitis, with special attention to appropriate diagnostic and treatment modalities, including rehabilitation, physical therapy, and injury prevention. Regional syndromes are addressed in more detail in subsequent chapters of this section.

PATIENT EVALUATION

Elements of a Musculoskeletal History

A focused history is crucial in evaluating and treating a patient with a musculoskeletal complaint. A primary concern is to rule out a musculoskeletal emergency that requires immediate evaluation and/or referral, such as septic arthritis, acute myelopathy or spinal cord compression, deep vein thrombosis, anterior compartment syndrome, or tumor (1). The American College of Rheumatology has named "red warning flags" in the history that suggest more urgent evaluation: A history of trauma sufficient to cause mechanical derangement, a hot swollen joint, constitutional symptoms, focal or diffuse weakness, neurogenic pain patterns, or claudication pain patterns (Table 68.1). Details regarding current and baseline levels of function are essential in a musculoskeletal history, because it helps one estimate the severity of the problem and establish appropriate therapeutic goals. Because treatment will often necessitate drug therapy and occasionally surgery, the clinician should review the patient's current chronic and active conditions, medications, and surgical history. Musculoskeletal injuries usually impact functional and work status; for this reason, an understanding of the patient's work requirement and support resources is important in developing a treatment strategy.

Pain and Discomfort

Pain, discomfort, and loss of function are the reasons most patients seek medical attention. The patient should be asked to localize the pain as precisely as possible and with one finger if possible. Answers to the following questions help define the problem:

- Did the pain begin suddenly or has it had a chronic course?
- What was the patient doing before the pain occurred?
- Was there a history of trauma?
- Did the patient twist a joint or extremity?
- Does the patient recall the position of the limb at that time?
- If the lower extremity is involved, could the patient bear weight immediately after or shortly after the injury?

The stability of the injured area can be inferred by the level of the activity the patient had after the injury. The ability to bear weight or continue with the activity often rules out substantial ligamentous injury, fractures, and dislocations.

- What is the character of the pain?

Night pain is typical with worsening osteoarthritis and tumors. Aching pain is more typical of muscle or joint problems. Sharp and, especially, radicular pain is typical of peripheral nerve or nerve root problem. Referred pain must always be considered; an example of this is knee pain, which can often be the presenting symptom for ankle or hip problem.

- What factors aggravate or lessen the pain?
- Has the patient taken any over the counter medications such as nonsteroidal anti-inflammatory drugs (NSAIDs) and have they helped the pain?

Baseline Activity and Fitness Levels

Because lack of fitness often increases the probability of injury, understanding the patient's baseline level of activity and fitness enables one to assess the patient's risk for specific sports-related injuries, sprains, strains, stress fractures, and overuse syndromes. Answers to

Table 68.1. Red Warning Flags Suggesting the Need for Urgent Evaluation of Musculoskeletal Problems

Feature	Differential Diagnosis
History of significant trauma	Soft tissue injury, internal derangement, or fracture
Hot swollen joint	Infection, systemic rheumatic disease, gout, pseudogout
Constitutional signs and symptoms (e.g., fever, weight loss, malaise)	Infection, sepsis, systemic rheumatic disease
Focal weakness	Focal nerve lesion (compartment syndrome; see Chapter 72), entrapment neuropathy, mononeuritis multiplex, motor neuron disease, radiculopathy
Diffuse weakness	Myositis, metabolic myopathy, paraneoplastic syndrome, degenerative neuromuscular disorder, toxin, myelopathy, transverse myositis
Neurogenic pain (burning, numbness, paresthesia), asymmetric	Radiculopathy, reflex sympathetic dystrophy, entrapment neuropathy
Neurogenic pain (burning, numbness, paresthesia), symmetric	Myelopathy, peripheral neuropathy
Claudication pain	Peripheral vascular disease, giant cell arteritis (jaw pain), lumbar spinal stenosis

Adapted from American College of Rheumatology. Guidelines for the initial evaluation of the adult patient with acute musculoskeletal symptoms. Arthritis Rheum 1996;39:1, with permission.

the following questions will help in this evaluation:

- What is the frequency and intensity of physical activity?
- Has there been a recent increase in the intensity or level of activity?
- Does the patient engage in frequent repetitive activities?
- Has the patient had a similar injury in the past?

For athletes or exercise enthusiasts, a history of a recent substantial increase in the distance jogged, weights lifted, or repetition of a particular training activity is a common reason for injury. For example, in a prospective study of 583 runners, the following factors were noted to predict musculoskeletal injury in the 12 months of follow-up: Running 40 miles or more per week, having a previous injury, and having been a runner less than 3 years (2). The clinician should determine if the patient routinely stretches before and after exercising and whether appropriate sporting or exercise equipment is used. One should also ask about the routine use of orthotics, braces, and other devices; for example, the use of tape or braces has been shown to reduce the incidence and decrease the severity of ankle sprains (3).

Physical Examination

Inspection

The area of pain should be inspected for any abrasions, lacerations, deformity, swelling, effusion, or erythema. If the patient is able to ambulate, the gait should be evaluated for asymmetry of movement of upper and lower extremities, imbalance, ease and amount of weight transferred to each leg, and velocity. Several characteristic gait abnormalities have been described (4). With an *antalgic gait,* the patient tries to limit the amount of weight-bearing on the affected leg. With stiffness or contracture of a hip or knee, the patient will lift the involved leg higher to clear the ground, producing the typical circumduction gait pattern. With *Trendelenburg gait,* the stabilizing effect of the hip abductor muscles is reduced or absent; thus, an excessive lateral list or shift of the thorax is demonstrated to keep the center of gravity over the weight-bearing leg.

Palpation

The area of pain, bony prominences, involved and surrounding joints, and areas of swelling should be palpated, noting any crepitus, joint laxity, swelling or effusion, or superficial signs of trauma. Then the muscular compartments of the affected limb should be palpated for a potential compartment syndrome, fascial hernia, and defect of a tendon or ligament (all discussed in Chapter 72).

Inspection and palpation should not be limited to the area of symptoms but should include the joints above and below the site of pain for potential referred pain. The contralateral limb should be examined for comparison.

Evaluation of Range of Motion and Muscle Strength

Range of motion evaluation and motor strength testing are often areas of confusion (5), in part because there are great disparities among clinicians in reporting their findings. One can avoid this confusion by measuring the range of motion of a joint from its normal anatomic position. The zero position for most joints is in the extended anatomic position. For example, in the case of the knee joint, the zero position is with the knee fully extended, and any degree of flexion is measured as a positive number from it (i.e., 0 to 130 degrees of knee flexion). However, if the knee has a flexion contracture (i.e., it cannot be extended completely), the amount of this contracture is noted (e.g., 10 degrees of a flexion contracture). Flexion is then recorded, as it normally would be, from the zero position and not the contracted position (i.e., range of motion, 10 to 130 degrees of flexion, signifying a 10-degree flexion contracture) (Fig. 68.1). It is preferable not to describe range of motion as a percentage of the contralateral limb because it may also be abnormal.

Muscle strength should be quantified on a scale of 0 to 5 (see Chapter 86). Each muscle group should be tested separately and documented and compared with the contralateral limb where appropriate. In the case of severe injury such as with an obvious fracture or dislocation, range of motion and strength testing should not be done because they would cause pain and discomfort and could worsen the injury.

Vascular and Sensory Evaluation

The distal neurovascular status of the affected limb should be assessed. The sensory examination should evaluate sharp or dull discrimination and light touch

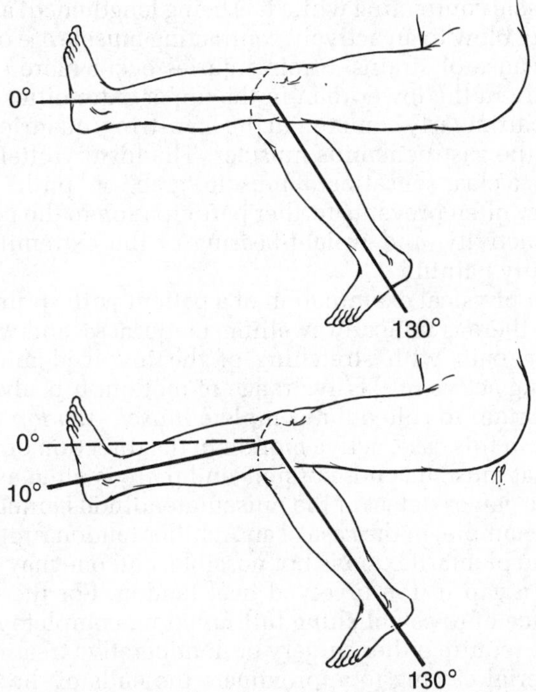

Figure 68.1. Evaluation of range of motion. Range of motion is determined from the normal anatomic extended position. Positive numbers denote the amount of flexion. **A:** The knee has normal range of motion from full extension (0 degrees) to 130 degrees. **B:** The knee has a flexion contracture of 10 degrees, so its final range of motion is 10 to 130 degrees.

sensation in a dermatomal pattern. Vascular evaluation, including palpation of pulses and an assessment of degree of capillary filling, will help define an associated problem. Comparison with the contralateral limb is valuable in assessing acute symptoms. Chapters 86 and 94 provide further information on vascular and sensory examinations of the extremities.

Imaging Evaluation

Imaging evaluation of the musculoskeletal system includes using any of many modalities such as plain x-rays, computed tomography (CT), magnetic resonance (MR) images, ultrasound, bone scans, and arteriograms. These studies often can help establish a diagnosis or narrow the differential diagnosis. The selection of the most valuable imaging technique is important. If one is uncertain as to what imaging evaluation to order, a radiologist or an orthopedist could be consulted by telephone.

Plain x-rays are the most commonly used imaging technique in the evaluation of musculoskeletal injuries. In evaluating a patient with injury, one should request x-rays if there is any bony tenderness, swelling, or deformity. Standard x-rays should include anteroposterior and lateral views, because some fractures are not seen in one plane; other views (e.g., stress views) can also be helpful. A stress view, obtained with the joint of interest in varus (distal bone bent toward midline) and/or valgus (distal bent away from midline) stress, can demonstrate abnormal openings or joint instability due to ligamentous injury, for instance (6). A useful principle is always to examine by x-ray the bones above and below any joint injury and/or the joints above and below any bone injury.

The use of CT, MR images, ultrasound, bone scans, and invasive imaging tests should be limited to situations in which the clinician suspects a specific diagnosis for which the imaging study would alter the treatment plan. These secondary imaging techniques are usually considered further to investigate an abnormality seen on plain films, and each offers qualitatively different information. CT better defines bony anatomy in cross-section. MR imaging is especially valuable in the evaluation of soft tissues and bone marrow. Ultrasound is of value for studying soft tissue lesions that are thought to be cystic or other collections of fluid. Bone scans define the extent of many skeletal lesions, such as metastatic or infectious diseases, and suggest whether the lesion is metabolically active or not. Arteriograms and venograms use contrast dye to define or rule out abnormalities of a vessel. In general, the use of these secondary imaging modalities is better deferred to an orthopedic surgeon, a vascular surgeon, or a sports medicine specialist. The specialist is often able to obtain the same information by a more focused physical examination and ultimately spare the patient additional discomfort, expense, and time. For example, in one study of meniscal injuries using arthroscopy as the gold standard, the accuracy of the clinical examination performed by orthopedists was 82% for medial meniscal tears, 76% for lateral meniscal tears, and 99% for complete tears of the anterior cruciate ligament; whereas the accuracy of MR imaging was 75%, 69%, and 98%, respectively (7).

SPRAINS AND STRAINS

The words sprain and strain are often used incorrectly and interchangeably. These are two distinct clinical entities.

Sprain is the stretching or tearing of a ligament and/or a joint capsule. The ankle is the most frequently involved joint in an athlete (8); nevertheless, any joint can be affected. A sprain usually occurs in adolescents and young to middle-aged adults when a sudden traumatic force or chronic repetitive stress is placed on a ligament. The force vector is directed in one or more directions that stretch the ligament to its limits. The history may reveal a twisting or pivoting injury to the joint. With the ankle, eversion and inversion injures are common. With the knee, the injury often occurs when the foot is planted and knee is pivoted internally or externally. On physical examination, patients with sprains typically have swelling, ecchymosis, and focal tenderness over the area of ligamentous injury. Stretching the ligament with either passive and/or active range of motion is painful. It is important to rule out a bony injury with x-rays.

Sprains are graded on a three-level continuum (Table 68.2). Grade I sprains entail stretching or microscopic tearing of the ligament with no clinical

Table 68.2. Severity of Ligamentous Sprains

Grade	Examination and Underlying Pathology	Recommended Treatment
I	No joint instability or laxity; minor ligamentous stretch without tear	NSAID, RICE protocol (see text), progressive weight-bearing
II	Moderate joint instability Partial ligamentous tear	Immobilization for 4–6 wk
III	Marked joint instability, loss of control of muscle is unable to bear weight Complete rupture of ligament	Immobilize and refer to orthopedist

NSAID, nonsteroidal anti-inflammatory drug.

evidence of joint instability or laxity on physical examination. These are minor injuries that resolve usually in a few days to weeks with minor symptomatic treatment such as brief periods of immobilization, NSAID use, and progressive weight-bearing and use as tolerated. The protocol of *r*est (period of no to partial weight-bearing), *i*ce (applied for 10 to 15 minutes several times a day), *c*ompression (with an ace wrap), and *e*levation (i.e., the RICE protocol) is used for relieving symptoms and expediting recovery.

Grade II sprains are partial tears of the ligament with mild to moderate instability and laxity of the joint. To prevent additional injury in a patient with grade II sprains, the affected area should be immobilized. The best modality for immobilization depends on patient reliability and the extent of injury. Options include prefabricated braces (either soft or hard), moon boots (large ski boot-like shoes), and a fabricated cast. If the lower extremity is involved, a brief period (usually 1 to 2 weeks, although the length of time required varies) of no to partial weight-bearing with crutches is followed by gradual progressive weight-bearing as tolerated. Even when progressive weight-bearing is allowed after 2 weeks, some patients may still require the use of a brace or splint for added protection and stability. NSAIDs to control pain and inflammation and physical therapy for muscle strengthening and preservation of function can expedite the clinical course.

A grade III sprain is a complete rupture of the ligament(s), and presents with obvious signs of joint instability and laxity. If the injury is in the lower extremity, a patient is often unable to bear weight. X-rays usually show lack of congruency of the articular surfaces of the bones of the joint or opening of the joint with varus or valgus stress (see above). A patient with such an injury should have the area immobilized with a splint and should be referred to an orthopedic surgeon. The orthopedist may consider prolonged immobilization, ligament repair, or reconstruction. Occasionally, depending on the severity of the injury and the effect of the problem on the patient's baseline function, these options may also be applicable for patients with severe grade II injuries or those for whom nonoperative methods have failed.

A *strain*, on the other hand, is not a ligamentous injury but rather a stretching or tearing of *muscle fibers* at a musculotendinous junction. Eccentric contraction (muscle contracting while it is being lengthened) and a direct blow to an actively contracting muscle are often the cause of strains. Strain injuries occur more commonly in the lower than in the upper extremities and are particularly common in the hamstring, quadriceps, and the gastrocnemius muscles. The history often reveals a clear sensation of muscle "grab" or "pull." The injury often prevents further participation in the physical activity, and weight-bearing of the extremity is usually painful.

On physical examination of a patient with strain injury, there is typically swelling, tenderness, and worsening pain with stretching of the involved muscle during active or passive range of motion. It is always important to rule out a complete *muscle–tendon rupture*. In this case, active motion in the direction of pull of that muscle is not possible and there is often a palpable gap or defect at the musculotendinous junction. For example, in the case of an Achilles tendon rupture, active plantarflexion is not possible, and one may palpate a gap in the involved heel tendon. For the best chance of re-establishing full function, complete ruptures require either surgery or nonoperative treatment by serial casting to approximate the ends of the tendon and allow time for muscle and tendons to heal (see Chapter 72).

When the stress has not resulted in complete rupture, the treatment is similar to that for sprains using the RICE protocol (see above). In the later stages, heat may also be effective. Muscle strengthening and careful stretching are crucial in preventing reinjury.

An important component in the treatment and prevention of sprains and strains is adequate conditioning. Fitness has been shown to be more important than stretching in predicting athletic injury risk (9). Stretching and warmups are believed to increase muscle flexibility and ability to extend when stressed during exercise. To be effective, stretching exercises, when performed, should be done correctly. Movements should be slow and graduated to allow for slow stretching of muscle fibers; bouncing is especially to be avoided, because it will increase the injury. The position of ultimate reasonably comfortable stretch should be held for 15 to 20 seconds and then repeated (Fig. 68.2). To minimize the chance of injury, any rigorous sport or exercise activity should immediately follow a slow, gentle warm up, and, on completion, be followed by a cool-down period (e.g., a slow jog after running). The cool-down allows gradual recovery from peripheral vasodilatation that occurs during exercise and removal of lactate from muscles. After a period of recovery from a strain (usually 2 to 4 weeks or until symptoms and signs are fully cleared), strengthening exercises of the strained muscle group will help decrease the likelihood of recurrence of injury.

PHYSICAL THERAPY

Physical therapy is an integral part in the treatment plan of most patients with musculoskeletal injury. Physical therapists are able to offer patients

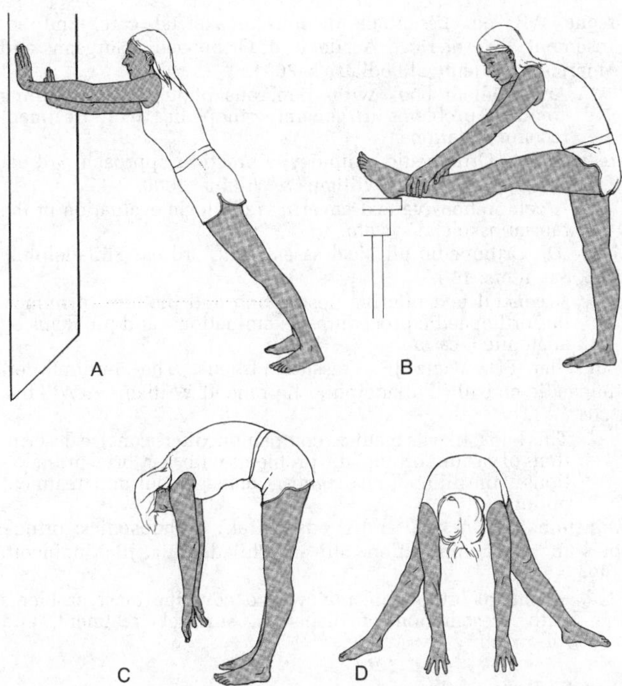

Figure 68.2. Stretching exercises. **A:** Stretch the Achilles tendon by leaning forward with the feet flat and placed at least 4 feet from the wall. **B:** Stretch the hamstring and gastrocnemius muscle groups by elevating the leg and bending forward as much as possible. **C:** Stretch the hamstring and back muscles by bending forward to touch the toes slowly while keeping the knees extended. **D:** Stretch the adductor muscles by gradually spreading the legs as far apart as possible while placing the fingers on the floor for support. With all stretching exercises, the motion should be slow and steady and bouncing should be avoided.

therapeutic and functional exercises, interventional treatment modalities such as ultrasound, and education to help the patient understand the problem, its course, its treatment, and prevention.

The major goals of a physical therapy consultation are to prevent disability, restore function, relieve pain, and educate the patient to minimize the chance for recurrence (10). Therapeutic exercises are essential in achieving the first two goals and are aimed at improving range of motion, strengthening weak muscles, and increasing endurance. Functional activities provided by a physical therapist include gait training (e.g., in using a crutch with certain weight-bearing restrictions), transfer to and from bed mobility, and activities of daily living with the current musculoskeletal injury. Physical modalities, such as heat and ultrasound (see below), help relieve pain and may decrease inflammation. Patient education by means of one-on-one teaching sessions, home exercise program, videos, and brochures can help prevent injury recurrence.

In the acute stage of musculoskeletal injury, the goals are to control inflammation, minimize loss of function, and maintain range of motion. These goals are accomplished using passive and active assisted range of motion exercises. In the subacute phase, the focus of the therapist is to improve range of motion and maintain strength; goals that are accomplished with active range of motion and strengthening exercises. In the chronic stage of the injury, the therapeutic focus is on increasing range of motion, strength, and endurance via active range of motion and aerobic exercises.

Physical modalities or agents that are used in physical therapy include the application of hot or cold packs, hydrotherapy, ultrasound, massage, electrical stimulation, and mechanical traction. Heat is generally prescribed to relieve pain and muscle spasm, whereas cold application is more appropriate for decreasing swelling and acute inflammatory reactions. Hydrotherapy, such as whirlpool, is helpful for relief of muscle spasms, improving range of motion of a joint, and decreasing the pain secondary to weight-bearing due to the buoyancy of the body in water. Ultrasound uses high-frequency sound waves to induce deep heat that can relieve spasm of deep muscles. Massage is often helpful in relieving soft tissue tightness and muscle spasms. Electrical stimulation is used to re-educate and contract muscle by direct stimulation. It also helps to overstimulate nerves, thus promoting pain relief, and it may improve circulation. Finally, an important role of a physical therapist is to teach patients appropriate strengthening and stretching exercises to perform on their own.

NONSTEROIDAL ANTI-INFLAMMATORY DRUGS

NSAIDs are a group of medications commonly prescribed to treat inflammatory conditions, such as those resulting from injury or overuse, in the musculoskeletal system. The inflammatory process in these conditions is mediated in part by prostaglandins, and NSAIDs inhibit the enzyme cyclooxygenase, thereby preventing prostaglandin production. NSAIDs are discussed fully in Chapter 77.

GENERAL APPROACH TO PATIENT AND REFERRAL GUIDELINES

With the history and physical examination described above, most patients with musculoskeletal complaints or injuries can be divided readily into acute or chronic musculoskeletal problems. The acute problems include patients with problems related to trauma, recent overuse syndromes, sprains and strains, stress fractures, joint infections, recent peripheral nerve or nerve root impingement, and compartment syndrome. The chronic problems include osteoarthritis, chronic overuse syndromes, bursitis, bony infections, bone and soft tissue tumors, chronic peripheral nerve or nerve root problems, and claudication. A precise time distinction between acute and chronic problems cannot be made. Nevertheless, it is a common presumption for one to consider any problem that persists for more than 3 months as a chronic condition. There can always be an element of acute on chronic injury as, for example, one may have a recent meniscal injury in the setting of knee osteoarthritis or an athletic injury may be the presenting complaint that brings attention to a joint affected by rheumatoid arthritis.

Table 68.3. Guidelines for Referral of Patients with Musculoskeletal Problems to a Specialist

Fractures
Acute dislocations
Grade III or severe grade II sprains
Suspected joint infections
Suspected compartment syndromes
Suspected cauda equina syndrome or acute myelopathy
Severe or progressive loss of function or work productivity
Problems that fail a reasonable trial of nonoperative treatment

In managed care environments, generalists are faced with the challenge of being the "gatekeepers" for referrals to specialists and other allied health professionals. Therefore, knowing when to and not to refer a patient is important. Table 68.3 provides a general criteria for referral to an orthopedic surgeon (1). Problems such as major fractures, open injuries, dislocations, compartment syndromes, and septic joint infections require immediate referral to an orthopedist for evaluation and treatment. Red flags warning of a serious problem in the history and physical examination of a patient include evidence of severe trauma, night pain, fever, chills, joint instability, gross deformity, locked joints, and marked restriction of joint motion. Patients with one or more of these manifestations should be referred urgently to a specialist. On the other hand, the generalist can comfortably treat without referral patients with most other musculoskeletal injuries using the conservative measures discussed above. If such measures fail after a reasonable period, then referral to an orthopedist is appropriate.

General References*

Canale ST, ed. Campbell's operative orthopaedics, 9th ed. St. Louis: CV Mosby, 1998.

A general orthopedic reference text oriented toward surgical procedures and their indications.

Garrett WE Jr, Speer KP, Kirkendall DT, eds. Principles and practice of orthopaedic sports medicine. Philadelphia: Lippincott Williams & Wilkins, 2000.

A comprehensive orthopedic reference text oriented toward diagnosis and treatment of sports medicine problems.

Greene WB, ed. Essentials of musculoskeletal care, 2nd ed. Rosemont, IL: American Academy of Orthopaedic Surgeons and American Academy of Pediatrics, 2001.

An excellent book with numerous photographs outlining common problems in general orthopedics with treatment recommendations.

Greenspan A. Orthopedic radiology: a practical approach. 3rd ed. Philadelphia: Lippincott Williams & Wilkins, 2000.

A comprehensive text covering radiologic evaluation of the musculoskeletal system.

Magee DJ. Orthopedic physical assessment. 3rd ed. Philadelphia: W.B. Saunders, 1997.

A general text offering description and pictures of numerous orthopaedic procedures, examinations, and problems by anatomic location.

Sponseller PD, Wenz JF, Frassica FJ, eds. The 5-minute orthopaedic consult. Philadelphia: Lippincott Williams & Wilkins, 2001.

This book, like its medical companion, offers concise descriptions of various orthopedic problems with very brief presentations of the differential diagnosis, management, and treatment options.

Weinstein SL, Buckwalter JA, eds. Turek's orthopaedics: principles and their application. 5th ed. Philadelphia: JB Lippincott, 1994.

A general orthopedic review text covering most problems with presentation of diagnosis, surgical treatment, and follow-up.

Specific References

1. American College of Rheumatology. Guidelines for the initial evaluation of the adult patient with acute musculoskeletal symptoms. Arthritis Rheum 1996;39:1.
2. Macera CA, Pate RR, Powell KE, et al. Predicting lower-extremity injuries among habitual runners. Arch Intern Med 1989;149:2565.
3. Verhagen EA, van Mechelen W, De Vente W. The effect of preventive measures on the incidence of ankle sprains. Clin J Sport Med 2000;10:291.
4. Magee DJ. Orthopedic physical assessment. 3rd ed. Philadelphia: W.B. Saunders, 1997.
5. Lea RD, Gerhardt JJ. Range-of-motion measurements. J Bone Joint Surg 1995;77A:784.
6. Senall JA, Kile TA. Stress radiography. Foot Ankle Clin 2000; 1:165.
7. Rose NE, Gold SM. A comparison of accuracy between clinical examination and magnetic resonance imaging in the diagnosis of meniscal and anterior cruciate ligament tears. Arthroscopy 1996;12:398.
8. Liu SH, Nguyen TM. Ankle sprains and other soft tissue injuries. Curr Opin Rheumatol 1999;11:132.
9. **9.** Pope RP, Herbert RD, Kirwan JD, et al. A randomized trial of pre-exercise stretching for prevention of lower-limb injury. Med Sci Sports Exerc 2000;32:271.
10. Ganz SB, Harris LL. Physical therapy. In: Paget SA, Gibofsky A, Beary JF III, eds. Manual of rheumatology and outpatient orthopedic disorders. 4th ed. Philadelphia: Lippincott Williams & Wilkins, 2000:431.

*Bold print (general references) and bold numerals (specific references) denote published controlled clinical trials, meta-analyses, or consensus-based recommendations.

CHAPTER 69

Shoulder and Elbow Pain

DAVID E. KERN, MD, MPH

SHOULDER PAIN

Shoulder pain is common. Its prevalence ranges from 8% to more than 20% in the population age 30 and older; it is most prevalent in middle and older age (1–4). It represents the 17th and 29th most common reasons why patients consult their internist and family physician, respectively (5). It is often associated with impairment of function (4,6). Persistent and recurrent symptoms are common (6–8).

Usually the primary care practitioner can establish the correct diagnosis and direct appropriate therapy without orthopedic or rheumatologic consultation. This section of the chapter reviews the major causes of shoulder pain and provides a basis for diagnosis and treatment of these conditions.

ANATOMY AND FUNCTION

To enable accurate diagnosis and treatment of disorders of the shoulder, it is necessary to understand the anatomy and function of the shoulder structures (Figs. 69.1 and 69.2; Table 69.1). Normal shoulder motion depends on the smooth, integrated movement of the glenohumeral, acromioclavicular, and sternoclavicular joints and the scapulothoracic articulation.

The shoulder structures themselves are organized in four layers (Fig. 69.1).

1. The most superficial layer of the shoulder consists of the deltoid (abducts the shoulder), pectoralis major and minor (adduct the shoulder), and trapezius muscles (elevate and rotate the scapula). The acromion, coracoacromial ligament, and deltoid muscle form a roof overlying the deeper structures.
2. Beneath the superficial layer is the *subacromial or subdeltoid bursa,* which assists free movement of underlying structures in relation to the roof.
3. Beneath the bursa lies the *rotator cuff,* a group of muscles and their tendons, which consists of the supraspinatus superiorly, the infraspinatus and teres minor posteriorly, and the subscapularis anteriorly. The rotator cuff muscles stabilize the humeral head in the glenoid fossa. *Abduction* of the shoulder is accomplished by the coordinated action of the deltoid (which initially elevates, or shrugs, the glenohumeral joint, then abducts the arm at the glenohumeral joint) and the rotator cuff muscles, especially the supraspinatus (which hold the humeral head in the glenoid fossa while abducting). In addition, the rotator cuff muscles assist in internal and external rotation of the shoulder. Repetitive impingement of these structures between the acromion or coracoacromial ligament and the greater tuberosity of the humerus during abduction is thought to lead to inflammatory and degenerative changes within the cuff that are the most common cause of nontraumatic shoulder pain.
4. Beneath the rotator cuff are the ligamentous capsule and the glenohumeral *joint space.* The tendon of the long head of the biceps runs through the joint capsule and along the bicipital or intertubercular groove of the humerus on its way from its origin on the superior aspect of the glenoid fossa to its muscular attachment on the proximal radius; its major function is to supinate the flexed forearm and to

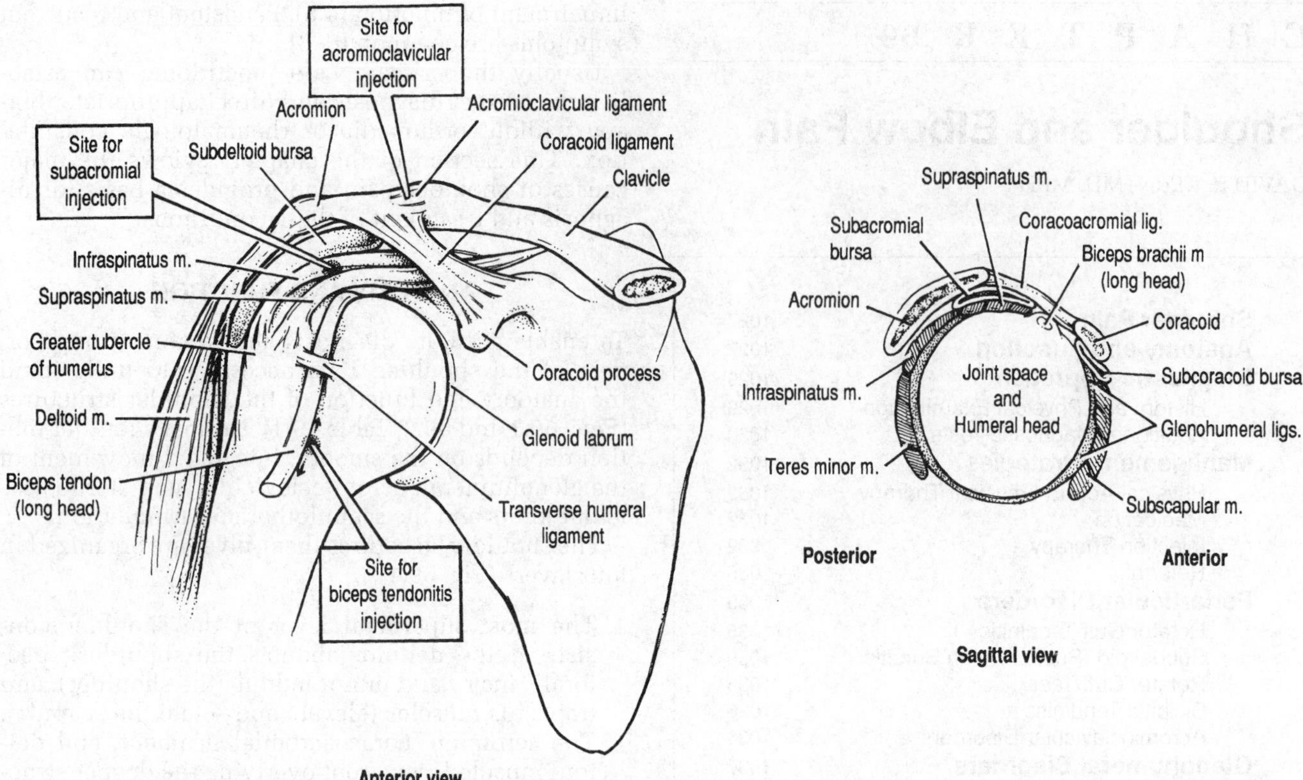

Figure 69.1. Structures of the shoulder and their relationships. Note that the subdeltoid bursa lies next to the supraspinatus tendon but separate from the shoulder joint. Note the acromion and coracoacromial ligaments, which may impinge on the supraspinatus tendon on abduction of the arm. Note the location for subacromial injection into the bursa and about the rotator cuff tendons. (Sagittal section adapted from Pansky B. Review of gross anatomy. New York: Macmillan, 1979.)

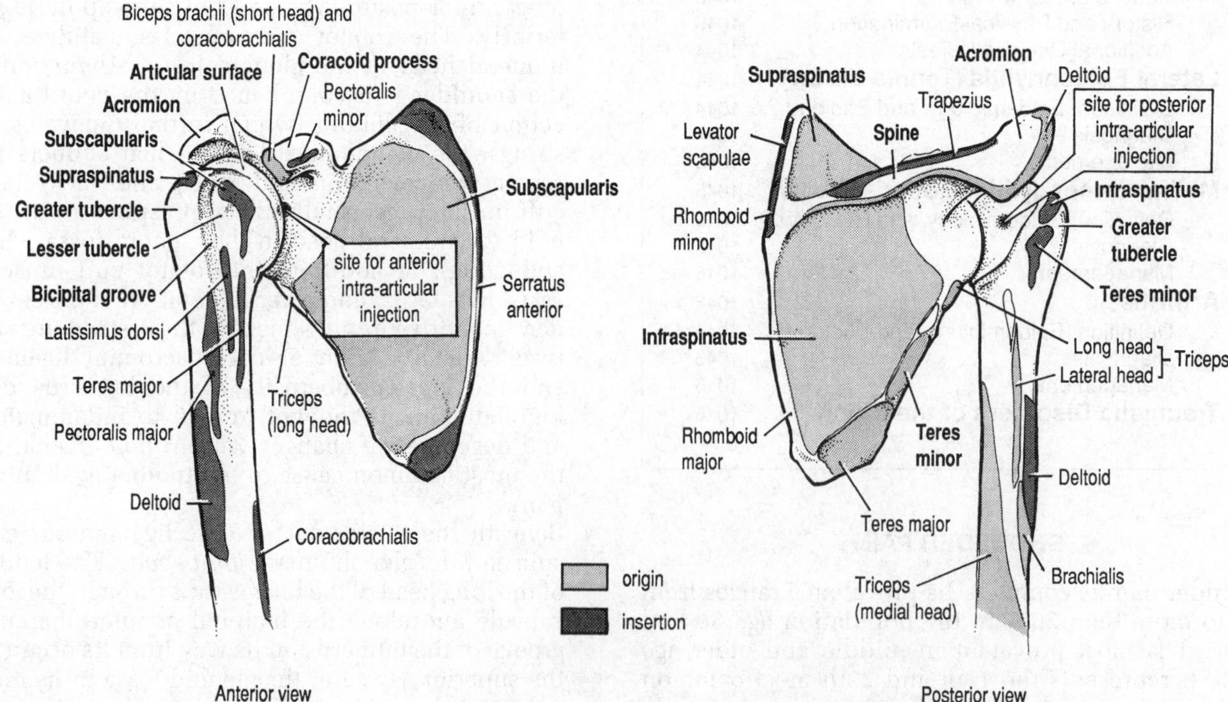

Figure 69.2. Humerus and scapula showing attachments of muscles. The distal attachments of the triceps and biceps onto the ulna and radius, respectively, are not shown. (Adapted from Agur AMR, Lee MJ, eds. Grant's atlas of anatomy. Baltimore: Williams & Wilkins, 1991.)

Table 69.1. Muscles Acting on the Shoulder Joint

Flexion	Extension	Abduction	Adduction	Medial Rotation	Lateral Rotation
Pectoralis major (clavicle head) Deltoid (anterior fibers) Coracobrachialis Biceps[a] (long head)	Latissimus dorsi Teres major Deltoid (posterior fibers) Triceps (long head)	Deltoid (as whole) Supraspinatus[a]	Pectoralis major (as whole) Latissimus dorsi Teres major Subscapularis Triceps (long head)	Pectoralis major (as whole) Latissimus dorsi Teres major Subscapularis[a] Deltoid (anterior fibers)	Infraspinatus[a] Teres minor Deltoid (posterior fibers)

[a]Muscles (rotator cuffs and biceps) most commonly associated with shoulder pain.
Modified from Pansky B. Review of gross anatomy. 4th ed. New York: Macmillan, 1979.

flex the supinated forearm. Also, it has a modest involvement in flexion of the arm at the shoulder.

The joint is formed by the articulation of the humeral head with the shallow glenoid fossa of the scapula, the diameter and depth of which are increased by the fibrocartilaginous glenoid labrum. The shallowness of the fossa enables nearly hemispheric motion of the arm, but this wide range of motion (ROM) is achieved at the price of joint stability. Stability of the shoulder joint depends primarily not on bony structures, but on the integrity of supporting soft tissue structures including the labrum, capsule, and rotator cuff.

DIAGNOSTIC APPROACH

Pain about the shoulder usually originates from one of three sites: periarticular structures (e.g., the rotator cuff), the glenohumeral joint, or sites distant from the shoulder. The causes of shoulder pain arranged by their relative frequencies are listed in Table 69.2.

History and Physical Examination

The history and physical examination are usually sufficient to establish a working diagnosis and direct effective treatment. The history is less useful than the physical examination in establishing the anatomic problem, but it is nevertheless helpful. *Perceived location* of the pain usually is not helpful, because most sources of pain (e.g., rotator cuff tendon, subdeltoid bursa, glenohumeral joint space) share a fifth (or sixth) cervical derivation and cause pain in the upper arm only. More severe lesions tend to cause pain radiating down the arm and forearm, usually along the anterolateral aspect. Pain confined to the point of the shoulder suggests a lesion of the acromioclavicular joint, which has a fourth cervical derivation. Involvement of other joints suggests a generalized arthritic process.

Asking about recent trauma and briefly reviewing the patient's problem list, medication list, and past medical history may be helpful in raising the suspicion for certain less common causes of shoulder pain, such as dislocation (e.g., from trauma), neoplasm (e.g., a history of breast or lung cancer), or osteonecrosis (e.g., from corticosteroid use). Dislocation of the glenohumeral joint should be suspected with major injuries to the arm, especially if the shoulder is abducted and externally rotated at impact, whereas injury to, or separation of, the acromioclavicular joint usually results from a direct blow to the acromion. Asking *what precipitates or makes the pain worse* is also helpful. Pain referred to the shoulder from a distant site should not be exacerbated by movement of the shoulder. In contrast, pain with active or passive movement of the shoulder suggests a shoulder or periarticular problem. A history of *occupational* (9) *and sports activities,* such as working with hands elevated, lifting heavy

Table 69.2. Differential Diagnosis of Shoulder Pain in Primary Care Adult Patients

Most Common
Rotator cuff tendinitis (supraspinatus, infraspinatus–teres minor, subscapularis)

Common
Rotator cuff tears (partial more common than complete)
Subdeltoid/subacromial bursitis

Intermediate
Acromioclavicular arthritis/strain
Adhesive capsulitis/frozen shoulder

Occasional
Biceps (long head) tendinitis
Cardiac (referred pain)
Carpal tunnel syndrome (referred pain)
Cerebrovascular accident with hemiparesis (see Chapter 91)
Cervical/neck disorders (referred pain)
Degenerative/osteoarthritis (often posttraumatic)
Dislocation
Fracture (neck of humerus, greater tuberosity)
Glenohumeral instability/subluxation
Glenoid labral tears
Neoplasm (local or referred pain)
Rheumatoid arthritis

Rare
Arthritis, other causes (e.g., gout, pseudogout, psoriasis, neuropathic, ankylosing spondylitis)
Infection (intra-articular or extra-articular)
Nerve entrapment: suprascapular, axillary, long thoracic, or spinal accessory nerves (referred pain)
Osteonecrosis (avascular or aseptic necrosis)
Polymyalgia rheumatica
Reflex sympathetic dystrophy/shoulder–hand syndrome
Sickle cell crisis
Thoracic outlet syndrome (referred pain)
Visceral—referred from sources other than neck or heart (e.g., pleural irritation by lung cancer or other cause; irritation to phrenic nerve or diaphragm by pathologic process such as subdiaphragmatic abscess, ruptured viscus, or disease of the mediastinum, pericardium, liver, spleen, or gallbladder; dissecting aortic aneurysm)
Other traumatic or periarticular soft tissue problems

Data from references 3, 6, 8a, and 9a and Cyriax (see General References).

objects, carrying loads supported by the shoulders, hand–arm vibration, pitching baseballs, swimming, or serving tennis balls, can identify exacerbating factors that may both suggest a cause and direct the attention of the clinician to an activity of the patient that should be modified as part of the treatment plan, especially in a patient with chronic or recurrent shoulder pain.

The physical examination is usually successful in identifying the source of the pain. The uninvolved shoulder should be used as a control to confirm any questionable abnormality found on examination of the symptomatic shoulder. *Inspection* is the least helpful part of the examination, but it may reveal evidence of atrophy or displacement of bony landmarks. A popular approach that is most useful and widely accepted, for the rest of the examination appears in Cyriax (General References). First, the *location of pain origin* is surveyed through a brief examination of the neck, scapula, shoulder, elbow, and wrist, usually involving a combination of active and resisted movements. The suspected abnormal site is then examined in depth. If the shoulder appears normal but another site is abnormal on the survey, the shoulder pain is probably referred from the abnormal site. If the survey reveals no abnormalities, the pain may be referred or an abnormality in the shoulder may still be present. The shoulder is examined in the following way.

Active motion is studied by having the patient perform a few simple maneuvers. The patient is asked to elevate the arm as far as possible (normal is 180°). External (lateral) and internal (medial) rotation is assessed with the elbow at the patient's side and the forearm held at a right angle in the anteroposterior (AP) plane (normal values are 40° to 45° and 55° to 60°, respectively). Internal rotation is usually limited by the patient's body and can be further evaluated by having the patient touch his or her back from below. Alternatively, external and internal rotation can be assessed with the patient's arm in 90° abduction. Adduction is assessed by placement of the patient's hands on the opposite shoulders.

Passive range of motion is then examined and compared with the active range. About 90° of arm elevation is accomplished through abduction at the glenohumeral joint, 60° by rotation of the scapula by the serratus anterior and upper half of the trapezoid, and 30° by adduction and external rotation, which increases the articulating surface of the humeral head and turns the surgical neck away from the tip of the acromion. Glenohumeral abduction can be isolated by immobilizing the scapula or observing for scapular movement with one's fingers on the inferior angle of the scapula.

Next, *resisted movements* are examined, because this helps elicit pain from the deep muscles of the rotator cuff. These tests are accomplished without movement of the shoulder joint, with the elbow at the patient's side, and with the forearm at a right angle in the AP plane. Abduction is tested by having the patient press outward at the elbow against the examiner's braced hand so that movement does not occur. Adduction is tested by having the patient press in, flexion forward, and extension backward at the elbow against the examiner's hand. External rotation is tested by having the patient press laterally and internal rotation medially at the wrist against the examiner's braced hand, again without movement and with the elbow kept at the side. Resisted flexion and supination of the elbow are assessed with the arm in the same position in order to test for a lesion of the biceps tendon. Strength and the elicitation of pain are noted.

Finally, *palpation* is performed. Palpation is less useful than the combination of active movements, passive ROM, and resisted movements because pain from palpation is common and nonspecific and because some structures are difficult or impossible to palpate. However, differential tenderness, compared with the control side, can help confirm disorders at the acromioclavicular joint, the bursa, or the biceps tendon in the bicipital groove.

Interpretation of the physical examination is addressed in Table 69.3. Both articular and periarticular disorders can cause pain and limitation on active movements. If both active and passive ROMs of the shoulder are limited, a disorder of the glenohumeral joint, adhesive capsulitis, or bursitis should be suspected. Limited ROM with a *capsular pattern* (lateral rotation more impaired than abduction, internal least impaired) suggests adhesive capsulitis or glenohumeral arthritis. A *noncapsular pattern* (abduction limited with little limitation to either rotation) suggests subdeltoid bursitis. If passive ROM is normal or exceeds the active range and passive movements are not painful or are less painful than active ones, a *periarticular cause* is likely. Pain on resisted movements identifies the anatomic location of the disorder (i.e., some element of the muscle or adjacent tissue, such as a bursa, that is being tensed). Weakness on resisted movements suggests a muscle or tendon tear or neurologic compromise. Sometimes strength cannot be accurately assessed because of pain, unless the shoulder is examined after the appropriately placed injection of a local anesthetic.

Additional Diagnostic Tests

Additional diagnostic tests should be used selectively to confirm or further define, for therapeutic purposes, a diagnosis suspected on the basis of history and physical examination. Depending on the circumstances, additional diagnostic tests may include a complete blood cell count, erythrocyte sedimentation rate, serologic tests for rheumatologic disorders, diagnostic arthrocentesis, plain radiographs of the shoulder or neck, and further imaging modalities. All have important roles in selected patients. Acute episodes of shoulder pain caused by rotator cuff tendinitis, bursitis, or biceps tendinitis usually should be managed without any additional testing.

Plain shoulder radiographs usually should be ordered in the presence of significant trauma, suspected

Table 69.3. Interpretation of the Physical Examination

L = Limited
P = Pain
W = Weak
( ) = Variably present

	Rotator Cuff Lesions							
	Supraspinatus tendinitis	Supraspinatus tear	Infraspinatus tendinitis	Subscapularis tendinitis	Subacromial/subdeltoid bursitis	Adhesive capsulitis/arthritis	Biceps tendinitis/arthritis	Acromioclavicular joint
Active range of motion	(L)[a]	(L)[a,c]	(L)[a]	(L)[a]	L[d] P	L[e] P		P[f]
Passive range of motion					L[d] P	L[e] P		P[f]
Painful arc	P[b]	P[b]	P[b]	P[b]	P			
Resisted *ab*duction	P	(P)[b,c] W						
Resisted external rotation			P					
Resisted internal rotation				P				
Resisted flexion/ supination of elbow							P	
Full passive *ad*duction								P[f]

[a]Range of motion may be limited by pain.
[b]Pain may be absent in deep or musculotendinous lesions.
[c]When the tear is complete, initiation of abduction may be impossible and pain may be absent.
[d]Limitation is in a noncapsular pattern, with marked limitation of abduction and little restriction of external rotation.
[e]Limitation is in a capsular pattern, with limitation of external rotation greatest, abduction intermediate, and internal rotation least.
[f]Pain is usually felt at A–C joint or point of shoulder (C4). For all other lesions, pain is usually felt in anterolateral aspect of upper arm (C5), with or without radiation to the forearm.

arthritis (limited ROM in the capsular pattern on physical examination), suspicion of neoplasm, suspicion of osteonecrosis, or chronic, recurrent, or unexplained symptoms. Standard views consist of AP films in external and internal rotation. In external rotation, the humeral head is club shaped and overlaps the glenoid; its greater tuberosity is seen in profile. In internal rotation, the humeral head is rounded. Failure to see this distinction, in the absence of anatomic abnormality, suggests significant limitation in rotational movement. Additional views can be helpful in specific circumstances. An axillary lateral view (which permits accurate evaluation of the glenohumeral articulation but requires that the arm be held in abduction) or a scapular "Y" view (a lateral view that displays the scapula on end) can detect a posterior dislocation, which may not be noticed on routine AP views. A caudal tilt view can help identify subacromial spurs, which may contribute to a chronic impingement or rotator cuff syndrome. A true AP view, in which the patient is turned 40° to 45° toward the symptomatic shoulder, provides a tangential view for evaluation of the glenohumeral joint space in a patient with arthritis. Plain radiographs, although useful in detecting fracture, dislocation, bone destruction, advanced osteonecrosis, calcific tendinitis, and arthritis, are insensitive in the diagnosis of early osteonecrosis and are, at best, only suggestive in the diagnosis of rotator cuff tear and other soft tissue disorders. For all of these reasons, a detailed explanation of the reason for the radiograph will guide the radiologist to obtain the appropriate views.

Further imaging studies are best ordered in consultation with a specialist when referral or the possibility of surgery is being considered. *Ultrasonography* (about 1.2 to 4 times more expensive than plain radiographs) can demonstrate even partial rotator cuff tears, but skilled interpretation is required. Reported sensitivities and specificities (compared with arthrography, magnetic resonance imaging [MRI], or direct visualization at surgery) are variable, ranging from 58% to more than 90% and from 50% to 96%, respectively. The diagnostic accuracy of ultrasonography for tendon tears ranged from 77% to 95% in recent reports (9a). *Arthrography* (3 to 8 times more expensive than plain radiographs) is both sensitive (approximately 92%) and specific (approximately 98%)

for detecting rotator cuff tears (10), but it causes patient discomfort and may miss partial tears, particularly those on the bursal side. Communication of dye between the glenohumeral joint and the subacromial space unequivocally confirms a full-thickness tear. Arthrography can also confirm a diagnosis of adhesive capsulitis when clinical findings are equivocal. *Arthrography combined with computed tomography (arthro-CT)* is of value in detecting soft tissue lesions (e.g., partial tendon tears) and intra-articular pathology (e.g., labral tears, capsular tears, loose bodies, chondral defects), especially in cases of recurrent subluxation/dislocation (11). *CT* (4 to 8 times as expensive as plain radiographs) and *MRI* (7 to 17 times as expensive) are noninvasive but costly techniques for the evaluation of soft tissue lesions. MRI better defines capsule anatomy, supraspinatus tendon integrity, the site of impingement, and bursal anatomy than does CT. MRI is equal to arthrography and superior to ultrasonography in detecting rotator cuff tears (sensitivity, 75% to 100%; specificity, 84% to 100%) (10,12). MRI is the imaging technique of choice in the diagnosis of early osteonecrosis (11).

MANAGEMENT STRATEGIES

Specific management varies depending on the disorder responsible for the pain. However, some management strategies are broadly applicable.

Physical Activity/Physical Therapy

In the treatment of acute pain, the patient may benefit from a brief period (2 to 3 days) of rest with the arm in a sling. Many patients can begin ROM movements immediately to maintain mobility, while avoiding aggressive exercise or overuse. Prolonged immobilization of the shoulder should be avoided whenever possible, because contracture of the shoulder capsule and periarticular structures, known as adhesive capsulitis or frozen shoulder, may result. When glenohumeral ROM remains restricted after the acute pain has diminished, specific exercises, such as pendular and wall-climbing exercises (Fig. 69.3), should be prescribed for 5 to 10 minutes two to four times per day to maintain joint mobility. Patients with impingement disorders (e.g., rotator cuff lesions, subdeltoid bursitis) should avoid repetitive tasks with their arms overhead or their elbows above midtorso height, especially if the condition is recurrent or chronic. A program of balanced isometric or isotonic exercise of the shoulder abductors, adductors, flexors, extensors, and internal and external rotators, to strengthen the rotator cuff musculature, may also help prevent recurrences. However, there is insufficient evidence from randomized controlled trials to draw conclusions about the efficacy of these recommendations (13,14).

The efficacy of adjunctive physical therapy measures, such as heat or ultrasound, has also not been adequately demonstrated (15–17). Nevertheless, on empiric and theoretical grounds, local cooling is generally recommended after acute injury to relieve pain and to limit hemorrhage and edema. Similarly, local superficial heat or ultrasound is often recommended to decrease pain and promote tissue extensibility in the subacute and chronic stages, respectively (18).

Referral to a physical therapist is recommended for patients who require a supervised exercise program after surgery or when satisfactory understanding of prescribed exercises or improvements in ROM have not been achieved after counseling by the health care practitioner.

Medication

Nonsteroidal anti-inflammatory drugs (NSAIDs) appear to be more effective than placebo but somewhat less effective than steroid injections in decreasing pain and restoring function in periarticular disorders (13,14,19–22). Generally, a 2-week course of one of these agents is prescribed for acute disorders (see Chapter 77 for a full discussion of NSAIDs). The effectiveness of NSAIDs for this purpose, compared with analgesics such as acetaminophen, has not been adequately studied (21), although NSAIDs have a theoretical advantage because of their anti-inflammatory properties. Concern has been expressed regarding possible gastrointestinal (peptic disease with bleeding or perforation) or renal (proteinuria and failure) toxicity, particularly in the elderly (23). The efficacy of topical treatments has been insufficiently studied in patients with shoulder pain.

Injection Therapy

Based on studies using injections of lidocaine only, placebo oral drugs, NSAIDs/analgesics, heat, ultrasound, exercise, and acupuncture, injections of depo corticosteroid appear to reduce pain and speed functional recovery in patients with rotator cuff tendinitis/bursitis and are probably more effective than NSAIDs/analgesics (19,20,24–27). A second or even third injection is sometimes required. Based on controlled and uncontrolled studies (28–37), steroid injections (often several), combined with an exercise program that is designed to increase ROM, may be more effective than analgesic or no therapy (38,39) in reducing pain and speeding the recovery of patients with adhesive capsulitis. A meta-analysis of numerous interventions for shoulder pain criticized the methodology of most studies and concluded only that subacromial injections of glucocorticosteroids or NSAIDs may be superior to placebo in improving range of abduction in rotator cuff tendonitis, but that the combination had not been proven more effective than either treatment alone (13,14).

A 60% to 90% success rate can be expected after steroid injections for the treatment of bursitis and tendinitis of the shoulder. In one study, injection, after diagnosis by the physical examination strategies

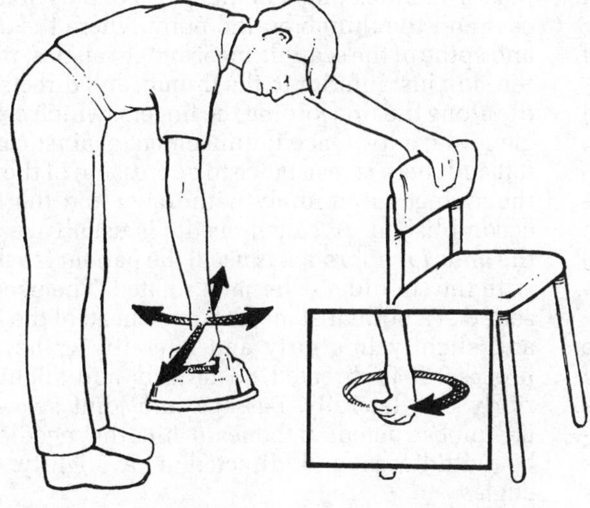
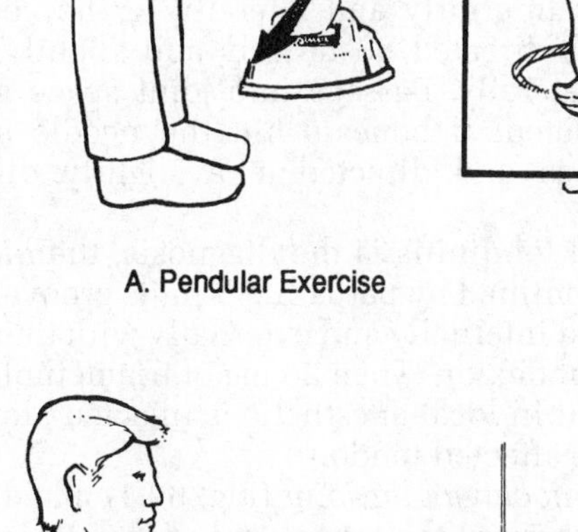
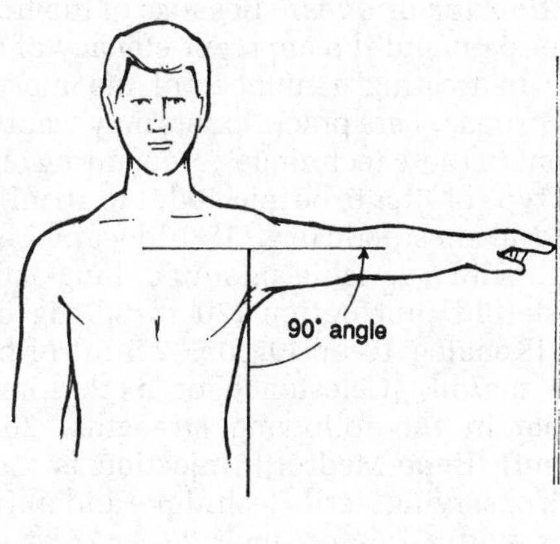

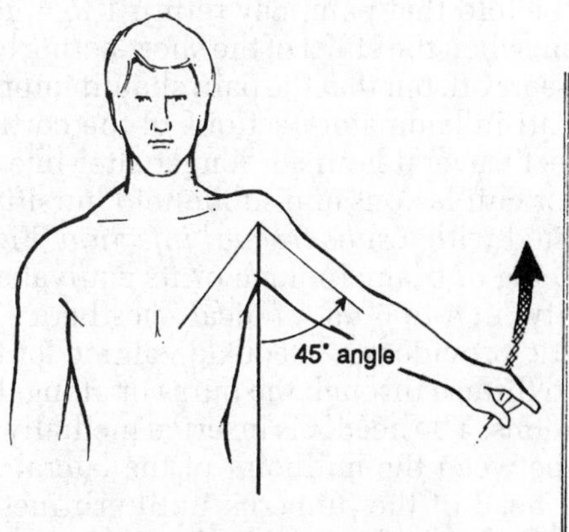

A. Pendular Exercise

B. Normal Abduction

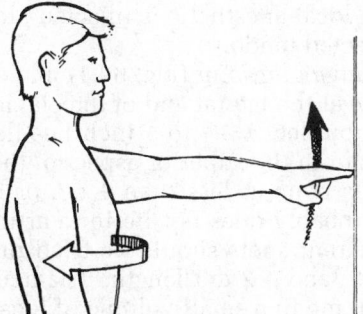

C. Correct Wall-Climbing Exercise

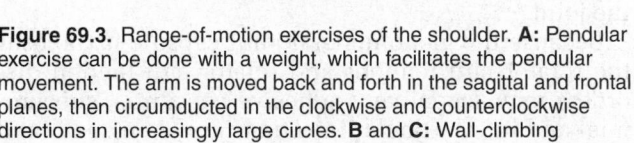

D. Incorrect Wall-Climbing Exercise

Figure 69.3. Range-of-motion exercises of the shoulder. **A:** Pendular exercise can be done with a weight, which facilitates the pendular movement. The arm is moved back and forth in the sagittal and frontal planes, then circumducted in the clockwise and counterclockwise directions in increasingly large circles. **B** and **C:** Wall-climbing exercise done correctly. The wall climb can be started facing the wall. The body is then turned until the patient is at a right angle to the wall. The shoulder movement is at the glenohumeral joint. **D:** Wall-climbing exercise done incorrectly, with shrugging of the scapula. (Redrawn from Cailliet R. Shoulder pain. Philadelphia: FA Davis, 1981.)

described earlier, was shown to be much more effective than tender or trigger point injections (20% success rate) (40). Serious complications of treatment (infection, degenerative changes after multiple injections, weakening or rupture of tendons) are rare (less than 0.1%) (41). They can be minimized by using sterile technique, observing contraindications to intra-articular injection (Table 69.4), following the procedures for injection described in Chapter 74, limiting the number of injections into an area over a given period, and avoiding the injection directly into tendons. Instead, the diluted steroid can be injected around the length of the affected tendon. Subcutaneous tissue atrophy occasionally occurs and may be caused by inappropriately superficial injections. Postinjection flares of pain are uncommon (approximately 2% of injections), begin 6 to 12 hours after injection, last up to 72 hours, and can be treated with local cooling and

Table 69.4. Contraindications to Arthrocentesis or Injection into the Shoulder or Periarticular Structures

Diagnostic and therapeutic
Overlying soft tissue infection
Bacteremia
Clotting disorder (relative)
Therapeutic (corticosteroid injection)
Septic arthritis
Unstable joint
Osteonecrosis
Neurotrophic joint
Marked juxta-articular osteoporosis
Intra-articular fracture

analgesics or NSAIDs. Systemic absorption of locally injected steroid does occur and may cause transient suppression of the hypothalamic–pituitary–adrenal axis; this possibility must be considered in certain situations, as in a diabetic patient in whom the blood sugar could become unusually elevated.

Injection Techniques. Because of the frequency of shoulder pain and the apparent efficacy of steroid injections in treating a number of the most common causes, primary care practitioners may want to become proficient in these techniques. Depending on the number and type of sites to be injected, 1 to 10 mL of a short-acting local anesthetic (e.g., 1% lidocaine) is mixed in a syringe with a variable amount of long-acting (depo) corticosteroid preparation (20 to 80 mg of triamcinolone [Kenalog 10 or 40], 0.5–2.5 ml of betamethasone (6 mg/ml) [Celestone], or methylprednisolone (available in the following strengths: 20, 40, and 80 mg/ml) [Depo-Medrol]). Injection is then accomplished, observing sterile technique and universal precautions, with a 1.5- to 2-inch, 22- or 25-gauge needle; an 18- or 20-gauge needle is used if joint aspiration is required. For patient comfort, the steroid injection may be preceded by superficial and deep infiltration of a local anesthetic using a 25- to 30-gauge needle. Patients should be told that pain may return 1 to 4 hours after injection, when the effect of the short-acting local anesthetic wears off, but that the pain should improve again as the anti-inflammatory actions of the corticosteroid take effect (several hours or longer after injection).

Rotator cuff lesions and subdeltoid bursitis are usually treated with a *subacromial injection* (Fig. 69.1) of 20 to 40 mg of triamcinolone or its equivalent (italics for clarity) in 4 to 6 mL of local anesthetic. The local anesthetic provides an adequate volume for the medication to diffuse through the bursa or along the rotator cuff tendons. The needle is inserted medially along the groove between the midpoint of the lateral acromion and the head of the humerus until grittiness and resistance to depression of the plunger are appreciated as the needle enters the rotator cuff tendon. The needle is then slowly withdrawn while the plunger is depressed lightly, until resistance lessens and some of the solution can be injected. The needle is then partially withdrawn and redirected anteriorly and then posteriorly to deposit the remaining solution. This technique probably results in deposition of solution both in the subacromial portion of the bursa and along the rotator cuff tendon. If bursitis is the predominant finding and there is marked tenderness over the lower portion of the bursa, the injection should be directed toward this area as well. One can describe (see Cyriax, General References) techniques for injecting around the insertion of the specifically involved tendons, but the therapeutic trials described previously generally used the subacromial fan distribution for injection.

Adhesive capsulitis is treated with *intra-articular injection* of 20 to 40 mg of triamcinolone or its equivalent in local anesthetic. A posterior or anterior approach may be used (Fig. 69.2). If the *posterior approach* is used, the patient should rotate the shoulder medially, which turns the articular surface posteriorly and presents a larger target. This position can be fixed, if necessary, by having the patient lie prone, with the forearm under the upper abdomen. The practitioner places an index finger on the point of the coracoid process and the thumb on the point where the acromion and spine of the scapula meet at right angles, punctures the skin just inferior to the thumb, and directs the needle along the line joining the fingers, which crosses the glenoid cavity. Once impingement against cartilage is felt and there is resistance to depression of the plunger, the syringe is minutely withdrawn and the injection accomplished. A 2-inch needle is usually required. If the *anterior approach* is used, the patient is asked to sit with the shoulder externally rotated. The needle is inserted at a point just medial to the head of the humerus and slightly inferiorly and laterally to the coracoid process. It is directed posteriorly and slightly superiorly and laterally. Passage into joint space should be unobstructed. If bone is hit, the needle should be withdrawn and directed at a slightly different angle.

If bicipital tendinitis is the diagnosis, the *bicipital tendon* is identified by palpating it in its groove as the arm is rotated internally and externally with the elbow held in 90° of flexion. Then 20 mg of triamcinolone or its equivalent in local anesthetic is injected along the length of the affected tendon.

The *acromioclavicular joint* (Fig. 69.1) may be palpated as a groove at the lateral end of the clavicle just medial to the shoulder. A ⅝- to 1-inch needle is directed inferiorly from the superior aspect of the joint. If the needle hits bone at less than 1 cm or ⅜-inch depth, the tip probably does not lie intra-articularly, and slightly different spots should be tried until the needle slips in to about 2 cm length. Triamcinolone (Kenalog) 4 to 10 mg in a small volume of local anesthetic is then injected about the joint space. Alternatively, the needle can be inserted from an anterior approach, with the tip of the needle slightly inferior to the joint.

Because the glenohumeral joint capsule juxtaposes the rotator cuff tendons and rotator cuff tendon disorders may accompany adhesive capsulitis, subacromial and intra-articular injections are often combined at the same time. This is particularly true for the treatment of adhesive capsulitis. Because intra-articular injections are not consistently successful in entering the joint space, the posterior and anterior approaches are sometimes used sequentially at the same or separate sessions.

Use of a short-acting local anesthetic with or without steroid allows the practitioner to assess immediately after injection the accuracy of the injection by asking the patient whether the pain is gone and by repeating the examination. Also, strength and ROM, now uninhibited by pain, may be assessed more accurately if the injection was effective.

Because pain may be completely relieved, patients may be tempted to resume full activity of their shoulder immediately after injection. Common sense suggests that the patient should rest the arm briefly after injection in the case of periarticular disorders, avoid heavy use (or use of the type that may have precipitated the disorder) for several weeks while healing occurs, and take appropriate precautions to prevent recurrence.

Referral

Occasionally, a patient needs to be referred to an orthopedist, rheumatologist, or physical medicine and rehabilitation specialist. Indications for referral include dislocation, fracture, functionally significant rotator cuff tear or rupture, suspected neoplasm, inability to perform indicated steroid injection therapy, nonresponsiveness to therapy, chronic or recurrent symptoms despite appropriate management, and uncertainty regarding the diagnosis or treatment.

PERIARTICULAR DISORDERS

Rotator Cuff Tendinitis

Rotator cuff tendinitis is the most common cause of shoulder pain (3,9a,26,40,42,43). The tendinous fibers of the rotator cuff muscles undergo degenerative changes with advancing age. The tendons, particularly the supraspinatus, which is the most superior, are thought to be worn down by repetitive excursion between the greater tuberosity of the humerus and the acromion and acromioclavicular ligament. Edema, hemorrhage, and inflammation associated with repeated trauma cause pain that may lead the patient to seek medical attention. Inflammation of the subacromial bursa may also occur in this manner. The *impingement syndrome* and *pericapsulitis* are less specific terms that are applied to these degenerative and inflammatory disorders of the tendons and bursa. Risk factors for rotator cuff tendinitis include repetitive overhead work or activities and increasing age.

In addition to the history noted previously (see Diagnostic Approach), patients often complain of night pain and difficulty sleeping on the involved side. The physical examination is characterized by pain on resisted abduction (supraspinatus, most common), lateral rotation (infraspinatus), and/or medial rotation (subscapularis, least common). In the most common lesions, which involve the superficial distal end of the tendons, there is a *painful arc*; that is, pain occurring between 60° and 120° of shoulder abduction (or 60° to 90° of glenohumeral abduction), where the impingement occurs, but resolving with further elevation as the shoulder is flexed, externally rotated, and adducted and the impingement is relieved. An impingement sign (pain) can also be elicited by forcibly flexing/elevating the arm to 130° while depressing the scapula (*Neer impingement sign*), or by elevating the shoulder to 90°, flexing the elbow to 90°, and internally rotating the humerus (*Hawkins impingement sign*). In isolated rotator cuff tendinitis, muscle strength is normal; passive ROM is normal or exceeds active ROM, which may or may not be limited by pain.

The indications for obtaining radiographs were stated previously. If rotator cuff tendinitis is the only problem, the radiographs are normal. However, periarticular calcification in the supraspinatus tendon or subacromial bursa is occasionally seen. Its clinical significance is uncertain, because the majority of patients with this radiographic finding do not have symptoms; calcium deposits may disappear spontaneously and usually require no specific treatment (44). However, in a randomized controlled trial in patients with calcific tendinitis, ultrasound therapy helped resolve the calcium deposits and resulted in clinical improvement (in pain, ROM, and quality of life) at 6 weeks but not at 9 months (15). In another trial, extracorporeal shock wave therapy resulted in disintegration of calcium deposits and improvements in a pain/function score in more treated than control patients (45). If calcium deposits are associated with chronic or recurrent symptoms and do not respond to conservative treatment, removal of the deposit by lavage and aspiration or surgery may occasionally be successful. An orthopedist should be consulted in this situation for consideration of the performance of these procedures.

Treatment of most patients with rotator cuff tendinitis was described previously (see Management Strategies). Most patients improve over the course of a few weeks. Relief usually occurs immediately after injection therapy. However, recurrences and eventually the development of chronic symptoms are common (2,6,7,46), underscoring the importance of a preventive exercise program and of preventive counseling based on a careful history of occupational and other activities (see above). Persistent symptoms despite appropriate treatment suggest the possibility of a continued impingement, a tear, or instability (see later discussion).

Subdeltoid (Subacromial) Bursitis

Bursitis may involve the subacromial or subdeltoid portion of the bursa and may accompany rotator cuff tendinitis. Its onset is often abrupt. The disorder is characterized by pain, often severe, with a noncapsular limitation (described earlier) of both active and passive ROMs. Active ROM is usually more limited than passive ROM. Abduction is significantly more limited than lateral or medial rotation. The bursa is tender to palpation; the area of tenderness may be used to direct the injection of corticosteroids. A painful arc may not be demonstrable until the patient recovers sufficient ROM. Treatment was described earlier (see Management Strategies).

Rotator Cuff Tear

By the sixth decade, degenerative changes in the rotator cuff are seen almost universally and are thought to be secondary to diminished blood flow. Tears and ruptures of the cuff may then occur even in the absence of significant trauma. In younger patients, trauma (e.g., falling on an outstretched hand), injuries with subluxation or dislocation, and overuse are usually involved.

Most tears occur just proximal to the insertion of the supraspinatus tendon. A small tear may be indistinguishable from rotator cuff tendinitis on physical examination. Larger tears are characterized by weakness on resisted abduction. In complete tears (ruptures), the patient is unable to initiate abduction or to lower the arm to the side smoothly *(drop arm test)* because the supraspinatus is necessary to stabilize the humeral head and to assist the deltoid in the initial phase of abduction.

Radiographs are indicated when symptoms are recurrent or persistent, despite treatment (see Diagnostic Approach). An uncommonly seen radiologic sign, narrowing of the space between the acromion and humerus (5 mm or less is abnormal), suggests a tear, as does proximal subluxation of the humeral head and erosive changes in the anterior aspect of the acromion. The techniques of arthrography, CT, ultrasonography, and MRI are more useful than radiography in confirming partial or complete tears (see Diagnostic Approach); an orthopedic surgeon should be consulted at least by telephone to discuss the approach to establishing the diagnosis.

In general, minor tears can be treated conservatively in the manner described for rotator cuff tendinitis. ROM movements, followed by strengthening exercises, are usually part of the rehabilitation program. The decision to treat a patient with a large tear medically or surgically depends on the severity of symptoms, the functional disability, and the functional demands of each patient. The patient, the family, the primary care practitioner, and an orthopedist are optimally involved in making decisions. Indications for surgery remain somewhat unclear because of uncertainty about short- and long-term benefits versus risks in the absence of well-designed controlled trials. However, if a complete tear is diagnosed, early surgical intervention seems to be preferable to delayed intervention (47). The traditional surgical approach involves the resection of the anterior acromion (acromioplasty) and repair of the rotator cuff tendon. The recovery period is more protracted after surgery (6 to 9 months of painful or restricted movement) than after conservative therapy (typically 8 weeks of painful or restricted movement). Arthroscopic repair may shorten the recovery period compared with open surgical techniques (48). Because immobilization of the shoulder joint after surgery can lead to adhesive capsulitis, early and regular postoperative passive ROM exercises under orthopedic or physical therapy supervision must be done. Complete pain relief and return to full function are uncommon after surgery.

Bicipital Tendinitis

With aging, the biceps tendon, like the rotator cuff tendons, is subject to inflammation, erosion, and rupture. Because the biceps tendon runs through the joint space and next to the rotator cuff and subacromial bursa, bicipital tendinitis can coexist with inflammation of these structures. However, attrition or chronic subluxation of the tendon in the bicipital groove of the humerus is more often responsible for symptoms.

Pain on resisted supination *(Yergason test or sign)* and flexion of the elbow are the characteristic findings on physical examination. If the glenoid origin is involved, the pain may be felt purely under the acromion. More often, pain is elicited in the upper arm, and the biceps tendon of the involved arm is tender to palpation in the bicipital groove. If bicipital tendinitis is isolated, active and passive ROM movements of the shoulder are painless and full. Radiographs are not necessary or diagnostic, but, if done for other reasons, they may show degenerative changes in the wall of the bicipital groove on tangential views.

Treatment was described earlier (see Management Strategies). Subacromial or intra-articular injection should suffice when this portion of the tendon is involved; otherwise, injection is directed along (but not into) the tendon in the bicipital groove. To diminish the chance of rupture, it is advised that injections be repeated no more than once or twice and separated by an interval of at least 4 to 6 weeks. For the same reason, injection is usually followed by a few days to 1 week of resting the tendon, and avoidance of fully loading the tendon for a few weeks.

Rupture of the biceps tendon, which occurs rarely, is evident on physical examination as a mass of contracted muscle midway between the shoulder and elbow *(Popeye sign).* Rupture is accompanied by a sudden painful popping sensation, usually during a lifting effort. The upper arm remains painful and tender for several days after the rupture. Surgical repair, if desired (e.g., in an athlete, if an occupation demands maximal biceps function), is best accomplished within 7 days; otherwise the tendon is likely to be contracted or fibrosed, precluding effective repair. Conservative management is an acceptable alternative. With regular exercise, the strength of forearm flexion and supination gradually returns; however, a 5% to 10% deficit in these movements usually persists.

Acromioclavicular Disorders

The acromioclavicular joint is formed by the articulation of the distal part of the clavicle with the acromion. Osteoarthritis is common in this joint during middle age and later life. Subluxation or dislocation may result from trauma, such as a fall on or a direct blow to the shoulder or acromion, which forces the scapula down and applies stress to the acromioclavicular and coracoclavicular ligaments. Laborers who lift heavy objects overhead or carry weights on their shoulders and athletes who compete in contact sports or weight lifting often sustain repetitive trauma to this joint. Injuries are classified as grade I, injury without subluxation; grade II, subluxation; and grades III to VI, complete dislocation. In grade III separation, there is modest superior displacement of the clavicle relative to the acromion. Types IV through VI are less common; they are characterized by posterior as well as superior, severe superior, and inferior dislocation of the clavicle, respectively.

Pain is usually localized to the exact site of the acromioclavicular joint or to the point of the shoulder (acromial area). There is little or no radiation of pain into the upper deltoid area. On physical examination, active and passive ROM are usually normal. Pain may be felt at the extreme limits of passive motion. *Full passive adduction* of the arm across the front of the upper thorax is often the most painful movement. Local tenderness is present when the superior ligament is involved. In grades III through VI dislocation, the acromion is displaced on palpation. Routine plain radiographs are indicated in situations of severe trauma. A 15° caudal tilt view of the acromioclavicular joint at 50% penetrance may be helpful in defining joint anatomy and pathology. Osteoarthritic changes are commonly seen on radiographs, but they also are often present in asymptomatic patients. Osteolysis of the distal clavicle may be seen as a posttraumatic change or in association with diseases such as rheumatoid arthritis, hyperparathyroidism, or sarcoidosis. Alleviation of pain after injection of a short-acting anesthetic directly into the acromioclavicular joint may be helpful in confirming this site as the source of pain. If a severe injury is suspected, the radiologic technician can be asked to obtain AP radiographs with the patient holding weights in both hands to help reveal grade II and grade III separations. However, one study suggested that weighted radiographs may miss acromioclavicular separations (49). Ultrasound, CT, and MRI may also be used when it is desirable to define acromioclavicular joint pathology. The choice of methods is best done in consultation with a radiologist, rheumatologist, or orthopedic specialist.

Treatment of pain caused by degenerative arthritis was discussed earlier (see Management Strategies) and includes the use of NSAIDs or nonnarcotic analgesics. Local injection of corticosteroid/anesthetic solution may relieve symptoms in arthritic or low-grade traumatic conditions. If subluxation or complete dislocation is suspected after acute trauma and pain cannot be controlled with conservative measures over a few days, referral to an orthopedist should be obtained for consideration of surgery. However, one caveat should be considered before surgery is contemplated: Several prospective studies of grade III injuries that compared conservative management with strapping or a sling versus open reduction and internal fixation failed to demonstrate improved results from surgical treatment. Therefore, conservative treatment of shoulder separations of grade I, II, or III lesions is currently recommended by most orthopedists (50–52). Conservative management consists of treatment with an analgesic and a sling until the acute pain subsides. The patient should be aware that there will be a permanent prominence of the distal clavicle in grade III separations and a 5% to 10% loss of shoulder strength, which for most people is functionally insignificant. Surgery may be considered in the rare person whose occupation depends on continuous overhead activity (e.g., painters, some athletes) and in whom conservative treatment has failed to control pain. Type IV through VI lesions are usually evaluated for operative repair (52).

GLENOHUMERAL DISORDERS

Adhesive Capsulitis

Adhesive capsulitis, or *frozen shoulder,* is a condition of unknown (but likely multiple) causes in which progressive restriction of shoulder motion occurs. It is commonly seen in diabetic patients. Often, an underlying painful condition of the shoulder, such as rotator cuff tendinitis or subdeltoid bursitis, precedes the development of adhesive capsulitis. However, this disorder may also occur in association with a cerebrovascular accident (especially hemiparesis, in which case it affects the paretic side), myocardial infarction, cervical radiculopathy, thyroid disorders, local or lung tumors, or Parkinson disease. A common underlying factor in most of these diverse conditions appears to be immobility of the arm. Eventually, the adhesive capsulitis may represent a greater disability than the initial cause of immobilization. Thickening of the joint capsule and capsular adhesions to the underlying humeral head develop. However, inflammatory findings in the capsule or synovial lining of the joint are not constant findings. It remains unclear, therefore, whether contracture of the shoulder capsule is a passive process related to lack of motion or an active process caused by inflammation.

Adhesive capsulitis is somewhat more common in women than in men, and it most frequently occurs between the ages of 40 and 60 years. The patient characteristically complains of the insidious onset of diffuse pain and limitation of motion in the shoulder. In particular, the patient notes difficulty in performing tasks that require overhead arm motion, such as combing the hair and grasping objects from high shelves. Physical examination reveals pain at the extremes of motion and markedly reduced active and passive ROMs of the glenohumeral joint, usually in a *capsular pattern* (see Diagnostic Approach). Injection of an anesthetic agent into the glenohumeral joint may reduce the pain, but it does not result in an improved ROM. If adhesive capsulitis is the only problem, a plain radiograph (see earlier discussion for indications) is usually normal and can help rule out arthritis, osteonecrosis, loose bodies, and other local pathology. Additional studies are rarely indicated. MRI with gadolinium, if done, may reveal thickening of the capsule and synovium. Arthrography, if performed, usually reveals a markedly reduced joint capacity, increased filling pressure, intact tendons, and an absence of inflammatory arthritic changes. If an arthrogram is done, corticosteroid injection and capsular distention by the orthopedist or radiologist can be accomplished at the same time, with accurate placement of solution.

The primary aims of treatment of adhesive capsulitis are pain relief, restoration of motion, and correction of any contributing cause. Treated only with analgesics, most patients recover within 2 to 3 years (38,39), but residual slight restriction of movement is common and severe restriction occasionally is present at 3 to 4 years (38,39,53). In controlled and uncontrolled trials, intra-articular and periarticular corticosteroid injection, usually combined with a progressive exercise program designed to increase ROM, has been associated with shortened recovery periods of 4 to 8 weeks (28–37). Typically, injections are repeated weekly for several weeks until the patient's pain is controlled and progress in mobility is being made. Capsular distention or rupture with 10 to 30 mL of fluid may actually speed recovery (30,36,54). An exercise program should be started as soon as the acute pain subsides. This may be limited initially to passive ROM exercises, performed at home with a trained family member. Active ROM can often begin after injection, with pendular and then wall-climbing exercises (Fig. 69.3). Too aggressive mobilization may actually be associated with less satisfactory outcomes (53). Referral to a physical therapist is usually indicated to increase motivation, to ensure patient understanding of the exercise program, and to train family members. If pain is a limiting factor, consideration may be given to suprascapular nerve block. Two studies have provided some evidence of its effectiveness in reducing pain in patients with frozen shoulder (55,56). In the past, referral to an orthopedist for manipulation of the shoulder under anesthesia to free capsular adhesions was recommended for patients who did not improve with conservative management. The efficacy of this treatment has not been studied in a controlled fashion. It is no longer generally recommended and should be considered only in recalcitrant cases.

Trauma

Because of its instability, the shoulder is the joint most commonly dislocated. Dislocation occurs most often in active young to middle-age adults. *Anterior dislocation* (95% of shoulder dislocations) usually results from a fall on an outstretched hand with forceful abduction, extension, and external rotation of the shoulder. On physical examination, the arm is held in the neutral position, and movement is avoided because of pain. The contour of the shoulder, which is normally convex below the acromion because of the humeral head, is flattened. The tip of the acromion is now the most lateral point of the shoulder region, and a noticeable prominence, caused by the displaced humeral head, is seen and felt inferior to the clavicle. Standard AP radiographs confirm the diagnosis.

Posterior dislocation (5% of shoulder dislocations) is less obvious and more likely to be overlooked on examination and radiography. It results from direct or indirect trauma that forces the humeral head posteriorly out of the glenoid fossa, and it may occur after an electrical shock or convulsion. On physical examination, the arm is held adducted and fixed in internal rotation. Anteriorly, there is flattening of the shoulder contour and prominence of the coracoid process. Posteriorly, there is prominence and rounding of the shoulder. The findings on standard AP radiographs are subtle (slight increase in space between the anterior glenoid rim and the medial humeral head; failure on the external rotation view [described earlier] to see the normal club-shaped humeral head, with its greater tuberosity prominent at the superolateral margin, because the shoulder is locked in internal rotation). An axillary lateral or scapular "Y" view (see Diagnostic Approach), however, reveals the posterior displacement of the humeral head relative to the glenoid fossa.

Treatment of dislocations requires prompt reduction and usually involves immediate referral to an orthopedist or emergency department. Postreduction management includes a 2- to 6-week period of immobilization in a sling (less time for older patients), with removal a few times per day to extend the elbow, followed by an intensive physical therapy program to restore ROM and strengthen the appropriate anterior or posterior muscle groups in the hope of preventing recurrence. Dislocations may be accompanied by rotator cuff injury, neurovascular compromise (commonly the axillary nerve in anterior dislocation), or fracture, so pretreatment and posttreatment physical examination and radiographic studies should be done to evaluate these complications and to ensure the adequacy of the reduction.

Recurrent dislocation may follow the acute dislocation. It is especially common in younger patients (more than 50% incidence in patients 25 years of age or younger) (57,58). Each subsequent dislocation may require less force; eventually dislocation may occur even during routine tasks such as combing the hair. A variety of surgical procedures are available to treat this condition.

A syndrome of *glenohumeral instability, with subluxation* with or without recurrent dislocation, is often seen in athletes, particularly in the dominant arm of baseball pitchers, racket sport players, and swimmers. Instability can be anterior, multidirectional, posterior, or inferior; the first two are most common. Patients with multidirectional instability are more likely to have joint laxity. *Anterior instability with subluxation* and secondary impingement can be an additional cause of rotator cuff tendinitis. In addition to pain, patients may describe a sense of instability, weakness, or even radicular symptoms. This syndrome can be difficult to diagnose. Physical examination should include an *apprehension test* for anterior instability. The arm is placed in 90° abduction and full external rotation; patients with a positive test experience apprehension and a sense of impending dislocation. Inferior instability may be detected by inferior traction on the patient's arm, revealing a *sulcus sign*, or subacromial indentation. Posterior instability is tested with a *jerk test*. With the shoulder and elbow in 90° of flexion and the shoulder in full internal rotation, the arm is adducted across the body while pushing the humerus posteriorly. A positive test is characterized by posterior subluxation or dislocation. In the case of dislocation, the humeral head can be felt to clunk back into the joint as the arm is abducted. *Joint laxity* is tested by having the patient try to touch a thumb to the volar surface of the forearm and by having the patient bend back the fingers at the metacarpophalangeal joints. Plain radiographs are usually normal, but they may show subluxation with the patient holding a weight while relaxing the shoulder musculature. Special radiographs may demonstrate a *Bankart lesion* (avulsion of the anterior inferior glenoid rim) or a *Hill–Sachs lesion* (compression fracture of the posterior humeral head) apparently caused by recurrent subluxation of the humeral head in front of the anterior glenoid rim. An arthrogram–CT or MRI may demonstrate a glenoid labral tear, laxity of the glenohumeral ligaments, or a Hill–Sachs lesion. Treatment for anterior instability often requires surgery. The mnemonic, *TUBS*, applies to anterior instability: *T*rauma, *U*nidirectional, *B*ankart lesion, *S*urgery. Treatment for multidirectional instability involves a program of shoulder strengthening exercises, with a good to excellent response to treatment in about 80% of patients (59). The mnemonic, *AMBRI*, applies to multidirectional instability: *A*traumatic, *M*ultidirectional, *B*ilateral signs of laxity, *R*ehabilitation as the preferred treatment, and *I*nferior capsule tightening if surgery becomes necessary. If conservative treatment fails or if help is needed in making the diagnosis, referral to an orthopedist is appropriate. Surgery is directed toward tightening the capsular structures and stabilizing the joint.

Glenoid labral tears most commonly result from a fall on an outstretched arm with the shoulder in abduction and forward flexion. They also occur in people involved in throwing sports, racket sports, and swimming. The torn labral fragment can catch between the glenoid and humeral head, causing a sensation of catching, locking, and slipping that has been called "functional glenohumeral instability." The diagnosis may be confused with rotator cuff tendinitis or bicipital tendinitis. It can be confirmed by arthro-CT, double-contrast arthrotomography, arthro-MRI, or arthroscopy. If the diagnosis is suspected, referral to an orthopedist is indicated. If the tear is associated with instability, the conservative or surgical treatments described earlier may be required. Treatment may involve arthroscopic debridement or stapling.

Fractures of the proximal humerus occur most commonly in elderly persons, usually after a fall, although they may accompany traumatic dislocation in patients of any age. The neck and the greater tuberosity are most often involved. Pain, swelling, and deformity are characteristic of displaced fractures. Extensive bruising of the upper and middle arm may appear 1 to 2 days after fracture of the neck. Plain radiography establishes the diagnosis. If fracture is suspected, true AP and axillary lateral (or scapular "Y") views, in addition to standard AP views, are recommended. Because radial nerve injuries are often associated, the practitioner should assess nerve as well as vascular function distal to the fracture site.

Shoulder injuries may also result in fractures of the clavicle or of the scapula. *Claviular fractures* usually result from a fall or direct impact to the clavicle. The patient experiences pain at the fracture site on attempted raising of the arm. *Scapular fractures* usually result from high-impact trauma, such as falls from a height or motor vehicle crashes. They may involve the glenoid, acromion, or coracoid process or the scapula proper. Often there are associated injuries, such as rib fractures, lung contusion, pneumothorax, and brachial plexus or spine injuries. The patient characteristically holds the arm at the side and experiences pain with any attempted movement of the arm. Referral to an emergency department or orthopedist is generally advised for definitive treatment, which varies depending on the type of fracture and the presence or absence of displacement of the segments.

Arthritic and Other Conditions

Arthritic conditions are distinguished by pain and limitation in a capsular pattern on active and passive ROM (see Diagnostic Approach). Plain radiographs may show chronic arthritic changes, but they may be normal in early or acute arthritis. Radiologic changes must always be interpreted with the clinical information on hand. Monoarticular arthritis uncommonly is the cause of shoulder pain. *Primary osteoarthritis* of the shoulder is uncommon, although secondary osteoarthritis may occur as a result of recurrent dislocation, complete rotator cuff tear (cuff tear arthropathy), fracture, neuropathy (Charcot joint), osteonecrosis, hemoglobinopathy, or inflammation (see Chapter 75). In chronic *inflammatory arthritides,* such as rheumatoid arthritis, the shoulder is usually involved as part of a constellation of articular complaints (see Chapter 77). A septic (usually gonococcal or staphylococcal, less commonly streptococcal or gram-negative) or microcrystalline (see Chapter 76) process should be suspected if the shoulder is the site of monoarticular arthritis of acute onset. Joint aspiration should be performed promptly to obtain fluid for culture and fluid analysis, including cell count and examination for crystals by polarization microscopy (see Table 74.2 in Chapter 74 and Table 76.1 in Chapter 76). The patient with a septic arthritis should be hospitalized and treated with intravenous antibiotics and drainage, usually by percutaneous but occasionally by surgical means.

Osteonecrosis (also called avascular or aseptic necrosis) of the humeral head should be suspected in the patient with a history of fracture of the humeral head, prolonged corticosteroid therapy, or sickle cell disease. Its incidence is also increased in patients with diabetes, alcohol abuse, or a variety of less common disorders. Diagnosis is confirmed by plain radiography or, if necessary, by a bone scan or an MRI (see Diagnostic Approach). Patients are staged from 0 to 4: 0, with all imaging studies normal, diagnosis by histology; 1, plain radiographs and CT normal, MRI and biopsy positive; 2, radiographs positive, no collapse; 3, subchondral radiolucency and early flattening dome; 4, flattening of head with joint space narrowing. The disease is often progressive. Treatment includes ROM exercises, analgesics or NSAIDs, and limitation of stress, as discussed previously (see Management Strategies). There is noncontrolled evidence that core decompression, which appears to be of benefit in hip osteonecrosis, may also be of assistance for grades 1, 2, or 3 disease of the humeral head (60); it is a reasonable option in patients with no response after a few months of conservative therapy. Patients with significant loss of function or severe pain whose condition does not respond to conservative management should be referred to an orthopedist for consideration of core compression, humeral head replacement, or total joint replacement. Total joint replacement is the treatment of choice for stage 4 lesions.

REFERRED PAIN

Occasionally, pain in the shoulder area is referred from other regions of the body. Referred pain should be suspected when (a) the initial physical examination reveals another source for the pain; (b) active, passive, and resisted movements and palpation of the shoulder fail to elicit or exacerbate pain; or (c) the pain is in an atypical distribution (see Diagnostic Approach). The common causes of referred pain are discussed here.

Visceral sources of referred pain may be suggested by a review of the patient's problem list or medical history and the absence of another cause for the referred pain. Irritation of the phrenic nerve or diaphragm may arise from pathologic processes abutting these structures, such as subdiaphragmatic abscess, ruptured viscus, or disease involving the mediastinum, pericardium, liver, spleen, or gallbladder. In addition, ischemic heart disease, apical or superior sulcus tumor of the lung (Pancoast tumor; see Chapter 61), and dissecting aortic aneurysms all may be causes of referred pain (usually acute) to the shoulder.

Reflex sympathetic dystrophy, or *shoulder–hand syndrome,* now designated *complex regional pain syndrome,* is a poorly understood condition that may be a cause of referred shoulder pain. It is characterized by stiffness, swelling without pitting edema, warmth and erythema, vasomotor instability, and patchy bone demineralization of the hand. The syndrome may occur in association with trauma or surgery of the involved extremity, acute myocardial infarction, or cerebrovascular accident. It is discussed further in Chapter 91.

Nerve compression or irritation that is manifested clinically by shoulder pain may originate at the level of the cervical spine, wrist, or shoulder. In addition to pain, the patient may occasionally complain of paresthesias, numbness, muscular weakness, or atrophy. Neurologic examination often delineates the nerves or nerve roots affected. *Cervical nerve root* irritation is a common cause of shoulder pain. The pain is often felt above the shoulder, rather than in the upper arm, and it may or may not be accompanied by neck pain. Characteristically the pain is exacerbated by movement of the neck but not of the shoulder. The diagnosis and management are discussed in Chapter 70. Compression of the median nerve in the carpal tunnel of the wrist, known as *carpal tunnel syndrome,* is occasionally associated with pain about the shoulder. Usually, the pain originates in the wrist and radiates to the upper arm or shoulder. This condition is discussed in Chapter 92. Irritation or compression of the *suprascapular nerve* at the suprascapular or spinoglenoid notch can occur as a result of direct compression from a space-occupying lesion such as a ganglion or lipoma or from nerve entrapment, often seen in athletes involved in excessive overhead activity. Patients experience deep posterior shoulder pain without sensory loss, and weakness on external rotation (infraspinatus) with or without weakness on abduction (supraspinatus). MRI, nerve conduction studies, and electromyograph can help confirm the diagnosis. In the absence of a space-occupying lesion, 6 months of conservative treatment is recommended, which includes a balanced muscle-strengthening program and use of NSAIDs and/or gabapentin or a tricyclic antidepressant. Surgery may be required for a space-occupying lesion or to decompress the nerve if conservative treatment fails. Damage to the *axillary nerve,* usually resulting from shoulder dislocation, humeral fracture, or blunt trauma, is characterized predominantly by deltoid weakness but may also be accompanied by a patch of sensory loss and pain over the outer shoulder. Other muscles innervated by C5 are not affected. Axillary nerve entrapment, termed the *quadrilateral space syndrome,* can cause similar symptoms. Shoulder pain may also result from irritation, compression, or injury of the *long thoracic nerve,* which supplies the serratus anterior and results in winging of the scapula, or of the *spinal accessory nerve,* which supplies the trapezius muscle and results in weakness of shoulder shrugging and abduction, associated with abnormal movement of the scapula.

Thoracic outlet syndrome is an uncommon but serious condition in which pain in the shoulder is a common complaint. Neck pain may also be present. The thoracic outlet consists of a series of three narrow, fixed passages within which the neurovascular supply of the upper extremity (brachial plexus and subclavian vessels) can become compressed as it exits the neck and thorax to enter the axilla. These three channels are (a) the space between the scalene muscles and first rib; (b) the costoclavicular space, bordered by the clavicle, first rib, and scapula; and (c) the space under the pectoralis minor where it inserts on the corocoid process (Fig. 69.4). Compression of the neural or vascular structures results most often from mechanical traction caused by muscle weakness, obesity, heavy breasts or arms, poor posture, or the carrying of backpacks or heavy loads on one's shoulders. Symptoms may also develop from periods of prolonged overhead work or sleeping with the arms hyperabducted. Only a minority of cases are caused by anatomic abnormalities such as a cervical rib (enlargement of the transverse process of C7), anomalies of the clavicle or first rib, cervical bands, hypertrophy of the omohyoid or scalene muscles, or subclavian artery aneurysms. The presenting complaint depends on the predominant structure that is compressed. If it is neural in origin, the patient complains of pain, often extending from the neck or shoulder area to the forearm or hand and accompanied by paresthesias or numbness, usually along an

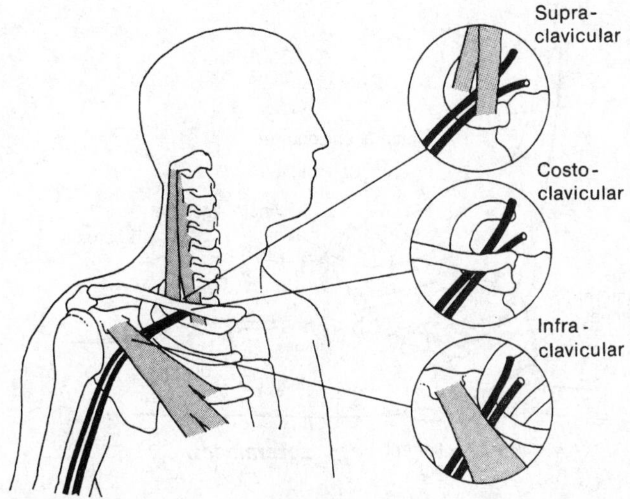

Figure 69.4. Points of neurovascular compression in the thoracic outlet syndrome. (From Steinberg GC, Akins CM, Baran DT, eds. Ramamurti's orthopaedics in primary care. Baltimore: Williams & Wilkins, 1992.)

ulnar distribution. Muscle weakness and atrophy may be noted on physical examination. If it is vascular in origin, the patient may complain of an alteration in color or temperature, swelling of the affected hand, or a Raynaud-like phenomenon. Neurologic complaints usually predominate.

On physical examination, the force of the patient's radial pulse is palpated during the following maneuvers:

1. The patient holds his or her breath in full inspiration while rotating the extended (posterior) neck toward the side that is being examined (*Adson test*), which constricts the scalene outlet; a modified Adson test also includes arm elevation and a Valsalva maneuver.
2. The patient assumes an exaggerated military posture with the shoulder braced posteriorly and inferiorly *(costoclavicular maneuver)*, which may constrict the neurovascular bundle in the costoclavicular space.
3. The patient abducts the arm 180° in external rotation *(hyperabduction maneuver)*, which constricts the neurovascular bundle beneath the pectoralis minor.
4. The patient repeatedly clenches and unclenches the fists for 3 minutes with the arms abducted to 90° and externally rotated (*Roos test*), which constricts the neurovascular bundle beneath the pectoralis minor.

Because a substantial percentage of normal patients manifest a decrease or obliteration of their radial pulse with these maneuvers (61), reproduction of symptoms in parallel with the change in arterial pulse at the wrist is necessary to properly interpret these physical findings. Only a minority of patients have discoloration, temperature changes, or edema as a result of arterial or venous compression. Plain films of the neck, chest, and shoulder should be obtained if referred pain is suspected. Noninvasive Doppler studies of the vascular structures of the upper extremity can be performed at rest and during the maneuvers listed if a vascular impingement is considered likely. Subclavian arteriography is occasionally needed to confirm stenosis, to identify an anatomic abnormality such as an aneurysm, or as a prelude to surgical intervention.

Management of the thoracic outlet syndrome depends on the underlying cause. For most conditions, conservative management is beneficial. This involves the identification and elimination (or reduction) of aggravating factors and the implementation of an appropriate exercise and postural program. Such conservative measures provide relief in 50% to 90% of patients according to Sheon et al. (General References). An occupational therapist (if functional guidance is necessary) or a physical therapist (if exercise guidance is necessary) should be consulted in initiating the exercise program. Occasionally, patients with severe or refractory pain may be helped by surgical intervention, which can involve resection of the first rib, a portion of the scalene muscles, or an abnormal constricting structure such as a cervical rib. Consultation with a surgeon should be considered in such situations.

ELBOW PAIN

Elbow pain, although less common than shoulder pain, is a problem not infrequently encountered by the primary care practitioner. It has a prevalence of a few percent in the adult population (1).

ANATOMY AND FUNCTION

The elbow, shown in Fig. 69.5, includes the distal humerus, the proximal ulna, and the proximal radius. The *elbow joint* consists of two articulations. The articulation between the trochlea of the humerus and the olecranon of the ulna, sometimes called the *humeroulnar joint*, enables flexion and extension. The articulation between the capitulum of the humerus and the head of the radius, sometime called the *humeroradial or radiocapitellar joint*, enables pronation and supination.

Movements at the elbow joint include flexion, extension, pronation, and supination. *Flexion* at the elbow is powered predominantly by the biceps and brachialis muscles, *extension* primarily by the triceps, *supination* primarily by the supinator and biceps, and *pronation* primarily by the pronators quadratus and teres. Importantly, the *wrist and finger extensors originate from the lateral epicondyle* of the humerus, the most common site of clinical symptoms, and the *wrist and finger flexors originate from the medial epicondyle* of the humerus, the second most common site of clinical symptoms at the elbow. Table 69.5 (pg. 1043) lists the function and innervation of the major muscles working across the elbow.

The *olecranon bursa*, a common site of bursitis, overlies the olecranon of the ulna and does not connect with the joint space.

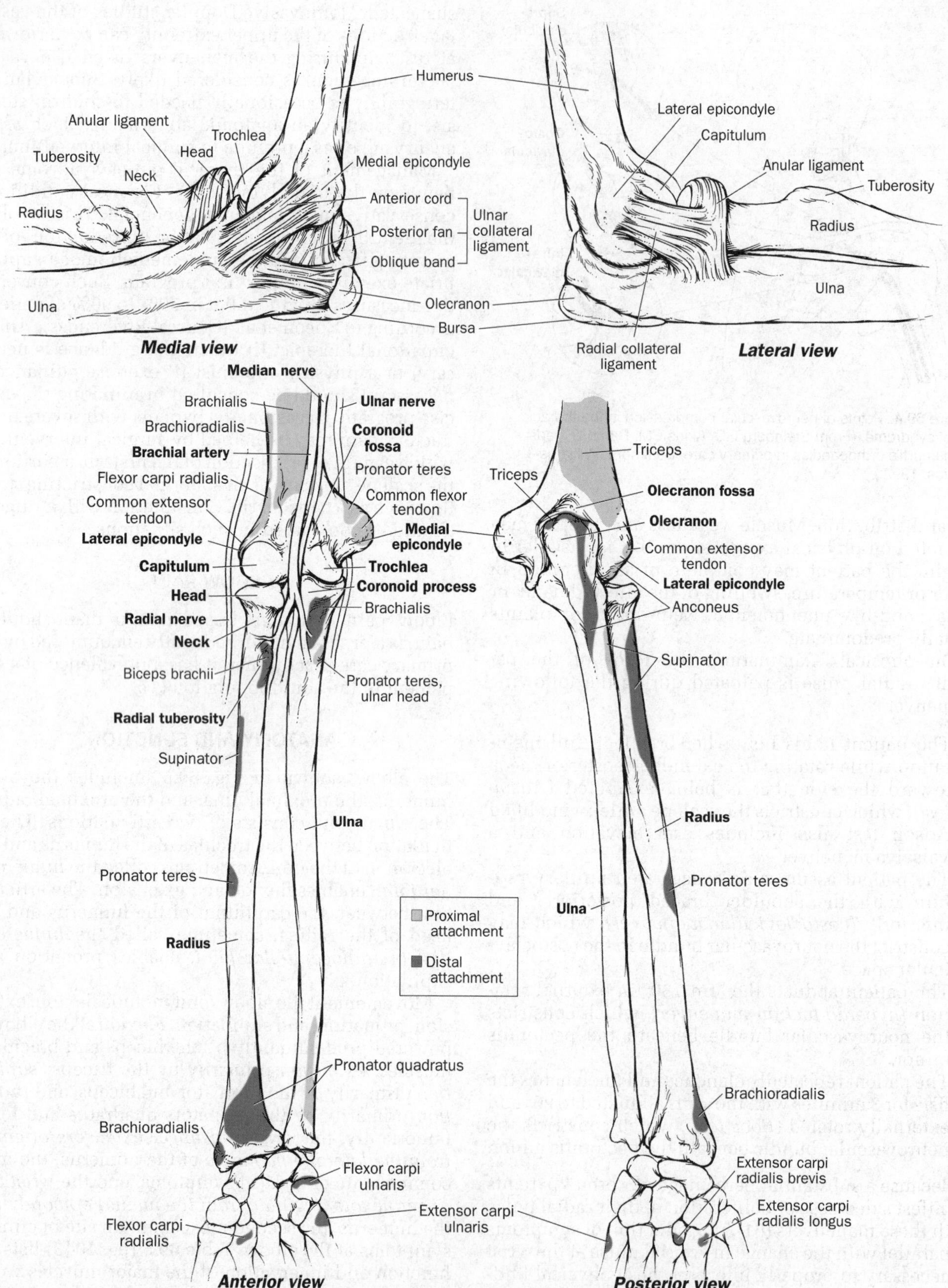

Figure 69.5. The elbow: bones, ligaments, arteries, nerves, and attachments of muscles acting on the elbow joint. The proximal attachments of the biceps brachii are shown in Fig. 69.2. Adapted from Agur AMR, Lee MJ, eds. Grant's Atlas of Anatomy, 9th ed. Baltimore, MD: Williams & Wilkins 1991; and Agur AMR, Lee MJ, eds. Grant's Atlas of Anatomy, 10th ed. Philadelphia: Lippincott Williams & Wilkins, 1999.

Table 69.5. Muscles About the Elbow: Actions and Nerve Supply

Action	Muscle	Nerve	Nerve Root[a]
Flexion of elbow	1. Brachialis	Musculocutaneous	C5, **C6**, (C7)
	2. Biceps brachii	Musculocutaneous	C5, **C6**
	3. Brachioradialis	Radial	C5, **C6**, (C7)
	4. Pronator teres	Median	C6, **C7**
	5. Flexor carpi ulnaris	Ulnar	C7, **C8**
Extension of elbow	1. Triceps	Radial	C6, **C7, C8**
	2. Anconeus	Radial	C7, C8, T1
Supination of forearm	1. Supinator	Deep branch of radial nerve	C5, **C6**
	2. Biceps brachii	Musculocutaneous	C5, **C6**
Pronation of forearm	1. Pronator quadratus	Anerior interosseus branch of median nerve	**C8**, T1
	2. Pronator teres	Median	C6, **C7**
	3. Flexor carpi radialis	Median	C6, **C7**
Flexion of wrist	1. Flexor carpi radialis	Median	C6, **C7**
	2. Flexor carpi ulnaris	Ulnar	C7, **C8**
Extension of wrist	1. Extensor carpi radialis longus	Radial	C6, C7
	2. Extensor carpi radialis brevis	Deep branch of radial nerve	**C7**, C8
	3. Extensor carpi ulnaris	Posterior interosseus nerve, branch of radial nerve	**C7**, C8

[a]Boldface type indicates main segmental innervation (from Agur AMR, Lee MJ. Grant's atlas of anatomy. 10th ed. Philadelphia. Lippincott Williams & Wilkins, 1999).
Modified from Magee DJ. Orthopedic physical assessment. Philadelphia: W.B. Saunders, 1997.

Unlike the shoulder, the elbow has considerable articular congruency, and joint instability is much less a problem with the elbow than with the shoulder. Stability is aided by various ligaments shown in Fig. 69.5.

DIAGNOSTIC APPROACH

Causes of Elbow Pain

Some causes of elbow pain are listed in Table 69.6. Lateral epicondylitis (tennis elbow) and medial epicondylitis (golfer's elbow) are discussed in detail in this chapter. General approaches to arthritis and traumatic injuries involving the elbow are also discussed. Olecranon bursitis is covered in Chapter 74. Compression and entrapment neuropathies are covered in Chapter 92.

History and Physical Examination

History

The history should include questions about the *onset and duration of symptoms; location and radiation of the pain and associated symptoms; precipitating, exacerbating, and relieving factors; and the patient's activities.* Acute onset suggests significant injury, whereas a subacute or gradual onset over days to weeks suggests an overuse syndrome. Pain well localized to the lateral or medial epicondyles suggest lateral and medial epicondylitis, respectively, whereas less well localized pain posterior to the lateral epicondyle is more suggestive of arthritis. Paresthesias or weakness distal to the elbow suggests nerve entrapment. Pain on flexion and extension of the elbow is characteristic of arthritis.

Activities that place individuals at risk include throwing, power gripping, using the elbow as a weight-bearing joint (e.g., gymnasts), and pronation–supination of the forearm, especially with an extended wrist. Particularly important are repetitive movements of these types, such as repetitive wrist turning, hand gripping or shaking, tool use, or twisting movements, and movements that exceed capacity or normal ROM. Individuals at particular risk include carpenters, gardeners, dentists, politicians, weight lifters, gymnasts, golfers, and racquet and throwing athletes, particularly novices.

Table 69.6. Differential Diagnosis of Elbow Pain in Adult Primary Care Patients

Most common
Lateral epicondylits (tennis elbow)

Second most common
Medial epicondylits (golfer's elbow)

Common to occasional
Olecrenon bursitis
Arthritis
Fracture
Dislocation
Median nerve compression
Radial nerve compression

Uncommon
Anterior capsule strain
Biceps tendinitis or tendon rupture
Loose body
Neoplasm
Olecranon impingement
Osteonecrosis
Radiocapitellar chondromalacia
Radial nerve compression
Referred pain, from neck, shoulder, wrist, or visceral organ
Triceps tendinitis
Ulnar collateral ligament sprain

Physical Examination

Physical examination includes inspection and palpation, ROM, and resisted movements.

Inspection. With the patient standing and facing the examiner, the *carrying angle* (the angle made by the axis of the humerus and forearm), which is normally 5° to 10° of valgus, can be assessed. An abnormal angle suggests previous or current injury. The presence of *ecchymosis* suggests trauma, whereas *swelling* (using the other elbow for comparison) may be seen in arthritis, bursitis, or trauma. Swelling over the posterior olecranon process is characteristic of olecranon bursitis; associated erythema suggests infection or gout, with overlying cellulitis.

Palpitation. In 90° of flexion the lateral epicondyle, medial epicondyle, and olecranon form a triangle, which becomes a straight line as the elbow is fully extended. Loss of this relationship suggests dislocation or displaced fracture. Small joint effusions may be detected by noting bulging in the triangular area that connects the lateral epicondyle, radial head, and olecranon in an area posterior and distal to the lateral epicondyle. Lateral and medial epicondylitis are characterized by tenderness over the respective condyles. Tenderness 4 to 5 cm distal to the lateral epicondyle suggests radial tunnel syndrome (posterior interosseus compression) (see Chapter 92). The swelling in olecranon bursitis feel cystic; associated warmth and tenderness suggest infection or gout, with overlying cellulitis.

Range of Motion. Normal *ulnarhumeral ROM* (flexion–extension) is 0° to 135° or 145°, with at least 30° to 130° being required for most normal activities of daily living. *Radiohumeral ROM* (pronation–supination) is tested with the elbow flexed at 90°; findings of 0° to 150° or 180° of total motion, and 70° to 90° each of pronation and supination from the sagittal plane, are normal. Most activities of daily living are accomplished with 50° each of pronation and supination. A limitation in the ROM suggests arthritis, joint effusion, or previous or current injury involving the joint. Locking suggests a loose body. Bursitis and epicondylitis rarely affect ROM, except when there is overlying cellulitis or the epicondylitis is severe.

Resisted Movements. With the elbow at 90° of flexion, the following six isometric movements are tested against counterpressure with no actual movement of the associated joint: elbow flexion, elbow extension, supination, pronation, wrist extension, and wrist flexion. Testing of wrist extension and flexion is indicated because, as noted previously, the wrist and finger extensors originate from the lateral epicondyle of the humerus and the wrist and finger flexors originate from the medial epicondyle. Pain on resisted movement that is localized to the tendon or other area of a muscle suggests an injury in the area of pain, such as tendinitis of the common extensor muscles of the wrists and fingers, commonly called lateral epicondylitis or tennis elbow. True weakness, rather than decreased resistance secondary to pain, suggests muscle or tendon rupture or tear. Soft tissue injuries (e.g., tendinitis) are characterized by normal, nonpainful ROM with pain, weakness, or both on resisted movements.

Check for Referred Pain. If referred pain is suspected, the physical examination should include the neck (e.g., nerve root impingement, described in Chapter 70), shoulder (discussed previously in this chapter), and/or wrist (e.g., carpal tunnel syndrome, covered in Chapter 92). In the case of referred pain, pain typically is not increased by testing ROM or resisted movements.

Additional Diagnostic Tests

The history and physical examination are usually sufficient to make a diagnosis in the patient with nontraumatic elbow symptoms. *Radiographs* are necessary in the presence of acute trauma to confirm a diagnosis of fracture or dislocation, and they may be useful in confirming and characterizing the type and severity of arthritis. Basic radiologic assessment includes an AP view of the extended elbow and a lateral view with the elbow flexed at 90° and the forearm supinated. Oblique views are used to help diagnose subtle fractures and when the elbow cannot be fully extended. *MRI* can help identify stress fractures; serious ligament, muscle, and tendon injuries; and nerve entrapment. *Neuroelectrodiagnostic studies* are helpful in diagnosing nerve entrapment syndromes (see Chapter 92). *Bursal or joint aspiration* is useful in distinguishing traumatic from infectious or other inflammatory etiologies and in diagnosing crystal-induced disease (see Table 74.2 in Chapter 74 and Table 76.1 in Chapter 76).

LATERAL EPICONDYLITIS (TENNIS ELBOW)

Definition, Epidemiology, and Etiology

The terms *tennis elbow* and *lateral epicondylitis* refer to injury in the region of the lateral epicondyle of the humerus at the origin of the common extensor muscles (Fig. 69.5, pg. 1042). The syndrome is the most common cause of elbow pain. It is associated with activities that involve excessive pronation and supination of the forearm, especially with an extended wrist, or with use of the common extensor muscles that exceeds capacity. Tennis, squash, and badminton players (especially novices), as well as throwers, bowlers, carpenters, gardeners, dentists, and politicians, are at risk. Case reports suggest a relationship with fluoroquinolone use (62). The pathogenesis of lateral epicondylitis has been shown in some studies to involve inflammation and injury (microtearing or microavulsion) of the common extensor muscles and tendons. It is unclear whether the aconeus muscle, radial collateral ligament, periosteum, radiohumeral synovium, or bursa is sometimes involved.

Diagnosis

The *history* is characterized by pain and tenderness localized in the *lateral* epicondylar area. It is more likely to be seen in the dominant arm. Sometimes the pain may radiate proximally into the arm or distally into the forearm. The onset is usually gradual but can be acute or subacute. Sometimes the patient complains of intermittent pain or weakness. The pain may be aggravated by lifting (especially with the *palm down*), by repetitive use of the forearm or wrist, or by shaking hands. On careful questioning, there is often a history of activities that predisposed the patient to this condition.

The *physical examination* characteristically reveals tenderness localized to the region of the *lateral* epicondyle and pain, similarly localized, on *resisted extension* of the wrist. Pain can also be elicited by stretching the wrist extensors through maximal *palmar flexing* of the wrist with the elbow fully extended and the forearm *pronated.* A tight handshake may also elicit pain. Sometimes there is pain on resisted radial deviation, supination, or pronation. ROM is normal.

The *differential diagnosis,* which includes arthritis, radial or posterior interosseus nerve entrapment (radial tunnel syndrome), trauma, osteochondral loose body, and referred pain, can usually be distinguished from the history and physical examination. In some cases, additional diagnostic tests are required to distinguish among potential causes (see Diagnostic Approach).

Management

A short course of *immobilization* with a sling or long arm splint with the wrist held in dorsiflexion may help to rest the tendons, although evidence supporting this approach is lacking (63). At least *temporary abstention* (usually a few weeks) from the type of overuse that may have precipitated the condition seems wise. *Analgesics, NSAIDs, ultrasound, iontophoresis with a steroid gel, or cryotherapy* may provide relief.

Corticosteroid injections are more efficacious than placebo and other conservative treatments in reducing symptoms during the first few weeks after treatment (about 80% to 90% efficacy, compared with 50% to 60% efficacy for placebo or NSAIDs) (64,65). However, long-term outcomes (e.g., at 12 months) are similar. A long-acting corticosteroid preparation (e.g., 10 mg of triamcinolone) with an equal volume of short-acting local anesthetic (e.g., 1% lidocaine) is injected, using a 22- or 25- gauge needle and sterile technique, in the area of maximal tenderness just superficial to the tendon. A painful reaction or resistance to injection suggests that the needle is at bone or within the tendon and should be withdrawn slightly. Contraindications and precautions are similar to those discussed previously for shoulder disorders (see Injection Therapy). The elbow should be rested for a few days after injection, and consideration should be given to having the patient wear a Velcro wrist brace for a few weeks.

Recurrence and prolonged minor discomfort that affects some activities are common (66). *Prevention of recurrence* may be aided by instituting an exercise program after the acute symptoms have subsided. These include grip exercises with a compressible ball or putty and stretch and isometric strengthening/toning exercises of the wrist extensors and flexors. Adjustment in activities that may precipitate or exacerbate symptoms is probably important. For example, changes in technique, racket handle, or frequency of use, combined with an exercise program, may help prevent recurrence in a novice tennis player. Alternating use of the left and right arms may be helpful for others. Referral to a physical therapist may be helpful in motivating patients, teaching them exercises, and analyzing and adjusting precipitating or exacerbating activities. Forearm bands, which theoretically reduce stress on the tendons, appear to help some patients during potentially exacerbating activities, although evidence of their efficacy is lacking (63).

If symptoms fail to respond to conservative treatment, orthopedic consultation should be considered. Surgery may occasionally be required, in which case MRI can be helpful in surgical planning by defining the degree of tendon degeneration and tear.

MEDIAL EPICONDYLITIS (GOLFER'S ELBOW)

Definition, Epidemiology, and Etiology

Medial epicondylitis (golfer's elbow) is caused by inflammation of the tissues in the area of the medial epicondyle, where the muscles that flex and pronate the wrist originate (Fig. 69.5, pg. 1042). It is caused by overuse of these muscles and is most commonly seen in persons who engage in such activities, including throwing athletes, golfers, swimmers, tennis players who pronate and flex during their serve, and individuals who engage in repetitive lifting, tooling, hammering, or tight gripping. Although medial epicondylitis is not uncommon, it is less common than lateral epicondylitis.

Diagnosis

The *history* is characterized by pain and tenderness localized in the *medial* epicondylar area. It is more likely to be seen in the dominant arm. Sometimes the pain may radiate proximally into the arm or distally into the forearm. The onset is usually gradual but can be acute or subacute. Sometimes the patient complains of intermittent pain or weakness. The pain may be aggravated by lifting (especially with the *palm up*), by repetitive use of the forearm or wrist, or by shaking hands. On careful questioning, there is often a history of activities that predisposed the patient to this condition.

The *physical examination* characteristically reveals tenderness localized to the region of the *medial* epicondyle and pain, similarly localized, on *resisted flexion* of the wrist. Pain may also be elicited by stretching the wrist flexors through maximal *extension* of the wrist with the elbow fully extended and the forearm *supinated.* A tight handshake may also elicit pain. Sometimes there is pain on resisted radial deviation, supination, or pronation. ROM is normal. The status of the *ulnar nerve,* which runs immediately posterior to the medial epicondyle, should be assessed (see Chapter 92).

The *differential diagnosis* which includes arthritis, ulnar nerve injury or compression (cubital tunnel syndrome), trauma, osteochondral loose body, and referred pain, can usually be distinguished from the history and physical examination. In some cases, additional diagnostic tests are required to distinguish among potential causes (see Diagnostic Approach).

Management

Management is similar to management for lateral epicondylitis, except that caution should be taken when injecting corticosteroids to avoid the ulnar nerve (Fig. 69.5, pg. 1042). As in lateral epicondylitis, steroid injection appears to have benefit in the short term (several weeks) but not in the long term (3 to 12 months) (67). Surgical outcomes are worse in patients who have concomitant ulnar neuropathy (68,69).

ARTHRITIS

Definition, Epidemiology, and Etiology

Arthritis refers to disease involving the synovium, cartilage or bone of the joint space. The most common types are rheumatoid arthritis (Chapter 77), posttraumatic arthritis, and crystal-induced arthritides (gout, pseudogout, or other; Chapter 76). Osteoarthritis (Chapter 75) is relatively uncommon and is most often seen in patients with a history of overuse (e.g., manual laborers, overhead throwing athletes). Infectious causes (e.g., due to local trauma or systemic infection) are occasionally seen.

Diagnosis

On *history*, the pain of arthritis is not as well localized as that of epicondylitis. Early in the course, it is often lateral, but posterior to the epicondyle. Later, it may be more diffuse. On questioning, the practitioner may discover patterns of pain and joint distributions characteristic of rheumatoid, degenerative, or crystal-induced arthritis (see Chapters 75 through 77).

On *physical examination*, there is usually a *limitation in the ROM.* Early on, there is a lack of full extension, which maximally reduces joint volume. Extension is usually more limited than flexion. Limitation of pronation and supination usually comes later, unless the arthritis was caused by injury to the radiohumeral area. Often there is *end-point stiffness or pain. Lack of smooth motion, catching, or locking* suggests the presence of a loose body, often seen in osteonecrosis. Soft tissue swelling or rheumatoid nodules suggest an inflammatory arthritis. Physical examination of *other joints* may reveal findings of degenerative arthritis (Chapter 75), inflammatory arthritis (Chapter 77), or crystal-induced arthritis (Chapter 76).

The *differential diagnosis* includes fracture of the radial head or distal humerus (including stress fractures), loose bodies, and osteonecrosis (avascular or aseptic necrosis or osteochondritis dissecans, most often seen in adolescent athletes with a repetitive overuse history), which often produces loose bodies.

AP and lateral radiographs (see Diagnostic Approach) can demonstrate patterns and characteristics of the various types of arthritides and reveal fractures or loose bodies. *MRI* may be required to reveal subtle fractures or loose bodies. If a septic effusion is suspected, joint aspiration is required for diagnosis. With the elbow resting at 90° flexion, the elbow joint is entered in the center of the triangle connecting the lateral epicondyle, radial head, and olecranon (i.e., inferior and posterior to the lateral epicondyle). Preparation is the same as for shoulder disorders (see Injection Therapy); fluid analysis is described in Table 74.2 in Chapter 74 and Table 76.1 in Chapter 76.

Management

Management of the various types of arthritis is discussed in Chapters 75 through 77. It usually involves a combination of specific medications, joint rest, and physical therapy. Occasionally intra-articular steroid injections are used in the management of rheumatoid arthritis, but this is probably best done in consultation with a rheumatologist. In the presence of disabling deformity or symptoms unresponsive to conservative treatment, the patient can be referred to an orthopedic surgeon for consideration of open or arthroscopic debridement or total joint replacement.

TRAUMATIC DISORDERS OF THE ELBOW

Traumatic injuries to the elbow include dislocation (posterior in more than 80% of the cases), fracture of the olecranon or coronoid process of the ulna, fracture of the radial head, and distal fracture of the humerus. Although patients usually present to the emergency room, they occasionally present to their primary care practitioner. The practitioner should, therefore, be aware of these injuries and have an approach to diagnosis and referral.

Dislocations and fractures of the radial head commonly result from falls on an outstretched hand with the arm in extension and adduction. Fractures of the olecranon usually result from a direct blow to or fall on the olecranon. Fractures of the coronoid process usually are preceded by sudden, strong resisted contraction of the brachialis muscle or occur in association with dislocation. Humeral fractures are relatively rare. Stress fractures of the olecranon usually are associated with overuse.

The *diagnosis* is suggested by acute and severe pain, swelling, ecchymosis, limited ROM, crepitus, and/or joint deformity. Physical examination should include palpation of the brachial, radial, and ulnar pulses and assessment of the distal vascular supply (warmth, color, and capillary refill). Median, radial, and ulnar nerve function should be assessed distal to the elbow. Radiographs of the elbow are always indicated and usually reveal the diagnosis. Dislocation is not infrequently accompanied by fracture (usually of the radial head or coronoid process). Stress fractures, usually of the olecranon, are characterized by a less dramatic history and physical examination and may require a bone scan or MRI for diagnosis.

Once a diagnosis has been made or seriously entertained, *referral* is usually made to an emergency department or orthopedic physician for treatment. In the case of vascular or neurologic compromise, dislocation, or displaced, open, or comminuted fractures, communication and transfer of care are urgent.

General References*

Anderson BC. Office orthopedics for primary care: diagnosis and treatment. 2nd ed. Philadelphia, WB Saunders, 1999.

Reader-friendly, practical approach to the diagnosis and treatment of specific musculoskeletal disorders, with sections on symptoms, physical examination, diagnostic testing, treatment (physical therapy, illustrated injection techniques, surgery options), recovery and rehabilitation, and prognosis for each disorder. Drug treatment is not covered.

Chumbley EM, Nirschl RP. Evaluation of overuse elbow injuries. Am Fam Physician 2000;61:691.

Review article provides expanded differential diagnosis of overuse syndromes.

Cyriax JH. Textbook of orthopaedic medicine. Vol. 1: diagnosis of soft tissue lesions. 8th ed. London: Bailliere-Tindall, 1982.

Source of most commonly accepted and useful approach to physical examination. Otherwise somewhat dated.

Cyriax JH. Textbook of orthopaedic medicine. Vol. 2: treatment by manipulation, massage and injection. 11th ed. London: Bailliere-Tindall, 1984.

Good quick reference to diagnosis and injection techniques.

Cyriax JH, Cyriax PJ. Cyriax's illustrated manual of orthopaedic medicine. 2nd ed. Oxford: Butterworth-Heinemann, 1993.

Abbreviated, well-illustrated but unreferenced version of the above two texts.

Gispen JC. Painful shoulder and the reflex sympathetic dystrophy syndrome. In: Koopman WJ, ed. Arthritis and allied conditions: a textbook of rheumatology. 14th ed. Baltimore: Williams & Wilkins, 2001:2095.

Comprehensive, up-to-date, well-referenced chapter with a large section on reflex sympathetic dystrophy.

Greene WB, ed. Essentials of musculoskeletal care. 2nd ed. Rosemont, IL: American Academy of Orthopaedic Surgeons, 2001.

Multiauthored text published by the American Academy of Orthopaedic Surgeon. It provides short sections on synonyms, definition, clinical symptoms, physical examination, additional diagnostic tests, differential diagnosis, adverse outcomes of the disease, treatment, adverse outcomes of treatment, and referral decisions, with red warning flags for each disorder or problem.

Martin SD, Thornhill TS. Shoulder pain. In: Ruddy S, Harris ED Jr, Sledge CB, eds. Kelley's textbook of rheumatology. 6th ed. Philadelphia: WB Saunders, 2001:475.

Comprehensive well-referenced chapter that includes discussions of surgical approaches to treatment.

Owen DS Jr. Aspiration and injection of joints and soft tissue. In: Ruddy S, Harris ED Jr, Sledge CB, eds. Kelley's textbook of rheumatology. 6th ed. Philadelphia: WB Saunders, 2001:583.

Good general source of injection technique.

Sheon RP, Moscowitz RW, Goldberg VM. Soft tissue rheumatic pain: recognition, management, prevention. 3rd ed. Philadelphia: Lea & Febiger, 1996:79.

Good source for advice on joint protection and for additional shoulder exercises.

Smith DL, Campbell SM. Painful shoulder syndromes: diagnosis and management. J Gen Intern Med 1992;7:328.

Well-referenced and practical.

Specific References

1. Allender E. Prevalence, incidence, and remission rates of some common rheumatic diseases or syndromes. Scand J Rheumatol 1974;3:145.
2. Bergenudd H, Lindegarde F, Nilsson B, et al. Shoulder pain in middle age: a study of prevalence and relation to occupational work load and psychosocial factors. Clin Orthop 1988;231:234.
3. Chard MD, Hazleman BL, King RH, et al. Shoulder disorders in the elderly: a community survey. Arthritis Rheum 1991;34:766.
4. Makela M, Heliovaara M, Sainio P, et al. Shoulder joint impairment among Finns aged 30 years or over: prevalence, risk factors and co-morbidity. Rheumatology (Oxford) 1999;38:656.
5. National Ambulatory Medical Care Survey, 1985. Hyattsville, MD: National Center for Health Statistics, 1989.
6. Vecchio PC, Kavanagh RT, Hazleman BL, et al. Community survey of shoulder disorders in the elderly to assess the natural history and effects of treatment. Ann Rheum Dis 1995;54:152.
7. van der Windt DAWN, Koes BW, Boeke AJP, et al. Shoulder disorders in general practice: prognostic indicators of outcome. Br J Gen Pract 1996;46:519.
8. Croft P, Pope D, Silman A. The clinical course of shoulder pain: prospective cohort study in primary care. BMJ 1996;313:601.
9. Hales TR, Bernard BP. Epidemiology of work-related musculoskeletal disorders. Orthop Clin North Am 1996;27:679.

9a. Smith DL, Campbell SM. Painful shoulder syndromes: diagnosis and management. J Gen Intern Med 1992;7:328.

10. Burk DL, Karasick D, Kurz AB, et al. Rotator cuff tears: prospective comparison of MR imaging with arthrography, sonography, and surgery. AJR Am J Roentgenol 1989;153:87.
11. Heron CW. Imaging the painful shoulder. Clin Radiol 1990;41:379.
12. Boorstein JM, Kneeland JB, Dalinka MK, et al. Magnetic resonance imaging of the shoulder. Curr Probl Diagn Radiol 1992;21:3.
13. **13.** Green S, Buchbinder R, Glazier R, et al. Systematic review of randomised controlled trials of interventions for painful shoulder: selection criteria, outcome assessment, and efficacy. BMJ 1998;316:354.
14. **14.** Green S, Buchbinder R, Glazier R, et al. Interventions for shoulder pain. Cochrane Database of Systematic Reviews. The Cochrane Library, Volume (Issue 3), 2001.
15. **15.** Ebenbichler GR, Erdogmus CB, Resch KL, et al. Ultrasound therapy for calcific tendinitis of the shoulder. N Engl J Med 1999;340:1533.
16. **16.** van der Heijden GJ, Leffers P, Wolters PJ, et al. No effect of bipolar interferential electrotherapy and pulsed ultrasound for soft tissue shoulder disorders: a randomised controlled trial. Ann Rheum Dis 1999;58:530.
17. **17.** van der Windt DAWN, van der Heijden GJMG, van der Berg SGM, et al. Ultrasound therapy for musculoskeletal disorders: a systematic review. Pain 1999;81:257.
18. Rocks JA. Intrinsic shoulder pain syndrome: rationale for heating and cooling in treatment. Phys Ther 1979;59:153.
19. **19.** Adebajo AO, Nash P, Hazleman BL. A prospective double blind dummy placebo controlled study comparing triamcinolone hexacetonide injection with oral diclofenac 50 mg TDS in patients with rotator cuff tendinitis. J Rheumatol 1990;17:1207.
20. **20.** Petri M, Dobrow R, Neiman R, et al. Randomized, double-blind, placebo-controlled study of the treatment of the painful shoulder. Arthritis Rheum 1987;30:1040.
21. **21.** van der Windt DAWM, van der Heijden GJMG, Scholten RJPM, et al. The efficacy of non-steroidal anti-inflammatory drugs (NSAIDs) for shoulder complaints: a systematic review. J Clin Epidemiol 1995;48:691.
22. **22.** White RH, Paull DM, Fleming KW. Rotator cuff tendinitis: comparison of subacromial injection of a long acting corticosteroid versus oral indomethacin therapy. J Rheumatol 1986;13:608.
23. **23.** Roth SH. Nonsteroidal anti-inflammatory drugs: gastropathy, deaths, and medical practice. Ann Intern Med 1988;109:353.
24. **24.** Berry H, Fernandes L, Bloom B, et al. Clinical study comparing acupuncture, physiotherapy, injection, and oral anti-inflammatory therapy in shoulder-cuff lesions. Curr Med Res Opin 1980;7:121.
25. **25.** Lee PN, Lee M, Haz AMMM, et al. Trial of treatments investigated by multivariate analysis. Ann Rheum Dis 1974;33:116.
26. Richardson AT. The painful shoulder. Proc R Soc Med 1975;68:731.

*Bold print (general references) and bold numerals (specific references) denote published controlled clinical trials, meta-analyses, or consensus-based recommendations.

27. Vecchio PC, Hazleman BL, King RH. A double-blind trial comparing subacromial methylprednisolone and lignocaine in acute rotator cuff tendinitis. Br J Rheum 1993;32:743.
28. Bulgen DY, Binder AI, Hazleman BL, et al. Frozen shoulder: prospective clinical study with an evaluation of three treatment regimens. Ann Rheum Dis 1984;43:353.
29. Dacre JE, Beeney N, Scott DL. Injection and physiotherapy for the painful stiff shoulder. Ann Rheum Dis 1989;48:322.
30. Jacobs LGH, Barton MA, Wallace WA, et al. Intra-articular distension and steroids in the management of capsulitis of the shoulder. BMJ 1991;302:1498.
31. Lloyd JA, Lloyd HM. Adhesive capsulitis of the shoulder: arthrographic diagnosis and treatment. South Med J 76:879, 1983.
32. Rizk TE, Gavant ML, Pinals RS. Treatment of adhesive capsulitis (frozen shoulder) with arthrographic capsular distension and rupture. Arch Phys Med Rehabil 1994;75:803.
33. Roy S, Oldham R. Management of painful shoulder. Lancet 1976;1:1322.
34. Steinbrocker O, Argyros TG. Frozen shoulder: treatment by local injections of depo corticosteroids. Arch Phys Med Rehabil 1974;55:209.
35. Weiss JJ, Ting YM. Arthrography-assisted intra-articular steroids in treatment of adhesive capsulitis. Arch Phys Med Rehab 1978;59:285.
36. Rizk TE, Pinals RS, Talaiver AS. Corticosteroid injections in adhesive capsulitis: investigation of their value and site. Arch Phys Med Rehabil 1991;7:20.
37. van der Windt DA, Koes BW, Deville W, et al. Effectiveness of corticosteroid injections versus physiotherapy for treatment of painful stiff shoulder in primary care: randomised trial. BMJ 1998;317:1292.
38. Grey RG. The natural history of idiopathic frozen shoulder. J Bone Joint Surg Am 1978;60:564.
39. Reeves B. The natural history of the frozen shoulder syndrome. Scand J Rheumatol 1975;4:193.
40. Hollingworth GR, Ellis RM, Hattersley TS. Comparison of injection techniques for shoulder pain: results of a double blind, randomized study. BMJ 1983;287:1339.
41. Gray RG, Gottlieb NL. Intrarticular corticosteroids: an updated assessment. Clin Orthop 1983;177:235.
42. Vecchio P, Kavanagh R, Hazleman BL, et al. Shoulder pain in a community-based rheumatology clinic. Br J Rheum 1995;34:440.
43. Deleted in page proofs.
44. Faure G, Daculsi G. Calcified tendinitis: a review. Ann Rheum Dis 1983;42[Suppl]:49.
45. Loew M, Daecke W, Kusnierczak D, et al. Shock-wave therapy is effective for chronic calcifying tendinitis of the shoulder. J Bone Joint Surg Br 1999;81:863.
46. Chard MD, Sattelle LM, Hazleman BL. The long-term outcome of rotator cuff tendinitis: a review study. Br J Rheumatol 1988;27:395.
47. Neviaser RJ. Ruptures of the rotator cuff. Orthop Clin North Am 1987;18:387.
48. Sachs RA, Stone ML, Devine S. Open vs. arthroscopic acromioplasty: a prospective, randomized study. Arthroscopy 1994;10:248.
49. Bossart PJ, Joyce SM, Manaster BJ, et al. Lack of efficacy of "weighted" radiographs in diagnosing acute acromioclavicular separation. Ann Emerg Med 1988;17:20.
50. Bannister GC, Wallace WA, Stableforth PG, et al. The management of acute acromioclavicular dislocation: a randomised prospective controlled trial. J Bone Joint Surg Br 1989;71:848.
51. Phillips AM, Smart C, Groom AF. Acromioclavicular dislocation: conservative or surgical therapy. Clin Orthop 1998;353:10.
52. Clarke HD, McCann PD. Acromioclavicular injuries. Orthop Clin North Am 2000;31:177.
53. Binder AI, Bulgen DY, Hazleman BL, et al. Frozen shoulder: a long-term prospective study. Ann Rheum Dis 1984;43:361.
54. Gam AN, Schydlowsky P, Rossel I, et al. Treatment of frozen shoulder with distension and glucocorticoid compared with glucocorticoid alone: a randomised controlled trial. Scand J Rheumatol 1998;27:425.
55. Jones DS, Chattopadhyay C. Suprascapular nerve block for the treatment of frozen shoulder in primary care: a randomized trial. Br J Gen Pract 1999;49:39.
56. Dahan TH, Fortin L, Pelletier M, et al. Double blind randomized clinical trial examining the efficacy of bupivacaine suprascapular nerve blocks in frozen shoulder. J Rheumatol 2000;27:1464.
57. Hovelius L, Augustini BG, Fredin H, et al. Primary anterior dislocation of the shoulder in young patients. J Bone Joint Surg Am 1996;78:1677.
58. Yu J. Anterior shoulder dislocations. J Fam Pract 1992;35:567.
59. Burkhead WZ Jr, Rockwood CA Jr. Treatment of instability of the shoulder with an exercise program. J Bone Joint Surg Am 1992;74:890.
60. Mont MA, Payman RK, Laporte DM, et al. Atraumatic osteonecrosis of the humeral head. J Rheumatol 2000;27:1766.
61. Rayan GM. Thoracic outlet syndrome. J Shoulder Elbow Surg 1998;7:440.
62. LeHuec JC, Schaeverbeke T, Chauveaus D, et al. Epicondylitis after treatment with fluoroquinolone antibiotics. J Bone Joint Surg Br 1995;77:293.
63. Struijs PAA, Smidt N, Arola, et al. Orthotic devices for tennis elbow (Cochrane review). In: The Cochrane Library, Issue 4, 2001. Oxford: Update Software.
64. Assendelft WJ, Hay EM, Adshead R, et al. Corticosteroid injections for lateral epicondylitis: a systematic overview. Br J Gen Pract 1996;46:209.
65. Hay EM, Paterson SM, Lewis M, et. al. Pragmatic randomised controlled trial of local corticosteroid injection and naproxen for treatment of lateral epicondylitis of elbow in primary care. BMJ 1999;319:964.
66. Binder AI, Hazleman BL. Lateral humeral epicondylitis: a study of natural history and the effect of conservative therapy. Br J Rheumatol 1983;22:73.
67. Stahl S, Kaufman T. The efficacy of an injection of steroids for medial epicondylitis: a prospective study of sixty elbows. J Bone Joint Surg Am 1997;79:1648.
68. Kurvers H, Verhaar J. The results of operative treatment of medial epicondylitis. J Bone Joint Surg Am 1995;77:1374.
69. Gabel GT, Morrey GT. Operative treatment of medial epicondylitis: influence of concomitant ulnar neuropathy at the elbow. J Bone Joint Surg Am 1995;77:1065.

CHAPTER 70

Neck Pain

FREDERICK A. LENZ, MD, PhD

Neck pain is a common problem. Nearly 50% of people over 50 years of age experience neck pain at some time. Because there are many structures in the neck that when diseased may cause pain, as well as multiple sources of referred pain, patients who complain of new or persistent neck pain should be systematically evaluated. This chapter provides a review of the skeletal structures of the neck, the method of evaluation for complaints of neck pain, a description of common problems and their treatment, and guidance for referral of selected patients with neck pain.

ANATOMY OF THE NECK AND SOURCES OF PAIN

The cervical spine consists of seven vertebral bodies connected by facet joints, interspinous ligaments, and an anterior and a posterior longitudinal ligament (Fig. 70.1). These ligaments provide stability when the neck is flexed and extended. The vertebral bodies are joined by intervertebral disks composed of a gel-like material (the nucleus pulposus) that absorbs increased pressure applied to the spine. The nucleus pulposus is contained within an annulus fibrosus, a fibrous structure ringing the outer margin of the disk. During the fourth decade of life, both the nucleus pulposus and the annulus fibrosus undergo progressive degeneration, seen microscopically as a loss of the fibrous pattern and the collagen alignment. As a result, the ability of the disk to absorb shocks is reduced. Facet joints are found between vertebral elements posteriorly, one on each side of the spine; they are apophyseal (projecting) joints with a synovium-lined capsule. It is within these small joints in the posterior spine that osteoarthritis, a breakdown of the articular cartilage within the joints, can occur. The intervertebral neural foramina, located on either side of the vertebral bodies, are the canals through which the nerve roots emerge from the spinal canal. The spinal canal and the foramina can be encroached on by a bulging intervertebral disk or an osseous proliferation (bony spur) originating in a vertebral body, by a facet joint, or from the bony margin of a neural foramen (Fig. 70.1). When the encroachment involves a nerve root, pain in the distribution of that root (radicular pain) may occur. The facet joint capsules and the intervertebral disk are innervated by fine nerves that have simple nerve endings. When these nerve endings are stimulated by degenerative disease within the disk or joint capsules, the patient may experience pain, which is referred to the posterior aspect of the neck at any level. The pain felt in the neck may not be at the cervical level from which the nerve is arising. In addition, stimulation of the nerves can cause pain to be referred to the interscapular area, superiorly and laterally over the shoulders. Spasm of any of the many muscles of the neck region is also a common source of pain.

EVALUATION OF THE PATIENT

History

The date of onset of the patient's symptoms and any associated trauma should be ascertained. Often, knowledge of the specific activity the patient was performing at the onset of pain is helpful in establishing the cause of the pain. Prolonged extension of the neck, as occurs in people doing overhead work, is a common occupational situation that can give rise to pain in the cervical region. Another common occupational cause of neck pain is prolonged sitting with the neck flexed in one position. This occurs commonly in computer operators or typists. The sustained position causes spasm of the neck muscles, which results in pain. Also, patients commonly sustain minor twisting injuries or trauma to the neck but do not experience neck pain within the first 24 hours, after which pain may begin to appear and progress. Reproduction or increase of pain by neck motion is helpful in localizing the problem to the cervical spine rather than to a referred source (Table 70.1). It is also important to know whether the pain is felt outside the neck as well, such as in the head, posteriorly between the scapulae, about the shoulder, down the arm, or in the hand. The patient should be asked about decreased sensation in the hands and, if possible, to say specifically which fingers are involved. If the pain and numbness are felt in a dermatome distribution (see dermatome map, Chapter 86), this indicates nerve compression (Table 70.2).

Muscle weakness in the shoulder, arm, and hand should be elicited to help identify potential nerve compression. Pain associated with motion of the shoulder is not characteristic of cervical spine disease and suggests that the problem is within the shoulder joint (see Chapter 69). Symptoms such as dizziness, visual changes, and ataxia brought on by neck motion (usually rotation) are not usually caused by nerve root compression or degenerative disk disease, but they may

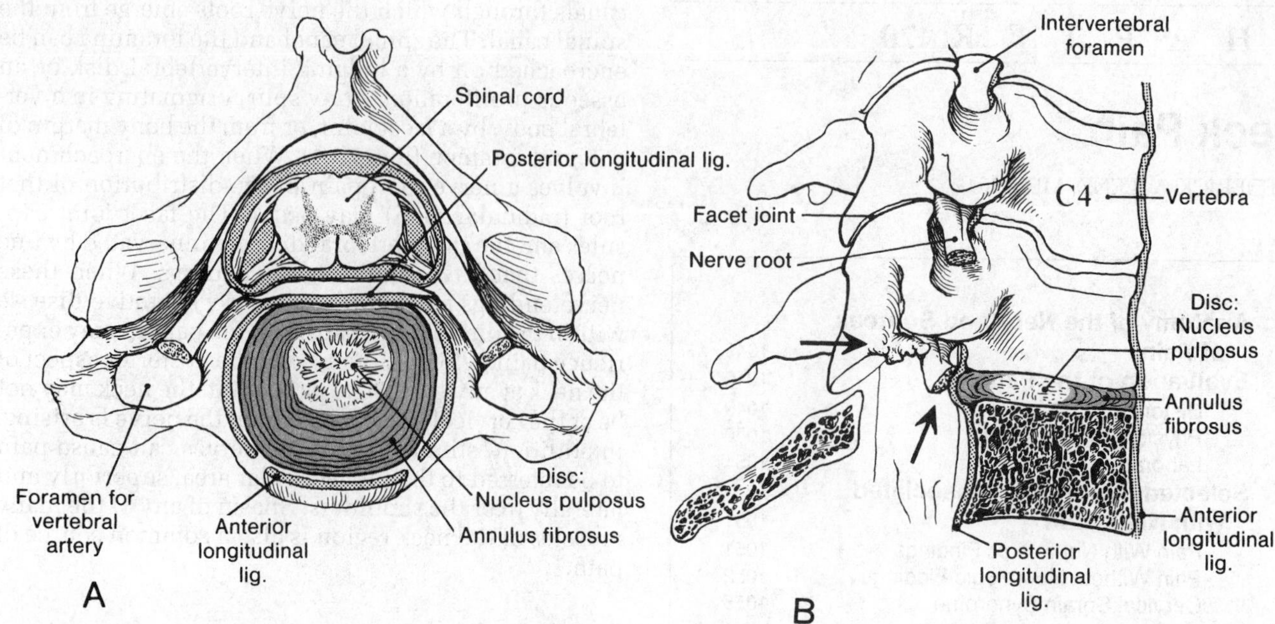

Figure 70.1. Anatomy of disk and ligaments of the cervical spine. **A:** Superior view. Note relationship of anterior and posterior longitudinal ligament to the intervertebral disk. **B:** Lateral view. Note relationship of the intervertebral foramen to the intervertebral disk and facet joint. Bulging of the intervertebral disk or bone spurs forming from the facet joint may cause compression of the nerve root within the intervertebral foramen (*arrows*).

Table 70.1. Sources of Referred Pain in the Neck[a]

Source	Referred Location
Disorders of the head	
Migraine or tension headache	Anterior or posterior
Sinus infection	Most often anterior but occasionally posterior
Temporomandibular joint problem	Usually anterolateral
Oral problems (see Chapter 112) such as a pharyngeal or tonsillar abscess	Middle of the neck
Distant lesions	
Irritation of the surface of the diaphragm innervated by the phrenic nerve (C-3, -4, and -5)	Often shoulder and low neck pain, but medial diaphragmatic lesion may be associated with neck pain
Shoulder problems (see Chapter 69) such as arthritis or periarticular inflammation	May be referred to the lateral part of the neck
Thoracic outlet syndrome from the compression of vascular and neural structures between the rib and the clavicle or between the scalene muscles	May be noticed in the lateral aspect of the neck
Lung problems such as superior sulcus tumor (Pancoast tumor)	Initially may be located in the lateral aspect of the neck and shoulder
Cardiovascular problems such as a heart attack or an aneurysm of the thoracic aorta	May be localized to the base of the neck

[a]The clue to referred pain is the absence of any tenderness in the neck or of exacerbation of symptoms with manipulation of the neck.

be found when bony spurs encroach on the vertebral foramina and compress the vertebral arteries. These rare symptoms usually occur when the neck is in a certain position, and they are usually of short duration.

Physical Examination

Anterior and posterior inspection of the head, neck, shoulders, and upper extremities should be done initially. Any abnormal posture such as torticollis (wry neck) or muscle atrophy will be noticed. Next, the patient should be asked to demonstrate active range of motion of the neck, including flexion to touch the chin to the chest, extension, rotation to touch the chin to the shoulder on both sides, and lateral bending to touch the ear to the shoulder on both sides. Normally, the chin can be placed easily upon the anterior chest and the neck can be extended so that the patient is looking directly above. Normally, there is almost 90 degrees of rotation of the neck to both sides. Simple hyperextension of the neck commonly exacerbates the pain caused by cervical disk degeneration. The patient should be asked to extend the neck and to maintain this position for 30 seconds to determine whether the pain is made worse. Putting direct compression on top of the head also may produce or exacerbate pain in the patient with degenerative disk disease, especially if the head is compressed while the neck is extended. The posterior neck muscles are palpated for muscle spasm, which may be asymmetric and may give the patient the appearance of torticollis (wry neck). Next, the shoulder should be subjected to a range of motion to see whether this elicits pain within the shoulder itself.

Selected neurologic tests (see Chapters 86 and 92) are important in the evaluation of the patient with neck pain whenever there is any suggestion of nerve root involvement or cord compression. These tests include reflex testing of the upper and lower extremities,

Table 70.2. Characteristic Findings at Individual Cervical Nerve Root Levels

Nerve Root	Disk Level	History	Examination[a]
C3	(C2–3)	Pain into the back of the neck to the pinnae and the angle of the jaw	No reflex changes
C4	(C3–4)	Pain into the back of the neck to the levator scapulae to anterior chest	No reflex changes
C5	(C4–5)	Pain into side of the neck to the superior lateral shoulder, numbness over the deltoid muscle	Deltoid muscle atrophy and weakness of shoulder abduction
C6	(C5–6)	Pain to the lateral aspects of the arm and forearm and into the thumb and index finger, with numbness of thumb and dorsum of hand	Weak biceps and brachioradial muscles and decreased biceps and brachioradial tendon reflexes
C7	(C6–7)	Pain into the midforearm to middle and ring fingers	Triceps muscle weakness with decreased triceps muscle reflex
C8	(C7–T1)	Pain to the medial aspect of the forearm into the ring and small fingers, with numbness of the ulnar border and small finger	Triceps weakness with weakness of intrinsic muscles of the hand

[a]Sensory testing usually shows abnormalities in the dermatome of the affected nerve root (see Chapter 86).

muscle strength testing of the upper extremities, and sensory testing of the upper extremities. The reflex testing should include the biceps, triceps, brachioradial, quadriceps, and gastrocnemius tendons and the plantar. Muscle strength in the upper extremities should include the biceps (flexion of elbow), triceps (extension of elbow), wrist extensors and flexors, hand and finger flexors, and intrinsic muscles of the hand. A sensory examination is then performed. An objective sensory deficit is one that conforms to a dermatomal distribution (see Chapters 86 and 92).

Cervical spine problems can cause cervical myelopathy when a bone spur forms posteriorly at the margin of an intervertebral disk and then impinges on the spinal cord, producing signs of cord compression: Increased reflexes in the upper and lower extremities with a positive Babinski sign. Intradural or other extradural lesions at this level could give similar findings.

Laboratory Assessment

If the history reveals severe progressive pain or an episode of recent trauma or if the neurologic examination reveals abnormalities, a complete set of cervical spine x-rays should be obtained. These films should include an assessment of levels C-1 through C7-T1 with oblique and open-mouth odontoid views. These x-rays will help in assessing the patient for fracture or metastatic disease. However, there is not a good correlation between clinical symptoms or signs and degenerative abnormalities on x-ray. In fact, in asymptomatic people after age 40, cervical degenerative changes (spondylosis) are common and are evident in more than 90% of people over age 50 (1). On the other hand, there may be serious cervical disease with minimal or no changes on x-ray.

Computed tomographic (CT) myelography is also useful in the evaluation of problems of the upper cervical spine. Magnetic resonance imaging (MRI) is especially useful when evaluating patients suspected of having abnormalities of the soft tissue such as metastatic cancer or a primary disk problem. CT myelography is more effective for assessment of abnormalities of bone such as osteophytes.

SELECTED SYNDROMES ASSOCIATED WITH NECK PAIN

Many problems of the neck may result in neck pain (Table 70.3). Because the most common problems—herniated cervical disk and cervical spondylosis (degenerative changes)—may have similar manifestations, they are discussed together based on the presence or absence of neurologic findings (see below).

Pain With Neurologic Findings

Diagnosis

Patients with neurologic findings can have either nerve root or spinal cord compression (upper motor neuron syndrome, see Chapter 86). The objective signs of nerve root compression are muscle weakness, a decreased deep tendon reflex, and decreased sensation in a dermatome distribution.

Patients with nerve root compression present with the acute or gradual onset of posterior neck pain that radiates to the shoulder and down one arm into the lower arm and often into the hand itself. The pain often radiates into a finger that corresponds to the dermatome of the nerve root involved. The pain may be made worse by movement of the neck and extreme neck positions. In addition, the patient may complain of decreased sensation and paresthesias in the arm and hand. A patient may have nerve root compression from the cervical spine but have little or no neck and arm pain and instead have arm weakness and loss of sensation. Nerve root compression can be caused by impingement of the nerve by a cervical disk—most common in younger patients—or by osseous proliferation that can impinge on the nerve as it exits through its foramen—most common in patients over age 50 (Fig. 70.1B). Also, the thoracic outlet syndrome may be confused with cervical disease associated with nerve root compression, and this syndrome should be ruled out (see Chapter 69).

Patients with spinal cord compression may have numb clumsy hands or spastic paraparesis. The complaint of neck pain does not need to be prominent, and radicular symptoms may be present. The presence

Table 70.3. Selected Problems of the Neck that May Result in Neck Pain

Problem	Comment
Arthritis	Especially rheumatoid (see Chapter 77) and degenerative joint disease (see text and Chapter 75).
Disk disease	See text.
Fibromyalgia	See Chapter 74.
Infection	Osteomyelitis or soft tissue infection; look for point tenderness (see Chapter 40).
Neoplasia	Myeloma or metastatic disease is associated with point tenderness and x-ray (or bone scan in the case of metastases) abnormalities.
Neuritis	Any nerve may be involved. A common one is the spinal accessory nerve. Look for tenderness over the nerve, lateral aspects of upper one-third of sternomastoid muscle.
Platybasia	A congenital disorder that may not manifest symptoms before age 40 or a complication of Paget disease; x-rays show characteristic changes (i.e., invagination of the base of the skull).
Sprain	Cervical sprain syndrome caused by whiplash and other forms of trauma (see text).
Structures in neck	Any organ or structure located in the neck may become a source of neck pain. Careful examination will detect abnormalities such as thyroiditis, lymphadenitis, pharyngitis, sialadenitis, or tender carotid artery (carotodynia).
Tendinitis	Any tendon may be involved but occipital and sternomastoid are particularly common. Local tenderness is a clue.
Torticollis (wry neck)	Diagnosis is usually obvious by observation. An underlying structural problem could produce reflex muscle spasm; therefore, with an initial episode an underlying problem (e.g., tumor or infection) should be considered.
Trauma	Because of the danger of cord injury, trauma associated with neck pain should be carefully evaluated.
Vascular	Arteritis or dissection may cause neck pain.

of radicular findings of weakness and fasciculations raises the possibility of motor neuron disease. In a younger patient, medical causes of myelopathy, such as multiple sclerosis, must be excluded.

Management

Patients with evidence of *myelopathy* (i.e., involvement of the spinal cord) must be referred to a neurologist or neurosurgeon to establish the cause. Investigation usually includes MRI or CT myelogram. If the myelopathy is secondary to a cervical disk or cervical spondylosis, surgery is often indicated—either laminectomy or anterior cervical fusions. Symptoms of myelopathy, particularly chronic myelopathy, may not remit after decompression, so the goal of surgery is to prevent progression.

Patients with *nerve root compression* leading to muscle weakness and sensory impairment should be referred to an orthopedist or to a neurosurgeon for more complete examination and follow-up. If the neurologic deficit would be unacceptable if permanent, the consultant will evaluate these patients further with CT, MRI, or myelography. If the neurologic deficit would be acceptable if permanent, conservative therapy is an option and has a good chance of success (2).

If the pain is severe, bed rest may be necessary. A *cervical collar* may be beneficial. It is helpful to place a small pillow under the nape of the neck to provide proper positioning. If muscle spasm is present, moist or dry heat applied to the neck may give symptomatic relief. Analgesia using a nonsteroidal anti-inflammatory drug (NSAID) (see Chapter 77) or acetaminophen may help. If a stronger analgesic becomes necessary, immediate-acting oxycodone, 5 to 10 mg orally three or four times daily, may be added. Although not a first-line agent, a muscle relaxant may be helpful (see Chapter 71) if symptoms persist after 3 or 4 days.

The acute phase usually lasts only 1 or 2 weeks. When symptoms become recurrent or chronic (lasting more than 2 to 3 weeks) *cervical traction* may provide relief. This is performed initially by a physical therapist, after x-rays of the cervical spine have been shown to rule out instability. For 30 minutes, 15 to 20 pounds of chin halter traction are applied to the neck. The neck must be positioned in slight flexion; extension, which could worsen symptoms, must be avoided. After several sessions, the patient can be instructed in the use of a home cervical traction unit that can be applied for 30 minutes at a time, up to three times a day, for several months. If symptoms persist for more than 2 or 3 weeks, a brief course of steroids may also be beneficial. Prednisone 60 mg/day is administered for 3 days followed by a 4-day taper. Even when symptoms and signs subside, there is a high rate of recurrence of symptoms. It is therefore important to educate the patient in activities or positions that should be avoided and in exercises that may help relieve muscle spasm (Figs. 70.2 and 70.3).

If the acute symptoms do not subside or if new signs develop, referral to a neurosurgeon is necessary for confirmation of the diagnosis and consideration of surgery (usually discectomy and anterior interbody fusion). The current standard of care is that surgery should be performed to relieve compression of neural structures as demonstrated by symptoms, signs, and radiologic findings (3). A trial of conservative therapy is indicated in all cases except those with evidence of myelopathy, functionally significant weakness, or instability. In some patients, neurologic deficits can take months to resolve postoperatively and may never resolve, particularly in the case of myelopathy.

Pain Without Neurologic Findings

Diagnosis

Most patients with neck pain have no objective neurologic findings. The patient may present either with an acute onset of pain (most of the time a disk herniation)

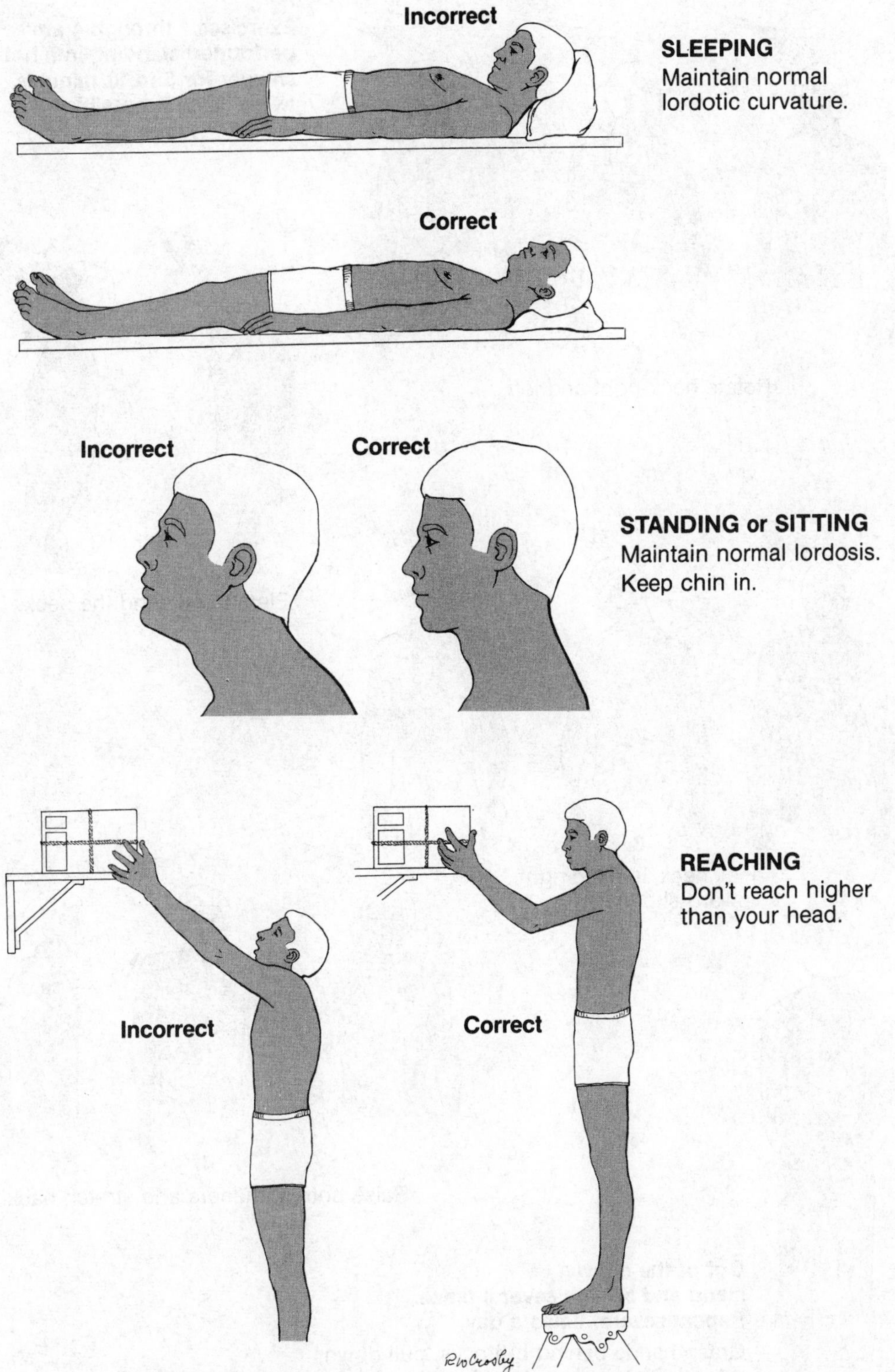

Figure 70.2. Positions to prevent recurrence of neck pain.

or with a slowly progressive discomfort (most often from osteoarthritis) that has been building over several months. In the acute disk herniation syndrome, the patient experiences sudden onset of neck pain that is associated with decreased range of motion of the cervical spine, bilateral muscle spasm, or occasionally asymmetric muscle spasm that produces torticollis (wry neck). The patient may have pain in the shoulder or arm but have no objective weakness or sensory findings on examination.

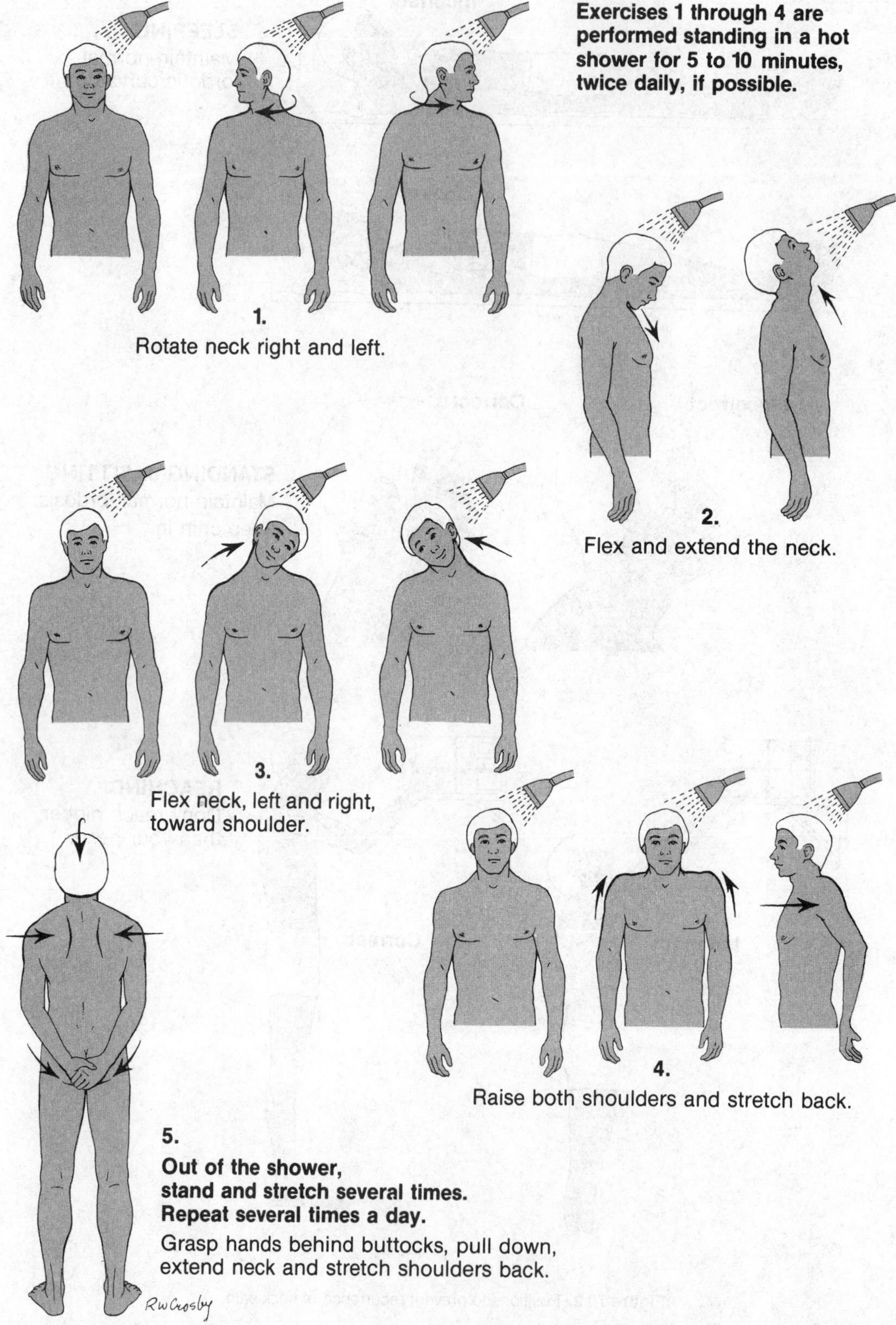

Exercises 1 through 4 are performed standing in a hot shower for 5 to 10 minutes, twice daily, if possible.
1.
Rotate neck right and left.
2.
Flex and extend the neck.
3.
Flex neck, left and right, toward shoulder.
4.
Raise both shoulders and stretch back.
5.
Out of the shower, stand and stretch several times. Repeat several times a day.
Grasp hands behind buttocks, pull down, extend neck and stretch shoulders back.
RwCrosby

Figure 70.3. Exercises to rehabilitate the neck.

Treatment

Initial treatment is basically the same as that outlined above for patients with neurologic findings. The neck may be "immobilized" with a cervical collar (4); several cervical collars are available, but a soft collar is often prescribed first, although it may serve only as a reminder to the patient not to move the neck too quickly or too far. Local heat and analgesics or NSAIDs (see Chapter 77) also may give symptomatic relief. Muscle relaxants (see Chapter 71) may be tried if symptoms persist after 3 or 4 days of initial treatment. In patients who have a chronic more insidious onset of pain, it is helpful to examine the patient's occupational situation more closely to see whether there are exacerbating circumstances (5). Any activity that creates a prolonged extension of the neck, such as overhead work (e.g., painting), or prolonged flexion of the neck, such as sitting at a computer or typewriter, may aggravate a pre-existing problem. If after initial treatment pain lasts more than 2 or 3 weeks, x-rays of the cervical spine should be obtained. The treatment is based on the severity of the symptoms. An oral rapidly acting agent, such as ibuprofen, 400 mg three times a day, may be tried over a course of 2 or 3 weeks. (Alternative NSAIDs, including aspirin, may be tried also; see Chapter 77.) When cost is a factor, generic NSAIDs should be prescribed. The patient should be informed that symptoms often may be chronic or recurrent and should be advised about how to avoid recurrences (Fig. 70.2).

If an acute severe episode of neck pain does not respond to treatment within a few weeks, the patient should be referred to a specialist. When the symptoms are more mild and chronic, a trial of treatment for several months would be reasonable before referral. In the absence of neurologic signs or symptoms, the symptomatic level is difficult to define. Provocative discography is sometimes used in this situation in an attempt to define the levels producing the patient's neck pain. Provocation of the patient's pain by injection of saline into the disk space and relief of the pain by injection of local anesthetic is assumed to implicate a particular level in producing the patient's pain. Anterior cervical fusions carried out on the basis of positive discograms are sometimes effective in treating patients with neck pain without neurologic symptoms.

Cervical Sprain Syndrome

Mechanism

Cervical sprain syndrome is a term given to acute injuries of the neck caused by sudden extension of the cervical spine *(whiplash)*. Patients involved in rear-end automobile accidents may have such acute hyperextension injuries to the neck. In experiments, monkeys subjected to acute hyperextension forces can show tearing of sternocleidomastoid and longus colli muscles in the absence of injuries to the anterior longitudinal ligament or disk. Thus, there may be physical causes for this syndrome (6), although psychological causes are also important (7).

Neck pain from more mild forms of injury that result from repeated hyperextension, such as movements associated with painting a ceiling, usually resolves in a day or two and is not known to be associated with pathologic changes. The reason that this syndrome can become persistent is unclear. A recent prospective study found that the presence of stress unrelated to the accident was a better predictor of persistent symptoms than clinical findings (8), suggesting that psychologic variables are important.

Diagnosis

Although patients usually have pain after the accident, it is not uncommon for the patient to be without discomfort initially. The patient experiences pain in the posterior or anterior region of the neck. It commonly radiates to the occipital aspect of the head, and it may radiate to the shoulders. Occipital headaches often occur. Disk herniation, fracture, or subluxation can occur in this setting. Therefore, it is essential to visualize the cervical spine radiologically down to C7-T1. If plain x-rays are normal, flexion extension x-rays should be obtained. Any patient with neurologic findings in this setting should be immobilized in a hard collar and seen urgently by a neurosurgeon or orthopedic surgeon before flexion–extension x-rays are taken.

Treatment

If muscle spasm or limitation of motion is present without neurologic findings, the patient may be placed in a cervical collar (see above). Analgesics such as acetaminophen or NSAIDs (or occasionally, for short periods, a narcotic), at adequate dosages, should be given. The patient should be warned that extension of the neck will exacerbate the pain. Heat applied to the cervical spine, either moist or dry, may give symptomatic relief but does not speed healing. Patients may seek manipulation for treatment of this condition and should be aware that the value of this modality is uncertain (9). The patient should be encouraged to perform daily work and activities as much as possible. If the patient has severe pain and muscle spasm at the initial injury, the clinical course will probably last 4 to 6 weeks. When the patient's pain subsides and he or she has full range of motion without muscle spasm, the collar can be gradually discontinued, and the patient should also be advised of the methods of relieving muscle spasm and preventing recurrent symptoms (Figs. 70.2 and 70.3). If there are no symptoms of nerve root compression, the patient with persistent symptoms should be considered for further workup.

General References*

Carette S. Whiplash injury and chronic neck pain. N Engl J Med 1994;330:1083.

This editorial outlines succinctly the magnitude of the problem of whiplash injury and reviews the treatment of chronic neck pain, which may follow.

*Bold print (general references) and bold numerals (specific references) denote published controlled clinical trials, meta-analyses, or consensus-based recommendations.

Hoving JL, Gross AR, Gasner D, et al. A critical appraisal of review articles on the effectiveness of conservative treatment for neck pain. Spine 2001;26:196.
An appraisal of articles on conservative treatment for neck pain.

Kalkanis SN, Borges L. Neck and back pain in the elderly. Curr Treat Options Neurol 2001;3:215.
A thorough review of conservative and surgical treatments.

Levy HI. Cervical pain syndromes: primary care diagnosis and management. Compr Ther 2000;26:82.
A review of the treatment and of the common cervical pain syndrome.

Nachemson AL, Jonsson E. Neck and back pain. Philadelphia: Lippincott Williams & Wilkins, 2000.
A comprehensive text.

Nakano KK. Neck pain. In: Ruddy S, Harris ED, Sledge CB, eds. Kelly's textbook of rheumatology. 6th ed. Philadelphia: W.B. Saunders, 2001.
An excellent discussion of the anatomy and biomechanisms and the diagnosis, treatment, and differential diagnosis of common cervical spine problems.

Specific References

1. Elias F. Roentgen findings in the asymptomatic cervical spine. NY J Med 1958;58:3300.
2. Saal JS, Saal JA, Yurth EF. Nonoperative management of herniated cervical intervertebral disc with radiculopathy. Spine 1996;21:1877.
3. Rothman RH, Simeone FA, eds. The spine. Philadelphia: W.B. Saunders, 1992.
4. Johnson RM, Hart DL, Simmons EF, et al. Cervical orthoses. J Bone Joint Surg 1977;59:332.
5. Dryer SJ, Boden S. Nonoperative treatment of neck and arm pain. Spine 1998;23:2746.
6. Bogduk N. Whiplash: the evidence for a organic etiology. Arch Neurol 2000;57:590.
7. Berry H. Chronic whiplash syndrome as a functional disorder. Arch Neurol 2000;57:592.
8. Karlsborg M, Smed A, Jespersen H, et al. A prospective study of 39 patients with whiplash injury. Acta Neurol Scand 1997;95:65.
9. Koes BW, Assendelft WJ, van der Heijden GJ, et al. Spinal manipulation and mobilization for back and neck pain: a blinded review. BMJ 1991;303:1298.

CHAPTER 71

Low Back Pain

DAVID G. BORENSTEIN, MD

Low back pain is one of the most common human afflictions. Between 70% and 80% of the population experience back pain some time during their lives. The prevalence of back pain ranges, in reports, from a low of 10% of adults during a 2-year period to a high of 20% of the population of a Western industrial society during a 2-week period (1,2). Although as many as 30% of people with back pain do not seek medical evaluation, the remainder eventually request medical advice. The office is the appropriate setting for the evaluation of these patients. A review of three time periods (1980–1981, 1985, and 1989–1990) studied by the National Ambulatory Medical Care Survey revealed mechanical low back pain (defined below) as the fifth most common reason for all physician office visits. Nonspecific low back pain was the most common diagnosis, accounting for 56.8% of these cases (3). Most patients with low back pain have underlying conditions that can be diagnosed and treated in the ambulatory setting. Most patients do not require hospitalization or surgery. The task is to separate the few who require more aggressive assessment from those who will recover with only office evaluation and conservative management.

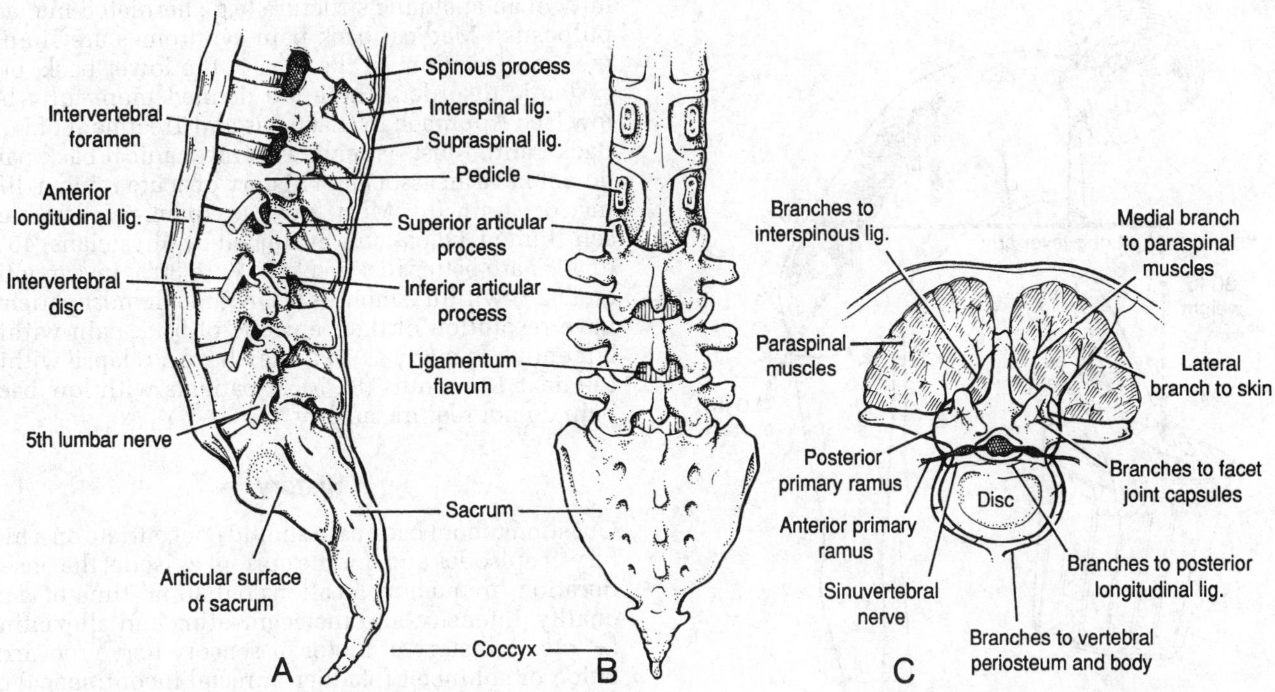

Figure 71.1. Anatomic relationships of the lumbosacral spine. **A:** Lateral view. **B:** Posterior view. **C:** Cross-sectional view.

ANATOMY AND BIOMECHANICS OF THE LUMBOSACRAL SPINE AND ASSOCIATED STRUCTURES

The structure of the lumbosacral spine is complex (Fig. 71.1, A–C). The lumbar spine is composed of five vertebrae with interposed intervertebral disks that consist of a gelatinous nucleus pulposus and a surrounding annulus fibrosus. The vertebrae and disks are supported by strong ligamentous structures and paraspinous muscles. The posterior aspects of the vertebrae surround the spinal canal, form the neural foramina, and interlock to form apophyseal joints (facet joints) whose main purpose is motion (Fig. 71.1, A and B). The sacrum is the part of the spine that interdigitates with the iliac bones to form part of the pelvis.

An understanding of the nerve supply to the lumbosacral spine is essential in recognizing the patterns of pain associated with disease processes that affect components of the back (4). The *sinuvertebral nerve* (Fig. 71.1C) is the major sensory nerve supplying structures in the lumbar spine. The nerve arises from the corresponding spinal nerve before it divides into anterior and posterior branches. The nerve enters the intervertebral foramen and divides into ascending, descending, and transverse branches that anastomose with the contralateral side and with sensory nerves at adjacent levels above and below. The sinuvertebral nerve supplies the posterior longitudinal ligament, superficial annulus fibrosus, epidural blood vessels, anterior dura mater, dural sleeve, and posterior vertebral periosteum. The posterior rami of the spinal nerves supply the apophyseal joints above and below the nerve and the paraspinous muscles at multiple levels. The complex innervation of lumbar spine structures helps explain the diffuse nature of pain associated with a wide variety of disorders.

A number of organs are situated in the retroperitoneum, anterior to the lumbar spine. The kidneys, ureters, aorta, inferior vena cava, pancreas, and periaortic lymph nodes are retroperitoneal organs. Diseases that affect these organs may result in referred pain that is localized to the lumbar spine.

In the upright position with a normal spinal curvature (lordosis), the ligamentous structures maintain the position of the spine with little need for contraction of the paraspinous muscles or for weight-bearing by the apophyseal (facet) joints (Fig. 71.1A). However, if the normal curve is flattened or accentuated, the paraspinous muscles contract and the apophyseal (facet) joints become weight-bearing. This change in body mechanics results in pain.

The lumbar vertebrae are exposed to tremendous forces. This is caused principally by the magnification of stresses that result from the lever effect of the arm in lifting and by vertical forces associated with the human upright position. Figure 71.2 demonstrates how lifting an object away from the body introduces the lever magnification phenomenon, resulting in a marked increase in forces on the vertebral bodies and disks. Because each intervertebral disk is a fluid system, hydraulic pressure is created whenever a load is placed on the axial skeleton. This hydraulic pressure magnifies three to five times the force that occurs on the annulus fibrosus. This force is akin to the hoop stress that occurs in a barrel when pressure

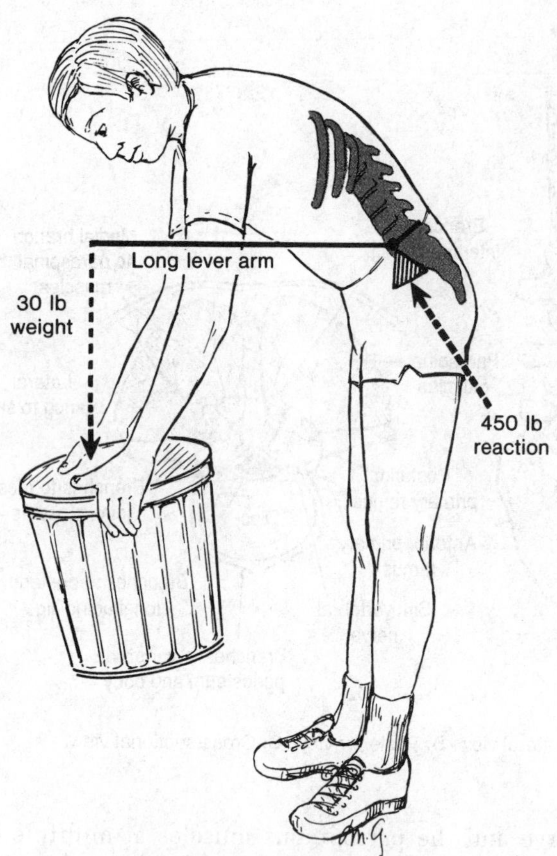

Figure 71.2. Forces in the lumbar area.

is applied to its liquid content. A study using a pressure transducer placed *in vivo* in the nucleus pulposus of an asymptomatic 45-year-old man documented highest intradiscal pressures associated with lifting a 20-kg weight. The lowest intradiscal pressures were associated with the prone position (5). The ability of the annulus fibrosus to withstand stress in any position decreases significantly with age, and by age 60 years many people have only 50% of the strength in these fibers that they had at age 30.

However, the lumbar spine is not just an isolated structure. Much support is obtained by the muscles and ligaments of the spine and by the muscles of the thoracic and abdominal cavities. These latter structures act as a sort of muscular cylinder that helps decrease the load on the axial skeleton by as much as 30% in the lumbar area and 50% in the thoracic spine.

EVALUATION OF PATIENTS WITH LOW BACK PAIN

Certain facts pertaining to the causes and natural history of back pain influence the evaluation and treatment of patients with this symptom. Back pain is most often associated with a mechanical cause, although it sometimes has a nonmechanical (called medical or systemic in this text) cause. Mechanical low back pain may be defined as pain secondary to overuse of a normal anatomic structure (e.g., muscle strain) or deformity of an anatomic structure (e.g., herniated nucleus pulposus). Medical back pain syndromes are simply the manifestation, in the area of the lower back, of a systemic disorder. These are defined more fully below (see Approach to Diagnosis and Treatment of Low Back Pain). Most patients with mechanical back pain do not have an associated history of acute trauma, lifting, or strain (6). Most low back pain problems are self-limited. Of patients evaluated by physicians, 40% to 50% are better in 1 week, 51% to 86% in 1 month, and 92% within 2 months (7). Although most patients have resolution of their episode of back pain within 2 months, as many as 75% may have a relapse within the next 12 months (8). Most patients with low back pain do not require surgery.

History

Questions about back pain should concentrate on a history of episodes and, for the current episode, the onset, duration, frequency, location, radiation, time of day, quality, intensity, and the aggravating and alleviating factors. A history of motor or sensory nerve root irritation or sphincter (bladder or rectal incontinence) or sexual dysfunction is important in identifying patients with *cauda equina compression* (see below). Occupational history may reveal predisposing factors associated with recurrent episodes of back injury.

Patients should also be questioned about systemic symptoms that are indicative of a medical (systemic) cause of their back pain. Patients with fever, weight loss, pain with recumbency, extended morning stiffness, acute bone pain, or viscerogenic pain should be evaluated for a systemic illness. Patients who are over 50 years of age are also at greater risk of a medical (systemic) cause for their pain. A history of cancer is a "red flag" for a medical cause of low back pain (9).

Physical Examination

Physical Examination of the Lumbosacral Spine and Associated Musculoskeletal Areas

Abnormalities of the spine may be discovered while the spine is stationary or in motion. The patient should be examined in an orderly fashion that evaluates the function of musculoskeletal and neurologic structures of the lumbosacral spine (10).

Initially, the patient is examined in a gown while *standing* barefoot or wearing only socks. The spinal column is examined from all directions to check for excessive kyphosis, lordosis, or scoliosis. The presence of scoliosis is best determined by having the patient flex at the waist with arms extended in front. Any asymmetry of the height of the shoulders can be appreciated. Any deviation of a spinous process from the midline is noted. Firm palpation of the paravertebral muscles and of each vertebral spine is performed. Isolated tenderness over a bone suggests a localized problem such as tumor, infection, or compression fracture. Firm paraspinous muscles result from spasm secondary to local injury or referred pain.

Mobility of the spine is assessed by having the patient bend forward and attempt to touch the toes (normal is about 50 to 80 degrees). However, the hip joints also participate in the movement. Range of flexion can be determined by quantifying the expansion of a 10-cm line measured from the lumbosacral junction superiorly during maximal flexion (*Schober test,* see Chapter 78) or noting the distance of the fingertips from the floor. During this movement the normally smooth rhythm of the reversal of the lumbar lordosis is noted. If the rhythm is interrupted or hesitant, an abnormality of the apophyseal joints or of paraspinous structures may be present.

Lateral flexion (normal is to about 30 degrees) and extension (normal is to about 30 degrees) are then assessed. Lateral flexion is usually preserved in disk disease but may be limited in patients with a spondyloarthropathy (i.e., a joint problem of the spine). Increased discomfort with extension suggests disease of the apophyseal joints or spinal stenosis.

The patient is then examined *bent forward* over the examining table. In this position, the inferior portion of the sacroiliac joints, ischial tuberosities, and sciatic notch are more easily palpated.

The *gait of the patient* should be observed. Patients with back pain may walk in a stiff guarded fashion or may favor one leg if a radiculopathy is present.

The patient is next examined *sitting with the legs dangling.* The deep tendon reflexes of the knees (L-4) and ankles (S-1) are elicited to test the integrity of the reflex arcs. An absent reflex may signify nerve root impingement secondary to a herniated nucleus pulposus. While seated, the patient extends each knee. The flexion of the hip and extension of the knee stretch the lumbar nerve roots. Radicular pain that radiates from the back to below the knee is associated with nerve root impingement. The origin of the pain from the nerve root can be confirmed by lowering the leg just to the point where the pain disappears and then reproducing the pain by dorsiflexing the foot. This sign, if positive, suggests a herniated intervertebral disk or, less commonly, bony impingement of a nerve root caused by arthritis affecting the apophyseal joints, lumbar stenosis, or, rarely, a tumor of the spinal cord or surrounding structures. This *distracted straight leg raising* (SLR) test helps confirm the organic source of pain and identify patients who may exaggerate their symptoms. Patients with functional complaints have no discomfort with a distracted SLR test but may describe excruciating pain when the SLR test is done in the supine position. Not all patients with a herniated disk have a positive SLR test. A patient, especially over age 30 years, may have a herniated disk that is too small or in the wrong location to irritate the nerve roots.

Next, the patient assumes the *supine* position, so that a *standard* SLR test can be performed. The examiner fully extends the knee and slowly flexes the lower extremity at the hip. Normally the hip can be flexed to 80 degrees without pain, except for discomfort in the thigh or behind the knee secondary to hamstring muscle tightness. A positive test is manifested by radicular pain that radiates below the knee on the affected side or bilaterally. The nerve root and surrounding dura do not move in the neural foramen until an elevation of 30 degrees or greater of the lower extremity has been reached. Therefore, radicular pain that is elicited at an elevation less than 30 degrees is suspect. The SLR is sensitive but nonspecific for the presence of a herniated intervertebral disk causing sciatica (11). After the SLR test, the unaffected lower extremity should be raised, thus performing the *crossed SLR test* (12). This procedure causes tension and stretch of the nerve roots of the opposite (affected) lower extremity and reproduces the radicular pain caused by SLR in that lower extremity. Although uncommonly positive (11), when it is so, there is a strong, but not absolute, correlation with disk herniation (13,14).

Next, *sensory assessment* of the buttock, perineum, and lower extremities should be performed. Chapter 86 shows the relevant sensory dermatomes that can be evaluated by pinprick and touch. Abnormalities help localize a lesion and help one determine the need and urgency of an orthopedic or neurosurgical consultation. An important component of the sensory assessment is the search for signs compatible with a *cauda equina syndrome* (a syndrome of neurologic dysfunction from compression of the nerves at the L4–5 level and inferior to the spinal cord proper, often secondary to a central disk herniation). The signs of compression of the cauda equina include saddle anesthesia, loss of anal sphincter tone (assessed by rectal examination), bilateral *sciatica* (pain in the distribution of the sciatic nerve), lower extremity motor weakness, and a history of bowel, bladder, or sexual dysfunction. This syndrome, if present, is an indication for immediate referral to a neurosurgeon or orthopedic surgeon for hospitalization and surgical decompression of the spinal cord. The best neurologic outcome occurs when decompression occurs in the first 48 hours after the onset of cauda equina compression (CEC) signs (15).

A detailed assessment of *motor function* of the lower extremities also helps localize a lesion in the patient in whom neurologic involvement is suspected (see Chapter 92). This assessment can be done while the patient is supine, sitting, or standing. Muscles tested include hip flexors (L2–3) and extensors (L4–5), the knee extensors (L3–4), the dorsiflexors of the foot (L4–5), the knee flexors (L5–S1), and the plantar flexors of the foot (S1–2). Subtle weakness may be elicited by having the patient walk on his or her toes (gastrocnemius muscle group, S1–2) and heels (tibialis anterior muscles, L4–5).

While the patient is in the supine position, an assessment of the hip, sacroiliac, and knee joints is done. The hip and knee joints are assessed by moving these joints through a normal range of motion when they are unweighted. Pain with motion suggests an articular cause of leg pain. The *sacroiliac joint* is tested by the Patrick or FABER (flexion, abduction, external rotation) test. The test is done by positioning the lateral malleolus of the tested leg on the patella of the opposite leg. Downward pressure is then placed on the medial aspect of the knee while stabilizing the pelvis by placing a hand on the contralateral anterior superior iliac spine. Pain associated with a quick pulse or downward pressure is usually localized to the lateral aspect of the lumbar spine and originates in the sacroiliac joint. Slow pressure may elicit groin pain indicative of hip joint dysfunction.

In the *lateral* position, the sacroiliac joint and muscles of hip abduction (L2–3) are tested. Pressure is applied to the iliac wing, compressing the sacroiliac joints. Pain felt in the sacroiliac joint suggests an intra-articular process or a strain of the posterior sacroiliac ligaments. The muscles of hip abduction are tested as the patient elevates the upper leg against downward pressure applied below the knee by the examiner.

In the *prone* position, the symmetry of the buttocks is assessed (gluteus maximus, L-5, S1–2). A femoral stretch test (i.e., extending the hip joint) elicits pain in the anterior thigh (L2–3) or the medial aspect of the leg (L-4) in patients with corresponding herniated intervertebral disks.

To evaluate the rare patients suspected of *malingering* or of a psychiatric origin for their back pain, Waddell et al. (16) identified five physical signs associated with functional disorders. First, overreaction during examination was found to be the single most important sign indicating a nonorganic cause. Overreaction may take the form of collapsing, sweating, tremor, muscle tension, bizarre facial expression, or disproportionate verbalization. Second, simulation testing may be used to elicit nonorganic pain. Two useful examples are axial loading and rotation. In the first example, with the patient standing, low back pain is reported in overreactors (but not in others) on vertical loading by pressing down on the patient's head. Neck pain is common during this examination in all and does not constitute a positive sign. In the hip rotation test, the patient stands with feet together and arms fixed firmly to the lateral sides of the body at the hip level by the examiner's hands. In this manner, the torso (and the spine) is passively rotated on the hips. Because the units of the spine itself are not moved, reports of low back pain are a positive sign of a nonorganic cause. However, in the presence of true radiculopathy, leg pain may be produced because there is movement at the hip joint and nerve roots may be stretched. Third is the use of distraction testing. This consists of observing the patient during the course of the examination for variable findings when the patient is unaware of being observed or tested, such as during the *distracted SLR* (see above). Fourth, superficial, nonanatomic, or variable tenderness is also a nonorganic sign. A useful technique is the Magnuson test, in which tender areas are subtly marked and later examined again for reproducibility. Fifth, motor or sensory findings that are not explained by an anatomic lesion provide clues that the problem is psychiatric in origin. Also, sudden giving away or flaccidity of a muscle during strength testing of the symptomatic area supports a nonorganic problem. A finding of three or more of the five types of signs is clinically significant.

Examination of Other Regions

Patients with constitutional symptoms or with symptoms not attributed to a local process in the back (e.g., abdominal pain) should undergo a focused physical examination. The physical examination, including pelvic and rectal and breast examinations in women, is particularly important in patients who describe new back pain and are 50 years of age or older.

Common origins of metastatic cancer to the spine are the breast, lung, prostate, thyroid, kidney, and rectum. Referred pain from cancer or other lesions may also be felt in the back. For example, pancreatic tumors or duodenal ulcers cause pain to be referred to the high lumbar or low thoracic vertebral region. Bowel or urinary tract cancer may cause pain to be referred to the mid- or low lumbar region, and a disease process located in the pelvis may cause lower lumbar or sacral pain. Also, neoplasia primarily affecting the bones, especially multiple myeloma, is an important consideration in the elderly.

Important also is the assessment of the adequacy of the arteries of the lower extremities. Vascular abnormalities may cause pain due to ischemia in the back, buttock, or lower extremities during exertion. In addition to diminished pulses and bruits over arteries, cutaneous signs of ischemia (ulcers, loss of hair or nails) should be sought in the legs or feet (see Chapter 94). Sudden change in a pain pattern associated with an abdominal aneurysm or an episode of hypotension should alert one to the possibility of impending extension or rupture of the aneurysm.

Although the physical examination adds essential information for the evaluation of low back pain, the reproducibility of findings can vary widely among examiners and at different times. In one study of the physical examination of patients with low back pain, McCombe et al. (17) evaluated the reproducibility of a number of signs. They conclude that precise examination, careful measurement of locations of pain and tenderness and degrees of movement of the back and legs, and careful documentation of this was most important to accurately reproduce a patient's findings. Certain caveats relevant to this examination were developed. The most important among these were as follows:

- Bony tenderness is more reproducible and of greater diagnostic significance than soft tissue tenderness;
- Pain on hip flexion and external rotation is reproducible and valuable;
- Heel and toe standing are not an accurate method of assessing muscle strength;
- SLR is reliable and reproducible if there is precise measurement and documentation of the extent of pain radiation;
- Measurements of the range of flexion and lateral bend are reliable.

A study by Jensen (18) of the accuracy of certain signs in predicting a precise cause and location of a problem showed a reasonable but imperfect correlation of disturbed sensory and motor function with anatomic abnormalities confirmed at surgery in 52 patients with lumbar disk herniations. The time of day of the examination also may have an effect on physical findings. Ensink et al. (19) reported the measured lumbar spine motion in 29 patients with chronic back pain in the morning and afternoon. Flexion was increased to the greatest degree at the end of the day and extension was independent of time of measurement. The sum of all these studies is that careful examination and precise measurements of dysfunction and pain location are important in evaluating back pain. However, no sign is absolutely diagnostic or perfectly reproducible and some signs are frankly unreliable. The entire constellation of findings must therefore be considered in developing a proper approach to a patient.

With information obtained from the history and physical examination, a working diagnosis may be generated based on first defining the pain as mechanical or nonmechanical (medical or systemic) in nature. Patients with mechanical disorders may be treated without additional laboratory or radiographic tests during the initial visit. On the other hand, those believed to have a nonmechanical (medical or systemic) problem should undergo further diagnostic testing.

Laboratory Evaluation

Radiographic Assessment

A *plain x-ray of the lumbar spine* is not a necessary part of the initial evaluation of patients with back pain unless they have a history of recent major trauma or acute constitutional symptoms. Patients with back pain of a mechanical origin often have normal x-rays. In addition, many patients with abnormal x-rays may be entirely asymptomatic (20). By age 50, 67% of normal people have evidence of disk disease characterized by narrowing of one or more disk spaces or disk calcifications; an additional 20% of people have lumbar osteophytes. In fact, only 13% of 50 year olds have normal x-rays. Two-thirds of patients with roentgenographic evidence of lumbar disk degeneration are asymptomatic. Osteoarthritis of the apophyseal (facet) joints is not correlated with symptoms (21). In addition, plain films may not be sensitive enough to identify bony lesions unless 50% of the medullary portion of the bone has been destroyed (22). Therefore, plain x-rays of the lumbar spine should be obtained only in patients who have failed a course of conservative therapy, persist with pain, have reflex asymmetry, have point vertebral tenderness, or are elderly and have new onset pain (because of the higher incidence of a fracture or a systemic cause of their symptoms) (23).

Other radiographic techniques that are useful in the evaluation of patients with back pain include *bone scan* (infection, tumor [but multiple myeloma is notoriously missed], arthritis, fracture), *computed tomography* (CT; disk herniation, spinal stenosis, myeloma, retroperitoneal structures), and magnetic resonance imaging (MRI; disk herniation, intraspinal tumors). Each should be highly selected on the basis of the history and physical examination and often a consultation from a radiologist, neurosurgeon, or orthopedist is helpful in deciding the approach. *MRI* can detect specific anatomic lesions in the lumbar spine with greater sensitivity than any other radiographic technique (24,25). MRI detects degenerative intervertebral disk disease and spinal stenosis and is an excellent method for detecting medical disorders affecting the lumbar spine, including primary and metastatic malignancies and osteomyelitis (26). Contrast MRI with gadolinium differentiates scar tissue from recurrent disk herniations in individuals who have undergone surgical discectomies. CT is especially valuable for the definition of trabecular architecture of bone. Benign and malignant tumors and infectious lesions may be differentiated by CT. Radiographic findings become significant only when the history, physical examination, and radiographic findings agree. These more expensive imaging techniques are confirmatory, not diagnostic, tests. Nearly one-third of asymptomatic patients have identifiable abnormalities that are of no significance (27–30).

Other Laboratory Evaluations

Most patients with low back pain do not require laboratory studies with their initial evaluation. Patients who are elderly, have constitutional symptoms, or have failed conservative therapy may benefit from a laboratory evaluation (see above). The laboratory evaluations that may be useful include complete blood count and erythrocyte sedimentation rate (inflammatory and neoplastic disorders), serum calcium concentration and alkaline phosphatase activity (diffuse bone disease), serum and urine electrophoresis (multiple myeloma), prostate-specific antigen (metastatic prostate cancer), urinalysis (renal disease), and occult blood in the stool (ulcers, gastrointestinal tumors). All such evaluations should be based on distinct diagnostic possibilities based on the history and physical examination.

APPROACH TO DIAGNOSIS AND TREATMENT OF LOW BACK PAIN

In describing various conditions that result in back pain, it is useful to place them into two categories: regional (mechanical) and medical (systemic or nonmechanical). Both are defined above (see Evaluation of Patients with Low Back Pain). Differentiating medical back pain syndromes from a mechanical cause can be difficult when the back is the only anatomic area in which symptoms are manifest. This difficulty is most commonly experienced when evaluating elderly patients. Systemic conditions that typically affect the low back region, including infections and tumors, are discussed below.

Most patients with an acute onset of low back pain have a regional (mechanical) cause for their symptoms. Up to 90% of these patients respond to a course of conservative medical therapy. A significant number of back pain patients may be resolved in as little as 2 weeks (31). Serial observation is very important in management of patients with back pain. If on reassessment there are symptoms or signs of progression or of an incomplete response to treatment, evaluation for an alternative diagnosis is indicated. The follow-up contact should occur 3 to 4 weeks after the initial visit for all patients because by this time most patients with nonserious disorders causing their symptoms are markedly improved. The follow-up visit is also important for patients whose back pain has resolved so that they have an opportunity to be educated in regard to recurrent symptoms and advised regarding prophylactic measures.

COMMON REGIONAL (MECHANICAL) BACK SYNDROMES

Lumbosacral Strain Syndrome

Lumbosacral strain is the most common cause of low back pain. The cause of back strain is not always clear but may be related to muscular, ligamentous, or fascial strain secondary to either a specific traumatic episode or continuous mechanical stress. People between the ages of 20 and 40 years are at greatest risk of developing muscle strain. Predisposing factors include failure to use good techniques in lifting, obesity, abnormal forward pelvic tilt (accentuated lordosis, most usually an acquired posture resulting from abdominal obesity), and leg length discrepancy (32).

Diagnosis

The patient complains of pain that may be severe in the back, buttock, or one or both thighs. Usually symptoms follow a recent increase in physical activity for that patient, such as gardening, lifting, or an infrequently played sport. Usually the patient experiences no (or minimal) discomfort during or immediately after the activity. Within the next 12 to 36 hours, as the soft tissues swell, pain develops and is associated with a feeling of muscular stiffness. The patient complains of pain that is accentuated by standing and bending and alleviated by lying. Table 71.1 provides information useful in the differential diagnosis of mechanical low back pain.

Examination of the back may show nonspecific signs of muscle spasm and loss of lumbar lordosis, but characteristically there is no evidence of nerve root impingement. Pain radiating to the low back from an inflamed ischial or trochanteric bursa is occasionally seen, but marked tenderness over the inflamed bursa should reveal the correct diagnosis (see Chapter 74).

Management

In December 1994, the Agency for Health Care Policy and Research (now the Agency for Healthcare Research and Quality) published a Clinical Practice Guideline booklet concerning the diagnosis and management of acute low back pain (33). The booklet included the recommendations of a 23-member panel that critically reviewed 3,918 published scientific articles. The recommendations are listed in Table 71.2. The reviewed articles related to management were rated from A to D, ranging from studies with strong research-based evidence to studies in which the design did not meet inclusion criteria. The final recommendations were based on the strength of evidence, risk-to-benefit ratios, and cost of each intervention. In the absence of controlled trials, the potential benefit of an intervention had to outweigh its possible risks to be considered cost-effective.

In general, the guidelines encourage early return of function. The recommended medications have mild toxicities and little abuse potential. Invasive therapies are limited to patients who fail to improve over 4 to 12 weeks. The guidelines do have limitations: The recommendations are options and not the sole method for treating low back pain; they are based on a small number of studies (although many were reviewed), and they are made for acute low back pain and do not apply to patients with chronic low back pain.

The conservative therapy of low back pain from lumbosacral strain includes controlled physical activity (low stress, gradually increasing aerobic and back-strengthening exercises), physical therapy, nonsteroidal anti-inflammatory drugs (NSAIDs), and muscle relaxants. In a study of medical therapy for low back pain with or without leg pain, the combination of an NSAID and a muscle relaxant was associated with the greatest number of individuals with improvement at 1 week (34). To minimize back motion and provide support, the bed should be firm but comfortable. A bed board cut from 5/8-inch or plywood placed between the mattress and box spring is usually effective. Avoiding strenuous activity for most patients is appropriate, and even for those with severe pain, a minimal period

Table 71.1. Information Useful in the Differential Diagnosis of Mechanical Low Back Pain

Characteristics	Lumbosacral Strain	Herniated Nucleus Pulposus	Osteoarthritis	Spinal Stenosis
Age (yr)	20–40	30–50	>50	>60
Pain characteristics				
Location	Back (unilateral)	Back and leg (unilateral)	Back (bilateral)	Leg (bilateral)
Onset	Acute	Acute (prior episodes)	Insidious	Insidious
Standing[a]	+	−	+	+
Sitting[a]	−	+	−	−
Bending[a]	+	−	−	−
Straight leg raising test	−	+	−	+ (stress, i.e., after walking)
Plain x-ray	−	−	+	+

[a] +, Exacerbating; −, alleviating.

Adapted from Borenstein DG, Wiesel SW. Low back pain: medical diagnosis and comprehensive management. Philadelphia: W.B. Saunders, 1989, with permission.

Table 71.2. AHCPR Guidelines for Management of Acute Low Back Pain

I. Patient education
   Patients with acute low back problems should be given accurate information about the following (strength of evidence = B):
   A. Expectations for both rapid recovery and recurrences of symptoms based on natural history of low back symptoms.
   B. Safe and effective methods of symptom control.
   C. Safe and reasonable activity modifications.
   D. Best means of limiting recurrent low back problems.
   E. The lack of need for special investigations unless danger signs are present (see text).
   F. Effectiveness and risks of commonly available diagnostic and further treatment measures to be considered should symptoms persist.

II. Medications
   Acetaminophen and nonsteroidal anti-inflammatory drugs (NSAIDs)
   A. Acetaminophen is reasonably safe and is acceptable for treating patients with acute low back problems (strength of evidence = C).
   B. NSAIDs, including aspirin, are acceptable for treating patients with acute low back pain (strength of evidence = B).
   C. NSAIDs have a number of potential side effects. The most common complication is gastrointestinal irritation. The decision to use these medications can be guided by comorbidity, side effects, cost, and patient and provider preference (strength of evidence = C).

III. Physical treatments
   Spinal manipulation
   A. Manipulation can be helpful for patients with acute low back problems without radiculopathy when used within the first month of symptoms (strength of evidence = B).
   B. A trial of manipulation in patients without radiculopathy with symptoms longer than a month is probably safe, but efficacy is unproven (strength of evidence = C).

IV. Activity modification
   Activity recommendations for bed rest and exercise
   A. A gradual return to normal activities is more effective than prolonged bed rest for treating acute low back problems (strength of evidence = B).
   B. Prolonged bed rest for more than 4 days may lead to debilitation and is not recommended for treating actue low back problems (strength of evidence = B).
   C. Low-stress aerobic exercise can prevent debilitation due to inactivity during the first month of symptoms and thereafter may help to return patients to the highest level of functioning appropriate to their circumstances (strength of evidence = C).

Ratings for strength of evidence: A, strong research-based evidence (multiple relevant and high-quality studies); B, moderate research-based evidence (one relevent, high-quality or multiple adequate studies); C, limited research-based evidence (one adequate scientific study); D, studies did not meet inclusion criteria.

of strict bed rest as short as 2 days has been shown to be adequate in relieving back pain (35). Controlled physical activity allows injured tissues to rest, permitting a greater opportunity for healing without reinjury. Pushing this concept further, Malmivaara et al. (36) reported on the efficacy of ordinary activity as tolerated in comparison with efficacy of bed rest for 2 days and back-mobilizing exercises. Better recovery, improved function, and fewer missed work days were associated with ordinary activity. Also, Faas et al. (37) showed the absence of significant benefit in the resolution of low back pain from exercise taught and monitored by a physiotherapist. In this study of 473 patients, flexion and stretching exercises were only minimally better at decreasing the duration of low back pain recurrences and had no other benefit compared with placebo interventions, which consisted of ultrasonography by a physiotherapist and usual care. The important lesson is that one should encourage the patient to do gentle activity as tolerated early in the course of acute low back pain when the cause is believed to be secondary to lumbosacral strain.

Physical therapy modalities, in the form of cold (ice massage) initially or heat subsequently, may decrease pain and diminish muscle spasm. The application of dry heat by a heating pad for 20 to 30 minutes several times a day (on low or medium setting with a protective towel between skin and pad to prevent burns) is preferred by some patients. Others prefer moist heat, which is accomplished by using hot towels, or a heat pack, which produces sustained heat for up to 30 minutes (available at pharmacies).

Nonnarcotic analgesics such as NSAIDs are helpful in making patients comfortable while their injury heals. NSAIDs with a rapid onset of action (such as aspirin, 600 mg four times a day; ibuprofen, 400 to 800 mg three times a day; diflunisal, 500 mg twice a day; ketoprofen, 25–50 mg 3–4×/day; diclofenac, 50 mg three times a day; or naproxen 250–500 mg twice a day) are most appropriate. In general, all nonsteroidal analgesics should be used for a limited time (e.g., 2 to 6 weeks) in treating patients with mechanical back pain. The choice of any of these nonsteroidal drugs must be made in consideration of both patient and drug characteristics. For example, some patients prefer twice a day drug administration, whereas a few prefer more frequent dosing. In general, NSAIDs are effective for short-term symptomatic relief of low back pain but are less effective for sciatica (38). Some groups of patients are especially vulnerable to the side effects of these drugs. Particularly important are the gastrointestinal and renal toxicity that occur often in elderly patients, especially women, who take NSAIDs. These drugs must be used with great caution or avoided in this population.

The new cytochrome cyclooxygenase-2 (COX-2) inhibitors decrease the risk for gastrointestinal toxicities in older patients or those with a history of gastrointestinal ulcers. For the older patient who is sensitive to NSAIDs, pain control with acetaminophen alone (or occasionally with small doses of a narcotic for a short time) is generally preferred. NSAID use is described in detail in Chapter 77. *Muscle relaxants* are not first-line therapeutic agents but should be considered for the patient with significant muscle spasm on physical examination. Cyclobenzaprine is more efficacious than placebo in the treatment of intractable pain syndromes associated with muscle spasm (39). Most patients have a beneficial response to the drug at a dosage of 10 mg once a day. The dosage may be increased up to 10 mg three times a day, but this is associated with a greater frequency of drowsiness and dry mouth. Taking the drug 2 hours or more before bedtime may limit early morning drowsiness. This efficacy of cyclobenzaprine may be judged after a 7- to 10-day trial. Other muscle relaxants that may be useful, if cyclobenzaprine is ineffective, include methocarbamol 750 mg four times a day, chlorzoxazone 500 mg four times a day, or orphenadrine citrate 100 mg twice a day (40). Drugs used for muscle spasticity, Tizanidine 1 mg or 2 mg at night, may also be helpful in some patients. Diazepam is no more effective than placebo in improving back spasm (41). This drug should not be used for patients with low back pain. Neither biofeedback nor acupuncture is recommended by the Agency for Health Care Policy and Research (33) for the treatment of patients with acute low back pain.

During the recovery period, the patient should be advised to avoid activities that greatly increase the forces applied to the lower spine (e.g., lifting, pushing, force on outstretched upper extremity, as in making beds or vacuuming, lurching, or bending). If the patient fails to respond or pain recurs, the patient should be reexamined 3 to 4 weeks later to investigate the possibility of a medical (systemic) cause of back pain. If a mechanical cause remains the most likely diagnosis, a modification in drug therapy (prescribing an alternative nonsteroidal and, if needed, muscle relaxant drug) is indicated.

For the patient who is recovering satisfactorily, various exercise programs have been advocated. One simple back strengthening exercise program combines isometric gluteal and abdominal muscle contractions and pelvic tilt (Fig. 71.3). These exercises, which are performed standing with the back against a wall, should be recommended as soon as tolerated (see above).

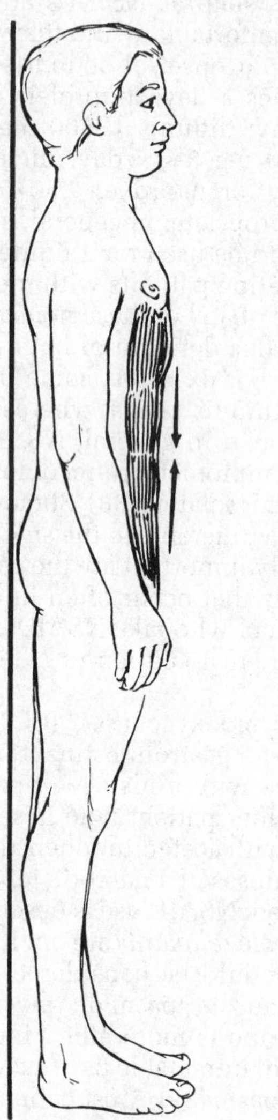

CONTRACT the abdominal muscles (pull umbilicus toward spine as hard as possible). Relax.

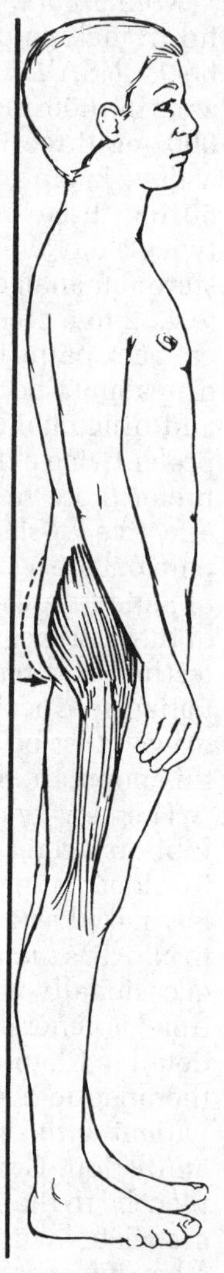

CONTRACT the gluteal muscles. Relax.

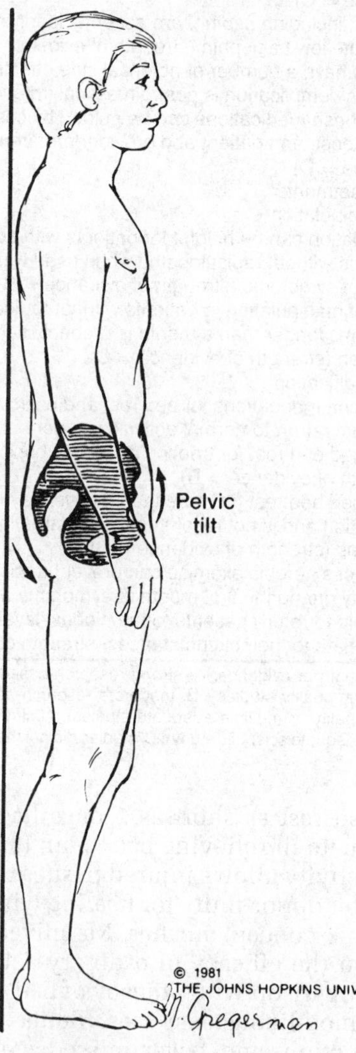

COMBINE abdominal and gluteal contractions, (produces a pelvic tilt with flexion of the lumbar spine). Relax.

Figure 71.3. Exercises: abdominal muscles and pelvic tilt.

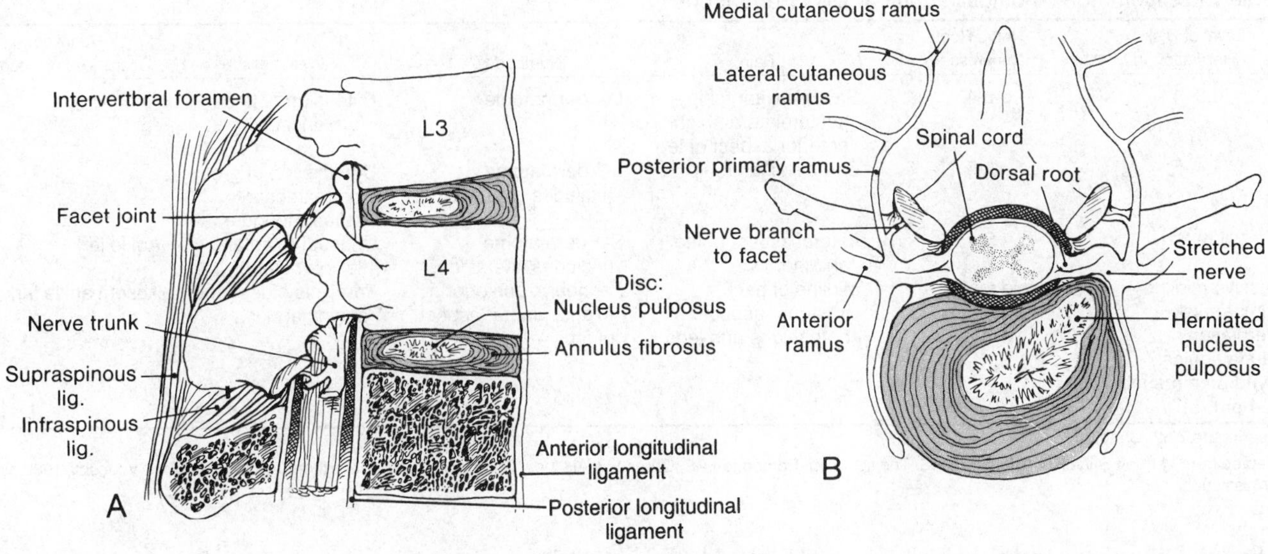

Figure 71.4. Normal disk. **B:** Herniated disk.

These exercises strengthen the muscles that support the spine and may relieve current symptoms and help prevent future episodes of back pain. The exercises should be performed for a few minutes four to six times a day. Exercises designed to strengthen the abdominal musculature, such as sit-ups with the knees flexed or STL, increase intradiscal pressure, may exacerbate symptoms, and are not recommended (however, see below for management of intercritical period).

Braces are reserved for the occasional patient with persisting back pain who must remain active while healing continues. However, only limited data support their use. Lumbosacral supports theoretically help relieve back pain by increasing intra-abdominal pressure, which results in greater support of the vertebral column, allowing paraspinous muscles to relax. The lumbosacral support may be a cloth corset fitted with metal stays posteriorly or a smaller cloth brace with a molded plastic insert. The patient should be provided a prescription for the corset or brace which will be fitted by an orthotist or physical therapist. The patient should use the support while working and then remove the appliance. The use of a lumbosacral support weakens supporting back muscles, so patients should be weaned gradually but steadily from their supports. It is important for this group of patients to return gradually to full activity because an abrupt return may cause a recurrence of low back pain. Although the use of a prophylactic lumbar brace will not prevent the onset of low back pain, the use of such a device seems to decrease the degree of pain workers experience while continuing to work (42).

Herniated Intervertebral Disk

The intervertebral disk is composed of the annulus fibrosus and the nucleus pulposus. The annulus fibrosus maintains pressure on the contents of the nucleus pulposus, allowing the intervertebral disk to cushion the forces placed on the spine. Tears in the annulus fibrosus allow the contents of the nucleus pulposus to herniate beyond their normal confines. Tears in the annulus may be associated with transient episodes of low back pain. Herniation of the nucleus may result in sudden severe pain if neural elements are compressed and inflamed by the nuclear contents (Fig. 71.4). A sudden pressure placed on the lumbar spine that may occur with flexion (e.g., bending over to lift a heavy object, lifting with the arms extended away from the body, a sudden lurch, or even a sneeze or cough) can precipitate the rupture. However, many patients who have a herniated disk do not give a history of injury or of a sudden increase in pressure. Lumbar disk disease is most common at the L4–5 and L5–S1 levels and is less common between the other vertebral bodies.

Diagnosis

Patients with herniated intervertebral disks complain of sharp lancinating pain. The pain radiates from the back down the leg in the anatomic distribution of the affected nerve root. The pain may be so severe that the patient resists examination and splints the back in an awkward position of lateral lumbar flexion and hip flexion. Patients with bilateral sciatica (pain in the distribution of the sciatic nerve L5–S1 roots [buttocks, posterior thighs, and extending below the knees]), progressive muscle weakness, or bladder or bowel incontinence should be evaluated for cauda equina compression (see above). The diagnosis of acute intervertebral disk herniation is most likely when physical examination reveals signs of nerve root compression with either a loss of motor function, loss of deep tendon reflexes, or a localized sensory deficit. Specific disk herniations may result in well-defined motor, sensory, and

Table 71.3. Common Findings in Lumbar Disk Herniations

Level of Disk Herniation	Nerve Root Compressed	Pain	Numbness[a]	Weakness	Reflexes (Decreased or Absent)
L3–4	L-4	Sacroiliac joint, hip, posterolateral thigh, anterior aspect of leg	L-4 dermatome	Extension of knee (quadriceps)	Knee jerk
L4–5	L-5	Sacroiliac joint, hip	L-5 dermatome (includes great toe)	Dorsiflexion of great toe (extensor hallucis longus)	
L5–S1	S-1	Lateral aspect of leg and foot	S-1 dermatome (includes lateral toes)	Unusual (plantar flexion of foot)	Ankle jerk
Massive midline lumbar disk herniation Cauda equina syndrome (usually L-4 or L-5)	Multiple roots in dural sac	Midline of back, posterior aspect of both thighs and legs	Perineum, posterior thighs, plantar aspect of feet	Paralysis of feet and sphincters	Absent ankle jerk

[a]See Figure 78.2, Chapter 78.

Adapted from Vanden Briuk KD, Edmonson AS. The spine. In: Edmonson AS, Crenshaw AH, eds. Campbell's operative orthopaedics. St. Louis: CV Mosby, 1980, with permission.

reflex deficits that aid in their diagnosis (Table 71.3). Patients with progressive neurologic deficits, particularly muscle weakness, should be referred to an orthopedist or neurosurgeon for close observation. These patients may benefit from early surgical intervention before a course of conservative therapy.

Documentation of the anatomic abnormality associated with radicular pain is necessary for patients who have continued pain despite a 3- to 4-week course of conservative therapy. A number of radiographic techniques may be useful for demonstrating disk herniation. In the past, CT and myelography were the preferred techniques to identify herniated disks. MRI readily identifies the location of herniated disks without the need for myelographic dye or radiation exposure (43). Therefore, in most circumstances, MRI examination has replaced the myelogram as the current preferred test by most surgeons for documenting disk herniation. Preliminary studies suggest that the uptake of MRI contrast (gadolinium) by sequestrated disks may identify abnormalities that will resorb spontaneously without the need for surgical excision (44). *Electromyography* is occasionally necessary for demonstrating the nerve root level associated with denervation of leg muscles. Electromyography may also be able to differentiate by the pattern of muscle involvement patients with herniated disk and those with peripheral sciatic nerve abnormalities secondary to another problem such as trauma or tumor. Its use is recommended only after consultation with an orthopedist, neurosurgeon, or neurologist.

Management

The treatment for most patients with a herniated disk is nonoperative because 80% of them respond to conservative therapy (see below) and are completely free of pain within 2 months. In patients whose pain and other neurologic abnormalities remit without surgical reduction of the disk, an adjustment of the annulus and posterior longitudinal ligament to the presence of the herniated disk fragment is the most likely reason for the diminution of edema, inflammation, back pain, and leg pain. Also, desiccation of the fragment may play a role in resolution of symptoms.

Conservative therapy consists of limiting physical activity with the patient at bed rest in the semi-Fowler position (hips and knees flexed, supported by pillows) for 2 days. Nonsteroidal anti-inflammatory analgesics and muscle relaxants, as described above, and narcotic analgesics (if the pain is severe) should be prescribed. However, patients whose symptoms are so pronounced that narcotics are required beyond 2 to 3 days and the individuals is unable to ambulate should be hospitalized until pain control is satisfactory, and an orthopedist or neurosurgeon should be consulted. Physical therapy is usually unnecessary in treating patients with acute disk herniations. Active exercise programs may intensify acute symptoms and should be avoided. Therapy such as ultrasound, short wave, diathermy, heat, or cold packs may provide short-term pain relief only (as they do in lumbosacral pain) but do not alter disk lesions or have any long-term effect on symptoms. Lumbar traction has not been shown to be more effective than bed rest in the treatment of lumbar disk disease and low back pain and is not indicated (45,46). Patients should be prescribed such a conservative regimen for 3 to 4 weeks, and if this fails they should consider epidural corticosteroid injection performed by a neurosurgeon, orthopedist, or rheumatologist. A series of three injections over 3 to 6 weeks may improve back and leg pain (47). Epidural injections can be helpful for reducing pain and improving sensory function early in the course of sciatica secondary to a herniated disk (48). Surgical decompression of the appropriate disk space is indicated for persistent pain resistant to conservative therapy. The size of the disk herniation does not correlate with a lack of response to conservative management. Large herniated disks are more likely to decrease in size as documented by CT and by contrast MRI (44,49). New minimally invasive techniques are being used for the removal of accessible disk fragments. These surgeries are associated with less damage to paraspinous soft tissues. Further investigation is needed to determine the efficacy of these techniques, such as arthroscopic discectomy, in comparison with standard discectomies (50). For management of the intercritical period, see Management of the Intercritical Period, below.

Osteoarthritis and Spinal Stenosis

The lumbar spine is one of the common locations for osteoarthritis. This joint disease is associated with joint pain, stiffness, deformity, and limitation of motion. Alterations over time secondary to osteoarthritis result in loss of disk volume, increased pressure on apophyseal joints, and hypertrophy of soft tissue and bony structures, resulting in a decrease in the size of the spinal canal. Osteoarthritis is discussed fully in Chapter 75.

Diagnosis

Initially, patients may complain of pain after repeated episodes of hyperextension that traumatizes the apophyseal (facet) joints, resulting in a stretching or tearing of the ligamentous capsule of the apophyseal joint. Typically, back flexion (bending forward) relieves the pain, whereas hyperextension (e.g., a painter working overhead) exacerbates it. Patients may also experience back pain related to gradual degeneration of the intervertebral disk or the development of osteophytes, either of which may impinge on a nerve root. Patients with lumbar osteoarthritis or degenerative disk disease describe back, buttock, or unilateral lower extremity pain. Examination usually reveals evidence of irritation of a specific nerve root, resulting in loss of a localized motor or sensory neurologic function or of an absent deep tendon reflex (L5–S1 disk, ankle or L3–4 disk, knee). The SLR may be positive. Many of these patients respond to conservative therapy because the anti-inflammatory action of the nonsteroidal drugs is effective in diminishing the swelling of the soft tissues, which causes nerve impingement.

As patients grow older, particularly during the fifth to seventh decade, back symptoms become suggestive of impingement of multiple nerve roots at different levels on both sides of the spinal cord. Spinal stenosis occurs most commonly in men, who complain of chronic low back pain with unilateral or bilateral lower extremity discomfort, exacerbated by extension of the spine while standing. They also may develop frank hyperesthesia or dysesthesias (Table 71.1). There also may be a history of disk surgery. Many patients with spinal stenosis have symptoms of claudication mimicking those of peripheral vascular insufficiency (51). These patients develop lower extremity pain while standing or walking or hyperextension of the spine in the absence of any evidence of peripheral vascular disease. Painful paresthesias are present in the feet or legs and may radiate to the hip girdle or lower trunk. Patients may experience lower extremity numbness and weakness. These symptoms are relieved by rest or flexion of the spine (the patient may report relief by bending forward as if to tie shoelaces). Physical examination may show no abnormalities until the patient is asked to walk. In this regard, the patient suspected of having spinal stenosis should be walked until pain develops—sometimes this requires many minutes—and then examined in the sitting position; abnormal motor or sensory deficits may be present only after such increased activity.

Plain x-rays show degenerative changes in the apophyseal joints (facet joints) and decreased anteroposterior canal diameter. CT is the best diagnostic radiographic technique for spinal stenosis (52). CT shows the narrowed canal or the impingement of osteophytes on the intervertebral foramina.

Management

Most patients with spinal stenosis can be treated nonsurgically. Activities that bring on pain should be discouraged. Patients may respond to NSAIDs or a course of epidural corticosteroid injections (administered by a consulting rheumatologist, neurosurgeon, anesthesiologist, or orthopedist). Operative therapy for spinal stenosis is reserved for patients who are severely incapacitated by their condition. Surgery for spinal stenosis requires decompression of the bony impingement of the spinal cord and nervi erigentes. If vertebral instability is documented before surgery, fusion of the vertebral bodies is accomplished also. Postoperative relief of pain is seen within a week or so and full recovery, when surgery is successful, within a month. Patients treated successfully with surgery have a more rapid and greater improvement in neurogenic claudication than medically treated patients. However, only two-thirds of patients describe improvement with initial decompressive surgery (53). Also, medically treated patients have no severe deterioration of neurologic function. Therefore, medical treatment for 2 to 3 years before considering surgery seems to be a good approach for most patients with spinal stenosis (54). Another study reported that 80% of individuals experienced immediate postsurgical improvement of neurogenic claudication. At 4-year follow-up, 70% of the surgical group continued with improved symptoms compared with 52% of patients treated nonsurgically (55).

MEDICAL (SYSTEMIC) BACK PAIN SYNDROMES

Spondyloarthropathies

Patients with spondyloarthropathies (ankylosing spondylitis, reactive arthritis, psoriatic spondylitis, enteropathic spondylitis) often complain of low back, buttock, or leg pain. These patients have morning stiffness as a major component of their symptom complex. Although back pain is the first symptom in a number of young patients, it is often associated with other symptoms and signs of the specific disorder (iritis, conjunctivitis, or skin rash). A clue to the presence of a spondyloarthropathy on physical examination is tenderness with percussion over the axial skeleton or sacroiliac joints. The sacroiliac joints may be painful when stressed while the patient is in the prone or supine position. Conditions affecting the axial skeleton and sacroiliac joints are discussed in Chapter 78.

Infections

Although rare, infection of the axial skeleton (osteomyelitis, discitis, or septic arthritis) must be considered in any patient with back pain (56). Osteomyelitis is an infection of the vertebral bodies. Discitis is an infection of the intervertebral disk (57). Septic arthritis of the back is an infection of the sacroiliac joints. These conditions are discussed in detail in Chapter 40.

Vertebral Fractures

Vertebral compression fractures are common, especially among the elderly, and usually the result of a flexion injury when the spine is abruptly flexed as it is, for example, during jumping. Fractures conceivably could be classified as a regional (mechanical) cause of back pain. It is arbitrarily classified as a medical (systemic) cause of low back pain because it most typically occurs in the elderly and often it is a manifestation of a systemic disorder such as osteoporosis. The thoracic spine is most commonly involved. The force needed to compress a vertebral body in healthy bone is considerable. However, when the bone is diseased, as it is with osteoporosis, multiple myeloma, metastatic cancer, or hyperparathyroidism, the injury may be insignificant. Pain is usually localized and immediate, although it may be delayed for several days after the fracture. Often tenderness over a single vertebra indicates the presence of a fracture, but an x-ray is necessary to confirm the diagnosis.

Other radiographic techniques are useful for identifying the locations of fractures that may not be detected by plain x-rays. A bone scan is often useful in demonstrating whether there are single or multiple fractures. CT, MRI, or myelography (the selection determined in consultation with an orthopedist and radiologist) is indicated for patients with compression fractures who also have neurologic deficits. These techniques can localize abnormalities associated with nerve impingement. Not all processes that weaken bone are detected by bone scan (e.g., multiple myeloma). Blood chemistries, including the concentration of serum proteins, and the serum and urine electrophoretic pattern of proteins are helpful in identifying patients with myeloma.

With lumbar or thoracic vertebral compression fractures, management includes rest, adequate analgesia, and gradual ambulation when the patient is free from severe pain. A lumbosacral support or, for the patient with a thoracic vertebral fracture, a chair-back or hyperextension brace may be helpful in alleviating pain. These may be obtained by prescription from an orthopedic appliance shop. The pain from a vertebral fracture may persist for several months, although the severe and incapacitating component is usually of only 2 to 3 weeks' duration.

Tumors

Tumors of the lumbar spine are unusual causes of back pain; however, these diseases are associated with the highest morbidity, mortality, and dysfunction. Patients with tumors of the lumbar spine usually have back pain as their initial complaint. Commonly, patients with tumor-associated pain have increased discomfort with recumbency. Physical examination demonstrates localized tenderness and neurologic dysfunction if the spinal cord or a nerve root is compressed. Although laboratory evaluation often yields nonspecific results, radiographic evaluation is useful in identifying the location and type of neoplastic lesion. In general, benign tumors are located in the posterior elements of vertebrae (spinous, transverse process), and malignant (both primary and metastatic) tumors are located in the anterior components of vertebrae (body). The definitive diagnosis of a tumor must be derived from histologic examination of biopsy material obtained from the lesion. The most effective therapy for both benign and malignant tumors is removal of the lesions that are accessible to surgical excision. When excision is impossible, partial resection, radiation therapy, corticosteroids, or chemotherapy may be indicated to control symptoms and compression of the spinal cord and nerve roots.

Referred Pain

Disease processes that affect organs in the retroperitoneum not only may cause pain locally but may refer pain in the distribution of the sensory nerve supplying the diseased tissue. Diseases of the vascular, genitourinary, and gastrointestinal systems may refer pain to the lumbar spine. Characteristically, referred pain is unaffected by the physical position of the patient. Patients usually have symptoms in the affected organ, raising the possibility of a medical cause of the patient's back pain (Tables 71.4 and 71.5).

MANAGEMENT OF THE INTERCRITICAL PERIOD

Although most patients with low back pain have a complete remission of symptoms within 3 to 4 weeks, many patients experience a recurrence (8). Patients should return to the physician's office even if they have had a resolution of their pain. The purpose of these visits is to discuss ways to prevent recurrent attacks of back pain by focusing education on posture, weight control, exercise, and work activities.

Figure 71.5 shows some correct and incorrect postures and practical advice that may be useful to give to patients who have experienced low back pain. Weight reduction is desirable in the obese patient, because excessive weight directly increases the load on the lower vertebral column and its supporting structures. Exercise initiated as soon as the acute pain subsides (usually 2 to 4 days after its onset) improves function and decreases pain (58). At a minimum, such

Table 71.4. Medical Causes of Low Back Pain

Systemic: Constitutional symptoms, severe localized pain, morning stiffness are clues suggestive of generalized disorder.
- Rheumatologic: spondyloarthropathies, polymyalgia rheumatica, fibromyalgia
- Infectious; vertebral osteomyelitis, Pott disease (tuberculosis of spine), discitis, septic arthritis, epidural abscess, herpes zoster
- Neoplastic:
  - Benign: osteoid osteoma, osteochondroma, giant cell tumor
  - Malignant: metastatic, multiple myeloma, chondrosarcoma, chordoma, lymphoma, retroperitoneal sarcoma, neural tumor
- Neurologic-psychiatric: neuropathic (Charcot) joints, femoral neuropathy, depression, hysteria
- Miscellaneous: vertebral sarcoidosis, Paget disease, retroperitoneal fibrosis

Referred pain: The absence of any tenderness, limitation of motion, or aggravation of pain or spasm during the physical examination is suggestive of referred pain (see Table 71.5 for dermatome to which pain from various visceral structures may be referred).
- Lower thoracic and upper lumbar pain from an upper abdominal disease process (e.g., pancreas)
- Low lumbar pain from a lower abdominal disease process (e.g., aortic aneurysm)
- Sacral pain from a pelvic problem (e.g., endometriosis, prostate cancer)

Table 71.5. Dermatome to Which Pain from Various Visceral Structures May Be Referred

Dermatome[a]	Viscera
L-1	Kidney, ureter, body of uterus, abdominal aorta, small intestine
L-2	Bladder, abdominal aorta, ascending colon
L-3	Abdominal aorta
L-4	Abdominal aorta
L-5, S-1, S-2	—
S-3	Rectum, anus, lower portion of bladder, cervix, upper vagina, prostate
S-4	Rectum, anus, base of bladder, cervix, upper vagina, prostate
S-5	—

[a]See Figure 78.2, Chapter 78, for cutaneous pattern of dermatomes.

Modified from Borenstein DG, Wiesel SW. Low back pain. Philadelphia: W.B. Saunders, 1989;33, with permission.

exercises alert patients to their back problem, which increases the likelihood of performing daily activities in a way that may allow them to avoid reinjury. Certainly, prolonged bed rest weakens back muscles and should be avoided. Furthermore, certain advice to the patient regarding lifting is prudent. Sudden loading of the spine when the back is flexed and the knees are straight markedly increases forces placed on the lumbar spine (Fig. 71.2) compared with when the knees are bent and the back is straight. Exercises that strengthen the quadriceps (extend knees) are theoretically sound for anyone who may have to lift at all. These exercises include swimming, cycling, or jogging on a flat even surface. The patient should be advised to exercise only if it does not initiate or increase back pain. In addition, because the abdominal muscles are important in supporting the spine when a weight is brought to bear on it, exercises that strengthen the abdominal muscles (Fig. 71.3) are helpful. Patient education is an effective component in the treatment of all patients who have experienced back pain. Education about such matters may improve a patient's life-style and the likelihood of returning to work (59). So-called back schools have been organized in many worksites. These are generally conducted by physical therapists. However, a large controlled trial of an educational program to prevent low back injuries organized as a back school for postal workers failed to prevent work-associated back injury in employees with or without a history of back injury, although the knowledge of safe behavior was increased by the training (60).

Complementary therapies are used frequently for a variety of medical problems, including low back pain (61). A wide variety of therapies has been promoted for the therapy of low back pain. These therapies have included spinal manipulation, massage, acupuncture, and magnets, among others. Acupuncture and chiropractic are discussed in Chapter 5.

Spinal manipulation seems to help many patients and has been recommended by the practice guidelines published by the Agency for Health Care Policy and Research (33). These guidelines do not specifically recommend that manipulation is done by a chiropractor. Initial evaluation of low back pain by a *chiropractor* may not include screening evaluation with history and physical examination for systemic disorders. Also, chiropractors generally do not offer additional therapies beyond those offered by an experienced physical therapist. Patient satisfaction with chiropractors seems to be related to the chiropractor's willingness to spend more time with the patient and listen to his or her concerns (62,63). Too often physicians and physical therapists do not show such a level of concern and may even minimize the patient's problems. Studies of manipulation of the back do not define precisely what is a standard manipulation or what it accomplishes physiologically, making comparisons of it with other treatments impossible.

Therapeutic massage has benefit for many individuals with chronic low back pain. This therapy given once a week over 10 weeks has demonstrated benefit months after the last treatment. The efficacy of this form of treatment is limited to the availability of experienced massage therapists (64). This same study failed to identify significant benefit of acupuncture for chronic low back pain. Acupuncture techniques can vary, and this may have an effect on the outcome of a clinical trial. Anecdotally, patients have described benefit of additional analgesia associated with acupuncture treatments. Additional trials are warranted to determine the efficacy of this treatment.

Magnets have also been suggested as effective for the treatment of low back pain. A pilot double-blind placebo-controlled trial using magnets for low back pain demonstrated no significant difference between study groups (65).

The patient may need to modify *work or athletic activities* once an episode of back pain occurs. It should be noted, however, that there is no convincing

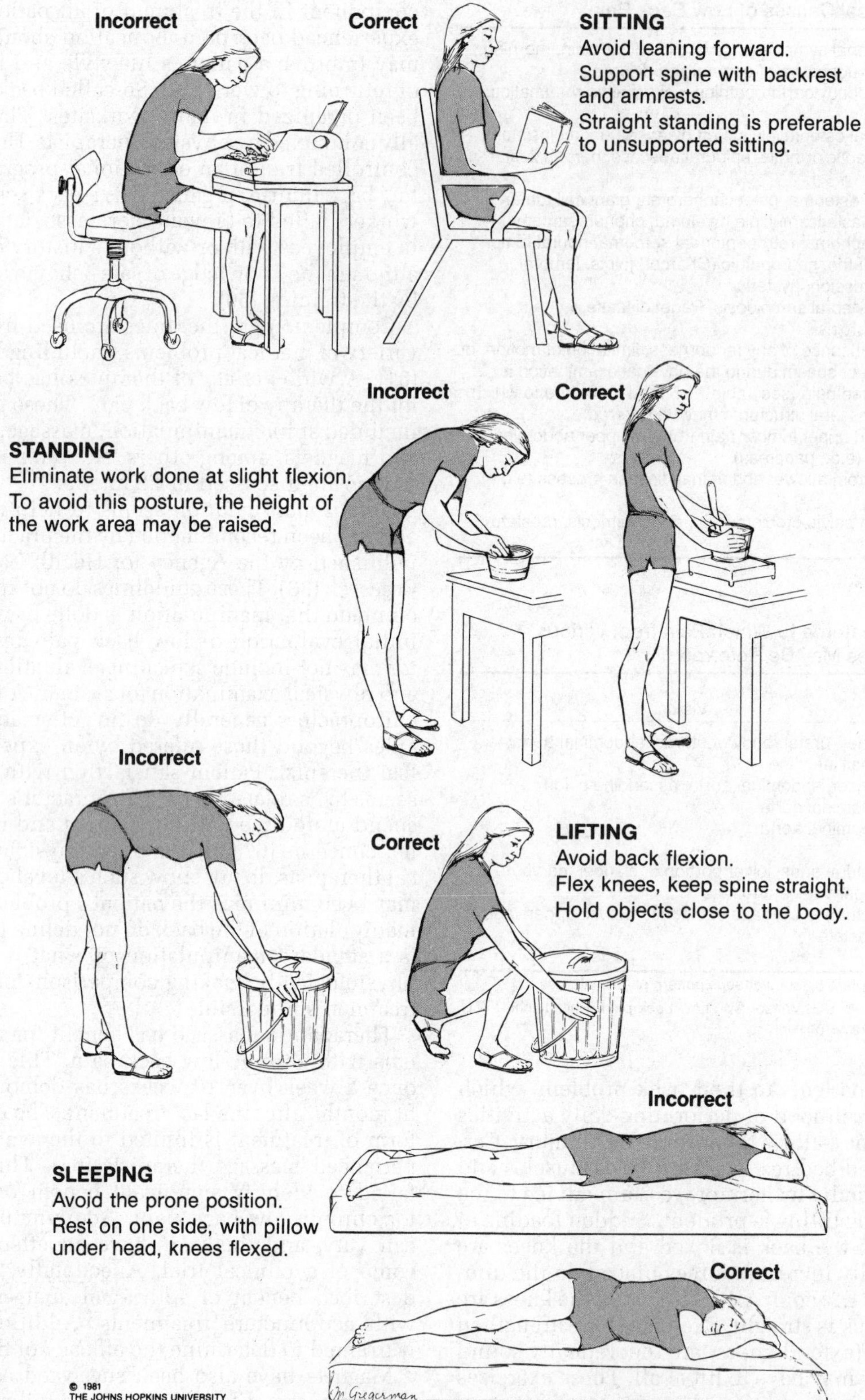
Incorrect
Correct
SITTING
Avoid leaning forward.
Support spine with backrest and armrests.
Straight standing is preferable to unsupported sitting.
Incorrect
Correct
STANDING
Eliminate work done at slight flexion.
To avoid this posture, the height of the work area may be raised.
Incorrect
Correct
LIFTING
Avoid back flexion.
Flex knees, keep spine straight.
Hold objects close to the body.
Incorrect
SLEEPING
Avoid the prone position.
Rest on one side, with pillow under head, knees flexed.
Correct
© 1981
THE JOHNS HOPKINS UNIVERSITY
M. Gregerman

Figure 71.5. Incorrect and correct postural attitudes.

evidence to support the concept that heavy labor or lifting predisposes to the development of the initial episode of back pain (66). Certain factors do predispose patients to injury, including improper technique in lifting, sitting for prolonged periods or not at all during the workday, and sudden maximal physical activity (e.g., participation in an occasional vigorous game without conditioning). Furthermore, back pain occurs more often in people who consider their occupation to be physically hard and in those who believe their work to be stressful to the spine or who are dissatisfied with their work (67–69).

General References

Borenstein DG, Burton JR. Lumbar spine disease in the elderly. J Am Geriatr Soc 1993;41:167.

A clinical review of back pain as commonly encountered in the elderly.

Borenstein DG, Wiesel SW, Boden SD. Low back pain: medical diagnosis and comprehensive management, 2nd ed. Philadelphia: W.B. Saunders, 1995.

A reference for all causes of low back pain.

Deville WLJM, van der Windt DAWM, Dzaferagic A, et al. The test of Lasegue: systematic review of the accuracy in diagnosing herniated disc. Spine 2000;25:1140.

Deyo RA, Weinstein JN. Low back pain. N Engl J Med 2001;344:363.

A good review of diagnosis and management of low back pain

Macnab I, McCulloch JA. Backache, 2nd ed. Baltimore: Williams & Wilkins, 1989.

A well-illustrated monograph of mechanical disorders of lumbar spine.

Nordin M, Anderson GBJ, Pope MH, eds. Musculoskeletal disorders in the workplace: principles and practice. St. Louis: CV Mosby, 1997.

A well-referenced encyclopedic text with a very good section on low back pain.

Steinberg GG, Akins CM, Baran DT, eds. Ramamurti's orthopaedics in primary care, 2nd ed. Baltimore: Williams & Wilkins, 1992.

An orthopedic-focused text that is practical and helpful.

Von Korff M, Moore JC. Stepped care for back pain: activating approaches for primary care. Ann Intern Med 2001;134:911.

A suggested method of approaching patients with back pain so that functional and fear aspects will not be overlooked.

Specific References

1. Frymoyer JW, Pope MH, Costanza MC, et al. Epidemiologic studies of low back pain. Spine 1980;5:419.
2. Nervill RLM, Turner JG. Orthopaedic disorders in general practice. Boston: Butterworth, 1985:35.
3. Hart LG, Deyo RA, Cherkin DC. Physician office visits for low back pain: frequency, clinical evaluation, and treatment patterns from a US national survey. Spine 1995;20:11.
4. Edgar MA, Ghadially JA. Innervation of the lumbar spine. Clin Orthop 1976;115:35.
5. Wilke H, Need P, Caimi M, et al. New in vivo measurements of pressures in the intervertebral disc in daily life. Spine 1999;24:755.
6. Hult L. Cervical, dorsal and lumbar spinal syndromes. Acta Orthop Scand 1954;17[Suppl]:1.
7. Dillane JB, Fry J, Kalton G. Acute back syndrome: study from general practice. BMJ 1966;3:82.
8. Van den Hoogen HJM, Koes BW, van Eijk JTM, et al. The prognosis of low back pain in general practice. Spine 1997;22:1515.
9. Deyo RA, Rainville J, Kent DL. What can the history and physical examination tell us about low back pain? JAMA 1992;268:760.
10. Hall H. Examination of the patient with low back pain. Bull Rheum Dis 1983;33:1.
11. Vroomen PC, de Krom MC, Knottnerus JA. Diagnostic value of history and physical examination in patients suspected of sciatica due to disc herniation: a systematic review. J Neurol 1999;246:899.
12. Hudgins WR. The crossed-straight leg-raising test. N Engl J Med 1977;297:1127.
13. Vaz M, Wadia RS, Gokhale SD. Another cause of positive crossed-straight-leg-raising test. N Engl J Med 1978;295:779.
14. Woodhall B, Hayes GJ. The well-leg raising test of Fajersztajn in the diagnosis of ruptured lumbar intervertebral disc. J Bone Joint Surg 1950;32A:786.
15. Shapiro S. Medical realities of cauda equina syndrome secondary to lumbar disc herniation. Spine 2000;25:348.
16. Waddell G, McCulloch JA, Kummel E, et al. Nonorganic physical signs in low-back pain. Spine 1980;5:117.
17. McCombe PF, Fairbank JCT, Cockersole BC, et al. Reproducibility of physical signs in low back pain. Spine 1989;14:908.
18. Jensen OH. The level-diagnosis of a lower lumbar disc herniation: the value of sensitivity and motor testing. Clin Rheumatol 1987;6:564.
19. Ensink F, Saur PMM, Frese K, et al. Lumbar range of motion: influence of time of day and individual factors on measurements. Spine 1996;21:1339.
20. Witt I, Vestergaard A, Rosenklint A. A comparative analysis of x-ray findings of the lumbar spine in patients with and without lumbar pain. Spine 1984;9:298.
21. Lawrence JS, Bremmer JM, Bier F. Osteo-arthrosis. Prevalence in the population and relationship between symptoms and x-ray changes. Ann Rheum Dis 1966;25:1.
22. Ardan GM. Bone destruction not demonstrable by radiography. Br J Radiol 1951;24:107.
23. Frazier LM, Carey TS, Lyles MF, et al. Selective criteria may increase lumbar-sacral spine roentgenogram use in acute low-back pain. Arch Intern Med 1989;149:147.
24. Albeck MJ, Hilden J, Kjaer L, et al. A controlled comparison of myelography, computed tomography, and magnetic resonance imaging in clinically suspected lumbar disc herniation. Spine 1995;20:443.
25. Modic MT, Ross JS. Magnetic resonance imaging in the evaluation of low back pain. Orthop Clin North Am 1991;22:283.
26. Alexander AR. Magnetic resonance imaging of the spine and spinal cord tumors. Spine State Art Rev 1988;2:499.
27. Boden SD, David DO, Dina T, et al. Abnormal magnetic resonance scans of the lumbar spine in asymptomatic subjects: a prospective investigation. J Bone Joint Surg 1990;72A:403.
28. Jensen MC, Brant-Zawadski MN, Obuchowski N, et al. Magnetic resonance imaging of the lumber spine in people without back pain. N Engl J Med 1994;331:69.
29. Wiesel SE, Tsourmas N, Feffer H, et al. A study of computer assisted tomography. 1. The incidence of positive CAT scan in an asymptomatic group of patients. Spine 1984;9:49.
30. Weishaupt D, Zanetti M, Hodler J, et al. MR imaging of the lumbar spine: prevalence of intervertebral disk extrusion and sequestration, nerve root compression, end plate abnormalities, and osteoarthritis of the facet joints in asymptomatic volunteers. Radiology 1998;209:661.
31. Coste J, Delecocuillerie G, Cohen de Lara A, et al. Clinical course and prognostic factors in acute low back pain: an inception cohort study in primary care practice. BMJ 1994;308:577.
32. Turek S. Orthopaedics: principles and their application. Philadelphia: JB Lippincott, 1984:1483.
33. Bigos SJ, Bowyer O, Braen G, et al. Acute low back problems in adults. Clinical Practice Guideline No. 14. AHCPR Publication No. 95-0642. Rockville, MD: Agency for Health Care Policy and Research, Public Health Service, U.S. Department of Health and Human Services, December 1994.
34. Cherkin DC, Wheeler KJ, Barlow W, et al. Medication use for low back pain in primary care. Spine 1998;23:607.
35. Deyo RA, Diehl AK, Rosenthal M. How many days of bed rest for acute low back pain? N Engl J Med 1986;315:1064.

36. Malmivaara A, Hakkinen U, Aro T, et al. The treatment of acute low back pain: bed rest, exercises, or ordinary activity? N Engl J Med 1995;332:351.
37. Faas A, Chavannes AW, van Eijk JTM, et al. A randomized, placebo-controlled trial of exercise therapy in patients with acute low back pain. Spine 1993;18:1388.
38. Koes BW, Scholten RJPM, Mens JMA, et al. Efficacy of nonsteroidal anti-inflammatory drugs for low back: a systematic review of randomized clinical trials. Ann Rheum Dis 1997;56:214.
39. Brown BR Jr, Womble J. Cyclobenzaprine in intractable pain syndromes with muscle spasm. JAMA 1978;240:1151.
40. Elenbaas JK. Centrally acting oral skeletal muscle relaxants. Am J Hosp Pharmacol 1980;37:1313.
41. Basmajian JV. Cyclobenzaprine hydrochloride effect on skeletal muscle in the lumbar region and neck: two double blind controlled clinical and laboratory studies. Arch Phys Med Rehabil 1978;59:58.
42. van Poppel MNM, Koes BW, van der Ploeg T, et al. Lumbar supports and education for the prevention of low back pain in industry: a randomized controlled trial. JAMA 1998;279:1789.
43. Boden SD. The use of radiographic imaging studies in the evaluation of patients who have degenerative disorders of the lumbar spine. J Bone Joint Surg 1996;78A:114.
44. Komori H, Okawa A, Haro H, et al. Contrast-enhanced magnetic resonance imaging in conservative management of lumbar disc herniation. Spine 1998;22:67.
45. Deyo RA. Conservative therapy for low back pain. Distinguishing useful from useless therapy. JAMA 1983;250:1057.
46. Beurskens AJ, de Vet HC, Koke AJ, et al. Efficacy of traction for nonspecific low back pain: 12-week and 6-month results of a randomized clinical trial. Spine 1997;22:2756.
47. Spaccarelli KC. Lumbar and caudal epidural corticosteroid injections. Mayo Clin Proc 1996;71:169.
48. Carette S, Leclaire R, Marcoux S, et al. Epidural corticosteroid injections for sciatica due to herniated nucleus pulposus. N Engl J Med 1997;336:1634.
49. Thelander U, Fagerland M, Friberg S, et al. Straight leg raising test versus radiologic size, shape, and position of lumbar disc hernias. Spine 1992;17:395.
50. Hermantin FU, Peters T, Quartararo L, et al. A prospective, randomized study comparing the results of open discectomy with those of video-assisted arthroscopic microdiscectomy. J Bone Joint Surg 1999;81A:958.
51. Karayannacos PE, Yashon D, Vasko JS. Narrow lumbar spinal canal with vascular syndromes. Arch Surg 1976;111:803.
52. Modic MT, Masaryk T, Boumphrey F, et al. Lumbar herniated disk disease and canal stenosis: prospective evaluation by surface coil MR, CT, and myelography. Am J Neuroradiol 1986;7:709.
53. Herno A, Airaksinen O, Saari T, et al. Surgical results of lumbar spinal stenosis: a comparison of patients with or without previous back surgery. Spine 1995;20:964.
54. Johnsson K, Uden A, Rosen I. The effect of decompression on the natural course of spinal stenosis: a comparison of surgically treated and untreated patients. Spine 1991;16:615.
55. Atlas SJ, Keller RB, Robson D, et al. Surgical and nonsurgical management of lumbar spinal stenosis: four-year outcomes from the Maine Lumbar Spine Study. Spine 2000;25:556.
56. Alamin TF, Hanley EN. Profiles of patients with spine infections. Semin Spine Surg 2000;12:212.
57. Zimmernman B, Lally EV. Infectious diseases of the spine. Semin Spine Surg 1995;7:177.
58. Estlander AM, Mellin G, Vanharanta H, et al. Effects and follow-up of multimodal treatment program including intensive physical training for low back pain patients. Scand J Rehabil Med 1991;23:97.
59. Rainville J, Ahem DK, Phalen L, et al. The association of pain with physical activities in chronic low back pain. Spine 1991;16[Suppl]:S198.
60. Daltroy LH, Iversen MD, Larson MG, et al. A controlled trial of an educational program to prevent low back injuries. N Engl J Med 1997;337:332.
61. Eisenberg DM, Davis RB, Ettner SL, et al. Trends in alternative medicine use in the United States, 1990-1997: results of a follow-up national survey. JAMA 1998;280:1569.
62. Cherkin DC, MacCornack FA. Patient evaluations of low back pain care from family physicians and chiropractors. West J Med 1989;150:351.
63. Kane RL, Leymaster C, Olsen D, et al. Manipulating the patient. A comparison of the effectiveness of physician and chiropractor care. Lancet 1974;1:1333.
64. Cherkin DC, Eisenberg D, Sherman KJ, et al. Randomized trial comparing traditional Chinese medical acupuncture, therapeutic massage, and self-care education for chronic low back pain. Arch Intern Med 2001;161:1081.
65. Collacott EA, Zimmerman JT, White DW, et al. Bipolar permanent magnets for the treatment of chronic low back pain: a pilot study. JAMA 2000;283:1322.
66. Rowe ML. Low back pain in industry. J Occup Med 1969;11:161.
67. Bigos SJ, Battie MC, Spengler DM, et al. A prospective study of work perceptions and psychosocial factors affecting the report of back injury. Spine 1991;16:1.
68. Dehlin O, Hedenrud B, Horal J. Back symptoms in nursing aides in a geriatric hospital. Scand J Rehabil Med 1976;8:47.
69. Krause N, Ragland DR, Fisher JM, et al. Psychological job factors, physical workload, and incidence of work-related spinal injury: a 5-year prospective study of urban transit operators. Spine 1998;23:2507.

CHAPTER 72

Knee and Leg Pain

RONALD P. BYANK, MD
ALI MOSHIRFAR, MD
SIMON C. MEARS, MD, PhD
JAMES F. WENZ, MD

A general knowledge of diagnosis and treatment options for various knee and leg problems is invaluable to the clinician. The joints of the lower extremity are constantly stressed with weight-bearing and at times experience joint reaction forces several times body weight. Overuse syndromes such as tendinitis, bursitis, and stress fractures are common in the lower extremity. This chapter presents a thorough overview of the anatomy of the knee, leg, and ankle and from this presents a common sense approach to the diagnosis, treatment, and prevention of knee and leg orthopedic problems.

PROBLEMS OF THE KNEE

Knee Anatomy

The knee is the largest joint in the body. It has both hinge-like and rotary motion (of the tibia on the femur) during flexion and extension. The principal anatomic components and their functions are as follow (Fig. 72.1):

- The knee joint is comprised of three articulations by the tibia, femur, and the patella: the lateral and medial tibiofemoral articulations and the patellofemoral articulation.
- The menisci are fibrocartilaginous buffers between the medial and lateral tibiofemoral joints. These structures act to distribute the weight borne by the joint and to absorb shock.
- Several muscles control the motion of the knee. Flexors are the hamstring muscles, which arise from the ischium and diverge to form the tendons that insert on the tibia (semimembranosus and semitendinosus muscles) and fibula (biceps femoris muscle), and the gastrocnemius muscle, which arises from the distal posterior femur and inserts on the calcaneus via the Achilles tendon. The extensors are the quadriceps muscles (rectus femoris, vastus medialis, vastus lateralis, and vastus intermedius) that originate from the ilium and femur and converge distally to form the common quadriceps tendon. The quadriceps tendon then attaches to the superior aspect of the patella, continuing as the patellar tendon to insert onto the tibial tubercle. The quadriceps muscles, quadriceps tendon, patella, and patellar tendon comprise the extensor mechanism, which allows for active extension of the knee joint.
- The collateral ligaments provide medial and lateral stability to the knee joint. The medial collateral ligament (MCL) arises from the medial femoral condyle and attaches to the medial proximal surface of the tibia. It resists valgus (medially directed) stresses applied to the knee. The lateral collateral ligament (LCL) attaches the lateral femoral condyle to the fibula and resists varus (laterally directed) stresses applied to the knee.
- The cruciate ligaments are intraarticular ligaments that stabilize the joint primarily in the anteroposterior plane. The anterior cruciate ligament (ACL) arises from the intercondylar eminence of the tibia and attaches posterosuperiorly to the medial aspect of the lateral femoral condyle. It resists anterior translation of the tibia on the femur. The posterior cruciate ligament (PCL) is attached posteriorly to the intercondylar fossa of the tibia and lateral meniscus and anterosuperiorly to the lateral aspect of the medial femoral condyle. The PCL resists posterior translation of the tibia with respect to the femur.
- The bursae of the knee, which provide lubrication between the many dynamic components of the knee, consist of the suprapatellar, prepatellar, superficial patellar tendon, retropatellar tendon, and pes

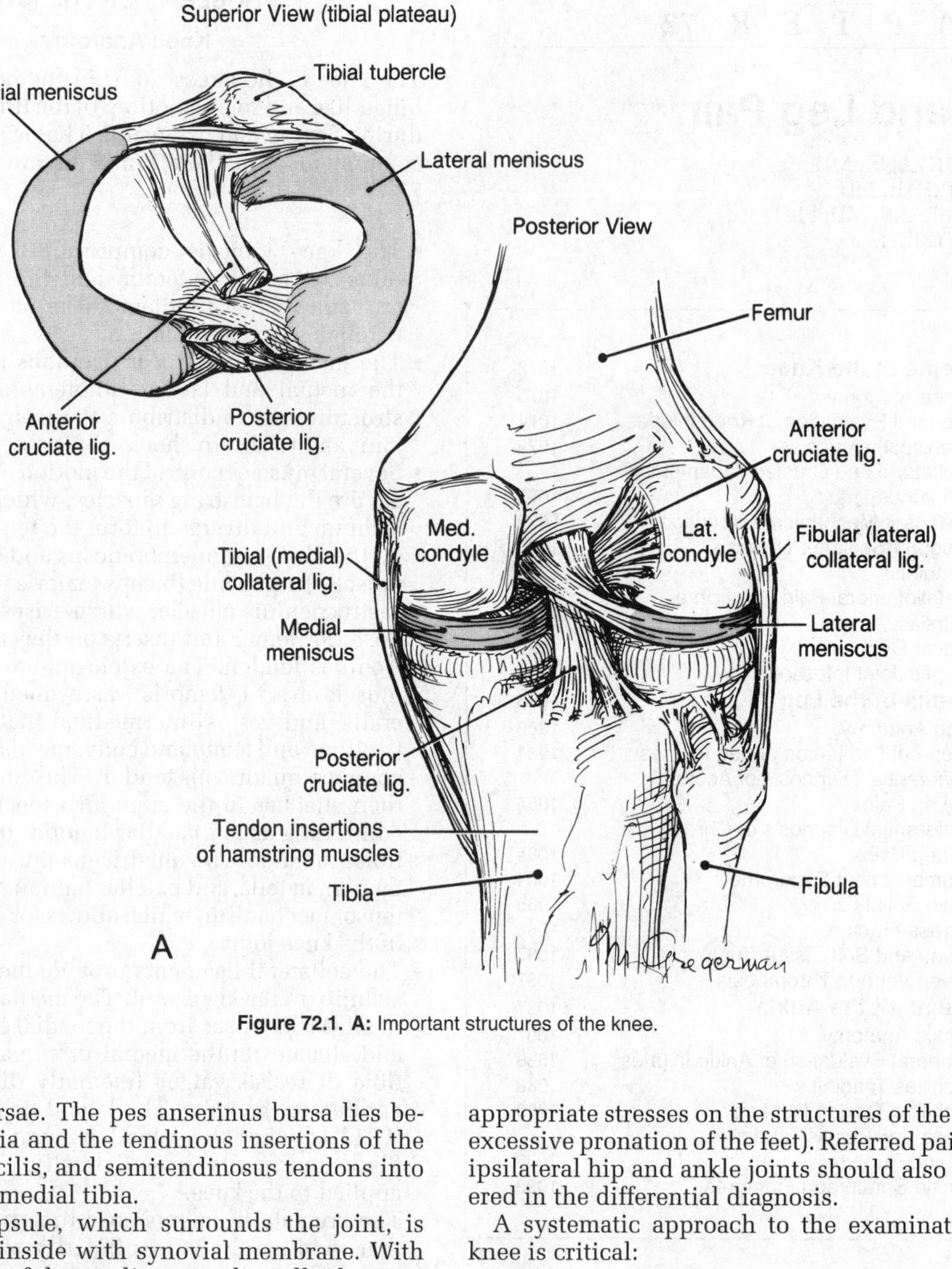

Superior View (tibial plateau)

Medial meniscus
Tibial tubercle
Lateral meniscus
Anterior cruciate lig.
Posterior cruciate lig.

Posterior View

Femur
Anterior cruciate lig.
Med. condyle
Lat. condyle
Fibular (lateral) collateral lig.
Tibial (medial) collateral lig.
Medial meniscus
Lateral meniscus
Posterior cruciate lig.
Tendon insertions of hamstring muscles
Tibia
Fibula

A

Figure 72.1. A: Important structures of the knee.

anserinus bursae. The pes anserinus bursa lies between the tibia and the tendinous insertions of the sartorius, gracilis, and semitendinosus tendons into the proximal medial tibia.

- The joint capsule, which surrounds the joint, is lined on the inside with synovial membrane. With the exception of the popliteus tendon, all other tendons lie outside the joint. The capsule is thickened medially and laterally around the patella. These areas are known as the medial and lateral patellar retinaculum.

General Evaluation of Knee Injuries

A traumatic knee injury may be caused by a single event in which the knee is suddenly stressed or by chronic or repetitive stress. When there is no history of sudden trauma, identification of three features is especially helpful in evaluating knee pain: Any recently initiated physical activities, a sudden change in the type or intensity of physical activities, and problems elsewhere in the lower extremity that may cause inappropriate stresses on the structures of the knee (e.g., excessive pronation of the feet). Referred pain from the ipsilateral hip and ankle joints should also be considered in the differential diagnosis.

A systematic approach to the examination of the knee is critical:

- The knee should be *inspected* in the extended supine position and in a seated 90-degree flexed position for any swelling, effusion, erythema, laceration, or wounds. The best reference for this is the contralateral normal knee. An effusion can usually be detected by asymmetry and the presence of a bulge on either side of the patellar tendon.
- Bony contours should be *palpated*, including the entire border of the patella for any tenderness or discontinuity in the quadriceps or patellar tendons. The tibiofemoral joint lines should be palpated for tenderness. The MCL and LCL should be stressed and palpated for tenderness. Most importantly, one should assess for knee effusion by patellar ballottement (Fig. 72.2). With the patient in the supine

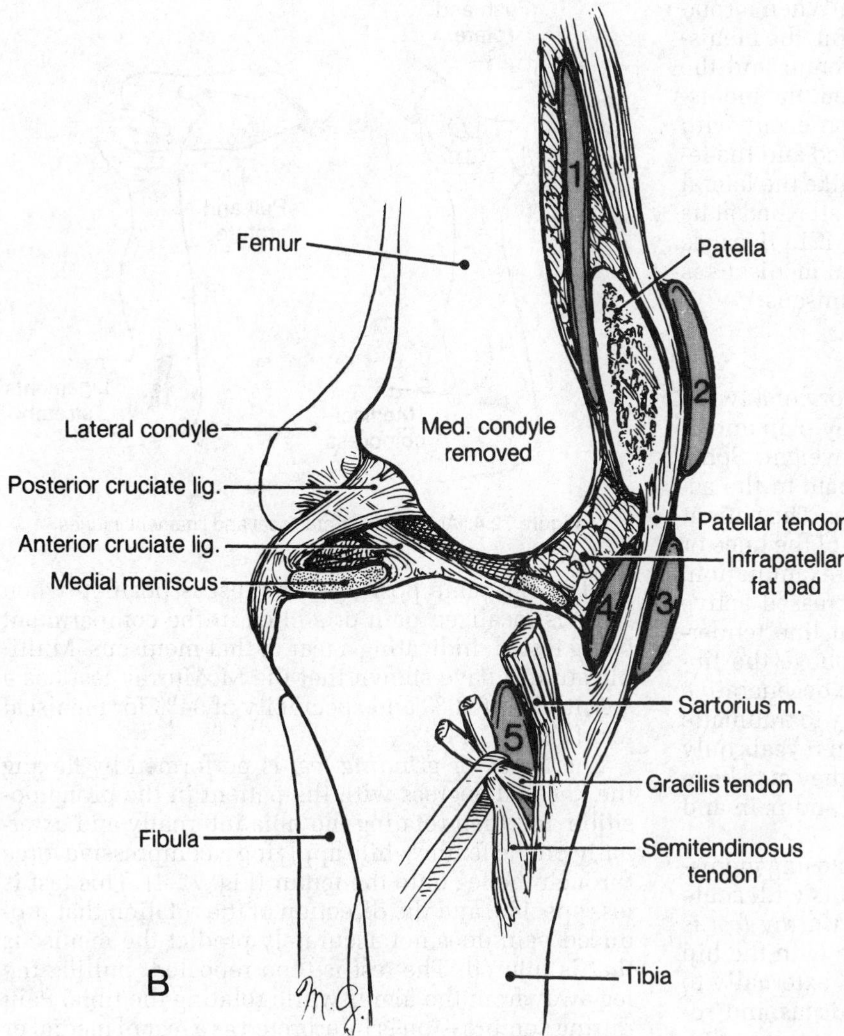

Figure 72.1. *(Continued)* **B:** Five bursae of the knee: suprapatellar, prepatellar, superficial patellar tendon, retropatellar tendon, and pes anserinus.

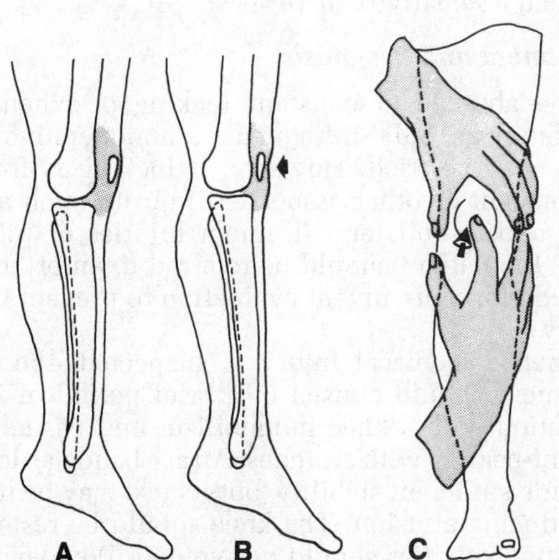

Figure 72.2. Examination for knee joint effusion in a patient in the supine position. **A:** The patella is forced away from the femur by effusion. **B:** The patella is forced down into the femur by the ballottement maneuver (lateral view). **C:** Anterior view of the ballottement maneuver.

position and the knee fully extended, the knee is compressed above and on either side of the patella to localize any fluid under the patella; then the patella is pressed down against the femur with a finger. If it is ballotable, an effusion exists.

- The knee should be placed through a *range of motion* of flexion and extension. The normal range of motion is from 0 degrees (or full extension) to 135 degrees of flexion (see Chapter 68 for a more detailed discussion of standard measurements of joint motion). Active and passive ranges of motion should be evaluated.
- The *strength* of the knee flexors and extensors should be assessed. This is quantified on a 0- to 5-point scale.
- Specific *provocative tests* to assess for particular injuries are discussed where appropriate below.

Meniscal Injuries

Definition and Mechanism of Injury

The medial and lateral menisci of the knee are fibrocartilaginous pads of tissue that function as shock absorbers between the tibia and femur. Meniscal tears commonly occur in young active patients and in older patients with more sedentary life-styles. When a rotatory force is applied to the flexed knee joint, the meniscus may become trapped between the femur and the tibia and then, when the knee is extended, the meniscus may be torn (1). The injury can also occur with pivoting activities when the foot is planted and the femur rotates with respect to the tibia. Unlike the lateral meniscus, the medial meniscus is firmly attached at its periphery to the joint capsule and the MCL. Because of its relative lack of mobility, the medial meniscus is torn more frequently than the lateral meniscus.

Signs and Symptoms

The patient usually presents with a history of a twisting flexion injury of the knee followed by pain and at times inability to flex the knee or bear weight. Some patients are able to continue to participate in the activity and then experience symptoms later. The patient may also report the feeling of instability of the knee or occasional locking of the knee joint. On examination, one can appreciate a knee effusion, decreased active and passive ranges of motion, and joint line tenderness along the meniscus (located just above the tibial plateau). An older patient may have a degenerative meniscal tear rather than a tear secondary to traumatic event. Examination of such patients often reveals only minimal joint line tenderness; however, they may have quadriceps muscle atrophy from disuse and pain and crepitus with range of motion.

Certain maneuvers are helpful in diagnosing meniscal injury, although more often for patients with acute rather than chronic symptoms. The *McMurray test* is performed with the patient lying supine with the hip and knee fully flexed; the foot is rotated externally to its full capacity to test the medial meniscus and rotated internally to test the lateral meniscus (Fig. 72.3). The knee and hip are then extended, with the foot

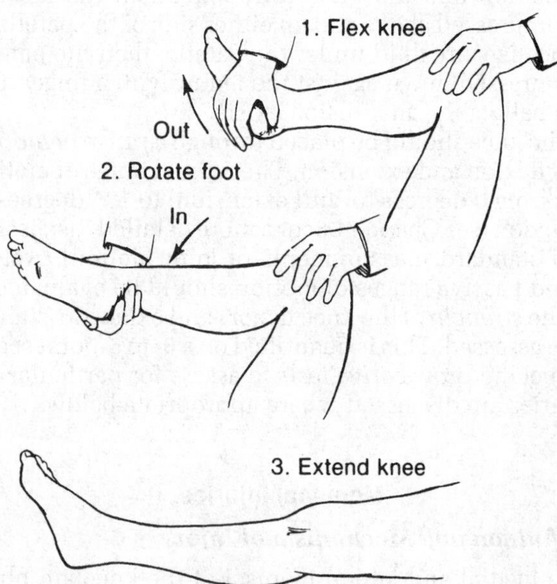

Figure 72.3. McMurray test for meniscal injuries.

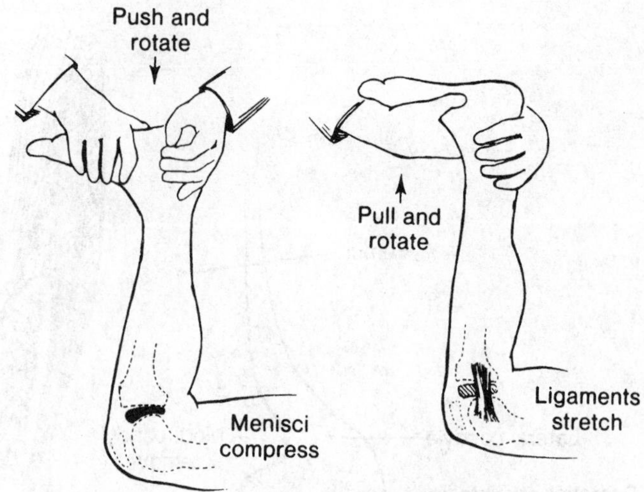

Figure 72.4. Apley test for meniscal and ligament injuries.

held in the same position. The test is positive when there is localized pain or a click in the compartment being tested, indicating a tear of that meniscus. Multiple studies have shown that the McMurray test has a sensitivity of 26% and specificity of 94% for meniscal tear (2).

The *Apley* or *grinding test* is performed by flexing the knee 90 degrees with the patient in the prone position and then rotating the tibia internally and externally on the femur while applying a compressive force through the leg onto the femur (Fig. 72.4). This test is less specific, and the direction of the rotation that produced pain does not accurately predict the meniscus that is injured. The test is then repeated, pulling the leg away from the femur while rotating the tibia. Pain during compression is interpreted as a tear of medial or lateral meniscus, whereas pain while the leg is pulled is interpreted as a ligamentous injury. In one study using arthroscopy as a control, the Apley compression test had a sensitivity of 16% (3).

Treatment and Prognosis

In the absence of constant locking or when locking happens only infrequently, nonoperative treatment may be tried. However, if locking is frequent or constant or other associated injuries such as cruciate and/or collateral ligament injuries or fractures exist, the patient should be referred to an orthopedic surgeon for more urgent evaluation to prevent further injury.

When a meniscal injury is suspected, the initial treatment should consist of a brief period of immobilization with a knee immobilizer and partial to no weight-bearing with crutches. An ace bandage does not provide sufficient stability, but its use may be helpful in reducing effusion. The knee should be rested and sporting activities should be avoided. Whenever possible, the knee should be elevated and ice packs should be applied to the knee for 15 minutes several times a day in the early recovery phase. To avoid the rapid onset of quadriceps atrophy, isometric quadriceps

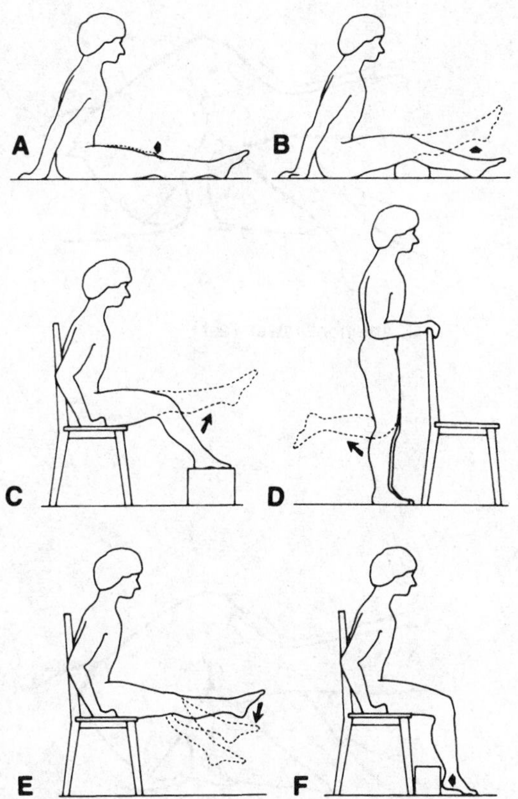

Figure 72.5. Restorative knee exercises. A: Isometric quadriceps exercise. B and C: Isotonic quadriceps exercises. D: Gravity-resisted isotonic hamstring (knee flexion) exercise. E: Gravity-assisted isotonic flexion exercises. F: Isometric knee flexion exercise.

strengthening exercises (Fig. 72.5) should be recommended as soon as the patient can do these comfortably. During this period, the patient should be placed on nonsteroidal anti-inflammatory drugs (NSAIDs) to help reduce inflammation. Symptoms often subside within 10 to 14 days. If symptoms resolve, the prognosis is variable. A small tear in a vascularized area may heal with fibrous tissue with no further symptoms. A larger tear, however, may result in recurrent symptoms after initial improvement. An orthopedic referral is justified if symptoms persist beyond 2 weeks despite nonoperative treatment.

A x-ray should be obtained if a fracture is suspected. Anteroposterior, lateral, and patellofemoral views are needed to rule out a fracture definitely. Magnetic resonance imaging (MRI) has sensitivity and specificity in the 90% range for detecting meniscal pathology (4,5). The ordering of MRI may be best deferred to the orthopedist, however, who may not even need it to treat the patient.

Arthroscopy is now the standard in evaluating and treating meniscal injuries. Depending on the location and the size of the tear, the surgeon may be able to repair the lesion or perform a partial meniscectomy. Every effort is made to conserve as much of the meniscus as possible to delay early osteoarthritis of the knee (6).

Prevention

Participation in sports that involve pivoting motion places one at risk for sustaining a meniscal tear. Unfortunately, muscular strengthening and condition cannot prevent this injury. The effectiveness of certain knee braces to prevent recurrent injury in at-risk individuals is controversial (7,8). The best prevention remains being aware of the mechanisms of injury and instructing athletes in efforts to avoid situations that could subject a fixed stance to twisting forces.

Collateral and Cruciate Ligament Injuries

Definition and Mechanism of Injury

The MCL and LCL provide stability against varus or valgus stresses (see above) in the knee joint. The cruciate ligaments provide anterior and posterior translational stability of the tibia with respect to the femur. Thus, injury to any one of these four ligaments can cause abnormal motion of tibia with respect to the femur when certain stresses are applied. Sprains and tears of the cruciate or collateral ligaments are caused by a combination of angulating and rotational forces at the knee joint. For example, an individual tackled from the side undergoes a valgus force to the lateral aspect of the knee, which can typically produce a tear of the MCL, ACL, and possibly PCL. Cruciate ligaments can also be torn secondary to dashboard injuries in motor vehicle crashes when the tibia is forced back against the femur. Hyperflexion and hyperextension injuries can sprain these ligaments as well.

Signs and Symptoms

The patient can often identify the mechanism by recalling how he or she was tackled or injured. The patient may even remember an audible "snap" or "pop" at the time of injury. The patient is usually unable to continue to bear weight or participate in the sporting activity. Immediate knee swelling and pain may be observed.

On physical examination a knee effusion, decreased active and passive range of motion, and increased laxity with provocative tests will be observed in the affected knee as compared with the contralateral normal knee. With ligamentous injuries, the sprain should be quantified by a three-level grading system (see Chapter 68). Briefly, a grade I sprain is a stretching of the ligament, a grade II sprain is a partial tear of the ligament fibers with some joint laxity, and a grade III sprain is a complete tear of the ligament with joint instability.

When injury to any ligament is suspected, the joint should be carefully evaluated for any instability (Fig. 72.6). Because the degree of ligamentous laxity varies tremendously between patients, assessment should be based on comparison with the uninjured knee. Examination can often be difficult, however, because of pain, swelling, and guarding by the patient. The stability of the collateral ligaments should be tested with the knee in about 20 degrees of flexion. Varus stress is applied to test the LCL (Fig. 72.6A), and valgus stress is

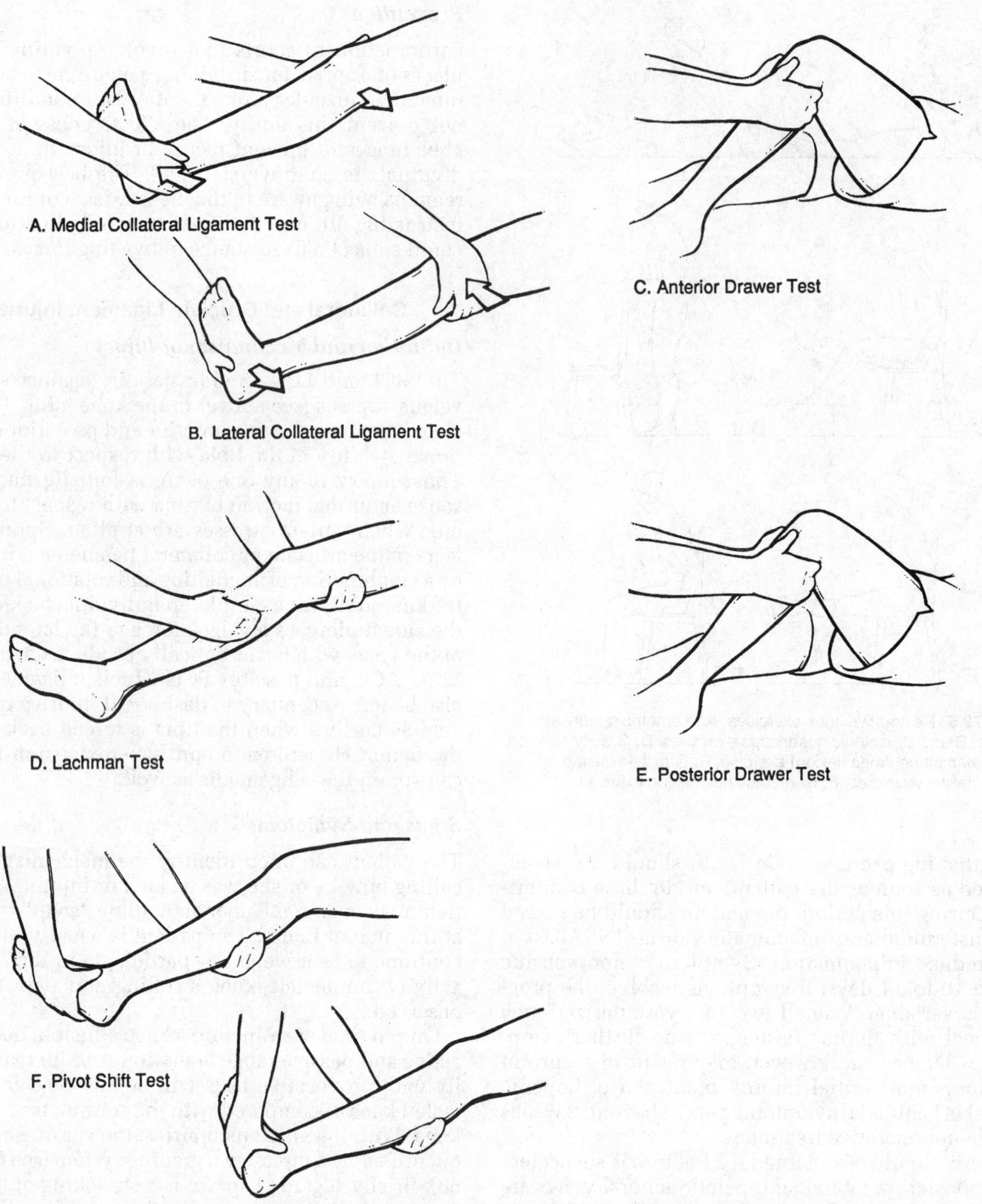

Figure 72.6. Examination for collateral and cruciate ligament injuries. **A:** Medial collateral ligament test. **B:** Lateral collateral ligament test. **C:** Anterior drawer test for anterior cruciate ligament. **D:** Lachman test for anterior cruciate ligament. **E:** Posterior drawer test for posterior cruciate ligament. **F:** Pivot shift test. (Modified and redrawn from Schott WN, Nisonson B, Nicholas JA, eds. Principles of sports medicine. Baltimore: Williams & Wilkins, 1984, with permission.)

applied to test the MCL (Fig. 72.6A). With grade I injuries, there is pain but no instability. With grade II and grade III injuries, however, the lateral or medial joint spaces of the knee joint widen when stress is applied. The integrity of the ACL and PCL is tested with the knee at 90 degrees and 15 degrees of flexion with the *anterior/posterior drawer tests* and *Lachman test,* respectively (Fig. 72.6, C–E). With the anterior and posterior drawer tests, the knee is flexed 90 degrees and the examiner exerts anterior or posterior pressure to the proximal tibia. Instability in the direction of the pressure indicates a tear of the respective cruciate ligament. The most sensitive test for the ACL is the Lachman test, in which the knee is flexed to 15 degrees and

Table 72.1. Accuracy of Physical Examination Maneuvers in Diagnosing Ligamentous and Meniscal Injuries

Maneuver	Sensitivity	Specificity	Positive LR (95% CI)	Negative LR (95% CI)
		ACL tear		
Composite[a]	82%	94%	25.0 (2.1–306)	0.04 (0.01–0.48)
Anterior drawer sign	62%	67%	3.8 (0.7–22.0)	0.30 (0.05–1.5)
Lachman test	84%	100%	42.0 (2.7–651.0)	0.1 (0.0–0.4)
Lateral pivot shift	38%	Not reported	—	—
		PCL tear		
Composite[a]	91%	98%	21.0 (2.1–205.0)	0.05 (0.01–0.50)
Posterior drawer test	55%	Not reported	—	—

[a]Composite is a combination of physical examination items.
ACL, anterior cruciate ligament; LR, likelihood ratio; CI, confidence internal; PCL, posterior cruciate ligament.
Adapted from Solomen DH, Simel DL, Bates DW, et al. Does this patient have a torn meniscus or ligament of the knee? JAMA 2001;286:1610, with permission.

the tibia is pulled anteriorly with respect to the femur. The test is considered positive when there is increased laxity with no firm end point. Another important test for determining ACL instability is the *pivot shift test* (Fig. 72.6F). With the foot internally rotated and knee flexed more than 40 degrees, the proximal tibia subluxes anteriorly with knee extension in the 20-degree to 40-degree range.

The accuracy of these diagnostic maneuvers was studied in a systematic review of the literature, which concluded that a composite examination, using several maneuvers, performed better than specific maneuvers alone (Table 72.1) (9). The composite examination for an ACL tear performed by orthopedic physicians was highly predictive, with a positive likelihood ratio of 25.0 and a negative likelihood ratio of 0.04. Similarly, the composite examination for a PCL tear had a positive likelihood ratio of 21.0 and a negative likelihood ratio of 0.05.

Treatment and Prognosis

As with any injury, x-rays should be obtained to rule out bony injuries. A complete series of anteroposterior, lateral, and patellofemoral views are required. If a large joint effusion is present, it should be aspirated for two reasons: removal of the fluid results in relief of discomfort and if a hemarthrosis is present, it may indicate a more serious injury such as osteochondral fracture and/or an ACL tear, and the patient should be referred to an orthopedic surgeon. At the time of aspiration, the joint may also be injected with a local anesthetic agent such as bupivacaine or lidocaine for some pain relief.

The joint should be rested by immobilization during a period of partial to no weight-bearing with crutches. The knee should be treated with the RICE (Rest, Ice, Compression, Elevation) protocol several times a day to decrease swelling and pain, and the patient should be placed on a course of NSAIDs. Most patients with minor grade I or II sprains improve markedly in 2 weeks and can be permitted to increase their activities gradually. However, patients with severe grade II or III injuries are not likely to have substantial improvement with this regimen and should be referred for additional tests or treatment. The specialist may often choose to obtain stress x-rays or MRIs to delineate the extent of the ligamentous injury. Treatment may consist of a longer period of immobilization with physical therapy and/or surgical reconstruction (tendon autografts or allografts). Chronic instability should be addressed early and thoroughly because, left untreated, it can lead to rapid onset of early osteoarthritis.

Prevention

Ligamentous injuries can be prevented to some extent with proper conditioning and muscle strengthening, but some mechanisms of injury (such as rotation) are hard to avoid in certain sports. Although some patients have the subjective feeling of more stability with prophylactic braces, such devices are rarely used because their clinical effectiveness is controversial (10,11). In one study of collegiate football players, the incidence of knee injuries was higher in a period when braces were worn compared with a period when braces were not worn (12). It is generally believed that there is insufficient evidence at this time to recommend prophylactic braces for prevention of ligamentous and cruciate injuries (7).

Extensor Mechanism Disruption

Definition and Mechanism of Injury

As discussed previously, the extensor mechanism consists of the quadriceps muscles, the quadriceps tendon, the patella, and the patellar tendon (with its ultimate insertion onto the tibial tubercle proximally). This mechanism is responsible for allowing active extension of the knee joint. Complete or partial disruption of any part of this mechanism results in the complete or partial inability to actively extend the knee (13). Injury to the extensor mechanism can occur in both young active individuals and more sedentary adults. It typically occurs after jumping (in which the sudden contraction of the quadriceps results in a tear of the quadriceps or patellar tendons), from a direct traumatic event such as a blow to the patella (which causes it to fracture and displace), or from a fall onto a partially flexed knee (in which there is forced flexion of the knee with concurrent quadriceps contraction).

Signs and Symptoms

The patient may give a history of immediate pain and knee swelling, inability to bear weight, inability to extend the knee actively, and the subjective feeling of knee instability. Physical examination shows knee effusion and asymmetry. When asked to extend the knee from a fully flexed position, the patient is unable to comply. With some injuries, because the medial and lateral patellar retinacula (see anatomy above) may still be intact, the patient may be able actively to extend the knee from 20 to 30 degrees of flexion; therefore, it is important to test for active knee extension from a fully flexed position. There may be a palpable defect in the quadriceps or patellar tendons or even the patella.

Treatment and Prognosis

Knee x-rays should be obtained to assist in ruling out a patellar fracture or tibial tubercle avulsion fracture as the possible cause of the extensor mechanism injury. On the lateral x-ray, a high riding patella (*patella alta*) may be appreciated secondary to rupture of the patellar tendon and the pull of the quadriceps tendon. MRI is not necessary in the diagnosis of this problem.

A knee immobilizer should be applied and appropriate pain medication should be prescribed. Regardless of the extent of the tear, patients with extensor mechanism injuries should be referred urgently to an orthopedic surgeon because they require long-term follow-up and extensive rehabilitation. Partial tears may be treated with a prolonged period of immobilization in an above the knee cast, cylinder cast, or splint. Complete or very large partial tears, however, require open surgical repair. Ideally, repair should be carried out within 1 week to prevent muscle and tendon retraction. After repair, the knee is immobilized for 6 weeks in full extension to relieve any tension on the repaired tissue and allow for complete healing. Afterward, the goals are restoration of full knee range of motion and strength with physical therapy. Potential complications can include knee stiffness and rerupture of the tendon.

Osgood-Schlatter Disease

Definition and Mechanism of Injury

Osgood-Schlatter disease is a form of apophysitis that affects the tibial tubercle (where the patellar tendon attaches). An apophysis is a secondary ossification center that ultimately fuses with the main bone during maturity. In Osgood-Schlatter disease, there is repetitive trauma to the patellar tendon insertion with microscopic tears and avulsions, yielding prominence of the tibial tubercle. This condition, common in active adolescents, is usually self-limited (14).

Signs and Symptoms

Typically, there is no clear history of trauma but rather one of overuse. Patients complain of pain and prominence over the tibial tubercle. In severe cases one may observe quadriceps atrophy secondary to disuse of the extensor mechanism. Physical examination reveals focal tenderness and prominence at the tibial tubercle.

Treatment and Prognosis

Appropriate series of x-rays, including anteroposterior, lateral, and patellofemoral views, should be obtained to rule out a fracture. The main form of treatment is activity modification, NSAIDs, the RICE protocol, and perhaps a brief period of immobilization. Active resisted knee extension activities such as climbing, running, and kicking should be avoided in the acute phase. Isometric exercises are useful to reverse quadriceps atrophy (Fig. 72.5). As symptoms improve, the patient should undergo a course of quadriceps and hamstring stretching exercises. The prognosis is usually very good with compliant patients. Refractory cases may be referred to an orthopedic surgeon, who may consider excising any heterotopic ossification in this area or pinning the apophysis, although these procedures are performed only rarely (15).

Tendinitis

Definition and Mechanism of Injury

Tendinitis of the patellar and quadriceps tendon is a common cause of anterior knee pain. It is thought to be secondary to chronic irritation and scarring within the tendons at their sites of origin or insertion. Patellar tendinitis occurs more commonly and is often referred to as a *jumper's knee* (16).

Signs and Symptoms

These forms of tendinitis present as anterior knee pain exacerbated by physical activities. Sports such as basketball and volleyball that involve jumping and running place one at risk for these conditions. In the case of quadriceps tendinitis, patients have localized pain and even clicking at the insertion of the quadriceps tendon into the superior pole of the patella. With patellar tendinitis or jumper's knee, patients have localized tenderness and swelling at the inferior pole of the patella. X-rays, although not necessary to diagnose the condition, may show calcification within the tendons, but this is not a specific finding.

Treatment and Prognosis

Treatment is aimed at reducing the stress on the tendon and avoiding activities that create microtrauma in this region. Initially, patients are treated with the RICE protocol and activity modification. A brief period of immobilization to rest the patellar and quadriceps tendons may also be useful. For refractory cases, referral to an orthopedist is appropriate for consideration of excision of the scarred and necrotic tendon fibers and calcification, although this procedure is rarely performed.

Prevention

Avoiding activities that require frequent jumping and running will likely reduce the recurrence of these conditions. Orthotics and braces are rarely useful, and their prescription is not recommended (17).

Patellofemoral Pain Syndrome

Definition and Mechanism of Injury

Patellofemoral joint disorders include problems of instability and alignment of the patella and distal femoral articular surfaces. This syndrome encompasses a great variety of problems ranging from

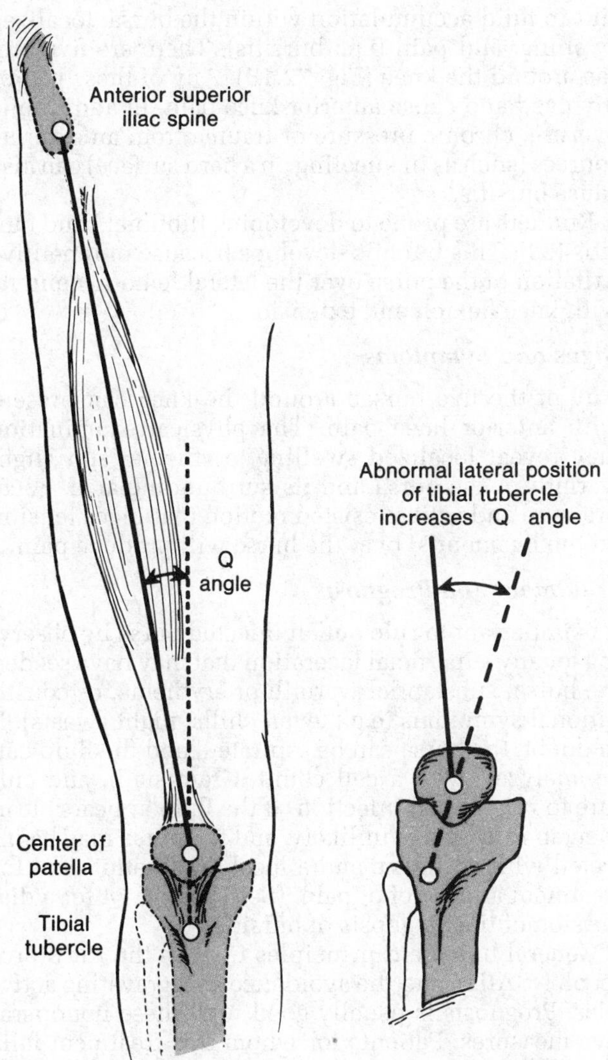

Figure 72.7. The Q angle is constructed by a line connecting the anterior superior iliac spine with the center of the patella to a second line connecting the center of the patella with the tibial tubercle (**left**). The normal angle is up to 20 degrees. **Right,** abnormal Q Angle.

abnormal motion of the patella as it moves over the femoral condyles to recurrent subluxation or dislocation of the patella. The instability usually occurs in the lateral direction. Patellofemoral malalignment is usually present and can be seen as a lateral tilt to the patella in the trochlea of the femur on the patellofemoral x-ray. This malalignment creates an incongruent articulation within the femoral condyles, which often leads to osteoarthritis in the patellofemoral joint. In time, the cartilage will become soft and degrade, causing crepitus and pain. This condition of softened articular cartilage is called chondromalacia.

Patellar instability and subluxation is often due to an increased angle between the quadriceps and patellar tendon (Q angle), a high riding patella (*patella alta*), or muscle and bony imbalances in the lower extremity. The normal Q angle (Fig. 72.7) is measured by a line connecting the anterior superior iliac spine to the center of patella and a second line connecting the center of the patella to tibial tubercle. A Q angle greater than 20 degrees may indicate lateral displacement of the patella; however, many studies have shown the Q angle is not reliably predictive of patellofemoral pain syndrome and is one of many potential associations (18,19). Patella alta is an anatomic variant in which the patella rests more proximally than usual, thereby allowing it to be more mobile and less constrained by the femoral condyles. Patella alta can be identified on a lateral x-ray if the distance from the inferior pole of the patella to the tibial tubercle exceeds the length of the patella by 25%. Normally these two distances are equal.

Patella subluxation can also be the result of altered anatomy at the hip or ankle joints. Patients with a variation in normal hip joint anatomy that results in compensatory external tibial torsion (external rotation of the lower leg) can have lateral displacement of the patella. Patients with excessive pronation of the feet and loss of the medial arch of the foot can have an abnormal Q angle secondary to rotation of the tibia.

Signs and Symptoms

Regardless of the cause of patellofemoral pain syndrome, patients typically complain of anterior knee pain. The pain is aching and chronic in nature and located around or under the patella. The discomfort is aggravated by running or walking up inclined surfaces, climbing or descending stairs, kneeling, or hyperflexing the knee. Often, there is a subjective feeling that the patella will dislocate as it subluxes laterally (Fig. 72.8).

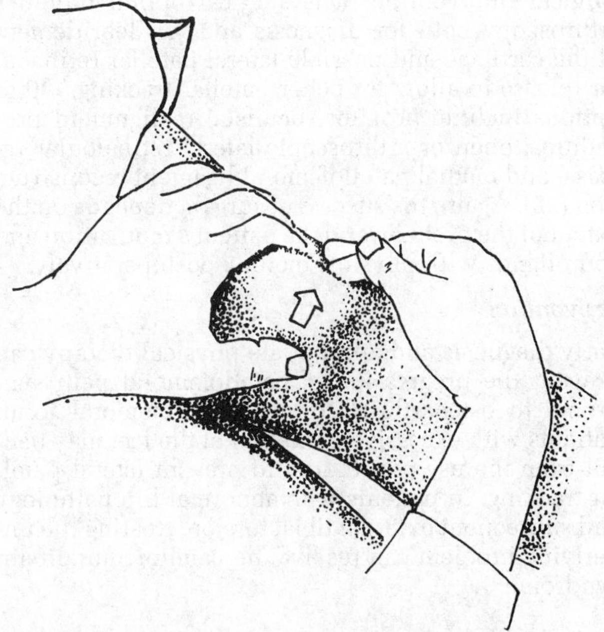

Figure 72.8. Patients with patellofemoral syndrome exhibit a positive apprehension sign when the patella is pushed laterally. They may also have focal tenderness under the lateral facet of the patella. (From Hobbs B. Patellofemoral syndrome. In: Sponseller PD, Wenz JF, Frassica FJ, eds. The 5-minute orthopaedic consult. Philadelphia: Lippincott Williams & Wilkins, 2001:241, with permission.)

Physical examination reveals pain or crepitus with patellofemoral manipulation or palpation of the articular surface of the patella. Attempts to push the patella laterally may cause pain and involuntary contracture of the quadriceps, the so-called apprehension sign. A mild knee effusion may be present. X-rays should be obtained. The patellofemoral view is the most diagnostic because it shows the lateral tilt of the patella.

Treatment and Prognosis

Generally, the knee should be rested by avoiding activities that aggravate the patellofemoral joint. NSAIDs, the RICE protocol, and immobilization should be prescribed (20). A brief period of crutch use may be helpful in resting the knee, but physical therapy is the mainstay of treatment. Therapy is directed at strengthening the quadriceps muscles with closed chain exercises (i.e., those in which the foot is in contact with the ground at all times). Such exercises allow for strengthening of multiple muscle groups and minimize patellofemoral shear forces. Orthotics may be helpful for some patients. For patients with severe foot pronation, shoe orthotics that restore the normal arch of the foot may alleviate the patellofemoral problem. A knee brace with a horseshoe-shaped pad to stabilize the patella may be beneficial to correct patellar-tracking problems (21).

The success of the treatment depends on the extent of the problem and the patient's motivation and compliance with therapy. Patients whose symptoms are refractory to nonoperative treatment should be referred to an orthopedic surgeon. Patients with recurrent dislocation or malalignment may require early surgical intervention. One surgical option includes arthroscopy both for diagnosis and for debridement of the cartilage and possible lateral patellar retinacular release to allow for better patellar tracking. Other options include proximal or distal realignment procedures, open or arthroscopic lateral retinalcular release, and medial patellofemoral ligament reconstruction (22). Again, the success of surgery depends on the extent of the problem and the patient's motivation and compliance with physical therapy postoperatively.

Prevention

Early diagnosis and appropriate physical therapy can prevent the progression of patellofemoral pain syndrome to osteoarthritis of the patellofemoral joint. Patients with excessive pronation of the feet may benefit from the use of orthotics to prevent lateral patellar tracking. In patients with abnormal hip pathology and subsequent external tibial torsion, treating the underlying problem can resolve the patellofemoral pain syndrome.

Bursitis

Definition and Mechanism of Injury

A bursa is a synovial-lined tissue that lies between adjacent structures such as a bone and a tendon to decrease friction. Chronic friction or overuse can result in fluid accumulation within the bursa, localized swelling, and pain (i.e., bursitis). There are five bursae around the knee (Fig. 72.1B). Any of these can be involved and cause anterior knee pain. In addition to overuse, chronic pressure or trauma from an external sources (such as in kneeling on a hard surface) can also cause bursitis.

Runners are prone to developing iliotibial band bursitis (23). This bursitis develops because of repetitive irritation of the bursa over the lateral femoral condyle with knee flexion and extension.

Signs and Symptoms

Any of the five bursae around the knee can present with anterior knee pain. The physical examination may reveal localized swelling, erythema, and slight warmth in the bursa and its surrounding area. Focal pressure and active resisted motion that place tension on the ligament(s) over the bursa will produce pain.

Treatment and Prognosis

It is important to rule out an infected bursa by observing for any superficial laceration that may have seeded the bursa, substantial warmth or erythema, or constitutional symptoms (e.g., fever, chills, night sweats). If in doubt, the bursa can be aspirated, and the fluid can be analyzed with a cell count, Gram stain, and culture to rule out an infection. If the fluid appears clear, then an infection is unlikely, and the bursa may be injected with cortisone and a local anesthetic agent for treatment and relief of pain. (See Chapter 74 for a discussion of the diagnosis of bursitis.)

General treatment principles involve the RICE protocol, NSAIDs, and the avoidance of aggravating activities. Prognosis is usually good with these nonoperative measures. Patients for whom this treatment fails should be referred to an orthopedic surgeon for possible resection of the bursa.

Prevention

Avoiding repetitive trauma and overuse can prevent bursitis. Activity modification such as avoiding kneeling is very important. Knee pads and some braces may also prevent recurrence.

Baker Cyst

Definition and Mechanism of Injury

A Baker or a popliteal cyst is a synovial cyst that develops in the popliteal bursa posterior to the knee joint. The popliteal bursa normally communicates with the knee joint; it can become more cystic when excessive fluid accumulation within the joint tracks into the popliteal bursa (24). This excessive fluid accumulation can be secondary to almost any problem affecting the knee, including osteoarthritis, trauma, synovitis, a meniscal tear, and so on.

Signs and Symptoms

Patients typically complain of swelling and pain in the popliteal fossa. On physical examination, there is local tenderness and fullness in the popliteal region.

Larger cysts can dissect inferiorly into the posterior calf musculature. Rupture of these dissecting cysts can cause severe pain in the calf, and this presentation can be confused with thrombophlebitis. Depending on the course of the inciting problem, the cysts can wax and wane in size and symptoms.

Whenever one examines a knee with a Baker cyst, the underlying cause should be sought. The physical examination should include a thorough evaluation of all the collateral and cruciate ligaments, menisci, and the patellofemoral joint.

Treatment and Prognosis

MRI and x-rays are not necessary, unless these studies are being obtained to diagnose other problems that might be causing the Baker cyst. X-rays frequently show evidence of osteoarthritis because this is the most common cause of a Baker cyst. Aspiration provides only transient relief, and the fluid generally reaccumulates because the Baker cyst communicates with the knee joint. The cyst will often resolve by treating the underlying cause. If the patient has pain in the posterior calf, an ultrasound can be obtained to rule out thrombophlebitis and to quantify the size and location of the Baker cyst.

Prevention

As discussed above, a Baker cyst can be caused by numerous problems within the joint that lead to increased fluid accumulation. Treating the underlying problem can lead to resolution of the cyst.

Septic Joint Infection

A septic knee is an infection of the synovial lining of the joint with microorganisms. This infection, which can occur in any age group, can occur via direct inoculation of the joint, seeding the joint hematogenously from a distant source, or via local spread from adjacent tissue (25,26). Predisposing factors include arthritis, gout, intravenous drug abuse, alcoholism, diabetes, systemic steroids, or immunosuppression.

In the management of septic arthritis of the knee joint, an emergent orthopedic referral is necessary for debridement. Debridement can be carried out via an open arthrotomy or arthroscopically. Most surgeons prefer an open technique to allow for a more thorough procedure. Depending on the extent of infection, a subsequent irrigation and debridement procedure may be indicated. Postoperative physical therapy is started as soon as possible for passive and active range of motion of the knee.

PROBLEMS OF THE LEG

Leg Anatomy

The principal anatomic components of the leg and their function are as follows (Fig. 72.9):

- The bony structures are composed of the tibia medially and the fibula laterally. The tibia is the main weight-bearing bone.

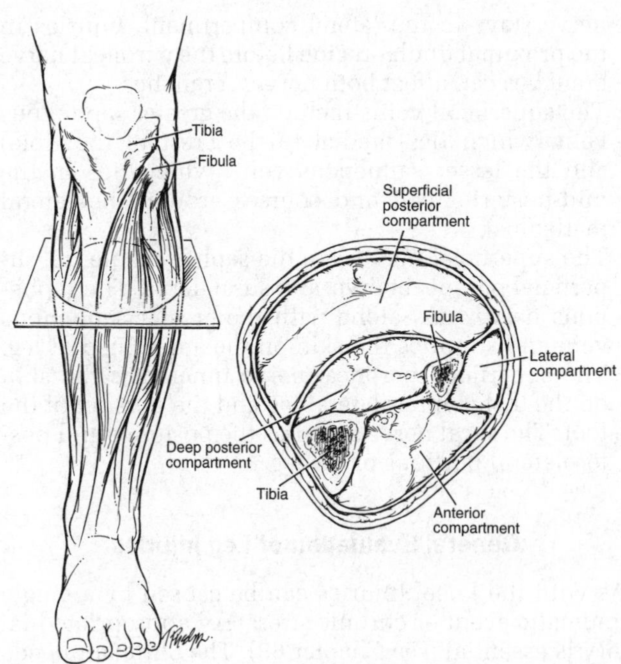

Figure 72.9. Leg anatomy. **A:** Coronal view. **B:** Cross-sectional view showing compartments.

- The leg has four fascial compartments: anterior, lateral, superficial posterior, and deep posterior compartments.
- The anterior compartment contains the tibialis anterior, extensor hallucis longus, extensor digitorum longus, and peroneus tertius muscles. The neurovascular supply to this compartment is via the deep peroneal nerve and anterior tibial artery.
- The lateral compartment contains the peroneus longus and brevis muscles. These muscles are innervated by the superficial peroneal nerve. This compartment does not contain an artery, but the peronei muscles receive their blood supply via branches of the peroneal artery, a tributary of the posterior tibial artery.
- The superficial posterior compartment contains the soleus and gastrocnemius muscles and the plantaris tendon. These two muscles merge distally to form the Achilles tendon. The tibial artery and posterior tibial nerve supply these muscles.
- The deep posterior compartment contains the tibialis posterior, flexor hallucis longus, and the flexor digitorum longus muscles. This compartment is innervated by the posterior tibial nerve and vascularized by the posterior tibial and peroneal arteries.
- The interosseus membrane is a fibrous connection between the lateral border of the tibia and medial border of the fibula. The membrane runs almost the complete length of each bone, separating the anterior and deep posterior compartments.
- The common peroneal nerve courses along the proximal neck of the fibula under the peroneus longus and then branches into its deep and superficial branches. The deep peroneal nerve then enters the anterior compartment, whereas the superficial peroneal

nerve stays in the lateral compartment. Injuries in the proximal fibular region before the peroneal nerve branches can affect both nerves' branches.

- The superficial veins include the greater saphenous vein (which lies medial to the crest of the tibia) and the lesser saphenous vein (which lies in the mid-posterior calf and courses around the lateral malleolus).
- The superficial nerves are the saphenous nerve, superficial peroneal nerve, and sural nerve. The saphenous nerve runs along with the greater saphenous vein and supplies the skin on the anteromedial leg. The superficial peroneal nerve innervates the skin on the distal anterolateral leg and the dorsum of the foot. The sural nerve supplies the posterior and posterolateral portions of the leg.

General Evaluation of Leg Injuries

As with the knee, injuries can be caused by a single traumatic event or chronic stress. An appropriate history is essential (see Chapter 68). The clinician needs to define the mechanism of injury. If there has been no acute trauma, then stress injury from chronic repetitive activity or increase in the frequency or duration of the activity is the likely cause. As with the knee, the general principles of inspection, palpation, and evaluation of range of motion and strength are addressed:

- One should *inspect* the leg for any gross deformity or swelling, observe for any superficial abrasion or laceration, and compare it with the normal contralateral limb.
- The entire medical crest of the tibia from the plateau to the medial malleolus and the fibular head proximally and its distal extension (the lateral malleolus) should be *palpated*. The common peroneal nerve wraps around the proximal fibula before it branches, and injury to this area can affect both the superficial and the deep peroneal nerves.
- All fascial compartments should feel soft during palpation. If any compartment feels tense or swollen in the setting of trauma, one must rule out a compartment syndrome by physical examination and the measurement of compartment pressures (see below).
- The *strength* of the muscles in each compartment should be tested. The anterior compartment is responsible for dorsiflexion of the ankle and extension of the toes. The lateral compartment everts the ankle joint. The deep posterior compartment inverts the ankle and plantarflexes the toes. The superficial posterior compartment plantarflexes the ankle. Each motion should be graded on a 0- to 5-point muscle strength scale.
- *Sensory examination* should be carried out over the appropriate dermatomes and superficial nerve distributions.

Differential Diagnosis of Acute Leg Pain

Trauma is the most common cause of acute pain. If the physical examination or history suggests the possibility of a fracture, biplanar full-length x-rays should be obtained. On the x-rays, the soft tissues should also be examined for the presence of a foreign body or swelling. Acute pain can also be a product of stress fractures (although they are usually associated with chronic injury) or sciatica from a herniated disk. In addition, nonorthopedic causes of acute leg pain, such as deep venous thrombosis (see Chapter 57), vascular insufficiency (see Chapter 94), acute monoarthritis (see Chapter 76), myopathy and neuropathy (see Chapter 92), and cellulitis (see Chapter 32) should be considered.

Differential Diagnosis of Chronic Leg Pain

Chronic pain is often more difficult to diagnose than acute pain. Defining the characteristics of pain is very important. Chronic night pain is often suggestive of a neoplasm. Bony tumors, soft tissue tumors, and infections often have insidious onsets. Chronic low back pain can present with chronic radicular nerve root pain such as sciatica. Stress fractures and shin splints can present in a chronic way in that pain is present only with activities and is relieved by rest. This scenario also occurs with vascular claudication in older patients with arteriosclerosis.

Compartment Syndrome

Definition and Mechanism of Injury

Compartment syndrome is a devastating injury and one of the most common reasons for medical malpractice lawsuits in orthopedics. A compartment is a group of one or more muscles and the associated neurovascular structures surrounded by an unyielding fibrous fascia. Compartment syndrome occurs when the pressure within a compartment rises to a point that prevents vascular supply to the compartment (27) that leads to ischemia and eventual necrosis of the compartment's contents. Compartment syndrome is a surgical emergency that requires immediate treatment to prevent irreversible muscle damage.

A common misconception is that if there is no fracture, then a compartment syndrome cannot exist. Arterial injury (e.g., intracompartmental hemorrhage from the fracture site) is a common etiology for the development of compartment syndrome in a trauma patient. A compartment syndrome also can develop secondary to muscle swelling from overexertion or overuse of muscles (28). Unlike a compartment syndrome caused by trauma, this form is usually transient. The lateral and anterior compartments are prone to this condition (Fig. 72.9). Activity can cause muscles to hypertrophy and repeated contraction can cause tissue edema. This scenario can occur in long-distance runners, military recruits, or in an individual who has experienced a substantial change in activity level. Exercise-induced compartment syndrome is usually not a surgical emergency.

Signs and Symptoms

In trauma-induced compartment syndrome, the prognosis worsens with time. Passive toe stretch (dorsiflexion and plantarflexion) causes severe pain. The pain is very severe, even at rest, and seems out of proportion to the injury. Often the compartment feels tense and swollen on palpation. The patient may experience paresthesia distally over the dorsum of the foot or toes. The distal aspects of the limb that depend on the blood supply from vessels within the compartment may feel cooler. Eventually, compartment syndrome may lead to pulselessness when the pressure within the compartment exceeds the systolic blood pressure, but this scenario is quite rare and occurs only very late in the course of the condition. Paralysis is also a very late finding, and usually by this stage irreversible damage has taken place. In exercise-induced compartment syndrome, the syndrome is reproducible with activity and the pain usually abates after the activity is stopped. Exercise-induced compartment syndrome can also be confused with thrombophlebitis or vascular insufficiency.

Although compartment syndrome is a clinical diagnosis, one (if experienced in the procedure) can obtain objective data by measuring the intracompartmental pressures. Measurements can be obtained via a commercially available compartment pressure measurement kit or one that is made with an 18-gauge needle connected to a manometer or arterial pressure monitoring line via intravenous tubing. A small amount of saline (1 mL) is injected into the compartment and the equilibrated pressure is then recorded. Some clinicians believe that a pressure reading higher than 30 mm Hg or within 30 mm Hg of diastolic blood pressure is indicative of a compartment syndrome and almost always requires fasciotomy. However, this "cutoff" measurement continues to be a subject of controversy. Others recommend decompression only if the differential pressure is more than 30 mm Hg (29).

Treatment and Prognosis

The treatment of acute traumatic leg compartment syndromes requires immediate referral to an orthopedist for emergent fasciotomy. Typically, all four compartments are released via medial and lateral leg incisions. If the diagnosis is recognized and treated in a timely fashion, then muscle necrosis can be avoided. However, delay in diagnosis or treatment can lead to the devastating results of necrosis of the entire contents of the compartment, kidney failure from rhabdomyolysis, potentially with contractures, and permanent motor and sensory deficits.

In the case of exercise-related compartment syndrome, activity modification, muscle strengthening, and stretching exercises are recommended. Initially, ice should be applied for 15 minutes several times a day, and the patient must rest from the aggravating exercises for 3 to 4 weeks. NSAIDs may also be helpful to reduce inflammation. Once symptoms subside, the patient should begin a conditioning program before returning to full exercise. Pre-exercise stretching is very beneficial. The patient should use well-designed and cushioned running shoes and avoid toe running or steep inclines. In refractory cases, stress fracture should be ruled out by x-ray, bone scan, or MRI. Patients for whom nonoperative modalities fail may be candidates for elective fasciotomy of the involved compartment (30).

Prevention

In the case of trauma-induced compartment syndrome, there is no prevention. Rapid diagnosis and fasciotomy are the only hope for avoiding severe complications (see above). Exercise-induced compartment syndrome can be prevented by adequate muscular conditioning, preactivity stretching, appropriate shoe wear, and running on level surfaces.

Shin Splints

Definition and Mechanism of Injury

Shin splints commonly refer to anteromedial mid to distal leg tenderness secondary to the pull and overuse of the muscles in this region. Such tenderness frequently occurs with activities such as running, jogging, or sustained walking. There is usually no history of trauma. The pain is thought to result from tendinitis of the posterior tibial tendon and periostitis from the pulling of this muscle from its bony attachments along the medial aspect of the tibia, interosseous membrane, and fibula. This condition typically develops in patients who are not properly conditioned, do not warm up or stretch properly before the activity, and run on hard or uneven surfaces with improper shoe wear.

Signs and Symptoms

Patients with shin splints typically complain of pain localized to the anteromedial mid to distal leg (Fig. 72.10). The onset of pain is typically gradual but occasionally can be abrupt; it occurs during or just after exercise. Occasionally, the pain is so severe that the activity has to be stopped. On physical examination, there is tenderness only along the medial aspect of the tibia. All compartments are usually soft.

X-rays occasionally show irregular bone formation on the surface of the tibia or fibula as a result of periostitis. A radionuclide bone scan is more sensitive than plain x-ray and may show increased isotope activity in the distal anteromedial tibia and fibula from periostitis. In a comparison of diagnostic imaging studies in patients with lower leg pain, MRI was found to have similar sensitivity as bone scans, but both had low specificity (31). Further diagnostic studies can often be avoided in the setting of a well-directed history and physical examination (32).

Treatment and Prognosis

Treatment involves ice packs applied several times a day to reduce swelling, NSAIDs to reduce inflammation, and avoidance of the precipitating activity. Acute shin splints should resolve with rest within 3 weeks; after this, conditioning is necessary before the patient can return to competitive sports. Stretching exercises are effective and should be routinely advised.

In refractory cases, one should rule out other possible causes of anteromedial distal tibia pain. Occasionally, fascial hernias, tenosynovitis, or tears of the

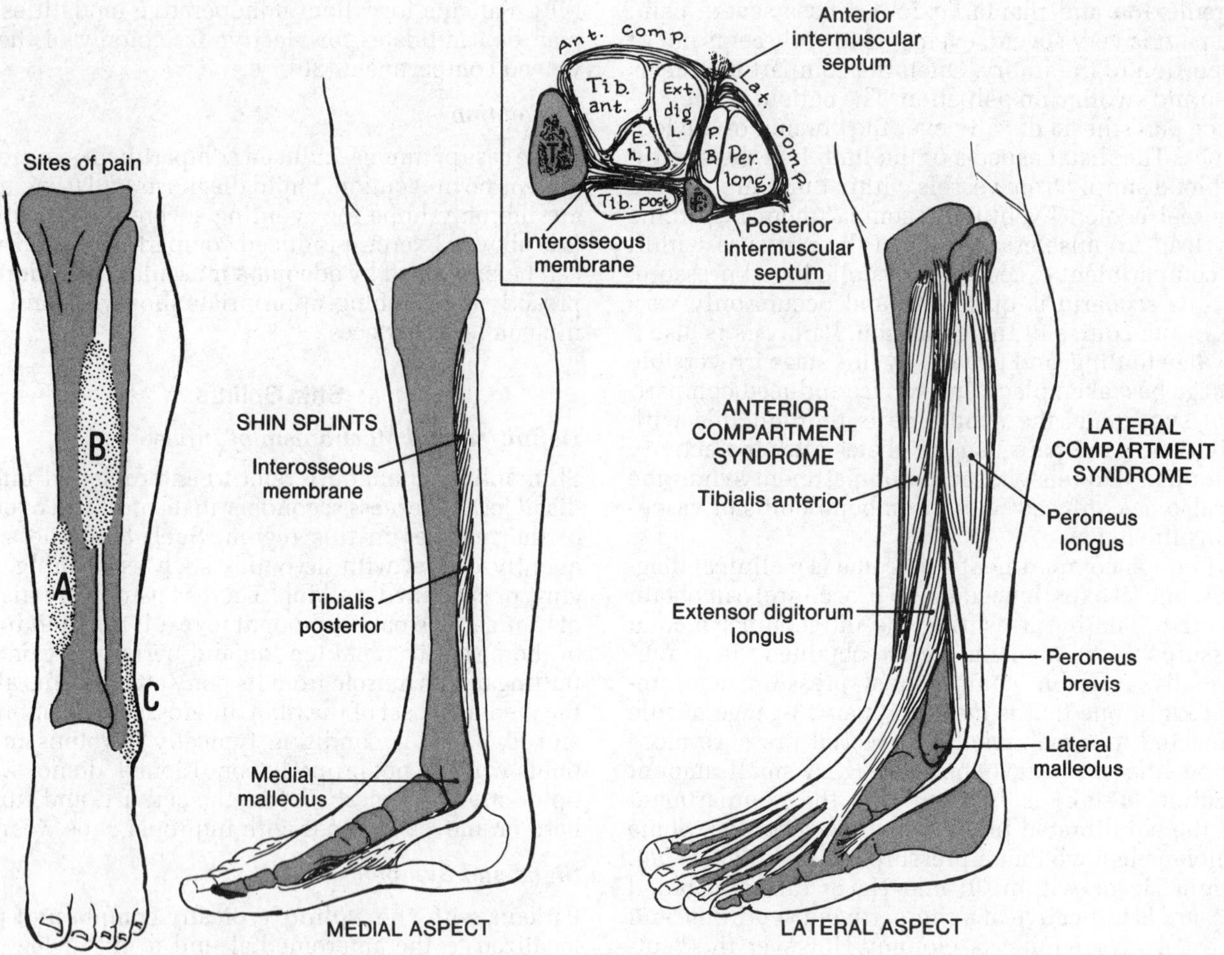

Figure 72.10. Sites of pain and relevant anatomy for **(A)** shin splints, **(B)** anterior compartment syndrome, and **(C)** lateral compartment syndrome.

interosseous membrane may produce symptoms suggestive of shin splints. Stress fracture should be ruled out with plain x-rays, even though with this condition, pain is present at the onset of the activity. If there is a high suspicion for a stress fracture but plain x-rays are negative, an MRI can be obtained. Exercise-induced compartment syndrome produces a similar pain, but the location is anterolateral to the crest of the tibia (Fig. 72.10).

Prevention

To help prevent shin splints, the patient should try stretching exercises before physical activity, avoid running on hard steep surfaces, and use proper shoes (see Chapter 73). These modifications will reduce the tendinitis and pull from the attachment site of the tibialis posterior muscle.

Stress Fracture

Definition and Mechanism of Injury

A stress fracture may occur in normal bone that is subjected to repetitive and unusual stress or in weakened bone (e.g., osteoporosis) that is subjected to normal stress (33). The bone remodeling process cannot keep pace with the mechanical stress, and ultimately the bone breaks. Often there is no history of acute trauma, but one should inquire about a recent change in the amount or duration of athletic activities. In studies of athletes, bone mineral density, biomechanical factors such as high longitudinal arch of the foot, leg-length inequality, and excessive forefoot varus, as well as high weekly training mileage, increased risk of recurrent stress fractures (34).

Signs and Symptoms

Typically, a patient complains of pain during the activity. Later, the pain can be present with normal daily activities or even at rest. Often, the patient will admit to a recent change in level, duration, or intensity of athletic activity. On physical examination, there is local tenderness and mild swelling, but this swelling may be more appreciable after a few weeks secondary to callus formation. There is usually no gross instability. In addition to the tibia and fibula, stress fractures are also common in the metatarsals, calcaneus, and femoral neck.

Treatment and Prognosis

Anteroposterior and lateral x-rays of the tibia should be obtained. Often, in the early stages (within the first 2 to 3 weeks) of the stress fracture, no fracture line is visible on x-rays. A bone scan, however, will show a stress fracture as an area of increased radionuclide activity 48 hours after injury. MRI, the most sensitive diagnostic procedure, can show the fracture within the first 48 hours and therefore is recommended when one is suspicious and the plain x-ray is negative (35). The patient with a stress fracture should be referred to an orthopedic surgeon for fracture care. Patients are placed on crutches with limited to no weight-bearing for 4 to 6 weeks. X-rays are obtained periodically during this time to document healing. After the initial period of immobilization and limited or no weight-bearing, the leg is typically placed in a below the knee cast or a specialized prefabricated boot. Pain relief is usually adequate with NSAIDs. Smoking should be discontinued (see Chapter 27) to promote bone healing. There is both experimental and clinical evidence that smoking slows healing of bone fractures and increases the frequency of nonunion (36,37). Most stress fractures heal with no complications, and patients are able to return to their baseline activity level within 2 to 3 months.

Prevention

The best way to prevent stress fractures of the tibia and fibula is to avoid overexertion and repetitive trauma and to prevent conditions that lead to intrinsic bone weakness such as osteoporosis. It is best to avoid suddenly increasing duration, intensity, and frequency of jogging or running. The use of shock-absorbing insoles in footwear appears to reduce the incidence of stress fractures (38).

Bone and Soft Tissue Tumors

Patients with a primary bone tumor typically complain of constant, deep, aching pain. Night pain is a common feature of malignant tumors. Osteoid osteoma is a benign bony tumor that can cause night pain, which is often relieved by NSAIDs. A sudden increase in pain after mild trauma should raise the possibility of a pathologic fracture and an underlying malignancy. On the other hand, pain is not the typical presenting complaint of soft tissue tumors. Rather, a growing mass is the usual presentation of a soft tissue tumor. Constitutional symptoms such as fever, malaise, weakness, and recent weight loss are also important symptoms that might be associated with a malignant bone tumor.

The patient should be examined for any local masses, focal tenderness, pain with palpation or weight-bearing, and any peripheral nerve deficit secondary to entrapment. Plain x-rays and other imaging modalities, if needed, should be obtained. Computed tomography is useful for bone tumors, and MRI is useful for soft tissue tumors. Laboratory studies include a complete blood cell count, calcium, magnesium, phosphorus, alkaline phosphatase, and erythrocyte sedimentation rate. Although the results of these tests are nonspecific, they may offer clues regarding bone turnover, an increased inflammatory state, and systemic illness. Patients suspected of having a bone tumor should be referred to an orthopedic surgeon.

Deep Venous Thrombosis

Deep venous thrombosis often presents in a nonspecific manner but is an important potential explanation for lower extremity pain. See Chapter 57 for a full discussion of the management of deep venous thrombosis.

PROBLEMS OF THE ANKLE

Ankle Anatomy

The ankle joint consists of articulations of the distal tibia and fibula with the talus. The principal anatomic components and their function are as follows (Fig. 72.11):

- The distal tibia and fibula, with their distal bony extensions, form the medial and lateral malleolus, respectively. The medial and lateral malleolus, along with the distal flat articular surface of the tibia (the tibial plafond), form an arch or mortise that articulates with the dome of the talus.

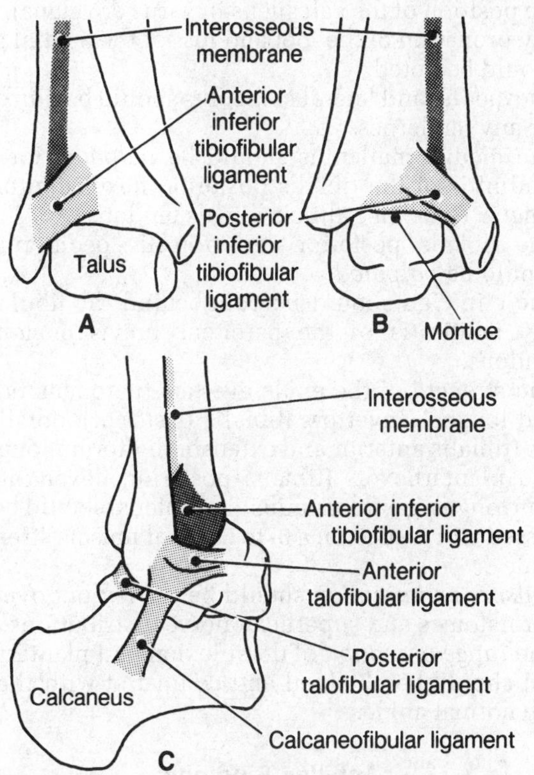

Figure 72.11. Ankle joint. **A:** Anterior view. **B:** Posterior view. **C:** Lateral view. (From Ramamurti CP, Tiner RV. Orthopedics in primary care. Baltimore: Williams & Wilkins, 1979, with permission.)

- The interosseous ligament runs almost completely along the length of the tibia and fibula. This ligament, along with the anterior inferior and posterior inferior tibiofibular ligament, stabilize the distal tibiofibular joint.
- The talus is stabilized within the mortise by the medial and lateral ligamentous structures. The lateral complex consists of anterior and posterior talofibular ligaments and the calcaneofibular ligament. The medial complex consists of the superficial and deep deltoid ligament connecting the medial malleolus to the talus and calcaneus.

General Evaluation of Ankle Injuries

A focused history is essential (see Chapter 68). As with the knee, injuries can be caused by a single traumatic event or by multiple and chronic stresses, and the clinician will need to define the mechanism of injury to effect a satisfactory outcome. If there has been no acute trauma, then stress injury from chronic repetitive activity or increase in the frequency or duration of the activity is the likely cause of injury. As with the knee, the general principles of inspection, palpation, and evaluation of range of motion and strength are addressed.

- The ankle should be *inspected* for any gross deformity or swelling and for any superficial abrasion or laceration. It should be compared with the normal contralateral limb. The resting position of the ankle, the presence of hindfoot varus or valgus (i.e., the position of the calcaneus in varus or valgus), and any pronation of the foot and loss of the medial arch should be noted.
- The medial and lateral malleolus should be *palpated* for any tenderness.
- The medial malleolus should be *palpated* for any tendinitis of the tibialis posterior, flexor digitorum longus, or flexor hallucis longus tendons.
- The tibialis posterior and dorsalis pedis pulses should be *palpated.*
- The clinician should *palpate* behind the fibula for any tendinitis of the peroneus brevis or longus tendons.
- The *strength* of the ankle everters (peroneus brevis and longus), invertors (tibialis posterior), dorsiflexors (tibialis anterior and extensor digitorum longus), and plantarflexors (tibialis posterior, flexor digitorum longus, gastrocnemius, and soleus) should be assessed and graded on a 0- to 5- point muscle strength scale.
- *Sensory examination* should be carried out over all dermatomes and superficial nerve distributions.
- The *range of motion* of dorsiflexion and plantarflexion should be obtained and compared with that of the normal ankle.

Achilles Tendinitis

Definition and Mechanism of Injury

Achilles tendinitis refers to chronic irritation of the Achilles tendon and its sheath secondary to repetitive use and trauma (39,40). The Achilles tendon is the terminal tendinous attachment of the soleus and gastrocnemius into the calcaneus. Achilles tendinitis is commonly seen in active individuals (adolescents to middle-aged adults) engaging in athletic activities without proper conditioning. However, Achilles tendinitis can occur even in well-conditioned athletes who run on hills or wear shoes with excessively rigid soles. Furthermore, structural abnormalities such as tibia vara (bowlegged deformity), tight hamstrings and calf muscles, a cavus foot (high arched foot, often with claw toes), and varus (inverted) heel deformity predispose to Achilles tendinitis. Initially, the peritenon (loose soft connective tissue surrounding the tendon) is inflamed, but in chronic cases the tendon itself undergoes mucoid degeneration with formation of longitudinal fissures in the tendon. This condition can increase the risk of a tendon rupture.

Signs and Symptoms

The patient typically complains of a burning type pain at the site of tendon insertion onto the calcaneus. The onset of pain usually coincides with the start of the activity; however, it may lessen or disappear completely as the activity continues. The discomfort often recurs after completion of the activity or early in the morning.

On examination there is local or diffuse tenderness of the Achilles tendon. A chronic tender nodule may be present in the substance of the tendon with crepitus and swelling. The patient experiences pain with passive stretch of the tendon.

Retrocalcaneal bursitis involving the bursa that lies between the calcaneus and Achilles tendon may produce symptoms similar to those of Achilles tendinitis. It also affects runners. On examination of a patient with retrocalcaneal bursitis, there is focal tenderness confined to the calcaneus.

Treatment and Prognosis

The general treatment protocol is like that for any other tendinitis condition. The inciting activity or sport should be stopped initially, and the patient should use the RICE protocol and should be placed on a trial of NSAIDs to reduce the inflammation. Runners should not run for several days, then reduce running mileage and avoid hills until symptoms have been completely absent for 10 to 14 days. If symptoms persist after this short rest period, the exercises that aggravate the condition may need to be stopped for 3 to 4 weeks or longer.

A physical therapy referral is beneficial for refractory cases of Achilles tendinitis, because ultrasound and other modalities can be highly effective. A removable heel lift inserted into the shoe may also provide some relief. If the syndrome is severe, splinting or casting the ankle joint and using crutches may be necessary to immobilize the Achilles tendon. In mild cases, the prognosis is excellent. Patients with conditions that do not respond in 2 weeks should be referred for an orthopedic consultation. Surgery is usually not necessary, but for some cases, operative options include open debridement and repair of the tendon (41). The patient with retrocalcaneal bursitis is best advised to rest from stressful activity, obtain properly fitted athletic shoes that are not tight around the Achilles tendon, and use a heel pad in regular shoes.

Prevention

Exercises that gently stretch the tendon may help condition runners and prevent recurrences. The use of good shoes is also important. Shoes should have flexible soles, a well-molded Achilles pad, and a rigid heel wedge.

Achilles Tendon Rupture

Definition and Mechanism of Injury

An Achilles tendon rupture is a disruption of the tendon usually 2 to 6 cm proximal to its insertion into the calcaneus. It typically occurs in middle-aged adults, usually during athletic activities that require rapid active plantarflexion of the ankle. Patients with Achilles tendinitis are at risk for tendon ruptures, as are patients with systemic inflammatory diseases, such as lupus and rheumatoid arthritis, and a history of systemic steroids (42). Achilles tendinitis and tendon rupture have also been associated with fluoroquinolone therapy (43). The rupture can be acute or chronic, complete or incomplete.

Signs and Symptoms

A patient with an acute rupture usually recalls a sudden snap and pain in the area of tendon insertion. A patient with a chronic rupture may not recall a particular event but generally has pain in this area. Depending on how complete the rupture is, the patient may not be able to actively plantarflex the ankle or may do so with weakness and pain. On examination, there is local pain and swelling. A palpable defect may be present in the tendon. The *Thompson test* (44) is positive. This test is performed by squeezing the mid to proximal muscular section of the calf. If the tendon is intact or not completely torn, the ankle will plantarflex. If the tendon is completely ruptured, no plantarflexion will occur.

X-rays should be obtained to rule out an avulsion fracture at the tendon insertion site. If the diagnosis is still not clear, MRI will delineate the degree of the tear and its location. Patients with acute or painful chronic tears or those with avulsion fractures should be referred to an orthopedic surgeon for definitive treatment. For a patient with an acute rupture, referral should be made urgently because delay in treatment beyond a few days may result in retraction of the proximal portion of the tendon.

Treatment and Prognosis

There is some controversy regarding the management of Achilles tendon ruptures (45,46). Both operative and nonoperative options are available. In the case of operative repair, primary anastomosis at the site of rupture is followed by a period of immobilization to allow for tendon healing. Nonoperative treatment entails immobilizing the ankle joint in plantarflexion to approximate the two ends of the tendon. This position is held for 4 weeks in a below the knee cast. Then the foot is brought into more dorsiflexion with another below the knee cast, and this process is repeated until the tendon is healed. Most surgeons recommend surgical repair of acute complete ruptures in young active patients. The prognosis of Achilles tendon ruptures is varied. Most patients are able to return to routine daily activities, but some may not be able to return to preinjury levels of sporting activities. Generally, compared with nonoperative modalities, surgical repair has a higher success rate of returning patients to preinjury sports levels with a lower chance of recurrence.

Prevention

Proper conditioning can prevent a tendon rupture. Appropriate stretching exercises should be performed before and after sporting activities. Also, appropriate treatment of Achilles tendinitis should be sought to decrease the potential chance of a rupture.

Posterior Tibialis Tendinitis and Rupture

Definition and Mechanism of Injury

Tendinitis of the posterior tibialis tendon is common. This tendon courses posterior to the medial malleolus, inverts the ankle joint, and plantarflexes the foot. Chronic irritation from the malleolus, along with a tenuous blood supply, place this tendon at risk for tendinitis and subsequent rupture. Patients with a history of trauma or previous surgery to the medial aspect of the foot, diabetes, obesity, or local steroid injection are at risk for dysfunction and tearing of this tendon.

Signs and Symptoms

Patients frequently complain of medial foot and ankle pain. The onset of the pain is usually gradual. Examination reveals tenderness along the course of the tendon behind the medial malleolus. Additionally, patients with a torn tendon may have gradual loss of the medial arch of the foot and, eventually, a flatfoot deformity. With complete tendon rupture, the foot abducts and the pain can move laterally in the region of the sinus tarsi or beneath the fibula where bony impingement can occur secondary to the loss of the medial arch. The hindfoot assumes a valgus position, allowing more of the toes to be visible when viewed from behind the patient (the "too-many-toes" sign). In the early stages, when only tenosynovitis is present, the tendon is intact and the patient is able to perform a single-heel rise. In more advanced stages of tendon attenuation or tear, however, the patient is unable to perform a heel rise. In advanced stages, x-rays show osteoarthritis in the ankle. MRI is valuable in showing posterior tibial tendon attenuation or tear.

Treatment and Prognosis

In the presence of an intact posterior tibial tendon with tendinitis, the standard RICE protocol with NSAIDs can be followed. The ankle joint should be immobilized for a period of 6 weeks with a rigid below the knee cast or boot to allow the inflammation to resolve. Subsequently, the patient can progress to a stiff-soled shoe with a medial heel wedge. Patients for whom such nonoperative measures fail may require surgical debridement of the tendon. For patients with incompetent or torn posterior tibial tendons, nonoperative treatment tends to be less effective and does not prevent progression to flatfoot deformity. Surgical options include reconstruction of the tendon, flexor tendon transfer, medial calcaneal osteotomy to displace the calcaneus medially, lengthening the lateral aspect of the foot, and ankle arthrodesis, or a combination thereof (47,48). The prognosis for this form of tendinitis tends to be good, but it may recur. The prognosis for posterior tibial tendon rupture varies and depends in part on the extent of the acquired flatfoot deformity.

Prevention

The best prevention for posterior tibial tendon rupture is to halt the progression of tibialis posterior tendinitis. Often early treatment of posterior tibial tendinitis with NSAIDs, immobilization, activity modification, and the use of orthotics is successful. Once the tendon is ruptured, the foot can develop a flatfoot deformity, and major surgical reconstruction may be necessary.

Ankle Sprain and Fractures

Definition and Mechanism of Injury

Ankle sprains and fractures occur when there is sudden stress on one or more of the supporting ligaments and bony structures. Numerous mechanisms have been described, but supination or pronation combined with internal or external rotation of the ankle joint are the main mechanisms (49) (Figs. 72.12 and 72.13).

The most frequently sprained ligament is the anterior talofibular ligament. All sprains are graded using a ligament grading system (see details in Chapter 68).

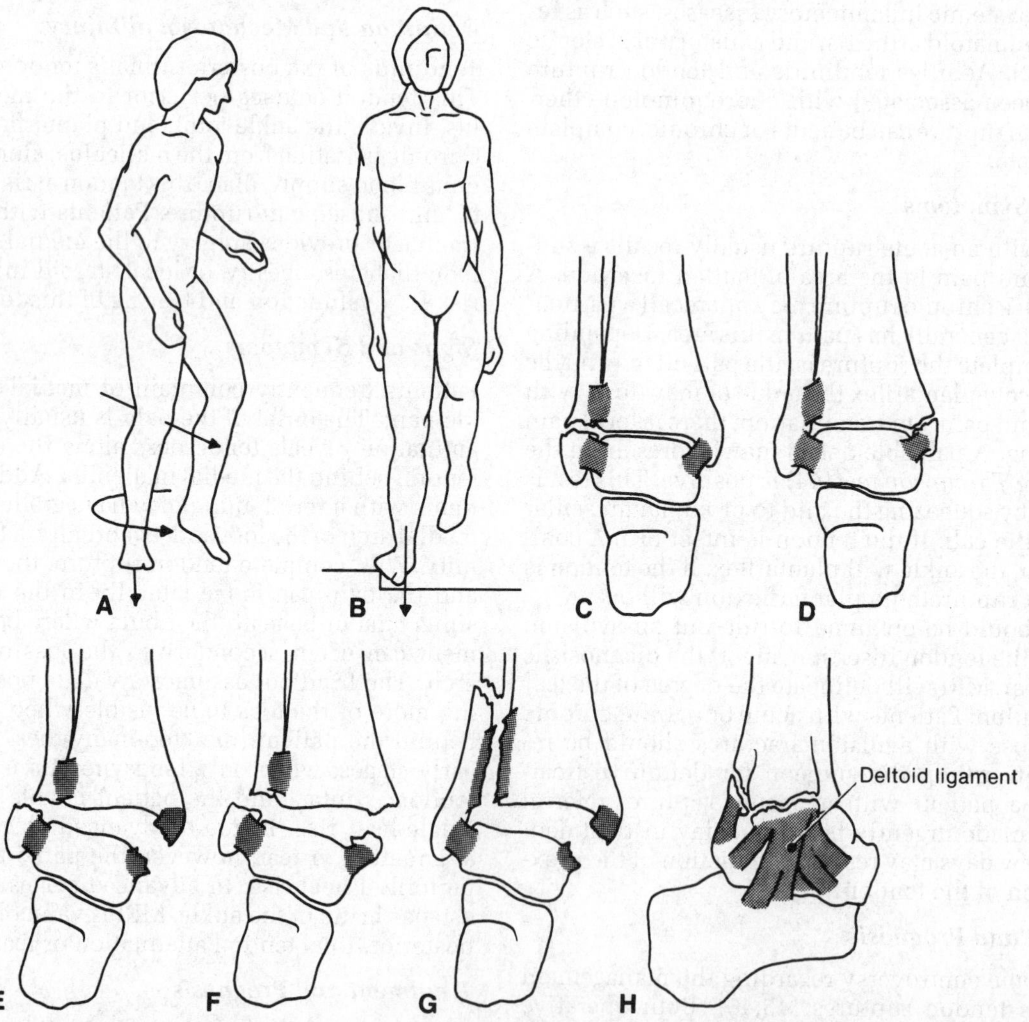

Figure 72.12. Pronation injuries of the ankle. **A:** Extremity rotates internally on the fixed foot. **B:** The foot is forced into pronation by weight taken on the lateral aspect of the forefoot. **C** and **D:** Forces of lesser severity may fracture a malleolus without tearing a ligament. **E, F,** and **G:** Forces of greater severity with different combinations of ligament and bony injury. **H:** When forward displacement of the tibia accompanies severe pronation forces, the posterior margin of the tibial articular surface may also be fractured. This injury is called a posterior malleolus fracture.

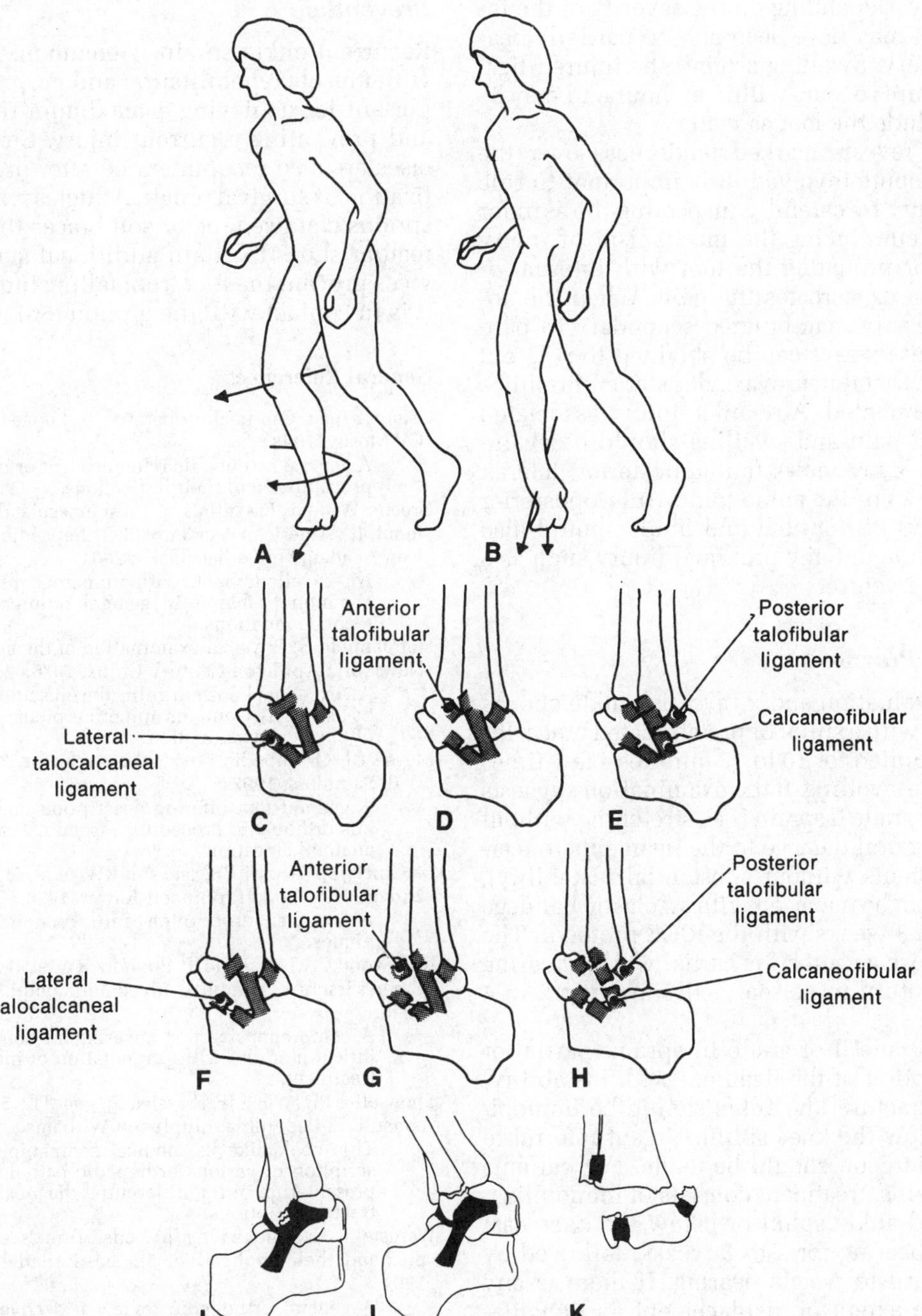

Figure 72.13. Supination injuries to the ankle. **A:** The extremity rotates externally on the fixed foot. **B:** The plantarflexed foot is forced into supination. **C–E:** In this sequence of injuries, the lateral talocalcaneal ligament **(E)** is injured before the anterior talofibular (D) ligament, which is injured before the calcaneofibular (E) ligament. **F–H:** When the injuring force is sufficient, the ligaments tear completely and in the same sequence. **I–K:** With sufficient force, the injuring force may avulse a flake of the fibula (I), fracture the end of fibula (J), or fracture both the medial and lateral malleolus (K) rather than tear the lateral ligaments.

Fractures are defined by their mechanism and particular bony and ligamentous injuries and are described as involving the medial or lateral malleolus, bimalleolar, trimalleolar (medial and lateral malleolus, and the posterior articular surface of the tibia), or bimalleolar equivalent (when the lateral malleolus is fractured and the deltoid ligament is torn medially with tenderness on palpation but no medial fracture on radiographs). Fractures may also cause injury to the syndesmotic ligament between the tibia and fibula, producing diastasis between the distal tibia and fibula.

Signs and Symptoms

The patient is usually able to recall the position of the foot at the time of injury and whether there was a sensation or sound of tearing of ligaments. Pain often is felt immediately. Depending on the severity of the injury, the patient may have been able to partially bear weight after injury. Swelling around the injured ligaments and fractures occurs within an hour and may be diffuse and include the foot as well.

Examination reveals marked tenderness over the bones and ligaments involved. It is important to rule out an open injury by carefully inspecting the skin for any wounds. Reproducing the mechanism of injury by supinating or pronating the foot with internal or external rotation exacerbates the pain. When the ankle cannot be easily manipulated secondary to pain or swelling, stress x-rays can be obtained to rule out joint instability. Distal neurovascular status should be tested and documented. Any ankle injury associated with substantial pain and swelling should be evaluated with three x-ray views (anteroposterior, lateral, and mortise view) of the ankle joint. Anteroposterior and lateral views of the tibia and fibula should also be obtained to rule out any proximal injury such as a proximal fibula fracture.

Treatment and Prognosis

After prompt evaluation and x-rays, the ankle should be immobilized with a splint or prefabricated brace. Ice packs may be applied for 10 to 15 minutes a few times a day to decrease swelling. If the examination suggests a mild grade I or grade II sprain (i.e., stretching without substantial structural damage to the ligaments to tearing of the ligaments without substantial instability), then the ankle can be managed with an elastic bandage or brace for 1 to 3 weeks with the RICE protocol. The patient should use a crutch for partial weight-bearing and gradually return to normal activities over 2 to 4 weeks.

For a severe grade II or grade III sprain (partial or complete disruption of the ligament with instability) or any type of fracture, the ankle should be immobilized with a below the knee splint. Urgent referral to an orthopedic surgeon should be made. For patients with severe sprains, treatment consists of immobilization with a rigid ankle splint or below the knee cast and no weight-bearing for 2 to 3 weeks, followed by progressive return to weight-bearing. If there is any bony injury, the extent of displacement and angulation, along with any ligamentous injury, needs to be defined because most of these fractures require open surgical reduction and fixation with plates and screws. After surgical fixation, a patient is placed in a below the knee splint for 6 weeks with no weight-bearing allowed.

Prognosis depends on the severity of the ligamentous and bony injury and the timing of intervention. Most patients with grade I and mild grade II sprains have a good prognosis with early return to preinjury levels of activity. For patients with severe grade II and grade III sprains and injuries with fractures, the prognosis is worse. Early referral to a physical therapist for range-of-motion and proprioception exercises is often useful and may improve the prognosis.

Prevention

Recurrent ankle sprain is common. Physical therapy with muscle rehabilitation and proprioception are important for achieving a maximum return to function and preventing recurrent injury. Strengthening exercises are also recommended after prolonged immobilization or surgical repair. Athletes with frequent ankle sprains can use tape or soft braces that are worn with regular shoes to attain additional stability. These devices prevent the foot from falling into inversion when it is in contact with the ground (50).

General References*

Canale ST, ed. Campbell's operative orthopaedics, 9th ed. St. Louis: CV Mosby, 1998.

A general orthopedic reference text oriented toward surgical procedures and their indications.

Greene WB, ed. Essentials of musculoskeletal care, 2nd ed. Rosemont, IL: American Academy of Orthopaedic Surgeons and American Academy of Pediatricians, 2001.

An excellent book with numerous photographs outlining common problems in general orthopedics with treatment recommendations.

Hoppenfield S. Physical examination of the spine and extremities. New York: Appleton-Century-Crofts, 1976.

An excellent book outlining the musculoskeletal examination by body part. Contains numerous pictures detailing the points of physical examination.

Magee DJ. Orthopedic physical assessment, 3rd ed. Philadelphia: W.B. Saunders, 1997

A general text offering description and pictures of numerous orthopedic procedures, examinations, and problems by anatomic location.

McGinty JB, Caspari RB, Jackson RW, et al. Operative arthroscopy, 2nd ed. New York: Lippincott-Raven, 1996.

An excellent description of arthroscopic indications and techniques.

Rockwood CA Jr, Green DP, Bucholz RW, et al., eds. Rockwood and Green's fractures in adults, 4th ed. Philadelphia: Lippincott-Raven, 1996.

A comprehensive text covering all bony and soft tissue injuries in adults with presentation of history, diagnosis, and treatment.

Sponseller PD, Wenz JF, Frassica FJ, eds. The 5-minute orthopaedic consult. Philadelphia: Lippincott Williams & Wilkins, 2001.

This book, like its medical companion, offers concise description of various orthopedic pathologies with very brief presentation of the differential diagnosis, management, and treatment options.

Weinstein SL, Buckwalter JA, eds. Turek's orthopaedics: principles and their application, 5th ed. Philadelphia: JB Lippincott, 1994.

A general orthopedic review text covering most problems with presentation of diagnosis, surgical treatment, and follow-up.

Specific References

1. Fadale PD, Noerdlinger MA. Sports injuries of the knee. Curr Opin Rheumatol 1999;2:144.
2. Stratford PW, Binkley J. A review of the McMurray test: definition, interpretation and clinical usefulness. J Orthop Sports Phys Ther 1995;22:116.
3. Fowler PJ, Lubiner JA. The predictive value of five clinical signs in the evaluation of meniscal pathology. Arthroscopy 1989;5:184.

---

*Bold print (general references) and bold numerals (specific references) denote published controlled clinical trials, meta-analyses, or consensus-based recommendations.

4. Cues JV III. Ryu R, Morgan FW. Meniscal pathology. The expanding role of magnetic resonance imaging. *Clin Orthop* 1990;252:80.
5. Jackson DW, Jennings LK, Maywood RM, et al. Magnetic resonance imaging of the knee. Am J Sports Med 1988;16:29.
6. Aagaard H, Verdonk R. Function of the normal meniscus and consequences of meniscal resection. Scand J Med Sci Sports 1999;9:134.
7. Martin TJ, Committee on Sports Medicine and Fitness. American Academy of Pediatrics: Technical report: knee brace use in the young athlete. Pediatrics 2001;108:503.
8. Requa RK, Garrick JG. A review of the use of prophylactic knee braces in football. Pediatr Clin North Am 1990;37:1165.
9. Solomon DH, Simel DL, Bates DW, et al. Does this patient have a torn meniscus or ligament of the knee? JAMA 2001;286:1610.
10. Rovere GD, Haupt HA, Yates CS. Prophylactic knee bracing in college football. Am J Sports Med 1987;15:111.
11. Johnston JM, Paulos LE. Prophylactic lateral knee braces. Med Sci Sports Exerc 1991;23:783.
12. Sitler M, Ryan J, Hopkinson W, et. al. The efficacy of a prophylactic knee brace to reduce knee injuries in football. A prospective, randomized study at West Point. Am J Sports Med 1990;18:310.
13. Haas SB, Callaway H. Disruptions of the extensor mechanism. Orthop Clin North Am 1992;23:687.
14. Krause BL, Williams JP, Catterall A. Natural history of Osgood-Schlatter disease. J Pediatr Orthop 1990;10:65.
15. Flowers MJ, Bhadreshwar DR. Tibial tuberosity excision for symptomatic Osgood-Schlatter disease. J Pediatr Orthop 1995;15:292.
16. Duri ZA, Aichroth PM, Wilkins R, et al. Patellar tendonitis and anterior knee pain. Am J Knee Surg 1999;12:99.
17. Yeung EW, Yeung SS. Interventions for preventing lower limb soft-tissue injuries in runners (Cochrane review). Cochrane Database Syst Rev 2001;3:CD001256.
18. Caylor D, Fites R, Worrell TW. The relationship between quadriceps angle and anterior knee pain syndrome. J Orthop Sports Phys Ther 1993;17:11.
19. Biedert RM, Warnke K. Correlation between the Q angle and the patella position: a clinical and axial computed tomography evaluation. Arch Orthop Trauma Surg 2001;121:346.
20. Juhn MS. Patellofemoral pain syndrome: a review and guidelines for treatment. Am Fam Physician 1999;60:2012.
21. Greenwald AE, Bagley AM, France EP, et al. A biomechanical and clinical evaluation of a patellofemoral knee brace. Clin Orthop 1996;324:187.
22. Bellemans J, Cauwenberghs F, Witvrouw E, et al. Anteromedial tibial tubercle transfer in patients with chronic anterior knee pain and a subluxation-type patellar malalignment. Am J Sports Med 1997;25:375.
23. Rouse SJ. The role of the iliotibial tract in patellofemoral pain and tibial band friction syndrome. Physiotherapy 1996;82:199.
24. Handy JR. Popliteal cysts in adults: a review. Semin Arthritis Rheum 2001;31:108.
25. Goldenberg DL, Reed JI. Bacterial arthritis. N Engl J Med 1985;312:764.
26. Gupta MN, Sturrock RD, Field M. A prospective 2-year study of 75 patients with adult-onset septic arthritis. Rheumatology 2001;40:24.
27. Mubarak SJ, Pedowitz RA, Hargens AR. Compartment syndromes. Curr Orthop 1989;3:36.
28. Abramowitz AJ, Schepsis AA. Chronic exertional compartment syndrome of the lower leg. Orthop Rev 1994;23:219.
29. McQueen MM, Court-Brown CM. Compartment monitoring in tibial fractures. The pressure threshold for decompression. J Bone Joint Surg 1996;78B:99.
30. Swain R, Ross D. Lower extremity compartment syndrome. When to suspect acute or chronic pressure buildup. Postgrad Med 1999;105:159.
31. Batt ME, Ugalde V, Anderson MW, et al. A prospective controlled study of diagnostic imaging for acute shin splints. Med Sci Sports Exerc 1998;30:1564.
32. Hester JT. Diagnostic approach to chronic exercise-induced leg pain. A review. Clin Podiatr Med Surg 2001;18:285.
33. Taylor D, Kuiper JH. The prediction of stress fractures using a "stressed volume" concept. J Orthop Res 2001;19:919.
34. Korpelainen R, Orava S, Karpakka J, et al. Risk factors for recurrent stress fractures in athletes. Am J Sports Med 2001;29:304.
35. Manaster BJ, Dalinka MK, Alazraki N, et al. Stress/insufficiency fractures (excluding vertebral). American College of Radiology. ACR Appropriateness Criteria. Radiology 2000;215[Suppl]:265.
36. Raikin SM, Landsman JC, Alexander VA, et al. Effect of nicotine on the rate and strength of long bone fracture healing. Clin Orthop 1998;353:231.
37. Schmitz MA, Finnegan M, Natarajan R, et al. Effect of smoking on tibial shaft fracture healing. Clin Orthop 1999;365:184.
38. Gillespie WJ, Grant I. Interventions for preventing and treating stress fractures and stress reactions of bone of the lower limbs in young adults (Cochrane review). The Cochrane Library, Issue 4. Oxford: Update Software, 2001.
39. Clain MR, Baxter DE. Achilles tendinitis. Foot Ankle 992;13:482.
40. Myerson MS, McGarvey W. Disorders of the insertion of the Achilles tendon and Achilles tendinitis. J Bone Joint Surg 1998;80A:1814.
41. Paavola M, Orava S, Leppilahti J, et al. Chronic Achilles tendon overuse injury: complications after surgical treatment. An analysis of 432 consecutive patients. Am J Sports Med 2000;28:77.
42. Kao NL, Moy JN, Richmond GW. Achilles tendon rupture: an underrated complication of corticosteroid treatment. Thorax 1992;47:484.
43. Ribard P, Audisio F, Kahn MF, et al. Seven Achilles tendinitis including 3 complicated by rupture during fluoroquinolone therapy. J Rheumatol 1992;19:1479.
44. Thompson TC. A test for rupture of the tendo Achilles. Acta Orthop Scand 1962;32:4861.
45. Cetti R, Christensen SE, Ejsted R, et al. Operative versus nonoperative treatment of Achilles tendon rupture. A prospective randomized study and review of the literature. Am J Sports Med 1993;21:791.
46. Jarvinen TA, Kannus P, Paavola M, et al. Achilles tendon injuries. Curr Opin Rheumatol 2001;13:150.
47. Weil LS Jr, Benton-Weil W, Borrelli AH, et al. Outcomes for surgical correction for stages 2 and 3 tibialis posterior dysfunction. J Foot Ankle Surg 1998;37:467.
48. Feldman NJ, Oloff LM, Schulhofer SD. In situ tibialis posterior to flexor digitorum longus tendon transfer for tibialis posterior tendon dysfunction: a simplified surgical approach with outcome of 11 patients. J Foot Ankle Surg 2001;40:2.
49. Beynnon BD, Renstrom PA, Alosa DM, et al. Ankle ligament injury risk factors: a prospective study of college athletes. J Orthop Res 2001;19:213.
50. Handoll HHG, Rowe BH, Quinn KM, et al. Interventions for preventing ankle ligament injuries (Cochrane review). The Cochrane Library, Issue 4. Oxford: Update Software, 2001.

CHAPTER 73

Common Problems of the Feet

BRUCE S. LEBOWITZ, DPM
DAVID E. KERN, MD, MPH

The primary care practitioner is often called on to treat patients who complain of problems with their feet. Although disorders of the feet are not life threatening, they should not be taken lightly. Any patient with a painful foot attests that the pain takes the joy out of living.

STRUCTURE AND FUNCTION

The abnormal foot cannot be understood unless the structure of the foot and its function during gait are understood.

Normal Gait

The bones and joints of the feet facilitate walking and running in an upright position (Fig. 73.1). The foot and leg function together to allow a smooth, even transfer of weight as one extremity moves ahead of the other. During gait, the foot first adjusts to a variable terrain and then acts to propel the body's weight forward.

In the *first stage of gait,* the heel strikes the ground and body weight begins to move distally over the lateral aspect of the foot. The foot is in a pronated position, meaning that the arch is flattened. In effect, the foot resembles a loose bag of bones during this stage, permitting it to adapt to the terrain and to act as a shock absorber when body weight strikes the ground.

In the *second stage of gait,* as weight moves distally to the ball of the foot and the body is propelled forward, the foot must convert to a rigid lever. This conversion, or supination, takes place in the subtalar and midtarsal joints. Supination serves to heighten the arch, pushing the bones and joints of the foot together rigidly enough to propel body weight forward efficiently.

For the lower extremity to function normally, certain structural criteria must be met; if they are not met, compensation occurs. Ideally, the leg should be in a plane perpendicular to the foot and ground, as in a stick figure drawing. The forefoot should be in a plane parallel to the rear foot, but various congenital factors may act to prevent this normal angulation. Varus (toward the midline or inverted) or valgus (away from the midline or everted) positions of the forefoot or hindfoot are the most common of these congenital factors.

Excessive Pronation

Excessive pronation (pronation extended through too much of the gait cycle) is the most common compensating mechanism when structural abnormalities are present. When the foot remains pronated during gait and does not resupinate in time, or at all, the condition known as *flatfoot* exists. The degree of this flatfoot position reflects the degree of pronation that is present. A number of problems may evolve from excessive pronation during gait, including bunions, calluses, and hammertoes. As pointed out in the discussion that follows, assessment of the mechanical basis for the condition is important in planning appropriate treatment for it.

Shoes

Shoes clearly play a role in the way feet function. Shoes protect feet from the elements, cushion the effect of walking on hard flat surfaces, and provide some support to the bones and ligaments. Unfortunately, many people favor short narrow shoes, high heels, and pointed toes. Obviously, squeezing a basically rectangular foot into a triangular shoe with the heels elevated from 2 to 5 inches creates significant stress for the foot. Most of the disorders of the foot discussed in this chapter are intensified by these demands of fashion.

Most people, in fitting themselves for shoes, do not take into account the variations in their foot size throughout the day and the variation in shoe size from manufacturer to manufacturer. Therefore, the following advice is often helpful: Buy shoes in the late afternoon when any swelling that might occur is already present; lightweight shoes are preferable to heavy

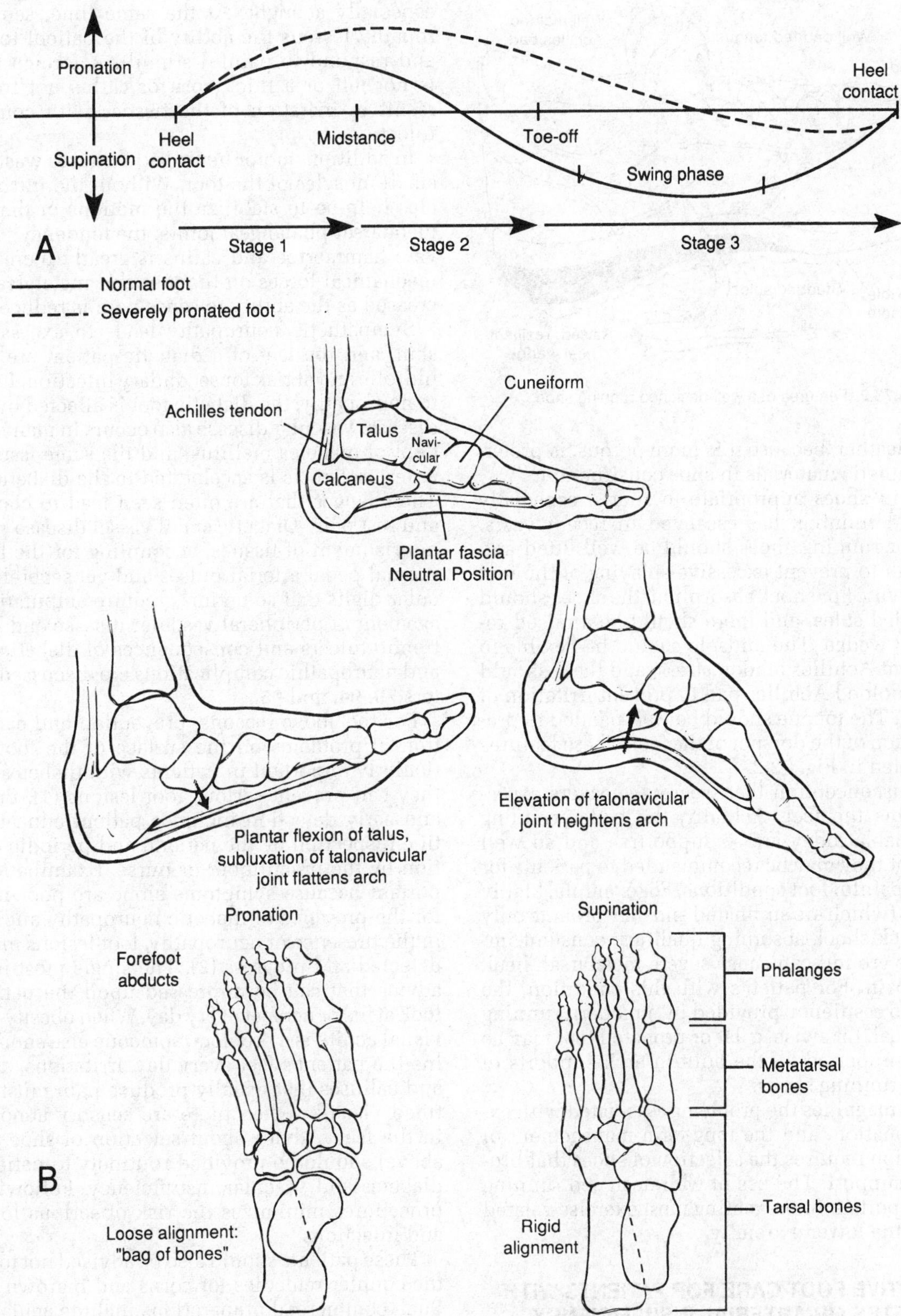

Figure 73.1. A: Schematic representation of the gait cycle for a normal foot and for a foot with excessive pronation. **B:** Schematic illustration of foot structure during pronation and supination during gait cycle.

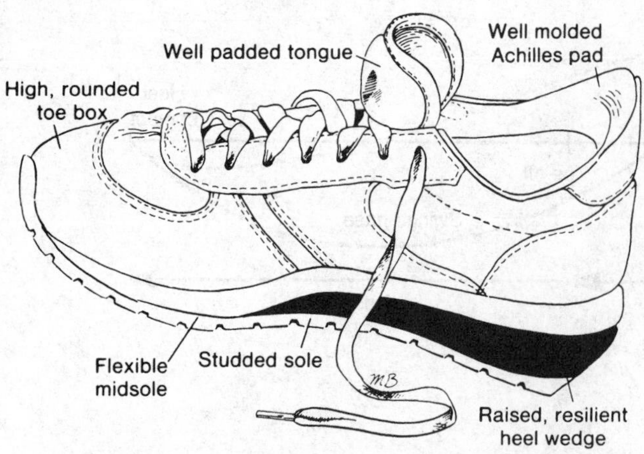

Figure 73.2. Features of a well-designed running shoe.

ones; and leather, because it is more porous, is preferable to synthetic materials in shoe construction.

Interest in shoes appropriate to sports, especially jogging and running, has escalated in recent years. Sneakers or running shoes should be well fitted and firm enough to prevent excessive splaying of the foot during activity. For shock absorption, the shoes should have studded soles, and there should be a raised resilient heel wedge. The midsole should be flexible to help prevent Achilles tendon stress, and there should be a well-molded Achilles pad to prevent irritation of the tendon. The tongue should be well padded to prevent irritation of the dorsum of the foot. These features are illustrated in Fig. 73.2.

It is a misconception that wearing sneakers excessively harms the feet. Actually, the better running shoes available today are so supportive and so well padded that they may be recommended to patients for numerous painful foot conditions. For example, highly arched feet (which are supinated and may pronate only slightly) lack shock-absorbing qualities; constant impact on the ground can cause severe metatarsal, heel, and arch pain. For patients with this condition, the support and resiliency provided by a modern running shoe are ideal. Likewise, a flat or pronated foot may be very well supported by the built-in arch supports of well-made running shoes.

Running magnifies the problems associated with excessive pronation, and the long-term management of this condition requires the selection of shoes that provide good support. The use of well-designed running shoes is important in preventing most exercise-related injuries of the lower extremity.

PREVENTIVE FOOT CARE FOR PATIENTS WITH DIABETES OR ARTERIAL INSUFFICIENCY

To understand the need for professional diabetic foot care, one must consider the special devastating effect diabetes mellitus has on the feet. The most important podiatric problem of diabetes is neuropathy (see Chapter 79). Sensory neuropathy may cause burning and sometimes unbearable pain in the feet and legs, especially at night. At the same time, sensory neuropathy lessens the ability of the patient to interpret and respond to painful stimuli. A foreign body that is not felt or a thick corn or callus not treated can result in irritation of the tissues with complicating infection.

In addition, motor neuropathy causes wasting of the small muscles of the foot. Without the intrinsic muscles helping to stabilize the motions of the toes and metatarsal phalangeal joints, the tendency to form severe hammertoe and callus is greatly increased. The mechanical forces on the toes and metatarsals are increased as the ability to sense pain is reduced.

Sympathetic neuropathy leads to excessively dry skin, and the feet of a diabetic patient are often anhidrotic and at risk for secondary infection. In addition to neuropathy, the diabetic foot is affected by vascular disease. Vascular disease also occurs in many independent of diabetes mellitus, and the same issues apply. Arteriosclerosis is accelerated in the diabetic patient. The changes that are often seen lead to claudication and rest pain. Diabetic small vessel disease affects the nourishment of tissues, accounting for the finding of normal pedal arterial pulses and yet severely dysvascular digits that sometimes require amputation. Management of peripheral vascular disease and lower extremity ulcers and consequences of diabetic vascular and neuropathic complications are discussed in Chapters 79, 94, and 95.

For the above reasons, prevention and early detection of problems on the surface of the foot are particularly important in patients with diabetes, because they can prevent serious foot lesions (1). Prevention and early detection includes patient education, routine inspection by the patient, and periodic examination by the practitioner or nurse. Examination is important because symptoms alone are poor indicators for the presence of diabetic neuropathy and because, in the presence of neuropathy, foot lesions may go undetected and progress (2). The single most important advice that can be impressed upon the patient is to look at his or her feet every day. When obesity or lack of visual acuity is a problem, someone else should examine the patient's feet every day. Irritations, abrasions, and calluses that usually produce pain must be identified visually when there are sensory abnormalities in the feet. Advice about selection of shoe gear (see above) should be provided routinely to patients with diabetes and vascular insufficiency. Following these procedures minimizes the risk of serious foot ulcers and infections.

These patients should also be advised not to use over the counter remedies for corns and ingrown toenails. Such commercial preparations include acids and tanning agents that can seriously injure the tender skin of these patients. Normal toenails should be allowed to grow past the end of the fleshy part of the toe; thick nails are best trimmed by a podiatrist, as are corns and calluses (see below). Soft cotton should be worn between toes that tend to rub each other, and talcum powder should be used to prevent interdigital moisture and maceration. Lanolin should be applied to dry and thickened skin to prevent fissuring, especially common in the heels of diabetic patients with anhidrosis from sympathetic neuropathy. Prescription-strength moisturizers such as ammonium lactate cream (Lac Hydrin 12%) are beneficial in neutralizing the drying effects of neuropathy. Tinea pedis should be treated (see Chapter 117) to prevent breaks in the skin, which could be sources of infection. In-shoe orthotics, which cushion and redistribute pressure, have been shown to be effective in preventing and treating diabetic ulcers (3).

A final note on prevention: Patients should be encouraged to shake out their shoes before putting them on as a simple obvious way to prevent foreign body penetration.

BUNIONS

Definition and Pathogenesis

Bunion (literally *turnip*) is a term used to describe the collective deformities of the first metatarsophalangeal joint (Fig. 73.3). These deformities include enlargement of the medial, medial–dorsal, or dorsal aspect of the first metatarsophalangeal joint and lateral deviation of the great toe. The enlargement of the joint may consist of bone or soft tissue or a combination of the two.

For many years, tight-fitting shoes were mistakenly considered to be the cause of bunions. It is known now that, although the pressure of tight shoes on an existing bunion can certainly result in pain that calls attention to the problem, bunions are not caused by poorly fitted shoes. The chief cause of the deformity is a hypermobile first metatarsal bone, most often related to excessive pronation (see above). The first metatarsal and great toe, which help propel body weight forward, should be stable during the final stage of gait when a tight, rigid, bony structure is needed. The intrinsic and extrinsic musculature should help to hold the metatarsal tight at this point. When there is excessive pronation, the entire foot remains loose and unstable. One result of such laxity in this stage of gait is hypermobility of the first metatarsal and buckling of the first toe; intrinsic and extrinsic muscles cause the first metatarsal to deviate medially and the great toe to deviate laterally. The combined deformity is called *hallux abducto valgus.* Eventually, arthritic hypertrophy of the head of the first metatarsal bone develops.

Symptoms

The presenting complaint of a patient with a bunion is pain localized to the first metatarsophalangeal joint. Pressure of the shoe on the enlarged metatarsal head, with or without pressure on adventitious bursa, can cause pain that is severe and even disabling; pain can also result from the joint motion itself. Often, crepitus can be felt within the joint. Sometimes the patient seeks help not because of pain, but because he or she is unable to wear shoes as a result of the deformity.

In evaluating a patient, the practitioner must be certain that the symptoms are a result of the bunion alone. Gout (see Chapter 76) may not only produce acute pain in the first metatarsophalangeal joint but may also aggravate a chronically painful joint. Therefore, gout should always be considered, especially in patients with bilateral bunion deformity and acute nonarticular pain in a foot.

Management

Acute symptoms caused by a bunion should be managed with rest, elimination of pressure on the bunion, soaks in warm water, and a nonsteroidal anti-inflammatory drug such as naproxen 250 to 500 mg every 8 to 12 hours or a cyclooxygenase-2 (COX-2) nonsteroidal anti-inflammatory drug when indicated; aspirin 600 mg every 4 to 6 hours may also be used, but the onset of action is slower. After the acute symptoms have subsided, the patient should be started on a program of long-term management.

Conservative long-term management of a bunion involves accommodating the deformity and attempting to arrest its progress. This is achieved by the use of molds and protective shields (Fig. 73.3, B and C). A mold, usually called an arch support, may be made from various types of materials to accommodate the plantar aspect of the foot. Protective shields are made of latex rubber.

Full foot molds or protective shields made by a podiatrist from a plaster impression are preferable to commercially made devices found in pharmacies and shoe stores. Commercial devices are manufactured to fit average shoe and foot sizes and do not take into account the shape of the individual patient's foot. The mold should be in place during the fitting of all new shoes. Occasionally, if the mold makes conventional shoes too tight, a specially built shoe, called an extra depth-inlay shoe, may be used. These enlarged shoes have a removable insole, for which one may substitute the patient's mold. The mold and shoes should minimize pressures against the bunion. In addition, the mold acts to reduce excessive pronation, thereby reducing the deforming forces in the forefoot.

Patients whose symptoms are not adequately controlled with conservative measures should be considered for surgery. The surgical management of a bunion must be individually planned for each patient, and in fact for each foot, to correct the specific deformity. Correction might involve resection of the bony protuberance of the first metatarsal head with or without metatarsal osteotomy for angular correction. In occasional patients with severe degenerative joint disease, surgical management involves removal of all or part of the joint and insertion of a titanium joint replacement (Fig. 73.3D). Depending on locale, referral for surgical correction of a bunion may be made to a general, orthopedic, or podiatric surgeon. (This surgery, like most podiatric surgery, is done on an ambulatory basis in most states.) A patient should expect to return to most of his or her preoperative activities within 6 to

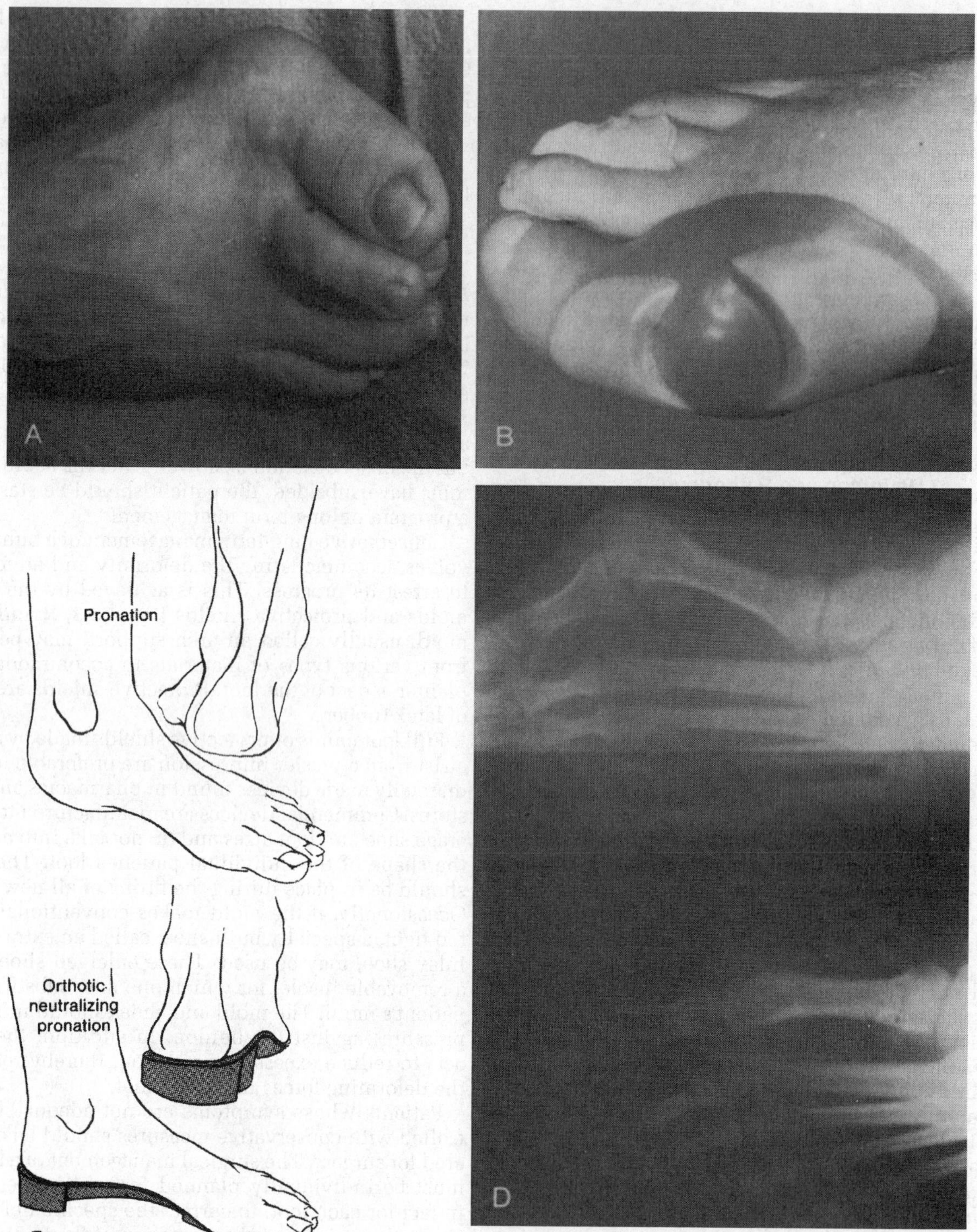

Figure 73.3. Bunions: appearance, orthotic compensation, and surgical repair. A: Bunion deformity. B: Bunion protected by latex shield. C: Leather orthotic arch support. D: Bunion deformity shown radiologically before and after surgical correction.

8 weeks after surgery; the interval may be somewhat longer after bilateral surgery. A tendency for the foot to swell postoperatively may persist for many months, however. Excessive pronation, the primary cause for bunion, persists after surgery. Therefore, a major determinant of the long-term results of surgery is follow-up foot care with orthotic appliances such as those described above.

Care for bunions is best individualized and negotiated with the consultant, because there is insufficient evidence from randomized controlled trials to determine which methods of either conservative, operative or postoperative treatment are the most appropriate (4,5). Surgical complications and continuing symptoms are not uncommon (5). Surgical treatment of diabetic patients with neuropathic and vascular disease may be complicated by infection, slow healing, or failure to heal. In these patients, therefore, a conservative approach is usually preferable.

Prevention

It is possible that the annoying symptoms of bunion deformity may be prevented if the deformity is recognized early (usually in the second or third decade) and the patient is referred for conservative management by a podiatrist.

CALLUSES AND CORNS

Definition and Pathogenesis

A *callus* is a thickening of the epidermis as a result of chronic intermittent trauma (Fig. 73.4). When there is intermittent irritation of an area of skin, the initial response is vasodilation; this is followed by increased production of corneum and hyperkeratosis. This process is normal and protective to skin and underlying tissue. When the process continues until there is buildup of excessive or highly concentrated callus, resulting in a corn, problems may develop. Skin lines may remain visible in callused tissue, but they usually do not pass through the highly concentrated center of a corn. Corns are most often located overlying the proximal interphalangeal joints of the lesser toes and centrally within plantar calluses. A number of processes not related to chronic trauma can produce focal calluses as well, namely *verruca plantaris* (plantar wart), *foreign body granuloma,* and *porokeratosis plantaris discreta.* These lesions are discussed below.

The primary cause for most symptomatic calluses is excessive pronation (see above), not restrictive shoes or walking on unyielding surfaces. During excessive pronation, the long flexor and extensor tendons pull on the distal phalanges, the toes appear to hammer, and a retrograde force pushes down on the metatarsal heads, increasing pressure on the plantar skin. Other

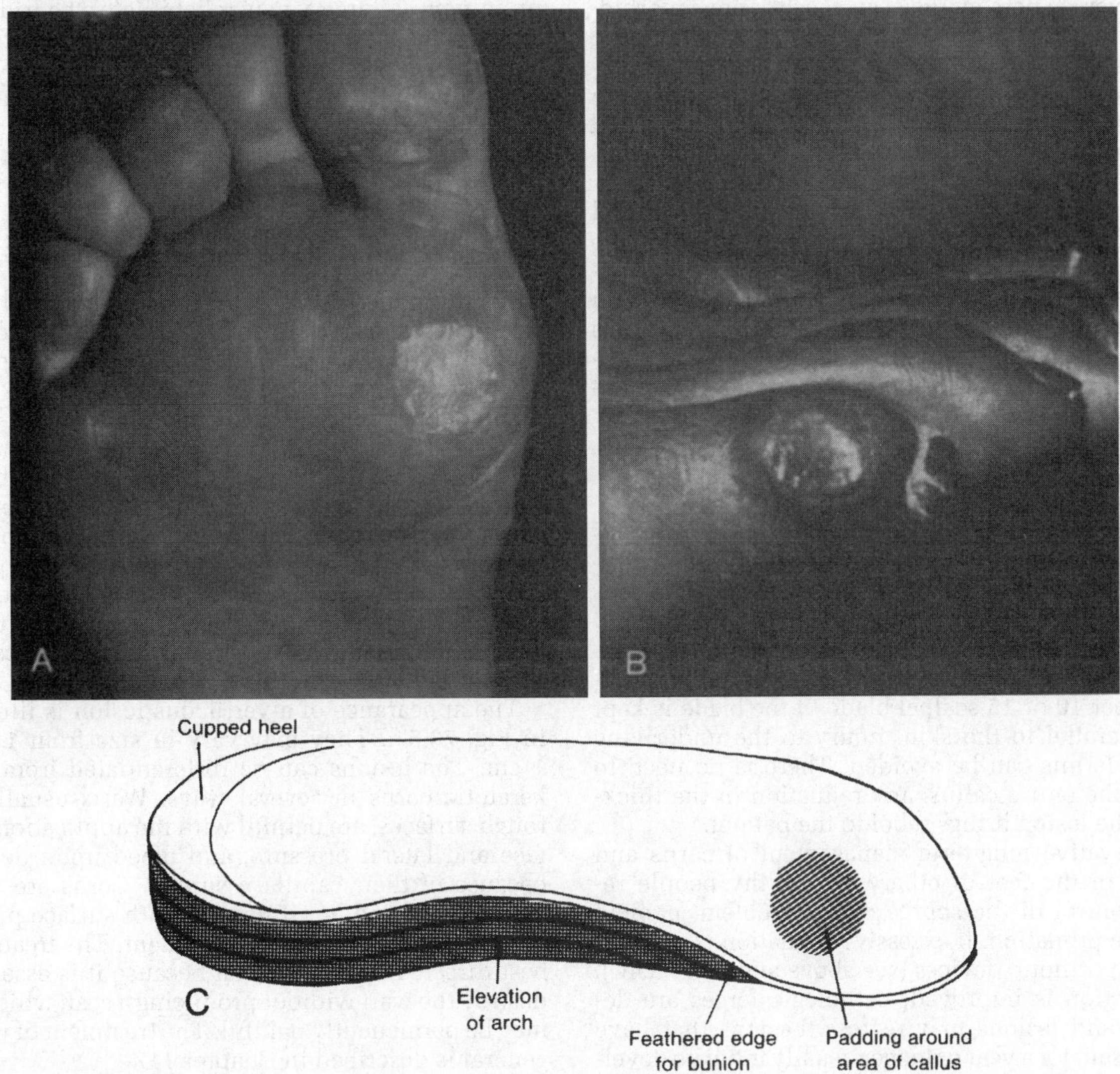

Figure 73.4. Calluses and corns. **A:** Typical plantar callus. **B:** Corn on the fifth digit. **C:** Orthotic device designed to shift weight from area of callus formation. (Photographs courtesy of Max Weisfeld, DPM.)

conditions that may promote this increased pressure are excessive supination (highly arched foot) and imbalance of the peroneal and tibial muscles caused by weakness, arthritis, or other conditions affecting one or both legs.

Symptoms

Diffuse callus is usually asymptomatic and easily controlled by the patient with pumice stones and cleansing agents readily available in pharmacies. Both calluses and corns produce pain. Thick accumulation of callus tends to cause a burning sensation in the foot. A corn located within a plantar callus gives the sensation of walking on a sharp pebble. Corns that occur dorsolaterally on fifth toes (Fig. 73.4B) often cause exquisite pain, especially with tight-fitting shoes. Such corns often have adventitious bursae associated with them and may produce symptoms of both bursitis and the discomfort of the corn pressing down on subcutaneous tissues.

Although corns and calluses can cause discomfort for the average person, they can cause serious morbidity in a diabetic patient (see above). A discrete lesion on the foot produces constant pressure on the underlying dermis. In a diabetic patient, this pressure often results in local breakdown of tissues, ulceration, and infection. Diabetic patients have the additional medical and mechanical problem of neurotrophic joints. In patients with the tendency to develop hammertoe and plantar-flexed metatarsal heads, these changes (and the calluses and corns that accompany them) may be accelerated by the loss of normal proprioception and pain sensation of a neurotrophic joint. Corns and calluses can be a serious problem also for patients with conditions other than diabetes that impair arterial circulation to the lower extremities (see Chapter 94).

Treatment

Treatment of corns and calluses depends on the location, severity, and type of lesion and on the physical condition of the patient. Occasionally, one sees patients who complain of severely painful corns and calluses. Dramatic relief may be obtained from the simple debridement of these painful lesions, using a sterile number 10 or 15 scalpel blade. If the blade is kept nearly parallel to the skin, injury to the underlying healthy dermis can be avoided. There is no need to debride the entire callus; any reduction in the thickness of the lesion brings relief to the patient.

Conservative long-term management of corns and calluses in the feet of otherwise healthy people requires control of the source of the problem, namely excessive pronation. If excessive pronation is neutralized with orthotic devices (see above and Fig. 73.4C), foot function is improved, pathologic forces are decreased, and lesions may regress. Lesions that have been present for a year or longer usually indicate developed structural changes in the bones and joints, with secondary histopathologic changes in the skin.

For patients whose symptoms are not controlled with conservative treatment, surgery may be helpful. A number of surgical procedures may be used to realign metatarsal heads or reduce hammertoe deformities. Often it is necessary to combine the surgical reconstruction of affected areas with control of pronation to achieve lasting resolution of symptoms. This may mean 6 to 8 weeks of convalescence (i.e., no weight-bearing for several days, then progression to partial, and then full weight-bearing, usually by 6 weeks) after foot surgery and the continued use of orthotics in shoes. The result is greater foot health and comfort.

For the patient with diabetes or peripheral vascular disease, conservative treatment involves frequent debridement of the hyperkeratotic areas, padding for protection, and the fabrication of molds (by a podiatrist or orthopedist) to shift weight away from problem areas and accommodate deformities (Fig. 73.4C). Extra-depth shoes are often prescribed in conjunction with such appliances. When refractory infection or ulceration occurs despite conservative management, surgical procedures may be performed to eliminate a bony prominence. Surgery may rehabilitate a bedridden patient or obviate future amputation. The risks of surgery include infection and failure to achieve the desired result; the risks must always be weighed against the hoped for goal. Management requires close collaboration between the patient's primary care practitioner and the consultant.

OTHER HYPERKERATOTIC LESIONS

Other discrete hyperkeratotic lesions commonly found on the foot include verruca plantaris, porokeratosis plantaris discreta, and foreign body granuloma. *Verruca plantaris,* or *plantar warts,* occur on the plantar aspect of the foot, usually on weight-bearing surfaces (Fig. 73.5A). They are discussed also in Chapter 117, but a brief account is provided here because of the importance of differentiating them from corns, calluses, and other hyperkeratotic lesions. Plantar warts can be asymptomatic or extremely painful. They are caused by a papilloma virus for which there is no specific treatment or prevention. Because they are benign and often resolve spontaneously, aggressive or untried therapies should be avoided.

The appearance of a verrucous lesion is illustrated in Fig. 73.5A. They may vary in size from 1 mm to 1 cm. The lesions can be differentiated from hyperkeratotic corns in several ways. Warts usually have rough surfaces, are painful with the application of surface and lateral pressure, and bleed upon debriding because of their capillary supply. Corns are usually smooth surfaced, most painful with surface pressure, and do not bleed upon debridement. The treatment is best directed by a podiatrist because it is essential to destroy the wart without producing a scar, which itself may be permanently painful. The treatment of warts in general is described in Chapter 117.

A *porokeratotic lesion* is a circumscribed discrete hyperkeratotic lesion on the plantar aspect of the foot

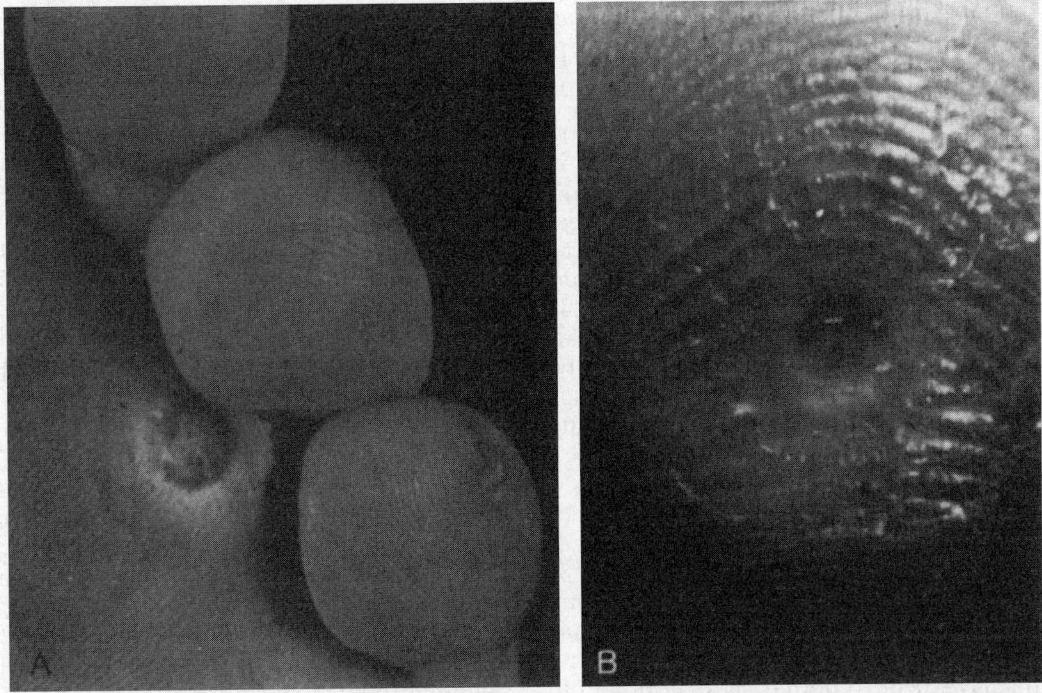

Figure 73.5. Hyperkeratotic lesions not caused by chronic trauma. **A:** Plantar wart. **B:** Porokeratosis on plantar surface. (Photographs courtesy of Max Weisfeld, DPM.)

that develops as a result of keratin occluding a sweat duct in the skin (Fig. 73.5B). The obstruction and resultant backup create a reaction in the skin similar to a deep large corn. This lesion need not be under a weight-bearing surface. It is usually painful, and after debridement there is characteristically even more distress. Treatment by the dermatologist or podiatrist is usually by local curettage.

Foreign bodies in the plantar surface of the foot can generate a local inflammatory reaction and thus create a hyperkeratotic lesion. One of the most common offending substances is hair (animal or human). For example, a dog hair, trapped in a carpet long enough to have dried out, can penetrate the skin rather easily. This lesion, although grossly resembling a simple callus, has a small aperture (entry wound) near the center, seen upon examination with a magnifying glass. The local reaction may or may not include infection. Treatment is simple excision of the foreign body.

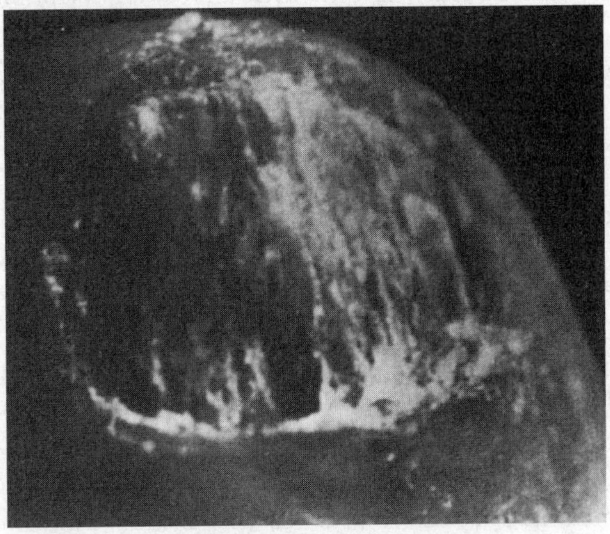

Figure 73.6. Myotic toenail.

NAIL CONDITIONS

Only two nail conditions are commonly brought to medical attention: onychomycosis (fungal infection) and ingrown toenails, with or without concomitant inflammation (paronychia).

Onychomycosis

Causes and Findings

The typical fungal infection of a toenail begins distally at the tip of the toe and moves proximally, subungually, and through the nail plate itself (Fig. 73.6). Etiologic agents are *Trichophyton mentagrophytes, Trichophyton rubrum,* or *Candida albicans.* The fungus produces yellowish discoloration and longitudinal striations in the nails and in the epidermis; the accompanying local inflammatory reaction stimulates hyperkeratosis under the nail. This hyperkeratotic accumulation tends to lift the nail up from the epidermis, facilitating further progression of the fungus. Eventually, the nail becomes mottled brownish yellow, thickened, and powdery. Usually, these infections are asymptomatic; patients are most concerned about the appearance of their nails, the possibility of spread of infection, and sometimes the inability to wear shoes when severe thickening of the nail plate is present.

Treatment

Fungus infections of toenails are difficult to eradicate medically. Oral medications are available to treat and resolve onychomycosis. Itraconazole is effective against dermatophytes such as *T. rubrum* and nondermatophytes such as yeasts and molds. Terbinafine is effective against most dermatophytes. Because not all dystrophic toenails are mycotic, treatment should be based on the results of nail fungal cultures. Both drugs are taken orally once a day for 3 months: terbinafine (Lamisil 250 mg) and itraconazole (Sporanox 200 mg). Although itraconazole is commonly prescribed as a pulsed dose for fingernail fungus, it is not approved for toenail fungus in pulsed form. (Pulsed doses refer to double dosing for 1 week followed by a 3-week respite.) Potentially serious adverse reactions include congestive heart failure (itraconazole) and hepatic toxicity (both medications). Rare incidents of leukopenia have been reported with terbinafine. White blood cell monitoring with terbinafine and liver function monitoring with both are recommended. An effective topical antifungal, ciclopirox (8% Penlac nail lacquer), is now available by prescription. Although it is not as effective as the oral medications, it requires no medical monitoring. Another effective topical agent, amorolfine (5% Loceryl nail lacquer), has not yet been approved for use in the United States.

When nail thickening is regarded as a problem by the patient, the process can be controlled by regular and thorough debridement. The debridement of mycotic or otherwise thickened toenails is a process generally performed by podiatrists. The debridement first involves soaking of the feet and cutting of the nails by heavy-duty cutters. Finally, the nails are thoroughly filed down with an electrically powered diamond-studded burr. These drills are fitted with vacuum extraction systems to protect the patient and podiatrist from breathing in the nail dust.

Another treatment is permanent removal of the nail, including matrixectomy. Because toenails serve no useful function, their absence causes no functional impairment. However, surgical correction should be reserved for patients whose nails are painful or for whom the appearance of the feet is a significant factor. The most common type of surgical correction of toenails performed by dermatologists, podiatrists, or surgeons is nail excision, followed by chemical destruction of matrix tissue and nail bed with 88% phenol. After a sterile dressing is applied to the toe, the patient may continue normal activities. The patient needs only to change bandages and soak the feet daily until healing is complete in 2 to 3 weeks. Skin formerly below the nail plate thickens. Anyone can disguise the fact that their nails have been removed by applying nail polish to this thickened skin.

Ingrown Toenails

Causes and Findings

Ingrown toenail, a painful condition in which the medial or lateral border of a toenail penetrates the flesh, is a common problem (Fig. 73.7). Ingrown toenails have been attributed to factors such as improper trimming, heredity, bony pathology, improper shoe fit, tight socks, obesity, and trauma. However, there is no clear-cut cause, and there are probably many contributing causes. The great toe is the one almost always involved, and the problem can be identified by inspection and by finding point tenderness upon pressing the margin of the toenail.

Treatment

There is a popular misconception that cutting a V in the center of a toenail causes the lateral borders to grow toward the center, thereby relieving the ingrown condition. This belief has no basis in fact because the nail plate is merely hornified keratin: nonliving fixed tissue in which growth no longer occurs.

Initial treatment of ingrown toenail depends on whether the patient's toe is infected (paronychia) or is chronically painful but not infected when the patient seeks care. The patient with an ingrown toenail often seeks help after attempting to excise the offending edge of toenail with whatever instruments are available; most of the nail edge may be removed in this way by the patient, but a small sharp piece of nail usually remains that pierces the skin with each step and promotes infection. The toe becomes red, swollen, and

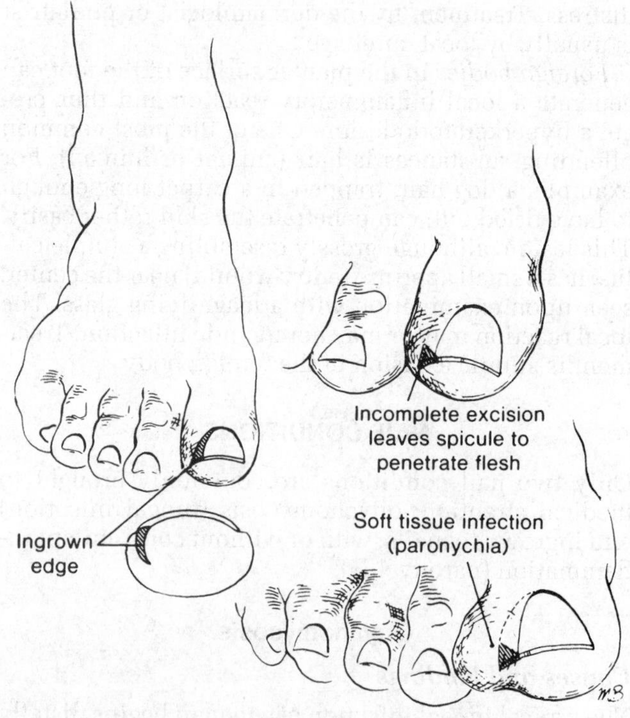

Figure 73.7. Schematic illustration of an ingrown toenail and complications that may occur.

exquisitely tender. The most vigorous soaking and the use of local and systemic antibiotics will not arrest such an infection as long as a nail spicule continues to penetrate the flesh. Therefore, the patient should be referred to a dermatologist, podiatrist, or surgeon for excision of the offending border of the nail; this procedure is done under local anesthesia and is curative. However, approximately 10% of patients have a recurrence, usually within 1 year. Systemic antimicrobials are rarely necessary. Definitive treatment of the ingrown nail itself varies according to the condition and needs of the patient.

For otherwise healthy patients, the procedure described above for removal of the entire toenail and for matrix destruction can also be used to eradicate permanently an ingrown border. After local anesthesia (obtained by injecting the base of the toe to create a full block, injecting a field on the medial surface from dorsal to lateral and on the lateral surface from dorsal to lateral), the offending edge of toenail is excised and then phenol and alcohol are applied to cauterize the matrix tissue. This procedure, followed by complete healing in 2 to 3 weeks, usually eliminates permanently this painful and sometimes dangerous condition. The use of phenol dramatically decreases the rate of recurrence of the ingrown nail and increases patient satisfaction but at the cost of an increased postoperative infection rate (6). Even with phenol ablation of the nail matrix, there is still a 20% to 30% chance of recurrence. It is not unusual to rephenolize a nail within a year of treatment.

Treatment of diabetic patients and patients with arterial insufficiency must be conservative because wound healing may be poor after surgical removal of the nail. In these patients, frequent and thorough debridement of ingrown borders is effective and safe. Treatment by a podiatrist or other practitioner who is skilled in this procedure may be needed every 3 to 4 weeks to prevent complicating soft tissue infection.

HEEL PAIN

Diagnosis

Heel pain is a common complaint. The most common pattern is pain that is localized to the medial plantar aspect of the heel. (Heel pain localized to the posterior aspect of the heel is discussed in Chapter 72, and heel pain as a manifestation of the tarsal tunnel syndrome is discussed in Chapter 92.) Characteristically, the first step in the morning is particularly painful. After 5 to 10 minutes of walking the pain eases, but during the course of the day's activities it becomes progressively worse. The reason that these symptoms appear, disappear, and reappear is not understood.

Examination of the foot reveals a tender area of the heel approximately 4.5 cm from the posterior margin of the plantar surface, corresponding to the medial condyle of the calcaneus. X-rays often reveal a calcaneal exostosis or spur at the point of tenderness (Fig. 73.8). These spurs are commonly found on x-rays of asymptomatic heels, and they are not the cause of pain in symptomatic heels. Because the attachment of the plantar fascia coincides with the point of greatest tenderness, it is believed that pain is caused by *plantar fasciitis*. One can picture the plantar fascia as an extension of the Achilles tendon, with the calcaneus acting as a fulcrum between fascia and tendon (Fig. 73.1B). Any condition that increases stress on the Achilles tendon may also stress the plantar fascia, such as overuse in running or jogging (especially with shoes having inflexible midsoles), excessive pronation (see above), or a sudden change to flat shoes after wearing high heels for prolonged periods. Heel pain may also be a manifestation of gout or Reiter syndrome, and these diagnoses should always be considered when evaluating such a patient (see Chapters 76 and 78).

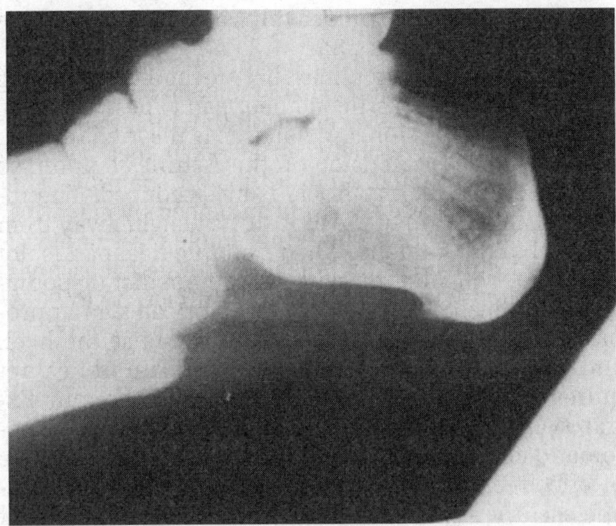

Figure 73.8. Radiologic view of a calcaneal exostosis (spur). (Photograph courtesy of Max Weisfeld, DPM.)

Treatment

Treatment should be aimed at both the local inflammatory process and the underlying mechanical problem. Initial treatment includes using an oral anti-inflammatory medication (see Chapter 77), resting, and soaking in warm water. An injection (using a 25-gauge 1-inch needle) of a corticosteroid and lidocaine (approximately 0.5 to 1 mL of suspension of a corticosteroid diluted with 1 to 2 mL of 1% to 2% lidocaine) into the tender area from the medial aspect of the heel usually brings short-term relief from pain that has not responded to other measures (7,8) (see also Chapters 69 and 74). The use of high dose repository steroids should be avoided because there is a risk of plantar fascial rupture after injection as some studies have indicated (8). The potential for fascial rupture may be minimized with the use of a combination solution such as Celestone/Soluspan, which combines a phosphate and acetate in one injection. Topical steroids delivered by iontophoresis may also be effective (7). In some cases stretching of the Achilles tendon will bring relief.

Spontaneous resolution of symptoms, over the course of months, is common (8).

Recurrent symptoms may be prevented by having the patient obtain a silicone heel pad. These pads are available in sport stores. When this is inserted into the shoes, it decreases tension on the Achilles tendon, so tension on the plantar fascia is also reduced. The increased angulation of the foot shifts weight away from the heel to the forefoot. When a simple heel pad is not sufficient, consultation with an orthopedist or podiatrist is indicated. The consultant fabricates an appropriate orthotic to minimize pronation, raise the heel, and protect the painful area. Rarely, a painful heel requires surgical fasciotomy and removal of the spur. Extracorporeal shock wave therapy is used in very symptomatic and resistant cases and has limited evidence of effectiveness (8). Extracorporeal shock wave therapy uses the same mechanism as lithotripsy but to treat heel spur pain. There is conflicting evidence regarding the effectiveness of dorsiflexion night splints, which stretch the Achilles tendon, in patients with chronic pain (longer than 6 months) (7).

METATARSALGIA

Definition and Pathogenesis

Metatarsalgia is pain in the forefoot. The most common condition causing metatarsalgia is *Morton neuroma.* This is a condition in which two interdigital plantar nerves between adjacent toes become compressed, inflamed, and ultimately painful. The compression of these nerves is enhanced by elevating the heel and compressing the forefoot. Therefore, women's fashionable, high-heeled, pointed-toe shoes are associated with this condition. In fact, 80% to 90% of patients with neuroma are female.

Symptoms and Signs

The symptoms of neuroma are specific and consistent. Typically, the patient describes a shooting, burning, or cramping pain in the foot involving two adjacent toes. The third and fourth toes are involved most commonly. However, the second and third toes often are affected also. The patient describes spontaneous pain during walking or running. Invariably, the patient instinctively removes the shoe and massages the affected area, thereby relieving the pain. Presumably, the swollen nerve (neuroma) has been pinched by the metatarsal bones, causing the pain that radiates to the toes. Stopping walking eliminates the trauma, and massage may change the position of the neuroma. All of these measures result in alleviation of the pain.

Examination of the foot reveals that the neurovascular status is normal unless another disease is present. Palpation between the metatarsal heads reveals marked tenderness. If the forefoot is compressed while the web space is palpated, the area may be exquisitely tender.

Stress fracture of a metatarsal bone should be suspected in the case of sudden severe pain localized to a metatarsal shaft. X-rays may be diagnostic but are often negative during the first few weeks of symptoms. Often the fracture will be apparent on repeat x-rays in 2 to 3 weeks. Bone scans and magnetic resonance images are more sensitive diagnostic tools and are often positive before the radiograph.

Treatment

The most effective treatment for metatarsalgia is the wearing of low, flat, wide, soft, leather shoes. Corticosteroid with lidocaine injections into the web space and reaching the plantar surface (0.5 mL of deposteroid with 1 mL of lidocaine using a 25-gauge 1-inch needle) may provide temporary relief. Nonsteroidal anti-inflammatory drugs are ineffective. Orthotics are helpful; however, if the patient is willing to wear wide enough shoes to accommodate them, the condition usually resolves, even without the orthotic. Surgical excision is successful in 80% to 90% of cases and is indicated if symptoms persist. For patients undergoing surgery, a recovery period of 4 to 6 weeks is necessary before they can return to full activity and wear their usual shoes. Surgical complications are rare. As with most surgery, the possibility of postoperative infection is less than 3%. Peculiar to neuroma surgery is the possibility of recurrence. Rarely symptoms are not reduced. Because neuroma is entirely a clinical finding, exploration for a neuroma will occasionally be fruitless. Fortunately, this is also an uncommon occurrence, but the possibility should always be told to the patient before surgery.

Metatarsalgia not caused by neuroma is more difficult to characterize, evaluate, and treat. Non-neuritic metatarsal pain may occur anywhere in the forefoot with or without radiation and may be exacerbated by high-heeled or, at times, low-heeled shoes. Palpation often reveals pain directly on a metatarsal head rather than between them. Rest, the application of ice, and elevation of the foot may help some patients, but most require referral to a podiatrist for padding, orthotics, or other treatment. Metatarsal stress fractures are another cause of metatarsalgia, usually characterized by sudden onset and pain on palpation over the involved metatarsal bone. Often there is no history of trauma. The use of shock-absorbing insoles in footwear has been shown to reduce the incidence of stress fractures in athletes and military personnel (9). Their diagnosis and management is discussed in Chapter 68.

General References*

Alexander I. The foot exam and diagnosis. Philadelphia: Churchill Livingstone, 1997.

Paperback book covering multiple foot issues aimed at the primary care practitioner.

Banks AS, ed. McGlamry's comprehensive textbook of foot surgery. 3rd ed. Philadelphia: Lippincott Williams & Wilkins, 2001.

*Bold print (general references) and bold numerals (specific references) denote published controlled clinical trials, meta-analyses, or consensus-based recommendations.

This two-volume text covers all aspects of foot care, including medical and surgical treatments.

Bowker JH, Pfeifer MA, eds. Levin and O'Neal's the diabetic foot. 6th ed. St. Louis: CV Mosby, 2001.

The most highly regarded resource for the care of the diabetic foot.

Robbins JM, ed. Primary podiatric medicine. Philadelphia: W.B. Saunders, 1994.

Intensive evaluation and management of foot diseases aimed at the specialist, but very readable.

Specific References

1. Litzelman DK, Slemenda Cw, Langefeld CD, et al. Reduction of lower extremity clinical abnormalities in patients with non-insulin-dependent diabetes mellitus: a randomized, controlled trial. Ann Intern Med 1993;119:36.
2. Franse LV, Valk GD, Heine RJ, et al. "Numbness of the feet" is a poor indicator for polyneuropathy in type 2 diabetic patients. Diabet Med 2000;17:105.
3. Spencer S. Pressure relieving interventions for preventing and treating diabetic foot ulcers. Cochrane Database of Systematic Reviews. Issue 1, 2001.
4. Ferrari J, Higgins JPT, Williams RL. Interventions for treating hallux valgus (abductovalgus) and bunions. Cochrane Database of Systematic Reviews. Issue 1, 2001.
5. Ferrari J. Hallux valgus (bunions). Clinical Evidence 2000;4:591.
6. Rounding C, Hulm S. Surgical treatments for ingrowing toenails. Cochrane Datatbase of Systematic Reviews. Issue 1, 2001.
7. Crawford F, Atkins D, Edwards J. Interventions for treating plantar heel pain. Cochrane Database of Systematic Reviews. Issue 1, 2001.
8. Crawford F. Plantar heel pain (including plantar fasciitis). Clinical Evidence 2000;4:664.
9. Gillespie WJ, Grant J. Interventions for preventing and treating stress fractures and stress reactions of bone of the lower limbs in young adults. Cochrane Database of Systematic Reviews. Issue 1, 2001.

C H A P T E R 74

Nonarticular Rheumatic Disorders

DAVID B. HELLMANN, MD

BURSITIS

General Considerations

Bursitis, the inflammation of a bursal sac, is a common problem. Bursal sacs are structures lined with a synovial membrane that secretes and absorbs liquid. The bursae thereby provide a lubricating mechanism between structures such as bones, ligaments, tendons, muscles, and skin. Although usually isolated, occasionally they are in communication with a joint space. There are more than 150 such structures in the body, but the number is not fixed and a new bursa may appear whenever there is friction between structures.

Bursitis is usually easy to diagnose and treat in the office. Occasionally, clinicians face the challenge of distinguishing bursitis from arthritis or other conditions. Also, it is important to quickly recognize and treat the few patients who have septic bursitis. When the diagnosis remains uncertain or the usual treatments are unsuccessful, referral to an orthopedist or rheumatologist may be necessary.

Causes

The most common cause of bursitis is minor trauma, as may occur to the subdeltoid bursa from repetitively throwing a baseball or to the prepatellar bursa from prolonged kneeling on a concrete floor. Because the development of bursitis is a function of both physical stresses and the condition of the bursa and surrounding tissues, bursitis is rare before the age of 20 and is particularly common in middle-aged and older people. Less often, bursitis is caused by systemic disorders such as rheumatoid arthritis, polymyalgia rheumatica, or gout. Septic bursitis after trauma is a special concern in patients with superficial bursitis (e.g., olecranon or prepatellar bursitis). Basic calcium phosphate crystals are known to be associated with calcific periarthritis, tendinitis, and bursitis, but little is understood about the exact mechanism of calcium crystal deposition.

Manifestations

Patients with acute bursitis experience abrupt onset of localized pain that is aggravated by any movement of the structures adjacent to the bursa. The pain is usually described as a deep aching discomfort. How well the patient can localize the discomfort depends on whether the bursa is superficial or deep to the skin and on whether the affected region has extensive or exiguous sensory nerve fibers. Thus, when asked "Where does it hurt?," the patient with anserine bursitis often uses a fingertip to pinpoint the location, whereas a patient with trochanteric bursitis usually waves the entire hand over the general region of pain.

Bursitis near the knee, hip, elbow, or shoulder can mimic arthritis of those structures. Features that suggest bursitis include sudden onset after some repetitive physical activity; swelling, redness, or tenderness localized to the bursa and not the joint (see below); absence of pain on passive motion of the joint; and, if necessary, a normal joint x-ray or magnetic resonance imaging.

Infection is suggested by fluctuant swelling of the bursa in association with redness and heat of the overlying skin (1–3). Fever should always suggest infection but can also complicate gouty bursitis. The absence of fever does not exclude infection; for example, only one-third of patients with olecranon septic bursitis demonstrate fever (1,2). A large bursal swelling can compress other structures or even rupture, thus explaining why bursitis around the knee or the hip can present as diffuse leg swelling (mimicking thrombophlebitis), an inguinal hernia, or a pelvic mass (4).

Aspiration of Bursae

Aspiration is usually easily accomplished by the generalist, especially when the bursa is superficial (Table 74.1). The chief indication for aspirating a bursa is to rule out infection. Analysis of bursa (or joint) fluid can also reveal whether the fluid is inflamed or contains crystals (usually from gout).

The laboratory tests performed on bursal (or joint) fluid depend on the clinical questions (Table 74.2). A bursal or joint fluid white blood cell count of greater than 1,000 indicates inflammation; fewer than 1,000 white blood cells is characteristic of traumatic fluid (Table 74.2). Bursal infection tends to give very high white blood cell counts, averaging approximately 75,000 for olecranon bursitis (2), but rheumatoid arthritis and gout can also occasionally produce markedly elevated bursal fluid white blood cell counts. Gram stains and cultures are the specific tests for infection. Similarly, examining the fluid with a microscope equipped with polarizing lenses is the only way to identify the crystals that are specific for gout (see Chapter 76). Therefore, most bursal fluid can be characterized by the white blood cell count, Gram stain plus culture, and the analysis for crystals. Glucose, protein, mucin clot, and other (e.g., enzymes, complement) determinations are not specific and are not needed.

Treatment

Treatment of septic bursitis requires administering antibiotics and draining the bursal sac. Gram stain of the bursal fluid (see below) should guide initial antibiotic choice. Most cases of septic bursitis are caused by *Staphylococcus aureus,* but Gram stain is positive in only 65%. If the Gram stain shows no bacteria or if gram-positive cocci are found, a penicillinase-resistant antistaphylococcal drug should be used. Vancomycin should be used initially if the patient has recently been in a facility where methicillin resistant *S. aureus* is prevalent. If gram-negative organisms are found, blood cultures should be obtained and an extrabursal site

Table 74.1. Technique for Aspiration of Superficial Bursae (or Joints) and Analysis of Bursal (or Synovial) Fluid

1. Determine by palpation the area of maximal tenderness or fluctuance and outline with indelible pen.
2. Clean the skin with iodine solution such as povidone (Betadine).
3. Anesthetize the skin with lidocaine in the area of planned aspiration.
4. Use an 18-gauge needle to aspirate.
5. Grossly inspect the fluid and analyze for the following:
   a. Cell count and differential; fluid must be in a tube containing heparin or ethylenediamine tetraacetate.
   b. Type of crystals (see Chapter 76).
   c. Gram stain and culture using transport media (even in the absence of a high white cell count).

Table 74.2. Patterns of Bursal (or Joint) Fluid Findings in Common Problems

	Normal	Trauma	Sepsis	Rheumatoid Inflammation	Microcrystalline Inflammation
Color of fluid	Clear yellow	Bloody, xanthochromic	Yellow to cloudy	Clear yellow to cloudy	Clear yellow to cloudy
WBC, RBC	0–200/0	<1,000/many	1,000–200,000/few	1,000–20,000[a]/few	1,000–20,000[a]/few
Crystals	~	~	~	~	+[b]
Culture	~	~	+	~	~

+, test positive; ~, not applicable or negative.

[a]Cell count in noninfected inflammatory fluid may sometimes be as high as it is with sepsis, thus the need for culture.

[b]Gout, negatively birefringent sodium urate. Pseudogout, positively birefringent sodium pyrophosphate (see Chapter 76).

WBC, white blood cell; RBC, red blood cell.

of infection should be sought. The antibiotic choice should be based on the most likely organism causing the extrabursal infection. The need for hospitalization depends on both the severity of the infection and the degree of compromise of the host. Patients with high fever and chills, intense surrounding cellulitis, deep bursal involvement, extrabursal infection, or suspicion of an uncommon organism should be hospitalized for parenteral antibiotics. Hospitalization should also be considered for patients who are compromised by age, alcoholism, diabetes mellitus, or immunosuppression, almost regardless of the intensity of bursal inflammation. Patients who are less ill and less frail can be treated as outpatients with oral antibiotics. Repeated bursal aspiration is also required until the fluid stops accumulating. On average, successful treatment of septic olecranon bursitis, for example, requires two to three aspirations over a week or two. The timing of these repeat aspirations is made solely on the clinical response (or absence thereof) of the patient. The duration of antibiotic therapy averages 3 to 4 weeks but should be individualized according to the clinical response and the character of aspirated fluid. Antibiotics should be continued for 5 additional days after the bursal fluid has cleared or has become sterile.

Gout, pseudogout, or rheumatoid arthritis should be treated with anti-inflammatory agents (see Chapters 76 and 77). Usually *traumatic bursitis* resolves spontaneously if the area of inflammation is rested. However, the spontaneous resolution requires several weeks and therapy shortens this period considerably. Therefore, if sepsis and gout are ruled out, the treatment outlined in Table 74.3 is indicated.

If there is no initial response to treatment with a nonsteroidal anti-inflammatory agent (see Chapter 77 for a description), the patient should be treated with an injection into the inflamed bursa of a mixture of lidocaine and depoglucocorticoid (Table 74.4). Immediate and dramatic but transient relief of pain secondary to lidocaine indicates that the proper site has been injected. The anti-inflammatory effect of the steroid injection is seen in approximately 72 hours. If a satisfactory response has not occurred, the bursa may be reinjected in approximately 2 weeks. Waiting 2 weeks before reinjection provides ample time to rule out iatrogenic sepsis, which rarely occurs after a steroid injection. Depending on the location, other modalities such as ultrasound, heat or cold application, and physical therapy may be used as adjuncts. If a bursitis does not respond to two steroid injections, rheumatologic consultation to rule out associated systemic disease may be necessary. Rarely, definitive treatment by surgical excision of the bursa may be necessary.

Table 74.3. Treatment of Bursitis

1. Splint where feasible (especially effective in the hand and fingers).
2. Application of heat or cold may be of benefit in some patients.
3. Anti-inflammatory agents: A nonsteroidal anti-inflammatory agent with rapid onset of action is preferred (see Chapter 77 for a full discussion of these agents).
4. Improvement is usual in several days, but the anti-inflammatory agent should be continued an additional 4–5 days to prevent recurrence.
5. If no significant response is noted in 5–7 days and sepsis has been ruled out, the bursa may be injected with lidocaine or a steroid preparation (see Table 74.4).

Table 74.4. Methods of Injection of Bursae or Joints with Lidocaine or Depoglucocorticoid Preparations

1. Be certain sepsis has been ruled out (Tables 74.1 and 74.2).
2. Prepare the skin carefully with an iodine-containing solution such as povidone (Betadine).
3. Anesthetize the skin with intradermal 1–2% lidocaine.
4. Mix 2–3 mL of 1–2% lidocaine with 20–40 mg of a depoglucocorticoid (such as Celestone, Aristocort, or Kenalog) and inject the bursa with 1–3 mL of this mixture using a 22-gauge needle.

Notes of caution: Injection into the skin will cause atrophy and thus should be avoided; the patient should understand that there is a possibility of this complication. Injection into tendons themselves may cause degeneration and, in time, rupture; these structures should be avoided by careful palpation.

Specific Forms

Several forms of bursitis are particularly common; their unique aspects are described here.

Olecranon Bursitis

This common form of bursitis—also called student's or miner's elbow—is characterized by a goose egg-like swelling located just behind the olecranon process of the ulna (see Chapter 69). An effusion of the elbow joint itself, in contrast, causes diffuse swelling. Another feature that distinguishes olecranon bursitis from elbow joint inflammation is that passive extension and flexion of the elbow are nearly painless when the only problem is olecranon bursitis. Important features of olecranon bursitis are that it is often associated with systemic disease, such as rheumatoid arthritis or gout; symptoms often are chronic, in that they have been present for 2 or 3 weeks before a patient sees a physician; and it is a common site for septic bursitis after trauma and may be associated with surrounding cellulitis. If rheumatoid arthritis or gout is present, it is important to realize that sepsis sometimes coexists. Traumatic olecranon bursitis is usually hemorrhagic, although xanthochromic fluid may be present.

Swelling in the area of the olecranon bursa should be aspirated if symptomatic (Tables 74.1 and 74.2). A Gram stain, culture, white blood cell count, and crystal identification with polarizing microscopy should be obtained.

Therapy. Therapy depends on the characteristics of the fluid (5). If monosodium urate crystals are present, specific therapy for gout is indicated (see Chapter 76). Traumatic bursitis responds to simple removal of fluid; however, if the fluid reaccumulates, a steroid injection (Table 74.4) should be given. If sepsis is identified, the patient should be treated with an antibiotic and bursal aspiration as outlined above. An x-ray of the elbow should be obtained to rule out osteomyelitis or a foreign body if the process has been present for more than 2 weeks.

Prepatellar Bursitis

Prepatellar bursitis (housemaid's or carpenter's knee) is a common form of bursitis, easily recognized by its location overlying the inferior portion of the patella (see Chapter 72). It is particularly common in carpet layers, plumbers, and carpenters. It is most often caused by trauma from kneeling, but it may also be a site of sepsis, and for this reason the bursa should always be aspirated, even if it feels dry.

Anserine Bursitis

The anserine bursa is fan shaped and lies between the confluence of tendons of the sartorius, gracilis, and semitendinosus muscles and the tibia at the anterior medial aspect of the knee just below the joint space (see Chapter 72) (6). Anserine bursitis is most often seen in patients with arthritis, especially overweight middle-aged women with osteoarthritis of the knee, and is recognized by its location; the pain is typically produced when the knee is flexed and is particularly troublesome at night. The patient often seeks comfort by sleeping with a pillow between the thighs.

If there is surrounding erythema or if the patient is febrile, aspiration should be attempted because sepsis, although uncommon, may be present. Therapy depends on the findings (Tables 74.2 and 74.3). When injection therapy is used, the solution should be injected in a fan-shaped pattern so that the entire bursa is treated.

Ischial Bursitis

The ischial bursa is located over the ischial tuberosity, close to the sciatic nerve and the posterior femoral cutaneous nerve. When a person is sitting, the ischial bursae are covered only with subcutaneous tissue and skin; when a person is standing, the gluteus maximus also covers the bursa.

The most common reason for inflammation of this bursa is trauma, as may occur in bicycling. It is rarely a site of sepsis. Usually, the inflammation results in an abrupt onset of pain, but occasionally the onset is more insidious. The patient often has exquisite pain when sitting or lying. Because of the close proximity of the sciatic nerve to the bursa, there may be an associated neuritis resulting from pressure on the nerve, which causes sciatic pain to radiate into the leg (see Chapter 71). Direct pressure over the ischial tuberosity causes sharp pain and the patient may hold the painful buttock elevated when sitting. In addition, the pain is intensified when the patient is supine and the hip is passively flexed. The patient has difficulty standing on tiptoe on the affected side.

The differential diagnosis of symptoms suggestive of ischial bursitis includes lumbar spine disease, thrombophlebitis, and inflammatory back disease or sacroiliitis (see Chapter 78). Localization of the pain over the ischial tuberosity and the finding of induration near the ischial tuberosity on rectal examination establish the diagnosis of ischial bursitis.

Aspiration of the bursa, even when it is inflamed, is discouraged because it is often difficult to localize, and the surrounding structures, especially the sciatic nerve, may be injured. If aspiration is indicated because there is associated fever and, therefore, the possibility of septic bursitis, the patient should be referred to an orthopedist for immediate evaluation.

The patient may obtain some comfort when sitting by using a pillow that allows pressure to be eliminated from the ischial tuberosity underlying the inflamed bursa. Standard therapy (Table 74.3) with a nonsteroidal anti-inflammatory agent usually provides dramatic improvement within 2 to 3 days; however, if there has been associated leg pain or weakness from sciatic nerve inflammation, those symptoms may persist for several months. Ultrasound therapy, administered by a physical therapist, may be effective and it should be considered if initial therapy has not relieved the symptoms within several days.

If the diagnosis is unclear, there is a question of sepsis, and the patient does not respond within a week to therapy, consultation with a rheumatologist or orthopedist is recommended. If the diagnosis is confirmed, the consultant may aspirate the bursa and, if sepsis is ruled out, inject it with lidocaine and depoglucocorticoid, which often results in dramatic improvement.

Semimembranosus Gastrocnemius Bursitis (Baker Cyst)

The semimembranosus gastrocnemius bursa, commonly called a cyst, lies in the posterior medial aspect of the knee behind the femoral condyle (see Chapter 72) and in 50% of patients is continuous with the knee joint. The cyst is best seen and palpated when the patient is standing. Swelling of this bursa is commonly associated with other knee problems such as internal derangements, rheumatoid arthritis, or degenerative arthritis. The bursa is rarely infected. Often, a Baker cyst is asymptomatic. With a large cyst the patient may note a vague discomfort or fullness behind the knee. Many Baker cysts produce symptoms only when they rupture, causing acute swelling, pain, and redness of the calf and lower leg (the syndrome of pseudothrombophlebitis). The possibility that a patient with acute calf swelling has pseudothrombophlebitis from a ruptured Baker cyst is strongly suggested by finding swelling of the knee joint. When in doubt, a study to exclude thrombophlebitis should be done (see Chapter 57). Sonography, magnetic resonance imaging, and arthrography can visualize a ruptured cyst but are usually not needed if the clinical picture is consistent and thrombophlebitis has been excluded (7). Rarely, an unruptured Baker cyst can compress deep veins and cause thrombophlebitis.

The differential diagnosis of a posterior knee fullness includes an aneurysm of the popliteal artery. Therefore, it is important to palpate any fullness for pulsations.

Management of an uncomplicated Baker cyst includes aspiration and instillation of a corticosteroid–anesthetic mixture. Usually, this can be accomplished by aspirating and injecting the joint space. Rarely, the cyst may need to be aspirated or injected from the posterior approach. Because of the important structures in the popliteal fossa (artery, nerve, and vein), aspiration of the bursa posteriorly should be done by an orthopedist. Weight-bearing should be minimized for several days. The response to this therapy is usually excellent. Management of a ruptured cyst consists of bed rest, heat, and elevation. Although no data confirm this recommendation, an elastic bandage around the knee when treating a Baker cyst is not recommended because it may cause the cyst to compress more severely the venous system, increasing the chance of a thrombophlebitis. Instillation of corticosteroids into the joint that has an effusion may be helpful. Nonsteroidal anti-inflammatory agents may also help; after symptoms have begun to abate, ambulation can slowly be increased.

Iliopectineal Bursitis

The iliopectineal bursa lies anterior to the hip joint, with which it communicates in approximately 15% of people. It lies between the inguinal ligament and the iliopsoas muscle just lateral to the femoral artery. It may be inflamed from running or other similar trauma. Pain in the anterior pelvis, groin, and thigh is the most common manifestation of iliopectineal bursitis; swelling may result in a bulge resembling a femoral hernia (see Chapter 97) below the inguinal ligament. Bursitis may be present in conjunction with intrinsic inflammatory joint disease such as rheumatoid arthritis. Extension of the hip (e.g., during walking) intensifies the pain, so the patient often limits the stride of the affected side. The anterior crural nerve (the largest branch of the lumbar plexus) lies just below the bursa and may be irritated from bursal inflammation; resulting neuritis causes pain in the thigh, which often is also intensified by walking, and there may also be weakness of anterior muscles of the thigh. When a bursa is enlarged it may compress the femoral vein, resulting in edema in the affected leg.

If a hernia can be ruled out (see Chapter 97), the bursa should be aspirated by an orthopedist. Aspiration and injection with lidocaine and usually a corticosteroid result in lasting improvement.

Trochanteric Bursitis

The trochanteric bursa lies in the lateral aspect of the thigh over the greater trochanter of the femur and is closely associated with tendons of the glutei muscles. The problem affects primarily older people. Most cases are of unknown cause, although many are thought to result from osteoarthritis. Infection of the bursa is rare. The onset of pain may be abrupt, subacute, or chronic. Patients with trochanteric bursitis often misinterpret their lateral buttock pain to be caused by hip arthritis (which more characteristically produces groin pain). At times, the discomfort mimics that of lumbar spine disease (see Chapter 71). Occasionally, trochanteric bursitis can cause pain that radiates to the knee or even to the groin. Discomfort is intensified by movement from the sitting to the standing position, going up and down stairs, or sleeping on the affected side.

On examination there is point tenderness over the bursa with reproduction of the pain. The Patrick test (external rotation of the hip combined with abduction) is often painful, whereas internal rotation, flexion, and extension of the hip are usually pain free. Any remaining concern about the knee or the lumbar spine causing the pain is eliminated by the normal physical examination of these structures. X-rays of the bursa, which sometimes reveal calcifications, are usually not necessary.

Therapy, as outlined in Table 74.3, is usually effective. In addition, it is important for the patient to sleep with a small pillow under the involved buttock to keep weight shifted off the bursa. Subdeltoid bursitis is discussed in Chapter 69.

TENOSYNOVITIS

As with bursae, there are many sites of potential tenosynovial inflammation. Tendinitis and tenosynovitis generally occur simultaneously. The synovial-lined tendon sheath is usually the site of maximal inflammation.

Inflammation of a sheath of a tendon is a common problem. For the most part, only long tendons have sheaths. Tenosynovitis most often occurs from exercise, especially when a tendon has been used repetitively in an improperly conditioned person (see Chapter 72). Tenosynovitis also may be part of a generalized inflammatory process. Sometimes tenosynovitis is the first manifestation of this process.

Tenosynovitis often affects the dorsal extensor tendons of the wrist. It is manifest most commonly by pain that is intensified with hand extension. In the acute stage, swelling and pain over the dorsal aspect of the wrist or over the dorsal radioulnar joint may occur. Occasionally, a friction rub is felt or heard when the appropriate muscle is contracted.

When tenosynovitis is identified in the absence of trauma, a systemic disease should be suspected. If present, specific therapy for that disease is obviously important. Gonorrhea should be suspected in sexually active people if inflammation involves the tendons of the ankle or wrist in the setting of a monarthritis, fever, and skin rash. Using Transgrow media, culture of the endocervical canal and rectum in women and of the urethra in men is indicated (see Chapter 37).

If the tenosynovitis has developed because of trauma, such as exercise or overuse, or for unknown reasons, nonspecific therapy with a nonsteroidal anti-inflammatory agent, as for bursitis (Table 74.3), is appropriate. The fingers should be splinted in the position of function. If symptoms persist after 3 or 4 days of conservative therapy, the peritenon (loose tissue surrounding the tendon) should be injected with lidocaine and a corticosteroid (e.g., Celestone, Aristocort, or Kenalog) (Table 74.4). To avoid injuring the tendon or causing skin atrophy, only small doses of depoglucocorticoid (i.e., about 0.5 mL of steroid mixed with an equal amount of lidocaine depending on the site) should be injected. To avoid injecting directly into the tendon, one should never inject if the syringe plunger cannot be depressed easily. Occasionally, symptoms are recurrent, in which case referral to a rheumatologist or orthopedist is indicated. Tenosynovitis and tendinitis involving specific tendons also are discussed in Chapters 68, 69, and 73.

STENOSING TENOSYNOVITIS

Stenosing tenosynovitis is not a complication of tenosynovitis; rather, it occurs primarily when trauma is severe and localized. In stenosing tenosynovitis, either a nodule forms on a tendon or an actual stenosis of a tendon sheath of a long tendon develops. This results in the affected part sticking in a fixed position that is sometimes painful. When this affects the flexor tendons of the fingers, it is called *trigger finger.* The patient is unable to flex a digit fully or, once it is flexed, the digit locks and literally must be straightened by external force until it suddenly snaps free. When stenosing tenosynovitis is present in the abductor or extensor tendon of the thumb, it is called *De Quervain disease,* the most common form of stenosing tenosynovitis. In this problem, the thumb usually still has motion and does not always lock like a trigger finger. To evaluate for De Quervain tenosynovitis, the patient should make a fist by curling the fingers over the flexed thumb, then passively deviate the fist in an ulnar direction. Exquisite pain over the base of the thumb with this maneuver *(Finkelstein test)* confirms the diagnosis. Stenosing tenosynovitis is usually caused by repeated trauma (e.g., prolonged use of a screwdriver), but it is occasionally seen in association with rheumatoid arthritis, amyloidosis, pregnancy, and myxedema.

The treatment is identical to that of bursitis as outlined in Tables 74.3 and 74.4. Splinting is especially helpful in the treatment of tenosynovitis of the hands and fingers. If the patient does not respond to several weeks of conservative therapy, surgical release may be necessary. When a nodule is palpable, it should be injected with a small amount of corticosteroid (e.g., 10 mg of Celestone, Aristocort, or Kenalog) and lidocaine. Often, the condition resolves in several days to weeks.

DUPUYTREN CONTRACTURE

The palmar fascia may undergo nodular hypertrophic fibroplasia of unknown cause. This results over many years in the development of a flexion contracture (Dupuytren contracture). The process causes the skin to be fixed to the underlying fascia by adhesive bands, resulting in a fixed puckered appearance. A Dupuytren contracture is almost always painless but may result in significant functional disability. Although all digits may be involved, the fourth and fifth are affected most commonly. The condition affects primarily middle-aged or older men and in nearly 40% is bilateral. It is more common in epileptics and alcoholics, but most affected patients have neither condition. Once the condition is present, passive extension of the fingers does not retard the process; in fact, it may accelerate it. If functional disability is present, the patient should be referred to an orthopedic surgeon for consideration for surgery. Oral anti-inflammatory agents and local cortisone injections are not effective in retarding the process.

GANGLIONS

Ganglions, cystic swellings arising from the synovium of a joint or tendon sheath, are the most common benign tumor of the hand. They tend to occur more often in women from the teens through age 50. Onset may be sudden or gradual and the cyst may change over time, sometimes disappearing and then recurring. The swellings are usually smooth, tense, and fixed to the deep tissues. The most common site is the dorsum of the wrist between the extensor tendon of the thumb and the extensor tendon of the index finger. They may also occur on the volar aspect of the foot (the tarsal area) and ankle. There may be associated aching or weakness of the involved area. Nonoperative treatment in symptomatic patients (generally asymptomatic ganglions are left untreated), consisting of aspiration or cortisone injection, may be successful. Recurrences may need to be treated by operative excision.

FIBROMYALGIA

Fibromyalgia (commonly called *fibrositis*) is a syndrome of widespread chronic musculoskeletal pain, chiefly affecting young women, that is unaccompanied by any objective findings except for increased tenderness at specific anatomic sites, known as tender points (8). The diagnosis is purely clinical; no laboratory tests establish the diagnosis of fibromyalgia. The cause of fibromyalgia is unknown, but speculations center on disturbances in rapid eye movement sleep, chronic viral infections, psychologic disorders, neuroendocrine abnormalities, and metabolic muscle defects (9). Usually fibromyalgia is primary, occurring in the absence of other medical conditions. Some patients have secondary fibromyalgia, which is diagnosed when the syndrome accompanies another disorder, most commonly hypothyroidism or rheumatoid arthritis.

Fibromyalgia is important to recognize for three reasons. First, fibromyalgia is common, affecting 3% to 10% of the general population and accounting for 20% to 30% of all patients referred to rheumatologists. Second, fibromyalgia responds, albeit imperfectly, to treatment. Third, failure to diagnose and treat fibromyalgia often subjects the patient to multiple consultations and needlessly expensive laboratory testing.

Manifestations

Ninety percent of patients with fibromyalgia are women. Most experience the gradual onset of symptoms between the ages of 20 and 45. The cardinal features of fibromyalgia are widespread soft tissue aching and stiffness, essentially daily, although varying in severity, often involving the axial skeleton and the shoulder and pelvic girdles, of more than 3 months' duration. Typically the pain is chronic, persisting for

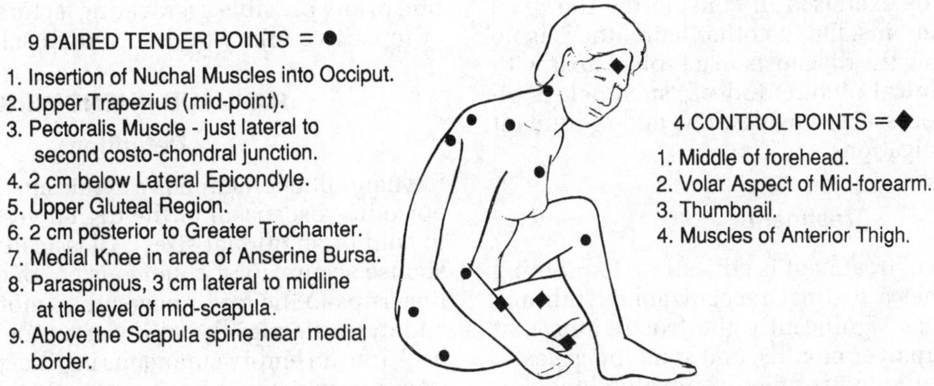

9 PAIRED TENDER POINTS = ●

1. Insertion of Nuchal Muscles into Occiput.
2. Upper Trapezius (mid-point).
3. Pectoralis Muscle - just lateral to second costo-chondral junction.
4. 2 cm below Lateral Epicondyle.
5. Upper Gluteal Region.
6. 2 cm posterior to Greater Trochanter.
7. Medial Knee in area of Anserine Bursa.
8. Paraspinous, 3 cm lateral to midline at the level of mid-scapula.
9. Above the Scapula spine near medial border.

4 CONTROL POINTS = ◆

1. Middle of forehead.
2. Volar Aspect of Mid-forearm.
3. Thumbnail.
4. Muscles of Anterior Thigh.

Figure 74.1. The tender point locations in fibromyalgia are remarkably constant from patient to patient. Multiple locations have been described; the nine paired tender points shown represent frequently occurring points in a wide distribution. Most patients with fibrositis usually have 11 or more tender points. Control points are not unduly tender; their examination should be interspersed with that of the tender points. (Modified from Bennett RM. The fibromyalgia syndrome. In: Kelly WN, Harris ED, Ruddy S, et al., eds. Textbook of rheumatology, 5th ed. Philadelphia: W.B. Saunders, 1997, 2001: 513.)

years. The condition may be aggravated by fatigue, tension, excessive work, immobilization, and changes in the weather. Although pain is the predominant symptom, most patients with fibromyalgia have many other symptoms, including fatigue, recurrent headaches, sore throat, depression, fitful sleep, difficulty concentrating, alternating constipation and diarrhea, numbness, swollen glands, and subjective sense of fever or joint swelling. In fact, a careful history to rule out depression (see Chapter 24) and somatization (see Chapter 21) is important.

Characteristically in fibromyalgia, the rich history of complaints contrasts starkly with the poverty of physical findings. Objective adenopathy, weakness, and joint inflammation or weakness are notably absent. Indeed, the only physical finding in fibromyalgia is tender points. Although the exact number and location of these tender points are somewhat controversial, nine paired tender points most commonly found, along with four control points, are illustrated in Fig. 74.1. Nearly 90% of patients with fibromyalgia have tenderness at least 11 of the 18 (nine paired) tender point sites (10).

Laboratory tests in primary fibromyalgia are normal. The purpose of the laboratory tests and physical examination is to exclude other causes of diffuse musculoskeletal pain, which include polymyalgia rheumatica (a condition of elderly people), Parkinson syndrome, polymyositis, endocrine disorders (especially hypothyroidism, but also hyperthyroidism, Addison disease, hyperparathyroidism, and panhypopituitarism), cancer, renal tubular acidosis, and chronic fatigue syndrome (considered by many experts to be a variant of fibromyalgia). Laboratory testing does not need to be extensive. Basic laboratory tests should include complete blood cell count, erythrocyte sedimentation rate, thyroid function tests, and muscle enzyme levels. By definition, all these studies are normal in patients with primary fibromyalgia, so any abnormalities should warrant a further search for an underlying disorder.

Table 74.5. Initial Examination of a Patient with Possible Fibromyalgia Syndrome

Diagnostic Step	Finding
Consider diagnosis	In any patient with chronic, poorly defined, generalized musculoskeletal pain; most patients have been studied previously, with normal test results; most often women, aged 20–50 yr; rule out depression and somatization by careful history.
Obtain positive response to most of the following	Chronic fatigue; chronic neck, shoulder, hip, and back pain; disturbed sleep; feeling unrefreshed and stiff in morning; hypersensitivity to cold, heat; history consistent with tension headaches, irritable bowel syndrome; subjective paresthesias and swelling of hands and feet without objective abnormalities.
Confirm presumptive diagnosis with physical examination	General physical examination findings normal and no evidence of arthritis or myositis (unless coexistent illness such as rheumatoid arthritis or hypothyroidism is present); tender point examination demonstrates multiple tender points at characteristic locations; associated diffuse muscle spasm and skin hypersensitivity may be present.
Laboratory tests	Complete blood cell count, erythrocyte sedimentation rate, thyroid function tests, and muscle enzyme levels should be normal.

From Goldenberg DL. Fibromyalgia syndrome. An emerging but controversial condition. JAMA 1987;257:2782, with permission.

The approach to the diagnosis of fibromyalgia is summarized in Table 74.5. The two criteria for the diagnosis—widespread pain and mild or greater tenderness in 11 or more of 18 tender point sites—are 88% sensitive and 81% specific. The diagnosis of fibromyalgia should not be made too quickly or too slowly. Because the diagnosis depends on excluding objective abnormalities, it is rarely wise to diagnose primary fibromyalgia on the patient's first visit. Documenting the absence of fever, weight loss, or any other abnormality takes time and increases the certainty of the diagnosis. Because fibromyalgia rarely begins after age 50, great caution should be exercised in considering the diagnosis in older patients. On the other hand, there is no benefit to delaying the diagnosis in a typical host with a compatible clinical picture. Indeed, such delays often prompt unnecessary consultations and redundant laboratory investigations.

Treatment

The cornerstone of treatment is education. Explaining to the patient that a distinct recognizable syndrome is present reduces significantly the frustrations that may have built up over months, and sometimes years, of previously unproductive medical evaluations. Patients also take solace in learning that fibromyalgia does not shorten life or cause crippling deformities and that the cause and treatment of fibromyalgia are under active investigation.

Patients should know that symptoms of fibromyalgia, although chronic, can be improved. The medications shown to be somewhat effective (approximately one-third of patients showing moderate to marked improvement) are the tricyclic antidepressants, amitriptyline (e.g., Elavil, Endep, or generic, 10 to 50 mg at bedtime), and cyclobenzaprine compounds, structurally related to the tricyclic antidepressants (e.g., Flexeril or generic, 5 to 30 mg at bedtime) (11). Fluoxetine (Prozac), a selective serotonin reuptake inhibitor, has also been demonstrated to be effective at 20 mg a day (12). Nonsteroidal anti-inflammatory medications are generally not effective. Corticosteroids and narcotics have no role in the treatment of fibromyalgia. Because of the modest efficacy of pharmacologic therapy, treatment may often include other modalities as well. These include physical therapy (relaxation, heat, massage) and a graded exercise program to maintain a good general level of aerobic fitness (13). Attempts should also be made to modify other aggravating factors such as mechanical, physical, and psychologic stresses.

MYOFASCIAL PAIN SYNDROMES

Related problems, possibly distinct from fibromyalgia, are the myofascial pain syndromes (MPS), characterized by the presence of deep tender points also. However, in MPS, the tender point is termed a *trigger point* because firm palpation of the point produces pain in a referred distribution. A second feature distinguishing MPS from fibromyalgia is the presence of just one or a regional clustering of points in MPS in contrast to the widespread distribution of symptoms and tender points in any given patient with fibromyalgia. A wide array of clinical syndromes in many different anatomic areas have been ascribed to MPS.

The pathogenesis of MPS is unknown. Patients with MPS may be helped by passive stretching of involved muscles after injection of the trigger point with a local anesthetic or use of a vapo-coolant spray (e.g., ethyl chloride). Attention should also be directed to elimination of any possible aggravating factors such as overuse or repetitive injury to involved muscle areas.

RAYNAUD PHENOMENON

Definition

Raynaud phenomenon is a syndrome characterized by episodic vasospasm of the digital vessels in response to cold or emotional stress. Classically, a triphasic response occurs. First cutaneous pallor extends from the fingertips to the mid-fingers; then mottling of the skin and cyanosis rapidly follow as venous blood refluxes back into an empty cutaneous capillary bed (this pallor or cyanosis persists until rewarming of the digits). Finally, the recovery phase occurs over 15 to 20 minutes, resulting in intense hyperemia (14,15). Vasospasm is usually triggered by an abrupt change in ambient temperature, so it may occur even in the summer when a patient moves into air-conditioned or refrigerated areas. One or two digits may have more intense vasospasm, but generally the episodes are bilateral and symmetric. Also, the feet and other acral parts (e.g., the ears or nose) may be involved. Patients often do not describe spontaneously the classic phases of Raynaud phenomenon but commonly note deep cyanosis associated with numbness, a pins-and-needles sensation, or frank pain on cold exposure.

Causes and Prevalence

Raynaud phenomenon most commonly occurs in an idiopathic or primary form, Raynaud disease, in which no underlying abnormality can be defined. Raynaud phenomenon may also occur secondary to a defined vascular abnormality or in association with a specific disease process (Table 74.6). Primary Raynaud phenomenon is thought to be common, occurring principally in women aged 20 to 30 years. The true prevalence of Raynaud phenomenon is unknown, but it has been estimated to be 2% to 6% of the general population and up to 20% of the selective population of young women. Patients with primary Raynaud phenomenon are otherwise healthy, generally have infrequent attacks (one to four episodes weekly), and rarely develop local cutaneous complications, such as digital pitting, ulcerations, or loss of hand function. Patients with primary Raynaud phenomenon usually have an uncomplicated course with gradual decrease over a number of years in the frequency of episodes. Estimates suggest that 8% to 19% of patients believed initially to have the primary form will develop a defined secondary form (usually a connective tissue disease).

In approximately 40% of patients who present to a general physician with Raynaud phenomenon, it is secondary to an underlying condition, the most common being a connective tissue disease (Table 74.6). Raynaud phenomenon occurs in more than 90% of patients with systemic sclerosis and may be the initial symptom, preceding the other features of the disease by years. Approximately 40% of patients with

Table 74.6. Classification of Raynaud Phenomenon

A. Primary: idiopathic Raynaud, Raynaud disease
B. Secondary: Disorders associated with Raynaud phenomenon

	Percentage of patients with stated disorder who also have Raynaud phenomenon
1. Connective tissue diseases	
a. Systemic sclerosis	90
b. Systemic lupus erythematosus	20
c. "Mixed" connective tissue disease	75
d. Dermatomyositis/polymyositis	20
e. Rheumatoid arthritis	10
2. Neurovascular compression	
a. Thoracic outlet syndrome (e.g., cervical ribs, scalenus anticus syndrome)	
b. Carpal tunnel syndrome	
3. Arterial disease	
a. Arteriosclerosis	
b. Arteritis (thromboangitis obliterans)	
4. Hematologic disorders	
a. Paraproteinemia	
b. Cryoglobulinemia	
c. Polycythemia	
d. Hyperviscosity syndrome	Unknown
5. Occupational	
a. Vibratory tools (white finger syndrome)	
b. Polyvinyl chloride exposure	
6. Drugs	
a. Ergot-containing drugs (such as ergotamine)	
b. Beta-adrenergic blockers	
c. Sympathomimetic agents (such as Actifed)	
d. Methysergide (Sansert)	
e. Chemotherapy (bleomycin, vinblastine)	
7. Miscellaneous	
a. Primary pulmonary hypertension	30
b. Migraine headache	10

systemic lupus erythematosus and 10% of patients with rheumatoid arthritis may also have associated Raynaud phenomenon. Raynaud phenomenon may be a presenting feature in patients who have a systemic vasculitis. Disturbances of the axillary or cervical neurovascular bundle also can lead to Raynaud phenomenon. Patients with neurovascular compression syndromes (cervical rib, scalenus anticus syndrome) and proximal vascular lesions (atherosclerosis) may present with unilateral Raynaud phenomenon. Hematologic abnormalities, such as cryoglobulinemia, paraproteinemia, or cold hemagglutinins, may present as typical Raynaud phenomenon. Ergot-containing drugs, such as ergotamine, and beta-blocking agents may be causative or potentiating agents. Occupational injury (vibration white finger syndrome) causing the syndrome occurs in a high proportion of workers operating vibratory tools (e.g., lumberjacks, shipyard workers, or meat cutters).

Initially, it may be difficult to determine whether a patient has a primary or secondary form of Raynaud phenomenon. Clues that suggest a secondary form include onset during childhood, male sex, onset in a woman after age 30, unilateral Raynaud, Raynaud affecting a single digit, fingertip ulcers, digital gangrene, or symptoms or signs of a systemic disorder.

Evaluation

Every patient with Raynaud phenomenon should have a focused history (including a drug review) and physical examination looking for diseases associated with Raynaud phenomenon. An extension of the examination, evaluation of the nail bed with an ophthalmoscope (using approximately a 20+ diopter), may reveal small telangiectasias or abnormal cutaneous capillary loops; these small vessel changes may be the earliest findings in an associated underlying connective tissue disease, primarily systemic sclerosis (16). The presence of ulcers on the digits indicates that the Raynaud is very severe and that the patient is likely to have a secondary form of Raynaud phenomenon. Patients with unilateral Raynaud phenomenon should be carefully evaluated for a local vascular lesion, including bilateral blood pressure determination, auscultation over major vessels to determine the presence or absence of vascular bruits, and assessment of the peripheral pulses. Special testing for possible neurovascular compression syndrome (see Chapter 69) and consideration for chest x-ray and a noninvasive evaluation of the peripheral circulation (Doppler studies or digital plethysmography) are appropriate when only unilateral Raynaud phenomenon is present. Angiography may be necessary in cases in which a correctable occlusive vascular lesion is strongly suspected. Carpal tunnel syndrome has been implicated in both unilateral and bilateral Raynaud phenomenon, and nerve conduction studies may be appropriate when the history and physical examination suggest this nerve compression syndrome (see Chapter 92).

If the patient is a woman with onset between the ages of 20 and 30 who has mild bilateral Raynaud, does not have nail fold capillary changes, and exhibits no other manifestations of a connective tissue disease, primary Raynaud is the likely diagnosis (15). For such a patient, the laboratory evaluation can be limited to verifying a normal complete blood count and testing renal and liver function to screen for collagen disease affecting these organs. If the patient is suspected of having secondary Raynaud, antinuclear antibody screen, cryoglobulins, Westergren erythrocyte sedimentation rate, and serum protein electrophoresis are indicated. Referring the patient to a rheumatologist for any additional evaluation is appropriate. Even when a systemic illness is not identified, the patient should be followed expectantly because an underlying illness may emerge several years later.

Treatment

The principal mode of treatment in patients in which a correctable cause cannot be found is to avoid the cold and stay warm (14). This includes wearing mittens or

Table 74.7. Nonpharmacologic Management of Patients with Raynaud Phenomenon

Education and reassurance
- Establish precipitating factors (e.g., refrigerator/freezer, air conditioning, emotional stress).
- Provide emotional support (e.g., assurance of the mild nature of the disease in most patients may reduce some of the stress that can precipitate attacks).

Avoidance of precipitating factors
- Wear gloves before reaching into refrigerator or freezer.
- Wear warm body clothing to avoid cold exposure when dressing.
- Keep head covered to avoid heat loss.
- Keep extremities warm and body well covered in cool weather or in air-conditioned environments.
- Be aware that stress can cause Raynaud attacks.

Avoidance of certain drugs that precipitate attacks
- Beta-blockers (e.g., propranolol)
- Ergot-containing drugs (i.e., ergotamine)
- Sympathomimetic agents (e.g., isoproterenol, Actifed, or other cold remedies)
- Nicotine (smoking)
- Oral contraceptives

gloves and avoiding a general chill of the body by wearing a hat and loose-fitting warm clothing in winter months. Smoking aggravates Raynaud phenomenon and should be stopped (see Chapter 27). Drugs that promote vasoconstriction (Table 74.6) should be stopped or avoided. Emotional stress should be assessed and controlled by appropriate measures (see Chapter 20). Patients with mild Raynaud phenomenon often improve with education about the cause and nature of these episodes. Unfortunately, temperature biofeedback therapy is ineffective. The nonpharmacologic treatment of patients with Raynaud phenomenon is summarized in Table 74.7. Most patients, particularly those with primary Raynaud phenomenon, do not need and should not be treated with drugs. Rather, pharmacologic treatment should be limited to patients with repeated attacks who limit their daily activities or who have developed digital ulceration or other ischemic changes. There is no evidence that decreasing the number of episodes of Raynaud phenomenon will alter the progressive changes that may occur in patients with scleroderma or another connective tissue disease.

A wide variety of vasoactive agents has been used in patients with Raynaud phenomenon, but few agents have been proven of definite benefit. Many of these patients are young women who have child-bearing potential; therefore, unproven treatment that may have a teratogenic effect should be avoided.

Calcium channel blockers are the cornerstone of drug therapy for Raynaud (17). Nifedipine has been most extensively used and its efficacy best documented, but other preparations (including amlodipine, isradipine, nicardipine, and felodipine) may also be effective (18). These agents relax smooth muscle, reduce peripheral vascular resistance, and increase peripheral blood flow. Patients with primary Raynaud respond better than patients with Raynaud phenomenon secondary to a connective tissue disease, especially systemic sclerosis. The major side effects of these agents are secondary to their vasodilatory activity and include hypotension, dizziness, headache, and peripheral edema. Approximately 40% to 50% of patients experience some light-headedness caused by hypotension and flushing on initiation of the calcium channel blockers; however, these side effects are usually transient, can be minimized by starting with low doses, and do not require the discontinuation of the medication. For this reason, the orthostatic blood pressure should be periodically measured. Calcium channel blockers should never be used during pregnancy or in a patient planning to become pregnant because they have been shown in animal models to be teratogenic.

As noted, the calcium channel blocker that has been most extensively studied, and the drug of first choice, is nifedipine. The initial dosage is usually 30 mg of a sustained-released preparation once daily. The patient should be encouraged to assume usual activities and to keep a diary of the number and intensity of Raynaud attacks. The patient should be monitored for important orthostatic hypotension (a symptomatic decrease in systolic pressure of 20 mm Hg or greater below baseline or a fall below 90 mm Hg). If needed to improve control of Raynaud phenomenon, the dosage of nifedipine can be increased by 30 mg sustained release every 2 weeks to a maximum of 90 mg sustained release daily. Thereafter, monitoring every 2 to 4 months is important because the initial response may be transient and side effects, such as esophageal reflux, may limit the usefulness of the drug. If nifedipine fails or is not tolerated, diltiazem at a dosage of 30 mg four times a day may be tried as an alternative calcium channel blocker. The dosage may be advanced by 30 mg/day every 3 to 4 days until the symptoms improve or a maximum of 120 mg four times a day is reached. Patients generally have resolution or a dramatic reduction in the intensity and number of episodes of Raynaud phenomenon in the summer. For this reason, medication should be discontinued unless repeated cold exposure or active Raynaud phenomenon is documented.

Other drugs have been used for the treatment of Raynaud phenomenon. Intravenous iloprost has been shown to be moderately effective for severe Raynaud in patients with scleroderma (19). The efficacy of an oral formulation has not been established. Losartan, an angiotensin II type 1 receptor antagonist, has shown promise in treating primary and secondary forms of Raynaud phenomenon. Topical nitroglycerin paste applied to the digits or nitroglycerin patches have been used with some success, but their indications are not established and consultation with a rheumatologist is suggested before prescribing them. Prazosin (Minipress) (20) may occasionally be of benefit if tolerated (2 to 8 mg/day in two or three divided doses). Nutritional antioxidants have not been shown to be effective.

Surgical sympathectomy was once popular for the treatment of Raynaud phenomenon but is now rarely performed, primarily because of the high relapse rate (40% to 50%) and frequency of significant postural hypotension. Selective digital sympathectomy may be done in centers where microsurgery is available; however, long-term controlled studies of this procedure are lacking. Sympathectomy should be considered only for short-term relief from an intractable course complicated by digital ulceration that has failed medical treatment. All patients who have had such a severe course or who have ulcers on their digits should be seen in consultation by a vascular surgeon or a rheumatologist. Local digital block performed by a vascular surgeon or rheumatologist has been used for temporary treatment of patients with significant digital tissue compromise; also, a good response may predict which patient may have a good effect from digital or cervical sympathectomy. A patient who has severe disease with digital ulcers is susceptible to developing secondary soft tissue infection. Local debridement and antimicrobial treatment may be necessary if ischemic ulcerations become infected. Whirlpool treatment is the most effective method of ulcer debridement. In instances of secondary complications, consultation with a vascular surgeon or a rheumatologist is advised.

General References*

Clauw DJ. Fibromyalgia. In: Ruddy S, Harris ED, Sledge CB, eds. Kelley's textbook of rheumatology, 6th ed. Philadelphia: W.B. Saunders, 2001.

Hellmann DB, Stone JH. Arthritis and musculoskeletal disorders. In: Tierney LM, McPhee SJ, Papadakis MA, et al., eds. Current medical diagnosis and treatment. Norwalk, CT: Appleton & Lange, 2001.

Owen DS Jr. Aspiration and injection of joints and soft tissues. In: Ruddy S, Harris ED, Sledge CB, eds. Kelley's textbook of rheumatology, 6th ed. Philadelphia: W.B. Saunders, 2001.

Schumacher HR. Synovial fluid analysis and synovial biopsy. In: Ruddy S, Harris ED, Sledge CB, eds. Kelley's textbook of rheumatology, 6th ed. Philadelphia: WB Saunders, 2001.

Specific References

1. Ho G, Mikolich DJ. Bacterial infection of the superficial subcutaneous bursae. Clin Rheum Dis 1986;12:437.
2. Ho G, Tice AD, Kaplan SR. Septic bursitis in the prepatellar and olecranon bursae: an analysis of 25 cases. Ann Intern Med 1987;89:21.
3. Zimmerman B III, Mikolich DJ, Ho G Jr. Septic bursitis. Semin Arthritis Rheum 1995;24:391.
4. Underwood PL, McLeod GA, Ginsburg WW. The varied clinical manifestations of iliopsoas bursitis. J Rheumatol 1988;15:1683.
5. Smith DL, McAfee JH, Lucas LM, et al. Treatment of nonseptic olecranon bursitis: a controlled, blinded prospective trial. Arch Intern Med 1989;149:2527.
6. Larsson L-G, Baum J. The syndromes of bursitis. Bull Rheum Dis 1986;36:1.
7. Pathria MN, Zlatkin M, Sartoris DJ, et al. Ultrasonography of the popliteal fossa and lower extremities. Radiol Clin North Am 1988;26:77.
8. Millea PJ, Holloway RL. Practical therapeutics. Treating fibromyalgia. Am Fam Physician 2000;62:1575.
9. Wolfe F. Fibromyalgia. The clinical syndrome. Rheum Dis Clin North Am 1989;15:1.
10. Wolfe F, Smythe HA, Yunus MB, et al. The American College of Rheumatology 1990 criteria for the classification of fibromyalgia. Arthritis Rheum 1990;33:160.
11. Carette S, McCain GA, Bell DA, et al. Evaluation of amitriptyline in primary fibrositis: a double-blind, placebo controlled study. Arthritis Rheum 1986;29:655.
12. Goldenberg D, Mayskiy M, Mossey C, et al. A randomized double-blind crossover trial of fluoxetine and amitriptyline in the treatment of fibromyalgia. Arthritis Rheum 1966;39:1852.
13. McCain GA, Bell DA, Mai FM, et al. A controlled study of the effects of a supervised cardiovascular fitness training program on the manifestations of primary fibromyalgia. Arthritis Rheum 1988;31:1135.
14. Block JA. Raynaud's phenomenon. Lancet 2001;357:2042.
15. Wigley FM, Flavahan NA. Raynaud's phenomenon. Rheum Dis Clin North Am 1996;22:765.
16. Fitzgerald O, Hess EV, O'Connor GT, et al. Prospective study of the evaluation of Raynaud's phenomenon. Am J Med 1988;84:718.
17. Rodeheffer RJ, Rammer JA, Wigley F, et al. Controlled double-blind trial of nifedipine in the treatment of Raynaud's phenomenon. N Engl J Med 1983;303:880.
18. Thompson AE, Shea B, Welch V, et al. Calcium-channel blockers for Raynaud's phenomenon in systemic sclerosis. Arthritis Rheum 2001;44:1841.
19. Wigley FM, Wise RA, Seibold JR, et al. Intravenous iloprost infusion in patients with Raynaud phenomenon secondary to systemic sclerosis: a multicenter placebo-controlled, double-blind study. Ann Intern Med 1994;120:199.
20. Wollersheim H, Thien T, Fennis J, et al. Double-blind, placebo-controlled study of prazosin in Raynaud's phenomenon. Clin Pharmacol Ther 1986;40:219.

---

*Bold print (general references) and bold numerals (specific references) denote published controlled clinical trials, meta-analyses, or consensus-based recommendations.

CHAPTER 75

Osteoarthritis

ALEXANDER S. TOWNES, MD

The common occurrence, chronic nature, and lack of definitive treatment of osteoarthritis in the past generated a sense of apathy and disinterest in this disease on the part of many clinicians and in the research community. A common attitude among patients often has been one of acceptance of the slow progression of symptoms as a part of aging. Certainly these attitudes are no longer valid in light of the great strides that have now been made in further understanding the high prevalence, the economic costs, basic mechanisms involved in pathogenesis, and new methods of diagnosis and potential prevention of the disease. The increasing awareness of the importance of this diagnosis prompted a National Institutes of Health (NIH) Conference for a comprehensive review and progress report on new insights into the disease (1,2).

Osteoarthritis is particularly important to those who see ambulatory adult patients. It is the most common form of arthritis (3). Osteoarthritis accounts for approximately half of all visits to the office for joint disease and is the most common arthritis diagnosis in general practice (4). Osteoarthritis engenders major economic costs estimated to be $15.5 billion (in 1994 dollars) annually, including work loss and medical expenses (5,6). It accounts for as much physical disability in the lower extremity as any other disease diagnosis (7).

PREVALENCE

Prevalence of osteoarthritis increases with advancing age, beginning perhaps as early as the third decade of life and being almost ubiquitous as detected by radiography or biochemical changes in articular cartilage in the seventh and eighth decades and beyond. It is fortunate and important, however, that clinical symptoms are not necessarily associated with structural changes or an inevitable accompaniment of aging. Symptoms and findings are uncommon below age 35 and are more common above age 65, with perhaps as much as 30% to 40% of the population aged 65 and above having some symptoms related to this diagnosis. Symptoms related to the knee and hip are the most prevalent in both sexes with symptomatic involvement of the hands more common in women beginning at the menopause (8). A survey of osteoarthritis of the knee in subjects aged 63 to 94 indicated an increasing prevalence of radiographic evidence of osteoarthritis with age to the level of 44% of subjects aged 80 or older and a higher proportion of symptomatic disease in women (11%) than in men (7%) (9). New onset of radiographic and symptomatic osteoarthritis of the knee continued to develop in elderly patients at the rate of 1% to 2% per year, again more in women than in men (10).

PATHOPHYSIOLOGY

The pathogenesis of osteoarthritis is multifactorial (11); however, the final common pathway is believed to be injury to articular cartilage, which then undergoes a sequence of changes resulting eventually in progressive depletion of the collagen and proteoglycan matrix and proliferation of underlying bone with osteophyte formation. Under normal conditions, chondrocytes regulate the extracellular matrix with a balance between the synthesis of its structural components and their degradation (12). In osteoarthritis there is disequilibrium between the degradation and repair processes in a complex milieu of cross-talk between inflammatory cytokine mediators (13), growth factors, and degradative enzymes involved in chondrocyte apoptosis (14) so that the structure is weakened and damage occurs. Susceptibility to cartilage damage increases with age and may be the result of abnormal biomechanics leading to excessive stress or defective matrix components and alteration of the normal structure. Impact loading and torsional, shear, and repetitive stress are more important than frictional wear (15). Changes are most severe in or may be confined entirely to areas of maximal stress on the articular cartilage, most striking in weight-bearing areas of the large joints. Synovitis is usually minimal in the early stages but may contribute to joint damage in advanced disease. Change in the hardness of bone and loss of ability of cartilage to absorb stress as a primary mechanism in osteoarthritis has also been proposed (16,17). The role of bone in the progression of the disease has also been suggested by observations that higher bone density predisposes (18) and osteoporosis mitigates against osteoarthritis (19). The increased prevalence of disease in women, the progression sometimes seen after menopause, and the apparent beneficial effect of estrogen replacement therapy (20) also suggest the possibility of hormonal influences that are as yet poorly understood. Crystalline deposits of calcium pyrophosphate, hydroxyapatite, or basic calcium salts may play a role in the synovial inflammatory response (21) or destructive arthropathy (22) in certain patients, especially those with more advanced osteoarthritis (see Chapter 76).

Because there are no nerve fibers in articular cartilage, no symptoms are caused by early changes in the joints. There are multiple sources of pain, however, as the disease progresses. Periosteal irritation as a result of proliferating bone, denuded bone, compression of soft tissues by osteophytes in confined spaces, microfractures of subchondral bone, stress on ligaments as a result of loss of cartilage and joint incongruity, low grade synovitis, effusion, and spasm of surrounding muscles are all potential sources of pain in osteoarthritis. A recent study has demonstrated correlation of knee pain or aching with bone marrow edema as detected by magnetic resonance imaging (MRI) in patients with mild to moderate osteoarthritis (23).

Table 75.1. Factors Contributing to Development of Osteoarthritis

Aging
Diminished proteoglycan aggregation
Diminished resistance of cartilage to fatigue fracture (?defective collagen network)
Decreased resiliency of soft tissues and bone
Loss of normal anatomic relationship (hip)
Heredity
Heberden nodes
Primary generalized osteoarthritis (female gender)
Postural or developmental defects (e.g., scoliosis, slipped capital femoral epiphyses, Legg-Clavé-Perthes disease)
Procollagen gene (*COL2A1*) defects
Abnormal distribution of mechanical stress
Postural or developmental defects
Joint instability or hypermobility
Local incongruity of joint surfaces posttraumatic, after meniscectomy, prolonged immobilization
Obesity
Excessive repetitive stress
Occupational
Sports related
Associated with neuropathy
Crystalline deposit disease
Calcium pyrophosphate
Hydroxyapatite
Previous inflammatory joint disease
Metabolic abnormalities
Ochronosis
Wilson disease
Acromegaly

CAUSES AND PREDISPOSING FACTORS

The precise cause of osteoarthritis is unknown. It is likely that multiple causes and many factors may influence disease expression, some of which are listed in Table 75.1.

Because of multiple etiologic mechanisms in the pathogenesis of osteoarthritis, the history should seek to determine specific factors that may be implicated in each patient. Heredity is clearly important, with influence on some patterns of disease development more evident than others, for example, in the hands (24) and knees of women (25) but not in the hips (26). A family history of onset in the fourth or fifth decades of osteoarthritis in the proximal and distal interphalangeal (DIP) joints is often associated with the development of generalized osteoarthritis. However, development of distal joint involvement (Heberden nodes) in older patients is likely to be benign and result in little functional impairment in the aging hand (27). Drawing attention of patients with the new appearance of bony enlargements of the distal joints to the occurrence of this abnormality in elderly family members and its benign course may reassure them.

Hereditary abnormalities in structural components of cartilage have also been implicated in the development of osteoarthritis. One syndrome, inherited as mendelian dominant, is related to a single base mutation in the type II procollagen gene (*COL2A1*) resulting in mild chondrodysplasia and premature osteoarthritis, often in the fourth decade (28). Type II collagen is a major structural protein in articular cartilage and important in maintaining its integrity during mechanical stress. Further studies indicate that this is probably a rare cause of osteoarthritis (29,30). Although osteoarthritis may dominate the clinical picture, evidence of mild often late-onset spondyloepiphysial dysplasia is evident. Whether heterogeneity or polymorphisms of alleles of the *COL2A1* gene (31,32) or others (33) involved in cartilage metabolism may play a role in the common forms of osteoarthritis remains to be determined. One study has implicated a defect in the gene for type IX collagen, another collagen important in cartilage structure, as a risk factor for lumbar disk disease (34).

Obesity is an obvious risk factor for osteoarthritis, but its extent and duration are important in assessing potential damage to weight-bearing joints, especially the knees. The association of obesity with osteoarthritis of the hands suggests the possibility of influences other than mechanical factors (35). Preceding trauma may be important in subsequent development of degenerative arthritis in a joint damaged by ligamentous instability or meniscal tear in the knee joint. Traumatic episodes with sufficient damage to induce these abnormalities are likely to be severe enough to be recalled, for example, as severe sprains with swelling lasting several days or longer after a sports-related or other injury. Jogging without preceding injury or joint pain does not significantly predispose to osteoarthritis (36). Moreover, people regularly engaging in vigorous running or other aerobic activities have lower mortality rates and slower development of disability than the general population (37). Studies in elite female athletes indicate a mild increase in prevalence of radiographic osteoarthritis in hips and knees (38).

Males engaging in mixed sports and power sports were more at risk than those in endurance sports and at an earlier age (39,40). Quadriceps muscle weakness (41) or other sensorimotor dysfunction (42) predispose to joint damage and disability in osteoarthritis of the knee. Postural defects with abnormal distribution of stress (e.g., valgus or varus knee deformities) induce osteoarthritic changes at the site of weight-bearing. Prior surgical removal of a meniscus in the knee is also a predisposing factor to osteoarthritis of the knee, with age over 35 at the time of surgery a major risk factor (43). Occupational-related repetitive stress and minor trauma may predispose to osteoarthritis (44, 45) and account for occurrence at sites not commonly affected (e.g., elbows of baseball pitchers and upper limbs of air hammer operators). Because abnormalities such as varus or valgus deformities of the knees may also occur as a result of osteoarthritic damage to the joint, the history is important in determining which came first.

Osteoarthritis may also be associated with other disease states: Preceding inflammatory arthritis; metabolic diseases, such as ochronosis, with deposition of metabolites in cartilage; diseases predisposing to chondrocalcinosis, such as hemochromatosis and hyperparathyroidism; and acromegaly.

GENERAL CLINICAL FEATURES

History

Characteristically, one or a few joints are involved in osteoarthritis and symptoms are localized to the affected joints. Joints commonly affected and those usually spared are shown in Table 75.2. Because the presentations of patients may differ, depending on the pattern of joints involved and predisposing factors, some of these presenting symptoms are highlighted separately after a general discussion of the symptoms and findings in this disease.

Table 75.2. Distribution of Joint Involvement in Osteoarthritis

- Commonly affected
  - Hands
    - Distal interphalangeal (Heberden nodes)
    - Proximal interphalangeal (Bouchard nodes)
    - Carpometacarpal of the thumb (joints between first metacarpal and greater multangular and between greater multangular and navicular)
  - Knees
  - Hips
  - Spine
    - Cervical
    - Lumbar
    - Thoracic
  - Feet
    - Metatarsophalangeal (especially first)
- Usually spared
  - Ankles
  - Hands
    - Metacarpophalangeal
    - Carpometacarpal (except first)
  - Wrists
  - Elbows
  - Shoulders

Osteoarthritis usually begins insidiously and progresses slowly. Aching discomfort early in the course characteristically increases in severity with use of the joint; therefore, it tends to reach a peak after the activity of the day and is relieved by rest. Pain is often aching in character and may be difficult for the patient to localize precisely. It is usually felt in the areas surrounding the involved joint. However, hip pain may be referred to the medial aspect of the thigh, the lateral portion of the buttock, or the knee. Morning stiffness and stiffness after rest (so-called gelling) may be absent or if present may last only 15 to 20 minutes or less, in contrast to a longer duration in inflammatory joint disease such as rheumatoid arthritis. However, in advanced disease, stiffness may be more profound and pain may occur at rest. When joint destruction is marked, the patient may be kept awake at night by the pain. As the disease progresses, large pieces of degenerated cartilage may shed into the joint, producing loose bodies that may cause the joint to lock or give way.

There are no systemic symptoms in osteoarthritis. This is an important negative feature of the history that helps differentiate this disease from other forms of arthritis.

The influence of psychologic factors on the level of pain and disability is an important consideration in evaluation and treatment of the patient with osteoarthritis. A study of patients with symptoms and objective clinical findings of osteoarthritis of the hip and knee demonstrate that psychologic variables account for a far greater percentage of the variation observed in both functional impairment and severity of pain than do objective estimates of disease severity (46). Thus in osteoarthritis, as in other chronic diseases in which chronic pain may occur, it is essential in taking the history to learn as much as possible about the patient and his or her environment to appropriately interpret findings and plan the most effective approach to treatment.

Physical Findings

Early in the disease there may be no physical findings. Most patients who have symptoms have some pain on passive motion of the involved joints or on motion against resistance. There is often a sense of crackling or crepitus as the joint is moved, probably caused by joint surface incongruities and irregularities of opposing cartilaginous or bony surfaces. Crepitus may be exaggerated by movement with weight-bearing or by manual compression of the joint during movement (e.g., compression of the patella against the condyle of the femur when patellofemoral arthritis is present). In patients with painful knees, crepitus transmitted to the tibia during a stress maneuver, although not a sensitive test, was able to localize the affected compartment of the joint with surprising specificity in disease of the medial and lateral compartments of the knee as assessed by direct observation with needle arthroscopy (47). In more advanced disease, joint motion may be limited and gross deformities may develop. Tenderness along the joint line is common but may be mild or absent. In contrast to most inflammatory joint diseases, soft tissue swelling is usually absent or minimal in osteoarthritis except in its most advanced stages. Bony enlargement and irregularity are common, especially in the hands at the DIP joints (*Heberden nodes*) and less commonly in the proximal interphalangeal (PIP) joints (*Bouchard nodes*). Joint effusions are uncommon compared with more inflammatory forms of joint disease. However, they may occur, especially in the knees. There is usually no detectable heat or redness over involved joints, although some warmth may be present as the disease progresses and chronic synovitis develops. With involvement of the hip or knee, gait may be altered and patients may be noted to have a noticeable limp.

Physical examination of the patient with osteoarthritis should always include a careful evaluation of the anatomically relevant components of the neurologic system, peripheral vascular system, and soft tissues because disease in these systems may produce pain or limited motion in an extremity that may be erroneously attributed to osteoarthritis (see below, Diagnosis and Differential Diagnosis). Because most of these patients are older, they often have other diseases concomitantly that may influence the interpretation of findings and influence decisions of management.

Laboratory Findings

Osteoarthritis is characterized by normal laboratory tests unless it is associated with some other disease process. In particular, acute phase reactants, including the erythrocyte sedimentation rate and the C-reactive protein, as usually measured, are characteristically normal, in contrast to the inflammatory arthritides. Mild and transient elevation of erythrocyte sedimentation rate may occasionally be associated with the acute inflammatory events described below or may be caused by intercurrent disease elsewhere. Recent extensive efforts to develop biologic markers to measure products of bone or cartilage breakdown to serve as a marker of disease activity or progression have not yet reached a degree of specificity to be clinically useful (48). Long-term studies are required, which are difficult to accomplish (49).

Examination of synovial fluid is helpful when effusion is present in a large joint. Synovial fluid in osteoarthritis is usually of the noninflammatory type (i.e., white blood cells below 2,000/mm^3 and, if performed, a protein content below 4 g/dL and glucose concentration approximately equal to a simultaneous serum glucose concentration; see Chapter 74). A more inflammatory fluid with elevated white cell count may occur especially when crystals of calcium pyrophosphate or hydroxyapatite are present (see Chapter 76).

Imaging

Radiographic findings are important in the diagnosis and differential diagnosis of osteoarthritis because certain abnormalities are characteristic of this disorder. Therefore, plain x-rays of the affected joints are indicated in the evaluation of patients who have persistent symptoms to confirm the diagnosis and determine the extent of abnormalities present. An x-ray is always indicated if an effusion is present (e.g., in the knee) to be certain that an injury is not present. However, in early disease, x-rays may be normal, and even with characteristic findings of joint narrowing and proliferation of subchondral bone with spur formation, symptoms may be absent. Hence, the importance of relating radiographic findings to the history and physical examination cannot be overemphasized. Standard x-rays are commonly used as a measure of prevalence of disease or progression over time. A set of standard criteria of the degree of radiologic disease graded on a scale of 1 to 4 was developed by Kellgren and Lawrence (50) and remains widely used in clinical and epidemiologic studies. In general, the more severe the radiographic changes, the more likely the patient is to have symptoms and findings of osteoarthritis. Radiographic findings from the earliest to the most advanced changes are listed in Table 75.3, and examples of x-rays are shown in Fig. 75.1.

For evaluation of hands, a single anteroposterior view of both hands is sufficient in most cases. Both hips can be visualized on a single anteroposterior film of the pelvis; more specific films including laterals and obliques may be required if an abnormality is detected or if findings do not correlate with the clinical picture. Anteroposterior and lateral films are required for adequate evaluation of the knee joint. Films made with the patient standing may better demonstrate advanced changes. Special views of the patella (skyline view) may also be required to demonstrate the extent of patellofemoral arthritis. In evaluating the spine, anteroposterior, lateral, and oblique views are needed, the latter to visualize the neural foramina and the localization of nerve root compression by bony spurs.

In patients with degenerative disease of the spine, computed tomography (CT) or MRI may demonstrate encroachment of osteophytes or disk material on nerve

Table 75.3. X-Ray Findings in Osteoarthritis

Earliest
No abnormality
Early
Slight loss of articular cartilage thickness (narrowing of radiologic joint space)
Moderate
Marginal osteophyte formation
Late
Loss of cartilage space (often focal in weight-bearing joints)
Sclerosis of subchondral bone
Subchondral cyst formation
Loose bodies
Subluxation or deformity

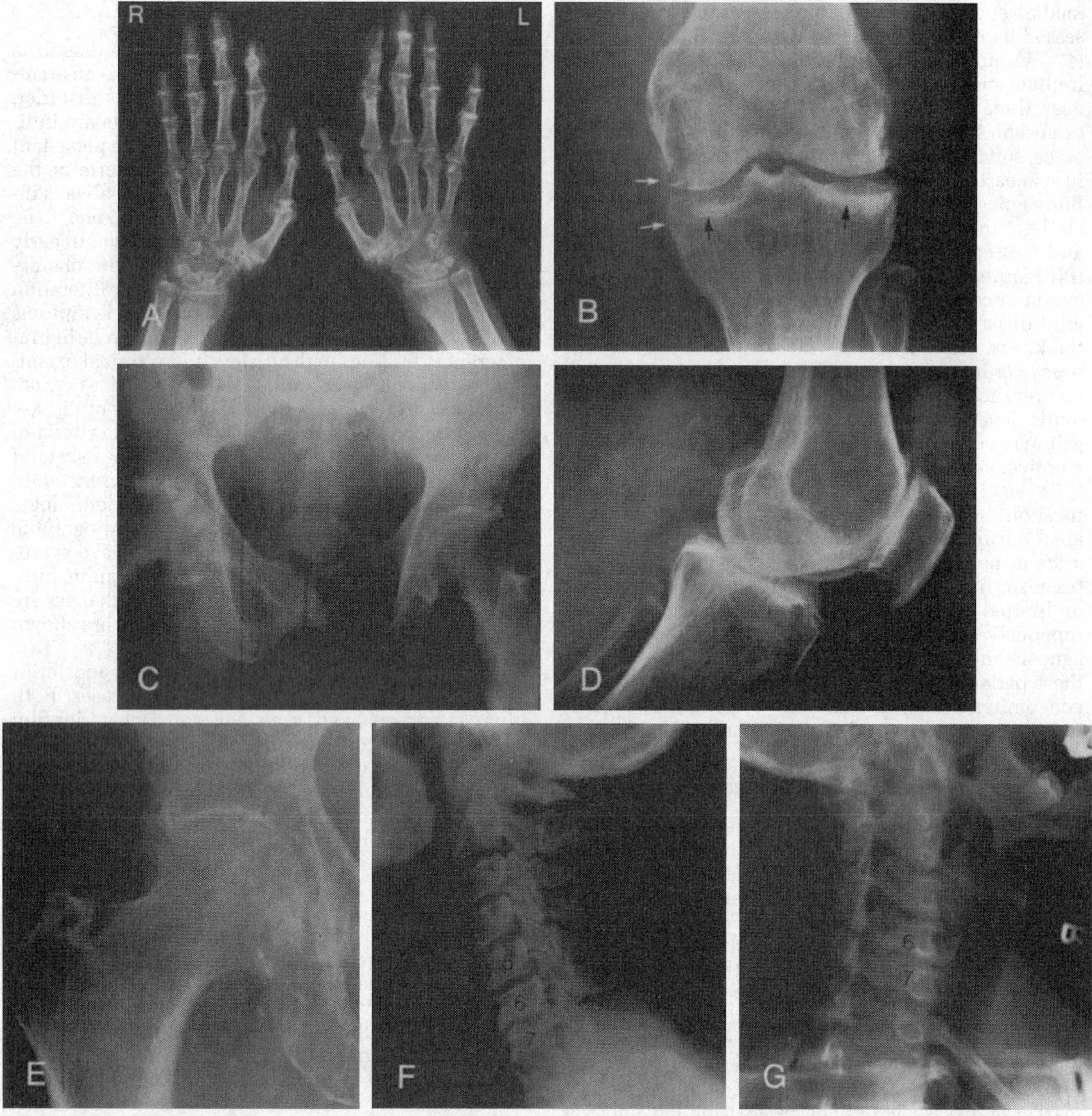

Figure 75.1. A: Hands of patient with degenerative joint disease. Note soft tissue enlargement on right over the second distal interphalangeal (DIP) joint (Heberden node); the loss of joint space and bony proliferation of all DIP joints, especially 2 and 3 in the right hand and 3 in the left hand; involvement of carpometacarpal joint of both thumbs with narrowing and increased density of subchondral bone; and normal metacarpophalangeal joints and wrist joints. **B:** X-ray of knee showing degenerative joint disease with loss of joint space (cartilage), especially in medial compartment, sclerotic subchondral bone, subchondral cysts, and early marginal spurs especially on lateral side. **C:** Pelvic film of a patient with advanced degenerative joint disease in the right hip. Notice the joint space narrowing and proliferation of subchondral bone. The left hip shows the minimal change of marginal sclerosis. **D:** Lateral x-ray of same knee in B illustrating the involvement of patellofemoral joint with narrowing and spur formation superiorly. **E:** X-ray of a hip showing early degenerative joint disease. Notice the narrowed joint space and spur formation of femoral head at upper margin of acetabulum **F:** X-ray of the lateral cervical spine showing degenerative joint disease. Note narrowing of C5–6 and, especially, C-7 interspace with anterior lipping and spur formation. **G:** Oblique x-ray view of cervical spine of same patient (F) showing osteophytes encroaching on neural foramina C5–6, C6–7.

roots. MRI is particularly useful in delineating soft tissue detail (e.g., in differentiating the annulus fibrosus from the nucleus pulposus of the intervertebral disc), whereas CT is useful for bone detail and calcifications. However, abnormal findings on CT and MRI in the absence of symptoms or equivocal findings despite significant symptoms and signs occur commonly. Thus, as with plain x-rays, careful correlation of findings with clinical symptoms is imperative. In general, CT and MRI and myelography are reserved for patients in whom conservative management has failed and in whom surgery or alternative causes of pain or radiculopathy are being strongly considered.

CT and MRI can also demonstrate lesions in peripheral joints but should be used only as an adjunct to conventional radiography. CT offers little advantage over plain radiographs or tomograms other than providing axial views and imaging of trabecular bone. MRI has all but replaced CT in specialized imaging of peripheral joints because it avoids CT radiation exposure and is particularly helpful in demonstrating soft tissue structures, including cartilage not shown on conventional x-rays. On the other hand, MRI may not show small calcific densities. Despite continued advances in MRI techniques, methods are complex and are not generally standardized so that performance and interpretation of these procedures requires considerable experience and expertise (51,52). Use of MRI to measure the volume of articular cartilage, to observe chondral defects, and to follow the course and progression of osteoarthritis holds promise for the future (53). MRI is most useful as an adjunct to arthroscopy to evaluate traumatic soft tissue injury such as ligamentous or meniscal tears (54). In moderate to severe osteoarthritis, physical examination and routine x-rays provide sufficiently sensitive and specific information. For this reason and because of the expense of MRI procedures and the complexity of available techniques, they are best reserved for the rheumatologist or orthopedic consultant for patients referred because of uncertain diagnosis or for consideration of arthroscopy or surgery after careful evaluation, including standard x-rays.

CLINICAL PATTERNS OF OSTEOARTHRITIS

Heberden Nodes

These bony enlargements of the DIP joints occur more often in women and commonly begin to appear in the fifth or sixth decade of life. They are often asymptomatic but a source of concern on the part of many patients, who may view them as an outward sign of aging or the beginning of a more serious and disabling arthritic disorder. This has been documented in two studies of elders in whom there was no correlation of osteoarthritis of the hands with objective measures of hand function, yet there was a definite correlation with subjective perception of functional limitation (55). Thus, one must be aware of and prepared to deal with the emotional investment of the patient who may focus concerns about declining functions on an obvious change in physical appearance, such as Heberden nodes. With a curt dismissal, no explanation of the true significance of this abnormality, and no opportunity for the patient to ventilate personal concerns, the clinician misses an important therapeutic opportunity.

Primary Generalized Osteoarthritis

The term *primary generalized osteoarthritis* was applied by Kellgren and Moore (56) to a group of patients whom they characterized as having osteoarthritis involving the DIP and PIP joints and the carpometacarpal joint of the thumb in addition to multiple other joints (hips, knees, metatarsophalangeal, and apophyseal joints of the spine). The term is often applied to patients with at least three areas of involvement with osteoarthritis. The radiologic appearance of the involved joints is similar to the usual changes of osteoarthritis, but the pattern suggests this syndrome. This pattern of osteoarthritis affects mostly middle-age women who have a positive family history of a similar disorder of joint involvement (57). Occasionally, in early phases they have had some inflammatory symptoms with an elevated erythrocyte sedimentation rate and an episodic course. It is suggested that these patients constitute a subgroup of patients with a heritable form of osteoarthritis that involves multiple joints and perhaps has some distinctive radiologic features. Some of these patients may also have autoimmune diseases such as hypothyroidism, or Sjögren syndrome (58). It is important to recognize the syndrome clinically, primarily to differentiate it from rheumatoid arthritis and other polyarticular diseases (59).

Erosive Osteoarthritis of Hands

The term *erosive osteoarthritis* has been applied to patients with severe osteoarthritis of the hands (DIP and PIP joints) in which extensive erosion of subchondral bone occurs, with eventual deformity and some limitation of motion of the finger joints. These patients also may have episodes of acute inflammation in these joints and their surrounding tissues. Some of these patients will also have generalized osteoarthritis with involvement of knees and feet. X-rays reveal the extensive bony erosion and subchondral cyst formation that may be interpreted incorrectly as rheumatoid or gouty erosions. The distribution of involvement in DIP and first carpometacarpal joints, sparing the metacarpophalangeal joints and wrists, should easily establish the true nature of the process. From the clinical view, this syndrome is important because of the severity of symptoms and physical findings, which are uncommon in milder forms of osteoarthritis of the hands. Functional status is not as favorable as in patients with nodal disease without erosions but is still surprisingly little affected (55).

Hip

Hip involvement is potentially the most painful and disabling joint abnormality in osteoarthritis. It is more often unilateral. Developmental defects in the structure of the hip, including congenital hip dysplasia, slipped capital femoral epiphysis, or unrecognized avascular necrosis, may have gone undetected but may have predisposed the patient to develop osteoarthritis; with age, disturbance of the normal anatomic relationship between femoral head and acetabulum may also predispose to osteoarthritis. Obesity is not a major causal factor in osteoarthritis of the hip but may predispose to bilateral rather than unilateral disease.

Pain, which early in the disease is associated with weight-bearing and movement, may become severe even at rest, and night pain is common in advanced disease. Pain may be referred to the ipsilateral groin or knee. Patients may walk with a limp or abnormal gait. Pain and limitation of motion during internal rotation and extension are early physical signs, and subsequently all motions may be painful and restricted. Clear identification of pain on motion of the hip is important in differentiating hip disease from bursitis (trochanteric and ischial; see Chapter 74), peripheral neuropathy (see Chapter 92), and other causes of pelvic pain. Flexion and adduction contracture and shortening may occur as disability progresses. Most patients who are symptomatic have characteristic changes of osteoarthritis on radiographic films of the hip. MRI may be useful to detect and differentiate early aseptic necrosis from osteoarthritis. Progression of osteoarthritis is variable but perhaps more likely to occur rapidly in the hip than in other joints.

Knee

The knee is the most common symptomatic joint in osteoarthritis. Chronic and slowly progressive pain with ambulation is the hallmark. There is a definite relationship to obesity, and the weight-bearing areas of the medial compartment are most often involved. Patellofemoral joint involvement is also common. The causative role of obesity in the development of osteoarthritis of the knee has been clearly shown in multiple epidemiologic studies (60). The association of obesity with osteoarthritis of the knee is stronger in women than in men, and the relative risk of osteoarthritis of the knee in obese African-American women is twice that of white women. In addition, evidence indicates that osteoarthritis of the knee is a consequence of and not a risk factor for obesity. Quadriceps muscle weakness was found to be a risk factor for knee osteoarthritis in both men and women over age 65 in both overweight and average-weight subjects (41).

Knee pain (especially with activities performed in flexion such as running or stair climbing) is a common symptom of *patellofemoral dysfunction.* This may arise from one or more factors resulting in abnormal knee mechanics (61) and may eventually lead to chondromalacia patellae (see Chapter 72). One technique is useful in treating this problem. Forcing the patella medially with strong taping to hold it in place for a few days resulted in better tracking of and thereby relief of pressure on the lateral aspect of the patella with movement. This produced pain relief in a short-term study of patients with patellofemoral arthritis with predominant changes in the lateral facet (62). Chondromalacia patellae usually occurs in younger people (second, third, and fourth decades), probably resulting from trauma and shearing forces against the patella as it contacts the femur in midflexion. Knee effusion is often associated with this syndrome. In younger patients with knee effusion who do not respond to rest or palliative aspiration, arthroscopy (see details in Chapter 72) may be indicated and shows characteristic changes. The relationship of this rather common syndrome to osteoarthritis is not entirely clear. Osteoarthritis of the patellofemoral joint may eventually develop in some cases. In patients below age 50 with the patellofemoral pain, the long-term outlook is good (63).

Spinal Syndromes

Osteoarthritis can result in neck or back pain that may be acute or chronic (see Chapters 70 and 71). Particularly in cervical spine involvement, symptoms may be more related to referred pain than to neck pain. These syndromes can also result in pain without obvious nerve root compression or neurologic abnormalities (64). Low cervical spine involvement can cause pain that is usually aching or burning in quality and referred to the upper anterior chest, to the lower border of the scapula, and radiating down the arm to the elbow. Confusion with anginal pain may occur, but the history usually makes it clear that pain is localized to one side and occurs at rest, particularly during the night or in the early morning after sleep (probably caused by positioning of the head during sleep). Although it may also be exacerbated by activity during the day, pain related to cervical arthritis does not subside rapidly with rest and is not related to specific exertion. Physical examination usually can reproduce the pain on extremes of movement of the neck or with manual compression of the cervical segments in hyperextension, rotation, or lateral flexion. Impingement by osteoarthritis of the cervical spine on the spinal cord itself rather than nerve roots is uncommon. *Central disk protrusion* or extensive anterior osteophyte formation (especially when associated with cervical kyphosis, which may cause additional narrowing of the spinal canal) is an occasional cause of cord compression with neurologic sequelae of weakness or spasticity from impingement on centrally located cerebrospinal tracts. Degenerative arthritis of the thoracic spine also can cause radicular pain in the thoracic area, but this is surprisingly uncommon in contrast to frequent radiologic findings of spur formation in the thoracic spine, probably because of the anterior position of most of these bony abnormalities. *Lumbar stenosis* caused by osteoarthritis is strongly suggested by a history of lower extremity pain with standing or walking that is considerably relieved or absent when seated. It is often associated with a

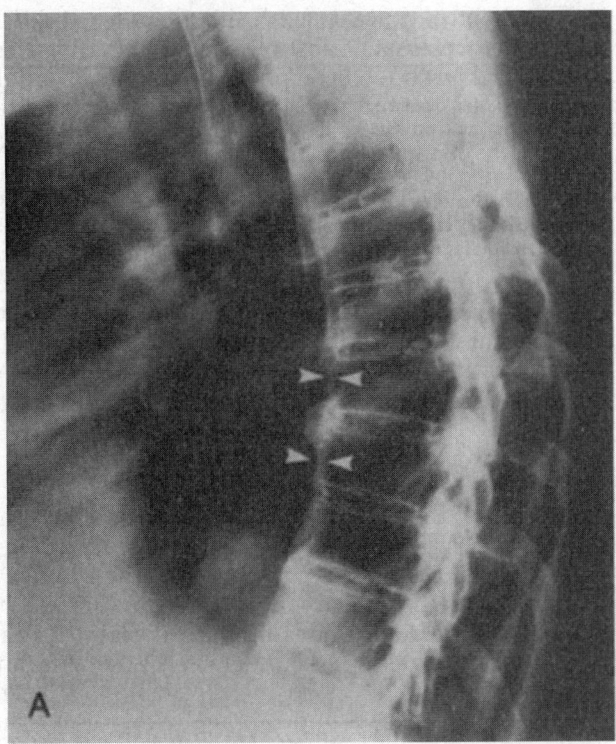

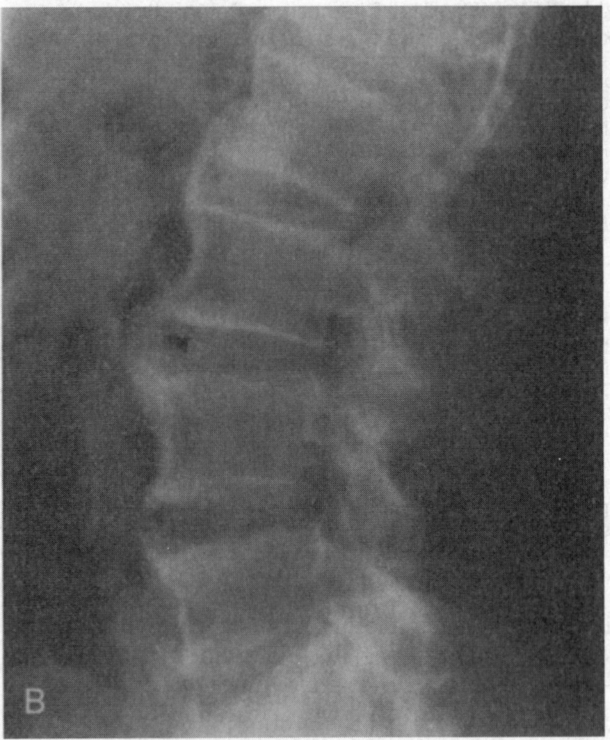

Figure 75.2. A: Lateral x-ray of thoracic spine of patient with diffuse idiopathic skeletal hyperostosis. **B:** Lateral x-ray of lumbar spine of patient with diffuse idiopathic skeletal hyperostosis. Prominent bony fusion and lipping anteriorly are seen.

slightly wide-based gait, no pain on flexion, and thigh pain within 30 seconds of lumbar extension (65).

Another spinal syndrome, the relationship of which to osteoarthritis is unclear, is *diffuse idiopathic skeletal hyperostosis.* Differing from the usual findings in osteoarthritis, the intervertebral disk height is relatively preserved despite extensive hyperostosis and osteophytic bony bridging between the vertebral bodies. In contrast to ankylosing spondylitis, motion and function may be less impaired because the apophyseal joints are usually spared. This syndrome is chiefly important because of its impressive radiographic appearance (Fig. 75.2), the diffuse bony changes with hyperostosis, and the importance of distinguishing it from ankylosing spondylitis (see Chapter 78).

Acute Exacerbations of Osteoarthritis

Some degree of synovial membrane inflammation is common in osteoarthritis. It is usually mild and focal as compared with rheumatoid arthritis but may be more extensive in advanced disease with release of inflammatory mediators that play a role in joint effusion and progression of damage to the articular cartilage (11). Patients with osteoarthritis may occasionally have acute or subacute painful episodes with swelling and exacerbation of the inflammatory process in the affected joint. These episodes are usually superimposed on more typical preceding symptoms and signs of osteoarthritis, but they may precipitate an initial visit to the primary care provider. In these patients there may be evidence of inflammation with pain, swelling, warmth, and some erythema on occasion. When the knee is involved, there is usually a joint effusion. The episodes, which are often precipitated by minor trauma, may be caused by sudden release into the joint of cartilaginous debris or microcrystalline deposits contained therein. In one study (21), calcium pyrophosphate or hydroxyapatite crystals were found in a high proportion of knee effusions of patients with such episodes, but these were also found in a significant proportion of unselected patients with osteoarthritis of the knee with effusion. Thus, the concurrence of crystalline deposit disease and osteoarthritis seems to be well established, although the relationship of cause and effect is unclear. From the clinical standpoint, however, this relationship provides one mechanism to explain these acute inflammatory episodes that punctuate the course of otherwise typical osteoarthritis (see Chapter 76). Sepsis may occasionally complicate an osteoarthritic joint, but it is a much less common event than occurs in a rheumatoid arthritic joint.

For these reasons a patient with established osteoarthritis who develops an acutely swollen painful joint should have the joint aspirated and the fluid analyzed because of the possibility of a complicating microcrystalline-induced or septic arthritis.

DIAGNOSIS AND DIFFERENTIAL DIAGNOSIS

The diagnosis of osteoarthritis is based on the history and physical findings related to the joints, the absence of systemic signs, and typical radiologic findings.

Table 75.4. Differential Diagnosis of Osteoarthritis: Extra-Articular Causes of Pain or Restricted Movement

Bone disease
- Osteopenia or osteoporosis (see Chapter 103)
- Malignancy: myeloma, metastatic
- Paget disease
- Osteomyelitis (see Chapter 40)

Periarticular soft tissue abnormalities
- Soft tissue contractures (Dupuytren, postcerebrovascular accident, or debilitating disease with disuse)
- Tendinitis or bursitis (see Chapter 74)
- Ligament strain (see Chapter 68)
- Reflex sympathetic dystrophy

Neuromuscular diseases
- Neuropathy (diabetes, alcoholism, B_{12} deficiency) (see Chapter 79)
- Parkinsonism (see Chapter 90)
- Tardive dyskinesias (see Chapters 25 and 90)
- Senile dementia with rigidity (see Chapters 26 and 90)

Vascular diseases (see Chapter 94)
- Atherosclerosis
- Diabetes
- Vasculitis

Differentiation from other forms of arthritis is usually easy, with the possible exception of some of the more unusual diffuse or inflammatory patterns of involvement described above. Consideration of the age of the patient, the distribution of the joints involved, and the radiologic findings usually lead to the correct diagnosis. Criteria for classification and reporting of osteoarthritis of the hip (66) and knee (67) have been reported by an expert panel of rheumatologists.

The most common errors in differential diagnosis occur in attributing symptoms of pain or restricted movement to osteoarthritis when the problem is not the joints. This is a particularly common mistake in the evaluation of knee pain (ligament injury; see Chapter 72), hip pain (bursitis; see Chapter 74), and shoulder pain (periarticular problem; see Chapter 69). Because x-rays may demonstrate changes of osteoarthritis in asymptomatic or mildly symptomatic patients, one must rely on a careful history and physical examination to localize the disease to the joints. Table 75.4 lists other disorders, also common in older patients, that often give rise to pain and to painful or restricted movement and that may be erroneously attributed to osteoarthritis unless a careful examination is done.

MANAGEMENT

Recent advances in understanding mechanisms involved in the occurrence and pathogenesis suggest that new methods of treatment directed toward the specific pathology of cartilage degeneration may soon be on the horizon (68). Although there is no cure for the disease, much can be done to relieve symptoms, minimize disability, and perhaps delay progression of the disease. Certainly a nihilistic approach to therapy is not justified. Objective studies to establish therapeutic efficacy of interventions require large numbers of patients and long-term follow-up, so that one must often rely on subjective and incomplete data in deciding the best management of patients with this disorder (49). The necessity to evaluate traditional and alternative treatments that have often been popular with the lay public has led to more objective studies of these modalities (69). Although evidence-based decisions are now possible for many therapeutic alternatives, one must still rely to some extent on subjective information, incomplete data, or the reviews and opinions of a panel of experts for guidance (2,70). All observers, however, agree on and strongly emphasize the fundamental importance of treatment measures other than pharmacotherapy as the first step in management of the patient with osteoarthritis (2,70).

General Measures

Patient Education

Explaining to the patient the nature of the disease, that other joints are not likely to be involved, that progression of disease is slow, and that preservation of function is likely reassures most patients. For the patient with Heberden nodes or mild disease in other joints, this reassurance and understanding are the most important therapeutic step in management. The importance of education and rapport with patients has been emphasized in studies that demonstrated improved clinical outcomes associated with mail (71) or telephone (72) interventions and group support (73). These strategies were also cost effective (74). Improvement in pain and functional status occurred in patients who had this added contact with providers. These observations reinforce the usefulness of a team approach in caring for patients with osteoarthritis and indicate an important role in management in the ambulatory care setting for office staff, nurses, therapists, and others as well as the primary care provider. In addition, the patient has an essential role in managing his or her disease. Self-management education is widely available through local chapters of the Arthritis Foundation as the Arthritis Self-Help Course, a 6-week course conducted by both lay leaders and professionals. Reinforcement by the clinician and his or her staff of the value of self-management is an important step in therapy (75). Useful patient reading for self-management is available for example in The Arthritis Help Book (76), which is used as a companion to the Self-Help Course.

Pain and discomfort of osteoarthritis are often exacerbated by use, especially continuous use or weight-bearing. Furthermore, excessive use of joints already damaged by osteoarthritis may accelerate cartilage degeneration. Therefore, rest is an important treatment modality for osteoarthritis. Short periods of rest through the day are usually more effective than are less frequent longer periods. With weight-bearing joints, rest is particularly important. Many patients, especially elderly ones, believe that use of a joint becomes limited if it is rested too much, so needless overuse is common. When an understanding of the value of rest balanced with appropriately directed exercise and reassurance about function are given, patients often quickly learn to live within their own limitations without undue restrictions of activity and with improvement in symptoms.

Use of Canes, Crutches, and Walkers

In more severe disease, rest from weight-bearing and stability when walking may be partially achieved by the use of a crutch, cane, or walker. The patient's attitude about the use of such assistive devices is an important consideration here because some interpret their cane as a sign of infirmity and fail to use it, whereas others carry it proudly as a badge of dependency even when it is not needed. Instruction in proper use of a cane, crutch, or walker should be given by the clinician or a physical therapist. The object is to take some of the weight off the affected limb; thus, a cane or a crutch should be used on the opposite side and used simultaneously with the affected limb for weight-bearing. Also, a cane of the proper length (e.g., from the floor to the bend of the wrist) should be held tightly and close to the body. Proper use is ensured by pressing the handle against the good hip. To completely prevent bearing weight on an affected limb, a crutch is required; it is used on the affected side, or two crutches are used. A walker does not provide this type of unilateral support, but it may be needed in patients with bilateral knee pain or in patients whose instability requires more support than that provided by a cane or a crutch.

Correction of Postural or Mechanical Strain

This is an important consideration in patients with poor body mechanics. Thus, patients with pronated feet (see Chapter 73) have excessive stress on the knees and low back. Genu varus or valgum stresses the lateral or medial compartment excessively. The use of a wedged insole to compensate for valgus stress in mild knee disease in an uncontrolled trial was effective in relieving pain and improving function (77). In patients with unicompartmental tibiofemoral disease, such a device may postpone the need for joint replacement (78). Instruction in proper lifting and avoidance of unnecessary strain on certain joints or muscles by occupational or other activities may also need attention, such as use of a cervical pillow in the patient with neck involvement (see also Chapters 70 and 71).

Physical Therapy

Simple measures can be prescribed for home use without the need for referral to a physical therapist in patients with mild disease. However, one must be sure that the patient understands directions. Reinforcement on subsequent visits is also important to ensure compliance. Patients with more advanced disease, especially those with functional limitations, should be referred to a physical or occupational therapist for more extensive instruction in an exercise program, joint protection maneuvers, use of assistive devices, gait training, and similar measures.

Heat. No controlled trials establish beneficial effects of the external application of thermal therapy. However, experience and precedent suggest that application of heat often provides symptomatic relief of pain, reduces muscle spasm, and facilitates performance of an exercise program. Most patients prefer moist heat, which can be applied for 15 to 20 minutes via bathtub, hot towels, or commercially manufactured packs. Dry heat using electric heating pads may also be used. Paraffin wax baths (available from large pharmacies) may be useful in patients with extensive hand involvement. With all modalities of heat therapy, temperatures that are very hot (above 110°F [43°C]) and prolonged or uninterrupted use should be avoided to prevent skin damage. This is especially important with electric heating pads, and patients should always be instructed to use the low temperature setting and place a towel between the skin and pad. Use of diathermy, ultrasound, heat cabinets, and other modalities offers little additional benefit but increases cost, and generally is not recommended. Cold packs may be more effective in relieving pain and reducing swelling, especially after minor trauma or after exercise to relieve muscle soreness. Limiting application to no more than 20 to 30 minutes is again important.

Exercise. Goals of an exercise program are to maintain or improve function by preserving range of motion and improving muscle strength. The latter is important to help stabilize the joint and by maintaining soft tissue cushioning of stress to reduce the stress applied to the joint. Gradual conditioning is important so that muscle pain and soreness are not aggravated. Pain is often relieved as strength is gained and mechanical advantage is restored. Exercise should be graded according to the ability of the patient and carried out regularly for optimal effect. In general, if muscle soreness or joint pain is worse after exercise, the intensity of the exercise should be reduced or progression halted until symptoms subside. Although walking may induce knee pain in patients with symptomatic osteoarthritis, supervised fitness walking accompanied by light stretching and strengthening exercises and educational sessions improves pain and physical fitness while reducing medication requirement (79). Aerobic exercise is highly desirable to maintain strength and general fitness. In a randomized trial in patients over 60 with knee osteoarthritis, improvement in pain and disability was observed both with a resistance exercise program and aerobic exercise (80). Exercise in a pool is a valuable means of aerobic exercise that does not involve weight-bearing stress.

Maintenance of quadriceps strength is particularly important in osteoarthritis of the knee (81). Weakness, proprioceptive impairment, and function can be improved with an exercise program (82), whether carried out in a formal physical therapy setting (83) or at home (84). This can be accomplished by beginning with slow full extension of the knee against gravity and then, as symptoms and progress allow, by extension against progressively increasing resistance. In patients whose pain prevents active quadriceps strengthening, isometric exercises are useful. With the knee extended the patient is instructed to tighten the quadriceps maximally so that the patella becomes fixed, hold for

10 to 15 seconds by count, release, and repeat. For patients who have difficulty rising from a seated position because of hip or knee disease, standing exercise from a high to a progressively lower stool may be useful in restoring function. The importance of maintaining muscle strength and conditioning is emphasized by studies measuring the energy expenditure of walking in patients with symptomatic arthritis of the hip or knee (85). The markedly increased energy requirement results in excessive fatigue that discourages mobility and may begin a cycle of progressive functional impairment in the frail elderly patient. Because of the importance of proper exercise in patients with arthritis, continued reinforcement by the clinician is needed.

Other Measures. Other nonmedicinal treatments occasionally have been shown to be useful in treatment of osteoarthritis, particularly in relieving pain. These include *transcutaneous nerve stimulation, acupuncture, low-energy laser,* and *pulsed electrical stimulation* (69). In most studies of these therapies, small numbers of patients are involved, pain relief rather than functional status or progression of disease have been assessed, with only modest short-term benefit as compared with control subjects. The use of topical capsaicin cream (0.025%) applied four times a day was effective in pain relief in a double-blind trial in knee osteoarthritis (86). Continued application for 2 to 4 weeks is necessary to achieve benefit. Initial discomfort from the application tends to disappear with continued use. Use of a stronger preparation (0.25%) applied twice daily was somewhat more effective but with more discomfort, especially at the initiation of treatment (87). Many patients report relief of stiffness and discomfort with a sense of joint protection through the use of elastic supports around the joint. Such devices used at the knee, however, should be fitted appropriately to avoid obstruction of venous circulation in the leg. Splints may be useful when the first carpometacarpal joint is involved or with finger deformities caused by erosive disease. Wearing nylon stretch gloves (e.g., Isotoner gloves, available in department stores) at night may provide relief for some patients with extensive hand involvement (88).

Nutrition and Diet

The lay public often seeks to implicate diet in the cause, exacerbation, or treatment of a chronic disease such as osteoarthritis. However, there are few well-controlled studies to establish such relationships, and patients should be warned against food fads and unwarranted claims of benefit. Obesity has been a well-established risk factor for osteoarthritis, but only recently have well-controlled studies been published that demonstrate improvement in pain and functional status with weight loss. Sustained weight loss with diet and exercise was shown to result in improvement in pain, disability, gait, and performance in patients with knee osteoarthritis (89,90).

A possible role for vitamin D deficiency in the development of radiographic joint space narrowing but not osteophyte development was reported in elderly women in a longitudinal study (91). Low levels of vitamin D also correlated with progression but not incidence of osteoarthritis of the knee (92). Although there are theoretical reasons for possible benefit of vitamin E and C as antioxidants in cartilage metabolism, no studies that show clinical benefit are available. Patients should be advised to follow a generally nutritious and healthful diet to maintain normal weight and include adequate amounts of fruits and vegetables to obtain appropriate vitamins and nutrients. If supplements are needed due to uncertainty of dietary intake, a once daily multivitamin or low doses (400 IU) of vitamin D, 200 to 400 IU of vitamin E, and 250 to 500 mg of vitamin C are sufficient.

Dietary supplements available in health food stores have not been well studied and are of doubtful value with the possible exception of glucosamine and chondroitin sulfate, two important constituents of articular cartilage. Numerous reports reviewed in a meta-analysis suggest that they are about as effective as nonsteroidal anti-inflammatory drugs (NSAIDs) in relieving the pain of osteoarthritis (93). There are theoretical reasons and biochemical evidence that glucosamine or chondroitin may favorably influence cartilage metabolism (94–96). One controlled study in patients with mild to moderate osteoarthritis also indicated that in addition to pain relief, some patients on glucosamine had slowing of progression of joint space narrowing by radiography (97,98). However, the conclusion that the small degree of reduction in joint space narrowing indicates improvement in the basic process of cartilage destruction needs further study and confirmation because radiographic joint space narrowing is difficult to measure with consistency and is contributed to by meniscal extrusion rather than thinning of articular cartilage in early osteoarthritis (99). Although well tolerated in studies to date, the long-term side-effect profile of glucosamine and chondroitin also need further evaluation. A large NIH-sponsored multicenter trial of glucosamine is currently underway and is much needed to more firmly establish the role of glucosamine and sulfated glycosaminoglycans in the management of osteoarthritis. Patients seeking glucosamine or chondroitin should be warned that as dietary supplements, they are not regulated by the Food and Drug Administration. Quantities of some preparations may not be standard and some may contain other unwanted substances. Established pharmaceutical firms have recently begun to market preparations in the United States of glucosamine (Aflexa) and a mixture of glucosamine and chondroitin (Flexagen). Glucosamine at the usual dose of 1,500 mg daily will cost about $25 to $40 a month.

Drug Therapy

There has been a minor revolution in the use of drugs in osteoarthritis with the addition of new therapeutic alternatives. Although the past dictum has been that no drugs will alter the course of osteoarthritis, the concept of chondroprotective drugs acting over the long term to modify the basic mechanism of disease (disease-modifying osteoarthritis drugs) are currently topics of discussion and research. As information about cartilage metabolism in osteoarthritis continues to develop, the promise of such agents may become closer to reality, but none has yet been proven clinically effective with certainty.

Currently, one needs to consider a hierarchy of treatment choices. The first efforts should always be to modify known risk factors (e.g., obesity) to establish a well-designed program of education and exercise to relieve pain and maintain maximum function. These measures may be sufficient in themselves without pharmacotherapy. For pain that is not adequately relieved by these general measures, the first drugs to consider adding are analgesics. Acetaminophen in doses up to 4 g/day often provides effective relief of pain and should be the first choice because of its low cost and low incidence of adverse effects. Because it may increase the half-life of warfarin, caution should be taken to monitor patients also receiving this agent, and acetaminophen should be avoided in patients with liver disease or chronic alcohol abuse. Nonacetylated salicylates or nonopioid analgesics are also acceptable alternatives. Opioids may be used occasionally on a short-term basis as an adjunct to other analgesics but in general are not appropriate for long-term use in this chronic disease.

Acetaminophen appears not to be as effective as NSAIDs in reducing inflammation, relieving moderate to severe pain, and improving functional status (100), and the current wisdom now favors NSAIDs for the treatment of osteoarthritis but with a strong hope for more scientific study (100a) in these and other treatments. The choice of NSAID therapy has been altered by the recognition of serious side effects and risks of gastrointestinal bleeding with previously standard agents, especially in the elderly. The availability of new NSAIDs more specifically inhibiting the cyclooxygenase-2 (COX-2) enzyme has clearly reduced the incidence of serious gastrointestinal bleeding, obstruction, or perforation compared with those primarily affecting COX-1 (101). However, concomitant use of low dose aspirin for its cardiovascular effects reduced the benefit in gastrointestinal risk reduction of the COX-2 inhibitor, celecoxib, to approximate that of ibuprofen or diclofenac (100). In another large trial with rofecoxib versus naproxen in which aspirin use was prohibited, the incidence of serious gastrointestinal events was significantly reduced with a relative risk of 0.6 per 100 patient years versus 1.4 for naproxen (102). Unfortunately, in this trial the risk for myocardial infarction, although small (0.4%), was significantly higher in the rofecoxib group. These findings can perhaps be explained by the fact that the COX-2 inhibitors unlike aspirin and standard NSAIDs do not block platelet thromboxane but may affect endothelial prostaglandins. In patients with established risk factors for arterial and venous thrombotic events, the COX-2 inhibitors may actually increase the risk for thrombosis (103). Thus, in the patient at risk for myocardial infarction or thrombotic events, a trade-off between the gastrointestinal protective effect of the COX-2–specific drugs and the antithrombotic action of aspirin or COX-1–inhibiting NSAIDs has been suggested (104). The overall clinical significance of these observations needs further study.

In selecting therapy with NSAIDs, one should weigh the complex interplay of risks and benefits and consider the patient's comorbid conditions and demographics. In the patient under age 65 with no serious comorbid conditions, no prior history of peptic ulcer disease, upper gastrointestinal bleeding, and not on steroids or anticoagulants, a low dose of a nonselective NSAID is a reasonable choice with relatively low risk and low cost. If a higher dose is required, the addition of misoprostol 200 μg three times a day (105) or a proton pump inhibitor (106) may further reduce the risk. Histamine-2 blockers are less effective (107). In the patient with a higher risk of gastrointestinal complications (e.g., elderly with comorbid conditions), a COX-2–selective NSAID is a safer choice (70). Celecoxib is effective at a dose of 100 mg twice a day or rofecoxib 25 mg daily. Celecoxib is contraindicated in patients with a history of an allergic reaction to a sulfonamide. In the patient who requires low dose aspirin, NSAID should be avoided or misoprostol or a proton pump inhibitor added. The effects of COX-2 inhibitors on renal function are similar to those of nonselective NSAIDs so that caution must be used with all these drugs in patients with mild to moderately impaired renal function and prohibited in patients with significant renal insufficiency (108). A full discussion of NSAIDs is also found in Chapter 77.

Nutritional supplements glucosamine and chondroitin sulfate have been dubbed "nutraceuticals" (109) since data from a controlled trial have indicated that they may have a pharmacologic role in therapy of osteoarthritis (97,98). Because of their apparent low toxicity profile they may offer an alternative to NSAIDs in relief of pain in patients with mild to moderate osteoarthritis. Of note is that pain relief did not occur until after 1 month of use in some reported trials. The potential of these compounds as chondroprotective agents remains to be firmly established *in vivo*. In view of the lack of firm assurance of the validity of earlier trials, it is prudent to await the outcome of an NIH-sponsored multicenter controlled trial and more long-term studies before recommending these agents.

Intra-articular and Invasive Measures

Corticosteroids. Intra-articular injection of corticosteroids has been a time-honored alternative for treatment of osteoarthritis (110), especially of the knee when there is an effusion present. Removal of joint fluid without corticosteroid injection usually does not improve symptoms unless microcrystalline arthritis is superimposed (see Chapter 76). Intra-articular steroid provides pain relief for variable periods of time and is often short lived. Presumably effective because of its anti-inflammatory properties, evidence to demonstrate an effect on inflammatory mediators in the joint is lacking (111). Multiple injections may enhance joint destruction or predispose to infection so that three to four injections per year in a joint is the maximum that should be used.

Hyaluronate. Another intra-articular therapeutic alternative (so-called viscosupplementation with hyaluronate) has been shown in randomized controlled trials to relieve pain in some patients with osteoarthritis of the knee (112). Two preparations are available: A very high molecular weight cross-linked hyaluronate (Hylan GF-20) requires one intra-articular injection per week for 3 weeks and a lower molecular weight sodium hyaluronate (Hyalgan) requires five weekly injections (113). Both have been found to be better than placebo but perhaps equal to NSAID therapy. One study suggested that the higher molecular weight product had a higher response rate (114). However, comparison with placebo in trials is difficult to interpret because of the obvious difference in the viscosity of the active agents and the invasive nature of the procedure. Also some of the evidence supporting the conclusion reached in the principal clinical trials has been questioned (115). In a survey of Hylan use in Canada, 76% improved with the mean duration of response of 8 months. Local inflammatory reactions developed in 8%, and patients with more advanced radiographic damage had a less favorable response (115a).

It is not clear whether the mechanism of action of this therapy is simply on mediation of pain or on some mechanical or metabolic process within the joint. More studies are needed to evaluate the long-term effects of these agents. Because this mode of therapy is invasive, expensive, and likely, at most, only equal in effect to NSAID therapy, it should probably be reserved for patients who have not responded to analgesics and a vigorous nonpharmacologic program or in whom NSAIDs are contraindicated (116).

Tidal Irrigation and Debridement. Tidal irrigation of the knee has been reported to provide relief of pain for up to 1 year in some patients with osteoarthritis of the knee (117). Using an intra-articular injection of corticosteroid and saline placebo as controls, lavage relieved pain significantly better than placebo and was comparable with the intra-articular steroid (118). However, the corticosteroid effect lasted only 4 weeks, and the lavage improvement was still significant at 24 weeks. Neither affected functional status. Problems in achieving adequate controls to critically evaluate this procedure, its invasiveness, and expense led to withdrawal at present of its former recommendation for its use in management (69). Arthroscopy with debridement was superior over the long term to lavage (119), but adequate control again is difficult. Arthroscopy with debridement is useful principally in patients with meniscal injury, loose bodies, or perhaps large osteophytes (117).

Orthopedic Surgery

An orthopedist should be consulted in the treatment of patients with osteoarthritis who have a problem of malalignment or major instability in weight-bearing joints, for symptoms or findings of loose bodies in the joint, and for intractable pain with advanced disease of the hips or knees. Osteotomy may correct malalignment. When pain or disability is refractory to treatment and joint destruction of a hip or a knee is advanced, consideration should be given to total joint replacement. Disabling pain and the progressive limitation of activities of daily living are the principal indications for this procedure. Contraindications include neuromuscular or sensory deficits, severe peripheral vascular disease, marked obesity, dementia, and lack of motivation or inability to cooperate with a postoperative rehabilitation program. Results of joint replacement in osteoarthritis of the hip are generally excellent. In patients with functionally significant osteoarthritis undergoing hip replacement, evaluation of function and short-term and long-term costs indicate that the procedure improved quality-adjusted life years and was cost effective (120). Total knee arthroplasty is also highly effective in reducing pain and disability with good to excellent results in most patients (121). Arthrodesis (i.e., surgical fusion of the joint) is usually reserved for patients with failed joint replacement. Major complications of joint replacement are postoperative thrombophlebitis and infection. Elimination of potential foci of infection is important preoperatively, and prophylactic antibiotics are advocated by some after joint replacement surgery and during dental or urinary tract procedures that might produce bacteremia. Although the continued improvement in synthetic materials and surgical techniques has prolonged the durability of an artificial joint, most rheumatologists do not refer patients with hip or knee arthritis for surgery until symptoms are pronounced or functional impairment is considerable enough to impair quality of life. Because prostheses wear out and must be replaced after 10 to 15 years, surgery is usually reserved for patients in their sixth decade or beyond.

New advances in culturing chondrocytes and transplanting cartilage tissues have shown promise in repairing chondral defects (122). Although potentially promising for the future in and correcting traumatic cartilage damage, there is currently no applicability of these techniques to the treatment of osteoarthritis.

PREVENTION

Because the cause of osteoarthritis is uncertain, so is its prevention. However, recognition of predisposing factors and elucidation of normal physiology of articular cartilage suggest certain prudent steps that can be recommended (60).

Immobilization with avoidance of joint stress gives rise to biochemical changes in cartilage similar to early lesions in osteoarthritis. Thus, normal stress and functioning of joints are important in maintenance of normal cartilage physiology. Perhaps one can abstract from this that a sedentary and inactive life-style is not good for the integrity of articular cartilage. Furthermore, because strong periarticular muscles lend stability and help absorb stress applied to joints, it seems logical that physical conditioning to maintain muscle strength and a lean habitus may be important in prevention of osteoarthritis. Because quadriceps weakness is a risk factor for osteoarthritis of the knee, strengthening this muscle group is especially important to prevent or halt progression of osteoarthritis of the knee. That weight loss reduces the risk for symptomatic knee osteoarthritis in women has been demonstrated (89,90). Soft tissues tend to lose mobility with advancing age, and such changes have been shown to increase impact stress of joints. Physical activity may retard this loss of mobility and therefore should be encouraged.

At the same time it is evident that repetitive stress, especially when abnormally applied or when resulting in injury or structural damage, is a strong predisposing factor to osteoarthritis. Thus, correction of abnormal mechanical forces from developmental or postural defects, avoidance of unusual occupational stress, and avoidance of traumatic injury to joints are important in prevention of osteoarthritis and preservation of good muscle strength and tone. Maintenance of good nutrition with adequate intake of vitamin D in elderly patients may be of benefit (91,92). Theoretically important in cartilage metabolism, whether antioxidants such as vitamin C and E are of benefit remains to be shown. Because epidemiologic studies indicate a role for estrogen in osteoarthritis in postmenopausal women and estrogen receptors have been demonstrated in adult articular cartilage (123), hormonal replacement therapy needs to be further evaluated as a preventive measure. New genetic or biochemical markers of susceptibility may eventually aid in identifying patients at increased risk of disease, and new therapeutic agents to prevent cartilage breakdown by inhibiting metalloproteinases or inflammatory mediators such as interleukin-1 hold promise for the future in prevention and treatment.

General References*

American Geriatrics Society Panel on Exercise and Osteoarthritis. **Exercise prescription for older adults with osteoarthritis. Pain: consensus practice recommendations.** J Am Geriatr Soc 2001;49:808.

An evidenced-based review of this subject with practical strategies and guidelines for the clinician.

Brandt KD, ed. Osteoarthritis. Rheum Dis Clin North Am 1999;25.

A compilation of authors discussing recent advances and issues.

Dieppe P, Altman R, Lequesne M, et al. Osteoarthritis of the knee: report of a task force of the International League of Associations for Rheumatology and the Osteoarthritis Research Society. J Am Geriatr Soc 1997;45:850.

*Bold print (general references) and bold numerals (specific references) denote published controlled clinical trials, meta-analyses, or consensus-based recommendations.

Current status referable to diagnosis, therapy, and outcomes.

Fitzgerald GA, Patrono C. The coxibs, selective inhibitors of cyclooxygenase-2. N Engl J Med 2001;345:433.

This article reviews the evidence that supports the theory that these agents would be less toxic in the gastrointestinal track compared to nonselective NSAIDs.

Harris ED, Ruddy S, Sledge CB, eds. Kelley's textbook of rheumatology. 6th ed. Philadelphia: W.B. Saunders, 2001.

Koopman WJ, ed. Arthritis and allied conditions, 14th ed. Baltimore: Williams & Wilkins, 2001.

These are two excellent multiauthored textbooks of rheumatology, with sections on osteoarthritis providing more detailed presentation of the topic and extensive bibliographies.

Ling SM, Bathon JM. Osteoarthritis in older adults. J Am Geriatr Soc 1998;46:216.

A good review of osteoarthritis in the elderly.

Moskowitz RW, Howell DS, Altman RD, et al., eds. Osteoarthritis, diagnosis and medical/surgical management. 3rd ed. Philadelphia: W.B. Saunders, 2001.

Peter JB, Pearson CM, Marmnor L. Erosive osteoarthritis of the hands. Arthritis Rheum 1966;9:365.

The original description of this concept.

Resnick D, Niwazama G. Diagnosis of bone and joint disorders. 4th ed. Philadelphia: W.B. Saunders, 2002.

A five-volume set with extensive coverage of radiography of all forms of arthritis.

Specific References

1. Felson DT, Lawrence RC, Dieppe PA, et al. Osteoarthritis: new insights. Part 1: the disease and its risk factors. Ann Intern Med 2000;133:635.
2. Felson DT, Lawrence RC, Hochberg MC, et al. Osteoarthritis: new insights. Part 2: treatment approaches. Ann Intern Med 2000;133:726.
3. Lawrence RC, Helmick CG, Arnett FC, et al. Estimations of the prevalence of arthritis and selected musculoskeletal disorders in the United States. Arthritis Rheum 1998;41:7789.
4. Marsland DW, Wood M, Mayo F. Content of family practice. I. Routine order of diagnostic frequency. II. Diagnosis by disease category and age/sex distribution. J Fam Pract 1976;8:37.
5. Yelin E. The economics of osteoarthritis. In: Brandt K, Doherty M, Lohmander LS, eds. Osteoarthritis. New York: Oxford University Press, 1998:23.
6. Gabriel SE, Crowson C, O'Fallon M. Costs of osteoarthritis: estimates from a geographically defined population. J Rheumatol 1995;43[Suppl]:23.
7. Guccione AA, Felson DT, Anderson JJ, et al. The effect of specific medical conditions on the functional limitation of elders in the Framingham study. Am J Public Health 1994;84:351.
8. Oliveria SA, Felson DT, Reed JI, et al. Incidence of symptomatic hand, hip and knee osteoarthritis among patients in a health maintenance organization. Arthritis Rheum 1995;38:1134.
9. Felson DT, Naimark A, Anderson J, et al. The prevalence of knee osteoarthritis in the elderly. The Framingham osteoarthritis study. Arthritis Rheum 1987;30:914.
10. Felson DT, Zhang Y, Hannan MT, et al. The incidence and natural history of osteoarthritis of the knee in the elderly. The Framingham osteoarthritis study. Arthritis Rheum 1995;38:1500.
11. Poole AR. An introduction to the pathophysiology of osteoarthritis. Frontiers Biosci 1999;4:662.
12. Goldring MB. The role of the chondrocyte in osteoarthritis. Arthritis Rheum 2000;43:1916.
13. Attur MG, Dave MN, Clancy RM, et al. Functional genomic analysis in arthritis-affected cartilage: yin-yang regulation of inflammatory mediators by alpha 5 beta 1 and alpha V Beta 3 integrins. J Immunol 2000;164:2684.
14. Lotz M, Hashimoto S, Kuhn, K. Mechanisms of chondrocyte apoptosis. Osteoarthr Cart 1999;7:389.
15. Setton LA, Elliott DM, Mow VC. Altered mechanics of cartilage with osteoarthritis: human osteoarthritis and an experimental model of joint degeneration. Osteoarthr Cart 1999;7:214.

16. Radin EL, Burr DB, Caterson B, et al. Mechanical determinants of osteoarthritis. Semin Arthritis Rheum 1991; 21[Suppl 2]:12.
17. Dequeker J, Luyten FP. Bone mass and osteoarthritis. Clin Exp Rheumatol 2000;18[Suppl 21]:S21.
18. Zhang Y, Hannan MT, Chaisson CE, et al. Bone mineral density and risk of incident and progressive radiographic knee osteoarthritis in women. J Rheumatol 2000;27:1032.
19. Dequeker J. Inverse relationship of the interface between osteoporosis and osteoarthritis. J Rheumatol 1997;224:795.
20. Wluka AE, Davis SR, Bailey M, et al. Users of estrogen replacement therapy have more knee cartilage than non-users. Ann Rheum Dis 2001;60:332.
21. Huskisson EC, Dieppe PA, Tucker AK, et al. Another look at osteoarthritis. Ann Rheum Dis 1979;38:423.
22. Dieppe P, Doherty M, McFarlane DG, et al. Apatite associated destructive arthritis. Br J Rheumatol 1984;23:84.
23. Felson DT, Chaisson CE, Hill CL. The association of bone marrow lesions with pain in knee osteoarthritis. Ann Intern Med 2001;134:541.
24. Doherty M. Genetics of hand osteoarthritis. Osteoarthr Cart 2000;8[Suppl A]:S8.
25. Spector TD, Cicuttini F, Baker J, et al. Genetic influences on osteoarthritis in women: a twin study. BMJ 1996;312:940.
26. Villiaumey J. Is the hip involved in generalized osteoarthritis? Br J Rheumatol 1993;32:85.
27. Pattrick M, Aldridge S, Hamilton E, et al. A controlled study of hand function in nodal and erosive osteoarthritis. Ann Rheum Dis 1989;48:978.
28. Ala-Kokko L, Baldwin CT, Moskowitz RW, et al. Single base mutation in the type II procollagen gene (COL2A1) as a cause of primary osteoarthritis associated with mild achondroplasia. Proc Natl Acad Sci USA 1990;87:6565.
29. Ritvaniemi P, Kokko J, Bonaventure J, et al. Identification of COL2A gene mutations in patients with chondrodysplasias and familial osteoarthritis. Arthritis Rheum 1995;38:999.
30. Loughlin J, Irven C, Fergusson C, et al. Sibling pair analysis shows no linkage of generalized osteoarthritis to the loci encoding type II collagen, cartilage link protein or cartilage matrix protein. Br J Rheumatol 1994;33:1103.
31. Uitterlinden AG, Burger H, VanDuijn CM, et al. Adjacent genes for COL2A1 and the vitamin D receptor are associated with separate features of radiographic osteoarthritis of the knee. Arthritis Rheum 2000;43:1456.
32. Vikkula M, Nissila M, Hirvensalo P. Multiallelic polymorphisms of the cartilage collagen gene: no association with osteoarthrosis. Ann Rheum Dis 1993;52:762.
33. Moos V, Rudwaleit M, Herzog V, et al. Association of genotypes affecting the expression of interleukin-1beta or interleukin-1 receptor antagonist with osteoarthritis. Arthritis Rheum 2000;43:2417.
34. Paassilta P, Lohiniva J, Goring HH, et al. Identification of a novel common genetic risk factor for lumbar disc disease. JAMA 2001;285:1843.
35. Carman WJ, Sowers MF, Hawthorne VM, et al. Obesity as a risk factor for osteoarthritis: a prospective study. Am J Epidemiol 1994;139:1199.
36. Panush RS, Hanson CS, Caldwell JR, et al. Is running associated with osteoarthritis? An eight-year follow-up study. J Clin Rheumatol 1995;1:35.
37. Fries JF, Singh G, Morfeld D, et al. Running and the development of disability with age. Ann Intern Med 1994;121:502.
38. Spector TD, Harris PA, Hart DJ, et al. Risk of osteoarthritis associated with long term weight-bearing sports. A radiologic survey of the hips and knees in female ex-athletes and population controls. Arthritis Rheum 1996;39:988.
39. Kujala UM, Kaprio J, Sarna S. Osteoarthritis of weight bearing joints of the lower limbs in former elite male athletes. BMJ 1994;308:231.
40. Buckwalter JA, Lane LE. Athletics and osteoarthritis. Am J Sports Med 1997;25:873.
41. Slemenda F, Brandt K, Heilman DK, et al. Quadriceps weakness and osteoarthritis of the knee. Ann Intern Med 1997;127:97.
42. Hurley MV, Scott DL. Improvements in quadriceps sensorimotor function and disability of patients with knee osteoarthritis following a clinically practicable exercise regime. Br J Rheumatol 1998;37:1181.
43. Neyret P, Donnell ST, Dejour H. Osteoarthritis of the knee following meniscectomy. Br J Rheumatol 1994;33:267.
44. Hadler NM, Gillings DB, Imbus HR, et al. Hand structure and function in an industrial setting. Influence of three patterns of stereotyped repetitive usage. Arthritis Rheum 1978;21: 210.
45. Coggon D, Croft P, Kellingray S, et al. Occupational physical activities and osteoarthritis of the knee. Arthritis Rheum 2000;43:1443.
46. Summers MN, Haaley WE, Reveille JD, et al. Radiologic assessment and psychosocial variables as predictors of pain and functional impairment in osteoarthritis of the knee or hip. Arthritis Rheum 1988;31:204.
47. Ike RW, O'Rourke KS. Compartment directed physical examination of the knee can predict articular cartilage abnormalities disclosed by needle arthroscopy. Arthritis Rheum 1995;38:917.
48. Garnero P, Rousseau JC, Delmas PD. Molecular basis and clinical use of biochemical markers of bone, cartilage and synovium in joint diseases. Arthritis Rheum 2000;43:953.
49. Herman JH, Hess EV. Therapeutic impasse in osteoarthritis. Br J Rheumatol 1994;33:1098.
50. Kellgren JH, Lawrence JS. Atlas of standard radiographs: the epidemiology of chronic rheumatism. Oxford, UK: Blackwell Scientific, 1963.
51. Waldschmidt JG, Braunstein EM, Buckwalter KA. Magnetic resonance imaging of osteoarthritis. Rheum Dis Clin North Am 1999;25:451.
52. McNicholas MJ, Brooksbank AJ, Walker CM. Observer agreement analysis of MRI grading of knee osteoarthritis. J R Coll Surg Edinb 1999;44:31.
53. Burstein D, Bashir A, Gray ML. MRI techniques in early stages of cartilage disease. Invest Radiol 2000;35:622.
54. McCauley TR, Disler DG. Magnetic resonance imaging of articular cartilage of the knee. J Am Acad Orthop Surg 2001;9:2.
55. Baron M, Dutil E, Berkson L, et al. Hand function in the elderly: relation to osteoarthritis. J Rheumatol 1987;14:815.
56. Kellgren JH, Moore R. Generalized osteoarthritis and Heberden's nodes. BMJ 1952;1:181.
57. Felson DT, Couropmitree NN, Chaisson CE, et al. Evidence for a Mendelian gene in a segregation analysis of generalized radiographic osteoarthritis. The Framingham study. Arthritis Rheum 1998;41:1064.
58. Pattrick M, Manhire A, Ward AM, et al. HLA-A, B antigens and alpha 1-anatitrypsin phenotypes in nodal generalized osteoarthritis and erosive osteoarthritis. Ann Rheum Dis 1989;48:470.
59. Buchanan WW, Park WM. Primary generalized osteoarthritis: definition and uniformity. J Rheumatol 1983;10[Suppl 9]:54.
60. Felson DT, Zhang Y. An update on the epidemiology of knee and hip osteoarthritis with a view to prevention. Arthritis Rheum 1998;41:1343.
61. Post WR, Fulkerson, JP. Anterior knee pain. A symptom, not a diagnosis. Bull Rheum Dis 1993;42:5.
62. Cushnagan J, McCarthy C, Dieppe P. Taping the patella medially: a new treatment for arthritis of the knee joint? BMJ 1994;308:753.
63. Kannus P, Natri T, Jarvinen M. An outcome study of chronic patellofemoral pain syndrome. Seven year follow-up of patients in a randomized controlled trial. J Bone Joint Surg Am 1999;81:355.
64. Weinstein JN. The role of neurogenic and non-neurogenic mediators as they relate to pain and the development of osteoarthritis. Spine 1992;17:S356.
65. Katz JN, Dalgus M, Stucki G, et al. Degenerative lumbar spinal stenosis: diagnostic value of the history and physical examination. Arthritis Rheum 1995;38:1236.
66. Altman R, Asch E, Black D, et al. Development of criteria for the classification and reporting of osteoarthritis of the knee. Arthritis Rheum 1986;29:1039.

67. Altman,R, Alarcon G, Applerouth D, et al. The American College of Rheumatology criteria for classification and reporting of osteoarthritis of the hip. Arthritis Rheum 1991;35:505.
68. Pelletier JP, Marcel-Pelletier J, Abramson SB. Osteoarthritis, an inflammatory disease. Potential implication for the selection of new therapeutic targets. Arthritis Rheum 2001; 44:1237.
69. Puett DW, Griffiths MR. Published trials of nonmedical and noninvasive therapies for hip and knee osteoarthritis. Ann Intern Med 1994;121:133.
70. American College of Rheumatology Subcommittee on Osteoarthritis. Recommendation for medical management of osteoarthritis of the hip and knee. Arthritis Rheum 2000; 43:1905.
71. Fries JF, Carey C, McShane DJ. Patient education in arthritis: randomized controlled trial of a mail delivered program. J Rheumatol 1997;24:1378.
72. Weinberger M. Telephone-based intervention in outpatient care. Ann Rheum Dis 1998;57:196.
73. Weinberger M. Improving functional status in arthritis: the effect of social support. Soc Sci Med 1986;23:899.
74. Cronan TA, Groessl E, Kaplan RM. The effects of social support and education interactions on health care costs. Arthritis Care Res 1997;10:99.
75. Brady TJ, Sniezek J, Conn DL. Enhancing self-management in clinical practice. Bull Rheum Dis 2000;49.
76. Lorig K, Fries JF. The arthritis help book, 5th ed. Reading, MA: Perseus Book, 2000.
77. Sasaki T, Yasuda K. Clinical evaluation of the treatment of osteoarthritic knees using a newly designed wedge insole. Clin Orthop 1987;221:181.
78. Keating EM, Faris PM, Ritter MA, et al. Use of unilateral heel and sole wedges in the treatment of medial osteoarthritis of the knee. Orthop Rev 1993;22:921.
79. Kovar PA, Allagrante JP, McKenzie CR, et al. Supervised fitness walking in patients with osteoarthritis of the knee. Ann Intern Med 1992;116:529.
80. Ettinger WH Jr, Burns R, Messier SP, et al. A randomized trial comparing aerobic exercise and resistance exercise with a health education program in older adults with osteoarthritis. The Fitness Arthritis and Seniors Trial. JAMA 1997;277: 25.
81. O'Reilly SC, Jones A, Muir KR, et al. Quadriceps weakens in knee osteoarthritis: the effect on pain and disability. Ann Rheum Dis 1998;57:588.
82. Hurley MV. The role of muscle weakness in the pathogenesis of osteoarthritis. Rheum Dis Clin North Am 1999;25:283.
83. Deyle GD, Henderson NE, Matekel RL, et al. Effectiveness of manual physical therapy and exercise in osteoarthritis of the knee. A randomized controlled trial. Ann Intern Med 2000;132:173.
84. O'Reilly SC, Muir KR, Doherty ME. Effectiveness of home exercise on pain and disability of patients with osteoarthritis of the knee. A randomized controlled trial. Ann Rheum Dis 1999;58:15.
85. Waters RL, Perry J, Conaty P, et al. The energy cost of walking with arthritis of the hip and knee. Clin Orthop 1987;214:278.
86. Deal CL, Schnitzer TJ, Lipstein E, et al. Treatment of arthritis with topical capsaicin: a double blind trial. Clin Ther 1991;13:383.
87. Schnitzer TJ, Posner M, Lawrence ID. High strength capsaicin cream for osteoarthritis pain: rapid onset of action and improved efficacy with twice daily dosing. J Clin Rheumatol 1995;1:268.
88. Ehrlich GE, DiPiero AM. Stretch gloves: nocturnal use to ameliorate morning stiffness in arthritic hands. Arch Phys Med Rehabil 1971;52:479.
89. Messier SP, Loeser RF, Mitchell MN, et al. Exercise and weight loss in obese older adults with knee osteoarthritis: a preliminary study. J Am Geriatr Soc 2000;48:1062.
90. Huang MH, Chen CH, Chen TW, et al. The effects of weight reduction on the rehabilitation of patients with knee osteoarthritis and obesity. Arthritis Care Res 2000;13:398.
91. Lane NE, Gore LR, Cummings SR, et al. Serum vitamin D levels and incident changes of radiographic hip osteoarthritis. A longitudinal study. Arthritis Rheum 1999;42:854.
92. McAlindon TE, Felson DT, Zhang Y, et al. Relation of dietary intake and serum levels of vitamin D to progression of osteoarthritis of the knee among participants in the Framingham study. Ann Intern Med 1996;125:353
93. McAlindon TE, LaValley MP, Gulin FP, et al. Glucosamine and chondroitin for treatment of osteoarthritis; a systematic quality assessment and meta-analysis. JAMA 2000;283:1469.
94. Bassleer C, Rovati L, Franchmont P. Stimulation of proteoglycan production by glucosamine sulfate in chondrocytes isolated from human osteoarthritic cartilage in vitro. Osteoarthr Cart 1998;6:427.
95. Gouze JN, Bordji K, Gulberti S, et al. Interlukin-1 beta downregulates the expression of glucuronyl transferase I, a key enzyme priming glycosaminoglycan biosynthesis. Influence of glucosamine on interlukin-1 beta mediated effects in rat chondrocytes. Arthritis Rheum 2001;44:351.
96. Shikhman AR, Kuhn K, Alaaeddine N, et al. *N*-acetylglucosamine prevents IL1-beta-mediated activation of human chondrocytes. J Immunol 2001;166:5155.
97. Reginster JY, Deroisy R, Rovati LC, et al. Long term effects of glucosamine sulfate on osteoarthritis: a randomized, placebo controlled clinical trial. Lancet 2001;357:251.
98. McAlindon T. Glucosamine for osteoarthritis: dawn of a new era? Lancet 2001;357:247.
99. Adams JG, McAlindon T, Dimasi M, et al. Contribution of meniscal extrusion and cartilage loss to joint space narrowing in osteoarthritis. Clin Radiol 1999;54:502.
100. Pincus T, Koch GG, Sokka T, et al. A randomized, double-blind, crossover clinical trial of diclofenac plus misoprostol versus acetaminophen in patients with osteoarthritis of the hip or knee. Arthritis Rheum 2001;44:1587.
100a. Felson DT. Editorial. The verdict favors nonsteroidal antiinflammatory drugs for treatment of osteoarthritis and a plea for more evidence on other treatments. Arthritis Rheum 2001;44:1477.
101. Silverstein FE, Faich G, Goldstein JL, et al. Gastrointestinal toxicity with celecoxib vs non-steroidal anti-inflammatory drugs for osteoarthritis and rheumatoid arthritis. The CLASS study: a randomized controlled trial. JAMA 2000;284:1247.
102. Bombardier C, Laine L, Raicin A, et al. Comparison of upper gastrointestinal toxicity of rofecoxib and naproxen in patients with rheumatoid arthritis. N Engl J Med 2000;343:1520.
103. Crofford LJ, Oates JC, McCune WJ, et al. Thrombosis in patients with connective tissue diseases treated with cyclooxygenase 2 inhibitors: a report of four cases. Arthritis Rheum 2000;43:1891.
104. Boers M. NSAIDs and selective COX-2 inhibitors: competition between gastroprotection and cardioprotection. Lancet 2001;357:1222.
105. Raskin JB, White RH, Jackson JE, et al. Misoprostol dosage in the prevention of nonsteroidal antiinflammatory drug-induced gastric and duodenal ulcers: a comparison of three regimens. Ann Intern Med 1995;123:344.
106. Hawkey CJ, Karrasch JA, Szezepanski L, et al. Omeprazole compared with misoprostol for ulcers associated with nonsteroidal antiinflammatory drugs. N Engl J Med 1998;338:727.
107. Yeomans ND, Tulassay Z, Jukaz L, et al. A comparison of omeprazole with ranitidine for ulcers associated with nonsteroidal antiinflammatory drugs. N Engl J Med 1998;338:719.
108. Swan SK, Rudy DW, Lassiter KC, et al. Effect of cyclooxygenase-2 inhibition on renal function in elderly persons receiving a low salt diet. A randomized controlled trial. Ann Intern Med 2000;133:1.
109. Deal CD, Moskowitz RW. Nutraceuticals as therapeutic agents in osteoarthritis. The role of glucosamine, chondroitin sulfate and collagen hydrolysate. Rheum Dis Clin North Am 1999;25:379.
110. Friedman DM, Morre ME. The efficacy of intraarticular steroids in osteoarthritis: a double blind study. J Rheumatol 1980;7:1850.
111. Young L, Katrib A, Cuello C, et al. Effects of intraarticular glucocorticoids on macrophage infiltration and mediators of

joint damage in osteoarthritis synovial membrane. Findings in a double-blind placebo controlled study. Arthritis Rheum 2001;44:343.
112. Adams ME, Atkinson MH, Lussier A, et al. The role of viscosupplementation with hylan GF-20 (Synvisc) in the treatment of osteoarthritis of the knee: a Canadian multicenter trial comparing hylan GF-20 alone, hylan GF-20 with nonsteroidal anti-inflammatory drugs (NSAIDs) and NSAIDs alone. Osteoarthr Cart 1995;3:213.
113. Altman RD, Moskowitz R, Hyalgan study group. Intraarticular sodium hyaluronate in the treatment of osteoarthritis of the knee: A randomized clinical trial. J Rheumatol 1998;25:2203.
114. Wobig M, Bach G, Beks P, et al. The role of elastoviscosity in the efficacy of viscosupplementation for osteoarthritis of the knee: a comparison of hylan GF 20 and a lower molecular weight hyaluronan. Clin Ther 1999;9:1549.
115. Brandt KD, Smith GN Jr, Simon LS. Intraarticular injection of hyaluronan as treatment for knee osteoarthritis. What is the evidence? Arthritis Rheum 2000;43:1192.
115a. Lussier A, Cividino AA, McFarlane CA, et al. Viscosupplementation with hylan for treatment of osteoarthritis: findings from clinical practice in Canada. J Rheumatol 1996;23:1579.
116. Brandt KD, Smith GN Jr, Simon LS. Response to letters to the editor regarding reference 115. Arthritis Rheum 2001;44:1473.
117. Chang RW, Falconer J, Stilberg D, et al. A randomized controlled trial of arthroscopic knee surgery versus closed needle joint lavage for patients with osteoarthritis of the knee. Arthritis Rheum 1993;36:289.
118. Ravaud P, Moulinier L, Giraudeau B, et al. Effects of joint lavage and steroid injection in patients with osteoarthritis of the knee. Results of a multicenter randomized controlled trial. Arthritis Rheum 1999;42:475.
119. Hubbard MJS. Articular debridement versus washout for degeneration of the medial femoral condyle. J Bone Joint Surg 1996;78;217.
120. Chang RW, Pellisier JM, Hazen GB. A cost effective analysis of total hip arthroplasty for osteoarthritis of the hip. JAMA 1996;275:858.
121. Dieppe P, Basler HD, Chard J, et al. Knee replacement surgery for osteoarthritis: effectiveness, practice variations, indications and possible determinants of utilization. Rheumatology 1999;38:73.
122. Buckwalter JA, Mankin HJ. Review: articular repair and transplantation. Arthritis Rheum 1998;41:1331.
123. Richmond RS, Carlson CS, Register TC, et al. Functional estrogen receptors in adult articular cartilage. Estrogen replacement therapy increases chondrocyte synthesis of proteoglycans and insulin-like growth factor binding protein 2. Arthritis Rheum 2000;43:2081.

CHAPTER 76

Crystal-Induced Arthritis

ALEXANDER S. TOWNES, MD

Gout was the first form of arthritis that was recognized to be caused by the deposition of (urate) crystals in the joints and periarticular tissues. It is now known that other crystalline substances—most commonly calcium pyrophosphate dihydrate (CPPD), hydroxyapatite, and basic calcium phosphates—also are implicated in the pathogenesis of certain kinds of arthritic disease. Although disorders associated with these various crystals differ in cause and specific characteristics, they have in common the deposition of crystals in and around joints, the propensity to episodes of acute inflammatory arthritis, and sometimes the development of a chronic destructive arthropathy. It is therefore appropriate to consider these varied clinical disorders together under the unifying concept of crystal-induced arthritis.

MECHANISMS OF CRYSTAL-INDUCED ARTHRITIS

Crystals such as monosodium urate and CPPD, when experimentally injected into joints, produce an acute inflammatory response. The mechanisms involved in this response are complex but perhaps are as well studied as any of the stimuli that produce arthritis. By the nature of their electrostatic surface characteristics and mechanical properties, crystals are capable of binding to plasma proteins including fibronectin, immunoglobulin G, C-reactive protein, and complement (1,2) as well as to cell surface receptors (3). Binding of crystals to macrophage-like synovial cells under certain conditions results in cellular activation and intracellular signal transduction (4) with release of cytokines, including tumor necrosis factor (TNF)–alpha (5), interleukin-1 (IL-1), IL-6 (6), and IL-8 (4). IL-8 production is a dominant chemotactin for the influx of neutrophils, the major inflammatory cell in the synovial fluid during an acute episode of gout or pseudogout (7,8). Neutrophils phagocytose crystals with release of IL-8, TNF-alpha (9), leukotrienes, prostaglandins, and lysosomal enzymes, further intensifying the inflammatory response. The mechanisms of crystal-induced stimulation and release of inflammatory mediators are for the most part similar with both monosodium urate (in gout) and with CPPD crystals (in pseudogout). The dissemination into the circulation of cytokines including IL-1, TNF-alpha, and IL-6 is probably responsible for the systemic effects of fever, leukocytosis, and acute phase reactants sometimes observed in acute crystal-induced arthritis (10,11).

Crystals may be identified in synovial fluid and synovial membrane in the absence of an acute inflammatory response (12,13) and can be helpful in the diagnosis between acute attacks (14). There is usually a paucity of neutrophils in this circumstance, with low levels of phagocytosis, mostly by mononuclear cells. Phagocytosis of crystals by mature monocytes has been reported to occur *in vitro* without secretion of proinflammatory cytokines and with the possible elaboration of anti-inflammatory substances (15). The events which then trigger acute inflammation are not entirely clear. A sudden increase of crystals within the joint as a result of change of temperature or pH with precipitation from the fluid phase or release from soft tissue deposits may initiate the cycle of increased phagocytosis and inflammation. In patients with gout, there is an association of acute attacks with rapid changes in serum urate concentration, as may occur with initiation of drugs that lower serum urate, or with alcohol ingestion, dietary indiscretion, or rapid weight loss. Rapid fall in serum calcium (16) and hypomagnesemia (17) may also precipitate CPPD-induced inflammation. The frequent development of acute gout or pseudogout after acute infection, trauma, surgery, or myocardial infarction suggests that the arrival of systemically generated cytokines may alter the balance within the joint toward a proinflammatory response and an acute clinical attack (18). In CPPD deposition disease, release of crystals from tissue deposits in cartilage or soft tissues may result from trauma or enzymatic digestion of matrix.

The invariable association between phagocytosis of crystals and the acute inflammatory response is important clinically, because demonstration of crystals within leukocytes from synovial fluid is a convenient method of making a definitive diagnosis in patients with acute inflammatory crystal-induced arthritis.

The acute inflammatory response in crystal-induced arthritis is self-limited. The complex mechanisms that terminate the attack are not well understood but may involve transforming growth factor (TGF)–beta and lipoproteins. TGF-beta, present in gouty effusions (19), markedly inhibited the leukocyte response in an *in vivo* model (20). Lipoproteins that coat crystal surfaces during the subsiding phase of inflammation displace immunoglobulin G (21), reduce their adherence to cell membranes, and inhibit phagocytosis and thereby may blunt or terminate the inflammatory response (21).

Although gouty arthritis and other crystal-induced diseases are usually characterized by symptoms and signs of acute inflammation, the persistence of crystals in the joint with mild chronic inflammation may contribute to chronic joint damage eventually. Sometimes a progressive destructive arthropathy occurs with little evidence of inflammation. In these patients (a few with CPPD and others with mixed CPPD, hydroxyapatite, and other basic calcium phosphate crystals), the polymorphonuclear response is for some reason markedly reduced, but extensive destruction of bone and soft tissues occurs. Release of protease and collagenase enzymes was demonstrated and was postulated to produce disruption of additional crystal deposits into the joint with continuation of the cycle of destruction (22). Others have not found collagenase (23) and have proposed other bone-resorbing agents, including prostaglandin E_2 (24).

Crystal Identification

The identification of crystals in synovial fluid or periarticular tissue is fundamental to the diagnosis and treatment of patients with crystal-induced arthritis. Crystals of monosodium urate are best identified by placing a drop of aspirated tissue fluid directly on a glass slide and examining the wet preparation through a microscope under polarized light (25). Although specialized equipment is ideal, crystals can be demonstrated adequately in the office by placing a plastic polarizing lens (e.g., made from an old pair of sunglasses) between the light source and the microscopic stage, and by placing another lens in the body or the eyepiece of the microscope. When one lens is rotated so that the field becomes dark, the negatively birefringent urate crystals (i.e., crystals capable of bending light rays in two planes—the notation of negativity is an arbitrary term used by physicists to describe the direction of bend), dimly seen in ordinary light, stand out brightly and can be identified within the cytoplasm of polymorphonuclear leukocytes. If a red plate compensator is placed between the light source and the stage of the microscope (one can be fabricated by wrapping a glass slide longitudinally with two or more layers of transparent tape) (26), the crystals are even more easily identified because the field turns red and crystals parallel to the axis of the compensator appear yellow, whereas those perpendicular to the axis appear blue. Monosodium urate crystals are usually needle or rod shaped. The size varies, but some large crystals equal to or larger than the diameter of the leukocyte are usually seen. A wet slide of joint fluid prepared in this manner may be kept for a few hours at room temperature; however, once the cells die and lyse, evaluation is less valid. If the aspirated fluid cannot be examined immediately, urate crystals may be preserved overnight by refrigeration in a plain test tube. However, CPPD crystals may dissolve within a few hours even at refrigerator temperatures (27). Methods useful for later examination include gram-stained smears (28) (Fig. 76.1C) and cytospin-stained smears (29). These methods function well for preservation of specimens for evaluation by light and polarized light microscopy, with sensitivity approximating that of wet mount preparations.

Monosodium urate crystals (which are usually present in abundance) are pathognomonic of gout (Table 76.1 and Fig. 76.1). Absence of crystals in an inflamed joint is strong evidence against the diagnosis, and in such cases, especially if leukocytosis is significant, infection or another diagnosis should be considered.

Monosodium urate is usually easily distinguished from CPPD on the basis of morphology and characteristics of the crystals under polarized light (Table 76.1 and Fig. 76.1). CPPD crystals vary much more in size and shape, from rod-like to rhomboid and irregular forms; they are usually much shorter than monosodium urate crystals, and they are never needle-like. They are usually refractile without polarized light and do not increase appreciably in brilliance when the light is polarized. They are weakly positively birefringent and change color in the opposite direction to urate when the red plate compensator is placed between the polarizing lenses (i.e., blue when parallel to the axis and yellow when perpendicular).

Because CPPD crystals are small and do not stand out in polarized light, they are overlooked more often by the occasional observer. The necessity to use ordinary light microscopy as well as polarized light has been emphasized by the observation that the majority of CPPD crystals (80% in one study) are not birefringent and could be missed if only polarized light is used (30). Use of 100× oil immersion (difficult for wet preparations) was useful in identifying small CPPD crystals in stained smears (28). Routine reports from nonspecialized clinical laboratories are often falsely negative. It is therefore important to be familiar with the expertise available and the operating characteristics of the particular laboratory called upon for crystal identification. Even with presumed knowledge of synovial fluid examination, discrepancies between laboratories in crystal identification occur (31). Appropriately prepared slides for quality control should be available (28,29,32,33). The clinician needs to alert the pathology laboratory if microcrystals are suspected in a tissue or biopsy specimen, because tissues for microscopy require alcohol fixative rather than formalin to preserve crystals of monosodium urate.

Other crystalline materials that may be seen include those from previously injected corticosteroids (which appear as crystals of varying and unusual configuration) and occasionally cholesterol crystals, which are easily distinguished from all of the others mentioned (resembling a folded envelope). Contaminating crystalline or refractile substances, such as ethylenediaminetetraacetic acid (EDTA) anticoagulant and talc, can be avoided by use of careful technique.

Table 76.1. Identification of Crystals in Synovial Fluid

Monosodium urate
Morphology
- Rod or needle shaped
- Length often approaches diameter of polymorphonuclear (PMN) leucocyte

Polarized light
- Stand out brightly when field is dark
- Strongly negative birefringent

Red plate compensator
- Yellow crystals parallel and blue crystals perpendicular to axis

Calcium pyrophosphate dihydrate
Morphology
- Rhomboid, rod, or irregular rhomboid shape
- Length variable, often smaller than one lobe of a PMN nucleus

Polarized light
- No increase in refractile appearance when field is dark
- Weakly positively birefringent (up to 80% non-birefringent and best seen with ordinary light)

Red plate compensator
- Blue crystals parallel and yellow crystals perpendicular to axis

Hydroxyapatite and basic calcium phosphates (BCP)
Not usually seen with ordinary or polarized light microscopy except as large aggregates that are not birefringent.
- Aggregates of BCP may occasionally be seen as "shiny coin" refractile bodies.

Stain nonspecifically with alizarin red S (available in histology laboratories) as clusters of crystalline material. Useful as a screening test.
Requires electron microscopy, x-ray diffraction, or microprobe analysis for more definite identification.

Calcium oxalate
Morphology
- Polymorphic, irregular squares, short rods, bipyramidal; may appear in clumps

Polarized light
- Variable, most not birefringent, some strongly positively birefringent

GOUT

Pathophysiology

Gout is a word derived from Latin meaning "a drop." It is applied to this form of arthritis because of the false belief, in ancient times, that the disease was caused by drops of bad humor. Gout is caused by an alteration in purine metabolism, the end product of which is uric acid. This alteration results in hyperuricemia and the deposition of urate crystals in various tissues. Periodic attacks of acute inflammatory arthritis, characteristic of gout, are caused by the deposition of urate crystals in and around joints. Primary gout is caused by an inborn error in the production or excretion of uric acid. Secondary gout is caused by an increased breakdown of nucleic acids in association with one of a variety of acquired diseases or by impaired excretion of urate as a consequence of acquired renal disease (Table 76.2).

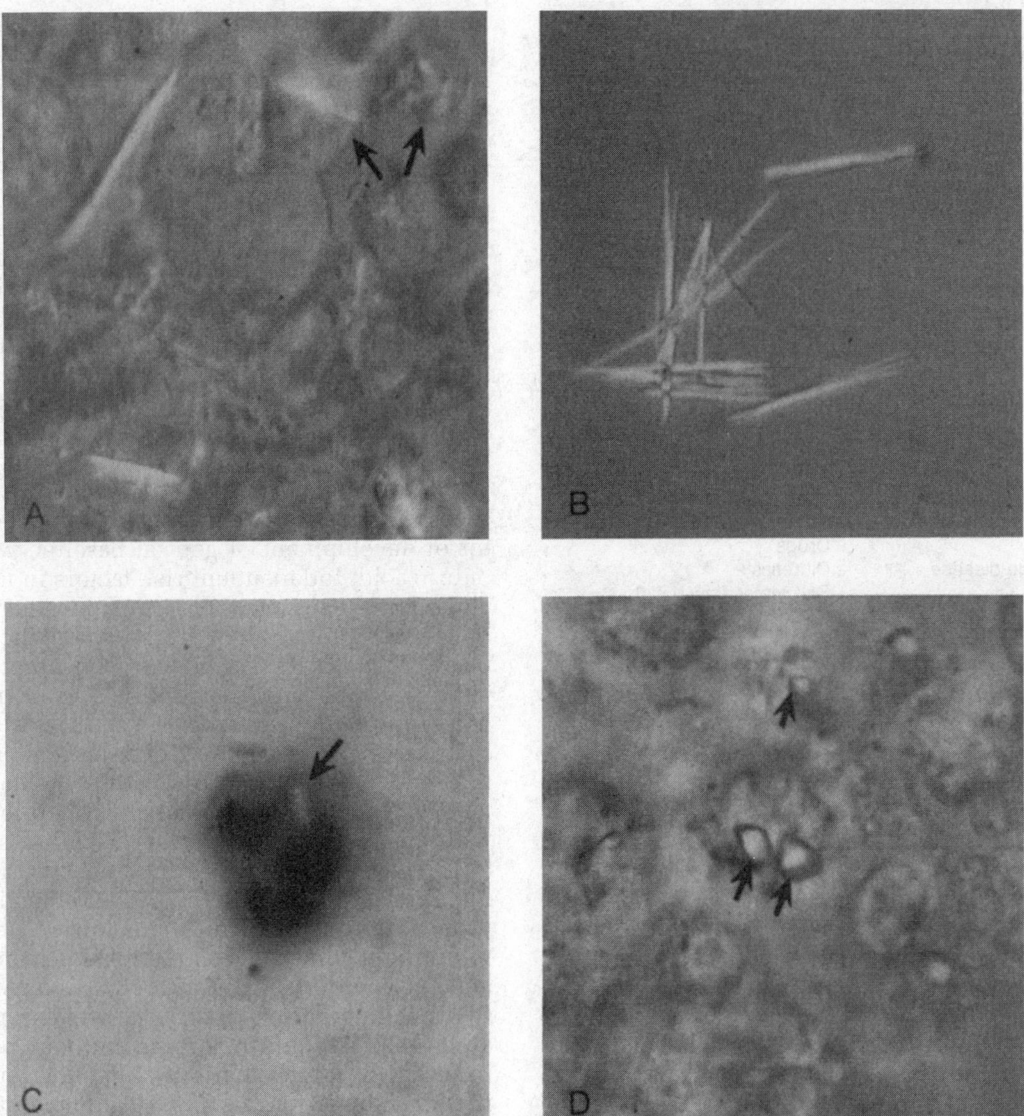

Figure 76.1. **A:** Urate crystals in synovial fluid examined by polarized light microscopy. Note the needle shape and variable size *(arrow)*, but many have larger diameter than white blood cells *(arrow)* (100 × oil immersion). **B:** Urate crystals from tophus examined by polarized light with red plate compensator (100 × oil immersion). **C:** Calcium pyrophosphate dihydrate (CPPD) crystals in white blood cell found on Gram staining (100 × oil immersion). Note the shape and size relative to nucleus and cytoplasm. **D:** Wet preparation of synovial fluid demonstrating varied size and shape of CPPD crystals phagocytized by white blood cells (100 × oil immersion lens, polarized light). Size and shape vary from squat rhomboid to rod shaped. Note several crystals in some cells.

Although there is frequently a family history of gout, few specific genetic defects responsible for hyperuricemia have been identified. In a segregation analysis of serum uric acid, the heritability factor was 0.399, supporting the hypothesis that hyperuricemia is a multifactorial trait influenced by complex hereditary and environmental factors (34). Therefore, in patients with primary gout due to overproduction of urate (only about 10% of patients), the specific cause usually is not identified. Overproduction of urate in primary gout can occur as the result of an X-linked dominant defect in hypoxanthine-guanine phosphoribosyl transferase, an important enzyme in purine metabolism, (35) or from overactivity of 5′-phosphoribosyl-pyrophosphate synthesis (36). An hereditary nephropathy with tubulointerstitial renal damage and early appearance of hyperuricemia and gout is an example of primary gout, with underexcretion of urate caused by an autosomal dominant gene (37,38). A positive family history and onset of gout before 35 years of age should suggest the possibility of a primary condition causing overproduction or underexcretion of urate. To assess production and excretion of urate, measurement in a 24-hour sample of urine may be indicated. Normal urinary uric acid excretion is less than 600 mg/day if the diet for 5 days has been free of foods rich in purines. Because this diet is impractical for most patients, a reasonable estimate can be made on a regular diet. Urinary excretion exceeding 1,000 mg/day is clearly abnormal, and 800 to 1,000 mg/day is borderline (39). An alternative method to screen for increased urate excretion on a regular diet is to measure urate and creatinine in serum and in

Table 76.2. Causes of Hyperuricemia

With Increased Urinary Urate	With Normal or Low Urinary Urate
10% of primary gout (defects usually unknown)	90% of primary gout (defects usually unknown)
	Familial juvenille hyperuricemic nephropathy
Specific enzyme defects	
HGPRTase deficiency, partial	
PP-Ribose-P synthetase variants	
Secondary causes	Secondary causes
Myeloproliferative disease	Decreased Renal function
	Inhibition of tubular urate excretion (competetive anions)
	Enhanced tubular urate absorption (fasting, dehydration)
	Insulin resistance
	Ethanol abuse
	Hypoxemia and tissue underperfusion
Lymphoproliferative disease	Lead nephropathy
Hemolytic diseases	
	Drugs
Glycogen storage disease	Diuretics
Psoriasis	Salicylates (low dose)
	Cyclosporine
Severe muscle exertion	
	Pyrazinamide
	Ethambutol
	Nicotinic acid
	Didanosine
	Others
	Obesity
	Hyperparathyroidism
	Sarcoidosis

Modified from Primer on the Rheumatic Diseases, Edition 11, copyright 1997, the Arthritis Foundation.

midmorning urine, calculating the urate excretion normalized to a glomerular filtration rate of 100 mL/minute (40). This may be calculated simply by using the formula, (Uu × Sc) ÷ Uc, where Uu (urine urate) is in mg/minute, Sc (serum creatinine) is in mg/minute, and Uc (urine creatinine) is in dl/minute (40). A value greater than 0.7 mg/dL is defined as overexcretion. Because overproduction related to a genetic defect is an uncommon cause of primary gout, the measurement of urinary urate is unnecessary for the management of most cases of gout unless a secondary cause of hyperuricemia is suspected or uric acid stones have developed.

Normal levels of serum urate vary widely in the population, with a range of 3 to 8 mg/dL; also, there may be spontaneous variation within an individual patient. The upper limit of normal for serum urate measured by the uricase method usually is considered to be 7.0 mg/dL for adult men and 6.0 mg/dL for adult women. Ranges may be higher by 1 mg/dL or more if automated colorimetric methods are used.

Epidemiology

Gout is estimated to occur at a lifetime frequency of 3 cases per 1,000 population in the United States. The prevalence of gout in the United States has been estimated to be 8.4 per 1,000 persons of all ages and both sexes, corresponding to a total of 2.1 million persons (1.5 million men and 550,000 women) (41). Because this figure is based on self-reported data, it is likely to be somewhat of an overestimate. A study in England suggested an increase in prevalence to perhaps 10 per 1,000 people (42). Obesity and excessive weight gain were important risk factors for the development of gout in a prospective study of white men (43). The incidence of gout in African American men was significantly higher than in white men, and gout was associated with systolic blood pressure at baseline and subsequent development of hypertension (44). Gout in all of its forms is ten times more common in men, and it is rare in premenopausal women. Gout is rare before 30 years of age and increases in frequency to a plateau at about age 60 years. Age at onset is probably related to the duration and severity of preceding hyperuricemia. In a prospective study of 223 men in Taiwan with asymptomatic hyperuricemia, the 5-year cumulative incidence of gout was 19% (45). The only predictor of development of gout at baseline was the level of uric acid. Independent risk factors in follow-up included further increase of serum urate, persistent alcohol consumption, use of diuretics, and increased body mass index. Excessive alcohol consumption was the most important independent risk factor in this group of hyperuricemic men (45).

Hyperuricemia due to decreased renal clearance of uric acid (46) is a constant feature of a complex cluster of metabolic and clinical abnormalities associated with insulin resistance, the so called syndrome X (47). These abnormalities include hyperinsulinemia, impaired glucose tolerance, dyslipidemia with elevated fasting triglycerides and lowered high-density lipoprotein cholesterol, hypertension, central obesity, and coronary artery disease (48). As a result of longstanding hyperuricemia, gout is often seen in middle-aged men with this syndrome and may be one of the initial clinical presentations (49). Management of gout in such patients may be difficult and requires attention to the other features of the syndrome. Although the etiology involves both genetic and environmental factors, increased visceral fat accumulation (43,50) and alcohol consumption (45,51) are risk factors that contribute to the abnormalities observed and to the development of clinical gout.

Use of thiazide diuretics is a risk factor for gout (52) and complicates the observed association of gout with hypertension. Diuretic use is often a factor in the occurrence of gout in elderly women (53). Gout is often a complication in patients who have undergone renal or cardiac transplantation, in part because of the hyperuricemic effect of cyclosporine (54). In a study of 225 patients after cardiac transplantation, 23 patients developed acute gout, complicating therapy, within 50 months of follow-up (55). A possible relationship of gout to hypothyroidism, especially in women, has also been reported (56).

Clinical Features

Acute Arthritic Attack

The acute arthritic attack is the hallmark of gout (Table 76.3). It is characterized by pain, swelling, and

Table 76.3. Clinical Features of Gout

Epidemiology
Sex: Males 10 to 1; rare in premenopausal women
Age: Usually middle age or older (peak age, 60 yr)

Acute Gout
History
- Acute attacks, recurrent, with disease-free intervals
- Rapid progression to peak severity within 24 h

Physical findings
- Usually monoarticular with swelling, tenderness, erythema, and intense inflammation
- Big toe metatarsophalangeal joint commonly involved (podagra)
- Forefeet, heels, ankles, knees, wrists, fingers, elbows, and other joints may be affected
- Occasionally polyarticular
- Fever may occur

Laboratory
- Joint aspiration where possible (see text) with leukocytosis and identification of urate crystals is diagnostic

Intercritical Gout
No symptoms or findings except hyperuricemia and crystals in synovial fluid from previously involved joints

Chronic Gout
Often polyarticular
Symptoms may persist between attacks
Tophi are common (approximately 90%–95%)
Joint damage and deformities may develop

discomfort that progress rapidly to a peak level of intensity within 24 to 36 hours after onset. The pain is often severe enough to prevent use of the affected joint or even for the patient to bear the weight of bed clothing. The metatarsophalangeal joint of the great toe is the most commonly affected joint, followed by the forefoot, heel, ankle, knee, wrist, fingers, and elbow. The great toe is affected at some time during the course of perhaps 90% of gouty subjects. Usually a single joint is involved early in the course of the disease, but pauciarticular arthritis (two or three joints) may occur; polyarticular (more than three joints) onset is rare. Polyarticular gout is more common in late disease associated with soft tissue tophi. Recurrent acute arthritis is more common in previously affected joints.

Several events may trigger an acute attack of gout: trauma, an acute illness such as an acute myocardial infarction, dietary indiscretion, overuse of alcohol, fasting, and recent administration of drugs that lower the serum urate concentration (see Pathophysiology).

A family history of gout may be present in patients with primary gout, and especially in patients who excrete excessive amounts of uric acid, in whom a specific enzyme defect may be suspected. However, a positive family history is obtained in fewer than half of gouty subjects, so a negative history is of no differential diagnostic value.

On physical examination of the patient with acute gouty arthritis, there is often erythema overlying or adjacent to the affected joints, especially when small joints are involved. The erythema often involves only a localized area rather than the entire joint. The intensity of the inflammatory reaction often results in a mistaken diagnosis of cellulitis, a diagnosis that may appear to be supported by a fever that may reach 101°F (38°C), although temperature in this range or higher is uncommon in acute gout. Joint swelling usually is marked, and joint effusion is also common. Tenderness on palpation or motion of the affected part usually is marked.

The intensity and severity of these classic acute signs and symptoms may vary from one attack to another. Early in the disease, milder episodes lasting only a few days may be passed off by the patient as being caused by minor trauma. The outward evidence of inflammation also may be less evident when a large joint such as the knee is involved, especially in elderly patients and in patients with polyarticular gout. However, the history almost always indicates rapid progression to a peak intensity within 24 to 36 hours, an important feature in differential diagnosis. A history of episodes of similar events is also helpful.

Laboratory findings may include a mild leukocytosis and an elevated erythrocyte sedimentation rate. Serum uric acid almost always is elevated, but this finding is of limited diagnostic value because of the frequency of hyperuricemia in the absence of gout and because the acute attack, which is related principally to the concentration of tissue urate, may occur at a time when the serum urate is normal as a result of previous drug administration or spontaneous variation. Examination of the synovial fluid provides diagnostic findings in almost all instances in which it can be obtained. There is a leukocytosis in the joint fluid with polymorphonuclear leukocytes that, when examined under polarized light, can be seen to contain phagocytized urate crystals (see Crystal Identification). The technique of aspiration of joint fluid is described in Chapter 74. One should be experienced in this technique before attempting it or the patient should be referred to a rheumatologist. The first metatarsophalangeal joint is a particularly painful joint to tap, especially during an acute attack, and this is not recommended without considerable experience. A dorsal approach with the toe in maximally tolerated plantar flexion is usually recommended.

The acute attack is self-limited, and even without treatment it subsides in several days to weeks. Early in the disease, once the acute attack subsides or is treated, there are no residual joint symptoms—another important point in the differential diagnosis.

Recurrent acute attacks are usual: Approximately 75% of patients have a second gouty attack within 2 years after their first, in most cases within the first year; occasionally, 10 years or longer may elapse between attacks (57).

Intercritical Gout

Between acute attacks of gout, patients are totally asymptomatic, with no abnormal physical findings unless tophi are present or unless the disease has progressed to the chronic phase. If the patient's first visit is at this stage, a presumptive diagnosis can be made on the basis of a history of a typical attack, especially if there have been multiple attacks, and hyperuricemia (58). Aspiration of the great toe during intercritical gout demonstrates urate crystals in about 70% of patients with gout, but crystals rarely may be found in patients with asymptomatic hyperuricemia or renal failure (13,59,60). Knee joint aspiration has also yielded urate crystals in patients with intercritical nontophaceous gout. In a study of 101 asymptomatic joints that had previously been inflamed, samples were obtained from 90 (90%) of attempts (91% knees, 86 % metatarsophalangeal joints). Crystals were found in all joints of patients who were not receiving urate-lowering therapy and in 53% of the patients receiving therapy, although 27% of those patients still had an elevated serum urate concentration (14). Therefore, in the patient who has a prior history of acute gout, especially within the past year, and who is not receiving urate-lowering therapy, aspiration of the affected joint where possible and synovial fluid analysis for crystals is a reasonably sensitive and highly specific test for the diagnosis of intercritical gout.

Chronic Gout

Chronic gout is uncommon, especially since the advent of effective therapy to control hyperuricemia. Patients with chronic gout often have some persistent symptoms (e.g., morning stiffness) and manifest signs of synovial tissue thickening and some joint deformity. Acute exacerbations are still common and are often polyarticular. Tophi (soft tissue deposits of sodium urate) are present in 90% to 95% of patients with chronic gout. The rate of formation of tophi seems to be a direct function of the level and duration of hyperuricemia. Tophi are chalky or pinkish, gritty, usually superficial deposits that are palpable in joints or over tendons, in pressure points, or in the pinnae of the ears. Tophi in fingerpads were found in 30% of a small group of patients with tophaceous gout attending hospital outpatient clinics (61). They are usually painless, but after palpation they may be tender. Large tophi may look like bulbous swellings of the joints or, when they are located over the extensor surface of the forearm or in the ulnar bursa, they may be mistaken for rheumatoid nodules. The distribution of tophi may be different in women, with elbows and feet less common sites than in men (62). The coincident occurrence of proven gout in distal interphalangeal joints associated with nodal osteoarthritis, especially in elderly patients receiving diuretic therapy for hypertension, has been reported (53,63). In patients with chronic gout who have radiographic changes of bone erosion, deformity of the fingers, and ulnar bursal nodules due to tophi, rheumatoid arthritis may also be suspected (64). In these patients, aspiration of joints or biopsy of tophi (65) with demonstration of urate crystals confirms the diagnosis of gout. The actual occurrence of gout and rheumatoid arthritis in the same patient is extremely rare (66).

Extra-articular Manifestations

It has long been known that gout may be associated with renal disease in three forms: Chronic urate nephropathy, nephrolithiasis, and acute uric acid nephropathy.

Chronic urate nephropathy develops after many years of hyperuricemia and results from the deposition in the interstitial medullary tissue of sodium urate crystals that cause, ultimately, an interstitial nephritis. In patients with asymptomatic hyperuricemia regardless of the level, the risk of developing nephropathy does not warrant treatment to lower the serum urate as a prophylactic measure. At one time, the frequency of the complication of chronic urate nephropathy in gouty subjects was assumed to be high. However, controlled studies indicate that the incidence of renal insufficiency caused solely by gout and hyperuricemia is low and renal dysfunction is usually mild; most often, renal failure in patients with gout can be attributed to other causes, such as vascular disease or primary renal disease (67). Renal insufficiency from primary gout and hyperuricemia is usually silent and suspected only because of the identification of a mild abnormality of the blood urea nitrogen or serum creatinine concentration. Some patients have slight proteinuria; only a few are found to have peripheral tophi. The evaluation and management of patients with renal failure are discussed in Chapter 52.

Uric acid nephrolithiasis accounts for only a small number of patients who have urinary calculi (see Chapter 51). However, approximately 20% of patients with gout develop calculi, although the stones may antedate acute gouty arthritis by years. From a different perspective, approximately 25% of patients with uric acid calculi have an abnormal serum urate concentration. The prevalence of uric acid calculi increases proportionately to the concentration of serum urate or the excretion of uric acid, whether or not gout is present. In one study, in which a cohort of men was followed for 12 years, serum levels of urate of 7 to 8, 8 to 9, and more than 9 mg/dL were associated with renal stones in 12.7%, 22%, and 40% of subjects, respectively (68). In gouty patients, urinary excretion rates of less than 300, 301 to 700, 701 to 1,100, and more than 1,100 mg uric acid per 24 hours were associated with an incidence of renal stones of 11%, 21%, 35%, and 50%, respectively (69). The development of uric acid calculi is related not only to uric acid excretion but also to urinary pH and concentration. An effective scheme for ambulatory evaluation of nephrolithiasis is presented in detail in Chapter 51 (70).

Acute uric acid nephropathy is associated with a sudden increase in urate production and a marked rise in uric acid excretion, which results in the formation of microcrystals in the renal tubules. This most often occurs in patients with lymphoproliferative or myeloproliferative disorders, especially during treatment. It occasionally is a complication of vigorous administration of potent uricosuric drugs such as Anturane. Preventive measures to lower urate production are effective, and acute uric acid nephropathy is rarely encountered in ambulatory practice.

Differential Diagnosis

During the acute attack, gout must be differentiated principally from acute infectious arthritis, bursitis related to a bunion (see Chapter 73), and other forms of crystal-induced arthritis. Therefore, it is important to aspirate joint fluid for smear and culture (see Chapter 74) as well as for crystal identification. If inexperienced in the aspiration technique of the joint in question, one should refer the patient to a rheumatologist. Infectious arthritis is associated with a very low synovial fluid glucose concentration, not found in gouty fluids. Rarely, acute gout and infectious arthritis coexist. Fever greater than 101°F (38°C) or lack of prompt defeverescence in response to anti-inflammatory drugs should raise suspicion of infection or an alternative diagnosis.

Radiographic Studies

In the early course of gout, radiographs are normal except for acute soft tissue swelling. As the disease progresses, lucent areas of urate deposits may be seen in bone adjacent to the joints (Fig. 76.2). These lesions may be mistaken for the erosions that are seen in rheumatoid or other arthritides, but osteoporosis and bony sclerosis, which are common in other erosive diseases, are not present. Overhanging margins of bone are said to be characteristic of gouty erosions but are not often found. Therefore, only occasionally are radiographic studies indicated as an aid to diagnosis or differential diagnosis of patients with suspected gout. Tophi appearing as capsular or intra-articular opaque masses were identified on computed tomographic scans of the knee in 5 of 16 patients with advanced crystal-proven gout, sometimes in the absence of subcutaneous tophi (71).

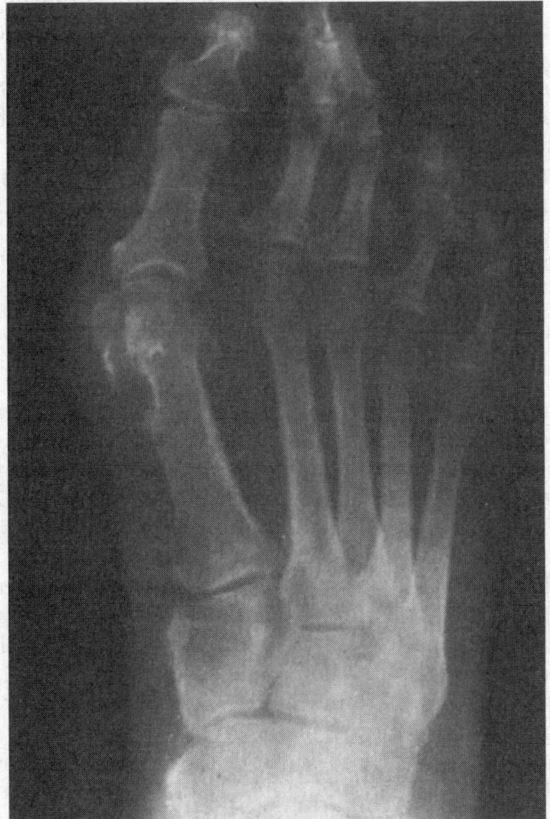

Figure 76.2. Radiograph of the foot in a patient with gout, showing soft tissue swelling over the first metatarsophalangeal joint and typical gouty erosion: away from joint margin, punched out with overhanging edge, and no osteoporosis.

Management

If the diagnosis of gout can be established with certainty by the demonstration of urate crystals, the treatment is generally straightforward. Unless there is a complicating illness, hospitalization is not required. Even the most severe case can be effectively managed on an ambulatory basis. The key elements in management are control of the pain of the acute attack and patient education. Patient education ensures compliance with therapy administered to reduce the serum urate concentration, which will prevent recurrent attacks and progression to chronic tophaceous gout. Lack of understanding of the disease and lack of compliance with therapy are major deterrents to effective management. Adapting an analogy of crystals to matches, as described by Wortman (72), is a useful way to explain to patients how drugs are used in treatment: early use of anti-inflammatory drugs, or occasionally colchicine, to "put out the fire" of an acute attack; colchicine prophylaxis between attacks to keep the "matches wet"; and urate-lowering drugs to "get rid of the matches." There are few randomized controlled trials in the Cochrane Collection addressing specific therapies in the treatment of gout (73). Empiric therapy as addressed here is based on available literature and experience and is effective for most cases of gout.

Management of the Acute Attack

If the diagnosis of acute gout is established or if gout has been diagnosed previously by the identification of urate crystals in the affected joints, rapid relief can be obtained in almost all cases by the administration of nonsteroidal anti-inflammatory drugs (NSAIDs) in appropriate dosages. The best studied NSAD in acute gout is indomethacin. Indomethacin (Indocin) 50 mg (two 25-mg capsules) every 6 hours for six to eight doses is dramatically effective in reducing pain, often within a few hours. In the absence of moderate to severe compromise of renal function, there are few side effects if the dosage is quickly reduced to 25 mg every 6 to 8 hours after the pain and inflammation begin to wane and maintained at that level until the attack is completely resolved, usually no more than 5 to 7 days. Alternatively, other NSAIDs, including cyclooxygenase 2 (COX-2)–specific inhibitors, may be used (see Chapter 77) and are apparently equally effective if comparable doses are used, although few comparative studies are available. The plasma concentration and therapeutic effect of indomethacin (and of naproxen, but apparently not of other NSAIDs) are potentiated by an unknown mechanism by the simultaneous administration of probenecid (see later discussion). Although the clinical significance of this interaction is unclear, especially with short-course therapy, the manufacturer recommends that the dosage of the NSAID be reduced in patients who also are taking probenecid. Caution should also be used in patients with impaired renal function or reduced renal blood flow caused by cardiovascular disease, because NSAIDs may acutely reduce renal function and precipitate acute renal failure or hyperkalemia. This is especially important in frail elderly patients with low muscle mass, in whom the degree of renal impairment may not be immediately evident from the level of serum creatinine.

Colchicine is the time-honored drug for treatment of acute gout, but its efficacy is limited by side effects that are almost invariable if an adequate dosage is administered orally. The usual regimen is 0.6 mg every 1 to 2 hours for up to a maximum of 10 doses in 12 hours, until relief is obtained or until side effects, usually diarrhea, nausea, or vomiting, develop. The total dosage should be reduced in patients with impaired renal or hepatic function. Currently, however, it is no longer necessary to subject a patient to severe diarrhea when he or she already has a very painful joint, so oral colchicine has largely been replaced by other agents that are as effective and have fewer side effects. The exception is in the well-instructed patient who, immediately after recognizing the onset of an acute attack of gout, can institute oral colchicine and in doing so can abort the attack with a few doses and minimal side effects.

Intravenous administration of colchicine rapidly provides a therapeutic plasma level of the drug and does not cause gastrointestinal side effects. It is useful in the treatment of acute gout when the patient cannot take medication by mouth, has peptic ulcer disease, or has another contraindication to the use of nonsteroidal agents or corticosteroids. Although generally this is a treatment restricted to inpatient hospital use, it conceivably could be used in an office or outpatient setting. Two milligrams of colchicine (available in ampules containing 1 mg in 2 mL) diluted with isotonic saline to 20 mL and given over 10 minutes intravenously usually provides relief within 6 to 8 hours and, if necessary, may be followed by one or two doses of 1 mg in 20 mL isotonic saline intravenously in 12 to 24 hours, not to exceed 4 mg in 24 hours. Reduced dosage is imperative in patients with impaired renal or hepatic function, in frail elderly patients with apparently normal renal function, and in patients with neutropenia. Care must be used to prevent extravasation of colchicine into the soft tissues, because it can cause necrosis. Intravenous colchicine should not be used if the patient has recently received a course of oral colchicine or if there is combined renal and hepatic disease, creatinine clearance less than 10 mL/ minute, or extrahepatic biliary obstruction. No additional colchicine should be given by any route for 7 days after a full intravenous dose. Because of the potentially serious toxicity of intravenous colchicine (74,75), its rare indication, and lack of knowledge by practitioners about its use and limitations, some medical centers have proscribed its use.

Production of a therapeutic response to oral colchicine of a typical attack of gout in the great toe has often been advocated to make a presumptive diagnosis of gout in the absence of crystal identification. Such a trial has limited value, however, because acute gout of several days' duration may not respond rapidly to colchicine and because pseudogout caused by CPPD-induced arthritis or occasionally by other forms of arthritis may affect this joint and respond.

Because the patient or the inexperienced clinician may be wary of attempting aspiration of the first metatarsophalangeal joint when it is exquisitely painful with acute inflammation, a presumptive diagnosis of gout is often made on clinical grounds and the patient is treated with nonsteroidal or other agents. A raised serum uric acid would further support the diagnosis of gout, but is neither specific nor always present. A strong suspicion of infection would mandate a diagnostic aspiration.

Corticosteroids provide another therapeutic alternative for acute gout in the patient who has a contraindication to therapy with NSAIDs (76). Aspiration and intra-articular injection of corticosteroid suspension (e.g., 40 mg of triamcinolone in the knee joint), is useful when a single large joint is involved. For patients requiring parenteral therapy, intramuscular or intravenous injections of adrenocorticotrophic hormone (ACTH) or soluble corticosteroid preparation is effective. Intramuscular ACTH, 40 to 80 units every 6 to 12 hours for up to 3 days; intravenous methylprednisolone, 100 to 150 mg repeated as needed; and triamcinolone acetonide, 60 mg intramuscularly per day for 2 to 3 days, are equally effective (77). Moderately high initial dosages of oral corticosteroids (30 to 60 mg/day of prednisone tapered slowly over 7 to 10 days) usually are required for complete resolution without recrudescence (77).

Drugs administered to lower serum urate have no place in the treatment of the acute gouty attack. In fact, these agents may exacerbate acute attacks by the associated changes in plasma urate concentration (see earlier discussion).

Intercritical Gout

The efficacy of colchicine in dosages of 0.6 mg given one, two, or rarely three times daily (dosage frequency depends on control; most patients tolerate two doses a day without side effects) in reducing the frequency of acute attacks of gout has been well established (57,78). Therefore, prophylactic colchicine is indicated for patients who have had more than one episode of acute gout in a single year or when therapy to lower urate is initiated (see later discussion). Caution again is required in patients with impaired renal function. Reversible myopathy and neuropathy have been observed in some patients whose serum creatinine was higher than 1.6 mg/dL even with two tablets per day (79). In elderly patients without tophi (nontophaceous gout), with infrequent acute attacks, and only mild hyperuricemia (i.e., less than 8 mg/dL), prophylactic colchicine may be all that is required. Some patients who have nontophaceous gout with infrequent attacks of arthritis (e.g., fewer than one or two a year) and mild hyperuricemia (less than 8 mg/dL) may elect not to take regular colchicine prophylaxis; in this instance, the episodic use of an NSAID such as indomethacin (Indocin, discussed earlier) is appropriate to control acute attacks. However, in most patients with gout and with persistent hyperuricemia of 8 mg/dL or higher, the serum urate concentration should be reduced to prevent recurrent gout and to reverse the accumulation of urate in the tissues. In this instance, colchicine prophylaxis should be continued until the patient has been free of attacks for at least 1 year after return of the concentration of serum urate to normal. As an alternative in patients intolerant of colchicine, NSAIDs can be used for prophylaxis, but they may have more serious toxic effects than colchicine. Omitting prophylactic therapy and treating acute attacks early if they occur is an alternative for some patients with infrequent attacks.

Two classes of drugs that lower serum urate concentration are available: *Uricosuric agents* promote urinary excretion of urate by blocking tubular urate resorption, and *allopurinol* (Zyloprim) decreases production of urate through inhibition of purine metabolism. Indications for the use of allopurinol are a history of urinary calculi or the presence of mild to moderate renal dysfunction, chronic tophaceous gout, or excessive basal urinary uric acid excretion (i.e., more than 750 mg/24 hours), or of high levels of serum urate associated with secondary gout. Uricosuric agents are most effective in patients with nontophaceous gout who have good renal function (creatinine clearance of at least 60 to 80 mL/minute) and normal uric acid excretion (less than 750 mg/24 hours). The terms *uric acid* and *urate* are sometimes used interchangeably, but the correct terminology uses uric acid where it is the dominant moiety in the uric acid—urate equilibrium. Uric acid is dominant only in very acid situations, such as the distal renal tubule. In blood and the usual tissue pH, the dominant moiety is urate. In most patients, clinical evidence identifying one of the causes of impaired urinary excretion rather than overproduction of urate (Table 76.2) is obvious. When there is uncertainty, evaluation of urinary uric acid excretion is important not only as a clue to the mechanism of hyperuricemia (Table 76.2) but in the choice of therapy.

Probenecid (Benemid) is the uricosuric agent of choice because of its well-established safety and its long duration of effect. An initial dosage of 0.5 g twice daily should be increased to 1.5 g daily or to a maximum of 2 g/day (in two or three divided doses) to achieve a serum urate concentration consistently lower than 6.5 mg/dL, the level required to produce a urate gradient from tissue to plasma and to prevent further deposition of urate. To minimize the chance of precipitating a recurrent arthritic attack, the uricosuric agent should not be initiated until at least 1 week after an acute attack of gout has subsided and only after colchicine prophylaxis (described earlier) has been initiated for 3 or 4 days. The principal side effect of probenecid is gastrointestinal distress (which is uncommon), but there is a risk of formation of uric acid calculi in the renal tubules during the first week of therapy, especially when there is a large basal uric acid excretion (i.e., 600 to 800 mg/day); this risk can be minimized by starting at a dose of 250 mg twice daily and gradually increasing the dose over 2–3 weeks. The patient may also be advised to drink 2 to 3 L of fluid daily and takes an alkalinizing agent such as sodium bicarbonate or citrate salt (polycitrate), 0.5 to 1 mEq/kg of body weight in five or six doses a day, to keep the urine pH (measured from time to time with pH paper) higher than 6.0 or 6.5 for the first few weeks of uricosuric therapy. Small dosages of aspirin (2.4 g/day), but not a single low-dose enteric tablet as used for cardiac prophylaxis (80), block the effect of probenecid on renal excretion of urate and should be avoided. Probenecid may reduce the excretion of other drugs, including NSAIDs and penicillin, and prolong their half-life. Probenecid may also cause a false positive test for glucose in the urine.

Sulfinpyrazone (Anturane) is a more potent uricosuric agent but has more potential for adverse effects, including renal toxicity and nephrolithiasis. It can be given beginning with 50 mg twice daily and increased gradually to 600 mg/day, if required, to achieve the desired serum urate level (i.e., less than 6 mg/dL). Sulfinpyrazone is available in 100 and 200 mg strengths. This agent, which is an analog of phenylbutazone, can cause gastric ulceration and platelet dysfunction. It can also interact with sulfonamides or sulfonylureas to increase their hypoglycemic effect. For these reasons, it should be used principally when probenecid or allopurinol is not tolerated.

Allopurinol (Zyloprim) is a potent agent that reduces the concentration of serum urate. Because it blocks urate production by inhibition of xanthine oxidase, it is particularly useful in patients with renal dysfunction or with uric acid calculi and in patients with longstanding gout with tophi. Serious side effects of rash, fever, leukopenia, hepatitis, and occasionally a generalized vasculitis occur in fewer than 2% of patients. These symptoms are most likely to occur within the first 2 months after initiation of therapy, so patients should be kept under close surveillance during this period. Toxicity is enhanced in patients with severe renal compromise or when the drug is administered concomitantly with ampicillin or thiazide diuretics (81). Allopurinol (Zyloprim, available in 100- and 300-mg tablets) should be started at a dosage of 200 mg/day and increased over 2 or 3 weeks until the serum urate concentration is consistently lower than 6.0 mg/dL; no more than 300 mg should be administered as a single dose. Prolonged use of dosages in excess of 300 mg twice a day increases the risk of toxicity; however, dosages of 400 to 600 mg/day may be required initially for effective control of serum urate and reduction of the tissue urate load. Careful monitoring of the dose in patients with renal insufficiency is mandatory (81). In patients with renal insufficiency and in those who have undergone renal or cardiac transplantation and are receiving cyclosporine, adverse drug reactions are common with allopurinol as well as with colchicine and NSAIDs (55).

Concomitant use of allopurinol and probenecid has been advocated for patients with chronic tophaceous gout. These agents seem to have an additive effect in lowering the serum uric acid concentration. However, use of a single agent, if possible, is preferred.

Compliance is the major factor in the effective treatment of intercritical gout. Patients feel well between attacks, and continued compliance with medications requires reinforcement in patient education and follow-up visits to ensure maintenance of normal serum levels of urate (72). The duration of treatment to lower serum urate is uncertain and depends significantly on the severity of the disease, the presence or absence of tophi, the frequency of acute attacks, and compliance with drug dosage. In one study, patients who were able to achieve a serum level of 6 mg/dL or less had a reduction in gout attacks and in the finding of crystals on knee joint aspiration, compared with patients whose serum urate concentration was higher (82). Continued treatment with drugs to lower serum urate was estimated to be cost-saving if the patient had two attacks per year and cost-effective if one attack per year occurred (83).

Dietary advice to patients with gout should be kept simple. High-purine foods (organ meats, seafood, all meats, meat gravies and extracts, lentils, peas, asparagus, yeast, and beer) are common in Western diets, and strict avoidance is neither practical nor necessary in the treatment of most patients with gout. Patients should be aware of these high-purine foods and avoid excesses of intake. More important dietary advice is to avoid alcohol (beer especially, because it also adds to the purine load) and to avoid fasting beyond 24 hours, because both these situations may be associated with an acute increase in the serum urate concentration, which may precipitate an attack of gout. Obese patients should have calorie reduction for weight loss, but a severe restriction may precipitate acute attacks. In a pilot study of patients with gout associated with elevated serum triglycerides and obesity, weight loss with moderate calorie and carbohydrate restriction and a proportionate increase of unsaturated fat and protein intake resulted in an improved lipid profile, a reduction of serum urate, and a decrease in acute attacks of gout (84). Possibly helpful as a nonpharmacologic management strategy, this diet, which addresses both the complicating factor of dyslipidemia and hyperuricemia, deserves further study with a larger number of patients.

Chronic Gout

Compliance with appropriate therapy should eliminate this phase of gout except in a few patients with severe disease who are intolerant of one or more drugs used in treatment. Continuous or intermittent use of NSAIDs may be required in some of these patients for adequate control of inflammation and chronic symptoms. Effective reduction in serum urate for months or years results in dissolution of tophi and general improvement. However, very large tophi may require surgical removal. After prolonged therapy and resolution of tophi, consideration has been given to discontinuation of therapy with urate-lowering drugs. However, acute attacks and tophi are likely to recur (85), so stopping therapy is generally not recommended.

Patients with chronic tophaceous gout and moderate renal insufficiency present a difficult problem in management. Uricosuric drugs usually are not effective, with the possible exception of benzbromarone (86), which is not available in the United States. NSAIDs, including the new COX-2–specific drugs, may further impair renal function. Withdrawal of NSAIDs produced a significant improvement in renal function in patients, with an average creatinine clearance of 60 mL/minute after control of hyperuricemia was achieved (87). The incidence of adverse reactions to colchicine and allopurinol is increased in patients with renal disease, requiring lower doses and careful monitoring (81). For patients with tophaceous and polyarticular gout whose renal function makes uricosuric drugs ineffective, there are few alternative agents to lower uric acid when a cutaneous reaction to allopurinol requires withdrawal of this therapy. Success was reported in desensitizing some patients by administering small, gradually increasing doses of allopurinol on a careful protocol beginning with 50 μg/day. A follow-up study indicated successful continuation of allopurinol and control of hyperuricemia in 78% of patients. Some developed a pruritic skin eruption that responded to withdrawal of allopurinol and dosage adjustment (88). It is important to note that patients with severe reactions, such as toxic epidermal necrolysis, hepatitis, or acute interstitial nephritis, were excluded from this study.

Asymptomatic Hyperuricemia

Hyperuricemia (more than 7 mg/dL in men or 6 mg/dL in women) is a common laboratory finding in asymptomatic patients evaluated in a variety of clinical settings. In most patients, clinical findings point to an obvious cause and no other therapy is required unless gout or nephrolithiasis develops. If the cause is unclear or the level of serum urate is near 11 mg/dL, further evaluation to estimate urinary excretion and identify secondary causes of excessive urate production (Table 76.2) should be initiated. Although serum urate is often markedly elevated in patients with end-stage renal disease, clinical gout is rare. Monocytes from these patients were found to be significantly suppressed in their ability to secrete proinflammatory cytokines after stimulation with monosodium urate crystals (89). This may be a factor in the low incidence of acute gout in these patients.

Hyperuricemia Secondary to Diuretics

The renal tubular handling of urate is complex: Complete glomerular filtration is followed by tubular resorption, tubular secretion, and further tubular resorption. The resorption of urate is in part modulated by the volume of extracellular fluid (expansion increases excretion and contraction decreases excretion). Diuretics modify the renal handling of urate and uric acid by their effect on volume, and some diuretics may directly affect urate transport. Thiazides regularly cause a dosage-related rise in the serum urate level. This elevation is reversed on withdrawal of the agent. The increase in concentration averages 1 to 2 mg/dL but occasionally may be 4 to 5 mg/dL. Furosemide also is often associated with a rise in concentration of serum urate; less commonly, ethacrynic acid, acetazolamide, and rarely triamterene are associated with hyperuricemia. Spironolactone is not associated with hyperuricemia.

The incidence of gout after the initiation of a diuretic is a complex issue. Other factors that affect the incidence of gout, such as hypertension and obesity, are often present in patients treated with diuretics. Approximately 10% of hypertensive patients with hyperuricemia secondary to diuretic therapy develop gout. This risk increases in patients with known gout and in patients with diseases associated with elevation of the serum urate concentration, such as myeloproliferative disorders or psoriasis. With diuretic therapy, uric acid excretion is diminished and there is no increase in the incidence of urinary calculi. The risk of developing urate nephropathy is minimal (see earlier discussion). For these reasons, expectant management of patients with asymptomatic hyperuricemia secondary to diuretics is appropriate.

Should acute gout develop, the treatment described previously may be initiated. Intercritical gout is managed similarly to primary gout, and prophylactic colchicine and uricosuric therapy with probenecid (if there is no renal failure) or allopurinol to decrease production of urate may be used. Reducing the dosage or stopping the diuretic is usually associated with a slight fall in the plasma urate concentration, but many patients continue to have attacks of gout. Therefore, if a patient develops gout while taking diuretics and the need for the diuretic continues, it is best to treat the gout as described previously and to continue use of the diuretic at the minimally effective dosage. In the management of hypertension, the use of beta-blockers, angiotensin-converting enzyme inhibitors and long-acting calcium channel blocking agents, which have no effect on urate excretion, may allow discontinuation of diuretics in some patients.

CALCIUM PYROPHOSPHATE DIHYDRATE–INDUCED ARTHRITIS

Pathophysiology

CPPD deposition disease occurs as a result of alteration of metabolism of inorganic pyrophosphate (iPP), which causes deposition of CPPD crystals in articular cartilage, fibrocartilage, ligaments, tendons, bursae, and synovia. This may occur as an accompaniment or consequence of aging, often in association with osteoarthritis, or as a result of genetic defects or certain systemic metabolic diseases (Table 76.4). The precise mechanisms by which these deposits develop are not clear and are likely to be multifactorial. Most of the research toward an understanding of this process has involved alterations of iPP metabolism in articular cartilage. With aging and cartilage degeneration chondrocytes proliferate, become hypertrophic, and undergo apoptosis, with an increased production of iPP and calcification (90). TGF-beta-1, activated through the action of transglutaminase (91), may play an important role in these changes. Upregulation of enzymes of the nucleotide triphosphate pyrophosphohydrolase family increase iPP production (92). TGF-beta also stimulates chondrocyte elaboration of matrix vesicles capable of greater precipitation of iPP with calcification (93). Once formed, calcium crystals may activate signal induction pathways with upregulation of metalloproteinases and enhancement of degenerative changes in articular cartilage (94). Once released in sufficient quantity into the joint, CPPD crystals induce an acute inflammatory response similar to that of monosodium urate and an acute arthritis, the syndrome of pseudogout.

Table 76.4. Diseases Associated with Calcium Pyrophosphate Dihydrate Deposition Disease

Osteoarthritis	Hereditary hypophosphatasia
Hemochromatosis–hemosiderosis	Hypothyroidism
Gout	Neurogenic arthropathy
Hyperparathyroidism	Osteochondrodysplasia
Hypomagnesemia	Synovial chondromatosis
	Gitelman syndrome

Epidemiology

Chondrocalcinosis increases in frequency with age; it is present in approximately 5% of the adult population at the time of autopsy and in 20% to 30% of people older than 80 years of age, most of whom are asymptomatic. The exact prevalence of CPPD deposit disease is unknown. In one series of consecutive patients with newly diagnosed crystal-induced arthritis, CPPD deposit disease accounted for about one third of the cases. Men are probably affected more than women, with a male/female ratio of 1.5:1 (95).

Causes

Familial cases with an autosomal dominant inheritance have been described (96) in which chondrocalcinosis appears at an earlier age. These families are uncommon, and many of these patients remain asymptomatic for many years. Although genetic defects in the nucleotide pyrophosphohydrolase enzymes have been suspected, the metabolic defect or defects have not been specifically identified. Early onset of osteoarthritis and chondrocalcinosis has been linked to chromosome 8q (97). Linkage to chromosome 5p has also been described (98), suggesting genetic heterogeneity. Most cases of CPPD deposit disease are sporadic and idiopathic; a few are associated with one of a variety of metabolic diseases (99). Many of the diseases associated with deposits of CPPD involve metabolic abnormalities in connective tissues, but the precise mechanisms of CPPD crystallization are unknown. A list of these associated diseases is presented in Table 76.4. There is a strong association with osteoarthritis (see Chapter 75).

Clinical Features

Patients are usually middle aged to elderly at the time of onset of arthritic symptoms (Table 76.5). There are several possible patterns of presentation. About one quarter of the patients have *self-limited, acute, goutlike attacks (pseudogout)* predominantly affecting the knees and wrists, but occasionally involving other joints, including rarely the first metatarsophalangeal joint. Monarticular attacks are the rule, but involvement of symmetric joints and polyarthritis may occur rarely. Symptoms are often less intense than they are in gout, but the presentation is variable and some attacks may be severe. Systemic symptoms, including fever to 101°F (38°C) or more, may occur as in gout, and patients are often misdiagnosed as having infection. In some elderly patients, fever is the dominant symptom and the joint abnormalities are subtle and may be overlooked (100). Attacks are often exacerbated by trauma or acute illness. Long intervals (sometimes years) between attacks are common.

In about half of the patients, and especially in women, the presentation resembles that of osteoarthritis with bilateral involvement, especially of the knees. The wrists, metacarpophalangeal joints, hips, shoulders, elbows, or ankles also may be affected. Acute exacerbations occur in about half of these patients, with features that resemble those of osteoarthritis, except that the disease is more progressive and destructive. Varus or valgus knee deformities are common, and extensive calcification around the patella may be seen on radiography. Flexion contractures may occur also. The relationship to ordinary osteoarthritis is still unclear, except that the involvement of joints not usually affected in osteoarthritis (metacarpophalangeal joints, wrists, shoulders, elbows) suggests a different pathogenesis. However, this is controversial. Use of a new, sensitive technique to measure calcium crystals along with light and electron microscopy allowed CPPD or basic calcium phosphate crystals to be demonstrated in 11 of 12 patients with typical osteoarthritis of the knee when they were not always detected by usual methods (see Chapter 75) (101).

In a few patients, persistent subacute inflammation with fatigue, morning stiffness, and synovial swelling in multiple joints lasting weeks or months resembles rheumatoid arthritis.

A few patients also have been reported with severely *destructive arthritis* that resembles the Charcot joints of neuropathic arthropathy but is associated with a normal neurologic examination. CPPD deposit disease may also be associated with a true neuropathic arthritis caused by tabes dorsalis.

Table 76.5. Clinical Features of Calcium Pyrophosphate Dihydrate Deposition Disease

Epidemiology
Age: middle aged or elderly

Site
Knee and wrist most common joints involved
Metacarpophalangeal joints, hips, shoulders, elbows, ankles may be affected
Arthritis usually monoarticular

Pattern
Acute goutlike attacks with symptom-free intervals in 25%
Osteoarthritislike disease in 50%, with superimposed acute attacks in half of these patients
Rheumatoidlike polyarthritis in 5%
Neuropathiclike arthritis without neurologic damage (rare)
Asymptomatic chondrocalcinosis in 20% (found on radiography)

Laboratory
Synovial fluid shows leukocytosis and characteristic CPPD crystals

Laboratory Findings

Patients may have peripheral leukocytosis and an elevated erythrocyte sedimentation rate in association with acute or subacute attacks of arthritis. The synovial fluid shows polymorphonuclear leukocytosis that may exceed 50,000/mm^3 in acute pseudogout but is more commonly in the range of 15,000 to 25,000/mm^3. Crystal identification is the key to diagnosis (see earlier discussion). In the absence of acute or subacute inflammation, leukocyte counts may be low (less than 2,000/mm^3) and crystals may be largely extracellular.

Because of the occasional association with other potentially treatable disorders (Table 76.4) and the ease of these determinations, the patient's serum calcium, phosphorus, magnesium, alkaline phosphatase, and uric acid (actually urate, as discussed earlier) concentrations should be measured, although they usually are normal (95). Chondrocalcinosis is a frequent manifestation of a rare genetic disorder, the Gitelman variant of Bartter syndrome (102). The findings of hypomagnesemia, mild hypokalemic alkalosis, and hypocalciuria lead to the correct diagnosis. The defect is an abnormality in the sodium chloride transporter in the distal convoluted tubule of the kidney. A striking reduction of chondrocalcinosis over a 10-year period (103) and a good prognosis (104) are seen if hypomagnesemia and hypokalemia can be reversed with potassium and magnesium supplementation, sometimes aided with spironolactone. Because pseudogout may be the presenting manifestation of hemochromatosis and because of the importance of early diagnosis in this disorder, measurement of serum ferritin is also indicated if there is any suspicion of this diagnosis (99).

Radiographic Findings

The typical radiographic findings of CPPD deposit disease are punctate and linear calcifications (chondrocalcinosis), seen most often in the fibrocartilage of the menisci of the knee, usually bilaterally (Fig. 76.3). Other fibrocartilages may show similar changes, including the disc in the distal radioulnar joint, the symphysis pubis, the lip of the acetabulum, the glenoid

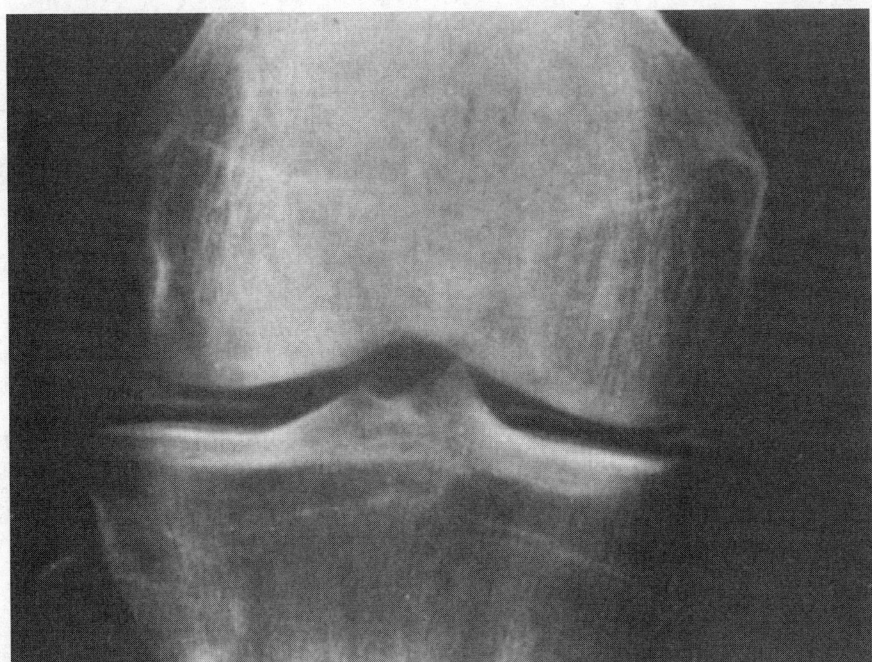

Figure 76.3. Radiograph of the knee in a patient with chondrocalcinosis. Stippled calcification of the medial and lateral menisci is easily identified.

fossa, and intervertebral discs. Hyaline cartilage may also be involved, with similar punctate linear calcifications that may be identified as a dense line parallel to the subchondral bone in the midzone of the articular cartilage. Calcification in the soft tissues of the joint capsule and occasionally in ligaments and tendons may also be seen but is less characteristic. In patients with the type of CPPD deposit disease that resembles osteoarthritis, subchondral cyst formation with bony collapse may be prominent. Osteophyte formation is variable and inconsistent.

These radiographic findings may be helpful in suggesting or confirming the diagnosis of CPPD deposit disease. However, it may not be possible to visualize the extent of deposits radiographically, and their absence does not exclude the diagnosis if typical crystals can be demonstrated in synovial fluid or in biopsy material. A detailed review with multiple illustrative examples of radiographic changes in CPPD deposition disease is available (105).

Management

No therapy influences the deposition or resolution of tissue deposits of CPPD in idiopathic CPPD deposition disease. In the acute pseudogout episode, diagnostic aspiration of synovial fluid (see Chapter 74) with removal of crystals and leukocytes may provide significant clinical improvement. Local injection of depo corticosteroid (see Chapter 74) is often effective and avoids potential side effects of systemic drug therapy. Efficacy of colchicine has been debated; although it is sometimes effective, the use of indomethacin (Indocin) or other NSAIDs is generally preferred, as described previously for acute gout. Because many of these patients are elderly (and may therefore have an impaired glomerular filtration rate), caution regarding renal toxicity of these agents should be exercised (see Chapter 52). As in the treatment of acute gout, a brief course of systemic corticosteroids is an alternative, but, because a single large joint is usually affected, intra-articular steroid administration is preferred. In patients with only recurrent acute attacks, no therapy is indicated between attacks, but early administration of anti-inflammatory agents on exacerbation may minimize or abort attacks. Therapy for patients with more subacute inflammation or for those with osteoarthritis-like disease is similar to that described for osteoarthritis (see Chapter 75), except that anti-inflammatory levels of drugs may be required for optimal symptomatic control.

HYDROXYAPATITE-INDUCED ARTHRITIS

The capacity of hydroxyapatite crystals to induce an inflammatory response was first appreciated in some patients with acute tendinitis (106). More recently, hydroxyapatite crystals were identified in patients with osteoarthritis, especially in association with acute inflammatory episodes (107), and in patients with destructive arthropathy of the shoulder joint (108). The latter, called *Milwaukee shoulder*, is associated with painful limited shoulder motion, complete disruption of the rotator cuff, and extensive degenerative changes in the bone. In these conditions (see Chapter 69), crystals of other basic calcium salts, including octacalcium phosphate and tricalcium phosphate in addition to hydroxyapatite, have sometimes been identified. This has prompted the use of the term *basic calcium phosphate (BCP) deposit disease* to describe these syndromes (108). The capacity of the various crystals to induce inflammation varies according to crystal type, surface area, and calcium/phosphate ratio (109). CPPD crystals may also be found in addition to BCP crystals in these syndromes and in some familial cases (110). Alizarin red S dye (available from scientific supply houses) may be used to stain wet preparations of synovial fluid to screen for the presence of hydroxyapatite crystals, which appear with ordinary light microscopy as red-stained clumps of crystalline material (111). Because all other calcium-containing crystals and even noncrystalline calcium salts stain with this dye, specific identification of BCP crystals requires techniques that are not usually available, such as electron microscopy, microprobe analysis, or x-ray diffraction. It is now clear that BCP crystals alone or in combination with CPPD are broadly associated with calcinosis in soft tissue, tendons, and bursae as well as in joints. These deposits may be secondary in some instances to trauma, neurologic injury, collagen disease, or chronic renal failure. In any of these locations an acute gout-like inflammation or a more chronic and sometimes destructive tissue response may ensue (112). One need only be aware of the potential inflammatory properties of this crystalline material and consider its implication in the these various clinical situations. The patient may be treated with aspiration, from a joint or soft tissue, of the crystalline material and subsequent local injection of a lidocaine/corticosteroids solution (see Chapter 74) or with an NSAID (see Chapter 77). These modalities should provide symptomatic relief in acute inflammatory arthritis or tendinitis associated with BCP crystal deposits. If symptoms become chronic or extensive destructive arthropathy is present, rheumatologic or orthopedic referral is indicated.

ARTHRITIS ASSOCIATED WITH CALCIUM OXALATE

Another crystal-associated arthritis has been demonstrated in patients receiving long-term dialysis therapy (usually hemodialysis, but also seen with peritoneal dialysis) for end-stage renal disease. Extensive deposits of calcium oxalate in soft tissues occur in this setting, and these deposits can cause acute arthritis, destructive arthropathy, tenosynovitis, or bursitis (113,114). These patients are difficult to treat because of the presence of extensive and continuing deposits and incomplete response to colchicine, nonsteroidal agents, and corticosteroids.

General References*

Emmerson BT. Drug therapy: the management of gout. N Engl J Med 1996;334:445.

A thorough and cogent exposition of the topic with extensive bibliography.

Reginato AJ, Reginato AM. Diseases associated with deposition of calcium pyrophosphate or hydroxyapatite. In: Ruddy S, Harris ED Jr, Sledge CB, eds. Kelley's textbook of rheumatology. 6th ed. Philadelphia: WB Saunders, 2001.

An excellent review.

*Bold print (general references) and bold numerals (specific references) denote published controlled clinical trials, meta-analyses, or consensus-based recommendations.

Schumacher HR. Crystal-induced arthritis: an overview. Am J Med 1996;100[Suppl 2A]:46S.

A brief review with good color photographs of urate and pyrophosphate crystals.

Schumacher HR Jr, Reginato AJ. Atlas of synovial fluid analysis and crystal identification. Philadelphia: Lea & Febiger, 1991.

Steinbach L, Resnick D Calcium pyrophosphate deposition disease: Imaging perspectives. Curr Probl Diagn Radiol 2000;29:209.

Detailed review with excellent reproduction of multiple radiographs.

Wortman RL, Kelley WN. Gout and hyperuricemia. In: Ruddy S, Harris Jr ED, Sledge CB, eds. Kelley's textbook of rheumatology. 6th ed. Philadelphia: WB Saunders, 2001.

Probably one of the most thorough reviews available on purine metabolism, hyperuricemia, and gout, with extensive bibliography.

Specific References

1. Kam M, Perl-Travis D, Addadi L. Antibodies against crystals. FASEB J 1992;6:2608.
2. Ortiz-Bravo E, Sieck MS, Schumacher HR Jr. Changes in the proteins coating monosodium urate crystals during active inflammation: Immunogold studies of synovial fluids from patients with gout and of fluid obtained using the rat subcutaneous air pouch model. Arthritis Rheum 1993;36:1274.
3. Barabe F, Gilbert C, Liao, N, et al. Crystal-induced neutrophil activation. VI: involvement of Fc gamma RIIIB (CD16) and CD11b in response to inflammatory microcrystals. FASEB J 1998;12:209.
4. Liu R, O'Connell M, Johnson K, et al. Extracellular signal-regulated kinase 1/extracellular signal-regulated kinase 2 mitogen-activated protein kinase signalling and activation of activator protein 1 and nuclear factor kappa B transcription factors play central roles in interleukin-8 expression stimulated by monosodium urate monohydrate and calcium pyrophosphate crystals in monocytic cells. Arthritis Rheum 2000;43:1145.
5. Di Giovine FS, Malawista SE, Mercer E, et al. Urate crystals stimulate production of tumor necrosis factor alpha from human blood monocytes and synovial cells: cytokine messenger RNA and protein kinetics and cellular distribution. J Clin Invest 1991;87:1375.
6. Guerne PA, Terkeltaub R, Zuraw B, et al. Inflammatory microcrystals stimulate IL-6 production and secretion by human monocytes and synoviocytes. Arthritis Rheum 1993;32:1443.
7. Terkeltaub R, Zachariae C, Santoro D, et al. Monocyte-derived neutrophil chemotactic factor/interleukin-8 is a potential mediator of crystal-induced inflammation. Arthritis Rheum 1991;34:894.
8. Terkeltaub R, Baird S, Sears P, et al. The murine homolog of the interleukin-8 receptor CXCR-2 is essential for the occurrence of neutrophil inflammation in the air pouch model of acute crystal-induced gouty synovitis. Arthritis Rheum 1998;41:900.
9. Matsukawa A, Yoshimura T, Maeda T, et al. Analysis of the cytokine network among tumor necrosis factor alpha, interleukin-1 beta, interleukin-8, and interleukin 1 receptor antagonist in monosodium urate crystal-induced rabbit arthritis. Lab Invest 1998;78:559.
10. Gordon TP, Terkeltaub R. Gout: crystal-induced inflammation. In: Gallin JI, Goldstein TM, Synderman R, eds. Inflammation: basic principles and clinical correlates. New York: Raven Press, 1988.
11. Malawista SE, Duff GW, Atkins E, et al. Crystal induced endogenous pyrogen production: a further look at gouty inflammation. Arthritis Rheum 1985;28:1039.
12. Agudelo CA, Schumacher H R Jr. The synovitis of acute gouty arthritis: a light and electron microscopic study. Hum Pathol 1973;2:265.
13. Roualt T, Caldwell DS, Holmes EW. Aspiration of the asymptomatic metarsophlangeal joint in gout patients and hyperuricemic controls. Arthritis Rheum 1982;25:209.
14. Pascual E, Batlle-Gualda E, Martinez A, et al. Synovial fluid analysis for diagnosis of intercritical gout. Ann Intern Med 1999;131:756.
15. Yaznik DR, Hillyer P, Marshall D, et al. Noninflammatory

phagocytosis of monosodium urate monohydrate crystals by mouse macrophages. Arthritis Rheum 2000;43:1779.
16. Malnik SD, Arliel-Romen S, Ervon E, et al. Acute pseudogout as a complication of pamidronate. Ann Pharmacother 1997;31:499.
17. Perez-Ruiz F, Testillano M, Gastoca MA, et al. "Pseudoseptic" pseudogout associated with hypomagnesemia in liver transplant patients. Transplantation 2001;71:696.
18. Terkeltaub RA. Pathogenesis and treatment of crystal-induced inflammation. In: Koopman WJ, ed. Arthritis and allied conditions. Philadelphia: Lippincott Williams & Wilkins, 2001:2335.
19. Fava R, Olsen N, Keski-Oja, et al. Active and latent forms of transforming growth factor beta activity in synovial effusions. J Exp Med 1989;169:291.
20. Liote F, Prudhommeaux F, Schlitz C, et al. Inhibition and prevention of monosodium urate monohydrate crystal-induced inflammation in vivo by transforming growth factor beta 1. Arthritis Rheum 1996;39:1192.
21. Terkeltaub R, Smelzer D, Curtiss LK, et al. Low density lipoprotein inhibits the physical interaction of phagocytic crystals and inflammatory cells. Arthritis Rheum 1986;29:363.
22. McCarty DJ, Halverson PB, Carrera GF, et al. "Milwaukee shoulder": association of microspheroids containing hydroxyapatite crystals, active collagenase and neutral protease with rotator cuff defects. I: clinical aspects. Arthritis Rheum 1981;24:464.
23. Dieppe PA, Cawston T, Mercer E, et al. Synovial fluid collagenase in patients with destructive arthritis of the shoulder joint. Arthritis Rheum 1988;31:882.
24. Alwan WH, Dieppe PA, Elson CJ, et al. Hydroxyapatite and urate crystal induced cytokine release by macrophages. Ann Rheum Dis 1989;48:476.
25. Phelps P, Steele AD, McCarty DJ Jr. Compensated polarized light microscopy. JAMA 1968;203:508.
26. Fagan TJ, Lidsky MD. Compensated polarized light microscopy using cellophane adhesive tape. Arthritis Rheum 1974;17:256.
27. Kerolous G, Clayburne G, Schumacher HR Jr. Is it mandatory to examine synovial fluids promptly after arthrocentesis. Arthritis Rheum 1989;32:271.
28. Petrocelli A, Wong AL, Swezey RL. Identification of pathologic synovial fluid crystals on gram stains. J Clin Rheumatol 1998;4:103.
29. Selvi E, Manganelli S. Catenaccio M, et al. Diff Quick staining methods for detection and identification of monosodium urate and calcium pyrophosphate crystals in synovial fluids. Ann Rheum Dis 2001;60:194.
30. Ivorra J, Rosas J, Pascual E. Most calcium pyrophosphate crystals appear as non-birefringent. Ann Rheum Dis 1999;58:582.
31. Schumacher HR Jr, Sieck MS, Rothfuss S, et al. Reproductibility of synovial fluid analyses: a study among four laboratories. Arthritis Rheum 19886;29:770.
32. Schumacher HR Jr, Sieck M, Clayburne G. Development and evaluation of a method for preservation of synovial fluid wet preparations for quality control testing of crystal identifications. J Rheumatol 1990;17:1369.
33. McGill NW, McGill VG. Quality assurance for synovial fluid examination for crystals: an improved method. Ann Rheum Dis 1997;56:504.
34. Wik JB, Djousse L, Boreski I, et al. Segregation analysis of serum uric acid in the NHLBI Family Heart Study. Hum Genet 2000;106:355.
35. Wilson JM, Young AB, Kelley WN. Hypoxanthine-guanine phosphoribosyl transferase deficiency: the molecular basis of the clinical syndrome. N Engl J Med 1983;309:900.
36. Sperling O, Elam G, Pinsky-Brosch S, et al. Accelerated 5′-phosphoribosyl-pyrophosphate synthesis: a familial abnormality associated with excessive uric acid production and gout. Biochem Med 1992;6:310.
37. Puig JG, Miranda ME, Felicitas A, et al. Hereditary nephropathy associated with hyperuricemia and gout. Arch Intern Med 1993;153:357.
38. Kamatani N, Moritani M, Yamanaka H, et al. Localization of a gene for familial juvenile hyperuricemic nephropathy causing underexcretion-type gout to 16p12 by genome-wide linkage analysis in a large family. Arthritis Rheum 2000;43:925.
39. Wortman RL, Kelley WN. Gout and hyperuricemia. In: Kelley's textbook of rheumatology. Philadelphia: WB Saunders, 2001:1339.
40. Simpkin PA, Horner PL, Paxon CS, et al. Uric acid excretion quantitative assessment from spot midmorning serum and urine samples. Ann Intern Med 1979;91:44.
41. Lawrence RC, Helmick CG, Arnett FC, et al. Estimates of the prevalence of arthritis and musculoskeletal disorders in the United States. Arthritis Rheum 1998;41:778.
42. Harris CM, Lloyd DC, Lewis J. Prevalence and prophylaxis of gout in England. J Clin Epidemiol 1995;48:1153.
43. Roubenoff R, Klag MJ, Mead LA, et al. Incidence and risk factors for gout in white men. JAMA 1991;266:3004.
44. Hochberg MC, Thomas J, Thomas DJ, et al. Racial differences in the incidence of gout: the role of hypertension. Arthritis Rheum 1995;38:628.
45. Lin KC, Lin HY, Chou P. The interaction between uric acid level and other risk factors on the development of gout among hyperuricemic men in a prospective study. J Rheumatol 2001;27:1501.
46. Facchini F, Chen I, Hollenbeck CB, et al. Relationship between resistance to insulin-mediated glucose uptake, urinary uric acid clearance and plasma uric acid concentration. JAMA 1991;166:3008.
47. Reaven GM. Syndrome X. Clin Diabetes 1994;12:32.
48. Davidson MB. Clinical implications of insulin resistance syndromes. Am J Med 1985;99:420.
49. Emerson B. Hyperlipidemia in hyperuricemia and gout. Ann Rheum Dis 1998;57:5090.
50. Takahashi S, Moriwaki Y, Tsutsumi Z, et al. Increased visceral fat accumulation further aggravates the risks of insulin resistance in gout. Metabolism 2001;50:393.
51. Ginsberg H, Olefsky J, Farquhar JW, et al. Moderate ethanol ingestion and plasma triglyceride levels: a study in normal and hypertriglyceridemic persons. Arch Intern Med 1974;80:143.
52. Scott JT, Higgins CJ. Diuretic induced gout: a multifactorial condition. Ann Rheum Dis 1992;51:259.
53. McFarlane G, Dieppe PA. Diuretic induced gout in elderly females. Br J Rheumatol 1985;24:155.
54. Lin HY, Rocher LL, McQuillan MA. Cyclosporine-induced hyperuricemia and gout. N Engl J Med 1989;321:287.
55. Wluka AE, Ryan PF, Miller AM, et al. Post cardiac transplantation gout: incidence of therapeutic complications. J Heart Lung Transplant 2000;19:951.
56. Erickson AR, Enzenauer RJ, Nordstrom DM, et al. The prevalence of hypothyroidism in gout. Am J Med 1994;97:231.
57. Yu TF, Gutman AB. Efficacy of colchicine prophylaxis in gout: prevention of recurrent gouty arthritis over a mean period of five years in 208 gouty subjects. Ann Intern Med 1961;55:179.
58. Wallace SL, Robinson H, Masi AT, et al. Preliminary criteria for the classification of the acute arthritis of primary gout. Arthritis Rheum 1977;20:895.
59. Wall B, Agudelo CA, Tesser JRP, et al. An autopsy study of the prevalence of monosodium urate and calcium pyrophosphate dihydrate crystal deposition in the first metatarsophalangeal joints. Arthritis Rheum 1983;26:1522.
60. Weinberger A, Schumaker HR Jr, Agudelo CA. Urate crystals in asymptomatic metatarsophalangeal joints. Ann Intern Med 1979;91:56.
61. Holland NW, Jost D, Beutler A, et al. Finger pad tophi in gout. J Rheumatol 1996;23:690.
62. Puig JG, Michan AD, Jiminez ML, et al. Female gout: clinical spectrum and uric acid metabolism. Arch Intern Med 1991;151:726.
63. Fam AG, Stein J, Rubenstein J. Gouty arthritis in nodal osteoarthritis. J Rheumatol 1996;23:684.
64. Schapira D, Stahl S, Izhak OB, et al. Chronic tophaceous gout mimicking rheumatoid arthritis. Semin Arthritis Rheum 1999;29:56.
65. Rege J, Shet T, Naik L. Fine needle aspiration of tophi for crystal identification in problematic cases of gout: a report of two cases. Acta Cytologica 2000;44:433.
66. Wallace SL, Klinenberg JR, Moshaim D, et al. Coexistent gout

and rheumatoid arthritis: case report and literature review. Arthritis Rheum 1979;22:81.
67. Yu TF, Berger L. Renal function in gout: its association with hypertensive vascular disease. Am J Med 1982;72:95.
68. Hall AP, Barry PE, Dawber TR, et al. Epidemiology of gout and hyperuricemia. Am J Med 1967;42:27.
69. Yu TF, Gutman AB. Uric acid nephrolithiasis in gout: predisposing factors. Ann Intern Med 1967;67:1133.
70. Levy FL, Adams-Huet BA, Pak CYC. Ambulatory evaluation of nephrolithiasis: an update of a 1980 protocol. Am J Med 1995;98:50.
71. Gerster JL, Landry M, Duvoisin B, et al. Computer tomography of the knee joint as an indication of intra articular tophi in gout. Arthritis Rheum 1996;39:1406.
72. Wortman RL. Effective management of gout: an analogy. Am J Med 1998;105:513.
73. Schlesinger N, Baker DG, Schumacher HR Jr. How well have diagnostic tests and therapies for gout been evaluated. Curr Opin Rheumatol 1999;11:441.
74. Wallace SL, Singer JZ. Systemic toxicity associated with IV colchicine: guidelines for use. J Rheumatol 1988;15:495.
75. Putterman C, Ben-Cherit E, Caraco Y, et al. Colchicine intoxication, risk factors, features and management. Semin Arthritis Rheum 1991;3:143.
76. Fam AG. Current therapy of acute microcrystalline arthritis and the role of corticosteroids. J Clin Rheumatol 1997;3:35.
77. Groff GO, Frank WA, Raddatz DA. Systemic steroid therapy for acute gout: a clinical trial and review of the literature. Semin Arthritis Rheum 1990;19:329.
78. Paulus HE, Schlosstein LH, Godfrey RG, et al. Prophylactic colchicine therapy of intercritical gout: a placebo controlled study of probenecid-treated patients. Arthritis Rheum 1974;17:609.
79. Kuncl RW, Duncan G, Watson O, et al. Colchicine myopathy and neuropathy. N Engl J Med 1987;316:1562.
80. Harris M, Bryant LR, Danaker P, et al. Effect of low dose daily aspirin on serum urate levels and urinary excretion in patients receiving probenecid for gouty arthritis. J Rheumatol 2000;27:2873.
81. Hande KR, Noone RM, Stone WJ. Severe allopurinol toxicity: description and guidelines for prevention in patients with renal insufficiency. Am J Med 1984;76:47.
82. Li-Yu J, Clayburne G, Sieck M, et al. Treatment of chronic gout: can we determine when urate stores are depleted enough to prevent attacks of gout? J Rheumatol 2001;28:577.
83. Ferraz MB, O'Brien B. A cost effective analysis of urate lowering drugs in non-tophaceous recurrent gouty arthritis. J Rheumatol 1995;22:908.
84. Dessein PH, Shipton EA, Stanwix AE, et al. Beneficial effects of weight loss associated with moderate caloric/carbohydrate restriction and increased proportional intake of protein and unsaturated fat on serum uric and lipoprotein levels in gout. Ann Rheum Dis 2000;59:539.
85. Van Lieshout-Zuidema MF, Breedveld FC. Withdrawal of long term anti-hyperuricemic therapy in tophaceous gout. J Rheumatol 1993;22:1383.
86. Perez-Ruiz F, Alonzo-Ruiz A, Calabozo M, et al. Efficacy of allopurinol and benzbromarone for the control of hyperuricemia: a pathogenetic approach to the treatment of primary chronic gout. Ann Rheum Dis 1998;57:545.
87. Perez-Ruiz F, Calabozo M, Herrero-Beites AM, et al. Improvement of renal function in patients with chronic gout after proper control of hyperuricemia and gouty bouts. Nephron 2000;86:287.
88. Fam AG, Dunne SM, Iazetta J, et al. Efficacy and safety of desensitization to allopurinol following cutaneous reactions. Arthritis Rheum 2001;44:231.
89. Schreiner O, Himmelsbach F, Galli PR, et al. Reduced secretion of proinflammatory cytokines of monosodium urate crystal stimulated monocytes in chronic renal failure: an explanation for infrequent gout episodes in chronic renal failure patients? Nephrol Dial Transplant 2000;15:644.
90. Lotz M, Hashimoto S, Kuhn K. Mechanisms of chondrocyte apoptosis. Osteoarthritis Cartilage 1999;7:389.
91. Rosenthal AK, Gohr CM, Henry LA, et al. Participation of transglutaminase in the activation of latent transforming growth factor beta 1 in aging articular cartilage. Arthritis Rheum 2000;43:1729.
92. Johnson K, Hashimoto S, Lotz M, et al. Upregulated expression of the phosphodiesterase nucleotide pyrophosphohydrolase family member PC-1 is a marker and pathogenic factor for knee meniscal cartilage matrix calcification. Arthritis Rheum 2001;44:1071.
93. Derfus BA, Carmacho NP, Olmez U, et al. Transforming growth factor beta-1 stimulates articular chondrocyte elaboration of matrix vesicles capable of greater calcium pyrophosphate precipitation. Osteoarthritis Cartilage 2001;9:189.
94. Cheung HS. Calcium crystals' effects on the cells of the joint: implications for pathogenesis of disease. Curr Opin Rheumatol 2000;12:223.
95. McCarty DJ. Pseudogout and pyrophosphate metabolism. Adv Intern Med 1980;25:363.
96. Reginato A, Valenzuela F, Martinez V, et al. Polyarticular and familial chondrocalcinosis. Arthritis Rheum 1970;13:197.
97. Baldwin CT, Farrer LA, Adair R, et al. Linkage of early-onset osteoarthritis and chondrocalcinosis to chromosome 8q. Am J Hum Genet 1995;56:692.
98. Andrew LJ, Brancolini V, Serrano de la Pena L, et al. Refinement of chromosome 5p locus for familial calcium pyrophosphate deposition disease. Am J Hum Genet 1999;64:136.
99. Jones AC, Chuck AJ, Arie EA, et al. Diseases associated with calcium pyrophosphate dihydrate deposition disease. Semin Arthritis Rheum 1992;22:188.
100. Rahman M, Schenberger KN, Schumacher HR Jr. Initially unrecognized calcium pyrophosphate dihydrate deposition disease as a cause of fever. Am J Med 1990;89:115.
101. Swan A, Chapman B, Heap P, et al. Submicroscopic crystals in osteoarthritis synovial fluid. Ann Rheum Dis 1994;53:467.
102. Punzi L, Calo L, Schiavon F, et al. Chondrocalcinosis is a feature of Gitelman's variant of Bartter's syndrome: a new look at the hypomagnesemia associated with calcium pyrophosphate dihydrate deposition disease. Rev Rheum Engl Ed 1998;65:571.
103. Smilde TJ, Haverman JF, Schipper P, et al. Familial hypokalemia/hypomagnesemia and chondrocalcinosis. J Rheumatol 1994;21:1515.
104. Barakat AJ, Rennert OM. Gitelman's syndrome (familial hypokalemia-hypomagnesemia). J Nephrol 2001;14:43.
105. Steinbach L, Resnick D. Calcium pyrophosphate dihydrate deposition disease: imaging perspectives. Curr Probl Diagn Radiol 2000;29:209.
106. Pinals RS, Short CL. Calcific periarthritis involving multiple sites. Arthritis Rheum 1966;9:566.
107. Huskisson EC, Dieppe PA, Tucker AK, et al. Another look at osteoarthritis. Ann Rheum Dis 1979;38:423.
108. Halverson PB, McCarty DJ, Cheung HS, et al. Milwaukee shoulder syndrome: eleven additional cases with involvement of the knee in seven (basic calcium phosphate crystal deposition disease). Semin Arthritis Rheum 1984;14:36.
109. Prudhommeaux F, Schlitz C, Liote F, et al. Variation in the inflammatory properties of basic calcium phosphate crystals according to crystal type. Arthritis Rheum 1996;39:1319.
110. Pons-Estel BA, Gimenez L, Sacnun M, et al. Familial osteoarthritis and Milwaukee shoulder associated with calcium pyrophosphate and apatite crystal deposition. J Rheumatol 2000;27:471.
111. Paul H, Reginato AJ, Schumacher HR Jr. Alizarin red staining as a screening test for calcium compounds in synovial fluid. Arthritis Rheum 1983;26:191.
112. McCarthy GM, Westfall PR, Masuda I, et al. Basic calcium phosphate crystals activate osteoarthritic fibroblasts and induce matrix metalloproteinase-13 in adult porcine chondrocytes. Ann Rheum Dis 2001;60:399.
113. Reginato AJ, Kurnick BRC. Calcium oxalate and other crystals associated with kidney diseases and arthritis. Semin Arthritis Rheum 1989;18:198.
114. Rosenthal AK, Ryan LM, McCarty DJ. Arthritis associated with calcium oxalate crystals in an anephric patient treated with peritoneal dialysis. JAMA 1988;260:1272.

CHAPTER 77

Rheumatoid Arthritis

ALAN K. MATSUMOTO, MD

Rheumatoid arthritis is a chronic inflammatory systemic disease of unknown cause that has a predilection for involvement of the peripheral joints. The articular inflammation has a variable course, but the primary clinical problem is an additive, progressive, symmetric polyarthritis leading to joint destruction, deformity, and loss of function. Extra-articular features and systemic symptoms are recognized as an integral part of the disease and may antedate the onset of inflammatory arthropathy.

In the past several years, a confluence of discoveries from many areas of research has greatly affected our approach to the treatment of rheumatoid arthritis. Recognition that joint destruction begins early in the course of disease and functional disability occurs quickly has led to more aggressive treatment regimens. Advances in immunology and biotechnology have yielded more effective and better-tolerated agents. More than ever, it is imperative for clinicians to efficiently make the diagnosis, identify patients with poor prognosis, and institute an appropriate and effective therapeutic plan.

EPIDEMIOLOGY

Population surveys have used somewhat different criteria for the diagnosis of rheumatoid arthritis, making accurate assessments of prevalence difficult. Most agree that it has a worldwide distribution with important geographic and ethnic/racial variations. In Caucasian populations, it has an estimated prevalence of 1% to 2%. Native Americans have a high prevalence of 3.5% to 5.3%, and in rural South African blacks and Japanese the prevalence is 0.1% (1).

Prevalence increases with age, approaching 5% in women older than 55 years of age. The average annual incidence in the United States is about 70 per 100,000 people (1). Both the incidence and the prevalence of rheumatoid arthritis are two to three times greater in women than in men. Although rheumatoid arthritis may manifest at any age, it most commonly affects patients in the third to sixth decades. Women tend to have a more severe articular disease, whereas extra-articular features are more common in men.

Genetic influences on disease frequency and severity are suggested by an increased incidence of the human class II histocompatibility antigens HLA-DR4 and HLA-DR1 in patients with rheumatoid arthritis, compared with a matched control population (2). The HLA-DR molecule consists of an α and a β chain, with the various HLA-DR specificities determined by heterogeneity at the three hypervariability regions of the HLA-DRβ chain. The molecular basis for the HLA association is defined by the presence of a shared amino acid sequence, amino acids 70 through 74 in the third hypervariable region of the DRβ chain, in patients with rheumatoid arthritis. The presence of this shared structural element or "susceptibility cassette" increases the risk for development of rheumatoid arthritis and correlates with greater disease severity (3).

PATHOGENESIS

Normal joint architecture consists of a fibrous capsule that surrounds a one- to three-cell-layer lining of synovial cells. Synovial cells bear markers of fibroblast and macrophage lineage and, among many functions, secrete joint lubricants such as hyaluronic acid. The area beneath the synovial lining cells is acellular. The pathologic hallmark of rheumatoid arthritis consists of infiltration of the subsynovia of affected joints by lymphocytes, plasma cells, and macrophages and hypertrophy of synovial lining cells and blood vessels into a tumor-like structure called the *pannus* (4). The event or factor triggering the recruitment of inflammatory cells to the joint remains unknown. Local production of rheumatoid factor–containing immune complexes activates complement and attracts inflammatory cells. The predominance and persistence of CD4-positive T cells in the rheumatoid synovium suggest an antigen-driven, cell-mediated inflammatory process. The inflammatory process is amplified by a number of macrophage- and fibroblast-derived cytokines found in large quantities in the rheumatoid joint, including tumor necrosis factor-alpha (TNF-alpha), interleukin 1 (IL-1), IL-6, and platelet-derived growth factor (5). These cytokines drive the recruitment of additional inflammatory cells and subsequent release of destructive enzymes. Enzymes such as collagenase and stromelysin destroy cartilage and bone, leading to loss of normal joint architecture.

HISTORY

The presentation of the disease (Table 77.1) varies from situations in which the diagnosis is obvious to ones in which the presentation is so atypical that it suggests other conditions. The typical case of rheumatoid arthritis begins insidiously, with the slow progressive development of signs and symptoms over weeks to months. Occasionally, patients experience an explosive polyarticular onset occurring over 24 to 48 hours. Sometimes an acute presentation appears to be associated with either emotional or physical stress, such as loss of a loved one or a recent injury.

Arthritic signs and symptoms provide the definitive clues to the diagnosis of rheumatoid arthritis. Often the patient first notices stiffness (see later discussion) in one or more joints, usually accompanied by pain on movement and by tenderness in the joint. Unlike a patient with gout (see Chapter 76), a patient with rheumatoid arthritis can bear weight and move the inflamed joint but has a persistent, deep, gnawing discomfort. Severe pain in a patient with established rheumatoid arthritis, particularly if limited to one joint, should suggest a superimposed infection or an acute structural problem. The number of joints involved is highly variable, but almost always the process is eventually polyarticular, involving five or more joints. Rheumatoid arthritis is an additive polyarthritis, with the sequential addition of involved joints, in contrast to the migratory or evanescent arthritis that can be seen in systemic lupus erythematosus (SLE) or the episodic arthritis seen in gout. The American College of Rheumatology criteria for the diagnosis of rheumatoid arthritis (6) emphasizes the importance of persistent symmetric swelling or fluid in the joints lasting longer than 6 weeks. Any joint may be involved, but there is a predilection for peripheral joints with a sparing of the axial skeleton. The joints involved most often are the proximal interphalangeal (PIP) and metacarpophalangeal (MCP) joints of the hands, the wrists (particularly at the ulnar–styloid articulation), shoulders, elbows, knees, ankles, and metatarsophalangeal (MTP) joints. Involvement of non–weight-bearing joints—shoulders, elbows, and wrists—should raise suspicion for rheumatoid arthritis. The distal interphalangeal (DIP) joints are usually spared.

Morning stiffness may be a feature of any inflammatory arthritis but is especially characteristic of rheumatoid arthritis. Virtually all patients complain of morning stiffness, and its duration is a useful gauge of the inflammatory activity of the disease. Significant morning stiffness is defined as stiffness, predominantly over joints, that persists for longer than 1 hour, often several hours. Similar stiffness can occur after long periods of sitting or inactivity (gel phenomenon). In contrast, patients with degenerative arthritis complain of stiffness that is often severe but lasts for only a few minutes (see Chapter 75).

Nonspecific systemic symptoms, primarily fatigue, malaise, and depression, are common but not invariable and may precede other symptoms of the disease by weeks to months. Usually the patient does not feel tired on awakening but complains of severe fatigue 4 to 6 hours later. Fever occurs occasionally and is almost always low grade (37° to 38°C; 99° to 100°F). A higher fever suggests another illness, and infectious causes must be considered.

It is typical of patients with rheumatoid arthritis that their symptoms wax and wane, especially at the beginning of the illness. Because of this and because objective signs may not be present at first, it is not unusual for the diagnosis to be delayed for months. Diagnosis may be complicated by the fact that patients with rheumatoid arthritis may present with nonspecific complaints or with signs and symptoms that mimic other musculoskeletal disorders. Atypical presentations include intermittent joint inflammation that can be confused with gout or pseudogout (see Chapter 76), proximal muscle pain and tenderness mimicking polymyalgia rheumatica, and diffuse musculoskeletal pain as seen in fibromyalgia (see Chapter 74).

During the time of diagnostic uncertainty, the physician can best serve the patient by providing reassurance, taking careful interval histories, performing periodic physical examinations (see later discussion), and, if appropriate, performing selected tests (discussed later). Symptomatic treatment with anti-inflammatory

Table 77.1. Symptoms and Signs of Rheumatoid Arthritis

Symptoms		Signs	
Extra-articular	Articular[a]	Extra-articular	Articular
Fatigue Depression Malaise Anorexia	Morning stiffness Pain and tenderness Swelling	Rheumatoid nodules Lymphadenopathy Splenomegaly Ocular disease Entrapment neuropathies	Pain on passive motion Tenderness Swelling Heat Typical deformity

[a]Persistence (6 weeks or longer) and symmetric nature of signs and symptoms are important, but not invariable, diagnostic features.

drugs may be instituted during this period (see later discussion).

PHYSICAL EXAMINATION

Patients with suspected rheumatoid arthritis should undergo an initial complete physical examination and then a limited examination every 3 to 6 months. The physical examination is important not only to make the diagnosis but to establish a baseline against which to assess the possible later development of both articular and extra-articular disease.

However, the primary focus of examinations in the physician's office is the joints. Serial joint examinations should be performed with careful records of the status of affected joints, as determined by history and previous examinations.

Joints

Swelling is the most measurable change that occurs in a joint affected by rheumatoid arthritis. Symmetric joint swelling, although not invariable, is characteristic of rheumatoid arthritis. The first change is usually periarticular soft tissue swelling. Eventually, increased amounts of fluid and synovial hypertrophy within the joint space produce more readily recognizable and often persistent changes. In the hands, where the disease is often first manifested, typical fusiform swelling of the PIP joints commonly occurs (Fig. 77.1). The MCP joints and the wrists swell even more often and are more specific for an inflammatory arthropathy. Careful palpation of the joints can help to distinguish the swelling of joint inflammation from the bony enlargement seen in osteoarthritis. The elbows, knees, ankles, and MTP joints are other common sites of disease where swelling may be readily apparent.

In contrast to gout (see Chapter 76) or septic arthritis, redness of affected joints is not a prominent feature of rheumatoid arthritis.

Pain on passive motion, although not specific for rheumatoid arthritis, is the most sensitive indicator of joint inflammation. When examining a joint, it is important to apply gentle but firm pressure at the

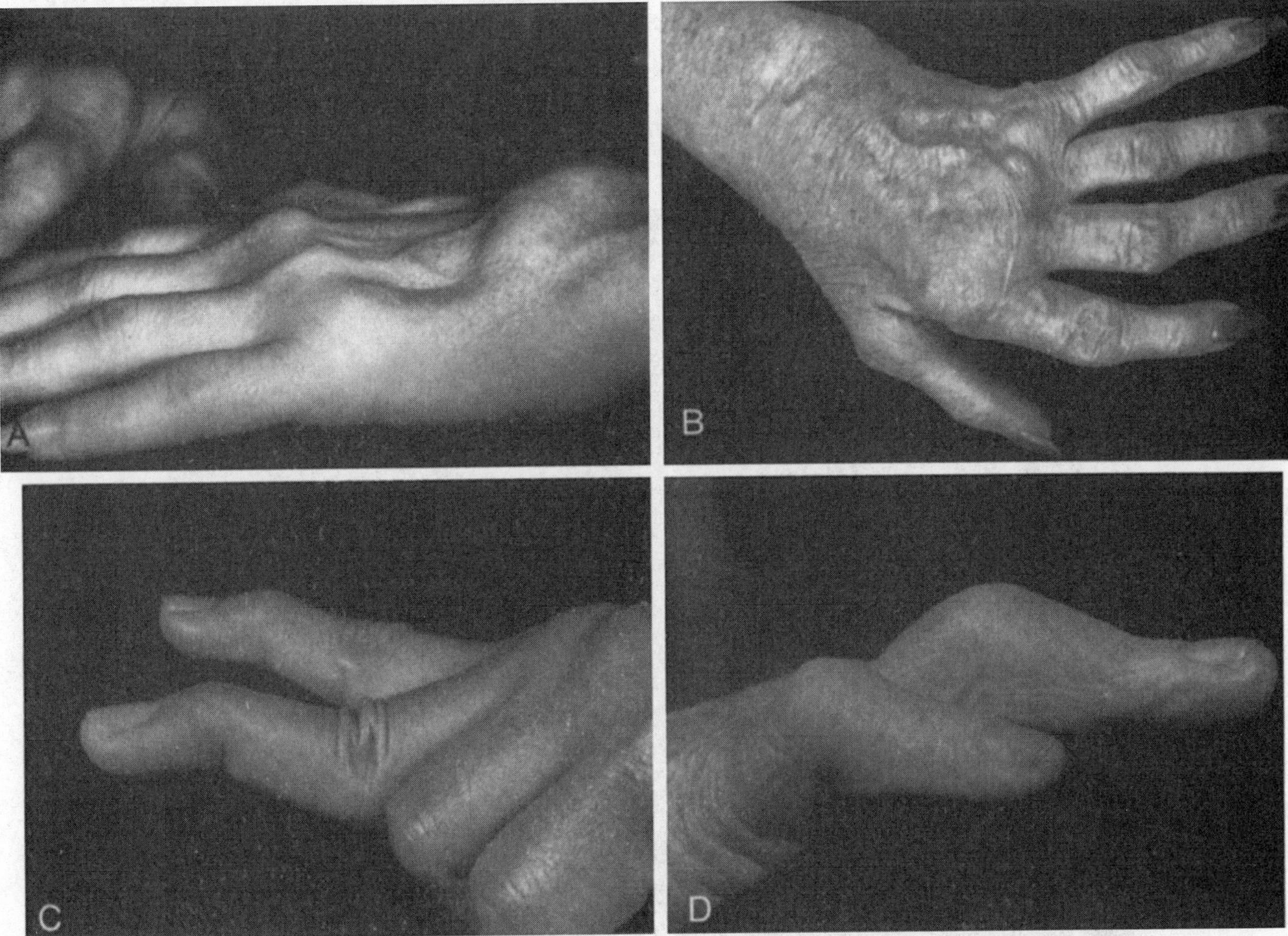

Figure 77.1. Hand deformities in rheumatoid arthritis. **A:** Typical fusiform swelling of the proximal interphalangeal (PIP) joints; note also the synovial swelling of the wrist and metacarpophalangeal joints. **B:** Ulnar deviation of the fingers. **C:** Swan-neck deformity (hyperextension of the PIP joint). **D:** Boutonniere deformity (flexion contracture of the PIP joint).

joint line so that tenderness caused by inflammation is elicited, but not so much pressure that a normal joint is inappropriately deemed symptomatic. Inflamed joints are also usually warmer than normal joints. Temperature of the joint is easier to assess by feeling them with the back of the fingers.

The *range of motion* of the joint may be limited by inflammation, structural deformity, or both. To institute proper therapy (see later discussion), it is important to determine which of these processes is the major factor limiting joint function.

Weakness is a common feature of patients with rheumatoid arthritis, but, like range of motion, it is difficult to assess. Patient perception of weakness and objective testing are influenced by pain that limits movement of the joints. The fatigue produced by the illness may contribute to an overall sense of weakness. Chronic, uncontrolled joint inflammation can have systemic effects, mediated by inflammatory cytokines, that result in a marked decrease in lean body mass (7). Weakness of one or more extremities may be caused by muscle atrophy, a result of joint deformity and disuse.

Permanent deformity is a consequence of the inflammatory process. Joint damage occurs at the level of the bone, cartilage, and periarticular soft tissues. Persistent tenosynovitis and synovitis leads to the formation of synovial cysts and to displaced or ruptured tendons. Extensor tendon rupture at the dorsum of the hand is a common and disabling problem. Cartilage damage and joint space narrowing occur early in the disease. Bony erosions seen at the margins of the joint, at the attachment of the synovium, are the hallmark of rheumatoid arthritis. Erosions occur rapidly within the first 2 years of the disease (8). These anatomic changes result in limitations in range of motion, flexion contractures, and subluxation (incomplete dislocation) of articulating bones. Typical visible changes (Fig. 77.1) include ulnar deviation of the fingers at the MCP joints, hyperextension or hyperflexion of the MCP and PIP joints, flexion contractures of the elbows, and subluxation of the carpal bones. Ankylosis (fusion) of the carpal and tarsal joints can occur, but ankylosis of other joints is rare. Commonly, displacement of the toes (cocked-up) with hallux valgus formation (angulation of the great toe laterally) leads to prominence of the metatarsal heads at the plantar aspect of the foot, resulting in pain with ambulation and ulcer formation.

Synovial cysts are common in patients with rheumatoid arthritis and can be readily seen and palpated overlying the joints with which they communicate. Synovial cysts of the popliteal space (Baker cysts) may develop secondary to chronic knee effusions from a variety of disorders but are especially prevalent in patients with rheumatoid disease (Fig. 77.2). If popliteal cysts rupture, the signs and symptoms mimic those of acute thrombophlebitis, with calf swelling, tenderness, and a positive Homan sign. A magnetic resonance imaging (MRI) scan or ultrasound of the popliteal

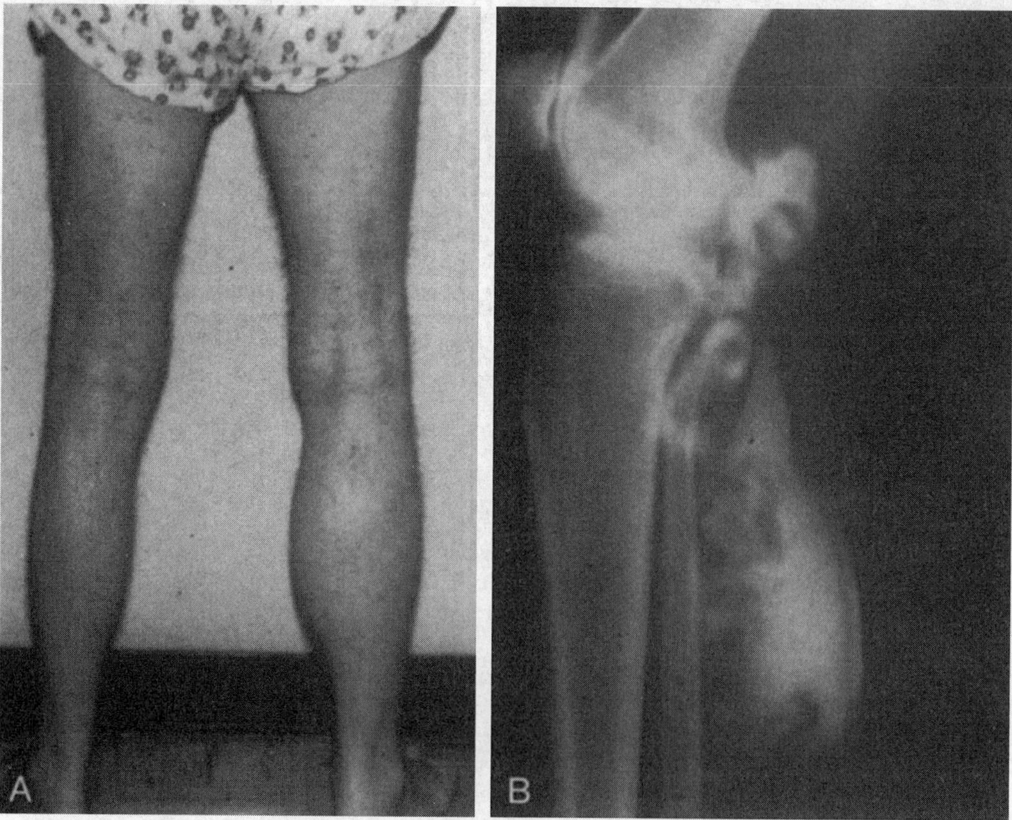

Figure 77.2. Baker cyst. **A:** Swelling of the calf secondary to dissection of the cyst. **B:** Arthrogram of the knee demonstrating the cyst.

space is a noninvasive technique that can be used to confirm the diagnosis. Noninvasive vascular studies of the lower extremities (see Chapter 57) are recommended to rule out deep vein thrombosis if the diagnosis is unclear. Symptoms can be relieved by decompression of the cyst through aspiration of synovial fluid from either the joint or the cyst and injection of a corticosteroid into the joint (see later discussion).

LABORATORY TESTS

Baseline diagnostic laboratory information in patients with suspected rheumatoid arthritis should include a complete blood count (CBC) and differential, erythrocyte sedimentation rate (ESR) or C-reactive protein (CRP), urinalysis, and rheumatoid factor titer. Except when it is caused by adverse drug reactions, renal disease is rare in rheumatoid arthritis, and an abnormal urinalysis should alert the clinician to alternative diagnoses. Baseline values of electrolytes, creatinine, and liver function tests should also be obtained before drug therapy is initiated. In selected patients, synovial fluid analysis, additional serologic studies, and appropriate radiographs are also important (see later discussion).

Hematology

A mild anemia, with hematocrit values in the range of 30% to 34%, occurs in approximately 25% to 35% of patients with rheumatoid arthritis. In most cases, the reduced red cell mass is caused by the anemia of chronic disease (see Chapter 55), a normocytic–normochromic process characterized by a low concentration of serum iron, a low serum iron-binding capacity, and a normal or increased serum ferritin concentration. However, true iron deficiency anemia occasionally develops secondary to intercurrent blood loss. The inflammation of rheumatoid arthritis inhibits erythropoiesis, making it difficult to differentiate anemia that is secondary to chronic blood loss from the anemia of chronic disease without an iron stain of the bone marrow. Nonsteroidal anti-inflammatory drugs (NSAIDs) increase the risk of gastrointestinal (GI) bleeding from peptic ulcer disease and gastritis, particularly in the elderly. In patients older than 40 years of age, it is especially important to monitor for GI blood loss and to consider other causes of blood loss, such as colonic lesions (see Chapter 42).

The leukocyte count is usually normal in patients with rheumatoid arthritis, but it can be mildly elevated secondary to inflammation. Similarly, the platelet count is usually normal but thrombocytosis can occur in response to inflammation. Drug reactions and Felty syndrome are rare causes of leukopenia or thrombocytopenia (see later discussion).

The ESR and CRP are usually elevated in patients with rheumatoid arthritis. In some patients, these tests are useful indicators of the degree of inflammatory disease activity. They should be obtained when changes in therapy are contemplated or to monitor response to therapy. Because the ESR is dependent on the age of the blood sample, CRP is generally favored unless ESR testing can be done promptly after the blood is drawn.

Serology

Rheumatoid Factor

Rheumatoid factors are antibodies directed against the Fc portion of immunoglobulin G (IgG). Although these antibodies may be any subclass (IgG, IgM, IgA), rheumatoid factors measured for clinical purposes are IgM. A positive test for rheumatoid factor is by no means pathognomonic of rheumatoid arthritis, but it is present in 70% to 90% of patients with the disease (9). A significant titer of rheumatoid factor is 1:80 or greater by the latex fixation method and more than 40 IU/mL by the enzyme-linked immunosorbent assay (ELISA) method. In early disease, the rheumatoid factor may be negative, but it becomes positive within the first 6 months of active disease. The titer does not correlate with the activity of disease, but patients with a high titer rheumatoid factor are more likely to have erosive joint disease, nodules, extra-articular manifestations, and greater functional disability over time.

Rheumatoid factors are also detectable in the serum of many patients without rheumatoid arthritis. Most of these patients have had chronic antigenic stimulation, such as prolonged infection (bacterial endocarditis, tuberculosis, cytomegalovirus, human immunodeficiency virus, viral hepatitis), collagen vascular disease, chronic lung disease (pulmonary fibrosis, sarcoidosis, asthma), or dysproteinemia (myeloma, macroglobulinemia, mixed cryoglobulinemia). Positive rheumatoid factors may occur transiently in normal individuals without rheumatoid arthritis after vaccination or after a self-limited viral infection. Finally, low titers of rheumatoid factors may be detected in the serum of apparently normal people, especially those older than 70 years of age, where their prevalence is anywhere from 10% to 25% (10).

Antinuclear Antibodies

Antinuclear antibodies (ANAs), measured by immunofluorescence techniques, are present in approximately 20% to 30% of patients with rheumatoid arthritis. ANAs are more common in patients with extra-articular manifestations of disease and in patients with a high titer of rheumatoid factor. In comparison with SLE, the titer of ANAs is lower in patients with rheumatoid arthritis, and antibodies to native deoxyribonucleic acid (DNA) or other specific nuclear antigens are unusual. The ANA test is usually unnecessary in a patient with typical rheumatoid arthritis unless the diagnosis is in doubt or other systemic symptoms are noted.

Serum Complement

Serum hemolytic complement (CH_{50}) and complement components C3 or C4 are usually normal or increased in patients with rheumatoid arthritis. Complement levels may be low in some patients with severe

Table 77.2. Synovial Fluid Findings in Various Arthritides[a]

Synovial Fluid Finding	Normal	Rheumatoid Arthritis	Noninflammatory Arthritis	Septic Arthritis
Color	Clear	Yellow	Clear-yellow	Variable
Clarity	Transparent	Turbid	Transparent	Opaque
Leukocytes (per mm^3)	<150	2,000–75,000	<2,000	>75,000
Polymorphonuclear leukocytes (%)	<25	>70	<25	>75

[a]See Chapter 74 also.

disease or systemic vasculitis. The test is most useful in helping distinguish early rheumatoid arthritis from immune complex–mediated diseases (e.g., SLE), in which serum complement components are often markedly decreased.

Synovial Fluid

Synovial fluid should be analyzed (Table 77.2) in a patient with monarthritis or with polyarthritis and fever, or in any patient with a joint effusion in whom the diagnosis is in doubt. Also, patients with known rheumatoid arthritis who develop disproportionate pain and swelling of one joint should have fluid aspirated from that joint to rule out infection. If the physician is unfamiliar or uncomfortable with arthrocentesis (see Chapter 74), the patient should be referred to a rheumatologist or an orthopedic surgeon.

There is increased susceptibility of the rheumatoid joint to infection. Streptococcal or staphylococcal organisms are most common. Whenever a single joint flares up, or when the flare-up is accompanied by fever or follows a recent invasive procedure, synovial fluid examination is essential to rule out infection.

Recommended studies on fluid aspirated from the joint include cell count and differential, Gram stain, culture, and crystal examination. Joint fluid should be added immediately to a tube containing ethylene diamine tetra-acetic acid (EDTA, purple top) or heparin to prevent clotting and cell lysis. If the quantity of fluid is limited, priority is given first to culture, then to Gram stain, and finally to crystal examination. There is considerable variation in the total leukocyte count and in the neutrophil count in the synovial fluid of rheumatoid joints, but in general the total count in an inflamed joint exceeds 2,000 cells/mm^3 and consists predominantly of neutrophils. Occasionally, the leukocyte count exceeds 75,000 cells/mm^3, but values in this range should raise concern about infection. Other analyses, such as protein, glucose, enzymes, complement, immune complexes, rheumatoid factor, ANA, viscosity, turbidity, and mucin clot, are not recommended, because they are neither specific nor sensitive.

Radiology

X-rays are occasionally necessary to exclude diseases that mimic rheumatoid arthritis (gout, pseudogout, sarcoidosis). However, x-ray changes require sufficient time (months) to evolve into a characteristic pattern, limiting their usefulness early in the course of the disease. Significant cartilage damage caused by inflammation occurs before radiographic changes can be observed. Radiographic studies should be obtained if there is suspicion of structural or traumatic damage to the bone or joint. They are of value also in determining the course of the erosive process (Fig. 77.3). However, it is recommended that the primary care physician seek the counsel of the rheumatology consultant when using serial radiographs to guide therapeutic decisions.

X-ray findings vary in rheumatoid arthritis depending on the duration and severity of the illness. Early in the disease, radiographs may show nothing other than soft tissue swelling. Thereafter, periarticular osteopenia may develop, most noticeably in the small joints of the hands, wrists, and feet. With progression of the disease, loss of cartilage causes narrowing of the joint space and juxta-articular erosions appear at the point of attachment of the synovium. In end-stage disease, large cystic erosions of bone may be seen. Bony proliferation may occur because of degenerative changes that follow inflammation. These changes are in contrast to the bony hypertrophy (osteophytes), sclerosis, and fusion seen in patients with osteoarthritis (see Chapter 75).

Special x-ray studies are helpful in certain situations. *MRI* is useful to define possible internal joint derangement or injury to a supporting structure, such as a torn rotator cuff of the shoulder or meniscal tears of the knee. MRI has largely replaced arthrography for the diagnosis of these problems. Computed tomography (CT) or MRI is important in the evaluation of cord compression secondary to atlantoaxial (C1/C2) subluxation.

Biopsies

Synovial biopsy is rarely necessary in the diagnosis of rheumatoid arthritis. Similarly, biopsy of a nodule (described later) is indicated only to distinguish it from another process (e.g., a tumor).

EXTRA-ARTICULAR DISEASE

Although the joints are almost always the principal focus of the rheumatoid arthritis, other organ systems may also be involved (11). Extra-articular manifestations of rheumatoid arthritis (Table 77.3, p. 1156) occur most often in seropositive patients with more severe joint disease. Extra-articular manifestations can occur in later stages of the disease, when there is little active synovitis ("burnt-out" disease). In contrast to the predilection of rheumatoid arthritis for women,

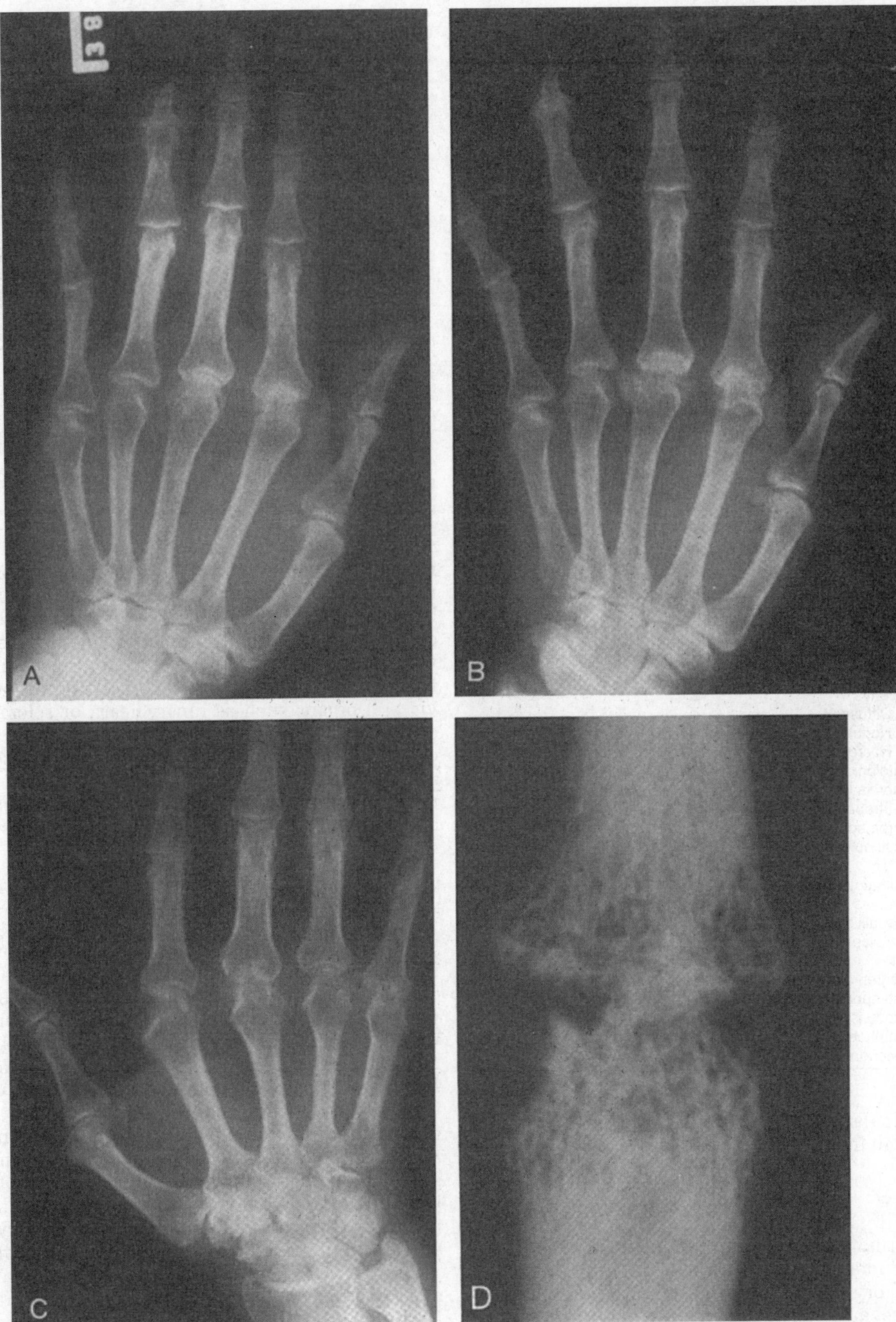

Figure 77.3. Radiographic changes in rheumatoid arthritis. **A:** Early joint space narrowing in the second and third metacarpophalangeal (MCP) joints. **B:** Cystic changes, erosions, and further bony proliferation in the second and third MCP joints. **C:** Periarticular osteoporosis, most noticeable in the interphalangeal joints, and numerous marginal erosions and cysts in the carpal bones and metacarpal heads. **D:** Juxta-articular erosions in a proximal interphalangeal joint.

Table 77.3. Systemic Manifestations of Rheumatoid Arthritis (Rheumatoid Disease)

- I. General
  - A. Fever
  - B. Fatigue, malaise, diffuse stiffness
  - C. Adenopathy
  - D. Splenomegaly
- II. Pulmonary
  - A. Pleuritis (± effusion)
  - B. Intrapulmonary nodules
  - C. Interstitial pneumonitis
  - D. Rheumatoid pneumoconiosis (Caplan syndrome)
  - E. Pulmonary fibrosis
  - F. Arteritis (rare)
- III. Cardiovascular
  - A. Heart
    - 1. Pericarditis, effusion, tamponade, constriction
    - 2. Myocarditis
    - 3. Endocarditis, including valvulitis
    - 4. Rheumatoid nodule (conduction defects)
  - B. Peripheral
    - 1. Vasculitis or arteritis
- IV. Nervous system
  - A. Peripheral neuropathy (mononeuritis multiplex)—sensory, motor, or both
  - B. Central nervous system
    - 1. Spinal cord lesion
      - a. Vascular thrombosis
      - b. Rheumatoid nodule
    - 2. Intracranial
      - a. Arteritis (rare)
      - b. Rheumatoid nodule (rare)
- V. Ocular
  - A. Keratoconjunctivitis (Sjögren syndrome)
  - B. Episcleritis (simple or nodular)
  - C. Scleritis
    - 1. Diffuse
    - 2. Nodular (scleromalacia perforans)
    - 3. Necrotizing
- VI. Hematologic
  - A. Anemia (chronic disease)
  - B. Neutropenia (Felty syndrome)
  - C. Thrombocytosis
  - D. Eosinophilia
- VII. Skin
  - A. Palmar erythema
  - B. Nodules
  - C. Vasculitic lesions
  - D. Leg ulcers (Felty syndrome)
- VIII. Others
  - A. Sjögren syndrome
  - B. Osteoporosis
  - C. Hyperviscosity
  - D. Lymphoma
  - E. Secondary amyloidosis (controversial)

extra-articular manifestations of the disease are more common in men.

Rheumatoid Nodules

Although not specific for rheumatoid arthritis (nodules with identical pathology may be seen in patients with SLE or rheumatic fever), the subcutaneous nodule is the most characteristic extra-articular lesion (Fig. 77.4). Nodules occur in 20% to 30% of cases, almost exclusively in seropositive patients. They vary in size from a few millimeters to several centimeters and are either fixed to surrounding tissue or freely movable beneath the skin. They are located most commonly on the extensor surfaces of the arms and elbows but are also prone to develop at pressure points on the feet and knees. Rheumatoid nodules may arise within tendons or ligaments and can cause joint dysfunction or tendon rupture. Rarely, nodules arise in visceral organs such as lungs, heart, or sclera of the eye. Wherever their location, nodules usually persist even with a remission in joint inflammation. Occasionally nodules regress spontaneously. Although the are usually asymptomatic, nodules can become painful, erode underlying bone, or ulcerate, requiring surgical excision.

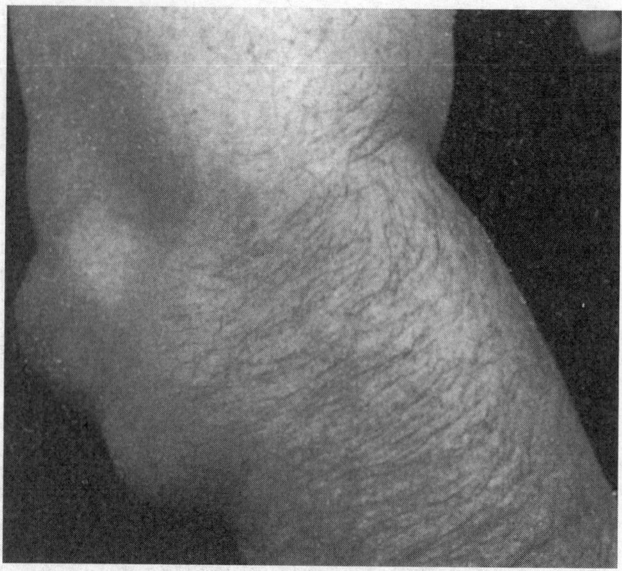

Figure 77.4. Rheumatoid nodules along the extensor surface of the forearm.

Pleuropulmonary Disease

There are several pulmonary manifestations of rheumatoid arthritis, including pleurisy with or without effusion, intrapulmonary nodules, rheumatoid pneumoconiosis (Caplan syndrome), diffuse interstitial fibrosis, and, rarely, bronchiolitis obliterans, pneumothorax, or pulmonary arteritis (12). On pulmonary function testing, there commonly is a restrictive ventilatory defect with reduced lung volumes and a decreased diffusing capacity for carbon monoxide. Although the issue is controversial, most rheumatologists believe that rheumatoid arthritis does not cause intrathoracic obstructive airway disease. Extrathoracic upper airway obstruction may occur secondary to involvement of the cricoarytenoid joints of the larynx.

Pulmonary involvement may precede by months the onset of arthritis. Pleurisy, the most common problem, is clinically apparent in 5% of patients, but pleural thickening and inflammation is found in 50% of autopsy cases. Pleural effusions, either unilateral or bilateral, are usually exudates. Even in transudates the glucose concentration of the fluid is usually low (less than 30 mg/100 mL), a finding otherwise seen only in pleural space infections. The first approach to the management of a pleural effusion includes a diagnostic aspiration and pleural biopsy to exclude infection and malignancy.

Rheumatoid nodules in the lung are usually asymptomatic, but cavitation simulating cancer or infection may occur. Therefore, appropriate diagnostic steps should be taken to ensure that an isolated pleural or pulmonary nodule is in fact rheumatoid in origin.

Interstitial pneumonitis or a fibrosing mononuclear alveolitis precedes progressive pulmonary fibrosis, the most severe form of rheumatoid lung disease. Fine dry rales are heard on auscultation of the lung, and reticulonodular infiltrates are seen on chest radiographs. This process is more common among patients who smoke.

Case reports have reported success in treating rheumatoid lung with glucocorticoids and a variety of immunosuppressive regimens including methotrexate, cyclosporin, cyclophosphamide, and azathioprine. There is no information, however, from controlled clinical trials. Patients with symptomatic pleural or pulmonary manifestations of rheumatoid arthritis should be monitored in consultation with a rheumatologist and pulmonologist.

Cardiac Disease

Pericarditis is the most common cardiac manifestation of rheumatoid arthritis (13). Echocardiographic studies demonstrate pericardial effusion in 55% of patients with subcutaneous nodules and 15% of patients who do not have nodules. Patients with symptomatic pericarditis usually present with fever, chest pain, and a pericardial rub that resolve spontaneously. Recurrent or persistent pericardial disease, complicated by tamponade or constriction, is rare. Other unusual cardiac manifestations include nonspecific valvulitis, nodule formation in a valve cusp, myocarditis, and conduction abnormalities secondary to nodule formation in the heart. The treatment of patients with symptomatic cardiac disease is best done in consultation with a rheumatologist and cardiologist.

Ocular Disease

Keratoconjunctivitis of Sjögren syndrome is the most common ocular manifestation of rheumatoid arthritis (see later discussion and Chapter 109). Episcleritis occurs occasionally and is manifested by mild pain and intense redness of the affected eye. Ordinarily, episcleritis is a self-limited process of a few weeks' duration. Scleritis and corneal ulcerations are rarer but more serious problems. Unlike episcleritis, scleritis is a slowly progressive, often bilateral process that may lead to perforation and loss of vision. It is characterized by nodularity, intense redness, and often severe pain. The distinction between episcleritis and scleritis is difficult (see Chapter 109), and all patients with a red, painful eye should be referred to an ophthalmologist.

Neurologic Disease

The most common neurologic manifestation of rheumatoid arthritis is a mild, primarily sensory *peripheral neuropathy* that usually is more marked in the lower extremities. Entrapment neuropathies (e.g., carpal tunnel syndrome, tarsal tunnel syndrome) sometimes occur in patients with rheumatoid arthritis because of compression of a peripheral nerve by inflamed, swollen tissue (see Chapter 92). Cervical myelopathy secondary to atlantoaxial subluxation is an uncommon but particularly worrisome complication potentially causing permanent, even fatal neurologic damage. Approximately 30% of patients with rheumatoid arthritis in a referral practice had atlantoaxial subluxation without symptoms, but very few of them developed neurologic dysfunction (see Ruddy, et al., in General References). Specific studies of the cervical spine (e.g., CT, MRI) are not indicated unless symptoms (pain, paresthesias, weakness) or neurologic signs are present. However, cervical spine studies and neurosurgical consultation should be sought at the first sign of cord compression. A patient with rheumatoid arthritis who may have sustained cervical injury or is at risk for a neck manipulation (e.g., during general anesthesia) should have flexion/extension cervical spine radiographs so that special caution can be exercised if subluxation, even without symptoms, is present.

Lymphoid Hyperplasia

Lymphadenopathy, either local or generalized, occurs in 25% or more of patients with rheumatoid arthritis. The nodes are nontender, firm, and freely movable. Although the diagnosis of lymphoma is sometimes considered, the process almost always proves to be benign. When examined by biopsy, the nodes show a proliferation of normal plasma cells. Splenomegaly occurs more rarely (5% to 10% of patients), usually in association with lymphadenopathy.

Felty Syndrome

Felty syndrome is characterized by rheumatoid arthritis, splenomegaly, and leukopenia–predominantly granulocytopenia (14). Patients with this syndrome usually are older, have a high titer of rheumatoid factor and ANA, have severe arthritis, and have other extra-articular manifestations of the disease. Recurrent bacterial infections and chronic refractory leg ulcers are the major complications. Patients with suspected Felty syndrome should see a rheumatologist urgently, because therapy is difficult and must be aggressive (see later discussion).

Rheumatoid Vasculitis

Evidence of vasculitis is found in 10% to 25% of autopsy patients with rheumatoid arthritis. The most common clinical manifestations of vasculitis are small digital infarcts along the nailbeds. In fewer than 1% of patients, a syndrome of accelerated vasculitis is seen. It is characterized by distal cutaneous ulcerations, gangrene, peripheral polyneuropathy, and visceral (intestinal, renal, cardiac, cerebral) ischemia. The abrupt onset of an ischemic mononeuropathy (mononeuritis multiplex) or progressive scleritis is typical of rheumatoid vasculitis. The syndrome ordinarily emerges after years of seropositive, persistently active rheumatoid arthritis; however, vasculitis may occur when joints are inactive. Immediate consultation with a rheumatologist and immunosuppressive therapy (discussed later) are usually indicated.

Sjögren Syndrome

Approximately 10% to 15% of patients with rheumatoid arthritis, mostly women, develop Sjögren syndrome, a chronic inflammatory disorder characterized by lymphocytic infiltration of lacrimal and salivary glands. This leads to impaired secretion of saliva and tears and results in the *sicca complex*: dry mouth (xerostomia) and dry eyes (keratoconjunctivitis sicca). Patients should use lubricating eye drops, be monitored by an ophthalmologist to prevent corneal ulcerations, and be monitored closely by a dentist to prevent dental caries. Artificial saliva preparations are available but are often disliked by patients because of their taste. Oral pilocarpine derivatives (Salagen, Evoxac) are also available for xerostomia but carry the troublesome side effect of hyperhidrosis.

Other exocrine glands can be affected, manifested clinically as dry skin, decreased perspiration, dry vaginal membranes, or a nonproductive cough. Commonly, there is also a polyclonal lymphoproliferative reaction, characterized by lymphadenopathy and occasionally splenomegaly. This can mimic and, rarely, transform into a malignant lymphoma. Sjögren syndrome may also be associated with a number of other systemic manifestations, including vasculitis, peripheral neuropathy, and thyroiditis.

COURSE

The course of rheumatoid arthritis, like that of most chronic diseases, cannot be predicted in a given patient. Several patterns of activity have been described: a spontaneous remission, particularly in the seronegative patient; recurrent explosive attacks followed by periods of quiescence, most commonly in the early phases; and the usual pattern of persistent and progressive disease activity that waxes and wanes in intensity.

A self-limited course with spontaneous remission is thought to occur in fewer than 10% of patients and is unlikely to occur after 6 months of active disease. Rarely, the inflammatory process is rapidly destructive, leading to early loss of function and disability. A few patients have a course that is characterized by remissions and exacerbations, often with months or even years during which they are asymptomatic. Most patients develop a more typical sustained, progressive course with persistent symptoms that vary in intensity. Paradoxically, patients who have an abrupt onset of their disease have a better prognosis than those with an indolent presentation. Patients almost always go into remission during pregnancy, but usually disease activity returns several weeks after childbirth. Although current medications are helpful to control the inflammatory process, fewer than 2% of patients demonstrate a sustained remission attributable to drugs. Patients with persistent signs of inflammation develop radiologic signs of joint damage within a 2-year period.

Significant morbidity from rheumatoid arthritis has long been recognized. Approximately 60% of the patients with rheumatoid arthritis were unable to work 10 years after the onset of their disease (15). Only recently, however, have studies demonstrated an increased mortality rate in rheumatoid patients. Median life expectancy was shortened by an average of 7 years for men and 3 years for women, compared with control populations, and in more than 5,000 patients with rheumatoid arthritis from four centers the mortality rate was two times greater than in the control population (16). Patients at *higher risk* for shortened survival are those with systemic extra-articular involvement, low functional capacity, low socioeconomic status, low education, and long-term prednisone use.

DIFFERENTIAL DIAGNOSIS

The difficulty of diagnosing early rheumatoid arthritis emphasizes the importance of a systematic approach to patients with arthritis (Table 77.4). Age, sex, ethnic background, and family history of the patient influence the likelihood of disease. Therefore, a clear definition of host features forms a framework to begin the evaluation of the patient with arthritis. Table 77.5 outlines examples of the differential diagnosis of polyarthritis based on age and sex. Other important factors include the patient's occupation, habits, drug usage, and medical history (Table 77.6). Finally, the characteristics of the arthritis itself provide important clues to the differential diagnosis (Tables 77.7 and 77.8).

Table 77.4. Outline of a Diagnostic Approach to Polyarthritis

A. Define the host features
   1. Age, sex, and ethnic background
   2. Family history
   3. Environmental factors
B. Describe the joint involvement
   1. Number
   2. Patterns
   3. Specific joints
   4. Intensity of pain
   5. Course
C. Characteristics of extra-articular features
D. Supporting laboratory studies
E. Response to therapeutic trial

Table 77.5. Differential Diagnosis of Polyarthritis Based on Age and Sex

Age (yr)	Male	Both Sexes	Female
Childhood (1–15)	Juvenile ankylosing spondylitis (Chapter 78) Kawasaki syndrome[a] Hemophilia (Chapter 56)	Juvenile rheumatoid arthritis, systemic onset (Still disease)[a] Rheumatic fever[a] Leukemia[a]	Juvenile rheumatoid arthritis[a] Pauciarticular arthritis[a] Juvenile rheumatoid arthritis, polyarthritis onset[a]
Young adult (15–30)	Ankylosing spondylitis (Chapter 78) Reiter syndrome (Chapter 78) "Reactive" arthritis[a] (Chapter 76) Behçet syndrome[a]	Psoriatic arthritis (Chapter 116) Lyme disease (Chapter 38) Inflammatory bowel disease (Chapter 46)	Systemic lupus erythematosus[a] Gonococcal arthritis (Chapter 37) Scleroderma[a]
Middle years (30–60)	Gout (Chapter 76) Palindromic rheumatism[a] Whipple disease[a]	Seronegative polyarthritis (Chapter 77) Hypersensitivity reactions (Chapter 30) Vasculitic syndromes[a] Relapsing polychondritis[a]	Rheumatoid arthritis Sjögren syndrome Sarcoidosis[a] Polymyositis[a] Erosive osteoarthritis (Chapter 75)
Elderly (60+)	Diffuse idiopathic skeletal hyperostosis (DISH) (Chapter 75) Hypertrophic pulmonary osteoarthropathy (HPO) (Chapter 61)	Pseudogout (Chapter 76) Polymyalgia rheumatica (Chapter 74) Tumor-related syndromes Secondary osteoarthritis (Chapter 75) Metabolic disorders	Primary generalized osteoarthritis (Chapter 75)

[a]These conditions are not discussed in this book. Information about them is contained in the General References at the end of this chapter.

Table 77.6. Examples of Environmental Factors in Diagnosis of Arthritis

Factor	Disease
Occupation	
Bartender	Gout (Chapter 76)
Health worker	Hepatitis (Chapter 47)
Athlete	Secondary osteoarthritis (Chapter 75)
Outdoor worker	Lyme disease (Chapter 38)
Gardener	Sporotrichosis[a]
Deep sea diver	Aseptic necrosis of bone[a]
Habits	
Alcohol abuse	Gout (Chapter 76), aseptic necrosis[a]
"Moonshine" ingestion	Saturnine gout (Chapter 76)
Smoking	Hypertrophic osteoarthropathy (Chapter 61)
Intravenous drug abuse	Septic arthritis, hepatitis, vasculitis
Sexual promiscuity	Gonococcal arthritis (Chapter 37) hepatitis (Chapter 47), Reiter syndrome (Chapter 78)
Drugs	
Diuretics	Gout (Chapter 76)
Corticosteroids	Aseptic necrosis[a]
Hydralazine, procainamide	Systemic lupus erythematosus[a]
Any drug	Hypersensitivity reactions (Chapter 30)

[a]These conditions are not discussed in this book. Information about them is contained in the General References at the end of this chapter.

MANAGEMENT

General Principles

Rheumatoid arthritis is a chronic disorder for which there is no known cure. It therefore requires a comprehensive program that combines medical, social, and emotional support for the patient. An understanding of each patient's specific problems is essential. Serial observations (Table 77.9) and in-depth investigation of the impact of the disease on both the patient and the patient's family provide the basis for effective management.

The major goals of treatment of the arthritis are to reduce pain and discomfort, prevent deformities and loss of joint function, and maintain a productive and active life. To achieve these goals, an understanding of the cause of pain and joint destruction is important. In rheumatoid arthritis, pain and dysfunction are caused by acute inflammation and subsequent mechanical and structural joint abnormalities. Acute inflammation is always the major problem in early disease. Mechanical and structural abnormalities do not ordinarily develop until later in the course of the disease. Each of these processes warrants a different therapeutic approach. Often both are present, although, depending on the stage of disease, one process may predominate.

Management begins with effective communication between physician and patient. It is essential that the patient and the patient's family be educated about the nature and course of the disease; the specific causes of the pain; and the goals, problems, and expectations of treatment. Chronic arthritis is a major emotional and physical stress that often requires a major change in lifestyle. Misunderstanding about the disease and the setting of inappropriate goals lead to frustration and depression. Clinical trials of education in rheumatoid arthritis have documented improved functional ability, reduction in tender joint counts, and improved patient compliance with effective patient education (17,18).

In addition to laboratory testing and physical examination, a simple self-report questionnaire has been shown to be an effective, inexpensive method to assess the patient's status and response to treatment (19) (Fig. 77.5, p. 1161). The questionnaire can assess functional status, which reflects both mechanical and inflammatory problems.

Treatment options include reduction of joint stress, physical and occupational therapy, drug therapy, and surgical intervention.

Reduction of joint stress is accomplished by a number of practical measures that do not depend on the use of drugs. Because obesity stresses the musculoskeletal system, ideal body weight should be achieved and maintained. Rest, in general, is an important feature of

Table 77.7. Assessment of Joint Involvement

Number		
Monarthritis	***Oligoarthritis* (2–4 joints)**	***Polyarthritis* (≥5 joints)**
Septic arthritis	Reiter syndrome	Rheumatoid arthritis
Gout	Inflammatory bowel disease	Systemic lupus erythematosus[a]
Pseudogout	Psoriatic arthritis	Serum sickness
Other crystals	Rheumatic fever[a]	Psoriatic arthritis
Local tumor[a]	Juvenile rheumatoid arthritis[a]	Tophaceous gout
Patterns		
Symmetric	***Asymmetric***	
Rheumatoid arthritis	Psoriatic arthritis	
Serum sickness	Reiter syndrome	
Systemic lupus erythematosus[a]	Gout, pseudogout	
Intensity of Pain		
Severe	***Moderate***	
Septic arthritis	All others, including rheumatoid arthritis	
Microcrystalline arthritis		
Course		
Acute	Infection, gout, pseudogout	
Chronic	Psoriatic arthritis, rheumatoid arthritis, ankylosing spondylitis	
Additive	Rheumatoid arthritis	
Migratory	Rheumatic fever,[a] systemic lupus erythematosus[a]	
Evanescent	Systemic lupus erythematosus,[a] viral[a]	
Episodic	Gout, pseudogout, palindromic rheumatism[a]	

[a]These conditions are not discussed in this book. Information about them is contained in the General References at the end of this chapter.

Table 77.8. Diagnostic Clues Provided by Arthritis of Specific Joints

First metatarsal (podagra)	Gout
Knee (acute, episodic)	Pseudogout
Distal Interphalangeal	Psoriatic arthritis Osteoarthritis
Metacarpals, wrist, metatarsals	Rheumatoid arthritis
Sausaged digits	Reiter syndrome Psoriatic arthritis Sarcoidosis
Sacroiliac	Ankylosing spondylitis Reiter syndrome Psoriatic arthritis Inflammatory bowel disease
Sternoclavicular	Septic arthritis Polymyalgia rheumatica
Heel/ankle	Reiter syndrome

Table 77.9. Observations to be Made Serially in Patients with Rheumatoid Arthritis

Duration of morning stiffness
Degree of fatigue
Limitations of function
Patient assessment of pain
Number of joints that are painful on passive motion or tender
Degree of swelling of affected joints

management (20). Eight to nine hours' sleep at night and a 2-hour rest period in the middle of the day are reasonable recommendations for everyone with active disease. When the joints are actively inflamed, vigorous activity (heavy work, brisk exercise) should be avoided because of the danger of intensifying joint inflammation or causing traumatic injury to structures weakened by inflammation. On the other hand, patients should be urged to maintain a modest level of activity to prevent joint laxity and muscular atrophy. Splinting of acutely inflamed joints, particularly at night, and the use of walking aids (canes, walkers) are all effective means of reducing stress on specific joints. Specially designed furniture and household utensils can help not only to relieve stress on joints but also to maintain independent function. Such aids are provided on recommendation of the consultant rheumatologist, orthopedist, physiatrist, physical therapist, or occupational therapist and are obtained from an orthotics appliance store.

A consultation with a *physical therapist* and an *occupational therapist* is recommended early in the course of treating a patient with rheumatoid arthritis. These therapists can effectively design a program of balanced rest and activity that is appropriate for the stage of the disease. Passive exercise (moving the joints through a full range of motion) is used when inflammation is active and poorly controlled. An active exercise program, when tolerated, can be designed to prevent contractures and muscular atrophy. The application of local heat, the use of various supporting aids, education in joint protection, and maintenance of good joint function are all part of the therapist's role.

Wet or dry local heat gives transient symptomatic relief of pain and stiffness, particularly to patients with chronic synovitis. A hot shower in the morning, coupled with passive warm-up exercises, may relieve stiffness and help the patient to get the day started.

Drug Treatment

Three general classes of drugs are commonly used in the treatment of rheumatoid arthritis: NSAIDs,

	Without Any Difficulty	With Some Difficulty	With Much Difficulty	Unable to Do
A. Dress yourself, including tying shoelaces and doing buttons?	______	______	______	______
B. Get in and out of bed?	______	______	______	______
C. Lift a full cup or glass to your mouth?	______	______	______	______
D. Walk outdoors on flat ground?	______	______	______	______
E. Wash and dry your entire body?	______	______	______	______
F. Bend down to pick up clothing from the floor?	______	______	______	______
G. Turn regular faucets on and off?	______	______	______	______
H. Get in and out of a car?	______	______	______	______

Figure 77.5. Self-report questionnaire used to quantitatively assess the functional capacity of the patient to accomplish activities of daily living.

corticosteroids, and disease-modifying antirheumatic drugs (DMARDs). NSAIDs and corticosteroids have a short onset of action, whereas DMARDs can take several weeks or months to demonstrate a clinical effect. Commonly used DMARDs include hydroxychloroquine, sulfasalazine, methotrexate, leflunomide, and the TNF inhibitors, etanercept and infliximab.

In the past, these drugs were prescribed in a stepwise fashion, starting with less toxic, generally less potent agents and moving to more toxic and potent agents. However, because NSAIDs appear to have little effect on the progression of the disease and because cartilage damage and bony erosions often occur early (within the first 2 years), rheumatologists now move more aggressively to a DMARD soon after the diagnosis is secure. Low-dose corticosteroids (less than 10 mg/day of prednisone) are used for patients who are disabled or significantly symptomatic while DMARD therapy is initiated. However, the physician should always try to lower the dosage of prednisone to the minimum consistent with control of synovitis.

The inflammatory process of rheumatoid arthritis involves complicated interactions of immunologic and inflammatory mediators. No single therapeutic agent currently exists to interrupt these interactions permanently. Only approximately 2% of patients have an initial remission of rheumatoid arthritis in response to a DMARD, and only approximately 10% of those patients stay in remission for longer than 3 years. For an individual patient, response to therapy can be variable and even the most successful therapies can become ineffective over time. Many patients with long-standing disease have had multiple unsuccessful trials of DMARDs, which is frustrating for both patient and physician.

Rheumatoid arthritis has a major impact on earning, functional capacity, and life span (see earlier discussion). Each therapeutic decision must be weighed in light of the potential risks and benefits, in both the long and the short term. Consultation with a rheuma-

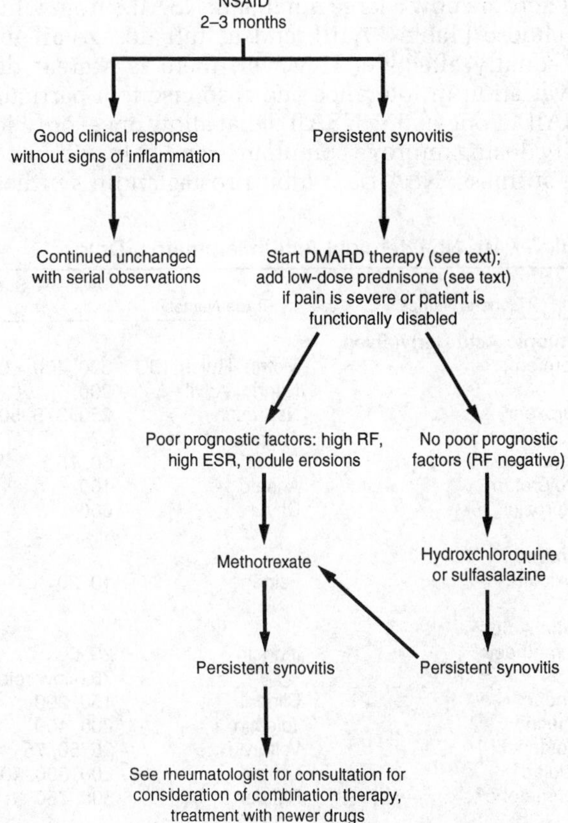

Figure 77.6. Suggested approach to drug treatment in rheumatoid arthritis.

tologist is important so that an appropriately aggressive drug treatment program can be established in the early phases of the disease (Fig. 77.6). Decisions must be made jointly with the patient and must incorporate patient expectations, comorbid medical problems, and the preservation of function. Detailed reviews of all drugs used in treating patients with rheumatoid arthritis are available (see Ruddy, et al., in General References).

Nonsteroidal Anti-inflammatory Drugs

In the presence of acute or chronic inflammation, it is appropriate first to prescribe NSAIDs. These drugs should always be used in conjunction with the general modalities of rest, heat, and joint protection. The major effect of these agents is to reduce acute inflammation, thereby decreasing pain and improving function. All of these drugs have mild to moderate analgesic properties independent of their anti-inflammatory effect.

Aspirin is the oldest drug of the nonsteroidal class. However, because of its higher rate of GI toxicity, the narrow window between toxic and anti-inflammatory serum levels, and the inconvenience of multiple daily doses, aspirin has largely been replaced by newer NSAIDs. Nonacetylated salicylates (Disalcid, Trilisate) are less potent anti-inflammatory agents but have the advantage of less GI toxicity, lack of inhibition of platelet aggregation, and decreased incidence of NSAID-induced angioedema reactions.

There are now a large number of NSAIDs from which to choose (Table 77.10), and at full dosage all may be equally effective. However, there is a great deal of variation in tolerance and response to a particular NSAID. Long-acting NSAIDs that allow once- or twice-daily dosing improve compliance and help with morning stiffness. NSAIDs inhibit prostaglandin synthesis by blocking cyclooxygenase enzymes. Prostaglandins are important mediators of pain and inflammation. There exist two isoforms of cyclooxygenase, COX-1 and COX-2. COX-1 is expressed under basal conditions in the stomach, platelets, and kidney. Because of its tissue localization, COX-1 is thought to play physiologic roles in gastric cytoprotection, platelet aggregation, and sodium and water balance. COX-2 expression is highly restricted under basal conditions and is induced in inflammatory cells by inflammatory or noxious stimuli. Prostaglandins produced by COX-2 mediate symptoms of pain, inflammation, and fever. The selective COX-2 inhibitors (celecoxib, rofecoxib) have been shown to be equally as efficacious as the older, nonselective NSAIDs, with less GI toxicity and without effect on platelet aggregation (21,22).

Dosage. If there is active inflammation, a full dosage of an NSAID should be prescribed (Table 77.10). A lower dosage should initially be used if inflammation is mild, mechanical pain is the major problem, the patient is elderly, or the patient suffers from conditions that increase the risk for toxicity (discussed later). If a particular preparation is ineffective after a 4-week trial or is not tolerated, another NSAID can be initiated. An individual patient's response to NSAIDs in both tolerance and effectiveness is unpredictable and varied. One should become familiar with a few of these agents rather than trying to master all available NSAIDs. Combinations of NSAIDs should be avoided,

Table 77.10. Nonsteroidal Anti-Inflammatory Drugs

Generic Names	Trade Names	Available Strengths (mg)	Recommended Dosage and Schedule	Maximal Daily Dosage (mg/day)
Propionic Acid Derivatives				
Ibuprofen[a]	Motrin, Rufen, IBU	300, 400, 600, 800	600–800 mg t.i.d.–q.i.d.	3,200
	Nuprin, Advil	200		
Naproxen[a]	Naprosyn	250, 375, 500	500 mg b.i.d	1,000
	Anaprox, Aleve	275		
Ketoprofen[a]	Orudis	50, 75	50 mg t.i.d.–q.i.d. or 75 mg t.i.d.	300
Flurbiprofen[a]	Ansaid	100	100 mg b.i.d.–t.i.d.	300
Oxaprozin[a]	Daypro	600	600–1,200 mg q.d.	1,200
Oxicams				
Piroxicam[a]	Feldene	10, 20	10–20 mg/day	20
Acetic Acids				
Indomethacin[a]	Indocin	25, 50	50 mg t.i.d.–q.i.d.	150–200
		75 (slow release)	q.d.– b.i.d.	
Sulindac[a]	Clinoril	150, 200	150–200 mg b.i.d.	400
Tolmetin[a]	Tolectin	200, 400	400 mg t.i.d.–q.i.d.	2,000
Diclofenac[a]	Voltaren	25, 50, 75	50 mg b.i.d.–t.i.d. or 75 mg b.i.d.	150
Etodolac[a]	Lodine	200, 300, 400, 500	200–400 mg t.i.d.	1,200
Nabumetone[a]	Relafen	500, 750	1,000–2,000 mg q.d.	2,000
Pyrazoles				
Ketorolac tromethamine	Toradol	10	10 mg q4–6h	Use only short periods
Nonacetylated Salicylates				
Diflurisal	Dolobid	250, 500	250–500 mg b.i.d.	1,000
Magnesium choline salicylate[a]	Trilisate	500, 750, 1,000	1,500 mg b.i.d.	3,000
Salsalate[a]	Disalcid	500, 750	1,500 mg b.i.d.	3,000
Cyclooxygenase-2 Inhibitors				
Celecoxib	Celebrex	100, 200	100–200 mg b.i.d.	400
Rofecoxib	Vioxx	12.5, 25, 50	12.5–25 mg b.i.d., 50 mg q.d. for acute pain	25

[a]Approved for use in rheumatoid arthritis.

Table 77.11. Side Effects of Nonsteroidal Anti-Inflammatory Drugs

	Approximate Incidence
Gastrointestinal	10%–20%
Epigastric pain, nausea	
Anorexia, dyspepsia, peptic ulceration	
Overt or occult bleeding	<1%
Hypersensitivity Reactions	1%–5%
Rashes, rarely Stevens–Johnson syndrome	
Very rarely, anaphylactoid reactions	
Aggravation of Allergic Rhinitis or Asthma	10% of sufferers
Renal Effects	>5%
Transient renal failure	
Water and salt retention	
Hypokalemia, inhibit diuretic action	
Interstitial nephritis, nephrotic syndrome	>1%
Hepatic Effects	5%–15%
Cholestatic hepatitis	
Central Nervous System	>5%
Tinnitus/deafness	Primarily aspirin
Headache, vertigo, confusion	Higher with indomethacin
Others	
Diarrhea	10%–15% (mefenamic acid, other fenamates)
Aggravation of congestive heart failure, angina	>1%
Toxic amblyopia	<1% (ibuprofen)

because studies show that combinations do not increase effectiveness but toxicities are additive.

Usual Time to Maximal Effect. Although these agents have therapeutic blood levels and analgesic effect within hours after the first dose, anti-inflammatory effects may take 2 to 4 weeks. In the absence of side effects, a reasonable trial period is 1 month.

Side Effects. The most common toxicity of NSAIDs is gastrointestinal (GI) disturbance (23–25) (Table 77.11). The term *NSAID gastropathy* describes a variety of gastric lesions, including mucosal erythema, gastric erosions, and frank ulcerations. NSAIDs also increase the risk of bleeding from the lower GI tract. Life-threatening bleeding may occur and does so more commonly in elderly patients (26). The gastropathy is caused by dose-related direct damage to the gastric mucosa and the blocking of locally produced protective prostaglandins. The patient should be carefully monitored for GI symptoms and evidence of GI blood loss. Patients at risk for NSAID gastropathy should be started on lower doses of NSAIDs and titrated to an effective dose.

A selective COX-2 inhibitor should be used in patients who are at increased risk for NSAID-induced gastropathy. Included in this group are patients with a history of peptic ulcer disease, patients with a history of GI bleeding, patients with bleeding diatheses, patients taking prednisone, and, perhaps, the elderly. COX-2 therapy might also be considered for patients taking warfarin who require an NSAID. In large studies, by comparison with nonselective NSAIDs, patients receiving COX-2 agents had roughly half the rate of GI perforation, symptomatic ulceration, and bleeding (21,22). It should be noted that the gastropathy is not completely eliminated with the use of the COX-2 agents, and continued caution needs to be exercised in patients at risk for GI bleeding. The advantage of lesser GI toxicity seen with the COX-2 inhibitors is diminished in patients who are taking low-dose aspirin for cardiovascular prophylaxis. Because COX-2 agents lack antiplatelet effects, low-dose aspirin should be taken concomitantly with a COX-2 inhibitor in patients who require cardiovascular prophylaxis. In clinical trials, higher rates of cardiovascular morbidity were seen when low-dose aspirin was discontinued (27). Alternatives to the use of a COX-2 inhibitor in patients who are at greater risk of GI morbidity include the use of a nonselective NSAID together with misoprostol (Cytotec), a prostaglandin analog, which has been shown to decrease endoscopic NSAID gastropathy (28). However, the drug is often associated with abdominal cramping and diarrhea. Use of a proton pump inhibitor may also decrease the risk of NSAID gastropathy (29). Although they improve GI tolerance and decrease dyspepsia, sulcrafate and histamine-2 blockers do not appear to significantly decrease the risk of GI bleeding.

Renal Side Effects. Because prostaglandins play a role in the regulation of renal blood flow and maintenance of glomerular filtration, NSAIDs can impair renal function in certain patients. Patients at highest risk are those with fluid imbalances or compromised renal function (e.g., heart failure, diuretic use, cirrhosis, dehydration, renal insufficiency) (30). If NSAIDs are prescribed for such patients, renal function should be monitored beginning soon after NSAID therapy is started with serial measurements of serum creatinine. Urinalysis is usually normal. The drugs should be stopped if there is a rise in serum creatinine or increased edema. Usually, the creatinine level returns to normal within 1 or 2 weeks. Rarely, an interstitial nephritis develops in association with a sustained rise in serum creatinine and eosinophiluria. The selective COX-2 inhibitors appear to have renal side effects similar to those of nonselective NSAIDs.

Fewer than 5% of patients develop a hypersensitivity reaction, usually a rash, to an NSAID. This reaction is usually specific to a particular drug, so another NSAID of a different class can be substituted. Rarely, an anaphylactoid reaction or worsening asthma can occur (see Chapter 30) that can be intrinsic to the mechanism of prostaglandin inhibition. If anaphylaxis or worsening asthma occurs with NSAID therapy, subsequent exposure to all classes of NSAIDs (including aspirin) is contraindicated. If NSAID therapy is deemed essential in the case of anaphylaxis, an allergy consultation is recommended for evaluation and possible desensitization. Although, on a theoretical basis, a selective

Table 77.12. Nonsteroidal Anti-Inflammatory Drugs: Drug Interactions

Antacids	Reduce rate and extent of absorption of NSAIDs; variable effect.
Anticoagulants	Aspirin, and potentially all NSAIDs, increases the risk of bleeding of an anticoagulant patient.
Oral hypoglycemic drugs	NSAIDs may potentiate the activity of sulfonylurea drugs.
Digoxin	NSAIDs may increase serum concentration.
Antihypertensive/ diuretics	NSAIDs may attenuate the effect of diuretics, β-blockers, hydralazine, prazosin, angiotensin-converting enzyme inhibitors.
Lithium	Elevation of plasma lithium level may occur, particularly with indomethacin and diclofenac.
Methotrexate	Salicylate inhibits the renal clearance of methotrexate, and toxic levels may occur.
Phenytoin	NSAIDs may displace phenytoin from albumin and increase the concentration of free drug.
Probenecid	Inhibits renal clearance of several NSAIDs.
Combination of NSAIDs	Should be avoided.

NSAIDs, nonsteroidal anti-inflammatory drugs.

COX-2 inhibitor might be safe in these instances, this has not been conclusively proven.

Significant drug interactions can occur with any of the NSAIDs (Table 77.12).

Corticosteroids

In a meta-analysis of ten clinical trials using short-term low-dose corticosteroids versus placebo and NSAID therapy, daily prednisolone of 15 mg (prednisone and prednisolone are equivalent in strength) or less was found to be highly effective in controlling pain and joint tenderness (31). It is controversial, however, whether such drugs can induce actual remission (32). They can be given systemically or injected intra-articularly, depending on the clinical situation. If patients continue to have active inflammation and functional disability despite the use of an NSAID, a low dosage of a corticosteroid (e.g., prednisone less than 10 mg/day orally) can be started at the same time a DMARD is begun (see earlier discussion and Fig. 77.6). Although prednisone can be started at higher dosages (15 to 20 mg/day), attempts should be made to taper the dosage over a few weeks to less than 10 mg/day. Once started, corticosteroid therapy is difficult to discontinue, even at low dosages. Tapering of prednisone should be done slowly over a few weeks; symptoms may reoccur with small reductions in dosage. At low dosages of prednisone, patients often notice a worsening of symptoms with reductions of 1 to 2 mg/day.

Weight gain and a cushingoid appearance are a common problem and a source of patient complaints. Recent studies have raised concern over the increased cardiovascular risk and accelerated osteoporosis associated with prednisone, particularly at dosages greater than 10 mg/day (33). Because osteoporosis is more common in both men and women with rheumatoid arthritis, patients with and without osteoporosis risk factors who are receiving prednisone should undergo bone densitometry to assess fracture risk. Hormone replacement therapy (in women) and bisphosphonates (in men and women) are recommended to prevent osteoporosis (see Chapters 84 and 103). A DMARD should be added if prednisone cannot be tapered to less than 10 mg/day, if concern exists about the morbidity of low-dose prednisone, or if significant poor prognostic factors (nodules, high-titer rheumatoid factor, radiographic erosions) are present.

Higher dosages of prednisone are rarely necessary unless there is a life-threatening systemic disease, and their use for prolonged periods leads to unacceptable steroid toxicity. Although a few patients can tolerate every-other-day dosing of corticosteroids, which may reduce side effects, most require corticosteroids daily to avoid symptoms. Once-daily dosing of prednisone in the morning is associated with fewer side effects than the equivalent dosage given two or three times a day. Repetitive short courses of high-dose corticosteroids, intermittent intramuscular injections, adrenocorticotropic hormone injections, and the use of corticosteroids as the sole therapeutic agent are all to be avoided. The use of pulse therapy (methylprednisolone, 100 mg intravenously daily on three consecutive days) for management of very difficult cases is controversial and should be reserved for patients for whom other therapy has failed and those who are experiencing a great deal of functional disability. Pulse therapy should always be initiated in conjunction with a rheumatologist, because other treatment modalities should be initiated concurrently. Clinical trials show no advantage to dosing with 1 g of intravenous methylprednisolone compared with 100-mg pulse treatments (34).

Intra-articular corticosteroids (e.g., 40 mg triamcinolone in a knee, 20 mg in a shoulder, or 2 mg in a finger) are effective for controlling a local flare in one or two joints without changing the overall drug regimen. Intra-articular injections of steroids into symptomatic joints (see Chapter 74) can help limit systemic side effects. If present, joint fluid should be obtained. Based on the clinical situation, if the suspicion of infection is high, injection should be delayed until culture results become known. The injection should be administered by a rheumatologist or orthopedist if the primary physician is inexperienced with the techniques. Generally, the same joint should not be injected with steroid more than twice a year because of the danger of causing deterioration of intra-articular cartilage, although it must be recognized that uncontrolled joint inflammation can also cause rapid deterioration of cartilage.

Disease-Modifying Antirheumatic Drugs (Agents with Delayed Onset of Action)

Although both NSAIDs and DMARDs improve symptoms of active rheumatoid arthritis, DMARDs may alter the disease course and improve long-term outcomes. In recent studies, sulfasalazine, methotrexate, leflunomide, etanercept, and infliximab all significantly slowed the development of radiographic changes, joint space narrowing, and erosions. Once the diagnosis of rheumatoid arthritis is established and

Table 77.13. Toxicities and Monitoring of Commonly Used Disease-Modifying Antirheumatic Drugs

Drug	Common Toxicities	Monitoring
Hydroxychloroquine	Macular damage	Ophthalmology examination every 6 mo
Sulfasalazine	Myelosuppression, hepatotoxicity	CBC, LFTs every month for first 3 mo, then every 3 mo
Methotrexate	Myelosuppression, hepatotoxicity, interstitial pneumonitis, alopecia, oral ulcers	CBC, LFTs, creatinine every 2–3 wk until dosage is stable then every 4–8 wk
Cyclophosphamide	Myelosuppression, hemorrhagic cystitis, alopecia, secondary malignancy (bladder cancer, myeloproliferative disorders), premature ovarian failure	CBC every 1–2 wk until dosage is stable then every 1–2 mo. Urinalysis every 1–2 mo. Urinalysis and urine cytology every 6–12 mo after cessation.
Lefuonomide	Myelosuppression, hepatotoxicity	CBC, LFTs every mo
Etanercept	Infection, injection site reactions	CBC, chemistries every 3–6 mo
Infliximab	Infection, infusion reactions	CBC, chemistries every 3–6 mo

CBC, complete blood count; LFTs, liver function tests.

patients experience persistent joint pain and swelling for 2 to 3 months despite NSAID therapy, a DMARD should be started (Fig. 77.6). The development of erosions or joint space narrowing on radiographs of the involved joints is a clear indication for DMARD therapy, but one should not wait for radiographic changes to occur. The decision to use a DMARD is difficult because of the need for frequent monitoring, expense, and potential toxicity related to drugs of this class (Table 77.13).

Choice of Disease-Modifying Agent

Hydroxychloroquine and sulfasalazine have the advantage of low toxicity and therefore are generally the first DMARDs used. Although these agents are well tolerated, most patients have a modest beneficial response, and very few have a complete remission. Therefore, hydroxychloroquine and sulfasalazine are most useful in patients with mild disease who are rheumatoid factor negative and lack other poor prognostic risk factors. Either drug is usually used in combination with an NSAID, corticosteroids, or another DMARD.

Methotrexate is the most widely prescribed DMARD because of its efficacy, ease of administration, and high patient tolerability (35). Despite the introduction of the newer agents (leflunomide, etanercept, infliximab), methotrexate remains the DMARD of first choice, particularly in patients with persistent, active disease who may have poor prognostic factors such as the presence of rheumatoid factor, rheumatoid nodules, poor functional status, young age, or erosions on radiography. If patients have active disease despite sulfasalazine or hydroxychloroquine, methotrexate is often added to the regimen. In clinical trials, methotrexate has compared favorably with the new agents in efficacy, tolerability, and ability to retard radiographic changes. Because of its widespread use over many years, methotrexate holds the advantage of greater long-term safety experience. The lower cost of methotrexate provides another significant advantage.

In patients with active joint inflammation despite methotrexate therapy, consideration should be given to one of the newly approved agents—leflunomide, etanercept, or infliximab. Because these agents have not been compared against one another in controlled trials, there is little evidence to guide choice of therapy. Trials have shown that all three agents provide significant benefit for patients for whom methotrexate therapy has failed (36–38).

Leflunomide is an oral agent that inhibits pyrimidine biosynthesis. It is well tolerated and effective and has been shown to retard radiographic progression. It should be considered in patients for whom methotrexate therapy has failed (36,39).

The TNF inhibitors etanercept and infliximab are the first biologic agents approved for the treatment of rheumatoid arthritis. TNF-alpha is found at high concentrations in the rheumatoid joint and is central to the chronic inflammatory response. Produced primarily by macrophages, TNF-alpha and IL-1 stimulate synovial fibroblasts to secrete matrix-degrading proteases, as well as IL-6 and IL-8, resulting in the influx of inflammatory cells into the synovium. These activities make TNF-alpha an attractive therapeutic target in rheumatoid arthritis (40). Etanercept is a bioengineered soluble receptor for TNF-alpha that is given by self-administered subcutaneous injection. Infliximab is a chimeric monoclonal antibody directed against TNF-alpha. Both agents inhibit TNF-alpha by binding it in the circulation, preventing binding of TNF-alpha with its cellular receptors. In clinical trials, both agents were highly efficacious and well tolerated without major organ toxicity (38,40).

The role of TNF-alpha in host defense against infection is well recognized. Despite concerns, there were no increases in serious infections in the clinical trials of etanercept and infliximab. Of unclear significance are scattered reports collected by the U.S. Food and Drug Administration (FDA) postmarketing reporting system of infections (including tuberculosis, *Listeria monocytogenes*, herpes, and *Pneumocystis carinii* pneumonia) in patients treated with these agents (41). Clinicians need to be vigilant for signs and symptoms of systemic infection. The TNF inhibitors are contraindicated in immunocompromised patients and in patients with recurrent or chronic infections. All patients should be evaluated for latent TB by tuberculin skin testing and chest radiographs. Latent TB should be treated with isoniazid therapy for 6 months before anti-TNF therapy is initiated (42).

The immune system has an important role in the surveillance for malignancy, and increased risk of malignancy is a theoretical concern with chronic long-term TNF-alpha inhibition. Short-term clinical trials of TNF-alpha inhibitors have not shown an increased frequency of malignancy compared with a matched control population, but definitive answers await information being collected in registries.

Azathioprine, cyclophosphamide, intramuscular gold, oral gold, cyclosporine, and D-*penicillamine* are drugs rarely used because of their greater toxicity or inferior efficacy in comparison with other DMARDs. Cyclophosphamide continues to be used with caution in patients with severe systemic manifestations of rheumatoid arthritis (e.g., vasculitis, interstitial lung disease). Serious risks associated with cyclophosphamide therapy include premature ovarian failure, bladder cancer, hemorrhagic cystitis, and secondary hematologic malignancies. These drugs should only be used in consultation with a rheumatologist.

Combinations of DMARDs are being used with increasing frequency either initially or, more commonly, as added agents when monotherapy is ineffective. Multiple studies support the use of combination therapy over single agents. The combination of methotrexate, sulfasalazine, and hydroxychloroquine was found to be superior to methotrexate alone in a controlled trial (43). Methotrexate combinations with leflunomide, etanercept, and infliximab have all proved to be effective and well tolerated. Despite the success of these trials, questions remain whether all patients require combination therapy and the potential for increased toxicities. Patients with newly diagnosed rheumatoid arthritis are often reluctant to embark on an aggressive program with multiple medications. Combination therapy should be directed only with the consultation of a rheumatologist.

Analgesic Drugs

Pain caused by inflammation is best treated by improving the anti-inflammatory drug regimen (see earlier discussion). Short-term or occasional use of opioid therapy is acceptable to maintain function during acute flares or while therapy is being adjusted. Chronic opioid therapy is often poorly tolerated owing to side effects such as diminished mental status, hypersomnolence, and constipation, particularly in the elderly. Dependency and addiction occur infrequently, but the clinician must be alert to these behavior patterns and avoid opioid therapy in patients who have a history of substance abuse. Mechanical pain secondary to structural joint damage, including joint space narrowing, subluxation, muscle atrophy, and weakness, is best approached through nonpharmacologic modalities such as splints, joint protection, and surgery.

Characteristics of Individual Drugs

Hydroxychloroquine. Originally designed as an antimalarial agent, hydroxychloroquine is a rapidly absorbed, safe, well tolerated, and often effective DMARD in the treatment of rheumatoid arthritis. It is particularly useful as a single agent in mild to moderate disease or in combination with other DMARDs (e.g., methotrexate) in more severe disease.

Mechanism. The mechanism of action of hydroxychloroquine in the treatment of patients with rheumatoid arthritis is unknown.

Dosage. The initial dosage is 400 mg/day (6 mg/kg) and should not be exceeded. Normally it is prescribed as a single nighttime dose to avoid gastrointestinal (GI) symptoms. If a good clinical response is noted, the dosage can be lowered to a maintenance dosage of 200 mg/day.

Usual Time to Maximal Effect. A period of 3 to 6 months is usual. A 6-month period without clinical effect should be considered a drug failure.

Side Effects. The most important toxicities are ocular: corneal deposits, extraocular muscular weakness, loss of accommodation, and a retinopathy that may progress to irreversible visual loss. At the dosage recommended, these toxicities are rare, but a baseline ophthalmologic examination and a follow-up examination every 6 months are recommended during the period of treatment. GI upset, pigmentation changes, leukopenia, and a variety of neurologic side effects can also rarely be seen.

Sulfasalazine. Sulfasalazine offers an option for mild disease. Sulfapyridine is linked to salicylic acid to create salicylazosulfapyridine, the currently used agent.

Mechanism. The mode of action is unknown. Studies comparing sulfapyridine (sulfonamide) with 5-aminosalicylic acid (anti-inflammatory) suggests that the active moiety in rheumatoid arthritis is the sulfonamide.

Dosage. Toxicities are dose related, with most occurring at the higher dosages of sulfasalazine. It is suggested to begin at 500 mg/day (available in 500 mg tablets) and to increase the dosage every week in evenly divided intervals to 2 g/day. The maximal dosage of the enteric-coated preparation is 2 to 3 g/day.

Usual Time to Maximal Effect. Clinical trials show improvement within 2 months after reaching full maintenance dosages. A 4- to 6-month trial is suggested.

Side Effects. Approximately 30% of patients receiving this drug experience side effects. These may be lessened by slow upward dosing. The most common side effects are GI effects, including nausea, vomiting, anorexia, heartburn, and epigastric distress. These symptoms can be reduced by stopping the medication and adjusting the dosage downward. The enteric-coated preparation is better tolerated. GI symptoms are often accompanied by central nervous system symptoms, including headache and dizziness. Rare but more serious side effects may occur in the first 3 months of treatment, including bone marrow suppression, mucocutaneous eruptions, and hepatotoxicity. Reversible infertility can occur secondary to oligospermia. Hypersensitivity reactions can be violent, and the drug should not be used in patients with known sulfa allergy.

Monitoring should include CBC and liver function tests at 2- to 4-week intervals for 3 months, then every 6 to 12 weeks for 6 months, and thereafter every 3 months.

Methotrexate. Methotrexate is a folic acid antagonist and is the best tolerated and most efficacious DMARD available. Methotrexate therapy should be considered in patients who have active disease with risk factors for poor prognosis (see earlier discussion). Rheumatology consultation is suggested to help with the decision to start methotrexate, to guide dosage titration, and to establish a monitoring schedule.

Mechanism. Although the immunosuppressive and cytotoxic effects of methotrexate are caused by the inhibition of dihydrofolate reductase, the anti-inflammatory effects in rheumatoid arthritis appear to be unrelated to this mechanism of action. This is evidenced by the continued efficacy despite supplementation with folic acid (44). The anti-inflammatory mechanism remains unclear but may be caused by increases in extracellular adenosine, a potent inhibitor of inflammation.

Dosage. Methotrexate (available as a 2.5-mg tablet) is prescribed in an initial dosage of 7.5 mg once weekly. Some patients prefer to use 2.5 mg every 12 hours for three doses to reduce GI side effects. If no effect is noted in 4 to 6 weeks, then the dosage can be increased to 15 mg once weekly. In elderly persons and partial responders, the dosage can be increased to 10 to 12.5 mg weekly. The maximal dosage is 25 mg weekly. Some patients who experience intolerable GI side effects can be changed to self-administered intramuscular injections (methotrexate is available as a 25-mg/mL solution). Contraindications to therapy include renal insufficiency, acute or chronic liver disease, alcohol abuse, leukopenia, thrombocytopenia, and untreated folate deficiency. Obesity, diabetes, and a history of hepatitis B or hepatitis C are factors that have been suggested but not confirmed to increase methotrexate hepatotoxicity. Salicylates (and probably other NSAIDs) and trimethoprim (Bactrim, Septra) block the renal excretion of methotrexate and lead to higher serum levels and potential toxicity. If alternatives exist, concomitant use of methotrexate and trimethoprim is to be avoided. NSAIDs and methotrexate are often used together, but methotrexate toxicity monitoring should be done more often when NSAIDs are added or changed while the patient is on methotrexate therapy.

Usual Time to Maximal Effect. The onset of action is 3 to 6 weeks, with 70% of patients having some response (4). A trial of 3 to 6 months is suggested.

Side Effects. The most serious complications of methotrexate therapy (hepatic cirrhosis, interstitial pneumonitis, and severe myelosuppression) are rare (45). *Stomatitis,* mild alopecia, and GI upset may occur; they are related to folic acid antagonism and can be improved with folic acid supplementation (44). Folic acid 1 mg/day has been shown not to diminish the efficacy of methotrexate. Before starting methotrexate, baseline studies should include a CBC, liver chemistries, serum creatinine, hepatitis B and C serologies, and chest radiography. Routine toxicity monitoring should include a CBC, liver transaminases, serum albumin, and serum creatinine every 4 to 8 weeks.

Hepatotoxicity is not significant if patients with pre-existing liver disease, alcohol abuse, or hepatic dysfunction are excluded from treatment. Patients are advised to limit alcohol consumption to one to two alcoholic beverages per week. Baseline or surveillance liver biopsies are not indicated unless pre-existing liver disease is suspected. Elevated liver enzymes do not directly correlate with toxicity, but therapy should be stopped if transaminases are elevated to three times the upper limit of normal. Liver biopsy should be done if elevated liver enzymes persist or if methotrexate therapy is to be continued (46).

Interstitial pneumonitis is rare (2%), but the clinician should be alert to symptoms of cough or shortness of breath that may herald the onset of this severe complication. Methotrexate pneumonitis can occur at any time during therapy and is not dose related. A baseline chest radiograph is useful for comparison. Patients with poor pulmonary reserve from other causes may be excluded from therapy over concerns of increased morbidity if methotrexate pneumonitis occurs.

Myelosuppression is also rare at the low dosages of methotrexate used for treatment of rheumatoid arthritis. Increased renal insufficiency from other causes, as well as use of trimethoprim (Proloprim, Trimpex), often raises methotrexate levels and causes myelosuppression.

In the absence of leukopenia, no conclusive information links methotrexate use in rheumatoid arthritis with increased risk of infection. The exception is a slight increased risk of localized herpes zoster infection.

Although there are case reports of lymphoma associated with methotrexate therapy, including a case in which the lymphoma resolved after cessation of therapy (47), increased occurrence of malignancy has not been found in large population-based studies (48), nor have there been noted effects on sperm production or ovarian function. Women of childbearing potential and men with partners of childbearing potential must understand that methotrexate has potential for teratogenesis and should practice effective birth control. Women must discontinue methotrexate for one ovulatory cycle before attempting conception, and men should wait 3 months.

Leflunomide

Mechanism. Leflunomide selectively inhibits *de novo* pyrimidine ribonucleotide biosynthesis and *in vitro* potently inhibits lymphocyte proliferation. The primary mechanism of action of leflunomide is thought to be cell cycle arrest of pathogenic T cells in the joint by depletion of nucleotide pools and inhibition of DNA synthesis.

Dosage. Leflunomide is a prodrug that is converted in the liver to an active metabolite. It is excreted equally in the kidney and the gut and must be used with caution in patients with hepatic or renal insufficiency. Because of its long elimination half-life of

15 to 18 days, therapy with leflunomide (available in 10, 20, and 100 mg preparations) is initiated with a loading dose of 100 mg daily for 3 days, followed by a maintenance dose of 20 mg daily. The maintenance dose should be decreased to 10 mg daily in patients who do not tolerate the higher dose. When necessary, as in the case of side effects, the elimination half-life can be decreased to 1 to 2 days by the administration of cholestyramine, 8 g three times daily for 11 days.

Time to Maximal Effect. Improvement should be seen at 6 weeks. A 3-month trial is usually warranted.

Side Effects. In clinical trials, the most commonly reported adverse events were liver transaminase elevation, alopecia, rash, and gastroenterology complaints, especially diarrhea. Occurring in roughly 25% of patients, the diarrhea is self-limited and rarely results in discontinuation of the drug. As with methotrexate, alanine aminotransferase and aspartate aminotransferase elevation (two to three times the upper limits of normal) occurs in 6% of patients taking leflunomide. Liver enzyme abnormalities normalize with cessation of the drug. Alopecia occurs in roughly 10% of patients (36,39).

Monitoring should include a CBC and liver enzyme testing monthly.

Etanercept. Etanercept is a fusion protein created by linking extracellular binding regions from two TNF-RII (p75) receptors to the Fc portion of a human immunoglobulin IgG1 molecule. The resultant molecule is a dimeric soluble TNF receptor that binds both TNF-alpha and lymphotoxin with high affinity and specificity.

Mechanism. Etanercept binds TNF-alpha in the circulation, blocks binding of TNF-alpha to its receptor on the surface of cells, and prevents activation of inflammatory cells. TNF-alpha probably is cleared from the circulation through Fc binding by the reticuloendothelial system.

Time to Maximal Effect. Although the clinical response can be dramatic in some patients, even after the first dose, the maximal effect was seen in 3 months in the clinical trials (37).

Dosage. The half-life of etanercept is 72 hours, allowing it to be given as a single 25-mg subcutaneous injection twice weekly. Currently, this is the only FDA-approved dose. Recommended dosing in patients with renal failure and hepatic insufficiency has not been established.

Side Effects. Injection site reactions occur in approximately 40% of patients treated with etanercept and consist of raised urticarial lesions limited to the injection sites. Reactions occur early after initiation of treatment, are generally mild and self-limited, decrease, and then resolve completely with repeated dosing. The injection site reactions are not associated with other features of hypersensitivity, and no specific therapy is generally required (37).

The concerns about increased risk of infections and malignancy were discussed earlier. TNF-alpha mediates many of the cardinal signs and symptoms of infection, such as fever and malaise, and clinicians must take this into account when evaluating a patient who is taking etanercept for possible infection. Etanercept should be stopped if a patient experiences fever or a systemic infection is suspected.

Several case reports of demyelinating syndromes in patients starting etanercept therapy have been published. Clinical trials of both etanercept and infliximab for the treatment of multiple sclerosis demonstrated possible worsening of the disease with drug therapy. However, the association of etanercept with these events in patients with rheumatoid arthritis is unclear.

No specific routine monitoring for etanercept has been established, but a CBC and chemistry profile every 3 to 6 months would seem to be prudent.

Infliximab. Infliximab is a chimeric mouse–human monoclonal antibody composed of human IgG1-kappa coupled to the variable regions of a high-affinity neutralizing murine anti–human TNF-alpha antibody.

Mechanism. Infliximab binds TNF-alpha with high affinity and specificity. Like etanercept, infliximab prevents binding of TNF-alpha to its cellular receptor.

Dosage. Infliximab therapy is initiated at 3 mg/kg by intravenous infusion at weeks 0, 2, and 6, followed by maintenance dosing every 8 weeks. For patients with an incomplete response, dosing may be increased to a maximum of 10 mg/kg every 4 weeks. Because a significant portion of the infliximab molecule is of mouse origin, patients may develop human anti-mouse antibodies with repeat dosing, which limits response duration between doses. Methotrexate decreases the frequency of these human anti-mouse antibodies, and current recommendations are for infliximab to be administered concomitantly with methotrexate (38).

Time to Maximal Response. Patients often experience rapid improvement, with maximal response seen after the 6-week initiation period.

Side Effects. Infusion reactions occur in approximately 20% of patients and consist mainly of mild headache, nausea, and flushing. The reactions are transient and can be controlled by slowing the rate of infusion or by pretreatment with antihistamines or acetaminophen. Infusion reactions do not increase over time.

The potential for increased frequency of malignancy and infection has already been discussed. Of unclear etiology and clinical significance is the development of low titers of anti–double-stranded DNA (anti-ds-DNA) antibodies in patients treated with infliximab or, with lesser frequency, in those treated with etanercept. Anti-ds-DNA antibodies are generally specific for SLE and do not develop in drug-induced syndromes. There has been only one reported case of a patient's developing a drug-induced lupus syndrome characterized by fever, rash, and pericarditis in the setting of the development of anti-ds-DNA antibodies.

Treatment During Pregnancy

Rheumatoid arthritis therapy during pregnancy is complicated by the fact that *none of the drugs discussed previously has been shown to be safe in pregnant women* with adequate, controlled studies. Although joint symptoms often remit during pregnancy, this effect is not universal. Treatment decisions require careful consideration of the risks and benefits to the mother and fetus and should be made together with obstetric consultation.

If possible, all DMARD therapy should be stopped in women who are planning to conceive and in pregnant and lactating women. Infliximab and etanercept are pregnancy category B, whereas hydroxychloroquine is category C (49). Methotrexate and leflunomide, because of evidence of potential teratogenicity, should be stopped in men and women who are planning conception; these drugs are category X. In the case of leflunomide, cholestyramine must be given to speed elimination (see earlier discussion).

Although safety has not been proven in controlled trials, no evidence exists for risks to the fetus from low-dose *prednisone* (less than 20 mg/day) or NSAIDs used in the first two trimesters. If necessary, joint symptoms are best managed with the lowest possible dosage of prednisone. Potential prednisone complications include worsening of maternal gestational diabetes, hypertension, and intrauterine growth retardation. NSAIDs should be avoided in the third trimester because of the potential for premature closure of the ductus, prolonged labor, and peripartum hemorrhage. Although both NSAIDs and prednisone are excreted in the breast milk, both are considered compatible with breast-feeding by the American Academy of Pediatrics.

Treatment of Felty Syndrome

The treatment of patients with Felty syndrome is especially complicated, and management should be coordinated with a consulting rheumatologist. These patients should be treated with a remittive agent; methotrexate is the most commonly used agent. If patients develop Felty syndrome while taking a DMARD, another DMARD should be tried. Asymptomatic patients who remain neutropenic despite DMARD therapy should be monitored closely for infection, but with no further therapy prescribed. The treatment benefits of splenectomy and granulocyte colony–stimulating factor are mixed and consist largely of uncontrolled case reports. Therefore, these therapies should be reserved for patients with persistent neutropenia and recurrent or severe infections.

Surgery

Although rheumatoid arthritis is generally an inflammatory process of the synovium, structural or mechanical derangement is a common cause of pain and loss of joint function. Pain and joint mobility may be improved by a surgical approach. The primary physician, the rheumatologist, and the orthopedist all help the patient understand the risks and benefits of the surgical procedure. The decision to have surgery is a complex one that must take into consideration the motivation and goals of the patient, the patient's ability to undergo rehabilitation, and the patient's general medical status.

Synovectomy is ordinarily not recommended for patients with rheumatoid arthritis, primarily because relief is only transient. However, an exception is synovectomy of the wrist, which is recommended if intense synovitis persists despite medical treatment over 6 to 12 months. Persistent synovitis involving the dorsal compartments of the wrist can lead to extensor tendon sheath rupture, resulting in severe disability of hand function.

Total joint arthroplasties, particularly of the knee, hip, wrist, and elbow, are highly successful. Arthroplasty of the MCP joints also can reduce pain and improve function. Other operations include release of nerve entrapments (e.g., carpal tunnel syndrome), arthroscopic procedures, and, occasionally, removal of a symptomatic rheumatoid nodule.

Table 77.14. Indications for Referral of Patients with Rheumatoid Arthritis for Consultation

To a Rheumatologist
If there is any question about the validity of the diagnosis
During the early phase of the disease to develop a management program
If the therapeutic regimen requires the use of DMARDs (see text)
If there are severe manifestations of extra-articular disease
If arthrocentesis is indicated and the primary physician is not comfortable performing the procedure (an orthopedist can also do this procedure)
For advice about splinting (an orthopedist can also provide this advice)
If there is any consideration of corrective surgery (an orthopedist can also provide this advice
To an Orthopedist
For advice about splinting
If there is any consideration of corrective surgery
To a Physical or Occupational Therapist
Soon after diagnosis to advise and institute appropriate physical therapy

Summary of Indications for Referral

The indications for consultation are listed in Table 77.14.

General References*

American College of Rheumatology Ad Hoc Committee on Clinical Guidelines. **Guidelines for the management of rheumatoid arthritis.** 2002 update. Arthritis Rheum 2002;46:328.

*Bold print (general references) and bold numerals (specific references) denote published controlled clinical trials, meta-analyses, or consensus-based recommendations.

Canoso JJ. Rheumatology in primary care. Philadelphia: WB Saunders, 1997.

A well-illustrated and practical text covering rheumatoid arthritis and many other important and common forms of arthritis and nonarticular rheumatic conditions.

Harris ED Jr. Rheumatoid arthritis. Philadelphia: WB Saunders, 1997.

Kippel JH, Weyand CM, Wortmann RL, eds. Primer on the rheumatic diseases. 11th ed. Atlanta: Arthritis Foundation, 1997.

Koopman WJ, ed. Arthritis and allied conditions. 13th ed. Philadelphia: Lea & Febiger, 1997.

Ruddy S, Harris ED Jr., Sledge CB, et al., eds. Kelley's textbook of rheumatology. 6th ed. Philadelphia: WB Saunders, 2001.

Sjögren's syndrome. Rheum Dis Clin North Am 1992;18:507.

Weisman MH, Weinblatt ME, Loouie JS, eds. Treatment of the rheumatic diseases: companion to Kelley's textbook of rheumatology. Philadelphia: WB Saunders, 2001.

Specific References

1. Hochberg MC, Spector TD. Epidemiology of rheumatoid arthritis: update. Epidemiol Rev 1990;12:151.
2. Ollier W, Thomson W. Population genetics of rheumatoid arthritis. Rheum Dis Clin North Am 1992;18:741.
3. Weyand CM, Hicok KC, Conn DL, et al. The influence of HLA-DRB1 genes on disease severity in rheumatoid arthritis. Ann Intern Med 1992;117:801.
4. Harris ED Jr. Rheumatoid arthritis: pathophysiology and implications for therapy. N Engl J Med 1990;322:1277.
5. Firestein GS, Alvaro-Garcia JM, Maki R. Quantitative analysis of cytokine gene expression in rheumatoid arthritis. J Immunol 1990;144:3347.
6. Arnett FC, Edworthy SM, Bloch DA, et al. The American Rheumatism Association 1987 revised criteria for the classification of rheumatoid arthritis. Arthritis Rheum 1988;31:315.
7. Roubenoff R, Roubenoff RA, Cannon JG, et al. Rheumatoid cachexia: cytokine driven hypermetabolism accompanying reduced body cell mass in chronic inflammation. J Clin Invest 1994;93:2379.
8. van der Heijde DMFM, van Leeuwen MA, van Riel PLCM, et al. Biannual radiographic assessments of hands and feet in a three year prospective followup of patients with early rheumatoid arthritis. Arthritis Rheum 1992;35:26.
9. Wolfe F, Cathey MA, Roberts FK. The latex test revisited: rheumatoid factor testing in 8287 rheumatic disease patients. Arthritis Rheum 1991;34:951.
10. Schmerling RH, Delbanco TL. The rheumatoid factor: an analysis of clinical utility. Am J Med 1991;91:528.
11. Hund ER. Extraarticular manifestations of rheumatoid arthritis. Semin Arthritis Rheum 1979;8:151.
12. Hyland RH, Gordon DA, Broden I, et al. A systematic controlled study of pulmonary abnormalities in rheumatoid arthritis. J Rheumatol 1984;10:395.
13. Lebowitz WB. The heart in rheumatoid arthritis (rheumatoid disease): a clinical and pathological study of sixty-two cases. Ann Intern Med 1963;58:102.
14. Rosenstein ED, Kramer N. Felty's and pseudo-Felty's syndrome. Semin Arthritis Rheum 1991;21:129.
15. Yelin E, Meenan R, Nevitt M, et al. Work disability in rheumatoid arthritis: effects of disease, social, and work factors. Ann Intern Med 1980;93:551.
16. Wolfe F, Mitchell DM, Sibley JT, et al. The mortality of rheumatoid arthritis. Arthritis Rheum 1994;37:481.
17. Superior-Cabuslay E, Ward MM, Lorig KR. Patient education interventions in osteoarthritis and rheumatoid arthritis: a meta-analytic comparison with nonsteroidal anti-inflammatory drug treatment. Arthritis Care Res 1996;9:292.
18. Hill J, Bird H, Johnson S. Effect of patient education on adherence to drug treatment for rheumatoid arthritis: a randomized controlled trial. Ann Rheum Dis 2001;60:869.
19. Pincus T, Callahan LF, Brooks RH, et al. Self-report questionnaire scores in rheumatoid arthritis compared with traditional physical, radiographic, and laboratory measures. Ann Intern Med 1989;110:259.
20. Mills JA, Pinals RS, Ropes MW, et al. Value of bedrest in patients with rheumatoid arthritis. N Engl J Med 1971;284:453.
21. Silverstein FE, Faich G, Goldstein JL, et al. Gastrointestinal toxicity with celecoxib vs non-steroidal anti-inflammatory drugs for osteoarthritis and rheumatoid arthritis. The Class Study: a randomized controlled trial. JAMA 2000;284:1247.
22. Bombardier C, Laine L, Reicin C, et al. Comparison of upper gastrointestinal toxicity of rofecoxib and naproxen in patients with rheumatoid arthritis. Vigor Study Group. N Engl J Med 2000;343:1520.
23. Allison FC, Howatson MD, Torrance MB, et al. Gastrointestinal damage associated with the use of nonsteroidal anti-inflammatory drugs. N Engl J Med 1992;327:749.
24. Simm LS. Nonsteroidal anti-inflammatory drug toxicity. Curr Opin Rheumatol 1993;5:265.
25. Soll AH, Weinstein WM, Kurata J, et al. Nonsteroidal anti-inflammatory drugs and peptic ulcer disease. Ann Intern Med 1991;114:307.
26. Griffin MR, Ray WA, Schaffner W. Nonsteroidal anti-inflammatory drug use and death from peptic ulcer disease in elderly persons. Ann Intern Med 1988;109:359.
27. Mukherjee D, Nissen SE, Topol EJ. Risk of cardiovascular events associated with selective COX-2 inhibitors. JAMA 2001;286:954.
28. Silverstein FE, Graham DY, Senior JR, et al. Misoprostol reduces serious gastrointestinal complications in patients with rheumatoid arthritis receiving nonsteroidal anti-inflammatory drugs. Ann Intern Med 1995;123:241.
29. Hawkey CJ, Karrasch JA, Szcepanski L, et al. Omeprazole compared with misoprostol for ulcers associated with nonsteroidal antiinflammatory drugs. Omeprazole versus Misoprostol for NSAID induced Ulcer Management (OMNIUM) Study Group. N Engl J Med 1998;338:727.
30. Whelton A, Hamilton CW. Nonsteroidal anti-inflammatory drugs: effects on kidney function. J Clin Pharmacol 1991;31:588.
31. Gotzche PC, Johansen HK. Short-term low-dose corticosteroids vs. placebo and nonsteroidal anti-inflammatory drugs in rheumatoid arthritis. (Cochrane Review). Cochrane Database Syst Rev 2001;2:CD000189.
32. Kirwan JR. The effect of glucocorticoids on joint destruction in rheumatoid arthritis. N Engl J Med 1995;333:142.
33. Saag KG, Koehnke R, Caldwell JR, et al. Low dose long term corticosteroid therapy in rheumatoid arthritis: an analysis of serious adverse events. Am J Med 1994;96:115.
34. Iglehart IW, Sutton JD, Bender JC, et. al. Intravenous pulsed corticosteroids in rheumatoid arthritis: a comparative study. J Rheumatol 1990;17:159.
35. Wolfe F, Hawley DJ, Cathey MA. Termination of slow acting antirheumatic therapy in rheumatoid arthritis: a 14-year prospective evaluation of 1017 consecutive starts. J Rheum 1990;17:994.
36. Smolen JS, Kalden JR, Scott DL, et al. Efficacy and safety of leflunomide compared with placebo and sulphasalazine in active rheumatoid arthritis: a double blind, randomised, multicentre trial. Lancet 1999;353:259.
37. Moreland LW, Schiff MH, Baumgartner SW, et al. Etanercept therapy in rheumatoid arthritis: a randomized controlled trial. Ann Intern Med 1999;130:478.
38. Lipsky PE, van der Heijde DMFM, St. Clair EW, et al. Infliximab and methotrexate in the treatment of rheumatoid arthritis. N Engl J Med 2000;343:1594.
39. Strand V, Cohen S, Schiff M, et al. Treatment of active rheumatoid arthritis with leflunomide compared with placebo and methotrexate. Arch Intern Med 1999;159:2542.
40. Choy EHS, Panayi GS. Cytokine pathways and joint inflammation in rheumatoid arthritis. N Engl J Med 2001;344:97.
41. Gershon S, Wise RP, Niu M, et al. Postlicensure reports of infections during use of etanercept and infliximab. Presented at the American College of Rheumatology 64th Annual Scientific Meeting. October, 2000.

42. Amerian Thoracic Society, Centers for Disease Control and Prevention. Targeted tuberculin testing and treatment of latent tuberculosis infection. Am J Respir Crit Care Med 200;161:S221.
43. O'Dell JR, Haire CE, Erikson N, et al. Treatment of rheumatoid arthritis with methotrexate alone, sulfasalazine and hydroxychloroquine or a combination of all three medications. N Engl J Med 1996;334:1287.
44. Morgan SL, Baggott JE, Vaughn WH. Supplementation with folic acid during methotrexate therapy for rheumatoid arthritis. Ann Intern Med 1994;121:833.
45. Weinblatt ME, Kaplan H, Germain BF, et al. Methotrexate in rheumatoid arthritis: a five year prospective multicenter study. Arthritis Rheum 1994;37:1492.
46. Kremer JM, Alarcon GS, Lightfoot RW Jr, et al. Methotrexate for rheumatoid arthritis. Arthritis Rheum 1994;37:316.
47. Kamel OW, van de Rijin J, Weiss LW, et al. Reversible lymphomas associated with Epstein Barr virus occurring during methotrexate therapy for rheumatoid arthritis and dermatomyositis. N Engl J Med 1993;328:1317.
48. Moder KG, Tefferi A. Hematologic malignancies and the use of methotrexate in rheumatoid arthritis: a retrospective study. Am J Med 1995;99:276.
49. Janssen NM, Genta MS. The effects of immunosuppressive therapy and anti-inflammatory medications on fertility, pregnancy and lactation. Arch Intern Med 2000;160:610.

CHAPTER 78

Sacroiliitis, Ankylosing Spondylitis, and Reactive Arthritis

FRANK C. ARNETT, Jr., MD

SACROILIITIS

Chronic inflammation of the sacroiliac joints, *sacroiliitis,* may occur as an isolated clinical syndrome or a component feature of several other chronic rheumatic disorders, which are classified within a family called *spondyloarthropathies* (1,2). Osteoarthritis may affect the sacroiliac joints in older people, but these are radiologic changes that are usually readily differentiated from inflammatory sacroiliitis and are typically unassociated with symptoms. Sacroiliitis is considered the *sine qua non* for early *primary ankylosing spondylitis*; however, this latter diagnosis should be applied only when symptoms or signs indicate progression of inflammation into additional segments of the axial skeleton. *Secondary forms of sacroiliitis* or spondylitis may complicate the clinical course in 10% of patients with inflammatory bowel disease (ulcerative colitis and Crohn disease), 20% of those with psoriatic arthritis, and 20% of those with reactive arthritis (formerly termed *Reiter syndrome*). The dominant clinical problems that bring the patient with primary spondylitis to a clinician and require careful management over many years are pain, limitation of motion, and deformity of the spine. In secondary spondylitis the same principles of diagnosis and management of the axial problem apply but must be accompanied by attention to the cutaneous, gastrointestinal (GI), genitourinary,

Table 78.1. Classification of Spondylitis and Frequency of HLA-B27[a]

Classification	HLA-B27 Positive
Primary	
Isolated sacroiliitis	70–90%
Ankylosing spondylitis	>90%
Secondary	
Spondylitis of inflammatory bowel disease	50%
Psoriatic spondylitis	50%
Reactive arthritis with spondylitis	90%
Infectious	
Sacroiliitis	Not increased
Discitis	Not increased
Osteomyelitis	Not increased
Degenerative spondylosis	Not increased

[a]Found in 8% to 10% of normal white subjects and 2% to 4% of blacks.

ocular, and peripheral articular manifestations of the primary disorders.

The pathogenesis of spinal inflammation is unknown; however, there is a strong hereditary component marked by the histocompatibility antigen HLA-B27 (3,4). This genetic marker is strongly associated with sacroiliitis and spondylitis regardless of clinical setting (Table 78.1). More than 90% of patients with primary ankylosing spondylitis have HLA-B27. Conversely, if normal subjects with HLA-B27 are carefully assessed, clinical or radiographic evidence of disease can be found in only 2% (5). Transgenic rats possessing the human HLA-B27 gene develop nearly all the clinical features of spondyloarthropathies and have confirmed the direct participation of this gene in disease pathogenesis (6). In addition to genetic predisposition, certain environmental agents appear to be associated with these diseases in the B27-positive host. There is evidence that normal bacterial flora in the GI tract participate in the pathogenesis of primary ankylosing spondylitis, as well as in the disease seen in HLA-B27 transgenic animals (6). Reactive arthritis is known to be triggered by certain specific GI, genitourinary, or other infections (7) (see Reactive Arthritis, below).

ANKYLOSING SPONDYLITIS

Prevalence

The prevalence of ankylosing spondylitis parallels the frequency of HLA-B27 in different populations in the United States and in other regions of the world. This gene occurs in 8% to 10% of white Americans, and the disease occurs in 0.1% to 0.2% of the white population (4,5). African Americans have a much lower frequency of both disease and the HLA-B27 gene. On the other hand, there is a high frequency of spondylitic disease and of HLA-B27 in certain Native American and Eskimo groups. Ankylosing spondylitis is common in Europeans and most Asian groups but is found rarely in African blacks and in Japanese, again reflecting the relative frequency of the B27 marker.

Histopathology

The spondylitic diseases are characterized by chronic inflammation of *synovial* joints, especially those in the axial skeleton; *fibrous* joints such as sacroiliacs and symphysis pubis; and nonarticular bony areas where tendons and fascia have their insertions *(enthesopathy)* (2,8). The chronic inflammatory infiltrates are nonspecific and histologically indistinguishable from those of rheumatoid arthritis. On the other hand, unlike the rheumatoid process in which there is cartilaginous and bony destruction, this inflammatory process tends to promote new bone formation across previous articulations. This ossification of the articular and ligamentous structures of the spine results in eventual fusion and gives rise to the characteristic radiographic findings.

History

The typical patient with sacroiliitis or ankylosing spondylitis is a young white man under the age of 40 years (Table 78.2). Occasionally, the diagnosis of ankylosing spondylitis is made in older patients, but careful questioning often reveals that symptoms began years earlier. However, the impression that women are affected less often than men (ratio, 1:3) may be caused by under-recognition of the disease in women. The initial symptoms of the disorder in women may be peripheral or cervical joint arthritis, and low back involvement may be absent or overshadowed by these complaints. Some are misdiagnosed and labeled seronegative rheumatoid arthritis (9) (see Chapter 77). Therefore, one should be mindful of these differences between men and women and must consider an emerging spondylitic process in young women who present with a seronegative arthritis. Similarly, children with ankylosing spondylitis are also more likely to develop a peripheral oligoarticular lower extremity arthropathy, including severe hip disease, and symptoms in the axial skeleton may not develop for many years, if ever. Their illness is often inappropriately labeled juvenile rheumatoid arthritis (5,9).

The usual presenting symptoms of sacroiliitis or ankylosing spondylitis are pain and stiffness in the low back or buttocks. These symptoms begin insidiously, and the patient has usually noticed them for at least 3 months before seeking medical advice. Unlike mechanical low back syndromes, the pain and stiffness of inflammatory disease are usually worsened by rest and improved by exercise. The patient is unable to rest at night or sit for prolonged periods and must arise and stretch to obtain relief. As in discogenic disease, however, symptoms of shooting pains into the buttocks and down the posterior or lateral thighs may mimic sciatica. These pains are usually transient and not associated with any demonstrable neurologic deficits. Often,

Table 78.2. Clues to Early Ankylosing Spondylitis

- A young man (less often a woman)
- Pain/stiffness in buttocks, low back, chest wall
  - Worse with rest
  - Better with exercise
- Sciatic-like pains
- Family history of spondylitis
- History of iritis

patients already have been treated conservatively or surgically for presumed disc disease.

With time, the disease progresses into the lumbar and thoracic regions. Chest wall radicular pain occurs often and may mimic pleuritic, pericardial, or anginal pain syndromes. Progressive limitation of spinal movements ensues, and patients may note more difficulty in bending forward, the development of a stooped posture, and actual loss of height. Finally, the disease process reaches the cervical spine, and if appropriate preventive measures are not taken, the neck may become fused in a flexed position. Although peripheral joints are uncommonly affected, the root joints (hips and shoulders) eventually become involved in 50% of patients. Occasionally, fusion of the back may be entirely asymptomatic, and the patient develops complaints only when the disease reaches the cervical spine, hips, or shoulders.

Additional important historical facts should be sought in the assessment of the patient. In 16% of patients, the family history is positive for a first-degree relative with spondylitis (5). The history should seek prior episodes of peripheral arthritis, perhaps beginning in childhood, or even an episode of reactive arthritis. Acute anterior uveitis (iritis) may have been a harbinger of the articular syndrome, and at least 25% of patients will have iritis at some time before or during their course of illness. The review of systems and family history should seek symptoms or diagnoses of psoriasis or inflammatory bowel disease in the patient or in family members. Patients with spondylitis may have relatives with psoriasis or inflammatory bowel disease but may never manifest these disorders themselves.

Physical Examination

A physical examination initially and every 4 to 6 months is important in patients with suspected spondylitis. Although the primary focus of examinations is the musculoskeletal system, especially the axial skeleton, shoulders, hips, and peripheral joints, additional attention must be directed toward the eyes, heart, skin, and GI tract. This practice ensures the diagnosis and provides the baseline with which the clinician can assess future articular or extra-articular complications or the superimposition of unrelated systemic or musculoskeletal disorders. It must be emphasized that ankylosing spondylitis is a disease that requires management over decades, and each new complaint cannot necessarily be ascribed to the basic disease process.

Articular Features

There are few measurable abnormalities in patients with early spondylitis (Table 78.3). In fact, the patient with sacroiliitis may have an entirely normal physical examination, despite significant symptoms of pain and stiffness in the low back region. At most, there may be tenderness on direct palpation of these joints in the buttocks or upon compression of the pelvis. Stressing the sacroiliac joint to elicit pain (see Chapter 71) may also be useful.

Table 78.3. Physical Examination in Ankylosing Spondylitis

Sacroiliac joints	Thoracic spine
Tenderness	Increased kyphosis
Pain with compression/stress	Tenderness
Lumbar spine	Pain with rib cage compression
Tenderness	Decreased chest expansion (<3 cm)
Paravertebral muscle spasm	Cervical spine
Loss of lordosis	Tenderness
Decreased flexion: Schober test (<5 cm) (see text)	Pain on motion
Abnormal finger-floor	Muscle spasm
Decreased lateral motion and extension	Decreased motion
Hips, shoulders	Kyphosis, decreased lordosis
Pain on motion	Occiput to wall movement (see text)
Decreased range	

Abnormalities that eventually appear in the patient with progressive disease relate to loss of range of motion and deformity in mobile structures. After evaluation of the sacroiliac regions the clinician should direct attention to the lumbar spine. The patient with lumbar involvement has often lost the normal lordosis, and there is flattening of that segment of the back. In addition, there is loss in range of motion when the patient attempts to bend forward and touch toes. It should be recalled that hip motion accounts for 90 degrees of the flexion of the trunk on the lower extremities and that the lumbar spine provides the remaining stretch by reversing its lordosis and becoming kyphotic. Serial measurements of the distance between the patient's fingertips and the floor with maximal forward bending should be obtained (because of variation between individuals, isolated measurements are not interpretable). Another objective measurement of lumbar motion is the *Schober test.* With the patient standing erect, a horizontal line is drawn at the L5–S1 region and another line 10 cm above that. With forward flexion, the distance between these two points should increase to 15 cm in the normal lumbar spine. This test is best applied and interpreted in the young patient because lumbar motion normally decreases with age. Lateral bending and extension of the lumbar spine should also be assessed at the same time.

Involvement of the *thoracic spine* is determined subjectively by the patient's complaints of pain or stiffness in that region and by demonstrable tenderness along the vertebral column and paravertebral muscles. Compression of the rib cage laterally and over the sternum may also elicit pain. Objective determination of fusion of the costovertebral joints is obtained by measuring the chest expansion. A tape measure is placed around the patient's chest wall at the nipple line or fourth intercostal space, and the change in circumference from full expiration to full inspiration is measured. Less than 3 cm is considered abnormal. Chest expansion in normal people also decreases with increasing age.

The range of motion of the cervical spine should be determined for extension, right and left rotation, lateral flexion, and forward flexion. Loss of extension is usually the earliest abnormality, and as the disease progresses, the patient tends to develop fixed deformity in the forward flexed position. Therefore, another rough estimate of developing cervical kyphosis is the occiput-to-wall measurement. This is obtained with the patient placing both heels against the base of the wall and attempting to extend the neck fully to touch the wall with the back of the head. This is normally readily accomplished.

Examination of the range of motion and elicitation of any pain on motion of both shoulders and hips is important because one-third to one-half of patients develop involvement of these joints some time during the course of the disease. Less often, peripheral joints become inflamed, but usually only transiently. The joints most commonly involved are the knees, ankles, and wrists. Approximately 10% of patients with ankylosing spondylitis complain of pain in the heels either at the Achilles tendon insertion or over the attachment of the plantar aponeurosis in the sole of the foot (enthesopathies). Swelling is usually not apparent in these areas, but tenderness to direct palpation is found.

Extra-Articular Features

Cardiac abnormalities occur in less than 5% of patients with ankylosing spondylitis (Table 78.4) (10). The most common, first-degree atrioventricular block, can be determined only electrocardiographically. A history of palpitations or syncope and the finding of a slow or irregular pulse on examination should alert one to higher degrees of atrioventricular block. At times a cardiac pacemaker is required for serious arrhythmias or complete atrioventricular dissociation. Aortic regurgitation caused by inflammatory thickening of the aortic valve and root is another serious cardiac complication. Once the diastolic murmur becomes apparent, there is usually cardiac decompensation requiring valve replacement in 1 to 2 years.

Iritis occurs in approximately 25% of patients with ankylosing spondylitis and does not necessarily parallel the course of the articular disease. It may occasionally be the sentinel symptom. Its onset is usually abrupt and unilateral, with intense pain, redness, and photophobia as the cardinal symptoms. Immediate ophthalmologic attention is required to prevent serious damage to the anterior chamber of the eye. Local corticosteroids are usually successful in abating an acute episode; however, frequent slit-lamp examinations determine the response and help determine whether systemic steroids are required.

Table 78.4. Extra-Articular Manifestations and Complications of Ankylosing Spondylitis

Cardiac	5%
First-degree AV block	
Second- and third-degree AV block	
Aortic regurgitation	
Ocular	25%
Acute iritis	
Chronic iritis	
Neurologic	Rare
Cauda equina syndrome	
Cord injury caused by fractures	
Renal	Rare
IgA nephropathy	
Amyloidosis	4%
Pulmonary fibrosis	Rare

The *cauda equina syndrome* is a rare but serious neurologic complication of spondylitis (see Chapter 71). It is believed to be related to entrapment of exiting lumbar and sacral nerves through the inflamed spinal column; however, compressive inflammatory lesions within the spinal column may be found in some cases and are surgically remediable. Patients with ankylosing spondylitis should be questioned regularly about paresthesias and pain or weakness in the legs and about symptoms of bladder or bowel sphincter dysfunction. Other neurologic sequelae of the disorder include injuries to the spinal cord from fracture dislocation of a rigid and brittle spine. The neck is especially prone to fracture, and paraplegia or quadriplegia may result (11).

Secondary amyloidosis can be found in approximately 4% of patients with ankylosing spondylitis, usually after many decades of persistent inflammatory disease. Proteinuria and nephrotic syndrome indicate renal involvement, which is usually the most serious manifestation of amyloidosis. *IgA nephropathy* has been reported as another cause of proteinuria and renal insufficiency in this disease.

Apical pulmonary fibrosis, sometimes with cavity formation, is rare and usually of no clinical consequence. This radiographic abnormality may mimic tuberculosis, and vice versa.

Laboratory Evaluation

Radiographic evaluation of the sacroiliac joints is the single most specific test for this disorder. Although a diagnosis of sacroiliitis/spondylitis can be suspected based on the history and physical examination, definitive diagnosis cannot be established without radiographic findings. A single anteroposterior view of the pelvis may be adequate to define sacroiliitis; however, at times Ferguson or oblique views are necessary to evaluate fully the integrity of the sacroiliac joints (2,12). The earliest radiographic change is usually bony sclerosis on the iliac sides of the joint margins. Thereafter, bony erosions occur (Fig. 78.1). There is eventual fusion across the joint space with subsequent loss of the early sclerotic changes (Fig. 78.2). Sacroiliitis is often confused with the radiographic anomaly *osteitis condensans ilii,* in which there is symmetric sclerosis on the iliac side of each sacroiliac joint without any erosions. This finding is most common in young women who have borne children.

An early radiographic finding on lateral lumbar spine films is squaring of the vertebral bodies. This phenomenon may also be seen in the thoracic and cervical regions. The apophyseal joints of the spine become fused and, presumably because of immobility, diffuse osteoporosis ensues. Calcification and ossification of the ligamentous structures between vertebral bodies result in the characteristic syndesmophytes seen on x-ray (i.e., the bamboo spine) (Fig. 78.2). Large "flowing" syndesmophytes, typically

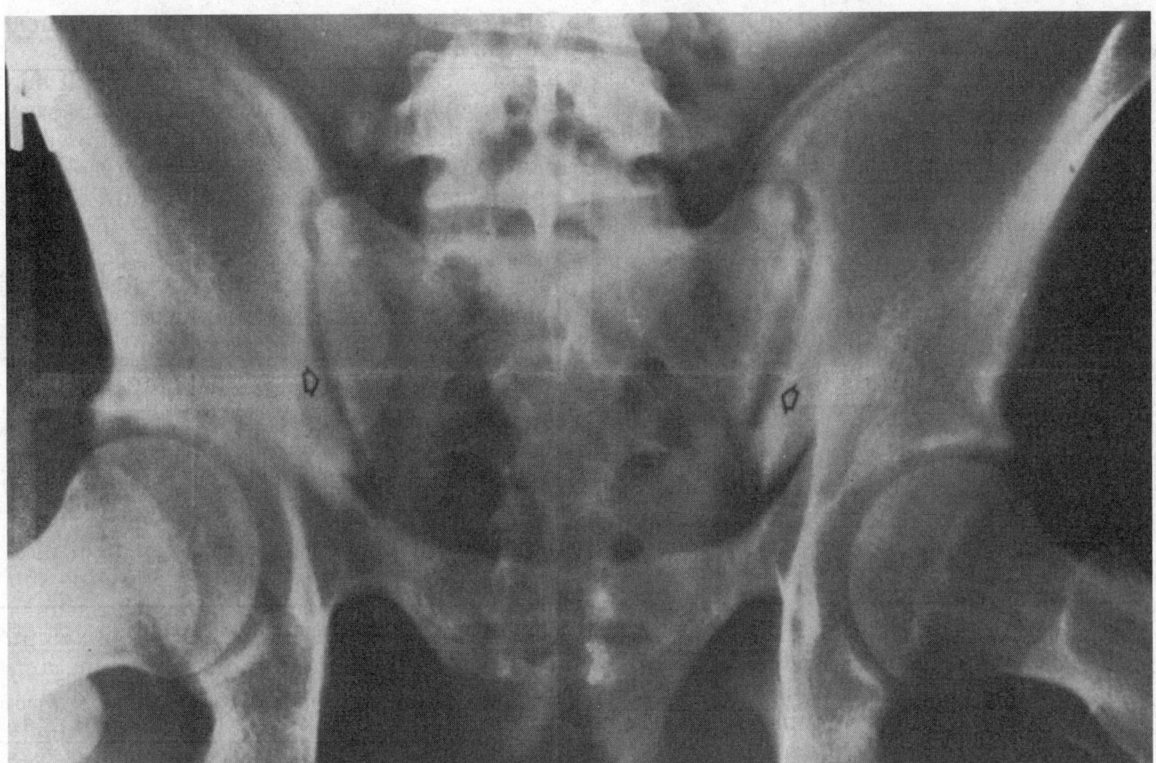

Figure 78.1. Early radiographic changes of sacroiliitis indicated by bony sclerosis on both sides of the joint margins, especially on the left *(arrows)*. Joint space erosions, a later manifestation of the disease, are present on both sides also.

most prominent in the right thoracic spine but also common in the lumbar and cervical areas, are seen in another disease, diffuse idiopathic skeletal hyperostosis, which may clinically and radiographically mimic ankylosing spondylitis. Such patients can usually be discriminated by disease onset in late middle age and the absence of sacroiliitis.

Radionuclide scanning (scintigraphy) of the sacroiliac joints is not useful if there is bilateral disease and is probably of most value in localizing pyogenic infections in the sacroiliac joints and other spinal structures. Computed tomography and magnetic resonance imaging of the sacroiliac joints are more sensitive than conventional x-rays in early disease but are also more expensive (12). Typing for HLA-B27 may be a more practical diagnostic approach when x-rays are not definitively abnormal (3) (see below).

Hematologic studies are usually normal. In patients with severe disease, however, there may be a mild normocytic–normochromic anemia reflective of chronic disease. The white blood cell count is usually normal, as is the platelet count, although patients with highly inflammatory disease may demonstrate mild thrombocytosis. The erythrocyte sedimentation rate is usually elevated. *Serologic studies* for rheumatoid factor and antinuclear antibodies are negative, and serum complement levels are normal.

On tissue typing, HLA-B27 occurs in more than 90% of patients with sacroiliitis or spondylitis. This genetic marker also occurs in 8% to 10% of the normal white American population. Recently, HLA typing by many commercial laboratories has become widely available and, when properly used, may be a helpful diagnostic aid in the assessment of a patient with low back symptoms or seronegative peripheral arthritis (3). It must be emphasized, however, that indiscriminate HLA typing cannot be substituted for a thorough clinical and radiographic evaluation of the patient. In fact, determination of B27 is rarely needed in making the diagnosis of spondylitis (see above). There are unusual circumstances, however, in which the patient gives a strong history suggestive of inflammatory axial skeletal disease but the x-rays are not yet diagnostic of sacroiliitis. In such situations, HLA typing may be helpful, as well as in children and women with early or atypical disease (9). Even then, a positive B27 does not establish a diagnosis of sacroiliitis but only provides supporting data for the diagnosis when the most specific finding (radiographic sacroiliitis) is not present.

Many patients already know their B27 status or wish to have the test performed because of the hereditary impact of disease on their family. In these circumstances, one must offer proper genetic counseling. The facts should be simply presented to the patient as they are currently known. It should be emphasized that spondylitis is not usually a life-threatening or crippling disorder and that symptoms can be controlled medically in most patients. The likelihood that a family member will develop inflammatory back disease is low. Because HLA antigens, including B27, are inherited in a mendelian dominant fashion, the risk of inheriting this tissue antigen type is 50% for each of a

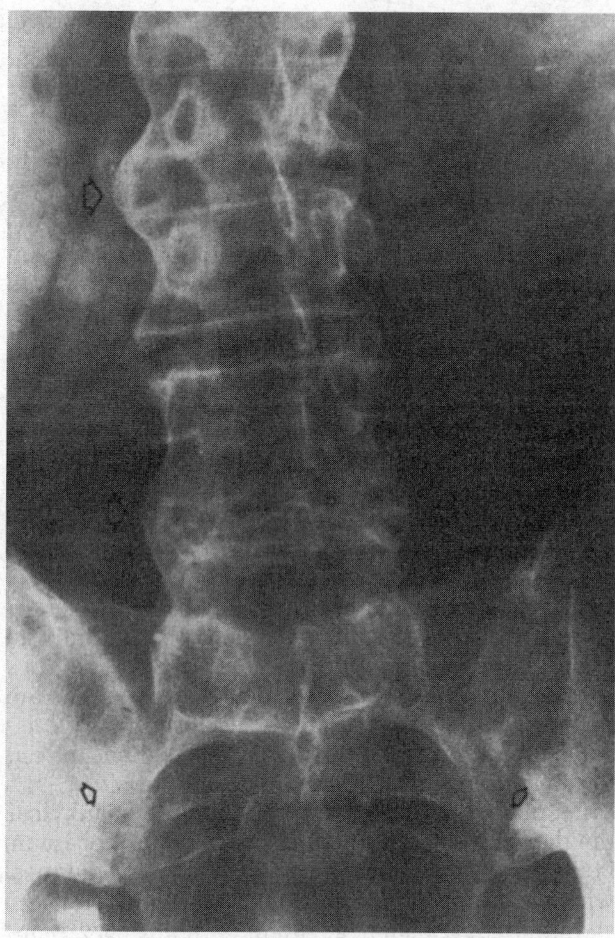

Figure 78.2. Late radiographic changes of sacroiliitis showing complete bony fusion of the joint spaces *(small arrows)*. Bridging syndesmophytes also are present in the lumbar spine *(large arrows)*.

patient's children (this assumes that the patient is heterozygous and the other parent is negative for B27). Even if a child inherits this tissue antigen type, the likelihood of developing arthritis is only around 20% (5). Therefore, without any knowledge of HLA status, every child of a patient with B27-positive spondylitis has roughly a 10% (50% times 20%) chance of developing spondylitis. The 90% probability of never developing this form of arthritis must be emphasized to patients concerned about this hereditary factor.

Diagnostic Criteria

The diagnostic criteria for ankylosing spondylitis are summarized in Table 78.5.

Course

It is impossible to predict the ultimate course of any patient with sacroiliitis. The inflammatory process may remain confined to these isolated joints or may progressively ascend into the lumbar, thoracic, and cervical spinal segments. Likewise, the duration of time from onset of symptoms to fusion of higher spinal segments is highly variable (13). Thus, each patient should understand the nature of this illness and the need for *continued medical surveillance,* as well as the principles of physical and pharmacologic management of the disorder (Table 78.6).

Table 78.5. New York Diagnostic Criteria for Ankylosing Spondylitis[a]

Clinical
Limitation of motion of the lumbar spine in all three planes: anterior flexion, lateral flexion, and extension
History of presence of pain at the dorsolumbar junction or in the lumbar spine
Limitation of chest expansion to 2.5 cm (1 inch) or less, measured at the level of the fourth intercostal space
Radiographic
Sacroiliitis: grade 3 (sclerosis and erosions of the joint margins) or grade 4 (fusion across the joint)

[a]Definite ankylosing spondylitis = grade 3 or 4 bilateral sacroiliitis with at least one clinical criterion *or* unilateral grade 3 or 4 or bilateral grade 2 (sclerosis or joint margins) sacroiliitis with clinical criterion 1 *or* with both clinical criteria 2 and 3.

From Bennet PH, Burch TA. New York symposium on population studies in the rheumatic diseases: new diagnostic criteria. Bull Rheum Dis 1967;17:453, with permission.

Table 78.6. Principles of Management in Ankylosing Spondylitis

Ensure patient understanding of disease process and objectives in management.
Alleviate pain and stiffness with anti-inflammatory drugs.
Use physical measures to maintain posture and range of motion in affected areas.

Management

Pharmacologic

Nonsteroidal anti-inflammatory drugs (NSAIDs) are used to relieve the pain and stiffness of the disease and to promote the patient's ability to perform the physical exercises so important to maintaining a good posture. It is unclear whether these drugs actually affect the natural history of the disease because no long-term controlled studies are available. It seems likely, however, that they do alter and improve overall functional capacity. Most often their use is required throughout the patient's life, but occasionally when symptoms completely remit, the NSAID may be tapered over several weeks and reinstituted if symptoms recur. Silent progress of the disease may occur; therefore, the clinician should closely monitor these patients even when they are not taking medication.

Indomethacin (Indocin) is especially effective therapy in many patients in dosages up to 75 to 150 mg/day. A number of side effects are important to consider, and these are discussed in detail in Chapter 77. Additional NSAIDs such as tolmetin (Tolectin), sulindac (Clinoril), and naproxen (Naproxyn) are also useful in those intolerant of indomethacin. Other NSAIDs may be tried when these drugs are ineffective. Newer cyclooxygenase 2 (COX-2) inhibitors such as celecoxib and rofecoxib may be equally effective in some patients and are less likely to cause major GI complications (see Chapter 77). Aspirin is usually ineffective. Low-dose prednisone (10 mg/day or less) may occasionally be necessary, especially in patients with peripheral arthritis or enthesopathy, but should not be used in the long term.

Sulfasalazine (Azulfidine), a drug used for inflammatory bowel disease, has recently been found to be effective therapy for ankylosing spondylitis, especially early in the disease, and it may have disease-modifying potential (14). Its mechanism of action is unknown but is presumed to be anti-inflammatory or antimicrobial. An enteric-coated preparation should be given starting at 500 mg/day for 1 week and gradually increased thereafter to total dosages of 2 to 3 g/day (1 g two to three times a day). Adverse reactions are common and include anorexia, headache, nausea, vomiting, gastric distress, and reversible oligospermia in men. Serious blood dyscrasias (aplastic anemia, agranulocytosis, thrombocytopenia), hypersensitivity reactions, hepatic or renal damage, and central nervous system reactions occur occasionally, and complete blood counts and urinalyses should be monitored. Absorption of folic acid and digoxin are both reduced by sulfasalazine. Consultation with a rheumatologist is suggested before using this agent.

Newer biologic agents, such as tumor necrosis factor antagonists (etanercept, infliximab), are currently undergoing clinical trials in this disease. Preliminary reports are encouraging (15,16).

Radiation therapy to the spine was once an effective means of relieving pain. This form of treatment is no longer recommended because of the risk of subsequent leukemia.

Physical Measures

Although anti-inflammatory agents relieve the pain and stiffness of spondylitis, an equally important function is their promotion of the patient's ability to perform the physical therapy necessary to prevent spinal deformity and loss of motion in the joints. In fact, such a program usually cannot be instituted until symptoms have been brought under control. The natural history of the disease should be explained so that the patient understands the rationale for the exercise program that must be followed (and that the clinician must reinforce) over many years. An erect posture when sitting or standing should be encouraged. The patient's bed should be firm or should be supported by a bed board. Use of a pillow should be avoided, or the smallest possible pillow should be used to prevent flexion of the neck. Sleeping in the prone position is most efficacious in promoting spinal extension, but the supine position is adequate if there is good support. The patient should refrain from sleeping on the side in a curled up position.

An active exercise program to promote extension of the back and increase range of motion of the axial and peripheral joints, as well as breathing exercises to maintain chest expansion, should be performed two to three times a day. Referral to a physical therapist to provide specific instructions and determine that the patient is performing well is a good investment. Swimming is an excellent recreational exercise for the patient with ankylosing spondylitis.

If spinal structures undergo complete ankylosis, the danger of spinal fracture after even minor trauma is increased. This is especially true in the neck, where whiplash types of injury occur. Thus, the spondylitic patient should take special precautions to prevent injury, including the use of a soft cervical collar when riding in an automobile or walking on slippery surfaces.

Prognosis

The prognosis for patients with ankylosing spondylitis is excellent. Most patients can be treated successfully by pharmacologic and physical means. Most continue to lead productive lives and change in vocational plans is usually not indicated. The morbidity from articular and extra-articular complications is low, and lifespan is not reduced significantly, if at all. In many instances pain in an affected area of the spine disappears after that segment has fused, and often disease halts at a particular segment and does not proceed to others. Although these facts should be optimistically presented to the patient, they are not cause for laxity in following the postural and exercise program and in maintaining close medical surveillance.

REACTIVE ARTHRITIS

Definition

Reactive arthritis (formerly termed Reiter syndrome) is a disorder that occurs after certain genitourinary or GI infections (7). Recently, studies have demonstrated bacterial antigens from the triggering microbe in the synovial fluid and tissue of patients with reactive arthritis. Moreover, there is increasing evidence for persistence of dormant microorganisms known to be associated with reactive arthritis (see below) in the gut, genitourinary tract, and even the joints in patients with this disease (17,18).

Unlike ankylosing spondylitis, reactive arthritis is primarily a peripheral arthritis. However, it shares with ankylosing spondylitis a predisposition to affect young people and a tendency for sacroiliitis or spondylitis, inflammation of tendon and fascial attachments, uveitis, the same cardiac complications, and a strong association with HLA-B27 (60% to 75% positive). Although it was classically defined as the triad of nongonococcal urethritis, conjunctivitis, and arthritis, it has been found that most patients do not express the classic triad and that approximately 40% of patients have arthritis as the only feature. Diagnosis depends on recognition of the typical pattern of arthritis, the presence of mucocutaneous lesions, and other features that are discriminating (7). The diagnosis and management of the disease focus primarily on symptoms and signs referable to the joints and nonarticular musculoskeletal structures. The diagnosis is made on clinical grounds based on a constellation of symptoms and signs. Typing for HLA-B27 may be a useful diagnostic aid in the incomplete or atypical case (3).

History and Examination

The principal clues to the diagnosis of reactive arthritis are summarized in Table 78.7. The patient with reactive arthritis is usually a young white person between puberty and age 40. Rarely it occurs in older patients. African Americans and Japanese (but not other Asians) are affected far less commonly, presumably because of the low frequency of HLA-B27 in these groups.

The disorder occurs in two main settings. First, the disease may follow an episode of diarrhea caused by *Shigella, Salmonella, Yersinia,* or *Campylobacter* (see Chapter 35). Second, the endemic form results primarily from venereal exposure, and *Chlamydia trachomatis* (see Chapters 37 and 102) is the most common causative agent. The sex ratio is equal in the postenteric form, but men appear to acquire the venereal form more often than women, although women with the disease are being recognized more often. The prevalence of postvenereal reactive arthritis has probably fallen over the last decade because of safer sexual practices.

In the classic form, urethritis, usually painless or with mild dysuria and a mucopurulent discharge, is usually the first symptom. It generally lasts only 1 to 2 weeks. *Conjunctivitis* usually follows shortly. This is most often mild with redness, weeping, and morning crusting. Generally, the conjunctivitis lasts only a few days. Photophobia is unusual, and its presence suggests uveitis (see below). Arthritis is usually the last feature of the triad to appear, usually from several days up to 1 month after the onset of urethritis. The *arthritis* is typically in the lower extremities, involving only one to four joints, most commonly the knees, ankles, and small joints of the feet. The patient notes pain, swelling, heat, and erythema over the joints. In addition to arthritis, more than 50% of patients have *nonarticular musculoskeletal pain* caused by inflammation of the insertion of tendons or fascia (enthesopathy). Heel pain caused by inflammation of the plantar aponeurosis or of the Achilles tendon insertion is one of the most prominent symptoms of the disease and may be one of the most disabling. Diffuse swelling of digits (sausaging), especially the toes, also occurs in more than 50% of patients and indicates involvement not only of the joints but of tendons and periosteal structures.

Table 78.7. Clues to the Diagnosis of Reactive Arthritis

A young person with arthritis
Symptoms
- Preceding diarrhea, urethritis, or conjunctivitis
- Lower extremity oligoarthritis (knee, ankle, foot)
- Heel pain or sausaging of digits
- Rash on soles, penis; painless oral ulcers; dystrophic nails
- Fever, weight loss, leukocytosis

HLA-B27 antigen

The *mucocutaneous features* of reactive arthritis are often asymptomatic and must be sought on physical examination. These include painless shallow oral ulcers, usually on the tongue and palate; circinate balanitis (Fig. 78.3) manifested by shallow moist painless ulcers on the glans penis in uncircumcised men or a dry scaling eruption on the glans in the circumcised; keratoderma blennorrhagica, a papulosquamous skin eruption usually beginning on the palms or soles (Fig. 78.4) and closely resembling pustular psoriasis; and onychodystrophy (Fig. 78.5). These lesions last for a highly variable period (several days to several months).

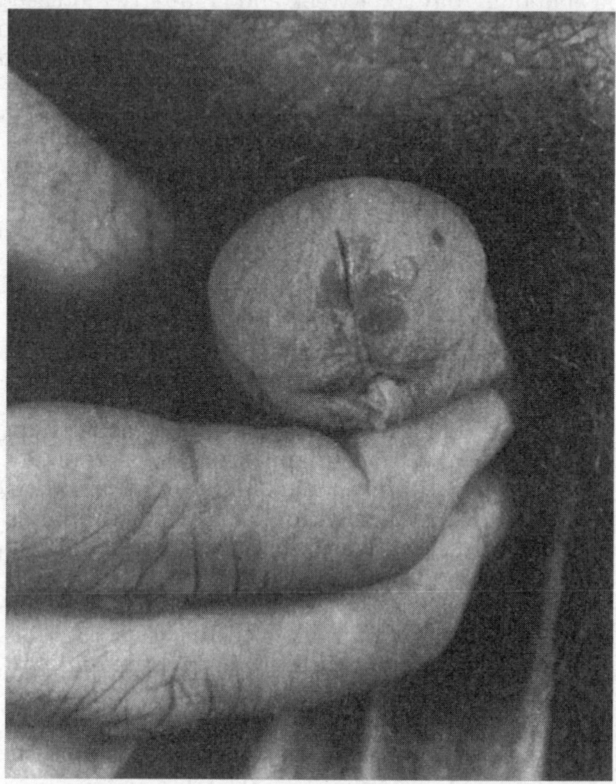

Figure 78.3. Moist, shallow, circular lesions on the glans penis characteristic of circinate balanitis.

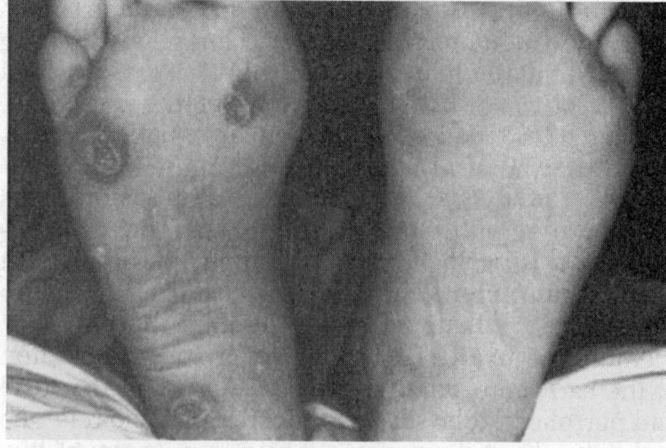

Figure 78.4. Typical keratoderma blennorrhagica involving the sole.

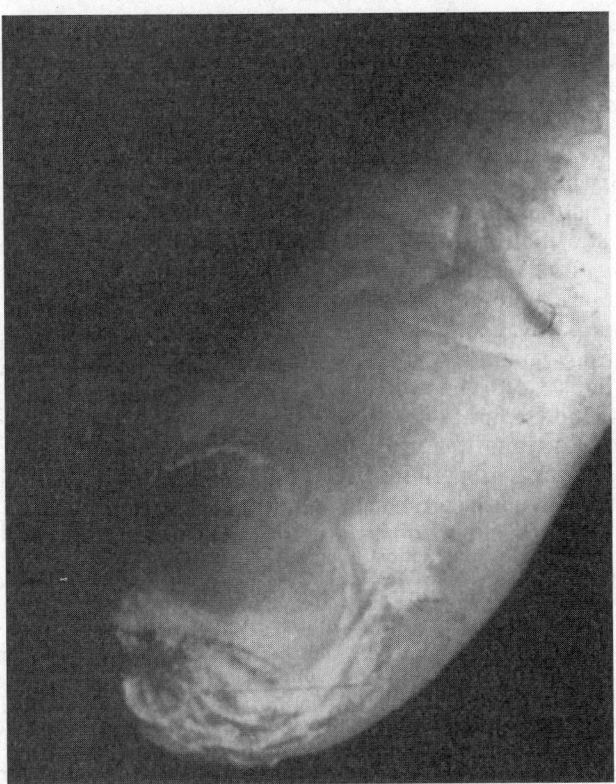

Figure 78.5. Opacification and onychodystrophy of a fingernail in reactive arthritis. (From Arnett FC. Reiter's syndrome. In: Fitzpatrick TB, Eisen AZ, Wolf K, et al., eds. Dermatology in general medicine, 3rd ed. New York: McGraw-Hill, 1985, with permission.)

Additional features include fever in approximately one-third of patients, weight loss, and uveitis. The disease may begin abruptly and run a toxic course or begin insidiously and pursue an indolent one. Often, heel pain (see Chapter 73) is the first symptom, and this complaint should raise the question of reactive arthritis.

Laboratory Evaluation

Hematologic studies usually demonstrate a mild normocytic–normochromic anemia characteristic of chronic disease. The hematocrit value rarely falls below 30%. A modest leukocytosis in the range of 10,000 to 15,000/mm^3 with a mild shift to the left is common in those with an acute toxic presentation. Thrombocytosis with platelet counts in the range of 400,000 to 600,000/mm^3 is found in approximately one-third of patients. The erythrocyte sedimentation rate and C reactive protein level are usually elevated.

Serologic studies for rheumatoid factor and antinuclear antibodies are negative. Serum complement is typically normal or elevated as an acute phase reactant. HLA typing reveals the B27 antigen in 60% to 75% of cases but is rarely required in diagnosing the disease. *X-rays* are typically normal early in the course of the disease; however, over time, periostitis may be seen involving the calcaneus or along the shafts of swollen digits. If sacroiliitis appears (it does in approximately 20% of cases), it is more likely to be unilateral in this disease than in ankylosing spondylitis. This may be detected by examination (see above) and confirmed by x-ray if there is doubt. In severe disease cartilage may be lost in joint spaces, and bony ankylosis may ensue.

Synovial fluid has the characteristics of a moderate inflammatory process with a poor mucin clot, white blood cell counts ranging from 5,000 to 50,000/mm^3, elevated protein, and normal glucose. Routine bacterial cultures are negative, but newer methods, such as polymerase chain reaction, have detected bacterial DNA or RNA in synovial fluid (17,18). Synovial biopsy demonstrates an acute and chronic inflammatory process that is nonspecific and indistinguishable from that of many other inflammatory synovitides, and therefore it is not usually necessary. A urinalysis performed on the first voided specimen in the morning which shows pyuria is a useful way to identify asymptomatic urethritis. *Urethral stains* and cultures are negative for gonococci in the majority, although the concurrence of gonococcal urethritis with reactive arthritis has been documented. Therefore, this culture should not be overlooked. *Chlamydia trachomatis* infection by urethral cultures or molecular probes or serum antibodies can be found in 30% to 50% of cases. It is mandatory that human immunodeficiency virus infection is considered in patients with sexually transmitted disease and, when appropriate, excluded by serologic testing (19) (see Chapter 37).

Course and Prognosis

Reactive arthritis follows a self-limited course and completely resolves in 3 months to 1 year in most cases, although annoying arthralgias may persist for many years. Approximately 15% of patients have relapses, and it is unclear whether these are caused by reinfection. Less commonly, a chronic progressive course ensues, resulting in articular destruction and fusion of peripheral and usually axial skeletal joints. Disability results primarily from severe heel pain, deformities of the feet, visual loss caused by uveitis, and, less commonly, cardiac complications. Approximately 10% of patients become permanently disabled and unable to work.

Management

Treatment is directed toward suppressing the inflammatory process in joints and tendon insertions, preventing deformity, and managing the extra-articular manifestations. In addition, recent studies support the rationale for eradicating a persisting microorganism with the use of antibiotics (14,20). When it appears that the disease was caused by *C. trachomatis* (positive urethral cultures/probes or serum antibodies), a 3-month course of tetracycline (or doxycycline 100 mg twice a day) has been shown to shorten the course of reactive arthritis (20). In those with a postdysenteric onset, identification of the initiating organism is often impossible because stool cultures are usually negative and serologic detection of the specific enteric pathogen often is unreliable. In such cases, a course of sulfasalazine is a rational approach (14). Patients who have had reactive arthritis who plan travel to areas endemic for the GI pathogens should receive prophylactic antibiotics. Even early antibiotic therapy for gastroenteritis does not appear to prevent the subsequent reactive arthritis.

Indole NSAIDs (indomethacin, tolmetin, or sulindac) are effective in suppressing inflammation and relieving pain in most cases of reactive arthritis. COX-2 inhibitors are more expensive but safer and may be beneficial in some patients. Aspirin is helpful in some patients. Systemic corticosteroids may be necessary to treat severe uveitis or inflamed joints that have been unresponsive to NSAIDs, and in these instances consultation with a rheumatologist also is suggested. At times, intra-articular corticosteroid injection (usually performed by a rheumatologist) may be useful when systemic therapy has not completely suppressed the inflammatory process. Tumor necrosis factor antagonists are showing encouraging early results in patients so treated (15,16). Only occasional patients with extensive cutaneous or articular disease require more radical therapy with cytotoxic drugs, and consultation with a rheumatologist should be sought in these circumstances. Anti-inflammatory agents are generally continued for as long as inflammatory signs, pain, and stiffness persist.

Physical measures are important adjuncts in the management of this disorder, as they are in ankylosing spondylitis. There is a tendency for fusion of affected peripheral and axial joints. During acute inflammatory episodes, rest is important, and severely inflamed joints should be splinted to ensure comfort for the patient. As soon as inflammation can be brought under control with drugs, the affected joints should be exercised to maintain their ranges of motion. At first, passive range of motion should be encouraged in all affected joints. Later, more active range-of-motion and strengthening exercises should be prescribed as the patient improves.

Painful feet, especially heels, may be helped by shoe inserts that shift weight-bearing to nonaffected areas (see Chapter 73).

Urethritis does not require specific therapy unless *C. trachomatis* (or gonococci) are identified. Patients should be counseled about ways to prevent reinfection with venereal and enteric pathogens (e.g., use of condoms and treatment of conjugal partner). Conjunctivitis responds to compresses or astringent drops (see Chapter 109). Uveal tract involvement, if present, requires close follow-up by an ophthalmologist to prevent permanent visual loss. The skin lesions are usually self-limited and require no therapy or only the use of local corticosteroid creams. Rarely, extensive psoriasis-like lesions or even erythroderma develop and require more intensive management by a dermatologist.

General References*

Arnett FC. Spondyloarthropathies. In: Rich RR, ed. Clinical immunology: principles and practice. St. Louis: CV Mosby, 2001.

Yu D, ed. Spondyloarthropathies. Rheum Dis Clin North Am 1998;24:663.

Specific References

1. Burgos-Vargos R, Pineda C. New clinical and radiographic features of the seronegative spondyloarthropathies. Curr Opin Rheumatol 1991;3:562.
2. Braun J, Sieper J. The sacroiliac joint in the spondyloarthropathies. Curr Opin Rheumatol 1996;8:275.
3. Khan MA, Khan MK. Diagnostic value of HLA-B27 testing in ankylosing spondylitis and Reiter's syndrome. Ann Intern Med 1982;96:70.
4. Gonzales-Roces S, Alvarez MV, Gonzales S, et al. HLA-B27 polymorphism and worldwide susceptibility to ankylosing spondylitis. Tissue Antigens 1997;49:116.
5. van der Linden S, Valkenburg HA, DeJongh BM, et al. The risk of developing ankylosing spondylitis in HLA-B27 positive individuals. A comparison of relatives of spondylitic patients with the general population. Arthritis Rheum 1984;27:241.
6. Taurog JD, Maika SD, Satumtira N, et al. Inflammatory disease in HLA-B27 transgenic rats. Immunol Rev 1999;169:209.
7. Keat A. Reactive arthritis. Adv Exp Med Biol 1999;455:201.
8. McGonagle D, Khan MA, Marzo-Ortega H, et al. Enthesitis in spondyloarthropathy. Curr Opin Rheumatol 1999;11:244.
9. Arnett FC, Bias WB, Stevens MB. Juvenile-onset chronic arthritis: clinical and roentgenographic features of a unique HLA-B27 subset. Am J Med 1980;69:369.
10. Bergfeldt L. HLA-B27-associated cardiac disease. Ann Intern Med 1997;127:621.
11. Hunter T, Dudo HI. Spinal fractures complicating ankylosing spondylitis. A long-term followup study. Arthritis Rheum 1983;26:751.
12. Ryan LM, Carrera GF, Lightfoot RW Jr, et al. The radiographic diagnosis of sacroiliitis. A comparison of different views with computed tomograms of the sacroiliac joint. Arthritis Rheum 1983;26:760.
13. Gran JT, Skomsvoll JF. The outcome of ankylosing spondylitis. Tissue Antigens 1997;49:116.
14. **14.** Dougados M, van der Linden S, Leirsalo-Repo M, et al. Sulfasalazine in the treatment of spondyloarthropathy. A randomized, multicenter, double-blind, placebo-controlled study. Arthritis Rheum 1995;38:618.
15. Brandt J, Haibel H, Cornely D, et al. Successful treatment of active ankylosing spondylitis with the anti-tumor necrosis factor alpha monoclonal antibody infliximab. Arthritis Rheum 2000;43:1346.
16. Van den Bosch F, Kruitkof E, Baeten D, et al. Effects of a loading dose regimen of three infusions of chimeric monoclonal antibody to tumor necrosis factor alpha (infliximab) in spondyloarthropathy: an open pilot study. Ann Rheum Dis 2000;59:428.
17. Gèrard HC, Branigan PJ, Schumacher HR, Jr, et al. Synovial *Chlamydia trachomatis* in patients with reactive arthritis/Reiter's syndrome are viable but show aberrant gene expression. J Rheumatol 1998;25:734.
18. Gaston JSH, Cox C, Granfors K. Clinical and experimental evidence for persistent *Yersinia* infection in reactive arthritis. Arthritis Rheum 1999;42:2239.
19. Winchester R, Bernstein DH, Fisher HD, et al. The co-occurrence of Reiter's syndrome and acquired immunodeficiency. Ann Intern Med 1987;106:19.
20. **20.** Lauhio A, Leirisalo-Repo M, Luhdevirta J, et al. Double blind, placebo-controlled study of three-month treatment with lymecycline in reactive arthritis, with special reference to chlamydia arthritis. Arthritis Rheum 1991;34:6.

*Bold print (general references) and bold numerals (specific references) denote published controlled clinical trials, meta-analyses, or consensus-based recommendations.

SECTION

11

Metabolic and Endocrinologic Problems

CHAPTER 79

Diabetes Mellitus

ROBERT I. GREGERMAN, MD

DEFINITION AND CLASSIFICATION

Classically, diabetes mellitus has been considered to be present when an individual exhibits an abnormal elevation of blood sugar in the fasting state or glucose intolerance upon glucose challenge. However, diabetes is not a single distinct disease entity as can be seen from the classifications below.

Until recently, the 1979 classification and terminology proposed by the National Diabetes Data Group of the National Institutes of Health (based on insulin dependence) (1) were widely followed. In 1997, the Expert Committee on the Diagnosis and Classification of Diabetes Mellitus of the American Diabetes Association (ADA) developed a new classification (2) (Table 79.1), followed in this chapter, that is based on etiology. However, there has been some modification of this classification, as new subtypes have been identified (see below).

Type 1 Diabetes Mellitus (Formerly Insulin-Dependent Diabetes Mellitus) and Its Slowly Progressive Form

Type 1 diabetes, which is said to account for approximately 10% of cases in the United States, generally has its onset in childhood, as early as infancy but more often near puberty, and was once called juvenile-onset diabetes mellitus. However, that designation was misleading because this type of diabetes also can develop in adulthood (3 and below). Its essential characteristic is that insulin dependence is eventually absolute; at this stage, without replacement insulin therapy, ketosis–acidosis ensues within hours. Type 1 diabetes mellitus is now considered a chronic autoimmune disease (4), characterized by destruction of beta cells in pancreatic islets and eventual failure to synthesize sufficient insulin. A variety of autoantibodies (e.g., to islet cells [see below], their enzymes, and to insulin) have been identified early in the course of the illness. There is clearly a genetic susceptibility to this process (see below), but environmental influences also play a role. Those influences are not yet well defined. There have been claims, for example, that viral infection (5) or antibodies to bovine albumin (6) may be important triggers, but the precise pathogenesis of type 1 disease has not been established.

Table 79.1. Classification and Clinical Characteristics of Diabetes Mellitus

Type of Diabetes	Former Terminology	Clinical Characteristics
Type 1	Insulin-dependent diabetes mellitus Juvenile diabetes Juvenile onset type diabetes Ketosis-prone diabetes Brittle diabetes	Onset usually in youth but occurs at any age. Insulin deficiency requires exogenous insulin to prevent ketosis–acidosis. Non–insulin-dependent phases may occur during natural history. 10%–12% of all cases.
Type 2	Non–insulin-dependent diabetes mellitus Adult-onset diabetes, maturity onset diabetes; stable diabetes, nonketosis-prone diabetes; in young people called maturity onset diabetes of youth	Onset generally after age 40, but may occur in young; not insulin dependent or ketosis prone, but may need insulin for control of persistent hyperglycemia; periods of ketosis-acidosis may occur during stress or illness; weight control of obese subtypes may ameliorate disease. 80%–90% of all cases.
Other types		
Diabetes mellitus associated with	Secondary diabetes	Diagnosis demands usual abnormalities of glucose handling and documentation of associated condition.
Pancreatic exocrine disease		
Hormone excess caused by endocrine disease or hormone treatment (steroids of glucocorticoid type)		
Drug use (e.g., thiazide diuretics nicotinic acid)		
Insulin receptor abnormalities		Usually associated with acanthosis nigricans; rare, familial.
Genetic syndromes		
Gestational diabetes mellitus	Gestational diabetes	Glucose intolerance has onset during pregnancy; does not include diabetic who becomes pregnant: increased risk of perinatal complications and future diabetes.

Modified from Expert Committee on the Diagnostic and Classification of Diabetes Mellitus. Report. Diabetes Care 1997;20:1183, with permission.

Classification of individual patients into type 1 and type 2 categories on strictly clinical criteria is unreliable. Either type can mimic the other at onset, and sometimes several years pass before the precise diagnosis is made (7–9). For example, it is now recognized that type 1 diabetes can develop over years, with a prolonged period of hyperglycemia before the onset of ketoacidosis. As a result, the World Health Organization proposed a new subgroup of diabetes that it designated "slowly progressive autoimmune type 1 diabetes," perhaps better known as *latent autoimmune diabetes in adults (LADA)* (10). This group has been estimated to account for nearly 10% of all cases of diabetes. If this estimate is correct, type 1 may account for as much as 20% of the diabetic population, 10% with onset in children and 10% as LADA.

Up to 80% of type 1 diabetics have islet cell antibodies (10); as stated, a variety of other autoantibodies may be present as well. Type 1 diabetics who do not have such antibodies have identical presentations to those who do. However, young diabetic patients who are antibody negative may have maturity onset diabetes of the young (MODY), a variant of type 2 diabetes, with a distinct genetic profile (see below) (11).

Inheritance

The genetics of type 1 diabetes are incompletely understood, and prediction of the occurrence of diabetes in offspring of diabetic parents is presently impossible. Even statistical estimates are crude. The prevalence of overt diabetes in offspring of conjugal type 1 diabetic parents is remarkably low, ranging from 3% to 12% in most reports (12). Only 2.5% of siblings of type 1 diabetic patients develop diabetes; when tested initially, these people may show only impaired glucose tolerance (IGT).

If expression of disease in type 1 diabetes was based entirely on genetics, one would expect 100% concordance for diabetes in monozygotic twins. However, this is not the case: Both members of pairs become diabetic only about one-third of the time (13). Thus, environmental factors must be important as well (14).

Parents who have an insulin-dependent diabetic child often wish to know the risk to future offspring. Prenatal HLA typing of fetal cells obtained at amniocentesis could be compared with that of the diabetic sibling. A fetus with the same HLA identity would have an increased risk, but the accuracy of the prediction would still be only approximately 50%. The imprecise nature of this assessment is in contrast to the nearly 100% certainty of predicting Tay-Sachs disease or Down syndrome. Thus, even with an accurate family history and pedigree, together with chemical assessment of diabetes (glucose tolerance testing), only crude predictions can be made for a couple who wish to know their own chances of developing diabetes and the risk for their offspring.

At this point, only a few generalities seem safe. Prospective parents should not be told to avoid procreation merely because one parent is diabetic. Even when both parents are diabetic, the risk of having a child likely to develop diabetes is relatively low.

Type 2 Diabetes Mellitus (Formerly Non–Insulin-Dependent Diabetes Mellitus or Maturity Onset Diabetes)

Type 2 diabetes is often only one component of a complex of abnormalities variously termed the *metabolic syndrome, syndrome X,* the *metabolic syndrome X,* or the *insulin resistance syndrome* (15). Hyperinsulinemia with or without obvious hyperglycemia is present and denotes the presence of insulin resistance. Other components of the syndrome are obesity (central type), hypertension, fasting and postprandial hyperlipidemia, abnormal concentrations of blood coagulation factors, and premature cardiovascular atherosclerosis. Its pathogenesis remains unclear.

Obesity may be the first manifestation of the metabolic syndrome. Only after some years does an obvious diabetic state emerge in which all or most of the various features of the metabolic syndrome also become apparent. As the condition evolves, insulin resistance progresses to glucose intolerance and finally to diagnosable type 2 diabetes.

Type 2 diabetes is the most common form of diabetes mellitus and accounts for approximately 80% of patients presenting with an overt abnormality of glucose metabolism. More than 10 million people in the United States are affected. Patients with type 2 disease are ordinarily neither absolutely dependent on treatment with insulin nor ketosis prone. Nonetheless, some patients being treated with oral hypoglycemic drugs (see below) may require insulin to control hyperglycemia or ketoacidosis during stress. Most are over age 40 at the time of diagnosis, but this type of disease is also seen in young people, and it is for this reason that older terms such as *maturity onset diabetes* have been abandoned.

A current concept of the evolution of the common form of type 2 disease is that obesity-related insulin resistance is superimposed on an individual with a limited ability to secrete sufficient insulin (i.e., beta cell dysfunction, presumably genetic) to compensate for the insulin resistance. In this scenario, obesity-related insulin resistance is the immediate cause of the glucose intolerance (hyperglycemia). Without obesity, an overt diabetic state would presumably not develop (16). However, 10% to 15% of type 2 patients are not obese. Some of these individuals are also insulin resistant, presumably secondary to other causes, perhaps genetic as well, but not all of the cases are in fact insulin resistant. At this point, the scenario becomes more speculative, because longitudinal data on individual patients are not available. Long-standing hyperinsulinemia may eventually diminish, the result of progressive impairment in the patient's ability to secrete insulin possibly, as a result of the accumulation in pancreatic islets of an amyloid-like protein, amylin. The degree of beta cell "exhaustion" is related in part to the duration of the illness. Some patients ultimately develop insulinopenia to the point that they become totally dependent on exogenous insulin and are at risk of developing ketoacidosis if stressed.

Included in the group of type 2 diabetic patients are those who develop the disease before they reach adulthood (known as *maturity onset diabetes of the young,* or MODY). These young adults (or older children) have what was once considered to be a "variant" of type 2 diabetes shown to be a heterogeneous genetic disorder; they are not ordinarily obese (11). MODY is relatively rare in most populations, accounting for about 2% of all cases of type 2 disease (17), but may be increasing in prevalence. MODY should not be confused with a more common problem: An increasing number of children and young adults are becoming obese and developing "ordinary" type 2 diabetes, a problem considered to be of epidemic health proportions in the United States (18) and is now also seen worldwide, mostly in children over the age of 10. Fifty percent to 90% will have a body mass index more than 27 kg/m^2. When diabetes is diagnosed, most prove to have a strong family history of type 2 diabetes. Nonobese young diabetic individuals should be tested for autoantibodies and C peptide to exclude type 1 diabetes and if these are negative or low, respectively, MODY should at least be considered.

A variant of type 2 diabetes has been called *atypical* diabetes, first described in adults who seemed to have type 2 but developed ketoacidosis during stress and required control with insulin. Adult African-American patients exhibit this response with some regularity, and it has recently been seen in obese African-American children. When the ketoacidosis is seen in a child, the issue of type 1 disease is raised, but obesity is the clinical clue that "atypical diabetes" is the correct diagnosis. MODY does not need to be considered in African Americans; it has to date been described only in whites, in Japanese, and, rarely, in Chinese.

Behavioral and possibly environmental factors appear to be involved in the onset of type 2 diabetes. Especially prominent is the role of excessive caloric intake and subsequent obesity in most cases. Although it is clear that obesity somehow aggravates the underlying genetic predisposition for the development of the metabolic abnormalities of the diabetic state and that weight loss often ameliorates them (above), it is also clear that the factors driving the development of obesity are themselves multifactorial. In type 2 diabetes, association with certain histocompatibility antigen (HLA) subtypes and with antibodies to islet cells has not been found. Blood insulin levels vary depending on the stage of the disease and may be supranormal in the early years and subnormal later in the disease. Insulin resistance is the rule, but measurement of insulin concentration has no clinically diagnostic or therapeutic usefulness. Measurement of insulin C peptide is sometimes useful, along with antibody determinations (see type 1, LADA).

Inheritance

Type 2 diabetes mellitus is genetically and clinically heterogeneous (17,19) with a much more obvious familial pattern of expression than type 1 disease (see below). Impaired first-phase insulin secretion is the earliest detectable abnormality in type 2 and is commonly abnormal in the first-degree relatives of patients with type 2 disease even when their conventionally measured oral glucose tolerance is normal. In contrast to type 1 diabetes mellitus, there is essentially complete concordance for type 2 diabetes in monozygotic twins (20).

Studies of ethnic groups show distinctive patterns of inheritance of type 2 diabetes and superimposed geographic (environmental) effects on these patterns. The most easily apparent correlate is obesity. Certain Native American tribes (e.g., Pima, Navajo) show a remarkably high prevalence of diabetes, with about one-half of the adults having the disease; obesity appears to be the major factor in expression of diabetes in these groups. The Hispanic population (Mexican American) of the southwestern United States also shows similar but less frequent expressions of obesity and diabetes. In nonnative populations in the United States, no such distinctive ethnic or racial patterns in the pathology of type 2 diabetes have been recognized to date.

Other Types of Diabetes

Sometimes diabetes is associated with another disease (Tables 79.1 and 79.2); usually the association is infrequent but more common than in the general population. This heterogeneous group includes some disorders in which there is a clear relationship between the associated disease and the diabetes (e.g., chronic pancreatitis) and many others in which an association has been noted but is not well understood (e.g., primary hyperaldosteronism).

Problems in Classification of Individual Patients

On occasion, classification may be difficult. For example, an adult with ketoacidosis may be erroneously classified as a type 1 diabetic when in fact the diabetes is type 2, with insulin dependence having been precipitated by the temporary stress of infection or trauma (see type 2, "atypical diabetes," above). Similarly, the process of distinguishing between a patient with type 1 diabetes and a thin patient with type 2 disease for whom insulin has been prescribed may require diagnostic procedures to exclude the possibility that the diabetes is one of the "other types" (Table 79.2).

Table 79.2. Diseases Associated with Diabetes Mellitus

Obesity	Autoimmune disorders
Endocrine disorders	Adrenal insufficiency (Addison disease)
Acromegaly	Thyroid disease
Aldosteronism	Hypoparathyroidism
Glucocorticoid excess (Cushing syndrome; iatrogenic)	Myasthenia gravis
Pheochromocytoma	Pernicious anemia
Thyrotoxicosis from any cause	Polyglandular failure (adrenals, gonads, thyroid)
Somatostatinoma	Primary hypothyroidism
	Graves hyperthyroidism

CLINICAL PRESENTATION

Most diagnoses of diabetes mellitus are now made at an asymptomatic stage of the disease as a result of routine blood tests that reveal elevation of plasma glucose (PG) concentration. When the diagnosis is actively sought, oral glucose tolerance tests (OGTT) reveal additional cases because up to one-fourth of patients with a diagnostic OGTT have a normal fasting plasma glucose (FPG) concentration. Unless the fasting glucose is elevated, patients do not have enough glucosuria to become symptomatic. Of patients with overt hyperglycemia who are symptomatic at time of diagnosis, most complain of increased frequency of urination (polyuria), due to the osmotic diuresis induced by the glucosuria; excessive thirst with compensatory increased fluid intake (polydipsia); and, if the disease is very severe, increased appetite and increased food consumption (polyphagia), often associated with weight loss if the increased food intake falls short of full compensation for the caloric loss that results from heavy glucosuria. All these symptoms are manifestations of excessive blood sugar and secondary glucosuria. Other symptomatic manifestations include blurred vision (osmolality-related changes in the shape of the lens of the eyes), vaginitis (usually caused by monilial infection), and skin infections. Furuncles and carbuncles, once common, are now rarely seen, but intertriginous candidiasis is common in the obese, and oral candidiasis (thrush) is common in patients with poor oral hygiene or poorly fitting dentures.

Usually, these symptoms are present for weeks or months before medical attention is sought. The onset of symptoms is often insidious and may be attributed by the patient, or even by the clinician, to emotional factors or a common problem such as a urinary tract infection. Indeed, the diagnosis may be missed for a time because the clinician, failing to consider the evolving character of the disease, believes that the patient is not diabetic on the basis of previous evaluation.

Many patients with type 2 diabetes present with minimal or no symptoms of hyperglycemia and glucosuria but have already developed complications such as neuropathy or, more commonly, vascular disease. Also, it is common to encounter patients who believe that their long-standing diabetes is "mild" only to find themselves with severe complications of the disease. Occasionally, a patient may be completely unaware of having diabetes and yet present with retinopathy or nephropathy.

DIAGNOSIS

Elevation of blood sugar concentration is the hallmark of diabetes mellitus. Glucosuria alone is not a pathognomonic finding because rare patients may have a renal tubular glucose leak (renal glucosuria) at normal concentrations of blood sugar. Often, patients show diagnostically elevated blood sugar levels (fasting; post-glucose load in a glucose tolerance test or postprandially) before glucosuria develops.

Criteria For Diagnosis of Diabetes Mellitus

The following revised criteria were established in 1997 by the Expert Committee of the ADA (see above) (2): (a) unequivocal elevation of PG concentrations associated with classic symptoms of diabetes mellitus, or (b) elevation of FPG on more than one occasion (see below), or (c) elevation of PG after an oral glucose challenge (standardized OGTT) on more than one occasion (see below). A *single* elevated FPG or a *single* OGTT never establishes the diagnosis (Table 79.3).

The ADA's decision (2) to promote the FPG, with a new and lower cut point (see below) rather than the OGTT as the primary basis for a diagnosis of diabetes, was based in part on the practical consideration that few physicians were performing glucose tolerance tests in any event and that the OGTT would best be reserved for research purposes. They further argued that, because of its simplicity, careful attention to the FPG would in fact result overall in a larger number of diagnoses of diabetes than was being made with the cumbersome OGTT. The diagnostic cut point of 126 mg/dL (7.0 mM) (see below) is not arbitrary; it is the level in several studies at which the risk begins for the development of diabetic retinopathy, whereas 110 mg/dL is the point above which acute-phase insulin secretion is lost in response to intravenously administered glucose, the hallmark of early diabetes. The ADA did not completely abandon the OGTT or modify its long-time cut points in the OGTT; a diagnosis of diabetes is established by *either* an elevated FPG *or* the OGTT. Nonetheless, a number of studies of different populations have shown that many fewer diagnoses of diabetes will be made when the ADA's fasting glucose limit is used, even though the new fasting diagnostic level is lower than the old one of 140 mg/dL. These studies clearly show that ADA's criteria for diagnosis are less sensitive than the OGTT (10). There is also poor correlation between the new category of impaired fasting glucose (IFG, see below) and impaired glucose tolerance (IGT), the latter term applying only to the values obtained using the OGTT (Table 79.3). The diagnostic significance of elevated postglucose load blood levels in the elderly is not clear, because increased cardiovascular risk attributable to these values has not been clearly demonstrated in this age group (21), unlike the situation in middle-aged persons.

In modern laboratories in the United States, glucose is determined in plasma or serum. Plasma and serum values are identical, but both are 5% to 15% higher than those obtained in whole blood from which they are derived. Portable devices for measuring blood glucose are not sufficiently accurate to be used in diagnosis.

Fasting Plasma Glucose

The latest ADA cut point for making a diagnosis of diabetes is a FPG of 126 mg/dL (Table 79.3), which is a lower value than that previously accepted (140 mg/dL). Two values of 126 mg/dL (7.0 mM) or greater obtained on different days are needed for a definitive diagnosis. Values above 110 and less than 126 mg/dL designate *impaired fasting glucose* (see below). It should be remembered that FPG may be elevated transiently by stress or illness.

Table 79.3. Interpretation of Values for Plasma Glucose

Test	Value (mg/dL)	Interpretation
Fasting PG (no caloric intake for at least 8 h)	<110	Normal
	110–125	Impaired fasting glucose (see text)
	≥126	Provisional diagnosis of diabetes mellitus[a]
Oral glucose tolerance test[b] (OGTT), 2-h PG	<140	Normal
	140–199	Impaired glucose tolerance (see text)
	≥200	Provisional[a] diagnosis of diabetes mellitus

[a]The diagnosis must be confirmed on another day according to the criteria described in the text.

[b]OGTT is performed in fasting patients by administration of 75 g of glucose dissolved in water following the standards of the World Health Organization (see text).

PG, plasma glucose.

Oral Glucose Tolerance Test

The OGTT, for many years an accepted diagnostic standard for the diagnosis of type 2 diabetes, is no longer recommended by the ADA for routine clinical use (see above). It is less convenient, more costly, and more variable than the FPG. However, as stated above, it is more sensitive for establishing a definitive diagnosis. It may have some utility, as for example when there is a need to prognosticate for a sibling of a diabetic the chances of developing diabetes. The test still has a place in diagnosis during pregnancy (see below).

Diagnostic criteria for the OGTT are listed in Table 79.3. The test may be falsely abnormal in people who have had a recent stressful illness, have had a reduced food intake (less than 150 g carbohydrate/day), or who have been taking one of a variety of drugs (e.g., glucocorticoids, most diuretics). Even smoking or caffeine or performance of the test in the afternoon can cause an abnormal test result. Also, the values in the OGTT tend to increase with age; that is also true of the FPG, but the latter increase with age is very small. Although the increase is of interest for research purposes, it has no place in the evaluation of individual patients (see below).

Measurement of a random 2-hour postprandial blood sugar should never be done for screening purposes; it has low sensitivity, specificity, and reliability.

Previous and Potential Abnormalities of Glucose Tolerance

According to the currently accepted scheme, people with a normal OGTT who previously showed either IGT or overt diabetic hyperglycemia should be classified as having a "previous abnormality of glucose tolerance." These people should not be considered diabetic and should not be labeled with the terms *prediabetic* or *latent diabetic*. Terms such as *subclinical, preclinical, chemical,* and *borderline diabetes* should also be avoided.

Impaired Fasting Glucose and Impaired Glucose Tolerance

Patients whose FPG levels or whose glucose levels obtained during an OGTT fall between normal and diabetic (Table 79.3) are now classified by the ADA into a group having *impaired fasting glucose.* The term *impaired glucose tolerance* separates those with glucose intolerance during an OGTT from those who meet the diagnostic criteria for diabetes mellitus.

Significance of Impaired Fasting Glucose or Impaired Glucose Tolerance for Development of Diabetes and Cardiovascular Disease

Both IFG and IGT are risk factors for the development of diabetes. In this combined group, one can expect 1% to 5% per year to develop diagnosable diabetes mellitus. On the other hand, many patients eventually show normalization of glucose tolerance, and still others remain in the IFG or IGT range. The higher the blood sugar within the range of IGT, the greater the tendency to progress to diabetes (22).

Perhaps some of the most convincing evidence on IGT progression has come from long-term studies of Pima Indians (23). The risk of progression to overt diabetes in this group is clearly related to the level of glucose within the range of 160 to 200 mg at 2 hours (three times the risk of that of people with lower values). In this group, however, the rate of decompensation to overt diabetes is still only 3% per year.

Studies of treatment of patients with IFG or IGT with oral antidiabetic (hypoglycemic) agents to prevent or delay the eventual development of diabetes are in progress. Recently, metformin has been shown to have a modest effect (see Prevention of Diabetes Mellitus, below).

However, IFG and IGT are generally conceded to be risk factors for cardiovascular disease (see below). Moreover, even the level of fasting blood glucose within the normal range clearly predicts cardiovascular death in nondiabetic men. The top glucose quartile had a relative risk of 1.4, even after adjusting for other risk factors (24). There is no risk of *microvascular* complications (retinopathy or nephropathy) in people with IFG or IGT unless they develop diabetes as defined above.

PREVENTION OF DIABETES MELLITUS

Prospective studies have shown that altering "lifestyle" can prevent or delay the development of diabetes in high risk patients showing IGT (25). Reduction of progression from IGT to diabetes ranged from 31% to 58% over 3 to 6 years. Whether similar results could be obtained under nonstudy conditions is problematic. Modest weight reduction (mean about 4 kg or 5% to 7% of body weight) and exercise (widely variable but about 2 to 4 hours per week) seem to be the most important contributors to success. Consumption of fiber from cereals and a low glycemic index also have been identified in other studies as contributors to prevention. Total fat intake and type do not seem to relate to the development of diabetes.

A large multicenter randomized prospective study in the United States (Diabetes Prevention Program) included a group who were treated with metformin but did not receive the other interventions (26). These individuals showed a lesser modest decrease in the rate at which diabetes developed over the 3 years of study. Metformin is not at this time approved for such preventive use.

TREATMENT OF DIABETES MELLITUS

Patient Education

Of the chronic conditions that are common in ambulatory practice, diabetes stands apart because of the broad scope and the critical importance of patient education and long-term management. For all diabetic patients, the following factors are important: the impact of diet and patterns of eating on diabetes, the implications of having diabetes on ordinary activities and of ordinary activities on diabetes, recognition of the signs of worsening diabetes, the importance of proper foot care and of regular eye examinations, and the clarification of misconceptions about diabetes. For patients receiving insulin, the following additional factors are important: correct administration of insulin, the unique constraints that insulin therapy places on dietary management and changes of activity, recognition of the symptoms of hypoglycemia, and adjustment of insulin dosage during intercurrent illness.

The patient's response to being informed of a diagnosis of diabetes varies widely. Many patients have already suspected the diagnosis as the result of previous observations of similar symptoms in family members. These patients are often aware of the complications of the disease (loss of vision, amputations) and the use of the needle (insulin self-administration). Transient or even prolonged anxiety or depression is common and should be anticipated by the caregiver. Similar problems at this time are commonly seen in close relatives or friends of the patient. Management of these minor mood disturbances is described in Chapter 20.

Many patients are reluctant to accept the need for self-injection of insulin, and many clinicians are unwilling to press the issue. The result is poor control, inappropriate use of oral hypoglycemic drugs, or both. Reluctance of both patient and clinician may stem from unfamiliarity with the techniques of insulin injection. In fact, insulin injection is simple and almost without discomfort. A firm attitude on the part of the clinician and input from nurses and, if necessary, other diabetic patients can overcome patient reluctance in almost all cases. The use of disposable syringes has eliminated the inconvenience of sterilization, and the modern thin, very sharp, plastic-hubbed, or syringe-attached needles render the injections practically painless. Aspects of technique are described below.

A substantial proportion of new diabetic patients have difficulty making the behavioral changes required for optimal management of their illness. Hence, a multifaceted approach is required, which often involves a diabetic educator, a nutritionist, the primary caregiver, and an endocrinologist. The ADA is a useful resource as well for educational material (see General References). General principles and strategies for educating, motivating, and empowering patients and for helping them make desired behavioral changes are discussed in Chapter 4.

Diet Therapy

Different diet strategies guide therapy for diabetes, depending on whether one is dealing with an obese type 2 diabetic patient or a patient of appropriate weight who has type 1 disease. For the obese type 2 diabetic, the immediate and long-term goal is weight reduction (see Chapter 83). In type 1 patients, timing of meals must be matched to the administration of insulin to prevent excessive postprandial hyperglycemia and to avoid hypoglycemia. In type 2 patients, timing of meals is not critical unless insulin is being used. Diet composition is shown in Table 79.4 and discussed below.

Most obese type 2 diabetic patients are not severely symptomatic and do not require immediate therapy with insulin or oral hypoglycemic agents for control of symptoms; rather, diet therapy is instituted for correction of hyperglycemia and weight. The blood sugar may fall rapidly on initiation of a diet (i.e., within a few days). This effect is caused by caloric restriction and occurs before significant weight loss is seen. Oral agents, if used along with diet, have the advantage that they do not usually produce hypoglycemia, but simultaneous institution of a weight reduction program and treatment with insulin can lead to hypoglycemia and must be done cautiously. No attempt at tight control should be made until active efforts to lose weight have ended. Some, perhaps 10%, of type 2 patients are not overweight. Such patients should not be advised to lose weight.

Population studies indicate that most type 2 diabetes is either made manifest by obesity in genetically predisposed persons or is actually caused by obesity. Overt diabetes in obese patients is potentially preventable or can be ameliorated by weight reduction; sometimes loss of even 5 or 10 pounds has a salutary effect. However, most patients are unable to achieve or maintain a weight that will reverse overt diabetes. In one study, a group of patients with IGT were shown to lose weight over a 1-year period using a reduced-fat diet (average weight loss 3.3 kg); this reduced the number of patients who progressed to diabetes. Over the following 4 years, however, weight was generally regained to baseline and glucose tolerance deteriorated (27).

A guiding principle for formulating diabetic diets should be the recognition that individual food preferences must be respected whenever possible. The dietitian should obtain the patient's preferred dietary history and then should attempt to construct the diet around these preferences. Such an approach is demanding for the dietitian, but the issuance of a standardized "American" diet to a diabetic from an ethnic minority is unlikely to be helpful. Chapter 83 on obesity and Chapter 4 on patient education deal with these principles in greater detail.

Prevention of Atherosclerosis

A goal of diet therapy, beyond weight reduction, is the prevention of atherosclerotic disease. This problem is both more prevalent and accelerated in all types of diabetes and accounts for approximately 25% of deaths among type 1 diabetic patients with onset before age 20. Without treatment adults with type 2 diabetes are two to four times as likely as those in the general population to die from coronary artery disease. A large portion of this excess mortality is undoubtedly caused by the abnormalities of lipids that are so common in diabetes mellitus.

The evidence that atherosclerosis in the diabetic may be preventable is based to a large degree on comparisons of the prevalence of atherosclerotic disease in different populations with widely varying diets (28,29). The diabetic subjects in the United States who followed conventional, widely used, high-fat, low-carbohydrate diabetic diets—at least until about 1970—had the highest rate of coronary disease seen anywhere in the world (three times the rate of the general population). For this reason and because of the evidence from population studies, the ADA

Table 79.4. Distribution of Major Nutrients in Diabetic Diets (United States)

	Nutrients (Percentage of Total Calories)						
				Fat			
	Starch and Other Complex Polysaccharides	Sugars and Dextrins	Total Carbohydrates	Total	% Monounsaturated or Polyunsaturated	Protein	Alcohol
Typical American diet	25–35	20–30	45–50	35–45	30	12–20	1–10
Current diabetic diets[a]	40[b]	10	50	30	50	20	—
Diet suggested by recent research	30	5	35	50	40 (monounsaturated or polyunsaturated) ≥10 (saturated)	15–20	1–10

[a]The recommended diet of the American Diabetic Association also provides < 100 mg cholesterol and 28 g dietary fiber.

[b]Even higher levels of starch and lower levels of fat might be desirable but are seldom possible in Western societies because they differ too much from the traditional diets of these cultures.

recommended that its old standard diabetic diets should be abandoned. Ironically, no strong evidence exists to support the notion that only the high-fat diets used for diabetes were responsible for the high rate of coronary atherosclerosis (see below), although they sometimes contained up to 70% of calories as fat. Type 2 diabetes is now recognized to be part of a syndrome that includes hyperlipidemia and a propensity to the development of atherosclerosis, probably regardless of diet (see Definition and Classification, the metabolic syndrome, above). Currently the ADA recommends that diet should be individualized to accommodate individual preferences along ethnic lines but also advocates a diet high in carbohydrates (50% of calories) and relatively low in fat (30%), a diet similar to that recommended by the American Heart Association for nondiabetic people (Table 79.4).

The ADA nutritional recommendations are in general but not completely followed in this chapter. For details, the reader is referred to their position paper (30). Although such diets have been successfully used in diabetic patients studied on metabolic wards, their reported beneficial effects on blood lipids may result from other factors: control of caloric intake with concomitant weight reduction, very low cholesterol content, high fiber content, and absence of sucrose. Several studies in which patients with type 2 diabetes received such diets resulted in unchanged low density lipoprotein (LDL) cholesterol, lowered high density lipoprotein (HDL) cholesterol, and increased triglyceride levels (31,32), as well as in accentuated postprandial lipemia with accompanying potential for increased atherogenicity. In contrast, another study used a high monounsaturated fat diet (50% of calories) low in carbohydrates (35%) that resulted in improved PG, triglycerides, and HDL cholesterol compared with the ADA diet (33). A later report comparing a high-carbohydrate (60% of calories) with a high-fat diet (40% of calories) rich in monounsaturates saw no differences in lipid profiles between these regimens (34). It is unclear whether seemingly small differences of carbohydrate and monounsaturated fat are critical or whether other factors are involved in this apparent discrepancy. The optimal diet for the control of blood lipids and glucose in the diabetic must still be considered unsettled, but it is reasonable currently to recommend up to 50% of calories from fat, provided that it is high in monounsaturates, and 35% of calories from carbohydrates.

Role of Alcohol (Ethanol)

Objective discussion of the role of moderate amounts of alcohol (ethanol) in the diet is confounded by cultural, social, and religious considerations and by concern for potential abuse and addiction. Moderate alcohol use in men is associated with decreased development of type 2 diabetes (35) and in diabetic women, with a reduced risk of atherosclerotic heart disease (36). Therefore, given the diabetic's high risk of atherosclerosis, it is reasonable, until evidence to the contrary is presented, for clinicians to tolerate if not encourage moderate amounts of alcohol in the diet, especially if the patient is already a user of alcohol. In nondiabetics up to two to three drinks per day for men and one to two for women seem to be optimal for reducing cardiovascular risks, although the dose response is difficult to define (37). On the other hand, alcohol, especially when ingested in the fasting state, can readily produce hypoglycemia in both nondiabetic and diabetic individuals. Diabetics receiving oral agents and/or insulin are probably especially vulnerable to this effect of alcohol. Although alcohol generally increases HDL, which appears to be at least part of its mechanism in preventing cardiovascular disease (see Chapter 82), it may also induce hypertriglyceridemia. If lipid control proves difficult with ordinary therapy in a particular diabetic, attention should be paid to a possible contributing role of excessive alcohol consumption, which may be unreported. Alcohol can also induce or worsen hypertension, another major problem in diabetics.

Role of Hyperglycemic Control in Control of Hyperlipidemia. Before hypolipidemic drug therapy is considered, efforts to control hyperlipidemia in diabetic patients should include at least an attempt at near normalization of the fasting blood glucose (along with initiation of the standard American Heart Association diet [see above] for at least 3 months). At present, no evidence is available that favors insulin or oral hypoglycemic drugs to achieve this goal in type 2 diabetes, although a theoretical advantage for glipizide (see below) has been suggested (38). Treatment of coexisting diseases that can cause hyperlipidemia (e.g., hypothyroidism) is also necessary.

It is inappropriate and usually ineffective to introduce hypolipidemic drug therapy (see below and Chapter 82) if hyperglycemia is not controlled. However, gross elevations of triglycerides (above 1,000 to 1,500 mg/dL) can predispose to acute pancreatitis. Early institution of drug therapy (gemfibrozil or another fibric acid) is indicated under these circumstances (i.e., even before glucose control is achieved).

Glycemic Index

The magnitude of the increase in blood glucose in the 3 hours after a meal is determined not only by the carbohydrate content of the meal but by the carbohydrate type(s) consumed. By comparing the percent increase of the blood glucose to a reference food, usually white bread or potato with the equivalent carbohydrate content, an index can be calculated to predict the glucose elevating effect of the food. Diets incorporating foods with low glycemic indices do reduce postprandial hyperglycemia. When combined with a high fiber content, which probably acts by slowing absorption, meals with low glycemic indices can be beneficial in terms of the total period of postprandial hyperglycemia. Adopting an optimal diet in terms of the glycemic indices and content of fiber may be quite effective and even comparable with the effect of an oral diabetic drug in a type 2 diabetic, but this approach requires a highly motivated patient and the services of a skillful dietitian (39).

Fiber

It is now recommended that most of the carbohydrate in the diet of both type 1 and type 2 diabetics is in the form of high-fiber foods (fruits and vegetables, especially legumes). The ADA currently recommends 25 g of such foods should be eaten each day, but there is evidence that 40 g/day may be preferable (40). A high-fiber diet results in lower mean blood glucose levels and may allow the administration of lower doses of hypoglycemic agents. There is often a modest reduction in LDL concentrations as well (see Chapter 82). In many patients these diets produce a variety of unpleasant side effects, including increased frequency of stools, diarrhea, abdominal pain, and flatulence. The formulation of fiber-rich diets (see Chapter 46) is difficult, and most patients do not accept the major alterations of diet that are necessary to produce the desired effects on blood glucose levels.

Estimation of Caloric Needs

Caloric requirements for maintenance of weight vary considerably from person to person and are influenced by activity level. Required calories are approximately 40 kcal/kg or 20 kcal/lb per day for an adult with normal activity. Thus, a person of 70 kg may require 2,800 kcal, although some lean men performing ordinary activities may require as much as 3,000 to 3,500 kcal/day. Individuals who perform manual labor may need 4,000 or more kcal, whereas sedentary people may need only 2,000 kcal or less.

In prescribing diets, caloric requirements are often underestimated. Clinicians commonly prescribe a 1,800-kcal diet for maintenance even if it is grossly inadequate for a particular patient's caloric needs. Prescription of such a diet leads to frustration and noncompliance. Overzealous decreases of calories for weight reduction may be equally defeating. When maintenance of weight is the goal, a careful dietary history by a skilled dietitian may be a good starting point for establishment of a patient's needs; the prescribed diet should then become simply a modification of that patient's ordinary pattern.

Diet During Conventional Insulin Therapy

Any patient who receives insulin faces a special problem. Unlike patients who are not receiving insulin, who require no special timing of meals, and whose total intake can vary from day to day, patients receiving standard therapy with insulin require rigid patterns of food intake; greater flexibility is possible with intensive conventional therapy (see below). Total caloric intake must be distributed among the meals of the day, which usually include mid-afternoon and bedtime snacks as well. Occasional patients strive to reduce insulin dosage by senseless restriction of intake, incorrectly reasoning that disease severity will somehow be less if they can treat their diabetes with less insulin. Needless to say, they must be dissuaded from such practices.

The exact composition of the diet for the patient with type 1 diabetes is less important for blood sugar control than is the constancy of distribution of the amount of food at each meal from day to day. Insulin effect (duration, intensity), even for a particular type of insulin, varies from patient to patient. Accordingly, avoidance of extremes of blood sugar concentration (hypoglycemia and hyperglycemia) requires some adjustment of food apportionment for each patient. However, one should attempt to simulate as closely as possible the patient's usual and preferred pattern of food intake. The main modification is usually to add between-meal snacks. Once an acceptable food pattern has been established and insulin dosage adjusted to that pattern, the patient must adhere to the program if extremes of blood sugar are to be avoided. Patients learn by trial and error how much latitude they can tolerate. Problems, not easily solved, are encountered in individuals who engage in strenuous sports or work that varies from day to day. Such people may have to eat more on some days than others or make frequent adjustments of their insulin dosage. Rigid control of blood sugar by use of conventional insulin therapy is not possible in such cases. Intensive therapy (see below) actually allows for better control of blood sugar and greater variation in diet and in the level of physical activity.

The major adaptive problem with diet in patients treated with conventional insulin therapy (see below) is the need for most of them to eat in a programmed fashion (i.e., "by the clock"). No longer can the person wait for hunger to prompt a meal, nor can dining out at a restaurant be approached with indifference to the time the meal will be served. To do so is to court a major hypoglycemic episode. However, delay of a meal may be unavoidable. To prevent hypoglycemia in this circumstance, about 10 g of carbohydrate per half hour should be ingested. This can be provided by 4 to 6 oz (180 mL) of a sugar-containing soda (soft drink) or 4 oz orange juice, palatable premeal alternatives to glucose tablets or candy (see Hypoglycemia During Insulin Therapy, below).

Exchange Lists and Special Foods. After a dietitian estimates the constituents that will be acceptable to a patient, joint discussion should be held with the spouse or other involved family members. Cooperation and participation of a spouse in the process may be essential for successful adaptation, which, for practical reasons, may require that both partners participate in the diet modifications.

The intelligent use of diet exchange lists (food equivalents) is helpful for many patients. Such lists are available from the ADA, the American Dietetic Association, and most hospital dietetic units.

Special diabetic or dietetic foods are expensive and usually are unnecessary. Some such foods do contain less simple sugar than is ordinarily the case, but sucrose has no worse a glycemic index than bread or potatoes. The patient must read the labels carefully to avoid deception.

Exercise as Therapy

Historically, exercise was recommended for control of hyperglycemia as part of a basic program of diet and insulin for type 1 patients, but conclusive data indicating such a benefit are not available. Although diabetics, like others, derive health benefits from regular exercise, the complexities of avoiding hypoglycemia during exercise in type 1 patients makes blanket recommendations tenuous (see, Exercise During Insulin Therapy, below). The case for exercise is better in type 2 diabetes. Regular exercise may actually help prevent the emergence of type 2 diabetes (41). The conditioning effect of regular exercise also decreases insulin resistance and can improve hyperglycemia. In patients with type 2 diabetes who receive sulfonylurea drugs, the likelihood of provoking hypoglycemia by an exercise program is not great, but obese patients on low-calorie weight-reduction diets who exercise at high intensity may be severely limited by lack of muscle glycogen unless they consume additional carbohydrates immediately before exercising. Walking or cycling may be the least threatening form of exercise for these patients; attention to a period of adaptation is vital. All patients must avoid exercise that aggravates latent or existing problems (e.g., foot trauma that can lead to ulceration). It should be assumed that patients with long-standing diabetes who may have occult cardiac disease must be especially cautious when initiating an exercise program. A stress electrocardiogram is a prudent but minimal measure in such patients (see Atherosclerotic Heart Disease and Diabetic Cardiomyopathy, below). The clearest rationale for exercise as therapy is as an adjunct to weight reduction programs. With weight loss, sensitivity to endogenous insulin may be restored in obese insulin-resistant patients and normoglycemia may ensue, sometimes obviating the need for oral agents or insulin. The blood sugar-lowering effect of exercise often antedates significant weight loss. Approaches to exercise therapy in healthy people and in patients with heart disease are described in Chapters 16 and 63, respectively.

Exercise During Insulin Therapy

Exercise-related hypoglycemia is a potential problem, because exercise has an insulin-like but insulin-independent effect on blood glucose that can be as strong as the maximal effect produced by insulin. The glycemic response to exercise is dependent on the exercise's intensity and duration. Exercise-related hypoglycemia can range from minimal and asymptomatic, requiring little or no therapy, to severe symptoms that need to be treated with intravenous glucose or injected glucagon. Some patients require an anticipatory reduction of insulin dose to prevent hypoglycemia. Others may need or prefer only additional food before moderate activity. In some patients, especially those who exercise sporadically, prolonged exercise may result in severe hypoglycemia some 6 to 15 hours after cessation of exercise. Modest exercise (walking 3.5 miles in 1 hour) may use 350 extra calories, but only 10 to 20 g of carbohydrates, a fraction of these extra calories, may be sufficient to prevent hypoglycemia. Similar considerations guide management of more vigorous exercise. Recent guidelines for type 1 diabetes are based on the assumption that the patient will be receiving a basal-bolus (e.g., ultralente-lispro) insulin regimen (42). Such an insulin program provides about as much flexibility of dosing as one can presently achieve and rivals that of a pump. At 30 minutes of exercise at levels 25%, 50%, and 75% of VO_{2max}, reductions of preprandial (breakfast) doses of lispro of 25%, 50%, and 75% were needed to avoid most episodes of hypoglycemia. Obviously, if a patient is to avoid hypoglycemia, any regular exercise program must be designed on an individual basis and must be reproducibly performed.

The hypoglycemic effect of exercise may be greater if the insulin has been injected into an extremity that is being exercised. Many patients ordinarily prefer to inject insulin into the thigh, but some who engage in vigorous exercise (jogging, other sports, manual labor) may have to use abdominal or arm injection sites to avoid excessive insulin effect caused by exercise-induced overly rapid absorption.

Selection of Patients for Insulin Therapy or Oral Hypoglycemic Drugs

Type 1 Diabetes

Many patients with type 1 diabetes are started on insulin during an episode of ketoacidosis. By the time the patient is seen in an ambulatory mode, he or she will have been switched from short-acting insulin, used in the treatment of the acute phase, to an intermediate- or long-acting preparation. The insulin dependence has been established by the occurrence of the acute episode. Unless this acute event was precipitated by stress in a type 2 diabetic patient, insulin dependence is usually absolute and permanent. Occasionally in adults (more often in children), the insulin requirement may decrease or even disappear over several months, but relapse is the rule in such cases. Many nonobese adults were in the past considered to have type 2 disease when first diagnosed because they had not developed ketoacidosis on presentation. It is now understood that such patients may have LADA (see page 1184). Conversely, patients presenting with ketoacidosis and thought to have type 1 may prove to have type 2 (see Definition and Classification, above). The presence of type 1 diabetes can be suspected from the lack of obesity, lack of response to sulfonylurea, an unequivocally low level of insulin C peptide (a marker for endogenous insulin secretion), and appropriate antibody determinations.

Type 2 Diabetes

There is no direct relationship between the level of glycemia and the type of pharmacologic therapy to be used. Although it is true that the magnitude of the hyperglycemia suggests which patients are likely to respond to oral agents, the glycemic goal of therapy should determine the selection of the agent(s) to be used. Obviously, if a single oral agent can achieve the glycemic objective, it is the simplest if not always the least expensive route. Other factors, including age of the patient, life expectancy, and the presence of comorbid disease(s), are important considerations in selecting a therapeutic regimen. As noted, the initial approach to the obese non–insulin-dependent patient should be caloric restriction and weight reduction. Such therapy, if successfully followed, can be expected to reduce if not normalize the blood sugar within a few weeks. However, significant caloric restriction may induce a marked fall in the blood sugar within a few days, well before significant weight loss has occurred. If FPG is less than 200 to 250 mg/dL, hyperglycemia and glucosuria will not ordinarily produce enough symptoms to be troublesome during this period and no additional drug therapy (oral hypoglycemics or insulin) is needed. Even an FPG of 300 may be tolerated. These patients are not prone to ketosis; no urgency exists for instituting drug therapy. On the other hand, symptomatic hyperglycemia or glucosuria, persisting for weeks despite efforts at (or actual) weight loss, should not be ignored. In this case, drug therapy is indicated for symptomatic relief of polyuria and thirst and can be discontinued if weight reduction is successful. Most patients with symptomatic type 2 diabetes are treated initially with oral hypoglycemic drugs, although some require insulin or a combination of oral agents or oral agents plus insulin (see below).

The imperative for use of insulin in patients with asymptomatic type 2 diabetes whose blood sugar cannot be controlled with oral agents is no longer in question. The evidence is clear that modest elevations of blood sugar do indeed relate to at least the microvascular complications of diabetes. The United Kingdom Prospective Diabetes Study (UKPDS) data (43) plus other studies and experimental observations have settled this issue. Patients with type 2 diabetes who do not respond to initial treatment with oral hypoglycemic agents are termed primary failures. Others, adequately controlled by oral hypoglycemic drugs for a time, become unresponsive to these agents (secondary failures). Insulin therapy may become essential in such cases. Other patients with type 2 disease develop grossly uncontrolled hyperglycemia during stress (trauma, infection, surgery, glucocorticoid therapy). Whether or not ketosis ensues, the gross hyperglycemia may produce severe osmotic diuresis and its sequelae. Such patients require control of hyperglycemia with insulin therapy, which may be discontinued as soon as the situation warrants. Occasional adults, usually not obese and not necessarily exhibiting much glucosuria, may exhibit unexplained weight loss and lack of well-being. Such patients may show dramatic improvement with insulin.

Some patients receive insulin therapy needlessly. Typically these are obese often elderly patients with type 2 diabetes who have already developed an array of medical problems, usually cardiovascular. The goals of therapy in these patients should be carefully defined. The blood sugar control, even with large amounts of insulin (e.g., 100 units a day), may be poor. Although aggressive use of insulin (200 or more units per day) will certainly normalize blood glucose, hypoglycemia becomes a risk in such people. On the other hand, abrupt discontinuation of insulin at doses of 100 or more units often results in no worsening of control and reveals that no significant insulin effect was manifest at the prescribed dosage. Such patients may do better with combination therapy (see Oral Hypoglycemic Drugs, below).

Determination of hemoglobin A_{1c} (HbA_{1c}) in cases of modest elevation of blood sugar is an important guide to therapy (see below). Using the best available methodology for measurement, the normal mean HbA_{1c} is approximately 5% and the upper limit of normal is 6.5% (3 standard deviations). A near-normal value (e.g., below 7.0%) might deter a recommendation for drug or insulin therapy, whereas an elevated value would suggest that long-term benefit might outweigh the possible risks or inconvenience of treatment. Recommendations for or against therapy under these circumstances are currently determined not only by the clinical circumstances, including lipid abnormalities, but by the long-term deleterious effect of hyperglycemia (see Normoglycemia as a Goal of Therapy, below).

Normoglycemia as a Goal of Therapy

Type 1 Diabetes Mellitus

The results of a National Institutes of Health-sponsored multicenter study, the Diabetes Control and Complications Trial (DCCT), were released in 1993 (44). The study's definitive results have profoundly altered the goals of clinical practice in patients with type 1 diabetes and have provoked new efforts to control blood glucose in type 2 diabetes. The DCCT enrolled only patients with minimal evidence of complications at entry, and the beneficial results were striking. The following is excerpted and minimally modified from the policy statement (44a) of the ADA on the implications of the DCCT results.

The DCCT was designed to test the proposition that the complications of diabetes mellitus are related to elevation of the PG concentration. Previous studies, for example, of patients who had received pancreas or islet cell transplants suggested that the incidence of renal disease could be reduced in euglycemic patients. In the DCCT trial, 1,441 patients with type 1 diabetes were studied; no patients with type 2 diabetes were included. Two groups of patients were followed long term: One treated conventionally (two injections of insulin daily, with a goal of clinical well-being, called standard treatment group) and another treated intensively (with a goal of normalization of blood glucose, called intensive treatment group). The intensive treatment group was clearly distinguished from the standard treatment group in terms of glycated hemoglobin levels and capillary blood glucose values throughout the study. Normalization of glucose values could not be achieved in every individual in the intensively treated group: Mean glucose values for the group were approximately 40% above normal limits. Nevertheless, over the study period, which averaged 7 years, there was approximately a 60% reduction between the intensive treatment group and the standard treatment group in the incidence of diabetic retinopathy, nephropathy, and neuropathy. Intensive therapy resulted in a delay in the onset and major slowing of the progression of these three complications. The benefits of intensive therapy were seen in all categories of subjects regardless of age, gender, or duration of diabetes, although all patients were under age 30.

A computer model that used the DCCT data projected considerable gains for patients with type 1 diabetes who maintain over their lifetimes a near-normal blood sugar: an extra 5 years of longevity, 8 years of sight, and 6 years' delay of renal failure, amputations, and neuropathy. The cost of the required intensive therapy is about $4,500 per patient per year (vs. $1,700 for conventional therapy). The DCCT is the longest and largest, though not the only, prospective study showing that lowering blood glucose concentration slows or prevents the development of diabetic complications. As such, it has major therapeutic implications for health care providers and their patients. However, strictly speaking, its results apply only to type 1 diabetes; relevance to type 2 diabetes is discussed below. Many questions remain unanswered, but the following conclusions appear warranted.

A primary treatment goal in type 1 diabetes should be blood glucose control at least equal to that achieved in the intensively treated cohort of the DCCT. This goal may not apply to all patients with type 1 disease and its pursuit must be based on sound clinical judgment. Of importance, intensively treated patients had a threefold greater risk of hypoglycemia than did patients in the control group. Because serious hypoglycemia is dangerous and is not entirely avoidable, the goal of near normalization of blood sugar may, after an initial effort, have to be abandoned for some patients.

There is no favored form of treatment to achieve tight control of blood glucose levels in type 1 diabetes. However, the goal is certainly not achievable in type 1 diabetic patients by use of single-dose or even two-dose insulin regimens. The decision to use multiple injections of insulin versus an insulin pump (see below) depends on patient preference and the ability of the health care team to provide the necessary resources and support, but even with these regimens normoglycemia can be achieved in only about half of the patients (DCCT results, above). The improvement seen in some of the others may, nonetheless, be worthwhile.

Young patients with type 1 diabetes in the early years of their disease stand to gain the most from normalization of blood sugar (tight control) because prevention of complications is the goal. Patients with type 1 disease who already have advanced complications of diabetes will not benefit at all because such complications are irreversible and probably cannot even be stabilized.

At what point in the course of type 1 diabetes should clinicians consider initiation of intensive therapy? After an initial period of conventional therapy for several months (see below), the issue of intensive therapy should be considered and discussed with patients who are suitable candidates. In those to whom tight control is suggested, the clinician must explain the current view that maintained normoglycemia prevents the long-term complications of diabetes mellitus. The magnitude of the effort that is necessary to maintain normoglycemia must also be explained, including the need for self-monitoring of blood glucose (SMBG). One of the frequent-dose intensive insulin therapy schemes (basal-bolus or multidose) or its alternative, infusion pump delivery of insulin, must also be presented (see below). If the patient understands and accepts the problems and effort required, the clinician may consider a program of tight control. However, serious consideration should be given to referral of the patient to an endocrinologist familiar with such a program because the process is difficult, very demanding of the clinician's time, and usually requires a team approach using a specially trained physician's assistant or nurse. The demands on the patient and the clinician are greatest at onset of intensive therapy. The effort should be made only when the schedules of all parties permit the undertaking.

When is conventional glycemic control rather than intensive therapy appropriate in type 1 diabetes? Often intensive therapy proves to be less than intensive, regardless of the initial intent. Conventional therapy attempts to achieve near normalization of *fasting* PG, as opposed to near normalization of blood sugar throughout the day (see below). Even this degree of control is simply not possible using conventional therapy. Many clinicians, failing to realize the limitations of one- or two-dose schedules, nonetheless still go through an agonizing trial of conventional therapy with such patients, only to have the effort end in failure and produce frustration for all involved. In such futile efforts, several types and mixtures of insulin are often tried along with both one- and two-dose schedules. At this point, the options include acceptance of a simplified treatment scheme that merely avoids excessive symptomatic glucosuria with resultant symptoms and prevents development of ketoacidosis (minimal therapy) or reconsideration of intensive therapy, perhaps under the direction of a specialist team.

Type 2 Diabetes Mellitus

The major conclusion of the DCCT that control of hyperglycemia prevents microvascular complications in type 1 diabetics (44) has since been proven valid for type 2 diabetics as well. The UKPDS, the largest of the studies of type 2 diabetes, reported on 5,102 patients studied for an average of 10 years (43,45,46). UKPDS produced some clear results. With intensified therapy with either insulin, a sulfonylurea, or metformin, a decrease of HbA_{1C} was accompanied by a decrease of microvascular complications (retinopathy, nephropathy, and possibly neuropathy) of 25%. For every percentage point decrease of HbA_{1C} (e.g., from 9% to 8%), there was a 35% decrease in the risk of these complications.

Thus, young or even middle-age patients with type 2 diabetes stand to gain as much from tight control as do young patients with type 1 disease. On the other hand, in patients whose life expectancy is limited by age, complications of diabetes, or concurrent disease, the problems associated with intensive insulin therapy should temper the clinician's approach to glucose control.

A major problem in type 2 diabetes is *macrovascular (atherosclerotic) disease.* Whereas hyperglycemia per se may directly contribute to the development of atherosclerosis, the clinical evidence is weak. Although the DCCT trial produced a favorable trend for type 1 diabetes, the data were not statistically significant. In fact, DCCT was so small and was conducted in such young patients (less than age 30) that it could not have been expected to yield useful information on slowing atherosclerosis through control of glycemia. The UKPDS did not demonstrate a significant effect on the development of cardiovascular complications except in a subgroup of obese patients treated with metformin (46).

Insulin Therapy

Insulins sold in the United States today are listed in Table 79.5. Until about 10 years ago, insulins were prepared from the pancreas of animals (cattle and pigs). Only a few of these preparations are still available. Most insulin is now made by recombinant methodology and has the amino acid sequence of the human or is modified from that sequence. Thus, so-called human insulin is actually produced in bacteria and purified for clinical use.

Except for the rapidly acting insulins, which are clear solutions, most preparations now in use are suspensions of insulin that have been modified by complexing the insulin with the protein protamine (neutral protamine Hagedorn [NPH]) or precipitated from solution (Lente) to prolong their action by delayed absorption after subcutaneous injection. However, some of the newest preparations have modified sequences so that they are clear solutions with altered durations of action related to their physicochemical properties, which in turn has been tailored to ensure delayed absorption (e.g., insulin glargine, see below). The characteristics and uses of these insulins are summarized below.

Rapidly Acting Insulins

Regular Insulin (Crystalline Zinc Insulin). Regular insulin is a completely dissolved (clear) preparation that has long been used intravenously in hospitalized patients for acute therapy of ketoacidosis. In the treatment of ambulatory patients, regular insulin is used subcutaneously, often in mixtures with other insulins. The onset of action of subcutaneously injected regular insulin is 20 minutes; peak action is at 2 to 4 hours, and the duration of action is 4 to 6 hours. Regular insulin also is used for continuous subcutaneous

Table 79.5. Insulins Sold in the United States as of October 2001

Trade Name	Manufacturer	Form	Cost Index[a]
Rapid acting (regular and analog)			
Humulin-R	Lilly	Human (rDNA)	1.0
Humulin-R Regular U-500[b] (concentrated)	Lilly	Human (rDNA)	0.7
Humalog (Lispro)	Lilly	Human (rDNA)	1.7–6.2[c]
Iletin II Regular	Lilly	Pork	2.0
Novolog (Aspart)	Novo-Nordisk	Human (rDNA)	—
Novolin R	Novo-Nordisk	Human (rDNA)	1.0
Novolin R Penfill and Prefilled	Novo-Nordisk	Human (rDNA)	1.7–2.1
Velosulin BR (for use with pumps)	Novo-Nordisk	Human (rDNA)	1.4
Intermediate acting (NPH, Lente and analog)			
Humalog Mix 75/25	Lilly	Analog (rDNA)	2.0
Humulin L (Lente)	Lilly	Human (rDNA)	1.0
Humulin N (NPH)	Lilly	Human (rDNA)	1.0
Lente Iletin II	Lilly	Pork	4.8
Novolin L (Lente)	Novo-Nordisk	Human (rDNA)	1.0
Novolin N (NPH)	Novo-Nordisk	Human (rDNA)	1.0
Novolin N Penfil and Prefilled	Novo-Nordisk	Human (rDNA)	1.7–2.1
NPH Iletin II	Lilly	Pork	4.8
Long acting (insulin zinc suspension)			
Humulin U (Ultralente)	Lilly	Human (rDNA)	1.0
	Novo-Nordisk	Human (rDNA)	1.0
Lantus (Glargine)	Aventis	Analog (rDNA)	2.0
Mixtures (NPH/regular and analog)			
Humulin 70:30	Lilly	Human (rDNA)	1.7
Humulin 50:50	Lilly	Human (rDNA)	1.7
Novolin 70:30	Novo-Nordisk	Human (rDNA)	1.7
Novolin 70:30 Penfil and Prefilled	Novo-Nordisk	Human (rDNA)	1.7

[a]Cost Index (relative prices) based per unit of insulin.

[b]All insulins are now marketed in a single strength (100 units per mL, U100) with the exception of Humulin-R Regular (500 units/mL U500).

[c]1.5- and 3.0-mL sizes for injection devices.

[d]Humalog Mix contains 25% or 50% insulin lispro. The remaining 75% or 50% is a protamine-lispro crystalline complex that provides a prolonged effect. Mix 75/25 approximates the action of NPH.

NPH, neutral promatine Hagedorn.

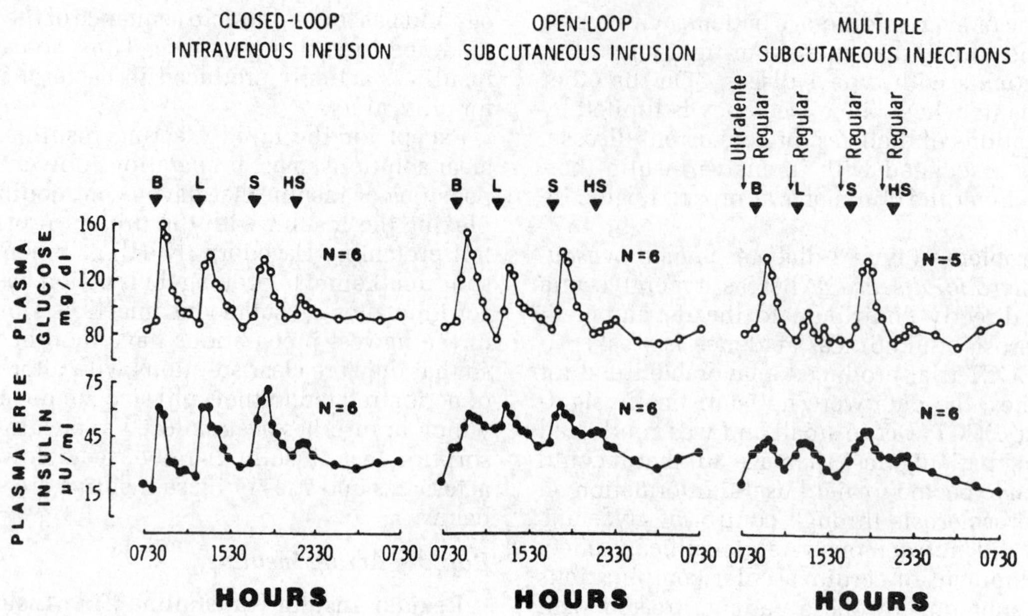

Figure 79.1. Plasma glucose and free insulin levels in patients with type 1 diabetes treated by three methods: closed-loop intravenous infusion (plasma glucose sensor-controlled apparatus), open-loop subcutaneous injections (insulin pump), and multiple subcutaneous injections (intensive conventional therapy). *B,* Breakfast; *L,* lunch; *S,* supper; *HS,* bedtime snacks. Note that the results are essentially the same with all methods used. (Modified from Rizza R, Gerich JE, Haymond MD, et al. Control of blood sugar in insulin-dependent diabetes; comparison of an artificial endocrine pancreas, continuous subcutaneous insulin infusion, and intensified conventional insulin therapy. N Engl J Med 1980;303:1313; Schade DS, Santiago JV, Skyler JS, et al. Intensive insulin therapy. Garden City, NY: Medica Examination Publishing, 1983:138, with permission.)

injection with portable infusion pumps and is increasingly used in combination with Ultralente insulin or insulin glargine in intensive control schemes; the long-acting component provides the equivalent of background activity provided by the basal infusion rate of a pump, whereas additional subcutaneous injections before meals are equivalent to the bolus injections of the pump (see below) (Fig. 79.1). Regular insulin is available as mixtures with NPH to provide a more rapidly acting component (Table 79.5).

Insulin Lispro. Insulin lispro, an amino acid-modified recombinant human insulin, when given subcutaneously has a more rapid onset of action (5 to 10 minutes) than ordinary regular insulin and a somewhat shorter duration of action, both resulting from its more rapid absorption. Lispro's main usefulness is in multidose programs involving intensive therapy (see below) and in insulin pumps.

Intermediate Acting Insulins

Neutral Protamine Hagedorn Insulin. NPH insulin is a standardized neutral crystalline suspension prepared from an excess of regular insulin and protamine zinc insulin. NPH is the most commonly used intermediate-acting insulin in the United States. NPH exhibits rather rapid onset of action and a duration of action that begins to wane after about 12 hours but may last up to 20 hours. When a single injection of NPH is given in the morning, the short-acting component provides insulin effect during the day or to a lesser extent into the evening when meals are elevating the blood glucose, whereas the long-acting protamine zinc insulin component provides background insulin that lasts into the night. NPH can be given in the evenings and in multidose schemes described below. For most patients the achieved ratio of insulin effects is inadequate. Nonetheless, in the United States, many physicians continue to prescribe a single daily injection of NPH, a practice that has long been discontinued in Europe, where NPH is almost always given in two doses. Recently, NPH has been increasingly used in combination with sulfonylureas (see below). Mixtures of NPH and regular insulin (e.g., 70:30; Table 79.5) are now marketed (see Mixtures of Insulin, below) and are useful in some patients in controlling the postprandial increase in blood sugar.

Lente Insulin. The Lente insulin series was devised to avoid the use of the foreign protein protamine. Controlled addition of zinc is used to prepare an amorphous, rapidly absorbed, and rapidly acting material, Semilente insulin, and a crystalline product with much slower absorption and longer action, Ultralente insulin. Lente insulin is a mixture (30:70) of amorphous (Semilente) and crystalline (Ultralente) insulins. Although commonly thought to be equivalent to NPH, Lente is slower in onset and its duration of action is significantly longer, usually exceeding 24 hours. If a single daily dose of insulin is the treatment goal, Lente may be appropriate and a better choice than NPH.

Long-Acting Insulins

Ultralente insulin of beef origin has a duration of action exceeding 24 hours but is no longer marketed in the United States and has been replaced by the human form. It may occasionally be used alone. Ultralente insulin (beef or human) until recently was the backbone of intensive therapy by the basal-bolus technique. The prolonged effect of this preparation provides the basal (background) activity equivalent to that of an insulin pump (see below). It is important to note that unlike the beef product, Humulin U (human recombinant ultralente) has a duration of action shorter than 24 hours and may not be the best choice for use as a source of basal activity in multidose intensive therapy schemes, although human ultralente has been successfully used for this purpose.

Insulin glargine (Lantus; formerly HOE 901), a new recently approved recombinant long-acting insulin analog, is a completely soluble preparation that lasts longer than 24 hours. Glargine is comparable in its duration of action with beef Ultralente, but glargine is promoted as providing a more constant blood level and more predictable in its absorption than either beef or human ultralente. Glargine is becoming the agent of choice for basal-bolus schemes. It is twice as expensive as Ultralente insulin and its long-term safety has not been established (47).

Mixtures of Insulins

A frequent goal of conventional insulin therapy is a single injection once daily. This goal is inferior to a multidose program for control of glycemia (see below) and should only be used if the patient refuses to take insulin at least twice daily. If a single dose is to be used, insulin effect must be prolonged sufficiently to produce normoglycemia in the morning and at the same time provide adequate daytime control of the increases of blood glucose that occur postprandially. However, the duration of action of NPH is usually too short for this goal, and Lente, although sometimes a better choice, is often unsatisfactory as well. One of two scenarios is observed. First, the excessive daytime hyperglycemia dictates the need for additional rapidly acting insulin. Thus, regular insulin is added to NPH or Lente. Second, the single injection of NPH or Lente controls daytime hyperglycemia but the total duration of action is inadequate, resulting in hyperglycemia at the beginning of the next day. Under these circumstances, an additional long-acting component is needed. If Lente is used, Ultralente can be added. However, most diabetologists in the United States use NPH; their only option is to give an additional dose before dinner or at bedtime. A two-dose scheme was long called a "split-dose program" (see below). A predinner or bedtime dose of NPH can also be added to a sulfonylurea regimen (see below).

Regular and NPH insulins can be mixed in the same syringe in all proportions without affecting the onset and duration of action of the separate components. In the United States, 70:30 and 50:50 mixtures of NPH and regular are now sold; in Europe a series of such mixtures (e.g., 90:10, 80:20) have long been available. Regular and Lente insulins cannot be mixed and allowed to stand for more than a few minutes before injection; delay of injection results in blunting of the action of the rapidly acting regular insulin.

Commercial Insulin Preparations

A number of products are available; the various types, species of origin, and the producers are listed in Table 79.5. Clearly, no clinician needs to memorize this ever-changing list. However, even though most clinicians write prescriptions for insulin without specifying the brand, it is important to recognize the product that the pharmacist has dispensed. Not all preparations are available in a given region; pharmacies often supply the products of particular manufacturers according to local profit considerations. At present, two companies market most of the insulin used in the United States: Lilly and Novo-Nordisk. Both produce reliable clinically comparable products within a particular category. A third company, Aventis, recently introduced insulin glargine.

Most problems caused by impurities in insulin in the past disappeared with the introduction of the highly purified animal insulins several decades ago. Allergic reactions and lipoatrophy were the two most troublesome events; both appear to have been related to impurities and now are rarely seen, except that lispro insulin used in a pump has recently been reported to produce lipoatrophy. *Purified animal insulin* of pig origin (the only animal insulin available now in the United States) is about as expensive as human insulin and is of a comparable degree of purity.

In the past, insulin resistance was often ascribed to antibody formation, but little evidence exists to document significant immunogenic differences or clinical improvement as the result of switching insulins. Human insulin is certainly immunogenic in humans. Some types of human insulin do differ from the products of animal origin by having somewhat more rapid onset and peak of action and shorter duration of effect. Given the variability of onset and duration shown under clinical conditions, these differences may not be particularly important, especially in multidose programs.

Trade Names, Unit Designations, and Syringes

All insulin (Table 79.5), regardless of type or source, is standardized at a specific concentration per milliliter. The symbol *U* refers to the insulin concentration in units per milliliter. All insulins are marketed at a concentration of 100 units/mL (U100). Human regular (Humulin R, concentrated, Lilly) also is marketed in a preparation that contains 500 units/mL. Although long-term storage is best done by refrigeration, insulin is stable for at least weeks at room temperature, and vials do not need to be refrigerated after opening. When insulin is used during travel, extremes of temperature should be avoided, as in a sun-exposed automobile or next to a stove or heating element.

Several sizes of syringes are available for use with U100. A 1-mL syringe can be used for all doses up to 100 units, but most accurate dispensing of less than 30 units is made when syringes of 0.5-mL (50 units) capacity are used. The bores of these syringes are smaller and the scales are consequently expanded. Some patients require more than 100 units for a single injection. For such use, 2-mL syringes (200-unit capacity) are manufactured, but these are in short supply and are difficult to obtain. No syringe is calibrated for use with U500.

The use of disposable plastic syringes with attached needles has greatly simplified use of insulin and is preferred by almost all patients. Many patients reuse disposable syringes without obvious harm, but the practice should be discouraged. Reusable glass syringes requiring detachable needles are also available. Special syringes are available for use by patients with severe impairment of vision that prevents them from accurately measuring a dose. However, a simple solution to this problem is often possible. Disposable syringes can be prefilled with ordinary sterile precautions by an able person (relative, friend, pharmacist) and safely stored in a refrigerator for at least a week.

Insulin Injection Technique

After initial instruction the patient should be observed during self-administration of insulin to be certain that the correct volume is being drawn into the syringe and that the proper injection technique is used. Sterilization of the skin with an alcohol wipe is not necessary, although the injection site should be clean. If the injection is made through skin that is wet with alcohol, unnecessary burning discomfort is produced. Injections with disposable needles are essentially painless. Repeated punctures of the rubber diaphragm of vials of insulin with the same needle dulls the point and leads to painful injections.

In ambulatory patients, insulin preparations should always be given subcutaneously. Most needles in present use are one-half inch in length. Unless the patient is very thin, the best technique involves insertion of the needle at 90 degrees to the skin surface. If the patient is very thin, the needle is 5/8 inch in length, or if the site is covered by thin skin, the needle may be inserted at approximately 45 degrees to avoid intramuscular injection. After injection, the area should not be massaged because that may accelerate absorption.

The choice of injection region is important because the rate of insulin absorption, and hence the duration and magnitude of insulin effect, varies considerably between anatomic locations. Absorption is slowest from the thigh, fastest from the anterior abdominal wall, and intermediate from the arm. In addition, absorption from an exercising extremity is accelerated (see above). The long-used technique of rotation of sites is unwise and may contribute to erratic control. On the other hand, the repeated use of precisely the same spot within a region should be avoided.

Insulin Injection Devices

A variety of devices is available to facilitate the injection of insulin. Button-like injection ports are devices that can be left in place, usually over the abdomen, all day and decrease the number of skin punctures when multiple injections are being given. Needleless injectors that use a high-pressure jet are used by some patients, but they are not always painless, and absorption may be more rapid than with ordinary injections. Fountain pen–shaped injectors use a cartridge containing insulin; the needle does not need to be changed for several days. Delivery is with a push button or a preset dial. These devices are especially useful for diabetic patients taking more than one injection daily, who are eating meals in a restaurant, or who are traveling. The cost of the insulin in the cartridges used with these devices is high (Table 79.5).

Initiation of Insulin Therapy: Setting the Goal

Type 1 Versus Type 2 Patients. Typical type 1 patients are almost always started on insulin during an initial acute episode of ketoacidosis that was treated during a hospitalization, and when encountered on an ambulatory basis, most will be receiving at least two injections of NPH insulin and a total dose of between 30 and 50 units per day. Adjustments of dosage must be made on knowledge of at least premeal and pre-bedtime self-monitoring of blood glucose (SMBG). Type 2 patients who require insulin will usually have received oral agents that have failed to control the blood sugar. The following section refers to insulin monotherapy; combination therapy using insulin plus oral agent(s) is described below.

At the time of initiation of therapy with insulin (or other agents), the clinician should establish a clear goal for the degree of control of glycemia. The blood glucose ranges that can be considered are the following: (a) hyperglycemia that is sufficient to avoid gross symptoms (minimal therapy), (b) approximation of a normal FPG with the expectation that postprandial blood sugar will be elevated (conventional therapy), and (c) near normalization of glucose over the entire day (intensive therapy). The choice of the terms minimal, conventional, and intensive therapy may not conform precisely to the use of these or similar terms by others, and no standard nomenclature currently exists. Obviously, many intermediate gradations of blood glucose may be achieved, but the goals are important for avoiding many management difficulties.

Some have taken the position that anything less than intensive (maximal) therapy is inappropriate, given the demonstration that microvascular disease can now be avoided or reduced if near normoglycemia is achieved. In this view, conventional therapy should now always be intensive (maximal) therapy.

Minimal Therapy. In this approach, the goals are (a) avoidance of the extremes of symptomatic hyperglycemia and hypoglycemia; (b) use of the least amount of insulin that is effective, usually in a single a.m. or p.m. dose; and (c) minimal testing of blood or urine, usually urine, with the first morning urine specimen negative to two plus, and a blood HbA_{1c} that corresponds to an average blood sugar of 230 to 310 mg/dL, or 9.5% to 12% (nondiabetic mean, 5%; range, 3.8% to 6.3%). Diet is prudent (less than 30%

as calories from fat, less than 10% from saturated fat, less than 300 mg of cholesterol). Exercise is according to patient preference.

Conventional Therapy. An attempt is made to approach a nearly normal fasting (prebreakfast) blood sugar, using one or more, usually two, doses of intermediate-acting (NPH) insulin, usually mixed with added regular insulin. The prebreakfast blood sugar should range from 70 to 140 mg/100 mL and the daily mean glucose 160 to 230 mg/100 mL, corresponding to an $HgbA_{1c}$ of 7.5% to 9.5%. SMBG is necessary, usually daily, but sometimes up to three times a day.

Institution of insulin therapy coincides with or follows the establishment of a diet (see above). As pointed out earlier, relative constancy of food intake is essential. If such modest dietary compliance cannot be ensured, the goal of insulin therapy should be changed to minimal (i.e., the avoidance of symptomatic hyperglycemia and ketoacidosis). Attempts to manipulate insulin dosage when the diet is fluctuating is likely to result in hypoglycemic episodes nor will insulin therapy achieve normoglycemia when the diet is varying greatly.

First attempts at blood sugar control in almost all ambulatory patients treated by the conventional approach should be done with an intermediate-acting insulin (NPH or Lente) given 30 to 45 minutes before breakfast. However, use of NPH usually requires two doses (see below, Evolution to a Two-Dose Insulin Program). Although initial dosages are often calculated as units per kilogram, the range of requirements is so large that one might just as well begin with the following dosages, ignoring the weight: A safe initial dosage for a diabetic who has not received previous insulin therapy is 15 units for a nonobese patient and 25 units for an obese patient. Many experts recommend adding 5 to 10 units of regular insulin to the NPH or Lente to help normalize the postbreakfast blood sugar during the morning. Because of this common practice, several manufacturers market mixtures of insulin (ratio of NPH to regular, 70:30).

Continuing to Adjust Insulin Dosage. The patient can be instructed to increase the initial dosage of insulin (see above) by 5 units every 3 days until satisfactory control is approached. Usually, such a program brings the patient under control within a few weeks. Increments of 10 units every 3 days are also safe as long as the patient is not markedly symptomatic or if no effect is apparent within a week. During this time the patient should at least monitor urine glucose, although blood glucose monitoring is preferred (see Monitoring Insulin Therapy, below). A telephone call to the physician, nurse, physician's assistant, or diabetes educator should be made every week (more often if the patient is insecure), but at least when a single-dose program is being established, the patient should be encouraged to proceed with the dosage adjustments as planned and should not require or expect a physician's instructions at every dosage increment. Unnecessary dependence is thus discouraged, and the patient's involvement in management is enhanced.

When glucosuria begins to subside, or when aglucosuria begins to be seen in the first morning specimen, the dosage of insulin should be held constant until the FPG can be obtained. Sometimes glucosuria first subsides during the day rather than in the morning. If this pattern develops, the dosage of insulin should be held constant until both FPG and the PG at the aglucosuric time are measured. When the PG is measured, a double-voided urine sample should be obtained and urine glucose should be measured simultaneously. A few such determinations allow an estimate of the patient's renal threshold; thereafter, the clinician can approximate elevations of the PG for that particular patient from the glucosuria. Progressing from the point of development of aglucosuria during some portion of the day to the eventual targeted level of PG control requires continued adjustment of insulin dosage, almost always upward, and adjustment of the patient to the diet and the routine of monitoring. During this time the patient should be reassured that the period of close dependency on the caregiver will soon come to an end. Every effort must also be made to avoid rigidly scheduled visits to the clinician's office or the clinical laboratory that interfere with the patient's livelihood or important personal affairs. Such intrusions only discourage the patient and promote future noncompliance. On the other hand, achievement of the targeted level of control should not be prolonged and should be accomplished within a few weeks. If months pass and the patient's control remains irregular, seems to follow no pattern, or is marked by many hypoglycemic episodes, the problem is either noncompliance (see Chapter 4), usually dietary, or improper prescription or administration of insulin. Noncompliance in the use of insulin can sometimes be ascertained by the equivalent of a pill count, by comparison of the volume of insulin used with the predicted volume of insulin use. For example, a 10-mL vial of U100 insulin contains 1,000 units; if the patient was supposed to receive 50 units daily, a vial should last 20 days (1,000/50).

Evolution to a Two-Dose Insulin Program. Most patients cannot be controlled with a single dose of intermediate-acting insulin (NPH or Lente; see Table 79.5 and page 1196). In these patients, a single dose will improve hyperglycemia and glucosuria; the late morning or afternoon glucose measurements are the first to show a tendency to normalize. However, the effect of the insulin is insufficient to ensure normoglycemia in the fasting state (i.e., in the early morning). Several maneuvers can be tried (depending on the type of diabetes): two doses of NPH, another type of insulin with longer action, insulin plus sulfonylurea and/or metformin, or evening insulin with or without an oral agent. A predinner or bedtime dose of the same intermediate-acting insulin can be added, sometimes requiring a concomitant reduction of the morning dose. For example, if such a patient is receiving 60 units of NPH prebreakfast daily, up to 15 units may instead be given in the evening—usually before dinner—and the morning dose can be reduced to 50 to 55 units. Additional increments of 5 units may then be made to either dose, depending on whether the fasting or postprandial glucose is too high. The evening dose will have its greatest effect on the fasting glucose. Patients using such a split-dose schedule often receive 40 units or more daily, with 50% to 70% of total daily dose in the morning and the remainder in the evening. A two-thirds morning, one-third evening split is common.

An alternative approach is to increase only the long-acting component. In this case, the Lente insulins are preferred (see Table 79.5 and page 1196, above). If the patient is already receiving NPH, a switch to the same dosage of Lente is made. Ultralente insulin may then be mixed with Lente in increments of 5 to 10 units. Because Lente insulin is already a mixture of Semilente and Ultralente in a proportion of 30:70, addition of Ultralente merely alters this ratio in favor of the longer acting component, thus providing a greater likelihood that early morning PG will be controlled without producing midday hypoglycemia. To some extent, addition of a more long-acting component effects a lowering of glucose even during the day and may prompt a decrease of the morning dosage. In any case, some patients can be controlled on a single injection of mixed insulins in this way. For the patient who refuses a second daily injection this approach is worthwhile; in fact, most patients readily accept a two dose program. Once the FPG is normalized, efforts to attain normalization during the day with these approaches are rarely successful and often end in unacceptable hypoglycemic episodes.

Evening Insulin Therapy for Type 2 Diabetes, Alone or in Combination With Sulfonylurea And/Or Metformin. Over the last 10 years, a number of investigators have reported improved control of hyperglycemia using intermediate-acting insulin (NPH) given in the evening (before dinner or at bedtime) rather than as conventionally used, in the morning. The insulin can be given alone or added to a sulfonylurea if insulin alone is inadequate. Part of the rationale includes a need for increased insulin action during the night to suppress the normal tendency for hepatic glucose output to increase during the early morning. Even patients with severe obesity are candidates for this type of therapy. Improved metabolic control has been claimed for this approach (48). If the patient is insulin naive and is receiving a sulfonylurea at maximal dose, NPH is generally given at bedtime with the aim of achieving a normal FPG; improved daytime control will usually follow. If the patient is receiving sulfonylurea plus metformin, the sulfonylurea is discontinued and the metformin continued before adding the NPH, a maneuver designed to avoid nocturnal hypoglycemia, usually mild, but a risk if the sulfonylurea is continued. Although a glitazone (see below) could be one of the components of this scheme, no studies of this type of combined therapy are yet available.

Intensive Therapy. The term intensive therapy has had different meanings over the years. At one time two doses of NPH was considered "intensive." Currently, this approach is an attempt to normalize not only FPG but also preprandial and postprandial levels. Much evidence suggests that the elevation of $HbA1_C$ is a function not only of the FPG or the height of postprandial glucose excursions but the mean 24-hour glucose or the integrated glucose concentration ("area under the curve") over the entire 24 hours of the day. Intensive therapy requires a maximal effort by the patient, the caregiver, and a team of support personnel (diabetes trained nurse and dietitian).

Intensive therapy uses an insulin pump (below) or, alternately, three or four daily doses of rapidly acting insulin are given preprandially in addition to a long-acting form of insulin to provide background insulin activity. Approximately 50% to 60% of the total daily dosage of insulin is given as the long-acting depot injection in the morning or before bed; the remainder is divided and given before meals as bolus injections of rapid-acting insulin (regular or lispro). Regular insulin can be mixed with the long-acting form before breakfast. The term basal-bolus is often used to describe multidose intensive therapy.

Other regimens have been developed that use three or four doses of short-acting insulin in combination with one or more doses of intermediate-acting NPH and sometimes an oral agent (sulfonylurea) (49). Regardless of the exact scheme, frequent smaller doses of insulin at equivalent or somewhat lower total daily amounts appear to produce better overall control than single larger doses, as evidenced by HbA_{1C} (44,50).

Lispro, although more expensive than regular insulin (Table 79.5), can be taken immediately before eating instead of 20 to 40 minutes before a meal. Also, because of its shorter duration of action, it is less likely to cause postprandial and nocturnal hypoglycemia. It is often given mixed with NPH, sometimes before each meal, and has been shown to achieve superior glucose control. Preprandial Lispro can also be used to advantage without NPH when insulin glargine is given as a single daily dose to provide peakless basal (background) insulin activity.

The goal for *pre*prandial sugars should be 70 to 120 mg/dL. Occasional *post*prandial blood sugars are measured and should not exceed 180 mg. Weekly, three morning levels should be determined to detect nocturnal hypoglycemia. Diet must be optimized and contain as close to a constant total of calories from carbohydrate at each meal as possible. SMBG must be practiced before any program of intensive therapy with insulin is initiated.

On such a program one can expect a daily mean glucose of 155 mg/dL and a HbA_{1c} of 7.2%. These values compare with a normal daily mean blood glucose of 110 mg/dL and HbA_{1c} of less than 5.0%. Thus, even with the best possible motivation and supervision, the mean blood glucose will still be on average 40% greater than normal, yet severe hypoglycemic attacks can be expected to occur about three times more often than during conventional therapy.

These numbers are mean (average) glucose values for the treatment groups of the DCCT. Some patients fare better in terms of the degree of control, and others do not do as well; the same is true of the frequency of hypoglycemia. For patients who can achieve the mean (or lower) values, the benefits in terms of prevention of complications are significant. However, these patients must decide whether the effort is personally worthwhile; the caregiver's role is that of a supportive advisor. A significant number of patients who try intensive therapy are not able to achieve a satisfactory degree of control because of lack of motivation or skill, but for others, despite maximal cooperation, the goal is not attainable, presumably because of their particular metabolic makeup.

Insulin Pumps for Intensive Therapy

Continuous subcutaneous insulin infusion using a pump was first reported in 1978. In the past two decades, many reports attest to the efficacy and advantages of this approach and have defined the complications and risks of this method of therapy. Not as generally appreciated is the demonstration that identical success at normalization can be achieved by multiple-dose programs (see above) (Fig. 79.1 and Table 79.6).

If a clinician decides to institute therapy with a pump, referral to a specialist familiar with one of these devices is usually necessary. Selection of a suitable current model of pump (cost of $1,500 to $3,000) and initiation of therapy are best made by a team active in this specialized field, although if necessary the continuation of therapy can be supervised by the general clinician.

Current pumps have fail-safe devices and alarms to guard against runaway pump action, power (battery) failure, empty insulin reservoir, and inadvertent turnoff. The insulin is administered through a 25-gauge scalp-vein needle attached to the pump via a piece of plastic tubing and inserted into the subcutaneous tissue of the abdomen. The needle is replaced every day or 2. Insulin reservoirs vary greatly in size and can accommodate 1 to several days' supply. Pumps must be worn almost continuously, being removed for only short periods (15 to 30 minutes) to allow showering, bathing, or swimming. Some patients need a respite from the pump (e.g., in anticipation of sexual activity); in that case a dose of intermediate-acting insulin can be used at bedtime and the pump used during the day. Other physical activities, including sports, are often performed with the pump in operation.

Table 79.6. Algorithm for Multidose Intensive Insulin Therapy

Target: Blood glucose 70–125 mg/dL AM fasting, before meals, at bedtime, and not below 50 mg/dL at 3 AM.

Insulin regimen

Insulin	Before B	Before L	Before D
Regular	10	6	8
Ultralente	10	0	10

Algorithm

Blood Glucose Before Meals (mg/dL)	Inject Regular Insulin as Below
60 or less	2 units less
70–140	Usual dosage
141–200	2 units extra
201–250	4 units extra
251–300	6 units extra
Over 300	8 units extra

All dosages are illustrative and must be adjusted as appropriate for each patient. B, Breakfast; L, lunch; D, dinner.

Initiation of therapy can be expected to take about 2 weeks, generally during at least a brief hospitalization in which the patient becomes familiar with pump operation as the dosage schedule is adjusted. Despite the apparent inconvenience of wearing the device, acceptance of the pump is remarkable. Many patients have continued pump therapy for 10 years or more. Patients, observing the improved blood glucose levels, are gratified by a sense of control of their destinies. In addition, they experience a normalization of activities by being freed from the tyranny of a clock-oriented existence because meals no longer need be taken at fixed times but can be taken at will without great concern over the possible development of hypoglycemia. However, hypoglycemia does occur even in the best-managed cases.

A number of problems with pump therapy have become obvious. Failure of the pump or clogging of its infusion line sometimes occurs. Diabetic ketoacidosis rapidly ensues, often overnight, when the insulin infusion is interrupted. Local infection at the needle site also predisposes to ketoacidosis caused by poor absorption of insulin from the infected area, and it may be severe enough to require antibiotic therapy and hospitalization. The approximate frequency of diabetic ketoacidosis has been estimated at one episode per 100 patient months, infection at one per 40 patient months, and severe hypoglycemia at one per 30 patient months.

Multidose Insulin (Basal-Bolus) Versus Pump for Intensive Therapy

As stated above, multidose insulin therapy and the insulin pump are equally effective in normalizing blood sugar (Fig. 79.1). Multidose intensive insulin therapy has the advantage over the pump approach of lower initial cost and freedom from the hazards of diabetic ketoacidosis and local infection but has the disadvantage of multiple injections. In crossover studies, an equal number of patients prefer one or the other form of therapy. Both forms of intensive therapy require extraordinary commitment by the patient, the family, and the clinician's team.

Hypoglycemia During Intensive Therapy. Intensively treated patients lose their early warning system of adrenergic symptoms of hypoglycemia and develop neuroglycopenic symptoms instead and at a lower level of blood sugar (a phenomenon termed "hypoglycemia unawareness"). Indeed, the 1980s saw an epidemic of frequent and severe hypoglycemia, a byproduct of the then-new popularity of intensive therapy. So far, intensively treated adults subject to repeated episodes of hypoglycemia have not shown decreased cognitive or psychomotor function, although this was a problem in children and in young adults in earlier studies of frequent severe hypoglycemic episodes.

Obstacles to Successful Intensive Therapy. Even with renewed efforts at tight control triggered by the DCCT, one must recall that considerable experience

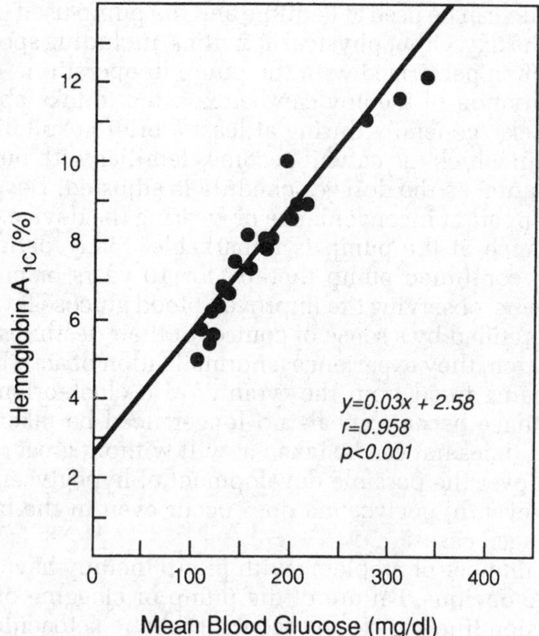

Figure 79.2. Relationship between hemoglobin A_{1c} and mean blood glucose. Twenty-one subjects performed self-monitoring of blood glucose four to six times per day for 8 weeks. The arithmetic mean of those values as compared with the hemoglobin A_{1c} value determined at the end of the 8-week period. (From Nathan DM, Singer DE, Hurxthal K, et al. The clinical information value of the glycosylated hemoglobin assay. N Engl J Med 1984;310:341, with permission.)

with intensive therapy programs has been available for some time. Initial enthusiasm that diabetic complications could be prevented or stabilized has often given way to discouragement as patients and families realize the intense demands of such therapy. The logistics and mechanics of multiple blood sampling, wearing a pump, cost, and the constant reminder of the presence of chronic illness all cause many patients eventually to abandon pump therapy. Moreover, in some patients blood sugars vary widely despite meticulous adherence to the rules of the intensive therapy program. Sometimes patients assume that they are at fault and stop reporting the truth about their glycemic control. Periodic monitoring with HbA_{1c} measurement is useful in defining the true state of control (see below and Fig. 79.2).

Monitoring Insulin Therapy

The rational approach to day to day monitoring depends on whether the treated patient has type 1 or type 2 diabetes and whether conventional or intensive therapy is being used. Frequent monitoring of blood glucose is not essential—or even desirable—in type 2 patients receiving minimal therapy. The simplest approach is to use urine glucose monitoring supplemented by SMBG. On the other hand, patients with type 1 diabetes receiving conventional therapy should be monitored by frequent SMBG. Unless insulin dosage is being adjusted as a function of the results of SMBG, multiple daily measurements are unnecessary.

Efficacy of treatment in the conventionally treated ambulatory patient should be monitored, if possible, by measuring fasting glucose levels. Near normalization of the fasting (overnight) PG represents the basic or coarse adjustment of insulin dosage. Preprandial and postprandial normalization can be viewed as fine adjustments, both of which are difficult to attain. No useful purpose is served by attempts to adjust preprandial glucose levels before normalization of the fasting level is achieved; only thereafter should blood glucose be monitored at mid-afternoon or before the evening meal. The availability of techniques for SMBG (see below) have made blood glucose much easier to track.

Urine Glucose Monitoring. Urine glucose monitoring is no longer advocated and is even disdained by most diabetologists. Yet it is a simple inexpensive procedure and provides considerable information. In some socioeconomic circumstances, it may be all that is available. As a sole technique for monitoring, it is inadequate but clearly preferable to no monitoring at all or to inaccurately performed blood monitoring. Two drawbacks are the variability among patients of the renal threshold (normal range, 160 to 250 mg/dL) and the inability to detect hypoglycemia. The first drawback can be ameliorated by multiple simultaneous determinations of blood and urine glucose to determine the renal threshold for an individual patient. Even two daily determinations of urine glucose can be a useful guide and may be complementary to blood monitoring.

Double-voiding technique should be used when possible. In this technique, the patient voids and empties the bladder, discards the sample, and voids again as soon as possible, using this specimen for testing. When heavy daytime glucosuria is still present, no useful purpose is served by additional frequent monitoring of PG. On the other hand, when glucosuria has cleared, PG determination becomes essential to determine whether the PG has reached or is approaching hypoglycemic levels.

Upward titration of insulin to the point of abolishing morning glucosuria can be accomplished without risk of hypoglycemia if the dosage escalation is stopped when glucosuria first disappears. The patient almost always is still hyperglycemic at this point. Further reductions of glycemia require blood glucose determinations. Monitoring blood sugar in the poor or homeless diabetic patient is often impossible, but urinary glucose measurement may still be practical and helpful.

The optimal frequency of SMBG or of urinary glucose must be determined for each patient. During initiation of therapy, determination of the degree of glucosuria four times daily (first voided morning specimen, prelunch, predinner, and at bedtime) is essential if insulin is to be varied (increased) as described above. Typically, fasting blood glucose must be determined every week or 2 while the insulin dosage is being adjusted and thereafter less often, perhaps only monthly or even every 2 to 3 months.

In ketosis-prone patients with type 1 diabetes, the urine should also be monitored for ketonuria. This can be accomplished using Acetest tablets or one of the combination "stix." Ordinarily, monitoring for ketones is not necessary as a routine procedure, even in type 1 patients. Some experts recommend monitoring for ketones whenever the PG exceeds 350 mg/100 mL or remains persistently elevated. Type 2 patients do not require monitoring for ketonuria unless a severe intercurrent illness develops.

Self-Monitoring of Blood Glucose. If glycemic control to a degree that approaches normoglycemia is the goal, SMBG is mandatory (see below). In the patient with type 2 diabetes, complete absence of glucosuria can often be achieved safely (i.e., with avoidance of most episodes of hypoglycemia) even without the need for frequent determinations of fasting blood glucose, but this is not possible in patients with type 1 diabetes or with intensive insulin therapy. Other indications for SMBG include patients with unusually low or high renal threshold for glucose, many patients with type 1 diabetes treated conventionally, all patients prone to hypoglycemic episodes, pregnant patients, and some patients with type 2 diabetes who, despite an inability to master effective therapy, seem to find SMBG more satisfying than the simpler and less expensive procedure of testing urine with occasional determination of fasting blood glucose or PG.

The process of SMBG should be initiated as a prelude to tight control because unless the patient is able to master the technique and accept it as an ongoing necessity, the effort at tight control will fail. SMBG does not eliminate the need for dietary compliance. Recent studies indicate that within the wide range of what is grossly considered normal, neither intelligence, socioeconomic status, nor personality type has any predictive value for success with intensive therapy. Patients of limited financial means may drop out of such a program simply because of its high cost (approximately $100 per month; but see below).

With programs of intensive therapy blood glucose may need to be monitored up to seven times daily: 1 hour before and after breakfast, lunch, and dinner and before bedtime. Testing may be reduced to four times daily once a pattern of normalization is achieved. Patients who monitor less than four times daily are unlikely to maintain near normalization of blood glucose.

The basis for all SMBG methods is a paper strip impregnated with an enzyme reagent (glucose oxidase) and suitable dyes. When placed in contact with a drop of capillary blood, the change of color intensity indicates the glucose concentration. Some strips are read only visually (without a reflectance meter) (e.g., Chemstrip bG), others either visually or with a reflectance photometer (e.g., Glucostix), and still others only with a photometer (e.g., Glucofilm). Accuracy of strips properly examined visually is adequate for monitoring control, except when the goal is intensive therapy with normalization of the blood sugar. For many patients a meter is not necessary, but most feel more secure with machine readings.

In the United States several meters are in widest use. Accu-Check, which uses Chemstrips bG, and Lifescan are particularly popular. All machines are reliable, portable, battery operated, and cost between $10 and $50 with rebates, depending on whether they have memory for previous determinations. The manufacturers have reduced the prices to promote sale of the matching strips, the retail cost of which is approximately $0.70 each. If four are used daily, the monthly cost is more than $80. Medicare now pays all costs of monitoring in eligible patients (over age 65), and many companies now provide all necessary paraphernalia through on-line orders.

Capillary blood is most commonly obtained from the tip of the finger, although some patients prefer the earlobe. The required drop of blood is obtained almost painlessly using a spring-triggered device such as the Autolet (about $30). Disposable Monolet lances are used to produce the puncture. At a current cost of $0.10 per Monolet, the monthly cost is approximately $12. Recently, a new device, said to be essentially painless, has been marketed that allows patients to obtain blood for testing from less sensitive areas (e.g., abdominal or forearm skin).

Blood flow from the finger can be enhanced before puncture by holding the hand in warm (not hot) water for 30 seconds. The skin should be quickly dried. Puncturing the thumb is least painful, but the ring finger has the best blood supply. Puncturing the lateral aspect of the fingertip (distal phalanx) is less painful than puncturing the ball. Pain is also less when sufficient pressure to produce erythema is applied to the palmar surface (ball) of the distal phalanx; an opposing digit of the same hand is used to apply the pressure. The first drop of blood produced suffices; the presence of extravascular fluid does not affect the result. The finger is inverted and the drop of a size recommended by the manufacturer is transferred to the strip according to the manufacturer's directions; then timing is begun. The strip usually is blotted or wiped, following directions of the supplier, and the glucose level is read. If the earlobe is used, a second or third sample can subsequently be obtained on the same day without repuncture if the site is rubbed with an alcohol wipe and allowed to dry, and the earlobe is flipped with the finger. This procedure is preferred by some patients.

Glycosylated Proteins, Hemoglobin A_{1C}. Chronic elevation of blood glucose results in an increase in the concentration of glycosylated hemoglobins, a major component of which is HbA_{1C}. Determination of the level of either the total glycosylated hemoglobin or HbA_{1C} gives essentially the same information, an integrated estimate of the degree of hyperglycemia over 5 weeks to 2 months (Fig. 79.2). The normal range of HbA_{1C} is 3.8% to 6.3% of total hemoglobin (normal range of total glycosylated hemoglobin is slightly higher, e.g., 5.3% to 7.9%) and may rise to 15% with chronic hyperglycemia postprandially. Values of less than 7.5% suggest excellent control with fasting and 1-hour postprandial sugars in the range of 70 to 120 and 100 to 140 mg/100 mL, respectively. With 120 to 140 mg/100 mL fasting and 141 to 160 mg/100 mL postprandial, one might see HbA_{1C} at 7.5% to 9%. At 140 to 160 mg/100 mL fasting and 160 to 200 mg/100 mL postprandially, values of

9.1% to 11% are common, whereas minimal control gives values of greater than 11%. Glycosylated hemoglobin levels fall slowly with reduction of mean glucose because circulating red blood cells containing high levels of glycosylated hemoglobin disappear normally in approximately 120 days. If euglycemia is established, glycosylated hemoglobins subsequently normalize in 4 to 6 weeks. Conversely, persistent hyperglycemia must be present for 1 to 4 weeks before elevated levels of glycosylated hemoglobins are seen. Short periods of hyperglycemia (6 to 24 hours' duration) may result in disproportionate elevations because some methods include measurement of unstable glycosylated derivatives. Other conditions render interpretations of glycosylated hemoglobin values uncertain, including any in which red cell lifespan is low (bleeding; hemolysis) or in which hemoglobin F is increased (some hemoglobinopathies).

The measurement of glycosylated hemoglobins is a useful clinical adjunct in the assessment of the efficacy of control of hyperglycemia. It is important to realize that glucose is not an inert substance but one that can produce postsynthetic modification of many proteins in addition to the one that is easily monitored as an index of glycemic control. Many proteins other than hemoglobin that also undergo glycosylation exist in nerve, retina, ocular lens, kidney, and cell membranes. Some of these alterations may produce harmful effects and provide a possible biochemical mechanism by which hyperglycemia per se may result in deleterious alterations of tissue structure and function and produce long-term complications of the diabetic state.

HbA_{1C} should, in theory, be usable not only for monitoring glycemic control but in the diagnosis of diabetes (chronic hyperglycemia) or in screening. The objections to such uses have been based on lack of standardization of methodology. Although this is no longer the situation, sensitivity and specificity barriers remain that are population (ethnicity) based (51). HbA_{1C} has also been found to be remarkably nonreproducible in healthy adults, in contrast to the situation in diabetics. To explain the variability of the HbA_{1C} in normal subjects, it has been postulated that the process of hemoglobin glycation varies from one erythrocyte generation to the next (52). The limitation on the use of HbA_{1C} for diagnosis and screening, therefore, is not technical or analytical but rather biological variability.

Fructosamine is the name applied to the ketoamines formed from glycosylated proteins other than hemoglobin. It can be measured accurately, quickly, and relatively cheaply, but because it varies with the concentration of albumin in the serum and because the turnover of albumin is much shorter than that of hemoglobin, measurement of HbA_{1C} is the preferred test in the evaluation of long-term control of blood glucose.

Factors Affecting Insulin Requirement

Insulin Resistance. Classically, the term *insulin resistance* referred to a state in which the requirement for insulin exceeds 200 units daily. This extreme type of insulin resistance is only occasionally caused by the development of antibodies to insulin (see below). Ordinarily, resistance to insulin occurs independently of antibodies to insulin. This resistance—or decreased sensitivity to insulin—is most apparent in type 2 diabetes that is associated with obesity. Even nondiabetic (often destined to eventually become overtly diabetic) obese patients who maintain normal levels of blood sugar do so by secreting supranormal amounts of insulin (i.e., they are in a state of compensated insulin resistance).

Although obese diabetic patients are insulin resistant in terms of their glucose homeostasis and certain aspects of lipoprotein metabolism, their metabolic state is not so deranged that it allows ketoacidosis to develop. In most insulin-resistant diabetic patients, weight reduction at least partially reverses the insulin resistance. Glucose tolerance often improves to (or toward) normal, and the need for insulin to control hyperglycemia may decrease or disappear, only to reappear when weight is regained, as is almost always the case.

Insulin Resistance Caused by Insulin Antibodies. Most cases of insulin resistance are related to the presence of the metabolic syndrome, not to insulin antibodies. However, in rare cases a slow increase of insulin requirement occurring over months may be related to development of insulin antibodies of the IgG type. Usually, the patient may be stabilized at a new higher dosage. Under these circumstances, the duration of action of short-acting insulin is often prolonged, whereas that of intermediate- or long-acting insulins may be shortened. Insulin requirement may exceed 200 units/day, and administration may become a problem. In patients who develop resistance while taking beef or beef–pork insulin, a switch to purified pork or human insulin may result in up to a 30% decrease in requirement. Occasionally, a short course of glucocorticoid therapy is necessary to effect reduction in insulin dosage. Prednisone (40 to 60 mg/day), rather than producing an increase in insulin requirement, usually produces a dramatic fall in insulin requirement after 7 to 10 days, although the response may occur after only a few days. Hospitalization should be considered after several days of such therapy in anticipation of development of hypoglycemia and rapid decrease of insulin dosage. When the decrease occurs, glucocorticoid therapy can be abruptly discontinued. Recurrence of the resistant state is infrequent but may occur after months or years.

Mechanisms of Insulin Resistance in Type 2 Diabetes Mellitus. Insulin resistance is a hallmark of type 2 diabetes, but the mechanisms are still being elucidated. Free fatty acids (FFA) have long been shown to interfere with glucose utilization. Because obesity and diabetes are often associated with elevations of plasma FFA, a major role in insulin resistance for FFA was suspected. Indeed, a specific role for increased FFA flux from the central body (intra-abdominal) fat depots has been postulated to result in increased hepatic glucose output and elevation of blood sugar (53).

In addition to the FFA hypothesis, recent work linking obesity and insulin resistance has focused on the secretion by adipose tissue of the cytokine tumor necrosis factor-alpha as a metabolic messenger that induces insulin resistance. The inhibitory effects of tumor necrosis factor-alpha on insulin action and experiments in animals support this concept, but when obese diabetic patients were given antagonists to tumor necrosis factor-alpha, no effect was seen (54). Nonetheless, the secretion of anti-insulin factors from fat cells remains an active area of research.

Changes in Insulin Requirement Caused by Stress and Other Factors. The stress of infection (or another inflammatory disorder) or trauma may increase insulin requirements quickly. Usually the site of any infection that is severe enough to produce this effect is obvious, or at least there is good evidence of an infectious process (fever, leukocytosis). The mechanisms by which infections increase insulin requirement are not understood completely but appear to relate to the interference of insulin action by cytokines (e.g., tumor necrosis factor-alpha). In addition, stress hormones such as cortisol may also increase insulin requirement by increasing insulin resistance.

Only rarely does a search for a hidden focus of infection provide an explanation for changing insulin requirements or even for the development of ketoacidosis. Although most type 2 diabetic patients are not prone to the development of overt ketoacidosis during metabolic stress, occasional patients, usually African-American type 2 diabetics, seem especially prone to this type of response (see Definition and Classification, atypical diabetes and LADA, above). After the acute episode is over, they may return to their baseline state. These patients may have been controlled by diet, oral agents, or insulin.

In type 1 patients many episodes of ketoacidosis that are not related to obvious stress are not caused by an increased insulin requirement. Rather, such episodes are usually related to noncompliance, although this may be unintentional, as when the patient mistakenly omits insulin.

Illness that produces anorexia may lead the patient to fear hypoglycemia if insulin use is continued when food intake has been decreased. Rather than omitting insulin completely, patients need to reduce its dosage, perhaps by one-third to one-half, but only as appropriate and as guided by SMBG. Insulin requirement tends to increase after the end of the first trimester of pregnancy (see below).

Decreases of Insulin Requirement. Vigorous exercise reduces blood glucose, and in anticipation of such activity, the dosage of insulin often needs to be reduced (see above). During *pregnancy,* insulin requirement drops during the first trimester, rises and may double during the second and third trimesters, and falls suddenly at delivery (see below). Diabetic patients who develop *nephropathy* often show a decreased insulin requirement. Patients receiving long-term dialysis may develop severe hypoglycemia, even after insulin is discontinued, an ominous prognostic sign, presumably caused by failure of gluconeogenesis. A tendency to normoglycemia or even hypoglycemia develops occasionally in patients previously requiring insulin who develop *chronic congestive heart failure.* Development of *adrenal* or *pituitary insufficiency* in a diabetic patient results in a decreased insulin requirement, but such cases are rare.

Effect of Anorexia. When a patient with type 1 diabetes develops anorexia because of mild short-term illness (cold, flu, gastroenteritis), insulin should not be discontinued, but a reduction of the normal dosage by one-third to one-half may be needed. More severe illness (e.g., a marked febrile state) may require continuation of the usual dosage or even an increase in the dosage despite decreased intake of food. Every effort should be made to ensure intake of 50 g of carbohydrate in every 8-hour period to prevent starvation ketosis and hypoglycemia. Careful monitoring of urine or blood ketones (and blood glucose) during such periods with prompt adjustment of insulin dosage may prevent a hospitalization for ketoacidosis.

Hypoglycemia During Insulin Therapy

Hypoglycemia is, of course, an inevitable effect of excessive insulin dosage. However, hypoglycemia also occurs in even the best managed patients, especially when intensive therapy is being used. The clinical problem is to recognize that hypoglycemia is occurring and then to respond to the problem in an appropriate fashion. Hypoglycemic episodes are usually not catastrophic, but inexperienced clinicians are likely to overreact when they occur or to fail to use sufficient insulin because of fear of inducing an episode.

When severe, hypoglycemia causes central nervous system symptoms (neuroglycopenic symptoms) ranging from headache or subtle disturbances of mental function, to confusion, visual disturbances, and personality change, or, rarely, to seizures, unconsciousness, and transient hemiparesis. More commonly, when hypoglycemia occurs during waking hours and is accompanied by the usual symptoms of epinephrine release (tremor, sweating, tachycardia, and palpitations), there is no problem in recognizing the condition. However, in some poorly controlled diabetics, as in some normal people, even mild reductions of blood glucose to levels (50 to 70 mg/100 mL) not clearly identifiable as hypoglycemia can sometimes produce epinephrine release with its resulting symptoms (see Chapter 81). Under these circumstances, documentable hypoglycemia is not present and the clinical situation may be confusing.

The most common cause of hypoglycemia in the diabetic patient receiving conventional insulin therapy is failure of the patient to eat at normal times. Skillful questioning usually reveals the problem (see Chapters 3 and 4).

Diabetic patients often develop defects in mechanisms that normally counterregulate hypoglycemia (55–59). This pathophysiologic state may occur within a few years of onset of the disease. Absolute deficiency of glucagon secretion is common in type 1 diabetes and sometimes occurs in type 2 diabetes as well. Defective endogenous glucagon responsiveness to hypoglycemia in type 1 diabetes is not normalized (reversed) by establishment of tight control (55). Defective counterregulation caused by impaired secretion of epinephrine is also common early in type 1 disease and may become marked in patients with autonomic (adrenergic) neuropathy late in the course of the illness. Other patients may have defective counterregulation caused by impairment of epinephrine action as a result of treatment with beta-adrenergic blocking drugs. In addition, such agents may mask many of the symptoms of epinephrine excess. Regardless of their precise mechanisms, these defective counterregulatory responses undoubtedly contribute in many diabetic patients to their high risk of developing severe hypoglycemia during therapy with insulin.

Many intensively treated patients appear to develop tolerance to hypoglycemia and remain asymptomatic despite markedly subnormal concentrations of glucose, a state called *hypoglycemia unawareness* (60).

Nocturnal or Early Morning Hypoglycemia. Excessive insulin action often occurs during the night or early morning hours. The hypoglycemia-induced release of epinephrine and other counterregulatory hormones (cortisol, growth hormone, glucagon) then causes rebound hyperglycemia, glucosuria, and ketonuria (*Somogyi phenomenon*). If the clinician notes an elevated blood sugar and prescribes still more insulin, the result is further hypoglycemia, perpetuation of the cycle, and possible serious consequences.

To detect this phenomenon, all insulin-receiving patients should be questioned carefully for clues to the presence of nocturnal hypoglycemia (e.g., nightmares, night sweats, and headache during the night or on arising), although these symptoms may not be present and hypoglycemia is revealed only by routine SMBG during the night (see below). The point at which epinephrine release is secreted and produces sweating and other symptoms is quite variable; some diabetic patients trigger secretion at glucose concentrations as high as 50 mg/dL, others do not have counterregulatory release until the blood sugar falls to as low as 30 to 40 mg/dL, and still others have defective counterregulation (see above) and only neuroglycopenic symptoms.

Increasing the intake of carbohydrate in the late evening or reducing insulin dosage by 10% in type 1 diabetes and up to 20% to 30% in type 2 diabetes often corrects the situation. In the latter patients, such a brief and substantial reduction in insulin dosage can be made with impunity.

The classic Somogyi phenomenon must be distinguished from two other possibilities: Waning of insulin action and the dawn phenomenon. *Waning of insulin action* occurs when the patient is receiving an insufficient amount of intermediate- or long-acting insulin; either a single morning dose is not carrying into the next day or the second dose, given before dinner or at bedtime, is inadequate. The *dawn phenomenon* is

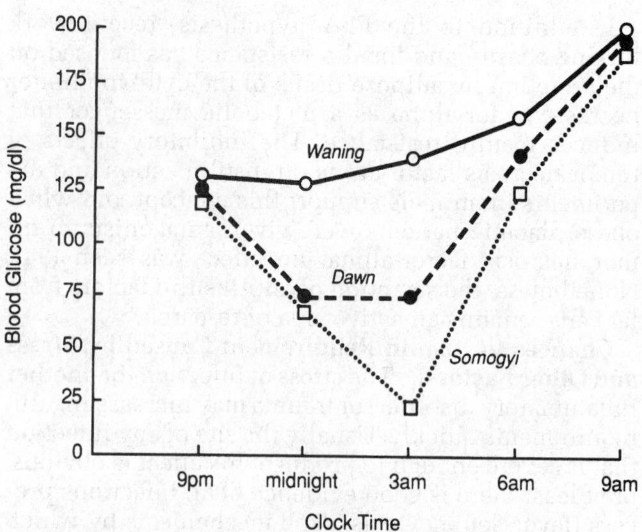

Figure 79.3. Idealized patterns of blood glucose concentrations during the night. The three patterns represent waning insulin action, the dawn phenomenon, and the classic Somogyi effect. All result in fasting hyperglycemia but are distinguished by the patterns of blood glucose concentration in the preceding hours.

an increase of blood sugar between 3 and 7 a.m. that occurs despite continuous subcutaneous infusion or background insulin action from a long-acting insulin. An increased amount of insulin is necessary to overcome the glucose raising action of growth hormone, which is secreted in pulsatile fashion during the night with considerable interindividual variation and, unfortunately, variation from day to day as well. Because of this variation, an amount of insulin that is sufficient one day may be inadequate or excessive on the next.

Obviously, patients with waning insulin action or the dawn effect need more insulin, whereas the Somogyi effect requires that less be given or dosing times adjusted. The simplest way to distinguish these is by SMBG, often for several nights, with samples at 9 p.m., midnight, 3 a.m., and 7 a.m. More frequent sampling may be needed. The differing patterns are shown in Fig. 79.3. Constantly rising glucose indicates waning insulin. A plateau followed by a rise indicates the dawn phenomenon. A drop during the night to a clearly hypoglycemic level points to the Somogyi effect. If SMBG cannot be done, cautious reduction of the dosage of (evening) insulin should be attempted. Although the existence of the Somogyi phenomenon has been repeatedly challenged (61), other evidence convincingly points to its contribution to the problem of glucose regulation (62).

Treatment of Hypoglycemia. The immediate therapy of daytime hypoglycemia in a conscious patient is ingestion of food, preferably sugar. Patients should carry a ready carbohydrate source, such as candy, and must realize that a tiny piece of such material will not suffice. Five or six Life Savers provide the minimum necessary 10 g of carbohydrate, as does a piece of fruit. Glucose tablets (5 to 10 g glucose/tablet) are now available. Also, 4 to 6 oz of sweetened fruit juice or of a nondiet soft drink are most satisfactory. A tablespoon of ordinary table sugar (sucrose) may be added to fruit juice or dissolved in one-half cup of water. Relief of symptoms should be seen in 10 to 20 minutes. Family members or friends should be instructed in the treatment of such an emergency and should not waste time attempting to reach medical assistance before administering sugar. Emergency medical care may be sought after sugar is given, but the problem is usually resolved by the time medical assistance can be obtained. If no obvious cause is apparent for the episode of hypoglycemia—such as a missed meal that is subsequently eaten—the patient should be on guard for recurrence over the next few hours, during which time repeated ingestion of sugar, at hourly intervals, may be advisable.

Occasional patients cannot be treated by the simple means described. Either because of a hypoglycemia-related alteration of mental status resulting in an uncooperative state or because of unconsciousness, some patients cannot take oral sugar. A safe and effective emergency therapy is administration of 1 mg of glucagon subcutaneously by a person instructed in this technique (glucagon promotes the breakdown of hepatic glycogen to glucose). Glucagon is readily available in single-dose form (1-mg vial) and should be kept available during initiation of insulin therapy and in hypoglycemia-prone patients. About 10 to 15 minutes are required for an obvious effect on the sensorium. As soon as possible, oral sugar should then be given. An effort should always be made to identify the cause of the hypoglycemic episode and to reduce insulin dosage or take other appropriate action to prevent recurrence.

Miscellaneous Factors Contributing to Hypoglycemia. Although defects of counterregulatory responses undoubtedly contribute to recurrent episodes of hypoglycemia in many patients, other factors in their daily lives also contribute. Noncompliance with diet may be deliberate or accidental. The need to consume small snacks can be unappreciated or forgotten. Meals are often taken off schedule, upsetting the effort to adjust insulin dosage to preferred time of meals. Amounts of food, if greatly varied, adversely affect insulin dosage. Emotional upset, difficult to evaluate as a cause of varying control, is nonetheless a significant factor in some circumstances. Injudicious use of alcohol is always a concern. Patients may have trouble measuring their insulin or may reverse the ratio of mixtures. Undocumented hypoglycemic reactions may be improperly treated and unreported. Techniques of blood monitoring are often at fault; patients misread directions or introduce variations that lead to errors of measurements. Not to be ignored is the effect of exercise (see above).

Allergic Reactions to Insulins

Allergy to insulin is rare. When it occurs, it is most commonly a local reaction at the site of injection. Local redness, swelling, heat, and itching occur within minutes to an hour after injection and persist for a few hours to a day, often with formation of an area of induration. Such reactions, no longer common, occur during the first few weeks of therapy and usually disappear as therapy is continued. Similar reactions can develop many hours or up to a day after injection (delayed hypersensitivity). Local reactions, misinterpreted as allergic, may also be caused by improper injection technique, the presence of preservatives in a particular brand, or even the injection of cold insulin.

Systemic allergic reactions, with or without a local reaction, are vanishingly rare; they are manifest by urticaria, angioedema, and even anaphylactic shock (IgE mediated; see Chapter 30). Such reactions seem to occur most often in patients who have previously received insulin and appear during reinstitution of therapy after a lapse of months or years. Local reactions may progress to systemic ones; if this seems to be occurring, one should treat the patient before anaphylaxis occurs. The first maneuver involves a trial of highly purified insulin. If this approach fails, drugs such as antihistamines and glucocorticoids are helpful, but persistent insulin allergy is best treated by *desensitization.* With the patient receiving no antihistamines or steroids and no insulin in the preceding 12 to 24 hours, the procedure involves injection of 0.1-mL volumes of insulin that have been diluted 1:100 in 0.1% human serum albumin to prevent adsorption losses onto glass. An initial dose (0.001 unit) is given intradermally. Subsequent doses of 0.1 mL contain doubling amounts (units). After several intradermal injections at 30-minute intervals, the subcutaneous route is used. If a reaction occurs, epinephrine may be administered; the dosage of insulin is reduced, but the process is continued. This procedure requires a series of solutions of insulin. These may be prepared by the clinician or pharmacist but are also available by telephone request to Eli Lilly Co. (Indianapolis, IN). Special kits and instructions for desensitizing patients who have delayed hypersensitivity reactions are also available from the same source.

Lipoatrophy and Lipohypertrophy

Insulin lipoatrophy is now an uncommon event. Harmless but disfiguring localized atrophy of subcutaneous fatty tissue occurs around the site of insulin injections and is sometimes seen simultaneously with insulin allergy. The process may be related to impurities in insulin preparations rather than to insulin itself because preparations of high purity are much less likely to produce this problem. However, even insulin lispro, used in an insulin pump, has been reported to produce this phenomenon.

Insulin lipohypertrophy is even less common than insulin atrophy. This phenomenon is probably caused by an intrinsic action of insulin and has not been improved by use of purer insulins. Repeated injections into the same area do appear to predispose to lipohypertrophy.

Oral Hypoglycemic Drugs

Sulfonylureas

Within a few years after their introduction nearly 50 years ago, sulfonylureas came into wide use for the treatment of type 2 diabetes. The acute hypoglycemic effects of the sulfonylureas appear to be mediated through insulin release. However, in chronic administration, during which blood glucose has been lowered or even normalized, no increase of plasma insulin is apparent. Studies of the mechanisms of action of these drugs show both an increase in the number of insulin receptors and a potentiation of insulin action. Effects other than the desired hypoglycemic action of the sulfonylureas have been studied in connection with drug interactions of these compounds (see below).

Current Place in Therapy. Although sometimes used to good purpose for treatment of symptomatic hyperglycemia, sulfonylureas were often administered to patients with type 2 diabetes who should have been treated initially with diet (i.e., by caloric restriction and weight reduction). Many patients with minimal fasting or simply postprandial hyperglycemia or impaired glucose tolerance on OGTT were also treated.

A multicenter cooperative study (the UGPD study), published in 1970 (63), suggested that tolbutamide was no more effective than placebo and might even increase the risk of death from cardiovascular disease. That study is now considered flawed. The recent UKPD study followed a much larger number of patients than did the UGPD and established unequivocally the value of sulfonylureas in the treatment of type 2 diabetics (43,45,46).

Candidates for Therapy With a Sulfonylurea. Obese type 2 diabetic patients who have not responded to a weight reduction diet within 3 to 4 months or who, having started on a diet, need interim symptomatic relief from hyperglycemia that is producing osmotic diuresis (polyuria, polydipsia) may benefit from an oral hypoglycemic drug. Typically, these patients are over age 40 and are more likely to respond if their diabetes has been present for only a few years. Other candidates are those who are unwilling to accept insulin therapy or in whom the risks of insulin-induced hypoglycemia seem unacceptable. The latter might include patients with occupations involving hazardous conditions (vehicle or dangerous equipment operators). Still others include nonobese patients in whom insulin therapy is unacceptable but for whom persistent hyperglycemia is a risk factor for microvascular disease.

Oral agents should not be prescribed for certain patients: those with a history of ketoacidosis, unless the latter has developed in relation to stress (see below); those with a history of severe toxic reaction to a sulfonylurea; and those with severe hepatic or renal disease, although correct choice of an agent may make such therapy possible.

Effectiveness. In optimally selected patients, about one-half can be expected to experience normalization of fasting blood sugar and about one-third do not respond. In others, some drug effect is evident, perhaps to a degree that permits symptomatic relief. Maximal drug effect can be expected within a few days to a week. Those who do not respond during initial therapy are considered to be primary sulfonylurea failures. In other cases, after a month or more of good response, the drug seems to become ineffective (secondary sulfonylurea failure). The frequency of this response has been estimated at 3% to 10% per year. Some apparent secondary failures are in fact caused by noncompliance. Only rarely in secondary failure is a switch from a maximal dosage of one sulfonylurea to another successful.

Dosing. In initiating therapy, an average dosage is usually appropriate. A single adjustment upward or downward by a factor of 2 may then be made as indicated by the blood sugar response after a suitable interval (see below). When switching from insulin to an oral agent, initial dosage can usually safely be at the maximum recommended level for the particular oral agent or at least in its mid-dosage range. Before switching from one sulfonylurea to another or from one type of oral agent to another, the first should have been tried at a maximal recommended dosage for at least 1 week; trials of more than 2 weeks are not indicated. In changing from a first- to a second-generation sulfonylurea, similar time intervals pertain.

Therapeutic Effects Versus Side Effects. No doubt exists that short-term symptomatic relief of hyperglycemia and its sequelae can be obtained in most type 2 diabetic patients treated with sulfonylureas. This result can be gratifying in properly selected patients. For example, patients who may have difficulty in self-administering insulin because of visual or other physical disabilities may benefit symptomatically from use of sulfonylureas. On the other hand, the use of sulfonylureas is not totally without risk because of their intrinsic pharmacologic action in lowering blood glucose and because of a number of potential toxic effects. Hypoglycemia can occur and may be both severe and protracted, especially in the elderly or in patients with decreased hepatic or renal function. Other complications of these drugs in elderly patients are described below.

Choice of Sulfonylureas

First-Generation Sulfonylureas. For patients with normal hepatic and renal function, there is little to lead one to choose among the first- or second-generation agents (Table 79.7) except for cost and convenience of dosing in that the longer acting drugs do not need to be taken as often. The frequency of toxicity with any of these drugs is very low. *Chlorpropamide* should never be used at a dosage greater than 500 mg/day, above which hepatic toxicity becomes common and additional therapeutic effect is not seen. Because of the ability of chlorpropamide to produce a syndrome of drug-induced water intoxication (SIADH), this drug should be avoided in the elderly (see above), in whom this effect has been seen almost exclusively. *Tolazamide* was introduced 30 years ago but has never been marketed vigorously.

Table 79.7. Oral Agents for Type 2 Diabetes

Drug	Brand Name	Generic	Tablet Size (mg)	Dosage Range (mg/dL)	Doses/day	Route of Inactivation
Sulfonylureas						
First generation						
Acetohexamide	Dymelor	+	250, 500	250–1,500	1–2	Liver, kidneys
Chlorpropamide	Diabinese	+	100, 250	100–500	1	Liver, kidneys
Tolazamide	Tolinase	+	100, 250, 500	250–1,000	1–2	Liver, kidneys
Tolbutamide	Orinase, Tol-Tab	+	500	1,000–3,000	2–3	Liver
Second generation						
Glipizide	Glucotrol; Glucotrol XL	+	5, 10 (tabs) 2.5, 5., 10 (XL)	2.5–40	1–2	Liver
Glyburide	DiaBeta, Micronase	+	1.5, 2.5, 6	1.25–20	1–2	Liver + 50% unmetabolized
	Glynase, Pres Tab		1.5, 3, 4.5, 6 (micronized)	0.75–12		
Glimeperide	Amaryl	–	1, 2, 4	1–8	1	Liver
Biguanide						
Metformin	Glucophage,	–	500, 850, 1,000	1,000–2,500	2 (3 for 2,500 mg)	Kidneys
	Glucophage XR		500	500–2,000	1	
Meglitinides						
Nateglinide	Starlix	–	60, 120	360	3	Liver, kidneys
Repaglinide	Prandin	–	0.5, 1, 2	1.5–16	3–4	Liver
Alpha-glucosidase inhibitors						
Miglitol	Glyset	–	25, 50, 100	75–300	3	Excreted intact by kidneys
Acarbose	Precose	–	25, 50, 100	75–300	3	Gastrointestinal tract
Thiazolidinediones ("Glitazones")						
Pioglitazone	Actos	–	15, 30, 45	15–45	1	Liver
Rosiglitazone	Avandia	–	2, 4, 8	4–8	1–2	Liver

The drug is remarkably safe and has never been associated with drug-induced SIADH.

Second-Generation Sulfonylureas. Second-generation sulfonylureas have been in wide use in the United States and abroad for many years. *Glyburide* (Micronase, Diabeta) and *glipizide* (Glucatrol) are both safe agents. Although all sulfonylureas improve the second phase of insulin secretion, claims have been made that only glipizide in response to glucose stimulation improves both first- and second-phase responses. The second-generation sulfonylureas are more potent on a per milligram basis but only rarely, if ever, are effective when a first-generation agent fails. Slow-release forms of glipizide (Glucotrol-XL) and glyburide (Glynase Prestab) are heavily marketed but are not a major advance. The latest entry to the U.S. market is *glimepiride* (Amaryl); the drug has no advantage over older agents and is much more costly. Glibenclamide and other sulfonylureas are widely used outside the United States.

Transfer from Insulin to a Sulfonylurea. Type 2 diabetics receiving insulin can be abruptly switched, provided that they do not need more than 40 units of insulin a day. Patients who require such large dosages are unlikely to respond well to a sulfonylurea. Patients with a history of ketoacidosis are ordinarily not candidates for a transfer from insulin. If the patient has manifested ketosis in the past (e.g., during stress) but is otherwise thought to be a candidate for a switch to an oral agent, the dosage of insulin may be cut in half as the drug is started. Subsequent monitoring over the next few days will show whether the oral agent can control hyperglycemia or must be abandoned. A history of hyperosmolar nonketotic coma does not preclude a successful change from insulin. Patients with no tendency to ketosis but whose diabetes is so severe that it has produced weight loss may not respond to sulfonylureas given as initial therapy but may respond after hyperglycemia has been controlled for a short time with insulin.

Comparative Cost. At present, the approximate monthly retail cost of therapy with these drugs has a wide range, depending on the dosage and the agent used. All the drugs, except glimepiride and the extended release products, are currently available in their generic forms at one-half to one-third the price of the trade name products.

Instruction to the Patient. The obese patient must be made to realize that weight reduction is the mainstay of therapy and is not simply a general health measure; weight loss has a specific beneficial effect in diabetes. Drug therapy is an adjunct, not a substitute, for weight reduction. The possible risks and goals of therapy should be clearly outlined. Although hypoglycemia is uncommon with the sulfonylureas, when it does occur, it is likely to be both severe and prolonged. Chlorpropamide and glyburide are the two drugs most likely to produce this problem. The symptoms of hypoglycemia should be clearly described to the patient and to whomever is in close contact with the patient, usually family or friends, and corrective measures outlined and understood (see Insulin Therapy, above). The possibility of drug interactions (see below) should be mentioned lest another clinician prescribe a drug that potentiates or decreases the effectiveness of the sulfonylureas, or vice versa. The sulfonylureas are most effective when administered about 30 minutes before breakfast or dinner.

Monitoring Therapy With Sulfonylureas. The frequency and type of monitoring (see above) should be determined by the severity of the diabetes and the goal of treatment. For patients whose FPG becomes normal or reaches an acceptable level, monitoring can be simple because patients receiving sulfonylurea drugs are not ketosis prone and have fairly stable diabetes. Similar considerations apply to patients being treated with diet alone. No compelling indication exists for SMBG (see above) in most such patients. Patients who have FPG in or near the normal range exhibit little or no fasting glucosuria but may show glucosuria in the postprandial state. If clinically stable, such patients can check their overnight (early morning) urine samples for glucose as infrequently as once a week or even every 2 weeks. More important, they should understand that development or worsening of glucosuria where none was evident is an indication for prompt contact with a clinician. Similarly, these patients must be taught that if they develop symptoms and signs of uncontrolled hyperglycemia (heavy glucosuria, polyuria, polydipsia, blurred vision), prompt advice from a clinician is absolutely necessary. Routine testing for urinary acetone is unnecessary unless the patient has new onset of persistent glucosuria or at some earlier time had an episode of ketoacidosis, perhaps during stress.

FPG should be determined every few months in most patients, but the best means of monitoring sulfonylurea-treated patients who respond to treatment with normalization of blood sugar is by determination of glycosylated hemoglobin. Development of frank hypoglycemia or excessive lowering of FPG below 70 mg/dL (which may be detected before symptoms develop) is an indication for downward adjustment of drug dosage. When dosages are changed or when drugs are added or removed, monitoring should be done more often, perhaps daily, with SMBG.

Special Considerations in Treatment of the Geriatric Patient. Many elderly patients are best treated with oral agents. Simple symptomatic therapy may be the foremost consideration for these patients. Insulin therapy may present special problems for elderly diabetics (because of poor vision or poor manipulative skill) that make self-administration of insulin difficult. On the other hand, many elderly patients can manage insulin therapy, especially of the type that is not excessively aggressive, and age alone should not deter the clinician from instituting insulin therapy. As noted earlier, insulin syringes can be prefilled and stored in the refrigerator for 1 to 2 weeks; this plan is useful for the older person who cannot accurately draw up the correct amount of insulin. The elderly are especially likely to have multiple diseases and to use multiple drugs. The risk of drug interactions in this group is therefore greater than in younger people (see below); insulin therapy avoids this problem. A study of various insulin regimens in the elderly, as well as of insulin–sulfonylurea combinations concluded that twice-daily insulin administration was the simplest, most effective, and most cost-effective regimen (64).

The elderly are also especially prone to development of severe and prolonged hypoglycemia with use of the sulfonylureas, which may be related, in part, to the decrease of renal function that normally accompanies aging and may be worse in the diabetic. Decreased renal function (glomerular filtration rate, creatinine clearance) is often present in the elderly even when the serum creatinine is normal because creatinine production decreases with age as muscle mass decreases. Thus, sulfonylureas that are disposed of exclusively by excretion (acetohexamide) or in part by this route (chlorpropamide, tolazamide) might be expected to be more likely to produce hypoglycemia when renal function decreases. In fact, no data are available to support this notion. Clinically, chlorpropamide and glyburide appear to be responsible for most instances of hypoglycemia in the elderly.

Chlorpropamide is also capable of inducing enhanced endogenous antidiuretic hormone action and inducing a water intoxication syndrome and was the first drug recognized to produce this syndrome (65). This phenomenon is seen almost exclusively in elderly diabetic patients. Tolazamide has not been associated with this problem, but the second-generation sulfonylureas can be. Tolbutamide only rarely produced this problem; it and tolazamide are probably the safest first-generation sulfonylureas for use in the elderly. Initial dosages should be low, and increases should be made cautiously. Second-generation drugs are prescribed much more often than first-generation drugs, probably because of intense marketing (although most are now available as generic products).

Drug Interactions. Various drugs enhance the hypoglycemic action of sulfonylureas, and others decrease their effect. Among the more commonly used drugs, salicylates, some sulfonamides, chloramphenicol, phenylbutazone and its derivatives, and warfarin all enhance the hypoglycemic action of the sulfonylureas. Nonspecific beta-blockers may mask the hypoglycemia-induced release of epinephrine and thus prolong and intensify hypoglycemic reactions. Beta-blockers may also block insulin release. Clonidine (Catapres), like beta-blockers, may mask the signs and symptoms of hypoglycemia. Acute ingestion of alcohol can enhance hypoglycemia; chronic alcohol use accelerates metabolic disposal of sulfonylureas and antagonizes their hypoglycemic action. Sulfonylureas, especially chlorpropamide, interfere with the metabolism of alcohol and may produce a disulfiram-like (Antabuse) effect (see Chapter 28). Diuretics (the thiazides, chlorthalidone, and loop diuretics) may produce hyperglycemia even in normal people and antagonize the sulfonylureas. Another commonly used drug, the anticonvulsant phenytoin (Dilantin), also has an antagonist action. Numerous other drugs may enhance or negate the effect of the sulfonylureas; equally important, the sulfonylureas themselves produce numerous alterations of drug action. These problems should not be overstated, but the clinician should be aware of these possibilities and interactions, especially in the elderly, who may be receiving many drugs. Therapy with insulin prevents these problems. A pharmacist with access to a computerized system for monitoring drug interactions can be of great assistance.

Biguanides

Metformin (Glucophage), a biguanide, was approved for use in the United States several years ago, after decades of use elsewhere (Table 79.7). The drug's lowering of blood sugar is probably the result of multiple actions; it does not enhance insulin secretion. Another biguanide, *phenformin,* was at one time in wide use in the United States but was withdrawn because of occasional cases of fatal lactic acidosis and other problems. Metformin causes lactic acidosis much less often (see below). The drug is effective as monotherapy, producing a 50 to 60 mg/dL fall of PG (decrease of HbA_{1C} of 1% to 1.5%). Currently, metformin is preferred by many as the initial oral agent over a sulfonylurea, although no consensus exists on this issue. The main advantages over sulfonylureas are that metformin does not produce hypoglycemia and is less likely to be associated with weight gain. The main disadvantage is that nearly 25% of patients cannot tolerate the gastrointestinal side effects of metformin, whereas sulfonylureas are very well tolerated. Data on overall efficacy are scarce; primary failures occur in 10% to 15% of patients and secondary failures in about 5%. Metformin is often used in combination with a sulfonylurea, as an add-on after failure of the latter. If the combination is effective, an attempt to reduce or withdraw the sulfonylurea can be made after a month. After another month, the need for readministration of the sulfonylurea can be determined. Small decreases of LDL cholesterol and triglycerides are common, as is minimal weight loss (1 to 3 kg). Metformin is not well tolerated by all patients: Nausea, anorexia, and diarrhea are fairly common side effects. These symptoms can be minimized by starting at a once-daily dose (500 mg) and increasing the dosage at weekly intervals until a maximum dosage of 2,500 mg in divided doses is reached. Lactic acidosis is very rare in younger patients, but if the patient has renal or cardiopulmonary disease with hypoxia, a significant risk is present. Metformin is not metabolized and is disposed of by renal excretion. It should not be used if renal function is decreased (serum creatinine above 1.5 mg/dL). The drug should be used with great caution in the elderly because their renal function is often compromised even when the serum creatinine is normal, the result of age or disease related diminution of muscle mass that causes decreased endogenous creatinine production.

Thiazolidinediones ("Glitazones")

Pioglitazone (Actos) and Rosiglitazone (Avandia) are the currently available drugs of this class (Table 79.7). The term "insulin sensitizers" has been applied to this group of drugs, but the term is misleading in that it implies specificity of action. To the contrary, although their effect on glucose metabolism is indeed to facilitate insulin's action, they also affect many other cellular processes through their action as specific activators of gene transcription factors of the PPAR family. These factors are involved in a myriad of cellular processes. Thus, widespread effects, possibly toxic, might be expected. Clinically, these drugs appear to be safe, although the first one marketed, troglitazone (Rezulin), was withdrawn from the market because of hepatic toxicity resulting in deaths. At present, the two agents marketed in the United States are probably less effective than the sulfonylureas or metformin when used as monotherapy. Limited experience in combination therapy has revealed that drug effects are additive to sulfonylurea or metformin (see Combinations of Oral Agents, below). Long-term experience is not available. Side effects include fluid retention and plasma volume expansion, a concern in patients with cardiac disease—certainly in patients with congestive heart failure, in whom this problem is sometimes exacerbated. Other disadvantages include weight gain, a delayed onset of action (1 to 3 weeks), a prolonged time to reach a full effect (4 to 12 weeks), and increases in LDL cholesterol. The glitazones should not be used as first-line therapy for type 2 patients.

Alpha-Glucosidase Inhibitors

Acarbose (Precose) is a relatively recently introduced agent for treatment of type 2 diabetes (Table 79.7). Monotherapy can be expected to produce only a minimal effect on the FPG (15 to 20 mg/dL) and then only in patients with no more than modest hyperglycemia. A greater effect is seen on postprandial than on fasting glucose (a reduction of 30 to 60 mg/dL), not a surprising finding because the drug is a nonabsorbable alpha-glucosidase inhibitor that acts by inhibition of the enzymes in the mucosal cells of the small intestine that digest complex carbohydrates. Abdominal fullness, flatulence, and, less commonly, diarrhea are the side effects, all of which tend to abate with time. Acarbose should be considered as an expensive adjunctive drug ($50 to $70 per month), which is only occasionally useful as monotherapy. The drug (50 to 100 mg) is taken at the beginning of each meal.

Meglitinides

Repaglinide (Prandin) and *nateglinide (Starlix)* act by rapidly stimulating the secretion of insulin from pancreatic beta cells by a mechanism different from that of the sulfonylureas (Table 79.7). The drugs are given shortly before meals, have a short duration of action, and are not prone to producing hypoglycemia. Repaglinide has been recommended for treatment of the elderly, a group in whom hypoglycemia is especially hazardous. In patients with moderate hyperglycemia, repaglinide has been reported to produce, on average, a reduction of FPG of about 60 mg%/dL and of HbA_{1C} of 1.7%. When substituted for metformin in patients whose response to metformin as monotherapy had become unsatisfactory, repaglinide produced only a minimal response, but when given in combination, the mean response of glucose was nearly 40 mg%/dL and HbA_{1C} 1.4%.

Combinations of Oral Agents

The increasing number of available oral agents and the relative ineffectiveness of monotherapy for control of glycemia have led in the last few years to a proliferation of combination therapies. A significant number of type 2 patients do initially reach glycemic targets with monotherapy but within several years require more than a single drug to maintain satisfactory levels of PG. The phenomenon is well known for the sulfonylureas and metformin and will probably occur with the newer agents.

Metformin plus a sulfonylurea is probably the most commonly used combination therapy at present. A glitazone plus either a sulfonylurea or metformin may also be used. In one study, patients received metformin (2,500 mg) plus 4 or 8 mg of rosiglitazone, all given together once daily. Only 28% of these patients reached an HbA_{1C} level of 7% or less. At the end of 26 weeks, patients receiving the combination had a mean FPG of about 180 mg% (66). Whereas this was 40 to 50 mg% lower than the metformin only group, these results fall far short of optimal control.

Pancreas and Islet Cell Transplantation

Pancreas Transplants

With the advent of more effective immunosuppressive regimens, the survival of transplanted patients and of the transplants themselves has improved considerably. Currently, graft survival approaches 90% at 5 years (67,68). Most transplantations have been simultaneous cadaveric pancreas–kidney transplantations in type 1 diabetics with end-stage renal disease. Alternatively, many patients have received renal transplants, either from cadavers or living related donors, followed at a later time with a cadaveric pancreas transplant. Pancreas transplantation alone, in patients without renal failure, has been done much less often because survival of the graft is considerably worse (67), perhaps because of a protective effect of the transplanted kidney.

The best candidates for transplantation are unstable diabetics with end-stage renal disease. There is no role currently for pancreas transplantation in type 2 diabetics. The best results are seen in relatively young patients (age 45 or less) with no cardiac risk factors (69): Both older age and heart disease are associated with poorer graft and patient survival (69).

When successful, pancreatic transplantation removes the need for exogenous insulin administration, protects the transplanted kidney from the noxious effects of hyperglycemia, and improves the recipient's quality of life. It does not appear to reverse diabetic retinopathy. Evaluation of patients for transplantation requires the collaborative efforts of an endocrinologist, usually a nephrologist, and a transplant surgeon.

Islet Cell Transplants

Islet cell transplantation has been generally unsuccessful in eliminating the need for exogenous insulin in type 1 diabetics (70). There is, however, one recent report from a group using a new glucocorticoid-free immunosuppressive regimen and relatively large numbers of cells (from two to three donors) that indicates an excellent outcome in seven of seven patients for at least an average of 1 year after transplantation (71).

Treatment of Other Types of Diabetes Mellitus (Secondary Diabetes)

Drug-induced diabetes (e.g., diabetes induced by high-dose thiazides) and diabetes associated with the use of glucocorticoids are usually not characterized by ketosis and ordinarily resemble type 2 diabetes. Treatment with a sulfonylurea may be tried, but insulin is often necessary. Withdrawal of the offending agent does not always ameliorate the diabetic state. The possibility of precipitating diabetes in patients with a strong family history should not deter the physician from the judicious use of diuretics or glucocorticoids when these agents are clinically indicated. Similarly, a diabetic who is already receiving insulin should not be denied diuretic therapy (e.g., when hypertension develops) or glucocorticoids for fear of aggravating the diabetes. If such aggravation occurs, usually only an increase of insulin dosage is necessary to reestablish the previous state of glycemic control.

Diabetes secondary to chronic pancreatitis or pancreatectomy should be treated with insulin. The insulin requirement is usually 20 to 40 units/day. The patients should be instructed to follow the dietary strategy outlined in Table 79.4. Alcoholic patients with this form of diabetes are particularly difficult to manage if they continue to drink heavily and to eat erratically.

COMPLICATIONS OF DIABETES MELLITUS

Diabetes mellitus is associated after many years with two distinct types of vascular damage in various organs (Fig. 79.4). Hyperglycemia produces microvascular (capillary) disease that affects the eyes, kidneys, and nerves. The blood lipid abnormalities of diabetes produce accelerated and extensive atherosclerosis of the cardiovascular and peripheral vascular systems. Coronary artery atherosclerosis and renal failure account for most of the deaths attributable to diabetes. Although considerable progress has been made over the past four decades in the understanding and treatment of this disease, diabetes remains a leading and increasing cause of death and enormous morbidity. In the United States and worldwide, the disease is showing a relentless increase.

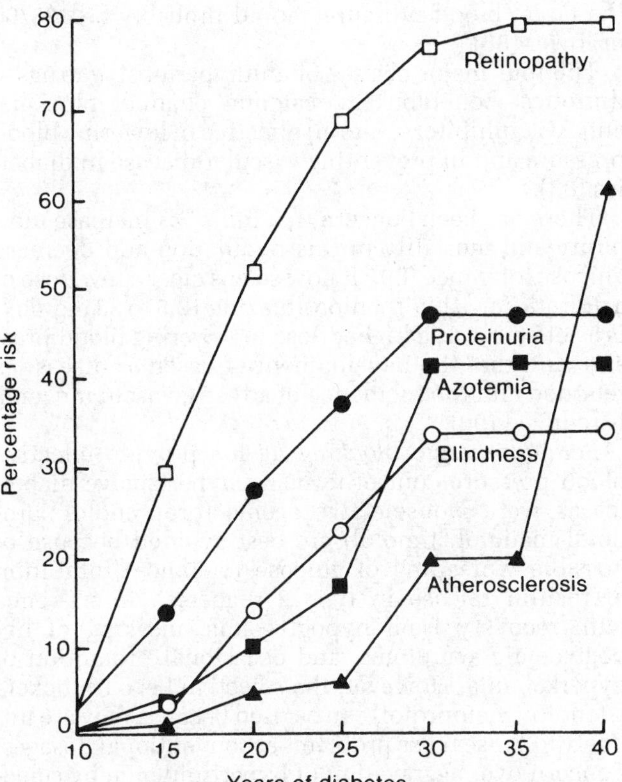

Figure 79.4. Complications of diabetes mellitus as a function of duration of the disease. (From Davidson MB. The continually changing "natural history" of diabetes mellitus. J Chronic Dis 1981;34:5, with permission.)

Atherosclerotic Vascular Disease

Diabetics experience two to four times the coronary artery disease of nondiabetics, and when myocardial infarction does occur, the morbidity and mortality in diabetics is twice that of nondiabetics (72). Early attention should be paid to complaints of chest pain and, even in its absence, diaphoresis, dyspnea, or nausea, because these may be anginal equivalents. In addition, diabetics have silent myocardial ischemia more frequently than nondiabetics (73,74). These considerations have led to guidelines for screening for cardiac disease in diabetics in the hope of improving outcomes (75). Because coexistent hypertension, diabetic cardiomyopathy, and autonomic neuropathy may alter the sensitivity and specificity of screening tests, more sophisticated studies, such as sestamibi imaging, may be necessary.

Because of the prevalence and severity of cardiac disease in diabetics, aggressive management of the risk factors (e.g., smoking cessation, blood pressure control, management of hyperlipidemia) is important (see Hypertension and its Therapy and Hyperlipidemia, below, and Chapters 62, 67, and 82).

Cardiovascular thrombotic events contribute to the morbidity and mortality of diabetes no doubt in part because of increased atherosclerosis, but probably also because of a variety of demonstrated alterations of platelet function and of the blood fibrinolytic system. Plasma plasminogen activator inhibitor type 1 and fibrinogenase are often elevated in type 2 patients, especially in the metabolic syndrome, and are correlated with elevated triglycerides and hyperinsulinemia (76). Although diabetes is considered to be a state of hypercoagulability, to date the relationship of these abnormalities to practical therapy is unclear.

Given the high cardiovascular risk of diabetic patients and the proven usefulness of aspirin therapy in nondiabetic patients, it is not surprising that antiplatelet therapy has been shown to be beneficial. The routine use of aspirin in type 2 diabetes is supported by at least six studies that attest to its safety and effectiveness (77). The recommended dose is 81 to 325 mg/day as an enteric-coated preparation, a recommendation sanctioned by the ADA (77). Aspirin does not increase intraocular bleeding in diabetic retinopathy and can be safely used in this condition. Studies of other antiplatelet agents (e.g., clopidogrel [Plavix]) in diabetics are not available, but their use may be considered in aspirin-allergic patients.

Diabetics are also more likely than nondiabetics to develop peripheral vascular disease (up to 30-fold increase in incidence) and cerebrovascular disease (a 2- to 6-fold increase in the incidence of stroke and cerebrovascular deaths).

Diabetic Cardiomyopathy

The Framingham study demonstrated that the risk of heart failure is increased 2.4-fold in diabetic men and 5-fold in diabetic women (78). This risk is associated with an increased mortality rate, even higher than the increased mortality rate of nondiabetics in heart failure. Although heart failure in diabetics is often associated with ischemic cardiomyopathy, a consequence of the accelerated atherosclerosis that is so often associated with diabetes (see above), it also may occur without clear-cut evidence of coronary artery disease. Increased left ventricular mass and primarily diastolic dysfunction are characteristic of this condition. Treatment should include an angiotensin-converting enzyme (ACE) inhibitor (see Hypertension and its Therapy, below, and Chapter 66).

Hyperlipidemia

Hypercholesterolemia in diabetics, as in nondiabetics, is a major risk factor for atherosclerotic disease. The kinds of lipid (lipoprotein) abnormalities in type 1 and type 2 diabetic patients differ. The term "diabetic dyslipidemia" embraces both of these patterns, but it is usually used to denote the pattern seen in type 2 diabetes (79). In patients with type 1 diabetes whose blood sugar is well controlled and who have normal renal function, the serum lipoproteins are not very different from those in normal subjects: LDL is usually normal, and HDL may even be higher than normal. Oxidized LDL, the formation of which is facilitated by glycation, is not ordinarily measured but is more atherogenic than normal LDL and is often increased.

In contrast, patients with type 2 disease have increased levels of intermediate-density lipoproteins (beta-very low density lipoprotein, intermediate-density lipoprotein), and HDL is often low. Glycated and oxidized LDL are increased. A direct contribution of hyperinsulinemia to the atherogenic process is also suspected but remains controversial. Current guidelines (see Chapter 82) consider diabetes mellitus equivalent to a cardiac risk factor and dictate treatment should be instituted to lower serum LDL if it exceeds 100 mg/dL.

Management

The gross hyperlipidemia of type 1 diabetes usually responds to conventional control of hyperglycemia. LDL cholesterol also is usually normalized. Triglycerides are usually not elevated after hyperglycemia is controlled. In patients with type 2 diabetes as part of the metabolic syndrome, hyperlipidemia may improve somewhat with effective lowering of hyperglycemia, but even euglycemia does not abolish the problem.

The serum lipid abnormalities that persist after the best achievable control of hyperglycemia in both type 1 and type 2 diabetes should be treated aggressively (80,81). At any given level of cholesterol, the type 2 diabetic has two to four times the risk of coronary artery disease of the nondiabetic. It is currently recommended that diabetics with LDL levels above 100 mg% should be treated with lipid-lowering agents (see Chapter 82). Using this criterion, 80% of diabetics will be candidates for treatment of hyperlipidemia.

Hypertension and Its Therapy

Hypertension is a common complication of diabetes. Type 1 diabetics have an increasing incidence of hypertension with time (5% by 10 years, 33% by 20 years [82]). In type 2 diabetes, hypertension is often part of the metabolic syndrome at onset, which also includes insulin resistance, obesity, and hyperlipidemia (see above).

The risk of microvascular and macrovascular complications is nearly doubled in hypertensive compared with normotensive diabetics (82,83), independent of the risk of microvascular complications imposed by hyperglycemia. In both type 1 and type 2 diabetics, therefore, control of hypertension is critical. A number of sizable prospective controlled studies support this statement (84–86).

Nonpharmacologic Treatment

In type 2 diabetes the same general measures that are important in the treatment of the diabetes itself—exercise and weight reduction–are important as well in the control of hypertension. In addition, sodium restriction is important to avoid volume expansion that is part of the syndrome (87).

Pharmacologic Treatment

If blood pressure cannot be reduced to 130/85 or lower, antihypertensive drugs should be prescribed (83) for both type 1 and type 2 diabetics. If patients already have evidence of renal disease (see below), the target blood pressure should probably be 125/80 or lower (88).

The four major classes of antihypertensive drugs—diuretics, beta-blockers, calcium channel blockers, and ACE inhibitors—are all effective in lowering blood pressure and in preventing vascular disease in diabetics (83).

There has been concern that *diuretics* increase morbidity and mortality in this population and decrease glucose tolerance (89). It now seems clear a low dose of a diuretic (e.g., hydrochlorothiazide 12.5 to 25 mg/day) is as effective as a higher dose in lowering blood pressure and that the development of vascular disease is retarded and the incidence of adverse vascular events is reduced (90).

Beta-adrenergic blocking agents provide effective blood pressure control in many hypertensive diabetics as well. Nonselective agents (propranolol, pindolol, nadolol, timolol) are best avoided because of possible worsening of glucose tolerance (inhibition of insulin release in type 2 diabetes), interference with recovery from hypoglycemia, masking of hypoglycemic symptoms, and occasional promotion of hyperkalemia. However, the selective beta-1-blockers (atenolol, metoprolol) can be used because they are unlikely to cause these problems at conventional dosages. Concern over aggravation of hyperlipidemia by selective beta-blockers is unwarranted because, unlike the nonspecific propranolol, which gave rise to these concerns, the more selective agents actually have only trivial effects on blood lipids.

As with diuretics there has been concern about the adverse effects of *calcium channel blockers* in the treatment of hypertensive diabetics (91). However, a number of studies have shown that these drugs, too, effectively reduce the risk of macrovascular disease in this population (85,92,93). Both nondihydropyridine blockers (e.g., verapamil) and dihydropyridine blockers (e.g., nifedipine) appear to be effective. Whether calcium channel inhibitors retard the development of microvascular disease remains to be seen (92).

ACE inhibitors have become the antihypertensive agents of choice in the treatment of hypertensive diabetics. They reduce the risk of macrovascular complications at least as well as other classes of hypotensive drugs (94–96) and have the best risk-to-benefit ratio (see Chapter 67). In type 1 diabetics, ACE inhibitors have the added advantage of retarding the development of renal microvascular disease (97). In type 2 diabetics, the effect of ACE inhibitors on the development of nephropathy has not been as clearly demonstrated, but recent studies have shown that *angiotensin receptor blockers* do have such an effect (98–100). The accumulated evidence, therefore, supports the preferential use of drugs that inhibit the renin–angiotensin system as primary agents in the treatment of both type 1 and type 2 hypertensive diabetics (101). As for now, the major difference between ACE inhibitors and angiotensin receptor blockers is cost. (ACE inhibitors are considerably cheaper than receptor blockers and will become cheaper still as the patents on them expire.)

Because of the need to lower blood pressure aggressively in hypertensive diabetics with even early evidence of renal disease, *combinations* of hypotensive agents often need to be prescribed. In such circumstances, adding a diuretic to an ACE inhibitor is probably the first thing to do. If optimum pressures are not reached, a beta-blocker and/or a calcium channel blocker can be added sequentially.

Other problems with antihypertensive drugs that may be especially troublesome in diabetic patients are erectile dysfunction (diuretics, alpha- or beta-adrenergic blockers) and hyperkalemia (triamterene, ACE inhibitors), possibly in relation to the subclinical hyporeninemic hypoaldosteronism often present in these patients.

Neuropathy

The precise prevalence of neuropathy in diabetic patients is unknown, although it is clear that neuropathy is common and that in most patients the occurrence and severity of involvement are related to duration of the disease. Usually, many years pass before the process becomes obvious, but occasionally even severe neuropathy can have an early onset (see Chapter 92 for a general discussion of peripheral neuropathy).

The most commonly appreciated abnormality is that which affects peripheral sensory nerves. Several types of sensation are involved (pain, proprioception, vibration, light touch) and can lead to unsteadiness, ataxic gait, and such uncommon but striking disorders as neuropathic arthropathy. Less well appreciated are the autonomic disorders that give rise to disturbances of cardiovascular function (postural hypotension, resting tachycardia), genitourinary function (impotence, bladder dysfunction), and gastrointestinal function (nocturnal diarrhea, fecal incontinence). Motor deficits are much less common but may occur with striking suddenness. Weakness is distal (neuropathic) rather than proximal (myopathic), although a specific type of myopathy also occurs in diabetic patients (see Amyotrophy, below). Some authors use the term *distal symmetric sensorimotor polyneuropathy* to describe the most common form of diabetic polyneuropathy.

Peripheral Sensory Neuropathy

Classically, the deficit is distal, with the lower extremities affected first, followed by the upper extremities. The term *stocking–glove distribution* is appropriate. The disorder is a symmetric polyneuropathy with a proximal–distal gradient of dysfunction. In severe cases, even the sensory innervation of the trunk is involved; in this instance, the most distal fibers are those of the anterior abdomen and lower thorax. Rarely, even the distal portions of the cranial nerves are affected (e.g., the distal sensory portion of the trigeminal nerve). The patterns of loss are not specific for diabetes mellitus and can be seen in such diverse states as amyloid neuropathy and toxic (e.g., lead) neuropathies.

The nerve damage may at first be asymptomatic, although subtle symptoms may be revealed with careful questioning of the patient. Alternatively, the patient may first complain of hyperesthesia and dysesthesia, including tingling and burning sensations. Later, various symptoms are experienced, including sensations of numbness or heaviness. Patients often complain that their feet feel dead or that they have a sensation of walking on a soft or nonexistent surface. Loss of ability to perceive temperature and firmness gives rise to these complaints. Severe, spontaneous, short-lived, stabbing leg pains and cramps are common. Often, these pains are most troublesome at night.

On neurologic testing, skin hypesthesia is the most common finding (pinprick, two-point discrimination, light touch). The hypesthesia and loss of temperature perception lead to unappreciated skin trauma and predispose to infection. Sensory loss in the fingertips can prevent the blind diabetic from learning Braille. Deep tendon reflexes, especially that of the Achilles tendon, are lost, often in the early stages of the neuropathy.

Peripheral Motor Neuropathy

Much less common and less well recognized are the motor function abnormalities that occur as part of diabetic neuropathy. The intrinsic muscles of the feet are those most commonly involved. Interosseous atrophy produces inability to separate toes but, more important, allows the foot to assume abnormal positions. When claw or hammer toe develops, new pressure points appear at the tips of the toes and along the dorsal aspects; hyperkeratosis, callus formation, and ulceration follow. The interosseous atrophy that may affect the hands does not lead to total loss of function but does result in weakness of grip. Diffuse weakness of the legs and upper extremities may also occur.

Therapy of Painful Peripheral Neuropathies

Until recently, medical therapy was limited to the acute and chronic treatment of pain with analgesics such as codeine. Although this approach will no doubt continue to be needed, relief of pain and discomfort can now be offered by use of amitriptyline and desipramine, shown to be effective in several well-designed trials (102). Amitriptyline may have more side effects than desipramine and may be less desirable for use in elderly diabetic patients. The mean effective dosage of drug is 100 mg/day. Recently, yet another antidepressant, venlafaxine, was noted in a small uncontrolled series to produce remarkable relief (103). The mechanism of action of these drugs in the relief of pain does not appear to be an effect on mood.

Capsaicin (Zostrix) applied to the skin as a cream three to four times a day has been shown to be effective in some patients in the treatment of painful diabetic neuropathy, including radiculopathy, and results in improvement in daily activities. The agent is well tolerated.

A number of other drugs (phenytoin, carbamazepine, gabapentin, and diphenhydramine) have been recommended for treatment of pain in peripheral neuropathy, but there have been no controlled trials to test their efficacy (see Chapter 92 for additional details). Transcutaneous electrical nerve stimulation has been said to be useful. Vitamin therapy is often given but is almost certainly useless for this purpose, although vitamin E has been shown to have some beneficial effect on nerve conduction velocity. The aldose reductase inhibitor aminoguanidine, long under investigation, has not proven effective prophylactically or therapeutically.

Mononeuropathies

Mononeuropathy (mononeuritis simplex and multiplex) may occur in any superficial nerve (simplex) or asymmetric simultaneous combination (multiplex). The lower extremities are more commonly involved (femoral, lateral femoral cutaneous, sciatic, peroneal) than are the upper (e.g., ulnar, radial). Onset is usually sudden with intense often cramping and lancinating pain (see Chapter 92). Typically, the pain is worse at night and, when the lower extremities are involved, may be relieved by pacing about. When the pain is radicular (trunk or abdomen), intrathoracic or intraabdominal disease may be misdiagnosed.

At onset, diagnosis can only be surmised, although tenderness along a nerve trunk is suggestive. Herpes zoster may be suspected, especially when hyperesthesia occurs, but when no vesicles appear and muscle weakness and atrophy are eventually evident, the diagnosis becomes obvious. The prognosis is good; complete recovery within a few months is the rule.

Cranial and Oculomotor Neuropathies

Cranial and oculomotor neuropathies are distinguished from other mononeuropathies mainly by their location. Pain and headache may be present. The most common nerves involved are III (palpebral ptosis, pupillary function undisturbed), VI (inward deviation of eye, diplopia), and IV (inward and upward deviations, diplopia). Recovery within 3 months is almost universal. When the facial nerve is involved, distinction from Bell's palsy is impossible (see Chapter 92), although the diabetic variety tends to be less severe and recovery is usually complete.

Autonomic Neuropathy

Abnormal Sweat Production. Almost always associated with other evidence of diabetic autonomic neuropathy, this complication in its typical form produces heat intolerance and increased sweating (hyperhidrosis) of the upper half of the body with decreased or absent sweating (anhidrosis) below the midtrunk. In other cases, anhidrosis is generalized, and recognition of the complication may be difficult. In women the condition may be confused with menopausal sweats.

Affected patients have decreased thermoregulatory reserve and are predisposed to hyperthermia and heat stroke. Another consequence of impaired sweating includes failure to recognize hypoglycemia (see Hypoglycemia During Insulin Therapy, above). This is a serious problem because one of the warning signals of insulin reaction is lost. Many elderly patients, including those without diabetes mellitus, already have impaired sympathetic responses as a result of aging rather than diabetes.

Cardiovascular Autonomic Neuropathies. In addition to abnormalities of innervation that result in abnormal cardiovascular reflexes (see below), diabetic cardiac denervation apparently accounts for the phenomenon of painless myocardial infarction, which is said to occur in more than 30% of diabetic patients who experience an acute event. Diagnosis is difficult unless acute electrocardiographic changes are present. Precipitation of unexplained ketoacidosis or myocardial failure may direct attention to these secondary events.

Resting Tachycardia. Heart rates of 90 to 100 beats/min are common in patients with autonomic neuropathy; occasionally even higher rates are observed. Normal sleep-related bradycardia is absent. Parasympathetic damage is the apparent explanation; the sympathetics appear to be less affected. A beta-blocker is useful if therapy is needed. In severe cases, the tachycardia "improves" over the years as denervation becomes more complete and the sympathetics are also lost.

Several noninvasive tests are available to assess the presence of autonomic cardiovascular dysfunction. These include the Valsalva maneuver, beat-to-beat heart rate variation, and the lying-to-standing heart rate response. Such assessments are more subtle indicators of the presence of autonomic dysfunction than is postural hypotension. These tests are rarely of use clinically but do allow objective assessment. The consequences—or at least the associations—of these abnormal cardiovascular reflexes in diabetic patients are important. Once they have developed, there is a marked decrease in 5-year survival. Sudden death, not attributable to myocardial infarction, has been described in many such patients (104).

Postural Hypotension. The most readily recognized troublesome cardiovascular abnormality is postural hypotension (see Chapter 89). The patient may complain merely of dizziness or faintness on standing, or the problem may be more severe, with visual disturbances and syncope. These symptoms may be confused with episodes of hypoglycemia. Remarkably, some patients with fairly marked postural hypotension are asymptomatic.

On initial examination, every diabetic patient should be checked for a postural decrease in blood pressure. In addition, a check for postural hypotension should be made whenever a potentially aggravating condition occurs. The onset or aggravation of postural hypotension is often associated with the beginning of therapy with a variety of drugs often used in diabetic patients such as antihypertensive drugs, including diuretics; vasodilators/antispasmodics, such as nitroglycerin (glyceryl trinitrate); antidepressants (tricyclic); and phenothiazines. Occasional diabetic patients may be unable to tolerate effective dosages of these drugs because of this problem.

The mechanism of this disorder is thought to reside in the efferent limb of the baroreceptor arc secondary to damaged sympathetic vasoconstrictor fibers in the splanchnic bed, muscles, and skin. Diminished plasma renin responses to postural change have been noted in such patients, as have abnormalities of plasma norepinephrine, but the role of these defects is unclear.

Various mechanical maneuvers, including the use of antigravity or space suits, have been recommended but are not useful. Drug therapy with clonidine, vasopressors such as phenylephrine, or combinations of tyramine or amine-containing cheeses and monoamine oxidase inhibitors have had their advocates, but none of these has been consistently effective. For patients with severe postural hypotension, the most useful drug has been the mineralocorticoid fludrocortisone (Florinef). In dosages of 0.1 to 1.0 mg/day, the drug is often helpful, but because one of its actions is to expand fluid volume, it can precipitate cardiac failure or produce severe hypertension in the recumbent state. Hypokalemia is common, requiring monitoring of electrolytes and appropriate management (K^+ sparing agents, supplements). Refractoriness may eventually occur. The beta-adrenergic agonist midodrine (ProAmatine) has been marketed for the treatment of orthostatic hypotension caused by a variety of causes, including diabetes. The drug requires careful dosing (starting at 2.5 mg twice a day) but seems useful (105). In mild cases, the simple advice that the patient assume upright positions slowly by sitting on the edge of the bed after recumbency may help avoid syncopal episodes; continuing postural hypotension, although readily documented, may not be especially symptomatic and may not warrant therapy (also see Chapter 89).

Foot Problems

A number of common foot problems (e.g., bunions, calluses, corns, fungal infections, and ingrown toenails) are problems in diabetic patients and can lead to devastating complications. Prevention through proper foot care and early recognition and treatment are important considerations in the long-term care of every diabetic patient. These problems are discussed in detail in Chapter 73.

Neuropathic Foot Ulcers

Epidemiology And Etiology. Diabetic foot ulcers and lower extremity amputations occur in some 15% of diabetics. The problem is multifactorial. Enormous morbidity and expense are involved. A major technical review of preventive foot care and the ADA position paper that followed have been published (106,107), as have the conclusions of a consensus conference on Diabetic Foot Wound Care (108).

Foot ulcers are typically plantar and occur at the point where weight-bearing is greatest. They are now considered to be primarily the manifestations of diabetic neuropathy, but high plantar pressures and low tissue oxygen tension and blood pressure at the toe are other independent factors (109). Other risk factors include hammer/claw toe and other acquired foot deformities. Although the diabetic is certainly prone to vascular (arterial) insufficiency and neuropathy and although the presence of vessel disease often contributes, the origin of the problem is primarily the sensory deficit. Neuropathy often is asymptomatic until an ulcer develops. Because the patient does not perceive pain normally, unappreciated trauma occurs, for example from new or poorly fitting shoes that produce pressure points that go unrelieved and end in penetrating abrasions. Wounds can also result from skin penetration by foreign materials or from accidents during self-trimming of toenails. In addition to the sensory deficit, simultaneous motor weakness of extensor or flexor muscles together with proprioceptive defects can also contribute to anatomic deformity that in turn produces pressure points and ulceration.

Altered motor nerve function leads to muscle atrophy and tendon shortenings, which result in chronic toe flexion and finally hammertoe deformity. This anatomic change shifts weight from the padded ball of the foot to the metatarsal heads, where calluses form and contribute to the formation of new pressure points. The calluses themselves may develop fissures, which further promote ulceration. A recently recognized contributor to the problem is diabetes or age-related loss of adipose tissue from the submetatarsal "padded" areas of the foot. This adipose padding normally distributes weight of the foot; loss of this tissue is a major anatomic destabilizer.

Management. Prevention is the mainstay of management. A simple nylon filament touch perception test allows detection of the sensory impairment, which is a major predictor of the risk of foot ulceration. Patients who cannot feel the filament are at about 10 times greater risk of ulceration and 17 times greater risk of amputation. Identification of such patients and institution of preventive measures may be useful in avoiding amputations. When an ulcer is present, decreased weight-bearing ("off loading") is an essential part of treatment. This is best accomplished with a total contact cast, the exact nature of which is best left to the treating practitioner's preference based on experience and technical expertise. Infection is not invariably present but when present is almost always a mixture of aerobic, facultatively anaerobic, and anaerobic organisms (110). In the presence of infection, a total contact cast is contraindicated. Antibiotics of choice and their method of administration are discussed under Infections, below. Intravenous antibiotics and hospitalization have been standard therapy for many years, but recently oral antibiotics in a home-based setting have been shown to be effective for most patients. Because callus formation aggravates the tendency to increase local pressure and worsens ulceration, regular debridement is essential. Some patients can be taught debridement techniques, which may at least delay the intervals between visits to the caregiver for this purpose, but usually periodic professional assistance is essential. Such care is often best provided by podiatrists (see Chapter 73). Fitting of custom-made molded shoes is helpful and is essential in some cases for prevention of ulceration or its recurrence. Remarkably, with proper treatment the ulcer may heal completely and not recur. However, recurrence is likely as long as the anatomic distortion or continued point pressure is left unmodified. Plantar injection of silicone reduces risk factors for ulceration but has yet to be shown in clinical trials to be effective in preventing actual ulceration (111).

Neuropathic Arthropathy (Diabetic Charcot Foot)

Neuropathic arthropathy, a complication of diabetes, is often unrecognized or misdiagnosed. The disorder, preceded by a sensory neuropathy, is a progressive degenerative change of the bony structure of the foot, most often involving the tarsal and tarsometatarsal joints (60%) but also the metatarsophalangeal joints (30%) and the ankle (10%). The prevalence has been estimated at 1 in 680 cases, but the disorder is probably more common. The patient presents with a swollen foot, often attributed to or associated with recent trauma. The foot may be painful or may be remarkably free of pain, considering the appearance. Examination shows moderate to gross deformity of the foot with rocker-bottom subluxation of the midtarsal region or subluxation of the metatarsophalangeal joints. Usually, the foot is erythematous and warm to the touch. An infected neuropathic ulcer may be present. More often than not, the pulses are intact. Clinicians unfamiliar with this presentation are likely to diagnose some other type of inflammatory arthritis or osteomyelitis, and their impression may be apparently verified by radiographic findings. In these early stages, the x-rays often show severe osteoarthritis, but as the disease progresses, there is complete destruction of the involved joints with resorption of the metatarsal heads and phalangeal diaphyses. Various other bony changes occur, including fractures, joint effusions, and subluxations. When these changes are at the maximal stage (i.e., when soft tissue involvement is most prominent), the diagnosis of osteomyelitis is often entertained, especially when there is an associated, often infected, ulcer. Synovial biopsy showing a thickened synovium containing osseous debris may provide the correct diagnosis and avoid the necessity of embarking on a prolonged and difficult course of antibiotic therapy for suspected osteomyelitis.

Diabetic Charcot foot may also be confused with the changes associated with osteoarthritis and gouty, rheumatoid, and psoriatic arthritis. Consultation by an orthopedic surgeon, rheumatologist, or podiatrist to confirm the diagnosis and assist with therapy is almost always indicated.

Treatment is based on the cessation of further trauma to the affected area, which is best accomplished by elimination of weight-bearing. Hospitalization may be necessary for this purpose. Reduction of edema and signs of inflammation may take several weeks. Immobilization with a cast may be helpful but should not be undertaken in the acute stage and, if used, should be done with great care to ensure the integrity of the areas covered by the cast. Simpler boot-like devices may also be used. Crutches can be used at this point, followed eventually by a walking cast. Up to 4 months of treatment may be required. Thereafter, molded or contoured shoes are essential to proper long-term management. Surgical intervention is inadvisable, although occasionally a stabilization procedure may be required if conservative therapy fails. Amputation is not indicated unless osteomyelitis unequivocally coexists or the entire process fails to respond to prolonged conservative efforts. Despite the discouraging appearance of the foot at its worst stages, sufficient healing and stabilization to produce a useful foot can be anticipated.

Digestive System Dysfunction

Most disorders of the gastrointestinal tract in diabetes are related to disturbances of motility. Esophageal motor dysfunction can be demonstrated on testing but is usually not a clinical problem.

Gastroparesis (atony of the stomach) is often asymptomatic but may be troublesome. Symptoms include anorexia, early satiety, postprandial fullness and bloating, and, occasionally, vomiting. Delayed and unpredictable emptying of the stomach may produce irregular diabetic control in already difficult to manage patients with type 1 diabetes. Diagnosis is apparent—sometimes as an incidental finding—on barium radiograph of the upper gastrointestinal tract. Scintigraphy is the most sensitive method to detect the presence of atony. Gastroparesis has long been thought to be a late complication associated with poor prognosis for survival, but a recent study found no evidence to support this notion (112). Metoclopramide (Reglan) 10 mg three times daily may be helpful (see Chapter 43). In intractable cases, gastrectomy may be needed.

Small bowel dysfunction is common and symptomatic, leading to diabetic diarrhea. Typically the diarrhea is nocturnal. Fecal incontinence, a result of impaired sensation of rectal distension, may occur and is very distressing. The disorder tends to be episodic, with attacks lasting from a few days to weeks or rarely months. Watery brown diarrhea, usually without steatorrhea, is typical. On barium radiograph of the small bowel, the findings are those of disturbed motility. Despite the distressing symptoms, the patient appears well; weight loss is uncommon. When steatorrhea occurs, pancreatic exocrine insufficiency and sprue syndrome, more common in diabetic patients than in the general population, should be considered. Fully developed sprue is associated with gross evidence of malabsorption. A trial of antibiotic therapy (e.g., tetracycline, 250 mg four times a day for 2 weeks) may improve the diarrhea and the malabsorption if the latter is caused by small bowel stasis and bacterial colonization. Symptomatic treatment with antispasmodics (e.g., Imodium) may be useful, especially when attacks of diarrhea are short lived.

Large bowel complaints, especially of constipation, are common in the elderly. It does not appear that diabetic patients are especially prone to any additional problems in this regard.

Patients with poorly controlled diabetes may develop *fatty changes of the liver.* Hepatomegaly or elevations of liver enzymes may occur and prompt a fruitless search for other diseases. Effective control of blood sugar results in disappearance of these abnormalities if diabetes is the cause. However, diabetes and obesity often coexist; fatty liver is also common in uncomplicated obesity.

Bladder Dysfunction (Neurogenic Bladder)

The symptoms of bladder dysfunction in diabetic patients are often overlooked. Onset is insidious and occurs over many years. Most patients (80%) have clinical evidence of neuropathy affecting other systems. The first clinical manifestation of bladder dysfunction is an increase in the interval between voiding until urine is passed only twice or even once daily. A need to strain, slow stream, dribbling, and sensation of incomplete voiding may be present. These symptoms should be routinely solicited from diabetic patients, especially when there are symptoms or signs of peripheral neuropathy.

Demonstration of residual urine is the hallmark of clinically symptomatic cystopathy, but many diabetic patients, when studied by cystometric techniques, have objective evidence of neurogenic involvement and a grossly enlarged bladder well before symptoms are evident. At this stage, residual urine is not present and other urinary tract abnormalities (recurrent infections) are not evident. If large volumes of residual urine do develop, patients become prone to infection (see Chapter 36) and incontinence (see Chapter 12). Patients suspected to have cystopathy should be referred to a urologist for evaluation and recommendations about treatment.

Erectile and Sexual Dysfunction

The frequency of erectile dysfunction, formerly termed impotence, is high in diabetic men, perhaps 50% to 60% overall. This complication, like many others in diabetic patients, is related to duration of disease. The problem is usually caused by a type of autonomic neuropathy involving the pelvic parasympathetic nerves, but impaired blood flow is the cause in some cases.

The problems leading to *erectile dysfunction* must be included in the differential diagnosis in the diabetic. Psychogenic factors probably account for a significant fraction of nondiabetic cases, but there is no evidence that psychogenic problems are more common in diabetic patients. The onset of erectile dysfunction in diabetics usually is slow (6 months to several years), often associated with retrograde ejaculation; impotence eventually becomes complete. Despite this, libido is characteristically retained. Although patients with psychogenic impotence often report nocturnal erections and emissions, these are absent in patients with diabetic impotence.

An important point on clinical examination is that testicular sensitivity to pressure sufficient to cause pain is retained in men with psychogenic impotence but is often greatly diminished or lost in the diabetic in whom accompanying sensory neuropathy is common.

Endocrinologic causes of impotence (see Chapters 6 and 85) should be considered because they are potentially treatable, but it is rare to find an endocrine basis for impotence in the diabetic. Testosterone production, easily verified by plasma testosterone measurement, is almost always normal in diabetic patients; therefore, as one would expect, testosterone therapy is useless in such patients.

A variety of drugs, especially ones that are often used in diabetics, may cause erectile dysfunction. The most common offenders are said to be the nondiuretic antihypertensives (mechanism unknown) (see Chapter 67) and the SRI class of antidepressants (see Chapter 24).

Several studies report that sexual function in diabetic women appears to be unaffected by the disease. Others assert that many diabetic women lose the ability to achieve orgasm (113).

The differential diagnosis and therapy of impotence are discussed in detail in Chapter 6. Considerable success was achieved in diabetic patients by the implantation of prosthetic devices that cause erection, but these operations have become much less popular than they once were because of recently introduced pharmacologic therapies. Self-administered intrapenile (intracavernal) injections of papaverine, papaverine plus phentolamine, or prostaglandin E plus phentolamine are also effective in many cases. Self-administration of intraurethral prostaglandin E (alprostadil; Muse) has been reported to be an effective, albeit expensive, therapy (about $20 per dose) for erectile dysfunction in diabetic and nondiabetic men (114). The overall success rate is claimed to be approximately 70% but is probably closer to 20%. Sildenafil (Viagra) is effective in over 50% of diabetic men (115). It has also been suggested that a combination of intraurethral prostaglandin plus oral sildenafil is effective for patients who wish to avoid penile injections (116). Because of their simplicity, these forms of therapy should probably be tried first, before initiating an extensive workup and certainly before proceeding to implantation of a prosthetic device.

Amyotrophy (Proximal Asymmetric Motor Neuropathy), Neuropathic Cachexia, and Myopathy

Amyotrophy is a rare but devastating complication of diabetes mellitus that is probably a proximal motor neuropathy. Severe asymmetric proximal muscle weakness and pain usually affect the pelvic girdle and thigh muscles, although upper truncal musculature can also be involved. The typical patient is a middle-aged or elderly type 2 diabetic with mild disease. Men are affected more often than women. Onset may be fairly rapid, and low-grade fever and elevated erythrocyte sedimentation rate may be present. Cerebrospinal fluid protein may be very high. Muscle biopsy shows fiber degeneration. Electromyography shows a pattern typical of motor denervation. Weight loss of moderate degree is common but may be severe

(20 to 30 kg). Prognosis for spontaneous improvement over 2 to 6 months is good, but complete recovery often requires 24 months or longer and significant residual effects are common.

Nephropathy

Progressive renal failure is a major life-threatening complication of diabetes. The relationship between hyperglycemia and the development of microangiopathy with eventual nodular glomerulosclerosis (Kimmelstiel-Wilson disease) is unequivocally established, as strong clinical and experimental evidence has accumulated in favor of such a relationship. One of the earliest indications of incipient diabetic nephropathy is proteinuria, first manifest as microalbuminuria. The detection and significance of proteinuria and of microalbuminuria in diabetic patients are discussed in Chapter 48. The critical role of control of blood pressure in retarding the development of diabetic neuropathy is described above (see Hypertension and its Therapy).

Diabetic patients with even minimal elevations of serum creatinine above 1.1 mg/dL, but not those with normal renal function, are at increased risk of acute renal failure from contrast media used in various radiographic procedures. Although the risk is only moderately increased (approximately 10% to 15% in the highest risk patients vs. 5% in low risk patients and less than 2% in those with no renal disease and in nondiabetic subjects), these procedures can often be replaced by others with less risk (magnetic resonance imaging, sonography). If contrast media are to be used, the dosage should be minimal and the patient well hydrated. Diuretics and/or ACE inhibitors should be reduced or briefly withheld. The clinical course of diabetic nephropathy and the impact of failing renal function on insulin requirement and on the dosage of oral hypoglycemic drugs are discussed in Chapter 52.

Skin Lesions

An uncommon abnormality known as *necrobiosis lipoidica diabeticorum* occurs in perhaps 0.3% of all diabetics, seemingly unrelated to glycemic control. Typically, lesions occur on the anterior legs but also on the arms, trunk, or face. The lesions, described as atrophic plaques, are sharply demarcated, orange or red, and often ulcerate. On biopsy, diagnostic findings include destruction of collagen fibers. Until recently no agent seemed to be useful, but several reports now indicate that these lesions respond rapidly to tretinoin-containing creams; pentoxifylline (Trental), 400 mg twice a day, also seems to be effective.

Infections

It is a long-time clinical observation that diabetic patients are more prone to infections than are nondiabetics. Clinicians often encounter patients who have experienced repeated bacterial or fungal skin infections (carbuncles, furuncles, external otitis, moniliasis) or gastrointestinal moniliasis at some time before the diagnosis of diabetes was made or in association with uncontrolled hyperglycemia. Once established, infections in the diabetic are difficult to treat and patients are prone to develop complications. Elevated blood glucose appears to be a major cause of this problem. Experimentally, hyperglycemia (blood glucose levels above 250 mg/100 mL) inhibits the phagocytic activity of granulocytes and the immune function of lymphocytes, factors that may contribute to lowered host resistance. Control of blood sugar, therefore, should be part of any treatment program for an infection. This conclusion is supported by recent studies of perioperative infections in diabetic patients undergoing coronary artery bypass surgery (117).

Urinary tract infections are an especially troublesome problem in diabetic patients. Although infections are not clearly increased in incidence, a greater prevalence of complications is obvious. Half of all cases of papillary necrosis occur in diabetics. Diabetic patients also seem prone to develop infections with unusual pathogens. However, no statistical case has been made for the desirability of suppression of asymptomatic bacteriuria in diabetics. Development of pyelonephritis is an indication for immediate hospitalization and vigorous antibiotic treatment; the risk of a renal abscess is a special hazard for the diabetic.

Skin infections caused by *Candida* are common in diabetics, especially those with type 2 disease who are obese. These infections require therapy with a local antifungal agent (see Chapter 117) and control of hyperglycemia.

Major soft tissue infections in diabetic patients require prompt hospitalization and treatment with parenteral antibiotics. However, most infections encountered involve the lower extremities, usually the feet, and are not complicated by serious conditions such as osteomyelitis or gangrene (see Neuropathic Foot Ulcers, above). Until several years ago such uncomplicated infections were treated by hospitalization and a combination of systemic antibiotics, often for several weeks. Such an approach could be expected to cost $10,000 to $20,000 per hospitalization. It is now clear that most of these less severe infections can be treated just as well with an oral antibiotic and without hospitalization (118).

Most *infections of the feet* (over half) are acute, with concomitant skin ulceration; others are acute infection of a previously uninfected chronic foot ulcer, whereas a lesser number are abscesses (often paronychias) or cellulitis. Although cultures of such lesions are of limited usefulness, they can be obtained by swab, aspiration, or curettage, the latter being more likely to reveal anaerobes. Aerobic gram-positive organisms are present in more than 50% of lesions, and aerobic gram-negative organisms in 15% to 25%. On average, slightly more than two organisms are isolated, and anaerobes are present in 15% of cases. *Staphylococcus* is the most common organism, followed by *Streptococcus* and the common gram-negative organisms (*Klebsiella, Pseudomonas, Proteus*). *Corynebacteria* should not be considered as merely contaminants; they are the only organism present in many cases.

Clindamycin or cephalexin given orally cures 75% of these infections clinically and bacteriologically, even when treatment is without reference to culture results. Another 15% to 20% of infections are greatly improved, and some 5% to 15% are treatment failures (118). Other antibiotic regimens yield similar results (110). The value of topical antibiotic preparations (povidone–iodine; silver sulfadiazine) is controversial (119).

It must be emphasized that such results can be expected only in these less severe infections. Gangrene, severe ischemia, crepitus, and persistent fever are indications for hospitalization. Also to be emphasized is the need for proper adjunctive local care of the foot: elevation of the affected extremity, limitation of ambulation, proper foot hygiene, and, of course, surgical drainage, if appropriate. Because diabetics may be at increased risk from influenza and its complications, it is recommended that they receive yearly influenza vaccinations (see Chapter 14).

Retinopathy

Diabetic retinopathy has become one of the leading causes of blindness in the United States. In type 1 diabetic patients, some degree of retinopathy can be detected by the most sensitive technique, angiography, after as little as 1 to 2 years in 10% of patients. By 10 years, retinopathy is evident in 50% of cases by ophthalmoscopy, with a 70% prevalence by angiography. At 25 years, nearly all patients can be shown to have some degree of retinopathy. By the time diabetes has been present for 15 to 20 years, about one-third of patients have severe disease and another one-half have obvious but lesser degrees of progressive retinal involvement. Remarkably, not all cases of early retinopathy are progressive. These figures represent the pre-DCCT era.

Type 2 diabetic patients also develop retinopathy, apparently with less frequency, but clearly related to duration and severity of the hyperglycemia. Hyperglycemia, as indirectly measured by glycosylated hemoglobin, clearly predicts the incidence and progression of diabetic retinopathy in type 2 diabetes (120,121).

In patients with retinopathy in whom intensive therapy is initiated, a paradoxical worsening of the retinopathy can be seen. Patients whose retinopathy is mild to moderate usually have no associated visual loss, and long-term intensive treatment of glycemia counterbalances the early worsening (122).

Blindness in Diabetic Retinopathy

The visual loss in diabetic retinopathy is potentially even more severe than in blindness due to other causes. Many people who are legally blind (defined as visual acuity less than 20/200 in both eyes) from causes other than diabetes have slow onset of visual loss, thus allowing time for adaptation. In addition, they often retain reasonably full visual fields and visual acuity at or close to the legal limit. Such patients can see well enough to ambulate independently and perform a variety of common activities (self-care, housework). With the aid of special devices they may even be able to read newsprint and to engage in some occupations. In contrast, the visual loss from diabetic retinopathy is often caused by sudden hemorrhage or retinal detachment and often leaves the patient with only light perception. In addition, the diabetic often already has other complications of the disease when blindness develops. Although total blindness afflicts only some diabetic patients, a larger number have some degree of loss of visual acuity caused by macular edema, the most common cause of visual loss in diabetics (see below).

Ocular Symptoms

Diabetic patients who experience symptoms of visual disturbance are not necessarily experiencing a catastrophic complication and deserve reassurance along these lines. Like others, diabetic patients develop changes of visual acuity such as a change in refractive error and astigmatism. In addition, they can experience decreased visual acuity as a result of marked changes in blood sugar (e.g., as the lens swells during acute normalization of blood sugar after prolonged hyperglycemia). However, sudden or persistent change of visual acuity requires examination by an ophthalmologist, especially when advanced retinal disease, proliferative diabetic retinopathy (PDR), is present. A common cause of visual loss in PDR, macular edema, is not readily detectable by the direct ophthalmoscopy available to internists and requires binocular slit lamp or stereoscopic fundus photography by an ophthalmologist.

Sudden painless loss of vision in PDR demands urgent ophthalmologic consultation. This symptom is often caused by hemorrhage from proliferating new vessels or from retinal detachment. Lesser degrees of hemorrhage may cause floaters or cobwebs. Another complication in PDR is outflow obstruction of the aqueous humor produced by fibrous scar tissue extending into the angle of the anterior chamber, causing a marked rise in intraocular pressure and acute (neovascular) glaucoma with severe pain. Loss of vision occurs unless emergency therapy is given.

Types of Retinal Disease in Diabetic Patients

The current classification of diabetic retinal disease is nonproliferative (or background), preproliferative, and PDR. The latter more advanced stage is the point at which sudden and massive visual loss becomes a problem.

Nonproliferative and Preproliferative Retinopathy. The earliest lesions—readily visible with an ordinary ophthalmoscope—are in the region of the macula: microaneurysms, punctate retinal hemorrhages, hard exudates, soft exudates (cotton wool), and so-called intraretinal microvascular anomalies (IRMAs). Both *microaneurysms* and *small dot intraretinal hemorrhages* appear as red dots, and both tend to fade within months. *Blot hemorrhages* are larger. Distinction can best be made by fluorescein angiograms, in which only microaneurysms light up. This procedure, performed by an ophthalmologist, often identifies extensive intraretinal disease when only a few abnormalities are evident by ophthalmoscopy.

Hard exudates are glistening yellow or white lipid deposits located in the outer retinal layers. If they are greater than one disk diameter from the macula, they are not ominous. *Soft exudates* are areas of ischemia or infarction of the nerve fiber layer; they disappear within a few months. *IRMAs* are dilated hypercellular vessels that are thought to represent either dilated capillaries or intraretinal vascular proliferation. These abnormal vessels are identifiable using the green filters of an ordinary ophthalmoscope but are best seen in the secondary phase of fluorescein angiograms, during which they leak dye into the retina. IRMAs occur adjacent to areas of capillary closure. Their identification is not essential in the routine examination.

Whereas changes of background retinopathy indicate capillary damage and leakage, preproliferative changes (many soft exudates, extensive hemorrhages, IRMAs, and venous bleeding from enlarged dilated [beaded, sausage-link] retinal veins) indicate areas of intraretinal vascular occlusion with resulting nonperfusion. Eyes with retinal ischemia and moderate to severe preproliferative changes have a 50% chance of developing new vessel proliferation (neovascularization) within 1 year.

Macular Edema. It is not usually appreciated by the general clinician that even without proliferative disease, macular edema may result in visual loss as severe as the 20/200 level. Spontaneous improvement is not common but may occur. Visual acuity can also become poor because of lack of proper perfusion of the perifoveal capillaries. In this instance, visual acuity may be as low as 20/200 in the absence of macular edema. Fluorescein angiography reveals the cause of poor visual acuity to be due to the lack of perfusion of the perifoveal capillaries. In the absence of accompanying proliferative disease, patients at this stage can usually ambulate freely and can engage in some occupations. Ability to read a newspaper, except with a vision aid, is unlikely, and the patient will have to stop driving.

Proliferative Retinopathy. At this stage of retinal disease, new vessels and accompanying fibrous tissue extend from the retinal substance and grow along the inner retinal surface and the posterior surface of the vitreous gel, often causing contraction of the gel and traction on the vessels and the retina. This process creates the conditions for retinal detachment and hemorrhage into the vitreous.

In addition, in advanced PDR, growth of new vessels and scar tissue into the angle of the eye may cause acute glaucoma (see Ocular Symptoms, above). When the new blood vessels grow out of the surface of the optic nerve heads, they are called new vessels on the disk; elsewhere in the retina, usually extending from large vessels, they are called new vessels elsewhere.

The National Diabetic Retinopathy Study (123) not only established the efficacy of photocoagulation therapy (see below) but also defined high-risk characteristics as follows: new vessels on the disk greater than 25% of the optic disk area, any new vessels on the disk with preretinal or vitreous hemorrhage, or new vessels elsewhere equal to or exceeding 50% of the disk area with preretinal or vitreous hemorrhage. The presence of high-risk characteristics increases the chance of blindness to 30% to 50% within 3 to 5 years unless appropriate photocoagulation therapy is given.

Treatment of Diabetic Retinopathy

Two forms of surgical therapy are now available for the treatment of proliferative retinopathy and its complications. Photocoagulation is of proven value in the prevention of visual loss caused by proliferative disease, and vitrectomy restores and appears to stabilize vision after hemorrhage and/or retinal detachment.

Photocoagulation Therapy. Argon laser therapy reduces severe visual loss by nearly 60% over 5 years in patients with proliferative disease. Multiple (1,200 to 1,600) 500-μm burns are placed in the retinal periphery. The Early Treatment Diabetic Retinopathy Study (124) evaluated panretinal photocoagulation (and laser photocoagulation using 450- to 650-μm widely spaced burns) to determine whether such therapy affects the course of disease in eyes with high-risk characteristics or preproliferative diabetic retinopathy. Considerable benefit has been shown.

Diabetic *macular edema* is also treated with photocoagulation therapy. Leaking microaneurysms and other lesions in the macula are treated with 50- to 100-μm burns. The Early Treatment Diabetic Retinopathy Study showed a reduction of visual loss due to macular edema of 50% over 3 years.

Patient Experience. Photocoagulation therapy is an office procedure, usually performed in several sessions. Ordinarily only topical (corneal) anesthesia is necessary. Occasionally, some pain is experienced, in which case a local anesthetic is injected into the retro-orbital tissues to allow a completed pain-free procedure.

Vitrectomy. Hemorrhage into the vitreous is the usual indication for vitrectomy, a procedure that removes old blood and opaque vitreous and can be combined with cataract extraction. Retinal detachment resulting from traction bands that are formed in the vitreous is another indication for vitrectomy. Other repair procedures can be attempted. The results of vitrectomy can be dramatic in restoring sight after vitreous hemorrhage. Currently, however, vitrectomy is used only in severely diseased eyes. Recovery of near-normal vision is the exception rather than the rule, but the results are definitely worthwhile in many patients.

Every effort should be made to control hypertension in an attempt to prevent retinal hemorrhages. Lifting of heavy objects, jarring exercise, and exposures to high altitudes may also increase the risk of hemorrhages and should be avoided in patients with PDR, but commercial airline travel presents no increased risk. The use

Table 79.8. Reasons for Referral of Patients with Diabetes Mellitus to an Ophthalmologist

High-risk patients
Neovascularization covering more than one-third of optic disk
Vitreous or preretinal hemorrhage with any neovascularization, particularly on optic disk
Macular edema (suspect from hard exudates in macula)
Symptomatic patients
Blurry vision persisting for more than 1–2 days or not associated with a change in blood glucose; suspect macular edema
Sudden loss of vision in one or both eyes
Black spots, cobwebs, or flashing lights in field of vision
Asymptomatic patients
Yearly examinations (an optometrist can check pressures if no retinal changes or if only BDR is present)
Hard exudates near macula
Any preproliferative or proliferative characteristics
Pregnancy

BDR, background diabetic retinopathy (see text).

Modified from ADA physician's guide to non–insulin-dependent (type II) diabetes. Diagnosis and treatment, 2nd ed. Alexandria, VA:ADA,1988, with permission.

of aspirin therapy does not increase the risk or severity of intraocular hemorrhage and is *not* contraindicated in PDR (122).

Role of the Primary Care Physician/Internist Versus That of the Ophthalmologist: Indications for Referral

If there is no evidence of retinal disease, diabetics should have yearly examinations of their eyegrounds, with their pupils dilated. If that cannot be done for any reason or if there is concern about the validity of the examination, referral to an optometrist or ophthalmologist is indicated (Table 79.8). Because most diabetic retinopathy occurs within several disk diameters of the macula, most lesions are visible by examination with the direct ophthalmoscope after dilation of the pupils. Nonophthalmologists often defer this examination out of concern over precipitating acute angle-closure glaucoma. Such reluctance is not warranted because this complication is rare at any age and is hardly ever seen before age 40. A drop of dilating solution (2.5% phenylephrine or 1% tropicamide) in each eye is sufficient and causes only sensitivity to bright light (requiring dark glasses) that lasts but a few hours.

If only minimal nonproliferative diabetic retinopathy is present, the patient does not need to be referred immediately if visual acuity is normal. Early preproliferative changes (see above) warrant prompt referral to a general ophthalmologist, whereas more extensive changes and proliferative changes should be followed by an ophthalmologist who is also expert in photocoagulation. In addition to examining the retina, the condition of the lens should be evaluated during the examination of the eye because senile cataracts occur prematurely in diabetic patients and metabolic cataracts result from chronic elevation of blood glucose levels.

Periodic checks of intraocular pressure to detect glaucoma, which is more prevalent in diabetics, should also be part of routine health maintenance. These evaluations can be made either by an optometrist or an ophthalmologist (see Chapter 108). Recommendations for follow-up are given in Table 79.8 and in detail elsewhere (125).

TRACKING AND COORDINATING CARE IN THE DIABETIC PATIENT

Because management of the diabetic patient is complex and multidimensional and because numerous interventions improve health care outcomes (see above), it is important for the primary care practitioner to have a systematic approach to monitoring and coordinating the various aspects of longitudinal care of the diabetic patient. A *flow sheet* that tracks treatment and treatment changes, critical laboratory and physical examination parameters, and key referrals is highly recommended (see Chapter 1, Fig. 1.2). Items that should be included on the flow sheet include serum glucose and HbA_{1C}, serum lipids, urine protein and renal function, foot examinations, and eye examinations. Prominent display of a *primary care front sheet* that includes a *problem list* (see Chapter 1, Fig. 1.1) is particularly important in diabetic patients, because diabetics are likely to have a plethora of associated conditions (see Complications of Diabetes Mellitus, above). Finally, a preventive care profile and flow sheet (see Chapter 14, Fig. 14.3) is important in the diabetic as in other patients. Some preventive care recommendations are more aggressive in the diabetic patient, such as recommendations for yearly influenza vaccinations and more aggressive lipid management. Knowledge of smoking status and smoking cessation counseling (see Chapter 27) are particularly important in the diabetic patient, whose risk of atherosclerotic disease is very high.

DIABETES DURING PREGNANCY AND GESTATIONAL DIABETES

Gestational Diabetes

The term *gestational diabetes mellitus* (GDM) refers only to women who meet the diagnostic criteria (Table 79.9) during pregnancy (see Diabetes During Pregnancy, below). Women who are known to have diabetes and who become pregnant are not included. Most gestational diabetic patients return to a state of normal glucose tolerance postpartum. GDM occurs in 1% to 14% of all pregnancies, depending on the prevalence of diabetes in the population. Such patients are at increased risk (approximately 30%) for developing diabetes within 5 to 10 years after parturition.

Table 79.9. Diagnosis of Gestational Diabetes by the OGTT

	Venous Plasma[a] (mg/dL)
Fasting	105
1 h	190
2 h	165
3 h	145

See text for indications.

[a]Test positive for diabetes mellitus: two or more of the values must be met or exceeded.

Diagnosis During Pregnancy

The ADA recommends that all pregnant women are screened for diabetes between the 24th and 28th weeks of pregnancy using a 50-g oral glucose load and a single blood sample 1 hour later. If the value exceeds 140 mg/dL, a glucose tolerance test is performed using 100 g of glucose. (The World Health Organization recommends a 75-g dose of glucose for the OGTT; no validation of this test through outcomes studies is available.) Criteria for a diagnosis of gestational diabetes are given in Table 79.9; they were not changed by the Expert Committee that promulgated new standards for diagnosis of diabetes (see above). The screening procedure identifies 80% to 90% of diabetic patients but has 15% to 20% false positives.

Overt diabetes (grossly elevated fasting and postprandial blood sugars) already under therapy with insulin in type 1 diabetics or untreated in type 2 diabetics has long been associated with adverse outcomes for both mother and fetus. No question remains that such patients should be treated with insulin in a fairly intensive manner; the result is a great reduction in perinatal mortality and morbidity. However, the implications of what is called gestational diabetes (i.e., elevated levels of blood sugar during pregnancy that meet standard diagnostic criteria in the nonpregnant state) are uncertain (see below). In populations that have a high prevalence of IGT and type 2 diabetes (e.g., Mexican Americans), gestational diabetes is clearly associated with increased perinatal morbidity and mortality, which can be reduced with treatment. In other populations, an adverse influence of gestational diabetes is much less obvious. The contrasting outcomes in different populations account for some of the differences of clinicians' attitudes toward treatment. The issues involved in initiating therapy with insulin are important and still not completely resolved: great emotional impact, expense, inconvenience, and potential adverse events (including low birth weight babies), especially with intensive insulin therapy.

Implications for Pregnancy of Oral Glucose Tolerance Test-Diagnosed Glucose Intolerance

A study of the effect of glucose intolerance, not overt diabetes, diagnosed by the glucose tolerance test reported significant stepwise increases of macrosomia, congenital abnormalities, perinatal mortality, prematurity, toxemia, and cesarean section as the OGTT 2-hour PG increased from 100 to 164 mg/dL (126). These observations have been challenged (127). However, on the basis of this report and others, obstetricians may initiate therapy with insulin that is designed to maintain fasting and postprandial blood sugars that are normal for pregnancy (i.e., lower than the nonpregnant state). At the very least, it is argued, normoglycemia prevents macrosomia and is therefore a worthwhile undertaking (128). Such an approach of course demands careful SMBG. Many practitioners remain skeptical of this approach as overly aggressive. Large studies of such intervention are not available. However, one can be certain that such therapy will be attended by many episodes of hypoglycemia.

In numerous earlier studies, the prognosis for the pregnant state and the perinatal morbidity of infants born of mothers with an abnormal OGTT but with essentially normal FPG did not differ from normal. This has led some to advocate diet therapy alone, as long as maternal fasting and postprandial glucose levels remain within the higher range of normal for the nonpregnant state. Fifteen years ago an authoritative view was that pregnant women with abnormalities of blood glucose should probably be vigorously treated. More recently, a more conservative and well-tempered view has emerged that takes into account severity of the glucose intolerance, population characteristics, and the long-term medical impacts on mothers and their children (129).

Contraceptive Methods in Diabetic Women

Use of high-dose estrogen-based contraceptives may be unwise because of possibly increased risk in the diabetic of vascular thrombosis and hyperlipidemia. Low-dose estrogen or progestogen alone would theoretically be safer. Intrauterine devices may produce infection more often in a diabetic. Thus, mechanical means of contraception such as the diaphragm or condom seem to be the safest methods (see Chapter 100).

Pregnancy in the diabetic woman presents a major challenge to the clinicians involved in the care of the mother and the fetus. Ideally, the medical team should include an experienced practitioner experienced in the care of diabetics, a perinatologist, and an obstetrician who cooperate actively in the management of the pregnancy. Others in the team may include an experienced diabetes teaching nurse and, ultimately, a pediatrician/neonatologist.

Most experts are now convinced that modern optimal management of diabetes during pregnancy has reduced perinatal infant mortality to that of nondiabetic women. However, the treatment of most pregnant diabetic women is in fact less than optimal. It is the exceptional baby that is conceived in a mother whose diabetes is under rigorous control by intensive therapy, whose physical and emotional health is uncompromised by the diabetes, and whose caregivers always provide unerring exemplary advice and care.

The possibility of diabetes in the newborn or young child is often of great concern; this issue has already been discussed (see Inheritance under Definition and Classification, above). Other questions concern maternal and fetal mortality. Although the diabetic woman without overt complications carries little or no increased risk to herself, the fetal risks must be presented with candor. Of special importance beyond that of fetal survival is the problem of an increased risk of congenital abnormalities (see below) and long-term neurologic abnormalities in children of diabetic mothers (130). Therefore, preconception patient education and intensive therapy are extremely important for diabetic women who plan to become pregnant. As women elect to have pregnancies at older ages, more type 2 patients are likely to be seen. Many, probably most, of these women should expect to require insulin therapy and should be switched to glyburide if already on a sulfonylurea (see below).

The course of the pregnancy in a diabetic woman and its impact on the fetus depend on the type of diabetes and the stage of the disease at which the pregnancy occurs. Thus, when pregnancy occurs in the type 1 diabetic without diabetic complications who is already under close medical supervision and is practicing intensive insulin therapy, management of the diabetes consists of continuation of therapy, perhaps with institution of even lower limits for blood glucose and special attention to avoidance of nocturnal hypoglycemia (see below). When pregnancy occurs in a diabetic woman with vascular disease, the mother is in danger of an adverse outcome. Nephropathy may worsen, at least temporarily, especially if hypertension is present. Premature delivery and smaller than normal infants occur with even modest increases of serum creatinine (above 1.5 mg/dL) and with proteinuria. Diabetic retinopathy, especially if already proliferative or if hypertension is present, may progress rapidly and result in loss of visual acuity. The long-term survival of the diabetic with microvascular disease is already significantly compromised and an honest prognosis in this regard may deter pregnancy, not necessarily because of concern over acceleration of the diabetic complications but out of concern for the future welfare of a child born to a mother whose health may be poor and whose survival is threatened. Under these circumstances, various questions must be asked. Does the woman fully understand the risks of continuing the pregnancy? Should an abortion be considered?

Fetal Mortality and Congenital Malformations

The view that the more severe the diabetic state, the worse the perinatal survival of the infant was definitively substantiated by a multicenter study (131) that showed that overtly diabetic women with nearly normal blood glucose levels are at no greater risk of having a spontaneous abortion than are nondiabetic women (83% successful outcome). In contrast, those with elevated blood glucose and elevated glycosylated hemoglobin in the first trimester have additional risk, estimated to be increased by 3% for each elevation of HbA_{1c} of approximately 0.5% above the upper limit of the normal range (approximately 6.5%). In contrast to earlier reports, patients classified according to the severity of diabetes based on age at onset, duration of disease, and presence of complications showed no difference between groups (127). Ketoacidosis occurs in 2% to 10% of diabetic pregnancies and is associated in these cases with fetal losses of 80% to 100%.

The incidence of significant congenital abnormalities in nondiabetic women is approximately 2% to 3% but rises to 8% to 12% in infants born to type 1 diabetic patients and reaches 25% when control is poor, as evidenced by grossly elevated glycosylated hemoglobin. Almost all authorities now agree that hyperglycemia during the early weeks of pregnancy (gestational weeks 3 to 7 when embryogenesis occurs) appears to account for the increased incidence of congenital malformations. Near normalization of blood sugar before conception and continued normalization through the critical first weeks have been reported to reduce this increased incidence to normal.

Maternal Mortality and Morbidity

Maternal mortality during pregnancy is definitely increased in diabetic women and at 0.5% is about 20 times that in nondiabetics. Most deaths are caused by ketoacidosis or hypoglycemia, the latter usually occurring in the first trimester or immediately postpartum, times at which insulin requirements often decrease. Optimal management could eliminate most or all of these deaths. Some deaths that may not be preventable include infections after cesarean section or hemorrhage after traumatic delivery of a large infant. Diabetics with overt heart disease (ischemic heart disease, congestive heart failure) have a high mortality (75%) when allowed to go to term. Such patients should never become pregnant or should have an abortion if pregnancy occurs.

Maternal morbidity also increases during the diabetic pregnancy. Polyhydramnios occurs in 25% of pregnancies (10 times greater incidence than expected). Asymptomatic bacteriuria (20%) and frank pyelonephritis (7%) occur three times more often than in the general population. Pyelonephritis is said to occur in 25% of bacteriuric diabetic patients and is associated with a high rate of fetal loss.

Management of Overt Diabetes During Pregnancy

Insulin Therapy: Monitoring Control

Patients with overt diabetes, including gestational diabetes, who are receiving insulin therapy must be carefully monitored (see SMBG) to establish safe and optimal control of blood sugar. Some obstetricians still favor hospitalization with frequent daytime blood sugar determinations (glucose panel) as an aid to establishment of optimal control, but patient compliance after hospitalization is critical, in any case.

There is as yet no good evidence that aggressive control of blood sugar is beneficial to the pregnant diabetic or her fetus (132). The goal of insulin and diet therapy should be the closest approximation of normalization of blood sugar that is possible using SMBG while avoiding therapeutic heroics (i.e., multiple and prolonged hospitalizations solely for the purpose of blood sugar control). Normal fasting blood sugar (not exceeding 90 mg/dL), preprandial blood sugar less than 105 mg/dL, and 2-hour postprandial blood sugars that do not exceed 120 mg/dL are considered tight control. However, some obstetricians using *conventional* therapy with insulin strive for blood sugar levels *averaging* 100 mg/dL through the day, a goal probably impossible to achieve without prolonged hospitalizations and excessively frequent and severe hypoglycemia. If near normalization of blood sugar is attempted, either *intensive therapy* using multiple daily doses of insulin or an insulin pump should be used in conjunction with SMBG (see Monitoring During Intensive Insulin Therapy, above). Intensified therapy is probably preferred because ketoacidosis and infection are significant risks with pump therapy; either complication could be lethal to the fetus.

Most patients managed with *conventional therapy* require at least two doses of intermediate-acting insulin or mixtures of intermediate- and short-acting insulin. A few patients with type 2 diabetes may have satisfactory control on a single dose of long-acting insulin. No particular insulin has any special advantage in the pregnant patient. Human insulin has been claimed to be less antigenic than animal insulins, a finding of no established clinical significance. Lispro insulin is said to be comparable with human insulin in terms of antigenicity and is claimed to produce less hypoglycemia when used appropriately.

It should be kept in mind that insulin requirements often decrease in the first trimester, only to increase during the third trimester by up to 50% and to fall again after delivery. Patients on intensive therapy should monitor their glucose in the fasting (overnight) state, before each meal, and possibly 2 hours after meals. In addition, monitoring during the night (2 to 3 a.m.) may be necessary because nocturnal hypoglycemia is common during pregnancy, especially in the first and third trimesters. Frequent monitoring of glucosuria and especially ketonuria remains an invaluable adjunct to ambulatory management, but only SMBG with frequent determinations can provide optimal management. Because of the disastrous effect of ketoacidosis during pregnancy, daily monitoring of urine for ketones is strongly advised. Minor ketonuria caused by carbohydrate lack is common but can usually be distinguished from ketoacidosis by rough quantitation of the ketonuria, minimal or absent glucosuria, and measurement of the blood sugar at less than 200 mg/dL. Determination of plasma bicarbonate and plasma ketones (negative when ketonuria is caused by carbohydrate lack) should be made if any doubt still exists. The development of ketoacidosis is an indication for immediate hospitalization.

Use of Oral Antidiabetic Drugs During Pregnancy in Type 2 Patients With Gestational Diabetes

Until recently, use of oral agents in the therapy of pregnant type 2 diabetics was considered to be contraindicated. First-generation sulfonylureas and metformin were known from animal studies to cross the placenta and to produce a number of problems, including fetal macrosomia, a result of hypersecretion of insulin by the fetus. However, a recent study using glyburide, known *not* to be transported into the fetus, showed that this sulfonylurea is safe and effective for controlling glycemia in women with gestational diabetes. Glucose control and maternal–fetal outcomes were the same in patients treated with up to 20 mg of glyburide daily as with the insulin group that received a mean of 85 units of insulin daily. Diagnosis of GDM was made by oral glucose tolerance testing and control was excellent in both groups, at a mean daily glucose level of 105 mg/dL and mean HbA_{1C} of 5.5%. Only 4% of patients randomized to glyburide eventually required insulin.

Although this study opens the way to use of glyburide for GDM, a number of caveats remain. Drug therapy was started at 11 weeks, thus beyond the period when teratogenicity issues were of concern. The study does not address the issue of whether women with type 2 diabetes being treated with glyburide who became pregnant should continue to take the drug through the critical period of organogenesis. Very little clinical information deals with metformin or other sulfonylureas, and no information is available for the glitazones. These drugs should still be considered to be contraindicated for treatment of GDM.

Diet Therapy

Diet therapy is often modified slightly to include increased protein intake. Weight gain of about 25 lb (11.5 kg) is expected and acceptable in both normal and diabetic pregnancies. Severe weight control, previously advocated by some, has been abandoned.

Timing of Delivery

This issue is decided by the obstetrician (and neonatologist) and has been argued for decades, since it was recognized that the incidence of stillbirths in diabetic women increases beyond the 36th week. However, attempts to deliver infants early (before 40 weeks) resulted in a high rate of cesarean section and a high rate of neonatal loss caused by neonatal respiratory distress syndrome. Currently, if fetal surveillance is normal, delivery is delayed to term when it is induced if the cervix is favorable or if spontaneous labor occurs. However, if the pregnancy has been complicated by vascular disease or poor control of glucose or if there are other adverse factors such as a prior stillbirth, delivery may be performed at 38 weeks in an effort to prevent late fetal death. Such early delivery is predicated upon finding suitable values for amniotic fluid phospholipids (lecithin/sphingomyelin ratio and the presence of phosphatidylglycerol), biochemical markers of fetal pulmonary maturation. Respiratory distress syndrome is highly unlikely if the lecithin/sphingomyelin ratio is greater than 2.0. Delivery despite fetal pulmonary immaturity may be necessary if the pregnant patient worsens (preeclampsia, renal failure) or there is evidence of fetal distress.

General References

Textbooks

Kahn CR, Weir GC, eds. Joslin's diabetes mellitus, 13th ed. Philadelphia: Lea & Febiger, 1994.

A classic major textbook, multiauthored, badly outdated but still useful; heavy with accumulated information and references. If one wishes to find much of the old material of the field, this is the book.

Pickup JC, Williams G, eds. Textbook of diabetes, 2nd ed. Cambridge, MA: Blackwell Science, 1977.

A multiauthored, two-volume, beautifully printed, authoritative book with a predominantly British and European viewpoint.

Porte D Jr, Sherwin RF, Ellenberg M, et al., eds. Ellenberg & Rifkin's diabetes mellitus, 5th ed. East Norwalk, CT: Appleton & Lange, 1997.

Another classic multiauthored major textbook by the some of most prominent people in the field. Well-printed, well-edited, and up-to-date clinical material. However, drug therapy of type 2 diabetes mellitus is already out of date.

Books For Physicians

American Diabetes Association (ADA). A series of authoritative, multiauthored, mini-textbooks in paperback, approximately $30 to $40 each. Can be ordered at 800-232-6733; or at the ADA website. Topics include: medical management of non-insulin dependent (type II) diabetes; medical management of insulin-dependent diabetes mellitus (type I); medical management of pregnancy complicated by diabetes; therapy for diabetes mellitus and related disorders; intensive diabetes management; the health professional's guide to diabetes and exercise.

The ADA also sells slides and CD-ROMS for teaching lectures and books on the vital statistics and costs of diabetes.

Journals For Professionals

Diabetes (monthly; includes both clinical and laboratory research); Clinical Diabetes (quarterly), Diabetes Care (monthly; title misleading, contains much clinical research), and Diabetes Spectrum (nurses, dietitians, educators; quarterly).

Primarily For Educators And Patients

The American Diabetes Association publishes many first-rate materials in English and Spanish at nominal prices: Practical psychology for diabetes clinicians; Life with diabetes; Facilitating lifestyle change: A resource manual; Diabetes education goals; Single-topic diabetes resources, reproducible handouts on a variety of topics; Right from the start; Gestational diabetes; and many small books on nutrition, exercise, and costs of care. Call 800-232-6733 or fax 770-442-9742; write to American Diabetes Association, Order Fulfillment Department, P.O. Box 930850, Atlanta, GA 31193-0850; or visit their website at www.diabetes.org

Milner-Fenwick, Inc. specializes in video materials for patient education (approximately $20 per tape). Spanish versions are available. Production is with the American Association of Diabetes Educators. Call 800-432-8433 or fax 410-252-6316; write to Milner-Fenwick, Inc., 2125 Greenspring Drive, Timonium, MD 21093; or visit their website at www.milner-fenwick.com.

Specific References*

1. National Diabetes Group. Classification and diagnosis of diabetes mellitus and other categories of glucose tolerance. Diabetes 1979;28:1039.
2. Expert Committee on the Diagnosis and Classification of Diabetes Mellitus. Report. Diabetes Care 1997;20:1183.
3. Karjalainen J, Salmela P, Ilonen J, et al. A comparison of childhood and adult type I diabetes mellitus. N Engl J Med 1989;320:881.
4. Eisenbarth GS. Type I diabetes mellitus. A chronic autoimmune disease. N Engl J Med 1986;314:1360.
5. Yoon JW. Role of viruses in the pathogenesis of IDDM. Ann Med 1991;23:437.
6. Karjalainen J, Martin JM, Knip M, et al. A bovine albumin peptide as a possible trigger of insulin-dependent diabetes mellitus. N Engl J Med 1992;327:302.
7. Niskanen LK, Tuomi T, Karjalainen J, et al. GAD antibodies in NIDDM. Ten-year follow-up from the diagnosis. Diabetes Care 1995;18:1557.
8. Turner R, Stratton I, Horton V, et al. UKPDS 25: autoantibodies to islet-cell cytoplasm and glutamic acid decarboxylase for prediction of insulin requirement in type 2 diabetes. UK Prospective Diabetes Study Group. Lancet 1997;350:1288.

*Bold print (general references) and bold numerals (specific references) denote published controlled clinical trials, meta-analyses, or consensus-based recommendations.

9. Tuomi T, Carlsson A, Li H, et al. Clinical and genetic characteristics of type 2 diabetes with and without GAD antibodies. Diabetes 1999;48:150.
10. Alberti KGMM, Zimmet PZ. Definition, diagnosis and classification of diabetes mellitus and its complications. Part 1. Diagnosis and classification of diabetes mellitus. Provisional report of a WHO consultation. Diab Med 1998;15:539.
11. Fajans SS, Bell GI, Polonsky KS. Molecular mechanisms and clinical pathophysiology of maturity-onset diabetes of the young. N Engl J Med 2001:345:971.
12. Atkinson MA, Maclaren NK. The pathogenesis of insulin-dependent diabetes mellitus. N Engl J Med 1994;331:1428.
13. Olmos P, A'Hern R, Heaton DA, et al. The significance of the concordance rate for type 1 (insulin-dependent) diabetes in identical twins. Diabetologia 1988;31:747.
14. Kumar D, Gemayel NS, Deapen D, et al. North American twins with IDDM. Genetic, etiological, and clinical significance of disease concordance according to age, zygosity, and the interval after diagnosis in first twin. Diabetes 1993;42:1351.
15. Reaven GM. Role of insulin resistance in human disease. Diabetes 1988;37:1595.
16. Gerich JE. Insulin resistance is not necessarily an essential component of type 2 diabetes. J Clin Endocr Metab 2000;85:2113.
17. Almind K, Doria A, Kahn CR. Putting the genes for type II on the map. Nat Med 2001;7:277.
18. Rosenbloom AL, Joe JR, Young RS, et al. Emerging epidemic of type 2 diabetes in youth. Diabetes Care 1999;22:345.
19. Kahn CR, Vicent D, Doria A. Genetics of non–insulin-dependent (type II) diabetes mellitus. Annu Rev Med 1996;47:509.
20. Barnett AH, Eff C, Leslie RDG, et al. Diabetes in identical twins: a study of 200 pairs. Diabetologia 1981;20:87.
21. Jarrett RJ. The cardiovascular risk associated with impaired glucose tolerance. Diabet Med 1995;13:S15.
22. Edelstein S, Knowler WC, Bain RP, et al. Predictors of progression from impaired glucose tolerance to NIDDM. An analysis of six prospective studies. Diabetes 1997;46:701.
23. Knowler WC, Saad MF, Pettitt DJ, et al. Determinants of diabetes mellitus in the Pima Indians. Diabetes Care 1993;16:216.
24. Bjornholt JV, Erikssen G, Aaser E, et al. Fasting blood glucose: an underestimated risk factor for cardiovascular death. Diabetes Care 1999;22:45.
25. Tuomilehto J, Lindström J, Eriksson JG, et al. Prevention of type 2 diabetes mellitus by changes in lifestyle among subjects with impaired glucose tolerance. N Engl J Med 2001;344: 1343.
26. Tataranni PA, Bogardus C. Changing habits to delay diabetes. N Engl J Med 2001;344:1390.
27. Swinburn BA, Metcalf PA, Ley SJ. Long term (5-year) effects of a reduced-fat diet intervention in individuals with glucose intolerance. Diabetes Care 2001;24:619.
28. West KM. Diet therapy of diabetes: an analysis of failure. Ann Intern Med 1973;79:425.
29. West KM. Diet and diabetes. Postgrad Med 1976;60:209.
30. American Diabetes Association. Nutrition recommendations and principles for people with diabetes mellitus. Diabetes Care 2000;23:543.
31. Chen Y-DI, Swami S, Skowronski R, et al. Effect of variations in dietary fat and carbohydrate intake on postprandial lipemia in patients with noninsulin dependent diabetes mellitus. J Clin Endocrinol Metab 1993;76:347.
32. Coulston AM, Hollenbeck CB, Swislocki ALM, et al. Deleterious metabolic effects of high-carbohydrate, sucrose-containing diets in patients with non–insulin-dependent diabetes mellitus. Am J Med 1987;82:213.
33. Garg A, Bonanome A, Grundy SM, et al. Comparison of a high-carbohydrate diet with a high monounsaturated-fat diet in patients with non–insulin-dependent diabetes mellitus. N Engl J Med 1988;319:829.
34. Bonanome A, Visona A, Lusiani L, et al. Carbohydrate and lipid metabolism in patients with non–insulin-dependent diabetes mellitus: effects of a low-fat, high-carbohydrate diet vs a diet high in monosaturated fatty acids. Am J Clin Nutr 1991;54:586.

35. Ajani UA, Hennekens CH, Spelsberg A, et al. Alcohol consumption and risk of type 2 diabetes mellitus among US male physicians. Arch Intern Med 2000;160:1025.
36. Solomon CG, Hu FB, Stampfer MJ, et al. Moderate alcohol consumption and risk of coronary heart disease among women with type 2 diabetes mellitus. Circulation 2000;102:494.
37. Gaziano JM, Gaziano TA, Glynn RJ, et al. Light-to-moderate alcohol consumption and mortality in the Physician's Health Study enrollment cohort. J Am Coll Cardiol 2000;35:96.
38. Stolar MW. Atherosclerosis in diabetes: the role of hyperinsulinemia. Metab Clin Exp 1988;37[Suppl 1]:1.
39. Rendell M. Dietary treatment of diabetes mellitus. N Engl J Med 2000;342:1440.
40. Nuttall FQ. Dietary fiber in the management of diabetes. Diabetes 1993;42:503.
41. Helmrich SP, Ragland DR, Leung RW, et al. Physical activity and reduced occurrence of non–insulin-dependent diabetes mellitus. N Engl J Med 1991;325:147.
42. Rabasa-Lhoret R, Bourque J, Ducros F, et al. Guidelines for premeal insulin dose reduction for postprandial exercise of different durations in type 1 diabetic subjects treated intensively with a basal-bolus insulin regimen. Diabetes Care 2001;24:625.
43. American Diabetes Association. Implications of the United Kingdom prospective study. Diabetes Care 1998;21:2180.
44. Diabetes Control and Complications Trial Research Group. The effect of intensive diabetes treatment on the development and progression of long-term complications in insulin-dependent diabetes. N Engl J Med 1993;329:977.
44a. American Diabetes Association. Implications of the diabetes control and complications trial. Diabetes Care 2002;25:S25.
45. Intensive blood-glucose control with sulphonylureas or insulin compared with conventional treatment and risk of complications in patients with type 2 diabetes (UKPDS 33). UK Prospective Diabetes Study (UKPDS) Group. Lancet 1998;352:837.
46. Effect of intensive blood-glucose control with metformin on complications in overweight patients with type 2 diabetes (UKPDS 34). UK Prospective Diabetes Study (UKPDS) Group. Lancet 1998;352:854.
47. Insulin glargine (Lantus), a new long-acting insulin. Med Lett 2001;43:65.
48. Garrison CR, Riddle MC. Evening insulin therapy for type II diabetes. Pract Diabetol 1990;9:1.
49. Bastyr EJ III, Stuart CA, Brodows RG, et al. Therapy focused on lowering postprandial glucose, not fasting glucose, may be superior for lowering HbA_{1C}. Diabetes Care 2000;23:1236.
50. Ohkubo Y, Kishikawa H, Araki E, et al. Intensive insulin therapy prevents the progression of diabetic microvascular complications in Japanese patients with non-insulin dependent diabetes mellitus: a randomized prospective 6-year study. Diabetes Res Clin Pract 1995;28:103.
51. Rohlfing CL, Little RR, Wiedmeyer H-M, et al. Use of GHb (HbA_{1C}) in screening for undiagnosed diabetes in the U.S. population. Diabetes Care 2000;23:187.
52. Simon D, Senan C, Balkau B, et al. Reproducibility of HbA_{1C} in a healthy adult population. Diabetes Care 1999;22:1361.
53. Bjorntorp P. Visceral obesity: a "civilization syndrome." Obesity Res 1993;1:206.
54. Paquot N, Castillo MJ, Lefebvre PJ, et al. No increased insulin sensitivity after a single intravenous administration of a recombinant human tumor necrosis factor receptor: Fc fusion protein in obese insulin-resistant patients. J Clin Endocrinol Metab 2000;85:1316.
55. Amiel S. Glucose counter-regulation in health and disease: current concepts in hypoglycemia recognition and response. Q J Med 1991;80:707.
56. Amiel SA, Tamborlane WV, Simonson DC, et al. Defective glucose counter-regulation after strict glycemic control of insulin-dependent diabetes mellitus. N Engl J Med 1987;316:1376.
57. Cryer PE. The metabolic impact of autonomic neuropathy in insulin-dependent diabetes mellitus [Editorial]. Arch Intern Med 1986;146:2127.
58. Cryer PE, Gerich JE. Glucose counterregulation, hypoglycemia, and intensive insulin therapy in diabetes mellitus. N Engl J Med 1985;313:232.
59. Cryer PE, White NH, Santiago JV. The relevance of glucose counterregulatory systems to patients with insulin dependent diabetes mellitus. Endocrinol Rev 1986;7:131.
60. Boyle PJ, Kempers SF, O'Connor AM, et al. Brain glucose uptake and unawareness of hypoglycemia in patients with insulin-dependent diabetes mellitus. N Engl J Med 1995;333:1726; Bolli GB, Fanelli CG. Unawareness of hypoglycemia [Editorial]. N Engl J Med 1995;333:1771.
61. Tordjman KM, Havlin CE, Levandowski LA, et al. Failure of nocturnal hypoglycemia to cause fasting hyperglycemia in patients with insulin-dependent diabetes mellitus. N Engl J Med 1987;317:1552.
62. Perriello G, DeFeo P, Torlone E, et al. The effect of asymptomatic nocturnal hypoglycemia on glycemic control in diabetes mellitus. N Engl J Med 1988;319:1233.
63. The University Group Diabetes Program. A study of the effects of hypoglycemic agents on vascular complications in patients with adult onset diabetes. Diabetes 1970;19[Suppl]:789.
64. Wolffenbuttel BH, Sels J-PJE, Rondas-Colbers GJ. Comparison of different insulin regimens in elderly patients with NIDDM. Diabetes Care 1996;19:1326.
65. Weissman PN, Shenkman L, Gregerman RI. Chlorpropamide hyponatremia: drug-induced inappropriate antidiuretic-hormone activity. N Engl J Med 1971;284:65.
66. Fonesca V, Rosenstock J, Wardham P, et al. Effect of metformin and rosiglitazone combination therapy in patients with type 2 diabetes mellitus. JAMA 2000;283:1695.
67. Gruessner A, Sutherland DER. Pancreas transplants for United States (US) and non-US cases as reported to International Pancreas Transplant Registry (IPTR) and to the United Network for Organ Sharing (UNOS). In: Cecka M, Terasaki P, eds. Clinical transplants 1997. Los Angeles: UCLA Tissue Typing Laboratory, 1998.
68. Sudan D, Sudan R, Stratta R. Long-term outcome of simultaneous kidney-pancreas transplantation: analysis of 61 patients with more than 5 years follow-up. Transplantation 2000;69:550.
69. Gruessner RW, Dunn DL, Gruessner AC, et al. Recipient risk factors have an impact on technical failures and patient and graft survival rates in bladder-drained pancreas transplants. Transplantation 1994;57:1598.
70. International Islet Transplant Registry, Vol 6, No. 1, Dec. 1996.
71. Shapiro AMJ, Lakey JRT, Ryan EA, et al. Islet transplantation in seven patients with type 1 diabetes mellitus using a glucocorticoid-free immunosuppressive regimen. N Engl J Med 2000;343:230.
72. Haffner SM. Coronary heart disease in patients with diabetes. N Engl J Med 2000;342:1040.
73. Nesto RW, Phillips RT, Kett KG, et al. Angina and exertional myocardial ischemia in diabetic and nondiabetic patients: assessment by exercise thallium scintigraphy. Ann Intern Med 1988;108:170.
74. Nesto RW, Watson FS, Kowalchuk GJ, et al. Silent myocardial ischemia and infarction in diabetics with peripheral vascular disease: assessment by dipyridamole thallium-201 scintigraphy. Am Heart J 1990;120:1073.
75. Consensus development conference on the diagnosis of coronary heart disease in people with diabetes: 10–11 February 1998, Miami, Florida. American Diabetes Association. Diabetes Care 1998;21:1551.
76. Joki R, Colwell JA. Clotting disorders in diabetes. In: Alberti KGMM, DeFronzo RA, Alberti KG, et al., eds. International textbook of diabetes mellitus. 2nd ed. Chichester, Sussex, England: John Wiley & Sons, 1997:1543.
77. Colwell JA. Aspirin therapy in diabetics (position statement). Diabetes Care 1997;20:1767.
78. Kannel WB, Hjortland M, Castelli WP. Role of diabetes in congestive heart failure: the Framingham study. Am J Cardiol 1974;34:29.
79. Goldberg IJ. Diabetic dyslipidemia: causes and consequences. J Clin Endocr Metab 2001;86:965.

80. Goldberg RB, Mellies MJ, Sacks FM, et al. Cardiovascular events and their reduction with pravastatin in diabetic and glucose-intolerant myocardial infarction survivors with average cholesterol levels. Circulation 1998;98:2513.
81. Haffner SM. Management of dyslipidemia in adults with diabetes. Diabetes Care 1998;21:160.
82. Epstein M, Sowers JR. Diabetes mellitus and hypertension. Hypertension 1992;19:403.
83. Grossman E, Messerli FH, Goldbourt U. High blood pressure and diabetes mellitus. Are all antihypertensive drugs created equal? Arch Intern Med 2000;160:2447.
84. UK Prospective Diabetes Study Group. Tight blood pressure control and risk of macrovascular and microvascular complications in type 2 diabetes: UKPDS 38. BMJ 1998;317:703.
85. Hansson L, Zanchetti A, Carruthers SG, et al. Effects of intensive blood-pressure lowering and low-dose aspirin patients with hypertension: principal results of the Hypertension Optimal Treatment (HOT) randomised trial. HOT Study Group. Lancet 1998;351:1755.
86. Heart Outcomes Prevention Evaluation Study Investigators. Effects of ramipril on cardiovascular and microvascular outcome in people with diabetes mellitus: results of the HOPE study and Micro-HOPE substudy. Lancet 2000;355:253.
87. National High Blood Pressure Education Program Working Group report on hypertension in diabetes. Hypertension 1994;23:145.
88. Agarwal R. Treatment of hypertension in patients with diabetes: lessons from recent trials. Cardiol Rev 2001;9:36.
89. Warram JH, Laffel LM, Valsania P, et al. Excess mortality associated with diuretic therapy in diabetes mellitus. Arch Intern Med 1991;151:1350.
90. Curb JD, Pressel SL, Cutler JA, et al. Effect of diuretic-based antihypertensive treatment on cardiovascular disease risk in older diabetic patients with isolated systolic hypertension. Systolic Hypertension in the Elderly Program Cooperative Research Group. JAMA 1996;276:1886.
91. Furberg DC, Psaty MB. Should dihydropyridines be used as first-line drugs in the treatment of hypertension? The con side. Arch Intern Med 1995;155:2157.
92. Birkenhager WH, Staessen JA. Treatment of diabetic patients with hypertension. Curr Hypertens Rep 1999;1:225.
93. Mason RP, Mason PE. Calcium antagonists and cardiovascular risk in diabetes. Diabetes Care 1999;22:1206.
94. Estacio RO, Jeffers BW, Hiatt WR, et al. The effect of nisoldipine as compared with enalapril on cardiovascular outcomes in patients with non-insulin-dependent diabetes and hypertension [ABCD trial]. N Engl J Med 1998;338:645.
95. Yusuf S, Sleight P, Pogue J, et al. Effects of an angiotensin-converting-enzyme inhibitor, ramipril, on cardiovascular events in high-risk patients. The Heart Outcomes Prevention Evaluation Study Investigators. N Engl J Med 2000;342:145.
96. Messerli FH, Grossman E, Goldbourt U. Antihypertensive therapy in diabetic hypertensive patients. Am J Hypertens 2001;14:12S.
97. The EUCLID Study Group. Randomised placebo-controlled trial of lisinopril in normotensive patients with insulin-dependent diabetes and normoalbuminuria or microalbuminuria. Lancet 1997;349:1787.
98. Lewis EJ, Hunsicker LG, Clarke WR, et al. Renoprotective effect of the angiotensin-receptor antagonist irbesartan in patients with nephropathy due to type 2 diabetes. N Engl J Med 2001;345:851.
99. Brenner BM, Cooper ME, de Zeeuw, et al. Effects of losartan on renal and cardiovascular outcomes in patients with type 2 diabetes and nephropathy. N Engl J Med 2001;345:861.
100. Parving HH, Lehnert H, Brochner-Mortensen J, et al. The effect of irbesartan on the development of diabetic nephropathy in patients with type 2 diabetes. N Engl J Med 2001;345:870.
101. Editorial. Prevention of end-stage renal disease due to type 2 diabetes. N Engl J Med 2001;345:910.
102. Max MB, Lynch SA, Muir J, et al. Effects of desipramine, amitriptyline, and fluoxetine on pain in diabetic neuropathy. N Engl J Med 1992;326:1250.
103. Davis JL, Smith RL. Painful diabetic neuropathy treated with venlafaxine HCl extended release capsules. Diabetes Care 1999;22:1909.
104. Ewing DJ, Campbell IW, Clarke BF. Assessment of cardiovascular effects in diabetic autonomic neuropathy and prognostic implications. Ann Intern Med 1980;92:308.
105. Low PA, Gilden JL, Freeman R, et al. Efficacy of midodrine vs placebo in neurogenic orthostatic hypotension. A randomized, double-blind multicenter study. JAMA 1997;277:1046.
106. Mayfield JA, Reiber GE, Sanders LJ, et al. Preventive foot care in people with diabetes. Diabetes Care 1998;21:2161.
107. American Diabetes Association. Preventive foot care in people with diabetes. Diabetes Care 1998;21:2178.
108. American Diabetes Association. Consensus development conference on diabetic foot wound care. Diabetes Care 1999;22:1354.
109. Kalani M, Brismar K, Fagrell B, et al. Transcutaneous oxygen tension and toe blood pressure as predictors for outcome of diabetic foot ulcers. Diabetes Care 1999;22:147.
110. Wheat LJ, Allen SD, Henry M, et al. Diabetic foot infections. Bacteriologic analysis. Arch Intern Med 1986;146:1935.
111. Van Schie CHM, Whalley A, Vileikyte L, et al. Efficacy of injected liquid silicone in the diabetic foot to reduce risk factors for ulceration. Diabetes Care 2000;23:634.
112. Kong MF, Horowitz M, Jones KL, et al. Natural history of diabetic gastroparesis. Diabetes Care 1999;22:503.
113. Ellenberg M. Sexual dysfunction in diabetic patients. Ann Intern Med 1980;92:331.
114. Padma-Nathan H, Hellstrom WJ, Kaiser FE, et al. Treatment of men with erectile dysfunction with transurethral alprostadil. Medicated Urethral System for Erection (MUSE) Study Group. N Engl J Med 1997;336:1.
115. Rendell MS, Rajfer J, Wicker PA, et al. Sildenafil for treatment of erectile dysfunction in men with diabetes: a randomized controlled trial. Sildenafil Diabetes Study Group. JAMA 1999;281:421.
116. Lepore G, Nosari I. Efficacy of oral sildenafil in the treatment of erectile dysfunction in diabetic men with positive response to intracavernosal injection of alprostadil. Diabetes Care 2001;24:409.
117. Golden SH, Peart-Vigilance C, Kao WHL, et al. Perioperative glycemic control and risk of infectious complications in a cohort of adults with diabetes. Diabetes Care 1999;22:1408.
118. Lipsky BA, Pecoraro RF, Larson, SA, et al. Outpatient management of uncomplicated lower-extremity infections in diabetic patients. Arch Intern Med 1990;150:790.
119. Caputo GM, Cavanagh PR, Ulbrecht JS, et al. Assessment and management of foot disease in patients with diabetes. N Engl J Med 1994;331:854.
120. Emanuele N, Klein R, Abraira C, et al. Evaluations of retinopathy in the VA Cooperative Study on Glycemic Control and Complications in Type II Diabetes (VA CSDM). A feasibility study. Diabetes Care 1996;19:1375.
121. Klein R, Klein BE, Moss SE, et al. Glycosylated hemoglobin predicts the incidence and progression of diabetic retinopathy. JAMA 1988;260:2864.
122. Ferris III FL, Davis MD, Aiello LM. Treatment of diabetic retinopathy. N Engl J Med 1999;341:667.
123. The Diabetic Retinopathy Study Research Group. Photocoagulation treatment of proliferative diabetic retinopathy. Clinical application of diabetic retinopathy study (DRS) findings, DRS report number 8. Ophthalmology 1981;88:583.
124. Early Treatment Diabetic Retinopathy Study Research Group. Early photocoagulation for diabetic retinopathy. ETDRS report number 9. Ophthalmology 1991;98:766.
125. Diabetic retinopathy. A booklet prepared by the Retina Panel, Quality of Care Committee, the American Academy of Ophthalmology, 1989. P.O. Box 7424, San Francisco, CA 94120-7424.
126. Tallarigo L, Giampietro O, Penno G, et al. Relation of glucose tolerance to complications of pregnancy in nondiabetic woman. N Engl J Med 1986;315:989.
127. Mills JL, Knopp RH, Simpson JL, et al. Lack of relation of increased malformation rates in infants of diabetic mothers to glycemic control during organogenesis. N Engl J Med 1988;318:671.

128. Jovanovic-Peterson L, Bevier W, Peterson CM. The Santa Barbara County Health Care Services program: birth weight change concomitant with screening for and treatment of glucose-intolerance of pregnancy: a potential cost-effective intervention? Am J Perinatol 1997;14:221.
129. Dornhorst A, Girling JC. Management of gestational diabetes mellitus [Editorial]. N Engl J Med 1995;333:1281.
130. Haworth JC, McRae KN, Dilling LA. Prognosis of infants of diabetic mothers in relation to neonatal hypoglycemia. Dev Med Child Neurol 1976;18:471.
131. Mills JL, Simpson JL, Driscoll SG, et al. Incidence of spontaneous abortion among normal women and insulin-dependent diabetic women whose pregnancies were identified within 21 days of conception. N Engl J Med 1988;319:1617.
132. Walkinshaw SA. Very tight versus tight control for diabetes in pregnancy (Cochrane Review). In: The Cochrane Library, Issue 4. Oxford: Update Software, 2001.

CHAPTER 80

Thyroid Disorders

ROBERT I. GREGERMAN, MD

Disturbances of thyroid growth and function are among the most common endocrinologic disorders encountered in ambulatory practice. Excessive production of the iodine-containing thyroid hormones thyroxine (T_4) and triiodothyronine (T_3) (Fig. 80.1) results in *hyperthyroidism* or *thyrotoxicosis;* decreased hormone production results in *hypothyroidism*. Generalized enlargement of the thyroid, regardless of cause, is termed *goiter*. Focal enlargement of the thyroid is termed a *nodule* and is usually benign. Either goiter or focal enlargement may be associated with abnormal thyroid function. Goiter can produce anatomic changes ranging from simply cosmetic to obstruction of contiguous structures such as the trachea and esophagus. *Thyroiditis* is a term that encompasses a diverse group of disorders characterized by acute, subacute, or chronic inflammation of the thyroid gland.

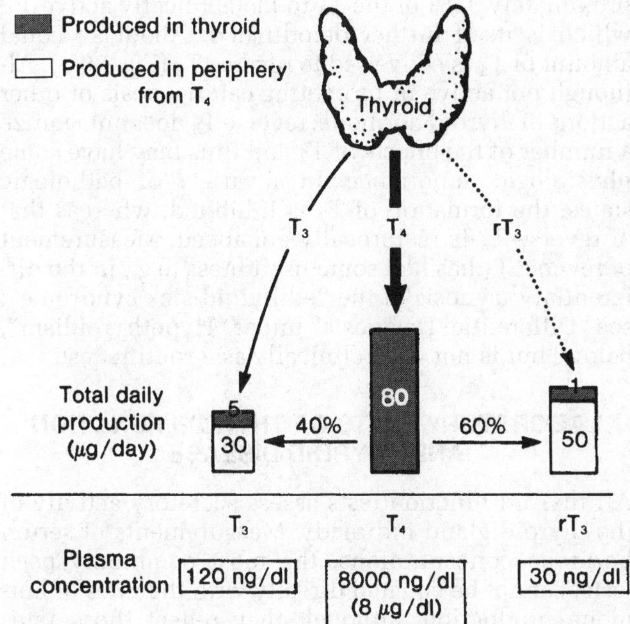

Figure 80.1. Production rates by the thyroid and in the periphery of thyroid hormones and their mean concentrations in the plasma.

THYROID PHYSIOLOGY

Thyroid Regulatory Mechanisms

The principal regulatory mechanism of the thyroid is the hypothalamic–pituitary–thyroid negative feedback control system. The hypothalamus secretes thyrotropin-releasing hormone (TRH), which travels via the hypophyseal portal system to the pituitary, where it stimulates release of thyroid-stimulating hormone (TSH). TSH stimulates many aspects of thyroid activity, including hormone synthesis, thyroid growth, and the release of thyroid hormones. Secretion of TSH by the pituitary is inhibited by the thyroid hormones—thus the term *negative feedback loop.*

The thyroid hormones are unique because they are the only substances in the body that contain the trace element iodine. Iodide from plasma is concentrated by an active process (iodide "pump") that can maintain a thyroid/plasma iodide ratio as high as 500:1. Iodide is thereafter converted through a series of enzymatic steps resulting in the formation of T_4 and T_3 within the thyroglobulin sequence. The iodide pump transports a number of anions other than iodide, a phenomenon that has been exploited diagnostically and therapeutically. As examples, the pertechnetate anion, TcO_4^-, as the radioactive isotope ^{99m}Tc, has been widely used for thyroid imaging (although ^{123}I is now preferred) and the perchlorate anion (ClO_4^-) has a rare use as a therapeutic agent (see below).

The minimal daily requirement of iodide is only about 100 to 200 μg, an amount that is determined by obligatory loss, mainly through the kidney. In the United States and in most developed countries, the minimal daily requirement is enormously exceeded by dietary intake because of the addition of iodide to dietary salt ("iodized salt"); for example, iodized salt provides about 1,000 μg in a normal 10-g daily intake. Thus, iodide deficiency and its consequence, iodide-deficiency goiter, is no longer common in the United States but is still a major problem in many parts of the world (1) (see also Goiter and Iodide Deficiency, below).

Any chemical substance that interferes with thyroid hormone function or release may lower blood hormone concentration and induce compensatory hypertrophy of the gland (goiter) via stimulation of TSH secretion. Certain substances are known to prevent iodide accumulation by impairment of the iodide pump. Other substances interfere with hormone synthesis or inhibit hormone release. Clinically useful agents that have been used for therapeutic effects in states of excess hormone production (hyperthyroidism) are known to act at one or another of these points. Perchlorate, now used therapeutically only occasionally, inhibits the iodide pump. The thiocarbamide "antithyroid" drugs (e.g., propylthiouracil and methimazole) interfere with hormone synthesis by blockade of incorporation of iodide into the tyrosines (organification) and with coupling reactions in iodothyronine formation, but they have more effect on coupling than on organification. Lithium ion (currently in wide use for the treatment of affective disorders, see Chapter 24) interferes with thyroglobulin proteolysis and hormone release and may result in goiter and, occasionally, hypothyroidism. Lithium also interferes with the action of TSH on the thyroid, and therefore some cases of hypothyroidism caused by lithium are not associated with goiter. Iodide itself in pharmacologic amounts interferes with hormone formation and release and in some individuals is a goitrogen.

Metabolic Effects of Thyroid Hormone

The thyroid hormones exert their actions through a variety of mechanisms. A classic thyroid hormone effect is on metabolic rate. Measurement of *basal metabolic rate* (BMR) was the basis for the first laboratory method for clinical assessment of thyroid status. The numerous known actions of thyroid hormones range from specific stimulation of mitochondrial oxidative metabolism to the nuclear regulation of protein synthesis. Thyroid hormones also exert specific regulatory effects on membrane function (e.g., potentiation of catecholamine effects). This action of thyroid hormones explains the signs of exaggerated sympathetic activity in hyperthyroidism and the effectiveness of the therapy of this condition by beta-adrenergic blockade.

Hormone Transport

The thyroid hormones in the blood are T_4 and T_3. Both hormones are tightly but reversibly bound to several plasma proteins, mainly thyroxine-binding globulin (TBG). In the normal person, 65% to 70% of the thyroid hormones are bound to TBG; approximately 15% to the secondary carrier, transthyretin (TTR), formerly called thyroxine-binding prealbumin; and approximately 15% to albumin. Variations of TBG occur in many clinical states and account for most of the changes in T_4 concentration seen in a variety of diseases, including hypothyroidism and hyperthyroidism. Small quantities of T_4 (0.03%) and T_3 (0.3%) are not protein bound but are free and in rapid equilibrium with the protein-bound fraction ("free T_4" and "free T_3").

The concentrations of free T_4 and T_3 in serum are thought to reflect the bioactive hormones exerting an effect on the tissues. Clinical status in a number of conditions correlates with free T_4 rather than with total hormone in serum. A good example of this correlation is the normal pregnant state in which total T_4 is high but in which there is no clinical or laboratory evidence of free thyroid hormone excess. The elevation is due to increased glycosylation (sialation) and binding capacity of TBG and to estrogen-mediated increase in the protein's concentration in serum.

In some pathologic states that affect the quantity of TBG in serum (Table 80.1), and hence the total T_4, the absolute concentration of free T_4 may not adjust to a normal value. During a variety of nonthyroidal illnesses, undefined factors in serum other than the concentration of TBG and TTR appear to determine the free hormone concentration, presumably by decreasing the affinity of the interaction of binding proteins with T_4 (see below).

Metabolism and Interconversion of Thyroid Hormones

Practically all tissues metabolize and degrade the thyroid hormones, but the liver is quantitatively most important as a site at which regulation of hormone degradation occurs. T_4 metabolism is the major source (80%) of circulating T_3 in the normal individual. The normal thyroid secretes mainly T_4 and only a small amount of T_3 (Fig. 80.1). Only in hyperthyroidism, iodine deficiency, and certain other pathologic circumstances is T_3 sometimes the predominantly secreted hormone.

Approximately 85% of the T_4 secreted is ultimately deiodinated and further degraded. The physiologically most important pathway involves conversion of approximately 35% of the T_4 to metabolically active T_3, which is itself further deiodinated. About an equal amount of T_4 is converted to reverse T_3 (Fig. 80.1). Although not active in promoting calorigenesis or other actions of thyroid hormone, reverse T_3 does antagonize a number of the effects of T_3 and thus may have some physiologic importance. In a variety of pathologic states, the formation of T_3 is inhibited, whereas that of reverse T_3 is reciprocally enhanced. Measurement of reverse T_3 has had some usefulness (e.g., in the differential diagnosis of the "euthyroid sick syndrome"; see "Differential Diagnosis" under "Hypothyroidism", below) but is not used clinically as a routine test.

Table 80.1. Factors Affecting Thyroxine-binding Globulin (TBG)

TBG Increased	TBG Decreased
Estrogens	Androgens
Exogenous	Anabolic steroids
Pregnancy	Cirrhosis
Hypothyroidism	Glucocorticoids
Acute hepatitis	Nephrotic syndrome
Cirrhosis	Severe chronic nonthyroidal illness
Genetic TBG excess	Cushing syndrome
Acute Intermittent porphyria	Genetic TBG deficiency
Perphenazine (Trilafon)	

LABORATORY TESTS OF THYROID FUNCTION AND THYROID DISEASE

All thyroid function tests assess secretory activity of the thyroid gland indirectly. Measurements of serum hormone concentrations, the most commonly used tests, cannot be equated directly with the rates of hormone production, although they reflect those rates when serum binding of hormones is normal. However, various illnesses, drugs, and alterations of physiologic state affect serum binding. Accordingly, proper interpretation of serum hormone concentrations demands concomitant assessment of serum binding. Thyroid gland function can be assessed somewhat more directly by measurement of thyroidal iodide accumulation ("uptake"; radioiodide uptake [RaIU]) using isotopes of iodide (^{131}I, ^{123}I) or other anions that are concentrated by the thyroid. These tests also must be properly interpreted because uptake of tracer amounts of these substances is only an approximation of the accumulation of stable iodide and of hormone synthesis. Methods are available to obtain such data more precisely for research purposes, but they are too cumbersome for ordinary clinical use.

Other useful laboratory tests include measurements of the integrity of the physiologic feedback control system (e.g., serum TSH concentration before and after stimulation by administered TRH) and of various serum immunoglobulins. Some immunoglobulins are associated with destructive autoimmune thyroid disease and others interact with the TSH receptor to stimulate thyroid overactivity in Graves disease or block the action of TSH in at least one type of hypothyroidism (see below).

Thyroid-Stimulating Hormone (Thyrotropin)

The serum TSH is an indicator of the functional state of the hypothalamic–pituitary negative feedback system. An elevated TSH implies that subnormal concentrations of thyroid hormones are present in the circulating blood; a low ("suppressed") TSH implies that excessive amounts of thyroid hormone are being produced and are inhibiting the pituitary's output of TSH. However, these considerations apply only under more or less normal physiologic conditions. In severe illness, TSH levels can be suppressed by circulating cytokines, and in the recovery phase of such illness, TSH may be clearly elevated (see Hypothyroidism Versus the Euthyroid Sick Syndrome, below).

Serum TSH is invariably elevated in primary hypothyroidism because of reduced feedback inhibition by the decreased concentrations of thyroid hormones produced by a failing thyroid gland. The measurement of serum TSH is important both in the diagnosis of primary hypothyroidism and in monitoring the adequacy of thyroid hormone replacement therapy (see below). Elevation of serum TSH is the most sensitive indicator of hypothyroid status, but not every elevated TSH indicates hypothyroidism (see below).

Elevations of TSH were for many years reliably measured by radioimmunoassay, but the available assays were not sufficiently sensitive to measure the *suppression* of TSH that occurs in hyperthyroidism. However, newer immunoradiometric (second generation) and chemiluminescent (third generation) assays are available that quantitate TSH within the normal and subnormal range. As a result, the determination of TSH has become the most commonly used thyroid "function" test. Recent evidence indicates that suppression or even modest elevation of TSH may be seen in or during the recovery phase of a variety of nonthyroidal illnesses, at least in hospitalized patients. Thus, caution should be exercised in interpreting this test (including third-generation assays) in patients who are seriously or chronically ill (see below) (2).

Although measurement of serum TSH is the most sensitive of the thyroid function tests in the detection of thyroid dysfunction, the specificity of the TSH as an indicator for diagnosis and therapy is quite low. The newer assays for TSH are widely and often inappropriately used as single tests for the diagnosis of hypo- or hyperthyroidism. However, the results of TSH assays must be interpreted in the context of the clinical circumstances and along with simultaneous measurements of the circulating thyroid hormones (see Subclinical Hyperthyroidism, Subclinical Hypothyroidism, and Screening for Thyroid Disease in Healthy Patients, below) (3).

Serum Thyroxine and Triiodothyronine

Measurements of the concentration of T_4 ("total T_4") and T_3 in serum, as determined by protein binding (T_4) or radioimmunoassay or other specific methods are commonly used and important tests of thyroid function. However, interpretation of a given value of T_4 must consider whether its binding to serum proteins is normal. Accordingly, T_4 must be measured in conjunction with some separate test that assesses its binding to serum protein carriers, including TBG, the major binding protein for the thyroid hormones. In routine practice this is done by determining the free T_4 or the free T_4 index (FTI; see below). In uncommon situations in which hyperthyroidism is suspected, the free T_3 should also be measured, but it is not a routine test (see below). Normal values of the common tests are given in Table 80.2.

Free T_4 Index, Free T_4, and Free T_3

The free (non–protein-bound) T_4 of serum is reported as a single number but is determined by separate measurements of (a) the percentage of non–protein-bound T_4 (best performed by equilibrium dialysis using a tracer amount of isotopic T_4, added to the serum) and (b) the total T_4. Their arithmetic product equals and is reported as the free T_4 (expressed as ng%, ng/dL, or pmol/L). The dialyzable (non–protein-bound) T_4, which normally approximates only about 0.03% of the total, is not ordinarily reported but is used by the laboratory to calculate the free T_4 in absolute units. Free T_4 can also be measured directly, by a sensitive assay. Equilibrium dialysis, though an expensive technique, is the gold standard for free T_4 determinations. Regrettably, less expensive methods that purport to determine the free T_4 are in wide use but are usually inaccurate.

The free T_4 hypothesis (see above) has been helpful as a physiologic concept. Determination of the free T_4 for clinical purposes is also often useful and sometimes essential. In some clinical states, such as during estrogen therapy, both T_4 and TBG are elevated and thyroid status is accurately reflected by the free T_4: The dialyzable fraction is decreased by the increased TBG, but because the total T_4 is elevated, the free T_4 is normal. In hyperthyroidism, free T_4 reflects thyroid status better than total T_4 because the altered metabolic state of hyperthyroidism itself lowers TBG; in some cases of hyperthyroidism, therefore, a normal or borderline elevation of total T_4 is associated with a clearly elevated free T_4. In hypothyroidism the opposite may be true; TBG is often elevated and the free T_4 is decreased more than is the total T_4. Under any of these circumstances

Table 80.2. Thyroid Function Tests[a]

	Serum T_4 (μg/dL)	Serum T_3 (ng/dL)	T_3 Resin Uptake (T_3U) (%)	T_3 Resin Uptake Ratio (T_3UR)	TSH (μU/mL)	Free T_4 (FT_4) (ng/dL)	Free T_4 Index (FTI)[b]
Normal mean	8	120	30	1		1.5	8.0
Normal range	5–12	80–160	25–35	0.85–1.15	0.3–5	1.0–2.0	5.8–10.6
Confidence limits	±1	±20	±2	±0.05		±0.3	

[a]See the text for limitations of interpretation of normal ranges. Confidence limits (95%) of a single value are approximate and depend on both the laboratory and the level within the range.

[b]The FTI on any sample is calculated as $T_4 \times T_3UR$, but the normal range for the FTI is determined empirically. The units of the FTI depend on whether the percentage T_3 resin uptake or the T_3 resin uptake ratio is multiplied times T_4.

T_4, thyroxine; T_3, triiodothyronine; TSH, thyroid stimulating hormone.

the free T_4 is a more sensitive test of thyroid status than the total T_4.

Problems of interpretation of the free T_4 arise in many seriously ill patients. A variety of nonthyroidal diseases ranging from acute infections to liver disease can result in elevation of the free T_4. In these situations, the patient is usually euthyroid with a normal T_4; the free T_4 is elevated only because the dialyzable fraction is increased. An explanation for this phenomenon is not available. Altered concentrations of neither TBG nor TTR account for the increased free T_4. The appearance of a factor in serum that interferes with protein binding of T_4 has been demonstrated. Thus, an elevated free T_4 is not a specific finding related solely to thyroid status. Moreover, the test is several times more expensive than the free T_4 index, which is preferred as the single most effective screening test of thyroid function (see below).

Free T_3

The T_3 in serum, like T_4, is mainly protein bound, also to TBG, but that fraction that is not bound is termed the free T_3. The measurement is made by equilibrium dialysis (see free T_4, above.) Free T_3 is not a routine test, but cases of very rare "free T_3 toxicosis" can be diagnosed with this test (see below).

Free T_4 Index

This test is a much simpler and less expensive alternative to the free T_4 and in most instances should be done routinely along with the total T_4 so that the latter can be properly interpreted. In most, but not all, cases, FTI closely parallels free T_4. In the laboratory the FTI involves simple measurement of the binding of tracer T_3 (T_3 uptake) to an inert material plus separate measurement of the total T_4 in the sample (see below for technical aspects of the test).

The T_3 uptake is often not reported as a separate test or value (as a percent) but is incorporated into the FTI calculation. T_3 uptake (T_3U) is not to be confused with the concentration of T_3 in serum. The T_3U measurement is not a thyroid function test at all but merely provides an indirect estimate of the concentration of serum TBG. To a smaller extent, T_3U is influenced by the quantity of T_4 in serum (i.e., by the degree of saturation of the T_4 [and T_3] binding sites on TBG). Although direct quantitation of TBG is now available, T_3U is much simpler. Technically, the T_3U is measured by adding a tracer quantity of T_3 and a nonspecific T_3 binding absorbent (resin) to a sample of serum to be tested. The tracer distributes itself between nonspecific binding sites on the resin and specific binding sites on TBG. Resin-bound tracer is inversely related to the quantity of TBG in the serum; the more TBG to bind the T_3, the less available to be bound to resin. The test result is expressed either as a percentage uptake of tracer into the resin or as a ratio of the test sample to that of the laboratory's control serum ("T_3U ratio"). Tracer T_4 has been used as an alternative to T_3; the results are similar, but T_3 is used for technical reasons.

The usefulness of the T_3U is in interpreting a given level of T_4. A high (or low) T_4 can be interpreted as reflecting increased (or decreased) T_4 secretion only if the serum binding of T_4 is normal (i.e., only if the TBG [T_3U] is normal); the FTI value corrects for the level of TBG, providing a more accurate assessment of thyroid function. For convenience, the T_4 and T_3U have been combined to give the FTI by simply multiplying one number times the other. The index is also sometimes confusingly designated the "T_7" or "T_{12}").

In severely ill patients of the type more likely to be hospitalized than to be ambulatory, the FTI may be misleading. In such cases the resin uptake is elevated, not necessarily because TBG is low but as the result of the appearance in serum of a nonspecific inhibitor of hormone binding that affects the distribution of tracer T_3 between sites in serum and sites on the resin. Both the free T_4 and FTI tests must be interpreted with caution in any patient with severe nonthyroidal illness.

Thyrotropin-releasing Hormone (TRH) Test

Parenterally administered TRH produces release of TSH from the pituitary. Response to TRH is abnormal in several clinical circumstances.

The TRH test occasionally is useful in the diagnosis of primary hypothyroidism. In minimal clinical hypothyroidism, the serum T_4 may be within the lower part of the normal range and the TSH may be borderline or only minimally elevated, even after repeated testing. In such cases an exaggerated serum TSH response to TRH is seen. In normal people the increment of TSH after TRH administration does not usually exceed 30 μU/mL, but elevations several times this amount may be seen in cases of borderline hypothyroidism. The test might be useful in cases of "subclinical hypothyroidism" (see below), but no systematic studies have yet been done to test this hypothesis.

For many years, the most common use of the TRH test was in the diagnosis of suspected hyperthyroidism. The advent of sensitive assays for TSH (see above) makes the TRH test usually unnecessary for this purpose. In the absence of severe illness, a suppressed TSH suggests hyperthyroidism. However, if hyperthyroidism is suspected and a second- or preferably third-generation TSH assay is not available or is equivocal, a TRH test can be done. The TRH test is also occasionally useful in the differential diagnosis of severely ill patients with low serum T_4 (see Hypothyroidism Versus the Euthyroid Sick Syndrome, below).

The TRH test has been used to determine the fine adjustment of T_4 replacement therapy, although sensitive second- or third-generation assays for TSH have largely replaced it for this purpose. When the basal TSH was in the normal range, in one study, all patients were within 25 μg of the "optimal" replacement. In 95% of all cases where the basal TSH was below the lower limit of normal, the patients were receiving at least 25 μg more than the "optimal dosage" (4). In elderly patients, suppressed TSH is a common occurrence. The TRH test is confirmatory in showing a blunted TSH response. Some of these individuals are thought to have "mild thyroid overactivity" (5), that is, "free T_3 toxicosis."

The TRH test is performed by injecting 500 μg of TRH intravenously. Serum TSH is measured before injection and at 20 and 30 minutes after injection. There may be a transient urge to urinate. A significant response is an increase in TSH of more than 1 μU/mL. The general practitioner can easily perform the TRH test in the office. (TRH [Thypinone] can be bought through any commercial pharmacy.)

Thyroidal Radioiodide Uptake (RaIU) Tests

These tests were introduced before measurements of serum hormones were available and are now only occasionally needed in ordinary clinical practice. The rate of tracer iodide accumulation (^{131}I, ^{123}I) in the thyroid can be measured by using times ranging from a few minutes to the plateau of accumulation (24 hours). The diagnostic usefulness of the RaIU in the United States is also seriously limited by the high iodide content of the diet from the iodization of table salt. This has resulted in RaIU values that are usually too low to discriminate normal function from hypofunction, so the test is now useless for the diagnosis of hypothyroidism. It is still of occasional diagnostic usefulness in hyperthyroidism, but because results are normal in up to 50% of cases of proven hyperthyroidism, a normal RaIU does not exclude the diagnosis. One important use of the test is in patients with hyperthyroidism associated with thyroiditis (see below). If this condition is suspected, an RaIU is important; a low value helps deter inappropriate therapy. Determination of the RaIU is sometimes used in the selection of dosage in RaI therapy. The RaIU is subject to interference by various chemical agents, especially iodide-containing drugs and the radiographic media used in pyelograms, cholecystograms, and in computed tomography (CT) contrast imaging.

Immunologic Tests

Assay of antibodies to thyroidal constituents (thyroglobulin, microsomes), so-called thyroid autoantibodies, is useful in determining the presence of autoimmune thyroiditis, in the differential diagnosis of goiter, and in predicting the significance of elevations of TSH (see Hypothyroidism and Goiter and Iodide Deficiency, below). The term *microsomal antibodies* is synonymous with thyroid peroxidase antibodies. Assays for thyroid-stimulating immunoglobulin (TSI) (see Graves Disease, below) are becoming readily available. TSI measurements are useful in the pregnant hyperthyroid patient because high levels are associated with an increased likelihood of neonatal hyperthyroidism due to placental transfer of the stimulator. The original test for TSI, a bioassay called the long-acting thyroid stimulator test, still performed in some laboratories, is not useful.

Other Tests: Fine-Needle Aspiration, Needle Biopsies, and Imaging

Fine-needle aspiration (FNA) for cytologic examination or biopsy of the thyroid is now routine in most centers. Although the procedure often failed to distinguish benign adenomas from well-differentiated follicular carcinomas, it appears that new immunologic methods will eliminate this deficiency (6). *FNA* (by use of a 25-gauge needle) with cytologic examination is simple, virtually painless, and without complications (see Thyroid Nodules, below). The procedure is ordinarily performed by an endocrinologist or a pathologist. A few centers use *needle biopsy* (aspiration or cutting), usually performed only if the simpler FNA is not sufficiently informative. In the hands of an appropriate operator, needle biopsy is probably more definitive and, because it is performed with local (cutaneous) anesthesia, is ordinarily painless. The only significant complication is local hemorrhage, but this is an uncommon, usually minor, problem. Ultrasound is often used to guide FNA and may lead to additional information, especially when cystic lesions are present.

Various *imaging techniques* are available to delineate the anatomy of the thyroid and to distinguish functional from nonfunctional nodules, a consideration in the differential diagnosis of thyroid neoplasms. The two commonly used techniques are radioisotopic scanning (scintiscan) and ultrasonography. CT and magnetic resonance imaging are not useful for evaluating nodules, although they have a place in evaluating substernal extension of goiter and in localizing metastatic lesions, as does F-18-fluorodeoxyglucose positron emission scanning (see Thyroid Carcinomas, Postoperative Therapy and Its Monitoring, below). The isotope most widely used in scintiscanning is ^{99m}Tc pertechnetate (TcO_4^-), but ^{123}I is the isotope of choice. (Rarely, tumors that would not take up ^{123}I do accumulate pertechnetate, thereby giving misleading information on the functional state of a nodule and obscuring the diagnosis.) Ultrasonography, now often the initial imaging procedure, is the best technique for determining the size of the thyroid; the number, size, and characteristics of nodules; and whether a nodule is cystic or solid, an important point in differential diagnosis of these lesions. Ultrasonography also provides an objective basis for evaluation of changes in the size of nodules with medical therapy. Both isotopic imaging and ultrasonography can determine whether a nodule is truly single or is in fact one of many in a multinodular gland.

Nonspecificity of Thyroid Function Tests in Nonthyroidal Illness

Thyroid function tests are frequently nonspecifically altered in many nonthyroidal diseases and by drugs and hormones (7–10); that is, these tests are not specific for thyroid disease when severe illness is present (Table 80.3). Moreover, a variety of drugs and hormones affects both thyroid function and the function tests (Tables 80.1 and 80.4). T_4, free T_4, FTI, T_3, and TSH can all be affected. Although much of the information on this subject comes from studies of hospitalized patients, in whom up to 30% will show one or more abnormalities on admission, ambulatory patients are probably also affected. Some examples are presented below.

Table 80.3. Nonthyroidal Illness: Effects on T_4, Free T_4, TBG, and TSH in Plasma[a,b]

	T_4	Free T_4	TBG	TSH
Liver disease				
Active hepatitis	↑	↔↑	↑	
Cirrhosis, other chronic diseases	↑↓	↔↑	↑↓	↔↑
Cholangitis	↑	↔↑	↑	
Renal disease				
Nephrotic syndrome	↔↓	↔	↔↓	
Uremia, chronic	↔↓	↔↓	↔↓	
Infections	↓	↑	↔	
Malnutrition	↔↓	↔↑	↔↓	
Severe acute illness[c]	↑↓	↔↑	↔	↑↓

[a]Most illnesses and even such minor alterations of physiologic state as decreased food intake will produce a decrease of plasma T_3.

[b]Changes of TSH not likely in ambulatory patients.

[c]Not likely to be seen in ambulatory patients.

T_4, thyroid hormone thyroxine; TBG, thyroxine-binding globulin; TSH, thyroid stimulating hormone.

Table 80.4. Drug and Hormone Effects on T_4, Free T_4, TBG, and TSH

Gonadal Hormones	T_4	Free T_4	TBG	TSH
Estrogens	↑	↔↓	↑	
Exogenous				
Pregnancy				↓
Androgens	↓	↔		
Testosterone		↑		
Anabolic steroids				
Glucocorticoids	↓	↔	↓	
Cushing syndrome				
Pharmacologic uses				
Psychotropic Drugs				
Perphenazine (Trilafon)	↑	↔	↑	
Amphetamines	↑	↑	↔	
Anticonvulsants				
Phenytoin (Dilantin)	↓	↔↓	↔	↔↑
Carbamezapine	↓	↔↓	↔	↔↑
Heparin	↔	↑	↔	
Adrenergic blockers				
Propranolol (Inderal)	↔ (↓T_3)	↔	↔	
Antiarrhythmic drugs				
Amiodarone	↑	↑	↔	
Gallbladder dyes				
Iopanoic acid	↑↔ (↓T_3)	↔↑	↔↑	↔↑
Ipodate	↑↔ (↓T_3)	↔↑	↔	↔↑
Opiates	↑		↑	
Miscellaneous				
Clofibrate	↑		↑	
5-Fluorouracil	↑		↑	

T_4, thyroxine; TBG, thyroxine-binding globulin; TSH, thyroid stimulating hormone.

Effects of Gonadal and Adrenal Hormones on Thyroid Function Tests

Estrogens (pregnancy, contraceptives) raise and androgens lower T_4, but not free T_4 or FTI, by altering serum TBG. Glucocorticoids inhibit thyroid activity acutely by interfering with TSH secretion, lowering TSH levels, and affecting the pituitary's responsiveness to TRH. The serum T_4 is lowered during chronic glucocorticoid therapy, mainly because of a decrease of TBG.

Liver Disease

Various alterations of thyroid function tests are produced by liver disease. Early in infectious hepatitis, the T_4 level is elevated secondary to an increase of TBG. Chronic liver disease produces many abnormalities in an unpredictable fashion. T_4 may be increased or decreased in parallel with TBG and the T_3U. Free T_4 is often elevated with no obvious relationship to the TBG. T_3 is usually low. A frequent and unexplained abnormality is elevation of TSH, although the response to TRH is not exaggerated as it is in hypothyroidism. RaIU is often elevated in acute alcoholic hepatitis with or without cirrhosis and in some cases of cholangitis. These changes have been attributed to both iodide depletion and acceleration of T_4 metabolism.

Renal Disease

The nephrotic syndrome is often associated with depressed T_4 and TBG, but the decrease of the T_4 is not always explained by a lowering of the TBG. In chronic renal disease, the average T_4, TBG, and the FTI are not significantly different from normal, but the range is greater and values may exceed the usual normal limits. Some patients with severe chronic renal failure receiving long-term dialysis show a progressive decrease of T_4; the mechanism is not known but the prognosis for survival in such patients is poor (see Hypothyroidism Versus the Euthyroid Sick Syndrome, below). As expected in any chronic illness, the serum T_3 is often depressed.

Infections, Malnutrition, and Drugs

The T_4 may drop early in the course of acute infection and free T_4 may rise. Neither change is accounted for by an alteration of TBG. During starvation or severe caloric restriction, serum T_3 falls. Free T_4 is often increased without relation to the TBG. Serum T_3 is often decreased in the elderly, a change that has been attributed to aging but may in large part be caused by diminished food intake and nonspecific illness (11). Closely correlated alterations of T_3U and serum TBG have been reported in protein-calorie malnutrition. Some pharmacologic agents affect the thyroid hormone levels (Table 80.4). Phenytoin (Dilantin) and carbamezapine lower T_4 and free T_4 into the hypothyroid range, but the TSH is normal. The apparently low free T_4 is an artifact of routine methodology and is an excellent example of how misleading this test can be in some circumstances (12). Heparin acutely elevates the free T_4; the mechanism of this change is unknown. Beta-adrenergic blockers decrease serum T_3 by inhibition of the normal T_4 deiodination route; reverse T_3 is increased. A similar decrease of T_3 through reduced hepatic metabolism of T_4 is produced by propylthiouracil, dexamethasone, amiodarone, and the radiopaque contrast media used for visualization of the gallbladder. In the case of the latter agents, additional mechanisms are operative because these compounds may also elevate T_4 and TSH, an effect attributed to their differential inhibition of conversion of T_4 and T_3 in the pituitary and the periphery. Amphetamine abuse may increase serum T_4, presumably by central stimulation of TSH release (7).

Altered Serum Thyroxine Caused by Inherited and Other Abnormalities of Protein Binding

In addition to those diseases or drugs that alter T_4 levels by affecting binding of the hormone to TBG, altered protein binding also occurs in inherited disorders of TBG excess, TBG deficiency, increased concentration of thyroxine-binding prealbumin, and increases in the number of T_4 binding sites on an albumin variant (familial dysalbuminemic hyperthyroxinemia). The first two conditions are X-linked. The latter two conditions, inherited as autosomal dominants, are rare. All these conditions can produce diagnostic difficulties, however, because they are not detected by the T_3 resin uptake, and the free T_4 index is accordingly elevated, although the free T_4 is normal (7), if measured by equilibrium dialysis. If a nonequilibrium dialysis method of measurement of free T_4 is used, the value may be spuriously elevated.

Alterations of Serum Thyroxine in Nonthyroidal Illness Not Caused by Abnormalities of Protein Binding

Elevations of T_4 that are unexplained by changes in thyroxine binding are common. These situations are difficult to distinguish from hyperthyroidism. Included are the elevation of T_4 seen in acute nonthyroidal illness, in psychiatric disease, and as the effect of some drugs. The stress of serious illness may also lower T_4 and simulate hypothyroidism (see Hypothyroidism Versus the Euthyroid Sick Syndrome, below), but such severe illness is rarely encountered in ambulatory patients. An exception may be seen in patients receiving dialysis for chronic renal failure. Abnormal thyroid hormone levels in these situations and diseases that are regularly associated with such changes (7–9) are described briefly below.

Increase of Serum Thyroxine During Nonspecific Illness: Euthyroid Hyperthyroxinemia. Although the phenomenon of decreased serum T_4 during severe illness is now widely recognized (see above), the frequent occurrence of *increased* T_4 (and FTI) caused by illness is not generally appreciated. The increase of T_4 is modest, and the T_4 generally does not exceed about 15 μg. This problem is, however, commonly seen in severely ill elderly patients in whom it raises the issue of hyperthyroidism (11). Similar findings have been reported in hyperemesis gravidarum.

Acute Psychiatric Illness. Restlessness, hyperactivity, tachycardia, and tremor are often seen as part of severe *acute* psychiatric illness. Clinical suspicion of hyperthyroidism (because of tachycardia, tremor, sweating) leads to thyroid function tests and laboratory results consistent with this diagnosis. Such patients may have elevated T_4, FTI, and T_3. The TSH may not be suppressed (13). In some series, up to one-third of acutely hospitalized psychiatric patients have an elevated T_4. Although the phenomenon is documented only in hospitalized patients, it may be encountered in any severely disturbed person. The T_4 returns to normal within 1 to 2 weeks of clinical improvement of the psychiatric disturbance. This phenomenon may represent a form of centrally driven hyperthyroidism (13).

Increased Serum Thyroxine Caused by Resistance to Thyroid Hormones. Rare but well-recognized cases of increased T_4 unaccompanied by binding protein abnormalities are seen with peripheral resistance to thyroid hormones. Originally described as a familial syndrome of increased T_4, goiter, deaf mutism, and some degree of hypothyroidism with delayed bone maturation and epiphyseal stippling, the most common situation is actually that of elevated T_4 in a phenotypically normal person without evidence of hyperthyroidism. The abnormality occurs both sporadically and in familial form and is probably part of a heterogeneous group of disorders with variable inheritance (14). Most cases are due to abnormal (mutant) thyroid hormone receptors.

Statistical Considerations in the Clinical Interpretation of Thyroid Function Tests

No single numerical value divides normal from abnormal in any thyroid function test. The upper and lower limits of normal for serum T_4, FTI, and T_3 are arbitrarily set as they are for most tests at ± 2 standard deviations from the mean. By definition, therefore, 2.5% of an apparently normal population will have abnormal values at each end of the distribution. To complicate the issue, a small number of hyperthyroid or hypothyroid patients have values that fall clearly within the normal range. In addition to the statistical overlap, both biologic (i.e., day to day) variation and unavoidable analytical error further obscure the dividing line between normal and abnormal. For example, 95% confidence limits for the analytic variation of a single T_4 test are ± 1 μg/dL at the upper and lower limits of the normal range. For all these reasons and because of the occasional instance of laboratory or reporting error, a single determination should not be relied on to establish or exclude a diagnosis with anything more than reasonable statistical certainty. Therefore, all abnormal values should be confirmed before therapy is undertaken, and borderline values should be repeated several times before diagnostic conclusions are drawn.

Premature institution of therapy may obscure the diagnosis.

HYPERTHYROIDISM AND THYROTOXICOSIS

Thyrotoxicosis is defined as any condition in which the cells of the body are exposed to excess amounts of circulating thyroid hormone. *Hyperthyroidism* is any condition in which thyrotoxicosis is attributable to hyperfunction of the thyroid gland. Often the terms are used interchangeably, although they do not mean precisely the same thing.

Essentially, the same presentation may result from any of several different pathologic processes (Table 80.5), and selection of proper therapy demands that the correct underlying diagnosis is established. The most common cause of hyperthyroidism is *Graves disease*, an autoimmune process also known as *diffuse toxic goiter*. Only slightly less common is hyperthyroidism caused by a hyperfunctioning multinodular goiter (toxic nodular goiter). Occasionally, hyperthyroidism is caused by a *solitary hyperfunctioning adenoma* ("hot nodule"). Thyrotoxicosis also has been seen with increasing frequency as a transient phenomenon in the evolution of *thyroiditis* (15,16). In addition, the induction of thyrotoxicosis by iodide and iodide-containing drugs (e.g., amiodarone) and contrast media should be considered for those patients who have had such exposures (17). The other causes of hyperthyroidism listed in Table 80.5 are rare and are not usually encountered in ordinary practice.

Table 80.5. Causes of Thyrotoxicosis[a]

Common
Graves disease
Toxic nodular goiter
Multinodular
Uninodular
Thyrotoxicosis in association with thyroiditis
Postpartum thyrotoxicosis
Iodide induced (iodide, iodine-containing drugs, and contrast media)
Rare to vanishingly rare
Thyrotoxicosis caused by TSH or TSH-like stimulator
Choriocarcinoma or hydatidiform mole
Embryonal cell carcinoma of testis
Pituitary tumor with TSH excess
Idiopathic TSH excess
Toxic thyroid carcinoma
Thyrotoxicosis caused by exogenous thyroid hormone
Factitia
Medicamentosa (iatrogenic)
Toxic struma ovarii

[a]Listed in approximate decreasing order of frequency.
TSH, thyroid stimulating hormone.

Graves Disease

Graves disease is a complex disorder comprising toxic goiter, ophthalmopathy, and occasionally dermopathy. At any given time during the course of the disease, one of these manifestations may be an isolated finding. Graves ophthalmopathy and Graves dermopathy can occur independently of thyroid hormone excess. It is generally accepted that ophthalmopathy and dermopathy are closely related but separate and overlapping immunologic disorders.

Various abnormal immunoglobulins are found in the serum of patients with Graves disease. Some of these immunoglobulins have TSH-like activity and are designated TSIs; they are antibodies to the normal receptor sites for TSH. The reasons for development of abnormal immunoglobulins in Graves disease are not clearly understood. Recent thinking views Graves disease as a failure of T-cell surveillance rather than as a response to thyroid antigens released from a thyroid damaged by unknown causes.

Clinical Presentation and Diagnosis of Thyrotoxicosis

Clinical History

The presentation of patients with thyrotoxicosis is highly variable (Table 80.6). The severity of the thyrotoxic aspect is determined not only by the degree of hormone excess but also by its rapidity of onset, its duration, and the age of the patient. The "typical" thyrotoxic patient has one or more of the following spontaneous complaints: nervousness, weight loss, palpitations (which at first may be intermittent), enlarging neck mass (goiter), change in appearance of eyes (Graves disease), or symptoms of heart failure. These symptoms usually have been present anywhere from a few weeks to up to a year or longer. Careful questioning often reveals other symptoms (below).

Table 80.6. Signs and Symptoms of Thyrotoxicosis

Organ or System	Signs and Symptoms
Adrenergic manifestations	Excess sweating, heat intolerance, palpitations, tachycardia, tremor, lid lag, stare, nervousness, and excitability
Hypermetabolism and catabolism	Increased appetite, weight loss
One system predominance	
Eyes[a]	Periorbital edema, exophthalmos (proptosis), chemosis, ophthalmoplegia, papilledema
Cardiac	Arrhythmia, congestive heart failure
Muscle	Fatigue and weakness, muscle wasting, proximal myopathy, periodic paralysis
Gastrointestinal	Increased frequency of bowel movements, pernicious vomiting
Bone	Acropachy, osteoporosis, hypercalcemia
Reproductive	Infertility, abortion, scanty menses, testicular atrophy, gynecomastia
Mental	Anxiety, irritability, psychosis, insomnia
Skin	Onycholysis, "pretibial" myxedema, hyperpigmentation

[a]Graves disease only.

The so-called nervousness in thyrotoxicosis is often irritability, inability to concentrate, restlessness, or overt emotional lability, but it is a tremor of the hands that most often leads the patient to express this complaint. Impairment of normal sleep pattern with frequent wakening is common. Some patients with *anxiety* may experience tachycardia, tremor, irritability, and weakness simulating thyrotoxicosis. The "anxiety" of thyrotoxicosis is more likely to appear as irritability and hyperkinesis than as an expressed feeling of being anxious. Primary anxiety disorders are either related to identifiable stresses, coexist with symptoms of depression, or have distinctive characteristics that make them recognizable (see Chapter 22). In depression, weight loss is invariably accompanied by anorexia, a relatively unusual symptom of thyrotoxicosis (see above).

Weight loss classically occurs in the face of increased appetite, although often no obvious change in appetite is noticed or there may actually be anorexia, especially in elderly patients. The only prominent gastrointestinal symptom is increased frequency of bowel movements, but actual diarrhea is not seen.

The *heat intolerance* of hyperthyroidism is often apparent only on questioning. Commonly the patient admits to having reduced the number of covers used on the bed at night or to the development of new and unusual habits, such as sleeping in the nude or with feet extended from under the blankets. Sweating is increased but is not usually a spontaneous complaint and may be denied.

As the disease progresses in severity, *skeletal muscle wasting* occurs, which tends to involve especially the limb girdle musculature, producing a proximal myopathy. This process results in weakness, expressed, for example, as great difficulty in climbing stairs or, on examination, in arising from a squatting position. Exertional dyspnea without evidence of cardiac failure is common and may be related to the myopathy.

Skin changes are hardly ever noticed by the patient, and "silky skin" or hair (a "classic" symptom) is only occasionally seen on examination. Hair loss is common, usually noticed as thinning of the scalp hair by women. Other skin changes include occasional cases in light skinned people of diffuse hyperpigmentation with darkening noted mostly over extensor surfaces of elbows, knees, and small joints. In African American patients, darkening of the skin is common, but its occurrence is discovered only by questioning.

Physical Findings

The thyroid is visibly or palpably enlarged in almost all young patients with hyperthyroidism, but in the elderly, the thyroid may not be enlarged. Asymmetric enlargement is common, especially in patients with toxic nodular goiter. Extreme vascularity of the gland in Graves disease may result in palpable or audible blood flow; a bruit is usually heard over the enlarged lobes but occasionally best heard more rostrally over the superior thyroidal arteries. A bruit over the thyroid of a hyperthyroid patient is usually diagnostic of Graves disease; this finding is not present in patients with toxic nodular goiter.

Cardiovascular findings include sinus tachycardia, systolic flow murmurs, wide pulse pressure commonly, and atrial fibrillation occasionally. It is a common belief that most patients with hyperthyroidism at least have a tachycardia, but in fact only 50% of patients, regardless of age, have an increased heart rate. The apex impulse is often prominent and forceful. Cardiac failure may develop in severe cases of long duration, especially in the elderly.

The *eye findings* can be separated into those that occur as a result of thyroid hormone excess and those that are part of the ophthalmopathy of Graves disease (18). Excessive thyroid hormone enhances sympathetic tone and the innervation of the eyelids is partially under sympathetic control. Lid retraction with increased scleral visibility above and below the iris (prominent "whites" of the eyes), along with infrequent blinking, leads to the striking "stare" so commonly seen. Failure of the lid to follow movements of the globe ("lid lag") is another manifestation of the same process. When Graves ophthalmopathy is present, there is forward protrusion of the globe. This process may be unilateral at first and is often asymmetric. The protrusion represents true proptosis and contributes an additional component to the stare produced by increased sympathetic tone. Extraocular muscle weakness may occur and results in limitation of ability to converge and to perform extreme movements of gaze; strabismus and diplopia are its more severe manifestations. The most serious complications of Graves ophthalmopathy are infiltrative disease and optic neuritis (see below).

Dermopathy, a unique, albeit unusual, finding in Graves disease, consists of more or less circumscribed areas of mucopolysaccharide deposition, typically over the shins—hence the term *pretibial myxedema*. This unfortunate designation unjustifiably suggests a relationship between the very different type of generalized mucopolysaccharide deposition in severe hypothyroidism (myxedema) and the localized deposition in Graves disease. No relationship exists between these processes. The lesions usually have sharp raised margins and may have an orange peel-like appearance. The affected area is often intensely pruritic.

Clubbing of the fingers and toes is rare (thyroid acropachy) and is distinguishable radiographically from that seen in pulmonary disease. A common sign is separation of the distal portion of one or more fingernails from their nail bed (onycholysis; "dirty fingernail" sign). A fine rapid tremor, usually of the hands, is a common physical finding (see Chapter 90).

In some patients, particularly elderly ones, the clinical picture may not suggest thyrotoxicosis. Such patients may have only unexplained weight loss or weakness. Occult neoplasm may first be suspected, and the diagnosis of hyperthyroidism may be missed entirely or considered only after extensive evaluation fails to yield a diagnosis. These are the patients with severe but not clinically obvious disease, termed in the past *apathetic hyperthyroidism.* The term was used to describe patients who did not have obvious activation of the sympathetic nervous system (e.g., tachycardia, lid retraction, tremor, etc.). Apathetic hyperthyroidism is only rarely encountered today probably because of increased awareness on the part of clinicians and because of modern diagnostic techniques that have led to earlier diagnosis of hyperthyroidism.

Congestive heart failure, atrial fibrillation, or new-onset or worsening *angina pectoris* may be the presenting manifestation of thyrotoxicosis. The notion that such patients are refractory to conventional doses of drugs for cardiac failure or to digitalis for control of ventricular rate in atrial fibrillation is incorrect most of the time.

Laboratory Diagnosis

Recognition of Graves disease in a typical case is not difficult, but because of its frequently insidious onset, an absence of eye findings, or of an overtly enlarged thyroid or because of involvement of one or relatively few organ systems, the diagnosis may be missed for months or years.

When prominent symptoms are present, the usual thyroid function tests substantiate the diagnosis in almost all cases: An increase in serum T_4 and FTI and a suppressed TSH. If these results are borderline or normal, the serum T_3 must be measured, because hyperthyroidism may be due to elevation of T_3 alone. However, so-called T_3 toxicosis (see below) occurs in less than 5% of all cases.

Perhaps the rarest and most difficult case to diagnose is the patient whose TSH is suppressed and who otherwise has normal blood tests, including the serum T_3. This finding is not specifically diagnostic of hyperthyroidism but should alert the clinician to the possibility of that diagnosis.

Occasionally, all tests of thyroid hormone levels are borderline. Sometimes, this is because the patient is seen relatively early in the evolution of hyperthyroidism. If the clinical suspicion of thyrotoxicosis is strong, serial determinations of T_4, T_3, and TSH should be done over weeks or months. It is sometimes reasonable to treat the symptoms with a beta-adrenergic antagonist (see below) while following the laboratory measurements, which may become diagnostic only after months. Antithyroid drugs should be avoided in this situation.

Hyperthyroidism Caused by Thyroid-stimulating Hormone Hypersecretion

A rare form of hyperthyroidism is due to excessive production of TSH by the pituitary (see Chapter 81).

Factitious Hyperthyroidism

When clinical hyperthyroidism is found in a patient without goiter or true exophthalmos (proptosis), suspicion of *factitious hyperthyroidism* may be warranted. As in true hyperthyroidism, the TSH will be suppressed and the T_4 will be elevated. However, the RaIU test will be very low, and the thyroid will be normal-sized on sonogram. Such findings suggest either the presence of thyroiditis with hyperthyroidism (see below) or ingestion of thyroid hormone. Some years ago, an epidemic of hyperthyroidism occurred in the United States when a change in a meat processing method resulted in the mass ingestion of cattle thyroid glands, inadvertently included in lean ground beef.

Therapy

Hyperthyroidism caused by Graves disease may be a self-limited process that terminates within a year or two in perhaps one-third of patients. In a few of these individuals, the disease recurs decades later. This natural history strongly influences selection of therapy. Other therapeutic considerations relate to the age of the patient and the presence or absence of complications of the hyperthyroidism, its severity, and the presence of comorbid conditions.

Because there is currently no means of controlling the underlying cause of the disease, presumed to be TSI production, therapy is designed to interfere with thyroid hormone synthesis by drugs or by ablation of thyroid tissue by radioiodide or surgery. Opinions differ on approaches, but the views expressed here closely approximate those of conservative medical opinion in the United States. Each form of therapy has advantages and disadvantages. None provides a simple definitive solution and none is truly curative, although the process is certainly treatable in all cases. The objective of therapy is to ensure minimal morbidity from both the therapy and the disease. The therapy of hyperthyroidism attributable to causes other than Graves disease is discussed separately. It is clear that any of the three forms of therapy described below when properly exercised results in a satisfactory outcome as shown in a prospective randomized trial (19).

Antithyroid Drugs

Antithyroid drugs predictably control excessive production of thyroid hormone in essentially all cases, although in only about 20% to 40% will a permanent remission of the hyperthyroidism be seen upon drug withdrawal. Males are much less likely to achieve remission (20%) than females (40%), and younger patients (less than age 40) are less likely (33%) than older patients (48%) (20). Relapses may occur within 6 months to a year or longer after apparent remission, but late relapses are uncommon except in postpartum patients. It is not generally appreciated that about half of the patients who have a permanent remission will become hypothyroid at between 15 and 20 years after successful treatment.

Restoration of the clinically euthyroid state with only antithyroid drug administration requires at least 4 to 8 weeks, although clinical improvement is usually seen within a week or two. Adjunctive therapy can be used concomitantly to afford more rapid symptomatic relief while the antithyroid drug is restoring a euthyroid state (see below). Antithyroid drugs are ordinarily the preferred initial treatment for children, some young adults without complications or other medical problems, and pregnant patients. The antithyroid drugs are also routinely used as preliminary therapy in patients who are to be treated by surgery (see below). The objective in these cases is to ensure euthyroid status at the time of operation. Patients who are to be treated with radioiodide (see below) are also commonly treated with an antithyroid drug before and/or after ablation. Radioiodide in less than thyroid-ablating doses is slow in producing its effect and may have to be given repeatedly; use of an antithyroid drug before or after such therapy is therefore a temporary, but useful, adjunct.

In the United States, only two thiocarbamide (thionamide) drugs are available: Propylthiouracil and methimazole (Tapazole). Other equally effective thiocarbamides are used in other countries. Methimazole may have an advantage when speed in restoration of euthyroid status is an urgent consideration. *Propylthiouracil*, unlike methimazole, in addition to its effects in inhibiting thyroid hormone synthesis, also inhibits conversion of T_4 to T_3 in peripheral tissues. On the other hand, *methimazole* is longer acting than propylthiouracil and may be given on a less frequent dosage schedule, thus facilitating compliance. In most adults with hyperthyroidism, 100 to 150 mg of propylthiouracil (available in 50-mg tablets) every 8 hours or 15 to 30 mg of methimazole (available in 5- and 10-mg tablets) every 24 hours usually suffices as initial therapy, whereas maintenance is often possible with 50 to 100 mg of propylthiouracil twice daily or 5 to 10 mg of methimazole once a day. The T_4 level (not the TSH) should be measured after about 2 weeks of treatment, at 1 month and every 2 to 3 months thereafter. If at these relatively low maintenance dosages of antithyroid drug the serum T_4 falls below normal, efforts to titrate the dosage downward are often tedious and unsuccessful and should be avoided. A euthyroid state can be achieved under these circumstances by the addition of oral T_4, usually at somewhat less than full replacement dose.

A simple treatment program that requires minimal follow-up is to initiate treatment with methimazole alone and, when the T_4 has become normal, to institute maintenance with a single daily dose of 40 to 60 mg of methimazole (an amount that completely halts thyroid hormone formation in almost all patients) *plus* 0.10 mg of thyroxine, full replacement for 80% of individuals. Small upward or downward adjustment of T_4 dosage can subsequently be made as needed. This type of combined therapy was long advocated by some for both convenience and simplicity and a belief that lasting remission was more likely with this program than with antithyroid drugs alone (21). There is, to date, no convincing evidence that the latter notion is valid. Moreover, it should be recalled that antithyroid drug therapy never induces permanent remission in patients with toxic nodular goiter (see below), which is the diagnosis in about half the thyrotoxic patients over age 55 years.

Although the recommended dosages of antithyroid drugs control the disease in most cases, some individuals may need higher dosages. Severely ill patients should be given larger doses from the beginning. The risk of an adverse drug effect (see below) may be increased, but this is not established and should not be a consideration under such circumstances. To achieve total blockade of hormone synthesis, as much as 200 mg of propylthiouracil every 4 hours may be necessary. Because methimazole has a longer duration of action, it need not be given so often, but 30 to 40 mg three times daily may be needed in rare cases.

Duration of Therapy

Therapy should continue for 12 to 24 months before discontinuation of the drug is considered, although conflicting clinical evidence suggests that lasting remission may not be related to duration of therapy beyond the point at which the patient becomes euthyroid. Patients who have continued to require large doses of drugs are almost certain not to have achieved remission. On the other hand, reduction of thyroid size during therapy is thought by some clinicians to be predictive of lasting clinical remission. If on clinical grounds, or as a result of testing, continued disease activity seems to be present, permanent discontinuation of antithyroid drug therapy without RaIU (or surgical) therapy is inadvisable and almost certainly will result in clinical relapse and needless morbidity. Measurement of titers of TSI may be useful in predicting that remission has occurred, but such measurements are not widely available and also are not highly accurate predictors.

If it appears that remission may have been reached, antithyroid drug therapy is stopped and the patient is observed. Routine determination of serum T_4 every 3 to 4 weeks for 3 to 6 months allows early recognition of the return of thyroid overactivity. If the situation is ambiguous and especially if there is evidence of continued disease activity, the antithyroid drug dosage may be reduced to one half the maintenance level for 3 to 6 months in the expectation that if recurrence occurs, it will still be detectable but blunted. Prophylactic use of a beta-adrenergic blocking drug (see below) during withdrawal of antithyroid drugs is a useful maneuver that prevents emergence of symptoms of overt hyperthyroidism if relapse occurs.

If the hyperthyroid state recurs, treatment with an antithyroid drug may be reinitiated for another year or other therapy may be undertaken (^{131}I or surgery). A second course of antithyroid drug has a significant chance of inducing remission. In selected patients, prolonged or even indefinite drug therapy is reasonable, but with most patients such an approach is undesirable.

Minor side effects of drug therapy occur in 1% to 5% of patients. Skin rashes, the most common side effect, are usually seen in the first months of therapy and often disappear even if therapy is continued. Antihistamine drugs are useful in controlling these rashes and the associated urticaria and pruritus that sometimes occur. Neutropenia is not uncommon but is usually not severe and is dose related. If the absolute number of polymorphonuclear neutrophils falls below 2,000, the dosage should be reduced, but the drug need not be immediately discontinued. The white blood cell count should be monitored after several weeks of therapy and after increases of drug dosage. If the side effects are not tolerated, a switch to the other thiocarbamide allows continuation of therapy in about half of the cases. Major complications of drug therapy occur in less than 0.1% of cases. *Agranulocytosis* is the most dreaded complication. Unlike neutropenia, thiocarbamide-induced agranulocytosis from antileukocyte antibodies is not dose related and is of such sudden onset that routine blood counts are of no help in prevention. However, the patient should be instructed to contact the physician promptly if severe sore mouth or sore throat and fever occur. Immediate hospitalization is probably indicated. Most patients with agranulocytosis eventually recover, albeit after a stormy course. Other toxic reactions include drug fever, arthralgias, and hepatitis. *Elevations of aminotransferase activity* are commonly seen in patients receiving propylthiouracil. If other liver enzymes are normal, the drug may be continued, but persistent laboratory evidence of hepatocellular damage indicates a need to discontinue therapy. Aminotransferase activity should be measured every 3 to 6 months. Methimazole is rarely a cause of cholestatic jaundice in patients taking the drug; hepatic enzymes (including serum alkaline phosphatase) should be measured at baseline and, as indicated, thereafter. (However, thyrotoxic patients often have elevations of serum hepatic enzyme activity at onset of their disease, particularly alkaline phosphatase activity.)

Adjunctive Drug Therapy

Iodide (Nonradioactive). Nonradioactive (stable) iodide (I^{127}) for the treatment of hyperthyroidism should be reserved for patients with severe illness or for patients with significant comorbidity. Occasionally, iodide therapy produces severe dermatitis. Use of iodide may preclude for many weeks the use of radioactive iodide, the uptake of which by the thyroid will be greatly diminished.

However, iodide is the best agent available for inhibiting hormone release and is useful in patients who need rapid correction of the hyperthyroid state. Iodide also has a time-honored place in preoperative preparation (see Chapter 93) for thyroidectomy to reduce vascularity of the gland. When given for several weeks after radioiodide therapy, iodide seems especially effective in accelerating restoration of euthyroid status. When given in this setting, some endocrinologists advocate initiating antithyroid drug therapy for at least 2 days before starting iodide therapy and continuing combined therapy for 2 months.

The standard dosage of iodide is one drop of a saturated solution of potassium iodide (40 mg) diluted in several ounces of water or juice once daily; higher dosages are often given but are unnecessary because a dose of only 5 mg produces a maximal effect. Lugol solution is an obsolete pharmacologic concoction, containing iodine and iodide, and has no virtue over iodide alone.

Adrenergic Antagonists. Many symptoms and signs of thyrotoxicosis are related to sensitization of the sympathetic nervous system and are in large measure abolished by beta-adrenergic blocking drugs. The indications for use of a beta-blocker in hyperthyroidism are severe tachycardia, tremor, sweating, and agitation. Although beta-blockers are effective for relief of these manifestations of hyperthyroidism, they do not appreciably affect excessive metabolic rate or reverse the catabolic state of severe cases. Beta-1-selective agents (e.g., atenolol, nadolol, metoprolol) are probably preferable to avoid unwanted side effects in susceptible individuals (e.g., asthmatics). Other uses for beta-blockers are in the prevention of symptoms during a trial of withdrawal of an antithyroid drug when blood hormone levels can be used to assess the progress of therapy and while awaiting the effects of ^{131}I therapy. Most patients require a beta-blocker in a dose equivalent to atenolol, 100 mg a day. The drug should be discontinued as soon as the patient is rendered euthyroid (T_4 normal).

Iopanoic Acid Therapy

This drug, an oral cholecystogram contrast agent, is a potent inhibitor of the conversion of T_4 to T_3. Some experts believe it is a useful clinical adjunct for the rapid correction of hyperthyroidism (see Thyrotoxicosis or Hypothyroidosis Caused by Iodide, below).

Radioactive Iodide Therapy

Radioactive iodide (^{131}I) is uniformly effective therapy; it is simple to administer and inexpensive. In the United States, unlike common practice in Japan and to a lesser degree Europe, it is the preferred form of therapy for most adults with Graves disease and has essentially replaced surgery for this disorder. The rapidity of response is dependent on dose and on the size of the gland, but improvement is often apparent in a few weeks and euthyroidism (or hypothyroidism, see below) is achieved on the average within a few months. Single dose radioiodide produces a euthyroid state in some 47% of males and 74% of females (20).

For many years, concern was expressed over the possibility of producing carcinoma of the thyroid, leukemia, or genetic damage in future offspring of women in their child-bearing years. Over the nearly 50 years that radioactive iodide has been used therapeutically, all these concerns have been shown to be groundless. Although low dosages of external radiation or radioiodide can produce carcinoma of the thyroid, particularly in children, the higher dosages used for treatment of hyperthyroidism do not. Long-term follow-up of treated patients over the past 30 years has failed to substantiate any such risk or any increased risk of leukemia. The amounts of radiation to the ovaries from therapeutic doses of radioiodide used for therapy of hyperthyroidism are lower than those delivered by diagnostic radiographic procedures and can be expected to produce no genetic effects. Thus, radioiodide therapy for hyperthyroidism can be considered without fear for any adult patient, including nonpregnant women of child-bearing age who plan to have children.

The single disadvantage of radioactive iodide is that hypothyroidism is a common consequence. Hypothyroidism follows radioiodide therapy in the immediate few months after therapy in a more or less dose-related fashion. Small single doses produce hypothyroidism within a year in approximately 10% of cases. Furthermore, of the patients rendered euthyroid, 3% to 4% per year develop hypothyroidism over the ensuing 20 years.

The high frequency of posttreatment hypothyroidism should be weighed against the advantages of radioiodide therapy. For most of those who become hypothyroid, replacement therapy with thyroxine is a trivial inconvenience. Unfortunately, a few patients discontinue their required lifelong replacement therapy and suffer the consequences of hypothyroidism.

Some endocrinologists, including the author, advocate the use of deliberately ablative doses of ^{131}I. This approach to therapy simplifies patient management, accelerates restoration of the euthyroid state, and is reasonable in view of the high probability of eventual posttherapy hypothyroidism regardless of dose. Nonetheless, many endocrinologists do not advocate deliberate ablation unless the patient is elderly, has experienced a major complication of hyperthyroidism (e.g., severe heart disease), has complicating medical problems that demand prompt control, or has severe ophthalmopathy (22). In young patients who are tolerating their disease reasonably well, some physicians prefer to use small doses of ^{131}I, repeated if necessary, until the patient is euthyroid. Such an approach does not, of course, guarantee that hypothyroidism will be avoided. As discussed below, larger doses of ^{131}I are appropriate initially in the treatment of toxic nodular goiter.

In the past, elaborate schemes have been used to estimate the required dose of ^{131}I. Unfortunately, none has proven helpful because the variability of the thyroid's sensitivity to radiation—the most important determinant of effect—is not measurable. Currently, in a typical low-dose treatment scheme, patients with small glands are given 3 to 5 mCi, whereas those with moderately enlarged to large glands are given 7 to 10 mCi (1 mCi equals 37 mBq). Ablative doses approximate 15 mCi. Because of the unpredictable response with nonablative doses, antithyroid drugs are often used initially to render the patient euthyroid. Antithyroid therapy is then interrupted for 48 hours before the ^{131}I is given and can be reinstituted 24 hours afterward. Alternatively, an antithyroid drug can be initiated 24 to 48 hours after therapy with ^{131}I, although recent evidence suggests that this maneuver does not hasten recovery from the hyperthyroid state. Similar approaches combining antithyroid drug and ^{131}I are almost routinely used in patients with severe or complicated hyperthyroidism (e.g., thyrocardiac disease).

Radioactive iodide can be administered only by an appropriately licensed physician—usually a nuclear medicine physician or an endocrinologist. A few precautions are necessary. In women of child-bearing age, a negative test for pregnancy must be obtained by the therapist immediately before the therapy dose is given because exposure of a fetus to radiation is unacceptable. In the United States, women who have a young child at home are given no more than 8 mCi and are instructed to avoid prolonged close contact (e.g., sharing a bed) for a week. Lactating women should not nurse for a month after therapy.

The undocumented notion has long persisted that radiation thyroiditis may produce excessive release of thyroid hormones 7 to 14 days after therapy, with the possibility of consequent worsening of the clinical state. This complication, if it occurs at all, must be rare. Nonetheless, prudence dictates a conservative approach in precarious patients (e.g., those in congestive heart failure) who are best brought to euthyroid status or who are at least significantly improved by antithyroid drug therapy before ablation with ^{131}I. At 3 months after ^{131}I therapy, when the short-term radiation effect becomes maximal, the antithyroid drug can be discontinued or tapered, provided that the laboratory and clinical evidence indicates return to euthyroid status. Adjunctive therapy with a beta-blocker is useful during this period to ameliorate possibly emerging symptoms if the dose of ^{131}I proves to have been inadequate. If the laboratory evidence indicates continuing hyperthyroidism, another dose of ^{131}I is required.

Therapy with ^{131}I is always successful if enough ^{131}I is given. "Failure" after one or more doses is never an indication for surgery or indeterminate therapy with antithyroid drug. Rather, additional ^{131}I should be given to complete the process.

Surgical Therapy

For many years surgical ablation of the thyroid (e.g., subtotal thyroidectomy) was the main therapy for hyperthyroidism. This procedure still has its advocates, especially for young adults and for children who cannot be treated successfully with antithyroid drugs. In the hands of experienced surgeons, subtotal thyroidectomy is effective therapy, attended by minimal morbidity. However, complications include the small but real risk of anesthetic and operative mortality, recurrent laryngeal nerve damage with vocal cord paralysis, permanent hypoparathyroidism, and, most commonly, hypothyroidism. The latter two complications are unavoidable to a certain extent and are not merely the consequence of poor surgical technique. In addition to about a 10% occurrence of immediate postsurgical hypothyroidism, 2% to 3% of patients become hypothyroid each year after surgery, a figure only slightly lower than that after therapy with ^{131}I. A higher complication rate must be expected when the operation is performed by surgeons with limited experience in thyroid surgery. Surgery is also followed by a significant (5%) rate of recurrent hyperthyroidism, sometimes occurring many years later. In this case, even the most enthusiastic supporters of surgical treatment agree that recurrent hyperthyroidism should *never* be treated by a second operation because the frequency of major complications rises to an unacceptable level.

Treatment of Hyperthyroidism During Pregnancy

Hyperthyroidism complicates about one to two pregnancies per thousand. However, the disease is almost always easily controlled in the mother, and when this is the case, the infants are unaffected and there is not any obvious increase in the incidence of congenital anomalies. In contrast, uncontrolled hyperthyroidism leads to preeclampsia, low birth weight, a high percentage of stillbirths, and congestive heart failure in the mothers. If hyperthyroidism is suspected, free T_4 and TSI assays are the preferred tests. (Alterations in TBG make total T_4 and T_3 assays difficult to interpret, and TSH levels may be low in euthyroid pregnant women.)

Although there have been no prospective clinical trials, opinion on this topic is essentially uniform: Hyperthyroidism should be treated with an antithyroid drug regardless of whether it is due to Graves disease or toxic nodular goiter (23,24). Surgery has been used successfully during pregnancy but has no advantage and may be associated with increased fetal losses. Radioactive iodide is contraindicated.

There is little to choose between the two available drugs, although in the United States propylthiouracil is favored. Methimazole may be associated with an increased incidence of the infrequent congenital skin anomaly, aplasia cutis (one in 2,000 normal births), a small (up to 3 cm) hairless patch on the head or neck that usually disappears spontaneously after a few years.

Therapy with antithyroid drugs during pregnancy is guided by the consideration that both drugs freely cross the placenta and, in large doses, can produce goiter and hypothyroidism in the infant. The dosage of antithyroid drugs should therefore be the minimal amount adequate to control the hyperthyroidism. A dose of drug that totally blocks hormone synthesis given along with a replacement amount of thyroxine is a scheme that is inappropriate during pregnancy, because it may lead to the use of larger doses of antithyroid drug than are absolutely necessary. When ordinary doses of antithyroid drug are used, the fetus is usually born euthyroid and without a goiter, but as a precaution, some experts reduce the dosage during the last 2 months of pregnancy and, if clinical circumstances permit, discontinue the drug entirely in the last month. This is often possible, because hyperthyroidism during pregnancy tends to ameliorate spontaneously as the pregnancy progresses, although exacerbation in the postpartum period is not unusual. Iodide as an adjunct should not be used during pregnancy because the fetal thyroid is especially susceptible to the goitrogenic effect of iodide.

Conventional thionamide drug therapy (i.e., propylthiouracil and methimazole are used in the United States, see below) does not preclude nursing. Infants show no effects from the small amounts of the drug that do get into breast milk, at least at daily doses of up to 20 mg of methimazole or 750 mg of propylthiouracil. Intellectual and somatic development is normal in the children of mothers who are receiving an antithyroid drug who are breast feeding their infants.

Concern has been expressed over the adverse effects of maternal thyroid hormone deficiency in hypothyroid women receiving T_4 replacement therapy during pregnancy on the subsequent neuropsychological development (I.Q.) of the child (25). Obviously, overtreatment of the pregnant hyperthyroid woman can also impair fetal development, and even a minor degree of maternal hypothyroxinemia may be harmful to the development of the fetal brain. This issue has been carefully reviewed and a strong case made for the avoidance of any T_4 deficiency in the mother during pregnancy, especially in the critical early phase of fetal brain development (26). Dependence on a low maternal TSH as an indicator of thyroid hormone adequacy in the first trimester is unreliable. Free T_4 (or FTI) and not total T_4 is the measurement necessary for assessing adequacy of thyroxine dosage, given the elevation of TBG in pregnancy. Moreover, free T_4 should be measured by equilibrium dialysis, because in the presence of elevated TBG other methods can yield spuriously high and therefore misleadingly reassuring values (27).

TSIs (see above) of Graves disease cross the placenta and enter the fetal circulation. Occasionally, the newborn infant is hyperthyroid at birth as a result of this passive transfer of stimulating antibodies. The clinician who will care for the newborn should always be alerted to this possibility.

Ophthalmopathy of Graves Disease

The serum of some patients with Graves *ophthalmopathy* contains a factor (exophthalmos-producing substance) that produces exophthalmos and other abnormalities of orbital tissues in test animals. In Graves ophthalmopathy, the extraocular muscles show interstitial edema, increased connective tissue, fatty infiltration, and infiltration with lymphocytes (18). Eventually, gross degenerative changes such as fibrosis may occur.

The exact frequency of ophthalmopathy in Graves disease is unknown, but most patients have either no obvious infiltrative eye involvement or show only minimal to moderate proptosis, which generally stabilizes at a tolerable level. Severe exophthalmos occurs in no more than a few percent of cases of Graves disease.

Graves ophthalmopathy and thyroid hyperactivity often coincide; in 85% of cases, the two occur within 18 months of each other. However, the ophthalmopathy may occur years before or after the onset of hyperthyroidism. Even if the patient is euthyroid (normal T_4 and T_3), the thyroid can frequently be shown to be autonomous, as demonstrated by a nonsuppressible

RaIU and a suppressed TSH. In this phase of the disease, the thyroid's activity is driven by TSIs rather than TSH, but the serum thyroid hormones are within the range of normal. Without evidence of either thyroid hyperfunction, disturbance of the negative feedback system (suppression of TSH), or dermopathy, the diagnosis of Graves ophthalmopathy cannot always be made with absolute assurance. Indeed, other diseases of the orbit or retro-orbital space must be considered. CT of the skull and the orbital contents and/or high-resolution sonography are useful diagnostic tools. These procedures can visualize the enlarged extraocular muscles typical of Graves ophthalmopathy, although such enlargement is also seen in pseudotumor. In many cases of Graves ophthalmopathy without overt hyperthyroidism, other aspects of Graves disease usually become apparent eventually, but several years may elapse before that occurs.

Proptosis becomes more than a cosmetic concern when the eyelids fail to close, especially when the patient is sleeping, setting the stage for exposure keratitis or corneal ulceration. This problem may be relieved by the application of liquid tears (available over the counter) and the wearing of eye patches at night and sunglasses in bright sunlight or on windy days. Paresis of the extraocular muscles producing diplopia can also be troublesome and may require use of an eye patch or corrective surgery. The most disturbing but fortunately uncommon eye involvement is severe chemosis (marked inflammation and edema) of the conjunctivae and periorbital soft tissues. Ophthalmopathy of this severity is termed malignant or infiltrative exophthalmos. Rarely, optic neuritis leading to blindness occurs.

Treatment of severe ophthalmopathy is best provided by an ophthalmologist who has experience with the problem, working in close collaboration with an endocrinologist. Corticosteroids (e.g., prednisone, 60 mg a day for 1 to 2 weeks, tapered over 6 to 8 weeks) are useful for patients with severe periorbital and conjunctival edema and inflammation. Other therapy, if warranted, includes low-dose orbital radiation, an established and useful therapy (28), and radioactive-iodide ablation of the thyroid (with or without orbital radiation), a less well proven therapy. Surgical decompression is only rarely needed and is reserved for patients with severe proptosis. There is considerable controversy about which therapy is optimal (22).

Despite claims to the contrary, no form of treatment of hyperthyroidism has been shown to have any consistent advantage for control of the ophthalmopathy. However, recent evidence supports the long-held belief that induction of hypothyroidism may aggravate exophthalmos. Development of clinical hypothyroidism should therefore be avoided if possible, especially when exophthalmos is present.

Thyrotoxicosis Associated With Thyroiditis

Classic subacute thyroiditis (see below) may be associated occasionally with short-lived self-limited thyrotoxicosis. The explanation for this phenomenon has been that the destructive inflammatory process causes release of preformed thyroid hormone. The thyrotoxicosis invariably disappears within a few months.

Lymphocytic thyroiditis is another apparently distinct variant of the thyroiditis–thyrotoxicosis syndrome. Such patients have a modestly enlarged nontender thyroid gland. No history of viral illness can be obtained. The RaIU is very low, as it is in subacute thyroiditis, whereas the T_4 and T_3 levels are high and the TSH level is low. About half of the cases have significant elevations of thyroid antibodies, and about half of these high titers subside within a few months. A propensity of the condition to occur in the postpartum period has been noted, sometimes in successive pregnancies and sometimes followed by the development of hypothyroidism (see Postpartum Thyroid Dysfunction, below). On biopsy (not ordinarily recommended) the changes seen differ from those of the peak phase of classic subacute thyroiditis, but the latter, in its late stage of evolution, may be indistinguishable from that of lymphocytic thyroiditis. Whether lymphocytic thyroiditis with spontaneously resolving thyrotoxicosis (silent thyroiditis) is a new disease, as has been suggested by some, or is a newly recognized variant of subacute thyroiditis is a matter of debate (16).

An RaIU measurement should be obtained in all patients with thyrotoxicosis who do not clearly have Graves disease (i.e., who do not have associated eye findings) or toxic nodular goiter. A very low RaIU establishes the diagnosis of hyperthyroidism associated with thyroiditis and allows the physician to avoid inappropriate therapy (radioiodide or surgery). Amiodarone-induced thyrotoxicosis should be considered as well (see below) in patients taking this drug. Treatment with an antithyroid drug may be useful; propranolol (see above) affords symptomatic relief and may be all the treatment that is necessary.

Long-term follow-up studies of these patients show that about half persist in having some degree of thyroid abnormality: antithyroid antibodies or goiter, recurring bouts of thyrotoxicosis, elevation of TSH (decreased thyroid reserve), and, occasionally, hypothyroidism (16).

Hyperthyroidism Associated With Multinodular Goiter (Toxic Nodular Goiter) or With a Solitary ("Hot") Nodule

Toxic nodular goiter is usually seen in adults in midlife or in the elderly. Although the typical patient with Graves disease usually relates symptoms extending over a few months to a year, the history in toxic nodular goiter is often much longer, and many years usually pass before a diagnosis is made. Because of the typical patient's age and the duration of illness, severe cardiac or musculoskeletal involvement is common.

Toxic nodular goiter appears to arise in the pathologic evolution of some cases of nodular goiter. Most nodular goiters (see below) are initially TSH dependent (i.e., RaIU is suppressible with exogenous thyroid hormone). Eventually, some of these goiters develop autonomous areas, with other regions of relatively decreased activity. Nodular goiters at this stage of evolution do not secrete enough hormone to produce clinical hyperthyroidism, but 20% of cases nevertheless can be shown to have nonsuppressible function. Some of these autonomously functioning goiters evolve to a stage in which excessive production of hormone and subclinical (see below) or clinical hyperthyroidism (low TSH, elevated T_4 and T_3, with or without overt clinical symptoms) ensues.

Therapy of toxic nodular goiter is best accomplished with ^{131}I. Rather large doses, in the range of 15 to 30 mCi, are usually necessary and may have to be repeated more than once. Hypothyroidism occurs much less commonly after ^{131}I therapy for nodular goiter than for Graves disease. If the clinical situation demands prompt relief of the hyperthyroidism, an antithyroid drug can be used after the therapeutic dose of ^{131}I because the response to radioiodide is often slow or multiple doses may be needed. Otherwise, ^{131}I given alone is simple therapy, without side effects, and easily monitored by measurements of serum T_4. With ablative therapy (large doses), thyrotoxicosis may be controlled in several weeks or with smaller doses, in several months. Other therapeutic considerations including the use of adjunctive therapy follow those outlined for the therapy of Graves disease with one exception: In hyperthyroidism due to toxic nodular goiter, antithyroid drugs alone, although effective while administered, will not produce a lasting remission. The same is true for hyperthyroidism due to a hot nodule (see Thyroid Disorders, below).

Hyperthyroidism Caused by Excessive Secretion of T_3

Triiodothyronine Toxicosis

In most cases of hyperthyroidism, the thyroid secretes excessive quantities of both T_4 and T_3. However, in perhaps 5% of all cases, T_3 is the predominant hormone secreted. So-called T_3 toxicosis may occur in hyperthyroidism due to Graves disease, toxic multinodular goiter, or autonomous adenoma. The patient who appears clinically hyperthyroid but whose T_4 is normal or low should have serum T_3 measured. T_3 toxicosis sometimes occurs early in the course of hyperthyroidism due to Graves disease and can develop during therapy with an antithyroid drug, in which case the dosage should be increased. Continuing clinical findings of hyperthyroidism during such therapy—despite a normal or low T_4—raise the possibility that T_3 toxicosis is now present and that more, rather than less, antithyroid drug is needed. The treatment of T_3 toxicosis is the same as is that of other forms of hyperthyroidism.

Free T_3 Toxicosis

On very rare occasions hyperthyroidism is suspected on clinical grounds and yet the only clue is a low TSH. T_4, free T_4, FTI, and serum T_3 (total) are all normal. Such patients may have the entity of "free T_3 toxicosis". Only a few cases have been reported. These patients may have some anatomic thyroid abnormality or thyroid autonomy (e.g., nodule, multinodular goiter) but the condition can apparently occur without such abnormalities. The only biochemical abnormality of serum hormones in these individuals, aside from a low TSH, is an elevation of their serum free T_3. T_3, like T_4, is mainly protein bound, but T_3 is much less tightly bound than T_4. Free T_3 is measured, like free T_4, by equilibrium dialysis. The metabolic effects of an elevation of free T_3 are clinically identical to that of an increased free T_4. Such patients are considered to have "free T_3 toxicosis" (29), an entity distinct from "T_3 toxicosis," which is far more common. Whether such patients need therapy should be determined by an endocrinologist.

Thyrotoxicosis or Hypothyroidism Caused by Iodide

Excess iodide from a variety of sources can induce hyperthyroidism, if the patient ingesting it was previously iodide depleted. If that is the case, a toxic nodular goiter may be produced or, less often, "latent" Graves disease. This phenomenon is called the Jod-Basedow effect in Europe. It is not seen often in the United States. In parts of the world where there is adequate iodine in the diet, excess iodide may cause hypothyroidism, especially if a patient has underlying thyroid disease, such as autoimmune thyroiditis.

Amiodarone (an antiarrhythmic agent; see Chapter 64) contains about 40% iodine and, in the United States, is the most likely source of excess iodide, released when the drug is metabolized. The intact drug also can exert a number of effects upon the thyroid and upon thyroid hormone metabolism: It markedly inhibits peripheral conversion of T_4 to T_3 and coincidentally increases the serum concentration of T_4 and free T_4.

There are two mechanisms by which amiodarone induces thyrotoxicosis. The first is by the Jod-Basedow phenomenon (type I amiodarone-induced thyrotoxicosis) and the second, much more common in this country, is from direct drug toxicity that results in thyroid cell destruction with release of preformed thyroid hormones that cause thyrotoxicosis (type II amiodarone-induced thyrotoxicosis) until the gland is depleted of its hormonal stores (1 to 3 months). The RaIU (or early phase 99m-pertechnetate uptake) is very low. Treatment includes methimazole and perchlorate and, if the clinical state is severe, glucocorticoids, which appear to accelerate recovery. Iopanoic acid can be used to inhibit T_4 to T_3 conversion if the amiodarone is to be discontinued. Amiodarone can be continued, if clinically indicated by the cardiovascular status. Transient and occasionally permanent hypothyroidism may follow. Treatment of amiodarone-induced thyrotoxicosis should be supervised by an endocrinologist.

In the United States, hypothyroidism due to amiodarone (20% of all patients) is more common than thyrotoxicosis. Most cases are presumably iodide induced in persons with subclinical autoimmune thyroiditis.

Subclinical Hyperthyroidism

The term *subclinical hyperthyroidism* has been applied to the clinical state in which the TSH is suppressed but the free T_4 and free T_3 concentrations are within the normal range (30–32). By definition, the patients are asymptomatic. This condition can occur in the absence of thyroid hormone administration or during treatment with T_4 for replacement or TSH suppression. In one large series, subclinical hyperthyroidism *was* associated with a threefold increased risk in people 60 years or older of developing atrial fibrillation (but *not* overt hyperthyroidism) over 10 years (31). In that study there were no other adverse outcomes, and in fact the condition may spontaneously abate (i.e., the TSH normalizes) (32) (see Screening for Thyroid Disease in Healthy Patients, below). Very few patients with only a low TSH subsequently develop clinical hyperthyroidism with elevation of T_4 or T_3 concentrations. Thus, the term *subclinical hyperthyroidism,* which is based only on a suppressed TSH, may be misleading.

Thyroid Storm (Thyrotoxic Crisis)

Thyroid storm, a severe exacerbation of hyperthyroidism, is rarely encountered. When thyroid storm does occur, it is usually in the setting of severe medical or surgical stress imposed on a patient with uncontrolled or unrecognized hyperthyroidism. Clinical features of full-blown thyroid storm include fever, sometimes to the level of extreme hyperpyrexia; marked tachycardia; great irritability; diarrhea; hypotension; and cardiovascular collapse. Thyroid storm often progresses rapidly to delirium and coma. Any severe exacerbation of hyperthyroidism demands immediate hospitalization and urgent consultation with an endocrinologist.

Surgery in the Patient With Hyperthyroidism

This problem is discussed in Chapter 93.

HYPOTHYROIDISM

Hypothyroidism, the metabolic state resulting from an inadequate level of circulating thyroxine, is common. Most cases can be diagnosed even when symptoms and signs are minimal, provided that the clinician considers the diagnosis and seeks appropriate laboratory confirmation. The manifestations of hypothyroidism are varied and to a large measure age dependent. *Myxedema* is the term for a severe form of hypothyroidism that results in deposition of mucopolysaccharides in the skin and other tissues, producing a characteristic appearance and a constellation of physical findings. The term *myxedema* is commonly but incorrectly used interchangeably with *hypothyroidism*. *Primary hypothyroidism* is the term used to indicate that the hormone deficiency results from a disease or other process within the thyroid gland. *Secondary hypothyroidism* or *central hypothyroidism* is much less common and results from lack of thyrotropin (TSH) secretion, a consequence of pituitary or, rarely, hypothalamic disease. The thyroid is usually smaller than normal and is not palpable. Serum TSH, using a second- or third-generation assay, may be low, but TSH assay in this situation can be misleading. Biologically inactive but immunoreactive TSH is often produced so that the measured TSH can be normal or even elevated. Abnormal TSH glycosylation accounts for this phenomenon. Almost invariably the hypothyroidism is part of a decrease in pituitary function involving trophic hormones in addition to TSH with concomitant hypogonadism or adrenal insufficiency. Causes include postpartum necrosis, pituitary tumor, pituitary apoplexy, and granulomatous disease or sometimes an autoimmune process involving failure of other endocrine glands. Some cases occur without identifiable cause and are termed idiopathic (see also Chapter 81).

Etiology

Worldwide, the most common cause of hypothyroidism remains dietary *iodide deficiency.* In the United States, iodide deficiency no longer exists because iodide, for over half a century, has been added to dietary salt to prevent goiter. Most cases of hypothyroidism in this country are due to *autoimmune destruction* of the thyroid, either with or without goiter (see below). Goitrous autoimmune thyroiditis is also called *Hashimoto thyroiditis.* At a later stage, the gland atrophies and a goiter is no longer palpable. Almost all remaining cases are iatrogenic, the result of therapy of hyperthyroidism, although it should be recalled that hypothyroidism also seems to be a late outcome of Graves disease, regardless of treatment (see above). *External radiation of the neck* (e.g., for nonthyroidal neoplastic disease) can also cause thyroid atrophy and subsequent hypothyroidism.

Autoimmune destruction of the thyroid may occur in association with other autoimmune glandular disorders, especially adrenal insufficiency (Schmidt syndrome) and autoimmune ovarian failure (polyglandular failure) and with diseases such as pernicious anemia. High titers of antibodies to thyroid antigens (thyroglobulin, microsomes) are seen in 90% of cases. An easily overlooked form of hypothyroidism is that which occurs *postpartum* (see Postpartum Thyroid Dysfunction, below). A classification of the causes of hypothyroidism is given in Table 80.7.

Drug-Induced Hypothyroidism

Although a variety of drugs can produce hypothyroidism, invariably associated with goiter formation, only a few in current use have such an effect. Lithium, widely used for the treatment of manic-depressive illness (see Chapter 24), is one such agent. If goiter occurs, lithium need not be stopped; addition of thyroxine relieves the hypothyroidism and causes regression of the goiter. Overtreatment of hyperthyroidism with an antithyroid drug will, of course, produce

Table 80.7. Clinical Classification of Hypothyroidism[a]

Hypothyroidism without goiter (decrease of thyroid tissue mass)
Postablative for hyperthyroidism (radioiodide therapy or surgery)
Autoimmune atrophy
Postpartum
External radiation
Developmental defect (congenital)
Pituitary or hypothalamic disease
Hypothyroidism with goiter
Autoimmune (Hashimoto disease)
Postpartum
Drug induced (e.g., antithyroid drugs, iodide, lithium[b])
Iodide deficiency (many geographic areas)
Genetic biosynthetic defects

[a]Hypothyroidism in the United States is now most commonly the consequence of therapy for hyperthyroidism. Hypothyroidism from idiopathic atrophy of the thyroid is second in frequency. Developmental defects (e.g., lingual thyroid) are rare. Hypothyroidism with goiter is nearly always caused by Hashimoto thyroiditis, rarely by a drug. Genetic biosynthetic defects are rare and usually become manifest in childhood.

[b]Hypothyroidism from chronic lithium therapy may occur without goiter.

hypothyroidism. Iodide in pharmacologic amounts is an antithyroid drug and also occasionally produces goiter and hypothyroidism (also see above). However, most adults who are susceptible to the antithyroid action of iodide have an underlying thyroid abnormality, such as Hashimoto thyroiditis (see below) or radioiodide-treated Graves disease. Amiodarone, an antiarrhythmic agent, contains iodine and can produce hypothyroidism in up to 20% of patients treated with this drug (see Thyrotoxicosis or Hypothyroidism Caused by Iodide, above).

Clinical Features

Hypothyroidism in the adult is highly variable in presentation. Usually, onset is insidious, often occurring over many years, with the result that the symptoms go unappreciated by patient and clinician alike. The nonspecificity of the symptoms also contributes to the delayed diagnosis. No predictable progression of symptoms is apparent, but easy fatigability, lethargy, increased sleep requirement (and, sometimes, sleep apnea; see Chapter 7), cold intolerance, muscle aching, and stiffness are perhaps the most common early symptoms. The skin is dry and may show scaling. Hair loss is common. The eyebrows become sparse, and the face is "puffy" (i.e., full) because of cutaneous deposition of mucopolysaccharides, with edema of the periorbital areas. The voice often becomes low pitched and rough. Constipation is common and may be severe enough to produce megacolon. Diminished hearing, especially in older persons, is easily overlooked or is attributed to aging. Ordinarily, the affected individual becomes abnormally placid, but agitation or frank psychosis may occur. In the elderly, depression is the most common psychiatric accompaniment of hypothyroidism. Despite common medical belief, the few available studies demonstrate that dementia caused by hypothyroidism is rare, if it occurs at all. Coexistence of the two processes in the elderly is, however, not uncommon. Paresthesias and pain in the hands from carpal tunnel syndrome may occur. Diminished sexual function is the rule. Women often experience menorrhagia. Rarely, galactorrhea may be seen in women of child-bearing age. Fertility is diminished, but pregnancy may occur and normal delivery is possible. The newborn is euthyroid, unless the mother's hypothyroidism is drug related or the hypothyroidism is of the rare familial athyrotic variety.

Subclinical Hypothyroidism

The most common stage of hypothyroidism likely to be encountered in ambulatory patients is mild hypothyroidism, commonly termed subclinical hypothyroidism. By definition, such an individual has an elevated TSH but serum thyroid levels that, although within the normal range, are presumably lower than they should be for that person (33). This condition is strongly age and gender dependent (8% of women and 4% of men 60 years and older) (11). The condition is characterized by a paucity of nonspecific but suggestive symptoms and few clinical findings. One study suggests that some of these patients improve after therapy with L-thyroxine (34). Many older women often show minimal elevations of TSH (6 to 10 μU) despite normal levels of T_4 (see Screening for Thyroid Disease in Healthy Patients, below). Only those with elevated thyroid autoantibodies are likely to develop overt clinical or laboratory hypothyroidism (50% over 5 years). The significance of minimal TSH elevation in the remainder of this group is unclear. The possibility that the immunoreactive TSH may not reflect its bioactivity has not been excluded in such patients.

Severe Hypothyroidism With Myxedema

In spontaneous cases of hypothyroidism, only with severe long-standing disease does extensive deposition of mucopolysaccharide occur, producing the clinical state of myxedema. Rarely, myxedema may develop rapidly (1 to 2 months) after radioiodide or surgical ablation of the thyroid for hyperthyroidism or after abrupt withdrawal of thyroxine replacement therapy.

In myxedema, a variety of manifestations can be appreciated on physical examination, and of course they vary with the severity and duration of the disease. The skin, in addition to being dry and scaling, is typically cool. The scaling may be extensive, and large flakes may be shed from the elbows and knees. The subcutaneous tissues may be infiltrated by mucopolysaccharides so the skin appears to be "thickened" or "doughy." In the elderly, atrophy of the epidermis may occur simultaneously, producing a stiff, translucent, parchment-like appearance. Yellow-orange discoloration of the skin from carotene deposition may be evident, especially in the palms. The presence of edema is not obvious because pitting is not noted except in extreme cases complicated by hypoproteinemia. An exception is the collection around the eyes of "bags of water" (lymphedema). This finding is not, however, specific for hypothyroidism. The tongue is sometimes enlarged. The heart rate is usually slow (sinus bradycardia). The heart may appear enlarged, because of either dilation of the myocardium or pericardial effusion. Pleural effusions and ascites may also be present, sometimes even in cases that are otherwise not clinically severe. Indeed, such effusions may be erroneously attributed to malignancy. Hyponatremia, clinically indistinguishable from the syndrome of inappropriate antidiuretic hormone (ADH) excess, may be present. Recent evidence suggests that this phenomenon is not ADH dependent; it disappears slowly as the patient is treated with T_4. The deep tendon reflexes characteristically show a delay in their relaxation phase, the so-called hung-up reflex. This is a highly suggestive finding but may be seen occasionally in other diseases. Mental functioning is slowed, as reflected in the characteristically slow speech. The reading speed may be greatly reduced. Hearing loss may be severe or of a degree apparent only on audiometric testing. Cerebellar dysfunction, if present, is usually evident only on extensive neurologic testing but in rare cases is grossly apparent as ataxia.

Myxedema Coma

Myxedema coma is a severe, often fatal, state that is a rare complication of long-standing disease and is typically seen in an elderly patient. Myxedema coma is often associated with or precipitated by pneumonia, peritonitis, or some other serious infection, the presence of which may not be immediately apparent. Severe respiratory failure is a major feature and can be due to a variety of factors ranging from upper airway obstruction to impaired chest wall mechanics. Because elderly patients often become hypothermic on exposure to cold or during sepsis, the diagnosis of myxedema coma is more commonly considered than actually confirmed. However, if myxedema coma is suspected, the patient should be hospitalized.

Laboratory Findings

In primary hypothyroidism, the combination of low serum T_4, FTI index (or free T_4), and high TSH is diagnostic. Difficulties in diagnosis are encountered only in occasional cases. The serum T_3 is usually low, but because T_3 decreases in a variety of nonthyroidal illnesses ranging from malnutrition to liver disease, its measurement is not useful for diagnosis of hypothyroidism. Furthermore, the T_3 is normal in many patients with mild hypothyroidism. In hypothyroidism caused by pituitary or hypothalamic disease, the TSH may not be low (see above). However, TSH may be low in severely ill patients with nonthyroidal illness also (see above). The TRH test is ordinarily unnecessary for diagnosis of primary hypothyroidism but can be helpful when the T_4 and TSH are borderline. In this situation, an exaggerated response to TRH may be seen (TSH increment greater than 30).

In addition to the definitive diagnostic tests, various other laboratory abnormalities are encountered, although they serve no useful diagnostic purpose. A common laboratory finding is elevation of serum enzymes that originate in skeletal muscle: creatine kinase and to lesser extents serum aspartate aminotransferase, serum alanine aminotransferase, and lactic dehydrogenase. Fractionation studies show that when these enzymes are elevated in hypothyroidism, they do not originate in cardiac muscle. Virtually all phenotypic abnormalities of hyperlipoproteinemia have been observed in hypothyroid patients and are reversible when thyroid hormone is replaced (see Chapter 82). Other abnormalities include electrocardiographic changes (e.g., flattened or inverted T waves, minor ST-segment depressions, and low amplitude QRS complexes) and abnormalities of blood gas measurements caused by hypoventilation. Anemia (see Chapter 55), usually normocytic and normochromic, may be present, as may macrocytic anemia of coexistent vitamin B_{12} deficiency (pernicious anemia). An abnormality of red cell shape (spiculation) also has been described in hypothyroidism.

Differential Diagnosis

The most difficult problem in diagnosis is the simple clinical appreciation of the possibility that the patient may be hypothyroid. Once suspected, the subsequent history, physical examination, and, particularly, laboratory findings will easily establish the diagnosis in all but a few cases. However, some special problems may be encountered. Any elderly patient who is sick, pale, and puffy faced becomes a suspect for the diagnosis, especially if an adequate history cannot be obtained. A patient with atypical chest pain, nonspecific electrocardiographic abnormalities, and elevated creatine kinase, aspartate aminotransferase, or alanine aminotransferase is occasionally labeled as having ischemic heart disease and myocardial infarction; the proper diagnosis may be hypothyroidism. A patient with the nephrotic syndrome might be mistaken for one having hypothyroidism. Although the serum T_4 may be low in nephrotic patients (because the TBG is low), the FTI (or free T_4) is normal, as is the TSH. More important, the patient with the nephrotic syndrome has features characteristic of that disorder (i.e., massive proteinuria and hypoalbuminemia and gross hyperlipidemia) (see Chapter 48).

Diagnosis of Hypothyroidism in Patients Already Receiving Thyroid Hormone Therapy

Patients are often encountered who, having been diagnosed as hypothyroid at some time in the past, are receiving replacement therapy when first seen. Lack of documentation may lead one to question the original diagnosis. Alternatives include continuation of therapy despite an uncertain diagnosis or discontinuation of therapy, a maneuver that will confirm or refute the need for continued treatment. In many instances, continuation of therapy may be simpler, less expensive, and more appropriate than an attempt to resolve the issue, but this can often be easily accomplished, even after many years of treatment, by abrupt discontinuation of hormone therapy. After 5 weeks, determination of serum T_4 (and FTI) is made. If the value is normal, the patient is considered euthyroid and the original diagnosis is discarded. In contrast, a low T_4 (and a subsequently determined high TSH) verifies a diagnosis of hypothyroidism.

Occasional euthyroid patients who are inappropriately treated with thyroid hormone for long periods, and most hypothyroid patients, become grossly symptomatic toward the end of the 5-week period of withdrawal. An occasional inappropriately treated patient can show a delay of several additional weeks for return of normal thyroid function. If the practitioner wishes to avoid the possibility of symptoms as a result of withdrawal, a rapid but expensive way to determine thyroid status while the patient continues to receive full hormone replacement is to administer human recombinant TSH followed 18 to 24 hours later by an RaIU test (see above). A normal or elevated RaIU post-TSH injection indicates normal thyroid function and a previously inappropriate diagnosis of primary hypothyroidism. Although no reports of the use of human recombinant TSH for this purpose are as yet available, bovine TSH, when it was available in the past, was routinely used in this fashion.

Hypothyroidism Versus the Euthyroid Sick Syndrome

The diagnosis of hypothyroidism in severely ill patients presents special problems (8,9). Patients with the euthyroid sick syndrome are usually elderly and often have sepsis. The T_4 and T_4 index are low; TSH may be low, normal, or moderately elevated, depending on the stage of the illness (2); and response to TRH is normal or blunted. Serum reverse T_3 is often elevated.

To date, the euthyroid sick syndrome has been clearly recognized only in hospitalized severely ill patients, but it probably also occurs in less dramatic form in chronically ill nonhospitalized people (9). Many patients with chronic renal failure undergoing hemodialysis appear to fall into this group. The mechanisms underlying this phenomenon appear to involve a combination of factors, including accelerated T_4 metabolism, impairment of TSH secretion (2,9), and impairment of T_4 binding to serum proteins. Most of these pathophysiologic abnormalities are probably due to excessive amounts of circulating cytokines (interleukin-1beta, tumor necrosis factor, and others) that are produced during severe illness.

Treatment

It has been clear for many years that T_4 is the best preparation for ordinary use. T_4 (levothyroxine, sodium L-thyroxine, and the U.S. brand names—Synthroid, Levothroid, Levoxy, Thyrox, Unithroid, Levotabs) is available in color-coded tablets of 25, 50, 75, 88, 100, 112, 125, 137, 150, 175, 200, and 300 μg. T_3 (liothyronine, Cytomel) is available in 5-, 25-, and 50-μg tablets. T_3 is also effective. However, it has no special advantage for routine therapy of hypothyroidism and has the distinct disadvantage that one cannot monitor the serum T_4 or T_3 to determine adequacy of replacement (because T_4 levels remain low and T_3 levels may fluctuate). Thyroglobulin preparations and desiccated thyroid ("thyroid extract") should no longer be used. Combination therapy using T_4 plus T_3 is discussed below.

Rate of Replacement With Thyroxine

Traditionally, initiation of thyroid hormone replacement therapy has been cautious and has used dosage schedules that ensure slow restoration of the patient to a normal metabolic state. Although this principle is conservative and rational, the practice is often unnecessary. Therapy must be adjusted to the individual case, with several points in mind. If the patient is not elderly and has never had overt cardiac disease, overcautious initiation of therapy will result only in needless prolongation of the hypothyroid state. If the patient has evidence of pre-existing cardiac disease or is frail and elderly, therapy should be started at low dosage: 12.5 to 25 μg of T_4 a day initially, with 25-μg increases at 4-week intervals, as tolerated. Only rarely will serious heart disease, such as angina pectoris, prevent at least partial replacement therapy, which is sufficient to eliminate myxedema, and most, if not all, unpleasant symptoms of hypothyroidism.

The usual hypothyroid patient, without complicating medical problems, may be started on full daily replacement dosage. Even with this therapeutic approach, the clinical response will be slow. One can expect several months to pass before restoration of a normal metabolic state.

The objective of therapy should be to restore the clinically euthyroid state if at all possible. Enough T_4 is given daily to maintain the serum T_4 at the mid to upper range of normal or, ideally, to the lowest level of T_4 at which the TSH is restored to normal (see below). The variability between individuals of optimal dosage is too great to rely on weight-based formulas (μg/kg). Most people need about 125 μg (0.125 mg) per day; only rarely is as much as 200 μg (0.2 mg) necessary, and more than that is rarely, if ever, needed. If a larger dose seems to be needed, noncompliance should be suspected (see Chapter 4). A single weekly dose of T_4 can be used; the dosage is slightly more than seven times the daily dosage (35). Once a week dosage has the advantage that it can be more easily supervised, if the circumstances warrant. Elderly patients may require only 100 μg/day or less for maintenance; often as little as 50 or 75 μg may suffice. The T_4 requirement during pregnancy is increased by about one-third (23).

Thyroid Hormone Replacement With Thyroxine Versus a Combination of Thyroxine and Triiodothyronine

Thyroid hormone replacement therapy has evolved from the use of crude extracts or powdered preparations of thyroid gland (desiccated thyroid) to that of two thyroid synthetic hormones, T_4 and T_3. When T_4 is given alone, hypothyroid patients are rendered clinically and biochemically euthyroid (normal) as measured by serum levels of T_4, T_3, and TSH. Serum T_3 is derived from T_4 by deiodination in nonthyroidal (peripheral) tissues, as is the case in normal persons, in whom secretion of T_3 from the thyroid amounts to only a tiny amount, about 6 μg/day. Nonetheless, for some time clinicians have noted that a significant minority of patients who are receiving only T_4 for replacement report a greater sense of well-being when taking approximately 50 μg of T_4 more than that which restored their TSH to the normal range (3). In a small study a number of patients were switched from T_4 alone to a combination of T_4 and T_3; they had significantly improved mood and neurologic function on extensive neuropsychological testing (36). However, the available information does not yet support a routine switch from T_4 monotherapy to a combination of T_4 and T_3 (37).

For patients on routine thyroid hormone replacement therapy, judicious use of small amounts of T_3 along with T_4 (10 μg per 100 μg of T_4) may be symptomatically beneficial for occasional patients and productive of possible minor side effects in a few others (37).

Importance of Avoiding Overtreatment During Thyroxine Replacement Therapy

Considerable concern has been expressed about whether T_4 replacement therapy or overtreatment with T_4 can lead to osteoporosis, because bone demineralization is a known complication of hyperthyroidism. Several studies have shown that T_4-treated patients, except for those with a history of hyperthyroidism, do not have decreased bone mineral density (38,39). In keeping with those conclusions, a recent study of women 65 years of age and older treated with T_4 showed no increase in fracture rate for those whose TSH was maintained in the normal range (0.5 to 5.5 mU/L) or even for those in the "borderline to low" range (0.1 to 0.4 mU/L). However, women whose TSH was suppressed below 0.1 mU/L had a threefold increased risk of hip fracture and a fourfold increased risk of vertebral fracture. Unfortunately, neither measurements of serum T_4 nor the dosages of T_4 were presented. Thus, the possibility exists that only women with overly elevated levels of thyroid hormone were subject to elevated risk of fracture (40), in which case these women may simply have been inadequately monitored. It should also be recalled that the elderly often need substantially less T_4 for replacement than younger persons; failure to appreciate this fact could have contributed to these fractures. Moreover, elderly women with already compromised age-related decreases of bone mineral density may be an especially high-risk group for the effects of overtreatment. The same concerns could be raised with respect to cardiovascular risk.

Monitoring

Determination of the T_4 alone is the least expensive way to follow the titration phase of replacement; use of the TSH is unnecessary at this stage. It is usually not helpful to measure the T_4 any sooner than 6 to 8 weeks after a change of dosage. When the T_4 reaches the middle to the upper part of the normal range, the TSH can be measured along with the T_4 and free T_4 (or FTI). The TSH serves as a fine adjustment in determining the final (maintenance) dose of T_4 (but that adjustment should not be overly emphasized; see below). Once the plateau of the desired dose of T_4 has been reached (i.e., that producing a T_4 level at which the TSH is satisfactory), repeat measurements of T_4 alone at yearly intervals should suffice, although some experts advocate routine use of the TSH alone. A third-generation TSH assay is not necessary for routine follow-up; its cost exceeds that of a T_4 measurement by 8- to 10-fold ($100 for a third-generation TSH is not unusual; sensitive second-generation assays are usually much cheaper). The advantage of the TSH is to avoid overtreatment and its consequences (see below).

The "ideal" laboratory goal of replacement therapy is thought by most experts to be a TSH that is within the normal range (0.5 to 4.5 mU/L in most laboratories). However, attaining such a precise target is expensive and probably unnecessary (41). As an example, a patient receiving a replacement dose of 0.1 mg of T_4 who has reached a serum T_4 of 9 μg% may have at this point a TSH that is slightly elevated at 7 μU/mL (normal up to 4.5). It is unlikely that such a patient will derive any clinical benefit if the dosage of T_4 is increased slightly (e.g., by 12 or 25 μg so that the T_4 reaches 10 or 11 μg% and the TSH falls to normal at 4 μU/mL). Similarly, if the TSH is found to be low (e.g., 0.2 μU/mL [lower limit of normal 0.5]), with a T_4 within the normal range, it is unlikely that any clinically useful result will follow from a minor downward adjustment of the replacement dosage of T_4. However, much effort and expense is frequently expended in such fine tuning, the clinical benefits of which are presently unproved and for which the evidence is rather unconvincing (see Subclinical Hypothyroidism, above). Moreover, the variability (error) of analytical measurement is usually not considered. Determination of serum T_3 during therapy with T_4 is unnecessary.

Experts have different opinions concerning the merits of generic versus brand names of T_4 for use in replacement therapy (41). Concern has been expressed over the bioavailability of hormone in certain generic preparations and even lack of standardization of certain brands of T_4, but clinically significant problems are not likely to be encountered with any of the preparations available in the United States.

Surgery in the Hypothyroid Patient

Patients with grossly evident hypothyroidism who require surgery are poor risks until their thyroid status is at least partially corrected (see Chapter 93), a process that requires 3 to 4 weeks with ordinary oral therapy. Elective surgery is best delayed in such patients. In an urgent situation, an intravenous dose of T_4 is probably warranted to prepare the patient for surgery in a few days. The increased susceptibility of severely hypothyroid patients to respiratory depression by conventional doses of many central nervous system active drugs should be borne in mind. This increased drug sensitivity has been responsible for precipitation of myxedema coma. On the other hand, patients with minimal hypothyroidism appear to tolerate ordinary surgical stress (e.g., elective cholecystectomy) well.

POSTPARTUM THYROID DYSFUNCTION

Postpartum thyroid dysfunction is common, occurring in some 17% of women in one study (42). Because of its high frequency, a good case has been made for routine screening (43). Both hyperthyroidism and hypothyroidism can occur; in some individuals one state follows the other. The hypothyroid variation may be transient, lasting only 1 to 4 months, and is most likely to occur in the first 8 months postpartum. However, in 30% of cases the hypothyroidism is permanent. Many cases that are not permanent are caused by the transient occurrence of thyroid-blocking antibodies. Most cases show antimicrosomal (thyroid peroxidase) antibodies; antithyroglobulin antibodies are uncommon. In the United States, the hyperthyroid variety has been associated with postpartum lymphocytic thyroiditis (see Thyrotoxicosis Associated with Thyroiditis, above). Postpartum hypothyroidism is often misdiagnosed as postpartum depression, and the two conditions are common and can coexist. Some women have repeated bouts of postpartum thyroid dysfunction with successive pregnancies. The disease also has other long-term implications as a risk factor for later development of both Graves disease and especially permanent hypothyroidism (17% of patients over 5 to 16 years in one series; 23% in 2 to 4 years in another [44]). Of special interest is the increased incidence (25%) in women with type 1 diabetes, a threefold increase over nondiabetic patients. Because of this high incidence, a 3-month follow-up (TSH and thyroid peroxidase antibodies) is recommended postpartum for all type 1 diabetic patients (45). The disorder is often familial.

SCREENING FOR THYROID DISEASE IN HEALTHY PATIENTS (HYPERTHYROIDISM AND HYPOTHYROIDISM)

Because thyroid diseases are common and clinical diagnosis can be difficult (see also Subclinical Hyperthyroidism and Subclinical Hypothyroidism, above), a rational argument can be made in favor of attempting to detect clinically inapparent thyroid disease by laboratory tests in individuals without overt symptoms (46,47). Modest degrees of hypothyroidism or hyperthyroidism are difficult to detect by routine clinical means, and several careful studies have confirmed this impression (48). However, the screening of asymptomatic populations by laboratory testing may not to be cost effective. Some experts now favor a case-finding approach—that is, testing only patients who are seeing a practitioner for symptoms—although there is not uniform agreement (49,50). In patients who exhibit any clinical findings that could conceivably be attributable to thyroid disease, laboratory testing should be done, but this approach should probably not be termed screening. Some success has been achieved by presenting a list of thyroid-related symptoms at the time of the patient's visit (51,52).

Most studies that have attempted to detect thyroid disease during screening have focused on evaluation of "sensitive" (second-generation) assays for TSH (see above) and their use as a single screening test. These are 10 times more sensitive than earlier assays (first generation) and, unlike the earlier assays, can recognize low (suppressed) values—those below the lower limit of the normal range (0.5 to 4.5 μU/mL). In these assays, the TSH is undetectable in patients with hyperthyroidism. Unfortunately, this finding is sensitive but not specific; many sick people and even "normal" elderly patients are found to have low levels of TSH (53,54). Thus, used alone, second-generation assays *cannot establish* a diagnosis of hyperthyroidism, whether in community populations or in sick patients at any age. A normal TSH *can* be useful in *excluding* a diagnosis of hyperthyroidism, but so can a normal T_4 (or FTI), at lower cost. Third-generation TSH assays are no more specific in this regard (2).

The results of screening for thyroid disease, using second-generation TSH tests and appropriate follow-up of abnormal values, are remarkably consistent in various populations (47,48,54,55). Approximately 1% of apparently healthy individuals, all ages included, are found to be hypothyroid. Many fewer individuals are shown to be hyperthyroid (0.1% to 0.2%). Women over 40 have the most thyroid disease; young men have essentially none. Asymptomatic patients with elevated or depressed levels of TSH may have subclinical hypothyroidism or subclinical hyperthyroidism (see above), respectively.

GOITER

A goiter is a thyroid gland that has undergone generalized enlargement. The term goiter should not be applied to a gland that is enlarged by a single nodule, although many continue to do so. The term implies nothing about the functional state of the gland. Goiter is the most common thyroid abnormality. *Diffuse goiter*, also called simple goiter, is a gland that, on gross examination, is uniformly and symmetrically enlarged without apparent irregularities. Most goiters are in fact multinodular, as revealed by palpation, sonography, or scan.

In some areas of the world, thyroid enlargement is so prevalent that it is termed *endemic goiter*. Before the widespread introduction of iodized salt, endemic goiter was common in the United States, but this is no longer the case. Endemic goiter, a term that for practical purposes is synonymous with *iodine deficiency goiter*, is now found principally in geographically isolated areas of the underdeveloped world, but some of these areas are vast, such as much of China, central

Asia, and Africa. Moreover, some parts of Europe such as Germany—which never iodized its salt supply—and parts of Italy, Switzerland, Denmark, and other countries are still areas of low iodide intake and, therefore, of goiter. The term *sporadic goiter* refers to thyroid enlargement as now encountered in the United States and other developed areas where iodide intake is adequate. Sporadic goiter is now seen in a small percentage of the U.S. population and increases in frequency with age. Its cause is unknown, but it is clearly not iodide deficiency.

The burden of iodide deficiency extends far beyond the development of enlarged thyroid glands in a large proportion of a population. Gross anatomic enlargement of the thyroid may be unsightly or produce mechanical obstruction for breathing and is certainly undesirable, but more devastating is the effect of iodide deficiency on brain development. Cretinism is the state of gross mental and physical retardation that results from hypothyroidism during fetal and early development. In iodide sufficient countries, great concern exists that even minor degrees of maternal hypothyroxinemia may be detrimental to *optimal* development of intelligence (26), reflecting the other end of the range of this problem.

Any process that prevents the synthesis of normal quantities of thyroid hormones, including iodide deficiency, produces goiter. If impairment of hormone synthesis is severe enough, goiter formation is associated with reduction of serum T_4 (but not T_3), eventually to be followed by clinical hypothyroidism. The mechanism of the thyroid enlargement in this situation is increased pituitary TSH secretion via activation of the negative feedback system. The resulting increased thyroid mass is a compensatory mechanism that may allow sufficient hormone synthesis to occur so that the patient remains euthyroid.

Drugs that interfere with thyroid hormone synthesis (e.g., thiocarbamides [thionamides, antithyroid drugs], lithium, iodides, etc.) can also lead to goiter. Withdrawal of a goitrogenic drug may result in regression of the goiter, as will simultaneous administration of enough T_4 or T_3 to suppress endogenous TSH secretion. The degree of regression depends on how long the goiter has been present. Long-standing goitrous enlargement is associated with the development of multiple large nodules, which are less likely to regress or to do so only incompletely.

Only one well-defined naturally occurring "goitrogen" is known: l-5-vinyl-2-thiooxazolidone. This substance, with a mechanism of action much like that of the thiocarbamides, is in cabbage, turnips, soybeans and soy products, and several other vegetables. Indeed, the recent advocacy of soy products (e.g., tofu) as a healthy source of protein has been reported to produce goiter. From time to time other poorly characterized goiter-producing substances have been detected in the food and water supplies of some areas. No specific environmental factor has been widely incriminated, however, as a cause of sporadic goiter, the etiology of which remains obscure.

Recognition

A visible or easily palpable mass in the base of the neck is the usual mode of presentation of goiter. Occasionally, especially in the elderly, an enlarged thyroid is neither visible nor readily palpable but is incidentally found by x-ray of the chest or esophagus when either a retrosternal mass is noted or the trachea or esophagus is found to be deviated. Confirmation of the nature of a neck mass as an enlarged thyroid gland and precise determination of its size are now most economically and accurately performed by ultrasound examination (sonography). Although radionuclide scintigraphy ("scanning") was previously used for this purpose, it is not as accurate as ultrasound, fails to show nodularity with comparable clarity, and cannot provide precise measurement of size or volume of the gland or of individual nodules. CT is accurate in delineating the relationship of a goiter to contiguous structures but is much less useful in defining the thyroid itself. The high iodide content of the sporadic goitrous thyroid enhances its x-ray density and identity.

Except in subacute thyroiditis, pain is not a usual symptom with a goiter but can develop during cyst formation or hemorrhage, a fairly common event, usually accompanied by rapid and sometimes painful enlargement of a portion of the gland. Obstruction of the trachea or esophagus can be produced by goiter, but dysphagia should not be readily attributed to minor degrees of thyroid enlargement. Hoarseness may occur because of involvement of the recurrent laryngeal nerve, but this is rare in patients with benign enlargement and its occurrence is suggestive although not diagnostic of thyroid malignancy.

Differential Diagnosis

Confronted with a goiter, the clinician's first thought should *not* be cancer. Most goiters (some 95%) represent benign disease (56). The frequency of carcinoma in multinodular goiter has been debated for years. Unwarranted concern has resulted in countless unnecessary operations (see below). The diagnosis of malignancy in a multinodular goiter is discussed below (see Thyroid Nodules and Thyroid Carcinomas). The assessment of goiter as a benign condition assumes, however, that malignancy has been excluded (see below).

Clinical and laboratory assessment of thyroid function should be made in all cases of goiter. Although most goiters are associated with normal serum thyroid hormone levels and a euthyroid state, either hypothyroidism or hyperthyroidism may be present. Tests should include serum TSH, FTI (or free T_4), and thyroid autoantibodies. Both the tissue and the functional status of the gland change with time, sometimes rather rapidly, and hence a precise diagnosis may not be possible at a single examination. Goiter in association with hyperthyroidism suggests Graves disease or toxic nodular goiter. Hypofunction in association with goiter is likely to represent goitrous autoimmune (Hashimoto) thyroiditis (see Hypothyroidism, above). If the clinical and laboratory assessments indicate normal thyroid function, as is usually the case, a diagnosis of *euthyroid goiter* is made. Possibilities such as drug ingestion may have to be excluded. Rarities such as an infiltrative process (amyloid disease, metastatic neoplasm) and the inherited defects of hormone synthesis (organification or coupling defects) also should be kept in mind (Table 80.7).

Multinodular enlargement almost always indicates a process of many years' standing. Differentiation of diffuse enlargement from nodular enlargement often requires ultrasound examination because small nodules are missed on physical examination, whereas ultrasound detects nodules as small as 0.5 cm in diameter. In contrast, an optimally performed scintiscan may show only irregular ("patchy") uptake of tracer, but even the best isotope technique can delineate nodules of only about 0.5 cm or more in size and is less sensitive than ultrasound. A goiter composed of many small nodules may appear on scintiscan to be homogeneous and non-nodular. Antithyroglobulin or antimicrosomal (thyroid peroxidase) antibodies in serum are readily determined commercially and should be routinely sought in all cases of goiter. Titers of such antibodies are elevated in the blood of 90% of patients with goiters caused by autoimmune (Hashimoto) thyroiditis. A goiter plus a high titer of antibody is essentially diagnostic of this disorder, which often leads to a hypothyroid state (see above). A proper history will point to possible drug-related goiter. Rapidity of enlargement may help differentiate benign from malignant lesions. The presence of pain will help identify fairly common subacute thyroiditis and exceedingly rare anaplastic carcinomas (see below).

Treatment of Sporadic Goiter: Suppression Therapy With Thyroxine

Although the cause of thyroid enlargement in sporadic goiter is unknown, its development nevertheless depends on the presence of TSH. Administration of a physiologic quantity of thyroid hormone results in suppression of TSH release. When TSH secretion is chronically suppressed in this manner, an enlarged thyroid may regress, if only partially, or at least cease to enlarge and form new nodules. The larger and more long-standing the goiter, the less likely is regression to occur. Only occasionally does a sporadic nodular goiter regress significantly (56). This has led some to suggest that small sporadic goiters should not be treated with suppression but treated expectantly or offered surgery or ^{131}I therapy (see below).

Suppression therapy is often and properly performed for cosmetic reasons. Suppression therapy is also clearly indicated for individuals with many years of life expectancy during which time mechanical obstructive problems may develop. However, little is to be gained by treatment of patients whose glands are relatively small and not a cosmetic problem or are known not to have changed in size over many years.

Until recently, a clear and unequivocal indication for therapy was the patient who had already had surgery for goiter (subtotal or lobe resection) (57). Recurrence of goiter was believed to be common in such people and thought to be predictably prevented with suppression therapy; however, this idea has been challenged (58).

Dosage of Thyroxine (or Triiodothyronine) for Suppression

Suppression therapy should be accomplished with T_4. The dosage should not be excessive lest subclinical or iatrogenic hyperthyroidism (see below) be produced. T_4 at an initial dose of 125 μg/day is usually ample. T_3 (Cytomel), 25 μg/day (q.d. at bedtime or twice as day) may also be used for suppression but has no clear-cut advantage over T_4.

Monitoring of Suppression Therapy With Thyroxine (or Triiodothyronine)

To avoid iatrogenic hyperthyroidism, suppression therapy must be monitored by periodic determination of *both* the serum TSH (by use of a second- or third-generation assay) *and* the T_4. The importance of monitoring is not only to establish that the dose of T_4 is adequate and that the TSH is lowered only to the proper level but that the production of T_4 by the gland is suppressible. Older literature clearly indicated that 20% of nontoxic nodular goiters are autonomous, that is, their function as measured by RaIU cannot be suppressed with doses of T_4 that should have completely suppressed TSH production. These studies antedate the era of sensitive TSH measurements. Systematic studies are not available, but one would expect that in most of these cases TSH would be low before suppression (subclinical hyperthyroidism), and therefore if suppression were attempted, the T_4 could rise into the hyperthyroid range as exogenous T_4 is added to that being produced by the thyroid.

At one time T_3 was more popular as suppression therapy than it is today. When T_3 is given, the serum T_4 falls to a level below normal if the thyroid is indeed suppressible.

Time Course of Therapeutic Response to Suppression

If the treated gland is diffusely enlarged and nonnodular or micronodular, obvious regression by 6 months can be expected in about one-half of cases. Glands with larger nodules are less likely to respond, and a second year of treatment will probably be needed before regression is apparent. Even if significant regression is not accomplished, prevention of further glandular enlargement is a reasonable goal and may make the undertaking worthwhile. A baseline ultrasound examination with determination of gland volume and repeat examinations at follow-up visits at 6-monthly or yearly intervals provide objective assessment of a therapeutic response.

Several years are usually necessary to discern regression of a long-standing multinodular goiter, and during that time, one or more of the larger nodules may become more easily palpable as the relatively normal portions of the gland regress. Some confusion may occur if this is interpreted as a progression of the disease or as the development of a malignant nodule. Serial ultrasound examinations will help avoid this error.

Once started, suppression therapy is usually continued indefinitely but can be terminated or withdrawn if regression occurs. Most goiters recur if treatment is discontinued, but therapy can be reinstituted. Suppression therapy does not lead to permanent loss of TSH secretion, even after decades of thyroid hormone administration, although occasional individuals may manifest a brief period of hypothyroidism when prolonged suppression therapy is discontinued.

Treatment of Goiter With Surgery

Suppression therapy is slow and produces a significant response in less than half of cases. The efficacy of suppression is much clearer in patients with single nodules (59) than in those with multinodular goiters. Some also believe that the risks of inadvertent overtreatment and the need for careful monitoring make suppression an unattractive mode of therapy (56). Goiters large enough (more than 150 mL in volume) to produce not only tracheal deviation but also significant tracheal compression, as assessed by plain x-ray views, by CT of the trachea, or by flow-loop respirometry (see Chapter 60), or large enough to interfere with swallowing are now uncommon in the United States. In these significantly symptomatic cases, surgery, although attended by significant morbidity, may be considered if an experienced surgeon is available.

Radioiodide Therapy for Benign Goiters

In recent years many endocrinologists have used RaI^{131} to treat patients with goiters (56). This approach is preferable, especially in the elderly or in patients with other serious medical problems (60)—even in patients with relatively large goiters (61).

Doses of 25 to 125 mCi are necessary. Although the response is slow, useful reduction in the size of the goiter over 1 year can be achieved (61). Nearly half of the patients develop hypothyroidism after therapy (60).

THYROID NEOPLASMS

Thyroid Nodules

One of the most common abnormalities of the thyroid is a localized area of enlargement commonly known as a nodule. The approach to evaluation and treatment of a nodule is not standardized among thyroidologists. In evaluating a thyroid nodule, the possibility of malignancy is the main concern. However, current data indicate that at least 95% are benign adenomas or cysts; the remaining ones are lesions of varying degrees of malignancy, almost all of low grade. Even those that are termed malignant on histologic grounds almost always behave clinically as benign lesions, and clinically aggressive thyroid carcinoma is unusual.

Nodules are usually discovered by the patient as a visible or palpable lump or incidentally by a clinician or dentist during a physical examination. As with most newly discovered masses, the patient's concern is whether the lump is a cancer. Immediate reassurance of the patient by the practitioner is the correct response for the following reasons: First, the lump is unlikely to be a cancer (5% chance) and, second, even if it is a cancer, it is very unlikely to require either urgent or intensive therapy or involve a fatal outcome because most thyroid "cancers" simply do not behave at all like the frequently lethal varieties of cancer familiar to most patients. Thyroid cancer is one of the least common causes of cancer death (see below). Having been reassured, the patient will still need a workup (below) and additional information.

Most truly solitary nodules are benign adenomas and are encapsulated. The growth of most benign adenomas, hypofunctional although they may be, seems to depend on endogenous TSH, but other poorly defined factors are now thought to be involved (62). Although usually relatively hypofunctioning, follicular adenomas may exhibit normal or greater than normal function (i.e., they take up iodine and elaborate and secrete thyroid hormone, sometimes enough to produce hyperthyroidism). Adenomas that are functional but independent of TSH are termed autonomous.

Benign thyroid nodules are present in up to 50% of the population, depending on age and on how they are detected (62). Whether a relatively small nodule (less than 1.5 cm diameter) is detected by palpation reflects in turn the skill and effort of the examiner, the self-awareness of the patient, and the anatomy of the individual's neck. In a group of more than 200 patients with thyroid nodules (4% of 5,000 patients examined only by palpation, ages 30 to 60) followed for 15 years, none developed clinically evident malignancy. In that population, "new" (palpable) thyroid nodules continued to appear at a rate of about 1 in 1,000 people per year, about twice as frequently in women as in men (63).

Management

General Considerations. The major concern with most nodules is malignancy. The diagnostic workup and therapeutic approach to these lesions should be determined by a number of considerations, including the biologic potential of the nodule and the age of the patient (64). In the elderly, even more than in the young patient, a conservative approach is necessary because thyroid nodules are so common in older persons (62) (see above).

Because most "cold" nodules (nonfunctioning on scintiscan)—variously estimated at 75% to 95% of all nodules encountered—are benign lesions, the overall risk of malignancy is small. The risk is smaller still when it is realized that the remaining lesions are almost always clinically nonaggressive papillary or follicular carcinomas. These lesions are usually nonlethal (see below) and slow growing, so a conservative plan is always reasonable. Nonetheless, many patients become extremely anxious when faced at this point with even the possibility of cancer and may wish to proceed directly to excision. Such patients should be strongly dissuaded from this course of action because immediate and indiscriminate excision of all thyroid nodules is irrational and cannot be justified (see above).

Once the "solitary" nodule has been discovered, there are four diagnostic options: FNA, ultrasound, scintiscan, or suppression therapy with T_4. All are equally acceptable (65). The choices are described below, along with their advantages and limitations.

The issue of whether to perform an immediate biopsy (FNA) of nodules or to treat them conservatively with initial suppression has been subjected to decision analysis. The conclusion is that *no best approach exists*. The decisions to operate, suppress, or aspirate have equal validity from the point of view of outcome and depend in the individual case on such subjective factors as psychologic disability, relative cost, and attitudes toward operative risk and long-term medical therapy (65).

Solitary nodules that are not unsightly and have not rapidly enlarged may be followed by periodic physical examination (palpation) or serial sonograms. On the other hand, the possibility of *cancer*, no matter how indolent that cancer might be, is usually extremely anxiety provoking for most patients or their caregivers; thus, some action is usually thought to be required. Moreover, follow-up alone would not be considered the standard of practice in most communities.

Choosing Between Fine-Needle Aspiration, Scintiscan, or Ultrasonogram. In most cases, no palpable lymph nodes are present, thyroid function is normal, and the nodule is not part of autoimmune (Hashimoto) thyroiditis (antibodies are negative; see above). Until about 30 years ago, the next step would have been immediate surgical excision or, in a more conservative mode, radionuclide scanning to determine whether the nodule was functioning. Although a hyperfunctioning ("hot") nodule would be found in only a small percentage of cases, hot nodules are almost invariably (99.8%) benign. In contrast, a hypofunctioning, or "cold," nodule would be considered suspect and in the past was an indication for immediate surgery to rule out carcinoma. Immediate surgery is certainly obsolete, and a thyroid scan is probably not as useful initially as ultrasonography. This approach has been supported by a study that has shown that the management of about 60% of patients evaluated initially by ultrasound is significantly altered (66).

Ultrasonography as the First Step. The main advantage of obtaining a sonogram as the first diagnostic maneuver after discovery of a nodule is that, even in expert hands, many solitary nodules turn out to be only one of many in a multinodular goiter (66). Obviously, the expertise of the examiner in palpating the thyroid will strongly influence the results, but most practitioners are not expert in the examination of nodular thyroids. The sonogram is objective and excludes the need for further workup when the solitary nodule turns out to be a multinodular gland. Although some may still believe that "dominant" nodules in a multinodular gland should be suspect, the chance that one is dealing with clinically significant thyroid carcinoma in a multinodular gland is low (see above) (56). Thus, the workup may be terminated upon identification of a multinodular goiter. Cysts will also be discovered by sonogram, another advantage, because again further workup is unnecessary. Of course, many cysts are also identified when FNA is the first procedure. If, with ultrasound, the nodule is truly solitary and is not cystic, one can proceed to FNA, suppression therapy with T_4, or, if the patient insists, surgical excision.

Fine-Needle Aspiration as the First Step

Patient Experience. FNA with a 25-gauge needle is essentially painless, but cutaneous anesthesia is preferred by some. Multiple aspirations are made, often through a single skin puncture. No significant bleeding is likely to occur, although ecchymoses often result.

Some clinicians believe that all newly discovered nodules should be excised. For such circumstances FNA helps to avoid unnecessary operations. However, when clinicians have an initial approach that is conservative, universal institution of FNA may *increase* the number of unnecessary operative excisions. Reasons include frequently indeterminate cytopathologic findings and discovery of papillary carcinomas that might have been adequately treated by suppression (see Therapeutic Consideration in Thyroid Carcinoma, below). Nonetheless, recent surveys indicate that FNA (with measurement of TSH) is the diagnostic procedure of choice of the majority of endocrinologists in the United States when faced with a patient with an apparently solitary thyroid nodule (67,68).

FNA with cytologic examination, because of its simplicity and safety, has largely replaced biopsy with a conventional cutting needle in the evaluation of a solitary thyroid nodule. It is possible under optimal conditions to make an accurate diagnosis (concerning possible malignancy) in more than 90% of cases with FNA, although it is difficult or impossible to distinguish benign adenomas from many well-differentiated follicular carcinomas (64), an important limitation of the technique. Multiple aspirations (six have been recommended as ideal) should be obtained to ensure adequate sampling for cytology (64). If inadequate material is obtained, the FNA should be repeated. However, it must be stressed that the most important consideration in the use of needle aspiration is the expertise of the pathologist who examines the biopsy material. If a specifically trained cytopathologist *who regularly examines such specimens from the thyroid* is not available, FNA should be avoided. Slides can be sent, regardless of geographic distance, to a trained person with ongoing experience. Similarly, if the patient is reluctant to have FNA, one of the other approaches can be taken, including suppression therapy with thyroxine (see below).

If FNA reveals a cancer (papillary or follicular), no further diagnostic studies are indicated and treatment should be instituted (see below). If the aspiration yields cystic fluid (clear or "chocolate" brown, indicating old hemorrhage) and no troublesome cosmetic issue remains, follow-up physical examination in 6 to 12 months is adequate. If FNA reveals a benign adenoma and if thyroid function tests are normal (see Autonomous (Hot) Nodule, below), no treatment is necessary unless the nodule increases in size. Of course, suppression therapy can be used for cosmetic considerations.

Scintiscan as the First Step: Hot, Warm, and Cold Nodules. Most patients will be evaluated initially by FNA or ultrasound, but a scintiscan may be done as the first step. It will identify a hot, warm, or cold nodule and, sometimes, a multinodular goiter (although ultrasonography is a better technique to demonstrate multinodularity). The scan does not need to be combined with a measurement of thyroidal RaIU, a procedure that adds no useful information but increases the cost of the workup.

Autonomous (Hot) Nodule. If uptake of isotope is exclusively concentrated in the nodule (hot), the nodule is considered to be autonomous (69). When an adenoma produces an amount of hormone equal to or greater than that of the output of the normal gland, TSH becomes suppressed; the remaining normal tissue then becomes relatively inactive and may not be visible, or may be only poorly visible, by scintiscan.

Management of a hot nodule depends on whether an excessive amount of thyroid hormone is being produced. If the amount of hormone produced by the adenoma considerably exceeds normal, thyrotoxicosis may be clinically apparent, at least in retrospect. Usually T_4 and T_3 are produced in excess, although hyperthyroidism caused by T_3 alone (T_3 toxicosis) is fairly common with such hyperactive nodules (15). If TSH is suppressed and if the T_4 (or free T_4 or FTI) is normal, the T_3 should be determined and, if this is normal, the free T_3.

The natural history of the hot nodule is variable. Over a 10-year interval, about one-third show little change, one-third become frankly hyperactive, and the remainder become cold, sometimes with obvious hemorrhagic infarction and cystic degeneration. Treatment of the hot nodule that is producing hyperthyroidism can be satisfactorily accomplished with surgery or radioactive iodine, although hypothyroidism may result with the latter. Several studies have shown that hot nodules can be safely and effectively ablated nonsurgically by injection with ethanol. The advantage over radioiodide is that hypothyroidism does not occur (70). Prophylactic ablative therapy is not indicated if hyperthyroidism is not present. Suppression therapy with thyroid hormone will, of course, be ineffective and lead to iatrogenic hyperthyroidism. An antithyroid drug will control the excessive thyroid hormone production but must be continued indefinitely and is a poor choice.

Warm Nodule. On the initial scan, some nodules are not unequivocally cold or hot; instead, they appear to take up some tracer, but not to the exclusion of the remainder of the gland. Their status can be further defined by repeating the scan after several weeks of suppression. Some prove to be autonomous and can be managed as a hot nodule; others prove to be cold and should be managed as described below.

Cold Nodule. If the scan shows no accumulation ("uptake") of isotope in the nodule (located by a marker), it is considered to be nonfunctional (i.e., "cold"); most nodules fall into this category. Although most cold nodules are benign, these are the lesions that are considered suspect and thus need to be subjected to FNA or ultrasound or treated with suppression.

Thyroid Hormone Suppression Therapy for Benign Nodular Disease

Efficacy of Suppression Therapy. The current consensus is that suppression therapy is often effective for treatment of benign nodular disease (59). Single nodules, simple (non-nodular) goiters, and multinodular glands do respond to suppression therapy, but the reported response rates are variable; approximately 25% show complete regression; another 25%, moderate regression; and the remainder, no apparent response (59). Studies that purport to show no responses at all may be the result of inadequate duration of therapy or inadequate dosage. Experienced clinicians have observed that the regression of nodular disease can be slow and may take years; studies using 6-month trials are simply too brief. The notion that the TSH should be suppressed only to the lower limits of normal (57) in "sensitive" assays (second or third generation) is unsupported. No data indicate that this degree of suppression is sufficient to induce regression. Additional studies are needed to determine the optimal degree of suppression required to effectively treat benign disease and to determine whether this differs from that required for the treatment of malignant lesions. Concerns about overtreatment are discussed below.

Safety of Suppression Therapy: Concerns Over Iatrogenic Bone Demineralization (Osteoporosis) and Heart Disease. The extensive experience of many thyroid experts does not suggest that adverse cardiac consequences are likely to occur (71). Also fears of inducing demineralization of bones are unfounded provided that suitable monitoring can be assured. Only patients with a history of overt hyperthyroidism show demineralization (see Hypothyroidism, Importance Of Avoiding Overtreatment During Thyroxine Replacement Therapy, above).

Course. Regression of a nodule over a 6-month period of suppression of TSH with T_4 indicates clinically benign disease; such nodules can be followed indefinitely with continued suppression therapy. Some endocrinologists are satisfied that benign disease is present when a nodule at least does not grow larger during suppression therapy over the initial 6 months, after which suppression can continue. Regression of some undetected TSH-dependent histologically malignant nodules will also no doubt occur. Clinicians should not be dismayed by this statement, implying as it does that some carcinomas are being "missed" by this approach. Suppression therapy is the mainstay of postoperative therapy of such lesions, and there is little reason to believe that the delay in diagnosis—if the diagnosis is ever made—will be harmful, although the data on this point are available only for 1 year of follow-up (65).

Treatment of Thyroid Cysts. If a predominantly cystic nodule is identified on sonogram, aspiration or suppression therapy, or both, can be considered. Some cystic nodules require several aspirations, but most eventually disappear with this approach. Sclerosing solutions have been used for recurrent cysts. Suppression therapy after aspiration is rational because most cysts arise in degenerated benign adenomas, but its usefulness is not established. The sonogram provides an objective and accurate measurement of the size of cysts for follow-up.

Thyroid Carcinomas

General Considerations

Approximately 75% to 85% of thyroid carcinomas are of the papillary variety; 5% to 15% are follicular carcinomas. Anaplastic and medullary carcinomas probably account for no more than 5% of the total. The relative frequency of the various types of thyroid carcinomas is markedly age dependent (see below).

Occult thyroid carcinoma (defined as a lesion with the histologic appearance of carcinoma but less than 1.5 cm in diameter) is found at autopsy in 5% to 10% of U.S. and European populations and in 30% of Japanese samples. Death from thyroid carcinoma is as rare in Japan as in the United States. Clearly, occult carcinoma behaves as a benign disease and does not warrant aggressive management.

In the United States, over 10,000 new cases of thyroid carcinoma are seen each year, but only about 1,500 persons die of this disorder. Most of these deaths result from anaplastic tumors (50%) or from unusually aggressive follicular carcinomas. A few deaths are attributable to aggressive papillary tumors and medullary carcinomas.

Papillary Carcinoma

Available information supports a middle-of-the-road initial approach, one that falls between thyroid hormone suppression therapy without surgery and radical surgery alone. Long-term observations have also reasonably defined the role of radioiodide ablation therapy (62,72).

Regarding surgery for papillary carcinoma, follow-up at 10 years indicates a recurrence rate of approximately 20% for subtotal resection versus 10% for total removal of the gland. Deaths caused by carcinoma are 1.5% and 0.5%, respectively. This small difference was statistically significant in one retrospective study and currently strongly influences the surgical approach. However, the complication rate for total thyroidectomy (hypoparathyroidism, vocal cord paralysis) remains high. As a result, many surgeons have now adopted a modified or near-total thyroidectomy. In this procedure the affected side is completely removed; most of the contralateral lobe is also removed but the posterior capsule is left, together with the tip of the upper pole. Whether this approach will succeed in reducing complications remains to be established. Conservative surgeons generally support more limited surgery (73). Visibly involved lymph nodes are always removed, but radical neck dissection is not justified even in the presence of obviously involved nodes (62,72). The presence of cervical node metastases at operation or the extent of lymphadenectomy does not seem to influence either recurrence or death rate. The death rate in lesions under 2.5 cm without local invasion and without evident distant metastases at the time of surgery is less than 1% in 10 years and is 4% to 8% in the less favorable categories (62,72).

Postoperative Therapy and Its Monitoring: Thyroid-stimulating Hormone Suppression, Thyroglobulin in Serum, and Residual Thyroid Tumor Ablation With Radioiodide

Thyroid-stimulating Hormone Suppression. Suppression of TSH after surgical treatment of differentiated thyroid cancer is of proven benefit, definitely lowering recurrence and mortality rates. However, supraphysiologic doses of T_4 for long-term TSH suppression therapy can result in iatrogenic hyperthyroidism, usually asymptomatic, but in some instances leading to cardiac hypertrophy, atrial fibrillation, and bone demineralization (see Hypothyroidism, above). The consensus view, nonetheless, is that long-term post-thyroidectomy TSH suppression is essential. Unfortunately, the optimal level of suppression is not known. In practice, a sensitive second- or a third-generation TSH assay should be used to monitor the suppression dose of T_4. During replacement/suppression therapy T_4 dosage is titrated by some experts to at least the minimal amount necessary to keep the TSH below the limit of normal (0.4 to 0.5 mU/L) but above 0.1 mU/L. At this level, the development of echocardiographic abnormalities is avoided and normal bone metabolic parameters are maintained. Others, however, titrate T_4 dosage to the limit of detection of TSH in a third-generation assay (0.01 mU/L) and believe that the minimal effect on cardiac function is not clinically significant (74).

Serum Thyroglobulin. Adequacy of the suppression dose of T_4 can be monitored not only by the level of TSH but by measurement of serum thyroglobulin, a marker that is a sensitive indicator of the post-thyroidectomy residual tumor burden. If the thyroglobulin is below 2 ng/mL with the TSH in the normal range, it has been suggested that no tumor remains and that the TSH can be allowed to remain in the normal range (i.e., that T_4 dosage can be at normal replacement levels).

Radioiodide Ablation of Residual Tumor. Postoperative therapy with full replacement doses of T_4 (see above) suppresses endogenous TSH, reduces recurrence, and is routine in all cases. In addition, postsurgical ablative therapy with radioactive iodide has a role, although not all cases of localized disease need to be treated. The patient with a minimal papillary lesion needs no such therapy, but the patient with a large locally invasive lesion should receive ablative therapy with ^{131}I. In cases with an intermediate-size lesion, without invasion of the thyroid capsule, and without lymph node metastases, the recurrence rate is greatly reduced by treatment with radioiodide, and deaths from recurrent disease may be completely abolished. The hesitation to use radioiodide routinely stems from the fear of radiation-induced leukemia, a problem that is a significant risk at high (cumulative) dosage of RaI^{131}.

Therapy with RaI^{131} after surgery requires that the patient's residual tumor is stimulated by TSH to take up a maximal amount of the dose of isotope. Until recently, this was accomplished by withdrawal of T_4 replacement/suppression therapy for 3 to 4 weeks, thus allowing endogenous TSH to rise. However, during the last week or 2 of this interval, many individuals experience the distressing symptoms of rapidly developing hypothyroidism, which then continues for several weeks even after reinstitution of T_4 therapy. Fortunately, it is no longer necessary to withdraw T_4. This period of discomfort can now be avoided, because recombinant human TSH has become available for routine use. Given by injection as two or three doses over 2 to 7 days, respectively, the recombinant human TSH primes the residual thyroid tissue and tumor as effectively as endogenous TSH after T_4 withdrawal. Two doses seem as effective as three (75). Use of recombinant human TSH is a significant advance for reducing morbidity in this situation. The first course of post-TSH RaI^{131} therapy is usually given several months after recovery from initial surgery with additional courses at approximately yearly intervals until post-therapy scans show that no residual functioning tissue in the thyroid bed or metastatic tumor tissue can be detected.

Ambulatory RaI^{131} Therapy. A dose of RaI^{131} greater than 30 mC, given for any purpose in the United States, requires isolation of the patient for several days in a suitable hospital room; lower doses can be used in an ambulatory setting. Some experts use the ambulatory approach, favoring a larger number of low doses, if necessary, over the traditional higher ones (100 to 150 mC) to avoid the need for hospitalization and isolation. No systematic comparisons of the two approaches have been made, but in low risk patients with no evidence of spread of tumor beyond the regional area, the results appear to be comparable. When a patient has evidence of distant metastatic disease, rigorous treatment with high dose RaI^{131} is indicated (76).

Follicular Carcinoma

Well-differentiated follicular carcinomas have until recently been very difficult or impossible to distinguish from benign follicular adenomas on cytopathologic grounds, but a new immunologic marker approach appears to have largely eliminated this limitation of FNA (6). This technique is not yet in wide use. In the past, even excised lesions were occasionally thought to be benign on histopathologic examination, only to declare themselves as malignant by developing metastases.

Follicular carcinoma can be more aggressive than papillary carcinoma, tends to be angioinvasive, and may metastasize to bones and lungs. The tumor may bypass regional lymph nodes, a marked difference from papillary disease. The most important prognostic feature is invasion of tumor, either through the tumor capsule or into blood vessels. At least one report suggests that, unlike papillary carcinoma, primary tumor size at presentation does not appear to influence prognosis (77). In contrast, in another series not a single patient died who was under 45 and who had an intrathyroidal tumor less than 2.5 cm in diameter (78).

The clinical presentation may be very different from that of papillary disease; the patient may already have metastatic disease involving lungs, bone, brain, or spinal cord at the time of initial diagnosis. In these cases, the primary tumor may be relatively small and initially overlooked. Only rarely do the metastases produce sufficient thyroid hormones to cause thyrotoxicosis.

The surgical approach to follicular carcinoma should be that taken for papillary carcinoma. Suppression therapy with thyroid hormone replacement is routine. Postoperative ablative therapy with radioiodide appears warranted (78), especially for those patients with overtly invasive disease. However, the case for *routine* postoperative use of ^{131}I ablation therapy (see above) in the treatment of follicular carcinoma is not statistically established (72).

Anaplastic Carcinoma

Fortunately, anaplastic carcinoma is distinctly uncommon; its frequency depends on the age of the population. Anaplastic carcinoma is rare in children and in adults under the age of 35. By age 50, as many as 10% of cases of thyroid carcinoma are due to anaplastic disease, and by age 80, by which time the overall incidence of thyroid carcinoma has fallen markedly, nearly half of the cases that do occur are of this variety. The disease is locally invasive in a highly aggressive fashion and quickly produces pain, dysphagia, hemoptysis, and hoarseness. Death usually occurs within 6 to 12 months. However, surgically resectable disease without evidence of metastases, even if it has extended outside the thyroid capsule, can be associated with long-term survival (20% to 30%). It is important to distinguish the small cell type of anaplastic carcinoma from lymphoma of the thyroid. This rare disease, unlike anaplastic carcinoma, is radiosensitive and amenable to chemotherapy.

Medullary Carcinoma

Medullary carcinoma accounts for 1% to 2% of all thyroid cancers. The tumors arise from the parafollicular or C cells and produce thyrocalcitonin. Both sporadic and familial varieties are known. The sporadic case typically presents as a solitary nodule, whereas the familial variety is often multifocal and part of a multiple endocrine adenomatosis syndrome. Diarrhea occurs in some patients. Thyrocalcitonin in serum is elevated in the basal state or after stimulation with calcium or pentagastrin infusion. Some authorities advocate obtaining at least a basal (unstimulated) serum thyrocalcitonin level as part of the initial evaluation of all nonfunctional thyroid nodules (79,80). Although such routine measurement of thyrocalcitonin is not ordinarily done in the United States, it is common practice in Europe. When surgical excision is performed before regional nodes have become involved, 90% of patients survive for 10 years. Once the nodes are involved, only 40% survival can be expected. Medullary carcinoma does not appear to respond to suppression therapy with thyroid hormone.

The Question of Carcinoma in the Multinodular Thyroid

For many years, occult thyroid carcinoma was defined as any lesion (nodule) 1.5 cm or less in diameter that on histologic examination appeared malignant. Most of these were undetectable by palpation or scan and were incidental findings at thyroid surgery or at autopsy (see Thyroid Carcinomas, General Considerations, above). Much evidence suggested that these lesions were not of clinical significance. Sonography (or occasionally palpation) now frequently identifies a lesion of 1 to 1.5 cm that is then subjected to FNA and reported by the cytopathologist as a thyroid carcinoma. Subsequently, without consideration of its size, the lesion is surgically removed without regard for its clinically innocuous character. Yet no new concepts or data have evolved in recent years to suggest that these small lesions now need surgical removal when previously they were properly ignored. The new reality is that identification of these small lesions, cytopathologically, is likely to lead to thyroidectomy.

The risk of *clinically significant* carcinoma in a nodular goiter is low. Recent evidence suggests that overall one can expect about 5% of multinodular glands to harbor such a lesion, about the same as for single nodules (56), a figure that has decreased from a high of about 20% only a few years ago. It seems clear that the true incidence is probably closer to the lower number and may be even less than 5% (81). It seems clear that therapy should be as conservative as possible, consistent with the patient's and clinician's levels of comfort (see above).

Radiation-Associated Thyroid Carcinoma

Low-dose irradiation of the thyroid is a stimulus to thyroid carcinogenesis, with a latency period of one to several decades (82). The radiation may be from an external source or from radioiodide as has occurred after nuclear bomb fallout or the nuclear reactor accident at Chernobyl. Public health authorities recommend stockpiling stable iodide for distribution to exposed persons in case of a nuclear plant accident. A single dose of 50 mg of sodium iodide would suffice to protect the thyroid in such an event.

In recent years, papillary and follicular thyroid carcinomas have been reported to occur in increased incidence in patients who received radiation therapy years earlier for conditions such as enlarged tonsils or adenoids, or an enlarged thymus, or for acne. A distinction must be made between treatment with penetrating external radiation and local irradiation with point sources (radium rod and plaque treatment). It has not been possible to relate thyroid carcinoma to the limited exposure that occurs with point sources of radiation.

No relationship has been seen between radiation and the development of medullary or anaplastic carcinoma, but radiation-induced cancers appear to present more often with dissemination than those occurring spontaneously, an argument for early detection (72). Accordingly, high-resolution thyroid scintiscans or sonograms should be part of the follow-up of patients previously exposed to radiation, because nonpalpable lesions can be detected. The only blood test of value is determination of serum thyroglobulin, elevation of which predicts the development of nodules (83).

The approach to the patient with a history of irradiation to the head and neck is not currently standardized. Examination of the patient at 2- to 3-year intervals should suffice. Routine isotopic scintigraphy or sonographic examination of the thyroid to detect patients with nonpalpable lesions is probably indicated. Many nonpalpable lesions (0.5 to 1.0 cm) can be detected by these methods. Thyroid suppression with T_4 is recommended even for patients with nodules detected only by scintigraphy or sonography. If careful follow-up reveals an increase in the size of the nodule despite suppression, surgery should be performed.

Surgical therapy should involve the same approach as that for nonirradiated patients (i.e., near-total thyroidectomy), although the earlier practice of lobectomy still has its advocates (73). All patients who have had surgery for benign or malignant nodules should receive suppression therapy with thyroid hormone. Recurrence of benign nodules, but not malignant ones, is greatly reduced (84).

Radiation of the head and neck predisposes patients not only to thyroid cancer but to salivary gland tumors with a ratio of benign to malignant lesions similar to that of nodules in the thyroid. The incidence of benign neural tumors (neurilemomas, acoustic neuromas) and parathyroid adenomas is also increased. External radiation can also ablate thyroid tissue and produce hypothyroidism. This has been seen, for example, in mantle irradiation for Hodgkin's disease and can occur after combined surgery and irradiation for head and neck cancers such as those of the larynx.

THYROIDITIS

Pyogenic (Suppurative) Thyroiditis

Pyogenic or suppurative thyroiditis, also known as acute thyroiditis, is rare, and most clinicians will never encounter a case. The thyroid infection usually follows bacteremia but can occur as an isolated primary event. The gland shows typical signs of an acute inflammatory process.

Riedel Thyroiditis

Riedel thyroiditis is another rare but indolent and painless form of thyroiditis. The intense induration associated with this process makes the clinical differentiation from infiltrating neoplasm difficult.

Hashimoto Thyroiditis

Hashimoto thyroiditis is common (see Hypothyroidism and Goiter and Iodide Deficiency, above, and Table 80.7). The process is painless and usually produces only modest enlargement of the thyroid. Nodularity is the rule, and the consistency on palpation is classically rubber-like. Distinction from other nontoxic nodular goiters is made by the presence of high titers of thyroid autoantibodies in the serum of approximately 90% of patients with Hashimoto thyroiditis.

Subacute Thyroiditis

Subacute thyroiditis, also known as granulomatous or de Quervain thyroiditis, is common. Many mild cases are probably never diagnosed. The term *subacute* is often deceiving and sometimes inappropriate. Although the onset may be insidious, it is perhaps just as often acute over several days. Many patients give a history of recent antecedent upper respiratory tract infection.

The earliest symptoms may be referred pain, usually to the ear, but pain can appear to originate in the jaw or occiput. This phase may last a few hours or days before tenderness and discomfort in the thyroid area become apparent. Rarely, the patient is concerned only with the referred pain and is unaware of thyroidal tenderness until examination makes it apparent. When the onset is acute, the symptoms and signs are more likely to be severe. Initially, pain and swelling of the thyroid are often unilateral, but the process usually does not remain localized for more than a few days. Systemic symptoms include fever, especially in acute cases, and a sensation of intense fatigue and malaise. The course may be protracted with symptoms persisting for months, although usually they subside within a week or 2.

The erythrocyte sedimentation rate is elevated. Early in the disease, the thyroidal RaIU is depressed, and serum T_4 may be elevated. Mild cases have no or only borderline abnormalities of the tests. Significant titers of thyroid autoantibodies are not common but can be seen. The RaIU test is not likely to be useful diagnostically because in many normal people the uptake is low (see above).

Clinical hyperthyroidism is occasionally seen with subacute thyroiditis (see above). Rarely, hypothyroidism occurs and lasts for several months. Permanent hypothyroidism is unusual. A variant of this syndrome has been described in which neither hypothyroidism nor hyperthyroidism is present but symptoms of severe systemic illness with fever and weight loss dominate (85). Blood tests of thyroid function are normal except for minimal elevation of free T_4 in a few. Thyroidal RaIU is low. Thyroid autoantibodies are not present. The thyroid is modestly enlarged and nontender in most cases, but even this clue is absent in some. Biopsies are typical of lymphocytic thyroiditis. Patients respond to anti-inflammatory therapy (see below).

Therapy

Therapy of subacute thyroiditis is symptomatic. The patient should be strongly reassured concerning the benign self-limited character of the disorder. No controlled studies of drug efficacy for symptom relief are available. Widespread practice indicates that thyroid tenderness often responds within several days to aspirin in doses sufficient to maintain therapeutic (anti-inflammatory) blood levels with prompt relapse if the dose is reduced to analgesic levels. Published experience with nonsteroidal anti-inflammatory agents is minimal but suggests that these agents may be as effective as aspirin. Codeine should be added if neck discomfort is severe. In less than 10% of cases, the process may be severe enough to require glucocorticoid therapy (30 to 60 mg of prednisone daily or equivalent). A glucocorticoid produces prompt relief of pain and tenderness but, if the disease is severe enough to require its use, will usually be necessary for weeks to several months. Relapse is common when glucocorticoid therapy is discontinued, and retreatment may be necessary.

Lymphocytic Thyroiditis (Silent Thyroiditis)

Lymphocytic thyroiditis is an important process that occurs in association with both hyperthyroidism and hypothyroidism and is discussed earlier, under Thyrotoxicosis Associated with Thyroiditis and with Postpartum Thyroid Dysfunction.

General References*

Braverman LE, Utiger RD, eds. Werner and Ingbar's The Thyroid, 8th ed. Philadelphia: JB Lippincott, 2000.

Comprehensive textbook on all aspects of the subject.

Felig P, Baxter JD, Frohman LA, eds. Endocrinology and Metabolism. 4th ed. New York: McGraw-Hill, 2001.

Williams RH, Wilson J, Foster D, et al., eds. Williams' textbook of Endocrinology, 9th ed. Philadelphia: Harcourt Brace, 1999.

Standard textbooks containing excellent chapters on the thyroid.

Hamburger JI. The Thyroid Gland: A Book for Thyroid Patients, 7th ed privately published by Dr. Hamburger, 1991. Available through The Thyroid Foundation of America, Inc. (Telephone: 617-726-8500; e-mail: www.tsh.org).

Wood LC, Cooper DS, Ridgeway EC. Your Thyroid: a home reference, 3rd ed. New York: Random House, 1996.

These two books are written for patients with thyroid disease.

Ross DA, ed. Assessment of Thyroid function and disease. Endocrinol Metab Clin North Am 2001;30.

Specific References

1. Laurberg P. Iodine intake—what are we aiming at? J Clin Endocrinol Metab 1994;79:17.
2. Franklyn JA, Black EG, Betteridge J, et al. Comparison of second and third generation methods for measurement of serum

*Bold print (general references) and bold numerals (specific references) denote published controlled clinical trials, meta-analyses, or consensus-based recommendations.

thyrotropin in patients with overt hyperthyroidism, patients receiving thyroxine therapy, and those with nonthyroidal illness. J Clin Endocrinol Metab 1994;78:1368.
3. Wardle CA, Fraser CA, Squire CR. Pitfalls in the use of thyrotropin concentration as a first-line thyroid-function test. Lancet 2001;357:1013.
4. Carr D, McLeod DT, Parry G, et al. Fine adjustment of thyroxine replacement dosage: comparison of the thyrotrophin releasing hormone test using a sensitive thyrotrophin assay with measurement of free thyroid hormones and clinical assessment. Clin Endocrinol 1988;28:325.
5. Stott DJ, McLellan AR, Finlayson J, et al. Elderly patients with suppressed serum TSH but normal free thyroid hormone levels usually have mild thyroid overactivity and are at increased risk of developing overt hyperthyroidism. Q J Med 1991;285: 77.
6. Bartolazzi A, Gasbarri A, Papotti M, et al. Application of an immunodiagnostic method for improving preoperative diagnosis of nodular thyroid lesions. Lancet 2001;357:1644.
7. Borst GC, Eil C, Burman KD. Euthyroid hyperthyroxinemia. Ann Intern Med 1983;98:366.
8. Wartofsky L, Burman KD. Alterations in thyroid function in patients with systemic illness: the "euthyroid sick syndrome." Endocrinol Rev 1982;3:164.
9. Wehmann RE, Gregerman RI, Burns WH, et al. Suppression of thyrotropin in the low-thyroxine state of severe nonthyroidal illness. N Engl J Med 1985;312:546.
10. Marquesee E, Haden ST, Utiger RD. Subclinical thyrotoxicosis. Endocrinol Metab Clin North Am 1998;27:37.
11. Gregerman RI, Katz MS. Thyroid diseases. In: Hazzard R, Bierman EL, Blass JP, et al., eds. Principles of geriatric medicine. 3rd ed. New York: McGraw-Hill, 1994:807.
12. Surks MI, DeFesi CR. Normal serum free thyroid hormone concentrations in patients treated with phenytoin or carbamazepine. JAMA 1996;275:1495.
13. Roca RP, Blackman MR, Ackerly MB, et al. Nonsuppression of serum TSH during hyperthyroninemia among acute psychiatric inpatients. Endocrine Res 1990;16:415.
14. Wortsman J, Premachandra BN, Williams K, et al. Familial resistance to thyroid hormone associated with decreased transport across the plasma membrane. Ann Intern Med 1983;98: 904.
15. Hamburger JI. Pitfalls in the laboratory diagnosis of atypical hyperthyroidism. Arch Intern Med 1979;139:96.
16. Nikolai TF, Coombs GJ, McKenzie AK. Lymphocytic thyroiditis with spontaneously resolving hyperthyroidism and subacute thyroiditis. Long-term follow-up. Arch Intern Med 1981;141:1455.
17. Daniels GH. Amiodarone-induced thyrotoxicosis. J Clin Endocrinol Metab 2001;86:3.
18. Bahn RS, Heufelder AE. Mechanisms of disease: pathogenesis of Graves ophthalmopathy. N Engl J Med 1993;329:1468.
19. Torring O, Tallstedt L, Wallin G, et al. Graves' hyperthyroidism: treatment with antithyroid drugs, surgery, or radioiodine—a prospective randomized study. J Clin Endocrinol Metab 1996;81:2986.
20. Allahabadia A, Daykin J, Holder RL, et al. Age and gender predict the outcome of treatment for Graves' hyperthyroidism. J Clin Endocrinol Metab 2000;85:1038.
21. Hashizume K, Ichikawa K, Sakurai A, et al. Administration of thyroxine in treated Graves' disease. Effects on the level of antibodies to thyroid-stimulating hormone receptors and on the risk of recurrence of hyperthyroidism. N Engl J Med 1991;324: 947.
22. DeGroot LJ, Gorman CA, Pinchera A, et al. Radiation and Graves' ophthalmopathy. J Clin Endocrinol Metab 1995;80:339.
23. Roti E, Minelli R, Salvi M. Management of hyperthyroidism and hypothyroidism in the pregnant woman. J Clin Endocrinol Metab 1996;81:1679.
24. Mandel SJ, Cooper DS. The use of antithyroid drugs in pregnancy and lactation. J Clin Endocrinol Metab 2001;86:2354.
25. Haddow JE, Palomaki GE, Allan WC, et al. Maternal thyroid deficiency during pregnancy and subsequent neuropsychological development of the child. N Engl J Med 1999;341:549.
26. Smallridge RC, Ladenson PW. Hypothyroidism in pregnancy: consequences to neonatal health. J Clin Endocrinol Metab 2001;86:2349.
27. Wang R, Nelson JC, Weiss RM, et al. Accuracy of free thyroxine measurements across natural ranges of thyroxine binding to single proteins. Thyroid 2000;10:31.
28. Kahaly GJ, Rösler H-P, Pitz S, et al. Low-versus high-dose radiotherapy for Graves' ophthalmopathy: a randomized, single blind trial. J Clin Endocrinol Metab 2000;85:102.
29. Figge J, Leinung M, Goodman AD, et al. The clinical evaluation of patients with subclinical hyperthyroidism and free triiodothyronine (free T_3) toxicosis. Am J Med 1994;96:229.
30. Sawin CT, Geller A, Kaplan MM. Low serum thyrotropin (thyroid-stimulating hormone) in older persons without hyperthyroidism. Arch Intern Med 1991;151:165.
31. Sawin CT, Geller A, Wolf PA, et al. Low serum thyrotropin concentrations as a risk factor for atrial fibrillation in older persons. N Engl J Med 1994;331:1249.
32. Utiger RD. Subclinical hyperthyroidism—just a low serum thyrotropin concentration, or something more? N Engl J Med 1994; 331:1302.
33. Cooper DS. Subclinical hypothyroidism. N Engl J Med 2001; 345:260.
34. Cooper DS, Halpern R, Wood LC, et al. L-Thyroxine therapy in subclinical hypothyroidism. A double-blind, placebo-controlled trial. Ann Intern Med 1984;101:18.
35. Grebe SKG, Cooke RR, Ford HC, et al. Treatment of hypothyroidism with once weekly thyroxine. J Clin Endocrinol Metab 1997;82:870.
36. Bunevicius R, Kazanavicius G, Zalenkevicius R, et al. Effects of thyroxine as compared with thyroxine plus triiodothyronine in patients with hypothyroidism. N Engl J Med 1999;340: 424.
37. Toft AD. Thyroid hormone replacement—one hormone or two? N Engl J Med 1999;340:469.
38. Baran DT. Detrimental skeletal effects of thyrotropin suppressive doses of thyroxine: fact or fantasy? J Clin Endocrinol Metab 1994;78:816.
39. Marcocci C, Golia F, Bruno-Bossio G, et al. Carefully monitored levothyroxine suppressive therapy is not associated with bone loss in premenopausal women. J Clin Endocrinol Metab 1994;78:818.
40. Bauer DC, Ettinger B, Nevitt MC, et al. Risk for fracture in women with low serum levels of thyroid-stimulating hormone. Ann Intern Med 2001;134:561.
41. Oppenheimer JH, Braverman LE, Toft A, et al. Thyroid hormone treatment: when and what? J Clin Endocrinol Metab 1995;80:2873.
42. Fung HYM, Kologlu M, Collison K, et al. Postpartum thyroid dysfunction in Mid Glamorgan. BMJ 1988;296:241.
43. Amino N, Tada H, Hidaka Y, et al. Screening for postpartum thyroiditis. J Clin Endocrinol Metab 1999;84:1813.
44. Premawardhana LDKE, Parkes AB, Ammari F, et al. Postpartum thyroiditis and long-term thyroid status: prognostic influence of thyroid peroxidase antibodies and ultrasound echogenicity. J Clin Endocrinol Metab 2000;85:71.
45. Alvarez-Marfany M, Roman SH, Drexler AJ, et al. Long-term prospective study of postpartum thyroid dysfunction in women with insulin dependent diabetes mellitus. J Clin Endocrinol Metab 1994;79:10.
46. Bagchi N, Brown TR, Parish RF, et al. Thyroid dysfunction in adults over age 55 years: a study in an urban US Community. Arch Intern Med 1990;150:785.
47. Helfand M, Crapo IM. Screening for thyroid disease. Ann Intern Med 1990;112:840.
48. Eggertsen R, Petersen K, Lundberg PA, et al. Screening for thyroid disease in a primary care unit with a thyroid stimulating hormone assay with a low detection limit. BMJ 1988;297: 1586.
49. Danese MD, Powe NR, Sawin CT, et al. Screening for mild thyroid failure at the periodic health examination. A decision and cost-effectiveness analysis. JAMA 1996;276:285.
50. Goldmann DR. Subclinical hypothyroidism revisited. When is not enough really not enough? J Gen Intern Med 1996;11:771.

51. Helfand M, Redfern CC, Sox HC. Screening for thyroid disease. Ann Intern Med 1998;129:141.
52. Helfand M, Redfern CC. Screening for thyroid disease: an update. Ann Intern Med 1998;129:144.
53. Ehrmann DA, Sarne DH. Serum thyrotropin and the assessment of thyroid status. Ann Intern Med 1989;110:179.
54. Parle JV, Franklin JA, Cross KW, et al. Prevalence and follow-up of abnormal thyrotrophin (TSH) concentrations in the elderly in the United Kingdom. Clin Endocrinol 1991;34:77.
55. Finucane P, Rudra T, Church H, et al. Thyroid function tests in elderly patients with and without an acute illness. Age Aging 1989;18:398.
56. Samuels MH. Evaluation and treatment of sporadic nontoxic goiter—some answers and more questions. J Clin Endocrinol Metab 2001;86:994.
57. Bistrup C, Nielsen JD, Gregersen G, et al. Preventive effect of levothyroxine in patients operated for non-toxic goitre: a randomized trial of one hundred patients with nine years follow-up. Clin Endocrinol 1994;40:323.
58. Hegedus L, Nygaard B, Hansen JM. Is routine thyroxine treatment to hinder postoperative recurrence of nontoxic goiter justified? J Clin Endocrinol Metab 1999;84:756.
59. Zelmanovitz F, Genro S, Gross JL. Suppressive therapy with levothyroxine for solitary thyroid nodules: a double-blind controlled clinical study and cumulative meta-analyses. J Clin Endocrinol Metab 1998;83:3881.
60. Wesche MT, Tiel-v Buul MMC, Lips P, et al. A randomized trial comparing levothyroxine with radioactive iodine in the treatment of sporadic nontoxic goiter. J Clin Endocrinol Metab 2001;86:998.
61. Bonnema SJ, Bertelsen H, Mortensen J, et al. The feasibility of high dose iodine 131 treatment as an alternative to surgery in patients with a very large goiter: effect on thyroid function and size and pulmonary function. J Clin Endocrinol Metab 1999;84:3636.
62. Mazzaferri EL. Management of a solitary thyroid nodule. N Engl J Med 1993;328:553.
63. Vander JB, Gaston EA, Dawber TR. The significance of nontoxic thyroid nodules. Final report of a 15-year study of the incidence of thyroid malignancy. Ann Intern Med 1968;69:537.
64. Hamburger JI. Diagnosis of thyroid nodules by fine needle biopsy: use and abuse. J Clin Endocrinol Metab 1994;79:335.
65. Molitch ME, Beck JR, Dreisman M, et al. The cold thyroid nodule: an analysis of diagnostic and therapeutic options. Endocrinol Rev 1984;5:185.
66. Marqusee E, Benson CB, Frates MC, et al. Usefulness of ultrasound in the management of nodular thyroid disease. Ann Intern Med 2000;133:696.
67. Singer PA, Cooper DS, Daniels GH, et al. Treatment guidelines for patients with thyroid nodules and well-differentiated thyroid cancer. Arch Intern Med 1996;156:2165.
68. Feld S. AACE clinical practice guidelines for the diagnosis and management of thyroid nodules. Endocr Pract 1969;2:78.
69. Hamburger JI. The autonomously functioning thyroid nodule: Goetsch's disease. Endocrinol Rev 1987;8:439.
70. Lippi F, Ferrari C, Manetti L, et al. Treatment of solitary autonomous thyroid nodules by percutaneous ethanol injection: results of an Italian multicenter study. J Clin Endocrinol Metab 1996;81:3261.
71. Ladenson PW. Thyrotoxicosis and the heart: something old and something new. J Clin Endocrinol Metab 1993;77:332.
72. Samaan NA, Schultz PN, Hickey RC, et al. The results of various modalities of treatment of well differentiated thyroid carcinomas: a retrospective review of 1599 patients. J Clin Endocdrinol Metab 1992;75:714.
73. Baker RR, Hyland J. Papillary carcinoma of the thyroid gland. Surg Gynecol Obstet 1985;161:546.
74. Shapiro LE, Sievert R, Ong L, et al. Minimal cardiac effects in asymptomatic athyreotic patients chronically treated with thyrotropin-suppressive doses of L-thyroxine. J Clin Endocrinol Metab 1997;82:2592.
75. Robbins RJ, Tuttle RM, Sharaf RN, et al. Preparation by recombinant human thyrotropin or thyroid hormone withdrawal are comparable for the detection of residual differentiated thyroid carcinoma. J Clin Endocrinol Metab 2001;86:619.
76. Maxon HR 3rd, Smith HS. Radioiodine-131 in the diagnosis and treatment of metastatic well differentiated thyroid cancer. Endocrinol Metab Clin North Am 1990;19:685.
77. Young RL, Mazzaferri EL, Rahe AJ, et al. Pure follicular carcinoma: impact of therapy in 214 patients. J Nucl Med 1980;21:733.
78. DeGroot LJ, Kaplan EL, Shukla MS, et al. Morbidity and mortality in follicular thyroid cancer. J Clin Endocrinol Metab 1995;80:2946.
79. Dunn JT. When is a thyroid nodule a sporadic medullary carcinoma? J Clin Endocrinol Metab 1994;78:824.
80. Pacini F, Fontanelli M, Fugazzola L, et al. Routine measurement of serum calcitonin in nodular thyroid diseases allows the preoperative diagnosis of unsuspected sporadic medullary thyroid carcinoma. J Clin Endocrinol Metab 1994;78:826.
81. Aghini-Lombardi F, Antonangeli L, Martino E, et al. The spectrum of thyroid disorders in an iodine-deficient community: the Pescopagano survey. J Clin Endocrinol Metab 1999;84:561.
82. Schneider AB, Recant W, Pinsky SM, et al. Radiation-induced thyroid carcinoma. Clinical course and results of therapy in 296 patients. Ann Intern Med 1986;105:405.
83. Schneider AB, Shore-Freedman E, Ryo UY, et al. Prospective serum thyroglobulin measurements in assessing the risk of developing thyroid nodules in patients exposed to childhood neck irradiation. J Clin Endocrinol Metab 1985;61:547.
84. Fogelfeld L, Wiviott MBT, Shore-Freedman E, et al. Recurrence of thyroid nodules after surgical removal in patients irradiated in childhood for benign conditions. N Engl J Med 1989;320:835.
85. Rotenberg Z, Weinberger I, Fuchs J, et al. Euthyroid atypical subacute thyroiditis simulating systemic or malignant disease. Arch Intern Med 1986;146:105.

C H A P T E R 81

Selected Endocrine Problems: Disorders of Pituitary, Adrenal, and Parathyroid Glands; Pharmacologic Use of Steroids; Hypocalcemia and Hypercalcemia; Disorders of Water Metabolism; Hypoglycemia; and Hormone Use of Unproven Value

ROBERT I. GREGERMAN, MD

PITUITARY DISEASES

Clinical Presentation

Disorders of the pituitary gland are manifest by disturbance of function (hypersecretion or hyposecretion of trophic hormones), by pituitary enlargement with anatomic encroachment on adjacent structures (enlargement of tumors), or by a combination of these processes. Many of the cases of hormone hypersecretion are due to benign tumors—often clinically inapparent microadenomas.

When a patient presents with evidence of decreased endocrine function, routine evaluation must include consideration of whether the process is primary (i.e., in the end organ) or is due to pituitary disease (i.e., secondary gland failure). For example, in most patients with hypothyroidism, thyroid-stimulating hormone (TSH) is elevated because of failure of normal inhibition of the negative feedback loop. However, if TSH is not elevated in the face of hypothyroidism, the possibility of hypopituitarism must then be further evaluated. Similarly, in patients with hypogonadism an easy differential diagnosis can usually be made because levels of follicle-stimulating hormone (FSH) and luteinizing hormone (LH) are almost always elevated when there is primary end-organ failure. However, there are exceptions to these statements. For example, TSH may be "normal" in hypothyroidism of pituitary origin (secondary hypothyroidism, see Chapter 80), and LH may not be elevated in the male gonadal failure that occurs in the elderly (see Chapter 85). Moreover, in patients with adrenal insufficiency, the serum adrenocorticotropic hormone (ACTH) does not always clearly differentiate primary from secondary disease. In cases of persistent endocrine hyperfunction, pituitary function may need to be evaluated but not necessarily routinely (see Graves Disease, Chapter 80, and Adrenocortical Hyperfunction, below).

Not infrequently, the possibility of pituitary disease is raised inadvertently. For example, radiologic examination of the head because of headaches, suspected sinusitis, injury, or other reasons may reveal an enlarged or an abnormal sella turcica. The issue then arises concerning further evaluation of this incidental finding, a so-called pituitary incidentaloma (1).

Evaluation of the Sella Turcica

The sella turcica as seen in plain films of the skull may appear deceptively normal or may appear abnormal when it is not. Magnetic resonance imaging (MRI) has almost totally replaced older techniques for evaluating the sella. MRI is most sensitive when the image is enhanced by gadolinium; computed tomography (CT) is less expensive but is less sensitive than MRI in the detection of intrasellar microadenomas. In a few centers, venous sampling techniques for ACTH can lateralize many of the nonvisualizable adenomas that are the cause of Cushing disease, thus facilitating pituitary hemisectioning at surgery. In addition, if suprasellar extension is present, the patient should be referred for ophthalmologic examination of the visual fields, preferably with a red dot, the most sensitive technique for detection of field defects produced by suprasellar masses.

Empty Sella Syndrome

An enlarged sella does not always mean that a pituitary tumor is present. Evaluation commonly leads to demonstration of an empty sella turcica (i.e., one not completely filled by the pituitary gland). Empty sellas are often discovered during evaluation of skull x-rays obtained for reasons other than suspected hypopituitarism—usually headache—and usually are not associated with clinical endocrine disease. The cause of the empty sella syndrome is unknown, but open communication of cerebrospinal fluid through a defect in the diaphragma sellae and a ruptured cyst have been postulated. In most cases, a rim of nonvisualizable normal pituitary tissue remains, and pituitary function, which should be routinely evaluated (e.g., measurement of TSH, follicle-stimulating hormone, and LH), is normal; in some there is minimal hypopituitarism or a visual field defect for reasons that are not clear but that could represent a previous cyst. The diagnosis can be made definitively by MRI. Angiography should be done only if surgical intervention is a consideration.

Pituitary Tumors

When a pituitary tumor is large enough to produce increased pressure within the sella turcica, enlargement and erosion of the bony walls of that structure either produce no symptoms or may cause headache. Tumor enlargement superiorly leads to encroachment on the adjacent optic chiasm and may produce visual field defects. Pituitary tumors large enough to be anatomically apparent are often associated with failure of hormone secretion (hypopituitarism), a process that results in selective or multiple end-organ failure (hypoadrenalism, hypogonadism, and/or hypothyroidism). The pituitary may also be affected by a wide variety of systemic illnesses, including granulomatous, infectious, vascular, and neoplastic processes, but all are extremely uncommon causes of hypopituitarism.

A related problem is that of *craniopharyngioma*. This developmental abnormality may simulate pituitary tumor. The lesion is usually outside the pituitary and presents as a suprasellar mass lesion readily evident on CT or MRI. Most cases are manifest during childhood.

Chromophobe Adenomas

Chromophobe adenomas, the most common of the pituitary tumors, account for approximately 85% of cases; most occur between ages 30 and 60, often in association with parathyroid or pancreatic islet cell adenomas and, sometimes, with the Zollinger-Ellison syndrome (see Chapter 43). These associations constitute the syndrome of multiple endocrine adenomatosis (type I). When the pituitary is not involved, but pheochromocytoma, medullary thyroid carcinoma, and occasionally parathyroid adenomas occur together, the syndrome is termed multiple endocrine adenomatosis type II.

Chromophobe adenomas are usually noninvasive but may infiltrate local structures and, on rare occasions, even behave as locally malignant lesions. Long thought to be functionless, many are now known to be prolactinomas (see below). A few produce growth hormone (GH) and, even fewer, gonadotropins. The term *chromophobe adenoma* belongs to the era in which pituitary tumors were classified by their histologic staining characteristics (chromophobe, eosinophile, and basophile). A more precise classification based on the secretory product of the tumor (e.g., somatotrope tumor, GH producing) can now be constructed, but the old terms persist.

Pituitary function remains clinically normal until more than 75% of the normal pituitary has been destroyed by the adenoma. Hypogonadism is usually the earliest evidence of a hormone deficiency state (60% to 80% of cases), but hypothyroidism as an initial manifestation is almost as common. Adrenal insufficiency is usually the last problem to develop and is often inapparent except on laboratory testing. In approximately 10% of cases, diabetes insipidus develops.

Prolactinomas: Prolactin and Galactorrhea. In the female, unilateral or bilateral galactorrhea may be the first clue to the presence of a prolactin-secreting adenoma (prolactinoma). In many cases, discharge from the breast is minimal and may be apparent only on physical examination when a few drops of milk may be expressible. Breast enlargement may occur in the male, but prolactin excess is an uncommon cause of gynecomastia (see Chapter 85). Galactorrhea in the male, a rare event, is diagnostic of a prolactinoma. Prolactin secretion appears to inhibit the secretion of gonadotropins and hence may also be associated with evidence of hypogonadism, including impotence and amenorrhea (see Chapter 85).

However, most cases of galactorrhea in women are not caused by a tumor but by functional disturbance of prolactin secretion, which in turn is either spontaneous or related to the use of certain drugs. In either case, the hallmark of galactorrhea is an increase of the concentration of prolactin in serum. Accurate radioimmunoassays for prolactin are widely available. The drugs most commonly incriminated in the production of galactorrhea are estrogens (oral contraceptives), phenothiazines, tricyclic antidepressants, and haloperidol. Rarely, galactorrhea occurs secondary to hypothyroidism.

The degree of prolactin elevation is strongly suggestive of the cause of the disorder. Levels of prolactin greater than 200 ng/mL are essentially diagnostic of tumor, even in the absence of changes in the sella. Elevated levels of prolactin less than 50 ng/mL are much more likely to be due to a functional disorder or a drug, but in many cases differentiation is impossible by quantification of the prolactin level.

Treatment. Most cases of galactorrhea, with or without microadenoma, can be treated successfully with bromocriptine (Parlodel), which often lowers the prolactin level, abolishes the galactorrhea, and restores normal menses. Bromocriptine not only reduces prolactin secretion but in many cases causes the tumor to shrink so dramatically that even visual field defects can be reversed. A favorable response occurs in 80% of cases. The drug is now commonly given preoperatively, even when a large tumor is present, because surgical removal is thereby facilitated. Long-term drug therapy is an alternative to surgery in most cases (2). Treatment with bromocriptine can be undertaken by the nonspecialist provided that tumor is unlikely. The drug is available as 2.5-mg tablets and 5-mg capsules; the initial dosage is 1.25 to 2.50 mg/day. The dosage may be increased by 2.5 mg every 3 to 7 days until an optimum response is achieved—usually 5 to 7 mg/day. Adverse effects—especially nausea, headache, dizziness, and fatigue—are common. If prolactin levels are very high, if radiographic evidence of tumor is present, or if the patient is intolerant of, or unresponsive to, bromocriptine, an endocrinologist should be consulted. An alternative drug that can be useful in bromocriptine intolerant or refractory cases is cabergoline, which has the advantage over bromocriptine of a need for much less frequent dosing (0.25 to 1 mg twice a week) (3); the adverse effects of the 2 drugs are similar.

Prolactin-secreting tumors in men tend to be diagnosed at a much later stage (i.e., as macroadenomas) than in women and to be associated with hypogonadism. Drug therapy is successful in about 80% of these cases (4).

Until recently the indications for surgical intervention (transsphenoidal; see Acromegaly, below) were mainly related to the size of the tumor. Visual field impairment has in the past been the major indication for urgent surgery, but extensive experience indicates that even patients with significant visual loss can be successfully treated with bromocriptine. With transsphenoidal surgery, microadenomas can often be removed successfully and normal pituitary function restored. With marked suprasellar extension, a transfrontal surgical approach may be needed. This is a much more formidable procedure. In many cases a large tumor cannot be completely removed; postoperative radiation therapy prevents clinical recurrence in these instances.

Acromegaly

Pituitary tumors that produce an excess of growth hormone (GH) result in the clinical state termed acromegaly. If the GH excess occurs before cessation of growth, gigantism occurs. When GH excess begins in the adult, the most common clinical feature suggesting the presence of acromegaly is insidious alteration of facial appearance over many years. Old photographs may be useful in helping to identify such changes. Physical findings include enlargement (lengthening) of the mandible, sometimes with separation of the teeth; coarsening of facial features because of both overgrowth of frontal, malar, and nasal bones and soft tissue overgrowth producing widening of the nose and protrusion of the lips; enlargement of the hands and feet, often noted by increasing glove and shoe size; and dermatologic changes that include skin thickening and sebaceous gland enlargement (hydradenitis). Commonly, patients present with a nerve entrapment (carpal tunnel) syndrome. Osteoarthritis and diabetes mellitus, although often seen in this disorder, are too common to provide a clue to the presence of acromegaly. Tumors large enough to produce sellar enlargement may lead to headache; suprasellar extension may result in visual field defects.

The laboratory diagnosis is simple in overt cases but may be difficult in mild cases. GH varies rapidly during the day in the serum of acromegalic patients, so single samples of blood may not be helpful. The best test for screening is probably the determination of *serum insulin-like growth factor I*. This product of GH action varies little and correlates well with the 24-hour integrated serum GH level, arguably the most definitive test. Unfortunately, the accurate laboratory determination of insulin-like growth factor I cannot be assumed. If GH is measured directly in screening, elevation of serum GH in the fasting basal state to values consistently greater than 10 ng/mL strongly suggests the diagnosis. However, stress and physical activity may also elevate the GH levels. Elevated values must therefore be confirmed with a test of the ability of glucose to suppress the GH. During a standard glucose tolerance test (see Chapter 79), the GH—determined simultaneously with the glucose—should normally fall to a value less than 2 ng/mL. Most acromegalics show no fall of GH, and a few exhibit a paradoxical rise during the test. Laboratory evidence of elevated and nonsuppressible GH warrants referral to an endocrinologist, as does the presence of equivocal clinical or laboratory findings.

Treatment of Acromegaly. Treatment should be directed by an endocrinologist (5). *Irradiation of the* *pituitary,* usually by external high-voltage techniques, has been standard treatment for years. Such therapy is effective but is usually extremely slow in its effect and may take several years to produce maximal suppression of hormone production. Surgery is indicated when rapid reduction of the elevated GH is needed (e.g., for cosmetic reasons in a young woman with early disease, visual field loss, or intractable headache). *Transsphenoidal operation* is now standard for most cases and should, if at all possible, include an attempt at selective removal of a microadenoma. The transsphenoidal operation involves minimal morbidity, a very low rate of complications, and essentially no mortality, but recurrences are common, leading some authorities to continue to advocate radiation therapy as the first approach for uncomplicated cases. The somatostatin analog, *octreotide* (a potent GH antagonist), is effective long-term medical therapy but should only be prescribed by an endocrinologist. The parent drug requires multiple subcutaneous injections each day, but long-acting depot preparations are now available and can be given every 4 weeks (6).

Cushing Disease

When evidence is obtained for overproduction of glucocorticoids and testing suggests the presence of adrenal hyperplasia (see Adrenal Diseases, below), evaluation of the sella turcica is in order. Most cases of Cushing disease with adrenal hyperplasia are caused by a basophilic microadenoma of the pituitary that can be visualized preoperatively, in 80% of cases, with an optimal MRI examination (see below).

Other Secretory Pituitary Tumors

Although quite rare, pituitary tumors that secrete thyrotropin (TSH) and produce hyperthyroidism do occur. Even rarer are cases of hypersecretion of TSH without demonstrable tumor. Patients with tumors have been successfully treated with a somatostatin analog (7). Tumors that produce excessive amounts of gonadotropins are very rare.

Pituitary Failure (Hypopituitarism)

Idiopathic Causes

Patients are occasionally encountered in whom pituitary failure occurs without evidence of pituitary tumor or of another demonstrable anatomic defect. Some are eventually found to have infiltrative processes (sarcoidosis, histiocytosis, lymphoma, benign lymphocytic infiltration [hypophysitis]). Hypopituitarism is diagnosed by the demonstration of end-organ failure that occurs in the absence of the expected elevation of trophic hormone. Isolated deficiencies of trophic hormones also occur but are rare. Among these, the most likely to be encountered is hypogonadotropic hypogonadism in the male, sometimes associated with anosmia *(Kallmann syndrome).* In these patients, no anatomic basis is apparent.

Sheehan Syndrome (Postpartum Pituitary Failure)

Massive uterine hemorrhage occurring at delivery occasionally results in pituitary infarction and panhypopituitarism. In this syndrome, failure of postpartum lactation and absence of menses are attended by development of debility and other evidence of end-organ failure. Because of improvements in obstetric care (prompt treatment of hemorrhage), such cases are now rare.

Pituitary Hemorrhage and Infarction

Rarely, hemorrhage into the pituitary gland (pituitary apoplexy), usually into an adenoma, leads to severe headache and/or signs of a rapidly expanding intracranial abnormality. Radiographic examination of the sella turcica is abnormal. Another rare phenomenon is that of pituitary infarction occurring during the course of a febrile illness, presumably viral. Intense headache lasts for days and is usually, but not always, severe enough to require hospitalization. The acute febrile illness subsides with symptomatic therapy and without specific clinical or radiographic findings, only to be followed later by the development of hypopituitarism. Both men and women can be affected.

Hormone Replacement Therapy for Hypopituitarism

Pituitary insufficiency, regardless of the cause, is treated with thyroid hormone (thyroxine, see Chapter 80), adrenal glucocorticoid (cortisol, see below), and gonadal hormone (testosterone [see Chapter 85] or an estrogen [see Chapter 106]). Except for GH, other pituitary trophic hormones are not used routinely (see below). Occasionally, young women may be candidates for therapy with gonadotropins to produce ovulation and restore fertility. Such therapy may be effective but is available at only a few centers. In men, normal libido and sexual performance consistent with age can be ensured with testosterone therapy. Restoration of fertility in the male is also possible with the use of a combination of gonadotropins, but such therapy is not generally available.

Growth Hormone Deficiency. The name "growth hormone" had its historical roots when it was found to be essential for normal growth and development in children. However, it has been known for over half a century that GH is a metabolic regulator, even in the adult. Except during aging (see below), GH deficiency in the adult is invariably a result of pituitary disease, and although most patients with pituitary disorders do reasonably well when end-organ hormones are replaced (adrenal, thyroid, gonadal), the inadequacy of replacement has only been recognized relatively recently (8).

The clinical state of the *adult* human with isolated GH deficiency (i.e., patients receiving replacement therapy only with end organ hormones) has been designated a deficiency "syndrome" only within the last 10 years (9). The abnormalities attributed to GH deficiency are a reduction in lean body mass and in muscle strength, an increase in body fat—especially abdominal fat—and alterations in mood (depression, emotional lability, anxiety) and energy level. Obviously, these features are not specific. However, treatment of GH-deficient adults improves psychological wellbeing, muscle strength, and exercise tolerance. Objective evidence validating these changes is available from psychological testing and measurements of lean body mass (body composition studies showing increased muscle, decreased fat) and exercise performance testing.

During normal aging, about one-half of the elderly develop a low GH state. In the past few years, small numbers of such patients have been studied during GH replacement therapy, alone or in combination with sex steroids, in an effort to ameliorate some of the effects of aging, especially the loss of muscle mass (sarcopenia) and strength. The results of such studies are encouraging of further research but do not suggest that GH will be a panacea for the adverse changes that accompany aging.

The diagnosis of GH deficiency in the adult is not simple. The gold standard is the insulin-tolerance test (ITT), that is, secretion of GH provoked by insulin-induced hypoglycemia. Various stimulatory tests have been proposed, using a variety of agents, alone and in combination. These tests are best left to a consulting endocrinologist, as is the advisability of using GH over the long term as part of a replacement program (a recombinant product is now available). The potential benefits are considerable, as is the cost at about $5,000 per year (10).

Hypopituitarism Secondary to Head Trauma

Head trauma has long been thought to account for only a tiny fraction of all cases of hypopituitarism, but recent observations indicate that head trauma, usually a result of a road accident (i.e., one involving a motor vehicle or bicycle), accounts for many cases. Patients may not recall such an occurrence until helped to remember (11). Careful questioning of relatives often reveals a positive history that would otherwise remain obscure. The trauma may not have seemed severe; neither skull fracture nor loss of consciousness need occur, although most cases have had both. Laboratory findings are highly variable and range from panhypopituitarism to selected hormone deficiencies. The typical case is a young male who develops end-organ failure within a year of the traumatic episode, although many years may pass before a diagnosis is made. Pituitary imaging may show an empty sella, pituitary atrophy, and/or areas of hypodensity, cysts, or microcysts. Spontaneous recovery or pituitary function may occur as late as 10 or more years after the event. Contrary to long-held belief, posterior pituitary dysfunction need not be present at any time.

Disturbances of Pituitary Function Caused by Nonendocrine Disease

Much more common than decreased pituitary function resulting from intrinsic pituitary disease is altered gonadotropin secretion on a functional basis. Many illnesses can affect the functional integrity of the hypothalamic–pituitary–end-organ axis. This phenomenon is most obvious as a disturbance of menstruation in women and, less often, impotence in men (see Chapter 85). Any disease that results in *malnutrition* can produce decreased gonadotropins and (secondary) amenorrhea or impotence. *Alcoholism* is an outstanding example. Liver disease does not need to be present in alcoholics to produce amenorrhea or impotence, but various liver diseases are themselves associated with loss of menses. The common factor seems to be malnutrition. In recent years, some individuals have undertaken caloric restriction in an attempt to extend lifespan. Although such persons maintain that they are not malnourished but rather are undernourished, they share many of the symptomatic features described here.

The classic example of nonendocrine illness that simulates an endocrine disturbance is *anorexia nervosa* (see Chapter 11). In this psychiatric disturbance, which results in severe malnutrition with resultant weight loss, the most marked disturbance of endocrine function is cessation of menses resulting from a decrease of gonadotropins. Other trophic hormones are not affected. Thyroid function is usually normal. Axillary and pubic hair are retained, giving important clinical evidence for the preservation of adrenal function. Although cortisol secretion is low (urinary steroid excretion is decreased), this results from slow metabolic disposal of cortisol rather than decreased ability to increase ACTH secretion appropriately; plasma cortisol is normal. GH concentration may be elevated, a consequence of starvation due to any cause. The diagnosis of anorexia nervosa should be based on the association of psychiatric abnormalities and obvious decrease in food intake. The tests described will serve merely to support the diagnosis.

Other diseases may also result in secondary amenorrhea because of failure of gonadotropin secretion. These include such diverse conditions as severe emotional disturbances, marked obesity, poorly controlled diabetes mellitus, and severe chronic infections.

ADRENAL DISEASES

Adrenocortical Insufficiency (Addison Disease)

In ambulatory patients the clinical presentation of adrenocortical insufficiency is related to a number of chronic complaints that are nonspecific in character. A high index of suspicion will result in far more tests than positive diagnoses, but detection of this rare problem is important to prevent morbidity culminating in acute hospitalization for full-blown disease (i.e., vascular collapse with Addisonian crisis).

Etiology and Association with Other Autoimmune Diseases

Adrenocortical insufficiency is now most commonly the result of *autoimmune disease* and is associated with the presence of antibodies to adrenal tissue. Most other cases are secondary to *pituitary disease*.

Many cases of autoimmune adrenocortical insufficiency are associated with autoimmune thyroiditis, although the two problems may develop years apart. The simultaneous occurrence of autoimmune thyroid and adrenal disease is termed *Schmidt syndrome*. Rarely, autoimmune adrenocortical insufficiency, autoimmune hypothyroidism, and autoimmune gonadal failure occur in the syndrome of *polyglandular failure*. There is also an association of autoimmune adrenocortical insufficiency with pernicious anemia and Sjögren syndrome and probably with systemic lupus erythematosus. *Tuberculosis,* once a common cause, now only rarely produces adrenocortical insufficiency in the United States and other developed countries, probably because of a relatively decreased incidence of tuberculosis in the Western world and because of effective therapy. Other rare causes of adrenocortical insufficiency include histoplasmosis, paracoccidiomycosis (in Central and South Americans), and sarcoidosis. Human immunodeficiency virus infection and diseases associated with the acquired immunodeficiency syndrome (e.g., cytomegalovirus, histoplasmosis, mycobacterial infection; see Chapter 39) often cause asymptomatic adrenal dysfunction, but symptomatic adrenal insufficiency is uncommon. Although infectious causes of adrenal insufficiency are not likely to be encountered in the United States, they should still be excluded, especially in the absence of evidence for coexistent autoimmune disease.

Clinical Presentation

Chronic symptoms include anorexia, weight loss, weakness, and decreased physical endurance. Vomiting may occur, and abdominal pain, sometimes resembling that of peptic ulcer disease, can be a presenting feature. Other symptoms include mental sluggishness, irritability, and symptoms of either postural hypotension or of hypoglycemia. In primary adrenal insufficiency, increasing pigmentation (white patients) or further darkening of skin (African American patients) may be noted. Loss of axillary and pubic hair—an important finding when present—may occur in women. Such hair loss is commonly overlooked on physical examination and is rarely volunteered as part of the history.

Physical examination often shows postural hypotension. Pigmentation is diffuse but is especially evident in the creases of the hands, the areolae, over pressure areas (knuckles, elbows), and in new scars. Pigmentation of buccal mucous membranes is a pathognomonic finding in white patients but is a normal finding in blacks. Lymphadenopathy is occasionally seen. When the adrenal insufficiency is secondary to pituitary disease, additional findings may relate to the manifestations of a pituitary tumor (headache, visual loss; see above), to hypothyroidism (see Chapter 80), or to hypogonadism (see Chapters 85 and 101).

Laboratory Evaluation

Classically, hyponatremia associated with hyperkalemia and some degree of azotemia provided the clues to the diagnosis. These abnormalities are manifestations of severe disease and are usually absent in the less severe cases that are likely to be encountered in ambulatory practice. Various other nonspecific abnormalities occur occasionally, including anemia, lymphocytosis, and eosinophilia.

Laboratory diagnosis of adrenal insufficiency depends on determination of serum cortisol. Determinations of serum cortisol made without prior adrenal stimulation by injected ACTH have many limitations. In this regard both the normal diurnal rhythm of cortisol and the high degree of variability of plasma cortisol in normal people must be kept in mind. Serum cortisol can be initially measured at any time of the day, and a robust normal value (15 to 25 μg/dL) will exclude the diagnosis. However, afternoon determinations may be low simply because of the normal evening drop, and even the fasting morning cortisol is highly variable. Values lower than 5 μg/dL at any time are highly likely to be due to adrenal insufficiency. Intermediate values (5 to 10 μg/dL) may be seen in less severe cases and may overlap those of normal subjects. Thus, measurement of unstimulated serum cortisol is useful and sometimes even definitive, especially in excluding the diagnosis, but may fail to detect mild cases or may yield indeterminate values.

Further evaluation of low or borderline values of serum cortisol should always be made by administering exogenous ACTH and then measuring cortisol again. The ease with which such testing is performed—and the common failure of unstimulated serum cortisol values to give definitive information—provides a cogent argument for use of ACTH stimulation as the preferred screening procedure for adrenal insufficiency. Many variations of *ACTH stimulation tests* have been advocated. The bolus intravenous injection of 0.25 mg of synthetic ACTH (Cortrosyn) (see below) has been used for years as a simple and reliable procedure in the diagnosis of adrenal insufficiency. The serum cortisol obtained 1 hour after injection will normally rise above the upper normal baseline range (to at least 18 to 20 μg/dL). Patients with adrenocortical insufficiency do not show a response. More recently, a 1-μg dose has been demonstrated to yield more accurate results and is used preferentially in many centers (12). Patients' responsiveness should be referred urgently to an endocrinologist for confirmation of the diagnosis and additional testing, including measurement of serum ACTH, in an attempt to distinguish primary from secondary adrenal insufficiency. An elevated ACTH level (above 100 pg/mL) is seen in primary adrenal insufficiency.

Other Tests. Tests of adrenal function based on *urinary excretion of steroid metabolites* (17-ketogenic steroids [17-KGS] or 17-hydroxysteroids [17-OHCS]) should be avoided in screening for adrenal insufficiency. These tests offer no advantage over plasma cortisol measurements and often yield artificially low values because of incomplete collection of urine. The adrenal response to ACTH is slow in secondary adrenal insufficiency and requires stimulation for up to 3 days. In the past, 2- to 3-day infusions were used to discriminate between primary and secondary adrenal insufficiency. However, other tests of pituitary function are available (e.g., serum ACTH—see above; follicle-stimulating hormone, LH, and GH) and serve better to distinguish between primary and secondary adrenal disease (13).

Although the adrenal mineralocorticoid *aldosterone* may be low in adrenal insufficiency, the hormone is secreted by the zona glomerulosa rather than the more central portion of the adrenal cortex and may be relatively unaffected by processes that destroy much of the glucocorticoid producing zone of the gland. Therefore, measurements of plasma and urinary aldosterone have no place in routine diagnosis of adrenocortical insufficiency. Routine radiographic studies should include a chest x-ray and, if appropriate (e.g., suspicion of adrenal hemorrhage or metastases), CT or MRI of the adrenals.

Treatment of Established Adrenal Insufficiency

The Addisonian patient should be helped to realize the importance of taking hormone therapy regularly, of self-care (dose adjustment) during situations of stress, and of the necessity of continuing to take replacement therapy for life.

Glucocorticoid (Steroid) Replacement Therapy. Replacement dosage for cortisol was established empirically decades ago; the ordinary recommended doses are probably higher than necessary. Secretion rates determined by stable isotope dilution suggest that 24-hour cortisol secretion is in the range of 5 to 15 mg/day (14), although older studies using radioactive labels gave somewhat higher values. Large or obese persons need more, but too much individual variation exists to make dose/weight calculations meaningful. Recommended dosage schemes vary. Under normal circumstances patients are given 15 to 20 mg of cortisol (or its equivalent) daily (20 mg of cortisol is equivalent to 25 mg of cortisone, 5 mg of prednisone, and 0.25 mg of dexamethasone). The simplest and least expensive scheme is 12.5 mg of cortisone (one-half of a 25-mg cortisone acetate tablet) twice daily; alternately, 10 mg of cortisol (hydrocortisone) is used on the same schedule. Some authorities prefer to simulate the normal diurnal rhythm of cortisol secretion, although no evidence indicates that this scheme is of any special benefit. In this approach, 10 to 15 mg of cortisol is taken on arising and 5 to 10 mg in the evening. Some physicians still prescribe as much as 30 mg of cortisol (hydrocortisone) per day, an amount that exceeds physiologic replacement for most persons and should be avoided.

Hydrocortisone is not readily available in pharmacies; as a result, noncompliance is more likely to result than with the use of other glucocorticoids (cortisone acetate, prednisone, dexamethasone) that are routinely kept in stock. Equivalent doses of prednisone or another glucocorticoid (Table 81.1) may be used but have no advantage. Their use may, indeed, dictate a requirement for additional mineralocorticoid therapy because glucocorticoids such as prednisone and dexamethasone have much less mineralocorticoid activity than does cortisol (or cortisone).

Table 81.1. Commonly Used Glucocorticoids[a]

Generic Name	Common Trade Name(s)	Equivalent Potency (mg)[b]	Sodium Retention Relative to Cortisol
Cortisol (hydrocortisone)	Cortef	20	—
Cortisone[c]	—	25	1
Prednisone	Deltasone, Meticorten, Delta Cortef	5	0.1
Prednisolone	Meticortelone, Sterane	4	0.1
Methylprednisolone	Medrol	4	0
	Aristocort, Kenacort	4	0
Dexamethasone[d]	Decadron	0.75	0
Betamethasone[d]	Celestone	0.6	0
For parenteral use			
Cortisol	Solu-Cortef		
Methylprednisolone	Solu-Medrol		
Triamcinolone	Aristocort		
Dexamethasone	Decadron		
Betamethasone	Celestone		
For topical use			
Triamcinolone	Aristocort, Kenalog		
Fluocinolone	Synalar		
Methamethasone	Valisone		
For inhalation and intranasal use			
Beclomethasone and others (see Chapters 30 and 60)	Vanceri		

[a]Most of the compounds listed are available in generic forms. All are marketed as ester derivatives or salts of esters (e.g., cortisol sodium hemisuccinate [Solu-Cortef]). For practical purposes, only cortisol and cortisone have significant salt-retaining (mineralocorticoid) action.

[b]Also equivalent to daily physiologic replacement when given in divided doses.

[c]Cortisone acetate has long been given parenterally (intramuscular route) as well as orally; however, this compound is unpredictably absorbed from injection sites and cannot be relied on to produce adequate blood levels.

[d]This compound has a relatively long duration of action and should not be used for alternate day glucocorticoid therapy.

Overtreatment with glucocorticoids should be avoided. Frequently increasing the dosage for treatment of nonspecific complaints is a common practice but should be avoided because iatrogenic subclinical Cushing syndrome (or at a minimum, hypertension) is a real hazard to the long-term well-being of patients with Addison disease. The response to replacement therapy varies: Weakness and lassitude ordinarily abate within hours to days, but other symptoms may diminish somewhat more slowly.

The requirement for glucocorticoids (cortisol) is increased during stress. In the ambulatory patient, minor stress (common "cold" without fever; simple dental extraction under local anesthesia) can be handled by a properly instructed and motivated patient. On many such occasions, no increase in dosage is needed, or at most an additional 5 or 10 mg of cortisol would be adequate. Telephone contact with the caregiver is also useful—or even essential—on many such occasions, especially in the early months of therapy before the patient's ability to deal with these episodes has been demonstrated. The most common stress for the ambulatory patient is an infection, often a viral febrile illness. Ordinarily, a febrile response to approximately 101°F (38°C) that is unaccompanied by vomiting or diarrhea can be handled by simply increasing the cortisol dose to 50 to 75 mg/day in divided doses. A more severe episode (e.g., bronchitis) may require 100 mg for a few days. The occurrence of vomiting or significant diarrhea requires contact with a physician and may demand the use of parenteral glucocorticoids.

The need for hospitalization during stress must be determined by the caregiver and depends on the circumstances. It is obviously prudent to be cautious, but in this long-term chronic illness, frequent and precipitous hospitalizations should be avoided. Many minor events can be handled by judicious increase of steroid dosage. Perioperative management is described in Chapter 93.

Although not all patients with fully developed adrenal insufficiency require mineralocorticoid therapy in addition to cortisol replacement, such therapy is usually started when the diagnosis is first made. The initial dose is 0.1 mg of fludrocortisone daily (Florinef, 0.1-mg tablets). Aldosterone is not available for therapy of Addison disease. Only rarely will patients require more than 0.1 mg of fludrocortisone. In the early days of replacement therapy, dosages as high as 0.2 mg/day were used, but hypertension and edema were common. A maintenance dosage of 0.05 mg is average, and some individuals require as little as 0.05 mg every other day. Adequacy of therapy can be judged by determinations of serum sodium and potassium levels and clinical observations, including normalization of blood pressure without postural hypotension. When, during stress, the dosage of cortisol is increased beyond 50 to 75 mg/day, fludrocortisone therapy becomes unnecessary, indeed undesirable, because the mineralocorticoid activity of cortisol is sufficient to maintain salt balance when taken in greater than baseline physiologic amounts.

The *patient and members of the patient's household should be educated* about the symptoms of Addisonian crisis and how to respond in emergencies. In addition, the patient should carry an identification document or wear an inscribed bracelet that identifies the Addisonian state and contains instructions for therapy. Appropriate information in addition to name, address, and telephone number should read approximately as follows:

> I am a patient with adrenal insufficiency (Addison disease). If I am seriously injured, found unconscious, or am vomiting, I should be given an injection of dexamethasone, as emergency treatment for Addisonian crisis. A filled syringe is with my belongings. Notify my health care giver (name, telephone number) or other medical authority immediately.

Syringes containing dexamethasone phosphate (4 mg in 1 mL of water) are available for patients and can be carried conveniently.

All patients with Addison disease should consume a liberal quantity of sodium (100 to 150 mEq [6 to 9 g NaCl]/day), regardless of whether mineralocorticoids are used. In the event of intercurrent diarrhea or profuse sweating, additional salt above the normal intake should be consumed. Electrolytes should be checked periodically (every 3 to 4 months during the critical first year of therapy). Mineralocorticoid therapy should be cautiously reduced if edema, hypertension, or hypokalemia is noted, and salt or mineralocorticoid should be increased if postural hypotension, hyponatremia, or hyperkalemia appears. Overtreatment with glucocorticoids should be carefully avoided. Over the long term, it should be borne in mind that if the Addison disease is idiopathic (i.e., autoimmune), related diseases and their own manifestations may appear at any time (hypothyroidism, hypoparathyroidism, hypogonadism).

Adrenocortical Hyperfunction: Cushing Syndrome

The adrenal glands produce several steroid products: glucocorticoids (chiefly cortisol), mineralocorticoids (chiefly aldosterone), and so-called adrenal androgens (a group of steroids collectively termed 17-ketosteroids [17-KS]). Clinical disorders may affect predominantly the secretion of one or other of these hormones. Table 81.2 lists these disorders of adrenal hyperfunction. Most are rather uncommon or rare, but some essentially functional disorders are commonly encountered. The approach presented here is predominantly oriented to the recognition—or exclusion—*and initial evaluation of these diseases in ambulatory patients*. Once the practitioner is reasonably certain that a problem exists, detailed evaluation often requires consultation with an endocrinologist and sometimes hospitalization for special procedures. However, many relatively simple tests to define the situation can and

Table 81.2. Adrenocortical Hyperfunction

Glucocorticoid excess predominates
- Adrenal hyperplasia (60%–70% of all cases)
    1. Pituitary microadenoma secreting ACTH (most cases of adrenal hyperplasia)
    2. Endocrine tumor (pheochromocytoma, medullary carcinoma of thyroid, others secreting ACTH in addition to other hormones [rare])
    3. Nonendocrine tumor secreting ACTH (rare)
- Adrenal neoplasm (30%–40% of all cases)
    1. Adrenal adenoma
    2. Adrenal carcinoma (about equal in frequency)

Adrenal androgen excess predominates (hirsutism/virilism)
- Some adrenal adenomas
- Some adrenal carcinomas
- Partial adrenogenital syndrome[a]

Aldosterone excess
- Primary aldosteronism
    1. Adrenal adenoma
    2. Adrenal nodular hyperplasia
- Secondary aldosteronism
    1. Salt and volume depletion, including diuretic use and various disease states causing increased production of renin
    2. Juxtaglomerular cell hyperplasia or tumor (rare)

[a]Complete enzymatic defects in steroid synthesis are rare and are invariably manifest early in life as adrenal insufficiency and abnormalities of genital development. In ambulatory adults, partial defects of synthesis of cortisol lead to compensatory adrenal hyperplasia with production of excessive quantities of adrenal steroids with weak androgenic activity. Hirsutism, with or without virilism, ensues (see Chapters 85 and 101).

should be performed on an ambulatory basis. It must be appreciated that details of diagnostic workups vary widely even among specialists and are in constant evolution as new hormone assays and tests emerge.

Differential Diagnosis of Cushing Syndrome (Glucocorticoid Excess of Any Cause)

Etiology. In this syndrome a supraphysiologic amount of glucocorticoid (cortisol) is secreted along with varying amounts of adrenal androgens. Most cases are due to *hypersecretion of ACTH from the pituitary* with resultant varying degrees of adrenal hyperplasia. The term *Cushing disease* refers to this particular variety of Cushing syndrome. In recent years it has become apparent that almost all of these cases (perhaps 90%) are caused by *pituitary microadenomas* that produce excessive amounts of ACTH (see Pituitary Diseases, above). A smaller number are caused by *adrenal adenomas* or, rarely, *carcinomas*. Cushing syndrome may also occasionally be caused by *ectopic production of ACTH* by a variety of malignant tumors. When a tumor causes Cushing syndrome, the malignancy is usually obvious, although small neoplasms may be inapparent by conventional CT and MRI when the evidence of glucocorticoid excess first appears (see below).

Cushing Disease (Adrenocorticotropic Hormone-Dependent Adrenal Hyperfunction)

ACTH-dependent hypercortisolism is due either to Cushing disease or the ectopic ACTH syndrome. MRI of the pituitary is relatively insensitive, identifying only 50% of pituitary microadenomas. The significant incidence of pituitary "incidentalomas" (see above) further lowers the accuracy of MRI in establishing the pituitary as the source of ACTH hypersecretion. Other tests, such as low and high dose dexamethasone tests, peripherally administered ovine corticotropin-releasing hormone (CRH), and metyrapone stimulation tests have all been used to identify the 5% to 10% of cases of ACTH-dependent Cushing syndrome that are due to ectopic ACTH production. If radionuclide scintigraphy or positron emission tomography fail to identify an ectopic cause of ACTH production (see below), cavernous sinus sampling by retrograde catheterization or inferior petrosal sinus sampling with ovine CRH stimulation is likely to make the distinction but, of course, cannot be of help in localizing the ectopic lesion. Such invasive sampling is performed in only a few centers (15). Once a diagnosis of hypercortisolism is made or strongly suspected, referral to an endocrinologist for further workup is essential.

Clinical Presentation of Cushing Syndrome

The severity of the signs and symptoms in Cushing syndrome depends on the magnitude of the steroid excess, the rapidity with which it develops, and the degree to which androgen production is increased. The signs and symptoms of glucocorticoid excess are familiar to all clinicians who have seen the entire picture of this disease emerge as the result of long-term treatment of patients with pharmacologic amounts of prednisone and similar drugs. Glucocorticoid excess produces increased deposition of subcutaneous fat in the face *(moon facies)* and in the upper body *(buffalo hump* and *truncal obesity)*. Skin changes include *telangiectasia* over the face, atrophy and thinning of the skin with easy or spontaneous bruising, ecchymoses, and development of purplish *abdominal striae*. Hyperpigmentation is sometimes seen. *Muscle weakness* results from so-called steroid myopathy (often associated with elevated serum creatine kinase) and is especially prominent in the shoulder and pelvic girdle areas. The extremities become thin as muscle wasting occurs. Bone mineral loss occurs, producing *osteoporosis* with its resultant back pain. Crush fractures of the vertebrae are common and often spontaneous, and hip or wrist fractures may occur after minimal trauma. *Hypertension* and diabetes mellitus are common. Hypokalemia may occur. Probably less well recognized are the *psychiatric disturbances* that result from chronic glucocorticoid excess. Lability of mood, depression, mania, and frank psychoses may all be precipitated by glucocorticoid excess.

Androgenic effects occur from both the intrinsic properties of the glucocorticoids and the associated production of adrenal androgens. With glucocorticoid excess alone, only mild signs are usually evident: hirsutism (facial, extremities, truncal) and acne. More profound androgenic effects that include virilization suggest adrenal tumor. These include frontal baldness in women, oligomenorrhea, increase in muscle mass, and enlargement of the clitoris. Androgenic effects cannot, of course, be appreciated in men.

Ectopic Adrenocorticotropic Hormone Syndrome

Small cell lung cancer, bronchial and other carcinoids, gastrinomas, nonsecreting islet cell tumors, insulinomas, glucagonomas, somatostatinomas, and even metastatic medullary carcinomas of the thyroid all are known to produce this syndrome. ^{111}In-pentetreotide scintigraphy and single photon emission tomography are current localization techniques that are being successfully used, but the localization can be unsuccessful even with these methods. These cases are challenges for even the most skillful endocrinologists and nuclear medicine experts (16).

Cushing Syndrome Due to Bilateral Adrenocortical Nodular Hyperplasia

ACTH-independent Cushing syndrome is an uncommon cause of hypercortisolism. Occasionally, a single adenoma is the cause. More often the adrenals contain multiple functioning macronodules. In rare cases, the abnormal adrenal tissue is hyperresponsive to gastrointestinal inhibitory peptide or to other hormones or cytokines (e.g., vasopressin, LH, interleukin 1-beta, etc.), apparently because of aberrant expression of increased numbers of receptors for these messengers. When gastrointestinal inhibitory peptide receptors are involved, the increased output of cortisol by the adenomatous tissue is increased even further by eating, which normally triggers gastrointestinal inhibitory peptide release. The term *food-dependent Cushing syndrome* has been given to such cases (17).

Cushing Syndrome Versus Pseudo-Cushing States

Patients With Obesity, Hirsutism, Hypertension, and/or Type 2 Diabetes Mellitus. In women, obesity is often associated with hirsutism, hypertension, and type 2 diabetes mellitus. When weight gain is rapid, striae may appear, and a truncal supraclavicular fat pad and a buffalo hump can be seen. These findings often raise the possibility of Cushing syndrome and provoke laboratory screening for this disorder. Few such patients are found to have Cushing syndrome. In recent years conditions that resemble Cushing syndrome have come to be called pseudo-Cushing states (see below).

Fifty percent of obese people do have increased cortisol production, which is a phenomenon of unknown mechanism resulting from the obese state. In these people the urinary excretion of steroid metabolites is increased, reflecting increased cortisol production, and may fall into the range of that seen in Cushing syndrome. However, in contrast to Cushing syndrome, such obese people have serum cortisol concentrations that are normal rather than elevated. The urine free cortisol is usually normal also. Furthermore, the suppressibility of the pituitary–adrenal axis in obesity is also normal (see Diagnosis, below). The obesity-related increase of urinary steroid metabolite excretion is one of several reasons why such measurements should be avoided for screening purposes.

Psychiatric Illness. Psychiatric symptoms are common in Cushing syndrome. However, it has also been appreciated that major depressive illness may be associated with excessive production of glucocorticoids and lack of suppressibility with dexamethasone (see below). These patients do not appear clinically to have full-blown Cushing syndrome, but some clinical features often suggest the diagnosis and may lead to laboratory investigation. Differentiation from true Cushing syndrome by laboratory tests may be difficult at first, but the differential diagnosis eventually becomes clear because remission of the psychiatric disturbance results in disappearance of the abnormal laboratory findings.

Other Pseudo-Cushing States. In addition to obesity and psychiatric disease, pseudo-Cushing states are seen in some patients with alcoholism, the alcohol-withdrawal syndrome, and the polycystic ovary syndrome.

Diagnosis

The tests of adrenal and pituitary function fall into two groups: Static measurements of blood or urine steroids or dynamic testing after stimulation or inhibition of the pituitary–adrenal axis. Both approaches are useful and may be combined. With regard to the measurements themselves, in blood both serum cortisol and ACTH can be assayed. In urine, assays are available for cortisol (free cortisol), two different groups of cortisol metabolites (17-OHCS and 17-KGS), and the adrenal androgens (17-KS), which also include some cortisol metabolites. The goal of the primary caregiver should be to use reliable relatively simple screening test(s) to evaluate suspected cases in ambulatory patients and to refer equivocal cases to an endocrinologist for more extensive evaluations.

Screening Tests for Suspected Cushing Syndrome. Cushing syndrome is relatively uncommon and its manifestations are quite nonspecific. Many patients with common nonendocrine disorders show similar or identical clinical findings to those seen in patients with Cushing syndrome. Typical cases of Cushing syndrome have clearly abnormal laboratory findings, but patients with evolving (early) Cushing syndrome or mild disease may have laboratory results that overlap with those of the pseudo-Cushing states. There is no gold standard for the diagnosis of mild-to-moderate Cushing syndrome. Currently used screening tests will be able to discriminate readily between patients with Cushing syndrome and those with pseudo-Cushing syndrome 80% of the time, although several observations (clinical and laboratory) are often required.

Suppression Tests Based on Plasma Cortisol. Many patients with Cushing syndrome have mild disease. Steroid production in such individuals is not greatly increased and there is considerable overlap with normal values. Accordingly, determination of plasma cortisol or urinary steroid excretion is not likely to be helpful.

An overnight dexamethasone test has long been advocated as a screening test. A single oral dose of 1 mg is given between 11 p.m. and midnight, and the serum cortisol is measured at 8 to 9 a.m. The sensitivity of the test depends on the diagnostic cut point for the suppressed cortisol level chosen. At 100% specificity, a plasma cortisol value above 7.5 μg/dL has been shown to distinguish Cushing syndrome from pseudo-Cushing syndrome with a sensitivity of 96% (18). If the test is abnormal, a more complicated but more reliable suppression test is performed in which dexamethasone is given orally at a dosage of 0.5 mg every 6 hours for 2 days. Plasma cortisol, urinary 17-OHCS, or both can be monitored during this test. The plasma cortisol at the end of the suppression period should be suppressed to less than 3 μg/dL. Urinary 17-OHCS during the second 24 hours should not exceed 2.5 mg.

Urinary Free Cortisol. Only small amounts of non–protein-bound cortisol ("free cortisol") are normally excreted in the urine, but as more cortisol is produced and the serum binding globulin for cortisol is increasingly saturated, a sharp rise in urinary free cortisol excretion occurs. This test, performed on a 24-hour collection of urine, is popular but subject to many methodologic pitfalls. Sensitivity of the test is close to 100% but specificity is relatively low (19). Normal upper limits vary, depending on the laboratory, from 100 to 200 μg per 24 hours and on the method used, with the least specific methods giving the highest values.

Plasma Cortisol and Its Diurnal Variation. The normal diurnal rhythm of plasma cortisol tends to be obliterated in Cushing syndrome. In normal individuals, the 4-p.m. cortisol is on an average 50% of that obtained in the early morning. Although widely advocated for diagnosis, determination of this rhythm by measurement of morning and evening (usually midnight) cortisol is an unreliable screening procedure in distinguishing Cushing and pseudo-Cushing syndrome (19). The values overlap too much with normal ones to be useful or reliable discriminators for clinically questionable cases.

Other Tests. All of the following have had their advocates (19): the standard low-dose (48-h, 2 mg/day) dexamethasone suppression test measuring urine 17 OHCS, high-dose dexamethasone tests measuring free cortisol, and the CRH test with dexamethasone pretreatment. Recently, a promising study was reported of the use of 1-deamino-8D-arginine vasopressin (or desmopressin). Desmopressin stimulates the release of ACTH (and cortisol) in patients with Cushing syndrome. The test seems to discriminate quite well between normal subjects, patients with pseudo-Cushing syndrome, and patients with Cushing syndrome (20).

Interpreting Tests and Additional Diagnostic Maneuvers. If Cushing syndrome is clearly established or if the tests are equivocal and the clinical features strongly suggestive, referral to an endocrinologist is appropriate. In expert hands, a variety of maneuvers can usually establish or exclude the diagnosis and differentiate among the causes of Cushing syndrome, but familiarity with the specialized test procedures is essential. Often a degree of laboratory precision is required that is not always achieved by ordinary commercial laboratories. Useful tests in such consultations, in addition to those described, include multiple samplings of plasma cortisol throughout the day and night (integrated blood levels), determinations of urinary excretion of steroids on multiple occasions, variations of the dexamethasone suppression test with the use of different doses of the steroid, and plasma ACTH measurements.

Until strong laboratory evidence is at hand to indicate that steroid production is abnormal, procedures such as CT or MRI of the sella turcica and of the adrenal areas are not justified. These procedures are not useful in screening, although they are important in determining the locus and cause of steroid excess once evidence for the presence of Cushing syndrome has been obtained.

Treatment of Cushing Syndrome

Unilateral adrenalectomy is the treatment of Cushing syndrome caused by an adrenal adenoma, and bilateral adrenalectomy is the treatment of Cushing syndrome caused by bilateral adrenal macronodular hyperplasia. Although surgical removal of the adrenals (bilateral adrenalectomy) was accepted for years as the most effective therapy for Cushing disease (adrenocortical hyperfunction caused by ACTH excess) as well, this treatment has been abandoned. Induction of permanent adrenal insufficiency, the risk of development of an enlarging pituitary adenoma accompanied by hyperpigmentation (*Nelson syndrome*), and significant operative mortality and morbidity are drawbacks of adrenalectomy for this condition. It is now appreciated that most cases of Cushing disease can be treated by transsphenoidal surgical removal of a pituitary microadenoma, and this has become the preferred therapy (21). However, a significant number (estimates range from 5% to 25%) of patients treated in this manner experience recurrence within a short time despite apparently successful removal of the tumor. Medical therapy with an inhibitor of adrenal steroid synthesis is effective for these cases, either alone or in combination with pituitary irradiation. The current drug of choice may be ketoconazole (600 to 800 mg/day), but older inhibitors (mitotane *o,p'*-DDD, metyrapone, and aminoglutethimide) are also effective. The selection of the therapeutic approach for the individual patient should be made by an endocrinologist.

Adrenal Androgen Excess

If evidence of Cushing syndrome coexists with signs of androgen excess, the 24-hour excretion of 17-KS should be measured along with 17-OHCS or 17-KGS. However, the 17-KS measurement is of no use in routine screening for Cushing syndrome. Elevated values do occur but do so less often than the other indices of cortisol production. When an adrenal tumor is the cause of the syndrome, measurement of urinary 17-KS may be the most abnormal test. Some adrenal tumors (benign adenomas or carcinomas) produce enormous amounts of 17-KS. In suspected cases of adrenal tumor, such as an abnormal CT or MRI of the adrenal gland, measurement of 17-KS is specifically indicated. Serum testosterone may be elevated in women but not in men (see Adrenal Mass Lesions, below).

Hirsutism

Hirsutism without virilism (androgen-dependent hirsutism) is common (see Chapter 101). The combination of hirsutism plus virilism, which is rare, is invariably associated with elevated urinary 17-KS. When such a patient is encountered, referral to an endocrinologist is the most appropriate course. In adults, most cases prove to be caused by adrenal tumors. Other causes, such as congenital adrenal hyperplasia (female pseudohermaphroditism, isosexual precocity in men, hypertension, and salt loss), become apparent in childhood. Only a few cases (due to 21-hydroxylase deficiency) have been seen in adults.

Other Adrenal Diseases

Mineralocorticoid Excess

The classic condition resulting from mineralocorticoid excess is primary aldosteronism due to a benign adrenocortical adenoma (Conn syndrome). Clinical features include hypertension and the manifestations of hypokalemia. A significant number of cases are due to bilateral adrenocortical nodular hyperplasia.

The evaluation of this condition is described in Chapter 50.

Mineralocorticoid Deficiency

Aldosterone deficiency is part of classic adrenal insufficiency (Addison disease) but may also occur as a selective functional deficiency state in the syndrome of hyporeninemic hypoaldosteronism. The identifying feature is hyperkalemia. The syndrome is described in Chapter 52.

Pheochromocytoma

Pheochromocytoma is a rare catecholamine (epinephrine, norepinephrine)-producing tumor that is usually considered in relationship to the evaluation of hypertension. This tumor is described in Chapter 67.

Adrenal Mass Lesions, Incidentally Identified (Adrenal Incidentalomas)

Adrenal masses are now commonly recognized during CT of the abdomen. When such a lesion is discovered, consideration should be given to the possible presence of Cushing syndrome, of mineralocorticoid or catecholamine excess producing intermittent or sustained hypertension (pheochromocytoma, aldosteronism), of hirsutism and virilization, and of feminization. Biochemical testing should be initiated as appropriate.

Most lesions incidentally encountered during CT are benign clinically silent adenomas, but a major concern is whether the mass represents a carcinoma. Three considerations are relevant in attempting to make this distinction: biochemical activity, size of the lesion, and the very low incidence of adrenal carcinoma. Most carcinomas produce biochemically measurable products (e.g., an excess of 17-KS), a few produce 17-KGS but produce normal 17-KS, and rarely only testosterone or aldosterone levels are increased. Benign adenomas may also produce excess quantities of steroids. Nevertheless, tumors producing biochemical products generally should be removed.

If no biochemical abnormality is demonstrable, the size of the lesion gives some indication of whether it is benign or malignant. When discovered, most adenomas are small (less than 6 cm diameter), and most carcinomas are large (more than 6 cm diameter). However, a conservative approach to all such biochemically silent lesions is warranted because even with tumors over 6 cm, more than 60 operations would be necessary to remove one carcinoma, and more than 4,000 operations would be needed to remove a single carcinoma if one considers all lesions of diameter greater than 1.5 cm.

Occasionally, the adrenal mass is cystic. Large cystic masses can be aspirated by needle puncture; clear fluid indicates a benign lesion, but bloody fluid is indeterminate and cytology is not helpful. Similarly, needle aspiration biopsy is usually not useful in distinguishing benign from malignant cystic lesions.

In follow-up of biochemically silent adrenal masses, CTs at 2, 6, and 18 months are indicated. Lesions that are stable at 18 months can be considered benign and should not be removed (22). A few cases develop a new contralateral mass; a few others emerge as hormone producing tumors (23). Subtle hypercortisolism in several standard tests of the hypothalamic–pituitary–adrenal axis may develop; in this setting these lesions have come to be termed "subclinical Cushing syndrome" and probably should be removed (24).

Pharmacologic Uses of Steroids as Anti-Inflammatory and Immunosuppressive Drugs

Most steroid (glucocorticoid) use is related to treatment of diseases other than adrenal insufficiency. The dosages used exceed those of physiologic output and are best termed supraphysiologic or, simply, pharmacologic. The anti-inflammatory and immunosuppressive properties of these drugs constitute an invaluable part of the modern therapeutic armamentarium, but such uses, at least when prolonged, are invariably associated with side effects. Short-term uses are much safer, if not entirely innocuous. Although the glucocorticoid and mineralocorticoid actions of steroids have been chemically dissociated, no such separation has been possible for other desired versus undesired effects. All available glucocorticoids share these properties to an equal degree, although potency (effectiveness per milligram) varies widely (Table 81.1). Despite this fact, certain glucocorticoid compounds have become associated with the treatment of particular conditions (e.g., dexamethasone for treatment of cerebral edema, methylprednisolone for hepatic disease). Often no pharmacologic basis exists to support such practices. On the other hand, differences between available preparations do exist that include different rates of absorption, metabolic disposal, and solubility. Exploitation of such properties is seen in dermatologic use. Triamcinolone and fluocinolone acetonides appear to be much more effective than hydrocortisone for topical use, a phenomenon apparently related to properties of absorption. Another example is the use of beclomethasone as an aerosol in the treatment of asthma (see Chapter 60) and allergic rhinitis (see Chapter 30).

Adverse Effects

Untoward effects of glucocorticoids are listed in Table 81.3. These problems are related to dose and, equally important, to duration of therapy. No contraindication exists to a single dose of glucocorticoid, regardless of the size of that dose. Thus, treatment of an allergic reaction with one or a few doses carries no risk. Long-term therapy, however, should be instituted only after consideration of the risks and benefits.

Adverse effects of steroids are related not only to duration of therapy but also to the dosage used. Obviously, the minimally effective dosage should be used. Nonetheless, some people seem especially vulnerable to unwanted side effects. Poorly nourished, debilitated, and elderly patients are more prone to the muscle-wasting effects of steroids (steroid

Table 81.3. Untoward Effects of Chronic Glucocorticoid Therapy

Acute
Fluid/electrolyte disturbances
Sodium retention
Fluid retention
Potassium depletion
Hypokalemic alkalosis
Gastrointestinal
Peptic ulcer (hemorrhage, perforation)
Ulcerative esophagitis
Endocrine
Precipitation of diabetes mellitus
Ophthalmic
Glaucoma
Neurologic
Mood swings
Acute psychosis
Convulsions
Chronic
Fluid/electrolyte disturbances
See above, plus hypertension
Musculoskeletal
Muscle weakness
Muscle atrophy
Steroid myopathy
Osteoporosis/pathologic fractures
Aseptic necrosis of femoral or humeral heads
Tendon rupture
Gastrointestinal
Pancreatitis
Dermatologic
Impaired wound healing
Atrophy of skin (fragility)
Ecchymoses
Increased sweating
Neurologic
Convulsions
Increased intracranial pressure
Insomnia
Euphoria
Depression
Endocrine
Menstrual irregularities
Carbohydrate intolerance/diabetes mellitus
Adrenal atrophy/disruption of normal response to stress (iatrogenic Addison disease)
Ophthalmic
Cataracts
Glaucoma
Hematologic
Thromboembolism
Other
Weight gain
Increased susceptibility to infections

myopathy). Postmenopausal women (already prone to develop osteoporosis) are especially vulnerable to the demineralization that accompanies steroid use. Biophosphonate inhibitors of bone resorption (e.g., alendronate) should be considered for such patients (see Chapters 84 and 103). Genetically predisposed individuals or patients in the early phase of the metabolic syndrome (see Chapter 79) may develop overt diabetes mellitus when given glucocorticoids. Peptic ulcer disease may be reactivated, and complications such as bleeding or perforation may be precipitated. Prophylactic use of antiulcer therapy should be considered in patients with a history of peptic ulcer disease. Dormant tuberculosis, clinically inapparent except for a positive tuberculin test, may reactivate. The role of isoniazid prophylaxis in this situation is described in Chapter 34. A gamut of psychiatric problems may be seen in patients who receive corticosteroids—emotional lability, depression, euphoria—which may necessitate adjustment of the dosage.

Topical Therapy

When steroids can be used locally, such use is preferred, especially when long-term treatment is involved. Although absorption may be complete from a local site, the amount of steroid required is often far less when use is local. This avoids, to some extent, systemic effects, side effects, and pituitary–adrenal suppression. In addition to dermatologic use of topical steroids, treatments of some ophthalmologic conditions, allergic rhinitis, asthma, and localized joint disease are examples of this principle.

Intermittent Therapy

Usually, severe disease requires initiation of steroid therapy given as multiple daily doses. When the disease intensity has waned (e.g., 1 to 2 weeks), conversion to alternate-day therapy can be made. Intermittent therapy of this type should always be considered when long-term use is contemplated. Such therapy is to be preferred because pituitary–adrenal suppression is not likely, and the adverse effects of glucocorticoids are minimized. When initiating intermittent therapy, the daily divided dose is given as a single morning dose. After this dose has been shown to be tolerated for several days, the single daily dose may be doubled and given as a single dose every other day. Thereafter, the dose given every other day can be reduced slowly, as clinically indicated. The patient may be symptomatic on the off day, particularly when alternate-day therapy is first started. To handle this situation, small doses of glucocorticoid may be given on this day. Nonsteroidal anti-inflammatory agents may also be helpful in ameliorating symptoms during transition.

Use of Adrenocorticotropic Hormone

The clinical indications for use of ACTH rather than a glucocorticoid are practically nonexistent. The practice continues, however, because ACTH was available for clinical use even before cortisone was. It is clear that in sufficient amounts (100 units), long-acting preparations (gel or zinc suspensions) given once daily are capable of stimulating adrenal secretion of up to 300 mg of cortisol daily. However, disadvantages are multiple: The route is parenteral, magnitude of response is unpredictable, mineralocorticoid effects (salt and fluid retention, potassium wasting) are considerable, and response in patients previously treated with glucocorticoids is slow and unpredictable. The only advantage is that adrenal responsiveness is maintained during therapy. Combined ACTH–glucocorticoid therapy has been advocated for this reason, as has the occasional injection of ACTH to prevent adrenal atrophy. However, the advantage of such an approach over that of intermittent glucocorticoid therapy is unclear. When ACTH is used alone at high dosages for a prolonged period, pituitary suppression occurs even though adrenal suppression does not. Another disadvantage of ACTH therapy is failure to produce more than the equivalent of 300 mg of cortisol (60 mg of prednisone) despite maximal stimulation of the adrenals. Such a dosage, although considerable, may be insufficient to produce the desired clinical effect. The only current fairly widespread (but diminishing) use of ACTH is in the treatment of acute exacerbations of multiple sclerosis.

Withdrawal from Acute or Chronic Glucocorticoid Therapy

Treatment with glucocorticoids (e.g., cortisone, hydrocortisone, prednisone) produces suppression of the hypothalamus–pituitary–adrenal axis; the output of ACTH falls, and there is subsequent adrenal atrophy and an inability to respond to stress with increased cortisol output. The time required for initial suppression is highly variable (see Recovery from Hypothalamus–Pituitary–Adrenal Suppression, below). Patients receiving daily pharmacologic doses of glucocorticoids (5 mg or more of prednisone or its equivalent daily) for more than 1 week should be presumed to have a suppressed response to stress (25). If stressed by surgery, trauma, or severe infection, these patients should be treated with replacement glucocorticoids as if they had Addison disease. On the other hand, glucocorticoids may be discontinued abruptly after 2 to 4 weeks of pharmacologic steroid therapy provided that the patient is not under stress, because baseline—as opposed to stress related—adrenal function is almost always adequate. Patients who have been treated with alternate-day steroid therapy are not at risk because pituitary–adrenal function seems well preserved in these individuals.

When it becomes desirable to terminate glucocorticoid therapy, the question arises of how to accomplish this goal while avoiding adrenal insufficiency. In the presence of active underlying disease, for which the glucocorticoids may have been given in the first place, a dilemma quickly becomes apparent. The nonspecific symptoms of adrenal insufficiency may be similar or identical to those of the disease that was under treatment. In addition, the occurrence of the "steroid withdrawal syndrome" (see below) may further compound the issue.

Withdrawal Schedule. No single scheme can solve this difficult clinical problem, although many have been proposed. However, a few general points can be made. First, even after prolonged therapy, in the absence of active underlying systemic disease, symptoms of true adrenal insufficiency will not occur until the daily dose of glucocorticoid drops below physiologic replacement (20 mg of cortisol, 5 mg of prednisone, or equivalent; see Table 81.1). Symptoms similar to those of adrenal insufficiency may occur as the daily dose is being reduced (see Steroid Withdrawal Syndrome, below), although most patients will not be symptomatic if they take a single 20- to 30-mg daily dose of cortisol (or 5 to 7.5 mg of prednisone). Continuation of 20 mg of cortisol daily for 2 months should ensure some degree of recovery of pituitary–adrenal function. Further withdrawal begins to re-establish the normal pituitary–adrenal relationship. Additional reductions of 5 mg of cortisol can be made every 2 to 3 weeks over the next 2 months or, alternatively, an every other day program can be tried over the same period; the glucocorticoid can then usually be stopped without producing symptoms. A laboratory assessment of the functional status of the patient's adrenals at this point is described below (see Recovery from Hypothalamus–Pituitary–Adrenal Suppression, below).

Steroid Withdrawal Syndrome: Distinction from Acute Adrenal Insufficiency. Abrupt withdrawal of pharmacologic doses of glucocorticoids, even after months of therapy, does not always produce chemical evidence of adrenal insufficiency. Nonetheless, the patient may experience many of the symptoms of adrenal insufficiency (e.g., lethargy, malaise, anorexia, nausea, vomiting, myalgias, fever, and, in severe cases, desquamation of skin in a manner resembling exfoliative dermatitis). Less than abrupt withdrawal may result in similar but not as severe symptoms. Such patients may be found to have normal or elevated levels of cortisol. This phenomenon is not simply adrenal insufficiency but rather is a pharmacologic withdrawal syndrome. Symptoms subside promptly with reinstitution of glucocorticoid therapy.

Recovery from Hypothalamic–Pituitary–Adrenal Suppression: Limitations of Testing With Adrenocorticotropin Hormone. Recovery of the hypothalamus–pituitary–adrenal axis after 1 week of "steroid burst therapy" (e.g., 40 mg of prednisone for 3 days, followed by a 4-day taper) appears complete within 1 additional week (25), but the rate of recovery is unpredictable after withdrawal from longer courses of therapy. After long-term glucocorticoid therapy (pharmacologic doses for a year or more), recovery of normal pituitary–adrenal responsiveness does not occur for at least several months, even if the patient receives no exogenous steroid therapy during that time. In the first month after withdrawal, both pituitary and adrenal function remain depressed (low plasma ACTH and low plasma cortisol). Over the following 4 months, pituitary function recovers first (plasma ACTH is elevated), but adrenal function remains subnormal (plasma cortisol is lower than normal). Eventually, adrenal function recovers (plasma cortisol levels normalize) and elevated plasma ACTH returns to normal. The entire process may require up to 9 months. During this interval the patient may fare well, provided there is no stress, but replacement therapy with glucocorticoids may become necessary at any time. Accordingly, no patient should be considered to have normal pituitary–adrenal function unless at least 1 year has elapsed after complete withdrawal of chronic glucocorticoid therapy. Occasional patients seem never to recover normal responsiveness. Ideally, therefore, all patients with a history of long-term steroid therapy, if they are to be tested for normality of the axis, should be tested 1 year after withdrawal. It is not clear, however, whether any practical test is available (see below).

Assessment of a glucocorticoid-treated patient's adrenal function under baseline conditions is easy. Both plasma cortisol measurements and urinary excretion of steroid metabolites give a reasonable estimate of such baseline function. However, predicting the response to stress is more difficult. Because hypothalamic–pituitary function usually recovers first, followed by adrenal function (see above), a normal response to exogenous ACTH would seem to indicate recovery of the entire axis but in fact does not do so with a reasonable degree of reliability (see also below). An accurate assessment of the integrity of the axis can be made by induction of hypoglycemia with insulin (insulin tolerance test, or ITT). Hypoglycemia triggers ACTH release and the cortisol secretory response of the adrenal. A normal ITT essentially ensures that if the patient is subjected to stressful circumstances, replacement therapy with steroids will not be necessary. However, the ITT must be done in a metabolic laboratory with careful monitoring and is considered to be dangerous and therefore inappropriate in patients over age 60.

Administration of CRH rather than ACTH has been advocated as an alternative to the insulin-induced hypoglycemia test. The end point is the plasma cortisol response. This procedure is easier and is completely safe. However, the correlation between the CRH and ITT is only fair, and the magnitude of the response is only a 1.5-fold mean increase in plasma cortisol, requiring a laboratory with optimal accuracy. Ideally, a CRH stimulation test should be done only by an endocrinologist.

As a practical matter, empirical short-term corticosteroid administration ("coverage") during stress is probably the simplest, safest, and cheapest way to manage patients in whom the status of the adrenal–pituitary axis is uncertain.

HYPOCALCEMIC STATES

Hypocalcemia is an uncommon problem in ambulatory patients. The classic cause of hypocalcemia is hypoparathyroidism, but most cases encountered are a consequence of inadvertent surgical ablation of the parathyroids during thyroidectomy or as a result of a metabolic disturbance such as renal failure. The causes of hypocalcemia are listed in Table 81.4.

Clinical Manifestations of Hypocalcemia

The symptoms of hypocalcemia are primarily neuromuscular and are not usually evident until the serum calcium falls below about 8 mg/dL, and often considerably lower. Mild but real symptoms are nonspecific and include psychologic manifestations (irritability, mood changes, lassitude, depression) and neuromuscular symptoms (paresthesias and muscle cramps [spasms]). More severe symptoms are seen at extremely depressed serum calcium levels (e.g., 5.5 to 6 mg%) and include delirium, psychosis, tetany (including laryngeal stridor), and seizures. Neuromuscular irritability can often be demonstrated by the twitching that can be induced by tapping or rubbing the face (e.g., during shaving) over the facial nerve just anterior to the ear. A positive response to this maneuver is contraction of the facial muscles around the lip *(Chvostek sign)*. Another clinical test is compression of the upper arm by a blood pressure cuff with the pressure elevated above the systolic pressure. A positive response is spasm of the hand induced within 3 minutes *(Trousseau sign)*. Signs of chronic hypocalcemia include patchy hair loss, scaling of skin, atrophy and brittleness of fingernails, and cataract formation. Candidiasis is common. Calcification of the basal ganglia may be seen on radiographic examination of the skull. Either osteosclerosis or osteopenia may occur depending on the cause of the hypocalcemia.

Table 81.4. Causes of Hypocalcemia

Hypocalcemia with high serum phosphate
Renal failure
Postablative hypoparathyroidism (post-thyroidectomy)
Idiopathic hypoparathyroidism
Pseudohyperparathyroidism
Hypocalcemia with low or normal serum phosphate
Malabsorption (vitamin D deficiency)
Magnesium deficiency (alcoholism)
Renal rickets (renal tubular acidosis; phosphate diabetes; cystinosis; Fanconi syndrome; vitamin D–resistant rickets)
Medullary carcinoma of thyroid

The serum alkaline phosphatase activity is elevated when severe metabolic bone disease is present. Parathyroid hormone levels are depressed in magnesium deficiency. Parathyroid hormone levels are regularly elevated in renal failure and in pseudohypoparathyroidism. Urine calcium is depressed in most hypocalcemic states, except when the rare renal tubular calcium-wasting syndromes are responsible for the hypocalcemia.

Laboratory Findings

Hypocalcemia can be defined as a serum calcium level below 8.5 mg/dL. However, because almost half of serum calcium is protein bound, reduction of serum albumin by 1 g/dL lowers the serum calcium by about 0.8 mg/dL. The level of serum calcium therefore must always be evaluated in the context of the serum albumin concentration; the serum magnesium concentration should also be evaluated at the same time (see Other Causes of Hypocalcemia from Causes Other than Parathyroid Disease, below). Plasma parathyroid hormone (PTH) levels are low or nondetectable in idiopathic or postablative hypoparathyroidism and in some cases of hypocalcemia due to magnesium deficiency, but they are elevated in pseudohypoparathyroidism, renal failure, malabsorption, and vitamin D deficiency. The interpretation and indications for determination of PTH levels are discussed below.

Hypoparathyroidism

Hypoparathyroidism is rare. Although most patients are diagnosed in childhood, some do not exhibit the disorder until adult life. Occasionally familial, the condition is often autoimmune, associated with high titers of antibodies to parathyroid tissue, and may be seen in association with other autoimmune endocrine diseases (adrenal insufficiency, Hashimoto thyroiditis) and pernicious anemia (see below).

The term "hypoparathyroidism" designates a group of conditions, all of which manifest hypocalcemia, and is thus a generic term for one of the many "hypoparathyroid disorders." Functional hypoparathyroidism (i.e., with hypocalcemia) arises from a defect in either PTH production (i.e., PTH deficiency), a defect in the PTH receptor, or insensitivity to PTH as a result of postreceptor (downstream) molecular defects. In recent years these various conditions have been shown to arise from distinct abnormalities of molecular genetics (26). An understanding of these and other defects has also explained the autosomal dominant syndrome of combined hypocalcemia and hypercalciuria (below). Mutations in the PTH gene, the transcription factors involved in PTH action, and the PTH receptor gene have also been identified. The entities pseudohypoparathyroidism (type Ia) and pseudo-pseudohypoparathyroidism (below) have been shown to involve inactivating mutations in the stimulatory G protein (Gsα). The gene for the calcium-sensing receptor of the cell membrane of parathyroid cells undergoes mutations that increase or decrease its normal function, regulation of the transcription of the PTH gene. Loss of function of the calcium-sensing receptor results in familial benign hypercalcemia with hypocalciuria; increased function leads to hypocalcemia with hypercalciuria. The pluriglandular (multiglandular) autoimmune syndrome, also known as the autoimmune polyendocrinopathy syndrome or the candidiasis–ectodermal dystrophy syndrome, includes hypoparathyroidism, Addison disease, candidiasis, and two or three of the following: type 1 diabetes, primary hypogonadism, autoimmune thyroid disease, pernicious anemia, chronic active hepatitis, malabsorption, alopecia, and vitiligo. The polyglandular autoimmune syndrome is yet another specific genetic defect.

Precise diagnosis of "hypoparathyroid" patients is important for avoiding inappropriate therapy. For example, patients with hypocalcemia and hypercalciuria were in the past treated with vitamin D. These individuals, who were usually asymptomatic at diagnosis, then developed massive hypercalciuria, nephrocalcinosis, and renal failure. Hypocalcemic individuals need referral to an endocrinologist.

Postthyroidectomy Hypoparathyroidism

Hypoparathyroidism was, in the past era of frequent surgical therapy of thyroid diseases, a complication of thyroidectomy. The hypocalcemic state could become evident immediately after surgery but often took many years to develop, presumably because of slowly progressive interference with the blood supply to the parathyroids. Routine screening of serum calcium in patients who have had a thyroidectomy reveals many asymptomatic mildly hypocalcemic patients. Most of these individuals seem to need no therapy, but in view of the subtle neuromuscular changes that can result from hypocalcemia, careful consideration should always be given to this issue. Hypoparathyroidism is rare after radioiodide therapy of thyroid disease; only a very few cases have been reported.

Pseudohypoparathyroidism

Pseudohypoparathyroidism (see Hypoparathyroidism, above) is a rare genetic disorder (X-linked dominant trait). In addition to hypocalcemia and its manifestations, there are associated skeletal developmental defects that result in short stature, shortening of metacarpals and metatarsals, and round face. Clinical manifestations attributable to hypocalcemia may not appear until adult life. The biochemical basis of the hypocalcemia is end-organ resistance to the action of PTH. The combination of hypocalcemia, an elevated level of PTH, and typical skeletal abnormalities is virtually diagnostic.

Treatment of Postsurgical Hypoparathyroidism

A few patients with minimal PTH deficiency can be managed by increasing dietary calcium by 1 to 2 g/day. Instruction by a dietitian is important.

Severely symptomatic patients should be hospitalized to receive intravenous calcium and for initiation of chronic therapy with oral calcium supplements and with vitamin D. Symptomatic patients who do not require hospitalization should also be prescribed calcium supplements and vitamin D. Calcium supplementation usually requires 1,500 to 2,000 mg/day of elemental calcium.

Because calcium gluconate and lactate contain only approximately 10% elemental calcium, one must administer 10 to 20 g of these salts; numerous tablets must be taken, and patient compliance is a common problem. Calcium carbonate contains approximately 40% elemental calcium, so fewer tablets are necessary, but this salt is insoluble at neutral pH and requires that gastric acidity is present for absorption to occur. Calcium citrate (21% elemental calcium) is now available in 950-mg tablets and is probably the best choice (8 to 10 tablets a day). Every effort should be made to work out an acceptable, palatable, and economic program with a consistently available preparation for what is invariably lifelong therapy.

The second mainstay of therapy is *vitamin D.* The most commonly used preparation in the past has been *ergocalciferol* (vitamin D_2, Calciferol). The dosage is usually 50,000 or 100,000 units daily, although higher doses may be necessary. The compound is available in 50,000-unit (1.25-mg) capsules. The sole advantage of ergocalciferol is cost; it is by far the least expensive form of vitamin D therapy. The disadvantage of ergocalciferol is its somewhat unpredictable toxicity with resultant hypercalcemia and all its manifestations (see below). Because vitamin D is fat soluble, toxicity may last for many weeks or even months after discontinuation of therapy. Glucocorticoids are effective therapy for hypercalcemia caused by vitamin D toxicity.

A preferable vitamin D preparation is its synthetic analog *dihydrotachysterol* (Hytakerol). The dosage varies from 0.2 to 2 mg/day. The compound is available as tablets and as a solution. The advantage of therapy with dihydrotachysterol is more rapid onset of action than D_2 and more rapid reversal of toxicity on withdrawal of the drug. The only disadvantage of dihydrotachysterol is its relatively high cost. Yet another effective compound is *1,25-dihydroxyvitamin D_3* (calcitriol, Rocaltrol), the natural active form of vitamin D. This compound is more rapid than dihydrotachysterol in onset and has a shorter duration of effect but has the disadvantage of even greater cost. The dosage is 0.25 to 1.0 μg/day.

Vitamin D, in whatever form selected, is given simultaneously, with calcium tablets with adjustments of dosage at weekly or biweekly intervals depending on the serum calcium level. The goal of therapy is a serum calcium concentration of 8.5 to 9.5 mg/dL. Hypercalcemia is to be avoided. Once a stable level of serum calcium is reached (1 to 2 months), the patient can be monitored at monthly intervals and eventually every 3 to 4 months. The possibility of toxicity from hypercalcemia must always to be kept in mind. Even mild hypercalcemia predisposes to nephrocalcinosis and nephrolithiasis in these patients.

Hypocalcemia from Causes Other Than Parathyroid Disease

When hypocalcemia is related to malabsorption, efforts to correct that situation should be undertaken, but simultaneous treatment with vitamin D and calcium may be indicated. One common cause of hypocalcemia is alcoholism with resultant *magnesium deficiency.* Overt malnutrition does not need to be present. The mechanisms by which alcohol abuse produces magnesium depletion include decreased dietary intake and alcohol-facilitated renal excretion of magnesium. Magnesium depletion results in both impaired secretion of PTH and impaired PTH action. Such patients usually require hospitalization. Intramuscular magnesium therapy normalizes the serum calcium within hours.

Other diseases associated with hypocalcemia include osteomalacia (vitamin D or calcium deficiency) (see Chapter 84) and variants of Fanconi syndrome (a spectrum of renal tubular abnormalities). The hypocalcemia associated with renal failure is described in Chapter 52.

HYPERCALCEMIC STATES

Because many routine automated blood analyses include determinations of serum calcium, many cases of hypercalcemia (in most laboratories, serum calcium greater than 10.5 mg/dL) are detected, most of them mild and asymptomatic. The demonstration of hypercalcemia always requires investigation.

Table 81.5. Causes of Hypercalcemia

Condition	Comment
Common causes	
Thiazide drugs	Mild elevation (not >12.5 mg/dL); requires 2 weeks or more to subside
Hyperparathyroidism	Often asymptomatic; commonly discovered on routine blood test
Malignancy (including myeloma)	Most common cause in hospitalized patients; may lead to initial encounter in ambulatory patients
Spurious	Inappropriate technique while drawing blood (venous stasis produces hemoconcentration)
Rare causes	
Milk alkali syndrome	Requires use (abuse) of both alkali ($NaHCO_3$) and large quantities of milk or calcium salts
Hypervitaminosis D	Usually 50,000 units or more daily
Thyrotoxicosis	Severe disease is evident
Paget disease of bone	Immobilization is necessary
Immobilization	Body cast in adolescent males; patients with Paget disease of bone; quadriplegia
Sarcoidosis	Hyperglobulinemia usually present
Chronic renal failure	Uncommon; may exacerbate after transplantation or during hemodialysis
Adrenal insufficiency	Hemoconcentration present
Idiopathic elevation	Mild elevation in postmenopausal women; may revert to normal with physiologic estrogen therapy

Etiologies

The causes of hypercalcemia are listed in Table 81.5. In an ambulatory setting the most common cause of hypercalcemia (80 to 90% of cases) is *hyperparathyroidism* due to a small indolent parathyroid adenoma (27). *Malignancy,* either due to bony metastases or to elaboration of a parathormone related protein (PTH-rh) or of calcitriol, is probably the second most common cause of hypercalcemia (the most common cause in hospitalized patients) (28) but usually is obvious at presentation and also often presents with associated ominous symptoms (e.g., weight loss and anorexia).

Nonmetastatic tumors associated with hypercalcemia, in the main, do so by generating excess PTH-rh (29); calcitriol production is mostly limited to some patients with lymphoma (both Hodgkin disease and non-Hodgkin lymphoma) (30). In times past, the use of thiazide diuretics also was a relatively common cause of mild hypercalcemia. Furthermore, thiazide therapy may unmask underlying hyperparathyroidism (see below). The problem is encountered less often now that dosages of thiazides are generally lower than in the past, but in any case, hypercalcemia is fully reversible upon withdrawal of the drug. If hypercalcemia persists despite thiazide withdrawal, another cause of hypercalcemia should be sought.

Diagnosis

Symptoms of hypercalcemia (Table 81.6) may be vague and difficult to interpret, especially when the serum calcium is only slightly to moderately elevated (10.5 to 12 mg%). More severe symptoms are experienced

Table 81.6. Symptoms and Signs of Hypercalcemia

Short term (readily reversible)
- General: weakness, anorexia, weight loss, fatigue
- Gastrointestinal: nausea, vomiting, constipation
- Genitourinary: polyuria, azotemia
- Musculoskeletal: bone aches
- Neurologic: lethargy, sleepiness, difficulty concentrating, confusion, psychosis
- Cardiovascular: bradycardia, electrocardiographic abnormalities (short QT, arrhythmias)
- Ophthalmologic: difficulty focusing
- Dermatologic: pruritis

Long term (irreversible or slowly reversible)
- Gastrointestinal: peptic ulcer, pancreatitis
- Genitourinary: renal calculi (colic, hematuria); nephrocalcinosis; polyuria
- Skeletal: bone loss (osteopenia); subperiosteal resorption, bone cysts, pseudogout
- Neuromuscular: muscle atrophy
- Ophthalmologic: band keratopathy; conjunctival calcifications (usually require slit-lamp examination)

when the serum calcium level is higher and, sometimes, when it is of relatively long duration.

Determination of PTH concentration is the critical test in elucidating the cause of hypercalcemia (see also Primary Hyperparathyroidism, below). Older PTH assays did not reliably distinguish hypercalcemia of hyperparathyroidism from that of malignancy. Current assays are much more precise so that the clinician should be certain that the laboratory is using a modern assay. The aforementioned PTH-rh produced by some malignant tumors can also be measured accurately; the specificity and the sensitivity of the test are in the range of 90% (29).

Primary Hyperparathyroidism

The term *primary hyperparathyroidism* refers to autonomous hyperfunction of one or more parathyroid glands. Hypercalcemia is the hallmark of this disorder. Secondary hyperparathyroidism, on the other hand, is a physiologic or pathophysiologic homeostatic response to situations that lower blood calcium.

The most common cause of primary hyperparathyroidism is a solitary benign adenoma (85% of patients). In a small proportion of patients, more than one adenoma is present, and in the remainder, the cause is idiopathic hyperplasia. Carcinoma of the parathyroid is rare (less than 1% of patients). Hyperparathyroidism may be familial and may occur as part of the syndrome of multiple endocrine adenomatosis (see Chromophobe Adenomas, above).

Diagnosis

Most cases are now detected by routine automated analysis of blood electrolytes. The symptoms (Table 81.6) or sequelae of hypercalcemia may also alert the physician to the diagnosis, but unlike the situation in the past, symptomatic hyperparathyroidism is now a rarity, except for a history of kidney stones in perhaps 20% of cases (31). Once the diagnosis is suspected, however, the presence of hypercalcemia must be established beyond a doubt. Multiple determinations of serum calcium should be made. Because of spontaneous fluctuations of the serum calcium and because of analytic error, values that are only minimally elevated (10.5 to 11.5 mg/dL) must be repeated several times. The resulting *mean* level should be used for diagnostic purposes, not the last—sometimes normal—value obtained.

Once hypercalcemia is established (greater than 10.5 mg/dL on multiple determinations), the next (or simultaneous) step is to determine the likelihood of the presence of other causes of hypercalcemia (Table 81.5). Finally, assay of PTH in blood should be performed (see below).

Other laboratory findings may include low serum phosphorus concentration and, very rarely in severe cases with bone involvement, elevation of serum alkaline phosphatase activity. Other abnormalities in laboratory tests occur but are not useful for screening or in differential diagnosis because they occur nonspecifically. Patients with hypercalcemia, regardless of cause, usually show hypercalciuria, but hypercalciuria may also occur without hypercalcemia. Increased excretion of hydroxyproline-containing peptides occurs, as it does in other bone diseases.

In severe cases of long duration, radiographic studies of various bones reveal a variety of changes suggestive but not diagnostic of hyperparathyroidism. Demineralization (osteopenia) and subperiosteal resorption are most obvious in the clavicles and the hands, and the lamina dura of the teeth may be resorbed. Cystic changes occur in skull and long bones (osteitis fibrosa cystica). None of these changes is seen in cases with minimal hypercalcemia (10.5 to 11.5 mg/100 mL). Radiographic studies are not useful for screening purposes.

Parathyroid Hormone Assays. Radioimmunoassays are useful but have several limitations. Specificity of the assays varies among laboratories because of the use of different antibodies. Some laboratories offer several different PTH assays, each of which has its own advantages and limitations. The most commonly used procedure until recently, the so-called C-terminal assay, measures a peptide fragment derived from PTH. This assay, as performed on peripheral venous blood (plasma or serum), may be the most sensitive test for detecting hyperparathyroidism, but it is also elevated by impaired renal function, partly because of decreased peptide fragment excretion, and is often elevated in normal elderly patients, especially women over age 65. The elevations seen in primary hyperparathyroidism are often only modest (e.g., 50% greater than the upper limits of normal). Accordingly, at least two or three assays should ordinarily be obtained. The assay also measures PTH-like materials produced by tumors.

Several other widely available assays measure intact hormone or N-terminal fragments. Although these assays are more specific and less likely to be elevated in cases of ectopic (tumor) production of PTH, they are also less sensitive in detecting primary hyperparathyroidism, being normal in nearly half of cases, albeit inappropriately so for the degree of hypercalcemia. In patients with chronic renal failure, in whom secondary hyperparathyroidism is invariably present, the intact hormone assays are not artificially raised by retention of PTH fragments, as are the C-terminal assays, and more or less reflect the degree of secondary hyperparathyroidism.

Recently introduced double antibody immunoradiometric and immunochemiluminescent assays are replacing the older radioimmunoassays. Both have improved sensitivity and appear to be superior for detecting hyperparathyroidism; frankly elevated levels are seen in 85% to 90% of hyperparathyroid cases. In some patients, the values are not overtly elevated (i.e., although normal, they are inappropriately so in the setting of hypercalcemia). Moreover, the assays show a high degree of specificity and do not detect the PTH-like peptides produced by tumors. Assays for PTH are now available that directly measure the tumor-produced PTH-like peptides but not PTH. The evaluating clinician is obliged to know the specificity and, especially when dealing with minimal abnormalities, the accuracy of the assay used in the laboratory. Endocrinologists are more likely than generalists to be familiar with these important details.

Steroid Suppression Test. Although most cases of hyperparathyroidism and of other hypercalcemic states can be diagnosed by the means described, the cause of occasional cases of hypercalcemia remains in doubt. In these, a short course of prednisone therapy (30 to 40 mg/day for 10 to 14 days) may help diagnostically. The hypercalcemia of hyperparathyroidism does not respond to such therapy. Although only about half of cases of hypercalcemia due to malignancy respond, hypercalcemia from diseases that are not always apparent, such as sarcoidosis and vitamin D intoxication, responds consistently. Determinations of blood calcium should always be obtained for several consecutive days before and daily during such a test.

Further Evaluation. Having established the presence of hypercalcemia and elevation of PTH and having excluded by appropriate means malignancy, impaired renal function, and other conditions listed in Table 81.5, the diagnosis of hyperparathyroidism is reasonably well established. However, the urinary excretion of calcium should be determined at this point because patients with *benign familial hypercalcemia* from parathyroid hyperplasia do not have hypercalciuria or other complications of minimal hypercalcemia and do not need surgical intervention. In most cases of hyperparathyroidism, referral to an endocrinologist should be made if the diagnosis is in doubt or if surgery is contemplated.

Preoperative Localization of Parathyroid Adenoma. A variety of imaging methods has been used, but none has been more successful than the technetium-sestamibi scan. Other techniques include ultrasound and CT and, in previously operated patients, selective venous sampling, but as yet none of these has been shown to improve primary surgical results. The importance of preoperative localization will probably be greatest when parathyroidectomy is performed by relatively inexperienced surgeons. Parathyroidectomy is an operation in which the outcome is clearly related to the surgeon's experience. The most successful surgeons have performed 100 or more parathyroidectomies, often 25 to 50 per year (32).

Apparently Asymptomatic Patient With Hypercalcemia

A common dilemma in demonstrated hyperparathyroidism with mild hypercalcemia is the so-called asymptomatic patient (33). Some experts are convinced that 80% of patients are, in fact, asymptomatic (34). Others believe that nonspecific but real symptoms may be present in 90% of patients with mild to moderate hypercalcemia (35). This view is based on studies of preoperative and postoperative symptom questionnaires. A National Institutes of Health Consensus Development Conference in 1990 (33) concluded that many patients over age 50 could be safely followed without surgery and outlined a plan for those for whom surgery should be recommended (see below). The issue was not resolved, however, and reports advocating surgery for all diagnosed patients have appeared. These widely discrepant views have led to a thoughtful recommendation for a new National Institutes of Health consensus conference. In the meantime, most would agree that clearly symptomatic patients or those with major complications should seriously consider surgery as an option and that asymptomatic patients without complications can be followed safely most of the time (34–36).

Complications of Hyperparathyroidism

Nephrolithiasis. Renal calculus disease (nephrolithiasis) develops in up to 20% of patients in some series and is related to the degree of hypercalcemia and hypercalciuria. Classic cases of hyperparathyroidism are no doubt at risk for progressive renal failure, but in minimal disease, this problem is not usually seen. Nonetheless, recurrent renal calculi are worth preventing, if possible, and surgical cure of the hyperparathyroidism would logically prevent recurrent stones. Unfortunately, no good data are available to support this course of action.

Bone Disease. Loss of bone mineral is a well-known effect of hyperparathyroidism and is often termed "osteoporosis." Successful parathyroidectomy results in rapid remineralization, especially of the lumbar spine and femoral neck with a mean post-parathyroidectomy rise of 12% in bone mineral (35). In postmenopausal patients improvement in bone density may reach 20%. Interestingly, although bone is demineralized in hyperparathyroidism, the rate of fractures is not known. The demineralization of PTH excess is associated with bone remodeling, and in animals given PTH, struts and connections among trabeculae are increased in association with increased tensile strength of bone. Human recombinant PTH has recently been shown to increase bone mineral density and to decrease bone fractures in women with "ordinary" osteoporosis. Clearly, PTH has effects on both bone mineral deposition and its resorption; the latter appears to dominate at higher doses and/or in relationship to its mode of administration (37).

Hypertension and Cardiovascular Disease. Hyperparathyroidism has been associated with hypertension, left ventricular hypertrophy, arrhythmias, and calcification of the coronary arteries, myocardium, and heart valves. Furthermore, increased mortality rates were reported in several large series. However, these observations represented the overt hypercalcemia of older series. In more recent studies, the cardiovascular death rate in minimal disease (serum calcium elevation not more than 1 mg% above the upper limits of normal) was reduced, as was overall death rate (38). Clearly, the severity of the hyperparathyroidism accounts for these differences. However, the association of hypertension and hyperparathyroidism remains unclear, because successful parathyroidectomy does not improve hypertension in these cases.

Therapy

In diagnosed patients the main question is whether surgical intervention is warranted. The rate of development of complications (neuromuscular disease, bone disease, decreased renal function) in patients with minimal asymptomatic hypercalcemia is low, with the exception of nephrolithiasis, which develops in approximately 20% of patients (31). Conditions classically associated with hyperparathyroidism, such as hypertension, peptic ulcer disease, and pancreatitis, may not be associated with it at all (31). However, the decision for or against surgery will obviously be based not only on the presence of complicating problems, but on such factors as patient age, associated medical illness, and the presence or absence of neuropsychiatric dysfunction. In many patients, medical management of the hyperparathyroidism may be indicated (see below).

Surgical versus Conservative Therapy. In 1990, the National Institutes of Health convened a Consensus Development Conference on the Management of Asymptomatic Primary Hyperparathyroidism (33). The Conference established guidelines for consideration of surgical treatment: (a) serum calcium concentration greater than 12 mg/100 mL; (b) hypercalciuria, greater than 400 mg/24 hr; (c) nephrolithiasis, cystic bone disease, or overt neuromuscular disease; (d) markedly reduced cortical bone density; (e) reduced renal function as determined by creatinine clearance in the absence of other causes; and (f) age less than 50 years. Whether all these guidelines (e.g., age) are equally important is unclear (31).

A major concern is whether conservative medical management permits progression of bone disease as measured by longitudinal changes in bone mineral density or biochemical indices. When a group of 66 patients were followed for 7 years (24 met guidelines for surgical intervention), no progressive changes were seen (39). Thus, conservative medical management appears safe.

If a decision is made to treat the patient surgically, referral to a surgeon experienced in parathyroid/thyroid exploration is essential. In experienced hands, an adenoma, if present, will be located and easily removed in perhaps 98% of cases (32). Parathyroid hyperplasia, which accounts for 10% of cases of hyperparathyroidism, is usually easily identified. In such cases, the surgeon should be prepared to perform a nearly total parathyroidectomy. Second neck explorations are technically difficult and may result in unnecessary morbidity (e.g., damage to the recurrent laryngeal nerve). Accordingly, any hyperplastic parathyroid tissue that is left behind should be identified with clips. As an alternative, many surgeons are now removing all parathyroid tissue from the neck and transplanting a portion of one hyperplastic gland to an accessible location, usually a sternocleidomastoid muscle or into the forearm.

Failure to identify an adenoma and absence of hyperplasia may require partial thyroidectomy—the adenoma may be embedded in the thyroid—or exploration of the anterosuperior mediastinum. This procedure may be performed at the time of initial surgery or at some time later. Such details obviously involve the surgeon's preference and experience but should be considered and discussed before surgery. If the neck has already been explored unsuccessfully, a selective venous catheterization study with sampling of PTH levels is a useful procedure for preoperative localization of the tumor. Only a few major medical centers can perform this procedure, but it is probably worthwhile to avoid unnecessary morbidity when a second operation is performed. Such localization studies are not indicated before initial surgery.

Medical Therapy. The medical therapy of hyperparathyroidism with phosphate is ordinarily limited to those patients in whom surgery is not desirable but who require therapy. Although intravenous phosphate therapy carries the risk of soft tissue calcium deposition, this problem is much less likely when phosphate is given orally. *Sodium–potassium phosphate salts* given orally (K-Phos, Neutra-Phos) may produce diarrhea. Dosage should be titrated upward as tolerated. A sodium-free preparation is also available (Neutra-Phos-K) for use in patients whose sodium intake should be restricted. Asymptomatic patients with mild hypercalcemia probably should not be treated with phosphate.

Estrogen is an effective alternative to surgery for uncomplicated hyperparathyroidism, as shown by improvement in bone mineral density (40). The effect on serum calcium usually does not exceed 0.5 mg%. Because many patients with asymptomatic hyperparathyroidism are postmenopausal women, this approach has considerable appeal. Unfortunately, not all patients respond and even in those who do, some abnormalities of bone persist. Norethindrone, a progestogen, has a similar effect to that of estrogen in occasional patients. The use of other potent antiresorptive agents (selective estrogen receptor modulators [e.g., raloxifene] or bisphosphonates) has not been evaluated.

Therapy of Hypercalcemia

The treatment of hypercalcemia due to hyperparathyroidism is discussed above (see Primary Hyperparathyroidism). Therapy to control hypercalcemia that results from a cause other than hyperparathyroidism is not commonly initiated in ambulatory patients. Most often the hypercalcemia or its underlying cause has required initial therapy in a hospital. However, when the acute symptoms of hypercalcemia have been controlled during hospitalization, long-term palliative therapy may be needed for the ambulatory patient.

Treatment of hypercalcemia of malignancy is usually begun in the hospital; the current drug of choice is the *bisphosphonate* pamidronate (Aredia). Once the problem is controlled, therapy may be continued on an ambulatory basis by administration of intravenous pamidronate, 60 to 90 mg, over a 2- to 4-hour period every 2 weeks. (If this dosage is inadequate or if severe hypercalcemia—calcium above 12.5 mg/100 mL—occurs, the patient may need to be hospitalized again.) Alternatively, the oral bisphosphonate alendronate may be prescribed, but it is not yet approved for this purpose by the Food and Drug Administration (FDA) and is associated with considerably more toxicity (e.g., oral and esophageal ulcers) than is pamidronate. Other drugs (e.g., glucocorticoids, mithramycin, calcitonin) that have been used in the treatment of malignancy are less effective or potentially more toxic than pamidronate and are prescribed less often today. If possible, the hypercalcemia of malignancy is best dealt with by an oncologist.

Glucocorticoids are often effective in lowering hypercalcemia caused by sarcoidosis and vitamin D intoxication. Mild hypercalcemia in elderly postmenopausal women may sometimes respond to physiologic amounts of estrogen (40). Treatment of hypercalcemia with phosphates administered orally is sometimes possible, especially in mild hyperparathyroidism (see above). Often, partial control of hypercalcemia is sufficient to relieve symptoms; complete normalization of calcium level is often not necessary.

DISORDERS OF WATER METABOLISM

Causes

The combination of excess thirst, increased intake of water, and increased output of urine is a common clinical presentation of a number of conditions (Table 81.7). In most of these, the symptoms are related to some event that results in excessive loss of fluid via the kidney. For example, *hyperglycemia* results in a large solute load (glucose) being presented to the renal tubules; an obligatory loss of water (osmotic diuresis) ensues. *Hypercalcemia* produces abnormalities of renal tubular function that result in impaired ability to concentrate urine. *Lithium,* widely used for treatment of bipolar affective disorders (manic–depressive illness), impairs the action of antidiuretic hormone (ADH) and thereby produces water loss.

Table 81.7. Causes of Polyuria[a]

Disorder	Mechanism
Glucosuria (diabetes mellitus)	Osmotic diuresis
Excessive intake of water	Psychogenic
Various drugs	Often due to anticholinergic effects producing dryness of mouth; possible central effects
Decreased ADH effect	Deficiency of ADH secretion (idiopathic diabetes insipidus or due to pituitary–hypothalamic disease); nephrogenic diabetes insipidus
Renal disease, plus renal effects of potassium depletion, hypercalcemia, and lithium therapy	In all of these disorders, impairment of renal concentrating ability is present
Hyperthyroidism	Impairment of urinary concentrating ability; decreased salivary flow

[a]Disorders associated with increased urine volume.
ADH, antidiuretic hormone.

A noteworthy disorder of water metabolism in ambulatory patients is that of *psychogenic water drinking.* In this disorder, the patient's psychiatric state alters normal behavior in such a way as to produce compulsive water drinking. Many of these patients have poorly defined psychiatric disorders, but some are overtly psychotic (41). Studies in these patients have identified unequivocal defects in urinary dilution, the osmoregulation of water intake, and the secretion of vasopressin, but the precise causes of these abnormalities remain unexplained (42). Occasional people begin excessive water intake in the mistaken impression that drinking large quantities of water is healthful. Regardless of the cause, once such behavior is started, a compulsive pattern tends to persist and is reinforced by a pathophysiologic mechanism. Whatever the cause, large urine output, if it persists for a long time, produces a reversible impairment of urine-concentrating ability due to washout of renal medullary solutes. Thus, the behavior pattern, although basically of psychogenic origin, may become self-perpetuating. Attempts to have the patient restrict water intake when urinary concentrating ability is impaired under these conditions lead to continued water loss, and the resulting hyperosmolality leads to intense thirst. Weaning from excessive water intake may be difficult.

A rare disorder of water metabolism in ambulatory patients is *diabetes insipidus,* a deficiency of ADH (arginine vasopressin). This condition is either idiopathic—in which case it is unassociated with other evidence of pituitary–hypothalamic disease—or, more commonly, is secondary to pituitary disease (tumor) or other disease in the hypothalamic–pituitary stalk-pituitary area (craniopharyngioma, aneurysm). Other rare causes include a variety of infiltrative diseases (sarcoidosis, tuberculosis), head trauma—especially with basal skull fracture or neurosurgical procedures—and central nervous system infections. The most common illness mimicking diabetes insipidus is the drug-related disorder that results from use of *lithium* for bipolar affective illness. Another rare condition resembling lack of ADH results from an inherited renal tubular resistance to ADH, *nephrogenic diabetes insipidus.*

Approach to the Patient with Polydipsia and Polyuria

The history should be corroborated by family or friends if possible. Important historical points are rapidity of onset of symptoms, a preference for use of iced water, and nocturnal drinking habits. Sudden onset and preference for iced water are classic features of diabetes insipidus. Numerous spontaneous awakenings at night to drink and urinate also strongly suggest this diagnosis, whereas absence of such events is in favor of functional disease. A careful psychiatric and pharmacologic history is important.

Initial laboratory workup should be simple. A morning serum glucose, sodium, or osmolality determination should be made along with serum potassium, calcium, urea nitrogen, and creatinine determinations.

Normal serum calcium and potassium concentrations exclude several metabolic problems, whereas abnormalities of calcium, potassium, or renal function make it clear that the problem is not primarily one of water metabolism (Table 81.7). Unless considerable glucosuria is present, the patient's problem is not caused by uncontrolled diabetes mellitus, even if blood glucose concentration is incidentally elevated.

The patient should collect all urine over one or two 24-hour periods. The sample should be examined to determine the volume, osmolality, total urine glucose excretion, and total creatinine excretion, the latter serving as a marker for completeness of the collection. Measurement of urine specific gravity is obsolete and should not be done. Normal urine volume ranges up to 2,500 mL; urine osmolality is decidedly low when the value is well below that of serum (less than 300 mOsm/kg; the urine is maximally dilute at 50 to 70 mOsm/kg).

The presence of a normal serum sodium or osmolality indicates only that the process is not severe enough to have overwhelmed the ability to excrete water or the homeostatic (thirst) mechanism. Elevated serum osmolality strongly suggests diabetes insipidus; reduced osmolality indicates psychogenic water drinking. In both diabetes insipidus and psychogenic water drinking, urine volume usually exceeds 4 L/day. Values less than 5 to 6 L/day do not distinguish between these possibilities but do indicate less than complete diabetes insipidus, in which urine volumes approach 10 to 12 L/day, as they may also in cases of severe psychogenic water drinking. If the serum sodium/osmolality is low and the urine volume is large with low osmolality, a diagnosis of psychogenic water drinking is essentially established.

If there is a large urine volume of low osmolality and normal serum electrolyte concentrations, additional testing is necessary to establish a diagnosis. Referral to an endocrinologist or nephrologist is appropriate, although under optimal conditions, further efforts to establish the diagnosis in the ambulatory patient may be undertaken before referral (see below). Hospitalization for testing under metabolic conditions is nearly always to be preferred in these cases.

Treatment

The treatment of *psychogenic water drinking* involves psychiatric counseling. These patients are difficult to manage, especially if they become severely hyponatremic. Weaning such patients from water may also be a slow process, not only because of the profound nature of their psychiatric disturbance but because of their acquired inability to concentrate urine, a process that is only slowly reversible.

The treatment of *diabetes insipidus* involves use of ADH in some form. For many years, pitressin tannate in oil given intramuscularly was the preferred agent, but it is no longer available. For ambulatory patients, ADH is available in a nasal spray solution as the synthetic analog desmopressin (1-deamino-8D-arginine vasopressin). A single dose acts for 12 hours or longer. Nasal absorption may be impaired by rhinitis or respiratory tract infections, during which treatment with injectable ADH (Pitressin) may be necessary. Patients with partial diabetes insipidus can sometimes be managed with chlorpropamide (Diabinese, 250 to 500 mg/day), a drug that potentiates endogenous ADH. However, hypoglycemia is a significant hazard. Nephrogenic diabetes insipidus, both idiopathic and secondary to lithium, is partially responsive to thiazide diuretics.

Syndrome of Inappropriate Secretion of Antidiuretic Hormone

The clinical manifestations of the syndrome of inappropriate secretion of antidiuretic hormone (SIADH) are due to hyponatremia and the diagnosis is based on that finding. There are multiple causes. Classically, the disturbance was related to ectopic production of ADH by a neoplasm. The tumor most likely to produce this syndrome is a small cell (oat cell) carcinoma of the lung, but many other tumors have also been shown to produce the same syndrome. The presence of a tumor is usually obvious but occasionally may be clinically occult. In addition, a variety of acute and chronic diseases of the central nervous system can produce SIADH. Centrally acting drugs may also produce ADH hypersecretion (e.g., morphine, barbiturates [43]). The first and best described drug-related SIADH is that due to chlorpropamide (Diabinese) during the therapy of diabetes mellitus (see Chapter 79). In this case, the disturbance is due to potentiation of ADH action, although increased ADH release may also be involved. Drug-related SIADH should always be considered; many drugs have now been implicated.

Treatment

The treatment of SIADH is usually that which is related to the underlying disease or involves withdrawal of drug therapy. Water restriction and/or increased salt intake (usually in addition to a loop diuretic, such as furosemide, 20 mg/day) is effective but is difficult to maintain in an ambulatory setting. Lithium and demeclocycline, a tetracycline analog, block the effect of ADH and are effective in some cases but rarely are needed in an ambulatory setting. Selective ADH receptor antagonists have been developed and offer promise for therapy (44), but none is yet available for clinical use.

HYPOGLYCEMIA

Because many of the symptoms of hypoglycemia are nonspecific, it is more often suspected than present. Chemical hypoglycemia, defined as a serum glucose concentration of less than 50 mg/dL (some now use 40 mg/dL as the cut point), may not be symptomatic, although levels less than 30 mg/dL are nearly always associated with symptoms. Hypoglycemia produces symptoms by two mechanisms: by triggering the release of epinephrine, one of several homeostatic responses that tend to normalize a low blood sugar, and by deprivation of the nervous system of glucose, its essential energy source.

Causes

There are numerous causes of hypoglycemia (Table 81.8), but by far the most common is due to an excess effect of insulin or of sulfonylureas in the treatment of diabetes mellitus (45). Rarely, some other drug produces hypoglycemia (Table 81.8). A few other conditions that produce hypoglycemia are associated with insulin overproduction, the rarest of which is an insulinoma. So-called postprandial hypoglycemia (within 2 to 4 hours of eating), it is now generally agreed, has been considerably overdiagnosed (46). The attribution of postprandial hypoglycemia to gastrectomy or early diabetes mellitus has not been well established; if symptomatic hypoglycemia does occur in these settings, it must be uncommon. Idiopathic postprandial hypoglycemia also appears to be quite rare (46,47).

Table 81.8. Causes of Hypoglycemia in Ambulatory Adults

Postprandial state
Reactive (idiopathic)
Early diabetes mellitus
Ethanol ingestion
Postgastrectomy state
Fasting state
Insulin excess
1. Insulin injection
2. Sulfonylurea ingestion[a]
3. Miscellaneous drugs and poisons[b]
4. Insulinoma
5. Autoimmune hypoglycemia (very rare)
Alcohol ingestion
Hormonal deficiencies
1. Glucocorticoid
2. Growth hormone
Fasting in normal young women (24–48 h)
Malnutrition
Liver disease
Extrapancreatic tumors
Renal failure (chronic end stage)
Congestive heart failure

[a]Many drugs, including such diverse compounds as anti-inflammatory agents, antibiotics, and lipid-lowering agents, potentiate the effects of sulfonylureas and may cause hypoglycemia.

[b]Haloperidol, propoxyphene, salicylates, etc.

Diagnosis

In some patients, the history suggests to the clinician that the patient is experiencing periodic hypoglycemia. Other patients will themselves suggest to their caregiver that hypoglycemia accounts for the symptoms. Much has been written in the lay literature about hypoglycemia, and many books attribute the entire range of human miseries to this disorder. Needless to say, the case has been overstated. The caregiver encountering such a patient may find mere reassurance ineffective, so convincing is some of the lay literature on this subject and so obsessed are some patients. Verification of the presence of hypoglycemia can be attempted by instructing the patient in the use of a glucose oxidase strip (e.g., Chemstrips bG). The strip can be brought or sent to the caregiver or laboratory within 1 week for confirmation of the reading. Unfortunately, failure to document the presence of hypoglycemia may not dispel the issue, and the generation of dubious or equivocal results with a glucometer may merely serve to prolong the preoccupation, initiate useless diets, or even delay diagnosis of serious but unrelated disease.

Defining Hypoglycemic Symptoms

Because laboratory confirmation may be difficult in some cases, an extraordinarily careful history is essential. The degree to which the history is convincing determines the vigor with which a rather nebulous diagnosis is to be pursued. Two issues guide the process. First, what exactly are the symptoms? Second, do the symptoms occur postprandially or in the fasting state?

Adrenergic versus Neuroglycopenic Symptoms. Two groups of symptoms and signs are associated with hypoglycemia. Many of the symptoms of hypoglycemia relate to stimulation by low blood glucose of the release of epinephrine. These comprise the first group and are termed adrenergic or sympathetic. Usually, these symptoms are of rapid onset, and more than one is ordinarily present. Typically, they last only 15 to 30 minutes and include sweating, tremor (shakiness), a sensation of hunger, and anxiety. Irritability and palpitations are often mentioned but are rarely spontaneous or prominent complaints.

The second group of symptoms is related to glucose deprivation of the central and, to a lesser extent, peripheral nervous systems. These symptoms are termed neuroglycopenic and, when severe, mimic those of central nervous system hypoxia. Minimal symptoms are headache, mental dullness, and sudden fatigue. Confusion and visual disturbances (blurring, dimming of vision) are associated with moderate to severe hypoglycemia, whereas unconsciousness and seizures are indications of very severe hypoglycemia.

An accurate history is essential to identify the time at which hypoglycemia occurs. In general, symptoms of true hypoglycemia do not occur within hours of eating a meal unless insulin or sulfonylurea has been prescribed in excess. There are exceptions to this statement, however, both in rare patients with an insuloma and in patients who have a disorder that causes true postprandial hypoglycemia.

Inquiry concerning the patient's dietary habits may be revealing. Some patients restrict carbohydrate intake intermittently. When this is done and a large carbohydrate meal follows, hypoglycemia may be precipitated. A history of previous gastrointestinal surgery (gastrectomy) is also important. The amount of alcohol consumed should be noted because ethanol ingestion may precipitate hypoglycemia, even in the nonfasting patient (see below). Often the patient may recall milder symptomatic episodes experienced over a long period because the intensity of postprandial hypoglycemia tends to wax and wane over the years. A family history of diabetes mellitus should be sought. Postprandial hypoglycemia can be an early manifestation of type 2 diabetes mellitus (see Chapter 79). Although symptoms and signs of anxiety or depression may be present, they have no diagnostic usefulness.

General physical examination can be expected to be negative. Even when early diabetes mellitus is found by glucose tolerance testing to be the cause of the hypoglycemia, complications of diabetes that can be found on physical examination (retinopathy, neuropathy) will not be present.

Nonhypoglycemia

The frequency with which self-diagnosis of hypoglycemia occurs depends on the patient population (48). The condition has been termed *nonhypoglycemia* and extends the concept of "nondisease," as it originates from misattribution by the clinician, such as misinterpretation of laboratory values, or misattribution of the patient. Identification of such individuals is important, as is their re-education. The ready acceptance by patients of hypoglycemia as a diagnosis is perhaps related to its social acceptability, the comfort received from attributing vague symptoms (e.g., fatigue, mental fogginess) to a real disease, the satisfaction of an escape into dietary rituals, and possibly relief from the anxiety that serious disease may be present.

The recognition of nonhypoglycemia requires a careful history that fails to demonstrate the legitimate symptoms of hypoglycemia as well as a clear demonstration that glucose metabolism is normal (see below). Exclusion of other organic disease is important (Table 81.8). Distinction from the rare idiopathic postprandial syndrome must be made (see below). Finally, psychiatric disease must be considered, based on positive findings rather than merely on an exclusion of organic illness.

If the evaluation fails to establish the presence of bona fide hypoglycemia, the issue of the therapy of nonhypoglycemia remains. This difficult problem includes at least three steps that have been termed disattribution, explanation and ventilation, and reattribution (48). *Disattribution* involves confrontation of the patient with the results of the test procedure. For some patients the mechanics or ritual of the procedure itself is impressive and therefore helpful. If the patient clings to the diagnosis of hypoglycemia despite strong evidence to the contrary, an attempt should be made to explore the reason for the patient's need to do so. During this process, an effort should be made to have the patient fully explain his or her notions about hypoglycemia and verbalize what might happen if those notions are challenged. Finally, an alternate explanation must be provided for the symptoms—reattribution—along with a treatment plan or a willingness to assist the patient in accepting an uncertain and ambiguous situation. Unless grossly apparent psychosocial problems become evident during this process, psychiatric referral may not be necessary. (Chapters 19 and 20 describe in detail interviewing and psychotherapeutic techniques for working with patients such as these.)

Laboratory Evaluation

As discussed above, an attempt can be made to determine the presence or absence of hypoglycemia by instructing the patient in the use of a glucose measuring strip. If the results are normal or equivocal and the diagnosis is still suspected, determination of serum glucose concentration needs to be done in a controlled setting. Blood sugar should be low at the time symptoms are experienced, and the symptoms should abate when the patient is fed carbohydrate. The glucose tolerance test has been largely abandoned as a diagnostic procedure in this situation because of its unreliability in establishing the diagnosis. If it is done, it should be modified to include more frequent sampling (30-minute intervals) and a longer period (5 hours). The patient should be observed during the entire test. Again, correlation of blood sugar values with symptoms is essential.

Assuming that the symptoms are not so profound as to have caused coma, in which case hospitalization is mandatory during the testing, an overnight (12-hour) fast followed by determination of serum glucose is the next simplest screening procedure. This test may have to be repeated several times. If hypoglycemia cannot be documented in this way, the period of fasting may have to be extended to 24, 48, or 72 hours. Ninety-five percent of patients with fasting hypoglycemia will be diagnosed by 48 hours (49). Hospitalization and close monitoring are necessary under these circumstances.

A sex difference in response to fasting is well established. Normal men may fast for up to 72 hours and will not show fasting plasma glucose below 50 mg/ dL. In contrast, women often exhibit a progressive fall in the concentration of plasma glucose during prolonged fasting. At 72 hours, most premenopausal women have a concentration of glucose less than 50 mg/dL and some as low as 25 mg/dL. Thus, prolonged fasting to establish the diagnosis of fasting hypoglycemia is not always useful because so many normal women become hypoglycemic.

Selected Specific Entities Causing Hypoglycemia

Insulinoma

This pancreatic tumor occurs with equal frequency in men and women and at any age. Symptoms of headache on arising, confusion before breakfast, or nocturnal or early morning seizures may be present for years before the diagnosis is suspected. Hyperinsulinism may produce abnormal hunger, weight gain, and obesity (although insulinoma is a very rare cause of obesity). Neuropsychiatric symptoms may lead to neurologic or psychiatric evaluations or to hospitalizations. In some of these cases, permanent neurologic deficits have been seen and are presumably related to long duration of symptomatic hypoglycemia before diagnosis.

Diagnosis. In addition to the demonstration of hypoglycemia, the simultaneous determination of plasma insulin activity remains the most definitive diagnostic test (50). During fasting in normal people, both glucose and insulin levels decline and the ratio of immunoreactive insulin (IRI) to glucose is maintained at less than 0.3 (milliunits of IRI/mg of glucose/dL). In many patients with insulinoma, an abnormally high IRI-to-glucose ratio is apparent after overnight fasting. These determinations should be made repeatedly because fasting hypoglycemia and an abnormal IRI-to-glucose ratio often occur only intermittently even in patients with subsequently proven insulinomas. In addition, a single abnormal ratio never establishes the diagnosis. Insulin-to-glucose ratios may be misinterpreted if the glucose concentration is not at hypoglycemic levels. The clinician should be cautious in accepting the accuracy of IRI values obtained from commercial laboratories. Proinsulin levels are elevated in 85% of patients with insulinoma and can be a useful adjunct, especially in those whose insulin levels are low.

A variety of other useful procedures should, if deemed necessary, be conducted by an endocrinologist. If fasting for 48 hours fails to provoke hypoglycemia (see above), the fast can be continued to 72 hours or the patient can be exercised as vigorously as tolerable. Up to 2 hours of exercise should be completed with sampling of plasma glucose every 15 to 20 minutes before concluding that hypoglycemia has not developed. An exercise bicycle, jogging, or vigorous calisthenics may be used. Exercise raises glucose levels in normal people but lowers plasma concentration further in patients with insulinoma. Provocative tests of insulin secretion (tolbutamide, leucine, glucagon) can be used with appropriate caution. Suppression of endogenous insulin C peptide is another useful procedure in difficult cases, but it requires induction of hypoglycemia by infusion of insulin under controlled conditions, a procedure that must be performed by an endocrinologist in a hospital.

The localization procedure of choice is ultrasonography of the pancreas. CT and MRI are apparently not useful. Celiac axis arteriography may be useful for localizing lesions smaller than 2 to 3 cm (i.e., those that can be expected to be seen with sonography) (51). These procedures must not be used as alternatives to the tests described above but should be performed after demonstration of abnormal secretion of insulin.

Treatment. The definitive treatment of an insulinoma is surgical.

Noninsulinoma Pancreatogenous Hypoglycemia Syndrome

A small number of adults (52) have recently been reported to have an unusually severe form of exclusively postprandial hypoglycemia. Their 72-hour fasts are negative for insulinoma. Partial pancreatectomy seems to be curative.

Insulin and Sulfonylurea Self-Administration

Occasional nondiabetic patients, usually family members of diabetics or people with medically related occupations, engage in surreptitious insulin administration. Examination may reveal needle marks. Other clues can be provided by the presence of antibodies to insulin, which are present only in persons given insulin or by the measurement of insulin C peptide. In people who are secreting insulin, C peptide is also produced concomitantly, but C peptide is not present in commercial insulin and will be present in very low concentrations or will be absent in the serum of patients whose hypoglycemia is induced by exogenous insulin.

Oral hypoglycemic drugs (sulfonylureas; see Chapter 79), like insulin, may occasionally be abused and cause fasting hypoglycemia. In the experience of one group, these agents produce the greatest difficulty in the diagnosis of factitious hypoglycemia (49). The first-generation sulfonylureas can be detected by analysis of the blood for the drugs, but the new sulfonylureas are not detected by currently available assays.

Alcohol Abuse

Alcohol abuse probably produces hypoglycemia more commonly than any other single cause. As stated above, ingestion of ethanol can produce postprandial hypoglycemia in normal well-nourished people who engage in social drinking. However, fasting hypoglycemia related to ethanol ingestion occurs in chronic alcohol abusers and especially in those who are malnourished. The situation most likely to provoke hypoglycemia is cessation of food intake and continued ingestion of ethanol over the ensuing 10 to 20 hours. Under these circumstances, ethanol intoxication (i.e., drunkenness) may mistakenly be thought to be responsible for the symptoms.

Liver Disease, Chronic Congestive Heart Failure, and Renal Disease

Although hypoglycemia can be seen in the course of severe acute hepatitis or as a result of chronic passive congestion in long-standing congestive heart failure, liver disease does not usually produce hypoglycemia. Patients with severe cirrhosis may occasionally have fasting hypoglycemia, but the development of hypoglycemia in such a patient should suggest the presence of a hepatoma. In patients with well-differentiated hepatoma, hypoglycemia may be an early symptom. Diabetic patients with renal insufficiency may become hypoglycemic because of a reduced requirement for hypoglycemic therapy (see Chapter 79).

Endocrine Disease

Glucocorticoids and GH are important regulators of glucose metabolism. Thus, either pituitary insufficiency or adrenal insufficiency (primary or secondary to hypopituitarism) can result in hypoglycemia as a presenting manifestation. The diagnosis of these disorders is described elsewhere in this chapter.

Autoimmune Hypoglycemia

There are rare conditions in which autoantibodies develop to insulin receptors. Patients have no history of insulin use. The hypoglycemia is often severe and refractory. These conditions are unlikely to be encountered in a nonspecialty setting.

HORMONE USE OF UNPROVEN VALUE

The lay press and the media regularly carry news of the use of various hormones for common problems. Health food stores are allowed to sell these substances as food additives, the term used by this industry, which is unregulated by the FDA under current law. Although most of these substances are relatively innocuous, they do pose some risk because they are not subjected to the rigorous drug testing that attends the approval of ordinary pharmaceuticals.

Dehydroepiandrosterone

Dehydroepiandrosterone (DHEA) and its metabolite, DHEA sulfate, are produced in amounts (25 to 50 mg/day) that far exceed daily secretion of any other adrenal steroid. It is not, however, classified as a hormone by the FDA and so it can be sold as an uncontrolled substance. Its physiologic function is uncertain. Because its secretion rate falls off dramatically with increasing age in many people and because of evidence, primarily in aged rodents but also in older humans, that it improves cellular immunologic function, a belief has taken hold in the lay population that DHEA can retard and perhaps even reverse the aging process (53). There is no evidence to support this belief (54) nor is the safety of DHEA established. Because it is metabolized to androgens and estrogen, it could conceivably exacerbate benign prostatic hypertrophy, prostate cancer, sleep apnea, and hyperlipidemia in men and heart disease and breast or gynecologic cancer in women.

Melatonin

Melatonin, a secretory product of the pineal gland, has been touted to be a regulator of circadian rhythms and so has been used to induce sleep and prevent or facilitate recovery from time-zone changes (jet lag). The agent is also promoted to slow aging and to enhance libido and as an antioxidant. No controlled studies are available to support any of these claims nor have dosages or toxicity been studied (see also Chapter 41).

Testosterone

Although long promoted as a libido and sex-performance enhancer, little if any evidence supports its usefulness in men with normal endogenous circulating levels. Some evidence supports a role for this agent in some men who at advanced age show decreased circulating levels, especially in regard to treatment of osteoporosis (see Chapter 84). The drug and other androgenic anabolic agents (synthetic steroids) have been widely used also to enhance muscle mass in male and female athletes and are probably effective for this purpose but could also have adverse effects (e.g., hepatic toxicity, exacerbation of prostatic cancer or of coronary artery disease). Erythrocytosis is also a "side effect" of parenteral testosterone, probably the result of grossly pharmacologic levels achieved with this route. The relatively new patches and gel do not create this problem.

Growth Hormone

Human recombinant GH (rhGH) is readily available but not approved for purposes other than enhancing the height of GH-deficient children. Like testosterone, or in combination with it, rhGH has been used to enhance muscle mass in athletes. Its effectiveness for this purpose is not established, and its long-term toxicity has not been studied. Because GH levels are low in at least half of elderly patients, rhGH has been used in clinical trials with the hope that it will restore muscle mass and reduce adiposity in the elderly. So far, the results are not encouraging. Complications have included pseudotumor cerebri, carpal tunnel syndrome, and peripheral edema. This hormone is clearly no panacea for the problems of aging (55). On the other hand, a role for GH as replacement therapy in panhypopituitarism has gained acceptance recently (see above).

General References*

DeGroot LJ, Jameson L, eds. Endocrinology, 4th ed. Philadelphia: WB Saunders, 2001.
A comprehensive multivolume text.

*Bold print (general references) and bold numerals (specific references) denote published controlled clinical trials, meta-analyses, or consensus-based recommendations.

Felig P, Frohman LA, eds. Endocrinology and metabolism, 4th ed. New York: McGraw-Hill, 2001.

An authoritative textbook of manageable size.

Wilson JD, Foster DW, Larsen PR, et al., eds. Williams' textbook of endocrinology, 9th ed. Philadelphia: WB Saunders, 1998.

The longtime standard textbook for the field.

Specific References

1. Molitch ME. Evaluation and treatment of the patient with a pituitary incidentaloma. J Clin Endocrinol Metab 1995;80:3.
2. Molitch ME, Thorner MO, Wilson C. Management of prolactinomas. J Clin Endocrinol Metab 1997;82:996.
3. Verhelst J, Abs R, Maiter D, et al. Cabergoline in the treatment of hyperprolactinemia: a study in 455 patients. J Clin Endocrinol Metab 1999;84:2518.
4. Pinzone JJ, Katznelson L, Danila DC, et al. Primary medical therapy of micro- and macroprolactinomas in men. J Clin Endocrinol Metab 2000;85:3053.
5. Melmed S, Ho K, Klibanski A, et al. Recent advances in pathogenesis, diagnosis, and management of acromegaly. J Clin Endocrinol Metab 1995;80:3395.
6. Robbins RJ. Depot somatostatin analogs—a new first line therapy for acromegaly. J Clin Endocrinol Metab 1997;82:15.
7. Kuhn JM, Arlot S, Lefebvre H, et al. Evaluation of the treatment of thyrotropin-secreting pituitary adenomas with a slow release formulation of the somatostatin analog lanreotide. J Clin Endocrinol Metab 2000;85:1487.
8. Gibney J, Wallace JD, Spinks T, et al. The effects of 10 years of recombinant human growth hormone (GH) in adult GH-deficient patients. J Clin Endocrinol Metab 1999;84:2596.
9. Cuneo RC, Salomon F, McGauley GA, et al. The growth hormone deficiency syndrome in adults. Clin Endocrinol 1992;37:387.
10. Bengtsson BA, Johannsson G, Shalet SM, et al. Treatment of growth hormone deficiency in adults. J Clin Endocrinol Metab 2000;85:933.
11. Benvenga S, Campenní A, Ruggeri RM, et al. Hypopituitarism secondary to head trauma. J Clin Endocrinol Metab 2000;85:1353.
12. Tordjman K, Jaffe A, Trostanetsky Y, et al. Low-dose (1 microgram) adrenocorticotrophin (ACTH) stimulation as a screening test for impaired hypothalamo-pituitary-adrenal axis function: sensitivity, specificity and accuracy in comparison with the high-dose (250 microgram) test. Clinical Endocrinol 2000;52:633.
13. Grinspoon SK, Biller BM. Laboratory assessment of adrenal insufficiency. J Clin Endocrinol Metab 1994;79:923.
14. Samuels MH, Brandon DD, Isabelle LM, et al. Cortisol production rates in subjects with suspected Cushing's syndrome: assessment by stable isotope dilution methodology and comparison to other diagnostic methods. J Clin Endocrinol Metab 2000;85:22.
15. Graham KE, Samuels MH, Nesbitt GM, et al. Cavernous sinus sampling is highly accurate in distinguishing Cushing's disease from the ectopic adrenocorticotropin syndrome and in predicting intrapituitary tumor location. J Clin Endocrinol Metab 1999;84:1602.
16. DeHerder WW, Lamberts SW. Tumor localization—the ectopic ACTH syndrome. J Clin Endocrinol Metab 1999;84:1184.
17. Pralong FP, Gomez F, Guillou L, et al. Food-dependent Cushing's syndrome: possible involvement of leptin in cortisol hypersecretion. J Clin Endocrinol Metab 1999;84:3817.
18. Papanicolaou DA, Yanovski JA, Cutler GB Jr, et al. A single midnight serum cortisol measurement distinguishes Cushing's syndrome from pseudo-Cushing states. J Clin Endocrinol Metab 1998;83:1163.
19. Newell-Price J, Grossman AB. The differential diagnosis of Cushing's syndrome. Ann Endocrinol 2001;62:173.
20. Moro M, Putignano P, Losa M, et al. The desmopressin test in the differential diagnosis between Cushing's disease and pseudo-Cushing states. J Clin Endocrinol Metab 2000;85:3569.
21. Lamberts SW, van der Lely AJ, deHerder WW. Transsphenoidal selective adenomectomy is the treatment of choice in patients with Cushing's disease. Considerations concerning medical treatment and the long-term follow-up. J Clin Endocrinol Metab 1995;80:3111.
22. Copeland PM. The incidentally discovered adrenal mass. Ann Intern Med 1983;98:940.
23. Barzon L, Scaroni C, Sonino N, et al. Rick factors and long-term follow-up of adrenal incidentalomas. J Clin Endocrinol Metab 1999;84:520.
24. Rossi R, Tauchmanova L, Luciano A, et al. Subclinical Cushing's syndrome in patients with adrenal incidentaloma: clinical and biochemical features. J Clin Endocrinol Metab 2000;85:1440.
25. Carella MJ, Srivastava LS, Gossain VV, et al. Hypothalamic-pituitary-adrenal function one week after a short burst of steroid therapy. J Clin Endocrinol Metab 1993;76:1188.
26. Thakker RV. Genetic developments in hypoparathyroidism. Lancet 2001;357:974.
27. Lafferty FW. Differential diagnosis of hypercalcemia. J Bone Miner Res 1991;6:S51.
28. Mundy GR, Guise TA. Hypercalcemia of malignancy. Am J Med 1997;103:134.
29. Ratcliffe WA, Hutchesson AC, Bundred NJ, et al. Role of assays for parathyroid-hormone-related protein in investigation of hypercalcaemia. Lancet 1992;339:164.
30. Roodman GD. Mechanisms of bone lesions in multiple myeloma and lymphoma. Cancer 1997;89:1557.
31. Silverberg SJ, Bilezekian JP. Evaluation and management of primary hyperparathyroidism. J Clin Endocrinol Metab 1996;81:2036.
32. Bone HG, Talpos GB. Therapeutic controversies in primary hyperparathyroidism: who needs parathyroid surgery? The case for parathyroidectomy in nonclassical primary hyperparathyroidism. J Clin Endocrinol Metab 1999;84:2278.
33. NIH Conference. Diagnosis and management of asymptomatic primary hyperparathyroidism: Consensus Development Conference Statement. Ann Intern Med 1991;114:593.
34. Silverberg SJ, Bilezikian JP. Therapeutic controversies in primary hyperparathyroidism: to treat or not to treat: conclusions from the NIH consensus conference. J Clin Endocrinol Metab 1999;84:2275.
35. Chan AK, Duh QY, Katz MH, et al. Clinical manifestations of primary hyperparathyroidism before and after parathyroidectomy. A case-control study. Ann Surg 1995;222:402.
36. Utiger RD. Treatment of primary hyperparathyroidism. N Engl J Med 1999;341:1301.
37. Neer RM, Arnaud CD, Zanchetta JR, et al. Effect of parathyroid hormone (1-34) on fractures and bone mineral density in postmenopausal women with osteoporosis. N Engl J Med 2001;344:1434.
38. Silverberg SJ. Cardiovascular disease in primary hyperparathyroidism. J Clin Endocrinol Metab 2000;85:3513.
39. Silverberg SJ, Gartenberg F, Jacobs TP, et al. Longitudinal measurements of bone density and biochemical indices in untreated primary hyperparathyroidism. J Clin Endocrinol Metab 1995;80:723.
40. Selby PL, Peacock M. Ethinyl estradiol and norethindrone in the treatment of primary hyperparathyroidism in postmenopausal women. N Engl J Med 1986;314:1481.
41. Goldman MB, Robertson GL, Luchins DJ, et al. The influence of polydipsia on water excretion in hyponatremic, polydipsic, schizophrenic patients. J Clin Endocrinol Metab 1996;81:1465.
42. Goldman MB, Luchins DJ, Robertson GL. Mechanisms of altered water metabolism in psychotic patients with polydipsia and hyponatremia. N Engl J Med 1988;318:397.
43. Miller M, Moses AM. Drug-induced states of impaired water excretion. Kidney Int 1976;10:96.
44. Saito T, Ishikawa S, Abe K, et al. Acute aquaresis by the nonpeptide arginine vasopressin (AVP) antagonist OPC-31260 improves hyponatremia in patients with syndrome of inappropriate secretion of antidiuretic hormone (SIADH). J Clin Endocrinol Metab 1997;82:1054.
45. Hart SP, Frier BM. Causes, management and morbidity of acute hypoglycaemia in adults requiring hospital admission. Q J Med 1998;91:505.
46. Service FJ. Hypoglycemia and the postprandial syndrome. N Engl J Med 1989;321:1472.

47. Palardy J, Havrankova J, Lepage R, et al. Blood glucose measurements during symptomatic episodes in patients with suspected postprandial hypoglycemia. N Engl J Med 1989;321:1421.
48. Yager J, Young RT. Non-hypoglycemia is an epidemic condition. N Engl J Med 1974;291:907.
49. Hirshberg B, Livi A, Bartlett DL, et al. Forty-eight-hour fast: the diagnostic test for insulinoma. J Clin Endocrinol Metab 2000;85:3222.
50. Gordon P, Skarulis MC, Roach P, et al. Plasma proinsulin-like component in insulinoma: a 25-year experience. J Clin Endocrinol Metab 1995;80:2884.
51. Service FJ. Clinical review 42. Hypoglycemias. J Clin Endocrinol Metab 1993;76:269.
52. Service FJ, Natt N, Thompson GB, et al. Noninsulinoma pancreatogenous hypoglycemia: a novel syndrome of hyperinsulinemic hypoglycemia in adults independent of mutations in Kir6.2 and SUR1 genes. J Clin Endocrinol Metab 1999;84:1582.
53. Baulieu EE. Dehydroepiandrosterone (DHEA): a fountain of youth? J Clin Endocrinol Metab 1996;81:3147.
54. Wolf OT, Neumann O, Hellhammer DH, et al. Effects of a two-week physiological dehydroepiandrosterone substitution on cognitive performance and well-being in healthy elderly women and men. J Clin Endocrinol Metab 1997;82:2363.
55. Marcus R, Reaven GM. Growth hormone—ready for prime time? J Clin Endocrinol Metab 1997;82:725.

CHAPTER 82

Disorders of Lipoprotein Metabolism

ANNABELLE RODRIGUEZ, MD
DAVID E. KERN, MD
MARC R. BLACKMAN, MD

Interest in plasma lipids, lipoproteins, and apoproteins stems from their strong relationship to the development of atherosclerosis (1–3). At a time when it is possible to reduce the frequency of premature death and disability from atherosclerotic disease, the clinician should be knowledgeable about, and capable of, diagnosing and treating the major abnormalities of lipoprotein metabolism.

LIPOPROTEIN NOMENCLATURE AND COMPOSITION

Lipids are insoluble in the aqueous plasma medium. They circulate in plasma as component parts of macromolecules that consist of a nonpolar hydrophobic lipid core of cholesterol esters and triglycerides and a polar hydrophilic monolayer surface coat of protein, phospholipid, and unesterified cholesterol (Fig. 82.1). These macromolecules, which are made miscible in plasma by their surface coat, are called lipoproteins.

Lipoproteins have traditionally been classified as a family of molecules containing the same basic constituents but in different proportions (Table 82.1). The major classes of lipoproteins can be separated from each other by differences in density (ultracentrifugation), net surface charge (electrophoresis), size, and composition. Ultracentrifugation, which has been the traditional method of classification, separates lipoproteins into five principal classes: *chylomicrons, very-low-density lipoproteins* (VLDLs), *intermediate-density lipoproteins* (IDLs), *low-density lipoproteins* (LDLs), and *high-density lipoproteins* (HDLs) (4).

Each lipoprotein contains characteristic proportions of lipids and type-specific apoproteins (apos) such that, with increasing lipoprotein density, the relative amount of lipid decreases and that of apoprotein increases (Table 82.1). For example, triglyceride is the major lipid component in chylomicrons and VLDL, whereas cholesterol is the major component of LDL. Intermediate-density or remnant lipoproteins are catabolic products of chylomicrons and VLDLs and contain similar amounts of both lipids and apos (see Normal Physiology of Lipoprotein Transport). The HDLs are the most dense lipoproteins; they contain proportionally the most apos and ordinarily consist of 15% to 25% cholesterol with a small amount of triglyceride in the core. HDLs are further subdivided into HDL_2 and HDL_3. The former is more buoyant, as reflected by its higher lipid-to-protein ratio and richer apo A–I and apo C and E content, relative to the more dense HDL_3, which has a lower lipid-to-protein ratio and a higher apo A–II than A–I composition. There is a strong inverse relationship of coronary risk to plasma concentrations of HDL_2 and apo A–I, related to the heightened capacity of the latter molecules to transport cholesterol from cells (5) (see later discussion).

A LIPOPROTEIN PARTICLE

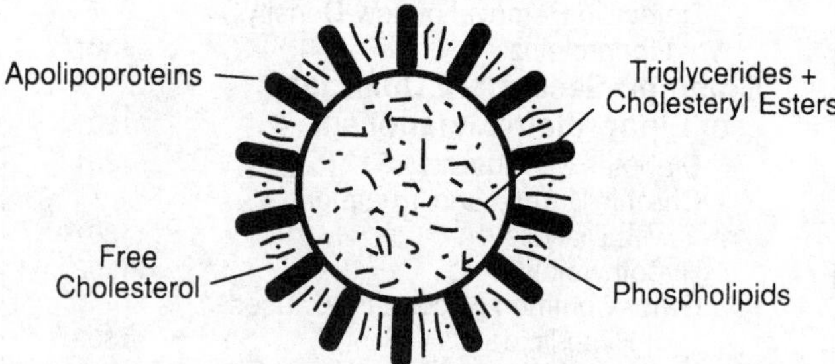

Figure 82.1. Structure of the lipoprotein macromolecule with the nonpolar lipids, cholesterol ester, and triglyceride in the lipoprotein core surrounded by a monolayer composed of specific apolipoproteins, proteins, and the polar lipids, unesterified cholesterol and phospholipid. (From The Johns Hopkins Physicians Lipid Education Program. 2nd ed. Baltimore: The Johns Hopkins University, 1988:11.)

NORMAL PHYSIOLOGY OF LIPOPROTEIN TRANSPORT

Plasma lipoproteins arise from both exogenous dietary sources and endogenous hepatic sources (Fig. 82.2). They carry lipids in three distinct but interacting pathways: The *exogenous pathway* consists primarily of chylomicrons; the *endogenous pathway* consists mostly of VLDL, IDL, and LDL; and the *reverse cholesterol transport pathway* consists mostly of HDL activity.

After the ingestion of fat, dietary triglycerides are hydrolyzed in the gut and absorbed by intestinal enterocytes. Triglyceride-containing chylomicrons, formed in these cells, are secreted into lymphatic vessels and subsequently enter the venous system via the thoracic duct. Chylomicrons function as a system of high-energy caloric transport, allowing the calories ingested in excess of the immediate needs of the body to be transferred to sites of storage between meals. Absorbed dietary cholesterol is also esterified and transported in chylomicrons.

Table 82.1. Classification of Plasma Lipoproteins by Physical and Chemical Characteristics

Lipoprotein Fraction (Ultracentrifugation)	Density (g/mL)	Migration (Electrophoresis)	Composition as Percentage of Total Mass			
			Cholesterol	Triglyceride	Apoprotein	Phospholipid
Chylomicron	0.95	Origin	2–7	80–90	2 (A, B-48, C, E)	3
Very low density (VLDL)	<1.006	Pre-β	10–22	50–70	6 (B-100, C, E)	14
β-Very low density (β-VLDL or $VLDL_2$)	<1.006	β	30–40	45	12 (B-100, B-48, C, E)	15
Intermediate density or remnant (IDL)	1.006–1.019	Slow pre-β	30–40	40	18 (B, E)	22
Low density (LDL)	1.019–1.063	β	45–50	5–10	21 (B-100)	22
High density (HDL)	1.063–1.21	α	15–25	3–5	50 (A, C, E)	28

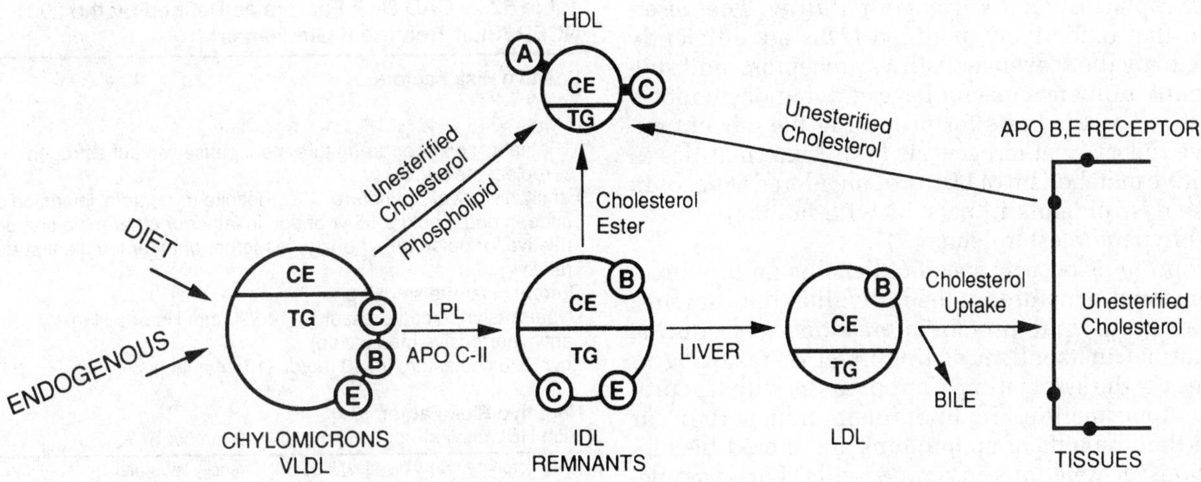

Figure 82.2. The normal physiology of lipoprotein transport is illustrated schematically.

Other triglyceride-rich lipoproteins are synthesized from endogenous sources by the liver and intestine. Cholesterol synthesis from acetate also occurs in the liver and is regulated by the enzyme hydroxymethylglutaryl coenzyme A (HMG-CoA) reductase. Triglycerides synthesized in the liver combine with cholesterol ester and are enveloped in a lipoprotein monolayer before being secreted into the hepatic venous outflow system as endogenous triglyceride-rich VLDLs.

Chylomicrons and VLDLs are transported to adipose tissue and muscle for storage and utilization. The uptake and storage of triglyceride are regulated by *lipoprotein lipase* (LPL). LPL hydrolyzes triglyceride and surface components from chylomicrons and VLDL to transform them into *remnant lipoproteins* (Fig. 82.2). The fatty acids released during this reaction migrate to muscle cells for combustion or to adipose cells for resynthesis and storage as triglyceride (6). The remnant lipoproteins are smaller, denser, and relatively enriched in cholesterol, apo B, and apo E compared with the chylomicrons and VLDL from which they are derived. They are taken up by apo B–E (LDL) receptors in the liver. The chylomicron remnants are further degraded, and the VLDL remnants are processed into IDL and cholesterol-rich LDL (Fig. 82.2). Apo C–II and apo C–III, and the phospholipids and free cholesterol released during the LPL reaction, are transferred to HDL for utilization. The surface material generated by LPL-mediated removal of core triglyceride from VLDL and chylomicrons is the substrate (apo A–I is the cofactor) for the enzyme *lecithin-cholesterol acyl transferase* (LCAT), which converts nascent HDL to mature spherical HDL and plays a major role in reverse cholesterol transport (see later discussion).

The LDLs are the principal carriers of cholesterol in plasma. Cholesterol is a major structural component of all cell membranes and is a precursor for steroid hormone synthesis by the adrenal glands and gonads. The LDL cholesterol-rich particles are derived mainly from VLDL and their catabolic remnants via the action of LPL and hepatic lipase. The principal removal of LDL occurs in the periphery by cells having a specific cell surface receptor (1) that recognizes all forms of apo B; this is currently referred to as the apo B–E (LDL) receptor (Fig. 82.2). After specific cell receptor binding, LDLs are internalized by receptor-mediated endocytosis and carried to lysosomes, where apo B is irreversibly degraded to amino acids and LDL cholesterol ester is hydrolyzed to free cholesterol. The free cholesterol is transported to an intracellular cholesterol pool, where it regulates, by a cellular feedback pathway, the resynthesis of cholesterol, cholesterol ester, and apo B–E (LDL) receptors (7).

The cholesterol content of the cell is also regulated by a removal system involving HDL as a vehicle for cholesterol transport from peripheral to hepatic cells for catabolism and excretion into bile directly or after conversion to bile acid (7,8). This process, termed *reverse cholesterol transport*, is thought to be one of the mechanisms for the antiatherogenic effect of HDL. It provides an efficient mechanism for the transfer of esterified cholesterol to LDL and VLDL, the absorption of free cholesterol from vascular endothelial cells, and the removal of cholesterol arising from cell membrane turnover and cell death. An apparent antiatherogenic alteration in both the lipoprotein and apoprotein composition of HDL, the formation of HDL_2, occurs during high-cholesterol feeding and represents one pathway by which the body can enhance its capacity to clear excess cholesterol from cells (7). HDL is also thought to be cardioprotective by acting as an antioxidant and endotoxin scavenger. The identification of the HDL receptor, SR-BI, has shown that it plays a major role in reverse cholesterol transport, with a key role in the selective uptake of cholesteryl esters in hepatocytes and gonadal cells (9,10). Research is currently underway to better define the role of SR-BI in atherosclerosis and to determine whether it might be a useful target for pharmacologic intervention.

Continued LDL catabolism in excess of that performed by hepatic and other parenchymal cells occurs in macrophages via a *scavenger pathway*. The observation that oxidatively modified LDLs are efficiently taken up by the scavenger pathway receptors, and subsequently influence macrophage and monocyte motility, served as the basis for proposing the current oxidative theory of atherogenesis (11). Abnormalities in oxidative metabolism of LDL are considered to account for the dyslipidemia in persons with homozygous familial hypercholesterolemia (11).

Apoproteins occupy specific domains on the three-dimensional structures of the individual lipoproteins. Alterations in lipid–protein interactions occur during the normal metabolism of lipoproteins, resulting in changes in the association of apoproteins with lipoproteins. Abnormalities in lipoprotein transport occur when the domains of apoproteins are altered by substitutions or deletions in amino acids. For example, the abnormal recognition of beta-VLDL by the apo B–E receptor on cells occurs because of an abnormality in apo E in dysbetalipoproteinemia (see Pathophysiology of Lipoprotein Disorders), and abnormalities in the apo B–E receptors are responsible for the defect in familial hypercholesterolemia (1,12).

Table 82.2. CAD Risk Factors as Defined by the 2001 NCEP Adult Treatment Guidelines[a]

Positive Risk Factors
Age
Male ≥ 45 yr
Female ≥ 55 yr or premature menopause without estrogen replacement therapy
Family history of premature CAD (definite myocardial infarction or sudden death before 55 yr of age in father or other male first-degree relative, or before 65 yr of age in mother or other female first-degree relative)
Current cigarette smoking
Hypertension (blood pressure ≥140/90 mm Hg or taking antihypertensive medication)
Low HDL cholesterol (<40 mg/dL [1.0 mmol/L])
Negative Risk Factor
High HDL cholesterol (≥60 mg/dL [1.6 mmol/L])

CAD, coronary artery disease; HDL, high-density lipoprotein.

[a]Diabetes mellitus is now considered a CAD risk equivalent (i.e., equivalent to having CAD) and has been removed from the risk factor table. This designation emphasizes the need to be aggressive in the lipid management of patients with diabetes mellitus.

Modified from the Executive Summary of the Third Report of the National Cholesterol Education Program (NCEP) Expert Panel on Detection, Evaluation, and Treatment of High Blood Cholesterol in Adults (Adult Treatment Panel III). JAMA 2001;285:2486.

PLASMA LIPOPROTEINS AS RISK FACTORS FOR ATHEROSCLEROSIS

The risk factor concept, which developed as an outgrowth of the Framingham study and other large epidemiologic studies, is based on the strong association between certain characteristics in people and the increased likelihood of developing cardiovascular disease (13). Among the risk factors for atherosclerotic vascular disease, the most clearly established ones are plasma total cholesterol levels (and plasma LDL and HDL content), hypertension, cigarette smoking, family history of premature coronary artery disease (CAD), and age. Diabetes mellitus is considered a risk equivalent (i.e., equivalent to having CAD). Each factor has been clearly implicated and makes a sizable independent contribution to the overall risk for development of CAD (Table 82.2). Other identified risk factors that have more modest associations with cardiovascular disease include central obesity and physical inactivity.

Evidence from several large prospective and retrospective epidemiologic studies among diverse populations has demonstrated that variations in plasma levels of certain lipids and lipoproteins are associated with an increased likelihood of developing or having CAD. *Hypercholesterolemia*, for example, is strongly associated with the subsequent development of CAD. The relationship is uniformly consistent, dose related, and independent of gender. The predictive value of the plasma level of total cholesterol is somewhat limited, however, by the fact that it reflects the opposing influences of LDL and HDL cholesterol. Levels of LDL correlate positively, whereas those of HDL, in general, are inversely related to CAD risk. The negative correlation between HDL levels and CAD depends mainly on its subfraction, HDL_2, which may provide, along with its major protein component, apo A–I, a better index of risk than the total plasma level of HDL (5). Over the range of total and HDL cholesterol plasma levels found in an average American population, the risk of CAD varies roughly fivefold. Although the impact of cardiovascular risk factors declines after 75 years of age, they are still predictive of CAD in older people. The relative risks of CAD associated with any particular risk factor (e.g., cholesterol levels) decrease with aging because of the increased prevalence of multiple risk factors; however, the absolute risk of morbidity and mortality increases markedly (14). Most, but not all, studies indicate that plasma levels of total cholesterol retain predictive value in the "old old"—that is, in men age 75 to 95 years (15–18). Moreover, HDL cholesterol levels and the ratio of LDL to HDL cholesterol remain useful predictors in this age group.

The relationships of plasma levels of total, LDL, and HDL cholesterol with CAD are independent ones, in that the associations remain significant even after statistical adjustment for other risk factors. A low concentration of HDL cholesterol is a stronger independent risk factor for CAD than is either total cholesterol or LDL cholesterol (3).

Increased fasting levels of plasma *triglyceride* and of its major lipoprotein transporter, VLDL, also correlate with an increased risk of atherosclerotic disease. There has been uncertainty about whether the association is independent of other risk factors (19,20). Recent analyses suggest that plasma triglyceride levels are a risk factor for CAD and are independent of HDL cholesterol levels (21,22). Treatment of hypertriglyceridemia depends on the causes and degree of elevation and on the presence or absence of other risk factors (Table 82.2; see Treatment). Hypertriglyceridemia may be especially important prognostically in patients with diabetes mellitus (23) or end-stage renal disease (24).

Not only do these lipoprotein and apoprotein abnormalities seem to increase one's predisposition to CAD, but there also is a parallel increased risk for cerebrovascular disease (13,25) and peripheral vascular disease as well (25).

A number of lipid fractions are even more strongly related to CAD than are total, LDL, and HDL cholesterol or apo A–I, and measurements of these fractions may become more useful in cardiovascular and cerebrovascular risk factor assessments (3). Elevated plasma concentrations of LDL apo B appear to discriminate between patients with and without atherosclerosis of the coronary and peripheral vasculature, even in the presence of normal total and LDL plasma cholesterol levels (2,26). The determination of the plasma LDL apo B concentration may also prove useful in assessing risk in hypertriglyceridemic patients (2,22). It is known that LDL consists of several lipoprotein subclasses that differ in size and core lipid content, and that LDL subclass pattern B, characterized by small, dense LDL particles, is associated with a threefold increased risk of myocardial infarction (MI), independent of age, gender, and body weight (27).

In addition, MI, the progression of angiographically documented CAD, postangioplasty restenosis, and cerebrovascular disease are strongly associated with the lipoprotein (a) [Lp(a)] blood pattern, particularly in patients with increased levels of LDL cholesterol (28). Current evidence (29) suggests that Lp(a) (distinct from apo A) consists of a circulating complex of LDL and apo(a) that is more atherogenic than LDL. Apo(a) exists in more than 30 isoforms and accounts for the great interperson variability in the plasma concentrations of Lp(a). Moreover, Lp(a) is structurally similar to plasminogen and inhibits the conversion of plasminogen to plasmin, thus attenuating fibrinolysis. Finally, Lp(a) appears to be directly involved in the formation of atherosclerotic plaques, perhaps because of its susceptibility to oxidative alteration in the arterial wall. However, at present there is no evidence from clinical trials to support routine measurement of Lp(a).

A number of investigations have demonstrated that tissue oxidative damage to LDL, and the subsequent interactions between damaged LDL and vascular endothelium, smooth muscle, macrophages, and monocytes, elicit more atherogenic activity than occurs with native LDL (11). Research in animals indicates that use of exogenous antioxidants retards the progression of experimentally induced atherogenesis by 30% to 80%. Although there have been epidemiologic reports that antioxidants (e.g., vitamin E) protect hyperlipidemic patients from the development or worsening of atherosclerotic heart disease (30,31), several prospective randomized trials have shown no benefit in this regard (32,33).

In *familial dysbetalipoproteinemia*, a genetic disorder characterized by elevated plasma concentrations of IDL and an abnormally migrating beta-VLDL (12), there is an increased risk of both peripheral and coronary atherosclerotic disease. In contrast, *fasting chylomicronemia* is associated with recurrent episodes of abdominal pain and pancreatitis but not with the early development of atherosclerosis.

In several epidemiologic studies, plasma total cholesterol levels lower than 180 to 195 mg/dL were associated with an increased risk of cancer, especially cancer of the colon. The evidence does not, however, suggest a significant causal link, because (a) in most studies the association was strongest in the first year of follow-up, then attenuated and disappeared in subsequent years, suggesting that preclinical cancer might have lowered levels of plasma cholesterol rather than vice versa; (b) studies comparing populations have shown a positive association between dietary fat intake and risk for major cancers such as breast, prostate, and colon cancer; and (c) the relationship was generally weak, was present in a minority of studies, and demonstrated no consistent relation between cholesterol level and cancer risk (34).

RATIONALE FOR DIAGNOSIS AND TREATMENT

Despite the fact that many risk factors linked with coronary and other atherosclerotic vascular disease have been identified and targeted for intervention, atherosclerotic disease constitutes the leading cause of death and disability in Western industrialized societies. In the United States, approximately 725,000 individuals die annually from atherosclerotic disease, 550,000 of them from CAD. The economic costs are formidable, with more than $80 to $100 billion being spent annually in direct health care costs, lost wages, and decreased productivity.

To control this problem, major risk factor identification and prevention programs, primarily targeting hyperlipidemia, hypertension, and smoking, have been promulgated during the past 20 years, and mortality from CAD has fallen steadily during this time (35).

The "lipid (or cholesterol) hypothesis," based on the data described, also postulates that favorable alterations of plasma lipoprotein levels by diet, drugs, or other therapy reduce the risk of atherosclerosis in humans. Indeed, randomized primary prevention trials have shown that lowering LDL cholesterol in asymptomatic hyperlipidemic middle-aged men significantly reduces their risk of death from coronary artery disease and of nonfatal MI (36–39). The relative risk reduction over 5 years is approximately 30%, and the absolute risk reduction is approximately 2% (the number needed to treat to avoid an adverse event is 50).

Recent results from the Air Force/Texas Coronary Atherosclerosis Prevention Study (AFCAPS/TexCAPS) have lent greater support to the rationale for primary prevention treatment (39). A total of 5,608 men and 997 women with average total and LDL cholesterol levels (221 and 150 mg/dL, respectively) and below-average HDL cholesterol levels (36 and 40 mg/dL, respectively) were studied for an average follow-up period of 5.2 years. The vast majority of the enrolled subjects were not candidates for active treatment based on the 1993 National Cholesterol

Education Program (NCEP) guidelines. This study compared the effects of placebo and lovastatin on the primary end points of unstable angina, fatal and nonfatal MI, and sudden cardiac death in middle-age patients (men age 45 to 73 years and postmenopausal women age 55 to 73 years). For study subjects receiving lovastatin treatment, the relative risks were significantly reduced for first acute coronary events, MI, unstable angina, coronary revascularization procedures, coronary events, and cardiovascular events. Lovastatin lowered LDL cholesterol levels by 25% to 115 mg/dL and increased HDL cholesterol levels by 6% to 39 mg/dL.

These results have not yet been shown definitively to be achievable in women or in men younger than 35 or older than 74 years of age. Also, the overall mortality rate was not affected by the interventions. Nevertheless, the evidence is strong enough to have led the U. S. Preventive Services Task Force (USPSTF) and the NCEP to recommend screening guidelines (see later discussion) and to recommend consideration of treatment of hyperlipidemic individuals (see Treatment).

Secondary prevention trials also have conclusively shown that cholesterol-lowering drugs can decrease CAD progression as well as the incidence of new and recurrent CAD-related events in patients with known atherosclerotic vascular disease (40–42). There is a consensus that treatment should be more aggressive in these populations (see Treatment). Relative risk reductions of 20% to 40% have been reported, with absolute risk reductions of 3% to 4% over 5 years of treatment. In these studies, all-cause mortality was also reduced by approximately 20%.

The importance of targeting HDL cholesterol levels, particularly in patients with known CAD, was highlighted in the recent report from the Veteran's Affairs High Density Lipoprotein Cholesterol Intervention Study (VA-HIT) (42). In this study, 2,531 men with known CAD, low HDL cholesterol levels (mean, 32 mg/dL), and "desirable" LDL cholesterol levels (mean, 111 mg/dL) were treated with placebo or gemfibrozil 600 mg twice daily for a mean follow-up period of 5.1 years. Gemfibrozil was chosen as the pharmacologic agent because of its relatively neutral effects on LDL cholesterol levels. The results showed significant relative risk reductions for nonfatal MI, CAD death, transient ischemic attack, angioplasty, carotid endarterectomy, stroke, and hospitalization for congestive heart failure. These beneficial effects of gemfibrozil treatment were associated with significant reduction in plasma triglyceride levels (24%) and increased HDL cholesterol levels (8%).

HYPERLIPOPROTEINEMIA

Definition

The diagnosis of hyperlipoproteinemia historically has been based on plasma levels of lipids or lipoproteins above the 95th percentile of those found in a reference population. Over the last 14 years, the Adult Treatment Panel (ATP) of the NCEP has evolved criteria for the diagnosis of hyperlipoproteinemia based on prognostic significance (Table 82.3) (43,44).

Table 82.3. Adult Treatment Panel III Criteria for the Classification of LDL, Total, and HDL Cholesterol (mg/dL) Based on Prognostic Significance

LDL Cholesterol	
<100	Optimal
100–129	Near or above optimal
130–159	Borderline high
160–189	High
≥190	Very high
Total Cholesterol	
<200	Desirable
200–239	Borderline high
≥240	High
HDL Cholesterol	
<40	Low
≥60	High

HDL, high-density lipoprotein; LDL, low-density lipoprotein.
Modified from the Executive Summary of the Third Report of the National Cholesterol Education Program (NCEP) Expert Panel on Detection, Evaluation, and Treatment of High Blood Cholesterol in Adults (Adult Treatment Panel III). JAMA 2001;285:2486.

Table 82.4. Causes of Secondary Lipoprotein Disorders

Exogenous	Alcohol, oral contraceptives, estrogens, androgens, corticosteroids, diuretics (thiazides, chlorthalidone), β-adrenergic–blocking agents, isoretinoin, obesity, nutrition (diet high in cholesterol/saturated fat)
Endocrine-metabolic	Diabetes mellitus, hypothyroidism, Cushing disease, Addison disease, acromegaly, hypopituitarism, growth hormone deficiency
Hepatic	Obstructive or parenchymal disease, hepatoma
Renal	Nephrotic syndrome, chronic renal failure, hemodialysis
Acute stress situations	Acute myocardial infarction, sepsis, burns
Pregnancy	
Pancreatitis	
Dysgammaglobulinemias	Multiple myeloma, macroglobulinemia
Systemic lupus erythematosus	
Gout	
Viral infections, including AIDS	
Other	Glycogen storage disease, lipodystrophies, progeria, acute intermittent porphyria, anorexia nervosa, Klinefelter syndrome

Classification

Primary versus Secondary

For clinical purposes, hyperlipoproteinemic states should be classified as primary (hereditary or sporadic genetic disorders of metabolism), secondary, or both. Secondary hyperlipoproteinemia is associated with an identifiable disease or condition and is reversible with control or eradication of that disease or condition. The major causes of secondary hyperlipoproteinemia are listed in Table 82.4.

Phenotypic versus Genotypic and Pathophysiologic

In the 1960s, it was popular to classify the various hyperlipidemic states *phenotypically*, based on specific concentrations of lipids and lipoproteins and electrophoretic patterns (Table 82.5). Although the phenotypic classification describes in abbreviated fashion the plasma lipoproteins that are present in elevated or low concentrations, it does not reflect the genetic mechanisms or pathophysiology of the lipoprotein disorders. It is desirable to classify patients *pathophysiologically* and *genotypically* (Table 82.5) to diagnose and treat lipoprotein disorders accurately. Because apoproteins, enzymes, and cellular receptors are the major regulators of lipoprotein metabolism, it is appropriate to categorize lipoprotein disorders whenever possible in terms of pathophysiologic defects in the structure, function, and metabolism of these molecules, rather than by using a rigidly fixed phenotypic classification. Often, the pathophysiologic and genotypic classification can be surmised from a patient's phenotypic pattern, medical history, family history, and physical examination. Sometimes family members must be studied or more sophisticated laboratory analyses performed, necessitating referral to a specialist in endocrinology and metabolism.

PATHOPHYSIOLOGY OF LIPOPROTEIN DISORDERS

The abnormal accumulation of lipoproteins in plasma results from their excessive production, defective removal, or both. Lipoprotein disorders may be primary (usually genetic); they may be secondary to certain diseases (especially diabetes mellitus, chronic renal disease, hypothyroidism, dysglobulinemia) or drugs (corticosteroids, estrogens, thiazide diuretics); or they may represent an interaction between primary and secondary factors. Abnormalities can occur in triglyceride-rich lipoprotein synthesis, LPL-mediated triglyceride catabolism, remnant lipoprotein catabolism, cholesterol-rich lipoprotein catabolism, or cholesterol-rich lipoprotein (LDL cholesterol) synthesis and absorption.

Increased Triglyceride Synthesis

Most triglyceride input is from the diet in normal individuals. However, abnormalities in the regulation of the endogenous production of triglyceride-rich VLDLs are fairly common and are the most common causes of hypertriglyceridemia. They are associated with an increase in plasma levels of VLDL (type IV) or VLDL plus chylomicrons (type V). The underlying metabolic cause for endogenous hypertriglyceridemia is usually related to hyperinsulinemia and insulin resistance, due most often to obesity, diabetes mellitus, the ingestion of excessive calories or alcohol, or the use of estrogens or corticosteroids.

The primary forms of endogenous hypertriglyceridemia are familial hypertriglyceridemia and primary familial combined hyperlipidemia. *Familial hypertriglyceridemia* results in an increase in the endogenous synthesis of large triglyceride-rich VLDLs. Many such patients are obese and exhibit mild glucose intolerance, hyperinsulinemia, and clinical evidence of diabetes mellitus, conditions that contribute to the excessive hepatic production of VLDL triglyceride.

In contrast, patients with *familial combined hyperlipidemia* (multiple lipoprotein–type hyperlipidemia) exhibit an increase in the production of apo B, which can appear in VLDL, LDL, or both. Various lipoprotein types (IIA, IIB, or IV) are found in patients with familial combined hyperlipidemia, and the presenting sign can be an increase in either VLDL triglyceride, LDL cholesterol, or both. The clinical expressions of this disorder vary among individual patients depending on diet, degree of obesity, level of physical activity, and concomitant use of other drugs.

Familial hypertriglyceridemia and familial combined hyperlipidemia are inherited as separate autosomal-dominant disorders, each occurring in approximately 1% of the general population. Familial hypertriglyceridemia is not associated with xanthomas unless hyperchylomicronemia supervenes. Basal concentrations (after a 12-hour fast) of total triglycerides and VLDL triglycerides are characteristically elevated, but plasma levels of total and LDL cholesterol are normal or low unless levels of VLDL cholesterol are also increased. Familial hypertriglyceridemia is not associated with an increased incidence of premature CAD; however, patients with familial combined hyperlipidemia are at high risk, primarily because of their increased plasma levels of apo B as well as abnormalities in the composition of HDL and reduced levels of apo A–I and HDL_2 (2). Familial combined hyperlipidemia may be present in as many as 10% of survivors of MI who are younger than 60 years of age and thus represents a common and important risk factor for atherosclerosis.

The diagnosis of these disorders of lipoprotein metabolism and their exact definition can be established only by family studies. A strongly positive family history of atherosclerosis favors the diagnosis of familial combined hyperlipidemia in hypertriglyceridemic patients in whom secondary causes for hyperlipidemia have been excluded. Differentiating between these two disorders of lipoprotein metabolism is important in the evaluation of a patient with hyperlipidemia, particularly with regard to deciding whether therapeutic intervention is warranted for the prevention of CAD and its complications.

Occasionally, patients have marked *hypertriglyceridemia* and *hyperchylomicronemia* (triglyceride levels greater than 1,000 mg/dL), pancreatitis, eruptive xanthomas, and lipemia retinalis. Coexistence of familial hypertriglyceridemia or familial combined hyperlipidemia with either obesity, uremia, untreated diabetes mellitus, chronic alcoholism, or the use of corticosteroids, thiazide diuretics, or estrogens can result in this syndrome. The chylomicronemia syndrome requires immediate treatment with elimination of

Table 82.5. Classification of Lipoprotein Disorders by Phenotypes and Genotypes and Corresponding Clinical Manifestations

Phenotype	Lipoprotein in Excess	Plasma Lipid Levels		Plasma Appearance[a]	Genotype	Age at Onset (Primary Form)	Xanthomas[b]	Other Clinical Manifestations
		Cholesterol	Triglyceride					
I	Chylomicrons	Normal or ↑	↑↑↑ Lipemia	Clear plasma, creamy supernatant	Familial lipoprotein lipase deficiency, apo C–II deficiency	Infancy or childhood	Eruptive, tuberoeruptive	Recurrent abdominal pain, other gastrointestinal symptoms, lipemia retinalis, hepatosplenomegaly
IIA	LDL	↑↑↑	Normal	Clear	Familial hypercholesterolemia Familial combined hyperlipidemia Polygenic and sporadic hypercholesterolemia	Childhood for homozygous FHC, late childhood to middle age for heterozygous FHC, adulthood for others	Tendinous, xanthelasma, tuberous; planar (homozygous)	Premature CAD, arcus corneae, aortic stenosis (homozygous FHC), arthritic symptoms
IIB	LDL + VLDL	↑↑	↑	Clear	Familial combined hyperlipidemia Familial hypercholesterolemia			
III	β-VLDL, IDL	↑↑	↑↑	Slightly turbid	Familial dysbetalipoproteinemia	Adulthood (occasionally late adolescence)	Planar (especially palmar), tuberous	Premature CAD and peripheral vascular disease, male > female, obesity, abnormal glucose tolerance, hyperuricemia; aggravated by hypothyroidism, good response to therapy
IV	VLDL	Normal or ↑[c]	↑↑	Turbid	Familial hypertriglyceridemia Familial combined hyperlipidemia Sporadic hypertriglyceridemia	Early to late adulthood	Usually none; rarely eruptive, or tuberoeruptive	CAD and peripheral vascular disease, obesity, abnormal glucose tolerance, hyperuricemia, arthritic symptoms, gallbladder disease
V	Chylomicrons + VLDL	Normal or ↑	↑↑↑	Turbid plasma, creamy supernatant	Homozygous familial hypertriglyceridemia	Childhood to middle age, usually adulthood	Eruptive, tuberoeruptive	Recurrent abdominal pain, other gastrointestinal symptoms, lipemia retinalis, hepatosplenomegaly, peripheral paresthesias, abnormal glucose tolerance, hyperuricemia

FHC, Familial hypercholesterolemia; CAD, coronary artery disease.

[a]Plasma obtained after 12 hr of fasting, left undisturbed in refrigerator overnight.

[b]Seen only in a minority of patients, but the frequency increases as plasma lipid levels rise.

[c]Cholesterol normal if triglycerides are less than 400 mg/dL.

dietary fat, nasogastric suction, and treatment of the secondary causes. Prevention is the primary means to avoid recurrences, and patients with primary hypertriglyceridemia often receive lipid-lowering agents prophylactically (7).

Decreased Lipoprotein Lipase–Mediated Triglyceride Catabolism

LPL is the rate-limiting enzyme for the uptake and storage of triglyceride by adipose or muscle tissue and for the processing of triglyceride-rich lipoproteins to chylomicrons and VLDL remnants. In patients with the autosomal-recessive trait of *apo C–II deficiency*, LPL activity is normal but marked hypertriglyceridemia is present. In contrast, in the more commonly encountered (yet also rare) autosomal-recessive syndrome of *familial LPL deficiency*, marked hypertriglyceridemia and chylomicronemia are both evident and LPL activity is absent. The type I phenotypic pattern is more likely to occur in patients with the familial form of LPL deficiency, rather than in those with apo C–II deficiency; yet both conditions manifest in childhood with episodes of eruptive xanthomas and with the acute abdominal pain of pancreatitis.

Most adult patients who have an acquired impairment in LPL function have moderately severe type 1 diabetes mellitus, hypothyroidism, end-stage renal disease, or dysgammaglobulinemia or are receiving corticosteroids or thiazide diuretics. The severity of the lipoprotein abnormality seems to be directly related to the decrease in LPL activity in postheparin plasma and adipose tissue.

The hypertriglyceridemia can be controlled by restriction of dietary fat and substitution of carbohydrates or medium-chain triglycerides as energy sources. Effective treatment of diabetes mellitus with diet, insulin, or an oral agent usually normalizes LPL activity and plasma triglyceride levels within several months. Similar beneficial changes are seen after appropriate treatment of hypothyroidism with thyroxine or of uremia with renal transplantation.

LPL also plays a role in the formation of HDL_2 (see Normal Physiology of Lipoprotein Transport). LPL appears to mediate the increase in HDL_2 seen in endurance-trained athletes (45) and in patients with primary hypercholesterolemia treated with colestipol. Hence, diseases associated with abnormalities in LPL often have concomitant reductions in HDL cholesterol.

Defective Remnant Lipoprotein Catabolism and Dysbetalipoproteinemia

Excessive accumulation of lipoprotein remnants in plasma is usually caused by a defect in their removal due to an autosomal-recessive derangement in the structure of apo E (12). *Apo E3*, the predominant form of apo E in the normal population, is absent in patients with the classic form of dysbetalipoproteinemia (type III hyperlipoproteinemia). The mutation causing this syndrome results in the occurrence of an abnormal form of apo E. Of the 1% of people who are homozygous for this condition, only 1% to 2% exhibit hyperlipoproteinemia clinically.

Dysbetalipoproteinemia (remnant removal disease or broad-beta disease) has served as a prototype for the study of remnant lipoprotein metabolism. It appears that several defects in lipoprotein metabolism are required before excessive accumulation of IDL and of cholesterol-enriched beta-VLDL can occur. The diagnosis is suggested by the initial findings of increased levels of beta-VLDL (rather than prebeta-VLDL) and similarly elevated plasma concentrations of cholesterol and triglyceride. It is made more likely by the finding of an abnormally cholesterol-rich VLDL fraction (ratio of VLDL cholesterol to VLDL triglyceride greater than 0.42). The presence of tuberous and planar xanthomas (Fig. 82.3) is highly characteristic of the disorder. Definitive diagnosis, however, requires analysis of VLDL to demonstrate the absence of apo E3. A strong association between this lipoprotein disorder and atherosclerosis of the coronary arteries and peripheral vessels has been reported, and vasculopathy appears to diminish during treatment.

The accumulation of remnants in plasma is also found in certain patients with hypothyroidism, end-stage renal disease, or liver disease. The latter disorders are associated with an increase in the activity of the enzyme hepatic lipase, suggesting that a relationship may exist between this enzyme and the catabolism of remnant lipoproteins by the liver.

Increased Cholesterol Synthesis

The accumulation of cholesterol-rich LDL can occur as a result of an increased input of cholesterol into the plasma from dietary or endogenous sources. The latter occurs because of an increase in HMG-CoA reductase activity and enhanced synthesis of cholesterol, or as a consequence of a primary genetic increase in the hepatic synthesis of apo B and cholesterol. The presence of apo B–enriched VLDL suggests a genetic disorder of overproduction of apo B, compared with the overproduction of VLDL triglyceride in familial hypertriglyceridemia.

The overproduction of apo B–containing LDL and VLDL leads to an increased propensity for the development of atherosclerosis (2). Moreover, the coexistence of obesity promotes the overproduction of apo B–enriched VLDL and cholesterol in these individuals. Finally, the augmented intake of dietary cholesterol usually contributes to the hypercholesterolemia that is characteristic of these patients.

Primary (sporadic) forms of hypercholesterolemia, with a genetic defect in the steps controlling the rate of hepatic synthesis of cholesterol from acetate, lead to an overproduction of cholesterol and resultant hypercholesterolemia. Usually, dietary therapy involving an increase in polyunsaturated fat and a reduction in

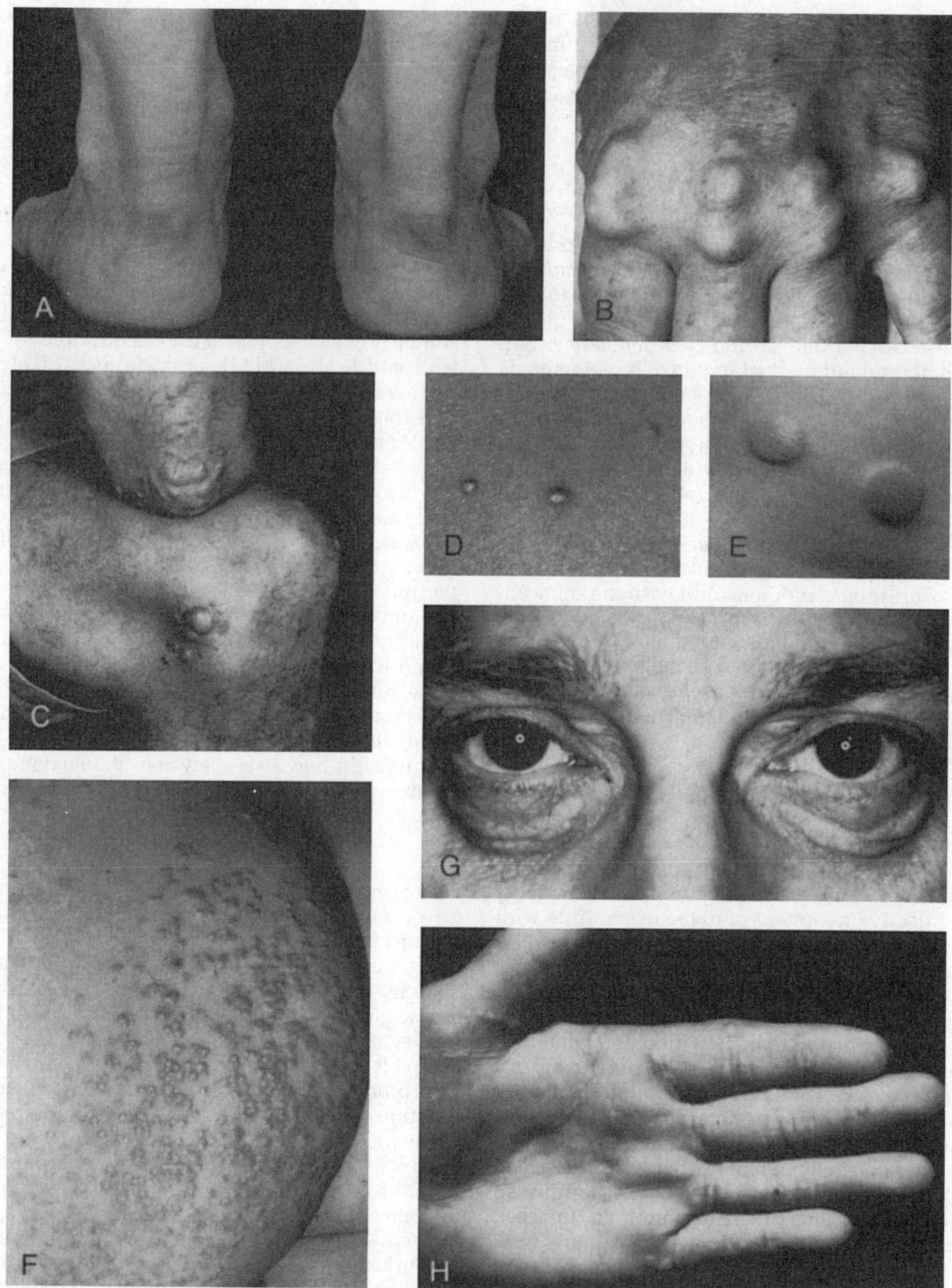

Figure 82.3. Dermatologic manifestations of lipid disorders. **A:** Tendinous xanthomas. **B:** Tuberous xanthomas. **C:** Tuberous xanthomas. **D:** Eruptive xanthomas. **E:** Planar xanthomas. **F:** Eruptive xanthomas. **G:** Planar xanthomas on eyelids (xanthelasma). **H:** Planar xanthomas confined to palm creases (xanthoma striata palmaris).

sucrose and simple carbohydrates is helpful in the treatment of these disorders; less often, drugs are required. Hypercholesterolemia in obese hyperinsulinemic patients with type 2 diabetes mellitus is decreased by hypocaloric diets and the return of body weight toward normal. In patients who are noncompliant with dietary measures, therapy with cholestyramine, nicotinic acid, or HMG-CoA reductase inhibitors (commonly known as statins) are usually effective in lowering plasma cholesterol levels.

Defective Removal of Low-Density Lipoproteins

Isolated primary elevations of plasma LDL or combined elevations of LDL and VLDL can be seen in affected members of families with familial hypercholesterolemia (1). Although the cells of some homozygous patients may be totally lacking in identifiable LDL (apo B–E) receptors, in other patients these receptors are present but are functionally defective. Individuals who are heterozygous for familial hypercholesterolemia exhibit more than a 50% reduction in LDL receptor number or a 50% defect in receptor-mediated catabolism; commonly their plasma levels of LDL cholesterol are greater than 400 mg/dL regardless of their level of cholesterol synthesis. In homozygous patients, plasma levels of LDL cholesterol may reach 1,000 mg/dL (7). Documentation of abnormal receptor binding in cultures of skin fibroblasts is necessary for the precise diagnosis of individuals with familial hypercholesterolemia.

Although primary causes (including familial combined hyperlipoproteinemia) predominate, secondary causes of increased concentrations of LDL cholesterol occur in patients with hypothyroidism, nephrotic syndrome, multiple myeloma, obstructive liver disease, or porphyria and in patients who have ingested excessive amounts of dietary cholesterol. The primary forms are associated with marked susceptibility to CAD and a high frequency of complications associated with early mortality, such as MI, stroke, and peripheral vascular disease. The hallmark of these disorders is the tendon xanthomas that often affect the Achilles tendon or the extensor tendons of the forearm and hand (Fig. 82.3). Patients with secondary hypercholesterolemia appear not to develop atherosclerosis at as high a rate as people with the primary disorders.

COMMON SECONDARY DISORDERS OF LIPOPROTEIN METABOLISM

Several disease states are commonly associated with increased plasma levels of VLDL, increased levels of both VLDL and LDL, or decreased levels of HDL cholesterol.

Diabetes Mellitus

Abnormalities in fat transport are often noted in patients with diabetes mellitus and are related to abnormalities in insulin action or insulin availability that lead to increased production or decreased removal of plasma lipoproteins. For example, patients with type 2 diabetes mellitus who are often obese, hyperinsulinemic, and insulin resistant exhibit both an enhanced production and reduced plasma clearance of triglycerides. These patients also have abnormalities in HDL cholesterol. In contrast, the hypertriglyceridemia that occurs in patients with insulin-dependent (type 1) diabetes mellitus is caused by markedly reduced levels of LPL activity, because insulin is required for normal synthesis of the enzyme (7). The diabetic lipemia syndrome is characterized by low or absent levels of LPL in the plasma and tissues of these patients. Although the underlying enzyme deficiency can be reversed after insulin repletion, normalization of the lipoprotein abnormalities can take several months.

In the treated diabetic patient, variability in plasma levels of lipoprotein lipids is primarily related to dietary factors, the amount and distribution of body fat, physical activity, and the degree of glycemic control. If glucose tolerance deteriorates because of inadequate insulin administration or increased insulin resistance, severe hypertriglyceridemia may ensue and alter the concentrations of other classes of lipoproteins. In well-treated type 1 diabetic patients, plasma levels of HDL cholesterol are increased; in contrast, even patients with well-treated type 2 diabetes usually have low HDL cholesterol levels. Regardless of the specific treatment or type of diabetes mellitus, women ordinarily exhibit higher plasma levels of VLDL triglyceride and LDL cholesterol, and lower levels of HDL cholesterol, than do diabetic men (23). This may explain the increased prevalence of atherosclerosis in diabetic women and the disappearance of the usual preponderance of atherosclerotic disease in men compared with premenopausal women (13).

Hypercholesterolemia, with increased plasma concentrations of LDL cholesterol and apo B, also can occur in patients with either type 1 or type 2 diabetes mellitus and is usually induced by diet. Intensive therapy with diet, exercise, and insulin usually normalizes lipoprotein levels unless a genetic lipoprotein disorder coexists.

Hyperlipidemia in the patient with diabetes mellitus increases the risk for the major complications of atherosclerosis, CAD, cerebrovascular disease, and peripheral vascular disease. The severity of peripheral vascular disease has been associated with the lipoprotein abnormalities in diabetic women. Whether treatment of the lipid abnormalities in diabetic patients will decrease their risk for CAD and other arteriosclerotic complications remains to be proved, but it can be recommended based on the known efficacy of treatment in other populations (see later discussion).

Chronic Uremia and Treatment with Dialysis

Many patients with chronic uremia have increased plasma levels of VLDL triglycerides and decreased levels of HDL cholesterol (24). These abnormalities persist during maintenance hemodialysis or peritoneal dialysis. The accelerated atherosclerosis observed in white versus African American men undergoing long-term hemodialysis appears to be related to the abnormal composition of HDL_2 cholesterol in the plasma of white men. A sedentary lifestyle, obesity, high-fat diets, or treatment with corticosteroids, beta-blockers, or androgens worsens the lipoprotein profiles in these patients, whereas effective reversal of these secondary causes improves the lipid profile (24).

Hypothyroidism

Adequate levels of thyroid hormone appear to be necessary for the homeostatic maintenance of lipoprotein physiology. Decreases in LDL receptor function, abnormalities in LPL and hepatic lipase-mediated metabolism of triglycerides and HDL, and reduced LCAT activity have been demonstrated in some patients with hypothyroidism. Consequently, increased plasma levels of VLDL, IDL, and LDL and reduced levels of HDL cholesterol have all been reported in patients with this disease. Treatment with thyroid hormone improves LDL receptor function, increases the activity and function of LPL and LCAT, and normalizes lipoprotein profiles.

Other Common Secondary Causes of Hyperlipidemia

Patients with the *nephrotic syndrome* commonly lose apo C–II in the urine, thus decreasing LPL-mediated triglyceride clearance. The hypoalbuminemia that accompanies the nephrotic syndrome increases hepatic VLDL synthesis, thereby elevating plasma levels of VLDL triglyceride and LDL cholesterol. Treatment of the primary disease causing the nephrotic syndrome usually corrects the lipoprotein abnormalities, but drug and diet (low-fat) therapy may be required. Reports suggest that statin therapy can ameliorate the nephrosis independently of its benefit in lowering LDL cholesterol levels (46).

Hypercortisolemia of endogenous or exogenous origin increases hepatic synthesis of VLDL, LDL, or both. Kidney transplant recipients treated with high dosages of corticosteroids often exhibit increased plasma levels of both VLDL and LDL as well as reduced levels of HDL cholesterol. The atherosclerosis that develops in such patients is probably related to these lipid abnormalities, which should be treated accordingly.

Obesity, alcohol ingestion, and *androgen administration* tend to increase hepatic lipoprotein synthesis but have different effects on levels of HDL cholesterol and LDL cholesterol. In obese people, plasma levels of VLDL triglyceride and LDL cholesterol are increased, whereas those of HDL are decreased. Mild alcohol ingestion (up to 2 oz/day) increases levels of VLDL triglyceride and HDL cholesterol but lowers levels of LDL cholesterol. Exogenous androgens raise levels of LDL cholesterol and lower HDL cholesterol levels.

Diseases affecting the liver, such as hepatitis or cholelithiasis, alter lipoprotein metabolism. Diseases causing an obstruction in the hepatobiliary system tend to elevate plasma LDL, IDL, and remnant lipoproteins and cause abnormal lipoproteins (Lp X) to accumulate in plasma.

Table 82.6. Factors that Affect High-Density Lipoprotein Cholesterol Levels

Increase	Decrease
Exercise	Androgens (male sex, drugs)
Oral estrogens (female sex)	In males, puberty
Alcohol (moderate)	In females, menopause
Familial (hyperalphalipoproteinemia)	Obesity
Leanness	Hypertriglyceridemia
Antihyperlipidemic drugs: nicotinic acid, colestipol, clofibrate, statins, gemfibrozil	Type 2 diabetes mellitus
Insulin	Familial hypoalphalipoproteinemia (Tangier disease)
Intravenous heparin	Cigarettes
	Sedentary lifestyle
	Probucol
	Uremia
	Vegetarian diet
	Progestogens

Inflammatory processes usually lower levels of HDL and LDL cholesterol and raise VLDL, depending on the nutritional state of the patient.

Drugs used to treat hypertension, particularly thiazide diuretics and beta-adrenergic blockers, raise levels of VLDL and LDL and lower levels of HDL cholesterol. Weight loss or discontinuation of these drugs usually normalizes lipoprotein profiles.

Hyperlipidemia occurs in patients with *systemic lupus erythematosus* or *dysgammaglobulinemia*. This may be related to interactions among amyloid protein, certain immunoglobulin fractions, and various steps in the lipoprotein cascade.

Table 82.6 lists several exogenous and endogenous factors that affect plasma levels of HDL cholesterol.

CLINICAL MANIFESTATIONS OF LIPOPROTEIN DISORDERS

Adverse clinical sequelae of the lipoprotein disorders most commonly manifest as disorders of the vascular, dermatologic, and gastrointestinal systems. The clinical manifestations associated with each of the major disorders of lipoprotein metabolism are outlined in Table 82.5.

Vascular

As discussed previously, increased levels of total cholesterol, LDL cholesterol, apo B–enriched lipoproteins, oxidized LDL, and Lp(a) and decreased levels of HDL cholesterol, HDL_2, and apo A–I contribute to the development of atherosclerotic disease. The earlier the onset of symptomatic disease of the coronary, cerebral, or peripheral vasculature, the more likely it is that a lipoprotein abnormality or another major risk factor (cigarette smoking, hypertension, diabetes) is present (13). In the most severe form of hypercholesterolemia, *homozygous familial hypercholesterolemia*, plasma levels of total cholesterol vary from 600 to 1,200 mg/dL, CAD generally develops in childhood, and very few patients survive past 30 years of age. In *heterozygotes*, plasma levels of total cholesterol vary from about 270 to 550 mg/dL and the time of onset of CAD varies between early adulthood and late middle age, with approximately 50% of men becoming symptomatic by age 50 years and 50% of women by age 60. Patients with *monogenic familial combined hyperlipoproteinemia* exhibit increased levels of VLDL, LDL, or both, as well as abnormalities in HDL, apo A-I, and apo B; most patients manifest symptoms of CAD by age 60 years. Individuals with *familial dysbetalipoproteinemia* develop premature peripheral vascular disease and CAD at about equal rates, with the mean age at onset in both men and women being about 40 years. Such patients seem to be especially responsive to therapy. Individuals with *monogenic familial hypertriglyceridemia* or with *fasting chylomicronemia* do not appear to be at increased risk for CAD unless other risk factors for atherosclerosis are also present.

Dermatologic

Xanthomas may occur in any of the hyperlipidemias; however, they are present in a minority of hyperlipidemic patients. They occur with increasing frequency as the plasma lipid levels rise. They are present predominantly in the primary forms of hyperlipoproteinemia: familial hypercholesterolemia, familial dysbetalipoproteinemia, and familial LPL deficiency. Xanthomas are cutaneous or subcutaneous papules, plaques, or nodules characterized histopathologically by localized collections of lipid-laden histiocytes (foam cells). The presence or absence of xanthomas should always be noted. If present, their appearance (see later discussion) can provide useful information about the nature of the underlying lipid disorder (Table 82.5). Unless tendons (especially the Achilles tendon) are palpated, the tendon thickening that is characteristic of tendon xanthomas may be missed. Xanthomas are divided morphologically into several types:

1. *Tendinous* (Fig. 82.3A)—firm subcutaneous masses that arise in tendons and occasionally in ligaments, fascia, or periosteum. They characteristically move in concert with the associated tendon and can appear as diffuse thickenings of the tendon. They most often occur on the Achilles tendons and the extensor tendons of the hands, knees, and elbows. The overlying skin is normal in color.
2. *Tuberous* (Fig. 82.3B and C)—soft cutaneous and subcutaneous nodules that may harden with age and increasing fibrosis. Occasionally, they occur as superficial extensions of tendon xanthomas. They can also form from the confluence of eruptive xanthomas, and an intermediate stage is called tuberoeruptive xanthomas. They occur most often on extensor surfaces and areas subjected to trauma, such as the elbows, the knees, the dorsa of the hands, the heels, and the buttocks. The overlying epidermis can be normal in color or have a yellow or orange hue.
3. *Eruptive* (Fig. 82.3D and F)—small (1 to 4 mm) cutaneous papules, that tend to appear in crops, often coincident with an abrupt rise in plasma triglyceride levels. Compared with the other types of xanthomas, they contain more inflammatory cells, free fatty acids, and triglycerides and fewer foam cells and cholesterol esters. They most often occur over pressure areas, such as the buttocks, parts of the trunk, elbows, and knees. They often have a yellow center and red halo. The lesions will disappear in concert with the reduction of triglyceride levels (generally when values are lower than 1,000 mg/dL).
4. *Planar* (Fig. 82.3E, G, and H)—flat, slightly elevated cutaneous lesions that occur most often in skin folds and scars but can be more widely distributed. When present on the eyelids, they are called *xanthelasma*. When located on the palms, they are called palmar xanthomas, and when confined to the palmar creases, *xanthoma striata palmaris*. They tend to be yellow or yellow-brown.

Hypercholesterolemia is associated with tendinous, planar, and tuberous xanthomas. Severe hypertriglyceridemia and chylomicronemia are associated with eruptive and occasionally tuberoeruptive or tuberous xanthomas. Palmar xanthomas are characteristic of familial dysbetalipoproteinemia and florid obstructive liver disease. Planar xanthomas on the body or palms in the presence of a type II lipid profile suggest homozygous monogenic familial hypercholesterolemia. The presence of tendinous or tuberous xanthomas or premature xanthelasma with a type II lipid profile suggests either heterozygous or homozygous monogenic familial hypercholesterolemia, as opposed to the polygenic or nongenetic forms. Tendon xanthomas are found in one third to one half of heterozygotes, whereas tuberous xanthomas are seen most often in patients with familial dysbetalipoproteinemia.

Occasionally, xanthomas appear in the absence of a hyperlipidemic state. For example, xanthelasma occur commonly in normolipidemic older individuals and in nonwhites, and planar xanthomas can occur in patients with lymphoma, leukemia, or myeloma. Studies in normolipidemic individuals with xanthelasma have revealed abnormalities in apo B and E suggestive of familial dysbetalipoproteinemia and/or increased levels of LDL apo B (47), suggesting that these individuals may be at an increased risk of developing atherosclerosis.

Differences exist in the responses to treatment of the various hyperlipidemia-associated xanthomas. Tendon xanthomas are the most resistant to treatment and, in practice, seldom disappear. In contrast, eruptive and planar xanthomas can disappear within a few weeks after plasma lipid levels return to normal.

Gastrointestinal

As many as 35% to 55% of patients with fasting chylomicronemia experience episodes of recurrent abdominal pain. Symptoms are ordinarily associated with marked elevations of plasma triglyceride concentrations (greater than 1,000 to 2,000 mg/dL).

Abdominal pain may be so severe that it prompts unnecessary surgery, particularly if the lipid disorder is not suspected. The pain is often associated with pancreatitis, although the responsible pathogenetic mechanism is not well understood. Routine serum amylase determinations are often subject to technical artifacts when hyperlipidemia is present because of the presence of an amylase-inhibiting factor that may or may not be triglyceride. In such cases, a more reliable estimate of the serum amylase value can be obtained by determining amylase levels on serial dilutions, until the value obtained no longer changes with further dilution. Another cause of abdominal pain may be rapid hepatic or splenic enlargement with capsular distension from triglyceride deposition in reticuloendothelial cells. Often the cause is unclear. Gastrointestinal symptoms other than abdominal pain, such as nausea, vomiting, borborygmi, and diarrhea, also occur.

Other Clinical Associations

Other clinical concomitants of hyperlipidemia include the following: premature arcus corneae (grayish-white corneal ring caused by lipid droplets) in hypercholesterolemia (elevated LDL); aortic stenosis in homozygous monogenic familial hypercholesterolemia; Achilles tendinitis in heterozygous monogenic familial hypercholesterolemia; obesity, glucose intolerance, hyperinsulinemia, hyperuricemia, and perhaps cholelithiasis in association with hypertriglyceridemia and elevated VLDL; recurrent polyarthralgias, arthritis, tenosynovitis, and sicca-like syndromes in hypertriglyceridemia (elevated VLDL) or hypercholesterolemia (elevated LDL); and lipemia retinalis (cream-colored retinal vessels) in chylomicronemia (evident when plasma triglycerides rise above 3,000 mg/dL; obvious when they exceed 10,000 mg/dL).

DIAGNOSIS

Indications for Evaluation

Over the years there has been disagreement about the optimal, cost-effective approach to the identification of hyperlipidemic patients at high risk for CAD (48–50). Some authorities believe that routine screening of healthy young adult men and women who have no CAD risk factors, family history, or clinical evidence of CAD is unwarranted because the benefits of case finding may be outweighed by the long-term risks of treatment. There is, however, a general consensus that screening is important, although there is some disagreement still about which populations should be targeted. The most widely used guidelines for case findings are those issued by the *ATP-III of the NCEP*, which updated for the third time its recommendations for the detection, evaluation, and treatment of high blood cholesterol in adults in 2001 (44). As in previous reports (43), the NCEP continues to emphasize LDL as the primary target of cholesterol-lowering therapy, the role of the clinical approach to primary prevention of CAD, and dietary therapy as the initial treatment, with hypolipidemic drug therapy reserved for patients at high risk for CAD. The new guidelines, however, emphasize CAD risk status as a major determinant for the type and intensity of treatment, pay more attention to HDL as a risk factor, and underscore the importance of including physical activity and weight loss as components of dietary therapy. With regard to assigning risk factor status, the revised NCEP report places patients with existing CAD and those with diabetes mellitus or other atherosclerotic disease at highest risk, maintaining lower target levels of LDL cholesterol in these patients. The report uses Framingham projections to predict CAD risk (see later discussion) over a 10-year span and targets patients with the metabolic syndrome for aggressive intervention. The panel also continues to recommend that HDL cholesterol greater than 60 mg/dL be considered a negative risk factor and that HDL cholesterol levels be used in the decision-making for drug therapy.

The panel continues to recommend that levels of total cholesterol should be measured in all adults 20 years of age or older at least once every 5 years, assuming that blood cholesterol levels are lower than 200 mg/dL, and that HDL should be measured at the same time if accurate results are available (see later discussion). An HDL level of less than 40 mg/dL is considered to be a low value. Measurements of total cholesterol and HDL for screening purposes can be obtained from nonfasting people. However, final classification of abnormal lipid profiles requires lipid determinations in subjects who have been fasted overnight (discussed later). The NCEP classifies individuals by serum levels of total, LDL, and HDL cholesterol (Table 82.7). In this schema, serum levels of total cholesterol less than 200 mg/dL are considered to represent a *desirable blood cholesterol*; levels between 200 and 239 mg/dL, a *borderline-high blood cholesterol*; and levels of 240 mg/dL or higher, a *high blood cholesterol*. Data from numerous epidemiologic studies reveal that the relationships between serum levels of total (or LDL) cholesterol and CAD risk are continuous and that CAD risk at a cholesterol value of 240 mg/dL is almost double that at 200 mg/dL and rises rapidly at levels above 240 mg/dL. Total cholesterol levels of 240 mg/dL or more correspond to the uppermost 20% of cholesterol values in the entire population 20 years of age and older. Patients with levels of total serum cholesterol between 200 and 239 mg/dL and either an HDL cholesterol concentration lower than 40 mg/dL, known CAD or diabetes mellitus, or two or more known risk factors for CAD (Table 82.2) are considered to have high blood cholesterol values.

Although there is a consensus on targets for lipid values and intervention in those with CAD risk (e.g., diabetes mellitus) or known CAD, there does exist an honest difference of opinion regarding when to begin screening for lipid disorders in the adult population. The USPSTF recommends that screening begin at age 35 years for men and age 45 years for women and that individuals age 20 years and older need be screened

Table 82.7. Comparison Between Recommendations of the Adult Treatment Panel III (ATP III) of the National Cholesterol Education Program and those of the U.S. Preventive Services Task Force (USPSTF) and the American College of Physicians (ACP)

	ATP III (2001)		USPSTF (2001)		ACP (1996)	
Parameter	Men	Women	Men	Women	Men	Women
Age to initiate screening						
Without risk factors	20	20	35	45	35	45
With risk factors	20	20	20	20	<35	<45
Frequency of screening (yr)	5	5	5	5	5	5
Measurements	Fasting total cholesterol, triglycerides, HDL, LDL[a]		Nonfasting total cholesterol, HDL[b]		Nonfasting total cholesterol[b,c]	

HDL, high-density lipoprotein; LDL, low-density lipoprotein.
[a]Fasting triglycerides and HDL are measured to enable calculation of the LDL.
[b]Triglyceride measurements are not recommended.
[c]HDL cholesterol measurements are not recommended.
From references 44 (ATP III), 50 (USPTF), and 51 (ACP) and U.S. Preventive Services Task Force, 2001.

only if they have associated risk factors for CAD (50) (see USPSTF, 2001, in General References). The USPSTF limits screening to measurement of total cholesterol and HDL (it finds no evidence supporting the routine measurement of triglycerides and, by extension, LDL for screening purposes). An older American College of Physicians (ACP) report does not support routine screening in young adult men (age 20 to 35 years), premenopausal women (age 20 to 45 years), or persons older than 65 years of age (51). It should be noted that the NCEP guidelines have been endorsed by more than 40 medical and health care organizations, including the American College of Cardiology, American Academy of Family Physicians, American Medical Association, American College of Preventive Medicine, and American Heart Association (AHA) (52,53).

Table 82.7 compares the recommendations of the NCEP, USPSTF, and ACP. The practitioner must decide, in consultation with his or her patients, which recommendations to follow. It is clear, however, that screening is indicated and that most patients with hyperlipidemia should be treated.

Evaluation of the Patient with Hypercholesterolemia

Once a patient is found to have a high blood cholesterol level or physical stigmata of hypercholesterolemia (e.g., dermatologic signs), decisions regarding possible diet, drug, or other therapy are made after a more detailed lipoprotein analysis, including measurements of triglyceride levels on a blood specimen obtained after an overnight fast, calculation of the LDL cholesterol level (discussed later), and determination of other CAD risk factors. The updated NCEP guidelines adjust the classification for LDL cholesterol levels as follows: LDL cholesterol levels greater or equal to 190 mg/dL are considered very high; 160 to 189 mg/dL, high; 130 to 159 mg/dL, borderline high; 100 to 129 mg/dL, near or above optimal; and less than 100 mg/dL, optimal. In patients with known CAD, diabetes mellitus, or two or more major CAD risk factors (Table 82.2), LDL cholesterol levels between 130 and 159 mg/dL are considered *high risk.* The NCEP considers an HDL level lower than 40 mg/dL to be an independent risk factor for CAD. Therefore, decisions regarding both the implementation and the goals of therapy are based not on ratios of LDL (or total) cholesterol to HDL cholesterol but on absolute levels of LDL and HDL cholesterol. Such decisions are also influenced by the presence or absence of other CAD risk factors.

Triglycerides. The current NCEP guidelines classify fasting triglyceride levels lower than 150 mg/dL as normal levels, those between 150 and 199 mg/dL as *borderline high,* those between 200 and 499 mg/dL as high, and those greater than or equal to 500 mg/dL as very high. There is a complex link between hypertriglyceridemia and CAD, which is explained in part by the association between high triglycerides and low HDL and/or unusually atherogenic forms of LDL. Moreover, elevated triglycerides often reflect increased triglyceride-rich remnant lipoproteins that have atherogenic potential. There is disagreement about the usefulness of measurement of triglyceride levels in the screening of healthy people (Table 82.7).

Measurement of plasma levels of total cholesterol, HDL cholesterol, and fasting triglyceride concentrations and calculation of the level of LDL cholesterol (see later discussion) are desirable when abnormalities are detected on screening or conditions coexist that could cause secondary abnormalities in lipoprotein metabolism (Table 82.4). Although the frequencies with which certain drugs (e.g., thiazide diuretics, antihypertensives, oral contraceptives) adversely affect lipoprotein metabolism are unknown and direct causal interrelationships between such drug-associated lipid abnormalities and premature atherosclerosis are unproved, it seems prudent also to consider the more complete evaluation before therapy is initiated with these drugs.

Laboratory Evaluation

Plasma or serum levels of total cholesterol are not appreciably influenced by acute dietary intake and therefore can be obtained from patients in the nonfasting state and at any time of the day. There is considerable biologic variability (6%) and laboratory variability (3%) in repeated measurements of total cholesterol in a given individual (50,54). Therefore, to be within 10% of the true value, two measurements are necessary. It is also important to obtain blood for cholesterol measurements from a nonstressed patient and to send the blood for analysis to a reliable laboratory.

Levels of total (and LDL) cholesterol fall during the first few days after an MI (55), so cholesterol determinations either should be made within 24 hours after a severe acute MI (when they are still valid) or should be postponed until 3 to 4 weeks after recovery. Fasting triglyceride (and VLDL) levels tend to rise slowly after an MI, peaking at 3 to 4 weeks and returning to baseline by 8 to 12 weeks. Therefore, triglyceride levels should be obtained either within 24 hours after the acute event or after 8 to 12 weeks.

The *determination of HDL cholesterol* is the measurement most subject to laboratory error. Again, there is considerable biologic variability (7.5%) and laboratory variability (6%) in repeated measurements of HDL in a given individual (50,54). To be within 10% to 15% of the true value, two to three measurements of HDL are necessary. Such measures to enhance validity are important because there is a relatively narrow range of HDL cholesterol values within which even small differences are prognostically important. For example, a reduction in HDL cholesterol of 5 mg/dL—from 40 to 35 mg/dL—increases the risk for CAD by approximately 25%. HDL levels are unreliable when triglyceride concentrations exceed 400 mg/dL. Under such circumstances, the plasma or serum should be ultrafiltered. If this is required, the physician should consult the laboratory.

In the nonfasting state, HDL levels are 5% to 10% lower than in the fasting state and therefore may slightly overestimate the risk of CAD. However, for screening purposes, nonfasting levels are acceptable.

Because *triglyceride levels* are 25% to 30% higher in the nonfasting state, it is important that triglyceride measurements be made only in fasting patients.

Calculation of LDL Level. Measurements of HDL and triglyceride levels allow one to calculate the LDL cholesterol level (provided the triglyceride concentration is less than 400 mg/dL) by the following formula: $\text{LDL-C} = \text{TC} - (\text{TG}/5 + \text{HDL-C})$, where LDL-C is the LDL cholesterol level, TC is the plasma level of total cholesterol, TG is the fasting plasma triglyceride level, and HDL-C is the level of HDL cholesterol.

Observation of a fasting plasma sample that has been left undisturbed overnight in a refrigerator at 4°C is indicated in the presence of a significantly elevated fasting plasma triglyceride level. Increased levels of total (or LDL) cholesterol do not affect the appearance of plasma, whereas hypertriglyceridemia associated with increased levels of VLDL imparts uniform turbidity to plasma, and hypertriglyceridemia associated with chylomicronemia is characterized by a creamy supernatant fraction that floats on the top of plasma.

A marked abnormality in plasma lipid concentrations, especially marked hypertriglyceridemia (greater than 2,000 mg/dL), can affect the validity of other laboratory tests. Marked hypertriglyceridemia has an inhibitory effect on the plasma amylase assay, interferes with the measurement of liver enzymes (aspartate aminotransferase, alanine aminotransferase) and calcium by autoanalyzer, and causes artifactual reductions in the serum concentration of molecules restricted to the aqueous phase (e.g., sodium). Ultracentrifugation of plasma, with the removal of chylomicrons, permits these measurements to be performed accurately; but sometimes serial dilutions of the plasma are necessary, particularly for the measurement of amylase.

Clinical Evaluation

Clinical data contribute substantially to the diagnosis of specific lipoprotein disorders and to decisions about treatment when abnormalities are found. History, physical examination, and indicated laboratory evaluation are required to rule out secondary causes of hyperlipidemia (Table 82.4). A positive family history, the presence of premature atherosclerotic disease, and the presence of specific dermatologic manifestations may permit the diagnosis of a primary form of hyperlipoproteinemia (Table 82.5). Assessment of the patient's family history and cardiovascular status is also important for risk stratification.

Referral

If laboratory and clinical evaluations do not result in a clear-cut diagnosis of a lipoprotein disorder, referral to a specialist in endocrinology and metabolism is indicated. Such specialists can perform (or readily obtain) and interpret more sophisticated tests, such as ultracentrifugal quantification of lipoprotein levels, apoprotein measurement, receptor analysis, and determination of LPL activity. They may also assist in the evaluation of family members, so that the presence of a genetic disorder can be accurately diagnosed. Referral should also be considered for patients who are refractory to the lifestyle and pharmacologic management strategies described previously.

TREATMENT

General Approach

The first step in the management of a lipoprotein disorder is accurate diagnosis. Causes of secondary lipoprotein disorders should be identified (Table 82.4) and treated. If the cause of a secondary disorder is not reversible or a primary disorder exists, treatment may be required that is specifically directed at the abnormal lipoprotein pattern.

Such treatment should be part of the comprehensive management of other coexisting CAD risk factors (e.g., cigarette smoking, hypertension, diabetes mellitus, obesity, inactivity). It will probably require behavioral change on the part of the patient and lifelong management, emphasizing the need for a positive patient–clinician relationship, appropriate patient education, and skill on the part of the clinician in promoting patient compliance (see Chapters 3 and 4). Long-term follow-up and monitoring of various parameters in such patients are necessary to enhance compliance, to assess the effectiveness of therapy, and to detect drug toxicity or the effect of concomitant therapy (e.g., diuretics, other antihypertensive agents) on plasma lipids.

Patients without CAD who are classified as having a *desirable total cholesterol level* (less than 200 mg/dL) and an HDL cholesterol level higher 40 mg/dL are usually instructed on the principles of a prudent diet and healthy lifestyle, educated about CAD risk factors (Table 82.2), and advised to have their total cholesterol level rechecked at least once every 5 years.

Patients with CAD, diabetes, secondary causes of lipid disorders, a total cholesterol level higher than 200 mg/dL, an HDL cholesterol level lower than 40 mg/dL, or risk factors (Table 82.2) should have a fasting lipid panel performed (fasting total cholesterol, triglycerides, and HDL cholesterol, and calculation of LDL—see previous discussion). *Treatment is then based primarily on LDL cholesterol levels* according to guidelines provided by NCEP (Table 82.8). The guidelines also emphasize the need to assess CAD risk for patients with more than two risk factors and an LDL cholesterol level between 130 and 159 mg/dL (see National Heart, Lung and Blood Institute website in General References for instructions on how to calculate risk according to the Framingham scoring system). Drug therapy is suggested for such patients who have a 10-year risk of developing ischemic heart disease of more than 10% (Table 82.8).

For patients with a *borderline high total cholesterol* of 200 to 239 mg/dL, HDL cholesterol greater than 40 mg/dL, and fewer than two risk factors, it is also reasonable to provide education about diet, exercise, and other lifestyle modifications and to recheck the total and HDL cholesterol in 1 to 2 years, in the absence of a fasting lipid profile.

Patients with isolated reductions in HDL cholesterol (less than 40 mg/dL) should be instructed in the value of weight loss, aerobic exercise, and discontinuation of cigarette smoking (see later discussion). Although certain drugs used for treatment of increased levels of LDL cholesterol or of triglycerides may also raise HDL levels, at present no data support their use in the healthy patient whose only lipid abnormality is a reduction in the level of HDL.

Management of hypertriglyceridemia must be individualized. When familial combined hyperlipidemia or familial dysbetalipoproteinemia is diagnosed, specific treatment is required. Patients with fasting triglyceride levels greater than 500 mg/dL sometimes accumulate chylomicrons and develop pancreatitis. The risk becomes substantial when triglyceride levels exceed 1000 mg/dL. The plasma triglyceride level should therefore be lowered in these patients. For patients with fasting triglyceride levels in the 200- to 499-mg/dL range, control of LDL cholesterol remains the primary goal but control of triglyceride level becomes a secondary goal. Diet, weight control, and regular exercise should be encouraged. Drug therapy should also be considered if treatment goals are not reached through lifestyle change, especially when CAD, diabetes, or coexistent risk factors (see Table 82.2) are present. The presence of the *metabolic syndrome*, which is associated with a very high risk of CAD, should probably also sway the clinician toward the use of drug therapy if treatment goals cannot be achieved by lifestyle change. The metabolic syndrome (also called metabolic syndrome X or insulin resistance syndrome) is characterized by abdominal obesity (see Chapter 83), low HDL cholesterol (less than 40 mg/dL in men, 50 mg/dL in women), hypertension (130/85 mm Hg or higher), fasting plasma glucose concentration 110 mg/dL or higher, and fasting triglycerides 150 mg/dL or higher. *Treatment goals are defined by a non-HDL cholesterol concentration* (i.e., total cholesterol minus HDL cholesterol) that is 30 mg/dL greater than the treatment goals for LDL cholesterol—that is, less than 190 mg/dL for one or no risk factors, 160 mg/dL for two or more risk factors and 10-year risk greater than 20%, and less than 130 mg/dL for CAD or CAD risk equivalent.

Table 82.8. LDL Cholesterol Goals and Cutpoints for Therapeutic Lifestyle Changes (TLC)[a] and Drug Therapy in Different Risk Categories

Risk Category	LDL Goal (mg/dL)	Level at Which to Initiate TLC (mg/dL)	Level at Which to Consider Drug Therapy (mg/dL)
CAD or CAD risk equivalents (10-year risk >20%)	<100	≥100	≥130 (100–129; drug optional)[b]
2+ Risk factors (10-year risk ≥20%)	<130	≥130	10-year risk 10%–20%: ≥130 10-year risk <10%;≥160
0–1 Risk factor[c]	<160	≥160	≥190 (160–189: LDL-lowering drug optimal)

CAD, coronary artery disease; LDL, low-density lipoprotein.

[a]Therapeutic lifestyle changes include diet, weight control, increased activity, and smoking cessation.

[b]Some authorities recommend use of LDL-lowering drugs in this category if an LDL cholesterol level of <100mg/dL cannot be achieved by therapeutic lifestyle changes. Others prefer use of drugs that primarily modify triglycerides and high-density lipoprotein (e.g., nicotinic acid, fibrate). Clinical judgment also may call for deferring drug therapy in this subcategory.

[c]Almost all people with 0–1 risk factor have a 10-year risk of CAD that is <10%; therefore, the 10-year risk assessment in people with 0–1 risk factor is not necessary.

Modified from the Executive Summary of the Third Report of the National Cholesterol Education Program (NCEP) Expert Panel on Detection, Evaluation, and Treatment of High Blood Cholesterol in Adults (Adult Treatment Panel III). JAMA 2001;285:2486.

Table 82.9. Nutrient Composition of the Therapeutic Lifestyle Changes (TLC) Diet

Nutrient	Recommendation
Saturated fat[a]	<7% of total calories
Polyunsaturated fat	Up to 10% of total calories
Monounsaturated fat	Up to 20% of total calories
Total fat	25%–35% of total calories
Carbohydrate[b]	50%–60% of total calories
Fiber	20–30 mg/day
Protein	Approximately 15% of total calories
Cholesterol	<200 mg/day
Total calories[c]	Balance energy intake and expenditure to maintain desirable body weight, prevent weight gain

[a]Trans fatty acids are another low-density lipoprotein–raising fat that should be kept at a low intake.

[b]Carbohydrates should be derived predominantly from foods rich in complex carbohydrates including grains, especially whole grains, fruits, and vegetables.

[c]Daily energy expenditure should include at least moderate physical activity (contributing approximately 200 kcal/day).

From the Executive Summary of the Third Report of the National Cholesterol Education Program (NCEP) Expert Panel on Detection, Evaluation, and Treatment of High Blood Cholesterol in Adults (Adult Treatment Panel III). JAMA 2001; 285:2486.

Nonpharmacologic Therapy

Diet

It is now well established that plasma lipid levels can be altered by dietary manipulations (Tables 82.9 and 82.10). Under strictly controlled conditions (e.g., in a metabolic unit), increased plasma levels of total (or LDL) cholesterol may be reduced by as much as 30% or more, and levels of triglyceride or VLDL (in the presence of marked elevations) by as much as 80% or more. Fasting chylomicronemia can also be eliminated. Under ambulatory conditions, in which diets tend to be less restrictive and noncompliance more common, reductions in lipid levels are less dramatic. For example, among prospective studies of cholesterol-lowering diets, the decrease in plasma cholesterol averaged 15% (range, 8.5% to 22%).

Single-Diet Approach. The third report of the ATP-III of the NCEP (see General References) continues to highlight dietary therapy as the first line of treatment of elevated blood cholesterol levels (Table 82.9). In primary prevention trials to date, dietary therapy has not been associated with decreased all-cause mortality. There is insufficient evidence to support treatment of healthy normolipidemic individuals with restrictive diets. Studies have shown little change in the lipid profiles of healthy subjects with intake of either a high- or a low-cholesterol diet (55a). Dietary therapy has more impact in those who are dyslipidemic and have risk factors for CAD. It is now appreciated that one diet can be used to treat all of the common forms of hyperlipoproteinemia (Table 82.9). The classification of diets as Step 1 and Step 2 has been eliminated and replaced with the Therapeutic Lifestyle Changes (TLC) diet. Using the principle of graduated regimen implementation (see Chapter 4), the diet can be introduced in a step-wise fashion. If severe chylomicronemia is present, dietary fat must be more severely restricted (see later discussion).

The AHA and other organizations publish useful booklets on this diet for the patient, physician, and nutritionist. Most patients with hyperlipoproteinemia benefit from referral to a suitably trained dietitian. The TLC diet actually incorporates several nutritional strategies, each of which tends to have a selective effect on plasma lipoprotein levels. It is helpful to consider each strategy separately.

Cholesterol Reduction. The TLC diet to lower serum cholesterol levels (Tables 82.9 and 82.10) is characterized by a restriction of dietary cholesterol to less than 200 mg/day and reductions in daily total and saturated fat intake to less than 35% and 7% of caloric intake, respectively. The total fat allowance can range from 25% to 35% as long as the intake of saturated fats and trans fatty acids is low. The other feature of the TLC diet is encouragement of the consumption of plant stanols/sterols (2 g/day) and soluble fiber (10 to 25 g/day). Caloric allowance is adjusted to ensure loss of excess weight or maintenance of ideal body weight (see Chapter 83). Restrictions in dietary cholesterol and saturated fats independently contribute to the reduction in plasma cholesterol levels. A modest increase in dietary polyunsaturated fat results in further, although less marked, reduction in plasma cholesterol level.

The two major categories of *polyunsaturated fatty acids* are the omega-6 and omega-3 types. Linoleic acid is the principal *omega-6 fatty acid*; when consumed in large amounts, it can decrease levels of total cholesterol. Lecithin, a phospholipid derived from soybeans, is a widely publicized popular remedy for hypercholesterolemia and is commonly sold in health food stores. Because it is not absorbed as such from the gastrointestinal tract, any hypocholesterolemic effect probably derives from its high content of linoleic acid. Vegetable oils rich in linoleic acid, such as safflower oil, soybean oil, sunflower oil, and corn oil, are the preferred dietary sources of the omega-6 fatty acids.

The major sources of the *omega-3 fatty acids* are the fish oils. Taken as dietary supplements, high dosages of fish oil lower elevated triglyceride concentrations but do not reduce levels of total or LDL cholesterol. Nevertheless, epidemiologic studies have shown an inverse relationship between the consumption of fish and the risk of adverse cardiac and other cerebrovascular events, in persons with and without ischemic heart disease (56,57). Also, several randomized controlled trials have demonstrated a modest reduction in cardiac events (1% to 3% absolute risk reduction) in patients with documented CAD who were prescribed omega-3 fatty acids (32,58). Side effects are predominantly gastrointestinal (nausea, bloating, flatulence, eructation, diarrhea, fishy aftertaste). Concerns that fish oil supplements may worsen hyperinsulinemia and increase insulin resistance were diminished by a meta-analysis that showed no adverse effects of these supplements on glycosylated hemoglobin levels (59).

The typical North American diet has an unfavorable polyunsaturated-to-saturated fat (P/S) ratio of 0.4. On

Table 82.10. Dietary Guidelines to Lower Blood Cholesterol

Food	Recommended	Avoid or Use Sparingly
Fish, Shellfish, Poultry, Shrimp, Lean Red Meats		
Up to 6 to 7 oz are recommended per day (limit shrimp to 3 oz)	Fish; skinless chicken, turkey, Cornish hen; very lean cuts of beef, lamb, pork and veal; low-fat lunchmeats with 3 g fat or less per oz. Dry beans or tofu may be used as a substitute for fish, poultry, and meat.	Any fatty cuts of meat; lunchmeats; sausages; scrapple, bacon; hot dogs; caviar, fish roe; deep-fried meats, fish, and poultry; organ meat; duck; goose
Fats and Oils		
Up to 6 to 7 tsp may be used per day, including fat used in cooking	Unsaturated oils: safflower, sunflower, corn, soybean, sesame, rapeseed (canola); soft margarine with first ingredient a liquid unsaturated oil listed above; 4 to 6 nuts or 3 olives count as 1 teaspoon of oil. Mayonnaise; salad dressing made with unsaturated oils listed above (2 teaspoons count as 1 teaspoon oil).	Butter; lard; palm kernel oil; meat fat; salt pork; bacon fat; coconut oil; palm oil; hydrogenated or solid shortenings; gravy; cream sauce; salad dressing made with cream, cheese, or sour cream
Milk and Yogurt		
2 or more cups recommended per day	Skim or 1% milk, including evaporated and powdered milk; buttermilk; nonfat and low-fat yogurt.	Whole milk, including evaporated and condensed milk; eggnog; yogurt; cream; sour cream; half and half; coconut milk
Cheese		
1 oz of recommended cheese or ¼ cup cottage cheese may be substituted for 1 oz of fish, poultry, or lean red meat	Low-fat cottage cheese; low-fat cheese with 4 g of fat or less per oz.	High-fat cheeses containing more than 4 g of fat per oz
Eggs		
Egg yolks should be limited to 2 per week, including those used in cooking	Egg whites (2 egg whites will substitute for 1 whole egg in recipes); cholesterol-free egg substitutes.	Egg yolks in excess of 2 per week
Vegetables and Fruits		
5 or more servings are recommended per day. Include at least 1 serving of citrus fruit or other source of vitamin C per day	Fresh, frozen, canned, or dried.	Vegetables in cream, cheese, or butter sauces, deep-fried vegetables, french fries
Breads and Cereals		
6 or more servings recommended per day	Loaf bread and bagels (except egg); English muffins, pita bread; most sandwich and dinner rolls; Melba toast; water crackers; soda crackers; rice cakes; rye crisp; matzo, pretzels, breadsticks (made without cheese). All cereals except as noted. Pasta (except egg); all grains, including rice, barley, buckwheat, bulgur, com, millet, rye, and oats.	Croissants, biscuits, and other rich rolls; pastries; doughnuts; egg breads; commercial baked products; high-fat crackers; cereals with added oils and coconut, such as granola-type; egg pasta
Desserts and Sweets		
Foods high in sugar are best used in small amounts. They should be used infrequently by persons with high triglycerides or excess weight.	Fruit; sugar, jelly; cocoa powder, gelatin, Italian ice; frozen fruit bars; frozen low-fat yogurt; pudding made with skim milk; angel food cake; sherbet; sorbet; low-fat cookies; homemade baked products made with skim or low-fat milk, egg whites, and small amounts of unsaturated fat.	Chocolate; ice cream; coconut; cream desserts; egg custard; commercial baked products
Miscellaneous	Fat-free broths. Air-popped popcorn or popcorn made with small amounts of unsaturated oil; pretzels, nuts (e.g., walnuts) vinegar, spices, herbs, mustard, fat-free salad dressing.	Cream or other fatty soups; high-fat snack foods such as potato chips, corn chips, granola bars, microwave popcom, nondairy creamers, and whipped toppings made with coconut or palm oil

Modified from The Johns Hopkins Physicians Lipid Education Program. 2nd ed. Baltimore: The Johns Hopkins University, 1988.

the other hand, there is no historical precedent that attests to the safety of diets that are very rich in polyunsaturated fats (e.g., P/S ratio of 1.5 or more). It does appear that the latter diets can promote the formation of lithogenic bile and actually increase the incidence of symptomatic biliary tract disease. Although there was a concern that such diets are associated with an increased risk of malignant disease, this finding was not supported when data from several trials were pooled (60). Another disadvantage to substantially increasing dietary intake of polyunsaturated fat is that the resultant high caloric intake might promote obesity. Finally, it should be noted that diets with very high P/S ratios (e.g., 3 or more) may decrease HDL levels and lead to an unfavorable increase in the LDL/HDL ratio. For all of these reasons, a P/S ratio of about 1.0 is recommended in most hypocholesterolemic diets.

Monounsaturated fatty acids, principally oleic acid, found in canola oil, olive oil, and certain forms of safflower and sunflower seed oil, lower levels of LDL cholesterol as effectively as do polyunsaturated fatty acids such as linoleic acid. Therefore, it is now recommended that the TLC diet contain approximately 20% monounsaturated fatty acids, derived mainly from these vegetable oils.

The influence of *dietary fiber* on plasma cholesterol levels is complex, dependent on the type of fiber, and somewhat controversial. Guar, pectin, and unprocessed high-fiber foods, such as legumes and oats, lower plasma total cholesterol levels, whereas other fibers, such as wheat bran, do not. Effects on levels of HDL cholesterol and triglyceride are minimal. In the amounts consumed in a palatable diet, fiber plays a minor role compared with control of dietary fats and cholesterol.

Although *garlic* supplements are effective in reducing total cholesterol, LDL cholesterol, and triglyceride concentrations modestly (about 5%) (61), reductions may not persist. The impact on clinical outcomes is unknown. Proven side effects are malodorous breath and body odor; there may also be gastrointestinal side effects such as abdominal pain, fullness, anorexia, and flatulence.

Margarines enriched with *plant sterols* (sitostanol and campestanol in Benecol, sitosterol and campesterol in Take Control) have been shown in a few studies to lower total and LDL cholesterol by about 10%. They are very poorly absorbed and probably act through the inhibition of cholesterol absorption. Their impact on cardiovascular outcomes is unknown. Although short-term studies have not demonstrated adverse clinical effects, the absorption of fat-soluble vitamins may be affected. A long-term safety profile has not been established. Because of this, the AHA does not recommend their consumption by the general population, but recommends reserving their use for secondary prevention and for patients with moderate to severe hypercholesterolemia (62). Margarines enriched with plant sterols are several times more expensive than ordinary margarines.

Soy proteins, which are found in tofu and soy milk, lower total cholesterol, LDL cholesterol, and triglyceride by about 10% (63) and may contribute to the lower risk of heart disease in Asian compared to Western societies. An advisory from the Nutrition Committee of the AHA concluded that 25 to 50 g/day of soy protein is both safe and effective in modestly reducing LDL cholesterol by 4% to 8% (64). The impact of such a diet on health has not been established.

Monitoring and Adjusting Diet. Results of the TLC diet should be monitored after 4 to 6 weeks and again at 3 months, when the effects should be maximal. In general, formal consultation with a dietitian is not required during implementation of the TLC diet, and the physician and other health care providers should serve as the primary sources of education, compliance monitoring, and encouragement for the patient. It is important to emphasize to all patients that dietary treatment of hypercholesterolemia implies permanent, rather than temporary, changes in eating behavior. If the goals of diet therapy are not met after 3 months, it is recommended that the patient continue on the TLC diet and that consideration be given to initiating drug treatment. Patients should also be referred to a dietitian for formal nutritional counseling. For patients with known CAD and for those with diabetes mellitus, it is recommended that pharmacologic and dietary therapy be initiated simultaneously.

Dietary and Drug Therapy. Dietary therapy alone is effective in lowering cholesterol levels in many of the almost 85% of hypercholesterolemic patients with polygenic or nonhereditary forms of hypercholesterolemia. However, numerous studies indicate that dietary therapy alone is less effective in lowering total or LDL cholesterol levels than is the combination of dietary therapy plus drug treatment. For example, in a multicenter trial comparing the separate and combined effects of intensive dietary therapy and low-dose lovastatin in outpatients with moderate hypercholesterolemia, a low-fat diet alone reduced LDL cholesterol by 5%, lovastatin alone lowered LDL by 27%, and lovastatin plus dietary therapy reduced LDL by 32% (65). In elderly patients with hypercholesterolemia, the benefits of diet therapy should be weighed against the possibility of inadequate nutrition.

Triglyceride Reduction. Diets designed to reduce plasma triglyceride and VLDL levels emphasize the loss of excess weight by total caloric restriction. Plasma triglyceride levels usually fall, often to normal, after a few days of caloric restriction. The reduction is maintained as long as weight loss continues at a rate of 1 to 2 lb (0.5 to 1 kg) per week. If normal weight is attained and maintained, further therapy may not be necessary. If hypertriglyceridemia persists or occurs in individuals of normal weight, a cholesterol-lowering diet, as outlined earlier, may be effective. Alcohol intake should be restricted, because it can cause a striking rise in triglyceride levels in some patients with hypertriglyceridemia. Although extreme increases in the carbohydrate content of a diet can cause transient and, rarely, sustained hypertriglyceridemia, there is no firm evidence to suggest that total carbohydrate restriction is helpful in the treatment of hypertriglyceridemia. There are conflicting data regarding the effect on plasma triglyceride level of excessive intake of sucrose (common sugar) and simple sugars. In most studies, especially in patients who are already hypertriglyceridemic, they do raise plasma levels of triglycerides and lower those of HDL cholesterol, but the effect is small. The rationale for dietary restriction of sugar is based more on the need to avoid excessive caloric intake (and to prevent caries) than on any direct effect on plasma lipids. Like alcohol, sucrose provides empty calories in that it contains none of the valuable nutrients (e.g., protein, fiber, minerals, vitamins). Therefore the substitution of complex carbohydrates (e.g., starches) for simple carbohydrates in the diet is recommended. A triglyceride-lowering diet should favorably affect plasma HDL cholesterol levels in most individuals, because obesity and triglyceride concentration are inversely correlated with the level of HDL cholesterol and plasma HDL usually rises during weight reduction. Plasma levels of total (and LDL) cholesterol often fall with loss of excess weight; if they rise, familial combined hyperlipoproteinemia may be present.

Chylomicron Reduction. Treatment of fasting chylomicronemia (type I) involves the restriction of dietary fat intake to 5% to 20% of total calories (0.5 g of fat per kilogram of body weight is a reasonable starting point). The fat deficit should be corrected predominantly by substitution of complex carbohydrates. Because medium-chain triglycerides (available as MCT oil) are transported directly from the intestine to the liver in the portal circulation without incorporation into chylomicrons, they may be added to the diet to provide calories. The recommended dose of MCT oil (available at most pharmacies) is 1 tablespoonful three to four times daily, mixed with foods. Five grams of vegetable fat rich in polyunsaturates should be included to prevent essential fatty acid deficiency.

Dietary fat is severely restricted until fasting chylomicronemia is eliminated and clinical symptoms are prevented or reduced in frequency; dietary fat is then chronically restricted to whatever degree is necessary to prevent fasting chylomicronemia. The efficacy of fat restriction in preventing recurrent abdominal pain is supported by clinical observations in individual patients.

If fasting chylomicronemia is accompanied by increased VLDL triglyceride levels, therapy is initiated with restriction of dietary fat intake and correction of coexistent secondary causes for the disorder. Once chylomicronemia has been eliminated, a triglyceride-lowering diet with a modest reduction in total fat intake (to approximately 30% of total calories) is all that is usually required to prevent recurrence. Total abstinence from alcohol is usually necessary.

Diets to Raise the HDL Level. Some studies have reported that low-fat, low-cholesterol diets have resulted in decreased levels of HDL cholesterol (66), whereas others have found increased HDL values (67). The dietary approach to the patient with an HDL cholesterol level lower than 40 mg/dL should incorporate loss of excess weight with an aerobic exercise program. Although moderate alcohol consumption (2 to 3 oz/day) is positively correlated with HDL cholesterol concentration and negatively correlated with CAD, it is discouraged for three reasons: Excessive use (more than two or three drinks per day) increases the overall risk of morbidity and mortality; its use may interfere with attempts to control obesity and hypertriglyceridemia; and evidence is not conclusive that modest intake results in an overall health advantage.

Exercise

During the past decade, evidence has accumulated that regular isotonic exercise enhances fatty acid oxidation and glycogen storage, thus increasing HDL formation, triglyceride clearance, and insulin sensitivity. These metabolic changes favorably affect plasma lipid levels. Most of the exercise programs that have been evaluated, including jogging, rapid walking, swimming, bicycling, cross-country skiing, and mountain climbing, have involved 30 minutes or more of continued effort at 70% to 85% of maximal heart rate at least three times weekly. In most studies, levels of HDL cholesterol have been shown to rise (approximately 20%) and triglyceride levels to fall (approximately 25%) with exercise (45). Although levels of LDL cholesterol usually do not fall in normal subjects, reductions of as much as 10% may occur in individuals with increased concentrations of total and LDL cholesterol.

Resistive training programs conducted in normolipidemic individuals have resulted in increases in HDL cholesterol of 10% to 15% and decreases in LDL cholesterol of 5% to 39% (68). In contrast, in one well-controlled prospective study of resistive training in subjects at risk for CAD (69), no changes in lipid profiles were observed after 20 weeks. Both aerobic and resistive exercise training improve glucose tolerance and insulin sensitivity, reduce blood pressure, and improve body composition (70,71).

To date, most prospective exercise studies have been performed in men. A meta-analysis of the existing longitudinal exercise investigations in women revealed an overall decrease in levels of total cholesterol and triglycerides with little or no change in values of HDL or LDL cholesterol (72). Gender-related differences in the lipoprotein response to exercise may reflect the generally higher endogenous levels of HDL cholesterol in women or differences in metabolic factors such as levels of sex steroids or regulatory enzymes.

It has been demonstrated in both cross-sectional and longitudinal epidemiologic studies that people who exercise regularly have a reduced risk for CAD. Exercise also improves glucose metabolism, assists in weight reduction, and may reduce blood pressure (73,74).

Therefore, exercise counseling (see Chapters 16 and 63) is an important part of the management of patients with abnormalities in lipoprotein metabolism.

Smoking Cessation

Plasma levels of HDL cholesterol have been found to be lower and levels of VLDL triglyceride higher in people who smoke cigarettes than in nonsmokers or ex-smokers. Moreover, an inverse relationship exists between the number of cigarettes smoked daily and the level of HDL cholesterol. Smoking cessation has been associated with a modest rise in plasma HDL concentration. It is not known how much of the increased risk of CAD associated with smoking is mediated through alteration in the plasma lipids and how much via other mechanisms. There is, however, substantial evidence that smoking cessation reduces CAD risk. There is also evidence that counseling of patients increases cessation rates. Therefore, all patients who smoke cigarettes should be counseled, regardless of their lipoprotein profile (see Chapter 27).

Drugs

The recommendations for drug therapy for primary prevention were updated by the ATP-III (44) and are discussed here. Candidates for drug therapy should always continue dietary intervention (described earlier), because the effects of each mode of treatment are often additive. For all patients, additional lifestyle changes such as weight control, habitual exercise, and cessation of cigarette smoking should be maximized. Information on lipid-lowering drugs is provided in Table 82.11.

Hypercholesterolemia

In general, the NCEP guidelines suggest a need for drug therapy (Table 82.8) when, despite 3 months of dietary intervention, the LDL level is still higher than the desired range. Patients with marked elevations of LDL cholesterol, in whom dietary therapy alone is unlikely to normalize LDL cholesterol levels, may be considered for drug therapy simultaneously with the initiation of dietary modification. After drugs have been started, LDL cholesterol levels should be checked at 4 to 6 weeks and at 3 months. Once target levels have been achieved, patients should be evaluated with measurement of LDL cholesterol every 4 to 6 months.

Drug therapy should be delayed in the following groups of patients: men younger than 35 years of age (with the exception of smokers whose LDL levels are between 160 and 189 mg/dL and all patients whose LDL levels are 190 mg/dL or higher) (44), premenopausal women without other risk factors whose LDL cholesterol levels are between 190 and 220 mg/dL, patients with fewer than two other risk factors and LDL cholesterol levels between 160 and 190 mg/dL, and patients with two other risk factors and LDL cholesterol levels in the range of 130 to 160 mg/dL on adequate dietary therapy.

Cholesterol-lowering drugs are categorized into two groups: (a) first-choice agents, such as HMG-CoA reductase inhibitors, bile acid sequestrants, and nicotinic acid, which are effective in lowering total and LDL cholesterol levels, reduce CAD risk, and are generally safe for long-term use; and (b) other drugs, such as gemfibrozil and probucol.

HMG-CoA Reductase Inhibitors. The *statins* (lovastatin, simvastatin, pravastatin, fluvastatin, atorvastatin) are specific, potent, competitive inhibitors of HMG-CoA reductase, the rate-limiting enzyme in cholesterol biosynthesis. These drugs increase hepatic LDL receptor activity and LDL clearance from the circulation and, in addition, decrease production of LDL (75). More than 15 years of clinical experience with this class of drugs has confirmed their effectiveness in reducing levels of total and LDL cholesterol by 20% to 50%, in decreasing triglyceride levels slightly, and in modestly increasing the levels of HDL cholesterol in some patients (75,76). They appear to be equally effective in individuals with familial and nonfamilial hypercholesterolemia. When compared with bile acid sequestrants and nicotinic acid in the treatment of patients with type IIa hyperlipidemia, statins induce a greater reduction in LDL cholesterol concentrations and better compliance.

A 5-year study demonstrated lovastatin to be comparable in safety to the other major cholesterol-lowering drugs (77). The safety profiles are similar for the other statins, with drug-related adverse events occurring in approximately 2% to 3% of patients. Side effects include increase in aminotransferase activity, myopathy, insomnia, myalgia, arthralgia, and gastrointestinal disturbances. No study has shown a significant increase in the development of lens opacities; therefore, routine ophthalmologic monitoring is not required. Periodic tests of liver function are now suggested before initiation of therapy, at weeks 6 and 12, and then semiannually. If the patient develops myalgia, the serum creatinine kinase level should be measured.

Bile Acid–Sequestering Resins. The bile acid–binding resins *cholestyramine* and *colestipol* are among the oldest agents used to treat hypercholesterolemia. They are useful for primary prevention therapy in young men and premenopausal women without other risk factors who have moderately increased LDL cholesterol levels. They enhance LDL catabolism and excretion and prevent intestinal absorption by diverting cholesterol and bile acids into the feces. They also increase levels of triglycerides and HDL, particularly HDL_2. At dosages of 20 to 24 g/day, a 20% to 30% reduction in LDL cholesterol may be achieved. Although the resins may be the safest of all of the hypolipidemic drugs, compliance with the older agents was a problem because taste and gastrointestinal side effects prevented many patients from taking a full dose. As many as 30% of clinical trial participants admit to taking less than half of the prescribed dosage of bile acid–binding resins (36). Gradual increase of dose, continuation of therapy, and concomitant symptomatic management of constipation may diminish side effects. The resins are better tolerated when used at lower dosages in combination with other lipid-lowering agents. They should not be overlooked as adjuvant therapy when other lipid-lowering agents fail to achieve the desired results. A newer bile acid resin is now available for prescription: Colesevelam (WelChol), is available in tablet form (625 mg, three tablets given twice a day with meals, or six tablets once a day with a meal) and is more palatable and has fewer drug interactions than the older bile acid resins. It can be given concurrently with statins and does not interfere with the absorption of vitamins A, D, E, or K (78). A 30-day supply costs approximately $141.00.

Nicotinic Acid (Niacin) *Nicotinic acid* (3 to 6 g/day) significantly lowers plasma levels of LDL and VLDL while raising the level of HDL cholesterol. It

Table 82.11. Commonly Used Lipid-Lowering Drugs[a]

HMG-CoA Reductase Inhibitors (Lovastatin, Pravastatin, Simvastatin, Fluvastatin, Atorvastin)

Efficacy: Decreases total cholesterol (20%–37%), LDL cholesterol (20%–48%), LDL apo B (20%–37%), VLDL cholesterol (27%–40%), and triglycerides (7%–27%). Provides variable and modest increases in HDL cholesterol (4%–12%) and apo A–I and A–II.

Pharmacokinetics: Incompletely absorbed (average 30%); extensive first-pass extraction by liver with less than 5% reaching systemic circulation; inactive lovastatin converted to several active metabolites; peak plasma concentrations of active metabolites within 2–6 hr; steady-state concentrations of total inhibitors achieved within 2–3 d; 83% of radiolabeled dose eliminated in feces (represents unabsorbed drug and active and inactive metabolites excreted in bile) and 10% in urine (as inactive metabolites).

Side effects: (a) Generally well tolerated, discontinuation required in 1%–2% of patients because of adverse effects; reasonable safety well established; (b) occasional: headache (9% of patients), gastrointestinal (flatulence, abdominal pains or cramps, diarrhea, constipation, nausea, dyspepsia—usually mild and transient [4%–6%]); elevation in liver aminotransferases, and, uncommonly, alkaline phosphatases usually within 3–16 mo ($\geq$3 times increase in 2%), reverses over several weeks after discontinuation of drug; mild increase in creatinine kinase (11%); myalgias (3%); rash and pruritis (5%); (c) uncommon: gastrointestinal (heartburn, dysgeusia), dizziness, insomnia, malaise, fatigue, myopathy (0.5%, but up to 30% in patients taking immunosuppressant drugs or gemfibrozil—also reported in patients taking nicotinic acid or erythromycin), renal failure from rhabdomyolysis.

Administration: Lovastatin (Mevacor, 20, 40 mg)—20–80 mg/d once daily with evening meal or twice daily with meals (administration with food results in 50% higher plasma concentrations of total inhibitors, effectiveness greater when given as evening dose, perhaps because cholesterol synthesis occurs mainly at night). Pravastatin (Pravachol, 10 and 20 mg)—10–40 mg once a day at bedtime. Simvastatin (Zocor, 5, 10, 20, and 40 mg)—5–40 mg once a day in the evening. Fluvastatin (Lescol, 20, 40 mg)—20–40 mg once a day at bedtime; 40 mg twice daily if no response; absorption not affected by food. Atorvastatin (Lipitor, 10, 20, 40 mg),—10 mg once a day; up to 80 mg once a day if no response. Obtain baseline liver function tests, then at 6, 12 weeks, and semiannually. Discontinue if aminotransferase rise more than 3 times normal.

Clinical use: First-line drugs, effective and well tolerated drugs for the treatment of hypercholesterolemia. When response to a single drug is inadequate, statins are effective in combination with a bile acid sequestering agent or nicotinic acid. Each drug contributes separately to reductions in lipoprotein concentrations.

Cost[b]: $41–112.00/mo.

Bile Acid–Sequestering Resins (Cholestyramine, Colestipol Colesevelan)

Efficacy: Decreases total and LDL cholesterol up to 25%–40% (onset 4–7 d, maximal effect within 1–3 wk. Mean reductions in total and LDL cholesterol of 13.4% and 20.3% (Lipid Research Clinics trial). Apo B level falls, while HDL level rises slightly. VLDL is unchanged or increased.

Pharmacokinetics: Not absorbed, but may bind other drugs (e.g., thiazides, digitalis preparations, anticoagulants, phenobarbital, thyroxine, phenylbutazone, propranolol, iron).

Side effects: (a) Common: unpleasant sandy/gritty preparations, gastrointestinal (e.g., constipation in 10%–20%, nausea, heartburn, abdominal discomfort, flatutence) often resolve with continued therapy or treatment of constipation), lowered serum folate levels; (b) uncommon: gastrointestinal (steatorrhea), hyperchloremic acidosis (small patients on high dosages), fat-soluble vitamin deficiency; increased alkaline phosphatase and amino transferase (usually transient) activity.

Administration: Cholestyramine—12–32 g/d given two to four times daily before or during meals; supplied as Questran 9-g packets each containing 4 g of active drug. Colestipol—15–30 g/d given two to four times daily before or during meals; supplied as Colestid in 5-g packets or 500-g bottles. Colesevelom—3 [wel Chol, 625 mg] tablets, twice a day with meals or 6 tablets once a day with a meal. Preparations should be taken with water or juice to prevent esophageal irritation or blockage. Other medicines should be taken 1 hr before or 4 hr after dosage. Monitor serum folate levels and consider supplemental multivitamins with folic acid.

Clinical use: Drugs of first choice in the treatment of hypercholesterolemia, because of their relative safety and efficacy. Well tolerated in combination with niacin or lovastatin. Contraindications include marked hypertriglyceridemia and severe constipation. Poor compliance limits use.

Cost[b]: Cholestyramine (generic) $22.00/mo; Colestipol, $50.00/mo; Colesevelan, $141.00/mo.

Nicotinic Acid (Niacin, and Preparations such as Nicobid (Time-released)

Efficacy: Decreases VLDL triglycerides within 1–4 d (mean 26% in Coronary Drug Project, range, up to 80% depending on pretreatment levels); decreases LDL cholesterol, onset 5–7 d, maximal effect 3–5 wk (mean decrease of 10% in total cholesterol in Coronary Drug Project, range up to 30%). Favorable impact on total and LDL cholesterol, triglyceride, VLDL, HDL (increases up to 35%), apos A–I and B.

Pharmacokinetics: Absorbed by mouth; peak concentrations in 20–70 min; at the high dosages used it is partially metabolized in liver and partially excreted unchanged in urine; plasma half-life is about 45 min.

Side effects: (a) Common: cutaneous flushing and pruritus, which diminish after several weeks of therapy; gastrointestinal (nausea, diarrhea, abdominal pain, abnormal liver function); (b) less common: dermatologic disorders (e.g., increased pigmentation); activation of peptic ulcer; anhythmia; gout; urinary frequency and dysuria; glucose intolerance. Sustained-release forms are associated with irreversible chronic liver disease and fulminant hepatic failure.

Administration: (50-, 100-, 250-, 300-, 400-, and 500-mg tablets). Gradual increase over 1–3 wk from 100–200 mg/d to 2–9 g/d; given in two to three times daily; give with meals to diminish side effects. Flushing may be ameliorated by pretreatment with aspirin, one-half to one 325-mg tablet 30 min before each dose. Extended-release forms may pose an increased risk of hepatic toxicity.

Clinical use: First-line (despite side effects) effective drug in the treatment of elevated LDL cholesterol or VLDL triglyceride or low HDL. Well tolerated in combination with bile acid binding resins and statins. Contraindications include peptic ulcer disease, arrhythmia, liver disease, diabetes mellitus, hyperuricemia, and gout.

Cost[b]: Generic $13.00/mo; time-release, $49.00/mo.

Fibric Acid Derivatives (Gemfibrozil, Fenofibrate)

Efficacy: Lowers triglycerides and raises HDL but may raise LDL. In familial combined hyperlipoproteinemia, use of any fibric acid analog is likely to raise LDL cholesterol.

Pharmacokinetics: Gemfibrozil and fenofibrate: completely absorbed; peak concentration within 2hr: half-life 1.5 hr; undergoes enterohepatic circulation; metabolized in liver and excreted in urine. May enhance action of oral anticoagulants, phenytoin, and hypoglycemic agents, and of furosemide by displacing them from albumin-binding sites.

Table 82.11. —*continued.* Commonly Used Lipid-Lowering Drugs[a]

Side effects: (a) Usually well tolerated; (b) occasional: (sixfold) increase in the incidence of cholelithiasis (may be less with gemfibrozil and newer analogs); other gastrointestinal (nausea, abdominal pain, diarrhea, weight gain); reduced libido, impotence; unusual flulike syndrome; (c) uncommon: rash, alopecia, breast tenderness, reversible abnormality in liver function, hepatomegaly, myositis, increased plasma glucose, etc; (d) unknown: (?)thromboembolism, (?)intermittent claudication, (?)arrhythmia, (?)neoplasia.
Administration: Gemfibrozil (Lopid, 600 mg)—600 mg twice daily (30 min before meals). Fenofibrate—300 mg/d in three divided doses taken with meals. Dosage reduction required in renal failure patients. Some recommend periodic monitoring of aminotransferase activity and creatinine kinase.
Clinical use: Gemfibrozil is the drug of choice in the treatment of elevated VLDL triglyceride; it can also be used to lower total and LDL cholesterol and to raise HDL cholesterol, of particular utility in type III. Fenobrate is more effective in lowering LDL. Use with caution in the presence of hepatic or renal insufficiency.
Cost[b]: $85.00/mo.

Probucol
Efficacy: Lowers LDL (8%–15%) and HDL (20%–25%). No effect on triglycerides.
Pharmacokinetics: Limited, variable absorption; steady state not reached for 3–4 mo and levels fall slowly over several months when treatment is stopped. Excreted in the bile.
Side effects: (a) common (10%): diarrhea, abdominal pain, nausea, dizziness; (b) cardiac: increases the Q-T interval moderately and should not be given to patients with a long Q-T, patients with arrhythmias, or patients who are taking other drugs that might prolong the Q-T (e.g., tricyclics, some antiarrhythmics—see Chapter 64).
Administration: (250, 500 mg tablets): 500 mg twice a day with meals.
Clinical use: Second-line drug in treatment of hypercholesterolemia.
Cost[b]: $30/mo.

apo, apoprotein; HDL, high-density lipoprotein; HGM-CoA, hydroxymethylglutaryl coenzyme A; LDL, low-density lipoprotein; VLDL, very-low-density lipoprotein.
[a]Mechanisms of action are described in the text.
[b]Costs are approximate, wholesale as of November, 2001.

is therefore the drug of first choice for patients with concomitant elevations in LDL cholesterol and triglycerides. It is the first lipid-lowering drug shown to lower levels of Lp(a) (26), and it is also one of the most potent agents in elevating HDL cholesterol levels. There is evidence in secondary prevention trials that nicotinic acid may reduce total mortality. Its use is often limited, however, by unpleasant side effects and the frequent presence of coexisting contraindications. Therapy should be discontinued if gout, hyperglycemia, or hepatotoxicity develops. By starting at a very low dosage of 100 to 200 mg/day and gradually increasing the dosage of the drug and adding aspirin, increased tolerance often develops to the common side effects of cutaneous flushing, rashes, hives, and pruritus. Sustained-release forms of nicotinic acid were initially thought to produce fewer side effects than immediate-release forms. However, because of reports of irreversible chronic liver disease and fulminant hepatic failure with sustained-release nicotinic acid, immediate-release forms are strongly preferred (79,80).

Fibrates *Gemfibrozil* is the most commonly used drug in this class in the United States. *Clofibrate*, rarely used since the World Health Organization Cooperative Trial reported significantly increased all-cause mortality in patients taking the drug (81), and *fenofibrate* are also available in the United States, whereas bezafibrate and ciprofibrate are available in Europe. Although gemfibrozil is approved for the treatment of hypertriglyceridemia, data from the Helsinki Heart and VA-HIT studies (37,42) reveal it to be effective in raising HDL cholesterol and reducing morbidity and mortality from CAD. In general, gemfibrozil is not considered as useful for secondary prevention as other drugs such as the statins, because it does not achieve maximal reductions in LDL cholesterol. Diabetic patients with elevated triglycerides and patients with type III hyperlipoproteinemia are excellent candidates for treatment with this drug. The VA-HIT study showed that gemfibrozil is associated with significant risk reductions for stroke, nonfatal MI, and CAD death in patients with known CAD and low HDL cholesterol levels (42). However, in patients with primary hypertriglyceridemia gemfibrozil may increase LDL cholesterol levels, whereas in patients with elevations of both cholesterol and triglycerides this drug can cause either an increase or a decrease in LDL cholesterol levels. The newer fibrates may lower LDL cholesterol more effectively than gemfibrozil does (82). A significant side effect of gemfibrozil is its tendency to increase bile lithogenicity.

Probucol. Probucol remains a second-line drug for the treatment of hypercholesterolemia. It appears to lower LDL cholesterol levels by a receptor-independent mechanism and by an increase in LDL catabolism. In addition, it inhibits the oxidative metabolism and tissue deposition of LDL. Probucol use leads to a reduction in total and LDL cholesterol levels of 8% to 15% and a concomitant reduction of HDL cholesterol levels by as much as 25%. The significance of the consequent reduction in the LDL/HDL ratio remains uncertain. To date, there are no reported studies of its efficacy in reducing CAD risk or of its long-term safety. The electrocardiogram (ECG) should be monitored in patients taking probucol, because the drug can cause prolongation of the Q-T interval (at which point the drug should be discontinued). Because it lowers HDL cholesterol levels, probucol is rarely used in clinical practice.

Combination Drug Therapy. If the response to one of the first-line drugs proves to be inadequate, combined therapy with two drugs should be considered. In general, one should choose drugs with complementary or synergistic mechanisms of action and should consult with a specialist in lipid disorders. The use of a bile acid sequestrant in combination with either nicotinic acid or a statin can lower levels of LDL cholesterol by 45% to 60% in patients with hypercholesterolemia and normal triglyceride levels (83). These regimens have been well tolerated, with synergistic effects on LDL cholesterol without an additive effect on drug-related toxicity. Probucol or gemfibrozil may also be used in combination with a bile acid–sequestering resin, although these regimens are less effective. The combination of a statin and gemfibrozil causes an increased risk of myopathy, and rhabdomyolysis has been reported with the combination of lovastatin and nicotinic acid (84).

Two placebo-controlled studies of intensive lipid-lowering therapy using combined colestipol and niacin therapy or combined lovastatin and niacin treatment for men with documented CAD showed reduced frequency of progression of coronary lesions, increased frequency of regression, and reduced incidence of cardiovascular events in the active drug groups, without cases of rhabdomyolysis (85,86). Patients with homozygous familial hypercholesterolemia may respond less well to treatment with drugs and diet than do patients with heterozygous monogenic, polygenic, or nonhereditary hypercholesterolemia.

Obviously, it is prudent to carefully monitor patients treated with combination therapy. This requires frequent follow-up visits and advising patients to call the office should they experience excessive muscle aches or weakness.

Other Hypocholesterolemic Drugs. The use of *estrogen replacement therapy* (ERT) in postmenopausal women has a number of effects on cholesterol metabolism (see Chapter 103 and 106). Treatment with oral estrogens usually lowers levels of LDL cholesterol and raises those of HDL cholesterol, but the dosages required for these effects probably exceed those for physiologic replacement therapy. In contrast, administration of transdermal estrogens usually results in lower LDL cholesterol levels but unaltered levels of HDL cholesterol. Both oral and transdermal ERT have been shown to significantly lower Lp(a) levels (31% and 16%, respectively) in postmenopausal women. Concomitant use of the progestin medroxyprogesterone acetate (Provera) with either form of ERT appears not to influence either form of ERT adversely. The primary side effect of unopposed estrogen is the increased risk of endometrial cancer, a risk that is greatly attenuated by cotreatment with progestogens (see Chapter 106).

Phytoestrogens, plant-derived estrogens, are substances that have attracted the attention of the American population. These plant derivatives are comprised mainly of three classes: isoflavones, coumestans, and lignans (87). In most studies, phytoestrogens have been reported to exert a favorable effect in improving lipid profiles (87).

The results from the Heart and Estrogen/progestin (HERS) trial have dampened, somewhat, the enthusiasm for hormone replacement therapy in the treatment of women with known CAD. The participants were postmenopausal women younger than 80 years of age with known CAD and an intact uterus. Study participants were treated with either an estrogen/progestin preparation or placebo for an average follow-up of 4.1 years (88). The results showed no statistically significant difference between the occurrences of nonfatal MI and congestive heart disease death between the two groups. There was an increase in thromboembolic and gallbladder disease among study participants taking the hormone supplements. The authors of this study did not recommend initiating hormone treatment in postmenopausal women with known CAD but did think it was appropriate for those women who were already receiving treatment to continue the therapy.

Hypertriglyceridemia

Drugs that decrease hepatic production of VLDL and apo B, enhance VLDL clearance by stimulating LPL activity, or both are generally effective in treating hypertriglyceridemia. Fibrates and nicotinic acid do both.

Although *nicotinic acid* may be most efficacious, its use is limited by its side effects and the presence of coexisting contraindications. The fibric acid derivatives *gemfibrozil and fenofibrate* are therefore the drugs most commonly used. Although gemfibrozil is generally well tolerated, an acute myositis, which is occasionally associated with renal failure, may occur, particularly in patients with impaired renal clearance or hypoalbuminemia. Either the drug should not be used or the dosage should be reduced by 70% to 90% in azotemic patients. Periodic monitoring of muscle enzymes (creatine kinase, aldolase) is required to avoid toxicity. If the level of LDL cholesterol rises in a patient taking gemfibrozil, the diagnosis of familial combined hyperlipoproteinemia should be considered.

For compliant patients who remain hypertriglyceridemic with diet and a single drug, combined therapy with a fibric acid drug and nicotinic acid may be useful. Rarely, after consultation with a specialist in lipid disorders, the progestational agent norethindrone acetate or the androgenic anabolic steroid oxandrolone—in women or men, respectively—may be required to treat persistent hypertriglyceridemia plus chylomicronemia.

Dysbetalipoproteinemia

The decreased remnant catabolism characteristic of this clinically uncommon disorder can be corrected or improved by drug therapy. *Gemfibrozil* appears to normalize lipid levels and to enhance remnant clearance in patients with dysbetalipoproteinemia. It is the drug of choice in this disorder. *Ethinyl estradiol* has a similar and even more dramatic effect, but at dosages that greatly exceed those used for postmenopausal replacement therapy. Hence, its use requires careful monitoring for possible adverse estrogenic effects that would necessitate discontinuation of the drug. *Nicotinic acid* is the drug of second choice.

SURGERY AND OTHER THERAPIES

More experimental forms of therapy (e.g., ileal bypass, portacaval shunt, plasma exchange, extracorporeal hemoperfusion, liver transplantation) exist for the severely hypercholesterolemic patient who is resistant or only partially responsive to treatment with diet, exercise, and lipid-lowering drugs. Patients with drug-resistant nephrotic syndrome from focal segmental glomerulosclerosis have shown improvement in renal function and proteinuria when treated with LDL apheresis combined with pravastatin (89). These therapies should be implemented only in consultation with a specialist in lipid disorders.

Obtaining Consultation

Indications for referral to a specialist in lipoprotein disorders have been discussed. The Lipid Metabolism Branch of the National Heart, Lung and Blood Institute (National Institutes of Health, Bethesda, MD 20205) can provide the names of research centers in each geographic area where sophisticated evaluation of lipoprotein abnormalities, consultation services, and experimental forms of therapy are offered.

Additional information for the management of hyperlipoproteinemia and other risk factors for CAD is available from both regional and national offices of the AHA. This agency can provide information about diet, drugs, and exercise in the treatment of hyperlipidemia, hypertension, cigarette smoking, and obesity. Another important resource is the AHA website, available at http://www.americanheart.org (accessed February 4, 2002).

General References*

National Heart, Lung, and Blood Institute of the National Institutes of Health website. Available at: http://www.nhlbi.nih.gov/. Accessed February 4, 2002.

The NCEP report is available at this website, as well as an interactive tool and 10-year risk calculator that can be downloaded to a Palm Pilot to help in applying the guidelines in practice. The website also has useful information for patients.

Pignone MP, Phillips CJ, Atkins D, et al. **Screening and treating adults for lipid disorders.** Am J Prev Med 2001;20:77.

Excellent evidence-based review and recommendations by the U.S. Preventive Services Task Force.

U.S. Preventive Services Task Force. **Screening adults for lipid disorders: recommendations and rationale.** Am J Prev Med 2001;20:73.

Executive Summary of the Third Report of the National Cholesterol Education Program (NCEP) Expert Panel on Detection, Evaluation, and Treatment of High Blood Cholesterol in Adults (Adult Treatment Panel III). JAMA 2001;285:2486.

Updated recommendations, generally accepted, for the detection and management of patients with high levels of total and LDL cholesterol and/or with low levels of HDL cholesterol.

*Bold print (general references) and bold numerals (specific references) denote published controlled clinical trials, meta-analyses, or consensus-based recommendations.

Specific References

1. Brown MS, Goldstein JL. How LDL receptors influence cholesterol and atherosclerosis. Sci Am 1984;251:58.
2. Brunzell JD, Sniderman AD, Albers JJ, et al. Apoproteins B and A-1 and coronary artery disease in humans. Arteriosclerosis 1984;4:79.
3. Lavie CJ. Lipid and lipoprotein fractions and coronary artery disease. Mayo Clin Proc 1993;68:618.
4. Lindgren FT, Jensen LC, Hatch FT. The isolation and quantitative analysis of serum lipoproteins. In: Nelson GJ, ed. Blood lipids and lipoproteins: quantitation, composition, and metabolism. New York: John Wiley & Sons, 1972:181.
5. Maciejko JJ, Holmes DR, Kottke BA, et al. Apolipoprotein A-I as a marker of angiographically assessed coronary artery disease. N Engl J Med 1983;309:385.
6. Nilsson-Ehle P. Regulation of lipoprotein lipase: triacylglycerol transport in plasma. In: Carlson LA, Pernow B, eds. Metabolic risk factors in ischemic cardiovascular disease. New York: Raven Press, 1982:49.
7. Havel RJ, ed. Symposium on lipid disorders. Med Clin North Am 1982;66:319.
8. Oram JF, Brenton EA, Bierman EL. Regulation of high density lipoprotein activity in cultured human skin fibroblasts and human arterial smooth muscle cells. J Clin Invest 1983;72:1611.
9. Acton S, Rigotti A, Landschultz KT, et al. Identification of scavenger receptor SR-BI as a high density lipoprotein receptor. Science 1996;271:518.
10. Landschultz KT, Pathak RK, Rigotti A, et al. Regulation of scavenger receptor, class B, type I, a high density lipoprotein receptor, in liver and steroidogenic tissues of the rat. J Clin Invest 1996;98:984.
11. Steinberg D. Antioxidant vitamins and coronary heart disease. N Engl J Med 1993;328:1487.
12. Mahley RW, Angelin B. Type III hyperlipoproteinemia: recent insights into the genetic defect of familial dysbetalipoproteinemia. Adv Intern Med 1984;29:385.
13. Kannel WB, Schatzkin A. Risk factor analysis. Prog Cardiovasc Dis 1983;26:309.
14. LaRosa J. Dyslipidemia and coronary artery disease in the elderly. Clin Geriatric Med 1996;12:33.
15. Krumholz HM, Seeman TE, Merrill SS, et al. Lack of association between cholesterol and coronary heart disease mortality and morbidity and all-cause mortality in persons older than 70 years. JAMA 1994;272:1335.
16. Corti M-C, Guralnik JM, Salive ME, et al. Clarifying the direct relation between total cholesterol levels and death from coronary heart disease in older persons. Ann Intern Med 1997;126:753.
17. Sorkin JD, Andres R, Muller DC, et al. Cholesterol as a risk factor for coronary heart disease in elderly men. Ann Epidemiol 1992;2:59.
18. Zimetbaum P, Frishman WH, Ooi WI, et al. Plasma lipids and lipoproteins and the incidence of cardiovascular disease in the very elderly: The Bronx Aging Study. Arterioscler Throm 1992;12:416.
19. Criqui MH, Heiss G, Cohn R, et al. Plasma triglyceride level and mortality from coronary heart disease. N Engl J Med 1993;328:1220.
20. Castelli WP. The triglyceride issue: a view from Framingham. Am Heart J 1986;112:432.
21. Hokansan JE, Austin MA. Plasma triglyceride level is a risk factor for cardiovascular disease independent of high-density lipoprotein cholesterol level: a meta-analysis of population-based prospective studies. J Cardiovasc Risk 1996;3:213.
22. Ginsberg HN. Hypertriglyceridemia: new insights and new approaches to pharmacologic therapy. Am J Cardiol 2001;87:1174.
23. Walden CE, Knopp RH, Wahl PW, et al. Sex differences in the effect of diabetes mellitus and lipoprotein triglyceride and cholesterol concentrations. N Engl J Med 1984;331:953.
24. Goldberg AP. Lipid abnormalities in hemodialysis: prevalence, implications and treatment. Perspect Lipid Disord 1984;2:17.
25. Heiss G, Johnson NJ, Reiland S, et al. The epidemiology of plasma HDL cholesterol levels. The Lipid Research

Clinics Prevalence Study. Summary. Circulation 1980;62 [Suppl4]:116.
26. Carlson LA, Hamsten A, Asplund A. Pronounced lowering of serum levels of Lp(a) in hyperlipidemic subjects treated with nicotinic acid. J Intern Med 1989;226:271.
27. Austin MA, Breslow JL, Hennekens CH, et al. Low-density lipoprotein subclass patterns and risk of myocardial infarction. JAMA 1988;260:1917.
28. Rader DJ, Brewer HB Jr. Lipoprotein (a): clinical approach to a unique atherogenic lipoprotein. JAMA 1992;267:1109.
29. Wade DP. Lipoprotein (a). Curr Opin Lipidol 1993;4:244.
30. Rimm EB, Stampfer MJ, Ascherio A, et al. Vitamin E consumption and the risk of coronary disease in men. N Engl J Med 1993;328:1450.
31. Stampfer MJ, Hennekens CH, Manson JE, et al. Vitamin E consumption and the risk of coronary disease in women. N Engl J Med 1993;328:1444.
32. Dietary supplementation with n-3 polyunsaturated fatty acids and vitamin E after myocardial infarction: results of the GISSI-Prevenzione trial. Gruppo Italiano per lo Studio della Sopravvivenza nell'Infarto miocardico. Lancet 1999;354:447.
33. Collaborative Group of the Primary Prevention Project. Low-dose aspirin and vitamin E in people at cardiovascular risk: a randomized trial in general practice. Lancet 2001;357:89.
34. Levy RI. Consideration of cholesterol and nonvascular mortality. Am Heart J 1982;104:324.
35. Cooper R, Cutler J, Desvigne-Nickens P, et al. Trends and disparities in coronary heart disease, stroke, and other cardiovascular diseases in the United States: findings of the national conference on cardiovascular disease prevention. Circulation 2000;102:3137.
36. Lipid Research Clinics Program. The Lipid Research Clinics Coronary Primary Prevention Trial results: II. The relationship of reduction in incidence of coronary heart disease to cholesterol lowering. JAMA 1984;251:365.
37. Frick MH, Elo O, Haapa K, et al. Helsinki Heart Study: primary prevention trial with gemfibrozil in middle-aged men with dyslipidemia. N Engl J Med 1987;317:1237.
38. Shepherd J, Cobbe SM, Ford I, et al. Prevention of coronary heart disease with pravastatin in men with hypercholesterolemia. West of Scotland Coronary Prevention Study Group. N Engl J Med 1995;333:1301.
39. Downs JR, Clearfield M, Weis S, et al. Primary prevention of acute coronary events with lovastatin in men and women with average cholesterol levels: results of AFCAPS/TexCAPS. Air Force/Texas Coronary Atherosilerosis Prevention Studies. JAMA 1998;279:1615.
40. Brensike JF, Levy RI, Kelsey SF, et al. Effects of therapy with cholestyramine on progression of coronary arteriosclerosis: results of the NHLBI type II coronary intervention study. Circulation 1984;69:313.
41. Scandinavian Simvastatin Survival Study Group. Randomised trial of cholesterol lowering in 4444 patients with coronary heart disease: The Scandinavian Simvastatin Survival Study (4S). Lancet 1994;344:1383.
42. Robins SJ, Collins D, Wittes JT, et al. Relation of gemfibrozil treatment and lipid levels with major coronary events: VA-HIT: a randomized controlled trial. JAMA 2001;285:1585.
43. The Expert Panel. Report of the National Cholesterol Education Program Expert Panel on Detection, Evaluation and Treatment of High Blood Cholesterol in Adults. Arch Intern Med 1988;148:36.
44. The Expert Panel. Executive Summary of the Third Report of the National Cholesterol Education Program (NCEP) Expert Panel on Detection, Evaluation, and Treatment of High Blood Cholesterol in Adults (Adult Treatment Panel III). JAMA 2001;285:2486.
45. Dufaux B, Assmann G, Hollman W. Plasma lipoproteins and physical activity: a review. Int J Sports Med 1982;3:123.
46. Fuiano G, Esposito C, Sepe V, et al. Effects of hypercholesterolemia on renal hemodynamics: study in patients with nephrotic syndrome. Nephron 1996;73:430.
47. Bergman R. The pathogenesis and clinical significance of xanthelasma palpebrarum. J Am Acad Dermatol 1994;30:236.
48. Hulley SB, Newman TB, Grady D, et al. Should we be measuring blood cholesterol levels in young adults? JAMA 1993;269:1416.
49. Leaf A. Management of hypercholesterolemia: are preventive interventions advisable? N Engl J Med 1989;321:680.
50. Pignone MP, Phillips CJ, Atkins D, et al. Screening and treating adults for lipid disorders. Am J Prev Med 2001;20:77.
51. American College of Physicians. Guidelines for using serum cholesterol, high-density lipoprotein cholesterol, and triglyceride levels as screening tests for preventing coronary heart disease in adults. Ann Intern Med 1996;124:515.
52. Cleeman JI, Grundy SM. National Cholesterol Education Program recommendations for cholesterol testing in young adults. Circulation 1997;95:1646.
53. Cleeman JI. Adults aged 20 and older should have their cholesterol measured. Am J Med 1997;102:31.
54. Hegsted DM, Nicolosi RJ. Individual variation in serum cholesterol levels. Proc Natl Acad Sci USA 1987;84:6259.
55. Gore JM, Goldberg RJ, Matsumoto AS, et al. Validity of serum total cholesterol level obtained within 24 hours of acute myocardial infarction. Am J Cardiol 19984;54:722.
55a. Ramsay LE, Yeo WW, Jackson PR. Dietary reduction of serum cholesterol concentration. BMJ 1991;303:1551.
56. Daviglus ML, Stamler J, Orencia AJ, et al. Fish consumption and the 30 year risk of fatal myocardial infarction. N Engl J Med 1997;336:1046.
57. Oomen CM, Feskens EJ, Rasanen L, et al. Fish consumption and coronary heart disease mortality in Finland, Italy, and The Netherlands. Am J Epidemiol 2000;151:999.
58. Von Schacky C, Angerer P, Kothny W, et al. The effect of dietary omega-3 fatty acids on coronary atherosclerosis: a randomized, double-blind, placebo-controlled trial. Ann Intern Med 1999;130:554.
59. Friedberg CE, Janssen MJ, Heine RJ, et al. Fish oil and glycemic control in diabetes: a meta-analysis. Diabetes Care 1998;21: 494.
60. Ederer F, Leren P, Turpeinin O, et al. Cancer among men on cholesterol-lowering diets. Lancet 1971;2:203.
61. Stevinson C, Pittler MH, Ernst E. Garlic for treating hypercholesterolemia: a meta-analysis of randomized clinical trials. Ann Intern Med 2000;133:420.
62. Lichtenstein AH, Deckelbaum RJ. Stanol/sterol ester-containing foods and blood cholesterol levels: a statement for healthcare professionals from the Nutrition Committee of the council on Nutrition, Physical Activity, and Metabolism of the American Heart Association. Circulation 2001;103:1177.
63. Anderson JW, Johnstone BM, Cook-Newell ME. Meta-analysis of the effects of soy protein intake on serum lipids. N Engl J Med 1995;333:276.
64. Erdman JW Jr. Soy protein and cardiovascular disease: a statement for healthcare professionals from the nutrition committee of the AHA. Circulation 2000;102:2555.
65. Hunninghake DB, Stein EA, Dujovne CA, et al. The efficacy of intensive dietary therapy alone or combined with lovastatin in outpatients with hypercholesteremia. N Engl J Med 1993;328: 1213.
66. Dattilo AM, Kris-Etherton PM. Effects of weight reduction on blood lipids and lipoproteins: a meta-analysis. Am J Clin Nutr 1991;56:320.
67. Watts GF, Lewis B, Brunt JHN, et al. Effects on coronary artery disease of lipid-lowering diet or diet plus cholestyramine in the St. Thomas Atherosclerosis Regression Study. Lancet 1992;339:563.
68. Hurley BF. Effects of resistive training on lipoprotein-lipid profiles: a comparison to aerobic exercise training. Med Sci Sports Exerc 1989;21:689.
69. Hurley BF, Hagberg JM, Goldberg AP, et al. Resistive training can reduce coronary risk factors without altering VO_2 max or percent body fat. Med Sci Sports Exerc 1988;20:150.
70. Goldberg AP. Aerobic and resistive exercise modify risk factors for coronary heart disease. Med Sci Sports Exerc 1989;21:669.
71. Goldberg LE, Elliot DL, Shutz RW, et al. Changes in lipid and lipoprotein levels after weight training. JAMA 1984;252:504.
72. Tran ZV Weltman A. Differential effects of exercise on serum

lipid and lipoprotein levels seen with changes in body weight: a meta-analysis. JAMA 1985;254:919.
73. Hagberg JM. Exercise, fitness, and hypertension. In: Bouchard C, Shepard RJ, Stephens T, et al, eds. Exercise, fitness and health. Champaign, IL: Human Kinetics, 1990:455.
74. Paffenberger RS, Hyde RT, Wing AL, et al. A natural history of athleticism and cardiovascular health. JAMA 1984;252:491.
75. Grundy S. HMG-CoA reductase inhibitors for treatment of hypercholesterolemia. N Engl J Med 1988;319:24.
76. The Lovastatin Study Group II. Therapeutic response to lovastatin in nonfamilial hypercholesterolemia: a multicenter trial. JAMA 1986;256:2829.
77. Lovastatin Study Group I–IV. Lovastatin 5-year safety and efficacy study. Arch Intern Med 1993;153:1079.
78. Colesevelam (WelChol) for hypercholesterolemia. Med Lett 2000;42:102.
79. Etchason JA, Miller TD, Squires RW, et al. Niacin-induced hepatitis: a potential side effect with low-dose time-release niacin. Mayo Clin Proc 1991;66:23.
80. McKenney JM, Proctor JD, Harris S, et al. A comparison of the efficacy and toxic effects of sustained vs immediate release niacin in hypercholesterolemic patients. JAMA 1994;271:672.
81. World Health Organization Clofibrate Trial. WHO cooperative trial on primary prevention of ischaemic heart disease using clofibrate to lower serum cholesterol: mortality follow-up. Lancet 1980;2:379.
82. Schonfeld G. The effects of fibrates on lipoprotein and hemostatic coronary risk factors. Atheroclerosis 1994;11:161.
83. Illingsworth DR. Mevinolin plus colestipol in therapy for severe heterozygous familial hypercholesterolemia. Ann Intern Med 1984;101:598.
84. Reaven P, Witztum JL. Lovastatin, nicotinic acid and rhabdomyolysis. Ann Intern Med 1988;109:597.
85. Blankenhorn DH, Nessim SA, Johnson RL, et al. Beneficial effects of combined colestipol-niacin therapy on coronary atherosclerosis and coronary venous bypass grafts. JAMA 1987;257:3233.
86. Brown G, Albers JJ, Fisher LD, et al. Regression of coronary artery disease as a result of intensive lipid-lowering therapy in men with high level of apo lipoprotein B. N Engl J Med 1990;323:1289.
87. Murkies AL, Wilcox G, Davis SR. Phytoestrogens. J Clin Endocrinol Metab 1998;83:297.
88. Hulley S, Grady D, Bush T, et al. Randomized trial of estrogen plus progestin for secondary prevention of coronary heart disease in postmenopausal women. JAMA 1998;280:605.
89. Hattori M, Ito K, Kawaguchi H, et al. Treatment with a combination of low-density lipoprotein apheresis and pravastatin of a patient with drug resistant nephrotic syndrome due to focal segmental glomerulosclerosis. Pediatr Nephrol 1993;7:196.

CHAPTER 83

Obesity

ROSS E. ANDERSEN, PhD
MARC R. BLACKMAN, MD

Although attempts at weight reduction are common in the United States, the prevalence of obesity has increased at an alarming rate since the 1980s (1,2). In 1991, 12.0% of Americans were classified as obese. The *prevalence* increased to 18.9% by 1999, a 57.5% increase during that 8-year period. The increase was similar in men and women (Fig. 83.1). Moreover, increases were seen across age groups, races, and social classes. (The greatest increase in the prevalence of obesity occurred among Hispanic Americans, who experienced an 82.7% rise.) In 1999, 17.7% of Caucasian American adults, 27.3% of African Americans, and 21.5% of Hispanic Americans were classified as obese (Fig. 83.2).

In response to these alarming developments, the third Public Health Service (PHS) 10-year plan, *Healthy People 2010*, established a goal of reducing the prevalence of obesity—specifically, to reduce to 15% the proportion of U.S. adults with a body mass index (BMI) of 30 kg/m^2 or higher (2a). Another objective was to increase to at least 75% the proportion of primary care providers who provide or request weight reduction services for patients with diagnoses of cardiovascular disease or diabetes mellitus.

More than 12.4% of U.S. boys and 10.9% of U.S. girls are now obese (3). Of even greater concern is the fact

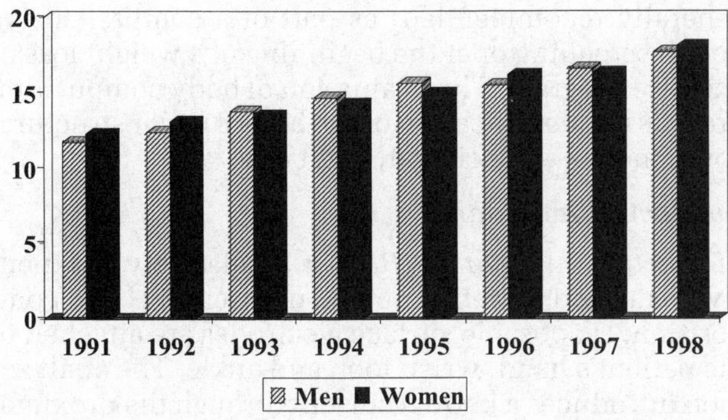

Figure 83.1. The spread of the obesity epidemic in the United States, 1991–1998. (Compiled from Mokdad AH, Serdula MK, Dietz WH, et al. The spread of the obesity epidemic in the United States, 1991–1998. JAMA 1999;282:1519.)

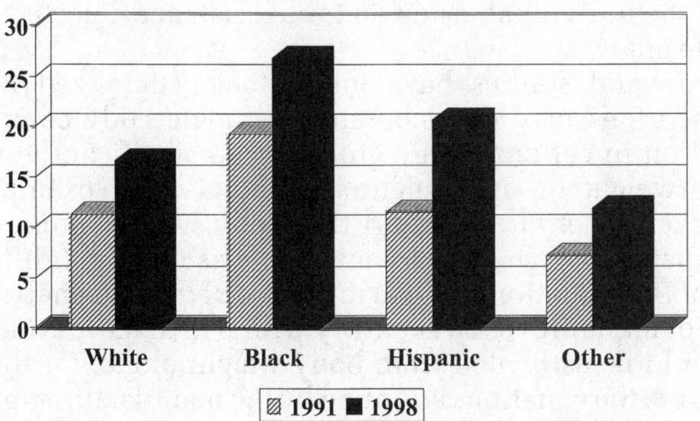

Figure 83.2. Race-specific changes in obesity prevalence in the United States, 1991–1998. (Compiled from Mokdad AH, Serdula MK, Dietz WH, et al. The spread of the obesity epidemic in the United States, 1991–1998. JAMA 1999;282:1519.)

that the prevalence of obesity in children in the United States has more than doubled in less than one generation and that 15% of non-Hispanic black children and 16.3% of Mexican American children are obese. These data mirror recent reports from Canada, Europe, and China (4).

Obesity is a major cause of mortality in the United States and throughout the world. It has been estimated that each year more than 300,000 Americans die from causes related to obesity. Overall, the direct costs of obesity account for approximately 9.4% of the annual health care budget in the United States (5).

MEASUREMENT

Obesity must be distinguished from overweight, which refers to an increase in body weight due to increased bone, muscle, or fat. Although the two terms are often used synonymously, errors do occur in equating obesity with overweight, as for example in the muscular athlete with normal or decreased body fat. Because body composition and, in particular, body fat normally vary with age, sex, diet, physical activity, and population group, it is important to compare measurements of body fat in individual patients with those derived from appropriate control groups.

Body Mass Index

The hallmark of obesity is an excess of body fat. An accurate assessment of body fat requires expensive equipment that is often not practical or necessary for clinicians to use. Body weight adjusted for stature is commonly used as a marker of adiposity in population studies and in clinical settings to evaluate the level of obesity. One such index is the *body mass index (BMI)*, calculated by dividing the subject's weight in kilograms by the square of the height in meters. Calculating BMI offers clinicians a simple, rapid, and inexpensive method to classify a patient's adiposity (Fig. 83.3). Population studies have consistently found that a BMI of 25 or higher is associated with an increased risk of cardiovascular and all-cause mortality. This increased risk appears to be modest until the BMI reaches 30 kg/m^2. The World Health Organization and the National Heart, Lung and Blood Institute (NHLBI)

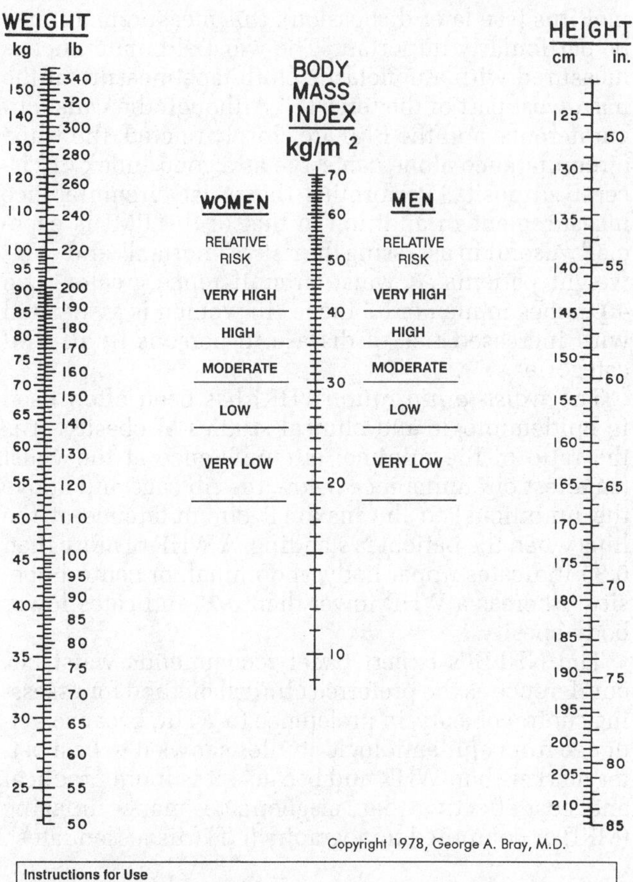

Figure 83.3. Nomogram for body mass index. (Copyright George A. Bray, 1978.)

Table 83.1. Classification of Underweight, Overweight, and Obesity by Body Mass Index

Classification	BMI (kg/m^2)	Obesity Class	Disease Risk[a]
Underweight	<18.5		Increased
Healthy weight	18.5–24.9		—
Overweight	25–29.9		Increased
Obesity	30–34.9	I	High
	35–39.9	II	Very High
Extreme morbid obesity	≥40	III	Extremely High

[a]Risk for type II diabetes and cardiovascular disease.

From National Institutes of Health, National Heart, Lung and Blood Institute. Obesity Education Initiative: Clinical Guidelines on the Identification, Evaluation, and Treatment of Overweight and Obesity in Adults. Rockville, MD: U.S. Department of Health and Human Services, 1998.

have created a classification of overweight and obesity based on BMI (Table 83.1) (6).

Waist Circumference and Waist-to-Hip Ratio

The *waist circumference* is a simple, low-cost anthropometric assessment that clinicians may use to inexpensively assess central adiposity. Because abdominal fat is associated with an increased risk for atherosclerotic heart disease, hypertension, and type 2 diabetes mellitus (see later discussion), this measurement may be particularly important. The waist circumference is measured with a nonelastic cloth tape measure at the narrowest part of the torso (7). Although the waist circumference and the BMI are closely related, the waist circumference alone can serve as a good index of visceral adiposity. Performing the waist circumference measurement in addition to that of the BMI is especially useful in assessing the risk of "normal" and overweight patients. A waist circumference greater than 40 inches in men or 35 inches in women is associated with increased risk of disease in persons in all BMI categories.

The *waist-to-hip ratio* (WHR) has been often used in epidemiologic and clinical studies of obesity. It is the ratio of the minimal circumference at the waist (smallest circumference below the rib cage and above the umbilicus) to the maximal circumference at the hips when the patient is standing. A WHR of more than 0.85 indicates upper body, abdominal, or central obesity, whereas a WHR lower than 0.75 indicates lower body obesity.

The NHLBI's expert panel recommends waist circumference as the preferred clinical method for assessing central obesity, in preference to WHR, because evidence from epidemiologic studies shows it to be a better marker than WHR and because it is more practical and cost-effective than magnetic resonance imaging (MRI) or computed tomography (CT) (discussed later).

Direct Measurement of Body Composition

Body composition assessments are performed primarily for research purposes and in special clinical settings, for example with athletes who are seeking to optimize their performance. An accurate assessment of body composition is sometimes included (but not generally recommended) as part of a comprehensive health screening or at the beginning of a weight loss or exercise program. The evaluation of body composition provides a quantification of the body's major structural components—muscle, fat, and bone.

Bioelectric Impedance

Bioelectric impedance (BIA) is a relatively inexpensive, safe, and portable method of assessing body composition. Disposable surface electrodes are attached to the patient's hand, wrist, foot, and ankle. The analyzer then introduces a known current through the proximal electrodes, which is detected by the distal electrodes and offers a measure of tissue resistance. Fat-free tissue is known to be a good conductor of electrical current, whereas adipose tissue is a poor conductor. The resultant measures derive from the significant relationships between both the fat-free tissue and total body water of the individual tested and the resistance detected by the analyzer.

Several studies have found that generalized BIA equations may not accurately estimate body composition in certain ethnic groups or in significantly underweight or overweight individuals. For example, Eckerson et al. (8) found that body weight alone estimated fat-free mass as accurately as did eight different BIA equations in lean men. Use of the BIA analyzer did not improve the accuracy with which fat-free mass could be estimated from body weight alone. Furthermore, the equations supplied by the manufacturer tend to *underestimate* body fat percentage in overweight women (7,9). When using BIA to assess overweight individuals, it is important to use fat- and gender-specific equations, which have been shown to significantly improve estimates of body composition in this group (10).

Near-Infrared Interactance

Near infrared interactance (NIR) applies the principal of light absorption and reflection to estimate body composition. This technique was developed with the use of very sophisticated and expensive computerized equipment in research and hospital settings. More recently, less expensive NIR equipment has been developed [e.g., Futrex (Futrex, Inc., Gaithersburg, MD)] for use in weight loss centers and other medical settings. Low-cost NIR instruments gather light-interactance information via an optic probe that is typically placed over the belly of the biceps muscle. The NIR data, height, weight, activity level, and frame size are entered into a prediction equation to estimate body composition.

There are significant problems with the single-site, less expensive NIR equipment. First, it does not predict body composition accurately. Second, the technique uses a generalized prediction equation that does not provide accurate predictions for significantly underweight or overweight individuals.

Research and Laboratory Methods

Field estimates of body composition simply divide the body into two components: fat and fat-free mass. Researchers and health care professionals are becoming increasingly interested in further compartmentalizing the body. For example, it is common for obesity researchers to examine the changes in fat, fat-free tissue, bone mass, and total body water that accompany weight loss. Two of the most commonly used methods that estimate body composition more precisely are *hydrodensitometry* and *dual-energy x-ray absorptiometry (DEXA)*.

Hydrodensitometry (Underwater Weighing). Hydrodensitometry is one of the oldest techniques for estimating body composition and for years was used as the "gold standard" against which new methods or equations to predict body composition were compared. This procedure allows the division of the body into two compartments: fat and fat-free mass. Underwater body weight is used in conjunction with weight measured on a conventional scale to estimate body density. Typically, individuals are immersed in a water-filled, heated tank into which a chair is suspended from a scale. While completely submerged, subjects completely exhale all of the air in the lungs and attempt to remain as still as possible while underwater. Most research laboratories also measure residual lung volume either during or before underwater weighing. A diver's belt is often secured to the chair or around the overweight person's waist to ensure that the individual does not involuntarily float to the surface during the procedure. Calculations of body density erroneously assume a constant density for fat-free mass, thus confounding the accurate measurement of body fat.

Dual-energy X-ray Absorptiometry. DEXA has become a popular method for quickly assessing body composition. The estimates offered by this method are very accurate, and the technique is much less cumbersome than hydrodensitometry. DEXA scans are especially useful in older people, in whom underwater weighing leads to an overestimate of total fat. The technique uses a very low x-ray dose to separate the body into three levels: fat, fat-free tissue, and bone mineral. Regional measurements of fat (e.g., arms, legs, trunk) are also possible with DEXA. Morbidly obese patients (i.e., those weighing more than 300 pounds) may exceed the size of the scan field of typical scanners, limiting the accuracy of this technique. DEXA systems are costly ($70,000 to $100,000), and in some states, a licensed X-ray technician is required to operate DEXA equipment.

Computed Tomography and Magnetic Resonance Imaging. Fat– and fat-free–regional tissue mass also can be quantified very accurately by the use of CT or MRI. Furthermore, these procedures are useful in distinguishing between visceral and subcutaneous fat in the abdominal region. Both of the procedures are costly and time consuming. In addition, CT scans involve exposure to radiation.

ETIOLOGY

The dramatic increases in the prevalence of obesity in both children and adults reflects a population shift toward a positive energy balance. Excessive body fat is a multifactorial trait that evolves from a complex interaction of molecular, cellular, physiologic, metabolic, behavioral, and social domains. Clearly, we become a fatter society when overall calories consumed exceed calories expended. Dietary intake and energy expenditure represent the two modifiable factors of this equation. It is apparent that there is an abundance of high-calorie, high-fat foods readily available throughout the world. However, the consumption of high-energy food alone does not completely explain the exponential increases in the prevalence of overweight persons detected in recent years.

Genetic Factors

With recent advances in molecular biology, both scientists and clinicians are excited by the possibility of identifying genes that are associated with the predisposition to obesity. It has long been known that BMI values are more similar among family members than among unrelated persons. Furthermore, obese children frequently have obese parents. Molecular biologists are currently searching for genes that are associated with satiety, nutrient preferences, fat distribution, metabolism, insulin sensitivity, and several other factors that may be associated with obesity. Most investigators now believe that the genetic influence on obesity is likely to be explained by a clustering of several genetic variants and not by a single major gene (11).

Some people are more prone to weight gain, and losing weight represents a lifelong battle; others are relatively protected from obesity. Bouchard et al. studied 12 pairs of identical twins who were fed a caloric surplus of 1,000 cal/day for 100 days. He detected three times more variance in response between twin pairs than within pairs for gains in fat and weight (12). Therefore, it is important for physicians to acknowledge that obesity cannot be explained by overeating alone. Patients who have a genetic tendency toward obesity should understand that it important to attempt to prevent weight gain.

Endocrine Factors

In both experimental animals and humans, certain primary endocrine disorders are important causes of obesity. These include hyperinsulinism, hypercortisolism, and deficiencies of growth hormone, thyroid hormone, or sex steroids. In each of these endocrinopathies, the excess fat accumulation is primarily distributed in the upper body and may contribute to enhanced cardiovascular risk. Moreover, the possible contribution to these syndromes of pathophysiologic alterations in an adipocyte-derived protein that inhibits appetite and increases energy expenditure, or its receptor in the hypothalamus, remains to be clarified.

The *metabolic syndrome* (obesity, hypertension, and insulin resistance) is the most common presentation of type 2 diabetes in the Western world (see discussion later in this chapter and in Chapter 79). *Hyperinsulinemia* also can result from appropriate or surreptitious use of exogenous insulin or from insulin hypersecretion by benign or malignant pancreatic neoplasms.

Hypercortisolism most often is iatrogenic, resulting from excess administration of exogenous glucocorticoids. Much less commonly, true Cushing disease or syndrome, or pseudo-Cushing syndrome caused by depression, is responsible (Chapter 81).

Because *growth hormone* exerts an influence on conversion of fat stores into energy for body growth and protein deposition, its absence, owing to pituitary dysfunction or removal, leads to increased adiposity that is reversible by administration of the hormone. Current research suggests that the normal age-related decline in growth hormone contributes to increased central adiposity in older people and that administration of growth hormone prevents or reduces this fat accumulation (13).

Although *thyroid hormones* directly modulate the overall basal metabolic rate (BMR), hypothyroidism *per se* is most often associated with modest or no weight gain. Morbid obesity (defined later) caused solely by hypothyroidism has not been documented, whereas moderate weight loss because of anorexia disproportionate to the decrease in BMR is occasionally seen.

The *polycystic ovary (Stein–Leventhal) syndromes*, a fairly common group of disorders in young women, are characterized by mild obesity, hirsutism, oligomenorrhea, and infertility in association with insulin resistance, glucose intolerance, and mild hypothalamic–pituitary–ovarian (and possibly adrenal) dysfunction. The obesity and the menstrual abnormalities are often ameliorated after ovarian wedge resection. The androgen excess may also be ameliorated with the use of various oral antidiabetic medications.

Hypothalamic obesity is a rare disorder associated most often with the presence of a craniopharyngioma or, less often, with other neoplastic or inflammatory diseases near the hypothalamic ventromedial nuclei, sites in the brain that appear to be involved in the control of normal feeding and satiety.

In addition to insulin and glucocorticoids, *other pharmacologic agents* induce increases in food intake and in body fat. The most commonly used of these agents are phenothiazines, tricyclic antidepressants, oral contraceptives, anticonvulsives (e.g., valproic acid), and the antihistamine cyproheptadine (Periactin). Weight gain associated with the latter drug probably results from its antiserotoninergic properties.

Most *chronic cigarette smokers* weigh less than age- and sex-matched nonsmokers but gain weight after they stop smoking. The weight gain often leads to resumption of smoking with its attendant risks for development of cardiovascular disease, emphysema, or cancer. Although the mechanisms responsible for weight loss during active cigarette smoking remain unknown, there is a strong positive correlation between the activity of the enzyme, adipose tissue lipoprotein lipase, in the fasting state and the amount of weight regained during the first 2 to 3 weeks after smoking cessation (14). Cigarette smoking also is associated with an increase in waist circumference, despite its tendency to decrease body weight and BMI (15).

Environmental Factors

In view of the obvious imbalance between energy input and expenditure in obese people, it is not surprising to find numerous clinical studies that document the relationship between poor nutritional habits, sedentary living, and the development of obesity. The adverse effects of an absolute or relative excess in total caloric intake, of a maldistribution of foodstuffs (especially too much fat or simple sugars), and of the general increase in sedentary lifestyles are particularly important.

Nutrition

One of the first things that people from foreign countries notice when they come to the United States is the large portions that are served in our restaurants. Supersized meals and portions have become the norm. We now have an unprecedented access to high-caloric foods that are widely available, low in cost, heavily promoted, and good tasting. Fast food restaurants are now appearing in service stations, schools, hospitals, and airports, and they may partially explain the increasing girth of Americans.

Socioeconomic Factors

Socioeconomic factors exert strong influences on the development and persistence of obesity in individuals as well as in population groups. In the United States, obesity is more common among children and adults from the lower socioeconomic groups, among African American and Hispanic women compared with white women, and among first-generation Americans compared with their descendants. Women born later in the 20th century are less heavy than women born in the early 1900s; the opposite trend appears true for men. The reason is unclear but may be related to the steadily increasing fashion consciousness and emphasis on exercise among American women.

Physical Inactivity

The prevalence of obesity reportedly doubled in England in a single decade (16); this trend was mirrored by the increase in the number of cars and television sets per household. In the United States, a strong relationship has been noted between television watching and fatness (17). Fully 26% of American children watch 4 or more hours of television each day, and the rate is much higher among Mexican American and African American children (30% and 43%, respectively) (17). Children who watch the most television are significantly fatter than those who watch less television. Moreover, boys and girls who are high television watchers and not regularly active are more obese than children who are low television watchers and highly active (17) (the influence of snacking on these outcomes was not measured).

Longitudinal and cross-sectional studies have consistently reported that physical activity is inversely related to weight. Lee et al. (18) examined the health benefits of leanness and the hazards of obesity while simultaneously considering cardiorespiratory fitness. They monitored 21,925 men, age 30 to 83 years. All participants had a baseline body-composition assessment and a peak treadmill exercise test. During an 8-year follow-up period, there were 428 deaths (144 from cardiovascular disease, 143 from cancer, and 141 from other causes). After adjusting for confounding variables, unfit lean men had twice the risk of all-cause mortality, compared with fit lean men (relative risk, 2.07; 95% confidence interval, 1.16 to 3.69; $p = .01$). Unfit lean men also had a higher risk of all-cause and cardiovascular disease mortality than did men who were fit and obese. The investigators concluded that the health benefits of leanness may be limited to fit men and that being fit may significantly reduce the hazards of obesity (18).

Simply increasing levels of exercise without restricting calories is a relatively ineffective way to lose weight. However, when combined with a healthy diet, increased physical activity may result in optimal changes in body composition by contributing to a negative energy balance and preserving lean body mass. Furthermore, most practitioners recognize that an active lifestyle plays an important role in long-term weight management. Although exercise is not consistently associated with weight loss in the short term, it is commonly cited as the strongest predictor of long-term success in weight management. Kayman et al. (19) reported that most women (90%) who lost weight and kept it off reported exercising on a regular basis. In contrast, only 34% of women who regained their lost weight reported participating in regular physical activity. A study of weight regain patterns in a group of women who had lost weight in a 16-week treatment program showed that, during the year after treatment, the most active third of patients actually lost an additional small amount of weight (20). The middle third reported meeting the current Surgeon General's recommendations for only 52% of the year after treatment, yet they maintained their full end-of-treatment weight loss. The least active third steadily gained weight through out the year after their treatment ended. These findings suggest that all patients should strive to incorporate regular physical activity into their lives daily but should realize that even irregular activity is much better than nothing at all.

Psychological Factors

Obese individuals carry an enormous psychological burden, because they must contend with discrimination and prejudice. In contemporary affluent societies, obesity is most often associated with behavioral and psychological determinants that affect both the circumstances and the substance of food intake. Although numerous studies have sought to identify the obese persona, it appears that no such diagnostic personality profile exists. Nonetheless, a major distinction between youth- and adult-onset obesity may reside in the distorted perception of body image that is commonly associated with obesity in childhood and adolescence. In the latter group, those affected often believe that their body habitus and weight are normal, a phenomenon rarely encountered in adult-onset obesity.

Binge-eating disorder is a psychological disorder that is occurring with increased frequency. People with this disorder report feeling out of control at times when they are eating. They may eat inordinate amounts of food, such as an entire bag of cookies or a full container of ice cream. Patients may report feelings of extreme guilt after bingeing. The disorder is relatively uncommon in the general obese population. However, it may afflict as many as 30% of patients who seek treatment for their weight. Obese binge eaters are more likely to stop their weight loss efforts early, to regain lost weight, and to respond poorly to generic weight management programs. Mental health professionals who specialize in the treatment of eating disorders are best equipped to help these patients.

Metabolic Concomitants

Although the exact roles of all organic and environmental factors in the pathogenesis of obesity remain to be elucidated, certain metabolic concomitants of excess adiposity, particularly upper body obesity, have been characterized. Numerous studies document the close association between obesity and diabetes mellitus and suggest that obesity *per se* is diabetogenic. Obesity leads to increased pancreatic insulin production and *hyperinsulinemia*, both basally and after stimulation by ingestion of glucose, amino acids, and so on. Evidence exists that the hyperinsulinemia and concurrent glucose intolerance are caused by *insulin resistance* at the tissue level (e.g., liver, adipose tissue, skeletal muscle), which results from a decrease in the number of cell surface receptors for insulin and/or from aberrant, insulin-dependent intracellular glucose metabolism (see Chapter 79). Finally, it has been proposed that chronic hyperinsulinemia leads to a further decrease in the number of cell surface insulin receptors (i.e., downregulation), the latter serving as an adipocyte response to prevent episodes of hypoglycemia.

There is also a significant association between obesity and the presence of *hyperlipidemia*, especially hypertriglyceridemia. This latter relationship probably results, at least in some patients, from the hyperinsulinemia-induced increase in hepatic triglyceride synthesis and formation of triglyceride-rich very-low-density lipoproteins (VLDL). Increased endogenous cholesterol synthesis is also more common in obese patients; it leads to increased circulating concentrations of total cholesterol and low-density lipoprotein (LDL) cholesterol and decreased concentrations of high-density lipoprotein (HDL and HDL_2) cholesterol and results in increased risk of coronary artery disease and, probably, cholesterol gallstones.

Many patients with adult-onset upper body obesity appear cushingoid. Simple obesity is associated with an *increased rate of cortisol production* that leads to increased hepatic steroid metabolism and increased urinary excretion of certain steroid conjugates. Such patients typically have increased urinary 17-hydroxycorticoids; however, results of plasma cortisol, urinary free cortisol, and overnight dexamethasone suppression tests usually are normal.

Salt and water retention is a common problem in obese patients, and it is in part mediated by increases in aldosterone secretion induced by dietary carbohydrate and, to a lesser extent, protein intake.

Onset of normal menarche does not occur until a critical body weight is reached (usually 40 to 45 kg), a finding that explains the earlier menarche in women with youth-onset obesity. *Menstrual abnormalities* such as dysfunctional uterine bleeding, amenorrhea, and infertility are also more common in obese women and are often associated with aberrant cyclical reproductive hormone function (subnormal levels of follicle-stimulating hormone in the follicular phase and of progesterone on the luteal phase).

Other important endocrine or metabolic sequelae of obesity include increased androgenicity, especially in women; augmented sympathoadrenal activity; decreased spontaneous and stimulated (e.g., by growth hormone–releasing hormone) growth hormone release; and hyperuricemia. In women with the polycystic ovary syndrome, hyperinsulinemia and insulin resistance contribute to obesity-related glucose intolerance and dyslipidemia and probably to the sympathoadrenal excess and hyperandrogenism. In patients with growth hormone deficiency, decreased availability of this lipolytic hormone permits excess accumulation of total body and intra-abdominal fat. The increased prevalence of hyperuricemia in obese individuals is responsible for their increased prevalence of gout.

RISKS

A large body of research and anecdotal data suggest that obesity and overweight are graded phenomena and that there is a strong positive correlation between the degree of excess adiposity and increased morbidity and mortality (24), the latter particularly from cardiovascular and cerebrovascular diseases. It now appears that this hypothesis must be somewhat modified.

Critical analysis of data derived from retrospective life insurance studies suggested that there was no significant increase in mortality until body weight rose to values greater than 30% above ideal body weight. Data from a large number of prospective studies also suggested that severe to extreme, but not mild to moderate, obesity is associated with decreased longevity. More recent reanalyses of data from various large-scale epidemiologic studies led several investigators to conclude that the "mortality-for-weight curves" are often J or U shaped, in that the highest mortality rates occur at both extremes of relative weight, and the lowest rates at intermediate weights (21). Andres demonstrated that the BMI associated with lowest mortality itself increases with advancing age, in both men and women, and therefore emphasized the need for age-specific weight–height tables (22). In this regard, Table 83.2 illustrates comparative weight-for-height data derived from the 1983 Metropolitan Height and Weight Tables (uncorrected for age) and from the Baltimore Longitudinal Study of Aging, conducted at the Gerontology Research Center of the National

Table 83.2. Comparison of the Weight-for-Height Tables[a] from Actuarial Data (*Build Study*, 1979): Non–Age-Corrected Metropolitan Life Insurance Company and Age-Specific Gerontology Research Center Recommendations

Height		Metropolitan 1983 Weights (lb)		Gerontology Research Center				
		Men	Women	Age-Specific Weight Range for Men and Women (lb)				
Feet	Inches	25–59 yr		25 yr	35 yr	45 yr	55 yr	65 yr
4	10		100–131	84–111	92–119	99–127	107–135	115–142
4	11		101–134	87–115	95–123	103–131	111–139	119–147
5	0		103–137	90–119	98–127	106–135	114–143	123–152
5	1	123–145	105–140	93–123	101–131	110–140	118–148	127–157
5	2	125–148	108–144	96–127	105–136	113–144	122–153	131–163
5	3	127–151	111–148	99–131	108–140	117–149	126–158	135–168
5	4	129–155	114–152	102–135	112–145	121–154	130–163	140–173
5	5	131–159	117–156	106–140	115–149	125–159	134–168	144–179
5	6	133–163	120–160	109–144	119–154	129–164	138–174	148–184
5	7	135–167	123–164	112–148	122–159	133–169	143–179	153–190
5	8	137–171	126–167	116–153	126–163	137–174	147–184	158–196
5	9	139–175	129–170	119–157	130–168	141–179	151–190	162–201
5	10	141–179	132–173	122–162	134–173	145–184	156–195	167–207
5	11	144–183	135–176	126–167	137–178	149–190	160–201	172–213
6	0	147–187		129–171	141–183	153–195	165–207	177–219
6	1	150–192		133–176	145–188	157–200	169–213	182–225
6	2	153–197		137–181	149–194	162–206	174–219	187–232
6	3	157–202		141–186	153–199	166–212	179–225	192–238
6	4			144–191	157–205	171–218	184–231	197–244

[a]Values in this table are for height without shoes and weight without clothes.

From Andres R. Mortality and obesity: the rationale for age-specific height-weight tables. In: Andres R, Hazzard WR, Bierman E, eds. Principles of geriatric medicine. New York: McGraw-Hill, 1985.

Table 83.3. Possible Medical Consequences of Obesity

Endocrine–Metabolic
Hyperglycemia, hyperinsulinemia, insulin resistance
Hypertriglyceridemia, hypercholesterolemia (↑ VLDL, ↑ LDL, ↓ HDL)
↑ Cortisol production but normal plasma cortisol, diurnal rhythm, urine free cortisol, and overnight dexamethasone suppression
Early menarche, menstrual abnormalities, hirsutism
↓ Sympathoadrenal activity
↓ SHBG and ↑ total or free androgens
↓ Growth hormone, basally and after provocative stimuli
Hyperuricemia, gout

Cardiovascular
Hypertension
Coronary artery disease
Congestive heart failure
Varicose veins
Cerebrovascular disease

Pulmonary
Hypoventilation (e.g., pickwickian) syndromes
Sleep apnea syndrome
Chronic respiratory infections

Gallbladder
Cholelithiasis (cholesterol gallstones)

Musculoskeletal
Osteoarthritis
Chronic orthopedic problems
↓ Ambulation

Renal
Nephrotic syndrome (normal or nonspecific biopsy)

Oncologic
Endometrial, breast carcinoma (postmenopausal women), prostate, colon

Dermatologic
Acanthosis nigricans
Chronic skin infections

Psychosocial
Depression, loss of self-esteem
↓ Employability

Pregnancy
Worsen underlying hypertension, diabetes mellitus
↑ Maternal mortality

Surgery (especially under general anesthesia)
Increased perioperative morbidity and mortality

HDL, high-density lipoprotein; LDL, low-density lipoprotein; SHBG, sex hormone–binding globulin; VLDL, very-low-density lipoprotein.

Institute on Aging. These data reveal that, for most of the heights reported, the Metropolitan optimal weights for men and women are similar to those for the age-adjusted weights of individuals in their thirties and forties. Therefore the Metropolitan tables overestimate the norms for younger adults but underestimate the corresponding norms for elderly people. In the age-adjusted data from the Gerontology Research Center, there is an increased weight allowance of about 10 lb per decade.

The risks of obesity, as noted previously, vary not only with the amount but with the topographic distribution of excess body fat. For example, studies from the Gerontology Research Center using various anthropometric ratios (including the WHR) have demonstrated an age-related increase in upper and central body adiposity. The ratios are independently influenced by BMI and are higher in men than in women despite a postmenopausal acceleration in the trend in women (23). Current evidence favors the view that hyperinsulinemia is the common pathogenetic mechanism by which upper body obesity influences known cardiac risk factors, such as hyperlipidemia, diabetes mellitus (25,26), and hypertension, although the significance of the hyperinsulinemia–hypertension link has been questioned (27).

The major physiologic and medical concomitants of moderate to extreme obesity are displayed in Table 83.3. A direct pathophysiologic link between obesity and each of these conditions has yet to be unequivocally established. In each instance, the morbidity associated with the condition is proportional to the degree of excess adiposity and may be partially or totally reversed with weight reduction. In addition, obesity, particularly when severe, often exacerbates or complicates the course of a variety of other conditions; for example, by delaying surgical procedures, enhancing perioperative risks, prolonging convalescence from many illnesses, and worsening pregnancy-associated problems.

EVALUATION

The history usually indicates whether the patient has youth- or adult-onset obesity, and it often provides important information regarding usual or unusual dietary practices as well as patterns of physical activity. It is particularly important to identify any medical or psychological factors that may motivate the patient to lose weight or that militate for or against certain treatment plans. The evaluation of the obese patient is outlined in Table 83.4.

Clinicians who work with obese individuals should have an accurate scale that is capable of measuring patients whose weight exceeds the limits of a typical balance beam scale. The physical examination should include measurements of the height and weight (and calculation of the BMI) and measurement of the waist circumference.

Resting blood pressure should also be assessed, because hypertension is common among obese persons. To ensure accurate measurements, it is important to use a cuff that is appropriate in size. Persons with

Table 83.4. Evaluation of the Obese Patient

Measure height and weight: calculate BMI[a]
Measure waist circumference (abnormal, >40 inches in men, >35 inches, in women)
Assess for causes of or contributors to obesity (see text)
Assess for comorbidities/complications (e.g., diabetes, hypertension, cardiovascular disease, hyperlipidemia)
Assess patient's desire to lose weight and willingness to make lifestyle changes

[a]Body mass index (BMI) = weight in kilograms divided by the square of the height in meters.

large-diameter arms should be assessed with a larger cuff designed for obese patients.

Although secondary obesity is rare, its importance lies in its reversibility after identification and specific therapy for the underlying medical or pharmacologic disorder. Special emphasis should therefore be placed on screening an obese patient for any contributing endocrine–metabolic process and on obtaining a history of medication use (see earlier discussion).

Evidence of glucose intolerance should be sought by obtaining fasting blood glucose levels. Hypercortisolemia should be suspected in any plethoric, hypertensive patient with upper body obesity, hypokalemia, and glucose intolerance. A normal overnight dexamethasone suppression test (1 mg of oral dexamethasone given at 11 p.m., followed by an 8 a.m. plasma cortisol value lower than 5 μg/dL) or a normal value for 24-hour urinary free cortisol excretion (less than 100 μg/24 hours) ordinarily eliminates the diagnosis of endogenous hypercortisolemia with a reasonable degree of certainty (see Chapter 81). Clinically significant hypothyroidism can usually be ruled out when the free thyroxine (T_4) index (i.e., serum $T_4 \times$ resin triiodothyronine [T_3] uptake) and the level of thyroid-stimulating hormone (TSH) are normal. The finding of menstrual irregularities, mild hirsutism (but not virilization), and central obesity in a young woman prompts suspicion of the polycystic ovary syndrome, a diagnosis made more likely by the additional findings of a mildly elevated serum testosterone level (60 to 100 ng/dL), flat basal body temperature curve (i.e., no ovulation), and palpable abnormalities on pelvic examination. Diseases of the hypothalamic–pituitary region should be considered in obese patients with otherwise unexplained neuroendocrine abnormalities. Certain rare syndromes, such as the Prader–Willi syndrome (obesity, short stature, hypogonadism, extreme appetite, and mental retardation), are typically recognized in childhood by their characteristic clinical presentations.

Fasting blood samples should be sent for determinations of triglyceride, total cholesterol, HDL cholesterol, and uric acid levels. Most patients with hyperlipidemia have acquired (secondary), not genetic (primary), hyperlipidemias and will respond to appropriate diet regimens (see Chapter 82). In patients with clinically apparent or suspected hypoventilation syndromes or sleep-disordered breathing, pulmonary function and polysomnographic profiles should be tested (Chapter 7).

A number of metabolic changes occur in obese persons that predispose them to gallstone formation. The motility of the gallbladder tends to decrease as body weight increases, which leads to less efficient emptying of the sac. This can lead to cholesterol stones, which also result in gallbladder inflammation.

In addition, patients should be asked about their mood and psychological well-being, because depression is more common among obese patients. Mental health professionals suggest that it is important to treat the depression before attempting to help patients reduce their weight.

One evaluation (28) of 234 obese women and 27 obese men led to detection of the following significant abnormalities: hypertension (16%), hypertriglyceridemia (25%), glucose intolerance (25%), hypercholesterolemia (11%), and hyperuricemia (7%). In 2 of 57 patients studied, T_4 values were abnormal: One was high and one low. Finally, the clinician should remember that physical examinations often are stressful experiences for obese persons, who may be ashamed of their bodies and worried that their healthcare provider will cast judgment on them.

MANAGEMENT

General Approach

There is a plethora of treatment options available to patients in today's weight-preoccupied society. With so many books, magazines, television shows, and Internet sites devoted to weight loss, it is often difficult for patients and clinicians to know where to begin.

Health professionals often tend to dismiss and criticize approaches that are offered outside the medical setting, particularly by profit-driven enterprises. In many cases, clinicians identify a single treatment method for all patients. For example, some clinicians believe that all overweight patients should use liquid meal replacements to assist them in their weight loss attempts. The recent *NHLBI obesity guidelines* (6) proposed a model that classified patients according to level of obesity, leading to a stepped-care decision based on potentially appropriate methods of treatment (Table 83.5). Final treatment selection

Table 83.5. Guidelines for the Treatment of Obesity[a]

Treatment	BMI Category				
	25–26.9	27–29.9	30–34.9	35–39.9	≥40
Diet, physical activity, and behavior therapy	With comorbidities	With comorbidities	+	+	+
Pharmacotherapy		With comorbidities	+	+	+
Surgery				With comorbidities	+

BMI, body mass index; +, use of indicated treatment regardless of comorbidities.

[a]Prevention of weight gain with lifestyle therapy is indicated in any patient with a BMI ≥ 25 kg/m² even without comorbidities, whereas weight loss is recommended for those with a BMI of 25–29.9 kg/m² or a high waist circumference only if they have two or more comorbidities. Combined therapy with a low-calorie diet, increased physical activity, and behavior therapy provide the most successful therapy for weight loss and weight maintenance. Consider pharmacotherapy only if a patient has not lost 1 lb/wk after 6 mo of combined lifestyle therapy.

Adapted from National Institutes of Health, National Health, Lung and Blood Institute. Clinical Guidelines on the Identification, Evaluation, and Treatment of Overweight and Obesity in Adults. Rockville, MD: U.S. Department of Health and Human Services, 1998.

should be based on a combination of client preferences, degree of obesity, comorbidities, and level of treatment.

It is common for clinicians to set lofty weight loss goals with patients based on height and weight tables. In many cases when such unrealistic goals are set, patients are left feeling a sense of failure when the "goal weight" is not met. Patients should be reminded that significant health improvements can be seen with even modest weight losses and that the major focus of most programs should be on maintenance of weight loss rather than achievement of an unrealistic "dream weight."

For most overweight people, attempts at weight management are assaults to their self-esteem. The majority of overweight people have lost and regained weight several times in full view of their coworkers, friends, and family members. Most feel a tremendous sense of shame and failure when they regain lost weight. Many studies have reported that obese patients feel that they are not treated respectfully by their health care professionals. Patients often report that their health care providers seem to feel that they are "weak willed" and "lazy."

Traditionally, the principal goal of obesity treatment has been to reduce body fat in order to manage medical problems such as hypertension, hypercholesteremia, or diabetes. Although these goals are important, clinicians should also try to reduce the emotional distress of obesity.

It is important to remember that overweight people are not all the same and that there are many reasons why people become overweight. Caregivers who involve their patients in the decisions about their weight loss goals are more likely to foster autonomy. Patients should feel that they are in a supportive relationship with their caregiver and that it is safe for them to discuss disappointment and frustration, particularly during periods of relapse.

Management of Mild to Moderate Obesity

Behavioral Change

No matter what approach to losing weight patients choose to follow, it is important to focus on changing behaviors that result in a negative energy balance. The goals should be to move from a traditional "weight loss" program to a "weight management" program. Typically this is done through a combination of increasing energy expenditure through sensible physical activity and reducing energy intake at the same time. Since the late 1960s, behavioral treatment programs have become increasingly intensive by focusing on changing eating habits, improving the quality of food consumed, increasing activity levels, managing hunger levels, and generally living a more healthy lifestyle. Treatment principles have been published in very "user-friendly" manuals such as the LEARN Program for Weight Control (29). Currently, it is believed that relapse prevention strategies should be a core part of any weight loss program with strong focus on the maintenance of weight loss.

Diet

Modification of food intake should play a key role in any weight management program. Clearly, a goal in any weight reduction program is to reduce energy intake in order to create an energy deficit. Dietary programs that suggest "quick and easy" results without effort or caloric restriction tend to be ineffective in the long run. In general, patients should be encouraged to reduce energy intake and, as much as possible, to eat a variety of foods. The food industry is selling supersize portions, and most people need to be taught to reduce the amount of food that they eat at each sitting. Many patients can benefit from meeting with a registered dietician, who can teach them proper meal planning, what constitutes a single serving of food, and who can work with them to tailor an approach that respects cultural preferences.

The Federal Government's Food Guide Pyramid can help patients meet dietary recommendations (see Fig. 15.1 and Table 15.1 in Chapter 15). People who want to reduce energy intake should be encouraged to avoid alcohol and to reduce the consumption of fatty foods as well as foods that are high in simple sugars. Smaller portions of lean meats and greater amounts of fresh fruits and vegetables should be encouraged. The Institute of Medicine suggests that energy intakes of less than 1,200 kcal/day may not meet nutrient requirements and could also result in the excessive loss of lean tissue (30).

General nutritional guidelines for reducing the risk of diet-related chronic disorders, including obesity, have been published by the National Research Council (Table 83.6). For most adults, a balanced diet containing 1,500 to 1,800 cal/day is necessary for maintenance of optimal body weight under conditions of basal activity. Therefore, modest caloric restriction to a diet containing 1,000 to 1,200 cal/day for women and 1,200 to 1,500 cal/day for men is appropriate, with small increases proportionate to increases in levels of physical activity. It is often useful to advise patients who are motivated to diet to purchase one of the readily available, inexpensive calorie counters and to use the information to limit their daily diet to a specific number of calories. In general, daily modest exercise programs should be tailored to the individual patient's ability and enjoyment. Regular physical conditioning facilitates weight loss and decreases or abolishes obesity-associated hyperinsulinemia, insulin resistance, glucose intolerance, hypertriglyceridemia, hyperuricemia, and systolic and diastolic hypertension; it also improves cardiovascular, respiratory, and musculoskeletal problems. A goal of a loss of 1 or 2 pounds (0.5 to 1 kg) per week is appropriate whenever a patient embarks on a weight reduction program.

Improved nutritional understanding often results from effective and practical dietary and behavioral counseling. As part of behavior modification, it is usually helpful to ask participants about their previous

Table 83.6. Recommended Dietary Guidelines

1. Reduce total fat intake to 30% or less of calories, saturated fatty acid intake to less than 10% of calories, and cholesterol intake to less than 300 mg/d. The intake of fat and cholesterol can be reduced by substituting fish, poultry without skin, lean meats, and low- or nonfat dairy products for fatty meats and whole-milk dairy products; by choosing more vegetables, fruits, cereals, and legumes; and by limiting oils, fats, egg yolks, and fried or other fatty foods.
2. Every day eat five or more servings of a combination of vegetables and fruits, especially green and yellow vegetables and citrus fruits. Also, include starches and other complex carbohydrates by eating six or more daily servings of a combination of breads, cereals, and legumes. An average serving is equal to one-half cup for most fresh or cooked vegetables, fruits, dry or cooked cereals or legumes; one medium piece of fresh fruit; one slice of bread; or one roll or muffin.
3. Maintain protein intake at moderate levels (<1.6 g/kg body weight for adults).
4. Balance food intake and physical activity to maintain appropriate body weight.
5. The committee does not recommend alcohol consumption. For those who drink alcoholic beverages, the committee recommends limiting consumption to the equivalent of <1 oz pure alcohol in a single day. This is the equivalent of two cans of beer, two small glasses of wine, or two average cocktails. Pregnant women should avoid alcoholic beverages.
6. Limit total daily intake of salt to 6 g or less. Limit the use of salt in cooking and avoid adding it to food at the table. Salty, highly processed salty, salt-preserved, and salt-pickled foods should be consumed sparingly.
7. Maintain adequate calcium balance (>1,000 mg/day; >1,500 mg/day in postmenopausal women).
8. Avoid taking dietary supplements in excess of the recommended daily allowance (RDA) in any one day.
9. Maintain an optimal intake of fluoride, particularly during the years of primary and secondary tooth formation and growth.

Adapted from Committee on Diet and Health, Food and Nutrition Board, Commission on Life Sciences, National Research Council. Diet and Health. Implications for reducing chronic disease risk. Washington, DC: National Academy Press, 1989.

efforts to lose weight and why they failed. Diet sheets and booklets that set forth recommendations that are easy to understand and follow, particularly when attuned to the sociocultural and economic characteristics of the patient, are especially valuable. Improved patterns of eating behavior should be encouraged. Specific suggestions should include smaller, more frequent, or regular meals, eaten more slowly, in defined surroundings, and avoidance of high-calorie, high-fat, nutritionally poor foods. Use of food diaries is especially helpful, particularly in assisting both patients and their physicians to identify specific and dietary behavioral patterns that contribute to obesity. For the patient who makes a significant effort, reinforcement of the improved eating behavior by his or her caregiver is important in maintaining weight reduction. Usually, formal consultation with a professional behavioral therapist is not required. Chapters 4 (on patient education and compliance-improving strategies), and 20 (psychotherapy in ambulatory practice) describe generic approaches to behavior modification that can be used in office visits.

The NHLBI, National Institute of Diabetes and Digestive and Kidney Diseases, and American Heart Association websites provide additional information that is useful to the clinician and patient (see General References). In addition, many commercial and self-help programs are available and can provide guidance and support to patients. Examples include Diet Workshop, Jenny Craig, The Solution, TOPS (Take Off Pounds Sensibly, an international nonprofit, noncommercial weight loss support group), and Weight Watchers. Most programs include a balanced weight reduction diet, exercise, and behavior modification. Overeaters Anonymous is a nonprofit international organization that provides support, patterned after the 12-step Alcoholics Anonymous program, for patients with eating disorders.

Physical Activity

Increasing physical activity levels should play a central role in all weight management programs. Appropriate physical activity may actually increase the rate of weight loss and also is critical in helping patients maintain weight loss after treatment is completed. Furthermore, an active lifestyle may help reduce the threat of many of the comorbidities that often accompany obesity, such as hypertension, dyslipidemia, and hyperglycemia (31).

Most obese persons are not as active as their leaner counterparts (32); therefore, it is important to increase levels of physical activity gradually in sedentary overweight patients. Patients often recognize that regular exercise is important from both a health and weight management perspective. Given this information, why do so few participate in regular activity? The top four barriers to exercise that obese patients cite are (a) lack of time, (b) embarrassment about being physically active, (c) inability to exercise vigorously; and (d) lack of enjoyment (33).

A lack of time has consistently been reported as the greatest obstacle to being active in sedentary adults. In response, new strategies to promote physical activity have moved away from the classic exercise prescription (e.g., 30 minutes of uninterrupted vigorous activity performed on three or more days per week). Lifestyle approaches to physical activity should encourage patients to look for opportunities to include short bouts of activity during their waking hours to increase energy expenditure (see Chapter 16). Increases in normal lifestyle activities, such as walking or climbing stairs, may be a suitable initial exercise program for an obese patient. This is especially true for those who do not have time for a traditional exercise program and for those who simply do not enjoy exercise. One study compared health outcomes in a group of obese women who were randomly assigned to a program of either diet plus lifestyle activity or diet plus aerobic exercise (20). After 16 weeks of treatment, similar and significant improvements were found in fitness, serum lipids profiles, blood pressure, and weight loss in the two groups. Interestingly, the trend to maintain lost weight during the year that followed active treatment was greater in the lifestyle group than in the aerobic group.

Epstein et al. examined the effects on weight change in children of reinforcing less sedentary behavior in their leisure time (34). Children who consciously reduced time spent in sedentary behaviors increased their liking for high-intensity activity and reported lower caloric intake than did children who participated in traditional exercise. This suggests that the goal of reducing time spent in sedentary activities is an important change for people attempting to lose weight.

It is important that physicians who counsel patients about their weight convey the message that "all lifestyle activity counts." Lifestyle activity may offer an exciting therapeutic option to overweight patients as they begin treatment, because most perceive that they could successfully comply with the exercise prescription.

Management of Morbid Obesity

Total Fasting

Significant weight loss (up to 5 to 6 kg/week) can be achieved by prolonged (4 to 8 weeks) starvation of motivated, hospitalized morbidly obese patients. Within 1 to 2 years after such treatment, however, few patients have maintained their initial weight loss, and in the long-term fewer than 5% attain and maintain their ideal body weight. A major hazard of such treatment is the extensive loss of lean body mass, and the consequent negative nitrogen balance, that occurs predictably within the first 1 or 2 weeks of starvation and continues at a somewhat lower rate thereafter. Other complications of this technique include orthostatic hypotension, ketoacidosis, electrolyte and vitamin deficiencies, weakness, decreased libido and impotence, menstrual irregularities, hyperuricemia and acute gout, renal uric acid calculi, emotional disturbances, and, rarely, sudden death. Given the need for hospitalization, the medical risks, and the high incidence of recidivism, this approach is not frequently used to treat morbid obesity.

Very-Low-Calorie Diets

Supplemented fasting techniques or very-low-calorie diets (VLCDs) remain a treatment option for significantly obese patients (i.e., those at least 30% overweight). They exploit in an ambulatory setting several of the advantages of total fasting, particularly those of significant short-term weight loss and high patient adherence. In general, patients consume 1.2 to 1.5 g of protein per kilogram of desirable body weight—enough to prevent loss of lean body mass in a hypocaloric diet (typically 400 to 800 kcal/day) supplemented by adequate hydration, potassium salts, and other vitamins and minerals. In one study of almost 1,200 patients who were monitored clinically and biochemically at frequent intervals (35), approximately 75% to 80% of the patients lost more than 40 lb (18 kg). Moreover, hypertension and glucose intolerance, as well as the need for appropriate medications, disappeared or diminished in most affected patients; other benefits, such as improved exercise tolerance, ambulation, pulmonary function, and psychosocial and employment status, also became evident. The disadvantages of the technique are similar to but of lesser magnitude than those described for total fasting. VLCDs are generally safe when combined with a visit to a practitioner every 2 weeks. These diets result in initial weight losses of approximately 20 kg in 16 weeks, but almost half of the patients regain their lost weight during the year after treatment. Success may be enhanced by combining this dietary approach with long-term behavioral modification techniques (36). Weight maintenance may be improved by adding a weight maintenance support group to the treatment plan for patients to attend after the initial treatment is completed.

Pharmacologic Therapy

Increasing interest in the use of medications for the treatment of obesity stems from the rapidly advancing state of knowledge regarding the biologic basis of obesity; from recognition that the aggregate impact of dietary, exercise, and behavioral therapies has not altered the increasing rate of weight gain in the United States and in many other populations; and from the consideration that obesity is a chronic disorder that requires long-term treatment. The initial, widely publicized report of safe and effective maintenance of weight loss for up to 3.5 years in some patients enrolled in a program of drug therapy combined with dietary and behavioral modification (37) further stimulated scientific, public, and commercial interests in the possible benefits of antiobesity drugs. Nonetheless, *to date there is no known pharmacologic agent for the treatment of obesity that is reliably effective, devoid of short- and long-term adverse effects, and inexpensive.* Therefore, pharmacologic therapy should have a very limited role in the management of obesity.

Concepts about drug therapy for obesity have changed considerably in recent years. These concepts are predicated on the recognition that the primary purpose for promoting weight loss and weight maintenance is to decrease adverse health risks and that obesity is a chronic disease. It is now believed that drug treatment should be used only in conjunction with a long-term weight loss and/or weight maintenance program that includes diet, physical activity, and behavior therapy, and that drugs should be started only after the aforementioned lifestyle interventions have failed to achieve significant weight loss (usually 1 lb/week) for at least 6 months. In general, drug therapy should be reserved for individuals with a BMI of at least 30 without, or a BMI of 27 with, obesity-related risk factors or disease. There is considerable interindividual variation in response to drug therapy. It has been found that those who lose at least 2 kg (4.4 pounds) within the first 4 weeks after starting treatment continue to lose weight in the long term, whereas those initially classified as nonresponders tend not to respond in the long term, even with escalating doses (38).

The agents currently approved by the U.S. Food and Drug Administration (FDA) for weight reduction are listed in Table 83.7. Most of the drugs used to promote weight loss have been anorexigenic agents or

Table 83.7. Pharmacologic Agents Approved for Weight Reduction by the U.S. Food and Drug Administration

Generic and Proprietary Names	Common Trade Names	Mechanism of Action	Dosage Forms (mg)	Administration (mg)	Comments and Cautions
Diethylpropion[a]	Tenuate, Propion	Amphetamine-like action; reduces appetite	25, 75	25 before meals (t.i.d.), 75 in morning	Schedule IV[b]; contraindications include MAO-inhibitor use within 14d, severe cardiovascular disease, hyperthyroidism, glaucoma, and history of drug use; use with caution in hypertensive patients; common side effects include restlessness, dry mouth, and constipation.
Mazindol[a]	Sanorex, Propion	Amphetamine-like action; reduces appetite	1, 2	1 before meals 2 in morning	Schedule IV; cautions as for diethylpropion; pulmonary hypertension has been reported.
Phentermine[a]	Ionamin, Fastin	Amphetamine-like action; reduces appetite	15, 30	15 t.i.d. 30 in morning	Schedule IV[b]; cautions as for diethylpropion, contraindications include moderate to severe hypertension; associated with valvular heart disease and pulmonary hypertension when used with fenfluramine; rare reports of pulmonary hypertension and heat stroke when used alone.
Sibutramine[c]	Meridia, Reductil	Inhibits norepinehrine, serotonin, and dopamine reuptake; reduces appetite	5, 10, 15	10 to 15 q.d.	Schedule IV[b], contraindications include MAO-inhibitor use within 14 d, coronary artery disease, congestive heart failure, dysrhythmia, stroke, severe renal or hepatic dysfunction; use with caution in hypertension, glaucoma, cholelithiasis, seizures; common side effects include headache, dry mouth, insomnia, dizziness, constipation, nausea, dyspepsia, increased appetite, nervousness, dysmenorrhea, rhinits/sinusitis
Orlistat	Xenicol	Inhibits gastric and pancreatic lipases; reduces fat absorption	120	120 t.i.d., during up to 1 h after meals, taken with meals containing fat	Contraindications includes chronic malabsortion syndromes and cholestasis; may decrease cyclosporin levels, may interfere with warfarin action through inhibition of vitamin K absorption; common side effects include diarrhea, fatty stools, abdominal pain, nausea, vomiting, flatulence, fecal urgency or incontinence; because orlistat reduces absorption of fat-soluble vitamins, patients should take a multivitamin supplement providing the fat-soluble vitamins and beta-carotene at least 2 hours before or after orlistat.

MAO, monoamine oxidase.

[a]Indicated as an adjunct (to diet, exercise, behavioral modification) for short-term use (less than 12–20 wk)

[b]The Federal Controlled Substance Act of 1970 places the prescription anorexiants into three of five schedule categories. Appetite suppressants in Schedule II are most likely to be abused (e.g., dextroamphetamine, methampehtamine) and are *not* recommended; those in Schedule IV have little risk of abuse or dependence.

[c]Indicated as an adjunct (to diet) for short- and long-term weight reduction, with efficacy up to 12 mo.

appetite suppressants. All affect brain neurotransmitters by influencing catecholamines (e.g., dopamine, norepinephrine), serotonin, or both. Some drugs may also increase energy expenditure, including certain of the classic catecholaminergic anorexigenic drugs, sibutramine (which blocks catecholamines and serotonin), and the new beta-3-adrenergic receptor agonists. Finally, some drugs primarily affect nutrient partitioning, such as orlistat, which reduces the absorption of one third of dietary fat by inhibiting gastric and pancreatic lipases.

The *anorexigenic derivatives of phenylethylamine* include the amphetamines, phenylpropanolamine, and other noradrenergic agents, such as fenfluramine and dexfenfluramine. All possess certain pharmacologic properties like those of epinephrine and norepinephrine; however, their various chemical modifications have led, to differing extents, to decreased cardiovascular and central nervous system toxicity and to preservation of anorexigenic properties. Despite their similarities in chemical structure, these agents exert their effects via different mechanisms of action and, consequently, exhibit different side effect profiles (see later discussion).

Phenylpropanolamine (Acutrim, Dexatrim) is an over-the-counter noradrenergic drug used as both an appetite suppressant and a decongestant. A review of placebo-controlled trials using this agent concluded that weight loss was less than that achieved with prescription noradrenergic agents but greater than that with placebo (39). However, in November of 2000, the FDA recommended that the drug be withdrawn from the market because of a small but significantly increased risk of hemorrhagic stroke in women.

In a prior detailed analysis of the safety and efficacy of the noradrenergic group of drugs and fenfluramine, the FDA examined clinical data from almost 10,000 patients reported in a large number of double-blind and two-drug comparison studies. At the end of 20 weeks, patients taking drugs and those taking placebo had equal dropout rates, whereas patients taking drugs averaged about 0.5 lb (0.25 kg) per week greater weight loss. There were no significant differences in weight loss when any drugs in this class were used. Intermittent therapy (2 to 4 weeks on, 1 to 2 weeks off) was often as effective as uninterrupted treatment, except with fenfluramine, which was sometimes led to depression after the drug was stopped.

Until September 1997, both *fenfluramine* (Pondimin) and *dexfenfluramine* (Redux) were available as nonscheduled prescription drugs. Their prior widespread use was based on early trials showing substantial efficacy with minimal side effects (38). The major obstacle to greater use was thought to be their potential for inducing neurotoxicity and psychobehavioral abnormalities, side effects that, although reported in animal studies, had yet to be documented in humans. However, these drugs were then reported to be associated with a number of severe adverse effects. The report that use of fenfluramine or its derivatives (especially dexfenfluramine) for longer than 3 months was associated with a 23-fold increase in the occurrence of primary pulmonary hypertension raised appropriate concern regarding one major possible side effect of this class of drugs (40). Subsequently, significant cardiac valvular dysfunction was reported, first in 24 women evaluated an average of 12 months after initiation of fenfluramine plus phentermine cotherapy (41). Both right- and left- sided functional valvular abnormalities were noted. Histopathologic findings were consistent with those reported in patients with carcinoid and ergotamine-induced valvular disease. Eight of the women also exhibited pulmonary hypertension. Based on these observations, subsequent similar reports (42), and the consequent public health implications of these findings, both fenfluramine and dexfenfluramine were removed from the U. S. market in September, 1997. This action did not limit use of phentermine, although it effectively ended further use of the popular, but non-FDA approved, "fen-phen" combination, for which there were more than 18 million prescriptions in 1996. The experience with fenfluramine and dexfenfluramine further underscores the need for caution in the pharmacotherapeutic management of obesity.

For the noradrenergic agents, the most common side effects are mild and consist primarily of insomnia, dry mouth, and restlessness, to which tolerance tends to develop after several weeks. Noradrenergic agents are contraindicated in patients taking monoamine oxidase inhibitors, in whom hypertensive crises may occur. They may be used in hypertensive patients whose blood pressure is controlled with medication.

It is evident that individual patients exhibit considerable variation in short- and long-term responsiveness to anorexigenic drugs and that patients often derive improved benefit, and avoid tolerance to the drug, after even small increases in dosage. Thus, there seems to be a role for the judicious use of these anorexigenic agents in carefully selected patients who are monitored in medically supervised, comprehensive, therapeutic programs that include diet and exercise. However, exact guidelines for the optimal use of these drugs remain to be determined.

Although the 2001 *Physicians Desk Reference* still lists several *amphetamines* with indications for their use in promoting weight loss, these drugs should not be used for treatment of obesity because of their high risk for abuse.

The therapeutic potential of the anorexigenic properties of the *antidepressant drugs fluoxetine* (Prozac) and *sertraline* (Zoloft) has been examined. These drugs exert their effects by blocking neuronal reuptake of serotonin in the central nervous system. Neither fluoxetine nor sertraline exerts any significant adverse effects on the heart. In addition, sertraline, unlike fluoxetine, does not significantly inhibit the hepatic microsomal enzyme system, so the frequency of drug interactions is minimized. Fluoxetine has been reported to be effective in reducing weight in obese, nondepressed patients, although the effective dose (60 mg/day) was substantially higher than that needed when the drug is prescribed as an antidepressant (20 mg/day), and the effect on weight reduction lasted only 6 to 12 months (43).

Sibutramine was approved by the FDA in November 1997, for the long-term management of obesity. Sibutramine blocks presynaptic reuptake of noradrenaline and serotonin and therefore may exert an effect on appetite regulation like that of combination drug therapy. Early trials revealed a dose-responsive reduction in weight in otherwise healthy obese patients, with oral dosages of 10 to 30 mg/day (5-, 10-, and 15-mg capsules), leading to average weight losses of 6 to 7 kg after 24 weeks (44). Side effects reported include dry mouth, constipation, and insomnia, as well as modest increases in heart rate and blood pressure. Subsequent studies revealed that sibutramine is effective in promoting or maintaining long-term weight loss, whether given continuously or intermittently (45,46), and that the short-term addition of orlistat does not influence the longer-term effects of the drug (47). However, there have been to date 29 deaths attributed to its use. Because of that, the advisability of using the drug has come under obvious question. As of this writing (March, 2002), there is petition before the FDA to ban its use (47a). Patients with a history of hypertension, coronary artery disease, congestive heart failure, and/or stroke definitely should not take sibutramine.

Orlistat was approved by the FDA in April, 1999, for the long-term management of obesity. Orlistat is a gastric and pancreatic lipase inhibitor that decreases intestinal triglyceride hydrolysis and blocks about one third of subsequent fat absorption. Reduction of body weight probably results from a dose-dependent fecal fat excretion and a decreased dietary fat intake (48).

At oral dosages of 180 to 360 mg/day for 12 weeks, modest weight loss was first reported in a short-term (49) study. The long-term effectiveness of orlistat was confirmed in multicenter studies using the same doses (50). Side effects included a mild decrease in absorption of fat-soluble vitamins, soft stools, and fecal soiling, of which the latter may limit its use. A multivitamin preparation should be recommended to patients taking this drug.

Further advances in the development of anorexigenic and other drugs for inducing weight loss may derive from increased understanding of the molecular basis of altered energy intake and expenditure in the obesity syndromes.

Surgical Interventions

The surgical treatment of obesity may be appropriate for severely obese patients who have failed to maintain a significant weight loss over a meaningful period with nonsurgical methods. *Gastric bypass surgery and its variants* (e.g., gastroplasty), currently more popular than jejunoileostomy, induce significant weight loss by promoting decreased oral food intake while preserving normal gastrointestinal absorptive and digestive function (51). In the gastric bypass procedure, the proximal 10% of the stomach is fashioned into a 15- to 30-mL pouch by anastomosis to the jejunum through a 0.9- to 1.2-cm channel, thus producing rapid gastric filling, slow emptying, and prolonged satiety. One year after surgery, weight loss in one review (51) of approximately 1,500 reported patients averaged 30% to 35% of baseline weight, with one third of patients losing 50 kg or more. Although carbohydrate and bile acids are absorbed normally after gastric bypass, glucose intolerance and hyperlipidemia (especially hypertriglyceridemia) are nonetheless substantially improved; in addition, liver function does not worsen, and malabsorption and kidney stones do not occur. Deficiencies of calcium or of iron and B_{12} hypovitaminosis occur occasionally. By taking frequent small feedings of high-calorie foods, it is possible for patients to "outeat" the bypass (the soft-calorie syndrome). Within the first postoperative month, vomiting occurs two to three times weekly in 65% to 70% of patients. However, this complication becomes progressively less frequent, so that by 2 years after surgery it occurs in fewer than 10% of patients. Other complications of the procedure include channel ulcers or obstruction, bile reflux, and the dumping syndrome. In centers with experienced personnel, the overall mortality rate has been reduced from 3% to 1%, but it remains as high as 8% to 10% in patients older than 50 years of age. Reoperation, necessitated either by surgical complications or by unsatisfactory weight loss, appears to be uncommon, and takedown of the gastric bypass has been described in fewer than 1% of patients.

The common *gastric restrictive operations*, such as vertical banded gastroplasty, create a 10- to 15-mL stapled proximal gastric pouch that limits receptive capacity. The opening between this pouch and the remainder of the stomach is externally banded to create an inner diameter of about 1 cm to delay emptying of solid food. Thus, the distal 80% to 90% of the stomach is no longer excluded from the flow of nutrients, and gastrointestinal continuity is maintained. Difficulties with gastric restrictive operations include distention of the wall of the proximal pouch, rupture of the staple line, and erosion of the band into the stomach. As with the gastric bypass procedures, postoperatively some patients exhibit the soft-calorie syndrome or vomiting.

Although more research is needed to determine the long-term efficacy and safety of gastric bypass surgery and its variants, it appears that these procedures may be of considerable benefit in the treatment of selected morbidly obese patients. Currently patient mortality associated with obesity surgery is less than 1% when the procedure is performed by a skilled surgeon. In contrast, the striking complication rates associated with jejunoileal bypass procedures militate strongly against use of this technique in all but the most extreme instances.

A National Institutes of Health Consensus Development Panel recommended that gastric bypass or restrictive procedures could be considered for well-informed and motivated severely obese patients in whom the operative risks were acceptable; that patients who are candidates for surgical procedures should be selected carefully after evaluation by a multidisciplinary team with medical, surgical, psychiatric, and nutritional expertise; that surgery should be performed by a surgeon who has substantial experience in the particular procedure and who works in a clinical setting with adequate support for all aspects of management and assessment; and that patients should undergo lifelong medical, psychologic, and nutritional surveillance after surgery.

PREVENTION OF OBESITY

The prevalence of obesity continues to increase at an alarming rate, despite the proliferation of low-fat foods, the physical fitness boom, and the multibillion-dollar dieting industry. It is clear that obese children are likely to become obese adults and that weight management becomes a lifelong struggle for most obese patients. Physicians must start to think about the importance of preventing obesity, especially in patients who are at risk for weight gain.

The sociocultural environment in which we live has contributed to the current epidemic of obesity. It seems reasonable, therefore, that changing the environment to one that is less injurious should become a top public health priority. Robinson et al. (52) showed that teaching children and their families to reduce television watching can attenuate weight gain in children. After-school sports and recreation programs could offer children opportunities to expend energy in safe environments. Improving the nutritional quality of school lunches should be a top priority for all school districts. Workplace educational programs can help to teach the public about the importance of healthy eating. King et al. (53) suggested that control of commercial advertising practices should be considered.

Much of the advertising directed toward children contains promotions for high-fat food items or fast food restaurants. An example of the value of this type of limitation can be seen in the reduced sales of tobacco products after advertising by the tobacco industry was controlled. Efforts to educate children about the importance of healthy eating and being active should be part of every school curriculum.

It is important for health care practitioners to express concern when patients have gained weight between office visits. Many individuals believe that weight is not important if their health care provider does not address their weight in an office visit (54). A weight goal should be set for each office visit and recorded in the patient's chart.

Obesity is a serious and common health problem. Health care regulators and providers must start to endorse broad-ranging changes in policy to address the situation. Efforts to prevent obesity would have a profound and positive impact on chronic disease and mortality.

General References*

Brownell KD. The LEARN program for weight control. Dallas, American Health Publishing, 1997.

Institute of Medicine. Weighing the options: criteria for evaluating weight-management programs. Washington, DC: National Academy Press, 1995.

National Heart, Lung and Blood Institute Obesity Education Initiative. Executive summary of the Clinical Guidelines on the Identification, Evaluation, and Treatment of Overweight and Obesity in Adults. Arch Intern Med 1998;158:1855.

Wadden TA, Wingate BJ. Compassionate treatment of the obese individual. In: Brownell KD, Fairburn CG, eds. Eating disorders and obesity: a comprehensive handbook. New York: Guilford Press, 1995:564.

National Heart, Lung and Blood Institute website. Available at http://www.nhlbi.nih.gov/guidelines/obesity/ob_home.htm. Accessed February 4, 2002.

Useful website with clinical guidelines full report, executive summary, practical guide, and a BMI calculator and obesity guideline that can be downloaded to a Palm Pilot.

American Dietetic Association website. Available at http://www.eatright.org/find2.html. Accessed February 12, 2002.

Database that allows you to locate registered dieticians in your area, by specialty focus.

Specific References

1. Kuczmarski RJ, Carrol MD, Flegal KM, et al. Varying body mass index cutoff points to describe overweight prevalence among U.S. adults: NHANES III (1988 to 1994). Obes Res 1997;5:542.
2. Kuczmarski RJ, Flegal KM, Campbell SM, et al. Increasing prevalence of overweight among US adults: The National Health and Nutrition Examination Surveys, 1960 to 1991. JAMA 1994;272:205.

2a. Healthy People 2010. Available at: http://www.health.gov/healthypeople. Accessed February 12, 2002.

3. Crespo CJ, Smit E, Troiano RP, et al. Television watching, energy intake, and obesity in US children: results from the third National Health and Nutrition Examination Survey, 1988–1994. Arch Pediatr Adolesc Med 2001;155:360.
4. Black AE, Goldberg GR, Jebb SA, et al. Critical evaluation of energy intake data using fundamental principles of energy physiology: 2. Evaluating the results of published surveys. Eur J Clin Nutr 1991;45:583.
5. Galuska DA, Serdula M, Pamuk E, et al. Trends in overweight among US adults from 1987 to 1993: a multistate telephone survey. Am J Public Health 1996;86:1729.
6. **6.** National Institutes of Health, National Heart Lung and Blood Institute. Obesity Education Initiative: Clinical Guidelines on the Identification, Evaluation, and Treatment of Overweight and Obesity in Adults. Rockville, MD: U.S. Department of Health and Human Services, 1998.
7. Andersen RE. Body composition assessment. In: Cotton RT, ed. Lifestyle and weight management consultant manual. San Diego, CA: American Council on Exercise; 1996:71.
8. Eckerson JM, Housh TJ, Johnson GO. Validity of bioelectrical impedance equations for estimating fat-free weight in lean males. Med Sci Sports Exer 1992;24:1298.
9. Heyward VH, Cook KL, Hicks VL, et al. Predictive accuracy of three field methods for estimating relative body fatness of nonobese and obese women. Int J Sport Nutr 1992;2:75.
10. Van Itallie TB, Segal KR. Nutritional assessment of hospital patients: new methods and new opportunities. Am J Hum Biol 1989;1:205.
11. Walston J, Seibert M, Yen C-J, et al. Tumor necrosis factor-a-238 and -308 polymorphisms do not associate with traits related to obesity and insulin resistance. Diabetes 1999;48:2096.
12. Bouchard C, Despres JP, Tremblay A. Genetics of obesity and human energy metabolism. Proc Nutr Soc 1991;50:139.
13. O'Connor KO, Stevens TE, Blackman MR. GH and aging. In: Juul A, Jorgensen JOL, eds. Growth hormone in adults. Cambridge, UK: Cambridge University Press, 1996:323.
14. Carney RM, Goldberg AP. Weight gain after cessation of cigarette smoking: a possible role for adipose-tissue lipoprotein lipase. N Engl J Med 1984;310:614.
15. Shimokata H, Muller DC, Andres R. Studies in the distribution of body fat: III. Effects of cigarette smoking. JAMA 1989;261:1169.
16. Prentice AM, Jebb SA. Obesity in Britain: gluttony or sloth? BMJ 1995;311:437.
17. Andersen RE, Crespo CJ, Bartlett SJ, et al. Relationship of physical activity and television watching habits among US children with body weight and level of fatness: results from the Third National Health and Nutrition Examination Survey. JAMA 1998;279:938.
18. Lee CD, Blair SN, Jackson AS. Cardiovascular fitness, body composition, and all-cause and cardiovascular disease mortality in men. Am J Clin Nutr 1999;69:373.
19. Kayman S, Bruvold W, Stern JS. Maintenance and relapse after weight loss in women: behavioral aspects. Am J Clin Nutr 1990;52:800.
20. Andersen RE, Wadden TA, Bartlett SJ, et al. Effects of lifestyle activity vs structured aerobic exercise in obese women. JAMA 1999;281:335.
21. Simopoulos AP, Van Itallie TB. Body weight, health, and longevity. Ann Intern Med 1984;100:285.
22. Andres R. Mortality and obesity: the rationale for age-specific height-weight tables. In: Hazzard WR, Bierman EL, Blass JP, et al., eds. The principles of geriatric medicine and gerontology. New York: McGraw-Hill, 1994:847.
23. Shimokata H, Tobin JD, Muller DC, et al. Studies in the distribution of body fat: I. Effects of age, sex, and obesity. J Gerontol 1989;44:M66.
24. Hubert HB, Feinleib M, McNamara PM, et al. Obesity as an independent risk factor for cardiovascular disease: a 26-year follow-up of participants in the Framingham Heart Study. Circulation 1983;67:968.
25. Kaplan NM. The deadly quartet: upper-body obesity, glucose intolerance, hypertriglyceridemia, and hypertension. Arch Intern Med 1989;149:1514.
26. Peiris AN, Sothmann MS, Hoffmann RG, et al. Adiposity, fat distribution, and cardiovascular risk. Ann Intern Med 1989;110:867.
27. Muller DC, Elahi D, Pratley RE, et al. An epidemiological test of the hyperinsulinemia-hypertension hypothesis. J Clin Endocrinol Metab 1993;76:544.

*Bold print (general references) and bold numerals (specific references) denote published controlled clinical trials, meta-analyses, or consensus-based recommendations.

28. Bray GA, Teague RJ. An algorithm for the medical evaluation of obese patients. In: Stunkard AJ, ed. Obesity. Philadelphia: WB Saunders, 1980.
29. Brownell KD. The LEARN program for weight control. Dallas: American Health Publishing, 1997.
30. Institute of Medicine. Weighing the options: criteria for evaluating weight-management programs. Washington, DC: National Academy Press, 1995.
31. Andersen RE. What can physicians do about obesity? Physician Sports Med 2000;28:15.
32. Andersen RE, Frankowiak SC, Snyder J, et al. Can inexpensive signs encourage the use of stairs: Results from a community intervention. Ann Intern Med 1998;129:363.
33. Andersen R, Franckowiak S. Obesity. In: Cotton RT, Andersen RE, eds. Clinical exercise specialist manual: ACE's source for training special populations. San Diego, CA: American Council on Exercise, 1999:158.
34. Epstein LH, Saelens BE, Myers MD, et al. Effects of decreasing sedentary behaviors on activity choice in obese children. Health Psychol 1997;16:107.
35. Genuth SM, Castro JH, Vertes V. Weight reduction in obesity by outpatient semistarvation. JAMA 1974;230:987.
36. Pi-Sunyer FX. The role of very-low-calorie diets in obesity. Am J Clin Nutr 1992;56:240S.
37. Weintraub M, Sundaresan PR, Cox C. Long-term weight control study: VI. Clin Pharmacol Ther 1992;51:619.
38. Guy-Grand B, Apfelbaum M, Crepaldi G, et al. International trial of long-term dexfenfluramine in obesity. Lancet 1989;26:1142.
39. Weintraub M. Phenylpropanolamine as an anorexiant agent in weight control: a review of published and unpublished studies. Clin Pharmacol Ther 1985;5:53.
40. Abenheim L, Moride Y, Brenot F, et al. Appetite-suppressant drugs and the risk of primary pulmonary hypertension. N Engl J Med 1996;335:609.
41. Connolly HM, Crary JL, McGoon MD, et al. Valvular heart disease associated with fenfluramine-phentermine. N Engl J Med 1997;337:581.
42. Bowen R, Glicklich A, Kahn M, et al. Cardiac valvulopathy associated with exposure to fenfluramine or dexfenfluramine: U. S. Department of Health and Human Services interim public health recommendations, November 1997. MMWR Morb Mortal Wkly Rep 1997;46:1061.
43. Goldstein DJ, Rampey AH, Roback PJ, et al. Efficacy and safety of long-term fluoxetine treatment of obesity: maximizing success. Obes Res 1995;3:481S.
44. Ryan DH, Kaiser P, Bray GA. Sibutramine: a novel new agent for obesity treatment. Obes Res 1995;3[Suppl 4]:553s.
45. Apfelbaum M, Vague P, Ziegler O, et al. Long-term maintenance of weight loss after a very-low-calorie diet: a randomized blinded trial of the efficacy and tolerability of sibutramine. Am J Med 1999;106:179.
46. Wirth A, Krause J. Long-term weight loss with sibutramine: a randomized controlled trial. JAMA 2001;286:1331.
47. Wadden TA, Berkowitz RI, Womble LG, et al. Effects of sibutramine plus orlistat in obese women following 1 year of treatment by sibutramine alone: a placebo-controlled trial. Obes Res 2000;8:431.
47a. URL:http://www.citizen.org/publications/release.cfm?ID=7160.
48. McNeely W, Benfield P. Orlistat. Drugs 1998;56:241.
49. Drent ML, Larsson I, William-Olssen T, et al. Orlistat (RO 18-0647), a lipase inhibitor, in the treatment of human obesity: a multiple dose study. Int J Obes 1995;19:221.
50. Sjöström L, Rissanen A, Andersen T, et al. Randomized placebo-controlled trial of orlistat for weight loss and prevention of weight regain in obese patients. Lancet 1998; 352:167.
51. Kral JG. Surgical treatment of obesity. Med Clin North Am 1989;73:251.
52. Robinson TN, Hammer LD, Killen JD, et al. Does television viewing increase obesity and reduce physical activity? Cross-sectional and longitudinal analyses among adolescent girls. Pediatrics 1993;91:273.
53. King AC, Jeffery RW, Fridinger F, et al. Environmental and policy approaches to cardiovascular disease prevention through physical activity: issues and opportunities. Health Educ Q 1995;22:499.
54. Bartlett SJ. Counseling, communications and group dynamics. In: Cotton RT, ed. Lifestyle and weight management consultant manual. San Diego, CA: American Council on Exercise; 1996:1.

CHAPTER 84

Metabolic Bone Disease: Osteomalacia, Male Osteoporosis, and Paget Disease of the Bone*

MICHAEL A. ANKROM, MD
MARC R. BLACKMAN, MD

OSTEOMALACIA

Definition

Osteomalacia is a disorder that is characterized by a defect in the mineralization of newly formed organic matrix of bone. In children it is popularly called rickets and is associated with deformities (e.g., bowing of the tibia, rachitic rosary of the ribs) that are attributable to the fact that the bones are still growing.

*Female osteoporosis is discussed in Chapter 103.

Osteomalacia in adults in the Western world is primarily a disease of elderly people and, for that reason, must be distinguished from osteoporosis (discussed later). The disorder is definitively diagnosed by bone biopsy, which shows an increased osteoid volume (more than 10%) and delayed mineralization when double-tetracycline labeling is done before the biopsy. However, if the disease is suspected, it can often be diagnosed without histologic confirmation (see later discussion).

Causes

The causes of osteomalacia are listed in Table 84.1.

Vitamin D deficiency is the most common cause. Vitamin D is an essential nutrient in the metabolism of calcium and phosphorus, the critical ingredients in mineralization of bone. It is provided in the Western world by ingestion of foods supplemented with vitamin D (ergocalciferol) and by synthesis of the vitamin (cholecalciferol) in skin exposed to sunlight. Vitamin D deficiency is a result in most cases of *poor diet* or *malabsorption*. Fortification of foods with vitamin D has made dietary deficiencies less common, but they still may occur in people who eat poorly, especially the frail elderly, some of whom also may have minimal exposure to sunlight (1). Dark-skinned people are at greater risk in this regard. Osteomalacia due to malabsorption of vitamin D has been associated most commonly with celiac disease, postgastrectomy syndrome, intestinal bypass or resection, and a variety of other intestinal disorders. Rarely, chronic hepatic or pancreatic disease may result in malabsorption of vitamin D as part of a generalized malabsorption of fat-soluble substances.

Osteomalacia associated with *congenital or acquired renal disease* may occur by a variety of mechanisms:

1. Phosphate wasting in, for example, renal tubular disorders. Rarely, patients with mesenchymal tumors waste phosphate (so-called oncogenic osteomalacia), apparently because of a toxic effect on the renal tubules by a product or products released by the tumors.
2. Chronic acidosis in patients with renal tubular acidosis or with chronic renal failure. The mechanisms are not entirely clear but seem to result primarily from an alteration in the milieu in which mineralization occurs.
3. Reduced synthesis of the most active form of vitamin D-1,25 dihydroxycholecalciferol (calcitriol) by the kidneys of patients with chronic renal failure.

Table 84.1. Causes of Osteomalacia

Vitamin D deficiency
Congenital rickets
Malabsorption
Renal disease
Medication associated
Anticonvulsants
Cyclosporin
Lithium
Fluoride
Aluminium (from hemodialysis)
Cancer associated
Genetic syndromes

A number of *medications*, with prolonged use, can cause osteomalacia, either indirectly because they inhibit vitamin D metabolism or directly because they inhibit mineralization of bone. These agents include anticonvulsants, lithium, fluoride, aluminum (historically, in dialysates), and cyclosporine (2). The first-generation bisphosphonates (e.g., pamidronate) developed for treatment of osteoporosis and Paget disease have been abandoned, except in rare instances, largely because they inhibit bone formation; the newer bisphosphonates (e.g., alendronate) do not.

Presentation

History

The clinical presentation of adult osteomalacia is quite variable: Affected people can be asymptomatic or can present with nonspecific musculoskeletal pain, weakness, or unprovoked or minimally provoked fractures (3). The practitioner who suspects osteomalacia should ask questions about the amount of sun exposure (at least 15 minutes/day is necessary for optimal synthesis of vitamin D), the amount of calcium and vitamin D consumed in the diet (through vitamin preparations and fortified milk products), the medications taken, and any history or symptoms of gastrointestinal or renal disease.

Physical Examination

Unlike the presentation in children, the physical examination in an adult may be unrevealing, although there may be objective evidence of weakness, especially of the proximal muscles. Also, there may be tenderness at the sites of otherwise inapparent fractures, typically in the lower spine or pelvis.

Radiography

Radiologic studies, including films of symptomatic bones and joints, should be part of the initial examination. Commonly, cortical thinning and reduced bone density are seen. *Looser lines*, although not common, are diagnostic of osteomalacia; they are pseudofractures ("milkman fractures") that occur typically in the femur, metatarsal bones, or pelvis, where they appear as symmetric, ribbon-like, radiolucent zones oriented perpendicular to the surface of the bone.

Laboratory Studies

Initial tests should include measurement of serum calcium, phosphate, albumin, creatinine, urea nitrogen, alkaline phosphatase, and 25-hydroxyvitamin D. However, vitamin D levels are low in a minority of patients, and serum calcium and phosphate levels are low in no more than half of the patients in whom they are measured (4). The serum alkaline phosphatase level is usually high. In one study, all patients had at least two abnormal tests when serum calcium, phosphate, and alkaline phosphatase were measured and radiographic findings were evaluated (4).

Bone Biopsy

As stated previously, bone biopsy is diagnostic of osteomalacia but ordinarily does not need to be done unless the diagnosis cannot be made noninvasively. In such circumstances, the distinction that must be made is between osteomalacia and osteoporosis.

Treatment

If medications are being given that interfere with vitamin D metabolism, they should be discontinued, if possible. Otherwise, 400 U/day of vitamin D_2 for 105 days has been recommended as appropriate therapy (5).

There is no standardized replacement regimen for patients with vitamin D deficiency. Dosing depends on the cause of the deficiency, the severity of the disease, and the preferences of the patient or, if the patient does not have the capacity to decide, the patient's caregiver. Pharmacologic vitamin D is available in several forms: D_2 (ergocalciferol, calciferol), vitamin D_3 (calcitriol [Rocaltrol]), the active form of the vitamin, and dihydrotachysterol (DHT [Hytakerol]), the synthetic analog of the vitamin. Nutritional deficiency of vitamin D can be treated with 50,000 IU of ergocalciferol (available in 50,000-U capsules) once or twice a week, orally or parenterally, until there is radiologically demonstrable healing of bone (usually by 6 to 12 months). Thereafter, the patient's diet should be supplemented by 400 to 800 IU/day (the higher dose is advisable in the elderly). DHT is costlier, but its effect is more rapid and its toxic effects (especially hypercalcemia) can be reversed more rapidly. It is given orally in doses of 0.2 to 2 mg/day. Calcitriol has the most rapid and most transient effect but is also the most expensive product; it is given in doses of 0.25 to 1.0 μg/day.

Patients with malabsorption require higher oral doses of vitamin D, the equivalent of 50,000 to 100,000 IU/day of Vitamin D_2.

The treatment of vitamin D deficiency in patients with renal disease is more complicated and is described in Chapter 52.

In addition to vitamin D supplementation, the diets of all patients should be enhanced by the addition of 1,000 to 1,200 mg of calcium per day (e.g., E-X Tums, two 600-mg tablets), but it is important to monitor serum calcium and urinary calcium excretion monthly and to modify the dose of vitamin D if hypercalcemia or hypercalciuria (see Chapter 51) occurs.

MALE OSTEOPOROSIS

Definition

Osteoporosis in men, as in women, is characterized by osteopenia (decreased bone mass) and a disruption of the normal architecture of bone. Osteoporosis in men and women is a disease of bone loss. The disease results in decreases in trabecular bone (e.g., vertebrae) and in cortical bone (e.g., hips, long bones) that weaken the overall structural support of the skeleton, predisposing it to fracture. The World Health Organization has defined osteoporosis as existing when bone mineral density as measured by bone densitometry (e.g., by dual-energy x-ray absorptiometry [DEXA scanning]) is more than 2.5 standard deviations below the gender-specific peak bone mass. Osteopenia is defined as existing when bone mineral density as measured by DEXA is between 2.5 and 1.0 standard deviations below the gender-specific peak bone mass.

Epidemiology

It has been estimated that more than 10 million people in the United States have osteoporosis, of whom more than 2 million are men (6). The most severe complication of osteoporosis in men is the development of a hip fracture. White men older than 50 years of age have lifetime risks of 6% and 5% for hip and vertebral fracture, respectively (7,8). The risks for African American men are less, probably because of their higher peak bone mass. With age, the risk of hip fracture for men increases (9–11). At age 80 years, the risk of hip fracture in men is one in six (17%) (12,13). A hip fracture is a medical emergency, and patients should be hospitalized immediately. Despite great improvements in surgical procedures and posthospital care and rehabilitation, the morbidity and mortality associated with hip fracture remain high, and are in fact higher in men than in women. Osteoporotic men are also at increased risk for vertebral fractures, which, with their potential for back pain, decreased mobility, and restrictive lung disease, are also significant contributors to morbidity.

Causes

Osteoporosis in men is caused primarily by the progressive loss of bone beginning at approximately 35 years of age, when the peak bone mass has ordinarily been achieved. The cause of such loss is unknown. Much less commonly, osteoporosis may be accelerated by a variety of pathologic conditions (Table 84.2), including endocrinopathies such as gonadal failure (see Chapter 85), hyperthyroidism (see Chapter 80), hyperparathyroidism (see Chapter 81), malabsorption syndrome, and hyperadrenalism (see Chapter 81); malignant disease (e.g., myelomas); and administration of certain drugs (especially corticosteroids, possibly the leading cause of osteoporosis in men). Genetic influences on the propensity to develop osteoporosis are poorly understood but probably reflect the interaction of multiple genes. Several well-defined genetic syndromes (osteogenesis imperfecta, Ehlers–Danlos syndrome, and Marfan syndrome) are associated with osteoporosis. The exact causes of age-related osteopenia in men are unknown but may include changes in

Table 84.2. Causes of Male Osteoporosis

Endocrine
Testosterone deficiency
Thyroid dysfunction
Hyperparathyroidism, primary or secondary
Growth hormone deficiency
Increased cortisol syndromes
Genetic
Osteogenesis imperfecta
Ehlers–Danlos syndrome
Other genetic syndromes
Renal causes
Chronic renal failure
Calcium loss syndromes
Drug induced
Steroid use
Anticonvulsants
Chronic heparin use
Oncologic
Myeloma and other malignancies that produce osteoclast activating factors
Malabsorption syndromes
Hepatic insufficiency
Immobility/disuse osteoporosis
Idiopathic

endocrine function, nutritional status, and physical activity that accompany normal aging.

Diagnosis

History

Osteoporotic men are usually asymptomatic until they fracture a bone, although backache, without fracture, is a frequent complaint. Fractures may be incurred after no apparent or minimal trauma, and loss of height after vertebral fracture is common. In a man with a recent fracture, a focused medical history to detect secondary causes of osteoporosis is important and should include an exploration of the chronic use of medications. In younger men, secondary conditions should be even more diligently sought, as should a family history compatible with osteoporosis (see earlier discussion).

Physical Examination

The patient's height and weight should be compared with his historical numbers and with normative standards. An examination of the spine (see Chapter 71) should be done, especially if the patient complains of backache or loss of height. A general examination should be performed to seek secondary causes of osteoporosis.

Radiography

Routine radiographs of the skeleton are often unrevealing, because a loss of 30% or more of bone mass must occur before osteopenia can be appreciated. Thinning of bone is usually seen first in the vertebrae, the pelvis, and the femoral heads.

The diagnosis of osteoporosis is made or confirmed by measurement of bone mineral density by DEXA scan or ultrasound (see Chapter 103). Multiple sites, including hips, lumbar spine, and forearms, are scanned according to standardized protocols.

Laboratory Studies

In contrast to osteomalacia (described earlier), levels of serum calcium, phosphate, and alkaline phosphatase are typically normal. If secondary causes of osteoporosis are under consideration, other tests (e.g., measurements of serum testosterone, thyroxine, thyroid-stimulating hormone, cortisol, parathormone) are indicated.

Bone Biopsies

The only reason to do a bone biopsy is if osteoporosis and osteomalacia cannot be distinguished on the basis of the rest of the evaluation (see Osteomalacia).

Treatment

There are multiple approaches to treatment. Dietary interventions include calcium supplementation of 1,000 to 1,500 mg/day and vitamin D_2 supplementation of 400 to 800 IU/day. These interventions are appropriate for all men at risk, including asymptomatic men older than 60 years of age and men taking corticosteroids or other osteoporosis-producing drugs chronically. Similarly, physical activity is important in maintaining bone mass. Resistance training and aerobic exercise, alone and in combination, have been effective in stabilizing bone density (14,15).

A number of drugs have been developed to increase bone mass, and one or more of them should be considered for all men with osteoporosis. (Men with osteopenia may be treated by diet supplementation and exercise alone and monitored by DEXA scanning—see later discussion).

Bisphosphonates are the primary drugs used in the treatment of men with osteoporosis. The protocols are similar to those used in the treatment of women with osteoporosis (Chapter 103). A typical regimen is alendronate, 5 mg orally every day, or, in a new preparation, 70 mg orally once a week. Alternatively, risedronate, a third-generation bisphosphonate, 5 mg a day or 30 mg a week, may be prescribed.

Bisphosphonates should be taken in the morning, while in the upright position, with a full glass of water, 30 minutes before eating breakfast to avoid esophagitis, the major complication of these drugs. If the oral preparations cannot be tolerated, pamidronate, an intravenously administered bisphosphonate, can be given (60 mg in saline, once every 3 months).

Calcitonin is an alternative for patients who cannot tolerate bisphosphonates. It is administered by nasal spray, one puff (200 IU) once a day, alternating nostrils. The major adverse effects are rhinitis and epistaxis. Calcitonin can have an analgesic effect after it is given for a few weeks.

Hydrochlorothiazide has been reported to be effective in increasing bone density, but less so than bisphosphonates or calcitonin (16), and it ordinarily is not prescribed unless the more potent drugs are not tolerated.

Because as many as 30% of men with osteoporosis have been found to be hypogonadal, the use of testosterone has been investigated in hypogonadal elderly men. In one study, testosterone administration increased vertebral bone mineral density in aged men with baseline serum testosterone levels lower than 200 μg/dL (17). The utility of testosterone supplementation in older men with low-normal or slightly reduced testosterone levels (200 to 400 μg/dL) has not been established.

A number of other therapeutic interventions are in the process of evaluation, including new bisphosphonates, slow-release fluoride (18,19), parathormone (20,21), growth hormone analogs (22), and selective androgen response modifiers (SARMS).

Follow-Up

The response to treatment of osteopenia (but not osteoporosis—see earlier discussion) should be assessed by DEXA scan every 12 months. The response to treatment of osteoporosis should be assessed by DEXA scan every 12 to 24 months.

The use of serum and urine biomarkers of bone metabolism to assess response to therapy is less reliable than DEXA scanning and is not recommended.

Patients receiving calcium and vitamin D supplementation should have serum calcium levels measured after 2 to 3 months, and then, if within normal limits, yearly thereafter to be sure that hypercalcemia does not develop.

PAGET DISEASE OF BONE

Definition

Paget disease is a focal skeletal disorder characterized by rapid absorption and subsequent formation of bone.

Epidemiology

Paget disease is a disorder of older individuals that increases in frequency with increasing age (23). It is the second most common disorder of bone in adults, after osteoporosis (24). In the United States, it occurs in approximately 3% of Caucasians older than 55 years of age; it appears to be less common among African Americans, although additional data are required to be certain of this impression (25). In the elderly it occurs almost equally often in men and in women. The epidemiology of Paget disease is unusual because of its distinctive geographic distribution throughout the world. Paget disease occurs commonly in England, North America, Australia, New Zealand, France, and Germany. By contrast, it is uncommon in Switzerland and rare in Africa and throughout Asia, including China, India, and the Middle East (26). This information is important because it points to factors, both genetic and environmental, that are essential to the occurrence of the disorder.

Pathogenesis

Normal bone remodeling depends on a coupled metabolic response of bone-forming osteoblasts and bone-resorbing osteoclasts. Paget disease is characterized by an initial phase of intense osteoclastic resorption followed by an increase in bone formation. As a result, the rate of bone remodeling is greatly enhanced, leading to the production of excessive, dense, but structurally deficient skeletal tissue. This weakened skeletal tissue is at risk for development of bony deformities and fracture. These changes are responsible for the signs and symptoms of the disease.

Etiology

In 1980, Rebel et al. (27) proposed that paracrystalline nuclear inclusion bodies observed in osteoclasts from patients with Paget disease were similar to the nuclear inclusions found in subjects with "slow virus" infections such as progressive multifocal leukoencephalopathy and subacute sclerosing panencephalitis. The inclusion bodies were subsequently identified, with the use of viral antisera, as nucleocapsids of the paramyxovirus family, with resemblance to both the measles and respiratory syncytial viruses (28). Both measles virus and respiratory syncytial virus nucleocapsids were identified in the same osteoclasts, suggesting the expression of antigen from an altered viral particle (29). However, attempts to isolate or pass an infectious agent from cultured surgical specimens or from cultured bone cells have been unsuccessful. Investigations into possible genetic or premalignant etiologies for Paget disease have been inconclusive (30,31).

Diagnosis

History

Early in the disease, patients are asymptomatic and are diagnosed only because a screening blood test has revealed an unexplained elevation of serum alkaline phosphatase (see later discussion).

Chronic pain is the most common complaint of patients with Paget disease of bone. Resulting from either direct pagetic involvement or osteoarthopathy, pain is the presenting complaint in two thirds of subjects older than 60 years of age (32). Bone pain or limitation of joint function points to the diagnosis in approximately 50% of patients with symptomatic Paget disease. Pagetic pain is typically increased at night and in the limbs with weight bearing (33). Pain in the extremities may result from expansion of bone with involvement of the periosteum. Lumbar spine pain may result from vertebral expansion, collapse, or microfractures. Facet enlargement, cord compression, or impingement of structures in the cauda equina or spinal nerve root may result in pain. The incidence of hip pain in Paget disease ranges from 30% to 50% (34). Pagetic coxopathy refers to involvement of both femur and acetabulum that may be associated with protrusio acetabuli. Involvement of the femur may be associated with coxa vara deformity (the angle between the neck and the shaft of the femur is decreased), with instability of gait and increased risk of fracture due to falling. Calcific periarthritis and calcium pyrophosphate deposition may affect joints in Paget disease and must be considered in the differential diagnosis of acute arthritis. Acute gouty arthritis can occur as a consequence of hyperuricemia. The dental complications of Paget disease can be severe and include osteolytic disease with loosening and loss of teeth as well as overgrowth of bone leading to spreading of teeth and malocclusion.

Neurologic symptoms and signs in Paget disease arise from three major sources. First, there can be a reduction in the size of neural foramina, leading to compression of the cranial nerves. Compression of the eighth cranial nerve causes one of the more common problems in patients with Paget disease—deafness—which occurs in more than one third of people with the disorder (35). Occasionally, various ocular and facial palsies also develop. Second, brain stem and cerebellar compression and/or hydrocephalus due to basilar invagination (so called platybasia) can occur. Third, spinal cord and nerve root compression occasionally occur. Rarely, ischemic brain disease may occur secondary to a vascular steal syndrome resulting from increased vascularity of the cranial vault. Myelopathy due to ischemic myelitis has also been reported in the presence of highly vascularized and hypermetabolic bone in the vertebral column or as a consequence of compression of the spinal arteries (36). Spinal stenosis may occur, depending on the level of vertebral involvement; symptoms vary from radicular pain to numbness, paresthesia, and, finally, progressive paraparesis with bladder and bowel involvement.

A history of repeated *unprovoked or minimally provoked fractures* is common in patients with Paget disease, especially fractures of the long bones of the lower extremities.

Physical Examination

Physical examination is normal early in the disease but later may reveal structural deformities of bone (e.g., sabre shins, frontal bossing of the skull), hearing loss, or signs of nerve root compression.

Laboratory Evaluation

Patients are often diagnosed after a screening blood test has revealed elevated serum alkaline phosphatase activity with normal serum calcium, phosphate, and parathormone concentrations and normal liver function tests. The alkaline phosphatase can be identified by the laboratory as originating in bone. The level of serum alkaline phosphatase generally correlates with the activity of the disease.

Other biologic markers of bone metabolism may be increased in patients with Paget disease. The high rate of skeletal turnover during the resorptive and mixed stages of the disease has resulted in the development of multiple assays to measure disease activity. Metabolic markers of bone disease, in addition to alkaline phosphatase, include osteocalcin, procollagen type I C-terminal peptide (PICP), and newer assays of nonmetabolized collagen peptides, including N-telopeptides and pyridinoline crosslinks.

The level of serum osteocalcin, a protein produced by osteoblasts, tends to be increased in states of high bone turnover. Osteocalcin levels are frequently, but not always, increased in Paget disease. PICP, although not specific for bone collagen turnover, is increased when bone turnover is elevated, and a rapid decline in serum levels has been observed after treatment of Paget disease with calcitonin and bisphosphonates (37). PICP, measured in urine, is a highly sensitive assay for the determination of tissue type I collagen breakdown and, consequently, measurement of the rate of bone resorption (37,38). Because pyridinoline crosslink excretion is increased overnight, specimens are collected as second voided urines over a 2-hour period during the morning (e.g., 7 to 9 a.m.). The N-telopeptides and PICP assays are believed to be the most sensitive markers of bone resorption and are readily available through commercial laboratories (39).

Radiology

The importance of radiologic evaluation in Paget disease cannot be underestimated. Only one third of patients have monostotic disease, with pelvic involvement in 72%, involvement of the lumbar spine in 58%, the thoracic spine in 45%, the femur in 55%, and the skull in 42% (40). The early radiologic lesions of Paget disease reflect severe localized osteolysis. These are typically "flame-shaped" osteolytic lesions that most commonly occur proximal to the distal epiphysis of a long bone. This resorptive lesion gradually progresses to the opposite end of the bone. As the disease evolves, an ingrowth of fibrovascular tissue and a high rate of bone remodeling may lead to deformity of the skull, enlarged dense vertebral bodies, and slowly progressive deformities of weight-bearing bones. Microfractures may occur on the convex side of the femur or tibia, increasing the degree of deformity and leading to the transverse or "banana" fracture that is typical of Paget disease. Pelvic involvement may be limited to the ilia and pubic rami but may involve the acetabulum or both the acetabulum and the femur, resulting in protrusio acetabuli.

For a complete evaluation, each patient should have a *bone scan* at the time of diagnosis to evaluate the extent of disease. Although scintigraphy is diagnostically less specific than radiography, bone scan identifies approximately 15% to 30% of lesions not visualized on radiographs (41). Alternatively, in 5% of cases the radiograph demonstrates diffuse pagetic involvement (e.g., of the pelvis) whereas the bone scan reveals little uptake of the isotope. In this circumstance, the alkaline phosphatase level may be normal or only slightly elevated, reflecting lesions that are sclerotic, relatively inactive, or "burned out."

Bone Biopsy

A bone biopsy is rarely needed to establish the diagnosis of Paget disease. However, a bone biopsy is indicated to rule out malignancy when mixed osteoblastic and osteolytic vertebral lesions are seen (see later discussion). The value of a vertebral needle biopsy is limited. An open biopsy of the involved bone is more likely to be diagnostic.

Complications

Apart from the orthopedic and neurologic problems that can occur in Paget disease, a few rarer complications may arise.

High-output heart failure may develop if a third or more of the bones are diseased; in addition, *calcific aortic stenosis, heart block, and left bundle branch block* appear to be more common than in the general population (42).

Osteosarcoma is a dreaded but unusual complication, sometimes multicentric; the tumors usually are detected because the patient complains of increased localized pain, sometimes associated with swelling. Radiologically, either osteolytic or osteoblastic lesions may be seen; computed tomography–directed biopsy can often make the definitive diagnosis and distinguish the malignancy from benign giant cell tumor of bone, the incidence of which is also increased in Paget disease.

Increased incidences of *primary hyperparathyroidism* and *hyperuricemia* have been reported in patients with Paget disease (23,43). *Urinary stones* (see Chapter 51) have been reported in 13% of patients (44).

Treatment

Effective medical therapy for Paget disease has been available for more than 20 years. The availability of newer and more potent agents suggests that treatment should be pursued more aggressively, both to control the disease and to decrease the risk of future complications. An asymptomatic patient without elevated markers of bone remodeling need not be treated. A general guideline is to treat if the serum alkaline phosphatase concentration is more than two to three times normal. Elevations of alkaline phosphatase indicate either a great deal of disease or an intense activity in a limited area. Such patients are at higher risk for future complications of their disease.

Bisphosphonates are the cornerstone of the treatment of Paget disease. Bisphosphonates bind to the surface of the hydroxyapatite crystal and decrease bone resorption by disrupting osteoclast recruitment and cellular activity. The effects of these agents may last several months. Because hypocalcemia can be induced by bisphosphonates, patients should have adequate intake of calcium (1,000 mg/day) and vitamin D_2 (800 IU/day). Of particular concern in the elderly are the most common side effects, epigastric pain, heartburn, and nausea due to esophagitis or gastritis. To avoid these symptoms, the drugs must be taken 30 to 60 minutes before breakfast, and the patient must stand for 30 minutes after dosing. Because it is less potent than newer agents and because it also inhibits bone formation, *etidronate* the first agent widely used to treat Paget disease, is used currently only if subjects have limiting side effects with newer agents (45).

Alendronate, the first of the third-generation oral bisphosphonates, is approved for the treatment of Paget disease at an oral dose of 40 mg/day (5-, 10-, 35-, 40-, 70-mg tablets). In one study, the drug caused a 71% fall in alkaline phosphatase levels, compared with 44% in patients treated with etidronate; osteolytic lesions improved; and no impairment of bone formation was seen on biopsy after 6 months of therapy (45,46). *Tiludronate* (200 to 400 mg/day, available in 200-mg tablets) and risedronate (30 mg/day, available in 5- and 30-mg tablets) are newer bisphosphonates approved for the treatment of Paget disease. They appear comparable to alendronate in potency (46–48). *Zoledronate* is a third-generation bisphosphonate currently in clinical trials (49,50).

Pamidronate, a potent second-generation bisphosphonate, is approved for intravenous administration only because of its low oral absorption. It is useful in refractory disease, producing disease remission for up to 3 years in up to 90% of patients (51–53). Infusions of pamidronate are then repeated at intervals based on the response of biochemical markers (see earlier discussion). Rare side effects of pamidronate therapy include a transient flu-like syndrome with leukopenia, anterior uveitis, episcleritis, and ototoxicity (54,55). Because the incidence of gastrointestinal side effects is less with pamidronate, this drug may be an acceptable alternative treatment for patients who are unable to tolerate oral bisphosphonate therapy.

Calcitonin is an alternative treatment to bisphosphonate therapy, although it may be less efficacious. The high doses used in subcutaneous administration often result in the development of nausea and transient flushing. Starting subcutaneous doses are in the range of 50 to 100 IU of salmon calcitonin or 50 IU of human calcitonin daily for 1 month; it is then continued three to four days per week thereafter (56). It also may be administered by intranasal spray in a dose of 200 to 400 IU daily. Nasal calcitonin causes less nausea, but 11% of patients develop rhinitis (57). Although prolonged remission may occur with calcitonin treatment, a partial or "plateau" response is more common: Biochemical parameters decline over a period of months but may not return to normal.

For patients with poor response to bisphosphonate or calcitonin therapy, second-line agents include *gallium nitrate* and *plicamycin (Mithramycin)*. Gallium nitrate, a potent antiresorptive drug, is currently an experimental therapy for Paget disease (58). In a multicenter trial, gallium nitrate was administered in doses of 0.05, 0.25 and 0.5 mg/kg per day by subcutaneous injection in two 14-day cycles; cyclical low-dose subcutaneous administration may be effective for patients with advanced disease that has been resistant to other agents (59).

Surgery

There are several skeletal problems that may require surgical intervention, but only after careful planning with an orthopedist or neurosurgeon. The operations are often complicated by infection and hemorrhage, in part because of the hypervascularity of pagetic bone.

For that reason bisphosphonate or calcitonin should be given for approximately 3 months before elective surgery, to decrease the risk of bleeding. To permit unhindered healing, however, it is best to stop treatment at the time of surgery and then resume it 8 weeks postoperatively.

Specific problems that may warrant surgical intervention include *basilar invagination and hydrocephalus* (which may require a ventricular shunt), *nerve compression syndromes* (sometimes reversible by medical therapy), *degenerative disease of joints* that may lead to joint replacement, and *pathologic fractures that require fixation.*

General References*

Osteomalacia

Reginato AJ, Falascia GF, Pappu, R, et al. Musculoskeletal manifestations of osteomalacia: report of 26 cases and a literature review. Semin Arth Rheum 1999;28:287.

Francis RM, Selby PL. Osteomalacia. Baillieres Clin Endocrinol Metab 1997;11:145.

Male Osteoporosis

Kaufman JM, Johnell O, Abadie E, et al. Background for studies on the treatment of male osteoporosis: state of the art. Ann Rheum Dis 2000;59:765.

Seeman E. The dilemma of osteoporosis in men. Am J Med 1995;98:76S.

Orwoll ES, Oviatt SK, McClung MR, et al. The rate of bone mineral loss in normal men and the effects of calcium and cholecalciferol supplementation. Ann Intern Med 1990;112:29.

Paget Disease

Ankrom MA, Shapiro JR. Paget's disease of bone (osteitis deformans). J Am Geriatr Soc 1998;46:1025.

Delmas PD, Meunier PJ. The management of Paget's disease of bone. N Engl J Med 1997;336:558.

Meunier PJ, Salson C, Mathieu L, et al. Skeletal distribution and biochemical parameters of Paget's disease. Clin Orthop 1987;217:37.

Hamdy RC. Paget's disease of bone: assessment and management. Eastbourne, East Sussex: Praeger Publishers, 1981.

Specific References

1. Gloth FM 3rd, Smith CE, Hollis BW, et al. Functional improvement with vitamin D replenishment in a cohort of frail, vitamin D-deficient older people. J Am Geriatr Soc 1995;43:1269.
2. Collins N, Maher J, Cole M, et al. A prospective study to evaluate the dose of vitamin D required to correct low 25-hydroxyvitamin D levels, calcium, and alkaline phosphatase in patients at risk of developing antiepileptic drug-induced osteomalacia. Q J Med 1991;78:113.
3. Reginato AJ, Falascia GF, Pappu R, et al. Musculoskeletal manifestations of osteomalacia: report of 26 cases and literature review. Semin Arthritis Rheum 1999;28:287.
4. Bringham CT, Fitzpatrick LA. Noninvasive testing in the diagnosis of osteomalacia. Am J Med 1993;95:519.
5. Christiansen C, Rodbro P. Initial and maintenance doses of vitamin D2 in the treatment of anticonvulsant osteomalacia. Acta Neurol Scand 1974;50:631.
6. Seeman E. The dilemma of osteoporosis in men. Am J Med 1995;98(2A):76S.
7. Ringe JD. Hip fractures in men. Osteoporos Int 1996;6[Suppl 3]:48.
8. Nguyen TV, Eisman JA, Kelly PJ, et al. Risk factors for osteoporotic fractures in elderly men. Am J Epidemiol 1996;144:255.
9. Francis RM. Male osteoporosis. Rheumatology (Oxford) 2000;39:1055.
10. Peris P, Guanabens N. Male osteoporosis. Curr Opin Rheumatol 1996;8:357.
11. Wishart JM, Need AG, Horowitz M, et al. Effect of age on bone density and bone turnover in men. Clin Endocrinol 1995;42:141.
12. Kelepouris N, Harper KD, Gannon F, et al. Severe osteoporosis in men. Ann Intern Med 1995;123:452.
13. Bendavid EJ, Shan J, Barrett-Connor E. Factors associated with bone mineral density in middle-aged men. J Bone Miner Res 1996;11:1185.
14. Snow-Harter C, Whalen R, Myburgh K, et al. Bone mineral density, muscle strength, and recreational exercise in men. J Bone Miner Res 1992;7:1291.
15. Jackson JA, Kleerekoper M. Osteoporosis in men: diagnosis, pathophysiology, and prevention. Medicine (Baltimore) 1990;69:137.
16. **16.** LaCroix AZ, Ott SM, Ichikawa L, et al. Low-dose hydrochlorothiazide and preservation of bone mineral density in older adults: a randomized, double-blind, placebo-controlled trial. Ann Intern Med 2000;133:516.
17. Medras M, Jankowska EA, Rogucka E. Effects of long-term testosterone substitutive therapy on bone mineral content in men with hypergonadotrophic hypogonadism. Andrologia 2001;33:47.
18. Balena R, Kleerekoper M, Foldes JA, et al. Effects of different regimens of sodium fluoride treatment for osteoporosis on the structure, remodeling and mineralization of bone. Osteoporos Int 1998;8:428.
19. Ringe JD, Dorst A, Kipshoven C, et al. Avoidance of vertebral fractures in men with idiopathic osteoporosis by a three year therapy with calcium and low-dose intermittent monofluorophosphate. Osteoporos Int 1998;8:47.
20. Reeve J, Meunier PJ, Parsons JA, et al. Anabolic effect of human parathyroid hormone fragment on trabecular bone in involutional osteoporosis: a multicentre trial. Br Med J 1980;280:1340.
21. Kurland ES, Cosman F, McMahon DJ, et al. Parathyroid hormone as a therapy for idiopathic osteoporosis in men: effects on bone mineral density and bone markers. J Clin Endocrinol Metab 2000;85:3069.
22. Valimaki MJ, Salmela PI, Salmi J, et al. Effects of 42 months of GH treatment on bone mineral density and bone turnover in GH-deficient adults. Eur J Endocrinol 1999;140:545.
23. Siris ES. Epidemiological aspects of Paget's disease: family history and relationship to other medical conditions. Semin Arthritis Rheum 1994;23:222.
24. Hamdy RC. Paget's disease of bone, assessment and management. Eastbourne, East Sussex: Praeger Publishers, 1981.
25. Perry HM III, Kraezle D, Miller DK. Paget's disease in African Americans. Clin Geriatr 1995;3:69.
26. Barker DJ. The epidemiology of Paget's disease of bone. Br Med Bull 1984;40:396.
27. Rebel A, Basle M, Pouplard A, et al. Viral antigens in osteoclasts from Paget's disease of bone. Lancet 1980;2:344.
28. Howatson AF, Fornasier VL. Microfilaments associated with Paget's disease of bone: comparison with nucleocapsids of measles virus and respiratory syncytial virus. Intervirology 1982;18:150.
29. Mills BG, Singer FR, Weiner LP, et al. Evidence for both respiratory syncytial virus and measles virus antigens in the osteoclasts of patients with Paget's disease of bone. Clin Orthop 1984;183:303.
30. Hoyland JA, Freemont AJ, Sharpe PT. Interleukin-6, IL-6 receptor, and IL-6 nuclear factor gene expression in Paget's disease. J Bone Miner Res 1994;9:75.
31. Price CH, Goldie W. Paget's sarcoma of bone: a study of eighty cases from the Bristol and the Leeds bone tumour registries. J Bone Joint Surg Br 1969;51:205.
32. Hamdy RC, Moore S, LeRoy J. Clinical presentation of Paget's disease of the bone in older patients. South Med J 1993;8610:1097.
33. Anonymous. Paget's disease and calcitonin. Br Med J 1977;3:505.
34. Altman RD. Articular complications of Paget's disease of bone. Semin Arthritis Rheum 1994;23:248.
35. Gold, DT, Boisture J, Shipp KM, et al. Paget's disease of bone and quality of life. J Bone Miner Res 1996;11:1897.

*Bold print (general references) and bold numerals (specific references) denote published controlled clinical trials, meta-analyses, or consensus-based recommendations.

36. Yost JH, Spencer-Green G, Krant JD. Vascular steal mimicking compression myelopathy in Paget's disease of bone: rapid reversal with calcitonin and systemic steroids. J Rheumatol 1993;20:1064.
37. Ebeling PR, Peterson JM, Riggs BL. Utility of type I procollagen propeptide assays for assessing abnormalities in metabolic bone diseases. J Bone Miner Res 1992;7:1243.
38. Alvarez L, Guanabens N, Peris P, et al. Discriminative value of biochemical markers of bone turnover in assessing the activity of Paget's disease. J Bone Miner Res 1995;10:458.
39. Rosen HN, Dresner-Pollak R, Moses AC, et al. Specificity of urinary excretion of cross-linked N-telopeptides of type I collagen as a marker of bone turnover. Calcif Tissue Int 1994;54:26.
40. Meunier PJ, Salson C, Mathieu L, et al. Skeletal distribution and biochemical parameters of Paget's disease. Clin Orthop 1987;217:37.
41. Fogelman I, Carr D. A comparison of bone scanning and radiology in the assessment of patients with symptomatic Paget's disease. Eur J Nucl Med 1980;5:417.
42. Hultgren HN. Osteitis deformans (Paget's disease) and calcific disease of heart valves. Am J Cardiol 1998;81:1461.
43. Lluberas-Acosta G, Hansell JR, Schumacher HR Jr. Paget's disease of bone in patients with gout. Arch Intern Med 1986;146:2389.
44. Harinck HI, Bijvoet OL, Vellenga CJ, et al. Relation between signs and symptoms in Paget's disease of bone. Q J Med 1986;58:133.
45. Siris E, Weinstein RS, Altman R, et al. Comparative study of alendronate versus etidronate for the treatment of Paget's disease of bone. J Clin Endocrinol Metab 1996;81:961.
46. Khan SA, Vasikaran S, McCloskey EV, et al. Alendronate in the treatment of Paget's disease of bone. Bone 1997;20:263.
47. Reginster JY, Colson F, Morlock G, et al. Evaluation of the efficacy and safety of oral tiludronate in Paget's disease of bone: a double-blind, multiple-dosage, placebo-controlled study. Arthritis Rheum 1992;35:967.
48. McClung MR, Tou CK, Goldstein NH, et al. Tiludronate therapy for Paget's disease of bone. Bone 1995;17[5 Suppl]:493S.
49. Arden-Cordone M, Siris ES, Lyles KW, et al. Antiresorptive effect of a single infusion of microgram quantities of zoledronate in Paget's disease of bone. Calcif Tissue Int 1997;60:415.
50. Buckler H, Fraser W, Hosking D, et al. Single infusion of zoledronate in Paget's disease of bone: a placebo-controlled, dose-ranging study. Bone 1999;24[5 Suppl]:81S.
51. DeLaRose RE. Intravenously administered pamidronate for treating refractory Paget's disease of bone. Endocrine Pract 1997;3:214.
52. Wimalawansa SJ, Gunasekera RD. Pamidronate is effective for Paget's disease of bone refractory to conventional therapy. Calcif Tissue Int 1993;53:237.
53. Anderson DC, Richardson PC, Brown JK, et al. Intravenous pamidronate: evolution of an effective treatment strategy. Semin Arthritis Rheum 1994;23:273.
54. O'Donnell NP, Rao GP, Aguis-Fernandez A. Paget's disease: ocular complications of disodium pamidronate treatment. Br J Clin Pract 1995;49:272.
55. Reid IR, Mills DA, Wattie DJ. Ototoxicity associated with intravenous bisphosphonate administration. Calcif Tissue Int 1995;56:584.
56. Singer FR, Keutman H, Neer RM, et al. Pharmacological effects of salmon calcitonin in man. In: Talmage RV, Munson Pl, eds. Calcium, parathyroid hormone and the calcitonins. Proceedings Amsterdam: 1972:89.
57. Silverman SL. Nasal calcitonin. Endocrine 1997;6:199.
58. Bockman RS, Wilhelm F, Siris E, et al. A multicenter trial of low dose gallium nitrate in patients with advanced Paget's disease of bone. J Clin Endocrinol Metab 1995;80:595.
59. Warrell RP Jr, Bosco B, Weinerman S, et al. Gallium nitrate for advanced Paget disease of bone: effectiveness and dose-response analysis. Ann Intern Med 1990;113:847.

CHAPTER 85

Problems in Male Reproductive Endocrinology

ADRIAN S. DOBS, MD, MHS
MARC R. BLACKMAN, MD

Relatively few caregivers are entirely comfortable investigating and managing sexual and reproductive problems. This is partly because medical school curricula and postgraduate training have generally not dealt adequately with reproductive medicine and partly because sexuality and gender identity are psychologically "loaded" issues, with the potential to produce acute feelings of embarrassment in both patient and clinician. Therefore, many clinicians regard complaints involving the reproductive system as esoteric, to be referred immediately to an appropriate specialist. However, sexual and reproductive dysfunction is far from rare. For example, almost 50% of men will experience some degree of erectile dysfunction (ED) between the ages of 20 and 50 years (1); up to 10% of married couples have trouble conceiving; and approximately 1 in 400 males is born with Klinefelter syndrome (XXY sex chromosomes). The constant outpouring of articles and programs dealing with human sexuality in the popular media has also led to a general expectation of "normal" sexual function as part of a healthy lifestyle. As a result, sexual dysfunction, even in the elderly, is likely to be perceived as a health problem. It is therefore important that generalists have adequate knowledge of reproductive and sexual disorders and of related history taking, physical diagnosis, and laboratory testing to allow them to distinguish patients who require only reassurance or simple treatment from those who should be referred to a specialist for more complex testing or therapy.

SEXUAL AND REPRODUCTIVE PHYSIOLOGY

Levels of Sexual Differentiation

Sexual differentiation can be viewed as two parallel continua, the first proceeding in time from conception to adulthood and the second in biological "depth" from genetic to psychological to social as follows: (a) *genetic sex* is determined at conception when the egg, bearing an X chromosome, is fertilized by a sperm bearing either a Y or an X chromosome, resulting in an XY male or an XX female, respectively. The Y chromosome contains a gene that specifies a product essential for differentiation of the primal gonad into a testis, but, because the X chromosome carries genes that regulate Y chromosome function, the testis differentiation genes are normally expressed only in the presence of a single X chromosome. Active function of two X-chromosomes, in the absence of a Y chromosome, must occur during fetal life in order to produce differentiation of the fetal gonad into an ovary. Thus, genetic sex determines (b) *gonadal (or somatic) sex*. The presence or absence of testicular function determines (c) *primary (or phenotypic) sex*, which is defined by the development of the genitalia. This is true because the embryonic testis produces two critical molecules. The first is *testosterone*, the major male sex steroid, which causes the development of the undifferentiated external genitalia into a penis and scrotum and of the wolffian (primitive mesonephric) duct system into epididymis, vas deferens, prostate, and seminal vesicles. The second is a peptide, *müllerian-inhibiting substance (MIS)*, which mediates the regression of the primitive müllerian duct structures. In the absence of MIS, the müllerian ducts develop into a vagina, uterus, and fallopian tubes; without the action of testosterone, female external genitalia (labia and clitoris) form. Therefore, normal infantile female genitalia will develop in the absence of both ovaries and testes.

It is the primary sex characteristics (appearance of the external genitalia) that identify an individual's apparent gender at birth. Further sexual development, defined as (d) *secondary sex,* occurs at puberty as a result of greatly increased secretion by the gonads of sex steroid hormones. In males, growth of male pattern body and pubic hair and beard, as well as increase in muscle mass, deepening of voice, and onset of male libido with ejaculations and increased frequency of erections, are characteristic effects of testosterone. In females, rounding of body contours with breast growth and subcutaneous deposition of fat in the hips and buttocks, and also the onset of menses, are effects of cyclic estrogen secretion, whereas growth of pubic and axillary hair (and probably libido) are manifestations of adrenal and, to a lesser extent, ovarian androgen secretion. Both sexes experience a period of accelerated increase in height at puberty, which is followed by closure of the epiphyses and cessation of growth of long bones. It is the hormone-dependent secondary sex characteristics that help define adult sexual identity and that stabilize the individual's (e) *tertiary (or psychological) sex*, which is the way in which a person identifies him– or herself. Only a handful of mammalian species (e.g., lions, baboons, gorillas) have a level of sexual dimorphism as overt as that of humans. The extent to which the physical differences between the sexes were reinforced by survival versus sexual "signaling" functions in our own and other species during evolution remains controversial. What is clear is that, in humans, identification as a man or a woman is crucial to balanced psychological and social function and is a critical component of self-image and quality of life. It should be borne in mind that any condition that alters a patient's perceived masculinity or femininity is felt as profoundly threatening, well beyond its biologic manifestations.

Male Reproductive Physiology

Activity of the male reproductive system is regulated by the neurosecretory cells contained in the hypothalamus. The axons of these cells end on capillaries of the median eminence, into which, at irregular intervals of 60 to 120 minutes, they secrete surges of a decapeptide, *gonadotropin-releasing hormone (GnRH).* Rather than returning blood directly to the heart, these vessels collect into the pituitary portal veins that ramify as sinusoidal capillaries within the pituitary gland. Thus, GnRH reaches the pituitary in high concentrations, where it stimulates gonadotropic cells to secrete luteinizing hormone (LH) and follicle-stimulating hormone (FSH). LH and FSH are large heterodimeric glycoprotein molecules, each of which consists of a common (identical for both hormones as well as for thyroid-stimulating hormone [TSH]) α subunit and a hormone-specific β subunit.

FSH acts directly on the Sertoli (support) cells of the seminiferous tubules to initiate and maintain early stages of maturation of the male germ cells (i.e., spermatogenesis). Induction of male fertility depends on the presence of FSH. FSH-stimulated Sertoli cells in turn secrete a peptide hormone called *inhibin* that downregulates pituitary production of FSH, forming a closed-loop negative feedback system (Fig. 85.1).

LH acts on the Leydig (interstitial) cells of the testis to stimulate testosterone secretion. Testosterone has effects within the testis to promote spermatogenesis and is also the major circulating steroid that produces and maintains male secondary sex characteristics (discussed earlier). In plasma, testosterone is partially bound to a protein, *sex hormone–binding globulin (SHBG)*, that decreases the testosterone clearance rate. SHBG-bound testosterone is not directly available to target cells but provides a circulating hormone reservoir in equilibrium with the free or bioactive fraction. The level of SHBG varies directly with the estrogen concentration, so that a hypogonadal man with relatively high estradiol may have a total testosterone level within the normal range. The free fraction correlates better than does total plasma testosterone with peripheral androgenic effects. Whether a cell responds to androgens depends on whether it contains androgen receptor protein. In the cells of hair follicles, pubic skin,

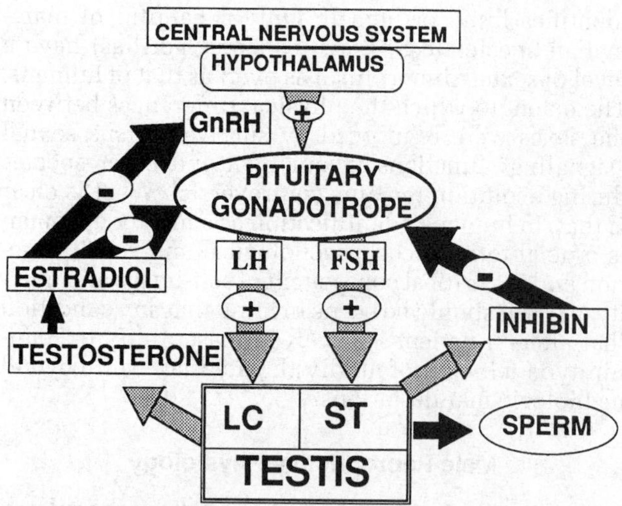

Figure 85.1. Reproductive endocrinology in the male. A variety of central nervous system inputs, from both exogenous (e.g., environmental stress) and endogenous (e.g., biorhythms) sources, act via neurotransmitters and neuropeptides to influence the amplitude and frequency of pulsatile hypothalamic neuronal output *(light gray arrows)* of gonadotropin-releasing hormone (GnRH) into the pituitary portal system. GnRH stimulates pituitary gonadotrophic cells to release luteinizing hormone (LH) and follicle-stimulating hormone (FSH). LH induces the Leydig cell (LC) compartment of the testis to secrete testosterone (T). FSH and T act together to stimulate spermatogenesis in the seminiferous tubule compartment (ST). T acts via negative feedback *(dark gray arrows)* to inhibit gonadotropin and GnRH secretion, probably after aromatization locally to estradiol. Inhibin, produced by the ST in response to FSH, also acts by negative feedback to decrease FSH release.

the prostate gland, and other male sex organs, testosterone is reduced by a cytoplasmic enzyme, 5-alpha-reductase, to 5-alpha-dihydrotestosterone (DHT). It is DHT that binds specifically to the androgen receptors of these organs. In certain other tissues (e.g., skeletal muscle), androgen action is mediated directly by testosterone without reduction to DHT. Similarly, testosterone can be aromatized to estradiol in peripheral adipocytes and, although there are androgen receptors in bone, it appears that estrogens may play a larger role in epiphyseal closure and the preservation of bone mineral density. Physiologic functions of testosterone include stimulation of growth and secretory activity of the prostate and seminal vesicles. Androgens also exert important systemic effects, such as promoting positive nitrogen and calcium balance (with increased muscle and bone formation) and augmenting function of apocrine and sebaceous glands of the skin, which may result in comedones and acne. Testosterone also exerts negative "feedback" at the hypothalamus and pituitary to inhibit secretion of gonadotropins. Thus, the reproductive hormones in men form a closed-loop autoregulated system (Fig. 85.1).

Male Hormones and Libido

Chapter 6 provides a description of the stages of the sexual response that characterize sexual physiology in men. Experimental evidence demonstrates that endogenous testosterone (2) stimulates sexual behavior in the male. Endogenous DHT has been shown to play a role as well (3). Observations on men acutely deprived of testosterone by inhibition of the hypothalamic–pituitary axis with a GnRH analog revealed variable degrees of loss of interest in sexual activity in as little as 2 to 4 weeks (4). Men who are chronically androgen deficient experience reduced arousal in response to sexual cues (e.g., female nudity) as well as less frequent erections and ejaculation. In a study of men with varying degrees of chronic hypogonadism (5), findings suggested the existence of two thresholds for serum testosterone: a level below which the sexual response to erotic stimuli is reduced but nocturnal erections remain intact, and a lower level below which erections are also impaired. In a rat model, testosterone administration to a castrated animal causes increased nitric oxide synthetase activity in genital skin, resulting in nitric oxide–induced vasodilatation and increased erectile function. Many hypogonadal men also report heightened emotional sensitivity, weepiness, and loss of aggressive interest, focus, and drive.

SEXUAL AND REPRODUCTIVE DYSFUNCTION IN MEN

Hypogonadism

Etiology

Failure of the testes to secrete adequate amounts of testosterone for development or maintenance of male secondary sex characteristics, body composition, and libido results in the syndrome of male hypogonadism. Although for purposes of diagnosis and classification, a level of 300 ng/dL of total serum testosterone or 120 ng/dL of free or "bioactive" testosterone is usually (depending on the assays employed) used as the cutoff point for diagnosis of hypogonadism, the clinician should bear in mind that these thresholds are derived from the 95% confidence limits around the mean for a population of young healthy men. Therefore, the definition of hypogonadism they provide is statistical rather than functional. There are no good experimental data that define the actual levels of total or free testosterone below which testosterone effect is suboptimal for various organ systems. For this reason, hypogonadism in a patient should be approached with the entire complex of signs and symptoms in mind and not rigidly defined by a threshold level of a single hormone.

It is helpful to classify male hypogonadism along each of the three axes shown in Fig. 85.2. These axes describe, respectively, the locus of the underlying lesion—*central, gonadal, or peripheral*; the type of underlying pathophysiology—*genetic or acquired,* and whether the onset of clinical manifestations occurs *before or after puberty.* Criteria for classification are shown in Table 85.1. Use of this system of classification narrows the range of possibilities and helps one to arrive more quickly at the correct diagnosis. Examples of classification of various hypogonadal conditions follow.

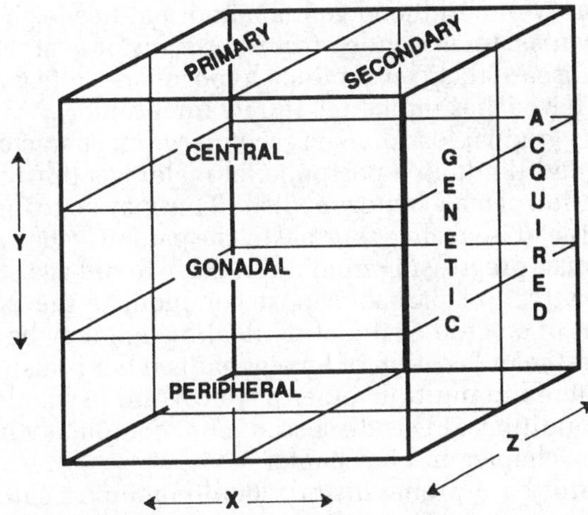

Figure 85.2. Each axis of the cube represents a different way of classifying hypogonadism. There are 12 possible categories and hence 12 "compartments" in the cube. The y-axis represents anatomic location (central, gonadal, peripheral); the z-axis etiology (genetic, acquired); and the x-axis time of onset (primary, secondary).

Table 85.1. Classification of Male Hypogonadism

Classification	Criteria
According to Location of Lesion	
Central (hypothalamic or pituitary)	Gonadotropins ↓ or → Testosterone ↓
Gonadal (testis)	Gonadotropins ↑ Testosterone ↓
Peripheral (failure of end-organ response)	Gonadotropins ↑ Testosterone ↑ or →
According to Etiology	
Genetic	History (especially family history) Buccal smear, karyotype
Acquired	History, physical examination, radiology Evidence of infection, trauma, neoplasia, etc.
According to Time of Onset	
Primary (failure of pubertal development)	History, physical examination
Secondary (loss of previously developed libido and secondary sex characteristics)	

Central. *Central* hypogonadism is dysfunction primarily at the level of the pituitary or the hypothalamus. It is characterized by deficient gonadotropin secretion. One example is *Kallmann syndrome,* which is associated with hyposmia or anosmia and is a result of defective forebrain development leading to absent hypothalamic GnRH secretion. Kallmann syndrome is also *genetic* (i.e., an inherited condition), and it may be caused by a mutation in a gene controlling a nerve secretory factor. The condition is expressed as a failure to mature sexually. *Acquired* hypothalamic failure can also occur, usually as a result of diencephalic tumors or granulomatous disease. Occasionally, pituitary hypogonadism is congenital (i.e., *genetic*), but more commonly it is acquired. The cause may be infectious (e.g., tuberculosis, systemic mycosis), traumatic, vascular (as in infarction with pituitary apoplexy), or, most commonly, neoplastic (usually either a nonsecreting adenoma or a craniopharyngioma). *Central* hypogonadism may also be associated with functioning pituitary tumors, including those that secrete prolactin (prolactinoma), growth hormone (acromegaly), or adrenocorticotropin (Cushing disease) (Chapter 81). Rarely, apparently nonsecreting pituitary adenomas produce a gonadotropin (usually FSH) or a β subunit thereof, leading to confusion of central with gonadal hypogonadism, which is characterized by elevated FSH levels.

Gonadal. The most common cause of *genetic, gonadal* hypogonadism in phenotypic males is Klinefelter syndrome, which, in its classic form, is caused by chromosomal nondisjunction producing XXY genetic sex. These patients have small, firm testes and gynecomastia. They usually enter puberty but fail to progress fully and present with a "eunuchoid habitus" (see later discussion). They typically have erectile dysfunction, a small phallus, and incomplete masculinization. Testosterone levels are generally in the low to low-normal range (200 to 350 ng/dL). Genetic, gonadal hypogonadism may also occur if one or more critical enzymes in the sex steroid synthetic pathway is missing or reduced in activity. Usually such defects involve enzymes common to the adrenal gland and testis and produce ambiguous genitalia or female phenotypic sex in XY individuals. *Acquired* causes of *gonadal* hypogonadism include trauma, cytotoxic agents (usually alkylating chemotherapy or radiation damage), infection (usually viral, such as mumps orchitis, or granulomatous, as in urogenital tuberculosis), and autoimmunity. Autoimmune damage to the testis may occur either alone or as part of a complex of multiple endocrine failure (Hashimoto thyroiditis, idiopathic Addison disease, adult-onset diabetes mellitus, hypoparathyroidism, or pernicious anemia). Occasionally, a varicocele produces partial hypogonadism. Whether these entities result in *secondary* or *primary* hypogonadism depends on the time of life at which the damage occurs.

Peripheral. *Peripheral* hypogonadism is always *genetic* and is caused by absence or dysfunction of androgen receptor protein. It is expressed as a continuum from complete androgen insensitivity (formerly called "testicular feminization"), in which the phenotype is female (affected patients have female external genitalia at birth and normal estrogenization at puberty but lack a uterus and menses); through varying degrees of partial androgen sensitivity, in which midline fusion of labioscrotal structures is highly variable (Reifenstein syndrome), producing gender-assignment confusion at birth; and ending with minor defects such as hypospadias and cryptorchidism, in which phenotypic gender is still clearly male. In all cases, the genetic sex is male (i.e., XY).

Numerous physiologic changes occur in men and women as they age. Although the timing of menopause in women is usually obvious because it is associated with the cessation of menses, the signs and symptoms of testosterone decline in aging men (the "andropause") are often subtle and nonspecific, and they do not occur in all men. Recent data from the Baltimore Longitudinal Study of Aging (6), as well as from other studies, suggest a progressive age-related decline in total testosterone, and a disproportionate decline in indices of unbound testosterone, in healthy aging men. In the Baltimore study, low levels of total testosterone occurred in 19%, 28%, and 49%, respectively, of men in their sixties, seventies, and eighties, whereas the corresponding prevalences of reduced free testosterone levels were 34%, 68%, and 91%. Deficient Leydig cell number and function is the principal cause of the age-related decline in testosterone in men, although numerous studies indicate that there are age-related derangements at all levels of the hypothalamic–pituitary–testicular axis. The decline in testosterone in aging men is hypothesized to contribute to loss of muscle and bone mass and strength and increased adiposity. However, to date it remains unclear whether the andropause represents a distinct clinical syndrome that requires treatment with androgens (see Aging).

Signs and Symptoms of Hypogonadism

Approach to the Patient. The approach to the patient with symptoms suggestive of hypogonadism should be directed first at determining whether hypogonadism truly exists, then at its classification as discussed earlier, next at discovering its specific cause, and finally at providing appropriate therapy and/or referral for the condition diagnosed.

Patient Presentations. Hypogonadism may manifest before puberty as genital intersexuality. A finding of hypospadias, cryptorchidism, or ambiguous genitalia in a patient with symptoms or signs of hypogonadism should lead to further diagnostic procedures. These patients are usually identified at birth and referred to an appropriate specialist, so they rarely present as a diagnostic problem for the primary care practitioner. However, boys are often brought to the attention of clinicians by parents who are concerned with failure of pubertal onset or progression (see Chapter 11).

Prepubertal development of hypogonadism is more commonly expressed as failure of secondary sex characteristics to appear at an appropriate age. It may stem from almost any of the causes cited previously and must be differentiated from constitutional delayed puberty, which is a common, idiopathic, self-limited, familial condition. A strong family history of late blooming and a finding of beginning enlargement of the testicles are reassuring in this regard. A set of standards for pubertal development of adolescent boys is available (see Chapter 11). In general, any boy who reaches 16 years of age without signs of pubertal onset (one of the first changes being an increase in testicular size) or who begins but does not complete puberty by age 18 years deserves further investigation. The index of suspicion should be heightened if the patient has a history of childhood genital abnormalities (e.g., hypospadias, undescended testes) or signs or symptoms of a disease that can produce hypogonadism (e.g., severe headaches indicating intracranial tumor).

The gradual loss of male secondary sex characteristics (and libido in a postpubertal male) is a third presentation of male hypogonadism. This may be so insidious that it is taken for normal by the patient, especially in a man progressing from middle age to old age.

Finally, and probably most common, is the complaint of erectile dysfunction (ED), which may be the earliest manifestation of hypogonadism but is also encountered in multiple other physical and psychological conditions. ED is discussed more completely later in this chapter and in Chapter 6.

History. A proper history should include a chronicle of pubertal progression, with time of appearance of pubic hair, beard growth, voice change, growth spurts, erections, and ejaculations. Of critical interest are loss or diminution of libido and erections or ejaculations, slowing of beard growth, thinning of body and pubic hair, changes in the breast (i.e., swelling or tenderness), and loss of aggressive impulse or drive. Severely hypogonadal men may report "hot flashes" and sweats similar to those associated with the menopause in women. The presence of headaches, double vision, or reduced peripheral vision may give clues to a pituitary tumor. Symptoms of hypothyroidism, adrenal failure, acromegaly, diabetes mellitus, anemia, pulmonary disease, or autoimmune disease (conditions dealt with in other chapters of this book) should be sought. A history of urologic problems, cryptorchidism, hypospadias, or episodes of orchitis is important. Finally, a family history of delayed puberty or of other endocrine abnormalities may suggest either hereditary late blooming in the case of prepubertal hypogonadism or familial autoimmune endocrinopathy in cases with postpubertal hypogonadism.

Physical Examination. The body habitus and facies should be evaluated first. Does the patient look mature or babyish? masculine or feminine? A lower body segment (femoral greater trochanter to floor) longer than the upper segment (femoral greater trochanter to crown) and an arm span greater than height defines "eunuchoid" proportions and suggests pubertal or prepubertal hypogonadism. Good muscle mass, axillary hair, and a palpable prostate on digital rectal examination militate against long-standing hypogonadism. Male pattern baldness is an androgen-dependent process. The presence of comedones, especially in the tragus of the ear, is a good sign of androgen activity. Complexion should be noted, because increased pigmentation suggests primary adrenal failure, and dry flaky skin suggests hypothyroidism. Vital signs should always be evaluated. The presence of hypertension may indicate an adrenal enzyme defect or Cushing disease, whereas postural hypotension may alert the clinician to Addison disease. Special attention should be paid to the eyes to look for limitation of extraocular movements, papilledema, or restriction of visual fields, all suggestive of an intracranial tumor. Examination of the male breast should include careful palpation for the subareolar thickening and nodularity that may be the only evidence of gynecomastia (see later discussion). Squeezing of the nipple may elicit galactorrhea, which, although rare in males, is highly suggestive of a prolactinoma.

Examination of the genitals is critical. Pubic hair pattern should extend up the linea alba to the umbilicus in a diamond shaped pattern (the so-called male escutcheon); a triangular pattern, cut off at the pubis, suggests androgen deficiency, as does sparse or excessively fine pubic hair. Penis size and location of urethral meatus, scrotal rugosity and pigmentation, and size and turgor of the testicles should all be noted. The normal adult testis should be no less than 15 mL in volume (approximately 4.0 × 3.0 cm) and should have the resistance to palpation of a firm, ripe plum. An "overripe," softer feeling is a sign of testicular atrophy. Careful palpation of the left side of the scrotum while the patient performs a Valsalva maneuver may reveal the presence of a varicocele, which is almost always on the left side. Approximately 5% of varicoceles are associated with reduced testosterone production from both testes (venous drainage from the left testis crosses over to the right). Rectal examination should assess prostate size, because the prostate shrinks with testosterone deficiency. Careful neurologic examination should include testing of the sense of smell to look for Kallmann syndrome.

Differential Diagnosis. The tests that give the most information about suspected male hypogonadism are serum testosterone and gonadotropin (LH and FSH) measurements. Table 85.1 shows the hormonal patterns typical of *central, gonadal, and peripheral* hypogonadism in males. These determinations are readily available from most commercial laboratories, and variability in results can be attributed to true biologic and/or assay differences. Ninety-five percent of adult men have morning serum testosterone levels between 300 and 1,200 ng/dL (with most between 450 to 700 ng/dL). Borderline values between 250 and 350 ng/dL should be considered suspicious. It is important that testosterone levels be determined in the morning, because the diurnal variation in testosterone concentration can produce an afternoon and evening decrement of as much as 200 ng/dL. Abnormal or ambiguous determinations should be repeated at least once for confirmation, because there is considerable variability both in radioimmunoassay determinations and, from time to time, in an individual patient. Total plasma testosterone is affected by variation in plasma SHBG levels in states such as aging, obesity, and liver disease. If testosterone levels are repeatedly in the borderline range, it may be helpful to obtain a measure of unbound testosterone. This can be done by assaying for either "bioactive" (non–SHBG-bound) or free (non–SHBG-, non–albumin-bound) testosterone. The latter should either be measured by dialysis methods or calculated from the values of total testosterone and SHBG using standard algorithms. Analog and radioimmunoassay methods for the direct measure of free testosterone should not be used, because they are unreliable.

In normal men, serum LH varies from 2 to 30 mIU/mL and FSH from 2 to 16 mIU/mL, but different assays have different ranges of normal. Low or normal LH and FSH in the presence of subnormal testosterone defines *central* hypogonadism. Increased gonadotropin levels with low testosterone indicate gonadal failure, except in rare cases of an FSH-secreting pituitary adenoma. Central hypogonadism caused by prolactin-secreting pituitary tumors (prolactinomas) is usually accompanied by plasma prolactin levels of 100 ng/mL or more. Impotence is an especially prominent symptom in hyperprolactinemic hypogonadism.

Peripheral hypogonadism (resistance to testosterone action) is a form of hypogonadism characterized by normal or increased testosterone levels. Gonadotropin levels are high or normal. Because, as noted earlier, these patients have some degree of intersexuality at birth, they rarely present a diagnostic problem. High gonadotropin and normal testosterone levels may also be seen in evolving central hypogonadism, especially that associated with age, when an increase in pituitary gonadotropin secretion is still able to compensate for the testicular failure.

Further investigation and initiation of treatment of proven hypogonadism should probably be undertaken by a specialist in endocrinology. Table 85.2 lists various investigative procedures and types of patients for whom they are pertinent.

Referral to a urologist for testicular biopsy may be helpful in diagnosing traumatic or infectious damage. Biopsy also shows a diagnostic form of shrinkage and hyalinization of tubules in Klinefelter syndrome. The procedure is rarely required and may cause hemorrhage and considerable pain. About 1 week is required for full recovery. Therefore, it usually should

Table 85.2. Additional Investigations That Are Useful in the Evaluation of Hypogonadism

Type of Failure	Radiologic Procedure	Hormone Measurements	Other Tests
Central	Skull film	Prolactin	Visual fields (formal)
	Computed tomography scan with contrast	Thyroxine (T_4)	Clomiphene test
	Magnetic resonance scan	Thyroid-stimulating hormone	Luteinizing hormone–releasing hormone test
	Cerebral angiogram	Cortisol (morning)	
		Growth hormone (with glucose tolerance test)	
Gonadal	Bone age (If primary)	T_4	Buccal smear
		Cortisol (morning)	Karyotyping Gonad biopsy

be undertaken only after consultation with an endocrinologist to confirm that the procedure is necessary to provide useful diagnostic information.

Hypogonadism Associated with Chronic Disease

It is now recognized that a variety of acute and chronic illnesses are often associated with male hypogonadism.

Severe acute illness is associated with dramatic declines in serum testosterone levels. The reason is not clear, but it is probably a combination of hypothalamic stress, anesthesia (when administered), and starvation. In most situations, the mechanism is central hypogonadism, suggested by the observation that serum FSH levels decline in postmenopausal women admitted to intensive care units, particularly if there has been any weight loss (7).

Before the widespread use of highly active antiretroviral treatment, nearly one third of men infected with the human immunodeficiency virus (HIV) were found to be hypogonadal. Multiple mechanisms appear to be responsible, including central abnormalities caused by granulomatous invasion of the hypothalamus or the pituitary gland and gonadal derangements resulting from prior use of cytoxan or other alkylating agents. Most often, the cause is central hypogonadism and is nonspecifically related to "stress." Similar observations have been made in men with other chronic diseases, such as cancer, heart disease, chronic renal failure, and diabetes mellitus (8,9). Investigations are ongoing to determine whether testosterone therapy would be beneficial in these disease states. There is evidence that HIV-infected men increase their weight, lean body mass, and muscle strength after 3 months of testosterone administration (10,11). It is not clear, however, whether these changes result in increased survival or decreased morbidity.

Therapy for Men with Hypogonadism

Therapy for central hypogonadism depends on the underlying cause and the patient's need for either virilization alone or virilization plus fertility. Central hypogonadism can be caused by a secretory or a nonsecretory tumor. An imaging procedure, usually magnetic resonance imaging with gadolinium, can detect a mass affecting the hypothalamus, the pituitary stalk, or the pituitary gland. Surgery is commonly required for tumors originating from the brain and affecting the hypothalamus. Similarly, tumors compressing the stalk or invading the pituitary gland and causing hypopituitarism or a visual field disturbance are also treated with a primary surgical approach, and possibly with postoperative radiation therapy. If, however, the tumor is secretory, usually a prolactinoma, then medical therapy is the first approach.

In patients with prolactinomas, treatment with synthetic dopamine agonists has proved effective not only in lowering serum prolactin, increasing gonadotropins and testosterone, and restoring libido but also in shrinking tumor mass and improving vision. Bromocriptine, the drug that has been used the longest, is associated with a high incidence of gastrointestinal side effects (dyspepsia, nausea, vomiting, cramping, or diarrhea in 10% to 15% of patients), some of which may be ameliorated by administration of the drug in divided doses with food or with an antacid. High dosages of bromocriptine have also been associated with depression and bizarre dreams or nightmares. Bromocriptine usually is started at a dosage of one 2.5-mg tablet/day and increased by one tablet/day each week up to a maximum of three tablets/day to obtain the desired effect. Dosages as high as 16 to 24 mg/day are sometimes necessary, but they are associated with frequent side effects. A long-acting dopamine agonist that is more specific for the D_2 receptor, cabergoline (Dostinex), is now available. The usual dosage is 0.5 mg twice a week (12). Cabergoline has a lower incidence of adverse effects than does bromocriptine (13) and may work well in patients in whom bromocriptine does not (14). Neurosurgery should be used only in circumstances in which dopamine agonists cannot be tolerated or are ineffective.

Once the underlying etiology is addressed, the next question is the specific treatment for the hypogonadism. If the patient is interested only in virilization and not in fertility, the aim of therapy is to replace deficient androgen, which may be necessary in patients with either central or gonadal hypogonadism (15). The reasons for replacing testosterone in male hypogonadism are multiple. The most pressing reason is to ameliorate or reverse the symptoms of testosterone deficiency (e.g., hot flashes, reduced libido, ED, emotional lability) and to restore male secondary sex characteristics (e.g., beard growth, pubic hair). Beyond this however, it has become increasingly apparent from a variety of clinical studies that testosterone deficiency in adults is associated with negative nitrogen balance, loss of lean body mass and muscle strength (16), loss of bone calcium with reduced bone mineral density (i.e., osteoporosis), and an increase in percent body fat with greater central fat distribution. The latter is, in turn, accompanied by deterioration of the serum lipid pattern (increased low-density lipoprotein cholesterol and triglyceride) and insulin resistance, and hence, presumably, by an increased risk of cardiovascular disease. Testosterone replacement can improve or reverse the hypogonadal changes in body composition and function (17,18). A third goal of treatment, correction of infertility, requires an alternative approach (see later discussion).

Testosterone Replacement Therapy. Options for testosterone replacement include transdermal patches (either scrotal or nonscrotal), topical creams, and implantable pellets (oral preparations are hepatotoxic and should not be used). The "tried and true" method is injection of testosterone enanthate (e.g., Delatestryl), cypionate, or other esters in oil. Effective therapy requires deep intramuscular injection at regular intervals. Therapy in usually started at 200 mg every 2 weeks. A lower dose or doses at greater intervals might be used in prepubertal males. The testosterone level should be measured at the midpoint between injections. This type of injection therapy inevitably produces unphysiologically high plasma testosterone levels immediately after injection that may fall to deficient levels before the next injection, depending on the dosage and interval. Another limitation is that the injections are moderately painful and necessitate regular visits to the caregiver's office or clinic.

Three forms of transdermal testosterone patches are now approved for use in the United States. All appear equally effective at mimicking the normal circadian rhythm (due to their slow release of testosterone) and at relieving the symptoms, improving body composition, and so forth in male hypogonadism. Testoderm is available as a 5-g scrotal or nonscrotal patch. It requires daily application of a single patch to the scrotal skin, which usually must be shaved. A potential limitation on use of this product is insufficient size of the scrotum in pubertal failure or long-standing hypogonadism. Serum DHT levels are usually elevated with this patch owing to the high concentration of 5-alpha-reductase in scrotal skin. The nonscrotal Testoderm patch is placed daily in the morning so that peak serum levels occur approximately 3 hours later. Whether this leads to increased growth of prostate tissue is currently unknown. Although it is well tolerated, the patch can dislodge with excessive sweating.

The 5-g Androderm patch results in peak serum testosterone levels 12 hours after application and can be applied to any skin surface that does not have underlying bony projections (e.g., back, thigh, chest, buttocks). Although the patch adheres fairly well, some men develop skin irritation and, occasionally, severe skin reactions. This can be prevented by use of triamcinolone ointment before application of Androderm.

The most recently approved form of testosterone replacement therapy is Androgel 1%, which is available in 2.5- and 5-g packets. This clear liquid is rubbed on the upper arms and abdomen every morning. The dose of 5 g results in mean serum testosterone levels of approximately 600 ng/dL. The gel is well tolerated with little or no skin irritation, but it is more expensive than the other forms of replacement. Because there can be some transference of gel within 1 hour after application, Androgel is not recommended in situations where the patient has regular skin-to-skin contact, such as frequent holding of infants.

It must be remembered that the replacement of testosterone may fail to restore sexual competence in hyperprolactinemic patients because of the antisexual effects of prolactin itself. In these cases, either surgery to remove the prolactinoma or a prolactin-lowering drug (see earlier discussion) may be required for potency to be restored.

Fertility. In addition to treating the underlying structural abnormality (e.g., by means of pituitary surgery) and testosterone replacement therapy, a third goal in hypogonadal patients may be to restore or improve fertility. Patients with gonadal hypogonadism may or may not be infertile, depending on the underlying lesion. Infertility that is primarily gonadal is usually resistant to medical intervention. Moreover, replacement of testosterone, by whatever means, suppresses LH and FSH, causing reduced sperm counts and testicular atrophy.

In patients with *central* hypogonadism (i.e., LH or FSH deficiency), infertility as well as deficient testosterone levels may be treated with gonadotropins. Human chorionic gonadotropin (hCG) may be used for its LH-like activity (human LH is unavailable). Injections of 2,000 IU of hCG (Pregnyl or Follutein) intramuscularly three times a week normalizes testosterone levels, usually within 1 month after initiation of therapy, and may also stimulate spermatogenesis. In patients with central failure, agents with both LH (hCG) and FSH-like activity may be required to initiate spermatogenesis. Because of the requirement for more frequent injections compared with testosterone, use of gonadotropin injections probably should be restricted to those patients with central hypogonadism who are concerned about fertility.

Safety of Testosterone Replacement. In general, testosterone replacement is a safe and effective treatment for male hypogonadism. Although testosterone therapy does not induce prostate cancer, it can cause such a cancer to grow and/or spread. The high prevalence of prostate cancer in older men necessitates that blood be obtained for measurement of prostate-specific antigen (PSA) and that a digital rectal examination be done before initiation of therapy. If either is abnormal, the patient should be referred to a urologist.

In addition, testosterone is a known stimulator of erythropoietin (Epo). In fact, testosterone is still occasionally used therapeutically as a safe and inexpensive alternative to Epo administration in patients with chronic anemia. However, testosterone replacement carries the risk of induction of erythrocytosis. In epidemiologic studies, hematocrit values greater than 45% were associated with an increased risk of stroke. Hematocrit values need to be monitored carefully in men who are receiving testosterone. Testosterone administration should not be started if the baseline hematocrit value is greater than 52%.

There are no definitive data to suggest that physiologic testosterone replacement alters glucose tolerance or serum high-density lipoprotein (HDL) levels, whereas supraphysiologic testosterone doses have been found to lower serum HDL.

Follow-Up for Men Treated with Testosterone Replacement Therapy. Follow-up of treated patients should include questions about sexual function as well as assessment of body habitus, beard growth, and, in patients with failure of pubertal development, growth in stature, growth of phallus, and depth of voice. Libido and potency usually return within a few weeks after initiation of treatment, whereas secondary sex characteristics improve gradually after 6 to 12 months. The patient should be evaluated for the possible development of gynecomastia or of prostate enlargement with symptoms of urethral obstruction as side effects of therapy. Hematocrit levels should be measured every 3 to 6 months, and the dose of testosterone should be reduced if the hematocrit rises to more than 52%.

Blood should also be obtained for the measurement of serum PSA. If the level rises above the normal range, the testosterone should be discontinued until a urologist can be consulted.

Gynecomastia

Importance

Significant enlargement of the male breast requires a clinician's attention so that those cases with a serious hormonal or neoplastic cause can be distinguished from the common benign idiopathic forms.

Etiology

During early adolescence, gynecomastia is common as plasma sex steroid hormone levels rise (occurring in up to 65% of boys age 14 years), but breast enlargement regresses spontaneously in most and is present in fewer than 15% of boys by age 17. Prevalence of gynecomastia increases again in the twenties, remains stable at around 25%, and increases gradually to approximately 60% of men age 50 years and older. This mild idiopathic gynecomastia is almost always less than 5 cm in diameter and causes no symptoms. Noticeable gynecomastia of greater than 5 cm in diameter may be the first clue to the presence of a benign or malignant adrenal or testicular neoplasm or a pituitary prolactinoma. In the case of adrenal tumors, there are usually associated symptoms and signs of Cushing syndrome. Malignancies of the testis, lung, stomach, and occasionally other cancers may secrete hCG, which can overstimulate testicular steroid production and thus lead, indirectly, to gynecomastia. Hypothyroidism and hyperthyroidism have also been associated with breast enlargement. The taking of exogenous estrogen, either purposely (by individuals with gender dysphoria or with prostate carcinoma) or accidentally because of estrogenic activity of various medications (e.g., diazepam, cimetidine, spironolactone, digitalis glycosides) should always be considered. Another iatrogenic cause is peripheral conversion to estrogens of excess androgens during testosterone or hCG therapy. Gynecomastia is also common in liver failure, in which hepatic metabolism of endogenous androgens is impaired. Finally, true gynecomastia must be differentiated from the "gynecoid" breast, seen in obesity and old age, which contains increased fatty tissue but not glandular breast tissue, and also from carcinoma of the male breast. Approximately 1% of all breast carcinomas occur in men.

Approach to the Patient

History. The duration and age at onset of breast swelling are important; for example, recent onset of breast swelling in a 30-year-old man would be of more concern than in an adolescent or than gradual breast enlargement in a 70-year-old man. The presence of tenderness or discharge and the quality of the discharge (clear, turbid, bloody) should be noted. Any symptoms of hypogonadism (see previous discussion) should be elicited, as should symptoms of hypothyroidism (see Chapter 80) or Cushing disease (see Chapter 81). A careful medication history and sexual history may reveal an exogenous cause.

Physical Examination. In general, the examination should be the same as for hypogonadism (described earlier), with the addition that signs of Cushing disease and thyroid disease should be emphasized. Deep palpation of the upper abdomen may reveal an adrenal tumor or downward displacement of the kidney by such a tumor. Careful bimanual palpation of the testicles may detect a secretory tumor (androblastoma). A useful formal system for staging of breast development was described by Marshall and Tanner in adolescent girls (see Chapter 11), but it is equally useful for staging of gynecomastia. Briefly, at stage I there is minimal proliferation of glandular tissue just beneath the areola. At stage II a flat pad of glandular tissue spreads beyond the bounds of the areola (i.e., greater than 5 cm). At stage III this pad rounds up, lifting the breast area forward from the chest wall in a cone shape with the nipple at the tip. At stage IV the areola spreads laterally as subareolar gland proliferation gives the breast a double-contoured appearance. Finally, further maturation with increase in fatty tissue results in the mature single contour of stage V. The examiner needs to differentiate among proliferation of glandular breast tissue (firm, slightly lobulated, and symmetrically distributed from the nipple outward with a limited boundary); fat (softer, diffusely distributed, and with no clear separation from surrounding subcutaneous adipose tissue); and tumor (hard, nodular, frequently tender, often fixed to skin or underlying muscle, and eccentrically located with regard to the nipple). Milky nipple discharge on firm squeezing suggests prolactinoma; clear or bloody discharge suggests breast cancer. Unilateral breast enlargement should increase the suspicion of neoplasia, but asymmetry occurs in 10% to 15% of patients with idiopathic gynecomastia. The decision whether further investigation is required depends on the age of the patient, the rapidity of enlargement of the breast, and the degree of such enlargement. Men between 18 and 45 years of age with recent onset of rapidly enlarging mammary glands, or with glandular breast tissue diameter greater than 5 cm, or with symptoms or signs suggesting hypogonadism, hypothyroidism, or Cushing disease, should receive further attention.

Diagnostic Procedures. Determinations of serum levels of estradiol, testosterone, gonadotropins (LH and FSH), serum prolactin, and hCG-β subunit are indicated. If the serum estradiol is greater than 50 pg/mL and if the testosterone/estradiol ratio is reduced to less than 100:1, the diagnosis of estrogen-secreting testicular tumor is strongly suggested. Elevation of 24-hour urinary 17-ketosteroids indicates an adrenal cause, in which case adrenal hyperfunction should be investigated with the diagnosis of adrenal neoplasm in mind (see Chapter 81). Gynecomastia in late adolescence or young adulthood accompanied by testicular atrophy (small, very firm testes) and low or low-normal testosterone levels with increased FSH and LH suggests the diagnosis of Klinefelter syndrome (XXY trisomy).

Elevated serum hCG should prompt a search for occult malignancy with particular attention to gonads, lungs, and gastrointestinal tract. Elevated prolactin concentrations could be associated with use of certain medications (especially major tranquilizers) or with a pituitary prolactinoma (see Chapter 81). The possibility of hypothyroidism should be evaluated by thyroxine (T_4), and TSH determinations. Finally, patients with firm, nodular, unilateral, or notably eccentric enlargement should be referred for mammography or surgical biopsy of the breast.

Therapy

Drug-induced gynecomastia remits gradually (in several months) if the drug is discontinued. Treatment of primary endocrine disease (e.g., prolactinoma, adrenal tumor, hCG-secreting carcinoma) should be undertaken by an appropriate specialist once the diagnosis is clear. Remission of the accompanying gynecomastia depends on the success of the treatment and the stage of advancement of breast development. If idiopathic gynecomastia is a cosmetic problem, plastic surgical excision of breast tissue is usually the therapeutic method of choice. It is important to bear in mind that breast development that has progressed beyond Tanner stage II (see Chapter 11) will never fully regress even if the proximate cause is corrected and therefore will require surgical intervention if complete cosmetic correction is desired.

Erectile Dysfunction

In this section, ED and loss of libido are considered only as they relate to endocrine disorders. For a more general treatment of sexual dysfunction, see Chapter 6. Briefly, ED is the inability to achieve or maintain erection satisfactorily enough to effect penetration and ejaculation. Transient or occasional ED is common and not necessarily evidence of a medical problem, but a pattern of repeated episodes (more than 25% of opportunities) lasting longer than 1 month should be investigated. ED may or may not be accompanied by loss of libido, depending on the cause.

Etiology

A disorder of any of the systems that maintain the sexual response and apparatus may lead to impotence. Causes may therefore be of several types: (a) *psychological* (see Chapter 6); (b) *vascular,* either of the arterial type, with diminished blood supply to the corpora cavernosa (e.g., congenital vascular anomaly, traumatic injury to vessels, large vessel atherosclerosis, disease of smaller peripheral vessels), or as a result of venous incompetence, in which partial erections occur but blood drains off because of "venous leak"; (c) *neuropathic,* involving damage to the peripheral pelvic autonomic nerves (e.g., diabetic neuropathy, heavy metal poisoning, nerve trauma) or disease of the spinal cord or brain (e.g., tumor, multiple sclerosis) that inhibits or obliterates the erectile response; (d) *toxic,* caused by substances of abuse (e.g., alcohol, opiates, major tranquilizers) that can acutely and chronically diminish sexual ability or any of a number of medications that affect the autonomic and central nervous system (e.g., tranquilizers, sympatholytic antihypertensives); (e) *debilitative,* related to various severe and chronic medical illnesses (e.g., malignancy, renal failure) that are accompanied by loss of sex drive and/or ED; and (f) *endocrine,* including hypogonadism and prolactinoma (see earlier discussion) as causes of ED.

Other endocrine diseases that commonly produce sexual dysfunction are hyperthyroidism and hypothyroidism, Cushing syndrome, and acromegaly. In one series of patients referred to a major diagnostic center for persistent symptoms without apparent psychiatric cause, 35% were found to have an endocrine disorder (19).

Approach to the Patient

History. The duration of symptoms, the frequency with which intercourse is attempted, and the percentage of attempts ending in erectile failure should be recorded to determine whether the ED is absolute or relative and whether it is progressing. ED unaccompanied by loss of libido suggests a neurologic or vascular problem, whereas loss of interest in sexual activity is consistent with either hypogonadism or a psychological cause. The history should include the patient's marital situation, whether there are sex partners other than the spouse, the perceived level of partners' desire, and a social and work history to determine whether there is excessive stress. Situational ED (i.e., experienced with one partner but not another) is good evidence of a psychological problem. Normal men often awaken in the morning with an erection. This is a local response to a full bladder; detumescence follows urination. Preservation of morning erections is good evidence against vascular or neuropathic disease; however, in the cited series (19), 14% of patients with an endocrine cause maintained morning erections. A history of medication use and substance abuse should be diligently sought. Heavy smoking is often associated with a peripheral vascular cause of impotence. The patient should be asked about symptoms of hypothyroidism or hyperthyroidism, Cushing disease, diabetes, peripheral neuropathy (paraesthesia, hyperesthesia, burning or shooting pains) or central nervous system disease, and vascular disease (claudication, angina, cold extremities, skin ulcers).

Physical Examination. The physical examination should be conducted with particular attention to the manifestations of hypogonadism described earlier, to signs of thyroid or adrenal disease (see Chapters 80 and 81), and also to signs of peripheral vascular disease (peripheral pulses, skin temperature, skin atrophy, hair loss) (see Chapter 94) and central or peripheral neuropathy (see Chapter 92).

Diagnostic Procedures. Hormone determinations should be used to investigate for hypogonadism or prolactinoma (see earlier discussion). If historical or physical findings lead to a suspicion of thyroid or adrenal disease, appropriate tests should be done (see Chapters 80 and 81). A fasting blood sugar measurement should always be obtained to screen for diabetes mellitus (see Chapter 79). Spontaneous erection during sleep (nocturnal penile tumescence) has been thought to absolutely exclude an organic cause of ED, but that impression is probably not valid.

Nocturnal penile tumescence may be tested by the patient at home using a "snap gauge," but, for definitive measurement, studies should be conducted with the use of quantitative instrumentation in a sleep laboratory. Definitive diagnosis of vascular disorders may require Doppler studies of penile blood flow or selective angiography, and venous incompetence may be revealed by dynamic cavernosography, all procedures used by urologists specializing in the diagnosis and treatment of ED. If peripheral neuropathy seems a likely cause, it can often be confirmed by referral to a urologist for bladder manometrics and to a neurologist for nerve conduction velocity measurements (see Chapter 92).

Therapy

Therapeutic efforts should be directed at the specific cause of the ED, whenever one can be found. Psychological ED may respond to various therapeutic modalities depending on its severity and associated problems (see Chapter 6). Vascular disease may respond to medication or to surgical revascularization. Caution should be exercised in this regard: Whereas good results are often obtained with surgery in young patients with traumatic or congenital abnormalities, results are almost always disappointing in older patients with atherosclerotic disease, perhaps because of the involvement of smaller peripheral vessels in the process. Neuropathic ED is occasionally reversible with removal of the inciting lesion (e.g., spinal cord tumor) or with aggressive diabetic control, but, if irreversible, it may also be treated with local measures (discussed later). Drug-induced ED is usually reversed if the offending agent can be discontinued. Treatment of hypogonadism has already been discussed. If sexual function does not improve within 6 weeks after specific therapy for an organic cause has been instituted, consideration should be given to the possibility that the experience and expectation of sexual failure are inhibiting the response (so-called performance anxiety) even though the primary cause is no longer present. Such secondary psychological ED may respond to psychological or behavioral therapy (see Chapter 6).

There are also approaches to therapy that may succeed in restoring sexual function despite an irremediable (e.g., vascular or neuropathic) cause. Sildenafil citrate (Viagra), an oral therapy for ED, is a selective inhibitor of cyclic guanosine monophosphate–specific phosphodiesterase type 5. The inhibition of this enzyme leads to increased concentrations of nitric oxide, resulting in vasodilatation and increased genital blood flow. Oral doses of 50 to 100 mg should be taken 30 minutes before the onset of sexual activity. Because there is some cross-reactivity with other phosphodiesterases, a side effect can include headaches and seeing a blue discoloration (due to retinal activation). Sildenafil is effective in approximately 60% of cases, but it is contraindicated in men who are taking nitroglycerin-type medications.

Other therapies generally require urologic consultation. Implantable penile prostheses have been used extensively but, because of local complications, are no longer as popular as they once were. Implants come in two basic types: those that are permanently stiff or semiflexible, and more complex devices that inflate by means of a pump and valve mechanism. Another option is the use of a device that draws blood into the penis by negative pressure, then retains it there with an occlusive ring applied to the base of the penis. A number of different types of suction devices are available. Although earlier reports stressed the satisfactory results obtained in selected patients, continuing experience with these devices has been less positive. For example, one retrospective study found that 81% of men using vacuum devices abandoned them because they "did not work," and that patients' attitudes toward the device were unfavorable overall (20).

For patients who cannot take sildenafil, injection of vasoactive agents directly into the corpus cavernosum is probably the most popular treatment. Various combinations have been used. Most effective is prostaglandin E_1 (PGE_1, alprostadil) or papaverine combined with phentolamine. One study concluded that papaverine plus phentolamine is about as effective as PGE_1, with similar rates of overly prolonged erections but significantly less pain (21). Cavernosal injection therapy usually produces erections lasting 30 minutes to several hours. Although it is highly effective, especially in the neuropathic ED of diabetes mellitus, injection therapy should be supervised by a urologist familiar with its use, because priapism is a potentially serious and fairly common (2% to 4%) acute complication. A long-term, but rare, complication is gradual fibrosis of the corpora cavernosa with loss of responsiveness. A promising newer modality, recently approved by the U.S. Food and Drug Administration, is alprostadil administered as a urethral suppository (MUSE). Studies show efficacy and adverse effect rates comparable to those of injection therapy (22,23), but experience with this method is still relatively limited.

Aging

Andropause–Epidemiology

A series of early investigations found that men's testosterone levels declined with age and that protein binding of testosterone to SHBG increased with age, resulting in a profound decrease in mean free (bioavailable) testosterone. In these same reports, the changes in androgens were generally accompanied by an increase in circulating estrone and estradiol and in gonadotropins. Decreases in free or bioactive testosterone remained disproportionate because of significant increases in SHBG. This decline could be observed even in studies in which older men were carefully selected to match younger men in terms of health, obesity, alcohol intake, and social class. Several longitudinal studies of the effects of age on sex steroids have demonstrated a significant decrease with age in both total testosterone and the free testosterone index (24). Although "male menopause" is a poor choice of words, "male andropause" is more appropriate, referring to age-related reductions in the production of testosterone and adrenal androgens. The clinical significance of the "male andropause" remains controversial. Independent of changes in levels of sex steroids, numerous studies in healthy men have revealed a steady decrease in both sexual interest and ability, with decreases in frequency of intercourse from an average of two to three events a week to fewer than two a month by age 70 to 75 (25). This decrease does not appear to be directly related to hypogonadism but probably reflects changes in other (i.e., nervous and vascular) systems that occur with age. There are no data to support a beneficial effect of administration of androgens to aging men whose testosterone levels are normal; however, there is improvement in sexual function, both libido and erectile function, in men with symptoms of hypogonadism, and men with free or total testosterone levels in the low-normal range appear to benefit from androgen replacement therapy. This benefit is usually more pronounced in younger men, compared with older men, because the latter commonly have comorbidities that complicate the mechanism of the sexual dysfunction. However, older men with abnormally low testosterone levels should be investigated in the same way as are other men with suspected hypogonadism and treated appropriately.

Even if an older man is not interested in sexual function, there are now several studies that suggest that there are other benefits of testosterone replacement therapy. Testosterone administration improves body composition, with increases in muscle mass and decreases in body fat, in aged andropausal men (26), as it does in frankly hypogonadal young and middle-aged men (27). In one recent investigation, testosterone supplementation of healthy aged men with low serum testosterone levels increased lumbosacral spine bone mineral density during a 3-year treatment period (28). However, men with low-normal testosterone levels did not benefit. Whether the increase in muscle mass is associated with improved functional status or with decreased morbidity or mortality remains to be determined.

The potential for testosterone therapy to improve cognitive function in older men, and perhaps to prevent or attenuate some of the symptoms of Alzheimer disease, is of great potential interest. Sex steroids exert multiple effects on brain function. Boys and men perform better than girls and women on neuropsychological tests of spatial relationships, whereas the opposite is true for tests of verbal fluency. Testosterone appears to exert some, if not all, of its effects on the brain after its conversion to estrogen. In one demographic survey, Barrett-Connor et al. (29) measured the association between baseline testosterone and neuropsychological performance in men between the ages of 59 and 89 years of age. After controlling for a number of possible confounding variables, higher bioavailable testosterone concentrations were observed in men who scored better on a measure of long-term verbal memory. In a recent randomized placebo-controlled clinical trial, testosterone replacement in older men was reported to improve visuospatial performance and verbal memory (30).

General References*

Roth J, Koch CA, Rother KI. Aging, endocrinology, and the elderly patient, In: DeGroot, eds. Endocrinology 4th ed, vol. 1. Philadelphia: WB Saunders, 2001:529.

Comprehensive review of effects of aging on hormone balance, including the male and female reproductive systems.

Santen RJ. The testis. In: Felig P, Baxter JD, Broadus AE, Frohman LA, eds. Endocrinology and metabolism. 3rd ed. New York: McGraw-Hill, 1995:885.

Excellent discussion of the physiology and pathology of the male reproductive system.

Specific References

1. Frank E, Anderson C, Rubinstein D. Frequency of sexual dysfunction in normal couples. N Engl J Med 1978;299:111.
2. Davidson JM. Hormones and sexual behaviour in the male. Hosp Pract 1975;10:126.
3. Mantzoros CS, Georgiadis EI, Trichopoulos D. Contribution of dihydrotestosterone to male sexual behaviour. BMJ 1995; 310:1289.
4. Loosen PT, Purdon SE, Pavlou SN. Effects on behavior of modulation of gonadal function in men with gonadotropin-releasing hormone antagonists. Am J Psychiatry 1994;151:271.
5. Carani C, Granata AR, Fustini MF, et al. Prolactin and testosterone: their role in male sexual function. Int J Androl 1996; 19:48.
6. Harman SM, Metter EJ, Tobin JD, et al. Longitudinal effects of aging on serum total and free testosterone levels in healthy men. Baltimore Longitudinal Study of Aging. J Clin Endocrinol Metab 2001;86:724.
7. Gebhart SS, Watts NB, Clark RV, et al. Reversible impairment of gonadotropin secretion in critical illness: observations in postmenopausal women. Arch Intern Med 1989;149:1637.
8. Baker HW. Reproductive effects of nontesticular illness. Endocrinol Metab Clin North Am 1998;27:831.
9. Nierman DM, Mechanick JI. Hypotestosteronemia in chronically critically ill men. Crit Care Med 1999;27:2418.
10. Bhasin S, Woodhouse L, Storer TW. Proof of the effect of testosterone on skeletal muscle. J Endocdrinol 2001;170:27.
11. Fairfield WP, Treat M, Rosenthal DI, et al. Effects of testosterone and exercise on muscle leanness in eugonadal men with AIDS wasting. J Appl Physiol 2001;90:2166.
12. Biller BM, Molitch ME, Vance ML, et al. Treatment of prolactin-secreting macroadenomas with the once-weekly dopamine agonist cabergoline. J Clin Endocrinol Metab 1996;81:2338.
13. Webster J. A comparative review of the tolerability profiles of dopamine agonists in the treatment of hyperprolactinaemia and inhibition of lactation. Drug Saf 1996;14:228.
14. **14.** Colao A, Di Sarno A, Sarnacchiaro F, et al. Prolactinomas resistant to standard dopamine agonists respond to chronic cabergoline treatment. J Clin Endocrinol Metab 1997;82:876.
15. Bhasin S, Bremner WJ. Clinical review 85: emerging issues in androgen replacement therapy. J Clin Endocrinol Metab 1997;82:3.
16. **16.** Griggs RC, Kingston W, Jozefowicz RF, et al. Effect of testosterone on muscle mass and muscle protein synthesis. J Appl Physiol 1989;66:498.

*Bold print (general references) and bold numerals (specific references) denote published controlled clinical trials, meta-analyses, or consensus-based recommendations.

17. Bhasin S, Storer TW, Berman N, et al. Testosterone replacement increases fat-free mass and muscle size in hypogonadal men. J Clin Endocrinol Metab 1997;82:407.
18. Brodsky IG, Balagopal P, Nair KS. Effects of testosterone replacement on muscle mass and muscle protein synthesis in hypogonadal men: a clinical research center study. J Clin Endocrinol Metab 1996;81:3469.
19. Spark RF, White RA, Connolly PB. Impotence is not always psychogenic: newer insights into hypothalamic-pituitary-gonadal dysfunction. JAMA 1980;243:750.
20. Earle CM, Seah M, Coulden SE, et al. The use of the vacuum erection device in the management of erectile impotence. Int J Impot Res 1996;8:237.
21. Bechara A, Casabe A, Cheliz G, et al. Comparative study of papaverine plus phentolamine versus prostaglandin E1 in erectile dysfunction. J Urol 1997;157:2132.
22. Hellstrom WJ, Bennett AH, Gesundheit N, et al. A double-blind, placebo-controlled evaluation of the erectile response to transurethral alprostadil. Urology 1996;48:851.
23. Padma-Nathan H, Hellstrom WJ, Kaiser FE, et al. Treatment of men with erectile dysfunction with transurethral alprostadil. Medicated Urethral System for Erection (MUSE) Study Group. N Engl J Med 1997;336:1.
24. Gray A, Feldman HA, McKinlay JB, et al. Age, disease, and changing sex hormone levels in middle-aged men: results of the Massachusetts Male Aging Study. J Clin Endocrinol Metab 1991;73:1016.
25. Martin CE. Sexual activity in the aging male. In: Money J, Musaph N, eds. Handbook of sexology. New York: Elsevier North Holland, 1977:813.
26. Snyder PJ, Peachey H, Hannoush P, et al. Effect of testosterone on body composition and muscle strength in men over 65 years of age. J Clin Endocrinol Metab 1999;84:2647.
27. Bhasin S, Storer TW, Berman N, et al. Testosterone replacement increases fat-free mass and muscle size in hypogonadal men. J Clin Endocrinol Metab 1997;82:407.
28. Snyder PJ, Peachey H, Hannoush P, et al. Effect of testosterone on bone mineral density in men over 65 years of age. J Clin Endocrinol Metab 1999;84:1966.
29. Barrett-Connor E, Goodman-Gruen D, Patay B. Endogenous sex hormones and cognitive function in older men. J Clin Endocrinol Metab 1999;84:3681.
30. Cherrier MM, Asthana S, Plymate S, et al. Testosterone supplementatiom improves spatial and verbal memory in healthy older men. Neurology 2001;57:80.

SECTION

12

Neurologic Problems

C H A P T E R 86

Evaluation of the Patient with Neurologic Symptoms

CONSTANCE J. JOHNSON, M.D.

This chapter describes the approaches to history taking, physical examination, and laboratory evaluation that are most useful in ambulatory patients with neurologic symptoms. One or more of these approaches is appropriate for patients with each of the neurologic problems discussed in subsequent chapters (headache, seizures, dizziness, vertigo, syncope, tremor, Parkinson disease, cerebrovascular disease, and peripheral neuropathy).

NEUROLOGIC HISTORY AND PHYSICAL EXAMINATION

General Principles

To proceed with appropriate diagnostic and therapeutic actions, one must localize the lesion in the nervous system and determine the probable cause of the signs and symptoms. This requires knowledge of the presentation, epidemiology, and temporal profile of neurologic diseases. For example, new-onset central paralysis of an arm in a 20-year-old could be caused by multiple sclerosis, whereas in a 60-year-old stroke is far more likely; if the pattern is peripheral, then traumatic nerve injury is likely in the young but tumor is an important consideration in the old. Figures 86.1 and 86.2 summarize facts that are often needed for anatomic localization. Additional details regarding the anatomic relationships of peripheral nerves are shown in Table 70.2 (cervical nerve roots) in Chapter 70, Table 71.3 (lumbar nerve roots) in Chapter 71, and Figs. 92.1 (upper extremity) and 92.2 (lower extremity) in Chapter 92.

Most individual neurologic symptoms or signs are not specific for a single functional or anatomic disturbance or for a single cause. For example, loss of a reflex is not necessarily caused by motor nerve damage, a hemiparesis is not necessarily a result of cerebrovascular disease, and a resting tremor is not necessarily a symptom of Parkinson disease. Nevertheless, the constellation of findings from the history and physical examination is often quite specific. Therefore, a thorough history and physical examination are adequate for making a working diagnosis for most neurologic problems encountered in office practice.

Depending on the hypotheses one is entertaining, a brief, general neurologic evaluation may be required; more often, only selected areas of the nervous system require evaluation.

Components of a General History

Higher Functions and Consciousness

Handedness. Is the patient right-handed or left-handed? Regardless of handedness, most people are left-hemisphere dominant for language; however, some left-handers are right- or mixed-hemisphere dominant. A knowledge of handedness is useful when localizing cortical versus subcortical lesions. A patient with right hemiparesis and intact language who is right-handed has a subcortical lesion. A patient with left hemiparesis and intact language who is left-handed may have a cortical or subcortical lesion.

Language. Has the patient had problems with thinking or speech? Minor difficulty in finding words is common in normal people, as are brief lapses of memory.

Memory. How is the patient's memory? What kinds of things are forgotten? (Ask the family whether any problems with the patient's concentration, memory, or general abilities have been noted.) Can the patient work, drive, and do usual chores?

Acute Cerebral Dysfunction. Has the patient ever fainted, lost consciousness, felt dizzy, or had a seizure (fit, convulsion)? Does the patient have frequent or disabling headaches? How often?

Mood. How are the patient's spirits? Does he or she feel depressed? Worry a great deal? How does the patient feel about the future? About self (confident, hopeless, helpless, guilty)?

Hallucinations/Delusions. Has the patient seen or heard things that are unusual or things that are not there? Does the imagination seem to play tricks? What feels wrong? Does he or she perceive being controlled by anything or anybody?

Cranial Nerves

Nerve I (Olfactory). Not tested in the brief history and physical examination unless patient specifically

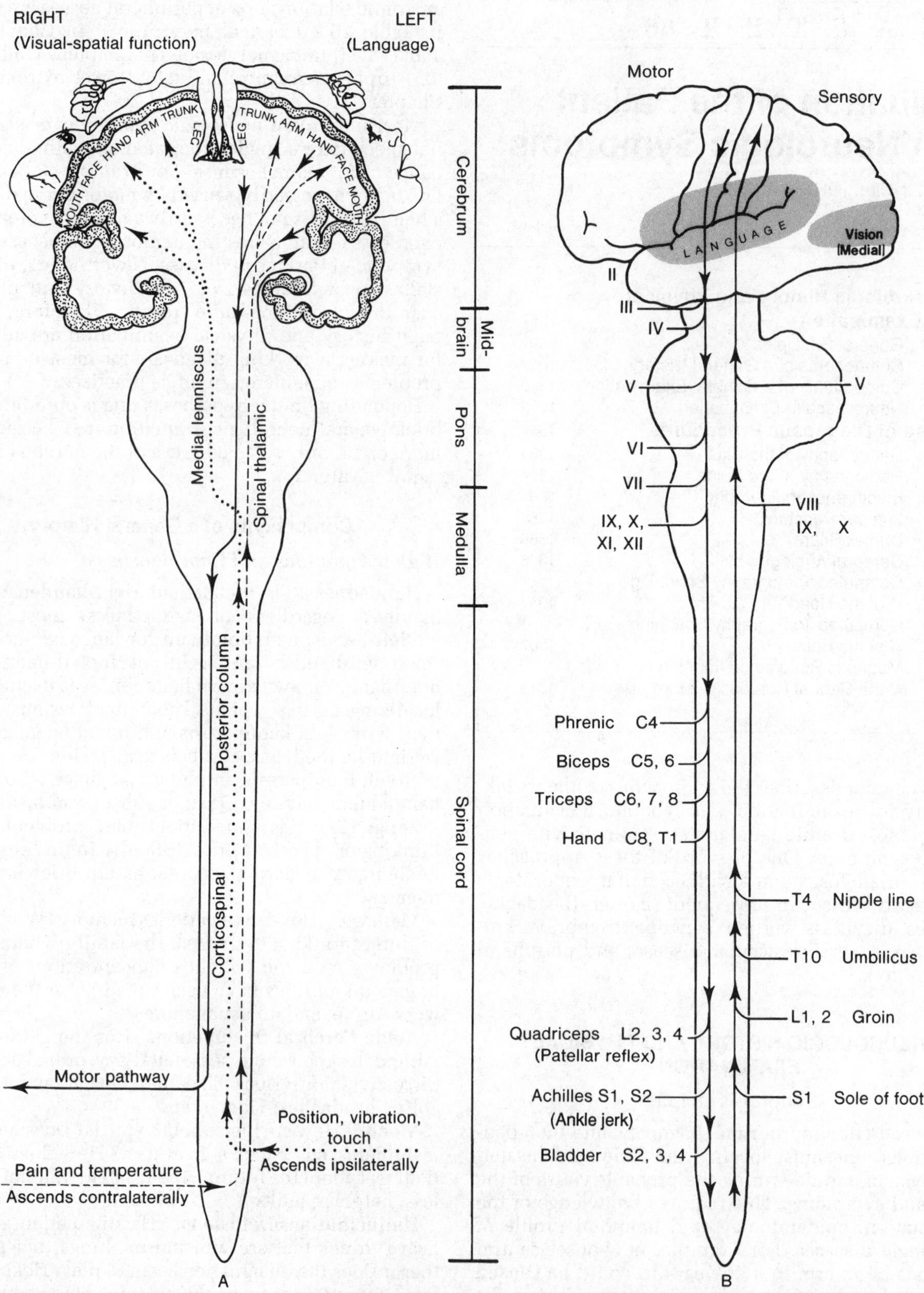

Figure 86.1. Schematic diagrams of neurologic localization—anterior **(A)** and lateral **(B)** views. Upper motor neuron signs and nonradicular sensory signs can define only the side of the lesion **(A)**; in general, they do not reveal the level of the lesion. The presence or absence of other neurologic signs or symptoms can help to specify the level of a localized neurologic problem **(B)**. (Courtesy of Barry Gordon, M.D., Ph.D.)

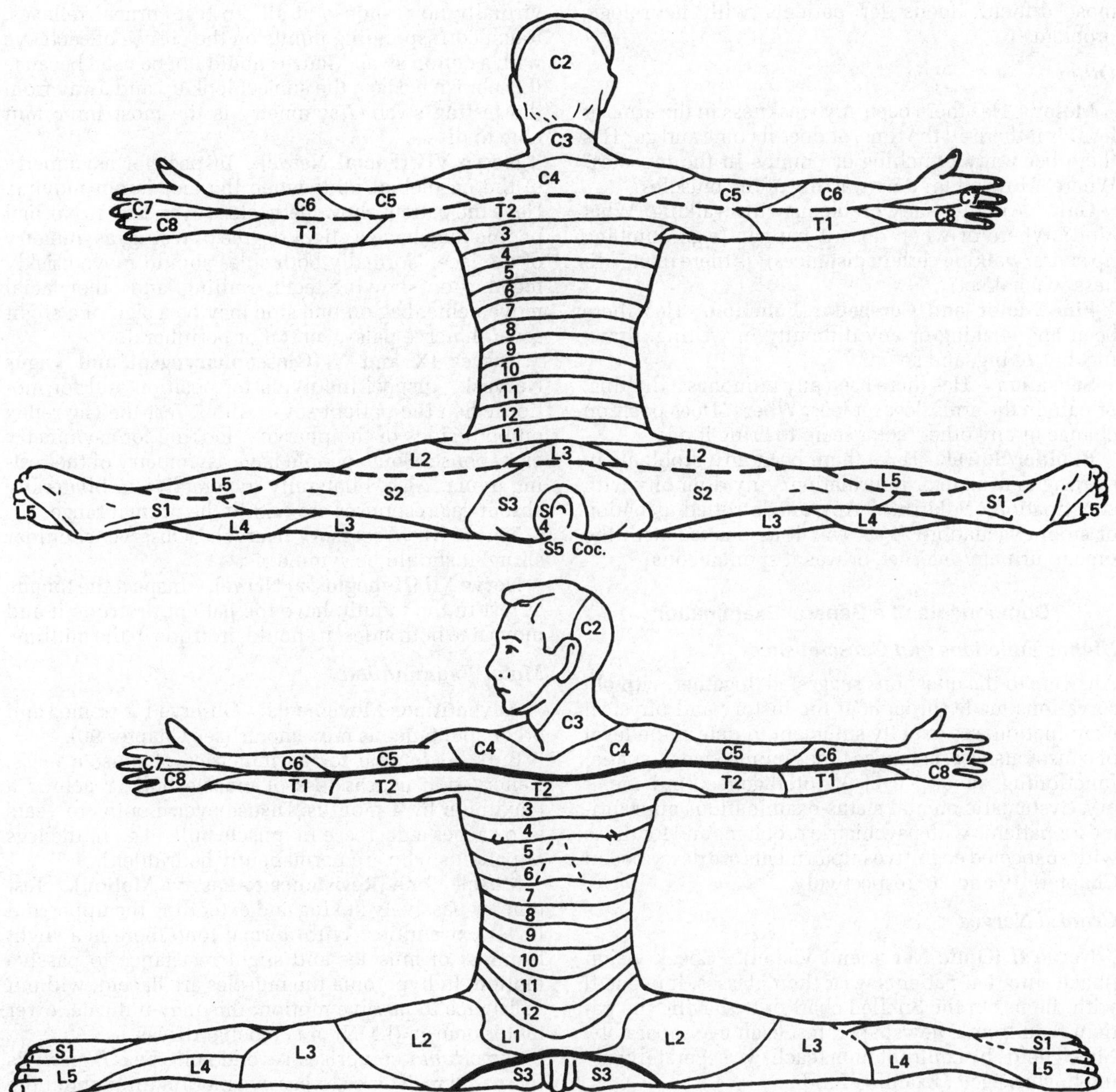

Figure 86.2. Cutaneous innervation areas of dermatomes. The numbers correspond to the spinal cord level of the dermatome. C, Cervical; T, thoracic; L, lumbar; S, sacral. (From Haymaker W, Woodhall B. Peripheral nerve injuries. 2nd ed. Philadelphia: WB Saunders, 1962.)

mentions a loss of smell or has a history of head trauma with loss of consciousness.

Nerve II (Optic Nerve and Vision). Is there impaired vision? Do things seem blurred, or are there patches where it is hard to see? Has vision ever been lost in one eye, or has the patient had trouble seeing out of one side or in one direction?

Nerves III, IV, and VI (Extraocular Motions). Has there ever been double vision?

Nerve V (Trigeminal Nerve). Has there been numbness over the face or difficulty chewing?

Nerve VII (Facial Nerve). Has there been any weakness in the face or paralysis of the face?

Nerve VIII (Auditory–Vestibular Nerve). How is the patient's hearing? Has there been any ringing in the ears or difficulty hearing out of one side? Any loss of balance, spinning sensations, or dizziness?

Nerves IX, X, and XII (Glossopharyngeal, Vagal, and Hypoglossal Nerves). Have there been any problems swallowing food? Does it seem to get caught anywhere? Where? What kinds of food has the patient had problems with? (Liquids are often the most difficult foods for patients with neurologic problems.)

Other

Motor. Has there been any weakness in the arms or legs? Is it there all the time, or does it come and go? Has there been any twitching or cramps in the muscles? Where? How often? Any wasting of the muscles?

Gait. Are there any problems with walking? What kind? Where or when does it happen (e.g., climbing up stairs, walking certain distances)? Is there unsteadiness when erect?

Fine Motor and Cerebellar Function. Has there been any shaking or any difficulty in writing, drawing, buttoning, and so on?

Sensation. Has there been any numbness, tingling, or pain in the arms, legs, or feet? Where? Does position change or any other factor seem to bring it on?

Bladder/Bowel. Have there been any problems in starting to urinate or in urinating? Any difficulty with constipation or diarrhea? Any uncontrolled urination or stool evacuation? If so, was it associated with the urge to urinate/defecate, or was it spontaneous?

Components of a General Examination

Higher Functions and Consciousness

Answers to the questions suggested, together with observations made throughout the history and physical examination, are usually sufficient to determine level of consciousness, language functioning, visual–spatial functioning, mood, level of intelligence, and memory. Systematic mental status examinations appropriate for patients with psychiatric problems and for those with suspected cognitive impairments are described in Chapters 19 and 26, respectively.

Cranial Nerves

Nerve II (Optic Nerve and Vision). Check vision (make sure that patients wear their glasses, if needed) with the use of the Snellen chart or by having the patient read from a newspaper; test each eye separately. Check fields by confrontation (each eye separately) using finger wiggle. Examine fundi.

Nerves III, IV, and VI (Extraocular Movement and Pupils). Have the patient move the eyes into all principal positions of gaze (horizontal, vertical, diagonal); observe for dysconjugate movements, and ask, while testing, about diplopia. Look for nystagmus, lid lag, and ptosis, and check pupils for size, symmetry, and reaction to light. The normal pupil size for young adults is 3 to 5 mm. In the elderly, normal pupils are often 2 to 3 mm. A slight degree of pupillary asymmetry, 1 mm or less, is present in about 5% of the normal population; it usually varies from hour to hour and day to day, and it decreases in bright light.

Nerve V (Trigeminal Nerve). With a pin, check for symmetry of perception over forehead, cheek, and chin. The corneal reflex is not routinely tested in the outpatient setting. There are wide variations in corneal sensitivity among normal individuals; some subjects, particularly those who have worn contact lenses, have virtually no response at all. To test corneal reflexes, touch corresponding points on the cornea of each eye with a cotton swab. Gauze should not be used because it is abrasive. Have the subject look up and away from the testing swab. Asymmetry is the most important clue to disease.

Nerve VII (Facial Nerve). Inspect for asymmetry of the nasolabial folds when the face is not moving. Have the patient show teeth, close eyes, frown. Normal people may have a slight degree of resting asymmetry of the face. Normally both sides should move briskly together on showing teeth, smiling, and other facial movements. Lag on one side may be a sign of a slight seventh nerve palsy, central or peripheral.

Nerves IX and X (Glossopharyngeal and Vagus Nerves). Inspect the uvula for position and for motion when the patient says “Ahh.” Test the gag reflex on both sides of the pharynx, looking for asymmetry of response. Some people have asymmetry of the resting uvula. Also, bilaterally hyperactive to bilaterally absent gag responses are within the normal range.

Nerve XI (Accessory Nerve). Observe shoulder shrug; it should be symmetric.

Nerve XII (Hypoglossal Nerve). Inspect the tongue at rest in the mouth; have the patient protrude it and move it to both sides. It should protrude in the midline.

Motor Examination

Adventitious Movements. Observe for tremor and other spontaneous movements (see Chapter 90).

Bulk. Examine for asymmetries of muscle mass. Denervation causes loss of muscle bulk, reaching a maximum by 4 months. Disuse over months to years also causes a decrease in muscle bulk (e.g., in the legs of patients who are permanently bedridden).

Muscle Tone (Resistance to Passive Motion). Test tone by passively flexing and extending the upper and lower extremities. With normal tone there is a slight firmness of muscles and slight resistance to passive motion. In hypotonia the muscles are flaccid, without resistance to passive motion; this may indicate lower motor neuron (LMN) or cerebellar disease.

Hypertonia comprises several subtypes. *Rigidity* is increased resistance to passive motion throughout the whole range of motion around a joint. In *spasticity,* the initial passive motion is easy, but then there is a tightening of the muscle (spastic catch), possibly followed by a sudden release (clasp-knife effect). Spasticity usually affects only one set of muscles around a joint (in the upper extremities, the biceps, forearm pronators, and finger flexors; in the lower extremities, the quadriceps, hamstrings, and plantar flexors). In *gegenhalten or paratonia,* resistance is present in all directions but varies with the examiner's force and speed. It often seems to be voluntary (fighting back). Gegenhalten is seen normally in infants, but it appears pathologically in adults with dementias or with frontal lobe disease.

Voluntary Strength. Test voluntary strength in several major muscle groups. Survey proximal and distal muscles in each extremity. An adequate screen includes testing of shoulder abduction, elbow extension and flexion, wrist and finger extension, grip strength, hip flexion, knee flexion and extension, and foot dorsiflexion. Observe the patient's gait (discussed later).

For precise documentation, the following rating scale can be used: 0, no movement; 1, flicker; 2, able to move with gravity eliminated (e.g., lateral motion of arm when recumbent); 3, able to move against gravity; 4, able to move against resistance; 5, normal strength.

In conversion reactions and malingering, strength on formal testing is usually jerky or giving. With sudden passive motions in the opposite direction, the examiner may find that the muscles produce normal resistive force. The examiner may find that the subject can do some voluntary activities (e.g., combing hair, reaching for objects, getting up or sitting down) with muscles that the he or she states are too weak to use for such motions on formal testing.

Reflexes. The most important reflexes to test are the biceps (C5–6), triceps (C6–8), patellar (L2–4), Achilles tendon (S1–2), and plantar flexion. Activity of the reflexes varies widely among patients and can vary depending on a patient's emotional state and ability to relax muscles. As in the rest of the examination, asymmetries between the two sides generally carry more weight than symmetric reflex changes; comparison must be made with the muscles relaxed to a similar degree and with the two extremities in identical positions. A decrease in the reflex is usually caused by disruption of the sensory or motor nerves of the reflex loop itself. Sometimes decreased reflexes are seen immediately after a cerebrovascular accident, in which case interpretation does not depend on the reflexes alone. Increased reflexes mean upper motor neuron (UMN) disease located anywhere from just above the anterior horn cell to the cerebral cortex.

A Babinski sign consists of dorsiflexion of the big toe after plantar stimulation; it may be associated with dorsiflexion and spreading of the other toes and dorsiflexion of the foot. The classic Babinski response is slow and deliberate. Nonspecific withdrawal may resemble the Babinski reflex, but it is usually rapid and the patient usually complains of subjective distress; a reliable Babinski sign should occur in the absence of any patient discomfort from the stimulus. A Babinski sign may be found as the sole indicator of UMN disease.

Sensation

The patient should be tested for symmetry and for differences in proximal and distal perception in all four extremities. Light touch (posterior columns) is not a well-delineated modality and can be normal when abnormalities of pinprick (lateral spinothalamic tract) or proprioception/vibration (posterior columns) are present; therefore, it should not be used as the sole screen of sensory function. Sensitivity to pinprick, proprioception, and vibratory sense should be tested. There are normal differences in pinprick perception over different areas of the body (e.g., it is decreased over the beard area), but patients usually ignore these differences. Particularly introspective or anxious patients can give very confusing responses and must be told to ignore small subjective differences. Repeated testing is often important to determine the reliability of a patient's response. Vibration sense should be tested with a 128-Hz tuning fork. Proprioception is tested in the most distal joint of the fingers and toes by moving the digit approximately 30° to 45° and then asking the patient to report the direction in which the digits have moved.

The Romberg test (patient stands with feet together and closed eyes while the ability to maintain balance is assessed) is a test of integrity of proprioception and the posterior columns through which proprioception is conveyed. The ability to stand with eyes closed must be interpreted with caution in patients with cerebellar ataxia. If the patient cannot stand steady with eyes open, the Romberg test may be altered to allow testing of posterior columns by having the patient stand with a wide base (to compensate for cerebellar ataxia) and then close the eyes. If the posterior columns are intact, the patient will not waver more than a slight amount.

Fine Motor and Cerebellar Function

The patient should be told to touch the thumb sequentially to each of the fingers of each hand separately; speed, effort, and rhythm of the movements should be observed. Finger-to-nose-to-finger movement should be tested (subject must touch examiner's moving finger, then touch his or her own nose, then touch the examiner's finger again, and so on) for speed, rhythm, intention tremor, and inaccuracy (dysmetria). The subject should be asked to tap each foot separately, and differences in speed, ease, and rhythm should be observed. In these tests, normal subjects show equal ability with either side or are slightly better on the side of their preferred hand. Slowness and subjective effort on repetitive movements, without a loss of rhythm, are characteristic of UMN lesions. Preserved speed with erratic movements and loss of rhythm may be seen in cerebellar disease. Finger–nose–finger testing may be affected by tremor of various types, as described in Chapter 90.

Station and Gait

Any tendency to list or any need for support while sitting, standing, or walking should be observed. The patient should be asked to walk normally and to walk on the heels and toes (to test strength and balance). Tandem gait testing (walking heel-to-toe) requires the patient to narrow the base of support and reveals abnormalities of balance in patients with ataxia not detected on normal walking.

In *cerebellar disease,* the patient exhibits a wide base (legs widely separated), unsteadiness, and lateral reeling. Lateral reeling can be evaluated by having the patient walk around a chair in both directions; the patient will tend to walk into the chair when it is on the affected side and to veer away from the chair when it is on the unaffected side. Because of fundamental abnormality of motor coordination, the patient with cerebellar disease affecting the lower extremities cannot participate in a standard Romberg test, which requires standing with the two feet together; a modified Romberg test for such patients was described earlier.

In *sensory ataxia* (loss of proprioception), there is uncertainty, slapping or stamping of the feet, and a positive Romberg test (the patient loses balance with eyes closed but can avoid falling when the eyes are open because of visually mediated vestibular or cerebellar compensation).

In a *spastic gait* (in UMN disease), the leg does not flex but circumducts, and there is foot dragging (the toe of the sole of the patient's shoe becomes disproportionately worn); there is also loss of arm swinging on the spastic side.

In a *parkinsonian gait,* there is unilateral or bilateral loss of arm swinging, the patient is bent forward, and there is rigidity, shuffling, and festination (the upper part of the body advances ahead of the lower extremities; gait becomes faster, as if to catch up).

In *lower motor neuron (LMN) paralysis* of the pretibial and peroneal muscles, foot-drop is seen; hip flexion is preserved, and the patient lifts the foot very high, advances it by swinging it forward, then slaps it down.

In *frontal lobe disease,* gait may be wide-based, shuffling, and slow, and turning is slow, but there is no weakness or loss of sensation.

Special Considerations in the Evaluation of Neurologic Symptoms and Signs

Neurologic signs are often subtle in ambulatory patients, compared with patients hospitalized for neurologic disease, and may be related to prior acute neurologic events. Two important considerations in the evaluation of ambulatory patients with neurologic symptoms and signs are the variability in performance over time and the difference between the manifestations of UMN and LMN lesions.

Variability over Time

In patients who have abnormalities of the peripheral nerves, spinal cord, and brainstem, symptoms and signs remain about the same after the basic problem has stabilized; later alterations of the findings usually reflect a change in the patient's disease. On the other hand, cognitive and language impairment can vary greatly from minute to minute, hour to hour, or day to day. The variability affects the psychomotor domain (e.g., performance of everyday tasks, memory, speech and language, and mood). For example,

- The patient may be able to dress, fix breakfast, and bring in the mail one morning, be incapable of these tasks the next morning, and perform them correctly on the third morning.
- The patient may remember his or her spouse's name in the morning but not in the evening of the same day.
- The aphasic patient may be able to say something one minute and unable to say it several minutes later.
- The stroke survivor's affect may vary from depressed to euphoric from hour to hour or day to day.

As a result of this type of variability, members of the patient's family may become confused and angry; they may inquire whether a change in behavior means that the disease is getting worse, or they may conclude that the patient is capable of doing certain tasks but is just not trying sometimes. When the pattern is clearly one of waxing and waning, the family should be reassured that, just as they have their good days and bad days, the patient does also, but in exaggerated and different ways. The evaluation and management of behavioral changes of patients with cerebral damage are discussed in more detail in Chapters 26 (dementia) and 91 (stroke).

Differences between Upper Motor Neuron and Lower Motor Neuron Symptoms

The manifestations and the course of UMN and LMN damage differ fundamentally. UMN lesions affect the pathways that bring a command from the cortex to the anterior horn cell. UMN function depends on integrity of the cortex and of the corticospinal and corticobulbar tracts. LMN lesions affect the final common pathway for muscle movements. LMN function depends on the integrity of the anterior horn cell in the spinal cord and its nerve fiber for carrying impulses to the muscle cell. A number of points are helpful in recognizing or distinguishing these two patterns of motor abnormality when they are not overt, which is often the case in patients seen in office practice.

Upper Motor Neuron Lesion Syndrome. If a UMN lesion is total, movements are absent. However, there may be preservation of involuntary movements, such as those associated with yawning, laughing, crying, or anger. When there is weakness (paresis) rather than paralysis caused by UMN damage, the following patterns of weakness are seen.

In the face, the lower muscles are usually involved. There is variable but often some involvement of the orbicularis oculi, producing a widened palpebral fissure and weakness of eye closure, but the forehead is completely spared. This is in contrast to LMN (peripheral) seventh nerve damage, in which both the upper and lower facial muscles are involved, although sometimes mild peripheral seventh nerve weakness (e.g., early Bell's palsy, an LMN lesion) can mimic a UMN pattern. One additional differential point is that the LMN lesion produces the same amount of weakness with both a voluntary and an involuntary movement (e.g., laughing). A UMN seventh nerve paresis (e.g., from stroke) may not be apparent when the patient is laughing or crying involuntarily and may be present only when the patient is asked to smile voluntarily.

In the arm and leg, distal muscles are affected by UMN lesions much more than proximal muscles are. In addition, some specific motor functions are affected more than others: in the arm, shoulder abduction and external rotation; in the forearm, extension and supination; in the wrist and fingers, extension; in the hip, flexion; in the knee, flexion; and in the foot and toe, dorsiflexion.

Whether or not the muscles are weak in a UMN lesion, voluntary movements are typically slowed and require greater effort than usual, and the ability to make fine movements with the affected limb is lost.

A patient with a very mild hemiparesis may be able to squeeze the examiner's hand with normal strength, but movements are slower and clumsier than usual; the patient may be unable to easily use fingers individually. Also, when the patient is asked to extend both arms with the eyes closed, there may be downward and inward drift of the weak arm (pronator sign). In the lower extremity, a patient with such a mild defect may be able to dorsiflex the foot voluntarily. However, the same patient may not be able to do this very rapidly (as revealed on attempted foot tapping), and the movement may not be automatically coordinated with walking, resulting in a foot-drop.

Typically (but not invariably), UMN lesions are accompanied by spasticity and hyperreflexia.

Lower Motor Neuron Lesion Syndrome. Weakness resulting from a permanent LMN lesion is fixed and unchanging. Only the muscles served by the involved spinal cord segment or peripheral nerve are weak. There are none of the widespread effects characteristic of a UMN lesion. Atrophy is usually apparent within several weeks after an LMN lesion, in contrast to UMN lesions, where atrophy is slight and late (many months). Pathologic fasciculations may be present in affected muscle groups, distinguishable from benign occasional muscle twitching by the fact that they are frequent and occur only in the denervated muscles. Muscles are usually flaccid and hyporeflexic or areflexic. If a peripheral nerve has been involved, there may be associated hypesthesia or anesthesia. In muscle disease (e.g., polymyositis, drug-induced myopathy), muscle tone, reflexes, and sensory function are normal. Weakness is typically proximal in the deltoids, iliopsoas, quadriceps, and neck flexor muscles. The patient complains of difficulty climbing steps or using the arms over the head.

In some situations, UMN and LMN lesions occur together. For instance, spinal cord injury typically gives signs of a LMN lesion at the level of the injury, caused by localized destruction of the anterior horn cells and their nerve roots; below the level of the injury, there may be a partial or complete UMN syndrome, with spasticity, hyperreflexia, and preserved involuntary reflexes. Likewise, amyotrophic lateral sclerosis, an idiopathic degenerative disease, affects both pyramidal tract cells and anterior horn cells. Along with LMN-type weakness, fasciculations, and wasting, these patients have hyperreflexia and may have Babinski signs.

Neurovascular Examination

This examination is especially important in patients in whom cerebrovascular disease or an increased risk of cerebrovascular disease is the problem (see Chapter 91). The examination includes an assessment of the heart and peripheral vasculature, with emphasis on the vessels of the head and neck.

Heart and Peripheral Vessels

The radial arteries should be simultaneously palpated at the wrists to determine any asymmetry in pulse amplitude or timing (pulse delay). The brachial arterial blood pressure should be measured in the supine, sitting, and standing positions. Blood pressure should be measured in both arms to check for asymmetry. Unequal blood pressure in the two arms (20 mm Hg or more difference in systolic pressure, more than 10 mm Hg in diastolic pressure) suggests a stenotic lesion of the subclavian or innominate artery on the side with the lower pressure. Orthostatic hypotension, defined as a fall in systolic pressure of more than 15 mm Hg on moving from a supine to an upright position, is common in autonomic neuropathy and may be important in explaining symptoms in patients with severe stenotic lesions of carotid or vertebral–basilar arteries.

A detailed cardiac examination can provide evidence of cardiomegaly, valvular disease, or arrhythmia, each of which may predispose a patient to a stroke. Finally, a complete assessment of the peripheral vasculature, for evidence of widespread atherosclerosis, should include palpation and auscultation of the femoral arteries and palpation of the arterial pulses in the feet.

Vessels of Head and Neck

Evaluation of the vessels of the head and neck may include inspection, palpation, and auscultation.

Inspection. Prominence of the superficial temporal artery with erythema and, occasionally, ulceration of the overlying skin in a patient with persistent malaise is suggestive of giant cell arteritis, an inflammatory process that can lead to retinal or cerebral infarction (see Chapter 87).

Dilation of the *episcleral arteries* of an eye can result from occlusion of the ipsilateral internal carotid artery; in this instance, the hemisphere on the side of the occlusion is being supplied in a retrograde fashion by the external carotid artery through dilated ophthalmic arteries. The funduscopic examination allows direct visualization of the retinal vessels, and changes resulting from atherosclerosis, hypertension, or diabetes mellitus can be detected. Moreover, the absence of an expected change can be informative, as in the case of the hypertensive patient with normal retinal vessels on the side of a severely stenosed carotid artery; in this instance, occlusive disease of the ipsilateral carotid artery protects the retina from the effects of chronic hypertension. A detailed funduscopic examination may also demonstrate emboli, seen as white or refractile elements in the retinal arterioles (see Fig. 91.1 in Chapter 91). These emboli may be composed of cholesterol, platelets and fibrin, or calcium and are suggestive of atherosclerotic carotid occlusive disease or cardiac valve disease.

Palpation. Reports of embolic stroke after firm palpation of a diseased carotid artery have left some clinicians with a sense of trepidation regarding manipulation of this vessel. The current consensus, however, is that gentle palpation of the carotid artery can be performed with limited risk and occasionally provides useful information about the status of the vessel. Perhaps more valuable, and without risk, is palpation of the superficial temporal and facial arteries, which are branches of the external carotid artery. A weak or absent pulse in these arteries on one side of the head is suggestive of ipsilateral occlusive disease of the external or common carotid artery. In contrast, an increase in pulsation in these vessels may result from stenosis or occlusion of the ipsilateral internal carotid artery that causes collateral flow through the external system. Finally, the finding of a tender superficial temporal artery with decreased pulsation may support other data consistent with the diagnosis of giant cell arteritis (see Chapter 87).

Auscultation. After auscultation of the heart to check for transmitted cardiac murmur, the examiner should proceed to the supraclavicular regions over the subclavian arteries and to the carotid arteries up to their bifurcation at the angle of the jaw; a cervical bruit is suggestive, but not diagnostic, of atherosclerotic occlusive disease. Auscultation may at times be useful over the occipital, temporal, and parietal regions of the cranium, and over the orbits. The finding of a cephalic bruit in an adult raises the possibility of an arteriovenous malformation; an orbital bruit suggests intracranial internal carotid artery disease.

USE OF DIAGNOSTIC PROCEDURES

Patients may be referred for any of a number of diagnostic procedures in the evaluation of a neurologic problem. The principles described in Chapter 2 are especially important in deciding which of these procedures to select. Costs of neurodiagnostic tests vary widely from region to region and within a region because fee profiles are individually determined. Charges for many of these tests are in the range of $200 to $2,000; however, practitioners should become aware of costs in their own regions. For most of the procedures currently available for ambulatory application, the definition, principal indications, limitations, and a description of the patient experience are provided here. Chapter 92 provides this information for nerve conduction tests and electromyography.

Radiography of the Skull

Definition of Procedure

The term *routine skull radiographs* refers to a set of films that include three standard views: lateral, anteroposterior (AP), and inclined AP. Many other views are possible and may be indicated in specific conditions (e.g., basal skull views for a patient with atypical trigeminal neuralgia).

Principal Indications

The principal indications are suspected skull fracture and problems involving the bones, such as metastatic tumor (osteoblastic or osteolytic), myeloma, or Paget disease.

Limitations

The skull radiograph has little value as a screening or diagnostic test for intracranial disease because few intracranial neurologic conditions are associated with bony changes.

Patient Experience. The patient will be asked to keep his or her head in several uncomfortable positions for short periods of time; accurate positioning might be impossible for elderly patients or for those who have neck problems.

Radiography of the Spine

Definition of Procedure

Standard spine films are usually AP and lateral views; oblique and flexion–extension views usually must be ordered specifically.

Principal Indications

The principal indications are suspected cervical spondylitic radiculopathy (in which case, oblique films are necessary to examine the intervertebral foramina through which the roots pass); suspected cervical or lumbar stenosis, spondylolisthesis, luxation, or subluxation; suspected vertebral fracture; and suspected metastatic tumor.

Limitations

Asymptomatic cervical spondylosis and interspace narrowing caused by disc degeneration are so common after 40 years of age (see Chapter 70) that their presence has limited usefulness in the absence of more specific findings from the history and physical examination. Negative films provide good evidence against spondylosis as the cause of radicular symptoms.

Radiographs do not show soft tissue, brain, spinal cord, or nerve roots. In patients with herniated intervertebral discs, films are usually normal or show only nonspecific intervertebral narrowing. However, patients with congenitally small bony canals (cervical or lumbar stenosis) are at risk for neurologic problems occurring secondary to degenerative changes in the disc and ligaments; the radiologist should be asked specifically about these possibilities if they are important diagnostic considerations.

Patient Experience. The patient must cooperate for several views. Patients with neck problems and those who are elderly may be unable to position themselves for adequate cervical spine films.

Electroencephalography

Definition of Procedure

The electroencephalogram (EEG) is a record of the (1- to 50-mV) electrical rhythms of the brain.

Principal Indications

One principal indication is known or suspected seizure disorder (see Chapter 88). Recording during sleep or after sleep deprivation significantly increases the chances of a useful diagnostic examination; for complex partial seizures, nasopharyngeal leads record from the medial temporal regions, where some of these seizures originate, and therefore can increase the yield of the study.

The procedure is also used for confirmation of focal brain lesions in the absence of other evidence (e.g., in the diagnosis and localization of stroke) and for confirmation of diffuse brain disease, such as dementia, delirium, cerebral vasculitis, or drug effect or withdrawal. The EEG may at times be helpful in differentiation of the dementia syndrome of depression from organic dementia (see Chapter 26). For sleep disorders (see Chapter 7), routine and special EEG recording techniques are often indicated.

Limitations

The EEG records cortical activity and, although it is sensitive for processes affecting the cortex, it is not useful for delineation of subcortical processes. However, this property can be useful in investigating vascular lesions when a cortical lesion is not identified on computed tomography (CT) or magnetic resonance imaging (MRI).

Negative Electroencephalogram. A single negative EEG is not evidence for the absence of a seizure disorder. For example, up to 50% of patients with known epilepsy have normal interictal records. Serial or repeated negative EEGs may be far more significant (see Chapter 88). A normal EEG in a patient with suspected delirium suggests psychiatric illness.

"Mildly Abnormal" Electroencephalogram. Depending on the reader and the classification scheme, some adult EEGs (5% to 30% or more) can be classified as minimally or mildly but nonspecifically abnormal. The relevance of these interpretations must be judged in the context of the patients' problems but should not be given undue weight because of the broad range of normal findings. This is particularly true in infancy, childhood, adolescence, and old age. For instance, temporal slow activity is present after 40 years of age in as many as 30% to 40% of subjects.

Patient Experience. Subjects are asked to lie down or recline while surface electrodes are attached with electrode paste. The total procedure takes an average of 40 to 60 minutes, with 20 to 30 minutes of actual recording time. For most of the actual recording, the patient is simply asked to lie calmly with eyes closed. Additional studies that most laboratories routinely perform include recording during hyperventilation (for 3 to 5 minutes) and during photic simulation with a repetitive flash. For many tracings, subjects are encouraged to fall asleep. Some laboratories induce sleep with oral chloral hydrate if permitted by the referring physician; if this is planned in advance, the patient should be told to bring someone who can drive the patient home.

The EEG is extremely sensitive to patient movement, sweating, and muscle tension, any of which can make a tracing uninterpretable.

For sleep-deprived EEGs, the patient is asked to stay up the night before, and the EEG is done in the laboratory first thing in the morning.

Nasopharyngeal leads are applied through the nostrils after local anesthesia of the nasopharynx by spray; they may interfere with nasal breathing and are mildly uncomfortable.

Lumbar Puncture

Definition of Procedure

Lumbar puncture is performed to obtain cerebrospinal fluid for analysis and to measure intracranial pressure. A normal opening pressure does not exceed 200 mm. Normal cerebrospinal fluid is crystal clear and contains no more than five mononuclear cells; the normal glucose concentration is two-thirds that of a simultaneously determined serum glucose level, and the protein concentration is less than 45 mg/dL. Xanthochromia is a yellowish discoloration of the spinal fluid that is present in red cell breakdown (indicating previous subarachnoid hemorrhage), in hyperbilirubinemia, and with extreme elevations of protein.

Principal Indications

Elevated intracranial pressure must be documented to diagnose benign intracranial hypertension (see Chapter 87). The low-pressure headache syndrome (see Chapter 87) can be documented by lumbar puncture but may be exacerbated by the procedure.

Lumbar puncture is used in the evaluation of patients with suspected meningitis; those with suspected or known chronic infection of the central nervous system, such as syphilis, acquired immunodeficiency syndrome (AIDS), Lyme disease, cryptococcus, or tuberculosis; those with subarachnoid hemorrhage; those with suspected demyelinating or inflammatory disease, such as multiple sclerosis or inflammatory neuropathy (e.g., Guillain–Barre syndrome); and those with undiagnosed central nervous system disease.

Limitations

The opening pressure depends on the intracranial pressure, which can be elevated by measures that increase venous pressure, such as straining and tightening of the abdominal musculature. A tense patient with an elevated opening pressure should be encouraged to relax, and pressure should be remeasured before fluid is removed. The closing pressure depends on the pressure/volume dynamics, which are influenced by the amount of fluid removed and the intracranial compliance. Abnormalities of cerebrospinal fluid are nonspecific; however, when they are interpreted in the context of the clinical presentation and further evaluation in the laboratory, diagnostic accuracy can be increased.

The procedure is completely safe if infection of the skin overlying the puncture site, an intracranial mass lesion, and bilateral brain edema are ruled out. Neurologic consultation and CT or MRI of the brain (see later discussion) before the lumbar puncture will eliminate the potential for complications caused by the latter two problems. If papilledema is present, an imaging study to rule out a mass lesion before lumbar puncture is always mandatory in an outpatient.

Patient Experience. Patients are often reluctant to undergo lumbar puncture, based on widespread belief that it is dangerous and very painful. The patient should be reassured that, after neurologic evaluation or an imaging study, the procedure is safe. Under adequate local anesthesia, the discomfort is mild. When lumbar puncture is done properly under aseptic conditions, the most common complication is a postprocedure headache (see Chapter 87). The probability of postprocedure headache can be decreased by using the smallest-gauge needle that is practical (20-gauge in most adults). Newer, blunt-tipped "atraumatic" lumbar puncture needles are postulated to result in a smaller dural hole and have been demonstrated to reduce headache after the procedure. The flow rate through the needle may be compromised with a needle of 22 gauge or higher, but it is adequate with the 20-gauge needle. For most patients, a 20-gauge atraumatic needle is ideal. Performing the tap with the patient in a sitting position also increases the likelihood of a first-pass nontraumatic tap; however, the lateral decubitus position is necessary to obtain a precise opening pressure measurement. After the lumbar puncture, the patient is instructed to lie flat for 5 to 60 minutes and to drink copious amounts of fluid over the ensuing 6 hours. A minority of patients complain of pain at the puncture site, which may be treated with nonnarcotic analgesics.

Duplex Scan

Definition of Procedure

Duplex scanning combines B-mode ultrasonic scanning of the carotid bifurcation with spectral analysis of a Doppler signal to assess plaque disease. The extent of plaque is classified into categories that vary among laboratories but usually approximate the following categories: 0 to 15%, 16% to 40%, 41% to 60%, 61% to 80%, 81% to 99%, and occluded. The percentage of stenosis approximates angiographic measurements; however, some discrepancy occurs because duplex scanning approximates area, whereas angiography is usually a linear measurement. Plaque characteristics such as calcification, hemorrhage, and ulceration can be determined. Plaque distribution in common, internal, and external carotid arteries is delineated.

Principal Indications

This noninvasive screening technique may be used in the evaluation of patients with asymptomatic carotid bruits, transient ischemic attacks (TIAs), or stroke. With use of this procedure, stroke-prone patients may be selected for arteriography (see Chapter 91).

Limitations

No more than 3 cm of the internal carotid artery can be imaged above the bifurcation. The proximal common carotid is imaged for a variable distance, depending on its tortuousity. This technique cannot distinguish complete occlusion from a very-high-grade stenosis. No information about intracranial disease is obtained.

Patient Experience. A comprehensive duplex examination of the carotid arteries takes approximately 45 minutes. The transducer head is held over the carotid bifurcation at the angle of the mandible. There is no appreciable discomfort or risk.

Cerebral Angiography

Definition of Procedure

Cerebral angiography provides imaging by intra-arterial injection of a contrast agent, by magnetic resonance technique (magnetic resonance angiography [MRA]), or by helical CT (see Computed Tomography.)

For intra-arterial angiography a flexible catheter is placed in an artery, usually the femoral artery, and passed to the aortic arch, where it is selectively advanced into the arteries of interest, including the common carotid or vertebral arteries, which are then injected with a contrast agent. Serial radiographs are taken.

MRA is a noninvasive procedure that uses radiofrequency signals to construct images of the cerebral vessels.

Principal Indications

Cerebral angiography can be used in the delineation of a number of intracranial processes. Since the advent of CT and MRI (discussed later), the principal indication for angiography has been the definitive diagnosis of cerebrovascular diseases including extracranial and intracranial arterial stenosis, vascular malformations, aneurysms, and vasculitis.

Limitations

Intra-arterial Angiography. Adequate renal function is a prerequisite. Serious complications (approximately 1% to 2% of patients) occur related to femoral puncture, manipulation of the catheter, and reactions to the contrast agent. Serious complications include femoral artery clot with embolization, stroke, and anaphylactic reaction to the contrast agent. The ionic load of the contrast agent may precipitate heart failure in susceptible patients.

Magnetic Resonance Angiography. Resolution with MRA is not yet as acute as with intra-arterial angiography; this limitation is related to disturbances of laminar flow and to the multiplanar course of cerebral vessels. The hazards associated with MRA are the same as those listed later for MRI. MRA may be used to noninvasively image the intracranial vessels and the carotid and vertebral arteries in the neck.

Patient Experience. For intra-arterial angiography, the patient lies on a radiography table and a femoral artery puncture is made after local anesthesia with lidocaine. The major discomfort is a burning sensation, which can be intense, that is felt with the injection of contrast material. Less stressful reactions are a metallic taste in the mouth, itching, and occasionally hives. Mild or severe bronchospasm, although uncommon, can occur. The patient must be able to lie still for the radiographs. After the procedure, patients are instructed to drink a large amount of fluid, limit activity, and monitor for signs of bleeding or obstruction at or distal to the site of arterial puncture. Instructions usually include limiting ambulation, no lifting or other strenuous activity for 24 hours, and no bathing for at least 12 hours. For MRA, the patient experience is the same as for MRI (see later section).

Computed Tomography Scanning of the Head

Definition of Procedure

CT uses narrow x-ray beams to exploit differences in x-ray absorption between different kinds of intracranial tissues. Without contrast, the CT scanner can distinguish the densities of bone, calcified tissue, blood, gray matter, white matter, cerebrospinal fluid, and air. Its resolving power is proportional to the differences in the densities of these tissues. Although CT scanning results are typically presented as horizontal slices through the brain, present technology allows slices to be reconstructed in the vertical plane or in any other plane to give a better perspective on abnormal findings. Helical CT reduces scanning time with some loss of resolution. It is useful for CT angiography.

Intravenous injection of contrast material is used to enhance the x-ray contrast of vascular lesions such as tumors and abscesses; contrast material diffuses into an area where the blood–brain barrier has broken down to increase the x-ray absorption density.

CT scanning is highly sensitive and often diagnostic; therefore, it has a place in both screening and specific investigations. Use of a contrast agent is not necessary for screening studies.

Principal Indications

CT is used in the evaluation of patients with intracranial problems when structural alteration is known or suspected, such as tumor, cerebrovascular disease, degenerative disease (Alzheimer disease, Huntington disease), hydrocephalus, subdural hematoma, or unexplained headache. CT is superior to MRI in identifying calcification and hemorrhage. CT is safe for patients with aneurysm clips, pacemakers, and implanted defibrillators. The imaging time and noise are much less than with MRI, which makes CT useful for uncooperative or confused patients. Many conditions can be assessed without the use of a radiographic contrast agent; this should be strongly considered for patients who have conditions for which the most common causes do not require contrast for visualization (i.e., dementia, remote stroke) and for elderly persons, in whom the risks associated with contrast studies are somewhat greater.

Limitations

A negative CT scan does not exclude a structural lesion or damage. The damage may not have caused enough change in local absorption density to produce contrast with its surroundings. This is not uncommon in cases of cerebral infarction within 1 week after the initial insult, when the original edema has cleared and new vessel formation and phagocytosis have not yet begun to affect brain density. A CT scan can also be negative because the damage is in an area of the brain that is poorly visualized, such as the brainstem or spinal cord. In addition, a CT scan is typically negative after transient ischemia, but this finding does not detract from the significance of the event and the need for further study. CT is less sensitive than MRI for stroke, vascular malformation, tumor, abscess, and demyelinating lesions.

When it is performed without contrast injection, CT scanning is essentially free of risk. When contrast material is used, the risk is that of the contrast agent itself—often a warm flush in the face, nausea, or sometimes vomiting. In approximately 1 case in 100,000 there is the possibility of death from anaphylaxis. The serum creatinine concentration should be measured before the infusion of contrast material. If it is abnormal, the risks and precautions related to renal insult from contrast media must be considered (see Chapter 52).

Patient Experience. The patient is asked to lie down with his or her head inside what looks somewhat like a large doughnut. Straps are usually applied over the forehead to prevent motion. The procedure takes 5 to 20 minutes, depending on the scanner. Contrast material may be given intravenously, by single bolus, or by intravenous drip.

Computed Tomography Scanning of the Spine

The definition of the procedure and the patient experience are the same as for CT scanning of the head.

Principal Indications

CT of the spine is the preferred technique for evaluation of acute fractures and bony impingement on the central canal. It does not visualize the spinal cord or nerve roots and has therefore been replaced by MRI for visualization of the spinal cord and disc disease. CT of the spine can be used for patients with aneurysm clips, pacemakers, and debrillators.

Limitations

If the spinal region to be studied spans three or more vertebrae, MRI is more practical than CT because MRI can visualize an entire region of the spine. Diagnostic accuracy of CT presupposes use of a localizer image for accurate selection of the plane and angle of the slice, as well as a thin slice for optimal resolution.

Magnetic Resonance Imaging of the Central Nervous System

Definition of Procedure

MRI is a noninvasive imaging technique that yields better contrast and sensitivity for most central nervous system lesions than does radiographic CT. It uses radio waves of a specific (resonance) frequency. No ionizing radiation is required. MRI studies usually are substantially more expensive than CT studies.

Principal Indications

The high tissue contrast achieved with MRI makes it the imaging technique of choice for most central nervous system diseases, including tumors (especially posterior fossa tumors), cerebral infarctions, vascular malformations, abscesses, white matter disease (e.g., multiple sclerosis), and spinal cord abnormalities including herniated nucleus pulposus.

In several aspects of brain imaging, MRI has been shown to be superior to CT. MRI provides better imaging of the posterior fossa than does CT because the surrounding bone causes no streak artifacts. Tissue contrast with MRI is superior to that obtained with CT. As a result, gray matter and white matter are better delineated and the extent of certain diseases is better appreciated. For example, MRI can reveal many more of the lesions of multiple sclerosis than can CT. Major blood vessels can be identified with MRI without the need for contrast media because the flowing blood, as a result of its velocity, appears dark. The common carotid, internal carotid, external carotid, and vertebral and basilar arteries are easily seen. Aneurysms of the internal carotid artery have been detected, and a thrombus in the lumen of the artery can be identified. Disc disease is easily evaluated without injection of contrast material, as is required for myelography.

Limitations

MRI has high sensitivity for disease detection in the central nervous system but is limited and may be less useful than CT in the evaluation of acute hemorrhages, calcified lesions, and bony structures, each of which is easily detected by CT. Because the scanning time is longer than that for CT studies, MRI studies are more subject to artifact caused by patient motion. Some claustrophobic patients cannot undergo the procedure without sedation.

The known hazards of MRI result from the force and torque exerted by the field on ferromagnetic objects brought into the vicinity of the magnet and on patients' prostheses, such as surgical clips, pacemakers, cochlear implants, metal in the eye, and joint replacements. Cardiac pacemaker and implanted defibrillator function can be disrupted and false signals produced. Ferromagnetic metal clips, such as those on cerebral aneurysms, may be dislodged.

Patient Experience. The patient lies supine on a table identical to the CT scanner, but the head holder consists of a plastic coil that passes very close to the patient's face. The entire table is then moved into a larger tunnel. The patient may experience claustrophobia. A loud knocking sound is heard during data collection, during which time the patient must remain absolutely still. The test lasts about 45 minutes.

General References

Baker AB, Baker LH, eds. Clinical neurology. 3 vols. New York: Harper & Row. Published since 1976, with yearly updates.

Contains excellent detailed reviews of the neurologic examination and neurodiagnostic tests.

Carson D, Serpell M. Choosing the best needle for diagnostic lumbar puncture. Neurology 1996;47:33.

Excellent discussion of pros and cons of various lumbar puncture needles.

Edelman RR, Warach S. Magnetic resonance imaging. N Engl J Med 1993;328:708.

Well-referenced review (this part covers the use of MRI for the nervous system).

Health and Public Policy Committee, American College of Physicians. Diagnostic evaluation of the carotid arteries. Ann Intern Med 1988;109:835.

Specific recommendations for the use of tests in screening and diagnosis.

Goetz CG. Textbook of clinical neurology. 1st ed. Philadelphia: W. B. Saunders, 1999.

Comprehensive description of neuroradiologic procedures, including all of the newer techniques covered in this chapter. Good background reading for a more thorough understanding of the technologic advances made in this field.

CHAPTER 87

Headaches and Facial Pain

CONSTANCE J. JOHNSON, MD

EPIDEMIOLOGY

Although epidemiologic surveys of headache are not always comparable or consistent with one another, all agree on the magnitude of the problem: 80% to 90% of U.S. adults report a history of recurrent headache, and in 30% to 50%, headaches are described as severe at times. Women suffer disproportionately from headaches, both in terms of numbers affected and in severity of headaches; the reported prevalence in women varies from slightly higher to three times higher than in men (1–3). In *surveys of visits to physicians,* headache was named by patients as the principal reason for approximately 2% to 4% of all visits to internists, general practitioners, and family practitioners (4). Most patients presenting to the office have a primary headache disorder that meets the criteria for tension-type headache, migraine, or cluster headache. A small percentage have a secondary headache disorder (temporal arteritis, acute sinusitis, or intracranial infection, tumor, or hemorrhage) (5). Most headache sufferers depend on self-care with over-the-counter remedies rather than on visits to their doctors to deal with their headache problems. Fewer than half of active migraine sufferers consult a physician for headache each year (6).

CLASSIFICATION

This chapter uses the diagnostic criteria for headache syndromes defined in 1988 by the *International Headache Society* (7). These criteria are widely used for clinical decisions as well as research. The term *muscle contraction headache* has been replaced by the term *tension-type headache.* Debate within the headache community continues about the practical difference between tension-type and migraine headache. Individual patients often have both types of headache. Some patients with frequent tension-type headache respond to drugs used for migraine, and some with mild migraine respond to regimens recommended for tension-type headache. Most patients presenting to the office have patterns that meet the criteria for one of these two types of headache. A small percentage have headache caused by drugs or toxins; infection (e.g., meningitis); traction on pain-sensitive intracranial structures (e.g., tumor, hemorrhage, edema); inflammatory disease (e.g., vasculitis); or diseases of the eye, ear, sinuses, teeth, or facial nerves and structures.

GENERAL APPROACH TO THE PATIENT WITH HEADACHE

History

The history provides the most useful information for evaluating headache, particularly a careful account by the patient of the current or most recent episode. The most useful aspects of the history in determining cause are the temporal profile, associated symptoms, disability, and family history; the least specific aspects are the character and location of the pain. Undue emphasis should not be placed on differentiating, for example, throbbing pain from pressure pain, because the subjective interpretation of headache pain is so variable. The following questions are helpful in the differential diagnosis of headache. (The interpretation of patients' answers to these questions is discussed in detail in later sections on specific headache syndromes.)

Associated Factors

Is there any warning of the attack (prodromal feeling, focal numbness or weakness, visual symptoms including the fortification hallucinations of migraine)?

Is the patient aware of any factors that can bring on these headaches (withdrawal from caffeine, alcohol ingestion, vasodilator use, psychosocial stress, perimenstrual period, foods, drug use, position, sexual orgasm, exertion, tobacco)? What drugs is the patient taking for other conditions? To what does the patient attribute the headache? Does the patient fear a dreaded cause such as a tumor?

Temporal Features

When did the patient first experience this type of headache? How does the headache begin (suddenly, or by building up slowly over a period of several hours or days)? When does the headache occur? Does it waken the patient from sleep or is it present on awakening? Does it recede after the patient has been up for several hours? What is the frequency of headaches? (Have the patient recount the past month's and the past year's pattern.) How long do the headaches last (maximum, minimum, average)? Have there been intervals of weeks or months without headache?

Character and Location of Pain

What kind of pain is the patient experiencing with the current headaches (band-like, squeezing, pressure, pounding, throbbing)? Where is the pain located (one side of the head, all over the head, in the eyes, radiating up the back of the neck)? Does the pain radiate anywhere or seem to spread during the course of an attack? How severe can the headaches be (on a scale of 1 to 10)? How does the patient rate this headache pain compared with the pain of other headaches or other situations (e.g., worst headache ever, worst pain in my life)? What is the average pain severity?

Aggravating and Alleviating Factors

Does anything make the headache pain worse (bending, standing, sneezing, straining, coughing)? What factors reduce the headache (lying down, ice packs, pressing on the temples, avoidance of work, simple analgesics, narcotics, other medications)? How is the patient currently treating the headache?

Environmental Exposures

Does the headache occur predictably after exposure to an environment that may have increased carbon monoxide levels (e.g., a closed room heated by a space heater)? Did the headache start after the patient began work (or activities at home) that entailed exposure to fumes or dust containing lead? These and other environmental exposures that can cause headache are listed in Table 8.2 in Chapter 8.

Associated Neurologic Symptoms

Does the patient have associated symptoms during the headaches, such as spots before the eyes (common in both tension and migraine headaches); inability to tolerate light, sound, touch, or movement; nausea or vomiting; focal numbness or weakness; or vertigo? Did the patient have motion sickness as a child? Does the patient note scalp tenderness? (All of these symptoms are common in migraine.)

Prior Evaluation

Has the patient been evaluated for the headaches, and what were the results of this evaluation? It is important to request previous records for all patients who give a history of severe, disabling headache, regardless of the reported duration of the present headache problem or the nature of the previous evaluation; sometimes just requesting the records reminds the patient of a 10- or 20-year history of severe headache and multiple visits, and sometimes the previous records confirm such a history despite poor recall by the patient. In either case, this information can be particularly valuable in evaluating a patient who describes recent onset of severe headaches.

Disability or Functional Impact

How are the headaches currently affecting the patient (work, social relationships)? How many days does the patient miss work/school or social/family events because of headache? How often does the patient have reduced productivity because of headache? How many days per month does the patient have headache?

Family and Household History

Is there a history of headaches in parents, siblings, children, or other people living in the patient's household? What type?

Physical and Laboratory Examination

In most cases the history suggests the probable basis for a patient's headache. Appropriate physical examination and laboratory studies are described for each type of headache in later sections. The appropriate extent of these objective aspects of the examination may vary from a limited physical examination (e.g., in a patient with headache after vasodilator therapy), to an examination focused on structures that may be the source of the headache (e.g., teeth), to a complete neurologic examination together with imaging studies or laboratory tests (as in the patient with new-onset or marked change in prior headache pattern, the patient with headache and a new focal neurologic abnormality such as weakness, or the patient whose presentation suggests giant cell arteritis).

The role of imaging studies for the patient with nonacute headache and a normal neurologic examination is addressed by a practice guideline issued by the American Academy of Neurology (AAN) (8). Based on a review of all relevant publications, there was sufficient information to be explicit in recommending *against* the routine use of imaging in such patients with migraine, including migraine with aura. Because of the meager amount of published evidence, the guideline makes no recommendations for patients other than those with migraine. To inform clinical decisions, however, the discussion that accompanies the guidelines cites one available study of a large health maintenance organization population in which it was estimated that a tumor would be found fewer than 1 in 10,000 patients who have headaches as their

Table 87.1. Abnormal Computed Tomography or Magnetic Resonance Imaging Findings in Migraine and Unspecified Headache

Finding	Migraine	Unspecified Headache
Total Scans	897 (100%)	1,825 (100%)
Tumor	3 (0.3%)	21 (1%)
Arteriovenus malformation	1 (0.1%)	6 (0.3%)
Hydrocephalus	—	8 (0.4%)
Aneurysm	—	3 (0.2%)
Subdural hematoma	—	5 (0.3%)
Total potentially treatable lesions	4/897 (0.4%)	43/1,825 (2.4%)[a] 3/725 (0.4%)[b]

[a]All studies.

[b]Without studies 9 and 10, which were done in the early computed tomography era and addressed any kind of headache at referral centers.

From Frishberg BM. The utility of neuroimaging in the evaluation of headache in patients with normal neurologic examinations. Neurology 1994;44:1191.

only symptom and a normal neurologic examination. Table 87.1 summarizes other information from the guideline that may be useful in decision-making about costly imaging studies for such patients.

For patients with *nonacute headache and an unexplained abnormal finding on neurologic examination*, the AAN guideline concluded that there is fair evidence to justify obtaining neuroimaging; it also concluded that the data are insufficient regarding the relative sensitivity of magnetic resonance imaging (MRI) or computed tomography (CT) scanning in the evaluation of headache (8). The properties of these two imaging techniques are described in Chapter 86.

Principles of Initial Treatment

Patients with a headache history consistent with tension-type headache or migraine and a normal examination can begin treatment as described later. A more extensive investigation should be carried out for patients who show either of the following situations after initial treatment: *failure to respond to treatment of the presumed condition* (and even in this situation, the extent of the evaluation should be tempered by the circumstances) or *significant changes in complaints or physical findings* that point to one of the less common causes of headache discussed later. The following are "red flags" suggesting that the headache is secondary: onset after 50 years of age, thunderclap onset, systemic illness, underlying malignancy or acquired immunodeficiency syndrome (AIDS), and a new-onset, steadily progressive headache.

Treatment Expectations

In studies on the issue of expectations of physicians and patients, the majority of physicians expected that their patients would demand pain relief and not care much about getting an explanation for their problem. In clinical studies, however, only 31% of patients stated that pain relief was most important, whereas 46% rated getting an explanation of their problem as their most important concern (9). Population studies of migraine sufferers have shown that they are both underdiagnosed and undertreated. The American Migraine Study, a comprehensive population survey, reported that only 29% of migraine sufferers were "very satisfied" with their treatment. Patients are dissatisfied with the time to onset and the degree of pain relief, and the majority are not using migraine-specific prescription medications (6).

When total relief of headache pain is not possible, the patient must be helped to understand the limitations of drug therapy. Selection of a treatment regimen is complicated by the high placebo response rate (20% to 40%) and the variable natural history of headaches. Because of this variability, a detailed baseline history of the patient's headache problems is important for subsequent assessment of the patient's response to treatment.

SPECIFIC HEADACHE SYNDROMES

Tension-Type Headache

Classification and Diagnostic Criteria

In the absence of any rigorous criterion or physiologic markers, the term *tension-type headache* has been applied to what is probably a heterogeneous group of headache syndromes. The 1988 international classification (7) delineated two subtypes of tension-type headache: *episodic headache* (fewer than 180 episodes per year) and *chronic headache* (more than 180 episodes per year, including continuous chronic headache) (10). Additional consensus criteria for *episodic tension-type headache* include the following:

1. Duration 30 minutes to 7 days
2. At least two of the following pain characteristics:
   a. Pressing/tightening (nonpulsating) quality
   b. Mild or moderate intensity
   c. Bilateral location
   d. No aggravation from walking stairs or similar routine physical activity
3. Both of the following:
   a. No nausea or vomiting (anorexia may occur)
   b. Photophobia and phonophobia are absent, or one but not the other is present

Recurrent tension-type headaches are usually similar in quality and location. Patients with *chronic tension headache* often have associated depression or anxiety. Occasionally a patient with chronic tension headache complains of headaches that have been unremitting for years.

Physical examination of the patient with tension headache is normal except for neck or scalp muscle tenderness in some patients.

Pathogenesis

Headache is widely accepted as a neurobiologic disorder. The symptoms of tension-type headache have been presumed to be a somatic consequence of psychosocial stress in the patient's life. Neither increased muscle tension nor precipitating stress is specific for tension-type headaches; both are also common in migraine, which is the prototype of a neurobiologic headache disorder (see later discussion). Table 87.2 summarizes the data on the frequency of several characteristics in a large number of patients and shows considerable overlap between tension-type and migraine headaches. The pathogenesis may be the same (see later discussion). Depression or anxiety, which can be masked, is usually associated with chronic tension headache. The causal relationship between headache and depression and anxiety is controversial; some believe these conditions to be causal, whereas others consider them to be secondary to headaches.

Treatment

Patients with intermittent headache that is not severe usually respond to simple over-the-counter analgesics. Most of these patients do not seek medical attention for their headaches but admit to headaches on review of systems. On the other hand, patients with continuous daily headache of months' or years' duration often seek medical attention. Many of them have depression or anxiety states. These patients describe constant headache that lacks any localizing characteristics and is refractory to analgesics and migraine prophylaxis with the exception of antidepressants. Some patients with chronic daily headache have medication overuse headache (rebound), caffeine withdrawal headache, or transformed migraine. The use of analgesic medications other than nonsteroidal anti-inflammatory drugs (NSAIDs) more than 3 to 4 days a week can result in chronic daily headache. Patients should withdraw from these medications for at least 1 month. NSAIDs do not appear to cause rebound and can be used during this time. If caffeine overuse and withdrawal seems to correlate with the complaint of chronic daily headache, patients should be counseled to restrict or eliminate caffeine intake.

Nonpharmacologic Treatment. It is usually helpful to explain to the patient that the mechanism of pain is unknown, and, when appropriate, that it may be related to stress. Emphasis on the benign nature of the headache is important to relieve patient concerns regarding more serious pathology such as a brain tumor. As explained elsewhere (see Chapter 20), concerned listening often helps to reduce somatic symptoms caused by stress, as does encouragement for any effort made by the patient to reduce stressful situations. For patients seeking nonpharmacologic relief of symptoms, massage of the scalp and neck muscles by another person or use of relaxation techniques (see Chapter 22) can be recommended. In addition, any other approach that the patient may have found helpful should be encouraged, including complementary and alternative treatment modalities (see Chapter 5).

Table 87.2. Characteristics of Migraine and Tension Type Headaches

Parameter	Migraine (%)	Tension (%)
Age at onset		
<20 yr	55	30
>20 yr	45	70
Premonitory symptoms	60	10
Frequency		
Daily	3	50
Less than once a week	60	15
Duration		
Constant, daily	0	20
1–3 days	35	10
Throbbing pain	80	30
Location		
Unilateral	80	10
Bilateral	20	90
Vomiting with attacks	50	10
Family history of headache	65	40

Adapted from Raskin NH, Appenzeller O. Headache. Philadelphia: WB Saunders, 1980; as modified from Friedman AP et al. Neurology 1954;4:773.

Pharmacologic Treatment. *Symptomatic* treatment with drugs is an important adjunct to the general measures just described. Most patients have used headache remedies containing acetaminophen, aspirin, or other NSAIDs before consulting their physician about treatment. For mild to moderate headaches, however, an additional trial of these mild analgesics should be recommended if they have not been taken at the usual effective dosage.

A number of drugs are widely prescribed for patients with moderate to severe episodic tension-type headaches that are unresponsive to acetaminophen, aspirin, or other NSAIDs. These drugs include codeine sulfate, propoxyphene (Darvon), and products that combine analgesics, sedatives, and caffeine (e.g., butalbital/caffeine plus aspirin or acetaminophen) or that include oxycodone plus aspirin or acetaminophen. Each of these drugs can lead to dependency. Therefore, it is unwise to initiate treatment with them unless there is a strict contractual agreement regarding the conditions for their use (see Chapter 29).

When disabling tension-type headache occurs in migraineurs, the triptan sumatriptan aborts the headache in a large proportion of patients (see later discussion).

Prophylaxis is warranted for the patient whose tension headaches are severe or frequent. A recent meta-analysis of placebo-controlled clinical trials concluded that tricyclic antidepressants greatly diminish headache suffering and analgesic use in at least one third of patients (10). One trial showed that when tricyclic antidepressants were used in conjunction with stress management techniques (relaxation and cognitive coping; see Chapters 20 and 22) the effectiveness of the two interventions was additive, producing greater than 50% reduction in headache index scores in 64% of patients, compared with 38% of those given tricyclics only, 35% of those given only stress management, and 29% of those given placebo (11). In some responders, the doses of tricyclics approached the levels used in the treatment of depression (amitriptyline 100 mg and nortriptyline 75 mg daily). A detailed discussion of the use of tricyclic antidepressants is found in Chapter 24.

Migraine

Classification and Diagnostic Criteria

The classification of migraine headache was revised in 1988 from the designations "common" and "classic" migraine to *migraine without aura* and *migraine with aura* (7).

Consensus criteria for the syndrome of *migraine without aura* include the following:

1. The patient has had at least five attacks fulfilling criteria 2 through 4.
2. Headache attacks last 4 to 72 hours (untreated or unsuccessfully treated).
3. Headache has at least two of the following characteristics:
   a. Unilateral location
   b. Pulsating quality
   c. Moderate or severe intensity
   d. Aggravation from walking stairs or similar routine physical activity
4. During headache, at least one of the following is present:
   a. Nausea or vomiting
   b. Photophobia and phonophobia

Head pain in a migraine attack usually increases gradually, reaching a peak after several hours and lasting for several hours to 1 day in typical cases. Attacks lasting 2 to 3 days are not uncommon, and some migraine attacks last 1 to 2 weeks. The pain may be described as pounding or throbbing, but the quality of the pain is variable and may be aching, pressing, or stabbing. Although headaches are typically unilateral at the beginning of a single attack, they may be bilateral or generalize. Most patients have attacks on both sides of the head; in a minority of patients, headaches are always on the same side.

The additional criteria for the syndrome of *migraine with aura* are the following:

1. The patient has had at least two attacks fulfilling criterion 2.
2. At least three of the following four characteristics are present:
   a. There are one or more fully reversible aura symptoms indicating focal cerebral cortical or brainstem dysfunction.
   b. At least one aura symptom develops gradually over longer than 4 minutes, or two or more symptoms occur in succession.
   c. No aura symptom lasts longer than 60 minutes; if more than one aura symptom is present, the accepted duration is proportionally increased.
   d. Headache follows aura with a free interval of less than 60 minutes. (It may also begin before or simultaneously with the aura.)

Headaches with aura are subdivided into the following categories: Typical, prolonged, familial hemiplegic, basilar, aura without headache, and acute-onset aura.

Migraine with typical aura (the most common form with aura) has one of the following types of aura symptoms:

- Homonymous visual disturbance
- Unilateral paresthesias or numbness
- Unilateral weakness
- Aphasia or unclassifiable speech difficulty

Fortification hallucinations are almost specific for migraine; these are slowly enlarging scotomata that are surrounded by luminous angles and that slowly change shape and appear to move across the visual fields (Fig. 87.1). Rarely, occipital lobe tumors or arteriovenous malformations produce the same effects.

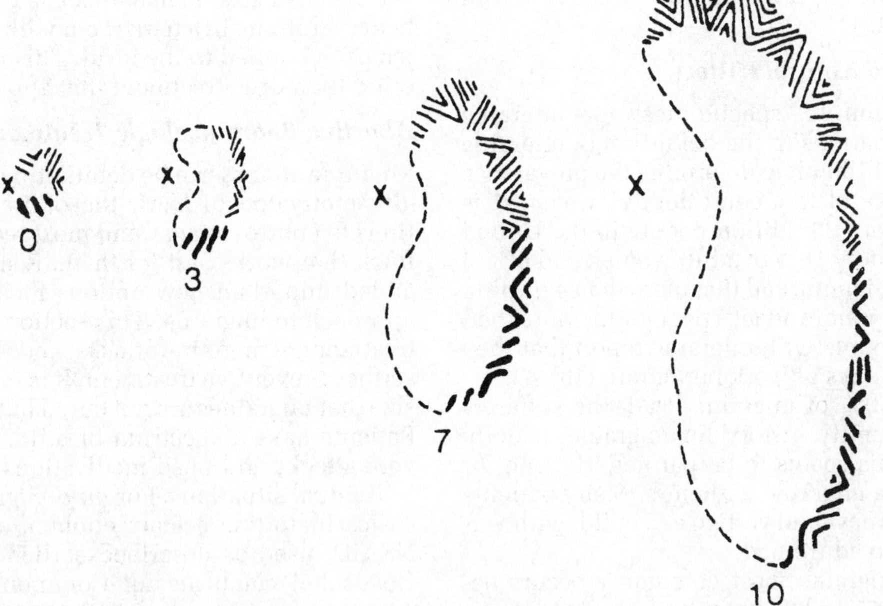

Figure 87.1. Lashley's maps of the progression of his own fortification spectra at varying time intervals after the onset of a migrainous attack. The X in each instance indicates the visual fixation point. The numbers represent minutes. (From Raskin NH, Appenzeller O. Headache. Philadelphia, W. B. Saunders, 1980; as appeared in Lashley KS. Arch Neurol Psychiatry 1941;46:331.)

Further types of migraine include ophthalmoplegic, retinal, childhood periodic syndromes, complications of migraine (infarction, status migrainosis), and unclassified.

Migraine is more common than is generally appreciated, and many patients with recurrent moderate to severe migraine headaches are misdiagnosed as having tension-type headaches. Failure of analgesics in a patient with recurrent, disabling headaches justifies a revised diagnosis of migraine.

In the *differential diagnosis of migraine,* the most important considerations are transient ischemic attacks (TIAs) or other cerebrovascular events, particularly in middle-age and older patients (see Chapter 91). *Migrainous ischemia* usually occurs in patients with a history of similar attacks, often in young adulthood. The family history tends to be particularly strong. Symptoms of migrainous ischemia typically last for one-half hour to several hours; TIAs usually last minutes to several hours. Headaches should be a prominent component of the migrainous ischemic event; although headache may occur in up to 25% of patients with TIAs, it is usually mild and transitory. Older patients with suspected migrainous ischemic events, particularly those with migraine equivalents (ischemic symptoms without headache), should be evaluated for TIA (see Chapter 91) before their symptoms are attributed to migraine.

Pathogenesis

Migraine is a neurobiologic disorder in which the trigeminovascular threshold is lowered, resulting in a cascade of events that includes activation of nociceptors of pain-producing structures and reduction in the normal mechanism of pain gating. Neuropeptides are released, and plasma protein extravasation occurs in the trigeminal ganglion. Positron emission tomographic studies during migraine reveal activation of brainstem areas (12).

Epidemiology and Natural History

The lack of a simple, specific test for migraine headache and variations in the definition of migraine headache make it difficult to determine the prevalence and natural course of this condition. However, it is estimated that about 28 million people in the United States (approximately 18% of adult women and 6% of adult men) have migraine and that more than 4 million of them have one or more attacks per month. More than half of working people with migraine report that they miss more than 2 days of work per month (13).

From 20% to 50% of migraine headache sufferers have a positive family history for migraine, usually in one parent. This seems to be particularly true for patients who have migraine with aura. Many patients report motion sickness and vertigo as a child, with vertigo persisting into adulthood.

The onset of migraine most commonly occurs between the ages of 15 and 25 years but can occur at any time throughout the adult life span. Episodic attacks are characteristic of migraine headache. Most migraine sufferers have several attacks each year; some have one or more episodes per week; and some have only rare episodes or even only a single typical episode in their lifetime. Migraine episodes usually become less frequent and less severe with age.

Possible Precipitating Factors. The perimenstrual period (particularly before the onset of bleeding, when levels of estradiol are falling), oral contraceptives (particularly off-days, presumably because of falling estrogen levels, or with use of triphasic pills), and menopause (estrogen deficiency) are associated with migraine headaches. The following substances may initiate headaches in susceptible subjects: vasodilators (nitrates and antihypertensives); alcohol; chocolate; cheeses, wines, and other foods containing tyramine; and monosodium glutamate. Withdrawal of caffeine or ergotamine can also cause headaches. An unusually long period of sleep (e.g., sleeping in on weekends) may provoke migraine. Attacks tend to occur also during periods of relaxation, such as weekends, holidays, or vacations. The patient should be asked about these associations and any others that may have been noted.

Nonpharmacologic Treatment

Most migraine sufferers can be helped by treatment, principally pharmacologic treatment. A number of nonpharmacologic measures may help also.

The most useful nonpharmacologic treatment is *avoidance of known trigger factors.* Common drugs that may trigger an attack are nitrates, vasodilators, and oral contraceptives. Other trigger factors that can be eliminated are alcohol, irregular sleep habits, excess caffeine use, and caffeine withdrawal. There are no consistently implicated dietary trigger factors; however, each patient should be encouraged to try eliminating any dietary component or other trigger factor that can be identified.

During an established attack, a patient usually feels better reclining in a dark room with a cool compress or ice pack applied to the head. This is the only practice other than drug treatment that appears to be helpful.

Abortive Pharmacologic Treatment

Migraine attacks can be debilitating. Sufferers are usually motivated to learn the optimal use of medications to control attacks and most readily learn the regimen that works best for them. Recent advances have added important new options for the pharmacologic approach to migraine. This section describes abortive treatment of migraine attacks, and the next section describes preventive treatment. It is important to emphasize that migraines are not cured but can be controlled. Patients have a spectrum of mild, moderate, and severe attacks and need medications stratified for their individual situations. For *mild migraine attacks,* analgesics including acetaminophen, aspirin, or another NSAID, used as described earlier (see Tension-Type Headache), can be useful. Commonly used agents and dosages of these and a number of products that combine analgesics, barbiturates, or caffeine are listed in Table 87.3.

Table 87.3. Drugs for Acute Migraine Attacks

Drug	Route	Trade Name	Dosage[a]
Nonprescription Analgesic			
Aspirin	Oral		650 mg q4h PRN
Acetaminophen	Oral	Tylenol	650 mg q4h PRN
Ibuprofen	Oral	Advil, Nuprin, etc.	200 mg 1 to 4 q4-8h PRN
Naproxen	Oral	Aleve	220 mg, one q6h PRN
Prescription Analgesics			
Naproxen (or other NSAID)[b]	Oral	Anaprox DS	550 mg q12h PRN
		Naprosyn	500 mg q12h PRN
Ketorolac	Oral, IM	Toradol	10-mg tablets: 2 initially then 1 q6h Prefilled syringes: 15, 30 mg 30–60 mg, then 30 mg q6h
Isometheptene, acetominophen and dichloralphenazone	Oral	Midrin	2 capsules, then 1 qh (up to 5 capsules/24 h)
Butalbital, acetaminophen	Oral	Phrenilin	1–2 q4h PRN (up to 6/day)
Butalbital, acetaminophen,	Oral	Fioracet, Esgic	1–2 q4h PRN
and caffeine	Oral	Fiorinol	1–2 q4h PRN (up to 6/day)
Butorphanol	Nasal spray	Stadol NS	1 mg (1 spray), may repeat this sequence in 3–4 h as needed
Prescription Nonanalgesics			
Ergotamine	Oral[c]	Cafergot Wigraine	2 mg at onset, 1 mg q0.5h (up to 6 tablets/day; 10 tablets/wk)
	Suppository[c]	Cafergot	2 mg at onset, may repeat in 1 hour (up to 5/wk)
	Sublingual	Ergostat	2 mg at onset and q0.5h (up to 3 tablets/day, 5/wk)
Dihydroergotamine	Intramuscular or Intravenous	D.H.E. 45	1 mg IM or IV and qh (3/day, IM, 2/day IV, 6/wk)
	Nasal spray	Migranol	0.5 mg spray: 1 spray in each nostril, followed by 1 spray in each nostril 15 min later
Triptans[d]			
Sumatriptan[f]	SC	Imitrex	6 mg may repeat in 1 hr (up to 2/24 h)
	Oral	Imitrex	50 mg or 100 mg. Repeat if no improvement after 2 h (max. cumulative dosage 200 mg/24 h)
	Nasal spray	Imitrex	5- or 20-mg spray may repeat in 2 h (up to 40 mg/24 h)
Zolmitriptan	Oral tablet and ZMT[e]	Zomig	2.5 or 5 mg[f] (max 10 mg/24 h)
Rizatriptan	Oral tablet and MLT[e]	Maxalt	10 or 5 mg[f] (max 30 mg/24 h)
Naratriptan	Oral tablet	Amerge	2.5 or 1 mg[g] (max 5 mg/24 h)
Almotriptan	Oral tablet	Axert	12.5 or 6.25 mg[f] (max 25 mg/24 h)

[a]Information given in quantities of available strengths unless otherwise described in parentheses.
[b]See list of NSAIDs and available strengths in Chapter 77.
[c]These ergotamine products also contain caffeine (100 mg per dose), which enhances gastrointestinal absorption.
[d]Usual adult doze listed first.
[e]Rapidly disintegrating form.
[f]Repeat at 2 hr if no improvement.
[g]Repeat at 4 hr if no improvement.

At the start of a *moderate to severe migraine*, a triptan, ergotamine tartrate, or an NSAID may be used. Triptans are highly effective, migraine-specific medications with a lower side effect profile than ergotamines.

Triptans. The triptans are selective serotonin 5HT1B/1D receptor agonists that are highly effective agents for treating migraine headaches (14). In the laboratory these agents have been shown to constrict extracerebral intracranial vessels and to inhibit activity in the peripheral trigeminal ganglion. All triptan compounds constrict the coronary arteries. Sumatriptan was the first agent introduced, followed by zolmitriptan, naratriptan, rizatriptan, and almotriptan. All triptans have similar efficacy and side effects. Triptans can be used at any time during a migraine, but they are more effective if taken early in the attack. The initial dose should be repeated after 2 hours for oral preparations and nasal spray, or 1 hour for injectable preparations, if the pain persists. Triptans can be combined with NSAIDs but not with ergotamine preparations in the same 24 hours (both are vasoconstrictors.) Although they are very safe medications in the healthy migraine patient, they should not be used by patients with coronary artery disease or uncontrolled hypertension.

Sumatriptan is available as tablets, injectable forms (stat dose self-injectable), and nasal spray. The second-generation triptans, which are similar to sumatriptan in efficacy, come only in tablet form. Two (zolmitriptan and rizatriptan) are available in usual and rapidly disintegrating tablet forms. Early controlled trials showed that 25, 50, or 100 mg of sumatriptan taken *orally* at the onset of aura or headache produced relief of headache symptoms within 2 hours in approximately 55% of patients and within 4 hours in about 70%

of patients. Similar responses to placebo occurred in no more than 20% of patients (6). In a more recent controlled trial, the 50-mg dose was comparable to the 100-mg dose, and both were superior to the 25-mg dose (15). *Nasal spray* is available as 5 and 20 mg. Placebo-controlled trials demonstrated some response with the 5-mg dose, but the 20-mg dose was superior to placebo and is the usual adult dose (16). Administration of a single 6-mg dose *subcutaneously* yielded symptom relief in about 75% of patients within 1 hour and in more than 80% within 2 hours (17). Sumatriptan also relieves nausea, vomiting, and other disabling symptoms of migraine with few side effects.

The unique advantage of sumatriptan and the other triptans compared with ergotamine is that the triptans are effective when taken at any time during a migraine headache, whereas ergotamine must be given at the beginning of an attack. The incidence of *recurrence of migraine* within the ensuing 24 hours is higher with the triptans than with ergotamine, although this has not been a significant limitation. The triptans are more expensive than ergotamine (e.g., sumatriptan costs $10 to $15 per pill, about $18 per spray dose, and about $35 per injected dose), but they may save on office visit or emergency room fees.

If a patient has *persistent headache after 2 hours,* the initial oral or spray dose should be repeated. For return of headache on the same day, treatment can be repeated up to the maximum doses shown in Table 87.3. The subcutaneous dose of sumatriptan may be repeated at 1 hour if the patient has had a partial response. Efficacy has not been demonstrated for a second dose in patients who did not respond initially.

When *tension-type headache* (see criteria listed earlier) occurs in migraineurs, sumatriptan 50 mg has been shown to be superior to placebo in producing a pain-free response at 4 hours after taking the medication (56% versus 36%) (18).

Practical information about available preparations and doses of sumatriptan and the second-generation triptans is presented in Table 87.3.

Side Effects. The most common side effects of the triptans are transient paresthesias, tingling, dizziness, and, after subcutaneous administration, injection-site reactions (pain, erythema lasting about 1 hour). One or more transient side effects occur in approximately 50% of patients after oral administration (25% with placebo) and in approximately 70% after injection (40% with placebo). Up to 5% of patients describe transient chest tightness. Many patients respond to a lower injected dosage (3 or 4 mg), which may be prescribed if side effects limit usefulness. This requires use of the multidose vial, which means that the patient must be instructed in sterile technique.

Contraindications. Because in large dosages sumatriptan is embryolethal in rabbits and because there has been no trial to establish the safety of sumatriptan in pregnant women, its use in pregnancy is proscribed. No adverse age-related effects have accrued in patients older than 60 years of age who participated in clinical trials. Triptans are not recommended for patients with hemiplegic or basilar artery migraine and are contraindicated for patients with coronary artery disease or uncontrolled hypertension.

Ergotamine. The action of ergotamine has traditionally been attributed to its vasoconstrictor properties; however, its effect may be related to its serotonin receptor agonist properties. Ergotamine is available in preparations that permit administration by multiple routes (Table 87.3). It provides effective symptom control in approximately 50% of migraine sufferers and is generally recommended as the most cost-effective first choice among the nonanalgesic agents. Dihydroergotamine, given intravenously or intramuscularly, is useful chiefly for treating refractory migraine in an emergency department or in hospitals.

The ideal route for administering ergotamine is one that is convenient, leads to prompt absorption of the drug, and is not affected by vomiting. Suppository and sublingual preparations meet these criteria. Ingested tablets can be vomited and are therefore less reliable. The traditional recommended schedules for ergotamine administration are summarized in Table 87.3. The objective of these schedules is to attain a total dosage that is effective but is below the dosage that produces nausea and vomiting. Traditionally this has been accomplished by taking additional doses at 30 and 60 minutes if the first dose is ineffective. An alternative strategy may increase the likelihood of prompt attenuation of headaches: Patients can determine the dosage that produces nausea for them (the nauseating dosage) by following the traditional schedule on a headache-free day. The cumulative dosage attained just before the nauseating dosage is the appropriate total therapeutic dosage (the subnauseating dosage) for that patient to take all at once at the onset of future attacks.

A number of points are important in instructing a patient about the use of ergotamine. The patient should understand that ergotamine is not a pain killer but is used to interrupt the events causing migraine pain, and that for maximal benefit one must take ergotamine at the onset of prodromal symptoms or headache (waiting for the headache to become well established is a common problem in patients who report no benefit from ergotamine). In order to ensure immediate access to their medicine, patients should be advised to carry some with them at all times. They should be informed that taking more than the recommended maximum daily dosage (Table 87.3) carries the risk of peripheral vasoconstriction in addition to nausea and vomiting. Because ergotamine preparations have a short shelf life, patients should obtain a new supply if they fail to obtain benefit from their medicine or if they have not used it for many months.

Side Effects. Occasionally a patient has side effects from ergotamine even when it is taken at the subnauseating dosage. These effects include abdominal cramps, vertigo, diarrhea, and distal paresthesia; less commonly, syncope, tremor, angina pectoris, and claudication may occur. However, most patients tolerate the drug well.

Serious adverse effects, including mental changes, edema, peripheral vascular occlusion, and distal gangrene, can occur if the daily dosage of ergotamine exceeds 6 mg or the weekly dosage exceeds 10 mg on a chronic basis. Patients should therefore be warned not to use ergotamine more than twice in the same week and no more than 10 mg in 1 week, to avoid both the aforementioned side effects and tolerance to the drug's effects.

Contraindications. The principal contraindications to ergotamine use are established angina, history of myocardial infarction, and symptomatic peripheral arterial disease. Ergotamine should not be used in combination with a triptan. Traditionally, hypertension has been named as a contraindication, but the risk has probably been overemphasized. If there is concern about the effect of ergotamine on the blood pressure of an individual patient, the blood pressure response to ergotamine can be measured in the physician's office, following the protocol for determining the subnauseating dosage of ergotamine outlined previously.

Nonsteroidal Anti-inflammatory Drugs. NSAIDs often help at the onset of an acute attack and should be used in full doses (Table 87.3). These drugs are generally more efficacious than simple analgesics (aspirin, acetaminophen) and narcotics (propoxyphene, low-dose codeine) and may be used for acute attacks alone or in conjunction with a triptan or ergotamine.

Narcotic Analgesics. For an established, severe migraine headache not responsive to NSAIDs, a triptan, or ergotamine, simple analgesics do not help. For this reason, reliable patients may be given small supplies of either codeine (60 mg) or an equipotent narcotic analgesic (see Table 13.1 in Chapter 13) to be taken as needed. This measure may save the patient unnecessary trips to the physician's office or an emergency department. Narcotic agents may be the only option for patients with coronary artery disease or for those patients who are unable to tolerate or are unresponsive to NSAIDs.

Nausea and Vomiting. These migraine symptoms can be treated with prochlorperazine suppositories (25 mg), which patients can easily self-administer. Because of the likelihood of vomiting, oral antiemetics are of limited usefulness but can be tried by patients who prefer not to take suppositories. Intravenous metoclopramide is also effective but is not practical for self-administration by patients.

Prophylactic Pharmacologic Treatment

Prophylactic drug therapy for migraine should be considered for patients who have two or more attacks per week or less frequent attacks that cannot be controlled with abortive therapy and that disrupt employment or social life. Known precipitating factors (described earlier) should be eliminated as the initial step in prevention.

The decision regarding prophylaxis must be made by the patient, after the distinction between abortive and prophylactic therapy has been explained clearly. Even a patient who has not had adequate relief from routine measures may forego prophylactic treatment because of the requirement that medicine be taken daily. For each of the drugs used prophylactically for migraine, a long trial period (2 to 3 months) may be necessary to assess effectiveness, and trials with a number of drugs may be necessary. Patients should understand that during the trial of prophylaxis they should continue their usual measures for treating migraine attacks.

Drugs that have been effective in migraine prophylaxis are listed in Table 87.4, which is adapted from the 2000 Practice Parameter of the American Academy of Neurology (see Silberstein, 2000, in General References). The table rates these drugs according to a mix of efficacy, strength of scientific evidence, and side effect profile. The anticonvulsant divalproex sodium (Depakote) is among the drugs receiving the best rating for migraine prophylaxis. Of patients taking divalproex sodium in dosages to achieve levels of 70 to 120 mg/L (500 to 1,500), 48% reported headache frequency reduced by 50%, compared to 14% of patients taking placebo (19). Despite this comparable efficacy profile, serious side effects are somewhat more likely than with the other drugs that received this rating. Patients who are not helped by prophylactic drugs can be referred to a neurologist or other specialist in migraine to learn of other options.

Table 87.4. Preventive Therapies for Migraine[a]

Group 1[b]	Group 2[c]	Group 3[d]
Amitriptyline	Beta-blockers	A: Antidepressants
Divalproex sodium	Atenolol/metoprolol/nadolol	Doxepine
Propranolol/timolol		Fluvoxamine
	Calcium-blockers	Imipramine
	Nimodipine/verapamil	Mirtazepine
		Nortriptyline
	NSAIDs	Paroxetine
	Aspirin/fenoprofen/flurbiprofen	Protriptyline
	Ketoprofen	Sertraline trazodone
	Mefenamic acid	Venlafaxine
	Neproxen	B: Other Cyproheptadine
	Naproxen sodium	Diltiazem
		Ibuprofen
		Tiagabine
		Topiramate
	Other	C: (side effect concerns)
	Feverfew	Methylergonovine (methylergometrine)
	Fluoxetine	
	Gabapentin	
	Magnesium vitamin B2	Phenelzine

[a]Does not include combination products.

[b]Medium to high efficacy, good strength of evidence, and mild-to-moderate side effects.

[c]Lower efficacy than those listed in first column, or limited strength of evidence, and mild-to-moderate side effects.

[d]Clinically efficacious based on consensus and clinical experience, but no scientific evidence of efficacy.

Modified from Silbserstein SD. Practice parameter: evidence-based guidelines for migraine headache—an evidence-based review. Report of the Quality Standards Subcommittee of the American Academy of Neurology. Neurology 2000;55: 754.

The following general conclusions can be drawn about migraine prophylaxis (17):

- At least 50% of treated patients report some improvement in their migraine syndrome during the first year, compared with 25% or less of control patients. During the second year of prophylaxis, the response rate may be lower.
- Most of the improvement consists of a decrease in frequency and severity of headaches and an increased responsiveness to abortive therapies; complete freedom from headaches occurs in only a minority of patients.
- Failure of a drug from one class does not predict response to another from that class or to a drug from another class. Therefore, a sequential trial of different drugs is reasonable.
- Comorbid conditions should be considered when selecting an agent. Patients with asthma or with athletic demands should not be given beta-blockers. Patients with mood disorders may benefit from divalproex or gabapentin.
- Failure to give an adequate dosage is a common reason for failure of migraine prophylaxis. Each class of drugs listed can be administered in the schedules and dose ranges found elsewhere in this book (antidepressants, Chapter 24; beta blockers and calcium antagonists, Chapter 67; NSAIDs, Chapter 77).
- To facilitate compliance, it is helpful to select agents that can be taken once per day.
- Each patient who chooses prophylactic therapy should be asked to keep a log in which to record the frequency and severity of headaches and the nature of any associated factors.

Alternative medicine to prevent migraine. Critical review of clinical trials have shown the following with regard to three popular nontraditional treatments for preventing migraine. The herbal remedy *feverfew* has not been shown convincingly to be superior to placebo (20). Acupuncture has been shown possibly to be superior to sham treatment (21). Homeopathic remedies have not been shown to be efficacious in the limited clinical trials available for review (22). Chapter 5 contains additional information about these nontraditional remedies.

Patients with Intractable Migraine Headaches

A small number of migraine sufferers have intractable and disabling headaches for which no effective regimen can be found despite trials of all available pharmacologic regimens. For a further assessment and consideration of other therapeutic options, these patients should be referred to a neurologist.

Cluster Headache

Classification and Diagnostic Criteria

Cluster headache is classified separately from migraine because of its distinct clinical characteristics and different therapy (7). It was previously designated by a number of names, such as *Horton's headache, histamine headache* (a misnomer), and *migrainous cranial neuralgia.* The 1988 international consensus criteria for the diagnosis of cluster headache include the following:

1. The patient has had at least five attacks fulfilling criteria 2 through 4.
2. There is severe unilateral orbital, supraorbital, or temporal pain lasting 15 to 180 minutes if untreated.
3. Headache is associated with at least one of the following signs, which must be present on the pain side:
   a. Conjunctival injection
   b. Lacrimation
   c. Nasal congestion
   d. Rhinorrhea
   e. Forehead and facial sweating
   f. Miosis
   g. Ptosis
   h. Eyelid edema
4. Frequency of attacks: from one every other day to eight per day.

Attacks occur in *clusters* extending over days to weeks, giving the syndrome its name. Most cluster episodes last 4 to 6 weeks and are followed by long pain-free intervals. The intervals between episodes range from 3 months to 5 years, and occasionally longer. However, most patients have one or two episodes per year. Permanent remission occurs in a minority of patients. In a small proportion of patients, the pattern converts from episodic to chronic or from chronic to episodic (23).

A typical attack begins with sudden stabbing or burning pain in the eye, orbit, and cheek on one side. The pain is usually excruciating. Unlike patients with migraine, patients with cluster headaches are usually agitated and often pace the floor during the attack. Characteristically, the patient describes at least one of the other symptoms listed. Usually the same side is involved during a cluster of attacks. Attacks may last from a few minutes to 3 hours (most often 30 to 40 minutes), and they tend to occur at the same time each day, most commonly at night after the patient has gone to bed. In some patients, alcohol is a potent trigger factor. Nitrates and vasodilator drugs may also induce attacks. Therefore, patients should be asked about concurrent use of alcohol and drugs.

The characteristics listed describe the diagnostic features for the typical syndrome of cluster headache. Some patients have less well-defined episodes, whereas other patients with chronic-pattern cluster headache have almost daily attacks of pain for a number of years.

Except during an attack, when the unilateral findings described are present, the physical examination in patients with cluster headache is unremarkable.

Differential Diagnosis

Cluster headache must be distinguished from tic douloureux (discussed later), acute glaucoma (by the presence of miosis, normal tonometry, and no lasting visual impairment), sinusitis (by lack of history of upper respiratory infection, lack of purulent rhinorrhea or sinus tenderness, and negative findings on radiography), peripheral dental abscess (by the absence of tenderness on tooth percussion), and atypical facial neuralgia (see later discussion).

Epidemiology

Cluster headache is much less common than migraine in the population. It occurs predominantly in middle-age men and is associated with being thin and smoking cigarettes. Onset usually occurs between the ages of 20 and 50 years. There is no evidence for a familial basis for cluster headache.

Treatment

Abortive. Because attacks can be short, lasting only 30 to 40 minutes, oral drug treatment may be ineffective in ameliorating an acute episode (24). When available, *100% oxygen,* administered for approximately 15 minutes at a flow rate of 7 L/minute, may abort an attack. In a double-blind trial, about half of the subjects were helped within 10 minutes by 100% oxygen but not by placebo (room air) given through a nonrebreathing face mask (25). The therapeutic effect of oxygen may result from its vasoconstrictor action. Injectable or nasal spray sumatriptan provides the most rapid onset of action of the triptans. *Subcutaneous sumatriptan,* used as described previously for migraine, was shown to decrease the severity of headache in approximately 75% of attacks as compared with placebo (26). *Ergotamine,* administered sublingually, may also be effective abortive therapy for cluster headaches. A sublingual preparation of ergotamine containing 2 mg (Table 87.3) may be given at the beginning of the attack and repeated twice at 30-minute intervals. No more than 6 mg should be taken in a 24-hour period, nor more than 10 mg/week.

Prophylactic. Other drugs, taken at the onset of a cluster episode and continued for several weeks, may be helpful for terminating an episode after the first headache occurs. Those drugs include verapamil, beta-blockers, and tricyclic depressants, in dosages similar to those described for migraine prophylaxis. *Prednisone,* beginning at 60 to 80 mg/day and tapering over 2 to 4 weeks, may shorten the duration of a cluster episode and decreases the severity and frequency of the attacks (24). A maximal effect occurs within 2 or 3 days after initiation of therapy. (See additional information on prescribing and tapering of corticosteroids in Chapter 81.)

For patients who suffer from almost *daily cluster headaches,* lithium carbonate has been used successfully. The use of this drug is described in detail in Chapter 24. Patients who respond to lithium seem to achieve control at serum levels lower than 0.8 mEq/L. If lithium fails to control daily cluster headache, the addition of ergotamine tartrate or methysergide (either alone or with ergotamine) may help.

The patient for whom neither treatment nor prophylaxis with the described regimens is effective should be referred for further empiric treatments to a neurologist or an internist with wide experience in headache management.

Sinus Headache

The pain of *acute sinusitis* may be described by the patient as headache. The diagnosis is based on the other manifestations of acute sinusitis and the reproduction or exacerbation of the patient's headache by applying pressure to affected sinuses (see Chapter 33).

Chronic sinusitis is often cited by patients as the reason for their headaches; it is actually an uncommon cause for recurrent headache. Chronic sinusitis can present diagnostic difficulties, particularly when it involves the sphenoid sinus (causing a dull, boring pain behind the eyes). The diagnosis of sinus headache is most likely when there is a history of preceding acute sinusitis, especially if there is not a long history of headache. The diagnosis and management of chronic sinusitis are discussed in Chapter 33.

Acute Exertional Headache (Orgasm, Cough, Sneeze)

The features of acute exertional headache are that it is of sudden (or almost instantaneous) onset and it is directly related to exertion of some kind (e.g., orgasm, coughing, sneezing, straining, bending, running, lifting). It may last from minutes to one-half hour, occasionally longer. The headache is presumed to be caused by transient intracranial–spinal pressure dissociations, and the course is benign. In about 10% of patients, significant organic disease is found (Arnold–Chiari malformation, hydrocephalus, tumor, or subarachnoid hemorrhage) (27).

Exertional headache must be differentiated chiefly from the headache of *subarachnoid hemorrhage.* The latter is usually far more persistent and is often associated with fever, stiff neck, progressive clouding of consciousness, syncope, and focal neurologic signs. Exertional headaches can be quite severe, but they are brief and recur with the trigger activity. Because it may be impossible to distinguish a first episode of exertional headache from a minor subarachnoid hemorrhage, and considering the 10% risk of another organic basis for the headache, CT, without and with contrast (because of the possibility of tumor or arteriovenous malformation), or an MRI scan (see Chapter 86) should be considered when patients initially report the problem. For a patient with a negative scan but a clinical presentation strongly suggestive of subarachnoid hemorrhage, a lumbar puncture should be done to rule out bleeding. If imaging findings and lumbar puncture results are normal, the benign nature of the condition should be explained to the patient. The patient usually finds ways to avoid some of the activities that produce headache. In addition, an NSAID (Table 87.3) or alpha-blocker (Table 87.4) can be tried for prophylaxis when the patient plans to engage in a headache-provoking activity.

Sudden-Onset Unprovoked Severe Headache

Sudden-onset, unprovoked severe headache is uncommon but alarming. In a single large prospective study based in general practice, 37% of patients with this presentation had serious central nervous system disease (25% had subarachnoid hemorrhage) (28). Fewer than 10% of those with subarachnoid hemorrhage had a history of "sentinel" severe headaches. In 1 year of follow-up, none of those with undiagnosed sudden headache experienced subarachnoid hemorrhage. Patients with sudden-onset headache (peak pain within 1 minute, duration at least 1 hour) should be evaluated promptly for intracranial disease (see Exertional Headache).

Headache Caused by Medications

Headache is a side effect of many drugs. Among the commonly used drugs for which headache is more than an occasional side effect are indomethacin (Indocin), nalidixic acid (NegGram), trimethoprim–sulfamethoxazole (Bactrim, Septra), oral contraceptives, and nitrates and other vasodilators. Therefore, as noted earlier, it is important to ask the patient routinely about new drugs when evaluating a headache of recent onset.

A throbbing vascular-type headache often occurs shortly after initiation of treatment (or a dosage increase) with a *vasodilator* drug. The most common offenders are the short- and long-acting nitrates, the dihydropyridine calcium channel blockers, and the vasodilators used to treat hypertension (hydralazine and minoxidil). The management of this problem depends on the indications for the drug and the severity of the headache. Some patients, if informed in advance of the possibility of headache, choose to take the drug anyway; this is particularly true of sublingual nitrates administered for angina. For the long-acting nitrates, dosage reduction may effectively reduce headache for some patients, whereas alternative antianginal treatment is needed for others (see Chapter 62). The headache associated with antihypertensive vasodilators can usually be prevented by treating the patient with a beta-blocker before the vasodilator is added (see Chapter 67).

Medication Overuse Headache (Rebound Headache)

Chronic daily or near-daily headache can be caused by overuse of analgesics such as acetaminophen, opiods, and analgesic combination medications. The patient typically has an escalating headache pattern for which increasing dosages of analgesics were taken, resulting in conversion to a daily headache pattern. Medication overuse can result in refractoriness to preventive medication. Patients often do not consider over-the-counter drugs as medications. A careful history of all treatments the patient has used for the headache should be elicited. Treatment consists of withdrawal from the analgesic.

Headache in Acute Febrile Illnesses

Acute febrile illnesses may cause vascular-type throbbing headaches that remit when the illness resolves. A febrile patient in whom the headache is the major symptom and in whom nuchal rigidity or other manifestation of meningeal irritation is present requires a cerebrospinal fluid (CSF) examination to exclude meningitis (see Chapter 86).

Giant Cell Arteritis and Polymyalgia Rheumatica

Giant cell arteritis (GCA) is a vasculitis that affects large arteries throughout the body. However, clinical manifestations are usually caused by involvement of extracranial branches of the carotid artery, and the most common syndrome is headache. GCA has also been called *temporal arteritis,* because temporal headaches and a positive temporal artery biopsy are the findings that are most typical of the disease. The cause of GCA is unknown.

Polymyalgia rheumatica (PMR) is a debilitating condition of older people that manifests with stiffness and aching of the neck and shoulder muscles and pelvic girdle. It precedes, accompanies, or follows the onset of GCA in approximately 50% of patients with GCA. In approximately 75% to 80% of patients with PMR in the United States and Europe, GCA does not occur (29). In patients who develop both GCA and PMR, the two syndromes may occur at the same time or GCA may begin months to years after the onset of PMR symptoms. In some patients, GCA precedes PMR.

Epidemiology

GCA and PMR are almost exclusively diseases of people older than 50 years of age; the average age at onset is 65 to 70 years. Both are uncommon among African Americans, Hispanics, and Asians. They are most common in people of northern European descent, and they are more common in women than in men. It is estimated that the prevalence of GCA is about 200 per 100,000 Americans older than 50 years of age (30). There are no population-based studies of frequency of PMR in the United States; however, it is estimated that the incidence and prevalence rates for PMR are about two or three times higher than the rates for GCA.

Manifestations

The headache of GCA does not have specific features that distinguish it clearly from other headaches (31). It is temporal in more than 50% of patients; however, it can be frontal, occipital, parietal, or holocephalic. The patient usually reports that it involves the surface and is not intracranial. It may be made worse by hair brushing, by resting the head on a pillow, or, at times, by exposure to cold. It usually is not described as throbbing. Because these symptoms are not specific,

Table 87.5. Clinical Features of Giant Cell Arteritis

Common Features	%[a]	Less Common but Characteristic Features
Headache	85	Raynaud phenomenon of limbs or tongue
Temporal artery tenderness	70	Tender scalp nodules
Jaw claudication	65	Thick, tender occipital arteries
Lingual, limb, or swallowing claudication	20	Necrotic lesions of scalp, tongue
Brachlocephalic bruits	50	Carotid artery tenderness
Thickened or nodular temporal artery	45	Swelling of the hands
Pulseless temporal artery	40	Taste, smell disturbances
Visual symptoms	40	Distended, beaded retinal veins
Fixed blindness, partial or complete	15	
Polymyalgia rheumatica	50	Diminished or absent radial artery pulses
Weight loss >6 kg	40	Mononeuropathy (median, peroneal, cervical root)
Erythrocyte sedimentation rate		
>50 mm/h	95	
>100 mm/h	60	
Fever (>37.7°C)	20	
Abnormal liver function	50	
Anemia (hematocrit <35%)	50	

[a]Approximate percentage of patients with common feature at initial evaluation.
Adapted from Raskin NH, Appenzeller O. Headache. Philadelphia: WB Saunders, 1980.

the most important factors suggesting the diagnosis of GCA are a number of associated findings, listed in Table 87.5. It is important to inquire specifically about pain (claudication) associated with chewing, swallowing, and arm or tongue motion, because these symptoms are highly suggestive of GCA. The combination of one or more of the findings listed in Table 87.5 with a new headache in an older patient is sufficient to suspect GCA.

PMR is insidious in onset. The chief complaints are aching and stiffness of the shoulder girdle and, less commonly, of the thigh muscles (31). These symptoms can make it particularly hard for the patient to get up in the morning. Associated low-grade fever, weight loss, and anorexia are common. On physical examination, there may be some tenderness of the shoulder and neck muscles, but there is no significant loss of muscle strength.

Diagnosis

If GCA or PMR is suspected, the erythrocyte sedimentation rate (ESR) measured by the Westergren method is the most useful screening test. The majority of patients have a markedly elevated ESR (often 100 mm/hour or greater). Because the upper limit of normal for people older than 60 years of age may be as high as 40 mm/hour, an ESR of 40 to 60 mm/hour is less informative than a very high ESR. Unlike other chronic inflammatory diseases, GCA and PMR are not associated with autoantibody production or abnormalities in complement factors or immunoglobulin levels.

Definitive diagnosis of GCA is made with a temporal artery biopsy. Because the typical histologic changes (inflammatory cells, edema, giant cells) are patchy in distribution, examination of serial sections of the resected segment of artery is essential. Occasionally, in patients with the clinical diagnosis of GCA, even extensive sampling of one temporal artery does not yield a positive biopsy and the other artery must also be examined by biopsy. In addition to a positive temporal artery biopsy, the American College of Rheumatology has designated four other features that may support the diagnosis of GCA: age of onset after age 50 years, new localized headache, Westgergren ESR greater than 50 mm/hour, and temporal artery tenderness or decreased temporal artery pulse. The presence of three of the five features is considered sufficient evidence to make the clinical diagnosis of GCA (32). In one retrospective study, it was found that the feature most predictive of a diagnostic temporal artery biopsy was the presence of either visual symptoms, a temporal artery that is abnormal on examination, or constitutional symptoms (33).

Patient Experience. A temporal artery biopsy can be done in an ambulatory surgery facility (by a general surgeon, ophthalmologist, vascular surgeon, plastic surgeon, or neurosurgeon). The local scalp hair is shaved, the skin is anesthetized with Xylocaine (lidocaine), and a large segment of artery (4 to 6 cm) is excised. The entire procedure requires about one-half hour. There are no serious sequelae.

The *diagnosis of PMR* is based on the combination of the typical symptoms, a high ESR, and exclusion of other explanations for the patient's symptoms. Normocytic anemia is common. Muscle enzyme levels, electromyography, and muscle histology are all normal. If a patient with typical PMR has manifestations suggesting GCA (Table 87.5), a temporal artery biopsy is indicated, because the recommended dosages of corticosteroids for the two conditions are different.

Course and Treatment

Both GCA and PMR are thought to be self-limited conditions in most patients, lasting up to 2 years. Treatment recommendations are based on comparisons of untreated patients with patients treated with corticosteroids. Treatment with corticosteroids appears to prevent almost entirely the most serious complication of GCA (unilateral or bilateral blindness caused by ischemic optic neuropathy, which occurs in 20% to 30% of untreated patients). Although the symptoms of both GCA and PMR may respond to aspirin and other NSAIDs, these agents have not been shown to prevent the progressive vasculitis in GCA that can lead to blindness.

Giant Cell Arteritis. If the diagnosis of GCA is strongly suspected, corticosteroid treatment should be initiated immediately and the temporal artery biopsy should be obtained within 3 to 4 days. If the patient has vision loss that is thought to be from GCA, it is recommended that treatment with steroids should be initiated intravenously (34). The initial oral treatment is prednisone (40 to 60 mg once per day) for 4 to 6 weeks. Within 1 to 3 days, symptoms usually remit entirely and there is a significant decrease in the ESR. After 4 to 6 weeks, the prednisone should be tapered every 1 to 2 weeks by approximately 10% until a dosage of 10 to 15 mg daily has been reached. Further tapering and duration of treatment depend on the clinical response and ESR (see Chapter 81). A 2-year course of prednisone is usually recommended. Some authors, who have documented GCA relapse after discontinuation of treatment, recommend lifelong maintenance treatment with low-dose prednisone, especially for patients who have no intolerable side effects from treatment (35). One controlled trial addressed to this issue found that combined prednisone and methotrexate treatment for 2 years reduced the frequency of relapse after discontinuation when compared to standard prednisone-only treatment (36).

Polymyalgia Rheumatica. If the patient has *isolated PMR,* the treatment is 10 to 20 mg of prednisone daily, tapered to a daily maintenance dosage of 5 to 7.5 mg after several weeks. Treatment is continued for approximately 2 years, with gradual discontinuation at the end of that time. The symptoms of PMR, as well as the ESR, respond to this regimen dramatically, often within the first 24 hours. In general, the ESR does not provide a useful guide to the activity of PMR, and it is reasonable to taper the prednisone without regard to the ESR. PMR recurs in some patients, within months to years after discontinuing prednisone; these patients usually respond to a second course of treatment.

Benign Intracranial Hypertension (Pseudotumor Cerebri)

Benign intracranial hypertension (BIH) is a condition of unknown cause characterized by headache, papilledema, and elevated intracranial pressure in the absence of a mass lesion or venous sinus thrombosis. Headache in this condition is presumably caused by stretching of the dura and the large vessels. Papilledema is a direct result of the increased pressure. The paucity of focal neurologic symptoms and signs is caused by the global increase in intracranial pressure. Those focal signs that do appear (e.g., sixth nerve palsies producing horizontal diplopia) are probably related to stretching of the involved structure.

This condition may occur *de novo,* or it may appear in association with a number of purported contributing factors (obesity, menstrual irregularity, steroid therapy or steroid withdrawal, oral contraceptives, nalidixic acid, and vitamin A intoxication).

Manifestations

The prototypical patient is an obese young woman who develops progressively more severe headaches, nausea, vomiting, dizziness, and transiently blurred vision. In approximately 50% of patients, onset is abrupt; the rest develop symptoms progressively over several weeks or months. The headache always precedes visual symptoms. It is usually generalized, constant, and often more severe in the morning, and it is aggravated by coughing, straining, or changing position. The diagnosis is suggested strongly by these historical characteristics coupled with a physical examination that shows papilledema without focal neurologic signs. Visual fields may be constricted and the blind spot enlarged. Rarely, the papilledema involves the macular area, resulting in blindness.

Differential Diagnosis

The diagnosis of BIH is always one of exclusion. The most important considerations in the *differential diagnosis* are intracranial mass lesion, hydrocephalus, hypertensive encephalopathy, and venous sinus thrombosis. To exclude an intracranial mass, venous thrombosis, or hydrocephalus, a CT or MRI scan (see Chapter 86) should be obtained. In BIH, the scan may show small ventricles, but there is no evidence of a mass lesion. After a negative scan, a lumbar puncture should be performed (see Chapter 86). In BIH, the CSF pressure is high (200 to 400 mm H_2O or more), the content of spinal fluid protein is normal or low, and the cell count is normal. The diagnosis of hypertensive encephalopathy should be made if the patient has the typical clinical features of BIH, severe diastolic hypertension (greater than 120 mm Hg), and a negative CT scan. In a very obese woman with a history of amenorrhea for many months, it is also important to consider pregnancy-induced hypertension (toxemia), which is ruled out by a negative pregnancy test (see Chapter 100).

For less clear-cut cases, such as a typical clinical presentation in an older male patient, or when the spinal fluid is abnormal, referral to a neurologist is indicated.

Treatment and Course

With treatment most patients recover completely from BIH within several weeks or months; however, some patients require ongoing therapy to control headaches and prevent visual loss. In a very obese patient, weight reduction is recommended, although this may not directly affect the course.

The goal of therapy is to reduce intracranial pressure in order to reduce the risk of loss of vision. At the time of the initial lumbar puncture, enough fluid should be removed to reduce the closing pressure to 100 mm H_2O or less (usually about 25 to 35 mL of fluid). Acetazolamide (Diamox), as 500-mg sustained-release capsules, is then begun on a twice-daily schedule with periodic checking of serum electrolytes. If the patient remains asymptomatic and the papilledema clears, acetazolamide can be tapered and discontinued. For patients with continued headache, visual impairment, and papilledema, repeated lumbar punctures should be performed with removal of adequate volumes of spinal fluid with each tap, and acetazolamide should be continued.

The use of corticosteroids to treat BIH is controversial. Should the patient remain symptomatic after repeated lumbar punctures and acetazolamide, CSF shunting via a lumboperitoneal shunt or surgical incision of the optic nerve sheath should be considered. Treatment of these patients is difficult and requires the consultation of neurologists and neurosurgeons experienced in handling this disorder.

Posttraumatic (Postconcussive) Headache

Manifestations

Head trauma, with or without loss of consciousness, may be followed by a number of symptoms that are collectively called the *postconcussive syndrome*: headache, vertigo (often positional; see Chapter 89), light-headedness or giddiness, poor concentration and memory, lack of energy, irritability, and anxiety. There is convincing evidence that these varied symptoms may be organic consequences of the injury, although their exact causal mechanism is not understood.

Headache is the most common and often the most troubling manifestation of this syndrome. It typically begins within 24 hours after the trauma as a dull, constant, generalized aching discomfort that may wax and wane throughout the day or become concentrated at different points on the head (bifrontal or unilateral). Headache may be worsened by sneezing, coughing, stooping, straining, or rapid head motions and changes in body position; it may be accompanied by nausea and vomiting.

Typically, these headaches worsen over days to weeks, then resolve over weeks or months; in some patients (roughly 15%), headache and other postconcussive symptoms continue for longer than 1 year. It is now appreciated that minor head trauma in patients with no headache history can lead to chronic recurrent headaches typical of migraine, with or without aura.

Differential Diagnosis

Subdural Hematoma and Other Expanding Mass Lesions. Although postconcussive syndrome is a far more likely explanation of posttraumatic headache and ill-defined intellectual impairments than is subdural hematoma, the seriousness of this possibility and the ease of ruling it out with CT scanning make it an important consideration.

Posttraumatic Dysautonomic Cephalgia. Predominantly throbbing headache pain associated with sweating of one side of the face, pupillary dilation, and, sometimes, carotid bifurcation tenderness may represent a lesion of the carotid sympathetic plexus produced by whiplash-like injury (37). This condition may respond well to propranolol (Table 87.4).

Preexisting Migraine or Chronic Tension Headaches. These must be excluded by history; furthermore, posttraumatic headaches may temporarily worsen a preexisting headache condition. (For details regarding cervical spine injury, see Chapter 70.)

Objective Tests

In addition to the neurologic history and examination, a number of objective tests may be helpful for confirming the diagnosis of postconcussive syndrome: electroencephalography, vestibular function tests, electronystagmography, and auditory and visual evoked potentials. Abnormal results, although indicative of organic disease, are nonspecific. Negative test results do not exclude an organic basis for the patient's symptoms.

Treatment

In most patients, the course of the illness is self-limited, albeit fairly lengthy. Treatment similar to that used for tension-type headache may be successful. Propranolol or amitriptyline, used alone or in combination (Table 87.4), dramatically reduces the frequency and severity of the headaches in some patients who develop typical migraine headaches after head trauma (38).

Low-Pressure (Post–Lumbar Puncture or Positional) Headache

Low-pressure headache from persistent leakage of CSF occurs most commonly after lumbar puncture. Less commonly, it results from a CSF fistula caused by blunt trauma to any part of the neural axis (i.e., closed head or spine trauma); occasionally, no causal event can be identified. The headache is markedly positional, brought on by sitting or standing, and relieved almost entirely by lying down. Nausea and dizziness are common nonspecific accompaniments. There are no focal neurologic symptoms or signs, and the patient is afebrile.

The majority of post–lumbar puncture and posttraumatic leaks close spontaneously, signified by resolution of the headache, within a few days; occasionally the problem does not resolve for several weeks. Appropriate management is essential for rapid healing of the leak: The patient is instructed to remain recumbent for several days, after which usual activities can be resumed. The rare patient with persistent, typical post–lumbar puncture headache should be referred to an anesthesiologist for epidural instillation of autologous blood; the blood will clot, forming a patch, at the site of the leak. Because of the risk of meningitis, any patient with a suspected persistent CSF fistula (i.e., a patient with a typical low-pressure headache that persists after blunt trauma) should be referred to a neurologist or neurosurgeon for complete evaluation.

Characteristics of Headache Caused by a Mass Lesion

For both the headache sufferer and the physician, concern about the possibility of a brain tumor often dominates the situation. The most important clue to the presence of an intracranial lesion is the simultaneous onset of headache and focal neurologic signs/symptoms, change in mental status, or a seizure. In a person older than 50 years of age, the onset of persistent headache for the first time is also a marker for a secondary headache disorder.

A number of nonspecific features may be clues to the presence of an intracranial mass lesion:

- Although the headache associated with a mass lesion can initially be intermittent, mild, and responsive to mild analgesics, typically it becomes more continuous and intense and, at the same time, less responsive to analgesics.
- The headache awakens the patient from sleep or is present on awakening every day, decreasing after the patient has been up for several hours.
- Coughing, sneezing, and straining aggravate a persistent headache caused by a mass lesion, presumably by transiently increasing intracranial pressure and accentuating the stretching of pain-sensitive structures.
- Anorexia, nausea, and vomiting are prominent features.

When one or more of these historical features are present or focal neurologic signs are found on examination, the patient should be evaluated for a mass lesion. A brain CT can be used if MRI is not readily available (see Chapter 86). If MRI or CT is positive for intracranial disease, the patient should be referred to a neurologist or neurosurgeon for definitive care.

FACIAL PAIN SYNDROMES

Idiopathic Trigeminal Neuralgia (Tic Douloureux)

Manifestations

Trigeminal neuralgia is seen almost exclusively in patients older than 40 years of age, most of them elderly. It has several distinguishing features: The pain is severe, paroxysmal, and lancinating, and it lasts only a few seconds to a minute. The patient's face usually contorts with the pain, and the patient may find it impossible to control his or her emotional response. Between attacks the patient is usually pain free, although some patients have a dull ache in the affected area. The interval between paroxysms is usually at least 2 or 3 minutes. The frequency of paroxysms is highly variable; some patients have hundreds each day.

The pain is usually felt in the structures innervated by the second and third divisions of the trigeminal nerve (lips, gums, cheek, chin). The pain is unilateral in a single attack, and in 95% of patients it remains unilateral. It is uncommon for attacks to involve both sides of the face simultaneously.

The patient often can identify trigger points on the face or in the mouth that, when touched (even by contact with a gust of cold air) or moved, precipitate pain.

A few patients with idiopathic trigeminal neuralgia have some areas of slightly decreased sensation that may be difficult to distinguish from normal; however, there is no objective decrease in sensation.

Other, less common syndromes with paroxysms of lancinating pain include glossopharyngeal neuralgia (pharynx pain) and occipital neuralgia (posterior head pain).

Differential Diagnosis

A syndrome identical or similar to idiopathic trigeminal neuralgia can be produced by a number of known conditions (i.e., secondary trigeminal neuralgia), such as multiple sclerosis, acoustic neurinoma, aneurysm, trigeminal neuroma, meningioma, and others. These conditions should be considered, particularly if the patient is younger than 40 years of age and has pain predominantly in the upper division of the trigeminal nerve (forehead and eye), bilateral pain, or evidence of bilateral sensory loss or associated motor signs (e.g., weak jaw, facial weakness, swallowing difficulty).

Treatment

In a patient with a typical clinical presentation, medical therapy (described later) can be initiated without further workup. Patients are in excruciating pain and should be seen promptly. If medical therapy is ineffective, or if there are any atypical features, referral to a neurologist is appropriate.

The initial treatment is *carbamazepine* (Tegretol, 200-mg tablets), one-half tablet (100 mg) twice daily, with meals, increasing every 2 to 3 days to a three-times-daily schedule and a total daily dosage of 300 to 600 mg. An few patients may need dosages as high as 1,200 mg/day; in these cases, blood levels should be monitored to confirm the adequacy of the drug trial. Most patients can expect excellent to satisfactory relief with carbamazepine. Benign side effects of the drug include nausea, vomiting, ataxia, vertigo, and transient leukopenia. The most serious side effects are persistent leukopenia and aplastic anemia. Patients must be informed of these possible risks, the frequency of which is unknown but appears to be quite low. Because of these risks, patients should have serial hemograms performed after 1 week, 6 weeks, 3 months, and on a periodic basis. Because trigeminal neuralgia can remit spontaneously after 6 to 12 months, discontinuation of drug therapy should be tried after treatment for 6 months to 1 year.

If the patient fails to improve with carbamazepine or fails to tolerate the drug, alternative medications can be tried: a *tricyclic antidepressant* (e.g., amitriptyline progressing over several weeks from 25 to 150 mg at bedtime) or the muscle relaxant *baclofen* (a trial of several weeks, progressing from 10 to 40 mg twice daily). A patient whose symptoms cannot be controlled with these medications should be referred for neurologic consultation.

Atypical Facial Pain

Atypical facial pain is a collective term for a variety of painful facial symptoms that do not meet the diagnostic criteria for a recognized entity. If untreated, most patients with this problem continue to complain of it for many years. The management of these patients involves excluding all reasonable possibilities; one-time referrals to a dentist and to an otolaryngologist should be part of this evaluation.

Most of these patients whose workup is negative improve on treatment with a tricyclic antidepressant.

Temporomandibular Joint Syndrome

On history and examination, some patients complaining of headache have the stigmata of this common syndrome: pain brought on by motion of the jaw and tenderness of the temporomandibular joint. The epidemiology, course, and management of this syndrome are described in Chapter 112.

General References*

Davidoff RA. Migraine: manifestations, pathogenesis, and management. Philadelphia: FA Davis, 1995.

Excellent up-to-date information on the science and practical issues of headache.

Delassio DJ, ed. Wolff's headache and other head pain. 5th ed. New York: Oxford University Press, 1987.

The most recent edition of the classic reference work on headache.

Silberstein SD. **Practice parameter: evidence-based guidelines for migraine headache (an evidence-based review). A report of the Quality Standards Subcommittee of the American Academy of Neurology.** Neurology 2000;55:754.

Evidence-based consensus on the efficacy of drugs and other modalities for the acute and preventive treatment of migraine headache.

American Academy of Neurology website. Available at: http://www.aan.com. Accessed February 4, 2002.

Easily assessed location for periodically-issued consensus guidelines on headache and other neurologic conditions.

Specific References

1. Cook NR, Evans DA, Funkenstein HH. Correlates of headache in a population-based cohort of elderly. Arch Neurol 1989;46:1338.
2. Linet MS, Stewart WF, Celentani DD. An epidemiologic study of headache among adolescents and young adults. JAMA 1989;261:2211.
3. Ziegler DK, Hassasein RW, Cough JR. Characteristics of life headache histories in a nonclinic population. Neurology 1977; 27:265.
4. Office visits to internists: National Ambulatory Medical Care Survey, United States, 1975. Advance Data, No. 16, February 7, 1978.
5. Dhopesh V, Anwar R, Herring C. A retrospective assessment of emergency department patients with complaint of headache. Headache 1979;19:37.
6. Lipton RB, Stewart WF, Simon D. Medical consultation for migraine: results from the American Migraine Study. Headache 1998;38:87.
7. Headache Classification Committee of the International Headache Society. Classification and diagnostic criteria for headache disorders, cranial neuralgias and facial pain. Cephalalgia 1988;8[Suppl 7]:1.
8. Frishberg BM, Rosenberg JH, Matchar DB, et al. Evidence-based guidelines in the primary care setting: neuroimaging in patients with nonacute headache. 2001 American Academy of Neurology. Available at: www.aan.com. Accessed February 4, 2002.
9. Packard RC. What does the headache patient want? Headache 1979;19:370.
10. Tomkins GE, Jackson JL, O'Malley PG, et al. Treatment of chronic headache with antidepressants: a meta-analysis. Am J Med 2001;111:54.
11. Holroyd KA, O'Donnell FJ, Stensland M, et al. Management of chronic tension-type headache with tricyclic antidepressant medication, stress management therapy, and their combination: a randomized controlled trial. JAMA 2001;285:2208.
12. Goadsby P. Pathophysiology of headache. In: Silbertstein S, Lipton R, Dalessio D, eds. Wolff's headache and other head pain. 7th ed. New York: Oxford University Press, 2001.
13. Lipton RB, Stewart WF, Diamond S, et al. Prevalence and burden of migraine in the United States: Data from the American Migraine Study II. Headache 2001;41:7.
14. Edmeads J. Advances in migraine therapy: focus on oral sumatriptan. Neurology 1995;45[Suppl 7]:S1.
15. Pfaffenrath VG, Cunin G, Sjonell G, et al. Efficacy and safety of sumatriptan tablets (25 mg, 50 mg, and 100 mg) in the acute treatment of migraine: defining the optimum doses of oral sumatriptan. Headache 1998;38:184.
16. Ryan RA, Elkind CC, Baker, et al. Sumatriptan nasal spray for the acute treatment of migraine: results of two clinical studies. Neurology 1997;49:1225.
17. Welch KMA. Drug therapy of migraine. N Engl J Med 1993; 329:1476.
18. Lipton RB, Stewart WF, Cady R, et al. Sumatriptan for the range of headaches in migraine sufferers: results of the spectrum study. Headache 2000;40:783.
19. Mathew NT, Saper JR, Silberstein SD, et al. Migraine prophylaxis with Divalproex. Arch Neurol 1995;52:281.
20. Pittler MH, Vogler BK, Ernst E. Feverfew of preventing migraine. Cochrane Database Syst Rev 2000;3:CD002286.
21. Melchart D, Linde K, Fischer P, et al. Acupuncture for idiopathic headache (Cochrane Review). Cochrane Database Syst Rev 2001;1:CD001218.
22. Ernst E. Homeopathic prophylaxis of headaches and migraine? A systematic review. J Pain Symptom Manage 1999;118: 353.
23. Pearce JM. Natural history of cluster headache. Headache 1993;33:253.
24. Dodick DW, Capobianco DJ. Treatment and management of cluster headache. Curr Pain Headache Rep 2001;5:83.
25. Fogan L. Treatment of cluster headache. Arch Neurol 1985; 42:362.
26. Sumatriptan Cluster Headache Study Group. Treatment of acute cluster headache with sumatriptan. N Engl J Med 1991;325:322.
27. Rooke ED. Benign exertional headache. Med Clin North Am 1968;52:801.
28. Linn FHH, Mijdicks EFM, Graaf Y, et al. Prospective study of sentinel headache in aneurysmal subarachnoid haemorrhage. Lancet 1994;344:590.
29. Hunder GG, Allen GL. Giant cell arteritis: a review. Bull Rheum Dis 1978–1979;29:980.
30. Lawrence RC, Helmick CG, Arnett FC, et al. Estimates of the prevalence of arthritis and selected musculoskeletal disorders in the United States. Arthritis Rheum 1998;41:778.
31. Weygaud CM, Gorozny JJ. Polymyalgia rheumatica and giant cell arteritis. In: Koopman WJ, ed. Arthritis and allied conditions: a textbook of rheumatology. 13th ed. Philadelphia: Lea & Febiger, 1997.
32. Hunder CG, Bloch DA, Michel BA, et al. The American College of Rheumatology 1990 criteria for the classification of giant cell arteritis. Arthritis Rheum 1990;33:1122.
33. Gonzalez-Gay MA, Garcia-Porrua C, Llorca J, et al. Biopsy-negative giant cell arteritis: clinical spectrum and predictive factors for positive temporal artery biopsy. Semin Arthritis Rheum 2001;30:249.
34. Neff AG, Greifenstein EM. Giant cell arteritis update. Semin Ophthalmol 1999;14:109.
35. Andersson R, Malmvall BE, Bengtsson BA. Long-term corticosteroid treatment in giant cell arteritis. Acta Med Scand 1986; 220:465.
36. Jover JA, Hernandez-Garcia C, Morado IC, et al. Combined treatment of giant-cell arteritis with methotrexate and prednisone: a randomized, double-blind, placebo-controlled trial. Ann Intern Med 2001;134:106.
37. Vijayan N, Dreyfus PM. Post-traumatic dysautonomic cephalgia. Arch Neurol 1975;32:649.
38. Weiss H, Stern BJ, Goldberg J. Chronic migraine after minor head trauma. Ann Neurol 1984;16:113.

*Bold print (general references) and bold numerals (specific references) denote published controlled clinical trials, meta-analyses, or consensus-based recommendations.

CHAPTER 88

Seizure Disorders

PETER W. KAPLAN, MBBS, FRCP

About 2 million people in the United States may have epilepsy. An even larger number seek medical advice for treatment of seizures, generating approximately 5% of visits to physicians and 20% of visits to neurologists (1). This chapter addresses the basic principles that should guide the diagnosis and management of seizures in office practice.

DEFINITION AND CLASSIFICATION OF EPILEPTIC SEIZURES

Any paroxysmal disturbance in consciousness, behavior, or motor activity may be called a spell, fit, or seizure, but this chapter addresses primarily *epileptic seizures.* These may be defined as the clinical manifestations of an abnormal, usually brief, excessive or hypersynchronous neuronal discharge in the cerebral cortex or deep limbic structures. A seizure has a definite start and finish. Seizures are associated with characteristic electrical abnormalities of the brain. Most patients are normal, and their electroencephalograms (EEGs) are often normal, between seizures (the interictal period).

The term *epilepsy* refers to a chronic neurologic condition that causes spontaneous, recurrent seizures. Therefore, single or even multiple seizures arising during transient systemic insult such as fever, infection, toxic causes (e.g., alcohol), or metabolic disturbances should not be labeled as epilepsy and are called *reactive seizures.*

The basic mechanisms underlying epileptic seizures are still uncertain, although much is known about predisposing conditions. The most widely accepted classification is based on behavioral and EEG aspects (Table 88.1) (2).

CLINICAL MANIFESTATIONS OF SEIZURE TYPES

The clinical manifestations of seizures vary according to the degree of maturity of the nervous system, the initial seizure focus, and the pattern of ictal spread. A seizure focus in the motor cortex produces jerking of the corresponding contralateral parts of the body; seizures in sensory regions result in abnormal sensations; and seizures in areas of higher cortical function may produce complex cognitive and behavioral manifestations (Fig. 88.1). Certain types of seizures manifest with sudden changes in vigilance or consciousness rather than with focal motor or sensory signs or symptoms.

Generalized Tonic–Clonic Seizures (Grand Mal)

Generalized tonic–clonic seizures (GTCSs) occur when ictal discharges involve most of the cortex. They may arise in the context of primary, *idiopathic generalized (genetic) epilepsies* (IGEs), in which seizure activity appears synchronously over both hemispheres, or they may result from *secondarily generalized seizure* discharges arising from a unilateral focus. GTCSs may be called *major motor seizures,* although the now-disused term *grand mal* referred to bilateral generalization of seizure activity.

Table 88.1. Classification of the Epilepsies

Primary Generalized Epilepsy (Idiopathic Generalized Epilepsy, IGE)
Tonic–clonic (grand mal) (GTC)
Absence (petit mal)
Myoclonic
Atonic, others

Secondarily Generalized Seizures

Partial (Focal) Epilepsy
With elementary symptomatology
  Focal motor
  Focal sensory
  Vegetative
  Psychic
  Mixed
With complex symptomatology
  Complex partial (psychomotor) (CPS)

Unclassifiable Seizures

Adapted from Dreifuss FE. Proposal for revised clinical and electroencephalographic classification of epileptic seizures. Epilepsia 1981;22:489.

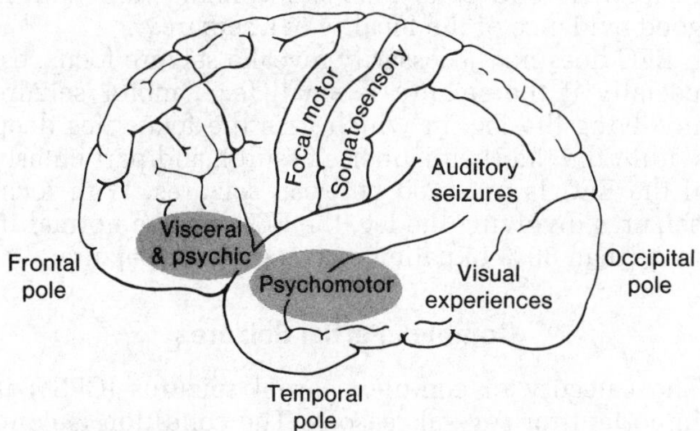

Figure 88.1. Relationship of local seizure phenomena to brain topography.

IGEs may appear at any age, although onset is rare after 35 years of age. Frequency may range from two seizures in an entire lifetime to several seizures a day. Symptomatic epilepsies giving rise to focal and secondarily generalized tonic–clonic seizures may occur throughout life, caused by developmental abnormalities, perinatal insults, infection and head trauma, and strokes, particularly in the elderly.

GTCSs typically begin with an arrest of activity and sudden loss of consciousness, followed by trembling, tonic extension of the arms and legs, and then clonic rhythmic but progressively slower limb jerking, followed by flaccidity, stupor, and labored, deep breathing. Seizures usually last less than 2 minutes and are followed by lethargy lasting minutes to hours. During the seizures, consciousness is always lost, so a history of the utterance of meaningful speech, the presence of purposeful eye movements, or a memory of the seizure itself excludes the diagnosis. Although malaise may precede GTCSs, a definite sensory, autonomic, psychic, or motor prelude suggests a *focal onset with subsequent generalization* (secondarily generalized tonic–clonic seizures). Tonic–clonic seizures may be accompanied by incontinence, sweating, tachycardia, elevated blood pressure, minor cardiac arrhythmias, and biting of the lip, cheek, and lateral aspect of the tongue.

The EEG that is typical in IGEs shows a pattern of bilateral synchronous spike-and-wave discharges, whereas patients with generalized seizures that arise from a lateralized focus may show focal epileptiform discharges over the affected cortical zone.

Generalized Absence Seizures (Petit Mal)

Typical absence seizures are also generalized seizures; they occur in *childhood absence epilepsy* (CAE), a type of IGE (3). Absence seizures may also occur in Lennox–Gastaut syndrome and in juvenile myoclonic epilepsy. CAE constitutes approximately 5% of childhood epilepsy. The onset is usually between 4 and 12 years of age. Most affected children (75%) have absence seizures that remit by the age of 20 years, although about half (especially those with atypical absence) may later develop tonic–clonic seizures.

Because of the previous classification of generalized seizures into "petit mal" and "grand mal" types, some patients incorrectly believe that these two entities represent different severities of the same seizure type (although both can occur with IGE). There is often confusion also between the staring component of absence seizures and the initial staring phase of partial complex seizures (see later discussion). Finally, the term "petit mal" was often incorrectly used by patients to refer to partial seizures with a motor component or to minor motor seizures. Such confusions in classification may lead to incorrect diagnosis, prognosis, and antiepileptic drug (AED) therapy.

Typical absence seizures in CAE, consisting of lapses of vigilance or awareness, usually last about 3 to 20 seconds. There is no tonic–clonic phase or loss of posture. Slight rhythmic twitching of the mouth and periorbital musculature or upgaze may be observed. With atypical absence seizures, duration may be prolonged, leading to confusion with complex partial seizures arising from the temporal or other lobes. In CAE, there is a rapid recovery of awareness after an absence seizure, but amnesia for events occurring during the seizure persists. Absence seizures typically occur up to 100 times per day. Children who have such frequent seizures may be labeled as being inattentive, daydreamers, or slow learners until the correct diagnosis is made.

Both clinical and EEG findings should be used to secure a diagnosis of CAE; neither alone is diagnostic. The EEG during an absence seizure shows a characteristic bilateral synchronous three-per-second spike-and-wave pattern; between seizures, the EEG may be normal, but brief 3-second bursts usually persist in the absence of AED therapy. Often, hyperventilation or stimulation with regularly flashing lights (intermittent photic stimulation) induces an absence seizure. Three-per-second spike-and-wave patterns on EEG may be seen in asymptomatic close relatives of patients with CAE as well as other seizure types (e.g., tonic–clonic seizures).

Myoclonus and Myoclonic Seizures

Myoclonus is the predominantly synchronous, involuntary, nonrhythmic jerking of limbs, trunk, or head. Epileptic myoclonus arises from paroxysmal discharges of the central nervous system above the brainstem. Conditions in which nonepileptic myoclonus (segmental myoclonus) may occur are conditions affecting the brainstem and the spinal cord.

Myoclonic seizures are most often seen after severe, diffuse cortical injury resulting from cerebral ischemia and anoxia; these seizures are difficult to suppress and carry a poor prognosis. When myoclonic seizures arise from hypoglycemia, severe renal or hepatic failure, or drug toxicity, they are often self-limited and resolve with correction of the underlying disturbance. Primary neurologic diseases, such as viral encephalitis, Jakob–Creutzfeldt disease, Huntington chorea, Wilson disease, and ceroid lipofuscinoses, may also include myoclonic seizures. Myoclonic seizures are also seen in IGEs, benign myoclonic epilepsy of childhood, juvenile myoclonic epilepsy, the Lennox–Gastaut syndrome (triad of multiple seizure types, psychomotor retardation, and a characteristic EEG pattern, seen mainly in children), progressive myoclonic epilepsies, and a wide variety of seizures from toxic and metabolic causes.

Myoclonic seizures consist of brief and violent muscular contractions, usually bilateral, that do not affect consciousness. Myoclonic contractions may be single or multiple, lasting for seconds to hours. Contractions may be rhythmic or irregular. When the upper limbs are involved, patients may drop or toss objects. When the legs or trunk are involved, the patient may suddenly fall. Myoclonic seizures may be spontaneous, or they may be induced by flashes of light, or more rarely by other triggering stimuli.

The usual EEG correlate of myoclonic seizures is generalized or multifocal spikes, polyspikes, and slow waves. Scalp-recorded EEG discharges may be seen in the case of cortical myoclonus but may not be seen in the case of subcortical myoclonus.

Localization-Related or Partial (Focal) Seizures without Impairment of Consciousness

Focal motor or sensory seizures may manifest at any age. The clinical manifestations depend on the brain region involved in the seizure.

The *motor cortex* is a common site of origin for focal seizures. Because the seizure discharges spread across the motor strip, clonus (alternating contraction and relaxation) may march up or down a limb and into the trunk or into another limb. Spread into a sensory area of the brain may cause numbness in the face, trunk, or limbs. *Sensory seizures* can also involve areas of special sensation such as sight or hearing. A focus in or near the visual cortex or its association areas may cause the patient to see spots, lights, or geometric shapes, similar to the experience of patients with classic migraine. Perception of buzzing, clicking, or ringing sounds may be generated from a focus in the superior and mesial temporal lobe. Gustatory and olfactory sensations, usually unpleasant, are components of partial seizures involving mesial temporal lobe structures. Seizures dominated by vestibular symptoms (e.g., dizziness, vertigo) are rare.

Retention of some degree of consciousness is characteristic of focal seizures, so that patients may, for example, walk and talk during a seizure—activities that would be impossible during a generalized seizure. However, a large focus in the dominant hemisphere may generate seizures that blunt awareness.

After a focal motor seizure, there may be *focal weakness of a limb, or Todd paralysis,* which usually resolves within a few hours or, rarely, after a few days. Distinction between cerebrovascular ischemic events with associated seizures and seizures with Todd paralysis may be difficult without clues from the patient's history. A Todd paralysis has localizing value and is good evidence of the focality of a seizure.

EEG does not necessarily reveal a seizure focus, especially if the seizure is small (e.g., motor seizure involving the leg, in which case the focus lies deep within the interhemispheric fissure), and particularly if the EEG is obtained between seizures. With focal seizures involving the leg, the EEG may be normal in more than 88% of patients even during a seizure.

Complex Partial Seizures

The category of complex partial seizures (CPSs) is important for several reasons: The condition is common in the adult population, the seizures are often misdiagnosed, and correct diagnosis leads to a search for potentially correctable lesions and effective AED therapy. CPSs are classified with focal or localization-related seizures because of clinical evidence linking these seizures with focal as opposed to generalized epileptiform discharges. CPSs are largely synonymous with the older term *psychomotor seizures,* but they are not synonymous with temporal lobe seizures because they can arise from any brain region. Although CPSs may begin at any age, the majority begin before age 20 years. An adult onset of CPS carries the same significance as does a new onset of any focal seizure; a treatable structural lesion should be sought. Patients with CPS who come to surgery or to postmortem examination may show either no histologic abnormality of the brain or tumor, infarct, granuloma, or infection; often with temporal lobe origin there is gliosis of the mesial temporal lobe. It is not known whether gliosis causes temporal lobe CPSs or results from them.

CPSs impair attention or consciousness through focal seizure activity. This is why they are called complex. The presentation of these seizures is more varied than that of the other seizure types and may include autonomic, psychic, visceral, sensory, or motor symptoms. Seizures often begin with an aura, which is, in fact, a simple partial seizure. The classic aura, usually consisting of an unpleasant olfactory or gustatory hallucination, is less common than is an aura of poorly described, unpleasant visceral sensations or malaise. In general, there is no clear boundary between the aura and the seizure itself, particularly when seizures feature distorted visual or auditory sensations, or vertigo or unsteadiness. Arrest of motor activity, rigid posturing of the head and eyes, and slow, repetitive limb movements may occur and are easily distinguished in most cases from the tonic–clonic sequence of convulsive attacks. Autonomic instability, including fluctuating heart rate or blood pressure, flushing, sweating, salivation, or changes in pupillary reactions, may occur in patients with CPSs. Patients often say that they feel strange or as if in a dream, or they experience inappropriate emotions such as intense dread or strange serenity. If they can talk during a CPS, patients may portray what appears to be a psychiatric disturbance. The distinction between CPSs and psychosis may be further obscured in patients who have psychological or psychiatric problems between seizures. Such patients can be misdiagnosed as schizophrenic.

In a condition whose presentation may range from apparent appendicitis to apparent schizophrenia, special efforts should be made to elicit a detailed history of a spell and, if possible, to observe one. CPSs should have a definite start and finish; they should be associated with some impairment in ability to register and process information during the seizure; and they should be stereotyped from episode to episode. Observations of automatic behavior, such as repetitive lip licking or smacking, raising and lowering of the arm, fidgeting or buttoning and unbuttoning of clothing, stroking or rubbing movements, or pacing in circles, may secure the diagnosis of a CPS, because such automatisms are common in CPS but uncommon in other seizure types.

The routine EEG is abnormal in fewer than half of patients with partial seizures, but positive tracings may be found in 80% to 90% of patients by recording EEGs during sleep and, in the case of temporal lobe origin, by using special electrodes positioned closer to temporal lobe structures.

Complex electrophysiologic mechanisms determine whether seizure discharges remain localized, spread along particular anatomic pathways, or involve much of the brain. AEDs can limit the spread of a focal seizure and prevent generalization. It is unknown how often tonic–clonic seizures are caused by spread from occult primary foci.

Unclassifiable Seizures

With an adequate history, most seizures should be classifiable by the scheme described. Often, however, the history is lacking. The event may not have been witnessed, or observers may report the patient's falling down and shaking but be unable to describe the full sequence of events. In these instances, it is best to list the seizure as unclassifiable or to use descriptive terms that are not otherwise used to classify seizure types, such as *jerks, convulsions,* or *staring spells,* until a specific seizure type can be identified.

CLASSIFICATIONS OF EPILEPSY SYNDROMES

Seizures are observable phenomena with symptoms or signs that last a finite time. An *epilepsy syndrome* is a cluster of signs and symptoms that occur together and constitute a chronic condition of recurrent seizures. There is no single known cause or pathology for epilepsy. Features of a particular epilepsy syndrome include cause, family history, age at onset, seizure frequency, typical course, precipitating factors, imaging studies, and the EEG. For example, damage to the temporal lobe may result in a condition of recurrent seizures characterized by an aura, unresponsiveness with automatisms, and tonic–clonic movements. This would represent a syndrome in which there is a progression of seizure types from simple partial to complex partial to secondarily generalized tonic–clonic seizures. If clinical data point to damage in the temporal lobe (EEG focus, imaging findings), the epilepsy syndrome is that of symptomatic temporal lobe epilepsy. This is also true with IGEs (previously called primary generalized epilepsies). For example, absence seizures may be seen in a number of epilepsy syndromes (e.g., CAE), each of which may have a different constellation of signs and symptoms and carry a different prognosis.

The importance of establishing a syndromic classification of epilepsy is that the particular prognosis in this chronic condition is tied to the epilepsy syndrome rather than the seizure type. Furthermore, success in the use of AEDs or even seizure surgery is also predicated more on the epilepsy syndrome classification than on the seizure type (4).

EPIDEMIOLOGY

The annual incidence rate of epilepsy is approximately 40 to 70 per 100,000 population, and the reported prevalence rates are between 1.5 and 57 per 1,000 (5). Partial epilepsies constitute about two thirds of the cases, one fifth are generalized, and the remainder are unclassified (6). In adults, CPSs constitute approximately 40%; GTCSs, about 40%; and simple partial (focal motor or sensory) seizures, approximately 15% (6). For younger age groups, partial seizures are less prevalent and generalized absence seizures are correspondingly more common.

NATURAL HISTORY AND PROGNOSIS

The natural course of epilepsy is difficult to determine because modern studies include a mixture of treated and untreated patients. Comparison of prevalence and incidence ratios suggests a crude mean for the duration of epilepsy of approximately 12 to 13 years (7), not taking into consideration the age at onset of epilepsy, the clinical type, or the response to treatment. *After a first unprovoked seizure, the cumulative risk of recurrence* at 3 to 5 years has been estimated to be 40% (8,9). Until further data are available, a 40% crude risk for recurrence within a few years after a spontaneous tonic–clonic seizure is a reasonable estimate. Of adults who have a recurrence of tonic–clonic seizures, approximately 60% have recurrence in the first year and 70% by 3 years (10). Risk factors that increase the risk of recurrence and decisions about treatment are discussed in a later section (see The Patient with a First Seizure). If a person has a second, unprovoked seizure, the risk for further seizures is higher, and after several unprovoked seizures it exceeds 75%.

Once two spontaneous seizures have occurred, epilepsy is considered to exist, and the epidemiologic focus switches to the possibility for remission. Before the development of AEDs, the spontaneous remission rate for all types of epilepsy was approximately 10% to 32%. Reported remission rates for epilepsy with or without treatment vary between 10% and 82% (11,12), according to when the study was done, retrospective versus prospective methodology, and the length of follow-up. Studies on prognosis have not yet clarified the role of treatment in the long-term outcome. The probability of going 5 years without a seizure is approximately 40% at 1 year and 50% at 2 years after diagnosis of epilepsy (11). From 50% to 82% of patients are in remission after 2 to 5 years (13,14). The probability of remission at 20 years is 80% to 85% for IGEs but only 65% for localization-related epilepsies. After being free from seizures for 5 years, almost 50% of patients relapse after tapering AEDs, usually in the first year and particularly in the first 6 months (15).

Prognostic factors include age at onset, severity of epilepsy, number of seizures before treatment, number of types of seizures, history of status epilepticus, number of medications required to control the disease, and length of time before attainment of seizure control. CPSs without secondary generalization are the most difficult seizure type to control (16,17).

Epilepsy that has not been controlled after 2 years of treatment represents a significant risk for chronic epilepsy. Some authorities believe that the long-term risk may be decreased by early treatment of seizures; however, this concept remains controversial. An abnormal EEG during AED withdrawal increases the chance of relapse in patients with CPSs (18), but a normal-EEG CPS does not exclude a relapse (83% versus 54%) (19). The presence of neurologic or psychiatric problems worsens the prognosis.

It is generally possible to reassure a person with epilepsy that the long-term prognosis for remission is good; however, except for CAE, which usually remits before young adulthood, the attainment of remission can be expected to require many years.

CAUSES OF SEIZURES

Classification of seizures requires clinical observation, and classification of an epilepsy syndrome often requires clinical, EEG, and imaging data. Because a seizure represents a symptom of cerebral dysfunction, a primary cause should be sought.

Epilepsy that arises from *definable causes* has also been called symptomatic, as opposed to essential or idiopathic. Symptomatic epilepsies often arise from identifiable brain lesions, as from infection, trauma, tumor, or stroke. With IGEs, however, patients have a normal examination, normal screening laboratory tests (discussed later), an EEG often showing a generalized spike-and-wave pattern, and a family history of similar seizures. Such patients would not be exhaustively studied for underlying causes.

Table 88.2 lists *specific causes* that should be considered for different types of seizures at various ages; the causes are listed from top to bottom in approximate order of frequency. It is worth emphasizing that many of the partial epilepsies display secondarily generalized seizures and that the focal onset may be obscured. Therefore, causes of focal seizures should be sought even in apparently generalized seizures.

Special issues are raised by *seizures that are manifested for the first time in the elderly.* First, most seizure disorders have onset in the first three decades of life, and onset of the IGE almost never occurs after this age. Second, cerebrovascular disease accounts for 30% to 60% of all new seizures in the elderly population. Tumors, the major cause of focal seizures in middle-age persons, have been found to be the cause of 2% to 30% of seizures in elderly patients (20); brain tumors in this age group are likely to be malignant. No cause is found in about half of elderly patients with seizures. When an elderly patient presents with seizures, a special effort should be made to find treatable conditions such as carotid artery stenosis, cardiac arrhythmias, infection, and toxic–metabolic derangements.

Posttraumatic Seizures

New-onset seizures after head trauma are usually partial (focal) in onset, and often secondarily generalized seizures occur after serious head injuries. There is little risk of seizures after mild head trauma with brief unconsciousness or amnesia, whereas severe injuries with intracranial hematomas, focal neurologic signs, and unconsciousness for longer than 24 hours result in epilepsy in about 10% of patients. Moderately severe injuries (skull fractures or unconsciousness for 30 minutes to 24 hours) impose an intermediate risk. Injuries over the vertex are more epileptogenic.

The value of *prophylactic therapy* to prevent the onset of posttraumatic seizures has not been firmly established. Until more data are available, the following approaches are recommended. Patients with minor scalp lacerations or brief loss of consciousness should not be considered to have a significantly increased risk of epilepsy. A single seizure occurring early (during the first 2 weeks after head injury), or while the patient is still experiencing the acute effects of injury, should not be an indication for long-term therapy; a second seizure in this setting might be grounds for treatment. Some patients with brain injuries should be considered for a 2- to 4-year course of prophylactic phenytoin, especially with severe, penetrating, or vertex injuries. A patient with a seizure occurring more than

Table 88.2. Causes of Seizures with Onset at Various Ages

Adolescent (12–21 yr)	Adult (21–65 yr)	Elderly (65+ yr)
	Common Causes	
Genetic (g or f) Mesial temporal sclerosis (f) Infection (m) Meningitis Viral encephalitis Abscess TORCHS[a] Parasites Psychogenic (m, usually g) Toxins or drugs (g)[a] Drug withdrawal (g)	Alcohol withdrawal (g) Toxins or drugs (g)[a] Drug withdrawal (g) Tumor (f) Trauma (f) Scar Subdural hematoma Mesial temporal sclerosis (f) Genetic (g) Psychogenic (m) Infection (m) Meningitis Viral encephalitis Abscess Syphilis Cerebrovascular (m) Thrombotic Embolic Hemorrhagic Cardiac arrhythmia	Cerebrovascular (m) Thrombotic Embolic Hemorrhagic Cardiac arrhythmia Trauma (m) Scar Subdural hematoma Tumor (m) Degenerative CNS disorders (e.g., Alzheimer's disease) Systemic infection
	Occasional Causes	
Metabolic (g, usually g) Hypoglycemia Hyponatremia Hypocalcemia Porphyria Trauma (f) Scar Subdural hematoma Tumor (f) Arteriovenous malformation (f) Subarachnoid hemorrhage (m) Eclampsia (m) Renal failure (g)	Metabolic (g) Hypoglycemia Hyponatremia Hypoxia (g) Renal failure (g) Eclampsia (m) Parasites	Alcohol withdrawal (g) Toxins or drugs (g)[a] Drug withdrawal (g) Hypoxia (g) Metabolic (g) Hypoglycemia Hyponatremia Hypocalcemia Infection (m) Meningitis Viral encephalitis Abscess
	Rare Causes	
Collagen disease (m) Hepatic failure (g) Multiple sclerosis (f)	Hypocalcemia Hypomagnesemia Collagen disease (m) Hypertensive encephalopathy (m) Hyperosmolar (m) Multiple sclerosis (f) Degenerative (m) Abscess Syphilis	Syphilis Parasites Hypertensive encephalopathy (m) Hyperosmolar (m) Renal failure (g) Hepatic failure (g) Degenerative (g) Factitious (m)
Idiopathic	Idiopathic	Idiopathic

f, Usually focal; g, usually generalized; m, often mixed; TORCHS, toxoplasmosis, rubella, cytomegalovirus, herpes, syphilis.
[a]See list of occupational exposures that may cause seizures, Table 8.3.

2 weeks after a head injury should be evaluated and managed as one would any other patient with new-onset seizures, and the seizure should not be attributed to a recent or remote episode of head trauma until other treatable causes have been excluded.

Alcohol-Related Seizures

Alcohol withdrawal is a common cause of seizures; almost all of them occur within the first 48 hours of abstinence or after marked reduction in alcohol intake, and most of them are generalized. In some series, up to 25% of withdrawal seizures have been focal, presumably because of an old cortical scar from trauma, infection, or vascular disease. The risk of epilepsy in the alcohol abuser is related to the amount of alcohol that was consumed (no longer being consumed at time of seizure) (21), but it may be increased by the higher likelihood of head trauma and intracranial infection in this population. If a known alcohol abuser has had a prior withdrawal seizure, presents a typical picture of a generalized seizure without focal features, and has a normal examination and no complications, then investigations may be limited. More often, the history is imprecise and findings are equivocal, or the patient has a fever or an elevated leukocyte count. In these instances, lumbar puncture, EEG, and continued observation are indicated. A computed tomography (CT) scan may be indicated with new-onset focal seizures, focal neurologic deficits, fever, neck stiffness, or signs of acute head trauma.

The use of AEDs to prevent alcohol withdrawal seizures is controversial. Some investigators recommend the use of AEDs for recent seizures or clusters of seizures during alcohol withdrawal (22), but others argue that alcohol withdrawal seizures are self-limited (23), and some studies show that treatment is usually ineffective (24). During alcohol withdrawal, hospitalized patients with a history of epilepsy may be given a 5-day course of phenytoin (300 mg/day) in an effort to prevent seizures and the attendant risks of aspiration pneumonia and falls. Long-term therapy with AEDs is not recommended.

Alcohol abusers may abuse other drugs. Concurrent benzodiazepine or barbiturate withdrawal can cause fulminant seizures. Occasionally, seizures occur during periods of alcohol consumption, as distinct from the period of alcohol withdrawal (25).

Seizures and Brain Tumors

Brain tumor is an uncommon cause of epilepsy, but epilepsy is a common symptom of brain tumors. About one third of intracranial and one half of intrahemispheric tumors are associated with seizures. Our present understanding of epilepsy secondary to tumor has been completely changed with the advent of CT and magnetic resonance imaging (MRI) head scanning (26). More and more often, tumors manifest with a single seizure, leading to early investigation and diagnosis with CT head scan or MRI. Between 1% and 16% of patients with epilepsy are found to have tumors. The probability varies according to age group: In adolescents it is approximately 1%; in young adults, 12% to 16%; and in older people, approximately 10% (27,28). *Young and middle-age adults with new onset of focal seizures* have the greatest chance of having a tumor (35%) (6). Nonetheless, CT or MRI scanning is not indicated in the investigation of patients with IGEs who have diagnostic EEG patterns and in previously investigated patients who present with repeated seizures of unchanged character.

Seizures may be generalized tonic–clonic or partial. Diverse and changing clinical features are highly indicative of neoplasia. The following features suggest that seizures may be associated with a brain tumor: Onset after 20 years of age, presence of persistent focal neurologic signs, signs of increased intracranial pressure, and focal unilateral slow waves on the EEG. Seizure frequency varies according to tumor location and histology: Frequent seizures are seen with supratentorial tumors, especially in the rolandic, temporal, or parietal cortical regions. Slow-growing tumors appear to be more epileptogenic.

Seizures and Cerebrovascular Disease

Cerebrovascular disease and epilepsy are the two most common causes of serious neurologic illnesses, and they often occur in the same patient. Ischemia damages brain and can lead to an epileptic focus. The incidence of early seizures (within the first 2 weeks after stroke onset) is approximately 5% in patients with nonembolic stroke (29). The seizures are more likely to be focal (80%) than generalized, and the distribution depends on stroke location. Only a small proportion of stroke patients develop recurrent seizures (i.e., epilepsy): 2.5% of those with intracranial hemorrhage and 3% of those with ischemic stroke (29). In ischemic stroke, although the highest incidence of seizures is shortly after stroke onset (30), epilepsy is most common (90%) in patients with late-onset seizures (more than 2 weeks after stroke) than in those with early-onset seizures (35%). Consequently, early seizures after stroke do not mandate AEDs; late recurrent seizures should be treated as epilepsy.

As previously mentioned, seizures in the elderly should raise the suspicion of cerebrovascular disease and may herald transient ischemia or impending stroke. In young patients, cerebral vascular disease is uncommon, but a seizure may lead to a diagnosis of an arteriovenous malformation, an aneurysm, collagen vascular disease, or a rare case of cortical thrombophlebitis.

Seizures and Infections

A seizure may be an early sign of bacterial meningitis, particularly in the very young and in the very old patient in whom the classic signs of meningitis may be lacking. Less fulminant forms of meningitis, such as cryptococcal or tuberculous meningitis, produce seizures that recur over weeks or months. Viral encephalitides, including herpes simplex encephalitis, the childhood exanthems, and the equine viruses, may also produce seizures. Human immunodeficiency virus (HIV) infection (see Chapter 39) is increasingly of concern as a cause of neurologic and systemic disease; most seizures associated with acquired immunodeficiency syndrome (AIDS) result from secondary complications such as cerebral toxoplasmosis, other atypical infections, or central nervous system lymphoma (31). Any meningoencephalitis can scar the cerebral cortex, resulting in an epileptic focus that can persist after resolution of the infection.

For reasons that are poorly understood, *systemic infections* may trigger seizures in susceptible patients, even if the infection does not directly involve the central nervous system. However, when a patient presents with a seizure and signs of infection, especially if the seizure is focal or if focal signs are detected on neurologic examination, the possibility of brain abscess must be explored with the use of head CT scanning or MRI, often with contrast.

EVALUATION OF A PATIENT WITH SEIZURES

In the evaluation of a patient with a history of one or more episodes of self-limited disturbance of consciousness or behavior, three questions must be addressed: First, were the events epileptic seizures? Second, if so, what type of seizures were they (Table 88.1)? Third, are there clues in the history, physical examination, or laboratory tests that point to a cause for the epileptic seizures (Table 88.2) or toward another cause?

Table 88.3. Differential Diagnosis of Seizure-like Behavior

Condition	See Chapters
Syncope	89
Cerebrovascular disease	91
Migraine	87
Narcolepsy	7
Fluctuating delirium	16
Paroxysmal vertigo	69
Breath-holding spells	
Episodic movement disorders	90
Malingering, factitious illness	21
Conversion disorder	21
Panic attack	22

Differential Diagnosis of Seizure-like Behavior

Determination of the nature of a seizure-like episode is often difficult (Table 88.3). Unless the physician has observed an attack, the patient or witnesses must be asked for information about the sequence of behavioral events with attention to specific signs of neurologic dysfunction. Inquiry should be directed at establishing whether there were tonic–clonic features, with or without biting of tongue, lip, or cheek; head and eye deviation; urinary or fecal incontinence; rhythmic face or limb jerking; or speech and motor arrest followed by automatisms. *Syncope* not caused by a seizure is characteristically associated with prodromal malaise, dizziness, and light-headedness, often with pallor, sweating, palpitations, and upright posture (see Chapter 89); if an observer notes sudden loss of consciousness and tone without convulsions and with brief postictal confusion, syncope is a much more likely diagnosis than is seizure. However, syncopal events can include some arrhythmic limb jerking, occasionally accompanied by incontinence and brief confusion. Transient numbness, weakness, speech or vision problems, or dizziness may occur with *cerebrovascular events* (see Chapter 91), including transient ischemic attacks, stroke, bleeding from an arteriovenous malformation or from an aneurysm, or a classic migraine (see Chapter 87). Precipitating factors such as postural changes, changes in antihypertensive medication, and the sequence of seizure characteristics may help distinguish epileptic seizures from cerebrovascular insufficiency. Particularly in the elderly, where the two conditions may be linked, a firm diagnosis may have to be deferred.

Hypoglycemia (see Chapter 81) is most commonly seen in alcoholics, diabetics, and patients who have had gastrointestinal surgery and often manifests with presyncopal symptoms.

Narcolepsy (see Chapter 87) is a rare disorder characterized by the sudden lapse into rapid eye movement (REM) sleep by episodes, when alert, of brief inhibition of muscle tone (cataplexy). These patients can be aroused from their sleep, often report that they dreamed during the attack, and deny postictal confusion.

In the elderly, a waxing and waning delirium with fluctuating agitation, lethargy, and occasional motor manifestations (see Chapter 26) occurring with intercurrent illness (e.g., renal failure, drug intoxication, infection) may superficially resemble a seizure but usually lacks both the stereotypical aspects of a seizure and a clear start and finish.

Vertigo, caused by disease of the inner ear, can present paroxysmally and may be confused with epilepsy (see Chapter 89).

Certain adults have *face or limb tics,* which, unlike most epileptic seizures, can be partially controlled by volition and often occur at predictable times.

Psychogenic Nonepileptic Seizures

In some patients, the greatest challenge is to distinguish between epileptic and psychogenic nonepileptic events. Misdiagnosis of an epileptic seizure may result in incorrect treatment of the actual underlying condition and the possible social stigma and consequences of being labeled an epileptic. *Panic attacks* can produce recurrent, fulminant, and moderately stereotyped symptoms, all of which may be seen in patients with partial complex seizures (see Chapter 22). Because epileptic seizures may have emotional concomitants (e.g., an aura of extreme fear) and may be triggered by stressful situations, the distinction can be difficult. If a diagnosis of psychogenic illness can be supported on other grounds, if the attacks are strongly linked to preceding anxiety, and if automatisms are lacking, a panic attack becomes a more likely diagnosis.

Patients with seizures caused by a *conversion disorder* may exhibit inattention, staring, deep unresponsiveness, and tonic and clonic movements that closely resemble epileptic events. These psychogenic seizures are involuntary events and must be differentiated from *malingering* and *factitious seizures,* which are produced deliberately by the patient. However, patients with nonepileptic events often also have epilepsy, and the management of epileptic events may be complicated by nonepileptic ones. Thrashing, asynchronous limb movements, crying, screaming, pelvic thrusting, and rapid side-to-side head turning have traditionally been ascribed to nonepileptic events but may also be seen with epileptic seizures. Observation of a generalized attack may reveal features that are atypical of an epileptic event, such as retention of protective reflexes (e.g., the blink reflex), a breathing effort when the airway is briefly occluded, coherent speech, or directed eye movements. Other features include the variability and nonstereotypy of each event, emotional precipitants, the usual presence of witnesses, recall after the event, biting of the tip of the tongue, forced eye closure, and the absence of postictal confusion (32). The motor activity may lack the organized tonic–clonic stages seen with generalized seizures, unless the patient is sophisticated and has observed seizures before. Psychogenic partial complex seizures may be the most difficult to diagnose.

As a general rule, purposeful, goal-directed behavior such as driving, shopping, talking in full sentences, or coordinated acts of violence should not be considered to be part of an epileptic seizure unless there is strong supporting evidence. Some of these features may be seen in the postictal state. Other features typical of a conversion disorder—presence of secondary gain, *la belle indifference,* inappropriate reactions to stress—may contribute to a correct diagnosis. Consultation among primary physician, neurologist, and psychiatrist may be required for proper diagnosis and management (see also Chapter 21).

Initial Determination of Seizure Type and Cause

The identification of seizure type (Table 88.1) should be made at the time of diagnosis of epilepsy. Features of the clinical onset should be especially addressed, because a brief focal onset or an aura may be the only indication that a seizure was secondarily rather than primarily generalized.

The history usually provides the main clues to the cause of the seizure. Contributory factors may include birth trauma or perinatal illness, head trauma, previous cerebral infarction or intracranial hemorrhage, encephalitis or meningitis, malignancies, and prior seizures. A family history of seizures may be pertinent because there is increased risk, particularly with IGEs, for seizures in relatives of people with epilepsy. There should be inquiry into the use of alcohol, benzodiazepines, barbiturates, and other proconvulsants such as cocaine, amphetamine, neuroleptic medications, tricyclic antidepressants, bupropion, and theophylline. Patients may volunteer accounts of precipitating events such as flashing lights or hyperventilation. In some epilepsies, patients identify particular stimuli such as games, music, eating, laughing, or the touching of certain regions of skin. These *reflex seizures* may be avoided by avoiding the offending stimulus.

A general physical examination and neurologic examination (see Chapter 86) may reveal asymmetries or provide evidence for a structural, metabolic, or other cause of the seizure disorder. Some findings (e.g., focal paralysis) may be postictal, indicating focal onset (Todd paralysis), or they conversely may be suppressed, warranting reexamination in a few hours or days.

Investigations in a Patient with Seizures

Laboratory tests are usually not very helpful in determining whether a seizure has taken place, but they may be useful in establishing an underlying cause, in epilepsy classification, and in patient management.

Laboratory Tests

Depending on one's diagnostic hypotheses, investigations may include a full blood count, blood urea nitrogen or serum creatinine concentration, serum glucose, and serum electrolytes. In evaluating test results, it should be remembered that *striking abnormalities may appear transiently immediately after a seizure* (e.g., metabolic acidosis, marked leukocytosis). If clinically indicated, blood gases, liver function tests, and a screen for proconvulsive drugs should be obtained. A baseline electrocardiogram may show arrhythmias or ischemia, although immediately after a seizure, these changes also may be results, rather than causes, of the seizure.

At times, measurement of a *serum prolactin level* helps in the evaluation of a patient with a suspected psychogenic seizure. Commonly, the prolactin level rises two- to threefold after an epileptic but not after a psychogenic tonic–clonic event. In a lesser percentage of patients (45%), CPSs may cause serum prolactin increases, as may syncope (33), but 85% of simple partial (epileptic) seizures cause no rise (34). Partial complex seizures of temporal lobe origin are more likely to cause prolactin increases than those from the frontal lobe (35). Because this transient rise is present for 10 to 60 minutes after the event, positive findings are helpful, but negative findings, especially if measured more than 1 hour after the event, are inconclusive.

Electroencephalography

The EEG is the most useful laboratory study in the diagnosis of seizure disorders. An EEG may show generalized or focal epileptiform activity, or, even in the absence of such activity, it may demonstrate asymmetries of basic rhythms, focal slow waves, or diffuse slowing, all of which may give direction to further investigation. The appearance of epileptiform discharges on an EEG performed within 1 week after a *first seizure* predicts an 83% recurrence rate within 2 years, compared with a 41% recurrence rate in patients without such findings (36). Usually, the EEG is obtained more than 48 hours after the seizure. About 50% of patients with epilepsy have a normal EEG first. In about 10% of patients with epileptic seizures, multiple EEGs are all normal (37). In general, the EEG should be relied on not to make a diagnosis of a seizure but to confirm a clinical impression derived from the history. When the history and EEG results are at variance, primacy should go to the history. Patients should not be treated for epilepsy because of an abnormal EEG alone, because interictal pattern epileptiform discharges may be seen in 0.4% of the healthy population, in 2.2% of patients with nonepileptic neurologic disease, and in 3.5% of asymptomatic relatives of people with epilepsy (38). Conversely, one should not be dissuaded from a clinical impression of a seizure disorder just because of a normal EEG.

If EEG confirmation of seizure activity is needed (e.g., the history is equivocal, seizures occur during sleep or drowsiness), a repeat study with sleep deprivation or sleep induction, hyperventilation or intermittent photic stimulation, use of other scalp or semi-invasive electrodes (nasopharyngeal or sphenoidal leads), or eventually the use of prolonged video monitoring with EEG recording may be indicated. Many hospitals have epilepsy monitoring units specializing in the diagnosis and treatment of epilepsy. Referral to such units is sometimes the most effective way to elucidate the nature of spells not delineated by more routine maneuvers.

Epileptiform EEG discharges can usually be observed in the presence of AEDs, although some generalized discharges may be suppressed. Therefore, medications should not be altered for the first EEG. If tracings are repeatedly negative and the diagnosis of epilepsy is suspect, then the patient can be admitted to a hospital for rapid tapering of AEDs and concurrent EEG and video monitoring to look for epileptic activity. However, abrupt withdrawal of barbiturates or benzodiazepines may precipitate seizures even in normal subjects. Among patients with epilepsy, the pattern of generalized EEG slowing without seizure discharges is fairly common, usually resulting from underlying diffuse cortical dysfunction, medication effects, or a postictal state.

Because EEGs can stay abnormal for several weeks after a tonic–clonic seizure, any findings should be reevaluated with repeated studies. An EEG is without risk (see Chapter 86), barring an injudicious interpretation.

Cerebrospinal Fluid Examination

Certain illnesses that lead to seizures may require examination of cerebrospinal fluid (CSF) to secure a diagnosis; examples are suspected acute or chronic meningitis or subarachnoid hemorrhage. The yield of CSF studies in patients with various seizure types is unknown, and the indication for these studies should be considered on a case-by-case basis. The CSF examination is not indicated in a normal child with classic absence epilepsy or with EEG evidence of focal rolandic spikes, and it is contraindicated in a patient in whom a mass lesion is strongly suspected. Most other patients with focal or generalized seizures of uncertain cause should undergo spinal fluid analysis (see Chapter 86).

After prolonged generalized seizures, the CSF may show a pleocytosis of up to 100 cells, presumably from a transient breakdown of the blood–brain barrier. Clearly, however, infection must be excluded or temporarily considered in this setting.

Cerebral Imaging

CT head scans (see Chapter 86) of patients with primary generalized seizures are abnormal (excluding nonspecific atrophy) in approximately 10% of instances. Scans of patients with focal motor or secondarily generalized seizures show a focal abnormality in 65%. Patients with CPSs show abnormalities about one third of the time. An abnormal and asymmetric neurologic examination has a high correlation with focal abnormalities on the head CT scan. Studies of patients with seizures show that MRI of the head (see Chapter 86) has a higher diagnostic yield than CT scanning and may show specific changes of mesial temporal sclerosis, various angiomas, neuronal migration disorders, or perisylvian polymicrogyria but is not a procedure needed for all patients (39).

Adults with new-onset focal or secondarily generalized seizures should have an MRI or CT scan with contrast if possible, unless the EEG shows a pattern of a genetic disorder. Patients with an abnormal neurologic examination should also be imaged. In patients with a normal examination and in children, this decision should be individualized. Subsequent imaging may also be indicated if there is a change in seizure pattern or neurologic examination.

Other Diagnostic Tests

Skull radiographs, radionuclide brain scans, pneumoencephalography, and arteriography have largely been replaced by newer imaging studies. Several techniques show promise for definition of seizure foci: Imaging of brain metabolism and chemistry by positron emission tomographic (PET) scanning; single-photon emission computed tomography (SPECT), which examines cerebral blood flow at particular time points; functional magnetic resonance imaging (fMRI); and magnetoencephalographic (MEG) recording of brain activity.

TREATMENT OF EPILEPSY

Except in unusual instances, epilepsy cannot be cured. In about three of four patients, it can be controlled so that the patient experiences few or no seizures. Much attention has been focused on the pharmacologic management of seizures, but the importance of a comprehensive approach cannot be overemphasized: A patient who is seizure free but so intoxicated by medicines that employment is impossible represents at best a dubious success. Employment problems and other social aspects of the management of epilepsy are considered in the following sections. General measures of therapy should not be neglected. Removal of precipitating factors for seizures, reduction of stress, and provision for adequate amounts of rest can all be important in the control of epilepsy and are also discussed here. Patients should be advised to wear *medical alert bracelets or medallions.*

The Patient with a First Seizure

In deciding whether to treat a first seizure, one should recall that a single seizure does not constitute epilepsy or necessarily require treatment. In patients with *"provoked"* or acute symptomatic seizures such as those that occur after alcohol withdrawal, cocaine intake, or overdose of tricyclics, identification and removal of the precipitating cause usually prevents further seizures, and AEDs are rarely indicated. In addition, single or early seizures (i.e., within 2 weeks) after head trauma or stroke do not require chronic AED therapy.

In about one third of patients with first seizures, the seizures are *unprovoked.* Such patients may be so frightened by the possibility of having another seizure, with potential repercussions on employment, social relations, and license to drive, that they are willing to accept the inconvenience and morbidity of chronic medication. Most patients first present to a physician after having had several unprovoked seizures. Of this group, more than three fourths may be expected to have further seizures. This contrasts with the finding from prospective studies that approximately 16% to 36% of patients who present after their first unprovoked seizure have a recurrence within 1 year, and that in the aggregate 27% to 50% have recurrent seizures within 3 years (8,9). Retrospective studies suggest higher recurrence rates.

Because for a given patient the probability of further seizures over a 5-year period may vary from 30% to 80%, it is important to consider the following *risk factors that increase the probability of additional seizures:* An identifiable cause for the first seizure, such as central nervous system infection or recent stroke or head injury; the presence of EEG epileptiform abnormalities; occurrence of the initial seizure at night; previous febrile seizures; status epilepticus or multiple seizures in the same day; Todd paralysis; and partial seizures (9,16). With genetic epilepsies, typically with childhood onset, in which the EEG shows epileptiform activity, there is an increased risk of seizure recurrence in the short term. Many of these epilepsy syndromes are age dependent and remit after several years.

In one prospective study, addressed to the issue of treatment after a first unprovoked tonic–clonic seizure, the rate of recurrence at 1 year in patients randomly assigned to AED treatment was 18%, compared with 38% for those who were not started immediately on treatment (40). Depending on the AED used, the incidence of side effects severe enough to warrant discontinuation of treatment ranges from less than 1% to approximately 6%. These figures usually are not used in deciding whether a patient should be offered a specific AED. Rather, the efficacy profile, the overall side effect profile, and the frequency with which the medication must be taken govern the institution of the drug (see later discussion).

General Principles of Drug Therapy

Many patients who have monthly or more frequent generalized seizures are probably undertreated; and the goal of therapy should be zero seizures. In contrast, other patients may be taking an unnecessary polypharmacy or incorrect regimens of AEDs. General principles for the planning of drug therapy are summarized in Table 88.4. Prospective observations show that, with adequate AED treatment, the prognosis for seizure control during the first 12 months varies according to seizure type: GTCS, 60% to 70%; mixed (predominately GTCS), 50% to 53%; CPS, 21% to 28% (16).

Selection of Drugs

To select the appropriate AED, it is important to know the type of epilepsy under consideration. Table 88.5 represents a general but not unanimous consensus on drugs of choice and alternatives for the principal types of seizures and epilepsy. Two large controlled clinical trials compared the effectiveness of several AEDs (carbamazepine, phenobarbital, phenytoin, and primidone) and valproic acid versus carbamazepine for the treatment of *partial seizures* or *secondarily generalized tonic–clonic seizures* (41,42). Both carbamazepine and phenytoin were highly effective and are recommended as drugs of choice for these two common types of seizures (42). Valproic acid is generally recommended as the drug of first choice for IGEs. *CAE* may be treated with either ethosuximide or valproic acid, although the former does not prevent concurrent tonic–clonic seizures. *Myoclonic seizures* are best treated with valproate, topiramate, or levetiracetam. A certain percentage of IGEs with GTCSs respond to monotherapy with carbamazepine (although absence seizures may worsen), and a certain percentage of partial seizures respond to valproic acid monotherapy. In several instances, more than one drug may be considered the drug of choice in terms of efficacy, in which case the selection can be made on the basis of personal familiarity with the drug, convenience of dose scheduling, or the relative risk and spectrum of side effects. For example, some practitioners prefer carbamazepine to phenytoin to avoid possible gum hyperplasia and hirsutism, even though these side effects are seen in only approximately 10% of patients. With phenytoin, the convenience of a simpler dosage regimen, lower cost, and availability of a parenteral preparation may offset these considerations. Several reviews and meta-analyses compared controlled trials of AEDs and revealed no significant differences in efficacy among AEDs in current use (43). Dosages, half-lives, serum levels, and principal side effects of the drugs are given in Table 88.6.

Table 88.4. Principles of Antiepileptic Drug Therapy

Decide whether to treat.
Select the proper drug for the particular form of epilepsy.
Start drugs slowly and build up levels gradually to avoid toxicity.
Start with one drug, and use it to effect or toxicity before adding another.
Choose the simplest regimen possible.
Suspect compliance problems in treatment failures.
Monitor blood levels in problem cases.
Withdraw medications gradually.
Decide how long to treat.

Dose Adjustment

The AED dosage should be increased over several weeks to avoid early side effects that might discourage the patient from continuing with treatment. Because some AEDs remain in the blood for some time, it may take several days to weeks before the effects of a dosage adjustment are manifested.

Although initial treatment *with more than one AED,* typically phenytoin and phenobarbital, was once common, there is little evidence that two drugs at subtherapeutic dosages are better tolerated or more effective than one drug at higher dosages. In fact, 90% of new-onset seizures that are controlled can be controlled with one drug. If one drug is unsuccessful, addition of a second helps in only approximately 36% of patients (44).

Compliance is a major factor in the success of drug therapy for epilepsy (see Chapter 4). Every effort should be made to simplify the dosage regimen and choose the best-tolerated drug. Phenobarbital and certain formulations of phenytoin can be given in a once-daily dose. The complexity of providing carbamazepine, primidone, valproate, or lamotrigine, which must be given in divided doses, should be offset by a better-suited profile of side effects for the

Table 88.5. Drugs of Choice[a] According to Seizure Type

Seizure Category or Epilepsy Syndrome	Drugs of Choice	Alternatives (Alphabetically)	Third Choice
Idiopathic generalized tonic–clonic seizures	Valproate Lamotrigine	Levetiracetam Phenytoin Topiramate Zonisamide	Phenobarbital Primidone
Idiopathic (primary) generalized absence seizures	Ethosuximide Valproate	Clonazepam Lamotrigine Levetiracetam	Acetazolamide Topiramate Zonisamide
Idiopathic generalized (juvenile myoclonic) epilepsy	Valproate Lamotrigine Clonazepam	Levetiracetam Topiramate Zonisamide	Phenobarbital Phenytoin Primidone
Partial simple and complex and secondarily generalized epilepsy	Carbamazepine Oxcarbazepine Phenytoin Valproate Lamotrigine	Gabapentin Levetiracetam Topiramate	Phenobarbital Primidone Tiagabine Zonisamide
Mixed seizure forms	Valproate Clonazepam Lamotrigine Topiramate	Carbamazepine Levetiracetam Phenytoin	Phenobarbital Primidone Zonisamide

[a]Not necessarily according to U.S. Food and Drug Administration approved indications.

individual patient. At each visit the patient (or other responsible person) should be asked to report on the exact medication regimen and encouraged to bring the most recent medicine bottles with them. All too often, inquiry indicates a need for clearer oral and written communication with the patient. If necessary, the drug regimen should be written out for the patient's use.

Familiarity with cost of medicines is important, because patients may be hesitant to buy an expensive medicine unless the need is clearly explained. *Generic brands* are less expensive, but for several AEDs, such as carbamazepine, primidone, phenytoin, and valproic acid, bioavailability is variable (45). Generally, generic brands should be avoided in patients with seizures that are difficult to control. If generic brands are prescribed, use of the same brand should be encouraged; drug levels may have to be checked more often if toxicity or seizures appear.

The optimal dosage of an AED may vary severalfold among different patients. Determination of serum levels (Table 88.6) is a reliable way to measure how much medication is circulating, but such measurements should not be ordered routinely. If a patient's seizures are controlled on the regimen that is initiated and there is no toxicity from that drug regimen, measurement of a drug serum level might lead one to alter a successful regimen inappropriately. If control is not optimal, drug levels can help detect inadequate compliance or absorption. They may also provide guidance for patients with symptoms that might be caused by drug intoxication. Ideally, blood specimens obtained to monitor side effects should be taken at times of peak serum concentrations, and specimens obtained to monitor drug efficacy should be taken at times of trough serum levels. It is important to know that for some AEDs, particularly phenytoin, drug dosage and drug level are not linearly related: A saturation point is reached above which small increments in daily dosage (e.g., increasing from 400 to 500 mg of phenytoin per day) may lead to marked increases in serum level and side effects. A serum level is most informative if measured in the steady state (Table 88.6), which requires a stable dosage for approximately five half-lives or longer before measurement.

Many patients with severe and long-standing epilepsy have endured a gradual increase in AED dosage. Excessive polypharmacy may be ineffective, may produce marked side effects, and may even limit the ability to increase a single potentially effective AED to the maximum dosage. In this circumstance, one should consider reduction in AED dosage or number of medications over several months. Other side effects may prompt discontinuation of AEDs.

Although several AEDs can cause modest rises in *liver enzyme levels,* only moderate to marked abnormalities (more than 2 times baseline) necessitate stopping the drug. Conversely, serious hepatotoxicity may not be heralded by changes in liver function tests. Symptoms may include anorexia, malaise, tiredness, and jaundice, usually appearing 2 to 16 weeks after starting treatment. Carbamazepine can cause mild *leukopenia and thrombocytopenia,* but a rapid, progressive leukocyte decline, typically to lower than 3,000 cells/mm^3 with a total neutrophil count of less than 1,000/mm^3, would warrant concern (32). *Nystagmus* should not be used as an indication of toxicity but rather as a marker of AED therapy. Conversely, ataxia, unacceptable somnolence, cognitive impairment, and malaise may indicate the need for modification of therapy.

Duration of Treatment

The determination of how long to maintain treatment with AEDs may be difficult, because seizures remit over time, and therefore freedom from seizures may not be the result of medication. About one half to two thirds of patients are entirely seizure free for 2 years with therapy. If an adult patient is seizure free for about 5 years on medication and then stops treatment by gradual taper, there is a 30% to 50% chance of

Table 88.6. Major Antiepileptic Drugs

Medication[a] (Brand Name)	Available Preparations and Strengths (mg)	Typical Adult Dose, Schedule, Range	Half-Life (hr)	Reference-Target Levels (mg/L)[b]	Major Side Effects
Carbamazepine[c] (Carbatrol)	200 mg, 300 mg capsules	Daily dose 200–800 mg, b.i.d.	10–25	4–12	Same as Tegretol
Carbamazepine (Tegretol)	200 tablets (100 chewable) 100/5 mL suspension	200 mg t.i.d. or q.i.d. (400–1,600 mg)	10–25	4–12	GI distress Ataxia Blurred vision Blood changes Hepatotoxicity
Carbamazepine extended release (Tegretol XR)	100, 200, 400 mg tablets	200–800 mg in two divided doses			Same as Tegretol
Clonazepam[c] (Klonopin)	0.5, 1, 2 mg tablets	2 mg t.i.d. (2–20 mg)	20–40	0.05–0.7	Drowiness Ataxia Behavior changes
Ethosuximide (Zarontin)	250 mg capsules 250 mg/mL syrup	250 mg b.i.d. to q.i.d. (500–1,500 mg)	30	50–100	Dizziness GI distress Sedation Headache
Felbamate (Felbatol)	400, 600 mg tablets 600/5 mL suspension	2,400–3,600 mg/d in 3 or 4 divided doses	20–23	30–50	Dizziness Nausea Vomiting Aplastic anemia Acute liver failure ↑ ALT Insomnia Headache Dizziness Weight loss
Fosphenytoin IV sodium (Cerebyx)	IV preparation 2 mL (100 mg PE) and 10 mL (500 mg PE)	150 mg PE/min diluted in 0.9% saline or 5% dextrose before infusion	15 min Converts to phenytoin with half-life of 22 h	10–20	Pruritis Paresthesia Dizziness Headache Somnolence Ataxia Nystagmus
Gabapentin (Neurontin)	100, 300, 400, 600, 800 mg capsules	600–1,200 t.i.d.	5–7	>4	Somnolence Ataxia Dizziness Fatigue Nystagmus Tremor Weight gain
Lamotrigine (Lamictal)	5, 25, 100, 150 and 200 mg tablets	75–250 mg b.i.d.	12–14 when added to enzyme-inducing AEDs 25-33 as monotherapy	4–18	Rash Dizziness Ataxia Somnolence Headache Blurred vision Nausea Vomiting
Levetiracetam (Keppra)	250, 500, 750 mg scored tablets	500–1,500 b.i.d.	6–8	3–37	Somnolence Asthenias Dizziness
Oxcarbazepine (Trileptal)	150, 300, 600 mg scored tablets	Starting dose 150–300 mg/d Total: 900–2,400 mg/day, given in two daily doses; 300 mg/5 mL (60 mg/mL) oral suspension	MHD 9.3 ± 1.8	MHD 50–200 mmol/L or 10–35 mg/L	Fatigue Dizziness Headache Sedation Ataxia Hypersensitivity Reactions Hyponatremia
Phenobarbital[c] (Luminal)	15, 30, 60, 100 mg tablets	100–200 mg q.d.	72	15–40	Sedation Hyperactivity Confusion Mood change
Phenytoin[c] (Dilantin)[c]	30, 100 mg capsules 50 mg chewable "Infatabs" 125 mg/5 mL suspension	300 mg q.d.[d,e] (200–500 mg)	22[e]	10–20	Ataxia Cosmetic changes (gum hyperplasia, hirsutism) Sedation Osteoporosis

Table 88.6.—*continued.* Major Antiepileptic Drugs

Medication[a] (Brand Name)	Available Preparations and Strengths (mg)	Typical Adult Dose, Schedule, Range	Half-Life (hr)	Reference-Target Levels (mg/L)[b]	Major Side Effects
Primidone[c] (Mysoline)	50, 250 mg scored tablets and suspension 250 mg/5 mL	250 mg t.i.d. or q.i.d. (500–1,500 mg)	3–12[f] 72[g]	6–12[f] 15–40[g]	Sedation Hyperactivity Mood change
Tiagabine (Gabritril)	2, 4, 12, 16 mg tablets	32–56 mg in two to four divided doses	12–15 with other AED 21–24 as monotherapy	Unknown	Dizziness Confusion Tiredness GI upset Headache Depression Tremor
Topiramate (Topamax)	25, 100, 200 mg tablets 15, 25 mg sprinkles	100–400 mg/day in two divided doses	12–15 with other AED, 21–24 as monotherapy	6.5–30	Somnolence Dizziness Ataxia Psychomotor slowing Paresthesias Weight loss Anorexia Fatigue Kidney stones Glaucoma
Valproate IV (Depacon)	IV preparation 5 mL single-dose vials equal to 100 mg/mL	60-min infusion but not >20 mg/min	16 ± 3	50–100	Same as valproic acid
Valproic acid[c] (Depakene)	250 capsules 250 mg/5 mL syrup	250 mg b.i.d. to q.i.d. (500–4,000 mg)/d	8–12	50–100	GI distress Drowiness Ataxia
Valproic acid; divalproex sodium (Depakote)	125, 350, 500 mg tablets 125 mg sprinkles	Same as above	8–12	50–100	Alopecia Tremor Blood changes Rare liver toxicity Rare pancreatitis
Zonisamide (Zonegran)	100 mg capsules	Starting dose 100 mg/d; increase by 100 mg/2 wk as tolerated	63	10–40	Fatigue Headache Somnolence Ataxia Agitation Anorexia Nausea Confusion Paresthesias Kidney stone (1%–2%) Mental slowing Hypersensitivity reaction Oligohydrosis

ALT, alanine aminotransferase; GI, gastrointestinal; MHD, 10-monohydroxy metabolite of oxcarbazepine; PE, phenytoin equivalents.
[a]Although generic products are available, there have been reports of bio-inequivalence between brand name and generic products.
[b]Laboratory may report same figures as micrograms per milliliter.
[c]Generic product available.
[d]These doses are usually attained gradually over days to weeks. The ranges are relatively rough guidelines; because absorption varies, serum levels are better guides to dosage.
[e]Only for Dilantin capsules (Kapseals).
[f]For primidone.
[g]For phenobarbital.

relapse during the next 5 years (45,15). Approximately 80% of relapses occur within 4 months after starting the taper, and 90% within the first year (46,47).

As with the decision to initiate therapy, the decision to terminate AED therapy must be individualized. A patient with seizures that were initially very difficult to control who has an underlying structural lesion or a persistently abnormal EEG may benefit from lifelong therapy. In contrast, a patient with idiopathic epilepsy who has been seizure free for 2 to 5 years and is willing to accept an increased risk of having a seizure may be a candidate for drug withdrawal. Certain patients who have attained seizure control over a long period do not wish to stop treatment. In these instances, potential benefits and risks of medication reduction should be discussed, but patients should not be forced off medications for the sake of principle. If more than one drug has been prescribed, the medications should be tapered one at a time, each over a period of several months, and reinstated rapidly if seizures recur.

The least effective medication or the most toxic may be chosen as the candidate for initial reduction.

An example of a cautious tapering schedule for a patient who has been taking carbamazepine 400 mg (two 200-mg tablets) three times daily would be reduction by one tablet per day every 2 weeks. During tapering and in the first few months after the tapering of all AEDs, it is prudent for the patient to refrain from driving.

Ambulatory Follow-Up

Seizure frequency, medication side effects, and social factors determine the pattern for outpatient follow-up. Patients who are free from seizures for longer than 1 year and who have no intercurrent problems may be seen yearly. Conversely, patients with frequent seizures, significant side effects, or social problems may need to be seen every few weeks during problem periods. Visits may be necessary every 2 to 4 weeks during adjustment of the drug regimen. For appropriate management and monitoring of therapeutic changes, a patient should be evaluated no sooner than five AED half-lives after the change is initiated.

Specific Antiepileptic Drugs

Carbamazepine (Tegretol, Carbatrol)

Carbamazepine has been used for more than two decades for the treatment of seizures and chronic neuropathic pains. Carbamazepine is one of the drugs of choice for CPSs, but it may worsen absence seizures. Studies comparing carbamazepine with other AEDs for the treatment of partial seizures showed that carbamazepine resulted in the highest rate of complete remission (although mean seizure frequency was similar for patients taking carbamazepine, phenytoin, or phenobarbital) (41). The adult dosage of carbamazepine is 400 to 1,600 mg/day with dosing guidelines for carbatrol and tegretol given in Table 88.6. It is advisable to initiate therapy with no more than 200 to 400 mg/day, increasing to the full dosage over 1 or 2 weeks. The half-life is about 10 to 25 hours, and dosage should be divided into three- or four-times-a-day regimens. A newer long-acting preparation, Tegretol XR, is available in 100-, 200-, and 400-mg tablets, with ports that allow slow release. This form can be taken twice daily. It is now the preparation indicated for all patients treated with Tegretol. Total daily dosage remains the same, meaning that conversion to the more convenient form is simple, but more even blood levels are obtained. Patients should be warned that the tablet shell may appear in the stool, but this does not represent inadequate release of contents. Patients must be instructed not to chew XR tablets but to swallow them whole. Another long-acting preparation, carbatrol, also has a long half-life and produces more constant blood levels. Recommended target serum levels with all preparations of carbamazepine are 4 to 12 mg/L. In 2001, a typical 1-month supply of generic carbamazepine cost about $20, versus $69 for Tegretol-XR and $209 for Trileptal (oxcarbazepine). Because of erratic absorption of the generic preparation, it should not be continued in any patient who takes it and continues to have seizures.

Because carbamazepine in tablet form may lose one third or more of its effectiveness if stored in humid conditions, patients should be advised to keep their tablet containers in a dry location, away from the bathroom. Recently, manufacturers have been asked by the U.S. Food and Drug Administration (FDA) to package carbamazepine in moisture-proof containers.

The *side effects* of carbamazepine include fatigue, nystagmus, diplopia, dizziness, ataxia, dysarthria, rash (including, rarely, Stevens–Johnson syndrome), inappropriate secretion of antidiuretic hormone, occasionally abnormal liver function tests, and an infrequent lupus-like syndrome. Gastrointestinal distress is the most common side effect, particularly if the medication is initiated too rapidly. Reversible leukopenia or thrombocytopenia is seen in 5% to 10% of patients, so blood counts may be monitored weekly for the first few weeks after the start of therapy. This drug has had a reputation for causing aplastic anemia, based largely on six cases of this complication that were reported in the 1960s (even though a causal relationship to carbamazepine was not established). The actual incidence of aplastic anemia is unknown, but it is thought to be very small (the warning provided by the manufacturer reports a general population incidence of potentially fatal blood dyscrasia of 8 per 1,000,000 and an incidence associated with carbamazepine of about 40 per 1,000,000).

Phenytoin (Diphenylhydantoin, DPH, PHT, Dilantin)

Since its introduction in 1938, phenytoin has been one of the major drugs used to treat seizures. It is most useful in IGEs and in epilepsies with simple and complex partial seizures, with or without secondary generalization. Phenytoin may make absence seizures worse.

Without a loading dose, a full week is required to reach therapeutic levels, but a load equal to three times the daily maintenance dose, given on the first day, achieves immediate therapeutic levels. This rapid dosing scheme is likely to induce transient side effects and is useful chiefly for initiating treatment in a patient who has seized repeatedly (e.g., in an emergency department) and remains unconscious.

The mean half-life of phenytoin is 22 hours, with a range from 7 to 42 hours. It is 90% protein bound, so *low serum albumin* can lead to an increased concentration of the free agent and consequently to increased toxicity. The drug is metabolized in the liver and is not excreted by the kidney. In renal failure, drug-binding proteins may be deficient, resulting in a low measured total serum level with an adequate free drug serum level. Dosage should be lowered only in renal failure to compensate for a decrease in serum protein, and then a reduction of approximately 25% usually suffices. Phenytoin is partially removed by hemodialysis.

The usual starting dosage of phenytoin is 100 mg/day for 3 to 5 days, increasing by 100 mg at similar intervals to 300 mg/day. If seizures are not controlled at this dosage, it is prudent to increase by increments of 50 mg/day, because small increases in dosage may cause large increases in serum levels. Phenytoin (as Dilantin) comes in 30- and 100-mg capsules, suspension (30 mg and 125 mg/5 mL), and chewable 50-mg tablets. This medication can be given once a day if it is given as Dilantin Kapseals, because this preparation is manufactured as a slow-release form. Other of phenytoin preparations are fast-release capsules; they are less expensive but must be given in divided doses (100 mg three times a day). A parenteral formulation of phenytoin is fosphenytoin sodium injection (Cerebyx), which can be given intramuscularly or intravenously. It is dosed in phenytoin equivalents (PEs) and can be given more rapidly intravenously at up to 150 mg/minute. A target range for phenytoin is generally between 10 and 20 mg/L (toxicity usually occurs at levels greater than 20 mg/L, but patients show fairly wide individual susceptibility to side effects). The lethal dose may range from 2 to 20 g.

A number of drugs elevate phenytoin plasma levels—disulfiram and isoniazid commonly. Amiodarone increases phenytoin 1.5 times, while fluconazole and miconazole increase phenytoin 2 to 4 times. Warfarin, chloramphenicol, methylphenidate, phenothiazines, benzodiazepines, propoxyphene, fluoxetine, omeprazol, propoxyphene, thioridizine, haloperidol, cimetidine, and erythromycin less often increase phenytoin plasma levels. Other drugs may lead to *decreased phenytoin* levels: Alcohol, folic acid, pyridoxine, theophylline, and occasionally carbamazepine, oral contraceptives, sulfonamides, ticlopidine, trazodone ciprofloxacin, and antacids. Phenytoin may decrease cyclosporin levels. These potential drug interactions may be managed best by patient and physician awareness and by observation of serum drug levels during times of medication changes.

There are many potential *undesirable effects of phenytoin*. Dose-related *acute effects* include ataxia (usually beyond 25 to 30 mg/L), lethargy, depression, paradoxic tendency to increase seizures at higher toxic levels (usually greater than 10 mg/L), and allergic reactions. *Chronic side effects* of phenytoin are generally manifested after a few months to several years of daily ingestion. Chronically progressive cosmetic changes can be vexing in young women. Gum hyperplasia occurs in approximately 10%; it may be forestalled by good oral hygiene, but once established it may regress only partially. Hirsutism is seen in 5% overall but in 30% of young women. Even more disconcerting are facial changes caused by thickening of subcutaneous tissue about the nose and eyes, the so-called leonine facies. Skin rash occurs in 2% to 10% of users of phenytoin, with a peak incidence about 2 to 8 weeks into the course. Stevens–Johnson syndrome occurs rarely. Lymphadenopathy develops in 2% to 5%, sometimes in association with fever, arthralgia, eosinophilia, and hepatosplenomegaly, presenting a picture of pseudolymphoma and, rarely, true lymphoma. Hepatitis and a variety of blood dyscrasias have been reported. Megaloblastic anemia may occur, which responds to folate. Many patients develop measurable antinuclear antibodies in the serum; a tiny minority of this group progress to symptomatic systemic lupus erythematosus, which remits entirely within days to weeks after discontinuation of phenytoin. The rare instances of pulmonary infiltrates and fibrosis have given rise to the term *Dilantin lung*. Phenytoin can induce liver enzymes, thereby secondarily affecting metabolism of numerous hormones and drugs. Induced inactivation of vitamin D leads to radiologic or biochemical evidence of bone disease in one of every three chronically treated patients. Teratogenic effects of phenytoin are strongly suspected (see later discussion).

Sodium Valproate (Depakote)

The antiseizure effect of valproic acid was discovered in 1963. Its effectiveness is broad, but it is thought to be particularly valuable for absence seizures and CAE, for idiopathic and symptomatic generalized epilepsies, and as a first- or second-line agent for partial epilepsies (47).

Valproic acid is a fatty acid, structurally dissimilar from all other common AEDs. It is usually prescribed as sodium valproate/valproic acid (Depakote), purported by the manufacturer to cause less gastrointestinal upset than pure valproic acid (Depakene). It is available in 125-, 250-, and 500-mg tablets and in 125-mg sprinkle capsules. Valproic acid is also available in generic form. Peak serum levels are reached in 1 to 4 hours after ingestion, and the half-life is about 8 to 12 hours. The drug is metabolized in the liver and excreted in the urine in modified form. The approximate target range is 50 to 100 mg/L. The manufacturer suggests initiation of therapy with a dosage of about 10 to 15 mg/kg per day, to be increased at weekly intervals by about 5 to 10 mg/kg per day to a maximal dosage of 60 mg/kg per day. A common final regimen is 250 to 500 mg orally, two to four times per day.

About one in five patients taking valproate has significant side effects, commonly gastrointestinal upset, drowsiness, rash, reversible hair loss, weight loss or gain, ataxia, tremor, or hyperactivity. A limited number of studies suggest that valproate inhibits platelet aggregation and may prolong the bleeding time, but this effect is poorly documented. Less commonly, valproate can produce frank thrombocytopenia. The health risk from use of valproate that has received the greatest attention is *hepatic toxicity*. Thirty-seven fatalities from hepatic failure associated with use of valproate were reported in the United States between 1978 and 1984 (48). Among patients receiving valproate as monotherapy, the calculated rate of fatality from hepatic injury was 1 per 37,000. This rate was much higher for children younger than 2 years of age and for children receiving polytherapy. These two risk factors together resulted in a fatality rate from hepatic injury of 1 per 500 children. In contrast, no fatalities from hepatic injury were reported in patients older than 10 years of age who were receiving monotherapy. Several patients have developed serious episodes of pancreatitis while taking valproate. Because of these recently discovered toxicities, and because of its high cost, valproate has not yet replaced ethosuximide as the drug of choice for absence epilepsy unless there are concurrent atypical absence attacks or tonic–clonic seizures. There may be drug interactions with aspirin, warfarin, cimetidine, phenothiazines, antacids, the benzodiazepines, and other AEDs such as lamotrigine.

Phenobarbital

In past decades, phenobarbital was a drug of choice for GTCSs. It is now a drug of last resort for a variety of seizure types. Phenobarbital has been used in the pediatric age group, where it may be better tolerated than phenytoin because it does not cause cosmetic side effects; however, it can cause significant behavioral side effects (hyperactivity in up to 40% of children).

Phenobarbital is a long-lasting drug. The gastrointestinal absorption is slow, so it takes 10 to 12 hours for levels to reach their peak after an oral dose, compared with 20 minutes after an intravenous dose. The drug is detoxified by the liver and excreted by the kidney, but the dosage need be only slightly reduced in renal failure. The serum half-life is about 72 hours, ranging from 37 to 96 hours. Therapeutic levels are 15 to 40 mg/L. Phenobarbital is a potent inducer of liver enzymes and leads to rapid tolerance, as well as to alteration of kinetics of numerous other medications. The dosage of phenobarbital is 1 to 3 mg/kg per day, or about 100 mg/day for the average adult. Little justification can be made for giving it in divided doses. Available tablet strengths are 15, 30, 60, and 100 mg.

The main *acute side effect* of phenobarbital in adults is sedation. After a few weeks, partial tolerance to the sedation usually develops. In elderly patients, phenobarbital can cause confusion and respiratory depression. Subtle or overt personality changes caused by phenobarbital probably occur more often than is generally recognized, especially in the elderly. Ataxia and nystagmus are common in all patients at high dosages. Occasionally, there is idiosyncratic allergy, with accompanying dermatitis or gastrointestinal symptoms. Connective tissue problems may occur. Phenobarbital must be administered with caution to potential drug or alcohol abusers or to unreliable patients who might precipitously discontinue their medicine. There are drug interactions with warfarin, beta-blockers, and corticosteroids, and possible interactions with acetaminophen, chloramphenicol, chlorpromazine, cimetidine, cyclosporine, desipramine, furosemide, haloperidol, meperidine, methadone, methyldopa, phenacemide, prochlorperazine, propoxyphene, rifampicin, thioridazine, tricyclic antidepressants, verapamil, and other AEDs.

Primidone (Mysoline)

Primidone is a barbiturate used for treatment of CPSs and other partial epilepsies (usually as a drug of last resort). It has also been used in place of phenobarbital for treatment of GTCSs or focal seizures and epilepsies, when the latter drug has failed, but it should not be a drug of first choice for these conditions. Primidone is in part excreted unchanged and in part metabolized to phenobarbital and to phenylethylmalonic acid (PEMA). Serum levels of primidone and PEMA can be ascertained, but it often suffices just to confirm that a therapeutic steady-state level of phenobarbital is present. To benefit from the short-lived primidone and PEMA, each of which has some antiepileptic action, primidone must be given in three or four divided doses. A therapeutic dosage is usually about 250 mg orally three or four times a day, but the initial dosages should be much lower to avoid inducing extreme sedation. It is reasonable to start with 125 to 250 mg daily, with increments each week, until therapeutic effect, therapeutic levels, unacceptable sedation, or the maximal dosage of 2 g/day is reached. If patients are taking other AEDs, it is better to start with a dosage of 100 to 125 mg/day. The dosage should be reduced by about half in patients with significant renal failure. Strengths available are 50- and 250-mg tablets and suspension.

Side effects and drug interactions of primidone parallel those of phenobarbital, except that primidone tends to be more sedating.

Ethosuximide (Zarontin)

Ethosuximide is the drug of choice for treatment of absence epilepsy in children (CAE) when there are concerns for potential hepatotoxicity from valproic acid and absence seizures are the only seizure type. It is as effective as valproate in controlling absence seizures. It has little efficacy in other types of seizures, and patients with mixed seizure types may respond better to valproate. Peak plasma levels are reached 3 to 7 hours after oral ingestion in children and 2 to 4 hours after ingestion in adults. It is only minimally protein bound, with a volume of distribution of 70% of body weight; it has minimal interaction with other AEDs. The half-life is about 30 hours in children, rising to 60 hours in adults, and 6 to 12 days, respectively, is required to reach steady state. Elimination is primarily by metabolism, with urinary excretion of the metabolites. Absence seizures appear to be controlled by blood levels of about 25 to 165 mg/L, with an average of about 60 mg/L. Levels of 150 mg/L may be needed and tolerated. Dose-related side effects include anxiety, depression, behavioral and psychiatric disturbances, nausea, vomiting, anorexia, fatigue, headache, lethargy, and dizziness. Liver function tests and complete blood counts are recommended monthly for 6 months by the manufacturer and occasionally thereafter. Ethosuximide is supplied as syrup (250 mg/5 mL) and as capsules (250 mg).

Clonazepam (Klonopin)

Clonazepam is a benzodiazepine, closely related to diazepam, that is used principally for treatment of myoclonus. It is not approved for treatment of partial seizures but has been used effectively for these conditions in Europe. Clonazepam is an oral medicine, with a serum half-life of 20 to 40 hours. Serum levels vary from 0.05 to 0.7 mg/L and correlate only very roughly with clinical effect. Because of the sedative effect of the medicine, therapy is usually initiated very gradually, beginning with 0.01 to 0.15 mg/kg, and increased every third day to clinical effect or to maintenance at 0.1 to 0.2 mg/kg per day. In adults the daily maximal dosage is 20 mg. Clonazepam commonly produces drowsiness, ataxia, and behavioral changes and can also cause dizziness and decreased muscle tone. Strengths available are 0.5-, 1-, and 2-mg tablets.

AED Formulations for Rapid Administration

In the acute treatment of seizures, fosphenytoin and intravenous valproate (both mentioned previously) are used when rapid intravenous AED supplementation is indicated. A new rectal diazepam gel has been formulated in prefilled, unit-dose, rectal delivery systems containing 2.5, 5, 10, 15, or 20 mg of diazepam with specialized applicators for children and adults. This product overcomes many of the problems associated with rectal administration by non–health professional caregivers. Rapid plasma concentrations are reached within 15 minutes, and multicenter studies have shown the safety and efficacy of this formulation for reducing seizure frequency in children and adults with acute repetitive seizures, thus forestalling the otherwise necessary admission of the patient to an emergency department.

Newer Antiepileptic Drugs

After more than a decade without new AEDs on the market, several new agents have become available in the United States. Experience with these medications has been gained predominantly in European and American trials. These drugs are likely to be recommended when a patient requires consultation for difficult-to-control epilepsy, but they are gaining popularity for use earlier in the treatment of epilepsy because of their *lower side effect profiles.* They are usually more expensive.

Felbamate (Felbatol)

Felbamate (FDA approved in 1993) is a drug that has been tested as add-on therapy for drug-resistant CPSs with or without secondary generalization and in patients with Lennox–Gastaut syndrome in several European and American trials.

An oral dose has a half-life of about 20 hours as monotherapy, or 14 hours in patients receiving polypharmacy, and a volume of distribution of 0.8 L/kg.

Typical dosing regimens vary from 2,400 to 3,600 mg/day. Felbamate may increase phenytoin levels but decrease carbamazepine levels. Little effect has been noted on valproate levels.

Side effects include mild problems such as weight loss, nausea, blurred vision, diplopia, headache, and ataxia, as well as severe problems including aplastic anemia (more than 30 reported cases, with 10 deaths) and primary hepatotoxicity (liver failure reported in about 20 cases, with some deaths). At present the drug is largely restricted to use for patients who have epilepsy that cannot be controlled by other AEDs, and in whom the morbidity from epilepsy is believed to outweigh the morbidity risk from felbamate.

Gabapentin (Neurontin)

This GABA analog (FDA approved in 1994) was developed and used as an AED based on the GABAergic theory of epileptogenesis; however, it probably does not directly enhance GABA, although whole-brain GABA levels may be increased. Gabapentin is not protein bound, does not alter other AED levels, and is not metabolized. The half-life is 5 to 7 hours.

Clinical trials so far have been as an add-on AED in refractory partial epilepsies with or without secondary generalization. There are usually few if any side effects (Table 88.6), although limb edema has been reported.

Lamotrigine (Lamictal)

Lamotrigine is structurally unrelated to any other AED in current use. Its antiepileptic action is probably related to its inhibitory effect on glutamate release and stabilization of neuronal membrane voltage-sensitive sodium channels.

It appears to be effective in patients with intractable CPSs with or without secondary generalization; patients with primary GTCSs, atypical absences, or nonconvulsive status epilepticus; and some patients with Lennox–Gastaut syndrome (see earlier discussion). It has also recently been approved for monotherapy when a patient who is already on an enzyme-inducing AED such as phenytoin or carbamazepine or an enzyme-inhabiting drug such as valproate is then weaned off that medication and maintained on lamotrigine.

The pharmacokinetics in normal human subjects show complete bioavailability, a very long plasma half-life (24 ± 5 to 7 hours), linear kinetics, and approximately 60% protein binding when used as monotherapy.

Enzyme-inducing AEDs reduce its half-life; valproate increases it, sometimes two-fold; but lamotrigine does not appear to alter other AED levels. The drug is well tolerated and side effects are few. Skin rashes, sometimes severe but reversible, occur in about the same percentage of patients as for those starting phenytoin or carbamazepine, if drug escalation is gradual, following new labeling guidelines. The incidence of skin rashes falls the more gradually the drug is started. Diplopia, dizziness, nausea and vomiting, drowsiness, and headache also occur in a small percentage of users. It may be used by women taking an oral contraceptive without altering the contraceptive's function.

The drug may be started at 50 mg each night for 2 weeks, 50 mg twice daily for 2 weeks, then 100 mg twice daily, increasing in steps of 50 mg every 2 weeks until seizure control, clinical toxicity, or a maximum dosage of 600 to 700 mg/day is encountered. In patients who are also taking valproate, lamotrigine should be started at 25 mg every other day, increasing by 25 mg every 2 weeks so as to minimize the incidence of rash. Lamotrigine serum levels do not clearly correlate with clinical response ("therapeutic level") but may be used as markers of patient compliance.

Topiramate (Topamax)

Topiramate was approved in early 1997 for use as *adjunctive therapy* in adults with partial seizures. It probably has multiple mechanisms of action, including modulating sodium channels, enhancing the effect of GABA, and decreasing the excitability of brain cells. More than 1 million patients have taken it, with a greater than 50% reduction in seizures in 35% to 44% of patients taking 400 mg/day in clinical trials. Topiramate has a time to maximum concentration of about 2 hours, a bioavailability of approximately 88% unaffected by food, and little plasma protein binding (13% to 17%). It has linear pharmacokinetics, is not extensively metabolized, and is predominantly excreted by the kidneys. It has limited pharmacokinetic interactions, and its half-life makes it suitable for twice-daily dosing. Clinical studies show that it has no effect on carbamazepine but may increase phenytoin levels in some patients. The side-effect profile is similar to those of most other AEDs, and most side effects are not serious. They occur in the first weeks of therapy and usually resolve by the fourth month. Side effects are predominantly central nervous system related, including dizziness, drowsiness, and problems with coordination. There is a 1.5% incidence of kidney stones. Oral contraceptive effectiveness may be affected. The medication is available in 25-, 100-, and 200-mg tablets. Therapy should be initiated at a dosage of 25 mg/day and gradually increased over several weeks to a recommended dosage of 200 mg to 400 mg/day in two divided doses.

Tiagabine (Gabitril)

Tiagabine was approved in late 1997 for adjunctive therapy for partial-onset seizures in adults and children 12 years and older. Tiagabine was specifically designed to inhibit the uptake of GABA and prolong its action after synaptic release. Clinical trials have shown it to be effective as an *add-on drug* for patients with intractable focal seizures; 26% of patients have a 50% or greater reduction in focal seizures (49). A reduction of 50% or more of CPSs was seen in 20% to 30% of patients. Tiagabine should be started at 4 mg once daily and increased by 4 mg the first week and 8 mg weekly thereafter to 32 to 56 mg/day. It should be taken with food, in divided doses (two to four times per day), with the largest dose at bedtime. Tablets are available in 2-, 4-, 12-, and 16-mg strengths. Side effects include dizziness, confusion, tiredness, gastrointestinal upset, encephalopathy, and nonconvulsive status epilepticus.

Oxcarbazepine (Trileptal)

Oxcarbazepine is a 10-keto analog of carbamazepine and is active as a prodrug, having similar efficacy but purportedly lower side effects than carbamazepine. It is effective against partial seizures.

Oxcarbazepine is metabolized to the pharmacologically active 10-monohydroxy metabolite (MHD). Protein binding is relatively low. The drug does not autoinduce and does not produce an epoxide that normally accounts for most side effects seen with carbamazepine. It is a less potent cytochrome P-450 enzyme inducer, and when patients are switched from carbamazepine to oxcarbazepine, levels of phenytoin, lamotrigine, and topiramate may rise.

In trials at the highest dose of 2,400 mg/day, 50% of patients had a 50% reduction in seizures, compared with 13% in the placebo group. Lower does may be better tolerated as adjunctive therapy.

Oxcarbazepine has been approved for initial monotherapy in adults and children with partial seizures. The side-effect profile is the same as for carbamazepine, but side effects reportedly occur less frequently and neutropenia is not seen. However, hyponatremia occurs in 2.5% of treated patients. Hypersensitivity and rash reactions are less common than with carbamazepine.

Initial doses are 150 to 300 mg/day in monotherapy, increasing to clinical effect, usually at about 900 to 2,400 mg/day. As adjunctive therapy, initiation is recommended at 150 mg. twice daily, with weekly increments of 600 mg/day or less for better tolerability. Serum levels of MHD are available with a target range of 50 to 200 mmol/mL.

Levetiracetam (Keppra)

This drug has a unique preclinical profile with an efficacy in various animal models of seizures. Levetiracetam absorption is not affected by food. It has very low protein binding and is not hepatically metabolized. Two thirds of the drug is excreted renally, unchanged. There are no known drug interactions, and levetiracetam is neither an inducer nor an inhibitor of cytochrome P-450 enzymes. It has no effect on oral contraceptives, digoxin, warfarin, or other AEDs. No dosage adjustment is needed for hepatic impairment, but adjustments are needed for renal impairment with creatinine clearance less than 50 mL/min. Therefore, the dosage may need to be adjusted in elderly patients. Trials have shown a 50% reduction in 23% to 42% of patients with levetiracetam dosages of 1,000 to 3,000 mg/day, compared with 10% to 17% for placebo. At the higher dosage, 8% of patients became seizure free.

The drug is well-tolerated with few adverse events, including somnolence, dizziness, anorexia, which are usually mild to moderate. Of the 100,000 individuals exposed to date, no serious hepatic, renal, cardiovascular, or other serious adverse events have been found. Rash is rare.

Levetiracetam is started at 500 mg twice daily, or more gradually, and increased as tolerated to 1,000 mg or 1,500 mg orally twice daily. More recently, fatigue and irritability have been noted.

Zonisamide (Zonegram)

Preclinical studies have suggested a similar profile to phenytoin, but with some action at other channels. The drug is reduced via a cytochrome P-450 (CYP 3A4) and by N-acetylone, with about one third excreted unchanged in the urine. The half-life is about 60 hours, and therefore steady state is reached in about 2 weeks. Hepatic metabolism of zonisamide is increased by enzyme-inducing drugs, but protein binding is relatively moderate (40%). Zonisamide neither induces nor inhibits hepatic enzymes; does not affect levels of phenytoin, carbamazepine, or valproate; and does not autoinduce. However, phenytoin and carbamazepine decrease the half-life of zonisamide to about 27 and 38 hours, respectively. Therefore, after enzyme-inducing AEDs are withdrawn, zonisamide levels may increase. Because of its renal excretion, adjustments should be made in renally compromised and elderly patients. With dosages between 100 and 600 mg/day, seizure reductions in up to about one third of patients were seen after exclusion of a placebo response. Zonisamide may be particularly effective in progressive myoclonus epilepsies. Side effects include dizziness, somnolence, headache, anorexia, nausea, and irritability, particularly with more rapid uptitration.

Zonisamide is a sulfonamide and may exhibit similar hypersensitivity reactions, occasionally with Stevens–Johnson syndrome. Rash may occur early in treatment. Aplastic anemia and agranulocytosis have been reported. About 1% of patients have renal stones, possibly because of the drug's effect as a carbonic anhydrase inhibitor. Initial dosing is 100 mg/day, with uptitration by 100 mg/day every 2 weeks as tolerated. Treatment may be once or twice daily, and dosages as low as 100 mg/day have been reported to be effective. Optimal plasma zonisamide levels for seizure therapy are reported to be 10 to 40 mg/mL, but evidence is scant.

Other Antiepileptic Drugs

Practitioners often use diazepam, clorazepate, or chlordiazepoxide to treat seizures under certain circumstances. Benzodiazepines (other than clonazepam and clorazepate) have drawbacks for long-term therapy; AED effects tend to diminish as sedative effects accumulate.

Vagal Nerve Stimulation for Refractory Seizures

Vagal nerve stimulation (VNS) is a recent treatment for refractory seizures; it provides a programmed, regular stimulus via coiled electrodes from a chest-implanted generator to the left cervical vagal nerve. The pulse generator is powered by a lithium battery connected to a helical bipolar lead, which is, in turn, attached to the midcervical portion of the left vagal nerve, delivering a biphasic current continuously cycling between on and off periods. Animal data suggest that VNS stimulates small unmyelinated C fibers, with the locus ceruleus playing a crucial role in the mechanism of VNS, because chemical lesioning reduces the anticonvulsant effect of stimulation. VNS inhibits seizures in multiple animal models, including maximum electroshock, pencillin, and pentylenetetrazol models. It also measurably alters cerebral blood flow in the thalamus, cerebellum, and cortex and activates inhibitory structures in the brain.

Several clinical studies using active-control, parallel-blinded formats revealed a substantial reduction in seizure frequency. Long-term studies have shown a sustained reduction of 50% or more in 37% of patients, with a 43% responder rate at 2 and 3 years. Common side effects include voice change and hoarseness. Reductions compared to baseline were about 35% at 1 year, increasing to 44% at 2 and 3 years. Other side effects included parasthesias, headache, and shortness of breath.

Careful patient selection and evaluation by epilepsy centers are optimal techniques for the choice of VNS for refractory epilepsy.

REFERRAL TO A NEUROLOGIST

The role of a consulting neurologist to help with the evaluation and management of epilepsy depends on the experience of the primary physician. Common problems for which referral may be helpful are listed in Table 88.7.

HOSPITALIZATION

Few general statements can be made about the need for hospital admission for seizure patients, because the availability of monitoring systems, emergency room holding rooms, and inpatient beds varies from locale to locale. A set of reasonable guidelines is shown in Table 88.7. Patients brought to offices or emergency rooms after a first seizure are usually admitted to facilitate the diagnostic workup and to observe the patient in case a serious underlying cause (e.g., meningitis, subdural hematoma) is present. This principle has exceptions. A young patient with a normal examination and a reliable family may be evaluated in an ambulatory setting. Any patient with new focal

Table 88.7. When to Refer or Hospitalize the Patient with Seizures

Diagnostic Issues for Referral
Question about whether a seizure took place
Abnormal physical examination
Questionable focal neurologic findings
Focal seizures
Focality on the EEG
Need for special diagnostic investigations (e.g., lumbar puncture, CT or MRI scan)
Uncertainty about cause

Therapeutic Issues for Referral
Complex medication adjustments
Patient does not respond to a drug of choice
Patient has significant medication side effects
Patient wishes to become pregnant
Patient wishes to taper off medication
Significant change in the pattern of seizures

When to Hospitalize
Most new-onset seizures
New focal signs on examination
Obtunded or prolonged postictal patients
Febrile patients
Crescendo pattern of seizures
All cases of status epilepticus
Barbiturate and benzodiazepine withdrawal seizures
Possibility of rapidly expanding mass lesion
Seizures after recent head trauma
Need for special inpatient studies
Consideration for neurosurgery
Monitoring of compliance

CT, computed tomography; EEG, electroencephalogram; MRI, magnetic resonanse imaging.

signs on examination should be admitted, as should obtunded patients, febrile patients, and those whose postictal lethargy persists for longer than 30 minutes. A patient with a crescendo pattern of seizures, with several in one day, especially if they are tonic–clonic seizures, should be admitted to a hospital immediately. *Status epilepticus,* a condition in which continuous or back-to-back seizures occur without intervening return of consciousness, is a medical emergency and requires immediate hospitalization. Barbiturate withdrawal seizures may become fulminant; therefore, patients having seizures in this setting should be admitted. If the possibility exists of a rapidly expanding mass lesion, such as tumor, abscess, or possible hematoma after head trauma, then admission should not be delayed. Reasons for elective admission include a need for special inpatient studies (arteriography, continuous monitoring), evaluation for possible neurosurgical procedures for intractable epilepsy, and, lastly, trials of supervised drug management to check for noncompliance as a factor in treatment failure.

Admission usually is not needed for patients who are known to have chronically recurrent seizures, whose pattern of seizures is stable, whose cause is established or is thought to be idiopathic on the basis of a prior thorough workup, who have fully recovered from recent seizures, who have normal examinations (or static documented old deficits), and who are reliable enough to return for follow-up.

SOCIAL ISSUES AND PATIENT EDUCATION

Once a serious underlying cause has been ruled out, there is a tendency for physicians to view epilepsy as a benign disease. From the viewpoint of the patient, this is often far from the case. Seizures are distressing for every patient and for the patient's family. Fear of having a seizure can cause people with epilepsy to withdraw from society, and those who are willing to compete may be faced with nearly insurmountable discrimination.

The Commission for the Control of Epilepsy and Its Consequences (1977) found that the unemployment rate among people with epilepsy is twice the national average, and the underemployment rate is even higher. Suspension of a driver's license (discussed later) may make it almost impossible to get to work. Children may be denied participation in sports or moved unnecessarily to special sections in school. Persons with epilepsy marry less often than matched subjects without epilepsy. A significant fraction of the public believe that people with epilepsy are likely to be physically unattractive. Because of these and other social stigmata associated with epilepsy, it is important to focus on the patient's overall functioning rather than simply on seizure control. The patient and family should be counseled regularly to help them address the concerns that limit full participation in society.

Patients should be told that epilepsy is a medical illness, because too many believe that it is a punishment for some past abuse. Whereas a single seizure should not be labeled as epilepsy, definite epilepsy should not be mislabeled as something else in an attempt to avoid facing the diagnosis. The patient should know that individual seizures usually do not cause measurable brain damage and that the condition does not lead to mental deterioration. Unfortunately, sudden unexpected death in epilepsy (SUDEP) does occur. Numerous historical figures, including Julius Caesar, Holy Roman Emperor Charles V, Fyodor Dostoyevsky, Gustave Flaubert, Napoleon Bonaparte, Jonathan Swift, George Frederick Handel, and President William McKinley achieved high stations while suffering from frequent seizures. The prognosis for most patients with epilepsy is good.

Restrictions of Activity

Patients often ask for guidelines about what they can and cannot do. Clearly, if identifiable precipitants such as sleep deprivation, flashing lights, alcohol, or particular medicines can be avoided, the patient should be so advised. Maximal activity consistent with avoidance of risk of personal injury should be the goal. The specifics must be formulated by a physician familiar with the individual patient and the patient's pattern of seizures. Patients with nocturnal seizures need not be restricted during the day. Contact sports are safe for people with infrequent seizures. Common sense dictates limits on activities during which a seizure could be fatal—for example, piloting an airplane, rock climbing, or scuba diving. Some potentially hazardous activities, such as swimming, may be acceptable if provisions can be made for proper supervision. Seizures are not contraindications to strenuous activities, including sex. Alcohol consumption (in moderation) can be enjoyed by most patients with impunity (5,19,50).

Driving a Motor Vehicle

Overall, motor vehicle accident rates for people with epilepsy are about twice the rates in control subjects. The actual proportion of all traffic accidents caused by people with epilepsy has been estimated at 1/10,000 accidents (5,19,51). It is estimated that 6/10,000 of all deaths at the wheel are from natural causes, including epilepsy, and that 5,000/10,000 are caused by alcohol use. Approximately 12% to 20% of accidents involving people with epilepsy occur with the patient's first seizure. As indicated by these statistics, seizures at the wheel do occur and can represent both personal and public dangers. The key element of increased risk is blunting or loss of consciousness. Seizures without this element (e.g., partial simple motor seizures) do not affect the risk of driving, and affected patients are usually exempted from restrictions, although in some, determining momentary loss of consciousness is problematic.

Some states require that physicians directly report occurrence of seizures to the Department of Motor

Vehicles; others require only documentation in the medical record that the patient has been informed of the risks for traffic accidents and has been instructed to contact the Motor Vehicle Department for a hearing (see requirements for each state at the website of the Epilepsy Foundation, in General References). Patients and physicians should be honest in their communications; both are potentially liable for consequences of inaccurate or incomplete information. In general, the physician should address the medical facts of a case and leave the final determination of licensing to the state authorities. Often, if an applicant has regular lapses of consciousness, the license will be suspended until a period of 3 months to 2 years without seizures has elapsed (depending on the state); the recent national trend has been to consider shorter periods of suspension.

Employment

It is illegal to discriminate against handicapped people, including people with epilepsy, in the job market. If a person with seizures is unemployed or dissatisfied with work, one should consider prompt referral to a vocational rehabilitation agency for possible retraining, patient and employer education, or advice on legal action. *The Epilepsy Foundation* (4351 Garden City Drive #406, Landover, MD 20785, telephone 301-459-3700; www.efa.org) is a central nonprofit organization that can serve as a source for information and action on social and occupational aspects of epilepsy; at least one chapter exists in each state. Their training and placement service has been effective in training people with epilepsy for work and in finding them employment, either in the general work pool or in sheltered workshops. The same local organizations may further aid patients with regular group counseling for those who cannot live independently, or by providing for regular home visits by visiting nurses and other medical personnel.

Some patients with difficult-to-control seizures should be advised to apply for *Social Security medical disability compensation* (see criteria in Chapter 9).

Pregnancy

Special problems are raised by a woman with epilepsy who is, or wishes to become, pregnant (52). Approximately 0.4% of all pregnancies occur in mothers with seizures. In women with epilepsy, child-bearing carries an above-average risk for eclampsia, vaginal hemorrhage, and complicated labor. The rates of premature birth and perinatal death are increased. Seizures become more difficult to control during pregnancy in approximately 30% to 50% of cases, easier to control in approximately 10% to 30%, and unchanged in the rest. Rarely, pregnancy can induce a new onset of recurring idiopathic seizures. AEDs—phenytoin, carbamazepine, valproic acid, and, to a lesser extent, most of the other agents—are believed to be *teratogenic.* The teratogenic effects of the newer AEDs are unknown. Studies suggest that the incidence of congenital abnormalities, particularly cleft lip, cleft palate, and cardiac defects, is two to six times higher in offspring of drug-treated mothers with epilepsy. Valproate and carbamazepine have specifically been associated with a 1% to 2% risk of neural tube closure defects for valproate and 0.5% to 1% for carbamazepine.

Authorities agree that tonic–clonic seizures can produce anoxic, ischemic, or traumatic damage to a fetus and that this risk must be balanced against the teratogenic potential of medication. The best solution to this dilemma is *careful planning.* Physicians should ask their patients not only to plan pregnancies but also to alert the physician to the plan months in advance. Before pregnancy, special efforts can be made to taper medications or to switch to phenobarbital or carbamazepine, which may be less teratogenic than phenytoin or valproate. However, most authorities agree that the AED to be used in pregnancy should be the one best suited for the patient and her epilepsy. Switching drugs after conception (i.e., when the patient discovers that she is pregnant) usually is not recommended, partly because the greatest vulnerability of the developing fetus is early in the pregnancy. Brief CPSs or absence seizures pose no known risk to a fetus, and a decision may be made by the patient to tolerate them during pregnancy rather than take medication. If pregnancy is unexpected, an ongoing successful regimen of AEDs should probably be continued, to avoid the possibility of fulminant withdrawal seizures during a critical obstetric stage. Ultimately, all of these relative risks must be discussed among primary and specialist physicians, the patient, and her partner, so that a mutually satisfactory plan can be derived. The problems of child-bearing are increased for mothers with epilepsy, but not greatly, and only the severely disabled epileptic woman should be flatly discouraged from having children.

Mothers taking AEDs who wish to breast-feed may do so, because the amount of AEDs excreted in breast milk is low, and the developing baby was exposed to even higher doses while *in utero.*

Potential parents wonder about the *likelihood that their child will have epilepsy* if they or one of their children have epilepsy. Although there are methodologic problems in performing studies to answer this question, it can generally be said that there is a risk of about 1 in 40 of transmitting IGE from the mother. When seizures result from head trauma, tumor, drug withdrawal, or other identified causes, then the risk of heritability is not increased.

Family Education

Families must be told how to *behave during a seizure*; too often, frantic efforts to treat the seizure result in extreme anxiety and broken teeth. Seizures should be allowed to run their course; unless convulsions become continuous or nearly continuous (status epilepticus) they are not dangerous, and no first aid can shorten them. The mouth should not be forced open so that matchbooks, pencils, or other objects can be pushed in. The family should be informed that it is impossible to swallow the tongue. The person undergoing a seizure should be moved away from sharp corners and heights and turned on his or her side to decrease the risk of aspiration. Forcible restraint during a tonic–clonic phase is of no value, and during the automatisms of CPSs restraints may increase agitation. There is little need to fear behavior during automatisms, because directed violence is extremely rare.

Concerned family members may be very helpful in *promoting improved seizure control*. They should be encouraged to discuss compliance, the cost of a pharmaceutical regimen, and how the seizures or drug toxicities affect school, work, and social relations. Patients should be encouraged to keep a log of their seizures, medication times, side effects, and possible precipitating stresses. Perfect control of epilepsy with no toxicity is an ideal attained in only a minority of cases; in the remainder, patient, family, and physician can decide in concert how to balance the inconvenience of seizures against the unpleasant side effects of medication and thereby achieve the best possible results.

Medicolegal Issues

In addition to conducting discussions of the diagnosis, management, and prognosis of epilepsy, it is important to document in the patient's record the principal points that have been addressed with the patient and the family. One should offer patients written information advising them of driving laws and warning them to avoid dangerous activities and occupations. They should also have full written records of medications and their side effects, in lay terms, and instructions to contact the physician for any worrisome side effects. In addition, all women of child-bearing age should be counseled regarding fetal teratogenicity, possible change in maternal seizure frequency, and the need or lack of need for AED therapy (see previous discussion). Many of these essential facts are covered well in patient education literature available from the Epilepsy Foundation (see previous discussion).

Attention to these aspects of patient and family education and a close, compassionate, and open doctor–patient relationship are sound ways to limit malpractice exposure.

General References*

Epilepsy Foundation website. Available at: http://www.efa.org. Accessed February 4, 2002.

Excellent resource of societal issues related to epilepsy.

Browne TR, Holmes GL. Epilepsy. N Engl J Med 2001;344:1145.

Well-referenced and practical review article.

Dam M, Gram M, ed. Comprehensive epileptology. New York: Raven Press, 1990.

A comprehensive review of epilepsy.

Greenberg MK, Barsan WG, Starkman S. Neuroimaging in the emergency patient presenting with seizure. Neurology 1996;47:26.

The use of imaging in patients with new-onset seizures.

Kaplan PW, Loiseau P, Fisher RS, et al. Epilepsy A to Z: a glossary of epilepsy terminology. New York: Demos Vermande, 1995.

One- to two-page condensed information, with references, on most practical aspects of epilepsy.

Kaplan PW, Schachter SC. The role of neurologist in the management of epilepsy: guidelines and tools for patient care. Neurologist 1996;2:302.

Comprehensive approach to longitudinal care of epileptic patients with special attention to patient education.

Levy RH, Dreifuss FE, Mattson RH, et al., eds. Antiepileptic drugs. 4th ed. New York: Raven Press, 1995.

A compendium of antiseizure medications.

Temkin O. The falling sickness: a history of epilepsy from the ancient Greeks to the beginnings of modern neurology. Baltimore: Johns Hopkins University Press, 1971.

The definitive history of epilepsy from ancient to modern times.

Wyllie E, ed. The treatment of epilepsy: principles and practice. Baltimore: Williams & Wilkins, 1997.

An excellent textbook of epilepsy.

Specific References

1. Annegers JF. Epidemiology of epilepsy. In: Wyllie E, ed. The treatment of epilepsy: principles and practice. 2nd ed. Baltimore: Williams & Wilkins, 1997:165.
2. **Commission on classification and terminology of the International League Against Epilepsy. Proposal for revised classification of epilepsies and epileptic syndromes. Epilepsia 1989;30:389.**
3. Berkovic SF. Generalized absence seizures. In Wyllie E, ed. The treatment of epilepsy: principles and practice. 2nd ed. Baltimore: Williams & Wilkins, 1997:451.
4. Benbadis SR, Luders HO. Epileptic syndromes: an underutilized concept. Epilepsia 1996;37:1029.
5. Sander JWAS, Shorvon SD. Epidemiology of the epilepsies. J Neurol Neurosurg Psychiatry 1996;61:433.
6. Treiman DM. Seizure types and causes of epilepsy. Semin Neurol 1981;1:65.
7. Anderson DW, McLaurin RL. The national head and spinal cord injury survey. J Neurosurg 1980;53[Suppl S]:S1.
8. Annegers JF, Shirts SB, Hauser WA, et al. Risk of recurrence after an initial unprovoked seizure. Epilepsia 1986;27:43.
9. Hauser WA, Rich SS, Annegers YF, et al. Seizure recurrence after a first unprovoked seizure: an extended follow-up. Neurology 1990;40:1163.
10. Hopkins A, Garman A, Clarke C. The first seizure in adult life: value of clinical features, electroencephalography, and computerized tomographic scanning in prediction of seizure recurrence. Lancet 1988;1:721.
11. Annegers JF, Hauser WA, Elveback LR. Remission of seizures and relapse in patients with epilepsy. Epilepsia 1979;20:729.
12. Shorvon SD. The temporal aspects and prognosis in epilepsy. J Neurol Neurosurg Psychiatry 1984;47:1157.
13. Delgado-Escueta AV, Treiman DM, Wahs GO. The treatable epilepsies (second of two parts). N Engl J Med 1983;308:1508.
14. Goodridge DMG, Shorvon SD. Epileptic seizures in a population of 6,000: 1. Demography, diagnosis, and classification, and role of the hospital services. BMJ 1983;287:641.
15. **MRC Antiepileptic Drug Withdrawal Study Group. Randomised study of antiepileptic drug withdrawal in patients in remission. Lancet 1991;337:1175.**
16. Mattson RH, Cramer JA, Collins JF, et al. Prognosis for total control of complex partial and secondarily generalized tonic clonic seizures. Neurology 1996;47:68.
17. Reynolds EH, Elwes RCD, Shorvon SD. Why does epilepsy become intractable: prevention of chronic epilepsy. Lancet 1983;2:952.
18. Schmidt D. Prognosis of chronic epilepsy with complex partial seizures. J Neurol Neurosurg Psychiatry 1984;47:1274.

*Bold print (general references) and bold numerals (specific references) denote published controlled clinical trials, meta-analyses, or consensus-based recommendations.

19. Tinuper P, Avoni P, Riva R, et al. The prognostic value of the electroencephalogram in antiepileptic drug withdrawal in partial epilepsies. Neurology 1996;47:76.
20. Schold C, Yarnell PR, Earnest MP. Origin of seizures in elderly patients. JAMA 1977;238:1177.
21. Hauser WA, Ng SKC, Brust JCM. Alcohol, seizures and epilepsy. Epilepsia 1988;29[Suppl 2]:S66.
22. Sampliner R, Iber FL. Diphenylhydantoin control of alcohol withdrawal seizures: results of a controlled study. JAMA 1974;230:1430.
23. Victor M, Brausch V. The role of abstinence in the genesis of alcoholic epilepsy. Epilepsia 1967;8:1.
24. Alldredge BK, Lowenstein DH, Simon RP. Placebo-controlled trial of intravenous diphenylhydantoin for short-term treatment of alcohol withdrawal seizures. Am J Med 1989;87:645.
25. Ng SK, Hauser WA, Brust JC, et al. Alcohol consumption and withdrawal in new-onset seizures. N Engl J Med 1988;319:666.
26. Morris HH, Estes ML, Gilmore R, et al. Chronic intractable epilepsy as the only symptom of primary brain tumor. Epilepsia 1993;34:1038.
27. Aicardi J. (ed.). Epilepsies as a presenting manifestation of brain tumors. In: Epilepsy in children. New York: Raven Press, 1986.
28. Luhdorf K, Jensen LK, Plesner AM. Epilepsy in the elderly: etiology of seizures in elderly. Epilepsia 1986;27:458.
29. Sung CY, Chu NS. Epileptic seizures in thrombotic stroke. J Neurol 1990;237:166.
30. Gupta SR, Naheedy MH, Elias D, et al. Postinfarction seizures: a clinical study. Stroke 1988;19:1477.
31. McArthur JC. Neurologic manifestations of AIDS. Medicine (Baltimore) 1987;66:407.
32. Engel JE Jr. Seizures and epilepsy. Philadelphia: FA Davis, 1989.
33. Oribe E, Rohullah A, Nissenbaum E, et al. Serum prolactin concentrations are elevated after syncope. Neurology 1996;47:60.
34. Wyllie E, Luders H, MacMillan JP, et al. Serum prolactin levels after epileptic seizures. Neurology 1984;34:1601.
35. Meierkord H, Shorvon S, Lightman S, et al. Comparison of the effects of frontal and temporal lobe partial seizures on prolactin levels. Arch Neurol 1992;49:225.
36. van Donselaar CA, Schimsheimer R-J, Geerts AT, et al. Value of the electroencephalogram in adult patients with untreated idiopathic first seizures. Arch Neurol 1992;49:231.
37. Browne TR, Holmes GL. Epilepsy. N Engl J Med 2001;344:1145.
38. Gastant H, Tassinari CA. Epilepsies. In: Remand A, ed. Handbook of EEG and clinical neurophysiology, vol.13, part A. Amsterdam: Elsevier, 1975.
39. Garcia-Herrero D, Fernádez-Torre, Barrasa J, et al. Abdominal epilepsy in an adolescent with bilateral perisylvian polymicrogyria. Epsilepsia 1998;39:1370.
40. Bleck TP. Recurrence of tonic–clonic seizures after antiepileptic drugs. Neurology 1993;43:478.
41. Mattson RH, Cramer JA, Collins JF, et al. Comparison of carbamazepine, phenobarbital, phenytoin, and primidone in partial and secondarily generalized tonic–clonic seizures. N Engl J Med 1985;313:145.
42. Mattson RH, Cramer JA, Collins JF. Department of Veterans Affairs Epilepsy Study No. 264 Group. A comparison of valproate with carbamazepine for the treatment of complex partial seizures and secondarily generalized tonic-clonic seizures in adults. N Engl J Med 1992;327:765.
43. Marson AG, Kadir ZA, Chadwick DW. New antiepileptic drugs: a systematic review of their efficacy and tolerability. BMJ 1996;313:1169.
44. Shorvon SD, Chadwick D, Galbraith AW, et al. One drug for epilepsy. BMJ 1978;1:474.
45. Browne TR, Le Duc B. Phenytoin: chemistry and bioinformation. In: Levy RH, Mattson RH, Meldrum BS, eds. Antiepileptic drugs. 4th ed. New York: Raven Press, 1995:235.
46. Buna DK. Antiepileptic drug withdrawal—a good idea! Pharmacotherapy 1998;18:235.
47. Practice parameter: a guideline for discontinuing antiepileptic drugs in seizure-free patients. Summary statement report of the Quality Standards Subcommittee of the American Academy of Neurology. Neurology 1996;47:600.
48. Dreifuss FE, Santilli N, Langer DJ, et al. Valproic acid hepatic fatalities: a retrospective review. Neurology 1987;37:379.
49. Richens A. Chadwick DW, Duncan JS, et al. Adjunctive treatment of partial seizures with Tiagabine: a placebo-controlled trial. Epilepsy Res 1995;21:37.
50. Mattson RH, Sturman JK, Gronowski ML, et al. Effects of alcohol intake in non-alcoholic epileptics. Neurology 1975;25:361.
51. van der Lugt PJ. Traffic accidents caused by epilepsy. Epilepsia 1975;16:747.
52. Morrell, MI. Seizures and epilepsy in women. In: Neurologic disease in women, part III, chap.14. New York: Raven, 1998: 189–206.

CHAPTER 89

Dizziness, Vertigo, Motion Sickness, Syncope and Near Syncope, and Disequilibrium

STEPHEN D. SISSON, MD
MARK F. WALKER, MD

DIZZINESS

Dizziness is the ninth most common chief complaint in ambulatory settings (1). However, the word *dizzy* is a very inexact term. It can refer to impending loss of consciousness or spatial disorientation. On the other hand, some patients use "dizziness" to refer to less specific subjective states such as fatigue, dysphoric mood, or disequilibrium or other subjective states. Occasionally, patients use the word *dizzy* to mean sick. A correct diagnosis for a patient's complaint of dizziness is often possible on the basis of the history and physical examination. A limited number of diagnostic studies can aid the evaluation of selected patients, but these can be interpreted properly only in the light of information gained from the patient.

Categorizing a Patient's Dizziness

Evaluation of the dizzy patient starts with categorizing the patient's symptoms. Categorization of symptoms can indicate what system is involved and give focus to the differential diagnosis. The major categories of dizziness are *vertigo,* the illusion that the patient or the environment is moving or rotating; *near syncope or syncope,* a sensation of impending faint or actual loss of consciousness; and *disequilibrium,* a sensation of impaired balance or ataxia (2). When a patient has ill-defined dizziness that cannot be readily classified, the patient should be asked to *use words more specific than dizziness* and should be asked to *describe a discrete recent episode.* Typical words they may use and potential categories are listed in Table 89.1. If the patient's initial account is too vague, the following questions may help:

- Is there actually the sensation of movement or rotation of you or the environment? (Positive response favors vertigo.)
- Is it a sensation that you might black out? (Positive response favors near syncope.)
- Is it a sensation of unsteadiness on your feet? A sensation that you are not sure where your hand or body is and that you cannot quite keep your balance? (Positive response favors disequilibrium.)

Questions about associated auditory, neurologic, or cardiac symptoms may help classify the patient's problem more specifically.

Table 89.1. Categorization of Terms Used by Patients to Describe Dizziness

Vertigo	Syncope or Presyncope	Disequilibrium
Spinning of self	Fainting	Imbalance
Spinning of environment	Light-headedness	Tilting
Swaying	Woozy	Poor equilibrium
Twisting	Blackout	Impeding fall
Moving	Pass out	Unsteady
Weaving	Spells	Staggering
Rocking	Fall-out	Drunk
Rolling		Listing
Tilting Spells		Spells

The patient who claims to be dizzy "right now" while sitting before the physician should be checked for hypotension, first while seated and then while standing, observed for hyperventilation (slow hyperpneic breathing, not overt tachypnea), and examined for nystagmus (see below). A patient who produces dizziness by turning his or her head should be asked to elaborate on the symptoms; vertigo (positional) and near syncope (caused by compromise of cerebral blood flow) are the two problems most likely to be described.

In some cases, *asking whether the patient can reproduce the symptoms* may be more efficient than exhaustive questioning. If the patient reports typical dizziness on rising from a chair, orthostatic hypotension (or possibly benign paroxysmal positional vertigo [BPPV]) is likely; hypotension can be confirmed by measuring supine and standing blood pressure. If the patient demonstrates gait ataxia (see Chapter 86) or reports dizziness on turning while walking (as opposed to turning their head while sitting), the problem may be disequilibrium rather than vertigo.

As part of the preliminary inquiry, it is important to ask the patient whether dizziness has interfered with usual activities, especially driving a motor vehicle. This information will be important in management regardless of the cause of dizziness.

DISORDERS OF THE VESTIBULAR SYSTEM

The purpose of the vestibular system is to sense movement of the head and, through the vestibulo-ocular reflex (VOR) and vestibulospinal reflex, to maintain stable gaze and posture during movement. Thus, the symptoms of vestibular dysfunction include an inappropriate sense of motion (vertigo), imbalance, and gaze instability (oscillopsia) when the head is moving.

Basic Principles of Vestibular Function

To understand disorders of the vestibular system and their symptoms and signs, it is helpful to keep in mind basic vestibular anatomy and function. The peripheral organs of the vestibular system are the labyrinths. The cochlea is the portion of the labyrinth responsible for hearing (see Chapter 110). The vestibular labyrinth consists of three semicircular canals (horizontal or lateral, anterior or superior, and posterior) and two gravity-sensitive structures (utricle and saccule) (see Fig. 110.1). The semicircular canals sense angular rotations of the head, and the otoliths sense linear motion (translation) and the orientation of the head relative to gravity. Attached to the utricle and saccule are calcium carbonate crystals termed otoconia; these are important in the pathophysiology of BPPV.

When the head is not moving, each vestibular nerve has an equal resting discharge rate, with no net difference in the inputs from the two sides. Rotation of the head excites one labyrinth and inhibits the other, disturbing this balance. This signals the brain that the head is moving and generates the appropriate compensatory eye movement to maintain steady gaze (*vestibulo-ocular reflex*). For example, when the head rotates to the right, there is a net increase in firing from the right horizontal canal. This causes the eyes to rotate to the left in the orbits, so that they remained fixed in space. This compensatory eye movement is called the VOR slow phase. If the head continues to rotate, these slow phases will be interrupted by rapid saccade-like movements in the opposite direction, termed quick phases. The combination of slow and quick phases is called *nystagmus. The direction of nystagmus is usually given by the direction of its quick phases,* even though it is the slow phases that reflect vestibular activity. Thus, prolonged rotation of the head to the right generates a right-beating nystagmus. This physiologic nystagmus maintains clear vision during head rotations.

Pathologic vestibular nystagmus results when one labyrinth or vestibular nerve is lesioned, removing the spontaneous discharge from that side and leaving the tonic input from the other side unopposed. The resulting imbalance creates a nystagmus, in which *slow phases are directed toward the side of the lesion and quick phases toward the intact side.* Thus, an acute left vestibular lesion causes a right-beating nystagmus. With time, the brain readjusts central vestibular tone to compensate for the peripheral imbalance, sometimes leaving only minimal residual symptoms and signs.

VERTIGO

Vertigo is a sense of illusory movement, either of oneself or of the surrounding environment. Patients may report feelings of spinning, tilting, or tumbling. Vertigo generally indicates an imbalance in the vestibular system. This may result either from a peripheral lesion, involving one of the labyrinths or vestibular nerves (e.g., vestibular neuritis), or from a central lesion (e.g., infarction) within the vestibular pathways of the brainstem and cerebellum. It is important to keep in mind that bilateral labyrinthine lesions, such as from aminoglycoside ototoxicity, often do not cause vertigo because the lesion is symmetric, thus creating no net imbalance. Vestibular schwannomas (acoustic neuromas) and other slowly growing tumors affecting the vestibular nerve also do not commonly produce vertigo, because the resulting vestibular imbalance is compensated centrally as it develops. The most severe vertigo occurs with an acute unilateral loss of peripheral input.

Evaluation of the Undiagnosed Patient

History

In taking a history from a patient with vertigo, there are several questions that are particularly helpful:

- *Is the vertigo episodic or has it occurred only once?*
- *How long does each episode last?* Episodes of BPPV last less than 1 minute, whereas transient ischemic attacks (TIAs) commonly last at least several minutes. Vertigo from migraine, Ménière disease, vestibular neuritis, or infarcts often lasts longer (hours to days).
- *Is there anything that consistently provokes vertigo?* BPPV is provoked by head movement. Other possible provoking factors include loud noise and Valsalva maneuvers (coughing, sneezing, and straining during defecation).
- *Are there any accompanying symptoms?* Auditory symptoms (such as hearing loss or ear pain, pressure, or fullness) suggest a peripheral lesion, whereas symptoms such as double vision, slurred speech, facial numbness, weakness, or limb incoordination should raise the suspicion of a brainstem or cerebellar lesion.

Physical Examination

When examining patients with vertigo, the goals are to look for signs of vestibular hypofunction and to distinguish peripheral from central lesions. It is always important to perform a basic neurologic examination, with particular attention to the cranial nerves, cerebellar function, and walking and balance (see Chapter 86) and to do a basic office assessment of hearing (see Chapter 110). Specific tests of the vestibular system involve looking for static imbalance and impairment of the VOR and testing for positional nystagmus.

As explained above, the hallmark of a static vestibular imbalance is a *spontaneous nystagmus.* However, it is important to remember that *a peripheral vestibular nystagmus is suppressed by vision.* Thus, except in the most acute stage of a peripheral lesion, nystagmus is not commonly seen during bedside examination. Techniques must be used to remove the subject's visual fixation while still allowing the examiner to view the eyes. In the vestibular clinic, this is done using specialized goggles with high magnification lenses (Frenzel lenses). An alternative method is to observe the optic disk carefully during direct ophthalmoscopy, while occluding the opposite eye with the hand. A nystagmus can be seen as alternating slow and quick movements of the optic disk. When doing this, it is important to remember that the apparent direction of nystagmus is reversed. This is because the optic disk is at the posterior pole of the eye. Thus, a right-beating movement of the optic disk is really a left-beating nystagmus. *A spontaneous nystagmus that is easily seen in the light is more often a sign of central disease.* Other features indicating a central lesion are a purely vertical (e.g., downbeat) nystagmus and a direction-changing (gaze-evoked) nystagmus.

Often more helpful in identifying a vestibular deficit are tests of dynamic vestibular function, that is, of the VOR. The most important of these is the *head thrust test.* The patient is asked to fixate a target (usually the examiner's nose) during rapid, low-amplitude, horizontal rotations of the head. If the VOR is working normally, gaze will remain stable and the patient will still be looking at the examiner at the end of the rotation. If the function of one or both labyrinths is impaired, rotation toward the affected ear(s) will fail to produce a normal excitatory stimulus, leading to a deficient VOR. The eyes will move with the head, and after the rotation, there will be a corrective rapid eye movement (saccade) to bring the eyes back to the point of original fixation. For example, in the case of a right vestibular lesion, when the head is turned to the left, the response will be normal and the eyes will remain stable in space. However, when the head is turned to the right, the eyes will move to the right with the head and a leftward corrective saccade will be seen. The head thrust test is the best bedside test to identify a peripheral vestibular lesion.

Another useful test of the VOR is *dynamic visual acuity* (3). This is based on the fact that a normal compensatory VOR is required to maintain clear vision when the head is moving. Thus, patients with an impaired VOR (particularly if bilateral) will have reduced visual acuity during head movement. To test dynamic acuity, first determine the patient's baseline visual acuity, using an eye chart or near vision card with appropriate correction (including reading glasses, if the near card is used). This is compared with the best acuity when the head is rotated back and forth (by the examiner) at a frequency of about once per second. A loss of more than one line of acuity is abnormal. Patients with bilateral vestibular loss will often have dramatic loss of acuity during head rotation.

Patients with recurrent episodes of vertigo should undergo *Dix-Hallpike positional testing* to look for evidence of BPPV. This is discussed below in the section on BPPV.

Formal Vestibular Testing

Several ancillary tests are helpful in the evaluation of patients who are referred for problematic vestibular disorders. Formal *audiometry* is used to identify evidence of hearing loss, particularly asymmetric (see Chapter 110). *Electronystagmography* consists of a battery of tests of eye movements and vestibular function. Eye movements are measured using either electro-oculography or video-oculography. Electro-oculography uses surface electrodes to detect the corneoretinal potential; as the eyes move, the position of these potential changes, altering the signal in the electrodes. With video-oculography, eye position is recorded by cameras attached to a mask or helmet worn by the patient. The electronystagmography typically includes a recording in the dark to look for spontaneous nystagmus, recordings of saccades and smooth pursuit, recordings of positional nystagmus, Dix-Hallpike testing, and caloric testing. Caloric testing measures the nystagmus generated when one of the external ear canals is irrigated with warm or cold water (or air). Warm water provides an excitatory stimulus to the horizontal canal of the irrigated ear, and cold water provides an inhibitory stimulus. A comparison of responses to irrigation of each ear is used to determine if there is a relative reduction of vestibular function on one side.

Rotatory chair testing uses the natural vestibular stimulus (head rotation) to test the functions of the labyrinths and VOR pathways. The patient is seated in a chair that is rotated in the dark, either at constant velocity or sinusoidally. Unlike caloric testing, rotational testing does not stimulate each labyrinth independently: Rotation in each direction affects both sides, exciting one and inhibiting the other simultaneously. Thus, it is more difficult to identify and localize a unilateral lesion using rotational testing. However, rotational testing is of particular benefit in identifying bilateral vestibular loss.

DISORDERS CAUSING VERTIGO

Common causes of vertigo are listed in Table 89.2 and discussed in this section. Causes are categorized according to the temporal pattern that emerges when the patient gives the history: acute onset, prolonged vertigo, or acute/subacute onset recurrent vertigo.

Acute Prolonged (Hours to Days) Vertigo

A single episode of prolonged (hours to days) vertigo may be due to either a peripheral or a central lesion. The primary questions to be answered are whether the lesion is in the vestibular periphery or in the brain and whether it is a stroke. It is important to remember that a peripheral lesion can be a stroke.

The symptoms of an acute unilateral vestibular lesion are severe vertigo (from the sudden imbalance of tonic vestibular input), nausea, and vomiting. Some patients will also have a loss of hearing in the affected ear, if the cochlea or auditory nerve is affected. Patients prefer to lie still with the eyes closed, because any head

Table 89.2. Causes of Vertigo According to Temporal Pattern

Temporal Pattern of Vertigo	Cause
Acute prolonged (hours to days) vertigo	
Peripheral	Vestibular neuritis labyrinthitis (if hearing loss present)
	Labyrinthine infarction
	Syphilis
	Autoimmune disease
	Bacterial labyrinthitis
	Ramsay-Hunt syndrome (herpes zoster oticus)
	Posttraumatic
Central	Infarct (brainstem, cerebellum)
	Cerebellar hemorrhage
	Multiple sclerosis
	Other inflammatory/autoimmune disorders
Recurrent vertigo	
Seconds	Benign paroxysmal positional vertigo (provoked by changes in head position)
	Perilymph fistula/superior canal dehiscence (provoked by loud noise/Valsalva)
Minutes	Transient ischemic attack
	Migraine (aura)
	Anxiety/Panic
Hours	Migraine
	Ménière disease
	Otosyphilis
	Autoimmune

movement makes the symptoms worse. They will have difficulty walking, and on Romberg testing they may fall toward the affected side.

Vestibular neuritis is a common cause of acute unilateral vestibulopathy. When hearing loss is present, the term *labyrinthitis* is often used, although the exact localization is not always certain. By simple office testing, the hearing loss is usually sensorineural, not conductive (see Chapter 110). Vestibular neuritis is generally thought to result from a viral infection of the labyrinth or vestibular nerve or a postinfectious inflammatory process. Bacterial labyrinthitis is more rare but may be a complication of mastoiditis or bacterial meningitis.

The acute severe symptoms of vestibular neuritis usually subside over the first several days with gradual continued improvement over the next several weeks to months, as the brain compensates for the peripheral lesion. If compensation is incomplete, there may be a lingering imbalance that never fully recovers. Once the acute stage has passed, examination findings may be minimal, with no spontaneous nystagmus in the light. The most consistent finding is a head thrust sign when the head is rotated toward the affected side (see above). A reduced caloric response confirms the unilateral pathology.

A *labyrinthine infarct* may be difficult to distinguish clinically from labyrinthitis. Thus, older individuals, particularly those with vascular risk factors, should be evaluated for cerebrovascular disease affecting the posterior circulation (see Chapter 91). The main concern is that a patient with vertebrobasilar disease could go on to have a second, and potentially more life-threatening, infarct in the brainstem or cerebellum. Other important diagnoses to consider are otosyphilis, vasculitis, and autoimmune inner ear disease, either isolated or as part of a systemic autoimmune process. Thus, patients should have serologic testing for syphilis (RPR/FTA; see Chapter 37), sedimentation rate, and specific tests for connective tissue disease or vasculitis, when suspected.

Symptoms that should raise suspicion of a central (brainstem or cerebellar) lesion include double vision, facial or limb numbness or weakness, slurred speech, and limb incoordination. A direction changing (gaze-evoked) or vertical (e.g., downbeat) nystagmus indicates central disease, as generally do other cranial nerve or cerebellar signs. Infarction in the territory of the anterior inferior cerebellar artery may produce a combination of both central and peripheral signs (4). A cerebellar or brainstem stroke is a medical emergency.

Some patients with peripheral disease will have ipsilateral facial weakness when there is a combined lesion of cranial nerves VII and VIII. In these cases, the facial weakness should have a peripheral pattern (the forehead is not spared). Ramsey-Hunt syndrome is a reactivation of herpes zoster virus that produces facial paresis, hearing loss, vertigo, and ear pain, with vesicular lesions in the external auditory canal. Early treatment with acyclovir is important.

Treatment of acute peripheral vertigo is largely aimed at explaining the cause and likely course to the patient and ameliorating the symptoms. Vestibular suppressants include antihistamines (e.g., promethazine, meclizine) and benzodiazepines (e.g., diazepam or lorazepam). Practical information about these drugs is summarized in Table 89.3. These should be used only in the acute stage (the first several days), when vertigo is severe, because they may impede the process of central vestibular compensation. Antiemetics may be helpful when nausea and vomiting are present. Ondansetron may have fewer side effects than antidopaminergic agents (e.g., prochlorperazine, chlorpromazine, metoclopramide). Patients should be encouraged to resume activity when possible, because this may facilitate the compensation process. For patients with troublesome persistent symptoms, referral for formal vestibular rehabilitation therapy may also help recovery.

Recurrent Vertigo

Recurrent attacks of vertigo can be distinguished by several features, including their duration, provoking factors, and associated symptoms. There are many underlying etiologies (Table 89.2); some common causes include BPPV, endolymphatic hydrops (Ménière syndrome), migraine, psychiatric disease, and TIAs.

Benign Paroxysmal Positional Vertigo

BPPV is a common cause of episodic vertigo (5). It consists of brief attacks of vertigo, provoked by changes in head position relative to gravity. The typical features of BPPV are listed in Table 89.4.

BPPV results from the accumulation of otoconial debris in one of the semicircular canals, usually the posterior. Otoconia are particles consisting of calcium carbonate crystals that are normally adherent to the membrane of the utricle (see above). If these particles are dispersed, either spontaneously or by trauma or inner ear injury, they may coalesce into a small clot and become free floating in the endolymph fluid. This

Table 89.3. Drugs for Symptomatic Treatment of Vertigo

Type of Action	Generic (Trade Name)	Available Preparations	Dosage and Schedule
Labyrinthine suppressants			
Antihistamines	Meclizine (Antivert, Bonine)	12.5 and 25 mg	12.5–25 mg b.i.d.–q.i.d.
Benzodiazepines	Clonazepam (Klonopin)	0.5 mg	0.25–0.5 mg q.d.–t.i.d
Antiemetic	Prochlorperazine (Compazine)	5-, 10-mg tablets	5–10 mg q4h p.r.n.
		10-, 25-mg suppositories	10 mg q.i.d., 25 mg b.i.d.
	Odansetron (Zofran)	4-, 8-mg tablets	8 mg b.i.d.

Table 89.4. Characteristic Features of Benign Paroxysmal Positional Vertigo

Predisposing factors
Head trauma
Labyrinthine lesion (e.g., labyrinthitis, Ménière disease)
Migraine
Prolonged supine or head back positioning (e.g., dental work)
Age
Vertigo provoked by
Lying down
Rolling to affected side in bed
Putting the head back to look up
Bending over and standing back up
Onset
Latency of several seconds from head movement before vertigo and nystagmus begin
Duration
Seconds (<1 min)
Other
Most common in the morning, after prolonged supine positioning
Symptoms (and nystagmus) fatigue with repeated positioning

clot of particles may fall into one of the semicircular canals, most commonly the posterior canal, due to its orientation. Then, when the head moves, this clot may move within the canal, causing pressure changes in the endolymph and deflecting the cupula. This leads to excitation of the canal, as if the head were rotating.

BPPV *is diagnosed* by the Dix-Hallpike positioning maneuver, illustrated in Fig. 89.1. The head is first turned 45 degrees to one side. This will place the posterior canal on that side in the plane of rotation. Then, the subject is brought quickly from a sitting to a head-hanging position. A patient with BPPV will describe vertigo when the affected ear is stimulated (i.e., when the head is turned to that side). While supporting the head, the examiner watches the eyes for any nystagmus to indicate excitation of the posterior canal. The expected nystagmus has both vertical and torsional (rotatory) components: *The eyes beat upward and the upper poles of the eyes beat toward the affected (down) ear* (Fig. 89.2). There is usually a latency of several seconds from the initial positioning until the vertigo and nystagmus begin, and the duration is less than 1 minute (commonly about 15 to 30 seconds). It is important to keep in mind that not all positional vertigo and nystagmus is due to BPPV. For example, patients with cerebellar disease or craniocervical junction abnormalities (e.g., Chiari malformation) may have positional nystagmus. In these cases, the nystagmus is usually sustained rather than transient. Common patterns are positional downbeat or horizontal, sometimes direction-changing, nystagmus.

Treatment of BPPV consists of the canalith repositioning (Epley) procedure shown in Fig. 89.3, which begins with the Dix-Hallpike maneuver, with the head turned to the affected ear (6). The purpose of the maneuver is to relocate the free-floating particles in the utricle. The four-step maneuver is repeated until no nystagmus is observed at the end of the several steps. After a treatment session, patients should be advised to keep their heads relatively upright for 48 hours so that canaliths will stay re-located and will not tend to gravitate back into the posterior canal. This approach

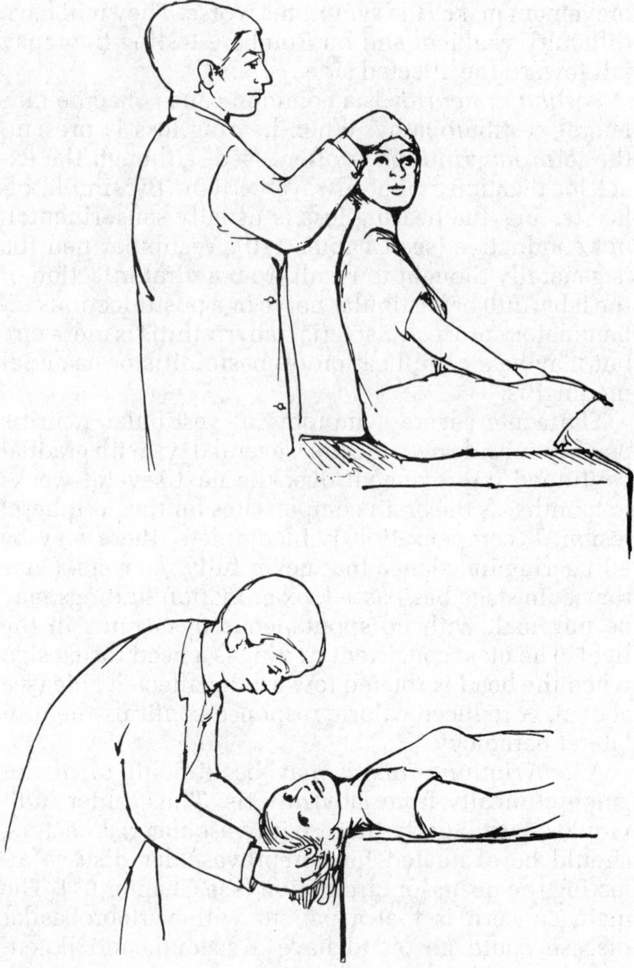

Figure 89.1. Dix-Hallpike maneuver for testing a patient for positional vertigo and nystagmus.

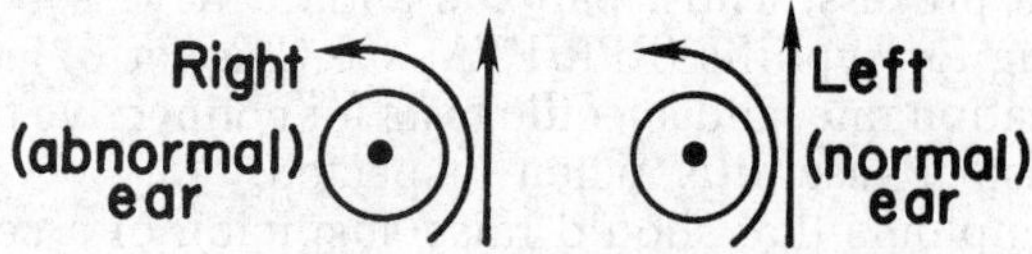

Figure 89.2. Pathognomonic nystagmus of benign paroxysmal positional vertigo. The pathognomonic nystagmus consists of quick phases directed upward (with respect to the head) and torsionally toward the abnormal ear. In this example, the torsional element is counterclockwise toward the abnormal right ear.

to treating BPPV is effective after one session in most patients (7). Contraindications to the Epley maneuver are severe disease of the neck and high-grade carotid stenosis. In refractory or recurrent cases, patients can be taught to perform a modification of the maneuver at home, in which the head rests on the bed but with pillows under the shoulders to simulate a head-hanging position (8). Brandt-Daroff physical therapy exercises may also be helpful (9). Making the diagnosis of BPPV quickly and accurately is important, because of the effectiveness of treatment and to avoid an unnecessary and expensive diagnostic workup for other causes (e.g., TIAs). Because BPPV may be a complication of labyrinthine injury, it may coexist with

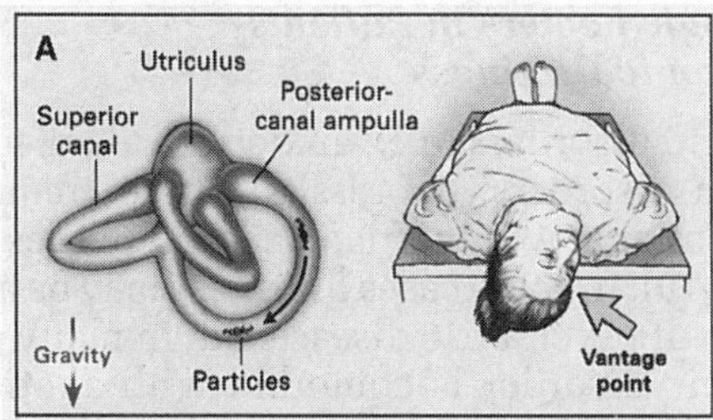

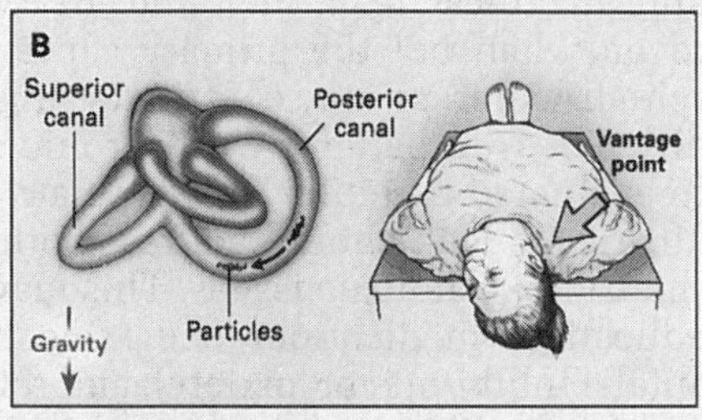

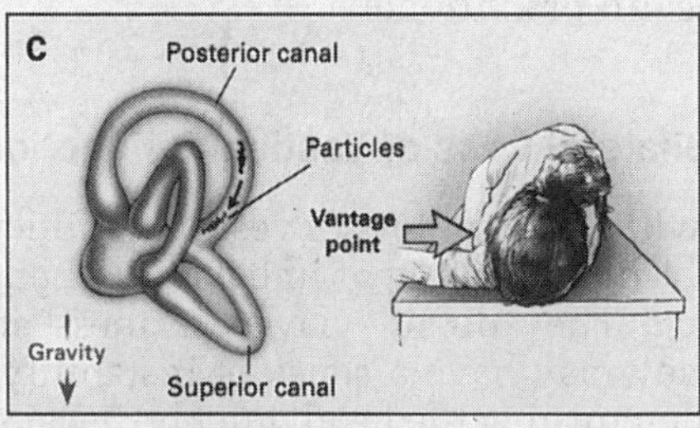

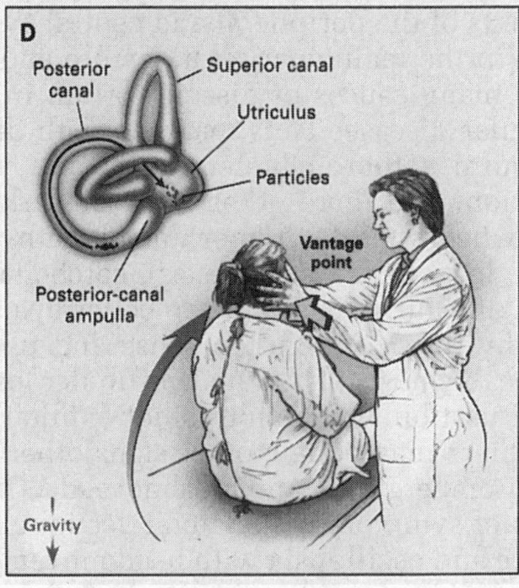

Figure 89.3. Bedside maneuver for the treatment of a patient with benign paroxysmal positional vertigo affecting the right ear (Epley maneuver). The presumed position of the debris within the labyrinth during the maneuver is shown in each panel. The maneuver is a four-step procedure. First, a Dix-Hallpike test is performed with the patient's head rotated 45 degrees toward the right ear and the neck slightly extended with the chin pointed slightly upward. This position results in the patient's head hanging to the right **(A).** Once the vertigo and nystagmus provoked by the Dix-Hallpike test cease, the patient's head is rotated about the rostral-caudal body axis until the left ear is down **(B).** Then the head and body are further rotated until the head is face down **(C).** The vertex of the head is kept tilted downward throughout the rotation. The maneuver usually provokes brief vertigo. The patient should be kept in the final face-down position for about 10 to 16 seconds. With the head kept turned toward the left shoulder, the patient is brought into the seated position **(D).** Once the patient is upright, the head is titled so that the chin is pointed slightly downward. (From Furman JM, Cass SP. Benign paroxysmal positional vertigo. N Engl J Med 1999;341:1590, with permission.)

other inner ear diseases (10). Vestibular suppressant drugs (Table 89.3) may reduce the intensity of a patient's symptoms, but they do not reduce the frequency of attacks.

Perilymph Fistula

A perilymph fistula is a relatively uncommon cause of recurrent vertigo and is sometimes difficult to diagnose (11). However, it is helpful to keep in mind because it may be amenable to surgical treatment. It results from a defect in the bony labyrinth or the round or oval window, creating a communication between the inner ear and either the middle ear or the intracranial space. Causes include barotrauma, erosion by a tumor (e.g., cholesteatoma), or head trauma. Vertigo is provoked by loud noises, tragal pressure, or Valsalva, with transmission of middle ear or intracranial pressure into the labyrinth through the communicating defect. Surgical exploration and repair may be necessary. *Superior semicircular canal dehiscence* is a recently described form of perilymph fistula, in which there is a defect in the bone overlying the superior canal, creating a communication with the middle cranial fossa (12). In these cases, there is likely a congenitally thin bony roof to the superior canal that may be disrupted by minimal trauma, creating the defect.

Transient Ischemic Attacks

Vertigo may be a symptom of TIAs involving the posterior circulation. Vertigo due to TIAs usually lasts for minutes. Repeated episodes of vertigo on an ischemic basis are unusual in the absence of other posterior circulation symptoms, such as visual field disturbances, double vision, slurred speech, or facial or limb weakness or numbness. However, occasional patients will have isolated vertigo (13). Patients suspected of having TIAs should be evaluated as described in Chapter 91.

Vestibular Migraine

Migraine is another common cause of recurrent dizziness (14,15). Patients with migraine may have a variety of symptoms that include both discrete attacks of vertigo and prolonged episodes of disequilibrium and motion sensitivity. Migrainous vertigo typically lasts minutes to hours. It may occur as an aura, preceding headache, or may be present simultaneously with headache. In many cases, headache and vertigo occur independently, and occasional patients thought to have vestibular migraine only rarely, if ever, have headache. Thus, the absence of headache does not rule out migraine as a cause of dizziness, although it should raise suspicion for other causes. Only a small fraction of patients with migrainous vertigo meet criteria for *basilar migraine*; in these patients, vertigo occurs as part of the aura, and there must be at least one other posterior circulation symptom.

The treatment of vestibular migraine is similar to that of migraine headaches. Patients with rare episodes can be given antiemetics and vestibular suppressants (Table 89.4) to be taken at the time of an attack. For those with more frequent and more debilitating attacks, prophylactic therapy is often helpful. Suggested prophylactic medications include antidepressants (tricyclics, serotonin selective reuptake inhibitors, venlafaxine), beta-blockers, valproate, calcium channel blockers, and acetazolamide. In an individual patient, several agents may need to be tried before finding one that works well without unacceptable side effects. With any of these medications, a low initial dose should be used, titrating upward as necessary, with dose increases about once weekly.

Patients with chronic refractory migraine are more likely to have comorbid psychiatric disease, including affective and anxiety disorders (see below) (16). These are very important to recognize and must also be addressed in the treatment plan. Chapter 87 provides a detailed account of migraine management.

Ménière Disease (Endolymphatic Hydrops)

The classic presentation of Ménière disease (see also Chapter 110) is recurrent attacks of vertigo, nausea, and vomiting; a transient decrease in hearing in the affected ear; ear pain, pressure, and/or fullness; and tinnitus, usually low pitched and described as "roaring" or "rushing." Less commonly, patients may also have drop attacks, in which they feel suddenly thrown to the ground. These are called otolithic crises of Tumarkin. The pathophysiology of Ménière disease is thought to be increased endolymph pressure within the labyrinth (hence the name, endolymphatic hydrops).

The differential diagnosis of Ménière disease includes a variety of inflammatory and infectious causes, such as otosyphilis, Lyme disease, connective tissue diseases, and autoimmune inner ear disease. Thus, all patients suspected of having Ménière disease should have serologic testing for these disorders. Those with positive syphilis serologies should undergo lumbar puncture. If the cerebrospinal fluid is abnormal (pleocytosis, elevated protein, positive VDRL), patients should be given a full neurosyphilis treatment regimen (see Chapter 37); treatment may be warranted even if cerebrospinal fluid is normal, when the suspicion is high. Sometimes it is also difficult to distinguish Ménière disease from vestibular migraine, especially if auditory symptoms are less prominent.

If possible, patients suspected of having Ménière disease should have an audiogram at the time of an attack. The classic finding is a predominantly low-frequency hearing loss in the affected ear that may improve when the attack resolves. The finding of a fluctuating low-frequency hearing loss on serial audiograms is helpful in making the diagnosis.

Treatment of Ménière disease includes sodium restriction (1 g/day) and diuretics (e.g., acetazolamide, hydrochlorthiazide/triamterene). In cases refractory to diuretics, intratympanic steroid or gentamicin injections may be helpful. The goal of gentamicin therapy is to ablate vestibular function partially to eliminate attacks of vertigo with minimal effects on balance. Surgical ablation (labyrinthectomy or vestibular nerve section) is reserved only for the most severe cases, after all other treatments have failed.

Psychologic Factors in Patients with Chronic Dizziness

Psychiatric disorders (e.g., anxiety/panic disorder, somatoform disorders, depression) are extremely common in patients with vertigo and other types of dizziness (17–19). In some cases dizziness may be a primary symptom of psychiatric disease, but in many cases the psychiatric disorder is comorbid with another problem causing dizziness (e.g., migraine, BPPV). When present, even when not the primary cause of dizziness, psychiatric disease may contribute substantially to disability. Thus, all patients with chronic dizziness should be evaluated carefully for psychiatric illness, and the treatment plan should address both medical and psychiatric/psychologic issues. This may include patient education, medications (e.g., selective serotonin reuptake inhibitors for anxiety), and referral to a mental health practitioner.

Bilateral Loss of Vestibular Function

Patients with bilateral loss of vestibular function have disequilibrium, a feeling of imbalance when standing or walking. They do not have dizziness at rest, although they may have a sense of instability or oscillopsia when turning the head quickly. Because several components of the peripheral and central systems are involved in the maintenance of posture and balance, there are many causes of disequilibrium in addition to vestibular disease. Thus, patients with disequilibrium require a thorough neurologic and vestibular examination. Are there other signs of parkinsonism (e.g., cogwheel rigidity, tremor), myelopathy (spasticity in the legs, increased reflexes), cerebellar disease (limb ataxia, slurred speech, cerebellar eye signs), or neuropathy (loss of vibration sense and proprioception)? The diagnosis of bilateral vestibular loss may be missed if vestibular function is not explicitly tested, because there may be few other signs other than gait ataxia, a Romberg sign, and an abnormal VOR.

The chief symptoms of bilateral vestibular loss are imbalance and oscillopsia with head movement (such as when walking or riding in a car, particularly on a bumpy road). These are due to the loss of the vestibulospinal reflex and VOR, respectively. Patients do not have vertigo because the lesion is symmetric, yielding no net imbalance in the inputs from the two labyrinths. Typical findings on examination include a marked loss of dynamic visual acuity (see above), bilateral head thrust signs, and a Romberg sign. Reduced rotatory chair responses confirm the diagnosis. The degree of disability depends both on the severity of vestibular loss and the extent of compensation. Some younger patients who are otherwise healthy may compensate well, with limited disability. Others, particularly those with superimposed neuropathy (causing proprioceptive loss) or poor vision, may be left with more substantial disability.

The most common identified cause of bilateral vestibular loss is *ototoxic drugs,* such as aminoglycosides and cisplatin (20,21). Gentamicin ototoxicity may occur even in the absence of "toxic" levels, with once daily dosing, and with a normal cumulative dose. If recognized early, stopping the drug may theoretically limit the damage and allow for some recovery of function. In many cases, however, the vestibular loss is not discovered until the course of treatment has been completed. Early symptoms of disequilibrium may be attributed to a general weakness arising from the patient's underlying systemic illness. Only after recovery from the acute illness, when the patient is more active, is the true balance impairment noted. For this reason, it is important to monitor vestibular function during gentamicin treatment, when possible. This can be done by measuring dynamic acuity with a near card, looking for head thrust signs, and checking for a Romberg sign, if the patient can stand.

Many cases of bilateral vestibular loss are idiopathic. Other causes include hereditary vestibular loss (22), bilateral sequential vestibular neuritis, combined cerebellar and vestibular degeneration, autoimmune disease, meningitis, sarcoidosis, metabolic disease (e.g., vitamin B_{12} deficiency), bilateral vestibular nerve tumors (e.g., schwannomas), and bilateral Ménière disease (23,24).

MOTION SICKNESS

Motion sickness is a feeling of nausea and dizziness evoked by excessive or prolonged vestibular or optokinetic stimulation (25). Other symptoms include diaphoresis, yawning, light-headedness, and malaise. Susceptibility to motion sickness varies among individuals; migraineurs are particularly motion sensitive. Most individuals adapt to continued motion (e.g., cruise), although some remain persistently motion sick. Individuals with bilateral vestibular paresis are insensitive to motion.

Several medications may assist in the prevention or reduction of motion sickness, when used occasionally during exposure to a provocative stimulus. Antihistamines such as meclizine (25 to 50 mg), dimenhydrinate (50 to 100 mg), or promethazine (25 mg) may be taken orally about 1 hour before travel. The major adverse effect is sedation, most prominently with promethazine. Transdermal scopolamine is an anticholinergic agent that is effective in preventing motion sickness. The 1.5-mg patch is designed to deliver 0.5 mg of scopolamine over 3 days. It should be applied at least 4 hours before travel. Adverse effects include dry mouth and sedation. Older individuals may be more sensitive to central nervous anticholinergic effects such as confusion and hallucinations. Occasionally, withdrawal symptoms occur, particularly after prolonged use.

After prolonged exposure to motion, such as returning to land after a cruise, many individuals have a feeling of continued motion ("landsickness") that usually resolves within 1 to 2 days. However, in some individuals these symptoms persist for months to years. This has been termed *mal de debarquement syndrome* (26). Typical features are a constant feeling of rocking or swaying when still. In contrast to motion sickness, these individuals feel best when moving and worse when motion stops. Mal de debarquement syndrome has been reported much more commonly in women, usually in their 40s. A history of migraine or other headaches is common. The etiology is uncertain; a failure of the vestibular system to readapt to the land-based environment has been suggested. Treatment with amitriptyline or benzodiazepines may help somewhat. It is not certain whether medications such as benzodiazepines can prevent mal de debarquement syndrome in susceptible individuals.

SYNCOPE AND NEAR SYNCOPE

Definitions and Pathophysiology

Syncope is "a sudden transient loss of consciousness associated with a loss of postural tone, with spontaneous recovery" (27). Syncope typically lasts from seconds to minutes; longer episodes are classified as stupor or coma. *Unconsciousness* implies that both cerebral hemispheres have become impaired or that certain critical structures in the brainstem have failed. In general, unilateral diseases of the cerebral hemispheres do not lead to unconsciousness unless the brain becomes more generally affected.

There are three major pathophysiologic mechanisms of syncope (28):

- *Acute decrease in cerebral blood flow.* This may be caused by cardiac disorders, pulmonary vascular disorders, failure of venous return, cerebrovascular disease, loss of peripheral vascular tone, and vasodepressor syncope, commonly referred to as vasovagal syncope. This last mechanism is thought to result from a triggering of a neural reflex resulting in an episode of hypotension in the setting of bradycardia and peripheral vasodilation. It is the most common diagnosed cause of syncope and carries a good prognosis (see details below).
- *Chemical aberration of blood flowing to the brain.* Examples include hypoglycemia, hypocapnia, and hypoxia.
- *Neural or psychologic causes.* These include nonconvulsive seizures and psychogenic syncope.

Syncope must be differentiated from presyncope and other disorders that may, on initial history taking, sound similar to syncope. *Many types of "spells" are not syncope;* a spell is "a sudden onset of a symptom or symptoms that are recurrent, self-limited, and stereotypic in nature" (29). Such spells are not necessarily syncope and may be caused by endocrine, cardiovascular, psychologic, pharmacologic, neurologic, or other miscellaneous disorders. Carcinoid syndrome and pheochromocytoma are classic examples of disorders in which patients describe spells that are distinct from syncope.

Presyncope, or near syncope, is the sense of imminent loss of consciousness without frank syncope. It may be a prelude to true syncope or it may be related to a spell or to unexplained dizziness.

Incidence and Mortality

In the longitudinal community-based Framingham study, one or more episodes of syncope per year was reported in 3% of adult men and 3.5% of adult women. Framingham subjects ranged in age from 30 to 62; the mean age of an initial episode of syncope was 52 in men and 50 in women (30). The incidence of syncope increased with increasing age, and in patients aged 65 or older, syncope occurred at an annual rate of 6%. Thirty percent of men and 27% of women who experienced syncope had more than one episode of syncope. Approximately one million medical evaluations are done annually on patients with syncope (31).

Morbidity and mortality in patients with syncope differ according to the underlying cause of the syncopal event. Studies of patients with syncope report a 1-year mortality of 18% to 33% for patients with a cardiovascular cause of syncope, 0% to 12% for patients with a known noncardiovascular cause, and 6% for patients with an unknown cause of syncope (32). A study of patients with inducible ventricular tachycardia showed that they are the subgroup with the highest mortality; those taking a drug that effectively suppressed ventricular tachycardia did slightly better (33). Patients with underlying heart disease who have a history of syncope do not have a higher mortality than patients with the same extent of heart disease who do not have a history of syncope (34).

Differential Diagnosis

The vasovagal faint is thought to be the most common cause of syncope, especially if there is no evidence of a cardiovascular cause. Vasovagal syncope may account for up to 40% of all syncopal events evaluated in the ambulatory setting. However, the differential diagnosis of disorders presenting as syncope is broad. Table 89.5 lists causes, classified as hypotension, cardiac disease, metabolic conditions, intracranial conditions, or psychiatric disorders. The list of medications that may cause syncope continues to expand. Any patient with dizziness or syncope should have all medications, including over the counter medications, reviewed in light of the patient's presenting complaint. Polypharmacy is a particularly common cause of syncope in the elderly. Depending on the diagnostic criteria used, *an underlying cause will not be found for approximately 38% to 42% of patients evaluated for syncope* (27). In a recent study of psychiatric illnesses in patients with syncope, of patients who did not have an underlying medical explanation found for their syncopal episode, 20% met diagnostic criteria for at least one psychiatric disorder (35). In this same study, approximately half of the psychiatric disorders were not recognized by the patient's physicians. Generalized anxiety, panic disorder, major depression, and alcohol dependence were prevalent in this group of patients

Table 89.5. Differential Diagnosis of Syncope/Near Syncope

Hypotension
- Vasovagal or neurocardiogenic syncope
- Vasodilating drugs
  - Angiotensin-converting enzyme inhibitors
  - Angiotensin receptor blockers
  - Alpha blockers
  - Calcium channel blockers
  - Nitroglycerine preparations
  - Vasodilator antihypertensives
- Drugs affecting autonomic function
  - Sympatholytic antihypertensives
  - Neuroleptics
  - Tricyclics and monoamine oxidase inhibitors
  - Levodopa
  - Cholinergic agents
  - Antihistamines
- Autonomic neuropathy
  - Peripheral neuropathy
  - Postsympathectomy
  - Tabes dorsalis and diabetic pseudotabes
  - Parkinsonism (Shy-Drager syndrome)
  - Idiopathic
- Decreased blood volume
  - Hemorrhage
  - Salt and water deficit
  - Fasting
  - Adrenal insufficiency
  - Hypoalbuminemia
  - Diuretics
- Venous pooling
  - Prolonged Immobility while standing
  - Severe varicose veins
  - Late pregnancy
  - After exercise
- Mobilization after bed rest
- Orthostasis of aging
- Valsalva maneuver
  - Tussive
  - Micturition
  - Defecation (with straining)
  - Intermittent positive-pressure breathing
- Compromise of cerebral blood flow caused by cervical osteoarthritis or subclavian steal
- Carotid sinus hypersensitivity
- Pulmonary embolism

Cardiac disease
- Arrhythmia (heart block, bradyarrhythmias, and tachyarrhythmias)
- Drugs associated with torsade de pointes
  - Quinidine
  - Procainamide
  - Disopyramide
  - Flecainide
  - Encainide
  - Amiodarone
  - Sotalol
  - Terfenadine
  - Astemizole
- Outflow obstruction
  - Aortic stenosis
  - Idiopathic hypertrophic subaortic stenosis
  - Aortic dissection
  - Myxoma
- Acute myocardial infarction
  - Mitral valve prolapse
  - Cyanotic congenital heart disease
  - Cardiac tamponade

Metabolic conditions
- Hypoglycemia or hyperglycemia (consider drugs causing hypo- or hyperglycemia)
- Hyponatremia, hypokalemia, or hypocalcemia
- Hypocapnia (hyperventilation)
- Hypoxia
  - Anemia
  - Airway obstruction
  - Carbon monoxide
  - Change to moderate/high altitude
- Hyperviscosity
- Drug overdose (sedatives and ethanol)

Intracranial conditions
- Seizure disorder
- Subarachnoid hemorrhage
- Cerebral embolism or thrombosis
- Migraine
- Acutely increased intracranial pressure
  - Tumor
  - Trauma
  - Ventricular obstruction
  - Hypertensive encephalopathy
- Brainstem compression
  - Cervical or odontoid fractures
  - Metastasis
  - Cysts or anomalies of the posterior fossa
  - Platybasia

Psychiatric disorders
- Panic disorder
- Generalized anxiety disorder
- Major depression
- Somatization disorder
- Conversion disorder
- Alcoholism

Modified from Lee JE, Killip T, Plum F. Episodic unconsciousness. In: Baron JA, ed. Diagnostic approaches to presenting syndromes. Baltimore: Williams & Wilkins, 1971, with permission.

Table 89.6. Diagnostic Studies that Demonstrated the Cause of Syncope in 107 of 204 Patients in Whom Exhaustive Study Established a Cause

Study	No. of Patients
History and physical	52
Electrocardiography	12
Electrocardiographic monitoring	29
Electrophysiologic studies	3
Cardiac catheterization	7
Cerebral angiography	2
Electroencephalography	1
Total	106[a]

[a]In one additional patient a diagnosis of aortic dissection was made at autopsy, 7 days after the patient presented with syncope.

From Kapoor WN, Karpf M, Wieand S, et al. A prospective evaluation and follow-up of patients with syncope. N Engl J Med 1983;309:197, with permission.

with unexplained syncope; these patients had higher rates of syncope recurrence during follow-up than patients with unexplained syncope who did not have underlying psychiatric disorders. This group of patients tends to be younger, without underlying heart disease.

Of patients for whom the cause of syncope is determined, hypotension is the cause in 20% to 50%, cardiac disease in 10% to 25%, metabolic disorders in less than 5%, intracranial disease in less than 5%, and psychiatric disorders in up to 30% (36). In many patients, no cause can be clearly discerned on initial evaluation. For patients with syncope of unknown origin, additional testing or prolonged follow-up may be necessary, but often a diagnosis is never established.

In a classic prospective evaluation of 204 patients presenting with syncope, 25% had the cause diagnosed on the basis of the history and physical examination. In this study population, in which approximately 50% of patients eventually received a diagnosis, the importance of the history and physical examination was well illustrated. Table 89.6 lists the diagnostic studies (including history and physical) that demonstrated the cause in patients for whom a cause was identified. This study was done before the widespread use of tilt-table testing (see below); recent studies suggest that tilt-table testing will demonstrate neurally mediated hypotension in one-half to two-thirds of patients with undiagnosed syncope (37).

General Approach to the Patient (38)

Most patients who come to a physician after an episode of syncope or near syncope do so after their symptoms have resolved. The history should be obtained both from the patient and from anyone who observed the episode. The inquiry should focus on the events immediately before and after the attack, associated problems that may have been present for days to weeks before the episode, and evidence of trauma, neurologic deficit, or aspiration complicating the current episode of syncope. The objectives of these initial steps are to reach a working diagnosis or decide what further evaluation is needed and to decide on initial management for the patient. Appropriate management may range from reassurance (e.g., the patient with vasovagal syncope), to volume expansion (e.g., the patient with a diarrheal illness), to hospital admission for observation, prompt diagnostic testing, and necessary treatment (e.g., the patient with a history suggesting life-threatening arrhythmias or the patient with a major fracture complicating syncope). Details regarding the critical features of many of the causes of syncope listed in Table 89.5 are described below.

History

Current Episode. The patient should always be questioned about his or her situation and body position immediately before the attack. If there was psychologic stress (e.g., an argument or fear about a medical procedure) or prodromal autonomic symptoms (nausea, pallor, diaphoresis), vasovagal syncope should be considered. If exercise preceded the attack, a number of cardiopulmonary abnormalities are possible, including aortic stenosis, hypertrophic cardiomyopathy, arrhythmia, and pulmonary hypertension. If syncope was associated with micturition, coughing, or defecation, the episode may have been caused by an associated Valsalva-induced decrease in venous return.

Syncope from most causes does not occur unless the patient is in the upright position. If the attack occurred when the patient first stood up, orthostatic hypotension caused by venous pooling, loss of intravascular volume, or autonomic failure should be considered.

Syncope that occurs when the patient is seated or recumbent suggests hypoglycemia, carotid sinus hypersensitivity, cardiac arrhythmia, hyperventilation, seizure, or a psychiatric disorder. Syncope or dizziness occurring with position change while recumbent should always be distinguished from BPPV (see above).

The patient also should be asked *whether consciousness was lost completely* and whether a fall or any injury occurred. Although patients with many different causes of syncope may recall feelings of dizziness, heaviness of the limbs, or dimming of vision before loss of consciousness, other associated symptoms may suggest a diagnosis. Nausea is characteristic of vasovagal syncope but may also occur with bradyarrhythmias, myocardial ischemia, and loss of intravascular volume. Palpitations may suggest an arrhythmia, whereas chest pain and diaphoresis suggest myocardial ischemia. Headache and characteristic visual changes suggest a migraine. Incontinence and tonic–clonic movements of the extremities suggest a seizure; a seizure may be the primary problem or may be secondary to another event, such as cerebral ischemia or cardiac arrhythmia. Hemiparesis, paraparesis, diplopia, and dysarthria may occur with transient occlusion of the basilar artery or vasospasm associated with migraine. The presence of multiple nonspecific associated complaints should raise suspicion of a psychiatric disorder.

Observations made by others who witnessed the period of unconsciousness. Particular attention should be paid to the duration of the spell, whether a convulsion occurred, the sequence of events, and how the patient seemed during the period of recovery. In general, recovery of consciousness is swift. If recovery of clear consciousness takes more than 5 minutes, one should suspect a seizure, hypoglycemia, or occluded intracranial vessel.

History preceding the current episode should be sought. Information about the patient during the hours, days, or weeks preceding syncope/near syncope is often helpful in the differential diagnosis. In particular, one should determine the frequency of any previous episodes of syncope or near syncope, as the frequency of episodes influences decisions regarding the urgency of obtaining diagnostic studies. Frequent episodes without injury, especially if the syncope typically is preceded by nonspecific prodromal symptoms, should raise suspicion of a psychiatric disorder. A history of dizziness in addition to syncope is a marker for a greater prevalence of psychiatric disorders, although cardiac arrhythmias may have a similar presentation (39). Other circumstances surrounding previous episodes of dizziness or syncope may help develop a working diagnosis for the current episode of syncope. For example, a patient may report that previous episodes of dizziness or near syncope occurred after taking a new antihypertensive or psychotropic medication. A patient convalescing from recent illness may relate the symptoms to being up and around after bed rest.

Some patients describe previous episodes of frank syncope, without prodromal near syncope. Most often, these patients have a history, often long-standing, of syncope caused by vasovagal attack brought on by psychologic or physical stress. A history of recurrent syncope without the features of vasovagal attacks warrants consideration of arrhythmia, transient cerebrovascular occlusion, or a seizure disorder.

A patient with known organic heart disease, especially a patient with depressed left ventricular function or a history of ischemic heart disease, is at high risk of syncope caused by an arrhythmia. Although uncommon, a family history of cardiomyopathy or arrhythmia (such as prolonged QT syndrome) should be sought while taking the history from the patient.

Physical Examination

General Examination. The physical examination should include a search for abnormalities that may confirm a diagnosis suggested in the history or may reveal an unexpected cause. As patients with organic heart disease may have life-threatening causes of syncope, the cardiovascular examination is particularly important in all patients who present for the evaluation of a syncopal event. The heart rate and blood pressure should be measured after the patient has been recumbent for a few minutes and again after standing for 1 to 2 minutes. Very different blood pressures in the two arms would raise the possibility of aortic dissection or subclavian steal. The strength and upstroke of the carotid pulses should be appraised, and any bruits should be noted. The pulse should be palpated for 1 to 2 minutes to look for irregularities. The heart should be examined for murmurs (particularly the murmurs of aortic stenosis and idiopathic hypertrophic subaortic stenosis), clicks, or gallops. Abdominal examination may reveal a large bladder or signs of a visceral catastrophe. If orthostatic hypotension has been found, a rectal examination should be performed to check the stool for occult or gross blood.

Carotid Massage. For patients with episodes suggestive of carotid sinus hypersensitivity (see below) or older patients with recurrent syncope and a nondiagnostic evaluation, carotid massage can be performed. However, it should be performed only if there are no carotid bruits and when there is intravenous access and electrocardiographic and blood pressure monitoring, with atropine at hand. When performed, carotid massage involves application of digital pressure over each carotid sinus separately, for up to 5 seconds. A resulting carotid asystole of more than 3 seconds or a systolic blood pressure drop of more than 50 mm Hg is considered abnormal.

Neurologic Examination. A brief examination of the major components of the nervous system (see Chapter 86) may reveal evidence of pre-existing neurologic disease or of an acute insult. One should note the patient's orientation, speech, memory (for general information and the episode itself), and judgment. The fundi may reveal microemboli (see Chapter 91, Fig. 91.1) or subhyaloid hemorrhages (a sign of subarachnoid hemorrhage). Involvement of the midbrain, pons, or medulla is suggested by nystagmus, ophthalmoplegia, and other abnormalities of the cranial nerves. Weakness, sensory abnormalities, and pathologic reflexes may indicate a lesion elsewhere in the central nervous system (CNS). Any neurologic abnormalities should raise the suspicion of cerebrovascular disease, intracranial mass, subarachnoid hemorrhage, seizure, or CNS infection. If trauma has occurred in the recent past or if a fall was sustained during the syncopal episode, subdural or epidural hemorrhage should be considered. A nonfocal neurologic examination makes an intracranial cause of syncope unlikely, whereas a focal neurologic examination should prompt imaging of the CNS.

Significance of Seizures and Neurologic Deficits. Seizure activity may occur after syncope with a variety of causes, including the simple faint, cardiac arrhythmias, hyperventilation, orthostatic hypotension, or venous pooling. This is not surprising because unconsciousness signifies a major disruption in normal brain function. A single tonic convulsion is the most common type of postsyncopal seizure; less often a focal seizure or a generalized convulsion may occur. In all three of these instances, the patient's evaluation should include routine tests for a seizure focus (see Chapter 88).

Minor neurologic signs, such as slight focal weakness, reflex asymmetries, or pathologic reflexes, may be found after syncope from any cause, particularly if the patient is examined immediately after recovering consciousness. Such findings rarely persist for more than a few minutes. If such signs persist, are more profound, or occur in a constellation that suggests a particular anatomic lesion, they warrant further pursuit. However, one should not be surprised if a source is not found because minor neurologic signs are not uncommon after general ischemic or metabolic insults to the brain.

Diagnostic Tests

The history and physical examination lead to a diagnosis in 25% of patients with syncope (37–39). For these patients, no additional diagnostic tests are necessary. For the remaining patients, however, several diagnostic tests should be considered.

Electrocardiogram. An electrocardiogram (ECG), with a rhythm strip, is indicated in all patients with syncope if the cause is not obvious from the history and physical examination. Although the ECG shows some abnormality in a large proportion of patients with syncope, it confirms a diagnosis in a much smaller number (Table 89.6). Specific diagnostic workups may be prompted by certain ECG abnormalities. For instance, sinus bradycardia in the absence of a beta-blocker should prompt concern for sick sinus syndrome or sinus arrest. Sinus tachycardia may be present in patients with dehydration, congestive heart failure, or pulmonary embolus. Left ventricular hypertrophy may be caused by aortic stenosis or hypertrophic cardiomyopathy, and a prolonged QT interval increases susceptibility to ventricular tachycardia. Left bundle branch block could be caused by cardiomyopathies or myocardial infarction, and bifascicular block is associated with increased risk for complete heart block (see details in Chapter 64). The noninvasive nature of the test and its low cost, with the potential to uncover a possibly life-threatening disorder, make the ECG a cornerstone of the evaluation of nearly all patients with syncope (38).

Electrocardiographic Monitoring. The *Holter monitor* is the most commonly used diagnostic test in patients with syncope, but it is nondiagnostic in more than 90% of patients with a history of syncope (40). The clinical significance of asymptomatic arrhythmias found on Holter monitoring is unknown. Holter monitoring is indicated particularly in patients whose history suggests a cardiac basis for syncope and in any older patient in whom the evaluation for syncope leads to an uncertain diagnosis. Table 89.7 lists the common diagnoses made on ambulatory monitoring in patients presenting with palpitations or syncope.

The value of Holter monitoring in patients with symptoms of dizziness or syncope was assessed in a meta-analysis of seven studies; Holter monitoring was nondiagnostic in 78% of cases (41). Interestingly, only one-fourth of patients with symptoms during monitoring had simultaneous arrhythmias, meaning that most patients (i.e., those experiencing symptoms without evidence of an underlying arrhythmia) undergoing Holter monitoring have the diagnosis of arrhythmia excluded by the findings.

The duration of Holter monitoring affects the diagnostic yield. In a study comparing the diagnostic yields of 24- 48-, and 72-hour Holter, a "major abnormality" was noted in 15% of patients within the first 24 hours, and 11% of patients who had a negative 24-hour Holter had a positive finding in the second 24 hours. Only 4.2% of patients with a negative 24- and 48-hour Holter had abnormalities documented in the third 24-hour period. None of the arrhythmias found after the first 24 hours was associated with symptoms (42).

Table 89.7. Rhythms that May Be Found with Ambulatory Monitoring in Patients Presenting with Palpitations or Syncope

Patients with Palpitations	Patients with Syncope
Sinus rhythm or tachycardia	Sinus bradycardia
Ventricular premature depolarizations	Sinus arrest
Atrial fibrillation	Second-degree or third-degree atrioventricular block
Supraventricular tachycardia	Ventricular tachycardia
Atrial premature depolarizations	Supraventricular tachycardia
Ventricular tachycardia	Pacemaker malfunction

Modified from Zimmetbaum PJ, Josephson ME. The evolving role of ambulatory arrhythmia monitoring in general clinical practice. Ann Intern Med 1999;130:848, with permission.

There are other methods to monitor patients for arrhythmias for longer periods, including an implantable device (43) and a simpler *loop recorder (event monitor),* which saves several minutes of rhythm retroactively when activated by a patient while symptoms are experienced. A study of 57 patients with unexplained syncope who underwent at least 24 hours of Holter monitoring without a diagnosis, who then underwent 1 month of monitoring with a loop electrocardiographic recorder, demonstrated a 25% diagnostic yield in this group (40). This type of testing may be useful in patients in whom arrhythmia is believed to be likely, who have a negative Holter monitor, and who have mild enough symptoms so that they can activate the recorder. Loop recorders may be of particular use in patients without organic heart disease who have frequent episodes of syncope (37). Loop monitors are less expensive than Holter monitoring. Typically, a 24-hour Holter with interpretation costs $200 to $300, whereas a 1-month loop recorder with interpretation costs approximately $100.

Arrhythmias detected during Holter monitoring but not accompanied by symptoms are difficult to interpret. Although some believe that these arrhythmias, even if unaccompanied by symptoms, may provide a working diagnosis, others disagree. Some arrhythmias, such as sinus arrest and nonsustained ventricular tachycardia, can be seen in normal people. Therefore, the results of the Holter must be interpreted with caution, with consideration paid to the severity of the detected arrhythmia and the presence of any underlying heart disease. Echocardiography may be of use in interpreting the significance of arrhythmias found on Holter monitoring. For instance, nonsustained ventricular tachycardia in a patient with a history of myocardial infarction or depressed left ventricular function is at increased risk for sudden death (40).

Electrophysiologic Testing. EP studies are considered the final step in the evaluation when arrhythmia is strongly suspected and noninvasive testing is nondiagnostic (i.e., in patients with organic heart disease and unexplained syncope). *Indications* (27) for EP testing include

- Structural or ischemic heart disease, congestive heart failure, valvular disease, or hypertrophic cardiomyopathy;
- Abnormalities on ECG such as bundle branch block or Wolff-Parkinson-White syndrome;
- Abnormalities on ambulatory monitoring, such as nonsustained ventricular tachycardia.

EP testing is most likely to produce abnormal findings in patients with underlying heart disease. In a study of 111 patients with *unexplained syncope* referred for EP testing, 50% of those with underlying heart disease had positive findings on EP testing, whereas 16% of those without underlying heart disease had positive findings (44). Because other studies have failed to identify clinical predictors that correlate with positive findings on EP studies (45) and because EP findings may lead to treatment that decreases episodes of syncope (33), there are no clear-cut guidelines for excluding EP testing for patients with unexplained syncope.

The most common abnormal finding in patients undergoing EP testing is ventricular tachycardia, followed by conduction disturbances and supraventricular tachycardia, with the percentage of patients with abnormal findings depending on the population studied. As with Holter monitoring, certain abnormalities detected, especially conduction abnormalities and even certain tachyarrhythmias, have questionable clinical significance.

Tilt-Table Testing. In the past 20 years, tilt-table testing has played an increasingly important role in the diagnosis and management of syncope. The most significant impact of tilt-table testing has been in patients without organic heart disease who have unexplained syncope. However, patients with organic heart disease and a negative evaluation for syncope (including EP testing) may also be evaluated with tilt-table testing (46). Tilt-table testing has dramatically reduced the proportion of patients with unexplained syncope.

The tilt-table test is a provocative test used to *document susceptibility to vasovagal syncope (see details below).* In vasovagal syncope that can be demonstrated by tilt-table testing, blood pooling in the lower extremities leads to central hypovolemia, which ultimately is associated with bradycardia in some individuals (the exact mechanism is a matter of debate). Resultant hypotension leads to decreased CNS perfusion, which leads to syncope. It is interesting to note that hypotension, and not bradycardia, is the cause of syncope. This conclusion is based on the observation that atropine, which prevents bradycardia, does not prevent syncope.

Patient Experience: The tilt-table test is performed by securing a patient to the tilt table in the supine position and then tilting the patient to a 60- to 80-degree angle within 10 to 15 seconds. (Many patients find this experience unpleasant, because it replicates the syncopal event. It is therefore important to discuss the test with the patient beforehand.) The patient is maintained at the tilted angle for up to 60 minutes, during which time blood pressure and heart rate are monitored. The mean time to syncope in patients with a positive test is 25 minutes (47).

A tilt-table test is deemed positive if syncope or presyncope with hypotension develops. If no event occurs, provocation with either isoproterenol or nitroglycerine may be tried, increasing sensitivity but losing specificity. Even without resorting to provocative testing, establishing susceptibility to vasovagal syncope does not guarantee this as the cause of the patient's event.

Although tilt-table testing is most commonly used to establish susceptibility to vasovagal syncope, other abnormal cardiovascular responses may be uncovered with the test. In the vasovagal response, both heart rate and blood pressure decline. However, in some patients, blood pressure may drop without significant changes in heart rate (termed the *dysautonomic response*). In others, heart rate may increase while blood pressure drops, termed the *postural orthostatic tachycardia syndrome* (48).

In 1996, the American College of Cardiology published a consensus document on indications for tilt-table testing in the assessment of patients with syncope (Table 89.8) (49). This consensus document, along with other studies on the evaluation of the patient with

Table 89.8. Summary of Principal Indications for Tilt-Table Testing for Evaluation of Syncope

Tilt-table testing is warranted
Recurrent syncope or single syncopal episode in a high-risk patient, whether or not the medical history is suggestive of neurally mediated (vasovagal) origin, and
No evidence of structural cardiovascular disease, or
Structural cardiovascular disease is present but other causes of syncope have been excluded by appropriate testing
Further evaluation of patients in whom an apparent cause has been established (e.g., asystole, atrioventricular block) but in whom demonstration of susceptibility to neurally mediated syncope would affect treatment plans
Part of the evaluation of exercise-induced or exercise-associated syncope
Conditions for which reasonable differences of opinion exist regarding utility of tilt-table testing
Differentiating convulsive syncope from seizures
Evaluating patients (especially the elderly) with recurrent unexplained falls
Assessing recurrent dizziness or presyncope
Evaluating unexplained syncope in the setting of peripheral neuropathies or dysautonomias
Follow-up evaluation to assess therapy of neurally mediated syncope
Tilt-table testing not warranted
Single syncopal episode, without injury and not in a high-risk setting with clear-cut vasovagal clinical features
Syncope in which an alternative specific cause has been established and in which additional demonstration of a neurally mediated susceptibility would not alter treatment plans
Potential emerging indications
Recurrent idiopathic vertigo
Recurrent transient ischemic attacks
Chronic fatigue syndrome
Sudden infant death syndrome

syncope, can be summarized as five indications for tilt-table testing:

1. Syncope presumed to be vasovagal, but the history or physical are inconclusive.
2. Recurrent syncope in a patient in whom organic heart disease has been excluded.
3. Syncope resulting in an accident or injury.
4. Syncope occurring in a high-risk setting.
5. When the establishment of a diagnosis of vasovagal syncope will impact management of syncope of another etiology.

Guidelines for Admission to a Hospital

Patients should be considered for admission to a hospital for initial evaluation and treatment if there is a high risk of injury from a recurrent event or a high risk of a life-threatening arrhythmia. Assessment of the risk of injury should be based on the degree of injury sustained in the current episode, the frequency of episodes, and the fragility of the patient. Assessment of the risk of an arrhythmia should be based on the status of any underlying heart disease and the presence of any current or previous ECG abnormalities.

Syncope from Hypotension or Circulatory Failure

Because of autoregulation, cerebral blood flow is protected over a wide range of systemic blood pressure. In normal people, a critical decrease in CNS blood flow (producing near syncope or syncope) does not occur until the mean blood pressure is below 50 mm Hg. Under a number of circumstances (e.g., sympatholytic drug treatment, cerebrovascular disease), however, the minimal tolerated blood pressure may not be this low. Thus, symptomatic failure of the systemic circulation may occur over a wide range of blood pressures.

Vasovagal (Neurocardiogenic, Vasodepressor) Syncope (Simple Faint)

The simple faint (vasovagal episode) has long been known to afflict young people; it is apt to occur in the setting of anxiety, fatigue, or pain and especially during venipuncture or other painful procedures. The simple faint is not just a disease of the young but can occur in older patients in identical settings. Improved understanding of the pathophysiology of vasovagal syncope has led to the term *neurocardiogenic or vasodepressor syncope.* Episodes are believed to be triggered when venous pooling or catecholamine release leads to increased ventricular contractions and activation of cardiac mechanoreceptors; this causes reflex increase in parasympathetic and decrease in sympathetic nervous system activity, resulting in symptomatic bradycardia or hypotension, termed the Bezold-Jarisch reflex. Vasovagal attacks nearly always occur while the patient is upright, but they may occur while seated; consciousness is nearly always regained promptly when the patient lies down. Typically, there is a prodromal warning period, lasting up to 5 minutes, when the patient feels dizzy or flushed, with mild nausea and occasionally palpitations or throat tightness. If the subject lies down during this stage, loss of consciousness may be avoided. An observer will note cold hands, pale skin, and tachycardia just before the patient loses consciousness. The absence of a prodrome, which may be a more common presentation in the elderly, does not exclude the diagnosis of vasovagal syncope (46). In addition, sudden loss of consciousness does not exclude the diagnosis of vasovagal syncope in any patient. After the faint, a flush replaces the pallor. If the patient is unable to lie flat, recovery may be prolonged; an occasional death has been noted if the person is held upright during the spell. Bradycardia may persist for up to 30 minutes after a simple faint. During this time the patient should remain lying down. The examination is otherwise normal unless there has been trauma or aspiration.

Vasovagal syncope is often selected as a diagnosis of exclusion because the history and physical examination are often nondiagnostic. As noted above (see Diagnostic Tests), standardized *tilt-table testing* can be used to confirm susceptibility to vasovagal syncope in patients for whom this information is needed to make a clinical decision.

In the *treatment of vasodepressor syncope*, education plays an important role. Merely lying down when a prodrome develops may abort a syncopal event. Increasing salt intake may also prevent recurrence. A high-salt diet with liberal fluid intake is commonly suggested, occasionally with the addition of compression stockings. Pharmacologic agents, including disopyramide, fludrocortisone, alpha-blockers, beta-blockers, and selective serotonin reuptake inhibitors, have all been used to treat vasodepressor syncope. The best studied class of drugs is beta-blockers (atenolol 50 mg daily or metoprolol 50 mg twice a day) (50,51). Despite concerns about worsening bradycardia with the addition of beta-blockers, these drugs have been well tolerated when used to treat patients with vasodepressor syncope. In one study, beta-blocker treatment prevented recurrent syncope in 90% of patients for two years or longer (51). Paroxetine (20 mg daily) is also well tolerated in patients with vasodepressor syncope and in one small controlled study decreased the recurrence of syncope over 25 months of treatment as compared with those receiving placebo by two-thirds (52). For patients with vasodepressor syncope and significant bradycardia, cardiac pacing showed promise in a preliminary study, but is undergoing further study for confirmation (53).

Autonomic Impairment

Syncope/near syncope caused by autonomic impairment is always associated with orthostatic hypotension. To document this problem, blood pressure must be taken while the patient is supine and again while standing. In some patients, exercise while standing (e.g., walking for a few minutes) may be required for a significant orthostatic drop (20 mm Hg systolic) to occur.

The most common cause of this problem is *antihypertensive drug use*; most syncope caused by these

Table 89.9. Four Phases of a Normal Valsalva Maneuver

Onset	*Phase I: A sharp rise* in systolic pressure caused by an abrupt increase in intrathoracic pressure and emptying of the pulmonary bed during forced expiration against a closed glottis.
(20–30 s) ↓	*Phase II: A gradual fall* in systolic pressure and a concomitant narrowing of peripheral pulse pressures caused by decrease in pulmonic and systemic venous return. *Heart rate increases* during this phase.
Release	*Phase III:* A sudden *further drop* in blood pressure occurs. Pulse pressure may be very narrow for the few beats during refilling of pulmonary venous reservoir.
	Phase IV (overshoot): Cardiac output increases with the increase in ventricular filling. Within 30 s of release of intrathoracic pressure, blood pressure *rises* above *its original level* because of reflex vasoconstriction initiated by small pulse pressure during phase III. The pressoreceptor stimulation in phase IV results in *transient bradycardia.*

drugs is preventable if the drugs are prescribed cautiously and the standing blood pressure, after exercise, is monitored routinely. Other drugs may also produce orthostatic hypotension (Table 89.5). The management of drug-induced orthostasis requires discontinuation or reduced dosage of the drug.

Orthostatic hypotension can also be caused by *autonomic neuropathy.* In patients suspected of having this problem, the integrity of the autonomic nervous system can be tested by noting the size and reaction of the pupils, the distribution of sweating, and the response to a Valsalva maneuver. The *Valsalva maneuver* is performed by having the patient expire against a closed glottis for 20 to 30 seconds and then release air from the chest (Table 89.9). This maneuver creates a sudden reduction in cardiac output, stimulating vagal (afferent) and sympathetic (efferent) responses. Absence of the reflex tachycardia (phase II) or absence of the blood pressure overshoot and reflex bradycardia (phase IV) indicate autonomic impairment. *Sympathetic failure* commonly occurs late in diabetic peripheral neuropathy (see Chapter 79) and may be the presenting feature of amyloidosis or the neuropathy associated with various neoplasms.

Shy-Drager syndrome, which occurs in late life, is caused by failure of central autonomic neurons and causes orthostatic hypotension, parkinsonism, and other autonomic symptoms in varying combinations. Sympathectomy, particularly when done bilaterally or in the lumbar segments, may be followed immediately by orthostatic hypotension and syncope, although usually venous tone recovers several weeks after the operation. Tabes dorsalis and more commonly diabetic pseudotabes may present with lightning pains and autonomic failure. The management of orthostasis caused by autonomic neuropathy is symptomatic and is summarized in Chapter 92.

Decreased Intravascular Volume

Decreased intravascular volume caused by hemorrhage or salt and water loss (e.g., from gastroenteritis, heat exposure, or diuretics) is recognized by the combination of orthostatic hypotension and an associated basis for the volume deficit. Hot weather and exercise predispose to volume depletion and thereby to syncope, particularly after vigorous exercise. Prolonged fasting, as in anorexia nervosa or with fad diets, also may produce syncope through volume depletion. Adrenal insufficiency caused by pituitary or adrenal disease may produce syncope through the combination of chronic volume deficit and a loss of vascular tone; the syncope is often precipitated by an intercurrent illness. Hypoalbuminemia caused by liver disease, enteropathies, or chronic disease can also lead to syncope/presyncope caused by intravascular volume deficit even though edema may be present. Volume expansion, either by increased salt and water ingestion or by intravenous fluids, is the initial treatment; the choice of ambulatory or hospital management and the planning of definitive treatment depends on the severity and cause of the volume deficit.

Venous Pooling

Venous pooling prevents return of blood to the heart, lowering cardiac output, at times sufficiently to produce near syncope or syncope. Symptoms may occur after prolonged standing in one position, particularly after exercise, as in recruits standing at attention. Severe dependent varicose veins or the compression of pelvic veins by a fetus or a large abdominal mass may produce symptoms through a similar mechanism. Syncope 15 to 30 minutes after exercise has been attributed to dilation of the splanchnic circulation before blood flow to the skeletal muscles has completely returned to normal. Management of these conditions involves chiefly avoidance of the precipitating factors. Supportive elastic stockings may be helpful for patients with marked pooling in varicose veins (see Chapter 95).

Orthostatic Syncope/Near Syncope After Bed Rest

This problem is caused by the combined effects of venous pooling, relative hypovolemia, and probably to some degree lowered sensitivity of the baroreceptor system. It is very common at all ages but is especially common among the elderly and should be anticipated in any person who has been at bed rest for more than a few days; moreover, it may persist for 1 or 2 weeks or longer after mobilization begins. Orthostatic symptoms may be minimized or prevented by having the patient gradually stand only after several minutes of sitting on the bed with the legs dependent. Practical exercises that may help convalescing or deconditioned patients in overcoming postural weakness and hypotension are illustrated in Fig. 89.4. These patients should be encouraged to be out of bed for at least 2 hours a day, including morning, afternoon, and evening.

Orthostasis of Aging

Transient orthostatic dizziness and hypotension occur in many healthy older people. A significant fall in systolic blood pressure also is common in elderly patients immediately after eating, even in a seated position

Leg Exercises
Starting position: Sitting in chair, exercise one leg at a time.

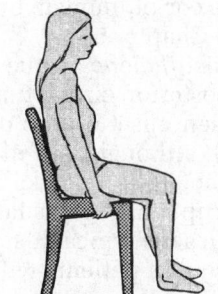

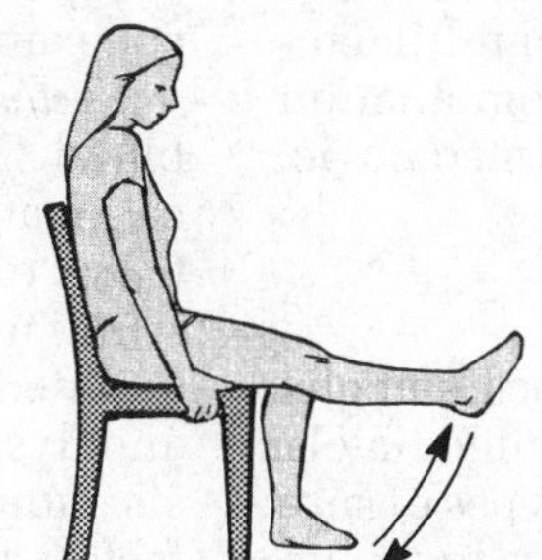

Raise leg up and down. Repeat 10 times.

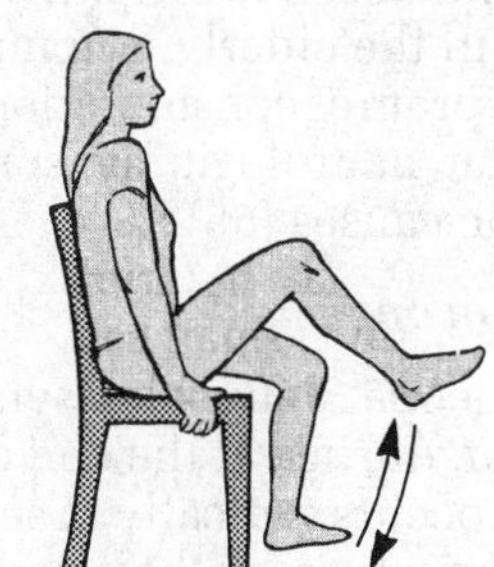

Keeping knee bent, raise leg up and down.
Arm Exercises: To increase effectiveness, hold a soup can in each hand for weight.

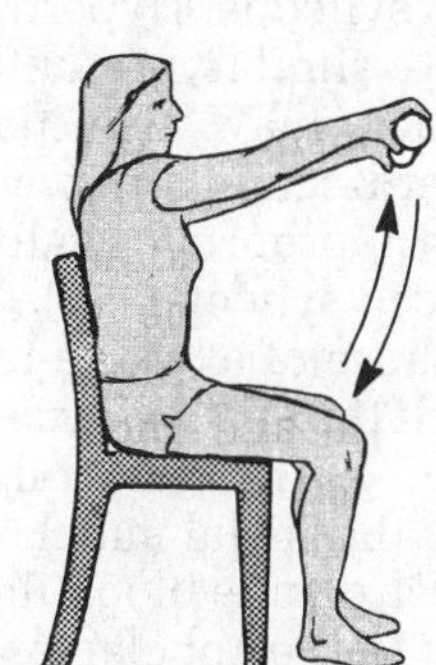

Start with arms straight out in front. Raise arms up and down, only to chin level. Repeat 10 times.

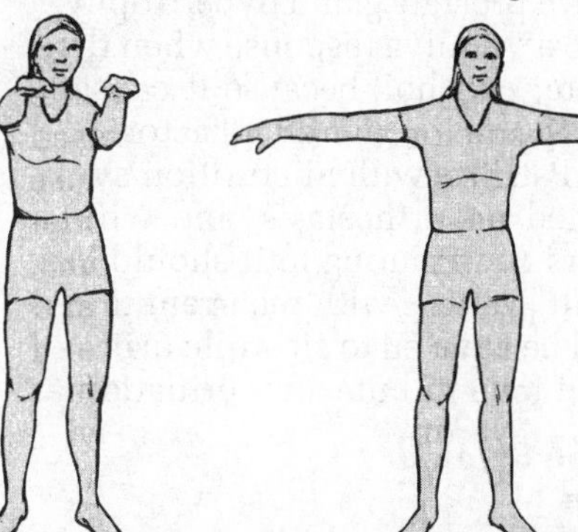

Start with arms straight out in front. Swing arms out to sides and return to front. Repeat 10 times.

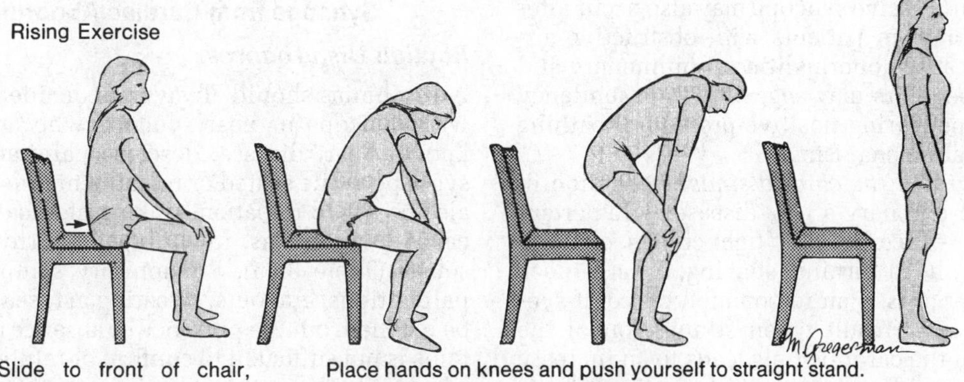

Rising Exercise
Slide to front of chair, keeping legs apart.
Place hands on knees and push yourself to straight stand. Sit down, using hands on knees to help.
Repeat 3–5 times using hands less and legs more each time. Repeat exercise without using hands to help.

Figure 89.4. Exercise for weakness and orthostatic hypotension after prolonged bed rest. Patient must be out of bed 2 hours a day, morning, afternoon, and evening. Exercises are done three times a day. (Courtesy of Karen Ryder, Registered Occupational Therapist.)

(54), which may make them especially susceptible to syncope when standing up after a meal. The physiologic basis for orthostatic symptoms in the elderly is often multifactorial and may be related not only to postural hypotension but also cerebral ischemia, vestibular dysfunction, visual impairment, and abnormal proprioception. The orthostasis of aging is important because it increases the risk associated with drugs that may cause orthostatic hypotension. Clearly, older patients should have their standing blood pressure checked whenever they complain of even mild orthostatic symptoms, and they should be monitored similarly whenever a drug in one of the groups listed in Table 89.5 is prescribed. Those who are troubled by orthostatic symptoms should be advised to follow the steps recommended above for patients rising after bed rest. Dizziness in the elderly is commonly multifactorial and should prompt consideration of a combination of cardiovascular, neurologic, sensory, pharmacologic, and psychologic causes (55).

Micturition Syncope

Micturition syncope, defined as syncope occurring at the beginning of, during, at the end of, or immediately after urination, occurs typically in several types of subjects: Young men who are otherwise healthy, in whom the Valsalva mechanism (see above) and direct vagal stimulation have been hypothesized as the basis for this form of syncope; older men and women, many of whom have baseline orthostasis related to drugs or to aging; and older men with prostate gland hypertrophy, which can predispose to a Valsalva response when the patient strains to urinate. Alcohol, because it causes venous pooling, may also be a predisposing factor, especially in young men. Patients with micturition syncope should be evaluated for orthostasis, and when this is found, any factors contributing to it should be modified. In addition, all patients with recurrent micturition syncope should be advised to sit while urinating and to remain seated for a minute after urination.

Other Forms of Syncope Related to Systemic Circulation

Tussive syncope may follow a prolonged bout of coughing in otherwise normal people or in patients with chronic cough (see Chapter 59), including cough due to gastroesophageal reflux (42). In these patients, the syncope is thought to be caused by the Valsalva mechanism (see above). Tussive syncope may also occur after only a slight cough in patients with obstructive airway disease because abnormalities of pulmonary and pleural vagal receptors may aggravate their tendency to faint. Syncope during positive-pressure breathing occurs by similar mechanisms.

Hypersensitivity of the carotid sinus is common in older men with coronary artery disease or hypertension and may be exacerbated by tight collars, cumbersome necklaces, head turning, shaving, or large neck masses; however, this is an uncommon cause of syncope. Syncope may result when stimulation of the baroreceptors in the carotid sinus leads to an increase in vagal activity with resulting bradycardia or leads to sympathetic relaxation with resulting hypotension (57). If carotid sinus syncope is suspected, one should consider performing a carotid massage (see above). Patients diagnosed as having carotid sinus syncope should be referred to a cardiologist for consideration of anticholinergic treatment or pacemaker insertion, if the symptoms are recurrent or severe.

Pulmonary embolism may cause sudden loss of consciousness in up to 10% of cases. In such cases, unconsciousness may be brief or prolonged and may be accompanied by a small seizure or minor neurologic abnormalities, even when paradoxic embolization has not occurred. The diagnosis of pulmonary embolism is suggested by the presence of dyspnea, hypotension, tachycardia, or acute cor pulmonale by ECG or physical examination (see Chapter 57).

Vertebrobasilar insufficiency, due to decreased blood flow to the posterior circulation of the brain, can lead to the sudden onset of loss of postural tone (i.e., "drop attacks"), although loss of consciousness is not necessarily seen. These attacks may also be associated with the abrupt onset of visual loss, diplopia, and dysarthria. Besides the typical history, the diagnosis should be suspected in patients with multiple risk factors for vascular disease.

Exercise-induced Syncope

Syncope that is brought on with exercise suggests cardiac or vascular causes. Aortic stenosis may limit cardiac output in response to increased demand (e.g., exercise) leading to syncope. Hypertrophic cardiomyopathy may have a similar presentation. Ischemia-induced arrhythmias may also be unmasked by exercise. An echocardiogram followed by exercise tolerance testing is the appropriate evaluation of patients with exercise-induced syncope (58).

An uncommon cause of exercise-induced ischemia is *subclavian steal.* If the subclavian artery is occluded proximal to the origin of the vertebral artery, increased oxygen demand by the distal subclavian artery territory may result in retrograde blood flow ("steal") from the vertebral artery to the subclavian artery. Exercise involving the arm is the typical activity that unmasks subclavian steal. Much more common on the left than on the right, subclavian steal should be associated with a decreased blood pressure on the affected side.

Syncope from Cardiac Abnormalities

Rhythm Disturbances

Arrhythmias should always be considered in patients with syncope or near syncope who are older, have known heart disease, describe palpitations, or have syncope while seated or recumbent. Suspicion should also be raised in patients taking medications that may cause arrhythmias, including antiarrhythmics themselves (Table 89.5). Premonitory symptoms such as palpitations, grayouts, sweating, nausea, and fear may be recalled, but the presence or absence of these symptoms is not sufficient to confirm or refute the diagnosis of an arrhythmia. Most patients with cerebral symptoms of arrhythmias have normal resting ECGs. In general, at least 24 hours of ECG monitoring should be performed to identify potentially important arrhythmias in patients with syncope that is not explained by the initial history, physical examination, and 12-lead ECG (see Electrocardiographic Monitoring above) and some should have EP testing (see above).

Outflow Obstruction

An obstruction to ventricular outflow caused by rheumatic or calcific aortic stenosis may lead to syncope. It nearly always follows exertion and is often associated with chest pain. Unconsciousness may be prolonged and may be followed by neurologic abnormalities. Similarly, hypertrophic cardiomyopathy may lead to syncope by outlet obstruction after exercise or by an arrhythmia at any time. The diagnostic approach to patients thought to have outflow obstruction is described in Chapter 65. A left-atrial myxoma (rare) may cause syncope by obstruction of blood flow when a patient leans over or undergoes exertion. Cyanotic congenital heart disease also leads to syncope after exercise or, rarely, during an airplane flight. Hypoxia and increased blood viscosity are contributing factors.

Myocardial Infarction

Acute myocardial infarction may present with syncope, which may result from an arrhythmia, low cardiac output, or severe pain. Embolization from a mural thrombus should be considered when syncope occurs during recovery from myocardial infarction.

Syncope from Metabolic Abnormalities

The initial history and physical examination should seek to identify any symptoms or signs of metabolic derangement, especially because some derangements may lead to lasting damage.

Hypoglycemia

Loss of consciousness may occur in hypoglycemic adults, although rarely in older patients, when the blood glucose level is below 40 mg/100 mL. Hunger, palpitations, sweating, and anxiety nearly always occur 5 to 15 minutes before the patient loses consciousness. Because the brain can survive for only about 10 minutes with a blood glucose of 20 mg/100 mL or less, the prophylactic administration of glucose is warranted in anyone who remains unconscious long enough for the physician to prepare the solution. Convulsions and incontinence commonly accompany hypoglycemic coma. The evaluation and management of hypoglycemia caused by exogenous insulin are described in Chapter 79. Reactive hypoglycemia and fasting hypoglycemia (which may be caused by insulinoma) may produce near syncope but only rarely unconsciousness. These problems are described in Chapter 81. Mild hypoglycemic symptoms may also occur postprandially in patients who have had ulcer surgery, as part of the dumping syndrome (see Chapter 43).

Hypocapnia (Hyperventilation)

Hypocapnia caused by hyperventilation leads to syncope, near syncope, or ill-defined dizziness by decreasing cerebral blood flow through vasoconstriction of small arterioles throughout the brain. A P_{CO_2} of 25 mm Hg is sufficient to lower cerebral blood flow to levels at which symptoms may occur; such a value may be produced in some people by a few very deep breaths. Athletes preparing to race, musicians playing wind instruments, or anyone who is fearful or anxious may develop transient symptoms in this way. Tetany or carpopedal spasm may or may not precede the cerebral symptoms. Recovery is prompt if ventilation is slowed. Hyperventilation may be a contributing factor in many patients with *chronic dizziness* (59). The diagnosis and management of hyperventilation related to anxiety, the most common cause of this problem, are described in Chapter 22.

Hypoxemia

Hypoxemia caused by any primary cause may predispose to syncope/near syncope. Severe anemia (see Chapter 55) may sufficiently deprive the brain of oxygen to lead to syncope after exercise; it may also predispose to syncope from any other cause. Asphyxiation caused by obstruction of the upper airway should be considered in small children, patients with bad teeth, or patients with masses in the neck. The "cafe coronary" caused by laryngeal aspiration of food is usually betrayed by sudden collapse at the table. However, patients with esophageal diverticula may choke hours after a meal. Poisoning with *carbon monoxide* is suggested by a history of exposure to products of combustion (e.g., poorly ventilated space heaters, gas-burning engines in closed spaces). Manifestations may include prodromal headache and confusion plus bright pink color and prolonged unconsciousness. Short-term exposure to moderate or *high altitude*, even in healthy young adults, may lead to syncope, possibly mediated by a decrease in arterial oxygen saturation (60).

Seizures are common in patients with acute hypoxemia, and neurologic sequelae are the rule after unconsciousness lasting more than 1 or 2 minutes. The management of hypoxemic syncope depends entirely on prompt and accurate diagnosis to prevent recurrence or worsening of the hypoxemia.

Drug Overdose

Overdose of some drugs may cause syncope/near syncope due to orthostatic hypotension. These drugs include sedatives, which may produce venous pooling (particularly chloral hydrate, paraldehyde, and ethanol and less often benzodiazepines and barbiturates), and all the drugs listed as potential causes of autonomic impairment in Table 89.5. However, overdose of most drugs is more likely to cause stupor or coma from their sedating effects than to cause syncope or near syncope from orthostatic hypotension.

Syncope from Intracranial Abnormalities

Seizure

Seizure as a cause of syncope is a diagnosis that is thought to be made easily from historical details. However, as noted above, brief clonic movements are seen in some patients who have syncope unrelated to seizure. In the prospective evaluation of patients presenting with syncope mentioned above, 50% of patients underwent EEG testing, and this confirmed an underlying seizure disorder in only 1.5% (37). It has been demonstrated that the best discriminating finding distinguishing seizure from syncope was orientation immediately after the event, as reported by an eyewitness. A seizure was found to be five times more likely if the patient was reported to be disoriented after the seizure. In the absence of an eyewitness, the age of the patient was the most useful discriminator; a seizure was three times more likely if the patient was younger than 45. Incontinence and trauma were not discriminative findings (61). The diagnosis and management of seizure disorders are described in detail in Chapter 88.

Subarachnoid Hemorrhage

A brief period of unconsciousness at the beginning of subarachnoid hemorrhage is the rule. This diagnosis is strongly suggested when the constellation of headache, confusion, and neck stiffness follows shortly after a syncopal episode. Any patient who is confused and develops headache during initial evaluation should be admitted for observation and evaluation, even if meningismus has not yet developed.

Embolism or Thrombosis

Cerebral embolism or thrombosis may cause brief (TIA) or prolonged (cerebrovascular accident) unconsciousness if the basilar artery is affected. Rarely, a carotid occlusion may cause unconsciousness initially, even if the remaining vessels are patent. A carotid occlusion likewise may cause loss of consciousness if the contralateral carotid is already occluded. In this instance, the period of unconsciousness is usually prolonged and seizures may occur; neurologic symptoms and signs are nearly always present. The diagnosis and management of cerebrovascular disease are described in Chapter 91.

Migraine

Migraine (see Chapter 87) may produce syncope or near syncope by spasm of the basilar artery or of the posterior cerebral arteries. Syncope that occurs with migraine is more often caused by hyperventilation or a vasovagal mechanism than by a central abnormality.

Increased Intracranial Pressure

Increased intracranial pressure, whether caused by a brain tumor, trauma, or an obstruction to the ventricular system, may result in syncope when a Valsalva maneuver is performed such as during straining at defecation or bending over. The hallmarks are pre-existing symptoms, papilledema, and neurologic signs.

Brainstem Compression

Rarely, brainstem compression caused by metastatic tumors, cystic anomalies, or a displaced fracture of C1 or of the odontoid process may lead to syncope with movement of the neck because of transient compression of critical structures of the brainstem. Patients with severe rheumatoid arthritis also may develop cervical instability leading to compression of the brainstem with neck motion (see Chapter 77). Associated neurologic abnormalities are often present. Patients thought to have this problem require prompt hospital admission for diagnosis and treatment.

Syncope from Psychiatric Disorders

As many as 25% of patients with syncope or near syncope may have a psychiatric diagnosis (36). The most common psychiatric diagnoses in patients with unexplained syncope are panic disorders and major depression. However, anxiety disorders, somatization, and conversion disorders also may be frequent causes of syncope or near syncope. The diagnosis and management of these disorders are described in Chapters 21, 22, and 24.

Selected Conditions that May Mimic Syncope

Hysterical Faint

Sudden dramatic fainting was said to be common in the 19th century, especially in women. Today, fainting caused by conversion disorder or other forms of somatization is more common. Usually the fainting occurs in a manner to avoid injury, an important distinguishing feature from true syncope. The patient crumples to the ground with a limp body and shallow respirations. Recovery is usually immediate. Often, the faint may be embellished with movements that resemble seizures, but more often voluntary movements are the rule. Hyperventilation or coaxing may reproduce the spell. Chapter 21 provides additional detail regarding the evaluation and management of such patients, whose physical symptoms are often caused by emotional factors.

Drop Attack

Older patients, especially men, may report sudden and unprovoked falls to the ground. Consciousness is not lost, and the patients can usually remember the entire episode. The history of maintenance of consciousness distinguishes drop attacks from syncope. Ischemia of the lower brainstem is thought to cause drop attacks, and occasionally patients report other concurrent symptoms that suggest vertebrobasilar ischemia. Management is identical to that of TIAs occurring in the posterior circulation (see Chapter 91).

Cataplexy

Cataplexy is a special kind of drop attack, not caused by ischemia that occurs as part of the syndrome of narcolepsy (see Chapter 7). The patient falls suddenly to the ground because of a loss of extensor muscle tone but without loss of consciousness. These spells are usually provoked by a sudden startle, a joke, laughing, or sneezing. They may be effectively managed by tricyclic agents. *Sleep paralysis* (paralysis of the limbs for a minute or 2 upon awakening) and peculiar visual hallucinations on awakening or before falling asleep may also accompany narcolepsy. (See Chapter 7 for additional details.)

DISEQUILIBRIUM OF MISCELLANEOUS ORIGINS

Some patients with persistent dizziness do not have manifestations that make it possible to classify their problem as vertigo or near syncope. Many of these patients have disequilibrium, or a sense of imbalance, that may be caused by cerebellar ataxia (see Chapter 86); multiple sensory deficits (e.g., partial hearing, visual, and proprioceptive impairment); lower extremity weakness (e.g., from an old stroke or from disuse after a period of bed rest); pain in a weight-bearing joint; recently initiated drugs, especially anxiolytics, hypnotics, or neuroleptics; or the onset of a progressive CNS disease such as parkinsonism (see Chapter 90), normal pressure hydrocephalus (see Chapter 26), or cerebellopontine angle tumor (see Chapter 110). These problems often occur in older patients, debilitated patients (particularly chronic alcoholics), or patients with long-standing diabetes mellitus. In these patients, cerebrovascular disease or autonomic neuropathy may cause periodic vertigo and near syncope to be superimposed on their day-to-day problem with imbalance.

The evaluation of patients describing imbalance consists chiefly of obtaining a history of the duration, progression, and day-to-day characteristics of the problem, focusing on the limitations imposed on their usual activities and on any falls or near accidents that may have occurred. In the physical examination, it is important to determine which of the many problems listed above may be contributing to the patient's symptoms.

Depending on the individual patient, management by the generalist may include referring the patient for correction of any impairment in hearing or vision (see Chapters 107 and 110), consulting a neurologist if unexplained progressive symptoms are found (e.g., cerebellar ataxia in an otherwise healthy person), consulting a physical therapist if weakness or the need for selecting a cane or walker is apparent, and discontinuing drugs that may be contributing to the patient's symptoms and avoiding drugs that may worsen symptoms (Tables 89.2 and 89.5).

CHRONIC DIZZINESS: GENERAL MEASURES IN MANAGEMENT

Patients with chronic dizziness, vertigo, syncope, or disequilibrium have a far better prognosis if their home environments are safe and others in their households are aware of risks that should be avoided and devices that may be helpful. A number of general measures to recommend include using night-lights, tacking down loose carpeting and floorboards, installing special railings in the bathroom, selecting proper footwear, and learning to assume an upright posture gradually. These measures can be accomplished most effectively if the physician or a visiting nurse evaluates the patient's home. In some patients with unsteady gait, a cane or a walker may be helpful; a physical therapist can be very helpful in selecting the best assistive device.

General References*

Baloh RW. Antiemetic and antivertigo drugs. In: Rowland LP, ed. Current neurologic drugs. Baltimore: Williams and Wilkins, 1998:184.

Baloh RW. Dizziness, hearing loss, and tinnitus. Philadelphia: F.A. Davis, 1998.

Brandt T. Vertigo: its multisensory syndromes, 2nd ed. London: Springer Verlag, 1999.

Furman JM, Cass SP. Benign paroxysmal positional vertigo. N Engl J Med 1999;341:1590.

Excellent review article.

Hotson JR, Baloh RW. Acute vestibular syndrome. N Engl J Med 1998;340:151.

Linzer M, Yang EH, Estes M III, et al. **Clinical guideline—diagnosing syncope. Part 1. Value of history, physical examination, and electrocardiography.** Ann Intern Med 1997;126:989.

The position paper from the American College of Physicians on the evaluation of the patient with syncope.

Linzer M, Yang EH, Estes M III, et al. **Clinical guideline—diagnosing syncope. Part 2. Unexplained syncope.** Ann Intern Med 1997;127:76.

The position paper from the American College of Physicians on the evaluation of the patient with unexplained syncope.

Specific References

1. Kroenke K, Mangelsdorff AD. Common symptoms in ambulatory care: incidence, evaluation, therapy and outcome. Am J Med 1989;86:262.
2. Warner EA, Wallach PM, Adelman HM, et al. Dizziness in primary care patients. J Gen Intern Med 1992;7:454.
3. Demer JL, Honrubia V, Baloh RW. Dynamic visual acuity: a test for oscillopsia and vestibulo-ocular reflex function. Am J Otol 1994;15:340.
4. Oas JG, Baloh RW. Vertigo and the anterior inferior cerebellar artery syndrome. Neurology 1992;42:2274.
5. Baloh RW, Honrubia V, Jacobson K. Benign positional vertigo: clinical and oculographic features in 240 cases. Neurology 1987;37:371.
6. Epley JM. The canalith repositioning procedure: for treatment of benign paroxysmal positional vertigo. Otolaryngol Head Neck Surg 1992;107:399.
7. Lynn S, Pool A, Rose D, et al. Randomized trial of the canalith repositioning procedure. Otolaryngol Head Neck Surg 1995;113:712.
8. Radtke A, Neuhauser H, von Brevern N, et al. A modified Epley's procedure for self-treatment of benign paroxysmal positional vertigo. Neurology 1999;53:1358.
9. Brandt T, Daroff RB. Physical therapy for benign paroxysmal positional vertigo. Arch Otolaryngol 1980;106:484.
10. Karlberg M, Hall K, Quickert N, et al. What inner ear diseases cause benign paroxysmal positional vertigo? Acta Otolaryngol 2000;120:380.
11. Friedland DR, Wackym PA. A critical appraisal of spontaneous perilymphatic fistulas of the inner ear. Am J Otol 1999;20:261.
12. Minor LB, Solomon D, Zinreich JS, et al. Sound- and/or pressure-induced vertigo due to bone dehiscence of the superior semicircular canal. Arch Otolaryngol Head Neck Sur 1998;124:249.
13. Gomez CR, Cruz-Flores S, Malkoff MD, et al. Isolated vertigo as a manifestation of vertebrobasilar ischemia. Neurology 1996;47:94s.
14. Neuhauser H, Leopold M, von Brevern M, et al. The interrelations of migraine, vertigo, and migrainous vertigo. Neurology 2001;56:436.
15. Dietrich M, Brandt T. Episodic vertigo related to migraine (90 cases): vestibular migraine? J Neurol 1999;246:883.
16. Swartz KL, Pratt LA, Armenian HK, et al. Mental disorders and the incidence of migraine headaches in a community sample:

*Bold print (general references) and bold numerals (specific references) denote published controlled clinical trials, meta-analyses, or consensus-based recommendations.

results from the Baltimore Epidemiologic Catchment area follow-up study. Arch Gen Psychiatry 2000;57:945.
17. Staab JP. Diagnosis and treatment of psychologic symptoms and psychiatric disorders in patients with dizziness and imbalance. Otolaryngol Clin North Am 2000;33:617.
18. Yardley L, Owen, N, Nazareth I, et al. Panic disorder with agoraphobia associated with dizziness: characteristic symptoms and psychosocial sequelae. J Nerv Ment Dis 2001;189:321.
19. Yardley L. Overview of psychologic effects of chronic dizziness and balance disorders. Otolaryngol Clin North Am 2000;33:603.
20. Halmagyi GM, Fattore CM, Curthoys IS, et al. Gentamicin vestibulotoxicity. Otolaryngol Head Neck Surg 1994;111:571.
21. Minor LB. Gentamicin-induced bilateral vestibular hypofunction. JAMA 1998;279:541.
22. Baloh RW, Jacobson K, Fife T. Familial vestibulopathy: a new dominantly inherited syndrome. Neurology 1994;44:20.
23. Brandt T. Bilateral vestibulopathy revisited. Eur J Med Res 1996;1:361.
24. Rinne T, Bronstein AM, Rudge P, et al. Bilateral loss of vestibular function: clinical findings in 53 patients. J Neurol 1998;245:314.
25. Takeda N, Matsunaga T. Neurochemical basis of motion sickness and its treatment and prevention. In: Baloh RW, Halmagyi GM, eds. Disorders of the vestibular system. New York: Oxford University Press, 1996:529.
26. Hain TC. Mal de debarquement. Arch Otolaryngol Head Neck Surg 1999;125:615.
27. Kapoor WN. Workup and management of patients with syncope. Med Clin North Am 1995;79:1153.
28. Savage DD, Corwin L, McGee DL, et al. Epidemiologic features of isolated syncope: the Framingham Study. Stroke 1985;16:626.
29. Young WF, Maddox DE. Spells: in search of a cause. Mayo Clin Proc 1995;70:757.
30. Farrehi PM, Santinga JT, Eagle KA. Syncope: diagnosis of cardiac and non-cardiac causes. Geriatrics 1995;50:24.
31. Fenton AM, Hammill SC, Rea RF, et al. Vasovagal syncope. Ann Intern Med 2000;133:714.
32. Hybels RL. Drug toxicity of the inner ear. Med Clin North Am 1979;63:309.
33. Bass EB, Elson JJ, Fogoros RN, et al. Long-term prognosis of patients undergoing electrophysiologic studies for syncope of unknown origin. Am J Cardiol 1988;62:1186.
34. Kapoor WN, Hanusa BH. Is syncope a risk factor for poor outcomes? Comparison of patients with and without syncope. Am J Med 1996;100:646.
35. Kapoor WN, Fortunato M, Hanusa BH, et al. Psychiatric illnesses in patients with syncope. Am J Med 1995;99:505.
36. Linzer M, Varia I, Pontinen M, et al. Medically unexplained syncope: relationship to psychiatric illness. Am J Med 1992;92[Suppl 1A]:18S.
37. Kapoor WN. Syncope. N Engl J Med 2000;343:1856.
38. Linzer M, Yang EH, Estes M III, et al. Clinical guideline—diagnosing syncope. Part 1. Value of history, physical examination, and electrocardiography. Ann Intern Med 1997;126:989.
39. Sloane PD, Linzer M, Pontinen M, et al. Clinical significance of a dizziness history in medical patients with syncope. Arch Intern Med 1991;151:1625.
40. Linzer M, Pritchett ELC, Pontinen M, et al. Incremental diagnostic yield of loop electrocardiographic recorders in unexplained syncope. Am J Cardiol 1990;66:214.
41. DeMarco JP, Philbrick JT. Use of ambulatory electrocardiographic (Holter) monitoring. Ann Intern Med 1990;113:53.
42. Bass EB, Curtiss EI, Arena VC, et al. The duration of Holter monitoring in patients with syncope. Arch Intern Med 1990;150: 1073.
43. Krahn AD, Klein GJ, Norris C, et al. The etiology of syncope in patients with negative tilt table and electrophysiological testing. Circulation 1995;92:1819.
44. Denniss AR, Ross DL, Richards DA, et al. Electrophysiologic studies in patients with unexplained syncope. Int J Cardiol 1995;35:211.
45. Denes P, Uretz E, Ezri MD, et al. Clinical predictors of electrophysiologic findings in patients with syncope of unknown origin. Arch Intern Med 1988;148:1922.
46. Sutton R, Bloomfield DM. Indications, methodology and classification of results of tilt-table testing. Am J Cardiol 1999;84: 10Q.
47. Fitzpatric AP, Theodorakis G, Vardas P, et al. Methodology of head-up tilt testing in patients with unexplained syncope. J Am Coll Cardiol 1991;17:125.
48. Grubb BP. Pathophysiology and differential diagnosis of neurocardiogenic syncope. Am J Cardiol 1999;84:3Q.
49. Benditt DG, Ferguson DW, Grubb BP, et al. Tilt table testing for assessing syncope. J Am Coll Cardiol 1996;28:263.
50. Mahanonda N, Bhuripanyo K, Kangkagate C, et al. Randomized double blind, placebo-controlled trial of oral atenolol in patients with unexplained syncope and positive upright tilt table test results. Am Heart J 1995;130:1250.
51. Cox MM, Perlman BA, Mayor MR, et al. Acute and long-term beta-adrenergic blockade for patients with neurocardiogenic syncope. J Am Coll Cardiol 1995;26:1293.
52. DiGirolamo E, DiIorio C, Sabatini P, et al. Effects of paroxetine hydrochloride, a selective serotonin reuptake inhibitor, on refractory vasovagal syncope: a randomized, double-blind, placebo-controlled study. J Am Coll Cardiol 1999;33:1227.
53. Connolly SJ, Sheldon R, Roberts RS, et al. The North American Vasovagal Pacemaker Study (VPS): a randomized trial of permanent cardiac pacing for the prevention of vasovagal syncope. J Am Coll Cardiol 1999;33:16.
54. Lipsitz LA, Nyquist RP, Wei JY, et al. Postprandial reduction in blood pressure in the elderly. N Engl J Med 1983;309:81.
55. Tinetti ME, Williams CS, Gill TM. Dizziness among older adults: a possible geriatric syndrome. Ann Intern Med. 2000;132: 337.
56. Puetz TR, Vakil N. Gastroesophageal reflux-induced cough syncope. Am J Gastroenterol 1995;90:2204.
57. Sugrue DD, Wood DL, McGoon MD. Carotid sinus hypersensitivity and syncope. Mayo Clin Proc 1984;59:637.
58. Linzer M, Yang EH, Estes M III, et al. Clinical guideline—diagnosing syncope. Part 2. Unexplained syncope. Ann Intern Med 1997;127:76.
59. Kroenke K, Lucas CA, Rosenberg ML, et al. Causes of persistent dizziness: a prospective study of 100 patients in ambulatory care. Ann Intern Med 1992;117:898.
60. Nicholas R, O'Meara PD, Calonge N. Is syncope related to moderate altitude exposure? JAMA 1992;268:904.
61. Hoefnagels WAJ, Padberg GW, Overweg J, et al. Transient loss of consciousness: the value of the history for distinguishing seizure from syncope. J Neurol 1991;238:39.

CHAPTER 90

Common Disorders of Movement: Tremor and Parkinson Disease

PAUL S. FISHMAN, MD, PhD

TREMOR AND OTHER ABNORMAL MOVEMENTS

Definition and Classification of Tremor

Tremor is defined as the involuntary rhythmic or oscillatory movement of a body part, resulting from alternating contractions of antagonistic muscle groups. Tremor is conveniently classified by its relationship to the conditions of rest, postural maintenance, and movement (kinetic or intention tremor) (1). Accurate classification of tremor type is important because each points to a group of specific underlying conditions (Table 90.1), with specific therapy.

Other Abnormal Movements

Tremor can usually be distinguished by its rhythmicity and the presence or absence of other neurologic signs but can be confused with other abnormal movements. The simplest abnormal movement is *myoclonus.* This is a brief twitch or jerk of a single muscle or fragment of a muscle. Such a movement can be normal, such as the myoclonic jerk associated with the early stages of sleep. When occurring repetitively throughout many muscle groups, they are frequently a sign of an underlying metabolic encephalopathy. In this setting they usually coexist with asterixis, (sometimes referred to as negative myoclonus). During *asterixis,* there is a sudden pause in muscle activity with a brief loss of posture. Myoclonus may be repetitive but is usually not rhythmic. The rare forms of repetitive myoclonus are more commonly confused with focal motor seizures with twitch-like quality. Patients who survive hypoxic/ischemic brain injury can also later develop myoclonic jerks with action or intention movements of the limb. This form of action, myoclonus, can be confused with an intention type tremor.

Chorea refers to brief rapid distal movements. These jerky movements are more complex than myoclonus, usually involving a small group of muscles in rapid succession. The speed and duration of chorea is variable, and these movements usually coexist with slower proximal writhing movements called *athetosis.* The best descriptions of choreoathetosis come from patients with Huntington disease, but these movements can occur with injury to the basal ganglia associated with other conditions such as stroke, acquired immunodeficiency syndrome, and systemic lupus erythematosis and after streptococcal infection (Syndeham chorea) and chronic neuroleptic exposure (tardive dyskinesia). Dramatic, vigorous, flinging movements are termed *ballismis* and can be viewed as an extreme form of chorea.

Sustained abnormal posture is referred to as *dystonia.* Dystonia can occur throughout the body (generalized), usually on an inherited basis, but is usually restricted to a specific body part (focal dystonia). *Cervical dystonia,* also called *spasmodic torticollis* or wry neck, is the most common focal dystonia characterized by intermittent or constant abnormal twisting of the neck. Tremor is commonly observed superimposed on a dystonic posture. Focal dystonia can also be provoked by specific movements (*action dystonia*). The involuntary muscle contraction of *writer's cramp* is the most common action dystonia.

Tics are repetitive rapid movements distinguished from chorea by their stereotyped pattern. They can be distinguished from tremor by their lack of rhythmicity, erratic appearance in different body parts, complexity of movement, and onset in childhood or adolescence. They often are associated with vocalizations and behavioral disturbances as in *Tourette syndrome.* Tics are often preceded by a buildup of inner tension that subsides after the tic. Patients may be able to temporarily suppress a tic, whereas most other abnormal movements usually lack such a degree of voluntary control.

EVALUATION OF THE PATIENT WITH TREMOR

The history and physical examination are fundamental in the diagnosis of tremor (Table 90.2), and in almost all cases no further workup is necessary. The differential diagnosis, in general practice, is almost always between Parkinson disease (PD) and essential tremor (ET). Most patients with tremor and other movement disorders do not have any specific abnormality on laboratory investigation (including imaging).

History

Important historical information includes the temporal onset of the tremor, associated neurologic symptoms, family history, a survey of medications and other medical illnesses, and whether the tremor is suppressed by alcohol. Almost all varieties of tremor increase in amplitude under stress, diminish with relaxation, and disappear during sleep. The impact of the tremor on the patient determines whether treatment is indicated. Some patients do not find their tremor disabling and seek medical attention only for diagnostic purposes. Young patients with ET may need only reassurance that their tremor is benign and that they do not have PD or another degenerative disorder. However, most patients find the tremor physically or emotionally problematic.

Emphasis should be placed on the *activities of daily living* (ADLs). Patients with tremor typically have trouble with tasks requiring fine motor control such as buttoning, feeding, shaving, brushing their teeth, writing, and cooking. Embarrassment is often an unvoiced source of disability, and patients should be questioned about social isolation caused by the tremor. The ADLs also provide objective parameters for judging the effectiveness of therapy.

Table 90.1. Conditions Associated with the Three Major Types of Tremor

- Resting tremor
  - Parkinson disease
  - Secondary parkinsonism: postencephalitic, toxic (neuroleptics, reserpine, carbon monoxide, manganese, carbon disulfide, MPTP),
  - Multisystem degenerative diseases with parkinsonian features
- Postural tremor
  - Exaggerated physiological tremor
    - Anxiety, fright, fatigue, exercise
    - Endocrine: thyrotoxicosis, hypoglycemia, pheochromocytoma
    - Drugs: any sympathomimetics, amiodarone, caffeine, theophylline, L-dopa, lithium, tricyclic antidepressants, neuroleptics, thyroid hormone, hypoglycemic agents, withdrawal from alcohol and sedative-hypnotic drugs
  - Essential tremor
    - Familial (autosomal dominant)
    - Sporadic
    - With other neurologic disorders: parkinsonism, torsion dystonia, spasmodic torticollis, neuropathy
- Kinetic or intention tremor (cerebellar dysfunction)
  - Cerebellar degeneration: inherited disease (spino-cerebellar atrophies), alcohol-abuse related, paraneoplastic syndromes
  - Cerebellar lesions due to stroke, hemorrhage, multiple sclerosis, or tumor
  - Drugs and toxins: phenytoin, barbiturates, lithium, alcohol, mercury, 5-fluorouracil, cyclosporin

MPTP, 1-methyl-4-phenyl-1,2,3,6-tetrahydropyridine.

Physical Examination

The objectives of the physical examination are to determine the frequency and conditions of maximal activation of the tremor and to search for associated neurologic signs. Patients should be examined with their hands resting on their laps, with their arms held outstretched, and while performing finger-to-nose and heel-to-shin maneuvers. Samples of handwriting and a drawing of a spiral should also be obtained as an objective means of following response to therapy. Observations while the patient is drinking from a cup or using a fork or spoon are also helpful in assessing functional impairment.

The *resting tremor of parkinsonism* is characterized by 3- to 6-Hz flexion–extension at the metacarpophalangeal joints, abduction–adduction of the thumb, and pronation–supination of the forearm; these produce the so-called pill-rolling tremor. Resting tremor is often brought out by having the patient walk or by distracting the patient with conversation or mental arithmetic. Early in its course, the parkinsonian tremor is almost always unilateral, which is one of the most helpful signs distinguishing it from ET. ET almost always begins bilaterally, although it may be asymmetric.

Table 90.2. Principal Features of Different Tremor Types

	Resting (Parkinsonian)	Postural (Essential)	Kinetic or Intention (Cerebellar)
History			
Age at onset	60 yr and older	All ages, more common after age 60	All ages
Family history	Negative	Often positive (autosomal dominant)	Occasionally positive
Response to alcohol	No effect	Often suppresses tremor	No effect or worsening
Physical examination			
Frequency	3–6 Hz[a]	6–12 Hz	3–5 Hz
Symmetry	Almost always begins unilaterally	Symmetric	Either symmetric or asymmetric
Body part(s) affected	Arms > legs	Hand > head > voice	Arms > legs > trunk/head
Associated signs	Bradykinesia, rigidity, postural instability	None	Dysarthria, nystagmus, broad-based gait

[a]Hz (Hertz), cycles per second.

Postural tremor is characteristic of ET and consists of 6- to 12-Hz symmetric flexion–extension at the wrists and shoulders. It is brought on by having the patient assume an antigravity posture of the upper extremities (i.e., outstretched arms), and it is not present when the arms are resting against the body or on a surface. ET may persist during finger-to-nose testing, leading to the misdiagnosis of a cerebellar tremor.

Kinetic tremor (also called *intention tremor*) is encountered most commonly in cerebellar disease and is characterized by 3- to 5-Hz irregular oscillations as the limb approaches a target. This type of tremor is often accompanied by inaccuracies in direction (dysmetria). In acquired cerebellar diseases, such as stroke and multiple sclerosis, kinetic tremors are often asymmetric, whereas heredofamilial and sporadic degenerative diseases involving the cerebellum produce bilateral symmetric tremor. Conditions that may mimic this aspect of cerebellar disease include marked ET (which may impair purposeful movements) and proprioceptive loss. Careful assessment of all the patient's signs and symptoms usually makes it possible to distinguish these conditions from true cerebellar dysfunction. Unlike patients with PD or ET, patients with cerebellar impairment rarely present complaining only of tremor. Additional signs pointing toward the cerebellum include gait ataxia, dysarthria, and nystagmus.

In general, it is difficult to estimate the rhythmic frequency of a tremor in a clinical setting. Tremors are commonly described as "fine" or "coarse"—a nonuseful composite of frequency and amplitude. Particularly for ET, it is useful to attempt to rate the severity of tremor by its peak to peak amplitude (severe, greater than 1 to 2 cm). This aspect is most clearly related to both disability and response to treatment.

PHYSIOLOGIC AND EXAGGERATED PHYSIOLOGIC TREMOR

Most people have a barely perceptible postural tremor, so-called physiologic tremor, that may be best appreciated by placing a piece of paper over the outstretched hands. Although asymptomatic, this tremor may be transiently exacerbated during systemic illness, metabolic derangements, stress, and by the use or withdrawal of certain drugs or alcohol (Table 90.1). The most important step in management is identification and removal of the offending cause; resolution of the tremor confirms the diagnosis of exaggerated physiologic tremor. Although discontinuation of tremorogenic drugs usually leads to prompt resolution of the tremor, it may take 1 to 2 weeks for the tremor to resolve after resolution of a systemic illness or a severe metabolic abnormality. It is difficult to distinguish an enhanced physiologic tremor from mild ET. The proof of this diagnosis rests on the resolution of the tremor. If the underlying condition cannot be eliminated (e.g., in patients requiring lithium for manic-depressive illness), the tremor can often be suppressed using medications for ET. For patients subject to situational anxiety manifested by exaggerated physiologic tremor, prophylactic treatment with propranolol (20 to 40 mg) taken 1 hour before an anxiety-producing situation (e.g., public speaking) may be helpful.

ESSENTIAL TREMOR

Characteristics

ET, the most common form of postural tremor, affects more than 1 million Americans (2). ET is synonymous with familial tremor, benign ET, and senile tremor when it occurs in the elderly. No neuropathologic abnormalities have been identified in ET, but physiologic evidence suggests that both the central and peripheral nervous systems are involved. The onset is insidious and may begin as early as childhood, but ET characteristically presents in adulthood, usually after age 50. Unlike the tremor of PD, which typically makes the patient seek medical attention within months of its onset, patients with ET often give a history of tremor going back many years. At least 50% of patients with ET give a positive family history; the inheritance is autosomal dominant. Patients with a positive family history are more likely to have a younger age at onset.

In its prototypical form, ET is characterized by a bilateral and symmetric tremor of the hands, but it may also affect other body parts either in isolation (commonly the head or voice) or combined with a hand tremor. At least half of patients with ET notice a beneficial effect from small amounts of alcohol (3). Although its regular use to suppress tremor should be discouraged, when used sparingly alcohol is an effective treatment for ET, particularly when exacerbated by situational stress. There does not seem to be an increased prevalence of alcoholism among patients with ET (4).

Treatment

When ET begins to interfere with the ADLs or causes significant embarrassment, treatment is indicated. Before starting medication, patients should be told that the goal of treatment is not to abolish the tremor, which is rarely possible, but instead to reduce its severity and allow them to function better. The patient's ADLs should be used as a gauge to determine the effectiveness of treatment. As with physiologic tremor, treatment begins with elimination of potentially exacerbating factors, including stimulant drugs and medication. ET also has a consistent relationship to exercise where education may help in its control (5). The tremor is worsened directly after vigorous physical exercise of the involved limb due to fatigue but is also more problematic if exercise is entirely avoided and the involved muscles become deconditioned. Some prosthetic devices, such as handwriting aids, are useful in reducing the disability of ET, particularly for patients who tolerate medications poorly.

The two medications most effective for ET are propranolol and primidone. The drugs are equally effective and may be synergistic (6). Surprisingly, despite its prevalence, none of the medications used in the treatment of ET is approved by the Food and Drug Administration (FDA) for this indication.

Propranolol is started at 10 mg twice per day in elderly patients and gradually increased, depending on the beneficial response and appearance of side effects, to a maximum of 320 mg/day. Once a stable dosage has been reached, patients can be converted to a long-acting form, because the once-daily administration is preferred by most patients (7). In younger patients, treatment can be started with the controlled release form (60 mg) with a gradual escalation of the dosage. Although other beta-blockers have also been shown to be effective for ET, none is superior to propranolol (8,9). Newer beta-blockers have the theoretical advantage of being beta-1 selective and therefore safer to use in patients with ET and asthma, but at the higher dosages usually needed, beta-1 selectivity is diminished. In general, beta-blockers should be avoided in the presence of bronchospastic disease, second- or third-degree heart block, or insulin-dependent diabetes.

Primidone, a barbiturate-like anticonvulsant, was found by serendipity to improve ET. The mechanism of action of primidone is unknown, but its effect does not appear to result from either of its metabolites, phenylethylmalonamide and phenobarbital (10). Primidone is available as scored tablets in two strengths, 50 and 250 mg. The starting dosage must be very low (e.g., 25 mg/day) because occasional patients (5% to 10%, especially the elderly) develop severe side effects after even a single small dose, known as the first-dose phenomenon. Symptoms include dizziness, lethargy, confusion, nausea, sedation, and ataxia, which usually diminish with continued use. The dose is initially given at bedtime and then gradually escalated to a maximum of 250 mg three times per day as tolerated. In general, if patients show no response to low dosages (250 mg/day), it is rare for higher dosages to be effective.

If there is a beneficial but suboptimal response to either propranolol or primidone used alone, the two should be combined beginning at low dosages and increasing in small increments, watching carefully for side effects, particularly in elderly patients. Blood levels of primidone or phenobarbital are not helpful (unless toxicity or noncompliance is suspected) because they do not correlate with its tremor-suppressing effect.

In general, patients who fail to respond to propanolol or primidone have a poor chance of success with other drugs. Although benzodiazepines have been widely prescribed for ET, the clinical trial experience with these drugs has been mixed at best. It has been difficult to assign an antitremor affect to these agents independent of their anxiolytic effect (11).

The most useful of the benzodiazepines is alprazolam, which has been shown to be effective in the treatment of ET (12). The maintenance dosage is 0.75 to 3.0 mg/day, in divided doses. Its rapid onset of action and intermediate half-life, in comparison with other benzodiazepines, allow for its intermittent use when situational stress temporarily exacerbates ET.

Stereotactic ablation of the ventral intermediate nucleus of the thalamus has long been accepted as the most effective treatment of severe or disabling ET (13). Effective to dramatic reduction of ET (80% to 90% decrease in amplitude) has also been demonstrated after ventral intermediate nucleus of the thalamus implantation of a high frequency stimulation device (14). These devices, usually termed deep brain stimulators (DBS), are FDA approved for control of tremor associated with either ET or PD. Implantation of thalamic DBS has a slightly lower risk of neurologic deficit but is a more extensive procedure requiring surgical placement of the pacemaker-like device in the chest and a continuing risk of device or lead malfunction (15,16). DBS placement is generally preferred over standard thalamotomy, although the older procedure may be more suitable for specific patients. Although the risk of serious morbidity is relatively low (less than 5%), patients referred for stereotactic surgery should first have an adequate trial of medication to control ET.

Intramuscular injection of *botulinum toxin,* the standard treatment of focal dystonia, has been used to treat ET as well. Most of the success of this therapy comes in patients with tremor localized to the head. Treatment of ET involving the hands is difficult to achieve without causing weakness of the involved muscles (17,18). Several other medications have shown benefit for ET in open-label studies that has not been verified in placebo-controlled trials, including clonidine, acetazolamide, and methazolamine. Studies of the anticonvulsant gabapentin for tremor have given conflicting results, whereas another new anticonvulsant, topiramate, has shown some effectiveness in small studies (19–21). These anticonvulsants appear to act by enhancing the action of the inhibitory neurotransmitter gamma-aminobutyric acid. The potential of this strategy has been demonstrated by reduction of tremor with intraoperative brain injection of gamma-aminobutyric acid agonists.

The atypical neuroleptic *clozapine* has also shown efficacy in otherwise refractory cases of ET. This drug is worth considering despite its potential to cause agranulocytosis, because its risk is lower than that of surgery for treatment of ET (22).

TREMOR CAUSED BY CEREBELLAR DYSFUNCTION (KINETIC OR INTENTION TREMOR)

Tremor is rarely the sole presenting sign of cerebellar dysfunction, and most often the underlying disease is already known or readily apparent (multiple sclerosis, stroke, drug intoxication, long-standing alcoholism, head trauma, inherited disease, or paraneoplastic syndrome). Occasionally, severe ET may be exacerbated with action, giving the impression of cerebellar disease, but the faster frequency, prominent postural component, and lack of associated cerebellar signs usually suffice to distinguish the ET from cerebellar dysfunction.

With the exception of drug-induced cerebellar tremor (Table 90.1), which should be managed by discontinuation or reduction of the dosage of the offending drug, a patient with newly diagnosed cerebellar tremor should be referred to a neurologist. Cerebellar tremors in general respond poorly to medication, which may also reflect the fact the tremor is intimately related to poor control of ballistic movements. Relatively small trials of clonazepam, carbamazepine, and isoniazid have shown some efficacy for cerebellar tremor. As with severe ET, there is a role for an occupational therapist. Weighted bracelets have had some benefit in dampening the tremor, and specialized devices to aid in writing and feeding are useful. Computer-controlled tremor damping gloves are under investigation to control severe ataxic tremor. As is the case with severe ET, stereotactic thalamotomy is a viable option for disabling cerebellar tremor (23).

PRIMARY WRITING TREMOR AND ORTHOSTATIC TREMOR

Two uncommon but distinct types of tremor are primary writing tremor (24) and primary orthostatic tremor (25,26). *Primary writing tremor* is one variant of a group of task-specific tremors. These are characterized by maximal activation during a specific task. Primary writing tremor occurs exclusively when patients attempt to write. It probably is related to ET but may share some features in common with focal action dystonias, such as writer's cramp. Writing tremor may respond to drugs used to treat ET (see above) or treatments of action dystonias such as anticholinergics or botulinum therapy. *Primary orthostatic tremor* is characterized by rapid shaking of the legs, only with standing, and may respond to clonazepam (0.5 to 3.0 mg/day).

PARKINSON DISEASE AND "PARKINSONISM"

Epidemiology

PD is one of the most common neurologic diseases in the ambulatory setting. Between 500,000 and 1 million persons are affected in the United States. The annual incidence of PD is about 18 per 100,000. In general, PD increases in incidence with age, with an average age at onset of 60. The incidence of PD appears to decline in the very old (27). This observation, along with the increasing incidence of tremor and other extrapyramidal symptoms in the elderly, makes the diagnosis of new-onset PD over age 80 somewhat suspect. Recently, there has been heightened awareness of young-onset PD; up to 5% of PD patients have an age at onset below 40 (28).

Pathogenesis

Premature dysfunction and death of *dopamine*-producing (and *neuromelanin*-containing) neurons of the substantia nigra is the basis for both the major motor symptoms of PD and its treatment. Along with neuronal loss, the pathologic hallmark of PD is an eosinophilic cytoplasmic inclusion called a Lewy body. Although the cause of PD in most cases is unknown, PD is emerging as the proving ground for theories of the interaction of environmental and genetic factors in neuronal aging and death. The evidence for an environmental basis of PD comes from two sources. In 1983, it was discovered that an impurity in the illegal production of meperidine, called MPTP (methyl-phenyl-tetra-pyridine), was capable of causing irreversible Parkinson symptoms in abusers who injected the drug (29). MPTP injection can cause similar symptoms in animals along with the death of dopaminergic nigral neurons. The mechanism of MPTP toxicity has been extensively studied and involves its metabolism within the brain by monoamine oxidase to a toxic metabolite that is taken up by dopaminergic cells. The final steps of toxicity involve impairment of mitochondrial energy generation, suggesting a role for oxidative injury. Dopamine and neuromelanin metabolism may also place nigral neurons at greater risk of oxidative injury (30). Epidemiologic studies also support a role for environmental factors in PD. An increased incidence of PD is found in farm workers with long-standing exposure to herbicides and pesticides (27,31).

Genetic factors clearly play a role in the development of PD. Five percent to 10% of PD patients have an affected first-degree relative. Two identified genes have been clearly associated with inherited forms of PD. Mutations in the gene for the protein *alpha-synuclein* lead to a form of PD, inherited on an autosomal dominant basis (32). Although families carrying these mutations are extremely rare, the role of alpha-synuclein in both inherited and sporadic PD is suggested by the observation that alpha-synuclein is a major component of Lewy bodies (33). Recessively inherited young-onset PD has been strongly associated with mutations in the gene for an enzyme termed *parkin* involved in the ubiquitin-proteasome pathway for degradation of aberrant cellular proteins (34).

Differential Diagnosis

The cardinal signs of PD include tremor at rest, bradykinesia, muscular rigidity, and postural instability. Common symptoms along with tremor include impaired handwriting (micrographia); difficulty walking; falling; poor coordination; difficulty arising from a deep chair, couch, or the toilet; drooling; and difficulty turning in bed. When the syndrome is fully developed, the diagnosis is straightforward. Patients where tremor dominates the clinical picture can be confused with ET, whereas patients without a resting tremor are difficult to distinguish from the other parkinsonian syndromes described below.

Although a discussion of each of the parkinsonian syndromes in Table 90.3 is beyond the scope of this chapter, three deserve special mention because the treatment and prognosis differ. Table 90.4 suggests clinical clues to these syndromes as well. *Neuroleptic-induced parkinsonism,* may be clinically indistinguishable from idiopathic PD and can be diagnosed only retrospectively when parkinsonian signs resolve after discontinuation of the offending drug. In some patients signs may take as long as 1 year to resolve completely, emphasizing the periodic need to reassess

Table 90.3. Differential Diagnosis of Parkinsonism

Toxins
- Manganese
- Carbon monoxide
- Carbon disulfide
- Cyanide
- Methanol
- MPTP

Drug induced
- Neuroleptics
- Metoclopramide (Reglan), Compazine

Multisystem degenerations
- Progressive supranuclear palsy
- Multisystem atrophy (includes the Shy-Drager syndrome, olivopontocerebellar atrophy, striatonigral degeneration)
- Cortico basal ganglionic degeneration

Primary dementing illnesses
- Alzheimer disease
- Creutzfeldt-Jakob syndrome
- Lewy body dementia

Heredofamilial diseases
- Wilson disease
- Juvenile Huntington disease
- Hallervorden-Spatz disease

Multi-infarct state: vascular parkinsonism

Trauma: dementia parkinsonism pugilistica

Senile gait disorder

Normal pressure hydrocephalis

Other structural lesions of the basal ganglia (tumor, arterioveacus malformation)

Table 90.4. Clinical Features Suggesting a Parkinsonian Syndrome Rather than Idiopathic Parkinson Disease

- Little or no response to L-dopa
- Bilaterally symetric involvement
- Early-onset dementia
- Rapid progression
- Early-onset dysarthria or dysphagia
- Prominent and early dysautonomia
- Early falling
- Impaired ocular motility
- Positive family history
- Lower motor neuron, cerebellar, or pyramidal signs

antiparkinsonian therapy. In patients whose signs never resolve, it is likely that the neuroleptic simply uncovered a case of latent PD.

Progressive supranuclear palsy is the most common nonpharmacologic mimic of PD. It is distinguished by impaired vertical eye movements, although early in its course ocular motility may be full with the only clinical clue being slow vertical saccades. Other distinguishing features include neck extension as opposed to the flexion seen in PD, early dysarthria and dysphagia, early and prominent balance and gait impairment with associated falls, greater axial than appendicular rigidity (axial dystonia), progression to severe disability in 5 to 10 years, and limited response to antiparkinsonian medications (35,36).

Wilson disease (hepatolenticular degeneration) is an autosomal-recessive condition characterized by copper accumulation throughout the body. Parkinsonian features in a young patient should prompt an investigation for this condition. Liver disease may be present at the onset of neurologic disease, but normal liver studies should not deter one from pursuing the diagnosis. The diagnosis is confirmed by demonstrating Kayser-Fleischer rings (green or golden deposits of copper in the Descemet membrane of the cornea), low blood ceruloplasmin, and elevated urinary copper excretion. Although a rare cause of abnormal movements, Wilson's disease is noteworthy as a potentially reversible cause of parkinsonism. Timely diagnosis and treatment with copper chelating agents such as penicillamine (1 to 2 g/day) can prevent progression and to some extent reverse neurologic signs and symptoms (37).

Manifestations

Resting Tremor

Tremor is the presenting complaint in at least 70% of patients with PD. The tremor is maximal when the limb is at rest and has a frequency of 3 to 6 Hz. It consists of flexion–extension at the metacarpophalangeal joints, abduction–adduction of the thumb, and pronation–supination of the forearm, producing the typical pill-rolling appearance. The tremor may affect the legs, lips, tongue, or chin but virtually never affects the head (a tremor of the head suggests ET). The parkinsonian tremor is accentuated by stress and distraction, diminishes with relaxation, and disappears during sleep. Although there may be an associated postural tremor in PD, typically the resting tremor suppresses with posture and movement, which helps to distinguish it from ET.

Rigidity

Rigidity is a form of abnormal muscular tone or resistance to passive movement. This feeling of resistance is present and unchanged when moving a patient's limb in flexion or extension, regardless of the speed of the movement, and is described as having a "lead pipe" quality. In this manner, rigidity can be distinguished from spasticity, the other major form of abnormal muscle tone. In spasticity, resistance is greater to extension than flexion and is particularly prominent at the onset of a rapid attempt to flex the arm or leg. This quality gives rise to descriptions of spasticity as "clasp knife" or having a "catch." When the limb of a PD patient is moved passively, there is also a regular ratchet-like quality to the resistance, which gives rise to the term cogwheel rigidity. Deep tendon reflexes are increased in patients with spasticity while they are normal or decreased in parkinsonism rigidity. Patients rarely complain of rigidity per se and instead notice stiffness or describe the abnormal tone as weakness. Cogwheel rigidity is best felt at the elbow, wrist, or neck and may be demonstrated or enhanced by having the patient perform a maneuver with the contralateral limb such as opening and closing the fist or drawing a circle in the air.

Bradykinesia and Akinesia

Patients with PD have difficulty initiating movements, and their movements are slow and performed with much greater conscious effort. Speech gradually becomes soft, slow, and monotonal (hypophonia). The blink rate is diminished, as is facial expression (hypomimia), producing the so-called masked face. Movements of PD patients are not only slowed but are reduced in amplitude. This is most prominent with repeated activity where the movements appear to collapse into a barely visible quiver.

Gait and Postural Abnormalities

Patients with moderate to severe PD are flexed at multiple joints (neck, hips, knees, elbows, and fingers), producing the typical stooped posture. Arising from a chair is often accomplished only with difficulty; patients may need to rock back and forth several times and eventually push off from arm rests. Early changes in gait include a reduction in stride length and diminished associated movements such as arm swing. The gait later becomes slow and shuffling. Turning is done *en bloc*, with the entire body moving as the feet slowly rotate. There is a tendency to progress involuntarily from walking to running (festination), seemingly in an attempt to catch up with the body's center of gravity thrown forward by the flexed posture. A patient may describe festination as like chasing your shadow. Patients have difficulty maintaining balance and are often unable to correct for a rapid postural displacement, particularly backward. The combination of the flexed posture, bradykinesia, freezing, festination, and impaired postural righting reflexes leads to one of the major problems in the latter stages of PD falling.

Other Associated Symptoms or Signs

Seborrhea and excessive perspiration and facial oiliness are both common, and although often attributed to inadequate hygiene caused by physical impairment, they are an intrinsic part of the disease process.

Dysphagia often surfaces in the latter stages of the disease where it contributes significantly to morbidity and mortality caused by inanition and aspiration pneumonia. Although not completely understood, swallowing abnormalities have been demonstrated at various levels: The voluntary muscles of the oral cavity plus the involuntary muscles of the pharynx and esophagus. Solids are usually more of a problem than liquids. If patients with advanced PD are unable to maintain sufficient caloric intake, a discussion of the pros and cons of tube feeding should be held with the patient and family.

Sialorrhea is probably the result of decreased initiation of swallowing rather than overproduction of saliva. This can be treated with a low dosage of an anticholinergic, but there is growing experience in the use of injection of the salivary glands with botulinum toxin in the treatment of sialorrhea (38).

Autonomic dysfunction may occur in PD itself and as a side effect of antiparkinsonian medication. When the clinical picture is dominated by severe dysautonomia, particularly when accompanied by cerebellar and lower motor neuron signs, with rapid progression and poor response to drugs for PD, this is known as the Shy-Drager syndrome (39). This syndrome is a reflection of the more widespread pathology of a form of atypical parkinsonism known as multisystem atrophy. Orthostatic hypotension and constipation are the most common autonomic signs in PD, but bladder dysfunction and impotence are also encountered. In each case, medications may be at fault, and a search for other causes should be carried out before the defects are ascribed to PD.

Natural History

PD patients can be viewed as having one of three forms of the disease with implications for both natural history and treatment:

- *Tremor predominant:* These patients have prominent tremor but little other signs and symptoms of PD. They have an earlier average age at onset but a more benign course. They may have little functional disability from bradykinesia or rigidity even years after the onset of tremor. The prominent tremor not only is cosmetically unacceptable and can lead to social isolation, but can also give a patient a misimpression of a poor prognosis. Frequently medications other than L-dopa are more useful in treatment. Such patients illustrate a poorly understood aspect of parkinsonian tremor. Although a true rest tremor (seen only at rest and suppressed with movement) is the most reliable diagnostic sign of PD, it does not correlate well with bradykinesia and rigidity. These other signs rather than tremor also more closely correlate with overall disease disability and dopaminergic cell loss on radionuclide scans (40). These patients account for approximately 20% of PD.
- *Classic PD:* These patients account for most cases (approximately 60% to 70%) and have all three of the cardinal features (tremor, bradykinesia, rigidity) at the time of diagnosis, frequently in the same body distribution. They generally have a good response to therapy for years after diagnosis. These are the patients who dominate most clinical trials of medications for PD.
- *Akinetic–rigid:* These patients lack a resting tremor, with stiffness and reduced movement dominating their clinical picture. Akinetic–rigid patients are in general poorly responsive to therapy. It is likely that the poor response of this group is due to its heterogenous nature, with many of these patients having more widespread neurodegenerative diseases than PD. Expert consultation is essential in evaluation in this group, looking for ocular movement abnormalities, behavioral and cognitive abnormalities, and autonomic and cerebellar dysfunction seen in the atypical parkinsonian syndromes.

Not only do these conditions have the abnormalities mentioned earlier, they have more rapidly progressive and disabling disease. Difficulties with speech, swallowing, and posture (with frequent falling) are seen relatively early in the course of many of these patients.

Table 90.5. Drugs Used for Parkinson Disease

Drug	Available Preparation (mg)	Schedule	Starting Dose (mg)	Maintenance Dose (mg)
Anticholinergic agents				
Trihexyphenidyl (Artane, generic)	Tablets: 2, 5 Elixir: 2 mg/5 mL	3–4 times daily	2	2–12
Benztropine mesylate (Cogentin, generic)	Tablets: 0.5, 1, 2	Once or twice daily	1	0.5–6
Dopaminergic agents				
Carbidopa L-dopa (Sinemet, generic)	Tablets: 10/100, 25/100, 25/250, 25/100 CR, 50/200 CR	2–4 times daily	50/200 in 2 divided doses	300–1,000 L-dopa
Bromocriptine (Pariodel)	Tablets: 2.5 Capsules: 5.0	2–3 times daily	1.25 daily	7.5–30
Pergolide (Permax)	Scored tablets: 0.05, 0.25, 1.0	3 times daily	0.05 daily	1–6
Pramipexole (Mirapex)	Tablets: 0.125, 0.25, 0.5, 1, 1.5	3 times daily	0.375 daily	4.5
Ropinirole (Requip)	Tablets: 0.25, 1, 2, 5	3 times daily	0.75 daily	3–15
Selegiline[a] (Eldepryl)	Tablets: 5.0	2 times daily	5 daily	10
Entacapone (Comtan)	Tablets: 200	Up to 8 times a day (along with carbidopa/L-dopa)	200	600–1,600
Anticholinergic or dopaminergic activity				
Amantadine (Symmetrel, generic)	Capsules: 100	2 times daily	200 daily	200–400

[a]Alternative generic name: deprenyl.

Treatment Overview

The problems facing PD patients vary throughout the course of this disease, which progresses over many years. Treatment strategies that consider both short- and long-term aspects of PD are useful in helping patients, families, and physicians in anticipating and preparing for new problems and maximizing functionality and quality of life.

Treatment of Early Parkinson Disease

Nonmedication Strategies

Education and counseling play a major role in newly diagnosed patients. Fear of disability and death are common but frequently are not voiced. Reassurance is needed that disease progression is in general slow and disability can be forestalled for many years. Patients also need to be reminded that both understanding and treatment of PD are among the most rapidly changing aspects of all of neurology. There is not only reason to be optimistic regarding treatment with current therapy, but therapy will clearly be improving over the patient's lifetime. Patient-oriented books and support groups are often helpful for both patient and families. However, support groups should not be allowed to become the sole source of information for newly diagnosed patients, because they tend to focus on the most severely affected patients. Exercise programs are useful both to reduce physical signs of PD but also in encouraging an active life-style. Restrictions in activity are only appropriate when activities pose a safety hazard (i.e., working at a height, with heavy machinery, bicycle riding, rollerblading) in early PD.

For tremor predominant patients, declining symptomatic medications remains a viable option. A resting tremor can be quite pronounced and still cause little or no functional impairment. Frequently, embarrassment caused by tremor is the major drive for seeking treatment.

Depression is common in PD (40% to 50% of patients) and frequently is present at the time of diagnosis (41,42). In general it is not closely related to physical disability (or fear of it), because the incidence of depression in PD is higher than in other disabling conditions. The diagnosis of depression is made more difficult by the presence of facial masking where outward expression of emotion may not be an accurate reflection of mood state. Treatment of depression is accomplished with standard antidepressants (such as the selective serotonin reuptake inhibitor group; see Chapter 24) rather than with anti-Parkinson drugs.

Medications

Table 90.5 lists the medications used for the treatment of early PD.

Anticholinergics. Patients with early PD, in whom tremor is the major aspect, can benefit from anticholinergics. In general, poor patient tolerance limits their use. Dry mouth (which may help sialorrhea), dry eyes, and mild visual blurring are common and dose related. Urinary retention, constipation, memory loss, and confusion are more serious problems, particularly in the elderly with a high prevalence of pre-existing dementia. Narrow angle glaucoma is a contraindication to these agents. Trihexyphenidyl and benzopine are the two most widely used of this class. Trihexyphenidyl is sometimes preferred because of its short duration of action (3 to 5 hours), because it allows a patient to target tremor control to desired situations. The recommended dose for trihexyphenidyl is 2 to 12 mg/day.

Selegiline. This drug is a selective MAO-B inhibitor with proven modest utility for symptoms of wearing off of L-dopa in more advanced disease. Its use in early PD remains controversial even after a major clinical study. Patients taking selegiline clearly were able to postpone use of L-dopa compared with those taking placebo (43). However, it remains uncertain if this reflected an actual neuroprotective effect on disease progression or was simply a reflection of a mild symptomatic effect (not anticipated at the time of the original study). At this time, no agent has shown a well-documented capacity to slow the rate of neuronal degeneration in PD. (Vitamin E failed to slow disease in the same large clinical trial.) Potential neuroprotection has been suggested for amantadine and for dopamine agonists. In view of the lack of any bona fide neuroprotectant, many physicians opt to use selegiline in young uncomplicated patients, where possible neuroprotection would be most beneficial. This should be done in the setting of a discussion with the patient regarding the controversy surrounding its use.

There have been two separate controversies over the use of selegiline. The first is whether or not it slows the rate of progression of PD. The consensus view of data flawed by selegiline's symptomatic effect is that it does not. A second controversy erupted from an open-label British study that found an increase in mortality among selegiline-treated patients. Examination of both previous and later studies with selegiline did not reveal any increased mortality. It is generally accepted that selegiline does not increase mortality in PD. Dietary restrictions usually recommended with MAOIs (see Chapter 24) are not necessary as long as the dose remains no more than the recommended 5 mg twice daily.

Amantadine. Although originally developed as an anti-influenzal drug, amantadine is an approved antiparkinsonian agent. Its effects are in general modest, but it is far better tolerated than anticholinergic drugs. It is useful for mild bradykinesia and rigidity as well as tremor. It has a stimulant effect in many patients, which may account for its use in the treatment of fatigue in multiple sclerosis and chronic fatigue syndrome. Dry mouth and insomnia are usually mild. Livedo reticularis on the legs with associated edema occurs in 5% to 10% of patients, leading to discontinuation of amantadine. Exacerbation of congestive heart failure has also been reported with amantadine use. A dose of 100 mg twice daily is usual in early PD.

Carbidopa/Levodopa (L-Dopa). Although the introduction of L-dopa for PD is one of the therapeutic highlights of neurology, its use in early PD remains controversial. Despite the introduction of new medications, L-dopa remains the most effective drug for overall relief of motor symptoms of PD. The controversy surrounding L-dopa use has both theoretical and clinical basis. As mentioned earlier, there is evidence that metabolism of dopamine generates oxidative injury, which may play a role in the progressive cell death in PD. This evidence comes mostly from cell culture studies with relatively little animal data, and no clinical studies support the concept that levels of L-dopa used in treatment of PD are toxic. Results of a major clinical study are in direct conflict with the belief that L-dopa treatment accelerates neuronal death in PD. Patients who had L-dopa treatment begun early in the course of their disease had less overall morbidity and mortality than patients where therapy was initiated at a later stage (44). L-Dopa therapy is, however, associated with a major complication of moderate to severe PD—a fluctuating response (45). Dose fluctuations take two forms:

- Loss of efficacy before the next dose of L-dopa (so-called wearing off).
- Involuntary choreiform movements called dyskinesias that usually occur at the peak effect of each dose. Dyskinesias in particular are associated with duration (in years) of L-dopa treatment.

A likely answer to the apparent conflict in clinical studies is that dyskinesias, although clinically important, are not as great a contributor to the overall severity of PD as the cardinal motor abnormalities. A practical approach is to defer initiating L-dopa until the patient's motor symptoms interfere with daily activities. L-Dopa therapy in early PD is initiated as carbidopa/L-dopa (Sinemet) at a dose one 25/100 tablet twice a day, although half of this dose is suggested for elderly patients.

The addition of carbidopa to L-dopa as a combination medication (Sinemet) dramatically improves its tolerability. Carbidopa inhibits the enzyme dopa-decarboxylase, preventing the conversion of L-dopa to dopamine outside of brain. This leads to marked reduction (10-fold) of the effective L-dopa dose with reduction in so-called peripheral side effects of nausea, gastrointestinal intolerance (cramps/diarrhea), and hypotension. Patients with refractory nausea on 25/100 combination tablets may benefit from additional carbidopa, available as 25-mg tablets (Lodosyn). Along with adjusting dose with timing of meals, nausea can be reduced with controlled-release preparations.

Although L-dopa is absorbed best on an empty stomach, this also usually leads to an increased incidence of nausea, so that it is initially prescribed with meals and, once tolerated, can be taken half an hour earlier. Although some patients have an immediate beneficial effect, it may take several weeks before a change is noticed. After that time, if there is no improvement, the dosage is gradually increased every few days to three to four times daily, using full or half-tablet increments, until the patient has shown significant improvement or a total daily dosage of 400 to 600 mg of L-dopa per day has been reached.

Although most patients tolerate carbidopa/L-dopa well, side effects are common, particularly in the elderly or in patients with dementia (see below). These include confusion, hallucinations, hypersexuality, and fluid retention. Orthostatic hypotension is common, particularly in patients with autonomic dysfunction related to their untreated PD. Standing and supine blood pressure measurements should be checked before and after initiating treatment.

Dopamine Agonists: Bromocriptine (Parlodel), Pergolide (Permax), Pramipexole (Mirapex), and Ropinirole (Requip). Medications from this group have been used as adjuvants to L-dopa for patients in the later stages of PD for many years. Recently there has been growing clinical experience with these agents as *initial therapy* of PD, particularly as an alternatives to L-dopa. All four dopamine agonists have been shown to be safe and effective as monotherapy for PD. The three newer agents appear to be somewhat more effective than bromocriptine, the first dopamine agonist introduced. The two newest agonists (pramipexole and ropinirole) have been shown to be virtually as effective as L-dopa in the treatment of mild PD patients (46,47). The major rationale for their use as initial therapy of PD is the significantly lower level of dose fluctuations—particularly dyskinesias—that occurs years later in patients initiated on agonist monotherapy other than L-dopa (48,49). As many as half of PD patients can be adequately treated with an agonist without L-dopa for 3 to 5 years. Many physicians choose these agents for theoretical reasons as well, because there is no possibility of oxidative injury (with possible neuroprotection) with these agents. Unlike L-dopa, dopamine agonists are not currently available as a combination pill with an agent to prevent dopamine-related side effects. Dopamine agonists have a higher incidence of nausea and gastrointestinal disturbances than carbidopa/L-dopa combinations. These side effects can be minimized by a very gradual titration schedule, allowing for tolerance to the drug to occur. The mantra for use of dopamine agonists is "start low, go slow, aim high," because starting doses are typically 1/10 of the therapeutic dose (Table 90.5). Patients need to understand both the schedule of dose escalation and its rationale. Overly slow escalation can lead to discontinuation by the patient due to a perceived lack of efficacy, whereas overly rapid escalation leads to discontinuation due to side effects (usually nausea). Once tolerance occurs these drugs can be used, with increasing efficacy, in doses well beyond their usual dosing guidelines. However, the cost of dopamine agonists is significantly higher than equivalent amounts of carbidopa/L-dopa, particularly in its immediate release generic from.

Domperidone is useful to relieve nausea caused by dopamine agonists (or levodopa) (50). Domperidone is a dopamine antagonist that does not cross the blood–brain barrier, and in contrast to the typical neuroleptics and related antinausea drugs does not worsen symptoms of PD. It is currently available through Canadian pharmacies as a stimulant for gastrointestinal motility (its indication worldwide).

Treatment of Moderate Parkinson Disease

Patients usually experience worsening motor symptoms of PD, requiring increasing amounts of medications (particular L-dopa) within the first 5 years after diagnosis. The most common new problem of patients in moderate stage of PD is a reduction in the duration of benefit of each dose of L-dopa, known as wearing off. Although patients with early PD may have uninterrupted benefit from taking L-dopa twice a day, patients with moderate PD may find that their symptoms may worsen at the end of a dose taken three or four times a day. Disease severity plays a major role in this change. L-Dopa has a very short serum half-life (90 minutes), but early PD patients appear to have a capacity for a sustained benefit well beyond its pharmacokinetic effect. As PD worsens, the duration of action of L-dopa approaches its short serum lifetime.

Addressing "Wearing Off" of L-Dopa

Several useful strategies reduce the wearing off of L-dopa. L-Dopa is available in a controlled-release form extending its duration of action by approximately 10% (51). Selegiline will inhibit the degradation of dopamine and extend the duration of action of L-dopa by approximately 10% to 15% (52). Selegiline is a virtually irreversible MAO inhibitor and is dosed twice a day regardless of a patient's L-dopa dose schedule. Selegiline is so long acting that when signs of dopamine excess occur with its use, L-dopa dose must be reduced along with discontinuation of selegiline. Inhibitors of the major dopamine degrading enzyme, catechol-*o*-methyl transferase (COMT), are also available. Tolcapone (Tasmar) was the first catechol-o-methyl transferase inhibitor released, and it remains the most potent drug to prolong the duration of action of carbidopa/L-dopa. Mild elevations of liver function tests were observed in clinical trials. After its release, reports of fatal hepatotoxicity mandated regular assessment of alanine aminotransferase levels, which has greatly limited its use. Entacapone (Comtan) has not been associated with hepatotoxicity. This catechol-*o*-methyl transferase inhibitor is more effective than selegiline in prolonging the duration of action of L-dopa and is used in a very different fashion (53). Entacapone is a short-acting medication that is given as a fixed dose (200 mg) along with each dose of L-dopa. Clinical trials are underway to develop a combined carbidopa/levodopa/entacapone preparation.

Use of the longer acting *dopamine agonists* along with L-dopa is another proven strategy to reduce wearing off and improve the duration of daily "on" time. All the dopamine agonists have shown significant improvement of PD patients when used along with L-dopa (54). For patients with severe wearing off, a combination of strategies to increase L-dopa action as well as the addition of agonist therapy is commonly used.

Management of dose fluctuations becomes more problematic when patients develop *both wearing off and clinically significant dyskinesias.* The overall strategy is to reduce the total amount of short-acting L-dopa and supplement therapy with a longer acting agent, usually a dopamine agonist. This strategy is based on the observation that most dyskinesias occur at the time of peak action of L-dopa (peak dose dyskinesia), although some dyskinesias may occur during rapid drop in L-dopa levels (wearing off dyskinesias). All forms of L-dopa extension therapy and agonist adjuvant therapy are associated with an increase in dyskinesias, particularly when these treatments are initiated. It is only through the reduction of the daily L-dopa dose that these dyskinesias can be controlled while maintaining an improved duration of "on" time.

Treatment of Severe Parkinson Disease

Drug Treatment of Motor Fluctuations

As PD worsens (usually at least 10 years after diagnosis), patients develop both wearing off and dyskinesias with increasing frequency and severity. The regimens of L-dopa extension drugs and dopamine agonists frequently make such motor fluctuations more unpredictable. Conflict between patients and their physicians over therapy are common in this period. Physicians view dyskinesias as the most medically refractory symptom and aim to reduce them by reducing total daily L-dopa. However, most PD patients do not view dyskinesias as their most significant problem and may even be unaware of mild dyskinesias. Patients usually view the intrusion of PD symptoms during a sudden "off period" as more distressing and functionally more important and seek increases in L-dopa. Direct discussions about both short- and long-term goals of therapy are needed to maximize both patient satisfaction and medication compliance.

Bioavailability of L-dopa is clearly influenced by dietary protein so that a *protein restriction/redistribution* diet is appropriate for patients with severe fluctuation in motor function (55). Consultation with a nutritionist is usually needed, because weight loss can occur in this population that is already below their ideal weight. Although daytime wearing off usually improves, evening dyskinesias may develop. Attempts at controlling daytime wearing off with drug therapy may also increase evening dyskinesias as L-dopa levels gradually rise over the day.

Sudden and unexpected wearing off can be treated with short-acting "rescue therapy." Immediate-release L-dopa can be precrushed and taken with water on an empty stomach to enhance rapidity of effect. Patients can prepare L-dopa in liquid form by dissolving tablets in water (with ascorbic acid as a preservative) and keeping the stock refrigerated. The short-acting dopamine agonist apomorphine is available in Canada as an injectable rescue therapy that acts within a few minutes and is in clinical trial in the United States (56). An advantage of rescue therapy for sudden unexpected wearing off is that these agents are short acting and usually do not require any further adjustment of a complex daily dosing regimen. Immediate-release L-dopa is also commonly used along with controlled release as the first daily dose to help quickly relieve morning stiffness and slowness.

Medical treatment of dyskinesias is extremely limited. The only agent that can be practically used is amantadine. At doses of up to 400 mg/day, this drug has been shown to significantly reduce L-dopa induced dyskinesias (57).

Surgery

Severe motor fluctuations despite optimal or tolerable medical therapy is the strongest indication for surgical treatment of PD. This is particularly true of patients who have L-dopa induced dyskinesias that are severe enough to impair function. Although stereotactic thalamotomy and thalamic DBS are effective for both essential and parkinsonian tremor, they are infrequently performed in PD patients (58). Thalamotomy has little effect on other signs of PD other than tremor. It is feared that if a PD patient has a thalamotomy for tremor and they develop other PD symptoms years later, they may require a second surgical procedure at a different brain location.

There are now two other brain locations where stereotactic surgery gives benefit for not only relief of tremor (although not as pronounced as thalamotomy) but of bradykinesia and rigidity as well. Pallidotomy, lesioning (or DBS) directed at the globus pallidum interna (GPI), has been the most widely used surgery for PD. Motor symptoms are particularly improved over the preoperative "off" state, along with a reduction in dyskinesias (59). This antidyskinesias benefit, although difficult to explain on a physiologic basis, is one of the strongest indications for pallidotomy. The elimination of dyskinesias also can allow the patient to tolerate higher doses of dopaminergic therapy, resulting in improvement of other motor symptoms. The most common complication of pallidotomy is a superior quadrant visual field cut (the lesion may extend into the optic radiations), but this usually is not functionally significant. Serious complications of PD surgery such as hemiparesis are seen in less than 5% of patients.

Another target for PD surgery that is approached with increasing frequency is the subthalamic nucleus. This small deep center is only approached with DBS, because of fear that a radiofrequency lesion could extend into the neighboring descending motor tracts, leading to a hemiparesis. Improvement in PD symptoms appear at least comparable with GPI surgery, although no large comparison studies have been published to date (60,61). Subthalamic nucleus surgery does not have the direct antidyskinesia effect of GPI surgery (dyskinesia can worsen in some patients), but unlike with GPI surgery PD medications can usually be reduced, with a concomitant reduction in dyskinesias. Benefits of surgery for PD appear to be detectable for at least several years.

There is a window of opportunity for PD surgery that cannot be reclaimed once it has passed. Stereotactic surgery for PD is very demanding on patients. For most of the hours of surgery the patient is awake and is an active participant as the target brain center is identified physiologically and test stimulation of the DBS unit is performed. Transient confusion can occur after surgery even in cognitively intact patients.

Dementia (see below), a common problem in severe PD, is a clear contraindication to this form of surgery. Poor postural stability, another problem of advanced PD, usually does not improve with surgery. In general, younger patients (less than 65) tolerate PD surgery better and have better outcomes.

Fetal brain tissue transplantation has also been performed to improved PD. In a recently reported placebo-controlled trial, only the younger patients received significant benefit (62).

Psychosis

Psychosis, including hallucinosis, can occur in any PD patient receiving dopaminergic therapy. Psychotic symptoms become more prevalent and serious in advanced cases. Age, presence of dementia, and dose of antiparkinsonian drugs are the major risk factors for psychosis in PD patients. Although all forms of PD therapy can cause psychotic symptoms, L-dopa appears to have a superior ratio of relief of motor symptoms of PD to induction of psychosis compared with the dopamine agonists. The most common useful strategy is to lower the dose of PD therapy. Anticholinergics in particular should be eliminated. However, many advanced PD patients will not be able to tolerate lowering the dose of their other PD medications. In the past, little could be done for these patients because typical neuroleptics worsened motor symptoms to the same extent as reducing a PD medication. The introduction of clozapine (Clozaril) has significantly improved the treatment of these patients. Relatively low doses (12.5 to 50 mg) of clozapine can successfully suppress hallucinations and delusions without worsening motor symptoms (63). Unfortunately, the most common serious side effect of clozapine (agranulocytosis) is an idiosyncratic event, so that regular monitoring of leukocyte count is needed even at these low doses. The newer atypical neuroleptics are also useful to treat psychotic symptoms in PD. At this time quetiapine (Seroquel) appears to be the most useful (25 to 75 mg/day), along with olanzapine (Zyprexa) (2.5 to 5mg/day) (64,65). Risperidone (Risperdal) appears to have a greater propensity to worsen motor symptoms in PD than other atypical neuroleptics.

Dementia

Dementia eventually occurs in at least 30% of PD patients. It is most strongly associated with age (as with virtually all dementing illnesses) but is also associated with duration and severity of motor signs of PD (42,66). Because dementia is not an invariable part of PD, an evaluation for a reversible cause is needed. The underlying basis for dementia in PD is controversial. Some of these patients have concomitant Alzheimer disease (see Chapter 26). Another group of demented PD patients may have the more widespread condition of Lewy body dementia where psychotic symptoms are common. Although experience with the anticholinesterase drugs developed for Alzheimer disease is limited for dementia in PD, this approach appears to hold promise (67). Cognitive responses appear to be similar to Alzheimer disease, and the behavior stabilizing effects of these drugs have been also shown in Lewy body dementia (68).

Autonomic Dysfunction

The most common serious form of autonomic dysfunction in PD is orthostatic hypotension, and it is usually worsened by dopaminergic therapy. Added dietary salt along with the mineralocorticoid fludrocortisone (Florinef) are useful to expand plasma volume. The limitations to this therapy are worsening of congestive heart failure and supine hypertension. Midodrine (ProAmantine) is an alpha-adrenergic agonist that is FDA approved for orthostatic hypotension due to autonomic failure (69). This short-acting agent can be dosed during the day (2.5 to 5 mg) every 4 hours to minimize recumbent hypertension. Poor esophageal and intestinal motility are also seen in advanced PD. Metoclopramide (Reglan) is, however, relatively contraindicated in PD because of its tendency to worsen motor symptoms.

SUPPORT GROUPS

American Parkinson Disease Association (APDA)
1250 Hylan Blvd.
Suite 4B
Staten Island, NY 10305-1946
(800) 223-2732
Fax: (718) 981-4399
www. apdaparkinson.org

International Tremor Foundation (ITF)
7046 West 105th Street
Overland Park, KS 66212-1803
(913) 341-3880
Fax: (913) 341-1296
www.essentialtremor.org

National Parkinson Foundation (NPF)
1501 NW 9th Avenue, Bob Hope Road
Miami, FL 33136-1494
(800) 327-4545
(800) 433-7022 (Florida)
www.parkinson.org

Parkinson's Disease Foundation (PDF)
William Black Medical Building
710 West 168th Street
New York, NY 10032
(800) 457-6676
www.pdf.org

Society for Progressive Supranuclear Palsy
Woodholme Medical Building
1838 Green Tree Road, Suite 515
Baltimore, MD 21208
(410) 486-3330
(800) 457-4777
Fax: (410) 486-4283
www.psp.org

WE MOVE
204 West 84th Street
New York, NY 10024, USA
(800) 437-MOV2 (in USA)
(212) 241-8567 (outside USA)
Fax: (212) 875-8389
E-mail: wemove@wemove.org
Website: http://www.wemove.org

General References*

Deuschl G, Raethjen, Lindeman M. Pathophysiology of tremor. Muscle Nerve 2001;25;716.

A review of the underlying basis of several forms of tremor.

Koller WC. Essential tremor. Neurology 2000;54:54.

A collection of reviews including epidemiology, treatment, and physiology.

Obeso JA, Benabid AL, Koller WC. Deep brain stimulation for Parkinson's disease and tremor. Neurology 2000;55:56.

Summaries of a 1997 meeting.

Olanow CW, Watts RL, Koller WC. An algorithm for management of Parkinson's disease (2001): treatment guidelines. Neurology 2001;56:S1.

A systematic contemporary treatment approach for the wide range of problems.

Waters CH. Diagnosis and management of Parkinson's disease. Caddo, OK: Professional Communications, 1998.

A clear, concise, and useful guide.

Weiner WJ, Shulman LM, Lang AE. Parkinson's disease. A complete guided for patients and families. Baltimore: Johns Hopkins University Press, 2001.

A comprehensive source for patients and families and a useful resource for practitioners as well.

Specific References

1. Hallett M. Classification and treatment of tremor. JAMA 1991;266:1115.
2. Begareche A, De La Puente E, Lopez De Munain A, et al. Prevalence of essential tremor: a door-to-door survey in Bidasoa, Spain. Neuroepidemiology 2001;20:125.
3. Growdon JH, Shahani BT, Young RR. The effect of alcohol on essential tremor. Neurology 1975;25:259.
4. Koller WC. Alcoholism in essential tremor. Neurology 1983;33: 1074.
5. Bilodeau M, Keen DA, Sweeney PJ, et al. Strength training can improve steadiness in persons with essential tremor. Muscle Nerve 2000;23:771.
6. Koller WC, Biary N, Cone S. Disability in essential tremor: effect of treatment. Neurology 1986;36:1001.
7. Koller WC. Long-acting propranolol in essential tremor. Neurology 1985;35:108.
8. Jefferson D, Jener P, Marsden CD. Beta-adrenoreceptor antagonists in essential tremor. J. Neurol Neurosurg Psychiatry 1979;42:904.
9. Larsen TA, Terlvainene H, Calne DB. Atenolol vs propanolol in essential tremor. A controlled, quantitative study. Acta Neurol Scan 1982;66:547.
10. Koller WC, Royce JL. Efficacy of primidone in essential tremor. Neurology 1986;36:121.
11. Thompson C, Lang A, Parkes DJ, et al. A double-blind trial of clonazepam in benign essential tremor. Clin Neuropharmacol 1988;7:83.
12. Huber SJ, Paulson GW. Efficacy of alprazolam for essential tremor. Neurology 1988;38:241.
13. Mohadjer M, Goerke H, Milios E, et al. Long-term results of stereotaxy in the treatment of essential tremor. Stereotact Funct Neurosurg 1990;55:125.
14. Pahwa R, Lyons KL, Wilkinson SB, et al. Bilateral thalamic stimulation for the treatment of essential tremor. Neurology 1999;53:1147.
15. Pahwa R, Lyons KE, Wilkinson SB, et al. Comparison of thalamotomy to deep brain stimulation of the thalamus in essential tremor. Mov Disord 2001;16:140.
16. Schuurman PR, Bosch DA, Bossuyt PM, et al. A comparison of continuous thalamic stimulation and thalamotomy for tremor. N Engl J Med 2000;342:461.
17. Jankovic J, Schwartz K, Clemence W, et al. A randomized, double-blind, placebo controlled study to evaluate botulinum toxin type A in essential hand tremor. Mov Disord 1996;11: 250.
18. Wissel J, Masuhr F, Schelosky L. Quantitative assessment of botulinum toxin treatment in 43 patients with head tremor. Mov Disord 1997;12:722.
19. Galvez-Jiminez N, Hargreave M. Topiramate and essential tremor. Ann Neurol 2000;47:837.
20. Gironell A, Kulisevsky J, Barbanoj M, et al. A randomized placebo-controlled comparative trial of gabapentin and propanolol in essential tremor. Arch Neurol 1999;56:475.
21. Pahwa R, Lyons K, Hubble JP, et al. Double-blind controlled trial of gabapentin in essential tremor. Mov Disord 1998;13: 465.
22. Ceravolo R, Salvetti S, Piccini P. Acute and chronic effects of clozapine in essential tremor. Mov Disord 1999;14:468.
23. Shazadi S, Tasker RR, Lozano A. Thalamotomy for essential and cerebellar tremor. Stereotact Funct Neurosurg 1996;65: 11.
24. Kachi T, Rothwell JC, Cowan JMA, et al. Writing tremor: its relationship to benign essential tremor. J Neurol Neurosurg Psychiatry 1985;48:545.
25. Heilman KM. Orthostatic tremor. Arch Neurol 1984;41:880.
26. Sander JW, Masdeu JC, Tavoulareas G, et al. Orthostatic tremor: an electrophysiological analysis. Mov Disord 1998;13: 735.
27. Tanner CM, Ben-Shlomo Y. Epidemiology of Parkinson's disease. Adv Neurol 1999;80:153.
28. Schrag A, Ben-Shlomo Y, Brown R, et al. Young-onset Parkinson's disease revisited—clinical features, natural history, and mortality. Mov Disord 1998;13:885.
29. Langston JW. The etiology of Parkinson's disease with emphasis on the MPT story. Neurology 1996;47[Suppl 3]:S153.
30. Jenner P. Oxidative mechanisms in nigral cell death in Parkinson's disease. Mov Disord 1998;13[Suppl 1]:24.
31. Lockwood AH. Pesticides and parkinsonism: is there an etiological link? Curr Opin Neurol 2000;13:687.
32. Polymeropoulos MH, Lavedan C, Leroy E, et al. Mutation in the alpha-synuclein gene identified in families with Parkinson's disease. Science 1997;276:2045.
33. Spillantini MG, Schmidt ML, Lee VM, et al. Alpha-synuclein in Lewy bodies. Nature 1997;388:839.
34. Kitada T, Asakawa S, Hattori N, et al. Mutations in the parkin gene cause autosomal recessive juvenile parkinsonism. Nature 1998;392:605.
35. Albers DS, Augood SJ. New insights into progressive supranuclear palsy. Trends Neurosci 2001;24:347.
36. Rehman HU. Progressive supranuclear palsy. Postgrad Med J 2000;76:333.
37. Schilsky ML. Treatment of Wilson's disease: what are the relative roles of penicillamine, trientine, and zinc supplementation? Curr Gastroenterol Rep 2001;3:54.
38. Pal PK, Calne DB, Calne S, et al. Botulinum toxin A as treatment for drooling saliva in PD. Neurology 2000;54:244.
39. Wenning GK, Seppi K, Scherfler C, et al. Multiple system atrophy. Semin Neurol 2001;21:33.
40. Benamer HT, Patterson J, Wyper DJ, et al. Correlation of Parkinson's disease severity and duration with FP-CIT SPECT striatal uptake. Mov Disord 2000;15:692.
41. Brooks DJ, Doer M. Depression in Parkinson's disease. Curr Opin Neurol 2001;14:465.
42. Giladi N, Treves TA, Paleacu D, et al. Risk factors for dementia, depression and psychosis in longstanding Parkinson's disease. J Neural Transm 2000;107:59.

*Bold print (general references) and bold numerals (specific references) denote published controlled clinical trials, meta-analyses, or consensus-based recommendations.

43. Shoulson I. DATATOP: a decade of neuroprotective inquiry. Parkinson's Disease Study Group. Deprenyl and tocopherol antioxidative therapy of Parkinsonism. Ann Neurol 1998;44: S160.
44. Markham CH, Diamond SG. Modification of Parkinson's disease by long-term levodopa treatment. Arch Neurol 1986;43: 405.
45. Ahlskog JE, Muenter MD. Frequency of levodopa-related dyskinesias and motor fluctuation as estimated from the cumulative literature. Mov Disord 2001;16:448.
46. Parkinson Study Group. Pramipexole vs levodopa as initial treatment for Parkinson disease: A randomized controlled trial. JAMA 2000;284:1931.
47. Rascol O, Brookes DJ, Korczyn AD, et al. A five-year study of the incidence of dyskinesia in patients with early Parkinson's disease who were treated with ropinirole or levodopa. N Engl J Med 2000;342:1484.
48. Shulman LM. Parkinson's disease: the proper use of dopamine receptor agonists. Curr Treat Options Neurol 1999;1:14.
49. Tuite P, Ebbitt B. Dopamine agonists. Semin Neurol 2001;21:9.
50. Jansen PA, Herings RM, Samson MM, et al. Quick titration of pergolide in cotreatment with domperidone is effective. Clin Neuropharmacol 2001;24:177.
51. Linazasoro G, Grandas F, Martinez Martin P, et al. Controlled release levodopa in Parkinson's disease: influence of selection criteria and conversion recommendations in the clinical outcome of 450 patients. Clin Neuropharmacol 1999;22:74.
52. Golbe LI, Lieberman AN, Meunter MD, et al. Deprenyl in the treatment of symptom fluctuations in advanced Parkinson's disease. Clin Neuropharmacol 1988;11:45.
53. Schapira AH, Obeso JA, Olanow CW. The place of COMT inhibitors in the armamentarium of drug the treatment of Parkinson's disease. Neurology 2000;55[Suppl 4]:S65.
54. Inzelberg R, Carasso RL, Schechtman E, et al. A comparison of dopamine agonists and catechol-O-methyltransferase inhibitors in Parkinson's disease. Clin Neuropharmacol 2000;23: 262.
55. Pincus JH, Barry K. Protein redistribution diet restores motor function in patients dopa-resistant "off" periods. Neurology 1988;38:481.
56. Poewe W, Wenning GK. Apomorphine: an underutilized therapy for Parkinson's disease. Mov Disord 2000;15:789.
57. Metman LV, Del Dotto P, LePoole K, et al. Amantadine for levodopa-induced dyskinesias: a 1-year follow up study. Arch Neurol 1999;56:1383.
58. Fox MW, Ahlsko JE, Kelly PJ. Stereotactic ventrolateralis thalamotomy for medically refractory tremor in postlevodopa era Parkinson's disease patients. J Neurosurg 1991;75: 723.
59. Hariz MI, Bergenheim AT. A 10-year follow up review of patients who underwent Leksell posteroventral pallidotomy for Parkinson disease. J Neurosurg 2001;94:552.
60. Limousin P, Krack P, Pollak P, et al. Electrical stimulation of the subthalamic nucleus in advanced Parkinson's disease. N Engl J Med 1998;339:1105.
61. Rodriguez-Oroz MC, Gorospe A, Guridi J, et al. Bilateral deep brain stimulation of the subthalamic nucleus in Parkinson's disease. Neurology 2000;55:S45.
62. Freed CR, Greene PE, Breeze RE, et al. Transplantation of embryonic dopamine neurons for severe Parkinson's disease. N Engl J Med 2001;344:710.
63. Parkinson Study Group. Low-dose clozapine for the treatment of drug-induced psycho Parkinson's disease. The Parkinson Study Group. N Engl J Med 1999;340:801.
64. Fernandez HH, Friedman JH, Jacques C, et al. Quetiapine for the treatment of drug-induced psychosis in Parkinson's disease. Mov Disord 1999;14:484.
65. Friedman JH, Goldstein S, Jacques C. Substituting clozapine for olanzapine in psychiatrically stable Parkinson's disease patients: results of an open label pilot study. Clin Neuropharmacol 1998;21:285.
66. Aarsland D, Andersen K, Larsen JP, et al. Risk of dementia in Parkinson's disease: a community-based, prospective study. Neurology 2001;56:730.
67. Hutchinson M, Fazzini E. Cholinesterase inhibition in Parkinson's disease. J Neurol Neurosurg Psychiatry 1996;61:324.
68. McKeith I, Del Ser T, Spano P, et al. Efficacy of rivastigmine in dementia with Lewy bodies: a randomised, double-blind, placebo-controlled international study. Lancet 2000;356: 2031.
69. Low PA, Gilden JL, Freeman R, et al. Efficacy of midodrine vs placebo in neurogenic orthostatic hypotension. A randomized, double-blind multicenter study. Midodrine Study Group. JAMA 1997;277:1046.

CHAPTER 91

Cerebrovascular Disease

CONSTANCE J. JOHNSON, MD

OVERVIEW

Epidemiology

Cerebrovascular disease is a major cause of disability and the third leading cause of death in the United States. According to 1997 American Heart Association estimates, the annual cost is greater than $18 billion and there are almost 4 million stroke survivors in this country (1). Approximately 80% of strokes are caused by thrombotic or embolic cerebral infarction, 12% by cerebral hemorrhage, and 8% by subarachnoid hemorrhage. Approximately 28% of strokes occur in people under age 65. The annual death rate from stroke is higher in African Americans (men, 52/100,000;

women, 40/100,000) than in whites (men, 27/100,000; women, 23/100,000) (1).

The death rate from stroke declined by 19.8% from 1984 to 1994 (1). Studies in the 1980s showed that stroke incidence had decreased nationwide and worldwide (2,3). Factors that may have contributed to the decline include more aggressive treatment of hypertension, more effective and early delivery of health care, and better management and recognition of the cardiogenic sources of cerebral embolization. Some community-based studies in the 1980s indicated a later stabilization of the decline; some also showed a possible increase in stroke incidence, a finding that may have resulted from the earlier detection of stroke because of the introduction of new imaging techniques such as computed tomography (CT) in the 1980s (4).

Ischemic cerebrovascular disease presents two major challenges in ambulatory practice: the prevention of stroke in the large number of people with risk factors that make them prone to stroke and the optimal care of the many stroke survivors in each community. Brain hemorrhage is an acute problem usually presenting to the emergency room and requiring hospitalization and is not covered in this chapter.

Risk Factors

A major goal of patient evaluation in ambulatory practice is the identification of the patient with an increased risk of stroke. Patients who have previously had a stroke are an important subgroup of this high-risk population. Community-based data on the natural history of stroke show that the first-year recurrence rate among survivors of a first stroke is approximately 10% and that the 5-year recurrence rate is approximately 20% (5). In addition to a history of stroke and aging, other factors that predispose a patient to stroke are transient episodes of focal cerebral dysfunction of vascular origin called transient ischemic attacks (TIAs), hypertension, certain cardiac disorders, cigarette smoking, diabetes mellitus, and hyperlipidemia.

Transient Ischemic Attacks

Approximately one-third of patients with a TIA subsequently develop a stroke, and the TIA provides a significant warning of impending infarction. The cause, natural history, and treatment of TIAs are discussed in detail later in this chapter.

Hypertension

Data accumulated during the Framingham study indicate that the risk of stroke is strongly related to hypertension. Atherothrombotic brain infarction occurred in hypertensive subjects (blood pressure greater than 160/95) four times more often than in normotensive subjects (6). Evidence from controlled trials shows that stroke risk and other cardiovascular disease risk is significantly reduced by the treatment of hypertension in all patients, including those with a history of cerebrovascular disease (7–9). Meta-analysis of nine randomized trials (62,605 hypertensive patients) revealed that calcium channel blockers and angiotensin-converting enzyme inhibitors reduced cardiovascular events including stroke due to reduction in systolic blood pressure. Although all antihypertensive agents were believed to have similar long-term efficacy and safety, there was a higher risk of stroke on captopril in one trial (10). The evaluation and long-term management of hypertension are discussed in detail in Chapter 67.

Cardiac Impairment

Patients with cardiac impairment are predisposed to stroke, either directly because of emboli from the heart that lodge in cerebral arteries and lead to cerebral infarction or indirectly because chronic atherosclerotic cardiac disease is associated with atherothrombotic cerebral disease. Cardioembolic stroke accounts for 15% to 30% of all ischemic strokes and is highly associated with cardiac arrhythmias, particularly atrial fibrillation with or without valvular disease; valvular disease; recent myocardial infarction; and dilated cardiomyopathy (11). Data from the Framingham study identified cardiac impairment as a significant risk factor in the occurrence of the more common nonembolic atherothrombotic brain infarction (12). Subjects with electrocardiographic evidence of left ventricular hypertrophy were nine times more likely to develop atherothrombotic brain infarction than those without this abnormality. Patients with coronary artery disease had five times the risk of atherothrombotic brain infarction, and those with radiographic evidence of cardiomegaly had three times the risk. When the contribution of concomitant hypertension was eliminated, left ventricular hypertrophy and coronary artery disease were each associated with a threefold increase in the risk of atherothrombotic brain infarction; the contribution of cardiomegaly on x-ray was not found to be significant when other variables were controlled. On the basis of these findings it was concluded that cardiac impairment, especially if associated with hypertension, significantly heightens the risk of stroke occurrence.

Lipids

Meta-analysis of three placebo-controlled randomized trials (19,768 patients) concluded that pravastatin 40 mg/day reduced ischemic stroke risk 23% across a range of lipid levels with no evidence for benefit in hemorrhagic stroke or stroke of unknown type (13).

Other Factors

A number of other factors have been associated with an increased incidence of stroke: family history of vascular disease, elevated serum glucose concentration, cigarette smoking, elevated blood hematocrit levels, and the presence of a cervical bruit. To date, definitive studies have not been done to establish whether modification of any of these risk factors reduces the likelihood of stroke. With regard to diabetes mellitus, prospective data from the Framingham study indicate an increased risk of cerebral infarction in subjects with even a modest abnormality of glucose tolerance (14). Cigarette smoking increases the risk of ischemic stroke and is a predictor of the presence of significant intracranial and extracranial vascular stenosis (11). The duration of cigarette smoking is predictive of extracranial carotid artery stenosis as detected by duplex scanning (15). Elevated blood hemoglobin and hematocrit levels have also been implicated as possible risk factors, but a cause-and-effect relationship has not been established (16). Oral contraceptive use is associated with a 5- to 10-fold increase in the risk of vascular diseases, including stroke (see details in Chapter 100). Although epidemiologic studies demonstrate a decreased risk of ischemic stroke for postmenopausal hormone replacement therapy users (17), the Heart and Estrogen-Progestin Replacement Study of 2,763 postmenopausal women with coronary disease revealed no significant effect on the risk for stroke (18). Finally, it is generally accepted that the presence of an asymptomatic cervical bruit correlates with an increased incidence of subsequent stroke, but there is controversy regarding the approach to patients with this finding (see below).

ASYMPTOMATIC CAROTID STENOSIS

Asymptomatic carotid stenosis is detected by the presence of a cervical bruit or because a vascular screening test was performed. Bruits occur in 4.5% of the population over 45 years of age (19). A bruit is not pathognomonic of underlying stenosis (see Table 91.1 for other causes). A duplex scan (see description in Chapter 86) can define which patients with bruits have carotid stenosis and require further evaluation. Stenosis exceeding 75% to 80% of the lumen is associated with an annual risk of ipsilateral stroke of 2% to 3% (20). A large controlled trial (ACAS) demonstrated that for asymptomatic patients with more than 60% stenosis of the carotid artery, the combination of medical management (risk factor reduction and 325 mg aspirin/day) and carotid endarterectomy (CEA) was superior to medical management alone (21). Over 5 years, the projected incidence of morbid events (perioperative death or stroke) was 5.1% for CEA patients, and the incidence of ipsilateral stroke was 11.0% for patients treated medically (an aggregate risk reduction of 53%). Patients to whom CEA is offered should be told that in ACAS there was approximately a 3% risk of perioperative stroke or death with CEA and that the benefit found in the ACAS trial accrued over 5 years.

Table 91.1. Possible Causes of Cervical Bruit

Physiologic murmur
Venous hum
Transmitted cardiac murmur
Atherosclerosis and stenosis of carotid, vertebral, subclavian, or innominate artery
Loops, kinks, inflammation, fibromuscular dysplasia of carotid artery
Arteriovenous fistula
Angiomatous malformation
Intracranial neoplasm
Paget disease of the skull

Patients with excess cardiac risk were excluded from the ACAS trial. Medical management alone would probably benefit the latter group. Information about the symptoms of TIA should be given to any patient with a cervical bruit so that the patient does not ignore warning symptoms. The American Heart Association has excellent patient education materials on TIA.

CLASSIFICATION OF CEREBROVASCULAR EVENTS

Type of Event

Symptoms and signs of vascular origin are characterized by the rapid onset of deficits in a vascular distribution. The following classification has been developed based on duration:

- A *transient ischemic attack (TIA)* is defined as a transient episode of focal cerebral dysfunction, rapid in onset (from none to maximal symptoms in less than 5 minutes), that usually lasts from 2 to 15 minutes but always resolves completely within 24 hours.
- A *reversible ischemic neurologic deficit (RIND)* is defined as an episode of focal cerebral dysfunction that lasts longer than 24 hours but resolves completely within 3 weeks. This type of event is sometimes called a minor stroke.
- A *completed stroke* is defined as an episode of focal cerebral dysfunction that has stabilized and may have improved but has not resolved completely after 3 weeks. The most characteristic pattern is the abrupt occurrence of a neurologic deficit that improves or worsens, sometimes repeatedly, over minutes to hours to days and then becomes a fixed deficit.
- The term *stroke in evolution* is used to describe a vascular syndrome that is acute in onset and progressively worsens during the period of observation.

Vascular Territory

Cerebrovascular events are also classified on the basis of the vascular territory involved. Symptoms and signs referable to the two major vascular territories are listed in Table 91.2. There is overlap in the symptoms that may make the distinction between carotid and vertebrobasilar disease difficult. The history alone often

Table 91.2. Clinical Features of Ischemia Involving the Major Vascular Territories

Carotid artery disease
Paresis (mono- or hemi-)
Sensory loss or paresthesias (mono- or hemi-)
Speech or language disturbances
Loss of vision in one eye or part of one eye (amaurosis fugax)
Homonymous hemianopsia
Cognitive impairment
Vertebrobasilar arterial disease
Vertigo, diplopia, dysphagia, or dysarthria when two occur together or when one occurs with any of the following:
Paresis (any combination of the extremities)
Sensory loss or paresthesias (any combination of the extremities)
Ataxia
Homonymous hemianopsia (unilateral or bilateral)

provides the evidence necessary to identify the arterial territory involved.

A subgroup of ischemic events, called *lacunar syndromes*, is caused by occlusion of penetrating nonanastomosing branches of the major cerebral arteries. The pathology of the involved vessels has been characterized; occlusion is caused either by miniature atherosclerotic plaques at the origin of vessels 400 to 1,000 μm in diameter or, more commonly, by a degenerative process called lipohyalinosis affecting vessels 200 μm or less in diameter. These changes correlate strongly with the presence of hypertension. At least 20 clinical lacunar syndromes have been described (22); lacunar infarctions may also be silent, identified only by CT or magnetic resonance imaging (MRI). The common syndromes are

- *Pure motor hemiparesis* (internal capsule or pons): hemiplegia or hemiparesis involving the face, arm, and leg without sensory deficit, dysphasia, or hemianopsia;
- *Pure sensory stroke* (thalamus): numbness of the face, arm, and leg on one side without weakness or hemianopsia;
- *Ataxic hemiparesis* (internal capsule or pons): cerebellar ataxia, weakness, and pyramidal signs involving the limbs on the same side, the lower extremity more than the arm;
- *The dysarthria or clumsy hand syndrome* (internal capsule or pons): dysarthria, facial weakness, clumsiness of the hand with little or no weakness, a slight imbalance, and a Babinski sign on the affected side;
- *Multi-infarct dementia*: a dementia syndrome characterized by stepwise progression (see description of dementia in Chapter 26).

SYMPTOMATIC PATIENTS

Transient Ischemic Attack and Stroke

Most TIAs and strokes are caused by artery-to-artery embolization, cardiogenic embolus, or small vessel (lacunar) disease. The distinction between TIA and stroke is becoming less important because a rigorous search for cause is indicated in both and many patients with TIA have evidence of brain infarction on imaging. Treatment is based on cause of the event regardless of whether the patient has had a TIA or stroke. Both events signal brain ischemia; stroke occurs when blood supply from collateral vessels is insufficient or the occluding thrombus is too large to be rapidly cleared.

For patients with TIA, other transient neurologic events described elsewhere, such as seizure (see Chapter 88), hypoglycemia (see Chapter 81), syncope (see Chapter 89), and migraine (see Chapter 87) must be considered. A Todd's paralysis (transient focal weakness after a focal motor seizure or secondarily generalized tonic–clonic seizure) is diagnosed when the primary event is a seizure. Transient episodes with altered consciousness are almost never vascular in nature. Migraine occurs primarily in younger patients, is associated with headache, and must conform to defined criteria (see Chapter 87). A mass lesion such as a tumor or subdural hematoma may present with transient neurologic symptoms; however, these patients usually have persistent signs and symptoms. CT or MRI (see Chapter 86) is diagnostic. Occasionally, an acute exacerbation of multiple sclerosis may mimic TIA; however, these patients are usually younger and have had multiple episodes with nonvascular localization (e.g., optic neuritis).

Evaluation

Initial evaluation of the patient with TIA or stroke may be in the hospital (the patient who presents within hours or days of the event) or in the ambulatory setting (the patient who presents within weeks of the event). A detailed history is essential to identify risk factors for cerebrovascular disease and to delineate and classify the focal symptoms (Table 91.2). The physical examination should include assessment for hypotension, hypertension, cardiac disease, cerebrovascular and peripheral vascular disease, and any persisting neurologic abnormality. The patient should also have a careful funduscopic evaluation to assess the status of the retinal vessels and to detect emboli (Fig. 91.1) that suggest atherothrombotic carotid occlusive disease or cardiac disease. A brain MRI or CT (see Chapter 86) can localize the event, demonstrate previous silent events, and rule out other causes of neurologic symptoms that mimic cerebrovascular disease.

If there is clinical evidence of *heart disease*, in particular a murmur, atrial fibrillation, or left ventricular dysfunction, a transesophageal echocardiogram should be obtained to look for a cardiac source of arterial emboli. Transesophageal echocardiogram can also evaluate the aortic arch as a source of embolism. In patients with heart disease, ambulatory cardiac monitoring to check for arrhythmias may be beneficial when the cause of the stroke remains unknown after duplex and transesophageal echocardiogram.

Screening tests to check for *treatable causes* of occlusive cerebrovascular disease include a serologic test for syphilis, hematocrit measurement (polycythemia), and erythrocyte sedimentation rate (vasculitis). If a hypercoagulable state is suspected, protein C and S, antithrombin III, anticardiolipin antibodies, factor V Leiden (or functional assay for activated protein C resistance), and homocysteine levels should be obtained (23).

Patients with carotid territory events should have a *noninvasive carotid evaluation*, using the available technique with the best performance characteristics. Decision analysis of the various available procedures shows that the preferred noninvasive technique is duplex ultrasonography (24). The characteristics of duplex ultrasonography and the patient experiences associated with it and other noninvasive diagnostic tests are described in Chapter 86.

Cerebral angiography (see description in Chapter 86) should be considered in patients who do not have a definite source of brain embolus identified in the heart,

Figure 91.1. Atheromatous debris embolus lodged in retinal arteriole (*arrow*) in patient with recurrent hemisphere transient ischemic attack and amaurosis fugax. These emboli persist for hours to weeks, and even permanently, whereas the platelet-fibrin emboli are fleeting and are gone within a few minutes. (From Meyer JS, Shaw T. Diagnosis and management of stroke and TIAs. Baltimore: Williams & Wilkins, 1982, with permission.)

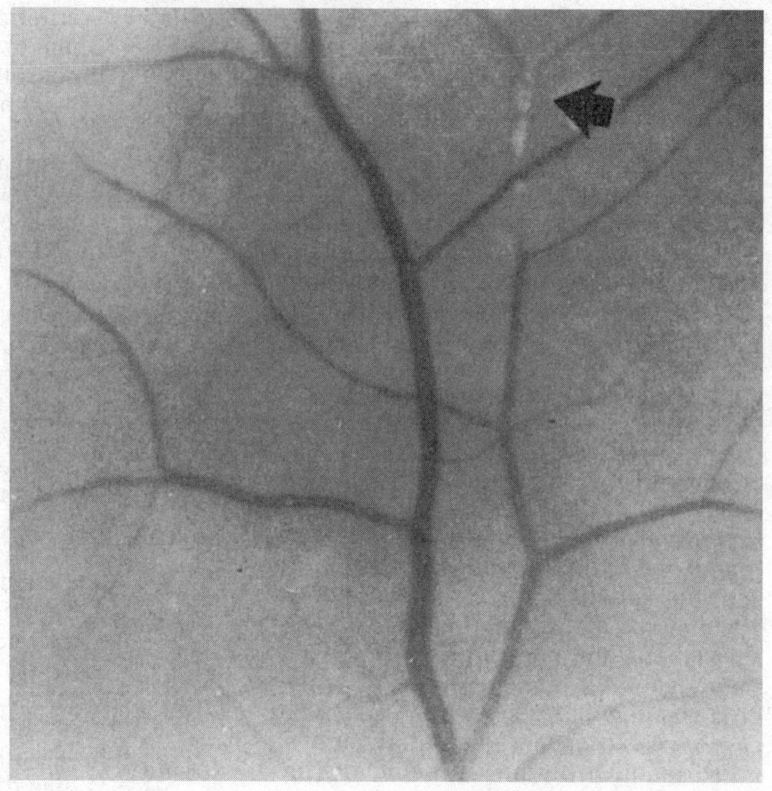

aortic arch, or carotid arteries. Although a duplex scan can rule out carotid stenosis, intracranial vascular disease cannot be identified conclusively by duplex. A limited (noninvasive) evaluation can be justified if the patient's event was so devastating that further evaluation and treatment are precluded.

Early Management

Atherothrombotic Events

Patients with atherothrombotic events, either cortical or lacunar, may be treated medically or surgically.

Medical Therapy. This aspect of management includes risk factor modification and anticoagulant and antiplatelet drugs.

Antihypertensive therapy after an acute ischemic stroke is usually deferred until the patient's neurologic deficit is stable. In a small controlled study of hypertensive patients who had sustained a nonembolic ischemic stroke, 44% of the untreated patients, compared with 20% of the treated patients, suffered another major stroke, and at the end of a 2- to 5-year follow-up period, 46% of the untreated patients and 26% of the treated patients had died (25). Although the number of recurrent strokes was small, the difference in mortality was statistically significant in favor of the treated group. A meta-analysis of nine trials of blood pressure lowering agents in hypertensive and nonhypertensive stroke survivors revealed a 28% reduction in stroke recurrence (26). The PROGRESS trial, a large, randomized, placebo-controlled trial of the angiotensin-converting enzyme inhibitor perindopril with and without the diuretic indapamide demonstrated a 43% decrease in recurrent stroke risk in both hypertensive and nonhypertensive stroke and TIA survivors who received both drugs. Perindopril alone lowered blood pressure without affecting stroke recurrence (27). Although questions remain about subgroups and specific medications, treatment of hypertension in stroke survivors appears beneficial. (See Chapter 67 for details on the treatment of hypertension.)

The *antiplatelet drugs* aspirin, aspirin and dipyridamole (28), ticlopidine (29), and clopidogrel (30) are effective in reducing the recurrence of TIA or stroke. Aspirin is the most widely studied and cheapest agent, with effectiveness in doses of 50 to 1,500 mg (31). Ticlopidine's side-effect profile (fatal neutropenia, diarrhea) outweighs its modest statistical advantage. Clopidogrel's efficacy in secondary stroke prevention was only evident as a combined reduction in myocardial infarction, stroke, or vascular death (30). In the European Stroke Prevention Study-II trial, aspirin plus dipyridamole (25 mg plus 200 mg twice daily) was compared with aspirin alone (25 mg twice daily), extended-release dipyridamole alone (200 mg twice daily), or placebo. There was a 23.1% reduction of stroke in those on combination therapy compared with aspirin alone. Side effects were minor: headache and gastrointestinal events with dipyridamole and bleeding and gastrointestinal events with aspirin, with the combination not significantly affecting side-effect incidence (28). Additional details regarding the use of and efficacy of antiplatelet drugs are in Chapter 57.

Anticoagulant therapy with warfarin [international normalized ratio (INR) 1.4 to 2.8) was compared with aspirin (325 mg/day) in a large, double-blind, randomized trial (Warfarin-Asprin Recurrent Stroke Study [WARSS]) in patients with prior noncardioembolic stroke, most with lacunar (55% in warfarin group, 56% in aspirin group) or cryptogenic (25% in warfarin group, 26% in aspirin group) stroke. Over 2 years of follow-up there was no difference in the rates of ischemic stroke, death, or major hemorrhage (approximately 17% in both groups) (32). Warfarin has been recommended for symptomatic patients (TIA or stroke) with known high-grade intracranial stenosis or preocclusive extracranial carotid bifurcation disease that cannot be addressed surgically (e.g., in patients who have cardiac disease precluding surgery). This approach is supported by a retrospective study of warfarin compared with aspirin in 151 patients with 50% or greater stenosis of an intracranial major artery, which showed a significant benefit from warfarin in reduction of stroke, myocardial infarction, or death (33). An ongoing prospective trial (Warfarin-Asprin Symptomatic Intracranial Disease [WASID]) is evaluating this group of patients (33a). Although patients with high grade intracranial disease were not excluded from WARSS, this group was not specifically studied, and the superiority of warfarin or aspirin in this group remains unsettled. Ongoing trials of higher on-treatment INRs and of warfarin in subgroups of patients will determine whether warfarin should be recommended for some patients (34). Based on all available data, aspirin appears superior in most patients with noncardioembolic strokes. Patients with significant intracranial disease could be treated with warfarin or aspirin until further data are available.

A role for *cholesterol lowering* in secondary stroke prevention was examined in a meta-analysis that included patients with stroke. Risk was reduced by 25% (35).

Surgical Therapy. *CEA* can be recommended to patients with hemispheric or retinal TIAs or nondisabling stroke with ipsilateral severe (70% or greater) stenosis at the carotid bifurcation. This recommendation is supported by a large clinical trial (NASCET) in which 9% of CEA patients versus 26% of patients receiving antiplatelet treatment experienced an ipsilateral stroke during the 2 years after initiation of treatment (36). For symptomatic patients with moderate (50% to 69%) stenosis, the rate of stroke (average follow-up of 5 years) was 15.7% in the surgical group compared with 22.2% in the medical group ($p = .045$.), a modest benefit compared with the benefit in patients with more severe stenosis. For stenosis less than 50%, there was no benefit (37). Patients who have undergone CEA are usually continued on long-term antiplatelet therapy.

In patients with *intracranial carotid and middle cerebral artery stenosis,* extracranial–intracranial bypass surgery has been shown in randomized controlled trials to confer no benefit beyond aspirin's effect (38). In patients with recurrent TIAs or strokes and arteriographic evidence of *severe vertebral or basilar artery stenosis,* bypass procedures, angioplasty, and stenting have been undertaken. The efficacy of these procedures has not yet been established. Because the guidelines for the treatment of patients with TIAs and survivors of stroke are still evolving, the advice of a neurologist who specializes in cerebrovascular disease should be sought.

Cardioembolic Events

Patients with cardioembolic events who benefit from anticoagulation with warfarin include those with atrial fibrillation (both valvular and nonvalvular disease), recent myocardial infarction, dilated cardiomyopathy, and rheumatic and prosthetic valves (11). Clinical trials consistently show an approximately two-thirds reduction in expected events in anticoagulated patients with atrial fibrillation; for those who have had a TIA or minor stroke the annual incidence of a new event is reduced from 12% to 4% and for those with no history of TIA or stroke the annual incidence is reduced from approximately 5% to 2% (39). Specific aspects of anticoagulant therapy to prevent cerebrovascular accident are described in Chapter 57 and in chapters that cover postinfarct mural thrombi (see Chapter 63), atrial fibrillation (see Chapter 64), and valvular heart disease (see Chapter 65). For patients with both a cardiac source and high-grade carotid stenosis (70% or higher) proximal to the territory of a TIA or stroke, CEA should be considered.

STROKE PROGNOSIS

Morbidity in Stroke Survivors

A number of studies have evaluated stroke survivors on the basis of the degree of neurologic, functional, and psychosocial impairment. Table 91.3 shows the spectrum and frequency of neurologic impairments found in stroke survivors in the Framingham study (40). Study subjects were living at home or in institutions at the time of functional evaluation. The interval between the stroke and the functional assessment ranged from 6 months to 33 years (mean, 7 years). It is notable that half of these patients (63 of 123) had no motor deficit. These findings are probably representative of the situation in other communities.

In a classic study of overall function, Katz et al. (41) found that of patients who survive a stroke,

Table 91.3. Prevalence of Neurologic Deficits in the 123 Survivors of Completed Stroke, Framingham Study (1972–1974)

		No. Surviving with			
Type of Peripheral Motor Deficit	Survivors	Sensory Deficit	Hemianopsia	Dysarthria	Dysphasia
No motor deficit	63	3	5	2	10
Left hemiparesis	28	13	6	3	2
Right hemiparesis	27	10	5	13	9
Bilateral motor deficit	4	4	3	2	1
No data	1	1	1	1	1
Total survivors	123	31	20	21	23

From Gresham E, Fitzpatrick TE, Wolf PA, et al. Residual disability in survivors of stroke: the Framingham study. N Engl J Med 1975;293:954, with permission.

approximately 50% are independent 2 years later and can ambulate and perform activities of daily living with minimal or no assistance. Spontaneous improvement is most rapid in the first few months after the stroke and is rarely noted after 2 years. Only a small percentage of stroke survivors remain bedridden and completely dependent. These findings were corroborated by results from the Mayo Clinic, where only 4% of the community-dwelling survivors of a stroke required total care at 6 months, 36% had some degree of neurologic deficit yet were able to work, and 29% were functioning normally (5). On the basis of the authors' assessment, 54% of their patients may have benefited from rehabilitative care, including the 10% who were aphasic.

The Framingham study provided information on the equally important *social and psychologic sequelae* of stroke (40). A significant decrease in the levels of vocational function and socialization outside the home was noted among stroke survivors compared with age- and sex-matched control subjects (Table 91.4), and the decrease exceeded that anticipated based on the levels of neurologic deficit. In a prospective study, the social and psychologic difficulties facing the stroke survivor were evaluated in more detail (42). Within the first 6 months after hospital discharge, 37% of the patients demonstrated moderate or severe depression, 32% anger or anxiety, 56% social isolation, 43% reduction in community involvement, 46% economic strain causing life-style alteration, and 52% disruption of normal family functions. Additional studies have confirmed the high incidence of moderate or severe depression in the first year after stroke and have shown that the risk of depression is particularly high in patients with damage in the left frontal hemisphere . Longitudinal studies show that poststroke depression lasts up to 2 years (43,44). Patients with poststroke depressive respond well to tricyclic antidepressants (see below). Recognition and treatment of the psychosocial problems of the stroke patient and family are discussed in more detail below.

Table 91.4. Prevalence of Four Types of Functional Disability in 119 Survivors of Completed Stroke and in 119 Controls, Framingham Study (1972–1974)

	Survivors		Matched Control Subjects[a]		
Type of Disability	No.	%	No.	%	*P* Value
All persons examined for functional disability	119	100	119	100	—
Dependent in activities of daily living	37	31	9	8	<0.0001
Dependent in mobility	24	20	6	5	<0.0001
Decrease in level of vocational function[b]	85	71	49	41	<0.0001
Decrease in socialization	74	62	37	31	<0.0001

[a]Matched for age and sex.

[b]Either stopped working or incomplete resumption of homemaking activities.

From Gresham E, Fitzpatrick TE, Wolf PA, et al. Residual disability in survivors of stroke: the Framingham study. N Engl J Med 1975;293:954, with permission.

Mortality in Stroke Survivors

The *death rate among stroke survivors* is significantly greater than that expected for the general population matched for age and sex. The 5-year cumulative mortality is approximately 50% to 60%, with the greatest number of deaths occurring in the first year. With time, however, the mortality rate approaches that of the general population, and in at least one study, the increased rate of death after a stroke subsided completely after 24 to 30 months (41). National data from the 1970s (Table 91.5) illustrate the dramatic impact of *age* on survival after stroke.

Studies that classified strokes on the basis of *type of vascular pathology* indicate that the early prognosis is much better for thrombotic or embolic disease than for hemorrhage (5). There is evidence that the type of pathology is a less reliable predictor of late prognosis. Eisenberg et al. (45) reported that patients with cerebral hemorrhage who lived 1 month had a 5-year survival equal to or better than patients with cerebral thrombosis.

The leading cause of death in stroke survivors is cardiovascular disease, with cardiac-related deaths exceeding deaths attributed to cerebrovascular disease by a factor of 2 to 1. Because cardiac disease is a major contributor to the cause of the stroke, stroke recurrence, and the survival from stroke, thorough evaluation and management of cardiac disease are of great importance in the care of stroke survivors.

LONG-TERM MANAGEMENT

Management of the patient who has survived a stroke involves the evaluation and treatment of physical and psychosocial sequelae and the selection of appropriate therapy to lessen the risk of recurrence. Once the patient has been discharged from the hospital, the patient's personal physician plays a critical role in coordinating care. Reduction in a patient's disability and

Table 91.5. Percentage Distribution of Stroke Survivors by Age Group

	Percentage Surviving									
		Days				Years				
Age Group	Onset	30	60	90	180	1	2	3	4	5
Under 65	100.0	73.7	71.1	69.4	65.9	63.2	57.6	57.6	52.0	49.2
65–74	100.0	75.6	69.5	65.2	63.1	59.4	52.9	46.1	42.7	34.5
75–84	100.0	68.1	62.1	57.6	52.4	45.7	37.2	30.0	23.1	21.9
85+	100.0	52.4	45.8	37.2	33.0	27.8	20.7	15.1	9.2	7.4

From National Survey of Stroke, U.S. Department of Health, Education and Welfare, Public Health Service, National Institutes of Health, NIH pub. no. 80-2069, January 1980, with permission.

dependency often requires the concerted efforts of the patient's family; physical, occupational, and speech therapists; and occasionally a psychiatrist. Patients with significant deficits persisting for 3 months or longer may qualify for *disability insurance under Social Security* (see Chapter 9).

Role of the Family

At the time of discharge from the hospital, appropriate education is especially important for the stroke survivor and the patient's family. At this juncture, patients are confronted with the full extent of their functional loss. By dispelling myths regarding stroke and supplanting them with accurate information, physicians and therapists can ensure that the actions of well-meaning family members do not foster the patients' feelings of inadequacy. The American Heart Association has produced a series of invaluable booklets that discuss stroke and its sequelae in lay terms and provide guidelines for the home management of the stroke patient. The titles of these publications are listed in Table 91.6.

The following general suggestions can be helpful for the family of a stroke patient with residual disability:

- Divide duties so that the full burden of care does not fall on one person.
- Help the patient take responsibility for exercising regularly.
- Allow the patient to take on responsibilities for self-care and other activities gradually and by easy steps. It calls for fine judgment to encourage independence and not to frustrate a patient with overly difficult tasks and to stimulate progress without encouraging unrealistic expectations.
- Praise any successful efforts that are made; do not be discouraged by failures. Recovery from stroke is a slow process.
- Have the patient participate in as many family activities and as much family planning as possible. Feeling useful is a tremendous morale builder.
- Help him or her keep in contact with the world.
- Do not relegate the patient to the sidelines and leave him or her with only television and radio. Encourage the patient to develop a hobby. Spend time with him or her and encourage visitors if warranted. Make him or her feel wanted and a part of the social picture.

Table 91.6. Booklets Published by the American Heart Association

Recovering from a Stroke is a booklet written for the patient and the patient's family on ways in which the patient can regain activities of daily living.

How Stroke Affects Behavior is a detailed booklet providing recommendations for the care of the patient who has completed most of his or her spontaneous recovery of higher functions and has major residual deficits (see Table 91.7).

Caring for a Person with Aphasia explains many of the problems in aphasia and suggests practical ways in which the family can help the aphasic patient.

Available without charge from local American Heart Association chapters.

- Get in touch with the doctor if things are not going as you believe they should.

Role of Rehabilitation

Success in stroke rehabilitation often depends on the extent of permanent damage and the patient's ability to use *alternative methods of function* to compensate for fixed deficits. As noted above, spontaneous improvement in the stroke survivor may continue to occur for the first 6 to 12 months after the stroke, yet the mechanisms underlying such gains remain obscure. In studies to determine whether intensive rehabilitation results in functional gains after the period of spontaneous improvement, it has been found that even significantly impaired patients admitted to a rehabilitation program 12 months after a stroke may show marked improvement in dressing skills, bladder and bowel function, and walking (46). These findings form the basis for the conclusion that a program of rehabilitation does improve the outcome of the stroke survivor. It is estimated that the savings derived in returning a patient to the family or to independent living more than equals the costs of rehabilitation (46).

It is clear that not all patients in a rehabilitation program show significant functional improvement. A number of patient characteristics correlate with poor rehabilitation results, including bowel and bladder incontinence, low self-care status on admission, right hemispheric involvement, intellectual and perceptual deficits, heart failure, signs of generalized arteriosclerosis, and lower educational levels (47,48). However, because none of these factors correlates strongly with poor outcome, the best approach is to offer rehabilitation services when possible to each stroke survivor with significant functional impairments.

It is generally agreed that, except for patients with evidence of subarachnoid bleeding, for whom bed rest and mild sedation are indicated, a *program of functional rehabilitation* should begin as soon as possible after a stroke occurs and the patient is stable. There are several reasons for the early initiation of a program of rehabilitation. First, it is generally accepted that patients who are provided with rehabilitation services early are likely to experience greater long-term functional improvement. Second, early transfer from bed to chair coupled with physical therapy reduces the complications that can develop in the immobile bedridden patient and that can subsequently limit the extent of functional recovery. Stretching of tight muscles, passive range of motion, and active or resistive exercises minimize the degree of muscle atrophy and prevent the development of contractures. In addition, even limited mobility of the patient reduces the risk of circulatory complications such as thrombophlebitis, postural hypotension, and pressure sores. Third, early rehabilitation is of particular benefit to the patient who demonstrates an impaired ability to communicate because of either aphasia or dysarthria. Approximately one-third of stroke patients exhibit some form of communication disorder, and many of these remain severely impaired beyond the period of spontaneous recovery (49). Such patients may feel desperately isolated because of their loss of ability to communicate. Therapists who specialize in speech and hearing are skilled in the evaluation and management of these problems and play an integral role in daily interactions with the patient and in recommending appropriate strategies to the patient's family and physician.

Everyone involved in the rehabilitation process must appreciate the significance of the functional losses sustained by the patient, so the losses must be viewed from the patient's perspective. This requires an awareness of the patient's usual activities before the stroke; this essential information should be obtained in conjunction with a social worker who can evaluate the patient's role at home before the stroke and can project how the stroke will alter that role when the patient returns home.

The rehabilitation initiated in the hospital can be continued after discharge. Most communities have physical, occupational, and speech therapists available for both home and ambulatory follow-up. For patients meeting eligibility criteria, these services are covered by third-party payers. The patient and family should be acquainted with the goals and plans for continued rehabilitation before discharge. Chapter 9 provides information about home health services. The comprehensive text of Brandstater and Basmajian (see General References) provides details about the many individualized approaches available for rehabilitation.

Management of Psychologic and Behavioral Sequelae

The high incidence of psychologic and behavioral problems among stroke survivors has been noted above. These problems often hinder rehabilitation efforts. Fear of a second stroke and depression caused by loss of functional ability are readily understandable in the context of the patient's predicament. Appropriate counseling of the patient and family (as outlined above), coupled with participation in an active rehabilitation program, are the best ways to minimize the adverse psychologic reactions to a stroke.

A number of stroke survivors experience *mood disturbances* that do not correlate with the level of functional disability, and there is evidence that for many patients the mood disorder is a specific complication of cerebral damage rather than a reaction to functional loss (43,44,50). This mood disorder may augment the cognitive impairment of the patient or on occasion may be expressed as an apparent cognitive impairment (pseudodementia of depression, described in Chapter 26). Response in such patients to antidepressant treatment may be dramatic. Earlier observations suggested that the type of mood disorder depends on the side of the brain affected by the stroke (51). Gainotti (52) reported that behavior denoting a catastrophic reaction (see Chapter 26) and anxious depressive orientation of mood (anxiety reactions, bursts of tears, provocative utterances, depressed renouncements, or sharp refusals to go on with the examinations) are more common among patients with *left* (dominant) hemisphere damage. Symptoms denoting an opposite emotional reaction (denial of illness, minimization, indifference reactions, and tendency to joke) and expressions of hate toward the paralyzed limbs are more common among patients suffering from a lesion of the *right* (nondominant) hemisphere. Most authorities agree, however, that both psychologic and physiologic factors contribute to the development of mood disorders after strokes. Tricyclic antidepressants have been shown to benefit patients with poststroke depression (43,44,51). Practical information about these and other antidepressant drugs is found in Chapter 24.

The American Heart Association booklet *How Stroke Affects Behavior* is particularly helpful for the family and for health care professionals caring for the patient who has survived a stroke. Table 91.7 contains summaries of the recommendations for dealing with permanent behavioral problems in these patients.

Management of Late Complications

A number of complications may occur during the months to years after a stroke.

Shoulder Problems

The painful shoulder is one of the most disturbing complications encountered in the patient with a residual hemiparesis. Shoulder pain is often caused by increased traction on the shoulder capsule secondary to abnormal positioning of the paralyzed arm. The normal alignment of the joint can be restored through the use of a sling and proper positioning of the arm at night. Physical therapy, after initial symptomatic treatment with analgesics and the application of heat, can limit the extent of permanent structural damage (see Chapter 69 for additional details).

The *shoulder–hand syndrome* occurs in approximately 5% of stroke patients. It is characterized by the occurrence of a painful shoulder associated with stiffness and swelling of the hand and fingers. Onset is acute or subacute (developing over 3 to 6 months) and may involve the hand and shoulder simultaneously or one followed by the other. Although a number of conditions can result in shoulder discomfort, the dystrophic changes in the hand are characteristic of the development of a complex regional pain syndrome. There is swelling below the wrist, and the intrinsic muscles of the hand atrophy with extension deformities in the metacarpophalangeal joints. At this stage radiographic examination of the hand often shows spotty demineralization of the carpal bones. The severe pain associated with this condition greatly hinders rehabilitation efforts. Therefore, early recognition and treatment are important. A nonsteroidal anti-inflammatory drug, local heat, and medications for chronic pain may be helpful.

Complications of Inactivity

The partially paralyzed stroke survivor often leads a sedentary existence, conducive to the development of

Table 91.7. Recommendations for Dealing with Behavioral Problems Associated with Permanent Loss of Higher Functions in Stroke Patients

Left hemisphere damage

Right hemiplegics often have difficulties with speech and language. They also tend to be somewhat cautious, anxious, and disorganized when attempting a new task. Keep in mind the following suggestions:

- Do not underestimate the patient's ability to learn and communicate even if he or she cannot use speech.
- If he or she cannot use speech, try other forms of communication. Pantomime and demonstration are often useful.
- Do not overestimate his or her understanding of speech and overload him or her with "static."
- Do not shout. Keep messages simple and brief.
- Do not use special voices.
- Divide tasks into simple steps.
- Give much feedback and many indications of progress.

Right hemisphere damage

If the patient is having difficulty with self-care activities, you can expect spatial–perceptual deficits. He or she will tend to talk better than he or she can actually perform. The patient may be impulsive or careless. Remember, when working with the patient who has significant spatial–perceptual deficits,

- Do not overestimate abilities. Spatial–perceptual difficulties are easy to miss.
- Use verbal cues if he or she has difficulty with demonstration.
- Break tasks into small steps and give much feedback.
- Watch to see what he or she can do safely rather than taking the patient's word for it.
- Minimize clutter.
- Avoid rapid movement around the patient.
- Highlight visual reference points.

One-sided neglect

One-sided neglect is a problem that involves more than a simple visual field cut or hearing loss. It can occur in both right and left hemiplegics but seems to be more common and more persistent among left hemiplegics. When dealing with a neglect problem, you should

- Keep the unimpaired side toward the action unless specifically working with neglected side.
- Avoid trapping the patient in an unnecessarily confined environment.
- Avoid nagging but give frequent cues to aid orientation.
- Provide reminders of the neglected side.
- Arrange the environment to maximize performance.

Memory problems

Some memory problems can be expected in most stroke patients. When working with memory deficits, you can often increase the patient's ability to perform if you

- Establish a fixed routine whenever possible.
- Keep messages short enough to fit retention span.
- Present new information one step at a time.
- Allow the patient to finish one step before proceeding to the next.
- Give frequent indications of effective progress; the patient may forget past successes.
- Train in settings that resemble, as much as possible, the setting in which the behavior is to be practiced.
- Use memory aids such as appointment books, written notes, and schedule cards whenever possible.
- Use familiar objects and old associations when teaching new tasks.

Adapted from How stroke affects behavior. Dallas, TX: American Heart Association.

vascular complications such as thrombophlebitis and pressure sores. Use of elastic stockings and frequent repositioning of the immobile patient by an informed family member minimizes these problems.

Neurologic Complications

Prolonged pressure on a paralyzed limb may lead to a peripheral nerve lesion, which may be difficult to recognize when superimposed on brain damage resulting from the stroke. An awareness of this potential complication can expedite its recognition, and electrodiagnostic studies can confirm the lower motor neuron damage (see Chapter 92). Once a diagnosis is made, prompt initiation of physical therapy limits the degree of functional loss resulting from this potentially reversible lesion.

Approximately 3% to 10% of stroke survivors develop *seizures* (epilepsy) as a late complication (53). Patients with damage to their sensorimotor cortex are the most likely to develop epilepsy, with the first seizure usually occurring 6 to 12 months after the stroke. Transient neurologic dysfunction after a seizure in a stroke survivor is often attributed to a second stroke. The rapid resolution of symptoms and electroencephalographic evidence of an epileptogenic focus point to seizure activity rather than ischemia as the cause. Recurrent seizures in the stroke survivor confirm the diagnosis of epilepsy. Seizure control can usually be achieved through the use of anticonvulsant medication (see Chapter 88).

Finally, *stroke-related deficits may transiently worsen* when the patient develops a major intercurrent illness such as pneumonia or myocardial infarction. In this instance, neurologic status returns to baseline after resolution of the intercurrent illness. (See discussion of upper motor neuron symptoms in Chapter 86.)

General Surgery

The approach to general surgery in patients who have a history of stroke is addressed in Chapter 93.

General References*

Brandstater M, Basmajian J, eds. Stroke rehabilitation. Baltimore: Williams & Wilkins, 1987.

A detailed, well-illustrated, and extensively referenced resource on all aspects of the rehabilitation of stroke patients.

Sacco RL. Extracranial carotid stenosis. N Engl J Med 2001;345:1113.

Well-referenced review article.

Welch KMA, Caplan LR, Reis DJ, et al., eds. Primer on cerebrovascular disease. New York: Academic Press, 1997.

An excellent source for clinicians with practical up to date information on diagnosis and treatment.

Specific References

1. American Heart Association. 1997 Heart and stroke facts statistical update. Dallas: American Heart Association, 1997.
2. Hachinski V. Decreased incidence and mortality of stroke. Stroke 1984;15:376.
3. Whisnant JP. The decline of stroke. Stroke 1984;15:160.
4. Broderick JP, Phillips SJ, Whisnant JP, et al. Incidence rates of strokes in the eighties: the end of the decline in stroke? Stroke 1989;20:577.

*Bold print (general references) and bold numerals (specific references) denote published controlled clinical trials, meta-analyses, or consensus-based recommendations.

5. Matsumoto N, Whisnant JP, Kurland LT, et al. Natural history of stroke in Rochester, Minnesota, 1955 through 1969: an extension of a previous study, 1945 through 1954. Stroke 1973;4:20.
6. Kannel WB, Wolf PA, Verter J, et al. Epidemiologic assessment of the role of blood pressure in stroke. JAMA 1970;214:301.
7. SHEP Cooperative Research Group. Prevention of stroke by antihypertensive drug treatment in older persons with isolated systolic hypertension. JAMA 1991;265:3255.
8. VA Cooperative Study Group on Antihypertensive Agents. Effects of treatment on morbidity in hypertension. Results in patients with diastolic blood pressures averaging 115 through 129 mm Hg. JAMA 1967;202:1028.
9. VA Cooperative Study Group on Antihypertensive Agents. Effects of treatment on morbidity in hypertension. II. Results in patients with diastolic blood pressure averaging 90 through 114 mm Hg. JAMA 1970;213:1143.
10. Staessen JA, Wang JG, Thijs L. Cardiovascular protection and blood pressure reduction: a meta-analysis. Lancet 2001;358: 1305.
11. Caplan LR. Stroke: a clinical approach. Boston: Butterworth-Heinemann, 1993.
12. Wolf PA, Kannel WB, McNamara PM, et al. The role of impaired cardiac function in atherothrombotic brain infarction: the Framingham study. Am J Public Health 1973;63:52.
13. Byington RP, Davis BR, White HD, et al. Reduction of stroke events with pravastatin: the Prospective Pravastatin Poolin (PPP) Project. Circulation 2001;103:387.
14. Kannel WB. Current status of the epidemiology of brain infarction associated with occlusive arterial disease. Stroke 1971; 2:295.
15. Whisnant JP, Homer D, Ingall TJ. Duration of cigarette smoking is the strongest predictor of severe extracranial carotid artery atherosclerosis. Stroke 1990;21:707.
16. Kannel WB, Gordon T, Wolf PA, et al. Hemoglobin and the risk of cerebral infarction: the Framingham study. Stroke 1972;3:409.
17. Paganini-Hill A. Estrogen replacement therapy and stroke. Prog Cardiovasc Dis 1995;38:223.
18. Simon JA, Hsia J, Cauley JA, et al. Postmenopausal hormone therapy and risk of stroke: the Heart and Estrogen-progestin Replacement Study (HERS). Circulation 2001;103:638.
19. Heyman A, Wilkinson WE, Heyden S, et al. Risk of stroke in asymptomatic persons with cervical arterial bruits: a population study in Evans County, Georgia. N Engl J Med 1980;302:838.
20. Hennerici M, Hulsbomer HB, Hefter H, et al. Natural history of asymptomatic extracranial arterial disease. Brain 1987;110: 777.
21. Executive Committee for the Asymptomatic Carotid Atherosclerosis Study. Endarterectomy for asymptomatic carotid artery stenosis. JAMA 1995;273:1421.
22. Fisher CM. Lacunar strokes and infarcts: a review. Neurology 1982;32:871.
23. Feinberg W, Coull B. Coagulopathies and stroke. In: Welch KMA, Caplan LR, Reis DJ, et al., eds. Primer on cerebrovascular diseases. New York: Academic Press, 1997.
24. American College of Physicians Health and Public Policy Committee. Diagnostic evaluation of the carotid arteries. Ann Intern Med 1988;109:835.
25. Carter AB. Hypertensive therapy in stroke survivors. Lancet 1970;1:485.
26. Gueyffier F, Boissel JP, Boutitie F, et al. Effect of antihypertensive treatment in patients already suffered from stroke. Gathering the evidence. The Indana (Individual Data Analysis of Antihypertensive Intervention trials) Project Collaborators. Stroke 1997;28:2557.
27. Progress Collaborative Group. Randomized trial of a perindopril-based blood-pressure-lowering regimen among 6105 individuals with previous stroke or transient ischemic attack. Lancet 2001;358:1033.
28. Diener HC, Cunha L, Forbes C, et al. European Stroke Prevention Study. 2. Dipyridamole and acetylsalicylic acid in the secondary prevention of stroke. J Neurol Sci 1996;143:1.
29. Hass WK, Easton JD, Adams HP. A randomized trial comparing ticlopidine hydrochloride with aspirin for the prevention of stroke in high-risk patients. N Engl J Med 1989;321:501.
30. CAPRIE Steering Committee. A randomized, blinded, trial of clopidogrel versus aspirin in patients at risk of ischemic events (CAPRIE). Lancet 1996;348:1329.
31. Johnson ES, Lanes SF, Wentworth CE 3rd, et al. A meta-regression analysis of the dose-response effect of aspirin on stroke. Arch Intern Med 1999;159:1248.
32. Mohr JP, Thompson JL, Lazar RM, et al. A comparison of Warfarin and aspirin for the prevention of recurrent ischemic stroke. N Engl J Med 2001;345:1444.
33. Chimowitz MI, Kokkinos MB, Strong J. et al. The warfarin-aspirin symptomatic intracranial disease study. Neurology 1955;45:1488.
33a. The Warfarin-Aspirin Symptomatic Intracranial Disease (WASID) Study Group. Prognosis of patients with symptomatic vertebral or basilar artery stenosis. Stroke 1998;29:1389.
34. Powers WJ. Oral anticoagulant therapy for the prevention of stroke [Editorial]. N Engl J Med 2001;345:1493.
35. Sirol M, Bouzamondo A, Sanchez P, et al. Does statin therapy reduce the risk of stroke? A meta-analysis. Ann Med Intern 2001;152:188.
36. North American Symptomatic Carotid Endarterectomy Trial Collaborators (NASCET). Beneficial effect of carotid endarterectomy in symptomatic patients with high-grade carotid stenosis. N Engl J Med 1991;325:445.
37. Barnett HJ, Taylor DW, Eliasziw M, et al. Benefit of carotid endarterectomy in patients with symptomatic moderate or severe stenosis. North American Symptomatic Carotid Endarterectomy Trial Collaborators. N Engl J Med 1998;339:1415.
38. EC/IC Bypass Study Group. Failure of extracranial–intracranial arterial bypass to reduce the risk of ischemic stroke: results of an international randomized trial. N Engl J Med 1985;313:1191–1200.
39. Anticoagulants for atrial fibrillation [Commentary]. Lancet 1993;342:1251.
40. Gresham GE, Fitzpatrick TE, Wolf PA, et al. Residual disability in survivors of stroke: the Framingham study. N Engl J Med 1975;293:954.
41. Katz S, Ford AB, Chinn AB, et al. Prognosis after strokes. II. Long-term course of 159 patients. Medicine 1966;45:236.
42. Feibel JH, Berk S, Joynt RJ. The unmet needs of stroke survivors. Neurology 1979;29:592.
43. Robinson RG, Starr LB, Kubos KL, et al. A two-year longitudinal study of post-stroke mood disorders: findings during the initial evaluation. Stroke 1983;14:736.
44. Robinson RG, Starr LB, Lipsey JR, et al. A two-year longitudinal study of post-stroke mood disorders: dynamic changes in associated variables over the first six months of follow-up. Stroke 1984;15:510.
45. Eisenberg H, Morrison JT, Sullivan P, et al. Cerebrovascular accidents: incidence and survival rates in a defined population. Middlesex County, Connecticut. JAMA 1964;189:883.
46. Lehmann JF, DeLateur BJ, Fowler RS, et al. Stroke: does rehabilitation affect outcome? Arch Phys Med Rehabil 1975;56:375.
47. Bourestom NC. Predictors of long term recovery in cerebrovascular disease. Arch Phys Med Rehabil 1967;48:415.
48. Lehmann JF, DeLateur BJ, Fowler RS, et al. Stroke rehabilitation: outcome and prediction. Arch Phys Med Rehabil 1975;56:383.
49. Sarno MT. Disorders of communication in stroke. In: Licht S, ed. Stroke and its rehabilitation. Baltimore: Williams & Wilkins, 1975.
50. Folstein MF, Maiberger R, McHugh PR. Mood disorders as a specific complication of stroke. J Neurol Neurosurg Psychiatry 1977;40:1018.
51. Robinson RG, Balduc PL, Price TR. Two-year longitudinal study of post stroke mood disorders: diagnosis and outcome at one and two years. Stroke 1987;18:837.
52. Gainotti G. Emotional behavior and hemispheric side of the lesion. Cortex 1972;8:41.
53. Lesser RP, Lauders H, Dinner DS, et al. Epileptic seizures due to thrombotic and embolic cerebrovascular disease in older patients. Epilepsia 1985;26:622.

CHAPTER 92

Peripheral Neuropathy

GARY J. ROMANO, MD, PhD
RALPH W. KUNCL, MD, PhD

DEFINITIONS AND PATHOPHYSIOLOGY

Peripheral neuropathies result from disease processes that involve the peripheral nervous system. The peripheral nervous system includes cranial nerves III through XII, dorsal and ventral spinal roots, dorsal root ganglia, spinal nerves, and most autonomic ganglia and nerves.

Peripheral nerves consist of a bundle of fibers called *axons;* the large and medium sized axons are normally covered with a layer of myelin. Most peripheral nerves are mixed nerves that carry both incoming sensory information (afferent fibers) and outgoing motor and autonomic impulses (efferent fibers). Large-diameter afferent fibers convey information about position and vibration; large-diameter efferent fibers innervate the muscles themselves. Small-diameter, often unmyelinated fibers convey pain and temperature sensation and autonomic information.

Based on the primary site of involvement of the peripheral nerves, peripheral neuropathies can be classified into three categories: neuronopathies, axonopathies, and myelinopathies. *Neuronopathies* result from processes affecting primarily the sensory cell bodies in the dorsal root ganglia or motor neuron cell bodies in the spinal cord. By convention, because motor neuron cell bodies are in the central nervous system, motor neuronopathies are not usually classified among the peripheral neuropathies. *Axonal neuropathies* result from processes affecting primarily the axon, whereas *myelinopathies* (also called demyelinating neuropathies) result from processes affecting primarily the myelin sheath. In some chronic disorders such as diabetes mellitus, irrespective of the primary pathologic process, the interdependence between axon and myelin produces secondary changes that, on biopsy, reveal a mixed pathologic picture. The etiologic diagnosis of peripheral neuropathies, therefore, depends on both the clinical features and the supportive laboratory and pathologic findings.

Three major anatomic patterns of peripheral nerve disease may be distinguished by clinical presentation: mononeuropathy, mononeuropathy multiplex (multifocal neuropathies), and polyneuropathy. *Mononeuropathies* are lesions of individual nerve roots or peripheral nerves; they usually are due to local causes such as trauma or entrapment (compression of a nerve by adjacent structures). *Mononeuropathy multiplex* refers to involvement of two or more named nerves, usually asymmetrically and not contiguously, either at the same time or sequentially. This less common pattern is usually caused by systemic diseases such as the necrotizing vasculitides (e.g., polyarteritis nodosa) or diabetes mellitus, which may affect several nerves focally. *Polyneuropathy* is the result of a generalized disease process affecting many peripheral nerves, often in a symmetric distribution.

In both axonal and demyelinating diseases, the longer larger nerves are generally involved earlier and more severely than the shorter nerves. In demyelinating neuropathies, this vulnerability of the longer axons may reflect the increased number of potential sites for demyelination; in axonal neuropathies, the longer axons require more metabolic support and therefore may be more susceptible to disruption of this support. As a result, symptoms of axonal and demyelinating types of neuropathies tend to appear first in the feet and then in the hands. Most polyneuropathies indiscriminately affect both the sensory and the motor nerve fibers (mixed polyneuropathies or sensorimotor neuropathies); some affect peripheral autonomic nerves. However, clinically (and occasionally pathologically) in some patients there is a predilection for the sensory nerves (sensory neuropathies), motor nerves (motor neuropathies), or autonomic nerves.

APPROACH TO THE PATIENT

History and Physical Examination

Symptoms of peripheral neuropathy include reduced sensitivity to stimuli (hypesthesia); spontaneous unusual sensations such as tingling, burning, or pain (paresthesias or dysesthesias); weakness; and muscle cramps. If autonomic nerves are involved, impotence, urinary retention or overflow incontinence, constipation or diarrhea, diminished sweating, and orthostatic hypotension are common symptoms. In patients with polyneuropathy, paresthesias in the feet are the most common presenting complaint. Often, patients are bothered by non-noxious sensory stimuli such as light touch perceived as pain (allodynia) and may report that symptoms are relieved by pacing the floor or by firm massage. Complaints of heaviness or coldness of the extremities are also common. Diminished joint position sense (proprioception) may be reported as unsteady gait, particularly on uneven surfaces or in the dark.

The *major signs of peripheral neuropathy* are sensory loss, weakness, muscle atrophy, diminished or absent tendon reflexes, and, if autonomic nerves are involved, trophic changes in the skin. The most common sensory modalities affected in polyneuropathy are pain and vibration, in a symmetric stocking–glove distribution. Thermal sensation is usually affected, but this is harder to document in the clinical setting. In polyneuropathies the weakness is most often distal, affecting the intrinsic muscles of the feet (e.g., inability to spread or extend the toes). In long-standing neuropathies the muscle imbalance causes high arched feet and hammer toes. Eventually, the shin may appear prominent because of atrophy of the tibialis anterior muscle (sharp shin sign), and there may be striking wasting of the small muscles of the hand. The skin of the lower extremities may appear shiny, scaling, and atrophic, although similar changes can be seen with vascular insufficiency. Marked loss of proprioception in the feet may be manifest as unsteadiness, ataxia, or a positive Romberg test (see Chapter 86 for additional details about neurologic signs).

Causes and Distinctive Features

Whereas a limited number of conditions produce mononeuropathy and mononeuropathy multiplex (Table 92.1), there are many causes of polyneuropathy (Table 92.2). Diagnosis often depends on obtaining a thorough history (e.g., of alcoholism or of occupational exposure to toxins) or finding a relevant systemic condition (e.g., diabetes mellitus). Table 92.3 lists the three features most useful in the differential diagnosis of a polyneuropathy—time course, selective functional involvement, and distribution—and the causes associated with these features.

Table 92.1. Common Causes of Mononeuropathy and Mononeuropathy Multiplex

Mononeuropathy
- Trauma: direct (occupational, recreational, e.g., ulnar or peroneal nerve), compression, and entrapment (e.g., carpal tunnel, root compression)
- Infection: herpes zoster
- Vascular: vasculitis, diabetes mellitus
- Neoplasm: neurofibroma, lymphoma

Mononeuropathy multiplex
- Diabetes mellitus
- Vasculitis

Table 92.2. Polyneuropathy: Causes and Modes of Predominant Involvement

	Predominant Involvement
Metabolic	
Diabetes mellitus	
Polyneuropathy	S, SM, A
Mononeuropathy	SM
Lumbar plexopathy (diabetic amyotrophy)	M > S
Alcohol with vitamin deficiency	SM
Uremia	SM
Porphyria	M > S
B_{12} deficiency	S > M
Toxic (see Table 92.5)	
Lead	M > S
Pyridoxine	S
cis-platinum	S
Most other drugs and toxic agents	SM
Infectious	
Diphtheria	M
Leprosy	S
Lyme disease	SM
Human immunodeficiency virus	S, SM, M
Inflammatory and collagen–vascular	
Guillain–Barré syndrome	M
Chronic inflammatory demyelinating polyneuropathy	M
Noncarcinomatous sensory neuropathy (e.g., Sjögren)	S
Systemic lupus erythematosus	SM
Polyarteritis nodosa	SM
Sjögren syndrome	SM, S
Rheumatoid arthritis	SM
Neoplastic	
Carcinomatous	S, SM
Paraproteinemia, plasma cell dyscrasias	S, SM, A
Benign monoclonal gammopathy	S, SM
Waldenström macroglobinemia	SM, M
Cryoglobinemia	SM
Hereditary	
Hereditary motor and sensory neuropathies	M > S
Amyloidosis	S > M, A
Dysautonomia (Riley–Day)	S, A
Tomaculous neuropathy	SM
Tangier (Bassen–Kornzweig)	S
Fabry	S

A, autonomic; M, motor; S, sensory.

Table 92.3. Polyneuropathy: Differential Diagnosis

- Time course
  - Acute (days)
    - *Guillain–Barré syndrome*
    - Porphyric neuropathy
    - Vasculitic neuropathy
    - Some toxins (e.g., triorthocresyl phosphate)
  - Subacute (weeks)
    - *Many toxins and drugs* (see Table 92.5)
    - *Nutritional neuropathies*
    - Carcinomatous neuropathies
    - Diabetic amyotrophy
    - Uremic neuropathy
  - Relapsing
    - Chronic inflammatory demyelinating polyneuropathy
    - Refsum disease
    - Porphyria
  - Chronic (many months or years)
    - *Diabetic motor and sensory neuropathy*
    - *Alcoholic neuropathy*
    - Chronic inflammatory demyelinating polyneuropathy
  - Very chronic (childhood onset)
    - Hereditary, motor and sensory neuropathies (e.g., Charcot–Marie–Tooth disease)
- Selective functional involvement[a]
  - Predominantly motor
    - Guillain–Barré syndrome
    - Chronic inflammatory demyelinating polyneuropathy
    - Acute intermittent porphyria
    - Lead neuropathy
    - Hereditary motor and sensory neuropathies (e.g., Charcot–Marie–Tooth)
    - Diphtheritic neuropathy
  - Predominately sensory
    - Global sensory loss
      - *Diabetes mellitus*
      - Carcinomatous sensory neuropathy (ganglioradiculitis)
      - Paraproteinemic and cryoglobulinemic neuropathy
      - Tabes dorsalis
    - Dissociated loss of pain and thermal sensibility
      - Diabetes (small fiber type)
      - Amyloidosis
      - Hereditary sensory neuropathies
      - Lepromatous leprosy
    - Dissociated loss of joint position and vibration sensibility
      - Subacute combined degeneration
      - Friedreich ataxia
  - Autonomic neuropathy
    - *Diabetes*
    - *Amyloid*
    - Acute, chronic, and relapsing pandysautonomia
    - Dysautonomia (Riley–Day)
- Distribution[b]
  - Proximal weakness
    - Guillain–Barré syndrome
    - Porphyria
    - Diabetic amyotrophy
    - Carcinomatous neuropathy with proximal weakness ("carcinomatous neuromyopathy")
  - Proximal sensory loss
    - Porphyria
    - Tangier disease (analphalipoproteinemia)
  - Temperature-related distribution
    - Lepromatous leprosy

The most common causes are set in Italic.

[a]Most polyneuropathies produce sensory and motor disturbances.

[b]Most polyneuropathies produce distal involvement.

Modified from Griffin JW, Cornblath DR. Peripheral neuropathies. In: Harvey AM, et al., eds. Principles and practice of medicine, 22nd ed. New York: Appleton & Lange, 1988, with permission.

Time Course

Mononeuropathies are often acute in onset; that is, the patient remembers the time of onset. The most common of the acute polyneuropathies, the Guillain-Barré syndrome, and other processes—metabolic, vasculitic, or toxic—may cause rapid onset of severe neurologic dysfunction, sometimes within hours. Most toxic neuropathies (e.g., lead poisoning) develop more slowly (within weeks), as do neuropathies associated with malnutrition (e.g., thiamine deficiency). The most common of the chronic neuropathies (gradual progression over months to years) are associated with diabetes mellitus (see Chapter 79) and alcoholism (see below); in an unselected population, these are the most common polyneuropathies.

Patients with *hereditary neuropathies* sometimes may be unaware that they have a long-standing progressive disorder. A history of a lack of athletic ability in school or problems fitting shoes may be useful clues. Irreducibly high-arched feet and hammer toes reflect long-standing disease occurring during foot development and may therefore suggest a hereditary process. *Mononeuropathy* usually produces both motor and sensory involvement in the distribution of the affected nerve root or peripheral nerve (see below and Tables 92.6 and 92.7).

Selective Functional Involvement

Most *polyneuropathies* produce both sensory and motor disturbances. Polyneuropathy with *predominantly sensory involvement* suggests diabetes mellitus, carcinoma, amyloidosis, and dysproteinemia. Occasionally, sensory losses are dissociated, that is, the patient has diminished pain and temperature sensation but preserved vibration and joint position sense; this pattern is typical of small fiber neuropathies. When position and vibratory sense are lost but pain sense is preserved, vitamin B_{12} deficiency (usually pernicious anemia) or, much more rarely, Friedreich ataxia should be considered. In polyneuropathy, *predominantly motor involvement* suggests inflammatory demyelinating neuropathy, hereditary neuropathies, lead intoxication, or acute intermittent porphyria. *Predominantly autonomic involvement* suggests diabetes mellitus, amyloidosis, familial dysautonomia, or dysproteinemia.

INVESTIGATIONS

Clinical Laboratory

The cause of a peripheral neuropathy must be identified because often neurologic dysfunction persists unless the underlying disease can be treated. The common causes of polyneuropathy (shown in italics in Table 92.3) may be obvious to a patient's physician, but sometimes even these require direct questioning (e.g., concerning alcoholism) or specific laboratory tests (e.g., measurement of glycosylated hemoglobin) before they are appreciated. If the cause of the neuropathy is not obvious, one should consider the following *screening tests* that may point to a cause: erythrocyte sedimentation rate, fasting blood glucose level, glycosylated hemoglobin, serum creatinine concentration, a complete blood count, serum B_{12} level, a chest x-ray, and a serum and urine immunofixation electrophoresis. Many unusual conditions may be associated with neuropathy, but an extensive screening program to rule out all these processes would be expensive and almost always unrewarding unless there is some clue in the history or physical examination to warrant a particular test (e.g., measurement of blood lead levels in a patient with a possible history of occupational exposure). If no cause of the process is identified on evaluation, consultation with a neurologist should be considered.

Nerve Conduction Studies

The measurement of nerve conduction is useful as an *initial diagnostic screen* because it can distinguish major categories of disease (axonal versus demyelinating) and can localize entrapments and other mononeuropathies. A baseline measurement makes it possible to differentiate progression of the peripheral neuropathy from other clinical conditions in the future.

Nerve conduction measurements involve stimulating a nerve at one point and recording the response, either at the muscle (motor nerve) or at some distance along the nerve (sensory nerve). The results of nerve conduction studies usually include latency of response, conduction velocity, and amplitude of response. The *latency of response* refers to the time elapsed between the start of the stimulus and the muscle response (muscle fiber depolarization) or nerve response (sensory nerve action potential). The *conduction velocity* between two points along the nerve is expressed in meters per second.

Conduction disturbances of the peripheral nerve may be localized, as in an entrapment syndrome, or may involve nerves more diffusely, as in polyneuropathies. In general, early axonal degenerations are associated with normal conduction and the presence of denervation on electromyography (EMG; see below), whereas early demyelination is characterized by slowing of nerve conduction and normal EMG studies. Nerve conduction velocities are normal, and sensory nerve action potentials are spared in cervical or lumbar disk disease with radiculopathy, because the potential site of nerve root compression at the neural foramina is proximal to the sensory cell body in the ganglion and therefore does not cause degeneration of the distal sensory nerve fiber. This is an important point because spondylitic radiculopathy is common and may mimic polyneuropathy (see Chapters 70 and 71).

The procedure has several *limitations*. First, nerve conduction studies test directly only the portion of the nerve between the stimulating and recording electrodes; they generally do not detect damage more distal than (e.g., intramuscular nerve) or more proximal to (e.g., nerve root) the segment tested. Long latency responses such as F waves or H reflexes can provide information about conduction over proximal nerve segments. Second, electrophysiologic studies measure the speed of conduction in the largest and fastest conducting fibers of peripheral nerves. Therefore, nerve conduction studies are most sensitive in diseases that involve such fibers but provide little information about processes affecting small fibers, such as a small fiber sensory neuropathy.

When ordering electrophysiologic studies, the clinical problem and question to be addressed should be specified as precisely as possible. Stating only "numbness in the upper extremities" or "test nerves in lower extremities" without any specific guidance is unlikely to be productive.

Patient Experience. With the patient comfortably positioned, surface electrodes are placed over the nerves and muscles to be tested. Nerves are stimulated with shocks applied to the skin. The shocks are mildly unpleasant. Nerves on both sides of the body may be compared. Testing takes approximately 20 to 60 minutes.

Electromyography

EMG involves the insertion of a needle electrode into a muscle to record muscle electrical activity. From the observation of muscle activity both at rest (spontaneous discharges) and during muscle contraction (volitional activity), much can be inferred about the integrity of motor nerves and the muscle itself.

Spontaneous *fibrillation potentials* are the action potentials of single myofibers that are twitching spontaneously. Fibrillation potentials and positive waves are usually, but not invariably, a good indication of denervation (they also occur in polymyositis and more rarely in other myopathic processes). *Fasciculations* are the spontaneous firings of whole motor units (all the muscle fibers innervated by a single motor neuron and its branches). Fasciculations may be seen in normal subjects, although they are more frequent and likely to be more polyphasic in states of denervation. Therefore, the presence of fasciculations is only moderately useful in diagnosing denervation.

Voluntary motor unit potentials are examined individually by asking the patient to contract a given muscle slightly. Long-duration, large-amplitude, polyphasic potentials suggest a denervating process. Brief, small-amplitude, polyphasic potentials are associated with myopathic processes. Graded increasing effort is used to analyze the orderly recruitment of motor unit potentials, including their number and firing rates. Recruitment of a reduced repertoire of large-amplitude motor unit potentials firing at rapid rates is indicative of denervation and reinnervation. Early recruitment of

Table 92.4. Electromyography: Patterns Typical of Nerve and Muscle Disorders

Disorder	Insertional Activity	Complete Rest (Spontaneous Activity)	Motor Unit Potentials	Recruitment
Neuropathic[a]	Increased	Fibrillations, positive sharp waves, fasciculations	Long duration, high amplitude, polyphasic	Reduced
Myopathic				
Myopathy	Normal	Normal or rare fibrillations	Brief duration, small amplitude, polyphasic	Early
Myositis	Increased	Fibrillations, positive sharp waves	Brief duration, small amplitude, polyphasic	Early

[a]Neuropathy or radiculopathy.

numerous brief small-amplitude motor unit potentials indicates a myopathic process.

One important use of EMG is to detect denervation in muscles that are clinically of normal strength. Due to the process of collateral reinnervation, significant numbers of motor axons may be lost before clinical muscle weakness is detectable. For example, in a slowly progressive chronic entrapment neuropathy such as carpal tunnel syndrome (CTS), more than 50% of the motor axons may be lost before thenar muscles become weak. By revealing such denervation changes, EMG studies help the clinician to determine the severity of the lesion and make informed decisions about prognosis and management. The EMG can also recognize denervation in muscles that are difficult to assess on physical examination. Another use of EMG is to help define entrapment neuropathies (e.g., radial nerve entrapment) and differentiate these from more proximal radicular compression (e.g., apparent CTS that is actually caused by C6 radiculopathy: normal NCV for the median nerve with abnormal EMG reflecting nerve root pathology). EMG is not as helpful in patients with diffuse peripheral neuropathy. However, it may detect the early denervation changes of axonal neuropathy before striking changes are recognized on nerve conduction studies. EMG can also help differentiate the muscle wasting of neuropathic or myopathic disorders from disuse atrophy. Table 92.4 summarizes the changes found in denervation and myopathic conditions.

The EMG electrodes mildly inflame the muscles into which they have been inserted (note that serum creatine phosphokinase activity is rarely altered substantially by this procedure). Thus, if there is a possibility that a muscle biopsy will be required, the muscle to be biopsied should not be tested by EMG. The need for EMG in patients with bleeding tendencies or at risk from recurrent infection should be carefully reviewed with a neurologist.

Patient Experience. There is usually discomfort with the initial insertion of the recording needles and during movement of the muscles when the needles are in place. Because the needles are very thin and penetrate only skin and muscle, the risks of infection or hemorrhage are almost nil. The procedure takes 30 to 60 minutes.

Nerve Biopsy

Nerve biopsy is a useful last step that should be reserved for patients in whom a specific histologic diagnosis and a management decision that may help the patient are possible (e.g., amyloidosis, demyelination, inflammation, or necrotizing vasculitis). Its use should be guided by the history and electrophysiology. The nerve studied by biopsy is almost always a sensory nerve (the sural) and sometimes may not reflect a disease process that appears to affect only the motor nerves. The biopsy always leads to a fixed numbness in the distribution of the excised nerve (usually the sural distribution on the lateral heel and ankle) but rarely may lead to painful sequelae such as neuroma formation. If a nerve biopsy is done, it should be done at a center where it is performed frequently, where plastic embedded nerve histopathology and electron microscopy are routinely available, and where a pathologist with special expertise in nerve morphology can interpret it, so that maximum information can result from this invasive procedure. Consultation with a neurologist is helpful in determining whether a nerve biopsy is indicated.

SPECIFIC CAUSES

Diabetic Neuropathy

Diabetic neuropathy is one of the most common neuropathies seen in primary care settings (1,2). The diabetic polyneuropathies have protean manifestations. They may present as a symmetric polyneuropathy or as a focal neuropathy. The former include sensory or sensorimotor polyneuropathy and autonomic polyneuropathy. The focal neuropathic syndromes include asymmetric lower limb mononeuropathy (diabetic amyotrophy), mononeuropathy multiplex, cranial neuropathy, entrapment neuropathies, and isolated trunk radiculopathies). The problem is discussed in detail in Chapter 79 and in the section on femoral neuropathy below.

Alcoholic Neuropathy

The neuropathy associated with alcoholism and related vitamin deficiencies is a sensorimotor polyneuropathy (3). The presenting symptoms are often pain and paresthesias in the feet and legs reflecting a distal symmetric sensorimotor axonopathy. Many patients are asymptomatic. Examination often shows diminished ankle jerks and a stocking–glove pattern of decreased sensation to all modalities. Autonomic features, including impotence, bladder dysfunction, and orthostatic hypotension, may rarely be seen. Electrodiagnostic studies commonly reveal reduced amplitudes of the sural sensory nerve action potentials and abnormal H reflexes. Sural nerve sections show primary axonal degeneration. Malnutrition and vitamin deficiencies (particularly thiamine deficiency) probably make a major contribution to the neuropathy, although there is evidence that alcohol has a direct toxic effect on peripheral nerves.

Treatment is aimed toward improved nutrition and vitamin replacement and effective treatment for the alcoholism (see Chapter 28). The paresthesias of a mild neuropathy can be expected to improve with good nutrition and abstinence from alcohol. However, with moderate to severe sensorimotor and autonomic neuropathy, significant residual symptoms and findings will persist.

Carcinomatous Neuropathies

The most common form of neuropathy associated with malignancies is a distal sensorimotor polyneuropathy. Compression or infiltration of nerves by tumor or a pure sensory neuronopathy occurs less commonly. Both the distal sensorimotor neuropathy and pure sensory neuronopathy are most often associated with carcinoma of the lung, and the onset of the neuropathic symptoms can either precede, follow, or coincide with the diagnosis of the malignancy (4,5).

Distal Sensorimotor Neuropathy

Distal sensorimotor neuropathy is primarily an axonal process with sensory loss and weakness appearing initially in the feet. It is more common in men, develops over weeks or months, and is generally progressive in its course. If the underlying cancer responds to treatment, the neuropathy may improve.

Carcinomatous Sensory Neuropathy

Carcinomatous sensory neuropathy has a distinctive pattern beginning subacutely, often with pain and paresthesias involving legs, arms, or, rarely, the face. Over many weeks a profound proprioceptive sensory loss develops, accompanied by pseudoathetosis (seemingly purposeless movements caused by loss of position sense). Areflexia is common. The patient may be unable to stand or walk unassisted despite normal strength. Nerve conduction studies may show reduced or unobtainable sensory potentials. It occurs more typically in women (4). The underlying tumor is most often small cell carcinoma of the lung, but this neuropathy also may accompany breast, ovarian, uterine, and gastrointestinal tract tumors. The neuropathy is usually progressive. A common chemotherapeutic agent for the treatment of ovarian cancer, *cis*-platinum, produces a similar picture.

Paraneoplastic Vasculitis of Nerve and Muscle

This disorder is a nonsystemic vasculitic neuropathy that usually affects older men, has a subacute onset, and is progressive. It may present as a painful symmetric or asymmetric sensorimotor polyneuropathy or, less commonly, as a mononeuritis multiplex. The tumors most frequently involved are lymphoma and small cell lung cancer. Electrodiagnostic studies reveal axonal degeneration affecting motor and sensory fibers. The erythrocyte sedimentation rate may be elevated, and the cerebrospinal fluid protein content is increased. Nerve biopsy reveals intramural and perivascular infiltrates without a necrotizing vasculitis. Muscle is often involved as well. It may respond to treatment of the tumor or to immunosuppression (6,7).

Paraproteinemic Neuropathies

An association between peripheral neuropathies and monoclonal gammopathies has been increasingly recognized. In patients with idiopathic peripheral neuropathy, a monoclonal gammopathy can be identified in nearly 10%. In half of these a plasma cell dyscrasia is diagnosed, whereas in the other half the monoclonal gammopathy is of undetermined significance and an association with the neuropathy is unclear (8). The malignancies associated with monoclonal gammopathies include multiple myeloma, osteosclerotic myeloma, Waldenström macroglobulinemia, B-cell lymphoma, and chronic B-cell lymphocytic leukemia.

Peripheral neuropathy may be the presenting symptom in plasma cell dyscrasias, such as in primary amyloidosis or the rare osteosclerotic form of myeloma. Patients with multiple myeloma may develop a mild distal sensorimotor neuropathy, a pure sensory neuropathy, or a subacute monophasic or relapsing and remitting neuropathy. Amyloid deposition may occur in these patients, usually causing a distal sensorimotor neuropathy, but may also present as CTS, multiple mononeuropathies, or autonomic dysfunction. Neuropathic symptoms typical in primary amyloidosis are prominent burning dysesthesias and autonomic dysfunction. Like the amyloidosis, the neuropathy generally does not respond to treatment.

Nearly 50% of patients with osteosclerotic myeloma have a neuropathy characterized as a symmetric, demyelinating, primarily motor neuropathy. All or some of the features of the POEMS syndrome (polyneuropathy, organomegaly, endocrinopathy, M component, and skin changes) may be present (9). Although the course is usually one of steady progression, improvement in the neuropathy occurred in nearly 50% of patients in one series in response to successful treatment of osteosclerotic myeloma.

Five percent to 10% of patients with Waldenström macroglobulinemia have a demyelinating sensorimotor polyneuropathy that predominantly affects large sensory fibers. Postural tremor and pseudoathetosis are common. Those patients with demyelinating neuropathy and IgM anti-MAG M protein may respond to therapy with plasma exchange or intravenous immunoglobulin, but most require chemotherapy.

Neuropathy Caused by Toxins and Drugs

Toxic neuropathies, including those caused by drugs, are becoming increasingly recognized. Toxic

Table 92.5. Toxins and Drugs Associated with Peripheral Neuropathies

Industrial[a]
Pesticides: organophosphates, dichlorophenyoxyacetate (2,4-D), Vacor rodenticide
Metal work: lead, arsenic, mercury, thallium, methyl bromide
Plastics, synthetic fabrics: *n*-hexane, methyl, *n*-butyl ketone, acrylamide, carbon disulfide, perchlorethylene, trichlorethylene, dimethylaminoproprionitrile
Gases: carbon monoxide, ethylene oxide
Euphorants
Glue sniffing: *n*-hexane, solvents
Nitrous oxide inhalation: whipped cream dispensers, dental offices
Pharmacotherapeutic agents
Antimicrobial: isoniazid, nitrofurantoin, metronidazole
Cardiovascular: hydralazine, procainamide, amiodarone
Other: phenytoin, colchicine, disulfiram, pyridoxine, vincristine, *cis*-platinum, taxol, thalidomide, pyridoxine (vitamin B_6)

[a]See also Chapter 8, Table 8.2.

neuropathies are potentially reversible if the toxin can be identified and the exposure to the toxin eliminated. The diagnosis may be made easily if there is a history of drug exposure (e.g., colchicine, isoniazid, hydralazine, vincristine) or industrial exposure (Table 92.5). Because these neuropathies have no distinguishing features on routine history or physical examination, a detailed history of exposure to drugs and the patient's occupation and recreational habits is important. Axonal involvement in the spinal cord may also occur and be masked by the toxic neuropathy. In these cases, a residual spastic paraparesis becomes apparent when the peripheral neuropathy has resolved. Toxic neuropathies are classically associated with chronic low-dose exposure (months to years), although they may appear within days to weeks with high-level exposure. The syndrome of proximal muscle weakness and axonal polyneuropathy caused by colchicine may appear after the patient has taken this drug for years, usually because of elevated drug levels caused by altered renal function. A delayed neuropathy associated with organophosphates develops 10 to 14 days after exposure, whereas Vacor, a rodenticide, produces an acute toxic neuropathy within 2 to 3 days.

Toxicity caused by megadose pyridoxine (vitamin B_6) consumption produces a gradually progressive sensory ataxia with profound distal limb impairment of position and vibratory sense (10). General public acceptance of vitamin B_6 therapy makes direct questioning about vitamin habits necessary. Neuropathy has been reported in patients consuming dosages as low as 200 mg/day.

Human Immunodeficiency Virus Infection

There are many peripheral nervous system manifestations of human immunodeficiency virus (HIV) infection (11). A *painful sensory neuropathy*, usually confined to the feet, affects 30% of patients with the acquired immunodeficiency syndrome, often late in the course. Nerve conduction studies show reduced or absent sensory potentials. Histologic studies demonstrate a reduction in the number of small unmyelinated fibers. Treatment is currently limited to symptomatic relief using tricyclic antidepressants such as amitriptyline (Elavil) or carbamazepine (Tegretol), described below.

Multiple *mononeuropathies* have been described, most often in HIV-infected patients who have not yet developed the acquired immunodeficiency syndrome. Both acute and chronic inflammatory demyelinating polyneuropathies (CIDPs) have been seen, usually in the early stages of HIV infection, in otherwise asymptomatic seropositive patients. Treatment has been tried with plasmapheresis, as in seronegative cases of demyelinating neuropathy.

Progressive polyradiculopathy is a cytomegalovirus infection-related syndrome that usually occurs late in the course of HIV disease and causes radiating pain and numbness in the cauda equina distribution. This is typically followed by progressive flaccid paraparesis, lower extremity areflexia, and sphincter dysfunction. Occasionally, there is an associated thoracic sensory level, hence the alternative term polyradiculomyelitis. Urinary retention occurs in most patients. Cranial nerves and the upper extremities are rarely involved. The mortality rate is nearly 100% if untreated, with a very rapid and progressive course (measured in days). Cerebrospinal fluid findings include a marked polymorphonuclear pleocytosis, and polymerase chain reaction for cytomegalovirus DNA is highly sensitive and specific. Treatment with ganciclovir is effective but must be initiated early (12,13). Chapter 39 provides a detailed account of the ambulatory care of patients with HIV infection.

COMPRESSION AND ENTRAPMENT NEUROPATHIES

When a peripheral neurologic abnormality occurs in one upper or lower extremity, the abnormality is usually caused by nerve entrapment or compression caused by anatomic abnormalities or trauma, although polyneuropathy and mononeuropathy multiplex may present initially as a focal deficit in one extremity. With clinical evaluation, it is usually possible to determine whether the patient's problem is caused by nerve root damage or damage to a peripheral nerve or one of its branches. Tables 92.6, 92.7, and 92.8 and Figs. 92.1 and 92.2 summarize the information needed to make this distinction: distribution of sensory, motor, and reflex deficits; common causative factors; and critical anatomic relationships.

Several common compression and entrapment neuropathies and specific approaches to treatment are discussed here. Working diagnoses and decisions regarding conservative management can usually be accomplished without costly electrodiagnostic studies. The latter are useful for unclear diagnosis and for supporting the decision to recommend surgery. Additional general aspects of prognosis and treatment are described in a later section (see Therapeutic Principles).

Table 92.6. Comparative Data on Root and Nerve Lesions in the Upper Extremity

Roots →	C5	C6	C7	C8	T1
Sensory loss[a,b]	Lateral upper arm	Dorsolateral forearm and thumb	Mid-dorsal forearm and middle finger	Medial forearm, ring and small fingers	Medial arm, axilla
Motor loss[b]	Deltoid, some biceps, infraspinatus and supraspinatus	Biceps, brachioradialis, some deltoid	Triceps, wrist and finger extensors	Thenar eminence and interossei of hand	Thenar eminence and interossei of hand
Tendon reflex	Biceps, brachioradialis	Biceps, brachioradialis	Triceps	Triceps, finger jerk	Finger jerk
Peripheral Nerves →	**Axillary**	**Musculocutaneous**	**Radial**	**Median (Carpal Tunnel)**	**Ulnar (Cubital Tunnel)**
Sensory loss	Over deltoid	Radial forearm	Dorsal lateral hand	First 3½ digits	4th and 5th digits
Motor loss	Deltoid	Biceps, brachialis	Triceps, wrist and finger extensors	Thenar: abductor pollicis brevis, opponens	Hypothenar: abductor digiti minimi, first dorsal interosseus
Tendon reflex	None	Biceps	Triceps, brachioradialis	Finger jerk	Finger jerk
Pain	Over deltoid	Lateral forearm	Dorsal lateral forearm and hand	Nocturnal in forearm, lateral hand, and first 3½ digits	4th and 5th digits and tenderness at elbow

[a]See dermatomal pattern, Fig. 86.2.
[b]Pain usually radiates from the neck to the distal area of sensory loss.

Table 92.7. Comparative Data on Root and Nerve Lesions in the Lower Extremity

Roots →	L2	L3	L4	L5	S1
Sensory loss[a]	Upper and medial thigh	Anterior thigh	Lateral thigh to medial leg	Lateral leg to dorsum of foot	Posterior leg to plantar foot
Motor loss	Iliopsoas (hip flexion)	Quadriceps (knee extension), adductor	Quadriceps, tibialis anterior (dorsiflexion of foot)	Great toe extensor, tibialis anterior, tibialis posterior	Gastrocnemius, gluteus maximus (hip extension)
Tendon reflex	Adductor	Adductor, knee jerk	Knee jerk	Medial hamstring	Achilles
Peripheral Nerves →	**Obturator**	**Femoral**	**Lateral Femoral Cutaneous (Meralgia Paresthetica)**	**Sciatic Peroneal Division**	**Sciatic Tibial Division**
Sensory loss, pain area	Medial thigh	Anterior medial thigh	Upper lateral thigh usually to 10–12 inches below the iliac crest	Dorsum of foot and lateral leg	Plantar foot (with burning pain), tips of toes
Motor loss	Adductors	Quadriceps (knee extension)	N/A	Tibialis anterior (dorsiflexion of ankle), extensor digitorum brevis (toe extension)	Gastrocnemius
Tendon reflex	Adductor	Knee jerk	N/A	None	Achilles

[a]See dermatomal pattern, Fig. 86.2.

Root compression symptoms caused by cervical and lumbar spine disease are discussed in Chapters 70 and 71.

Median Nerve (Carpal Tunnel Syndrome)

Causes

CTS is the most common of all the entrapment neuropathies. In CTS, symptoms and signs result from compression by neighboring anatomic structures on the median nerve as it passes from the forearm to the palm (Fig. 92.1). The median nerve and nine digital flexor tendons pass through the carpal tunnel, a rigid compartment formed by the concave arch of the carpal bones and roofed by the transverse carpal ligament. Conditions that cause a decrease in the size of the carpal tunnel (e.g., Colles fracture, rheumatoid arthritis, congenital carpal tunnel stenosis), enlargement of the median nerve (e.g., amyloid, neuroma, endoneural edema in diabetes mellitus), or increase in the volume of other structures within the tunnel (e.g., tenosynovitis, ganglion, lipoma, urate deposits in gout, hematoma, fluid retention in pregnancy) may all result in compression of the median nerve. Many cases previously classified as idiopathic are explained by occupational factors. CTS in the workplace is associated with occupations in which the wrist position deviates from the normal straight alignment and with occupations involving the use of greater hand force in all wrist positions (e.g., meat processing, fruit packing, upholstering, and waiting on tables). Median nerve compression can also be caused by tasks that require a sustained or repeated stress over the base of the palm, such as that caused by the use of tools such as screwdrivers, scrapers, paint brushes, and buffers. Vibration exposure (low frequency, 10 to 40 Hz) is another well-recognized risk factor for CTS (typically from air-powered tools). Repetitive wrist and hand movements

Table 92.8. Entrapment Neuropathies: Common Causative Factors

Nerve, Location	Causative Factors
Median	
At wrist	Meat processing, upholstering, knitting, painting, weight lifting, using vibrating tools, pregnancy, musical instruments
At forearm	Repeated pronation (e.g., screwdriver), weight lifting
Ulnar	
At wrist	Bicycling, leaning on a walker, using pliers, using palm as a hammer
At elbow	Injury to elbow, chronic flexion of elbow (e.g., sitting in wheelchair or lying in bed), leaning on elbow on tables and desks
Radial	
At forearm	Lipoma, tennis, trauma
At arm	Saturday night palsy, bridegroom's palsy, crutches, pneumatic tourniquets
Axillary	Fracture/dislocation of shoulder, deep injections into deltoid muscle
Musculocutaneous	Weight lifting, shoulder dislocations
Tibial	
At knee	Chronic, standing
At ankle	Trauma, weight gain, or edema
Peroneal	
At knee	Ankle sprains, crossed legs, after weight loss, squatting, kneeling
At ankle	Tight shoes, trauma
Femoral	Inguinal surgery, childbirth, psoas hemorrhage, dorsal lithotomy position
Lateral femoral cutaneous	Ascites, overweight, pregnancy, utility belts, blunt sports injury to anterior iliac spine
Obturator	Pelvic fracture, hip surgery, childbirth, retroperitoneal hematoma, malignancy
Sciatic	Hip surgery, pelvic fracture, injections, endometriosis, retroperitoneal hematoma, lipoma

in activities such as knitting, crocheting, hooking rugs, playing a musical instrument, painting, woodworking, gardening, lifting weights, or typing when the keyboard is too high may also lead to CTS.

Manifestations and Evaluation

The onset of symptoms of CTS is usually insidious and nocturnal because of sustained posture of wrist flexion during sleep. Symptoms in the hand may initially be described as episodic tingling and numbness with gradual progression to more severe symptoms, such as burning, aching, or a painful numbness in the fingers and deep in the palm. The fingers are sometimes described as feeling swollen, even though little swelling is apparent on inspection. Many patients have accompanying dull aching pain in the forearm, sometimes reaching the shoulder.

As CTS progresses, the nocturnal pain and tingling may begin to wake the patient after a few hours' sleep. Relief may be obtained by hanging the arm out of bed or shaking or rubbing the hand. At this stage episodic tingling may develop during the day, but the associated pain in the arm occurs less often during the day than at night. In addition to sensory symptoms, there is a subjective feeling of uselessness and clumsiness in the fingers with difficulty performing certain tasks, such as unscrewing bottle tops, turning a key, or crocheting.

Objective changes in sensation and strength may appear in the hand, but some patients may have severe attacks of pain for many years without developing neurologic signs. Sensory signs within the median nerve distribution (Table 92.6) are first evident and most pronounced in the fingertips. Occasionally, instead of decreased sensation, there is an overreaction to cutaneous stimuli in the median innervated lateral three and a half fingers. Isolated thenar wasting or isolated sensory impairment in the distribution of one of the lateral three digital (thumb and digits 2, 3, lateral half of 4) nerves may be unusual presenting features of median nerve lesions at the wrist. Mild weakness of the abductor pollicis brevis (to test, patient abducts thumb at right angle to palm, against resistance) or of the opponens pollicis muscle (to test, patient touches base of little finger with thumb, against resistance) is often present with no visually apparent atrophy. Prolonged hyperflexion of the wrist may reproduce sensory symptoms (*Phalen sign*). *Tinel sign,* consisting of shock-like pain and tingling elicited by percussion of the median nerve at the wrist, is a less specific finding. In a systematic review of the accuracy of the physical examination to diagnose CTS, hypalgesia in the median nerve territory, a classic pattern of pain with hand symptom diagrams, and weak thumb abduction were the strongest predictors of electrodiagnostic CTS (14).

For *electrodiagnostic studies*, see details above. Although abnormalities of the *nerve conduction studies* in CTS are more likely to be found when physical signs are evident on examination, a significant number of patients with typical symptoms have no findings other than those detected on electrodiagnostic testing. In addition, because central nervous system or root lesions can occasionally result in similar sensory symptoms, confirmation of a peripheral nerve lesion by electrophysiologic testing is important. The most common finding on nerve conduction studies in CTS is abnormality in the median sensory nerve studies, including a segmental reduction in conduction velocity across the wrist and a reduction in the action potential amplitude. Abnormalities of median motor nerve conduction studies, including prolonged distal motor latency, are less common but important findings. Needle electrode examination (EMG) is important to confirm localization of median nerve entrapment, to look for evidence of associated axonal degeneration and to rule out possible coexistent cervical radiculopathy (double crush syndrome).

Treatment

Immobilization of the wrist with a close-fitting *anterior splint* (extends from the upper part of the forearm to the metacarpophalangeal joints), which is worn by the patient at night or when resting, holds the wrist immobilized in a neutral position. This often alleviates all symptoms, but if symptoms persist after a few weeks, additional therapy is indicated. A trial of oral anti-inflammatory medication is often used but generally yields temporary relief at best.

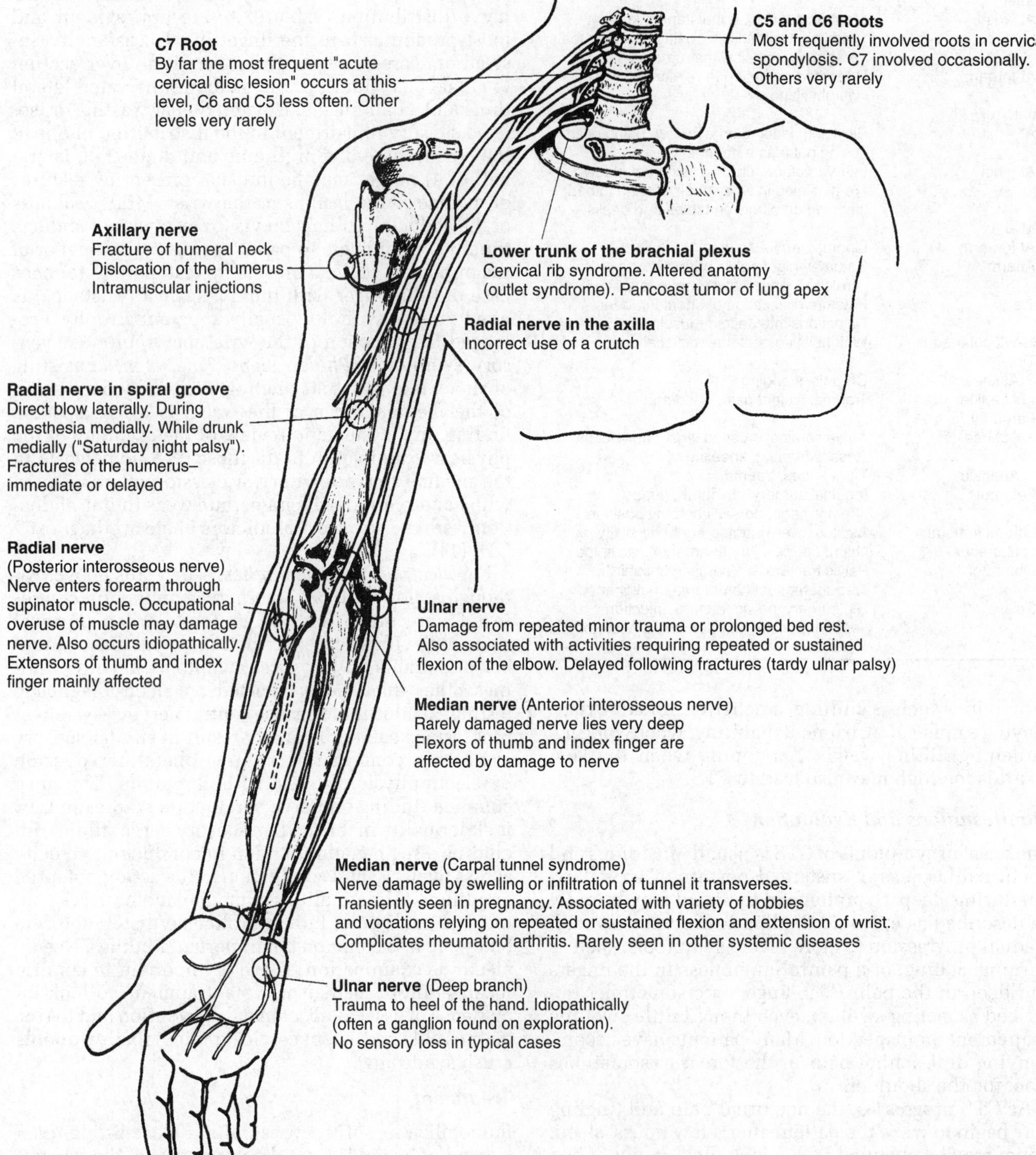

The most frequently encountered causes of damage at the various sites are indicated
C7 Root
By far the most frequent "acute cervical disc lesion" occurs at this level, C6 and C5 less often. Other levels very rarely
C5 and C6 Roots
Most frequently involved roots in cervical spondylosis. C7 involved occasionally. Others very rarely
Axillary nerve
Fracture of humeral neck
Dislocation of the humerus
Intramuscular injections
Lower trunk of the brachial plexus
Cervical rib syndrome. Altered anatomy (outlet syndrome). Pancoast tumor of lung apex
Radial nerve in the axilla
Incorrect use of a crutch
Radial nerve in spiral groove
Direct blow laterally. During anesthesia medially. While drunk medially ("Saturday night palsy"). Fractures of the humerus– immediate or delayed
Radial nerve
(Posterior interosseous nerve)
Nerve enters forearm through supinator muscle. Occupational overuse of muscle may damage nerve. Also occurs idiopathically. Extensors of thumb and index finger mainly affected
Ulnar nerve
Damage from repeated minor trauma or prolonged bed rest. Also associated with activities requiring repeated or sustained flexion of the elbow. Delayed following fractures (tardy ulnar palsy)
Median nerve (Anterior interosseous nerve)
Rarely damaged nerve lies very deep
Flexors of thumb and index finger are affected by damage to nerve
Median nerve (Carpal tunnel syndrome)
Nerve damage by swelling or infiltration of tunnel it transverses. Transiently seen in pregnancy. Associated with variety of hobbies and vocations relying on repeated or sustained flexion and extension of wrist. Complicates rheumatoid arthritis. Rarely seen in other systemic diseases
Ulnar nerve (Deep branch)
Trauma to heel of the hand. Idiopathically (often a ganglion found on exploration). No sensory loss in typical cases

Figure 92.1. Anatomic relationships of nerves to the upper extremity. (Modified from Patten J. Neurological differential diagnosis, 2nd ed. New York: Springer-Verlag, 1995, with permission.)

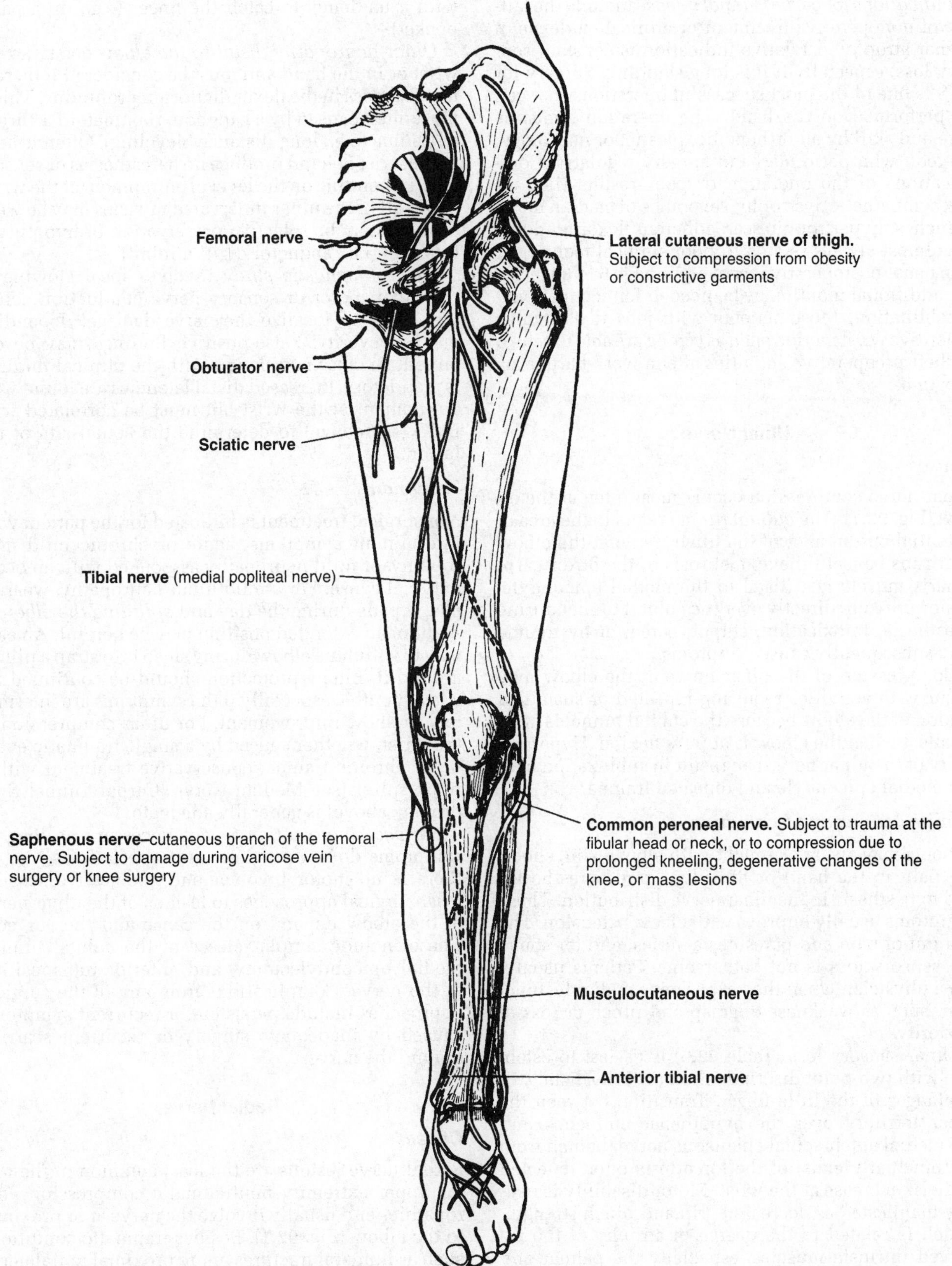

Figure 92.2. Anatomic relationships of nerves to the lower extremity. (Modified from Patten J. Neurological differential diagnosis. 2nd ed. New York: Springer-Verlag, 1995, with permission.)

Indications for carpal tunnel release include the failure of nonoperative treatment or clinical evidence of thenar atrophy. A relative indication is constant sensory loss, especially if it is long standing. Surgery for CTS is one of the most successful operations that can be performed on the hand. The operation demands care and skill by an orthopedic, plastic, or neurologic surgeon who performs hand surgery regularly. Complications of the operation or poor results (i.e., reflex sympathetic dystrophy, severance of median nerve branches, hypertrophic scar, adherent flexor tendons) are almost always related to poor surgical technique. The usual postoperative recovery time is 6 to 8 weeks. An additional month may be needed for occupational rehabilitation. Most patients with jobs that involve repetitive wrist motion such as typing are able to return to their preoperative activities after a work-hardening program.

Ulnar Nerve

Causes

Ulnar nerve compression occurs most often at the elbow (Fig. 92.1). The *cubital tunnel* refers to the area of potential entrapment of the ulnar nerve at the elbow as it runs beneath the aponeurosis of the flexor carpi ulnaris muscle just distal to the medial epicondyle. Minor pressure directly over the cubital tunnel during anesthesia, intoxication, stupor, coma, or by trauma may subsequently cause symptoms.

Compression of the ulnar nerve at the elbow may occur with activities requiring repeated or sustained flexion of the elbow because the cubital tunnel is at its smallest when the elbow is at 90% flexion. Hypermobility of the ulnar nerve can result in subluxation over the medial epicondyle and repeated trauma.

Manifestations and Evaluation

Patients may awaken at night with elbow pain, shooting pain in the hand or fifth digit, and paresthesias and hypesthesia in the ulnar nerve distribution. These symptoms usually improve with elbow extension. The amount of pain and paresthesia varies, and for some, the sensory loss is not bothersome. Patients usually see a physician when they experience motor dysfunction, such as weakness of grasp and pinch or loss of dexterity.

Ulnar sensory loss (Table 92.6) is easiest to establish with two-point discrimination over the distal two phalanges of the little finger. Transition between the ulnar territory over the hypothenar eminence and the medial antebrachial cutaneous nerve (branch from the brachial plexus) of the forearm is often detected at the skin crease at the wrist. Motor disability is usually manifested as decreased grip and pinch strength, which is related to the degree of atrophy of the involved intrinsic muscles, especially the palmar and dorsal interossei and flexor digitorum profundus to the fourth and fifth digits. One of the earliest signs of ulnar nerve entrapment is weakness of fifth finger adduction with a tendency to catch the finger (e.g., on a pants pocket).

Ulnar neuropathy distal to the elbow occurs at the wrist or in the hand and must be considered if there is no weakness in the flexor digitorum profundus. This is most often caused by a ganglion, rheumatoid arthritis, or trauma (e.g., long-distance bicycling). Often lesions in the wrist or hand produce no paresthesias or sensory loss. Depending on the level of entrapment at the wrist, either all of the ulnar innervated muscles may be weak or there may be selective preservation of hypothenar function (i.e., abductor digiti minimi).

Electrodiagnostic study involves focal slowing of the ulnar motor or sensory nerve conduction across the elbow to localize the nerve damage, depending on the severity. False-positive findings may be obtained, so close correlation with the clinical findings is mandatory. Increased distal latencies are found with entrapment at the wrist but must be correlated with EMG (see above) to determine the actual site of the lesion.

Treatment

Nonsurgical treatment is indicated for the patient with intermittent symptoms, acute or chronic mild neuropathy, or mild neuropathy associated with an occupational cause. For a mild ulnar neuropathy, wearing elbow pads during the day and *splinting the elbow* at night in an extended position may be helpful. An easy way to splint the elbow during sleep is to strap a pillow around it. Elbow protection should be continued for 2 to 3 months, especially if the symptoms are intermittent or show improvement. For ulnar compression at the wrist, whether caused by a single traumatic event or by chronic trauma, conservative treatment with a wrist splint (see Median Nerve [Carpal Tunnel Syndrome], above) is generally adequate.

Surgical intervention is not necessary as long as symptoms do not progress and especially as long as there is no motor involvement or objective sensory loss. Surgical approaches to lesions of the ulnar nerve at the elbow depend on the cause and the surgeon. These include simple release of the cubital tunnel, medial epicondylectomy, and anterior transposition of the nerve. Complications from any of the surgical approaches include persistent or recurrent symptoms caused by inadequate surgery or recurrent scarring around the nerve.

Radial Nerve

Causes

Radial nerve lesions are the least common of the major upper extremity nontraumatic compression neuropathies and usually involve the nerve at or proximal to the elbow (Fig. 92.1). Besides traumatic conditions such as humeral fractures, more proximal radial nerve injuries can occur when the arm has been held in a hyperabducted position that causes traction to the nerve, as in surgery or sleep. Proximal nerve injury may also follow axillary pressure caused by incorrect use of a crutch. The middle third of the nerve is compressed against the humerus in the so-called Saturday night palsy, as when an intoxicated person sleeps with the arm draped over a chair. Compression of the posterior interosseous nerve (branch of radial nerve in the forearm) can result from a variety of masses, such as lipomas, fibromas, or calluses from old fractures.

Manifestations and Evaluation

The radial nerve is predominantly a motor nerve. Depending on the location of a high radial compression, the triceps function (elbow extension) may or may not be affected. Elbow flexion and supination may be slightly affected by brachioradialis weakness. The most obvious finding in a radial palsy is wrist drop and digital extensor paralysis (finger drop). A lesion of the posterior interosseous nerve results in finger drop alone.

High radial nerve lesions may produce sensory loss over the dorsum of the hand. Pain and tenderness in the area of nerve damage may be present. Nerve conduction studies and EMG (see above) can be helpful in localizing and quantifying radial nerve compression. For example, acutely, a Saturday night palsy can cause focal slowing of conduction at the site of pressure injury but normal motor and sensory conduction below this lesion.

Treatment

The treatment of traumatic radial nerve compression is generally conservative and recovery of function occurs within a few weeks to months. To prevent flexor contractures, a *cock-up splint for the wrist joint* should be accompanied by a *spring-loaded extensor brace for the fingers* if the weakness is severe and long lasting. Individually constructed splints made by an occupational therapist are superior to those obtained from a surgical supply house. For compression of the posterior interosseus nerve with no obvious cause, imaging of the nerve should be performed to investigate for possible masses. If no mass is identified, surgical exploration is indicated if there has not been spontaneous recovery within 2 to 3 months.

Peroneal Nerve

Causes

The most common site of compression of the peroneal nerve is at the fibular head (Fig. 92.2). Such compression may result from improperly applied plaster casts or tight stockings and garters or from falling asleep with the side of the leg resting against a protruding object, as in a drug- or alcohol-induced stupor or in the weakened bedridden patient. Prolonged leg crossing, squatting, or kneeling may also result in peroneal compression. Entrapment of the peroneal nerve can also occur in the *fibular tunnel* formed by the peroneus longus muscle.

Manifestations and Evaluation

Symptoms of peroneal palsy consist of painless weakness of ankle dorsiflexion (foot drop) and foot eversion and sensory loss over the lateral calf and dorsum of the foot. *Electrodiagnostic studies* and nerve conduction studies can detect focal slowing or conduction block in the peroneal nerve segment across the fibular head. The superficial peroneal sensory potential may be absent. EMG may demonstrate denervation in peroneal innervated muscles with sparing of the short head of the biceps femoris muscle, the most distal of the peroneal innervated muscles above the fibular head. Peroneal palsy with loss of motor function and no clear history of trauma or external compression should be investigated with appropriate physical examination and imaging of the popliteal fossa to rule out a mass lesion.

Treatment

Mild compressive peroneal lesions can be treated conservatively. Patients should be advised to avoid potentially injurious positions for the nerve (e.g., leg crossing, squatting). A custom-fitted *ankle–foot orthotic* is recommended for increased ankle stability and prevention of plantar flexion contractures. Most patients with a transient compressive insult recover peroneal function within weeks to months. Surgical exploration should be considered in severe cases with no clear cause.

Tibial Nerve (Tarsal Tunnel Syndrome)

Causes

The *tarsal tunnel* is located at the inferoposterior margin of the medial malleolus (Fig. 92.2) and is formed by bones of the ankle and the flexor retinaculum (fibrous sheath from medial malleolus posteroinferior to the medial side of the calcaneus). In addition to the posterior tibial nerve, the tunnel contains the posterior tibial artery and three long flexor tendons (15).

Enlarged tortuous veins within the tarsal tunnel, fracture or dislocation at the ankle, and tenosynovitis may lead to compression of the tibial nerve trunk. Prolonged standing and walking often aggravate the pain, indicating that stasis or engorgement within the tunnel is likely to play some role. Also, sensory symptoms are made worse by the venous stasis and engorgement that occur at night during sleep. Except for a high prevalence in jockeys, no common occupational factors have been identified.

Manifestations and Evaluation

The primary symptom of tarsal tunnel syndrome is pain and dysesthesia in the sole of the foot. The burning pain (description by patient may vary, e.g., walking on knives or pins, sole feels very thick) worsens with rest after a day of activity. Nocturnal pain is characteristic. Any or all the three terminal divisions of the tibial nerve (medial plantar, lateral plantar, and calcaneal) may be affected, resulting in sensory disturbance over the entire plantar surface or only one portion of it.

Tinel sign, consisting of shooting pain to the plantar surface produced by gentle percussion over the tarsal tunnel, may be present. Sensory loss, if present, is localized to the plantar surface of the foot and over the tips of the toes (the sural and peroneal territories on the dorsum of the foot do not include the tips of the toes). Weakness in the intrinsic muscles of the foot may lead to a change in configuration of the foot and to instability of the phalanges, which impairs the pushing-off phase of walking. Tarsal tunnel syndrome is usually unilateral.

In the tarsal tunnel syndrome, sensory nerve conduction studies of medial and lateral plantar nerves are the most sensitive electrodiagnostic measures, showing reduced sensory nerve action potential amplitudes or absent responses. Reduced motor or sensory conduction velocities across the flexor retinaculum are found less commonly. EMG demonstrates chronic partial denervation in the tibial innervated intrinsic muscles of the feet (e.g., abductor hallucis and abductor digiti quinti).

Treatment

It is important to identify and remove any source of external pressure at the flexor retinaculum. Definitive treatment of tarsal tunnel syndrome is surgical release of the flexor retinaculum, which can result in dramatic relief of symptoms.

Femoral Nerve

Causes

The femoral nerve may be injured by stab wounds to the groin or hip, pelvic fractures, inguinal surgery (inguinal hernia, vascular repair, node resection), angiography, or retraction during pelvic surgery (Fig. 92.2). Stretch injuries can occur with prolonged lithotomy position or with hyperextension during gymnastics or dance. Pressure on the femoral nerve can also be produced at the psoas muscle by hematoma or abscess.

Manifestations and Evaluation

The patient often complains about buckling of the knee (quadriceps weakness), and falls are common. Pain in the groin radiating into the thigh may be severe. Sensory loss is present in the anterior medial thigh and medial leg. Weakness of the quadriceps (knee extension) and loss of the knee jerk are noted on examination. Weakness of hip flexors indicates a more proximal lumbar plexus or root lesion. EMG helps differentiate these problems.

Femoral neuropathy is to be distinguished from *diabetic lumbar plexopathy* (diabetic amyotrophy). The latter disorder, seen most commonly in diabetics over 50 years of age, begins abruptly with severe pain in the thigh and progresses over days to produce weakness, often most severe, in the femoral nerve distribution. With EMG a wider distribution of involvement can be appreciated. Sensory signs are mild. The prognosis for recovery over 2 to 6 months is good (see Chapter 79).

Treatment

Treatment depends on accurate diagnosis (e.g., discontinuation of anticoagulants when a psoas hematoma has been identified as the cause of the neuropathy). Physiotherapy may be required to maintain the mobility of the hip joint. The outcome and extent of rehabilitation measures are determined by the cause and extent of injury.

Saphenous Nerve

The saphenous nerve is one of three sensory branches of the femoral nerve (Fig. 92.2). It is most often injured at Hunter canal (10 cm proximal to the medial condyle of the femur). Vein stripping and knee surgery are common causes. A small medial nerve branch can be injured by knee surgery. The patient has pain and numbness at the medial aspect of the knee and leg. The pain may worsen with walking and climbing. Manual pressure over the Hunter canal produces pain that radiates. If the pain becomes chronic, local anesthetic can be injected to the area of injury.

Sciatic Nerve

Causes

The sciatic nerve is often injured as a complication of trauma involving structures that the nerve traverses (Fig. 92.2), including hip fractures, dislocations, and arthroplastic surgery. Compression of the nerve can occur in comatose or chronically bedridden patients or after sitting on a hard edge. Hematoma, endometriosis, lipoma, and aneurysms of the gluteal artery are other causes of compression. Injections into the buttock are now less common causes of sciatic nerve injury. Benzylpenicillin and diazepam are particularly potent damaging agents. Injections usually cause immediate dysfunction with poor recovery.

Manifestations and Evaluation

Symptoms of sciatic nerve compression may mimic L5–S1 radiculopathy caused by disk disease (see Chapter 71). The lateral trunk or peroneal division of the sciatic nerve is often affected more severely than the tibial division. Therefore, the distinction between a proximal sciatic injury and a more distal peroneal injury (e.g., after awakening from hip surgery) may be difficult. EMG studies may be particularly helpful in this clinical situation.

Lateral Femoral Cutaneous Nerve (Meralgia Paresthetica)

The lateral femoral cutaneous nerve may be compressed or stretched at the anterior superior iliac spine at the lateral end of the inguinal canal (see lateral cutaneous nerve of the thigh; Fig. 92.2), causing burning pain, paresthesia, and decreased sensation over the lateral thigh. The sensory involvement is more lateral than that in femoral neuropathy, which causes sensory loss in the anterior medial aspect of thigh, and there is no motor involvement or loss of patellar reflex. Point tenderness can usually be elicited at the passage of the nerve at the ipsilateral anterior iliac crest. Common causes include obesity, acute abdominal enlargement (ascites, pregnancy), external mechanical trauma (girdle, utility belt, climbing with body against utility pole), and diabetes mellitus. The nerve compression may be relieved by weight loss or correction of the aggravating condition. Pain may respond to medical management (see below), but generally resolves spontaneously over months. If the pain is severe, local injection of an anesthetic may provide relief for long periods; sectioning of the ligament over the canal or sectioning of the nerve is rarely needed. Paresthesias and pain usually disappear gradually, but a painless sensory loss in the lateral thigh may persist.

Bell's Palsy

Paralysis of the facial muscles caused by inflammation and swelling of the seventh (the facial) cranial nerve (Bell's palsy) is seen occasionally in a general medical practice. One large series reported an incidence of 23 cases per 100,000 population per year (16). There is no predilection for a particular sex, age group, or race. In most patients, the cause of the condition is unknown. Two specific causes for seventh nerve neuropathy that have been recognized in recent years are Lyme disease (17,18) (see Chapter 38) and HIV infection (see Chapter 39). Several small studies have suggested that asymptomatic reactivation of varicella zoster virus is responsible for a substantial proportion of cases of Bell's palsy (19).

Manifestations

Usually, patients note the sudden onset, within hours, of a unilateral paralysis of a facial nerve: the eyebrow sags, the eye cannot be closed, the nasolabial fold disappears, and the mouth is drawn to the unaffected side. Less commonly, there is loss of taste on the anterior two-thirds of the tongue and there is hyperacusis (an accentuation of sounds) in the affected ear. There may be pain behind the ear. Most patients recover spontaneously within weeks to a few months; approximately 15% recover incompletely, but severe residual weakness is rare (16). Patching of the unclosed eye may be needed to avoid corneal injury. In those who do not recover completely, there is a considerable risk of synkinesis (a contraction of all the facial muscles on the affected side when the patient attempts to move just one or a few of them) caused by aberrant reinnervation.

Management

Therapeutic trials of treatment for Bell's palsy have lacked sufficient power to be conclusive, but meta-analysis of several trials show that corticosteroid therapy early in the course improves facial outcomes (20,21). Combined acyclovir–prednisone was found to improve recovery over prednisone alone in one trial (22). The current standard of treatment when the palsy has been present less than 4 days is prednisone 60 to 80 mg/day for 1 week, and valacyclovir (because of improved oral absorption) 1 g three times day for 1 week (23).

LESS COMMON PROBLEMS

Hereditary Motor and Sensory Neuropathies

Of the heritable disorders affecting the peripheral nervous system, the hereditary motor and sensory neuropathies (HMSN) are the most common. HMSN are a heterogeneous group of neuropathy syndromes affecting an estimated 1 per 2,500 people (see General References). HMSN are classified into three types: HMSN type I, or Charcot-Marie-Tooth disease; HMSN type II, or the neuronal form of Charcot-Marie-Tooth disease; HMSN type III, or Dejerine-Sottas disease; HMSN IV, a rare childhood form; and CMT-X, an X-linked form. The most common type, HMSN type I, is characterized by slowly progressive distal weakness; muscle wasting; foot abnormalities, including pes cavus and hammer toe; and mildly diminished distal sensation. Symptoms are usually manifest by the fourth decade; however, many patients have few or no symptoms. Sensory symptoms are rarely the presenting complaint and when present suggest an acquired rather than inherited neuropathy.

Physical examination demonstrates a wide range of clinical severity and may include distal weakness, thin peroneal muscles, diminished deep tendon reflexes in the legs, characteristic abnormalities of the feet (see above), and mildly reduced distal sensation. Occasionally, enlarged nerves can be palpated. Electrophysiologic studies of sensory and motor nerves show diffuse involvement, with severely reduced conduction velocities uniformly along the nerve segment. Nerve pathology shows onion bulb formation composed of redundant Schwann cell processes resulting from recurrent demyelination and remyelination. Diagnosis is established by identifying a history of childhood onset and by physical examination, characteristic electrophysiologic findings, electrodiagnostic evaluation of family members, and genetic testing. In most families, HMSN type I is transmitted as an autosomal dominant pattern, and genetic mutations have been localized to chromosomes 1 and 17. The most common treatment required is the use of custom-fitted ankle–foot orthotics.

Guillain-Barré Syndrome

Guillain-Barré syndrome or acute inflammatory polyradiculoneuropathy is a rapidly progressive paralytic syndrome affecting all ages. Evidence is strong for an immune-mediated pathogenesis. Most cases of Guillain-Barré syndrome follow a mild viral illness (by 10 to 12 days) (24). The syndrome also may be associated with pregnancy, the postoperative period, recent influenza immunization, and HIV infection. A link between *Campylobacter jejuni* and Guillain-Barré syndrome is particularly strong; it is estimated that 20% of cases of Guillain-Barré syndrome follow *Campylobacter* infection (see Dyck et al., General References). More severe cases of Guillain-Barré syndrome are associated with *Campylobacter* infection. Diagnosis of *C. jejuni* infection is based on isolation of *C. jejuni* from stool. The *differential diagnosis* in patients with the rapid onset of a polyradiculopathy includes acute intermittent porphyria, botulism, diphtheria, poliomyelitis, Lyme disease, and toxic neuropathies (arsenic, thallium).

Manifestations

There is rapid progression of ascending symmetric weakness (usually moving from the lower extremities to the upper extremities) accompanied by loss of deep tendon reflexes. Although acute pain or paresthesias in the back and proximal limbs may be prominent early symptoms, objective evidence of sensory loss is generally limited to mild impairment of distal joint position sense and vibratory sensation. Cranial muscle weakness may be present, with bilateral facial nerve palsy in 40% of patients. Nerve conduction studies (see above) show changes of demyelination (prolonged distal motor and F-wave latencies and reduced motor conduction velocities). The cerebrospinal fluid may show an increased protein concentration with normal cell counts (cytoalbumin dissociation).

Management and Course

Because of rapid progression of the disease, patients suspected of having this disorder should be admitted to the hospital for close monitoring for potential respiratory failure and autonomic instability (hypotension, hypertension, cardiac arrhythmias, or hyperpyrexia occur in two-thirds of patients with Guillain-Barré syndrome). Treatment with either plasmapheresis or intravenous human immunoglobulin early in the course shortens the period of disability, and the combination is no better than either treatment alone (25). Recovery is complete in approximately 50% of patients (although it may take 6 to 18 months); most of the remainder have only mild residual deficits, but 10% have severe permanent disability. Splints (to prevent contractures) and physiotherapy should be used until the recovery period is complete.

Chronic Inflammatory Demyelinating Polyneuropathy

CIDP is an acquired motor and sensory neuropathy of unknown cause but with strong evidence for an immune-mediated pathogenesis. CIDP can occur in the absence of systemic disease or, less commonly, in association with such disorders as systemic lupus erythematosus, HIV infection, or dysproteinemias. Clinically, CIDP is a predominantly *motor polyneuropathy*. It may affect all ages and may have either a chronic progressive or relapsing course. Weakness typically develops over at least 2 months (distinguishing CIDP from acute inflammatory demyelinating neuropathy, so-called Guillain-Barré syndrome) and generally begins in the legs. Sensory involvement is variable. Most patients experience some degree of numbness or paresthesia; occasionally, there may be painful dysesthesias. On examination, weakness may be both proximal and distal, and the tendon reflexes are reduced or absent in all four limbs.

Electrodiagnostic studies demonstrate features of demyelination, including prolonged distal and F-wave latencies, reduced conduction velocities variably along nerve segments, abnormal temporal dispersion, and conduction block. Cerebrospinal fluid protein is often elevated. Sural nerve pathology may show evidence of demyelination and remyelination with onion bulb formation, subperineurial and endoneurial edema, and mononuclear cell infiltration.

Management

Common practice is to begin treatment with prednisone 1 mg/kg per day (26) and to use either plasmapheresis or intravenous human immunoglobulin as adjuvants (27). Each of these immunomodulating therapies has been demonstrated to be effective in randomized placebo-controlled trials, and most patients respond. Long-term corticosteroid therapy usually is effective but is limited by side effects. The effect of either plasmapheresis or human immunoglobulin is large and of equal likelihood, but for most patients is short-lived and requires continued intermittent treatment (27). For plasmapheresis, improved motor conduction velocities and reversal of conduction block predict improvement in motor function (28). Plasma exchange treatments should be given two to three times per week until improvement is established, then tapered in frequency; concurrent immunosuppressive drug treatment is usually required (28). Human immunoglobulin treatment is effective in about two-thirds of patients, most often in patients with acute relapse or disease duration less than 1 year (29). Improvement after a dose of 2 g/kg lasts a median 6 weeks and is reproducible, so that follow-up pulses of 1 g/kg as single infusions can maintain a stable benefit (29). Of the two adjuvants, both are extraordinarily expensive, but intravenous immunoglobulin infusion may be preferable because it does not require expensive medical devices and can be given at home (27).

Multifocal Motor Neuropathy

Patients with multifocal motor neuropathy have progressive, predominantly distal, asymmetric weakness that usually begins in the arms. Early in the disease course, multifocal motor neuropathy can mimic CIDP or the lower motor neuron presentation of amyotrophic lateral sclerosis. Nerve conduction studies show multiple areas of persistent partial motor conduction block, and many patients have high IgM anti-GM1 ganglioside antibody titers. Most patients with multifocal motor neuropathy respond to immunosuppressive therapy with human immune globulin or cyclophosphamide (Cytoxan) (30). Corticosteroids are ineffective.

THERAPEUTIC PRINCIPLES

General Measures that Improve Nerve Function

Treatment of peripheral neuropathies first requires identifying and treating any underlying cause, if possible. For type 1 diabetes mellitus, for example, it is now known that intense efforts at tight glucose control dramatically reduce the incidence of neuropathy (see Chapter 79). Efforts should be made also to prevent further damage; for example, patients with an underlying generalized polyneuropathy are more prone to pressure palsies, and it is important to educate them about habits that could be injurious (e.g., leaning on elbows or crossing legs). The daily administration of multivitamins is necessary only in patients whose nutrition may be poor. For entrapment and compression neuropathies, eliminating pressure on the affected nerve is the primary mode of treatment. Pain and paresthesias may be relieved rapidly within hours or days. The prognosis for recovery depends on the pathophysiology of the nerve injury. When little or no denervation is demonstrated by EMG, which suggests that the predominant pathophysiology is edema or demyelination, recovery of function over weeks is expected. In more severe cases with marked denervation indicating axonal injury, recovery is more prolonged (months).

The most important *prognostic indicators for traumatic nerve injuries* are the site, mechanism, and completeness of the injury. Traumatic injuries can occur at the level of the root, plexus, or peripheral nerve. Root avulsion has the worst prognosis. Electrodiagnostic studies are helpful in localizing the site of injury; however, because denervation may not be evident for at least 14 days, EMG studies should be done approximately 3 to 4 weeks after injury. Complete nerve transections caused by sharp penetrating injury, although rare, more often benefit from early primary anastomosis than do complicated nerve injuries such as gunshot wounds. Physical therapy, particularly range-of-motion exercises, should be initiated early after injury to prevent contractures. The onset of spontaneous recovery can vary from weeks to 6 months or more after injury. In cases of persistent loss of function or severe pain, surgical exploration should be considered.

Symptomatic Treatment for Irreversible Damage

Polyneuropathy is often irreversible and progressive. Symptomatic therapy and rehabilitative measures are therefore fundamental in helping these patients.

Motor Neuropathies

In most polyneuropathies, weakness usually affects ankle dorsiflexors early (causing foot drop); ambulation can be greatly improved by a custom-fitted ankle–foot orthotic, such as a rigid plastic splint worn in the shoe or a spring-loaded brace attached to the shoe. Fine motor weakness in the hands can be aided by special tools, such as large-handled utensils and other devices, provided by occupational therapists.

Sensory Neuropathies

Small hard objects (keys, faucet handles) can be built up with soft materials. Occupational therapists can make useful suggestions in this regard. Anesthetic limbs are vulnerable to repeated unrecognized trauma. The patient should always check the temperature of bath water, pot handles, and so on with parts of the body that have normal sensation. Meticulous care should be given to feet and toenails to prevent ulceration or infection (see Chapter 73). Moisturizing cream for dry insensitive skin will reduce serious abrasions.

Pain associated with sensory neuropathies is usually chronic and difficult to treat. Simple analgesics (aspirin), whirlpool, and massage may help relieve mild pain. Outside pain treatment centers, narcotics should probably be avoided because of the potential for addiction. Gabapentin (Neurontin) was initially developed as an anticonvulsant but its membrane stabilizing properties also render it quite effective at reducing neuropathic pain and dysesthesias. It is generally well tolerated but may be sedating in elderly patients. Therefore, it is usually best to begin gabapentin therapy with a small dose in the evenings (100 to 300 mg) and gradually increase the dose and the frequency to three or four times a day, reaching a maximum of 3,600 mg/day. Tricyclic antidepressants (e.g., amitriptyline or nortriptyline, 25 to 75 mg at bedtime) are often effective (for details, see Chapter 24). Mexiletine (Mexitil) is another membrane stabilizer (used most often in treatment of cardiac dysrhythmias) that is useful in this regard. These compounds (especially gabapentin) are so efficacious that their use has supplanted that of the more historical drugs carbamazepine and phenytoin for treatment of neuropathic pain. Carbamazepine (Tegretol) 200 to 1,000 mg/day in divided doses may provide relief of refractory pain and is worth a therapeutic trial. This drug is started at 100 mg two or three times a day and is increased slowly (200 mg every 4 days in divided doses), to yield a serum level of 8 to 12 μg/mL. Once a therapeutic daily dosage has been established, conversion to the sustained-release form of Tegretol allows a more convenient twice-daily schedule. Intolerance to carbamazepine (ataxia, drowsiness, and nausea) is especially likely in the older patient. Hematologic values and liver function tests must be checked periodically. If Tegretol has been maintained in the therapeutic range for 2 to 4 weeks and still proves unsuccessful, it should be discontinued, and phenytoin (Dilantin) 300 to 500 mg/day to yield a serum level of 15 to 20 μg/mL may be tried. Details regarding carbamazepine and phenytoin are found in Chapter 88.

Autonomic Neuropathies

Autonomic dysfunctions should also be approached symptomatically (31). The *hypotonic bladder* may

Table 92.9. Measures that May Help Patients with Orthostatic Hypotension Caused by Autonomic Neuropathy

Avoid sudden changes in position
Avoid excessive intake of alcohol
Avoid diuresis
Correct hypovolemia
Discontinue or reduce the dosage of drugs known to cause orthostatic hypotension:
Antihypertensive drugs
Nitroglycerin
Diuretics
Neuroleptics
Tricyclic antidepressants
CNS depressants (opiates, alcohol)
Levodopa
Prescribe mineralocorticoid (if no congestive heart failure or hypertension)
Supplement diet with salt
Tilt up the head of the bed (may stimulate renin release)
Use elastic support stockings

CNS; central nervous system.

be treated by drugs that increase bladder tone (Urecholine, 10 to 25 mg every 8 hours), by self-catheterization, or occasionally with surgery to decrease resistance to bladder emptying. Details regarding the evaluation and management of the hypotonic bladder are in Chapter 6. For *male sexual impotence,* penile prostheses and pharmacologic erections produced by intracavernous injection or intraurethral suppositories have represented significant advances (see Chapter 6). The knowledge that sexual dysfunction has a neurologic basis may relieve the anxiety that often accompanies the problem. A check for medications that may be contributing to impotence is important (see Chapter 6).

Orthostatic hypotension may be treated with salt supplementation and a volume-expanding mineralocorticoid (fludrocortisone 0.1 to 0.2 mg/day) in patients without congestive heart failure or hypertension. A recently released expensive alpha-$_1$-adrenergic agonist, midodrine (ProAmatine), has been shown to help patients with orthostatic hypotension. The dosage is 10 mg three times per day. Contraindications are the same as those for fludrocortisone (32). Support stockings with pressure gradients may be helpful to prevent venous pooling, but many patients do not tolerate these stockings well. Arising slowly from recumbent or sitting positions, maintaining active ambulation, and sleeping with the head of the bed elevated on blocks (to stimulate renin release) are other measures that may help. Table 92.9 summarizes the practical ways to manage orthostatic hypotension caused by autonomic dysfunction.

OTHER PROBLEMS

Restless Legs Syndrome

Restless legs syndrome is common, affecting perhaps 5% of the general population. It is an important cause of insomnia (see Chapter 7). Patients complain of an aching or painful crawling sensation deep inside the legs at rest, especially in the evening or in bed. Walking provides some relief, but the dysesthesias often return quickly upon resting (33,34).

The exact pathophysiology has not been elucidated; both peripheral and central mechanisms have been proposed. The syndrome has been related in some patients to the peripheral neuropathies of diabetes mellitus and uremia. An association has also been found with iron and folate deficiency anemias, calcium and potassium deficiency, pregnancy, postgastric surgery state, excessive caffeine, sedative drug withdrawal, and exposure to neuroleptic medication. An idiopathic form is associated with periodic movements during sleep and a positive family history.

These patients should be evaluated for associated conditions for specific treatment. Restricting caffeine use and performing regular exercise before bedtime may be helpful recommendations. Simple analgesics (aspirin, acetaminophen) at bedtime may help early symptoms. In other patients, nonsedating dosages of clonazepam (Klonopin, 0.5 to 2 mg) or triazolam (Halcion, 0.125 mg) may relieve nocturnal symptoms. The drug of choice for people with severe restless leg syndrome is Sinemet (a combination of L-dopa and carbidopa) at dosages of one-half to two 25-/100-mg tablets at bedtime. If the patient is typically awakened later during the night, the controlled-release form of Sinemet is preferable. Sinemet is generally well tolerated (see details in Chapter 90). Dopamine agonists such as ropinirole and pramipexole have also been reported to be useful in treating this disorder.

Muscle Cramps

Cramps are localized involuntary painful contractions of skeletal muscles that produce a visible, palpable, hard, and bulging muscle. They must be distinguished from the sensation of cramp such as that described with intermittent claudication; the latter is not associated with a palpable hard and bulging muscle.

Ordinary muscle cramps are common and may be stopped by stretching the affected muscles. Frequent cramps are most often associated with denervating diseases, fatiguing exercises, salt depletion, dehydration, pregnancy, hypothyroidism, alcoholism, uremia, or hypomagnesemia. Patients with frequent daytime cramps related to exercise or fasting should be referred to a neurologist for evaluation for one of the rare muscle enzymatic defects (e.g., myophosphorylase, phosphofructokinase, or carnitine palmityltransferase deficiency). If no correctable associated condition exists, these patients may be given a therapeutic trial of phenytoin, carbamazepine, or amitriptyline (see above for dosages).

Nocturnal cramps occur in 15% of healthy young adults and are even more common in the elderly. Regular passive stretching of leg muscles often prevents nocturnal cramps. If this is not effective, empiric trial of medicine can be considered. Meta-analysis of published and unpublished controlled trials showed that quinine, which requires a prescription (usual dose 325 mg at bedtime), reduced by about 21% the frequency of night cramps (35). Another drug reported to be effective is single-dose clonazepam, 0.25 to 0.5 mg at bedtime.

General References*

Dawson DM. Current concepts: entrapment neuropathies of the upper extremities. N Engl J Med 1993;329:2013.

Dawson DM, Hallett M, et al. Entrapment neuropathies, 3rd ed. Philadelphia: Lippincott-Raven, 1999.

Dyck PJ, Thomas PK, Asbury AK, et al. Diabetic neuropathy. Philadelphia: WB Saunders, 1987.

A thorough review of pathophysiologic and clinical aspects of diabetic neuropathy.

Dyck P, Thomas PK, Griffin JW, et al., eds. Peripheral neuropathy, 3rd ed. Philadelphia: WB Saunders, 1993.

An excellent comprehensive review.

Medical Research Council. Aids to the examination of the peripheral nervous system. London: Bailliere-Tindall, 1986.

Well-illustrated guide to the physical examination for testing all peripheral nerves.

Midroni G, Bilbao JM. Biopsy diagnosis of peripheral neuropathy. Stoneham, MA: Butterworth, 1995.

Schaumburg HH, Berger AR, Thomas PK. Disorders of peripheral nerves, 2nd ed. Philadelphia: FA Davis, 1992.

A short work organized by disease processes that involve peripheral nerves.

Stewart JD. Focal peripheral neuropathies, 2nd ed. New York: Raven Press, 1993.

Specific References

1. Ewing DJ, Clarke BF. Diabetic autonomic neuropathy: present insights and future prospects. Diabetic Care 1986;9:648.
2. Vinik A, Mitchell B. Clinical aspects of diabetic neuropathies. Diabetes Metab Rev 1988;4:223.
3. Behse F, Buchthal F. Alcoholic neuropathy: clinical, electrophysiological and biopsy findings. Ann Neurol 1977;2:95.
4. Horwich MS, Cho L, Porro RS, et al. Subacute sensory neuropathy: a remote effect of cancer. Ann Neurol 1977;2:7.
5. Wilkinson M, Croft PB, Urich H. The remote effects of cancer on the nervous system. Proc R Soc Med 1967;60:683.
6. Oh SJ Paraneoplastic vasculitis of the peripheral nervous system. Neurol Clin 1997;15:849.
7. Oh SJ, Slaughter R, Harrell L. Paraneoplastic vasculitic neuropathy: a treatable neuropathy. Muscle Nerve 1991;14:152.
8. Kissel J, Mendell JR. Neuropathies associated with monoclonal gammopathies. Neuromusc Disord 1996;6:3.
9. Miralles GD, O'Fallon JR, Talley NJ. Plasma-cell dyscrasia with polyneuropathy. The spectrum of POEMS syndrome. N Engl J Med 1992;327:1919.
10. Schaumberg H, Kaplan J, Windebank A, et al. Sensory neuropathy from pyridoxine abuse, a new megavitamin syndrome. N Engl J Med 1983;309:445.
11. Cornblath DR. Treatment of the neuromuscular complications of human immunodeficiency virus infection. Ann Neurol 1988;2:S88.
12. Eidelberg D, Sotrel A, Vogel H, et al. Progressive polyradiculopathy in acquired immunodeficiency syndrome. Neurology 1986;36:912.
13. De Gans JH, Portugies P, Tiessens G, et al. Treatment for cytomegalovirus polyradiculomyelitis in patients with AIDS: treatment with ganciclovir. AIDS 1990;4:421.
14. D'Arcy CA, McGee S. Does this patient have carpal tunnel syndrome? JAMA 2000;283:3110.
15. Goodgold J, Kopell HP, Spielholz NI. The tarsal tunnel syndrome. N Engl J Med 1965;273:742.
16. Hauser WA, Karnes WE, Annis J, et al. Incidence and prognosis of Bell's palsy in the population of Rochester, Minnesota. Mayo Clin Proc 1971;46:258.
17. Finkel M. Lyme disease and its neurologic complications. Arch Neurol 1988;45:99.
18. Halperin JJ, Little BW, Coyle PK, et al. Lyme disease: cause of treatable peripheral neuropathy. Neurology 1987;37:1700.
19. Furuta Y, Ohtani F, Kawabata H, et al. High prevalence of varicella zoster virus reactivation in herpes simplex virus-seronegative patients with acute facial palsy. Clin Infect Dis 2000;30:529.
20. Williamson IG, Whelan TR. The clinical problem of Bell's palsy: is treatment with steroids effective? Br J Gen Pract 1996;46:743.
21. Ramsey MJ, DerSimonian R, Holtel MR, et al. Corticosteroid treatment for idiopathic facial nerve paralysis: a meta-analysis. Laryngoscope 2000;110:335.
22. Adour KK, Ruboyianes JM, Von Doersten PG, et al. Bell's palsy treatment with acyclovir and prednisone compared with prednisone alone: a double-blind, randomized, controlled trial. Ann Otol Rhinol Laryngol 1996;105:371.
23. Grogan PM, Gronseth GS. Practice parameter: Steroids, acyclovir, and surgery for Bell's palsy (an evidence-based review): Report of the Quality Standards Subcommittee of the American Academy of Neurology. Neurology 2001;56:830.
24. Ropper AH, Wijdicks EFM, Truax BT. Guillain-Barré syndrome. Philadelphia: FA Davis, 1991.
25. Plasma Exchange/Sandoglobulin Guillain-Barré Syndrome Trial Group. Randomized trial of plasma exchange, intravenous immunoglobulin, and combined treatments in Guillain-Barré syndrome. Lancet 1997;349:225.
26. Dyck PJ, O'Brien PC, Oviatt KF, et al. Prednisone improves chronic inflammatory demyelinating polyradiculoneuropathy more than no treatment. Ann Neurol 1982;11:136.
27. Dyck PJ, Litchy WJ, Kratz KM, et al. A plasma exchange versus immune globulin infusion trial in chronic inflammatory demyelinating polyradiculoneuropathy. Ann Neurol 1994;36:838.
28. Hahn AF, Bolton CF, Pillay N, et al. Plasma-exchange therapy in chronic inflammatory demyelinating polyneuropathy: a double-blind, sham-controlled, cross-over study. Brain 1996;119:1055.
29. Hahn AF, Bolton CF, Zochodne D, et al. Intravenous immunoglobulin treatment in chronic inflammatory demyelinating polyneuropathy: a double-blind, placebo-controlled, crossover study. Brain 1996;119:1067.
30. Azulay JP, Rihet P, Pouget J, et al. Long term follow up of multifocal motor neuropathy with conduction block under treatment. J Neurol Neurosurg Psychiatry 1997;62:391.
31. McCleod JG, Tuck RR. Disorders of the autonomic nervous system. II. Investigation and treatment. Ann Neurol 1987;21:519.
32. Low PA, Gilden JL, Freeman R, et al. Efficacy of Midodrine vs placebo in neurogenic orthostatic hypotension: a randomized, double-blind multicenter study. JAMA 1997;277:1046.
33. Gibb WRG, Lees AJ. The restless leg syndrome. Postgrad Med J 1986;62:329.
34. Walters A, Hening W. Clinical presentation and neuropharmacology of restless legs syndrome. Clin Pharmacol 1987;10:225.
35. Man-Son-Hing M, Wells G, Lau A. Quinine for nocturnal leg cramps: a meta-analysis including unpublished data. J Gen Intern Med 1998;13:600.

*Bold print (general references) and bold numerals (specific references) denote published controlled clinical trials, meta-analyses, or consensus-based recommendations.

SECTION 13

Selected General Surgical Problems

C H A P T E R 93

Preoperative Planning for Ambulatory Patients

RICHARD J. GROSS, MD, SCM

PREOPERATIVE PLANNING: OVERVIEW

Preoperative evaluation for elective surgery is now done almost entirely in the ambulatory setting, because most surgery is now performed in outpatient surgical units. For inpatient surgery, most patients are admitted on the day of surgery. The primary care practitioner invests substantial time in establishing a diagnosis for the initial complaint, arriving at the decision to recommend surgery, and discussing the findings with the patient and family. The practitioner then evaluates the medical risks from factors unrelated to the primary surgical problem and consults on the care of the patient's medical problems in the perioperative period.

The *principal reasons for office-based preoperative assessment* are that health care insurers reimburse only for same-day surgery for many procedures, insurers do not reimburse for admission the day before surgery for preoperative assessment, office assessment eliminates the costs and inconvenience associated with unanticipated cancellation of surgery after the patient has been admitted, and better planning of care and higher patient satisfaction are often achieved.

In general, the surgeon expects the referring clinician to have made an independent assessment of the need for surgery and of the medical acceptability of the patient for surgery. Although the surgeon obtains the actual consent for the surgical procedure, the patient's decision is based in part on the counseling provided by the referring practitioner. The referral itself is usually understood by a patient and the family as an endorsement of the consulting surgeon and of the surgeon's opinion. For these reasons, it is important for referring practitioners to know the place of surgery in the management of a broad array of conditions. *General guidelines on eligibility for same-day ambulatory surgery,* based on the patient's medical status, are summarized in Table 93.1 (1,2).

Laparoscopic techniques, though more comfortable to the patient, do not necessarily carry a lower medical, anesthetic, or surgical risk. General, spinal, and epidural anesthesia carry similar mortality risks in terms of medical problems. Local and regional anesthesia presumably carry lower risk, although data to prove this impression are lacking (regional anesthesia is usually a block, such as an axillary block). Surgery involving the thoracic and abdominal cavities and vascular surgery

Table 93.1. General Guidelines on Patient Eligibility for Ambulatory Surgery Based on Medical Condition (Not Considering Type of Surgery)

American Society of Anesthesiologists (ASA) class[a] 1 or 2 (some class 3 for minor procedures):
- *Class 1:* There is no physiological, biochemical, or psychiatric disturbance. The pathologic process for which operation is to be performed is localized and not conducive to systemic disturbance. *Examples:* A fit patient with inguinal hernia; fibroid uterus in an otherwise healthy woman.
- *Class 2:* Mild to moderate systemic disturbance caused either by the condition to be treated surgically or by other pathophysiologic processes. *Examples:* Presence of mild diabetes mellitus, essential hypertension, or anemia.
- *Class 3:* Severe systemic disturbance from whatever cause, even though it may not be possible to define the degree of disability with finality. *Examples:* Severe diabetes mellitus with vascular complications, moderate to severe degrees of pulmonary insufficiency, angina pectoris or healed myocardial infarction.

Stable chronic medical problems well controlled by medicines; absence of acute medical problems.
No recent myocardial infarction or unstable cardiac disease.
No decompensated lung disease.
If diabetic, not taking insulin; if taking insulin; stable and capable of self-monitoring (diabetics should be operated upon in the morning).

[a]For explanation of ASA class see Grossman L. Anesthesia: risks, techniques and agents, organ effects and specific concerns. In: Gross RJ, Caputo GM, eds. Medical consultation: the internist on surgical, obstetric, and psychiatric services, 3rd ed. Baltimore: Williams & Wilkins, 1998:55, with permission.

Adapted from Gross RJ, Babbott SF. Evaluation of healthy patients and ambulatory surgical patients. In: Gross RJ, Caputo GM, eds. Medical consultation: the internist on surgical, obstetric, and psychiatric services, 3rd ed. Baltimore: Williams & Wilkins, 1998:37, with permission.

carry higher medical risks than other types of surgery with certain exceptions, such as radical head and neck surgery and hip replacement.

In counseling the patient and family, the patient's primary care practitioner and the consulting surgeon should explain clearly the objective, potential complications, and expected outcome of the operation. This is especially important for surgical procedures that are undertaken for asymptomatic conditions (e.g., elective cholecystectomy) and for procedures that may be disfiguring (e.g., mastectomy or amputation). Preoperative counseling should be documented in the patient's record, including any special issues raised by the patient and how they were resolved (e.g., obtaining additional consultations or providing supportive counseling).

Approximately 50% of adults who undergo surgery are ostensibly in good general health; the other 50% have various medical problems (the percentages vary depending on the age of the population). In perhaps 5% to 10% of patients, new medical problems are identified during preoperative evaluation; a small proportion of these problems have implications for the planning of surgery.

The role of the primary care practitioner in relation to the surgeon and anesthesiologist will vary depending on the setting. In many university hospitals, the anesthesiologist will be more involved in the preoperative evaluation and postoperative care and the surgeon more involved in the postoperative care of medical problems than in community hospitals, but there is wide variation in practices, even among physicians within one institution. The primary care practitioner should be sensitive to the roles of the anesthesiologist and surgeon, usually making recommendations as a consultant rather than mandating management. In some instances, especially areas where there are differences in specialty practices, the recommendations should be worded "consider" rather than recommend. Perioperative management works best when the primary practitioner, surgeon, and anesthesiologist agree on their individual roles and coordinate care.

Whenever surgery is planned, the patient's referring practitioner should complete an appropriate preoperative evaluation (see below), ensure existing medical conditions that may affect the outcome of surgery are optimally controlled, and communicate specific recommendations to the surgeon regarding the care of the patient's medical problems during the perioperative period, including recommendations for office or telephone follow-up. This chapter provides guidelines for these steps in the management of patients with common medical problems.

GENERAL PREOPERATIVE EVALUATION

There is no consensus on the makeup of a general preoperative evaluation. For adult patients undergoing general or spinal anesthesia, most practitioners perform a history and physical examination and order a number of laboratory tests (e.g., electrocardiogram [ECG] in patients over age 40 and hematocrit, electrolytes, glucose, measurement of serum urea nitrogen or creatinine, and dipstick urinalysis in most adults). This complete workup has been criticized for having a low yield and being unnecessarily costly (1). The large number of factors that influence the preoperative evaluation make a consensus unlikely. The patient's age, the nature of the planned surgery (major or minor), the type of anesthesia to be used (general, spinal, regional, or local), and the interval since the patient's last comprehensive evaluation are relevant in the preoperative evaluation of every patient. In addition, one or more of the following considerations are often pertinent: estimating operative risk, establishing a baseline for expected postoperative changes or possible complications, avoiding harm to other patients or medical personnel (e.g., hepatitis, tuberculosis, or human immunodeficiency virus [HIV] infection), documenting selected information for medicolegal reasons, determining drug dosage, and detecting rare but potentially catastrophic circumstances (e.g., thrombocytopenia in a patient scheduled for a craniotomy).

A practical approach for the individual patient is to select one of the two general types of preoperative evaluation as summarized in Table 93.2 (i.e., a limited or a comprehensive workup). Guidelines for choosing between these alternatives are summarized in Table 93.3. Additional tests are added as indicated by the individual patient's medical and surgical problems. Selected screening tests should be added to the workup to avoid potential catastrophes associated

Table 93.2. Two Types of General Preoperative Evaluation

Component of Workup	Limited Workup[a]	Comprehensive Workup[a]
History	HPI, past medical history, allergies, medications, brief ROS (heart, lungs, hemostasis/bleeding problems, endocrine, and new symptoms, especially upper respiratory infection), family history (of surgical/anesthesia problems, bleeding disorders, thromboembolic disease)	HPI, past medical history, social history, family history, allergies, medications, complete ROS
Physical examination	Vital signs, oral cavity, chest, heart, and abdomen	Complete physical examination
Laboratory[a]	Hematocrit, urinalysis (dipstick only), ECG (some cases > age 35), serum potassium concentration in some cases, pregnancy test[b]	Chest radiograph, ECG (> age 35), complete blood count, serum urea nitrogen or serum creatinine, serum glucose, serum electrolytes, urinalysis, pregnancy test[b]

[a]Basic evaluation for screening and baseline data. Other tests may be added to evaluate known disease in a patient or to follow up findings in the preoperative history and physical examination; see also Table 93.4.

[b]Women in child-bearing age group.

HPI, history of present illness; ROS, review of symptoms; ECG, electrocardiogram.

Table 93.3. Guidelines for Selecting the General Preoperative Evaluation

Limited Workup	Comprehensive Workup
Age < 40 yr	Age > 40 yr (especially >60 yr)
Recent comprehensive physical examination	No, old, or inadequate data base
Well patient	Patient with moderate or severe major organ disease
Local, or regional, anesthesia	General, spinal, or epidural anesthesia
Established patient; previously examined by practitioner	New patient, unknown to practitioner
Minor procedure	Major procedure (especially thoracic, abdominal, neurosurgical)

with certain high-risk situations (Table 93.4). Routine HIV screening of preoperative patients is currently not recommended; instead, the universal precautions described in Chapter 39 are recommended.

A common approach is to recommend fewer tests as part of the basic limited or comprehensive workup and to use a grid to select tests based on individual patient characteristics and type of surgery (3). A number of such grids have been published, but recommendations are not uniform (1). Most hospitals or surgical centers have their own grids, which either are sent by the surgical center with the request for preoperative evaluation or may be requested by the referring practitioner. Because of non-uniformity of recommendations, the primary care practitioner should review the grid. *Commonly overlooked aspects of evaluation* and planning in the assessment of the outpatient presurgical patient are listed in Table 93.5.

CURRENT MEDICATIONS AND KNOWN ALLERGIES

All prescribed and nonprescribed drugs that a patient is taking and any known drug allergies should be communicated to the responsible anesthesiologist, surgeon, or preoperative unit at the surgical center. This information is critical for optimal perioperative management (Table 93.6). Some drugs may have to be discontinued days to weeks in advance of surgery. Some are withheld immediately before surgery, whereas others are taken immediately preoperatively. Most medications have a duration of action between 6 and 12 hours. Sometimes, omission of one or more doses may precipitate symptoms. For many patients it is appropriate to give a dose of medication, with a small amount of water (1 ounce or less), in the morning before the induction of anesthesia and resume the medication orally 6 to 12 hours later. When important oral medications cannot be continued throughout the perioperative period, alternate medications or routes of administration are used.

In addition to the patient's list of current prescribed medications, the referring practitioner should remember to communicate important related information to the anesthesiologist, surgeon, or surgical center. The patient should be asked specifically about nonprescription drug use that, although common, is often not mentioned spontaneously (e.g. aspirin-containing compounds and nonsteroidal anti-inflammatory drugs [NSAIDs], which may potentiate postoperative bleeding, and sedatives, which may interact with anesthetic drugs). The use of recreational substances that may affect the patient's course during or after surgery (alcohol, tobacco, illicit drugs) should be documented. The following should also be noted: prior allergic reactions to local and general anesthetic agents (e.g., halothane) and to drugs used for medical conditions, prior reactions to blood products, and a family history of reactions to anesthesia or blood transfusions. Finally, chronic corticosteroid use at any time within the past year should be reported, because perioperative steroids may be required to cover the stresses of surgery.

PREOPERATIVE DONATION FOR AUTOLOGOUS TRANSFUSION

Donation of one or more units of autologous blood for transfusion for elective surgery is now widely practiced. The risks of autologous transfusion are lower than the risks with bank blood, but bacterial contamination and transfusion of the wrong unit remain small possibilities.

Current blood preservation methods limit autologous donation to about 3 units. Single units are donated beginning about 4 weeks before surgery, at weekly intervals. In preoperative planning, it is important to leave sufficient time for donation of the required

Table 93.4. Additional Preoperative Screening Tests for Common High-risk Situations

High-risk Situation	Screening Tests
Patient undergoing neurosurgical, cardiac, vascular, or major abdominal procedure	Tests of hemostasis: platelet count, prothrombin time, partial thromboplastin time
Patient on diuretics, with vomiting/diarrhea, other abnormal fluid loss, cardiac disease, renal disease	Electrolytes
Patient with increased risk of active liver disease (e.g., alcoholism, drug addiction, homosexuality, dialysis, high-risk medications) who is undergoing general or spinal anesthesia	Liver function tests: serum aminotransferases, alkaline phosphatase, bilirubin, serology for hepatitis B, C
Patient with increased risk of chronic pulmonary disease (e.g., smoker with ≥10 pack years) who is undergoing general anesthesia	Pulmonary function tests (spirometry)
Patient with increased risk of tuberculosis (e.g., known exposure, HIV positive, underprivileged population)	Chest x-ray, purified protein derivative skin test for TB
Patient with increased risk of coronary artery disease (i.e., smoker, hypertensive, strong family history, diabetic, hyperlipidemia)	ECG
Malnourished patient or prolonged inability to eat	Nutritional assessment

HIV, human immunodeficiency virus; TB; tuberculosis; ECG; electrocardiogram.

Table 93.5. Commonly Forgotten or Underestimated Items in the Office Evaluation and Management of the Surgical Patient

Evaluation
- One disease (review the problem list)
- The generally sick patient (patient sicker than any one disease alone)
- Inquiry about current medications (e.g. aspirin, other over the counter [OTC] medications)
- Blood tests indicated by specific medical disease or medications (e.g., drug levels, potassium for diuretics)
- Inquiry about abnormal bleeding problems or disorders
- Inquiry about history of transfusion or transfusion reactions
- Inquiry about current use of alcohol or illicit drugs
- Pregnancy test (serum qualitative human chorionic gonadotropin)
- Spirometry (indications given under chronic obstructive lung disease)
- Echocardiogram (to clarify the need for subacute bacterial endocarditis prophylaxis)

Management
- Telling patient to report even minor intercurrent illnesses between physical and day of surgery
- Telling patient to stop smoking, drinking alcohol, taking illicit drugs, OTC medications (and no new OTC medications)(see Table 93.6 for medications; smoking should stop 8 weeks before admission; alcohol and illicit drugs 1 or more weeks preoperatively)
- Perioperative management of medications (see Table 93.6): whether to take medications the morning of surgery and when to restart postoperatively. Discontinue certain medications (such as aspirin, coumadin). Coverage for corticosteroids if indicated
- Subacute bacterial endocarditis prophylaxis
- Informing patient (briefly) what to expect preoperatively and postoperatively; whom to call if unexpected problems arise
- Informing patient about, and planning several weeks in advance for, autologous transfusion

Adapted from Gross RJ, Caputo GM, eds. Medical consultation: the internist on surgical, obstetric, and psychiatric services, 3rd ed. Baltimore: Williams & Wilkins, 1998:38, with permission.

units but not so much time that the units expire if there is a minor delay in the scheduled surgery. Usually this is arranged by the surgeon, but the patient's primary care practitioner may want to discuss this option with the patient, including the time necessary (depending on the number of units needed) and any medical contraindications or limitations in autologous donations.

Medical problems that are potential contraindications or that limit the number of units donated (depending on the severity of the situation) include anemia, cardiovascular disease, hypertension and antihypertensive medication, lung disease with significant hypoxia, orthostatic hypotension, certain infectious diseases (including hepatitis and HIV infection), very frail or debilitated patients, and far advanced age. Despite this list of limitations, most patients are able to donate blood for autologous transfusion, including most elderly patients with chronic diseases. The patient's practitioner may want to plan for partial volume repletion with saline at the time of donation for some patients who may be very sensitive to the volume loss. Most patients are prescribed iron (see Chapter 55) beginning about 1 week before the first donation and continuing for 2 to 3 months after donation (depending on the number of units donated).

SURGERY IN THE ELDERLY PATIENT

Risk

The mortality risk associated with anesthesia and surgery is increased in the elderly. However, the risk in elderly patients has fallen substantially over the past 10 to 20 years. The overall mortality risk for major surgery in patients under 65 is approximately 1%; the risk is approximately 5% between ages 65 and 80. Patients over age 80 have a 10% risk, although mortality as low as 6% to 8% has been reported (1,4–6).

Several factors are more important than age itself in increasing surgical risk in older patients (6). The most important of these factors are general overall health, nutrition, type of surgery (body cavity versus non–body cavity; emergency versus elective), type of anesthesia, coexisting conditions (cardiac, infectious, renal, pulmonary, central nervous system), and psychosocial status (attitude toward surgery, will to live, cognitive level, social situation). Common *causes of death* include uncorrectable surgical lesions such as infarcted bowel or ruptured aneurysm, coexisting cardiac disease, infections (especially pneumonia), renal disease, and pulmonary disease. In the preoperative evaluation, attention should be focused on managing or preventing these conditions.

Certain common procedures can be performed at low risk in the elderly, often without general

Table 93.6. Recommended Perioperative Management of Medications[a]

Drug Class	Anticipated Problems	Recommended Perioperative Management
Analgesics		
Narcotics	Decreased cough reflex, increased CNS depression by anesthesia, hypotension	Inform anesthesiologist of use.
Aspirin compounds[b]	Increased bleeding	Discontinue 1–2 weeks before surgery.
NSAIDs	Gastrointestinal tract bleeding	Discontinue 1–2 weeks preoperatively.
Antibiotics		
Tetracycline	Risk of renal failure if given with methoxyflurane	Use alternative antibiotic or anesthetic.
Anticoagulants, antiplatelet drugs		
Warfarin[b]	Increased bleeding	Discontinue 4–7 days before surgery, vitamin K1 if needed, check prothrombin time before operation.
Aspirin, other NSAIDs, clopidogrel[b]		Discontinue aspirin and other NSAIDs 1 week before surgery; clopidogrel 2 weeks before surgery.
Bronchodilators		
Theophylline[b]	Inability to give orally	Switch to intravenous aminophylline.
Beta-2-sympathomimetics[b]	Inability to give orally	Switch to aerosolized or subcutaneous beta-2 agent.
Cardiovascular		
Antihypertensives[b]	Interaction with anesthetics, hypotension	Inform anesthesiologist of use.
	Inability to give orally	Plan postoperative regimen with alternative agents if needed.
Antiarrhythmics[b]	Inability to give orally	ECG monitor in operating room and postoperatively, use alternative parenteral agents.
Beta-blockers[b]	Myocardial depression, bradycardia	Continue intravenously, taper to lower dosage, or discontinue depending on circumstances.
Digitalis[b]	Toxicity	Obtain serum levels preoperatively.
	Inability to give orally	Give 75% of daily oral dosage of digoxin intravenously each day.
Long-acting oral nitrates[b]	Inability to give orally	Substitute transdermal nitroglycerine.
Corticosteroids[b]	Adrenal insufficiency	Plan coverage (with intravenous corticosteroids) adequate for the stress of surgery.
	Poor wound healing	Discuss with surgeon.
Diabetes		
Oral hypoglycemics[b] Sulfonylureas	Inability to give orally	Withhold a.m. of surgery; switch to insulin preoperatively in selected patients.
Thiazolidinediones Metformin[b]	Risk of lactic acidosis; inability to give orally.	Withhold 48 h pre- and postoperatively.
Insulin[b]	Risk of hyperglycemia or hypoglycemia	Give one-third to one-half of usual dosage preoperatively.
Diuretics	Electrolyte abnormalities, hypotension, inability to give orally	Obtain electrolytes and check blood pressure (lying, standing) within 24 h preoperatively, use intravenous furosemide if needed.
Gastrointestinal		
Antacids[b]	Inability to give orally	Intravenous H_2 blockers, nasogastric suction (if patient has active peptic ulcer disease).
Gout		
Benemid, allopurinol	Inability to give orally	Observe, treat acute gout with intravenous colchicine.
Lipid lowering		
Lovastatin, other hydroxymethylglutaryl CoA reductase inhibitors	Rhabdomyolysis	? Discontinue preoperatively.
Gemfibrozil	Rhabdomyolysis	? Discontinue preoperatively.
Neurologic		
Levodopa/carbidopa[b]	Interaction with anesthetics (hypertension or hypotension), inability to give orally	Inform anesthesiologist of use; check with anesthesiologist on whether can be given preoperatively, resume orally as soon as possible after surgery.
Barbiturates	Increased CNS depression by anesthesia, inability to give orally	Inform anesthesiologist of use; give daily dosage intramuscularly.
Dilantin	Inability to give orally	Give daily dosage slowly intravenously (or substitute phenobarbital before admitting patient for surgery).
Psychiatric		
Antidepressants[b]	Hypotension or hypertension, arrhythmias	Inform anesthesiologist of use; withhold monoamine oxidase inhibitors 2 weeks preoperatively; selectively withhold other agents 24 h preoperatively.
Neuroleptics (i.e., phenothiazines and haloperidol)[b]	Arrhythmias, enhancement of neuromuscular blocking agents, hypotension	Inform anesthesiologist of use; withhold 24 h preoperatively in some cases.

Table 93.6.—*continued.* **Recommended Perioperative Management of Medications**

Drug Class	Anticipated Problems	Recommended Perioperative Management
Benzodiazepines	Increased CNS depression by anesthesia	Inform anesthesiologist of use.
Lithium[b]	Myocardial depression, hypernatremia	Inform anesthesiologist of use: determine blood levels; withhold 24 h preoperatively; avoid diuretics and NSAIDs; follow electrolytes closely.
Recreational drugs		
Alcohol Illicit drugs Tobacco[b]	Affect drug metabolism, drug interactions, withdrawal syndrome, impaired respiratory function Increased bronchospasm, secretions	If possible, have patient discontinue use 1 or more weeks before admission for surgery; inform anesthesiologist and surgeon of recent use.
Thyroid therapy		
Thyroid hormone[b]	Inability to give orally	Usually can be discontinued for up to 7–10 days.
Antithyroid drugs[b]	Inability to give orally	Use parenteral iodides or propranolol if necessary.
Topical drugs for glaucoma		
Timolol	Systemic beta blockage	Notify anesthesiologist preoperatively.
Phospholine iodide	Prolonged muscle relaxant activity	Discontinued 7–10 days preoperatively.

[a]If the patient will be able to take medication orally within 12 h postoperatively, most maintenance drugs can be given at that time. If a shorter interval is crucial, a maintenance drug can be given with less than 1 oz of water, several hours before anesthesia (e.g., 6 a.m.), and the drug can be resumed orally after surgery.

[b]See additional details in subsequent sections of this chapter.

NSAIDs, nonsteroidal anti-inflammatory drugs; CNS, central nervous system; ECG, electrocardiogram.

anesthesia. These low-risk operations include cataract surgery, simple hernia repair, and transurethral prostate resection. The risks of some major surgical procedures in the elderly have fallen greatly over the past few years; examples include elective abdominal aortic aneurysm repair and repair of hip fractures. Laparoscopic surgery, such as for cholecystectomy, produces fewer medical complications but has not yet been shown to have a lower mortality than traditional surgery in the elderly.

Perioperative Management

The elderly patient undergoing major surgery should have a comprehensive preoperative evaluation (Table 93.2) because of the wide variety of coexisting, often unrecognized, medical conditions found in older patients. The workup should be reviewed specifically for the risk factors listed above. Any major preoperative risks must be weighed against the benefits of the operation, with attention to the fact that quality of life may be as important as longevity in this age group. An accurate estimation of average future longevity for the patient's age group is important; this is often underestimated (see Chapter 12, Table 12.1).

Preoperative cardiac evaluation is discussed below. Manifestations of infection (including simple upper respiratory infections) should be carefully sought because classic signs may not be present in the elderly. Spirometry should be performed in patients over age 65 if there is pulmonary disease, because of the increased incidence of pulmonary complications in older patients. It should be remembered that serum creatinine may be falsely low in elderly patients because of their reduced muscle mass; therefore, a creatinine clearance should be obtained if the state of the patient's renal function is not certain, because of the importance in determining drug dosages. Finally, a baseline mental status examination (see Chapter 26) should be completed because postoperative changes in mental status are common in the elderly. If there is hearing impairment caused by cerumen impaction preoperatively, this problem should be corrected.

Elderly patients often have limitations of understanding because of memory deficits and hearing problems. Because these are often known to the primary care practitioner, informing the surgeon, anesthesiologist, and surgical center of these limitations can improve communication and management at each of these levels. Explanation of what to expect during hospitalization and surgery is especially important in the elderly not only because of the above factors, but because elderly patients may be less likely to ask questions of the surgeon and may have outdated conceptions of the nature of surgery.

Simple measures planned before admission may help reduce the high incidence of *postoperative confusion* in older patients, including correction of reversible hearing or vision deficits, planning to allow family members to stay beyond visiting hours, avoiding placing the patient unnecessarily in an intensive care unit, returning the patient to the same room postoperatively, allowing the presence of familiar objects, leaving a night-light on, and avoiding unnecessary instrumentation. Early mobilization, uninterrupted sleep, and frequent orientation to time, place, and current events are also important. Tranquilizers, sedatives, hypnotics, and pain medications should be used in reduced dosages and for appropriate indications, not routinely.

Postoperative mobilization of the elderly patient should be planned and anticipated by the patient, preoperatively. In general, the patient should expect to resume ambulation as early as possible.

SURGERY IN THE PREGNANT PATIENT

Risk

Up to 2% of women require nonobstetric surgery during pregnancy. Risks posed to the mother and fetus include complications from the surgical problem, effects of anesthesia and medication (including teratogenicity), risks of x-rays and other diagnostic procedures, precipitation of premature labor, and fetal death. Because of these problems, women of child-bearing age who are not known to be pregnant should be screened for pregnancy before surgery. History and sensitive serum human chorionic gonadotropin pregnancy tests usually suffice, but very early pregnancy may still be missed. If it is uncertain whether a woman is pregnant, nonurgent surgery should be postponed for 2 to 3 weeks until the situation is clarified; more urgent surgery requires judgment on an individual basis.

Physiologic alterations in pregnancy that may complicate anesthetic and surgical management are listed in Table 93.7. Two common changes of pregnancy should be taken into account when evaluating the patient preoperatively: The normal serum creatinine concentration is lower in pregnancy and an S_3 gallop, systolic murmur, or edema is commonly present in the pregnant patient without cardiac disease.

Perioperative Management

Preoperative planning and perioperative management for the pregnant surgical patient involves a number of complex issues, considered below.

Urgency

Can the surgery be postponed until after delivery or is it urgent (e.g., acute appendicitis), when delay will increase fetal–maternal mortality? In general, emergency surgery should not be delayed because of pregnancy, but totally elective surgery should be postponed until the postpartum period. In intermediate situations, the duration and risk to the mother of waiting must be balanced against the risk of immediate surgery.

Testing

Tests should be carefully planned to allow a precise diagnosis with minimal risk, especially risk from x-ray exposure. Whenever possible, other tests should be substituted for radiologic procedures (e.g., gallbladder sonogram instead of oral cholecystogram in suspected cholelithiasis). Routine x-rays, such as chest films or flat abdominal films, should be avoided. When these x-rays are unavoidable, use of lead screening, collimated equipment with minimal exposure, and few films can minimize fetal exposure.

Medications

Drugs required during the perioperative period should be anticipated. The potential effects on the fetus should be ascertained from obstetric colleagues or available reference sources, and the least toxic alternative should be used. Routine drugs prescribed postoperatively should be avoided unless they are deemed to be necessary and risk to the fetus has been assessed.

Anesthesia

A decision on the type of anesthesia must be left to the anesthesiologist and obstetrician. Local or regional anesthesia would presumably be safer than general or spinal anesthesia, but no data exist to support this impression.

Table 93.7. Physiologic Alterations in Pregnancy and Their Relevance to the Surgical Patient

System	Change	Clinical Implications
Cardiovascular	Uterine compression of vena cava and aorta in supine position	Decreased cardiac output and uterine perfusion; avoid supine recumbency; tilt hips 15 degrees in perioperative period.
	Decrease in blood pressure in early to midgestation	Altered criteria for diagnosis of hypotension.
	Presence of dyspnea, third heart sound, and edema	No known increased risk, and such findings are not an indication for diuretic therapy or delay of surgery.
Respiratory	Decreased arterial Po_2 when patient is in the supine position	Avoid supine recumbency.
	Decreased pulmonary functional residual capacity and increased O_2 consumption	Increased risk of hypoxia perioperatively; avoid hypoventilation and increase inspired O_2 content before procedures inducing apnea (intubation or tracheal suctioning).
	Arterial Pco_2 and serum HCO_3 decrease to 30 mm Hg and 20 mmol/L, respectively	Maternal and fetal acidosis may occur in patient ventilated to "normal," nonpregnant values of arterial Pco_2; normal values for pregnancy should be used to guide diagnosis and therapy of acid-base disturbances.
Hematologic	Decreased venous flow in legs and increased levels of clotting factors	Increased risk of thromboembolism; avoid supine position and consider use of support stockings or pneumatic compression device.
	Proximity of fetal and maternal circulations	Risk of isoimmunization; Rh0(D) immune globulin should be considered when uterine trauma is likely.
Gastrointestinal	Decreased gastric motility and reduced competency of gastroesophageal sphincter	Increased risk of aspiration; preoperative antacids should be considered.
Renal	Dilation of urinary collecting system	Increased risk of urinary infection, so catheterization should be avoided when possible.
	30% to 50% increase in glomerular filtration rate and renal plasma flow with a concomitant decrease in serum creatinine and urea nitrogen to 0.5 and 9 mg/dL, respectively	Serum creatinine above 0.8 mg/dL may reflect impaired renal function; the clearance of many drugs is increased, and dosage schedules may require alteration.

From Barron WM. The pregnant surgical patient: medical evaluation and management. Ann Intern Med 1984;101:683, with permission.

Monitoring of Fetal Status

Monitoring of fetal status by the obstetrician should be planned throughout the perioperative period.

PROBLEMS AFTER DISCHARGE

Miscellaneous Problems

During the weeks and months after surgery, patients often have questions about incisional pain, various symptoms in the system that was operated on, restrictions of activity, and return to work. These questions are best answered by the surgeon. In addition, patients who have major surgery often complain of postoperative fatigue, a problem that can usually be handled by the patient's primary care practitioner.

Postoperative Fatigue

Patients with postoperative fatigue may describe a number of symptoms, including the need for increased sleep, weakness of the arms and legs when resuming usual activity, symptoms of orthostatic hypotension, and loss of interest in resuming usual activities (7). The symptoms of postoperative fatigue often last for 1 or more months. The physiologic changes responsible for these symptoms have not been well defined.

The primary care practitioner should also be aware of specific, often treatable, conditions that may contribute to or cause postoperative fatigue. Sleepiness may be related to sedatives, tranquilizers, or analgesics prescribed at the time of discharge and may improve with discontinuation of these drugs. The patient with orthostatic symptoms may have had a drug prescribed that can produce this problem (diuretics, antihypertensives, long-acting nitrates, antidepressants); because bed rest alone may cause orthostasis, these drugs should be resumed cautiously in a patient who has had recent major surgery and blood pressure should be checked in the lying, sitting, and standing positions. Dosage reduction or discontinuation of the drug should be considered where orthostatic hypotension is documented or orthostatic symptoms persist. Loss of interest may also be secondary to drugs prescribed after surgery (see Chapter 24 for a list of drugs that may cause a depressed mood). Alternatively, this symptom may represent a minor mood disturbance in a patient who has had similar problems at previous times of stress (see Chapter 21), or it may represent a reactive depression, similar to a grief reaction (see Chapter 24), that is related to disfiguring surgery. Because other medical problems related to surgery may occasionally cause postoperative fatigue, a hematocrit, serum urea nitrogen or creatinine, electrolytes, glucose, liver enzymes, and other tests indicated by clinical findings should be checked if the history suggests a problem that testing would identify or if fatigue is prolonged.

When evaluation of postoperative fatigue does not disclose contributing factors that can be treated, patients should be reassured that the problem will gradually resolve; they should also be given a rough timetable for a return to regular activities that is realistic in terms of both the surgical procedure and the fact that postoperative fatigue may take a number of months to resolve entirely. Simple exercises for patients convalescing from bed rest are illustrated in Chapter 89. For selected patients, these or similar exercises can be recommended during the period of recovery from postoperative fatigue.

PATIENTS WITH CARDIOVASCULAR DISEASE

Overview

Most forms of general anesthesia can cause cardiovascular stresses (decreased myocardial contractility, peripheral vasodilatation, arrhythmias, hypotension), and spinal or epidural anesthesia can cause hypotension. These factors and the stresses associated with surgery itself probably account for the greatly increased risk of surgery for patients with underlying cardiovascular disease (8).

Ischemic Heart Disease

Risk

Ischemic heart disease poses four major risks perioperatively in the patient undergoing general anesthesia: myocardial infarction (MI), ischemic pulmonary edema, life-threatening arrhythmias, and cardiac death. These risks depend on the patient's preoperative status. Overall, the risks for patients with arteriosclerotic heart disease are two or three times those of patients of the same age without cardiac disease.

The increased risk posed by ischemic heart disease is partially dependent on *preoperative cardiac status* (Table 93.8). Stable mild to moderate angina pectoris alone represents only a small increase in risk. The risk attending severe or unstable angina cannot

Table 93.8. Summary of Perioperative Cardiovascular Risk in Patients with Ischemic Heart Disease

Patient Status (Preoperative)	% Mortality (Range) Total	% Mortality (Range) Cardiac	Postoperative Myocardial Infarction (%)
No "cardiac disease"[a]	3 (0.2–10)	?[b]	0.8 (0.1–2)
"Cardiac disease" present[a]	11 (5–20)	?	5 (2–8)
Angina (stable)	4 (4–12)	?	4(?)
Past myocardial infarction			
All	5–15	5	7
Within 3 mo	25–40 } 15–25[c]	?	35
Between 3 and 6 mo	5–20 } 15–25[c]	?	17–25[d]
More than 6 mo	2.5	?	5
Unknown	?	?	10

[a]Cardiac disease data based mostly on patients with ischemic heart disease.

[b]?, data not available or uncertain.

[c]Recent figures show that postoperative mortality may be less.

[d]Recent studies indicate that current risk of reinfarction may be approximately 2%–6%, using modern hemodynamic monitoring and anesthesia.

From Kammerer WS, Gross RJ. Medical consultation: the internist on surgical, obstetric, and psychiatric services, 2nd ed. Baltimore: Williams & Wilkins, 1990, with permission.

be estimated accurately because of varying definitions and the small number of patients reported in the medical literature, but there is a significantly increased risk. An MI during the 6 months preceding surgery represents a high risk, particularly an MI 3 months or less before surgery. There is some evidence (8,9) that aggressive perioperative management may significantly lower cardiovascular risk (e.g., reduce recurrent MI risk from 30% to 4%). By 6 months after an infarction, the risk of a perioperative MI has plateaued but remains larger than the risk in a control population.

In addition to a recent MI, a number of factors contribute to the risk of perioperative cardiac complications or mortality. The most important of these factors are age greater than 70, decompensated congestive heart failure (CHF), arrhythmias, and other organ system disease (see Table 93.9). These and other factors were incorporated in 1986 into a Modified Cardiac Risk Index (Detsky) (Table 93.9; Fig. 93.1); and in 1999 into a Revised (Simple) Cardiac Risk Index (Table 93.10), all of which have been validated (10–13). A single prospective study found the Revised Cardiac Risk Index performed slightly to moderately better than the other indices (13). More recently, the *American College of Physicians published its "Guidelines for Assessing and Managing Perioperative Risk from Coronary Artery Disease"* (see General References) based on a critical review of the literature from 1977 to 1996. The guidelines use point scores from the Modified Cardiac Risk Index (Detsky) for stratification of patients into *three groups with different risks of perioperative cardiac events: low risk* (below 3%), *intermediate risk*

Table 93.9. Modified Cardiac Risk Index[§]

Variable	Points, *n*
Coronary artery disease	
Myocardial infarction <6 months earlier	10
Myocardial infarction <6 months earlier	5
Canadian Cardiovascular Society angina classification	
Class III	10
Class IV	20
Alveolar pulmonary edema	
Within 1 week	10
Ever	5
Suspected critical aortic stenosis	
Arrhythmias	
Rhythm other than sinus or sinus plus arterial premature beats on electrocardiogram	5
>5 premature ventricular contractions on electrocardiogram	5
Poor general medical status, defined as any of the following: Po_2 <60 mm Hg, Pco_2 >50 mm Hg, K^+ level <3 mmol/L, blood urea nitrogen level >50 mmol/L, creatinine level >260 μmol/L, bedridden	5
Age >70 years	5
Emergency surgery	10

[§]Class I = 0 to 15 points; class II = 20 to 30 points; class III = more than 30 points.

II Canadian Cardiovascular Society classification of angina: 0 = asymptomatic; 1 = angina with strenuous exercise; II = angina with moderate exertion; III = angina with walking 1 to 2 level blocks or climbing 1 flight of stairs or less at a normal pace; IV = inability to perform any physical activity without development of angina.

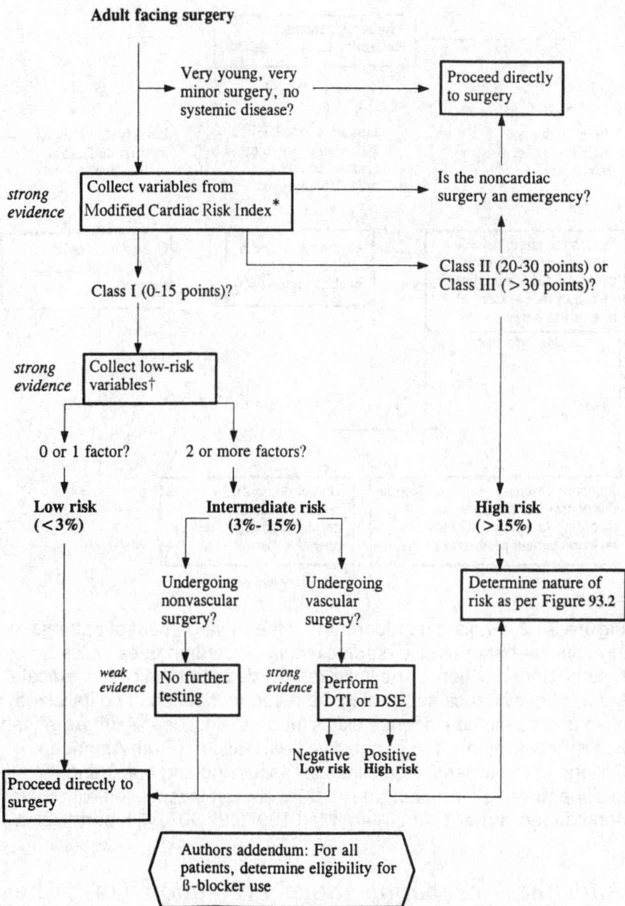

Figure 93.1. Suggested algorithm for the risk assessment and management of patients at low or intermediate risk for perioperative cardiac events, usually myocardial infarction and death. Boxed phrases indicate recommended actions. The italicized words beside the boxes indicate the level of evidence supporting the recommendation. If no italicized word is present, no evidence exists for or against use. See Table 93.9. *DTI,* dipyridamole thallium imaging; *DSE,* dobutamine stress echocardiography. (From American College of Physicians. Guidelines for assessing and managing the perioperative risk from coronary artery disease associated with major non-cardiac surgery. Ann Intern Med 1997;127:309, with permission.)

Table 93.10. Revised (Simple) Cardiac Risk Index[a]

Risk Factors	Points
History of ischemic heart disease	1
History of congestive heart failure	1
History of cerebrovascular disease	1
High risk type of surgery	1
Preoperative treatment with insulin	1
Preoperative serum creatinine >2.0 mg/dL	1

[a]Class I, 0 points; class II, 1 point; class III, 2 points; class IV, 3 or more points.

From Lee TH, Marcantonio ER, Mangione CM, et al. Derivation and prospective validation of a simple index for prediction of cardiac risk of major noncardiac surgery. Circulation 1999;100:1043, with permission.

(3% to 15%), and *high risk* (above 15%). They provide practical guidelines for management for each risk category, as shown in Figs. 93.1 and 93.2.

A joint *American College of Cardiology/American Heart Association Task Force also has issued*

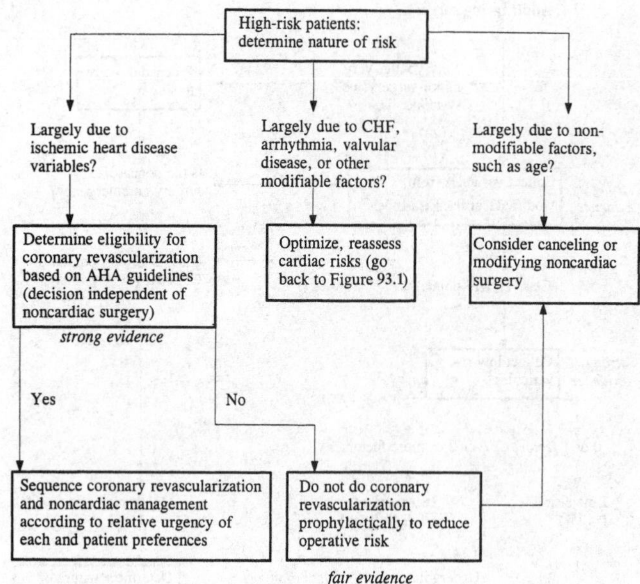

Figure 93.2. Suggested algorithm for the management of patients at high risk for perioperative cardiac events. Boxed phrases indicate recommended actions. The italicized words below the boxes indicate the level of evidence supporting the recommendation. If no italicized word is present, no evidence exists for or against use. *AHA,* American Heart Association; *CHF,* congestive heart failure. (From American College of Physicians. Guidelines for assessing and managing the perioperative risk from coronary artery disease associated with major non-cardiac surgery. Ann Intern Med 1997;127:309, with permission.)

guidelines for perioperative evaluation (14). They contain less quantitative information for risk stratification than the American College of Physicians' guidelines. They add the information in Table 93.11, which stratifies the *risk of cardiac death or MI according to type of noncardiac surgical procedure*; procedures are listed as high risk (above 5%), intermediate risk (below 5%), and low risk (below 1%).

Clinical assessment of the cardiac patient is approximately 75% sensitive for detecting high-risk patients. In intermediate- or high-risk *vascular surgery patients,* dipyridamole–thallium or other types of stress tests can accurately identify those with ischemia who have an increased operative risk. In nonvascular surgery patients, the usefulness of preoperative stress testing for risk assessment has not been definitely demonstrated (14) (see General References). Detailed discussion of the use of noninvasive testing for preoperative decision-making is contained in the American College of Physicians' guidelines and other publications (8,14).

Perioperative Management

Patients with established ischemic heart disease should have a comprehensive preoperative evaluation (Table 93.2). A *baseline ECG* should be obtained before surgery for all patients with known coronary artery disease and for all patients over approximately ages 35 to 40. Noninvasive tests of cardiac function, including echocardiography, nuclear scanning, and stress tests, should generally be reserved for situations where the evidence for the presence or severity of cardiovascular disease is questioned or in certain high-risk situations, such as vascular surgery, where precise information about the degree of severity is desired (see above).

Table 93.11. Cardiac Risk[a] Stratification for Noncardiac Surgical Procedures

High (reported cardiac risk often >5%)
Emergent major operations, particularly in the elderly
Aortic and other major vascular
Peripheral vascular
Anticipated prolonged surgical procedures associated with large fluid shifts or blood loss
Intermediate (reported cardiac risk generally <5%)
Carotid endarterectomy
Head and neck
Intraperitoneal and intrathoracic
Orthopedic
Prostate
Low[b] (reported cardiac risk generally <1%)
Endoscopic procedures
Superficial procedure
Cataract
Breast

[a]Combined incidence of cardiac death and nonfatal myocardial infarction.
[b]Do not generally require further preoperative cardiac testing.
From ACC/AHA Task Force. Guidelines for perioperative cardiovascular evaluation for noncardiac surgery. J Am Coll Cardiol 1996;27:910, with permission.

Based on the preoperative evaluation, the risk of general anesthesia and surgery should be estimated for each patient. For patients with recent MI (within less than 6 months), unstable angina, or less severe coronary artery disease and multiple other risk factors (Fig. 93.1 and Tables 93.9 and 93.10), only urgent lifesaving surgery should be undertaken until the risk is lowered. Surgery may be done 3 months after infarction when the risk of waiting the additional 3 months is thought to be significant (e.g., recurrent cholecystitis). Patients with stable angina or uncomplicated recovery from MI more than 6 months previously have a small increase in risk that does not decline further with time; thus, there is no need to postpone necessary operations.

Coronary artery bypass surgery or angioplasty should be considered before elective noncardiac surgery, in consultation with a cardiologist, in patients who have other indications for coronary revascularization (see Chapter 62). Although guidelines do not generally recommend bypass surgery or angioplasty prophylactically before noncardiac surgery without other indications, these interventions may need to considered in an occasional high risk patient. Routine *postoperative ECGs* need to be obtained only in high-risk patients (e.g., all patients with known coronary artery disease and any adults who develop hypotension during surgery) because the yield of useful information from them in low and intermediate risk patients is low.

For patients taking a long-acting oral nitrate for angina, the drug should be administered on the morning of surgery with a sip of water. If the patient is unable to take medications orally, nitroglycerin paste or a transdermal patch can be substituted. If there is no simple way to determine the paste dosage equivalent to the oral nitrate, an intermediate dose equivalent to 1 to 2 inches of Nitrol paste every 4 to 6 hours is recommended.

For patients taking a beta-blocking agent for angina, intravenous small dosages of propranolol (1 to 2 mg every 6 hours) can be substituted, given by a physician, while the patient is unable to take medications by mouth. This should protect the patient from the risk of acute cardiac ischemia, which occasionally follows abrupt cessation of beta-blocking agents. Patients able to resume oral intake within 12 to 24 hours usually can be observed without intravenous propranolol, particularly if a long acting beta-blocker was administered preoperatively.

For patients who are not already taking a beta-blocking agent, who have coronary artery disease, who are intermediate to high risk, and who are undergoing major surgery, a beta-blocker should be started preoperatively and continued during the perioperative period, based on a randomized controlled trial (15). Although only patients undergoing vascular surgery were studied, it is reasonable to extend the use of beta-blockers to other major surgery until data are available. The authors recommended a beta-blocker dose sufficient preoperatively to lower the heart rate to less than 70 beats/min and in the immediate postoperative period to less than 80 beats/min (15); this degree of beta-blockade may not be achievable in some patients. Beta-blockers should be initiated 1 to 2 weeks preoperatively and the patient's response evaluated in the office before surgery. Consideration should be given to chronic beta-blockers after surgery because of their efficacy in coronary disease (see Chapters 62 and 63). If beta-blockers are not going to be continued indefinitely for chronic indications, they should be continued for a minimum of 2 to 4 weeks postoperatively, longer if there are ongoing cardiac stresses, and then tapered.

Calcium blocking agents can usually be given on the morning of surgery. Another type of antianginal medication must be used postoperatively until the patient can resume oral intake. Diltiazem and verapamil are available in intravenous form, but maintenance regimens are not established.

Intensive intraoperative monitoring using Swan-Ganz and radial artery catheters should be planned in consultation with the anesthesiologist and surgeon for patients who are very sensitive to volume changes, such as those in CHF (see below); for operations when loss and replacement of large volumes of fluid are expected (e.g., aneurysm repair); and for patients with a recent MI (less than 6 months), severe unstable coronary disease, or with very high risk.

Hypertension

Risk

Controversy still exists about whether mild to moderate hypertension (diastolic 110 mg Hg or lower) increases anesthetic and surgical risks. The only prospective study showed no correlation between uncontrolled diastolic pressures in this range and the risk of perioperative cardiac, renal, or cerebrovascular events (16). Patients in this study often had other cardiac risk factors that did correlate with the incidence of perioperative cardiac morbidity (Tables 93.9 and 93.12).

Too few patients have been studied to define adequately the risk for patients operated on when their diastolic pressure exceeds 110 mm Hg, but there is probably an increased risk (16). Likewise, risk is probably increased in selected patients with significant cardiac, renal, or cerebrovascular disease.

Perioperative Management

The basic preoperative evaluation in the hypertensive patient should establish whether there is end-organ damage (renal: serum creatinine concentration and urinalysis; cerebrovascular: history, neurologic and neurovascular examination; cardiovascular: history, cardiac examination, chest x-ray, and ECG). Blood pressure and pulse measurements should be made with the patient lying or sitting and standing (after brief exercise, to identify the maximal orthostatic fall in patients taking antihypertensive drugs); the preoperative status of blood pressure control may then be classified as untreated, hypertensive despite therapy, or controlled.

Patients who are controlled or patients who are partially controlled and have diastolic pressures 110 mm Hg or lower should be continued on their prescribed antihypertensive medication. Three exceptions to this rule are reserpine, guanethidine, and monoamine oxidase inhibitors. A patient taking any of these infrequently used drugs should be switched to a different

Table 93.12. Risk of Perioperative Cardiac Complications in Patients with Mild to Moderate Hypertension

Preoperative Characteristics	Mean Point Total[a] (± SEM)	Patients with No Cardiac Complication (%)	Patients with Minor Complications Only[b] (%)	Patients with Major Nonfatal Complications[c] (%)	Patients with Cardiac Death[c] (%)
Normal blood pressure, no history of hypertension	4.3 ± (0.3)	89	9	2	0.2
Hypertension controlled, taking antihypertensive drug(s)	6.9 ± (0.6)	76	15	8	1
Hypertensive					
Taking antihypertensive drug(s)	4.4 ± (0.5)	93	8		1
Not taking antihypertensive drug(s)	5.5 ± (0.6)	88	9	1	1

[a]See Table 93.9.

[b]New or worse heart failure, supraventricular tachycardia, or intraoperative or postoperative ischemia (typical chest pain or electrocardiogram changes).

[c]Fatal events or life-threatening events (pulmonary edema, myocardial infarction, ventricular tachycardia).

Adapted from Goldman L, Caldera DL. Risks of general anesthesia and elective operation in the hypertensive patient. Anesthesiology 1979;50:285, with permission.

drug during the 2 weeks preceding surgery, because each of these drugs may cause markedly labile blood pressure during anesthesia.

Untreated patients with diastolic pressures 110 mm Hg or lower may undergo surgery, with institution of antihypertensive therapy after convalescence from surgery, if there are no other complicating cardiovascular risks. Alternatively, as long as adequate time is allowed to measure full effects of antihypertensive medication, there is no reason not to treat hypertension preoperatively. Because for most antihypertensive medications this requires several weeks, a decision may need to be made about delaying surgery versus instituting antihypertensives postoperatively.

Individual judgments must be made about patients with *diastolic pressures that are repeatedly above 110 mm Hg,* depending on the severity and duration of hypertension, the presence of end-organ damage, and the extent of planned surgery. Most patients with diastolic blood pressure above 110 mm Hg should have their blood pressure at least partly controlled before admission for nonurgent surgery, although there are no randomized studies proving that such control modifies risks. Attempts to control blood pressure too rapidly (e.g., rapid increases in diuretic treatment over several days) may result in volume depletion, hypokalemia, or hypotension at the time of surgery. Therefore, these patients should have their blood pressure stabilized during the 1 to 2 weeks before admission for surgery. There are no data on the perioperative risk of isolated systolic hypertension, but it seems reasonable to aim for a systolic pressure of 160 or below (see Chapter 67).

For all hypertensive patients, significant intravascular volume expansion or contraction should be avoided, because these conditions may either cause a significant rise in blood pressure (volume expansion) or fall in blood pressure (volume contraction, especially in the patient who is taking antihypertensive drugs).

Current antihypertensive medications should be continued through the morning of surgery (diuretics are usually withheld the morning of surgery) and resumed postoperatively when the patient is stable and can take oral medications. Because bed rest and inactivity during convalescence can lower blood pressure, some patients require less antihypertensive medication postoperatively and during the first few weeks after major surgery. Relatedly, because antihypertensive effects may be amplified when the postoperative patient's position changes from recumbent to sitting or standing, blood pressure should be measured in these positions postoperatively and after antihypertensive treatment has been instituted or resumed.

In some patients, the diastolic pressure exceeds 110 mm Hg postoperatively before oral medication can be resumed. When patients remain severely hypertensive despite control of secondary causes, such as pain, and the hypertension poses immediate health risks, the blood pressure can be controlled by the careful use of parenteral or transcutaneous agents. These include intravenous propranolol, hydralazine, transcutaneous clonidine (especially for patients who were taking clonidine before surgery who are at risk of rebound hypertension and tachycardia due to clonidine withdrawal), intravenous enalapril, intravenous labetalol, parenteral diuretics, parenteral methyldopa, intravenous nitroprusside, and intravenous or transcutaneous nitroglycerin.

Valvular Heart Disease

Risk

The risk of surgery in the patient with valvular heart disease varies with the valve affected (aortic versus mitral), the nature (stenosis versus insufficiency), and the severity of the lesion (8,11). The severity of valvular lesions as judged clinically by New York Heart Association classification (see Chapter 66) provides a reasonable indication of surgical risk except in patients with aortic stenosis.

Valvular heart disease poses *two major surgical risks: cardiac death and CHF.* The presence of aortic stenosis of any degree of hemodynamic significance poses a high risk of surgical mortality. Mild to moderate mitral lesions or aortic insufficiency pose only slightly increased risk of cardiac death; however, hemodynamically severe valvular disease (New York Heart Association class 3 or 4) caused by these lesions creates major risks. In addition to increasing the risk of perioperative mortality, significant valvular disease poses an increased risk of decompensated heart failure.

Little specific information exists regarding the risks associated with *prolapsed mitral valve* or *hypertrophic cardiomyopathy.* It is reasonable to assume that the risk in patients with prolapsed mitral valve depends on the degree of mitral regurgitation. Patients with hypertrophic cardiomyopathy may be very sensitive to volume contraction and are probably best managed with a Swan-Ganz catheter in place during major procedures associated with rapid volume changes.

Patients with artificial heart valves, patients with any evidence of valvular heart disease (including mitral prolapse and hypertrophic cardiomyopathy), and patients with congenital structural defects (e.g., patent ductus arteriosus, ventricular septal defect) have a small but definite risk of acquiring *bacterial endocarditis* when they undergo procedures in the oral cavity and upper respiratory, gastrointestinal, or genitourinary tracts (17).

Perioperative Management

The basic cardiac evaluation should delineate the nature and severity of the valvular disease and should identify any associated cardiac conditions. The uses of echocardiography and cardiac catheterization to evaluate valvular heart disease are described in Chapter 65. Patients with severe valvular disease should have corrective cardiac surgery followed by a period of convalescence before they undergo major elective noncardiac operations. The preoperative management of CHF, arrhythmia, or anticoagulant therapy (in patients with artificial valves) is described in subsequent sections of this chapter.

Patients undergoing procedures attended by a risk of *endocarditis* (Table 93.13) should receive *antimicrobial prophylaxis* (as summarized in Tables 93.13 and 93.14). The information in these tables was updated in the 1997 recommendations of the American Heart Association on the basis of an exhaustive review of the literature between 1936 and 1996. The information in Table 93.14 is available from the American Heart Association in a wallet-sized card for patients. The authors emphasize that these recommendations are not based on randomized controlled trials and that they should not be substituted for clinical judgment (17).

Table 93.13. Subacute Bacterial Endocarditis Prophylaxis: Recommendations for Procedures in the Respiratory, Gastrointestinal, and Genitourinary Tracts (See Recommended Antibiotic Regimens, Table 93.14)

- Endocarditis prophylaxis recommended
  - Respiratory tract
    - Tonsillectomy or adenoidectomy
    - Surgical operations that involve respiratory mucosa
    - Bronchoscopy with a rigid bronchoscope
  - Gastrointestinal tract[a]
    - Sclerotherapy for esophageal varices
    - Esophageal stricture dilation
    - Endoscopic retrograde cholangiography with biliary obstruction
    - Biliary tract surgery
    - Surgical operations that involve intestinal mucosa
  - Genitourinary tract
    - Prostate surgery
    - Cytoscopy
    - Urethral dilation
- Endocarditis prophylaxis not recommended
  - Respiratory tract
    - Endotracheal intubation
    - Bronchoscopy with a flexible bronchoscope, with or without biopsy[b]
    - Tympanostomy tube insertion
  - Gastrointestinal tract
    - Transesophageal echocardiography[b]
    - Endoscopy with or without gastrointestinal biopsy[b]
  - Genitourinary tract
    - Vaginal hysterectomy[b]
    - Vaginal delivery[b]
    - Cesarean section
    - In uninfected tissue
      - Urethral catheterization
      - Uterine dilation and curettage
      - Therapeutic abortion
      - Sterilization procedures
      - Insertion or removal of intrauterine devices
  - Other
    - Cardiac catheterization, including balloon angioplasty
    - Implanted cardiac pacemakers, implanted defibrillators, and coronary stents
    - Incision or biopsy of surgically scrubbed skin
    - Circumcision

[a]Prophylaxis is recommended for high-risk patients; optional for medium-risk patients.

[b]Prophylaxis is optional for high-risk patients.

From Dajani AS, Taubert KA, Wilson W, et al. Prevention of bacterial endocarditis. Recommendations by the American Heart Association. JAMA 1977;277:1794, with permission.

Congestive Heart Failure

Risk

Information on the risk of developing CHF perioperatively is limited because of the few studies available. However, the best prospective studies (11–14) closely correspond to general clinical experience. The most significant risk factors for postoperative CHF are decompensated failure preoperatively and, to a lesser extent, prior CHF that is clinically stable preoperatively (Table 93.15) (10–14). However, only 40% of patients who develop perioperative CHF have had prior failure. The best predictors for the other 60% of patients are age greater than 60, major surgery (especially abdominal aortic aneurysm repair or major abdominal surgery), and nonspecific ECG abnormalities.

Patients with postoperative pulmonary edema have a high total mortality (20% to 57%), most of which is cardiac. Patients who develop less severe postoperative CHF do not have an increased risk of postoperative cardiac death, although the overall mortality from all causes is increased. Most postoperative CHF occurs during or within several hours of surgery.

Perioperative Management

Patients with compensated CHF should have a comprehensive preoperative evaluation (Table 93.2). This evaluation should include an assessment of volume status (lying and standing blood pressures, inspection of neck veins, determination of whether edema is present) and examination for cardiac gallops and rales. Laboratory data should include blood urea nitrogen, creatinine, electrolytes, and a digoxin level if that drug is being administered. Noninvasive methods for assessing left ventricular function (see Chapter 66) may be useful when the degree of cardiac dysfunction is uncertain.

Although there are no definitive perioperative studies in this regard, it is prudent to administer digitalis to patients with a confirmed history of moderate or severe dilated congestive cardiomyopathy, ideally during the week before admission. Most controversy about preoperative digitalization has concerned the patient who has a history of no or minimal CHF yet has a risk of developing CHF because of an enlarged heart or because the surgery will involve major volume shifts. Most experts do not recommend digitalis in this situation (14).

Patients with decompensated CHF should have all but life-saving surgery postponed until the failure is controlled, either in the office or in the hospital. Patients with controlled CHF should be maintained on their usual oral regimen until midnight before surgery and maintained with intravenous diuretics and digoxin (75% of the oral dosage) during the immediate postoperative period. Perioperative monitoring with a Swan-Ganz catheter should be considered in advance in situations where large volume shifts are anticipated during surgery or the heart failure is severe or decompensated.

Table 93.14. Prevention of Bacterial Endocarditis in Patients with Valvular Heart Disease, Prosthetic Heart Valves, and Other Abnormalities of the Cardiovascular System

Situation	Agent	Regimen[a]
	Dental, Oral, Respiratory Tract, or Esophgeal Procedures	
Standard general prophylaxis	Amoxicillin	Adults: 2.0 g; children: 50 mg/kg orally 1 h before procedure
Unable to take oral medications	Ampicillin	Adults: 2.0 g i.m. or i.v.; children: 50 mg/kg i.m. or i.v. within 30 min before procedure
Allergic to penicillin	Clindamycin	Adults: 600 mg; children: 20 mg/kg orally 1 h before procedure
	or	
	Cephalexin or cefadroxil[b]	Adults: 2.0 g; children: 50 mg/kg orally 1 h before procedure
	or	
	Azithromycin or clarithromycin	Adults: 500 mg; children: 15 mg/kg orally 1 h before procedure
Allergic to penicillin and unable to take oral medications	Clindamycin	Adults: 600 mg; children: 20 mg/kg i.v. within 30 min before procedure
	or	
	Cefazolin[b]	Adults: 1.0 g; children: 25 mg/kg i.m. or i.v. within 30 min before procedure
	Genitourinary, Gastrointestinal (Excluding Esophageal) Procedures	
High-risk patients[c]	Ampicillin plus Gentamicin[d]	Adults: ampicillin 2.0 g i.m. or i.v. plus gentamicin 1.5 mg/kg (not to exceed 120 mg) within 30 min of starting the procedure; 6 h later, ampicillin 1 g i.m./i.v. or amoxicillin 1 g orally Children: ampicillin 50 mg/kg i.m. or i.v. (not to exceed 2.0 g) plus gentamicin 1.5 mg/kg within 30 min of starting the procedure; 6 h later, ampicillin 25 mg/kg i.m./i.v. or amoxicillin 25 mg/kg orally
High-risk patients allergic to ampicillin/amoxicillin[c]	Vancomycin plus Gentamicin[d]	Adults: vancomycin 1.0 g i.v. over 1–2 h plus gentamicin 1.5 mg/kg i.v./i.m. (not to exceed 120 mg); complete injection/infusion within 30 min of starting the procedure Children: vancomycin 20 mg/kg i.v. over 1–2 h plus gentamicin 1.5 mg/kg i.v./i.m.; complete injection/infusion within 30 min of starting the procedure
Moderate-risk patients[c]	Amoxicillin or ampicillin	Adults: amoxicillin 2.0 g orally 1 h before procedure, or ampicillin 2.0 g i.m./i.v. within 30 min of starting the procedure Children: amoxicillin 50 mg/kg orally 1 h before procedure, or ampicillin 50 mg/kg i.m./i.v. within 30 min of starting the procedure
Moderate-risk patients allergic to ampicillin/amoxicillin[c]	Vancomycin[c]	Adults: vancomycin 1.0 g i.v. over 1–2 h; complete infusion within 30 min of starting the procedure Children: vancomycin 20 mg/kg i.v. over 1–2 h; complete infusion within 30 min of starting the procedure

[a]Total children's dosage should not exceed adult dosage.

[b]Cephalosporins should not be used in individuals with immediate-type hypersensitivity reaction (urticaria, angioedema, or anaphylaxis) to penicillins.

[c]High risk: prothestic heart valve, history of endocarditis, complex cyanotic congenital heart disease. Moderate risk: Uncorrected congenital conditions (patent ductus, ventricular septal defect, coarctation, bicuspid aortic valve); rheumatic valve disease; hypertrophic cardiomyopathy; prolapsing or leaking mitral valve (i.e., audible click and murmurs or Doppler-confirmed mitral insufficiency).

[d]No second dose of vancomycin or gentamicin is recommended.

From Dajani AS, Taubert KA, Wilson W, et al. Prevention of bacterial endocarditis. Recommendations by the American Heart Association. JAMA 1997;277:1794, with permission.

Table 93.15. Risks of Developing CHF in the Perioperative Period

Patient Characteristics	Size of Risk: All CHF (%)	Size of Risk: Pulmonary Edema (%)
No prior CHF	4	2
Past CHF		
All—now compensated	16	6
Past pulmonary edema (regardless of current status)	32	23
Decompensated CHF preoperatively	21	16
Preoperative physical findings:		
S3 gallop	47	35
Jugular venous distension	35	30
NYHA class preoperatively (see Table 61.3)		
Class 1	5	3
Class 2	7	7
Class 3	18	6
Class 4	31	25

Table based on 1,001 consecutive patients undergoing general surgery, orthopedic surgery, or urologic surgery (transurethral resection of the prostate omitted because of existing evidence of its safety even in elderly patients).

CHF, congestive heart failure.

Adapted from Goldman L, Caldera DL, Southwick FS, et al. Cardiac risk factors and complications in non-cardiac surgery. Medicine (Baltimore) 1978;57:357, with permission.

Arrhythmias

Arrhythmias that are most common in ambulatory patients are described in detail in Chapter 64.

Risk

Patients with arrhythmias before surgery have significantly increased risks of cardiac morbidity and death. These risks have not been quantified for subgroups of patients with specific arrhythmias, except as indicated in the cardiac risk indices shown in Table 93.9. Patients with complete heart block, Mobitz type II second-degree block, and a few patients with sick sinus syndrome (see Chapter 64) have a significant risk of complications during anesthesia if a pacemaker is not inserted. On the other hand, there is little or no increased risk associated with bifascicular or trifascicular block on ECG in patients who are asymptomatic.

Arrhythmias do occur in approximately 20% or more of adult patients during general anesthesia; however, most of these patients do not have preoperative arrhythmias. Most intraoperative arrhythmias are supraventricular, transient, and related to specific anesthetic or surgical manipulation and do not require specific therapies. The number of arrhythmias that are detected clinically, without the use of continuous monitoring, is lower: Supraventricular arrhythmias are detected clinically in 4% of patients and other arrhythmias in 11% (11,18).

Perioperative Management

Patients with arrhythmias should have the comprehensive preoperative evaluation (Table 93.2) expanded in several ways. The probable cause of the arrhythmia should be delineated (see Chapter 64). If the arrhythmia is intermittent or control is uncertain, 24-hour Holter monitoring should be done. Levels of antiarrhythmic drugs that are being administered should be obtained. This evaluation should be accomplished before admission for surgery.

Patients with *supraventricular arrhythmias* should have their ventricular rates controlled or should be converted to more stable rhythms. Except for atrial fibrillation, this usually means conversion either to normal sinus rhythm or atrial fibrillation because other supraventricular arrhythmias are hemodynamically unstable or give an unpredictable ventricular response even with appropriate drug therapy. Patients with atrial fibrillation should have their rates slowed but should be able to accelerate their heart rate under stress as indicated by their ability to raise their pulse rate more than 10 points by mild exercise.

Established indications for *preoperative digitalis administration* in patients with arrhythmias are control of rate in atrial fibrillation and prophylaxis of supraventricular arrhythmias in selected patients (e.g., some patients with past histories of supraventricular arrhythmias who remain at high risk for recurrence). Patients with *ventricular arrhythmias* should be treated according to the criteria outlined in Chapter 64.

Antiarrhythmic drugs should be continued orally through the morning before surgery, after which the following intravenous treatment should be substituted until the patient can take oral medications again: intravenous digoxin (75% of the oral dosage) for patients taking digoxin and intravenous lidocaine or procainamide for patients taking quinidine, procainamide, or disopyramide for ventricular arrhythmias. Amiodarone is available in an intravenous preparation.

There is general agreement that patients undergoing general anesthesia should have a *prophylactic or therapeutic pacemaker* inserted for the following conditions:

- Symptomatic or significant dysfunction of the sinoatrial node;
- Idioventricular rhythm;
- Current or past history of third-degree or Mobitz type II second-degree atrioventricular (AV) block;
- Occasional instances of Mobitz type I (Wenckebach) second-degree AV block;
- Occasional patients with trifascicular block (right bundle branch block plus left anterior hemiblock plus first-degree AV block; alternating left and right bundle branch block; or left bundle branch block and first-degree AV block), especially in the presence of severe valvular disease, ischemic disease, CHF, or syncope;
- A history of Stokes-Adams attacks.

Patients with a history suggesting symptomatic bradyarrhythmias (especially a history of syncope or near syncope and an underlying ECG abnormality) probably should have a temporary pacemaker recommended if a full workup to evaluate the cause of the symptoms cannot be performed preoperatively. Isolated conditions for which a pacemaker is more controversial, but generally not indicated, include bifascicular block, bundle branch block, first-degree AV block, and asymptomatic sinus bradycardia.

PATIENTS WITH PULMONARY DISEASE

Overview

Patients with significant pulmonary disease have an increased mortality and morbidity during surgery. The increased risks are caused chiefly by the following physiologic changes produced by the effects of anesthesia, sedatives, and analgesics: abnormalities of pulmonary gas exchange, causing hypoxemia; depression of the cough reflex and decrease in clearance of respiratory tract secretions; respiratory depression; and loss of sighing and normal lung inflation. Each of these changes increases the risk of atelectasis and pneumonia. In addition, normal breathing and voluntary coughing are decreased after surgery because of pain and discomfort, especially after upper abdominal and thoracic surgery. Optimal preoperative treatment of pulmonary disease can reduce perioperative morbidity and mortality.

Chronic Obstructive Pulmonary Disease

Risk

The precise risk of perioperative death from pulmonary causes for patients with chronic obstructive pulmonary disease (COPD) is not known because of the lack of information regarding patients with mild lung disease. In patients with moderate to severe COPD, pulmonary deaths occur in approximately 4% (versus 0 to 2% of unselected patients) and pulmonary complications in 36% (versus 9% of unselected patients) (19–21).

A *smoking history, dyspnea, cough, or abnormal spirometry* increases the risk of minor postoperative pulmonary complications (i.e., atelectasis or infection without significant respiratory compromise). The risk of respiratory failure requiring vigorous postoperative respiratory therapy is increased in patients with a forced expiratory volume in 1 second (FEV_1) less than 1.5 L. An FEV_1 less than 1.0 L or a P_{CO_2} greater than 45 mm Hg predicts a substantial increase in perioperative pulmonary mortality and in the incidence of postoperative respiratory failure requiring prolonged mechanical ventilation. However, no study has definitively shown that any pulmonary function test, including FEV_1 or arterial blood gases, predicts major pulmonary complications (respiratory failure, need for mechanical ventilation, or death) with enough precision to establish a prohibitive criteria for surgery. The decision for surgery in the presence of pulmonary disease requires consideration of all clinical and laboratory data (19–23).

A number of *nonpulmonary factors* are helpful in predicting postoperative pulmonary complications in patients with COPD (Table 93.16). The greatest risks are in patients who are older than 60, who undergo upper abdominal and thoracic operations or operations under general anesthesia lasting more than 3 hours, or who have repeated operations within 1 year. A much lower risk is posed by operations on the extremities, back, breast, and central nervous system. Lower abdominal surgery represents an intermediate risk. Combining these factors with the pulmonary factors listed above increases the practitioner's ability to predict operative morbidity.

The *type of anesthesia* may affect the risk of pulmonary complications. Local anesthesia creates very little risk; if the patient is also sedated ("moderate sedation"), however, there may be temporary deterioration in respiratory control and there may be a suppression of the cough reflex. Spinal anesthesia has been reported to be associated with a low mortality rate in patients with COPD in some studies (21). However, because of the simultaneous use of sedation, lack of control of the airway, less ability to monitor (especially P_{CO_2}), and because the patient must ventilate in the supine position, spinal anesthesia creates a significant risk of intraoperative and postoperative respiratory complications; this is especially true of obese patients with chronic pulmonary disease. Because of these problems, general anesthesia, which permits control of ventilation and clearance of secretions, is often preferable to spinal anesthesia in patients with moderate or severe COPD.

Perioperative Management

Patients with known COPD should have a comprehensive preoperative evaluation (Table 93.2) and additional evaluation focused on the status of their pulmonary disease (22,23). If they are taking aminophylline, they should have measurement of the serum aminophylline concentration and adjustment of the dosage if it is above or below the therapeutic range. Any history of smoking, chronic or intermittent sputum production, recent upper respiratory infection, dyspnea on effort, or concomitant cardiovascular disease is particularly pertinent. Ideally, smokers should stop smoking 8 weeks before admission for surgery to be performed under general or spinal anesthesia, and patients with upper respiratory infections should have surgery postponed at least 2 weeks, regardless of how minor the episode.

Table 93.17 summarizes for patients undergoing general or spinal anesthesia the principal *indications for preadmission spirometry alone* (forced vital capacity and FEV_1) or for spirometry plus lung volumes and arterial blood gases. Unfortunately, major operations are often performed without pulmonary function testing, despite the fact that even experienced clinicians sometimes misjudge the severity of obstructive lung disease. Spirometry is indicated to clarify the presence and severity of lung disease in questionable cases, including patients without a prior diagnosis of pulmonary disease. However, the ability of pulmonary function testing to predict adverse outcomes for high-risk patients has not been clearly established (23). Pulmonary consultation should be obtained for patients whose FEV_1 is less than 1.0 L, those whose P_{CO_2} is above 45 mm Hg, and those with less severe pulmonary disease who are being evaluated for thoracic or upper abdominal surgery.

Preoperatively, the patient should be instructed on coughing and deep breathing exercises, as well as on the use of devices such as an incentive spirometer that will be used postoperatively. Patients already taking inhaled or oral bronchodilators and inhaled steroids should continue their regimen through the morning of surgery. Patients who have a history of intermittent airway obstruction should be started on an inhaled bronchodilator before surgery. To prevent bronchospasm, especially in the immediate postoperative period, inhaled (beta-2-sympathomimetics) and occasionally intravenous aminophylline should be administered (the serum aminophylline level should be kept

Table 93.16. Nonpulmonary Factors that Increase Pulmonary Risks During General Surgery

Most Important	Other
Age over 60	General anesthesia lasting more than 3 h
Upper abdominal or thoracic operation	Obesity
Repeat operations within 1 yr	Abnormal electrocardiogram
	Poor patient effort/cooperation
	Narcotic analgesics
	Upper respiratory infection

Table 93.17. Indications for Pulmonary Function Tests in Preoperative Patients with Pulmonary Disease

Spirometry only (FEV_1 and FVC)
Smokers (>10 pack years)
Any pulmonary symptoms (e.g., dyspnea, wheezing, cough, or sputum production)
Upper abdominal surgery
Age > 60
Repeat surgery within 1 yr
Multiple other risk factors (obesity, recent upper respiratory infections, narcotics abuse, abnormal ECG)
Spirometry, lung volumes, and arterial blood gases
Thoracic surgery
Upper abdominal surgery and pulmonary disease
Patients with restrictive lung disease
Patients with chronic obstructive pulmonary disease with FEV_1 <1.0 L

FVC, forced vital capacity; ECG, electrocardiogram.

in the therapeutic range [10 to 20 mg/L]) while the patient cannot take oral medications. Patients who have received corticosteroids for more than 2 weeks during the year before surgery should be appropriately covered for stress with parenteral steroids (see below); occasionally steroids may need to be reinstituted or the dose increased to control the pulmonary disease. Patients with chronic purulent sputum production should receive a 5- to 7-day course of broad-spectrum antibiotics (tetracycline, amoxicillin, trimethoprim–sulfamethoxazole, azithromycin, or clarithromycin) to decrease the quantity and purulence of secretions. Finally, arterial blood gases should be checked in patients with moderate to severe COPD before and, as needed, after surgery. Pulse oximetry is usually obtained pre- and postoperatively but does not measure PCO_2. There is some dispute about the efficacy of most of these individual measures. However, controlled trials show that the combination, preoperatively, of bronchodilators, antibiotics, lung expansion, and mobilization of secretions decreases the number of perioperative complications (21).

Lung Resection and Chronic Obstructive Pulmonary Disease

Overall mortality rates for lung resection are about 5% for lobectomy and approximately 15% for total pneumonectomy. The mortality and morbidity rates for lung surgery vary widely depending on patient factors (particularly age and pulmonary function), type of operation (pneumonectomy, lobectomy, segmental resection), and experience and skill of the surgical team.

Assessment of pulmonary function in the patient with COPD who has an indication for lung resection (usually a tumor) should be performed in the ambulatory setting. Use of the following criteria to select candidates for lung resection has reduced mortality for patients with COPD: *For pneumonectomy,* the major criteria for operability are FEV_1 of 2 L or more and forced vital capacity 50% of predicted or more. Patients with an FEV_1 below 2 L should have quantitative perfusion lung scanning to determine the FEV_1 that can be expected after pneumonectomy (e.g., if 30% of perfusion and ventilation goes to the affected lung, the patient's pulmonary function will be decreased by approximately 30% postoperatively). Those with a predicted postoperative FEV_1 as low as 0.8 to 1 L can undergo pneumonectomy, although their mortality risk is probably increased.

Patients not meeting the criteria for pneumonectomy may tolerate lobectomy or segmental resection. Most patients with a preoperative FEV_1 of 1.5 L or more can tolerate a lobectomy. The patient may undergo resection of the segment or lobe if the predicted postoperative FEV_1 is greater than 0.8 to 1 L by quantitative perfusion lung scanning. Other measures in preoperative planning for the patient with COPD undergoing pulmonary resection are similar to those described for such patients in the preceding section.

Asthma

Risk

Asthma affects approximately 3% of Americans, which makes it one of the most common pulmonary diseases (see Chapter 60). It is difficult to give a firm estimate of the operative risks posed by asthma, because in most reports data on asthma are pooled with results for other types of obstructive airway disease. The most dangerous period for the asthmatic is not usually the period during general anesthesia, because the anesthetic may be an effective bronchodilator, but is the immediate postoperative period. The major risks are severe bronchospasm and inspissation of thick secretions.

Perioperative Management

The asthmatic patient should have a comprehensive evaluation (Table 93.2) in the office before admission for surgery. This allows adequate time for changes in chronic management before admission. The patient should stop smoking 8 weeks before surgery. Spirometry (FEV_1 and forced vital capacity) should be performed on asthmatic patients before operation; peak flows (if normal) are adequate in mild stable asthmatics undergoing minor surgery. Arterial blood gases should be measured in decompensated or severe asthmatics, in asthmatics with substantial abnormalities of spirometry, and when there is clinical concern about hypoxia or hypercarbia. Pulse oximetry is useful where CO_2 retention is not a concern. Serum aminophylline levels should be measured in patients on this medication, because levels on standard doses are frequently subtherapeutic or toxic.

Beta-2-sympathomimetics and inhaled steroids can be continued as inhaled aerosols until the induction of anesthesia and can be resumed in the recovery room. Planning for the immediate preoperative period should include administration of oral and inhaled bronchodilators on the morning of surgery and scheduling of surgery early in the day. In very severe asthmatic patients who are taking aminophylline, a constant infusion of aminophylline may be used in the perioperative period when the patient cannot take medicine by mouth; most patients are adequately treated by resuming aminophylline, intravenously or orally, in the recovery room. Patients who have taken systemic corticosteroids for more than 2 weeks during the previous year should receive dosages of parenteral steroids sufficient to cover the stress of surgery (see below) (24). Some patients will require reinstitution of or increase in their oral corticosteroid dose to control asthma before surgery.

PATIENTS WITH RENAL DISEASE

Risk

The size of the operative risk for patients with chronic renal disease depends on the severity of their disease (see Chapter 52). The type of surgery also influences risk; high-risk surgery includes trauma, vascular, and some gastrointestinal surgery (e.g., when bleeding, jaundice, or infection is present preoperatively) (25). Other risk factors include advanced age, volume depletion, hypotension, sepsis, nephrotoxins (radiocontrast; medications, especially aminoglycosides), and CHF (25). Overall, the surgical mortality after major surgery in patients with severe renal disease (i.e., creatinine clearance less than 10 to 15 mL/min, including patients on dialysis) is approximately 2% to 4% when these cases are managed carefully. In patients not requiring dialysis, postoperative acute renal failure is the gravest complication (25).

The major complications associated with surgery in the patient with moderate to severe renal disease are worsened renal failure, electrolyte disturbances (especially acidosis and hyperkalemia), volume contraction, volume overload, toxicity caused by agents that are nephrotoxic or are excreted by the kidneys, anemia, and bleeding. Volume contraction, with the risk of ischemic cerebral, cardiac, or renal damage, is a particular risk in patients with the nephrotic syndrome; these patients usually have a slightly contracted intravascular volume at baseline and are at risk of hypovolemia if an effort is made to decrease their edema with potent diuretics preoperatively. Toxic renal damage may follow the use of two classes of agents that are often used in the perioperative period: radiocontrast materials and aminoglycoside antibiotics.

Perioperative Management

Before admission for surgery, patients with chronic renal failure should have the comprehensive evaluation outlined in Table 93.2, and current volume status should be documented. Weight and orthostatic blood pressure are important in assessing preoperative volume status. Baseline creatinine clearance should be documented. Radiocontrast studies should be avoided, if at all possible, in the preoperative workup of patients with significantly elevated serum creatinine concentrations or with other risk factors because of the risk of acute renal failure (25) (if radiocontrast studies are required, use of intravenous hydration and oral acetylcysteine may reduce this risk) (26).

The most important consideration in perioperative management of patients who do not require dialysis is avoidance of fluid imbalance. When the surgery carries a risk of significant volume shifts, Swan-Ganz catheterization may be considered to ensure close monitoring of the intravascular volume. Administration of drugs such as antihypertensives should follow the guidelines stated elsewhere in this chapter. Adjustments in the dosages of drugs should be appropriate for the patient's degree of renal insufficiency as outlined in Chapter 52 (27). Blood urea nitrogen, serum creatinine, and electrolytes should be monitored before and after surgery to detect hyperkalemia and deterioration of renal function. Patients with renal failure often have a metabolic acidosis compensated by hyperventilation; postoperatively, continued appropriate hyperventilation is necessary to avoid a potential precipitous fall in arterial pH. Preoperative prophylactic dialysis is not generally recommended in the patient not already on chronic dialysis. Patients with chronic anemia secondary to renal failure usually are well compensated and do not require preoperative transfusion unless they are symptomatic from the anemia or a large blood loss is expected during surgery; preoperative use of erythropoietin is a consideration to avoid transfusion.

In general, the nephrologist caring for patients on chronic dialysis should coordinate the medical management of these patients throughout the surgical episode. Although these patients have a very high postoperative complication rate (caused by hyperkalemia, bleeding, arteriovenous fistula thrombosis, pneumonia, wound infection, and arrhythmias), their risk of dying from surgery remains in the 2% to 4% range if complications are carefully managed (25).

PATIENTS WITH ENDOCRINE DISEASE

Diabetes Mellitus

Risk

Total surgical mortality for all diabetic patients is approximately 2% to 4%; less than 0.3% die as a result of poor control of their diabetes. Approximately 15% of diabetic patients have postoperative complications that may be related to diabetes, particularly wound infection.

Perioperative Management

Each diabetic patient should have the comprehensive preoperative evaluation outlined in Table 93.2, with particular attention to determining diabetes control and the presence of cardiovascular disease. Patients who are responsible can monitor their own glucose, and patients who are compliant are good candidates for outpatient surgery. Relative contraindications to outpatient surgery include significantly uncontrolled diabetes, the occasionally extremely labile diabetic, and noncompliant diabetic patients requiring insulin.

Measurement of fasting blood glucose electrolytes, blood urea nitrogen, and creatinine should be obtained at the time of the preoperative office evaluation. If the patient is monitoring glucose at home, these should be reviewed, as well as any recent glycohemoglobin A_{1C} measurements. The patient should be told to call if his or her home glucose measurements are higher or lower than predetermined values (specific values should be given to the patient in writing) between the time of the office medical evaluation and surgery and also postoperatively. The patient or nurse should do a bedside glucose determination on arrival at the hospital. The state of hydration should be determined to ensure that the diabetic is not significantly volume contracted. Elective surgery should not be undertaken until diabetes is at least reasonably controlled (fasting blood glucose at 250 mg/l00 mL or less).

The appropriate perioperative treatment of diabetes depends on the type of surgical procedure planned

Table 93.18. Management of Diabetes on Day of Surgery

Surgical Procedure	Treatment Required to Control Glucose Preoperatively		
	Diet Only	Oral Hypoglycemic Agent	Insulin
Minor	Observe	Withhold until after procedure	Withhold until after procedure or use "major" protocol
Major	Observe	Change to long-acting insulin (achieve control with insulin before operation)	*Preferred regimen:* One-half to two-thirds of total long-acting insulin dosage preoperatively; regular insulin only if needed *or* One-third of total long-acting insulin dosage preoperatively; one-third postoperatively; regular insulin only if needed *or* Continuous low-dose infusion of regular insulin *or* Regular insulin in each liter of dextrose 5% in water (D5W)

and the preadmission regimen, as summarized in Table 93.18. *Diabetic patients who are controlled by diet* can be monitored with daily fasting blood glucose levels throughout the operative episode and treated with insulin if unacceptable rises in glucose occur.

Treatment of patients taking oral agents varies because they represent a heterogeneous group. Patients with mild elevations of glucose who are undergoing minor procedures that will allow them to eat the same day can take their oral hypoglycemic drug on the day *before* surgery and resume it when they begin eating on the day of surgery. If the patient is to undergo a major procedure, oral agents (including thiazolidinediones) should be discontinued beginning on the morning of surgery and not continued postoperatively because they have relatively long half-lives, control is less predictable, and because the drugs cannot be given parenterally postoperatively. Therefore, such patients should be switched to management by diet only or to insulin. Human insulin is preferred for the patient who has not taken insulin previously An exception is the patient taking *chlorpropamide* (Diabinese), which should be withheld 2 to 3 days before surgery because of its particularly long half-life. *Metformin* should be withheld at least 48 hours before elective surgery. It should not be restarted (except for minor procedures) until 48 hours postoperatively, until the patient is stable and eating, and, for major procedures, until a postoperative serum creatinine has been measured. Metformin should also be withheld for 48 hours before and after any radiocontrast x-ray that is part of the preoperative evaluation. It is especially important to withhold metformin in major procedures with the risk of hypotension or renal failure (e.g., vascular surgery) because of the risk of lactic acidosis.

For the patient who is taking insulin before surgery, one of several strategies is recommended for the preoperative period (Table 93.18). Because of its simplicity and the small risk of hypoglycemia, the first regimen (giving one-half to two-thirds of the usual total daily dosage of long-acting insulin preoperatively) is preferred. Postoperative management is easiest with a single morning dose of long-acting insulin, with the dosage adjusted according to the metabolic status and calorie intake; supplemental regular insulin may be given as needed. Sliding-scale regular insulin alone (without long-acting insulin) is not recommended because it does not provide adequate control of blood glucose. Blood glucose measurement using a bedside technique is recommended; fasting glucose and electrolyte concentrations should be measured daily in the immediate postoperative period.

Adrenal Insufficiency and Chronic Steroid Therapy

Risk

It is generally agreed that patients who are currently taking a pharmacologic dosage of corticosteroids (more than the equivalent of 20 to 30 mg of hydrocortisone daily), have taken corticosteroids at a pharmacologic dosage for 2 or more weeks in the past year, or are receiving replacement dosages for adrenal insufficiency are at risk of developing adrenal insufficiency because of the stress of surgery. Patients in each of these groups should therefore receive extra corticosteroids in the perioperative period (see Chapter 81 for additional details).

Perioperative Management

These patients should have a comprehensive evaluation before admission (Table 93.2). For patients with adrenal insufficiency, the evaluation should include particular attention to factors that may reflect the adequacy of corticosteroid replacement (i.e., lying and standing blood pressure, concentration of serum urea nitrogen or serum creatinine, glucose, and electrolytes). Adrenocorticotropic hormone stimulation or insulin-hypoglycemia testing to determine the need for steroid coverage in patients previously on steroids is not recommended for routine use because there is not adequate evidence that a normal response precludes the need for steroid coverage during surgery.

Patients on chronic steroid therapy may receive the usual steroid dosage by mouth the day before surgery. On the day of surgery, hydrocortisone 100 mg should be administered intravenously at 6 a.m. A second 100-mg dose should be given intravenously during surgery and then a 100-mg dose should be given intravenously every 6 hours for the first 24 hours after surgery, followed by 50 mg every 6 hours for the second 24 hours after surgery, and 25 mg every 6 hours for the third 24-hour period. Alternatively, a continuous infusion of hydrocortisone after an initial bolus dose preoperatively may be given (28). The patient may then return to the preoperative medical regimen.

There are two exceptions to these guidelines. First, the regimen is based on the assumption that there is no prolonged stress after surgery; if this occurs, higher dosages of corticosteroids must be continued for a longer time postoperatively. Second, for minor procedures, patients may return to their usual dosage within 24 to 48 hours postoperatively. For outpatient surgery, equivalent dosages of oral prednisone may be given as an outpatient for the postoperative care (preoperative dosage should still be given intravenously).

Hypothyroidism

Risk

The major potential complications of surgery in hypothyroid patients are increased sensitivity to and prolonged half-life of anesthetic agents, hypoventilation and respiratory arrest in the immediate postoperative period, hyponatremia caused by decreased free water clearance, and myxedema coma. The risks of surgery in patients with mild to moderate hypothyroidism are probably not as high as once thought (29). Nonetheless, hypothyroid patients should delay elective surgery for 4 to 6 weeks and should be treated with thyroxine (see Chapter 80).

Perioperative Management

Hypothyroid patients should be evaluated carefully before admission for surgery. The patient should have the comprehensive evaluation outlined in Table 93.2, and the serum thyroid-stimulating hormone concentration should be checked (unless a value from the past 2 months is available) (see Chapter 80 for details).

Specific recommendations for preoperative management depend on the *status of the patient's hypothyroidism.* Patients with previously known and adequately treated hypothyroidism can undergo surgery. The half-life of administered thyroxine is about 7 days. Therefore, oral thyroxine can usually be omitted on the day of surgery and resumed when the patient is able to take oral medication. The stress of major surgery or severe infection may accelerate the turnover of thyroxine, occasionally necessitating daily treatment with intravenous thyroxine (50% of the oral dosage) in patients in either of these situations.

If the hypothyroidism has been effectively treated for a long period (as indicated by no or only minor symptoms or a normal or only a slightly increased thyroid-stimulating hormone), the patient can usually tolerate surgery and thyroid replacement can be adjusted postoperatively. For hypothyroid patients who have not been treated or who remain significantly hypothyroid because of inadequate replacement therapy, elective surgery should be postponed because of the risks listed above. Such patients should receive adequate thyroid replacement for a minimum of 1 to 2 months before elective surgery (4 to 6 months for patients with profound myxedema). Surgery required before this period in mild to moderately hypothyroid patients may be considered, especially if minor surgery under local anesthesia is being performed, if the patient can be started on a total replacement dosage immediately, and if there is prompt improvement in signs and symptoms of hypothyroidism (see Chapter 80 for additional details). When a patient with previously undiagnosed hypothyroidism requires immediate major surgery, an endocrinologist should be consulted regarding perioperative treatment and monitoring.

Hyperthyroidism

Risk

The major risk of operation in patients with uncontrolled hyperthyroidism is *thyroid storm* (see Chapter 80). In an old series, there were only 25 episodes of thyroid storm after 1,383 operations on thyrotoxic patients (30). However, surgery accounts for up to one-third of the cases of thyroid storm reported—probably in patients with unrecognized hyperthyroidism.

Perioperative Management

The patient with known hyperthyroidism should be reassessed clinically and with thyroid function tests before admission for surgery. In previously undiagnosed patients, the usual approach should be used in evaluation and management (see Chapter 80).

The treatment of the hyperthyroid patient during surgery depends on the patient's current thyroid status. Patients previously diagnosed and adequately treated should take their current treatment until midnight the night before surgery and should resume treatment when they can take substances by mouth again. Patients with new, known, or recurrent hyperthyroidism who are not euthyroid should be brought to a euthyroid state with thyroid blocking agents or iodides (see Chapter 80). Ideally, surgery should be postponed for several months in these patients until a consistent euthyroid state is attained. An endocrinologist should be consulted regarding the treatment and monitoring of any patient with uncontrolled hyperthyroidism who requires urgent surgery.

Obese Patients

Risk

Massive obesity significantly increases the risk of mortality associated with surgery. In one study, for example, women undergoing surgery for adenocarcinoma of the uterus had a 20% operative mortality if they weighed more than 300 pounds (136 kg), compared with a 1.5% mortality for obese women weighing between 200 and 240 pounds (91 and 110 kg) (31). Less severe obesity probably does not increase mortality risks.

Moderate or massive obesity also increases the risk of a number of perioperative problems, including difficult intubation, difficulty in ventilating the patient during anesthesia, the need for a large amount of anesthesia during induction, potential delay in anesthesia washout because of slow release of anesthetic agents from adipose tissue, postoperative atelectasis and pneumonia, thromboembolism, difficult postoperative mobilization, nosocomial wound infection (particularly when there is increased moisture caused by pannus adjacent to the surgical incision), wound dehiscence, and late incisional hernia.

Perioperative Management

For massively obese patients, a program of gradual weight reduction (see Chapter 83) should be planned, if the patient is amenable, before any elective operation; this may require up to 6 months. When prompt surgery is needed, these patients should have a comprehensive evaluation (Table 93.2). In particular, these patients should be checked for uncontrolled diabetes mellitus and significant hypoventilation, two common complications of obesity that increase the risk of surgery. Either of these two problems should be managed preoperatively, as discussed above.

Massively obese patients should be given preoperative instruction in deep breathing and in the use of the incentive spirometer or other devices designed to prevent pulmonary complications postoperatively. Prophylaxis of thromboembolic disease should be given (see Chapter 57). Other recommendations for perioperative management depend on obesity-associated conditions, such as diabetes, that the patient may have.

PATIENTS WITH GASTROINTESTINAL OR HEPATIC DISEASE

Peptic Ulcer Disease

Risk

Data are lacking on the risk and the management of surgery in patients with active peptic ulcer disease.

Perioperative Management

Patients with active ulcer disease should have elective nonulcer surgery postponed until the ulcer heals. The average time required for the healing of uncomplicated ulcers is 4 to 6 weeks for duodenal ulcer and 6 weeks for gastric ulcer (see Chapter 43). There is no consistent relationship between disappearance of ulcer symptoms, ulcer healing, and recurrence. Therefore, it is best to wait several weeks after all symptoms have disappeared and 6 weeks to 3 months from the beginning of an episode before admission for elective nonulcer surgery. If surgery cannot be deferred this long or if ulcer recurrence is suspected, endoscopy should be considered preoperatively. Before surgery, these patients should also have the comprehensive medical evaluation summarized in Table 93.2, and multiple stool samples should be checked to exclude active bleeding.

No empiric data confirm these guidelines or indicate whether surgery can be done safely as soon as an ulcer has healed (as shown by endoscopy). If urgent abdominal surgery must be performed in a patient with active ulcer disease, consideration should be given to whether surgical treatment is needed for the ulcer as well (see Chapter 43 for detailed discussion of indications for and types of surgery). Patients with remote or inactive ulcer disease require no special therapy preoperatively or postoperatively.

Patients with recently active ulcer disease should continue their current therapy until midnight the day before surgery. Because H_2 blockers (cimetidine, ranitidine, famotidine) can be given intravenously, one of these should be used throughout the period when the patient cannot take medications by mouth; nasogastric suctioning may also be recommended during this period. For patients unable to take medications by mouth, some proton pump inhibitors can be given by nasogastric tube (lansoprazole); alternatively intravenous H_2 blockers can be prescribed.

Hepatitis

Risk

General anesthesia and surgery during acute hepatitis are associated with a high mortality and morbidity (32). The major problem accounting for these risks is postoperative hepatic encephalopathy and its complications. The catabolic effects of surgery, hypotension during anesthesia, and hepatic toxicity from anesthetic agents are the principal factors that may precipitate hepatic encephalopathy.

Perioperative Management

Patients with a history of acute hepatitis should have a comprehensive evaluation (Table 93.2), and liver function tests (serum aminotransferases, bilirubin, alkaline phosphatase, albumin, and prothrombin time) should be obtained before admission for surgery. Serologic tests for hepatitis B antigen and hepatitis C antibody should also be performed (see Chapter 47), if they have not been done previously.

Ideally, surgery should be postponed for a minimum of 6 to 12 months after all laboratory evidence of active liver disease has returned to normal. This cautious approach is advised because there is a risk of exacerbating hepatic injury if surgery is performed earlier. Only urgent life-saving surgery should be performed during the acute phase of hepatitis, whatever its cause.

Anticipation of postoperative complications (particularly bleeding and encephalopathy) is important in the patient with active hepatitis who must undergo surgery. For the patient with an abnormal prothrombin time (less than 50% of normal), fresh frozen plasma can be given throughout the immediate perioperative period. When immunologic tests or epidemiologic information indicates infectious hepatitis (see Chapter 47), the surgical team should be notified in order to minimize the risk of spreading infection.

Cirrhosis

Risk

Most data regarding the risks of surgery in the cirrhotic patient have been collected in trials of portal–systemic shunts; therefore, these data may not accurately reflect the risks of surgery unrelated to the liver. The

Table 93.19. Child's Classification of Operative Mortality Risk in the Cirrhotic Patient

	Risk Group by Severity of Liver Disease		
	A (Minimal)	B (Moderate)	C (Advanced)
Bilirubin (mg/100 mL)	<2.0	2.0–3.0	>3.0
Serum albumin (g/100 mL)	>3.5	3.0–3.5	<3.0
Ascites	None	Controlled	Poorly controlled
Encephalopathy	None	Minimal	Coma
Nutrition	Excellent	Good	Poor ("wasted")
Operative mortality (%)	0	9	53

From Siefkin AD, Bolt RJ. Preoperative evaluation of the patient with gastrointestinal or liver disease. Med Clin North Am 1979;63:1309, with permission.

most widely used measure of the mortality risk from shunt procedures is the Child index, which incorporates measurements of serum bilirubin, albumin, ascites, encephalopathy, and nutrition (Table 93.19). The perioperative complications encountered in these patients are those associated with chronic cirrhosis: encephalopathy, jaundice, gastrointestinal hemorrhage, infection, and hepatorenal syndrome.

Regional and spinal anesthesia do not entirely eliminate the risks of complications in cirrhotic patients. For example, increased morbidity and mortality caused by liver disease have been associated even with hernia repair under local anesthesia in some patients. The stress of the procedure itself, decreased hepatic blood flow, and complications such as hypotension and wound infection may worsen hepatic function, even in the absence of toxic general anesthetics.

Perioperative Management

In addition to a comprehensive preoperative evaluation (Table 93.2), patients with cirrhosis should have liver function tests (serum amino transferase, bilirubin, alkaline phosphatase, albumin, and prothrombin time). Liver biopsy is indicated in selected patients to establish the presence of cirrhosis, provide an additional indicator of the severity of liver damage, or exclude active hepatitis. Computed tomography or sonogram is only occasionally needed to exclude other causes of hepatomegaly. In the history and physical examination, a search should be made for complications of cirrhosis, especially encephalopathy, bleeding, varices, and ascites.

The expected benefits of surgery must be weighed carefully against the risks in patients with cirrhosis. In general, risks are higher and only essential surgery should be performed. There are stable patients with mild cirrhosis, however, who have no ongoing injury (e.g., due to removal of a toxin or discontinuation of alcohol) and in whom standards may be liberalized.

A number of precautions should be emphasized in the cirrhotic patient who does require surgery. Local (or, as a second choice, spinal) anesthesia may be safer than general anesthesia, although data are lacking. Therapy to prevent complications of liver disease, such as postoperative bleeding (fresh frozen plasma for the patient with an abnormal prothrombin time or partial thromboplastin time) and encephalopathy (see Chapter 47), should be established and maintained throughout the operative period, and the patient should be repeatedly checked for evidence of these two problems. The occasional patient who is taking chronic corticosteroid therapy for liver disease should have the steroid dosage increased during the perioperative period as described above.

PATIENTS WITH IATROGENIC IMPAIRMENT OF HEMOSTASIS

All anticoagulants and platelet inhibitors increase the risk of intraoperative and postoperative bleeding and should be discontinued before any type of surgery. Patients receiving drugs in these classes should have a comprehensive preoperative evaluation (Table 93.2) before admission for surgery, and an appropriate plan for perioperative management of anticoagulation should be communicated to the surgeon, anesthesiologist, and/or surgical center.

Anticoagulants

On the basis of critical assessment of risks and benefits, recommendations for the perioperative management of patients taking oral anticoagulants have recently been revised (33). *Coumarin derivatives* should be stopped 4 to 7 days before surgery, depending on the patient's current international normalized ratio (INR). In patients maintained at a high INR, coumarin should be discontinued earlier. The INR should be measured the day before surgery. If the INR remains elevated, 1 mg of vitamin K_1 should be administered subcutaneously. Within 12 hours, this dose will usually normalize the INR of a patient who has been off coumarin for 4 to 7 days. The larger doses of oral vitamin K_1 previously recommended (e.g., 10 mg) are believed not to be necessary and to increase, possibly, the risk of thromboembolism (33).

The authors of a recent review (33) recommended preoperative use of intravenous heparin, while the INR is subtherapeutic, only for patients at very high risk of thromboembolism, such as those with recent (within 1 month) venous thromboembolism or arterial embolism. Postoperatively, intravenous heparin is also recommended in these high-risk patients and in patients who have had venous thromboembolism within the 3 months preceding surgery. An alternative to intravenous unfractionated heparin preoperatively is subcutaneous low molecular weight heparin in therapeutic or prophylactic doses depending on the underlying diagnosis. Intravenous heparin should be stopped about 6 hours before surgery; the last dose of low molecular weight heparin should be given at least 24 hours before surgery. An INR and, if the patient is taking unfractionated heparin, a partial thromboplastin time and a platelet count should be checked before surgery (33).

These recommendations for use of preoperative and postoperative heparin are much more limited than previous recommendations. Other authors recommend preoperative or postoperative intravenous or low molecular weight heparin for other high-risk patients, such as those with mechanical valves and multiple risks (e.g., mechanical valve, atrial fibrillation and/or history of embolization).

Preoperative placement of a vena caval filter is an option in patients with recent venous thromboembolism or patients for whom the risk of bleeding due to heparin is unacceptably high (33). Warfarin (Coumadin) ordinarily can be resumed 24 to 72 hours after surgery, at the preoperative dosage, *if* all surgical bleeding is controlled; the INR usually reaches 2.0 after 3 days. Patients who have undergone intracranial, spinal, or ophthalmologic operations probably should not be anticoagulated for 48 hours to several weeks after surgery. For patients with a high risk of thromboembolism (see above), continuous-infusion heparin can be reinstituted 12 to 24 hours postoperatively without a bolus, if the surgeon is confident that hemostasis is ensured, and continued until full anticoagulation with warfarin has been re-established (33).

Antiplatelet Agents

Aspirin prolongs the bleeding time and may increase blood loss during and after operation in some patients. Generally, if aspirin is not being used as a critical therapy, it should be discontinued 7 or more days before surgery because the effect of aspirin on platelets continues for this period of time. Discontinuation of aspirin is particularly important before procedures for which hemostasis is critical, such as neurosurgical operations or some ophthalmologic surgery. Aspirin may be continued when its indication is important (e.g., coronary artery disease) and the risk of bleeding is low (e.g., breast biopsy, some peripheral vascular surgery). Because *some NSAIDs other than aspirin* may impair platelet function also, it is prudent to advise patients to discontinue NSAID use 1 week before surgery, especially surgery for which increased bleeding would be especially harmful (Table 93.4). *Ticlopidine* (Ticlid) and *clopidogrel,* platelet aggregation inhibitors, should be discontinued at least 2 weeks before surgery to ensure that the bleeding time is not prolonged in the perioperative period.

PATIENTS WITH A CHRONIC INFECTION

Two types of chronic bacterial infection pose risks to the patient and to others in the operating room: staphylococcal skin infections and pulmonary tuberculosis. They require appropriate management before surgery.

Skin Infections

Chronic bacterial skin infections (usually caused by staphylococci) pose a high risk for wound sepsis and may be the source of infections in other patients (34). Therefore, they should be suppressed or eradicated before admission of the patient for an elective operation. Chapter 32 describes strategies for accomplishing this.

Tuberculosis

Active pulmonary tuberculosis poses a problem for the surgical patient because of the general debilitation it causes. It also creates the risk of infection for others in the operating room. Therefore, adult patients with a history of unexplained chronic cough or a history of tuberculosis should be evaluated for active tuberculosis before admission for surgery. Patients with active pulmonary tuberculosis should be stable and have negative sputum cultures before admission for elective surgery. The ambulatory treatment of tuberculosis is described in Chapter 34.

Human Immunodeficiency Virus Infection

Acquired immunodeficiency syndrome poses many problems in preoperative evaluation that are beyond the scope of this chapter but are addressed elsewhere (see General References and Chapter 39). Several important issues are summarized here.

The risk of transmission to health care workers is very small, but it does exist. Universal precautions are recommended in the care of all patients, not just known HIV-positive patients (see Chapter 39). Screening of all surgical patients for HIV infection is not currently recommended by expert consensus, but this issue continues to be controversial.

HIV-infected patients pose challenges in addition to the usual preoperative evaluation. Decision-making is complicated by the wide spectrum of morbidity in HIV infection, ranging from the lack of symptoms in the recently infected patient to the debilitation in the preterminal patient. Decision-making should balance the status and prognosis of the patient's HIV infection (asymptomatic, symptomatic), mean life expectancy, the patient's wishes, the increased risk for the specific operation posed by the HIV infection, and the indications for and expected benefit of the surgery during the patient's expected length of survival.

PATIENTS WITH NEUROPSYCHIATRIC DISEASE

Neuropsychiatric problems present ill-defined risks during surgery and the postsurgical period. The major concerns are worsening of mental status caused by both metabolic changes and psychologic stresses. The patient with psychiatric disease may decompensate postoperatively, making care difficult and jeopardizing wound healing.

Cerebrovascular Disease

Risk

Patients with recent strokes have a significant risk of worsening focal deficits during carotid artery surgery, but this risk cannot necessarily be extrapolated to other types of surgery. Patients with recent strokes (less than

6 weeks preoperatively) also have a risk of deterioration in their general mental status, regardless of the status of their focal deficits, if they undergo major surgery; however, firm data are lacking on the size of this risk.

Perioperative Management

Patients with recent strokes should have a comprehensive preoperative evaluation (Table 93.2), emphasizing documentation of the preoperative neurologic impairment and the detection of treatable underlying causes of the stroke. The data regarding the course of the patient's stroke should be reviewed, and additional testing (see Chapter 91) should be performed if necessary to exclude a treatable cause.

No specific perioperative therapy for the patient with a stable completed stroke is needed. In general, it is prudent to delay elective noncarotid surgery for at least 6 weeks after a completed stroke, although no firm data are available to support this practice.

Asymptomatic Cervical Bruit

Risk

Cervical bruits are present in approximately 4% of people over the age of 45. These bruits may be caused by a number of processes (see Chapter 91), including common or internal carotid stenosis. In the patient with an asymptomatic cervical bruit, there is slight or no increased risk of cerebrovascular accident during surgery (35).

Perioperative Management

Apart from a careful history and physical examination to exclude evidence of a prior stroke or transient ischemic attack related to the cervical bruit, no special approach is needed for these patients. Duplex carotid ultrasound can help establish whether the cervical bruit is caused by carotid stenosis and the degree of stenosis; its value has not been established for estimating risk of postoperative stroke. Hypotension and excessive neck manipulation should be avoided during surgery in patients known to have carotid bruits. The patient with a history of symptoms possibly related to the bruit should be evaluated as described in Chapter 91.

Data summarized in Chapter 91 show that patients with high-grade asymptomatic and symptomatic carotid stenosis have a lower long-term stroke rate if carotid endarterectomy is performed. When patients such as these require elective surgery for another condition, a decision must be made on which of the two surgeries to do first.

Parkinson Disease

Risk

The perioperative risks in patients with Parkinson disease are caused by musculoskeletal rigidity, which may impair voluntary postoperative ventilation, mobilization, and swallowing. These patients are also subject to postoperative delirium. The rigidity of patients taking antiparkinson medication may worsen after the patient has missed one or more doses (see Chapter 90). Despite this potential problem, most patients with Parkinson disease tolerate anesthesia and temporary omission of medications.

Perioperative Management

The patient should have a comprehensive preoperative evaluation (Table 93.2), and the antiparkinsonian regimen should be tailored to provide the best possible relief of symptoms (see Chapter 90). For patients taking an anticholinergic agent, the drug may be continued until midnight before surgery and resumed when the patient is able to take oral medications. L-Dopa or Sinemet (L-dopa/carbidopa) should be continued until induction of anesthesia, and the drug should be resumed as soon as possible after surgery. Postoperative physical therapy to maintain range of motion may help these patients until they are able to take oral medication. Parkinsonian patients should be observed for postoperative delirium and aspiration.

Dementia and Organic Brain Syndrome

Risk

Patients with dementia have an increased risk of mortality and morbidity during surgery. The increase in mortality is caused largely by lack of cooperation (e.g., with postoperative respiratory care). Much of the morbidity is related to the development of delirium caused by anesthesia, perioperative medications, and surgical stress. Because surgery is always a difficult process for a demented patient and because the degree of increased risk is ill defined, the potential benefits of surgery should be carefully reviewed before a final decision to operate is made.

Perioperative Management

The patient should have a comprehensive evaluation (Table 93.2) before admission for surgery. The patient should be checked for metabolic abnormalities that may worsen cerebral function before admission, just before surgery, and throughout the postoperative period. Emphasis should be placed on detecting and correcting hypovolemia, electrolyte abnormalities, and hypoxia. Before major surgery, it is advisable to document the patient's mental status formally (see Mini-Mental Status Examination, Chapter 26) so that mental states after surgery can be compared with baseline status. See Surgery in the Elderly Patient, above, for simple measures to decrease the incidence of postoperative delirium. When demented patients undergo major procedures, constant observation is recommended for the first 24 to 48 hours after surgery.

Other Psychiatric Problems

Risk

The major problems associated with general surgery in psychiatric patients are lack of cooperation with postoperative care, postoperative psychosis, and interactions between psychotropic medications and anesthetic agents. The degree of cooperation that can be expected postoperatively can generally, but not always, be predicted on the basis of the patient's past behavior and preoperative mental status. Obtaining informed consent is also an issue.

Perioperative Management

A careful history of the patient's past psychiatric illness should be obtained. The patient's *mental status* should be documented preoperatively (see Chapter 19) so that it can be compared with postoperative changes. The patient's *ability to give informed consent* should be evaluated (see Chapter 19); involvement of a designated decision-maker other than the patient may be required. A psychiatric consultation should be obtained in all patients with psychosis or other severe psychiatric problems. An additional issue that must be dealt with by the patient's primary care practitioner and surgeon is the likely effect of the patient's psychiatric state on the surgical evaluation and outcomes (e.g., evaluating symptoms in a patient with one of the somatoform disorders, described in Chapter 21, or evaluating the need for cosmetic surgery).

Careful explanation of the operation is especially crucial to management of patients with psychiatric disorders or with anticipated stress reactions to surgery. The procedure should be explained in language the patient can understand. After the explanation, the patient should be asked to express any concerns about the planned surgery, and the patient's comprehension of the planned surgery should be assessed and documented. The need to ventilate about anxiety associated with disfiguring surgery (e.g., mastectomy, amputation) and with the fear of not waking up is particularly common in both anxiety-prone patients and those who are usually free of anxiety.

Patients with severe *psychosis* should be in a stable manageable state before admission for elective surgery. This should be accomplished through close collaboration between the patient's primary care practitioner, the surgeon, and psychiatrist.

Patients with mild to moderate *anxiety or depression* can be managed by supportive counseling, use of support by family members, selective use of antidepressants or minor tranquilizers, and careful explanation of the procedure to the patient. These interventions should be initiated before hospital admission, not at the last minute before surgery.

The patient's use of *psychotropic drugs* should be communicated to the anesthesiologist. Neuroleptics and tricyclic antidepressants can interact with anesthetics to cause increased sedation, hypotension or hypertension, and arrhythmias. Small to moderate dosages of phenothiazines, haloperidol, and tricyclic antidepressants should be continued until about 12 hours before surgery. In the occasional patient taking a very high dosage of these agents, it is recommended that the drug is stopped about 24 hours before surgery, except in patients who have severely decompensated in the past when their medication has been changed. The dosage of benzodiazepines does not need to be changed unless it is very high.

Lithium carbonate can prolong the action of muscle relaxants and cause myocardial depression and hypernatremia. Lithium should be discontinued 24 hours preoperatively; however, the anesthesiologist should be aware that it has been administered recently. A blood lithium level and electrolyte measurements should be obtained before surgery as a guideline. Additional information about lithium is provided in Chapter 24.

Monoamine oxidase inhibitor antidepressants can enhance the effect of sympathomimetic agents and sympathetic responses to anesthesia and can decrease the rate of elimination of certain anesthetic agents. Because of these problems, monoamine oxidase inhibitors should be discontinued at least 2 weeks before surgery, and the anesthesiologist must be informed of their recent administration.

General References*

American College of Physicians. **Guidelines for assessing and managing the perioperative risk from coronary artery disease associated with major noncardiac surgery.** Ann Intern Med 1997;127:309.

Evidence-based clinical guidelines based on review of all literature from 1977 to 1996. Accompanying article contains details and more than 200 references.

Caputo GM, Gross RG. Medical consultation on surgical services: an annotated bibliography. Ann Intern Med 1993;118:290.

Gross RJ, Caputo GC, eds. Medical consultation: the internist on surgical, obstetric, and psychiatric services, 3rd ed. Baltimore: Williams & Wilkins, 1998.

A comprehensive multicontributor book, extensively referenced.

Specific References

1. Babbott S, Gross RJ. Evaluation of the healthy patient and the ambulatory surgery patient. In: Gross RJ, Caputo GC, eds. Medical consultation: the internist on surgical, obstetric, and psychiatric services, 3rd ed. Baltimore: Williams & Wilkins, 1998:25.
2. Gold BS, Kitz DS, Lecky JH, et al. Unanticipated admission to the hospital following ambulatory surgery. JAMA 1989;262:3008.
3. Roizen MF. Preoperative evaluation. In: Miller RD, ed. Anesthesia, 4th ed. New York: Churchill-Livingstone, 1994:827.
4. Djokovic JL, Hedley-White J. Prediction of outcome of surgery and anesthesia in patients over 80. JAMA 1979;242:2301.
5. Hosking MP, Warner MA, Lobdell CM, et al. Outcomes of surgery in patients 90 years of age and older. JAMA 1989;261:1909.
6. Gross RJ. Special topics. In: Gross RJ, Caputo GC, eds. Medical consultation: the internist on surgical, obstetric, and psychiatric services, 3rd ed. Baltimore: Williams & Wilkins, 1998:615.
7. Rose EA, King TC. Understanding postoperative fatigue. Surg Gynecol Obstet 1978;147:97.
8. Falcone RA, Ziegelstein RC. Cardiovascular disease and hypertension. In: Gross RJ, Caputo GC, eds. Medical consultation: the internist on surgical, obstetric, and psychiatric services, 3rd ed. Baltimore: Williams & Wilkins, 1998:149.
9. Rao Tadikonda LK, Jacobs K, El-Etr A. Reinfarction following anesthesia in patients with myocardial infarction. Anesthesiology 1983;59:499.

---

*Bold print (general references) and bold numerals (specific references) denote published controlled clinical trials, meta-analyses, or consensus-based recommendations.

10. Goldman L, Caldera DL, Nussbaum SR, et al. Multifactorial index of cardiac risk in noncardiac surgical procedures. N Engl J Med 1977;297:845.
11. Goldman L, Caldera DL, Southwick FS, et al. Cardiac risk factors and complications in non-cardiac surgery. Medicine (Baltimore) 1978;57:357.
12. Detsky AS, Abrams HB, McLaughlin JR, et al. Predicting cardiac complications in patients undergoing non-cardiac surgery. J Gen Intern Med 1986;1:211.
13. Lee TH, Marcantonio ER, Mangione CM, et al. Derivation and prospective validation of a simple index for prediction of cardiac risk of major noncardiac surgery. Circulation 1999;100:1043.
14. ACC/AHA Task Force. Guidelines for perioperative cardiovascular evaluation for noncardiac surgery. J Am Coll Cardiol 1996;27:910.
15. Poldermans, D, Boersma, E, Bax, JJ, et al. The effect of bisoprolol on perioperative mortality and myocardial infarction in high-risk patients undergoing vascular surgery. N Engl J Med 1999;341:1789.
16. Goldman L, Caldera DL. Risks of general anesthesia and elective operation in the hypertensive patient. Anesthesiology 1979;50:285.
17. Dajani AS, Taubert KA, Wilson W, et al. Prevention of bacterial endocarditis. Recommendations by the American Heart Association. JAMA 1997;277:1794.
18. Goldman L. Supraventricular tachyarrhythmias in hospitalized adults after surgery. Chest 1978;73:450.
19. Kroenke K, Lawrence VA, Theroux JF, et al. Operative risk in patients with severe obstructive pulmonary disease. Arch Intern Med 1992;152:967.
20. Lawrence VA, Page CP, Harris GD. Preoperative spirometry before abdominal operations: a critical appraisal of its predictive value. Arch Intern Med 1989;149:280.
21. Tarhan S, Moffitt ED, Sessler AD, et al. Risk of anesthesia and surgery in patients with chronic bronchitis and chronic obstructive pulmonary disease. Surgery 1973;74:720.
22. Tisi GM. Preoperative evaluation of pulmonary function: validity, indications, and benefits. Am Rev Respir Dir 1979;119:293.
23. Smetana GW. Preoperative pulmonary evaluation. N Engl J Med 1999;340:937.
24. Oh SH, Patterson R. Surgery in corticosteroid-dependent asthmatics. J Allergy Clin Immunol 1974;53:345.
25. Briefel G, Turer P. Renal disease. In: Gross RJ, Caputo GC, eds. Medical consultation: the internist on surgical, obstetric, and psychiatric services, 3rd ed. Baltimore: Williams & Wilkins, 1998:207.
26. Tepel M, van der Giet M, Schwarzfeld C, et al. Prevention of radiographic-contrast-agent-induced reductions in renal function by acetylcysteine. N Engl J Med 2000;343:180.
27. Bennett WM, Aronoff GR, Golper TA, et al. Drug prescribing in renal failure. Philadelphia: American College of Physicians, 1994.
28. Lamberts SWJ, Bruining HA, DeJong FH. Corticosteroid therapy in severe illness. N Engl J Med 1997;337:1285.
29. Ladenson PW, Levin AA, Ridgway EC, et al. Complications of surgery in hypothyroid patients. Am J Med 1984;77:261.
30. McArthur JW, Rawson RW, Means JH, et al. Thyrotoxic crisis: an analysis of the thirty-six cases seen at the Massachusetts General Hospital during the past twenty-five years. JAMA 1947;134:868.
31. Strauss RJ, Wise L. Operative risks of obesity. Surg Gynecol Obstet 1978;146:286.
32. Harville DD, Summerskill WHJ. Surgery in acute hepatitis. JAMA 1963;184:257.
33. Kearon C, Hirsh J. Management of anticoagulation before and after elective surgery. N Engl J Med 1997;336:1506.
34. Hiral D. Nasal *Staphylococcus aureus* and postoperative infection. Am Surg 1980;46:310.
35. Ropper AH, Wechsler LR, Wilson LS. Carotid bruit and the risk of stroke in elective surgery. N Engl J Med 1982;307:1388.

CHAPTER 94

Peripheral Arterial Disease and Arterial Aneurysms

RITA A. FALCONE, MD

The aging process is associated with the development of variable degrees of degenerative arterial disease. Longevity and quality of life may be improved by recognition, evaluation, and appropriate therapy of diseases that affect blood vessels (see, e.g., Chapters 62 and 91). The purpose of this chapter is to provide guidelines for recognition and management of the more commonly encountered problems of acute and chronic occlusive peripheral arterial disease (PAD) and of abdominal and peripheral arterial aneurysms.

ACUTE PERIPHERAL ARTERIAL OCCLUSION

Acute ischemia occurs when there is a sudden decrease in arterial perfusion of the lower extremities. It demands immediate recognition and management in an effort to minimize morbidity, including limb loss and death, because irreversible changes such as muscle necrosis, extensive arterial thrombosis, and neurologic deficits may occur in the affected extremity as early as 4 to 6 hours after acute arterials occlusion.

Causes

The two major causes of acute arterial occlusion are cardioarterial embolism and *in situ* thrombosis. Most large arterial emboli originate in the heart. Arrhythmias and mural thrombi are the major risk factors for embolization. Rare sources of emboli include proximal arterial lesions such as aortic aneurysms or large ulcerative aortic plaques, which are commonly associated with arterial *cholesterol microemboli.* These microemboli may cause the "blue toe syndrome" (the acute development of cyanosis of the toes or the distal feet, often in association with strong posterior tibial or dorsalis pedis pulses) (1). Left atrial myxomas, debris from prosthetic heart valves, paradoxical emboli (venous clots passing through a congenital cardiac defect into the arterial circulation), and foreign body emboli have also infrequently been associated with sudden arterial occlusion.

In situ thrombosis of an arteriosclerotic lesion accounts for approximately 85% of acute occlusive events (2). Such thrombotic complications are most likely to occur in segments of severe stenosis such as the aortic bifurcation, the iliac bifurcation, the common femoral bifurcation, and the superficial femoral artery just above the knee.

Upper extremity ischemia is usually secondary to arterial embolism. Acute thrombosis virtually never causes ischemia in the upper extremity because chronic arteriosclerotic lesions are uncommon and collateralization is excellent. Thoracic outlet compression may rarely give rise to subclavian or axillary arterial thrombosis. Concomitant problems such as hypovolemia from volume depletion or hemorrhage, congestive heart failure, erythrocytosis, or trauma all have profound influences on management.

Clinical Manifestations

More than 90% of the time, acute embolic occlusion may be distinguished from acute thrombotic occlusion on clinical grounds alone. In instances in which doubt exists about the cause, especially in the absence of atrial fibrillation and recent myocardial infarction, arteriography is essential to distinguish embolus from thrombosis (see Laboratory and Radiographic Studies, below).

Emboli lodge at arterial bifurcations, most often in the lower extremities. Multiple emboli can result from a "shower discharge" of clots from the heart. Therefore, although the legs are affected most often, there may also be symptoms and signs of ischemia elsewhere.

Clinical manifestations vary depending on the adequacy of pre-existing collateral circulation and the site of occlusion. If pre-existing collateral vessels, stimulated by underlying occlusive arterial disease, are present, acute ischemic symptoms may be mild. Total arterial occlusion of a previously normal arterial tree causes severe symptoms. The cardinal features of acute ischemia include the six *Ps* of arterial occlusion: Pulselessness, pallor, poikilothermia, pain, paralysis, and paresthesias. The latter three *Ps* reflect neurophysiologic sequelae of ischemia, and the former three result from mechanical occlusion of an artery. Three-fourths of patients complain of pain, but 20% note numbness as the first manifestation of sudden arterial occlusion. Initially, the pain may be mild, but as the ischemia progresses, pain worsens, only to subside later as anesthesia and paralysis develop.

Additional findings include absent or faint distal pulses, poor capillary filling, and collapsed or severely sunken veins on the dorsum of the foot. Pedal edema, if present, is not a result of arterial occlusion, but it may be secondary to heart failure or pooling of blood in the extremities of patients who attempt to relieve ischemic pain by maintaining their legs in a dependent position for long periods.

Cardiac examination may reveal atrial fibrillation, a diastolic rumble or the opening snap of mitral stenosis, the click of a prosthetic heart valve, or a third heart sound associated with congestive heart failure. A recent history of chest pain or electrocardiographic evidence of myocardial infarction also suggests a cardiac origin of acute leg ischemia.

Laboratory and Radiographic Studies

Laboratory studies usually are not helpful in making the diagnosis of acute arterial ischemia of the lower extremities. Arterial blood gas measurements and pH should be obtained to serve as baseline studies for subsequent comparative measurement and to identify metabolic acidosis secondary to muscle ischemia. Hyperkalemia may be noted, particularly if prolonged limb ischemia has occurred. An x-ray of the chest may document cardiac enlargement or congestive heart failure. An electrocardiogram and, if time permits, a transthoracic or transesophageal echocardiogram may be useful in delineating cardiac disease. All these studies should be obtained after the patient is hospitalized. Although noninvasive evaluation by Doppler ultrasonography or by plethysmography is often superfluous, the inability to obtain any arterial Doppler signal in the foot in a patient with an acute occlusion supports the decision for urgent revascularization.

Contrast arteriography is not performed routinely in patients with acute ischemia except in occasional instances of modest ischemia when it is needed to distinguish between thrombosis and embolus (see below). Evidence of generalized and severe arteriosclerosis, a tapered arterial occlusion, and well-developed collateral vessels suggest acute thrombosis. Normal-appearing arteries with scanty collateral circulation and an occlusion with an inverted meniscus configuration indicate embolic occlusion. (Magnetic resonance angiography is being done in some centers as a less invasive alternative technique, especially when there are contraindications to contrast angiography.) However, embolization can occur in patients who also have chronic occlusive disease, and the diagnosis is occasionally still in question after angiography. In any case, the decision for immediate surgery is based on the clinical status of the extremity, not on the arteriogram.

Differential Diagnosis

Every effort should be made to differentiate embolism from thrombosis because the therapy of the two conditions is different. History is often helpful in separating these two entities. A history of intermittent claudication or of rest pain suggests the acute ischemic event is thrombosis. Absence of a history of intermittent claudication usually indicates embolism. However, a minority of patients who suffer acute superficial femoral arterial occlusion secondary to thrombosis have never had symptoms of intermittent claudication before the sudden occlusive event. On physical examination, classic findings of chronic ischemia such as loss of hair on the toes and dorsum of the foot and the leg, along with nail, skin, and muscle atrophy, suggest arterial thrombosis rather than embolism. A laterally pulsatile abdominal mass suggesting an abdominal aortic aneurysm (AAA) from which a mural thrombus may have embolized to the distal arterial tree might be evident. Finally, if the acute ischemic episode involves only one leg, palpating the popliteal and femoral arteries may detect an aneurysm. If the contralateral vessel is vigorously pulsating and aneurysmal, a thrombosis of an aneurysm on the ipsilateral or symptomatic side may have occurred, especially if a nonpulsatile mass can be palpated.

An acute dissection of the thoracic and abdominal aorta may present as unilateral lower extremity ischemia. Under these circumstances, patients may relate a history of severe, searing, ripping thoracic back pain and may provide a history of long-standing hypertension. Chest x-ray may reveal a widened mediastinal silhouette, and a murmur of aortic insufficiency may be present if the dissection originates in the ascending aorta.

Treatment

Evaluation and therapy must proceed simultaneously in the management of acute arterial ischemia of the extremities. The cornerstone of early management is the immediate intravenous administration (in the clinician's office) of 100 to 150 units heparin sodium/kg body weight (3) (although no prospective controlled studies have established its efficacy) and then urgent vascular surgery consultation.

There may be a role for the interventional radiologist and for intra-arterial infusion of *fibrinolytic* agents directly into the site of the acute arterial occlusion (2–4). If that is the case, a multiple purpose polyethylene catheter is imbedded into the occluding clot after the arteriographic study is performed. Protocols may vary, but typically urokinase or tissue plasminogen activator is infused for 30 to 60 minutes and a second arteriogram is performed. Therapy is continued for 24 to 48 hours with clinical and angiographic reevaluation at 8- to 12-hour intervals. Such therapy is contraindicated when the extremity is in dire jeopardy because the time required for lysis to occur may be longer than the safe interval before necrosis occurs. In patients whose limbs are not immediately threatened, this therapeutic approach can be efficacious, particularly for high-risk patients in whom operation may be contraindicated. It is generally accepted that clots older than 7 to 10 days are resistant to lysis. Untoward bleeding is the major complication of fibrinolytic therapy and may result in significant morbidity. The duration of the infusion and the optimal dosage to be administered to restore circulation are not yet firmly established. Therefore, until further experience is gained with this modality, it should be reserved for highly selected patients who are cared for in centers specializing in management of vascular disease.

Surgical revascularization, (see below) can then be performed, if necessary, after blood flow to the ischemic extremity is restored. The introduction of the balloon-tipped embolectomy catheter by Fogarty et al. in 1963 revolutionized the management of acute embolic occlusion and converted a previously complex undertaking into a simple operative procedure that invariably can be performed under local anesthesia with improved survival and limb salvage rates.

After discharge from the hospital, patients are almost always maintained on therapeutic levels of oral anticoagulants for the rest of their lives, although only in patients with embolism associated with atrial fibrillation has efficacy been established (see Chapter 57). Furthermore, they must be evaluated several times a year to ensure that optimal cardiac function is maintained and for continued evaluation of their peripheral circulation.

Results

Despite improved diagnosis, preoperative care, operative management, and postoperative support, mortality from acute lower extremity ischemia continues to be discouraging. Early operative mortality rates still average 15% or more (2). Virtually all deaths are related to complications of cardiovascular disease, which reinforces the contention that recognition and correction of cardiovascular risk factors for arterial embolism or thrombosis are critical in the acute and long-term management of such patients (5).

The likelihood of successful limb salvage, which exceeds 95% in most series, is directly related to the time between arterial occlusion and restoration of blood flow. Therefore, it is improbable that a 100% limb salvage rate will ever be achieved.

CHRONIC PERIPHERAL ARTERIAL DISEASE

In contrast to the management of acute arterial occlusion, which requires emergent or urgent treatment, chronic peripheral arterial disease can usually be managed electively because of the presence of collateral channels that bypass slowly developing atherosclerotic lesions and maintain a viable extremity. A knowledge of the natural history (see below) of chronic peripheral arterial disease is necessary for the appropriate management of these patients.

Causes and Pathophysiology

The most common cause of chronic peripheral arterial disease (PAD) is atherosclerosis. Atherosclerotic risk factors for chronic PAD are similar to those for coronary artery and cerebrovascular disease: Age greater than 50 years, male sex, tobacco use, diabetes mellitus, hypertension, and hyperlipidemia. Many patients with PAD have associated coronary artery disease and 10% have associated cerebrovascular disease (6). Often patients will not succumb to complications of PAD but will present with fatal or nonfatal cardiovascular and cerebrovascular complications. Therefore, significant focus on risk factor modification is needed to reduce the risk of these associated events.

The prevalence of intermittent claudication in patients with PAD is 1% to 2% for those under the age of 50 and increases to 5% for those 50 to 70 (6,7). Men are affected 1.5 to 2 times more often than women until age 70, when prevalence rates for intermittent claudication for men and women are nearly equal (6).

Smoking is the single most important modifiable risk factor for the development of PAD (see below). Smokers develop PAD a decade earlier than age-matched nonsmokers, are at increased risk of amputation, and have less successful outcomes after lower extremity revascularization surgery (8). Tobacco use is synergistic with other risk factors for the development and progression of arterial disease (9).

Diabetic patients (see Chapter 79) manifest PAD a decade earlier than nondiabetic patients. In diabetics, PAD often develops in the more distal arteries of the leg earlier than it does in nondiabetics, and options for revascularization are therefore often limited. If a limb neuropathy is present, paresthesias and undetected infections and ulcerations can occur. Diabetics have a sevenfold higher rate of amputation than do nondiabetics (10,11).

Hypertension is a major risk factor for the development of PAD, especially in females (10,12). Observational studies support the practice of aggressive blood pressure control (see Chapter 67) in patients with PAD, although no prospective randomized trials have yet been done (see below).

Hyperlipidemia is prevalent in patients with PAD, but the direct association is controversial. Nevertheless, treating hyperlipidemia is important in atherosclerotic patients in any case and should be undertaken aggressively in this population as well (see Chapter 82).

Although atherosclerosis is a generalized disease, it has a remarkably segmental distribution. Arteriosclerosis is prone to develop at major arterial bifurcations, in areas of arterial fixation, and at points of marked arterial angulation such as the aortic, common iliac, and common femoral artery bifurcations; the infrarenal aorta; and the distal superficial femoral artery as it enters Hunter canal. With gradual development of such lesions, the formation of collateral vessels compensates for segmental obstructive processes. In many instances collaterals are sufficient to provide adequate blood flow even during moderate exercise, so symptoms are minimal. However, as progressive main arterial involvement occurs, collateral channels may become ineffective or occluded, and ischemic symptoms progress from exercise-induced discomfort in the muscles of the lower extremity to rest pain and finally to tissue necrosis (see Chapter 95).

Thromboangiitis obliterans, or *Buerger disease*, is a severe chronic panarteritis that leads to fibrosis and obliteration of small vessels at the tibial and pedal arterial levels. The arteries of the forearm and hand can be involved, and superficial phlebitis may be seen as well. Buerger disease is an uncommon cause of lower extremity arterial insufficiency in the United States. This entity affects young men in their twenties and thirties and is almost always associated with severe tobacco addiction. Successful management hinges on cessation of all forms of tobacco usage.

Natural History

Intermittent claudication reflects a relatively benign condition (13–15). Approximately one-third of patients improve, one-third remain stable and tolerate their symptoms, and one-third deteriorate and require revascularization. Relentless progression of the peripheral atherosclerotic process is unlikely in most nondiabetic patients, particularly if use of all tobacco products is discontinued. Less than 4% of patients will ultimately require amputation, although diabetics are at increased risk (8). On the other hand, patients with ischemic rest pain or gangrene are at very high risk for amputation if revascularization is not undertaken.

The overall 5- and 10-year survival rates among patients with intermittent claudication are approximately 70% and 40%, respectively, and the most common cause of death (in 75%) is coronary artery disease (16).

Clinical Manifestations

Symptoms

Many patients with PAD are asymptomatic. When symptoms begin they are often described as pain or discomfort that develops in the affected limb with exercise and is relieved within several minutes with rest (claudication). The discomfort is often localized to the calf, although it can also affect the buttocks and thigh as well. The distance a patient walks before developing claudication should be documented. When symptoms advance to pain or discomfort at rest or when supine, it may be assumed that blood flow to the lower extremity is marginal. Gravity can increase blood flow slightly, and patients often learn to alleviate the symptoms by dangling the affected leg over the side of a bed or by standing up.

Physical Examination

A complete vascular examination should routinely be performed, noting the status of all peripheral pulses, the presence or absence of bruits and peripheral aneurysms, and the blood pressure measurements in both upper extremities. In patients with mild intermittent claudication, the skin, hair growth, feet, and toenails may appear normal, and faintly palpable dorsalis pedis and posterior tibial pulses may be present. However, with progressive arterial involvement trophic changes may occur with hair loss and the development of thin parchment-like skin. Lack of pulses below the inguinal ligaments, blanching and pallor with elevation of the extremity, and dependent rubor all indicate advanced ischemia. Gangrenous areas may be evident on the toes. The typical locations of ischemic ulcers are the calcaneus, the lateral malleolus, and the dorsum of the foot (see Chapter 95).

Laboratory and Radiographic Studies

The distribution and severity of PAD can be determined objectively by noninvasive Doppler flow studies. Doppler signals from the dorsalis pedis, posterior tibial, peroneal, or lateral tarsal arteries are located, and a sphygmomanometer cuff is placed immediately above the malleoli and inflated to above systolic pressure to obliterate the Doppler signal. As the cuff is slowly deflated, Doppler signals return at the systolic opening pressure. The highest pressure recorded is compared with the brachial arterial systolic pressure. A resting ankle/brachial (ABI) index of 1 or greater is normal. For patients with intermittent claudication the mean index is 0.59; for those with rest pain, 0.26; and for those with impending gangrene, 0.05 (17). The accuracy of the measurement is quite high (18).

A Doppler study of lower extremity blood flow, although important, is not necessarily required in evaluating all patients with lower extremity arterial occlusive disease. However, noninvasive testing may be helpful in distinguishing vascular insufficiency from other causes of leg pain such as neurogenic claudication secondary to cauda equina compression from spinal stenosis. In the latter condition, Doppler ABI indices are normal at rest and after exercise. Doppler flow studies, with the patient at rest, are almost always sufficient to make the diagnosis of peripheral arterial occlusive disease (19). Rarely, the studies need to be repeated after exercise on a treadmill or even after simply walking the patient to the point of claudication. Noninvasive studies can also document the efficacy of nonoperative therapy and determine whether deterioration of the circulation is progressive (20). Also, comparison of preoperative and postoperative noninvasive data is useful in documenting the effectiveness of operative therapy.

The gold standard study, if it is determined the patient is a candidate for operation, is arteriography (see below). Although risks are very small in experienced hands, arteriography is used only when operation is indicated and agreed to by the patient. Finally, laboratory studies may also reveal hyperglycemia or hyperlipidemia that requires appropriate management.

Treatment and Results

Treatment for arterial insufficiency of the legs may be either operative or nonoperative. Indications for operation are shown in Table 94.1. Patients should usually be managed nonoperatively unless one of these indications is present and medical management has failed. Knowing the natural history of the occlusive process aids significantly in determining whether the patient's symptoms warrant operative intervention in view of associated risk factors and life expectancy. Except for patients who are not considered operative candidates, ischemic rest pain, nonhealing ulcers, pregangrenous changes, and gangrene are unequivocal indications for expeditious revascularization.

General Measures

An itemized list of recommendations written in nontechnical language should be given to and carefully reviewed with the patient (Table 94.2). Meticulous skin hygiene and avoidance of injury to the foot, however slight, cannot be overemphasized. An otherwise asymptomatic ischemic foot becomes symptomatic when trauma leads to a nonhealing ulcer that may require revascularization. If the patient's feet are cold, particularly at night, a warm pair of socks or a muffler is advised but not the use of heating pads or hot water bottles, which may cause tissue breakdown and ulceration. Patients should inspect their

Table 94.1. Indications for Operation for Arterial Insufficiency of the Legs

Claudication that is intolerable in a patient at low surgical risk
Ischemic rest pain
Impending gangrene
Nonhealing ulceration

Table 94.2. Advice that Should Be Given to Patients with Arterial Insufficiency

Quit smoking. Use *no* tobacco in *any* form.[a]
If overweight, lose weight.
Walk to the point of claudication at least 30 minutes a day.
Keep feet very clean. Bathe at least daily in lukewarm water.
Gently apply lanolin or mild hand cream to feet after bathing.
Wear clean, preferably cotton, socks daily (cotton does not retain moisture).
Avoid injury to feet. Wear properly fitting shoes to prevent calluses, corns, blisters. Avoid shoes made of synthetic material that does not "breathe." Wear slippers at night and use a night light after going to bed.
Place lamb's wool (available from pharmacies) between overriding toes.
Avoid extremes of temperature. Do no put feet in hot water or use heating pads on lower extremities. In cold weather, wear socks to bed to warm feet. Do not get feet cold or wet.
If feet hurt at night, raise head of bed 6–10 in. (15–25 cm) on blocks.
For any sudden change in symptoms such as prolonged pain, numbness or tingling, or inability to move foot or leg, consult your health care provider *immediately*.

[a]See Chapter 27 for ways to help patients to stop smoking.

feet every day and should bathe them at least once a day in lukewarm water and thereafter apply lanolin or hand cream to the skin to keep it soft and pliable and to avoid cracking and fissuring and subsequent skin breakdown.

Exercise is the cornerstone of therapy for symptomatic PAD. Supervised exercise rehabilitation programs (e.g., in cardiac rehabilitation centers; see Chapter 63) using a treadmill have been found to be the most successful at relieving intermittent claudication symptoms (10,18). Significant improvement in walking times before onset of intermittent claudication can occur when the program includes up to 30-minute sessions of intermittent treadmill exercise three times a week for 3 to 6 months. These programs require a motivated and compliant patient. During sessions, trained personnel may also reinforce the need for risk factor modification. Patients are also encouraged to continue a walking exercise program at home. Other measures that significantly affect outcome include maintaining satisfactory cardiac function (see Chapter 66).

Smoking cessation (see Chapter 27) is critical for patients with chronic PAD, and the decrease in mortality rates for patients who stop smoking is significant (18,20). Smoking cessation improves symptoms of intermittent claudication in up to 85% of patients and improves exercise tolerance by up to 300%. Patients must clearly understand that nicotine absorption occurs through the buccal mucosa with the use of chewing tobacco, pipes, cigars, and cigarettes and does not require inhalation of smoke.

Diabetic patients with PAD have a high risk of eventual amputation, and the general principles of foot care are especially important for them. In addition, diabetics should be seen by a podiatrist every 3 months for trimming of their nails and calluses and for close inspection for early signs of infection or ulceration. Intensive hypoglycemic therapy, of value in many diabetics, has not yet been demonstrated to affect the course of atherosclerotic peripheral vascular disease (10) (see Chapter 79).

Management of coexistent hypertension (see Chapter 67) is sometimes challenging, and one often may have to settle for less than ideal blood pressure control because the symptoms of the arteriosclerotic occlusive process may worsen if the patient is returned to a normotensive state. It now seems clear that beta-blockers, previously thought to be harmful to patients with PAD, may be used in the treatment of hypertension in this population unless the occlusive disease is severe (21). Angiotensin-converting enzyme inhibitors, may, however, be the antihypertensive agents of choice (22). In patients taking antihypertensive drugs, it is important to check at each visit for orthostatic drops in blood pressure and to adjust the treatment regimen accordingly if orthostatic hypotension occurs.

Pharmacologic Management

Antiplatelet Drugs. Aspirin, 81 to 325 mg/day, has been demonstrated to reduce the risk of vascular events in patients with atherosclerotic disease (see Chapters 57 and 62). It has not, however, been shown unequivocally to alter the progress of PAD (23). Nevertheless, its use in patients with PAD is reasonable, especially considering that most of these patients have systemic atherosclerosis. Ticlopidine and clopidogrel, two other drugs that inhibit platelet plug formation, are approved for treatment of patients with PAD. Ticlopidine is prescribed less often because of hematologic side effects (see Chapter 57). Clopidogrel has fewer side effects (although rare instances of thrombotic thrombocytopenic purpura have been reported [24]) and has been shown to be slightly more effective than aspirin in preventing progression of PAD (25). Nevertheless, aspirin at present is the more cost-effective drug.

Vasodilator Drugs. There is no objective evidence to suggest that vasodilating drugs are beneficial to patients with PAD. Blood vessels in ischemic tissue beds are already maximally dilated. When systemic vessels are dilated by these drugs, blood flow to the compromised extremity may actually decrease. Therefore, these drugs are not recommended for treatment of patients with PAD.

Pentoxifylline. This drug is a xanthine derivative that has been used for many years to treat patients with PAD. It decreases blood viscosity by a direct effect on the red blood cell membrane. Enough data have now accumulated to show that pentoxifylline (typically one 400-mg tablet three times a day) has little, if any, effect in reducing symptoms in patients with PAD and probably should not be prescribed (10).

Cilostazol. This drug is a phosphodiesterase inhibitor that has relatively recently been approved for treatment of PAD. Its mechanism of action is unknown, although it does affect platelet and endothelial function. A number of controlled trials have shown the drug to be effective in improving exercise tolerance in patients with PAD (10,26). A standard dosing schedule is 100 mg (50- and 100-mg tablets are available) twice a day. Because cilostazol inhibits several hepatic drug-metabolizing enzymes, its daily dosage should be lowered if drugs metabolized by those enzymes (e.g., erythromycin or omeprazole) are concomitantly prescribed. The major side effects reported by the manufacturer are headache (up to 34% of patients), diarrhea (up to 19% of patients), and palpitations (up to 10% of patients). Cilostazol is contraindicated in patients with congestive heart failure of any severity.

Anticoagulant Drugs. There is no evidence that heparin or warfarin has any beneficial effect in patients with PAD (27) except in reducing the incidence of embolization in patients with atrial fibrillation (see Chapters 57 and 64).

Operative Intervention

It is only upon failure of nonoperative therapy and among patients with clear indications for surgery that arteriographic studies are obtained. It must be understood that arteriography serves as a roadmap for the vascular surgeon when reconstructing the vascular tree. No characteristic arteriographic findings distinguish between patients with intermittent claudication, those with ischemic rest pain, and those with gangrene and ulceration. As a generalization, however, patients who have intermittent claudication usually have hemodynamically significant proximal arterial occlusive lesions affecting the iliofemoral or the femoral–popliteal system. Characteristically, such patients have reasonably good outflow with two or more tibial vessels patent. Patients with advanced ischemic changes are found to have diffuse multisegment involvement and none or only one patent tibial vessel in the lower leg or foot. However, there is considerable overlap between groups, and no single arteriographic finding consistently characterizes any one symptom complex.

Arteriography occasionally demonstrates a distribution of advanced arterial involvement without a reasonable runoff vessels for bypass. Under these circumstances, nonoperative therapy is all that may be offered, and there is a significant risk of subsequent amputation.

Indications for operation among patients with intermittent claudication relate mainly to the ability of the patient to tolerate the pain. Nonlimiting claudication and mild ischemic rest pain that is controlled by non-narcotic analgesics are not indications for operation, particularly in high-risk patients. A trial of conservative management is especially important if other risk factors, such as recent myocardial infarction, are present.

When it is determined that the condition of the patient warrants operative intervention and when arteriography documents adequate outflow vessels, a number of options for arterial reconstruction are open to the vascular surgeon, including autogenous vein or prosthetic graft bypass and endarterectomy. There is a definite preference for bypass surgery rather than endarterectomy. Direct reconstructive procedures include aortofemoral bypass, femoral–popliteal bypass, and femoral–tibial bypass. Extra-anatomic reconstruction includes axillounifemoral bypass, axillobifemoral bypass, and femoral–femoral bypass.

The operative mortality rate for aortofemoral bypass grafting is less than 5% with a patency rate of 80% to 90% at 5 years (8). Operative mortality for extra-anatomic reconstructions is slightly less than for aortofemoral bypass, but the outlook for graft patency is not as good. Operative mortality for autogenous vein femoral–popliteal and femoral–tibial bypass procedures ranges from 0.5% to 1% depending on the general condition of the patient (8,28). Five-year patency rates for such procedures vary between 60% and 70% (8,28), and it should be emphasized that patency varies directly with adequacy of the vein used and the extent of the disease in the vessel being reconstructed.

In general, in contrast to aneurysmal disease, arterial reconstruction for occlusive disease is palliative and does not significantly increase the patient's life expectancy because most patients have significant coincident coronary artery disease. However, the quality of life may be vastly improved by surgery, particularly for those who would have undergone amputation if successful arterial reconstruction had not been feasible.

Patients with aortofemoral arterial occlusive disease who do not have coronary artery disease or diabetes mellitus have survival rates that equal those of the normal age- and sex-adjusted population. It appears that the presence of coronary artery disease reduces life expectancy by approximately 10 years, and the presence of diabetes mellitus reduces life expectancy by an additional 15 years (29).

Balloon Angioplasty, Stents, and Laser and Mechanical Atherectomy

Percutaneous transluminal arterial dilation (angioplasty) is used as an alternative to surgical reconstruction for highly selected patients with arterial occlusive disease. It is a technique that uses a catheter with an attached balloon to dilate the stenosed artery. Advantages include lower morbidity, lower mortality, and possibly lower cost compared with arterial reconstruction. Patients who are not candidates for surgery, if subjected to percutaneous transluminal angioplasty, could conceivably require operation if complications occur after the percutaneous procedure. Therefore, a cooperative approach between the interventional radiologist and the vascular surgeon is mandatory.

Most authors agree that the best results with percutaneous transluminal angioplasty are obtained in patients with short segment stenoses of the iliac arteries, in which success rates range from 76% to 93% at 1 year and from 66% to 92% at 2 years. The reported results of angioplasty for femoropopliteal disease range from 51% to 80% at 1 year and from 46% to 75% at 2 years. There is general agreement that results are less satisfactory if the arteriographic runoff is poor. In the properly selected patient, the probability of early success of percutaneous transluminal angioplasty is high if the involved vessel is the iliac artery, there is a short segment of stenosis and not occlusion, and the runoff is good (30). Results are less satisfactory when multiple dilations are required. Results of angioplasty are improving with the advent of *metallic stents* placed at the time of initial balloon angioplasty or at repeat angioplasty in the event of restenosis.

Patients with longer stenoses and total occlusions have less favorable outcomes, but in very poor-risk patients, angioplasty may be the only alternative to operative reconstruction. Occlusions less than 5 cm long and stenoses less than 10 cm long appear to be the outer limits for successful percutaneous transluminal angioplasty.

Amputation

In debilitated patients with frank gangrene or unremitting ischemic rest pain in whom arterial reconstruction or transluminal angioplasty is not indicated or feasible, amputation is the only alternative. The goal of amputation is to relieve the patient of disabling pain, remove nonviable and potentially infected tissue, and select a level that will provide the greatest chance of healing with maximal prosthetic rehabilitation.

If the gangrenous process is dry and does not involve the great toe, autoamputation may be allowed to occur or formal surgical amputation may be performed. If pulses are palpable in the foot and the ischemic process affects the tips of the digits, primary healing usually occurs after toe amputation. Nonischemic neurotrophic ulcers on the plantar aspects of the foot in diabetic patients often heal if the head of the metatarsal is removed to relieve the pressure necrosis that occurs as a result of the diabetic neuropathy.

Mortality for amputation is directly related to the preoperative condition of the patient and to other complicating diseases. Mortality rates for amputations performed for occlusive arterial disease have been reported to be as high as 30%, with higher mortality rates recorded in the more proximal amputations.

After successful amputation, which includes primary healing that results in a stump amenable to prosthetic fitting, the most important aspect of therapy is rehabilitation. Prosthetic mobility requires almost twice as much energy with an above-knee amputation than with a below-knee amputation, and mobility is further inhibited by increased age, infirmity, obesity, and a poorly fitting prosthesis. It is difficult to predict successful rehabilitation in the atherosclerotic population, but cooperation between the surgeon and the rehabilitation team is pivotal to a satisfactory outcome.

ABDOMINAL AORTIC ANEURYSMS

An aneurysm, a blood-filled dilatation of a blood vessel, is generally defined as a 50% increase in diameter of a blood vessel. In the infrarenal abdominal aorta, a diameter of greater than 4 cm is also considered diagnostic of an aneurysm. The recognized incidence of abdominal aortic aneurysms (AAAs) has increased with the advent of sensitive and specific diagnostic noninvasive tests such as ultrasonography, computed tomography (CT), and magnetic resonance imaging (MRI).

The most common site of an arterial aneurysm is the abdominal aorta. AAA is encountered two to three times more often than the second most common type, the popliteal artery aneurysm, and has been found in almost 2% of consecutive postmortem studies (31).

Etiology and Natural History

An AAA is a disease of the media characterized by degeneration of extracellular matrix proteins, which maintain the integrity of the vessel wall. AAAs are most often infrarenal (75%). Only 5% involve the suprarenal aorta, and 25% involve the iliac arteries (32).

The highest prevalence of such aneurysms is in white males greater than 65 years old (33). Age-adjusted incidence is fourfold to sixfold higher in men than in women for both asymptomatic and ruptured AAAs.

The relationship between AAA and atherosclerosis is not clear. It is not known why some patients develop atherosclerosis and calcification of the abdominal aorta and some develop aneurysmal dilatation. Recently, genetic factors have been found to play a role (34). The prevalence of AAA is 1% in elderly siblings of subjects without AAA and increases fourfold in siblings of subjects who have AAA (35).

Tobacco use is the risk factor most strongly associated with AAA (36). Smokers with small AAAs (4 to 5.5 cm) have been found to have an increased risk of rupture (1.9%/yr versus 0.5%/yr for nonsmokers) and poorer long-term survival.

Our understanding of the *natural history* of AAA is clouded by early studies (37) that documented high risks of rupture but included more patients with large aneurysms than patients with smaller ones. This is important, because the risk of rupture is related to the size of the aneurysm (38). The advent of noninvasive screening techniques has allowed the detection of small asymptomatic aneurysms and improved our understanding of the rate of growth and risk of rupture of AAAs. Studies that have prospectively followed AAA size indicate that the average rate of expansion is 0.3 to 0.4 cm/yr, with a range of 0.24 to 0.9 cm/yr (39–41). The risk of rupture is negligible for AAAs less than 4.0 cm but increases significantly when the aneurysm reaches a size of 5.0 cm or more or when the rate of expansion is more than 0.5 to 1.0 cm in 6 to 12 months (42). Thus, whereas early studies demonstrated improved life expectancy with surgical treatment of AAA (41,43), more recent studies have suggested that early surgery may not offer a long-term survival advantage for patients with small asymptomatic aneurysms, who may be followed with serial ultrasound examinations (39) (see Treatment and Results, below).

Clinical Manifestations

History

The presentation of an AAA depends on whether complications have occurred. More than 50% are asymptomatic when first discovered during routine examination by a caregiver, by the patient who complains of a second heart in the abdomen upon palpating a pulsatile epigastric mass, or serendipitously during radiographic or ultrasonographic abdominal studies in the pursuit of another diagnosis. The patient may complain of abdominal, flank, or back pain as the aneurysm expands and becomes symptomatic, a harbinger of rupture.

Most aneurysms that *rupture* bleed into the retroperitoneal space, affording life-saving tamponade. Under these circumstances, the patient presents with a history of syncope or of flank or back pain in a hypovolemic, but not necessarily a hypotensive, state. On the other hand, the patient with an uncontained intraperitoneal rupture of an AAA typically presents in shock secondary to blood loss and requires immediate operative intervention. Aneurysms may rupture into adjacent structures and cause large arteriovenous fistulas, such as an aortocaval or aortorenal fistula with high-output cardiac failure, or into the gastrointestinal tract, usually the duodenum, causing an aortoenteric fistula with massive hematemesis or hematochezia.

Other complications. If aneurysms are large enough, they may produce symptoms due to compression of adjacent structures such as the ureter, duodenum, vena cava, or vertebral column. Dislodgment of laminated clots from the wall of the aneurysm occasionally may cause peripheral embolization to femoral, popliteal, or distal vessels. When emboli occur, patients may complain of symptoms of sudden leg ischemia as the first indication of AAA (see below). If emboli are small and distal vessels are patent, small areas of tissue necrosis in the toes or skin of the lower extremities are seen.

After seeking specific historical information regarding the aneurysm, the patient should be questioned about other symptoms so that an estimate of the extent of atherosclerotic involvement is obtained. This information often influences recommendations for or against surgical therapy (see Chapter 93). Symptoms of transient cerebral ischemia or previous stroke, angina pectoris or previous myocardial infarction, or cardiac decompensation such as significant severe shortness of breath, ankle edema, orthopnea, and paroxysmal nocturnal dyspnea are especially important in determining the risks in this group of patients.

Physical Examination

Abdominal palpation is only moderately sensitive and specific in the diagnosis of an AAA (44). As previously noted, most patients with asymptomatic AAAs are discovered on routine physical examination to have an epigastric or left upper quadrant pulsatile mass. However, a pulsatile mass may not be palpable in obese patients or in those with very small aneurysms. Typically, asymptomatic aneurysms may be discovered when x-rays are obtained to evaluate other intra-abdominal conditions.

It is important to palpate the epigastrium because the bifurcation of the abdominal aorta is at the level of the umbilicus. Only rarely when palpating inferior to the umbilicus will one identify an AAA unless both common iliac arteries are also aneurysmal. The laterally pulsatile nature of an aneurysm is a clue in differentiating it from the anteriorly transmitted aortic pulsation through viscera or from a mass overlying the aorta. Conditions confused with aneurysms include pancreatic pseudocyst, horseshoe kidneys, neoplasms of the stomach or transverse colon, and retroperitoneal soft tissue tumors. Often, a normal but prominently pulsatile abdominal aorta in a healthy person and an undilated but tortuous aorta in an elderly person may simulate an AAA. In this circumstance, the pulsatile mass is felt to the left of the midline but not to the right. One should palpate the abdomen by approaching the midline both from the right and from the left to identify the laterally pulsatile characteristic of an aneurysm. Risk of rupture correlates best with the size of the aneurysm as determined by ultrasonography and not by physical examination alone (see below).

One-fourth to one-third of patients have significant associated occlusive arterial disease as well as the AAA, so a systematic evaluation should be performed. Systemic blood pressure should be measured in both arms. Carotid bruits can be detected by listening with the bell of the stethoscope over the carotid bifurcations at the angle of the mandible with the patient supine and holding his or her breath. Examination of the lower extremities should be directed to the character of the femoral, popliteal, and pedal pulses and to the presence or absence of femoral and popliteal bruits and aneurysms. In less than 10% of patients with AAA, there may be coexistent peripheral aneurysms involving the popliteal or femoral arteries.

Laboratory and Radiographic Studies

The presence or absence of an AAA must be confirmed by ultrasonography. The accuracy of sonographic diagnosis of AAAs approaches 100% (45). Anteroposterior and cross-table lateral plain x-rays of the abdomen also document AAAs in 70% to 80% of cases because the aneurysm wall is often calcified. Ultrasonography is simple, safe, and cost effective and is recommended as the method of choice for verifying or excluding an AAA and for serial follow-up every 6 months to assess aneurysmal size for patients being treated nonoperatively.

CT and MRI are more expensive and should be used only as an adjunct to ultrasonography for confirming unusual situations, such as a suspected leak in an otherwise stable patient, extent of visceral artery involvement, inflammatory change, or the presence and characteristics of horseshoe kidney. Generally, the cost of a CT is about double that of a sonogram. The MRI costs twice as much as the CT and rarely provides additional information.

Objective measurement of peripheral pulses in the lower extremities and baseline Doppler blood flow studies are of value during long-term follow-up. Because atherosclerotic disease may be progressive, the patient should be followed on a yearly basis after convalescence from surgery.

Treatment and Results

Whereas patients with symptomatic AAAs require operative intervention, it is not clear that early surgery improves mortality in patients with small asymptomatic aneurysms in whom a strategy of "watchful waiting" may be reasonable. In one study, 1,090 patients aged 60 to 76 years with asymptomatic AAA between 4.0 and 5.5 cm in diameter were randomly assigned to undergo elective surgery or serial ultrasonographic surveillance every 6 months. Surgery was recommended to patients randomized to the surveillance strategy if the AAA diameter exceeded 5.5 cm. After an average of 4.6 years, there was no difference in mortality between the groups (39). The decision about when, and if, to recommend surgery to patients with asymptomatic AAA depends on the assessment of the risk of rupture compared with the risk of elective operative repair (46). The risk of rupture, in turn, is most closely related to AAA size and rate of expansion. Patients with an AAA less than 5.5 cm in diameter may be followed by serial ultrasound examinations performed at 6-month intervals. If the aneurysm exceeds 5.5 cm or if the rate of expansion exceeds 0.5 cm in a 6-month interval, the risk of rupture should be considered high and elective surgery should be strongly considered. When surgery is not recommended, therapy with beta-blockers should be considered in an effort to reduce the rate of AAA expansion. This recommendation is based largely on a single study of 121 patients with AAA (approximately two-thirds of whom received beta-blockers) who were monitored with serial ultrasound examinations approximately every 8 months for an average of 43 months. Among patients with AAA 5 cm or greater, beta-blockers significantly reduced the expansion rate from 0.68 to 0.36 cm/yr (40).

Controversy exists regarding the routine use of preoperative aortography among patients with AAAs. Although some surgeons routinely recommend aortography, most use aortographic studies selectively. Under certain circumstances abdominal aortography is helpful and even mandatory. Indications for aortography include the possibility of anomalous renal or visceral vasculature or occlusive disease involving these same vessels that would alter the operative approach. It is important to determine the extent of reconstruction necessary so that the anomalous vessels are not violated and the occlusive lesions are addressed. Drug-resistant renovascular hypertension is an indication for aortography to document renal artery stenosis that can be corrected at the time of abdominal aortic aneurysmectomy. Aortography is essential for delineation of the anomalous circulation of the rare horseshoe kidney initially detected by ultrasonography. Alternatively, spiral CT and three-dimensional reconstruction could be considered instead of aortography.

It is essential to inform the patient of various risks of operative versus nonoperative treatment. Equally important is explaining complications that may occur in the postoperative period. Although this is primarily the responsibility of the operating surgeon, it is appropriate for the primary clinician to discuss with the patient what is likely to occur. The patient should know that a Dacron or polytetrafluorethylene prosthesis will be used to replace the abdominal aorta and that such arterial grafts are very durable. Fortunately, complications are rare and include (but are not limited to) paraplegia from spinal cord ischemia, renal failure, amputation, graft infection, ischemic colitis, and aortoenteric fistula. It should be stressed to the patient that postoperative complications of abdominal aortic aneurysmectomy are magnified by the urgency of the operative procedure.

Endovascular stent-grafting of AAAs is a new investigative approach. This technique uses an endoprosthesis that is delivered percutaneously through the femoral artery and deployed in the area of the aneurysm. The endograft is secured with metallic expandable stents and thrombosis of the external surrounding aneurysm, in theory, reduces the risk of rupture. To date, the most common adverse long-term problem with the current devices is "endoleak," which represents persistent filling of the AAA from either the anastomotic site or through other collateral blood vessels (42). These devices remain investigational only. To date, there are no Food and Drug Administration-approved AAA endovascular stents in the United States.

If operation is not recommended or accepted, the patient should be evaluated every 3 to 6 months by interval history, physical examination, and ultrasonography. A patient with a rupturing or symptomatic aneurysm complains of steady dull abdominal, flank, or back pain. If such pain occurs or if a change in existing symptoms is noted in a patient being followed with an AAA, the patient should be instructed to seek surgical attention promptly.

PERIPHERAL ARTERIAL ANEURYSMS

Peripheral arterial aneurysms may involve the carotid, subclavian, brachial, iliac, femoral, and popliteal arteries. More than 90% of peripheral aneurysms involve either popliteal or femoral arteries. Popliteal arterial aneurysms predominate. Tortuous vessels presenting as serpiginous pulsations under the skin may be mistaken for peripheral aneurysms. The most noted example of this is a tortuous subclavian or common carotid artery in an elderly hypertensive patient that may be confused with a carotid or subclavian artery aneurysm. The pathogenesis of peripheral aneurysms is unknown. There is a male predominance (30:1 ratio, men versus women) and up to 50% are bilateral (47).

Most peripheral arterial aneurysms are arteriosclerotic in origin; mycotic, traumatic, and syphilitic aneurysms are rare. Peripheral arteriosclerotic aneurysms are localized manifestations of a generalized disease process. This is underscored by noting that among a group of 37 patients with common femoral aneurysms, 95% had another aneurysm elsewhere and 92% had associated aortoiliac aneurysms (48). Femoral aneurysms can be bilateral in up to 60% of cases. Similarly, among 36 patients with popliteal arterial aneurysms, almost 80% had an aneurysm elsewhere, two-thirds had aortoiliac aneurysms, and bilateral popliteal aneurysms occurred in 50% of these patients (48). Therefore, when a peripheral aneurysm is found, the clinician should be aware that they can be multiple and bilateral, and the popliteal, femoral, and aortoiliac areas should be carefully assessed by physical examination and ultrasonography.

Femoral and, particularly, popliteal arterial aneurysms are associated with a high incidence of distal thromboembolism and eventual limb loss. Untreated peripheral aneurysms may eventuate in limb loss approximately 75% of the time from either distal embolization or acute thrombosis. On the other hand, rupture with exsanguinating hemorrhage is not a major risk with femoral or popliteal arterial aneurysms as it is for AAAs.

Clinical Manifestations

Most patients with peripheral arterial aneurysms are elderly, and many are asymptomatic. Femoral arterial aneurysms are usually evident, particularly when they measure 4 or 5 cm in diameter. Similarly, popliteal aneurysms, if they are large, are easily identified. However, popliteal aneurysms may be overlooked because many clinicians do not routinely palpate the popliteal fossa during a physical examination. Approximately 50% of femoral and popliteal aneurysms present with limb-threatening complications of thrombosis, embolization, or rupture. Hence, the discovery of an asymptomatic aneurysm in these anatomic areas is a clear indication for timely repair. Once complications of peripheral aneurysms develop, there is a 25% risk of limb amputation.

An enlarged artery with a very prominent femoral or popliteal pulse to physical examination is characteristic of a femoral or popliteal aneurysm and should be confirmed by ultrasonography. Diagnosis of femoral aneurysm is easily made on clinical examination alone, but the diagnosis of popliteal aneurysm may be more difficult. When the popliteal fossa is palpated, the patient's leg should be relaxed while the examiner passively flexes the knee with the fingers, compressing the popliteal artery in the fossa, and the thumbs on the patella, giving counter-compression. If an unusually prominent popliteal pulsatile mass is palpated and the examiner suspects aneurysm, the patient may be placed in the prone position and the lower leg supported by the examiner's arm to facilitate popliteal arterial palpation. Ultrasonography should be obtained for anything remotely suspicious because diagnosis and treatment before the occurrence of complications are exceedingly important. Occasionally, the only manifestations of a popliteal aneurysm are small punctate necrotic areas of skin over the anterior tibial region or small gangrenous areas of the tips of toes. This "blue toe syndrome" is a result of microemboli from the aneurysm that have showered to the periphery.

Once the diagnosis of a peripheral arterial aneurysm is made, the patient should be referred to a vascular surgeon. Arteriography is mandatory to confirm the anatomy and patency of the femoral–popliteal and tibial arteries when planning operative intervention.

Treatment and Results

Treatment of symptomatic peripheral aneurysms is indicated in all instances. Because the natural history is one of eventual limb loss, it is important to offer surgical therapy in most cases to maintain or improve quality of life by avoiding amputation. Surgical correction includes replacement of femoral aneurysms with prosthetic or reversed autogenous saphenous vein grafts. Similarly, popliteal aneurysms are managed by bypassing the diseased segment with autogenous saphenous vein.

Operative mortality for management of peripheral aneurysms is approximately 1% to 3%. Limb salvage is obtained in more than 90% of cases and is related to the degree of arterial involvement peripheral to the aneurysm. In almost all series reporting repair of popliteal aneurysms, amputations in the postoperative period have been associated with severe occlusive arterial disease manifested by gangrene and rest pain preoperatively.

General References*

Boyd AM. The natural course of arteriosclerosis of the lower extremities. Angiology 1960;11:10.

This study of 1,440 patients with intermittent claudication, carefully evaluated and followed over 15 years, for the first time documented the natural history of intermittent claudication. This study provides the control database against which results of surgical and nonsurgical therapy are judged.

Crawford ES, Saleh SA, Babb JW III, et al. Infrarenal abdominal aortic aneurysm: factors influencing survival after operation performed over a 25-year period. Ann Surg 1981;193:699.

Experience of an outstanding vascular surgical group that evaluated 920 consecutive patients operated on for abdominal aortic aneurysm. This article is the gold standard against which the results of others are measured.

Ernst CB. Abdominal aortic aneurysm. N Engl J Med 1993;328:1167.

An excellent review.

Rutherford RB, ed. Vascular surgery. 5th ed. Philadelphia: WB Saunders, 2000.

The first comprehensive text of vascular surgery. Specific disease entities are extensively discussed, including nonoperative and operative aspects. Basic pathophysiologic concepts are lucidly presented. This work should be in the library of all interested in vascular diseases.

Wilt TJ. Clinical strategies in the diagnosis and management of lower extremity peripheral vascular disease. J Gen Intern Med 1992;7:87.

A well-referenced review.

Yao RST, Pearce WH, eds. Progress in vascular surgery. Stanford, CT: Appleton & Lange, 1997.

Excellent review of emerging diagnostic and therapeutic modalities.

Specific References

1. Kempczinski RF. Lower extremity arterial emboli from ulcerating atherosclerotic plaques. JAMA 1979;241:807.
2. Ouriel K, Veith FJ, Sasahara AA. A comparison of recombinant urokinase with vascular surgery as initial treatment for acute arterial occlusion of the legs. Thrombolysis or Peripheral Arterial Surgery (TOPAS) Investigators. N Engl J Med 1998;338:1105.
3. Jackson MR, Clagett GP. Antithrombotic therapy in peripheral arterial occlusive disease. Chest 2001;119:2835.
4. Results of a prospective randomized trial evaluating surgery versus thrombolysis for ischemia of the lower extremity. The STILE trial. Ann Surg 1994;220:251.
5. Braithwaite BD, Davies B, Birch PA, et al. Management of acute leg ischaemia in the elderly. Br J Surg 1998;85:217.
6. Vogt MT, Wolfson SK, Kuller LH. Lower extremity arterial disease and the aging process: a review. J Clin Epidemiol 1992; 45:529.
7. Dormandy J, Mahir M, Ascady G, et al. Fate of the patient with chronic leg ischaemia: a review article. J Cardiovasc Surg 1989;30:50.
8. Weitz JI, Byrne J, Clagett GP, et al. Diagnosis and treatment of chronic arterial insufficiency of the lower extremities: a critical review. Circulation 1996;94:3026.

*Bold print (general references) and bold numerals (specific references) denote published controlled clinical trials, meta-analyses, or consensus-based recommendations.

9. Kannel WB, McGee DL. Update on some epidemiologic features of intermittent claudication: the Framingham Study. J Am Geriatr Soc 1985;33:13.
10. Hiatt WR. Medical treatment of peripheral arterial disease and claudication. N Engl J Med 2001;344:1608.
11. Jonason T, Ringqvist I. Factors of prognostic importance for subsequent rest pain in patients with intermittent claudication. Act Med Scand 1985;218:27.
12. Hughson WG, Mann JI, Garrod A. Intermittent claudication: prevalence and risk factors. Br Med J 1978;1:1379.
13. Boyd AM. The natural course of arteriosclerosis of the lower extremities. Angiology 1960;11:10.
14. Imparato AM, Kim G-E, Davidson T, et al. Intermittent claudication: its natural course. Surgery 1975;78:795.
15. Juergens JC, Barker NW, Hines EA. Arteriosclerosis obliterans. Review of 520 cases with special reference to pathogenic and prognostic factors. Circulation 1960;21:188.
16. Criqui MH, Denenberg JO, Langer RD, et al. The epidemiology of peripheral arterial disease: importance of identifying the population at risk. Vasc Med 1997;2:221.
17. Yao JST. Hemodynamic studies in peripheral arterial disease. Br J Surg 1970;57:561.
18. Dormandy JA, Rutherford RB. Management of peripheral arterial disease (PAD). TransAtlantic Inter-Society consensus (TASC) Working Group. J Vasc Surg 2000;31[Suppl 1]:S1.
19. Pallerito JS, Taylor KJ. Doppler color imaging. Peripheral arteries. Clin Diagn Ultrasound 1992;27:97.
20. Quick CR, Cotton LT. The measured effect of stopping smoking on intermittent claudication. Br J Surg 1982;69:S24.
21. Radack K, Deck C. Beta-adrenergic blocker therapy does not worsen intermittent claudication in subjects with peripheral arterial disease: a meta-analysis of randomized controlled trials. Arch Intern Med 1991;151:1769.
22. Joint National Committee. The Sixth Report of the Joint National Committee on Detection, Evaluation, and Treatment of High Blood Pressure (JNC-VI). Arch Intern Med 1997;157: 2413.
23. Food and Drug Administration. Internal analgesic, antipyretic, and antirheumatic drug products for over-the-counter human use: final rule for professional labeling of aspirin, buffered aspirin, and aspirin in combination with antacid drug products. Federal Register 1998;63:56802.
24. Bennett CL, Connors JM, Cariwile JM, et al. Thrombotic thrombocytopenic purpura associated with clopidogrel. N Engl J Med 2000;342:1773.
25. CAPRIE Steering Committee. A randomized, blinded, trial of clopidogrel versus aspirin in patients at risk of ischaemic events (CAPRIE). Lancet 1996;348:1329.
26. Dawson DL, Cutler BS, Hiatt WR, et al. A comparison of cilostazol and pentoxifylline for treating intermittent claudication. Am J Med 2000;109:523.
27. Clagett GP, Graor RA, Salzman EW. Antithrombotic therapy in peripheral arterial occlusive disease. Chest 1992;102[Suppl 4]:516S.
28. Taylor LM Jr, Edwards JM, Porter JM. Present status of reversed vein bypass grafting: five-year results of a modern series. J Vasc Surg 1990;11:193.
29. Malone JM, Moore WS, Goldstone J. Life expectancy following aortofemoral arterial grafting. Surgery 1977;81:551.
30. Lally ME, Johnston KW, Andrews D. Percutaneous transluminal dilatation of peripheral arteries: an analysis of factors predicting early success. J Vasc Surg 1984;1:704.
31. Carlsson J, Sternby NH. Aortic aneurysms. Acta Clin Scand 1964;127:466.
32. Olsen PS, Schroeder T, Agerskov K, et al. Surgery for abdominal aortic aneurysms: a survey of 656 patients. J Cardiovasc Surg 1991;32:636.
33. Hallett JW Jr. Abdominal aortic aneurysm: natural history and treatment. Heart Dis Stroke 1992;1:303.
34. Marian AJ. On genetics, inflammation and abdominal aortic aneurysm. Circulation 2001;103:2222.
35. Baird PA, Sadovnick AD, Yee IM, et al. Sibling risks of abdominal aortic aneurysm. Lancet 1995;346:601.
36. UK Small Aneurysm Trial Participants. Smoking, lung function and the prognosis of abdominal aortic aneurysm. Eur J Vasc Endovasc Surg 2000;19:626.
37. Estes JE. Abdominal aortic aneurysm. A study of 102 cases. Circulation 1950;2:258.
38. Szilagyi DE, Smith R, DeRusso FJ, et al. Contribution of abdominal aortic aneurysmectomy to prolongation of life. Ann Surg 1966;164:678.
39. The UK Small Aneurysm Trial Participants. Mortality results for randomised controlled trial of early elective surgery of ultrasonographic surveillance for small abdominal aortic aneurysms. Lancet 1998;352:1649.
40. Gadowski GR, Pilcher DB, Ricci MA. Abdominal aortic aneurysm expansion rate: effect of size and beta-adrenergic blockade. J Vasc Surg 1994;19:727.
41. Nevitt MP, Ballard DJ, Hallett JW Jr. Prognosis of abdominal aortic aneurysm: a population-based study. N Engl J Med 1989;321:1009.
42. Hallett JW Jr. Management of abdominal aortic aneurysm. Mayo Clin Proc 2000;75:395.
43. Szilagyi DE, Elliott JP, Smith RF. Clinical fate of the patient with asymptomatic abdominal aortic aneurysm and unfit for surgical treatment. Arch Surg 1972;104:600.
44. Fink HA, Lederle FA, Roth CS, et al. The accuracy of physical examination to detect abdominal aortic aneurysm. Arch Intern Med 2000;160:833.
45. La Roy LL, Cormier PJ, Matalon TA, et al. Imaging of abdominal aortic aneurysms. AJR Am J Roentgenol 1989;152:785.
46. Katz DA, Littenberg B, Cronenwett JL. Management of small abdominal aortic aneurysms. Early surgery vs watchful waiting. JAMA 1992;268:2678.
47. Dawson I, Sie RB, Van Bockel JH. Atherosclerotic popliteal aneurysm. Br J Surg 1997;84:293.
48. Dent TL, Lindenauer SM, Ernst CB, et al. Multiple arteriosclerotic arterial aneurysms. Arch Surg 1972;105;338.

CHAPTER 95

Lower Extremity Ulcers and Varicose Veins

JAMES M. WONG, MD
ROBERT J. SPENCE, MD
CALVIN E. JONES, JR., MD

LOWER EXTREMITY ULCERS

Ulceration of the lower extremity, most often caused by either macrovascular or microvascular disease, is a common and important problem in ambulatory medical practice. Accurate diagnosis is based mainly on history and physical examination and is essential for appropriate treatment. Inappropriate therapy can lead to the loss of a toe or even a limb. Generally, it is necessary to give detailed instructions to the patient and to have a great deal of patience. Patient compliance with treatment has been shown to be critical in the success of therapy and the prevention of recurrent ulceration (1).

History

A complete general medical history is extremely important. Illnesses such as arteriosclerotic vascular disease or hypertension, diabetes mellitus, sickle cell disease, and collagen-vascular disease may be associated with ulcers of the lower extremities. A history of corticosteroid therapy may explain failure of ulcers to heal. A history of drug abuse or a psychiatric history may be pertinent in the explanation of factitious ulcers.

Specific attention should be paid to duration of ulceration and previous attempts at therapy; symptoms of peripheral arterial vascular disease, such as intermittent calf claudication, intermittent thigh or gluteal claudication, impotence, calf pain at rest, and feelings of coldness and tingling in the legs; a history of deep vein thrombosis, ulceration, or injury to the lower extremities; and a history of discomfort associated with footwear or of chronic swelling, and, if swelling has occurred, whether it has been alleviated by lying down.

Ischemic pain in the calf at rest is usually a symptom of advanced peripheral arterial disease, and it is characteristically alleviated if the patient dangles his or her feet over the edge of the bed or sits in a chair when awakened at night by ischemic pain. These symptoms must be differentiated from *nocturnal leg cramps* that occur in many people who have no evidence of peripheral vascular disease. Leg cramps are usually accompanied by palpable hardening of the calf muscles and involuntary muscle contraction of the flexor muscles of the toes. The cramps usually are relieved if the patient gets out of bed and walks around. Examination of the extremities in these patients (see below) is usually normal.

Physical Examination

A general physical examination of the patient is undertaken in conjunction with the examination of the lower extremities. The general examination should include a search particularly for abdominal aortic aneurysm and other intra-abdominal masses, lymphatic masses in the groin, and signs of long-standing hypertension and cardiac disease. Needle tracks and brawny indurated hands may indicate a history of drug abuse, as may skin ulcers in areas other than the lower extremities.

Examination of the Lower Extremities

Both lower extremities should be bared. Initial examination is performed while the patient is supine. Both legs are examined and compared. Particular points to be noted include the following:

1. The presence of *pitting or nonpitting edema*. Pitting edema is a sign of chronic venous obstruction or of an acute inflammatory process. Nonpitting edema is a sign of lymphatic obstruction. If edema is present, it is important to note whether it is unilateral, and if it is bilateral, whether it is asymmetric or symmetric. Very firm brawny edema suggests a long-standing process.
2. The presence of *hemosiderin* deposited in the skin of the ankles (a sign of venous insufficiency).
3. The *general appearance* and quality of the skin, including hair growth (hair loss may signify arterial insufficiency).
4. Evidence of *fungal infection* (scaling, apparently pruritic lesions).
5. The *status of the nails* (deformity and hypertrophy are associated with arterial insufficiency).

After inspection of the feet and legs, a vascular examination of the lower extremities is conducted. Femoral, popliteal, dorsalis pedis, and posterior tibial pulses are palpated and graded. The *capillary refill time* after pressure on the toes with the legs elevated 45 degrees is observed (normally less than 5 seconds). Auscultation from the mid-abdomen down to the popliteal regions is performed to detect bruits that are produced by narrowed atherosclerotic arteries. The temperature of the legs is felt with the dorsum of the hand, both descending from the thigh to the foot and comparing one side with the other. The patient is asked to sit up and to dangle his or her legs so that venous filling time and dependent rubor can be assessed. Evidence of *varicose veins* is best sought with the patient standing.

Inspection and Palpation of Ulcer or Ulcers

Ulcerated areas on the legs are often very tender; palpation, although necessary, should be done gently, with the gloved hand.

Site. An accurate description of the site of the ulcer, preferably with reference to an anatomic landmark (e.g., the medial or the lateral malleolus), should be recorded.

Size. The size of the ulcer must be documented. The vertical and horizontal diameter in millimeters should be noted in the patient's record in a reproducible fashion. This measurement is particularly important for future reference when the progress of healing and the efficacy of treatment are assessed. Only by measuring in millimeters can the often subtle changes be appreciated in future evaluations.

General Character. It should be noted whether the ulcer is regular or irregular in outline. The edges should be examined to determine whether they are raised, heaped, everted, or flat and whether they are undermined or there is any evidence of epithelial ingrowth from the edge of the ulcer toward the center (i.e., healing). The base should be examined to see whether it is clean or covered with exudate and to see the type of tissue of which it is constituted (e.g., clean fascia, granulation tissue, dirty exudate, debris). The vascularity of the base is the most critical characteristic to be noted when considering the potential of the ulcer for healing.

Tenderness. If the ulcer is tender, it should be determined whether it is very tender, such as in acute inflammation or ischemia, or only mildly tender, as in a neuropathy with loss of superficial sensation.

Changes in Adjoining Skin. It should be noted whether there are fluctuant areas of purulence near the ulcer, particularly on the sole of the foot; any callosities surrounding the ulcer; heavy deposition of pigment near the ulcer; or local edema.

When the examination of the ulcer is completed, the patient should stand, preferably on a stool, and face the examiner. Edema should now be looked for, as should the presence of varicose veins along the course of the short and long saphenous veins on the front and back of the legs (Fig. 95.1). In particular, the appearance of perforator varicosities (see Physical Examination, under Varicose Veins, below) should be noted, usually above the medial malleolus, and the relationship of these perforators to ulcerated areas should be sought.

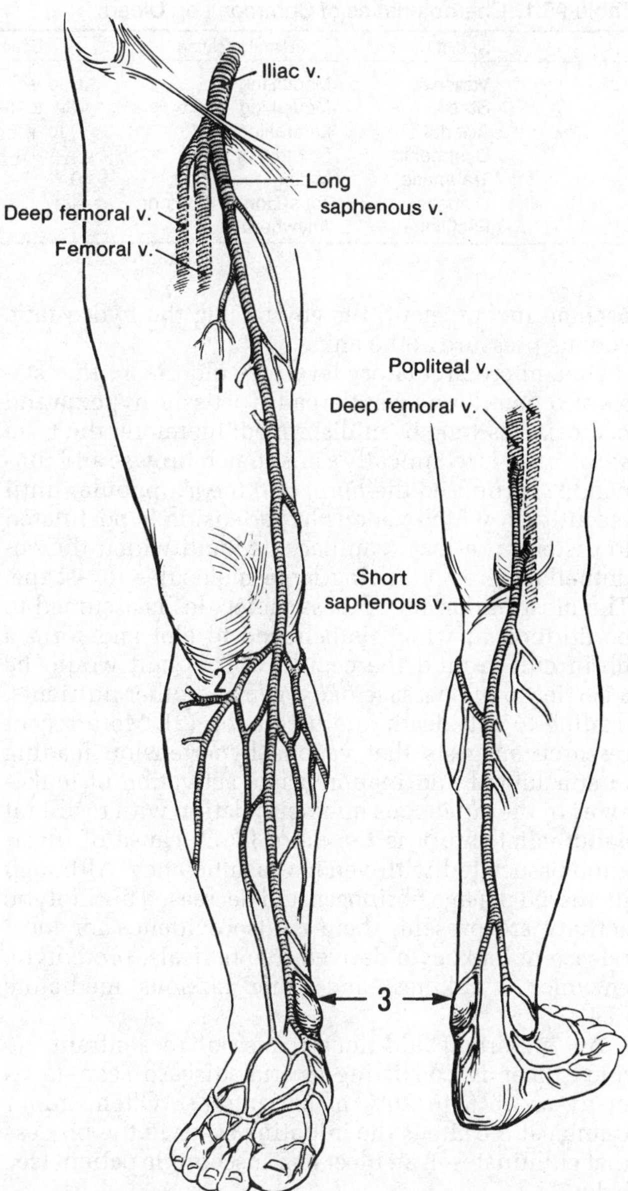

Figure 95.1. Venous circulation of the lower extremity. *1,* Hunter canal perforator; *2,* anterior communicating vein of the leg; *3,* ankle perforators.

Types and Characteristics of Leg Ulcers

The principal characteristics of common ulcers are shown in Table 95.1.

Ulceration Associated with Venous Insufficiency

Chronic venous insufficiency is the most common cause of leg ulcers. The disorder probably follows deep venous thrombosis with destruction of valves in the deep venous system and reversal of normal superficial-to-deep flow of blood in the perforating veins. The muscular action of the calf becomes ineffective, and blood flows to the superficial veins instead of in the usual centripetal direction through the deep venous system. Valves in the superficial (saphenous) system

Table 95.1. Characteristics of Common Leg Ulcers

Type of Ulcer	Usual Location	Edema	Pigmentation	Evidence of Arterial Insufficiency
Varicose	Medial leg	0 to +	0 to +	0
Stasis	Medial leg	++ to ++++	+++	0 to +
Arterial	Lateral leg, foot	0 to +	0	++++
Dystrophic	Sole, tip of toe	++	0	0
Traumatic	Midleg, toe	0	0	0 to ++++
Diabetic	Toes, dorsum, or foot	++	0	+ to +++
Factitious	Anywhere	+	0	0

become incompetent, thereby raising the hydrostatic venous pressure at the ankle.

On a microcirculatory level, the old theory that stasis of venous blood was the cause of tissue hypoxia and necrosis has long been disproved; therefore, the term *stasis ulcer* is technically a misnomer. Browse and Burnand (2) proposed the *fibrin cuff theory,* popular until recently, in which venous hypertension is postulated to distend the local capillary bed and widen the endothelial pores, allowing large molecules to escape. The most important of these molecules is assumed to be fibrinogen, which is believed to clot and form a fibrin cuff around the capillary. This cuff would be a barrier to the passage of oxygen and other nutrients, leading to cell death and ulceration (2). More recent research suggests that venous hypertension leading to attachment and inappropriate activation of leukocytes in the cutaneous microcirculation with resultant endothelial injury is the more likely cause of ulceration associated with venous insufficiency. Although increased plasma fibrinogen and decreased fibrinolytic activity are present, there is also evidence for local release of leukocyte-derived free radicals, proteolytic enzymes, cytokines, and other noxious mediators (3,4).

An important additional cause of recalcitrant venous ulcer is coexisting arterial disease seen in as many as 15% to 20% of patients (3). Often, minor trauma at the site is the initiating event in the process that culminates in an ulcer in a susceptible patient (see below).

The physical examination reveals edema, hemosiderin deposition, and ulceration, usually in line with the long saphenous vein, the short saphenous vein, or over a medial ankle perforator (Fig. 95.1). Arterial circulation in the leg may be entirely normal. Varicosities may or may not be present. The ulcer is usually fairly superficial and involves the skin, with irregular margins and with exudate covering the floor of the ulcer. The ulcer is usually movable with the skin and is tender. In grossly neglected cases, the ulceration may be massive and may involve most of the circumference of the leg. Occasionally, cellulitis may be evident, with erythema, tenderness, and fever secondary to superimposed bacterial infection (see Chapter 32).

Ulceration Associated with Arterial Insufficiency

Arterial insufficiency (see also Chapter 94) is the second most common cause of leg ulcers and, along with venous insufficiency, accounts for most leg ulcers. Ulcers associated with peripheral arterial occlusive disease usually begin with trauma and therefore appear at sites that are most subject to trauma (i.e., on toes, over the lateral or medial malleolus, at the base of the fifth metatarsal, at the head of the first metatarsal, on the heel or the ball of the foot, and in the distal pretibial region).

Ulcers secondary to occlusive arterial disease are characteristically painful, probably related to local inflammation and to ischemia. The foot may appear atrophic with shiny, fragile, transparent, hairless skin; the nails are often hypertrophied and deformed. Other hallmarks of arterial insufficiency (e.g., pulselessness and coolness) may be present. Because some patients are relieved of pain when they dangle the ulcerated leg, dependent edema may be present.

Dystrophic Ulcers

A neuropathic or dystrophic ulcer is usually associated with somatic or sympathetic neurologic dysfunction. The precise pathogenesis of these ulcers is unknown. Perhaps sympathetic dysfunction causes a reduction of arterial blood flow to local areas of skin that result in ulceration. Furthermore, hypesthesia or anesthesia renders the patient more susceptible to trauma. Dystrophic ulcers are most commonly associated with peripheral neuropathies (see Chapter 92) and the neuropathies of congenital or acquired disease of the spinal cord, such as Friedreich ataxia, syringomyelia, or multiple sclerosis. Peripheral neuropathies caused by vitamin deficiency or injuries may also result in ulcers. Ulceration almost always occurs in areas of pressure. The patient may complain of pain in the ulcer, but the ulcer is usually insensitive to light touch. There may be deformity in the foot associated with the neuropathy (*talipes calcaneovalgus* or *equinus,* deformities in which the anterior part of the foot is elevated and the heel is turned outward or in which the foot is plantar-flexed, respectively) or there may be a back deformity or surgical scar, as might occur in a patient with a meningomyelocele. Usually, neurologic examination of the lower extremity is abnormal, revealing decreased proprioception, decreased cutaneous sensation, and perhaps impaired movement. The ulcer may be undermined, and there may be subcutaneous tracking of infected material into adjacent tissues that, on pressure, exude loculated pus from the undermined border of the ulcer. If the neuropathy is severe, the patient may be ambulating without pain, yet show advanced ulceration of the sole of the foot.

Posttraumatic Ulcers

Posttraumatic ulcers are common and usually are associated with impairment in nerve or vascular supply of the leg. Minor injury to the toe of a patient with arteriosclerotic occlusive vascular disease or a leg injury in a patient with chronic venous insufficiency may lead to ulceration. However, such ulcers may develop in the legs of otherwise healthy people, particularly after major injuries such as fractures that involve areas where vascular supply is normally marginal. The most susceptible site is the junction of the middle and lower third of the subcutaneous surface of the tibia. In this situation, most traumatic ulcers, even in healthy youngsters, heal with some difficulty, and in older patients and in those with even minimal arterial insufficiency, injury at this site resolves with great difficulty. Posttraumatic ulcers may be accompanied by problems of chronic infection and present with tenderness and local cellulitis.

Diabetic Ulcers

Diabetic ulcers have features of dystrophic, traumatic, and arterial ulcers because all three factors contribute to their development. The characteristic location of such an ulcer is in an area of pressure, such as a corn or a callosity (see Chapter 73). The ulcer is fairly insensitive, often heavily infected, with undermined edges and tracks under the plantar fascia or proximally on the dorsum of the foot. Although usually patients are aware that they are diabetic, some are not, and a thorough evaluation upon suspicion of diabetes is mandatory because control of the ulcer depends to a large extent on control of the diabetes. Radiologic examination is important because the bone underlying the ulcer may be the site of chronic osteomyelitis that may necessitate surgical intervention (see example in Chapter 40).

Factitious Ulcers

Factitious ulcers are self-inflicted or self-maintained ulcers. Because they develop in the absence of any other local or systemic cause, diagnosis of factitious ulcers requires a high degree of suspicion. They most commonly occur in the legs of addicts who inject drugs into slightly varicose leg veins. The distribution of these ulcers is usually bizarre. They may be multiple and bilateral; if the history can be obtained, the diagnosis is easily made.

Factitious ulcers may also occur in patients with poor hygiene, psychiatric disorders, or disorders associated with pruritus, such as scabies, which has led to excoriation. The diagnosis should be suspected if the patient appears to derive some real or imaginary gain from having the ulcer. Any ulcer without a definite cause that fails to heal in an apparently healthy environment should lead to the suspicion that it is factitious.

Neoplastic Ulcers

Neoplastic ulcers of the leg are rare, but when they do occur, they are usually either basal cell or squamous cell carcinomas and have the usual characteristics of these tumors (see Chapter 114). They have elevated or rolled edges, are anesthetic, and are usually attached to deeper tissue. *Marjolin ulcer,* a rare form of squamous cell carcinoma that occurs in burn scars of long duration, also may be seen on the legs.

Hypertensive Ulcers

Another rare type of ulcer is associated with uncontrolled systemic arterial hypertension. It is thought that there is a progressive increase in the thickness of the arteriolar wall, decrease in the diameter of its lumen, progressive ischemia, and infarction of the skin (5). These ulcers are extremely painful and occur most often in women on the posterolateral aspect of the leg and ankle. Ordinarily there is no evidence of peripheral arterial or venous disease.

Miscellaneous

Ulceration of the legs may occur in *sickle cell disease, polyarteritis nodosa,* collagen-vascular diseases, and other systemic conditions (e.g., ulcerative colitis). In these instances, the diagnosis depends on accurate diagnosis of the systemic disorder.

Corticosteroid therapy, particularly if it is longstanding, can lead to atrophy of the skin, increasing its fragility and susceptibility to injury. Furthermore, the impairment by corticosteroids of wound healing may prevent some ulcers from healing.

A toxic cause of skin ulceration is the *brown recluse spider bite,* common in the southeastern United States. The poison of the brown recluse spider contains a necrotizing enzyme that causes a rounded sloughing ulcer of approximately 3 to 4 cm with an indurated edge. The patient may not be aware of having been bitten by a spider. These ulcers are refractory to healing by use of conservative measures and should be surgically excised and closed.

Cutaneous cytomegalovirus infection has become more common in association with the increased incidence of acquired immune deficiency from human immunodeficiency virus infection. Cytomegalovirus infection can cause lower extremity ulceration.

In the tropics, ulceration of the foot and leg may occur from *local mycoses* such as *maduromycosis* and *cutaneous leishmaniasis;* these conditions should be kept in mind when a patient has returned from a tropical climate.

Laboratory Aids in Diagnosis

Bacteriology

Leg ulcers are often infected and almost invariably contaminated, usually with enteric organisms. Infections are particularly hazardous in diabetic patients and those with chronic arterial insufficiency. Biopsy cultures of the ulcer bed may be useful, and cultures of obviously purulent ulcers are mandatory because antibiotic therapy is an important part of management, particularly when invasive infection is apparent (see Chapter 32). Viral culture of a small biopsy may be necessary to diagnose cytomegalovirus-induced cutaneous ulceration. If fungal infection is suspected (unusual degree of scaling and excoriation), unless the clinician is experienced in the scraping of lesions and the microscopic identification of fungi, dermatologic consultation is indicated.

Biopsy

Biopsy by a surgeon or a dermatologist is indicated if neoplastic or obscure fungal disease is suspected. Biopsy may be performed in the office under local anesthesia and should include a wedge-shaped section of the edge and floor of the ulcer. Any chronic ulcer that exists in a long-standing scar of any type should be biopsied to rule out squamous cell carcinoma. Sometimes only a biopsy of bone makes a definitive diagnosis of osteomyelitis that underlies a chronic ulcer.

Laboratory Tests for Systemic Disease

These tests are performed as dictated by the clinical diagnosis when the ulcer is suspected to be part of a systemic disorder (e.g., diabetes, polyarteritis nodosa, or sickle cell disease).

Noninvasive Vascular Testing

Noninvasive vascular testing can define the anatomy and function of the venous system of the lower extremities. Particularly in the case of persistent lower extremity ulceration, noninvasive testing may be helpful in determining the cause and determining whether surgery might correct the venous problem and help heal the ulcer. When ulceration is noted in a patient with occlusive arterial disease, the patient should be referred to a vascular laboratory for noninvasive arterial testing. Noninvasive vascular testing is discussed more fully later in this chapter.

Natural History and Management

Generally, chronic ulcers develop initially from skin trauma, which may be exceedingly minor (6). However, the insult may occur in a milieu of macrocirculatory or microcirculatory disease or other unfavorable local or systemic factors. Once the wound becomes inflamed, the local metabolic rate increases the demand for oxygen and nutrients, which leads to compromise and death of tissue when the demands are not met. The tissue then may become infected, resulting in more inflammation, propagating the cycle, making the ulcer enlarge and then become chronic. Treatment of the ulcer requires breaking this cycle.

Edema is commonly associated with lower extremity ulcers, particularly those related to chronic venous disease. When present, it retards healing and reduces the skin resistance to trauma and subsequent infection. This makes the treatment of edema a very important component of ulcer therapy and prevention.

Chronic open wounds are all colonized by microorganisms to a greater or lesser extent. As long as an ulcer is an open wound, invasion by organisms is rare, and the threat of invasive infection and systemic toxicity is minimal. Furthermore, because the bacteria are on the surface of the wound rather than in the tissue, and the tissue in the base of the ulcer is often poorly vascularized, systemic antibiotics do not affect the surface flora significantly. Topical antibiotics are generally more appropriate for open wounds, and systemic antibiotics are reserved for evidence of invasive infections.

Pus under pressure (i.e., an abscess) greatly increases the risk of invasive infection. When a collection of loculated pus exists, it must be adequately drained. Eschars that overlie ulcers may hide such loculated pus and should generally be debrided. Wet eschars can simply be lifted with a tweezer and snipped. Dry eschars must be cut with a scissors or a scalpel along the plane of necrosis to avoid incising healthy tissue.

Most ulcers of the lower extremities can be treated on an ambulatory basis (1,7). However, the presence of one or both of the following may be an indication for hospitalization:

- The extent of the ulcer and the associated edema is so great that a period of absolute bed rest and elevation is required that is not possible outside the hospital.
- The appearance of invasive infection is heralded by cellulitis, lymphangitis, and systemic symptoms.

Ensuring adequate nutrition is an important aspect of managing the patient with a leg ulcer. Identification and correction of nutritional deficiencies improves management: however, there is no evidence that supplementation in the absence of a specific deficiency accelerates healing (8).

Ulceration Associated with Venous Insufficiency

Probably no other form of ulcer taxes the patient or the practitioner as much as that associated with chronic venous insufficiency (1,6). The mainstays of therapy are elimination of necrotic tissue and infection, cleansing of the ulcer bed to facilitate healthy tissue growth, reduction of edema by elevation and compression, and ensuring adequate arterial perfusion. The patient should be at rest, and the ulcer should be treated with dressings and topical antibacterial agents if infected. Most of these ulcers heal by the use of nonoperative therapy.

The first step in managing these ulcers is to create an optimal environment. In the absence of other systemic factors, this step is primarily an attack on necrotic tissue, edema, and the bacterial colonization of the wound. Initial outpatient treatment consists of debridement of necrotic tissue and determination of the adequacy of arterial supply to the lower extremity in the office. Debridement can be performed safely using sharp scissors and forceps. Cutting within the necrotic tissue, leaving a thin layer above vascularized tissue, allows debridement without pain and bleeding. The residual necrotic layer resolves with further local debridement as performed during appropriate changes of dressings and through wound and bacterial autolysis. Arterial inflow is adequate if bounding foot pulses are present or the patient's ankle–brachial blood pressure index is greater than 0.8 (most accurately measured by a vascular laboratory).

Compression dressings can be used if arterial flow is adequate to reduce the edema and should be worn whenever the extremity is dependent. Patients at home should be placed at rest with the extremity elevated. Wounds will not heal with contamination greater than 10^5 organisms/g of tissue. After adequate bacteriologic cultures, a suitable topical antibacterial preparation such as silver sulfadiazine cream (e.g., Silvadene Cream 1%) or sodium oxychlorosene solution (Clorpactin 0.4% in water or isotonic saline) should be applied.

Invasive infection in the tissue surrounding the ulcer is uncommon but should be suspected in ulcers in which an eschar trapped pus under pressure before debridement and in those that exhibit erythema, tenderness, and swelling locally (i.e., cellulitis). Invasive infection should be treated with an appropriate systemic antibiotic.

Recent studies suggest that systemic medical treatment with pentoxifylline (400 mg three times a day) may be given as adjunctive therapy. The drug is thought to reduce leukocyte activation and enhance fibrinolysis along with its well-recognized rheologic effects on blood and blood flow. Use of other systemic medications is less well established (3).

With intensive therapy, edema and bacterial overgrowth can be controlled in 48 to 72 hours. Thereafter, these optimal conditions must be maintained; healing is encouraged by the use of any one of several different dressings and techniques. Edema is kept to a minimum with leg elevation and compression bandages or stockings. Antibacterial dressings can be discontinued in favor of dressings that provide an optimal wound healing environment and are more conducive to wound healing.

One of the following approaches can be used:

1. For *wet-to-dry dressing,* a sterile gauze pad moistened in normal saline (not soaking wet, because this can cause maceration) is secured over the ulcer (with a rolled bandage, not with an adhesive tape, which can damage the skin adjacent to an ulcer) and left to dry; necrotic tissue and other debris are removed when the dry dressing is removed, gently, at the end of each dressing interval. This procedure is appropriate early in ulcer management when there is substantial exudate and debris to remove and there has been little healing.
2. Cleaner ulcers may have a similarly moistened dressing *(wet-to-wet dressing)* applied and then moistened again before removing. This results in somewhat less vigorous debridement but protects the healing tissue of the ulcer.
3. The lower extremity may be wrapped with a zinc oxide–gelatin dressing (*Unna boot,* Dome paste boot) that has long been used successfully in the treatment of leg ulcers. If used, it is imperative that it is not wrapped tightly and that it is placed smoothly from the metacarpal–phalangeal joints to just below the tibial tuberosity, including the heel. This can be done best by keeping the bandage roll on the surface of the leg as the leg is wrapped. Wrinkles, failure to wrap the heel, and compression that is either too tight or too loose result in treatment failure and can result in further ulcerations. The Unna boot is then covered with an elastic wrap for gentle compression. When first applied it should be removed within 48 hours to ascertain that the compression is adequate and that further problems are not being created. The bandage may then be reapplied and changed weekly, and healing usually results. An Unna boot should not be applied if there is a suspicion of peripheral arterial disease because it could cause more ischemia. A similar type of dressing that has gained popularity is the *four-layer compression dressing.* This dressing works on a similar principle but has an absorptive layer that may be useful, particularly for more exudative wounds.
4. When the ulcer is clean, or if it is quite shallow, a good alternative is a *hydrocolloid dressing* (e.g., Duoderm, Mitraflex) under an elastic bandage. This dressing does not disrupt the growth of healing tissue and allows healing in a moist environment (9). Small amounts of residual necrotic debris in the ulcer are removed by fibrinolytic action of the fluid that builds up under the dressing. The ulcer usually requires a change of dressing every 48 to 72 hours. However, it requires changing more frequently if the fluid that develops leaks out the side of the dressing.

Many new dressings are currently being evaluated in the treatment of lower extremity ulcers. These include calcium alginate, hydrogels, and new types of debriding gauzes. Serial compression pumps to reduce edema are now available for home use. No conclusions can be drawn at this time regarding the efficacy of any of these new treatments.

Occasionally, diuretics may be helpful in managing edema even when no element of cardiac or renal failure exists. Elastic compression should always be used first to avoid the danger of volume depletion. Ultimately, if edema and bacterial colonization can be controlled, the ulcer will usually heal, although several weeks to months may be required. After the healing, the patient must be advised to keep the leg elevated, if possible, when sitting down and to wear some form of elastic compression permanently, preferably a made-to-measure elastic support garment. If the ulcer still fails to heal, skin grafting may be required along with venous ligation and stripping. This requires surgical consultation and hospitalization.

Ulceration Associated with Arterial Insufficiency

Arterial ulcers are very difficult to heal unless blood flow to the area can be improved. Therefore, if there is any suspicion of arterial insufficiency, the patient should be referred for noninvasive vascular testing and, possibly, surgical evaluation. If the patient's lesion is unsuitable for surgical correction or if the patient has already had an operation but ulceration persists, the ulcer can sometimes be healed with painstaking debridements every 2 or 3 days. However, this treatment requires expertise; if doubt exists, surgical referral should be made.

A pair of sharp scissors or a scalpel is used to remove the dry eschar that covers the ulcer and to remove the necrotic edges of the ulcer carefully without causing bleeding (see above). Wet-to-wet dressings are then applied, using a topical antibiotic solution such as sodium oxychlorosene or polymyxin–bacitracin 5% aqueous suspension. The patient is instructed to apply the bandage wet in the morning and to remove it in the evening after wetting it again. This has the effect of debriding the ulcer and promoting wound healing, consisting of wound contraction and reepithelialization.

Very tenacious residual necrotic debris after sharp debridement may be removed with a short course of a *proteolytic enzyme* applied three to four times a day followed by the application of a wet-to-dry dressing or by hydrocolloid dressings. In conjunction with these measures, meticulously compulsive foot protection, soft footwear, elevation of the extremity, and avoidance of weight bearing are mandatory.

Dystrophic Ulcers

Dystrophic ulcers are a real threat to the limb because infection often advances unnoticed by the patient until there is considerable spread of pus under the eschar or in the tissue around the ulcer. Treatment consists of bed rest, relieving pressure on bony prominences frequently, appropriate antibiotic therapy as indicated after culture (see Chapter 32), debridement of necrotic skin edges (which can be done without anesthesia in the office; see above), and wet-to-wet dressings as described above.

Once the ulcer has been rendered clean by debridement and dressings, slow healing may progress, often over several months. In patients with dystrophic foot ulcers, total contact casting (see Diabetic Ulcers, below) has been successful in relieving pressure on the ulcer and providing an environment conducive to healing. This technique has provided a new means of treating these patients while they remain ambulatory and has considerably reduced hospitalization rates for this condition.

Traumatic Ulcers

Traumatic ulcers usually heal by avoidance of weight bearing, elevation, topical antibiotic therapy when the ulcer is infected, and protection of the ulcer by dressings (see above). If no progress is made within 2 to 3 weeks, the patient should be seen by a surgeon for possible operative debridement and surgical closure of the wound.

Diabetic Ulcers

Infected diabetic ulcers impose such a serious risk of limb loss that most of these patients should be hospitalized. In the hospital, diabetes can be regulated more meticulously, any pockets of suppuration can be drained, proper debridement can be carried out, and bone biopsy can be done if osteomyelitis is suspected.

Once the ulcers are clean and uninfected, leg elevation and avoidance of pressure and shearing forces on the area of ulceration will allow healing. In patients with foot ulcers, *total contact casting* has been successful in alleviating these forces and in providing an optimal environment for healing while the patient remains ambulatory. The procedure involves the application of a plaster cast directly to the foot (without first wrapping the foot in gauze, as would be done for a fracture). The patient's weight is thereby distributed evenly over the entire foot, reducing pressure on the ulcer. Ordinarily, the cast is left in place for approximately a week. This technique is best provided by specialists experienced in its use because improper cast application can result in development of other skin problems or of worsening of the ulcer.

Factitious Ulcers

The key to the management of factitious ulcers is making the diagnosis. The diagnosis is made by maintaining a high degree of suspicion, particularly in ulcers that have no clear cause and occur in what appears to be an otherwise healthy environment. These ulcers usually heal if the cause can be found and controlled. Psychiatric consultation may be indicated if there is evidence of anxiety, depression, and so on (see Chapter 19). An ulcer suspected of being a factitious ulcer can often be diagnosed and treated simultaneously by placing an occlusive dressing that prevents the patient from manipulating the ulcer. These patients must be carefully followed to monitor progress and to avoid the development of problems under the occlusive dressing.

Hypertensive Ulcers

Control of the patient's chronic hypertension and education regarding the importance of long-term control are the two keystones in the management of hypertensive ulcers. Otherwise, the management follows the general principles applied to venous stasis ulcers.

Chronic Ulcers Associated with Corticosteroid Treatment

Systemic corticosteroids have an inhibitory effect on wound healing that can be partially reversed by vitamin A. Ulcers that fail to heal in patients being treated with corticosteroids may be treated with vitamin A 25,000 units/day orally; ointments containing vitamin A (e.g., A and D Ointment) may be used alone or in combination (e.g., with silver sulfadiazine cream) directly on the ulcer.

Neoplastic and Other Ulcers

Neoplastic and other unusual ulcers, such as that from the previously mentioned brown recluse spider bite, are a surgical problem; these patients should be referred promptly for consultation.

Growth Factor Therapy

Certain growth factors may be capable of reversing some or all the adverse effects caused by underlying local and systemic factors that contribute to the formation of ulcers in the lower extremities. *Platelet-derived growth factor* and *epidermal growth factor* seem to be the most effective (10). Only recombinant platelet-derived growth factor-BB (becaplermin) is approved by the Food and Drug Administration and only for the topical treatment of diabetic neuropathic ulcers; a 15-g tube, enough for a week or two, costs over $500. The use of cultured (Apligraf) or banked allograft skin as a biologic dressing in an effort to enhance local growth factor production has been established (11). Further research should identify other growth factors that may enhance wound healing. However, topical growth factor therapy should not be considered a substitute for proper wound care.

Prevention and General Foot Care in Susceptible Patients

Foot and leg ulcers from any cause often recur after healing because, with the exception of varicose veins, factitious ulcers, and surgically corrected occlusive arterial disease, the underlying disease is difficult to reverse. It is therefore mandatory to be familiar with the principles of foot care, and patients must understand and carry out instructions aimed at minimizing exposure to trauma. Patients with peripheral arterial disease or diabetes should wear very comfortable footwear, even if it is not fashionable (see Chapter 73). The front of the shoe should be broad so that the toes can spread. Areas of pressure caused by foot deformities should be corrected by orthopedic shoes with appropriate fittings (e.g., insoles or metatarsal bars); patients with these problems should be referred to an orthopedic surgeon or podiatrist.

Patients should be instructed to keep their feet very clean (i.e., at least once-daily showers or footbaths in tepid water). Patients with impaired cutaneous sensation should use a mirror to examine the undersurface of their feet daily.

Nails should be carefully trimmed, preferably with clippers; under no circumstances should sharp scissors be used to trim the sides of nails because they may injure the delicate nail fold and become a portal of entry for infection. Patients can protect their toes during walking by inserting small fluffy pieces of cotton wool between them. Lanolin or other emollient creams are useful in preventing cracking of hardened areas of skin and keeping the skin soft and supple. Patients should avoid extremes of temperature and should reduce exposure to trauma (e.g., a night-light in the bedroom to avoid stubbing a toe). With attention to these small details, recurring trouble can often be prevented.

VARICOSE VEINS

Causes

Varicose (swollen) veins of the lower extremities are common; they affect women more often than men and usually become symptomatic between the ages of 20 and 40. The prevalence of varicose veins varies widely, ranging from a low among women of lowland New Guinea of 0.1% to a high among the women of South Wales of 50%. In the United States, varicose veins affect 19% of men and 36% of women.

Varicose veins are caused by an incompetence of the valves of the long or short saphenous veins (Fig. 95.1), permitting retrograde or downward flow of blood or simply stagnation of the normal centripetal flow (12). In the perforator system, which is a system of veins communicating between the deep and the superficial veins, destruction of valves interferes with the unidirectional movement of blood from superficial to deep.

The disorder is aggravated, indeed may be caused, by conditions elevating intra-abdominal pressure, such as pregnancy, large intra-abdominal tumors, conditions causing chronic straining (e.g., prostatic obstruction, carcinoma of the sigmoid colon), and occasionally mechanical interference with venous return in the venous system itself, such as thrombosis of the pelvic veins.

Symptoms

The symptoms of uncomplicated varicose veins usually consist of heaviness and aching in the area of the veins or in the calves. The patient may complain of mild edema at the end of a long day's work. Occasionally, patients complain of varicose veins for cosmetic reasons and desire treatment. Patients with uncomplicated varicose veins do not complain of intermittent claudication or severe pain; in the presence of these symptoms, other causes must be carefully sought. Occasionally, thrombophlebitis supervenes in a varicose vein and causes severe pain; the vein is then palpable as an inflamed cord. After rest, elevation, application of local heat, and appropriate anti-inflammatory therapy (e.g., aspirin), the varix in the thrombosed vein disappears.

Physical Examination

It is useful to have some idea of the anatomy of the venous system of the leg (Fig. 95.1). This makes it possible to judge the patient's symptoms on the basis of an anatomic abnormality detected by physical examination. There are several types of varicose veins, which conform to the underlying anatomic arrangement of these veins.

Telangiectasia (Sunburst Varices)

These are not, in the true sense of the word, varicose veins but rather dilations of subcutaneous venous plexuses that have a spider-like arrangement and an unsightly purple color. These veins are often the object of cosmetic complaints by patients. Otherwise, they are essentially asymptomatic.

Varicosities of Long Saphenous System

Varicosities of the long saphenous system are the most common type of varicose veins. The long saphenous vein begins anterior to the medial malleolus at the ankle, courses superficially to the medial side of the knee, and then curves upward to enter the deep system just below the inguinal ligament medial to the femoral artery. The vein has several tributaries in the calf and in the thigh that are superficial, and it is also joined by several perforating veins from the deep venous system; the valves at these junctions can become incompetent and lead to focal varicosities (Fig. 95.1). There are three or four consistent perforators: three above the medial malleolus at a distance separated by approximately 3 cm and a fourth just above the knee joint. If varicosities appear in this situation, the perforator system is almost certainly incompetent. Varicosity of the long saphenous vein is clearly visible with the patient standing.

Varicosities of Short Saphenous System

The short saphenous vein arises behind the lateral malleolus and courses upward behind the calf to join the popliteal vein in the popliteal space (Fig. 95.1). Varicosities of this system are best seen with the patient standing with his or her back to the examiner.

Perforator Varicosities

As mentioned above, perforator incompetence is usually noticed in the long saphenous vein where the ankle perforators and the above-the-knee perforator join the vein; however, perforators join other superficial veins that, in turn, join the long and short saphenous system. Examination may reveal that there is no incompetence of the short or long saphenous veins, only of the perforators.

Clinical Testing to Determine Level of Incompetence

One or two easy clinical tests can be performed in the office that will aid in determination of the severity of the problem and selection of appropriate treatment.

Trendelenburg Test

The patient lies supine and raises the affected leg to empty the veins. A venous tourniquet is applied just below the saphenous opening about 3 inches (7.6 cm) below the inguinal ligament and the patient then stands up. Constriction is released; if the saphenofemoral valve is incompetent, the veins will fill immediately from above; if not, the veins fill slowly from below. If the veins fill rapidly before the release of the tourniquet, this indicates the presence of incompetent perforator veins allowing reflux from the deep system. This test is now repeated at successively lower levels in the leg so the location of incompetence may be mapped.

Perthes Test

The Perthes test is a test for deep venous thrombosis in association with varicose veins. A tourniquet is lightly applied below the inguinal ligament, as in the Trendelenburg test, and the patient is instructed to walk in place. If varicose veins are accompanied by a thrombosed deep femoral system, the varicose veins become prominent after this exercise.

Noninvasive Vascular Testing

The advent of the modern vascular laboratory has revolutionized the evaluation of varicose veins. Any patient who, by physical examination, is suspected of having venous incompetence at the saphenous femoral junction should be referred to a noninvasive vascular laboratory for evaluation before treatment is planned.

Effective treatment of lower extremity venous insufficiency is predicated on accurate localization of the problem. Various noninvasive vascular examinations and radiologic studies can be successfully used to define the anatomic extent of venous reflux (13). The utility and limitations of these modalities are based on the concept of systolic and diastolic closure of lower extremity venous valves. Venous valves close in response to two distinct physiologic actions. Coaptation of valve cusps occurs during muscular contraction and subsequent forward (toward the heart) flow of blood (systolic closure). These valves include side branches and perforator veins. Diastolic closure occurs immediately after relaxation of muscular contraction when valves proximal to that contraction close to prevent reflux of blood.

Ambulatory venous pressure (AVP) measurement is performed by cannulating a vein on the dorsum of the foot with a small gauge butterfly needle connected to a pressure transducer, amplifier, and recorder. Resting pressures are obtained with the patient standing still, supporting his or her weight on a frame. After the completion of 10 toe raises at one per second, another pressure reading is obtained. This is defined as the *AVP*. The *pressure recovery time* (PRT) is the time for the pressure to return to the resting baseline pressure. In practice, measurement of the time to return to 90% of resting pressure provides a more reproducible PRT. Application of a 2.5-cm-wide pneumatic cuff or occlusive elastic tourniquet above and then below the knee permits segregation of the superficial venous system from the deep system. Obliteration of the saphenous system in this manner permits differentiation of the level of reflux. An AVP in excess of 45 mm Hg signifies venous incompetence, as does a PRT of less than 18 seconds. If the AVP and PRT remain abnormal after the segregation of the saphenous (superficial) system by tourniquets, deep venous and perforator involvement should be suspected (14,15).

AVP measurement is highly sensitive in the detection of venous reflux and is a direct measure of venous pressure. Limitations of this test include inconsistent reproducibility, patient discomfort, and lack of efficacy as a screening test.

The simplest noninvasive test for lower extremity venous reflux is *continuous wave Doppler.* The examiner insonates the venous system with a Doppler probe and listens for venous reflux after provocative maneuvers, such as Valsalva maneuver or manual compression proximal to the transducer. The Valsalva maneuver and proximal compression normally result in the cessation of venous flow. The presence of venous signals during these maneuvers is indicative of venous reflux. Continuous wave Doppler samples any structure in the path of the emitted ultrasound and does not allow for discrimination of the vein being tested. Similarly, anatomic variations such as bifid veins will be unrecognized.

Photoplethysmography (PPG) can readily provide a noninvasive assessment of lower extremity venous valvular function. PPG venous testing is performed with the patient in a sitting or standing position. A PPG diode that emits infrared light is placed superior to the medial malleolus (16). The amount of attenuation of the emitted, and subsequently reflected light is related to numerous factors, which include the amount of blood in the tissues. Changes in the reflected light can be displayed qualitatively on a strip chart. After the establishment of a resting baseline recording, the lower extremity venous system is emptied by alternating plantar flexion and dorsiflexion of the foot or firm calf compressions. This results in a fall from the baseline on the strip chart. While the patient remains motionless, venous refill, which is displayed as a slow rise on the chart, is recorded. The time from completion of venous emptying to return of PPG reading to baseline represents the *venous recovery time.* A venous recovery time less than 23 seconds is considered abnormal. Similar to AVP testing, the saphenous system can be occluded with pneumatic cuffs or elastic tourniquets to permit differentiation of the level of disease. Normalization of a shortened venous recovery time after application of an above-knee tourniquet demonstrates superficial venous incompetence. The deep/perforator system is considered involved if the venous recovery time remains abnormal after constriction of the superficial veins.

Venous PPG has the advantage of being noninvasive and easily performed. Inconsistency of the effort of the patient to perform the necessary maneuvers and the inability to provide quantitative data are limitations of this modality. Similarly, PPG testing does not detect proximal valvular insufficiency in the presence of competent distal veins.

Vascular duplex scanning combines high-resolution ultrasonic imaging with pulsed-wave Doppler. This allows real-time visualization of vascular structures and precise placement of the Doppler sample. In addition to spectral waveforms, the Doppler information can be displayed in a color-coded format on the gray-scale image. The spectral waveforms and color coding obtained by Doppler depicts the velocity of the blood flow as defined by the Doppler equation. The Doppler-derived velocity is a vector that processes both magnitude and direction. Analysis of the Doppler data can therefore demonstrate the direction of blood flow relative to the transducer (15). The saphenofemoral and saphenopopliteal junctions can be imaged in the groin and popliteal space, respectively, and venous flow recorded by spectral analysis or color Doppler. Venous reflux in response to Valsalva maneuver or proximal limb compression can be observed as either waveforms that are inverted to the normal antegrade flow or color coding indicating retrograde flow. Duplex ultrasonography offers selective sampling of venous structures and precise localization of disease. A brief wisp of reflux is often observed after provocative maneuvers, and retrograde Doppler flow that lasts longer than 1 second is considered abnormal. The entire length of the deep and superficial systems can be interrogated. Careful duplex examination of the medial calf and thigh can demonstrate incompetent perforator veins. Not only is this diagnostic, but it can also be used to localize and mark perforators for surgical ligation. Deep venous thrombosis can also be readily identified by this modality.

Venous duplex scanning must be performed by a skilled operator and requires expensive ultrasound equipment (15). However, its noninvasive nature makes it acceptable to patients. Duplex scanning correlates with AVP and can be used to quantitate the volume of reflux, which correlates with the degree of venous stasis skin changes (13).

Treatment

Depending on the patient's presentation, four options are available.

Observation

Observation is an acceptable option in patients with mild to moderate asymptomatic subcutaneous varices with no history of postural edema, superficial phlebitis, stasis dermatitis, or pain. If the offending telangiectatic venous plexus is large enough to accommodate a 25-gauge needle, a sclerosing solution may be injected. The technique is described below. Other treatments such as freezing with carbon dioxide snow, cautery under local anesthesia, and even laser therapy have been advocated, but their use requires a great deal of skill, and unnecessary skin scarring may result that is, in the end, more unsightly than the original vein. Probably the safest treatment of this kind of vein is the use of masking cosmetic creams, together with reassurance.

Support Hose

Support hose maintain compression of subcutaneous varicose veins and prevent edema. Graduated compression hose in the 30- to 40-mm Hg range are available in most pharmacies in various ready-to-fit sizes, including knee, thigh, and panty hose configurations. The patient should be measured and fit early in the morning before any edema has developed to obtain maximal therapeutic benefit from the compression hose. They should be worn continuously, removed at bedtime, and reapplied immediately upon arising in the morning.

Sclerotherapy

Sclerotherapy is efficacious for segmental subcutaneous varicose veins that are not associated with significant greater or lesser saphenous valvular incompetence and for cosmetically unacceptable telangiectasia (17). The procedure can easily be performed in the office by anyone skilled with a needle; however, the patient should be warned that several sittings may be required for complete elimination of the veins.

The patient stands with a tight tourniquet around the thigh, just enough to make the vein prominent. The area of the vein is lightly prepared with a suitable antiseptic, and 0.5 mL of sclerosing solution is injected by use of a 2-mL syringe, after initial aspiration to make sure the needle is in the vein. Immediately after the end of the injection, the needle is withdrawn and the vein is gently compressed with a 2 × 2-inch gauze for 3 minutes, after which the tourniquet is released and compression is continued for 2 minutes more. The patient wears an elastic bandage on the area for approximately 4 hours. The sclerosant produces an inflammatory reaction in the intima, which obliterates the vein. Failure to use a tourniquet may release an unnecessarily large amount of sclerosant into the major veins of the leg and cause undesirable thrombosis at distant sites. The patient should be warned that extravasation of the sclerosant is a possibility and may cause skin necrosis. Several commercially available sclerosant solutions, morrhuate sodium and sodium tetradecyl sulfate (Sotradecol), are suitable for injection.

Surgical Therapy

Symptomatic patients should be referred for surgical consultation. Attempts to inject and compress veins associated with clear-cut varicosities of the major superficial systems are doomed to failure without surgical intervention; nevertheless, injection or primary treatment of saphenous varicosities is preferred in some centers, mostly in Europe.

Varicosities associated with incompetent greater or lessor saphenous systems require stab avulsion in conjunction with saphenous ligation and stripping, usually from the level of the groin to the knee in the case of greater saphenous incompetence. If an operation has been performed on the long or short saphenous system, there are often residual varicosities of a minor degree that require additional injection therapy, which may be performed in the office. The recurrence rate of major varicosities after operation is 10% to 20% in most large series.

When associated perforator incompetence is demonstrated, surgical treatment should include ligation of these communicating vessels at the fascial level. This may be accomplished through either multiple incisions or preferably with endoscopic techniques (18).

For varicosities accompanied by valvular incompetence in the iliac, femoral, and popliteal deep veins that has caused greater and lesser saphenous insufficiency, reconstructive approaches may include various methods of direct and indirect valvuloplasty (19–21). Excision and stripping of a long and a short saphenous vein should be the last treatment option.

Varicose veins should not be treated in patients who have an underlying cause associated with increased intra-abdominal pressure until the primary cause has been removed. However, the wearing of elastic stockings may give comfort during this time. Such stockings may be advisable for support in any patient with varicose veins in whom other treatment is undesirable or contraindicated. A further consideration in the selection of therapy is whether the patient has coronary artery disease; although veins that are severely varicose are not suitable for use in coronary bypass surgery, if patients have minimal varicose veins and may become candidates for a coronary artery bypass, these veins should be preserved, if possible, for potential use (22). Weight reduction in overweight patients is advisable for anyone with varicose veins, regardless of other modes of treatment.

General References*

Apelqvist J, Bakker K, van Houtum WH, et al. **International consensus and practical guidelines on the management and the prevention of the diabetic foot. International Working Group on the Diabetic Foot.** Diabetes Metab Res Rev 2000;16:S84.

Review of the consensus process and reprint of the Practical Guidelines.

Goldman MP, ed. Treatment of varicose and telangiectatic leg veins. St. Louis: CV Mosby, 1991.

A superb compendium of office sclerotherapy.

Goldman MP, Bergan JJ. Ambulatory treatment of venous disease: an illustrative guide. St. Louis: CV Mosby, 1996.

Kistner RL. Veins and lymphatics. In: Hardy JD, ed. Textbook of surgery. Philadelphia: JB Lippincott, 1988.

A good discussion of modern noninvasive vascular testing and of surgical techniques available for the treatment of varicose veins.

Rutherford RD, ed. Vascular surgery, 5th ed. Philadelphia: WB Saunders, 2000.

Several chapters of this excellent vascular surgery text are devoted to the diagnosis and treatment of lower extremity venous disease.

Sumpio BE. Foot ulcers. N Engl J Med 2000;343:787.

Tremblay S, Lewis EW, Allen PT. Selecting a treatment for primary varicose veins. Can Med Assoc J 1985;133:20.

A sensible discussion of options.

Walshe C. Living with a venous leg ulcer: a descriptive study of patients' experiences. J Adv Nursing 1995;22:1092.

Specific References

1. Erickson CA, Lanza DJ, Karp DL, et al. Healing of venous ulcers in an ambulatory care program: the roles of chronic venous insufficiency and patient compliance. J Vasc Surg 1995;22:629.
2. Browse NL, Burnand KG. The cause of venous ulceration. Lancet 1982;2:243.
3. Dormandy JA. Pharmacologic treatment of venous leg ulcers. J Cardiovasc Pharmacol 1995;25[Suppl 2]:S61.

*Bold print (general references) and bold numerals (specific references) denote published controlled clinical trials, meta-analyses, or consensus-based recommendations.

4. Smith PDC. The microcirculation in venous hypertension. Cardiovasc Res 1996;32:789.
5. Duncan HJ, Faris IB. Martorell's hypertensive ischemic leg ulcers are secondary to an increase in the local vascular resistance. J Vasc Surg 1985;2:581.
6. Douglas WS, Simpson NB. Guidelines for the management of chronic venous leg ulceration. Report of a multidisciplinary workshop. Br J Dermatol 1995;132:446.
7. Friedman SJ, Su WPD. Management of leg ulcers. Am Fam Physician 1983;27:219.
8. McClave SA, Finney LS. Nutritional issues in the patient with diabetes and foot ulcers. In: Bowker JH, Pfeifer MA, eds. Levin and O'Neal's the diabetic foot, 6th ed. St. Louis: Mosby, 2001.
9. van Rijswijk L, Brown D, Friedman S, et al. Multicenter clinical evaluation of a hydrocolloid dressing for leg ulcers. Cutis 1985;35:173.
10. Steed DL. The role of growth factors in wound healing. Surg Clin North Am 1997;77:575.
11. Spence RJ, Wong L. The enhancement of wound healing with human skin allograft. Surg Clin North Am 1997;77:731.
12. Goldman MP, Fronek A. Anatomy and pathophysiology of varicose veins. J Dermatol Surg Oncol 1989;15:138.
13. Vasdekis SN, Clarke GH, Nicolaides AN. Quantification of venous reflux by means of duplex scanning. J Vasc Surg 1989;10:670.
14. Nicolaides AN, Zukowski AJ. The value of dynamic venous pressure measurements. World J Surg 1986;10:919.
15. van Bemmelen PS, Bedford G, Beach K, et al. Quantitative segmental evaluation of venous valvular reflux with duplex ultrasound scanning. J Vasc Surg 1989;10:425.
16. Nicolaides AN, Miles C. Photoplethysmography in the assessment of venous insufficiency. J Vasc Surg 1987;5:405.
17. Weiss RA, Weiss MA, Goldman MP. Physicians' negative perception of sclerotherapy for venous disorders: review of a 7 year experience with modern sclerotherapy. South Med J 1992;85:1101.
18. Gloviczki P, Bergan JJ, Rhodes JM, et al. Mid-term results of endoscopic perforator vein interruption for chronic venous insufficiency: lessons learned from the North American Subfascial Endoscopic Perforator Surgery Registry. J Vasc Surg 1999;29:489.
19. O'Donnell TF, Mackey WC, Shepard AD, et al. Clinical, hemodynamic, and anatomic follow-up of direct venous reconstruction. Arch Surg 1987;122:474.
20. Raju S, Fredericks R. Valve reconstruction procedures for nonobstructive venous insufficiency: rationale, techniques, and results in 107 procedures with two to eight-year follow-up. J Vasc Surg 1988;7:301.
21. Wilson NM, Rutt DL, Browse NL. Repair and replacement of deep vein valves in the treatment of venous insufficiency. Br J Surg 1991;78:388.
22. Friedell ML, Samson RH, Cohen MJ, et al. High ligation of the greater saphenous vein for treatment of lower extremity varicosities: the fate of the vein and therapeutic results. Ann Vasc Surg 1992;6:5.

CHAPTER 96

Diseases of the Biliary Tract

ESTEBAN MEZEY, MD, FACS
JEFFREY S. BENDER, MD

Diseases of the biliary tract are commonly encountered in ambulatory practice. Many patients are discovered to have asymptomatic gallstones during the course of evaluation of another condition; others are found to have symptomatic chronic cholecystitis. Less commonly, patients present with an acute illness caused by acute cholecystitis or common bile duct obstruction. This chapter describes the cause, diagnosis, and treatment of these various conditions.

CHOLELITHIASIS

Epidemiology

Approximately 10% of the U.S. population has gallstones. In their lifetime, only 50% will ever be symptomatic, with 80% of them having chronic symptoms and 20% presenting with an acute illness. About 500,000 cholecystectomies are performed each year in the United States.

Ninety percent of gallstones found in patients in the United States are cholesterol gallstones; 10% are pigment (bilirubinate) stones. The prevalence of gallstones is greater in women than in men and increases with age. In the United States, 10% to 15% of men and 20% to 40% of women after age 60 are affected (1). The prevalence of cholesterol gallstones is particularly high in the Native Americans of the southwestern United States; for example, 70% of Pima women over age 25 have cholelithiasis (2).

Gallstone Formation

Bile is produced in the liver and excreted into the duodenum and contains bile acids (primarily cholic, deoxycholic, and chenodeoxycholic acid), phospholipids (primarily lecithin), and cholesterol. The solubility of cholesterol depends on its incorporation with bile and phospholipids into a micelle. In the intestinal tract, bile salts are necessary for the absorption of dietary fats; they solubilize fatty acids and monoglycerides into micellar solutions. The fatty acids are absorbed in the jejunum, whereas the bile salts are absorbed in the ileum and enter the enterohepatic circulation.

Three major types of gallstones form in human bile: cholesterol stones (more than 70% cholesterol), mixed stones (50% to 70% cholesterol), and pigment stones (12% cholesterol). These stones probably develop in three stages: first, the formation of a supersaturated bile; second, the crystallization or initiation of stone formation; and third, the growth of the stone to a certain detectable size before crystals in the bile are expelled into the intestine. It is likely, but not clearly established, that one of these stages is more important in the formation of certain types of stones than in others.

Cholesterol Stones

The hypersecretion of biliary cholesterol appears to be the real culprit in the pathogenesis of cholesterol stones, but this might not be true in all patients. Several mechanisms of increased cholesterol secretion have been identified (1). Cholesterol crystals form when the amount of cholesterol in bile exceeds the solubilizing properties of bile salts and phospholipid (supersaturated bile). The cholesterol crystals are caught in a film of mucin gel that lines the gallbladder and provides a nucleus for the formation of gallstones. Growth of these stones occurs, especially in a dyskinetic gallbladder, one in which contraction is impaired, as in diabetes mellitus and pregnancy. The mucin gel itself might decrease gallbladder motility and emptying.

Pigment Stones

Formation of pigment stones is probably initiated by supersaturation of unconjugated bilirubin in the gallbladder and common bile duct. Unconjugated bilirubin, like cholesterol, is insoluble in water. An increased concentration of unconjugated bilirubin in bile results either from its formation from conjugated bilirubin in the biliary tree through the action of a glucuronidase (perhaps of bacterial origin, in patients with infected bile; see below) or from increased production of unconjugated bilirubin by the liver (e.g., in patients with hemolytic anemia). A diseased gallbladder is probably not a factor in the formation of pigment stones.

Risk Factors

Because most patients with cholelithiasis are asymptomatic, it is difficult to evaluate risk factors precisely. Known risk factors for the development of cholesterol and pigment stones are listed in Table 96.1 (3).

Cholesterol Stones

The demography of cholesterol stones probably reflects both genetic predisposition and nongenetic ethnic characteristics. For example, it is known that obese people and nonobese people who eat a high-calorie diet secrete more cholesterol into their bile than the average person. Therefore, populations in whom obesity is common (e.g., the Native Americans of the American southwest) or who consume high-calorie diets (occidental societies in general) are more susceptible to cholelithiasis.

The reasons for the increasing incidence of gallstones in middle-aged and elderly people are unknown but may be related to the time that elapses between formation of supersaturated bile and formation of stones and between formation of stones and recognition of them. The enhancement by estrogens of the secretion of cholesterol in bile is reflected in the higher prevalence of gallstones in women (between puberty and menopause) than in men (see above) and in women who take estrogenic preparations compared with women who do not (see Chapters 100 and 106).

Finally, there are a number of ways by which the concentration of bile acids in bile is reduced, favoring the formation of gallstones: Drugs used to treat

Table 96.1. Risk Factors for Gallstones

- Cholesterol stones
  - Demography: Northern Europe, North and South America more than the Orient; Native Americans; probably familial predisposition
  - Obesity
  - High-calorie diet
  - Drugs used in the treatment of hyperlipidemia; clofibrate, cholestyramine, gemfibrozil, colestipol
  - Gastrointestinal disorders involving major malabsorption of bile acids; ileal disease, resection or bypass; cystic fibrosis, with pancreatic insufficiency
  - Female sex hormones: women more at risk than men, use of oral contraceptives and other estrogenic medications
  - Age, especially among men
  - Probable but not well established: pregnancy, diabetes mellitus, and polyunsaturated fats
- Pigment stones
  - Demography: oriental more than occidental; rural more than urban
  - Chronic hemolysis
  - Alcoholic cirrhosis
  - Biliary infection
  - Age

From Bennion LJ, Grundy SM. Risk factors for the development of cholelithiasis in man. N Engl J Med 1978;299:1161, with permission.

hyperlipidemia, such as clofibrate, cholestyramine, gemfibrozil, and colestipol (see Chapter 82), decrease bile acid secretion, and certain disorders of the gastrointestinal tract (ileal resection, Crohn disease of the ileum) reduce bile acid resorption.

Pigment Stones

The demography of pigment stones is entirely different from that of cholesterol stones. The propensity of oriental people to develop pigment stones is not entirely understood, but it may be attributable to the higher prevalence of bacterial infection of the bile (usually *Escherichia coli* infections) and of *Ascaris* infestation in the Orient compared with the Occident. In the United States, patients with pigment gallstones do not usually have infected or infested bile. The recognized risk factors in the United States are hemolysis and alcoholic cirrhosis. Like cholesterol stones, pigment stones are more common with advancing age, but endogenous and exogenous estrogens and obesity have no influence on their development.

Natural History

Many attempts have been made to study the natural history of gallstones among the 2 to 3 million people in the United States known to have them. Of these people, 50% are asymptomatic, having had gallstones discovered incidentally on abdominal radiography (10% to 15% are radiopaque) or another imaging study or during celiotomy for treatment of another condition. The other 50% are symptomatic (i.e., gallstones are discovered during evaluation of the typical or atypical abdominal pain of acute or chronic cholecystitis; see below).

Approximately 18% of people with silent gallstones develop symptoms in 15 to 20 years, and 3% develop complications of biliary tract disease: acute cholecystitis, pancreatitis, or obstructive jaundice (4). The risk of developing complications is unrelated to the severity of symptoms but does increase with the length of time symptoms have been present. Most complications occur only among symptomatic patients. However, 20% of the time acute cholecystitis is the first indication of cholelithiasis. Complications, if they occur, are usually experienced within 5 years of the discovery of gallstones.

Causes of death related to cholelithiasis among patients not having cholecystectomy are acute cholecystitis, cholangitis with liver abscess, necrotizing pancreatitis, gallbladder carcinoma, and gallstone ileus with mechanical small bowel obstruction. In Lund's study of the natural history of cholelithiasis, 2.7% of the deaths among patients not operated on were attributed to gallbladder disease (5).

Asymptomatic Patients

It cannot be predicted on the basis of the size or number of stones or the sex or age of the patient which asymptomatic patients are likely to become symptomatic. Whether asymptomatic patients should undergo elective cholecystectomy, therefore, depends largely on the bias of the primary clinician and the consulting surgeon. Approximately 18% of patients become symptomatic (see above), sometimes at a point in their lives when operation is more dangerous because of age, intercurrent illness, or the presence of acute cholecystitis. The risk of complications of cholelithiasis, other than acute cholecystitis, is negligible in the asymptomatic patient. Carcinoma of the gallbladder is more common among people with gallstones and the risk—0.3% to 1% over a lifetime—is approximately the same as the historic operative mortality from cholecystectomy. However, recent technologic changes have decreased the operative risk considerably. If the gallbladder is calcified, the risk of cancer is nearly 50%, however, and cholecystectomy should be performed. Likewise, prophylactic cholecystectomy is recommended for Native Americans with cholelithiasis, because they have a 3% to 5% risk of developing gallbladder cancer (6). Prophylactic cholecystectomy has also been recommended for children with gallstones, in whom symptoms almost always develop (7), and in patients with sickle cell anemia and cholelithiasis because the symptoms of either condition can easily be confused with the other. Otherwise, the current consensus at this point is not to recommend elective cholecystectomy in the asymptomatic patient. The legitimacy of this same approach in the diabetic patient has been endorsed (8). This recommendation is unchanged even with the emergence of laparoscopic cholecystectomy and its attendant lower morbidity and shortened convalescence (see below).

CHOLECYSTITIS

The hallmark of cholecystitis is abdominal pain (9), often epigastric at onset, but localizing within a few hours to the right upper quadrant. The pain is characteristically, but not always, severe and unremitting, with only slight variations in intensity. Use of the term *biliary colic*, therefore, is not precise because colic is defined as pain that waxes and wanes. Some patients describe the pain as heavy and aching and others as knife-like. Occasionally, it radiates into the right side of the back or, less often, into other parts of the abdomen. The pain, often accompanied by slight nausea, usually begins abruptly, within 1 to 3 hours of eating a meal. (The historical association of the pain with fatty food intolerance is unfounded [10].) Patients may also complain of being awakened in the middle of the night. A typical attack subsides spontaneously within 2 to 3 hours. The frequency of such attacks is extremely variable, from every day to only once or twice a year.

A patient who presents with this history is very likely to have gallstones. However, the degree of inflammation of the gallbladder cannot be determined from the history. There may be gallstones without any inflammation at all, there may be acute inflammation, or there may be chronic inflammation with fibrosis.

However, an attack lasting more than 6 hours generally heralds the onset of acute cholecystitis (i.e., acute inflammation). The severity of the symptoms and the presence or absence of signs of inflammation or biliary obstruction determine the clinician's response (see below).

Acute Cholecystitis

Pathophysiology

More than 90% of the time, acute cholecystitis is caused by a gallstone that obstructs the cystic duct. Acute acalculous cholecystitis occurs primarily in patients who have sustained major trauma, including major operations. Inflammation of the gallbladder in early acute cholecystitis is probably caused by irritation by concentrated static bile. As the process progresses, the bile often becomes infected; bile cultures are positive in only 20% to 30% of patients during the first few days of an attack, but by 7 to 10 days, almost 80% of biliary cultures are positive. In certain patients (e.g., diabetics and patients with acalculous cholecystitis), mural ischemia might also play a role. The difference between the presentation of acute and chronic cholecystitis (see below) is probably caused by the length of time the cystic duct has been totally obstructed and by the intensity of the inflammation.

Signs and Symptoms

The pain of classic acute cholecystitis is severe and persistent. It is usually accompanied by nausea and fever (99 to 102°F [37 to 39°C]) and, less often, by vomiting. Unless treated, the symptoms are likely to persist for up to a week.

The severity and persistence of the pain usually cause the patient to see his or her caregiver (see Chapter 45 for a general discussion of abdominal pain). On examination, the patient is restless. There is considerable right upper quadrant abdominal tenderness, associated with involuntary guarding of the abdominal wall. This guarding, indicative of early peritoneal inflammation, is particularly important to recognize. It is not a feature of less acute disease (see below). *Murphy's sign,* the sudden involuntary arrest of inspiration (because of pain) when the examiner palpates the right upper quadrant during inspiration, is caused by the abutment of the inflamed gallbladder against the examiner's fingers as it moves downward with expansion of the chest cavity. This sign is more often elicited after several days of inflammation. In one-third of patients, the gallbladder is palpable during an attack of acute cholecystitis if the right upper quadrant is probed very gently. Occasionally, patients are mildly jaundiced (see below).

Laboratory Tests

Leukocytosis (12,000 to 15,000 white blood cells/mm^3) caused by a neutrophilic granulocytosis is common. Serum amylase activity may be increased in the absence of other evidence of acute pancreatitis. Often, serum aminotransferases (aspartate aminotransferase and alanine aminotransferase) are increased as well. Twenty percent of patients have mild hyperbilirubinemia (less than 4 mg/100 mL).

Biliary scintigraphy is the test of choice in the diagnosis of acute cholecystitis. The imaging compounds are ^{99m}Tc-labeled derivatives of iminodiacetic acid (TcHIDA, PIPIDA, or DISIDA), which are concentrated in bile. The study requires injection of isotope intravenously and evaluation of uptake of the isotope by the gallbladder. If the cystic duct is obstructed, because of acute inflammation or because of a stone, uptake does not occur. The test takes 1 to 4 hours to complete. A positive study shows isotope in the biliary tree and in the duodenum but not in the gallbladder. A negative study shows isotope in the gallbladder as well. If isotope is not excreted, the test is uninterpretable, but if it is excreted, the sensitivity of the test is extremely high (essentially 100%). Specificity is also high (95%), but false positive results may occur in patients with chronic cholecystitis or acute biliary obstruction caused by pancreatitis.

Ultrasonography may also be used to diagnose acute cholecystitis in a patient with characteristic symptoms. If there are stones in the gallbladder, thickening or edema of the wall, or an "ultrasonic Murphy's sign" (produced by the pressure of the transducer on the inflamed gallbladder), the positive and negative predictive value of the test is greater than 92% (11).

Differential Diagnosis

The differential diagnosis must include disorders that might cause severe right upper quadrant abdominal pain and, usually, leukocytosis and slightly abnormal hepatic tests: acute pancreatitis, appendicitis, hepatitis, hepatic abscess, a perforated or penetrated peptic ulcer, acute pyelonephritis, myocardial infarction, and right lower lobe pneumonia or pleuritis. Because of the severity of the illness, these distinctions should be made in the hospital.

Treatment

The patient suspected of having acute cholecystitis should be hospitalized for observation, hydration, and further diagnostic procedures (see below and Chapter 45 for a discussion of these procedures as they pertain to ambulatory patients). If the pain is intolerable, the caregiver can administer a narcotic parenterally while arranging admission. The patient should be told that in the hospital intravenous rather than oral feeding will be given, that if there is vomiting a nasogastric tube will be passed, and that antibiotics will be administered. Because 30% to 40% of patients develop gangrenous or perforated gallbladders if cholecystectomy is delayed, urgent operation is generally indicated once the diagnosis is made, especially in diabetics and in the elderly (12,13), among whom rapid development of complications is more likely. A randomized prospective study that compared early and delayed cholecystectomy for acute cholecystitis concluded that the duration of hospitalization and the duration of disability were significantly reduced by early operation (14). The presence of emphysematous cholecystitis caused by gas-forming bacterial infection dictates emergency operation (air bubbles in the right upper quadrant on a plain film of the abdomen indicate the diagnosis). Laparoscopic choleciptectomy is ordinarily the operative procedure of choice (15). A discussion of surgery of the biliary tract and of the results and complications of operations is provided below.

Chronic Cholecystitis

Pathophysiology

Symptomatic chronic cholecystitis is associated with gallstones more than 95% of the time; the remaining cases are caused by other diseases of the gallbladder, such as cholesterolosis (the appearance of macrophages laden with cholesterol crystals in the wall of the gallbladder, often without stones). Recurring attacks of mild acute cholecystitis cause eventual fibrosis, so the gallbladder empties poorly. The symptoms of chronic disease, like those of acute cholecystitis, are caused by obstruction by a gallstone of the cystic duct. In chronic recurrent cholecystitis, obstruction of the cystic duct is short (probably no more than a few hours) compared with the length of time of obstruction in acute cholecystitis, so inflammation is less intense. Chronicity of symptoms may also be related to gallbladder dyskinesia secondary to mural fibrosis.

Signs and Symptoms

Many patients who complain of biliary pain for the first time probably already have chronic gallbladder inflammation. The character and location of the pain are identical to those of acute cholecystitis. Pain is variably associated with nausea and, occasionally, vomiting. Unlike classic acute cholecystitis, fever is unusual with chronic disease. Typically, pain occurs after eating, begins 1 to 6 hours after a meal (see above), and lasts for 2 to 3 hours. Nonspecific symptoms—postprandial pain, bloating, belching, flatulence, so-called fatty food intolerance—thought by many to suggest gallbladder disease, are extremely common in the general population and therefore are not helpful diagnostically (see Cholecystitis above).

The patient with chronic cholecystitis usually seeks care less urgently than does the patient with acute cholecystitis. On examination during the attack, although there is tenderness to deep palpation in the right upper quadrant of the abdomen, there is no muscle guarding, as there is in patients with acute inflammation. Murphy's sign (see above) is absent, the gallbladder is rarely palpable, and jaundice usually is not present. Between attacks, there is no abdominal tenderness.

Laboratory Tests

The white blood count, serum amylase, serum aminotransferases, and serum bilirubin are usually normal. Unlike patients with acute cholecystitis, patients with symptoms of chronic cholecystitis can be evaluated further in an ambulatory setting, but some are hospitalized early in an attack because of an inability to distinguish it from an episode of acute cholecystitis. If a TcHIDA scan is obtained to help in making that distinction, it may be positive, even in patients with chronic cholecystitis, because of transient obstruction of the cystic duct.

Ultrasound. Ultrasound has replaced oral cholecystography (at approximately the same cost) as the principal test for the detection of gallstones. The advantages of ultrasound are that it exposes the patient to no radiation, it is much quicker (5 to 10 minutes), and it has no side effects. It is not influenced by associated gastrointestinal or hepatic disease. The detection rate for gallstones 3 mm or greater in diameter is 89% to 96% by ultrasound with 93% to 97% specificity (3% to 7% false positive) (16).

Oral Cholecystogram. The oral cholecystogram documents whether the gallbladder is functioning and whether radiolucent stones are present. Currently, it is obtained only if ultrasound is equivocal. Approximately 75% of gallbladders are visible on the first dose, and another 15% become visible on the second dose. Oral cholecystogram is reliable only if the Telepaque is ingested at the proper time, retained in the gastrointestinal tract, absorbed from the small bowel, transported to the liver, esterified to glucuronide, and excreted by the liver into the bile. Therefore, gastrointestinal or hepatic disease may cause a false positive study. However, the specificity of the test is high (4% false positive) if radiolucent stones are present in an opacified gallbladder or if the gallbladder fails to concentrate contrast material after the second Telepaque dose. The sensitivity of the test is lower (10% false negative), one of the reasons it has been replaced by ultrasonography.

Computed Tomography. Computed tomography (CT) accurately identifies gallstones 80% of the time. Currently, it has no advantages over (and costs about twice as much as) oral cholecystogram and ultrasonography in the diagnosis of gallbladder disease. However, CT might be useful occasionally if both the oral cholecystogram and ultrasound are equivocal.

Treatment

The treatment of choice for symptomatic chronic cholecystitis is elective cholecystectomy in patients who can tolerate an operation (see below). Medical therapies for cholelithiasis such as gallstone dissolution with ursodeoxycholic acid (Actigall) or gallstone lithotripsy are no longer used because of low effectiveness and high recurrence rates. These medical therapies became obsolete with the advent of laparoscopic cholecystectomy (see below). Risks of not treating patients with chronic cholecystitis include gangrene and perforation of the gallbladder, choledocholithiasis (see below), pancreatitis, and, rarely, gallstone ileus (the obstruction of the small bowel by a large gallstone passed through an acute fistula that has formed between the gallbladder and the duodenum).

SYMPTOMATIC PATIENTS WHO HAVE NO DETECTABLE GALLSTONES

Adenomyomatosis of the Gallbladder

Adenomyomatosis of the gallbladder is often asymptomatic, but some patients have symptoms indistinguishable from those with chronic cholecystitis (17). The disease is caused by thickening of the gallbladder wall due to hyperplasia of the epithelium with the formation of glands and diverticula through the muscular wall. The diagnosis is often suspected during ultrasonography or cholecystography, but many cases are revealed by the pathologist after removal of the gallbladder. Adenomyomatosis is found in approximately 20% of patients who undergo cholecystectomy for biliary symptoms. It has been considered not to predispose to gallbladder cancer, but a report of a large number of cases from Japan shows a higher prevalence of gallbladder cancer in segmental adenomyomatosis, which is characterized by a concentric narrowing dividing the gallbladder into two segments (17). Cholecystectomy relieves the symptoms in most patients with symptomatic adenomyomatosis.

Biliary Dyskinesia

Some patients with symptoms suggestive of gallstones have a normal abdominal sonogram, a normal oral cholecystogram, and a normal abdominal CT. These patients may have *biliary dyskinesia,* a term used to denote abnormally decreased emptying of the gallbladder. The diagnosis is best made by cholecystokinin (Kinevac)-stimulated cholecystography with a ^{99m}Tc-iminodiacetic derivative (i.e., TcHIDA). Often, the patient's pain is reproduced after the Kinevac injection (it stimulates gallbladder contraction), and abnormally decreased emptying of the gallbladder can be documented as a markedly decreased ejection fraction (percentage of the isotope excreted) of less than 30% compared with a group of normal subjects. Such patients, if severely symptomatic, should be offered elective cholecystectomy, after which symptoms usually abate. At operation, many of these patients prove to have stones too small to identify by ultrasonography or they have biliary sludge.

Biliary Sludge

In some symptomatic patients who have no gallstones detectable by the standard techniques, the gallbladder reflects, on ultrasonography, echoes now recognized to be characteristic of biliary sludge. *Biliary sludge* is a term applied to excessively viscous bile that contains cholesterol crystals, calcium bilirubinate granules, and mucin. In such patients duodenal drainage, ordinarily done by a consulting gastroenterologist, may prove useful in identifying the cholesterol crystals or the bilirubinate granules.

Patient Experience. The test is performed by having the patient swallow a plastic double-lumen tube, weighted at the end by a mercury-filled bag. There are holes in the tube above the bag. When the bag has passed into the second portion of the duodenum (documented by fluoroscopy), magnesium sulfate is injected into one lumen of the tube to stimulate contraction of the gallbladder. Duodenal contents are then aspirated and the sediment is separated by centrifugation and examined under a microscope. The patient's experience during this procedure is similar to that of patients undergoing upper endoscopy (see Chapter 45).

Biliary sludge may be a precursor of gallstones and of pancreatitis (18), but in a given patient the course is entirely unpredictable. Nevertheless, as with biliary dyskinesia, severely symptomatic patients with biliary sludge should be offered elective cholecystectomy.

CHOLEDOCHOLITHIASIS

Epidemiology

Common duct stones occur in approximately 15% of patients with chronic cholecystitis, either before or after cholecystectomy. The incidence increases with age and the length of time symptoms of gallbladder disease have been present. There are three categories of common duct stones: concomitant gallbladder stones and common duct stones, retained stones found in the common duct soon after cholecystectomy or common duct exploration, and common duct stones identified long after cholecystectomy or common duct exploration. The incidence of common duct stones decreases exponentially in the first year after cholecystectomy only to rise again, reaching a peak at 3 years. In one study, 26% of symptomatic common duct stones occurred 10 or more years after cholecystectomy (19). Also, patients with congenital agenesis of the gallbladder have a 20% incidence of common duct stones. These observations support the concept that common duct stones originate in the gallbladder or in the intrahepatic or common bile ducts.

Signs and Symptoms

Approximately 6% of patients with common duct stones are asymptomatic. More typically, patients develop severe colicky right upper quadrant pain, often associated with jaundice, mild fever, and nausea and vomiting. The pain usually begins abruptly and lasts up to an hour. If nothing is done, attacks recur at variable periods. Eventually cholangitis develops, manifested by persistent malaise and anorexia and intermittent fever, chills, and jaundice, associated with persistently high serum alkaline phosphatase. Suppurative ascending cholangitis characterized by right upper quadrant pain, high fever, shaking chills, and jaundice (Charcot triad) is life threatening and constitutes an emergency.

Rarely, painless jaundice is the only presenting complaint of a patient with choledocholithiasis. In such a circumstance the diagnostic studies should be the same ones performed on the patient with more typical signs and symptoms (see below).

On physical examination, if the patient is asymptomatic, no abnormal signs are elicited. If the patient is symptomatic, right upper quadrant abdominal tenderness and muscle guarding are usually present, similar to the findings in patients with acute cholecystitis. The patient is usually mildly to moderately jaundiced.

Laboratory Tests

Because of the acute onset of symptoms and the severity of pain in patients with choledocholithiasis, laboratory studies in the ambulatory setting are usually not appropriate. If such studies are done, leukocytosis and increases in serum alkaline phosphatase, serum bilirubin, serum aminotransferases, and serum amylase are likely to be observed. The first diagnostic test is ordinarily *ultrasonography* (or CT—equally useful, but more expensive). If the common duct is dilated, the next test is cholangiography.

The preferred procedure is *endoscopic retrograde cholangiopancreatography (ERCP)* because it affords the best visualization of the common bile duct, intrahepatic bile ducts, and the pancreatic duct (20). It also allows diagnosis by cytology or biopsy and the opportunity of intervention, such as removal of a stone from the common bile duct. Percutaneous transhepatic cholangiography is most useful in visualizing obstruction of the intrahepatic bile ducts, which can be relieved by stenting in the case of strictures or removal of stones from the small bile ducts. In addition, percutaneous transhepatic cholangiography is used to visualize the bile ducts in patients who have had a gastrojejunostomy where the sphincter of Oddi is not accessible for ERCP. A newer procedure, magnetic resonance cholangiopancreatography, has the advantage that it is not invasive and is as accurate as ERCP in its diagnostic aspects, but it lacks the opportunity of therapeutic intervention (21).

Treatment

If common duct stones are discovered during cholecystectomy, they are removed. If the patient presents to the clinician with severe right upper quadrant pain, tenderness, guarding, or jaundice, hospitalization for further diagnostic studies and treatment should be arranged. If sonography or CT shows a dilated biliary tree with probable distal obstruction, ERCP should be performed. Common duct stones must be removed, either by operation (see below) or, if possible, at the time of ERCP by endoscopic sphincterotomy. ERCP is performed only in the hospital, usually in the radiology department because fluoroscopy and x-rays of the cannulated duct are required. The patient experience during the procedure is essentially the same as it is during other kinds of upper endoscopy (see Chapter 45), except that ERCP usually lasts for 30 to 60 minutes and may be complicated 5% to 10% of the time by postendoscopic infection, especially if the common duct is manipulated, and by pancreatitis. In an 8-year follow-up of patients after endoscopic sphincterotomy, papillary stenosis or recurrent bile duct stones occurred in less than 5% of the cases (22).

Cholangitis

Bacterial infection of the biliary tree generally occurs in association with bile duct obstruction caused by choledocholithiasis, tumor, or biliary strictures. The principal symptoms are fever, chills, and abdominal pain. Jaundice is often but not invariably present. On examination, there is abdominal tenderness and often rebound tenderness. Abnormal laboratory tests include leukocytosis and elevations of the serum bilirubin and alkaline phosphatase. Serum aminotransferases may also be moderately elevated. Blood cultures are often positive. The patient may deteriorate rapidly and develop hypotension and changes in mental status. Hospitalization is mandatory for therapy with antibiotics, followed by appropriate relief of biliary obstruction either surgically, by endoscopic sphincterotomy, or by placement of a biliary stent.

Primary sclerosing cholangitis (23,24) is a chronic inflammation of unknown cause of intrahepatic and extrahepatic bile ducts that leads ultimately to fibrosis and cholestatic liver disease. Most patients are men. There is a very high correlation with concomitant inflammatory bowel disease, most commonly ulcerative colitis. The course of the cholangitis is unpredictable, but patients with advanced disease develop jaundice, right upper quadrant abdominal pain, fever, pruritus, and weight loss and ultimately die of hepatic failure. Diagnosis is made most easily by the demonstration of typical cholangiographic changes during ERCP. Adenocarcinoma of the bile ducts is a common complication that occurs in at least 9% to 15% of patients (25). Patients with ulcerative colitis and primary sclerosing cholangitis are also at increased risk of colon cancer, beyond the risk imposed by ulcerative colitis alone (26,27). No specific treatment influences the outcome of affected patients (including those with inflammatory bowel disease) with the exception of liver transplantation (see Chapter 47).

BILIARY TRACT OPERATIONS

Primary caregivers should be aware of the mechanics of biliary surgical procedures so that they can inform and reassure patients who are to be referred to a surgeon.

Cholecystectomy

Laparoscopic cholecystectomy has replaced open cholecystectomy as the procedure of choice for the removal of the gallbladder for cholelithiasis and for acute and chronic cholecystitis. Laparoscopic cholecystectomy is performed under general anesthesia. A pneumoperitoneum is established, and a laparoscope and three additional cannulas are inserted through which instruments are placed to remove the gallbladder. Relative contraindications to laparoscopic cholecystectomy include a gangrenous or perforated gallbladder, peritonitis, cholangitis, previous upper abdominal surgery, and cirrhosis (28). Common duct stones are also a contraindication unless they can be extracted by endoscopic sphincterotomy before the cholecystectomy or unless the surgeon is experienced in laparoscopic common duct exploration. Laparoscopic cholecystectomy has the advantage over open cholecystectomy of a shorter hospital stay. In elective cases, the stay is approximately 24 hours, with a return to normal activity in 10 to 14 days. In one study, laparoscopic cholecystectomy needed to be converted to open cholecystectomy in only 4.7% of cases (29). The common reasons for conversion are severe scarring or acute inflammation that obscures the anatomy, adhesions related to prior surgery, aberrant anatomic features that make dissection difficult, and bile duct, bowel, or vascular injuries that occur during surgery. Common duct stones encountered during the procedure can sometimes be removed by laparoscopic choledochoscopy but otherwise require open common duct exploration or postoperative ERCP. In a reported series, complications occurred in 5.1% of cases (29). The most common complication is wound infection in 1.1% of cases, followed by bile duct injury in 0.5% of cases. Other complications are prolonged ileus, bowel injury, and operative bleeding. Mortality in elective cases is less than 0.1%

Elective open cholecystectomy has a mortality rate of 0.3% or less. Urgent or emergency operation for acute cholecystitis has a mortality rate of up to 10% depending on whether common duct stones are present. The morbidity of cholecystectomy is primarily related to superficial wound infection (less than 5% to 7%). Wound infection is more common if the operation lasts longer than 2 hours, the patient is obese or diabetic, and the patient has acute rather than chronic cholecystitis. Other possible but rare (less than 1%) immediate complications of cholecystectomy are postoperative bleeding, postoperative bile leak, injury to biliary ducts (0.1%), and retained common duct stones.

Cholecystostomy

Cholecystostomy may be required in the patient who is critically ill from acute cholecystitis and who has associated severe cardiac, pulmonary, or renal disease that contraindicates the use of general anesthesia or of a prolonged operation. Another less often cited indication for cholecystostomy is inability to detect normal biliary anatomy because of a severe inflammatory process near the main bile ducts. Rather than risk possible injury to structures in the porta hepatis, a cholecystostomy may be performed.

A cholecystostomy can be done through a small incision in the right upper quadrant. A large drainage tube is inserted into the gallbladder through a stab wound in the fundus. An attempt is made to remove stones. The tube is brought through the abdominal wall and allowed to drain freely. An attempt should be made to empty the gallbladder of stones before placing the tube. If a stone is impacted at the cystic duct, future cholecystectomy will be necessary or a mucous fistula will persist after the tube is removed. However, if all stones are removed, only 30% to 50% of patients will develop recurrent symptoms of cholelithiasis within 2 years after the tube is removed. The operative mortality is very high from cholecystostomy, not because of the operation but because the patient is critically ill.

Choledochotomy

Common duct exploration or choledochotomy, whether combined with cholecystectomy or as an isolated operation, has a higher morbidity and mortality rate than does simple cholecystectomy. The operation takes longer than cholecystectomy and patients are generally older, two factors important in determining morbidity and mortality. Generally the patient is hospitalized 3 to 5 days longer for common duct exploration than for cholecystectomy alone (see below). A drain (called a T-tube) is generally placed in the common duct at the time of operation. This is done to stent the repair and to allow postoperative imaging to rule out retained stones or other technical problems.

COURSE AFTER OPEN BILIARY SURGERY

Normal Course

The patient is usually discharged 5 to 7 days after an uncomplicated open biliary tract operation. Skin sutures or staples will have been removed, and the patient will be allowed to bathe. Usually patients are requested to avoid driving and sexual relations for 1 week from the day of discharge. Patients are generally advised to avoid heavy (approximately 15 pounds [7 kg] or more) lifting for 4 to 6 weeks. The incidence of incisional hernia (see Chapter 97) is low after a right subcostal oblique incision and slightly higher with a vertical midline or paramedian incision. The patient returns to the surgeon's office for evaluation at 1 and 6 weeks after operation. The wound and the drain sites, if present, should be healed unless there has been wound infection. If a common duct exploration was performed, the T-tube is removed at the first visit, assuming the postoperative cholangiogram is normal. The patient should be able to resume an unrestricted regular diet within a few days of operation without difficulty. Stools should be at preoperative frequency and of normal color. Immediate weight loss of 10 to 20 pounds is normal, even in uncomplicated cases. Ten percent of patients have diarrhea for up to 6 weeks but rarely longer than that.

The patient should be expected to complain about pulling sensations in the area of the incision because the right rectus muscle has been divided and resutured. If the subcostal incision was made close to the costal margin, the patient often complains also about discomfort on bending or sitting. The area just below a right subcostal incision is apt to be numb for several months because of interruption of a cutaneous sensory nerve to this area. Sensitivity does return, however, in most cases. It is not surprising to find patients gaining weight after cholecystectomy, especially if they had lost weight preoperatively.

Postcholecystectomy Syndrome

Approximately 90% of patients operated on for symptomatic biliary tract disease become asymptomatic or have trivial symptoms (e.g., occasional dyspepsia). The other 10% may continue to be symptomatic, either because they were treated for the wrong disease or because they have developed a postoperative complication. In the former category are patients who had gallstones but whose symptoms actually emanated from another disease (e.g., recurrent pancreatitis, peptic ulcer disease, angina, reflux esophagitis, or irritable bowel syndrome).

Postoperative problems associated with the operation itself include retained common duct stones, an excessively long cystic duct remnant, and common duct injury with eventual bile duct stricture and recurrent cholangitis. Sphincter of Oddi dysfunction is increasingly being recognized as one of the treatable causes of postcholecystectomy syndrome. The diagnosis is made by showing a decrease in the emptying of the biliary tree by cholecystokinin cholecystography with ^{99m}Tc-iminodiacetic derivatives (see above) and by demonstrating an elevated sphincter pressure by manometry during ERCP. Sphincterotomy in patients with elevated sphincter pressure results in pain relief in more than 90% of cases (30).

General References*

Kaplowitz N. Liver and biliary diseases. 2nd ed. Baltimore: Williams & Wilkins, 1996.
A comprehensive text.

Ransohoff DF, Gracie WA. Treatment of gallstones. Ann Intern Med 1993;119:606.
A comprehensive review of risks and benefits of therapy for patients with gallstones.

Specific References

1. Johnston DE, Kaplan MM. Pathogenesis and treatment of gallstones. N Engl J Med 1993;328:412.
2. Thistle JL, Schoenfield LJ. Lithogenic bile among young Indian women: lithogenic potential decreased with chenodeoxycholic acid. N Engl J Med 1971;284:177.
3. Bennion LJ, Grundy SM. Risk factors for the development of cholelithiasis in man. N Engl J Med 1978;299:1161.
4. Gracie WA, Ransohoff DF. The natural history of silent gallstones. The innocent gallstone is not a myth. N Engl J Med 1982;307:798.
5. Lund J. Surgical indications in cholelithiasis; prophylactic cholecystectomy elucidated on the basis of long-term follow-up on 526 nonoperated cases. Ann Surg 1960;151:153.
6. Lowenfels AB, Lindstrom CG, Conway MJ, et al. Gallstones and risk of gallbladder cancer. J Natl Cancer Inst 1985;75:77.
7. Pokorny WJ, Saleem M, O'Gorman RB, et al. Cholelithiasis and cholecystitis in childhood. Am J Surg 1984;148:742.
8. Friedman LS, Roberts MS, Brett AS, et al. Management of asymptomatic gallstones in the diabetic patient. A decision analysis. Ann Intern Med 1988;109:913.
9. Diehl AK, Sugarek NJ, Todd KH. Clinical evaluation for gallstone disease: usefulness of symptoms and signs in diagnosis. Am J Med 1990;89:29.
10. Mogadam M, Albarelli J, Ahmed SW, et al. Gallbladder dynamics in response to various meals: is dietary fat restriction necessary in the management of gallstones? Am J Gastroenterol 1984;79:745.
11. Ralls PW, Coletti PM, Lapin SA, et al. Real-time sonography in suspected acute cholecystitis. Prospective evaluation of primary and secondary signs. Radiology 1985;155:767.
12. Mundth ED. Cholecystitis and diabetes mellitus. N Engl J Med 1962;267:642.
13. Morrow DJ, Thompson J, Wilson SE. Acute cholecystitis in the elderly, a surgical emergency. Arch Surg 1978;113:1149.
14. Jarvinen HJ, Hastbacka J. Early cholecystectomy for acute cholecystitis: a prospective randomized study. Ann Surg 1980;191:501.
15. Bender JS, Zenilman ME. Immediate laparoscopic cholecystectomy as definitive therapy for acute cholecystitis. Surg Endosc 1995;9:1081.
16. Ferruci TJ. Body ultrasonography. N Engl J Med 1979;300: 538.
17. Ram MD, Midha D. Adenomyomatosis of the gallbladder. Surgery 1975;78:224.
18. Lee SP, Nicholls JF, Park HZ. Biliary sludge as a cause of acute pancreatitis. N Engl J Med 1992;326:589.
19. Thurston OG, McDougall RM. The effect of hepatic bile on retained common duct stones. Surg Gynecol Obstet 1976;143: 625.
20. Schofl R. Diagnostic endoscopic retrograde cholangiopancreatography. Endoscopy 2001;33:147.
21. Magneson TH, Bender JS, Duncan MD, et al. Utility of magnetic resonance cholangiography in the evaluation of biliary obstruction. J Am Coll Surg 1999;189:63.
22. Prat F, Malak NA, Pelletier G. Biliary symptoms and complications more than 8 years after endoscopic sphincterotomy. Gastroenterology 1996;110:894.
23. Lee YM, Kaplan MM. Primary sclerosing cholangitis. N Engl J Med 1995;332:924.
24. Angulo P, Lindor KD. Primary sclerosing cholangitis. Hepatology 1999;30:325.
25. Rosen CB, Nagorney DM, Wiesner RH, et al. Cholangiocarcinoma complicating primary sclerosing cholangitis. Ann Surg 1991;213:21.
26. Brentnall TA, Haggitt RC, Rabinovitch PS, et al. Risk and natural history of colonic neoplasia in patients with primary sclerosing cholangitis and ulcerative colitis. Gastroenterology 1996;110:331.
27. Shetty K, Rybicki L, Brezezinski A, et al. The risk for cancer or dysplasia in ulcerative colitis patients with primary sclerosing cholangitis. Am J Gastroenterol 1999;94:1643.
28. Gadacz TR. Laparoscopy cholecystectomy. In: Cameron JL, ed. Current surgical therapy, 4th ed. St. Louis: CV Mosby, 1992: 330.
29. Southern Surgeons Club. A prospective analysis of 1518 laparoscopic cholecystectomies. N Engl J Med 1991;324:1073.
30. Greenen JE, Hogan WJ, Dodds WJ, et al. The efficacy of endoscopic sphincterotomy after cholecystectomy in patients with sphincter-of-Oddi dysfunction. N Engl J Med 1989;320: 82.

*Bold print (general references) and bold numerals (specific references) denote published controlled clinical trials, meta-analyses, or consensus-based recommendations.

CHAPTER 97

Abdominal Hernias

MARK D. DUNCAN, MD, FACS
JEFFREY S. BENDER, MD, FACS

DEFINITIONS

A hernia is a protrusion of a viscus or part of a viscus from its normal location in the body. Clinically common hernias involve anatomic defects in the abdominal wall, typically in the inguinal, femoral, or umbilical regions or at the site of a previous surgical incision. The term *ventral hernia,* referring to an anterior abdominal wall hernia, is often used to denote an incisional hernia. A hernia is *reducible* if its contents can be pushed back into the abdominal cavity, and *incarcerated* if they cannot be pushed back. *Strangulation* of a hernia occurs when the blood supply to the herniated tissue is compromised. All strangulated hernias are incarcerated, but incarcerated hernias may not be strangulated.

This chapter describes the more common types of abdominal hernias and discusses the role of the general physician in their diagnosis and treatment.

HERNIAS OF THE GROIN

Inguinal Hernias

Inguinal hernias (Fig. 97.1) are classified as direct or indirect; about two thirds are indirect (1). *Direct hernias* are portions of the bowel or omentum that protrude directly through the floor of the inguinal canal to emerge through the external inguinal ring above the inguinal ligament (Fig. 97.2). *Indirect hernias* enter the inguinal canal through its internal ring, lateral to the inferior epigastric vessels, traverse the canal, and emerge also through the external inguinal ring (Fig. 97.2). Indirect hernias, as they get larger, have a propensity to extend into the scrotum.

Epidemiology and Causes

Inguinal hernia is a common problem in ambulatory practice and accounts for approximately 75% of all abdominal wall hernias. Inguinal hernia repair is one of the most common general surgical procedures performed in the United States (1). The majority of inguinal hernias occur in men (1); 5% to 10% of men in the United States develop an inguinal hernia during their lifetime. Although femoral hernias (discussed later) are much more common in women than in men, the most common groin hernia in women is an indirect inguinal hernia. Less than 10% of inguinal hernias in adults are bilateral when the patient is first seen, but a hernia may occur on the opposite side at some time in the future. The chance of developing a contralateral inguinal hernia is the same regardless of which side is affected first.

All *indirect inguinal hernias* are caused by a congenital defect in which the processus vaginalis remains patent. The processus vaginalis is a tract lined with peritoneum that extends from the peritoneal cavity into the scrotum in the male. With time this tract may enlarge, and abdominal contents may herniate into it. The combination of this congenital abnormality and a predisposing acquired condition that increases intra-abdominal pressure (e.g., obesity, chronic obstructive airway disease, ascites, chronic constipation with straining at stool, prostatism with straining at urination, hard physical labor) determines when an inguinal hernia develops. Occasionally, only intra-abdominal fluid gravitates into the scrotum, causing scrotal swelling when the patient is upright but draining back into the abdominal cavity when the patient is supine. Such a lesion is called a *communicating hydrocele*; it is more commonly seen in children than in adults. Indirect hernias, because they are associated with a congenital defect, develop in younger people but increase in incidence with advancing age; they are about four to five times more common after 50 years of age than before.

Direct inguinal hernias are acquired lesions and are influenced not only by changes in intra-abdominal pressure but also by progressive attenuation of the inguinal structures as part of the normal aging process. Rarely, inherited defects in collagen synthesis (e.g., Marfan syndrome) provide an obvious explanation for accelerated weakening of these structures. Direct hernias are predominantly problems of middle-aged and elderly people.

History

Most patients complain of a dull ache in the groin and a bulge, either localized to the groin or at times extending into the scrotum in men or the labia in women. Sometimes pain precedes discovery of the mass by some months (perhaps because, in early stages of herniation, the internal canal is stretched before omentum or bowel manifests as a bulge at the external inguinal ring). Occasionally, the patient recalls a sharp pain during a strenuous event, which represents the initial herniation. Often the patient or the clinician notices a herniated mass in the absence of pain or symptoms. Small reducible hernias may be noticed intermittently, at times of increased intra-abdominal pressure.

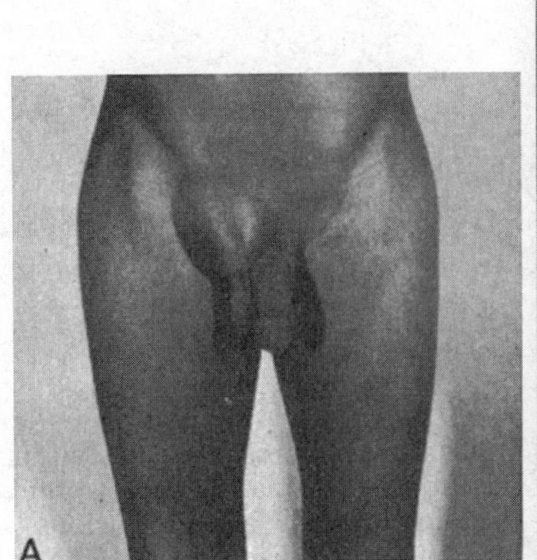

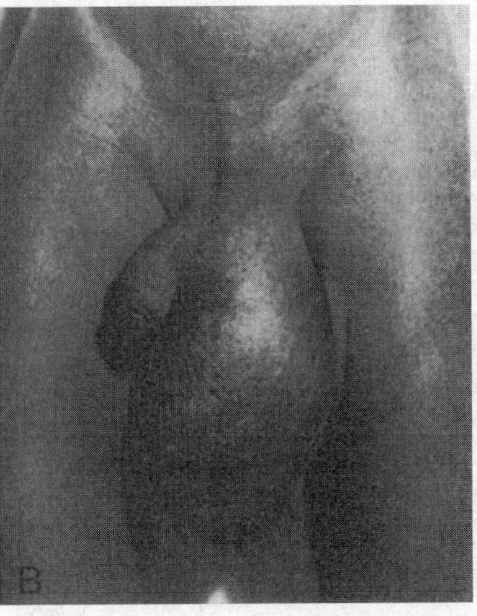

Figure 97.1. **A.** Right inguinal hernia in a young adult male patient. **B.** Left scrotal hernia. (From Zimmerman LM, Anson BJ. Anatomy and surgery of hernia. 2nd ed. Baltimore: Williams & Wilkins, 1967:1552.)

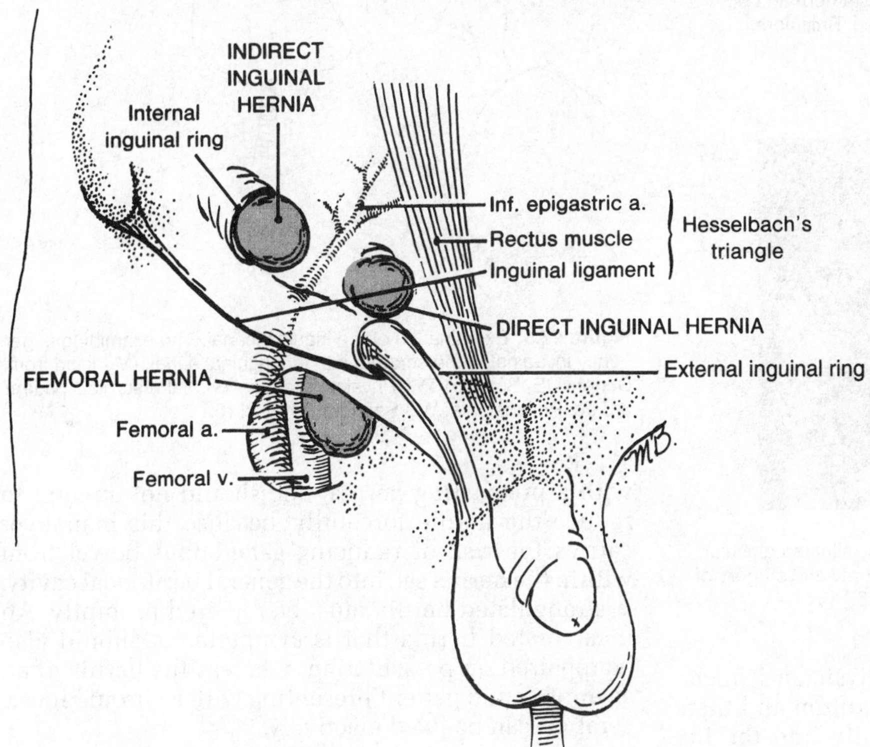

Figure 97.2. Artist's rendition of groin region, illustrating indirect and direct inguinal hernias and femoral hernia. (Modified from Dunphy JE, Botsford TW. Physical examination of the surgical patient. 3rd ed. Philadelphia: WB Saunders, 1964:118.)

If a hernia incarcerates, it may become more painful, although many patients with chronically incarcerated hernias are pain free. Indirect hernias have an approximately 10% chance of incarcerating; direct hernias incarcerate only rarely. Essentially all strangulated hernias are symptomatic: The hernia becomes extremely painful and tender, and nausea, vomiting, abdominal distention, constipation, and fever (with leukocytosis) are common.

Physical Examination

The examination should be performed with the patient standing and then again with the patient recumbent. An indirect hernia sometimes can be distinguished from a direct hernia by inspection: An indirect hernia, once it has entered the inguinal canal, manifests as an elliptical swelling descending toward or even into the scrotum (Fig. 97.3). A direct hernia manifests as an isolated oval swelling near the pubis; it rarely is found in the scrotum (Fig. 97.4). If the hernia is visible, an attempt should be made to push it back into the abdominal cavity. If the hernia cannot be reduced, the patient should be asked to lie down and another attempt should be made to reduce it. Approximately 10% of inguinal hernias are incarcerated when they are first diagnosed.

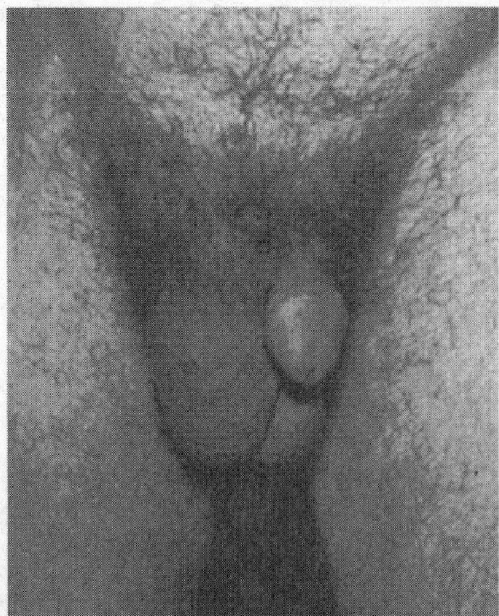

Figure 97.3. Indirect inguinal hernia. Swelling is oblique and cylindrical and extends into the scrotum. (From Zimmerman LM, Anson BJ. Anatomy and surgery of hernia. 2nd ed. Baltimore: Williams & Wilkins, 1967:155.)

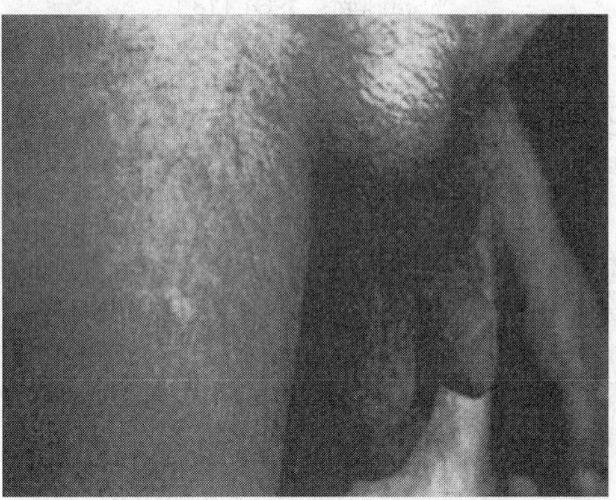

Figure 97.4. Direct inguinal hernia. Note medially situated globular swelling. (From Zimmerman LM, Anson BJ. Anatomy and surgery of hernia. 2nd ed. Baltimore: Williams & Wilkins, 1967:154.)

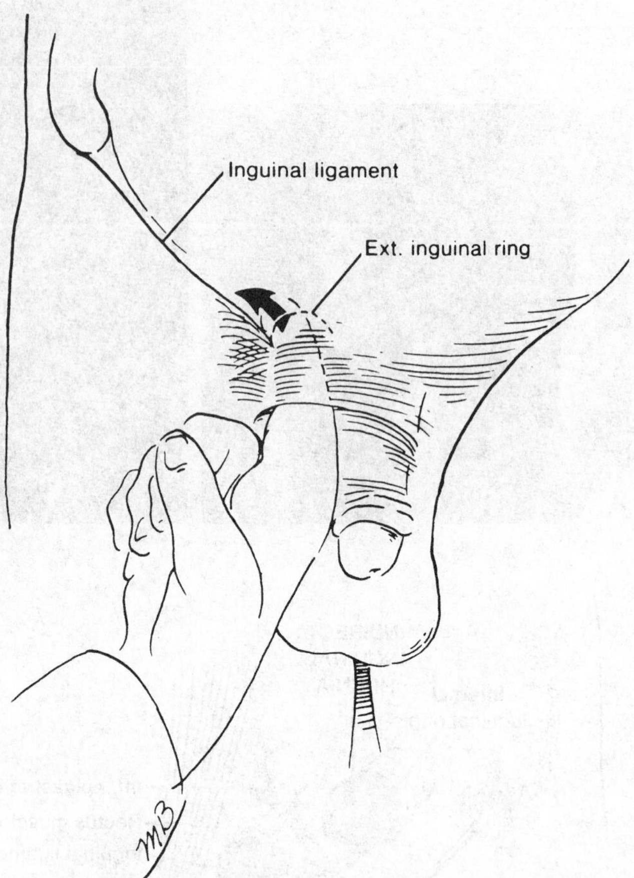

Figure 97.5. Examination of the inguinal canal. The examining finger gently invaginates the scrotum into the inguinal canal. (Modified from Dunphy JE, Botsford TW. Physical examination of the surgical patient. 3rd ed. Philadelphia: WB Saunders, 1964:116.)

If the hernia is not visible, the physician's finger should be placed at the base of the scrotum and then gently advanced cephalad and laterally into the inguinal canal (Fig. 97.5). The external ring can be examined without causing the patient a great deal of discomfort. The size of the ring, in itself, does not predict the presence of a hernia or the propensity to develop one, because the external ring is an opening in the aponeurosis of the external oblique muscle that does not contribute to the integrity of the floor of the inguinal canal. When the examining finger has been directed through the external ring, having the patient increase intra-abdominal pressure by coughing or straining causes a hernia to protrude and to be felt as an impulse or bulge at the tip of the examining finger.

An attempt should be made to reduce an incarcerated hernia; however, if strangulation is suspected, as when a patient presents with severe pain associated with a preexisting hernia, one should not attempt to reduce the hernia forcefully, because this maneuver carries the risk of reducing gangrenous bowel from within the hernia sac into the general peritoneal cavity. A strangulated hernia must be repaired promptly. An incarcerated hernia that is symptomatic should also be repaired on presentation, whereas the hernia of an asymptomatic patient presenting with a chronic incarceration can be fixed electively.

Differential Diagnosis

The most common cause of groin pain that is mistaken for a hernia is *strain of the adductor muscles* of the thigh at their attachment to the pelvis. Because, like groin hernia, the onset of this symptom is related to physical labor, both the patient and the clinician are convinced that a hernia must be present. In the absence of appropriate physical findings, the temptation to surgically explore the groin must be firmly resisted. As with other muscular injuries, groin strain can take months to resolve.

An incarcerated scrotal hernia must be distinguished from other scrotal lesions (Fig. 97.6). One of the most common of these is a *hydrocele*—a tense,

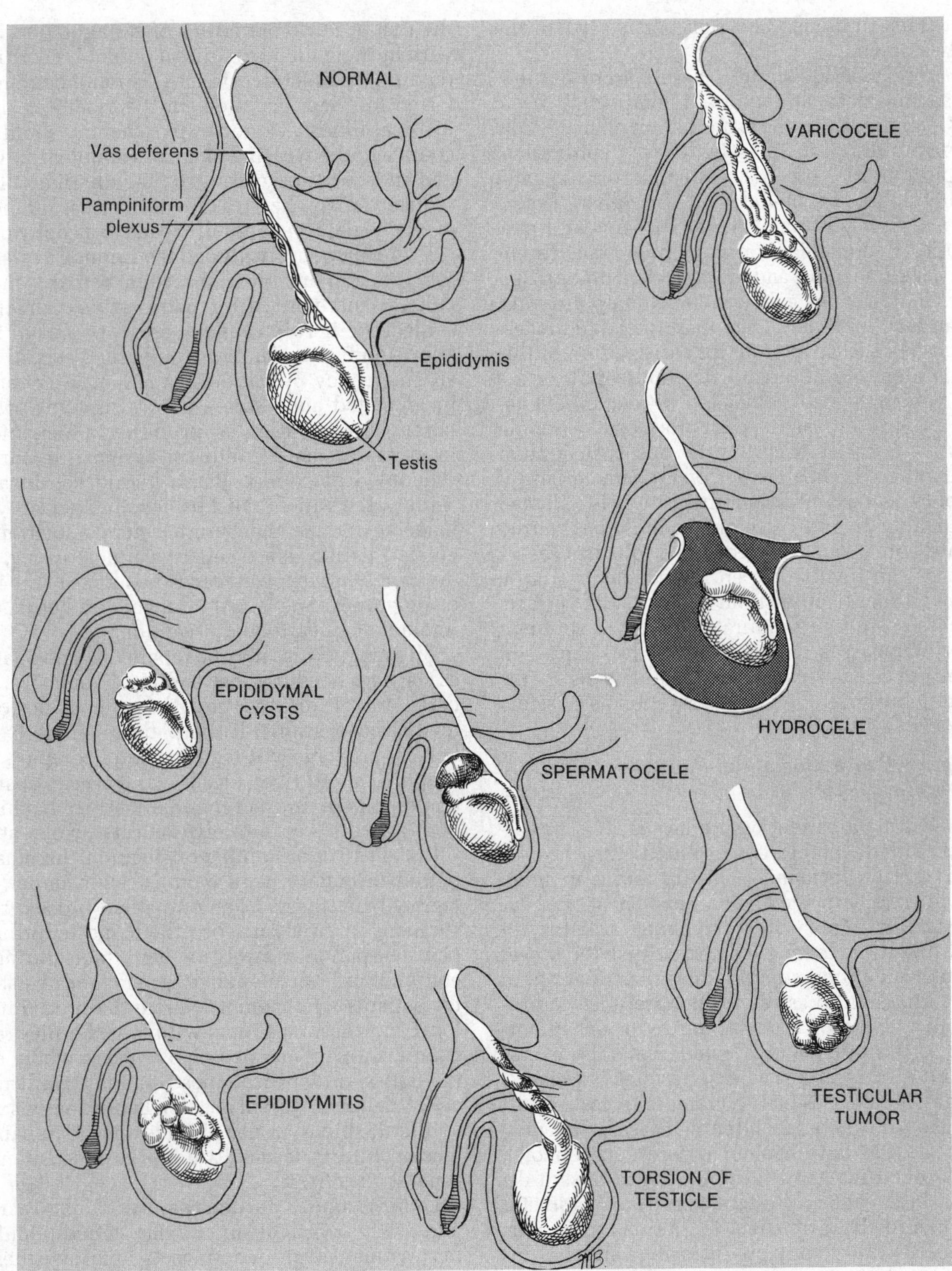

Figure 97.6. Lesions palpable in the scrotum. A correct diagnosis can usually be made if the normal anatomic relationships of the contents of the scrotum are borne in mind. (Modified from Dunphy JE, Botsford TW. Physical examination of the surgical patient. 3rd ed. Philadelphia: WB Saunders, 1964:111.)

slightly fluctuant mass that can be distinguished from a hernia or a solid mass by transillumination. Another common scrotal mass is a *varicocele*—an enlarged venous plexus that on palpation feels soft and worm-like and extends from the testicle up toward the spermatic cord. It does not transilluminate and, when the patient lies down, it collapses. If a varicocele is of recent onset in an adult, occurs on the left, and does not disappear in the supine position, one must consider obstruction of the left spermatic vein (which enters the left renal vein) by a retroperitoneal neoplasm. A *spermatocele* is a localized but vaguely circumscribed mass that also does not transilluminate and that persists when the patient lies down.

Apart from distinguishing a hernia from another kind of scrotal mass, an important component of the physical examination is the examination of the testicle and its surrounding structures. In that way, epididymal cysts, epididymitis, orchitis, testicular torsion, and testicular tumors can be detected. *Epididymal cysts* can occur in any portion of the epididymis and may be smooth or lobulated; some of them transilluminate; they are innocuous and require no treatment. *Epididymitis* manifests as a tender, swollen epididymis. The inflammation, if untreated, may spread to the testicle (orchitis); see Chapter 36 for a discussion of this problem. Often, elevation and immobilization of the scrotum relieve the pain associated with an inflammatory process. In contrast, the pain produced by *torsion of the testicle* is unremitting. Sudden onset of testicular pain in an otherwise healthy person is characteristic of this problem. On examination, the testicle is enlarged and exquisitely tender. The patient should be referred immediately to a general surgeon or urologist. *Testicular tumors* can involve the entire testicle or simply protrude as a small nodule from the testicular surface. These masses are more indurated than the common benign scrotal masses, and they usually lack the slight tenderness of the normal testicle. Patients with suspected tumors should be referred as soon as possible to a urologist.

Preoperative Evaluation of the Patient with a Hernia

When evaluating a patient with a hernia, it is important to consider whether coexistent disease has allowed the hernia to manifest at that point in time. Focused questions in the medical history should include a specific inquiry about smoking, a history of cough, difficulty urinating, or difficulty with bowel movements, including straining and constipation. A rectal examination, to assess for the presence of prostatic hypertrophy or a rectal mass, is an important part of the preoperative evaluation. The examiner should also ascertain whether ascites is present. Anything that increases intra-abdominal pressure will place tension on the endoabdominal fascia and may contribute to the development or presentation of a hernia. A practitioner would not want to miss a diagnosis of lung cancer, prostate cancer, or colorectal cancer when referring a patient for hernia repair. Furthermore, attention to any predisposing causes of increased intra-abdominal pressure may limit the effect these conditions have on hernia recurrence rates.

Management

Almost all inguinal hernias should be repaired. Severe coexistent illness is the only real contraindication to herniorrhaphy (see Chapter 93 for a discussion of anesthesia/surgery risks in patients with coexistent medical conditions). Although no sense of urgency is associated with elective repair, it should be recognized that the risk of incarceration or of strangulation is greater with indirect than with direct hernia. Accordingly, the repair of a direct hernia may be more confidently deferred, or even declined, in the face of a significant medical illness. Nonoperative therapy should be discouraged; the wearing of a truss is potentially dangerous and does not guarantee that a hernia will remain reduced. Also, the pressure of the truss on the margin of a large defect eventually leads to atrophy of the fascial and aponeurotic (broad tendinous) layers, causing the hernia to enlarge. Subsequent repair is more difficult and therefore carries a greater risk of recurrence.

Elective herniorrhaphy prevents acute incarceration (and strangulation) and the need to perform an emergency operation. If the hernia is chronically incarcerated and there are no symptoms of strangulation (strangulation is primarily a risk in acutely incarcerated, small, indirect hernias), repair may be scheduled electively. If the hernia has incarcerated acutely, the patient must be hospitalized and attempts made to reduce the hernia before operation. Strangulated hernia is a true surgical emergency, because delay in treatment can lead to gangrene of the intestine or omentum. Suspected strangulated hernias require immediate operative intervention.

Bilateral hernias may be repaired at one operation or as staged procedures, depending on their size, the type of repair required, the age of the patient, and coexistent medical conditions. If the patient is elderly and the hernias are large and require complex repair, herniorrhaphies should be staged 4 to 6 weeks apart. Bilateral repairs of indirect inguinal hernias in children or young adults are routinely done at one operation.

Currently, most unilateral inguinal hernias are repaired through a 6- to 8-cm incision under local or regional anesthesia as an outpatient procedure. Many surgeons routinely use prosthetic mesh during the repair. The patient is rarely uncomfortable during the operation. Epidural, spinal, or general anesthesia is used for patients who cannot tolerate the procedure under local anesthesia, patients with large hernias requiring complex repair, and obese patients, in whom repair of the hernia under local anesthesia is technically difficult. Bilateral inguinal herniorrhaphy may also require epidural, spinal, or general anesthesia. Repair of hernias in children is usually done with the patient under general anesthesia.

Laparoscopic Herniorrhaphy. Laparoscopic (or minimally invasive) surgery has gained popularity in the treatment of groin hernias. General anesthesia is required. A laparoscope and two or three instruments are introduced into the peritoneal cavity, usually through separate 0.5- to 1.0-cm incisions rather than one long incision. Under direct visualization, indirect hernia sacs can be dissected and even large defects can be repaired with the use of prosthetic mesh. Laparoscopic herniorrhaphy is an outpatient procedure. Advantages to the laparoscopic approach include lower levels of postoperative pain and shorter recuperative time than after the standard type of repair. Several large studies have documented the safety of the procedure with good short-term follow-up (2–5). It is perhaps particularly suited to recurrent groin hernias or bilateral hernia repair. The complication rate in experienced hands is now about the same as it is for anterior repair (about 10%) (2–4). Ilioinguinal neuralgia seems to occur more often after laparoscopic repair, but this may also be true of anterior repairs in which mesh is used. More significantly, data regarding long-term recurrence rates are lacking. The cost of laparoscopic repair at this time is significantly higher than that of open repair. As surgeons' familiarity with the laparoscopic approach to the groin improves, complication rates should decrease; if long-term review validates low recurrence rates, the postoperative benefits of laparoscopic repair will make it attractive for selected patients with groin hernias. Although laparoscopic repair is an accepted technique for recurrent or bilateral inguinal hernias, the predominant approach still remains the traditional open anterior repair.

Course and Recovery

No matter which anesthesia or technique is used, certain *complications of herniorrhaphy* are possible (in approximately 7% of patients): recurrence (the most common complication), urinary retention, wound infection, hydrocele formation, femoral or ilioinguinal neuralgia, scrotal hematoma, and, rarely, unilateral testicular atrophy. The general practitioner and the surgeon should discuss these complications with the patient before the operation and provide assurance that, except for recurrence of hernia (and testicular atrophy), they are usually transient problems.

When patients are discharged from the hospital, they are ambulatory but typically require narcotic analgesics for relief of pain. Patients are admitted to the hospital only if urinary retention or another complication (e.g., bleeding, hypotension) occurs. Patients with preexisting medical illnesses, particularly cardiac disease, may be admitted as needed for medical management perioperatively. For the first week, the patient is advised to avoid lifting or straining and to use a stool softener and a mild laxative (see Chapter 46). The patient can return to light work (and light activity such as long walks) within another 2 weeks, but an occupation that requires heavy lifting or considerable exertion requires a total convalescence of 6 weeks.

Driving a car during the first 2 weeks should be discouraged, not because it is a form of strenuous activity, but because the patient, fearing pain or injury, may not step on the brake vigorously enough or soon enough in a crisis to avoid a collision. Sexual activity is permitted if it is not uncomfortable to the patient. Resumption of normal recreational and work activities requires common sense. Most patients are fully rehabilitated and working less than 1 month after herniorrhaphy. Because recurrence may be related to premature untoward exertion, patients must be cautioned to avoid strenuous activity for 6 weeks.

Approximately 1% to 7% of indirect and 4% to 10% of direct inguinal hernias recur. More than 50% of the recurrences occur within 5 years after the initial repair. The recurrence rate after repair of a recurrent hernia is even higher, ranging from 5% to 35%. Most surgeons use mesh in the repair of recurrent hernias.

Femoral Hernias

Epidemiology and Causes

A femoral hernia is a protrusion of omentum or bowel through the femoral canal (Fig. 97.2). It is much more common in women than in men. The incidence increases with increasing age, presumably because of the degradation of collagen and attenuation of tissue that accompanies aging. It is likely, however, that a contributing cause of a femoral hernia is a congenitally large femoral ring. Preperitoneal fat, forced through the large ring, enlarges it further. Increased pressure produced by straining or pregnancy undoubtedly contributes to femoral herniation. Femoral hernias are bilateral in at least 15% of cases. The risk of incarceration, and particularly of strangulation, is especially high with this type of hernia.

History. The primary symptom of a femoral hernia is a bulge in the groin. A dull pain may be experienced, but less commonly than in patients with an inguinal hernia. Approximately 20% of femoral hernias incarcerate (twice the rate of indirect inguinal hernias). The symptoms of incarceration and strangulation are the same as in patients with inguinal hernias.

Physical Examination. A mass is often palpable, medial to the femoral vessels and inferior to the inguinal ligament. The mass is usually reducible, and occasionally it is tender. Despite careful examination, the hernia often is difficult to detect, especially in obese women, even if it is incarcerated or strangulated. Therefore, women with signs and symptoms of unexplained intestinal obstruction should be examined carefully for evidence of a strangulated femoral hernia.

Differential Diagnosis. A femoral hernia must be distinguished from an enlarged lymph node, a lipoma, a saphenous varix, and a direct inguinal hernia. The first three of these possibilities are not reducible. A *lymph node* or *lipoma* may not transmit an impulse to the examiner's finger when the patient coughs. A *saphenous varix* may simulate a hernia impulse, however, because increased venous pressure induced by the Valsalva maneuver is transmitted to the varix. A lymph node or lipoma is more movable than a hernia, and a varix can be collapsed by compression of the saphenous vein. The distinction between a femoral and other groin hernias sometimes can be made only at operation.

Management and Course. Femoral hernias should be repaired unless the patient is unable to tolerate an operation. The increased risk of incarceration and strangulation adds to the urgency of the recommendation. The operative and postoperative considerations of inguinal hernia (discussed earlier) apply to femoral hernias as well, except that, for technical reasons, a larger proportion of femoral hernias may have to be performed under spinal or general anesthesia, usually as outpatient procedures. Laparoscopy (see earlier discussion) can also be used in femoral hernia repair. Between 1% and 7% of femoral hernias recur and, as with inguinal hernias, 5% to 35% of repaired recurrent hernias also recur.

UMBILICAL HERNIAS

An umbilical hernia is a protrusion of omentum or bowel through the umbilical ring. These hernias are probably caused by congenital defects. Among adults, they appear most often in middle-age multiparous women, in patients with cirrhosis of the liver and ascites, and in frail elderly people. They are also common in infants, especially African American infants. Most umbilical hernias are obvious as an enlargement of the umbilical ring with protrusion of intra-abdominal contents through it. However, a few patients complain only of vague intermittent pain and tenderness in the region of the umbilicus. On examination, a small defect is usually found that contains a small piece of omentum, preperitoneal fat, or a knuckle of bowel. If patients are placed in the supine position and then asked to raise their head and cough, the hernia can be palpated.

The most common complication of umbilical hernia is incarceration with or without strangulation. Incarceration is more common with umbilical hernias than with groin hernias. For that reason, unless the patient cannot tolerate an operation, all umbilical hernias in adults should be repaired. Morbidity and mortality from such an operation are much lower if it is performed electively rather than in response to acute incarceration or strangulation. The only exception to this recommendation is umbilical hernias in infants. These tend to close spontaneously as the child gets older, and repair should be deferred until school age.

The repair may be done under local anesthesia if the hernia is small; otherwise, general or spinal anesthesia is preferred. The procedure does not require overnight hospitalization.

EPIGASTRIC HERNIAS

An epigastric hernia is a protrusion of fat or omentum through the linea alba between the umbilicus and the xiphoid cartilage. These hernias almost never contain a viscus. A congenital defect in the linea alba is probably the major disposing factor. Epigastric hernias most commonly appear between the ages of 20 and 50 years and are three times more common in men than in women. Most patients complain of a small, painless, subcutaneous mass, most often just to the left of the midline. Usually the hernia consists of preperitoneal fat or fat of the falciform ligament. Larger defects also contain omentum. Complications are more common in patients with small hernias because these are more likely to incarcerate. When this happens, there is usually local pain and tenderness and, less often, deep epigastric pain, abdominal distention, and nausea and vomiting. All epigastric hernias should be repaired, usually as outpatient procedures. The recurrence rate after epigastric herniorrhaphy is approximately 10% and usually can be attributed to failure to appreciate multiple defects in the linea alba at the time of the initial operation.

INCISIONAL HERNIAS

An incisional hernia is the protrusion of omentum or bowel through a fascial defect at the site of a prior surgical incision. Unlike the other types of abdominal hernia, a congenital weakness of the abdominal wall does not contribute to the development of the hernia. Any abdominal incision may be the site of a hernia. The major risk factors leading to the development of an incisional hernia are wound infection and obesity. With the increasing use of chronic ambulatory peritoneal dialysis to treat patients in chronic renal failure (see Chapter 52), it has become apparent that incisional hernias (as well as inguinal hernias) are particularly common in this group of patients.

The hernia usually manifests as a bulge through the incision that may enlarge if neglected (Fig. 97.7) and may even lead to intestinal obstruction. It should be repaired electively once the diagnosis is made to avoid the development of a larger defect that will complicate repair and be more likely to recur. If possible, an obese patient should lose weight before the operation (see Chapter 83). We do not advocate laparoscopic repair for these hernias because of the presence of a previous incision and adhesions, although the technique is used in some centers . Prosthetic mesh is commonly employed to repair incisional hernias. In using mesh, effort is taken to avoid exposure of the viscera to coarse textured mesh, which may lead to bowel obstruction or fistula. Instead, the surgeon interposes peritoneum or biodegradable mesh between permanent mesh and underlying viscera. Repaired incisional hernias have a much higher recurrence rate than do other kinds of abdominal hernias. Many patients with incisional hernia have significant comorbidity from underlying medical conditions, which must be taken into account when considering surgery.

DIASTASIS RECTI

Diastasis recti refers to wide separation of the rectus abdominus muscles in the midline, with attenuation of the linea alba. It is not a true hernia. Patients may present with an asymptomatic midline linear bulge that protrudes when the patient strains and is more predominant in the epigastrium. This is usually mistaken for a hernia and can be quite large. On examination, however, there is no scar indicating a prior incision, and there is no palpable fascial defect. Surgical correction of diastasis recti is not required, because this condition is rarely symptomatic and carries no risk of visceral incarceration because the fascia remains

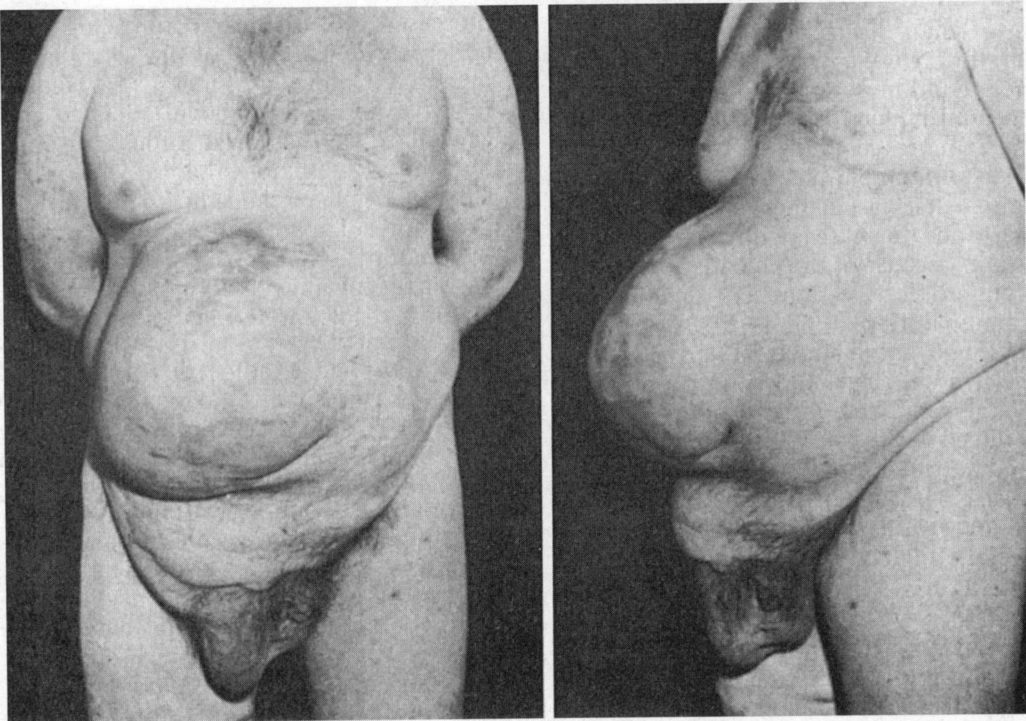

Figure 97.7. Large postoperative (ventral) hernia after cholecystectomy. (From Zimmerman LM, Anson BJ. Anatomy and surgery of hernia. 2nd ed. Baltimore: Williams & Wilkins, 1967:287.)

intact. Patients who are concerned about the appearance of the abdominal wall can be counseled or referred for cosmetic surgery.

General References*

Nyhus LM, Condon RE, eds. Hernia. Philadelphia: JB Lippincott, 1995.
A definitive text.

Rutkow IM, ed. Hernia surgery. Surg Clin North Am 1993;73.
Fourteen articles on various aspects of hernias.

*Bold print (general references) and bold numerals (specific references) denote published controlled clinical trials, meta-analyses, or consensus-based recommendations.

Specific References

1. Rutkow IM, Robbins AW. Demographic, classificatory, and socioeconomic aspects of hernia repair in the United States. Surg Clin North Am 1993;73:413.
2. Memon MA, Rice D, Donohue JH. Laparoscopic herniorrhaphy. J Am Coll Surg 1997;184:325.
3. Stoker DL, Spiegelhalter DJ, Singh R, et al. Laparoscopic versus open inguinal hernia repair: randomized prospective trial. Lancet 1994;343:1243.
4. Swanstrom LL. Laparoscopic herniorrhaphy. Surg Clin North Am 1996;76:483.
5. Webb K, Scott NW, GO PMNYH, et al., on behalf of the EU Hernia Trialists Collaboration. Laparoscopic techniques versus open techniques for inguinal hernia repair (Cochrane Review). In: The Cochrane Library, Issue 1, 2002. Oxford: Update software.

CHAPTER 98

Benign Conditions of the Anus and Rectum

JEFFREY S. BENDER, MD, FACS
MARK D. DUNCAN, MD, FACS

Anorectal disorders are often encountered in an ambulatory practice. The four most common—pruritus ani, anal fissure, hemorrhoids, and perirectal abscess/fistula—are discussed in some detail in this chapter. Also included, because of their importance to the primary care provider, are less common disorders such as proctalgia fugax and rectal prolapse. The final section addresses sexually transmitted diseases of the anus and rectum. Cutaneous disorders that involve the perianal area and perineum are discussed in Chapters 102 and Section 17. Other conditions that may affect the rectum are discussed in Chapters 35 and 45.

PRURITUS ANI

Definition

Pruritus ani, a distressing perianal itch, is more common in men than in women. It varies in intensity but usually is greatest at night. The itching often abates spontaneously, only to recur after variable asymptomatic periods.

Causes

Pruritus ani is a symptom, not a disease. Although 50% to 75% of the time the cause is unknown, the symptom may be a manifestation of a myriad of anorectal disorders (Table 98.1). Of these, anal neoplasia is the most serious cause that must be ruled out, especially in older adults. The itching is most often associated with macerated skin, often complicated by excoriation and secondary infection. These changes may be caused by fecal contamination or excessive cleansing efforts, exacerbated by scratching.

Diagnosis

When a patient complains of perianal itching, several specific historical points should be obtained and several observations should be made to aid in establishing a diagnosis.

History

Dietary history should include information on intake of milk, caffeine (coffee, tea, colas), chocolate, tomatoes, and spices; excessive consumption of any of these can lead to pruritus ani. Medications that cause gastrointestinal irritation (e.g., laxatives, colchicine) and certain antibiotics (especially tetracycline) can also cause perianal itching, as can chronic diarrhea from any cause. Any history of tissue protrusion or incontinence should be noted. Last, personal stress is a major contributing factor, and a careful personal history should be elicited.

General Physical Examination

The patient's skin should be examined for signs of a dermatologic problem, such as psoriasis or contact or atopic dermatitis, or a fungal infection (Table 98.1).

With the patient in the lateral decubitus or knee-chest position and the buttocks separated, the perianal area is inspected. During the inspection, the patient should be asked to strain or bear down. This maneuver may demonstrate prolapse or incontinence.

If skin lesions are identified, appropriate evaluation (e.g., a potassium hydroxide preparation) to establish a diagnosis (e.g., *Tinea, Candida*) should be done to initiate definitive therapy (see Chapter 117). In children up to age 14 years, and in adults who live in households with infected children, the evaluation should include several cellophane tape preparations in an attempt to demonstrate the ova of pinworms (see later discussion).

Table 98.1. Causes of Pruritis Ani

Diet
Milk
Caffeine
Chocolate
Tomatoes
Spices
Drugs
Oral antibiotics (e.g., tetracycline)
Colchicine
Laxatives
Dermatologic disorders
Psoriasis
Atopic dermatitis
Contact dermatitis
Lichen planus
Diarrhea
Fissures
Fistulas
Infections and Infestations
Fungi and yeast (especially in diabetic patients) (see Chapter 79)
Erythrasma
Scabies (see Chapter 117)
Pinworm (*Enterobius vermicularis*) infestation, more common in children
Vaginal infections (see Chapter 102)
Viral (condylomata, venereal warts, herpes simplex)
Obesity and excessive sweating
Poor anal hygiene
Rectal prolapse
Prolapsed hemorrhoids
Neoplasia

Rectal Examination

Digital rectal examination should always be performed using a well-lubricated, gloved finger. At initiation of the examination, the patient should be asked to bear down, which minimizes discomfort. Excessive pain localized to a specific area should alert the practitioner to the possible presence of an anal fissure (discussed later). All structures within reach of the finger should be assessed (anus, sphincter, distal rectum, prostate gland, and cervix).

Anoscopy

After rectal examination, and without enema or laxative preparation, an anoscopy should be performed. The usual disposable anoscope, although convenient, provides only a barely adequate view. A well-lubricated anoscope should be inserted gently while the patient bears down. The addition of a local anesthetic ointment does little if anything to decrease any discomfort. After removal of the obturator, the rectum should be inspected under adequate light. Visualization of the more distal anal structures is possible only through the side aspect of the instrument as it is slowly withdrawn. Rotation of the anoscope is often uncomfortable and may tear the anal mucosa. Therefore, for adequate inspection of all quadrants, the anoscope must be withdrawn and reinserted three or four times.

Cellophane Tape Examination for Pinworms

Cellophane tape examination is easily accomplished by the patient at home or by the practitioner in the office. Swabs are commercially available (Pinworm Diagnostic Tapes, Parke-Davis), but they are also easily made by folding clear cellophane tape, sticky side out, over a tongue blade. At night pinworms migrate from the anal canal to the perianal area, where they deposit eggs. Therefore the swab should be obtained on arising, before a bowel movement and before the perianal area is cleansed. The swab is placed at the anal verge and then the tape is mounted onto a glass microscopic slide. A specimen obtained in this way keeps for several days. The slides should be examined under the low-power (10×) objective of the microscope, searching for the typical ova of pinworm (Fig. 98.1).

Treatment

Most patients with pruritus ani can be diagnosed and treated adequately by the general practitioner. Evan if the evaluation is inconclusive except for the identification of excoriation, symptoms can be controlled by simple measures.

Counseling about the factors responsible for pruritus ani should ensure a clear understanding of the potential roles of stress, lifestyle, and diet.

Dietary change should eliminate potentially causative foods and beverages. It may take 2 weeks for the symptom to resolve after diet modification. It will then recur within 48 hours after resumption of the offending food.

Tepid sitz baths for 15 to 20 minutes provide excellent temporary relief (e.g., at bedtime). If possible, these should be used several times daily at the outset of symptoms.

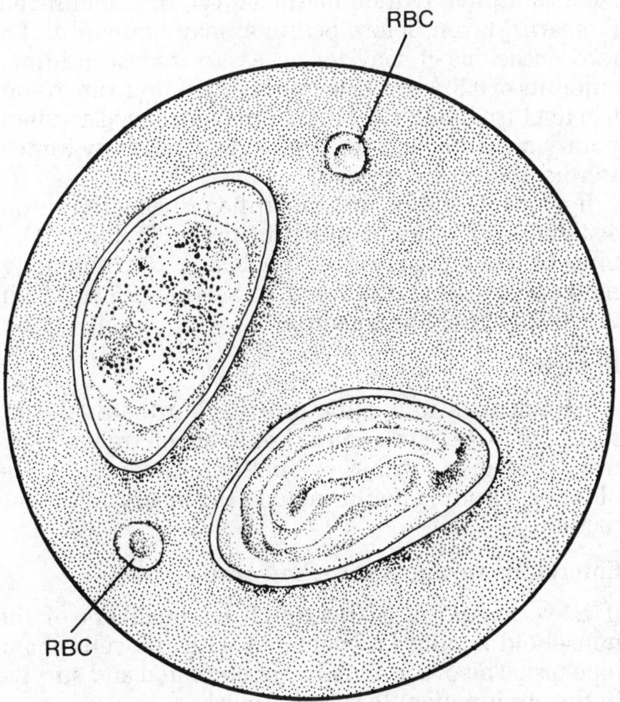

Figure 98.1. Appearance of the eggs of *Enterobius vermicularis* (pinworm). The egg is approximately 20 to 50 mm and typically has one flattened side.

Anal cleanliness and dryness are mandatory and must be gentle. Once or twice daily, and after each bowel movement, the perineal area should be cleansed with a plain mild soap such as Ivory and then rinsed with cotton swabs moistened with warm water. Glycerin–witch hazel wipes (Tucks) or diaper wipes may be used unless they cause irritation or burning. After cleansing, the area should be thoroughly dried by blotting, not rubbing, with soft, white, nonperfumed toilet paper (colored or perfumed tissues, which are potentially allergenic or irritating, should be avoided). A handheld blow dryer is a useful alternative.

The perianal area must be kept dry at all times. This is best accomplished by the application of cornstarch powder or plain talc (Johnson's Baby Powder). A thick layer of zinc oxide or A and D Ointment may be substituted but must be thoroughly and gently removed at the time of each cleaning.

Diarrhea or constipation should be controlled (see Chapters 45 and 46). Bulk laxatives such as Metamucil and stool softeners such as Colace or Peri-Colace are preferred. They are not irritating, and they tend to absorb mucus, a possible irritant to the sensitive perianal tissue.

The patient should wear cotton underwear to provide better ventilation and should avoid polyester clothing. Prolonged sitting, especially on synthetic materials (e.g., vinyl seats), which prevent proper ventilation, should be avoided.

In general, the use of all other creams, ointments, and medications should be discontinued.

For the occasional patient with symptoms severe enough to cause insomnia, an antipruritic sedative such as diphenhydramine (Benadryl) or trimeprazine (Temaril), taken before bedtime, may be helpful. On rare occasions it may be necessary to use minimal amounts of 0.5% or 1.0% hydrocortisone cream to control nocturnal itching. This should be viewed as a temporary measure, and the prolonged use of any topical steroid should be avoided.

If a specific problem is identified during the initial evaluation of a patient with pruritus ani (Table 98.1), it must be treated appropriately. Chapter 102 (nonmalignant vulvovaginal disorders), or Sections 15 and 17 in this book should be consulted.

Referral

A patient with idiopathic pruritus ani that is not responsive to these therapies should be referred to a gastroenterologist. Further evaluation, especially in the older age group, should include the entire colon and rectum.

Enterobius vermicularis *(Pinworm)*

If *E. vermicularis* is identified, all members of the household should be evaluated with the cellophane tape test. The ova are easily disseminated and survive in the environment for up to 3 weeks.

The drug of choice to eradicate this infestation is pyrantel pamoate (Pin-X). It is available as an oral suspension and is given as a single dose. An alternative drug, mebendazole (Vermox), is given as a single chewable tablet; it should not be used in infants or pregnant women. These agents approach 100% effectiveness in killing the worms, and symptoms usually subside within 48 hours. The patient is no longer infective once the deposited eggs are removed from the perianal area and clothing by cleaning. Both drugs are well tolerated but can cause mild, transient gastrointestinal distress. Pyrantel pamoate has been associated with transitory elevation of liver enzymes, and its use should be avoided in patients with known liver disease.

Clothing and bed linens should be laundered with detergent and hot water on the same day that oral treatment is given. All infected members of the household should be treated simultaneously. It should be understood that reinfestation is common and that retreatment may be necessary.

ANAL FISSURE

Definition

An anal fissure is an acutely painful, elliptical, mucosal tear extending from the anal verge to the pectinate line (Fig. 98.2). It is most often located in the posterior midline of the anal canal, less commonly anteriorly. The inciting factor is usually trauma secondary to the passage of a large, hard stool or, less commonly, anal intercourse. The underlying pathophysiology is diminished anodermal blood supply abetted by increased anal sphincter tone (1). This leads to an unremitting cycle of pain, reluctance to have a bowel movement, and then further tearing once the bowel movement occurs. The problem is a common one, occurring with equal frequency in men and women (it is uncommon in children). Most patients, and many clinicians, attribute the pain to hemorrhoids, especially when streaking of the stool with blood occurs. It is important to remember that hemorrhoids, unless acutely thrombosed, are not a cause of anal pain.

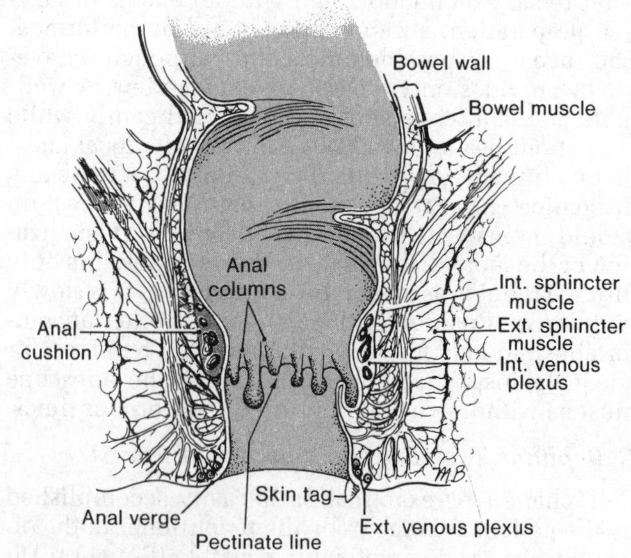

Figure 98.2. Important structures of the anal area.

As an anal fissure becomes chronic it looks more like an ulcer crater, with raised edges, scarring, and the exposed external sphincter at the base. These changes are usually associated with a prominent posterior skin tag known as a sentinel pile. This often resembles an external hemorrhoid, which helps further the confusion of these two diagnoses. Occasionally a chronic fissure, often in an atypical location, is caused by an inflammatory condition such as Crohn disease, syphilis, gonorrhea, or tuberculosis; iatrogenic scarring from local surgery or irradiation; or anal cancer.

Diagnosis

An acute anal fissure manifests with the sudden onset of sharp rectal pain that occurs during defecation and is followed by a dull aching discomfort that may persist for several hours. There may be associated minimal bright red bleeding, usually noticed just on the toilet tissue. Itching and mucus discharge can be additional complaints. As noted, the pain is so severe that patients avoid having a bowel movement, further aggravating the situation.

On examination, when the buttocks are gently retracted, most anal fissures can be readily visualized, usually at the posterior margin of the anal verge. It may help to ask the patient to strain. With more chronic fissures, a posterior sentinel pile may be appreciated. Once an anal fissure has been identified by inspection, usually no attempt should be made to perform a digital examination or anoscopy until treatment has alleviated the symptoms.

Treatment

Many patients with acute anal fissure can be made comfortable within a day or two, and cured within 3 weeks, by the use of conservative therapy. Stool softeners such as Colace or Peri-Colace or bulk laxatives such as Metamucil should be taken, and cathartics should be avoided. A high-fiber diet is recommended, along with the consumption of eight glasses of water daily.

Anal discomfort is relieved by the use of warm baths for 15 to 20 minutes two to three times per day and after each bowel movement (2). Local anesthetic creams (e.g., Balneol, Nupercainal Cream) are also useful in providing temporary relief of symptoms. Suppositories generally are not useful. This is because, to be held internally, they must be passed above the sphincter muscle (a process that causes much discomfort) and then above the area where their action is needed.

Nitric oxide (NO) mediates relaxation of the internal anal sphincter. NO donors, such as nitroglycerin, isosorbide dinitrate, or glyceryltrinitrate, are effective in the treatment of anal fissures. Most (3–5) but not all (6) studies have shown that the topical use of these agents results in early symptomatic relief and in cure of up to 80% of both acute and chronic anal fissures after 6 weeks of treatment. Recurrence rates are unknown. The major side effect has been headache. A similar positive therapeutic effect has been achieved by the local injection of botulin toxin (7,8), which should be done only by a surgeon or a gastroenterologist. It is conceivable that these approaches might obviate operation for at least some chronic fissures.

Once a fissure becomes chronic or if 6 weeks of conservative therapy has failed, the next step is surgical referral for a lateral anal sphincterotomy. This procedure is usually done on an ambulatory basis, often under local anesthesia. Postoperative complications (e.g., bleeding, abscess formation) occur in fewer than 5% of cases. There may be early problems with some degree of anal incontinence in up to 8% of cases, but this is a long-term problem in fewer than 1% of patients and is usually confined to difficulty controlling flatus or liquid.

Pain relief is noted within 48 hours, and the fissure is usually healed in 2 to 3 weeks. The recurrence rate is 1% to 8%, and 96% of patients have a lasting excellent or satisfactory result. Transient postoperative incontinence is common.

HEMORRHOIDS

Definition

A precise characterization of hemorrhoidal disease is impossible because, despite centuries of medical speculation, neither the pathogenesis nor the cause has ever been elucidated. Hemorrhoids are not varicosities of the rectal venous plexus. There are no certain data to prove any of the popular theories of causation, such as a low-fiber diet, constipation, straining at stool, venous hypertension, obesity, certain occupations, genetic predisposition, and many others.

The currently popular theory associates hemorrhoids with distal displacement of the anal cushions. Anal cushions are part of the normal anatomy of the anal canal (Fig. 98.2). These cushions, which consist of hemorrhoidal venous and arterial plexuses, smooth muscle, and connective tissue, lie under the mucosa. The cushions apparently permit the passage of variable-sized stools without disruption of the rectal mucosa. Three cushions are usually found, in the right anterolateral, right posterolateral, and left lateral portions of the anal canal (Fig 98.3), the common locations of internal hemorrhoids. This theory is consistent with an observed increase in hemorrhoidal disease in association with aging, groin hernias, and urogenital prolapse, all potentially caused by connective tissue degeneration.

Classification

Hemorrhoids are described as internal or external depending on whether they originate above or below the pectinate (dentate) line. External skin tags are commonly, and erroneously, referred to as hemorrhoids as well (Fig 98.2). Internal hemorrhoids are graded based on the degree of prolapse. *First-degree hemorrhoids* project into the anal canal but do not prolapse. *Second-degree hemorrhoids* prolapse with defecation and spontaneously reduce. At these stages the only

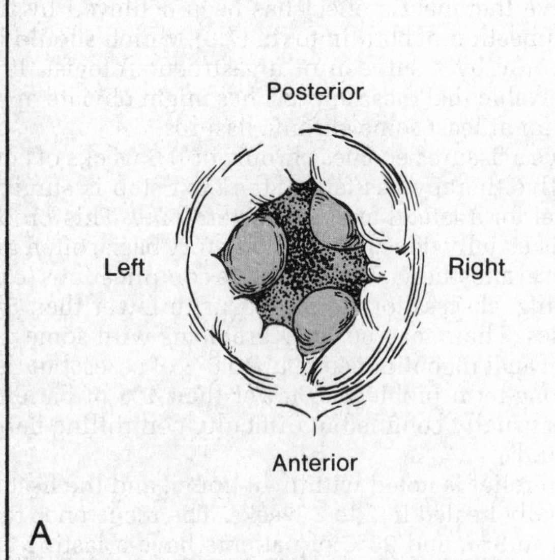

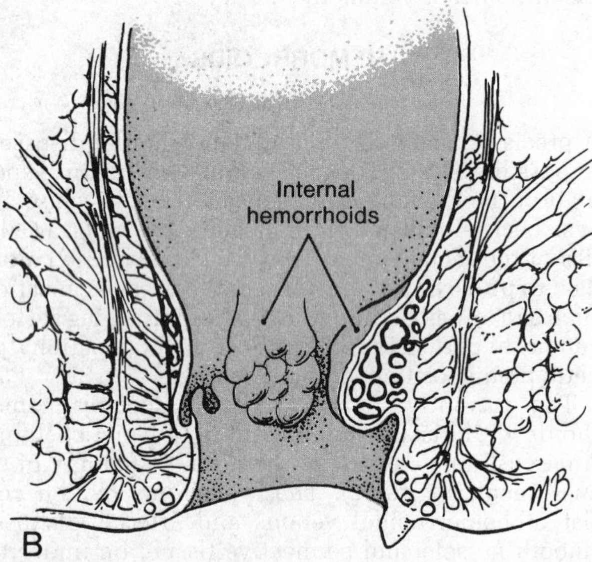

Figure 98.3. **A.** Common sites of hemorrhoids. **B.** Protrusion of anal cushions.

symptom is painless, bright red bleeding. *Third-degree hemorrhoids* protrude with straining and often require manual reduction. In addition to hematochezia, these are associated with discomfort and sometimes a mucus discharge. *Fourth-degree hemorrhoids* are irreducibly prolapsed through the anus. They can cause severe discomfort, bleeding, and mucus discharge. At this stage strangulation can occur, constituting an exceedingly painful and potentially lethal emergency. This classification of hemorrhoidal disease is summarized in Table 98.2.

Epidemiology

Asymptomatic hemorrhoids are said to be present in half of the population older than 50 years of age, but this figure is suspect because the definition of the diagnosis is uncertain. The prevalence of self-reported hemorrhoidal complaints was 4.4% (equivalent to about 10 million people) in a national health survey, but patients tend to attribute all anorectal symptoms to hemorrhoids (9). The prevalence is the same in both sexes, but women develop hemorrhoids earlier, often in association with pregnancy, and men more commonly seek treatment (9).

Table 98.2. Classification of Hemorrhoids

External hemorrhoids: Hemorrhoids arising from the inferior hemorrhoidal plexus exterior to the anal verge, covered by pain-sensitive skin. Thrombosis can cause acute and sometimes severe discomfort.

Internal hemorrhoids: Hemorrhoids arising from the anal cushions, normal structures lying above the anal verge, covered by pain-insensitive mucosa. Internal hemorrhoids may be classified further.

- *First-degree:* Hemorrhoids bulging into the lumen of the anal canal
- *Second-degree:* Hemorrhoids that prolapse during defecation but reduce spontaneously
- *Third-degree:* Prolapsed hemorrhoids that require manual reduction
- *Fourth-degree:* Hemorrhoids that are irreducibly prolapsed

Thrombosed internal hemorrhoids: An internal hemorrhoid may prolapse and strangulate, which leads to thrombosis, an excruciatingly painful condition. If swelling progresses, gangrene of the hemorrhoids with ulceration, local infection, or pyelphlebitis (septic phlebitis of the portal venous system) may result.

Diagnosis

Symptoms

External hemorrhoids manifest with pain, often exquisite, as a result of thrombosis in the external venous plexus. There is a tender lump, and the pain is exacerbated by defecation.

Asymptomatic hemorrhoids noticed incidentally during an examination should not be considered a problem and should not be treated. The symptoms associated with internal hemorrhoids were summarized in the classification scheme just presented and can be elaborated as follows:

Bleeding. Characteristically, the bleeding from hemorrhoids is mild, intermittent, and bright red. Occasionally it may drip into the commode or be sustained. Massive hemorrhage is rare. Rectal bleeding should never be attributed to hemorrhoids unless all other causes can be ruled out.

Prolapse. Prolapse of internal hemorrhoids produces the sensation of fullness in the anal canal, especially after defecation. This discomfort affects 80% of patients with symptomatic hemorrhoids, but it is not true pain.

Pain. The acute pain attributed to internal hemorrhoids usually is caused by a fissure (see earlier discussion). Pain caused by internal hemorrhoids indicates thrombosis or strangulation and if unresponsive to conservative management (see below), mandates referral to a surgeon. Thrombosis and strangulation occur when fourth-degree hemorrhoids are trapped by congestion and spasm of the anal canal. If ulceration ensues, localized infection may result, which rarely may spread to the portal venous plexus, leading to potentially lethal pylephlebitis.

Physical Examination

The patient is placed in the lateral decubitus or knee-chest position and the buttocks are gently separated. Skin tags are seen as soft, painless excrescences just beyond the anal verge. A thrombosed external hemorrhoid manifests in the anal canal as a firm, tender mass with a bluish discoloration. Internal hemorrhoids can sometimes be visualized as well, especially if the patient strains.

Digital rectal examination is performed principally to rule out other anal and distal rectal disease. Nonvisible internal hemorrhoids are rarely palpable.

Anoscopy is the definitive diagnostic procedure for internal hemorrhoids. It should be performed thoroughly and carefully, as described previously for the diagnosis of pruritus ani, with the use of a good side-viewing anoscope.

Sigmoidoscopy, using the flexible fiberoptic sigmoidoscope, should be performed for any patient older than 40 years of age with the recent onset of bleeding from internal hemorrhoids. This is a part of the assessment of gastrointestinal bleeding, as discussed more fully in Chapter 45.

Differential Diagnosis

Several other problems may be confused with hemorrhoidal disease. *Hypertrophied anal papillae* occur along the pectinate (dentate) line (Fig. 98.2) in association with an anal fissure (see earlier discussion), with Crohn disease, or without obvious cause. These papillae usually are asymptomatic and require no therapy unless they have become particularly large, eroded, or infected or unless they bleed. Hypertrophied anal papillae often have the appearance of a fibrous polyp and are easily differentiated from hemorrhoids by their location and consistency.

Rectal prolapse is more common in the elderly but can occur at any age. Prolapse is identified by the circumferential abnormal downward displacement, or herniation, of rectal mucosa or of the full thickness of the rectal wall. When mild, it is commonly mistaken for hemorrhoidal disease and may respond to similar methods of treatment.

Protruding tumors such as rectal polyps, anal carcinoma, and even low-lying rectal carcinoma can be confused with hemorrhoids. If there is suspicion about the diagnosis, referral to a surgeon or gastroenterologist for evaluation and biopsy is appropriate.

Course

Without treatment, symptoms of hemorrhoids usually resolve spontaneously or in response to self-treatment within several days to several weeks, even when thrombosis is present. However, most patients develop recurrent symptoms, although the asymptomatic intervals may be long.

Treatment

The aim of treatment (10) is to relieve symptoms, and only symptomatic hemorrhoids need treatment. Therapy does not necessarily reduce venous bulges, although often they do regress, Most patients respond to conservative therapy.

Skin tags rarely need treatment. If they are sufficiently prominent to cause true discomfort, the patient can be referred for surgical excision.

Thrombosed external hemorrhoids are often acutely and severely painful and may require surgical referral for management. If the patient presents more than 72 hours after the onset of pain and as the acute symptom is subsiding, conservative measures usually resolve the problem. These consist of the approach used for conservative treatment of symptomatic internal hemorrhoids. In addition, topical analgesics such as Nupercainal or 5% lidocaine ointment should be applied. If prolonged sitting is necessary, an inflatable ring is helpful.

Symptomatic internal hemorrhoids, even fourth-degree ones, in the absence of severe symptoms, deserve a trial of conservative management. The first step is to avoid constipation and straining by giving a bulk laxative such as Metamucil and stool softeners such as Colace or Peri-Colace. In conjunction, the patient should eat a high-fiber diet with bran cereals and whole wheat bread and drink at least eight glasses of water daily.

Swelling and prolapse often respond to warm sitz baths taken twice daily and after each bowel movement.

Topical preparations may relieve discomfort, and putatively reduce swelling as well. Corticosteroid-containing preparations such as Anusol-HC and ProctoFoam-HC may be used initially, but their use should be discontinued after 2 to 3 weeks and the non–steroid-containing versions substituted. These preparations come as creams, foams, and suppositories. All three forms are beneficial, and their use depends on patient and clinician preference.

Surgical Management

Patients should be referred to a surgeon for evaluation whenever there is doubt about the diagnosis, if there is no response within 3 or 4 weeks to conservative therapy, if pain is severe (as may occur with thrombosis); or if there is evidence of strangulation, ulceration, or perianal infection. When uncomplicated hemorrhoids are recurrently symptomatic, the patient should be referred to a surgeon for definitive treatment.

The surgeon evaluates the patient, confirms the diagnosis, and then considers several therapeutic options that are not normally provided by general practitioners.

External Hemorrhoids. The usual indication for the surgical treatment of external hemorrhoids is painful acute thrombosis, especially within 48 to 72 hours after onset. The procedure is surgical excision under local anesthesia on an ambulatory basis (the local anesthesia of choice for all anal and perianal procedures is bupivacaine 0.5% with epinephrine 1:200,000 and sodium bicarbonate). Incision and evacuation of the thrombus are not adequate treatment. The entire thrombosed portion of the external venous plexus should be excised along with a transverse elliptical wedge of overlying skin.

Sometimes external skin tags are sufficiently troublesome to warrant excision. This can be done as an office procedure under local anesthesia.

Internal Hemorrhoids

Injection of Sclerosing Agents. The submucosal injection of a symptomatic hemorrhoid with several milliliters of a sclerosing solution causes fibrosis and retraction of the hemorrhoid. This procedure is excellent therapy for small bleeding internal hemorrhoids (first- or second-degree; Table 98.2); it is simple, requires no anesthesia, and can easily be performed in the office in a few minutes. After this procedure the patient usually requires no recovery period and can return to work immediately. There may be a period of several days when the patient experiences a sensation of anal fullness. This symptom is usually well tolerated or is easily controlled by the use of sitz baths three to four times a day and by mild analgesics such as acetaminophen.

The clinician performing this procedure must be experienced with its use. With the proper technique there are essentially no complications. If the solution is improperly injected, severe pain, necrosis, and rectal stenosis can occur. Injection of sclerosing agents usually provides temporary relief, but recurrence is common. The procedure may be repeated several times, but persistent recurrence should lead to the consideration of another mode of therapy. This approach is most useful for symptomatic first-degree hemorrhoids that are so small that there is insufficient tissue for rubber band ligation.

Rubber Band Ligation. Rubber band ligation of hemorrhoids is a simple office procedure that is the initial treatment of choice for most symptomatic internal hemorrhoids of all degrees except the fourth (Table 98.2) (11,12). The patient requires no special preparation, and no anesthesia is necessary. Using an anoscope and a special instrument, one or two rubber bands are applied near the base of the hemorrhoid and at least 0.5 cm above the pectinate line. No more than two hemorrhoids should be treated at a single session, but all of the hemorrhoids should be banded ultimately. Constriction by the rubber band results in ischemic necrosis of the hemorrhoid, which sloughs and is passed in the stool 5 to 10 days later, usually along with a small amount of blood. Complications are very rare, but delayed massive bleeding and pelvic sepsis have occurred.

Usually, after rubber band ligation of hemorrhoids, the patient is not disabled and has only minimal discomfort characterized by a sensation of rectal fullness, a symptom that is usually well controlled by the use of sitz baths and a mild oral analgesic such as acetaminophen. Aspirin and nonsteroidal anti-inflammatory analgesics should not be used because of the risk of prolonged bleeding. If the discomfort is more severe, a mild relaxant such as diazepam (Valium) is helpful to relieve anal sphincter spasm. If the rubber band is improperly placed below the pectinate line, the patient will experience severe pain and the rubber band must be removed.

After rubber band ligation, the usual conservative measures for internal hemorrhoids should be practiced for 2 to 3 weeks until healing is complete. Further ligation is then performed if necessary. Banding provides good relief of hemorrhoidal disease approximately 70% to 90% of the time. Symptoms recur in 15% to 45% of patients after 18 months to 5 years.

Laser Therapy and Infrared Photocoagulation. Laser therapy and infrared photocoagulation are available as treatment modalities for first-, second-, and third-degree hemorrhoids (Table 98.2). Both require expensive equipment, and the carbon dioxide laser demands special expertise. Therefore neither modality is widely available.

Hemorrhoidectomy. Hemorrhoidectomy is indicated for large internal hemorrhoids after other forms of therapy have failed; for strangulated, ulcerated, or gangrenous third- or fourth-degree hemorrhoids; and when symptomatic hemorrhoids are present in conjunction with other benign anorectal conditions (e.g., fistulas, fissures) that require surgery (1). The procedure is usually done under general or regional anesthesia, although local anesthesia is possible. Patient preparation consists of taking a laxative the evening before the operation. The purpose of the operation is to remove hemorrhoidal tissue and to appose the skin and mucous membrane. The operation has a reputation for severe postoperative pain, especially when some perianal skin is also excised. Postoperative discomfort is best controlled by sitz baths, stool softeners, oral analgesics, and a muscle relaxant such as diazepam (Valium). Topical nitroglycerin may also be beneficial. Most patients can go home the same day.

Postoperative complications are urinary retention and bleeding. The former can be averted by adequate control of pain and muscle spasm. The incidence of significant bleeding is 1% to 2%, and infection is rare. Late complications of incontinence or anal stenosis should occur in fewer than 1% of patients. The late recurrence rate is less than 5%.

Special Considerations

Because of an increased risk of complications associated with operative procedures in patients with severe congestive heart failure or debilitating disease, the treatment of hemorrhoids in these patients should be as conservative as possible. Patients who have cirrhosis present a special risk because of the frequent association of hemostatic dysfunction. Hemorrhoidectomy should not be done in patients with Crohn disease and should be done in patients with ulcerative colitis only when they are in remission. Immunocompromised patients should not undergo anorectal surgery.

Hemorrhoids are common in pregnancy and are best managed conservatively. They often resolve spontaneously after delivery. Occasionally, development of strangulated hemorrhoids requires surgical intervention during the pregnancy.

ANORECTAL ABSCESSES AND ANORECTAL FISTULAS

Definition

An *anorectal abscess* is an abscess involving the perineum and perianal structures. Abscesses are classified by their anatomic location (Fig. 98.4). Low intramuscular or perianal abscesses are located in the subcutaneous tissue immediately surrounding the anus, which is the site of 40% to 50% of all anorectal abscesses. *Ischiorectal abscesses* are located in the ischiorectal fossa, a fat-filled space between the distal levator ani (external anal sphincter) and the ischial tuberosity, and account for 20% to 40% of anorectal abscesses. *Intersphincteric, high intermuscular (postanal), and pelvirectal (supralevator) abscesses* are far less common and account for approximately 10% of all abscesses. Anorectal abscesses are common, and the general physician should be familiar with their presentation, so if this problem is suspected, the patient can be promptly referred to a surgeon.

An *anorectal fistula (fistula-in-ano)* is a tract lined by granulation tissue that has an internal opening in the anal canal and an external opening in the perianal skin. The internal opening is usually located in one of the anal crypts at the upper end of the anal canal just above the pectinate line (Fig. 98.2).

Causes

Anorectal abscesses are more common in men. Most are associated with cryptoglandular infection. Occasionally, anorectal abscesses occur in association with other anal and perianal disorders (Table 98.3). Anal glands, thought to be diverticula of the anal canal mucosa, are located circumferentially around the anus at the level of the pectinate line. Many of these glands pass through the internal sphincter into the intersphincteric space. They normally drain into the anal crypts. Infection and abscess formation result when drainage of these glands is blocked. Bacterial cultures from the abscesses usually grow a mixed flora.

Most anorectal fistulas result from abscess formation in the anal glands and drainage through the perianal skin. Unless this is recognized and treated at the same time, the incidence of fistula formation after drainage of anorectal abscesses is about 50%. Some fistulas are not pyogenic in origin and are associated with inflammatory bowel disease or tuberculosis. Fistulas

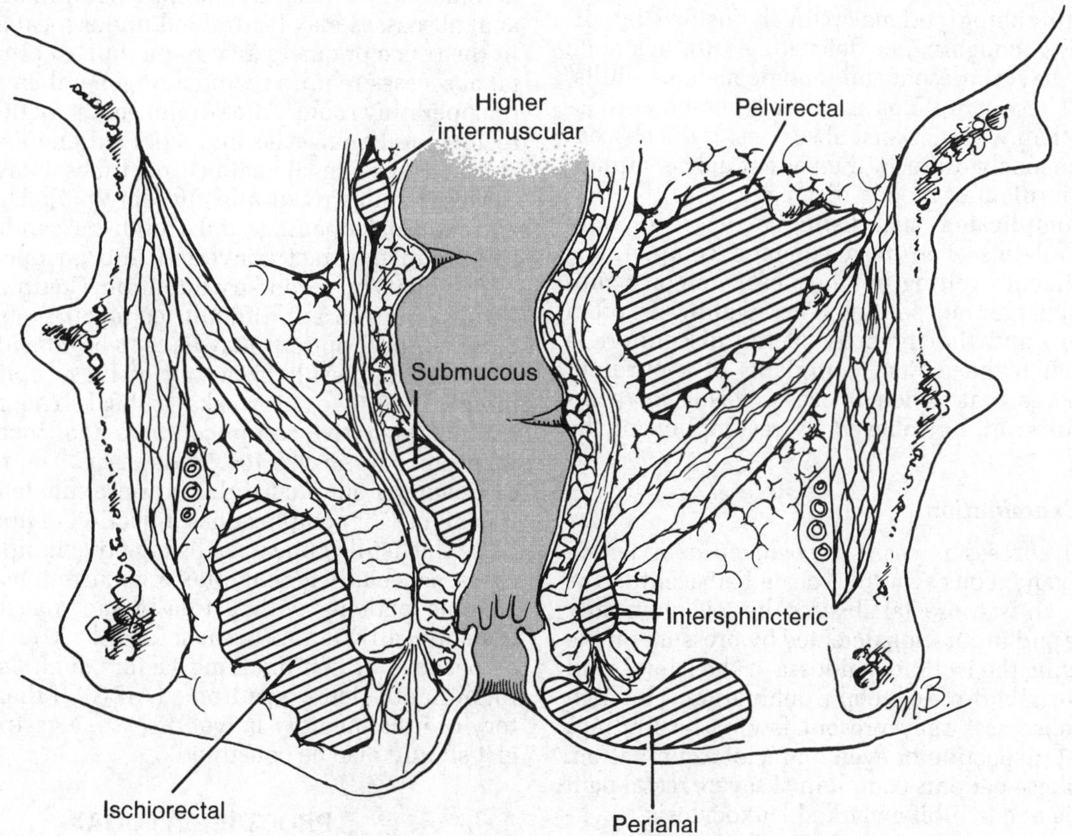

Figure 98.4. Anatomic classification of common anorectal abscesses.

Table 98.3. Conditions That May Be Complicated by Anorectal Abscess and Fistula-in-ano

Inflammatory bowel disease
Chronic infections (uncommon)
Actinomycosis
Tuberculosis
Lymphogranuloma venereum
Schistosomiasis (rare)
Amebiasis (rare)
Infection anatomically adjacent to the rectal area and presenting as anorectal abscess or fistula-in-ano
In women
Pelvic inflammatory disease
Bartholin gland abscess
In men
Infections of a Cowper gland (small periurethral glands)
Pilonidal sinus (occasionally occurs in females)
Foreign body (e.g., an ingested bone or a penetrating wooden splinter)
Trauma
Surgery (e.g., hemorrhoidectomy, prostatectomy)
Radiation
Laceration (e.g., from an enema)
Abnormalities of host defense (e.g., bone marrow aplasia, neutropenia, leukemia or lymphoma, diabetes mellitus)
Carcinoma of anus or rectum

that do not originate in anal glands may result from diverticular disease, neoplastic disease, or trauma.

Diagnosis

History

Most commonly, a patient with an anorectal abscess describes throbbing perianal pain intensified by sitting, walking, coughing, or defecating (13). Systemic symptoms may be present and include malaise, chills, and fever. These symptoms are more common with ischiorectal than with perianal abscesses. If the abscess has spontaneously drained, the patient may complain of a mucopurulent or bloody discharge.

An uncomplicated anal fistula may create only minor complaints. The most common complaint is painful perianal swelling, but the most common symptom is discharge and soiling. The swelling is often intermittent, and the intensity of the discomfort is variable. Often the patient complains of a purulent anal discharge that, when it ceases, leads to recurrent painful swelling relieved by resumption of the discharge.

Physical Examination

A perianal abscess is easily recognized as a warm, tender, subcutaneous swelling located adjacent to the anus. With an ischiorectal abscess there is often only tenderness and induration detected by pressure on the skin overlying the ischiorectal fossa or the lateral wall of the anal canal during rectal examination. The high anorectal abscesses may present few or no findings on perianal inspection or even on rectal examination. However, these patients complain of severe rectal pain and pyrexia and exhibit a marked leukocytosis.

The diagnosis of an anorectal fistula is established by inspection and palpation of the perianal area and performance of a digital rectal examination. Often the external opening of the fistula in the perianal area can be seen. Digital examination of the rectum may enable identification of the indurated tract of the fistula as it passes to its internal opening at the pectinate line. Often the location of the internal opening is facilitated by anoscopy. Gentle passage of a probe may be attempted, but care must be taken not to create a false passage. Occasionally, accurate localization must await surgical exploration. When complex perineal infection is present, especially if no internal opening is found, the possibility of hydradenitits suppurativa must be considered (see Chapter 115).

Treatment

Even the suspicion of an anorectal abscess should lead to urgent referral to a surgeon for drainage (13). Temporizing treatment with oral antibiotics and sitz baths simply increases the risk of complications, such as systemic infection. An anorectal abscess may also be associated with a rapidly spreading necrotizing infection that destroys large areas of skin, subcutaneous tissue, and fascia. Patients with coincident diabetes mellitus are particularly vulnerable to complicated and extensive perirectal involvement. Finally, spontaneous rupture can occur either externally or internally, resulting in a complex fistula that is difficult to manage.

Preoperative broad-spectrum antibiotics need be given only to patients with anorectal abscesses who have vulvular heart disease, diabetes, extensive inflammation or who are immunocompromised. Perianal abscesses may be drained under local anesthesia in the office or emergency room, but all other anorectal abscesses require regional or general anesthesia in the operating room. After drainage, the patient should receive oral analgesics and stool softeners and be instructed to begin sitz baths three times a day.

Most fistulas require fistulotomy (13). The internal and external openings must both be carefully identified and the tract converted into an open wound, which heals by secondary intention. Complex chronic fistulas can present difficult technical problems, and other surgical options may have to be considered. The wounds that result from any of these options commonly take 6 to 12 weeks to heal. The most serious postoperative complication is anal incontinence, which occurs in 3% to 7% of cases. The recurrence rate even for simple fistulas is approximately 5%, and it is higher for complex ones. Injection of fibrin glue to close the fistula appears to be effective in up to 60% of cases, especially for complex or recurrent fistulas (14).

Some patients with fistula-in-ano may be treated nonsurgically, either because of a lack of symptoms or because of complicating factors such as acquired immunodeficiency syndrome (AIDS). If there is a history of inflammatory bowel disease, a gastroenterologist should also be consulted.

PROCTALGIA FUGAX

Occasionally, healthy young adults develop the sudden onset of severe rectal pain, variably intermittent and usually lasting from less than 30 minutes to 1 hour: proctalgia fugax. It often awakens the patient at night. It is significantly more common in women than in men, and it can occur after sexual intercourse. The pain is described usually as a spasm or a cramp. The problem is not associated with systemic illness or other gastrointestinal diseases such as irritable bowel syndrome, and the cause is uncertain. There is often an association with psychiatric disturbances. Proctalgia fugax was long thought to result from spasm of a portion of the levator ani muscle, but it is now thought to be caused by paroxysmal hyperkinesis of the smooth muscle of the internal anal sphincter (15). Patients with proctalgia fugax may obtain relief by taking a hot sitz bath or applying pressure in the perianal area near the site of the discomfort. There are no proven pharmacologic remedies for this affliction. However, if the attacks are severe and frequent, some patients may find relief from the use of sublingual or cutaneous nitrates. There is also the possibility that nifedipine, a calcium channel blocker, decreases the frequency and intensity of attacks, and that the inhalation of albuterol shortens the duration of pain. The problem usually persists for many years but then disappears in later life.

RECTAL PROLAPSE

Definition

Prolapse is a protrusion of the rectum through the anus. The protrusion may contain only mucosa (a mucosal prolapse), or it may contain all layers of the bowel wall (a full-thickness prolapse, or procidentia). There can also be an internal prolapse, or internal rectal intussusception, which produces typical symptoms without any external protrusion. This is often associated with the solitary rectal ulcer syndrome.

Causes

Prolapse is more prevalent in women (approximately 80% of the cases), with a peak incidence between the ages of 60 and 80 years. In men the peak incidence occurs at about 40 years of age. The exact pathogenic mechanism in not known. Multiple factors are associated with this disease. Weakening of the fascial attachments of the rectum, attenuated muscles in the perirectal area and pelvic diaphragm, straining caused by chronic constipation, and even congenital fascial defects all lead to the development of rectal prolapse. Prolapse is often observed after severe chronic diarrhea.

Prolapse also occurs commonly in children, usually before 2 years of age. This is almost always a mucosal prolapse, and conservative treatment usually suffices until the condition spontaneously resolves.

Diagnosis

History

Patients have variable symptoms, depending on the degree of prolapse. Initially, the protrusion occurs only with defecation, and the patient can easily reduce it manually. At this stage there may be no associated incontinence and the condition is sometimes mistaken for symptomatic internal hemorrhoids. The patient may complain of a sensation of displaced tissue at the time of a bowel movement, and there is often a feeling of incomplete evacuation. With progression of the problem, prolapse occurs with any straining and, eventually, simply with walking or even standing. At this stage incontinence is almost invariably a problem. With more profound prolapse, the patient may complain of tenesmus and also may develop a continuous mucous discharge. The prolapsed rectum may become excoriated and ulcerated, leading many patients to complain of bleeding. In association with an advanced degree of prolapse, the patient may also have urinary incontinence, and in women there may be associated uterine prolapse. Patients with increasing degrees of prolapse experience considerable embarrassment and consequently may avoid social contact.

Physical Examination

The clinician can best recognize rectal prolapse by inspecting the anus when the patient strains in a squatting position or sits on a commode. It is wise to anticipate incontinence with this maneuver. If the prolapse is full-thickness (procidentia), concentric folds of the rectal mucosa are seen; in mucosal prolapse, only radial folds are seen. Digital examination almost always reveals a patulous and relaxed anal sphincter that often admits two to four fingers. Palpation of the protruding tissue between the examiner's finger provides the sensation of only mucosa in mucosal prolapse or of a double layer of bowel wall in full-thickness prolapse. The rectal examination in patients with prolapse is usually associated with minimal or no discomfort.

Occasionally, prolapsed hemorrhoids are confused with rectal prolapse, but the absence of concentric or radial folds of mucosa and the prominent location of prolapsed hemorrhoids in the left lateral, right anterior, or right posterior edges of the anus suggest the proper diagnosis (Fig. 98.3). On occasion, a prolapse is associated with a rectal tumor. For that reason, a flexible fiberoptic sigmoidoscopic examination should be performed for any patient with rectal prolapse. Other diagnostic studies are not usually required, but a defecatory videoproctogram (available in only a few centers) is useful, especially for identifying an associated rectocele or internal prolapse.

Treatment

If the prolapse is small and limited to the mucosa, the patient may benefit from taking stool softeners and using an irritant rectal suppository (see Chapter 46) to initiate defecation and thereby avoid straining at stool. If prolapse progresses despite this treatment, or if extensive mucosal prolapse is noted, it is appropriate to refer the patient to a surgeon. Redundant tissue may be treated either by rubber band ligation, as for internal hemorrhoids, or by sclerosis. Both procedures can usually be performed in the surgeon's office without anesthesia and are usually successful in preventing progressive degrees of rectal mucosal prolapse.

If procidentia (full-thickness prolapse) is present, only operative treatment is effective. Several procedures are available for the restoration of anal continence and reduction of prolapse. All of these operations require hospitalization, and most require general anesthesia. One important factor to consider before operation is whether incontinence will be improved. If a full preoperative assessment of anorectal function leads the gastroenterologist and surgeon to believe that incontinence is likely to persist, the alternative of providing the patient with a permanent diverting colostomy must be considered.

Both abdominal and perineal operations are available for the treatment of complete procidentia. The perineal approaches have usually been reserved for very elderly or high-risk patients because of perceived less-than-perfect results. However, published studies indicate that these operations may be satisfactory (16). Nonetheless, the most successful operative procedures for full-thickness rectal prolapse require an abdominal proctopexy, in which the rectum is secured to presacral fascia either by primary suture or by the use of synthetic mesh. This may or may not be accompanied by anterior resection of redundant sigmoid colon. Complications associated with the transabdominal surgical repair of prolapse are fecal impaction, presacral hemorrhage, stricture, infection, fistula formation, pelvic abscess, and intestinal obstruction. The complication rate is about 5%. However, fecal impaction can occur in up to 10% of patients after abdominal proctopexy. The complication rate for perineal repairs is low, and fecal impaction is rare. However, anastomotic leak with pelvic abscess, pelvic hematoma, and anastomotic stricture can occur. The operative mortality rate for abdominal operations is less than 3%, and for perineal procedures it is less than 1%.

Recurrence rates are in the range of 2% for the abdominal approaches and up to 30% for the perineal ones. However, of patients with preoperative fecal incontinence, 15% to 30% continue to have some degree of postoperative incontinence. This problem sometimes responds to biofeedback, which ordinarily is available only in specialized gastroenterology laboratories.

SEXUALLY TRANSMITTED DISEASE

Definition

In addition to the putatively more common sexually transmitted diseases such as gonorrhea and syphilis, proctitis characterized by rectal pain, tenesmus, and often anal discharge should raise suspicion of the so-called gay bowel syndrome. This syndrome and other anorectal diseases have become increasingly common as a consequence of the sexual practices of homosexual men, such as anal receptive intercourse and anilingus. Homosexuality is not, by itself, a risk factor for proctitis. However, promiscuity, failure to use condoms, and multiple contacts lead to a high risk for development of the syndrome, which can also occur in women who engage in the same practices.

Causes

Gay bowel syndrome is a generic term that refers to numerous types of anal and rectal diseases seen in homosexual men. Although the problem is often a nonspecific inflammation caused by trauma, this form of proctitis can be caused by a variety of pathogens (bacteria, viruses, spirochetes, and parasites) (17). The nature and prevalence of a number of specific causes of perianal disease and proctitis in this population are listed in Table 98.4. It should be noted that lymphogranuloma venereum (LGV) is caused by specific immunotypes of *Chlamydia*. Condylomata acuminata associated with certain human papillomavirus (HPV) types are particularly prone to result in high-grade anal dysplasia, or even invasive squamous carcinoma. This is a particular risk for patients with human immunodeficiency virus (HIV) infection.

Diagnosis

Perianal lesions are seen in association with condylomata acuminata, herpes simplex virus type 2 (HSV2), syphilis, chancroid, granuloma inguinale, and molluscum contagiosum. Perianal lesions in the form of abscesses, strictures, and fistulas are a late manifestation of LGV and granuloma inguinale.

Condylomata acuminata are recognized as a typical collection of venereal warts, often extending within the anal canal. There is no specific diagnostic test. *HSV2 infection* manifests initially as perianal or anal canal vesicles, but these have usually ruptured and coalesced into ulcerations before the patient is seen. Precise diagnosis requires either a direct fluorescent

Table 98.4. Sexually Transmitted Anorectal Diseases in Homosexual Men

Cause	Prevalence (%)
Bacterial	
Chlamydia trachomatis and lymphogranuloma venereum	15
Gonorrhea	45–55
Chancroid	5
Shigella	30–50
Granuloma inguinale	Uncommon
Viral	
Herpes simplex virus type 2	95
Condylomata acuminata	50–75
Molluscum contagiosum	Uncommon
Spirochetes	
Syphilis	Common
Protozoa	
Amebiasis	20–32
Giardiasis	4–18

monoclonal antibody technique or culture of the virus. A *perianal chancre* may suggest the diagnosis of primary syphilis, and the typical verrucous excrescence of a *condyloma latum*, although rare, is pathognomonic of primary or secondary syphilis. The diagnosis must be confirmed by dark-field examination for spirochetes. *Chancroid* is associated with anorectal ulcers and abscesses, and the diagnosis is confirmed by culture. *Granuloma inguinale* is a chronic granuloma that eventually causes red, hard, perianal masses; biopsy is necessary for diagnosis. *Molluscum contagiosum* causes self-limited, painless, round, umbilicated lesions that can be confused with cutaneous cryptococcosis in patients with AIDS.

Proctitis is a manifestation of gonorrhea, *Chlamydia* infection, HSV2, amebiasis, shigellosis, or occasionally rectal syphilis. All of these infections cause essentially similar and nonspecific symptoms of rectal discharge, pruritus, tenesmus, hematochezia, and constipation or diarrhea. Pain (odynochezia) is especially typical of HSV2, *Chlamydia* infection, and chancroid and may also accompany syphilis. The proctitis of amebiasis has a rather typical appearance on sigmoidoscopy, but the symptoms are principally those of colitis, as is also true of shigellosis. Constitutional symptoms accompany HSV2 infection and consist of urinary retention, impotence, and unexplained but disabling dysesthesias of the perineum, buttocks, and posterior thighs. Inguinal adenopathy is a common finding in conjunction with syphilis, LGV, or HSV2 infection.

Diagnosis of all of these lesions requires anoscopy and flexible sigmoidoscopy. Gonorrhea causes a nonspecific mucosal inflammation with erythema, friability, and an exudate. Gram staining of the exudate reveals gram negative intracellular diplococci, and a culture is confirmatory. Luetic proctitis is also nonspecific, and the diagnosis is made by dark-field examination of the exudate and serologic tests for syphilis (see Chapter 37). *Chlamydia* causes only a nonspecific proctitis, but LGV causes linear and aphthous ulcers extending up from the rectum to the distal colon as well. Histologically as well as clinically, these findings resemble Crohn disease, and the diagnosis of LGV requires culture of the organism, which commonly necessitates tissue culture inoculation. Rising acute convalescent antichlamydial serum antibody titers are confirmatory but usually are not manifested for 1 month. Although the warts of condylomata acuminata usually appear in the perianal area, anoscopy is necessary to look for involvement of the anal canal. HSV2 also causes predominantly perianal lesions, but anoscopy and sigmoidoscopy should be performed, because the anal canal can contain vesicular lesions or ulcers and the distal rectum may reveal proctitis with or without ulcers as well. Amebiasis often manifests with a characteristic sigmoidoscopic appearance of punched-out ulcers with a yellow base in addition to diffuse inflammation. The diagnosis is confirmed by stool examination for ova and parasites, as is that of giardiasis. A positive stool culture makes the diagnosis of shigellosis; proctitis with ulcerations are shown on proctoscopy.

It should be emphasized that none of these lesions is likely to be recognized unless an appropriate history is obtained. These patients rarely volunteer information regarding their sexual practices, so the clinician is obligated to ask the necessary questions or the diagnosis will be missed.

Treatment

Surgical referral is rarely appropriate for these diseases. When surgery is required, evaluation by a gastroenterologist should precede any operative approach except in the case of condylomata acuminata. Indeed, for most of these lesions, the differential diagnosis is sufficiently complex that gastroenterology consultation is usually appropriate. The exceptions are perhaps gonorrheal or luetic proctitis, because the diagnosis, if suspected, is easily made and treatment is usually successful (see Chapters 37 and 102).

Chlamydia infections (see Chapter 36) respond to doxycycline, azithromycin, ofloxacin, or erythromycin base. The duration and success of treatment depend first on a correct diagnosis (Crohn disease does not respond to antibiotics) and second on the severity and duration of the infection. LGV may progress to abscess, fistula, and stricture formation and may require surgical management, occasionally necessitating a colostomy.

Condylomata acuminata, if the lesions are small, may be treated by the topical application of podophyllin or bichloracetic acid (see Chapters 102 and 117). Larger warts require surgical treatment by a combination of excision and fulguration. The carbon dioxide laser is of no advantage in the treatment of these lesions. There is experimental interest in the use of an autologous vaccine and interferon, but there are no definitive clinical studies as yet. Recurrence is likely, whatever method is used (see also Chapter 102). Molluscum contagiosum is a self-limited disease, but it is also sometimes treated by local destruction to prevent spread.

There is no cure for HSV2 infection, but the use of antiviral agents (eg., acyclovir, famicyclovir, or valacyclovir) may shorten the clinical course.

Amebiasis is treated with metronidazole and, usually, with diiodohydroxyquin as well (see Chapter 35). Metronidazole is also the therapy for giardiasis.

Chancroid responds to ceftriaxone, azithromycin, or erythromycin base. The drug therapy for shigellosis is ciprofloxacin or double-strength trimethoprim-sulfamethoxazole. Granuloma inguinale responds to doxycycline or streptomycin.

General References*

Corman ML. Colon and rectal surgery. 4th ed. Philadelphia: JB Lippincott, 1998.

*Bold print (general references) and bold numerals (specific references) denote published controlled clinical trials, meta-analysis, or consensus-based recommendations.

Fazio VW, Tjandra JJ. The management of perianal diseases. Adv Surg 1996;29:59.
Janicke DM, Pundt MR. Anorectal disorders. Emerg Med Clin North Am 1996;14:757.
Nagle D, Rolandelli RH. Primary care office management of perianal and anal disease. Prim Care 1996;23:609.

Specific References

1. Schouten WR, Briel JW, Auwerda JJ, et al. Anal fissure: new concepts in pathogenesis and treatment. Scand J Gastroenterol Suppl 1996;218:78.
2. Dodi G, Bogoni F, Infantino A, et al. Hot or cold in anal pain? A study of the changes in internal sphincter pressure profiles. Dis Colon Rectum 1986;29:248.
3. Lund JN, Scholefield JH. A randomised, prospective, double-blind, placebo-controlled trial of glyceryl trinitrate ointment in treatment of anal fissure. Lancet 1997;349:11.
4. Kennedy ML, Sowter S, Nguyen H, et al. Glyceryl trinitrate ointment for the treatment of chronic anal fissure: results of a placebo-controlled trial and long-term follow-up. Dis Colon Rectum 1999;42:1000.
5. Zuberi BF, Rajput MR, Abro H, et al. A randomized trial of glyceryl trinitrate ointment and nitroglycerin patch in healing of anal fissures. Int J Colorectal Dis 2000;15:243.
6. Altomare DF, Rinaldi M, Milito G, et al. Glyceryl trinitrate for chronic anal fissure: healing or headache? Results of a multicenter, randomized, placebo-controlled, double-blind trial. Dis Colon Rectum 2000;43:174.
7. Maria G, Cassetta E, Gui D, et al. A comparison of botulinum toxin and saline for the treatment of chronic anal fissure. N Engl J Med 1998;338:217.
8. Jost WH, Schrank B. Repeat botulin toxin injections in anal fissure: in patients with relapse and after insufficient effect of first treatment. Dig Dis Sci 1999;44:1588.
9. Johanson JF, Sonnenberg A. The prevalence of hemorrhoids and chronic constipation: an epidemiologic study. Gastroenterology 1990;98:380.
10. Standards Practice Task Force, American Society of Colon and Rectal Surgeons. Practice parameters for the treatment of hemorrhoids. Dis Colon Rectum 1993;36:1118.
11. Murie JA, Sim AJW, Mackenzie I. Rubber band ligation versus haemorrhoidectomy for prolapsing haemorrhoids: a long term prospective clinical trial. Br J Surg 1982;69:536.
12. Nivatvongs S, Goldberg SM. An improved technique of rubber band ligation of hemorrhoids. Am J Surg 1982;144:379.
13. Standards Practice Task Force, American Society of Colon and Rectal Surgeons. Practice parameters for treatment of fistula-in-ano: supporting documentation. Dis Colon Rectum 1996;39:1363.
14. Venkatesh KS, Ramanujam P. Fibrin glue application in the treatment of recurrent anorectal fistulas. Dis Colon Rectum 1999;42:1136.
15. Rao SS, Hatfield RA. Paroxysmal anal hyperkinesis: a characteristic feature of proctalgia fugax. Gut 1996;39:609.
16. Agachan F, Pfiefer J, Joo JS, et al. Results of perineal procedures for the treatment of rectal prolapse. Am Surg 1997;63:9.
17. Goldberg GS,Orkin BA, Smith LE. Microbiology of human immunodeficiency virus anorectal disease. Dis Colon Rectum 1994;37:439.

SECTION

14

Gynecology and Women's Health

C H A P T E R 99

Approach to Women's Health

PATRICIA A. THOMAS, MD

Women's health is currently conceptualized as a holistic, multidisciplinary approach to the health care of women throughout the life span and, as such, is much evolved from its narrow origins in the biomedical approach to reproductive health (1). On a global scale, women's health embodies a variety of social and economic concerns that affect the lives of girls and women worldwide. Many forces converged to promote the development of this field, but perhaps the most compelling for clinicians was the evidence that previous models failed to deliver quality health care to a substantial proportion of women.

The Council on Graduate Medical Education's *1995 Report on the Status of Women* made several observations about the need for new clinical competencies in women's health (2). First, women have important health needs throughout their life spans, not just during the reproductive years. It is true that women live longer than men; in 1999, the age-adjusted death rate for the 15 leading causes of death combined was 58.2% higher for men than women (3). Although women enjoy longer life, they report poorer health status than men, suffer more chronic illness and mental illness than men, and experience more disability in later years (Figs. 99.1 and 99.2). Economic factors may explain some of these differences. In a 1999 national survey, 12% of women younger than 44 years of age reported having no health insurance coverage, and 9% of women overall reported that cost concerns had prevented their seeking care at least once in the previous year (4). Second, inadequate health insurance and fragmented delivery of primary care services have led to poorly coordinated care for many routine and comprehensive health concerns of women (Fig. 99.3, page 1559). There appears to be a bias in the provision of care that women receive, compared with men, for a number of chronic illnesses. Men are more likely to undergo noninvasive investigations for coronary artery disease, to undergo renal transplantation, and to receive zidovudine for human immunodeficiency virus infection and acquired immunodeficiency syndrome (5). The reasons for these gender inequalities are unclear and call for further research. Third, the aging population, an increasingly diverse ethnicity, and changes in family structure in the U. S. population are all expected to have significant effects on the health status of women in the years ahead.

Although women receive more health services than men, women are less satisfied with their care (Fig. 99.4, page 1559). The 1993 Commonwealth Fund Survey, a private foundation that supports independent research on health and social issues, found that 41% of women but only 27% of men had changed physicians in the previous year because of dissatisfaction with care (6). This may relate to the traditionally fragmented health care received, since women frequently see more than one clinician for routine care. Dissatisfaction has also been traced to gender differences in communication and lack of a sense of partnership with one's physician. In one report, women's overall satisfaction with care was more dependent than men's on informational content, continuity, and multidisciplinarity (7). The rising number of women in medical careers, as well as the lay women's health movement, have advanced the standard toward a woman-centered approach to communication and shared decision-making.

No situation highlights the pitfalls of the biomedical organ-based approach to health care more than the issue of hormone replacement therapy (HRT) in menopause. There is strong evidence for the efficacy of HRT in preventing postmenopausal osteoporosis, a disease with a significant burden of illness. Growing evidence of a long-term increase in breast cancer risk with this preventive strategy, however, became evident in the 1990s (8). Using conclusions from observational studies, physicians counseled women that there was significant risk reduction for cardiovascular disease with HRT, until a 1998 randomized clinical trial suggested otherwise (9). In making the decision whether to use HRT as a preventive medicine then, a woman often has to weigh her perceived risks of heart disease, breast cancer, and osteoporosis, as well as the side effects of medication, in the setting of incomplete evidence for efficacy. Most women overestimate their risk of breast cancer and, for a variety of sociocultural reasons, are most concerned about even a minimal increase in breast cancer risk. The clinician who is knowledgeable about the totality of a woman's health, her individual risks and her health belief systems, is ideally equipped to counsel the patient in this difficult decision.

What constitutes effective clinical practice of women's health? The field is still evolving, but a common approach is to consider prevention, risk assessment, and illness by stages of life. Many of the diseases that must be considered in the care of women are common to both men and women. Often the prevalence is higher in women (e.g., eating disorders, autoimmune disease), or the clinical presentation is different

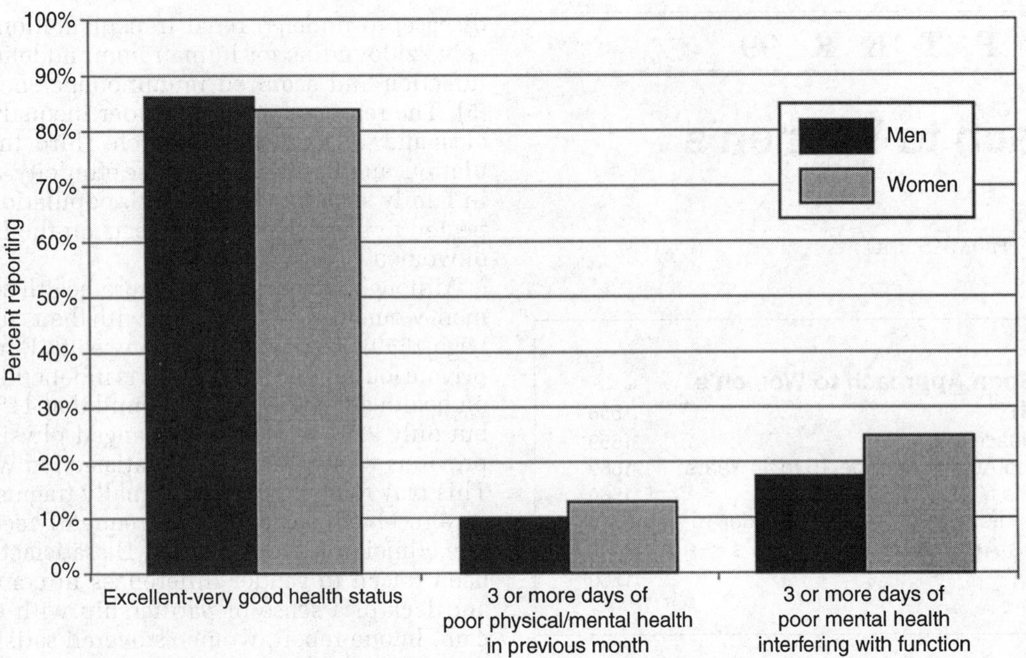

Figure 99.1. Self-reported health status by gender. (From Behavioral Risk Factor Surveillance System. 1999 Survey data. Atlanta, GA: National Center for Chronic Disease Prevention and Health Promotion, Centers for Disease Control and Prevention, U. S. Department of Health and Human Services, June 2000.)

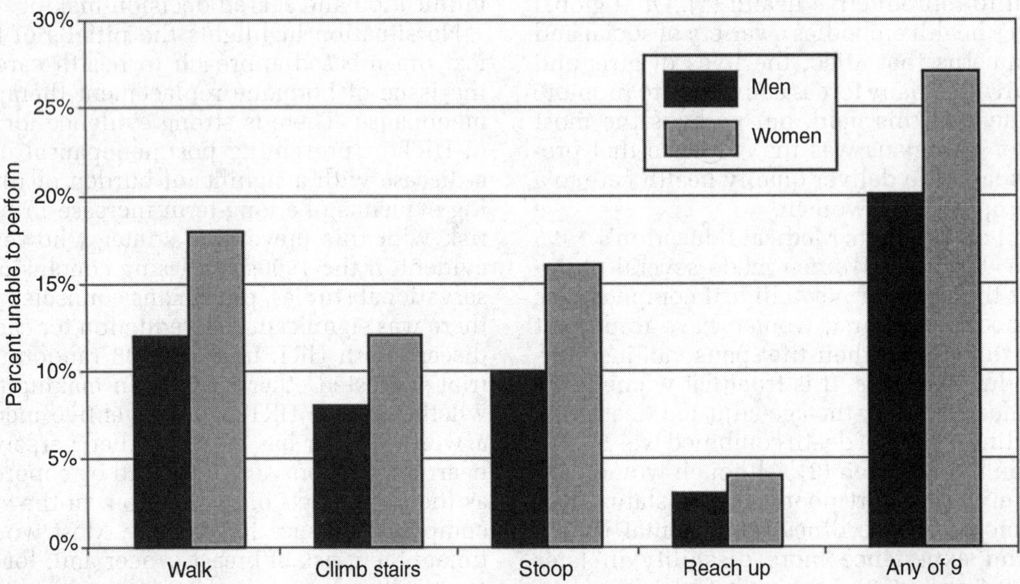

Figure 99.2. Chronic disability in women: self-report of functional disability in men and women. (From Federal Interagency Forum on Aging-Related Statistics. Older Americans 2000: key indicators of well-being. National Institute of Aging, National Center for Health Statistics. Washington, DC: U. S. Government Printing Office, August 2000. Available at: http://www.agingstats.gov. Accessed February 15, 2002.)

in women (e.g., coronary artery disease). An interwoven theme in women's health is that female patients may fail to respond to narrow biomedical approaches to illness, perhaps because of sex-specific biologic and gender-specific psychosocial factors. Throughout this textbook, authors have attempted to highlight these differences in their discussions, and readers are encouraged to use those chapters referred to here for more in-depth discussion of these topics.

A LIFE SPAN APPROACH TO WOMEN'S HEALTH

Most clinicians understand well that health and illness are the result not only of physiologic changes but also of social, cultural, and economic changes in the

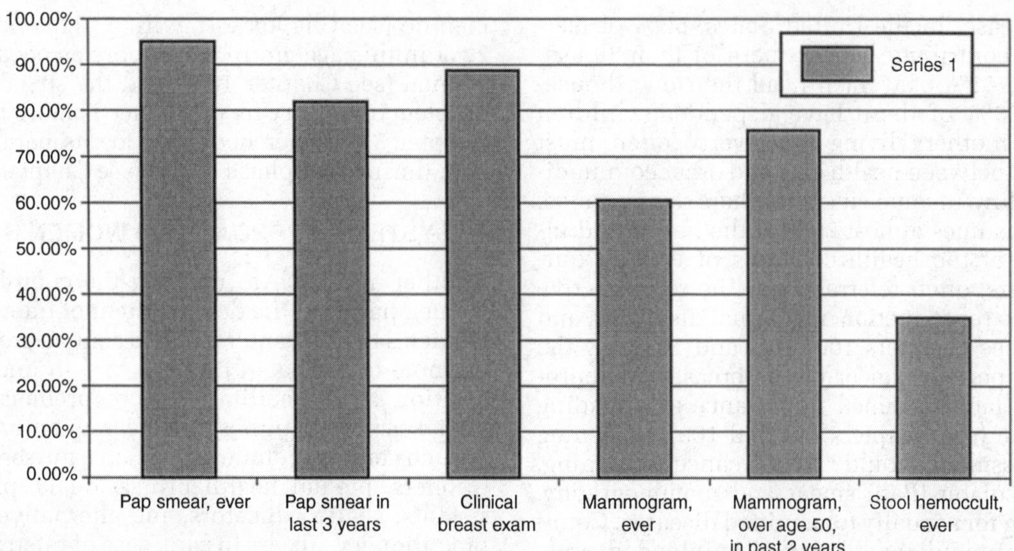

Figure 99.3. Delivery of primary care services to women. Percentage of women receiving primary care services by self-report. (From Behavior Risk Factor Surveillance System. 1999 Survey data. Atlanta, GA: National Center for Chronic Disease Prevention and Health Promotion, Centers for Disease Control and Prevention, U. S. Department of Health and Human Services, June 2000.)

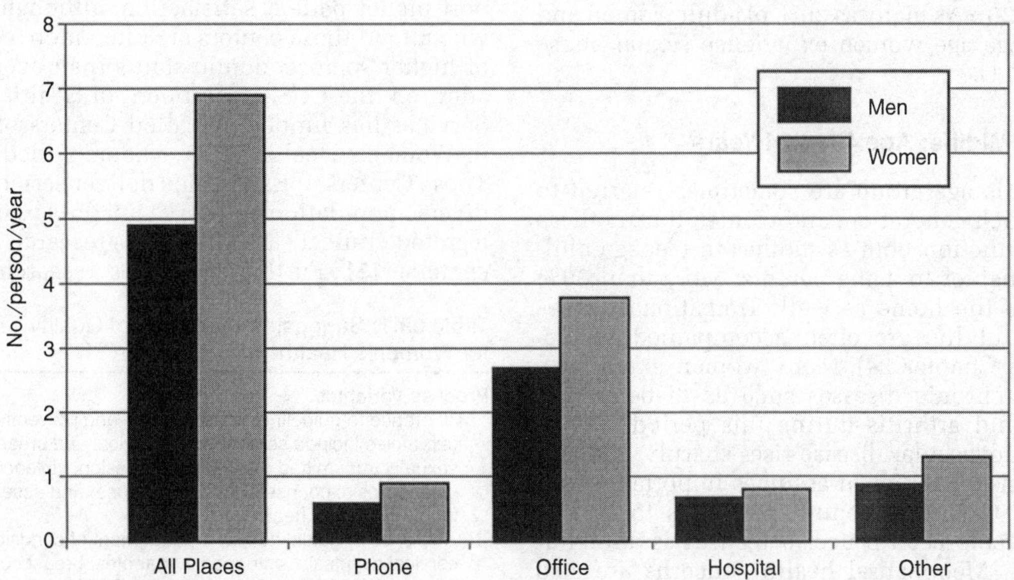

Figure 99.4. Use of health care services by gender. Annual health service contacts by gender and location. (From Division of Health Interview Statistics, National Center for Health Statistics. National health interview survey, Series 10, no. 199. 1995:109.)

patient's life. In the field of women's health, newer competencies call for the clinician to possess the knowledge and attitudes necessary to integrate biologic and psychosocial factors in the provision of comprehensive care of women. The following discussion provides some examples of how this integration could be applied over life stages.

Adolescence

Clinicians who care for adult women often care for adolescents also. In addition to issues of puberty and sexual differentiation, issues of gender identity and body image become manifest in these years (Chapter 6). Major causes of death in this age group are trauma and suicide. Many chronic adult diseases, such as autoimmune disease, first manifest at puberty. Eating disorders are becoming increasingly prevalent in this age group. The foundation of counseling for health risk behaviors begins in these years.

Young Adulthood: Age 15 to 44 Years

In early adulthood, women may be juggling career, social relationships, and family life. Economically, women often lose wage equity with men just as family burdens increase. In the United States, 52% of married women contribute half or more of their household income; 41% of women head their own households, and 28% of these have dependent children (10). Single mothers living in poverty often must make choices between health care and other commodities. Among low-income single mothers, for instance, childcare consumes almost 20% of the household income. Many of the health concerns of women during these years, often referred to as the reproductive years, relate to reproduction, menstrual disorders, and conception (see Chapters 100, 101, and 102). By the close of this period, cancer of the breast and reproductive tract have assumed importance as a leading cause of death (see Chapters 104 and 105). Screening and risk assessment should include cancer screening, with Papanicolaou (Pap) smear and mammography, and screening for sexually transmitted diseases. Counseling issues include avoidance of unintended pregnancy and sexually transmitted diseases, weight management, and smoking cessation (see Chapter 4). As with men, significant mortality and morbidity during these years is related to violence and injury; domestic violence is especially prevalent in this age group (see Chapter 28). As many as 20% of adult women and 15% of college age women experience sexual abuse and assault (11).

Midlife: Age 45 to 64 Years

Persons of this age group are sometimes referred to as the sandwich generation, and women during these years often function both as mother to teenage children and daughter to aging parents. More than 60% work outside the home as well. Transitional issues at this time of life are often accompanied by depression (see Chapter 24). Many women experience the onset of chronic diseases such as diabetes, hypertension, and arthritis during this period. Prevalence of cardiovascular disease rises sharply, and cardiovascular risk assessment assumes importance (see Chapter 62). Cancer screening continues to be important, and colorectal cancer screening is added at age 50 years. Menopausal health concerns are also important, beginning with perimenopausal symptoms and culminating with decisions regarding HRT (see Chapter 106).

Late Life: Age 65 Years and Older

At the age of 65 years, the average U. S. woman has 21 years of life ahead. More women than men will assume caregiver roles to sick spouses. In 1999, 41% of women older than 65 years of age lived alone, compared with 17% of men, accounting for the importance of social isolation in this group (12). After lifelong lower wages compared with men, the retirement years for women are also often years of economic deprivation. Older women have a higher poverty rate than older men (11.8% versus 6.9% in 1999) (13). Women have higher rates of severe depression than men do (see Chapter 24), with a frequency of 18% to 22% in this age group. Osteoporosis occurs earlier in women (see Chapter 103), and the socially disabling problem of urinary incontinence is more frequent (see Chapter 54). Other health concerns parallel those of men during this phase of life (see Chapter 12).

SYSTEMS APPROACH TO WOMEN'S HEALTH

Another approach to meeting the complex needs of women has been the development of interdisciplinary women's health centers. These centers are designed to promote coordinated clinical care in one geographic location and to facilitate the comprehensive delivery of that care. Disciplines that are frequently represented in such centers include physicians, nurses, nurse practitioners, mental health professionals, physician assistants, health educators, and alternative health care practitioners. Access to care, ease of referral, increased communication, and coordination of care among clinicians can be facilitated with such an integrated center. Many centers are hospital sponsored. A review of the experience of these centers noted that preventive services are delivered at higher rates and women report higher patient satisfaction, although the women who attend these centers are often more educated and of higher socioeconomic status than average (14). In addition, the U. S. Department of Health and Human Services has funded so-called Centers of Excellence in Women's Health in 18 academic medical centers. These Centers of Excellence deliver services to a more diverse population and serve not only as models of integrated clinical care but also as research and training centers (15). Further outcomes research is needed,

Table 99.1. Suggested Measures of Quality for Women's Health

Process Variables

- Adherence to guidelines for screening and preventive care (examples include screening for cervical and breast cancer, sexually transmitted diseases, depression, violence, and osteoporosis; counseling at menopause; and assessment of risk for diabetes and heart disease)
- Adherence to guidelines for management of conditions such as cervical dysplasia, osteopenia, diabetes, breast complaints, and chlamydial infection, including timely follow-up of positive screening tests
- Access to care
- Interpersonal aspects of care, such as the amount of information exchanged during an office visit and the active involvement of the patient in the decision-making process
- Utilization of health care resources in the ambulatory setting, including number of office visits, use of diagnostic tests, time spent with providers, and changes in source of care over time

Outcome Variables

- Functional status, including general health, mental health, and social functioning
- Clinical status, including condition-specific measures when available
- Changes in patient behavior, such as smoking cessation or initiation of exercise
- Patient satisfaction
- Professional satisfaction

From Carlson KJ. Multidisciplinary women's health care and quality of care. Women's Health Issues 2000;10:219, with permission.

however, to better understand the impact of this model on women's health (Table 99.1). Several measures of quality, such as patient satisfaction, are still in development.

The growth of women's health centers, coupled with the founding of the Office of Research on Women's Health at the National Institutes of Health and expanded funding of research initiatives, promises to continue the development of knowledge that will inform clinicians and patients about the delivery of health services to women in the decades ahead.

General References*

Allen KM, Phillips JM. Women's health across the lifespan: a comprehensive perspective. Philadelphia: Lippincott-Raven, 1997.

Women's health for the practitioner discussed in an environmental context, including sections on cultural diverseness, health policy and research, and extensive health promotion.

Council on Graduate Medical Education. Fifth report: women and medicine. Washington, DC: U. S. Department of Health and Human Services, 1995.

This advisory group of academic and medical communities addressed the health status of women and equity of women in the physician workforce, with summary recommendations, including delineation of competencies in women's health.

Falik MM, Collins KS, eds. Women's health: the Commonwealth Fund survey. Baltimore: Johns Hopkins University Press, 1996.

This is a detailed analysis of a 1993 national survey conducted by the Commonwealth Fund that explored women's health from the perspectives of care-seeking behaviors, lifespan and cultural issues, behavioral well-being, and socioeconomic circumstances.

Goldman M, Hatch M, eds. Women and health. New York: Academic Press, 2000.

Comprehensive resource in biomedical as well as environmental issues relating to the health of women. Includes chapters on international issues, women at work, and environmental exposures, as well as approaches to organ-based health problems.

Wallis LA, ed. Textbook of women's health. Philadelphia: Lippincott–Raven, 1998.

Comprehensive textbook, includes detailed approaches to care as well as discussion of social and cultural information, research and life-cycle transitions.

*Bold print (general references) and bold numerals (specific references) denote published controlled clinical trials, meta-analyses, or consensus-based recommendations.

Specific References

1. Hoffman E, Magrane D, Donoghue GD. Changing perspectives on sex and gender in medical education. Acad Med 2000;75:1051.
2. Council on Graduate Medical Education. Fifth report: women and medicine. Washington, DC: U. S. Department of Health and Human Services, 1995.
3. National Center for Vital Statistics. Health—United States, 2000. Hyattsville, MD: Public Health Service, 2000.
4. Behavioral Risk Factor Surveillance System. 1999 Survey data. Atlanta, GA: National Center for Chronic Disease Prevention and Health Promotion, Centers for Disease Control and Prevention, U. S. Department of Health and Human Services, June 2000.
5. Raine R. Does gender bias exist in the use of specialist health care? J Health Serv Res Policy 2000;5:237.
6. Falik MM, Collins KS, eds. Women's health: the Commonwealth Fund survey. Baltimore: Johns Hopkins University Press, 1996.
7. Weisman CS, Rich DE, Rogers J, et al. Gender and patient satisfaction with primary care: tuning in to women in quality measurement. J Womens Health Gend Based Med 2000;9:657.
8. Grodstein F, Stampfer MJ, Colditz GA, et al. Postmenopausal hormone therapy and mortality. N Engl J Med 1997;336:1769.
9. Hulley S, Grady D, Bush T, et al. Randomized trial of estrogen plus progestin for secondary prevention of coronary heart disease in postmenopausal women. JAMA 1998;280:605.
10. U. S. Department of Labor, Womens Bureau. Available at: www.dol.gov/dol/wb.
11. Tjaden P, Thoennes N. Prevalence, incidence and consequences of violence against women: findings from the National Violence Against Women Survey. National Institute of Justice, Centers for Disease Control and Prevention. Washington, DC: U. S. Government Printing Office, November 1998.
12. Federal Interagency Forum on Aging-Related Statistics. Older Americans 2000: key indicators of well-being. National Institute of Aging, National Center for Health Statistics. Washington, DC: U. S. Government Printing Office, August 2000. Available at: http://www.agingstats.gov. Accessed February 15, 2002.
13. Current Population Reports. Poverty in the United States: 1999. Publication no. P60-210 Washington, DC: U. S. Bureau of the Census, September 2000.
14. Carlson KJ. Multidisciplinary women's health care and quality of care. Women's Health Issues 2000;10:219.
15. Weisman CS, Squires GL. Women's health centers: are the National Centers of Excellence in Women's Health a new model? Women's Health Issues 2000;10:248.

CHAPTER 100

Contraception and Preconception Counseling

JEFFREY M. SMITH, MD, MPH
GEORGE R. HUGGINS, MD

Contraception provides a woman and her partner with the ability to determine the number and timing of pregnancies. In general, avoidance of unwanted pregnancies and continued consistent use of a contraceptive method are issues that require ongoing management and consultation rather than an isolated decision.

There are many contraceptive methods (1). It is important to understand the benefits and limitations of all of them to be able to educate the patient fully about her options. The physician should be prepared to deal with women who have varying knowledge and experience about contraception. Table 100.1 lists the percentage distribution of use of contraceptive methods by women in the United States. These most recent data, from 1995, do not include percentage distributions for levonorgestrel implants (Norplant) and medroxy progesterone acetate injectable suspension (Depo-Provera), each estimated to be less than 5%. In 1995, 64.2% of all women of reproductive age were using a contraceptive method.

The failure rates of various methods of contraception are shown in Table 100.2. Perfect use refers to the annual percentage of unexpected pregnancy among couples who use the method correctly and consistently, whereas typical use reflects common irregularities in use other than voluntary termination of the method. Clearly there is very little difference between the two failure rates with some methods, whereas others show a considerable difference. This information should be used in helping to educate the patient.

Once it is established that a woman desires fertility regulation, a focused medical history should be obtained, including information about past pregnancies, menstruation, smoking, and medical problems that may affect selection of one method over another. A physical examination with special emphasis on the pelvic examination is important. A cancer detection smear and, if indicated (e.g., in a woman with multiple sexual partners), a gonococcus culture and chlamydia smear of the endocervix (see Chapter 102) are

Table 100.1. Contraceptive Use Among U.S. Women at Risk for Pregnancy[a]

Contraceptive	% U.S. Women Age 15–44 Yr in 1995
Female sterilization	25.6
Oral contraceptive	24.9
Male condom	18.9
Male sterilization	10.1
No method	7.5
Withdrawal	2.9
Injectable	2.7
Periodic abstinence	2.2
Diaphragm	1.7
Progestin implant	1.3
Spermicide	1.3
Intrauterine device	0.7
Natural family planning	0.3
Others—each 1% or less[b]	0.1

[a]Those at risk for pregnancy are those who are either current contraceptive users or are nonusers who are exposed to unplanned pregnancy (not currently pregnant, not trying to achieve pregnancy, not having sex within 3 months of the interview, not noncontraceptively sterile).

[b]Includes douche, foam, cream/jelly alone, sponge, vaginal suppository, cervical cap, and female condom.

Modified from Abma J, Chandra A, Mosher W, et al. Fertility, family planning, and women's health: new data from the 1995 National Survey of Family Growth. National Center for Health Statistics. Vital Health Stat 23, no. 19, 1997 (2).

Table 100.2. Summary of Methods of Contraception, Their Mechanisms of Action, Failure Rates, and Major Adverse Effects

Method	Mechanism of Action	Failure Rate %[a] Typical Use	Perfect Use	Some Adverse Effects
No method		85	85	—
Spermicide alone	Inactivation of sperm	26	6	Irritation can occur
Withdrawal		19	4	—
Periodic abstinence	Avoidance of coitus during presumed fertile days	25	1–9	—
Diaphragm or cervical cap with spermicide	Mechanical barrier to sperm; inactivation of sperm	20–40	6–26	Increased risk of urinary tract or vaginal infection
Condom	Mechanical barrier to sperm	14	3	Allergic reactions
Oral contraceptives				
Combined	Suppression of ovulation, changes in cervical mucus and endometrium	5	0.1	Estrogen-related risk of thromboembolism, stroke; myocardial infarction in older smokers; hypertension
Progestin only	Changes in cervical mucus and endometrium, possibly suppression of ovulation	5	0.5	Irregular, unpredictable bleeding in some
Intrauterine device	Inhibition of sperm migration, fertilization, or ovum transport			Pelvic inflammatory disease; uterine perforation; increase in menstrual blood loss with copper
Levonorgestrel,		0.1	0.1	
Progesterone T		2.0	1.5	
Copper T 380A		0.8	0.6	
Medroxyprogesterone (Depo-Provera)	Changes in cervical mucus and endometrium, suppression of ovulation	0.3	0.3	Menstrual irregularities; headache; weight gain
Levonorgestrel subdermal implants (Norplant)	Same as medroxyprogesterone acetate	0.05	0.05	Menstrual irregularities; headache; weight gain
Sterilization				
Vasectomy	Vas deferens occlusion	0.5	0.5	Surgical procedure
Tubal ligation	Fallopian tube occlusion	0.15	0.10	Surgical procedure

[a]Percentage of accidental pregnancy during first year of use among women in the United States who are more likely (low failure rate) and less likely (high failure rate) than average to use the method correctly and consistently. (Harlap S, Kost K, Forrest JD. Preventing pregnancy, protecting health: a new look at birth control choices in the United States. New York: Alan Guttmacher Institute, 1991:33.) Perfect use refers to clinical trial data with highly motivated patients; typical use refers to usual clinical experience (see text).

Adapted from Hatcher RA, Trussell J, Stewart F, et al. Contraceptive technology. 17th ed. New York: Ardent Media, 1998.

suggested. After this evaluation, the physician and patient (and, sometimes, her partner) are ready to discuss the various contraceptive methods and develop a satisfactory plan.

A pelvic examination is not immediately necessary for the initiation or continuation of a hormonal method such as oral contraceptive pills, Norplant, or Depo-Provera. Although an annual pelvic examination is seen as a necessary step in preventive health care for women of reproductive age, the deferral of this examination should not preclude prescription of a safe contraceptive method and risk an unsafe or unwanted pregnancy.

CONTRACEPTION IN SPECIAL CIRCUMSTANCES

During the time leading up to the menopause, a woman's concern regarding unplanned pregnancy is heightened by abnormal menstrual cycles and episodes of amenorrhea. Although fertility declines with age, missing a period is disturbing to a woman in the perimenopause unless a very reliable method of contraception is being used. Some methods are particularly advantageous to women in the perimenopause.

The postpartum woman needs help in getting back on a contraceptive program, and usually her obstetrician has given her advice in this regard. Also, the woman wishing to use an intrauterine device (IUD) needs to wait for involution of the uterus—which usually occurs 4 to 6 weeks after delivery—and therefore is at risk for pregnancy until the IUD is inserted. The physiology of the female reproductive cycle, important to an understanding of the many contraceptive methods, is discussed in Chapter 101.

Occasionally, the physician is confronted with the need to provide emergency contraception for a patient, for example after sexual assault or current method failure. This is discussed fully later in this chapter.

ORAL CONTRACEPTIVES

Mechanism of Action

Oral contraceptires (OCs) prevent ovulation by inhibition of gonadotropin-releasing factors in the hypothalamus. The principal effect of this inhibition appears to be suppression of the surge in activity of luteinizing hormone at midcycle, thereby removing a major stimulus to ovulation. In addition, OCs make cervical mucus more viscus and therefore less easily traversed by sperm. They also have a direct effect on endometrial development in high doses, making the uterus less receptive to implantation of the fertilized ovum (3).

Preparations and Dosage Schedules

The combined OC was first introduced for use in the United States in 1960. In the ensuing years, significant changes were made in steroid dosages and some new steroids were introduced. Since 1970, all new OCs introduced in the United States have contained ethinyl estradiol as their estrogen. As their progestin, many OCs in current use contain levonorgestrel or norethindrone. In 1992, however, two new progestins, norgestimate and desogestrel, were introduced in the United States in an effort to decrease unwanted side effects of oral contraception. More recently, a lower-dose OC formulation was released that contained 20 μg of estrogen, again to decrease adverse effects and improve compliance.

There are three different preparations of OC pills:

- Monophasic—contains the same dosage of estrogen and progestin for 21 days each cycle.
- Multiphasic—contains one to two levels of estrogen and two to three levels of progestin, which vary through the cycle.
- Progestin only (mini-pill)—contains progestin only in a steady, continuous dosage.

The progestin-only preparations do not consistently inhibit ovulation, and unwanted pregnancy is three to five times more likely with them than with OCs that contain estrogen and progestogen. Therefore, they should be prescribed only for women who cannot be given estrogen (e.g., those with a history of thromboembolism). Few women are taking progestin-only preparations at present.

Conditions requiring precautions for the use of OCs are listed in Table 100.3.

If a woman chooses oral contraception and has no clinical contraindications, then the first choice should be a combination preparation containing between 20 and 35 μg of estrogen. Use of pills containing 50 μg of estrogen should be avoided, and the few women who may need them should be evaluated by an obstetrician-gynecologist if the clinician is not fully familiar with their use. The choice of progestin is less critical, and no progestin is clearly superior to another. The newer progestins (desogestrel and norgestimate) cause less hirsuitism, acne, and weight gain, as well as a more favorable lipid profile.

Table 100.3. Conditions Requiring Precautions for the Use of Oral Contraceptives

Known or suspected pregnancy
Breast-feeding mother (first 6 mo)
Non–breast-feeding mother (first 3 wk)
Undiagnosed, abnormal genital bleeding
Jaundice, known or suspected liver failure
Smoker and age 35 yr or older
Ischemic heart disease
Cerebral vascular or coronary artery disease (current or remote)
Hypertension (greater than 160/100 mm Hg)
Diabetes with vascular lesions
Thrombophlebitis or thromboembolic disorders (current or remote)
Migraine headaches with focal neurologic symptoms
Known or suspected carcinoma of the breast
Known or suspected estrogen-dependent neoplasia
Major surgery with prolonged bed rest

From World Health Organization. Improving access to quality care in family planning: eligibility criteria for initiating and continuing use of contraceptive methods. Geneva: WHO, 1996.

To suppress ovulation and yet allow periodic bleeding, the combination tablet is taken every day for 3 weeks. The woman starts the medication by the fifth day of her cycle, counting the first day of menstrual bleeding as day 1. An alternative is to start on the first Sunday after the onset of a menstrual period. This latter practice allows the packaging of the tablets to provide for the user a minicalendar, which minimizes missing a dose. The tablets are arranged in circles or rows, making it easier to use them regularly. In the 28-day formulation, the last seven tablets have no hormonal effect and are there to help the woman stay on schedule and thereby improve compliance. An exception to this is a combination pill that adds a small dose of estrogen to the pills taken on the last 5 days, instead of using inert pills, to prevent the estrogen withdrawal headache experienced by some women. The drop in hormone level after 21 days produces withdrawal bleeding, just as it does in the normal menstrual cycle. Women typically have their menses 2 to 3 days after finishing their active pills.

Postpartum women choosing an OC should wait 3 weeks because of the theoretical increased risk of thromboembolism after pregnancy, but no longer than 4 to 6 weeks, at which time ovulation typically resumes. Breast-feeding women rarely need additional contraception for the first 6 months after delivery. If contraception is believed to be necessary, combined OCs are usually avoided because they may decrease the quantity of breast milk. Women who have had a spontaneous or therapeutic abortion may start taking the drug on the first Sunday after the event.

Noncontraceptive Benefits

In the past few years, OCs have been found to be associated with a significant number of beneficial side effects. These involve decreased risks for benign breast tumors, functional ovarian cysts, acne vulgaris, anemia, pelvic inflammatory disease, endometrial carcinoma, and carcinoma of the ovary. Table 100.4 shows the estimated number of hospitalizations averted each year in the United States by OC use.

In the United States and other developed countries, a number of deaths are averted each year by the use of OCs because of their protective effect against ovarian and endometrial carcinoma. On balance, probably more deaths are averted than are caused by OC use in developed countries. In developing countries, where access to obstetric care may be limited, many maternal deaths are averted by the avoidance of pregnancy with OCs.

Recognition of these noncontraceptive benefits of OCs helps place them in a much more positive perspective for women and, indeed, puts the risk–benefit ratio of OCs in a more proper perspective.

Table 100.4. Noncontraceptive Health Benefits of Oral Contraceptives[a]

Disease	Hospitalizations Prevented per 100,000 OC Users per Year	Number of Hospitalizations Prevented per Year	Number of Deaths Averted per Year
Benign breast disease	235	20,000	—
Ovarian retention cysts	35	3,000	—
Iron deficiency anemia[b]	320	27,000	—
Pelvic inflammatory disease (first episodes)			
Total episodes[b]	600	51,000	100
Hospitalizations	156	13,300	—
Ectopic pregnancy	117	9,900	10
Endometrial cancer[c]	5	2,000	100
Ovarian cancer[c]	4	1,700	1,000

[a]Except where noted, figures refer to hospitalizations prevented among the estimated 8.5 million current users of oral contraceptives in the United States.

[b]Episodes prevented regardless of whether hospitalization occurred.

[c]Based on an estimated 39 million U.S. women who have ever used oral contraceptives.

Adapted from Ory HW. The noncontraceptive health benefits from oral contraceptive use. Fam Plann Perspect 1982;14:182.

Limitations

Thromboembolic Disease

In the late 1960s, the first epidemiologic studies conducted in Great Britain and the United States showed an increased risk of thromboembolic disorders and myocardial infarction among OC users. It was quickly determined that the risk of thrombophlebitis and other vascular accidents was related to the dosage of estrogen, the woman's age, and whether she was a smoker or nonsmoker (4,5). Decreasing the estrogen dosage in the OCs from 80 to 50 μg achieved a reduction of approximately 30% in the incidence of thromboembolic disease. A further reduction from 50 μg into the range of 30 to 35 μg further decreased the risk of venous thrombosis and other serious vascular complications.

However, the risk of thromboembolic disease must be kept in perspective. The general risk of thromboembolism in a nonpregnant woman of reproductive age is about 4 per 100,000. For women taking OC preparations the risk is about 10 to 15 per 100,000. However, for a woman who is pregnant the risk is 60 per 100,000 (6).

Approximately 10 million women in the United States use OCs. Cardiovascular problems, heart attack, stroke, thrombophlebitis, and pulmonary emboli are the main causes of serious morbidity and death associated with OC use (7,8). Therefore, women with a history of thromboembolism, stroke, or ischemic heart disease should not use combined OCs. Women who are older than 35 years of age and smoke should not use OCs owing to the risk of cardiovascular disease. Smokers who are younger than 35 years of age are not prohibited from using OCs if it is the best method for them; they should, of course, be encouraged to quit smoking (9).

Age and smoking play significant roles in determining the risk of serious cardiovascular events. An estimated 86% of deaths associated with OC use result from a combination of smoking and pill use by women 35 years of age and older (10). This form of contraception, therefore, should be avoided in women who continue to smoke. Because of the risk of thromboembolism, OCs should be discontinued 30 days before major surgery. They need not be discontinued before minor surgery (11).

Hypertension

With the older high-dose OCs, the risk of developing high blood pressure was approximately 7%. Clinical trials have shown that low-dose OCs (20 to 35 μg of estrogen) are responsible for only small changes in blood pressure. Therefore, if an OC user develops hypertension, the hypertension should be evaluated and not ascribed to contraceptive use. Women with preexisting mild hypertension and those who develop mild hypertension while taking OCs may safely use OCs if their blood pressure is monitored and controlled. Severe hypertension or hypertension with vascular changes is a contraindication to the use of OCs (9).

Neoplasia

After almost 35 years of contraceptive use, the data concerning the relationship between OC use and neoplasia are mostly reassuring (Table 100.5).

There is a relationship between the long-term use of OCs and the development of benign hepatic neoplasia (12). These lesions are rare, and although the increased relative risk in long-term users is high, the absolute incidence is very low. Long-term use of OCs has been associated with a significantly decreased incidence of endometrial and ovarian cancer (13–15). Compared with never-users, women who have used OCs for up to 4 years have a relative risk (RR) for development of ovarian cancer of 0.7; for 4 to 11 years of use, the RR is 0.4; and for 12 or more years, it is 0.2. A similar comparison for endometrial cancer shows an RR of 0.6 for women who used OC for 2 years and 0.4 for those with 4 or more years of use. This protective effect may persist for up to 10 years after discontinuation of OCs (15,16).

The data are inconclusive for malignant melanoma and cervical neoplasia. With regard to the development of cervical neoplasia, several studies show a slightly increased risk directly related to length of OC use (14,16,17). Nevertheless, no firm conclusions can be drawn at this time.

Table 100.5. Oral Contraceptives and Neoplasia Risk

Type of Neoplasia	Increased	No Effect	Decreased	Inconclusive Information
Hepatocellular adenoma	X			
Cervical neoplasia				X
Endometrial cancer			X	
Ovarian cancer			X	
Breast cancer		X		
Pituitary adenoma		X		
Malignant melanoma				X

Similarly, data regarding breast cancer and OC use are conflicting and no conclusions are currently possible (18). Although some data suggest that OCs may advance premenopausal breast cancer, this is a rare time for its occurrence. Epidemiologic evidence suggests a relative risk of 1.1 (confidence interval, 0.8 to 1.4) for ever-users versus never-users (16). The incidence of benign breast tumors and fibrocystic disease is reduced by the administration of high-progestin-dose OC hormones. Data on the newer, low-dose progestin contraceptive pills are inconclusive (19).

Altered Metabolism of Glucose or Lipids

With the OCs that contain more than 50 μg of estrogen, abnormal glucose tolerance tests can be seen after 3 months of use. However, this reduction in glucose tolerance is not seen with the low-dose preparations. Also, the new triphasic and low-dose forms do not appear to alter the lipid profile even in long-term users, whereas the high-dose preparations (more than 50 μg of estrogen) adversely affect the lipid profile (20,21).

Gallbladder Disease

The incidence of symptomatic gallbladder disease increases twofold within the first 1 to 2 years of OC use. An estrogen-associated increase in the concentration of cholesterol in the bile has been demonstrated in women taking OCs and may be the pathogenetic mechanism.

Headaches

Some women with a history of migraine headaches note a worsening of these headaches while taking OCs. The development or worsening of severe recurrent headaches is a reason to recommend another contraceptive method.

Birth Defects

The suggestion that hormonal ingestion during the first 3 months of pregnancy may result in the subsequent development of birth defects is unlikely. Although initial epidemiologic studies done in the 1960s and early 1970s seemed to favor an association with some cardiovascular and limb defects, more recent studies tend to refute this association. There is no evidence that prior use of contraceptives has any effect on the development of any birth defect. Establishing a pregnancy within one to two cycles after discontinuation of OCs is not associated with a higher incidence of birth defects (22,23), so no period of protection with another contraceptive method is needed when pregnancy is desired.

Other Side Effects

In general, minor side effects occur early in the course of taking OCs and may be transient. Thorough education by the physician increases the likelihood that the woman will tolerate these effects and continue taking the medication.

Alopecia. Alopecia is a rarely reported side effect (see Chapter 115). Most often it is transient; but if hair loss for longer than 3 months is reported, the drug should be discontinued and the woman should use some other form of contraception.

Nausea. Nausea occurs in approximately 5% of women, typically resolves within 3 months after initiation of OC use, and almost always can be eliminated by taking the contraceptive at bedtime.

Fatigue. Increased fatigability is occasionally described by OC users, but usually it is of short duration.

Change in Menstrual Flow. The most typical pattern is a reduction in the amount and duration of menstrual flow, which often is a welcomed effect. On occasion, there is no bleeding; if the woman has taken the OC regularly (so that pregnancy is not likely), she can be advised to continue the pills for another cycle. If she is again amenorrheic, a pregnancy test (discussed later) should be done. If pregnancy is ruled out, she can either select another contraceptive method, be placed temporarily on a 50-μg estrogen pill (which results in more menstrual bleeding), or be reassured that if she continues taking the method correctly she will remain amenorrheic.

Breakthrough Bleeding. Breakthrough bleeding is most common during the first three cycles after initiation of an OC. It is of no concern as long as the woman has not missed a dose. Failure to take daily doses increases the chance of breakthrough bleeding, particularly in the early part of the cycle. If breakthrough bleeding continues for several cycles, referral to a gynecologist is indicated to rule out an organic cause and to consider use of a higher dosage of estrogen.

Weight Gain. Approximately 5% of women show some weight gain, sometimes associated with fluid retention (24).

Vaginitis. It has been difficult to document a close relationship between OCs and vaginitis. The hormones do alter the vaginal milieu, but vaginitis develops in only a small proportion of women. Standard diagnostic methods and subsequent therapy (see Chapter 102) allows most women to continue to use the OC.

Skin Changes. Some women, especially dark-skinned ones, note chloasma (yellowish-brown discoloration of the skin) and a change in hair texture. Chloasma is unlikely to resolve with continued administration of the OC and is therefore a reason to discontinue it if the cosmetic effect is unacceptable.

Emotional Changes. Typically, OCs improve depression and premenstrual irritability. In some women, however, the progestin agent can cause or exacerbate depression. Women who have a history of depression should be monitored especially carefully for recurrence or exacerbation of this problem. If depression develops or worsens and is thought to be caused by the OC, the medication should be discontinued.

Effects on Laboratory Tests. OCs can alter the results of a number of laboratory tests (25). The alterations reflect physiologic changes in most instances but rarely signify clinically significant disease.

Drug Interactions. OCs may alter the effectiveness of a number of other drugs; conversely, a number of other drugs may alter the effectiveness of OCs. In general, concomitant use of antibiotics does not decrease OC effectiveness. Physicians should investigate the possibility of drug interaction before prescribing any other medication to a woman using an OC preparation. Table 100.6 lists drugs that may interact with OCs.

Instructions. Women should be instructed to begin the pills on the first Sunday (by convention) after her next normal menses. She should take the pills at the same time each day. If a single pill is missed, she should take the missed pill as soon as she remembers it. If two or more pills have been forgotten, she should take two pills a day until she has caught up and then continue the normal regimen but use a backup method (i.e., condoms) for 1 week.

Follow-Up. A woman taking OCs should see a physician once a year for a pelvic examination and a cervical smear for cytology, but inability to schedule these evaluations should not be a reason to withhold a contraceptive prescription. Screening for sexually transmitted diseases (see Chapter 102) may need to be done if the woman is at risk. OCs may be discontinued at any time if pregnancy is desired or another method of contraception is planned. The first few menstrual periods after withdrawal may be heavier than during the time OCs were used. There is no change in fertility after a course of OCs, regardless of duration of use. A pill-free or rest period is not advocated when switching to another method or in anticipation of becoming pregnant.

Table 100.6. Selected Drugs That May Interact with Oral Contraceptive Preparations (OCs)

Drugs That May Decrease the Effectiveness of OCs, Resulting in Breakthrough Bleeding, Pregnancy, or Both

Well-established, commonly occurring drug reactions
- Anticonvulsants: barbiturates, phenytoin (Dilantin), primidone (Mysoline)
- Antimicrobial: rifampicin

Reported Instances of Possible Drug Interactions

Antimicrobials
- Breakthrough bleeding only: neomycin, nitrofurantoin, phenoxymethylpenicillin (penicillin V)
- Breakthrough bleeding and pregnancy: ampicillin, chloramphenicol, sulfamethoxypridaxine (Kynex, Midicel)

Others: chlordiazepoxide (Librium), meprobamate, phenacetin (no longer available in the U.S.), and phenylbutazone (Butazolidin, not available in the U.S. at this time)

Drugs Whose Effectiveness May be Altered by OCs

Anticoagulants: effect may be reduced by simultaneous administration of OCs

Clofibrate (Atromid-S): control of cholesterol and triglyceride levels may be lost when OCs are simultaneously administered

Thyroid hormone in patients without a functioning thyroid gland: mostly a theoretical concern; however, increased dosage of thyroid hormone may be needed

Tricyclic antidepressants: higher dosages of estrogen may inhibit the effect of antidepressants, and tricyclic toxicity may be increased

Caffeine: metabolism of caffeine may be decreased; patients who take large amounts of caffeine (e.g., 4–8 cups of coffee per day) should be cautioned regarding symptoms of caffeinism

EMERGENCY CONTRACEPTION

Emergency contraception describes the use of a contraceptive method after intercourse to prevent pregnancy. This name is preferred to "morning-after pill," which suggests a very brief window of potential use after unprotected intercourse. Emergency contraception is indicated after intercourse without a method, current method failure (i.e., condom rupture), or rape. Access to emergency contraception can be increased by providing a patient with instructions and a prescription during a routine office visit or by making patients aware of how to access it urgently (1-888-NOT-2-LATE or *www.not-2-late.com*). Emergency contraception should *not* be used if a pregnancy test is positive.

Insertion of an IUD, possible up to 5 days following unprotected intercourse, is the most effective form of emergency contraception, with a pregnancy rate of approximately 0.1 per 100 women. Oral contraceptives are also highly effective as emergency contraceptive measures and are used up to 72 hours following unprotected sex. Progestin-only methods are more effective than combination pills, with pregnancy rates of 1.1% and 3.2%, respectively (26). Emergency contraception is ineffective at disrupting an already established pregnancy.

Method Use

Currently available methods of emergency contraception include OC pills or the copper IUD (see later discussion of indications and precautions). Possible combinations shown to be effective include two dedicated products, as well as alternative regimens of OCs.

Dedicated products:

- Plan B, 1 tablet containing 0.75 mg levonorgestrel each dose
- Preven, 2 tablets (each containing 50 μg ethinyl estradiol and 0.25 mg levonorgestrel)

Oral contraceptive regimens for emergency contraception:

- Progestin-only OCs containing 0.075 mg levonorgestrel (e.g., Ovrette), 20 tablets each dose
- Combined OCs containing 30 μg ethinyl estradiol and either 0.3 mg norgestrel (e.g., Lo/Ovral) or 0.15 mg levonorgestrel (e.g., Nordette), 4 tablets each dose
- Combined OCs containing 50 μg ethinyl estradiol and 0.5 mg norgestrel (e.g. Ovral), 2 tablets each dose

The first dose is taken within 72 hours (earlier administration increases effectiveness), and then repeated (second dose) 12 hours later. Antiemetics taken 1 hour before dosing increase the likelihood of adequate absorption for those women nauseated by the high estrogen dose. Neither a pelvic examination nor blood pressure measurement (asymptomatic women) is necessary before providing the method. The IUD can be inserted up to 5 days after unprotected intercourse.

Pregnancy testing is unnecessary before emergency contraception unless there is information to suggest that conception already occurred in a previous cycle. A woman should return for pregnancy testing if she does not get her menses within 3 weeks after taking emergency contraception. Women given emergency contraception should also receive counseling to help them choose an appropriate method for ongoing contraception.

SUBDERMAL CONTRACEPTIVE

The Norplant subdermal contraceptive method consists of six Silastic capsules (Dow Corning, Midland, MI), each containing 36 mg of levonorgestrel (a progestin) in crystalline form. The capsules are 34 mm long and 2.4 mm in diameter. They are inserted subdermally in the inner aspect of the upper arm. They provide contraceptive protection for at least 5 years, with a first-year failure rate of only 0.2 pregnancies per 100 users (27). Pregnancy rates range from 0.5 to 1.1 per 100 woman-years for the remaining 4 years. This level of effectiveness is much higher than that of any other form of reversible contraception except Depo-Provera and is similar to that seen in the first year after surgical sterilization (Table 100.2). The system contains no estrogen and therefore is useful in some women for whom combined OCs would be contraindicated. The system initially releases levonorgestrel at approximately the level seen with the mini-pill progestin-only oral medication (discussed previously). Over the first 12 to 18 months, this level falls by 50% and then remains constant for the remainder of the 5 years. This level is about one third that seen in women taking low-dose combined OCs. Thus, the Norplant system provides excellent protection from pregnancy with no estrogen component and a substantially reduced level of progestin. Norplant prevents contraception through thickening of the cervical mucus, disordered maturation of the endometrial lining, and suppression of ovulation. Approximately 50% of women after the first year resume normal ovulatory cycles. Therefore the main contraceptive effect is via the thickening of the cervical mucus.

Patient Experience. Worldwide, Norplant insertions and removals are performed by nurses, physician assistants, general physicians, and obstetricians. The insertion is done in an office setting using local anesthesia. Most insertions take 5 to 10 minutes. Removal takes somewhat longer and is likewise done under local anesthesia. Most women report minimal or no discomfort with either insertion or removal when it is performed by someone who is experienced and skilled in these techniques. Difficult removals are often caused by poor placement and have resulted in unwarranted negative impressions of the method. Initial claims of systemic effects due to the Silastic have not been borne out.

Contraindications

Because Norplant contains no estrogen, there are few absolute contraindications. Pregnancy, undiagnosed genital bleeding, and carcinoma of the breast constitute the only absolute contraindications. It should be used with great caution in women who have had breast cancer (and a 5-year disease-free interval) or active liver disease (e.g., severe decompensated cirrhosis, active viral hepatitis). The system can be used safely by women who have diabetes mellitus, hypertension, or migraine headaches. Effectiveness is lowered in women who are taking barbiturates, phenytoin, carbamazepine, primidone, phenylbutazone, or rifampicin.

Side Effects

Change in the menstrual bleeding pattern is the most common side effect associated with Norplant use, and women should be prepared for this when choosing the method. The change in pattern is one of unpredictability. Some women have prolonged spotting; others (10% to 15%) develop amenorrhea; only rarely do women develop prolonged heavy bleeding. In some studies, up to 75% of women experienced menstrual irregularities during the first year. Menstrual blood loss for women with Norplant is overall less than for women not using hormonal contraception. Therefore, no action need be taken to address prolonged spotting. If women are troubled by the spotting, they can be treated with 1 month of OCs in an effort to cause mild proliferation and controlled shedding of the endometrium.

Less common side effects are similar to those seen in OC users. Fewer than 10% of users experience headaches, nervousness, dizziness, abdominal cramping, nausea, acne, or weight gain. Only rarely do women complain of hair loss.

Removal and Return of Fertility

After removal (see Patient Experience) of the Norplant, serum blood levels of contraceptive hormone fall to undetectable levels within 2 weeks. The return of fertility among women who discontinue Norplant is considered immediate.

INTRAMUSCULAR INJECTABLE CONTRACEPTIVES

Progestin-only Injectables

Depo-medroxyprogesterone acetate (DMPA) (Depo-Provera, UpJohn, Kalamazoo, MI), a C-21–17 acetoxyprogestogen that is similar to natural progesterone, has been in use in the United States since 1992. Early issues and concerns regarding a relationship to breast cancer have been successfully resolved. DMPA is administered as an intramuscular injection of 150 mg that provides contraceptive efficacy for at least 14 weeks.

Administration every 12 weeks provides a margin of error should the woman fail to return at the exact appointed time. In this dosage, the failure rate is comparable to that of Norplant (28). Despite a large worldwide experience with this form of contraception, there are no data on its use by self-injection; accordingly, it should be administered by a health professional.

Mode of Action

Like other progestin-only contraceptives and combination OCs, DMPA acts by inhibiting ovulation, thickening cervical mucus, and altering the composition of the endometrium.

Side Effects

The most common side effect associated with DMPA is a disruption in the menstrual pattern. This disruption is unpredictable and can range from prolonged periods of amenorrhea (common) to episodes of heavy bleeding (rare). Approximately 50% of women using DMPA for 1 year develop amenorrhea, compared with 10% to 15% of Norplant users. Other side effects are similar to those seen with Norplant. After discontinuation of DMPA, women wishing to achieve a pregnancy experience a temporary delay in return to fertility lasting as long as 4 to 9 months after the last injection. By 2 years after the last injection, these women have essentially achieved the same fertility as those who discontinue other, nonhormonal methods.

Combined Injectables

In 2000, a new combined estrogen–progestin contraceptive was approved by the U. S. Food and Drug Administration (FDA) and marketed under the trade name Lunelle. The monthly injectable contraceptive combines 25 mg of medroxyprogesterone acetate and 5 mg of estradiol cypionate. The first-year failure rate is 0.1 to 0.4 per 100 women. Its mode of action is similar to that of combined OCs, as are the precautions for prescribing the method (29).

Side Effects

The side effect profile for the combined monthly injectable is similar to that of OCs, although spotting or bleeding is increased in the first month of use.

Method Use

The first injection should be given within 5 days after onset of menses. The first menses should be expected early. Subsequent injections should be given every 28 ± 5 days. There is a rapid return to fertility within 2 months after the last injection.

INTRAUTERINE CONTRACEPTIVES

Intrauterine contraceptives are one of the most effective methods of contraception. Pregnancy rates range from 0.14 to 3 per 100 women per year. The first modern IUDs appeared in the early 1960s and were made of a biologically inert plastic. The second-generation IUDs, copper- and progesterone-containing devices, have been available since the early 1970s (30,31).

During the late 1970s, serious concerns were raised regarding the safety of all IUDs. Studies showed a strong relationship between IUD use and the development of pelvic inflammatory disease. The Dalkon Shield specifically was removed from the market because of its link to spontaneous septic abortions and pelvic inflammatory disease. The clearly increased risk for infection with this product has been attributed to the multifilament tail (the string that hangs into the vagina), which seemed to act as a wick for bacteria. (Other IUDs used a monofilament tail.) Because of the publicity from the Dalkon Shield, distribution of other devices was discontinued by manufacturers because of low sales volume or concern regarding litigation costs. The ongoing concern over the relationship between IUD use and the development of pelvic inflammatory disease with resultant tubal infertility is valid. However, epidemiologic studies in the 1970s tended to overstate the risk of pelvic infection from IUD use, for the following reasons:

- In most early studies, the control group included women who were using diaphragms and OCs. These modalities are protective against pelvic inflammatory disease.
- The risks for specific IUDs were not analyzed separately. Dalkon Shield wearers, with substantially higher risk for infection, were included in most analyses.
- Most studies did not analyze for factors that significantly affect the risk of pelvic inflammatory disease, such as multiple sexual partners and previous history of pelvic infection.
- Recent epidemiologic studies adjusted the relative risks of tubal infertility by type of IUD used and number of sexual partners. They showed that women who had had only one sexual partner in their lifetime had no significantly increased risk of tubal infertility. However, women who had more than one sexual partner had a three to four times higher risk (31). At present, IUD use is recommended only for women who have had at least one child and who are in a mutually faithful, monogamous relationship.

Types

Two types of IUDs are available in the United States: progesterone-releasing and copper-bearing. All of the devices have a *monofilament string* attached, which allows for surveillance and removal (discussed later). Return to fertility is rapid for both types of IUD.

The copper IUD (ParaGard T380A), which contains no hormone, has a body of polyethylene wound with copper wire and a copper collar on each of its transverse arms. The copper inhibits sperm motility and capacitation, making them unable to penetrate the ovum. There is no evidence that IUDs work after fertilization as an abortifacient. Currently the ParaGard is approved by the FDA for at least 10 years of continuous use. It has an cumulative 10-year failure rate of 2.1% to 2.8%.

Two hormone-releasing intrauterine contraceptives are now available: The Progestasert IUD and the Mirena intrauterine system, approved by the FDA in 2001. The Progestasert is a plastic T-shaped device that contains a reservoir of 38 mg of progesterone that is released and exerts a local contraceptive effect. The progesterone reservoir is depleted after 12 months, and the device must then be removed and replaced by a new one.

The Mirena has a small, T-shaped frame with a steroid reservoir that releases levonorgestrel at the rate of 20 μg/day. It is currently approved for 5 years of continuous use and has an overall failure rate of 0.14 per 100 woman-years (32), comparable to that of sterilization. The levonorgestrel thickens cervical mucus and suppresses endometrial proliferation to inhibit passage of sperm, in addition to altering sperm transport as a result of the presence of the IUD in the uterine cavity. The progestin exerts a predominantly local effect; therefore, plasma concentrations of levonorgestrel are lower for Mirena users than for women using oral pills or implants.

Use and Insertion

If the clinician is not experienced in IUD insertion, the woman should be referred to a gynecologist. The IUD is best inserted at the time of a menstrual period. This provides assurance that the woman is not pregnant and permits easier insertion of the device because the cervix is slightly dilated. The usual small amount of bleeding associated with insertion becomes a part of the normal menstrual flow.

Women typically experience some cramps when the IUD is inserted; these can be limited by the administration of nonsteroidal analgesics before the insertion (e.g., ibuprofen 400 mg). If cramps persist beyond a few hours, this may be an indication that the device is not inserted properly and should be removed.

After insertion, the woman should feel the string of the IUD. She repeats this monthly, after each menstrual period, to ensure that the device is in place.

Bleeding Patterns

Copper IUD users typically note increased menstrual bleeding, and some experience cramping, which usually subsides within 3 months. Conversely, levonorgestrel IUD users experience a substantial decrease in their menstrual bleeding and cramping. The average number of bleeding days decreases from 5 in the first month to 1 in the sixth month; between 15% and 20% of women are amenorrheic by the end of the first year of use (33,34). This bleeding pattern has prompted the noncontraceptive use of this method for women with irregular bleeding.

Risks

Precautions for the use of an IUD are shown in Table 100.7. The most commonly encountered serious side effect is the development of pelvic inflammatory disease. Cumulative discontinuation rate for pelvic inflammatory disease are 2% to 3% for both types of IUD (35). The woman must be instructed to report any fever, pelvic pain, or discomfort promptly. Copper IUD users must also report any missed menstrual periods and be evaluated for pregnancy (including ectopic pregnancy); however, this does not hold true for levonorgestrel IUD users. Those users found to be pregnant should be promptly referred to a gynecologist for evaluation. Uterine perforation, a rare complication, is most likely to occur at the time of insertion. Finally, the use of the IUD by young, nulliparous women who have multiple sex partners is associated with a significantly increased incidence of uterine infection.

Table 100.7. Conditions Requiring Precautions for the Use of an Intrauterine Device (IUD)

Known or suspected pregnancy[a]
Genital bleeding of unknown cause
Abnormalities of the uterus resulting in distortion of the uterine cavity
Pelvic inflammatory disease (current or within the last 3 mo)
Postpartum or postabortion infection (current or within the last 3 mo)
Untreated acute cervicitis (until infection is controlled)
Patient or her partner has multiple sexual partners
Genital tract tuberculosis
Known or suspected genital tract cancer
Wilson disease or known allergy to copper (copper-containing IUDs)
History of ectopic pregnancy (requires evaluation)

[a]Except when being used for emergency contraception.

World Health Organization. Improving access to quality care in family planning: eligibility criteria for initiating and continuing use of contraceptive methods. Geneva: WHO, 1996.

Monitoring

There should be an annual follow-up that includes a review of any problems; a pelvic examination including cervical cancer smear, gonorrhea culture, and chlamydia culture (if either is indicated); and detection of the device. The follow-up is best done by a gynecologist if the clinician is not experienced in examining women with an IUD.

The IUD is easily removed by gentle traction on the string at or around the time of a menstrual period. Removal at this time allows the bleeding associated with removal to be part of the menstrual period. Also, the IUD is easier to remove during menstruation than later in the cycle (see earlier discussion).

As with other methods, if the woman terminates this form of contraception other than to attempt pregnancy, she will need help in choosing another form of contraception.

DIAPHRAGM

The diaphragm is a low-cost patient-dependent contraceptive device. It is a dome-shaped rubber device that is held open by a metallic band or spring. It is filled with a spermicidal cream or jelly before each use and placed in the vagina over the cervix to prevent sperm deposited during ejaculation from reaching the cervical os. As seen in Table 100.2, with typical use the failure rate is high, whereas correct or ideal use results in a lower failure rate, as is true of all barrier methods.

The diaphragm may be prescribed and fitted by the generalist or an assistant. For better effectiveness, the woman should be asked to insert the diaphragm in the office and have the provider check its placement. The device fits between the posterior fornix and the symphysis. The largest device that is comfortable is the proper one to use. Manufacturers of diaphragms have excellent booklets that are useful in helping a woman acquire the skill necessary for comfortable use of this form of contraception.

The woman applies spermicidal jelly to the inside of the dome and inserts the diaphragm in the vagina as long as 4 hours before intercourse. She should check for position with her finger and allow the device to remain in place for at least 6 hours after coitus. If repeated intercourse occurs within 6 to 8 hours, additional jelly should be placed in the vagina first, without removal of the diaphragm.

With care a diaphragm should last 2 years. The woman will need a new fitting if she gains or loses significant weight, has a baby, or has pelvic surgery.

The cervical cap has been approved by the FDA for use. Such devices come in several sizes, and they must be fitted by a health professional to go over the cervix. Proper fitting can be accomplished in approximately 80% of women. The cap may be used with or without spermicide. The spermicide may increase slightly the contraceptive effect. Generally, the cap is about as effective as the diaphragm and can be left in place for up to 48 hours.

Limitations

Restrictions on the use of the diaphragm or cervical cap include sensitivity to the rubber or to the spermicidal material that is used. Alterations in pelvic shape may also preclude proper fitting of the diaphragm. It is not suited for women who will not or cannot touch their vagina, such as those who are very obese and those who have a musculoskeletal disorder. Women who use fitted barriers and develop symptoms of toxic shock syndrome should be evaluated immediately.

Some women report discomfort while the diaphragm is in place. This discomfort is most often related to a wrong design or to improper fitting, and re-evaluation usually identifies the problem. A few women develop recurrent cystitis with frequent diaphragm use; this should lead to a discussion of alternative methods of contraception.

CONDOM

The *male condom* is a latex rubber sheath that is placed over the erect penis. It is the only reversible effective male method of contraception except for coitus interruptus. Condoms, when properly used, are an effective form of contraception, and their failure rate with experienced and strongly motivated couples is as low as 1 or 2 per 100 couple-years of exposure. However, rates during the first year of use or in less motivated couples may be considerably higher. Its effectiveness can be enhanced if it is combined with application of a spermicidal jelly or foam in the vagina. Some condoms are being manufactured in containers with a spermicidal lubricant. The condom, when used properly, provides considerable protection against sexually transmitted diseases, including gonorrhea, herpes, chlamydia, and human immunodeficiency virus (HIV) infection. Its only side effects are rare instances of sensitivity to the lubricating material or to latex and skin irritation from friction.

The *female condom* is a disposable, prelubricated polyurethane sheath between two rings of differing sizes. One ring is placed in the vagina, as with the diaphragm, and the larger ring rests exteriorly on the vulva. Studies show that it is impenetrable to the passage of HIV as well as other common sexually transmitted disease agents. Expected pregnancy rates are comparable to those seen with male condom use (1,36).

VAGINAL SUPPOSITORIES, FOAM, AND JELLY

Vaginal suppositories, foam, and jelly contain a spermicidal material combined with cream, jelly, or foam. The material is inserted in the vagina at least 10 to 15 minutes before intercourse. The spermicidal material is dispersed in the vagina and over the cervix. This creates a barrier around the cervical os to prevent sperm from entering the intrauterine cavity. All of these forms of contraception may be obtained without prescription. They are especially useful when additional protection is desired at midcycle with the condom or to increase the effectiveness of the diaphragm when repeated intercourse occurs. The side effects are minor and are related to sensitivity to the spermicidal material.

RHYTHM

The *rhythm method* or *periodic abstinence* requires avoidance of intercourse during a calculated fertile period. The human ovum probably is viable for only 12 to 24 hours after ovulation, whereas sperm retain the capability for fertilization for 48 hours to 5 days. Information suggests that conception is most likely during a 6-day interval ending on the day of ovulation (37). The development of a method of contraception that avoids intercourse at the fertile time is logical; however, the risk of pregnancy in women who use this method of contraception is high (Table 100.2). Three methods have been developed to calculate the fertile period.

The *calendar method* attempts to establish the portion of the cycle when intercourse is safe. The woman keeps a careful record for several months of the duration of each menstrual cycle beginning with the first day of bleeding. She then subtracts 18 days from the shortest cycle and 11 days from the longest cycle, representing the beginning and the end of the fertile time. Intercourse is avoided during this fertile period. Obviously, the more regular the woman's periods are, the shorter is this interval and the better the protection. For example, if the shortest cycle is 27 days and the longest is 33 days, then the client is possibly fertile from day 9 until day 22, an interval of 12 days. On the other hand, if she is regular and bleeds every 28 days, her fertile period is 7 days in duration, starting on day 10 of the menstrual cycle.

The *basal body temperature method* takes advantage of the slight drop in body temperature that is associated with ovulation and is followed by a rise in temperature of approximately 1°F (0.5°C). The woman takes her temperature each morning beginning at day 3 of the cycle. The fertile period begins on the day of the first drop or rise in temperature and continues for 3 to 4 days.

The *cervical mucus method* requires the woman to learn, over a number of cycles, the changes that indicate ovulation. She is taught to examine her cervical mucus for clarity. She learns to identify abdominal discomfort associated with ovulation and to use this information to avoid intercourse when conception is possible. This method requires effort and regular cycles, but it has been used effectively by many women.

STERILIZATION

Simple methods of permanent contraception are available to both men and women (38,39). At present in the United States, sterilization is the most popular method of contraception in persons older than 30 years of age. The total number of sterilizations is rising, and at present the rate of elective sterilization is somewhat higher for women than for men (40).

Individuals and couples considering sterilization need very careful education so that they understand the nature and risks of the procedure. Informed consent is required.

Vasectomy

Vasectomy, when properly performed, has a very low failure rate of 0.02% to 0.05%. The complication rate is approximately 4 in 1000, and, for the most part, complications are minor. They include infection, hematoma, epididymitis, and granuloma formation. Long-term serious side effects have not been reported among the very large numbers of men who have had the procedure performed. There was a transient concern, now known to be unwarranted (41), that antibodies to sperm that develop in some men after vasectomy predispose them to atherosclerosis. Before 1990, several studies examined the possible influence of vasectomy on the risk of developing prostate cancer. The results showed no statistically significant relationship. However, two studies published in early 1993 suggested that there is an increased risk of prostate cancer among men who have had a vasectomy. A consensus conference convened by the National Institutes of Health in March 1993 considered the available data and concluded that there were insufficient data to recommend changes in the current clinical practice concerning vasectomy (42).

Patient Experience. This procedure is done under local anesthesia in the urologist's office or outpatient surgical suite. There is minimal operative discomfort. Postoperatively, mild discomfort is common but is usually controlled with a mild analgesic, such as acetaminophen. Vigorous physical activity and sexual activity are restricted for 5 to 7 days until the wound has healed. Follow-up visits are necessary so that sperm counts can be performed. Usually, 6 to 12 weeks or approximately 20 ejaculations are required for the ejaculate to become free of sperm. Therefore, use of another contraceptive method is necessary until aspermia is confirmed.

Reanastomosis of the vas deferens can be accomplished surgically and results in patency in approximately 60% of cases. Nevertheless, vasectomy should not be undertaken unless the man genuinely wants permanent sterilization.

Tubal Ligation

Despite some sterilization failures with tubal ligation, it remains among the best methods of long-term contraception. Overall failure rates are 0.5% at 1 year and approximately 1.8% at 10 years (43). The major complication rate is approximately 4 per 1000. The complications are bleeding, infection, and bowel, bladder, or uterine trauma.

Patient Experience. Laparoscopy or minilaparotomy in the United States is usually performed with the use of general anesthesia. Uncomplicated tubal ligation is usually performed as an outpatient procedure and is very well tolerated. Mild abdominal discomfort, when present, usually lasts for only a few days, or rarely for a few weeks. Mild analgesics (e.g., acetaminophen) provide relief. The woman typically is able to return to her usual activities in 48 to 72 hours. Sterilization is immediate, and intercourse is permitted as soon as the wound is no longer painful.

Tubal ligation is performed in the first half of the menstrual cycle before ovulation has occurred. This avoids the possibility of fertilization of an ovum occurring a day or two before the surgical procedure. If the woman is using effective contraception, tubal ligation may be performed at any time.

Reanastomosis of the fallopian tubes can be accomplished surgically and results in a significant chance of fertility. The success of reanastomosis depends primarily on the type and extent of the initial ligation and is not related to the time between ligation and anastomosis. Nevertheless, a woman should not undergo tubal ligation unless she genuinely desires permanent sterilization.

The existence of a posttubal syndrome, characterized by heavier menstrual bleeding and more pelvic pain than in the unsterilized population, has been questioned. After sterilization, most women notice no significant change in symptoms associated with their menstrual periods.

OTHER CONTRACEPTIVE METHODS

Other hormonal methods are under investigation but are not yet available in the United States. A single-rod progestin-only subdermal implant would provide effective contraception for 3 years. Two other contraceptives combine ethinyl estradiol with progestin derivatives delivered as either a skin patch or a vaginal ring.

The sponge is a barrier contraceptive impregnated with nonoxynol 9 (a spermicidal agent) that is placed high in the vagina before intercourse. The sponge is no longer available in the United States.

DIAGNOSING PREGNANCY

Human chorionic gonadotropin (hCG) is a glycoprotein hormone that is produced by the blastocyst and the placenta. Its secretion begins very early and can be detected in the maternal blood as early as 6 days after fertilization. When fertilization occurs, the level of hCG is approximately 100 mIU at the time of the missed menses, and its concentration in serum approximately doubles every 48 hours during the first 10 weeks of a normal pregnancy. In the past, a number of conditions could give rise to a false positive result, such as the presence of foreign protein or cross-reaction with the luteinizing hormone (LH), follicle-stimulating hormone (FSH), and thyroid-stimulating hormone (TSH). The alpha-subunit for hCG is common to all of these hormones. However, the beta-subunit for hCG is unique, and the currently available pregnancy tests that use the monoclonal antibody methodology test only for the beta-subunit. A false positive reaction, even with home pregnancy detection kits, is extremely rare. There are four major types of pregnancy tests, each with its own characteristics; all are very accurate (see later discussion). The Icon, an enzyme-linked immunoassay, is the most commonly used test because of its simplicity, accuracy, and availability. Any clinician who may be asked to diagnose pregnancy should have a rapid pregnancy diagnosing kit in the office. There is no clinical situation in which one of these tests has a distinct advantage over another.

Radioimmunoassay

The radioimmunoassays are performed on serum samples. Tests include Chorio Quant, Beta Tec, and HCG Beta III. Their features are as follows:

- Accurate (almost 100% accuracy for positive result in normal pregnancy) when used at least 7 days after conception
- No LH cross-reaction
- Specific for hCG (detects the beta-subunit)
- Used for assessing abnormal pregnancy (ectopic, molar, threatened abortion)
- Requires that the specimen be sent to a laboratory, and the typical turnaround time is 1 day

Enzyme-linked Immunoassay

The enzyme-linked immunoassay tests (Icon, Confidot, Quest) are performed on urine or serum. Their features are as follows:

- Accurate when used at least 12 days after conception
- No LH cross-reaction
- Specific for hCG (detects the beta-subunit)
- Used for routine pregnancy confirmation
- Easy to use, and results are available in a few minutes

Radioreceptorassay

The radioreceptorassay pregnancy test (Biocept-G) is performed on serum. It has the following features:

- Accurate when used at least 14 days after conception
- LH cross-reaction possible
- Used for early confirmation of normal pregnancy
- Specimen usually is sent to a laboratory, and the turnaround time is typically 1 day

Immunoassay

The immunoassays (Neocept, Pregnosis) are performed on urine or serum. Their features are as follows:

- Accurate when used at least 28 days after conception
- LH cross-reaction possible
- Used for routine pregnancy confirmation
- Serum assay usually is sent to a laboratory, but urine assay can be done in the office

The biological half-life of hCG is approximately 1.5 days. The serum hCG result becomes negative approximately 10 days after delivery, artificial termination of pregnancy, or spontaneous or therapeutic abortion, if all trophoblastic tissue is expelled.

The hCG test may remain positive for weeks to months if small foci of functioning trophoblastic tissue remain. This could be seen after incomplete abortion, persistent hydatidiform mole, or choriocarcinoma.

UNPLANNED PREGNANCY

All contraceptive methods are associated with some failures, which may result in an *unplanned pregnancy.* Women with such a pregnancy are faced with the difficult decision of whether to carry or to terminate the pregnancy. Estimates are that almost 50% of the approximately 4 million births in the United States in 1992 were unplanned.

Currently, about 1.5 million *therapeutic abortions* are performed each year in the United States. The usual method of early termination of pregnancy in the United States is a surgical suction dilation and curettage performed in an outpatient center, free-standing clinic, or obstetrician's office, usually with the patient under local anesthesia. The *antiprogesterone compound,* mifepristone, was approved in 2000 for use in conjunction with misoprostol for the medical termination of early pregnancy. The current FDA-approved regimen provides 600 mg of mifepristone orally on day 1, followed on day 3 by 400 μg of misoprostol given orally in the provider's office. Other effective regimens using these medications are being studied.

PRECONCEPTION CARE

A variety of medical conditions, occupational situations, and social practices have consequences on early pregnancy. Because organogenesis begins about 17 days after conception, whereas traditional prenatal care may not commence for several weeks thereafter, there is ample reason to provide preconception care in an effort to optimize a woman's medical, social, and emotional readiness for pregnancy.

Preconception care should include a thorough history, a targeted physical examination, focused laboratory investigations, and specified counseling. The couple should be interviewed regarding family and genetic history, with appropriate carrier screening for inheritable conditions such as hemoglobinopathies, Tay-Sachs disease, or cystic fibrosis, among others. Existing medical conditions should be reviewed and medical therapy optimized, especially for patients with diabetes mellitus or hypertension. Women should discontinue, or be offered alternatives to, drugs known to be contraindicated in pregnancy, such as isotretinoin or coumadin. Infectious disease risks should be assessed (e.g., rubella, hepatitis B, HIV), and, if appropriate, vaccines should be offered for rubella and hepatitis B. In addition, screening should be offered for sexually transmitted diseases such as chlamydia, gonorrhea, and syphilis. Nutrition and eating habits should be evaluated. Although a multivitamin may be suggested, megavitamin supplementation should be avoided. Evidence suggests that daily intake of 0.4 mg of folic acid before conception significantly reduces the risk of neural tube defects.

Finally, a review of a couple's social readiness for pregnancy can help them focus on the upcoming responsibilities of pregnancy and childcare. Social habits of smoking and alcohol intake should be curtailed, and providers should take the opportunity to motivate substance abusers to seek counseling. Patients should consider domestic and economic readiness for pregnancy, and they should know their employer's policy regarding leave benefits for complicated and uncomplicated pregnancies (44).

General References*

World Health Organization. Improving access to quality care in family planning: eligibility criteria for initiating and continuing use of contraceptive method. Geneva: WHO, 1996.

A detailed consensus document from the World Health Organization on the use of contraceptives.

Colditz GA. Oral contraceptive use and mortality during 12 years of follow-up: the nurses' health study. Ann Intern Med 1994;120:821.

A very large study showing that the long-term use of oral contraceptives is safe.

Hatcher RA, Trussell J, Stewart F, et al. Contraceptive technology. 17th ed. New York: Ardent Media, 1998.

A regularly updated text covering all aspects of contraception. It is highly recommended.

Speroff L, Darney PD. A clinical guide for contraception. Baltimore, MD: Williams & Wilkins, 1992.

*Bold print (general references) and bold numerals (specific references) denote published controlled clinical trials, meta-analyses, or consensus-based recommendations.

Specific References

1. Choice of Contraceptives. Med Lett Drugs Ther 1995:37:941.
2. Abma J, Chandra A, Mosher W, et al. Fertility, family planning, and women's health: new data from the 1995 National Survey of Family Growth. National Center for Health Statistics. Vital Health Stat 23, no. 19, 1997.
3. Durand JL, Bressler R. Clinical pharmacology of the steroidal oral contraceptives. Adv Intern Med 1979;24:97.
4. Layde PM, McCarthy PS, Lord JAH, Smith CFC. Incidence of arterial disease among oral contraceptive users: Royal College of General Practitioners Oral Contraceptive Study. J R Coll Gen Pract 1983;33:75.
5. Stadel BV. Oral contraceptives and cardiovascular disease (two parts). N Engl J Med 1981;305:612, 672.
6. Nilsson S, Mellbin T, Hofvander Y, et al. Long-term follow-up of children breast-fed by mothers using oral contraceptives. Contraception 1986;34:443.
7. Hannaford PC, Croft PR, Kay CR. Oral contraception and stroke: evidence from the Royal College of General Practitioners' Oral Contraception Study. Stroke 1994;25:935.
8. Lowe GDO, Greer IA, Cooke TG, et al. Risk of and prophylaxis for venous thromboembolism in hospital patients. BMJ 1992;305:567.
9. World Health Organization. Improving access to quality care in family planning: eligibility criteria for initiating and continuing use of contraceptive methods. Geneva: WHO, 1996.
10. Ory HW, Forrest JD, Lincoln R. Making choices: evaluating health risks and benefits of birth control methods. New York: Alan Guttmacher Institute, 1983.
11. Coagulation and thrombosis with OC use: physiology and clinical relevance. Dialogues in Contraception. Little Falls, NJ: Health Learning Systems, 1996.
12. Edmondson HA, Henderson B, Benton B. Liver-cell adenomas associated with use of oral contraceptives. N Engl J Med 1976;294:470.
13. Centers for Disease Control. Cancer and steroid hormone study: oral contraceptive use and ovarian cancer. JAMA 1983;249: 1596.
14. Trussell J, Stewart F, Potts M, et al. Should oral contraceptives be available without prescription? Am J Public Health 1993;83:1094.
15. Harlap S, Kost K, Forrest JD. Preventing pregnancy, protecting health: a new look at birth control choices in the United States. New York: The Alan Guttemacher Institute, 1991.
16. Beral V, Hermon C, Kay C, et al. Mortality associated with oral contraceptive use: 25 year follow up of cohort of 46,000 women from the Royal College of General Practitioners' oral contraceptive study. BMJ 1999;318:96.
17. Brinton LA, Huggins GR, Lehman HF, et al. Long term use of oral contraceptives and risk of invasive cervical cancer. Int J Cancer 1986;38:339.
18. Rosenberg L, Palmer JR, Clarke EA, et al. A case-control study of the risk of breast cancer in relation to oral contraceptive use. Am J Epidemiol 1992;136:1437.
19. LiVolsi VA, Stadel BV, Kelsey JL, et al. Fibrocystic breast disease in oral-contraceptive users. N Engl J Med 1978;299:381.
20. Krauss RM, Burkman RT. The metabolic impact of oral contraceptives. Am J Obstet Gynecol 1992;167:1177.
21. Petitti DB, Sidney S, Bernstein A, et al. Stroke in users of low-dose oral contraceptives. N Engl J Med 1996;335:8.
22. Committee on Gynecologic Practice. Contraceptives and congenital anomalies: ACOG committee opinion no. 124, July 1993. Int J Gynecol Obstet 1993;42:316.
23. Linn S, Schoenbaum SC, Monson RR, et al. Lack of association between contraceptive usage and congenital malformation of offspring. Am J Obstet Gynecol 1983;147:923.
24. Moore LL, Valuck R, McDougall C, et al. A comparative study of one-year weight gain among users of medroxyprogesterone acetate, levonorgestrel implants, and oral contraceptives. Contraception 1995;52:215.
25. Effect of oral contraceptives in laboratory test results. Med Lett Drugs Ther 1979;21:54.
26. Task Force on Postovulatory Methods of Fertility Regulation. Randomised controlled trial of levonorgestrel versus the Yuzpe

regimen of combined oral contraceptives for emergency contraception. Lancet 1998;352:428.
27. Cullins VE, Remsburg RE, Blumenthal PD, et al. Norplant: welcome new contraceptive option. Contemp Obstet Gynecol 1992;37:46.
28. Cullins VE. Injectable and implantable contraceptives. Curr Opin Obstet Gynecol 1992;4:536.
29. Hall PE. New once a month injectable contraceptives, with particular reference to Cyclofem/Cyclo-provera. Int J Gynaecol Obstet 1998;62[Suppl 1]:S43.
30. Population Information Program. Population reports: intrauterine devices. IUDs: a new look. Series B, No. 5. Baltimore: Johns Hopkins University, 1988.
31. Luukkainen T, Toivonen J. Levonorgestrel-releasing IUD as a method of contraception with therapeutic properties. Contraception 1995;52:269.
32. Burkman RT. The Woman's Health Study: association between intrauterine device and pelvic inflammatory disease. Obstet Gynecol 1981;57:269.
33. Pakarinen PI, Suvisaari J, Luukkainen T, et al. Intracervical and fundal administration of levonorgestrel for contraception: endometrial thickness, patterns of bleeding and persisting ovarian follicles. Fertil Steril 1997;68:59.
34. Luukkainen T, Allonen H, Haukkamaa M, et al. Effective contraception with the levonorgestrel-releasing intrauterine device: 12-month report of a European multicenter study. Contraception 1987;36:169.
35. Sivin I, el Mahgoub S, McCarthy T, et al. Long-term contraception with the levonorgestrel 20 mcg/day (LNg 20) and copper T 380A intrauterine devices: a five-year randomized study. Contraception 1990;42:361.
36. The female condom. Med Lett Drugs Ther 1993;35:123.
37. Wilcox AJ, Weinberg CR, Baird DD. Timing of sexual intercourse in relation to ovulation. N Engl J Med 1995;333:1517.
38. Hulka JF. Current status of elective sterilization in the United States. Fertil Steril 1977;28:515.
39. Seiler JS. The evolution of tubal sterilization. Obstet Gynecol Surv 1984;39:177.
40. Peterson LS. Contraceptive use in the United States: 1982–1990. Public Health Service, Centers for Disease Control and Prevention, National Center for Health Statistics. Hyattsville, MD: U.S. Department of Health and Human Services, 1995.
41. Massey FJ Jr, Bernstein GS, O'Fallon WN, et al. Vasectomy and health: results from a large cohort study. JAMA 1984;252:1023.
42. Klitsch M. Vasectomy and prostate cancer: more questions than answers. Fam Plann Perspect 1993;25:33.
43. Peterson HB, Xia Z, Hughes JM, et al. The risk of pregnancy after tubal sterilization: findings from the U.S. Collaborative Review of Sterilization. Am J Obstet Gynecol 1996;174:1161.
44. American College of Obstetrics and Gynecology. Preconception care. ACOG Technical Bulletin no. 205. Washington, DC: ACOG, May 1995.

C H A P T E R 101

Menstrual Disorders and Other Disorders of Female Reproductive Endocrinology

MARIA ELENA SOLER, MD, MPH, MBA
CATHERINE S. TODD, MD, MPH
ADRIAN S. DOBS, MD, MHS

A normal menstrual cycle in a woman of reproductive age is an indicator of health. Absent or abnormal menses is not only a source of discomfort and anxiety but may also signify pathology in a wide variety of systems. Because there are a myriad of causes for abnormal vaginal bleeding, it is helpful to think of relevant etiologies during the various stages of a woman's reproductive life. This chapter reviews the evaluation and management of common menstrual disorders by age group to guide clinical care.

FEMALE REPRODUCTIVE PHYSIOLOGY

The female hypothalamus releases gonadotropin-releasing hormone (GnRH) rhythmically, stimulating intermittent peaks of release of luteinizing hormone (LH) and follicle-stimulating hormone (FSH) from the pituitary. Complex modulation of rates of hormone release in women results in a cyclic rather than a tonic secretory pattern. Estradiol nadir in the late luteal phase allows the level of FSH to increase. At the beginning of each cycle, FSH initiates the recruitment of 10 to 30 follicles from a cohort of small primordial follicles resident in the ovary from birth (1). Negative feedback from estradiol and inhibin suppresses FSH, leading to dominant follicle selection by day 6 or 7 of the menstrual cycle. LH stimulates the interstitial (thecal) cells that surround the follicle to make androgens and small amounts of estrogens (estradiol and estrone). The granulosa cells convert thecal androgens to estradiol. Estradiol, in concert with FSH, increases the expression and number of FSH receptors on granulosa cells. A dominant (graafian) follicle emerges in each cycle as the follicle with early robust aromatase activity that has higher estradiol production, leading to increased FSH receptor number, which further increases aromatase activity. As FSH drops in midcycle, only the follicle with the greatest number of FSH receptors survives, and adjacent follicles undergo atresia (degeneration). Rising estrogen secretion in this early or *follicular* phase of the cycle induces proliferation of the uterine endometrium. A small midcycle drop in FSH and progesterone triggers the LH surge, which causes the follicle to release the ovum (ovulation). LH then induces the follicle to become a functioning corpus luteum, producing both estradiol and progesterone during the latter half of the cycle (*luteal* phase). The luteal phase is relatively constant at 14 ± 2 days. Progesterone acts on the uterus to produce a secretory endometrium that is rich in glycogen and, in concert with estrogen, causes a negative feedback effect that gradually reduces the secretion of LH and FSH. With loss of gonadotropic stimulation, the corpus luteum involutes, steroid secretion diminishes, and the endometrium, left without estrogen and progesterone support, sloughs off as the menstrual flow. Breakdown of the endometrium is orderly and progressive, providing reproducible menstrual flow. Average blood loss is approximately 40 mL. At this point, with estradiol and progesterone negative feedback at low levels, FSH and LH begin to rise, a new cohort of small follicles is recruited, and the stage is set for the next cycle.

ABNORMAL BLEEDING PATTERNS

When evaluating abnormal vaginal bleeding, it is helpful to define various bleeding patterns. The normal intermenstrual interval is 28 ± 7 days (2). The normal duration of menstrual flow is 4 to 7 days, with a mean blood loss of 40 mL. Prolonged excessive bleeding of greater than 80 mL or lasting longer than 7 days is menorrhagia. *Metrorrhagia* is bleeding between periods. Menses less than 21 days apart is defined as *polymenorrhea*. *Oligomenorrhea* is menses greater than 35 days apart, of which the majority are anovulatory. *Amenorrhea* is defined as no menses for at least 6 months. *Dysfunctional uterine bleeding* is a clinical term referring to abnormal bleeding in premenopausal women that is not caused by identifiable gynecologic pathology. Postmenopausal bleeding must be investigated (see Chapter 106).

Anovulatory Bleeding

Endometrial breakdown and vaginal bleeding may occur without ovulation. This type of bleeding is most common at either end of the reproductive life span, due to disturbances in the pituitary–hypothalamic axis. This bleeding can manifest in a variety of ways, from chronic spotting to intermittent heavy bleeding. In one form of this phenomenon, extended unopposed estrogen exposure leads to proliferative or hyperplastic endometrium that subsequently disintegrates as a result of transient interruption in estrogen stimulation. Such bleeding, from estrogen withdrawal without secretory transformation of the endometrium by progesterone, is often prolonged, unduly heavy, or both. Bleeding may also occur from unstable endometrium produced by prolonged exposure to progestins. This occurrence is limited to circumstances in which progestins are administered for hormonal contraception, such as medroxyprogesterone acetate (MPA), or for induction of amenorrhea to control gynecologic disorders such as endometriosis.

Atrophic Bleeding

The most common form of postmenopausal bleeding is bleeding from atrophic endometrium. This bleeding often occurs after coitus or other mechanical trauma as a result of the thinning and subsequent fragility of nonestrogenized tissue. This diagnosis cannot be established, however, without first ruling out malignancy with endometrial sampling (see later discussion). All postmenopausal bleeding is abnormal, and gastrointestinal/urinary sources should be excluded, as should gynecologic malignancies.

Postcoital Bleeding

The cause of postcoital bleeding is usually mechanical trauma. The cervix in pregnant women and in women taking oral contraceptives (OCs) tends to be friable due to the exposure of the endocervix. This is visible on speculum examination and is termed an *ectropion cervix*. Postcoital bleeding may also occur as a result of local pathology. Lesions such as cervical polyps or vaginal or cervical malignancy may be friable and contribute to vaginal bleeding, whereas lesions such as submucous myomas may disturb the endometrium itself.

Bleeding from local pathology is usually superimposed on an underlying discernable menstrual pattern in premenopausal women, as erratic bleeding through the cycle and/or accentuated menstrual flow. A similarly erratic bleeding pattern may be seen in women using combination OCs for the first month, and the patient should be counseled that this effect is transient and is not an indication to discontinue contraception or change to another brand.

Amenorrhea

Amenorrhea is divided into two categories: primary and secondary. *Primary amenorrhea* is diagnosed in young women who are without onset of menses by age 16 years with development of secondary sexual characteristics, or without either secondary sexual characteristics or menstruation by age 14 years (see later discussion). *Secondary amenorrhea* is diagnosed in women with a previously normal cycle who have had no menses for 6 months or have missed three menstrual cycles. Any report of missed menses necessitates a pregnancy test, because this is commonly the cause of missed menses.

EVALUATION OF ABNORMAL BLEEDING

Diagnostic evaluation of a patient with abnormal bleeding is modified depending on the patient's age. A basic overview of the evaluation includes the following.

History

The history can help establish the likelihood that abnormal bleeding is associated with one of four common causes: pregnancy, bleeding due to abnormal endocrine control, bleeding due to gynecologic pathology, or menstrual disruption due to systemic disease. The key items to note are the patient's age, onset of menarche, prior menstrual cycle history, contraceptive and sexual history, and any symptoms of systemic disorders.

A chronicle of pubertal events should be recorded, including earliest budding of breast tissue (thelarche), pubic hair darkening and lengthening (pubarche), onset of menstrual flow (menarche), and time of onset and cessation of the growth spurt. A menstrual history includes the average interval between menses, their regularity, and when any irregularity developed; date of last period and previous period before that; duration of flow and its magnitude; and presence of ovulatory pain (mittelschmerz), premenstrual tension, and dysmenorrhea (the latter three findings suggest ovulatory cycles). A pregnancy and nursing history (mature and premature deliveries, abortions, success with and duration of lactation, and ages of living children) and a history of gynecologic surgery (including dilation and curettage) are pertinent. One should ask whether the patient is troubled by growth of excessive hair and, if so, the duration of symptoms, the location and severity of the problem, and any treatment used. Symptoms of estrogen deficiency (hot flushes, vaginitis, dyspareunia, breast atrophy) are important (see Chapter 106). A careful history of medication and drug use, including use of OCs, may be helpful. A further general history should include weight gain or loss; dietary habits (especially rigorous dieting); strenuous exercise (e.g., running, ballet, gymnastics); symptoms of diabetes mellitus, adrenal disease, or thyroid disease; and history of tuberculosis or hepatic, renal, or neurologic problems. A family history should include ethnic origin and familial occurrence of reproductive and other endocrine dysfunctions (e.g., hirsutism, oligomenorrhea, hypothyroidism, type 1 diabetes mellitus).

Physical Examination

Findings on the general physical examination can provide important clues to the diagnosis of anovulatory states. Examples of these include obesity, galactorrhea, hirsutism, and stigmata of nonreproductive endocrine disorders such as Cushing syndrome and thyroid dysfunction. Pelvic examination is of chief importance in identifying lesions of the external genitalia, vagina, or cervix and in delineating uterine size and shape. Clinically important lesions of the uterus affecting the endometrial canal are not reliably detected by physical examination, however.

On inspection one should note body habitus (obese or wasted, mature or child-like, masculine or feminine). The presence or absence of pubic and axillary hair; distribution of coarse dark hair on chest (periareolar, midsternal), abdomen, buttocks, and extremities; and the density of such hair must be noted. The quality of the patient's voice should be evaluated. Examination of breasts and pubic hair should include an estimate of their stage of maturity based on available standards. Nipples should be squeezed gently to assess for expressible galactorrhea. On pelvic examination it is important to look for clitoromegaly (greater than 2.0 cm in length), state of the vaginal mucosa (dry versus moist, thick and rugose versus thin and atrophic), discharge, presence or absence and size and mobility of cervix and uterus. Bimanual examination should be done to estimate the uterine size, presence of fibroids, and whether ovaries are enlarged. In primary amenorrhea without maturation, signs of Turner syndrome (wide-set eyes, shield chest, wide-set nipples, "webbing" of neck, short fourth metacarpal, and signs of aortic coarctation) should be sought. The remainder of the general physical examination should be as described, looking especially for signs of an intracranial mass lesion and thyroid or adrenal disease.

Laboratory Tests and Radiology

It is critical to exclude pregnancy in all women of reproductive age (Table 101.1). All women with secondary amenorrhea should be considered pregnant until proven otherwise (even if sexual activity is not admitted, as may be the case with adolescents). Specific human chorionic gonadotropin (hCG) assay is the most sensitive test for pregnancy. Screening for sexually

Table 101.1. Suggested Diagnostic Studies in the Evaluation of Abnormal Vaginal Bleeding

Laboratory or Diagnostic Study	Clinical Presentation	Diagnosis
Serum human chorionic gonadotropin (beta-subunit)	Amenorrhea or menorrhagia in a woman of reproductive age	Pregnancy
Complete blood count	Menorrhagia	Anemia, blood dyscrasias
Thyroid-stimulating hormone	Anovulatory pattern	Hypothyroidism
Prolactin	Anovulatory pattern	Prolactinoma
Follicle-stimulating hormone, luteinizing hormone	Secondary amenorrhea	Estrogen deficiency
Coagulation profile	Menorrhagia	Bleeding diathesis
Dihydroepiandrosterone (DHEAS)	Hyperandrogenism	Polycystic ovary syndrome (PCOS)
Serum testosterone	Hyperandrogenism	PCOS
Glucose, hemoglobin A1c, lipids	Hyperandrogenism	PCOS
Pap smear	Abnormal bleeding, amenorrhea	Malignancy, hormonal status
Endometrial biopsy	Menorrhagia	Malignancy or polyp

transmitted diseases (chlamydia, gonorrhea) is important (see Chapter 37), because cervicitis may be associated with vaginal bleeding.

In evaluating the endocrine status, serum estrogen radioimmunoassays have now improved to the point that one can generally distinguish low-normal from definitely low values (less than 40 pg/mL is suspect, and less than 25 pg/mL is severely deficient), but estrogen status may also be assessed by vaginal cytology or by the provocation of withdrawal bleeding. Cells for vaginal cytology should be obtained at the time of pelvic examination so that a maturational index can be estimated (see Chapter 102). A *progesterone withdrawal test* (7 days of 10 mg MPA [Provera] orally or a single 100-mg dose of progesterone in oil intramuscularly) results in withdrawal bleeding within a few days (2 to 5 days for oral drug, 7 to 10 days for intramuscular) if estrogen levels are adequate. If there is no bleeding, a 21-day course of estrogen (1.25 mg conjugated estrogen [e.g., Premarin] per day) with 5 to 10 mg of MPA (Provera) for the last 7 days should be administered. Absence of vaginal bleeding at that point indicates an absent or severely damaged endometrium, sometimes secondary to previous overvigorous dilation and curettage (Asherman syndrome).

Other systemic causes of abnormal bleeding include coagulopathies (see Chapter 56). Studies have demonstrated a wide variation in the prevalence of coagulation disorders, ranging from 5% to 20% of hospitalized adolescents with menorrhagia (3). Leukemia, idiopathic thrombocytic purpura, and severe liver or kidney disease can cause coagulopathy. A history of bleeding diathesis with prior surgery, trauma, or dental procedures should be elicited.

The routine laboratory studies done for the evaluation of abnormal uterine bleeding are the complete blood count, thyroid-stimulating hormone (TSH), and prolactin. The investigation of central hypogonadism should include a serum prolactin level, especially if galactorrhea is present. Prolactin values between 30 and 100 ng/mL are elevated and are consistent with a prolactinoma, but they may result from other causes such as hypothalamic (idiopathic) galactorrhea or drug effects. Values greater than 100 ng/mL almost always mean that a prolactinoma is present. If the physical examination suggests that the patient is hyperandrogenic, testosterone, dehydroepiandrosterone-sulfate (DHEAS), and serum 17-OH progesterone concentrations should be determined. It is important to identify chronic anovulation in hyperandrogenic patients early in life to help reduce future cardiovascular disease, endometrial cancer, and diabetes.

Papanicolaou Smear and Endometrial Biopsy

Evaluations to exclude malignancy include a recent Papanicolaou (Pap) smear, with colposcopy and biopsy if any cervical abnormalities are seen. Visible lesions of the external genitalia, vagina, and cervix require biopsy, because cytologic evaluation becomes less sensitive in the presence of inflammation and necrosis (4).

Endometrial biopsy is needed in all women older than 35 years of age who have abnormal vaginal bleeding and should be done in all patients with chronic anovulation even if they are younger (4). The principal use of endometrial biopsy is to exclude malignancy or premalignant states in the endometrium. Endometrial biopsy is indicated for evaluation of postmenopausal bleeding, abnormal bleeding in the perimenopausal woman, and less often, abnormal bleeding in younger women who are at risk for neoplasia owing to anovulation (5). Sampling of endometrial tissue by blind transcervical biopsy accurately reflects the histologic state of the endometrium to a remarkable degree, given the small portion of endometrial surface retrieved (6). The procedure is discussed more fully in Chapter 104. Numerous studies have validated the accuracy of histologic results achieved by biopsy using formal dilatation and curettage as a gold standard. The sensitivity of the technique in detecting endometrial carcinoma ranged from 85% to 95% in several series (7).

Imaging of the Reproductive Tract

The chief value of imaging procedures in the patient with abnormal bleeding is to identify lesions of the uterus, fallopian tubes, and ovaries and to assess the appearance of the endometrium. Transvaginal ultrasound provides high-resolution images that permit evaluation for endometrial thickness, endometrial contour, and presence of leiomyomas in the subadjacent myometrium. Simultaneous transcervical instillation of fluid (sonohysterography) can add sensitivity to detection of lesions affecting the endometrial canal (8,9). Transvaginal ultrasound is also a cost-effective complement to endometrial biopsy in the evaluation of abnormal bleeding (10). Clinicians should consider ultrasound evaluation of the endometrial thickness, particularly in older patients in whom biopsy may be difficult. Computed tomography (CT) and magnetic resonance imaging (MRI) have not been shown superior to these ultrasound techniques. During proliferation in the normal cycle, endometrial thickness may reach 1 cm or more and appears as distinct layers due to the stromal edema in the opposing anterior and posterior surfaces. Secretory endometrium appears homogenous and more echogenic. Excessive thickness, with or without irregularity, is consistent with hyperplasia or may belie the presence of endometrial polyps. Leiomyomas are easily distinguishable. Those that are subadjacent to, or that distort, the uterine cavity are more likely to be associated with abnormal bleeding. Sonohysterography is a particularly helpful adjuvant to standard vaginal sonography to identify submucosal fibroids and polyps.

The significance of endometrial thickness in the evaluation of postmenopausal bleeding has received considerable study. Malignancy or other abnormal proliferation is unlikely when the endometrial thickness is less than 4 mm (10,11). If endometrial biopsy in such patients yields insufficient tissue for histologic interpretation, as may commonly occur, malignancy is adequately ruled out if the endometrium is less than 5 mm thick on ultrasound evaluation. Further investigation should be done if tissue sampling is insufficient for diagnosis and endometrial thickness is 5 mm or more, depending on the entire clinical picture, including age, symptoms, and risk factors.

AGE-SPECIFIC GUIDELINES FOR EVALUATION OF ABNORMAL VAGINAL BLEEDING

Adolescent: 13–18 Years

The principal causes of menorrhagia in the young patient are anovulatory bleeding and bleeding diathesis. However, the possibility of pregnancy should never be overlooked in a young woman with bleeding complaints, even in the absence of a supporting history (3). The history provides important clues to the evaluation: erratic and unpredictable bleeding patterns suggest an ovulatory disturbance, whereas regular heavy menses associated with nongynecologic bleeding problems suggest bleeding diathesis.

Anovulatory bleeding at this age is a normal physiologic event; 85% of perimenarchal cycles are anovulatory. This is especially true in the first 2 years after menarche. If the history and examination are otherwise normal, symptomatic management and observation are preferable to endocrine evaluation over the short term. If evidence of ovulatory disturbance is present more than 1 year after menarche, endocrine evaluation should be undertaken. Endocrine assessment for persistent anovulation and anovulatory bleeding in the very young woman is sufficiently investigated with assessment for thyroid dysfunction (TSH) and hyperprolactinemia (serum prolactin). A pattern consistent with chronic anovulation is commonly revealed, and if this is the case it is likely that normal cycles will be established with further maturation. OCs may be used to regulate the menstrual cycle and help allay anxiety and possible concerns about pregnancy if the teenager is sexually active.

Anovulatory bleeding may be heavy and require emergency care. The risk of endometrial cancer in this group is extremely rare. Endometrial biopsy should be confined to those cases in which medical management has failed. In the young woman, it is important to rule out coagulopathy and leukemia with a complete blood count and coagulation profile. Acute episodes of menorrhagia related to anovulation can usually be arrested with high doses of oral progestational agents in the form of OCs or MPA, 10 mg daily, administered for 1 to 2 weeks, during which time bleeding tapers or ceases. After progestin treatment is stopped, "normal," self-limited, menstrual withdrawal occurs. Further episodes of anovulatory menorrhagia can be prevented by regular progestin-induced withdrawal with OC use. If bleeding is severe, it can be managed acutely with either intravenous conjugated estrogen, 25 mg every 4 hours for up to 24 hours, or 2.5 mg conjugated oral estrogen, up to 10 mg/day; 90% to 95% of patients respond to medical therapy within 1 to 2 days. Once bleeding has stopped, OCs are started in a taper regimen (3 pills/day for 3 days, then 2 pills/day for 3 days, then 1 pill/day for 4 weeks). Then a withdrawal bleed is allowed, and standard cyclic OCs are started. Endometrial curettage is almost never necessary.

Primary Amenorrhea

Primary amenorrhea is defined as absence of menses by age 16 years with development of secondary sexual characteristics, or absence of both development of secondary sexual characteristics and menstruation by age 14 years. It is not usually idiopathic, and an underlying cause must be sought. *Primary central amenorrhea* with maturational failure suggests idiopathic or genetic gonadotropin deficiency of pituitary or hypothalamic origin. A patient with primary *gonadal* failure is most likely to have Turner syndrome (XO sex chromosomes and no ovaries). *Primary amenorrhea with normal maturation* may be the result of peripheral causes as simple as imperforate hymen with obstruction of menses or as serious as congenital uterine agenesis.

The first component of the evaluation is to determine the presence or absence of normal secondary sexual characteristics. The presence of breasts confirms an intact hypothalamic–pituitary–ovarian axis and functional ovaries. Pubic and axillary hair indicate normal androgen and androgen-receptor function. Physical examination should include growth chart, Tanner staging (see Chapter 11), neurologic examination, galactorrhea and olfactory tests, and Turner stigmata.

If the patient has normal secondary sexual characteristics but no menses, she probably has an anatomic problem, usually one that is obvious on examination. If the uterus is present, it may be abnormal (Rokitansky–Küster–Hauser syndrome) or there may be an abnormality in the outflow tract (müllerian agenesis). An MRI or pelvic ultrasound examination helps confirm the diagnosis. These patients should be referred to a pediatric gynecologist for further evaluation and treatment.

The presence of normal breast development and height but no sexual hair suggests androgen insensitivity. Serum testosterone levels in the male range and XY karyotype confirm the diagnosis (see Chapter 85).

If the patient has no secondary sexual characteristics and no menarche, then an FSH level may be diagnostic. Elevated FSH indicates ovarian dysgenesis. If the FSH is low or normal, the diagnostic possibilities include hyperprolactinemia, thyroid disease, brain tumor, and Turner syndrome.

Amenorrhea Secondary to Weight Loss, Eating Disorders, or Exercise

Functional hypothalamic dysfunction is common in younger women, and if endocrine evaluation is inconclusive, attention should be given to the possibilities of stress at home or in school, adjustment problems, substance abuse, and eating disorders (see Chapter 11). Irregular menses, delayed onset of menarche, and secondary amenorrhea are not uncommon in women who are 10% to 12% less than their ideal body weight. With excessive weight loss, amenorrhea may last longer than 1 year after dieting ceases. This phenomenon arises from hypothalamic suppression with decreased GnRH secretion. There are many theories as to the exact mechanism by which the hypothalamus is suppressed; however, a significant determinant is amount of body fat. As body fat decreases, there is a measurable decrease in LH pulsatile frequency and amplitude before onset of irregular menses. According to Speroff et al. (12), the minimum level of body fat associated with menarche is 17%, with secondary amenorrhea associated with levels less than 22%.

The treatment for this phenomenon focuses on contraception and bone loss. It is still possible to ovulate with this condition and, in the presence of irregular or absent menses, it is difficult to gauge whether the cause is pregnancy or physical activity. It must be stressed to these patients that contraception is necessary to ensure that an undesired pregnancy is avoided. Those desiring conception should be advised to decrease their level of activity with the possibility of establishing a regular menstrual cycle or at least enough GnRH secretion to result in ovulation. Another issue raised by this condition is whether the decreased amount of estrogen results in increased rates of bone demineralization. Several studies have established a radiologically detectable decrease in bone mineral density in amenorrheic female athletes, despite a normal rate of bone turnover (13–15). Hetland et al. (14) noted a 10% decrease in lumbar bone density in amenorrheic runners, with a concomitant 25% to 44% decrease in circulating progesterone and estradiol (14). Prior et al. (15) reported increased bone mineral density after a year's treatment with cyclic progesterone, which occurred regardless of calcium supplementation and was significantly higher than with calcium alone. They also noted a significant decrease in bone mineral density in runners who were taking placebo for both estrogen and MPA. Based on this evidence, both contraception and osteopenia concerns can be addressed with hormonal contraception, preferably with combined OCs or, alternatively, with progestin-only contraceptives (see Chapter 100).

Anorexia nervosa, bulimia, and a host of other body image disorders that are distinguished by disordered perceptions of appearance and need for food have received a large amount of attention in the last decade. This class of disease conjures certain images, and most practitioners are able to name many of the features of the disease: overachieving personality type, social isolation, secretive eating habits, an obsessive concern with calorie content and exercise, and overwhelming fear of being perceived as fat. Despite this general knowledge, anorexia and other eating disorders are underdiagnosed, perhaps because of nondisclosure of worrisome symptoms and signs by patients or fear of social stigmata attached to the diagnosis by the patient, her family, or even the practitioner. Menstrual irregularity or amenorrhea occurs secondary to hypothalamic suppression and low GnRH secretion, similar to that of exercise-induced amenorrhea. Amenorrhea is a relatively benign symptom of the disease; other symptoms and signs that occur as the disease progresses are constipation (from low intake and laxative abuse), hypotension, hypothermia, lanugo formation, and possible cardiac arrhythmia (especially with hypokalemia and other electrolyte imbalances secondary to laxative abuse). This disease is associated with a 5% to 15% mortality rate.

Individuals with any of the risk factors listed should be asked about their behaviors with food and their family relationships, because abrupt changes may cause a tendency toward anorexia to become active disease. Patients with this type of amenorrhea should be referred to a multispecialty practice (psychiatry, behavioral therapy, nutrition, and internal medicine) that specializes in eating disorders with hospitalization as needed. The amenorrhea resolves in up to 70% of these women after normal body weight is attained (12). Pregnancy must be ruled out; the severe self-imposed malnutrition of eating disorders confers significant risk to the fetus, and also the weight gain associated with pregnancy further intensifies feelings of fatness. Contraception should be offered to all patients who are sexually active, with the possible beneficial effect of appetite stimulation with hormonal contraceptives. If hormonal contraceptives are not desired, the patient should be given hormone replacement therapy because she is at risk for bone loss due to lack of estrogen. A daily dose of conjugated estrogen 0.625 mg and progesterone 2.5 mg is adequate for bone protection but will not result in menstrual bleeding. A cyclic progesterone regimen with up to 1.25 mg daily estrogen is necessary for resumption of menstruation. Progesterone (at least 5 mg) may be given on the first 12 days of each cycle in the presence of continuous estrogen; withdrawal bleeding occurs 3 to 5 days after the progesterone is finished. Alternatively, estrogen may be given on days 1 through 25 each month, with progesterone given on days 14 and 25 and withdrawal bleeding occurring on day 29 to 30. Regularly menstruating women who begin strenuous exercise programs are unlikely to become amenorrheic unless significant weight loss is associated with the exercise. Stress and/or anorectic behavior may accompany athletic training (especially in dancers or gymnasts) and should be sought in the history.

Reproductive Adult: Up to 45 Years

The "reproductive adult female" (loosely, women between the ages of 18 and 45 years) fall into an age range in which many different conditions may surface. Some of the physiologic causes of irregular bleeding or amenorrhea in this age group are pregnancy (intrauterine, ectopic, or miscarriage) and lactation. Beyond these causes, there are various pathologic conditions that should be considered.

Polycystic Ovary Syndrome

Polycystic ovary syndrome (PCOS) is the most common endocrine disorder among women of reproductive age. Estimates suggest that 5% to 10% of premenopausal women have the full-blown syndrome of hyperandrogenism, chronic anovulation, and polycystic ovaries, the original constellation known as Stein–Levinthal syndrome (16). The associated decrease in ovulation rate in patients with PCOS causes varying degrees of infertility. In contemporary gynecology, PCOS is meant to include those patients with chronic anovulation who also exhibit hyperandrogenism clinically or biochemically. Therefore, although PCOS is named in relation to an ovarian morphologic abnormality, it is defined by functional abnormalities (described later) and not by ovarian morphology. The classic ovarian morphology of PCOS (enlarged, with numerous small subcortical follicles) is inconsistently present among patients with ovulatory dysfunction and is observed in some women without a disorder of ovulation (17,18). Ultrasound or laparoscopic evaluation of the ovaries is not useful in the evaluation of ovulatory disorders.

Women with this syndrome secrete excessive quantities of androgenic steroids from the ovaries and often from the adrenal glands as well. The initial impetus for increased androgen levels is not clear. Androgens are converted peripherally to estrone, resulting in increased LH secretion. LH elevation results in increased peripheral free estradiol and increased ovarian androgen secretion, leading to the development of a vicious cycle. FSH continues to be secreted at low levels, causing new cysts to form that persist for 2 to 6 months and contribute to the milieu of increased steroid secretion.

The clinical concerns with this process are anovulation and the effects of chronic estrogen stimulation. Women with this disorder are classically obese (40%) with some degree of hirsutism (70%) and acne (11%), although this is not always true, and usually present with the complaint of absent or infrequent heavy menses (80%) or primary infertility. The most consistent endocrine feature is ovarian hyperandrogenism. Unopposed estrogen production, inappropriate LH/FSH secretion, hyperinsulinemia, hyperprolactinemia, and decreased sex hormone–binding globulin (SHBG) may be present. Diagnostic evaluation should include a detailed history and physical examination with particular attention paid to the degree and distribution of hair, signs of virilization, acanthosis nigricans, and obesity. In approximately 50% of patients, hyperandrogenism is accompanied by carbohydrate intolerance and increased levels of insulin and insulin-like growth factor-I (19). Studies of patients with PCOS suggest that there are two etiologically distinct subpopulations (20). Insulin-resistant patients tend to be more obese, to have a greater waist-to-hip ratio, to be more hirsute, and to have higher levels of plasma testosterone and lower levels of SHBG. The finding that the drug troglitazone improves insulin sensitivity and also lowers free testosterone and SHBG levels in patients with insulin-resistant PCOS suggests that the insulin resistance may be the underlying cause of the gonadal dysregulation (21). Finally, a unique insulin receptor defect has been identified in approximately 50% of women with PCOS (16). In contrast, the non–insulin-resistant patients have higher LH/FSH ratios than do insulin-resistant patients, suggesting that the former group has a primary problem with neuroendocrine regulation.

The goals of laboratory evaluation are to assess hyperandrogenism and glucose resistance. Screening tests should include testosterone and DHEAS for those with hirsutism; prolactin and TSH for those with anovulation; fasting glucose, fasting insulin level, and hemoglobin A1c for obese women older than 35 years of age or with a family history of diabetes mellitus; and a lipid profile.

Therapeutic options depend on the patient's symptoms and her desire for fertility. Anovulation occurs as a result of impairment of the LH surge and can be diagnosed in a variety of ways, although irregular menses implies that ovulation is unlikely (17). A basal body temperature chart can be used to demonstrate the erratic pattern of bleeding to the patient or aid clinical diagnosis if the menses are somewhat regular. An elevated LH/FSH ratio in the presence of irregular menses is virtually diagnostic of this disorder. However, an LH/FSH ratio greater then 2.5:1 is found in only 60% of patients with PCOS. If the patient remains anovulatory, or for those patients with anovulation alone, clomiphene or gonadotropins may be useful to induce ovulation. Referral to a reproductive endocrinologist is indicated if the patient desires pregnancy.

Even if fertility is not immediately desired, the danger of unopposed estrogen secretion must be addressed. Women who have had an abnormal bleeding pattern for longer than 1 year should be referred to a gynecologist for endometrial biopsy to rule out endometrial hyperplasia or malignancy. Patients diagnosed in adolescence or in their early twenties with this disorder and those who have had 6 months or less of amenorrhea benefit from an immediate course of MPA (Provera), 10 mg daily for 10 to 12 days, to induce a withdrawal bleed and restore secretory endometrium. After this initial treatment, maintenance is best achieved with the use of combined OCs with low estrogen analog content for continuous ovarian suppression and also for contraception, because ovulatory cycles may occur after progesterone withdrawal (see Chapter 100). OCs increase SHBG and decrease free androgens and 5 alpha-reductase. Spironolactone may also be used as an antiandrogen to treat hirsutism (12) (see later discussion).

As noted, these patients tend to have impaired glucose metabolism with insulin resistance resulting in hyperinsulinemia and male-pattern lipid levels. These factors, in combination with the tendency to be overweight, put them at increased risk for diabetes and cardiovascular disease. Combination OCs are advantageous for adjustment of the lipid profile, although weight control has been demonstrated to be the most beneficial factor for preventing chronic disease. Therefore, patients with dyslipidemias or insulin resistance should be counseled on lifestyle changes, treated with insulin sensitizers if needed, and monitored closely for the rest of their lives (22) (see Chapter 79).

Secondary Amenorrhea

Secondary amenorrhea is diagnosed in women with previously normal cycles who have had no menses for a total of 6 months or have missed three menstrual cycles. There are many causes for this condition, although one of the most prevalent and most easily diagnosed is pregnancy, which must be ruled out before proceeding with the workup (Fig. 101.1). Feminized patients with *central secondary amenorrhea* may have a brain tumor or anorexia nervosa, but most commonly they have hypothalamic amenorrhea. Although this can have an *exogenous* cause (see later discussion),

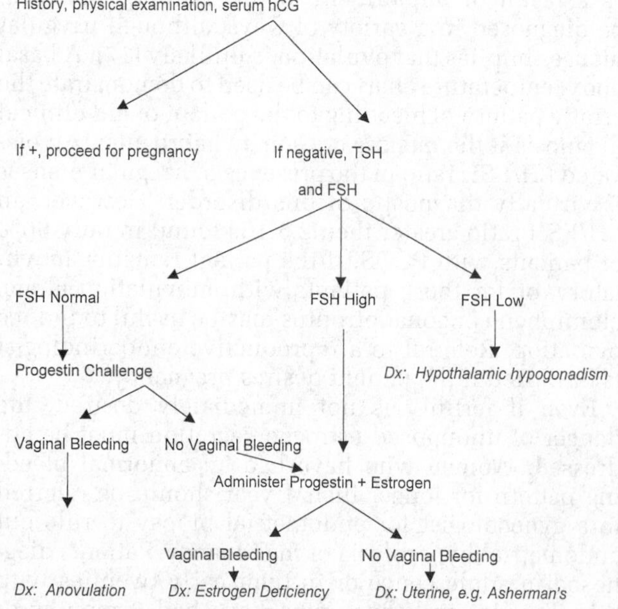

Figure 101.1. Approach to secondary amenorrhea.

it is often idiopathic with no explanation even after thorough examination. Pituitary amenorrhea is usually *acquired* and is often accompanied by deficiencies in other hormone axes (adrenal, thyroid).

The term *gonadal secondary amenorrhea* refers to loss of function of the ovary itself after puberty. This can be caused by infection (e.g., tuberculosis), neoplasm (e.g., Krukenberg tumor—metastasis of a gastrointestinal neoplasm to an ovary), trauma, surgery, or an autoimmune disorder. The latter category is often associated with a syndrome of polyglandular failure that may include disorders of the thyroid (Hashimoto thyroiditis) and adrenal (primary Addison disease), type 1 diabetes mellitus, and, rarely, autoimmune hypophysitis. Autoimmune ovarian failure is the most common cause of idiopathic premature menopause.

Exogenous amenorrhea can be caused by other systemic disease, such as hyperthyroidism or hypothyroidism, liver failure, renal failure, or other nonendocrine illness. *Hypothalamic (secondary, central, acquired) amenorrhea* is also often *exogenous* in that there is a proximate cause, such as weight loss (especially in anorexia nervosa), pathologic obesity, vigorous exercise (e.g., runners, ballet dancers), or severe stress, as in grief reactions or mental illness. Another form of *exogenous* interruption of menses may result from consumption of substances of abuse (opiates, alcohol) or prescribed medications (major tranquilizers, estrogens).

Serum or urinary gonadotropins are used to classify hypogonadism as *gonadal* (LH and FSH elevated) or *central* (LH and FSH low or normal). The investigation of central hypogonadism should include a serum prolactin level, especially if galactorrhea is present. Prolactin values between 30 and 100 ng/mL are elevated and are consistent with a prolactinoma, but they may be related to other causes such as hypothalamic (idiopathic) galactorrhea or drug effects. Values greater than 100 ng/mL almost always mean that a prolactinoma is present. Further testing should be undertaken by appropriate specialists and is similar to that outlined for patients with male hypogonadism (see Chapter 85). If hirsutism is present, the serum testosterone and urinary 17-ketosteroids should be measured.

A history of dilatation and curettage suggests a uterine cause for secondary amenorrhea. If TSH, FSH, and prolactin levels are normal, a *progestin challenge* should be done to evaluate estrogen production. A progestin challenge is done by prescribing oral MPA (Provera), 10 mg once a day for 5 days. Patients usually bleed 2 to 7 days after the last pill, although sometimes ovulation is triggered and they do not bleed until 14 days later. If the patient bleeds in response to progestin, then the diagnosis is anovulation. The underlying cause of anovulation should then be sought (e.g., stress, weight loss, anorexia, PCOS).

Patients who do not respond to progesterone challenge should be assessed for cessation of estrogen production with a combined estrogen plus progestin challenge (OCs). If the patient bleeds, then the problem is that she does not produce estrogen (i.e., gonadal secondary amenorrhea). The history is important in making the differential diagnosis and will implicate possible underlying causes as well as identify women in whom early menopause follows a clearly familial pattern. When the diagnosis is made in women who are younger than 30 years of age, a karyotype should be performed to exclude gonadal dysgenesis. Among the remainder, precise distinction between autoimmune and idiopathic causes is difficult. All patients with premenopausal estrogen deficiency should be screened periodically for evidence of associated autoimmune endocrinopathy affecting the adrenal, parathyroid, and thyroid glands and the gastric parietal cells. These patients are essentially menopausal and must be given hormone replacement therapy for bone protective effects (see Chapter 106). Future fertility is not possible from a native oocyte, although the patient may be referred to a reproductive endocrinologist to explore options of oocyte donation.

If the FSH is low or normal, then the diagnosis is hypothalamic amenorrhea. This is not common but is easily treated. Usually it is caused by stress or weight loss, although a head CT should be obtained to rule out a brain tumor, and the diagnosis of other rare central nervous system disorders should be entertained. This group is characterized by deficient gonadotropin secretion and mimics the endocrine state of the prepubertal girl. The low gonadotropin levels are not necessarily lower than those seen during parts of the normal cycle (particularly the luteal phase) and are of significance only in the context of concurrent diminished ovarian function. When fully expressed, these disorders are markedly hypoestrogenic: withdrawal bleeding does not occur after challenge with a progestational agent. Vasomotor symptoms such as hot flushes and night sweats may be present.

The differential diagnosis of hypothalamic amenorrhea includes conditions associated with destruction of hypothalamic and pituitary tissue such as ischemic necrosis (Sheehan syndrome), head trauma, and neoplasms such as craniopharyngioma and pituitary adenoma. Evaluation should consider both destructive and functional origins of hypogonadotropism through a careful history, physical examination, and, if a functional or nutritional cause is not evident, imaging of the pituitary and juxtapituitary structures. One of the more common intracranial lesions in women is a pituitary microadenoma or macroadenoma, which may be treated with bromocriptine and monitored with prolactin levels and imaging (see Chapter 81). Imaging of the sella turcica and determination of the prolactin level should be repeated annually to rule out or monitor pituitary adenoma, with the possibility of increasing this interval to every 2 to 3 years if results are stable for several years. Because all of these patients are hypoestrogenic and anovulatory, estrogen replacement must be prescribed (either combined OCs or hormone replacement therapy) and the patient reassured that ovulation induction is possible with GnRH analog injections when conception is desired. Treatment is given to remove the cause, restore normal menstrual function, or replace hormones. Patients desiring fertility will not respond to clomiphene and must be treated with gonadotropins for ovulation induction.

If no bleeding occurred with the combined estrogen/progesterone challenge, a uterine problem such as Asherman syndrome is indicated. A hysterosalpingogram or hysteroscopy will show intrauterine adhesions (Asherman syndrome). This diagnosis is usually suspected with a history of postpartum hemorrhage or menorrhagia requiring a dilatation and curettage. The treatment consists of resection of the adhesions, treatment with estrogens for several weeks postoperatively, and re-evaluation with a hysterosalpingogram. Successful pregnancies are achieved in 60% to 85% of patients, although they are at higher risk of abnormal placentation.

Menorrhagia or Intermenstrual Bleeding

Dysfunctional uterine bleeding (DUB) is a diagnosis of exclusion. Women presenting with menorrhagia (prolonged excessive bleeding) or metrorrhagia (bleeding between periods) need to be evaluated for organic, systemic, and iatrogenic causes for their abnormal bleeding (Table 101.2).

Organic Causes. The most common cause for abnormal bleeding in the reproductive age group are accidents of pregnancy. Miscarriage and ectopic pregnancy should be evaluated by performing a beta-hCG assay, as well as a pelvic ultrasound examination if indicated.

Prolonged excessive bleeding (menorrhagia) as a feature of otherwise normal cycles requires evaluation to exclude pathology affecting the endometrium. The most common reason is leiomyomas or "fibroids," which are a benign overgrowth of the smooth muscle that makes up the myometrium. Leiomyomas are present in up to 40% of women at the time of death (based on autopsy studies), are stimulated by estrogen, and typically become symptomatic in the age

Table 101.2. Causes of Abnormal Vaginal Bleeding in a Woman of Reproductive Age

Pregnancy
Local pathology
Leiomyoma
Endometrial polyp
Cervical polyp
Cervicitis
Endometritis
Malignancy
Foreign body
Systemic causes
Hypothyroidsim
Hyperprolactinemia
Polycystic ovary syndrome
Coagulopathy
Medications
Phenothiazines
Isoniazid
Opiates
Tricyclic antidepressants
Metoclopramide
Alpha-adrenergic antihypertensives

range of 30 to 40 years. A history of heavy, prolonged menses with possible clot passage and an enlarged, irregularly shaped uterus on pelvic examination most commonly suggests leiomyomas. In this circumstance, evaluation by an experienced examiner, endometrial biopsy in every patient older than 40 years of age, and imaging (pelvic ultrasound) are warranted to exclude another neoplasm masquerading as leiomyoma. Any patient with presumed leiomyomas exhibiting rapid uterine growth should be referred to a gynecologist for evaluation and hysterectomy, because leiomyomas do rarely undergo malignant degeneration (less than 1%). Leiomyomas may also undergo other types of degeneration (cystic, hemorrhagic), typically when blood supply is outgrown, and this may result in a significant amount of abdominal and pelvic pain.

Abnormal bleeding caused by leiomyomas may respond to hormonal management. Options include high-dose progestins (Depo-Provera, 150 mg or more, by intramuscular injection as frequently as monthly to control symptoms), OCs, or a GnRH agonist. GnRH agonists (leuprolide, goserelin, nafarelin) provide irreversible blockade of estrogen receptors and effectively induce a temporary menopausal state. These medications are not options for long-term therapy and may only be used for 6 months because of risks of bone depletion and adversely affected lipid profiles that result from estrogen depletion. However, these medications are useful for decreasing the size of the uterus or allowing the resolution of anemia before surgery. Surgical options are hysterectomy or myomectomy, depending on the patient's preferences for future fertility. Patients who are asymptomatic or who are not anemic and refuse hormonal or surgical therapy may be observed, because these tumors usually decrease in size when the menopause is reached. Leiomyomas should not be considered a contraindication to hormone replacement therapy.

The cause of menorrhagia accompanying otherwise normal cycles in the presence of a normal pelvic examination can be submucous leiomyomas or endometrial polyps, which usually are revealed by ultrasound, especially if it is performed with fluid contrast in the endometrial canal (sonohysterography) (5). The etiology of endometrial polyps is unknown. Because polyps are often associated with endometrial hyperplasia, unopposed estrogen may be the cause. These polyps rarely bleed enough to cause a clinically significant anemia. Occasionally a pedunculated endometrial polyp protrudes through the external cervical os and can cause intermenstrual or postcoital bleeding. The rate of malignant transformation in an endometrial polyp has been estimated to be as high as 0.5%. However, a case-controlled study from Sweden estimated that the increased risk of endometrial cancer in women with endometrial polyps is only twofold (23). Malignant change in an endometrial polyp, when found, is often of a low stage and grade and usually curable. The management of endometrial polyps consists of resection via the hysteroscope and examination of the endometrial lining.

Cervical lesions such as cervical polyps or cervicitis may cause irregular bleeding, particularly postcoital spotting. These lesions can be diagnosed by visualization of the cervix. In addition, traumatic vaginal lesions, severe vaginal infections, and foreign bodies have been associated with abnormal bleeding. Similarly, infections of the upper genital tract, such as endometritis, have been associated with intermenstrual spotting and may even manifest as prolonged menses. Malignancies of any portion of the genital tract may manifest as abnormal bleeding, particularly cervical and endometrial cancer. Less commonly, vaginal, fallopian tube, and ovarian cancer may produce abnormal bleeding. Careful physical examination and evaluation with cervical cytology, endometrial sampling, and ultrasound, when indicated, help to establish the diagnosis.

Systemic Causes. Hypothyroidism is frequently associated with menorrhagia as well as intermenstrual bleeding. The incidence of this disorder among women with menorrhagia is estimated to range between 0.3% to 2.5%. TSH should be measured and, if abnormal, appropriately treated (see Chapter 80). Although hyperthyroidism is not usually associated with menstrual abnormalities, hypomenorrhea, oligomenorrhea, and amenorrhea have been reported. Similarly, hyperprolactinemia and PCOS are most often associated with amenorrhea but can sometimes manifest as irregular menses.

Systemic disorders that produce abnormalities in coagulation or platelet abnormalities, such as von Willebrand disease, prothrombin deficiency, leukemia, severe sepsis, idiopathic thrombocytopenic purpura, hypersplenism, cirrhosis, and chronic renal disease, may all be associated with excessive or irregular bleeding (see Chapter 56).

Iatrogenic Causes. Foreign bodies in the uterus, such as an intrauterine device (IUD), frequently produce abnormal uterine bleeding. Several medications may interfere with the neurotransmitters responsible for releasing and inhibiting hypothalamic hormones, resulting in anovulation and abnormal bleeding. Medications typically implicated are phenothiazines, isoniazid, opiates, metoclopramide, tricyclic antidepressants, and alpha-blockade antihypertensives. Exogenous hormones such as danazocrine and OCs or MPA can cause irregular bleeding.

Dysfunctional Uterine Bleeding

After organic, systemic, and iatrogenic causes for the abnormal bleeding are ruled out, the diagnosis of DUB can be made. Treatment is age dependent and should be tailored to the patient, after reviewing all of her options. For adolescents, either expectant management or OCs may be appropriate. DUB during the reproductive years can usually be well managed with OCs, including the 20-μg pill, or with cyclic progestins (see Chapter 100). OCs offer several advantages, including ease of use and predictable menses. Cyclic progestins are a good option for women who cannot tolerate OCs and those in whom OCs are contraindicated.

A low-dose progestin, such as MPA (Provera) 2.5 mg, may be given 12 days during every second or every third month. Another option for some DUB patients is the use of a progestin IUD. DUB in women of late reproductive age to postmenopause can be treated with cyclic progestin, low-dose OCs, or cyclic combination hormone replacement. Treatment choice depends on the patient's symptoms and her need for contraception. Medical management generally offers excellent results for DUB management and should be the first line of treatment in the majority of cases. If medical management fails, surgical options include endometrial ablation, through a variety of techniques, or hysterectomy for definitive management.

Late Reproductive Age through Postmenopause: Greater than 45 Years

Perimenopause usually commences in the fifth decade, heralded by alterations in menstrual rhythm. Although the transition to the postmenopausal state can be brief and uncomplicated, the normal perimenopause is characterized in many women by the unpredictable occurrence of both shortened and lengthened ovulatory cycles as well as anovulatory episodes commencing well before menopause (24,25). The resulting menstrual chaos is a cause for inconvenience, frustration, and fear among affected women. It is in this age group that the term DUB is most commonly applied to the menstrual history. The clinician's focus must be to distinguish those patients whose symptoms are a result of the normal dysfunction of this transition from those who harbor gynecologic pathology. The perimenopausal woman is at increased risk for endometrial hyperplasia, endometrial polyps, and leiomyomas.

Patients approaching the end of the reproductive years often exhibit symptoms long before the manifestation of menopausal symptoms. Patients note bleeding patterns consistent with an anovulatory state, resulting from the decreased number of remaining oocytes. There is also an increased perception of premenstrual symptoms, which is probably secondary to increased levels of hormones resulting from elevated GnRH concentrations required to induce ovulation with limited numbers of recruitable oocytes. In addition to exclusion of pregnancy, many patients with abnormal patterns and amounts of flow require endometrial biopsy and ultrasound examination. These patients must undergo workup to exclude other causes of disordered bleeding, especially endometrial neoplasia.

Although there are several causes of bleeding after the menopause, it is the only symptom of many women with endometrial neoplasia, which must be ruled out first. The following section discusses endometrial hyperplasia and malignancy. This being said, there are several benign causes that should be considered in the differential diagnosis. Unexpected bleeding is common during hormone replacement therapy, with either cyclic regimens or continuous combined estrogen–progestin regimens, but it requires the same attention given to postmenopausal bleeding in a woman not receiving hormones (8,26) (see Chapter 106). Vaginal bleeding may also occur secondary to atrophic changes occurring after the menopause, in which the mucosal tissue has thinned due to lack of estrogen. This bleeding may occur after examination or coitus, and a tear will be clinically evident. Unless bleeding occurs regularly as a result of hormonal replacement therapy, vaginal bleeding in the postmenopausal woman should be regarded as a result of genital tract malignancy until proven otherwise. Careful clinical examination and endometrial biopsy are mandatory.

Endometrial Neoplasia

Endometrial carcinoma is the most common of the gynecologic malignancies and also one of the most treatable, because it is typically diagnosed at an early stage owing to the symptom of postmenopausal bleeding. Because of the possible underlying cause of carcinoma, such bleeding must be investigated further immediately. The approach to diagnosis of endometrial carcinoma is fully discussed in Chapter 104.

DYSMENORRHEA

Dysmenorrhea (painful menstruation) is a common problem. It is considered *primary* when it appears within 1 or 2 years after the menarche. If painful menstruation appears for the first time or suddenly intensifies in a mature woman, it is referred to as *secondary* dysmenorrhea and is almost always a result of a specific pathologic process, such as uterine myomas, endometriosis, pelvic inflammatory disease, or an intrauterine contraceptive device. Therefore, in secondary dysmenorrhea, one should seek an initiating cause. Patients with secondary dysmenorrhea usually should be referred to a gynecologist. Typical primary dysmenorrhea consists of the development within 1 or 2 days after the onset of menstruation of either crampy or sustained lower abdominal and pelvic pain that may radiate into the legs and that can be associated with nausea, vomiting, irritability, diarrhea, or abdominal distention. In a few patients, symptoms may be so severe that performance of usual daily activities is impaired or prevented. Usually the discomfort is most severe during the initial several hours of menstrual flow, fades gradually, and disappears within 2 or 3 days. The episodes tend to become less severe with increasing age and often disappear spontaneously within 5 or 10 years after the menarche or after the first pregnancy. Occasionally, idiopathic dysmenorrhea reappears (or makes its first appearance) during the perimenopausal period. The hormonal pattern leading to primary dysmenorrhea is not completely understood, but it requires ovulation and disappears if ovarian hormones are suppressed. The proximal cause of symptoms appears to be increased or sustained myometrial contractions, possibly from excess formation of uterine prostaglandins.

Mild forms of dysmenorrhea require only analgesic therapy, such as aspirin or acetaminophen, and reassurance from the physician. A number of preparations are available without prescription and are marketed for menstrual cramps. Most are combination tablets, and none is proven to be more effective than aspirin or acetaminophen alone. Examples of these combination tablets are Femcaps (aspirin, phenacetin, citrate, ephedrine, and atropine) and Midol (aspirin, caffeine, and cinnamedrine). Analgesics work best when taken promptly at or slightly before the onset of menses and continued regularly (every 4 to 6 hours), rather than only when pain is perceived.

When symptoms are more severe or incapacitating, nonsteroidal anti-inflammatory drugs (NSAIDs) that have antiprostaglandin activity greater than that of aspirin should be tried; they are effective in approximately half of the patients. Ibuprofen (e.g., Motrin 400 mg four times daily for 5 to 6 days), mefenamic acid (Ponstel 250 mg four times daily for 5 to 6 days), and naproxen (Naprosyn 500 mg two times daily for five doses) have been approved by the U. S. Food and Drug Administration (FDA) for use in dysmenorrhea. NSAIDs are most effective if given just before menstrual flow begins and continued for 2 to 3 days thereafter. However, because of the uncertainty of the effects of these agents in early pregnancy, it is suggested that their use be delayed until the beginning of menstrual flow in those patients who are sexually active and who are not using effective means of birth control. The patient should use one agent as a trial for three cycles, then discontinue the agent if there has been inadequate control of the symptoms. It is currently unknown whether one NSAID might be effective after another has failed.

Steroidal contraceptive agents, either oral or implantable (Norplant), suppress ovarian hormone production and therefore usually control dysmenorrhea; these agents occasionally may be necessary for management of the problem when it is severe. The use of OCs is discussed fully in Chapter 100. The unusual patient who does not respond to any of these therapies should be seen by a gynecologist for evaluation for an undetected problem causing secondary dysmenorrhea or to provide more experienced guidance in drug therapy for primary dysmenorrhea.

PREMENSTRUAL TENSION SYNDROME

The premenstrual tension syndrome is an ill-defined complex of signs and symptoms that occurs to some degree in approximately 30% of women of reproductive age. Symptoms include irritability and increased aggressiveness, cravings for sweet or salty foods, nervousness, depression, tearfulness, mood swings, difficulty concentrating, headaches, fullness and tenderness of the breasts, fatigue, and abdominal bloating. A significant minority of affected women find such symptoms severely disruptive to their lives. Any or all of the symptoms may be present, and the characteristic complaints vary among patients, but the hallmark of the syndrome is that these problems appear during the latter half (luteal phase) of the menstrual cycle, disappear with the onset of menstruation, and are absent during the first part (follicular phase) of the cycle.

Investigations of the cause of this entity have not been rewarding. Most studies have found no typical pattern of hormone or electrolyte changes that distinguishes symptomatic from asymptomatic women. Nonetheless, although progesterone supplementation does not eliminate symptoms, the suppression of ovarian cyclicity medically (e.g., with GnRH analogs) or surgically effectively eliminates premenstrual syndrome, and sex steroid hormone replacement in suppressed patients does not restore symptoms. It therefore seems most likely that the symptoms stem from an "abnormal" physical response to a more or less normal pattern of steroid hormone fluctuations during the menstrual cycle.

There is at this time no truly specific treatment for the premenstrual tension syndrome. Although pyridoxine, minor tranquilizers, and thiazide diuretics have all been tried, their effectiveness has not been substantiated in clinical trials, nor is there a definite rationale for the use of any of these agents. It is advisable to treat symptoms of mild premenstrual syndrome empirically, while reassuring the patient that she is not mentally ill but rather the victim of a common, hormonally related malady with no serious physical consequences. In severe cases, a trial of ovarian suppression with steroid hormone replacement may be warranted, but such treatment should be implemented only by a medical or gynecologic endocrinologist.

Galactorrhea

Galactorrhea refers to the production of milk (confirmed by demonstration of fat after staining of the fluid with Sudan stain) in a woman who is not recently postpartum or nursing a baby. *Secondary central amenorrhea* is often accompanied by galactorrhea (15% of cases). In approximately 40% of cases, galactorrhea/amenorrhea is caused by a prolactin-secreting pituitary adenoma that may or may not be readily detectable by imaging procedures (macroadenoma versus microadenoma). Other causes of galactorrheic amenorrhea include medication (isoniazid, phenothiazines), recent pregnancy, hypothyroidism, and idiopathic hypothalamic dysfunction. Occasionally, a woman who has nursed has mild persistent galactorrhea (without amenorrhea) for up to 5 years after weaning. In these cases, prolactin levels are usually normal (less than 30 ng/mL).

Hirsutism and Virilization

Growth of coarse dark hair (terminal hairs) in various body areas (besides the scalp and eyebrows) depends on the action of androgens. The pattern of hair growth reflects the relative sensitivity of various zones of the skin to androgen effect. Whereas pubic and axillary hair appears in both sexes, further hair growth diverges because of differing androgen levels. Although male patterns vary, maximum expression of androgen effect includes terminal hair development over the face, limbs, chest, superior pubic triangle, linea alba, and back. In those carrying genes for male-pattern baldness, high levels of androgens are also associated with loss of scalp hair, with hair receding first at the temporal hairline ("widow's peak") and later at the crown.

Hirsutism with Virilization

Most women (80%) develop some degree of dark hair growth over the legs and forearms but not much facial hair. About one third have small amounts of hair on the chest and abdomen (extending along the linea alba). Abnormally high levels of plasma androgens can result in male distribution of hair growth, the state of hirsutism. Over time, very high levels of androgen production also lead to virilization, defined as increased muscle mass, redistribution of fat from subcutaneous depots in hips and breasts to abdominal and intra-abdominal areas ("male habitus"), clitoral enlargement (greater than 2.0 cm), deepening of the voice, male-pattern baldness, development of acne, and increased perspiration odor from activation of sebaceous glands.

Excess body hair without signs of virilization is termed "simple hirsutism." Hirsutism with virilization is rare and is usually a result of diagnosable causes, the most common of which are adrenal or ovarian tumor, congenital adrenal hyperplasia, male pseudohermaphroditism, and use of exogenous androgen (e.g., female athletes and body builders). Truly virilized women usually should be referred directly to an endocrinologist for detailed diagnostic investigation.

Hirsutism without Virilization

Although simple hirsutism may be an early manifestation of Cushing syndrome or of an adrenal or ovarian neoplasm, most cases fall into a group termed "idiopathic" or "constitutional" hirsutism. The prevalence of simple hirsutism has been estimated to be as high as 10% in adult North American women. It typically develops during the late teens, although progression may be so slow that troublesome amounts of hair do not appear for 10 or more years after onset of menses.

In one half to two thirds of hirsute women, excessive ovarian production of androgens (testosterone or androstenedione) is demonstrable and is often associated with oligomenorrhea and decreased fertility. Ovarian structure may show hyperthecosis (overgrowth of interstitial tissue) or multiple cyst formation (PCOS; see earlier discussion).

In about half of all patients with simple hirsutism, elevated serum testosterone levels are not demonstrable. However, approximately half of patients with normal total testosterone have been shown to have increased plasma "free" (i.e., non–protein-bound) testosterone due to reduced SHBG. Increased hair follicle conversion of testosterone to the more potent dihydrotestosterone has been demonstrated in some of the remaining cases, and other causes of increased sensitivity of hair follicles to androgens have been postulated.

Racial and ethnic factors are also important determinants of hair growth. Women of Asian ancestry and Caucasian women of northern European origin usually have relatively little terminal hair on face, torso, or extremities. In contrast, Caucasian women of Mediterranean origin often develop mustache, beard, or sideburn hair and have dark hair on legs and arms. Constitutional hirsutism also tends to run in families. Therefore, a patient with moderate hirsutism who is of Mediterranean origin, who has a mother with excessive facial hair, and who has normal menses is unlikely to have identifiable endocrine disease. The timing of onset of hirsutism is also important. For example, sudden development of hirsutism many years after menarche is likely to be caused by a tumor of the ovary or adrenal rather than a functional cause.

Transitory hirsutism may occur during pregnancy and occasionally during menopause. A number of pharmacologic agents, including glucocorticoids, phenytoin (Dilantin), minoxidil, diazoxide, and phenothiazines, can produce hirsutism. Drug-induced hirsutism is characterized by increased hair growth that is not limited to the androgen-sensitive areas of the skin. Rare causes include chronic local skin trauma and porphyria cutanea tarda.

Besides PCOS, the other major cause of adult-onset simple hirsutism, sometimes with disturbance of menstrual pattern, is *congenital adrenal hyperplasia (CAH).* CAH is produced by a deficiency of one of the several enzymes in the steroid synthetic pathway. Although such defects are usually manifested in childhood as ambiguous genitalia with salt loss (21-hydroxylase deficiency) or salt-retaining hypertensive syndromes (11-hydroxylase deficiency), patients with partial 21- or 11-hydroxylase defects can manifest hirsutism with onset in puberty or in adult life without symptomatic disturbances of salt and water balance.

Approach to the Patient

A careful ethnic and family history is essential. The temporal evolution of the problem should be noted, including the menstrual history. On physical examination, one should carefully note the distribution and density of terminal hairs in the sideburn and mustache areas, the periareolar and midsternal regions, and over the back and buttocks. Particular attention should be paid to the pattern of pubic hair. In the female, the pubic hair forms an inverted triangle in the inferior pubic region only. The male escutcheon is a rhomboid space with terminal hairs filling the superior pubic triangle and extending up the linea alba to the umbilicus. A male type escutcheon in a female is a good presumptive sign of hyperandrogenism. Physical signs of virilization (discussed earlier) should be sought. Patients with virilism require urgent referral to an endocrinologist, whereas those with severe ovarian dysfunction may require the attention of a gynecologist for treatment of abnormal menstruation or impaired fertility. Finally, symptoms and signs of Cushing syndrome (in which hirsutism and even virilization may occasionally be more prominent than the classic "cushingoid" changes) should also be sought. Obesity with acanthosis nigricans is highly suggestive of the insulin-resistant variant of PCOS.

The decision to proceed with laboratory testing depends on the history and severity of the hirsutism. Laboratory studies can be performed sequentially if financial considerations are dominant or simultaneously if speed is of the essence. Serum testosterone, which is of ovarian and rarely of adrenal origin, is measured first. A normal serum testosterone level suggests idiopathic hirsutism and excludes major ovarian disorders. Not excluded are mild cases of ovarian hyperthecosis/polycystic ovaries with abnormal androstenedione production or decreased SHBG (increased free or bioavailable androgen). The uncovering of such borderline cases usually is not worthwhile because management would be unaffected. If the testosterone level is increased to between 85 and 200 ng/dL, a diagnosis of ovarian hyperthecosis or PCOS is most likely. Increased LH and low-normal or reduced FSH is highly suggestive of PCOS but does not occur in all patients. Pelvic sonography usually reveals multiple cysts or thickening of the cortex and enlargement of the ovaries. Levels of testosterone greater than 200 ng/dL suggest a diagnosis of ovarian neoplasm, and specialists should direct further diagnostic evaluation. This may include sonography, CT laparoscopy with ovarian biopsy, or ovarian vein catheterization.

If testosterone levels are normal, excess production of weak androgens (e.g., androstenedione, DHEAS) by the adrenal remains a consideration and can be confirmed by appropriate assays. In 21-hydroxylase deficiency, which is the most common type of CAH producing adult hirsutism, serum 17α-OH progesterone and urinary pregnanetriol may be elevated. However, in about half the patients with this syndrome, these steroid levels are significantly increased only after stimulation with exogenous adrenocorticotropic hormone (ACTH). Therefore, if CAH is suspected, endocrine specialty referral is appropriate. Large increases in serum DHEAS or 24-hour urinary excretion of 17-ketosteroids suggests adrenal neoplasia (adenoma or carcinoma) and should be evaluated by an endocrinologist.

Therapy

Treatment of hyperandrogenism and hirsutism has been reviewed (27). Therapy for simple hirsutism usually is local and essentially cosmetic, even if there is a hormonal abnormality, because medical reduction of androgen excess does not rapidly affect the presence of existing hair and is often incomplete.

Local measures include bleaching, wax stripping, shaving, plucking (tweezing), using hair removal creams (depilatories), and performing electrolysis. Contrary to popular belief, such measures do not accelerate the growth rate of remaining hair. Plucking can cause local infection. Wax applications and hair removal creams are effective but may be irritating and must be used with care. All of these procedures must be repeated at intervals. Electrolysis and thermolysis are effective procedures for permanent removal of hair, but they are expensive and uncomfortable. Effectiveness and safety (avoidance of burns, scarring, and infection) depend on the technique of the operator. Referral of the patient requires that the physician be familiar with the electrologist's skill. Under the best of circumstances, electrolysis is generally successful in destroying approximately 50% of the follicles treated at one time. Invariably, therefore, many repetitions are required.

Patients with hyperandrogenic hirsutism (PCOS or CAH) often respond to medical therapy. Such patients should be cautioned not to expect rapid results, because dedifferentiation of androgenized follicles may require 6 to 18 months, even if androgen excess is totally eliminated. The immediate benefit to be expected is prevention of progression of the hirsutism, with variable degrees of reversal occurring only as therapy is continued. Medical therapy is directed toward suppressing androgen production, blocking peripheral androgen action, or both. Although such therapy appears more rational when androgen excess is demonstrable, patients with idiopathic hirsutism may occasionally respond. Adrenal suppression with low dosages of dexamethasone, although introduced on the erroneous assumption that adrenal androgens were responsible for most cases of hirsutism, is nonetheless effective in about one third of cases. This seems to be so because of an accompanying reduction of ovarian androgen secretion, which is either directly dependent on ACTH or indirectly dependent via ovarian conversion of circulating adrenal steroids. Adrenal suppression is, of course, effective in cases of CAH. This form of therapy is simple and usually free from side effects. Dexamethasone can be given as a single dose of 0.1 to 0.3 mg (as a pediatric solution) orally at bedtime. At these low dosages, neither glucocorticoid excess (i.e., iatrogenic Cushing syndrome) nor chronic adrenal suppression with adrenal insufficiency is likely to occur, but levels of both plasma or urinary cortisol and adrenal androgen should be monitored, and the dosage of dexamethasone should be adjusted to keep both in the normal range. Side effects of dexamethasone therapy include occasional insomnia and appetite stimulation.

The most appropriate treatment for ovarian hyperandrogenism is suppression of ovarian androgen production. The first line of treatment is use of a cyclically administered estrogen–progestin combination (OC). This is effective in about half of the cases. Estrogens, especially when given orally, also increase the concentration of plasma SHBG, reducing the concentration of circulating free androgens. Because progestins have some intrinsic androgen-like activity on hair follicles, a combination that minimizes the content of progestational agent may be most appropriate. Agents containing 2 mg or less of norethindrone or 0.5 mg or less of norgestrel are acceptable. When used, OCs should be given on the usual schedule recommended for fertility control for the particular preparation (see Chapter 100).

Disadvantages of OCs include their potential for cardiovascular, thrombogenic, and other undesirable effects. These disadvantages have probably been overstated and are less often seen with the low-dose contraceptives of today than with their high-dose predecessors; nonetheless, possible adverse effects must be weighed carefully when they are to be prescribed for an essentially benign problem. Combined adrenal–ovarian suppression may be used if neither alone is effective.

Suppression of ovarian androgen production by OCs precludes pregnancy. Therefore, therapy must be interrupted when fertility is desired and the drug withheld until pregnancy is terminated. Spironolactone (Aldactone), at a generally well-tolerated dosage of 25 to 50 mg twice daily, suppresses ovarian androgen production and antagonizes androgen action at the hair follicle. Spironolactone is a well accepted and relatively safe drug, and the combination of spironolactone with an OC is often effective in more severe cases of hirsutism and in those that are unresponsive to ovarian and/or adrenal suppression alone. Contraindications to spironolactone include concomitant use of potassium supplements or renal insufficiency, either of which may predispose to hyperkalemia.

Cyproterone acetate and flutamide are competitive inhibitors of androgen that block peripheral androgen receptors and have been used successfully in the treatment of hirsutism. Finasteride (Proscar), which inhibits the enzyme (5-alpha-reductase) mediated conversion of testosterone to the active form, dihydrotestosterone (DHT), in prostate, also appears to be effective in skin and hair follicles (28). Studies of finasteride in the treatment of idiopathic hirsutism (27) and PCOS (29) have shown mixed results. Although none of the latter agents is currently approved by the FDA for the treatment of hirsutism in women, it is not unreasonable to try one of them alone or in combination with ovarian or adrenal suppression in resistant cases.

Finally, suppression of the reproductive system with the use of a GnRH antagonist such as buserelin has also been found to be effective in reducing severe ovarian hyperandrogenism with hirsutism (30). However, because of their attendant risks of osteoporosis or hot flushes, the usefulness of these agents is limited.

FEMALE SEXUAL DYSFUNCTION (FRIGIDITY AND DYSPAREUNIA)

Definition

As in the male, female hyposexuality can be divided into reduced sexual interest or appetite (inhibition of desire), failure of arousal (inhibition of excitement), and anorgasmia. For a more complete discussion, see Chapter 6. The discussion here is limited to physical and especially to endocrine etiologies.

Etiologies

Organic causes of female hyposexuality include diabetes mellitus with peripheral neuropathy, hyperprolactinemia, hypogonadism with estrogen deficiency, and organic disease of the vagina, uterus, fallopian tubes, or ovaries with resultant dyspareunia. Various endocrine (e.g., hyperthyroidism, hypothyroidism) and other systemic debilitating diseases can also cause loss of interest in sexual activity.

History

Questions should be the same as those asked of a woman with hypogonadism (see earlier discussion). Additional questions should be asked about dyspareunia. If there is pain or discomfort on intercourse, it is important to know whether it occurs with attempts at penetration (suggesting local vaginal or vulvar problems) or only after deep penetration (suggesting pelvic disease, such as leiomyoma, endometriosis, or salpingitis). The physician should determine whether there was a previous history of satisfactory sexual activity and, if so, the time and circumstances of onset of its deterioration. Careful questioning should reveal to what extent the problem is one of loss of interest, excitation (lubrication and heightened pelvic blood flow), or orgasm. A history of symptoms of diabetes mellitus, peripheral neuropathy, or thyroid, adrenal, or other serious systemic disorders should be obtained. Knowledge of medication use (tranquilizers, OCs) and substance abuse (opiates, alcohol) is also important.

Physical Examination

The physical examination should be conducted in the same way as for patients with female hypogonadism (see previous discussion). Careful attention should be given to the genitalia, uterus, and adnexa for evidence of infection, atrophy, or neoplasia. Endometriosis, a common cause of dyspareunia, is sometimes detected on rectovaginal examination by palpation of nodules in the space between the rectum and vagina (pouch of Douglas). Neurologic examination should include testing of peripheral sensation, position sense, and deep tendon reflexes.

Diagnostic Procedures

If evidence of hypogonadism exists, appropriate tests should be made (see earlier section) to classify the syndrome and diagnose the underlying condition. Measurement of the serum prolactin concentration may be helpful even in patients without apparent galactorrhea or amenorrhea (see earlier discussion). Patients with pelvic disease should be referred to a gynecologist for further evaluation and therapy.

Therapy

Therapeutic efforts should be directed at the specific organic cause whenever possible. Estrogen deficiency should be corrected, and hyperprolactinemia should be treated surgically or medically (see earlier section). If no organic cause is evident after careful examination, consideration of various modes of psychological diagnosis and treatment is appropriate (see Chapter 19).

General References*

American College of Obsterics and Gynecology. Bulletin 134: Dysfunctional Uterine Bleeding, 128 Amenorrhea. ACOG Compendium. Washington, DC: ACOG, 2000.

American College of Obsterics and Gynecology. Bulletin 14: Management of Anovulatory Bleeding. ACOG Compendium. Washington, DC: ACOG, 2000.

Mischell DR, Jr. Abnormal uterine bleeding. In Mischell DR, Stenchever M, Droegemueller W, Herbst A, eds., Comprehensive Gynecology, 3rd ed. St. Louis, Mosby-Year Book, 1997:1025–1042

An authoritative and comprehensive chapter in an excellent textbook.

Specific References

1. Erickson GF. An analysis of follicle development and ovum maturation. Semin Reprod Endocrinol 1986;4:233.
2. Lenton EA, Landren B, Sexton L, et al. Normal variation in the length of the follicular phase of the menstrual cycle: effect of chronologic age. Br J Obstet Gynecol 1984;91:681.
3. Kadir RA, Economides DL, Sabin CA, et al. Frequency of inherited bleeding disorders in women with menorrhagia. Lancet 1998;351:485.
4. Gay JD, Donaldson LD, Grellner JR. False negative results on cervical cytologic studies. Acta Cytol 1985;29:1043.
5. Ash SJ, Farrell SA, Flowerdew G. Endometrial biopsy in DUB. J Reprod Med 1996;41:892.
6. Youssif SN, McMillan DL. Outpatient endometrial biopsy: the pipelle. Hosp Med 1995;54:198.
7. Langer RD, Pierce JJ, O'Hanlan KA, et al. Transvaginal ultrasonography compared with endometrial biopsy for the detection of endometrial disease. Postmenopausal Estrogen/Progestin Interventions Trial. N Engl J Med 1997;337:1792.
8. O'Connell LP, Fries MH, Zeringue E, et al. Triage of abnormal postmenopausal bleeding: a comparison of endometrial biopsy and transvaginal sonohysterography versus fractional curettage with hysteroscopy. Am J Obstet Gynecol 1998;178;956.
9. Goldstein SR, Zeltser I, Horan CK, et al. Ultrasonography-based triage for perimenopausal patients with abnormal uterine bleeding. Am J Obstet Gynecol 1997;177:102.
10. Meuwissen JH, Oddens BJ, Klinkhamer PJ. Endometrial thickness assessed by transvaginal ultrasound insufficiently predicts occurrence of hyperplasia during unopposed oestrogen use. Maturitas 1996;24:21.
11. Weber AM, Belinson JL, Bradley LD, et al. Vaginal ultrasonography versus endometrial biopsy in women with postmenopausal bleeding. Am J Obstet Gynecol 1997;177:924.
12. Speroff L, Glass R, Kase N. Anovulation and polycystic ovary syndrome. In: Clinical gynecologic endocrinology and infertility. 6th ed. Philadelphia: Lippincott Williams & Wilkins, 1999:Chapter 12.
13. Warren MP. Effect of exercise and physical training on menarche. Semin Reprod Endocrinol 1985;3:17.
14. Hetland ML, Harbo J, Christiansen C, et al. Running induces menstrual disturbances but bone mass is unaffected except in amenorrheic female athletes. Am J Med 1993;95:53.
15. Prior JC, Vigne YM, Barr LS, et al. Cyclic medroxyprogesterone treatment increases bone density: a controlled trial in active women with menstrual cycle disturbances. Am J Med 1994;96:521.
16. Dunaif A. Hyperandrogenic anovulation (PCOS): a unique disorder of insulin action associated with an increased risk of non-insulin-dependent diabetes mellitus. Am J Med 1995;98:335.
17. Hull HGR. Epidemiology of infertility and polycystic ovarian disease: endocrinological and demographic studies. Gynaecol Endocrinol 1987;1:235.
18. Polson DW, Wadsworth J, Adams J, et al. Polycystic ovaries: a common finding in normal women. Lancet 1988;2:870.
19. Falsetti L, Eleftheriou G. Hyperinsulinemia in the polycystic ovary syndrome: a clinical, endocrine and echographic study in 240 patients. Gynecol Endocrinol 1996;10:319.
20. Meirow D, Yossepowitch O, Rosler A, et al. Insulin resistant and non-resistant polycystic ovary syndrome represent two clinical and endocrinological subgroups. Hum Reprod 1995;10:1951.
21. Dunaif A, Scott D, Finegood D, et al. The insulin-sensitizing agent troglitazone improves metabolic and reproductive abnormalities in the polycystic ovary syndrome. J Clin Endocrinol Metab 1996;81:3299.
22. American Society for Reproductive Medicine. Use of insulin sensitizing agents in the treatment of polycystic ovary syndrome. A Practice Committee Opinion. April 2000. Available at: http://www.asrm.org. Accessed February 15, 2002.
23. Pettersson B, Adami HO. Endometrial polyps and hyperplasia as risk factors for endometrial carcinoma. Acta Obstet Gynecol Scand 1985;64:653.
24. Santoro N, Brown JR, Adel T, et al. Characterization of reproductive hormonal dynamics in the perimenopause. J Clin Endocrinol Metab 1996;81:1495.
25. Prior JC. Perimenopause: the complex endocrinology of the menopausal transition. Endocr Rev 1998;19:397.
26. Ettinger B, Li DK, Klein R. Unexpected vaginal bleeding and associated gynecologic care in postmenopausal women using hormone replacement therapy: comparison of cyclic versus continuous combined schedules. Fertil Steril 1998;79:865.
27. Knochenhauer ES, Azziz R. Advances in the diagnosis and treatment of the hirsute patient. Curr Opin Obstet Gynecol 1995;7:344.
28. Castello R, Tosi F, Perrone F, et al. Outcome of long-term treatment with the 5 alpha-reductase inhibitor finasteride in idiopathic hirsutism: clinical and hormonal effects during a 1-year course of therapy and 1-year follow-up. Fertil Steril 1996;66:734.
29. Tolino A, Petrone A, Sarnacchiaro F, et al. Finasteride in the treatment of hirsutism: new therapeutic perspectives. Fertil Steril 1996;66:61.
30. Bertoli A, Fusco A, Magnani A, et al. Efficacy of low-dose GnRH analogue (Buserelin) in the treatment of hirsutism. Exp Clin Endocrinol Diabetes 1995;103:15.

*Bold print (general references) and bold numerals (specific references) denote published controlled clinical trials, meta-analyses, or consensus-based recommendations.

CHAPTER 102

Nonmalignant Vulvovaginal and Cervical Disorders and Chronic Pelvic Pain

ANNE E. BURKE, MD
JEFFREY M. SMITH, MD, MPH

Vulvovaginal symptoms constitute a significant proportion of problems presented to the primary care provider. The diagnosis and treatment of these disorders can be both satisfying and exasperating. Most diagnoses are readily made in one office visit. Treatment is usually easily rendered. However, the patient with recurrent or persistent symptoms presents special problems. Appropriate evaluation and treatment of both the easily treated patient and the patient with persistent symptoms require a knowledge of the anatomy, physiology, and pathology of the vulva and vagina.

ANATOMY AND PHYSIOLOGY

Vulva

The external genitalia of the female human is denoted the vulva (Fig. 102.1). The vulva consists of the labia majora, labia minora, vestibule, clitoris, prepuce, and mons pubis.

The mons pubis (mons veneris) is a cushion of fat covered by stratified squamous skin and its appendages (hair follicles, sebaceous and apocrine sweat glands). The mons is located superior to the clitoris and encompasses the triangular-shaped hair-bearing tissue situated in front of the symphysis pubis. The labia majora are composed of longitudinal folds of fat and connective tissue corresponding to the dartos of the male scrotum. When the labia majora are parted, the vaginal vestibule is seen. The vestibule begins at the hymenal ring and extends outward to the labia minora, upward to the frenulum of the clitoris, and downward to include the posterior fourchette. The vaginal orifice (introitus) and urethral meatus open in the midline of the vestibule. Ducts of the Skene glands (paraurethral glands), the Bartholin glands (major vestibular glands), and the minor vestibular glands also open in the vestibule. The hymen, a firm, often crescent-shaped membrane consisting of a double plate of stratified squamous epithelium, partially obscures the vaginal orifice (introitus) in virgins. Residual tags of the hymen, the carunculae hymenalis, are often noted at the inferior edges of the introitus. The fourchette, the most posterior boundary of the vestibule, is formed by the fusion of the inferior aspects of the labia majora. The clitoris, homolog of the penis, is located in the midline at the most superior aspect of the vestibule. The labia minora bifurcate anteriorly, forming the prepuce and frenulum of the clitoris.

Vulvar Glands

The major vestibular glands, or Bartholin glands, are paired glands whose ducts exit at the introitus, above the fourchette at the 5 and 7 o'clock positions. The minor vestibular glands are numerous small glands whose ducts exit laterally to the hymenal ring. These small glands may extend superiorly to the region of the urethra. Ducts from the Skene glands (paraurethral glands) open in the vestibule immediately beneath the urethral meatus.

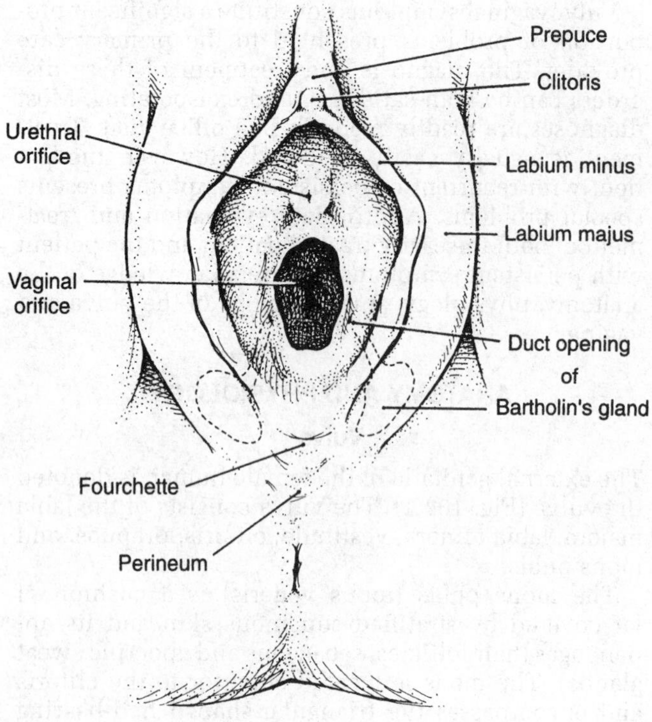

Figure 102.1. Anatomy of the vulva.

Vagina

The vaginal canal extends from the vestibule to the uterine cervix. The vaginal wall consists of an outer fibrous layer, a middle muscular layer, and an inner epithelial layer composed of nonkeratinizing, stratified squamous cells. No glands are present in the normal vagina.

When stimulated, the major nerve endings of the vagina cause the sensation of pain or light touch. Compared with the neural supply of the vulva, the vagina has few nerve endings. For this reason, vaginal infections are often asymptomatic until the discharge comes in contact with the vulva. The squamous epithelium of the vagina is hormone dependent. In the absence of estrogen, the vaginal epithelium is thin and fragile and consists of undifferentiated basal and parabasal cells. Progesterone leads to a decrease in superficial cells and a relative increase in intermediate cells. Pregnancy, lactation, and oral contraceptives produce the progesterone-dominant state. Normal vaginal discharge is composed of transudation through the vaginal wall, secretions of Bartholin and Skene glands, desquamated vaginal epithelial cells, cervical mucus, endometrial fluid, tubal fluid, and leukocytes.

Bacteria normally present in the vagina include lactobacillus, *Staphylococcus epidermidis, Corynebacterium* species, nonhemolytic streptococci, diphtheroids, peptostreptococci, *Bacteroides* species, and *Mycoplasma* species (1,2). Yeast are normal inhabitants of the vagina. The presence of *Gardnerella vaginalis,* also a normal inhabitant of many women's vaginas, is not diagnostic of vaginal pathology (3,4).

Physiologic vaginal discharge (pH, 3.8 to 4.5) is not malodorous or associated with pruritus. It varies in amount, is white or mucoid in color, and typically has a floccular consistency. The amount and consistency of the discharge depend on several factors: hormonal profile, presence of menstrual flow, frequency of coitus, use of antibiotics, and even stress (5,6). The *saline wet slide preparation* of normal discharge shows rare leukocytes, variable numbers of mononuclear cells, large gram positive rods, and vaginal epithelial cells with distinct borders (Table 102.1).

VULVOVAGINITIS

Abnormal vaginal discharge with associated vulvar irritation is the hallmark of vulvovaginitis. The most common vulvovaginal problems are vulvovaginal candidiasis, bacterial vaginosis (BV), and trichomoniasis infections. Atrophic vaginitis is a common problem among older women. Foreign bodies are a rare cause of vulvovaginitis in adults. Although they are not a cause of adult vaginitis, gonorrhea and chlamydial infections of the cervix (see Chapter 37) may initially manifest as an abnormal discharge and therefore may be misinterpreted as a vulvovaginitis.

Candida

Candida infection (Table 102.1) is an extremely common cause of adult vulvovaginitis, accounting for almost 30% of infections in symptomatic women (7). *Candida albicans* is a yeast that has no true mycelial form, and for this reason infection should be called *candidiasis* rather than *moniliasis* (a common term used in older literature), which implies infection by a mycelial form. The presence of *Candida* within the vagina is not sufficient for the diagnosis of vulvovaginitis; up to 20% of nonpregnant women of reproductive age are normally colonized with the yeast (6,7). Therefore, one should prescribe treatment only if the woman is symptomatic from vulvovaginal candidiasis; the presence of yeast in a Papanicolaou (Pap) smear or other examination is not in itself an indication for treatment.

The change in *Candida* from normal flora to a pathogen occurs when the organisms proliferate to the point that the normal microbiologic balance of the vagina is upset. Predisposing factors to infection include pregnancy, diabetes mellitus, immunosuppression, antibiotic or corticosteroid therapy, iron deficiency anemia, vaginal surgery, oral contraceptives, and infection with human immunodeficiency virus (HIV) (8–10). *Candida* may also proliferate in the setting of persistently moist and macerated skin, as can occur with the use of occlusive synthetic clothing. In many cases there is no identifiable predisposing factor.

Patients usually present with intense vulvar itching or burning associated with a thick, curd-like vaginal discharge. The vulva and vagina are typically inflamed. The vaginal mucosa may exhibit adherent white patches of exudate similar in appearance to

Table 102.1. Vaginal Discharge

	Physiologic	*Candida*	Bacterial Vaginosis	*Trichomonas*	Atrophic
Symptoms	None	Pruritus, burning	± Pruritus, burning	± Pruritus	± Vulvar, vaginal dryness
Malodor	None	Yeast smell	Fishy or musty	Variable	Variable
Increased mucosal erythema	None	Yes	±	Yes	±
Consistency	Floccular	Thick, curd-like	Thin, creamy	Copious, frothy	Mucoid, blood tinge
pH	3.5–4.1	3.5–4.5	5.0–6.0	6.0–7.0	As high as 7.0
Wet smear	Rare WBCs, large gram positive rods, squamous epithelial cells	Budding filaments, spores, pseudohyphae	Clue cells[a]	Copious WBCs, trichomonads	Copious WBCs, parabasal and intermediate cells, paucity of superficial cells
Potassium hydroxide preparation	—	Budding filaments, spores, pseudohyphae	Fishy odor, musty odor	—	—
Treatment of choice (see text for dosages)	None	Imidazole or triazole derivative	Metronidazole or clindamycin	Metronidazole	Estrogen cream

WBCs, white blood cells.
[a]See page 1595 and Fig. 102.4.

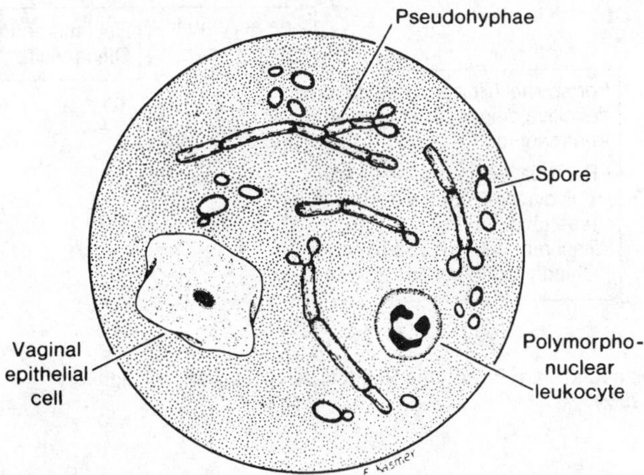

Figure 102.2. Potassium hydroxide preparation showing yeast and pseudohyphae of candidiasis.

oral thrush. Vulvar erosions with satellite pustules may be seen. Microscopic evaluation of an admixture of vaginal secretions with a 20% potassium hydroxide (KOH) solution typically supports the diagnosis. The KOH causes lysis of epithelial cells, leukocytes, and red blood cells, facilitating viewing of budding filaments, pseudohyphae, or spores (Fig. 102.2). Although up to one third of infected patients have negative findings on a KOH slide preparation, the presence of pseudohyphae and a normal vaginal pH in a woman with symptoms of vaginitis is quite helpful for diagnosis. Although failure to identify yeast on microscopic examination should not preclude treatment in a woman with classic symptoms, repeatedly negative wet smears should prompt further evaluation of the patient's condition.

Treatment

Candida vulvovaginitis may be treated either topically or orally. Antifungal medications include imidazole derivatives, the triazole derivative gentian violet, and the antifungal polyene macrolide antibiotic nystatin. The imidazole derivatives, triazoles, and nystatin increase the permeability of the cell membrane of fungi. This alteration of permeability results in the loss of the selective barrier function of the cell membrane so that potassium and other cellular constituents are lost.

The U. S. Food and Drug Administration (FDA)–approved prescription treatment of *Candida* vulvovaginitis includes oral and topical regimens. Terconazole is a topical triazole effective against a broad spectrum of candidal strains, including *C. albicans, Candida glabrata,* and *Candida tropicalis* (11). Terconazole is prescribed as one 80-mg suppository or as one applicator full of 0.4% cream intravaginally at bedtime for 7 days, or one applicator full of 0.8% cream intravaginally at bedtime for 3 days. An oral treatment, fluconazole 150 mg in one dose, maintains therapeutic concentrations in vaginal secretions for 72 hours and appears to be as effective as topical therapy (9,12). Fluconazole may interact with other medications, including cimetidine, cyclosporine, hydrochlorthiazide, isoniazid, oral contraceptives, phenytoin, rifampin, sulfonylureas, theophylline, warfarin, and zidovudine. Although it is unlikely that one 150-mg dose will cause a serious adverse reaction, there is potential for arrhythmia when fluconazole is taken with a nonsedating antihistamine, or for idiosyncratic liver dysfunction, which could be more serious when it occurs in a patient with existing liver disease. The advantages of fluconazole include patient preference and compliance, which must be weighed against its contraindication in pregnancy and its drug interaction and side effect potential.

A number of imidazoles that were originally available only by prescription are now available over the counter. Topical miconazole, clotrimazole, butoconazole, and tioconazole are available as nonprescription medications. Regimens include butoconazole 2% cream, 5 g intravaginally for 3 days; clotrimazole 1% cream, 5 g (one applicator full) intravaginally for 7 days; miconazole 2% cream or 100 mg suppository, intravaginally for 7 days; and miconazole 200 mg suppository, intravaginally for 3 days (13). These over-the-counter imidazoles are effective primarily against

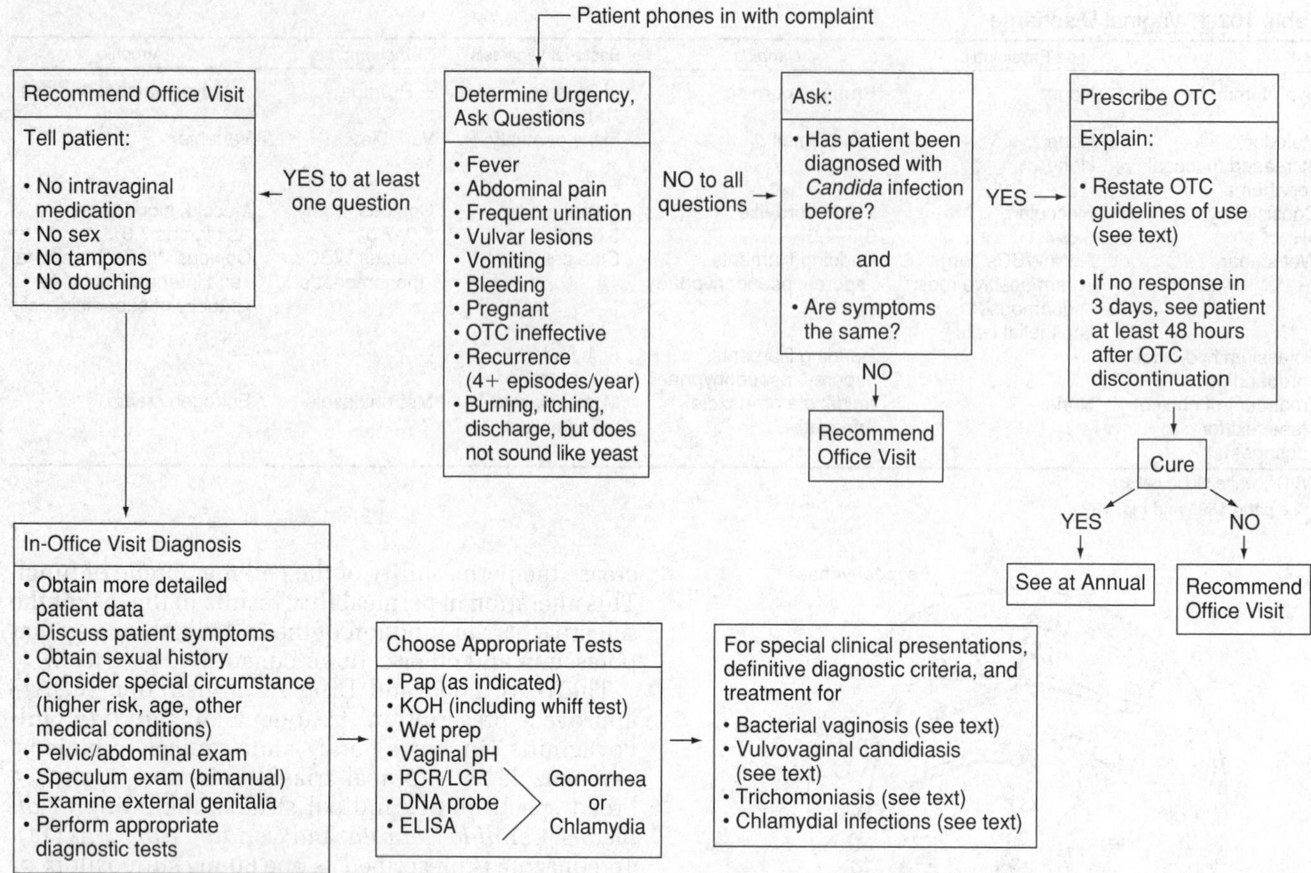

Figure 102.3. Telephone triage advice for patients with probable vulvovaginal candidiasis. (Modified from Vulvovaginitis: a practice protocol for the managed care clinician. National Association of Managed Care Physicians Roundtable Highlights 1:14, January 1996.)

C. albicans, which remains the most commonly isolated pathogen among women with vulvovaginal candidiasis. However, the number of infections caused by nonalbicans species may be increasing, in part because of the increased use of over-the-counter antifungal treatments. Currently, up to 20% of candidal vulvovaginitis is caused by nonalbicans strains (10,14,15). Therefore, it is prudent to prescribe a broad-spectrum antifungal agent when treating this vaginitis. Of particular note are studies that show enhanced *in vitro* or *in vivo* activity against *Candida* species with terconazole, butoconazole, and tioconazole (3,11).

Many women seek advice about an abnormal discharge via telephone, often after attempting self-medication (Fig. 102.3). However, because the reliability of self-diagnosis is poor (16), self-medication with over-the-counter antifungals is recommended only if

- The woman has had candidal vulvovaginitis previously diagnosed by a health care provider
- Her symptoms are consistent with the previous infection
- She does not have signs or symptoms suggestive of pregnancy, pelvic inflammatory disease (PID), or other condition requiring physical evaluation
- She agrees to be evaluated if there is no response in 3 days or no cure in 7 days.

If a pelvic examination is performed because of uncertainty of the diagnosis based on the telephone discussion, then certain precautions are necessary. Before being seen for pelvic examination, the woman should not have used any intravaginal medication for at least 48 hours, because intravaginal medication may mask the correct diagnosis.

With any effective antifungal regimen, symptoms typically diminish in 1 to 2 days. If a multiday regimen is prescribed, the physician should encourage patients to complete the treatment course. The 7-day regimen described previously is more effective during pregnancy, when the infection can be more resistant, and has also been shown to be more effective than oral fluconazole in severe infections (10).

All patients should be encouraged to wear cotton underwear that is nonconstricting. Excess vaginal moisture and heat associated with nylon or other synthetic materials and with tight-fitting pants may increase susceptibility to candidiasis.

Resistant or Recurrent Candidiasis

Candida infections of the vagina may persist or recur. Persistent vulvovaginal candidiasis is a consequence of inadequate treatment. Recurrent infections, defined as four or more symptomatic episodes annually, are caused by reintroduction of the organism and affect fewer than 5% of women with candidiasis (13). The only way to distinguish persistent from recurrent infection is by documenting eradication of the infection after a treatment course. This documentation, in practice, is not done commonly after an initial episode. However, if a second episode of *Candida* vulvovaginitis is experienced soon after the first, the physician should see the patient in follow-up within 1 to 2 weeks to re-examine the patient and determine by a KOH preparation (see previous discussion) whether the organism has been eradicated. Persistent infection should be treated with a 7-day course of a broad-spectrum antifungal agent. Recurrent infection requires more intensive treatment: 10 to 14 days of topical therapy, or additional doses of oral fluconazole (10). The diagnosis must also be confirmed, because contact dermatitis or infection with other organisms may cause similar symptoms. In certain instances, the inherent properties of *Candida* may be the cause of recurrent infection. *Candida* possesses the ability to change its surface antigens (17), which can alter its susceptibility to antifungal agents. Because each imidazole derivative has a distinct spectrum of activity against the various species of *Candida,* switching to a different imidazole derivative or triazole may effect a cure. If that fails, referral to a gynecologist is appropriate for confirmation of the diagnosis and consideration of an alternative therapy such as gentian violet, nystatin, boric acid, or suppressive therapy. Suppressive therapy should be initiated only after culture confirmation of the diagnosis.

The role of sexual transmission in vulvovaginal candidiasis is controversial. Treatment of male sexual partners with antimycotics can be considered if the partner is symptomatic. Although one study suggested a benefit from routine treatment of male sexual partners (9), other studies have failed to demonstrate a reduction in recurrences, and so routine treatment of male partners is not recommended (9,13).

The gastrointestinal tract is a natural reservoir for *Candida.* However, studies have failed to show an association between recurrences and the presence of intestinal *Candida.* Perineal contamination of the vulva through improper hygiene is thought to be another factor in the pathogenesis of recurrent infection. Therefore, patients with recurrent infections should be instructed to wipe from front to back when bathing and after urination or defecation. Eight ounces of lactobacillus acidophilus yogurt eaten daily for 6 to 12 months may decrease recurrences. If recurrences continue, a gynecologist should be consulted. Prolonged systemic antifungal maintenance therapy (for at least 6 months) may also be considered for recurrent infection. Options include ketoconazole 200-mg tablets, two times a day orally for 2 weeks, 100 mg (one-half tablet) per day for 6 to 12 months, or fluconazole 150 mg orally once a month for 12 doses (i.e., 1 year). There may also be a role for topical antimycotics in maintenance therapy (9). Ketoconazole and fluconazole should be restricted in pregnancy. Current data do not support the use of oral nystatin to prevent recurrence (18).

If recurrences are related predictably to specific events, such as menses, a prophylactic topical or oral antimycotic used for several days before onset of menses may be preventive. Sometimes recurrences are related to coitus, and for women in whom coital events can be predicted, prophylactic therapy is helpful.

Patients who continue to have recurrent infections despite the institution of these measures should be evaluated for diabetes mellitus (see Chapter 79) and HIV infection (see Chapter 39), although current recommendations of the Centers for Disease Control and Prevention (CDC) state that HIV testing can be reserved for patients who demonstrate other risk factors for infection. Many patients, however, experience recurrent vulvovaginal candidiasis in the absence of recognized predisposing factors. Some of these patients may be found to have a primary deficiency of cell-mediated immunity to *Candida* that often is temporary.

Bacterial Vaginosis

Bacterial vaginosis (*Gardnerella* vaginitis, nonspecific vaginitis, *Corynebacterium* vaginitis, anaerobic vaginosis, and *Haemophilus* vaginitis) (Table 102.1) is the most prevalent cause of vaginal symptoms among reproductive-age women. Because up to half of women with BV are asymptomatic, the infection is probably even more prevalent than is recognized (6).

In addition to *G. vaginalis,* an increased proportion of anaerobic bacteria such as *Bacteroides, Peptostreptococcus,* and *Eubacterium* is recovered from the vaginas of symptomatic women (2,19). Like *C. albicans,* most of these organisms are found in low concentrations in the vaginas of normal, asymptomatic women (3,4,6). Associated symptoms are caused by overgrowth of these bacteria and a decrease in the proportion of *Lactobacillus.*

Patients with symptomatic BV usually complain of thin, creamy, malodorous vaginal discharge with accompanying vulvar itching or burning. The vaginal mucosa and vulva may be mildly inflamed. The odor of this infection is usually described as fishy or musty and is commonly noted after coitus, when the alkaline seminal fluid has caused the release of volatile fatty acids and amines.

The diagnosis is confirmed through examination of the saline wet slide preparation (see previous discussion), production of the characteristic odor, and determination of the vaginal pH. With the use of nitrazine paper, vaginal pH can be determined easily. Vaginal discharge of women with BV typically has a pH between 5.0 and 6.0. The saline wet slide preparation is significant for vaginal squamous cells covered with *G. vaginalis* and other bacteria ("clue cells") (Fig. 102.4). Leukocytes usually are not abundant unless a mixed infection is present. The addition of a 20% KOH solution to the discharge causes the release

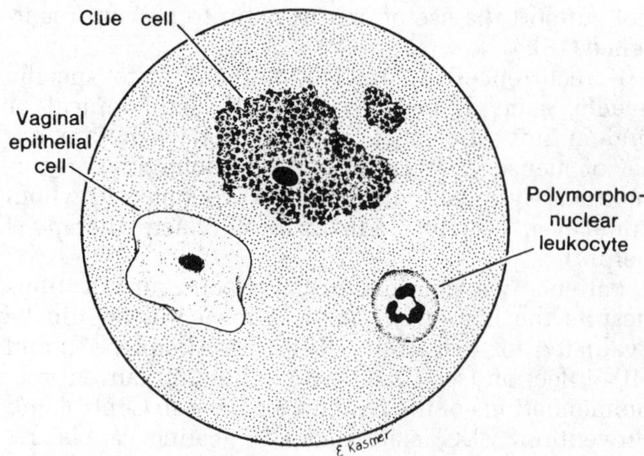

Figure 102.4. "Clue" cells.

of amines and volatile fatty acids that produce the fishy odor (whiff test).

The diagnosis of BV vulvovaginitis is made when at least three of the following four criteria are met (20):

- Vaginal pH greater than 4.5
- Thin, homogeneous vaginal discharge of variable amount
- Fishy odor after the addition of 20% KOH solution to the discharge (whiff test)
- Clue cells on saline wet preparation

Treatment

The treatment of choice for BV vaginitis is metronidazole 500 mg orally two times a day for 7 days, or 0.75% metronidazole gel intravaginally two times a day for 5 days, or 2% clindamycin phosphate cream intravaginally for 7 nights. Topical treatment is associated with a lower incidence of systemic side effects. Oral metronidazole may also be given as a single 2-g dose, and this effects an initial cure at least 80% of the time, although recurrence rates may be higher than with the longer regimen. (6) In addition, the higher oral dose is more likely to be associated with gastrointestinal side effects. Metronidazole is contraindicated in the first trimester of pregnancy. Because of the side effects that develop when the drug is taken with alcohol (disulfiram reaction), its use should be avoided in anyone using alcohol or anyone suspected of having severe hepatic disease. Alternative regimens that may be tried if metronidazole is contraindicated are clindamycin 300 mg orally two times a day for 7 days, or 2% clindamycin phosphate cream (see earlier discussion). Patients should be advised that the mineral oil in clindamycin cream can weaken condoms, diaphragms, and cervical caps. There is no role for sulfa-based vaginal cream or ampicillin in the treatment of BV.

The role of sexual transmission in the acquisition of BV has not been resolved completely. *G. vaginalis* can be recovered from most male contacts of infected women, yet *Gardnerella* also can be isolated from up to one third of women who have never been sexually active. In addition, recurrence rates for the infection are the same for women whose partners do or do not harbor *G. vaginalis* (21). Because of the possible role of sexual transmission, condoms should be used during therapy. Because there is no clear evidence that partner treatment improves recurrence rates (22), routine treatment of male partners is not currently recommended (13).

BV has been associated with preterm birth, and treatment of BV may reduce the risk of preterm delivery in high-risk women (23,24). However, treatment of asymptomatic BV in all pregnant women has not been conclusively shown to affect pregnancy outcome (25). Because of the association between BV and posthysterecomy vaginal cuff cellulitis, preoperative treatment should be given (26).

Trichomonas

Trichomonas infection (Table 102.1) is a common sexually transmitted disease (STD). It is caused by the motile, unipolar flagellated protozoan, *Trichomonas vaginalis.* Aside from sexual transmission, the organism can be acquired through close contact with contaminated water or clothing.

Patients usually have a copious and often frothy vaginal discharge accompanied by vulvar pruritus. Additional symptoms include vaginal burning, vaginal spotting, and symptoms of urethral irritation: Dysuria, frequency, and urgency. Pelvic discomfort may be experienced by some patients. Dyspareunia is common. On physical examination, variable amounts of vulvovaginal erythema may be seen. Typically, there is less erythema than is seen in *Candida* vulvovaginitis. The vaginal mucosa or cervix may exhibit a characteristic strawberry appearance (reddish color with punctation).

The diagnosis is established by assessing vaginal pH and examining the saline wet slide preparation (see earlier discussion). The vaginal pH is usually between 6 and 7. On the saline preparation (Fig. 102.5), a multitude of polymorphonuclear leukocytes are

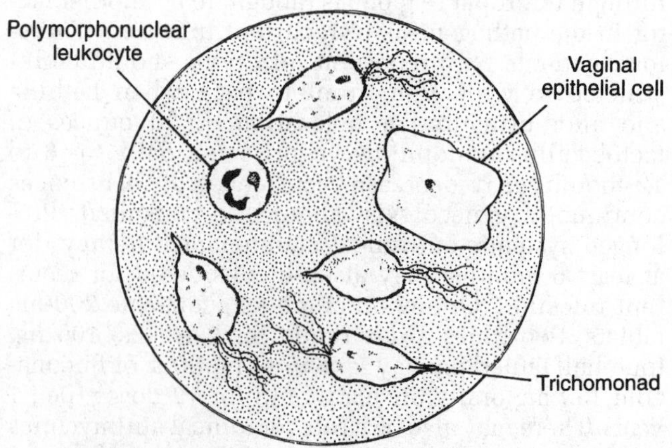

Figure 102.5. Saline preparation showing trichomonads.

seen. Among the white blood cells, trichomonads can be identified by the movement of their flagellae. Sensitivity of the wet mount may be examiner dependent. Because cold saline causes immobilization of the trichomonads, the solution should be at a comfortable room temperature. Atrophic vaginitis (discussed later) produces a discharge with a pH between 6 and 7 and copious white blood cells, but characteristically it does not contain mature squamous cells. Therefore, the presence of discharge containing numerous white cells and mature squamous epithelial cells, with a pH between 6 and 7, is presumptive evidence of trichomonas vulvovaginitis.

Treatment

Treatment consists of a single 2-g dose of oral metronidazole. Patients who do not respond to this therapy may be treated with metronidazole 500 mg, two times per day for 7 days, or 2 g per day for 3 to 5 days. Vaginal metronidazole may also be considered, although this regimen is less effective (13,27). Patients not responding to either of the oral regimens should be referred to a gynecologist for evaluation and treatment, which is likely to be difficult. Metronidazole is contraindicated in the first trimester of pregnancy, and it should be used cautiously in patients with severe hepatic disease. When taken within 24 hours of alcohol consumption, metronidazole causes severe reactions similar to those that occur when alcohol and disulfiram are consumed together. In these situations or when there is an intolerance to systemic metronidazole, metronidazole gel twice a day for 7 days may be tried as an alternative. The sexual partner or partners should be similarly treated, and it is usually pointless to attempt to recover the organism from the partner. Intercourse should be avoided or a condom used during treatment.

Atrophic Vaginitis

Atrophic vaginitis (Table 102.1) is a common disorder that affects 10% to 40% of postmenopausal women (28). Caused by estrogen deficiency, it may be seen in women who have undergone oophorectomy, have premature ovarian failure, or are breast-feeding. Rarely, atrophic vaginitis develops in girls who are premenarchal (i.e., have unestrogenized tissues) when an additional precipitant, such as wearing of occlusive clothing made of synthetic materials, is encountered.

Estrogen deficiency results in thinning and fragility of the vaginal and vulvar epithelium. Instead of the glycogen-rich superficial cells, the epithelium comprises primarily parabasal and intermediate cells. This altered vaginal environment is associated with an elevation of pH to as high as 7.0. In this milieu, pathogenic bacteria may flourish. The patient may complain of a thin, blood-tinged vaginal discharge and vulvar and vaginal dryness. Some patients also note urinary incontinence (see Chapter 54). Because symptoms may appear 10 years or longer after menopause, the condition is often underdiagnosed and undertreated (28).

Visual examination of the normal atrophic vagina reveals a pale vaginal mucosa with decreased or absent rugal folds. Vulvar examination demonstrates thin, often shiny skin with decreased subcutaneous tissue and variable loss of hair. In atrophic vaginitis, erythema and petechial hemorrhages may be superimposed on these findings.

Examination of a saline wet slide preparation (see earlier discussion) of the discharge of women with atrophic vaginitis typically shows numerous leukocytes mixed with immature, intermediate, and parabasal epithelial cells. Microorganisms seen on the slide are usually secondary invaders of the inflamed mucosa. Often, in the past, diagnosis was made by taking a smear of the vaginal wall and determining the maturation index; however, this test is no longer recommended because it has not proved to be reliable. Not all women with atrophy on vaginal examination have atrophic vaginitis. Treatment should be instituted only if symptoms are present and examination of the saline wet preparation reveals the findings described.

Estrogen replacement therapy is the treatment of choice for atrophic vaginitis and other manifestations of urogenital atrophy (29,30). Estrogen may be administered via oral, vaginal, or transdermal routes. The vaginal route seems to be associated with better symptom relief (28,31). However, beneficial systemic effects of estrogen replacement, such as prevention of osteoporosis, may be lost if the patient opts for vaginal treatment alone. Optimally, patients with this disorder should be provided both an oral treatment for systemic estrogen replacement therapy benefits *and* topical therapy for expeditious relief from atrophic vaginitis. One-half to one applicator of estrogen cream every night for 1 to 2 weeks is followed by application every other night for 1 to 2 weeks. The medication can then generally be discontinued, and most patients have only infrequent symptoms (e.g., every 1 to 2 months), for which an applicator full on 1 or 2 days when there are symptoms usually provides adequate control. Some patients, however, require up to 24 months of therapy, and the response may still be incomplete (31).

Local therapy may also be achieved through the use of an estrogen-containing vaginal ring. This ring is placed in the vagina and works continuously for 3 months (32,33). The ring does not require removal for intercourse. Absorption of estrogen to a level consistent with the early follicular phase of the menstrual cycle may occur with topically applied preparations. Therefore, if administration of a topical estrogen is prolonged (e.g., daily or every other day for more than 1 year), the patient will be at risk for complications of continuous unopposed estrogen therapy (see Chapter 106), including uterine cancer (see Chapter 104). Such patients should be monitored concomitantly by a gynecologist if the generalist is not experienced in screening for uterine cancer or so that a progestin can be prescribed (see Chapter 106). The physician should be certain that none of the contraindications for estrogens (e.g., breast cancer) is present and that the same precautionary surveillance (e.g., for hypertension) is provided to the patient using long-term topical estrogen preparations.

Some patients cannot or will not use topical vaginal preparations and refuse long-term systemic hormonal replacement therapy. In this instance, oral conjugated estrogen 0.625 mg/day may be prescribed for 1 month. Occasionally a repeated course of oral estrogens is necessary if symptoms persist. If retreatment courses become frequent, it is necessary to provide close surveillance for the complications of estrogen therapy (see Chapter 106). Generally a gynecologist should be consulted to participate in the care of the patient with frequently recurrent attacks of atrophic vaginitis.

Cytolytic Vaginosis and Desquamative Inflammatory Vaginitis

Cytolytic vaginosis and desquamative inflammatory vaginitis are uncommonly recognized *vulvovaginitides* that are often confused with other vaginal inflammatory conditions. Cytolytic vaginitis is caused by an overgrowth of long, serpiginous lactobacilli, rod-shaped organisms that causes shedding and cytolysis of vaginal epithelial cells. The vaginal discharge of cytolytic vaginosis usually increases during the luteal phase of the menstrual cycle and grossly resembles a candidal discharge; the discharge is thick and white, with an acidic pH. The patient usually experiences severe vulvar burning, dysuria, and dyspareunia. KOH preparation reveals an absence of fungi. The saline wet slide preparation reveals an abundance of lactobacilli, fragmented epithelial cells, and naked nuclei. Therapy has not been well established. Currently an intravaginal douche two to three times a week of 30 to 60 mg sodium bicarbonate in 1 L of warm water is recommended. Alternatively, the patient can take amoxicillin clavulanate 500 mg, three times a day for 7 days (34,35).

Desquamative inflammatory vaginitis is a disorder of unknown cause that usually is characterized by copious vaginal discharge and epithelial cell exfoliation. Patients experience intense vulvar pain and burning, severe dyspareunia, and dysuria. The vulva and vagina are usually very inflamed, with various stages of denudation. The discharge is seropurulent, with a pH of 6.0 to 7.0. The characteristic violaceous papules and gingival and buccal mucosal lesions of lichen planus may be seen if the patient has the form of desquamative inflammatory vaginitis that is associated with lichen planus (36,37). Saline wet slide preparation reveals parabasal cells, an absence of lactobacilli, a predominance of inflammatory cells, and fragmented epithelial cells. This entity is distinguished from atrophic vaginitis by nonresponse to topical estrogen. Treatment is with topical corticosteroids. One-half of a 25-mg rectal steroid suppository or one applicator of rectal hydrocortisone foam intravaginally should be used twice daily for 1 to 2 months; the dosage can then be reduced to once a day for an additional 2 months, followed by one- to three-times-a-week maintenance therapy. If there is no response, a gynecologist or dermatologist should be consulted for confirmation of the diagnosis and consideration of additional treatments, including systemic corticosteroids or antibiotics.

Foreign Body

An occasional cause of vaginal discharge in adults is a foreign body. Lost tampons, forgotten diaphragms, and other smaller objects are easily found by examination. Symptoms improve after removal of the foreign body. Because secondary bacterial infection is also present, use of metronidazole, or clindamycin as prescribed for BV, and a povidone douche once daily for 3 to 4 days may accelerate healing.

GONOCOCCAL AND CHLAMYDIAL INFECTIONS

In the United States, gonococcal and chlamydial infections are the most common STDs of the upper genital tract. These infections may initially manifest as an abnormal discharge that is the result of an associated cervicitis, not a vaginitis. However, the patient usually considers the discharge a sign of vaginal infection. Although a purulent discharge is classically associated with gonorrhea, a mucopurulent discharge is seen with chlamydia. For both infections, most patients do not recognize signs or symptoms until the disease affects the upper genital tract and causes PID. A full discussion of diagnosis and treatment of gonoccocal and chlamydial infections is presented in Chapter 37.

Chlamydia trachomatis Infection

Chlamydia trachomatis is believed to be the etiologic agent in a substantial number of cases of PID. In the United States, chlamydial infections are more common than gonorrhea. Routine screening is recommended for women who are younger than 25 years of age, have other STDs, have multiple sex partners, or have a male partner who has multiple sex partners (13).

Genital tract chlamydial infection is more indolent than is gonorrhea in both males and females, but the symptoms, when present, are similar: lower abdominal pain, dysuria, mucopurulent discharge, and fever. On examination the cervix may be red, edematous, and friable. Typically, the cervical discharge is less profuse than it is in patients with gonorrhea. Sequelae of chlamydial infection include ectopic pregnancy, PID (see later discussion), and infertility. Early treatment reduces the risk for these sequelae.

Although the traditional gold standard for chlamydia diagnosis is culture, newer laboratory procedures, ligase chain reaction (LCR) and polymerase chain reaction (PCR), are highly specific (greater than 99%) and sensitive (up to 96%) for chlamydia and can be applied to endocervical or first-catch urine specimens (38,39). Culture is not ordinarily done because it is expensive and not always reliable. LCR and PCR have been found

Table 102.2. Management of Gonococcal and Chlamydial Infections[a]

Uncomplicated Gonococcal Infection (Asymptomatic, Cervicovaginal, or Anorectal Symptoms; Pharyngitis): Dual Treatment for Possible Coinfection with Chlamydia is Recommended

1. Treat for gonoccal infection
   a. Cefixime 400 mg PO (once) *or*
   b. Ceftriaxone 125 mg IM once (or equivalent cephalosporin) *or*
   c. Ciprofloxacin 500 mg PO (once) or ofloxacin 400 mg PO (once; contraindicated in pregnancy and in those ≤16 yr of age) *or*
   d. Ofloxacin 400 mg PO (once) *or*
   e. Spectinomycin 2 g IM (once)
2. Treat for chlamydia with doxycycline or azithromycin (see below)
3. Treat partner(s)
4. Report to local health department

Chlamydia Cervicitis

1. Treat patient
   a. Azithromycin 1 g PO once *or*
   b. Doxycycline 100 mg b.i.d. for 7 d *or*
   c. Ofloxacin 300 mg PO b.i.d. for 7 d *or*
   d. Erythromycin 500 mg PO q.i.d. for 7 d
2. Treat partner(s)

Pelvic Inflammatory Disease

1. Ambulatory treatment
   a. Ofloxacin 400 mg PO b.i.d. for *14 d plus* metronidazole 500 mg PO b.i.d. for 14 d *or*
   b. Ceftriaxone 250 mg IM once (or cefoxitin 2 g IM once with probenecid 1 g PO) *plus* doxycycline 100 mg PO b.i.d. for 14 d
   c. Contact or observation within 72 hr to ensure improvement
2. Indications for hospitalization
   a. Diagnosis uncertain (to exclude appendicitis, ectopic pregnancy, nongonococcal pelvic inflammatory disease, pelvic abscess)
   b. Diagnosis is certain but patient is toxic or unable to follow ambulatory treatment reliably, or has nausea, vomiting, high fever (>38.3°C), or tubo-ovarian abscess
   c. Patient does not respond promptly to ambulatory treatment
   d. Pregnancy
3. Indications for parenteral therapy: same as indications for hospitalization plus one of the following
   a. A pelvic abscess is present
   b. Immunodeficiency is present
4. Inpatient treatment or ambulatory parenteral treatment
   a. Cefoxitin 2 g IV q6hr or cefotetan 2 g IV q12hr *and* doxycycline 100 mg IV q12hr *or*
   b. Gentamicin 2.0 mg/kg as an initial dose followed by 1.5 mg/kg q8hr *and* clindamycin 900 mg IV q8hr *or*
   c. Ofloxacin 400 mg IV q12hr and metronidazole 500 mg IV q8hr *or*
   d. Ampicillin/sulbactam 3 g IV q6hr and doxycycline 100 mg PO q12hr
   e. After hospital discharge or adequate clinical response from parenteral antibiotics, continue oral therapy with either doxycycline 100 mg b.i.d. or clindamycin 450 mg PO q.i.d. for at least 14 d total therapy

Gonococcal/Arthritis–Dermatitis Syndrome (Hospitalization is Recommended)

1. Initial treatment
   a. Ceftriaxone 1.0 g IM or IV q.d. for at least 49 hours or ceftizoxime 1 g IV q8hr for at least 48 hr
   b. For patients allergic to beta-lactam drugs, spectinomycin 2 g IM q12hr or ofloxacin 400 mg IV q12hr or ciprofloxacin 500 mg IV q12hr should be given
   c. Patients may be discharged 48 hr after clinical improvement, with close follow-up (see below)
2. If the infecting organism is proven to be penicillin-sensitive, parenteral treatment may be switched to ampicillin 1 g q6hr
3. Treat for potential coexistent chlamydial infection (see above)
4. The patient should complete 7 d of antibiotic therapy with either cefixime 400 mg PO b.i.d. a day or ofloxacin 400 mg PO b.i.d. or ciprofloxacin 500 mg PO b.i.d. (contraindicated in pregnancy and in those ≤16 yr of age)

[a] *Note:* Of the antibiotics listed use azithromycin, amoxicillin, gentamicin, clindamycin, spectinomycin, or cephalosporins in pregnant women. Ceftriaxone is effective against penicillinase-producing *Neisseria gonorrhoeae* (as well as many other organisms).

From Centers for Disease Control and Prevention. 1998 Sexually transmitted diseases treatment guidelines. MMWR Morb Mortal Wkly Rep 1998;47(RR-1):1.

to detect up to 40% more infections than culture (40). The fluorescent antibody staining technique, enzyme immunoassay, and DNA probe test are inexpensive and easy to use, although less sensitive than the amplification methods. For all of these laboratory procedures, the manufacturer-designated cotton swab should be used to obtain a sample of endocervical discharge.

If chlamydial infection is suspected, azithromycin or doxycycline is the drug of choice (Table 102.2). Treatment should be initiated before the results of the diagnostic assays are available: The recommended treatments are safe enough and, especially for doxycycline, inexpensive enough that empiric initiation of therapy is quite cost-effective, especially in patients who may not return for follow-up. Infected women should abstain from intercourse for 7 days after treatment begins, and all partners should be treated. Because the recommended treatments are extremely effective, routine follow-up is not necessary (13). Chlamydia, like gonorrhea, is a reportable disease.

PELVIC INFLAMMATORY DISEASE

PID is a clinical diagnosis. It refers to upper genital tract inflammation caused by ascending pelvic infection and can include endometritis, salpingitis, tubo-ovarian abscess, or peritonitis, singly or in any combination. Most cases are believed to be attributable to initial infection with gonorrhea or chlamydia, but vaginal flora (e.g. *G. vaginalis, Haemophilus influenzae,* anaerobes, and enteric gram negative rods) have also been implicated. *Mycoplasma hominis* and *Ureaplasma urealyticum* are also recent suspects. The sequelae of PID can be severe: a single episode of acute salpingitis causes infertility in approximately 8% of patients, and this complication rate can increase to 40% after three or more bouts with PID (41).

PID usually begins shortly after a menstrual period (which may be altered) and is typically characterized by fever, nausea, abdominal pain, and marked pelvic tenderness. Nonspecific symptoms such as dyspareunia, abnormal vaginal bleeding, and discharge may also be indicative of PID. The mildness of symptoms in many cases may delay diagnosis and increase the probability of inflammatory sequelae. Physical examination may reveal marked tenderness of the pelvic organs to touch or motion. The adnexa may also be enlarged. The leukocyte count is usually elevated. The CDC, in an attempt to reduce the number of unrecognized, untreated cases of PID, has simplified the minimum criteria necessary to initiate antibiotic treatment for probable PID. The minimum criteria are as follows (13,42):

- Lower abdominal tenderness
- Adnexal tenderness
- Cervical motion tenderness
- No evidence of competing diagnosis (e.g., ectopic pregnancy, appendicitis)

If all of these criteria are met, treatment should be started empirically. Additional criteria that increase the specificity of the diagnosis are the following:

- Fever greater than 101°F (38.3°C)
- Abnormal vaginal discharge
- Documentation of infection with *Neisseria gonorrheae* or *C. trachomatis*
- Increased erythrocyte sedimentation rate
- Increase in C-reactive protein

Treatment

In instances of uncomplicated PID, the recommended treatment is either ofloxacin plus metronidazole or an oral cephalosporin (e.g., cefoxitin, ceftriaxone) plus doxycycline (Table 102.2). Because PID is usually polymicrobial, broad-spectrum antibiotic coverage must be effective against chlamydia, gonorrhea, and anaerobes, the common organisms involved. Erythromycin, amoxicillin, or azithromycin should be used in pregnant patients because of the effect of tetracycline on fetal development and the possible effect on maternal liver function. Because the male sexual partner is often infected as well, he should be treated (see Chapter 37). Women receiving treatment for chlamydia or PID should either abstain from intercourse or ensure that their partners use condoms until completion of therapy.

Indications for hospitalization are included with treatment recommendations in Table 102.2. PID during pregnancy is rare. An obstetrician-gynecologist should be consulted promptly if this diagnosis is entertained during pregnancy.

The presence of a pelvic or tubo-ovarian abscess; pregnancy; poor compliance; immunocompromise; severe illness with nausea, vomiting, or high fever; or failure of outpatient treatment should also prompt hospital admission (13,42). The switch from intravenous to oral antimicrobial therapy should be based on clinical assessment and can be done 24 hours after the patient has shown clinical improvement.

All regimens used to treat PID should cover gonorrhea and chlamydia even if cultures are negative. Anaerobic coverage is also currently recommended. Intravenous treatment regimens include (a) cefotetan 2 g every 12 hours or cefoxitin 2 g every 6 hours with oral or intravenous doxycycline 100 mg every 12 hours or (b) clindamycin 900 mg every 8 hours with gentamicin 2 mg/kg loading dose followed by 1.5 mg/kg every 8 hours or gentamicin on a daily dosing regimen (13). Possible alternative intravenous regimens include (a) ofloxacin 400 mg every 12 hours or levofloxacin 500 mg daily with metronidazole 500 mg every 8 hours or (b) ampicillin/sulbactam 3 g every 6 hours with doxycycline 100 mg orally or intravenously every 12 hours (13). A review of the literature suggests that these regimens have clinical cure rates greater than 90% (42). After patients have demonstrated significant clinical improvement, oral therapy should be continued with doxycycline 100 mg orally twice daily or clindamycin 450 mg four times a day to complete a 14-day course. Adequate anaerobic coverage is likely of greater importance in patients with tubo-ovarian abscesses, concurrent BV, or HIV infection (42). If tubo-ovarian abscess is present, the use of clindamycin, clindamycin with doxycycline, or metronidazole with doxycycline should be considered.

Oral therapy and outpatient care are effective but should incorporate follow-up within 72 hours with abdominal and pelvic examination to assess response to treatment and to expedite admission, intravenous therapy, and further evaluation if no significant improvement has occurred. The CDC recommends a choice of several different outpatient PID regimens: (a) ofloxacin 400 mg orally twice a day with metronidazole 500 mg orally twice daily for 14 days or (b) ceftriaxone 250 mg intramuscularly once and doxycycline 100 mg oral b.i.d. for 14 days, cefoxitin 2 g intramuscularly with probenecid 1 g orally once and doxycycline 100 mg oral b.i.d. for 14 days, or another third-generation cephalosporin with doxycycline 100 mg orally twice a day for 14 days and optional metronidazole 500 mg orally twice daily for 14 days. Cefoxitin- and ofloxacin-based regimens have cure rates of at least 89%.

Any sexual partners of the patient within the 60 days preceding the diagnosis of PID should be treated empirically for gonorrhea and chlamydia even if the patient's cultures were negative. Some experts also recommend rescreening women for gonorrhea and chlamydia 4 to 6 weeks after diagnosis and treatment of PID (13).

VULVAR ULCERATIONS

Herpes Simplex

The most common cause of vulvar ulceration is herpes simplex, an enveloped DNA-containing virus specific for humans. Although both herpes simplex types 1 and 2 (HSV1 and HSV2) can cause genital ulceration, type 2 is implicated in most recurrent genital infections. This STD is characterized by exacerbations and remissions that are independent of repeated exposure to the virus. The seroprevalence of herpes virus type 2 has increased significantly over the past two decades, and is estimated at almost 25% among women in the United States (43). This may be an underestimate, because many cases of primary and some episodes of recurrent herpes are asymptomatic (44). The virus exists in latent form in pelvic nerve ganglia and within autonomic nerves along the uterosacral ligaments. Factors influencing recurrence of the infection are not well understood. It is thought that recurrences are correlated with stress and with the premenstrual period of the menstrual cycle. Recurrences are common, with about two thirds of infected women experiencing at least two recurrent episodes annually (45).

When the infection is initially contracted, the patient may develop a prodromal illness characterized by fever, malaise, and lymphadenopathy. Rarely, meningitis or encephalitis can develop. Before lesions appear, paresthesias and burning may occur. The initial formation of vulvar vesicles may be asymptomatic. These vesicles typically measure 1 to 10 mm in diameter. They are most commonly located on the labia minora, on the labia majora, and around the clitoris in a clustered, linear, or serpiginous arrangement (Fig. 102.6).

In the next stage of the process, the vesicles enlarge and rupture to form shallow, painful ulcerations. The ulcerations generally coalesce and are surrounded by an erythematous border.

Clinical suspicion of this diagnosis should be confirmed through a viral culture available through the health department (a special viral transport culture medium is required) or with a direct fluorescent antibody test. The culture or antigen detection test should be prepared from fluid obtained from an unroofed vesicle or the base of an ulcer. Viral identification via culture (findings are usually positive in 48 hours, but occasionally 7 days or longer is required) or antigen detection is most likely during the first 3 days of infection, and a negative test obtained after this period is not a guarantee of the absence of herpes. (Although presumptive treatment based on clinical symptoms is reasonable, the diagnosis should not be definitively made in the absence of laboratory confirmation.) The measurement of titers of serum antibodies to herpes virus is not generally helpful in the diagnosis of herpetic infection because of lack of specificity of the finding. Type-specific (HSV1 and HSV2) serologic testing is available and can be useful for partner testing as well.

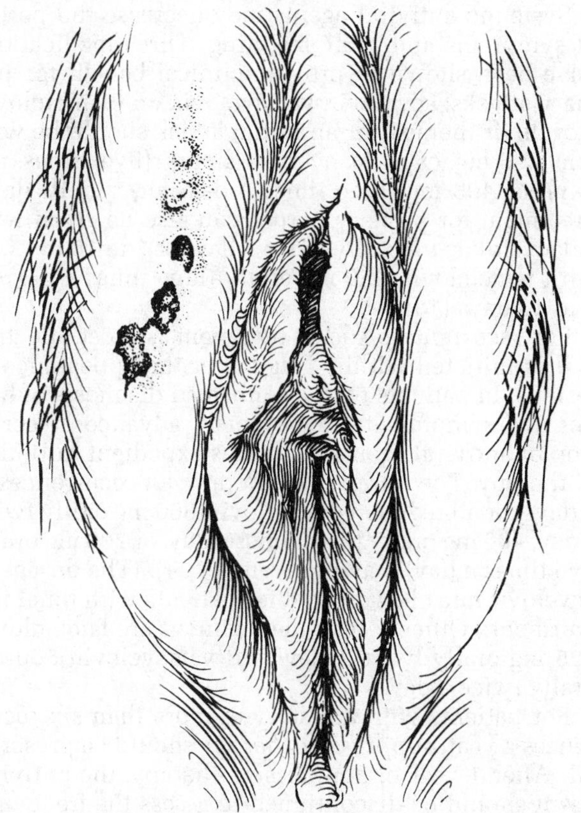

Figure 102.6. Herpes simplex.

Ulcerations in close proximity to the urethra may result in dysuria or urinary retention. Although the cervix and vagina are involved in more than 50% of cases, cervical and vaginal ulcerations may be asymptomatic because of the lack of free nerve endings in the vagina and cervix. With extensive cervical involvement, cervical motion tenderness may be elicited.

A honey-colored crust forms as the lesions heal. The ulcerations usually heal spontaneously in 1 to 3 weeks. Secondary bacterial invasion may prolong this healing process to 6 weeks or longer. Usually, there is no permanent scarring.

The symptoms of recurrences are generally milder than the initial attack and last for 8 to 10 days. Of patients with symptomatic recurrent herpes, 85% experience a prodrome of itching, tingling, burning, or tenderness.

Treatment

Therapy for herpes is aimed at palliation of symptoms and slowing viral replication. As yet, there is no means to eradicate the latent virus. (See Chapters 37 and 39 for additional discussion of treatment of genital herpes in the immunocompromised host.)

Systemic antiviral agents may decrease the period of symptoms and viral shedding. Three medications have been shown to provide clinical benefit for primary attacks: acyclovir, valacyclovir, and famciclovir. Acyclovir therapy for an initial attack should be with one 200-mg capsule every 4 hours (five times per day), or 400 mg three times a day, for 7 to 10 days. Treatment for primary herpes can also be given with valacyclovir, 1 g orally twice a day for 7 to 10 days, or with famciclovir, 250 mg orally three times a day for 7 to 10 days (13).

For *recurrent episodes,* treatment is most effective if it is initiated within 1 day after the appearance of lesions. In patients with a confirmed diagnosis of herpes and symptomatic recurrences, advance prescription of antiviral agents facilitates expedient initiation of therapy. The duration of therapy for recurrences is 5 days for all regimens. Acyclovir (800 mg orally twice a day, 400 mg orally three times a day, or 200 mg orally five times a day) may be given (13,44). (The dosage of acyclovir must be adjusted for patients with renal impairment.) Other acceptable regimens are famciclovir, 125 mg orally twice a day, and valacyclovir, 500 mg orally twice a day.

For patients with a history of more than six recurrences a year, *suppressive therapy* should be prescribed. After 1 year of suppressive therapy, the antiviral agent should be discontinued to assess the frequency of recurrence. Safety of up to 6 years of suppressive therapy has been documented. Recommended regimens for suppressive therapy include acyclovir, 400 mg orally twice a day; famciclovir, 250 mg orally twice a day; or valacyclovir, 250 mg orally twice a day, 500 mg once a day, or 1000 mg orally once a day (13,44).

Oral analgesics, topical anesthetics, compresses of Domeboro solution (available over the counter), witch hazel pads, warm tea bag compresses, and sitz baths may alleviate symptoms. Ten percent povidone–iodine applied twice daily for several days inhibits secondary bacterial infection and promotes drying of the lesions. A patient who also has dysuria from the infection may benefit from phenazopyridine, 100 to 200 mg three to four times a day for 3 to 4 days. For any topical therapies, patients should be instructed to use a finger cot or rubber glove when touching unhealed lesions to prevent autoinoculation. Finally, although topical acyclovir has been used often in the past for symptomatic relief of recurrent herpetic infection, it is ineffective and should not be used in this way (13,44,46).

Patients are often distressed by a diagnosis of herpes and should be reassured that, although the virus is not "curable," attacks are self-limited and will probably decrease in frequency over time. Because asymptomatic disease is more prevalent than previously thought, with subclinical viral shedding often occurring (47,48), symptoms do not necessarily indicate recent infection, and recent infection does not necessarily imply partner infidelity. Sexual contact should be avoided during symptomatic episodes, and condom use is recommended during all sexual exposures to partners not known to be infected.

Syphilis

Syphilis is an STD caused by the spirochete *Treponema pallidum.* Vulvar ulcerations can be seen in all stages of syphilis (see Chapter 37). The primary chancre appears approximately 3 weeks after the infection has been contracted (range, 10 to 90 days). It is a single, hard, painless lesion with an ulcerated central core. Often, multiple lesions occur that are painful and soft because of secondary bacterial invasion. Chancres are commonly found on the labia, fourchette, or cervix. These initial lesions usually heal spontaneously in 1 to 6 weeks. Between 3 and 4 days after the appearance of the chancre, inguinal adenopathy develops. With time, these firm, nontender lymph nodes become bilateral.

Secondary syphilis develops 2 to 8 weeks after the chancre in untreated patients. Because the chancre is usually painless, lack of treatment is more common in women than in men. Condylomata lata represent the classic vulvar, secondary syphilitic lesion. The plaques are multiple and commonly confluent. They are often grayish with a moist, necrotic appearance. The center of the lesion may be ulcerated. Other manifestations of secondary syphilis include malaise, a flulike syndrome, arthralgias, maculopapular rash, and lymphadenopathy.

Diagnosis and treatment of syphilis is fully discussed in Chapter 37.

Other Causes of Vulvar Ulcerations

Less common causes of vulvar ulceration include granuloma inguinale, lymphogranuloma venereum, chancroid, hidradenitis suppurativa, Behçet disease, Crohn disease, and tuberculosis. A synopsis of common findings, diagnosis, and treatment of vulvar ulcerations is found in Table 102.3. Any patient with an ulcer that is nonhealing, recurrent, or not easily diagnosed should be referred to a gynecologist or dermatologist.

MISCELLANEOUS LESIONS

Bartholin Cyst or Abscess

Obstruction of the major duct of the Bartholin gland (major vestibular gland) results in a Bartholin cyst (Fig. 102.1; Table 102.4). Infection and obstruction of the duct lead to a Bartholin abscess. Most Bartholin cysts occur because of mechanical blockage of the outflow of normal mucus secreted by the gland. If the cyst causes no symptoms and is only 1 to 2 cm in diameter, no treatment is necessary. Rapid enlargement, pain, hemorrhage, or secondary abscess formation requires the same therapy as a primary abscess. If a Bartholin cyst or abscess is suspected, to confirm the diagnosis and rule out carcinoma in an older woman and to initiate treatment, the gynecologist creates a fistula from the cyst or abscess to the vestibule by marsupialization, incision, and drainage, or, rarely, excision. A Bartholin abscess harbors *N. gonorrhoeae* in approximately 10% of cases. Therefore, culture for *N. gonorrhoeae* is

Table 102.3. Causes of Vulvar Ulcerations

Disease Entity	Cause	Appearance	Transmission	Symptoms: Other Manifestations	Diagnosis	Treatment
Herpes simplex (see text)	Herpes simplex type 2 Rarely herpes simplex type 1	Vulvar vesicle(s) Vulvar ulceration	Sexual	Fever, malaise, lymphadenopathy, burning, paresthesia, dysuria, urinary retention, painful ulcer	Viral culture or direct fluoroscent antibody test	Acyclovir Palliative treatment of lesions
Herpes zoster	Varicella zoster	Ulceration following the distribution of dermatome	Previous varicella zoster infection	Fever, malaise, lymphadenopathy, painful ulcer	Distribution of lesions Viral culture or direct fluoroscent antibody test	Acyclovir, valacyclovir, or famciclovir Palliative treatment of symptoms
Syphilis (see text and Chapter 37)	*Treponema pallidum*	*Primary:* Chancre (hard, painless lesions with central ulceration, lymphadenopathy) *Secondary:* Condyloma latum (multiple flat plaques, often confluent); rash (especially palm and soles, lymphadenopathy) *Tertiary:* Gummatous tumors or ulceration	Sexual	*Secondary:* Malaise, flu-like syndrome, arthralgias, lymphadenopathy *Tertiary:* Central nervous system signs and symptoms	Positive fluroscent treponomal antibody test Rising VDRL or rapid plasma reagin titers	Benzathine penicillin G, tetracycline, or doxycycline
Granuloma inguinale	*Calymmatobacterium granulomatis*	Painless, erythematous nodule that ulcerates (ulcers have irregular borders with a granulation base); lymphadenopathy in latter stages (scarring and lymphedema)	Sexual	Nonhealing ulcer that becomes painful after secondary bacterial infection	Donovan bodies (macrophages containing intracytoplasmic pleomorphic rods) on tissue crush preparation or biopsy	Trimethoprim/sulfamethoxazole (Bactrim, Septra) or doxycycline, alternatively ciprofloxacin or erythromycin with addition of gentamycin if improvement is inadequate with either in a few days
Lymphogranuloma venereum (LGV)	*Chlamydia trachomatis* serotype L1, L2, or L3	Vulvar papule that ulcerates in 4–6 wk; hallmark inguinal adenitis; nodes are unilateral and edematous; later bubo formation (enlarged, matted nodes held together by inflammatory reaction); fistula formation, vulvar fenestration	Sexual	Fever, malaise, initially painless	Titer of at least 1:64 on LGV complement fixation test	Aspiration of fluctuant buboes Doxycycline Erythromycin Surgical reconstruction
Chancroid	*Haemophilus ducreyi*	Soft, painful, chancre-like ulcer	Sexual	Painful ulcer Inguinal adenopathy	Culturing is difficult; diagnosis of exclusion	Azithromycin Ceftriaxone Erythromycin Ciprofloxacin
Hidradenitis suppurativa (see Chapters 32 and 115)	Inflammation/infection of apocrine sweat glands	Vulvar abscess formation with draining sinuses, scarring, and induration; fistula formation	Nontransmittable	Pruritus, burning	Appearance Biopsy	Surgical excision Occasionally systemic antibiotics Rarely systemic or intralesional corticosteroids
Behçet disease	? Autoimmune	Vulvar ulcerations with associated oral ulcerations and ocular inflammation		Arthritis, erthema nodosum, pyoderma, thrombophlebitis, acne, ulcerative colitis, neurologic symptoms	Diagnosis of exclusion	No definitive treatment High-dose oral contraceptives Intralesional corticosteroids Chlorambucil
Crohn disease	Unknown	Linear ulcerations similar to a knife cut; draining sinuses; fistulous tracts		Oral ulcerations Gastrointestinal symptoms	Biopsy	Corticosteroids Sulfones Metronidazole Surgical reconstruction
Tuberculosis (see Chapter 34)	*Mycobacterium tuberculosis*	Painless ulceration	Airborne Primary inoculation		Biopsy, acid-fast cultures	Antituberculous therapy

Table 102.4. Common Nonmalignant Vulvar Lesions

Disease Entity	Cause	Appearance	Symptoms	Complications	Diagnosis	Treatment	Other
Bartholin cyst	Obstruction of the duct of the gland	Discrete swelling of the inferior aspect of labium majorum	None or vulvar pain caused by enlargement	Infection, hemorrhage into the cyst; carcinoma, if age ≥40 yr	Visual inspection	None, unless symptomatic, infected, or hemorrhagic—then incision and drainage	
Bartholin abscess	Infection and obstruction of the duct of the gland	Discrete swelling of the inferior aspect of the labium majorum	Pain	Hemorrhage; carcinoma, if age ≥40 yr	Visual inspection	Incision and drainage Marsupialization; rarely, excision	Culture for gonorrhea
Condylomata acuminata	Human papillomavirus	Single or multiple, 2–3 mm in diameter and 10–15 mm high, fine, finger-like projections or flat-topped lesions; lesions may become confluent	Itching, vaginal discharge	Secondary ulceration and infection	Visual inspection, biopsy	Podophyllum 10%–25%; trichloracetic acid; liquid nitrogen or nitrous oxide or interferon injection	5-Fluorourucil for intravaginal lesions; laser surgery, excision, or electrodesica-tion; treat partner
Sebaceous cyst	Unknown	Discrete swelling, often 1 cm in diameter; firm, solid with a yellow color	Vulvar irritation caused by enlargement; pain, if infected	Infection	Visual appearance, biopsy	None; excision, if infected or bothersome	

indicated. Adequate drainage usually obviates the need for systemic antibiotics. Sitz baths provide temporary symptomatic relief until drainage can be performed.

To drain a Bartholin abscess, one should perform the following:

1. Inject lidocaine in a vertical line over the most fluctuant area of the abscess at the medial aspect of the labia majora.
2. With a scalpel, incise the anesthetized area to the abscess cavity.
3. Drain all purulent material.
4. Break up loculation within the abscess cavity with a clamp.
5. Irrigate copiously with a 1:1 solution of physiologic saline and hydrogen peroxide.
6. Pack the cavity with Nu-Gauze packing material or place a small catheter in the cavity.
7. Instruct the patient to take sitz baths three or four times a day.
8. Repeat irrigation and packing one or two times a week until the cavity has healed.

Condylomata Acuminata (Venereal Warts, Anogenital Warts, Genital Warts)

Condylomata acuminata are caused by human papillomavirus (HPV) and are transmitted sexually. This viral infection has a prevalence estimated at 10% to 20% among persons 15 to 49 years of age (49), with an estimated annual incidence of 1% (50). Importantly, nonacuminata HPV types may be related to the subsequent development of cervical and vulvar dysplasia (see Chapter 104). Most HPV infections are asymptomatic. Condyloma acuminata usually occurs during the reproductive years and is commonly seen in association with other vulvovaginal infections (including candidiasis, trichomoniasis, BV, gonorrhea, and syphilis). It may have a more active course in pregnant women.

The patient most often complains of a new growth on her vulva, perineum, or anus, and there is often associated itching and a vaginal discharge. These symptoms may be part of an associated vaginal infection, or they may represent infection in the crevices of the wart. Often, there is a history of warts on the penis of the sexual partner, who should also be evaluated.

The examination is characteristic and is almost always diagnostic. A nodule or wart of 1 to 2 mm usually first appears on the labia, often about the posterior introitus, but then spreads, with discrete or congruent lesions appearing on the perineum, anus, vagina, and cervix. They may coalesce into a cauliflower-like lesion that can become huge (Fig. 102.7). In the male, genital warts are often less conspicuous. Examination after swabbing the genitalia with a weak (e.g., 3%) acetic acid solution usually makes the lesions more visible. The presence of external warts should prompt examination of the vagina and cervix for additional lesions.

Treatment

Two patient-applied therapies are approved by the FDA: podofilox 0.5% solution or gel and imiquimod 5% cream. Neither has been proven safe in pregnancy. Patients must be shown how and where to apply the treatment. Podofilox is applied twice daily for 3 days, followed by 4 days of no therapy, and then repeated for a maximum of four cycles. Imiquimod is applied at bedtime three times a week for up to 16 weeks.

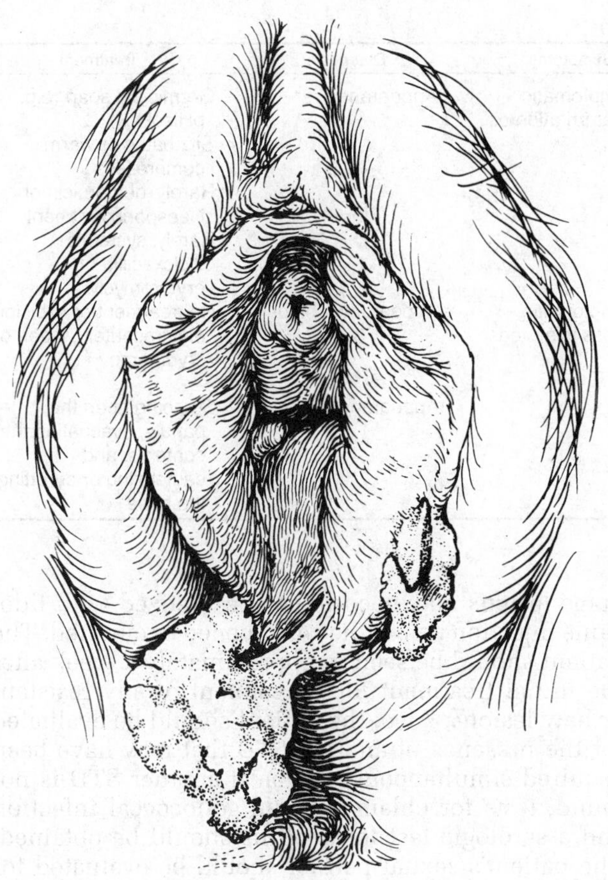

Figure 102.7. Condylomata acuminata.

Imiquimod must be washed off with soap and water within 10 hours after application.

Provider-administered treatment of the warts is accomplished by painting them carefully with a 10% to 25% tincture of podophyllin. This solution is irritating: it commonly causes transient discomfort and burns normal skin if applied to it. If such contamination does occur, the skin should be washed promptly with alcohol and then water. The podophyllin should be left on the warts for 8 to 12 hours and then removed with soap and water. During that time, the patient should not engage in sexual intercourse. The patient should be seen weekly for retreatment until healing occurs. If her sexual partner has warts, he should be treated also, and he should use a condom during intercourse until healing is complete.

If improvement has not occurred after the third treatment, one should switch to trichloroacetic acid (TCA) 80% or 90%. TCA may also be used as initial therapy (13). The TCA is applied sparingly to the warts at weekly intervals. The solution should be applied only to the warts and should be allowed to dry before the patient stands. A plain water and baking soda slurry is useful to neutralize the acid and remove any excess solution. Neither podophyllin nor TCA is suitable for eradication of large warts (greater than 2 to 2.5 cm) or of warts on the cervix or vagina. Also, podophyllin has been reported to cause fetal abnormalities and should not be used during pregnancy. In these instances, and if complete eradication has not occurred after six treatments, referral to a dermatologist or a gynecologist is suggested for evaluation and consideration of treatment with other modalities, such as cryosurgery, laser surgery, electrodesiccation, simple surgical excision, or intralesional interferon injection.

Sebaceous Cyst (Epidermal, Keratinous, or Inclusion Cyst) and Seborrheic Dermatitis

Sebaceous cyst is discussed in Table 102.4, and seborrheic dermatitis is discussed in Chapter 116.

Vulvar Papules

Folliculitis

Overgrowth of skin staphylococci and streptococci can result in vulvar folliculitis (Table 102.5). Predisposing factors for this disorder include immunosuppressive therapy, local trauma, poor hygiene, and occlusive (synthetic) clothing. Infection of the hair follicle is identified by erythematous papules or pustules with a central hair shaft. Treatment consists of cleansing the area with a germicidal soap. Warm sitz baths or compresses help relieve the discomfort. Gentamicin or bacitracin ointment may be prescribed to accelerate healing. If the lesions do not heal within 1 week, systemic dicloxacillin, cephalexin, or erythromycin should be prescribed. In a diabetic patient, the infection could become worse more rapidly; therefore, a systemic and a topical antimicrobial agent are usually prescribed at the time of diagnosis.

Acrochordon

Acrochordons, commonly known as skin tags, are sessile or pedunculated fibroepithelial polyps. Acrochordons are benign and should be removed only if they are large or annoying to the patient. A gynecologist or dermatologist should be consulted or a biopsy performed if there is doubt regarding the diagnosis.

Molluscum Contagiosum

Molluscum contagiosum is a benign lesion caused by a pox virus that is transmitted by close contact, including sexual intercourse. However, sexual intercourse is not necessary for transmission, because the disease can be spread via fomites or autoinoculation. Although trunk, face, and extremity lesions are common among schoolchildren, the lesions of adults are usually located on the genitalia. The adult patient characteristically sees a physician because of a painless new growth in the vulva, perineal area, or thighs. The lesions have a typical appearance, permitting diagnosis by inspection in most instances (Fig. 102.8). The individual lesions are wart-like papules varying from 1 to 10 mm in diameter. They have a smooth surface and a central umbilical depression containing keratin. There may be multiple separate lesions or one large, coalesced lesion. If there is any doubt about the diagnosis, the central cheese-like core may be expressed

Table 102.5. Common Vulvar Papules

Disease Entity	Cause	Appearance	Symptoms	Diagnosis	Treatment
Folliculitis (see Chapter 32)	Staphylococcus or streptococcus	Erythematous papules or pustules with a central hair shaft	Asymptomatic Vulvar irritation or pain	Appearance	Germicidal soap (e.g., pHisoHex) Sitz baths or warm compresses Rarely, gentamicin or Neosporin ointment Rarely, systemic dicloxacillin or erythromycin
Acrochordon		Soft, skin-colored, sessile or pedunculated tags of skin	Asymptomatic unless infarcted	Appearance; biopsy	No treatment or excision electrocautery, laser, or cryotherapy
Molluscum contagiosum	Pox virus Possibly sexually transmitted	Wart-like papules 1–10 mm in diameter with a central umbilical depression		Appearance; biopsy	Scraping open the papule, evacuating the contents, and cauterizing or curetting the base

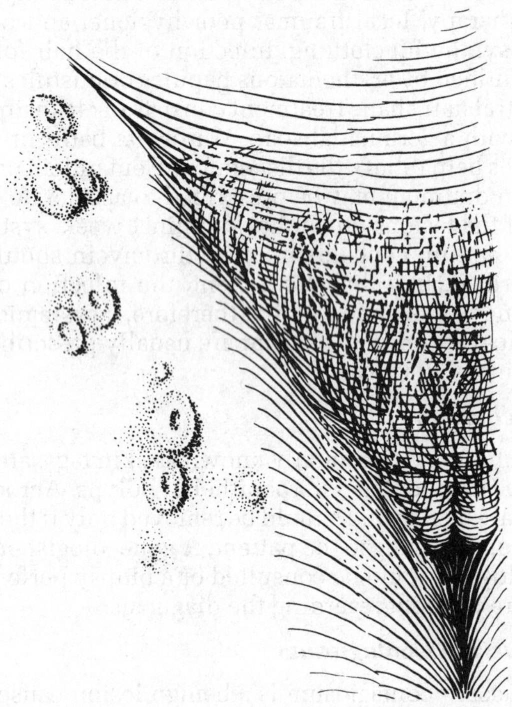

Figure 102.8. Molluscum contagiosum.

onto a slide and examined under a microscope using the low-power objective. Characteristic large inclusion bodies, which occupy most of the cytoplasm of the cells, are identified. Occasionally, the lesion resembles bacterial infection, such as folliculitis or furunculosis, but in these instances, the expression of pus (rather than a cheesy material) from the lesion permits differentiation. If doubt remains regarding the diagnosis, the patient should be referred to a dermatologist or gynecologist for confirmation.

Because spontaneous resolution can take months to years, treatment should be given. Therapy consists of scraping open the papule (with a scalpel blade), evacuating its contents, and curetting or cauterizing the base. Large lesions may need to be anesthetized with lidocaine injection before they are opened or curetted. The patient should be seen in approximately 1 week after the initial treatment for retreatment of any resistant or new lesions. Also, the patient should be evaluated for the presence of another STD that may have been acquired simultaneously. Even if another STD is not found, tests for chlamydia and gonococcal infection and a serologic test for syphilis should be obtained. The patient's sexual partner should be evaluated for lesions of molluscum contagiosum or evidence of another STD. A condom should be used until the patient's lesions have healed.

Hypopigmented and Hyperpigmented Lesions of the Vulva

Hypopigmented and hyperpigmented lesions of the vulva may range from nonmalignant to malignant disorders. Differentiation of the various processes is difficult by inspection alone. Biopsy must be performed to determine the diagnosis. Referral to a gynecologist or dermatologist is recommended when any such lesion is identified (see Chapter 104).

Intertrigo

Intertrigo, an important and common disorder, is discussed in Chapter 116.

Contact Dermatitis (Reactive Dermatitis)

Contact dermatitis is discussed in Chapter 116.

Vulvodynia

Vulvodynia is a syndrome of unexplained vulvar pain. The syndrome is often accompanied by sexual dysfunction and psychological disability. Vulvodynia may respond to a tricyclic antidepressant or a serotonergic reuptake inhibitor. Most patients with from this syndrome require a multidisciplinary approach from the primary care clinician, gynecologist, and psychiatrist or psychologist. Before the diagnosis of vulvodynia is made, other commonly misdiagnosed vulvar or vaginal conditions must be excluded. These conditions include vaginismus, cytolytic vaginosis, desquamative inflammatory vaginitis, pudendal neuralgia, vulvar dermatoses, vulvar allergic or reactive dermatitis, vulvar adenomas, and vulvar vestibulitis. If a woman continues to experience vulvar pain and burning despite treatment of recognized disorders, the physician should refer her to a gynecologist who is experienced in the diagnosis and treatment of vulvovaginal disorders.

Tampon-Related Ulceration and Toxic Shock Syndrome

Repetitive tampon use during periods of diminished or absent menstrual flow may result in vaginal ulceration. Typically, patients with this problem develop intermenstrual bleeding or abnormal vaginal discharge. The ulcers are usually located in one of the vaginal fornices. They are superficial, erythematous, and 1 or 2 mm in diameter (often they are mistaken for herpes). The ulcers heal spontaneously in a few days if tampon use is discontinued.

Toxic shock syndrome is caused by coagulase-positive *Staphylococcus aureus.* It is associated with fever greater than 102°F (39°C), severe headache, sore throat, vomiting, and diarrhea. Hypotension and shock may develop within 48 hours after the onset of the disorder. Other manifestations include palmar erythema, a sunburn-like rash with skin desquamation, myalgias, and conjunctivitis.

Pelvic examination typically reveals a purulent vaginal discharge. The vaginal walls are usually inflamed and may be ulcerated. Bimanual examination does not usually reveal any abnormal tenderness.

If a tampon is present at the time of the examination, it should be removed and cultured. Testing for gonorrhea and chlamydia (described previously) should be done to rule out either infection, which may occasionally be associated with symptoms that mimic the toxic shock syndrome.

The vagina should then be thoroughly cleaned with Betadine. The patient should be hospitalized for intravenous therapy with a therapy effective against betalactamase–resistant organisms and supportive care.

Cases of toxic shock syndrome must be reported to the state health department and to the CDC.

The patient should not use tampons for several subsequent menstrual cycles. In general, all patients using tampons should be encouraged to change them every 6 hours at least and to avoid tampons made of superabsorbent material (super tampons).

Pubic Lice

Pubic lice are discussed in Chapter 117.

Scabies

Scabies is discussed in Chapter 117.

Urethral Syndrome

Urethral syndrome is discussed in Chapter 36.

Psoriasis

Psoriasis is discussed in Chapter 116. The classic appearance of psoriasis is usually altered on the vulva. Because the vulva is moist, the psoriatic scale often is not present, and psoriasis may appear as a nonspecific dermatitis. It is rare for a patient to have psoriasis only on the vulva, so a general dermatologic examination should be performed. Patients with suspected psoriasis on the vulva should be referred to a dermatologist or gynecologist for confirmation of the diagnosis.

PSYCHOSEXUAL ASPECTS OF VULVOVAGINAL COMPLAINTS

A clinician should not suggest treatment for an organic vulvovaginal disorder unless its diagnosis is confirmed. The vulvovaginal region may be the focus of symptoms of a psychological disorder. Alternatively, a woman with chronic vulvar pain (e.g., vulvodynia) who has received no relief may develop psychological symptoms. A psychiatric diagnosis should be considered if a patient seeks repeated appointments and the physician finds no organic cause of the symptoms. Psychological support should be considered for any patient who experiences any form of chronic pain. Other chapters deal in detail with diagnosis and management of specific sexual psychological disorders (see Chapter 6) and other psychological disorders, particularly somatoform disorders (see Chapter 21), that may present with symptoms related to sexual function.

CHRONIC PELVIC PAIN

Chronic pelvic pain is a common clinical problem, with an estimated prevalence of 15% percent in women age 18 to 50 years (51). It is frustrating to patient and clinician alike: the symptoms are often poorly defined, diagnosis can take time, and often no cause is found. Further, there is no treatment that effects an easy cure. Despite these frustrations, however, chronic pelvic pain is treatable, and improvement is likely for many patients.

Pain is generally understood to be chronic if it is present for longer than 3 to 6 months. Chronic pelvic pain is a complex, multifactorial entity that can result from any number of causes. Diagnosis alone can require several visits and, once a treatment plan is established, frequent follow-up may be necessary to monitor improvement and provide continued support for the patient. Both the clinician and the patient must understand that a clear cause may not emerge and that complete resolution of symptoms may not occur (52).

Causes of Pelvic Pain

It should not be assumed that all pelvic pain is gynecologic in origin: gastrointestinal, genitourinary, and musculoskeletal conditions are often implicated. The list of potential causes is long and diverse. One common gynecologic cause is endometriosis, although not all patients with endometriosis suffer from pelvic pain. Other gynecologic diagnoses include pelvic adhesions and chronic infection. Bowel dysmotility disorders, especially irritable bowel syndrome, may be present in a majority of women with chronic pain complaints. Musculoskeletal and urologic disorders (e.g., interstitial cystitis) also account for a significant proportion of chronic pelvic pain diagnoses (53,54).

Evaluation of the Patient with Chronic Pelvic Pain

The most important components of the evaluation of the patient with chronic pelvic pain are a thorough history and physical examination. Imaging techniques and laboratory studies should be used judiciously, because their role in diagnosis is limited (52). Some investigators recommend that a complete blood count, urinalysis, and cervical cultures be performed in all patients, with the decision to perform additional tests individualized for each woman (55). Endoscopic studies, including laparoscopy, are not routinely recommended but can be valuable if a particular diagnosis is suggested by the results of the history and physical examination.

History

The goal of the history is to elucidate the nature of the pain. Questions must be asked regarding the character, intensity, and distribution of the pain, as well as the duration of symptoms. The woman should also be asked whether the pain demonstrates a cyclic variation, specifically in relation to the menstrual cycle, and whether the symptoms themselves have changed over the course of time. Asking the woman to maintain a pain diary can be extremely helpful and is recommended for all patients who present for evaluation of pain. The physician should also explore the impact that the pain has had on the patient's life events and relationships, as well as the possible effects these may have had on the pain. A comprehensive review of systems is useful in determining related gastrointestinal, urologic, or affective complaints. Mood disorders or depressive symptoms in particular may compound pain symptoms, and vice versa.

Direct inquiries should be made regarding a history of sexual abuse. Studies indicate that such a history is more common in patients with chronic pelvic pain (52,55). However, many patients with chronic pelvic pain do not have a history of sexual abuse, so it should not merely be assumed.

Physical Examination

A general physical and neurologic examination is indicated for any woman presenting for evaluation of chronic pelvic pain. At the start of the physical examination, the patient should be asked to point to the site of the pain: if one finger is sufficient, the pain is more likely to emanate from a specific source than if she uses her whole hand (53). The abdominal and pelvic examinations are important components of the evaluation, as is a thorough musculoskeletal examination. With the woman's permission, the clinician should attempt to reproduce her pain symptoms during the course of the examination.

Abdominal examination should begin with visual inspection for surface irregularities or scars. Palpation should include the back and inguinal region as well as the abdomen. Point tenderness ("trigger points"), which may be localizable by palpation with a single examining finger, should be noted, as should any deeper or more diffuse tenderness. Much of the musculoskeletal examination, including flexion and extension of the abdominal musculature and lower extremities, can also be incorporated into the abdominal examination. The pelvic examination should be comprehensive, including speculum examination, bimanual examination, and examination of the external genitalia and should also focus (with the woman's permission) on symptom reproduction (52).

Treatment

One should make an effort to treat any identifiable symptoms and to improve the woman's quality of life. Given the complex nature of chronic pelvic pain, this may involve a multidisciplinary approach. Mainstays of medical therapy (51) include oral analgesics, specifically nonsteroidal anti-inflammatory drugs, which are most effective if used on a round-the-clock basis. Some patients benefit from the use of psychotropic medications, specifically tricyclic antidepressants and selective serotonin reuptake inhibitors. Narcotics should be used with caution (55).

Treatment should also be targeted to the particular source of the patient's pain. Pain related to the menstrual cycle, for instance, can be treated with a trial of hormonal therapy, such as a monophasic oral contraceptive or a continuous progestin (oral or injectable). Bowel disorders may respond to medical treatment or dietary alteration, including fiber supplementation. Alternative modalities, such as injection with local anesthetics or acupuncture, may also be considered. Psychotherapy can be a useful adjunct to medical treatment. For women who do not respond to treatment, referral to a specialist may be indicated.

General References*

Black MM, Mckay M, Braude P. Obstetric and gynecological dermatology. London: Mosby–Wolfe, 1995.

*Bold print (general references) and bold numerals (specific references) denote published controlled clinical trials, meta-analyses, or consensus-based recommendations.

An excellent text with color photographs of a large variety of vulvar lesions.

Briggs GG, Freeman RK, Yaffe SJ. Drugs in pregnancy and lactation. 4th ed. Baltimore: Williams & Wilkins, 1994.

A compendium of drugs with fetal and neonatal risk assessments for each drug.

Drugs for sexually transmitted diseases. Med Lett Drugs Ther 1994; 36:1.

Kaufman RH, Friedrich EG Jr, Gardner HL. Benign diseases of the vulva and vagina. 3rd ed. Chicago: Year Book, 1989.

Although dated, this text is the classic reference for disorders of the vulva and vagina.

Lynch PJ, Edwards L. Genital dermatology. New York: Churchill Livingstone, 1993.

Easy to read, with excellent photographs.

McCormack WM. Pelvic inflammatory disease. N Engl J Med 1994;330:115.

A thorough and well-referenced review.

Sobel JD. Vaginitis. N Engl J Med 1997;337:1896.

An excellent review with good figures and summary tables covering all the common vaginitidies.

Tobin MJ. Vulvovaginal candidiasis: topical versus oral therapy. Am Fam Physician 1995;54:1715.

Easy-to-read review of topical and systemic therapy.

Specific References

1. Larsen B, Galask RP. Vaginal microbial flora: practical and theoretic relevance. Obstet Gynecol 1980;55:1005.
2. Keane FEA, Ison CA, Taylor-Robinson D. A longitudinal study of the vaginal flora over a menstrual cycle. Int J STD AIDS 1997;8:489.
3. American College of Obstetricians and Gynecologists. Vaginitis. ACOG Tech Bull 1996;226:1.
4. Eschenbach DA, et al. Influence of the normal menstrual cycle on vaginal tissue, discharge, and microflora. Clin Infect Dis 2000;30:901.
5. Friedrich EG Jr. Vaginitis. Am J Obstet Gynecol 1985;152:247.
6. Carr PL, Felsenstein D, Friedman RH. Evaluation and management of vaginitis. J Gen Intern Med 1998;13:335.
7. Sobel JD. Vulvovaginal candidiasis. In: Holmes KK, et al, eds. Sexually transmitted diseases. 3rd ed. New York: McGraw-Hill, 1999.
8. Galask RP. Vaginal colonization by bacteria and yeast. Am J Obstet Gynecol 1988;158:993.
9. Ringdahl EN. Treatment of recurrent vulvovaginal candidiasis. Am Fam Phys 2000;61:3306.
10. Sobel JD, et al. Vulvovaginal candidiasis: epidemiologic, diagnostic, and therapeutic considerations. Am J Obstet Gynecol 1998;178:203.
11. Cooper CR, McGinnis R. In vitro susceptibility of clinical yeast isolates to fluconazole and terconazole. Am J Obstet Gynecol 1996;175:1626.
12. Reef SE, et al. Treatment options for vulvovaginal candidiasis, 1993. Clin Infect Dis 1995;20[Suppl 1]:S80.
13. Centers for Disease Control and Prevention. 1998 Sexually transmitted diseases treatment guidelines. MMWR Morb Mortal Wkly Rep 1998;47(RR-1):1.
14. Horowitz BJ. Mycotic vulvovaginitis: a broad overview. Am J Obstet Gynecol 1991;165:1188.
15. Kent HL. Epidemiology of vaginitis. Am J Obstet Gynecol 1991;165:1168.
16. Ferris DG, Dekle C, Litaker MS. Women's use of over-the-counter antifungal medications for gynecologic symptoms. J Fam Pract 1996;42:595.
17. Soll DR. High-frequency switching in *Candida albicans* and its relations to vaginal candidiasis. Am J Obstet Gynecol 1988;158: 997.
18. Sobel JD. Pathogenesis and treatment of recurrent vulvovaginal candidiasis. Clin Infect Dis 1992;14[Suppl 1]:S148.
19. Spiegel CA, Davick P, Totten PA, et al. *Gardnerella vaginalis* and anaerobic bacteria in the etiology of bacterial (nonspecific) vaginosis. Scand J Infect Dis 1983;40[Suppl]:41.
20. Amsel R, Totten PA, Spiegel CA, et al. Nonspecific vaginitis: diagnostic criteria and microbial and epidemiologic associations. Am J Med 1983;74:14.
21. Vontver LA, Eschenbach DA. The role of *Gardnerella vaginalis* in nonspecific vaginitis. Clin Obstet Gynecol 1981;24:439.
22. Hamrick M, Chambliss ML. Bacterial vaginosis and treatment of sexual partners. Arch Fam Med 2000;9:647.
23. Hauth JC, Goldenberg RL, Andrews WW, et al. Reduced incidence of preterm delivery with metronidazole and erythromycin in women with bacterial vaginosis. N Engl J Med 1995;333: 1732.
24. McGregor JA, French JI, Parker R, et al. Prevention of premature birth by screening and treatment for common genital tract infections: results of a prospective controlled evaluation. Am J Obstet Gynecol 1995;173:157.
25. American College of Obstetricians and Gynecologists. Antimicrobial therapy for obstetric patients. ACOG Educ Bull 1998;245:1.
26. American College of Obstetricians and Gynecologists. Antibiotic prophylaxis for gynecologic procedures. ACOG Pract Bull 2001;23:1.
27. Forna F, Gulmezoglu AM. Interventions for treating trichomoniasis in women. Cochrane Database Syst Rev 2000;3:CD000218.
28. Cardozo L, Bachmann G. Meta-analysis of estrogen therapy in the management of urogenital atrophy in postmenopausal women: second report of the Hormones and Urogenital Therapy Committee. Obstet Gynecol 1998;92(4 Part 2):722.
29. Elia G, Bergman A. Estrogen effects on the urethra: beneficial effects in women with genuine stress incontinence. Obstet Gynecol Surv 1993;48:509.
30. Notelovitz M. Estrogen therapy in the management of problems associated with urogenital aging: a simple diagnostic test and the effect of the route of hormone administration. Maturitas 1995;22[Suppl]:S31.
31. Bachmann G, Nevadunsky NS. Diagnosis and treatment of atrophic vaginitis. Am Fam Physician 2000;61:3090.
32. Bachmann G. The estradiol vaginal ring: a study of existing clinical data. Maturitas 1995;22:S21.
33. Henriksson L, Stjernquist M, Boquist L, et al. A one-year multicenter study of efficacy and safety of a continuous, low-dose, estradiol-releasing vaginal ring (Estring) in postmenopausal women with symptoms and signs of urogenital aging. Am J Obstet Gynecol 1996;174:85.
34. Cibley LJ, Cibley LJ. Cytolytic vaginosis. Am J Obstet Gynecol 1991;165:1245.
35. Horowitz BJ, Mardh PA, Nagy E, et al. Vaginal lactobacillosis. Am J Obstet Gynecol 1994;170:857.
36. Kaufman RH, Friedrich EG Jr, Gardner HL. Benign diseases of the vulva and vagina. 3rd ed. Chicago: Year Book, 1989.
37. Oates JK, Rowen D. Desquamative inflammatory vaginitis: a review. Genitourin Med 1990;66:275.
38. Davis JD, Riley PK, Peters CW, et al. A comparison of ligase chain reaction to polymerase chain reaction in the detection of *Chlamydia trachomatis* endocervical infections. Infect Dis Obstet Gynecol 1998;6:57.
39. Puolakkainen M, et al. Comparison of performances of two commercially available tests, a PCR assay and a ligase chain reaction test, in detection of urogenital *Chlamydia trachomatis* infection. J Clin Microbiol 1998;36:1489.
40. Stamm, W. *Chlamydia trachomatis*. In: Holmes KK, et al, eds. Sexually transmitted diseases. New York: McGraw-Hill,1999.
41. Westrom L, et al. Pelvic inflammatory disease and fertility: a cohort study of 1844 women with laparoscopically verified disease and 657 control women with normal laparoscopic results. Sex Transm Dis 1992;19:185.
42. Rolfs RT. Think PID: new directions in prevention and management of pelvic inflammatory disease. Sex Transm Dis 1991;18:131.
43. Fleming DT, et al. Herpes simplex virus type 2 in the United States, 1976 to 1994. N Engl J Med 1997;337:1105.
44. American Medical Association. Genital herpes: a clinician's guide to diagnosis and treatment. Part I. In: Evans RM, Brakl MJ, eds. Chicago: AMA, 1997. (Available by writing to the Division of CME, Attention: Genital Herpes Education Program, American Medical Association, 515 N. State Street, Chicago, IL60610.)

45. Whitley RJ, Roizman B. Herpes simplex virus infections. Lancet 2001;357:1513.
46. Worrall G. Topical acyclovir for recurrent herpes labialis in primary care: critical appraisal. Can Fam Physician 1991;37:92.
47. Drake S, Taylor S, Brown D, et al. Improving the care of patients with genital herpes. BMJ 2000;321:619.
48. Wald A, Zeh J, Selke S, et al. Virologic characteristics of subclinical and symptomatic genital herpes infections. N Engl J Med 1995;333:770.
49. Koutsky L. Epidemiology of genital human papillomavirus infection. Am J Med 1997;102:3.
50. Fazel N, Wilczynski S, Lowe L, et al. Clinical, histopathologic, and molecular aspects of cutaneous human papillomavirus infections. Dermatol Clin 1999;17:521.
51. Mathias SD, Kuppermann M, Liberman RF, et al. Chronic pelvic pain: prevalence, health-related quality of life, and economic correlates. Obstet Gynecol 1996;87:321.
52. Steege JF. Office assessment of chronic pelvic pain. Clin Obstet Gynecol 1997;40:554.
53. Reinter RC. Evidence-based management of chronic pelvic pain. Clin Obstet Gynecol 1998;41:422.
54. Zondervan KT, et al. Chronic pelvic pain in the community–symptoms, investigations, and diagnoses. Am J Obstet Gynecol 2001;184:1149.
55. Scialli AR. Evaluating chronic pelvic pain: a consensus recommendation. J Reprod Med 1999;44:945.

C H A P T E R 103

Osteoporosis*

MICHELE F. BELLANTONI, M.D.

Osteoporosis is defined as a disease characterized by abnormalities in the amount and architectural arrangement of bone that lead to impaired skeletal strength and an undue susceptibility to fractures. Both men and women can develop osteoporosis, but women bear a disproportionate burden of this illness because of their lower peak bone mass in adulthood and the dramatic impact of menopause on bone mass. From the age of 50 years, the lifetime risk for any fracture of the hip, spine, or distal forearm is 39% in white women (1). Because late-life fractures significantly affect the duration and quality of life, risk assessment, prevention, and treatment of osteoporosis are important components of comprehensive primary health care in women.

EPIDEMIOLOGY

Using the World Health Organization (WHO) criteria, 30% of Caucasian postmenopausal women in the United States have osteoporosis, and 54% have osteopenia. The prevalence of low bone mass increases with age. Using the WHO definition of osteoporosis, the prevalence in the United States of osteoporosis in Caucasian postmenopausal women based on the lowest bone mass at any site is estimated to be 14% of women age 50 to 59 years, 22% of women age 60 to 69 years, 39% of women age 70 to 79 years, and 70% of women age 80 years or older (1).

Bone mass predicts fracture risk. For every 1 standard deviation (SD) below peak bone mass, the risk of vertebral fracture is two times that of normal bone mass, and for the hip the risk is 2.5 times greater (2). Vertebral fractures are the most common osteoporotic fractures. Although they are often asymptomatic, multiple vertebral fractures can result in spinal kyphosis, the so-called "dowager's hump," and chronic pain. Hip

*Male osteoporosis is discussed in Chapter 84.

fractures, however, result in institutionalization and excess mortality. The 1-year mortality rate according to age at hip fracture is estimated to be roughly 20% in individuals younger than 70 years of age; 30% for those age 70 to 79 years, and almost 40% for those age 80 to 89.9 years (3). More than half of hip fracture survivors fail to return to independent living (4).

RISK FACTORS

To assess a woman's risk for osteoporosis, the clinician should consider those factors that affect peak bone mass, which occurs by the early thirties, and those factors that are associated with accelerated bone loss. Fracture risk has also been shown to increase independently of bone mass for those women with (a) a maternal history of hip fracture, (b) greater height, and (c) increased likelihood of falling.

Genetic factors play the greatest role in determining peak bone mass. African American women have on average greater bone mineral density than Caucasian women do (5). There are clinically significant contributions to bone mass from nutrition, drug exposures, endocrine health after puberty, and weight-bearing status (Table 103.1). For example, most teenagers and young adults do not receive the Recommended Daily Allowance (RDA) for calcium of 1,200 mg. Beverages high in phosphate (e.g., carbonated sodas) and a high protein diet result in excessive urinary excretion of calcium. *Caffeine, alcohol, and smoking* are harmful to bone metabolism. The use of *systemic glucocorticoids* in dosages equivalent to prednisone 7.5 mg daily or greater impairs bone formation. *Phenytoin and other antiseizure medications* impair vitamin D metabolism. *Oligomenorrhea and amenorrhea* cause accelerated bone loss, as does *hyperthyroidism* or oversupplementation of thyroxine (see Chapter 80). *Immobility* is associated with thin bone, so any condition that limits daily activity can promote osteoporosis.

A slow loss of bone mass begins as a natural consequence of aging in the fourth decade of life. The menopausal transition has the greatest impact on bone health in women, with rates of bone loss that can exceed 4% per year and extend for 10 years or longer. There is individual variation in the rate and duration of bone loss. It appears that body fat, a nonovarian source of circulating estrogens, influences the rate of bone loss, with higher amounts of body fat protecting against menopausal bone loss. Studies of African American women have shown that, although on average they have higher peak bone mass than Caucasian women, they experience comparable rates of menopausal bone loss that are clinically significant for lean African American women (6).

Table 103.1. Determinants of Peak Bone Mass and Bone Loss

Peak Bone Mass	Bone Loss
Genetics	Menopause
Nutrition	Nutrition
Calcium	Calcium
Vitamin D	Vitamin D
Body mass	Body mass
Weight-bearing exercise	Weight-bearing exercise
Exposures	Exposures
Steroid medications	Steroid medications
Phenytoin	Phenytoin
Phosphate containing beverages	Phosphate containing beverages
Caffeinated beverages	Caffeinated beverages
Tobacco use	Tobacco use
Excessive alcohol intake	Excessive alcohol intake
Sex hormone deficiency	
Amenorrhea	
Pituitary disease	

Bone loss in women continues into older age: the Study of Osteoporotic Fractures showed clinically significant bone loss occurring in women 65 years of age and older (7). Factors contributing to this bone loss include inadequate intake of calcium and vitamin D, lack of weight-bearing exercise, and possibly age-related changes in endocrine functions beyond those of estrogen deficiency, including age-related decreases in circulating growth hormone and adrenal androgens (8).

The WHO has proposed a clinical definition of osteoporosis based on epidemiologic data that link low bone mass with increased fracture risk (discussed earlier). In study populations of Caucasian postmenopausal women, a bone mineral density that was more than 2.5 SD lower than normal peak bone mass was associated with a fracture prevalence of 50%, meaning that 50% of women with bone mass at this level had at least one bone fracture (9). Based on these data, the WHO defined osteoporosis as bone mineral density at least 2.5 SD lower than peak bone mass, osteopenia as bone mass between 1.0 and 2.5 SD lower than the peak, and normal as bone mineral density within 1.0 SD below the normal peak bone mass. However, the WHO criteria apply only to Caucasian, postmenopausal women and not men, premenopausal women, or women of ethnicity other than Caucasian. Clinically significant low bone mass is not yet classified in these populations.

SCREENING

Despite the prevalence and impact of osteoporosis, there is controversy about the effectiveness of screening populations for this disorder. One reason is that the cost-effectiveness of universal screening for osteoporosis has not been clearly demonstrated. Of course, counseling women for lifestyle modification, such as smoking cessation, exercise, and calcium intake, is recommended regardless of the results of testing. It is difficult to assess the impact of testing if a woman has decided to use postmenopausal estrogen replacement for other reasons. The results of several expert panels' recommendations for screening in postmenopausal women are listed in Table 103.2. One approach, as suggested by the U. S. Preventive Services Task Force, is to use screening in high-risk postmenopausal women if it would assist a woman's decision to take postmenopausal estrogen therapy (5). The National Osteoporosis Foundation guidelines recommend screening for women at menopause who have one additional

Table 103.2. Recommendations for Osteoporosis Screening

U. S. Preventive Services Task Force
High-risk postmenopausal women to assist with decision for hormonal therapy
National Osteoporosis Foundation Guidelines
Postmenopausal women <65 yr with additional risk factors
Women age 65 yr and older with no risk factors
Postmenopausal women <65 yr who present with fractures
Women who are considering therapy for osteoporosis
Women who have taken hormone replacement therapy for a prolonged period
Medicare Guidelines
Estrogen-deficient women at clinical risk for osteoporosis (includes estrogen users)
Individuals with vertebral abnormalities
Individuals receiving chronic glucocorticoid therapy
Individuals with primary hyperparathyroidism
Individuals being monitored to assess the response to an FDA-approved therapy

risk factor (10). The National Osteoporosis Foundation also suggests that bone densitometry is appropriate in the setting of a positive family history of osteoporosis, smoking, lean body habitus, chronic thyroxine or phenytoin use, height loss, vertebral deformity without radiographic confirmation, or any fracture for which the degree of trauma is disproportionate to the degree of injury. The American Academy of Family Physicians recommends screening in women age 40 to 64 years who have risk factors.

SCORE, a six-question screening questionnaire for osteoporosis, was shown to have 89% sensitivity and 50% specificity in an ambulatory population of postmenopausal women (11). This questionnaire (Fig. 103.1) can be used by caregivers to identify individuals for whom bone densitometry is warranted to confirm the clinical suspicion of osteoporosis.

Medicare guidelines for bone densitometry became effective July 1, 1998 (12). Criteria for the need for bone densitometry are as follows: (a) An estrogen-deficient woman at clinical risk for osteoporosis (the clinician can refer a postmenopausal woman who is receiving hormone replacement if there is concern that the therapy may not be preventing bone loss); (b) vertebral abnormalities demonstrated radiographically to be indicative of osteoporosis, osteopenia, or vertebral fracture; (c) chronic glucocorticoid use, defined as prednisone 7.5 mg/day or greater (or equivalent steroid) for 3 months or longer, or anticipated use of such therapy; (d) primary hyperparathyroidism; and (e) an individual being monitored to assess the response to, or efficacy of, an osteoporosis drug therapy approved by the U. S. Food and Drug Administration (FDA). Medicare will cover a bone mass measurement for a beneficiary once every two years. More frequent screening is covered if it is medically necessary, such as with steroid use or to confirm the findings of a screening study (e.g., ultrasound, peripheral bone densitometry). Medicare reimbursement for central bone densitometry (see later discussion) is roughly $140; peripheral densitometry and ultrasound studies are reimbursed at approximately $50.

It is now possible for patients to receive peripheral densitometry at locations such as pharmacies and health fairs. Again, because bone mass at peripheral sites changes more slowly with time and there is discordance in bone mass among various anatomic sites, a normal peripheral bone mass measurement in a patient with significant risk factors for osteoporosis should be confirmed with a bone mass measurement of the spine and hip.

Bone Densitometry

The current standard for assessing bone mass *is dual energy x-ray absorptiometry* (DEXA). Measurement of the bone mass of the lumbar spine and hip is currently used for diagnostic purposes and for monitoring of treatment. Measurement at peripheral sites (e.g., wrist, heel) can be a useful screening tool in older individuals; however, there is discordance among bone sites in rates of loss with aging. Many newly postmenopausal women have a normal bone mass of the heel and yet have clinically significant low bone mass of the spine. Falsely normal readings of the spine may occur in older women who have significant degenerative changes of the spine that result in calcification of the posterior structures of the vertebrae and adjacent soft tissues. Vertebral compression fractures also result in falsely elevated bone density measurements.

Currently, the different manufacturers of bone densitometers all use different reference populations from which the standard deviations from normal (T scores) are calculated. There are differences in calibration among companies as well, so that an individual patient's bone density reading can differ by as much as 12% from one machine to the next. Therefore, to monitor a patient's response to treatment, the same bone densitometer must be used. This is a challenge when patients are often referred to centers based on insurance coverage.

Whereas the T score is used to assess bone mass, diagnose osteoporosis, and predict fracture risk, the Z score, or comparison with age-matched individuals, is used to determine whether the patient's bone mass is unexpectedly low. A Z score of −2.0 or more is often used to determine whether a more extensive laboratory assessment should be done to assess for secondary causes of bone loss (e.g., myeloma, vitamin D deficiency, hyperparathyroidism).

The FDA has approved *ultrasound* techniques of the heel for use in screening tests for low bone mass (13). T scores of −1.8 or more are associated with significant risk of fracture, and T scores of −2.5 or more are considered to be diagnostic of osteoporosis for DEXA. Peripheral ultrasound is accurate, but there are insufficient data to access precision over time. Therefore, this technology is not currently used to monitor response to treatment, although this recommendation may change with more data. A positive screening result should be confirmed with DEXA of the spine and

Osteoporosis Evaluation: SCORE Sheet™

Name____ **Date**__________

1. How old are you? [|]

   ↑ **Multiply the number in this box by 3 and enter in the space at right**______

2. What is your race? ◯ African-American/Black American
   If checked, enter 0 at right ______

   ◯ Caucasian, Hispanic, Asian, Native American/American Indian, Other
   If checked, enter 5 at right ______

3. Have you ever been treated for or told you have rheumatoid arthritis? Yes ◯ No ◯
   If Yes, enter 4 at right/If No, enter 0 at right ______

4. Since the age of 45, have you experienced a fracture (broken bone) at any of the following sites?

   Hip Yes ◯ No ◯ **If Yes, enter 4 at right,/if No enter 0 at right** ______

   Rib Yes ◯ No ◯ **If Yes, enter 4 at right,/if No enter 0 at right** ______

   Wrist Yes ◯ No ◯ **If Yes, enter 4 at right,/if No enter 0 at right** ______

5. Are you now taking or have you ever taken hormone replacement therapy (for example: estrogen, Premarin, Estrace, Estaderm, or Estratab)?

   Yes ◯ No ◯ **If No, enter 1 at right/If Yes, enter 0 at right** ______

   Add scores from questions 1 – 5. ______
   SUBTOTAL

6. How much do you weigh now? [| |] (If weight is under 100, put 0 in the first box.)

   ↑ ↑

   Take the above numbers and enter in the space at right ______
   Then subtract from the subtotal.

   = ______
   TOTAL SCORE

If your score is 6 or higher, talk to you doctor about being evaluated further for osteoporosis.
If your score is less than 6, you should still talk to your doctor about osteoporosis and the risk factors associated with it.

This quiz is not a substitute for your physician's clinical judgment and consideration of any risk factors you may have.

™ **Bone Measurement Institute**

Figure 103.1. Osteoporosis screening questionnaire for postmenopausal women.

hip to obtain a baseline bone density measurement, from which treatments can be monitored for effectiveness. Also, because of discordance of bone loss with aging, a negative screening test result in the setting of significant risk factors should be confirmed with DEXA of spine and hip (Fig. 103.2).

A bone density study provides information on the patient's current bone mass but does not assess whether bone loss is accelerated. Blood and urine studies have been developed to assess bone turnover. Most of these measure markers that are breakdown products of proteins specific to bone, including n-telopeptide (NTX or Osteomark), C-telopeptide (CTX), and deoxypyridinoline crosslinks (Pyrilinks-D). The appropriate use of these markers in clinical practice is controversial (14). There are data to show that

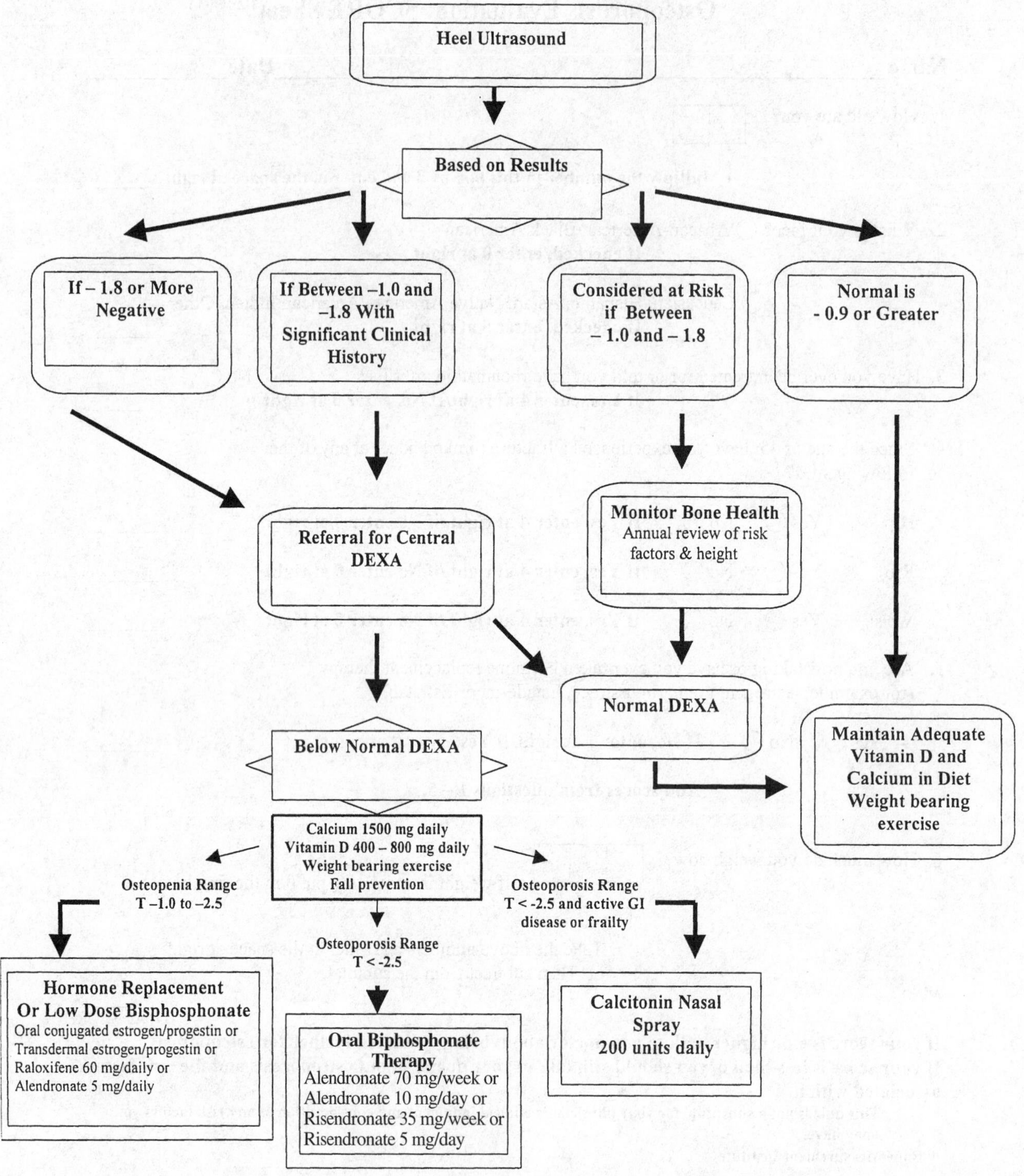

Figure 103.2. Algorithm for use of heel ultrasound as an osteoporosis screening test.

they predict perimenopausal bone loss as assessed by bone densitometry over 1 to 2 years. Small studies show that markers may be used to monitor response to treatments such as bisphosphonates and estrogen (15). Studies are repeated at 3 months after treatment. The variablity in measurements is estimated at 20%, and a decrease in value of 30% is considered a treatment response. Older women typically have low bone turnover at baseline, yet they respond to current osteoporosis treatments. Therefore, the utility of monitoring bone biomarkers in states other than high turnover ones such as perimenopause, hyperparathyroidism, hyperthyroidism, or Paget disease of the bone is not established.

Previous fractures predict future fractures. One vertebral fracture is associated with a fivefold increase in risk for subsequent vertebral fracture and a twofold increase in risk for hip fracture. Two or more vertebral fractures increase the risk of subsequent vertebral fracture by 12-fold (16). Almost half of frail elders admitted to an inpatient rehabilitation unit after a fracture had experienced a previous fracture. The majority of the earlier fractures were of minimal or short-term impact on functional state, whereas the more recent fracture greatly affected physical function. Yet, none of the earlier fractures resulted in an effective treatment program that may have prevented the more recent fracture.

The great majority of all fractures in older women result from falls (17). An elderly woman with a history of one or more falls should undergo a careful assessment of risk factors for falling and be helped to develop a strategy to prevent further falls (see Chapter 12).

Once osteoporosis is diagnosed, further laboratory studies to assess for metabolic bone diseases are needed based on the clinical history and the degree of osteoporosis. A serum calcium determination and measurement of the alkaline phosphatase level are recommended at the time of initial diagnosis; if these are normal, no further testing is routinely recommended. If the Z score is −2.0 SD below the peak or more negative, or if the history is relevant, other studies should be considered, including serum protein electrophoresis, serum thyroxine (T_4) and thyroid-stimulating hormone (TSH), serum parathyroid hormone, serum 25-hydroxyvitamin D, and 24-hour urinary calcium and cortisol excretion studies. Estrogen levels in blood or urine are not useful to predict bone loss.

PREVENTION

Primary health care should routinely address bone health (18). Young adults should be encouraged to achieve normal peak bone mass through adequate dietary calcium (1,000 mg daily), weight-bearing exercise, and maintenance of normal body weight and reproductive function. Young women who experience prolonged amenorrhea should receive hormone replacement, often in the form of estrogen-containing oral contraceptives.

For newly menopausal women at risk for accelerated bone loss from estrogen deficiency, the options for estrogen replacement are increasing, as is the information on risks and benefits of estrogen replacement therapy (Chapter 106).

Compliance with long-term estrogen therapy is enhanced by educating women that the risk of death from hip fracture is equal to the risk of death from breast cancer.

Selective *estrogen receptor modulators* such as *raloxifene*, 60 mg daily, offer a choice to women who are unable to take estrogen. The effects of raloxifene on bone and lipids are comparable to those seen after estrogen replacement (19). There appear to be no growth-promoting effects on breast or endometrium, thus reducing the risk profile of hormone replacement. The downside to raloxifene is that hot flushes are not improved over placebo, and the risk of thromboembolic disease (see Chapter 57) is at least comparable to that associated with estrogen replacement. Cost is also an issue, with estrogen/progestin therapy costing roughly $25 per month, whereas raloxifene is more than $60 per month. Because there are no long-term data on the benefits and risks of these newer pharmacologic agents, it is reasonable to recommend more traditional estrogen and progestin treatments as initial hormone replacement measures and to limit selective estrogen receptor modulator therapy to those who do not tolerate estrogen therapy or who are unwilling to use estrogen due to increased risk of breast cancer. For example, many women who have first-degree relatives with breast cancer will not consider estrogen, although there are no data to support an increased risk of breast cancer with estrogen therapy beyond that of the family history.

Tamoxifen, an older selective estrogen receptor modulator currently used to treat breast cancer, has estrogenic effects on bone. A study of tamoxifen use in older nursing home residents found that those who took 10 mg of tamoxifen daily had a lower rate of hip fracture than women not receiving such therapy (20). However, raloxifene, an FDA-approved drug for treatment of osteoporosis, is recommended over tamoxifen for women who are not being treated for breast cancer.

There is evidence to suggest that initiating estrogen therapy in older women may be of benefit to bone mass, although the maximum benefits are achieved through early menopausal hormone replacement and maintenance of the estrogen-repleted state for the long term. For example, the Study of Osteoporotic Fractures provided epidemiologic data that bone loss continues in older women and that estrogen may decrease this loss (21). The average rate of bone loss from the total hip in this study was sufficient to increase the risk of hip fracture by 21% per 5 years in women age 80 years or older. However, compared with nonusers, current estrogen users had a 33% lower age-adjusted mean rate of loss at the total hip. There are no completed long-term clinical trials of estrogen in older women; however the Women's Health Initiative is conducting a study to determine the risk–benefit ratio of estrogen use in older postmenopausal women. At present, the maximum benefit to bone is currently achieved with bisphosphonate therapy, so it appears that initiating estrogen therapy in women more than 10 years postmenopause may not be the optimal strategy except in the setting of mild osteopenia.

Nutritional supplements that contain *plant-derived estrogenic compounds* are under study for their potential to improve bone health. Currently, 50 mg per day of isoflavones is considered the minimum effective intake to prevent osteoporosis (22).

Bisphosphonates such as alendronate 5 mg daily, or a 35-mg tablet once weekly, have been shown to prevent accelerated bone loss in newly postmenopausal women and may be useful for women who are unable to take estrogen due to a history of estrogen-sensitive cancers or raloxifene due to clotting disorders (23). Bisphosphonate therapy is not recommended for women considering pregnancy, because the drug remains in bone for years after the last dose, and its potential to impair fetal bone development has not been adequately studied.

Calcium absorption declines with estrogen deficiency and aging. Postmenopausal women younger than 65 years of age who are not receiving estrogen, as well as all men and women older than 65 years of age, should receive 1,500 mg elemental calcium daily (24). Dietary sources are less constipating and include milk, yogurt, calcium-fortified fruit juices, and breakfast cereals. Chocolate chews that contain 500 mg elemental calcium and 100 to 200 units of vitamin D are a low-caloric dietary supplement. Tablets of calcium with and without vitamin D are available in chewable and nonchewable forms. No one source of calcium has been determined to be more effective clinically, although calcium citrate may be less constipating. Personal choice should be considered in planning strategies for calcium supplementation to achieve long-term compliance.

Vitamin D deficiency occurs when older individuals do not drink vitamin D–fortified milk, take a daily multiple vitamin that includes 400 units of vitamin D, or receive 15 minutes of daily sun exposure to the face. Vitamin D absorption declines with aging and with small bowel resection. Ideally, individuals older than 65 years of age should receive 800 units of vitamin D daily (see Chapter 84).

Weight-bearing exercise is recommended to maintain bone health with aging. Walking is excellent weight-bearing exercise for the hips. A weight-lifting program is recommended for the spine and arms under the guidance of an exercise physiologist to prevent neck and spine injuries due to excessive use of the weights. Strong muscles can absorb the physical forces associated with falls and reduce risk of bone fracture. Any physical activity that promotes muscle strength is helpful to bone, including swimming and water aerobics, both of which are well-tolerated forms of exercise, especially for women with osteoarthritis or other musculoskeletal conditions that limit their ability to walk or lift weights.

Other behavioral strategies to prevent osteoporosis include smoking cessation and limiting phosphate-containing, caffeine-containing, and alcoholic beverages to two per day.

TREATMENT

Osteoporosis management is evolving. There is consensus that calcium intake should be achieved through diet and supplements equal to 1,500 mg of elemental calcium daily. *Vitamin D* recommendations are 800 to 1,000 units daily. *Weight-bearing exercise* has been shown to increase bone mass, but weight lifting should be performed under the guidance of a trained professional to prevent vertebral fractures. The National Osteoporosis Foundation has developed an exercise video tape that focuses on abdominal and back muscle exercises and is recommended even in the setting of severe osteoporosis and frailty.

At present, there are three FDA-approved, non–sex-steroid treatments for postmenopausal osteoporosis, all of which act principally to inhibit bone resorption (Table 103.3). These include oral bisphosphonates, selective estrogen receptor modulators, and calcitonin.

Table 103.3. Comparison of Osteoporosis Treatments

Drug	Cost Per Month	Prevention Dose	Treatment Dose	Advantages	Disadvantages
Calcium	$4–$10	1,000 mg daily	1,500 mg daily Carbonate 500 mg/tab Citrate 325 mg/tab	Adjuvent to other treatments	Constipation
Vitamin D	$2–$5	400 I.U. daily	800–1,000 I.U.	Adjuvent to other treatments	
Alendronate	$67	5 mg daily 35 mg weekly	10 mg daily 70 mg weekly	Most effective class of antiresorptive agents	Gastrointestinal side effects of acid reflux and constipation
Risedronate	$60	5 mg daily 35 mg weekly	5 mg daily 35 mg weekly	Most effective class of antiresorptive agents	Gastrointestinal side effects of acid reflux and constipation
Estrogen				Effective for prevention; treats hot flushes; improves lipid profile	Vaginal bleeding, breast tenderness, increased risk of breast cancer in the long term
Conjugated					
Animal	$30	0.3–0.625 mg/d	0.3–0.625 mg/d		
Plant	$40–$60	0.3–0.625 mg/d	0.3–0.625 mg/d		
Estradiol					
Oral	$30–$60	1 mg daily	1 mg daily		
Transdermal	$40–$60	50 μg patch twice weekly	50 μg patch twice weekly		
Raloxifene	$60	60 mg daily	60 mg daily	Does not stimulate breast or endometrium	Hot flushes Blood clots
Intranasal calcitonin	$60	200 I.U. daily	200 I.U. daily	No gastrointestinal side effects	No effect on hip fracture risk

Oral Bisphosphonates

Alendronate, 10 mg daily (25), or risedronate, 5 mg daily (26), were shown in 3-year clinical trials to reduce the risk of new vertebral and hip fractures by about 50%. Gastrointestinal side effects are the most common, especially nausea, acid reflux symptoms, and constipation. To maximize absorption, the drug must be taken on an empty stomach with only water, and the patient must wait 30 to 60 minutes before eating or drinking. Adequate calcium and vitamin D (described previously) are essential for optimizing treatment response. There are data to show that alternative alendronate dosing of 70 mg once weekly results in increases in bone density at 1 year similar to those achieved with daily alendronate therapy, but with less gastrointestinal adverse reactions (27). The 70-mg tablet of alendronate is now available for once-weekly dosing. Risedronate, 5 mg daily, has been shown to significantly reduce vertebral fractures after just 12 months of therapy. Reanalysis of the alendronate database showed similar early reductions in vertebral fracture. Short-term studies showed less asymptomatic gastric erosions with risedronate than with alendronate (28). The clinical significance of these data is questioned given that most asymptomatic gastric erosions observed with nonsteroidal anti-inflammatory drugs healed without intervention in previous studies. There are not sufficient data to distinguish adverse effect profiles or the efficacy of postprandial dosing alternatives that have been approved outside the United States for risedronate dosing. Most likely, other oral bisphosphonates will receive FDA approval. Cycled etidronate is not recommended for use in menopausal osteoporosis, because studies have suggested that long-term etidronate may lead to impairment in new bone formation (29).

Data support the use of alendronate 10 mg or risedronate 5 mg daily in the prevention and treatment of steroid-induced osteoporosis in both women and men (30). Further data support the combination of estrogen and bisphosphonate as additive to increase bone mass at 1 year, but the burden and cost of two-drug therapy must be weighed against the modest increase of about 1% additional increase in bone density at 1 year (31).

Bisphosphonate therapy is possible via intravenous infusion. Although this therapy not approved by the FDA for treatment of osteoporosis, pamidronate 30 or 60 mg infused intravenously over 2 hours every 3 months for 2 years was shown to increase bone mineral density of the spine and the hip by roughly 11% and 5.5%, respectively (32). Ibandronate has been given by intravenous push rather than lengthy infusion, but this therapy is not yet available in the United States for clinical use (33).

Calcitonin

Calcitonin, given in a nasal spray (200 units) or one metered puff daily, alternating nostrils, is a second-line treatment for those who do not tolerate bisphosphonate therapy. This therapy has been shown to reduce the risk of vertebral fractures, but the effects on the hip appear to be less than that of bisphosphonate therapy (34). Calcitonin is considered second-line therapy to bisphosphonates for both postmenopausal and steroid-induced osteoporosis.

Other Treatments

Selective *estrogen receptor modulators* such as raloxifene and tamoxifen are considered less effective than bisphosphonates and are best employed for prevention or treatment of mild osteoporosis.

Parathyroid hormone, at low doses, increases new bone formation, but in excess it leads to bone loss, as seen in hyperparathyroid syndromes. Recently, nightly subcutaneous injections of parathyroid hormone were reported to increase bone density and to reduce vertebral fractures, similar to the effects that were found in previous studies of currently available oral bisphosphonates (35). Trials combining parathyroid hormone injections with bisphosphonates are ongoing.

Sodium monofluorophosphate plus calcium has been shown to reduce vertebral fractures; however, as with calcitonin, the effects on bone mineral density of the total hip were not significant (36). Fluoride therapy does not have approval of the FDA, and older studies in which it was taken without vitamin D supplementation resulted in osteomalacia.

Hormonal therapies such as testosterone, dihydroepiandrosterone (DHEA), and growth hormone have been tested, but none of these therapies is available for clinical use to treat osteoporosis. Growth factors that are specific to bone formation rather than systemic in effect are under clinical investigation.

An osteoporosis treatment program can often be implemented in the setting of new fracture, a time when many patients who were previously unwilling to consider osteoporosis management become interested. Calcium supplementation should be prescribed, although 1,500 mg daily may not be tolerated initially owing to constipation from narcotic pain medications prescribed for fracture pain. Vitamin D, 800 to 1,000 units, is recommended. Bisphosphonate therapy in this setting has been difficult to implement due to the high prevalence of gastroesophageal reflux and constipation, although once-weekly dosing may be tolerated. Calcitonin therapy has less adverse effects and is used routinely in the management of acute vertebral fractures.

General References*

Osteoporosis: review of the evidence for prevention, diagnosis, and treatment and cost-effectiveness analysis. Osteoporosis Int 1998;8[Suppl 4]:5007.

Miller PD. Management of osteoporosis. Adv Intern Med 1999;44:175.

*Bold print (general references) and bold numerals (specific references) denote published controlled clinical trials, meta-analyses, or consensus-based recommendations.

National Institutes of Health. Osteoporosis prevention, diagnosis, and therapy. NIH Consensus Statement 2001;285:785.

Eastell R. Treatment of postmenopausal osteoporosis. N Engl J Med 1998;338:736.

Specific References

1. Melton LJ III, Chrischilles EA, Cooper C, et al. Perspective: how many women have osteoporosis? J Bone Miner Res 1992;7:1005.
2. Melton LJ III, Atkinson EJ, O'Fallon WM, et al. Long-term fracture prediction by bone mineral assessed at different skeletal sites. J Bone Miner Res 1993;8:1227.
3. Miller PD. Management of osteoporosis. Adv Intern Med 1999;44:175.
4. Riggs BL, Melton LJ 3rd. The prevention and treatment of osteoporosis. N Engl J Med 1992;327:620.
5. National Institutes of Health. Osteoporosis prevention, diagnosis, and therapy. NIH Consensus Statement 2001;285:785.
6. Luckey MM, Wallenstein S, Lapinski R, et al. A prospective study of bone loss in African-American and white women: a clinical research center study. J Clin Endocrinol Metab 1996;81:2948.
7. Cummings SR, Black DM, Nevitt MC, et al. Bone density at various sites for prediction of hip fractures: The Study of Osteoporotic Fractures Research Group. Lancet 1993;341:72.
8. Anonymous. Consensus Development Conference: diagnosis, prophylaxis, and treatment of osteoporosis. Am J Med 1993;94:646.
9. The WHO Study Group. Assessment of fracture risk and its application to screening for postmenopausal osteoporosis. Geneva: World Health Organization, 1994.
10. National Osteoporosis Foundation. Physician's guide to prevention and treatment of osteoporosis. Belle Mead, NJ: Excerpta Medica, 1999.
11. Lydick E, Cook K, Turpin J, et al. Development and validation of a simple questionnaire to facilitate identification of women likely to have low bone density. Am J Managed Care 1998;4:37.
12. Health Care Financing Administration. Medicare Program. Medicare coverage and payment for bone mass measurements. Federal Register 1998;63(121):34320.
13. Cheng S, Tylavsky F, Carbone L. Utility of ultrasound to assess risk of fracture. J Am Geriatr Soc 1997;1382.
14. Garnero P, Hausherr E, Chapuy MC, et al. Markers of bone resorption predict hip fracture in elderly women: The EPIDOS prospective study. J Bone Miner Res 1996;11:1531.
15. Hamwi A, Ganem AH, Grebe C, et al. Markers of bone turnover in postmenopausal women receiving hormone replacement therapy. Clin Chem Lab Med 2001;39:414.
16. Ross PD, et al. Pre-existing fractures and bone mass predict vertebral fracture incidence in women. Ann Intern Med 1991;114:919.
17. Cummings SR, Nevitt MC, for the Study of Osteoporotic Fractures Research Group. Non-skeletal determinants of fractures: the potential importance of the mechanics of falls. Osteoporos Int 1994;1[Suppl]:657.
18. Eastell R. Treatment of postmenopausal osteoporosis. N Engl J Med 1998;338:736.
19. Ettinger B, Black DM, Mitlak BH, et al. Reduction of vertebral fracture risk in postmenopausal women with osteoporosis treated with raloxifene: results of a 3-year randomized clinical trial. JAMA 1999;282:637.
20. Breuer B, Wallenstein S, Anderson R. Effect of tamoxifen on bone fractures in older nursing home residents. J Am Geriatr Soc 1998;46:968.
21. Ensrud KE, Palermo L, Black DM, et al. Hip and calcaneal bone loss increase with advancing age: longitudinal results from the study of osteoporotic fractures. J Bone Miner Res 1995;10:1778.
22. Consensus Opinion. The role of isoflavones in menopausal health: consensus opinion of the North American Menopause Society. Menopause 2000;7:215.
23. McClung M, Clemmesen B, Daifotis A, et al. Alendronate prevents postmenopausal bone loss in women without osteoporosis. Ann Intern Med 1998;128:253.
24. Dawson-Hughes B, Harris SS, Krall EA, et al. Effect of calcium and vitamin D supplementation on bone density in men and women 65 years of age or older. N Engl J Med 1997;337:670.
25. Cummings SR, Black DM, Thompson DE, et al. Effect of alendronate on risk of fracture in women with low bone density but without vertebral fractures: results from the Fracture Intervention Trial. JAMA 1998;280:2077.
26. Harris ST, Watts NB, Genant HK, et al. Effects of risedronate treatment on vertebral and nonvertebral fractures in women with postmenopausal osteoporosis. JAMA 1999;282:1344.
27. Schnitzer T, Bone HG, Crepaldi G, et al. Therapeutic equivalence of alendronate 70 mg once-weekly and alendronate 10 mg daily in the treatment of osteoporosis. Aging Clin Exp Res 2000;12:1.
28. Lanza FL, Hunt RH, Thomson ABR, et al. Endoscopic comparison of esophageal and gastroduodenal effects of risedronate and alendronate in postmenopausal women. Gastroenterology 2000;119:631.
29. Sahota O, Fowler I, Blackwell PJ, et al. A comparison of continuous alendronate, cyclic alendronate, cyclical etidronate with calcitriol in the treatment of postmenopausal osteoporosis: a randomized controlled trial. Osteoporosis Int 2000;11:959.
30. Saag KG, Emkey R, Schnitzer TJ, et al. Alendronate for the prevention and treatment of glucocorticoid-induced osteoporosis. N Engl J Med 1998;339:292.
31. Bone HG, Greenspan SL, McKeever C, et al. Alendronate and estrogen effects in postmenopausal women with low bone mineral density. J Clin Endocrinol Metab 2000;85:720.
32. Thiebaud D, Burckhardt P, Melchior J, et al. Two years of effectiveness of intravenous pamidronate versus oral fluoride in postmenopausal osteoporosis. Osteoporos Int 1994;4:76.
33. Thiebaud D, Burckhardt P, Kriegbaum H. Three monthly intravenous injections of ibandronate in the treatment of postmenopausal osteoporosis. Am J Med 1997;103:298.
34. Gennari C, Camporeale A. Calcitonin in the treatment of osteoporosis. Osteoporos Int 1997;7[Suppl 3]:S159.
35. Neer RM, Arnaud CD, Zanchetta JR, et al. Effect of parathyroid hormone (1-34) on fractures and bone mineral density in postmenopausal women with osteoporosis. N Engl J Med 2001;344:1434.
36. Reginster JY, Meurmans L, Zegels B, et al. The effect of sodium monofluorophosphate plus calcium on vertebral fracture rate in postmenopausal women with moderate osteoporosis. Ann Intern Med 1998;129:1.

CHAPTER 104

Early Detection of Gynecologic Malignancy

CATHERINE S. TODD, MD, MPH
GEORGE R. HUGGINS, MD

The female reproductive organs are common sites for the development of malignancy. Roughly 14% of cancers in women arise from the genital tract (1). Women who have a gynecologic cancer discovered while it is still confined to the site of origin can expect a 60% to 90% 5-year survival rate. In contrast, more extensive cancers involving distant spread have a 5-year survival rate of 0% to 60%. If preinvasive lesions are detected and appropriate treatment is initiated, a 100% cure rate is expected. The vulva, vagina, and cervix all have well-characterized preinvasive lesions.

With the exception of the vulva and breast, the patient is unable to perform a satisfactory gynecologic self-screening examination. However, with the pelvic examination, all components of the genital system except the fallopian tubes may be inspected, palpated, and screened for cancer or its precursors. Therefore, practitioner-initiated screening is vital for women at risk for gynecologic malignancies.

VULVAR LESIONS

The vulvar skin is subject to disease similar to that of the skin elsewhere, but the prevalence of various conditions is modified in that the vulva does not receive direct sun exposure. The benign conditions are common, whereas the malignant conditions are uncommon, representing only approximately 2% of malignancies of the female genital tract (1). Squamous cell carcinoma comprises almost 85% of all vulvar cancers, followed by melanoma (5%) and sarcoma (2%). In contrast, basal cell cancer, common in sun-exposed skin, accounts for only 2% to 7% of vulvar malignancies (2–4).

Preinvasive lesions of the vulva are called *vulvar intraepithelial neoplasia* (VIN). This term is now used to include diseases that were once called *Bowen disease, erythroplasia of Queyrat, squamous cell carcinoma* in situ, *Paget disease, and condyloma acuminata.* The average age of women with preinvasive lesions is between 40 and 50 years. However, a disturbing trend in the last 20 years has been a doubling in the rate of VIN, with significantly younger age at presentation, primarily attributed to human papillomavirus (HPV) exposure (5). Most women with invasive vulvar cancer are diagnosed in the seventh decade of life, although the disease may occasionally develop in women younger than 40 years of age. This age differential supports the hypothesis that progression from preinvasive lesions to cancer of the vulva is an indolent process. An increased risk of vulvar cancer is associated with a history of condyloma acuminata, increasing number of lifetime sexual partners, immunosuppression, and smoking.

The pathognomonic lesion of VIN is a papular or maculopapular lesion with a roughened surface; however, VIN can have many different appearances, and the lesions often appear to be well defined and innocent. The lesions may vary from white to hyperpigmented. They may be sharply demarcated or generalized over the vulva and may even spread to adjacent regions. Some may resemble seborrheic keratoses, nevi, lentigo, intertrigo, condylomata acuminata, or condylomata lata. Because VIN and vulvar cancer can masquerade as many other disease entities, the diagnosis and definitive treatment are often delayed while treatment for an incorrectly diagnosed lesion is instituted. Some women with vulvar cancer note symptoms for up to 16 months before seeking treatment. Furthermore, medical management may have been used for up to 12 months before the definitive diagnosis was made (6).

One should be suspicious when any lesion is seen, especially if the lesions are chronic and not immediately responsive to topical treatment. The most common symptom of vulvar neoplasia is itching, which occurs in 70% of patients. Other symptoms include ulceration, bleeding, pain, or the presence of a mass.

No vulvar equivalent of the cervical Papanicolaou (Pap) smear is available; therefore the primary method of diagnosis of lesions is early recognition and prompt referral to a gynecologist for diagnosis by biopsy.

The treatment of VIN depends on the extent of the lesion. If the vulvar lesions grossly appear to be *condyloma acuminata* and are not extensive, they may be treated empirically without biopsy (see Chapter 102). If no decrease in size is apparent within 2 to 4 weeks, the suspected condylomata acuminata should be biopsied to confirm the diagnosis. The gynecologist and pathologist must be aware of prior treatment of the lesion, because podophyllin and 5-fluorouracil (two common topical agents used in the treatment of condyloma acuminata) can cause abnormal mitoses and bizarre cells that may lead an erroneous diagnosis of advanced VIN or cancer.

Small lesions may be excised entirely. Laser vaporization, ultrasonic ablation, or skinning vulvectomy is necessary for widespread disease.

Vulvar cancer can also masquerade as *vulvar dystrophy* (formerly known as *lichen sclerosus, atrophic vulvitis, or kraurosis vulvae*). Once these lesions are proven by biopsy, they may be treated safely by a general gynecologist by the application of a topical steroid with regular follow-up to prevent atrophic changes related to overuse of steroid cream.

Prevention of advanced disease requires that the patient be taught to examine her vulva periodically with the use of a mirror and to report any changes in the external genitalia. It is important that one examine the patient promptly if a change is noted and that a periodic examination, usually in conjunction with a routine gynecologic examination, be performed even when there are no complaints. Special sensitivity must be used in older women, who often are reluctant to complain of a vaginal or vulvar problem and who are resistant to a screening vaginal examination.

CERVICAL LESIONS

Epidemiology and Etiologic Factors

Invasive epithelial carcinoma of the cervix is the third most common malignancy of the reproductive organs after endometrial and ovarian carcinoma. Approximately 12,900 new cases of cervical cancer are diagnosed annually in the United States, with approximately 4,340 deaths annually (1). Significant reduction in mortality and morbidity has been achieved by vigorous promotion and acceptance of the annual pelvic examination in combination with the cancer detection smear (Pap smear) (7). The incidence of cervical cancer has increased in younger women. In 1981, women younger than 50 years old accounted for 21% of all cervical cancer deaths. By 1987 this figure had risen to 27%, and by 1997 it had risen further to 43.9% for women younger than 55 years of age (1,8). The increase in cervical cancer in this population parallels the increasingly early onset of sexual activity among women. In 1971, 28% of 15- to 19-year-old women reported that they had had sexual relations; by 1982, this figure was 42%, and by 1995, it was 50% (9).

HPV is a significant etiologic agent in the development of cervical cancer; HPV DNA is found in more than 90% of all cervical cancers (10). The virus is transmitted sexually, by autoinnoculation from condylomata elsewhere on the body, or from mother to neonate. More than 60 strains of HPV have been identified, at least 11 of which are tropic for the genital tract. HPV 6/11 are most often found in cervical condylomata and low-grade dysplasia. HPV 16 is found in approximately 55% of cervical cancers, HPV 18 is found in 15% to 20%, and HPV 31/33/35 are found occasionally (11). Women who become infected with HPV before 25 years of age are 40 times more likely to develop cervical cancer than those who are uninfected (12).

Infection with herpes simplex virus type 2 and with the Epstein–Barr virus correlates with the incidence of cervical cancer. The question remains whether these viruses are promoters, cocarcinogens, or solely an index of past sexual behavior. It is well documented, however, that human immunodeficiency virus (HIV) is a promoter of cancerous conditions resulting from HPV infection by allowing uncontrolled viral mutagenesis secondary to suppressed immune function (13). Decreased exposure to these agents through use of barrier contraception until a mutually monogamous relationship is established is a reasonable intervention.

Pap Smear

The mainstay of cervical cancer control is regular screening by means of Pap smears, with referral for colposcopy and biopsy whenever a significant abnormality is found. *Colposcopy* is an office procedure, done during a pelvic examination with the use of an instrument similar to a dissecting microscope. It illuminates and magnifies (8× to 10×) the cervix, vagina, and vulva. In spite of the popularity of the Pap smear, there are severe caveats about it that are often not appreciated. The efficacy of the Pap smear as a screening tool has never been tested in a prospective, blinded study. The typical false negative rate for a Pap smear in most laboratories is 20%, but reports cite values ranging from 3% to 60% (7). Despite this limitation, the widespread use of the Pap smear has been accompanied by a significant decrease in the incidence of invasive carcinoma of the cervix. Likewise, there has been a corresponding increase in the detection of preinvasive lesions (Fig. 104.1). The success of cytologic screening of the cervix has led many physicians to place an inordinate amount of faith in the Pap smear. Indeed, 25%

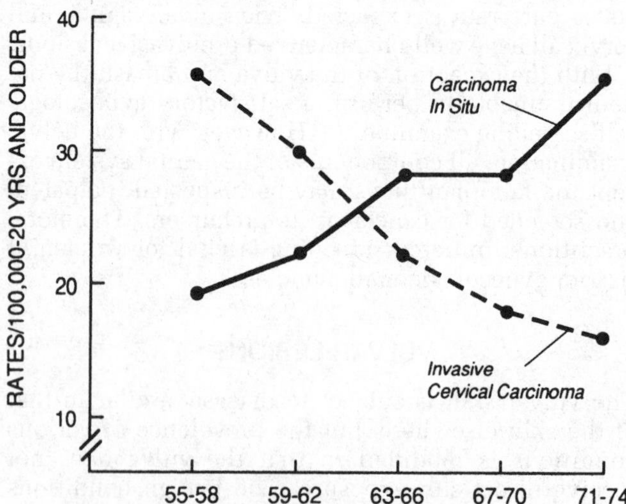

Figure 104.1. Average annual age-adjusted incidence rate trends for invasive carcinoma and carcinoma *in situ* of the cervix from the Toledo, Ohio, area. (Redrawn from Kim K, Rigal RD, Patrick JR, et al. The changing trends of uterine cancer and cytology: a study of morbidity and mortality trends over a twenty year period. Cancer 1978;42:2439.)

of all missed cervical cancers result from false negative screening results (14). Some new screening techniques have been introduced, most notably liquid suspension Pap test techniques. However, the improvement in test sensitivity is variable, and the cost is substantially increased for this method. The liquid suspension method is acceptable clinically, but whether it is preferable is controversial (14,15). It should never be considered a perfect diagnostic test. Any visible cervical lesions of uncertain origin may represent an early cancer, and patients with such lesions should be referred to a gynecologist for evaluation.

A screening Pap smear should not be obtained if a woman has douched or used vaginal medication or a tampon in the previous 24 hours. These activities may alter or remove cells completely and yield an erroneous interpretation. Lubricants may also interfere with cytologic interpretation. The speculum used in the examination should be unlubricated or, if necessary, lubricated only with water.

The most important area to be sampled is the squamocolumnar junction, because most cervical neoplastic processes arise at this site. The anatomic relationships of this junction are different in the adolescent, the sexually active woman, and the postmenopausal woman (Fig. 104.2). Once the cervix is visualized, the cervical spatula should be placed firmly against the cervix and rotated at least 360°, preferably 720°, in a continuous unidirectional sweep. A plastic brush (Endo-C, Milex Chicago) should be used to sample the endocervical canal. This increases the recovery of endocervical cells and decreases the number of inadequate Pap smears. Both specimens should then be smeared together onto a clean microscopic slide and immediately sprayed or immersed in fixative to prevent an air-drying artifact. An additional sample taken from the posterior vaginal fornix of perimenopausal or postmenopausal women may occasionally detect malignant cells that have exfoliated from the endometrium, fallopian tubes, or ovaries.

One should select a reputable cytology laboratory, use the proper fixative techniques required by the laboratory, and learn the reporting systems of the particular laboratory. In 1988, the National Cancer Institute Workshop recommended a revision in the manner of reporting the results of the Pap smear known as the Bethesda System (16). It is important to provide the laboratory with the patient's age and the date of her last menstrual period, and to comment on the presence or absence of infection. The laboratory report should state whether the sample was satisfactory or unsatisfactory. An unsatisfactory slide must be repeated. The Pap smear is unsatisfactory if no endocervical cells are present in a specimen obtained from a premenopausal woman with an intact cervix (7).

The Bethesda System is the method currently recognized for reporting cervical and vaginal cytology. There are four categories of squamous epithelial cell abnormalities: atypical squamous cells of undetermined significance (ASCUS), low-grade squamous intraepithelial lesion (LSIL), high-grade squamous intraepithelial lesion (HSIL), and squamous cell carcinoma. Patients with Pap smears showing HSIL or squamous carcinoma should be referred to a gynecologist for evaluation and management. Some patients with LSIL who are reliable and free of risk factors can be simply monitored, because approximately 60% of LSILs regress spontaneously. These women need Pap smears every 4 to 6 months for 2 years. If repeat Pap smears show persistent abnormalities, the patient should be referred for colposcopy and biopsy.

Pap smears showing ASCUS are further qualified as either reactive or suggestive of an intraepithelial lesion. Specific cervical or vaginal infections associated with an ASCUS-reactive report (see Chapter 102) should be treated and the smear repeated in 3 months. A few weeks after treatment, 90% of smears with atypia secondary to chlamydia revert to normal (17). ASCUS Pap smears favoring intraepithelial lesion should be treated as LSIL Pap smears, with careful follow-up or colposcopy and biopsy, especially if risk factors are present or follow-up is questionable (18).

A consensus panel convened in 1988 made recommendations regarding frequency of cervical cancer screening (16). Annual screening should begin once a woman is 18 years old or becomes sexually active and should continue into the postmenopausal years. After a woman has had three consecutive annual Pap smears that are satisfactory and normal, the interval may be reduced to every 1 to 3 years, at the provider's discretion, depending on the presence of risk factors for cervical cancer (Table 104.1). These include HPV infection, HIV infection, cigarette smoking, and multiple sexual partners. Additional risk factors for preinvasive lesions, which should be considered as well, include early age at first coitus, early age at first pregnancy, low socioeconomic status, and African American or Hispanic race.

After a patient has undergone treatment for a preinvasive lesion, there should be increased surveillance, preferably every 3 to 4 months, for 1 year. Cytologic smears may be performed yearly thereafter, if normal. Women who have undergone total hysterectomy (cervix removed) for malignant or premalignant disease should receive an annual smear from the vaginal apex to evaluate for local recurrence. The effectiveness of screening women whose hysterectomy was for benign indications has not been shown (19).

ENDOMETRIAL CARCINOMA

Epidemiology and Etiologic Factors

An estimated 38,300 cancers of the endometrium are detected each year. This is the most common gynecologic cancer, yet it has a relatively low mortality rate, with approximately 6,400 deaths annually, despite its high prevalence (1).

Unopposed estrogen stimulation has been firmly implicated in the genesis of this cancer, and several situations are associated with such exposure. Endogenous stimulation occurs in women who are anovulatory, such as patients with polycystic ovary disease,

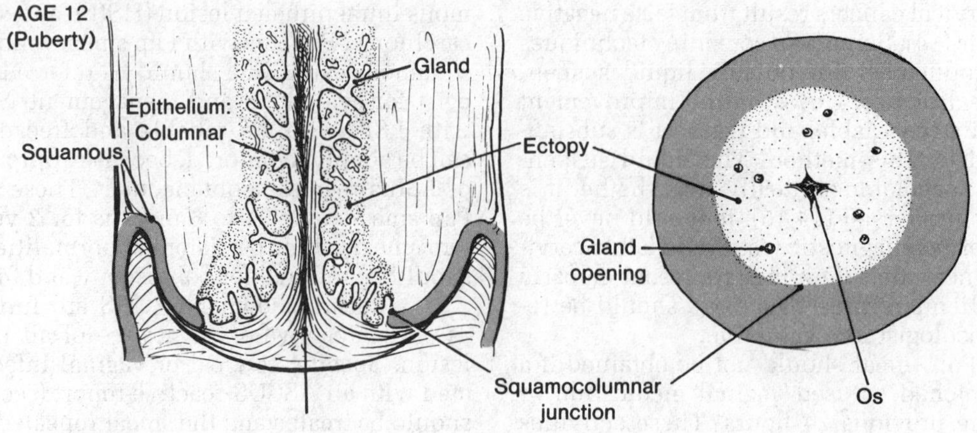

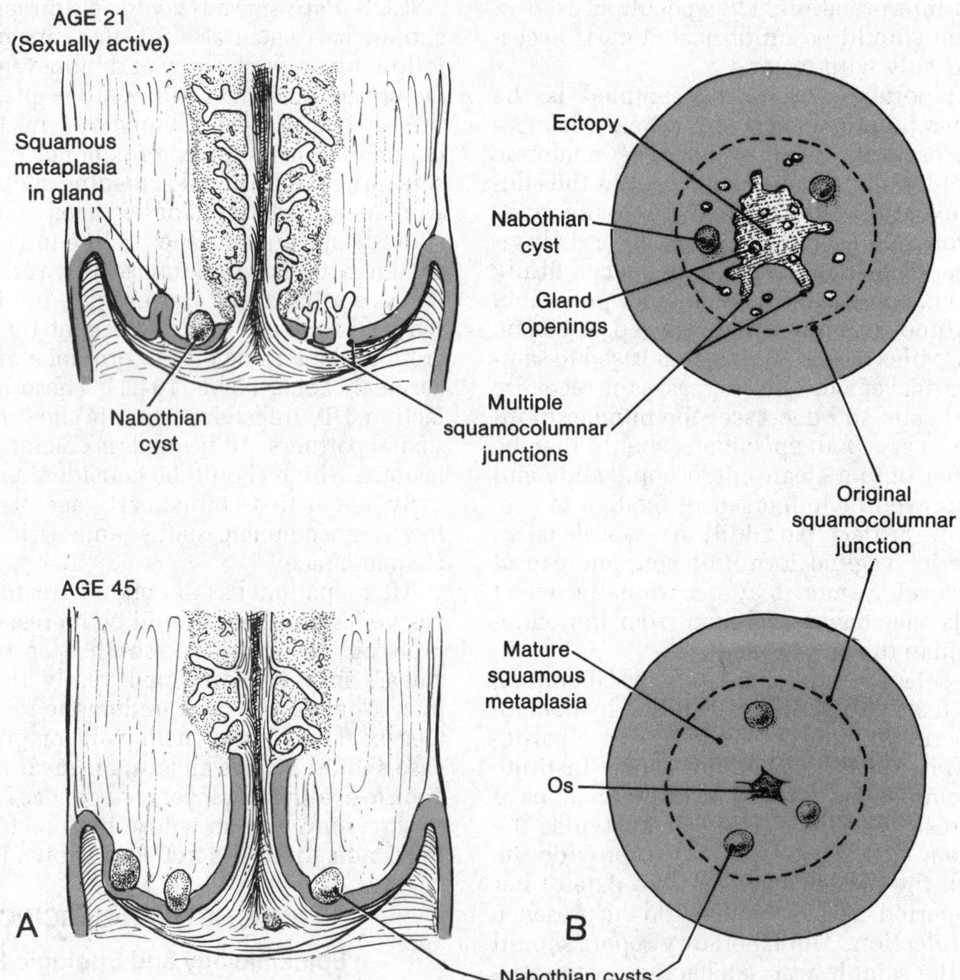

Figure 104.2. The uterine cervix in women of various ages. **A.** Coronal section of the cervix and vaginal vault. **B.** Vaginal view of the cervix. (Redrawn from Briggs RM. Dysplasia and early neoplasia of the uterine cervix: a review. Obstet Gynecol Surv 1980;34:70.)

diabetes mellitus, and extreme obesity. These women often have a history of infrequent menses and infertility. Factors that affect endometrial cancer risk are listed in Table 104.2.

Women who are extremely obese or who have diabetes mellitus metabolize sex steroids differently than do women with normal body weight. There is increased conversion of androstenedione to estrone, which stimulates the endometrium and predisposes it to cancer.

Long-term use of unopposed estrogen in postmenopausal women significantly increases the risk of

Table 104.1. Cervical Neoplasia Risk Factors

Epidemiologic Characteristics
Early intercourse
Multiple sex partners
Early marriage
Early child-bearing
Prostitution
Male factors: high-risk consort (see text)
Low socioeconomic status
African American or Hispanic race
Sexually transmitted infection
Other Potential Factors
Compromised immune status
Oral contraceptive use
Cigarette smoking
Prior radiation
Intrauterine exposure to diethylstilbestrol
Viral Associations
Papillomavirus
Herpesvirus
Cytomegalovirus

Table 104.2. Endometrial Carcinoma Risk Factors

Increased Risk	Diminished Risk
Unopposed menopausal estrogen replacement therapy	Ovulation
Menopause after 52 years of age	Progestin therapy
Obesity	Combination oral contraceptives
Nulliparity	Menopause before 49 years of age
Diabetes	Normal weight
Feminizing ovarian tumors	Multiparity
Polycystic ovary syndrome	
Tamoxifen therapy for breast cancer	

endometrial carcinoma. In the PEPI Trial, a longitudinal study looking at postmenopausal hormone replacement, 62.2% of women taking continuous unopposed estrogen developed abnormal endometrial histology during the 3 years of the trial. Of those who developed abnormal histology, one third did so during the first year of use (20). There is a 14-fold increase in risk of endometrial cancer among women who use unopposed estrogen replacement therapy for 7 years (21). This increased risk can be nullified by adding a progestin (e.g., Provera) to the estrogen regimen (see Chapter 106). In contrast, women who have used oral contraceptives and those who have had children have a reduced risk of endometrial cancer.

Screening Techniques

No population-based screening tools exist, but several methods for the early detection of endometrial cancer are suitable for office practice. To be broadly applied, such methods must be sensitive, specific, well tolerated, safe, and inexpensive, and they must lead to an effective intervention (22). The most accurate approach is to directly obtain a sample of endometrium for histologic examination. The most widely used instrument is the Pipelle endometrial suction curette (United International Marketing Resources, 475 Danbury Rd., Wilton, CT 06897; telephone 800-243-6608). The Pipelle is a flexible plastic tube 3.4 mm in external diameter with a small opening of 2.6 mm near the blunt tip. Suction is applied with an integral movable plastic plunger. Unfortunately, because of its flexibility, the Pipelle cannot always be inserted into a stenotic cervical os. This instrument produces minimal pain, and the specimen obtained is equivalent to that obtained with the Novak curette, but with less patient discomfort. The Pipelle biopsy is both sensitive and specific, although there have been reports of neoplasms residing solely in a polyp or covering less than 5% of the endometrial surface and not recovered by this method (23,24). For this reason, unexplained postmenopausal bleeding, even with negative Pipelle biopsy, should be investigated further.

All women with unexplained postmenopausal bleeding and those who are at high risk for endometrial cancer should undergo an evaluation. Additionally, some premenopausal women older than 30 years of age who have intermenstrual spotting, prolonged menses, or menorrhagia should be evaluated. Such an evaluation should consist of a pelvic examination and, if indicated, an endometrial biopsy. The size and consistency of the uterus should be noted. When observed over time, a rapid increase in uterine size may indicate malignancy rather than growth of fibroids. For women who are not bleeding but who are at increased risk for endometrial cancer (e.g., those with diabetes or obesity), transvaginal ultrasound may help determine the need for endometrial sampling. Those with an endometrial thickness greater than 5 mm who are not taking estrogen replacement (which increases the endometrial thickness) should undergo endometrial biopsy (25). Evaluation of postmenopausal bleeding or irregular bleeding in a patient at risk for endometrial carcinoma is typically managed by referral to a gynecologist.

The Pap smear obtained without an additional specimen from the vaginal pool is unreliable for the detection of endometrial cancer. When a sample is obtained from the vaginal pool, the recovery of abnormal endometrial cells may be as high as 65%. However, a normal Pap smear in a woman at risk for endometrial cancer should not delay further evaluation.

OVARIAN CANCER

Ovarian cancer is the most problematic gynecologic cancer. Most lesions are silent until they have reached a size large enough to produce symptoms from pressure of the mass and associated ascites. By this time, they have usually metastasized. The cure rate for advanced lesions is low. Approximately 23,400 new cases of ovarian cancer are discovered among American women each year, resulting in 13,300 deaths annually (1). Although ovarian cancer is the third most common gynecologic cancer, it has the highest mortality rate—50% of all deaths from gynecologic cancers. The cause of ovarian cancer is unknown, and little progress has been made in identifying the patient at

Table 104.3. Ovarian Carcinoma Risk Factors

Increased Risk	Decreased Risk
Older age	Multiparity
Late menopause	Oral contraceptive pills
Nulliparity	
Late child-bearing	
Breast-feeding	
Personal or family history of breast cancer	

risk, in early detection, or in improving the survival rate (26). The risk increases with increasing age and may affect 1% or 2% of women in their ninth decade. Factors that affect the risk of ovarian cancer are listed in Table 104.3.

The symptoms of ovarian cancer are nonspecific and are often ignored by both patient and physician until the tumor is far advanced. Most commonly, symptoms are referable to the gastrointestinal tract and consist of feelings of abdominal fullness, bloating, eructation, and pelvic pressure. Pain or constipation appears only very late. Abnormal uterine bleeding occurs only rarely in association with ovarian cancer.

The most common sign of ovarian cancer is an adnexal or abdominopelvic mass. The diagnostic evaluation of such a mass differs in each stage of a woman's life.

Premenarche Period

About two thirds of ovarian tumors are benign in this age group. The most common tumors are *benign cystic teratoma* (dermoid), *benign simple cyst,* and *cystadenoma.*

Malignant tumors in this age group arise from the germ cells or gonadal stromal cells in 80% to 90% of cases (27). Usually no risk factors are elucidated. The most common presenting complaint is pain, which is caused by rapid tumor growth. These neoplasms typically express a variety of serum tumor markers—lactate dehydrogenase, alpha-fetoprotein, human chorionic gonadotropin, and inhibin—which assist in making the diagnosis.

Reproductive Period

Most ovarian masses found during this period are functional cysts. The normal dimensions of the premenopausal ovary is 1.5 × 3 × 3.5 cm. If ovulation fails to occur, a unilocular cyst is formed and may reach 10 cm in diameter. When ovulation does occur, a corpus luteum forms that may occasionally become enlarged because of internal hemorrhage. Both of these ovarian cysts are often detected because of the frequent evaluation by pelvic examination of women in this age group. These cysts usually resolve spontaneously within 2 to 4 weeks.

If the ovarian enlargement is persistent after 2 to 4 weeks and if it is demonstrated to be truly cystic by ultrasound, a period of suppressive therapy and observation is warranted. Oral contraceptive pills containing 35 to 50 μg of ethinyl estradiol (see Chapter 100) may be prescribed for 3 months to suppress gonadotropins. This therapy prevents future cyst formation and provides a stable hormonal milieu for the existing cyst to regress. Estrogen blocks the pituitary gonadotrophins that are the stimulus for the formation and maintenance of ovarian cysts. If the ovarian cyst persists for longer than 90 days despite gonadotropin suppression, the diagnosis of ovarian neoplasia should be considered strongly and a gynecologist should be consulted.

In a classic study by Spanos observing persistent adnexal masses, 92% were benign neoplasms while 6.8% were malignant (28). Ultrasound is the best method to diagnose and monitor ovarian cysts. Any ovarian tumor that is irregular, septate, semisolid, solid, or larger than 8 cm in diameter on ultrasound evaluation should be strongly suspected to be malignant. For women with those findings, prompt arrangements for gynecologic consultation should be made.

Perimenopausal and Menopausal Periods

During this era of a woman's life the incidence of ovarian cancer is highest. In the American population, the annual incidence increases from 10 per 100,000 for women younger than 65 years of age to 55.3 per 100,000 after age 65 (1). This dramatic increase in incidence has led some investigators to propose aggressive means to manage minimal ovarian enlargement.

In 1973, Barber and Graber (29) proposed that any palpable ovary in a postmenopausal women is abnormal and requires laparotomy. They called this the *postmenopausal palpable ovary (PMPO) syndrome.* However, experience in recent years has proved that, although evaluation is essential, a more conservative approach to management of the PMPO syndrome is warranted. Fewer 10% of patients with the PMPO syndrome have an ovarian malignancy (30).

Although use of pelvic ultrasound and measurement of serum tumor markers (e.g., CA-125) is becoming more widespread for screening for ovarian cancer, the efficacy of these tests is controversial. The sensitivity of CA-125 as a single screening mechanism is low (particularly before menopause) (31); however, systems have been developed that combine patient age, ovarian volume on ultrasound, radiologic features of the mass, and possibly CA-125 values to predict the probability of malignancy. Two systems, the Risk of Malignancy Index (RMI) and the Ovarian Tumor Index (OTI), are best suited to determine the probability of malignancy in a known adnexal mass (32–34). Neither ultrasound nor computed tomography of the abdomen and pelvis is able to indicate the malignant potential of ovarian masses; nevertheless, these procedures are useful in determining the extent of the tumor. The determination of the concentration of tumor markers such as alpha-fetoprotein, human chorionic gonadotropin, and carcinoembryonic antigen may be helpful in the evaluation of an ovarian mass in a premenopausal woman and in monitoring the course of the patient after treatment. A newly identified tumor marker for ovarian cancer, lysophosphatidic acid (LPA), has a sensitivity and specificity superior to those of CA-125; however, the clinical application of this test has not yet been established (35).

Risk and Prevention

Ovarian cancer is one of the cancers that may be inherited, and such cases account for 10% of epithelial ovarian cancers. It has been linked to the BRCA1 and BRCA2 mutations and to the Lynch II syndrome (hMLH1 and hMSH2), and it is characterized by autosomal dominant inheritance. Genetic screening should be considered for any woman who has more than one first-degree relative with premenopausal breast cancer, a personal history of premenopausal breast cancer, or a family history of both premenopausal breast cancer and ovarian cancer at any age (36). If such a patient is identified, she should be referred to a gynecologic oncologist for further counseling and discussion of surveillance tactics. Generally, prophylactic oophorectomy after completion of child-bearing is recommended only for women with known familial cancer mutation. For patients who have not completed child-bearing and for any other woman of reproductive potential, the use of combined oral contraceptives significantly decreases the risk of ovarian cancer. The use of combined oral contraceptives can decrease the risk of ovarian by 10% to 12% with each year of use, with a 50% risk reduction after 5 years and 80% after 10 years of use. The protective effect appears to continue, regardless of the time of discontinuation of the combined oral contraceptives (37). This protection is also extended to women at risk for hereditary ovarian cancer, reducing their risk by 60% with less than 6 years and by 70% with more than 6 years of use (38).

The only available cost-effective method of screening for ovarian cancer is the periodic pelvic examination. Postmenopausal women should have periodic pelvic examinations if there are no mitigating factors that preclude aggressive therapy, such as very advanced age, chronic illness, or disability.

General References*

American College of Physicians. Screening for ovarian cancer: recommendations and rationale. Ann Intern Med 1994;121:141.

A thoughtful statement concerning the ineffectiveness of ovarian cancer screening in most women.

Berek JS, Hacker NF. Practical gynecologic oncology. 2nd ed. Baltimore: Williams & Wilkins, 1993.

Herbst AL, Mishell DR Jr, Stenchever MA, et al. Comprehensive gynecology. 2nd ed. St. Louis: CV Mosby, 1992.

Morow CP, Townsend DE. Synopsis of gynecologic oncology. New York: Wiley, 1987.

Sawaya GF, Brown AD, Washington AE, et al. Current approaches to cervical-cancer screening. N Engl J Med 2001;344:1603.

A case-based discussion of the current approaches to cervical cancer screening.

*Bold print (general references) and bold numerals (specific references) denote published controlled clinical trials, meta-analysis, or consensus-based recommendations.

Specific References

1. Ries LAG, Eisner MP, Kosary CL, et al. (eds). SEER Cancer Statistics Review: 1973–1998. Bethesda, MD: National Cancer Institute, 2001.
2. Mateus C, Fortier-Beaulieu M, Lhomme C, et al. [Basal cell carcinoma of the vulva: 21 cases]. Ann Dermatol Venereol 2001;128:11.
3. Piura B, Rabinovich A, Dgani R. Basal cell carcinoma of the vulva. J Surg Oncol 1999;70:172.
4. Nehal KS, Levine VJ, Ashinoff R. Basal cell carcinoma of the genitalia. Dermatol Surg 1998;24:1361.
5. Joura EA, Losch A, Haider-Angeler MG, et al. Trends in vulvar neoplasia: increasing incidence of vulvar intraepithelial neoplasia and squamous cell carcinoma of the vulva in young women. J Reprod Med 2000;45:613.
6. DiSaia PJ, Creasman WT, eds. Clinical gynecologic oncology. St. Louis: CV Mosby, 1989.
7. Koss LG. The Papanicolaou test for cervical cancer: a triumph and a tragedy. JAMA 1989;261:737.
8. Booth M, Beral V. Cervical cancer deaths in young women. Lancet 1989;1:616.
9. Abma J, Chandra A, Mosher W, et al. Fertility, family planning, and women's health: new data from the 1995 National Survey of Family Growth. Vital Health Stat 23, no. 19. National Center for Health Statistics, May 1997.
10. Bosch FX, Manos MM, Munoz N, et al. Prevalence of human papillomavirus in cervical cancer: a worldwide perspective. International Biological Study on Cervical Cancer (IBSCC) Study Group. J Natl Cancer Inst 1995;87:796.
11. Richard RM. Typing HPV DNA gains clues for therapy. Contemp Obstet Gynecol 1988;31:4.
12. Butler EB, Stanbridge CM. Condylomatous lesions of the lower female genital tract. Clin Obstet Gynecol 1984;11:171.
13. Cappiello G, Garbuglia AR, Salvi R, et al. HIV infection increases the risk of squamous intra-epithelial lesions in women with HPV infection: an analysis of HPV genotypes. DIANAIDS Collaborative Study Group. Int J Cancer 1997;72:982.
14. Sawaya GF, Grimes DA. New technologies in cervical cytology screening: a word of caution. Obstet Gynecol 1999;94:307.
15. Hutchinson ML, Berger BM, Farber FL. Clinical and cost implications of new technologies for cervical cancer screening: the impact of test sensitivity. Am J Managed Care 2000;6:766.
16. National Cancer Institute Workshop. The 1988 Bethesda system for reporting cervical/vaginal cytologic diagnoses. JAMA 1989;262:931.
17. Mecsei R, Haugen OA, Halvorsen LE, et al. Genital *Chlamydia trachomatis* infections in patients with abnormal cervical smears: effect of tetracycline on cell changes. Obstet Gynecol 1989;73:317.
18. Kurman RJ, Henson DE, Herbst AL, et al. Interim guidelines for management of abnormal cervical cytology. JAMA 1994;271:1866.
19. Cervical cytology: evaluation and management of abnormalities. ACOG Tech Bull 1993;183:1.
20. Writing Group for the PEPI Trial. Effects of hormone replacement therapy on endometrial histology in postmenopausal women. JAMA 1996;275:370.
21. Ernster VI, Bush TL, Huggins GR, et al. Benefits and risks of menopausal estrogen and/or progestin hormone use. J Prev Med 1988;17:201.
22. Pritchard KI. Screening for endometrial cancer. Is it effective? Ann Intern Med 1989;110:177.
23. Dijkhuizen FP, Mol BW, Brolmann HA, et al. The accuracy of endometrial sampling in the diagnosis of patients with endometrial carcinoma and hyperplasia: a meta-analysis. Cancer 2000;89:1765.
24. Guido RS, Kanbour-Shakir A, Rulin MC, et al. Pipelle endometrial sampling: sensitivity in the detection of endometrial cancer. J Reprod Med 1995;40:553.
25. Carter J, Carson LF, Byers L, et al. Transvaginal ultrasound in gynecologic oncology. Obstet Gynecol Surv 1991;46:687.
26. Smith LH, Oi RH. Detection of the patient at risk; clinical, radiological and cytological detection. Clin Obstet Gynecol 1977;20:607.

27. Breen JL, Marson WS. Ovarian tumors in children and adolescents. Clin Obstet Gynecol 1977;20:607.
28. Spanos WJ. Preoperative hormonal therapy of cystic adnexal masses. Am J Obstet Gynecol 1973;116:551.
29. Barber HRK, Graber EA. The PMPO syndrome (postmenopausal palpable ovary syndrome). Obstet Gynecol Surv 1973;28:357.
30. Goldstein SR, Sulramanyan B, Snyder JR, et al. The postmenopausal cystic adnexal mass: the potential role of ultrasound in conservative management. Obstet Gynecol 1989;73:8.
31. Eltabbakh GH, Belinson JL, Kennedy AW, et al. Serum CA-125 measurements >65 U/mL: clinical value. J Reprod Med 1997;42:617.
32. Twickler DM, Forte TB, Santos-Ramos R, et al. The Ovarian Tumor Index predicts risk for malignancy. Cancer 1999;86:2280.
33. Sassone AM, Timor-Tritsch IE, Artner A, et al. Transvaginal sonographic characterization of ovarian disease: evaluation of a new scoring system to predict ovarian malignancy [Review]. Obstet Gynecol 1991;78:70.
34. Jacobs IJ, Skates SJ, MacDonald N, et al. Screening for ovarian cancer: a pilot randomised controlled trial. Lancet 1999;353:1207.
35. Xu Y, Shen Z, Wiper DW, et al. Lysophosphatidic acid as a potential biomarker for ovarian and other gynecologic cancers. JAMA 1998;280:719.
36. Berchuck A, Carney M, Lancaster JM, et al. Familial breast-ovarian cancer syndromes: BRCA1 and BRCA2. Clin Obstet Gynecol 1998;41:157.
37. Hankinson SE, Colditz GA, Hunter DJ, et al. A quantitative assessment of oral contraceptive use and risk of ovarian cancer. Obstet Gynecol 1992;80:708.
38. Narod SA, Risch H, Moslehi R, et al. Oral contraceptives and the risk of hereditary ovarian cancer. Hereditary Ovarian Cancer Clinical Study Group. N Engl J Med 1998;339:424.

CHAPTER 105

Diseases of the Breast

MICHAEL J. PURTELL, MD
RODRIGO ERLICH, MD

One of every eight women in the United States will develop breast cancer. It is the second leading cause of cancer death among women, with 182,000 new cases seen each year and 44,000 deaths (1,2). Not surprisingly, the fear of breast cancer is prominent in the patient who has breast-related complaints, although most of these are secondary to benign causes. Many women view breast cancer as the leading threat to their health, although statistically it ranks near lung cancer and behind cardiovascular diseases as a cause of death in women. (3,4). The primary caregiver must have a rational approach to the diagnosis and treatment of breast complaints and breast masses. He or she carries out the screening program for cancer and supervises the patient's referral. If cancer is found, the primary caregiver is the one to whom the patient initially turns for information. A reassuring patient–caregiver relationship is critical in dealing with this emotionally charged area of medicine.

NORMAL ANATOMY AND PHYSIOLOGY OF THE BREAST

The breast is a modified sweat gland. An extension of breast tissue reaches toward the axilla. There are 12 to 20 acini arranged like a bunch of grapes, with draining ducts emptying into openings on the nipple. These ducts are lined by two layers of epithelium, one of which serves as a basement membrane and source of epithelial cell reproduction. This "reverse layer" can proliferate in certain pathologic conditions. Surrounding each duct is a specialized periductal fibrous layer, which is under hormonal influence.

With each menstrual cycle, a fall in hormonal activity at the menses results in the desquamation of duct lining, which proliferates again at the cessation of menses. Increases in periductal vascularity and lymphocytic infiltration accompany this proliferation. During pregnancy the ducts and acini proliferate maximally, often never returning to normal in the postpartum period. In many parts of the breast, the glandular hypertrophy remains until it involutes at menopause. At that time there is a loss of parenchyma and an increase in fat, especially in the periductal region. The lobular anatomy slowly disappears. Variations in hormonal balance result in various benign pathologic conditions occurring during the active menstrual child-bearing years and at menopause. It is important to realize that anatomic changes associated with normal hormonal fluctuations during a menstrual cycle do not occur to the same degree in all areas of the breast. This accounts for the asymmetric palpatory findings in the normal breast, which is often lumpy.

SCREENING PROCEDURES

Physical examination (see later discussion) and mammography are useful screening procedures for the detection of breast masses. Mammographic techniques have improved considerably, and the radiation exposure per examination has dropped to very low levels, so the risk of inducing breast cancer from routine screening mammography is almost negligible. Routine screening mammography in women older than 50 years of age (although poorly studied in those older than 74 years) has been proven in controlled studies to decrease deaths from breast cancer (5). All practitioners should encourage routine physical examination and screening mammography in women older than 50 years of age. Although mammography is the more sensitive of the two screening procedures, physical examination is also important because up to 15% of palpable breast cancers are not visualized on mammography (6) Self-examination of the breast is often advocated but there is no evidence that it is effective in lowering a woman's probability of dying from breast cancer (7), and it certainly should not substitute for examination by the practitioner and by mammography.

Routine screening mammography in women younger than 50 years of age remains controversial except for women with increased risk by virtue of a previous breast cancer, a strong family history or prior exposure of the breast to low-dose ionizing radiation (e.g., a patient who as a teenager received mediastinal radiation for Hodgkin disease) (8,9). The American Cancer Society, the American College of Radiology. The U.S. Preventive Services Taskforce (6,8,10) recommend a baseline mammography examination every 1 to 2 years, between the ages of 35 and 40 years and mammography thereafter. The Canadian Task Force on periodic health examination does not recommend routine screening mammography before the age of 50 years (10). In early 1997, the National Institutes of Health held a consensus conference devoted to breast cancer screening. It was concluded that there were not enough data to recommend routine mammographic screening for women before age 50 years. This statement stirred considerable public debate. The National Cancer Institute (NCI) subsequently distanced itself from this conclusion and issued an independent recommendation for screening beginning at age 40 years.

There are several reasons for this controversy. Mammography can certainly identify nonpalpable, highly curable breast cancers in young women. However, if reduction in deaths from breast cancer is the main goal, although some trials show a 40% reduction, others show no survival benefit for screened women in their forties (11). The trials showing no benefit have been criticized for lack of statistical power in the age range of 40 to 49 years owing to relatively low numbers and contamination of the control groups by participants undergoing mammographic screening. Many of the tumors found in the young are *in situ* cancers that may not become invasive for years, if ever. In addition most of the cancers found in women who began screening in their forties were not discovered until the women were in their fifties. This would suggest that perhaps if they had been screened after 50 years of age the results would have been unchanged. Of major concern is the lack of test specificity in young women, who often have dense breasts, complicating interpretation. This leads to a much higher benign-to-malignant biopsy ratio than that found in older women. In order to find cancer, lesions that are associated with cancer only 5% of the time or less are often biopsied (12). As a result, large numbers of normal women must undergo physical and psychological trauma to find the occasional woman potentially benefited by the diagnosis of an early cancer. The recommendation for early follow-up of a suspicious lesion is potentially more harmful than biopsy. The impact of this frequent recommendation on a young woman (usually with no disease) is poorly studied but is likely to be profound, especially if she has problems with anxiety, depression, or somatization. For the immediate future it will be up to the primary caregiver and his or her anxious patient to sort through the complex scientific and political considerations. Gail and Rimer have provided guidelines that may help the primary caregiver select patients in their forties who might best be served by screening mammograms (13).

As of this writing (4/02) controversy has erupted over a re-analysis of published reports on the efficacy of mammography (13a). The authors have questioned the validity of these reports and have suggested that mammography may be of no value for women of any age. However, rebuttals of this re-analysis have begun to appear (13b) and it seems prudent to continue to follow current guidelines (see above) for the time being.

Several new screening procedures are under review that may gain importance in the near future. Magnetic resonance imaging (MRI) has been shown to have increased sensitivity (virtually 100%) but reduced specificity when compared with routine mammography (14). At present it remains too expensive and nonspecific to be employed routinely. However, in situations in which there is a high clinical suspicion for breast cancer but no lesion is noted on the mammogram, it may be helpful. Ultrasonography to distinguish between solid or cystic lesions and sestamibi scanning are adjunct imaging procedures. For lesions larger than 1 cm noted on a mammogram and for palpable abnormalities, the sestamibi scan has an 80% probability of predicting whether the lesion will prove to be malignant (15). This information might assist in deciding whether to biopsy a mammographic abnormality or to monitor it with serial mammograms. The technique of ductal milking, in which the breast ducts are lavaged with fluid, which is then examined cytologically, is still in its infancy but may gain prominence in the future.

Whatever decision the primary caregiver makes about the usefulness of screening mammography in the young woman, it is important that an office interview be scheduled for anyone contemplating screening. A woman needs to understand her likely experience when she goes for testing, particularly if it is her first mammogram. Patients should know that mammography may be uncomfortable because of the need for breast compression. The postmammography plan of communication should be worked out ahead of time to minimize the anxiety of waiting for a telephone call. Young women in particular should understand the poor specificity of the test and the high likelihood of a recommendation for intervention (biopsy or early follow-up), especially with the first mammogram. The patient should know that if she receives that recommendation, in most instances, the chance of benign or no disease far outweighs the chance of cancer.

CLINICAL CHARACTERISTICS OF COMMON DISEASES OF THE BREAST

Benign Tumors

Fibroadenoma

Fibroadenoma is the most common cause of a unilateral discrete mass in the 15- to 35-year-old age group. The peak incidence is from 20 to 25 years of age. In 10% to 15% of cases, there are multiple tumors. The rapid growth seen during pregnancy, just before menopause, and in animals given estrogens all suggest that fibroadenomas are under hormonal control. The natural history of a fibroadenoma is that of a tumor growing rapidly in the pregnant patient and then growing old with the patient, perhaps calcifying in the postmenopausal woman.

A fibroadenoma has both fibrous and epithelial components. The tumor probably arises from terminal ducts and lobules, and the rare finding of lobular carcinoma rather than intraductal carcinoma within or in the vicinity of a fibroadenoma is consistent with such an origin.

The patient with a fibroadenoma usually complains only of the mass and denies pain, nipple discharge, or other breast changes. On physical examination, the lesion is usually firm but not rock hard; it is smooth and well circumscribed, nontender, and easily movable. It often rolls about in the breast, mimicking a very large marble. In some adolescents, giant fibroadenomas can be confused with virginal hypertrophy; however, they are usually more discrete than is diffuse hypertrophy. Mammography is often diagnostic, usually revealing a discrete, round, well-circumscribed lesion without associated calcium. In addition, a skilled cytopathologist can usually confirm the diagnosis with the sample from a fine-needle aspiration. However, because of the rare possibility of simultaneous lobular carcinoma or progression to cystosarcoma phylloides and the inability to definitely exclude carcinoma (present in 2% to 3% of cases), excisional biopsy sometimes may be recommended.

Cystosarcoma Phylloides

Cystosarcoma phylloides is a sarcomatous tumor of the breast that may arise from a fibroadenoma. The overgrowth of stroma mainly distinguishes it from a fibroadenoma. It has a malignancy rate of 20% to 30%, with 2% to 3% of cases having already metastasized at diagnosis. Benign tumors are treated with wide excision and malignant tumors by modified radical mastectomy.

Intraductal Papilloma

Intraductal papillomas often manifest with serosanguinous, spontaneous, recurrent, or persistent nipple discharge from a single duct. These small tumors are not palpable, but their location can usually be determined by applying pressure on various quadrants of the areolocutaneous margin and noting which quadrant produces the discharge. An intraductal papillary cancer is a possibility that must be excluded by excising a small, pie-shaped segment in the area producing the discharge.

Fibrocystic Disease

Fibrocystic changes of the breast are quite common and occur to some extent in most women. Because up to 90% of women have some degree of cysts and epithelial hyperplasia on biopsy or at autopsy, it may be reasonable to consider fibrocystic disease a normal variant rather than an actual pathologic entity. The patient with fibrocystic change usually complains of dull, aching pain in the area of most pronounced nodularity, and this pain is often more prominent just before the onset of menses. On physical examination the breast feels lumpy, with bilateral, diffuse, tender, easily movable ill-defined masses, usually in the upper outer quadrant of the breasts. At times, especially with a discrete cystic lesion, it is hard to distinguish cystic changes noted on examination or on a mammogram from cancer, making management of such cases difficult. Because of this uncertainty, many patients undergo at least one biopsy to rule out cancer. Most lesions are benign (16); usually, the histology is either normal (70%) or shows only epithelial hyperplasia (25%). These findings are of little concern; such patients are at low risk for development of breast cancer and do not require more vigilant follow-up than normal (16). In contrast, a report of hyperplasia with atypia (3% to 4% of benign biopsies) is significant, particularly if the mother or a sister of the patient has had breast cancer. In the absence of a positive family history, the finding of atypia increases the risk for breast cancer development 4-fold, and in association with a positive family history this risk is increased almost 11-fold (16). These patients require careful follow-up, with annual mammogram and biannual physical examinations, and in selected cases, even prophylactic bilateral mastectomies may be considered.

Sometimes fibrocystic disease is associated with *duct ectasia,* usually heralded by spontaneous discharge of thick, gray-green fluid from multiple dilated ducts. At other times duct ectasia and discharge may be present in the absence of palpable fibrocystic lesions. In the first instance, a biopsy should be done to rule out carcinoma; in the second, the administration of estrogen may stop the discharge. If it does not, mammography should be performed and then a biopsy should be considered.

Premature Hyperplasia

A concentric unilateral swelling can occur beneath the nipple before puberty in girls. This commonly occurs between the ages of 7 and 9 years. The lump can be 1 to 2 cm in diameter and is usually nontender. Within a year, a contralateral lump appears and often both lumps remain static until puberty. A biopsy is contraindicated and is equivalent to total mastectomy.

Gynecomastia

The main differential in male breast masses lies between gynecomastia (see Chapter 85) and male breast cancer. The latter is rare, accounting for approximately 1% of all breast cancers. Although gynecomastia has many causes, its physical characteristics are usually unvaried. Gynecomastia appears as a breast mass beneath the areola, is usually slightly tender, and is easily movable. It is never associated with ulceration or nipple retraction. If gynecomastia is ruled out, a breast mass in a male should be examined by biopsy.

Cancer

The increased practice of routine screening for breast cancer by mammography, using sensitive equipment, has resulted in a change in the presentation of breast cancer. A large percentage of cases (15% to 20%) are now detected by mammography alone, without an associated palpable mass (6). The remaining breast cancers are found by the patient or the practitioner, and 15% of these are clinically advanced. These advanced cases may be recognized by some of the following signs: skin changes (e.g., dimpling, peau d'orange, erythema), altered venous pattern, matted fixed axillary nodes, or a mass fixed to the chest wall. Less advanced cases may manifest with a painless, hard irregular mass, often (37%) located in the upper outer quadrant of the breast. These may be associated with subtle skin dimpling or nipple retraction. Palpable, movable axillary lymph nodes less than 2 cm in diameter about half of the time on biopsy only reactive changes in patients with breast cancer, without tumor involvement.

EVALUATION OF A BREAST MASS

History: Risk Factors and Symptoms

The chance of a woman's developing cancer increases with age (2,9,17). The risk to age 50 years is approximately 2.5%; to age 70, approximately 8% (and to age 110, approximately 12%). Many factors have been shown to alter these numbers (see later discussion). Women are becoming increasingly sensitive to their high risk of developing breast cancer and are more aware of factors that may modulate their risk (Table 105.1). Genetic testing for breast cancer susceptibility genes (BRCA1 and BRCA2) has now become commercially available. Women with worrisome family histories (18) and those who have developed breast cancer before menopause may inquire about undergoing such testing. It falls on the primary caregiver to guide the patient in understanding her own risk and to counsel her as to whether her risk may justify such actions as genetic testing or prophylactic mastectomy. Individual factors usually are expressed as relative risk—the increased risk when a factor is present relative to the risk when it is absent, all other factors being the same. Women sometimes incorrectly sum their various relative risks to achieve an overall estimated cumulative (absolute) risk that is several times higher than that observed in epidemiologic studies. They also may fail to realize that their risk of dying from breast cancer is one third of their chance of developing breast cancer. Probability curves have been developed to guide the practitioner in combining various risk factors to estimate a woman's chance of developing breast cancer over time and have been published (18–20). Genetic

Table 105.1. Risk Factors for Carcinoma of the Breast

Factors	Relative Risk
Positive family history	1–5 (see text)
Early menarche and late menopause (cyclic ovarian activity >40 yr)	Slight
Nulliparity	Slight
Previous breast cancer	5
Benign disease of the breast	1–4 (see text)
Radiation	Dependent on dosage

screening may be appropriate for a woman who has a strong family history (more then five relatives with a history of breast or ovarian cancer with onset before 50 years of age) or a personal history of breast cancer before 35 years of age, especially if she is of Jewish descent (21–23). It is recommended that such women receive expert genetic counseling before considering testing and that testing be done in an academic center. Guidelines for such testing have been published by the American Society of Clinical Oncology (24).

In ascertaining a woman's risk, the menstrual and reproductive history is important. Early menarche and late menopause (i.e., prolonged duration of ovarian activity, greater than 40 years) are associated with a slightly increased risk for development of breast cancer, whereas menopause before 35 years of age (normal or surgical) reduces the risk. The risk of breast cancer is increased in nulliparous women, whereas a full-term pregnancy before age 18 years offers some protective benefit. It appears unlikely that the use of oral contraceptives changes a woman's risk of breast cancer, but postmenopausal estrogen replacement therapy may increase the risk by 30% (see Chapter 106). A family history of breast cancer is a major risk factor (25). The occurrence of breast cancer in a first-degree relative (sister or mother) increases a woman's probability of developing cancer two- to fourfold. It is debatable to what extent this increase in risk depends on the relative's having been premenopausal when diagnosed or having developed bilateral cancers. For instance, some reports estimate that the lifetime risk of developing breast cancer for a daughter or sister of a premenopausal woman with bilateral disease is 50%, but that there is no increased risk if the relative was postmenopausal and had unilateral disease (25). Others suggest that these estimates are too high or too low. It is important to reassure patients that breast cancer in more distant relatives (e.g., aunts) has little or no effect on a woman's risk. The other major risk factor besides family history is a personal history of breast cancer, which increases the risk of contralateral breast cancer fivefold (26). An assessment tool developed by Gail for the NCI can be used to easily calculate a woman's relative risk for developing breast cancer. It is widely available, including on the World Wide Web at an NCI website (http://intouchlive.com/home/frames.htm?http://intouchlive.com/cancergenetics/gail.htm&3). This tool was used to select patients for the preventive trial discussed later in this chapter. Its limitations are discussed at the NCI website, but they stem from not including information about second- and third-degree relatives. It tends to be unreliable for patients with a strong family history, especially if they have not undergone routine mammographic screening. For such women, the risk assessment tool developed by Claus (18) (which can be accessed via a link at the same NCI website) is more appropriate.

The patient should be questioned about the presence of other symptoms (e.g., pain, discharge) related to a breast mass, the duration of those symptoms if present, and whether the discovery of the mass or onset of the other symptoms was associated with changes in the menses, injury to the breast, pregnancy, or changes in medication.

After the presence of a mass, *nipple discharge* is the second most common sign of breast cancer. Nonlactational nipple discharge can be unilateral or bilateral, spontaneous or evoked only by pressure and massage, and persistent or recurrent. If the discharge is associated with a mass on physical examination, the mass should be the primary concern. Nipple discharge in women older than 50 years of age must be viewed with more suspicion than in younger women, regardless of its presentation. Discharge evoked only by trauma, massage, or pressure has no clinical importance. Spontaneous, recurrent, or persistent discharge from one or two ducts not associated with a mass requires surgical exploration of the duct to differentiate benign papilloma from intraductal papillary carcinoma. Both are possible without a presenting mass, and the character of the discharge is not helpful (see Chapters 81 and 101 for a discussion of galactorrhea).

Physical Examination

The patient should be seated undressed to the waist on an examining table. Inspection and palpation of the nodal drainage areas (supraclavicular and axillary) should be performed. Inspection and palpation of the nipples, areolae, and breasts are done next. While the patient is sitting, her arm on the side being examined can be raised by the clinician to allow palpation high into the axilla. The examination should then be repeated with the patient in the supine position with her arm raised over her head so that the breast flattens on the chest wall. If the clinician cannot appreciate a mass noted by the patient, it is important to allow the patient sufficient time to find the lesion herself rather than to dismiss the complaint. If both the patient and the clinician cannot locate the mass, the patient should be reassured that benign fibrous masses often disappear spontaneously, as do menstrual-related cysts.

Initial Management

The three most common masses found in the breast are fibroadenoma, fibrocystic changes, and carcinoma. Each of these common lesions has a peak incidence at different ages, but there is considerable overlap. Because of this overlap and the inability of the clinician from history, physical examination, or radiographic studies to make a diagnosis with certainty, a biopsy usually is the only definitive test to rule out carcinoma.

Age 15 to 30 Years

An easily movable, nontender, smooth, marble-like mass in a woman younger than 30 years of age is most likely a fibroadenoma. The mass should be electively excised. This can be delayed up to several months if the mass is not growing rapidly and if there are no major risk factors (significant family history or prior breast cancer). A mammogram should not be routinely obtained in the evaluation of a discrete mass in this age group. The tissue is too dense to allow useful interpretation, and the radiation may slightly increase the risk for development of a neoplasm. Perhaps a patient who has large breasts that are difficult to examine, persistent symptoms, or a strong family history should have a mammogram.

Age 30 to 50 Years

A discrete mass noted during the reproductive years that feels cystic might be watched through one or two menstrual cycles. A sonogram can be useful in distinguishing a cystic from a solid mass. If the mass persists, a surgical consultation is probably necessary to allow histologic examination of the mass. A mammogram can be obtained before the consultation, especially if the patient has never had one. A persistent mass that is not seen on mammography should not be ignored; 10% to 15% of palpable breast cancers are not seen on mammography (6).

Age 50 Years or Older

A patient 50 years of age or older with a suspicious mass should be referred for possible biopsy. A mammogram should be obtained to search for other areas of disease that also may need to be biopsied.

All Ages

The usual evaluation of a persistent, palpable, discrete breast mass involves histologic examination even if the mammogram is not suspicious. An exception is a cystic mass that disappears after aspiration or menstruation. If the mass is larger than 2 cm, an incisional biopsy is usually performed; otherwise the mass should be removed *in toto*. *Fine-needle aspiration* for cytology is often performed first because it is easier and less traumatic than an open biopsy. Simultaneous biopsy, frozen section, histologic examination, and, if malignant, immediate mastectomy should be considered only in special cases at the wish of the patient and only after detailed discussion. Waiting for permanent sections allows detailed examination of the tissue and certainty of the diagnosis. In addition, the treatment of primary breast cancer has undergone many changes in recent years, with several treatment options now available to the patient. The one-step approach deprives a patient of her right to a second opinion in regard to treatment options for her breast cancer.

Needle Aspiration of a Palpable Mass

In the past, aspiration was limited to nodules thought to be cystic, with sonography used to help distinguish cystic from solid lesions. More recently, aspiration by the surgeon of solid lesions to obtain material for cytologic examination has allowed the diagnosis of carcinoma to be made in the office and perhaps can spare some patients a surgical biopsy. In the case of the cystic lesion, if the mass does not completely disappear, if the fluid is bloody, or the mass rapidly reoccurs, an open biopsy is necessary. (Cytologic examination of the fluid is usually of little use and need not be done routinely.) If the lesion disappears completely without recurrence, routine follow-up is sufficient. If the results of cytology obtained by needle aspiration of a solid lesion are negative, formal biopsy usually is required, because false negative findings are common.

Surgical Biopsy

The referring practitioner should not only inform the patient of the need for surgical consultation but also explain clearly the reasons why it is needed and that a biopsy may be recommended by the surgeon. The patient should be encouraged to ask questions. The consultation is stressful, and the patient is more likely to absorb information from her personal caregiver. In addition, the patient needs support from her personal caregiver and the reassurance of continued involvement in her care should a biopsy reveal cancer.

Preparation

Most biopsies can be done on an outpatient basis in an ambulatory surgery unit. Either local anesthesia with intravenous sedation (preferred) or general anesthesia can be used. The patient should not eat or drink after midnight on the night before the biopsy.

Operation. A 2.5- to 5.0-cm incision is used to allow an adequate biopsy that is cosmetically satisfactory. The incision site is selected very carefully to minimize the potential for disfigurement should cancer be found and should breast-conserving therapy subsequently be chosen. It should be explained to the patient that, in addition to a possible residual mass, a ridge of tissue secondary to sutures and scar often remains after the operation. Removal of a large mass might necessitate a small drain, which is withdrawn in the office 1 or 2 days after the biopsy.

If the mass is palpable, then the tissue of concern is easily located and biopsied. As noted previously, biopsies increasingly are being obtained for mammographic lesions found in the absence of a palpable mass. In these instances, the procedure is more complicated. Under mammographic guidance, a radiologist places thin needles or hooks into the breast, with the tips resting within 1 cm of the suspicious area on the mammogram. Methylene blue or some other color marker is then injected into the breast to mark the abnormal area noted on the mammogram. The patient then proceeds to the ambulatory surgery unit, where the surgeon excises the stained area. If the mammographic abnormality contains microcalcifications, radiography of the biopsy specimen is used to ensure that they have been removed with the biopsy specimen. Several weeks after the biopsy, the patient should have a mammogram to confirm that the suspicious area is no longer present.

An alternative procedure available at most imaging facilities uses stereotactic imaging to guide an automatic biopsy gun equipped with a core biopsy needle. In experienced hands, adequate tissue can be obtained almost 100% of the time with this technique, with a diagnostic sensitivity of 95% or better (27,28). The referring practitioner should ensure that the facility has digital equipment that allows rapid imaging. Otherwise the procedure can be quite prolonged and tiring for the patient. In addition in the absence of such equipment, time constraints will make it impractical to obtain multiple biopsies from separated suspicious areas. Stereotactic biopsy greatly simplifies the diagnostic process and may allow a preliminary diagnosis to be made on the day of the procedure. However, there are a few caveats: Because radiographic stereotactic biopsy shifts the diagnostic procedure from the surgeon to the radiologist, it must be made clear to all whether the primary caregiver or the radiologist is responsible for reporting the final results to the patient and arranging appropriate follow-up. Not all areas of the breast are easily accessable to stereotactic biopsies; for example, deep or very superficial lesions are not. These are better approached by surgery with needle localization. In addition, a negative result from a stereotactic core biopsy usually entails a subsequent surgical biopsy to ensure that the result was not falsely negative. The primary practitioner needs to work with the surgeon and radiologist so the patient undergoes the minimal number of procedures. For instance, stereotactic biopsy might be recommended for a patient with a suspicious microcalcification on the mammogram, because it is possible to check and ensure that it has been sampled by the core. On the other hand, a patient with a suspicious deep, spiculated mammographic finding might best be served with surgical biopsy.

Follow-up. Ecchymoses or hematoma (5% of patients) and wound infection (1% to 2% of patients) are the main complications of breast biopsy. A large hematoma may require evacuation, but this usually can be done in the office. Exercise and strenuous activities should be avoided for 7 to 10 days after a breast biopsy to guard against late bleeding. The long-term sequelae of breast biopsy are minimal; chronic scar formation may cause some difficulty with follow-up examinations and interpretation of mammograms. Detailed descriptions of the biopsy site should be noted in the patient's chart by caregivers on follow-up, and details of the biopsy should be conveyed to radiologists reading future mammograms.

Follow-Up Management of a Benign Breast Mass

Fibroadenoma

After excision of a fibroadenoma, the patient should have routine follow-up as defined by her risk factors for carcinoma and age. The patient should be reassured that there is no increased risk of malignancy because of the fibroadenoma.

Fibrocystic Disease

If on histologic examination the epithelium is normal, no special follow-up is necessary for the patient with a benign biopsy. Even if proliferative epithelial changes are noted, the increased risk is so minimal (less than twofold) that the patient should be reassured and no special follow-up is warranted. Only the finding of atypia, especially in a patient with a history of breast cancer in a sibling or mother, requires special consideration. Without such a family history, monthly self-examinations of the breasts, a physical examination twice yearly, and an annual mammogram should suffice. With a positive family history, the patient may consider the 40% lifetime risk of developing breast cancer sufficient to contemplate bilateral prophylactic simple mastectomy with reconstruction (16). Subcutaneous mastectomy with implants should not be considered as a compromise, because the 15% to 20% of the breast that is left behind with this procedure remains at risk.

As mentioned earlier, the pain associated with fibrocystic changes is often ameliorated once a cancer has been excluded. If pain continues, the patient should be advised to wear a brassiere both day and night. A number of pharmacologic and dietary strategies are said to be effective in the management of painful fibrocystic changes (e.g., vitamin E, primrose oil, avoidance of caffeine), usually without adequate supporting evidence. However, *danazol,* a weak androgenic steroid, has been shown to decrease pain and nodularity in up to 70% of patients with fibrocystic changes when used in dosages of 100 to 400 mg/day for 4 to 6 months (29). Side effects are minor, the most common being weight gain, acne, and amenorrhea. Tamoxifen (discussed later), 20 mg/day, is equally effective (29); its major side effects are hot flushes and vaginal discharge.

CANCER

If the biopsy reveals carcinoma, consultation with a medical oncologist and radiation oncologist should be considered. The treatment of breast cancer is complex and rapidly changing and involves the coordinated efforts of the surgeon, radiation oncologist, medical oncologist, and primary practitioner. The primary caregiver may not be knowledgeable in all of the details of treatment, but it is important to understand the general concepts discussed here because the patient will look to her caregiver for support and clarification as she struggles with difficult treatment decisions.

Staging

Several clinical staging systems have been devised for breast cancer, but none facilitates the management of individual patients. It is perhaps simplest to divide tumors into three main groups: clearly *resectable* tumors (not fixed to the chest wall and not associated with fixed matted axillary nodes); *locally advanced* tumors (fixed to the chest wall or associated with the presence of matted axillary nodes or inflammatory skin changes, but without signs of metastasis); and *metastatic* tumors.

In the absence of symptoms or physical findings, patients with resectable tumors require minimal further studies consisting of a chest radiograph, routine blood analyses (including liver function tests and determination of the serum calcium concentration), and, if not done before the biopsy, a mammogram to look for contralateral disease or multicentric lesions. In addition, the patient's history should be retaken to ensure that there are no musculoskeletal complaints suggestive of bony metastases. If there are, bone scanning and local radiographs of the symptomatic region should be obtained. In general, liver and bone scans should not be obtained routinely in patients with good prognoses, such as those having tumors less than 5 cm in diameter and uninvolved axillary lymph nodes. In the absence of symptoms, physical findings, or abnormal serum chemistries, these studies are more likely to produce confusing false positive results than to disclose unexpected metastases. Imaging might be considered for a patient who has a high risk for metastatic disease and whose treatment plan would be greatly altered in the presence of metastatic disease. An example would be a patient with more than three positive lymph nodes who is being considered for postlumpectomy radiotherapy; one might not proceed with radiation if a liver scan were highly suspicious for metastatic disease.

Surgery

Radical mastectomy, for years the standard procedure, is no longer performed. The modified radical mastectomy (removal of the breast and the ipsilateral axillary lymph nodes), which preserves the pectoral muscles, is of equal efficacy but is less disfiguring, allows easier reconstruction, and only occasionally leads to clinically significant arm edema (30).

A *modified radical mastectomy* requires general anesthesia and a short period of hospitalization, usually no more than 2 to 5 days. Most patients are ambulatory and eating normally within 24 hours after the operation. Occasionally, a patient is discharged with a drain, which is removed at the time of follow-up. Serous fluid may accumulate under the skin flap even after the drain is removed and may require aspiration in the office. In the early postoperative period, the patient may be inconvenienced by arm and shoulder discomfort, but usually she can use the arm normally within 2 to 3 weeks. Some patients experience shoulder and arm pain for a much more extensive period; it is important for these patients to continue arm exercises as prescribed by the surgeon. In 10% of patients, after modified radical mastectomy, lymphedema of the ipsilateral upper extremity develops. Usually swelling is minimal in the morning and increases during the day. Typically, the degree of swelling gradually becomes worse over several years. Management includes the following:

- Instruct the patient to sleep with the arm propped up on a pillow and to take special care not to sleep with the arm under her head.
- Minimize the amount of time that the arm is allowed to hang down (e.g., while sitting).
- Minimize trauma to the arm. This includes limiting the use of the affected arm for blood pressure determinations, phlebotomy, and insertion of intravenous catheters.
- Aggressively treat any infection of the arm. The patient should be instructed to see her practitioner as soon as signs or symptoms of infection (erythema, swelling, pain) are noted, no matter how minimal. (Cellulitis is the major complication of lymphedema.)
- If the degree of swelling is unsightly or uncomfortable, the patient can be fitted with a Jobst sleeve (available at Jobst outlets in most cities) to be worn during waking hours. A trial with a lymphedema pump (a pneumatic sleeve, sold by medical supply houses, that applies intermittent compression to the affected arm) can be considered for severe, refractory cases. Severe lymph edema is managed with the help of a physical therapist. Aggressive early intervention in patients with arm edema may delay or prevent the fibrosis and occult infections that make the process irreversible.
- The clinician should be attentive to sudden changes in the rate of edema formation, especially if it is associated with new arm pain. This may indicate recurrence of tumor in the axilla. Nevertheless, it should be noted that arm swelling can occur as a natural sequela years after the mastectomy.

It is most important to be sensitive to cosmetic and emotional needs of the patient after what most patients consider disfiguring surgery. Most hospitals have a representative from the American Cancer Society Reach for Recovery program or someone serving a similar role who can assist in this regard, and this person should make contact with the patient in the perioperative period to offer help. Within 3 to 6 weeks after the operation, most patients can be fitted with a breast form if skin healing is complete. These forms can be obtained from medical appliance stores.

Breast reconstruction after mastectomy should be discussed with the patient *before* the surgery to allow referral to a plastic surgeon *before* her scheduled mastectomy. The patient then can decide which of several reconstruction procedures she prefers. A common technique of breast reconstruction involves implantation of a tissue expander that is gradually inflated over several weeks to effect sufficient stretching of the chest tissues to allow the later insertion of a saline-filled implant after removal of the expander. Use of autologous tissue is gaining in popularity. A transrectus myocutaneous (TRAM) flap or a latissimus dorsi flap is most commonly used. Careful discussion of all the options with the plastic surgeon is critical for the patient's satisfaction with the surgical result. Reconstruction can be done at the time of mastectomy or later as a second operation. Immediate reconstruction has the advantage of avoiding a second operation and allows the patient the psychological benefit of awakening with some resemblance to her premastectomy appearance. A nipple complex, if desired, can be reconstructed or represented as a tattoo. A poor prognosis or the planned use of postoperative radiotherapy should not serve as contraindications for immediate reconstruction.

Radiotherapy Combined with Surgery

Radiotherapy alone as treatment for primary breast cancer has not been systematically studied. The National Surgical Adjuvant Breast Project (NSABP) has established, for patients with resectable primary tumors 4 cm in diameter or smaller, that complete excision of the primary tumor (lumpectomy, usually with removal of lymph nodes, unless the tumor is only intraductal; see later discussion), followed by breast irradiation five times a week for approximately 5 weeks, is as curative as a modified radical mastectomy (31). For larger lesions, the information is not as well established, but a certain number of these women, especially those with tumors smaller than 5 cm, might also be considered for excision and radiotherapy. The main considerations are cosmetic. These include the relative sizes of the tumor and the remaining breast and how close to the nipple complex the tumor lies. The larger the ratio of tumor size to uninvolved breast, the more likely it is that a poor cosmetic result will occur, because a larger percentage of the normal breast will be exposed to radiation dosages that lead to disfiguring fibrosis. Usually if a tumor is close to or involves the nipple complex, a better cosmetic result is achieved after mastectomy and reconstruction than after lumpectomy and radiotherapy.

The main purpose of radiation after lumpectomy is to reduce the local recurrence rate, which is 42% after lumpectomy without radiation (31), with little effect on overall survival. Even so, patients should be warned that there is a significant incidence of recurrent breast cancer in the irradiated breast, not only at the lumpectomy site, but also elsewhere in the breast (32). In most reported series, the incidence is about 20%, with recurrence occurring up to two decades after lumpectomy; in contrast, the local recurrence rate after mastectomy is 2% to 9%, with recurrence usually in the first 5 years (30–33). However, a local relapse after breast-conserving therapy does not appear to affect survival, unlike that after a mastectomy (31,33). Patients whose cancer recurs after lumpectomy, whether previously irradiated or not, can undergo a salvage mastectomy and survive as long as patients initially treated with a modified radical mastectomy. However, any prior radiotherapy would make reconstruction more difficult than if modified mastectomy were chosen initially. One argument for postexisional radiotherapy is that the reduced risk of suffering the psychological trauma of finding a lump at the surgical site in the future more than offsets the immediate side effects of radiation.

Of patients choosing lumpectomy and radiotherapy, more than 80% are satisfied with the cosmetic results. The treatment is accompanied by minimal, if any, postoperative breast lymphedema or impaired wound healing. The irradiated breast atrophies over a number of months and may remain tender during this period. For some patients, reduction mammoplasty of the opposite breast may need to be considered.

In summary, for most patients with tumors smaller than 5 cm that can be completely excised without affecting the nipple/areolar complex and leaving sufficient remaining breast tissue, there exists a choice between mastectomy and breast-conserving lumpectomy with radiotherapy. All patients should have their choices well outlined and be given information that clearly describes the benefits and disadvantages of the treatment options.

Intraductal Carcinoma

With the increased use of mammography, up to 20% of all new breast cancers are noninvasive *intraductal lesions* (34). The optimal treatment for these lesions has not been precisely defined. Mastectomy is curative 99% of the time, but it is probably an overly aggressive treatment. However, a simple lumpectomy may not be sufficient. The NSABP study compared local excision for patients with small (less than 2.5 cm), intraductal (noninvasive) carcinoma with and without breast irradiation (35). The results suggested that local excision for intraductal cancer without local radiation may prove to be unacceptable because of a high rate of relapse (16%) at or near the biopsy site. (Approximately half of the recurrences were invasive, and radiotherapy appeared to reduce their incidence by 70%.) This conclusion is not universally accepted. It is unclear to what degree radiotherapy prevented or merely delayed local recurrences. Other, albeit nonrandomized, studies suggest that with careful patient selection, a practitioner can identify women who may not need irradiation after removal of an intraductal lesion. The following features are associated with a better prognosis: a completely excised, well-differentiated tumor without comedonecrosis, smaller than 25 mm in diameter; a tumor found incidentally or detected by mammographic microcalcifications; and a tumor that occurs in an older woman. The recurrence rate in such cases can be as low as 3% (36). Many believe that patients whose tumors have these characteristics can be cured by simple excision without irradiation. Clinical trials are ongoing to define more clearly the selection criteria to identify those patients who may not require radiotherapy.

Multimodality Treatment

Patients with locally advanced unresectable disease or with inflammatory disease should be considered for treatment with initial systemic chemotherapy followed by surgery if sufficient tumor reduction occurs or by local irradiation, perhaps with further chemotherapy. For a select group, such an approach may allow long-term survival. Another group of patients who should be considered for preoperative therapy are those who desire breast-conserving therapy but have tumors too large for such as option. Several cycles of chemotherapy—or, for older, less fit patients with estrogen receptor–positive tumors, a short course of an oral antiestrogen or an aromatase inhibitor—has been shown to cause sufficient tumor regression to allow lumpectomy with negative margins in 80% of patients who otherwise would have required a mastectomy (37).

Prognosis, Further Therapy, and Follow-Up

Prognosis

Current estimates of survival are based mainly on tumor size, whether the tumor is wholly intraductal (noninvasive), and the results of axillary node sampling. The cure rate with mastectomy approaches 100% for women whose tumor consists only of intraductal carcinoma. (Axillary node involvement occurs in fewer than 3% of these patients, so node resection provides little further information and may be omitted.)

A special case is *lobular carcinoma in situ* (LCIS). This diagnosis should more accurately be classified as a premalignant lesion and not be considered a neoplasm. It should be viewed as a risk factor in a manner similar to the finding of hyperplasia with atypia on a biopsy. Although there continues to be some disagreement among experts about how significant a risk factor LCIS is, a reasonable estimate is that a woman with a finding of LCIS has a 15% to 30% lifetime risk of developing invasive cancer, or approximately 0.5% to 1% risk of cancer per year. It is important to realize that this risk applies to both breasts (as does any other risk factor). Recommendations vary for LCIS, but most oncologists recommend close mammographic follow-up, with prophylactic bilateral mastectomies reserved for women who are psychologically unable to deal with their increased risk of breast cancer. Such women should be considered for preventive therapy with tamoxifen (see later discussion).

For women with invasive cancer, the status of the axillary lymph nodes is the best indicator of prognosis (Table 105.2) (30,38). Survival at 10 years is approximately 65% with no node involvement, 37% with one to three positive nodes, and 13% with four or more nodes involved (39). The size of the tumor is also important.

Patients with tumors larger than 5 cm do somewhat worse, especially if there are positive nodes; patients with tumors smaller than 1.0 cm (especially if less than 0.5 cm) with uninvolved nodes do better. Within these subgroups, patients whose tumor is rich in estrogen receptors (and progesterone receptors) may do better than those whose tumor lacks significant receptor content (40). However, estrogen and progesterone receptor content is more properly to be considered as a predictor for response to hormonal treatments rather than as a prognostic indicator. The need to determine more accurately the prognosis of individual patients is important, because prognostic category is the basis for patient selection for adjuvant therapy after treatment of the primary tumor. Patients whose tumors appear well differentiated to the pathologist tend to survive better than those whose tumors appear poorly differentiated. Tumors from individual patients are now routinely characterized by molecular biologic analysis. The extent of aneuploidy, percent of tumor cells in S-phase (synthesizing DNA), and degree of HER-2/NEU receptor overexpression are routinely determined. There is a sense that patients whose tumors show aneuploidy, have more than 6% to 7% of their cells in S-phase, or are 3+ expressers of HER-2/NEU receptor do worse than predicted by the current criteria of node status. As yet, however, the data have not sufficiently accumulated to guide the clinician regarding how best to apply these newer measurements (41). Consequently, nodal status still remains the cornerstone in assessing a patient's prognosis.

From this discussion it is clear that axillary dissection serves mainly to obtain prognostic information and may not directly improve a patient's survival. Unfortunately, it is the disruption of the lymphatic drainage of the arm and nerve damage from this operation that result in the long-term sequelae of arm swelling, arm and shoulder pain, and hypoesthesia or hyperesthsia. In attempts to minimize this operation, techniques have been developed to identify intraoperatively the axillary lymph nodes to which a particular woman's breast cancer would first metastasize. Injection of the tumor with a radioactive colloid and/or dye (methylene blue) with diffusion of the tracer to the axilla allows the surgeon to identify the lymph nodes that initially drain the tumor. Removal and pathologic examination of these nodes can predict whether the remaining nodes will be involved with breast cancer. If the sentinel nodes prove negative, then the chance that no other nodes are involved is greater than 95% and the patient can be spared a formal axillary dissection with its consequences (42).

The primary caregiver needs to be mindful of two aspects of the sentinel node approach. First, there is a necessary learning curve for this procedure (43). The rate of false negative findings may be as high as 30% unless the surgeon has performed 10 to 20 procedures. Use of both tracers may facilitate and shorten the learning curve (44). Second, the limited number of nodes presented to the pathologist (1–3) allows detailed examination of them. Not only are thinner slices produced, but also the pathology department has the ability to stain the slides with antibodies to the cytokeratin of breast cancer cells. These detailed procedures greatly increase the sensitivity of the examination. Microscopic nests of tumor cells that would not have been found by a routine dissection can now

Table 105.2. Survival of Patients with Breast Cancer Relative to Status of the Axillary Lymph Nodes

Status of Nodes	Crude Survival (%) 5-Year	Crude Survival (%) 10-Year	5-Year Disease-Free Survival (%)
All patients	63.5	45.9	60.3
Negative axillary lymph nodes	78.1	64.9	82.3
Positive axillary lymph nodes	46.5	24.9	34.9
1–3 positive axillary lymph nodes	62.2	37.5	50.0
≥4 positive axillary lymph nodes	32.0	13.4	21.1

Constructed by use of data in Fisher B, Slack N, Katrych D, Wolmark N. Ten-year follow-up results of patients with carcinoma of the breast in a co-operative clinical trial evaluating surgical adjuvant chemotherapy. Surg Gynecol Obstet 1975;140:528.

be detected. Conflicting data have led to a controversy about whether a node containing a few tumor cells discoverable only through such detailed scrutiny should be considered positive or negative when making a decision concerning adjuvant therapy (45–47). Many, but not all, experts believe that such nodes should be viewed as negative until prospective trials examining this question have concluded (47). The primary caregiver may assume that the uncertainty of this situation will prove stressful for the patient. Therefore, if a patient chooses to undergo a sentinel operation, guidelines about how the nodes will be examined and the information interpreted need to be established before the operation. In addition, because no quantitative information is obtained, if decisions concerning adjuvant therapy are to be based not only on whether the nodes are positive but also on the number of positive nodes, examination of a single positive node would be inadequate (see later discussion).

Adjuvant Therapy

Adjuvant systemic therapy decreases the predicted death rate by approximately 30% (48,49). Therefore, the absolute degree of benefit from adjuvant therapy increases as the predicted prognosis worsens and, conversely, may be clinically insignificant in a woman whose cure rate with primary treatment alone is high. For example, a woman with one to three positive nodes has a 50% chance of her cancer returning. Adjuvant therapy can reduce this risk by 15% (0.3×0.5). However, a woman with a tumor smaller than 1.0 cm and no positive nodes has a cure rate of more than 90%. In this case, adjuvant therapy would improve her chances by only 3% (0.3×0.1). Most oncologists would urge adjuvant therapy in the former case but be less enthusiastic in the latter. It should be noted that in surveys women have stated that they would accept the short-term side effects of adjuvant chemotherapy for as little as a 1% improved probability of survival. Consequently, almost all patients, particularly those with poor prognoses, should have the benefits of further treatment with chemotherapy, hormonal therapy, and radiotherapy presented to them by the medical or radiation oncologist in an attempt to improve disease-free survival and cure (see Chapter 10).

Currently, patients are selected for various adjuvant therapies based on the number of axillary nodes involved, their menopausal status, and the estrogen receptor status of the tumor (48,49). Systemic chemotherapy is recommended to all premenopausal women with metastases to axillary nodes. For patients who opt for lumpectomy and radiotherapy, results seem to be better if the chemotherapy is delivered between the lumpectomy and the breast irradiation (50). For premenopausal women, a major shift in the paradigm for guiding adjuvant selection has been the realization that both premenopausal and postmenopausal women accrue the same benefit from tamoxifen, an estrogen receptor modulator (48). As little as a decade ago, it was believed that tamoxifen adjuvant therapy was inappropriate for premenopausal women, especially if combined with chemotherapy. Now it is standard to treat premenopausal women whose tumors are receptor positive with tamoxifen along with chemotherapy or, in selected patients with good prognoses (negative nodes and estrogen receptor–positive tumors smaller than 2 cm in size), to treat with tamoxifen alone. In addition, because the most recent meta-analysis of adjuvant therapies suggested that oophorectomy is as effective as chemotherapy in premenopausal patients with receptor-positive tumors, there is renewed interest in medical oophorectomy using luteinizing hormone–releasing hormone (LHRH) agonists combined with tamoxifen (51). Similarly, use of tamoxifen is recommended for postmenopausal women with axillary node involvement if their tumors contain significant estrogen receptors. The postmenopausal patient with positive nodes whose tumor is estrogen receptor positive may obtain a small increase in survival (less than 8%) by the addition of chemotherapy to tamoxifen (51). Whether such treatment is warranted, given the additional toxicity, is for the individual patient to decide. Postmenopausal patients whose tumors lack estrogen receptors can benefit from chemotherapy, especially if their axillary nodes contain tumor. Patients diagnosed with only ductal carcinoma *in situ* should also be considered for tamoxifen. A recent clinical trial demonstrated a 44% to 52% decrease in the occurrence of invasive breast cancer in the ipsilateral and contralateral breasts when tamoxifen was employed along with radiation (52).

Aromatase inhibitors are a class of drugs that have gained importance in the treatment of metastatic breast cancer in postmenopausal women with estrogen receptor–positive tumors. They show equal or improved efficacy compared with tamoxifen (53,54). Trials examining the use of aromatase inhibitors in the adjuvant setting are now concluding. It is likely that these agents may replace tamoxifen or be used in some combination with tamoxifen as adjuvant therapy in the near future.

Several adjuvant chemotherapeutic regimens are used. Among these, efficacy is probably equivalent but side effects and duration differ. Data from recent randomized trials suggested that high-dose chemotherapy with stem cell rescue benefits patients with poor prognoses no better than standard chemotherapies do. Hence, high-dose therapy should no longer be considered outside of a clinical trial (55).

Postmastectomy radiotherapy should be considered for all women with node-positive disease. Studies have shown not only a decreased local reoccurrence rate in women receiving postoperative radiotherapy but also an increased survival rate (56–58). Although these results are still controversial for women with less than four positive nodes, a recent NCI consensus conference recommended postmastectomy radiotherapy for women with four or more positive nodes (59).

There are uncommon long-term side effects of adjuvant therapy which must be recognized by the patient and the primary caregiver. Chemotherapy can cause premature menopause and a slight increase in the incidence of second neoplasms, mainly hematologic. Radiotherapy can lead to darkened skin, pulmonary damage, or later solid neoplasms (but not breast cancer in the unaffected breast). In 20% of patients, tamoxifen causes bothersome hot flushes that, if severe, can sometimes be ameliorated with low-dose progesterone, venlafaxine (Effexor), or one of the other selective serotonin reuptake inhibitors. There is an increased incidence of endometrial carcinoma in women treated with tamoxifen (annual rate, 1.7 per 1,000, or an approximately twofold increased risk). Therefore, all women taking tamoxifen should have annual gynecologic examinations and be instructed to report any spotting. More detailed follow-up, such as uterine sonography, is unwarranted. Because of possible rare ocular effects, periodic eye examinations are also recommended. Abnormal liver function tests are occasionally observed, but it is unclear whether the drug can induce hepatoma in humans (as opposed to its effects in rats). Tamoxifen does seem to decrease the risk of developing cancer in the unaffected breast (60), and it may have a bone-preserving effect in postmenopausal women.

The selection criteria for adjuvant systemic therapy are constantly being re-examined as new information is obtained. The NCI recently held a consensus conference to review the literature on the adjuvant therapy of breast cancer (59). It was concluded that it is acceptable to offer adjuvant chemotherapy to most women younger than 70 years of age who have tumors larger than 1 cm, regardless of nodal and receptor status, and tamoxifen to all women whose tumors are receptor positive. The optimal duration of tamoxifen therapy recommended was 5 years. Patients, especially those whose tumors are node negative, may paradoxically lose some of the benefit of tamoxifen if it is continued for longer than 5 years (61).

Follow-up

The patient with breast cancer has a fivefold greater risk for development of cancer in the other breast (26). Consequently, she should be screened with routine mammography and physical examinations, as would any woman with moderately increased risk. Patients choosing lumpectomy and radiotherapy should have a biannual mammogram and careful examination of the irradiated breast every 3 months to look for a local, potentially curable recurrence. Patients who have had a mastectomy should have the scar examined at regular intervals, because a small number (10%) of patients with recurrences in the scar may be cured with local resection followed by radiotherapy.

At present there is little evidence to support the concept that the asymptomatic patient is benefited by prompt diagnosis and initiation of treatment of recurrent systemic metastases (62). No studies have demonstrated that monitoring of patients with radiography, liver function tests, or breast cancer markers at regular intervals improves survival or minimizes the morbidity of a relapse. This probably is true because there is no curative salvage therapy. If these studies are normal, they serve to reassure the patient. However, if they are abnormal, they often initiate a series of difficult management issues that mainly provoke uncertainty in the caregiver and anxiety in the patient without clear benefit to either. Therefore, follow-up plans can be individualized. Most women, when apprised of the lack of benefit from detailed laboratory and imaging follow-up, are comfortable doing without these studies (62).

Given the data suggesting that estrogen replacement is beneficial in ameliorating many postmenopausal changes, especially the development of osteoporosis, the primary caregiver may well be asked about the risks of estrogen replacement therapy in a patient with a history of breast cancer. In the past the answer was simply that it is contraindicated. It now appears that this recommendation was not based on reliable data. In fact, it remains unknown what the effect of estrogen replacement will be on a woman's breast cancer. It may be that the risk is more theoretical than actual, and this question is currently under investigation. Many oncologists believe that, until further data are available, a practitioner could consider estrogen replacement in appropriate circumstances and with informed consent.

Prevention

A large trial in the United States examined the use of tamoxifen for 5 years in women who were without known breast cancer but were considered to be at high risk for development of cancer (63). The cohort receiving tamoxifen had a 50% odds reduction of developing breast cancer. This cohort also acquired a two- to threefold increased risk for development of a deep vein thrombosis or uterine carcinoma. The tumors that were prevented were receptor positive, suggesting that the effect may have been related more to early treatment than to prevention. Despite these results, many women at high risk are not receiving tamoxifen. One reason is that the absolute number of breast cancers prevented in the treated group was quite small. In addition, two smaller European studies failed to confirm the American findings (64,65). Because a trial examining the effect of another estrogen receptor modulator, raloxifene, on osteoporosis saw a reduction in breast cancers in the treated group (66), a clinical trial is being conducted in the United States examining the effect of tamoxifen or raloxifene on breast cancer development. The primary caregiver needs to keep abreast of this field and to be aware of the results as they become available. The current recommendation would be to discuss preventive therapy using tamoxifen with any woman younger than 60 years of age who has a 1.67 or greater risk of developing breast cancer as determined by the Gail tool (67), as well as any woman who is older than 60 years of age or who has LCIS (see p. 1635).

Breast Cancer in the Elderly

Fifty percent of all new breast cancers occur in women 65 years of age or older. In the year 2020, it is estimated that 20% of the U. S. population will be that old (68). In patients older than 68 years of age with breast cancer, 60% of the tumors are node negative and at least 58% are estrogen receptor positive (69). Several studies have shown that older women are less likely to receive postoperative radiation or adjuvant systemic therapy than are younger women (70–72). In healthier older women, such "undertreatment" may lead to poorer outcomes.

A major factor related to the ultimate benefits of adjuvant chemotherapy in older women is the effect of comorbidity on survival. In a study of almost 1,000 women (73), it was found that women with breast cancer who had three or more comorbid illnesses had a 20-fold increased risk of dying from a cause other than breast cancer, when compared with women who had no comorbid conditions, even after adjustment for disease stage, type of therapy, race, and social and behavioral factors.

It is clear that the benefits of adjuvant therapy decrease with increasing age and comorbidity. The effect of adjuvant treatment on overall life expectancy is small for the oldest patients. Women in their eighties who have estrogen receptor–positive tumors should be considered for adjuvant tamoxifen therapy if they have high-risk node-negative or node-positive tumors, provided they are in good general health with a life expectancy of at least 5 years. Chemotherapy is unlikely to benefit these patients unless they are in excellent health and have high-risk, estrogen receptor–negative, node-positive tumors. The greatest dilemma is for women in their seventies; comorbidity and risk of metastases must be carefully considered in each of these cases before final recommendations about treatment are made.

Older patients are clearly underrepresented in cancer clinical trials (74). Efforts are now underway to overcome this deficiency, with increasing focus on breast cancer research in older women.

General References*

Winer EP, Morrow M, Osborne CK, et al. Malignant tumors of the breast. In: DeVita VT Jr, Hellman S, Rosenberg SA, eds. Cancer: principles and practice of oncology. 6th ed. Philadelphia: Lippincott–Raven, 2001;1651.

An in-depth chapter on breast cancer.

Harris JR, Lippman ME, Morrow M, et al. Diseases of the breast. 2nd ed. Philadelphia: Lippincott–Raven, 1999.

An excellent and extensive reference.

Silva OE, Zurrida S, eds. Breast cancer: a practical guide. Amsterdam: Elsevier, 2000.

Handy paperback.

Specific References

1. Parker SL, Tong T, Bolden S, et al. Cancer statistics, 1997. CA Cancer J Clin 1997;47:5.
2. Ries LAG, Kosary CL, Hankey BF, et al. SEER cancer statistics review 1997–1993: tables and graphs. NIH pub. no. 96-2789. Bethesda, MD: National Cancer Institute, 1995.
3. Phillips KA, Glendon G, Knight J. Putting the risk of breast cancer in perspective. N Engl J Med 1999;340:141.
4. Black WC, Nease RF Jr, Tosteson AN. Perceptions of breast cancer risk and screening effectiveness in women younger than 50 years of age. J Natl Cancer Inst 1995;87:720.
5. Tabar L, Gad A, Holmberg LH, et al. Reduction in mortality from breast cancer after mass screening from mammography. Randomized Trial from the Breast Cancer Screening Working Group of the Swedish National Board of Health and Welfare. Lancet 1985;1:829.
6. Health and Public Policy Committee, American College of Physicians. The use of diagnostic tests for screening and evaluating breast lesions. Ann Intern Med 1985;103:143.
7. Thomas DB, Gao DL, Self SG, et al. Randomized trial of breast self-examination in Shanghai: methodology and preliminary results. J Natl Cancer Inst 1997;89:355.
8. U.S. Preventive Task Force. website: http://www.ahcpr.gov/clinic/3rduspstf/breastcancer.
9. Tabar L, Vitak B, Chen HH, et al. Beyond randomized controlled trials: organized mammographic screening substantially reduces breast carcinoma mortality. Cancer 2001;91:1724.
10. Miller AB, Baines CJ, To T, et al. Canadian National Breast Screening Study: 1. Breast cancer detection and death rates among women aged 40 to 49 years. Can Med Assoc J 1992;147:1459.
11. Hendrick RE, Smith RA, Rutledge JH 3rd, et al. Benefit of screening mammography in women aged 40–49: a new meta-analysis of randomized controlled trials. J Natl Cancer Inst Monogr 1997;22:87.
12. Moskowitz M. The predictive value of certain mammographic signs in screening for breast cancer. Cancer 1983;51:1007.
13. Gail M, Rimer B. Risk-based recommendations for mammographic screening for women in their forties. J Clin Oncol 1998;16:3105.
13a. Olsen O, Gotzsche PC. Cochrane review on screening for breast cancer with mammography. Lancet 2001;358:1340.
13b. Duffy SW, Tabar L, Smith RA. The mammographic screening trials: Commentary on the recent work by Olsen and Gotzsche. Ca. Cancer J Clin. 2002;52:68.
14. Weinreb JC, Newstead G. MR imaging of the breast. Radiology 1995;196:593.
15. Khalkhali I, Villanueva-Meyer J, Edell SL, et al. Diagnostic accuracy of 99mTc-sestamibi breast imaging: multicenter trial results. J Nucl Med 2000;41:1973.
16. Dupont WD, Page DL. Risk factors for breast cancer in women with proliferative breast disease. N Engl J Med 1985;312:146.
17. Miller BA, Feuer EJ, Hankey BF. Recent incidence trends for breast cancer in women and the relevance of early detection: an update. CA Cancer J Clin 1993;43:27.
18. Claus EB, Risch N, Thompson WD. Autosomal dominant inheritance of early-onset breast cancer: implications for risk prediction. Cancer 1994;73:643.
19. Benichou J, Gail MH, Mulvihill JJ. Graphs to estimate an individualized risk of breast cancer. J Clin Oncol 1996;14:103.
20. Vogel VG. Assessing women's potential risk of developing breast cancer. Oncology 1996;10:1451.
21. FitzGerald MG, MacDonald DJ, Krainer M, et al. Germ-line BRCA1 mutations in Jewish and non-Jewish women with early-onset breast cancer. N Engl J Med 1996;334:143.
22. Greene MH. Genetics of breast cancer. Mayo Clin Proc 1997;72:54.
23. Langston AA, Malone KE, Thompson JD, et al. BRCA1 mutations in a population-based sample of young women with breast cancer. N Engl J Med 1996;334:137.
24. Statement of the American Society of Clinical Oncology. Genetic testing for cancer susceptibility. J Clin Oncol 1996;14:1730.
25. Anderson DE, Badzioch MD. Risk of familial breast cancer. Cancer 1985;56:383.
26. Nielsen M, Christensen L, Andersen J. Contralateral cancerous breast lesions in women with clinical invasive breast carcinoma. Cancer 1986;57:897.
27. Gisvold JJ, Goellner JR, Grant CS, et al. Breast biopsy: a comparative study of stereotaxically guided core and excisional techniques. AJR Am J Roentgenol 1994;162:815.
28. Schmidt RA. Stereotactic breast biopsy. CA Cancer J Clin 1994;44:172.
29. Kontostolis E, Stefanidis K, Navrozoglou I, et al. Comparison of tamoxifen with danazol for treatment of cyclical mastalgia. Gynecol Endodcrinol 1997;11:393.
30. Fisher B, Redmond C, Fisher ER, et al. Ten-year results of a randomized clinical trial comparing radical mastectomy and

*Bold print (general references) and bold numerals (specific references) denote published controlled clinical trials, meta-analysis, or consensus-based recommendations.

total mastectomy with or without radiation. N Engl J Med 1985;312:674.
31. Fisher B, Redmond C, Poisson MD, et al. Eight-year results of a randomized clinical trial comparing total mastectomy and lumpectomy with or without irradiation in the treatment of breast cancer. N Engl J Med 1989;320:822.
32. Gage I, Recht A, Gelman R, et al. Long-term outcome following breast-conserving surgery and radiation therapy. Int J Radiat Oncol Biol Phys 1995;33:245.
33. Lichter A, Lippman M, Danforth D, et al. Mastectomy versus breast conserving therapy in the treatment of stage I and II carcinoma of the breast: a randomized trial at the National Cancer Institute. J Clin Oncol 1992;10:976.
34. Schnitt SJ, Silen W, Sadowsky NL, et al. Ductal carcinoma in situ (intraductal carcinoma) of the breast. N Engl J Med 1988;318:898.
35. Fisher B, Constantino J, Redmond C, et al. Lumpectomy compared with lumpectomy and radiation therapy for the treatment of intraductal breast cancer. N Engl J Med 1993;328:1581.
36. Lagios MD. Duct carcinoma in situ: pathology and treatment. Surg Clin North Am 1990;40:853.
37. Dixon JM, Renshaw L, Bellamy C, et al. The effects of neoadjuvant anastrozole (Arimidex) on tumor volume in postmenopausal women with breast cancer: a randomized, double-blind, single-center study. Clin Cancer Res 2000;6:2229.
38. Fisher B, Bauer M, Wickerham L, et al. Relationship of number of positive axillary nodes to the prognosis of patient with primary breast cancer: an NSABP update. Cancer 1983;52:1551.
39. Fisher B, Slack N, Katrych D, et al. Ten year follow-up results of patients with carcinoma of the breast in a cooperative clinical trial evaluating surgical adjuvant chemotherapy. Surg Gynecol Obstet 1975;140:528.
40. McGuire WL, Clark GM, Dressler LG, et al. Role of steroid hormone receptors as prognostic factors in primary breast cancer. NCI Monogr 1986;1:19.
41. Reed DN Jr, Johnson J, Richard P, et al. DNA flow cytometry does not predict 5- or 10-year recurrence rates for T1-2 node-negative breast cancer. Arch Surg 2000;135:1422.
42. Krag D, Weaver D, Ashikaga T, et al. The sentinel node in breast cancer: a multicenter validation study. N Engl J Med 1998;337:941.
43. Cody HS 3rd, Hill AK, Tran KN, et al. Credentialing for breast lymphatic mapping: how many cases are enough? Ann Surg 1999;229:723.
44. McMasters KM, Tuttle TM, Carlson DJ, et al. Sentinel lymph node biopsy for breast cancer: a suitable alternative to routine axillary dissection in multi-institutional practice when optimal technique is used. J Clin Oncol 2000;18:2560.
45. Clare SE, Sener SF, Wilkens W, et al. Prognostic significance of occult lymph node metastases in node-negative breast cancer. Ann Surg Oncol 1997;4:447.
46. Braun S, Cervatli BS, Assemi C et al. Comparative analysis of micrometastases to the bone marrow and lymph nodes of node-negative breast cancer patients receiving no adjuvant therapy. J Clin Oncol 2001;19:1468.
47. Rosser RJ. Safety of sentinel lymph node dissection and significance of cytokeratin micrometastases. J Clin Oncol 2001;19:1882.
48. Early Breast Cancer Trialists' Collaborative Group. Tamoxifen for early breast cancer: an overview of the randomized trials. Lancet 1998;351:1451.
49. Early Breast Cancer Trialists' Collaborative Group. Polychemotherapy for early breast cancer: an overview of the randomised trials. Lancet 1998;352:930.
50. Recht A, Come SE, Henderson IC, et al. The sequencing of chemotherapy and radiation therapy after conservative surgery for early-stage breast cancer. N Engl J Med 1996;334:1356.
51. Early Breast Cancer Trialists' Collaborative Group. Ovarian ablation in early breast cancer: overview of the randomized trials. Lancet 1996;348:1189.
52. Fisher B, Dignam J, Wolmark N, et al. Tamoxifen in treatment of intraductal breast cancer: National Surgical Adjuvant Breast and Bowel Project B-24 randomized controlled trial. Lancet 1999;353:1993.
53. Bonneterre J, Thurlimann B, Robertson JF, et al. Anastrozole versus tamoxifen as first-line therapy for advanced breast cancer in 668 postmenopausal women: results of the tamoxifen arimidex randomized group efficacy and tolerability study. J Clin Oncol 2000;18:3748.
54. Nabholtz JM, Buzdar A, Pollak M, et al. Anastrozole is superior to tamoxifen as first-line therapy for advanced breast cancer in postmenopausal women: results of a North American randomized trial. J Clin Oncol 2000;18:3758.
55. Peters WP, Dansey RD, Klein JL, et al. High-dose chemotherapy and peripheral blood progenitor cell transplantation in the treatment of breast cancer. Oncologist 2000;5:1.
56. Overgaard M, Hansen PS, Overgaard J, et al. Postoperative radiotherapy in high-risk premenopausal women with breast cancer who receive adjuvant chemotherapy. Danish Breast Cancer Cooperative Group 82b Trial. N Engl J Med 1997;337:949.
57. Ragaz J, Jackson SM, Le N, et al. Adjuvant radiotherapy and chemotherapy in node-positive premenopausal women with breast cancer. N Engl J Med 1997;337:956.
58. Anonymous. Favourable and unfavourable effects on long-term survival of radiotherapy for early breast cancer: an overview of the randomised trials. Early Breast Cancer Trialists Collaborative Group. Lancet 2000;355:1757.
59. National Institutes of Health Consensus Development Conference statement: adjuvant therapy for breast cancer, November 1–3, 2000. J Natl Cancer Inst 2001;93:979.
60. Fisher B, Constantino J, Redmond C, et al. A randomized clinical trial evaluating tamoxifen in the treatment of patients with node-negative breast cancer who have estrogen-receptor–positive tumors. N Engl J Med 1989;320:479.
61. Fisher B, Digman J, Bryant J, Wolmark N. Five years versus more than five years of tamoxifen for lymph node-negative breast cancer: updated findings from the National Surgical Adjuvant Breast and Bowel Project B-14 randomized trial. J Natl Cancer Inst 2001;93:684.
62. GIVIO Investigators. Impact of follow-up testing on survival and health-related quality of life in breast cancer patients: a multicenter randomized controlled trial. JAMA 1994;271:1587.
63. Fisher B, Costantino JP, Wickerham DL, et al. Tamoxifen for prevention of breast cancer: report of the National Surgical Adjuvant Breast and Bowel Project P-1 study. J Natl Cancer Inst 1998;90:1371.
64. Powles T, Eeles R, Ashley S, et al. Interim analysis of the incidence of breast cancer in the Royal Marsden Hospital tamoxifen randomised chemoprevention trial. Lancet 1998;352:98.
65. Veronesi U, Maisonneuve P, Costa A, et al. Prevention of breast cancer with tamoxifen: preliminary findings from the Italian randomized trial among hysterectomised women. Italian Tamoxifen Prevention Study. Lancet 1998;352:93.
66. Cummings SR, Eckert S, Krueger KA, et al. The effect of raloxifene on risk of breast cancer in postmenopausal women: results from the MORE randomized trial. JAMA 1999;281:2189.
67. Gail MH, Costantino JP, Bryant J et al. Weighing the risks and benefits of tamoxifen treatment for preventing breast cancer. J Natl Cancer Inst 1999;91:1829.
68. Yancik R, Ries LA. Aging and cancer in America: demographic and epidemiologic perspectives. Hematol Oncol Clin North Am 2000;14:17.
69. Diab SG, Elledre RM, Clark GM. Tumor characteristics and clinical outcome of elderly women with breast cancer. J Natl Cancer Inst 2000;90:550.
70. Ballard-Barbash R, Potosky AL, Harlan LC, et al. Factors associated with surgical and radiation therapy for early stage breast cancer in older women. J Natl Cancer Inst 1996;88:716.
71. Busch E, Kemeny M, Fremegen A, et al. Patterns of breast cancer care in the elderly. Cancer 1996;78:101.
72. Hillner BE, Penberthy L, Desch CE, et al. Variation in staging and treatment of local and regional breast cancer in the elderly. Breast Cancer Res Treat 1996;40:75.
73. Satarino WA, Ragland DR. The effect of comorbidity on 3-year survival of women with primary breast cancer. Ann Intern Med 1994;120:104.
74. Trimble EL, Carter CL, Cain D, et al. Representation of older patients in cancer treatment trials. Cancer 1994;74:2208.

CHAPTER 106

Menopause and Beyond

REDONDA G. MILLER, MD

Each year more than 31 million women in the United States experience menopause. These women frequently present to primary care clinicians with a number of symptoms related to estrogen deficiency, as well as the psychosocial issues related to midlife changes in family and social relationships. The average age is 51 years, but menopause may occur earlier in smokers (1). Given the increasing life expectancy in the United States, the average woman can expect to spend more than one third of her life in the postmenopausal years.

Because several chronic diseases associated with aging are first manifested at menopause, this is an opportune time for the primary care clinician and patient to assess risk and initiate preventive strategies for cardiovascular disease, osteoporosis, and cancer, in addition to addressing the symptoms of menopause. There are complex relationships among these diseases; for instance, the risk of osteoporosis seems to be inversely related to the risk of breast cancer (2). Hormone replacement therapy (HRT), the most effective treatment of menopausal symptoms, has been shown to affect the outcomes of these chronic diseases as well, which has made the decision to use HRT an increasingly complex one.

DEFINITION AND PHYSIOLOGY

The menopause is defined as the *last* menses. This is a clinical diagnosis that can be determined with certainty only when menses have been absent for 12 months. *Perimenopause* is the span of time that encompasses the period of initial menstrual irregularity, typically 2 to 8 years before menopause, the menopause itself, and the year subsequent to the menopause. Perimenopause usually begins in the forties, but it is not uncommon for women to experience symptoms as early as their thirties.

During perimenopause, a host of hormonal changes occur. Ovarian follicles undergo progressive atresia over the course of a woman's lifetime, with a consequent gradual fall in estradiol. There is also a loss of production of the glycoprotein inhibin by the ovaries. Inhibin provides negative feedback to the pituitary gland, and, in its absence, pituitary production of follicle-stimulating hormone (FSH) and luteinizing hormone (LH) increases. An FSH level greater than 30 mIU/mL may be supportive of menopause, but the level tends to fluctuate significantly throughout the perimenopause and is not reliably diagnostic. Routine measurement of FSH is not recommended. On the other hand, FSH measurement is useful in certain situations, such as in a hysterectomized woman without classic vasomotor symptoms or a woman who may be experiencing premature ovarian failure.

Because both estradiol and FSH have large fluctuations during this period, the diagnosis of perimenopause is often made clinically, with the onset of menstrual cycle irregularity in a woman with previously regular menstrual cycles. Menstrual irregularity can take the form of shortened cycles, missed cycles, or irregular spotting. Some patients have regular cycles up until the point of menopause. A perimenopausal woman should be cautioned that pregnancy is a possibility until she has been amenorrheic for more than 1 year or until FSH levels have consistently been greater than 30 mIU/mL.

Women may consult their primary care clinicians during this period for concerns about abnormal uterine bleeding or amenorrhea. Patients with abnormal vaginal bleeding (see Chapter 101) should be referred immediately for evaluation. Amenorrhea in women younger than 50 years of age should be evaluated with a pregnancy test. Thyroid dysfunction can also affect the menstrual cycle and should be assessed by screening tests in women who present with menstrual irregularities.

CLINICAL CONSIDERATIONS

Clinical guidelines (see General References) for management of menopause generally recommend that the office evaluation of the menopausal patient include a comprehensive risk assessment and screening, as well as attention to the common symptoms of estrogen deficiency (Table 106.1).

The severity of menopausal symptoms is highly variable and is related to both physiologic and cultural factors. Some women are quite debilitated, whereas others have minimal or no symptoms. As an example, a prospective study of 478 Australian women from premenopause to postmenopause found that the number of women reporting five or more symptoms increased by 14% from early to late menopause. Lower estrogen levels, smoking, and a history of no occupation predicted vasomotor symptoms. Insomnia, which

Table 106.1. Office Evaluation of the Perimenopausal Patient

Assess Current Symptoms
- Hot flushes
- Menstrual irregularity: abnormal bleeding, amenorrhea
- Symptoms of pelvic floor relaxation; bladder dysfunction
- Sexual function (e.g., loss of libido, dyspareunia)
- Sleep disturbances

Assess Risk of Osteoporosis, Breast Cancer, Endometrial Cancer, Cardiovascular Disease
- Reproductive history: menarche, parity, contraception, surgical history
- Physical activity, use of tobacco
- Dietary history (e.g., intake of vitamin D and calcium)
- History of hormone replacement therapy (HRT)
- Family history of osteoporosis, cancer, heart disease
- History of fractures, loss of height

Assess Psychosocial Status
- Mood changes, difficulty with concentration
- Expectations of menopause
- Family and work

Assess Chronic Medical Conditions That May Affect HRT Decision
- Hypertension
- Diabetes mellitus
- Hyperlipidemia
- Gallbladder disease
- Thromoboembolic disease

Physical Examination, to Include
- Weight, height, body mass index
- Posture
- Vision and hearing screens
- Breast examination
- Pelvic and rectal examination

Laboratory testing, to Include
- Lipid profile
- Serum thyroid-stimulating hormone, if indicated
- Serum follicle-stimulating hormone, if indicated (see text)
- Bone mineral density, if indicated (see Chapter 103)
- Screening protocols for mammography, colon cancer, and cervical cancer (see Chapter 1)

Counseling and Patient Education
- Exercise prescription
- Nutrition and weight management
- Vitamin D and calcium supplementation
- Avoidance of triggers for hot flushes
- Benefits and risks of HRT
- Alternatives to HRT therapy

increased throughout the menopause, was related not only to hot flushes but also to psychosocial factors (3).

Regardless of initial symptom severity, there are many long-term effects of estrogen deficiency on bone, heart, and breast, which should be evaluated in every patient.

Vasomotor Symptoms

Vasomotor symptoms are the most common reason women seek medical care during perimenopause. These symptoms are usually most common in the first 2 to 3 years of perimenopause and then taper off gradually. The prevalence varies by culture. Up to 75% of women in the United States and Europe experience hot flushes, whereas only 20% of Asian women do. In migration studies of Japanese women, the incidence of hot flushes approached the overall U.S. incidence within one or two generations, which implicates nongenetic factors, such as diet (4). The intensity and frequency of hot flushes are also variable and are usually more severe in women who undergo surgical menopause.

The hot flush is a sensation of heat that typically develops in the head and neck region and then slowly spreads down the arms and across the chest. Intense diaphoresis and visible flushing may accompany the hot flush. Occasionally women may experience a prodrome of nausea, light-headedness, or palpitations. The episode may end with chills and a feeling of coldness. The entire event usually lasts between 30 seconds and 5 minutes. Hot flushes frequently occur at night, leading to lack of sleep and subsequent daytime fatigue and irritability. Other triggers of hot flushes include spicy food, caffeine, alcohol, stress, humid environments, and sexual activity. In a study of African American and Caucasian women, significant predictors of hot flushes were higher FSH levels, anxiety, alcohol use, body mass index, and parity; there was no difference by race (5).

The exact cause of hot flushes is unknown, but they may be related to alterations in the hypothalamic thermoregulatory center that are precipitated by a lack of estrogen and increasing gonadotropin levels. Documented increases in skin conductance and peripheral temperature and a subsequent fall in core temperature coincide with the flush (6). Studies using an ingested telemetry pill found that the thermoneutral zone, that is, the range of core body temperature within which sweating, peripheral vasodilatation, and shivering do not occur, is virtually nonexistent in symptomatic women but normal in aysmptomatic women (7). Central sympathetic activation is increased in symptomatic women and also reduces the thermoneutral zone in animals. The beneficial effect of clonidine for hot flushes may relate to its reduction of central sympathetic activation.

Treatment

Simple measures can help women cope with hot flushes. Wearing layered clothing permits adjustments for temperature. Regular exercise and avoidance of known triggers can help with prevention. Table 106.2 lists common therapies for vasomotor symptoms, of which estrogen replacement is the most effective. It has been shown to decrease hot flushes and improve nighttime insomnia. Both oral and transdermal estrogens (see later discussion) are effective and work within 1 to 4 weeks. Most women respond to standard doses, but occasionally higher doses are required.

For women who are unable or unwilling to take estrogen, other alternatives are available, but none is as effective as estrogen. Progestins alone by oral, topical, or injectable routes may give some relief. The antihypertensive agents clonidine and methyldopa are moderately effective in controlling vasomotor symptoms, but side effects of drowsiness, constipation, and dry mouth may be limiting. Estrogen's interaction with serotonergic and dopamingergic neurotransmitters has led to the use of one class of antidepressants, selective serotonin reuptake inhibitors (SSRIs) (see Chapter 24)

Table 106.2. Therapies for Menopausal Vasomotor Symptoms

Agent	Dose	Side Effects
Estrogen	Variable (see Table 106.5)	Breast tenderness, vaginal spotting, headaches
Progestins		
Medroxyprogesterone acetate	Oral: 5–10 mg PO q.d. Depot: 50–150 mg every month Transdermal: 20 mg PO q.d.	Breast tenderness, irritability, depression, headaches
Clonidine	Oral: 0.1–0.3 mg PO t.i.d.	Fatigue, dizziness, dry mouth, constipation
Methyldopa	500 mg PO b.i.d.	Headache, somnolence, gastrointestinal upset
Serotonin reuptake inhibitors		
Paroxetine	10–20 mg q.d.	Somonolence, dry mouth, decreased appetite, nausea, constipation
Venlafaxine	37.5–150 mg q.d.	
Fluxetine	20 mg q.d.	
Veralipride	100 mg PO q.d.	Galactorrhea, increased prolactin levels
Tibolone	2.5 mg PO q.d.	Venous and leg disorders
Herbals	Variable	Gastrointestinal upset
Soy protein		
Black cohosh		

and veralipride, a dopamine agonist, for menopausal symptoms. Clinical trials of paroxetine, venlafaxine, and fluoxetine found a reduction in hot flushes of 60% to 80%, with associated improvement in sleep and depression (8,9). Veralipride eliminated hot flushes in 80% of treated patients in one controlled trial (10); it increases estradiol and prolactin levels, and some patients experienced breast discharge. There have been rare reports of movement disorders in patients taking veralipride.

Tibolone is a synthetic steroid analog with both estrogenic and androgenic properties. Side effects are similar to those of estrogen, but vaginal spotting is much less common (11). Both tibolone and veralipride seem to be safe for *short-term* use, but neither is available in the United States.

Finally, herbal preparations may provide a benefit in the treatment of vasomotor symptoms. Many women prefer herbals as a more natural alternative than prescription medication, and food supplements are being heavily marketed in the United States. The most studied agents are black cohosh and soy protein.

Black cohosh (*Actaea racemosa* L) is a North American herb used by Native Americans and thought to have estrogenic properties. As with many herbal preparations, issues of dose and bioavailability confound the literature regarding effectiveness (see Chapter 5). A 1998 review (12) of eight studies concluded that black cohosh is safe and effective, but one randomized controlled trial in breast cancer patients found no benefit of black cohosh over placebo for treatment of hot flushes (13). A standardized extract of black cohosh is marketed as Remifemin and frequently prescribed in Europe.

Phytoestrogens are plant steroids that bind to estrogen receptors, although with much less affinity than human estrogen. They exhibit both estrogenic and antiestrogenic effects. Isoflavones, one of three types of phytoestrogens, are thought to have the most estrogenic activity. Isoflavones are found in soy, chickpeas, lentils, and beans. There appears to be individual variation in the physiologic response to ingestion of isoflavones, but they are relatively well tolerated except for moderate gastrointestinal distress. Three placebo-controlled trials of soy protein found statistically significant reductions of hot flushes with supplementation (phytoestrogen, 17 mg twice daily; phytoestrogen, 45 mg once daily; and soy 60 mg once daily), but the clinical significance was small, approximately one hot flush per day (14–16). Isoflavones favorably affect the lipid profile, by increasing high-density lipoprotein (HDL) and decreasing low-density lipoprotein (LDL) cholesterol levels, but there are insufficient data regarding any effect on breast or endometrial cancer risk or on bone mass, suggesting caution in recommending these supplements (17). A review of more than 1,000 articles on phytoestrogens found only 74 that addressed human subjects and none that addressed primary or secondary prevention of cancer (18).

Urogenital Symptoms

After menopause, the urogenital tract undergoes significant changes and atrophy. Although the exact role of estrogen is unknown, estrogen receptors are located throughout the urogenital tract, and the decline in estrogen levels often correlates with the development of symptoms. Symptoms can be highly variable in character and onset. Some women experience vaginal dryness, itching, and burning. Dyspareunia and loss of libido may be sequelae. Up to one third of women develop urinary incontinence, usually with a stress pattern (see Chapter 54). Estrogen receptors are also found on the pelvic musculature and ligaments, and the decline in estrogen may lead to uterine and bladder prolapse. Other factors that further increase the risk of prolapse include advancing age and history of multiple births. Finally, estrogen plays a role in maintaining vaginal acidity by allowing lactic acid–producing bacilli to flourish. Without estrogen, the flora may shift to bacteria such as *Escherichia coli*, leading to more frequent urinary tract infections. All of these symptoms may occur within the perimenopause or may take up

Table 106.3. Therapies for Vaginal Dryness and Genitourinary Symptoms

Preparation	Estrogen (Brand)	Dose
Lubricants	No estrogen (Replens)	Use liberally as needed with intercourse
Cream	Conjugated estrogens (Premarin)	0.5–2.0 g q.d. for 3 weeks each month
	Estradiol (Estrace)	2–4 g q.d. × 2 wk then ↓ dose
	Estropipate (Ogen)	2–4 g q.d. for 3 wk each month
	Dienestrol (Ortho Dienestrol)	1–2 applicators q.d. for 1–2 wk then ↓ dose
Ring	Estradiol (Estring)	Insert and replace every 90 d
Tablet	Estradiol (Vagifem)	1 tablet vaginally q.d. × 2 wk, then 1 tablet twice weekly

to 10 years to manifest. Many women never approach their primary care provider owing to embarrassment or the misconception that these symptoms cannot be treated.

Treatment

Estrogen is effective in alleviating many of the urogenital symptoms. It improves vaginal dryness, atrophic vaginitis, and dyspareunia. Estrogen has also been shown to lessen the symptoms of urinary incontinence in perimenopausal women (19) (see Chapter 54). Postmenopausal women with recurrent urinary tract infections can prolong time to recurrence by using estrogen (20).

Lower doses of estrogen are needed for the relief of genitourinary symptoms than for vasomotor symptoms (Table 106.3). Local delivery of estrogen can result in high tissue levels and is often adequate. Numerous preparations of local estrogen therapy are available today. They include creams (conjugated equine estrogens, estradiol, and diethylstilbestrol), estriol pessaries, and estradiol rings and tablets. All seem comparable in effectiveness, so patient preference plays a large role in choice. Both creams and pessaries, however, can be messy to administer and result in discharge. On the other hand, the vaginal ring and estrogen tablets are well tolerated and only rarely result in mild leukorrhea. Given the low doses used, local estrogen administration is relatively safe and does not seem to result in endometrial hypertrophy. It does not, however, confer the added benefit on vasomotor symptoms, lipid profile, and bone density that systemic administration does.

Cognition and Depression

Women may experience many cognitive symptoms during the perimenopause. Many women describe difficulty with concentration, poor memory, and feelings of sadness or depression. It remains controversial as to whether these symptoms are truly related to menopause or perhaps related to the loss of sleep and fatigue associated with nocturnal hot flushes. Another possibility is that they are a reaction to the changes in a woman's cultural roles that may be associated with menopause. Data supporting these hypotheses are conflicting. One longitudinal analysis of more than 2,500 women found no relationship between menopause and depression (21), but another large, cross-sectional study suggested that postmenopausal women using estrogen alone were at decreased risk for depression (22). The second study, however, found no decrease in depression risk among women using *both* estrogen and progestin.

A loss of libido is another frequent concern described by perimenopausal and menopausal women. The lack of interest in sex is probably multifactorial. Depression and low self-esteem, vaginal dryness and dyspareunia, and a decline in testosterone levels may all play a role. Some experts promote the addition of androgens to estrogen therapy to improve libido (23). Testosterone can be delivered as methyltestosterone, 1.25 to 2.5 mg/day; as micronized testosterone, 2.5 to 5.0 mg/day; or with a transdermal patch, 150 to 300 μg/day. Androgens can prevent postmenopausal bone loss. The side effects of excessive androgen use include acne, hirsutism, alopecia, and voice deepening. Androgens may lower HDL levels, potentially worsening cardiovascular risk. The American Association of Clinical Endocrinologists practice guidelines (24) suggest four situations in which androgen plus estrogen therapy may be considered: (a) Oophorectomized women, (b) women who have experienced inadequate relief of vasomotor symptoms with estrogen, (c) women who are at risk for osteoporosis and unable to take other therapies, and (d) women with unsatisfactory sexual function, especially loss of libido. Large, randomized trials examining the benefits of adding androgen therapy to estrogen in postmenopausal women do not exist. Further research is under way.

Cardiovascular Changes

The leading cause of death among American women is coronary heart disease (CHD). Before menopause, the rate of myocardial infarction in women is much lower than in men, but by the eighth decade the rates have equalized. Much of the premenopausal protection from CHD in women has been attributed to estrogen.

There are several effects of estrogen on the cardiovascular system. The most obvious effect is on the lipid profile. Within 6 months of the menopause, total cholesterol and LDL cholesterol begin to increase. HDL cholesterol levels fall as a result of the estrogen deficiency. This is particularly important in women, because low HDL seems to be a stronger predictor of CHD death in women than in men. Other changes that take place with menopause are increased levels of plasminogen-activator inhibitor type 1 (PAI-1), lipoprotein(a), and homocysteine. Each of these is thought to be an independent risk factor for CHD.

Observational studies have demonstrated a protective effect of estrogen on cardiovascular disease. Estrogen appears to decrease the risk of CHD and CHD death in postmenopausal women by 40% to 60% (25,26). Estrogen may exert much of its protective effect through changes in the lipid profile. Oral estrogen increases HDL cholesterol by roughly 15% and decreases LDL cholesterol by up to 19% (27,28). Triglycerides are also increased, but usually not to a large degree. Addition of a progestin, such as medroxyprogesterone acetate, to estrogen attenuates the beneficial effects on lipid but does not eliminate them (28). With norethindrone acetate use, LDL is still lowered, but there does not seem to be a beneficial increase in HDL. Micronized progestin may be least detrimental on the lipid profile.

Estrogen may have other favorable effects on the cardiovascular system. Evidence suggests that it decreases levels of PAI-1, lipoprotein(a), and homocysteine. There is also literature to support a direct vasodilatory effect of estrogen on the coronary vasculature.

Conversely, estrogen has been shown to have unfavorable effects on the cardiovascular system. Estrogen use can increase triglyceride levels and activate coagulation factors. Recently, the role of estrogen replacement therapy in secondary prevention of CHD has become clouded. Observational data had shown a protective effect, but the first randomized, controlled trial, the Heart and Estrogen/Progestin Replacement Study (HERS), suggested otherwise (29). Postmenopausal women with established CHD had similar rates of myocardial infarction and CHD death whether they were treated with hormone replacement or not. Analysis of time trends in the study revealed an excess of events in the estrogen-treated group in year 1 but fewer events in years 4 and 5. This may represent a manifestation of the early prothrombotic effects of estrogen (with increased early events) followed by more long-term beneficial changes. Alternatively, high-risk women may have cardiac events early, leaving only lower risk women in the study. There are currently seven large ongoing clinical trials addressing the use of estrogen in primary and secondary prevention of cardiovascular disease, which have the objective of clarifying this controversial area. As of July 2001, the American Heart Association has concluded that HRT should not be initiated for the secondary prevention of cardiovascular disease and that there is insufficient evidence for its use in primary prevention (30).

Osteoporosis

Osteoporosis is a large health problem that remains underdiagnosed. An average 50-year-old white woman has up to a 50% chance of sustaining an osteoporotic fracture in her lifetime (31). Hip fractures alone are associated with a significant mortality rate of 20% at 1 year. Other sequelae of fracture include difficulty with ambulation, dependence on assisted living, chronic pain, and loss of quality of life. The most rapid loss of bone mineralization occurs in the years after menopause. After 30 years of age, most women experience a loss of approximately 0.5% to 1.0% of their bone density per year. In the first 5 years after menopause, the rate accelerates to 3% to 5% per year before returning to the baseline rate. Prevention of perimenopausal bone loss is therefore crucial. Serial yearly height measurements in the office may provide an early clue to the development of osteoporosis. The loss of 1 inch or more in height is highly suggestive of the disease.

All perimenopausal women should be counseled regarding proper dietary calcium intake. The National Osteoporosis Foundation recommends that women consume at least 1,000 mg/day, or 1,500 mg/day if frank osteoporosis is present. Women also should be encouraged to pursue weight-bearing exercise, because this has been shown to be helpful in bone density preservation. Osteoporosis and its management is discussed more thoroughly in Chapter 103.

THERAPEUTIC OPTIONS

Hormone Replacement Therapy

HRT is not for every woman. It has been associated with great benefits, but it also has significant drawbacks.

Advantages of Hormone Replacement Therapy

Many advantages of estrogen have been discussed. One of the most rapid benefits a woman taking HRT experiences is significant relief of vasomotor symptoms. Hot flushes diminish within days to weeks. Vaginal dryness improves, leading to improved ability to have intercourse. Urinary tract infections are less frequent as well.

Estrogen plays a significant role in modifying several chronic diseases. Use of estrogen at menopause allows a woman to preserve bone density and aids in the prevention of osteoporosis. In women who are already osteopenic or osteoporotic, estrogen serves to increase bone density and decrease the fracture rate by up to 40% to 60%. Estrogen may also have significant benefits on the cardiovascular system, particularly in primary prevention.

Estrogen may play a preventive function in several other chronic diseases. Estrogen receptors are widespread throughout the body, including the central nervous system. It has been proposed that estrogen may protect against Alzheimer disease. A published meta-analysis demonstrated that estrogen users had a 29% decrease in the risk of dementia (32), but two randomized clinical trials of estrogen replacement therapy in women with mild-to-moderate Alzheimer disease found no differences in cognitive performance between women taking estrogen and those taking placebo (33,34). Estrogen therapy has also been linked to a decreased rate of colon cancer (35). Other purported but not proven roles include prevention of macular degeneration, lens opacities, tooth loss, age-related hypertension, and skin aging.

Disadvantages of Hormone Replacement Therapy

Some of the more prevalent disadvantages of estrogen therapy are the non–life-threatening side effects. Menopausal women starting HRT may experience breast tenderness or vaginal spotting. These symptoms tend to resolve within 2 months in most women. Low-dose oral bromocriptine (2.5 mg twice daily) may be helpful in alleviating the breast tenderness on a short-term basis, as may prescribing an estrogen-free period a few days each month. Contrary to popular belief, postmenopausal doses of estrogen are not associated with weight gain.

The biggest fear shared by many women is that estrogen may cause breast cancer. These fears are not unfounded, and many studies have unsuccessfully attempted to put the issue to rest. Given the observational nature of most of these studies, they are confounded by selection and lead-time bias. Two studies are most often cited. The Nurses' Health Study monitored almost 70,000 postmenopausal women and found a relative risk for development of breast cancer of 1.3 to 1.4 among current users of estrogen (36). Duration of use greater than 10 years was highly correlated with the development of breast cancer, and former use was not. Conversely, the Iowa study of high-risk women with positive family histories showed no increased risk, even with use lasting longer 5 years (37). No study has definitively shown increased mortality due to breast cancer, leading some experts to postulate that estrogen use may result in "better-differentiated" and less aggressive tumors. Another possibility is that women who use estrogen are more compliant with mammography and more likely to have cancers detected earlier. Estrogen's exact role in the development of breast cancer, therefore, remains controversial.

Studies have repetitively linked endometrial adenocarcinoma to the use of unopposed estrogen in women with an intact uterus. The risk is roughly 2.3 times that of women who do not use estrogen. Risk is related to duration of use. In women using unopposed estrogen for longer than 10 years, the relative risk rises to 9.5 (38). If estrogen is combined with a progestin, the risk is not elevated above that of nonusers. Therefore, use of a progestin *with* estrogen in nonhysterectomized women should be considered the standard of care. The progestin may be given continuously or cyclically with the same protective benefit. Given that many women will experience some mild vaginal spotting with the institution of HRT, one must distinguish this fairly common side effect from a more serious problem. If vaginal bleeding is mild and occurs immediately in an otherwise healthy woman initiating HRT, watchful waiting is appropriate. Temporarily increasing the dose of progestin may help alleviate this bleeding. If the bleeding persists beyond 6 months, is particularly heavy, or starts months to years *after* the initiation of HRT, the patient should be further evaluated. A transvaginal ultrasound examination may be helpful in assessing the thickness of the uterine lining and detecting fibroids. Referral to a gynecologist and probable endometrial biopsy is also warranted.

Some concern has been raised about a possible link between estrogen and ovarian cancer. Earlier studies were inconsistent, but a recent cohort study of more than 200,000 women suggested that use for longer than 10 years conferred more than twice the risk of mortality from ovarian cancer, compared with no use (39). For former users, risk decreased with time. These results must be interpreted cautiously, because many study participants were taking unopposed estrogen; combination therapy is not well studied.

Estrogen replacement therapy has been linked to an increased risk of venous thromboembolic disease. Users tend to have 2.5 to 3.5 times the risk of nonusers (28,40). This is less than the risk associated with oral contraceptive use, probably because postmenopausal doses of estrogen are considerably lower than those in oral contraceptives. Estrogen also increases the risk of gallbladder disease in women, albeit only modestly (29). In the liver, estrogen can increase the metabolism and turnover of cholesterol, leading to increased excretion in the bile and subsequent stone formation. This side effect does not lead to any greater mortality.

The absolute contraindications to estrogen are relatively few. Most experts would agree that a personal history of breast cancer and acute thromboembolic disease fall into this category (Table 106.4). Many of the disadvantages listed previously must be taken in context with the patient's individual risks and may be considered relative contraindications, depending on the clinical setting. Some of the relative contraindications can be addressed by alternative delivery; transdermal estrogen avoids the first-pass effect and has some advantages in specific situations (see later discussion).

Available Formulations

HRT may be delivered by several different routes and formulations, each with unique characteristics (41) (Table 106.5). Deciding which to use is often a matter of individual choice and preference. After careful evaluation of the patient and discussion of her concerns, the primary care clinician is ideally suited to tailor a treatment regimen that will best meet the patient's needs (Table 106.6). In a woman without a uterus, estrogen

Table 106.4. Potential Contraindications to Hormone Replacement Therapy

Strong Contraindications	Cautious Use Advised
Personal history of breast cancer	Strong family history of breast cancer
Endometrial cancer within 5 yr	Past history of thromboembolic disease
Recent thromboembolic event (<1 yr)	Chronic liver disease
Unexplained vaginal bleeding	History of gallbladder disease and no cholecystectomy
Severe hepatic dysfunction, aspartate aminotransferase twice normal	Migraine headaches

Adapted from A decision tree for the use of estrogen replacement therapy or hormone replacement therapy in postmenopausal women: consensus opinion of the North American Menopause Society. Menopause 2000;7:79.

Table 106.5. Forms of Hormone Replacement Therapy (HRT)

Form of HRT	Dose	Comments
Estrogens	Conjugated: 0.625 mg PO q.d. Esterified: 0.625 mg PO q.d. Estradiol: 0.05–1 mg PO q.d. Estropipate: 0.625 mg PO q.d.	Use only in hysterectomized women Initial breast tenderness Benefits: improvement in vasomotor symptoms, relief of vaginal dryness, cardioprotection, osteoporosis prevention Escalate dose if hot flushes unrelieved
Cyclical estrogens and progestin combination	Estrogen: one of the above preparations on days 1–25 AND Medroxyprogesterone: 10 mg PO q.d. on days 16–25 OR Micronized progesterone: 200 mg PO q.d. on days 16–25	Monthly withdrawal bleeding Benefits comparable to estrogen alone Mild detriment on lipid profile
Continuous conjugated estrogens and progestin combination	Estrogen: one of the above PO q.d. AND Medroxyprogesterone: 2.5–5 mg PO q.d. OR Micronized progesterone: 100 mg PO q.d. OR Norethindrone acetate: 1 mg PO q.d.	Vaginal spotting Escalate dose or progestin for persistent vaginal spotting Benefits comparable to estrogen alone Mild detriment on lipid profile
Transdermal estrogen	Estradiol: 0.05–0.1 mg topically once or twice per week	Use only in hysterectomized women or must add a progestin Easier for compliance Less benefit on lipid profile Less risk in patients with liver disease
Estrogen and androgen combination	Esterified estrogens and methyltestosterone: 0.625/1.25 mg PO q.d.	? Benefit on libido Must add a progestin for women with a uterus

Adapted with permission from Miller RG, Chang KK. Management of the menopausal patient. Primary Care Reports 2000;6:39.

alone can be prescribed without a progestin, because there is no risk of endometrial hyperplasia. Estrogen can be delivered by several routes, including orally, transdermally, or vaginally. The doses used are much lower than those found in oral contraceptives, but they are adequate to restore physiologic status. Oral conjugated equine estrogens are the most widely used and studied type. Other preparations use esterified estrogens, ethinyl estradiol, or estropipate. Oral administration provides "first-pass" metabolism through the liver and thus offers the most benefit on the lipid profile. Transdermal estrogens are often more convenient, but they lack the metabolic effects in the liver, and consequently have less beneficial effect on cholesterol. In a woman with liver disease or high triglycerides, however, this may be desirable. Both oral and transdermal forms are very useful in relieving vasomotor symptoms. Young women experiencing surgical menopause often require higher doses of estrogen, as much as 1.25 to 2.5 mg conjugated estrogen per day. If the initial dose is ineffective, escalating the dose for a brief period may be helpful. Vaginal estrogens are very effective locally, providing relief of vaginal dryness and dyspareunia. They offer very little systemic absorption and therefore do not afford protection against osteoporosis or coronary heart disease, nor do they help with systemic hot flushes.

In a woman with a uterus, a progestin (synthetic progesterone) must be added to estrogen. Table 106.5 summarizes the ways to do this. The first is to cycle the estrogen and progestin so that monthly sloughing of the endometrium occurs; this is referred to as *cyclic combined therapy*. This is accomplished by giving the estrogen on menstrual cycle days 1 through 25 and the progestin on days 16 through 25. After day 25, the woman experiences a period. Most women do not like the inconvenience associated with continued menses. A useful alternative is to deliver both the estrogen and the progestin on a continuous daily basis (*continuous combined therapy*). This method may result in some initial vaginal spotting that usually resolves within 2 to 3 months. Vaginal spotting is most common in women within 1 or 2 years of menopause, and cyclic therapy may be preferable for these women. Increasing the dose of progestin for a period of 1 to 2 months may decrease the amount of bleeding. Many combination products containing various forms of both estrogen and progestin are available and offer the convenience of once-a-day dosing.

As with estrogen, the choice of progestin type is one of preference. All have some detrimental effect on the lipid profile. Micronized progesterone may affect the lipid profile least. Medroxyprogesterone acetate (MPA) is popular because of the potential for less androgenic activity and its availability in combination pills. Norethindrone acetate (also available in a combination preparation) results in the least amount of vaginal spotting and bleeding, but, as noted previously, may preclude the rise in HDL seen with other combinations.

For postmenopausal women with poor libido, some experts have recommended adding an androgen to the HRT regimen. Only limited data from small studies are currently available (23). Other potential benefits of androgen therapy include improved mood and added

Table 106.6. Suggested Hormone Replacement Therapy Regimens for Specific Patient Situations

Patient Situation	Suggested Regimen	Comments
Perimenopausal patient with menstrual irregularity	Low-dose oral contraceptive, containing 20 μg ethinyl estradiol (see Chapter 100)	No upper age limit in nonsmokers; can be used into menopause; if needed, check FSH level after day 2 placebo week
Menopausal, no uterus	Daily oral or transdermal estrogen	Side effect of breast tenderness; can add estrogen-free period at end of month
Menopausal, with uterus, within 1–2 yr after menopause	Cyclic estrogen + progestin	Advantage of predictable vaginal bleeding
Menopausal, with uterus, wishes to avoid vaginal bleeding	1. Continuous combined therapy 2. Cyclic therapy in 90-day cycles	1. Frequent spotting if recently menopausal (in first 6 mo)
History of hypertension	Transdermal estrogen	Avoids hepatic production of angiotensinogen
History of diabetes mellitus	Transdermal estrogen	Less hypertriglyceridemia, but less beneficial effect on lipids; may want to add lipid-lowering therapy (see Chapter 82)
History of gallbladder disease, chronic liver disease	Transdermal estrogen	—
Migraine headache	Transdermal estrogen	—
History of coronary artery disease	Initiation ERT currently not recommended	Increased risk of CV events
Increased risk of cardiovascular (CV) disease	ERT with micronized progestin	Best effect on lipid profile; no evidence to date of primary prevention of CV disease
Increased risk of osteoporosis	ERT	Requires lifelong therapy to maintain benefit; re-evaluate at 5–7 yr for alternative (e.g., SERM)
Increase breast cancer risk, wishes to avoid ERT	Progestin-only treatment of vasomotor symptoms; low-dose, topical therapy for vaginal/genitourinary symptoms; SERM, bisphosphonates, calcitonin for prevention of osteoporosis (see Chapter 103); modification of CV risk (see Chapter 57)	
Premenopausal, oophorectomized, with vasomotor symptoms and loss of libido	May require higher doses of estrogen, 1.25–2.5 mg q.d.	Consider addition of androgen (e.g., testosterone)
Elderly patient with osteoporosis	Start with 0.3 mg conjugated equine estrogens OR SERM or bisphosphonate (see Chapter 103)	May be intolerant of higher doses of estrogen

CV, cardiovascular; ERT, estrogen replacement therapy; SERM, selective estrogen receptor modulators.

increases in bone mineral density. However, HDL cholesterol decreases, in contrast to the increase seen with estrogen alone. This may have an impact on long-term primary cardioprotection. Other expected androgenic side effects, such as hirsutism, acne, and weight gain, have not been commonly described with the use of low doses of testosterone. In a postmenopausal woman with low libido, a 3- to 4-month trial of androgen therapy is a reasonable approach, keeping in mind that definitive data regarding effectiveness are not available. If this is successful, the patient may require the therapy indefinitely. Adding an androgen to estrogen does not negate the necessity for a progestin in a woman with a uterus.

Selective Estrogen Receptor Modulators

Selective estrogen receptor modulators (SERMs) are a relatively new class of drugs that have both estrogen receptor agonist and antagonist effects, depending on the target organ. Tamoxifen, one of the first SERMs, has been available since 1969. It is used primarily for prevention of breast cancer recurrence. There are several limitations to its use, including a worsening of hot flushes, an increased risk of endometrial hyperplasia and possible adenocarcinoma, and an increased risk of thromboembolic disease. A newer SERM, raloxifene, demonstrates estrogenic effects on bone, the lipid profile, and the coagulation system, and antiestrogenic effects on the breast and uterus. The approved dose is 60 mg once a day. At this dosage, there are several benefits to raloxifene therapy (Table 106.7). Perimenopausal women can expect to gain an average of 1% to 2% in bone mineral density at both spine and hip at 2 years (42). Regarding the lipid profile, total cholesterol declines by 6% to 7% and LDL cholesterol falls by 10% with treatment. In contrast to the effect with estrogen, however, HDL cholesterol also falls by about 3%. How this relates to long-term protection from cardiac events and mortality is currently unknown. Women taking raloxifene do not experience any thickening of the uterine lining or any increase in

Table 106.7. Estrogen versus Raloxifene for Hormone Replacement Therapy

	Estrogen	Raloxifene
Hot flushes	↓	0 or ↑
Breast tenderness	↑	0
Uterine hyperplasia and bleeding	↑	0
Cholesterol		
High-density lipoprotein	↑	0
Low-density lipoprotein	↓	↓
Bone mineral density	↑	↑
Venous thromboembolism	↑	↑

Reprinted from Miller RG, Chang KK. Management of the menopausal patient. Primary Care Reports 2000;6:39, with permission.

the incidence of uterine cancer (42). Finally, data from the 7,700 women in the Multiple Outcomes of Raloxifene Evaluation (MORE) trial suggest that raloxifene may play a role in breast cancer prevention, with the observation of a 76% reduction in the risk of invasive cancer in treated women (43). This was not a primary design of the study, however, and additional studies designed to clarify this point are pending.

Raloxifene is not without drawbacks. In many women, it leads to onset or worsening of hot flushes. There is also a threefold increase in the risk of thromboembolic disease, comparable to the risk with estrogen.

Despite the lack of a head-to-head comparison, raloxifene is considered a reasonable alternative for the woman who does not want to take estrogen or has a contraindication to its use but who still desires bone protection and lower LDL cholesterol.

OVERALL APPROACH TO HELPING WOMEN DECIDE ABOUT USING HORMONE REPLACEMENT THERAPY

Helping a women decide whether to pursue HRT for menopause is a complicated task. The controversy around the pros and cons of HRT seems to become murkier every day. In addition, each woman has a different risk profile for various diseases and certainly different preferences and fears about HRT. Women do not always openly express these preferences and fears. In fact, up to 20% of women prescribed estrogen for the first time discontinue it within 1 year, 10% use it only intermittently, and up to 30% never fill the prescription (44). The clinician should have an extensive and ongoing dialogue with the patient about HRT.

Women who wish to use estrogen predominantly for control of vasomotor symptoms are easier to counsel. Such short-term use of estrogen (less than 5 years) carries less risk from a breast cancer perspective. However, with the recent recognition of an early increase in cardiac events, special consideration should be given to women at high risk for CHD. The cases of women who are interested in using estrogen for long-term health benefits are more complicated. Those at high risk for osteoporosis may gain the most advantage from HRT use. Long-term cardiovascular benefits are less clear, although numerous observational studies support a trend toward protection with duration of use. Women with a personal or strong family history of breast cancer are probably better served by raloxifene.

Several authors have tried to weigh these advantages and disadvantages to aid physicians in counseling their patients. Data from the Nurses' Health Study demonstrated that users of estrogen had a significant reduction in all-cause mortality compared with nonusers, with a relative risk of 0.63 (45). Women with cardiac risk factors had the most benefit. The reduction in mortality attenuated with duration of use but still remained significant at more than 10 years. Other investigators used decision analysis to determine the effect of long-term HRT on life expectancy. Their model suggested that most women would experience increased life expectancy with HRT use. Only women who were without cardiac or osteoporosis risk factors but who have two first-degree relatives with breast cancer would not benefit (46).

HRT should not be a universal recommendation for all women. It must be tailored to the individual patient. Most current decision-making is done on the basis of observational evidence. Results from the large, randomized Women's Health Initiative, due in 2005, may provide more insight into which women should be targeted. For now, an open line of communication with the patient about menopause and its related issues will ensure a smooth transition into the postmenopausal years.

General References*

Nawaz H, Katz DL. American College of Preventive Medicine practice policy statement: perimenopausal and postmenopausal hormone replacement therapy. Am J Prev Med 1999;5:355.

A decision tree for the use of estrogen replacement therapy or HRT in postmenopausal women: consensus opinion of the North American Menopause Society. Menopause 2000;7:76.

American Association of Clinical Endocrinologists. AACE Medical Guidelines for Clinical Practice for Management of Menopause. Endocr Practice 1999;5:355.

North American Menopause Society. Clinical challenges of perimenopause: consensus opinion of the North American Menopause Society. Menopause 2000;7:5.

Mosca L, Collins P, Herrington DM, et al. Hormone replacement therapy and cardiovascular disease: a statement for healthcare professionals from the American Heart Association. Circulation 2001;104:499.

Specific References

1. McKinlay SM, Bifano NL, McKinlay JB. Smoking and age at menopause. Ann Intern Med 1985;103:350.
2. Cauley JA, Lucas FL, Kuller LH, et al. Bone mineral density and risk of breast cancer in older women: the study of osteoporotic fractures. JAMA 1996;276:1404.
3. Dennerstein L, Dudley EC, Hopper JL, et. al. A prospective population-based study of menopausal symptoms. Obstet Gynecol 2000;96:351.
4. Kolonel LW, Hankin JH, Nomura AMY. Multiethnic studies of diet, nutrition and cancer in Hawaii. In: Hayashi Y, Nagao M, Sugimura T, et al., eds. Nutrition and cancer. Tokyo: Japanese Science Society Press; 1986:29.
5. Freeman EW, Sammel MD, Grisso JA, et al. Hot flushes in the late reproductive years: risk factors for African-American and Caucasian women. J Womens Health Gend Based Med 2001;10:67.

*Bold print (general references) and bold numerals (specific references) denote published controlled clinical trials, meta-analyses, or consensus-based recommendations.

6. Tataryn IV, Lomax P, Meldrum DR, et al. Objective techniques for the assessment of postmenopausal hot flushes. Obstet Gynecol 1981;57:340.
7. Freedman RR. Physiology of hot flushes. Am J Human Biol 2001;13:453.
8. Loprinzi CL, Kugler JW, Sloan JA, et. al. Venlafaxine in management of hot flushes in survivors of breast cancer: a randomised controlled trial. Lancet 2000;356:2059.
9. Stearns V, Isaacs C, Rowland J, et al. A pilot trial assessing the efficacy of paroxetine hydrochloride in controlling hot flushes in breast cancer survivors. Ann Oncol 2000;11:17.
10. David A, Don R, Tajchner G, et al. Veralipride: alternative antidopaminergic treatment for menopausal symptoms. Am J Obstet Gynecol 1988;158:1107.
11. Hammar M, Christau S, Nathorst-Boos J, et al. A double-blind, randomised trial comparing the effects of tibolone and continuous combined hormone replacement therapy in postmenopausal women with menopausal symptoms. Br J Obstet Gynaecol 1998;105:904.
12. Lieberman S. A review of the effectiveness of *Cimicifuga racemosa* (black cohosh) for symptoms of menopause. J Womens Health 1998;7:525.
13. Jacobson JS, Troxel AB, Evans J, et. al. Randomized trial of black cohosh for the treatment of hot flushes among women with a history of breast cancer. J Clin Oncol 2001;19:2739.
14. Washburn S, Burke GL, Morgan T, et al. Effect of soy protein supplementation on serum lipoproteins, blood pressure, and menopausal symptoms in perimenopausal women. Menopause 1999;6:7.
15. Albertazzi P, Pansini F, Bonaccorsi G, et al. The effect of dietary soy supplementation on hot flushes. Obstet Gynecol 1998;91:6.
16. Murkies AL, Lombard C, Strauss BJG. Dietary flour supplementation decreases postmenopausal hot flushes: effects of soy and wheat. Maturitas 1995;21:189.
17. North American Menopause Society. The role of isoflavones in menopausal health: consensus opinion of the North American Menopause Society. Menopause 2000;7:215.
18. Glazier MG, Bowman MA. A review of the evidence for the use of phytoestrogens as a replacement for traditional estrogen replacement therapy. Arch Intern Med 2001;161:1161.
19. Fantl JA, Cardozo L, McClish DK. Estrogen therapy in the management of urinary incontinence in postmenopausal women: a meta-analysis. First report of the Hormones and Urogenital Therapy Committee. Obstet Gynecol 1994;83:12.
20. Eriksen B. A randomized, open, parallel-group study on the preventive effect of an estradiol vaginal ring (Estring) on recurrent urinary infections in postmenopausal women. Am J Obstet Gynecol 1999;180:1072.
21. Avis NE, Brambilla D, McKinlay SM, et al. A longitudinal analysis of the association between menopause and depression: results from the Massachusetts women's health study. Ann Epidemiol 1994;4:214.
22. Whooley MA, Grady D, Cauley JA, et al. Postmenopausal estrogen therapy and depressive symptoms in older women. J Gen Intern Med 2000;15:535.
23. Davis SR, McCloud P, Strauss BJ, et al. Testosterone enhances estradiol's effects on postmenopausal bone density and sexuality. Maturitas 1995;21:227.
24. AACE medical guidelines for clinical practice for management of menopause. Endocr Practice 1999;5:355.
25. Grodstein F, Stampfer MJ, Manson JE, et al. Postmenopausal estrogen and progestin use and the risk of cardiovascular disease. N Engl J Med 1996;335:453.
26. Nabulsi AA, Folsom AR, White A, et al. Association of hormone replacement therapy with various cardiovascular risk factors in postmenopausal women. N Engl J Med 1993;328:1069.
27. Walsh BW, Schiff I, Rosner B, et al. Effects of postmenopausal estrogen replacement on the concentrations and metabolism of plasma lipoproteins. N Engl J Med 1991;325:1196.
28. The Writing Group for the PEPI Trial. Effects of estrogen or estrogen/progestin regimens on heart disease risk factors in postmenopausal women. JAMA 1995;273:199.
29. Hulley S, Grady D, Bush T, et al. Randomized trial of estrogen plus progestin for secondary prevention of coronary heart disease in postmenopausal women. JAMA 1998;280:605.
30. Mosca L, Collins P, Herrington DM, et. Al. Hormone replacement therapy and cardiovascular disease. Circulation 2001;104: 499.
31. Chrischilles EA, Butler CD, Davis, CS, et al. A model of lifetime osteoporosis impact. Arch Intern Med 1991;151:2026.
32. Yaffe K, Sawaya G, Lieberburg I, et al. Estrogen therapy in postmenopausal women: effects on cognitive function and dementia. JAMA 1998;279:688.
33. Henderson VW, Paganini-Hill A, Miller BL, et al. Estrogen for Alzheimer's disease in women: randomized, double-blind, placebo-controlled trial. Neurology 2000;54:295.
34. Mulnard RA, Cotman CW, Kawas C, et al. Estrogen replacement therapy for treatment of mild to moderate Alzheimer's disease: a randomized controlled trial. JAMA 2000;283:1007.
35. Nanda K, Bastian LA, Hasselblad V, et al. Hormone replacement therapy and the risk of colorectal cancer: a meta-analysis. Obstet Gynecol 1999;93:880.
36. Colditz GA, Hankinson SE, Hunter DJ, et al. The use of estrogens and progestins and the risk of breast cancer in postmenopausal women. N Engl J Med 1995;332:1589.
37. Sellers TA, Mink PJ, Cerhan JR, et al. The role of hormone replacement therapy in the risk for breast cancer and total mortality in women with a family history of breast cancer. Ann Intern Med 1997;127:973.
38. Grady D, Gebretsadik T, Kerlikowske K, et al. Hormone replacement therapy and endometrial cancer risk: a meta-analysis. Obstet Gynecol 1995;85:304.
39. Rodriguez C, Patel AV, Calle EE, et al. Estrogen replacement therapy and ovarian cancer mortality in a large prospective study of US women. JAMA 2001;285:1460.
40. Daly E, Vassey MP, Hawkins MM, et al. Risk of venous thromboembolism in users of hormone replacement therapy. Lancet 1996;348:977.
41. Miller RG, Chang KK. Management of the menopausal patient. Primary Care Reports 2000;6:39.
42. Delmas PD, Bjarnason NH, Mitlak BH, et al. Effects of raloxifene on bone mineral density, serum cholesterol concentrations, and uterine endometrium in postmenopausal women. N Engl J Med 1997;337:1641.
43. Cummings SR, Eckert S, Krueger KA, et al. The effect of raloxifene on risk of breast cancer in postmenopausal women: results from the MORE randomized trial. Multiple Outcomes of Raloxifene Evaluation. JAMA 1999;282:2189.
44. Johannes CB, Crawford SL, Posner JG, et al. Longitudinal patterns and correlates of hormone replacement therapy use in middle-aged women. Am J Epidemiol 1994;140:439.
45. Grodstein F, Stampfer MJ, Colditz GA, et al. Postmenopausal hormone therapy and mortality. N Engl J Med 1997;336:1769.
46. Col NF, Eckman MH, Karas RH, et al. Patient-specific decisions about hormone replacement therapy in postmenopausal women. JAMA 1997;277:1140.

SECTION 15

Selected Problems of the Eyes

CHAPTER 107

Common Problems Associated with Impaired Vision: Cataracts and Age-Related Macular Degeneration

ANDREW P. SCHACHAT, MD

CATARACTS

A cataract is an opacification of the lens of the eye. Approximately 95% of people older than 60 years of age have some opacification of the lens, but most often these opacities are of no visual importance. A *significant cataract* results in interference with visual acuity. In the United States, cataracts are a common cause of diminished vision and may result in blindness. The incidence of diminished visual acuity from cataracts increases steadily after 50 years, reaching almost 50% in people older than 75 years of age. Cataracts are usually bilateral, and the progression is slow and may vary between eyes. The rate of progression is not individually predictable, and there is no treatment that retards the progression. When the cataract is advanced, the only therapy is surgery. A large clinical trial, the Age-Related Eye Disease Study, is investigating the role of vitamins in the progression of cataract and age-related macular degeneration. More than 4,000 patients are enrolled, and in late 2001 initial results were announced; vitamin and mineral supplementation did not alter cataract progression.

Anatomy and Physiology

The lens is derived entirely from the evagination of surface ectoderm in the fetus. It is located immediately posterior to the iris and is suspended there by radially attached zonular fibers from the ciliary body (see Fig. 108.1, page 1662, in Chapter 108). It is a biconvex, transparent structure with an elastic capsule whose shape is altered by ciliary body contraction, permitting images to be brought into sharp focus on the retina. The lens is acellular and avascular and lacks innervation. Nourishment is provided from the surrounding aqueous and vitreous humor, and metabolic byproducts are removed by diffusion into the aqueous humor. The continued transparency of the lens requires the active metabolism of the elastic capsular epithelium, so any insult to the epithelium may result in lenticular opacities. New lenticular fibers are produced throughout life, and, because none are lost, increasing density of the fibers of the lens develops with age, which also contributes to cataract formation.

Causes

There are many causes of cataracts (Table 107.1). Although senescent cataracts—the result of the aging process just described—account for the vast majority of cataracts, the generalist occasionally sees patients with congenital or traumatic lens opacities. The mechanism of opacification in all of these instances is thought to be direct trauma or interference with metabolic activity of the capsular epithelium and with continued fiber production.

Many of these types of cataracts have a distinctive appearance. The ophthalmologist may therefore suggest the possibility of an underlying disorder such as myotonic dystrophy (iridescent spots) or Wilson disease (sunflower cataract). Steroid therapy and radiation treatment are associated with posterior subcapsular cataracts, although these may also be idiopathic or related to numerous other conditions. Age-related cataract is significantly associated with dermatologic abnormalities and their treatment. Steroid use is particularly strongly associated (1).

Symptoms and Examination

The primary symptom of cataract is impaired vision; usually patients describe a constant fog over the eye. They may also see rings or halos around lights and objects. Objects appear more blue and yellow in color. With immature cataract formation, distant vision often is impaired to a greater extent than is near vision.

The location of the cataract within the lens determines the extent of the visual loss. Central opacities cause noticeable loss of vision and a distinct glare when the patient is in bright light. Bright light constricts the pupil so that the dense portion of the lens occludes and diffuses light. Therefore the patient who has central opacities finds that vision is better in low light, when the pupil is widely dilated. In selected cases, use of dilating drops (mydriatics) is helpful and delays the need for surgery. Because there may be contraindications to the use of mydriatics (e.g., narrow-angle glaucoma attacks may be precipitated), it is best

Table 107.1. Causes of Cataracts

Congenital
Autosomal-dominant inheritance (25% of congenital cataracts)
Maternal malnutrition
Maternal infections (rubella, syphilis)
Maternal metabolic disease (e.g., diabetes mellitus)
Maternal medication (corticosteroids)
Prematurity
Traumatic
Senescent
Secondary
Drug therapy (corticosteroids)
Degenerative eye disease (severe myopia)
Retinal dystrophy
Essential iris atrophy
Retinal detachment
Glaucoma
Intraocular neoplasia
Ocular ischemia (e.g., Takayasu disease)
Associated with metablic disease
Diabetes mellitus
Wilson disease
Hypoparathyroidism

to rely on an ophthalmologist to prescribe them. Peripheral opacities cause noticeable loss of vision only late in the development of the cataract.

Cataracts are easily identified by illuminating the lens with a slit lamp, but most general physicians find that they can see a cataract easily through a moderately plus lens (such as a +2 or +3 lens on the dial) of the direct ophthalmoscope. The lens appears cloudy. Similarly, a light from a small flashlight may be reflected off the opacity in the lens. Visual acuity should be tested in both eyes if cataracts are suspected. If the patient describes any visual symptoms or is measured, an impairment in visual acuity, the patient should be referred to an ophthalmologist. In adults, screening for cataracts is best done by a visual acuity examination with use of a Snellen chart. The *Snellen chart* is easy to use, and the result is a ratio of the distance a patient stands from the chart to the distance that a subject with normal vision would stand to read the line of images in question. Therefore, 20/100 means that the patient is seeing clearly at 20 feet an image that a person with normal vision would see at 100 feet. It is critical to check separately the visual acuity of each eye with the other eye covered and with the patient using his or her glasses.

Cataract Surgery

Indications

Before surgery is indicated, optical manipulations such as mydriatics to help the patient see around a central cataract (discussed previously) or new glasses for the progressive myopia associated with many nuclear cataracts may improve the vision of patients with cataracts. Also, visual aids, such as magnifying lenses and large-print materials, may be helpful (see Advice for the Visually Impaired). The decision to remove a cataract is determined by the visual needs of the patient, the degree of the cataract, and the presence of any other ocular abnormalities. The ophthalmologist performs a complete ocular assessment before advising the patient about surgery.

Each patient must determine his or her own visual need based on daily activities. The ability to read, drive, cross streets safely, and perform daily routines are clearly of prime importance. For example, a patient usually requires visual acuity of at least 20/40 in the better eye to operate a motor vehicle safely or to continue moderately active daily life. Blurred vision has an important impact on patients' functioning and well-being. The impact of blurred vision on role limitations caused by other health problems was found to be significantly greater than the impact of hypertension, history of myocardial infarction, type 2 diabetes, indigestion, trouble urinating, or headache (2). Because the impact of blurred vision is so significant and the success rate for cataract surgery so high, it is not surprising how often the procedure is performed.

Surgery

Cataract surgery should be performed only after considerable deliberation, because a number of complications might occur and vision after cataract extraction may still be a major problem (see later discussion). For patients with other health problems, the generalist and the ophthalmologist should plan cataract surgery together. Cataract extraction is an elective procedure, and the patient should be in the best possible condition at the time of operation.

Approximately 600,000 cataract extractions are performed in the United States every year, and cataract surgery is the most common major surgical procedure performed in the elderly in this country. Surgery involves removal of the opacified lens from the eye. The extraction may be intracapsular, involving complete removal of the lens, or extracapsular, leaving the posterior capsule of the lens intact. In the 1990s, the overwhelming majority of cataract surgeries were extracapsular. Microsurgical techniques have greatly improved the immediate outcome of surgery and have significantly shortened the period of disability. Extracapsular extraction is most commonly performed because it leaves the posterior capsule intact, permits easier lens implantation (see later discussion), and is associated with fewer postoperative complications. Both eyes usually require operation, but normally only one lens is extracted at a time, so that the patient has vision on the nonoperated side when the eye that has been operated on is covered by a patch for a few days after surgery. Some surgeons attempt to avoid the use of a patch, and so-called no-stitch surgery with very small incisions is in vogue. There is no proof that any particular extracapsular surgical approach is better than any other. For patients with bilateral cataracts, the second procedure is usually performed a few months after the first; once the visual result is known in the first eye, the patient and ophthalmologist again assess the visual needs, risks, benefits, and alternatives to surgery in the second eye.

Preoperative Evaluation. The current standard of care is a history and physical examination, but few if any laboratory investigations are required. Health service researchers are debating the extent of a preoperative evaluation. In the current climate of cost awareness, a minimalist approach is being phased in. The history should elicit clues about bleeding tendencies. If appropriate, aspirin should be discontinued for 7 to 14 days before the surgery, although some surgeons do not stop aspirin, given the low risk of bleeding with small-incision surgery. The ability of the patient to lie flat should be assessed. Diabetes mellitus and hypertension, if present, should be controlled. A recent myocardial infarction (within 6 months) should delay surgery. A randomized trial, the PORT-II study showed that routine preoperative testing before cataract surgery did not reduce the incidence of perioperative medical complications (3a). The testing evaluated in this study included ECG, CBC, and levels of electrolytes, urea, nitrogen, creatinine, and glucose.

Patient Experience. Cataract surgery is performed most often by use of local anesthesia supplemented with intravenous analgesia and sedation. Surgery is normally performed on an outpatient basis. The patient experiences moderate discomfort, but this lasts only a day or so and is controlled with analgesics. A hyperosmotic agent (e.g., glycerin, mannitol) or local pressure may be used to dehydrate and soften the eye in preparation for surgery.

After discharge from the surgical unit a patient must restrict his or her activities for several weeks to minimize the frequency of complications, although with small incisions and the newest microsurgical techniques the rehabilitation period is becoming shorter. These restrictions are listed in Table 107.2 and are rather conservative. Many ophthalmologists are much more liberal. There are no permanent restrictions; however, caution with steps or when walking and working with machinery may be necessary if perception is seriously altered by use of aphakic spectacles (see later discussion).

Complications

Complications occur in approximately 5% of patients who have cataract extraction, and 1 of every 5,000 eyes operated on is lost because of complications. Knowledge of the possible complications after cataract surgery aids one in educating patients. Because of the potential for complications, one must ensure that the patient keeps the scheduled postoperative appointments with the ophthalmologist.

Table 107.2. Temporary Restrictions After Cataract Surgery

Wear eye shield during sleep and wear glasses at other times; shields are usually worn for 1 month and then discontinued.
Minimize bending or stooping for 3 or 4 weeks.
Do not sleep on side of operated eye for 3 or 4 weeks.
Do not wash hair for 2 weeks.
No showers for 2 weeks, although a bath is allowed (but with assistance to prevent a fall).
No strenuous or excessive physical activity for 4 weeks and then only after approval of the ophthalmologist.

These measures are suggested to prevent inadvertent injury to the eye, diminish disruptive pressure on the wound, avoid a sudden rise in ocular pressure, and diminish the chance of infection. These recommendations are conservative. The ophthalmologist may prefer a more liberal set.

Optometrists are allowed under Medicare to receive reimbursement for postoperative follow-up care. It makes sense that follow-up during the postoperative period by the surgeon is preferable.

Inflammation and Infection. All postoperative patients have some degree of traumatic intraocular inflammation. This is usually controlled effectively with topical corticosteroids. Bacterial intraocular infection, endophthalmitis, is a dangerous postoperative inflammation that must be recognized early before it devastates the eye. If a patient complains of decreased vision, pain, discharge, and redness, endophthalmitis may be present and the patient should be seen immediately by an ophthalmologist. Most infections occur within a few days after surgery; however, an operated eye is predisposed to involvement from systemic infection, so a patient with an acute red eye occurring at any time after eye surgery should be seen urgently by an ophthalmologist. Low-grade chronic inflammation is common after cataract surgery, and resultant macular edema is one of the most common causes of postoperative visual loss.

Hemorrhage. The sudden occurrence of hemorrhage in the uveal tract (the iris, the ciliary body, and the choroid) can adversely influence the final visual outcome. Although this complication is usually seen intraoperatively, it may rarely occur postoperatively. The event is characterized by a usually painless but precipitous change in visual acuity. Postoperative hemorrhage from the iris or an inadequately closed corneoscleral wound is more common than is vitreous hemorrhage. In all instances of hemorrhage, urgent referral to an ophthalmologist is indicated. Although anticoagulation is not an absolute contraindication to cataract extraction, it probably does increase the risk of hemorrhage. For this reason, anticoagulants and antiplatelet agents such as aspirin are stopped, if possible, before and for 1 to 2 weeks after surgery.

Retinal Detachment. The incidence of retinal detachment after cataract surgery is approximately 1% to 3%. Retinal detachment may be characterized by suddenly decreased visual acuity, flashes of light, and the development of floaters, veils, or curtains in the visual field. Patients with symptoms of retinal detachment should be seen immediately by an ophthalmologist so that surgical reattachment of the retina may be accomplished.

Glaucoma. This secondary form of glaucoma is caused by several factors that lead to true or functional angle closure: the effect of the proteolytic agent chymotrypsin on the angular structures at the time of intracapsular operation (rare today), scarring caused by postoperative inflammation, or the misdirection into and subsequent trapping of the aqueous in the vitreous gel (see Fig. 108.1 in Chapter 108). Glaucoma may develop within a few days after surgery. Early glaucoma is usually transient, but it may become chronic. Glaucoma may appear as late as 1 to 2 years after surgery in 0.6% to 5% of patients, depending on the type of surgery. The patient who has developed secondary glaucoma usually complains of redness, tenderness, and pain in the eye. Furthermore, if the patient has been fitted with a temporary spectacle, he or she notices a decrease in visual acuity caused by corneal edema. A postoperative patient with suspected glaucoma should be seen immediately by an ophthalmologist. Additional information about glaucoma is provided in Chapter 108.

Delayed Opacification of the Posterior Capsule. Extracapsular extraction is performed more often than intracapsular extraction because it is associated with fewer complications. However, 20% to 50% of patients experience a gradual decrease in vision in the first few years after this technique because of opacification of the posterior lens capsule. This complication can now be treated effectively by a special laser instrument (yttrium–aluminum–garnet [YAG]) that opens the posterior capsule without the need for intraocular surgery. The procedure is painless and is performed in the office. However, it is performed only when the potential for visual improvement outweighs the risks, because retinal detachment and perhaps macular edema become somewhat more common (3). Clinical trials of an agent that may retard the development of opacification of the posterior capsule are underway.

Optical Correction after Cataract Extraction

The removal of a cataract improves light transmission to the retina, but vision remains blurred without corrective lenses. Three types of lenses are used: aphakic spectacles, contact lenses, and intraocular lenses. The last option is now the norm. Aphakic spectacles are discussed mainly for historical reasons. Contact lenses are used more than aphakic spectacles, but almost all patients, even children, are now candidates for intraocular lenses.

Aphakic spectacles are rarely used today. With aphakic spectacles there is a narrower field of vision, as well as considerable distortion of images, which appear rounded and three to five times larger than when the lens is present in the eye. Peripheral ring scotomata and loss of some depth perception also occur. Even modern aphakic spectacles are heavy and thick so that the patient often has considerable initial difficulty adjusting to them and needs support, understanding, and encouragement from family members. With experience, however, most patients can function acceptably and perform all of their necessary daily activities.

A unilateral cataract extraction results in a pronounced disparity in image size if an aphakic spectacle is used postoperatively; therefore, unilateral surgery is generally not advised unless the patient will be able to use a contact lens or is a candidate for an intraocular lens implantation (see later discussion). Indeed, because intraocular lenses are used so often, unilateral cataracts are operated on much more often than they were in early decades; also, under certain circumstances monolenticular extraction may be indicated to permit the ophthalmologist to monitor the course and treatment of ocular diseases such as diabetic retinopathy and macular degeneration.

The use of *contact lenses* after cataract extraction provides considerable improvement over spectacles. There is substantial distortion reduction and expansion of the field of vision. However, the patient must be motivated to use contact lenses, and this motivation must be considered before surgery is undertaken. Often elderly patients are concerned about being agile enough to insert contact lenses, although there are some long-wear lenses on the market. The patient must also be fitted with a pair of spectacles with one lens missing so that he or she can see well enough to place one contact lens. A regular set of aphakic spectacles is also necessary as a backup to the contact lens.

Because of the visual handicap experienced after cataract extraction, plastic *intraocular lenses* are inserted at the time of surgery in 95% or more of patients undergoing cataract extraction. They are even used successfully in developing countries. Long-term survival of these inert prostheses is very good. The insertion of intraocular implants adds a few minutes to the operative time beyond that required for lens extraction. If the eye is otherwise healthy, more than 90% of patients undergoing this technique experience an improvement in vision to 20/40 or better. New multifocal lenses (to replace bifocals) are under investigation.

AGE-RELATED MACULAR DEGENERATION

Age-related macular degeneration (AMD) is the leading cause of severe visual loss in people older than 50 years of age. The macula is the central area of the retina used for fine focus such as reading. There is no universally agreed definition of age-related macular degeneration. It is characterized by the development of drusen, retinal pigment epithelial changes, and in some cases abnormal choroidal vessels and hemorrhage. Drusen are excrescences that develop along Bruch membrane, which lies between the retina and choroid and appear, on ophthalmologic examination, as tiny discrete white or yellow deposits. They are at times difficult to visualize, and the ophthalmoscope must be in sharp focus on the retina. Most patients older than 50 years of age have a few drusen, and there is no consensus as to how many drusen and what degree of retinal pigment epithelial changes constitute AMD. Drusen formation alone almost never reduces visual acuity.

Epidemiology

The Framingham Eye Study found that AMD was present in one or both eyes of almost 6% of subjects age 52 years or older (4). The prevalence is strongly age related. Comparable rates were found in the Health and Nutrition Examination Survey (HANES) (5). In the Beaver Dam Eye Study, approximately 30% of adults age 75 years or older had early AMD and another 28% developed it over the next 5 years. Early signs were twice as common in women, and patients with early

AMD had significantly greater risk of developing advanced AMD (6). Risk factors identified in some series include hyperopia (far vision), decreased handgrip strength, light iris color, systemic hypertension, family history, cardiac hypertrophy, short height, history of previous lung infection, cigarette smoking, cardiovascular disease, chemical exposure, and sunlight exposure. The strength and validity of these associations are debated, and additional epidemiologic studies investigating risk factors are underway.

Clinical Features

There are two major forms of AMD. The nonneovascular or *atrophic form* is characterized simply by drusen formation and atrophic retinal pigment epithelial changes. It is the most common form of AMD. The *neovascular or exudative form* of AMD, in which subretinal choroidal neovascularization occurs, can lead to subretinal hemorrhage and fluid accumulation and, eventually, extensive scarring. Although it is the rarer form, it accounts for the majority of visual loss seen in patients with AMD.

Drusen vary in distribution, number, size, and shape. They may or may not have pigmentary alterations around them. Small drusen are difficult to see with the direct ophthalmoscope, but larger or so-called soft drusen should be apparent (Figs. 107.1 and 107.2). Atrophy associated with AMD may represent true atrophy of retinal pigment epithelium or simply loss of pigment from within retinal pigment epithelial cells. Clinically, the distinction is impossible to make (Fig. 107.3). If atrophy involves the macula (the aspect of the central retina that is temporal to and slightly below the optic disc), visual acuity is usually reduced.

Neovascular AMD is characterized by the accumulation of fluid, hemorrhage, or lipid beneath or within the retina (Fig. 107.4). Accumulation of fluid beneath the retinal pigment epithelium may lead to pigment epithelial detachment. Choroidal

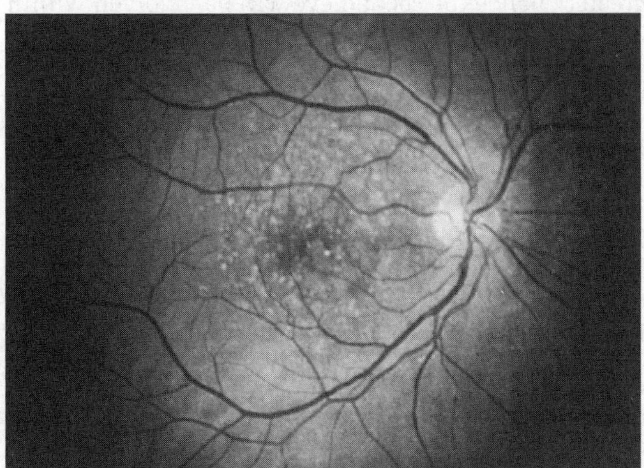

Figure 107.1. Hard drusen are the tiny dots in the central retina (macular area). They are minimally elevated and, when viewed in color, are yellow-white. The visual acuity is normal.

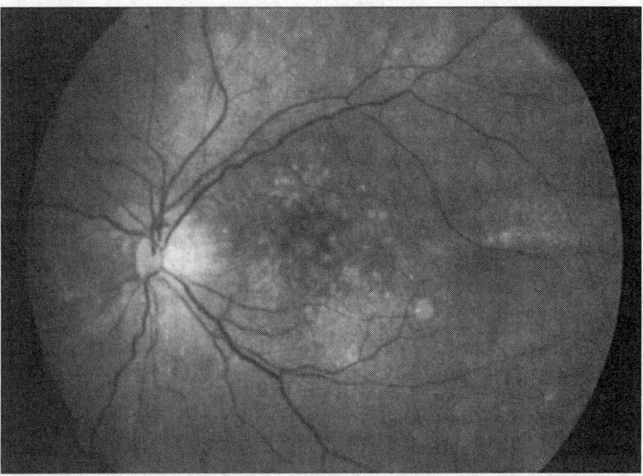

Figure 107.2. The larger blotches in the central retina are soft drusen. Patients with soft drusen are at increased risk of developing neovascular exudative macular degeneration. The visual acuity is normal.

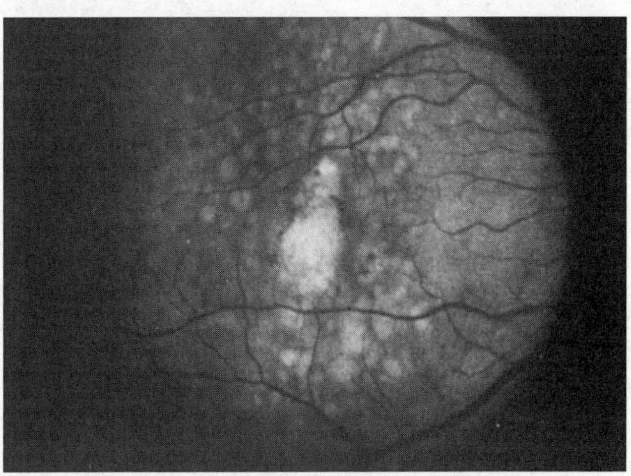

Figure 107.3. The patient with nonneovascular atrophic macular degeneration has hard and soft drusen. There is a zone of central atrophy, and, if the center of the macula is involved, vision is usually decreased.

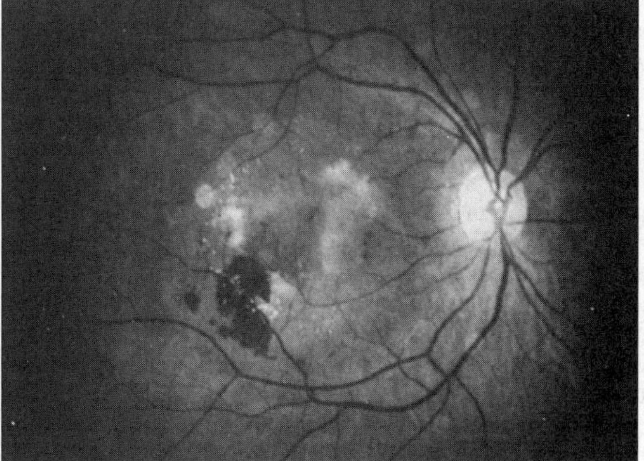

Figure 107.4. Neovascular macular degeneration. There is subretinal blood and lipid. Subretinal fluid can be seen on stereoscopic photographs (not shown). The patient has choroidal neovascularization.

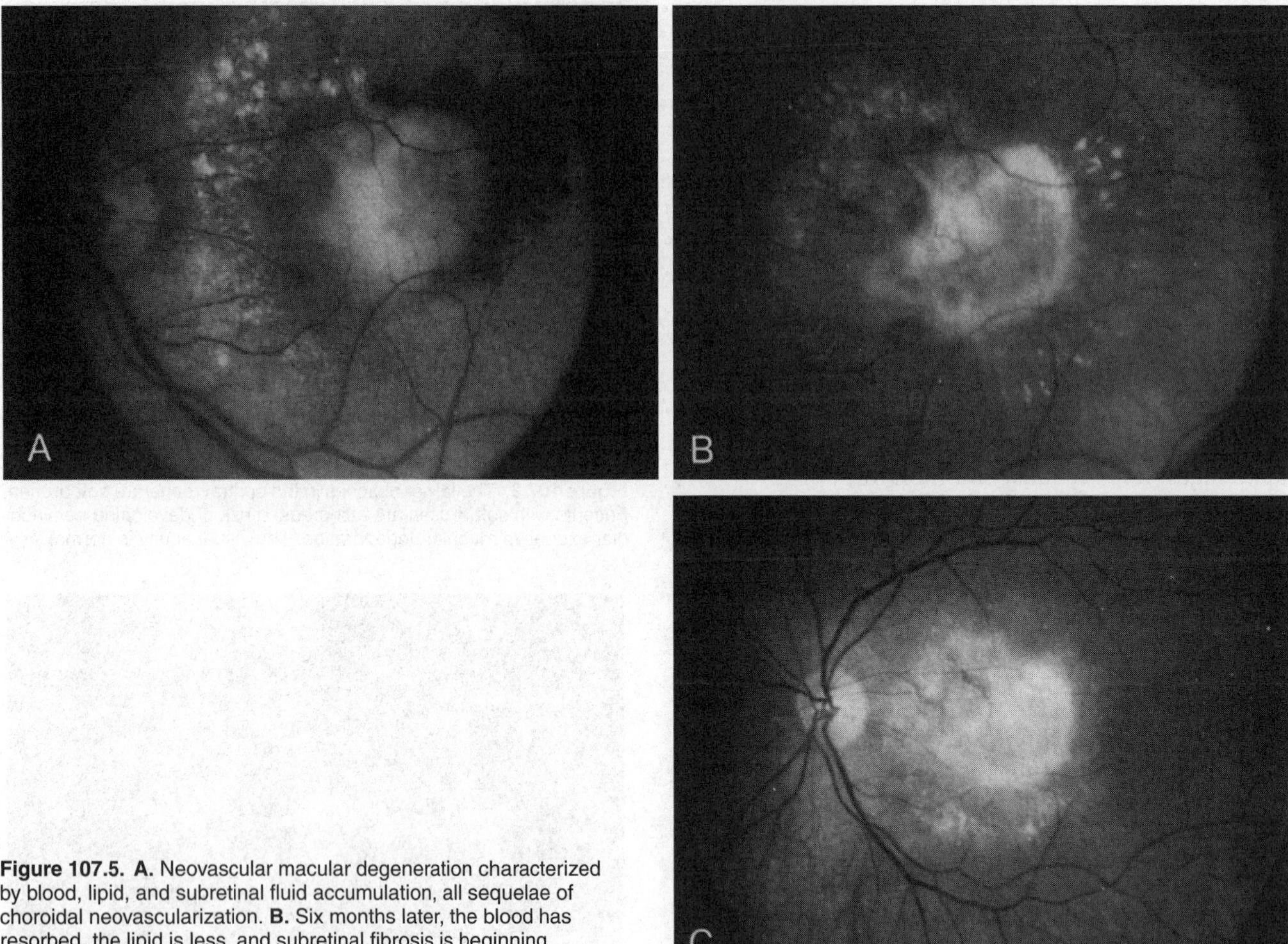

Figure 107.5. **A.** Neovascular macular degeneration characterized by blood, lipid, and subretinal fluid accumulation, all sequelae of choroidal neovascularization. **B.** Six months later, the blood has resorbed, the lipid is less, and subretinal fibrosis is beginning. **C.** One year later, a disciform scar has formed.

neovascularization may grow through or actually cause breaks in Bruch membrane. The new blood vessels beneath the retina are the cause of the hemorrhage and lipid accumulation (Fig. 107.5A). After the active phase, subretinal fibrosis or a so-called disciform scar is seen (Fig. 107.5B and C).

Although the subretinal new vessels are rarely directly visible, the technique of *fluorescein angiography* allows their diagnosis (Fig. 107.6). Intravenous fluorescein dye is injected in the antecubital fossa. Within 10 to 20 seconds, the dye can be photographed traversing vessels in the eye. The presence of increasing hyperfluorescence in certain patterns as the angiogram progresses is a marker for choroidal neovascularization. The interpretation of fluorescein angiograms is complex and requires the expertise of an ophthalmologist experienced in the procedure. For patients who are allergic to fluorescein, and perhaps in special situations, indocyanine green (ICG) angiography may be useful and is being used by some retina specialists. Because ICG contains iodine, the ophthalmologist may request that metformin be temporarily discontinued.

Natural History and Treatment

The natural history of bilateral drusen is uncertain. Patients who have exudative disease in one eye and drusen only in the second eye have a rate of 4% to 15% per year for development of exudative disease in the previously uninvolved eye. In high-risk non-neovascular disease (numerous large drusen and pigment changes), if the fellow eye already has choroidal neovascularization, there is approximately a 50% or greater chance the second eye will be involved within 5 years. Patients with AMD should be examined by an ophthalmologist at least annually or, in high-risk cases, perhaps twice annually.

Although numerous dietary and vitamin therapies have been recommended for patients with the atrophic form of the disease, widespread use of these therapies in patients with AMD is not yet warranted (7) except as indicated from the Age-Related Eye Disease Study (8). That randomized study investigated the role of vitamin supplementation over a 10-year period. Almost 4,000 patients participated, and the initial 5-year outcomes were reported in the fall of 2001 (8). The conclusion of this important investigation was that individuals older than 55 years of age should have a dilated eye examination to ascertain their risk of developing advanced AMD. Those showing predictive changes who have no contraindication (e.g., smoking) should consider taking a supplement of antioxidants (vitamin C, 500 mg; vitamin E, 400 IU; and beta-carotene, 15 mg) plus zinc (80 mg). Copper (2mg) is added to reduce

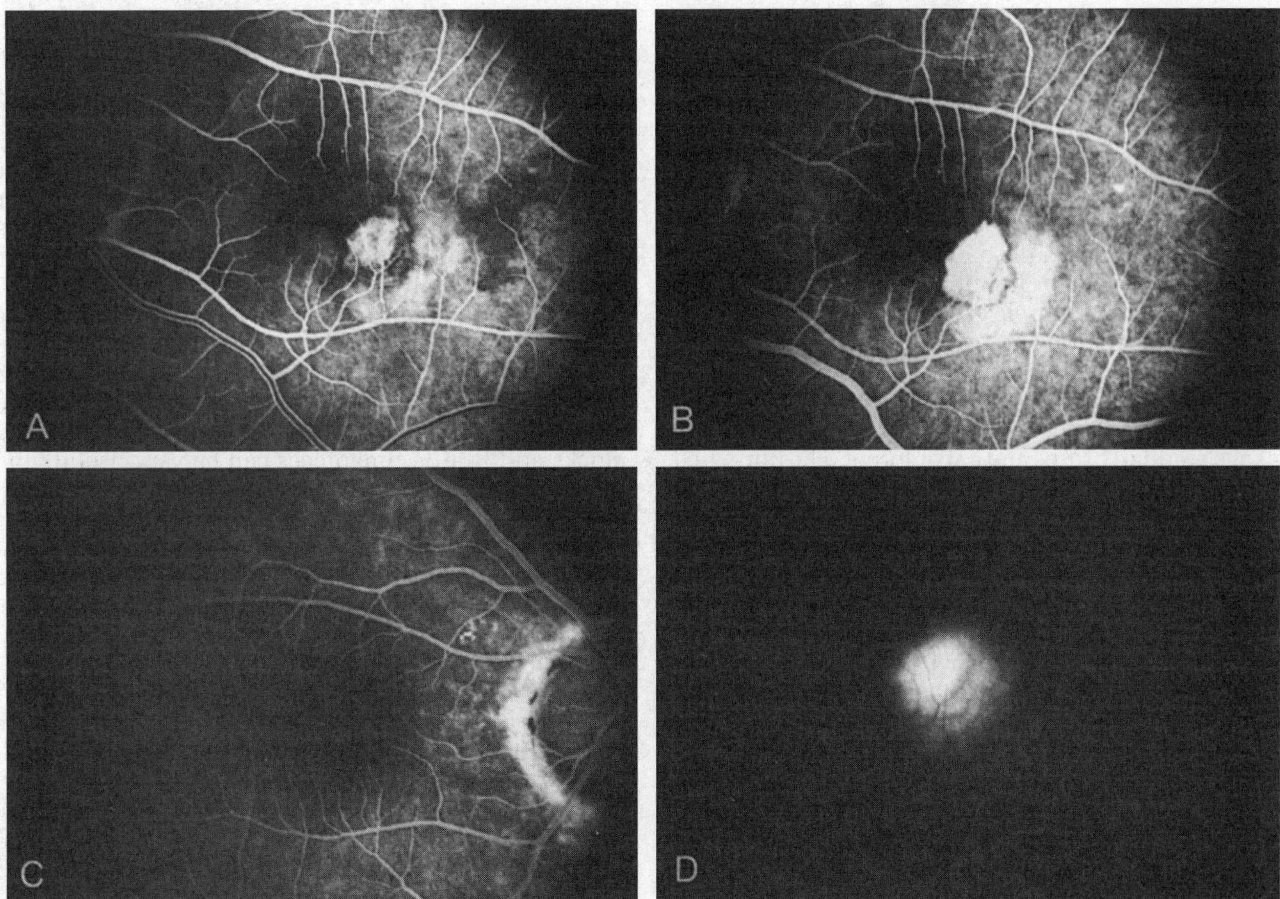

Figure 107.6. Fluorescein angiogram of choroidal neovascularization. **A.** In the early phase, 18 seconds after intravenous injection of dye, the fluorescein is seen filling retinal arteries and laminar venous filling is beginning. A zone of hyperfluorescence (brightness) is seen at the inferotemporal aspect of the macula. This is caused by dye leaking from abnormal choroidal vessels (choroidal neovascularization). **B.** The leaking is increased 10 seconds later. **C.** For comparison, a view of the normal fellow eye illustrates a normal angiographic pattern. **D.** A late frame, taken approximately 10 minutes after the injection, shows continued leakage of dye from the choroidal new vessels.

the theoretical risk of Zn-induced copper deficiency anemia. The combination is available in an over-the-counter supplement, Ocuvite preservision (Bausch and Lomb). The generalist will want to have an ophthalmologist involved in this risk assessment and in coming to a decision about and planning for preventive treatment in patients who are at risk.

Because chronic light toxicity may play a role in the pathogenesis of AMD, avoidance of sunlight has been considered. One review (9) concluded that no data exist to support the notion that any form of sunglasses can reduce chronic photic insult and thereby reduce a putative factor in the development of AMD. Nevertheless, the use of sunglasses is inexpensive and presumally without side effects and therefore should not be discouraged.

There is a treatment for some patients with neovascular disease, but because the clinical features are subtle and the treatment is beyond the scope of general practice, referral to an ophthalmologist is indicated. The Macular Photocoagulation Study (MPS) compared the value of laser photocoagulation with that of no treatment for patients with well-defined choroidal neovascularization outside the center of the macular area. After 3.5 years of follow-up, 62% of untreated patients had a loss of six or more lines of vision on a Snellen chart, compared with 47% of treated patients. The difference was statistically significant (10). Subsequent investigations by the MPS investigators extended the treatment recommendations to include lesions closer to the center of the macula (juxtafoveal lesions) as well as lesions in the macular center (subfoveal lesions). The "MPS" type of treatment allowed about 10% of patients to be treated, but with a resultant blank spot and, usually, reduced vision. In April 2000, a major advance in the treatment of neovascular AMD became available. Photodynamic therapy allows treatment of about twice as many patients, at least 20%, and with a chance for stabilization, whereas the "hot" laser used in the MPS usually reduced vision immediately.

Photodynamic therapy is a two-step procedure. The first step is to administer a photosensitizing drug that is allowed to circulate and bind to target tissues. In the second step, a low-power laser, about 1/100th the power of the hot laser, is used to irradiate the target tissue and activate the drug. Toxic intermediates are produced, damaging target tissues, and the damage is selective because at the treatment time selected there is more drug in target cells and less in adjacent cells. The drug carrier allows important selectivity as well.

Although other agents are under study, only one ocular drug has been approved by the U. S. Food and Drug Administration for photodynamic therapy: Verteporfin (Visudyne, Novartis). Verteporfin, a bromatoporphyrin derivative monoacid, is administered intravenously as a liposomal preparation with a dose of 6 mg/m^2 body surface area. After an infusion, 689-nm wavelength light from a diode laser is used to activate the drug. The liposomal drug in the bloodstream exchanges carriers with low-density lipoprotein (LDL) cholesterol, and the LDL–drug complex is taken up by target cells rich in LDL receptors. The new vessel endothelial cells preferentially take up the drug and thus are preferentially damaged. The new vessels tend to recur, but, with a series of about five treatments over 2 years, the leakage gradually stops and a scar forms. The untreated natural history leads to a larger scar. The Treatment of Age-Related Macular Degeneration with Photodynamic Therapy (TAP) study randomly assigned about 600 patients to study groups (11). The chance of stabilization with treatment was doubled with photodynamic therapy, and the chance for improvement was about 16%. Certain types of new vessels, so-called predominantly classic new vessels, respond best. A companion study, the Verteporfin in Photodynamic Therapy (VIP) study, demonstrated safety and efficacy for occult vessels and for new vessels complicating pathologic myopia (12). Verteporfin has a short half-life and clears quickly, so patients must remain indoors and out of sunlight for only a few days. Immediate severe vision loss is seen in only a few percent of eyes, compared with 95% or more with the older laser technique. Severe photosensitivity reactions develop in about 1%, and transient back spasms during the infusion, seen with other liposomal drugs, also occur in about 1% of patients.

A large randomized trial of interferon, a systemic agent with antiangiogenesis activity, showed no benefit (13). Other antiangiogenesis agents are under study. There are numerous reports concerning low-dose radiation therapy (14). Radiation has antiangiogenesis effects. The results are contradictory, but the treatment is of doubtful benefit. Surgery to remove the abnormal blood vessels from beneath the retina is being studied in a large, prospective, randomized trial (the Subfoveal Surgery Trial, or SST), and results are expected shortly after the completion of the study in 2002.

ADVICE FOR THE VISUALLY IMPAIRED

If vision cannot be improved or maintained at an acceptable level, it is important for the physician to aid the patient in finding resources that may provide some help in lessening the ever-increasing isolation and loss of mobility that result from blindness. Dr. DeWitt Stetten (see General References) wrote an essay describing his experience with progressive blindness and outlining a number of useful aids that he identified. He described the increasing availability of large-print books, journals, and newsprint (e.g., *The New York Times*). Many books are available on tape from the *Talking Books Program* of the Library of Congress. Most local libraries can provide information on the availability of these tapes. Some journals may be obtained on tape from *Recorded Periodicals* (919 Walnut St., Philadelphia, PA 19107). *Newsweek* magazine is available on disposable phonographic records (P.O. Box 6435, 1839 Frankfort Ave., Louisville, KY 40206). A variety of aids for the blind may be ordered from the catalog of SFB Products (Box 385, Wayne, PA 19087) or Lighthouse low-vision products (36-20 Northern Blvd., Long Island City, NY 11101, telephone 800-453-4923). A portable cassette tape recorder designed for the blind can be purchased through the American Printing House for the Blind, Inc. (General Office, P.O. Box 6085, Louisville, KY 40206). Talking clocks and Braille timepieces can be very useful, and information concerning these and other aids is available from the National Institutes of Health Volunteers for the Visually Handicapped (4405 East–West Highway, Bethesda, MD 20814). Several types of reading machines and magnifying devices are also available, although these are expensive (see Stetten in General References).

Visual Foundation, Inc. (770 Center St., Newton, MA 02158) is a self-help organization developed by people with impaired vision. They have published a handbook, *Coping with Sight Loss,* that provides information for the visually impaired on visual aids, devices, recreation, tax benefits, reading materials, and referral sources. The handbook is published in large print and on cassette tapes and is a useful resource for both patients experiencing loss of vision and physicians who are caring for these patients.

Dr. Schachat has no proprietary interest in Ocuvite. He does receive honoraria and/or travel expense reimbursement from Novartis, manufacturer of Visudyne.

General References*

Bressler NM, Bressler SB, Fine SL. Exudative age-related macular degeneration. In: Ryan SJ, ed. Retina. 3rd ed. St. Louis: CV Mosby, 2001:1100.

Jaffe NS, Jaffe MS, Jaffe GF. Cataract surgery and its complications. St. Louis: CV Mosby, 1990.

Liesegang TJ. Cataracts and cataract operation: two parts. Mayo Clin Proc 1984;59:556.

Sarks SH, Sarks JP. Age-related macular degeneration: atrophic form. In: Ryan SJ, ed. Retina. 3rd ed. St. Louis: CV Mosby, 2001:1064.

Stark WJ, Woethen DM, Holladay JT, et al. The FDA report on intraocular lenses. Ophthalmology 1983;90:311.

The standard reference regarding intraocular lenses.

Stetten D Jr. Coping with blindness. N Engl J Med 1981;305:458.

A concise description of aids to help cope with blindness, written by Dr. Stetten as he experienced progressive vision loss.

Straatsma BR, Foos RY, Horwitz J, et al. Aging-related cataract: laboratory investigation and clinical management. Ann Intern Med 1985;102:82.

This University of California, Los Angeles conference reviews all aspects of senescent cataracts and contains superb color photographs of a variety of common cataract patterns.

*Bold print (general references) and bold numerals (specific references) denote published controlled clinical trials, meta-analysis, or consensus-based recommendations.

Specific References

1. Phillips CI, Donnelly CA, Clayton RM, et al. Skin disease and age-related cataract. Acta Derm Venereol (Stockholm) 1996; 76:314.
2. Lee PL, Spritzer K, Hays R. The impact of blurred vision on functioning and well-being. Ophthalmology 1997;104:390.
3. Tielsch JM, Legro MW, Cassard SD, et al. Risk factors for retinal detachment after cataract surgery: a population-based case-control study. Ophthalmology 1996;103:1537.

3a. Schein OD, Katz J, Bass EB, et al. The value of routine preoperative medical testing before cataract surgery. N Engl J Med 2000;342:168.

4. Leibowitz H, Krueger DE, Maudner LR, et al. The Framingham Eye Study Monograph. Surv Ophthalmol 1980;24[Suppl]:335.
5. Klein BE, Klein E. Cataracts and macular degeneration in older Americans. Arch Ophthalmol 1982;100:571.
6. Klein R, Klein BEK, Jensen SC, et al. The five-year incidence and progression of age-related maculopathy. The Beaver Dam Eye Study. Ophthalmology 1997;104:7.
7. Newsome DA, Swartz M, Leone NC, et al. Oral zinc in macular degeneration. Arch Ophthalmol 1988;106:192.
8. Age-related Eye Disease Study Research Group. A randomized, placebo-controlled, clinical trial of high dose supplementation with vitamins C and E, beta-carotene and zinc for age related macular degeneration and vision loss. Arch Opthal 2001;119:1417.
9. Bressler NM, Bressler SB, Fine SL. Age-related macular degeneration. Surv Ophthalmol 1988;32:375.
10. Macular Photocoagulation Study Group. Argon laser photocoagulation for neovascular maculopathy: three-year results from randomized clinical trials. Arch Ophthalmol 1986;104:694.
11. Photodynamic Therapy of Subfoveal Choroidal Neovascularization in Age-Related Macular Degeneration with Verteporfin. Two-year results of 2 randomized clinical trials: TAP Report 2. Treatment of Age-related Macular Degeneration with Photodynamic Therapy (TAP) Study Group. Arch Ophthalmol 2001;119:198.
12. Verteporfin in Photodynamic Therapy Study Group. Verteporfin therapy of subfoveal choroidal neovascularization in age-related macular degeneration: two year results of a randomized clinical trial including lesions with occult with no classic choroidal neovascularization. Verteporfin in Photodynamic Therapy Report 2. Am J Ophthalmol 2001;131:541.
13. Pharmacological Therapy for Macular Degeneration Study Group. Interferon alfa-2a is ineffective for patients with choroidal neovascularization secondary to age-related macular degeneration. Results of a prospective randomized placebo-controlled clinical trial. Arch Ophthalmol 1997;115:865.
14. Fine SL, Maguire M. It is not time to abandon radiotherapy for neovascular age-related macular degeneration. Arch Ophthalmol 2001;119:275.

C H A P T E R 108

Glaucoma

DAVID S. FRIEDMAN, MD, MPH*

Glaucoma is a progressive disease of the optic nerve head with a characteristic appearance (and cupping). Although many persons with glaucoma have elevated intraocular pressure (IOP), virtually all population-based studies of glaucoma have found that half of those with glaucoma have IOPs in the normal range (i.e., less than 21 mm Hg). Furthermore, even in developed countries, fewer than half of those with glaucoma know they have the disease. Glaucoma is the second leading case of blindness in the United States, with almost 2 million Americans affected. The glaucomas are classified into primary and secondary groups (Table 108.1). Among African Americans, whites, and Hispanics, primary open-angle glaucoma accounts for 95% of all patients with glaucoma, but among other populations (e.g., Chinese and those from south India), angle-closure glaucoma accounts for almost half the cases (1–3).

ANATOMY AND PHYSIOLOGY

The eye continuously circulates *aqueous humor* that maintains the shape of the eye and provides nutrition to avascular intraocular structures such as the lens (Fig. 108.1). IOP is maintained in a steady state by ongoing production and removal of aqueous humor. Elevated eye pressure is in part caused by obstruction to the outflow of aqueous humor at the level of the trabecular meshwork.

The aqueous humor is a clear ultrafiltrate of the blood and occupies part of the posterior and anterior chambers of the eye. It is produced both by secretion and ultrafiltration at the level of the epithelium of the ciliary body. At least two enzymes have been implicated in aqueous formation: sodium/potassium-activated ATPase and carbonic anhydrase. Antagonists of these enzymes appear to reduce the rate of aqueous formation and thereby lower IOP. Once produced, the aqueous humor circulates from the posterior chamber into the anterior chamber of the eye. The trabecular meshwork, an intricate system of connective tissue

*Dr. Andrew Schachat contributed to this chapter in the last edition of this book.

fibers, is located in the periphery of the anterior chamber. The aqueous humor percolates through this meshwork to be reunited with the venous blood via canal of Schlemm.

TYPES OF GLAUCOMA

Table 108.1 outlines the major types and causes of glaucoma. However, only primary open-angle glaucoma and primary angle-closure glaucoma are discussed in this chapter because they are the types likely to be seen regularly. Open-angle glaucoma takes its name from the normal-appearing anterior chamber angle, a contrast to the narrow angle of angle-closure glaucoma, as shown in Fig. 108.2. Individuals with *normal-tension glaucoma* behave similarly to those with higher pressure open-angle glaucoma, and research has shown that IOP-lowering therapy can prevent progression of the disease in these individuals (4).

Table 108.1. Types of Glaucoma

Primary
Open angle: 90% of whites, Hispanics, and African Americans, 50% of Chinese and southern Indians
Angle closure: 10% of whites, Hispanics, and African Americans, 50% of Chinese and southern Indians
Congenital: infant and juvenile onset
Secondary
Open angle: Results from topical or systemic steroids, ocular inflammation, or obstructed venous return from the eye (e.g., carotid cavernous sinus fistula)
Angle closure: Results from trauma, neovascular change in the iris, ocular neoplasia, cataract surgery, and iris abnormalities

Primary Open-Angle Glaucoma

Prevalence and Risk Factors

Primary open-angle glaucoma is by far the most common cause of glaucoma in the United States; the prevalence increases after the age of 40 years and approaches 3% for whites over 75 years of age and 8% for blacks and Hispanics (1). Indeed, because open-angle glaucoma is so prevalent, is asymptomatic, and is treatable, open-angle glaucoma is the primary reason behind the recommendation for annual eye examination for people 65 years and older. Primary open-angle glaucoma causes 15% to 20% of all blindness in this country (see Chapter 107 for a discussion of blindness). Men and women are affected equally, but African Americans are affected at a higher frequency and at an earlier age, and open-angle glaucoma is the leading cause of blindness in African Americans. Recent research in Hispanics in Arizona indicates that Hispanics have rates similar to whites until their sixties, when rates increase dramatically and are closer to those of blacks.

Open-angle glaucoma is familial, but the pattern of inheritance is not yet known. Siblings of affected individuals are at 10 times the risk of having open-angle glaucoma (5). An association between open-angle glaucoma and both diabetes mellitus and elevated blood pressure has been proposed, but these hypotheses are

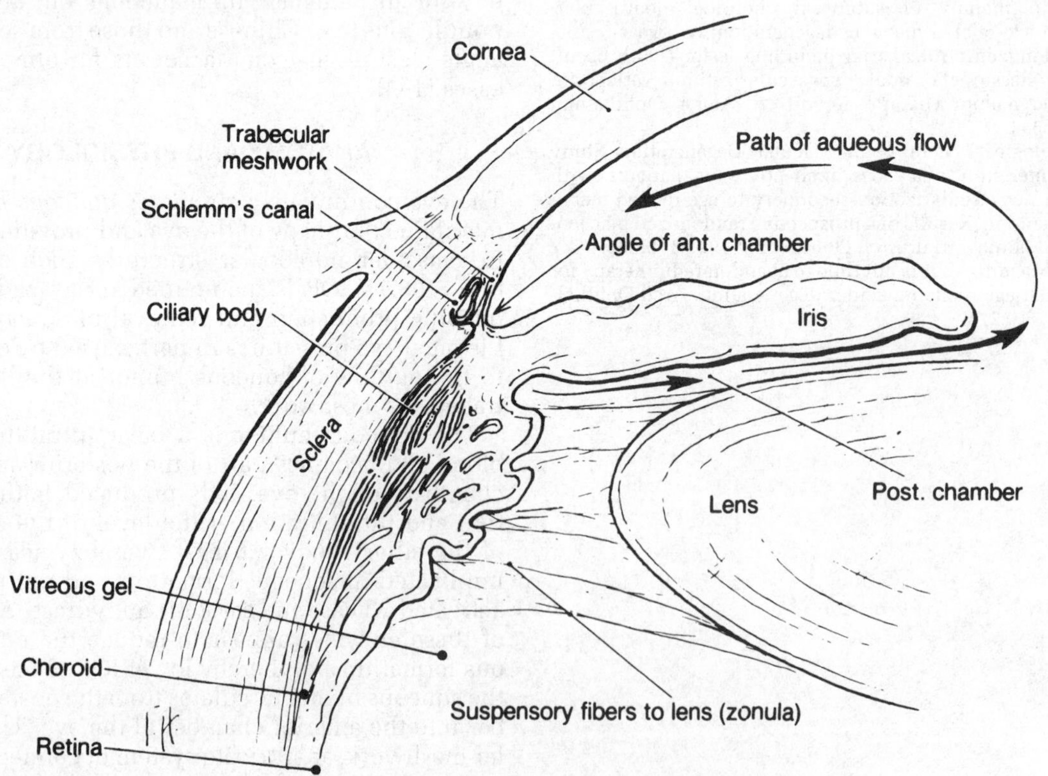

Figure 108.1. Anatomy of the eye: cross-section of the cornea. (From Basmajian JV. Grant's method of anatomy. 8th ed. Baltimore: Williams & Wilkins, 1971:543, with permission.)

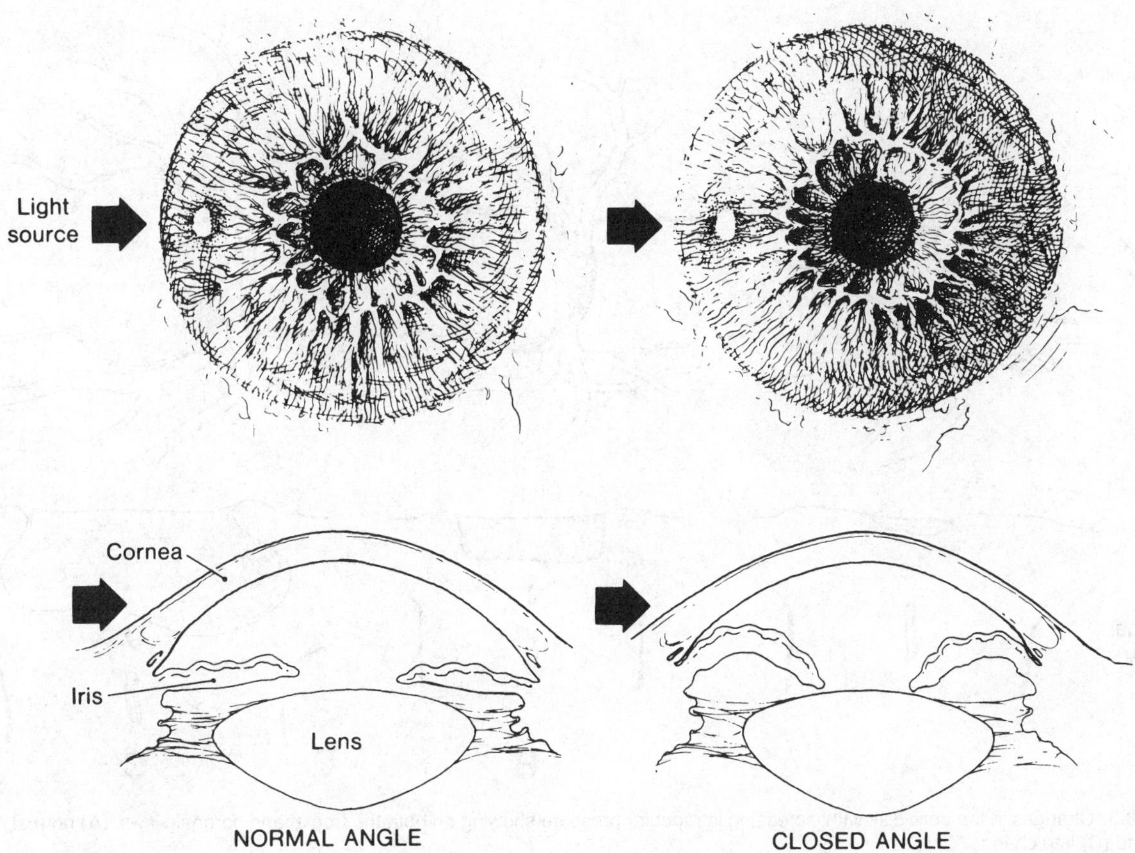

Figure 108.2. Illustration showing a shadow cast on the nasal side of the iris resultant from the bowed iris in angle-closure glaucoma (*right*). In open-angle glaucoma, the iris is not bowed, so the shadow is not cast (*left*).

uncertain and more research is necessary to define such relationships. Patients who have high degrees of myopia (near vision) likely are at higher risk of open-angle glaucoma, but this hypothesis is uncertain as well (6). Glaucoma risk may also be increased with prolonged use of oral and nasal glucocorticoid inhalers, especially in individuals with a family history of glaucoma (7,8).

Manifestations and Physical Examination

Open-angle glaucoma is typically asymptomatic until its latest stages. When symptoms do occur, damage to the optic nerve is present and may be substantial. Central vision and the ability to recognize forms on a vision test chart are preserved until very late. For this reason, testing of visual acuity is not a reliable method to screen for glaucoma. Occasionally, a patient with open-angle glaucoma may notice halos around lights and blurring of vision if there is a sudden rise in IOP. Patients with this history should be referred urgently to an ophthalmologist. Patients with open-angle glaucoma rarely complain of headache that can be attributed to increased IOP.

The ocular pressure may be elevated for years before any change in the optic disk is noted. The change in the optic disk is revealed by increasing excavation of the central physiologic disk cup, visible on funduscopic examination (Fig. 108.3). This is most easily seen by use of the direct ophthalmoscope. Over years the pink color of the disk fades and becomes pale, and vessels coursing over the disk show a sharp bend at the rim. Patients thought to have an enlarged optic cup (cup-to-disk ratio $\geq$0.7) should be referred to an ophthalmologist within a month.

One should assume that open-angle glaucoma has no symptoms until the patient is on the verge of blindness. Detection must be accomplished based on knowledge of risk factors (age, race, and family history) and examination findings. The diagnosis is then confirmed after referral to an ophthalmologist.

In evaluating the patient with increased IOP, the ophthalmologist performs tonometry to measure the eye pressure, gonioscopy (see below), funduscopy, and visual field examinations (see below). Characteristic visual field changes, called nerve fiber bundle defects, are seen in glaucoma.

Screening for Open-Angle Glaucoma

The ideal method for screening for primary open-angle glaucoma is controversial, and false positive and false negative detection rates are high. Population-based screening for glaucoma remains controversial because of the lack of an ideal screening device, the relatively high cost of screening and referral, and the limited data on treatment efficacy. However, recent developments have increased the evidence in support of wider

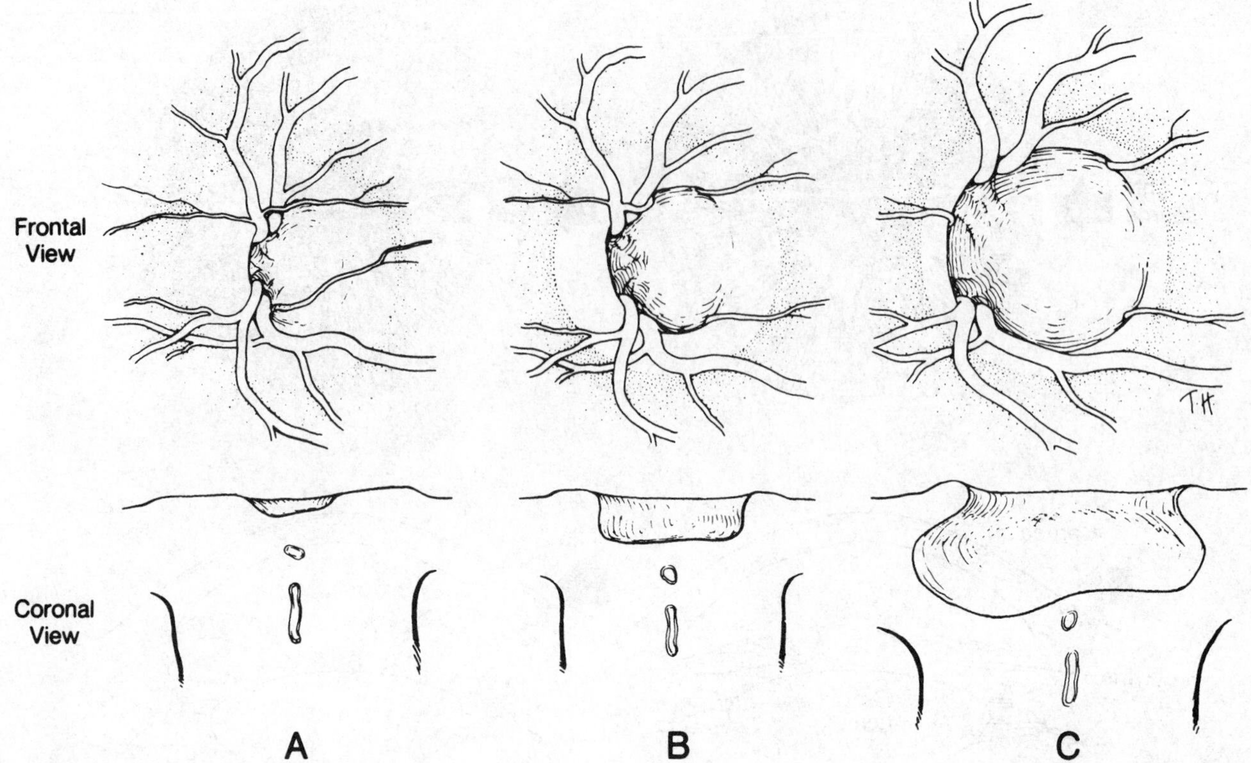

Figure 108.3. Changes in the optic disk with increasing intraocular pressure showing on both the frontal and coronal views: **(A)** normal, **(B)** early change, and **(C)** late change.

screening, and the Center for Medicare and Medical Services (formerly Health Care Financing Administration) recently added a benefit for glaucoma screening to Medicare beneficiaries with known risk factors. A new screening device, the frequency doubling technology perimeter, has demonstrated sensitivity and specificity over 90% in several recent reports (9,10). In addition, two publications indicate that lowering eye pressure is associated with slower progression of glaucoma (4,11).

Screening for glaucoma involves one of three different approaches: tonometry, funduscopic assessment of the optic cup through the dilated pupil, and visual field assessment. For years it has been recommended that primary care clinicians screen high-risk patients for glaucoma by measuring eye pressure directly with a Schiötz tonometer. This approach is now known to be too insensitive and nonspecific to be of value. IOP screening, even with ideal instruments, has poor screening characteristics, because half of all individuals with glaucoma have eye pressures in the normal range. New digital imaging devices show promise for detecting glaucoma by assessing the optic nerve head appearance. These instruments can collect data through an undilated pupil in under 1 minute and may be more widely used in the future (12). Finally, functional tests such as the perimeter described above show tremendous promise as screening devices. They obtain results in under 2 minutes per eye, are portable and inexpensive, and could conceivably be used in public settings such as departments of motor vehicles. More research is needed, however, to study the performance of each of these devices in community-based populations. Because ophthalmologists generally do all three evaluations, the ideal screening approach at present is a complete eye examination. Primary care clinicians are encouraged to advise white and Hispanic patients aged 65 and older (those at high risk) to be referred to an eye specialist every year or 2 for glaucoma screening, whereas African Americans should be referred at an earlier age, perhaps even age 40.

Patients referred to an ophthalmologist generally have an evaluation consisting of several observations: determination of the IOP by applanation tonometry; funduscopic assessment of the optic disk and retina through the dilated pupil; visual field assessment, usually with a computerized perimeter; and gonioscopic examination, which permits the ophthalmologist to visualize the angle of the anterior chamber by using an instrument containing a contact lens and mirror. The patient usually experiences minimal or no discomfort during these procedures.

Approximately one-fifth of patients found to have asymptomatic increased IOP on preliminary screening are shown to have glaucoma after thorough evaluation. Approximately 30% may be found not to have elevated pressures on reassessment, and about 50% have "ocular hypertension" without glaucoma. The ophthalmologist should follow this latter group of patients, with elevated IOP but with normal-appearing optic disks and normal visual fields, yearly. It is estimated that approximately 1% of these patients develop glaucoma each year, but a randomized clinical trial of these individuals is underway to determine whether or not early treatment is of benefit. Most glaucoma specialists today will observe an individual with an IOP less than 26 mm Hg and no evidence of disk or visual field damage.

Treatment

When the ophthalmologist establishes the diagnosis of open-angle glaucoma, treatment is prescribed based on the level of IOP, the degree of visual field loss, and the amount of optic nerve damage. As stated above, lowering IOP in individuals with open-angle glaucoma has recently been proven to slow the rate of progression of the disease. IOP lowering can be achieved by three different approaches: medical therapy, laser treatment, and surgical procedures.

Most ophthalmologists initially treat open-angle glaucoma with medicines, although the American Academy of Ophthalmology Preferred Practice Pattern recommends that all three approaches be discussed and considered as potential primary treatments.

The options for medical treatments have increased over the last several years with new effective medications available. IOP-lowering drugs work by one of three mechanisms: decrease aqueous production (beta-blockers, alpha agonists, and carbonic anhydrase inhibitors [CAIs]), increase outflow through the trabecular meshwork (miotics and prostaglandin α-agonists), or increase outflow through alternative pathways (uveoscleral outflow, prostaglandins).

The aim of therapy is to maintain the IOP at a level that does not lead to further optic nerve damage. Target pressures are chosen based on the IOP at which the patient sustained damage and the severity of the glaucoma. For example, an individual who presents with severe damage at a pressure of 20 mm Hg likely needs a pressure around 14 mm Hg to be safe, whereas an individual with mild disease and a pressure of 30 mm Hg can be followed at an IOP of 24. Patients are usually prescribed either a topical beta-blocker or a prostaglandin as initial therapy, although the U.S. Food and Drug Administration approval for prostaglandins is for second-line therapy. Alpha agonists and topical CAIs are also frequently prescribed. Combination drops are now available, with a combination beta-blocker and topical CAI widely used. Miotics, which were the mainstay of therapy for many years, are now rarely used because they cause miosis and dim vision. The movement toward prescribing prostaglandins as primary therapy has been driven by the excellent side-effect profile of these agents. No definite systemic side effects have been shown to be caused by prostaglandins. Ocular side effects include changing blue or hazel eyes to brown in a significant proportion of individuals. These agents also increase eyelashes in number and length. All other eye drops can have significant systemic side effects. Eye drops enter the bloodstream directly through the nasal mucosa without any first pass through the liver, resulting in relatively high levels of drug in the blood. Beta-blocking agents can exacerbate congestive heart failure, cause shortness of breath in otherwise healthy elderly individuals (13), lead to depression, and raise low-density lipoprotein cholesterol. Alpha agonists can cause dry mouth and, in about 10% of patients, significant lethargy. All individuals on these agents should be questioned about this side effect, because many may not identify the association with the eye drops they are taking. Alpha agonists can also lead to systemic hypotension. Topical CAIs are usually well tolerated with no reports of aplastic anemia or kidney stones caused by these agents since they were released over 5 years ago.

Oral CAIs are now rarely prescribed for glaucoma. Topical CAIs are used first, but in rare patients, oral CAIs can significantly drop the eye pressure when topical therapy is inadequate. Oral CAIs have myriad side effects (Table 108.2) and are therefore only used as a last resort.

Topical agents for glaucoma are tested in a one-eyed trial to see if they are effective for the patient. Once effectiveness and tolerability is determined, the agents are typically used bilaterally unless there is no evidence of disease in the contralateral eye. Once the target IOP has been attained, the ophthalmologist usually examines the patient two or three times per year for assessment of visual fields, measurement of IOP, funduscopic examination, and gonioscopy.

Argon laser trabeculoplasty is an alternative approach to lowering IOP for individuals with glaucoma and ocular hypertension and is considered a reasonable first-line therapy. This office procedure requires

Table 108.2. Systemic Effects of Medications Used to Treat Glaucoma

Considerable absorption of drug may occur through the nasal mucosa via flow through the lacrimal duct. Closing the eye for 2 minutes after instillation or pressing on the nasal lacrimal duct decreases the systemic uptake of eyedrops.

Beta-adrenergic blocking agents
- Pulmonary: bronchospasm (the incidence is decreased with selective beta-blockers such as betaxolol)
- Cardiovascular: bradycardia, hypotension, decreased cardiac contractility
- Central nervous system: fatigue, depression, memory loss, impotence

Miotics (e.g., Pilocarpine)
- Unstable refractive error, decreased night vision especially in those with cataracts, ciliary muscle spasms, ocular burning; long-acting agents such as phospholine iodide because of irreversible depletion of cholinesterase may make general anesthesia dangerous.

Alpha-agonists
- Systemic hypotension, somnolence, dry mouth, dizziness

Oral carbonic anhydrase inhibitor
- Malaise, fatigue, anorexia, depression, decreased libido, systemic acidosis (especially a risk in those with severe respiratory disease or those taking large dosages of salicylates), nausea, vomiting, diarrhea, alterations in taste of carbonated beverages. Topical carbonic anhydrase inhibitors do not appear to produce these side effects.

Reprinted from Everitt DE, Avorn J. Systemic effects of medications used to treat glaucoma. Ann Intern Med 1990;112:120, with permission.

only topical anesthesia and can result in a significant reduction in ocular pressure in close to 90% of patients. However, this effect is frequently transient, with about 50% of treatments still effective 5 years after initial treatment (14). The safety of this treatment is well documented in two large National Institutes of Health-sponsored clinical trials (14,15). The mechanism by which laser trabeculoplasty exerts its beneficial effects is uncertain but is most likely due to the release of growth factors at the time of therapy. A modification of this procedure using a different laser may allow for more repeat laser treatments than is currently possible using the argon laser.

Surgery in primary open-angle glaucoma is designed to construct outflow channels for the aqueous humor or, in the worst cases, to destroy the ciliary body in order to decrease aqueous production. Surgery lowers pressure more than medicines or lasers but has more potential adverse consequences. In the last few years, tremendous advances have been made in glaucoma filtering surgery. The major problem with the procedure, which makes a hole in the eye to allow aqueous drainage into the subconjunctival space, is the tendency for healing, which closes the hole in younger patients and certain other groups at high risk for filter failure. Topical antimetabolites used at the time of surgery are associated with an important increase in the success rate by retarding closure of the new channel. There is concern about late infections in all patients who have had glaucoma filtering surgery, and late infections may be more common in these antimetabolite procedures. Currently, unless results from new trials recommend otherwise, surgical procedures are reserved for patients in whom medical management fails. Medications may still be required after surgery. New nonpenetrating procedures, in which the aqueous fluid percolates through a very thin membrane of tissue that is left at the time of surgery, are under investigation and show promise. These may have a safer profile than standard filtration procedures. Another significant improvement on the horizon is the use of more specific agents to modulate wound healing. These drugs may lead to more healthy tissue after surgery and may reduce the likelihood of eye infections in operated eyes.

Monitoring

The patient with open-angle glaucoma must receive regular ophthalmologic follow-up, and the generalist should be alert to any side effects from the drugs prescribed by the ophthalmologist (Table 108.2).

There has been concern particularly about the use of systemic medications such as anticholinergics, adrenergics, hypnotics, and corticosteroids. Except for corticosteroids, none of these drugs is contraindicated in open-angle glaucoma. The concern raised by these medications is that they can cause acute angle-closure glaucoma in susceptible individuals, but this angle-closure glaucoma is relatively rare among most U.S. populations. Systemic corticosteroids (including inhaled steroids) and, in particular, corticosteroids applied to the eye may raise IOP and are relatively contraindicated in open-angle glaucoma.

Primary Angle-Closure Glaucoma

The basic defect in primary angle-closure glaucoma is the inability of aqueous humor to reach the filtration apparatus. When the pupil is in a mid-dilated position, the iris is bowed forward and blocks the outflow of aqueous humor (Fig. 108.2). The primary site of aqueous blockage is at the iris–lens interface. The iris moves forward as the pressure rises behind it, and there is blockage of the trabecular meshwork by the peripheral iris.

Although this form of glaucoma is far less common than open-angle glaucoma in the United States, it is important that one is aware of it because an attack may be precipitated by the use of mydriatics, sympathomimetics, and hypnotics; if this occurs, urgent recognition and treatment are mandatory to prevent damage to the eye and in several instances topiramate (an antiseizure medicine). In addition, all too often, cases of angle-closure glaucoma are misdiagnosed as possible neurosurgical or gastrointestinal conditions (because of symptoms such as headaches and nausea and vomiting) so recognition of the condition is important. Patients often have a positive family history, women are affected more than men, and the condition is far more common among Asians and those from the Indian subcontinent than among whites, African Americans, and Hispanics.

Patients who have smaller eyes with shallow anterior chambers are predisposed to primary angle-closure glaucoma. Patients with these predispositions can develop either acute attacks of angle-closure glaucoma, with extremely elevated eye pressure and pain, or can develop a silent form of the disease known as chronic angle-closure glaucoma. However, the probability of inducing acute angle-closure glaucoma in older blacks and whites is less than 1 in 3,000, so one should dilate individuals in need of a detailed examination of the eye whenever medically necessary. If an acute attack develops in such a circumstance, it can often be treated rapidly with minimal adverse sequelae.

Diagnosis

Early diagnosis of this problem is critical because blindness may ensue and virtually every case is surgically curable if diagnosed early. Cure is increasingly less likely if repeated attacks have occurred and have resulted in scarring of the trabecular meshwork. Although many acute attacks occur without any prodromal symptoms, some may experience episodes of ocular pain (usually located in the periocular or supraocular region), episodes of blurred vision, and seeing halos around lights at night before the initial attack. These symptoms occur because of corneal epithelial edema that has developed as a result of the increased IOP. Often patients find relief in well-lighted rooms or outdoors, where daylight causes constriction of the pupil and opening of the angle of the anterior chamber.

Examination during an acute attack usually reveals marked elevation of IOP, to 60 to 90 mm Hg. The eye is red and painful, although rarely the patient complains of abdominal pain or headache only. Frequently there is tearing and photophobia. Corneal edema is present during an acute attack, and the anterior chamber may appear cloudy because of inflammation.

In patients predisposed to angle-closure glaucoma, the anterior chamber is shallow. This may be seen by illuminating the eye with a flashlight from the side and showing a shadow resulting from the bowed iris over the nasal portion of the eye (Fig. 108.2). Examination of the anterior chamber angle with a gonioscopic lens may reveal scarring of the trabecular meshwork and peripheral anterior synechiae.

If the diagnosis of acute angle-closure glaucoma is suspected, an urgent referral to an ophthalmologist is indicated. The ophthalmologist will probably initiate treatment with immediate administration of acetazolamide (Diamox) 500 mg orally and instillation of pressure-lowering eye drops. If it will take hours to reach an ophthalmologist, one should initiate therapy. In severe cases, the ingestion of hyperosmotic glycerol—1 mL/kg mixed as a 50% solution with chilled juice—almost always interrupts an acute attack. Hyperosmotic agents such as glycerol or intravenous mannitol dehydrate the vitreous and lower eye pressure. Practitioners who use mydriatics for funduscopic examination or who have patients with narrow anterior ocular chambers may want to have an angle-closure kit consisting of glycerol (glycerin, available as generic), acetazolamide (Diamox), and a beta-blocker eye drop for use if an acute attack develops. Patients found to have a shallow anterior chamber even if they have not had a symptomatic attack of glaucoma should be referred to an ophthalmologist for evaluation, for education regarding specific manifestations of an acute attack, and for their initial treatment, usually prophylactic argon laser iridotomy.

Differential Diagnosis

The patient who has acute angle-closure glaucoma may present with an acute red eye. Initially, one will want to differentiate angle-closure glaucoma from acute iritis, acute conjunctivitis, and iridocyclitis. Chapter 109 discusses this differential diagnosis.

Course Without Treatment

Severe attacks of angle-closure glaucoma may cause blindness in 2 to 3 days or less depending on the level of IOP and the sensitivity of the ciliary body and optic nerve to ischemia. In some instances, ciliary ischemia stops aqueous production before blindness occurs. However, untreated acute attacks typically result in severe blinding glaucoma.

The treatment of acute primary angle-closure glaucoma is essentially surgical. If the diagnosis is made early enough in the course of the disease, a peripheral iridotomy can be done to relieve the pupillary block and allow the IOP to return to normal. In some acute cases, the trabecular meshwork remains permanently damaged or the filtering angle is scarred closed. Chronic medical therapy or even surgery may be required to prevent progressive optic nerve damage in these cases. Laser peripheral iridotomy under topical anesthesia has little risk and results in cure in most cases. Surgical iridectomy may also be performed. The laser iridotomy in the attack eye is performed as soon as the view is clear enough to do so. Generally, the contralateral eye is operated on prophylactically within a day or 2. Follow-up care by the ophthalmologist after laser iridotomy is necessary to make sure that IOP control has been achieved.

When one is aware that a patient has a shallow anterior chamber or is under treatment for angle-closure glaucoma, there should be concern about the use of certain medications. Systemic anticholinergics and adrenergic drugs may rarely precipitate an acute attack by causing dilation of the pupils. Hypnotics have also been implicated in causing acute attacks. Corticosteroids or vasodilating drugs are not contraindicated in patients with angle-closure glaucoma.

General References

American Academy of Ophthalmology Preferred Practice Pattern Committee. Primary *open angle* glaucoma preferred practice pattern. San Francisco: American Academy of Ophthalmology, 2000.

American Academy of Ophthalmology Preferred Practice Pattern Committee. Primary *angle-closure* glaucoma preferred practice pattern. San Francisco: American Academy of Ophthalmology, 2000.

Anderson DR, Patella VM. Automated static perimetry. 2nd ed. St. Louis: CV Mosby, 1998.

Explains the details of visual field testing.

Congdon N, Wang F, Tielsch JM. Issues in the epidemiology and population-based screening of primary angle-closure glaucoma. Surv Ophthalmol 1992;36:411.

Excellent review of the epidemiology of angle-closure glaucoma.

Everitt DE, Avorn J. Systemic effects of medications used to treat glaucoma. Ann Intern Med 1990;112:120.

A brief review of the important systemic manifestations of topical and systemic drugs used to treat glaucoma.

Fraunfelder FT, Roy FN. Current ocular therapy. 4th ed. Philadelphia: WB Saunders, 1995.

This text provides a brief review of many common eye problems. It gives excellent therapeutic guidelines and has some pertinent references.

Newell FW. Ophthalmology, principles and concepts. St. Louis: CV Mosby, 1996.

Quigley HA. Open-angle glaucoma. N Engl J Med 1993;328:1097.

Excellent summary of the disease.

Shields MB. Textbook of glaucoma. 4th ed. Baltimore: Williams & Wilkins, 1997.

Sommer A. Doyne lecture: glaucoma: facts and fancies. Eye 1996;10:295.

U.S. Preventive Services Task Force. Screening for glaucoma. In: Guide to clinical preventive services-report of the US preventive services task force. Baltimore: Williams & Wilkins, 1995.

Wilson MR. Epidemiological features of glaucoma. Int Ophthalmol Clin 1990;30:153.

This article provides a brief summary of the epidemiology of open-angle glaucoma.

Specific References

1. Tielsch JM, Sommer A, Katz J, et al. Racial variations in the prevalence of primary open-angle glaucoma. The Baltimore Eye Survey [see comments]. JAMA 1991;266:369.
2. Foster PJ, Oen FT, Machin D, et al. The prevalence of glaucoma in Chinese residents of Singapore: a cross-sectional

population survey of the Tanjong Pagar district. Arch Ophthalmol 2000;118:1105.
3. Dandona L, Dandona R, Mandal P, et al. Angle-closure glaucoma in an urban population in southern India. The Andhra Pradesh eye disease study. Ophthalmology 2000;107:1710.
4. Collaborative Normal-Tension Glaucoma Study Group. The effectiveness of intraocular pressure reduction in the treatment of normal-tension glaucoma. Am J Ophthalmol 1998;126:498.
5. Wolfs RC, Klaver CC, Ramrattan RS, et al. Genetic risk of primary open-angle glaucoma. Population-based familial aggregation study. Arch Ophthalmol 1998;116:1640.
6. Mitchell P, Hourihan F, Sandbach J, et al. The relationship between glaucoma and myopia: the Blue Mountains Eye Study. Ophthalmology 1999;106:2010.
7. Garbe E, LeLorier J, Boivin JF, et al. Inhaled and nasal glucocorticoids and the risks of ocular hypertension or open-angle glaucoma. JAMA 1997;277:722.
8. Mitchell P, Cumming RG, Mackey DA. Inhaled corticosteroids, family history, and risk of glaucoma. Ophthalmology 1999;106:2301.
9. Quigley HA. Identification of glaucoma-related visual field abnormality with the screening protocol of frequency doubling technology. Am J Ophthalmol 1998;125:819.
10. Patel SC, Friedman DS, Varadkar P, et al. Algorithm for interpreting the results of frequency doubling perimetry. Am J Ophthalmol 2000;129:323.
11. The AGIS Investigators. The advanced glaucoma intervention study (AGIS). 7. The relationship between control of intraocular pressure and visual field deterioration. Am J Ophthalmol 2000;130:429.
12. Wollstein G, Garway-Heath DF, Fontana L, et al. Identifying early glaucomatous changes. Comparison between expert clinical assessment of optic disc photographs and confocal scanning ophthalmoscopy. Ophthalmology 2000;107:2272.
13. Diggory P, Heyworth P, Chau G, et al. Unsuspected bronchospasm in association with topical timolol—a common problem in elderly people: can we easily identify those affected and do cardioselective agents lead to improvement? Age Ageing 1994;23:17.
14. Anonymous. The advanced glaucoma intervention study (AGIS). 4. Comparison of treatment outcomes within race. Ophthalmology 1998;105:1146.
15. Glaucoma Laser Trial Research Group. The Glaucoma Laser Trial (GLT) and glaucoma laser trial follow-up study. 7. Results. Am J Ophthalmol 1995;120:718.

CHAPTER 109

Diseases of the Eyelid, Conjunctiva, and Anterior Segment of the Eye

ROBERT S. WEINBERG, MD*

*Dr. Andrew Schachat contributed to this chapter in the last edition.

Patients with eye problems often present for care initially to their primary care provider. It is important, therefore, to recognize the nature and severity of a patient's ocular complaint and to formulate a logical approach the evaluation and treatment. A few problems require urgent ophthalmic attention, but most may be appropriately managed by the primary care provider.

With a systematic approach to the patient, beginning with the history and proceeding with examination of the parts of the eye suggested by the history, one should be able to recognize what external ocular problems may be safely managed. When referral to an ophthalmologist is indicated, one should understand whether that referral should be on an emergent, urgent, or routine basis and what should be expected from the consultation.

Often, discussions about eye problems for the generalist center around the *red eye,* a dramatic presentation, frequently causing a patient to seek medical attention. Although the topic of the red eye is covered in this chapter, it is only one of many presenting complaints.

APPROACH TO THE PATIENT

Even with a problem that appears limited to the eye and the visual system, obtaining an accurate history is most important in suggesting a diagnosis. History should include information about the duration and severity, whether or not there is any perceived change in vision, and whether the problem is unilateral or bilateral. Other complaints peculiar to the eye include photophobia, pain or foreign body sensation, and redness or discharge. The time of day that symptoms occur may be important because some conditions are worse on awakening whereas others worsen as the day progresses. Because there is a relationship between skin disease and eye disease, awareness of a previously diagnosed dermatologic problem such as acne rosacea or atopic dermatitis is important. Because there is a perception by lay people that eye drops are not medicines and because some eye preparations are available over the counter, one should ask the patient if they have tried to care for the problem using drops or ointments. Also, patients may not make the connection of current symptoms with recent or past ocular surgery, and therefore this history must be solicited. Because patients who wear contact lenses, even occasionally, may have specific related problems, that history too should be obtained.

EXAMINATION AND ANATOMY

All conditions discussed in this chapter involve the parts of the eye visible with normal room illumination or with the aid of a flashlight and without additional magnification.

Visual Acuity

Examination of the eye should always begin with a measurement of visual acuity. This should be done one eye at a time and with glasses, if the patient wears them. Although an eye chart may be used, simply having the patient cover one eye at a time and look at an object in the examination room will provide information about whether or not there is any subjective difference in vision between the two eyes. If the perceived change is new, ophthalmology referral is indicated without regard to the cause of the problem.

Structures of the External Eye

An overview of the pertinent anatomy of those parts of the anterior segment of the eye visible with room illumination or with a handheld light are shown in Fig. 109.1. (See Fig. 108.1, p. 1662.)

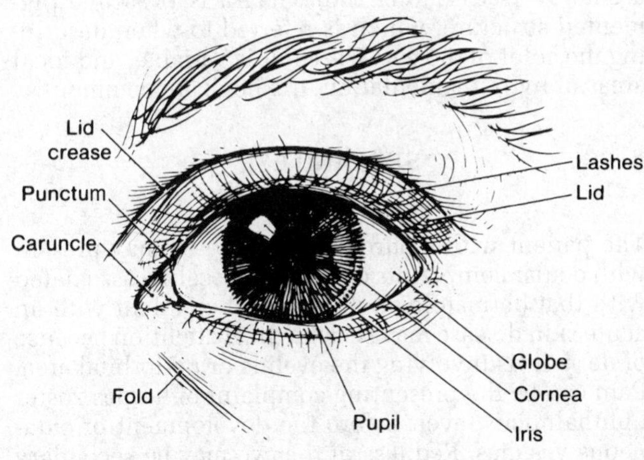

Figure 109.1. External landmarks of the eye.

Systematic Examination of the External Eye

The examiner should begin the evaluation by judging the patient's face for redness, scaling dermatoses, or telangiectasias on the cheeks, nose, and eyelids. Examination of the *eyelids* begins with an assessment of the position of the lids. Asymmetry of lid position, either ptosis or lid retraction, may suggest an orbital abnormality, such as thyroid ophthalmopathy. Periorbital edema, or swelling of the lids, may be present. The lids should be examined for lesions distorting the normal contour. Normal *eyelashes* are roughly parallel and of equal length, with none missing or broken and without discharge. Even without the aid of a slit lamp, the *tear film* is visible as a thin layer of liquid above the lower eyelid. Quantitative measurement of the tear film, *Schirmer's test,* usually done by an ophthalmologist, can confirm an impression of dry eye or tear dysfunction. Even without a Schirmer's test, close inspection of the external eye can provide an indication of a dry eye. Alternatively, tearing or epiphora may in itself be a presenting complaint or a secondary sign of ocular inflammation.

The *conjunctiva* is the mucous membrane lining the eyelids and covering the globe. The normal conjunctiva is lustrous, secondary to the moisture of the tear film. Small conjunctival vessels are present. Although the conjunctiva appears white, it is actually translucent, with the white color that of the underlying sclera. The *episclera* is vascularized connective tissue deep to the conjunctiva and superficial to the sclera. The *sclera,* relatively rigid connective tissue, is normally white to pale yellow in color. The sclera begins at the limbus, the peripheral margin of the cornea, and extends posteriorly to the optic nerve. Areas of scleral thinning or translucency may be seen normally within the palpebral fissure, anterior to the insertions of the horizontal rectus muscles. The *cornea* is thin, 500 to 600 μm, and transparent. The normal cornea is 11 mm in diameter. The *anterior chamber* is the optically clear space, filled with aqueous humor, between the cornea and the iris. Anterior chamber depth may be approximated by shining a hand light at the lateral limbus. If a shadow is seen on the nasal iris, the anterior chamber is shallow (see Chapter 108). The *iris* is a vascular pigmented structure, which is referred to when describing the color of the eye. Iris color is variable, and focal areas of hyperpigmentation, iris nevi, are common.

SKIN AND EYE

History

The patient with a chronic skin disease may present with ocular complaints of itching or scaling associated with that dermatologic disorder. The patient with an acute skin disease may seek medical attention because of dermatitis involving the eyelids or periorbital area. Pain can be the presenting complaint of herpes zoster ophthalmicus, even before the development of cutaneous vesicles. Redness of the eye may be secondary to eyelid disease.

Examination

Examination of the eyes should begin with a general observation of the skin of the face. Special attention should be given to the eyelids and eyelashes.

Common Conditions of the Skin About the Eyes

Scaling Dermatoses and Atopic Dermatitis

Patients complain of itching but may have pain if there is associated bacterial blepharitis. Examination usually reveals scaling and redness of the eyelids. Patients with atopic dermatitis may have a combination of staphylococcal blepharitis and herpes simplex blepharitis or keratitis. Atopic dermatitis is one of the few diseases associated with bilateral herpes simplex keratitis (1).

Seborrheic Dermatitis

Seborrheic dermatitis is extremely common. In addition to dandruff, there may be scaling of the nose and face and eyelids. Redness of the eyes and morning discharge often occurs. Seborrheic blepharitis with oily debris along the eyelid margin, scurf, is a sign of seborrheic blepharitis (Fig. 109.2, Color Plate section).

Acne Rosacea

Acne rosacea is a common cause of ocular problems. Ocular problems may actually be the presenting complaint for a patient with acne rosacea. A sty in an adult should prompt one to consider that that patient may have acne rosacea. Early in the course of acne rosacea, telangiectases on the cheeks and nose and eyelids may be difficult to see without magnification, perhaps the reason that an ophthalmologist, with the aid of a slit-lamp instrument, may suggest the diagnosis in an early stage (Fig. 109.3, Color Plate section).

Herpes Zoster

Herpes zoster may affect any dermatome. Between 9% and 16% of patients with herpes zoster have involvement of the skin innervated by the trigeminal nerve (2). Unilateral headache or eye pain may be the presenting complaint, hours to days before vesicles appear. Ocular involvement may be in the form of blepharitis, with swelling of the eyelids and vesicles on the skin, or as acute uveitis, with blurred vision, pain, redness, and photophobia (Fig. 109.4, Color Plate section).

Management

When a patient with an acute or chronic skin problem complains of eye problems, whether it is itching, discharge, or pain, urgent referral to an ophthalmologist is appropriate.

EYELIDS

Disorders of the eyelids are a frequent cause of ocular problems. Patients complain of redness of the eyes, with discharge and discomfort, but no change in vision. Blepharitis, inflammation of the eyelids, causes discharge, which tends to be worse in the morning upon awakening.

History

Eyelid disorders tend to become chronic. Symptoms often are worse in the morning upon awakening. If there is discharge, noting that the discharge occurs in the morning should strongly suggest the diagnosis of blepharitis.

Examination

Patients with blepharitis may notice redness of the eyes, with conjunctival injection secondary to inflammation of the eyelids. Redness of the eyes can be caused by irritation from the discharge on the eyelids or from changes in the tear film, associated with meibomian gland congestion. When there is meibomian gland congestion in blepharitis, there is less oil in the tear film, allowing for more rapid evaporation of the aqueous component of the tears and causing dryness of the eye. Tear dysfunction with an abnormality of the tear film occurs frequently in patients with blepharitis. Eyelid swelling and ptosis also may be present.

Edema

Systemic diseases may cause swelling of the eyelids. Patients with thyroid dysfunction can have eyelid swelling. Because the skin of the lids is especially thin, conditions with fluid retention, such as congestive heart failure or renal failure, may cause fluid to be retained in the eyelids. Allergic conjunctivitis (see below) is frequently associated with eyelid swelling.

Blepharitis

Blepharitis may be infectious or noninfectious. Infectious blepharitis is common and most frequently caused by coagulase-negative staphylococcal species. *Staphylococcus aureus* is perhaps the next most common bacterial cause of blepharitis. Other bacteria, such as *Streptococcus* species, and various gram-negative organisms, such as *Pseudomonas* species, *Klebsiella pneumonia,* and *Escherechia coli,* may also cause blepharitis. Specific signs in blepharitis caused by staphylococcal species include lid margin ulcerations, broken and missing eyelashes, and collarettes or fibrin on the base of lashes (Fig. 109.5, Color Plate section).

Seborrheic blepharitis, associated with seborrheic dermatitis, causes oily debris (i.e., scurf) on the eyelid margins. Mixed blepharitis refers to the simultaneous coexistence of staphylococcal blepharitis and seborrheic blepharitis. Viral blepharitis is less common than bacterial blepharitis but presents with vesicles on the eyelids (Fig. 109.6, Color Plate section). Herpes zoster and herpes simplex both can cause viral blepharitis. In the past, vaccinia vesicular dermatitis after smallpox vaccination was a more frequent cause of viral blepharitis, with inoculation of the eyelids by a patient's hands touching their recent smallpox vaccination site. Parasitic blepharitis occurs most commonly associated with infection by *Phthiris pubis.* Pubic hair and eyelashes are strong enough and far enough apart to allow the parasites to grow (Fig.109.7, Color Plate section). Patients with parasitic blepharitis complain of itching of the eyes. Adult lice and nits are visible on the eyelashes.

The lid margins, surrounding skin, conjunctiva, and cornea may be involved singly or collectively. The skin may also show changes of seborrheic dermatitis or it may be excoriated and macerated, especially at the lateral canthal margin. Crusting is noted at the bases of the eyelashes. The conjunctiva may show changes of papillary hyperplasia (multiple conjunctival mounds with a central single vessel). Corneal changes occur after months of inflammation and are manifest as fine discrete peripheral defects. There may also be ulceration, clouding, and vascularization of the margins of the cornea. The diagnosis of conjunctival involvement in blepharitis is made by examination and, in cases in doubt, by scraping the conjunctivae and the margins of the eyelids and by culturing the exudate.

Treatment should be continued for at least 3 weeks. Daily cleansing of the eyelashes with a neutral soap (e.g., dilute Johnson's Baby Shampoo) followed by the application of an antibiotic ointment (erythromycin, bacitracin, or sulfacetamide) to the eyelashes at bedtime for several weeks reduces the bacterial count, cleanses the lids, and minimizes recurrences. Patients with blepharitis are often best served by using an ophthalmologist to prescribe their long-term management.

Hordeolum

A hordeolum (Fig. 109.3, Color Plate section) is a common infection in the glands of the eyelid caused by *S. aureus.* It is characterized by the sudden onset of localized pain, swelling, redness, and often purulent discharge. The infected gland may be a meibomian gland just under the conjunctival side of the eyelid, and this is called an *internal hordeolum.* An internal hordeolum may be large and may point to either the skin or the conjunctival side of the lid. Also, a smaller gland associated with an eyelash follicle under the skin side of the lid may be infected, and this is called an *external hordeolum* or sty. A sty usually is smaller than an internal hordeolum but is easily recognized in that it always points to the skin side of the lid.

The differential diagnosis includes tumors of the lid margin (see below) and other localized inflammatory lesions of the eyelid, such as *Molluscum contagiosum* or herpes simplex, before vesicles develop. Patients with sties or hordeola have blepharitis, so the history of morning discharge and redness and the observation of irregular, missing, or broken eyelashes support the diagnosis. Many adult patients have acne rosacea with blepharitis and develop recurrent sties.

Management should not only be aimed at treating the acute problem, the hordeolum, but also at handling the pre-existing chronic problem, the blepharitis. Both types of hordeolum may be treated without obtaining a culture. Initial management consists of hot compresses, applied for 5 minutes or more at least two to four times a day, and topical ophthalmic antibiotic ointment, such as erythromycin, bacitracin, or sulfacetamide 10%, applied at bedtime. Systemic antibiotics are not indicated, unless there is evidence of cellulitis. Because most hordeola resolve with conservative management and to avoid initiating increased inflammation, incision and drainage by the ophthalmologist is generally not done for 3 or more weeks.

Chalazion

A chalazion is a sterile lipogranulomatous inflammation of a meibomian gland secondary to chronic inflammation (Fig. 109.8, Color Plate section). A chalazion can develop from an internal hordeolum that does not resolve. The swelling may appear anywhere on the eyelid (although the upper lid is a more common location), and it usually points toward the conjunctival side. Chalazia are frequently seen in patients with acne rosacea. The presence of blepharitis, with or without acne rosacea, confirms the diagnosis. The differential diagnosis includes various lid margin tumors. However, these are rare, whereas chalazia are common. A chalazion is not painful but may cause discomfort or a feeling of fullness in the lid. Visual acuity may rarely be affected if the chalazion is large enough to cause pressure on the cornea and induce astigmatism. Some chalazia do resolve over periods of months. Incision and drainage by the ophthalmologist is frequently recommended if the patient is not willing to wait for the possibility of gradual slow resorption over time. Therefore, an ophthalmologist should be consulted if there is doubt about the diagnosis or treatment.

Lid Margin Tumors

Sties and chalazia are very common, but they must be differentiated from lid margin tumors, which occur rarely. Lid margin tumors are usually slow growing, not painful, and not associated with underlying blepharitis. Chronic irritation of the eye with redness may be caused by lid margin tumors, which prevent complete lid closure. Both squamous and basal cell carcinomas can occur on the eyelids, as can malignant melanomas. Patients suspected of such lesions should be referred to an ophthalmologist.

Eyelashes

Examination of the eyelashes can be done with room illumination or with the use of a flashlight. Attention to the eyelashes may provide clues about the nature of a patient's ocular complaints. Normally, the lashes are roughly equal in length and have a uniform distribution, with no areas of the lid margin devoid of lashes. A history of loss of lashes, sparse lashes, or discharge on the lashes suggests blepharitis. Inwardly directed lashes, trichiasis, can be a cause of foreign body sensation, corneal irritation, and redness of the eye.

TEARS

The *tear film* provides nutrition and protection to the cornea and the conjunctiva. The terms "dry eye," decreased tear production, and keratitis sicca are synonymous but are more appropriately included in the term tear dysfunction. Tear dysfunction is a frequent cause of chronically red eyes.

The tear film consists of three layers. The outer layer of the tear film, the oily layer, is produced by the oil glands of the lids and serves to prevent evaporation of the aqueous layer. Patients with acne rosacea may actually have rapid evaporation of tears because the oily secretions of the meibomian glands are so viscous that there is insufficient oil in the tear film. The middle layer of the tear film, the aqueous layer, is produced by the lacrimal gland and accessory lacrimal glands. The aqueous layer of the tear film provides oxygen to the cornea. The inner layer of the tear film, the mucous layer, is produced by the goblet cells of the conjunctiva. The mucous layer allows the aqueous layer of the tear film to adhere to the cornea. Although patients with red eyes may have problems with any layer of the tear film, the term "dry eye" generally refers to a decrease in the aqueous component of the tear film. The term "tear dysfunction" means an abnormality of the tear film, whether causing rapid evaporation, insufficient mucus, or inadequate aqueous production in patients with, as examples, acne rosacea, pemphigoid, or a connective tissue disorder, respectively.

History

Patients with tear dysfunction usually have complaints of redness and burning, itching and foreign body sensation, or blurring and decreased vision. The redness and most other complaints associated with decreased tear production are generally worse as the day progresses, with normal activity allowing progressive evaporation of tears and more and more drying. Symptoms in patients with tear dysfunction tend to be less on awakening, because the eyes have been closed during sleep and drying does not occur when the eyes are closed.

Examination

Although it is easy for an ophthalmologist to assess the status of the tear film with the use of fluorescein staining and slit-lamp biomicroscopy, close inspection of the tear meniscus, the layer of tears above the lower lid margin, can be done with flashlight illumination. A layer of moisture, approximately 1 to 2 mm high, is normally visible above the lower lid. The normally lustrous cornea often appears dull or with certainly less luster in a patient who has dry eyes.

Ocular Conditions

Ocular conditions that cause tear dysfunction include blepharitis; acne rosacea; exophthalmos (with decreased blinking and a larger area from which tears can evaporate); and cicatrizing conjunctivitis (such as that seen with chemical burns), Stevens-Johnson syndrome, or mucous membrane pemphigoid (with loss of normal goblet cells).

Systemic Conditions

Many patients have tear dysfunction as part of a systemic disease. Sjögren syndrome with an associated dry mouth and dry eye is frequently seen with connective tissue disease or sarcoidosis.

Medications Causing Conditions

Both topical and systemic medications may alter tear production. Among the most commonly used medications that can cause tear dysfunction are beta-blockers, diuretics, and some psychoactive drugs.

Management

Although the initial treatment of tear dysfunction may simply involve the frequent use of artificial tears, routine nonurgent referral to an ophthalmologist often is indicated because of the chronic and often therapeutically frustrating nature of this problem. If systemic medications are implicated in causation of tear dysfunction, selection of medications that do not cause dry eye may be advisable.

CONJUNCTIVA

The conjunctiva is a mucous membrane, which is the inner lining of the eyelids, and the outer coating of the globe.

History

Patients with conjunctival disease complain of redness and usually discharge. There may also be irritation or foreign body sensation, but there is no pain (unless severe, e.g., in hyperacute forms, see Hyperacute Bacterial Conjunctivitis, below) nor change in vision with isolated conjunctivitis.

Examination

Color

Normally, the conjunctiva is translucent, allowing the color of the underlying white or off-white color of the sclera to be seen. Yellow coloration of the conjunctiva is seen in patients with jaundice or in patients who have had a subconjunctival hemorrhage in which the blood is being resorbed. Hyperemia of the conjunctiva has many causes such as polycythemia, acne rosacea, and conditions with venous obstruction (superior vena cava syndrome). Examination of the conjunctiva with a flashlight will show if a discharge is present. Conjunctivitis tends to cause diffuse conjunctival redness. Conjunctivitis is usually bilateral but may present initially in one eye.

Discharge

There are three main types of conjunctivitis: Bacterial, viral, and allergic. The type of discharge may help to determine the type of conjunctivitis: Bacterial has purulent discharge; viral, watery; and allergic, ropy.

Luster

The conjunctiva is normally lustrous, shiny, and reflecting light. Decreased conjunctival luster can be a sign of a dry eye and may be seen in patients with tear dysfunction, conjunctival cicatrization, or vitamin A deficiency (Bitot spot).

Conjunctivitis

The diagnosis and management of conjunctivitis can be confusing, considering the variety of ocular infections. Most instances of conjunctivitis in adults are not emergencies, and often they are self-limited. However, conjunctivitis may lead to serious complications such as corneal scarring, lid damage, or, in cases in which the patient has had previous glaucoma filtration surgery, endophthalmitis. If a conjunctival filtering bleb is present, indicating successful filtration surgery, bacteria may enter the eye through that scleral opening. In the normal eye, an intact sclera prevents access of bacteria to the vitreous of the eye.

Conjunctival Flora

Under normal conditions the conjunctival sac has a bacterial flora composed of several species. The most commonly encountered organism is *Staphylococcus albus,* followed by corynebacteria, *S. aureus,* and *Streptococcus* species. Some normal patients harbor *Pseudomonas* species and fungi. This complex flora complicates the establishment of a specific cause in a patient with infectious conjunctivitis and is the reason that routine culture of the conjunctival discharge is not recommended.

Presentation

Conjunctivitis is usually not painful, but often there is mild discomfort, burning, discharge, tearing, itching, and lid swelling. Vision is well preserved. Most often, infectious conjunctivitis is bilateral.

Laboratory Diagnosis

Occasionally, there may be doubt about the diagnosis of conjunctivitis. In this uncommon situation, a simple culture or staining by the laboratory of the conjunctival material helps in determining the cause and subsequent management of the condition. The eyes and conjunctivae are not sterile, and organisms, even pathogens, may be cultured from normal subjects (see above). A positive culture does not necessarily mean there is a clinical infection. Most often, however, an adequate diagnosis can be made from the appearance of the conjunctiva, and a culture is unnecessary. Immunologic tests are available and permit immediate diagnosis of some causes of infectious conjunctivitis, especially chlamydia. The availability of these tests varies from community to community. Therefore, one not familiar with their use should consult an ophthalmologist by telephone for a recommendation.

Culture

In the occasional instance that culture is initiated, specimens should be obtained with a sterile swab by everting the eyelid and wiping the conjunctival sac. This material should be obtained without topical anesthesia because the preservatives in the anesthetic solution inhibit the growth of organisms. The specimen must be transferred immediately into transport media or delivered immediately to the laboratory for culturing. Each eye should be cultured separately, even if there is only monocular involvement, so that the apparently uninfected eye provides information about the nature of the normal flora.

Scraping is recommended in the evaluation of patients with conjunctivitis only when the diagnosis is uncertain. Referral to an ophthalmologist in situations in which scrapings are considered is recommended if one is not experienced in this technique.

After culture (if done), a topical anesthetic (e.g., proparacaine [Ophthaine]) should be instilled, and scrapings of the conjunctiva, well away from the cornea, should be obtained. A sterile platinum spatula (available from medical supply stores) or the dull side of a sterile scalpel blade can be used to scrape the conjunctiva. The material obtained by this method is smeared on a glass slide and sent to the laboratory to be stained with Gram or Giemsa stain. The appearance of the cells found in these scrapings is helpful in determining the diagnosis. The differential findings are discussed below and are listed in Table 109.1.

Hyperacute Bacterial Conjunctivitis

The name of this condition reflects its onset and the very thick exudate associated with it (Fig. 109.9, Color Plate section). Typically, the discharge is so copious that it accumulates in the lashes or runs down the patient's cheek. One eye is usually involved before the other, but within several days the second eye becomes involved through autoinoculation. The infection quickly involves the surrounding structures and is associated with aching discomfort, swelling of the lid, and tenderness of the eye. Enlarged preauricular lymph nodes are often present. Early in the course of the infection the cornea is not involved, but as the conjunctival swelling and tissue reaction increase, a peripheral corneal ring ulcer may develop because of compression of the peripheral corneal circulation.

Neisseria gonorrhoeae or *N. meningitidis* is usually implicated in this hyperacute form of infection. Inoculation is a result of spread by autoinoculation from infected genitalia. The gonococcus has the ability to penetrate the intact corneal epithelium, so central corneal ulceration and endophthalmitis may also occur. Meningococcal conjunctivitis is indistinguishable from gonococcal conjunctivitis, although the former occurs more often in younger patients, may be bilateral at the onset, and can proceed to metastatic meningitis or meningococcemia.

If needed in establishing the diagnosis of hyperacute conjunctivitis, conjunctival scrapings reveal an overwhelming number of polymorphonuclear leukocytes and intracellular gram negative diplococci. Culture should be obtained on Thayer-Martin selective medium or should be sent to the laboratory on Transgrow medium. The differentiation between gonococcus and meningococcus requires special bacteriologic studies.

Therapy of hyperacute conjunctivitis must be prompt to avoid corneal damage or systemic spread and should include the administration of both systemic and topical antibiotics. Because of the seriousness of this condition, an ophthalmologist should be consulted immediately. Institution of appropriate antibiotics by the ophthalmologist should result in the disappearance of the discharge within 24 to 48 hours, although lid swelling and conjunctival reaction do not abate for several days. If a corneal ulcer occurs, it takes time, often weeks, to heal; if the cornea has been scarred, visual acuity may be affected. In rare cases endophthalmitis may occur, and blindness is possible.

Table 109.1. Diagnosis Based on Cells in Material Scraped from Conjunctiva

Cells	Significance
Polymorphonuclear leukocytes	Bacterial, fungal, chlamydial (inclusion conjunctivitis), trachoma, Stevens–Johnson syndrome
Mononuclear cells	Viral
Eosinophils	Allergy, ocular pemphigoid
Epithelial metaplasia (atypical, large cells)	*Chlamydia*, herpes simplex

Acute Bacterial Conjunctivitis

Acute bacterial conjunctivitis, like hyperacute bacterial conjunctivitis, has an abrupt onset but is characterized by a less thick often mucopurulent discharge. This form of conjunctivitis is often called catarrh or *pink eye* (Fig. 109.10, Color Plate section); it is seen at all ages and at any time of year. Pink eye is a nonspecific term applied to almost any minor infectious conjunctivitis, especially bacterial and viral forms. The most common cause of bacterial conjunctivitis is *S. aureus* infection. *Pneumococcus* and *Haemophilus* species also cause the problem, but infections with these organisms have a more restricted geographic distribution than do staphylococcal infections; pneumococcal infections occur primarily in the northern states during the colder months, and *Haemophilus infections* occur more commonly in the warmer regions of the United States throughout the year. Also, pneumococcal or

Haemophilus conjunctivitis is more common in younger patients than is staphylococcal conjunctivitis. Rarely, other bacteria, such as *Moraxella lacunata, Escherichia coli,* or *Proteus* species, cause this form of conjunctivitis.

Patients complain of eye irritation and watering, and typically the eyelids stick together after sleep. The infection starts unilaterally, but very often, because of autoinoculation, the contralateral eye becomes involved in 1 or 2 days. Examination reveals hyperemia of the palpebral conjunctiva (i.e., the conjunctival side of the eyelid); bulbar conjunctival petechiae, characteristic of *Haemophilus* infection, may be seen.

Acute bacterial conjunctivitis is usually self-limited and generally lasts 7 to 14 days, although *Haemophilus* infections may last somewhat longer. The diagnosis is suspected by the examination; however, with the unusual situation of doubt, the diagnosis could be confirmed by examination of the scrapings of the conjunctiva and by culturing the exudate.

Topical treatment usually results in the resolution of symptoms in a day or two. A number of effective topical antibiotics are available, and one should be used for 5 to 6 days. Sodium sulfacetamide (Sulamyd-10%)—either the solution (two drops in the eye every 3 hours while awake) or the ointment (a small amount applied to the lower conjunctival sac four times a day and at bedtime)—is generally satisfactory. If there is an allergy to sulfa drugs, erythromycin or bacitracin ophthalmic ointment, or a topical fluoroquinolone solution, four times a day and at bedtime may be used. Topical aminoglycosides occasionally may be indicated for a specific infection, but they may cause redness, irritation, and *conjunctivitis medicamentosa.* Therefore, topical aminoglycosides should be limited and generally left to an ophthalmologist to prescribe. Also, cool compresses several times a day may provide comfort and diminish matting.

Chronic Bacterial Conjunctivitis

S. aureus causes most cases of chronic bacterial conjunctivitis, but occasionally it is caused by other agents, such as *Staphylococcus epidermidis, Moraxella lacunata, Corynebacterium diphtheriae,* or *Streptococcus pyogenes. S. aureus* colonizes the margin of the eyelid and the follicles containing the eyelashes. Both *S. aureus* and *S. epidermidis* elaborate an exotoxin that injures the conjunctiva and cornea, and this toxin is responsible for the chronic inflammation.

Patients with chronic bacterial conjunctivitis complain of a sensation of a foreign body in the eye and redness and itching; often eyelids stick together after sleep. There is often a history of recurrent styes (see below) and loss of eyelashes. Examination shows erythema of the lid margin, and sometimes a minimal exudate is present. Occasionally, mucous strands may be found in the conjunctival fornices, and the eyelids may appear thickened and red.

The lid margins, surrounding skin, conjunctiva, and cornea may be involved singly or collectively. The skin may also show changes of seborrheic dermatitis or it may be excoriated and macerated, especially at the lateral canthal margin. Crusting is noted at the bases of the eyelashes. The conjunctiva may show changes of papillary hyperplasia (multiple conjunctival mounds with a central single vessel). Corneal changes occur after months of inflammation and are manifest as fine discrete peripheral defects. There may also be ulceration, clouding, and vascularization of the margins of the cornea. The diagnosis is made by examination and, in the occasional situation of doubt, by scraping the conjunctivae and the margins of the eyelids and by culturing the exudate or by referring the patient to an ophthalmologist.

Usually, a topical fluoroquinolone or sulfacetamide, one or two drops or a small amount of ointment every 4 hours while awake, or erythromycin ointment (Ilotycin ophthalmic ointment), every 4 hours while awake, is effective. Treatment should be continued for 2 weeks. Daily cleansing of the eyelashes with a neutral soap (e.g., Johnson's Baby Shampoo) followed by the application of an antibiotic ointment (e.g., bacitracin or erythromycin) to the eyelashes four times a day for several weeks reduces the bacterial count, cleanses the lids, and minimizes recurrences.

Viral Conjunctivitis

Viral conjunctivitis, also known as acute follicular conjunctivitis, is common. It is caused by a variety of agents. The onset is abrupt and unilateral, but contralateral involvement in a day or 2 from autoinoculation is very common. Excessive tearing is often the major complaint, and there is no purulent discharge. The conjunctiva nearly always shows hyperemia, which may be diffuse or segmental (Fig. 109.11, Color Plate section). Viral conjunctivitis may be accompanied by tender preauricular lymphadenopathy. Often, the lymphoid tissue of the eyelid becomes edematous in response to the infection and may appear as elevated palpebral and bulbar conjunctival lesions. When there is doubt about the diagnosis, examination of the conjunctival scrapings shows mononuclear cells. Viral cultures are expensive but are occasionally used by ophthalmologists in special circumstances.

The disease is self-limited, lasting only a few days, and treatment is therefore supportive. Vasoconstrictive drops (two drops four times a day for a few days) containing naphazoline (e.g., over the counter agents Albalon, Naphcon-A, or Vasocon-A) are helpful in relieving conjunctival congestion and hyperemia, and cool compresses as needed also provide relief. Sulfacetamide (Sulamyd) or erythromycin (Ilotycin), as described above, may be used if symptoms have not been controlled in a few days with topical vasoconstrictive drops; in this instance bacterial conjunctivitis may have developed.

Rarely, corneal inflammation may develop and cause an opacity in the cornea. When corneal opacification is noted, an ophthalmologist should be consulted urgently because loss of vision may occur. Some types of viral conjunctivitis *(epidemic keratoconjunctivitis)* are highly contagious. The examiner should take care not to become infected or to infect other patients; all instruments should be cleansed, and thorough hand washing is critical. The family should be instructed that disease transmission is via tear droplets, so towels and washcloths should not be shared. Because epidemic keratoconjunctivitis is so contagious, one should ask the patient to stay away, for about 10 to 12 days, from school or jobs where individuals are aggregated in one space. Often referral to an ophthalmologist is appropriate if there is doubt about the diagnosis or if there is concern about the spread of the disease to others.

Inclusion Conjunctivitis (Inclusion Blennorrhea)

Inclusion conjunctivitis is common in sexually active young adults. The disease is caused by a species of *Chlamydia* and is a result of contamination of the eye from the urethra after a sexual contact.

The problem is usually characterized by the abrupt onset of ocular discomfort, with varying degrees of diffuse conjunctival hyperemia and sometimes mucopurulent discharge that may result in matting of the eyelashes. The eyelids appear swollen, and inspection of the palpebral conjunctiva, especially of the lower lid, shows many small follicles (raised pale mounds of varying size) (Fig. 109.12, Color Plate section). Occasionally, preauricular lymphadenopathy develops. Without treatment, the disease becomes chronic and remitting, and in 2 or 3 weeks a superficial corneal inflammation (keratitis) may appear. This may be identified with the naked eye as dots or cloudy streaks on the superior portion of the cornea. Also at this stage, there may be an associated iritis manifested by photophobia and blurring of vision.

This syndrome may occur in association with urethritis in men or with cervicitis and a vaginal discharge in women. Most often, however, there are no genitourinary symptoms, although *Chlamydia* species can be cultured from the urethra in men or the endocervical canal in women. The culture is time consuming and expensive, however, and infrequently done (see Chapters 37 and 102). Two highly specific and sensitive direct slide tests for the detection of *Chlamydia* (see Chapter 37) are increasingly available commercially, and these appear to be diagnostic in patients with conjunctivitis. In some cases, reactive arthritis is present (see Chapter 78).

The diagnosis is suggested by the history and appearance, but if there is doubt it may be confirmed by the direct slide test of the conjunctiva or examination of the material obtained from conjunctival scraping. This material, when stained by the laboratory with Giemsa stain, shows large basophilic cytoplasmic inclusion bodies. Gram stain does not reveal these bodies but shows many polymorphonuclear leukocytes.

Therapy is effective but must be systemic. Oral tetracycline, 250 mg four times daily for 21 days, is the preferable regimen; when tetracycline cannot be given, good results may be achieved with erythromycin, 250 mg four times a day for 21 days, or trimethoprim–sulfamethoxazole (e.g., Bactrim DS or Septra DS), 1 tablet twice a day for 21 days. It may take several months for the follicular hyperplasia to resolve, but the patient should experience symptomatic improvement within several days. The application of cool compresses for 20 minutes several times a day also provides comfort in the first few days of treatment. Because this disease is difficult to diagnose, referral to an ophthalmologist is appropriate.

Because the disease must be assumed to be sexually transmitted, the sexual partner should be similarly treated. Other venereal diseases should be sought, and a condom should be used until therapy has been completed.

Allergic Conjunctivitis

Allergic conjunctivitis is a common and mild conjunctivitis often encountered in patients with allergic rhinitis (see Chapter 30). Often the patient describes a history of allergy to grasses, pollens, and other agents and usually complains of itching and tearing. Often, there is marked swelling of the conjunctiva and slight to moderate redness of the eye, and at times there is serous crusting in the morning.

When there is doubt about the diagnosis, conjunctival scrapings (see above) may be examined. A finding of many eosinophils is diagnostic. When conjunctivitis is associated with allergic rhinitis, it usually parallels the rhinitis in severity and duration. When it occurs as an isolated problem, it is short-lived and treatment is symptomatic. An over the counter topical astringent solution (e.g., Albalon, Naphcon-A, or Vasocon-A, using one to two drops four times 1 to 2 days) and cool compresses as needed are very effective. Occasionally, symptoms are severe, and oral antihistamines may relieve itching.

Topical antihistamine solutions (e.g., Naphcon-A, over the counter) and topical mast cell stabilizers (e.g., pemirolast [Alamast], requires a prescription) both are effective therapy for chronic or seasonal allergic conjunctivitis. Also corticosteroid eye drops (e.g., HMS Liquifilm or FML Liquifilm) are very effective for this condition, but they must be used cautiously because their use is associated with corneal ulceration and perforation in the presence of herpes simplex infection, the development of fungal infection, and, when used chronically, the development in some patients of open-angle glaucoma and, rarely, cataract formation. For these reasons, topical corticosteroids are not recommended without at least a telephone consultation with an ophthalmologist.

Chemical Conjunctivitis

Many agents may enter the conjunctiva and produce inflammation. Irritation from such agents as smoke, smog, sprays, chlorinated water, hairspray, makeup, and industrial dust is common. The history of the exposure makes the diagnosis obvious. The patient should thoroughly rinse the conjunctival sac with water as soon as contamination with a chemical has occurred. The patient will also benefit from cool compresses for 15 to 20 minutes several times a day, and occasionally the use of an over the counter topical vasoconstrictor solution (Albalon, Naphcon-A, or Vasocon-A) as necessary.

Conjunctivitis medicamentosa is conjunctival injection secondary to use of eye drops, which may be irritating to the conjunctiva. This condition can occur usually after several days to weeks of instillation of almost any type of eye drop. Patients complain of redness, discomfort and tearing, or itching. Generally there is no discharge. The history of eye drop or ointment use is essential to establishing the diagnosis. Topical aminoglycosides and some antiglaucoma agents are frequent causes of conjunctivitis medicamentosa. Treatment consists of stopping the inciting agent and using artificial tears for comfort. Because either the preservative or the active ingredient of the eye drop may be the inciting agent, preservative-free artificial tears may be indicated.

In the case of an injury from an acid or alkali, serious permanent damage may occur, and this problem is a true ophthalmologic emergency. Patients should be advised to irrigate the conjunctival sac with copious amounts of water and to see an ophthalmologist immediately. If the patient presents to one's office, irrigation should be repeated promptly and the patient should then be sent immediately to an ophthalmologist. Over-irrigation may increase irritation slightly, but under-irrigation may make blindness more likely. Therefore, when in doubt, one should always irrigate. Normal saline stings less than water, but one should use whatever is immediately available.

Subconjunctival Hemorrhage

The conjunctiva is thin and transparent. Subconjunctival hemorrhage is an accumulation of blood under the conjunctiva (Fig. 109.13, Color Plate section). Acutely, a subconjunctival hemorrhage presents as a localized, usually unilateral, bright red area within the palpebral fissure. Subconjunctival hemorrhages are not painful and do not affect vision. A patient may be unaware of a subconjunctival hemorrhage until looking in the mirror or until someone else notices that one eye is bright red. Subconjunctival hemorrhages may occur spontaneously, especially in older individuals with dry eyes, but can be associated with minor eye rubbing or trauma, or with Valsalva maneuver associated with straining at stool, vomiting, coughing, or sneezing. Subconjunctival hemorrhage may occur during uncomplicated eye surgery, especially if subconjunctival injections are given at the time of surgery. Anticoagulants may be associated with subconjunctival hemorrhages, especially if doses are excessive. Uncommonly, topical corticosteroid eye drops, causing increased capillary fragility, can be a cause of subconjunctival hemorrhage.

Only rarely a subconjunctival hemorrhage may be indicative of a bleeding diathesis. Therefore, workup is generally not indicated unless there are signs of bleeding or easy bruisability elsewhere. There is no specific treatment. Artificial tears may be recommended if there is discomfort.

Pterygium

A pterygium is localized fibrovascular tissue (Fig. 109.14, Color Plate section), which is most frequently present within the interpalpebral fissure, at the three or nine o'clock position. A pterygium begins with localized conjunctival swelling and is termed a pingueculum when it does not extend onto the cornea. Once fibrovascular tissue extends onto the cornea, the lesion is called a pterygium. Occasionally, both pingueculae and pterygia can become inflamed, causing local redness. There is no discharge or change in vision. Discomfort, if present, is minimal. Both pingueculae and pterygia are caused by chronic exposure to ultraviolet light. Long-term exposure to dust and wind may also be contributory. Acute conjunctival injection may be managed with lubrication with artificial tears. Rarely are topical anti-inflammatory agents necessary. Patients believed to have pterygia or pinguecula should be referred to an ophthalmologist for evaluation and continuing care.

Polycythemia

The appearance of the conjunctiva can be suggestive of a diagnosis of polycythemia. Dilation and engorgement of the conjunctival vessels can be present in primary or secondary polycythemia.

Conjunctival Scarring

Normally, there is no scarring of the conjunctiva. Conditions characterized by conjunctival cicatrization frequently present with shortening of the inferior fornix, seen as symblepharon, bands of scar tissue between the tarsal and bulbar conjunctiva. Such scarring can follow chemical conjunctivitis or Stevens-Johnson syndrome but may be the initial manifestation of mucous membrane pemphigoid, a systemic disease occurring in the elderly (see Chapter 117).

EPISCLERA

The episclera is vascularized connective tissue deep to the conjunctiva and above the sclera. Normally, episclera vessels are barely visible without the magnification of a slit-lamp biomicroscope.

History

Patients with episcleritis complain of the sudden or gradual onset of localized redness, with mild discomfort, but no change in vision. Although most patients with episcleritis have no underlying systemic disease, approximately 25% of patients do. Of these, connective tissue disease, rheumatoid arthritis, syndromes with HLA-B27 antigen (ankylosing spondylitis, inflammatory bowel disease, reactive arthritis, and psoriatic arthritis), systemic lupus erythematosus, and polyarteritis are the most common. In the patient with inflammatory bowel disease, acute episcleritis may be a problem, which heralds a flare-up of the bowel inflammation. Patients with acne rosacea may have episcleritis. Gout is a rare cause of episcleritis.

Examination

Episcleritis is characterized by localized redness, usually of one eye. There is no discharge. Tenderness may be present, but discomfort is generally mild and pain unusual.

Episcleritis

There are two main types of episcleritis: Diffuse and nodular. Diffuse episcleritis is more common and less frequently associated with systemic disease. Nodular episcleritis is characterized by localized swelling on the surface of the eye (Fig. 109.15, Color Plate section). This form of episcleritis is usually associated with connective tissue disease and may be either an initial or a late manifestation.

Management

Patients with episcleritis generally should be referred to an ophthalmologist for confirmation of the diagnosis and to be certain that scleritis is not present (see below). Episcleritis is not vision threatening. Because episcleritis tends to be self-limited, clearing spontaneously within 7 to 10 days, treatment may not be necessary. However, because episcleritis responds well to topical corticosteroid drops, they frequently are prescribed to shorten the course of the condition. The generalist in the care of patient's with episcleritis is usually focused on the search for a systemic cause for the condition.

SCLERA

The sclera is connective tissue deep to the conjunctiva and episclera and external to the retina. The sclera, composed of interlaced collagen fibrils, is similar in structure to cartilage, begins at the periphery of the cornea (the limbus), and extends circumferentially to the optic nerve.

History

Scleritis is inflammation of the sclera, and it may be unilateral or bilateral. Scleritis characteristically causes severe pain. That pain may be interpreted by the patient as ocular, but a history of severe unilateral headache, accompanied by nausea and vomiting is not unusual. Scleritis should be considered in a patient who has headache, nausea, and vomiting, and redness of the eyes. There is no discharge, but there may be complaints of decreased vision, photophobia, and pain on eye movement.

Examination

Ocular redness in scleritis may be diffuse or localized and unilateral or bilateral (Fig. 109.16, Color Plate section). The redness is darker than the bright red color of an acute subconjunctival hemorrhage and generally darker than the redness of episcleritis. There is no discharge, but tearing may be copious. Differentiation from episcleritis can be difficult without the use of a slit-lamp biomicroscope. However, the instillation by an ophthalmologist of 2.5% phenylephrine hydrochloride ophthalmic solution can blanch vessels in most instances of episcleritis but has no effect on the redness in scleritis.

Causes of Scleritis

Approximately 75% of patients with scleritis have an associated systemic disease. Systemic causes of scleritis are similar to those of episcleritis. Rheumatoid arthritis is the most common.

Management

Because of the severity of the pain experienced by patients with scleritis, urgent referral to an ophthalmologist is indicated. However, one may play an important role in directing the diagnostic search for an underlying systemic cause and in collaborating with the ophthalmologist in the medical management of the condition. The treatment of scleritis requires the use of systemic medications. Corticosteroids, frequently in high oral or intravenous doses, are the initial therapeutic choice. But for patients either unresponsive to high dose corticosteroids (doses greater than 60 to 80 mg/day of prednisone) or in whom high dose corticosteroids are contraindicated, oral Cytoxan is frequently necessary. Treatment of scleritis is aimed at control of pain and cessation of tissue destruction, and weeks or months of therapy may be necessary to control the disease. An ophthalmologist should be consulted urgently to confirm the diagnosis and help in the management.

CORNEA

The cornea is clear, compact, and highly innervated.

History

Corneal disease causes decreased vision, pain, foreign body sensation, and redness.

Acute Problems: Corneal Abrasion, Foreign Body, Ulcer, and Edema

If the symptoms are acute, the differential diagnosis includes corneal abrasions, corneal foreign bodies, and corneal ulceration. *Corneal injury* is usually recognized easily because of intense pain localized to the cornea after an injury and because of identification of a corneal lesion. If the injury is secondary to minor trauma (corneal abrasion) from a foreign body, the foreign body should be removed and a patch placed over the eye for 24 hours; the use of a topical antiprostaglandin agent without patching is also considered an acceptable treatment (see below). On the other hand, if an extensive epithelial defect (as revealed by fluorescein staining, see below) is present, urgent ophthalmologic referral is indicated.

Fluorescein staining is easily accomplished by moistening a sterile fluorescein strip in the lower conjunctival sac and waiting a moment for the fluorescein to diffuse into the tears. The epithelial defect stains a brilliant green. A penlight with a cobalt blue filter (e.g., Blu-Spot no. 2015, available from medical supply companies) is inexpensive and highlights fluorescein staining. Corneal ulcers also stain with fluorescein, but staining appears to be deeper, indicating subepithelial corneal involvement. Corneal ulceration can lead to blindness, and patients suspected of having this condition should see an ophthalmologist emergently.

Patients with *corneal abrasions* most often will provide a history of trauma. That trauma may be relatively minor, such as eye rubbing, or may be more severe, with a history of a scratch by a sharp object. Frequently, patients with corneal abrasions have difficulty keeping their eyes open and, in addition to redness of the involved eye, have copious tearing.

With *corneal foreign body* there is a history of the sudden onset of severe sensation of an object in the eye, accompanied by tearing, redness, and blurred vision. There is often a history of working with tools, especially those that are power driven, but there may be a history of exposure to wind or a dusty environment.

Foreign bodies often lodge in the conjunctiva or cornea. Most often they can be visualized with the naked eye; if not, sterile fluorescein staining (see above) may outline an area of corneal epithelial damage. Foreign bodies may be removed by irrigation of the conjunctival sac with a sterile solution of physiologic saline or eyewash. If they are not rinsed away, mechanical removal is indicated. This may be accomplished, when the object is in the cornea, by placing in the eye a drop of topical anesthetic (e.g., Ophthaine) and removing the foreign body with a sterile needle held carefully with the arm braced. A cotton swab should *not* be used to remove a foreign body from the cornea because often it is irritating to the structure and thus delays healing. Most generalists are reluctant to use a needle; therefore, most patients with corneal foreign bodies are referred. If the foreign body is not on the cornea, removal is easier and usually does not require anesthesia. After removal, it is wise to instill a drop of antibiotic (e.g., sulfacetamide 10% or bacitracin) and cover the eye with a patch for 24 hours. The eye patch should be applied tightly enough to prevent the eyelids from moving. If the patch falls off before the 24-hour period is up, the patient should not try to reapply it because often this may cause more irritation. Recently, ophthalmologists have begun using patching for corneal abrasions less often so that the patient can still see with the injured eye. When the eye is not patched, a topical antiprostaglandin, such as diclofenac or ketorolac, may be used for a day or 2 for comfort.

If the offending material is a piece of metal, rust rings surrounding the area of the epithelial defect may be observed. These rings are not harmful, and only the foreign body should be removed. In any instance when the foreign body is not easily removed or if symptoms persist beyond a day after removal of a foreign body, an ophthalmologist should see the patient urgently.

With *corneal ulcer,* often the patient who uses contact lenses will complain of the sudden onset of pain, redness, and discharge.

Corneal edema when acute is associated with blurred vision and conjunctival redness, sometimes associated with nausea and vomiting. This is usually caused by sudden and marked elevation of intraocular pressure. The edema is secondary to the aqueous humor being forced into the cornea. Angle-closure glaucoma is the usual cause; therefore, a positive family history, a past history of haloes around lights, and the presence of hyperopia or farsightedness often are present (see Chapter 108).

Examination

The cornea is normally crystal clear. Hand light examination can demonstrate irregularity of the corneal surface and may show a foreign body, corneal opacity, or corneal edema.

Chronic Problems

When there is a chronic history of blurred vision not accompanied by pain and associated with decreased corneal clarity, on examination there may be chronic corneal edema present.

Management

Corneal problems of any type should be referred to an ophthalmologist.

ANTERIOR CHAMBER

The anterior chamber is the optically clear space between the cornea and the iris.

History

Patients with anterior chamber inflammation complain of pain, redness, and sensitivity to light.

Symptoms may be acute. If there is a history of blunt trauma, bleeding into the anterior chamber (hyphema) or traumatic iritis should be suspected.

Examination

One should look for the depth and clarity of the anterior chamber.

Acute Iritis

Acute iritis presents with pain, photophobia, and redness. Although acute iritis may arise spontaneously, blunt trauma to the eye can cause iritis (traumatic iritis). There is no discharge, but vision may be blurred. The redness in acute iritis is diffuse. Slit-lamp biomicroscopy is necessary to fully evaluate the amount of anterior segment inflammation. Patients suspected of having acute iritis should be urgently referred to an ophthalmologist for diagnosis and management.

Hyphema

A hyphema is the accumulation of blood in the anterior chamber of the eye. A hyphema, if large enough, can be seen with room illumination or with a flashlight. Hyphemas are most often preceded by blunt trauma directly to the eye but can occur without trauma in rare patients with a bleeding disorder.

Hypopyon

A hypopyon is the accumulation of white blood cells in the anterior chamber of the eye. Corneal ulceration (see above) is the most common cause of hypopyon. Patients complain of severe pain, redness, decreased vision, and discharge. Other causes of hypopyon include endophthalmitis and severe iritis (see above).

Management

Patients suspected of having anterior chamber disorders should be referred emergently to an ophthalmologist.

THE RED EYE

A complaint by a patient of a red eye is common in an ambulatory practice. Many of the conditions discussed in this chapter can cause redness of the eye. A red eye is usually caused by an infection and most often is self-limited; however, there are serious considerations in the differential diagnosis of this infection that must be recognized so that an urgent ophthalmologic consultation can be obtained. *Hyperacute conjunctivitis, keratitis* (corneal inflammation), *iritis* or *uveitis* (inflammation of the uveal tract), *scleritis,* and *acute glaucoma* are important vision-threatening conditions that cause a red eye; patients suspected of having one of these conditions should be referred to an ophthalmologist (Table 109.2).

Table 109.2. Major Causes of a Red Eye

Conditions that require referral to an ophthalmologist
Acute glaucoma
Acute iritis
Acute corneal tear or infection (keratitis)
Acute scleritis or episcleritis
Bacterial conjunctivitis (hyperacute)
Conditions that usually can be managed by a generalist
Bacterial conjunctivitis (acute and chronic)
Viral conjunctivitis
Inclusion conjunctivitis
Allergic conjunctivitis
Chemical conjunctivitis
Foreign body
Subconjunctival hemorrhage

Several important features of the history and physical examination (Table 109.3) may suggest a specific diagnosis. The patient should be asked specifically whether treatment for an ocular disorder has been given, whether pain in one or both eyes has been experienced, and whether there is visual loss or photophobia (light sensitivity). When the eyes are examined, it is essential to evaluate the following features: Visual acuity, the nature of the discharge, the appearance of the cornea, the size and reactivity of the pupil, and the extent of the redness. When evaluating the extent of redness, an attempt should be made to determine whether there is simply conjunctival injection or whether there is ciliary injection as well. The ciliary vessels run in the sclera beneath the conjunctiva. Ciliary injection usually causes a purplish or violaceous zone of injection around the cornea. Unlike the conjunctival vessels, ciliary vessels do not constrict after the administration of a weak solution of a mydriatic such as 2.5% phenylephrine (Neo-Synephrine). The conjunctival vessels move with the conjunctiva when the conjunctiva is touched with a cotton swab. Ciliary vessels do not. Glaucoma, keratitis, and scleritis are characterized in most cases by ciliary injection. In selected patients special assessments, such as measurement of ocular tension or inspection of the eye after fluorescein staining, are necessary to establish a diagnosis.

Before making the decision to treat a patient without obtaining ophthalmology consultation, one should answer the following questions:

- Has a thorough ocular examination been performed?
- Is impaired vision present and, if so, has an explanation been identified?
- Is the natural history of the condition known or is the usual response to treatment known?
- Has the appropriate follow-up arrangement been made to confirm that the condition is self-limited and improving?

Conjunctival infections, allergies, eyelid inflammation, and irritation are the most common causes of red or irritated eyes, as discussed in detail above. Most

Table 109.3. Important Observations in Evaluation of a Patient with a Red Eye

	Glaucoma	Iritis	Corneal Injury	Scleritis	Episcleritis	Bacterial Conjunctivitis	Inclusion Conjunctivitis	Viral Conjunctivitis	Keratitis	Allergic Conjunctivitis
History of previous ocular disorder or condition predisposing to an ocular disorder	+/−	+/−	−	+	−	−	−	−	Often	Previous history of allergies
Pain[a]	+	+	+	+	+	Mild discomfort or burning	Mild discomfort or burning	Mild discomfort or burning	+	−
Visual acuity	Diminished and blurred	Blurred	Usually diminished	Normal	Normal	Normal	Occasionally blurred, if chronic	Normal	Diminished	Usually normal
Discharge	None	None	Usually none	None	None	Present: thick or thin	None or mucopurulent	Watery	Usually some	Mild or none
Appearance of cornea	May be hazy	Normal	May be streaky	Normal	Normal	Normal	Normal except if late when superior dots or streaking may be seen	Normal	Corneal opacity	Normal
Pupil	Often dilated, mid-dilated, or fixed	Small and different from opposite side	Normal	Normal	Normal	Normal	Normal	Normal	Normal	Normal
Redness	Around cornea	Around cornea	Localized or diffuse	Localized or diffuse	Localized	Diffuse	Diffuse (variable)	Segmental or diffuse	Around cornea	Diffuse
Selected evaluations	Ocular pressure[b] in eye is high (see Chapter 108)	Normal	Fluorescein stain[c] shows epithelial defect as brilliant green	A drop of phenylephrine 2½% on the conjunctiva will constrict superficial but not deep vessels (see the text)	None	None	None	None	A diagnostic scraping may be performed by an ophthalmologist	None

[a]Photophobia in addition to pain may be seen in varying degrees with nearly any of these conditions, but its presence is neither universal nor diagnostic.

[b]Should not be measured if a discharge is present or a corneal ulceration is seen.

[c]Use individually packaged sterile fluorescein strips.

patients with these problems can be managed without consulting an ophthalmologist.

General References

Fraundelder FT, Roy FH, eds. Current ocular therapy. 5th ed. Philadelphia: WB Saunders, 2000.
A valuable compendium.

Lebowitz HM. Primary care: the red eye. N Engl J Med 2000;343:345.
A well-referenced and easily accessible review.

Vaughan D, Asbury T, Riordan-Eva P, eds. General ophthalmology. 15th ed. Stamford, CT: Appleton & Lange, 1999.
A classic text.

Specific References

1. Pavan-Langston D. Viral disease of the cornea and external eye. In: Albert DM, Jakobiec FA, eds. Principles and practice of ophthalmology. 2nd ed. Philadelphia, WB Saunders, 2000:846.
2. Womack L, Liesegant T. Complications of herpes zoster ophthalmicus. Arch Ophthalmol 1983;101:42.

SECTION 16

Selected Problems of the Ears, Nose, Throat and Oral Cavity

CHAPTER 110

Hearing Loss and Associated Problems

JOHN K. NIPARKO, MD
HOWARD W. FRANCIS, MD

In the United States, an estimated one in nine people develops a permanent hearing impairment that diminishes the ability to carry out everyday communication. Hearing loss is especially common in the elderly, who account for 40% of the hearing impaired but only 13% of the population. In fact, the only chronic disorders that are more prevalent are hypertension and arthritis. Many causes of hearing impairment are preventable. Early detection and intervention can often ameliorate an acquired hearing impairment.

When evaluating a patient with hearing loss, the diagnostic strategy should determine the mechanism of loss (conductive or sensorineural), the likely cause, and the need for referral to an otolaryngologist for further evaluation. This chapter includes a brief review of the anatomy and physiology of the auditory system that will help in understanding auditory pathology and details strategies of diagnosis and early treatment.

EAR STRUCTURE AND FUNCTION

The *external ear* (Fig. 110.1) is composed of the auricle, the auditory meatus, and the external ear canal. The outer portion of the canal is cartilaginous and is covered by thick skin that contains hair follicles and the cerumen-secreting glands; cerumen protects the epithelium and captures foreign particles entering the canal. The inner portion of the canal is bony and is covered by squamous epithelium without hair follicles or cerumen glands.

The *middle ear* (Fig. 110.1) consists of the tympanic membrane, the air space behind it, and the three linked ossicles: the malleus, incus, and stapes. The malleus is attached to the tympanic membrane and is linked to the stapes by the incus. The stapes makes contact with the inner ear via the stapes footplate at the oval window. The middle ear is lined with a mucus-secreting epithelium similar to that which lines the nose. The middle ear communicates with the nasopharynx via the eustachian tube and posteriorly with the mastoid air cells. Intermittent opening of the eustachian tube ensures equal pressure on either side of the tympanic membrane, which facilitates the transmission of sound from the tympanic membrane to the oval window.

The *inner ear* (Fig. 110.1) lies within the temporal bone of the lateral skull base and is encased in the compact otic capsule and is fluid filled. It consists of sensory organs for hearing (*cochlea*) and balance (*vestibular labyrinth*). Nerves from the cochlea and vestibular labyrinth unite to form the eighth cranial nerve.

Cranial nerve VII (facial) traverses the temporal bone in close association with the middle and inner ear structures. For this reason, facial muscle paresis and paresthesias of the anterior two-thirds of the tongue and soft palate may manifest from pathologic processes of the middle and inner ear.

Sound is funneled through the auricle into the external ear canal, vibrating the tympanic membrane; the vibration is transferred across the ossicular chain. The large surface area of the vibrating tympanic membrane and the lever action of the ossicles improve sound transmission to the inner ear, where vibrations of the stapes footplate create a fluid wave in the cochlea. This wave stimulates the hair cells that translate vibratory energy into action potentials that trigger auditory neurons.

DETERMINING SEVERITY AND MECHANISM OF HEARING LOSS

Regardless of the specific cause of hearing loss, the approximate severity of the impairment and the probable cause can often be determined in the office. This determination can be made from a combination of the history, the patient's ability to hear the spoken voice, and testing with a tuning fork.

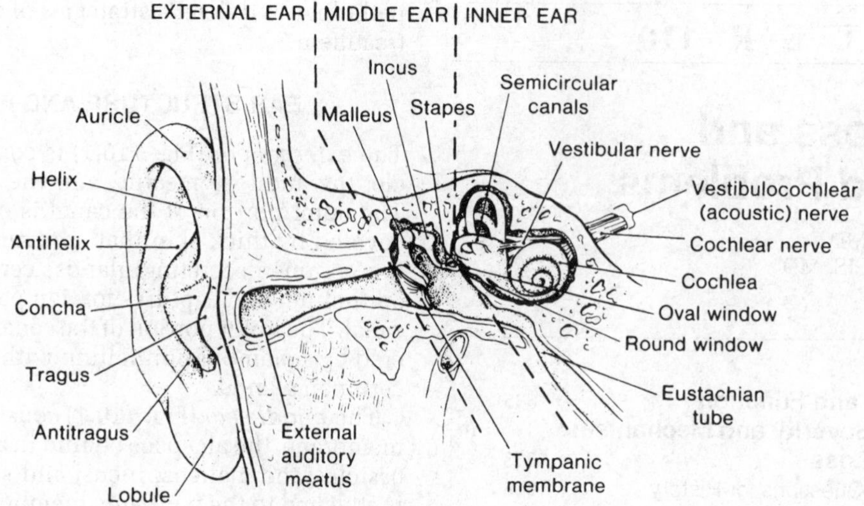

Figure 110.1. Normal structures of the ear.

Table 110.1. A Practical Method for Approximating the Severity of Hearing Loss in the Office

Severity of Hearing Loss	Social Difficulty	Office Voice Test	Pure-Tone Audiogram
Normal hearing	None	18 ft or more using normal voice	No loss over 10 dB
Slight hearing loss	Long-distance speech	Not over 12 ft using normal voice	10–30 dB loss
Moderate hearing loss	Short-distance speech	Not over 3 ft using normal voice	Up to 60 dB loss
Severe hearing loss	All unamplified voices	Raised voice at meatus	Over 60 dB loss
Profound hearing loss	Voices never heard	All speech and sound	Over 90 dB loss

Adapted from Mawson SP. Disease of the ear. Baltimore: Williams & Wilkins, 1974, with permission.

Suggested Questions for History

To help establish a differential diagnosis for the possible causes of hearing loss, the following information should be acquired:

- Is one ear involved or both? Is speech better understood on the telephone in one ear compared with the other?
- Was the onset of hearing loss abrupt or gradual? Has it progressed rapidly? Has hearing acuity fluctuated?
- Does the patient have associated tinnitus, vertigo, otalgia, otorrhea, or facial weakness?
- Is there a family history of hearing loss?
- Has the patient a history of noise exposure?
- Are there related causes of hearing loss such as syphilis, diabetes mellitus, hypothyroidism, head trauma, or autoimmune disease?
- Has the patient been exposed to ototoxic agents such as aminoglycosides, diuretics, aspirin, or chemotherapeutic agents?

Evaluating the Severity and Range of Hearing Impairment

A practical method for evaluating the *severity of hearing impairment* includes a historical estimate of speech recognition impairment in noisy settings and an assessment of response to voice testing in the office; these two findings can be equated with various levels of abnormality in the audiogram (Table 110.1). *Slight* impairment indicates difficulty in hearing distant speech in noise (e.g., group meetings, social gatherings, or the theater). *Moderate impairment* includes some difficulty with short-distance speech and conversation. *Severe impairment* indicates no understanding of the conversational voice but understanding of the amplified voice. Amplification may be achieved by raising the voice or electronically by use of a hearing aid (see below). *Profound* (or total) impairment indicates inability to hear and understand the spoken voice despite maximal amplification. This also may be summarized by recalling that a soft whisper is about 25 decibels (dB), a moderate whisper is about 40 dB, and conversational speech is about 60 dB. In the office, ambient sound can markedly affect the ability of a patient with hearing impairment to respond to this cursory assessment of audition. Therefore, as quiet an environment as possible is advised.

In the patient with significant hearing impairment, the *frequency range* can be approximated in the office by testing recognition of words containing the sound "ah" (low frequency, vowel sound), such as *apple, hot dog,* and *airplane,* and the sound "s" (high frequency, consonant), such as *ice cream, stairway, baseball,* and *sunset,* when these words are spoken in a medium voice about 2 feet behind the test ear, with the opposite ear covered.

Physical Findings

Otoscopy

Assessment of the External Canal and Tympanic Membrane. Complete inspection of the external ear canal and drum requires pulling the pinna in a posterosuperior direction to align the membranous and bony portions of the canal. The entire drum should be inspected (Fig. 110.2), particularly the posterosuperior aspect, where chronic inflammatory changes often occur. Cerumen accumulation in this region of the drum is unusual and may suggest an underlying problem (Fig. 110.3).

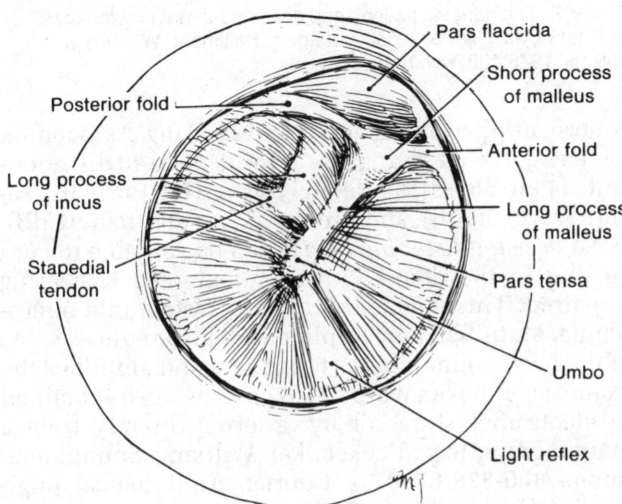

Figure 110.2. Right tympanic membrane, showing important landmarks.

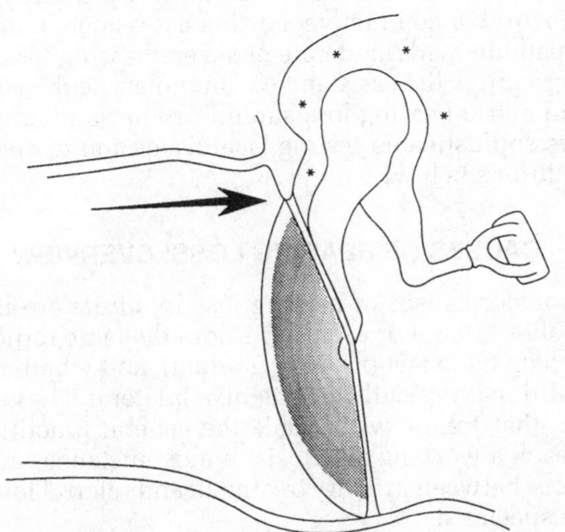

Figure 110.3. Cross-sectional drawing of middle ear depicted in Fig. 110.1. *Arrow* indicates the region of the tympanic membrane that may develop a retraction. Retraction pockets may accumulate desquamated debris and extend into regions of the epitympanum depicted by asterisks.

Membrane Mobility. During the otoscopic examination, it is important to assess tympanic membrane mobility with air insufflation. To do this, the examiner must seal the otoscope speculum tip with the ear canal. The absence of mobility suggests a pathologic condition such as negative pressure consequent to eustachian tube dysfunction, middle ear fluid, or a mass.

Preliminary Hearing Testing

Tuning Fork Tests

The mechanism of hearing loss can be classified as conductive or sensorineural through use of a 512-Hz tuning fork. Conductive losses result from external or middle ear disease, whereas sensorineural losses are caused by an inner ear or auditory neuronal problem.

Weber Test. For the Weber test, the tuning fork is held against a spot in the midline of the forehead and the patient is asked in which ear it sounds louder (Table 110.2). A unilateral conductive hearing loss with normal bilateral inner ear function produces a louder sound in the affected ear. A unilateral sensorineural hearing loss produces a louder sound in the normal ear.

Rinne Test. In the Rinne test, the vibrating tuning fork stem is placed against the mastoid bone and held in place until it becomes no longer audible and then it is held about an inch away from the external meatus (Table 110.2). The Rinne test can differentiate conductive from sensorineural hearing losses. Air conduction is perceived longer than bone conduction with normal hearing and with sensorineural hearing loss, whereas the reverse is true for conductive losses.

Speech Recognition Testing

In patients with sensorineural hearing loss, impaired understanding of speech may differentiate cochlear and neural (retrocochlear) deficits. In the latter condition, patients generally have a greater reduction of speech discrimination than do those who have cochlear disorders. Recruitment, a sense of ear discomfort

Table 110.2. Classification of Probable Mechanism of Hearing Loss Using Tuning Fork Tests

Classification	Rinne Test	Weber Test
Normal hearing		
Both ears	AC > BC	Midline
Conductive loss[a]		
Right ear	Right ear: BC > AC Left ear: AC > BC	Lateralized to right ear
Left ear	Right ear: AC > BC Left ear: BC > AC	Lateralized to left ear
Both ears	Right ear: BC > AC Left ear: BC > AC	Lateralized to poorer ear
Sensorineural loss		
Right ear	AC > BC bilaterally	Lateralized to left ear
Left ear	AC > BC bilaterally	Lateralized to right ear
Both ears	AC > BC bilaterally	Lateralized to better ear

[a]Because sound transmission by air is much more efficient than by bone, air conduction may remain greater than bone conduction in early or minimal conductive hearing loss.

AC, air conduction; BC, bone conduction.

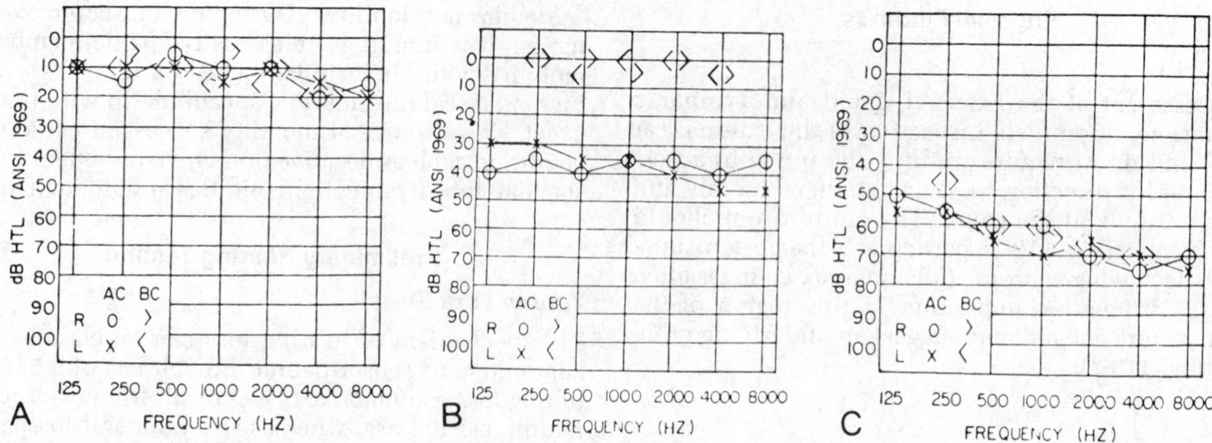

Figure 110.4. Examples of audiograms. **A:** Audiogram in a person with normal hearing. **B:** Bilateral conductive hearing loss (moderate). **C:** Bilateral sensorineural hearing loss (severe). (From Price L, Snider R. The geriatric patient: ear, nose and throat problems. In: Reichel W, ed. Clinical aspects of aging. Baltimore: Williams & Wilkins, 1978:489, with permission.)

with sudden increments in the loudness of a sound, is characteristic of cochlear dysfunction.

Audiometry

Whereas the office examination can only approximate the loss, audiometric evaluation establishes the precise level of hearing loss. Pure tone air conduction and bone conduction measurements are made for sounds of varying intensity (decibels) and frequency. Results are plotted on a graph called an audiogram in which the vertical axis shows the sounds heard in decibels and the horizontal axis shows the frequency of the stimulus in Hertz. Examples of audiograms showing normal hearing, conductive hearing loss, and sensorineural hearing loss are reproduced in Fig. 110.4. Speech audiometry measures the subject's ability to hear and understand the spoken word.

Audiometry is performed by audiologists, some of whom have their offices in association with an otolaryngologist. Many, however, are independent. Patients can be referred directly to an audiologist. The location of an accredited audiologist can be obtained by telephoning the action line of the American Speech-Language and Hearing Association at 800-638-8255 or www.ASHA.org.

An audiogram is easily accomplished when proper testing facilities are available. The patient is comfortably seated in a soundproof room and is asked to record the sounds heard. A series of pure tones are presented to the patient. The procedure takes only about 20 to 30 minutes.

Small hand-held audioscopes, costing about $500, are available for use in the office. These are useful as a rough screen of hearing impairment. Usually, four pure tones are emitted in sequence. Because of masking effects, background noise can adversely affect a patient's ability to respond to test signals and the examining room must be quiet.

The lowest audible intensity for normal ears is approximately 10 to 20 dB (Fig. 110.4). Conversational speech is typically delivered at 45 to 55 dB. The American Speech-Language and Hearing Association has categorized hearing loss as mild (26 to 40 dB), moderate (41 to 55 dB), moderately severe (56 to 70 dB), severe (71 to 90 dB), and profound (greater than 91 dB).

An *assisted listening device* can be valuable in conversing in the office with a patient who is hearing impaired. This device is simply a system of a microphone, amplifier, and earphones. It also reduces some of the background noise in the room and amplifies the examiner's spoken word. Such devices can be obtained in electronics stores or by ordering directly from a manufacturer (e.g., Pocketalker, Williams Sound, telephone 800-328-6190; or Chorus, Audiological Engineering Corp., 800-283-4601).

After this initial evaluation, the presence or absence of hearing loss should be established. If there is hearing loss, it should be determined whether it is primarily unilateral or bilateral and whether it is primarily sensorineural or conductive. Further assessment and care for patients with moderate or severe hearing loss usually requires the assistance of an otolaryngologist. An asymmetric hearing loss should prompt a referral for more sophisticated testing (see discussion of specific conditions below).

CAUSES OF HEARING LOSS: OVERVIEW

The major causes of hearing loss in adults are listed in Table 110.3. For each condition, the table indicates mechanism, onset (rapid or gradual), and whether the condition is typically unilateral or bilateral. The guidelines that follow will enable the general practitioner to reach a working diagnosis in most instances and to choose between primary treatment and referral for care by a specialist.

Conditions of the External Ear

Cerumen Impaction

The patient usually complains of intermittent fullness and hearing impairment on the affected side and

Table 110.3. Causes of Hearing Loss in Adults

Causes	Mechanism	Onset Rapid (Hours to Days) or Gradual (Months to Years)	Bilateral or Unilateral
External auditory canal			
Cerumen impaction	C	Either	Usually unilateral
Foreign body	C	Rapid	Unilateral
Otitis externa	C	Rapid	Unilateral
New growth	C	Gradual	Unilateral
Middle ear			
Serous otitis media	C	Either	Either
Acute otitis media	C	Rapid	Unilateral
Barotrauma	C or SN	Rapid	Unilateral
Traumatic perforation of tympanic membrane	C	Rapid	Unilateral
Chronic otitis media	C	Gradual	Unilateral
Cholesteatoma	C or SN	Gradual	Either
Ossicular chain problem			
Adhesive otitis media	C	Gradual	Unilateral
Tympanosclerosis	C	Gradual	Either
Traumatic injury	C or SN	Rapid	Unilateral
Otosclerosis	C and/or SN	Gradual	Bilateral
New growths	C or SN	Gradual	Unilateral
Inner ear			
Presbycusis	SN	Gradual	Bilateral
Acoustic trauma	SN	Gradual	Bilateral
Drug-induced	SN	Either	Bilateral
Ménière syndrome	SN	Rapid	Usually unilateral
Central nervous system infection			
Meningitis	SN	Rapid	Either
Syphilis	SN	Either	Either
Tuberculosis	SN	Either	Either
Acoustic neuroma	SN	Gradual	Unilateral
Mumps	SN	Rapid	Unilateral
Atraumatic sudden sensorineural hearing loss	SN	Rapid	Unilateral

C, conductive; SN, sensorineural.

may give a history of episodes. These symptoms may increase after showering or swimming, as moisture occludes the ear canal, or with cotton-tipped swab use. Diagnosis is made by otoscopy.

Several precautions should be kept in mind in considering cerumen removal. An only hearing ear, a postsurgical ear, and an ear that is prone to infection should not be irrigated. If the cerumen appears to be soft, it may be removed by irrigation with use of a rubber-bulb syringe and warm tap water, directing the water upward and backward against the wall of the canal. If painful, irrigation should be discontinued and the patient referred to an otolaryngologist. If the cerumen is impacted and difficult to remove, a few drops of hydrogen peroxide (or carbamide peroxide, Debrox) should be instilled twice daily for 1 week before irrigation. Alternatively, a ceruminolytic agent (Cerumenex) may be used. In general, ceruminolytic agents should be used only in the office because casual use by the patient at home increases the risk of allergic dermatitis. With the patient's head tilted laterally at 45-degree angle, the ear is filled with ceruminolytic drops. A cotton plug is inserted for 15 to 20 minutes; the ear is then irrigated with lukewarm water and a soft rubber syringe. After irrigation, the tympanic membrane usually shows some injection around the handle of the malleus. Hearing impairment should be relieved after removal of cerumen. The occasional patient with an impaction may not respond to the usual measures described above and should be referred to an otolaryngologist.

An impaction often follows vigorous efforts by the patient to remove wax with a cotton-tipped swab. The patient should be reminded that ear wax is secreted to protect the lining of the canal and that the swab should be used only to remove cerumen in the outer portion of the canal, for cosmetic purposes. Recurrent impactions are often caused by eczema of the skin of the external ear canal and may require regular irrigation and possibly topical therapy of the skin condition (see below).

Foreign Body

Foreign bodies in the ear canal are most often the result of accidental insertion or entrance of an insect, which is followed by fullness and hearing impairment. Foreign bodies can be removed by the use of alligator forceps or a wax spoon. Removal by irrigation should be avoided if the foreign body is a vegetable, as water causes further swelling. Insects should first be killed by instillation of mineral oil. Hearing impairment resolves promptly after removal of a foreign body. Great care must be taken to avoid damage to the eardrum, especially in children and patients in whom the foreign body is deeply imbedded. In difficult extractions, an otolaryngologist may suggest anesthesia, either local injection or general.

Otitis Externa (Swimmer's Ear)

Otitis externa is most common in the summer, when heat and moisture promote swelling and maceration of the stratum corneum of the skin. In the external canal, this process may at first cause pruritus. The patient may give a history of having scratched the ear for a few days before the onset of drainage and pain. The pain is aggravated by movement of the external ear and jaw motion. Hearing impairment occurs in patients with swelling or debris that occludes the canal. The characteristics of the skin of the canal and of the exudate may provide adequate clues to the cause, and cultures are needed only for patients who do not respond promptly to topical treatment. Copious or greenish exudate suggests *Pseudomonas aeruginosa,* the bacteria most often seen in otitis externa. Yellow crusting in the midst of a purulent exudate suggests *Staphylococcus aureus.* Canal skin that is scaling, cracked, and weeping indicates *secondary eczema.* Fluffy material resembling bread mold, varying in color from white to black, suggests a *fungal agent* (*Aspergillus* or *Candida*).

There are three general principles of treatment for all types of otitis externa: removal of all infected debris (with a suction cannula if available), acidification of the canal, and instillation of an appropriate topical antimicrobial (see below). Lavage with hydrogen peroxide, commonly done in the past, is not recommended because it may be irritating to the inflamed and sensitive tissues and it is not adequately cidal to microbes.

For *bacterial infections* the patient should instill an antimicrobial–corticosteroid preparation (e.g., Cortisporin Otic Suspension, containing polymyxin B–neomycin–hydrocortisone, three or four drops three to four times daily for 5 to 7 days). Alternative topical antimicrobial agents include ofloxacin otic solution (Daiichi) and ciprofloxacin hydrochloride with hydrocortisone (Bayer). Gentle daily irrigation of the canal by the patient with a solution of acetic acid (50:50 white vinegar in sterile water) either alone or with steroids has the dual benefit of debriding infected material and acidifying the canal.

For *fungal infections,* the canal should be thoroughly cleaned out and lightly dusted with sulfanilamide powder. A dispenser containing sulfanilamide powder for this use can be obtained from any pharmacy. The fungal infection usually resolves after a single dusting with this powder. Clotrimazole (Lotrimin) 1% solution, three drops twice a day for 14 days, is an effective alternative. Daily irrigations with an acetic acid preparation also provide benefit. Topical steroid creams may be needed if excessive desquamation is present.

For *eczema* without superimposed infection, a topical *steroid cream* is applied daily for 14 days (e.g., triamcinolone 0.1%). If satisfactory control has been achieved with the steroid, then chronic symptoms, which are very common, may be controlled by weekly and, eventually, monthly applications.

In some patients, the canal may be so swollen that topical medication does not enter the canal adequately. In this case, a cylindrical cotton wick (or a commercially available sponge wick, such as Oto-wick) should be inserted by gentle twisting into the canal until only the end is visible. The patient may then apply several drops of the medication to the wick three to four times daily, and the wick will carry it into the canal. The wick can usually be removed after 48 to 72 hours, and treatment can be continued as stated above.

Most episodes of otitis externa resolve completely after 5 to 7 days, and it is important to terminate topical treatment at this time. Topical medicines alter the canal environment, and persistent treatment often leads to atopic or chemical dermatitis or fungal colonization. As a precaution against overtreatment, the prescription for eardrops should be nonrefillable, and only a small amount (10 mL) should be dispensed.

During treatment of otitis externa, moisture must be kept from entering the ear canal. During bathing, the ear should be plugged with cotton impregnated with petroleum jelly. To prevent recurrence, the patient should be warned against the future use of cotton-tipped swabs or other objects in the ear. Hearing impairment caused by otitis externa should resolve promptly when swelling recedes.

In two situations, the patient with otitis externa requires prompt referral to an otolaryngologist: patients whose findings suggest *mastoiditis* (slow response of the otitis externa to treatment and tenderness over the mastoid process) and patients whose findings suggest *malignant otitis externa,* usually diabetic or immunologically impaired patients. Malignant otitis externa is an osteitis of the bone underlying the external auditory canal, caused by *Pseudomonas.* The distinguishing features are fever, excruciating pain, and the presence of friable reddish granulation tissue that fills a breach in the canal epithelium. Because of the propensity for rapid spread to contiguous structures, this condition is an emergency, requiring hospital admission for debridement and intravenous antibiotics.

New Growth

Malignancies of auricular and periauricular skin are both common and notoriously difficult to control (1,2), and any suspicion of a new growth should prompt urgent referral to an otolaryngologist. Cutaneous malignancies that commonly occur in these sites are *basal cell carcinomas* and *squamous cell carcinomas.* Moreover, multiple tissue planes and the topography of this region can confound cure (Fig. 110.5). If diagnosed late, cutaneous malignancies of the auricle, preauricular region, and external auditory canal often extend along embryologic planes to involve deep structures such as the parotid gland and may erode into the mastoid cortex en route to the skull base. The morbidity and mortality associated with such extensions underscore the importance of early complete initial removal of malignancies in this region. Malignancies of the external auditory canal commonly present with a history of chronic otitis externa, the prolonged treatment of which results in delayed diagnosis and treatment. Early referral of patients with suspicious ear lesions and refractory otitis externa is recommended.

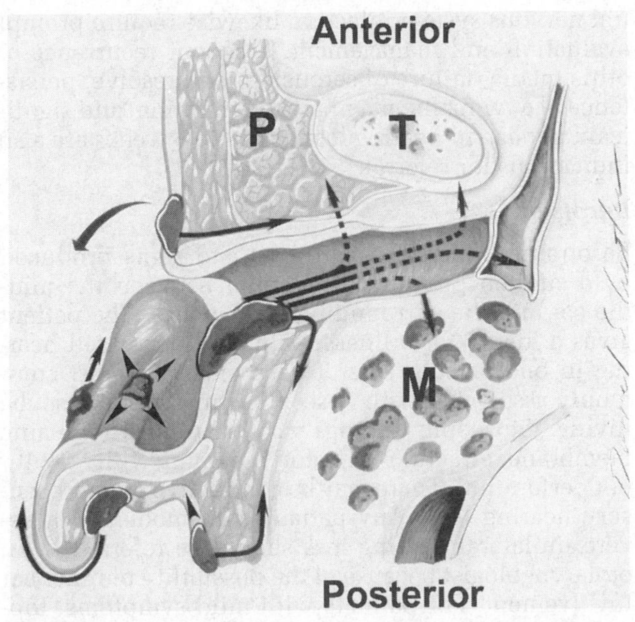

A

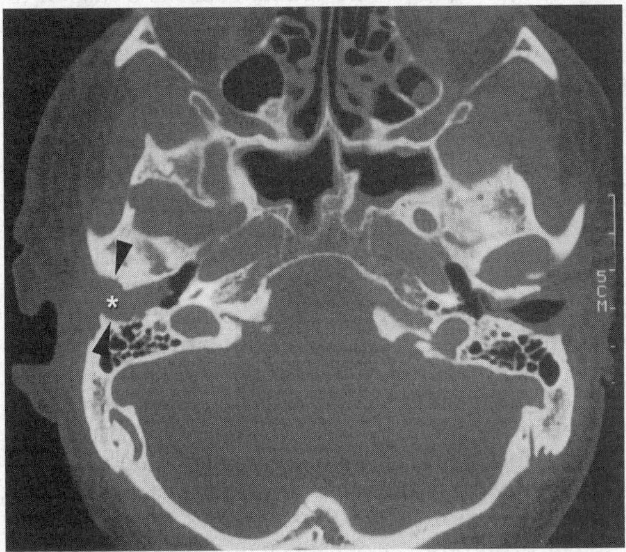

B

Figure 110.5. Cutaneous malignancies of the ear. **A:** Axial cross-sectional drawing of ear and temporal bone indicating potential paths of spread of cutaneous malignancies originating on the auricle, the preauricular region, and external auditory canal. *M,* mastoid; *P,* parotid gland; *T,* temporomandibular joint. **B:** Axial computed tomography of head, indicating soft tissue obliteration of the right ear canal (∗) and erosion of its bony walls (*arrowheads*).

Conditions of the Middle Ear

Conductive hearing loss is produced by conditions of the middle ear, tympanic membrane, and external ear canal. Most commonly, however, conductive hearing loss results from interference with the sound transformer mechanism of the tympanic membrane and middle ear ossicles. In addition to the history, the middle ear assessment includes otoscopic inspection for signs of acute inflammation (erythema, discharge, or bulging of the tympanic membrane), changes in the tympanic membrane not caused by acute inflammation (retraction, scarring, distortion of normal structures, perforation), cholesteatoma (squamous debris accumulation within the middle ear), and evidence of reduced middle ear aeration as indicated by diminished movement of the drum on pneumatic insufflation.

Serous Otitis Media

The patient usually complains of fullness and decreased hearing in one or both ears with minimal or no pain. There is often a history of recent viral upper respiratory infection, exacerbation of allergic or vasomotor rhinitis, or prior acute otitis media. Rarely, serous otitis media may be caused by nasopharyngeal carcinoma, and this possibility must be ruled out in adults with a new onset of serous otitis that does not resolve after appropriate management (see below). There is otoscopic evidence of eustachian tube closure and retraction of the tympanic membrane, failure of the membrane to move on pneumatic otoscopy (a crude test of eustachian tube patency, but not always abnormal in serous otitis), or a visible air–fluid level behind the membrane. Usually, the tuning fork test reveals a conductive hearing loss (see above).

Medical management consists first of using systemic antibiotics because chronic middle ear effusions are culture positive in up to 50% of cases. Recommended regimens include a 10-day course of amoxicillin alone or combined with clavulanate, cefuroxime axetil, cefaclor, or trimethoprim–sulfamethoxazole (3,4). Topical decongestants in the form of nasal sprays or drops are often used to relieve eustachian tube obstruction. Nasal sprays containing the sympathomimetics may be obtained over the counter (e.g., Neo-Synephrine 0.25% or 0.50% spray or drops). After 3 to 4 days of topical treatment, rebound nasal mucosal hyperemia may occur. Therefore, the patient should be instructed explicitly to discontinue spray (or drops) after 3 days. Systemic decongestants (e.g., pseudoephedrine) are probably not helpful (5). If serous otitis media coincides with symptoms of allergic rhinitis, eustachian tube function and middle ear aeration may be helped by the use of a nasal steroid spray for a few weeks or the duration of the seasonal allergy alone or in combination with an antihistamine (see Chapter 30).

All patients should be re-evaluated after 4 to 6 weeks. If conductive hearing loss persists beyond 6 weeks, the patient should be referred to an otolaryngologist, who will confirm and quantify the conductive hearing loss and check for other conditions that may be causing the hearing loss. Persistent effusion after 3 months of medical therapy is an indication for surgery, particularly when associated with hearing loss or tympanic membrane changes. Surgery consists of a myringotomy with placement of a ventilation tube. This procedure is usually done under local anesthesia in the office. The tube typically falls out spontaneously in several months. The results are excellent but the patient must keep moisture out of the ear (e.g., avoid swimming) until healing is complete, which usually takes 6 to 18 months.

Acute Otitis Media

Patients with acute suppurative otitis media complain of marked pain in the ear, and most give a history of a recent upper respiratory infection. Drainage of purulent material from the ear indicates probable tympanic membrane perforation or concomitant otitis externa. On examination, there is injection and loss of luster of the tympanic membrane, grayish-pink coloration of the entire membrane, and, eventually, bulging of the membrane and loss of landmarks. Some patients have a conductive hearing loss demonstrated by tuning fork tests (see above). There may be tenderness to palpation of the mastoid bone because the mucosa lining of the mastoid cells is continuous with that of the middle ear. Evidence of otitis externa is usually not present. The most common etiologic agents are *Streptococcus pneumoniae* (pneumococcus), *Haemophilus influenza,* and *Moraxella catarrhalis* (3,4). Although some cases are caused by viral pathogens, diagnosis of these cases is usually not practical and treatment should be the same for all patients with acute otitis media.

Medical treatment consists of systemic antimicrobials for 10 days. The antibiotic course should be completed to avoid recurrent or persistent infection and mastoiditis. Amoxicillin, 500 mg three times daily for 10 days, remains the drug of first choice. The growing prevalence of beta-lactamase–producing bacteria may necessitate the use of amoxicillin–clavulanate (Augmentin 250/125 or 500/125 tablets), cefuroxime axetil (Ceftin 250- or 500-mg tablets), or clindamycin (Cleocin 300mg tablets) as second-line antimicrobial choices. For penicillin-allergic patients, erythromycin, cefuroxime axetil, and trimethoprim–sulfamethoxazole (e.g., Bactrim, Septra, or generic) may be used. Aspirin, acetaminophen, or ibuprofen every 4 to 6 hours should be recommended for pain. If perforation with discharge occurs, Cortisporin otic suspension, four drops three times daily for 1 week, may be added to the treatment. If the tympanic membrane is bulging with pus and the patient describes severe pain or vertigo, myringotomy by an otolaryngologist is indicated to prevent extension of the infection and resultant complications.

Close follow-up is recommended within a week of starting therapy to ensure a normal response to treatment. Recovery from the pain of acute otitis media is usually prompt. Pain and fever should be absent by 3 days of therapy. If not, alternative antibiotics should be prescribed with follow-up within a few days. Within 1 to 4 weeks, hearing impairment should resolve and the tympanic membrane assumes its normal appearance. Serous otitis may be present after other signs and symptoms of acute otitis have resolved. In the patient who notes persistent otalgia, fever, or other signs of toxicity despite adequate antibiotics for 48 hours, subacute mastoiditis should be suspected, and prompt referral to an otolaryngologist is indicated. Facial nerve dysfunction, vertigo, and signs of central nervous system infection likewise require prompt evaluation and management. Frequent recurrence of otitis media, failure of serous otitis to resolve, persistence of a tympanic membrane perforation, and significant persistent hearing loss after 4 to 6 weeks are also indications for referral.

Barotrauma

Barotrauma refers to symptoms and signs produced by a sudden pressure differential between the middle ear and the surrounding atmosphere. The patient gives a history of fullness, pain, and decreased hearing in one or both ears. This problem is most commonly associated with descents while flying or scuba diving. Otoscopic findings vary from mild tympanic membrane retraction to hemotympanum, with or without perforation. There may be conductive or neurosensory hearing loss. Any patient with moderate or severe unilateral hearing loss should be referred to an otolaryngologist because of the possibility of inner ear involvement. For patients with mild symptoms, topical or oral decongestants may alleviate symptoms. Prophylaxis against barotrauma consists of use of the Valsalva maneuver and chewing gum or swallowing during descent in airplanes and management of allergic conditions involving the upper respiratory tract.

Temporal Bone Fractures

Traditional classification of the lateral skull base is based on the orientation of the fracture line in relation to the long axis of the temporal bone (petrous pyramid). Knowledge of the fracture line orientation predicts the extent of middle- and inner-ear damage and the pattern of cranial nerve injury. Eighty percent of temporal bone fractures are longitudinal, most often caused by blows to the lateral skull (6). The plane of fracture extends along the external ear canal to involve the ossicular chain (to produce a conductive hearing loss) and occasionally the facial nerve. Transverse temporal bone fractures extend perpendicularly to the long axis of the petrous pyramid, crossing the inner ear (to produce a sensorineural hearing loss) and often the facial nerve. Transverse fractures account for approximately 20% of temporal bone fractures. Evaluation of a temporal bone fracture requires a careful otoscopic and cranial nerve evaluation, supplemented by high-resolution computed tomography. Treatment is dictated by sequelae of the fracture.

Traumatic Perforation of Tympanic Membrane

A tympanic membrane perforation may be caused by a cotton-tipped swab or other object for removing wax, foreign bodies, forcefully directed water, and blast waves resulting from detonation of high explosives. Symptoms include decreased hearing, tinnitus, pain, and bleeding. Otoscopic examination reveals a perforation, commonly in the area of the pars tensa (Fig. 110.2). Air insufflation, which aids in the diagnosis, especially if a perforation is suspected but not seen, shows an immobile tympanic membrane.

The objective of treatment is the prevention of infection. Most linear tears and small perforations of the membrane heal spontaneously in several weeks. Large perforations may require grafting by an otolaryngologist. This procedure is usually done under general anesthesia as an outpatient procedure. A piece of temporal fascia is used for the patch. The results are highly successful with minimal postoperative discomfort. If there is a strong possibility that the middle ear has been contaminated at the time of injury, oral antibiotics (ampicillin or erythromycin 250 mg four times daily for 1 week) are indicated. Patients should prevent water or other contaminants from entering the ear by the insertion of a petroleum jelly-covered cotton plug. Swimming should be avoided altogether. Patients whose perforation was self-inflicted should be warned against future syringing and probing to remove cerumen.

After spontaneous closure or myringoplasty, the hearing loss caused by perforation usually resolves completely. Within a few months the perforation or surgical repair is no longer visible, although occasionally a thin area or a whitish scar remains. Tinnitus, sensorineural hearing loss, and vertigo are signs of inner ear injury and necessitate prompt referral to an otolaryngologist, who will evaluate the patient for a fistula, which requires prompt repair.

Chronic Otitis Media

Chronic otitis is present when a patient has otorrhea, either persistent or recurrent, and there is perforation of the tympanic membrane and usually some degree of conductive hearing loss. The management of this problem has two objectives: eradication of infection and restoration of hearing. When chronic otitis media is initially recognized, the patient should be referred to an otolaryngologist for evaluation (7).

Chronic otitis media can be divided into two major subgroups: inactive and active. The clinical characteristics of these two groups are summarized in Table 110.4. The fundamental difference in the active subgroup is the presence of, or potential for, bone destruction caused by invasion by squamous epithelium known as *cholesteatoma.* Cholesteatoma occurs when squamous epithelium of the auditory canal invades the middle ear through a pre-existing perforation (acquired cholesteatoma). The cholesteatoma appears as a mass of keratinaceous debris that accumulates at the site of invasion of squamous epithelium. As the mass enlarges, it carries the potential to erode bone and promote further infection. Facial paralysis caused by cranial nerve VII involvement, meningitis, and brain abscess may occur as a complication of active cholesteatoma.

The commonly performed surgical procedures for chronic otitis media are as follows:

- *Simple mastoidectomy* removes the mastoid cells and cholesteatoma, usually through a postauricular incision. The canal wall remains intact.
- In *modified radical mastoidectomy,* the mastoid cells are exteriorized to form a common cavity with the external auditory canal, draining and eradicating infection caused by cholesteatoma.

Table 110.4. Chronic Otitis Media: Features Distinguishing Inactive and Active (Cholesteatoma) Forms

Feature	Inactive	Active (Cholesteatoma)
Discharge	Mucoid or mucopurulent	Purulent, foul
Location of pathology	Middle ear; eustachian tube	Middle ear, attic, antrum, any part of temporal bone
Tympanic membrane perforation	Pars tensa (central)[a]	Pars flaccida[a] of marginal
Middle ear mucosa	Mucous membrane	Stratified squamous epithelium
X-rays	Normal; clouding of mastoid cells	Underdevelopment of sclerosis of mastoid cells; bone destruction
Cholesteatoma formation	No	Yes
Bone erosion	No	Yes
Treatment of infection	Medical/surgical (surgery if the perforation fails to heal spontaneously)	Surgical

[a]See Fig. 110.2.

- In *myringoplasty,* the tympanic membrane perforation is closed by use of a tissue graft.
- In *tympanoplasty,* the conductive mechanism, including tympanic membrane perforation and ossicular disruptions, is repaired.

These operative procedures are usually done as outpatient surgical procedures. General anesthesia is usually required for both types of mastoidectomy, whereas the plasty procedures can most often be done with only local anesthesia. There is moderate discomfort for 2 to 3 days. However, for 4 to 6 weeks after any of these procedures, the patient must avoid heavy lifting, strenuous exercise, or any similar activity that could result in a Valsalva maneuver, which results in the increase of air pressure in the middle ear and may disrupt the repair. The success rate of all these procedures is approximately 80%.

Acute or chronic suppurative otitis media may become complicated by extension of infection beyond the confines of the middle ear into bone and other surrounding structures. These complicating infections are mastoiditis, facial nerve paralysis (caused by cranial nerve VII involvement), petrositis (inflammation of the petrous portion of the sphenoid with diplopia, pain around the eye, and persistent otorrhea), labyrinthitis, brain abscess, extradural abscess, subdural abscess, lateral sinus thrombophlebitis, meningitis, and otitic hydrocephalus. Symptoms not attributable to the typical course of acute or chronic otitis media may signify the presence of one of these complications and require immediate referral and hospitalization.

Ossicular Chain Problems

The most common of these (adhesive otitis media and tympanosclerosis) occurs as sequelae to otitis media. Others (ossicular injury or otosclerosis) may affect the ossicular chain in the absence of a history of or signs of prior otitis media. Ossicular chain problems may be recognized by demonstrating conductive hearing loss (usually chronic, either unilateral or bilateral). Changes of the tympanic membrane indicative of prior otitis media may or may not be present, depending on the problem (see above). In some conditions, otoscopy may even be diagnostic. Each of these conditions requires referral to an otolaryngologist for accurate diagnosis and consideration of surgical management.

Adhesive Otitis Media. There is a history of ear infection, and the tympanic membrane is retracted and atrophic in areas of healed perforations. The eardrum is usually draped over the promontory and incudostapedial complex. Adhesive otitis media is usually a late complication seen in patients with persistent middle ear inflammation. Hearing loss is usually mild, although some patients may require ossicular reconstruction or a hearing aid (see below).

Tympanosclerosis. There is a history of infection, often bilateral. There is usually, but not always, a tympanic membrane perforation, and discrete plaques of dense collagen with calcified hyaline may be seen in the middle ear. In selected patients, tympanic membrane and ossicular reconstruction is necessary to improve hearing.

Traumatic Ossicular Injury. There is a history of trauma (e.g., temporal bone fracture and the causes of traumatic perforation listed above) followed by unilateral hearing loss, which may be conductive or mixed. A hemotympanum (blood behind the eardrum) is usually seen, although occasionally the tympanic membrane is normal. Hearing status after surgical exploration depends on the type of injury found at surgery.

Otosclerosis. Otosclerosis is a disease of the labyrinthine capsule in which sponge-like bone is laid down, causing fixation of the stapes and conductive hearing loss, usually bilateral. The history discloses a slowly progressive hearing loss, usually in adults in their second or third decades, more commonly in females, and often accelerated by pregnancy. History is key in establishing the diagnosis because examination of the tympanic membrane is usually normal. This is the most common cause of progressive conductive hearing loss in young adults. The results of surgery, consisting of stapedectomy or stapedotomy and prosthetic replacement, are excellent.

New Growths of Middle Ear

A number of benign and malignant growths may be seen on inspection of the tympanic membrane of patients with progressive unilateral conductive hearing loss. Malignant tumors most commonly present with a history of chronic discharge, occasionally bloody.

CHRONIC SENSORINEURAL HEARING LOSS

Presbycusis

A certain degree of hearing loss, beginning in the high-frequency range, is universal among elderly people. Most do not complain of deafness, and often a family member is the first to notice the hearing deficit. Clearly, social and psychologic factors are important in determining the level of reported disability. For this reason, in the general population of elderly, in whom hearing loss is common, screening of asymptomatic patients using an office audiogram is not usually recommended because obtaining a hearing aid (see below), the usual prescription, is expensive and cumbersome and most patients will not use one until they have perceived their hearing problem and seek a remedy on their own. When an older patient is first found to have moderate hearing loss, the patient and family should be counseled as outlined below, and the patient should be offered a referral for evaluation by an audiologist (see Audiometry, above) or by an otolaryngologist (8).

Noise-induced Hearing Loss

Noise-induced hearing loss is a form of sensorineural hearing loss commonly found in patients employed in high-noise industries or exposed to intense noise from power tools, firearms, and other sources (9). Loud rock music also may cause hearing loss, but because of the range of sound it is a slower process, often occurring 10 to 15 years after repeated exposure. Like presbycusis, it is initially a high-frequency hearing loss, eventually involving lower frequencies. Prophylaxis by wearing muffs and earplugs in high-noise settings and reducing noise levels are the best ways to prevent acoustic trauma. Established hearing loss caused by noise is usually irreversible, but progressive hearing loss can be prevented. Acute hearing loss caused by an acute episode of acoustic trauma, such as gunfire or cordless telephone ringer accidents (a loud sound or shock caused by electrical surge), is often reversible and referred to as a temporary threshold shift.

Drug-induced Hearing Loss

A number of drugs may produce bilateral sensorineural hearing loss, and the patient's personal clinician often is the first to learn of this problem (Table 110.5). For most of these drugs, ototoxicity is dose related; however, hearing impairment may occur even at therapeutic dosages. A mild hearing loss occurs in as many as 10% of patients whose serum levels of gentamicin and tobramycin are maintained within the therapeutic range (10).

The prognosis for drug-induced hearing loss varies according to the drug. Salicylates in high dosages and quinine usually produce temporary high-frequency deafness, but permanent deafness has been reported in patients surviving salicylate poisoning and in infants of mothers who received quinine during pregnancy. Aminoglycoside ototoxicity may occur suddenly after a few doses, may be permanent, and may progress after discontinuation of the drug. Diuretic-induced ototoxicity may be seen after extremely high dosages, usually in patients with renal insufficiency. Its onset may be

Table 110.5. Drugs that May Cause Sensorineural Hearing Loss

Antibiotics	Diuretics
Streptomycin	Ethacrynic acid
Neomycin	Furosemide
Gentamycin	Other Drugs
Tobramycin	Salicylates
Chloramphenicol	Quinidine
Vancomycin	Quinine
	Cisplatin

sudden, after intravenous (and rarely oral) administration, and the hearing deficit may be permanent.

Ménière Syndrome

Ménière syndrome is characterized by spells of a constellation of otologic symptoms. Symptoms are thought to be caused by endolymphatic hydrops manifested by excess fluid and pressure in the cochlea and vestibular labyrinth. Ménière attacks consist of fluctuant hearing loss, roaring tinnitus, aural fullness, and spontaneous peripheral-pattern vertigo (see Chapter 89). However, in many instances the disorder produces a nonclassic array of symptoms. An attack may last for minutes to an hour, often with nystagmus present on physical examination. Between attacks, tinnitus and sensorineural hearing loss often persist. Symptoms are unilateral in 70% to 80% of cases (11). The hearing loss and vertiginous episodes may occur simultaneously or in tandem. Vertigo may be accompanied by nausea and emesis. In severe episodes, other vagal symptoms may occur, including pallor and sweating and rarely bradycardia. Audiometry demonstrates sensorineural hearing loss, predominantly in lower frequencies in early stages of the disease.

The *differential diagnosis* of Ménière syndrome includes a number of conditions that may also present with hearing loss and vertigo unrelated to position change: viral labyrinthitis, acoustic neurinoma, syphilitic vertigo, labyrinthine fistula, vestibular granuloma, temporal bone fracture, or multiple sclerosis (see Chapter 89 for details regarding vertigo).

Patients with suspected Ménière syndrome should have prompt referral to an otolaryngologist to confirm the diagnosis and initiate *treatment*. Patients are placed on a low sodium diet (<2,000 mg/day) and are treated empirically with diuretics, 50 mg of hydrochlorothiazide daily or its equivalent, with attention to avoid hypokalemia (see Chapter 50). The antihistamine meclizine can be tried in a dosage of 25 mg three to four times daily, but often this fails to prevent attacks of vertigo. For nausea, the patient should take the antiemetic prochlorperazine either as a 5- or 10-mg capsule four times daily or as a 25-mg suppository twice daily. After the acute attack has subsided, the patient should continue diuretic treatment; after 1 year without recurrence, diuretic treatment can be discontinued. For the occasional patient with severe recurrent Ménière syndrome refractory to medical treatment, several surgical procedures offer high response rates.

ACOUSTIC NEUROMA

Acoustic neuroma, an uncommon benign tumor, usually arises from the vestibular fibers of nerve VIII. It grows slowly, expanding within the internal auditory meatus until it is large enough to extend into the posterior fossa and compress adjacent structures. Essentially all patients present with symptoms of eighth nerve impairment: Unilateral hearing loss is found in most patients, and chronic, usually mild, positional vertigo or sense of imbalance occurs in many patients. Audiometry usually demonstrates significant sensorineural hearing loss with poor discrimination. Neurologic examination (see Chapter 86) shows involvement of the following neurologic structures, in decreasing order of frequency: cranial nerves V, VII, VI, and cerebellum (ataxia, with tendency to fall toward the side of the lesion). Referral to an otolaryngologist for evaluation is essential whenever unilateral sensorineural hearing loss is initially found. Diagnosis of acoustic neuroma is based on a characteristic audiogram and computed tomography or magnetic resonance imaging (12). The results of surgical treatment generally permit the patient to resume usual activity, but often with permanent unilateral hearing loss (13). In a few patients with good hearing preoperatively, it may be possible to preserve hearing.

SUDDEN SENSORINEURAL HEARING LOSS

Sudden sensorineural hearing loss, usually unilateral, is an otologic emergency. The cause is often difficult to ascertain and may include viral cochleitis, arterial occlusion (especially in patients with other evidence of arterial occlusive disease, such as embolic transient ischemic attacks), inner ear fistula, autoimmune factors (14), sudden expansion of a cerebellopontine angle tumor (e.g., a meningioma or acoustic neuroma, discussed above), temporal bone fracture, and noise trauma. Symptoms, which occur over a matter of minutes to hours, include tinnitus or hearing loss. After prompt evaluation for conductive hearing loss (including simple cerumen impaction), these patients should be referred immediately for evaluation by an otolaryngologist. A number of empirical medical therapies (e.g., corticosteroids, vasodilators, membrane-deforming agents, or anticoagulants) have been tried with varying success. For patients with suspected inner ear fistulas, surgical exploration may be necessary. Most patients have permanent severe unilateral hearing loss, and they and their families should be instructed about adequate noise protection for the only hearing ear, preferential seating for optimal use of the good ear, and precautions when driving to compensate for missed sound cues.

TINNITUS

Tinnitus ("ringing") is the perception of sounds in the absence of a normal sound stimulus. Intermittent tinnitus is common in the general population. Persistent tinnitus may be caused by a number of identifiable problems. Occasionally, tinnitus may be experienced only at night, in bed, when ambient noise is reduced.

Subjective Tinnitus

The term *subjective tinnitus* is used when the subject complains of noises that cannot be heard by the observer. Subjective tinnitus may be subdivided into two types. *Tympanic* tinnitus usually arises as a result of a conductive lesion (all of the causes of conductive hearing loss). It is thought to be caused by removal of the normal masking effect of ambient noise, with emergence of otherwise subaudible tympanic, vascular, and muscular noises. The patient often describes the tinnitus as pulsating. *Petrous* tinnitus is caused by conditions affecting the cochlea or eighth nerve that lead to sensorineural hearing loss. It is attributed to recognition of auditory stimuli produced by mechanical cochlear deformation or hyperirritability of the acoustic nerve. It may be intermittent or continuous with varying intensity.

After the patient's primary otologic problem has been defined, the most important requirement in helping the patient with tinnitus is reassurance, because patients may believe that their tinnitus reflects a serious intracranial condition. Short-term bedtime sedation to ensure adequate sleep is important. Some patients also find that the sound of an FM radio (FM delivers a broader range of frequencies, particularly in the higher spectrum than AM) helps them get to sleep by competing with the more distressing sounds caused by tinnitus. For patients with severe tinnitus, *masking treatment* (an apparatus that externally generates white noise and is available from an audiologist) may be helpful. The distressing nature of severe and chronic tinnitus has resulted in the development of tinnitus clinics and support groups in most large cities (15,16).

Objective Tinnitus

Objective tinnitus is a noise audible to the examiner and originates from the region of the patient's ear. Causes include aneurysm of the internal carotid artery, benign vascular tumors of the middle ear, temporomandibular joint instability, and myoclonus of the palatal muscles. Although not audible by the examiner, a complaint of pulsatile tinnitus may also indicate benign intracranial hypertension. These patients should be referred to an otolaryngologist for a diagnostic workup. Also, patients with tinnitus that lateralizes to one ear should also be referred for further evaluation.

DEALING WITH THE PATIENT WITH PERMANENT HEARING LOSS

Communication

Counseling of the family and others who speak to the patient with moderate to severe hearing loss should emphasize the following points:

- Facilitate communication by consistently using the following adjuncts to speech: face patients, obtain their attention, use gestures, speak at a moderate pace and audibly, or move closer if the patient says that it helps. Most patients with significant hearing loss are most affected at high frequencies and have better preservation of their lower frequency hearing. Because speech frequencies are generally higher during shouting, the use of a full clear voice is more constructive.
- Ensure adequate lighting (to aide in lip reading and facial expressions) and minimize background noise, which confuses sound perception.
- Be patient and ask how you can facilitate communication.

For the patient with *profound* or *total hearing loss,* the principle governing all communication is that the patient must see the message. Most patients let the clinician know the mode of communication they prefer (lip reading or writing). Whenever there is any question about the effectiveness of lip reading, written exchange of information should be used. This can be facilitated by ensuring that paper and a pen or pencil are always available to the patient. The use of a word processor program with large font is particularly helpful in facilitating communication with deaf patients. When sign language is the preferred mode of communication, arrangements should be made in advance for an interpreter to be present at appointments. Also, various devices are now available, although they are moderately expensive, that make it possible for totally deaf people to receive telephone calls (messages are entered by the sender in code on a touch-tone unit and displayed visually for the deaf receiver) and to follow television programs. Many people who are totally deaf at an early age learn sign language, and programs for learning sign language are widely available. Valuable information to help people with any level of hearing impairment may be obtained from Self-Help for Hard of Hearing People, Inc., *www.SHHH.org,* and The A.G. Bell Association for Deaf and Hard of Hearing Children, *www.AGBell.org.*

Hearing Aids

Hearing aids (miniature battery-powered microphone–amplifier–loudspeaker units) can assist the patient with sensorineural hearing loss and patients with irreversible conductive loss (17). The currently available aids include in-the-ear, delicate, and behind-the-ear units. Older devices were incorporated into eyeglasses or carried in a pocket with a wire connection to the ear mold. Hearing aids can increase the intensity of a sound by up to 70 dB. Thus, a sound of about 60 dB (the level of average conversational speech) passing through an aid may enter the ear at a level of 130 dB. This represents the maximal usable gain of an aid because sounds above this level become painful.

Federal law now prevents the sale of hearing aids to people who have not been evaluated. Only trial and adjustment determine whether a patient referred for a hearing aid will benefit. Medicare and other third-party insurers do not pay for hearing aids, and they are expensive, typically costing over $600. Most hearing aid dealers allow a 30-day trial period during which the patient pays a rental fee; some states require this by law. Currently, only some people who would benefit from a hearing aid own one, usually because of the cost and the difficulty or embarrassment perceived in using it. Also, many who own units do not use them regularly because of difficulty in using them or the presence of irritating sounds, which often can be eliminated by adjustment of the device by an audiologist.

Patients may mention certain specific problems with the hearing aid. There may be irritation of the conchal cartilage, infection in the external canal, or an increase in cerumen accumulation. In each of these situations, the fitting audiologist should evaluate use of the aid. A better fitting mold is needed to avoid recurrence in some patients. Others may do well by removing the aid periodically during the day.

Amplification devices have evolved considerably in the past decade. Digital hearing aids convert electronic sound information from the microphone into a digitized code, which is then processed by an amplifier consisting of microchips instead of electronic circuitry. All adjustments are programmed using computer software. Substantially more expensive, the primary advantage of digital signal processing is the greater processing power than prior analog signal processors in the hearing aid. The greater processing power represents greater decision-making ability by the instrument, allowing many more adjustments and greater precision of adjustments for the listener to make according to the acoustic environment.

For selected patients, semi-implantable systems, including implantable bone conduction aids and cochlear implants, are now available (18). The cochlear implant is used in patients who are unable to derive significant benefit from the use of powerful hearing aids. Young deaf children who are appropriately managed with cochlear implants demonstrate an increased likelihood of gaining access to mainstream education opportunities (19). Deaf adults with previous experience with verbal language also enjoy significant changes in quality of life as a result of increased access to the spoken word (20).

General References*

Cummings C, Fredrickson J, Harker L, et al., eds. Otolaryngology: head and neck surgery. St. Louis: CV Mosby, 1998.

A good review focused on elderly patients.

Jerger J, Chmiel R, Wilson N, et al. Hearing impairment in older adults: new concepts. J Am Geriatr Soc 1995;43:928.

*Bold print (general references) and bold numerals (specific references) denote published controlled clinical trials, meta-analyses, or consensus-based recommendations.

A thorough review of the causes, evaluation, and treatment of hearing loss.

Nadol JB. Hearing loss. N Engl J Med 1993;329:1092.

Niparko J, Kemink J. Hearing loss: strategies in evaluation and management. Consultant 1987;27:39.

Rosenfeld RM. An evidence-based approach to treating otitis media. Pediatr Clin North Am 1996;43:1165.

Rosenfeld RM, Post JC. Meta-analysis of antibiotics for the treatment of otitis media with effusion. Otolaryngol Head Neck Surg 1992;106:378.

A thorough analysis of the treatment of otitis media with effusion.

Specific References

1. Niparko J, Swanson N, Baker S, et al. Local control of auricular and periauricular cutaneous carcinoma with Mohs surgery. Laryngoscope 1990;100:1047.
2. Gillespie MB, Francis HW, Chee N, et al. Squamous cell carcinoma of the temporal bone: a radiographic-pathologic correlation. Arch Otolaryngol Head Neck Surg 2001;127:803.
3. Bluestone CD, Klein JO. Otitis media, atelectasis and eustachian tube dysfunction. In: Bluestone CD, Stool SE, eds. Pediatric otolaryngology, 2nd ed. Philadelphia: WB Saunders, 1990:320.
4. Hoberman A, Paradise JL. Acute otitis media: diagnosis and management in the year 2000. Pediatr Ann 2000;29:609.
5. Bluestone CD, Mandel EM, Cantekin EI, et al. Evaluation of decongestant antihistamine therapy for otitis media with effusion. Ann Otol Rhinol Laryngol 1983;92:35.
6. Backous D, Minor L, Niparko J. Trauma to the external auditory canal and temporal bone. Otolaryngol Clin North Am 1996;29:5.
7. Kemink J, Telian S, Niparko J. Evaluation and treatment of the draining ear. Mod Med 1988;56:76.
8. Miller MH. Restoring hearing to the older patient: the physician's role. Geriatrics 1986;41:75.
9. Dobie RA. Noise-induced hearing loss: the family physician's role. Am Fam Physician 1987;36:141.
10. Smith CR, Lipsky JJ, Laskin OL, et al. Double-blind comparison of the nephrotoxicity and auditory toxicity of gentamycin and tobramycin. N Engl J Med 1980;302:1106.
11. Balkany TJ, Kires B, Arenberg IK. Bilateral aspects of Meniere's disease. Otolaryngol Clin North Am 1980;13:4.
12. Armington WG, Harnsberger HR, Smoker WR, et al. Normal and diseased acoustic pathway: evaluation with MR imaging. Radiology 1988;167:509.
13. Ojemann RG, Montgomery WW, Weiss AD. Evaluation and surgical treatment of acoustic neuroma. N Engl J Med 1972;287:895.
14. Stone JH, Francis HW. Immune-mediated inner ear disease. Curr Opin Rheumatol 2000;12:32.
15. Hawthorne MR, O'Connor S, Britten SR, et al. The management of a population of tinnitus sufferers in a specialized clinic. Part I. Description of the clinic organization and the population seen. J Laryngol Otol 1987;101:784.
16. O'Connor S, Hawthorne M, Britten SR, et al. The management of a population of tinnitus sufferers in a specialized clinic. Part II. Identification of psychiatric morbidity in a population of tinnitus sufferers. J Laryngol Otol 1987;101:791.
17. Department of Health, Education and Welfare. A report on hearing aid health care. Washington, DC: U.S. Government Printing Office, 1974.
18. Cohen N, Waltzman S. The Department of Veterans Affairs Cochlear Implant Study Group: a prospective, randomized study of cochlear implants. N Engl J Med 1993;328:233.
19. Francis HW, Koch ME, Wyatt JR, et al. Trends in educational placement and cost-benefit considerations in children with cochlear implants. Arch Otolaryngol Head Neck Surg 1999;125:499.
20. Palmer CA, Niparko JK, Wyatt JR, et al. A prospective study of the cost-utility of the multichannel cochlear implant. Arch Otolaryngol Head Neck Surg 1999;125:1221.

CHAPTER 111

Selected Disorders of the Nose and Throat: Epistaxis, Snoring, Anosmia, Hoarseness, and Hiccups

MARK F. WILLIAMS, MD

EPISTAXIS

Epistaxis is very common, with most individuals having at least one "nosebleed" during their lifetime. Most episodes of epistaxis do not require medical attention and are usually self-limited with inconsequential loss of blood. The overall goal in the management of epistaxis is to stop the bleeding and ultimately to correct any underlying pathology that precipitated the event. Rarely, severe uncontrolled epistaxis may cause aspiration and substantial blood loss and may be life threatening. Most patients with epistaxis can be managed by the primary care provider, with only some cases requiring otolaryngologic consultation for initial management.

Pathophysiology

Epistaxis is defined as bleeding emanating from the nose or nasopharynx. The blood may flow anteriorly through the nares or posteriorly and may be swallowed. The nasal mucosa has a rich anastomosis of vessels, arising from multiple sources. The blood supply to the lateral nasal wall is derived from the internal maxillary and facial arteries from the external carotid system. The nasal septum is supplied by the anterior and posterior ethmoid arteries from the internal carotid system.

The nasal mucosa is composed of a thin stratified columnar epithelium with goblet cells supplying the mucous blanket. The nasal secretions provide and protect the underlying epithelium. On the lateral nasal wall (i.e., on the turbinates), the submucosa is thickened with the presence of venous sinusoids and mucous glands. The submucosa of the nasal lining is quite thin with the blood vessels in close proximity to the mucosal surface. Dryness or irritation causes mucosal disruption and bleeding from underlying vessels. These vessels will not be fully protected from rebleeding until the overlying mucosa has healed. A cycle of rebleeding may occur as local infection and inflammation initiate the formation of granulation tissue, which remains quite friable and will cause persistent bleeding. The rebleeding cycle ceases only when the underlying epithelium is regenerated and the submucosal vessels are protected.

The anterior septum is particularly prone to environmental irritation (dry air, smoke, toxic inhalants); it is the site of approximately 90% of all episodes of epistaxis. Anterior epistaxis occurs more frequently when the weather is cold and humidity is decreased. More posteriorly, on the septum and in the lateral nasal wall, the vessels are of a larger caliber, and epistaxis from these posterior vessels is typically quite brisk. With increasing age and concomitant arteriovascular disease, posterior epistaxis becomes more prevalent. The presence of arterial disease in these vessels also compromises vascular contraction during acute epistaxis, which prolongs uncontrolled bleeding (1). The posterior nasal cavity is very difficult to access and evaluate, so posterior epistaxis can be quite difficult to control.

Etiology

The etiology of epistaxis usually can be readily determined (2). It is more important to ascertain the cause of the nasal bleeding in refractory and recurrent cases, as opposed to isolated episodes that are self-limited and not severe. Recurrent and refractory epistaxis may point to a significant underlying medical condition. Epistaxis often is caused by a combination of factors, so it is helpful when evaluating a patient with problematic epistaxis to consider both local factors and systemic factors (Table 111.1).

Local Factors

Conditions that alter the physiology of the nasal mucosa and environmental factors, such as decreased temperature and humidity, lead to disruption of the nasal epithelium and subsequent vascular injury and hemorrhage. For example, hospital admissions for epistaxis increase during the winter months, with up to two-thirds occurring during January and February

Table 111.1. Causes of Epistaxis

Cause
Local mucosal irritation
Trauma
Fracture
Surgery
Anatomic derangement
Septal deviation
Foreign body
Neoplasm
Hypertension (?)
Chronic renal failure
Defects of coagulation
Heredity
Medication

Adapted from Lepore ML. Epistaxis. In: Bailey BJ, ed. Head and neck surgery—otolaryngology, 1st ed. Philadelphia: JP Lippincott, 1993:8, with permission.

in the northern hemisphere (3). This may be related to low humidity in households with dry-air heating systems.

Local trauma is also commonly implicated in epistaxis. Any blunt force directed to the mid-face or adjacent regions can cause shearing of the nasal mucosa, which will be accompanied by brisk nasal bleeding. Perhaps more important is trauma from persistent nose picking. Patients with recent nosebleeds may perceive nasal obstruction due to crusting and promote rebleeding while trying to remove the crust. Local inflammation due to upper respiratory infections, chronic sinusitis, allergic rhinitis, or environmental irritants can also alter normal nasal physiology, leading to dryness and crusting with subsequent vascular exposure and bleeding.

Anatomical derangements such as nasal septal deviation are also common in patients with epistaxis (4). It is not clear how septal deformities promote epistaxis, except that septal deflections can cause disruption of laminar airflow, leading to local areas of dryness that are prone to mucosal disruption and bleeding. Intranasal foreign bodies are rare in adults but are an important cause of epistaxis in children. In adults, a nasal foreign body may be found in a victim of a recent motor vehicle accident who unknowingly had a piece of glass impacted in the nasal cavity that was not readily apparent on initial evaluation. Industrial chemical exposures, (e.g., to the fumes of chromates, ammonia, and sulfuric acid) have also been implicated in causing recurrent epistaxis (5). Cigarette smoke, including second-hand sources, is also an irritant that can promote epistaxis.

Epistaxis occasionally occurs subsequent to iatrogenic trauma (nasal and sinus surgery). Benign and malignant intranasal tumors are uncommon but may present with persistent epistaxis.

Systemic Factors

A variety of systemic factors related to either vascular fragility or clotting abnormalities may be a case of repeated epistaxis. Long-standing hypertension may be a factor in promoting epistaxis, but it remains controversial whether there is a higher rate of arterial hypertension in epistaxis patients versus normal control subjects (1). It appears that hypertensive patients on diuretics are more susceptible to epistaxis than those taking beta-blockers (6). Many patients have elevated blood pressure at the time of their treatment for epistaxis, but this may simply be a result of pain and anxiety. It is important to ascertain whether or not hypertension returns to normal after treatment, so that patients found to have underlying hypertension can receive appropriate treatment (7). Generalized vascular disease associated with hypertension may also be a factor, because underlying atherosclerotic vessels are known to have decreased elasticity and capacity to contract and assist in clot formation.

Patients with end-stage renal disease on hemodialysis are prone to recurrent epistaxis. This may be due to a decrease in platelet activity or frequent exposure to heparin (8,9). Septal perforation is noted in up to 8% of patients with chronic renal failure, and this perforation can precipitate turbulent airflow, local irritation and crusting, and recurrent hemorrhage. Alcohol abuse with associated poor nutrition and vitamin C and K deficiencies may lead to poor wound healing and clotting formation, respectively. Additionally, liver disease may also cause alterations in the normal clotting mechanism, thus setting the stage for persistent and recurrent epistaxis.

Patients with hereditary coagulation abnormalities, such as hemophilia or von Willebrand disease, can have problematic and persistent epistaxis. Acquired conditions, such as thrombocytopenia from a hematologic malignancy or chemotherapy, may also be significant. Osler-Rendu-Weber disease (hereditary hemorrhagic telangiectasia) very commonly presents with recurrent epistaxis. This inherited condition results in a lack of the contractile elements in the vessel walls with formation of telangiectasias on the nasal, oral, intraoral, and gastric mucosa. These patients often have recurrent gastrointestinal bleeding as well as epistaxis, and treatment is often problematic.

Numerous medications are also implicated in epistaxis. Nonsteroidal anti-inflammatory agents are commonly a factor, with as many as 75% of epistaxis patients having previously been on one of these drugs (10). It is important to determine by a careful history when these agents, including aspirin, have been used (11). These medications interfere with normal platelet function by inhibiting the cyclooxygenase pathway and arachidonic acid metabolism. Other agents that dry the nasal mucosa, such as tricyclic antidepressants, antipsychotic agents, and antihistamines, may promote mucosal disruption and bleeding. Nasal steroid sprays may also cause epistaxis, either due to the vehicle, the medication itself, or trauma from the nasal spray applicator.

Approach to Management

Management of a patient with epistaxis should proceed at a pace congruent with the severity of bleeding and acuity of the situation. Initially, patients should be assessed for stability and the severity of their blood loss. As always, the standard ABCs (airway, breathing, and circulation) need to be supported. Intravenous access should be established in all patients who are actively bleeding.

Fortunately, most epistaxis is not accompanied by massive blood loss, and the focus is on local control of the bleeding. It is important, though, not to take a casual approach to epistaxis because fatalities, although rare, are known to occur, especially in patients with existing comorbidities such as coronary artery disease or chronic pulmonary disease. The initial history should ascertain on which side the bleeding began and whether or not it was mostly isolated nasal bleeding or associated with excessive spitting up of blood, which would suggest a posterior bleeding site. The duration of the nosebleed and an estimation of blood loss are also pertinent. A history of previous epistaxis and how those episodes were treated may suggest the initial treatment in a given situation. A past medical history should ascertain whether or not hypertension, liver disease, alcoholism, cardiac disease, or renal insufficiency is present. A review of the patient's medications will determine if nonsteroidal anti-inflammatory agents, warfarin, or aspirin-containing products are contributing to clotting abnormalities.

At initial presentation, it is reasonable to obtain laboratory studies, including a complete blood count (to determine if anemia is present), prothrombin time/partial thromboplastin time and platelets (to assess for significant coagulopathy), and a type-and-screen to make blood available if the episode of epistaxis is intractable.

A brief general examination may suggest a bleeding diathesis. The next step is to examine the nasal cavity. It is important to have adequate lighting and suction available. Universal precautions for all health care personnel are important, because epistaxis management can be quite bloody. Appropriate protective gear should be worn, including eyewear and gowns. The patient should to be supplied with a handful of gauze or tissues and should be draped appropriately to allow comfortable examination. All clots should be removed from the nose, preferably through intranasal suctioning, and patients also may be asked to blow their noses to remove any clots. A headlight is helpful in performing intranasal examination. Intranasal examination may be aided by decongesting the nose. Topical decongestants (e.g., oxymetazoline 0.05%, two to three sprays in each nostril) will cause significant vasoconstriction and either decrease or stop the flow of blood (12). It is important that the decongestants are applied after removal of blood clots, so they may be most effective on the nasal mucosa.

Treatment

Because most nasal bleeding is anterior, local compression of the nose should be performed initially using the thumb and index finger to compress the cartilaginous portion of the nose. This can be initiated by instructing the patient to perform this maneuver while the other materials are being collected. Treatment of epistaxis should be performed in a step-like fashion to provide the least invasive means to control the episode. If the bleeding site is seen to be anterior, a cotton ball impregnated with a decongestant and lidocaine may be used to anesthetize and decongest the area of the bleeding vessel. Silver nitrate cautery may then be used to lightly cauterize the area around the vessel. The silver nitrate stick should be used from a peripheral to central fashion around the bleeding vessel, with the stick rolled over the mucosa lightly until a gray residue appears. This technique is difficult to perform during active bleeding and often will not be successful. It is important to avoid deep chemical cautery with silver nitrate, as well as bilateral septal cautery, to avoid injury to the underlying cartilage, which may subsequently lead to septal perforation. If the bleeding is controlled with this method, a cotton swab saturated with normal saline should be used to neutralize any residual silver nitrate and curtail the chemical cautery. After silver nitrate cautery, an antibiotic ointment should be applied to prevent crusting and subsequent local bacterial infection.

If the bleeding persists, the next level of intervention is anterior packing. Traditional anterior packing dictates placement of a layer of $\frac{1}{2}$-inch lubricated gauze coated in antibiotic ointment. This is a difficult technique to master, and presently there are available expandable nasal tampons (Merocel, Xomed Surgical Products, Jacksonville, FL) that are as effective and much easier to place. When using a nasal tampon, it is important to have a good idea where the site of bleeding is to determine the length of the nasal tampon to apply. The common length is up to 10 cm, which will pack the entire nose, including the posterior choanae. It is also important to understand that the floor of the nose slants caudally from an anterior to posterior direction and that the tampon should be directed somewhat inferiorly as opposed to cranially. In addition, the nasal tampon should be coated with an antibacterial ointment to prevent premature expansion of the tampon by blood during the insertion and to provide an impediment to bacterial overgrowth of the packing. The packing should be left in place from 3 to 5 days to allow clotting and healing of the bleeding area. If necessary, bilateral tampons or synthetic sponge packs can be placed. The success rate is high, and minimal experience is needed for placement. In addition, patient tolerance of this form of packing is superior to the classic layered gauze. After placing the pack, the oropharynx should be examined to determine if there is any residual bleeding. If there is bleeding noted posteriorly, the anterior tampons may be inadequate. After packing, an oral antibiotic such as a first- or second-generation cephalosporin (e.g., cephalexin 250 mg orally four times daily) or amoxicillin/clavulanate (Augmentin, 500 mg twice daily) with staphylococcal coverage should be used for 10 days to avoid bacterial overgrowth and to prevent toxic shock syndrome.

If this is ineffective, posterior nasal packing may be needed. The posterior vessels are difficult to visualize and are not affected by pressure from the usual anterior nasal packing. Posterior packing is necessary in cases of a posterior site of bleeding and in situations where nasal septal deflection prohibits adequate insertion of a tampon. Although only about 5% epistaxis originates from a posterior nasal source, it is these patients who are at most risk of complications and adverse sequelae (13). Posterior nasal packing is difficult to perform and requires a complex procedure to allow insertion of a nasal pack from the oropharynx into the nasopharynx. However, commercially available balloon intranasal catheters (Epistat) may be placed by otolaryngologists or other clinicians experienced in their use. Because insertion of the posterior packing is painful, the clinician should provide mild sedation before placement. In addition, any patient who undergoes posterior nasal packing should be admitted to the hospital for observation. Posterior packing universally will cause swallowing difficulty, so maintenance of hydration by administration of intravenous fluids is important. Posterior nasal packing is usually removed after about 48 to 72 hours. Often it is difficult to determine initially whether posterior packing is necessary, and it is reasonable to proceed with anterior packing first. If this fails to control bleeding, then posterior packing is indicated.

Consideration should be given as well to hospitalization of elderly and debilitated patients who require anterior nasal packing. An otolaryngologist should be consulted if there is doubt about the management of such a patient. Bilateral, as well as posterior, nasal packing will obstruct the nasal airway and may promote hypoxia or hypercapnia (14). Also, posterior packing and the mild sedation it requires can promote decreased arterial oxygenation and hypercapnia. Therefore, continuous pulse oximetry is indicated and admission to an appropriate care unit to ensure the necessary surveillance should be considered based on the patient's age and general health. These patients are at risk for a nasal vagal response, bradycardia, hypertension, apnea, dislodged packing, aspiration, persistent bleeding and significant hypoxia.

Surgical Interventions

If these packing procedures are ineffective, more invasive procedures may be performed by a consulting otolaryngologist, including extracranial arterial ligations, if necessary (15,16).

Special Cases

In patients with severe coagulopathy or thrombocytopenia, placement of intranasal packing can be problematic, because at the time of removal a raw nasal mucosa may continue to bleed. In these circumstances, the use of a porcine pack may be appropriate. This entails using a strip of ordinary salt pork to pack the nose. Homogenates of salt pork contain an activation factor that promotes platelet aggregation. In addition, the porcine packing is less irritating to the nose, and upon removal there is less nasal mucosal irritation to promote bleeding (17).

Nasal bleeding associated with significant facial or head trauma can be complicated by disruption of the cribriform plate in the anterior cranial base permitting displacement of packing material into the intracranial space. Therefore, in these situations, packing and nasal instrumentation, should be deferred and prompt otolaryngology consultation arranged. Arterial embolization is also an effective method for intractable nosebleeds, especially in patients who are not considered surgical candidates (18).

Follow-up and Patient Education

Most patients can be treated in an outpatient setting and return for packing removal. If the patient's epistaxis is recurrent and persistent, prompt otolaryngologic evaluation is appropriate, even if packing was unnecessary. Persistent and refractory epistaxis can be evaluated by testing for coagulopathy or any hematopoietic malignancies. Sinus x-rays or computed tomography (CT) can rule out an intranasal mass. Nasal endoscopy has revolutionized sinonasal evaluation, and this procedure is easy to perform in the otolaryngology office setting using topical anesthesia. The nasal endoscope allows a well-illuminated magnified view of the entire nasal cavity to assess for potential bleeding sites, anatomic abnormalities, or tumors.

Many patients with persistent epistaxis, even after determining there is no sinister underlying pathology, will have etiologic factors that cannot be modified. For example, patients may require warfarin or may have an underlying chronic medical condition that is unlikely to change. It is important to educate these individuals about conservative measures that can alleviate the cycle of epistaxis. Patients should be informed about the physiology of epistaxis, with a cycle of desiccation, crushing, mucosal disruption, and hemorrhage followed by crushing and rebleeding. It may be helpful to explain this phenomenon by analogy to a puddle of water that dries and one can then see the ground on the bottom caking and cracking. This exemplifies the nasal mucosa and its fragility and need for humidification. Patients should be instructed to avoid aspirin therapy within 2 weeks of their nosebleed to allow for a reasonable period of time for healing. In addition, humidification of the nose should be stressed with liberal use of nasal saline spray and application of a nasal emollient (Vaseline, Bacitracin) twice a day to the nasal vestibule. Room humidifiers should also be used to elevate the humidification of the household air.

Patients should be instructed what to do if subsequent nosebleeds occur. This includes instructing the patient in digital compression of the anterior nose. Application of pressure to the entire soft pliable portion of the nose with the thumb and finger should be demonstrated. It is important to stress that this maneuver should be performed for at least 5 minutes by the clock without peeking to see if bleeding is continuing. Patients prone to nosebleeds should keep oxymetazoline spray (0.05%) on hand, remove any intranasal clots by blowing, and spray each nostril generously two to three times. These self-administered treatments control simple epistaxis in about two-thirds of patients (12). If these methods fail, patients should be instructed to seek care from their provider or an emergency room for more definitive management.

Some patients who are prone to persistent and severe nosebleeds (e.g., those with hereditary hemorrhagic telangiectasias) have learned to self-apply anterior packing. In the situation of recurrent one-sided nosebleeds, certain anatomic abnormalities may respond to "nasal rest." This is achieved by having a patient take a small cotton ball impregnated with petroleum jelly and place it into the anterior nares to obstruct all airflow in the bleeding nasal cavity. This can be continued for several days at a time to prevent desiccation and allow for healing.

SNORING

Snoring is a significant behavioral and social problem with potentially important medical implications. Approximately 25% to 50% of men and 15% to 30% of women become chronic snorers (19). Chronic snoring may be a symptom of obstructive sleep apnea (OSA) syndrome (see Chapter 7). However, snoring is not a specific marker for OSA, although it is the cardinal symptom (20). Snoring without OSA is often designated benign snoring, but a better term may be nonapneic snoring, because the medical implications of benign snoring are still being elucidated. There is no clear evidence that nonapneic snoring is a significant risk factor for the more severe medical consequences of OSA. However, benign snoring may fragment sleep and result in daytime hypersomnolence and dysfunction. Clearly, the personal and social impact of snoring can be substantial, such as when bed partners require alternative sleeping arrangements (21). Primary care clinicians and otolaryngologists are often called on to evaluate and treat individuals with this symptom.

Pathophysiology

Snoring is a consequence of the elasticity of the soft tissues of the oropharynx. The snoring sound is thought to be generated by vibrations of the collapsing soft tissues of the pharynx, soft palate, and uvula. It is occasionally difficult to determine the exact anatomic site causing the snoring. Compared with nonsnorers, nonapneic snorers are noted to have smaller airways with higher airway compliances, but these changes are not as severe as in fully developed sleep apnea (20). Airway collapsibility is deterred by sustained pharyngeal muscle tone, which is absent during rapid-eye-movement sleep. Thus, snoring is significantly related to the stage of sleep (22).

One of the difficulties in studying snoring and assessing appropriate management interventions is that there are few objective measures of this phenomenon. Often the clinician has to rely on snoring assessment by the bed partner, because approximately 75% of snoring patients are unaware that they snore (21). Common risk factors for snoring are male gender, obesity, alcohol consumption, ingestion of sedatives or muscle relaxants, and smoking. Even small amounts of alcohol (e.g., one or two glasses of wine with dinner) can significantly aggravate snoring. The use of sedatives or muscle relaxants will also cause a relaxation of the pharyngeal musculature and promote snoring. Smoking may also contribute by increasing pharyngeal inflammation and edema due to the irritant effects of tobacco smoke, leading to pharyngeal narrowing and subsequent snoring. Nasal obstruction from chronic rhinitis or sinusitis may also be a contributing factor. There may also be a familial predisposition to snoring (23).

Evaluation

The office evaluation of patients with snoring should focus on their medical and sleep histories and include a general examination with emphasis on the head and neck. The main task of the evaluation is to determine how severe and disruptive the snoring is and whether further evaluation for OSA syndrome (as outlined in Chapter 7 and below) is indicated.

Sleep and Medical Histories

Patients should be queried about their awareness of snoring and whether they awake at night with a gasping or choking sensation. They should also be asked if they awake in the morning feeling rested or not and if they awake with a headache. Symptoms of daytime somnolence should be ascertained, especially interference with work, driving, or other tasks.

Because most snorers are unaware of their problem, it is helpful to talk to a bed partner or other close observer. This person should be questioned about the frequency, persistence, and severity of snoring and especially whether there are apneic periods, gasping, or choking. Initial assessment of the degree of personal and social disruption is also pertinent: for example, is the patient able to maintain a normal sleeping arrangement or must the bed partner leave the room for sleep. For the reasons indicated above, it is important to inquire about recent change in weight and its effects on the snoring pattern, as well as the use of alcohol, tobacco, and prescription and over the counter drugs. Finally, the patient should be questioned about nasal and sinus symptoms that may be associated with snoring.

Examination

Physical examination is directed at the head and neck. Careful nasal examination should be performed to look for nasal polyps, nasal septal deviation, turbinate hypertrophy, or any evidence of anatomic nasal airway obstruction (see Chapter 33). The oral examination should focus on identifying macroglossia and tonsillar hypertrophy. Sometimes the uvula may be elongated, swollen, and inflamed, secondary to trauma from the vibrations produced during snoring. It should also be determined whether hypertension is present and whether there is evidence of cardiopulmonary disease.

If snoring is severe or disruptive, referral to an otolaryngologist is indicated for airway assessment, usually with transnasal flexible fiberoptic laryngoscopy to rule out any obstruction. Flexible fiberoptic laryngoscopy can be performed easily with topical anesthesia, and it provides a useful evaluation of the entire upper airway.

Because OSA syndrome can have significant and preventable morbidity, it is important to consider whether it is present in patients who snore. Nevertheless, most snorers do not have OSA syndrome. There are as yet no validated clinical criteria for determining whether a patient who snores has sleep apnea. Important features associated with OSA syndrome include apneas reported by an observer; nocturnal gasping or choking reported by the patient or an observer; very loud or disruptive snoring; daytime somnolence; hypertension; nocturnal or early morning angina or palpitations; and headaches on awakening, which are characteristically brief (24). If some of these features are present, and especially if one or more are severe, further testing, such as overnight pulse oximetry or formal polysomnography (sleep study), is indicated (19) (see Chapter 7).

Treatment of Nonapneic Snoring

There are two therapeutic approaches to nonapneic snoring: low-risk conservative measures and surgery, commonly directed at the soft palate. If conservative measures do not produce satisfactory results, and surgical options are considered, the patient should undergo polysomnography to rule out OSA syndrome before referral to an otolaryngologist. This will prevent future masking of OSA symptoms by the surgical intervention and unanticipated perioperative complications of existing OSA.

Nonsurgical Treatment

Conservative measures aimed at decreasing upper airway resistance include improved overall muscle tone and weight loss. This can be achieved by instituting an exercise program. For some patients, weight loss is the only nonsurgical therapy that will relieve benign snoring. Although it is unclear how much weight loss is needed to provide symptomatic improvement, achievement of ideal body weight is not necessary (20). Addressing sleep posture is also helpful in some patients. Many patients achieve marked reduction in snoring when sleeping in the lateral decubitus or prone positions. The classic treatment of sewing a pocket in the back of the pajamas to place one or more tennis balls to force the patient to sleep on the side has anecdotal support. The use of over the counter nasal dilation devices, such as an external adhesive strip (e.g., Breathe Right), may provide relief in some patients, but studies are inconclusive (25). Internal nasal dilators are much less tolerated by patients. The use of various oromandibular splinting devices that advance the lower jaw (sleep splints) has been advocated by many dental professionals, and some efficacy has been reported (20,26). These devices, unfortunately, are often poorly tolerated and require customized fitting by a dentist or oral surgeon who is familiar with their application to achieve satisfactory results.

The use of phosphocholinamine, a tissue lubricant placed intranasally, has been found to reduce snoring frequency by about 25% in a small study (27). However, this is an oil-based agent, and there is the theoretical risk of aspiration and lipoid pneumonia. Protriptyline, a tricyclic antidepressant, has also been found to reduce snoring by as much as 30% (28) in most patients. The long-term efficacy, however, is unknown, and the anticholinergic side effects may be bothersome. If significant nasal obstruction is present, it is reasonable to treat with systemic decongestants (see Chapter 33) and intranasal steroids (see Chapter 30) to maximize the cross-sectional area of the nasal airway. Improving the nasal airway may be enough in some patients to obviate or reduce snoring. Continuous positive airway pressure (CPAP) administered via a nasal mask is commonly used to treat OSA. This device applies a pneumatic "splint" to the airway structures and almost invariably eliminates snoring. Nonapneic snorers are often hesitant to use the CPAP system and usually tolerate it poorly. It is not clear why nonapneic snorers are less tolerant of CPAP, but it may be due to the lack of significant symptomatic benefits compared with patient with OSA (29).

Surgical Treatments

When the snoring patient has an obvious anatomic abnormality that leads to upper airway obstruction (such as enlarged tonsils and adenoids, severely deviated nasal septum, or nasal polyps), surgical therapy may be recommended by an otolaryngologist. Objective evidence of the outcomes of such surgery in reducing snoring is not available, however.

Uvulopalatopharyngoplasty (UPPP) was first described in the early 1960s as a treatment for snoring (30). This technique was subsequently applied as treatment for OSA with some success. The technique entails removal of any existing tonsil tissue and partial resection of the soft palate, uvula, and anterior tonsillar pillars. The airway is thus opened, allowing for increased airflow and reducing the extent of vibratory tissue to generate snoring. Although UPPP is initially quite effective in snoring resolution, long-term success rates range only from 46% to 73% (31). UPPP is an aggressive procedure that requires an approximate 3-week postoperative convalescence. Patients often complain of severe odynophagia postoperatively, and because of this only 60% of patients indicate they would undergo the same treatment again (32). Another disadvantage of UPPP is nasopharyngeal incompetence, so that almost one-fourth of patients complain of intermittent nasopharyngeal regurgitation for up to 1 year after surgery (33).

Because of the limitations of UPPP, more effective and safer palatal procedures for benign snoring have been devised. Most notable is laser or cautery-assisted uvuloplasty, in which the uvula alone is truncated in the office setting under local anesthesia. Uvuloplasty is associated with fewer complications than UPPP, but the technique still entails significant postoperative pain. Uvuloplasty appears to be equally effective as UPPP for snoring treatment, but multiple office excisions are often required and up to 77% of patients abandon their course of uvuloplasty therapy because of pain (34). Uvuloplasty may rarely cause postoperative bleeding and temporary nasopharyngeal regurgitation.

Other forms of surgical therapies for snoring use laser or other modalities to produce palatal stiffening (19). A newer technique involves the delivery of radiofrequency energy with a needle electrode into various sites of the soft palate, resulting in fibrosis and stiffening (35). Radiofrequency ablation is generally safe, minimally invasive, and has few complications (36). Postoperative pain is minimal, because there is no mucosal disruption, and acetaminophen alone is often sufficient for analgesia. Radiofrequency ablation does require, like uvuloplasty, three to four treatments to achieve an appropriate level of snoring cessation. Currently, only a limited number of otolaryngologists perform this procedure. Large-scale trials or systematic reviews of surgical therapies for snoring are not yet available (19). The American Sleep Disorders Association has promulgated practice parameters for some of these techniques (37).

ANOSMIA

Chemosensory disorders affect up to 2 million adults in the United States (38). Unfortunately, the sense of smell is often ignored by clinicians and its disorder relegated to the level of an inconvenience. Anosmia can result in significant debility, especially in individuals who rely on the sense of smell for their occupation (e.g., chefs, police officers, florists). In addition, anosmia can be dangerous because affected individuals are unable to discern gas leaks, spoiled food, or smoke. Anosmia and its often accompanying decreased sense of taste can lead to poor nutritional intake and eating displeasure.

Pathophysiology

The sense of *smell* depends on olfactory chemoreceptors located high in the nasal cavity along the upper septum and cribriform plate, which underlies the anterior cranial fossa. These receptors process odorant molecules in a complex and as yet poorly understood process (39). The odorant molecules are dissolved in the nasal mucous and presented to the neurepithelium of the olfactory nerve for processing. It is not completely understood how the normally functioning olfactory system is able to process and differentiate the multitude of odors presented to it. The sense of *taste* is a more gross perception, which is mediated by taste buds located on the tongue, soft palate, and oropharynx. The sensation of taste generated by these receptors is limited to the basic qualities of salty, sour, sweet, and bitter. Most individual perceptions of flavor and taste are in fact olfactory sensations, classically evidenced by the fact that children are often convinced to take distasteful medicine by holding their nose and preventing any olfactory input. Thus, a patient who complains of a diminished taste may in fact have hyposmia or anosmia.

There is also a chemosensory sense mediated by the trigeminal nerve, which is triggered by pungent and irritant compounds, such as hot peppers, horseradish, mustard, and so on, and perceived as burning or irritating. This pathway is independent from the other modalities of taste and smell.

Dysfunction of smell is classified as complete or partial and is referred to, respectively, as anosmia or hyposmia. Another interesting variation of smell disturbance is phantosmia, in which spontaneous and distorted olfactory hallucinations are manifest. These phantosmias are often described in association in patients with seizure activity, psychiatric illness, and Alzheimer disease (40).

Evaluation

Patients are very sensitive to a decrease in their sense of smell if it occurs suddenly. However, with aging the sense of smell declines naturally, and it may not be as noticeable because of its gradual decrease. When evaluating a patient with diminished smell or taste, it is important to determine the duration of the complaint and whether the sensory loss acutely followed head trauma or an upper respiratory tract infection (a more gradual progression would accompany sinusitis, nasal polyposis, or an intracranial tumor). The patient's medication list should be reviewed because many medications alter the senses of taste and smell (41). Common medications that can impair the sense of smell are shown in Table 111.2.

Anosmia can be considered in two broad categories: sensorineural, in which the olfactory loss is constant, and conductive, whereby the patient may intermittently have olfactory function. *Sensorineural loss* signifies a loss of the neuroepithelium or damage to the olfactory nerves, resulting in the inability to smell.

Causes of sensorineural anosmia include upper respiratory tract infection and trauma. Postviral-induced anosmia is also quite common, accounting for up to a third of anosmia cases. Patients will typically report a very severe respiratory tract infection, and as their congestion resolves they do not regain their sense of

Table 111.2. Some Common Medications that Can Impair the Sense of Smell

Beta-blockers
Ciprofloxacin
Diltiazem
Docycycline
Enalapril
Methotrexate
Nifedipine

Adapted from Ackerman BH, Kasbekar N. Disturbances of taste and smell induced by drugs. Pharmacotherapy 1997;17:482, with permission.

smell. The etiologic factor is damage to the olfactory neurepithelium by the viral agent. These patients are often not rendered completely anosmic and have a reduced sense of smell. Additionally, these patients also tend to be older individuals, which may suggest that the anosmia may be related to a series of viral insults throughout life, resulting in progressive anosmia.

History of head trauma is another important factor. Up to 5% of patients suffering head injury will have olfactory loss, depending on the severity of the head injury (42). The mechanism of injury is typically a frontal or occipital blow, which results in stretching or sheering of the olfactory nerves as they exit the cribriform plate. A basilar skull fracture is not necessary to precipitate anosmia. These patients are typically younger and are often completely anosmic. Prior radiation therapy also often results in marked dysfunction of both smell and taste (43).

Conductive olfactory loss implies that the odorant is unable to reach the olfactory epithelium. Many disease processes, such as nasal polyps and nasal septal deviation, may precipitate this.

Many patients do not have evidence of the preceding causes and after a careful work up will be believed to have an idiopathic cause. Rare causes include endocrine disorders such as Kallmann syndrome (hypogonadotropic hypogonadism; see Chapter 81) and Turner syndrome (44).

Physical examination should focus on the nasal anatomy (see Chapter 33). Inspection of the anterior nasal cavities may not be adequate to completely evaluate potential causes of anosmia. If anterior anatomic abnormalities are observed or if the cause of anosmia remains unclear, referral to an otolaryngologist is indicated.

An appropriate next step in anosmia evaluation would be to determine if the smell disturbance is reversible. This can be done clinically by using a short course of high dose systemic corticosteroids in a tapered fashion (e.g., oral prednisone 60 mg daily for several days, followed by tapering doses to complete a 10-day course). If the olfactory deficit results from nasal inflammation, such as allergic rhinitis or chronic rhinosinusitis, then the olfactory deficit can be temporarily reversed. If the patient does not respond to this steroid challenge, imaging studies and consultation with an otolaryngologist may be warranted, especially if the history or examination do not suggest a cause. The best initial test is a CT of the sinuses. Sinus CT will completely delineate the nasal cavity and determine if there is adequate patency of the air passages and will evaluate for associated sinusitis. However, the CT is very poor for evaluating soft tissue and the anterior cranial fossa. When the cause of anosmia remains obscure, a magnetic resonance image may be needed to rule out anterior cranial fossa tumors, such as meningioma, or other soft tissue neoplasms.

Olfactory Testing

Olfactory testing may be performed by an otolaryngologist to determine threshold odor identification or odor intensity. Odor identification is often tested using the University of Pennsylvania Smell Identification Test. In this test, a patient releases 40 microencapsulated odorants by rubbing designated areas on a card and answers corresponding questions about the identities of the odors. The answers are graded using normative data based on gender and age.

Treatment and Management

Inflammatory nasal disease is quite common and can affect a patient's sense of smell. Some patients will have subacute sinusitis in which the nasal symptoms (congestion, facial pain, and nasal drainage) are subtle and not appreciated, and the primary complaint of the patient is anosmia or a distorted sense of smell. CT (see above) may show chronic sinusitis, and subsequent treatment of this sinusitis (see Chapter 33) can, in many cases, restore normal olfaction. Nasal polyp removal by an otolaryngologist may restore normal olfaction, although polyps often recur and olfaction may be compromised early as polyps regrow.

The prognosis for recovery of disorders of odorant conduction (polyps, septal deviation, rhinosinusitis) causing poor delivery of olfactants to the neuroepithelium is good if the underlying nasal pathology can be remedied. Sensorineural loss caused by damage to the olfactory neurons after trauma or viral infection has a much less favorable prognosis. Approximately 30% of patients with posttraumatic anosmia improve partially or completely within the first year, most within the first 12 weeks (45).

Vitamin A and zinc are commonly prescribed for anosmia; however, their efficacy is not well supported (46). Newer and not yet standardized approaches for disorders of olfaction, such as olfactory epithelial biopsy by an otolaryngologist, with histopathologic and electron microscopic evaluation, are being studied in some centers.

It is important to counsel patients who suffer persistent anosmia about coping maneuvers, such as having appropriate gas and smoke detectors in their home and having adequate assistance with food preparation and evaluation for spoiled foods. Detecting the need to change diapers for small children and cleaning up after pets may be problematic for patients with anosmia. In food preparation, care must be taken not to overuse salt and sugar to add flavor because these additives may precipitate other medical problems. The use of temperature (i.e., hot or cold), texture, and spices in food preparation can be helpful.

HOARSENESS

Because the voice is so important to interpersonal communication, hoarseness causes a great deal of patient distress. Hoarseness is an imprecise term used to describe any alteration in a patient's normal voice quality. Otolaryngologists and speech pathologists use the term *dysphonia* to more accurately portray abnormal voice quality and localize the disease process to the laryngeal structures. Simply put, hoarseness is the symptom and dysphonia is the corresponding sign. A dysphonic patient will have a breathy, strained, rough, raspy, tremulous, or weak voice. A complaint of hoarseness should be evaluated thoughtfully, because it may represent a significant underlying disorder. Appropriate referral to an otolaryngologist for direct visualization of the laryngeal structures is warranted if hoarseness persists longer than a few weeks.

Pathophysiology

The evaluation of hoarseness depends on an understanding of the pertinent anatomy and normal physiology involved with voice production. The vocal tract can be thought of in three separate compartments: the lungs, the larynx, and the oral cavity. The lungs are the power source for voice production. The larynx, most notably the true vocal folds, are the anatomic site for sound production. Sound is generated by airflow through closely approximated vocal folds. The establishment of a mucosal wave, or undulation of the laryngeal mucosa, generates sounds of varying pitch, quality, and volume. The quality of the sound produced is determined by multiple factors, including the degree of vocal fold opposition, the tension in the laryngeal musculature, and the properties of the vocal fold epithelium itself (47). In the oral cavity, sound produced in the laryngeal structures is further modified by the tongue, lips, and teeth. Strictly speaking, the laryngeal phase of sound production is the site of origin of true hoarseness and dysphonia. The pulmonary portion of vocal production will determine the strength of the sound produced, and the oral cavity is primarily involved in articulation and the refinement of the sound to produce speech. An alteration in the oral phase of vocal production is more appropriately described as dysarthria.

The larynx is comprised of a cartilaginous skeleton, including the epiglottis, thyroid cartilage, cricoid cartilage, and paired arytenoid cartilages. This cartilaginous framework provides for continuity of airflow from the trachea, through the glottis, to the oral tract. The soft tissue structures in the larynx are comprised of laryngeal musculature, including the vocal fold abductors, adductors, and tensors. These muscular structures adjust the coaptation and tension of the vocal folds, which is a major determinant of the quality of sound production. Any alteration in the innervation or function of the laryngeal musculature will result in dysphonia. The mucosal epithelium for most of the larynx is made up of columnar epithelium and mucous-secreting goblet cells, which promote a moist environment for efficient voice production. The true vocal folds are lined with squamous epithelium, which overlies a loose lamina propria (48). This histologic arrangement allows the subglottic airflow to traverse the larynx and produce a mucosal wave in the overlying epithelium, generating sound. Increased viscosity of the loose lamina propria of the vocal folds from dehydration, inflammation, or scarring will result in the need for an increase in the pressure of the airflow through the larynx to establish the vibratory phase of the vocal folds. Adequate hydration of this gelatinous lamina propria layer and the maintenance of a lubricated mucosa of the laryngeal structures is important in determining the quality of laryngeal sound production.

Many local and systemic disorders alter these important elements of the laryngeal environment. With the exception of the cricothyroid muscle, which provides some vocal fold tension, the laryngeal muscles are innervated by the right and left recurrent laryngeal nerves. It is an important anatomic consideration that the recurrent laryngeal nerves, after branching from the main trunks of the vagus nerves, travel in slightly different pathways to ultimately provide laryngeal innervation. The right recurrent laryngeal nerve loops around the right subclavian artery, whereas the left recurrent laryngeal nerve loops around the arch of the aorta, and both travel cephalad to enter the larynx below the thyroid cartilage. The left recurrent laryngeal nerve (but usually not the right one) during a portion of its course traverses the mediastinum and may be impacted by a variety of mediastinal lesions. Any lesion along the course of the recurrent laryngeal nerves may result in paralysis of the ipsilateral vocal fold. It is also important to know that the motor fibers of the vagus nerve originate in the nucleus ambiguous of the medulla, and any neurologic process at the brainstem level will also impact vocal function (49). Sound production also requires the coordination of efforts between the expiratory thoracic musculature and laryngeal musculature.

Differential Diagnosis and Evaluation

The differential diagnosis of hoarseness is broad, as shown in Table 111.3. A careful history and physical examination, and sometimes visualization of the laryngeal structures (see above), allows a diagnosis to be made in most cases.

Initial evaluation starts with characterizing a patient's voice complaints. A rough and raspy sound suggests a mucosal irregularity, whereas a breathiness or weakness of the voice suggests an incomplete closure of the true vocal folds (i.e., vocal fold paralysis or an endolaryngeal mass). It is also important to listen

Table 111.3. Common Problems That Can Cause Hoarseness

Laryngitis
Acute viral
Gastroesophageal reflux
Postnasal drip/sinusitis
Benign lesions
Vocal nodules
Vocal polyps
Laryngeal papilloma
Squamous cell carcinoma
Vocal fold paralysis
Functional dysphonia
Hypothyroidism

carefully to the patient to determine if the complaint of hoarseness is related to an articulation or resonance disturbance of the oral phase of speech or to a lack of speech volume resulting from an inadequate pulmonary phase of voice production. The duration of symptoms is important, because acute voice alteration may represent a self-limited process such as a viral upper respiratory tract infection, whereas chronic and progressive hoarseness is more concerning for an underlying condition. Fluctuation of the hoarseness implies that a fixed lesion (i.e., polyp, nodule, or tumor) is not present.

Any inciting event, such as recent voice abuse, neck trauma, or intubation, should be elicited. Recent *voice abuse* suggests that a vocal fold hemorrhage or nodules can be the cause of the persistent hoarseness. Hoarseness that develops after a single event of excessive vocal use or coughing often represents an acute vocal fold hemorrhage. Vocal fold polyps are usually pedunculated masses and are often associated with smoking. They are located on the free edge of the true vocal fold and are extremely common benign lesions causing hoarseness in the adult patient. *Neck trauma* can result in arytenoid dislocation, laryngeal fractures, or even recurrent laryngeal nerve paralysis. Recent *endotracheal intubation* can also produce persistent hoarseness from arytenoid dislocation, recurrent nerve paresis (or paralysis), and traumatic laryngeal granulomas.

Voice complaints that are worse in the morning and resolve during the day are suggestive of laryngeal irritation from *gastroesophageal reflux disease*. Patients with laryngeal manifestations of gastroesophageal reflux disease often do not have the classic symptoms of heartburn and indigestion (50). Associated symptoms should also be carefully investigated. Dysphagia or aspiration associated with hoarseness may indicate that a *laryngeal tumor* is present or that a neurologic process, such as *recurrent laryngeal nerve paralysis*, is the culprit. Persistent otalgia with a normal ear examination is also worrisome for referred pain from a supraglottic or glottic malignancy. Such pain is referred to the area of the ear via the vagus nerve, which, in addition to supplying the laryngeal structures, contributes to the innervation of the external ear canal. *Allergic rhinitis or chronic sinusitis* with postnasal drainage may also promote chronic laryngeal irritation and hoarseness. It is important to elucidate past surgical history, because an endotracheal intubation may damage the larynx, and many *surgical procedures* place the recurrent laryngeal nerve at risk (Table 111.4).

Hypothyroidism may produce significant hoarseness due to edema of the laryngeal submucosal lamina propria (51). Medications also may be implicated in voice disturbances. Aspirin, nonsteroidal anti-inflammatory agents, and anticoagulants may promote vocal fold hemorrhage. Antihistamines and diuretics may produce upper airway dryness, which also will adversely affect the voice (52).

Social history is also important in evaluating patients with hoarseness and dysphonia. Exposure to tobacco smoke, ethanol, or environmental pollutants directly causes laryngeal irritation and increases the risk for laryngeal carcinoma. Cigarette smoking and alcohol also contribute to the drying of secretions and chronic inflammation. An understanding of the patient's activities that involve the voice (e.g., a teacher, singer, or avid sports fan) is pertinent to diagnosis and to treatment. Patients who use their voice professionally often require early and aggressive intervention and specialized long-term care. Such patients should be referred to an otolaryngologist. The presence of a loud work environment or frequent contact with individuals who have hearing loss may require a patient to speak in an unnaturally loud voice, which can promote the formation of vocal fold nodules.

Table 111.4. Surgical Procedures with a Risk of Laryngeal Denervation

Carotid endarterectomy
Anterior cervical fusion
Thyroidectomy
Esophagectomy
Tracheal surgery
Skull base surgery
Thoracic aneurysm repair
Cardiac surgery

Physical Examination

A focused head and neck examination should be performed on patients who present with a complaint of hoarseness. Otoscopic examination helps to identify whether associated ear complaints are due to otologic pathology or may be referred from a laryngeal process. Nasal examination may demonstrate abnormal secretions, polyps, or purulence, suggesting chronic rhinitis or sinusitis. Oral cavity and oropharyngeal examination may reveal "cobblestoning" or lymphoid hypertrophy of the posterior pharyngeal wall suggestive of chronic postnasal drainage. The neck should be carefully palpated for thyroid masses, diffuse thyromegaly, or lymphadenopathy. Cranial nerve evaluation, to determine if abnormalities are present that may be associated with a vagal neuropathy, is also indicated. The presence or absence of manifestations of hypothyroidism (see Chapter 80) should be assessed.

When a current or recent upper respiratory tract infection is identified and hoarseness has been of a short duration (less than 2 weeks), it is reasonable to defer direct laryngeal examination. In this situation, hoarseness likely is a result of acute viral laryngitis, which should resolve in a few weeks. If it does not, referral to an otolaryngologist is appropriate.

Examination by an Otolaryngologist

A patient with hoarseness that has persisted for more than 2 to 3 weeks should undergo visualization of the laryngeal structures by an otolaryngologist. Any gross abnormality of the larynx, such as polyps, nodules, tumor, or vocal fold motion impairment, usually can be identified by indirect mirror examination. In approximately 10% to 15% of patients, the laryngeal structures are not fully visualized because of the patient's anatomy (e.g., an overhanging or retroflexed epiglottis) or an overactive gag reflex. If it is necessary for complete visualization of laryngeal structures, the otolaryngologist will use transnasal flexible fiberoptic laryngoscopy. This procedure is easy to perform, is well tolerated, and usually lasts less than 5 minutes. This endoscopic examination may be recorded and documented by video. Only occasionally will patients need to be taken to the operating room for direct laryngoscopy. This relatively brief procedure requires general endotracheal intubation but allows a very detailed microscopic examination of the entire larynx and biopsy of any suspicious lesion.

Ancillary Testing

Thyroid function tests should be done if hypothyroidism is suspected (see Chapter 80). Video stroboscopy is a specialized examination performed by an otolaryngologist that requires flash instrumentation that can be synchronized to the patient's voice (53). The larynx is visualized under a stroboscopic light source that displays slow motion and allows a very finely detailed examination of the mucosal wave of the true vocal fold. This examination may reveal subtle neurologic deficits with inadequate glottic closure, submucosal cysts, and mucosal abnormalities such as dysplasia or tumor. In the event that a vocal fold paralysis is noted and there is no previous surgical procedure that would put the recurrent laryngeal nerve at risk, an imaging study such as a CT or magnetic resonance image (preferably from the skull base through the entire course of the recurrent laryngeal nerve), should be performed to rule out a neoplastic process. It is important that evaluation of left true vocal fold paralysis include the aortic arch, because this represents the course of the recurrent laryngeal nerve. If dysphagia is present, a barium swallow or esophagoscopy may be pertinent to evaluate for an esophageal neoplasm, which also may be implicated in recurrent laryngeal nerve paralysis.

Management

Treatment for hoarseness depends on its cause (Table 111.3). Inflammatory processes and *acute laryngitis* are often self-limited. It is important to note that true vocal folds have no lymphatic elements so resolution of edema and restoration of a truly normal voice may take some time. The patient should maintain adequate hydration and avoid the use of antihistamines and decongestants, which may have a drying effect and delay recovery. If the symptom persists and there is an associated sore throat, treatment for chronic or relapsing pharyngitis may be indicated (see Chapter 33).

Laryngeal complications of *gastroesophageal reflux* are best managed by use of proton pump inhibitors in a higher dose than used for usual esophageal gastroesophageal reflux disease, because this is an atypical or extraesophageal manifestation of gastroesophageal reflux disease that requires more aggressive therapy (see Chapter 44). Patients will often improve after a 6- to 8-week course of proton pump inhibitor therapy, although it may take up to 6 months for these symptoms to resolve completely and the laryngeal examination to normalize. *Chronic laryngitis from toxic exposure* such as cigarette smoke is best treated by smoking cessation or the elimination of other inciting agents. Vocal hygiene measures are important adjunctive treatments for all causes of hoarseness (see below).

Anatomic Lesions

The treatment of *vocal fold polyps* is simple surgical excision by suspension microlaryngoscopy. *Vocal fold nodules* often occur on the free edge of the vocal fold secondary to voice abuse. These nodules often resolve with appropriate speech therapy and voice rest. Occasionally, they have to be excised surgically if they progress to a fibrotic stage, when resolution by conservative measures is unlikely. Postintubation lesions such as true *vocal fold granulomas* are present in the posterior glottis where the endotracheal tube was positioned. A granuloma can also form in the posterior glottis with gastroesophageal reflux or extreme vocal abuse or in patients with chronic and marked cough syndromes. These granulomas can usually be ameliorated by speech therapy or aggressive treatment for gastroesophageal reflux. These lesions, unless they are obstructing the airway, rarely require surgical treatment. Human papilloma virus can cause recurrent respiratory *papillomas* that affect the glottic larynx; although they are present in all age groups, they are usually seen in children. This viral illness has no curative medical therapy at present. The recommended therapy is frequent surgical excisions often using a carbon dioxide laser. These lesions will recur at an interval, and serial excisions are often required.

Neoplastic lesions, such as laryngeal tumors, cause hoarseness from the tumor mass itself, interruption of the normal mucosal wave or by contiguous spread, and true vocal fold paralysis. These lesions are often easily detected on laryngeal examination and require operative biopsy for a tissue diagnosis. Treatment often requires surgical excision, irradiation, or both. Vocal fold paralysis with no obvious etiology is suggested by a previous surgical procedure that placed the recurrent nerve at risk and requires workup (see above) to rule out an underlying neoplasm anywhere along the tract of the recurrent laryngeal nerve. If no lesions are found and the paralysis is accompanied by significant hoarseness with a harsh breathy voice or aspiration, a procedure can be performed to medialize this vocal fold toward the normal opposite side, either by an injection of Gelfoam into the true vocal fold or by operative introduction of a spacer (medialization laryngoplasty) (54).

Vocal Hygiene

Patients with any process causing hoarseness should be educated about voice abuse. They should be advised to avoid straining their voices by using a loud voice or harsh whispering. It is important for these patients to maintain adequate hydration (e.g., six or more large glasses of water each day). Caffeine and alcohol should be avoided because of their drying and diuretic effects. Antihistamines and drugs with anticholinergic side effects should also be avoided, because they cause excessive dryness. Guaifenesin (e.g., Robitussin) may also be helpful as a mucolytic.

HICCUPS

Hiccups are a common phenomenon that affects, at some time or another, most individuals. Usually, a bout of hiccups is a mild short-lived annoyance that resolves spontaneously. When hiccups are prolonged (more than 48 hours) or intractable (more than 1 month) it is important to rule out a serious underlying medical illness. Hiccups, sometimes referred to as *singultus,* involve the involuntary spasmodic contraction of the diaphragm. This spasmodic contraction of the diaphragm begins at inspiration, which is suddenly checked by closure of the glottis, giving the characteristic sound of hiccuping (55).

Pathophysiology

For unknown reasons, persistent hiccups in men are found to be caused by a specific organic etiology in over 90% of cases, whereas specific causes are less likely to be found in women after detailed evaluation (56). The afferent portion of the hiccup reflex arc arises from the phrenic and vagus nerves and the thoracic sympathetic chain. There is no discrete central connection for this reflex arc, although it appears to be located somewhere in the spinal cord, between segments C3 and C5. The phrenic nerve provides the efferent limb of the reflex arc. Fluoroscopy reveals that hiccups are most often unilateral, with the left diaphragm being more frequently involved than the right (57). The frequency of hiccups decreases as arterial P_{CO_2} rises, and this is the physiologic basis for the popular hiccup treatment of breathing into a paper bag. The etiology of self-limited hiccups appears to be related mostly to ingestion of food and alcohol and gastric distention. These self-limited hiccups are thought to result from peripheral irritation of the branches of the vagus and phrenic nerve in the upper abdomen (55). Local irritation of the vagus nerve and diaphragm (e.g., by pneumonia, aortic aneurysm, pericarditis, abdominal abscesses, and various thoracic and abdominal tumors) appears to be an important mechanism for development of intractable hiccups. In addition, central nervous system lesions, such as multiple sclerosis; meningitis; and central nervous system neoplasms can also provoke hiccups. Psychogenic factors also may be the cause of intractable hiccups. Stress, conversion reaction, anxiety states, and malingering may all be psychogenic factors in the etiology of hiccups.

Evaluation

A focused history to determine the onset, precipitating factors, and duration of the hiccups is important. Associated medical events, such as trauma, surgery, or recent acute illness, should be elicited. Weight loss, fatigue, or night sweats suggest an underlying malignancy. The presence of hiccups during sleep usually indicates an underlying organic cause, whereas if the hiccups cease during sleep a psychogenic or idiopathic etiology is more likely (56). Any previous bouts of hiccups and the response to therapy should be reviewed and may suggest precipitants and effective treatments.

The head and neck, chest, and abdomen should be examined. The ears should be examined for any external auditory canal abnormality, which may trigger hiccups by irritating the vagally supplied external auditory canal skin. Pharyngitis or oropharyngeal inflammation may also be a trigger for hiccups. A cervical process, such as a thyroid tumor or malignant lymphadenopathy along the course of the recurrent laryngeal nerve in the neck, may also provide a trigger for these episodes. Examination of the chest is important to assess for infection, thoracic aortic aneurysm, pericarditis, or pulmonary or mediastinal tumor. The abdomen should be evaluated for an acute process such as bowel obstruction or abscess or an underlying neoplasm. A detailed neurologic examination should be performed, because early multiple sclerosis is thought to be one of the most frequent neurologic causes of intractable hiccups in young adults (58).

A chest x-ray may be helpful in evaluating patients with hiccups by ruling out pulmonary, mediastinal, or cardiac sources of phrenic, vagal nerve, or diaphragmatic irritation (59,60). Because hyponatremia may cause hiccups, the serum sodium concentration should be measured (61). Other studies may be indicated based on the findings identified by the history and physical examination.

Management

The most important consideration in the management of prolonged and intractable hiccups is to determine the etiology and correct any underlying pathology if possible. Once the instigating cause has resolved, the hiccup bout should also abate. In cases where the cause is idiopathic or not immediately apparent, therapies should be initiated that are specifically directed at terminating hiccups.

Initial efforts to treat hiccups usually involve physical maneuvers. These are performed in an attempt to interrupt the reflex arc. Many of these are folk remedies, such as swallowing rapidly and sequentially small sips of water or inducing a startle reaction. The aforementioned breathing into a paper bag may also be tried. A more established maneuver that can be performed by the clinician is stimulation of the nasopharynx with a red rubber catheter; cessation rates of nearly 100% have been reported with this technique (57).

If physical maneuvers fail, then pharmacologic intervention should be attempted. Unfortunately, most studies related to the use of pharmacologic agents for hiccups have involved only small numbers of patients or relied on anecdotal clinical observations. Chlorpromazine hydrochloride is the most commonly used drug. The mechanism of action is unclear. However, a cure rate for intractable hiccups of almost 80% has been reported (62). Care must be taken when administering chlorpromazine intravenously (25 to 50 mg in 500 to 1,000 mL of normal saline over several hours) or intramuscularly (25 to 50 mg), because postural hypotension is common. If hiccup cessation is achieved with initial parenteral treatment, then 25 to 50 mg orally twice daily is recommended for 7 to 10 days (63).

Metoclopramide is the second drug of choice for intractable hiccups, with 10 mg given as an intravenous infusion over 1 to 2 minutes. If successful, an oral maintenance dose of 10 mg four times daily may be used for 7 to 10 days. Success rates of approximately 80% with metoclopramide have been reported (64). Many anticonvulsants also have been reported to be effective for treating hiccups, including phenytoin, phenobarbital, carbamazepine, and valproic acid. Phenytoin is the most efficacious in patients who have a central neurologic cause of their hiccups (65). In patients with multiple sclerosis, carbamazepine has been reported to be an effective agent for treating associated hiccups (66).

Less conventional therapies, such as hypnosis, psychotherapy, and acupuncture, may be tried if physical maneuvers and drug therapy fails (67,68). Surgical disruption of the phrenic nerve is considered only as a last resort. Before embarking on this mode of therapy, it is important for the otolaryngologist to identify which leaflet of the diaphragm is involved. An initial attempt at blocking the phrenic nerve with a local anesthetic usually should be performed to determine if phrenic nerve surgery ultimately would be fruitful.

General References*

Bailey BJ, ed. Head and neck surgery—otolaryngology. 3rd ed. Philadelphia: Lippincott Williams & Wilkins, 2001.
Standard textbook for nose and throat problems.

Bromley SM. Smell and taste disorders: a primary care approach. Am Fam Physician 2000;61:427.
Complementary specialty and primary care approaches to disorders of smell and taste.

Ossguthorpe JD, Ossoff RH, eds. Otolaryngology for the internist. Med Clin North Am 1999;83.
A useful compendium on ear, nose, and throat problems.

Rousseau P. Hiccups. South Med J 1995;88:175.
A useful update.

Seiden AM, Duncan HJ, Smith DV. Office management of taste and smell disorders. Otolaryngol Clin North Am 1992;25:817.
Specialty approach to disorders of taste and smell.

Simpson CB, Fleming DJ. Medical and vocal history in the evaluation of dysphonia. Otolaryngol Clin North Am 2000;33:719.
A framework for evaluation of hoarseness.

*Bold print (general references) and bold numerals (specific references) denote published controlled clinical trials, meta-analyses, or consensus-based recommendations.

Specific References

1. Jackson KR, Jackson RT. Factors associated with active, refractory epistaxis. Arch Otolaryngol Head Neck Surg 1988;114:862.
2. Alvi A, Joyner-Triplett N. Acute epistaxis: how to spot the source and stop the flow. Postgrad Med 1996;99:83.
3. Pollice PA, Yoder MG. Epistaxis: a retrospective review of hospitalized patients. Otolaryngol Head Neck Surg 1997;117:49.
4. O'Reilly BJ, Simpson DC, Dharmeratnam R. Recurrent epistaxis and nasal septal deviation in young adults. Clin Otolaryngol 1996;21:12.
5. Sessions RB. Nasal hemorrhage. Otolaryngol Clin North Am 1973;6:727.
6. Dhillons RS, East CA. Ear, nose and throat and head and neck surgery. London: Churchill Livingstone, 1994.
7. Herkner H, Laggner AN, Mullner M, et al. Hypertension in patients presenting with epistaxis. Ann Emerg Med 2000;35:126.
8. Milam SB, Cooper RL. Extensive bleeding following extractions in a patient undergoing chronic hemodialysis. Oral Surg Oral Med Oral Pathol 1983;55:14.
9. Simpson HK, Baird J, Allison M, et al. Long-term use of low molecular weight heparin tinzaparin in haemodialysis. Haemostasis 1996;26:90.
10. McGarry GW. Drug induced epistaxis? J R Soc Med 1990;83:812.
11. Akama H, Hama N, Amano K. Epistaxis induced by a nonsteroidal anti-inflammatory drug? J R Soc Med 1990;83:538.
12. Krempl GA, Noorily AD. Use of oxymetazoline in the management of epistaxis. Ann Otol Rhinol Laryngol 1995;104:704.
13. Viducich RA, Blanda MP, Gerson LW. Posterior epistaxis: clinical features and acute complications. Ann Emerg Med 1995;25:592.
14. Peretta LJ, Denslow BL, Brown CG. Emergency evaluation and management of epistaxis. Emerg Med Clin North Am 1987;5:265.
15. Shaw CB, Wax MK, Wetmore SJ. Epistaxis: a comparison of treatment. Otolaryngol Head Neck Surg 1993;109:60.
16. Small M, Moran AG. Epistaxis and arterial ligation. J Laryngol Otol 1984;98:281.
17. Carr ME, Gabriel DA. Nasal packing with porcine fatty tissue for epistaxis complicated by qualitative platelet disorders. J Emerg Med 1985;3:449.
18. Ernst RJ, Bulas RV, Gaskill-Shipley M, et al. Endovascular therapy of intractable epistaxis complicated by carotid artery occlusive disease. Am J Neuroradiol 1995;16:1463.
19. Jones TM, Ah-See KW. Surgical and non-surgical interventions used primarily for snoring. The Cochrane Database of Systematic Reviews. The Cochrane Library, http://www.cochranelibrary.com, 2001.
20. Hoffstein V. Snoring. Chest 1996;109:201.
21. Hoffstein V, Mateika S, Anderson D. Snoring: is it in the ear of the beholder. Sleep 1994;17:522.
22. Perez-Padilla JR, West P, Kryger M. Snoring in normal young adults: prevalence in sleep stages and associated changes in oxygen saturation, heart rate, and breathing pattern. Sleep 1987;10:249.
23. Teculescu DB, Mauffret-Stephan F. Familial predispositions to snoring [Letter]. Thorax 1994;49:95.
24. Loh NK, Dinner DS, Foldvary N, et al. Do patients with obstructive sleep apnea wake up with headaches? Arch Intern Med 1999;159:1765.
25. Breathe Right nasal strips to decrease snoring. Med Lett Drugs Ther 1994;36:100.
26. O'Sullivan RA, Hillman DR, Mateljan R, et al. Mandibular advancement splint: an appliance to treat snoring and obstructive sleep apnea. Am J Respir Crit Care Med 1995;151:194.
27. Hoffstein V, Mateika S, Halko S, et al. Reduction in snoring with phosphocholinamine, a long-acting tissue-lubricating agent. Am J Otolaryngol 1987;8:236.
28. Series F, Marc I. Effects of protriptyline on snoring characteristics. Chest 1993;104:14.
29. Rauscher H, Formanek D, Zwick H. Nasal continuous positive airway pressure for nonapneic snoring? Chest 1995;107:58.
30. Fujita S, Conway W, Zorick F, et al. Surgical correction of anatomic abnormalities in obstructive sleep apnea syndrome: uvulopalatopharyngoplasty. Otolaryngol Head Neck Surg 1981;89:923.

31. Littlefield PD, Mair EA. Snoring surgery: which one is best for you? Ear Nose Throat J 1999;78:861.
32. Katsantonis GP, Friedman WH, Rosenblum BN, et al. The surgical treatment of snoring: a patient's perspective. Laryngoscope 1990;100:138.
33. Croft CB, Golding-Wood DG. Uses and complications of uvulopalatopharyngoplasty. J Laryngol Otol 1990;104:871.
34. Astor FC, Hanft KL, Benson C, et al. Analysis of short-term outcome after office-based laser-assisted uvulopalatoplasty. Otolaryngol Head Neck Surg 1998;118:478.
35. Powell NB, Riley RW, Troell RJ, et al. Radio frequency volumetric reduction of the tongue: a porcine pilot study for the treatment of obstructive sleep apnea syndrome. Chest 1997; 111:1348.
36. Pazos G, Mair EA. Complications of radiofrequency ablation in the treatment of sleep-disordered breathing. Otolaryngol Head Neck Surg 2001;125:462.
37. Standards of Practice Committee of the American Sleep Disorders Association. Practice parameters for the use of laser-assisted uvulopalatoplasty. Sleep 1994;17:744.
38. Mott AE, Leopold DA. Disorders in taste and smell. Med Clin North Am 1991;75:1321.
39. Anholt RR. Molecular physiology of olfaction. Am J Physiol 1989;257:C1043.
40. Pryse-Phillips W. Disturbances in the sense of smell is psychiatric patients. Proc R Soc Med 1975;68:472.
41. Ackerman BH, Kasbekar N. Disturbances of taste and smell induced by drugs. Pharmacotherapy 1997;17:482.
42. Costanzo R, Becker DP. Smell and taste disorders in head injury and neurosurgery patients. In: Meiselman HL, Rivlin RS, eds. Clinical measurement of taste and smell. New York: Macmillan, 1986:565.
43. Ophir D, Guterman A, Gross-Isseroff R. Changes in smell acuity induced by radiation exposure of the olfactory mucosa. Arch Otolaryngol Head Neck Surg 1998;114:853.
44. Smith DV. Taste and smell dysfunction. In: Paperella MM, Shumrick DA, Gluckman JL, et al., eds. Otolaryngology—head and neck. 3rd ed. Vol. 3. Philadelphia: WB Saunders, 1990:1911.
45. Duncan JH, Seiden AM, Paik SI, et al. Differences among patients with smell impairment resulting from head trauma, nasal disease, or prior upper respiratory infection. Chem Senses 1991;16.
46. Schecter PJ, Friedewald WT, Bronzert OA, et al. Idiopathic hypogeusia: a description of the syndrome and a single-blind study with zinc sulfate. Int Rev Neurobiol Suppl 1972;1:125.
47. Jiang J, Lin E, Hanson DG. Vocal fold physiology. Otolaryngol Clin North Am 2000;33:699.
48. Hirano M. Morphological structure of the vocal cord as a vibrator and its variations. Folia Phoniatr (Basel) 1974;26:89.
49. Furstenburg AC, Magielski JG. A motor pattern in the nucleus ambiguus: its clinical significance. Ann Otol Rhinol Laryngol 1972;64:788.
50. Koufman JA. The otolaryngologic manifestations of gastroesophageal reflux disease (GERD): a clinical investigation of 225 patients using ambulatory 24-hour pH monitoring and an experimental investigation of the role of acid and pepsin in the development of laryngeal injury. Laryngoscope 1991;101[4 Pt 2 Suppl 53]:1.
51. Ritter FN. Endocrinology. In: Paparella M, Shumrick D, eds. Otolaryngology. Philadelphia: WB Saunders, 1973:727.
52. Sataloff RT, Hawkshaw M, Rosen DC. Medications: effects and side effects in professional voice users. In: Sataloff RT, ed. Professional voice. San Diego: Singular Publishing Group, 1997:457.
53. Sataloff RT, Speigel JR, Hawkshaw MJ. Strobovideolaryngoscopy: results and clinical value. Ann Otol Rhinol Laryngol 1991;100:725.
54. Wanamaker JR, Netterville JL, Ossoff RH. Phonosurgery: silastic medialization for unilateral vocal fold paralysis. Op Techn Otolaryngol Head Neck Surg 1993;4:207.
55. Haubrich WS. Hiccup. In: Bockus ML, ed. Gastroenterology. 4th ed. Philadelphia: WB Saunders, 1985:195.
56. Sovadjian JV, Cain JC. Intractable hiccups: etiologic factors in 220 cases. Postgrad Med 1968;43:72.
57. Salem MR, Baraka A, Rattenborg CC, et al. Treatment of hiccups by pharyngeal stimulation in anesthetized and conscious subjects. JAMA 1967;202:126.
58. Birkhead R, Friedman J. Hiccups and vomiting as initial manifestations of multiple sclerosis [Letter]. J Neurol Neurosurg Psychiatry 1987;50:232.
59. Nathan M, Leshner R, Keller A. Intractable hiccups. Laryngoscope 1980;90:1612.
60. Graham D. Esophageal motor abnormality during hiccup. Gastroenterology 1986;90:2039.
61. Jones J, Lloyd T, Cannon L. Persistent hiccups as an unusual manifestation of hyponatremia. J Emerg Med 1987;5:283.
62. Davignon A, Lauieux G, Genest J. Chlorpromazine in the treatment of persistent hiccough. Union Med Can 1955;84: 282.
63. Loft LM, Ward RF. Hiccups: a case presentation and etiologic review. Arch Otolaryngol Head Neck Surg 1992;118:1115.
64. Middleton RSW. The use of metoclopramide in the elderly. Postgrad Med J 1973;49[Suppl]:90.
65. Laing T, Marariu M, Malik G, et al. Intractable hiccups and a posterior fossa arteriovenous malformation: a case report. Henry Ford Hosp Med J 1981;29:145.
66. McFarling DA, Susac JO. Hoquet diabolique: intractable hiccups as a manifestation of multiple sclerosis. Neurology 1979;29: 797.
67. Smedley WP, Barnes WT. Postoperative use of hypnosis on a cardiovascular service. JAMA 1966;197:371.
68. Wensel LO. Acupuncture in medical practice. Reston, VA: Reston Publishing, 1980:200.

CHAPTER 112

Common Problems of the Teeth and Oral Cavity

DOUGLAS K. MACLEOD, DMD

The purpose of this chapter is to provide guidelines for recognizing, treating, and referring patients with acute dental and oral problems and to increase awareness of chronic dental and oral problems that may require referral and treatment. These types of problems are often neglected by the patient because of fear or ignorance about possible corrective treatment, anticipated pain from the procedure, or the anticipated cost of treatment.

ORAL EXAMINATION

The systematic examination of the oral cavity should include lips, cheeks (buccal mucosa), hard and soft palate, salivary ducts (parotid duct orifice in the buccal mucosa opposite the upper second molars and submandibular duct orifice beside the lingual frenulum), tonsillar area, tongue, floor of the mouth, gingiva, and teeth, noting the normal structures and any deviations from normal. A dental examination includes an evaluation of the number (20 in the primary dentition and 32 in the permanent dentition; Fig. 112.1), position, and arrangement of the teeth and a check for caries (see below), erosions, abrasions, and fractures. It is important to examine the gingiva completely. The normal healthy gingiva is firm, pink, and nontender and does not bleed on palpation or probing. The parts of a tooth and its adjacent structures are shown in Fig. 112.2.

ACUTE DENTAL AND ORAL PROBLEMS

Toothaches (Pulpitis)

Presentation

Patients with toothache have a large carious lesion (see Dental Caries, below), a large restoration (filling), or a combination of both. In the early stages, there is inflammation involving a portion of the pulp tissue (the central portion of the tooth, containing vital soft tissue; Fig. 112.2A).

There is severe pain in response to thermal stimuli, particularly cold, and this pain persists for longer than 15 seconds after the stimulus is removed. As the area of inflammation increases, the pain becomes more severe; it may radiate to the suborbital area, the side of the face, or the ear. When total necrosis of the pulp occurs, sensitivity to thermal stimuli is lost. If, at this point, the inflammatory exudate cannot escape into the oral cavity, the pressure is released via the root apex, and there is exquisite sensitivity to percussion of the crown of the tooth. The signs and symptoms of pulpitis may be confused with pericoronitis (painful wisdom teeth, see below) or periodontitis (see below), and without further diagnostic aids (i.e., dental x-rays) it may be difficult to differentiate between these conditions.

If pulpitis is not treated, complications may occur, ranging from a localized alveolar abscess (an abscess of the bony supporting structure of the teeth) to facial cellulitis. The rate and type of complication depends on the location of the affected tooth, host resistance, and virulence of the bacteria present.

Treatment

Depending on the situation when the patient is seen, one has three options. For patients who are afebrile and have no extraoral swelling (swelling that produces facial asymmetry) or intraoral swelling (swelling that disrupts the supporting alveolar bone and soft tissue), analgesics (acetaminophen 650 mg and/or codeine 30 mg or immediate-release oxycodone 5 mg every 4 hours) and referral within 24 hours are indicated. When slight extraoral or intraoral swelling or a low-grade temperature elevation is present, antibiotics (penicillin V 250 mg or, for patients allergic to penicillin, Clindamycin 300 mg every 6 hours) should be added, and the patient should be seen by a dentist within 12 to 24 hours. Patients with temperatures greater than 101°F (38.5°C) with intraoral or extraoral swelling causing facial asymmetry need immediate consultation and treatment by a dentist. Treatment of these types of problems varies from extraction of the affected tooth, root canal therapy (endodontics), or incision and drainage to hospital admission for intravenous antibiotics for facial cellulitis.

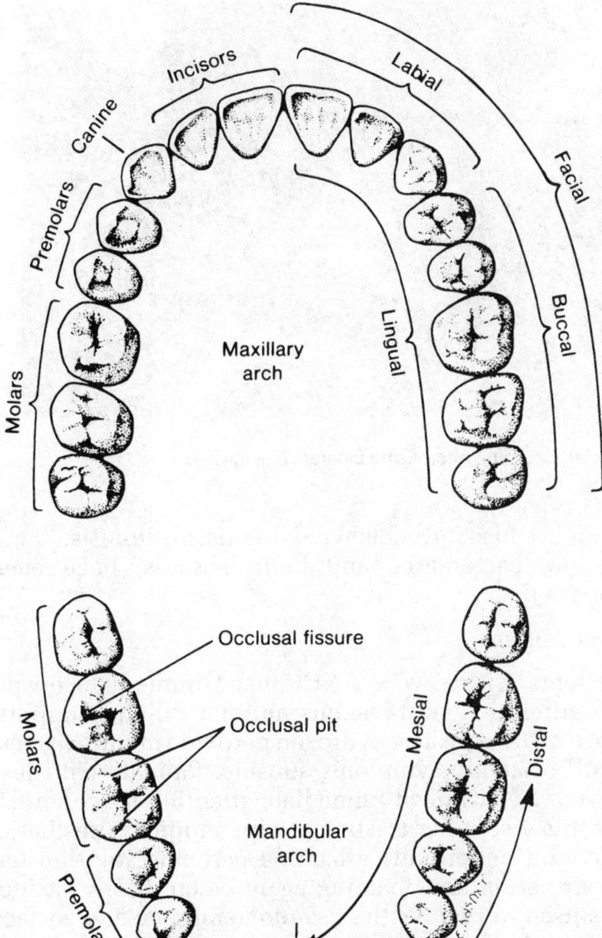

Figure 112.1. Permanent dentition.

Pericoronitis (Third Molar or Wisdom Tooth Pain)

Presentation

Pericoronitis is acute inflammation of the tissue around the crown of a partially erupted tooth. Patients with pericoronitis are usually between the ages of 15 and 25, although rarely the condition can be seen in older patients if they still have their third molars (see below). The patient may give a history of subacute episodes of pain of the gingiva that partially covers the crown of an incompletely erupted tooth. The tooth most often affected is the mandibular third molar (wisdom tooth). The space between the crown of the tooth and the overlying gingival flap is an ideal area for the accumulation of food and bacteria; this leads to inflammation. The flap is traumatized by contact with the tooth in the opposing jaw, usually the maxillary third molar, and the inflammation is aggravated.

The patient describes pain that radiates to the ear, throat, and floor of the mouth. He or she complains of a foul taste, and there is swelling of the affected area so that he cannot close the jaw properly. In severe cases, pain spreading to the oropharynx and base of the tongue makes it difficult to swallow. The gingival tissue is markedly red, swollen, and tender (Fig. 112.3A). Occasionally, tender lymphadenopathy and systemic manifestations (fever, leukocytosis, and malaise) are present. Peritonsillar abscess, cellulitis, and Ludwig angina (cellulitis of the floor of the mouth) are possible complications.

Treatment

In afebrile patients, one needs only to make a dental referral and prescribe analgesics. Febrile patients should be treated with antibiotics (penicillin V 500 mg or, for patients allergic to penicillin, Clindamycin 300 mg every 6 hours), moderate analgesics (acetaminophen 650 mg and/or codeine 30 mg or immediate-release oxycodone 5 mg every 4 to 6 hours), and chlorhexidine gluconate 0.12% oral rinse and brush with a soft toothbrush twice a day (Peridex or Periogard, by prescription); the rinse should be expectorated after use. All patients should be seen by a dentist within 24 hours. Depending on many factors, the dentist either excises or debrides the flap or removes the partially erupted lower tooth. The preferred treatment for third molars that are erupting in a position that produces poor occlusion is to remove the traumatizing maxillary third molar tooth and allow the infected flap to heal. The mandibular tooth is then removed 7 to 10 days later, after the acute infection has resolved. When

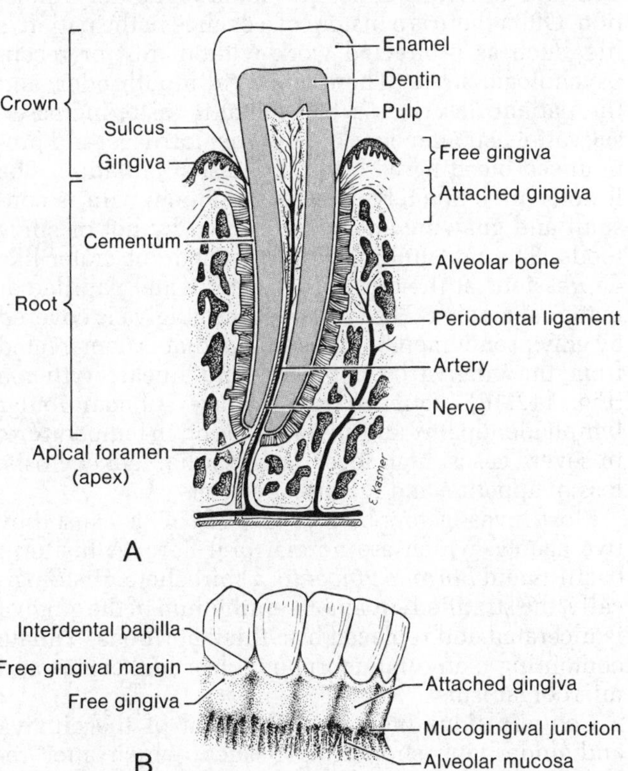

Figure 112.2. Structure of normal teeth and gingiva. A: A tooth and its parts. B: Teeth and gingiva.

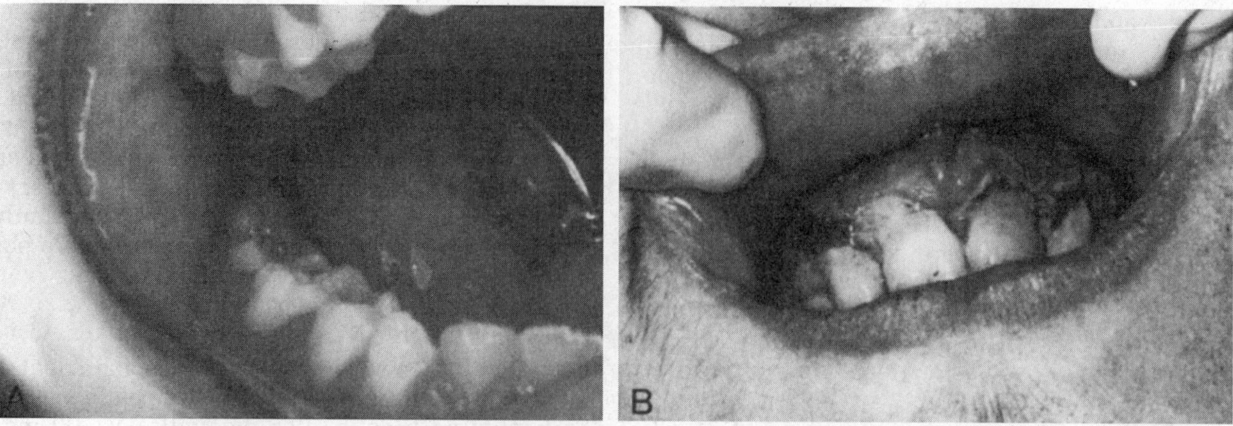

Figure 112.3. A: Pericoronitis of the mandibular third molar. **B:** Acute necrotizing ulcerative gingivitis.

pericoronitis involves eruption of third molars that are in good position for occlusion, the inflamed gingival flap is removed and the teeth are left in place.

Acute Necrotizing Ulcerative Gingivitis (Vincent Infection, Trench Mouth)

Acute necrotizing ulcerative gingivitis (ANUG) may occur at any age, but it is more common among young to middle-aged adults.

Presentation

ANUG has a sudden onset and is usually associated with a debilitating illness or acute respiratory infection. Often there is a history of a change in the patient's life, such as protracted work without rest or recent psychologic stress. There is a fetid mouth odor, and the patient describes a foul metallic taste, increased salivation, spontaneous gingival hemorrhage, and pronounced bleeding with the slightest stimulation. The lesions are extremely sensitive to touch; pain is constant and gnawing and is intensified by hot or spicy foods. The oral findings are punched-out crater-like depressions at the crest of the interdental papillae or marginal gingiva. The surface of the gingiva is covered by gray pseudomembranous slough that is demarcated from the gingiva by a pronounced linear erythema (Fig. 112.3B). Patients usually have submandibular lymphadenopathy and slight elevation in temperature; in severe cases, high fever, tachycardia, leukocytosis, loss of appetite, and malaise are seen.

Most investigators believe that ANUG is caused by two agents, which are normal oral flora: A fusiform bacillus and *Borrelia vincentii,* a spirochete. Histologically, the stratified squamous epithelium of the gingiva is ulcerated and replaced by a thick fibrinous exudate containing many polymorphonuclear leukocytes and microorganisms.

Complications include destruction of the gingiva and underlying supporting tissues, which after repeated episodes of ANUG can result in the loss of teeth. In rare cases, severe sequelae, such as noma (rapidly spreading gangrene of oral and facial tissue, which occurs in the debilitated and nutritionally deficient patient), fusospirochetal meningitis, peritonitis, pneumonia, bacteremia, and brain abscess, have been reported.

Treatment

Patients with severe ANUG need immediate hospital admission, intravenous antibiotics, and supportive care (analgesics, hydrogen peroxide mouthwashes) until systemic symptoms subside. Patients with less severe ANUG need immediate attention by a dentist. At this visit, after treatment with a topical anesthetic, a cotton pellet and carbamide peroxide solution (an oxygenating and foaming agent, such as Gly Oxide) are used to remove the pseudomembrane and surface debris. Antimicrobials are usually prescribed for a few days by the dentist. After irrigation with warm water, the superficial calculus is removed. Patients are instructed to avoid tobacco and alcohol, to rinse with warm water and chlorhexidine gluconate 0.12% twice daily, and to confine toothbrushing to the removal of surface debris. When these instructions are followed after effective removal of all irritants by the dentist, a patient usually improves markedly within 5 days. If after the acute phase the patient does not continue periodic dental care, ANUG may recur and lead to eventual tooth loss.

Recurrent Aphthous Stomatitis

Aphthous ulcers, also called *canker sores,* occur at some time in 20% to 50% of the adult population, are slightly more common in females, have familial tendencies, and occur most often during the winter and spring (1). Recurrent aphthous stomatitis (RAS) was once thought to be a recurrent infection by the herpes simplex virus (HSV), but that is not the case; the cause of the condition is still unknown.

Presentation

Aphthous stomatitis is characterized by superficial ulcerations on the mucous membranes of the lips, cheek, tongue, floor of the mouth, palate, and gingiva. This condition begins with a prodromal burning 1 to 48 hours before the appearance of discrete vesicles, which are approximately 2 to 5 mm in diameter and are painful. After 2 days, they rupture and form saucer-like ulcers that consist of a red or grayish red central portion and an elevated rim-like periphery. There may be a single lesion or multiple ulcers.

The lesions heal spontaneously within 7 to 10 days. As a rule, the lesions are larger than those seen in acute herpetic gingivostomatitis (see below) and do not exhibit the diffuse gingival involvement or systemic symptoms seen in that condition.

RAS occurs in the following forms:

- *Occasional aphthae:* a single lesion, at intervals from months to years, that heals uneventfully;
- *Acute multiple aphthae:* acute episode that persists for weeks, with lesions developing sequentially at different sites in the mouth, often associated with acute gastrointestinal disorders;
- *Chronic recurrent aphthae:* one or more lesions always present for years.

Treatment

Treatment of aphthae is symptomatic. A mouthwash containing equal parts of Benadryl suspension and Kaopectate (Benadryl 5 mg/mL mixed with an equal amount of Kaopectate, prepared by a pharmacist) is helpful in reducing the pain, as is viscous Xylocaine applied by cotton-tip applicator to painful lesions. Kenalog in Orabase (triamcinolone acetonide) can help limit the extent of ulceration that will develop. The Orabase aspect of this product is a paste specially designed to adhere to the surface of oral lesions.

In more severe cases, tetracycline has been successful in decreasing pain and duration of the ulcers; the patient should be instructed to empty a 250-mg capsule in 50 mL of water and to use this as a rinse, which is then swallowed, three or four times a day for 5 to 7 days. The patient should be encouraged to take sufficient amounts of nonirritating liquids or soft food to maintain hydration and nutrition. Intake may be facilitated by using a straw to prevent contact with the painful ulcers. Based on empiric experience, the amino acid L-lysine may also help reduce symptoms. The patient should be instructed to take orally 1,000 to 1,500 mg with each meal during prodromal symptoms and on the days lesions are present and then as a preventive measure, 500 mg with each meal indefinitely.

Acute Herpetic Gingivostomatitis

Acute herpetic gingivostomatitis occurs most often in infants and children below the age of 6 years, and it is equally common in males and females. It is caused by HSV, and most oral infections are caused by HSV type 1. However, it also occurs in older patients, including (rarely) the elderly. Most adults have developed immunity to HSV as a result of childhood infection, usually inapparent. Although recurrent acute herpetic gingivostomatitis has been reported, it does not usually recur unless immunity has been altered by a debilitating systemic disease.

Presentation

Acute herpetic gingivostomatitis appears as a diffuse, erythematous, shiny involvement of the gingiva and the adjacent oral mucosa, with varying degrees of edema and gingival bleeding. In the initial stage it is characterized by the presence of discrete spherical gray vesicles that may occur in the gingiva, labial and buccal mucosa, soft palate, pharynx, sublingual mucosa, and tongue. Within 24 hours the vesicles rupture and form small painful ulcers with a red, elevated, halo-like margin and a depressed yellowish or grayish white central portion. Regional lymphadenopathy, fever as high as 105°F (40.5°C), and generalized malaise are common. The course is limited to 7 to 10 days, and the ulcers heal without scarring. This condition is differentiated by the presence of diffuse gingival involvement and systemic symptoms, which are not present in RAS.

Treatment

The treatment is the same as that for RAS (see above). Antibacterial agents are not helpful, and corticosteroids are contraindicated. Idoxuridine has been used successfully in treating immunosuppressed patients with primary herpes infections, but because of toxicity, its use should be limited to such patients, in consultation with a specialist in infectious disease. The role of oral acyclovir in herpetic gingivostomatitis is uncertain. Its use is probably warranted in the management of severe infection, although this should be done in consultation with an infectious disease specialist or a dentist (see Chapter 102 for a discussion of acyclovir).

Herpes Simplex Labialis

Recurrent herpes simplex infections of the lips or perioral area occur in 20% to 40% of the adult population. Evidence suggests that recurrent herpes is not a reinfection but a reactivation of virus that remains latent in the nerve tissue.

Presentation

The natural history of this problem has been well delineated. Most affected subjects have several episodes during an average year. In approximately 60% of episodes, there is prodromal tingling for a number of hours before the appearance of the first vesicles. Pain is moderate to severe during the first 24 hours after appearance of vesicles and then rapidly diminishes. After 48 hours, vesicles are usually replaced by ulcer crusts. The process usually resolves after 7 to 9 days, but lesions may persist as long as 2 weeks. The therapy of this condition is discussed in Chapter 117.

Sialadenitis

Presentation

Sialadenitis is an inflammation of the salivary gland. Patients with sialadenitis experience pain and enlargement of the affected gland. In bacterial sialadenitis, the pain and swelling are not related to eating. The overlying skin may be red and tense, and the affected gland yields a purulent discharge at the duct orifice. Bacterial sialadenitis is more common in children than in adults. Obstructive sialadenitis is more common than bacterial infection of the salivary glands and is associated with salivary stones or a mucous plug. It occurs most often in middle-aged men. The involved gland is enlarged and painful, and the symptoms are more prominent before, during, and soon after eating. The submandibular gland is most often affected (75% of cases), whereas the parotid (20% of cases) and major sublingual glands (5% of cases) are less often involved. Mumps is more common in children but does occur in adults when it often is more severe. The parotid gland is swollen and tender, and there is usually no redness, heat, or discharge. Most often both parotids are involved and, often, other salivary glands. Systemic symptoms are common.

Treatment

Treatment of bacterial sialadenitis consists of heat application (external moist heat packs to the affected gland for 15 to 20 minutes and intraoral warm rinses), analgesics (acetaminophen 650 mg and/or immediate-release oxycodone 5 to 10 mg or codeine 30 mg every 4 to 6 hours), antibiotics (penicillin V 500 mg or, for patients allergic to penicillin, Clindamycin 300 mg every 6 hours for 7 days), and a liquid diet for the first 2 to 3 days.

The management of obstructive sialadenitis is more complex. When this diagnosis is suspected, the patient should be referred to a dentist or otolaryngologist. In cases in which the stone is lodged in the duct, the acute phase is managed in the same manner as is bacterial sialadenitis, and after resolution has begun a sialogram is obtained to determine the extent of the problem. Surgical removal of the stone from the duct is eventually performed to prevent recurrence. In chronic obstructive sialadenitis, surgical excision of the gland is often necessary. The likelihood of recurrence after the first episode is unknown.

Temporomandibular Joint Pain

Several studies of healthy populations have shown that symptoms of temporomandibular joint (TMJ) disorders are present at some time in 25% to 50% of people but are not considered a serious problem by most patients (2). Most (70% to 90%) patients who have these symptoms are women between the ages of 24 and 40. Multiple factors may lead to TMJ pain; there may be a history of stress, bruxism (grinding of teeth), external blows to the jaws, or whiplash injury. TMJ pain may be present at some point in 20% of patients with rheumatoid arthritis. Patients with osteoarthritis of other joints may complain of TMJ clicking and snapping, but pain is usually absent.

Presentation

TMJ disorders are characterized by pain and tenderness in the muscles of mastication and in the TMJ, by crepitus when the joint is moved, and by a decrease in range of motion. In some severe cases there is a noticeable incoordination on the opening and closing of the jaw. This appears as a unilateral shift of the chin upon opening or closing the mouth. Examination may show malocclusion caused by teeth that interfere with the normal movement of the mandible or tenderness of the muscles of mastication.

Treatment

Patients with acute TMJ pain should be managed with moderate analgesics (acetaminophen 650 mg and/or immediate-release oxycodone 5 to 10 mg or codeine 30 mg every 4 to 6 hours) and referral to a dentist within 24 to 48 hours to begin therapy. The dentist's goal is to make the patient aware of the cause of the problem through education. Depending on the severity of symptoms and the state of the patient's dentition, the dentist will prescribe one or a combination of the following: avoidance of excessive jaw motion, moist heat to affected muscles, soft diet, disengagement of upper and lower jaws with a night guard to separate the upper and lower teeth (a hard appliance constructed to fit the individual patient, which is quite costly), therapeutic exercises, and vapocoolant spray (ethyl chloride to decrease muscle pain). In atypical cases, trigger point injections of Xylocaine may be used to distinguish TMJ symptoms from trigeminal neuralgia (see Chapter 87). Once the acute episode has subsided (in about 7 to 14 days) the dentist can detect and eliminate any occlusal interferences and rule out any degenerative joint disease that may have predisposed the patient to TMJ symptoms. In the past, injections of sclerosing agents into the TMJ and condylectomy were tried, but with poor success. In a 10-year study, 97 of 100 patients treated conservatively improved. Of these, 83 had permanent improvement. Of the three patients who had intractable severe symptoms, two required prolonged psychotherapy and one developed systemic arteritis (3).

Local Alveolar Osteitis (Dry Socket)

Local alveolar osteitis (dry socket) is the most common complication of tooth extraction. It occurs in approximately 5% of all tooth extractions, but it is more common after the removal of an impacted third molar. This problem results from the loss of the blood clot located at the site of the extraction. Most often this occurs when the extraction has been difficult and has resulted in considerable trauma to the socket and gum.

Patients with this problem describe intense localized pain 2 or 3 days after an extraction. This pain is caused by irritation of the sensory nerves in the dry exposed bony socket. There is often a foul odor emanating from the socket, but no suppuration is present.

One should control the pain the patient is experiencing with immediate-release oxycodone, 5 to 10 mg or codeine 30 mg every 3 to 4 hours, and acetaminophen, 650 mg three to four times per day. The patient should be referred promptly to a dentist for irrigation and the placement of a dressing. The dentist needs to see the patient every day or 2 for approximately 10 days until the socket becomes reepithelialized. There are no long-term sequelae.

CHRONIC DENTAL AND ORAL PROBLEMS

Periodontal Disease (Pyorrhea)

Periodontal disease is a general term used to describe diseases that destroy the gingival and bony structures that support the teeth (Figs. 112.4 and 112.5). Periodontal disease is usually subdivided into *gingivitis* and *periodontitis*. The major difference between the two is that in periodontitis there is loss of the supporting bony apparatus of the teeth.

Two-thirds of young adults, 80% of middle-aged adults, and 90% of people in the United States over 65 suffer from periodontal disease (4). Poor oral hygiene, which permits plaque to accumulate on the teeth, is the major etiologic factor. Most periodontal disease, and therefore most loss of teeth, is preventable. Prevention consists of routine plaque control (see below).

Relationship of Calcium Channel Blocking Drugs to Gingival Overgrowth

Calcium channel blocking drugs are widely used for management of cardiovascular conditions. Nifedipine is one of the most often prescribed drugs in this group and the first to be associated with gingival overgrowth. Most other calcium channel blocking agents have been associated with gingival enlargement, although not to the same degree as nifedipine. The onset of gingival enlargement usually appears within 2 months after initiation of nifedipine therapy and is most pronounced in the anterior facial gingiva. The tendency for overgrowth occurs in approximately 15% to 20% of patients, and although it does not appear to be dose related, occasionally a decrease in enlargement after dosage reduction has been reported. The histologic, histochemical, and electron microscopic examinations of nifedipine-induced gingival enlargement closely resembles phenytoin- or cyclosporine-induced gingival overgrowth, suggesting a similar pathogenic mechanism. Chronic inflammation is always present, and an association between plaque accumulation and drug-induced overgrowth has been documented. Meticulous plaque control does not usually cause remission or consistently stop recurrence after surgical removal. Whenever gingival overgrowth develops, an alternative to nifedipine should be considered. If a calcium channel blocking agent is essential for the patient, an agent other than a dihydropyridine should be used. Examples of such agents that could be used in this situation are diltiazem, verapamil, or bepridil.

Patients who have had organ transplants may be taking cyclosporine, an immunosuppressant drug used extensively to suppress organ and bone marrow transplant rejection. The combination of cyclosporine and calcium channel blocking agents appears to have a synergistic effect on the gingiva. The hyperplasia produced is extreme and often recurs after surgical excision.

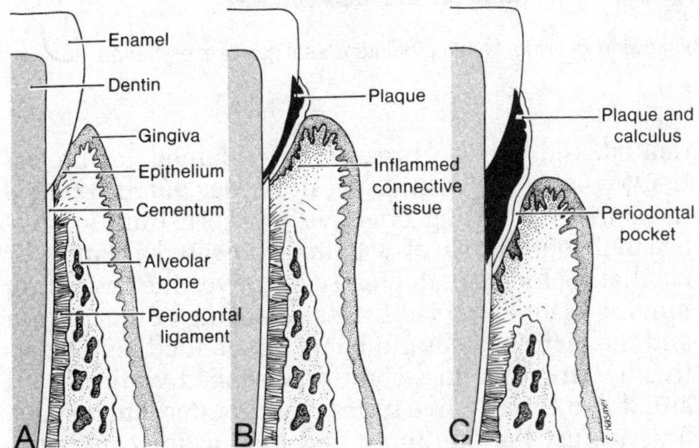

Figure 112.4. Dentogingival junction in health. **A:** Plaque free. **B:** Gingivitis resulting from plaque accumulation with inflammation of soft tissue. **C:** Periodontitis resulting from long-standing inflammation that has caused bone loss and tooth mobility.

Gingivitis

Presentation. Gingivitis is usually seen in one of four forms: *acute,* a painful condition that has a rapid onset and is of short duration; *subacute,* which is less severe than the acute condition; *recurrent,* which reappears after being eliminated by treatment or after disappearing spontaneously; and *chronic,* the most common form, which has a slow onset, is of a long duration, and is usually painless unless complicated by acute exacerbations (Fig. 112.5).

The early signs of inflammation of the gingiva, which precede frank gingivitis, are increased gingival fluid secretion and bleeding from the gingival sulcus upon gentle probing. Healthy gingiva is usually coral pink, whereas in gingivitis the gingiva becomes bright red secondary to increased vascularity and a decrease in keratinization. These changes start in the interdental papillae and free gingiva and spread to the attached gingiva. Both acute and chronic forms produce changes in the normally firm resilient consistency of the gingiva. In acute gingivitis the gingiva has a diffuse edematous appearance, whereas in the chronic form the tissue has a fibrous appearance that pits on pressure.

The development of gingivitis is a consequence of supragingival and subgingival plaque formation (Fig. 112.4). Plaque is a transparent deposit composed primarily of bacteria and their byproducts. Gram-positive filamentous rods, mainly *Actinomyces,* appear to be of major significance. Small amounts of plaque are not visible unless they are stained. As plaque accumulates, it becomes visible as a mass that varies in color from gray to yellowish gray to yellow. Measurable amounts of plaque may form within 1 hour after a thorough cleaning of the teeth, with maximal accumulation in 30 days or less. Bacterial plaque, if left undisturbed, mineralizes and forms calculus (tartar),

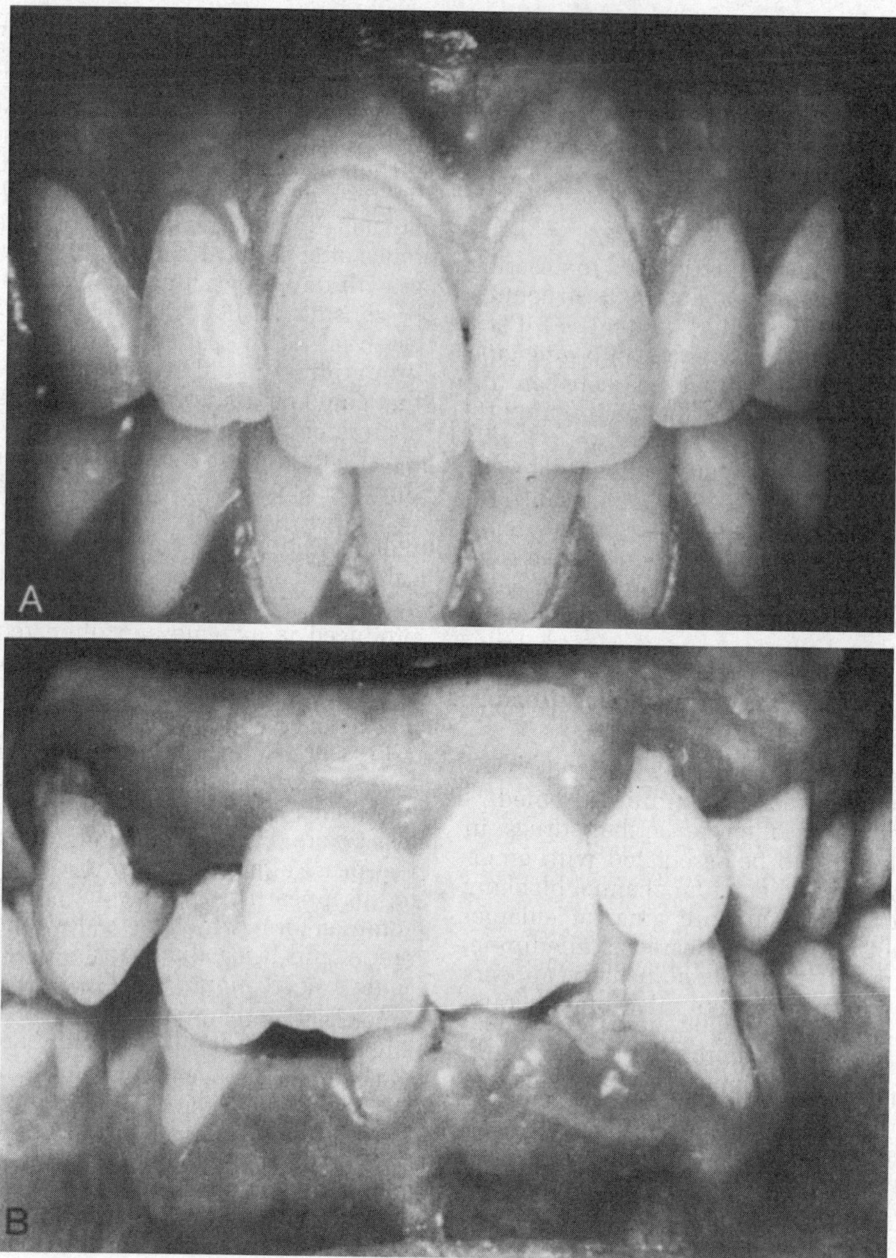

Figure 112.5. Normal gingiva **(A)** and chronic periodontal inflammation **(B)** showing swelling, blunting of interdental papillae, erythema, and bleeding.

as shown in Fig. 112.4C. This process usually starts between the 1st and 14th day after plaque formation. Calculus is always covered by plaque. When calculus is present, the gingival tissues are unhealthy by definition. The major complication of untreated gingivitis is periodontitis, that is, the extension of the inflammation to the supporting bony structures of the teeth (see below and Fig. 112.4C).

Treatment. Patients presenting with any one of the four forms of gingivitis usually require one to three dental visits (spread over about a 4-week period) for treatment. The mechanical removal of plaque and calculus from the affected areas of the teeth and gingiva is achieved with the appropriate instruments. After all the plaque and calculus have been removed by the dentist, the disease process is explained to the patient, who is then instructed in proper *plaque control measures,* including effective toothbrushing (a soft-bristled toothbrush or a battery-powered rotating or oscillating toothbrush greatly improves the ease of removing plaque and facilitates cleansing of the gingiva and the teeth and should be recommended) and effective flossing (the floss should be rubbed vertically up and down three to five times in each interdental space first against the one tooth and then against the adjacent one, once daily). Maintenance of the disease-free state is possible only by continued effective plaque control measures by the patient and by professional cleaning every 4 to 12 months (to remove plaque and calculus that may be missed by brushing and flossing).

Mouthwashes are available that help in the treatment of gingivitis (5). Chlorhexidine gluconate, 0.12% oral rinse twice daily (Peridex or PerioGard, available by prescription), has been shown to be microbicidal. The rinse should be expectorated after use. Complications from its use are common and include a brown stain of the teeth, possible taste alterations, and increase in calculus formation. For these reasons a patient should not use the material without consulting a dentist. Factors that usually result in recurrence are incomplete removal of plaque and calculus, inadequate plaque control because of insufficient patient instruction, premature dismissal of the patient before competence is demonstrated, and lack of patient cooperation.

Periodontitis

Presentation. A patient with periodontitis has red and bleeding gums and an unpleasant taste in his or her mouth but is usually free of pain unless there is an acute infection superimposed on the underlying chronic process. The principal physical findings are the signs of inflammation of the gingiva described above and periodontal pockets around the teeth, from which pus may often be expressed upon gentle pressure. As periodontitis advances, the teeth loosen and spread apart, creating unattractive spaces and exposing the roots of the teeth as the bony support is lost. Mastication is impaired, and spontaneous pain and acute abscess may occur. The most important consequence of periodontitis is the destruction of the alveolar bone, which deprives the teeth of their support and is responsible for the loss of the teeth. The essential steps leading to destruction of bone are gingivitis, degeneration of collagen bundles of the periodontal ligament, and conversion of the shallow (3 mm or less) physiologic gingival sulcus to a deepened periodontal pocket (more than 3 mm). As this pocket deepens, more debris accumulates in it. Inflammation progresses further inward, and the gums recede permanently. The apically progressing inflammation eventually reaches the alveolar crest, and bone resorption begins. This process continues, resulting in continued destruction of the alveolar bone.

Treatment. Most patients with periodontitis can be treated effectively, provided the diagnosis is made before a significant amount of supporting alveolar bone is lost. The aims of treatment are to preserve the teeth by eliminating the disease, restore effective function, and prevent recurrence. When treated in the early stages, the major consequence of periodontitis (loss of bone support for the teeth) can be prevented. If proper treatment is postponed, there may be insufficient bone support once treatment is undertaken, and the natural teeth may eventually be lost. Although some patients do not seem concerned with this problem, many are subsequently disappointed when they find dentures do not function as efficiently as natural teeth.

Treatment of periodontitis is divided into two phases. Phase I is similar to the treatment of gingivitis described above; that is, removal of local irritant (plaque and calculus) and institution of effective plaque control (continual removal of the plaque). This treatment allows resolution of the inflammation. The success of this phase of therapy depends largely on the patient's ability to maintain plaque-free teeth (see Gingivitis, above). Phase II is the surgical phase, in which the goal is to improve the gingival architecture that remains despite the disease. Experience shows that patients have difficulty preventing inflammation in periodontal pockets greater than 5 mm. Surgical treatment is therefore designed to decrease the depths of the pockets.

Denture Problems

Twenty million American adults are missing all their teeth. Of these, many have obtained dentures. In addition, many of the edentulous population have managed well without teeth, are content to remain as they are, and, regardless of the quality of dentures constructed, are unwilling or unable to adapt to using dentures.

Presentation

Often a patient who has had dentures for years, upon specific questioning, indicates the dentures are not satisfactory. The most common denture problems are looseness and discomfort. If the patient is followed at least yearly by his or her dentist, one can generally assume the present situation is the best that can be achieved. On the other hand, if the patient has tolerated the same set of loose or uncomfortable dentures without seeking help for a number of years, he or she should be encouraged to seek care promptly. Failure to remove dentures at night is the reason for denture problems in some patients. This practice can cause bony erosion with loss of conformity of the dentures to the supporting structures, mucosal ulceration, and oral candidiasis.

Treatment

Depending on the condition of the patient's oral cavity, the present dentures, and the edentulous ridges, a number of treatment modalities are available, including rebasing or relining the existing dentures (5 to 7 days), making a new set of dentures (2 to 5 weeks), and preprosthetic correction of soft and hard tissue (4 to 6 weeks of healing), followed by relining, rebasing, or remaking of dentures. In recent years, there have been marked improvements in dental implants for patients who have had trouble using dentures (especially lower dentures). The placement of implants is expensive (about $1,600 to $1,800 per implant, often with a reduction in price for multiple installations, and often five to six implants are used per arch) and time consuming (2 to 3 months) and requires that new dentures are made after placement of implants. The implants function as a replacement for the teeth roots the patient had previously lost through dental caries, periodontitis, or trauma. Most conservative dentists reserve implants for the patient missing at least all posterior teeth or all natural teeth.

Dental Caries

Dental caries is a disease of the calcified tissues of the teeth characterized by demineralization of the inorganic portion (enamel and dentin of the tooth; Fig. 112.2A). Dental caries is one of the most common diseases in humans. It affects all people regardless of race, location, or economic stratum, and it can occur at any age. Poor oral hygiene and a diet high in sugar promote caries, whereas routine oral hygiene and raw coarse foods tend to reduce caries. Ingestion of fluorides in drinking water reduces susceptibility to caries. The form of the tooth affects caries; that is, the deep pits and fissures on molars and premolars especially predispose these teeth to the disorder.

Presentation

Dental caries usually presents as a nonpainful, white, brown, or black spot on the enamel of a tooth. The most common location is the biting surface in conjunction with the pits and fissures of the tooth. Other locations include the smooth surfaces where the teeth come into contact with each other. Without the aid of special equipment (x-rays and hand instruments) and expertise of dental personnel, the best indicator of dental caries is the presence of brown or black spots in areas associated with lost portions of the tooth.

When a caries progresses rapidly to involve the pulp, as in children, the term *acute caries* is used. Slowly progressing caries seen in adults is called chronic caries. Occasionally, a carious lesion may cease to progress (arrested caries). This is caused by breakage of enamel walls, thereby exposing the lesion to the cleaning action of the toothbrush, saliva, fluoride, and mastication. The term *recurrent caries* is used for carious lesions that begin around the margins of defective restorations.

A carious lesion usually develops after bacterial plaque (see above) forms on the tooth surface. The primary bacteria involved in this process are *Streptococcus mutans* and *Lactobacillus acidophilus.* These bacteria metabolize dietary fructose to produce lactic acid, which results in decalcification of the enamel. The rate of development of caries depends on the susceptibility of the enamel.

Treatment

The treatment for most carious lesions is their removal, followed by a restoration (filling) that replaces the lost portions of the tooth. The goals are to remove the lesion, protect the pulp from irritants, and restore the tooth to function. With the advent of enamel and dentin bonding agents, a sealant (a thin plastic layer of resin) can be placed over a noncarious tooth in the deep fissures to prevent dental caries. In cases when caries involves a tooth already significantly affected by periodontal disease, the tooth must be removed.

The major *complication* that results from delaying treatment is acute pulpitis and its complications (see above). In addition, delaying treatment may result in a more difficult restoration or possible loss of the involved tooth. In cases in which the existing decay process is very close to the pulp, the heat generated by the rotary instruments used to prepare the restoration may result in a transient pulpal inflammation. This inflammation results in a dull ache in the tooth for 2 to 3 days, which is usually relieved by aspirin or ibuprofen or other NSAID. When the restoration process leaves only a paper-thin layer of dentin covering the pulp tissue, the transient pulpitis may be converted to acute pulpitis (irreversible), which then requires tooth extraction or root canal therapy for relief of pain. Root canal therapy consists of three parts: Removal of the infected nerve tissue, debridement and preparation of the nerve canal space, and obturation (filling) of the canal space with a biologically inert material.

Angular Cheilosis

Presentation

Angular cheilosis is characterized by a feeling of dryness and a burning sensation at the corners of the mouth. The epithelium at the commissures appears wrinkled and macerated. In time, the wrinkles deepen to fissures that appear ulcerated but do not bleed, although a crust may form. These lesions stop at the junction of the mucous membranes. They show a tendency for spontaneous improvement; only rarely do the lesions completely disappear.

There are several causes for cheilosis. A number of microorganisms may cause it in otherwise healthy people: *Candida albicans,* staphylococci, and streptococci. In addition, angular cheilosis caused by overclosure of the jaws may be seen in edentulous patients. Overclosure causes a fold to be produced at the corners of the mouth in which saliva tends to collect, inviting the growth of microorganisms. Angular cheilosis is also seen in riboflavin deficiency, which usually occurs in patients with multiple vitamin deficiencies. The lips show fissures, painful cracks, and scaling; these changes become severe at the corners of the mouth and are similar in appearance to angular cheilosis caused by overclosure of the mandible.

Treatment

Edentulous patients troubled by angular cheilosis should be referred to a dentist, who will evaluate them for mandibular overclosure, because correction of this problem (making or remaking of dentures) may lead to remission. Treatment is otherwise symptomatic and consists of applying petrolatum-containing ointment (e.g., Vaseline, Chapstick) to the scaling area to minimize discomfort.

Thrush (Oral Candidiasis)

Presentation

The typical lesions of oral candidiasis are white curdlike plaques on an erythematous mucosa (Fig. 112.6). These plaques are loosely attached and may be scraped off the oral mucosa. They begin as pinpoint spots.

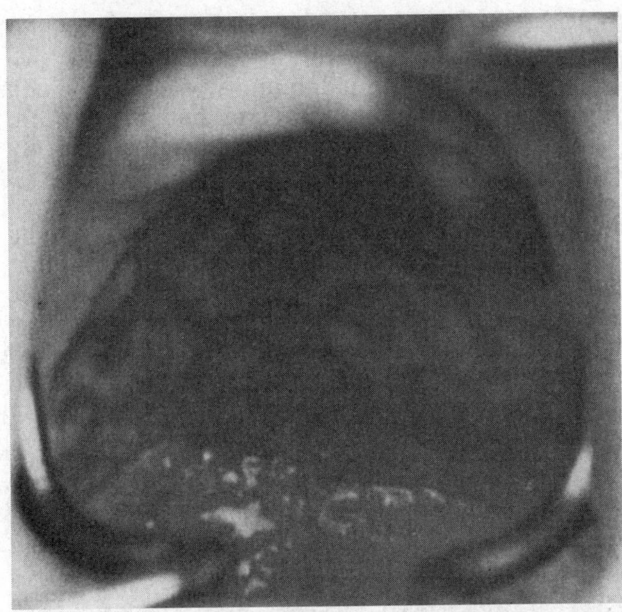

Figure 112.6. Candidiasis (thrush) of the hard palate.

Involvement may include the corners of the mouth, as noted in the previous section. The tongue is often reddened, and the patient describes a burning sensation.

Thrush may occur chronically in patients with poor oral hygiene and poor nutrition. It may also be brought on or exacerbated by debilitating systemic illness, antibiotic therapy, impaired immune system, use of steroids or antimetabolites, or dental extraction. Thrush does not appear to be more common in diabetic patients. It is common in patients with human immunodeficiency virus infection (see Chapter 39).

The white plaques of thrush may suggest hyperkeratosis or leukoplakia. In these instances, a scraping reveals pseudo-hyphae and budding spores when the condition is candidiasis.

Treatment

The patient should be advised to use good oral hygiene practices. Specific treatment consists of nystatin oral suspension, 4 to 6 mL held in the mouth for several minutes before swallowing, four times daily. Thrush usually resolves entirely after 1 to 2 weeks of treatment. Treatment should be continued for several days after visible lesions have disappeared. More intensive treatment is needed in patients with human immunodeficiency virus infection (see Chapter 39).

Halitosis

Presentation

Halitosis is a foul or offensive odor emanating from the oral cavity. Mouth odors originate from local or remote sites. The local causes can be retention of odoriferous food particles on or between the teeth, ANUG (see above), caries, chronic periodontal disease, dentures, tobacco smoking, and healing of surgical or extraction wounds or debris accumulated between the small papilla of the tongue. Extraoral causes of halitosis include infection in adjacent structures (rhinitis, sinusitis, tonsillitis), pulmonary infections, alcoholic breath, the acetone odor of the diabetic, or the uremic breath associated with renal failure.

Treatment

Local causes of this condition are treated by improvement in oral hygiene (brushing teeth and tongue) and by specific treatment of the underlying conditions by a dentist. If these measures are unsuccessful, pleasant-smelling mouthwashes or breath fresheners used frequently (every 2 to 4 hours) may greatly reduce the problem. Halitosis caused by remote factors may be masked with mouthwashes and fresheners until the remote problem has been resolved.

Xerostomia (Dry Mouth)

Presentation

Xerostomia, or dry mouth, results from a partial or complete lack of saliva. This defect results in cracking of the lips, difficulty in swallowing, or changes in the tongue texture. The patient often increases liquid consumption to eliminate the dryness. Xerostomia may be a secondary complication of salivary gland disease (e.g., Sjögren syndrome) or radiation treatment, but medication is the most common cause. Anticholinergic, decongestant, and antihistamine drugs are the most common offenders.

The loss of saliva results in a loss of the protective coating of the mucous membranes of the oral cavity. Infections, severe dental caries, and problems with dentures very commonly result from the loss of saliva.

Treatment

Treatment of xerostomia is symptomatic. Patients should be referred to a dentist for an evaluation to identify an underlying problem such as caries and for instruction in the use of daily topical fluoride to help prevent recurrence of caries. The dryness may be lessened if the patient regularly irrigates the mouth with topical methylcellulose or a saliva substitute (Glandosane, Oralube, MOI STIR, Salive Substitute [Roxane Laboratories] or Xerolube, all available without prescription). The saliva substitutes also decrease the risk of caries because they contain sodium fluoride.

Common Tongue Conditions

Geographic Tongue

Benign migratory glossitis, or geographic tongue, is an asymptomatic inflammatory condition consisting of multiple areas of desquamation of the filiform papillae of the tongue in an irregular pattern (Fig. 112.7A). The central portion of an affected area is usually denuded, and the border may be outlined by a thin yellowish white line or band. The fungiform papillae persist in the desquamated area as small, elevated, red dots. The areas of desquamation remain for a short time in one

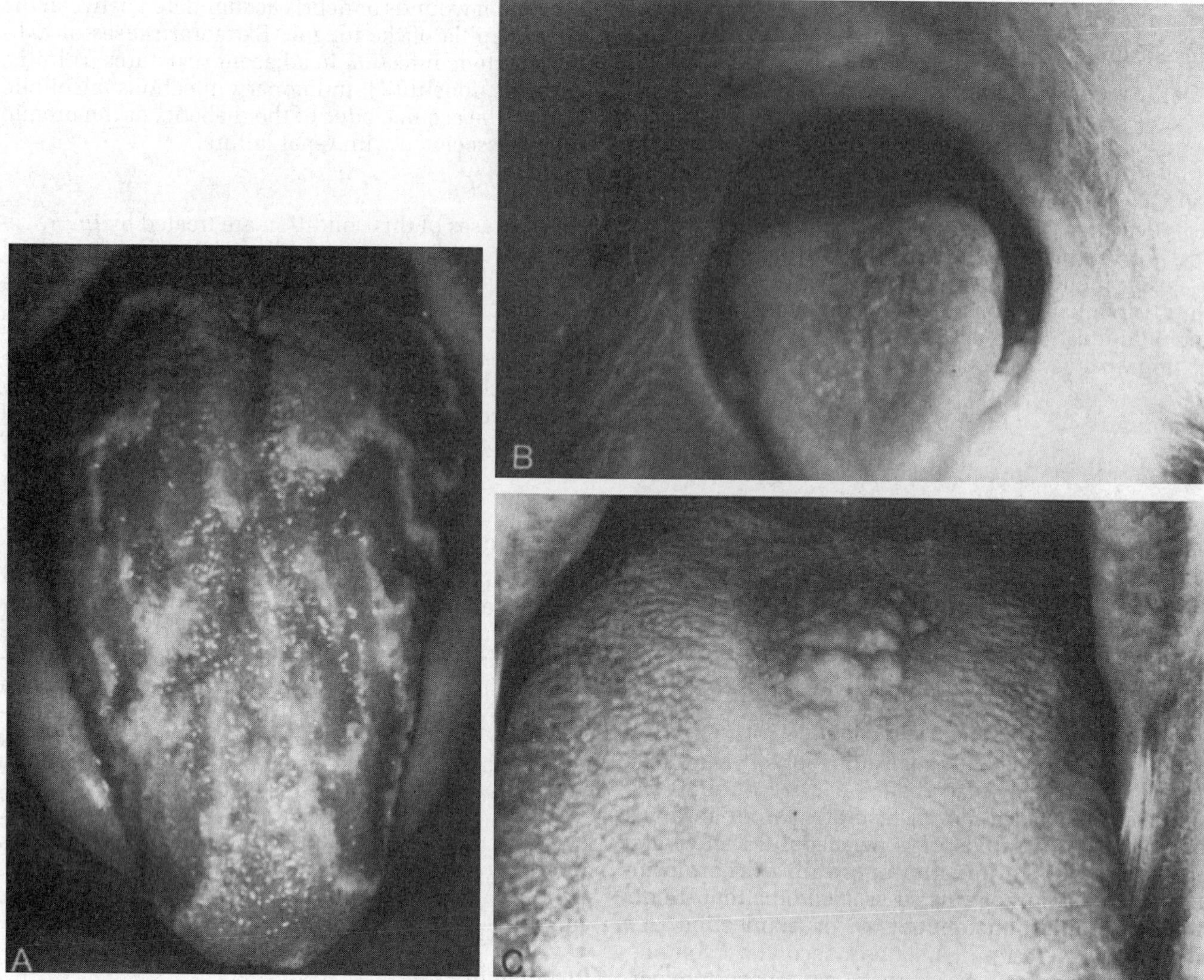

Figure 112.7. Common benign problems of the tongue. **A:** Geographic tongue. **B:** Hairy tongue. **C:** Median rhomboid glossitis.

location and then heal and reappear in other locations. The condition may persist for weeks or months and then regress, only to recur at a later date. Women are affected twice as often as men, and there is no racial difference. Because the cause is unknown and the condition is benign, management consists of reassurance. Large doses of vitamins are not effective.

Hairy Tongue

Hairy tongue is a condition characterized by hypertrophy of the filiform papillae of the tongue caused by the lack of normal desquamation of the keratin layer (Fig. 112.7B). This results in a thick matted layer on the dorsum of the tongue. The color of the papillae varies from yellowish white to brown or even black depending on their staining by extrinsic factors (tobacco, foods, or medications). The hypertrophied tissue may touch the palate and produce gagging in some patients. Most patients with hairy tongue are heavy smokers, but the cause is unknown. Treatment of this benign condition consists of brushing the tongue with a tongue blade or toothbrush to promote desquamation and remove debris.

Median Rhomboid Glossitis

Median rhomboid glossitis is a congenital abnormality of the tongue that appears clinically as an ovoid-, diamond-, or rhomboid-shaped reddish patch on the dorsal surface of the tongue. On examination, there is a slightly raised or flat area that is distinctive because there are no filiform papillae (Fig. 112.7C). Despite its name, this abnormality is not inflammatory; it is caused by failure of the tuberculum impar to retract before fusion of the lateral halves of the tongue, so that a structure free of papillae is interposed. The prevalence of the abnormality is less than 1%, and there are no sex or racial differences. The only clinical significance of this innocuous condition is that it is occasionally mistaken for a carcinoma; differentiation from cancer is aided by the presence of the lesion since childhood and the fact that a carcinoma rarely develops on the dorsum of the tongue. If one is unsure

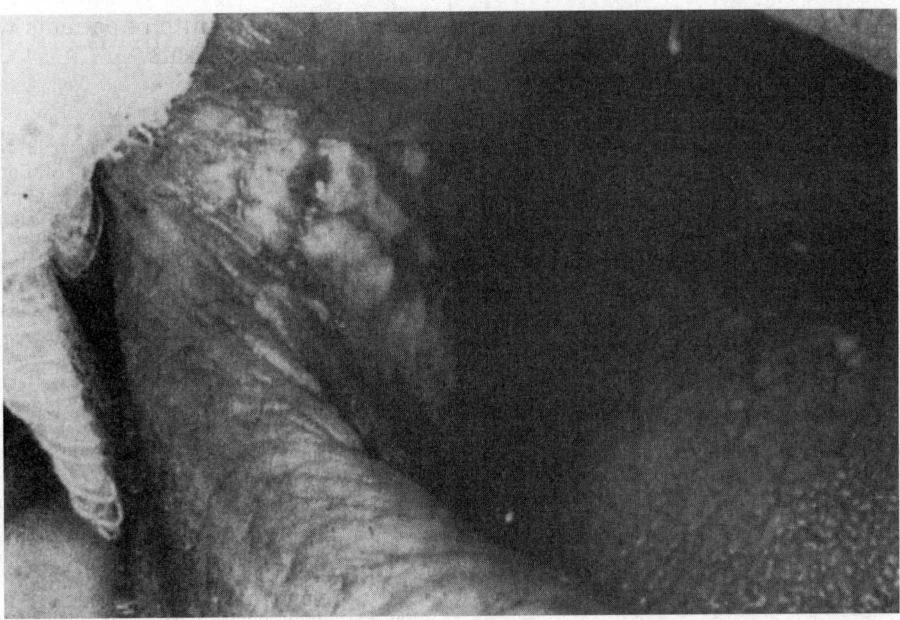

Figure 112.8. Leukoplakia showing early changes of epidermoid carcinoma.

of the diagnosis, the patient should be referred to a dentist.

Leukoplakia and Erythroplakia

Presentation

Leukoplakia and erythroplakia are asymptomatic conditions of the oral mucosa that may become malignant. *Leukoplakia* varies in appearance from a grayish white, flattened, scaly lesion to a thick irregularly shaped plaque (Fig. 112.8). Histologically, there is hyperkeratosis, acanthosis, and some degree of dyskeratosis. It is commonly associated with underlying inflammation caused by a chronic irritant (tobacco, alcohol, poorly constructed dentures). Leukoplakia may be found anywhere in the oral cavity but most often is found in the buccal mucosa, followed, in descending order, by the alveolar mucosa, tongue, lip, hard and soft palates, floor of the mouth, and gingiva. *Erythroplakia* refers to a lesion that is velvety red in appearance, small (2 cm or less), and with or without a hyperkeratotic component. It is found in the floor of the mouth, soft palate, and ventrolateral border of the tongue.

The significance of these lesions has been delineated in a longitudinal study of mucosal lesions (6). Of 200 white lesions examined by biopsy, only 4 were malignant. In the same study, an erythroplastic component was present in 90% of the 158 asymptomatic squamous cell carcinomas found, suggesting, but not proving, that erythroplakia may be an important precursor of squamous cell cancer.

Treatment

It is impossible to determine which lesion showing leukoplakia or erythroplakia will undergo malignant transformation. Discontinuance of chronic irritants is recommended, followed by a 14-day observation period to allow inflammatory lesions to heal. If the lesion persists, referral to a dental surgeon for a biopsy and regular follow-up surveillance, even if the lesion is benign, are indicated. The biopsy procedure is as simple as having a restoration (filling) or a tooth extraction.

Other conditions that may resemble leukoplakia or erythroplakia are lichen planus, chemical burns, candidiasis (thrush), psoriasis, lupus erythematosus, and syphilitic mucous patches. Each of these has characteristic histologic features.

Squamous Cell Carcinoma

More than 90% of all malignant tumors of the oral cavity are squamous cell carcinomas. They are four times more common in men than women and are most common after the fourth decade. In the United States, oral cancer is the 8th most common form of cancer in men and the 12th in women. Fifteen thousand new cases are found each year, and about 7,500 patients die of this disease annually. Of lip carcinomas, 95% occur on the lower lip and appear as an ulcer, wart, sore, or scale (7). This lesion is more common in fair-skinned patients. Of the intraoral carcinomas, 50% occur on the tongue (usually the ventrolateral border; Fig. 112.9) and 16% on the floor of the mouth; the remaining 34% are equally distributed between the gingival mucosa, palate, and buccal mucosa. Sixty percent of intraoral carcinomas present as ulcers, 30% as growths, and the remaining 10% as white lesions or other abnormalities of the mucosa (8). Carcinoma of the tongue and floor of the mouth metastasizes early and carries a poor prognosis.

The cause of oral carcinoma is unknown. Ill-fitting dentures, actinic radiation, tobacco, jagged teeth,

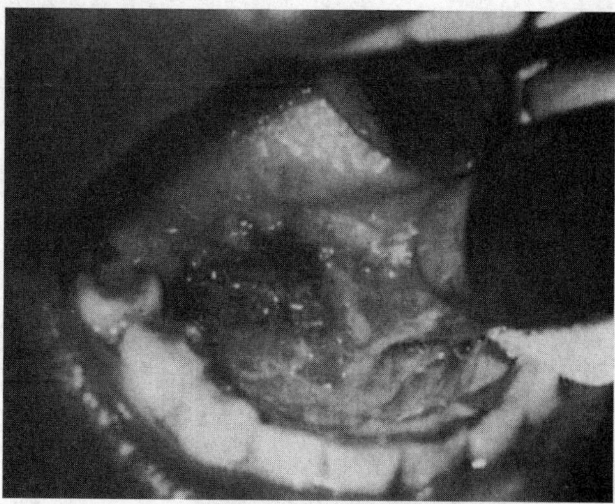

Figure 112.9. Squamous cell carcinoma of the floor of the mouth.

syphilitic glossitis, and alcoholism are believed to be risk factors.

Presentation and Evaluation

Patients usually give a history of knowledge of the lesion for 6 to 18 months when they first present; for many reasons they have not sought evaluation. All patients with suspicious lesions should be referred promptly to a dental surgeon for biopsy. Biopsy is a simple procedure, not very different from having a restoration or tooth extraction. Usually it is done under local anesthesia.

Treatment

Definitive surgery is a team effort between the otolaryngologist and the dentist. The dentist's role is to evaluate, for long-term prognosis, any teeth not to be removed in the surgical field and to remove any of these teeth affected with untreatable periodontitis. This is done to avoid osteoradionecrosis, a condition seen in the postradiation patient in whom the socket of an extracted tooth fails to heal as the result of diminished blood supply. Lip tumors have the highest success rate (10-year cure rate between 80% and 92%), whereas only one-fifth of patients with tongue cancer live longer than 5 years.

General References

Cummings CW, Fredrickson JM, Harker LA, et al., eds. Otolaryngology: head and neck surgery. 2nd ed. St. Louis: CV Mosby, 1998.
Volume 2 contains several excellent chapters on the oral cavity and the diseases affecting it. There are many excellent color photographs of common lesions.

Epstein JB, Stevensen, Moore P, et al. Management of xerostomia. J Can Dent Assoc 1992;58:140.

McDowell JD, Kassebaum DK. Diagnosing and treating halitosis. J Can Dent Assoc 1993;124:55.

Okeson JP. Management of temporomandibular disorders and occlusion. St. Louis: CV Mosby, 1998.

Thaller SR, Montgomery WW, eds. Guide to dental problems for physicians and surgeons. Baltimore: Williams & Wilkins, 1988.

Williams RC. Periodontal disease. N Engl J Med 1990;322:373.
A thorough review.

Wood NK, Goaz PW. Differential diagnosis of oral lesions. 5th ed. St. Louis: CV Mosby, 1996.
A well-referenced text.

Websites

Oral Pathology Image Base Data, *http://www.uiowa.edu/~oprm/AtlasHome.html*

Dermatology Online Atlas, *http://www.dermis.net/doia*

Specific References

1. Graykowski EA, Barile MF, Lee WB, et al. Recurrent aphthous stomatitis: clinical, therapeutic, histopathologic, and hypersensitivity aspects. JAMA 1966;196:637.
2. Franks AS. The social character of temporomandibular joint dysfunction. Dent Pract Dent Rec 1964;15:94.
3. Apfelberg DB, Lavey E, Janetos G, et al. Temporomandibular joint disease: results of a ten year study. Postgrad Med 1979;65:167.
4. U.S. Department of Health, Education and Welfare, Public Health Service. Research explores pyorrhea and other gum diseases: periodontal disease (PHS Publication 1482). Washington, DC: US Government Printing Office, 1970.
5. Briner WW, Grossman E, Buckner RY, et al. Effect of chlorhexidine gluconate mouth rinse on plaque bacteria. J Periodontal Res 1986;21[Suppl 16]:44.
6. Mashberg A, Morrissey JB, Garfinkel L. A study of the appearance of early asymptomatic oral squamous cell carcinoma. Cancer (Philadelphia) 1973;32:1436.
7. Mashberg A, Morrissey JB, Garfinkel L. A study of the appearance of early asymptomatic oral squamous cell carcinoma. Cancer 1973;32:1436.
8. Bhaskar SN. Synopsis of oral pathology, 4th ed. St. Louis: CV Mosby, 1973:463.

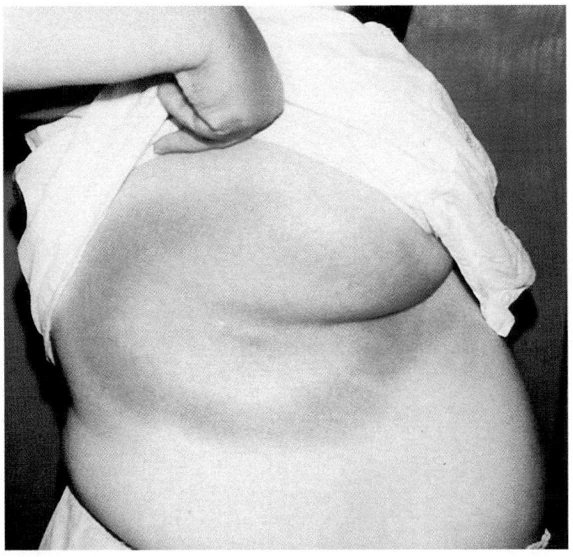

Figure 38.2. Classic erythema migrans rash of early Lyme disease with bright red border and partial central clearing, the so-called "bull's-eye" rash. (Photograph courtesy of Paul Auwaerter, M.D.)

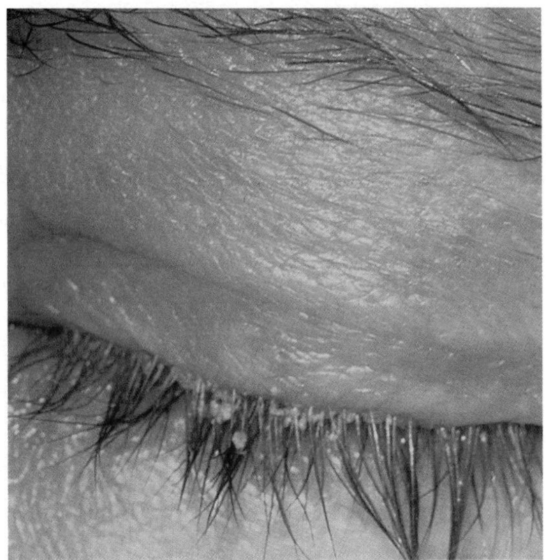

Figure 109.2. Seborrheic blepharitis. Note the oily debris, scurf on the lashes, but no broken or missing lashes.

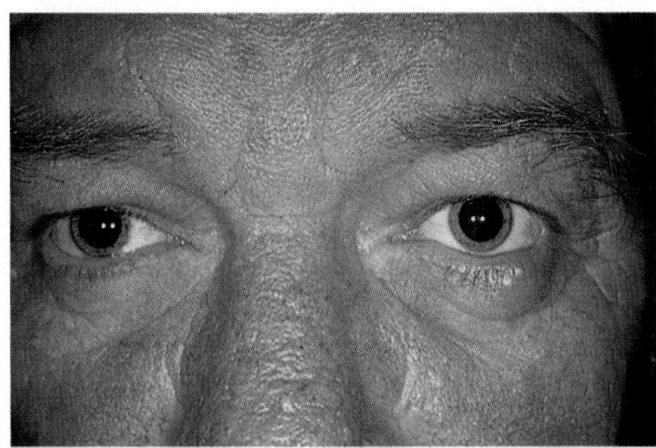

Figure 109.3. Acne rosacea with hordeolum. Man with rhinophyma, oily skin, and acute localized painful swelling (hordeolum) on the left lower eyelid.

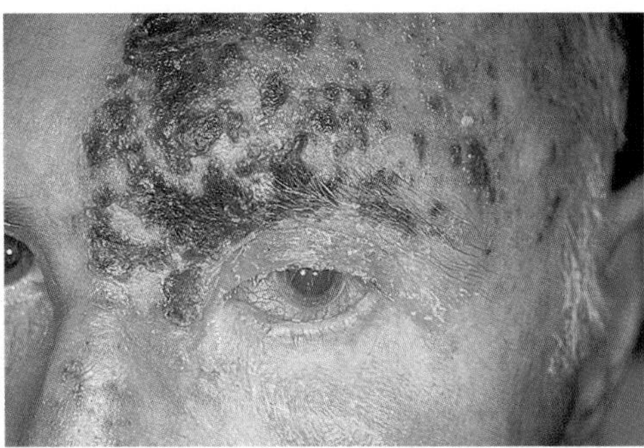

Figure 109.4. Herpes zoster. Note the crusting lesions on the forehead and scaling of the upper eyelid with conjunctival injection.

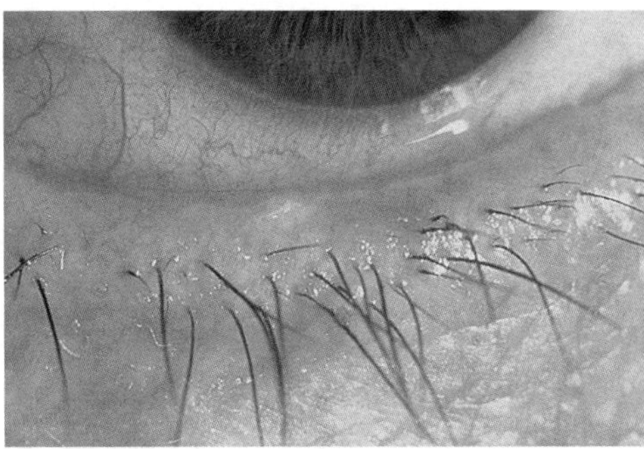

Figure 109.5. Staphylococcal blepharitis. Note that the lashes are sparse, misdirected, and of varying lengths. The lid margin shows ulceration.

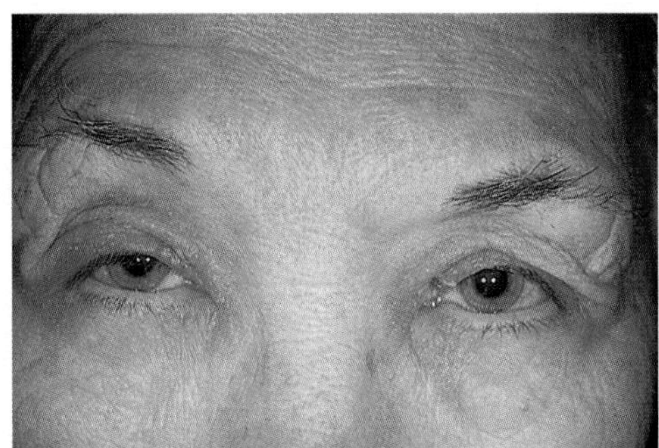

Figure 109.6. Blepharitis. Woman with morning discharge and crusting in both eyes. Note the redness and swelling of the eyelids.

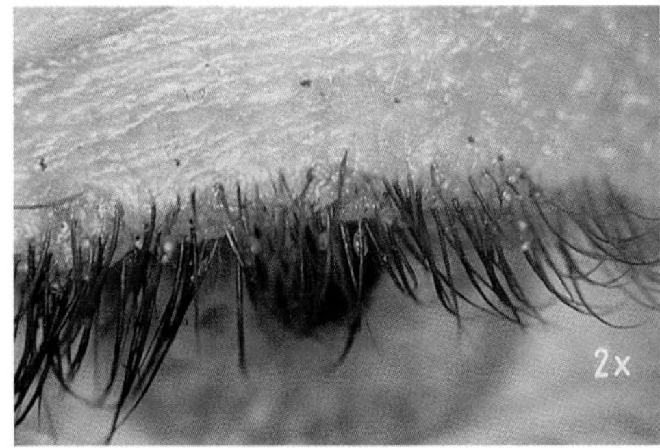

Figure 109.7. Parasitic blepharitis. Note the adult lice and nits on the lashes of a patient with *Pediculosis pubis*.

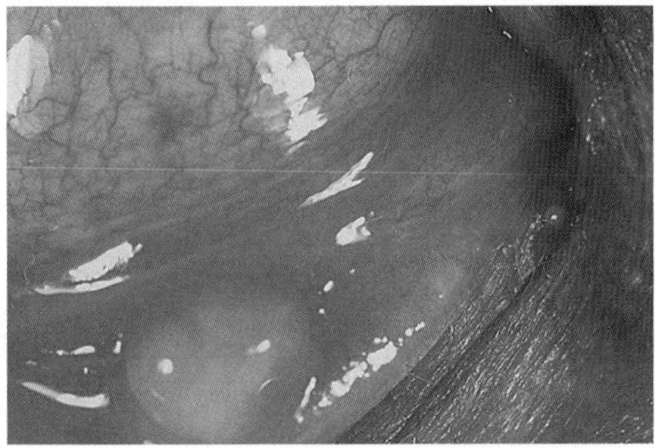

Figure 109.8. Chalazion. Note the localized swelling of the inferior tarsal conjunctiva in a patient with chronic blepharitis. The lower lid is retracted inferiorly.

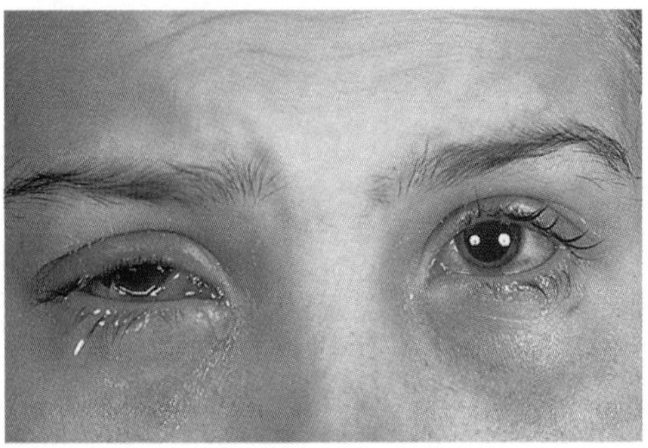

Figure 109.9. Hyperacute purulent conjunctivitis. Note the severe degree of injection, swelling, and purulent discharge.

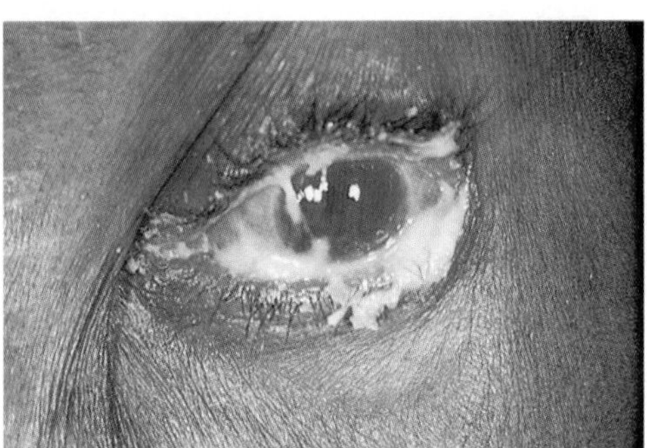

Figure 109.10. Acute bacterial conjunctivitis (severe example). Note the marked erythema, pus, and edema.

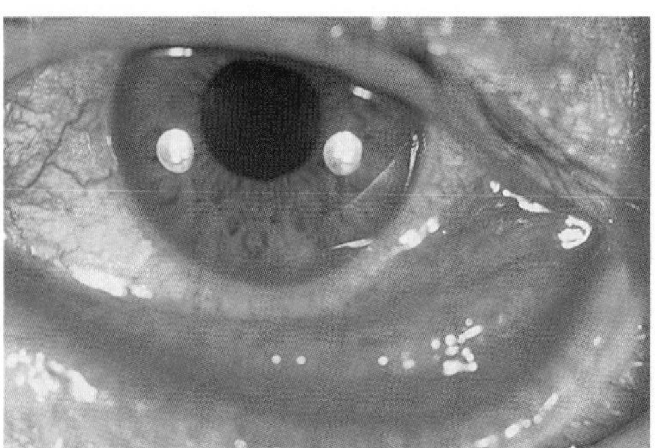

Figure 109.11. Viral conjunctivitis. Note the watery conjunctival discharge and conjunctival hyperemia. The lower lid is retracted inferiorly, demonstrating tarsal conjunctival edema and injection.

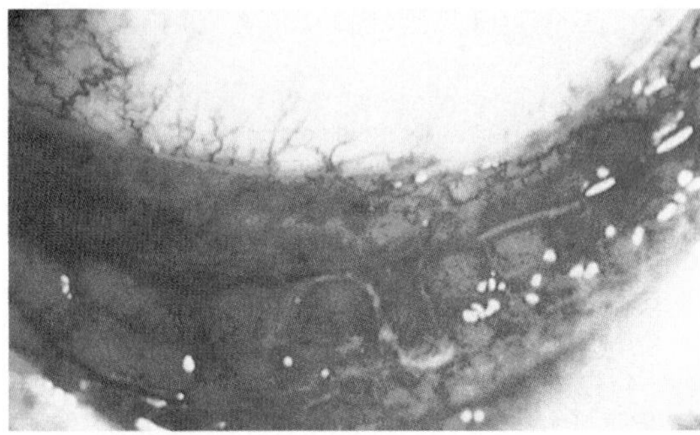

Figure 109.12. Inclusion conjunctivitis. Note the redness, edema of the lid and conjunctiva, and the many small follicles appearing as pale mounds.

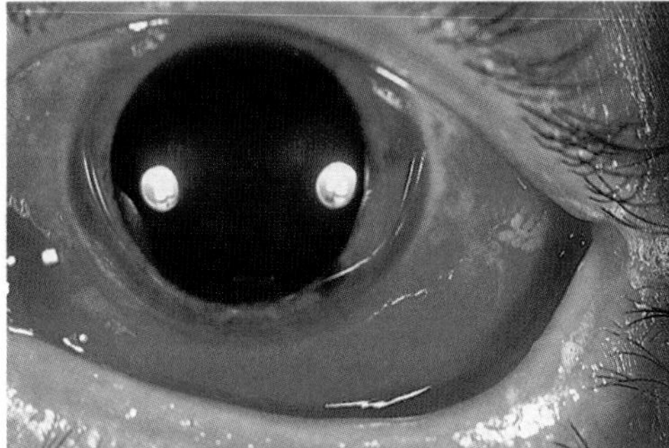

Figure 109.13. Subconjunctival hemorrhage (severe example). Note the diffuse conjunctival redness. (Pupil has been pharmacologically dilated.)

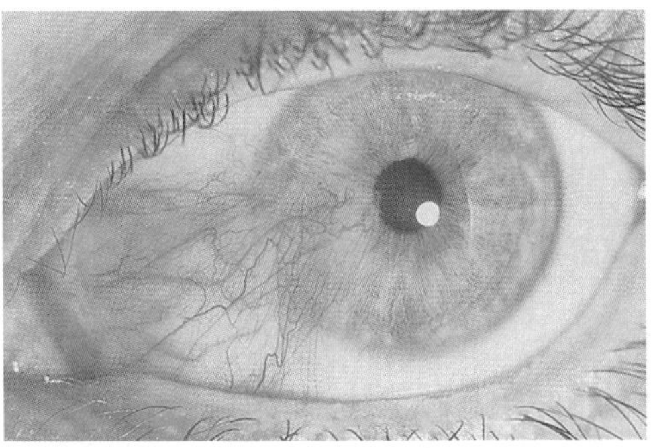

Figure 109.14. Pterygium. Note the localized conjunctival injection with extension of blood vessels into the cornea.

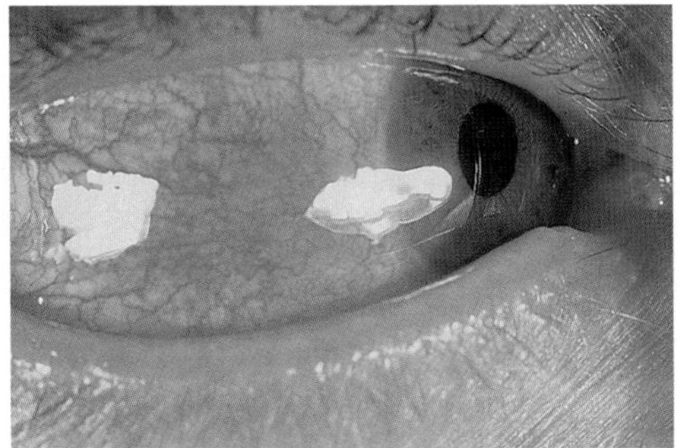

Figure 109.15. Episcleritis. Note the localized redness without discharge. (Light reflexes artifacts are present on the surface of the eye.)

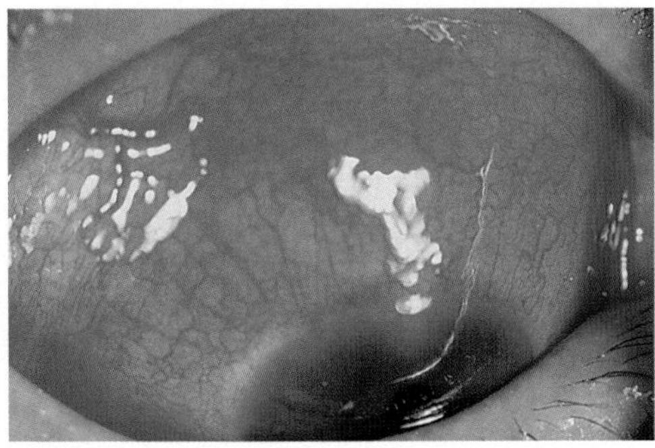

Figure 109.16. Scleritis. Note the diffuse intense redness without discharge. (Patient with rheumatoid arthritis.)

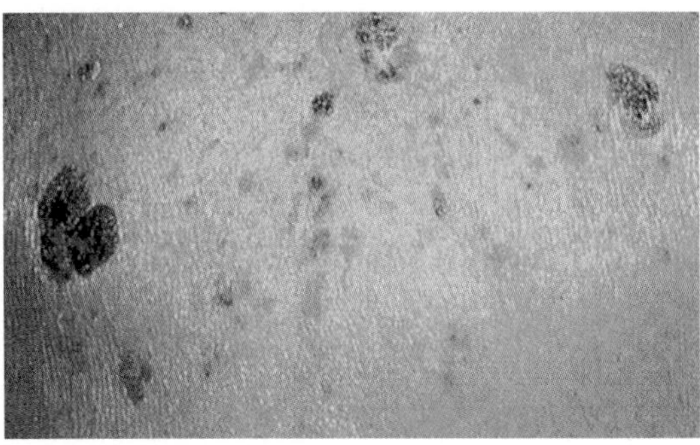

Figure 113.1. Multiple seborrheic keratoses (upper back). "Stuck-on," sharply circumscribed, tan to deep brown, finely papillated to verrucous flat-topped papules and plaques.

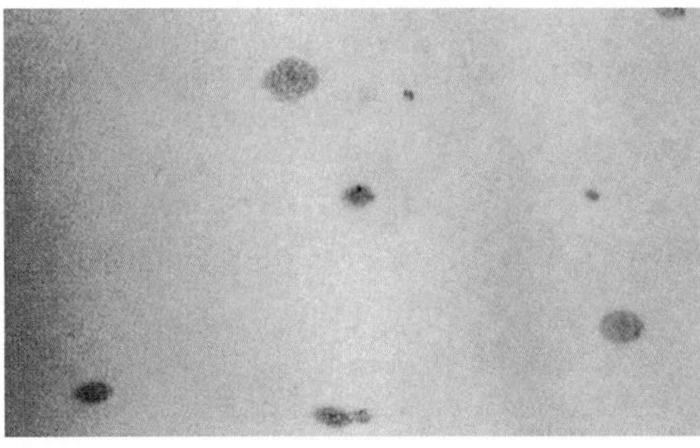

Figure 114.1. Atypical moles (dysplastic nevi). Multiple lesions, showing one to four of the ABCDs: asymmetry, border irregularity, color variegation, diameter 6 mm or greater.

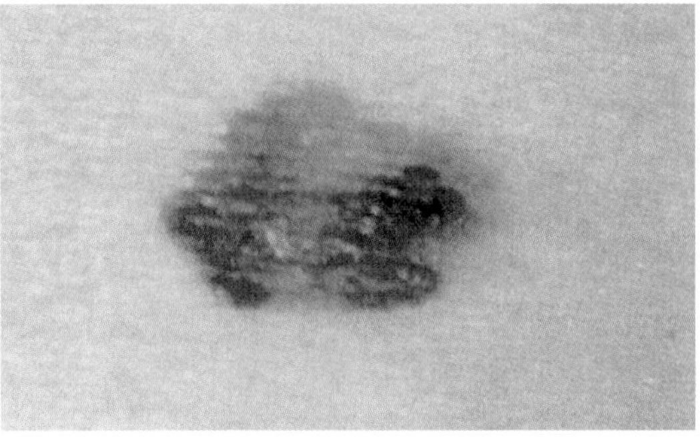

Figure 114.2. Superficial spreading malignant melanoma.

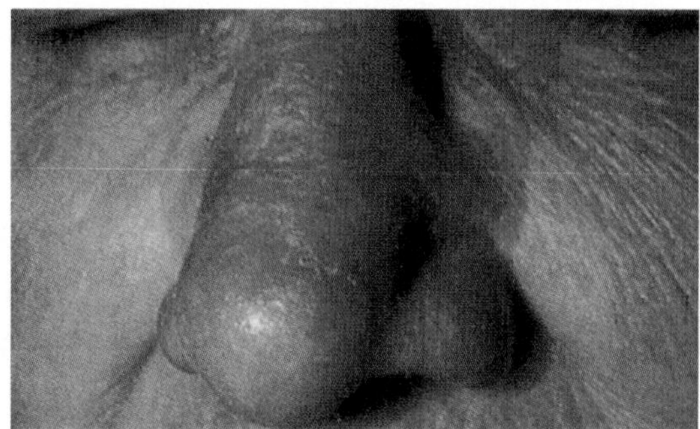

Figure 114.3. Actinic keratosis, nose.

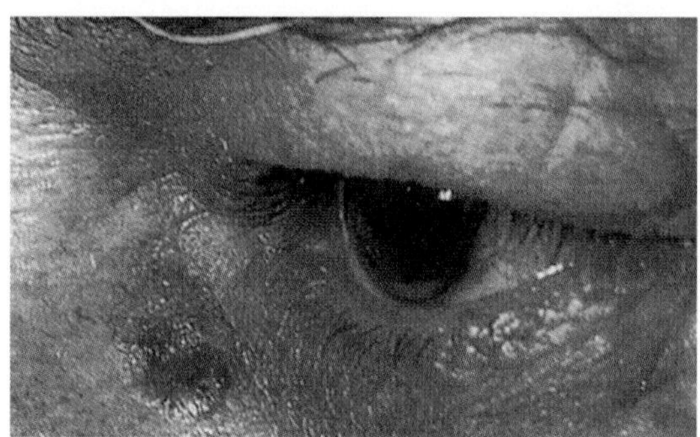

Figure 114.4. Basal cell carcinoma.

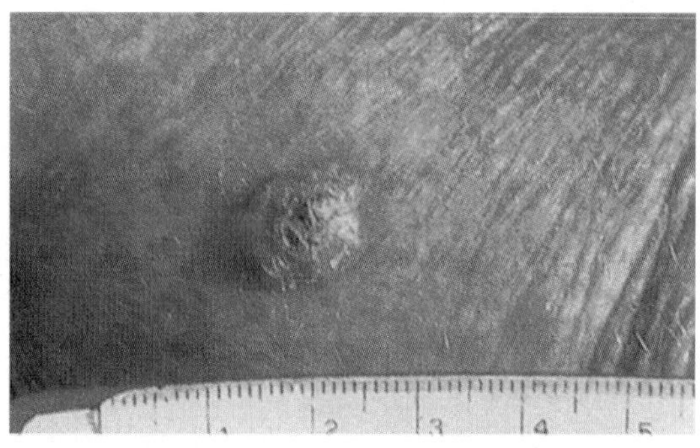

Figure 114.5. Squamous cell carcinoma.

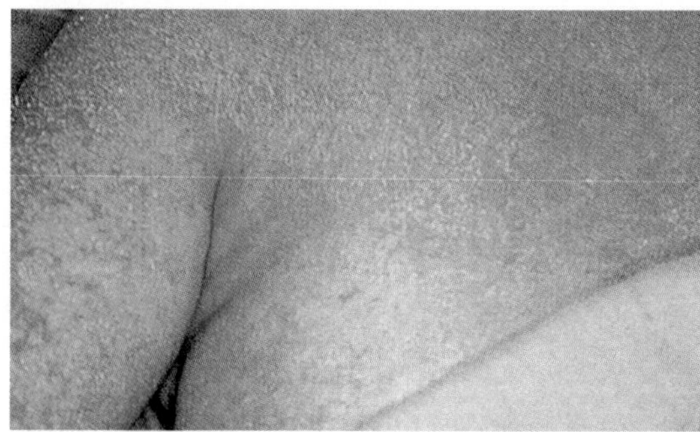

Figure 116.1. Asteatotic dermatitis (upper back and arm). Reticulate erythema highlighting minute cracks in the skin, diffuse dryness (asteatosis), and scale.

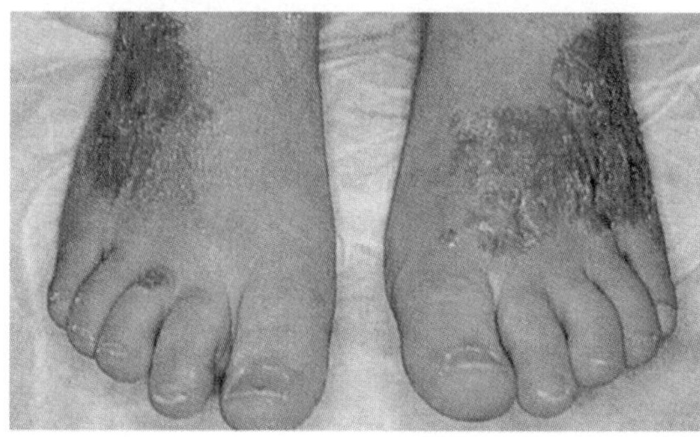

Figure 116.2. Acute contact dermatitis from shoes.

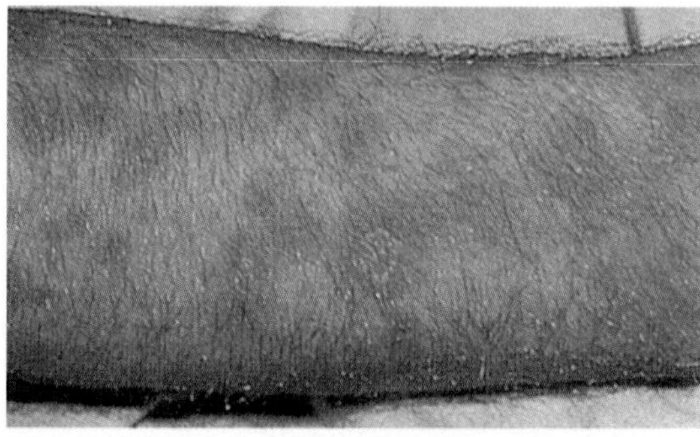

Figure 118.1. Erythema multiforme (extensor arm). Erythematous macules with dusky central area ("target") with focal areas of fine scale.

SECTION 17

Common Disorders of the Skin

CHAPTER 113

Diagnoses and Treatment of Skin Disorders

S. ELIZABETH WHITMORE, MD, ScM

SKIN EXAMINATION AND DEFINITIONS

The primary goal of the skin examination is to define the *morphology* (appearance) of the lesion and the extent of disease. The former allows the correct diagnosis to be made and the latter aids in the determination of prognosis and treatment. The examination of the lesion or eruption of concern is ideally followed by a complete skin examination. This latter may reveal findings helpful in diagnosis or may expose a previously unrecognized skin disease. The examination is most easily done in a systematic fashion, starting at the top with the scalp, face, and oral mucosa and then moving to the anterior then posterior aspect of the body. Good lighting is essential.

Mastering the definitions of commonly used dermatologic terms should aid in both diagnosis and communication with other physicians:

- *Atrophy:* Thinning of the epidermis or dermis causing fine wrinkling or depression of the skin (e.g., discoid lupus erythematosus, steroid-induced atrophy, normal aging).
- *Bulla:* A blister, similar to a vesicle but larger than 5 mm in diameter, filled with serous or serosanguinous fluid (e.g., friction blister, bullous pemphigoid).
- *Burrow:* A linear thread-like elevation of the skin, typically a few millimeters long (pathognomonic for scabies).
- *Comedone:* A plugged pilosebaceous follicle (e.g., a closed comedone or "whitehead" seen in acne).
- *Crust:* Yellowish-brown sticky debris consisting of dried serum, scale, and usually bacteria (e.g., impetigo, impetiginized eczema).
- *Cyst:* A circumscribed, firm, yet often slightly compressible, spherical lesion, fixed in the dermis (e.g., epidermal inclusion cyst).
- *Erosion:* A focal loss of a portion of the epidermis, nonscarring (e.g., candidiasis in the inframammary crease with a moist surface, impetigo).
- *Excoriation:* A self-inflicted disruption of the epidermis.
- *Fissure:* A vertical cut extending into the dermis (e.g., angular cheilitis or "cracks at the angle of the mouth" caused by *Candida,* salivary enzymes, or a vitamin deficiency).
- *Hive:* See *Wheal.*
- *Hyperkeratotic:* Heaped up or stacked scale (e.g., hypertrophic actinic keratosis, squamous cell carcinoma, wart).
- *Macule* or *macular:* A flat color change (e.g., freckle, cafe-au-lait spot, junctional nevus or "flat brown mole").
- *Morphology:* Shape of the primary lesion (e.g., stellate, linear, round, or diffuse).
- *Nodule:* A solid lesion up to 2 cm in diameter with an appreciable deep (dermal or subcutaneous) component (e.g., dermatofibroma, nodular melanoma, erythema nodosum, lipoma).
- *Papule:* An elevated often dome-shaped bump up to 10 mm in diameter, (e.g., intradermal nevus or "skin-colored mole," molluscum contagiosum).
- *Plaque:* A flat-topped elevated area of skin, the surface area of which is much greater than the thickness (e.g., psoriasis, cutaneous T-cell lymphoma, or "mycosis fungoides").
- *Pustule:* A circumscribed lesion visibly filled with purulent material (e.g., folliculitis, acne pustule, pustular psoriasis).
- *Scale:* Surface alteration resulting in a flaky surface, caused by abnormal proliferation or desquamation of the outermost epidermal layer, the stratum corneum (e.g., psoriasis, seborrheic dermatitis, tinea).
- *Sclerosis:* Scar-like induration (e.g., systemic sclerosis, localized scleroderma or "morphea").
- *Secondary changes:* Changes that occur as a result of the natural development or external manipulation of the primary lesion.
- *Telangiectasia:* A dilated superficial capillary or venule; may be linear, spider-like, or mat-like (e.g., starburst leg telangiectasias, telangiectasias in a basal cell carcinoma or in an area of steroid- or lupus-induced atrophy).
- *Tumor:* A large mass, greater than 2 cm in diameter, with significant thickness (e.g., neglected squamous cell carcinoma, cutaneous lymphoma).
- *Ulcer:* A loss of skin extending into the dermis that always heals with scarring (any loss that penetrates the dermal–epidermal junction scars; e.g., venous stasis ulcer, pyoderma gangrenosum).
- *Urticarial:* Adjective describing plaques that are edematous, erythematous, or blanched (e.g., urticaria or "wheals" or "hives," urticarial vasculitis, Sweet syndrome, or "acute febrile neutrophilic dermatosis").
- *Vesicle:* A blister up to 5 mm in diameter filled with serous or serosanguinous fluid (e.g., herpes simplex infection, vesicular hand dermatitis).

- *Wheal or hive:* An erythematous or blanched edematous plaque with no surface change, *present for no more than 24 hours* (i.e., urticaria, by definition).

Based on the morphology of the observed skin changes, a differential diagnosis or diagnosis of the skin lesion or eruption may be made, which may or may not require biopsy for confirmation. Table 113.1 provides a summary of selected disorders categorized by morphology and pathophysiology of disease. Those conditions that are common, diagnostically difficult, and therapeutically complicated are discussed in detail in the chapters that follow.

TOPICAL THERAPEUTICS

Topical Corticosteroids

Topical corticosteroids are categorized based on the degree of vasoconstriction produced upon application to the skin, with superpotent products producing the most vasoconstriction. Vasoconstriction correlates well with biologic activity, therapeutic efficacy, and undesirable side effects. The latter include local effects such as acne, rosacea, striae, atrophy (cigarette paper-like wrinkling of the skin), and increased risk of fungal infection. In addition, systemic effects, as evidenced by hypothalamic–pituitary–adrenal axis suppression, may occur with the use of potent corticosteroids over large areas.

Although there are over 20 different preparations, it is easiest to become familiar with and prescribe just 4 different corticosteroids based on the strength needed. All topical corticosteroids except 0.5% and 1% hydrocortisone are by prescription only. Examples include

- Low potency: hydrocortisone 1% or 2.5%;
- Mid-potency: triamcinolone (acetonide) 0.1%;
- High potency: fluocinonide;
- Super potency: clobetasol (propionate).

Generally, only low potency preparations should be used on the face and in areas of thin skin (e.g., folds and genitalia). Unless a drying effect is desired, ointments are preferred as they aid most in restoring the skin barrier.

An accurate estimation of the amount of corticosteroid needed is important because of the cost of these preparations. Dermatoses are generally treated until clear, and the application is repeated for recurrences. Acute and subacute dermatitis generally clear in 1 to 2 weeks; chronic dermatitis may require chronic intermittent therapy. One gram covers a 10 × 10-cm area: 2 g covers the hands, head, face, or anogenital area; 3 g covers the anterior or posterior trunk or an arm; 4 g covers a single lower extremity; and 30 g covers the entire skin surface. Therefore, for a 1-week two times daily application for each of these areas, 30 g, 45 g, 60 g, and 420 g, respectively, should be prescribed. Most corticosteroids come in 15-, 30-, 60-, and 120-g tubes. In addition, 1-pound jars of hydrocortisone or 0.1% triamcinolone cream or ointment may be requested.

Emollients (Skin Moisturizers)

Very simply, emollients may be classified as *oil in water* (mostly water), *water in oil* (mostly oil), and *oil* preparations. Because the purpose of emollients is to trap moisture after hydrating the skin with a warm bath or shower, occlusive substances are most efficient. Unfortunately, not all patients are amenable to putting petroleum jelly on their skin one or two times a day. A good compromise is Eucerin Original lotion or Nivea moisturizing cream (water in oil). Still lighter oil-in-water moisturizers include Lubriderm, Moisturel, Curel, Vaseline Intensive Care, and Keri lotions. Formulations that contain alpha-hydroxy acids aid in normal desquamation of the skin, making it softer and smoother (e.g., Am-Lacten, Eucerin Plus, and AquaGlycolic lotion). Although they are useful, patients who have "sensitive" or irritated skin may experience stinging and develop an irritant contact dermatitis from the added alpha-hydroxy acid. A good rule to follow is that if it burns or stings, it should not be used.

Topical Antifungal Agents

Several topical antifungal agents are available (see Chapter 117). *Polyenes* such as nystatin (cream, ointment, and powder, by prescription) are used only for candida. In contrast, topicals that may be used for both candida and dermatophytes include *imidazoles,* such as clotrimazole (Mycelex OTC and Lotrimin AF cream, lotion, and solution, all over the counter), sulconazole (Exelderm 1% cream or solution, by prescription), and ketoconazole (Nizoral cream or 2% shampoo, by prescription), which are fungistatic. Finally, for dermatophyte but not candida infections, *allylamines,* such as terbinafine, may be used and are fungicidal (Lamisil cream, lotion, or spray, over the counter).

Creams are applied one or two times per day and should be continued for 2 weeks after clinical resolution of the infection, and as needed for recurrences. Nizoral shampoo is intended for treatment of scalp seborrheic dermatitis, but it may also be used for tinea versicolor. For the former, it is lathered on the scalp and rinsed after 3 minutes, two or three times per week; for the latter, it is applied to the trunk from the neck to the waistline, left 5 minutes, then lathered and rinsed, daily for 10 to 14 days, with a single application repeated every 1 to 2 weeks to prevent recurrences.

Compresses and Baths

Compresses are used to dry and debride localized areas of acute dermatitis, characterized by moist, erythematous, edematous papules, plaques, and vesicles or bullae with serous discharge. Several solutions dry by precipitating protein (Burow's aluminum acetate solution, 1:20 dilution; Domeboro aluminum sulfate and calcium acetate solution, 1:20 dilution; Aveeno Colloidal Oatmeal Packet). Some act as germicidals

Table 113.1. Selected Skin Disorders Based on Morphology

Disorder	Description	Common Presentation	Possible Systemic Associations	Risks	Recommendations	Differential Diagnosis	Key to Diagnosis
Hypopigmented and Depigmented Macules and Patches							
Vitiligo	Depigmented patches caused by loss of melanocytes, immunologically mediated; favors periorificial and "tip" areas	New-onset stark white skin around the eyes, lips, fingertips, and penis	Autoimmune thyroiditis, pernicious anemia, Addison disease, diabetes mellitus	Skin cancer	Sunscreens	Postinflammatory hypopigmentation, albinism, chemical leukoderma	Acquired depigmentation without a history of exposure to phenolic compounds which may cause depigmentation
Idiopathic guttate hypomelanosis, "snowflakes"	Hypopigmented 3- to 8-mm macules caused by focal loss of melanin production	Asymptomatic whitish macules on the pretibial and extensor forearm surfaces	None	None	Sunscreens	Vitiligo	Small macules of hypopigmentation on sun-damaged skin
Tinea versicolor	See Chapter 117						
Halo nevus	Symmetric depigmented halo around a nevus	Small symmetric halo surrounding an evenly pigmented brown papule in a young individual	In adults and those with a history of melanoma, suspect melanloma or associated metastatic melanoma	Misdiagnosis	If halo is asymmetric or nevus is abnormal by the ABCDs, biopsy to rule out melanoma	Melanoma with regression, dysplastic nevus	Symmetric mole with symmetric halo of depigmentation
Hyperpigmented Macules and Patches							
Junctional nevus	Light to dark macule of uniform shape and brown color, may develop from early childhood to early thirties; formed by nests of melanocytes at the dermal–epidermal junction	2- to 6-mm sharply circumscribed, evenly pigmented, brown macule	None	People with >40 to 50 nevi have an increased risk of melanoma	Monthly self-examinations; intermittent physican examination	Lentigo simplex, freckle	May be difficult to clinically distinguish from lentigo and freckles; however, all three are benign
Solar lentigo	"Liver spot"; brown, 2-mm to 2-cm macule occurring on a background of chronic sun-damaged skin	Multiple hyperpigmented 3- to 8-mm brown macules on the face and dorsal hands	None	None	Prevention: sunscreen use; elective treatment: cryosurgery, laser surgery, hydroquinone fading creams	Lentigo simplex, lentigo maligna (i.e., melanoma *in situ*)	Homogeneous pigmentation on background of sun-damaged skin

Continued

Table 113.1.—*continued.* **Selected Skin Disorders Based on Morphology**

Disorder	Description	Common Presentation	Possible Systemic Associations	Risks	Recommendations	Differential Diagnosis	Key to Diagnosis
			Hyperpigmented Macules and Patches				
Cafe-au-lait spot	Evenly pigmented, light to medium brown, 1- to several cm macule; noted at birth or in early childhood	Tan brown macule	Neurofibromatosis: Presence of six cafe-au-lait spots greater than 1.5 cm often with axillary freckling; may have tumors, e.g., CNS neoplasms, pheochromocytoma Albright syndrome: large, unilateral, pigmented macule with an irregular border, polyostotic fibrous dysplasia and precocious puberty Tuberous sclerosis: cafe-au-lait spots, seizures, adenoma sebaceum (perinasal skin colored papules), and ash leaf macules (hypopigmented macules)		Lightening or removal may be attempted with laser surgery	Junctional nevus	Macular pigmentation with no surface change (i.e., no epidermal alteration)
Melasma	Irregular tan to brown pigmentation; favors cheeks, forehead and upper lip	Patchy brown discoloration on central forehead and cheeks	Pregnancy and exogenous estrogens	N/A	Sunscreens and avoidance of sun exposure, hydroquinone fading creams, or elective laser surgery	Hydroquinone induced in "pseudo-ochronosis"	Female, facial location, intensifies in the summer
Xanthelasma	See Chapter 82						
Xanthoma	See Chapter 82						
			Papules				
Warts, tumors	See Chapter 117						
Compound nevus	Tan to dark brown, 2- to 6-mm dome-shaped papule, formed by nests of melanocytes, both at the dermal epidermal junction and in the dermis	Stable brown "mole"	None	None	Patient self-examinations for changes, as with all nevi; biopsy if diagnosis is in question	Melanoma, intradermal nevus, dermatofibroma, neurofibroma	Soft, circumscribed, symmetric, evenly colored papule
Intradermal nevus	Skin color to light brown, generally 2- to 6-mm fleshy papule; consists of nests of melanocytes confined to the dermis	Dome shaped, skin-colored papule	None	None	Biopsy if diagnosis is in question	Amelanotic melanoma, dermatofibroma, neurofibroma	Soft, circumscribed, symmetric, skin colored papule

Seborrheic keratosis (Fig. 113.1)	"Stuck on" appearing tan, yellowish-brown to black-brown plaque with a friable, fine papulated, or smooth surface studded with tiny white flecks of keratin; caused by local proliferation of the epidermis; common after age 30 or 40	Tan to dark brown finely papulated "stuck on" flat topped papules over the trunk	"Sudden" eruption of many inflamed seborrheic keratoses; may herald a malignancy, most often with adenocarcinoma	None	Liquid nitrogen cryosurgery or curettage may be used on pruritic or troublesome lesions; biopsy, never destroy, if diagnosis is in question	Wart, squamous cell carcinoma, basal cell carcinoma, melanoma	Characteristic "stuck on" appearance
Cherry angioma	"Cherry red" 0.5- to 6-mm dome-shaped nonblanching papules which favor the trunk, formed by dilated capillaries; common after age 30 or 40	Minute to 4-mm red to purple dome-shaped papules	Hereditary hemorrhagic telangiectasia: autosomal dominant, punctate telangiectasias on the oral mucosa and fingers +/− AV malformations in the GI tract, lungs, and CNS CREST: sclerodactyly with punctate and matlike telangiectasias on the face and fingers	None	Cauterize if traumatized or if desired for cosmesis	Hemangioma	Characteristic size and cherry red appearance
Dermatofibroma	Smooth, circumscribed, 3- to 10-mm papule in the skin; feels like a "pea in the skin"; composed of fibroblasts, questionable reaction to earlier insect bite	Small, brownish ill-defined macule with underlying papule		None	Biopsy if diagnosis is in question	Nodular melanoma, nevus	Characteristic "pea-like" dermal papule without surface change
Condyloma acuminatum	See Chapter 117						
Molluscum contagiosum	See Chapter 117						
Basal cell carcinoma	See Chapter 114						
Squamous cell carcinoma	See Chapter 114						
Kaposi sarcoma	See Chapter 39						
				Plaques			
Psoriasis	See Chapter 116						
Seborrheic dermatitis	See Chapter 116						
Atopic dermatitis	See Chapter 116						
Nummular dermatitis	See Chapter 116						
Secondary syphilis	See Chapter 37						
Contact dermatitis	See Chapter 116						
Tinea	See Chapter 117						
Xanthoma	See Chapter 82						

Continued

Table 113.1.—*continued.* Selected Skin Disorders Based on Morphology

Disorder	Description	Common Presentation	Possible Systemic Associations	Risks	Recommendations	Differential Diagnosis	Key to Diagnosis
				Plaques			
Pityriasis rosea	Self-limited eruption, lasting several weeks, initial lesion: herald patch; >1-cm erythematous oval plaque with fine peripheral scale, usually on the chest, followed in 7–14 days by an eruption of smaller plaques over the trunk; variable pruritus	1- to 3-cm oval plaque, followed by a shower of 25–100 similar 3- to 15-mm papules and plaques on the trunk, with the long axes of the lesions oriented along the skin lines in a "Christmas tree" pattern	None	None	If pruritic, midpotency topical corticosteroids; if extremely pruritic, consider phototherapy	Secondary syphilis, primary HIV exanthem, tinea corporis, tinea versicolor, psoriasis	Herald patch, negative test for syphilis
Pityriasis alba	A mild form of dermatitis, in young patients; hypopigmented, slightly scaly, up to several cm macules or minimally elevated plaques; occasionally pruritic	Asymptomatic scaly patches over the arms and legs	More common in patients with atopy	None	Emollients, hydrocortisone; phototherapy	Tinea versicolor, hypopigmented mycosis fungoides, sarcoidosis	May be difficult to exclude other diagnoses without further evaluation (i.e., KOH +/– biopsy)
Mycosis fungoides	Cutaneous T-cell lymphoma most often affects patients over age 40; however, any age may be affected; erythematous to brawny patches, plaques, or tumors; may assume bizarre irregular shapes; asymptomatic or pruritic	Several-year history of scaly reddish plaques gradually increasing in number over the trunk	None	Although a lymphoma, evidence of systemic involvement with simple testing is usually absent unless the disease progresses; poor prognosis is associated with greater than 10% body surface area involvement, tumor, and lymphadenopathy (the latter requires biopsy to determine reactive vs. neoplastic)	Treatment varies with the stage of the disease and age of patient; PUVA, electron beam, topical nitrogen mustard, interferon γ, observation	Parapsoriasis, psoriasis, sarcoidosis, pityriasis alba	Biopsy required

Erythema nodosum	Hypersensitivity reaction to some antigen, erythematous, tender nodules most often on the pretibial legs; develop in crops and involute over 2–3 weeks, resolve with a local bruise, never suppurate and drain; caused by a localized inflammatory infiltrate in the septum surrounding fat lobules	Acute onset of erythematous nodules over the pretibial area associated with mild arthralgias	More common associations include streptococcal infection, vaginal candidiasis, tuberculosis, viral hepatitis, coccidioidomycosis, histoplasmosis, lymphogranuloma venereum, *Yersinia enterocolitica*; inflammatory bowel disease, or reaction to sulfonamides, barbiturates, various antibiotics, salicylates, oral contraceptives, or pregnancy	None	Evaluation to exclude possible associations; review of Rx and OTC medications, throat culture, ASO titer, chest x-ray, PPD; complete viral hepatitis screen; additional workup based on clinical findings; reassess chronic disease with a search for "occult infection" (dental, sinus, gallbladder, other gastrointestional, etc.)	Other forms of panniculitis and polyarteritis nodosa	Tender nodules on the pretibial legs that resolve over a few weeks without ever ulcerating
Lipoma	Benign fatty tumor, often solitary, on the trunk	Asymptomatic rubbery nodule, movable under the skin	None	None	Excision if desired or diagnosis is in question	Cyst, neurofibroma, soft tissue malignancies	Soft nodule, freely movable under the skin

CNS, central nervous system; AV, atrioventricular; GI, gastrointestinal; CREST, *c*alcinosis, *R*aynaud phenomenon, *e*sophageal motility disorders, *s*clerodactyly, and *t*elangiectasia; HIV, human immunodeficiency virus; OTC, over the counter; ASO, antistreptolysin; PPD, purified protein derivative of tuberculin.

(silver nitrate 0.1% to 0.5% solution, acetic acid 1% to 5% solution). All, including saline made by adding 2 teaspoons salt per 1 L of water, promote drying through evaporation and remove devitalized tissue through physical softening, allowing mechanical removal upon lifting the damp ("wet to damp") or dry ("wet to dry") dressing.

Compresses may be gauze or cotton sheeting. For the latter, a clean sheet should be cut and folded into six to eight layers to approximate the area of affected skin. This is immersed in the soaking solution and squeezed just short of dripping wet. It is placed on the site for 15 to 30 minutes, three or four times per day, and is rewetted every 15 minutes for a "wet to damp" dressing.

When more than one-third of the body surface area is affected by acute dermatitis or impetiginization, compresses are not only impractical but may cause hypothermia. Warm *baths* are used instead. Preferred drying and soothing additives include Aveeno Oatmeal Packet, sodium bicarbonate (baking soda, 3 cups), hydrolyzed starch (Lint, 4 cups mixed with water in a large mixing bowl and then added to the bath water), and a mix of half of each of the bicarbonate and starch mixtures.

Baths are also useful for generalized dry pruritic dermatoses such as atopic dermatitis, generalized psoriasis, morbilliform drug eruptions, and erythroderma. Instead of drying additives, oil (1/8 cup bath oil or Aveeno Oilated Oatmeal Packet) is added to the bath water to help trap moisture in the skin. Patients must be warned about oil making the bathtub slippery and should be advised to purchase secure bath mats for the tub and for the floor outside the tub. Unsteady or frail patients should not use bath oil. Baths should be taken three or four times a day for 20 minutes and a heavy moisturizer (e.g., Vaseline jelly, Aquaphor ointment, Eucerin Original Lotion) must be reapplied immediately after lightly patting dry, leaving some moisture on the skin.

SKIN BIOPSY

Skin biopsy for histologic examination of the skin is required to confirm the diagnosis of many skin conditions. Types of biopsies that may be used include *punch, ellipse,* and *shave.* They may be *incisional* (sampling a portion of the lesion) or *excisional* (removing the entire lesion). Skin biopsy is a simple and invaluable procedure that may be easily mastered with the help of a skilled instructor and practice.

General References

Ackerman BA, Kerl H, Sanchez J. A clinical atlas of 101 common skin diseases with histopathologic correlation. New York: Ardor Scribendi, 2000.

Fitzpatrick TP, Johnson RA, Wolff K, et al. Color atlas and synopsis of clinical dermatology. 3rd ed. New York: McGraw-Hill, 1997.

A concise disease discussion, with excellent photographs.

Habib TP, Quitadamo MJ, Campbell JL, et al. Skin disease: diagnosis and treatment. St. Louis: Mosby, 2001.

An excellent text of clinical diagnosis and therapy.

Kazin, RA, Lowitt NR, Lowitt MH. Update in dermatology. Ann Intern Med 2001;135:124.

Highlights 10 articles of interest to the generalist.

Lamberg SI. The little black book of dermatology. Malden, MA: Blackwell, 2000.

A comprehensive clinical handbook organized by chief complaint, body part affected, or associated condition.

Lookingbill DP, Marks JG Jr. Principals of dermatology. 3rd ed. Philadelphia, PA: WB Saunders, 2000.

Websites

www.cancer.org (American Cancer Society Website; also telephone 800-ACS-2345)

An excellent resource for educational materials on skin cancer for physicians and patients.

www.aad.org (American Academy of Dermatology Website)

www.psoriasis.org (National Psoriasis Foundation Website)

http://tray.dermatology.uiowa.edu/home.html

University of Iowa Website with over 300 clinical photographs; also resource for dermatology patient support group.)

http://www.med.jhu.edu/peds/dermatlas.

Also see review: Lamberg L. Internet dermatology atlas aids physicians and parents. JAMA 2001;25:2065.

CHAPTER 114

Atypical Moles and Common Cancers of the Skin

S. ELIZABETH WHITMORE, MD, ScM

ATYPICAL MOLES

Atypical moles (or dysplastic nevi) affect 10% to 30% of the general population. These acquired lesions have clinical and histologic features that differ from common moles (i.e., melanocytic nevi). The latter are tan to dark brown in color, sharply circumscribed, 2- to 6-mm macules or papules that develop in childhood or early adulthood; the average adult has 20 common moles. In contrast, *atypical moles or dysplastic nevi are often larger than 6 mm, irregular or ill-defined, variegated in color* (Fig. 114.1, Color Plate section), and *may continue to appear after age 35.* Because of these atypical features, biopsy may be required to exclude the possible diagnosis of melanoma.

Patients with a few nonfamilial atypical moles and no personal history of melanoma are at increased risk for melanoma when compared with the general population, with a relative risk somewhere between 2 and 8 (1). With the goal of detecting melanomas as early as possible, patients are asked to perform monthly self-examinations, looking for any change in the appearance of a mole, and to have physician skin examinations done every 6 to 12 months.

The *familial atypical mole and melanoma (FAMM) syndrome,* formerly called the dysplastic nevus syndrome, is associated with an extremely high risk of melanoma. Although the prevalence is probably greatly underestimated, it is said to affect at least 300,000 people. These individuals begin to develop atypical lesions at puberty and continue to develop new lesions throughout their lives. Patients with this syndrome have a family history of melanoma in at least one first- or second-degree relative and many nevi, often more than 50, some or many of which are atypical. Patients with the FAMM syndrome have a lifetime risk of developing melanoma approaching 100%. Patients with sporadic atypical mole syndrome with a mole pattern similar to that of the FAMM syndrome also have a significantly increased risk of developing melanoma. All these patients should perform monthly self-examinations, looking for any changes in the appearance of their moles. Additionally, they should be examined at 4- to 12-month intervals by a dermatologist so that appropriate biopsies or photographs can be taken. Patients should be counseled on methods of self-examination and means of sun protection (avoidance of exposure during peak sun intensity hours, use of high sun protection factor sunscreen, and appropriate protective clothing) because sun exposure increases the risk of malignancy. Also, it should be made clear that other family members may be similarly affected and advised, because early detection saves lives.

MELANOMA

Cutaneous malignant melanoma is the third most common type of skin cancer and the leading cause of death from skin disease (1–3). The incidence of melanoma in this country is increasing more rapidly than any other cancer. Amazingly, the risk has increased over 20-fold in the last 70 years (4,5). It is estimated that in the United States, 51,400 new cases of melanoma will be diagnosed and 7,800 persons will die with melanoma. The estimated lifetime risk of melanoma in American white males is 1 in 70. Melanoma is the most common and second most common cancer in women aged 25 to 29 and 30 to 34 years, respectively (6). Unfortunately, public knowledge of melanoma is poor; a recent survey demonstrated that 50% of men and 35% of women were unfamiliar with the term *melanoma* and only 31% of adults limit sun exposure, 28% use sunscreen routinely, and 28% wear protective clothing (3).

Although melanoma occurs with greatest frequency within a small subpopulation of persons having the FAMM syndrome or nonfamilial atypical moles, most patients who develop melanoma have neither of these relatively uncommon risk factors. Six much more common independent risk factors for melanoma include family history of melanoma, blond or red hair, marked freckling on the upper back, three or more blistering sunburns before age 20, three or more summers spent outside working as a teen, and the presence of actinic keratoses (see below). Having one or two of these risk factors increases risk by 3.5-fold and having three or more risk factors increases risk by 20-fold. Although rare in African Americans, melanomas are most often found on the hands and feet, where incidence is similar among various races. Although the cause of melanoma is unknown, ultraviolet radiation is an important risk factor. Evidence for this includes the greater incidence of melanoma found in persons living closer to the equator, persons having a history of blistering sunburns, and persons with a history of basal or squamous cell carcinoma (7).

As a general rule, all pigmented lesions should be scrutinized for atypical features that may suggest melanoma. These include the *ABCDs: asymmetry, border irregularity, color variegation* (variable degrees of brown, tan, black, red, white, or blue), and *diameter greater than 6 mm.* Although one or more of these features may be present in a given melanoma, they may be absent. For instance, a nodular melanoma usually presents as a symmetric, dome-shaped, deeply but evenly pigmented, rapidly growing papule or nodule, exhibiting none of the ABCDs. For this reason, excisional biopsy of *changing* or *atypical* moles should generally be performed, and ongoing close surveillance of patients with many remaining moles or the sporadic or familial atypical mole syndrome by a dermatologist or practitioner skilled in the area should be recommended. Finally, patient education is of key importance, with focus on the appearance of atypical moles and melanomas using the ABCDs, monthly or bimonthly self-examination, protection from the sun (sun avoidance, sunscreen use, and protective clothing), and awareness of the possible familial link (i.e., patients with atypical moles or melanoma should most certainly inform relatives of the possible genetic link and the need for skin examination).

There are four common subtypes of melanoma: superficial spreading, nodular, lentigo maligna, and acral lentiginous melanoma. Fortunately, the characteristically difficult to diagnose amelanotic melanoma, which is usually white, pink, or red, is relatively rare. The characteristics of these melanoma subtypes are outlined in Table 114.1.

Superficial spreading melanoma arises from a preexisting nevus in approximately 25% to 50% of cases. Typically, radial or outward growth occurs over a period of months to years. Clinical changes caused by this malignant transformation are generally seen as a change in diameter and border irregularity. With time, growth descends vertically from the epidermal–dermal junction and the surface becomes papular. This vertical growth creates the potential for metastasis. A superficial spreading melanoma is shown in Fig. 114.2 (see Color Plate section).

Nodular melanoma usually does not manifest any of the ABCDs of atypical pigmented lesions because it generally has no radial but only a vertical growth phase. This type of melanoma is usually a dome-shaped or polypoid, symmetric, deeply pigmented papule. It may develop *de novo* or arise within a pre-existing nevus. Nodular melanoma tends to grow rapidly over weeks to months.

Lentigo maligna melanoma occurs on sun-exposed skin, most commonly on the face. It arises from a pre-existing lentigo maligna, which is a tan, brown, or brown/black, typically irregularly outlined macule on a sun-exposed site, usually present for many years. In fact, the term lentigo means freckle. Lentigo maligna melanoma has a radial growth phase like that of superficial spreading melanoma and therefore commonly shows the ABCDs of atypical pigmented lesions.

Acral lentiginous melanoma occurs with equal frequency in both light and deeply pigmented persons. This is in contrast to all other types of melanomas, which are rare in deeply pigmented persons. It is the most frequent type of melanoma occurring in African Americans and Asians. It presents on the peripheral parts (hence the name), especially the palms, soles, or subungually (i.e., underneath the nail plate) within the nail unit, and usually displays some of the ABCDs of atypical pigmented lesions. Hutchinson sign marked by pigment extending onto the skin of the nailfold in association with a subungual pigmented lesion is highly suggestive of melanoma, and biopsy is mandatory. Acral lentiginous melanoma frequently has a poor

Table 114.1. Features of the Subtypes of Melanoma

Melanoma Subtype[a]	Approximate Frequency (%)	Clinical Appearance	Location	Age Group Most Often Affected	Differential Diagnosis
Superficial spreading	70	Usually brown but may be variably colored brown, black, blue, red, and white; flattish papule, plaque, or maculopapule, usually over 6 mm in diameter; usually showing 1 or more of the ABCDs[b] of atypical moles and melanoma	Anywhere, often on the back in men and on the legs in women	30–40 yr	Nevus, seborrheic keratosis
Nodular	16	Colored as above or amelantoic, dome-shaped or polypoid papule or nodule; typically symmetric and uniform	Anywhere	40–50 yr	Nevus, thrombosed capillary hemangioma, pyogenic granuloma
Lentigo maligna	5	Tan or brown, less often black, blue, or red, irregular macule with focal surface elevation; later may develop distinct papules and nodules within	Face most often; other sun-exposed surfaces	50–70 yr	Solar lentigo (liver spot)
Acral lentiginous	<5	Similar in appearance to lentigo maligna melanoma; when it occurs as a pigmented streak in the nail with extension onto the nail fold skin, it is called *Hutchinson sign* (see text); seen most often in African Americans and Asians	Palms, soles, phalanges	All ages	Nevus, postinflammatory or drug-induced hyperpigmentation, fungal infection-induced nail dystrophy; pyogenic granuloma

[a]Other rare types combined make up less than 5% of melanoma.
[b]ABCDs, see text p. 1735.

prognosis because diagnosis is often delayed. Up to 50% of patients with acral lentiginous melanoma give a history of preceding trauma of the skin in the area of the lesion. This history and the mistaken acceptance by the patient and physician that the pigment change or nail dystrophy is the result of trauma often contributes to a delay in biopsy and diagnosis.

Although the U.S. Preventive Service Task Force has not found sufficient evidence to recommend routine full body skin examination for melanoma, an argument can be made that early detection and excision is associated with a lower incidence of melanoma associated morbidity and mortality. With the latter in mind, our urgent aim is to detect melanoma as early in evolution as possible. At present, this seems best facilitated through public and professional education. A study involving 102 patients (47 male, 55 female) diagnosed with melanoma seen at one institution between 1995 and 1997 found that 55% of malignancies were self detected, whereas 24% were detected by the health care provider. Those detected by professionals were thinner than those detected by patients (0.23 mm versus 0.9 mm, $p < .001$). These data should motivate continued patient and professional education (8).

Patients with suspicious lesions should be referred to a dermatologist or surgeon for evaluation for possible melanoma. In contrast to patients with suspected basal cell carcinoma (BCC) or squamous cell carcinoma (SCC) in whom a delay of 4 to 6 weeks is acceptable, patients with melanoma should be seen within a week or two. The suspected lesion will likely be fully excised for diagnosis. When full excision of the lesion is not possible because of anatomic location or size, an incisional biopsy of the most atypical and elevated area of the lesion is performed. If the diagnosis of melanoma is confirmed histologically, reexcision with an appropriate margin of normal surrounding tissue, as dictated by the vertical thickness of the melanoma, is necessary (0.5 cm for melanoma *in situ*; 1 cm to 2 or 3 cm for invasive melanoma). Simultaneous sentinel lymph node excision or elective lymph node dissection in patients with melanoma clinically limited to the skin remains controversial. Although data are still being gathered regarding the use of sentinel lymph node biopsy, many centers routinely perform sentinel lymph node biopsies for melanomas over 1 mm in thickness (9–11).

Follow-up surveillance and testing in patients after melanoma excision is controversial. A noncon-current prospective study has addressed this issue: 261 patients having moderate or high risk for recurrent melanoma (thickness greater than 1.68 mm) were studied, undergoing examination monthly for 2 months, then bimonthly for the first year, and every 4 and 6 months for the second and third years, respectively. Evaluation included history, physical examination, complete blood count, chemistry, and chest x-ray. Of these patients, 161 developed recurrent melanoma; 145 were fully assessable. Recurrent disease most often occurred in the regional lymph nodes (45%) or skin (22%). Disease was detected by the patient or by history (68%), examination (26%), and chest x-ray (6%), suggesting that routine blood testing is not necessary for follow-up surveillance and chest x-ray yield is limited (12).

A more comprehensive follow-up regimen has been proposed based on data accrued on 373 patients at a large university melanoma center (13). Among the patients reported, 21% developed a recurrence with nearly 80% of these recurrences developing in the first 2 years. Five percent developed a second melanoma during the surveillance period. Of the melanoma recurrences, half were detected by the patient and half by the professional. Based on these data, the recommendations for follow-up visit frequency in patients with melanoma is as follows:

- Stage I (<1.5 mm thickness): annually;
- Stage II (≥1.5 mm thickness, localized disease only): every 6 months for 2 years, then annually;
- Stage III (local noda1 or in-transit metastases): every 3 months for 1 year, every 4 months for the next year, then every 6 months for 4 years, and annually thereafter (persons with stage III disease were all encouraged to undergo adjunctive systemic therapy).

Usually, the dermatologist or plastic surgeon will establish this follow-up schedule, but the generalist should reinforce the plan.

Further recommendations for each visit include a focused history and physical examination, complete blood count, liver function tests, and lactate dehydrogenase level, with abnormal results prompting further evaluation. Although some authorities recommend an annual chest x-ray, others recommend this only if the findings of history and physical examination suggest a problem (13,14).

The prognosis for a patient after excision of a primary cutaneous melanoma depends on the thickness of the melanoma and whether there is evidence of spread to lymph nodes or distant metastases. Ten-year survival rates, based on melanoma thickness, are as follows: ≤1 mm, 92%; >1 to 2 mm, 78%; >2 to 4.0 mm, 60%; >4 mm, 55%. If ulceration is present, 10-year survival rates decrease to 69%, 63%, 53%, and 36%, respectively. In patients with metastases to the regional lymph nodes, the 5-year median survival is less than 30%. When distant metastases are present, the median survival is 6 months.

Adjuvant therapy for persons at "high risk" for recurrence and mortality after definitive surgery is controversial. Although adjuvant interferon-alpha-2b is approved by the U.S. Food and Drug Administration for this, the benefit of this treatment is debated (11). Therapeutic melanoma vaccines hold promise but are still investigational (15).

ACTINIC KERATOSIS AND NONMELANOMA SKIN CANCER

Actinic Keratosis

Actinic keratoses are sun-induced precancers or focal areas of epidermal dysplasia (Table 114.2). Although

Table 114.2. Nonmelanoma Skin Cancers, Keratoacanthomas, and Actinic Keratoses

Neoplasm	Clinical Type	Presentation	Key Features	Differential Diagnosis
Actinic keratosis		Erythematous, scaly to hyperkeratotic macules; ill-defined border; usually multiple; always on sun-damage skin	Scaly, ill-defined lesion on sun-damaged skin	Bowen disease, superficial BCC, SCC, dermatitis, tinea
Keratoacanthoma		Firm to hard, volcano-like crater with a central keratin plug	Keratin-filled "crater"	SCC, prurigo nodularis
Basal cell carcinoma (BCC)	Noduloulcerative	Small, firm, waxy papule often with telangiectasias; may ulcerate, often on the face	Waxy papule	Intradermal nevus, fibrous papule, folliculitis, seborrheic keratosis
	Superficial	Erythematous, sharply circumscribed, scaly macule border or thin plaque with a fine thready border, often on the trunk	Thread-like border	Actinic keratosis, Bowen disease, nummular dermatitis, contact dermatitis, tinea
	Morpheaform	Spontaneous scar-like lesion; whitish yellow, smooth, shiny scar surface	"Spontaneous" scar	Scar, granuloma annulare, sarcoid, localized scleroderma
	Pigmented	Blue, brown, or black waxy papule; mostly found in deeply pigmented white, Asian, or African-American people	Pigmented waxy papule	Seborrheic keratosis, nevus, melanoma
Squamous cell carcinoma (SCC)	Common SCC	Firm to hard, erythematous, hyperkeratotic nodule, or ulcerated nodule; especially on the dorsal hands, forearms, and face	Firm/hard keratotic nodule	Keratoacanthoma, hypertrophic actinic keratosis, seborrheic keratosis, prurigo nodularis
	Bowen disease, SCC *in situ*	Erythematous, sharply circumscribed, scaly macule or thin plaque	Circumscribed scaly erythema	Actinic keratosis, superficial BCC, dermatitis, tinea

occasionally seen in teenagers, they generally begin to develop in the fourth or fifth decades of life in fair-skinned persons with other evidence of sun damage, such as freckling or solar lentigines (liver spots). Lesions appear as ill-defined erythematous, generally 2- to 8-mm scaly macules or minimally elevated hyperkeratotic papules on sun-exposed sites (Fig. 114.3, Color Plate section). They are most easily detected by gently running the fingertips over the area because they feel like islands of fine sandpaper. Although precancerous, less than 1% progress to invasive SCC.

Patients with actinic keratoses should be treated with topical 5-fluorouracil cream (Carac, Fluoroplex, Efudex) or cryotherapy using liquid nitrogen to destroy the abnormal epidermis. With cryotherapy, the treated area may blister, crust, and then heal in 1 to 2 weeks without scarring. However, postinflammatory hypopigmentation or depigmentation, leaving a whitish macule, is not uncommon. If one is unfamiliar with either of these forms of therapy, referral to a dermatologist is appropriate. New lesions are likely to occur, and patients with actinic keratoses should be examined every 6 to 12 months.

Nonmelanoma Skin Cancers

The two most common skin cancers and the most common cancers in humans, *BCC* and *SCC*, make up 95% of the estimated 1.3 million skin cancers expected in 2001 in the United States. The anticipated ratio of BCC to SCC is 4:1 (16–18).

The most important risk factors for nonmelanoma skin cancers (NMSCs) include cumulative sun exposure (for most Americans, over 80% of the lifetime sun exposure occurs before age 18), fair skin color, and older age. Less well-established and important risk factors for SCC include tobacco smoking and sunlamp or suntan parlor use.

Even though almost all NMSCs occur on sun-exposed surfaces, covered or usually covered sites such as the hair-bearing scalp, genitalia, or lower extremities may develop cancers. In these sites normally protected from sun exposure, other risk factors are usually involved, such as a distant history of scalp irradiation for treatment of tinea or a hemangioma, prior genital human papilloma virus infection, and chronic ulceration (e.g., hidradenitis suppurativa, chronic leg ulcer).

Patients who have undergone organ transplants are also at increased risk for NMSC, because of therapeutic immune suppression. The frequency of SCCs in these patients may reach 30% to 40% 10 years after transplantation. This represents a 4- to 21-fold increase in frequency of SCC (19).

In certain disorders, patients have early onset of innumerable skin cancers. The most common of these is *basal cell nevus syndrome,* an autosomal dominant inherited disorder in which patients develop palmar pits (ice pick-like indentations), jaw cysts, and calcification of the falx cerebri, in combination with multiple BCCs, usually beginning in the teens or twenties. A mutation in the Patched (*Ptc*) gene on chromosome 9 is believed to be responsible for this syndrome as well as some sporadic BCCs (20). Another disorder, *xeroderma pigmentosum*, is an autosomal recessive condition with childhood onset of SCCs, BCCs, and occasionally melanomas. Patients have a defect in excision or postreplication repair of ultraviolet radiation-induced DNA changes.

Basal Cell Carcinoma

Eighty percent of BCCs develop on the head and neck. Other commonly affected sites include the upper trunk in both sexes and the legs in women. Patients typically give a history of a new lesion or a lesion that repeatedly gets red, peels, or bleeds and then improves, only to repeat the cycle. BCC may be divided into subtypes based on clinical morphology: *nodular ulcerative, superficial, morpheaform or sclerosing,* and *pigmented.*

Nodular ulcerative BCC accounts for approximately half of all cases of BCC. Typically, the lesion is first noted as a firm, pink/white to semitranslucent ("opalescent") papule with telangiectasias. If allowed to progress to a nodule, the vascular supply may become insufficient and ulceration may occur forming the classic "rodent ulcer" (Fig. 114.4; see Color Plate). Before ulceration, the differential diagnosis includes an intradermal nevus, fibrous papule, inflamed follicle, and seborrheic keratosis. Several points may help distinguish these entities. A nevus is soft and typically present for many years, an inflamed hair follicle should resolve in no longer than a few weeks from onset, and a seborrheic keratosis has a stuck-on appearance and a fine papulated or pebbly surface. If the diagnosis of BCC cannot be excluded clinically, biopsy must be performed. Suspected BCCs should also be biopsied to confirm the diagnosis for definitive treatment.

Superficial BCC appears as a sharply circumscribed, erythematous, scaly, 3-mm to many centimeter macule or a slightly elevated plaque with a characteristic thread-like border. The differential diagnosis includes actinic keratosis, Bowen disease (SCC *in situ*), extramammary Paget disease, dermatitis (nummular or contact), psoriasis, and tinea.

Morpheaform or sclerotic BCC develops as a spontaneous, macular, slightly elevated or depressed scar. It has a white, faint pink, or yellow appearance, looking devoid of vessels and appendygeal structures (hair and sebaceous and eccrine glands). The differential diagnosis includes a traumatic or surgical scar, localized scleroderma (morphea), and, less often, granuloma annulare and cutaneous sarcoidosis.

Pigmented BCCs are similar in appearance to nodular or superficial BCCs but are pigmented. They occur most often on more deeply pigmented whites, Asians, and African Americans. The differential diagnosis includes melanoma, seborrheic keratosis, and nevus.

Squamous Cell Carcinoma

SCC may develop *de novo* or may arise from an actinic keratosis (16). It appears as a firm to hard erythematous to brawny nodule, often with central hyperkeratotic (stacked) scale or ulceration (Fig. 114.5; see Color Plate). The hyperkeratotic scale may form a horn (pointed surface protrusion). The differential diagnosis includes keratoacanthoma, wart, and seborrheic keratosis. *Keratoacanthoma* mimics SCC both clinically and histologically but is believed to be a benign self-healing tumor. It develops over several weeks, beginning as a rapidly enlarging papule with a central hyperkeratotic plug that spontaneously involutes over several weeks.

Pathogenesis of Nonmelanoma Skin Cancers

BCC and SCC are derived from keratinocytes; BCC specifically arises from basal keratinocytes of the epidermis and adnexa. It is believed that damage caused by ultraviolet B radiation (wavelengths 290 to 320 nm) to DNA in the form of cyclobutane pyrimidine dimers, inadequacy of DNA repair mechanisms, and suppression of the local immune surveillance system are all important in the development of NMSC.

Prognosis and Therapy of Nonmelanoma Skin Cancer

Although BCC rarely metastasizes (<0.03%), SCC may do so in approximately 3% of patients. Rates are greatest for SCCs developing on the lips, in scar tissue, and in areas of chronic inflammation. Sites of metastasis may include regional lymph nodes, liver, lung, bone, and brain. Metastatic SCC is associated with a 5-year survival rate of approximately 15% to 40%. People who have had one NMSC are at increased risk for future skin cancers. Within 5 years of one NMSC, a patient has a 50% chance of developing a second tumor (21). Patients with previous NMSC have a 17-fold increased risk of developing melanoma (7).

Patients suspected of having NMSC should have biopsy confirmation before definitive treatment. Treatment options for cancers include excisional therapy, *Mohs micrographic surgery* (a procedure in which the visible cancer is excised and the specimen immediately examined histologically to ensure that the margins are free of cancer; if cancer is still present, a deeper section is taken and examined; this is repeated until the resected tissue is free of cancer), electrodesiccation and curettage, cryosurgery, or radiation therapy. The treatment modality depends on the type of cancer (cell type, primary or recurrent), location, the patient's age and ability to tolerate a procedure, local availability of the procedure, and patient preference. Nonsurgical nonradiation therapies are under study and hold promise. For example, imiquimod cream, an immune response modifier that enhances local cutaneous cytokine production when applied topically, appears to be effective in the treatment of superficial BCC (22).

In patients who develop many NMSC, such as those with organ transplants or with basal cell nevus syndrome or xeroderma pigmentosum (see above), chemoprophylaxis with retinoids may be considered. At appropriate dosages of isotretinoin or acitretin, patients seem to develop fewer cancers. Unfortunately, the retinoid must be continued indefinitely to maintain the protective effect. Retinoids have many potential side effects; in addition to being teratogenic and often causing elevation of lipids, they may cause tendon calcification and vertebral hyperostosis with chronic administration (23). Such patients generally should be followed by a dermatologist.

Specific References*

1. Koh HK. Cutaneous melanoma. N Engl J Med 1991;325:171.
2. Perniciaro C. Dermatopathologic variants of malignant melanoma. Mayo Clin Proc 1997;72:273.
3. Su WPD. Malignant melanoma: basic approach to clinicopathologic correlation. Mayo Clin Proc 1997;72:267.
4. Greenlee RT, Hill-Harmon MB, Murrary T, et al. Cancer statistics, 2001. CA Cancer J Clin 2001;51:15.
5. Rigel DS, Carucci JA. Malignant melanoma: prevention, early detection, and treatment in the 21st century. CA Cancer J Clin 2000;50:215.
6. Rigel DS, Friedman RJ, Kopf AW. The incidence of melanoma in the United States: issues as we approach the 21st century. J Am Acad Dermatol 1996;341:839.
7. Marghoob AA, Slade J, Salopek TG, et al. Basal cell and squamous cell carcinoma are important risk factors for cutaneous malignant melanoma. Cancer 1995;75:707.
8. Epstein DS, Lange JR, Gruber SB, et al. Is physician detection associated with thinner melanomas? JAMA 1999;281:640.
9. Gadd MA, Cosimi AB, Yu J, et al. Outcome of patients with melanoma and histologically negative sentinel lymph nodes. Arch Surg 1999;134:381.
10. Gerhenwald JE, Thompson W, Mansfield PF, et al. Multi-institutional melanoma lymphatic mapping experience: the prognostic value of sentinel lymph node status in 612 Stage I or II melanoma patients. J Clin Oncol 1999;17:976.
11. Kanzler MH, Mraz-Gernhard S. Treatment of primary cutaneous melanoma. JAMA 2001;285:1819.
12. Weiss M, Loprinzi CL, Creagan ET, et al. Utility of follow-up tests for detecting recurrent disease in patients with malignant melanoma. JAMA 1995;274:1703.
13. Poo-Hwu WJ, Ariyan S, Lamb L, et al. Follow-up recommendations for patients with American Joint Committee on Cancer stages I-III malignant melanoma. Cancer 1999;86:2252.
14. Terhune MH, Swanson N, Johnson TM. Use of chest radiography in the initial evaluation of patients with localized melanoma. Arch Dermatol 1998;134:569.
15. Hsueh EC, Nathanson L, Foshog LJ, et al. Active specific immunotherapy with a polyvalent melanoma cell: vaccine for patients with in-transit melanoma metastases. Cancer 1999; 85:2160.
16. Alam M, Ratner D. Cutaneous squamous cell carcinoma. N Engl J Med 2001;344:975.
17. National Melanoma/Skin Cancer Detection and Prevention Month, May 1996. JAMA 1996;275:1537.
18. Preston DS, Stern RS. Nonmelanoma cancers of the skin. N Engl J Med 1992;327:1649.
19. Hoyo E, Kanitakis J, Euvrard S, et al. Proliferation characteristics of cutaneous squamous cell carcinomas developing in organ graft recipients. Arch Dermatol 1993;129:324.
20. Johnson RL, Rothman AL, Xie J, et al. Human homology of patched, a candidate gene for the basal cell nevus syndrome. Science 1996;272:1668.
21. Karagas MR, Stukel TA, Greenberg ER, et al. Risk of subsequent basal cell carcinomas and squamous cell carcinoma of the skin among patients without prior skin cancer. JAMA 1992;267:3305.
22. Marks RB, Gebauer K, Shumack S, et al. Imiquimod 5% cream in the treatment of superficial basal cell carcinoma: results of a multicenter 6-week dose-response trial. J Am Acad Dermatol 2001;44:807.
23. **23.** Bouwes Bavinck JN, Tieben LM, Van Der Woude FJ, et al. Prevention of skin cancer and reduction of keratotic skin lesions during acitretin therapy in renal transplant recipients: a double-blind, placebo-controlled study. J Clin Oncol 1995;13:1933.

*Bold print (general references) and bold numerals (specific references) denote published controlled clinical trials, meta-analysis, or consensus-based recommendations.

C H A P T E R 115

Disorders of the Pilosebaceous Unit: Acne and Related Disorders and Hair Loss

S. ELIZABETH WHITMORE, MD, ScM

ACNE VULGARIS

Definition and Pathogenesis

Acne vulgaris is a chronic disorder affecting the pilosebaceous units (hair follicles and sebaceous glands) of the face, chest, and back. *Four things must be present* for inflammatory acne to develop: androgen-stimulated sebum production; *Propionibacterium acnes*, an anaerobic diphtheroid of the normal follicular flora that proliferates in response to increased sebum; altered keratinization and desquamation of the cells lining the follicles; and a host inflammatory response.

Sebum production tends to be greater in people with acne than in those without acne. It is stimulated by *androgens*, primarily testosterone in males and testosterone and dehydroepiandrosterone in females. Sebum provides a favorable environment for proliferation of the *P. acnes,* which in turn metabolizes sebum, yielding glycerol and free fatty acids. These free fatty acids are believed to promote keratinization and *impaired desquamation* of the follicular epithelium, leading to *plugging*, seen clinically as comedones (i.e., white- and blackheads). *P. acnes* also causes inflammation directly, triggering the release of proteolytic enzymes, hyaluronidase, and neutrophil chemotactic factors, resulting in erythematous papules and pustules. If enough follicular damage occurs, the contents of the follicle spills into the dermis, causing an intense host response, seen as an acne cyst (pseudocyst).

Epidemiology

With an estimated 17 million people affected, acne is the most common skin disease in the United States. Acne not only affects over 85% of adolescents and young adults (aged 12 to 25 years) but often persists, develops for the first time, or recurs in the third, fourth, and fifth decades (1,2). A community-based study from the United Kingdom found that among 749 adults, the overall prevalence of clinical acne was 12% in women and 3% in men (3). Physiologic or minimal acne prevalence was 54% in women and 40% in men. Acne may contribute greatly to psychosocial problems such as depression, anxiety, self-imposed isolation, and a negative body image. Successful acne treatment usually corrects or significantly improves these problems.

Clinical Presentation

The earliest changes in acne may be seen in the prepubescent years with the appearance of closed and open *comedones* (white- and blackheads, respectively). As the disease progresses, *erythematous, follicular papules, pustules, and cysts* may develop on the face and upper trunk. Patients may be asymptomatic or complain of itching and soreness; they often find it impossible to resist physically manipulating (i.e., squeezing) the lesions.

Evaluation

Before one can determine the course of treatment for a patient, both the clinical severity of the disease and the impact of the disease on the patient must be appreciated. In some, acne may be extremely distressful, and unless asked, most remain silent on the issue.

A tragic suicide in a teen taking the acne medication isotretinoin (Accutane) raised concern about a possible association of isotretinoin depression and suicide risk. Although two large population-based cohort studies (in the United Kingdom and Canada) have not found any association between isotretinoin therapy and increased risk for suicide, depression, or other psychiatric disorders, the issue is still under study. Regardless, the clinician should be vigilant to recognize depression among patients with acne. Indeed, recognizing; and addressing the potential psychological impact that acne has in patients may be the most important part of acne therapy (4,5).

When patients present with acne, one should ask about past and present use of over the counter and prescription topical and systemic therapies. Poorly tolerated and ineffective medications should not be prescribed a second time. All over the counter and prescription medications should be reviewed. Drugs that may cause or aggravate acne include hormonal contraceptives, that have progestins with greater androgenic effects (e.g., levonorgestrel as in Norplant); corticosteroids; lithium; iodides; phenytoin; anabolic steroids; and high dosages of vitamins B_2 (riboflavin), B_6 (pyridoxine), and B_{12} (cyanocobalamin) (6).

Examination of the face, chest, back, and upper arms is done to determine the type of acne (e.g., comedonal, inflammatory, papular–pustular, or cystic/nodulocystic) and whether scarring has occurred (e.g., ice pick to soft undulations creating shadows). Although most patients with acne have normal androgen levels, females should be assessed for evidence of androgen excess with review of the menstrual and reproductive histories, evaluation of the scalp for possible androgenic alopecia, and examination of the face, presternal chest, upper abdomen, upper back, and trunk for evidence of hirsutism. Abnormal findings warrant evaluation beginning with serum testosterone and dehydroepiandrosterone sulfate (7). Chapter 101 provides a discussion of abnormalities in this hormonal axis.

Before proceeding with an individualized treatment plan, patients should be asked how acne affects their lives: whether there are any activities or interactions they avoid because of their acne; whether they worry, become anxious, distressed, or depressed about their acne; and whether there are other problems related to their acne. Additional screening for depression should be performed as indicated. Obviously, an individual whose self-image has been negatively affected by acne should be given more aggressive therapy than a teen who is unfazed by acne.

Therapy

Successful acne therapy (with the exception of isotretinoin therapy) is expected to control, not cure, acne (Table 115.1). A given treatment should be used for at least 6 to 8 weeks before assessing its effectiveness. If improvement is suboptimal or the acne is causing scarring, referral to a dermatologist is appropriate.

COMEDONAL ACNE

Comedonal (white- and blackhead) acne responds nicely to comedolytic agents. These agents essentially "unplug" comedones by promoting normal desquamation of the follicular epithelium. Available products include over the counter salicylic acid (Neutrogena Clear Pore gel, Clean and Clear Continuous Control Acne Wash, Neutrogena Acne Wash, and Neutrogena Skin Clearing Oil Free Foundation or Pressed Powder for females) and prescription topical synthetic vitamin A derivatives (retinoids), such as tretinoin (Retin A and Avita), adapalene (Differin), or tazarotene (Tazorac). Although all these agents work through a similar mechanism, they vary in their therapeutic effects and irritancy effects. A mild agent is tretinoin cream 0.025% and a very strong agent is tazarotene gel 0.1%.

When prescribing topical retinoids, patients should be instructed in the following fashion: carefully read

Table 115.1. Acne Therapy

Type of Acne	Clinical Appearance	General Hygiene	Initial Therapy	Re-evaluate	Therapy if Not Responding[b]	Therapy Change if Responding Nicely
Comedonal acne	Open and closed comedones (blackheads and whiteheads)	*Gently* wash face with fingertips two times/day using antibacterial soap	Retin A 0.01% gel or 0.05% cream daily	8 wk	Increase Retin A to twice daily or change to 0.025% gel or 0.1% cream	No change
Inflammatory acne	Comedones and inflammatory papules and pustules	As above	Retin A, p.m. Benzoyl peroxide (BPO) gel a.m. or as tolerated[c] or erythromycin 2% or clindamycin 1% solution or gel two times/day	8 wk	Add oral antibiotics; tetracycline 500 mg two times/day or erythromycin 250 mg three to four times/day; if no response after 8 wk, refer	Decrease oral antibiotics by one tablet each month; if flare occurs, increase by one tablet and hold for several months; then decrease again and re-evaluate
Cystic acne	As above plus cystic or nodular lesions	As above	Retin A and BPO or topical antibiotic,[d] plus oral antibiotics as above	8 wk	Accutane[e] (*cis*-retinoic acid) administered by a physician with experience using this teratogenic drug (see text)	
Scarring inflammatory acne[e]	Inflammatory acne with resultant scarring					

[a]A good review of acne therapy is provided in Leyden JJ. Therapy for acne vulgaris. N Engl J Med 1997;336:1156.
[b]If not responding, always review patient's regimen; the patient may be noncompliant or just unintentionally using medications incorrectly.
[c]BPOs (benzoyl peroxide), such as OTC Oxy or Rx Brevoxyl 4%, Benzac AC 5%, Desquam E 5%. The advantage of BPO over topical antibiotic is that BPOs are bacteriocidal for *Propionibacterium acnes*, so there is less chance for bacterial resistance. Patients should be instructed to use these drying medications as tolerated and as limited by irritation.
[d]Topical erythromycin such as A/T/S or EryMax; clindamycin such as Cleocin T gel.
[e]Scarring inflammatory acne is not an FDA-approved indication for Accutane; recommend referral to a dermatologist who is interested in treating this challenging form of acne to prevent further permanent disfiguring scarring.

and follow the medication instructions included with the product; expect mild irritation; and titrate to tolerance, that is, if daily application is excessively irritating, reduce the frequency of application to two, three, or four times per week, as tolerated. Patients need to know that dosing frequency is best left up to them and that it may vary over time (e.g., twice weekly application in the dry cold winter months versus daily application in the hot humid summer months). Because all retinoids are teratogenic, topical retinoids should not be used in persons presently pregnant or considering conception. Specifically, tazarotene is included with Pregnancy Category X medications (i.e., proper testing to exclude pregnancy when starting therapy and adequate birth control measures to prevent pregnancy must be used in conjunction with therapy), whereas the other topical retinoids are included in Pregnancy Category C. Caution is also recommended regarding use in lactating women. The clinician not familiar with these agents should read the manufacturers' summaries or Physicians' Desk Reference before prescribing topical synthetic vitamin A derivatives.

INFLAMMATORY ACNE

Mild inflammatory acne consisting of comedones and erythematous papules with or without pustules (usually up to 15 papules) may be treated with a combination of a comedolytic agent (see above) and a topical antibacterial directed at *P. acnes*. Appropriate antibacterial agents for this condition are topical benzoyl peroxide, which is bactericidal, or a bacteriostatic drug such as erythromycin or clindamycin. Benzoyl peroxide is a primary irritant, so low concentrations are best (2.5% to 5%) in all patients, except those with exceptionally excessive sebum, in whom a more concentrated gel (8% to 10%) is helpful because of its drying effect. Benzoyl peroxide as a leave-on gel or wash-off cleanser is available over the counter (e.g., Oxy Sensitive Skin Treatment 2.5% gel or Oxy 10 Acne Treatment 10% gel; Oxy Clean Moisturizing Face Wash or Medicated Cleansing Bar) and by prescription (e.g., Brevoxyl 4% or 8% Gel, Cleansing Lotion or Creamy Wash, Benzac AC 2.5%, 5%, or 10% Gel). Daily or less frequent use as tolerated is recommended, to be adjusted by the patient. Alternatively, topical erythromycin 2% (e.g., A/T/S, Em-Gel) or clindamycin 1% (e.g., Cleocin T Pledgets, Cleocin T Gel) may be used. Benzoyl peroxide and tretinoin should not be applied simultaneously because of resultant oxidation of the latter; therefore, one is used in the morning and the other at night. Topical antibiotics and tretinoin may be applied together. The patient may use medicated (as mentioned under comedonal acne) or nonmedicated makeup, as long as it is oil free.

If inflammatory acne does not improve in 6 to 8 weeks of treatment or if a patient *initially* presents with moderate or severe inflammatory acne or inflammatory acne of any severity that is negatively affecting self-esteem, treatment should include an oral antibiotic, such as tetracycline 500 mg two times a day (if nausea develops, a reduced dose of 250 mg two times a day may be tried), doxycycline 100 mg two times per day (patients must be cautioned about associated photosensitivity), or erythromycin 333 mg two to three times a day. Especially with extremely determined and/or compliant acne patients, it should be made clear that if the medication is making them feel nauseated, just "not so good," or depressed, the antibiotic should be stopped and another substituted. Although these antibiotics would not be expected to be associated with depression, idiosyncratic reactions are always possible; also, bringing up the issue of depression may open yet another door for a patient to discuss depression, if present. Oral antibiotics are always used in combination with topicals, in anticipation of tapering or discontinuing oral therapy after several weeks or months while continuing topicals alone (Table 115.1). Patients should be told that antibiotics only suppress and do not cure acne. Therefore, as long as a patient is still in his or her "acne years" (the duration of which is always difficult to predict), ongoing treatment is necessary. Patients on long-term oral or topical antibiotic therapy should be watched for the development of *P. acnes* antibiotic resistance, characterized by worsening or flaring of previously well-controlled acne (8).

CYSTIC ACNE

Cystic acne, characterized by deep-seated, inflammatory, nodular cysts, should always be treated aggressively to prevent permanent scarring. If patients do not respond to oral antibiotics in combination with topical agents in 6 to 8 weeks, referral to a dermatologist should be made. Although the dermatologist may prescribe an alternative nonretinoid therapy, it is likely that the systemic retinoid isotretinoin (13-*cis*-retinoic acid, Accutane) will be needed. Isotretinoin is "curative" in approximately 70% of patients, although the basis for this is unknown. Because of the side effects of this drug, one who is not very familiar with the drug and prescribing it regularly should refer the patient to a dermatologist who uses it frequently. The greatest concern with isotretinoin is its teratogenic potential. It may produce fetal anomalies involving the central nervous system, heart, bones, and thymus in 30% to 40% of exposed fetuses. All women of childbearing age must be counseled on the use of two concurrent forms of contraception (see Chapter 100). In the very unlikely event that pregnancy develops, an abortion should be strongly recommended. If a patient is morally against abortion, she must remain abstinent from sexual intercourse for the 20- to 28-week period of treatment, as well as for 1 month before and after treatment, or forego isotretinoin therapy. The maker of isotretinoin (Roche Dermatologics) has developed a patient instruction/consent form packet that is critical for both the clinician and the patient to review carefully.

Some side effects with isotretinoin therapy are essentially inescapable. These include dry skin, nose, and eyes. Mild elevations of triglyceride, cholesterol, and liver enzymes are seen in approximately 25% of patients. Infrequent or unusual side effects include hair loss, musculoskeletal aches, *Staphylococcus aureus* folliculitis and ocular keratitis, reduced night vision, marked elevation of triglyceride with the potential for an associated acute pancreatitis, marked elevation of cholesterol and liver enzymes, leukopenia, and pseudotumor cerebri.

Some patients developing triglyceride elevations may have an inherited familial lipid disorder (8a) and a useful summary regarding this unusual side effect of isotretinoin therapy is available (8b).

ROSACEA (ACNE ROSACEA)

Acne rosacea, usually referred to as *"rosacea"*, is a chronic inflammatory disorder favoring the central portion of the face. It occurs most commonly in fair-skinned whites with blue eyes. Affected patients usually develop initial signs of the disease in their twenties or thirties with central facial erythema, exaggerated flushing, telangiectasias, and intermittent erythematous follicular papules and pustules and edema. Rarely, patients may develop associated *rhinophyma;* this bulbous nose enlargement is seen more often in men than in women and is caused by hyperplasia of the sebaceous glands. Rosacea does not cause comedones and therefore can be differentiated from acne vulgaris. However, occasionally patients have both rosacea and acne.

Rosacea may also involve the eyes, causing a mild inflammation of the lid margins manifest by mild erythema and causing the sensation of dry or scratchy eyes. Other slightly or somewhat less common changes include conjunctivitis, blepharitis, episcleritis, and recurrent chalazion and hordeolum (see Chapter 109). Less than 5% of patients with rosacea develop a painful and vision-threatening condition of the cornea, *rosacea keratitis.*

Although the cause of rosacea remains unknown, the condition is characteristically so well controlled with antibiotics that lack of a clinical response should raise a question about the diagnosis. For patients with ocular symptoms, a moderate number of papules, or with burning and stinging, systemic treatment is preferred: tetracycline 500 mg or doxycycline (photosensitizing) 100 mg orally two times a day or erythromycin 333 mg orally two to three times a day. If a good response is seen, the dose may be reduced at 1 and 2 months and then the drug discontinued at 3 months, switching over to topical therapy. If a flare occurs, the oral antibiotic may be restarted and tapered again. Although some patients can discontinue therapy after several months, most flare without some therapy. For long-term treatment, topical therapies are generally preferred and include metronidazole gel, lotion, or cream (MetroGel, -Lotion, -Cream or Noritate Cream) applied to the central face two times a day (Noritate, once daily) after washing.

HIDRADENITIS SUPPURATIVA

Hidradenitis suppurativa is characterized by inflammation and occlusion of follicles in areas where apocrine glands are found. Onset is usually in the late teens or early adult years, and disease may persist for decades. Sites where apocrine glands are normally present or ectopic apocrine glands are sporadically present are affected. These sites include the axillae, perineum, inguinal folds, pubic region, and often the umbilicus, breasts, postauricular area, scalp, and back. Affected areas are studded with large comedones, inflammatory papules, pustules, and cysts. Sinus tracts form when cysts rupture and drain serum, blood, or purulent material. Patients may also have cystic facial acne and scarring scalp folliculitis.

Complications of and associations with hidradenitis suppurativa may include secondary amyloidosis, anemia of chronic disease, depression, and sacroiliitis. Finally, patients are at risk for episodes of acute bacterial cellulitis and, after many years, squamous cell carcinoma in this chronically inflamed tissue.

The differential diagnosis of hidradenitis suppurativa includes recurrent bacterial folliculitis and furunculosis (see Chapter 32), scrofuloderma (*Mycobacterium tuberculosis* infection with an ulcerated draining lymph node), granuloma inguinale (*Calymmatobacterium granulomatis,* a sexually transmitted disease characterized by genital and inguinal sinuses and hypertrophic scars), lymphogranuloma venereum (see Chapter 37), Crohn disease (see Chapter 46), and a pilonidal cyst. The diagnosis of hidradenitis suppurativa is made by recognizing comedones, which are not present in these other disorders. Skin biopsies for histopathology and tissue cultures may be required to exclude other diagnoses.

The pathogenesis of this disorder is not well understood. It is debated whether infection in these patients is a primary or secondary event. Treatment consists of short courses of antibiotics for acute secondary infection. Specific antibiotic therapy should be based on the results of culture taken from draining lesions. Chronic ongoing therapy includes oral tetracycline or erythromycin for anti-inflammatory and antibacterial effects and topical benzoyl peroxide in a regimen similar to that used in acne (see above). Surgical therapy ranging from tract marsupialization to deep wide excision should be considered for patients with severe disease. It is best to consult with a dermatologist early when dealing with the patient suspected of having this problem.

MILIARIA

Miliaria is a disorder of sweat retention caused by occlusion of the ducts of the eccrine glands. Unlike the sebaceous and apocrine glands, which secrete through the hair follicles to the skin surface, eccrine glands are separate from hair follicles. They are directly connected to the surface of the skin through eccrine ducts. Although it is not a follicular disorder, as are acne and folliculitis, it may mimic these disorders. Miliaria occurs most often in active people who are perspiring heavily and who are wearing occlusive clothing or are confined to bed for extended periods.

The eruption almost always occurs on the trunk. When the sweat duct is occluded very superficially, asymptomatic, noninflammatory, 1- to 2-mm vesicles that easily rupture are seen in the upper central chest or back (*miliaria crystallina*), creating a distinctive appearance. When the duct is occluded deeper in the skin, pruritic, nonfollicular, erythematous papules occur over the chest and back (*miliaria rubra*). Lesions may be few to many in number.

The differential diagnosis of miliaria rubra includes infectious and noninfectious folliculitis. These forms of folliculitis are distinguished by their involvement of hair follicles as opposed to just the eccrine ducts.

The treatment of miliaria includes providing a cool environment, removing occlusive clothing, and modifying positioning in bedridden persons. Cool baths and topical antipruritic lotions containing menthol or phenol (e.g., Sarna lotion) may reduce pruritus when present. Drying lotions (e.g., Zeasorb AF lotion/powder) may also be helpful.

NONINFECTIOUS ALOPECIA: NONSCARRING AND SCARRING

When assessing the chief complaint of hair loss, it is helpful to understand normal hair physiology. Every individual hair may be classified based on whether it is growing, transitional, or resting. These phases are *anagen* (lasting 2 to 6 years), *catagen* (lasting 2 to 3 weeks), and *telogen* (lasting 2 to 3 months), respectively (9). Scalp hair loss in excess or *alopecia* involving the scalp may be *nonscarring* or *scarring*; fortunately, nonscarring alopecia is far more common.

Nonscarring Alopecia

Nonscarring alopecia is so designated because the affected hair follicles are not permanently lost or damaged. Clinically, noninflammatory and nonscarring alopecia (hair loss without visible changes of erythema, scale, scarring) is characteristic of male and female pattern hair loss (i.e., androgenetic alopecia), alopecia areata (histologically inflammatory), telogen effluvium, anagen effluvium, and various systemic causes of diffuse hair thinning, including thyroid disease, systemic lupus erythematosus, and drug-induced hair loss.

Androgenetic alopecia is common in both men and women. Typically, men experience a frontal and vertex type of thinning, variably followed by confluence over the entire crown (top of the head); in contrast, women experience mild to moderate thinning over the entire crown with notable sparing of the frontal hair margin. In both sexes, the onset of androgenetic alopecia may be as early as the late teens. Rarely, women show a male pattern of hair loss. In all women with hair loss, regardless of the pattern, one should look for signs of virilization (e.g., facial, upper chest, upper back, and upper abdomen hair growth; clitoral hypertrophy; deepening voice; and muscular body habitus). Appropriate evaluation should be performed to exclude hyperandrogenemia caused by adrenal hyperplasia, polycystic ovary disease, insulin resistance (10) that is often accompanied by acanthosis nigricans, a velvety hyperpigmentation around the base of the neck and axillae (11), and various adrenal and ovarian tumors (see Chapter 101). Additionally, women who are taking testosterone (e.g., Estratest), progestational drugs with greater androgen effects (e.g., levonorgestrol), or over the counter dehydroepiandrosterone should be told that these agents aggravate androgenetic alopecia and should be avoided.

Treatment options in patients who desire more hair include oral finasteride (Propecia, 1-mg tablets) for men and topical *minoxidil, hair transplants,* and various *hair prostheses*, varying from woven-in individual hairs to full-scalp wigs, for both women and men. Each of these treatments has its disadvantages. Over the counter topical *minoxidil* 2% solution (Rogaine) produces significant hair growth in only approximately 20% of patients; however, a greater percentage of patients have a reduction in further hair loss. Rogaine Extra Strength for Men (minoxidil 5% solution) is also available over the counter and is said to grow 45% more hair than the 2% Rogaine. Oral finasteride or topical minoxidil therapy must be ongoing to maintain hair growth, at a cost of $20 to $60 per month. In contrast, hair *transplants* are permanent. The surgery is expensive and associated with discomfort; however, many patients are very pleased with the results. Hair weaves in which natural or synthetic hair is woven into the patient's own hair must be repeated as the hair grows out. Finally, although some people do well with a wig, they may be uncomfortable, difficult to manage, and costly.

Telogen effluvium is a common disorder in which patients experience shedding of telogen hairs diffusely over the scalp. The percentage of telogen or resting hairs may shift upward to approach 20% (versus normal 10%) of the scalp hair. This amount of hair loss is usually evident only to the patient, who notes excessive hair coming out on shampooing and combing. Telogen effluvium may begin 2 to 3 months after such events as childbirth, general anesthesia, and catabolic states such as high fever for many days, rapid weight loss, and protein malnutrition. This form of alopecia is self-limited; however, several months may elapse before hair loss stops and new anagen hair growth begins. Because (anagen) hair grows approximately 1 cm per month, depending on the individual's chosen hair length, return to the "pre-telogen effluvium" appearance may take a year or so. Reassurance of this expected ultimate outcome is extremely important.

Numerous nonchemotherapeutic drugs have been reported to cause hair loss through a variety of mechanisms, primarily affecting telogen hairs (10% to 20% of the scalp hairs), therefore producing a chronic telogen effluvium that is usually appreciable only to the patient. The most common of these drugs are anticoagulants, anticonvulsants and cholesterol-lowering agents. This hair loss is reversible with discontinuance of the causative medication.

Anagen effluvium may be caused by chemotherapeutic agents and ionizing irradiation. Patients have shedding of the actively growing hairs in the scalp, which constitute approximately 90% of the total scalp hair. Hairs are shed rapidly over a matter of days, and patients typically have no or only very sparse hairs left on the scalp (the remaining telogen hairs). With the occasional exception of ionizing radiation induced effluvium, this hair loss is temporary.

Alopecia areata is an immunologically mediated form of hair loss that typically presents with one to a few coin-shaped areas of hair loss. Although yet to be determined, it is believed that a certain genetic constitution and triggering factors are necessary for disease expression. Infrequently, patients may have total scalp hair loss (*alopecia totalis*) or total body hair loss (*alopecia universalis*). Most patients with just one or two patches of alopecia will have spontaneous hair regrowth within 1 year; however, recurrences in the same or new sites are common. Although *most* patients with alopecia areata do not have any associated disorders, alopecia areata is associated with an increased lifetime risk of autoimmune conditions, such as thyroid disease, pernicious anemia, and Addison disease. Initial treatment of patients with alopecia areata usually consists of topical corticosteroid solutions (e.g., clobetasol or fluocinonide solution, three to four drops applied to each quarter-sized area, including 0.5 cm of radially encircling normal scalp) or corticosteroid scalp injections. Other treatments (e.g., topical minoxidil, topical irritants, topical sensitizers, photochemotherapy) may be helpful in some patients, but, as with topical and intralesional corticosteroids, well-controlled studies demonstrating efficacy are limited or lacking.

Although still other disorders may cause variable degrees of nonscarring alopecia, the alopecia is merely secondary to the primary inflammatory process or due to trauma. Examples of the former include tinea capitis and seborrheic dermatitis and the latter include prolonged pressure-associated ischemia-induced alopecia (e.g., prolonged unrecognized unconscious state, prolonged surgery) and trichotillomania (self-inflicted alopecia).

Scarring Alopecia

Scarring alopecia is relatively uncommon. It is characterized by focal scarring with a loss of hair and visible hair follicles. One of the most common forms of scarring alopecia seen occurs primarily in African-American women (12). After years of chemical permanent solutions and traction, a resultant permanent hair loss favoring the crown and temporal scalp may develop. Similar to our paradigm for the development of nonmelanoma skin cancer with repeated sun exposures beginning in childhood eventuating in skin cancer after the third or fourth decade, the same model may be applied to this externally induced scarring hair loss. As with skin cancer, education to prevent disease must begin in school children.

Causes of scarring alopecia that are independent of external factors are discoid lupus erythematosus, folliculitis decalvans, cicatricial pemphigoid, lichen planopilaris, and pseudopelade (idiopathic scarring alopecia). Scarring alopecia is irreversible in most instances because the scarred follicles are incapable of producing new anagen hairs. Patients suspected of having scarring alopecia should be referred as early as possible to a dermatologist in hopes of preventing further permanent hair loss.

Specific References

1. Shalita AR, Pochi PE, Leyden JJ, et al. Acne therapy in the '90s. J Int Postgrad Med 1991;4:1.
2. Kligman AM. Postadolescent acne in women. Cutis 1991;48:75.
3. Goulden V, Stables I, Cunliffe WJ. Prevalence of facial acne in adults. J Am Acad Dermatol 1999;41:577.
4. Jick SS, Kremers HM, Vasilakis-Scaramozza C. Isotretinoin use and risk of depression, psychotic symptoms, suicide, and attempted suicide. Arch Dermatol 2000;36:1231.
5. Wysowski DK, Pitts M, Beitz J. Depression and suicide in patients treated with isotretinoin. N Engl J Med 2001;344:460.
6. Sherertz EF. Acneiform eruption due to megadose vitamins B_6 and B_{12}. Cutis 1991;48:119.
7. Lucky AW. Hormonal correlates of acne and hirsutism. Proceedings of a symposium, NICHD conference: androgens and women's health. Am J Med 1995;98:89S.
8. Eady EA, Jones CE, Tipper JL, et al. Antibiotic resistant propionibacteria in acne: need for policies to modify antibiotic usage. BMJ 1993;306:555.

8a. Rodondi N, Darioli R, Ramelet AA, et al. High risk for hyperlipidemia and the metabolic syndrome after an episode of hypertriglyceridemia during 13-cis retinoic acid therapy for acne: a pharmacogenetic study. Ann Intern Med 2002;136:582.

8b. Anonymous. An unusual "side effect" of an acne drug. Ann Intern Med 2002;136:I–38.

9. Price VH. Treatment of hair loss. N Engl J Med 1999;341:964.
10. Beatty OL, Harper R, Sheridan B, et al. Insulin resistance in offspring of hypertensive parents. BMJ 1993;10:92.
11. Stuart CA, Pate CJ, Peters EJ. Prevalence of acanthosis nigricans in an unselected population. Am J Med 1989;87:269.
12. Ackerman AB, Walton NW, Jones RE, et al. Hot comb alopecia/follicular degeneration syndrome in African-American women is traction alopecia! Dermatopathol Pract Concept 2000;6:320.

CHAPTER 116

Dermatitis and Psoriasis

S. ELIZABETH WHITMORE, MD, ScM

DERMATITIS

Dermatitis, or *eczema*, is a nonspecific term indicating inflammatory changes visible in the epidermal surface of the skin. No matter what the specific "subtype" of dermatitis, acute, subacute, and/or chronic changes may be seen. In *acute dermatitis*, changes consist of edema, papules, vesicles, serous discharge, crusting, scaling, and erythema. In *subacute dermatitis*, lesions are erythematous and scaly and may be edematous, but serous discharge and crusting are absent. In *chronic dermatitis*, changes consist of a scaly thickening of the skin, giving a washboard or tree bark appearance called *lichenification*. The phase, acute, subacute, or chronic, generally determines the prescribed treatment. Table 116.1 summarizes the features, treatment, and prognosis of several specific types of dermatitis. The different types of dermatitis are traditionally categorized based on associated manifestations, as with "atopic" dermatitis; mechanism, as with "contact" dermatitis; morphology, as with "nummular" dermatitis; and location, as with "hand" dermatitis. Dermatitis can be viewed as primarily caused by endogenous (e.g., atopy) or exogenous (e.g., external contact) factors, although both factors are eventually involved.

Atopic Dermatitis

Atopic dermatitis is considered an endogenous dermatitis. Affected patients will usually confirm the validity of the quote, "atopic dermatitis is the itch that rashes." Patients typically have associated atopic

Table 116.1. Summary of the Diagnostic, Therapeutic, and Prognostic Features of the Phases of Dermatitis

Phase	Typical Morphology	Primary Treatment of Dermatitis	Indicators of Colonization or Secondary Infection Requiring Therapy	Treatment of Infection	Second-Line Treatment for Unresponsive Dermatitis, or First-Line Treatment for Very Severe Dermatitis	General Prognosis
Acute dermatitis	Papules, papulovesicles, erythema, serous discharge, and crusting	Saline compresses four times/day, switching when dry to corticosteroid creams[a] two times/day (high potency) and emollients with antipruritic agents	Moderate to severe crusting representing impetiginization or erythema representing erysipelas or cellulitis	Oral antistaphylococcal antibiotics (dicloxacillin or cephalexin) except in cases of erysipelas or cellulitis, which typically require i.v. antibiotics (see Chapter 32)	Prednisone 0.7 to 1 mg/kg/day tapered over approximately 2 wk	Usually excellent
Subacute dermatitis	Erythema, edema, papules, and scale	Topical corticosteroid (high-potency) ointments[a] and emollients[b]	As above or numerous excoriations	As above	Phototherapy or photochemotherapy with UVB or PUVA, respectively	Usually good, but recurrences are not uncommon
Chronic dermatitis	Lichenified or thickened papules and plaques	As above	As above or nonhealing fissures	As above	As above	Treatment is difficult, recurrences very common

[a]Only low-potency corticosteroids should be used on the face; elsewhere, when using super-, high-, or mid-potency corticosteroids, side effects such as atrophy, telangiectasia, striae, or systemic absorption with hypercortisolism and hypothalamic–pituitary–adrenal axis suppression are possible.

[b]Corticosteroids and emollients are discussed in detail in "Topical Therapeutics," Chapter 113.

UVB, ultraviolet B.

diseases, such as allergic rhinitis or allergic asthma, and 70% give a family history of atopy. Atopic diseases are characterized by an imbalance in the normal T helper cell immune response, with T_H2 cells infiltrating the affected tissues. This dominant T_H2 response with a predominance of T_H2-derived cytokines (e.g., interleukin-4, -5, and -13) over T_H1 cytokines (e.g., interferon-gamma and interleukin-12) is believed to play a key role in the pathogenesis of disease (1). Other immunologic alterations, including elevated serum IgE levels, a reduced delayed hypersensitivity response, decreased numbers of T-suppressor lymphocytes, increased percentage of B lymphocytes with surface-bound IgE-1, and decreased number or activity of natural killer lymphocytes, may be seen. However, not all patients with atopic dermatitis express these abnormalities, and their role in the development of atopic dermatitis is unclear.

Atopic dermatitis may be divided into subsets based on age of onset: *infantile*, with onset between 2 months and 2 years; *childhood*, with onset between 2 years and adolescence, and *adult*, with onset in adulthood. Areas of involvement are typically those that patients can scratch. Therefore, affected sites include the cheeks and extensor surface of the arms and legs in infants; the flexural surface of the arms, legs, neck, wrists, and ankles in children; and these same sites and often also (or only) the hands or face in adults. The morphology of the lesions varies based on duration and external trauma (i.e., rubbing and scratching). *Acute lesions* consist of erythema, edema, papules, vesicles, erosions, crusts, and scale, whereas *chronic lesions* consist of scaly papules coalescing into lichenified plaques, often with focal excoriations.

Treatment depends on the patient's age and the location of the dermatitis. For all ages, facial dermatitis is usually treated with over the counter (0.5% or 1%) hydrocortisone ointment or cream. In children, hydrocortisone or slightly more potent prescription steroids (e.g., hydrocortisone butyrate) are used on nonfacial sites. In teens and in adults, fluorinated mid-potency (e.g., triamcinolone acetonide, betamethasone valerate) to high-potency (e.g., fluocinonide, betamethasone dipropionate) corticosteroids are used on nonfacial sites. Care must be taken to avoid local and systemic side effects. Corticosteroids applied to large body surface areas may produce hypercortisolism and hypothalamic–pituitary–adrenal axis suppression in the same way that orally administered steroids may. Topical corticosteroids should always be used in combination with emollients (i.e., simple oil or water and oil moisturizing creams and lotions; see Chapter 113). Emollients protect, hydrate, and permit the skin to repair, thereby restoring the barrier between the body and the environment. Topical steroid use should be discontinued as soon as the lesions have cleared and should be restarted as needed. An alternative nonsteroidal anti-inflammatory agent, tacrolimus, which for many years has been used systemically to prevent organ transplant rejection, is now available in a topical form, Protopic ointment, and can be tried if corticosteroids cannot be used or are ineffective (2). Not infrequently, patients with atopic dermatitis may require intermittent oral antibiotics for recurrent infection, or "dermatitis-triggering" colonization with *Staphylococcus aureus*.

For patients unresponsive to these therapies, a consulting dermatologist would consider in-office phototherapy using ultraviolet (UV)-B radiation or photochemotherapy with psoralen and UV-A radiation (i.e., PUVA). Because systemic corticosteroid therapy is associated with numerous long-term unacceptable side effects, it should be avoided in the treatment of atopic dermatitis. Alternative systemic immune modulating therapies, such as cyclosporine, interferon-gamma, mycophenolate mofetil, and various immune modulating monoclonal antibodies, are still under investigation in the treatment of recalcitrant atopic dermatitis.

The generalist should be familiar with the nonpharmacologic measures to aid patients with atopic dermatitis. Measures that reduce anxiety, such as adjunctive massage therapy administered by the parents, may be helpful in children with atopic dermatitis (3). Also, although most patients with chronic atopic dermatitis have discovered which products to use and which to avoid, review of exacerbating factors may be helpful (e.g., irritating harsh soaps, recurrent wetting and drying, and coarse fabrics).

As a point of information, the generalist should inform patients with respiratory allergies that although desensitization immunotherapy may be helpful for allergic rhinitis and conjunctivitis, it will have no effect on the course of their atopic dermatitis. In contrast, addressing food allergies with appropriate dietary elimination is helpful in some children (4). Dietary modifications, especially in children, should be supervised by a qualified dietitian. Occasionally, adults may find certain foods exacerbate their dermatitis (e.g., gluten, milk). In these instances, as long as a balanced diet is maintained, a trial elimination of suspected triggers for 6 to 8 weeks should be encouraged. An occasional patient thought to have atopic dermatitis may instead have dermatitis herpetiformis. This is an extremely pruritic papulovesicular eruption on the extensor surfaces and lower back. Affected individuals have a gluten sensitivity with antigliadin antibodies or antiendomysial antibodies. The diagnosis is made by skin biopsy for routine histology and direct immunofluorescence; the latter will reveal IgA deposited in the dermal papillae.

Nummular Dermatitis

Nummular dermatitis is an idiopathic dermatosis seen most often in adults. Lesions consist of pruritic, sharply circumscribed, 1- to 2-cm, vesicular (acute) to lichenified (chronic), erythematous plaques favoring the extremities. Lesions may be mistaken for tinea corporis or impetigo because of their annular shape. Tinea is ruled out with a negative potassium hydroxide preparation (see pg. 1756), and impetigo is excluded based on the lack of honeycomb-like surface crust.

Treatment for nummular dermatitis is similar to that for atopic dermatitis. Emollients in combination with mid- to high-potency corticosteroids generally clear the lesions; to prevent recurrences after clearing, the topical corticosteroid should be tapered over 2 weeks with one application every other or every third day. Patients with unresponsive dermatitis may have misunderstood the importance of the topical steroid application or instead may have a secondary staphylococcal infection that requires specific treatment (Table 116.1).

Asteatotic Dermatitis

Asteatotic, xerotic, or *dry skin* dermatitis is most often seen in the wintertime in people living in low-humidity environments. Factors associated with decreased sebum oil production such as slowly declining testosterone levels in men and women after the sixth decade, cholesterol lowering medications, and any medications that reduce the production or effects of androgens (e.g., chemotherapeutic drugs and antiandrogens that suppress gonadal function or block androgen effects) may predispose patients to asteatotic dermatitis. Diminished epidermal and sebaceous gland sebum production allows loss of normally retained moisture in the stratum corneum. Skin changes typically begin with dryness in the early fall, which then progresses to patches of faint erythema appearing *cracked* or superficially fissured (Fig. 116.1, Color Plate section). Patients complain of a stinging, tight feeling to their skin with or without associated pruritus.

Treatment involves hydration of the skin with warm baths or showers using oilated soaps (e.g., Oil of Olay Body Wash, Dove, Oilatum, or Aveeno Oilated Oatmeal Soap) followed by *patting dry*, leaving some moisture on the skin. A mid-potency corticosteroid ointment (as opposed to a cream) is then applied to the erythema, with a *top coat* of an emollient (see Chapter 113) to these and all areas of the skin. Extremely hot showers, which strip natural body oils; drying soaps; and stiff large-fiber clothing (e.g., wool) should be avoided. When the dermatitis has cleared, only the topical corticosteroid is discontinued; all other measures must be continued as long as the dry environmental exposure or sebum reducing medication continues.

Contact Dermatitis

Contact dermatitis may be either *irritant* or *allergic* in nature. Irritant contact dermatitis may develop in anyone, whereas allergic contact dermatitis occurs only in people immunologically capable of recognizing and reacting to a particular allergen.

Irritant contact dermatitis to harsh chemicals results in a scalded, erythematous, moist appearance of the skin with peeling of the most superficial epidermis, leaving a lacy border. This is often caused by substances with extremes of pH, such as harsh alkaline cleansers and strong acid solutions. In contrast, mild irritants produce macular erythema that, with chronic exposure, may evolve into scaly plaques. With all forms of contact dermatitis, the eruption is limited to the area of contact. It is often the localized distribution and shape of the lesion that suggests the diagnosis, for example, irritant contact dermatitis at the forearm site of a solvent spill and allergic contact dermatitis on the earlobes bearing gold-colored earrings.

Allergic contact dermatitis (Fig. 116.2, Color Plate section) is caused by a delayed hypersensitivity reaction. Sensitization, if and when it develops, takes place through cutaneous exposure and requires approximately 1 week. A substance containing an allergen (i.e., hapten) is applied to the skin; the hapten binds to a protein to form a complete allergen, which is processed by the Langerhans cell, the resident antigen-presenting cell in the epidermis. As sensitization proceeds, the Langerhans cell moves into the dermis and through the lymphatics to the local lymph nodes, where it stimulates a lymphocyte clone that recognizes the antigen. If the substance is still in the skin 1 week after initial application or when subsequent re-exposure takes place, the Langerhans cells within the epidermis present the allergen to the memory T cells. These T cells secrete cytokines and other soluble mediators, which lead to recruitment of additional inflammatory cells (e.g., monocytes, neutrophils), resulting in the clinical picture of an acute dermatitis.

The most common cause of allergic contact dermatitis is a *plant dermatitis,* caused by the *Rhus* genus, which includes *poison ivy, oak, and sumac.* In sensitized persons, a minute amount of the oleoresin (oil) from these plants will produce a vesiculobullous eruption in the areas of contact, beginning 6 to 72 hours after exposure. Patients often note that new blisters continue to develop over many days and assume that their scratching is causing the rash to "spread." However, this is not the case; once the allergen is flushed from the skin, spreading cannot occur. The reason that new lesions may continue to develop for many days is because lesions take longer to evolve on skin that is thicker and penetration is slower (e.g., the palm) or where lesser amounts of oleoresin have contacted the skin. Also, continued unrecognized exposure to the oleoresin that may persist on clothing, tools, sports equipment, or the fur of pets may lead to "chronic poison ivy." Allergens other than Rhus are less common sensitizers and typically produce a less pronounced dermatitis with erythema, edema, and mild or no vesiculation. Such allergens include nickel (commonly found in gold-colored costume jewelry); neomycin, benzocaine, and merthiolate in topical medicinals; fragrances and preservatives in cosmetics and personal products; and preservatives in ophthalmologic, otic, and dermatologic prescription and nonprescription medications. Various common *occupational exposures* may also cause allergic contact dermatitis. More common allergens include potassium dichromate in cement, dyes, or textiles; epoxy resins in adhesives, finishing products, and casings for electrical devices; natural rosin in adhesive materials; thiuram, mercaptobenzothiazole, and carbamates in rubber products; glyceryl monothioglycolate and paraphenylenediamine in hair wave and dye formulations; and acrylates in methylmethacrylate used in orthopedic surgery, dentistry, and nail sculpturing.

Allergic contact dermatitis characteristically develops unexpectedly, appearing "out of the blue" after months or years of unremarkable exposures. Evaluation for possible allergic contact dermatitis requires a detailed history of personal product use, occupational exposures, and avocational exposures followed by patch testing with standardized common and suspected allergens to confirm the diagnosis and identify the causative allergen. When the diagnosis appears to be allergic contact dermatitis but no direct exposure is uncovered, unrecognized exposures should be sought. For example, occasionally the allergen exposure occurs through contact with the "nonallergic" spouses' personal products or work clothes.

The prevention of irritant and allergic contact dermatitis involves the recognition of irritants or allergens and elimination or minimization of exposure. Topical treatment is similar to that used for atopic dermatitis with emollients in combination with mid- to high-potency topical corticosteroids (Table 116.1). In cases of vesiculobullous dermatitis or dermatitis involving the face, hands, or genitalia, oral corticosteroids may be administered if no contraindications exist. Treatment should begin with 0.7 mg/kg/day of prednisone tapered over 2 weeks (e.g., 40 to 60 mg for 4 days, 30 to 40 mg for 5 days, and 20 mg for 5 days).

Contact Urticaria

Contact urticaria, although not a form of dermatitis, is a contact reaction. It may be caused by a histamine releasing nonimmunologic substance or an allergen-induced IgE-mediated immunologic reaction. The most common cause of immune mediated contact urticaria is *latex protein* (5,6). It is estimated that 10% of health care workers have been sensitized to natural rubber latex. Latex is ubiquitous in our environment, being present in over 40,000 medical and nonmedical devices and products. Childhood exposure to latex during surgical procedures greatly increases the risk for development of latex allergy. In fact, in one study of children who have experienced at least three surgical procedures, the prevalence of latex allergy was 34% (7).

Health care workers with latex contact urticaria typically present with a history of itching and hives in areas of contact with gloves. Identification of this allergy is important because, in addition to local reaction, latex exposure may cause generalized urticaria and even anaphylaxis, depending on how much histamine reaches the systemic circulation. Anaphylaxis is more likely to occur with oral, vaginal, rectal, or invasive intracorporeal latex contact. Diagnosis is made by *in vitro* latex IgE radio allergosorbent testing (RAST) or *in vivo* patch, prick, or scratch testing. The former is preferred, because *in vivo* testing may cause anaphylaxis. However, RAST testing is not 100% sensitive; therefore, when allergy is strongly suspected and RAST testing is negative, referral to an allergist for skin testing is appropriate. Patients with latex allergy and all their health care providers must be educated about the potential life-threatening nature of this product and should be counseled on avoidance of all latex items, including latex gloves, balloons, condoms, and medical devices such as latex tubing, dental dams, surgeons' gloves, and catheters. A Medic Alert bracelet should be worn and an epinephrine-containing autoinjector (Epi-Pen) should be prescribed and carried by the patient at all times for an emergency (see Chapter 30).

Hand Dermatitis

Hand dermatitis is a very broad term encompassing conditions that affect the hands exclusively, such as *dyshidrotic hand dermatitis*, also known as *vesicular hand dermatitis*, and several forms of dermatitis that may affect any area, including the hands (e.g., atopic hand dermatitis, nummular hand dermatitis, and contact hand dermatitis). *Dyshidrotic or vesicular hand dermatitis* is an idiopathic condition in which pinpoint to 2-mm vesicles develop on the sides of the fingers and often the palms. The lesions are intensely pruritic and usually cycle over 1 to 2 weeks, with cycles recurring at variable intervals every several weeks to several months. As each cycle resolves, there is focal desquamation (peeling) of the affected skin.

Hand dermatitis is idiopathic. Although this disorder is called dyshidrotic, there is actually no consistently identified abnormality in eccrine gland function (sweating). Similarly, the inflammation is not due to a contact allergy. However, because allergic contact dermatitis may occasionally mimic this condition (depending on mode of contact), any suspicion of allergic contact dermatitis should be investigated with patch testing (see above). Treatment for vesicular hand dermatitis includes frequent emollient application and a high potency topical corticosteroid cream or ointment (e.g., fluocinonide) used for flares of disease. Follow-up visits should include examination for the steroid-induced side effect of skin atrophy (evidenced by shiny thin-appearing skin, loss of skin lines, or increased visibility of dermal vessels). Patients with recalcitrant dermatitis should be referred to a dermatologist for alternative therapies (e.g., phototherapy or photochemotherapy).

Infectious Eczematoid Dermatitis

Infectious eczematoid dermatitis is a secondary change within a primary form of dermatitis. Patients become infected with *S. aureus* and other organisms (usually gram-positive bacteria) and show extensive crusting and exudation within their primary dermatitis. Treatment includes systemic antistaphylococcal antibiotics (e.g., dicloxacillin or cephalexin 500 mg two to four times a day, depending on the severity of infection) and treatment of the primary dermatitis with soaks, topical corticosteroids, and emollients.

Intertriginous Dermatitis (Intertrigo)

Intertriginous dermatitis occurs in skin folds, such as the inframammary creases, abdominal folds, inguinal folds, gluteal cleft, finger and toe webs, and angles of the mouth. Patients develop moist erythema and, at times, fissures with weeping of serous fluid. Such skin changes provide a very hospitable environment for yeast and bacterial growth. The affected areas typically burn, sting, and itch.

The differential diagnosis of intertrigo includes primary *Candida* infection, *seborrheic dermatitis*, and *psoriasis*. *Candida* infection is diagnosed with a positive potassium hydroxide preparation (see page 1756) or, if unavailable, "swab" culturette submitted for fungal culture. Seborrheic dermatitis and psoriasis are usually diagnosed by identifying skin lesions elsewhere. When presumed intertrigo does not respond to therapy, unusual diagnoses such as *Bowen disease* (squamous cell carcinoma *in situ*), *extramammary Paget disease*, *Langerhans cell histiocytosis*, and *glucagonoma syndrome* must be considered and a biopsy should be taken.

Therapy for intertrigo is directed at keeping the affected areas dry. Gauze may be placed in skin folds where appropriate, and a powder (e.g., Zeasorb or Zeasorb-AF, which contains an antifungal agent) or plain talc or baby powder should be applied frequently to dry the skin and reduce yeast colonization or infection. If obesity is the cause of the problem (e.g., abdominal or inguinal folds), weight reduction should be discussed with the patient (see Chapter 83). A cool environment is also beneficial. In edentulous patients with intertriginous dermatitis at the angles of the mouth due to overlapping skin, appropriate treatment for possible oral candidiasis and denture refitting should be prescribed. If these measures are ineffective, referral to a dermatologist for consideration of collagen injections may be considered. Collagen is injected into the crease formed by the opposing folds of skin. Although collagen injections must be repeated every 6 to 12 months, they may be a very worthwhile treatment for this chronic painful fissuring.

Seborrheic Dermatitis

Seborrheic dermatitis is a common condition present in approximately 3% to 5% of the population. Onset of seborrheic dermatitis is usually in early adulthood, and the course is characterized by frequent spontaneous remissions and exacerbations. In this disorder, an inflammatory epidermal hyperproliferation affects the areas the body more heavily populated with sebaceous glands, favoring the scalp and facial hair-bearing areas, central face (glabellar area and nasal folds), ears, presternal chest, axillae, umbilicus, inguinal folds, gluteal cleft, and perianal skin. Pruritus is variably present. *Dandruff*, a term commonly used synonymously with seborrheic dermatitis, is generally considered a noninflammatory (nonerythematous) scaling of the scalp skin.

Although the cause of seborrheic dermatitis is unknown, several observations have been made and hypotheses proposed over the years. *Pityrosporum*, a lipophilic yeast normally present on the skin, has been suggested as the cause of seborrheic dermatitis in that the yeast stimulates an immune response with resultant cutaneous inflammation. Although seborrheic dermatitis may occur in any individual, it occurs for unknown reasons with increased frequency and severity in patients with acquired immunodeficiency syndrome and Parkinson disease.

The treatment of seborrheic dermatitis is directed at decreasing epidermal hyperproliferation, inflammation, and *Pityrosporum* yeast using, respectively, topical tars, hydrocortisone, and ketoconazole. For the scalp, ketoconazole, selenium sulfide, zinc pyrithione, or tar shampoos and clear nongreasy mid- to high-potency corticosteroid solutions are preferred. Specifically, treatment for the scalp may include a medicated shampoo used every other night for 1 month, followed by prophylactic use once to twice weekly. If this alone is not effective, a fluorinated corticosteroid solution (e.g., Cormax Scalp Application, Lidex Solution) applied after shampooing should be added (two to three drops massaged into each quarter-sized of the affected scalp). Once under control, the corticosteroid is discontinued and repeated for recurrences only. For facial and body seborrheic dermatitis, hydrocortisone 1% cream (solution for the beard, mustache, eyebrows, outer auditory canal) may be used up to two times a day to control redness and scaling. Alternatively, ketoconazole cream (e.g., Nizoral 2% cream) may be used twice daily in a similar fashion. However, unlike hydrocortisone, ketoconazole cream may be continued after clearance to prevent recurrences.

Perioral Dermatitis

Perioral and sometimes *periorificial dermatitis* is an eruption of minute papules and pustules on a background of erythema and scant scale in a perioral or periorificial (mouth, eyes, and nares) location. Although it may occur at any age, it is most common in young women. It is uncommon and may be differentiated from acne by the lack of comedones and from contact dermatitis by the fact that it always spares the vermilion border, beginning 2 to 3 mm from the lip margin. Unlike allergic contact dermatitis, the most common symptoms are burning and stinging but not itching. *Perioral/periorificial dermatitis*, especially in the perinasal area, is a frequent precursor of acne in adolescent children and also frequently overlaps with perinasal seborrheic dermatitis and rosacea in adults.

The cause of *perioral dermatitis* is not known, but it has been associated with topical and aerosolized inhaled fluorinated corticosteroids and fluorinated toothpastes. Initial treatment is similar to that used for acne rosacea, but medications can usually be stopped in 4 to 8 weeks, often without a recurrence. If recurrences do occur, treatment is simply repeated.

PSORIASIS

Definition and Prevalence

Psoriasis is an idiopathic benign epidermal hyperproliferation that affects 2% of the population (8,9). It is believed to be of multifactorial inheritance, with multiple genetic and environmental factors required for expression. Although the average age at onset of psoriasis is approximately 30 years, more than one-third of patients develop the disease before age 20, and the average age at onset is 27 years. Most patients who develop psoriasis have lifelong disease with periods of remission and exacerbation. Factors associated with exacerbation include sunlight/UV radiation deprivation (likely due to lack of beneficial UV radiation effects on psoriasis lesions but possibly also due to reduced serum levels of vitamin D), infections, certain drugs including lithium and antimalarials, local cutaneous trauma, alcohol ingestion, and physical and psychologic stress.

Psoriasis may have a significant negative impact on many important aspects of life. Unlike other chronic diseases that may be easily concealed, psoriasis may be obvious because of thickened crumbly nails, heavy scalp scale, or hand, elbow, or knee involvement. The effect of the disease on the quality of life in patients with psoriasis has been compared with patients having other chronic diseases. When asked how many years of life patients would be willing to give up or how willing they would be to risk their lives to be free of their disease, patients with moderate psoriasis responded similarly to patients having had a kidney transplant. Patients with severe psoriasis responded similarly to those undergoing hospital-based dialysis (8). Patients with psoriasis involving exposed areas may also experience social rejection by people who believe that the disease is contagious or represents a manifestation of a disease or disorder they irrationally fear, such as acquired immunodeficiency syndrome. Psoriasis may be a devastating financial burden also. It may cause physical and occupational disability, particularly when it affects the hands or feet or causes incapacitating psoriatic arthritis.

Clinical Presentation

Psoriasis may be divided into four major subtypes depending on the appearance of lesions: plaque, guttate, erythrodermic, or pustular. *Chronic plaque psoriasis* is the most common type of psoriasis. Patients exhibit one to many deeply erythematous, sharply demarcated, oval plaques several centimeters in diameter, with moderate to heavy silvery white surface scale, commonly on the scalp and over one or more extensor surfaces. Intertriginous plaques may also be present in the axillary, inframammary, umbilical, abdominal, inguinal, gluteal, and popliteal fossae. These fold area lesions have little or no scale and instead are moist and intensely erythematous. Patients who have numerous widespread plaques have *generalized plaque psoriasis*.

Guttate psoriasis is the next most common type of psoriasis. Approximately one-third of patients have a sibling or parent with psoriasis (versus about 8% of the general population with such a family history) (10). Guttate psoriasis is characterized by an acute exanthem-like eruption of guttate (drop-like)

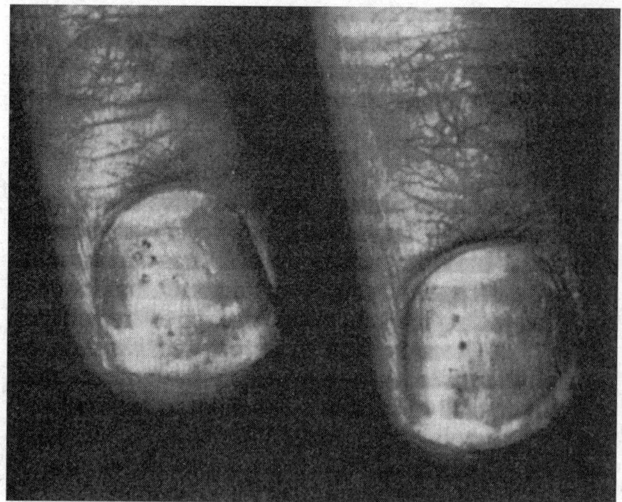

Figure 116.3. Minute pits are commonly seen on the surface of nails in patients with psoriasis.

erythematous, scaly papules, generally 1 mm to 1 cm in diameter. Although lesions are typically on the trunk and proximal extremities, the eruption may be widespread, involving the face, scalp, hands, and feet. Guttate psoriasis is often triggered by an infection, most often a streptococcal pharyngitis or a viral upper respiratory tract infection.

Erythrodermic psoriasis and *pustular psoriasis* are rare. In both types, a generalized exfoliative erythroderma (a scaly erythema) is present. In pustular psoriasis, crops of tiny, superficial, nonfollicular pustules develop, coalesce into "lakes of pus," and then desquamate in waves of lacy scale. Erythrodermic and pustular psoriasis are severe diseases, particularly in patients with other chronic illnesses. Potential complications include high-output congestive heart failure, sepsis, intravascular volume depletion, and vitamin and nutrient deficiencies caused by increased requirements and losses.

Nail involvement is seen in 30% of patients. Although not pathognomonic, the most commonly noted changes are pitting (ice pick-like marks in the nail plate, Fig. 116.3), *onycholysis* (separation of the nail plate from the nail bed, with resultant white color caused by air between the plate and bed), and *subungual hyperkeratosis* (crumbly scale between the plate and bed). The latter may be very distressing because it is both obvious on casual observation and often difficult to adequately treat.

Extracutaneous Disease

Arthritis has been said to affect less than 5% to nearly one-third of patients with psoriasis. Although it is generally believed that psoriasis and psoriatic arthritis are one disease involving two organ systems, it has been suggested that the two are separate entities occurring together by chance and that the activity of the psoriasis may modify or enhance the activity of simultaneously occurring joint disease (11). Regardless of cause, any patient with psoriasis and debilitating or destructive arthritis should be treated aggressively to prevent disease progression and disability.

Pathogenesis

Skin affected by psoriasis exhibits an accelerated rate of epidermal cell replication and a dysfunction of normal keratinocyte-to-keratinocyte inhibition of uncontrolled proliferation. Although not to the same degree, normal-appearing skin shows mildly accelerated proliferation. A basic issue that is still not fully understood is whether the primary defect triggering defective epidermal turnover resides in cytotoxic T cells, keratinocytes, locally produced cytokines, or other factors.

Treatment

Therapy for psoriasis depends on the degree of body surface area involvement and the clinical subtype of disease and prior response to therapy (9). One caveat should be noted by all clinicians prescribing any medications for patients with psoriasis, even mild psoriasis. Although systemic corticosteroids dramatically improve psoriasis acutely and in years past may have been used to treat psoriasis, systemic corticosteroids should be avoided. First, systemic corticosteroids would not be appropriate for psoriasis because it is a chronic disease requiring chronic therapy and, second, eventual corticosteroids withdrawal or dosage tapering may precipitate erythrodermic or pustular psoriasis.

Localized chronic plaque psoriasis is treated with bland emollients alone or combined with keratolytics (e.g., U-Lactin lotion, over the counter; AmLactin lotion, over the counter; Lac-Hydrin cream 12%, by prescription), topical corticosteroids, calcipotriene (Dovonex ointment or cream, a topical vitamin D derivative), or tazarotene (Tazorac 0.05% and 0.1% gel, a synthetic topical vitamin A derivative, *nota bene*: teratogen, Pregnancy Category X) applied twice daily. Although generic formulations of topical steroids tend to be relatively inexpensive, the vitamin D and vitamin A derivatives are very expensive. If these products made psoriasis vanish forever, patients would probably be happy to pay any price. But because this is not the case, patients who sacrifice to purchase them are likely to be disappointed. Topical steroids and vitamin D and vitamin A derivatives appear to be of similar efficacy in clinical trials; however, in a given patient one treatment may be much more effective than another. To achieve the best possible response, often some combination of a vitamin D or A topical and a corticosteroid is sought, requiring both a motivated patient and an empathetic clinician. A potential side effect of potent topical corticosteroids is atrophy (cigarette paper wrinkling or striae when severe). Side effects common to calcipotriene and vitamin A derivatives are irritation and stinging.

Generalized plaque psoriasis is difficult, time consuming, and expensive to treat with topical preparations. Also, the greater volume of topical corticosteroid needed to cover all the areas of psoriasis may ultimately produce effects similar to systemic corticosteroid administration. For these reasons, patients with generalized plaque psoriasis are frequently treated with phototherapy using UV-B radiation (UV radiation 290 to 320 nm wavelength) or photochemotherapy with the phototoxic agent 8-methoxypsoralen (Oxsoralen Ultra) orally in combination with controlled UV-A radiation (UV radiation 320 to 400 nm wavelength) given in a phototherapy light unit (PUVA). Patients are generally treated three times a week until clearance occurs and then may receive maintenance light treatments (PUVA only; UV-B maintenance should not be used because of the risk of sunburn) or may discontinue treatments until the next flare of psoriasis occurs. A patient should never be given 8-methoxypsoralen to be used with natural sunlight or in a suntan parlor because severe burns and even death may occur. Also, self-administered light treatment even without a phototoxic agent is best avoided because careful monitoring is difficult and severe burning may result. Over a long period, PUVA therapy increases a patient's risk of skin cancer, both nonmelanoma and likely also melanoma skin cancer. Therefore, patients treated with PUVA should be followed throughout their lives, preferably with yearly full skin examinations. Alternative therapies to phototherapy and photochemotherapy include methotrexate, acitretin, and cyclosporine (12), but these should only be used in consultation with a dermatologist.

Guttate psoriasis, particularly with the initial episode, is usually very responsive to most treatments. Sunlight or in-office UV-B phototherapy combined with emollients and low-potency topical corticosteroids often work well. In addition, because triggering infections, especially streptococcal pharyngitis, may precipitate guttate psoriasis, appropriate evaluation should be performed.

Erythrodermic and pustular psoriasis may cause severe and even life-threatening illness, particularly in elderly patients with cardiovascular disease. Depending on the severity of the psoriasis and underlying medical problems, patients may require hospitalization, warm baths, bland emollients, and systemic therapy with acitretin (a synthetic retinoid), weekly low-dose methotrexate, or cyclosporine. Patients without infection may have signs and symptoms identical to those seen with sepsis, with cyclic fevers up to 40°C and an increase in white blood cell count up to 40,000 cells/mm^3 with neutrophilia, tachycardia, and orthostatic hypotension, so that possible sepsis must be excluded with blood and urine cultures and other appropriate testing. The hemodynamic instability seen is caused by marked vasodilation and increased cardiac output and is particularly problematic in the setting of pre-existent cardiovascular disease or volume depletion. In addition, vitamin and nutrient deficiencies may result from the accelerated epidermal turnover rate. After all the acute cutaneous and systemic problems have been addressed and the patient's cutaneous disease is controlled, the systemic therapy for psoriasis generally must be continued or PUVA substituted to prevent severe flares.

Patients requiring systemic therapies for psoriasis are probably best cared for with the consultation of a dermatologist. Those receiving methotrexate, acitretin, or cyclosporine must be monitored closely. Methotrexate is an abortifacient and must not be taken by either men or women within 3 months of planned conception. The most important side effects of methotrexate are acute cytopenias and chronic hepatitis and cirrhosis. Acitretin is teratogenic. Women taking acitretin must abstain from alcohol and wait 2 years after drug cessation to begin to try to conceive. For this reason, it may be best to avoid this medication totally in women of child-bearing potential. Important potential side effects of acitretin include hypertriglyceridemia and hypercholesterolemia, hepatitis, pseudotumor cerebri, bony hyperostosis, hair loss, fragile skin, painful palmar and plantar desquamation, and arthralgias. Cyclosporine has many notable side effects, including hypertension, decreased renal blood flow, glomerular and tubular toxicity, paresthesias, and anergy (12,13). Whether cyclosporine is associated with an increased risk of cutaneous or lymphoproliferative malignancies in nontransplant patients is unclear (14).

Several investigational therapies may eventually prove useful. Among these are thiazolidinediones (e.g., pioglitazone), particularly attractive for patients also requiring oral hypoglycemic agents. Thiazolidinediones are insulin sensitizing agents that act as ligands for the peroxisome proliferator-activated receptor gamma, a member of the nuclear hormone receptor superfamily that includes the retinoic acid receptor and the vitamin D receptor (both of which are targets of presently available U.S. Food and Drug Administration-approved topical and systemic psoriasis therapies). The potential beneficial effect is believed to occur through inhibition of cell proliferation and promotion of cell differentiation (15,16). Various therapies involving monoclonal antibodies targeted at the T cells migrating into the skin are under investigation but are not yet recommended outside of a protocol study. Finally, a small subpopulation of patients with psoriasis, those who have serum antigliadin antibodies, may benefit from a gluten-free diet (17).

Specific References

1. Kay AB. Allergy and allergic diseases. First of two parts. N Engl J Med 2001;344:30.
2. Ruzicka T, Bieber T, Schöpf E, et al. A short-term trial of tacrolimus ointment for atopic dermatitis. N Engl J Med 1997;337:816.
3. Schachner L, Field T, Hernandez-Reif M, et al. Atopic dermatitis symptoms decreased in children following massage therapy. Ped Derm 1998;5:390.
4. Sampson HA, Picasco MC, Caskil CC. Food hypersensitivity and atopic dermatitis: evaluation of 113 patients. J Pediatr 1985; 107:669.

5. Bubak ME, Reed CE, Fransway AF. Allergic reactions to latex among health-care workers. Mayo Clin Proc 1992;67:1075.
6. Sussman GL, Tarlo S, Dolovich J. The spectrum of IgE-moderated responses to latex. JAMA 1991;265:2844.
7. Brehler R, Kütting B. Natural rubber latex allergy: a problem of interdisciplinary concern in medicine. Arch Intern Med 2001;161:1057.
8. Baughman RD. A 61-year-old man with psoriasis. JAMA 1996; 276:1421.
9. Greaves MW, Weinstein GD. Treatment of psoriasis. N Engl J Med 1995;332:581.
10. Naldi L, Peli L, Parazzini F, et al. Family history of psoriasis, stressful life events, and recent infectious disease are risk factors for a first episode of acute guttate psoriasis: results of a case-control study. J Am Acad Dermatol 2001;44:433.
11. Katz A. Psoriasis and arthritis. Cutis 1990;46:323.
12. Ellis CN, Fradin MS, Messana JM, et al. Cyclosporine for plaque type psoriasis. N Engl J Med 1991;324:277.
13. Bos JD. Use of cyclosporin A in psoriasis. Lancet 1989;2:8678.
14. Zacharie H, Kragballe K. Cyclosporine versus methotrexate toxicity in psoriasis. Lancet 1990;335:924.
15. Ellis CN, Varani J, Fisher GJ, et al. Troglitazone improves psoriasis and normalizes models of proliferative skin disease. Arch Dermatol 2000;136:609.
16. King AB. A comparison in the clinical setting of efficacy and side effects of three thiazolidinediones. Diabetes Care 2000;23:557.
17. Michaëlsson G, Gerden B, Hagforsen E, et al. Psoriasis patients with antibodies to gliadin can be improved with gluten-free diet. Br J Dermatol 2000;142:44.

CHAPTER 117

Primary Superficial Fungal and Viral Infections and Infestations

S. ELIZABETH WHITMORE, MD, ScM

DERMATOPHYTE INFECTIONS

Dermatophyte infections are caused by fungi that penetrate the hair, nails, and stratum corneum of the skin. Symptoms of fungal infections, regardless of location, are usually pruritus or stinging. Although transmission of infection may occur through direct contact, indirect transmission is more common with exposure to dermatophyte-laden caps, pillow cases, towels, and clothing, as well as baths, showers, pool decks, and gymnasium floors.

Tinea Capitis

Tinea capitis (scalp infection) is seen primarily in preadolescent children 4 to 12 years old. Rarely, healthy adults and occasionally immunosuppressed individuals develop this infection. In the United States, tinea capitis is caused usually by *Trichophyton tonsurans*. Within well-defined scaly patches of the scalp, broken hairs, flush with the scalp up to a few millimeters in length, are seen. In contrast to seborrheic dermatitis, lymphadenopathy is usually present (1). The most severe complication of tinea capitis is *kerion formation,* in which boggy, inflammatory, pustular plaques of potentially scarring hair loss develop. If this is not treated early and aggressively with antifungals in combination with intralesional or oral corticosteroids, it generally causes a disfiguring permanent scarring in the scalp. Tinea capitis is diagnosed with a positive potassium hydroxide (KOH) preparation (see page 1756) or fungal swab culture (2). With a kerion, the KOH preparation (see page 1757) and fungal culture may be negative because of the intense host response.

When the diagnosis of kerion is suspected, treatment should be given as soon as possible in an attempt to prevent irreversible scarring alopecia. This includes selenium sulfide or ketoconazole shampoo to reduce spore shedding and oral griseofulvin to eradicate the fungus. Griseofulvin is not only teratogenic but may also reduce the effectiveness of oral contraceptive pills. Young women who are sexually active must be instructed on the use of two forms of birth control when prescribed griseofulvin, and a pregnancy test must also be performed before institution of therapy if there is any question of pregnancy. Common side effects of griseofulvin include mild diarrhea and headache limited to the first several days of treatment. If these symptoms persist more than a few days, dosage reduction or initiation of another antifungal (e.g., fluconazole once weekly treatments for 2 months [3], itraconazole, or terbinafine [4]) may be substituted but it is best to consult, at least by telephone, with a dermatologist because newer drugs do not yet have U.S. Food and Drug Administration (FDA) approval and certain contraindications may exist. After 4 to 6 weeks of therapy, fungal culture is repeated; if results are negative 2 weeks later, treatment is stopped at that time.

Tinea Faciei

Tinea faciei is often misdiagnosed as rosacea or cutaneous lupus. Lesions tend to appear less "ringworm-like" (less sharp and clearly annular) than fungal infections elsewhere on the body. Patients often note that lesions flare with sun exposure, again suggesting diagnoses such as lupus erythematosus and acne rosacea instead of tinea. Lesions vary from erythematous, ill-defined, scaly plaques to the more classic sharply circumscribed plaques with leading edge scale and central clearing. Diagnosis may be made with a positive KOH preparation; however, on the face, false-negative KOH preparations are common with tinea faciei, and diagnosis may require culture or biopsy. Treatment is generally an oral antifungal (e.g., griseofulvin, itraconazole, fluconazole) because topical therapy may fail to clear this infection.

Tinea Corporis

Tinea corporis indicates a tinea infection outside of the head, face, groin, hands, and feet. Classic lesions are annular (ring-like) plaques that show a delicate scale at the advancing margin. KOH preparation from these lesions is usually positive. Treatment usually consists of topical imidazole antifungals (see Chapter 113) for 1 month with systemic therapy reserved for patients with a great number of lesions or unresponsive to prior topical treatment.

Tinea Cruris

Tinea cruris is predominantly seen in men. Lesions are semicircular scaly plaques on the superior medial thighs extending into the inguinal folds and onto the perineum. Diagnosis is based on a positive KOH preparation (see below). Treatment with topical imidazoles (see Chapter 113) for a few to several weeks is usually adequate to control the problem.

Tinea Pedis

Tinea pedis is exceedingly common, eventually affecting up to 80% of men. Patients may have interdigital and plantar involvement with absent or moderate erythema, scale, and focal maceration. Less commonly seen is acute onset "oozing and blistering" on the plantar feet. Occasionally, interdigital tinea pedis with interdigital fissures may provide a point of entry for *Streptococcus,* which may ascend and cause recurrent streptococcal erysipelas cellulitis of the leg (5). Diagnosis is made with a positive KOH preparation (see below), and treatment may be initiated with topical imidazoles. When plantar involvement is present, topical therapy may be unsuccessful and requires oral therapy for complete clearance. If treatment failure occurs in a patient at risk for leg cellulitis (e.g., history of prior leg erysipelas or cellulitis, venous stasis, or deep or superficial venous thrombosis), oral therapy should be prescribed to decrease the risk of recurrent ascending bacterial streptococcal cellulitis (6).

Tinea Manum

Tinea manum (tinea of the palmar skin) is uncommon. When seen, it often manifests as "two feet, one hand" syndrome, with areas of involvement as the name implies. The palm shows diffuse usually noninflammatory scaling, and the KOH preparation (see below) or fungal culture is positive. Treatment typically requires systemic therapy, but topical imidazoles (see Chapter 113) may initially be tried for 6 to 8 weeks. If topical therapy is unsuccessful or if nail involvement is present, oral itraconazole or terbinafine may be prescribed.

Tinea Unguium (Onychomycosis)

Tinea unguium of the toenails is very common, whereas fingernail infection is relatively rare. Although the incidence of tinea unguium is from 2% to 13% of the general population, the prevalence in the older male population is much higher. Tinea unguium represents approximately 30% of all mycotic infections of the skin and nails. Changes include white discoloration, subungual crumbly debris, and thickening of the nails. Patients are typically asymptomatic unless the toenails become ingrown or secondary bacterial infection occurs. Treatment is notoriously difficult. The recent addition of ciclopirox nail lacquer (Penlac) is a topical therapy available by prescription. However, cure rates are less than 50%.

When patients desiring systemic therapy understand the expense, potential side effects, and required laboratory studies (see below), itraconazole or terbinafine may be used. Cure rates several months after completion of a 3-month course of therapy vary from 50% to more than 70%. Because these drugs are retained in the nail for many months after drug discontinuance, patients should not be evaluated for clearance of an organism until several months after completion of therapy. If they are not clear, another 3-month course of therapy may be initiated. Both itraconazole and terbinafine may cause hepatotoxicity, so baseline and monthly liver function studies should be performed. After completion of systemic therapy, ongoing topical prophylactic antifungal preparations may help reduce recurrence rates (e.g., Penlac Nail Lacquer or an over the counter topical antifungal cream, lotion, gel, or powder).

YEAST INFECTIONS

Candidiasis

Candida albicans and other *Candida* species are yeast-like fungi that most often cause superficial cutaneous infections; however, in immunocompromised patients, *Candida* may cause systemic infections, including septicemia. *Candida* infection presents most often as a diaper rash in infants, summertime inframammary rash in women, vaginitis in premenopausal women, oral candidiasis in endogenously or exogenously immunosuppressed patients, and buttock and perineal rash in incontinent patients. The cutaneous changes are similar in most areas and appear as erythematous, slick, shiny patches with an irregular border of delicate scale and often satellite papules and pustules. The diagnosis can be confirmed with a KOH preparation or a swab culture (see below).

Candidiasis may be treated with topical nystatin cream or an imidazole cream (see Chapter 113). Topicals should be applied two times a day and are continued for 1 to 2 weeks after clearing is seen (i.e, commonly applied for up to a month in total). For infections unresponsive to topical therapy and when benefit outweighs risks, expense, and required testing, oral itraconazole or fluconazole for 10 to 14 days may be used. Pretreatment liver function tests are prudent in patients with multiple medical problems, and all patients should be instructed to report any signs or symptoms or hepatotoxicity during treatment. Topical nystatin powder or simple body powder may be helpful in preventing recurrences.

Tinea Versicolor

Tinea versicolor is a chronically recurring superficial yeast infection of the skin caused by *Pityrosporum orbiculare,* also known as *Malassezia furfur.* Tinea versicolor is seen most often in teens and young adults. It is common year round in tropical climates and during the warm months in temperate climates.

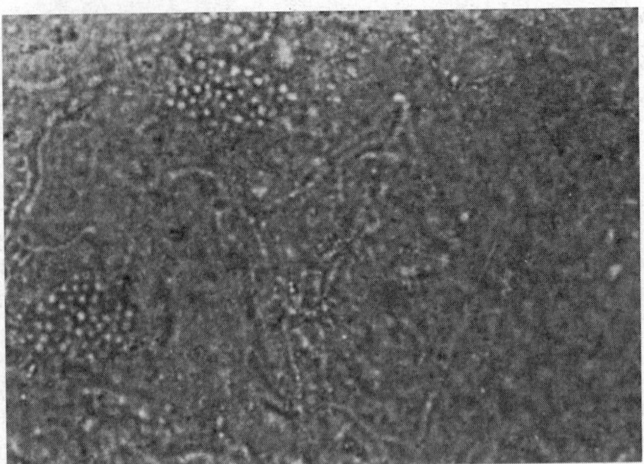

Figure 117.1. Short hyphae and spores of *Malassezia furfur* seen in tinea versicolor (potassium hydroxide preparation, ×400).

Tinea versicolor appears as round to oval, scaly hypopigmented, hyperpigmented, or salmon colored macules that coalesce to form large confluent patches over the upper trunk and shoulders and, less often, on the face, scalp, genitalia, arms, and thighs. Although usually asymptomatic, some patients may have significant pruritus, particularly when perspiring during and after exercising. Diagnosis is made with a positive KOH preparation (see below) showing pseudohyphae and spores (Fig. 117.1). A simple and usually effective 5-day therapy is daily ketoconazole shampoo (prescription Nizoral 2% or over the counter Nizoral AD 1%) applied undiluted as a lotion and left on for 5 minutes before being rinsed. Once-weekly applications may be useful in preventing recurrences. Although not yet an FDA-approved indication, oral itraconazole 200 mg daily for 1 week in a controlled trial appears effective (7); however, recurrence is common.

In contrast to the superficial "epidermal" fungal infections mentioned above, deep fungal infections of the skin involve the underlying dermis. Excluding sporotrichosis, cutaneous infection usually results from seeding of the skin from a distant visceral organ infection (e.g., pulmonary). Some of the more common deep fungal infections are summarized in Table 117.1.

Potassium Hydroxide Wet Mount Preparation

Dermatophyte and yeast infections of the skin are diagnosed with microscopic examination of surface skin scale. For this examination, scale is scraped from the advancing margin of an active lesion using a number 15 surgical blade held at a slightly less than 90-degree angle to the skin surface. The scale is placed on a glass slide, one to two drops of KOH 20% added, and a coverslip applied. This is gently heated with a low flame, avoiding boiling, which, if it occurs, will result in crystallization and invalidation of the procedure. With light microscopy, the slide is scanned with the

Table 117.1. Selected Deep Fungal Infections

Fungus	Endemic Area in the United States/Source	Usual Site of Primary Infection/Associated Cutaneous Hypersensitivity Reactions	Primary Cutaneous Inoculation[a]	Cutaneous Lesions Caused by Organisms
Blastomyces dermatitidis	Mississippi River basin, Great Lakes region, Southeast United States/bird excreta, wood	Pulmonary/rare erythema nodosum	Rare	Present in 70%; centrifugally enlarging plaques with a verrucous, pustular border; also, pustular ulcerations, subcutaneous abscesses, widespread or acral pustules
Coccidioides immitis	Southwest United States/soil	Pulmonary/50% of symptomatic infections with toxic erythema: diffuse exanthem, erythema multiforme, erythema nodosum	Rare	Verrucous plaque or granulomatous nodule (especially face); also, papules, pustules, nodules, subcutaneous
Histoplasma capsulatum	Central and southeast United States/bird and bat excreta, especially chicken coops	Pulmonary/rare erythema nodosum	Rare	Nasal or oral mucosal lesions in 50%; also, 6% with variable cutaneous lesions; ulcerating papules, nodules, plaques; ulcers, erythroderma[b]
Sporothrix schenckii	Ubiquitous, humidity favors growth/decaying vegetable matter, wood ("splinters")	Cutaneous (pulmonary possible)	Common	A papule that enlarges into an ulcerated nodule, usually with associated regional lymphangitis and lymphadenopathy
Cryptococcus neoformans	Ubiquitous/pigeon excreta, soil, some fruits	Pulmonary	Rare	Papules, pustules, ulcerating nodules, ulcers, abscesses, acneiform lesions, cellulitis, ecchymoses, vasculitis[b]
Candida albicans and *Candida tropicalis*	Ubiquitous	Oral mucosa, then esophagus most often	Rare	Erythematous to purpuric 0.5- to 1-cm papulonodules commonly on the trunk and proximal extremities, with associated fever and myalgia; also cellulitis, ecthyma gangrenosumlike eschar, nodular folliculitis and abscesses, purpura

[a]Nodule or chancriform ulcer with or without lymphangitis or lymphadenopathy.
[b]In human immunodeficiency virus–infected patients, may develop molluscum contagiosum–like lesions.

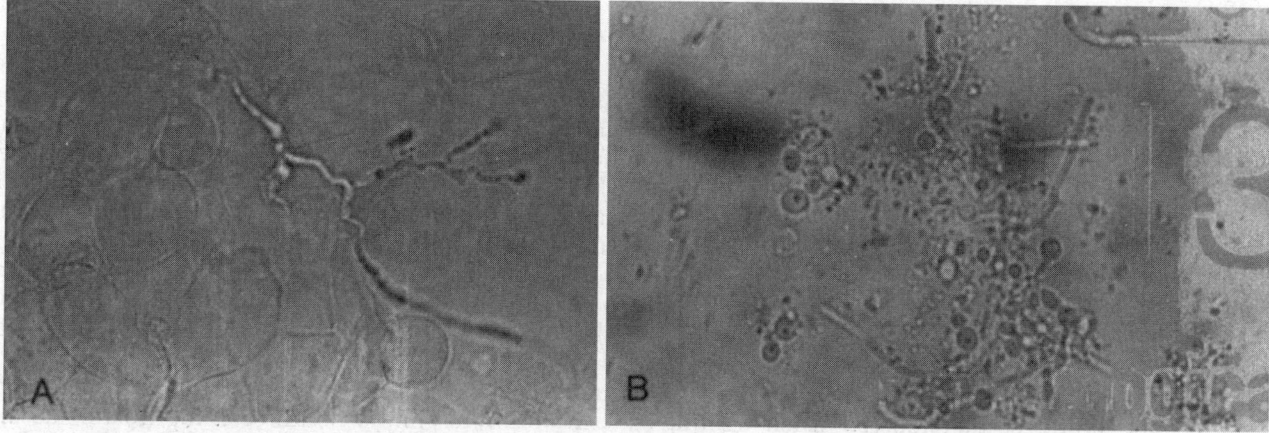

Figure 117.2. A: Hyphae of *tinea* (potassium hydroxide preparation, ×400). **B:** Pseudohyphae of *Candida* (potassium hydroxide preparation, ×400). (Courtesy of William G. Merz, PhD.)

10× objective and then examined more closely with the 40× objective. Dermatophyte hyphae are seen as refractile rod-shaped filaments of uniform width with characteristic branching (Fig. 117.2A). These hyphae traverse several normal cells and therefore can be distinguished from cell membranes. In contrast, *Candida* and *Pityrosporum* appear as nonbranching pseudohyphae and clusters of budding spores (Fig. 117.2B). Occasionally, *Candida* may show branching hyphae.

Fungal Culture

When the diagnosis of a fungal infection is strongly suspected despite a negative KOH preparation, when KOH examination is not available, and when the identification of a specific dermatophyte is important, a fungal culture should be done. Depending on the site of suspected infection, scale is taken from the advancing margin of the skin lesion, under the nail, or the scalp. The latter sample should also include several "broken off" hairs extracted with tweezers or forceps. Specimens may be placed between two glass slides, taped together, and sent in a sterile cup to the laboratory. Alternatively, particularly when the patient is not able to hold still and using a no. 15 blade may be dangerous, a culturette swab firmly rubbed over the area may be used.

LOCALIZED VIRAL INFECTIONS OF THE SKIN

Warts

Warts, also known as *verrucae,* are benign proliferations of the epidermis caused by human papilloma virus (HPV) infection. Warts are most common in children and immunocompromised patients. Three clinical features of all forms of warts include disruption of normal skin lines, surface pinpoint black dots (thrombosed capillaries), and appearance at sites of contact or trauma.

Common warts (*verrucae vulgaris*) may be noted initially as smooth, skin-colored, <1-mm papules that gradually enlarge to several millimeters with a rough, finely papulated, or hyperkeratotic (warty) surface. Warts may coalesce to form large plaques. Common warts are most often found on the hands.

Flat warts (*verrucae plana*) are skin-colored to pink flat-topped papules usually less than a few millimeters in diameter. They occur most commonly on the dorsal aspect of the hands, face, and, in women, the legs.

Genital warts (*condylomata acuminata*) begin as minute flat papules that often become verrucous on the external genitalia, vagina, cervix, perirectal, and/or anal canal. This HPV infection of the cervix or anorectal area predisposes to intraepithelial neoplasia. Immunosuppression, for example, from immunosuppressive therapy in an organ transplant recipient to a patient infected with human immunodeficiency virus (HIV), may increase the risk of anal intraepithelial neoplasia when genital warts are present.

Plantar warts (*verrucae plantaris*) appear as circumscribed, thickened, barely elevated papules with surface callous. Extensive infection with HPV may manifest as warts covering the entire heel or plantar aspect of the foot. Plantar warts are often confused with corns or clavi (see below). Warts can be distinguished by paring the surface with a number 15 surgical blade as minute black dots (thrombosed capillaries) should become visible. In contrast, paring of corns reveals a central core that is easily removed with the paring blade.

Treatment

Two precepts should be remembered when treating warts: There are no guarantees in the success of any treatment and the lesions themselves are benign and should not be treated with modalities that result in harm or scarring, such as ionizing irradiation, deep surgical excision, or deep destructive therapies (extending into the dermis).

Treatment of common, flat, and plantar warts is typically daily self-application of *topical 17% salicylic acid solution* (e.g., Occlusal or Duofilm) or a 40% salicylic acid patch (MediPlast), all available over the counter. Before application, the wart may be soaked in warm water for several minutes and then filed to remove the white macerated surface with a nail file or pumice stone (available in pharmacies). Because of the risk of infection transmission, whatever instrument is used it must not be used elsewhere or by others. If after 6 weeks of daily therapy the wart is still present, weekly or biweekly *liquid nitrogen cryotherapy* (usually done by a dermatologist) may be started. Patients should be warned that although liquid nitrogen should not cause scarring, it may cause blistering and, upon healing, permanent depigmentation of the skin, particularly important with face and hand warts, and, rarely, superficial nerve damage (usually on the lateral surface of the digits). If after several cryotherapy sessions warts are still present, other options should be considered, such as "watchful waiting," laser vaporization, and curette and desiccation. Patients should be warned that these latter treatments may cause scarring.

Initial treatment of condyloma acuminatum may be administered by the patient. Two options are available. Podofilox 0.5% (Condylox gel or solution) is a patient-applied podophyllin derivative that is applied two times a day for 3 consecutive days each week. After several weeks of treatment, clearance rates are 30% to 50%. Another patient-applied medication is imiquimod 5% cream (Aldara). This agent causes local endogenous cytokine release that is believed to lead to a host effected clearance of HPV. Imiquimod cream is applied three times per week for up to 4 months. Both of these medications require a prescription. If these medications are ineffective, liquid nitrogen cryotherapy may be used in the same manner as outlined for other warts (see above). Additional alternative therapies, which may be considered by a consulting dermatologist, include laser vaporization, curette and desiccation, and scalpel excision.

Molluscum Contagiosum

Molluscum contagiosum is common in young children and HIV-infected patients. Lesions are caused by the pox virus, a DNA virus. The lesions are umbilicated, skin-colored to whitish, 1- to 4-mm papules, typically on the neck, trunk, genital, and eyelid areas. The central umbilicated depression contains molluscum bodies, which are enlarged degrading keratinocytes, packed with viral material. The diagnosis is made by obtaining a curette of the molluscum for KOH preparation (see above). With light microscopy, the round, homogeneous, 25-μm molluscum bodies are easily seen.

In children, simple nonthreatening treatments are best. Scotch tape stripping (tape quickly and firmly applied and immediately removed a dozen times) once to twice daily for several weeks may suffice by unroofing the lesion and stimulating a host response through the mild local trauma. Alternatively, topical salicylic acid 17% preparations (as for warts; see above) or topical tretinoin (Retin-A 0.025% gel) applied directly to the lesion twice a day may be tried for 6 weeks. If lesions persist, either curettage or liquid nitrogen cryotherapy may be used, remembering that the latter may cause permanent depigmentation.

HERPES INFECTION

Herpes Simplex

Herpes simplex virus (HSV) infection may be caused by HSV type I or II, typically with type I causing *herpes labialis* and type II causing *herpes genitalis*. HSV is commonly present in asymptomatic individuals. For example, a study of randomly selected patients in a family medicine clinic found 56% seropositivity for HSV I, 23% seropositivity for HSV II, 12% seropositivity for both HSV I and II, and 33% seronegativity (8). Active infection results in a recurrent localized clustered (herpetic) blistering of the skin. After a primary infection has occurred, the virus remains dormant in the cranial nerve or dorsal root nerve ganglia innervating the region of cutaneous infection. Lesions may recur at any time, often being triggered by sun exposure, illness, menses, local trauma, and physical and psychologic stress. Transmission occurs through direct contact with an infected person actively shedding virus. The virus may live on fomites, but unlike HPV, HSV quickly dies on drying (30 minutes), making fomite transmission unlikely.

Primary herpes infection in the oral cavity causes the painful febrile illness acute herpetic gingivostomatitis (see Chapter 112). After healing the virus remains latent, and subsequent reactivation causes herpes labialis, manifest as clustered vesicles on or about the lips. Notably, most patients with recurrent herpes labialis have no history of primary acute herpetic gingivostomatitis or herpetic infection elsewhere and therefore are presumed to have had an asymptomatic primary oral infection. Lesions heal in approximately 1 to 2 weeks, with a typical sequence of rupture, crusting, and desquamation. The lesions are infectious as long as the skin is not intact. The importance of asymptomatic viral shedding in viral transmission, as is known to occur with genital herpes and with exceptionally high frequency in patients with acquired immunodeficiency syndrome (AIDS), is not known (8). Genital herpes, the most common cause of genital ulcers, is discussed in Chapter 102.

Herpes simplex infection may occur anywhere on the body; a common site in health care workers is on the finger (*herpetic whitlow*), acquired through exposure to a patient with active herpes infection. Viral transmission has been reported to occur through vinyl gloves, so one is wise to double glove if touching open herpes lesions is required during an examination.

Chronic herpetic infections in immunocompromised patients appear as chronic punched-out ulcers that may be solitary or multiple. The expanded AIDS surveillance case definition for AIDS diagnosis includes a chronic herpes simplex ulcer present for 1 month or longer in a patient infected with HIV.

Fortunately, *cutaneous complications* of HSV infection are rare. These complications include *cutaneous dissemination* in patients with generalized atopic dermatitis and *recurrent erythema multiforme* as a hypersensitivity response. A history of the latter is an indication for ongoing prophylactic antiviral therapy (see Chapters 102, 112, and 118). Ocular complications include *herpetic keratitis,* a primary or secondary infection that involves the cornea of the eye and is best managed emergently by an ophthalmologist because of the potential for permanent corneal scarring and loss of vision. Albeit rare, the most common systemic complication is Bell's palsy (9). Other serious and systemic complications that are rare complications of HSV include acute ascending necrotizing myelopathy and necrotizing lymphadenitis associated with herpes genitalis (10) and recurrent lymphocytic meningitis (11).

Treatment

Although no treatment is necessary for recurrent facial HSV, topical agents may be used to provide comfort and potentially shorten the symptomatic period. Topical penciclovir (Denavir cream), by prescription, may slightly speed lesion healing when applied every 2 hours for 4 days. Although systemic antiviral therapy is generally more effective, it is not recommended routinely except in patients with AIDS or other immunocompromised patients having chronic persistent infections, patients with atopic dermatitis and a history of cutaneous dissemination, and persons with HSV associated erythema multiforme. Finally, prophylaxis should be given when HSV recurrences may complicate procedures, such as facial cutaneous surgery, oral surgery, and dental work. Prophylaxis may also be welcomed by patients when recurrences may be anticipated, such as sun exposure (oral antiviral and topical high SPF sunscreen), or important social events in which recurrence would be devastating (12).

Novel treatments appear to have promise for HSV. In a randomized, double-blind, placebo-controlled, pilot study, stannous fluoride 0.4% gel applied twice daily at the onset of prodromal symptoms prevented blisters from developing in most individuals, and in those who developed lesions, it decreased their duration significantly (13). Also, aspirin initiated at the onset of recurrent HSV, at a dose of 125 mg, decreased the duration of lesions by almost 50%, whereas a dose of aspirin of 250 mg/day did not show this benefit (14).

Herpes Zoster (Shingles)

Herpes zoster represents a reactivation of the varicella–zoster virus. After initial varicella (chickenpox) infection, the virus resides in a dorsal root or cranial nerve ganglia. At any point thereafter, latent virus may be reactivated and produce multiple erythematous plaques surmounted by clustered vesicles, in a dermatomal or zosteriform distribution. In an immunocompetent patient, lesions begin with vesicles that become turbid in 3 days, dry and crust in 7 to 10 days, and clear within 2 to 3 weeks. New lesions may continue to appear for up to 1 week. Herpes zoster affects a thoracic dermatome in 50%, a cervical dermatome in 20%, the trigeminal dermatome in 15%, and a lumbosacral dermatome in 10% of patients. Of patients with herpes zoster, two-thirds are over 50 years of age and about 10% were less than 20 years of age (15).

Often, patients who have herpes zoster develop a prodrome of pain in the affected dermatome. Occasionally, this painful prodrome is misdiagnosed as an acute painful disease such as pleurisy, myocardial infarction, cholecystitis, appendicitis, renal colic, or a ruptured intervertebral disk. Rarely, patients may experience acute segmental neuralgia with a concurrent rise in varicella virus antibodies without developing skin lesions. This is called zoster sine herpete.

There are several very significant potential complications of zoster (16). When the trigeminal dermatome is affected, involvement of the second branch may be associated with involvement of the eye. Affected patients must be evaluated emergently by an ophthalmologist because keratitis, uveitis, secondary glaucoma, iridocyclitis, or rarely panophthalmitis may develop. *Ramsay-Hunt* syndrome is the constellation of herpes zoster affecting the facial and auditory nerves, causing facial palsy with cutaneous zoster of the external ear or tympanic membrane with associated tinnitus, vertigo, and/or hearing deficit. Among all patients with herpes zoster, motor nerve involvement occurs in only 5%. The incidence is probably understated because mild or partial deficits likely go undetected. Weakness or paralysis usually begins within weeks of the onset of the rash and may involve the muscle groups outside of the affected dermatome. Full recovery from this weakness or paralysis occurs spontaneously in only about half of patients who are so affected (17). Meningoencephalitis may develop with cranial nerve herpes zoster in immunocompromised patients, most often in association with cutaneous dissemination. *Granulomatous angiitis* of cerebral arteries is an unusual complication of ophthalmic zoster that may lead to a syndrome of delayed contralateral hemiplegia occurring weeks to a few months after an episode of zoster. Such patients are usually diagnosed as having a typical cerebrovascular accident, but arteriograms reveal segmental narrowing or occlusion of cerebral arteries ipsilateral to the site of the ophthalmic zoster. Finally, *disseminated herpes zoster,* defined as more than 20 vesicles at a distance from the primary dermatome, occurs almost exclusively in immunocompromised patients. Such patients should be hospitalized and isolated as appropriate to protect those not immune to the virus for intravenous acyclovir therapy. Approximately 10% of patients with disseminated cutaneous lesions develop widespread often fatal visceral infection, particularly of the lungs, liver, and brain (16).

The presumptive diagnosis of herpes zoster is made clinically. A *Tzanck smear,* done when there is doubt about the diagnosis, shows multinucleated giant cells (see below). Such a positive smear confirms that the eruption is herpes zoster or herpes simplex and rules out other blistering disorders such as impetigo, erythema multiforme, and pemphigus, which occasionally may be confused with herpes infection. Herpes simplex can occur in a dermatomal pattern, so any case of "recurrent" herpes zoster should be cultured because the correct diagnosis is more likely recurrent dermatomal HSV infection. It is important to confirm this infection because recurrent zoster (as opposed to HSV) raises the possibility of an associated illness causing immunosuppression and should prompt further evaluation of immune function.

The early treatment of acute herpes zoster reduces the severity, shortens the duration of the infection, and potentially reduces the incidence of post herpetic neuralgia. Kost and Straus (18) put forth a useful algorithm for treatment and prevention of acute herpes zoster and postherpetic neuralgia (PHN). Antiviral therapy affects the course of disease if initiated within 48 to 72 hours of its onset. A 1-week course of an oral antiviral (e.g., acyclovir [Zovirax] 800 mg five times a day, valacyclovir [Valtrex] 1,000 mg three times a day, famciclovir [Famvir] 500 mg three times a day) is used in immunocompetent patients. Acyclovir has been shown to reduce zoster-associated acute pain and new lesion formation, and both valacyclovir and famciclovir reduce acute pain and speed healing (19,20).

Topical therapy will ease the pain from open lesions. Wet to damp dressings promote drying of the lesions, and a topical ointment (e.g., plain petrolatum or antibiotic ointment with caution given the potential development of allergic contact dermatitis if Neosporin or bacitracin are used) generously applied promotes healing, prevents secondary infection, and reduces the pain caused by air contacting the denuded skin. If acute neuralgia is present, nonsteroidal anti-inflammatory drugs, amitriptyline (see below), or narcotics may be needed to provide comfort. These must be used with caution, particularly in persons living alone, those on multiple medications, and the elderly.

PHN, or pain after the cutaneous lesions have resolved, is most commonly seen in patients over 50 years. Other predictors of the development of PHN include a greater number of health care encounters in the 6 months before zoster, baseline conditions causing immunosuppression, treatment with steroids in the 6 months before zoster, zoster associated prodromal symptoms, discomfort severe enough to interfere with daily living, and prolonged time to crusting of skin lesions. However, in one study (21), treatment with acyclovir was not associated with a reduced risk of PHN. In contrast, other studies have found benefit with antiviral therapy given during the acute herpes zoster infection. Both valacyclovir and famciclovir have been shown to reduce the incidence and duration of PHN (19,20). Its been estimated that six patients need to be treated with antivirals to prevent one case of PHN (22). The utility of supplemental corticosteroids in the prevention of PHN remains controversial (23,24) and therefore is not recommended. A small study found that amitriptyline 10 to 25 mg nightly initiated at the time of diagnosis of acute zoster reduced the incidence of PHN by 50% (25). If larger studies ultimately show this same benefit, amitriptyline (with appropriate caution; see Chapters 12 and 24) would seem to be an ideal treatment for persons with painful acute herpes zoster.

Once developed, treatment of PHN may be very difficult. Some success has been reported with topical capsaicin cream (Zostrix 0.025% and Zostrix HP 0.075%), applied four times a day. Capsaicin depletes substance P in peripheral sensory nerves and may alleviate pain. Not infrequently, there is a delay of several weeks before an effect is appreciated. Patients must be cautioned that about four applications are needed to fully deplete the substance contributing to pain (substance P), so the first few applications (typically, three) when substance P is being released produce local burning and stinging. However, with subsequent *consistent* applications, the pain should not recur. Alternatively or in conjunction with capsaicin, anesthetic over the counter LidoDerm topical patches and over the counter ELA-Max cream may be tried. Unfortunately, both are quite expensive for long-term use. For some patients, systemic treatment with amitriptyline (as opposed to prevention; see above) is appropriate initial therapy for PHN. Oral amitriptyline in dosages of 12.5 to 150 mg/day (26) may decrease the discomfort of PHN (see Chapters 12 and 24). Gabapentin studied over a 2-month treatment period in a multicenter, double-blind, randomized, placebo-controlled study also was found to be effective in reducing pain and sleep disturbance and improving mood and quality of life (27). PHN most often remits spontaneously within 6 months; however, when this is the case and the pain cannot be controlled, referral to a pain specialist is appropriate. Although still investigational (28), intrathecal methylprednisolone may prove to be helpful for intractable PHN.

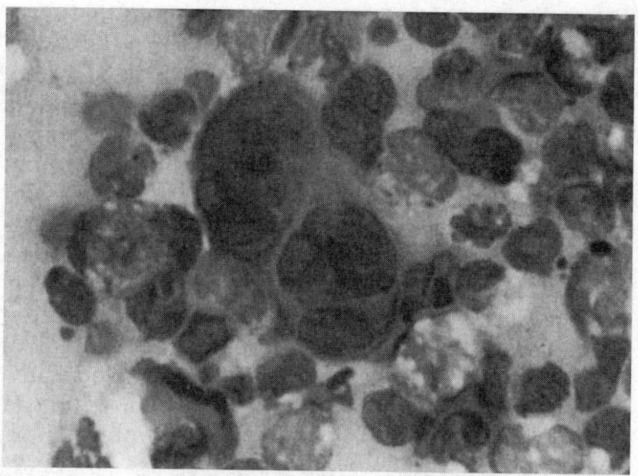

Figure 117.3. Tzanck smear: gentle scraping from the base of a vesicle and stained with Wright or Giemsa stain. Multinucleated cells from herpes simplex are shown (×400).

Tzanck Smear

The sensitivity of a *Tzanck smear* in detecting herpetic changes is greatest when a specimen is taken from the intact vesicle. A chosen vesicle is unroofed, and the base is firmly scraped with a number 15 surgical blade and smeared onto a glass slide. When vesicles are not present, an early crusted papule is sampled by removing the surface crust and scraping the base. Immediate tissue smear staining is performed with the commercially available Tzanck stain (Dif-Quik Stain, Baxter Scientific Products, McGraw Park, IL), which is a three-step immediate stain. Alternatively, a Giemsa stain may be done by combining 0.5 mL water with 0.5 mL Giemsa tissue stain in a small syringe and flooding over the specimen and then thoroughly rinsing with tap water after 30 seconds. Although the slide may be viewed directly, covering with mounting medium and a coverslip greatly improves resolution. The slide is searched for giant cells containing multiple syncytial nuclei (nuclei that mold together in a jigsaw puzzle-like fashion) (Fig. 117.3). The Tzanck smear preparation should be positive when performed on lesions of herpes simplex, varicella, and herpes zoster eruptions (Fig. 117.3). If the Tzanck smear is nondiagnostic, biopsy of a papule, vesicle, or crusted papule for routine histopathology (results available in 2 to 4 days) should reveal diagnostic herpetic changes of balloon cells and multinucleated giant cells.

INFESTATIONS

Scabies

Human scabies is caused by infestation with the mite *Sarcoptes scabiei* var. *hominis*. Infestation causes an intense intractable pruritus that is classically most disturbing at night, when competing external stimuli are minimal. The signs and symptoms of scabies infestation are caused by the host's immune response to the mite and its eggs and feces. Generally, this response is delayed, so patients become itchy approximately 10 days to 2 weeks after exposure and infestation. Scabies is seen most often in children, and the pathognomonic lesions are burrows, which are thread-like linear ridges a few millimeters in length with a minute black dot at one end. Burrows occur most often on the hands, wrists, soles, waist, penis, nipples, axillae, and gluteal cleft. Depending on the duration of infestation, patients may have few to innumerable scratches, excoriations, crusts, and eczematous papules and plaques. Less often, small nodules may develop, tending to favor the scrotum, axillae, and buttocks.

Scabies infestation is confirmed by identifying the mite, eggs, or feces in the superficial skin. This often can be done by scraping the black dot at one end of a burrow using a number 15 surgical blade. If a black dot is not seen, both ends of the burrow are scraped. The sample is prepared on a glass slide with a drop of mineral oil and a coverslip and then viewed with light microscopy. The mite is an approximately 0.2 mm with eight short legs; eggs are smaller and oval and feces are still smaller round pellets.

Patients and family members should be treated with an overnight application of prescription lindane lotion (Kwell lotion, 30 mL per single application) or permethrin cream (Elimite cream, 30 g per single application, 60-g tube). Either is applied from the neck down, using an old toothbrush to get under the finger and toenails and showered off 8 to 12 hours later. After this is completed, patients often require emollients and a mid-potency corticosteroid (e.g., triamcinolone 0.1% ointment) after using the scabicides to suppress the "hyperreactivity" caused by the mites (see Chapter 113). Although both lindane and permethrin are neurotoxins, systemic absorption of lindane is greater (29) so it should be avoided in infants, pregnant and lactating women, and patients with seizure disorders. It should also be avoided when enhanced systemic absorption is possible, such as in patients with extensive secondary excoriations and dermatitis or with widespread skin diseases (e.g., generalized

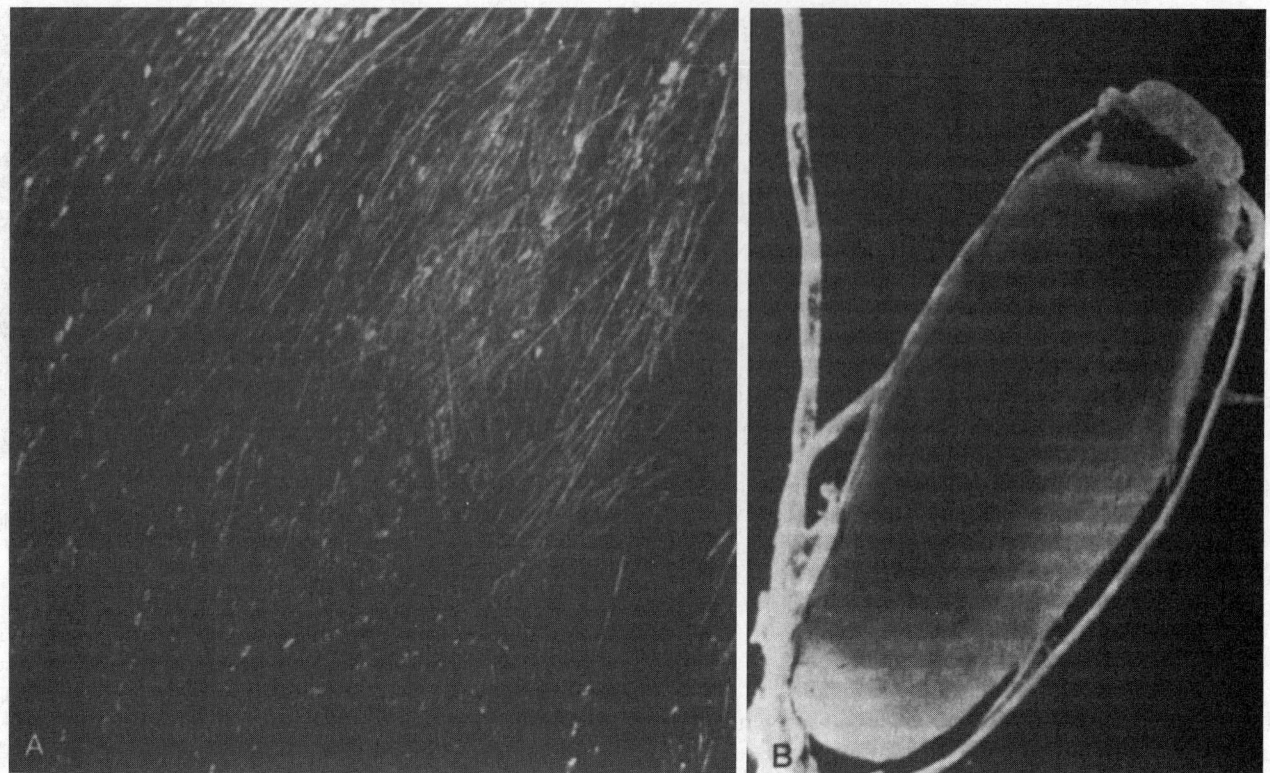

Figure 117.4. *Pediculus humanus* var. *capitis* (head louse). **A:** Gross appearance of nits on the hair shaft. **B:** Microscopic appearance (×100). (Courtesy of Reed and Carnrick, Kenilworth, NJ.)

atopic dermatitis, widespread psoriasis). All bed clothing, linens, unwashed clothing, and stuffed animals should be washed and dried in a hot dryer. The latter is necessary, because it is the temperature of the hot dryer that kills the mite. Alternatively, the mites and eggs may be killed by placing the items in airtight plastic bags for 2 weeks.

An alternative treatment now available in this country in patients resistant to topical scabicidal therapy is ivermectin (6-mg tablets). Although it is not FDA approved for this indication (30), successful therapy has been reported using a single dose of 0.2 mg/kg (e.g., a single dose of two tablets for a 60-kg adult) (31).

Pediculosis

Infestation with the human louse (*Pediculus humanus capitis* and *corporis, Phthirus pubis*) affects different areas of the body and is called *pediculosis capitis, corporis,* and *pubis. Pediculosis capitis* is most common in children. Patients with lice often have intense pruritus, scalp and posterior neck excoriations, and often secondary bacterial infection with pustules, crusting, and adenopathy. *Pediculosis corporis* is seen most often in patients exposed to others who, like themselves, are unable to maintain good hygiene. *Pediculosis pubis* (pubic lice) is usually a sexually transmitted disorder.

Patients with pediculosis usually have nits firmly attached to head, body, or pubic hairs (Fig. 117.4). Nits are less than 1-mm-long "shells" that may or may not still contain an egg. Lice hatch from these eggs and are visible, being less than 2 mm long with three pairs of legs that terminate in sharp claws. They are found in the hair or adjacent skin and, specifically in pediculosis corporis, in the seams of clothing. Treatment should be initiated with pyrethrin shampoo (e.g., RID, over the counter) or lindane shampoo (e.g., Kwell, by prescription) for pediculosis capitis and pubis and lindane lotion for pediculosis corporis. The shampoo is left on for 5 to 10 minutes and then washed off; the body lotion is left on overnight. Because no pediculicides are 100% ovicidal, nits that potentially contain living eggs and will remain attached to the hair after treatment must be removed with a fine-tooth comb after undiluted white vinegar is applied to the hair for 15 minutes. Close contacts should be treated in a similar fashion, and bed clothing and linens and unwashed clothes should be washed and put through a hot dryer cycle to destroy the lice and eggs. Alternatively, these items may be sealed in an airtight plastic bag for 2 weeks.

Specific References*

1. Hubbard TW. The predictive value of symptoms in diagnosing childhood tinea capitis. Arch Pediatr Adolesc Med 1999;153:1150.
2. Friedlander S, Pickering B, Cunningham BB, et al. The utility of the cotton swab method in the diagnosis of tinea capitis. Pediatrics 1999;104:276.

*Bold print (general references) and bold numerals (specific references) denote published controlled clinical trials, meta-analysis, or consensus-based recommendations.

3. Gupta AK, Dlova N, Taborda P, et al. Once weekly fluconazole is effective in children in the treatment of tinea capitis: a prospective, multicentre study. Br J Dermatol 2000;142: 965.
4. Haroon TS, Hussain I, Aman S, et al. A randomized double-blind comparative study of terbinafine for 1, 2 and 4 weeks in tinea capitis. Br J Dermatol 1996;135:86.
5. Semel JD, Goldin H. Association of athlete's foot with cellulitis of the lower extremities: diagnostic value of bacterial cultures of ipsilateral interdigital space samples. Clin Infect Dis 1996;23:1162.
6. Eriksson B, Jorup-Rönström C, Karkkonen K, et al. Erysipelas: clinical and bacteriologic spectrum and serological aspects. Clin Infect Dis 1996;23:1091.
7. Nickman JG. A double-blinded, randomized placebo controlled evaluation of short term treatment with oral itraconazole in patients with tinea versicolor. J Am Acad Dermatol 1996;34:785.
8. Oliver L, Wald A, Kim M, et al. Seroprevalence of herpes simplex virus infection in a family medicine clinic. Arch Fam Med 1995;4:228.
9. Murakami S, Mizobuchi M, Nakashiro Y, et al. Bell's palsy and herpes simplex virus: identification of viral DNA in endoneurial fluid and muscle. Ann Intern Med 1996;124:27.
10. Wiley CA, VanPatten PD, Carpenter PM, et al. Acute ascending necrotizing myelopathy caused by herpes simplex virus type II. Neurology 1987;37:1791.
11. Tedder DG, Ashley R, Tyler KL, et al. Herpes simplex virus infection as cause of benign recurrent lymphocytic meningitis. Ann Intern Med 1994;121:334.
12. Rooney JF, Strauss SE, Mannix ML, et al. Oral acyclovir to suppress frequently recurrent herpes labialis. Ann Intern Med 1993;118:268.
13. Embro WJ. Treatment of herpes simplex labialis with stannous fluoride gel. Cosmetic Dermatol 1999;39.
14. Karadi I, Karpati S, Romics L. Aspirin in the management of recurrent herpes simplex virus infection. Ann Intern Med 1998;128:696.
15. Oxman MN, Strauss SE. Varicella and herpes zoster. In: Freedberg IM, Eisen AZ, Wolff K, et al, eds. Fitzpatrick's dermatology in general medicine. 5th ed. New York: McGraw-Hill, 1999:2436.
16. Ragozzino MW, Melton LJ III, Kurland LT, et al. Population-based study of herpes zoster and its sequelae. Medicine 1982;61:310.
17. Akiyama N. Herpes zoster infection complicated by motor paralysis. J Dermatol 2000;27:252.
18. Kost RG, Straus SE. Postherpetic neuralgia: pathogenesis, treatment, and prevention. N Engl J Med 1996;335:32.
19. Tyring S, Barbarash RA, Nahlik JE, et al. Famciclovir for the treatment of acute herpes zoster: effects on acute disease and postherpetic neuralgia. A randomized, double-blind, placebo-controlled trial. Collaborative Famciclovir Herpes Zoster Study Group. Ann Intern Med 1995;123:89.
20. Valacylovir. Med Lett 1996;38:4.
21. Choo PW, Galil K, Donahue JG, et al. Risk factors for postherpetic neuralgia. Arch Intern Med 1997;157:1217.
22. Jackson JL, Gibbons R, Meyer G, et al. The effect of treating herpes zoster with oral acyclovir in preventing postherpetic neuralgia: a meta-analysis. Arch Intern Med 1997;157: 909.
23. Whitley RJ, Weiss H, Gnann JW, et al. Acyclovir with and without prednisone for the treatment of herpes zoster. A randomized, placebo-controlled trial. Ann Intern Med 1996;125:376.
24. Wood MJ, Johnson RW, McKendrick MW, et al. A randomized trial of acyclovir for 7 days or 21 days with and without prednisolone for treatment of acute herpes zoster. N Engl J Med 1994;330:896.
25. Bowsher D. The management of postherpetic neuralgia. Postgrad Med J 1997;73:62.
26. Max MB, Schafer SC, Culnane M, et al. Amitriptyline, but not lorazepam, relieves post-herpetic neuralgia. Neurology 1988;38:1427.
27. Rowbotham M, Hardern N, Stacey B, et al, for the Gabapentin Postherpetic Neuralgia Study Group. Gabapentin for the treatment of postherpetic neuralgia. JAMA 1998;280:187.
28. Kotani N, Matsuki A, Watson CPN. Correspondence regarding intrathecal methylprednisolone for intractable postherpetic neuralgia. N Engl J Med 2000;344:1019.
29. Meinking TL, Taplin D. Safety of permethrin versus lindane for the treatment of scabies. Arch Dermatol 1996;132:959.
30. Nightingale SL. From the Food and Drug Administration: ivermectin approved for strongyloidiasis and onchocerciasis. JAMA 1997;277:703.
31. Meinking TL, Taplin D, Hermida JL, et al. The treatment of scabies with ivermectin. N Engl J Med 1995;333:26.

CHAPTER 118

Autoimmune Blistering Diseases, Photosensitive Eruptions, and Drug Eruptions

S. ELIZABETH WHITMORE, MD, ScM

AUTOIMMUNE BLISTERING DISORDERS

Primary bullous dermatoses associated with autoantibodies to various components of the epidermis (1) include bullous pemphigoid, pemphigus vulgaris, bullous lupus erythematosus, acquired epidermolysis bullosa acquisita, linear IgA bullous dermatosis, vancomycin and other drug-induced linear IgA dermatoses, and paraneoplastic pemphigus. Patients with these conditions have flaccid to tense bullae, with or without an erythematous, urticarial base, distributed in a localized or generalized fashion on the skin and mucosal surfaces. Because some of these disorders may be associated with significant morbidity and mortality, patients suspected of having an autoimmune blistering disorder should undergo skin biopsy for routine histologic and special staining (direct immunofluorescence to identify the site of deposited immunoglobulin within the epidermis). Not infrequently, very aggressive therapies, including prednisone, cytotoxic agents, or plasmapheresis, may be required.

The various patterns of these disorders are described below.

Bullous pemphigoid typically includes mild asymptomatic oral involvement and tense skin blisters; affected patients are usually over age 60. Herpes gestationis is similar to bullous pemphigoid, but it occurs in association with pregnancy. *Pemphigus* vulgaris and *paraneoplastic* pemphigus (2) are associated with extensive oral lesions, and in pemphigus cutaneous blisters exhibit a positive *Nikolsky* sign in which pressure applied to a blister causes the blister to enlarge by spreading outward into the adjacent skin. Neoplasms accompanying "paraneoplastic" pemphigus may include lymphoma, chronic lymphocytic leukemia, poorly differentiated sarcoma, bronchogenic squamous cell carcinoma, and thymoma. *Bullous lupus erythematosus* occurs in the setting of systemic lupus erythematosus. Vancomycin and other drug-induced linear IgA dermatoses appear similar to bullous pemphigoid but usually clear upon withdrawal of the triggering drug. In general, one will want to consult with a dermatologist if there is any doubt about the diagnosis or treatment of a patient suspected of having a form of autoimmune blistering disorder.

PHOTOSENSITIVITY

Photosensitivity is an abnormal response to natural sunlight or artificial ultraviolet (UV) radiation or visible light. It manifests as a diffuse macular erythema (*phototoxic reaction*) or a papular or papulovesicular erythema (e.g., *photoallergic reaction*) on the exposed surfaces. The phototoxic or sunburn-like reaction is caused by phototoxic drugs such as sulfonamides, quinolones, doxycycline, phenothiazines, nonsteroidal anti-inflammatory drugs (NSAIDs), porphyrin precursors, and psoralens. Just like a sunburn, it is either asymptomatic or painful. This is a nonimmunologic toxic reaction that occurs in any patient who has a sufficiently high serum level of a photoactivated drug and sufficient UV-A (wavelength from 320 to 400 mm) radiation exposure. Besides the usual summer sunlight, other significant UV-A exposures should be remembered; wintertime sunlight, most intense on highly reflective snow covered high altitude places like ski slopes, sunlight passing through car windows (unlike UV-B, spanning wavelengths from 290 to 320 mm, longer wavelength UV-A does pass through glass), and tanning salon sessions. Although any of these drugs (see above) may cause severe phototoxicity, the most frightening reaction and outcome results when psoralen is taken before tanning salon or natural sunlight exposure. Indeed, death from burns has occurred with tanning salon exposure after taking psoralen. Patients may unknowingly receive a severe phototoxic reaction if they take any of these drugs and attend a tanning salon session or sun bathe.

Sun-exposed site pruritic, papular, or papulovesicular erythema may represent a *drug-induced photoallergic eruption*, *polymorphous light eruption*, or *cutaneous lupus erythematosus*. The drug-induced photoallergic eruption is a cell-mediated immune reaction that is most often caused by thiazides, NSAIDs, sulfonamides and sulfonylureas, oral contraceptives, and quinidine. *Polymorphous light eruption* is a common idiopathic disorder in which patients typically develop a pruritic papular eruption on the extensor surface of the arms and other sun-exposed sites, typically sparing the chronically sun-exposed ("hardened") face. The eruption typically occurs with each of the first several beach, pool, or picnic sun exposures in the late spring or summer months. After these two or three exposure-associated rashes, patients usually become hardened on the sites of the prior eruption, showing a tan, and have no further problems until the next spring or summer. When the diagnosis of photoallergic drug eruption or polymorphous light eruption cannot be made based on the patient's appearance and clinical course (photoallergy should resolve with drug withdrawal and polymorphous light eruption should resolve with continued sun exposure), further evaluation for possible lupus erythematosus, including *skin biopsy*, should be done. A dermatologist should be consulted if there is doubt about the diagnosis.

In all patients with photosensitive disorders, appropriate protective sun-blocking clothing and high sun protection factor (e.g., SPF 30) sunscreens should be used. These eruptions are caused primarily by UV-A radiation in the case of drug eruptions and UV-B and UV-A radiation in the case of polymorphous light eruption and lupus erythematosus. UV-A passes through window glass (see above) and patients who are photosensitive or on photosensitizing drugs should be made aware to avoid sunlight received through glass.

Sunscreens and Sunblocks

Sunscreens and sunblocks should be recommended not only for people with photosensitivity, but also for normal people spending time out of doors in sunny seasons. Sunburns may be treated with palliative oral analgesics and tepid water baths. Suntanning should be discouraged because both UV-B and UV-A are known carcinogens.

Sunscreens contain chemicals that absorb UV radiation. Adverse reactions to any sunscreen may occur. These chemicals are altered by radiation, and this is believed to be the cause of burning and stinging that may occur with higher SPF (see below) sunscreens, particularly when used on the face. Such reactions are most common in fair-skinned women especially if also using alpha-hydroxy acid or retinoic acid-based (e.g., Renova, Retin-A) facial creams. The alternative to sunscreens for people who experience either stinging or true allergic reactions are *sunblocks*. These block rather than absorb UV radiation and include plain zinc oxide (visibly white) and micronized zinc oxide and titanium dioxide (translucent when applied). Sunblocks tend to be less cosmetically acceptable because they have a chalky feel; however, they effectively block both UV-B and UV-A.

Sunscreens and sunblocks are given an *SPF* rating, which is the ratio of time needed for UV-B radiation to cause minimal erythema (redness) when using versus not using the sunscreen. In the laboratory, an SPF of 15 screens 92% of UV-B, and an SPF of 30 screens 96% of UV-B. However, most sunscreen users apply significantly less than 50% of the amount of lotion needed for this protection, turning an SPF 30 product effectively into an SPF 15 product, at best. For this reason, it is best to recommend an SPF 30 sunscreen, preferably waterproof. Alternatively, because sunscreens are expensive, sun protection can be provided with tight-weave clothing, hats, and avoidance of sunlight exposure during peak UV-B radiation times (10 a.m. to 3 p.m.). Finally, because some people may ordinarily obtain some or all of their vitamin D from the sun instead of through their daily diet or by taking supplemental vitamins, the recommendation for sunscreens and sun avoidance should also include a recommendation for adequate daily vitamin D ingestion (see Chapter 103).

DRUG ERUPTIONS

Numerous prescription and nonprescription medications may cause a wide array of cutaneous abnormalities and aggravate pre-existing dermatoses (Table 118.1). It has been estimated that in hospitalized patients, 2% to 3% have adverse cutaneous drug reactions and 2% of these reactions are severe, being associated with significant morbidity and potential mortality (3,4). A recent systematic review of the MEDLINE database from 1966 to 2000 identified nine large studies containing primary data on the rates of cutaneous reactions to drugs. Analysis of these studies revealed "remarkable agreement" between the studies on reaction rates to drugs, with antibiotics causing most reactions (5).

The common drug eruptions (e.g., exanthems), potentially life-threatening eruptions (e.g., toxic epidermal necrolysis [TEN] and vasculitis [4,6]), and poorly tolerated reactions (e.g., acne, alopecia, photosensitivity, psoriasis, and pigmentary changes) are discussed below. A Medic Alert bracelet indicating the drug and type of reaction should be recommended for all patients having severe drug eruptions.

Urticaria

Urticaria is discussed in Chapter 30.

Exanthems

The most commonly seen acute drug-induced eruption is a pruritic exanthem. This is usually macular and papular (morbilliform) but may be a purely macular erythema, exfoliative erythroderma, or scarlatiniform eruption. Although innumerable drugs may cause this eruption, the most commonly implicated drugs include penicillins and semisynthetic penicillins, cephalosporins, sulfonamides, quinidine, cimetidine, allopurinol, carbamazepine, phenytoin, isoniazid, and nitrofurantoin.

Although data suggest that patient reported history regarding drug allergy, particularly penicillin allergy, may be incorrect (7), it should always be presumed to be accurate, and if the decision is made to administer the drug, a reaction must be anticipated. When the question of possible immediate reaction (IgE, anaphylaxis) to penicillins and cephalosporins arises, testing may be done to confirm or exclude an IgE mediated allergy (see Chapter 30). Unfortunately, such testing is not available for other drugs or for other types of immune reactions.

Eruptions may begin at any time but usually occur at one of two periods of drug administration: after 2 to 3 days or after 9 to 10 days. The early form is seen in patients who have previously been sensitized to the drug. With this prior sensitization, an exanthem may or may not have occurred, depending on the timing of sensitization and how soon the drug was stopped. The more delayed reaction occurring 9 to 10 days after drug initiation occurs in patients not previously sensitized to the drug. Systemic manifestations of drug sensitivity such as associated fever, lymphadenopathy, and visceral hypersensitivity are usually absent. When visceral hypersensitivity occurs, it may involve the kidneys, liver (hepatitis, cholestasis), and gastrointestinal tract (bleeding). Systemic involvement is more common with certain drugs such as allopurinol, phenytoin, and isoniazid. Rarely, an exanthem may be complicated by the subsequent development of toxic epidermal neurolysis (see page 1767).

With uncomplicated nonbullous cutaneous eruptions, the suspected causative drug should be stopped if possible, and topical treatment begun to reduce pruritus. Such treatment includes frequent application of bland, topical, over the counter preparations containing menthol or phenol such as Sarna or Sarna HC (with 1% hydrocortisone) lotion or Aveeno Anti-Itch cream. In contrast, systemic drug hypersensitivity syndromes require immediate intervention with prompt discontinuation of all suspected drugs and close observation (4).

Erythema Multiforme

Erythema multiforme (EM) is a mucocutaneous hypersensitivity syndrome caused most commonly by a drug or infection. It is divided into EM minor and EM major, depending on whether it affects one or more than one mucosal surface, respectively (4,6). Although the pathogenesis of EM is unknown, it is believed that an infection or a drug leads to a cell-mediated cytotoxic reaction in the epidermis.

EM major, which accounts for approximately 20% of cases of EM, may cause morbidity and even mortality. It is associated with drugs more often than EM minor, but similar infections may cause both forms (see below). Patients usually have a prodrome of malaise, myalgia, fever, and sometimes upper respiratory symptoms. The eruption develops rapidly, is

Table 118.1. Adverse Cutaneous Drug Reactions and Some Common Causative Drugs

- Acne
  - Androgenic hormones
  - Corticosteroids
  - Halogens (bromides, iodides)
  - Anticonvulsants
  - Tuberculostatic drugs
  - Lithium
  - Cyclosporin
  - Vitamin B_{12}
  - Oral contraceptives
- Alopecia
  - Cytostatic drugs
  - Anticoagulants
  - Androgenic hormones
  - Phenytoin
  - Cholesterol-lowering agents
  - Colchicine
- Erythema multiforme and toxic epidermal necrolysis (see text)
  - Sulfonamides
  - Penicillins
  - Nonsteroidal anti-inflammatory drugs
  - Anticonvulsants
- Exanthematous eruptions (see text)
  - Penicillins
  - Sulfonamides
  - Barbiturates
  - Phenytoin
  - Carbamazepine
  - Allopurinol
  - Gold salts
  - Phenothiazines
- Fixed drug eruptions[a]
  - Phenolphthalein
  - Tetracyclines
  - Sulfonamides
  - Barbiturates
  - Penicillins
- Nonpigmenting fixed drug eruption[b]
  - Acetaminophen
  - Pseudoephedrine
  - Radiocontrast media
- Leukocytoclastic vasculitis
  - Sulfonamides
  - Phenytoin
  - Allopurinol
- Papulosquamous eruptions (psoriasislike eruptions or exacerbation of psoriasis)
  - Antimalarials
  - Lithium
  - Beta-blockers
  - ACE inhibitors
  - Sulfonamides
- Lichen planus-like eruptions
  - Gold
  - Captopril
  - Furosemide
  - Beta-blockers
  - Quinidine
  - Quinine
  - Sulfonylureas
  - Thiazides
- Pityriasis rosea-like eruptions (see Table 113.1; pityriasis rosea)
  - Barbiturates
  - Gold
  - Metronidazole
  - Bismuth
  - Captopril
  - Clonidine
  - Metoprolol
- Photosensitivity
  - Tetracycline
  - Demeclocycline
  - Doxycycline
  - Sulfonamides
  - Nonsteroidal anti-inflammatory drugs
  - Phenothiazines
  - Thiazide diuretics
  - Psoralens
- Porhyria cutanea tarda[c]
  - Estrogens
  - Androgens
  - Alcohol
  - Antimalarials
  - Sulfonamides
  - Sulfonylureas
  - Rifampicin
  - Quinidine
  - Quinine
- Acute intermittent porphyria[c]
  - Estrogens
  - Androgens
  - Alcohol
  - Antimalarials
  - Sulfonamides
  - Sulfonylureas
  - Barbiturates
- Urticaria/angioedema
  - Opiates
  - Penicillins
  - Sulfonamides
  - Aspirin
  - Quinine
  - Nonsteroidal anti-inflammatory drugs
  - ACE inhibitors
  - Radiocontrast media
  - Hyperosmolar solutions
  - Amphetamines
  - Azodyes and benzoates in drugs
- Eczematous eruptions
  - Beta-blockers
  - Diuretics
  - Sulfonylureas
  - Phenothiazines
  - Penicillins
  - Sulfonamides
- Pruritus
  - Opiates
  - Aspirin
  - Antidepressants
  - Belladonna alkaloids
  - Barbiturates
  - CNS stimulants
  - Estrogens
  - Hepatotoxic drugs

[a]One or more, 1–4 cm, asymmetrically distributed erythematous patches that resolve with hyperpigmentation and become acutely inflamed again with drug readministration.

[b]One or more, 1–4 cm, erythematous macules that fade completely and become acutely inflamed with drug readministration.

[c]Not described in this textbook.

ACE, angiotensin-converting enzyme; CNS, central nervous system.

generally widespread, and involves at least two mucosal surfaces, usually the conjunctiva and the oral mucosa. Cutaneous lesions evolve quickly from macules into target-like plaques with dusky centers (Fig. 118.1, Color Plate section), often surmounted by blisters and often confluent over large areas. Usually, the lips are covered with hemorrhagic crusts and the mucosa shows diffuse pseudomembranous denudation, and the eyes show conjunctival injection, erosions, or exudate. Less often the nasal, genital, esophageal, and, rarely, the respiratory mucosae are involved.

The most common and significant acute complication of EM major is secondary bacterial infection and sepsis; the most devastating long-term complication is ocular scarring and vision loss. Patients with EM major must be hospitalized and, depending on the extent of disease, may benefit from care in a burn unit. Ophthalmologic consultation should be obtained immediately.

EM minor causes 80% of all cases of EM. It is seen in patients of all ages but is more common in patients who are between the ages of 20 and 40 years. Most cases of EM minor are caused by a preceding herpes simplex virus infection. Most patients with recurrent EM minor, even those without a history of HSV infection, have detectable HSV DNA in the lesions. Causes of EM minor other than herpes simplex infection include other viral infections, *Mycoplasma pneumoniae*, other bacterial infections, and drugs (most commonly sulfonamides, penicillins, NSAIDs, and anticonvulsants).

EM minor begins with asymptomatic to tender erythematous to violaceous macules that evolve into papules with an expanding border, leaving a nonblanchable, dusky, slightly depressed center, creating an iris or target lesion. Lesions may coalesce into plaques or become bullous (*bullous EM*). The eruption favors the palms and soles, dorsal hands and feet, and knees and elbows, but may be widely distributed. Approximately 20% of patients have mucosal lesions with mild to extensive flaccid bullae and deep erosions of the lips, buccal mucosa, and gingiva. EM is occasionally limited to the mouth without cutaneous lesions. Patients may have associated fever and malaise. If the diagnosis cannot be made on clinical grounds, skin biopsy should be done and will show necrotic keratinocytes, epidermal and dermal edema, and a mononuclear cell infiltrate. The treatment of EM minor involves identification of the causative drug or infection and withdrawal of any suspected offending drug. Although necessary, treatment of a causative infection does not change the course of the EM. For symptomatic relief, the oral lesions may be treated with an oral suspension containing diphenhydramine and antacid (e.g., Benadryl Elixir and Maalox in equal parts; swish for 1 minute and expectorate, four to six times per day) or sucralfate (e.g., Carafate 16 g [16 tabs] in 60 mL water; add to 180 mL 70% sorbitol; paint on erosions with finger as needed) in combination with 3% hydrogen peroxide washes (swish for 15 seconds and expectorate or swab with dental sponge four to six times per day). Topical anesthetics (Xylocaine gel) may be applied to individual painful lesions before meals. The use of systemic corticosteroids is controversial, and consultation with a dermatologist is recommended. One should note that if used, corticosteroid therapy should be given early in the course of the disease. If given after the eruption has fully evolved, one would not be expected to alter the severity of EM and use of corticosteroids may increase the risk of secondary infection and even impair healing. In cases of recurrent EM minor triggered by HSV, prophylactic acyclovir should be given to prevent HSV recurrences (see above).

Toxic Epidermal Necrolysis

TEN, fortunately uncommon, is associated with a 25% to more than 40% mortality rate (6). Because it has many features in common with EM major, these reactions are believed to represent a continuum of one disease. TEN is most often caused by drugs, especially sulfonamides, anticonvulsants, NSAIDs, allopurinol, colchicine, cephalosporins, quinolones, and aminopenicillins (6).

Similar to a sunburn, TEN typically begins with a diffuse painful erythema, often first noted on the trunk. Rapidly, patchy, and then coalescing areas of dusky epidermal necrosis and skin sloughing develop. Oral and ocular manifestations are similar to the changes seen in EM major. Although the diagnosis is made presumptively and appropriate management initiated, biopsy should be done to confirm the diagnosis. This reveals epidermal necrosis with sloughing of the epidermis from the dermis and a sparse mononuclear perivascular dermal infiltrate.

Patients with TEN are critically ill and may develop a number of associated problems, including cytopenias, hepatitis, hypoalbuminemia, hypophosphatemia, prerenal azotemia, disseminated intravascular coagulation, and pancreatitis (4). These patients should urgently be admitted to a hospital and ideally to a burn unit. Urgent consultation with a burn unit or medical intensivist, a dermatologist or plastic surgeon, and an ophthalmologist should be obtained. Mortality is most often the result of sepsis, whereas chronic morbidity is most often caused by cutaneous and ocular scarring, with the latter potentially leading to severe vision loss.

Nonspecific Eruptions Secondary to Drugs

Toxicity in the Elderly

Drug toxicity is an important cause of cutaneous eruptions in patients with declining renal or hepatic function, particularly when they are on multiple drugs that compete for hepatic metabolism or renal secretion. Such situations are typical of the elderly, who are most at risk for drug reactions in general (see Chapter 12).

Toxic drug eruptions may occur at any time while the patient is taking a drug. When an eruption occurs months or even years after the start of a drug, a toxic drug reaction is often not considered. Such instances of toxicity after many months of drug administration may result in pruritus with an associated or resultant dermatitis and possibly exacerbation of previously existing skin diseases (e.g., psoriasis, atopic dermatitis) (8). Drug withdrawal in this situation usually leads to a slow improvement over several weeks. Toxic drug reactions should be considered in patients complaining of new usually symmetric dermatoses or exacerbation of previously stable skin conditions, even if a patient has been on a drug for months or years. Whenever possible, such drugs should be eliminated or reduced in dosage (8,9).

Specific References*

1. Helm KF, Peters MS. Subspecialty clinics: dermatology. Immunodermatology update: the immunologically mediated vesiculobullous diseases. Mayo Clin Proc 1991;66:187.

*Bold print (general references) and bold numerals (specific references) denote published controlled clinical trials, meta-analysis, or consensus-based recommendations.

2. Anhalt GA, Soo Chan K, et al. Paraneoplastic pemphigus. N Engl J Med 1990;323:1729.
3. Bigby M, Jick S, Jick H, et al. Drug-induced cutaneous reactions: a report from the Boston Collaborative Drug Surveillance Program on 15,438 Consecutive Patients, 1975–1982. JAMA 1986;256:3358.
4. Roujeau JC, Stern RS. Severe adverse cutaneous reactions to drugs. N Engl J Med 1994;331:1272.
5. Bigby M. Rates of cutaneous reactions to drugs. Arch Dermatol 2001;137:765.
6. Roujeau JC, Kelly JP, Naldi L, et al. Medication use and the risk of Stevens–Johnson syndrome or toxic epidermal necrolysis. N Engl J Med 1995;333:1600.
7. Salkind AR, Cuddy PG, Foxworth JW. Is this patient allergic to penicillin? An evidence-based study analysis of the likelihood of penicillin allergy. JAMA 2001;285:2498.
8. Gilleaudeau P, Vallat VP, Carter DM, et al. Angiotensin-converting enzyme inhibitors as possible exacerbating drugs in psoriasis. J Am Acad Dermatol 1993;28:490.
9. Carrington PR, Sanusi ID, Zahradka S, et al. Enalapril-associated erythema and vasculitis. Cutis 1993;51:121.

INDEX

Page numbers followed by *t* and *f* indicate tables and figures, respectively.

T